Pediatrics

ASSOCIATE EDITORS

Carol D. Berkowitz, MD
Professor of Clinical Pediatrics and Executive Vice Chair
Department of Pediatrics
Harbor-UCLA Medical Center
Torrance, California;
David Geffen School of Medicine at UCLA
Los Angeles, California
General Medical Care

Jeffrey R. Botkin, MD, MPH
Professor of Pediatrics
Associate Vice President for Research Integrity
Department of Pediatrics
University of Utah
Salt Lake City, Utah
Social Aspects of Care

Patricia K. Kokotailo, MD, MPH
Associate Professor, Director of Adolescent Medicine
Department of Pediatrics
University of Wisconsin–Madison Medical School
Madison, Wisconsin
Adolescent Care

Peter A. Margolis, MD, PhD
Professor of Pediatrics and Epidemiology
Co-director, North Carolina Center for Children's
Healthcare Improvement
The University of North Carolina at Chapel Hill
Chapel Hill, North Carolina
Health Promotion and Disease Prevention

Richard A. Molteni, MD
Clinical Professor and Associate Dean
Department of Pediatrics
University of Washington School of Medicine;
Vice President Medical Director
Children's Hospital and Regional Medical Center
Seattle, Washington
Newborn Care

Ardis L. Olson, MD
Associate Professor of Pediatrics
Dartmouth Medical School
Hanover, New Hampshire;
Attending Pediatrician
Department of Pediatrics
Dartmouth-Hitchcock Medical Center
Lebanon, New Hampshire
Chronic Medical Care

Kenneth B. Roberts, MD
Professor
Department of Pediatrics
The University of North Carolina School of Medicine
Chapel Hill, North Carolina;
Director
Pediatric Teaching Program
Moses Cone Health System
Greensboro, North Carolina
Fundamentals

Mark L. Wolraich, MD
CMRI/Shaun Walters Professor of Pediatrics
Department of Pediatrics
University of Oklahoma Health Sciences Center;
Department of Pediatrics
Oklahoma University Children's Hospital
Oklahoma City, Oklahoma
Mental Health Care

Pediatrics

Edited By

Lucy M. Osborn, MD, MSPH, FAAP
Professor Emeritus
Department of Pediatrics
University of Utah Medical School
Salt Lake City, Utah

Thomas G. DeWitt, MD, FAAP
Weihl Professor and Director
Division of General and Community Pediatrics
Associate Chair for Education
Department of Pediatrics
University of Cincinnati College of Medicine
Cincinnati Children's Hospital Medical Center
Cincinnati, Ohio

Lewis R. First, MD, MS, FAAP
Professor and Chair
Department of Pediatrics
Senior Associate Dean for Educational and Curricular Affairs
University of Vermont College of Medicine
Chief of Pediatrics
Vermont Children's Hospital at Fletcher Allen Health Care
Burlington, Vermont

Joseph A. Zenel, MD, FAAP
Associate Professor and Vice Chair
Department of Pediatrics
Oregon Health & Science University
Doernbecher Children's Hospital
Portland, Oregon

Illustrated by Nadine Sokol

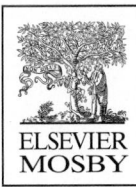

ELSEVIER
MOSBY

ELSEVIER
MOSBY

The Curtis Center
170 S Independence Mall W 300E
Philadelphia, Pennsylvania 19106

PEDIATRICS

ISBN 0-323-01199-3

NOTICE

Pediatrics is an ever-changing field. Standard safety precautions must be followed, but as new research and clinical experience broaden our knowledge, changes in treatment and drug therapy may become necessary or appropriate. Readers are advised to check the most current product information provided by the manufacturer of each drug to be administered to verify the recommended dose, the method and duration of administration, and contraindications. It is the responsibility of the treating physician, relying on experience and knowledge of the patient, to determine dosages and the best treatment for each individual patient. Neither the publisher nor the editors assume any liability for any injury and/or damage to persons or property arising from this publication.

Library of Congress Cataloging-in-Publication Data
Pediatrics/[edited by] Lucy M. Osborn ... [et al.]; illustrated by Nadine Sokol.—1st ed.
    p.; cm.
    ISBN 0-323-01199-3
    1. Pediatrics. 1. Osborn, Lucy M.
    [DNLM: I. Pediatrics. WS 200 P3729 2005]
RJ48.P429 2005
618.92—dc22

2004052407

Acquisitions Editor: Judith Fletcher
Developmental Editor: Marla Sussman
Editorial Assistant: Dana Lamparello
Cover Art: Madeleine Moore

Printed in the United States of America

Last digit is the print number: 9 8 7 6 5 4 3 2 1

*To our colleagues and patients who have taught us
and to our families who have supported us*

To Seth, Andrea, Jenny, and Anne
L.M.O.

To Florence, Keally, Will, and David
T.G.D.

To Sandy, David, and Rachel
L.R.F.

To Jeanette, Matthew, Alison, and Christine
J.A.Z.

CONTRIBUTORS

Henry T. Akinbi, MD
Assistant Professor, Department of Pediatrics, University of Cincinnati; Neonatologist, Divisions of Pulmonary Biology and Neonatology, Children's Hospital Medical Center, Cincinnati, Ohio
■ *Infants of Diabetic Mothers*

Olakunle B. Akintemi, MBBS
Associate Professor, Department of Pediatrics, The University of North Carolina, Chapel Hill, North Carolina; Attending Physician, Department of Pediatrics, Moses Cone Health System, Greensboro, North Carolina
■ *Principles of Decision Making*

Joshua Alexander, MD
Director, Pediatric Rehabilitation, Department of Physical Medicine and Rehabilitation, The University of North Carolina School of Medicine, Chapel Hill, North Carolina
■ *Physical Therapy* ■ *Occupational Therapy*

Paula Algranati, MD
Professor of Pediatrics, Director of Medical Student Education in Pediatrics, Department of Pediatrics, University of Connecticut School of Medicine, Farmington, Connecticut; Attending Physician, Department of Pediatrics, Connecticut Children's Medical Center, Hartford, Connecticut
■ *Physical Examination: Skills and Terminology, Normal Variations, and Implications of Deviations from Normal*

Craig A. Alter, MD
Associate Professor, Department of Pediatrics, University of Pennsylvania; Clinical Associate Professor, Department of Pediatric Endocrinology, The Children's Hospital of Philadelphia, Philadelphia, Pennsylvania
■ *Principles of Growth and Maturation*

Harold N. Amer, MD
Clinical Professor, Department of Pediatrics, University of California at Los Angeles; Medical Director, Pediatric Intensive Care Unit, Cedars-Sinai Medical Center, Los Angeles, California
■ *Acute Respiratory Failure*

Alice Ammerman, DrPH, RD
Associate Professor, Department of Nutrition, Schools of Public Health and Medicine, The University of North Carolina, Chapel Hill, North Carolina
■ *Promoting Healthy Nutrition*

Sudhir K. Anand, MD
Professor, Department of Pediatrics, UCLA School of Medicine, Los Angeles California; Chief, Pediatric Nephrology Division, Department of Pediatrics, Harbor-UCLA Medical Center, Torrance, California
■ *Hypertensive Crisis* ■ *Hematuria and Glomerular Disorders* ■ *Approach to the Child with Proteinuria* ■ *Acute Renal Failure* ■ *Disorders of the Renal Tubules* ■ *Urinary Tract Infections*

Barbara K. Ariue, MD
Clinical Instructor, Department of Pediatrics, Harbor-UCLA Medical Center, Torrance, California; Staff Physician, Department of Pediatrics, Huntington Memorial Hospital, Pasadena, California
■ *Anaphylaxis* ■ *Insect Allergies*

F. Daniel Armstrong, PhD
Professor, Associate Chair and Director, Mailman Center for Child Development, Department of Pediatrics, University of Miami School of Medicine; Chair, Pediatric Bioethics Committee, Department of Pediatrics, Holtz Children's Hospital at the University of Miami/Jackson Memorial Medical Center, Miami, Florida
■ *Conceptualizing Behavioral and Mental Health Issues in Pediatrics*

Robert D. Baker, MD
Professor of Pediatrics, Department of Pediatrics, State University of New York at Buffalo; Co-chief, Digestive and Nutrition Center, Department of Pediatrics, Women and Children's Hospital at Buffalo, Buffalo, New York
■ *Hyperalimentation*

Susan S. Baker, MD, PhD
Professor of Pediatrics, Digestive Diseases and Nutrition Center, Department of Pediatrics, State University of New York at Buffalo; Co-director, Digestive Diseases and Nutrition Center, Department of Pediatrics, Women and Children's Hospital at Buffalo, Buffalo, New York
■ *Hyperalimentation*

James F. Bale, Jr., MD
Professor and Vice Chair, Department of Pediatrics, University of Utah School of Medicine; Medical Staff, Primary Children's Medical Center, Salt Lake City, Utah
■ *Congenital Disorders of the Central Nervous System*

William F. Balistreri, MD
Dorothy M.M. Kersten Professor of Pediatrics, Department of Pediatrics, University of Cincinnati

Medical Center; Director, Department of Gastroenterology, Hepatology, and Nutrition, Cincinnati Children's Hospital Medical Center, Cincinnati, Ohio
■ *Inflammatory Bowel Disease* ■ *Liver and Biliary Tract Disorders* ■ *Liver Transplant*

Michael J. Bamshad, MD
Associate Professor, Departments of Pediatrics and Human Genetics, University of Utah, Salt Lake City, Utah
■ *Principles of Human Genetics* ■ *Presentation and Initial Evaluation of Genetic Disorders*

Steven Barnett, MD
Assistant Professor, Department of Family Medicine, University of Rochester School of Medicine and Dentistry, Rochester, New York
■ *Care of the Deaf Child*

Tammy DeShazo Barry, PhD
Assistant Professor, Department of Psychology, Texas A&M University, College Station, Texas
■ *Aggressive/Oppositional Behaviors (Oppositional Defiant and Conduct Disorders)*

Barry G. Baylen, MD
Clinical Professor of Pediatrics, Department of Pediatrics, University of California at Los Angeles; Chief, Division of Pediatric Cardiology, Department of Pediatrics, Los Angeles County Harbor-UCLA Medical Center, Los Angeles, California
■ *Cardiac Failure* ■ *Approach to the Child with a Heart Murmur* ■ *Acute Cardiac Rhythm Disorders*

Suzanne E. Beck, MD
Assistant Professor of Pediatrics, Department of Pediatrics, Drexel University College of Medicine; Attending Physician, Department of Pediatrics, Section of Pediatric Pulmonology, St. Christopher's Hospital for Children, Philadelphia, Pennsylvania
■ *Bronchoscopy*

Omer G. Berger, MD
Professor of Pediatrics, Department of Pediatrics, University of Cincinnati College of Medicine; Attending Pediatrician, Department of General and Community Pediatrics, Cincinnati Children's Hospital Medical Center, Cincinnati, Ohio
■ *Lead Poisoning*

Carol D. Berkowitz, MD
Professor of Clinical Pediatrics and Executive Vice Chair, Department of Pediatrics, Harbor-UCLA Medical Center, Torrance, California; David Geffen School of Medicine at UCLA, Los Angeles, California
■ *Craniofacial Disorders*

Frank M. Biro, MD
Professor of Clinical Pediatrics, Department of Pediatrics, University of Cincinnati; Associate Director, Division of

Adolescent Medicine, Cincinnati Children's Hospital Medical Center, Cincinnati, Ohio
■ *Male Genitourinary Disorders*

Elizabeth G. Blatt, MSW, ACSW
Social Worker, Main Street School, North Syracuse Central School District, North Syracuse, New York
■ *Child Advocacy*

Steven D. Blatt, MD
Associate Professor of Pediatrics, Director, ENHANCE Services for Children in Foster Care, Department of Pediatrics, SUNY Upstate Medical University; Attending Physician, Department of Pediatrics, University Hospital; Attending Physician, Department of Pediatrics, Crouse Hospital, Syracuse, New York
■ *Child Advocacy*

Linda S. Book, MD
Professor of Pediatrics, Chief, Pediatric Gastroenterology, Hepatology, and Nutrition, Department of Pediatrics, University of Utah; Medical Director, Pediatric Liver Transplantation, Department of Pediatrics, Primary Children's Medical Center, Salt Lake City, Utah
■ *Ascites and Peritonitis* ■ *Acute Hepatobiliary Disorders*

Nicole K. Boramanand, CPNP
Pediatric Nurse Practitioner, Electrophysiology, Section of Pediatric Cardiology, Yale University School of Medicine, New Haven, Connecticut
■ *Chronic Rhythm Disorders*

Carl Bose, MD
Professor and Division Chief, Department of Pediatrics, Division of Neonatal-Perinatal Medicine, The University of North Carolina at Chapel Hill; Attending Neonatologist, North Carolina Children's Hospital, Chapel Hill, North Carolina
■ *Stabilization and Transport of Ill Newborns*

David W. Boyle, MD
Associate Professor, Department of Pediatrics, Indiana University School of Medicine; James Whitcomb Riley Hospital for Children, Indianapolis, Indiana
■ *Delivery Room Management and Transitional Care*

Rebecca C. Brady, MD
Instructor, Department of Pediatrics, University of Cincinnati College of Medicine; Instructor, Department of Pediatrics, Cincinnati Children's Hospital Medical Center, Cincinnati, Ohio
■ *Serious Systemic Infections*

Susan Bratton, MD, MPH
Clinical Professor, Department of Pediatrics, University of Michigan at Ann Arbor; Pediatric Critical Care Medicine Staff, Department of Pediatrics, C. S. Mott Children's Hospital and the University of Michigan Health System, Ann Arbor, Michigan
■ *Approach to the Child with Respiratory Distress*

Maria Britto, MD, MPH
Associate Professor, Department of Pediatrics and Internal Medicine, University of Cincinnati; Associate Professor, Division of Adolescent Medicine, Cincinnati Children's Hospital Medical Center, Cincinnati, Ohio
■ *Chronic Illness in the Adolescent*

Donald C. Bross, PhD, JD
Professor in Pediatrics (Family Law), Department of Pediatrics, University of Colorado School of Medicine; Attorney Member, Child Protection Team, The Children's Hospital; Director of Education and Legal Counsel, Kempe Children's Center, Denver, Colorado
■ *Legal Aspects of Abuse and Neglect*

Carol S. Bruggers, MD
Associate Professor of Pediatrics, Pediatric Hematology-Oncology, University of Utah School of Medicine; Primary Children's Medical Center, Salt Lake City, Utah
■ *Management of the Child with Asplenia*

Karen F. Buchi, MD
Associate Professor, Department of Pediatrics, University of Utah; Active Staff, Department of Pediatrics, University Hospital; Active Staff, Department of Pediatrics, Primary Children's Medical Center, Salt Lake City, Utah
■ *Foster Care*

Silvia Buratti, MD
Fellow, Division of Pediatric Gastroenterology, Hepatology and Nutrition, University of California at San Diego; Children's Hospital and Health Center, San Diego, California; Resident, Department of Pediatrics, Università degli Studi di Genova and IRCCS G. Gaslii, Genoa, Italy
■ *Approach to the Child with Abdominal Pain*

Lisa D. Burrows-MacLean, PhD
Clinical Assistant Professor, Department of Pediatrics and Psychology, University at Buffalo; Clinical Director, Center for Children and Families, University at Buffalo, Buffalo, New York
■ *Behavior Modification* ■ *Mental Health Interventions: Evidence-Based Approaches*

Brenda Bursch, PhD
Associate Professor, Department of Psychiatry and Biobehavioral Sciences and Department of Pediatrics, David Geffen School of Medicine at UCLA; Director of Pain Services, Department of Psychiatry and Biobehavioral Sciences, UCLA Neuropsychiatric Hospital; Associate Director of Pediatric Psychiatry, Consultation Liaison, Department of Psychiatry and Biobehavioral Sciences, UCLA Neuropsychiatric Hospital, Los Angeles, California
■ *Chronic Functional Pain/Somatic Complaints and Associated Disability*

Sergio R. Russo Buzzini, MD, MPH
Assistant Professor of Pediatrics, Division of Adolescent Medicine, Medical University of South Carolina, Charleston, South Carolina
■ *Sexual Development, Sexual Orientation, and Gender Identity Issues*

Darlene A. Calhoun, DO
Rothman Associate Professor, Department of Pediatrics/Neonatology, University of South Florida College of Medicine/All Children's Hospital, St. Petersburg, Florida
■ *The Bleeding Circumcision* ■ *Neonatal Erythrocytosis (Polycythemia)*

Charles W. Callahan, DO, COL, MC
Professor of Pediatrics, Department of Pediatrics, Uniformed University of the Health Sciences, Bethesda, Maryland; Chief, Department of Pediatrics and Pediatrics Pulmonology, Tripler Army Medical Center, Honolulu, Hawaii
■ *Outpatient Asthma Management*

Kathleen M. Campbell, MD
Fellow, Department of Pediatrics, University of Cincinnati College of Medicine; Fellow, Division of Pediatric Gastroenterology, Hepatology, and Nutrition, Department of Pediatrics, Cincinnati Children's Hospital Medical Center, Cincinnati, Ohio
■ *Inflammatory Bowel Disease*

Samuel J. Casella, MD
Associate Professor of Pediatrics, Department of Pediatrics, Dartmouth Medical School, Lebanon, New Hampshire
■ *Disorders of the Thyroid and Parathyroid Glands*

Sara Chaffee, MD
Associate Professor of Pediatrics, Department of Pediatrics, Dartmouth Medical School, Hanover, New Hampshire
■ *Long-term Follow-up of Survivors of Childhood Cancer*

Gary M. Chan, MD
Professor, Department of Pediatrics, University of Utah; University Hospital; Primary Children's Hospital; LDS Hospital, Salt Lake City, Utah
■ *Metabolic Bone Diseases in Children*

Ruey-Kang R. Chang, MD, MPH
Assistant Professor, Department of Pediatrics, David Geffen School of Medicine at UCLA; Pediatric Cardiologist, Department of Pediatrics, Mattel Children's Hospital at UCLA, Los Angeles, California
■ *Approach to the Child with Chest Pain* ■ *Approach to the Child with Syncope*

Michael Chobanian, MD
Associate Professor of Pediatrics and Medicine, Department of Medicine, Dartmouth Medical School; Director of Transplantation, Renal Transplantation, Dartmouth-Hitchcock Medical Center, Lebanon, New Hampshire
■ *Renal Transplant*

Nedra K. Christensen, PhD, RD
Associate Professor, Nutrition and Food Sciences, Utah State University, Logan, Utah
▪ *Principles of Nutrition* ▪ *Nutrition in Children with Chronic Diseases*

Robert D. Christensen, MD
Lewis A. Barness Professor and Chairman, Department of Pediatrics, University of South Florida College of Medicine; Physician in Chief, All Children's Hospital, St. Petersburg, Florida
▪ *The Bleeding Circumcision* ▪ *Neonatal Erythrocytosis (Polycythemia)*

Edward Christophersen, PhD
Professor, Department of Pediatrics, University of Missouri at Kansas City School of Medicine; Staff Psychologist, Department of Pediatrics, Children's Mercy Hospital, Kansas City, Missouri
▪ *Soiling Problems (Encopresis)* ▪ *Day/Nighttime Wetting Problems (Enuresis)*

Joseph A. Church, MD
Professor, Clinical Pediatrics, Keck School of Medicine, University of Southern California; Head, Division of Clinical Immunology and Allergy, Director, Children's AIDS Center, Children's Hospital Los Angeles, Los Angeles, California
▪ *Human Immunodeficiency Virus Infection*

Sterling K. Clarren, MD
Head, Division of Hospital Medicine/Robert A. Aldrich Professor of Pediatrics, Department of Pediatrics, University of Washington School of Medicine; Director, Inpatient Medical Services, Children's Hospital and Regional Medical Center, Seattle, Washington
▪ *Prenatal Factors Affecting the Newborn*

George J. Cohen, MD
Clinical Professor, Department of Pediatrics, George Washington University School of Medicine; Attending Pediatrician, Department of General Pediatrics, Children's National Medical Center, Washington, DC
▪ *Divorce*

Valeria Cohran, MD
Pediatric Gastroenterology Research Fellow, Department of Pediatric Gastroenterology and Hepatology, Cincinnati Children's Hospital Medical Center, Cincinnati, Ohio
▪ *Liver Transplant*

Conrad R. Cole, MD, MPH
Assistant Professor, Department of Pediatrics, Health Policy, and Management, Emory University; Attending Pediatric Gastroenterologist, Children's Healthcare of Atlanta at Egelston, Atlanta, Georgia
▪ *Malabsorption Disorders*

William Coleman, MD
Professor of Pediatrics, Center for Development and Learning, Department of Pediatrics, The University of North Carolina School of Medicine; North Carolina Children's Hospital, Chapel Hill, North Carolina; Assistant Consulting Professor of Pediatrics, Department of Pediatrics, Duke University Medical Center, Durham, North Carolina
▪ *Family Focused Behavioral Pediatrics: A Primary Care Approach*

Stephen H. Contompasis, MD
Associate Professor, Department of Pediatrics, University of Vermont, College of Medicine; Attending Physician, Children's Health Care Service, Fletcher Allen Health Care, Burlington, Vermont
▪ *Special Education*

W. Carl Cooley, MD
Associate Professor of Pediatrics, Department of Pediatrics, Dartmouth Medical School, Hanover, New Hampshire; Medical Director, Crotched Mountain Rehabilitation Center, Greenfield, New Hampshire; Co-director, Center for Medical Home Improvement, Hood Center for Children and Families, Lebanon, New Hampshire
▪ *The Primary Care Medical Home for Children with Special Health Care Needs* ▪ *Down Syndrome*

David M. Coulter, MD
Associate Professor, Division of Neonatology, Department of Pediatrics, University of Utah School of Medicine; Attending Neonatologist, Department of Medicine, Primary Children's Medical Center; Attending Neonatologist, Department of Pediatrics, University of Utah Medical Center; Attending Neonatologist, Department of Pediatrics, LDS Hospital, Salt Lake City, Utah
▪ *Infectious Diseases in the Neonate*

Cori Daines, MD
Assistant Professor, Department of Pediatrics, University of Cincinnati Medical School; Assistant Professor, Department of Pediatric Pulmonary Medicine, Cincinnati Children's Hospital Medical Center, Cincinnati, Ohio
▪ *Disorders of the Bronchi*

Helen F. Deitch, MD
Staff Physician, Department of Obstetrics and Gynecology, Centre Medical and Surgical Associates, PC, State College, Pennsylvania
▪ *Gynecologic Disorders*

Judy T. Del Mundo, MD
Staff Physician, Department of Pediatrics, El Camino Hospital, Mountain View, California; Staff Physician, Department of Pediatrics, O'Connor Hospital; Staff Physician, Department of Pediatrics, Good Samaritan Hospital; Asthma and Allergy for Adults and Children, San Jose, California
▪ *Food and Drug Allergies* ▪ *Serum Sickness*

Gregory B. Di Russo, MD
Assistant Professor, Department of Cardiovascular Surgery, The George Washington University School of

Medicine and Health Sciences; Director of Cardiac Transplantation and Cardiovascular Care, Department of Cardiovascular Surgery, Children's National Medical Center, Washington, DC
- *Long-term Management after Cardiac Surgery*

Mary Beth Dinulos, MD
Assistant Professor of Pediatrics, Department of Pediatrics (Genetics and Child Development), Dartmouth Medical School, Hanover, New Hampshire; Assistant Professor of Pediatrics, Department of Pediatrics (Genetics and Child Development), Dartmouth-Hitchcock Medical Center, Lebanon, New Hampshire
- *Chromosome and Single Gene Disorders*

Tracy R. Dobbins, MA
Graduate Student, Department of Clinical Psychology, The University of North Carolina, Greensboro, North Carolina
- *Principles of Child Development and Developmental Assessment*

Mia Dodson, MD
Fellow in Developmental and Behavorial Pediatrics, Yale University School of Medicine, Department of Pediatrics, New Haven, Connecticut
- *Normal Variations: Personality and Temperament*

Ranjan Dohil, MBBCh, MRCP
Associate Professor, Department of Pediatrics, University of California at San Diego; Pediatric Gastroenterology, Children's Hospital, San Diego, California
- *Disorders of the Stomach*

Howard Dubowitz, MD, MS
Professor of Pediatrics, Chief, Division of Child Protection, Co-director, Center for Families, Department of Pediatrics, University of Maryland School of Medicine; University of Maryland Hospital, Baltimore, Maryland
- *Child Neglect: The Inadequate Promotion of Children's Health and Development*

Nanette C. Dudley, MD
Associate Professor, Department of Pediatrics, University of Utah; Attending Physician, Pediatric Emergency Medicine, Primary Children's Medical Center, Salt Lake City, Utah
- *Glucose and Electrolyte Disorders*

Cynthia Edstrom, MD
Attending Neonatologist, Department of Neonatoloy, St. Luke's Children's Hospital, Boise, Idaho
- *Thrombocytopenia, Bleeding Disorders, and Disorders of Coagulation in Newborn Infants*

Wendi Ehrman, MD
Assistant Professor of Pediatrics, Department of Pediatrics, Medical College of Wisconsin; Assistant Professor of Pediatrics, Department of Pediatrics, Children's Hospital of Wisconsin, Milwaukee, Wisconsin
- *Adolescents and Sexually Transmitted Diseases*

S. Jean Emans, MD
Professor of Pediatrics, Department of Pediatrics, Harvard Medical School; Chief, Division of Adolescent/Young Adult Medicine, Department of Medicine, Children's Hospital Boston, Boston, Massachusetts
- *Contraceptive Methods and Counseling*

Robert Englander, MD, MPH
Associate Professor, Department of Pediatrics, Connecticut Children's Medical Center, University of Connecticut School of Medicine; Director of Inpatient Services, Connecticut Children's Medical Center; Associate Director, Pediatric Residency Training Program, Connecticut Children's Medical Center, Hartford, Connecticut
- *Principles of Pathophysiology*

William A. Engle, MD
Erik T. Ragan Professor of Pediatrics, Department of Pediatrics, Indiana University School of Medicine, Indianapolis, Indiana
- *Delivery Room Management and Transitional Care*

Gregory M. Enns, MB, ChB
Assistant Professor of Pediatrics, Director, Biochemical Genetics Program, Department of Pediatrics, Stanford University, Stanford, California
- *Lysosomal Storage Disorders* ■ *Diagnosis and Treatment of Children with Suspected Metabolic Disease*

Heidi M. Feldman, MD, PhD
Professor of Pediatrics, Department of Pediatrics, University of Pittsburgh School of Medicine; Ronald L. and Patricia M. Violi Professor of Child Development, Department of Pediatrics, Children's Hospital of Pittsburgh, Pittsburgh, Pennsylvania
- *Speech and Language Skills and Language Disorders*

James Filiano, MD
Associate Professor of Pediatrics, Department of Pediatrics/Neurology, Dartmouth-Hitchcock Medical Center, Dartmouth Medical School; Director of Neurometabolism, Department of Pediatrics, Children's Hospital at Dartmouth (CHaD), Lebanon, New Hampshire
- *Neurodegenerative Diseases*

Patricia Flanagan, MD
Associate Professor of Pediatrics, Brown University; Director, Teens with Tots Program, Department of Pediatrics/Adolescent Medicine, Rhode Island Hospital/Hasbro Children's Hospital, Providence, Rhode Island
- *Prevention and Diagnosis of Pregnancy*

Kori Flower, MD, MS, MPH
Fellow, Robert Wood Johnson Clinical Scholars Program, School of Medicine, The University of North Carolina at Chapel Hill; Clinical Instructor, Department of Pediatrics, The University of North Carolina, Chapel Hill, North Carolina
- *Promoting Healthy Nutrition*

Kenneth L. Fox, Jr., MD
Assistant Professor of Pediatrics, Department of Pediatrics, Division of General Pediatrics, Boston University School of Medicine; Staff in Medicine, Department of Pediatrics, Boston Medical Center, Boston, Massachusetts
- *Effects of Poverty*

Gerri Frager, MD, FRCP
Assistant Professor—Pediatrics, Dalhousie University; Medical Director, Pediatric Palliative Care Service, IWK Grace Health Centre, Halifax, Nova Scotia, Canada; Faculty Scholar, Alumnus, Open Society Institute, Project Death in America
- *Bereaved Children*

Mary A. Fristad, PhD, ABPP
Professor, Department of Psychiatry and Psychology, The Ohio State University; Director of Research and Psychological Services, Division of Child and Adolescent Psychiatry, The Ohio State University Medical Center, Columbus, Ohio
- *Sadness and Depressive Disorders*

Paul Fu, Jr., MD, MPH
Assistant Professor, Departments of Pediatrics and Health Services, David Geffen School of Medicine at UCLA and UCLA School of Public Health, Los Angeles, California; Department of Pediatrics, Harbor-UCLA Medical Center, Torrance, California; Office of the CIO and Medical Director for Information Systems, Los Angeles County Department of Health Services, Los Angeles, California
- *Sports Medicine* ▪ *Presentation and Initial Evaluation of Disorders of White Blood Cells*

Marianne Gausche-Hill, MD
Professor of Medicine, Department of Medicine, Geffen School of Medicine at UCLA, Los Angeles, California; Director of EMS, Harbor-UCLA Medical Center, Department of Emergency Medicine; Director of Pediatric Emergency Medicine, Department of Emergency Medicine, Little Company of Mary Hospital, Torrance, California
- *Sudden Infant Death Syndrome (SIDS) and Apparent Life-Threatening Event (ALTE)*

Michael A. Gerber, MD
Professor of Pediatrics, Department of Pediatrics, University of Cincinnati College of Medicine; Attending Physician, Division of Infectious Diseases, Cincinnati Children's Hospital Medical Center, Cincinnati, Ohio
- *Serious Systemic Infections*

George Gershman, MD, PhD
Associate Professor of Pediatrics, Chief, Division of Pediatric Gastroenterology, Department of Pediatrics, Harbor-UCLA Medical Center, Torrance, California
- *Approach to the Child with Gastrointestinal Bleeding*
- *Gastroesophageal Reflux*

Ronald L. Gibson, MD, PhD
Professor, Department of Pediatrics, University of Washington School of Medicine, Seattle, Washington
- *Cystic Fibrosis*

Debora W. Goebel, MD
Pediatric Otolaryngologist, Children's Hospital, Omaha, Nebraska
- *Disorders of the Nose and Sinuses*

Melanie A. Gold, DO
Associate Professor of Pediatrics, Department of Pediatrics, University of Pittsburgh School of Medicine; Director of Family Planning Services and Director of Adolescent Medicine Research, Division of Adolescent Medicine, Children's Hospital of Pittsburgh, Pittsburgh, Pennsylvania
- *Sexual Development, Sexual Orientation, and Gender Identity Issues*

Robert E. Goldsby, MD
Assistant Professor, Department of Pediatrics, University of California, San Francisco, California
- *Leukemias* ▪ *Lymphomas*

Estherann Grace, MD
Associate Clinical Professor of Pediatrics, Department of Pediatrics, Harvard Medical School; Department of Medicine, Children's Hospital, Boston, Massachusetts
- *Eating Problems and Disorders*

Richard Grady, MD
Assistant Professor, Department of Urology, University of Washington; Director, Clinical Research, Department of Pediatric Urology, Children's Hospital and Regional Medical Center, Seattle, Washington
- *Disorders of the Genitourinary System in the Newborn*

Jeanne Greenblatt, MD, MPH
Clinical Associate Professor, Departments of Psychiatry and Pediatrics, University of Vermont, College of Medicine; Attending Physician, Department of Psychiatry, Fletcher Allen Health Care, Burlington, Vermont
- *Psychotropic Agents*

Geeta Grover, MD
Associate Clinical Professor, Department of Pediatrics, University of California, Irvine, College of Medicine; Attending Physician, Department of Developmental-Behavioral Pediatrics, Children's Hospital of Orange County, Orange, California
- *Disorders of the Lower Extremities*

Ann P. Guillot, MD
Professor of Pediatrics, University of Vermont, Department of Pediatrics, Vermont Children's Hospital; Director of Pediatric Nephrology and Residency Program, Vermont Children's Hospital, Burlington, Vermont
- *Fluids and Electrolytes*

Daniel T. Gustafson, PhD, Major (USAF)
Child Psychologist, 31st Medical Group, Aviano, Italy
- *Obsessive-Compulsive Disorder: Cognitive-Behavioral and Psychopharmacologic Treatments*

Stephen L. Guthery, MD, MSc
Assistant Professor of Pediatrics, Division of Pediatric
Gastroenterology and Nutrition, University of Utah
School of Medicine, Primary Children's Medical Center,
Salt Lake City, Utah
■ *Liver and Biliary Tract Disorders*

Joseph F. Hagan, Jr., MD, FAAP
Clinical Professor, Department of Pediatrics, University of
Vermont College of Medicine; Vermont Children's
Hospital at Fletcher Allen Health Care; Primary Care
Pediatrician, Hagan and Rinehart Pediatricians, Burlington,
Vermont
■ *Divorce*

Neal Halfon, MD, MPH
Director, UCLA Center for Healthier Children, Families,
and Communities, University of California; Professor,
Department of Pediatrics, Public Health, and Policy
Studies, University of California, Los Angeles, California
■ *Developmental and Behavioral Surveillance and
Promotion of Parenting Skills*

Jane N. Hannah, EdD
Lower School Head, Currey Ingram Academy, Brentwood,
Tennessee
■ *Learning Disabilities*

Janet K. Harnsberger, MD
Clinical Professor of Pediatrics and Family Practice,
Department of Pediatrics, University of Utah, Salt Lake
City, Utah
■ *Approach to the Child with Difficulty Swallowing*

Lisa Hartling, MSc
Research Associate, Department of Pediatrics, University
of Alberta, Edmonton, Alberta, Canada
■ *Principles of Clinical Epidemiology*

Jacinto Hernandez, MD
Professor of Pediatrics, Department of Neonatology,
University of Colorado Health Sciences Center;
The Children's Hospital, University Hospital,
Centura-Porter Adventist Hospital, Centura Littleton
Adventist Hospital, Centura Avista Adventist Hospital,
Centura–St. Anthony Central, Centura–St. Anthony
North, Denver Health Medical Center, Exempla/Lutheran
Medical Center, Exempla/St. Joseph's Hospital, Denver,
Colorado
■ *Routine Care of the Full-Term Newborn*

Mark Herron MD
Resident Physician, Department of Dermatology,
University of Utah School of Medicine, Salt Lake City,
Utah
■ *Approach to Dermatologic Disease and Eczematoid
Eruptions* ■ *Papulosquamous Disorders* ■ *Disorders of
the Sebaceous and Sweat Glands* ■ *Disorders of the Hair
and Nails* ■ *Disorders of Pigmentation* ■ *Cutaneous
Tumors* ■ *Dermatologic Manifestations of Systemic
Disease* ■ *Acne*

Harry R. Hill, MD
Professor, Departments of Pathology, Pediatrics, and
Medicine, University of Utah Medical Center; Professor,
Primary Children's Medical Center, Salt Lake City, Utah
■ *Complement Disorders* ■ *Phagocytic and Leukocyte
Abnormalities* ■ *T- and B-Lymphocyte Disorders*

Paula J. Adams Hillard, MD
Professor, Department of Obstetrics and Gynecology,
University of Cincinnati College of Medicine; Director of
Gynecology, Division of Adolescent Medicine, Cincinnati
Children's Hospital Medical Center, Cincinnati, Ohio
■ *Gynecologic Disorders*

Richard Hong, MD
Clinical Professor, Department of Pediatrics, University
of Vermont School of Medicine; Attending Physician,
Department of Pediatrics and Medicine, Fletcher Allen
Health Care, Burlington, Vermont
■ *Principles of Immunology*

Katharine Hopkins, MD
Associate Professor, Department of Diagnostic Radiology,
Oregon Health & Science University; Chief, Department
of Pediatric Radiology, Doernbecher Children's Hospital,
Portland, Oregon
■ *Diagnostic Imaging*

Kenneth Huff, MD
Professor, Department of Pediatrics and Neurology, UCLA
School of Medicine, Los Angeles, California; Chief,
Division of Neurology, Department of Pediatrics, Harbor-
UCLA Medical Center, Torrance, California
■ *Central Nervous System Failure* ■ *Approach to the
Child with Breath-Holding Spells* ■ *Approach to the Child
with Weakness or Paralysis* ■ *Approach to the Child with
Movement Disorders*

Christopher M. Hull, MD
Resident Physician, Department of Dermatology,
University of Utah School of Medicine, Salt Lake City,
Utah
■ *Approach to Dermatologic Disease and Eczematoid
Eruptions*

Laura M. Ibsen, MD
Assistant Professor, Department of Pediatrics, Oregon
Health & Science University; Medical Director,
Cardiovascular Intensive Care, Pediatric Intensive
Care Unit, Doernbecher Children's Hospital, Portland,
Oregon
■ *Approach to the Child with Respiratory Distress*
■ *Vascular Access*

Stanley H. Inkelis, MD
Professor of Pediatrics, Department of Pediatrics, David
Geffen School of Medicine at UCLA, Los Angeles,
California; Director, Pediatric Emergency Medicine,
Department of Emergency Medicine, Harbor-UCLA
Medical Center, Torrance, California
■ *Disorders of the Pharynx*

J. Craig Jackson, MD

Professor, Department of Pediatrics, University of Washington; Medical Director, Infant ICU, Children's Hospital and Regional Medical Center, Seattle, Washington

■ *Respiratory Disease in the Newborn* ■ *Aspiration Syndromes* ■ *Respiratory Distress Syndrome* ■ *Diagnosis and Management of Air Leaks* ■ *Persistent Pulmonary Hypertension of the Newborn* ■ *Atelectasis* ■ *Bronchopulmonary Dysplasia*

Alain Joffe, MD, MPH

Director, Student Health and Wellness Center, Johns Hopkins University; Associate Professor of Pediatrics, Johns Hopkins Medical Institutions, Baltimore, Maryland

■ *Legal and Ethical Issues in Adolescent Health Care*

F. Leonard Johnson, MD

The Robert C. Neerhout and Credit Union for Kids Professor of Pediatrics and Chairman, Department of Pediatrics, Oregon Health & Science University; Physician in Chief, Doernbecher Children's Hospital, Portland, Oregon

■ *Blood and Bone Marrow Transplantation (Hematopoietic Stem Cell Transplantation)* ■ *Blood Product Transfusions*

Jennifer Johnson, MD, MS

Associate Professor, Emeritus, Department of Pediatrics, University of California at Irvine, Orange, California

■ *Psychosocial Issues of Maturation*

Wendi A. Johnson, MD

Department of Pediatrics, St. Cloud Hospital; CentraCare Women and Children's Clinic, St. Cloud, Minnesota

■ *Sports and the Adolescent*

Troy Johnston, MD

Assistant Professor of Pediatrics, Department of Pediatrics, University of Washington; Seattle Children's Hospital and Regional Medical Center, Seattle, Washington

■ *Disorders of the Cardiovascular System in the Newborn*

Gary R. Jones, MD

Associate Professor, Department of Pediatrics, Oregon Health & Science University; Attending Physician, Division of Pediatric Hematology/Oncology, Doernbecher Children's Hospital; Medical Director, Childhood and Adolescent Bone Tumor Program, Shriners Children's Hospital, Portland, Oregon

■ *Antineoplastic Agents*

Kenneth Lyons Jones, MD

Professor of Pediatrics, Department of Pediatrics, UCSD School of Medicine, La Jolla, California; Professor, Department of Pediatrics, UCSD Medical Center, San Diego, California

■ *Principles of Dysmorphology*

Marilyn C. Jones, MD

Adjunct Professor, Department of Pediatrics, University of California at San Diego, La Jolla, California; Director,

Dysmorphology and Genetics, Children's Hospital and Health Center, San Diego, California

Principles of Dysmorphology

Nicholas Jospe, MD

Associate Professor of Pediatrics, University of Rochester; Golisano Children's Hospital at Strong, Department of Pediatrics, University of Rochester, Rochester, New York

■ *Disorders of Pubertal Development* ■ *Disorders of Sexual Differentiation* ■ *Disorders of the Adrenal Glands*

James J. Joyce, MD, FACC

Associate Professor of Clinical Pediatrics, Department of Pediatrics, Tulane University School of Medicine; Director of the Adult Congenital Heart Disease Program, Departments of Pediatrics and Internal Medicine, Tulane University Medical Center, New Orleans, Louisiana

■ *Approach to the Child with a Heart Murmur* ■ *Acute Cardiac Rhythm Disorders*

Amy H. Kaji, MD

Research and Disaster Medicine Fellow, Department of Emergency Medicine, Harbor-UCLA Medical Center, Torrance, California

■ *Sudden Infant Death Syndrome (SIDS) and Apparent Life-Threatening Event (ALTE)*

Karen Ann Kalinyak, MD

Professor of Pediatrics, Division of Hematology/Oncology, Medical Director, Division of Hematology/Oncology, Temple University School of Medicine, Philadelphia, Pennsylvania; Professor of Pediatrics, Medical Director, Department of Hematology/Oncology, Cincinnati Children's Hospital Medical Center, Cincinnati, Ohio

■ *Anemias and Other Disorders of Red Blood Cells*
■ *Chronic Anemia*

Lawrence C. Kaplan, MD, ScM, FAAP

Associate Professor of Pediatrics, Department of Pediatrics, Dartmouth Medical School, Hanover, New Hampshire; Director, Division of Genetics and Child Development, Department of Pediatrics, Children's Hospital at Dartmouth, Lebanon, New Hampshire

■ *Cerebral Palsy and Post-anoxic Disorders*

Lilah M. Katcher

Project Manager, Wisconsin Early Hearing Detection and Intervention Tracking, Wisconsin Division of Public Health, Madison, Wisconsin

■ *Care of the Deaf Child*

Murray L. Katcher, MD, PhD

Professor of Pediatrics, University of Wisconsin Medical School; Chief Medical Officer and State Maternal and Child Health Director, Wisconsin Division of Public Health, Madison, Wisconsin

■ *Care of the Deaf Child*

Anne E. Kazak, PhD, ABPP

Professor, Department of Pediatrics, University of Pennsylvania; Director, Department of Psychology, The

Children's Hospital of Philadelphia, Philadelphia, Pennsylvania
- *Adaptation in Childhood Chronic Illness: Risk and Protective Factors*

Kathi J. Kemper, MD, MPH
Caryl J. Guth Chair for Holistic and Integrative Medicine, Professor of Pediatrics and Public Health Sciences, Wake Forest University Baptist Medical Center, Winston-Salem, North Carolina
- *Principles of Integrative Pediatrics*

William A. Kennedy, MD
Assistant Professor of Pediatrics, Department of Pediatrics, University of California, Los Angeles, California; Harbor-UCLA Medical Center, Department of Pediatric Infectious Diseases, Torrance, California
- *Infections of the Central Nervous System* ■ *Disorders of the Lungs and Pleura*

Edward Kent, MD, FAAAI
Clinical Associate Professor of Pediatrics, University of Vermont School of Medicine, Burlington, Vermont; Allergy and Asthma Associates PC, Timberlane Medical Center, South Burlington, Vermont
- *Allergy and Skin Testing*

Perri Klass, MD
Assistant Professor, Department of Pediatrics, Boston University School of Medicine, Boston, Massachusetts; President and Medical Director, Reach Out and Read National Center, Somerville, Massachusetts
- *Literacy*

Terry P. Klassen, MD, MSc, FRCPC
Professor and Chair, Department of Pediatrics, University of Alberta; Clinical Leader, Stollery Children's Hospital, Edmonton, Alberta, Canada
- *Principles of Clinical Epidemiology*

Thomas S. Klitzner, MD, PhD
Professor, Department of Pediatrics, David Geffen School of Medicine at UCLA; Chief, Pediatric Cardiology, Department of Pediatrics, Mattel Children's Hospital at UCLA, Los Angeles, California
- *Approach to the Child with Chest Pain* ■ *Approach to the Child with Syncope*

Jane Knapp, MD, FAAP, FACEP
Professor of Pediatrics, Department of Pediatrics, University of Missouri; Children's Mercy Hospital, Kansas City, Missouri
- *Aspiration and Ingestion of Foreign Bodies*

Thomas Koch, MD
Professor, Department of Pediatrics and Neurology, Oregon Health & Science University; Director of Pediatrics Neurology, Department of Neurology, Doernbecher Children's Hospital, Portland, Oregon
- *Electrodiagnostics in Pediatrics* ■ *Antiepileptic Therapy*

Samuel A. Kocoshis, MD
Professor of Pediatrics, University of Cincinnati College of Medicine; Director, Nutrition and Intestinal Transplantation, Gastroenterology, Hepatology and Nutrition, Cincinnati Children's Hospital Medical Center, Cincinnati, Ohio
- *Congenital Anatomic Disorders of the Gastrointestinal Tract* ■ *Malabsorption Disorders*

Jeffrey L. Koh, MD, MBA
Director, Pain Management Center, Associate Professor, Department of Anesthesiology, Oregon Health & Science University, Portland, Oregon
- *Analgesics/Pain Medications/Sedation*

Alan Kohrt, MD
Clinical Associate Professor, Department of Pediatrics, University of Pennsylvania School of Medicine; Attending Physician, Diagnostic Center, The Children's Hospital of Philadelphia, Philadelphia, Pennsylvania; Pediatric Advisor, Educating Physicians in their Communities (EPIC) Immunization Education Program, Pennsylvania Chapter, American Academy of Pediatrics, Rosemont, Pennsylvania
- *Immunizations: A Systems Approach*

Lois Kohrt, BS
Director of Practice Management, Ambulatory Administration, The Children's Hospital of Philadelphia, Philadelphia, Pennsylvania; Practice Management Advisor, Co-author, Trainer, Immunizations Education Program, Pennsylvania Chapter, American Academy of Pediatrics, Rosemont, Pennsylvania
- *Immunizations: A Systems Approach*

Patricia K. Kokotailo, MD, MPH
Associate Professor, Director of Adolescent Medicine, Department of Pediatrics, University of Wisconsin–Madison Medical School, Madison, Wisconsin
- *Risk and Resilience* ■ *Alcohol, Tobacco, and Other Drug Use*

Dan Kovarik, MD
Director of Pediatric Anesthesia, Maine Medical Center, Portland, Maine; Assistant Clinical Professor of Anesthesia, Vermont College of Medicine, Burlington, Vermont
- *Analgesics/Pain Medications/Sedation*

Rekha Krishnankutty, MD
Fellow, Department of Pediatrics, Harbor-UCLA Medical Center, Torrance, California
- *Infections of the Skin*

Alan M. Lake, MD, FAAP
Associate Professor, Department of Pediatrics, Johns Hopkins University School of Medicine, Baltimore, Maryland
- *Disorders of the Gastrointestinal Tract and Liver*

Gregory L. Landry, MD
Professor, Department of Pediatrics, University of Wisconsin Medical School; Staff Physician, Department of

Pediatrics and Sports Medicine, University of Wisconsin Hospital; Head Medical Team Physician, Division of Intercollegiate Athletics, University of Wisconsin, Madison, Wisconsin
- *Sports and the Adolescent*

Kyle Landt, MD
Assistant Professor, Department of Pediatrics, Dartmouth Medical School, Hanover, New Hampshire; Assistant Professor, Department of Pediatrics, Dartmouth-Hitchcock Medical Center, Lebanon, New Hampshire; Staff, Department of Pediatrics, Elliott Hospital, Manchester, New Hampshire
- *Disorders of Growth and Stature*

Wendy Lane, MD, MPH
Instructor, Department of Pediatrics and Epidemiology and Preventive Medicine, University of Maryland School of Medicine, Baltimore, Maryland
- *Disease Screening and Surveillance*

Jason Lang, MD
Clinical Fellow in Pulmonary Medicine, Children's Hospital Boston, Harvard Medical School, Boston, Massachusetts
- *Blood Product Transfusion*

Carole Lannon, MD, MPH
Co-director, North Carolina Center for Children's Healthcare Improvement, The University of North Carolina at Chapel Hill; Clinical Associate Professor, Department of Pediatrics and Internal Medicine, The University of North Carolina School of Medicine, Chapel Hill, North Carolina; Senior Vice President, National Initiative for Children's Healthcare Quality (NICHQ), Boston, Massachusetts
- *Improving Preventive Services for Children*

Timothy R. La Pine, MD
Adjunct Assistant Professor of Pathology, Assistant Professor of Pediatrics, University of Utah; Adjunct Assistant Professor of Pathology, Assistant Professor of Pediatrics, University of Utah Medical Center; Assistant Professor, Primary Children's Medical Center, Salt Lake City, Utah
- *Complement Disorders* ▪ *Phagocytic and Leukocyte Abnormalities* ▪ *T- and B-Lymphocyte Disorders*

David Lawrence, MD
Fellow, Division of Neonatology, Cincinnati Children's Hospital, Cincinnati, Ohio
- *Infants of Diabetic Mothers*

Kenneth K. Lee, MD
Assistant Professor of Pediatrics, Department of Pediatrics, Division of Pediatric Gastroenterology, Medical College of Wisconsin; Attending Physician, Department of Pediatrics, Division of Pediatric Gastroenterology, Children's Hospital of Wisconsin, Milwaukee, Wisconsin
- *Endoscopy*

Peter Lee, MD
Department of Pediatric Gastroenterology, INOVA Fairfax Hospital for Children, Fairfax, Virginia
- *Congenital Anatomic Disorders of the Gastrointestinal Tract*

Corinne E. Lehmann, MD
Assistant Professor, Departments of General Internal Medicine and Pediatrics, University of Cincinnati College of Medicine; Assistant Professor, Division of Adolescent Medicine, Cincinnati Children's Hospital Medical Center, Cincinnati, Ohio
- *Male Genitourinary Disorders*

Richard S. Lemons, MD, PhD
Division Chief and Medical Director, Department of Pediatrics, Division of Pediatric Hematology-Oncology, University of Utah Medical Center; Medical Director, Department of Pediatric Hematology-Oncology, Primary Children's Medical Center, Salt Lake City, Utah
- *Bone Marrow Dysfunction* ▪ *Leukemias* ▪ *Lymphomas*

Claire O. Leonard, MD
Associate Professor, Department of Pediatrics, University of New Mexico, Albuquerque, New Mexico
- *Presentation and Initial Evaluation of Metabolic Disorders* ▪ *Disorders of Energy Metabolism* ▪ *Disorders of Protein Metabolism*

Nancy D. Leslie, MD
Associate Professor of Clinical Pediatrics, Division of Human Genetics, Cincinnati Children's Hospital Medical Center, Cincinnati, Ohio
- *Principles of Metabolism*

Marcia Levetown, MD, FAAP
Adjunct Associate Professor, Department of Internal Medicine, Baylor College of Medicine; Director, Department of Palliative Care, The Methodist Hospital; Independent Consultant, Palliative Care Education and Program Development; Pediatric Hospice Physician, Houston Hospice, Houston, Texas
- *Bereaved Children*

Charlotte W. Lewis, MD, MPH
Assistant Professor, Department of Pediatrics, University of Washington; Attending Pediatrician, Department of Pediatrics, Children's Hospital and Regional Medical Center, Seattle, Washington
- *Dental Disorders*

Paul F. Lewis, MD
Associate Professor, Department of Pediatrics, Oregon Health & Science University; Public Health Physician, Oregon Health Services, Acute and Communicable Disease, Portland, Oregon
- *Bacterial Infections* ▪ *Viral Infections*

Mary Ann Limbos, MD, MPH
Associate Professor of Clinical Pediatrics, Department of Pediatrics, USC Keck School of Medicine; Attending

Physician, Department of General Pediatrics, Children's Hospital at Los Angeles, Los Angeles, California
■ *Approach to the Child with Diarrhea* ■ *Approach to the Child with Constipation*

Gregory S. Liptak, MD, MPH
Professor, Department of Pediatrics, University of Rochester Medical Center; Attending Physician, Department of Pediatrics, Strong Memorial Hospital, Rochester, New York
■ *Spina Bifida*

Clive M. Liu, MD
Resident Physician, Department of Dermatology, University of Utah School of Medicine, Salt Lake City, Utah
■ *Vesiculobullous Disorders*

John E. Lochman, PhD
Professor and Saxon Chairholder in Clinical Psychology, Department of Psychology, University of Alabama, Tuscaloosa, Alabama; Adjunct Professor of Psychiatry and Behavioral Sciences, Department of Psychiatry and Behavioral Sciences, Duke University Medical Center, Durham, North Carolina
■ *Aggressive/Oppositional Behaviors (Oppositional Defiant and Conduct Disorders)*

Gillian Lockitch, MB, ChB, MD, FRCPC
Professor, Department of Pathology and Laboratory Medicine, University of British Columbia; Director, Department of Pathology and Laboratory Medicine, Children's and Women's Health Centre of British Columbia, Vancouver, British Columbia, Canada
■ *Laboratory Testing of Infants and Children*

Joan MacCracken, MD
Emeritus Associate Clinical Professor, Department of Pediatrics, Tufts University Medical School, Boston, Massachusetts; Emeritus Staff, Departments of Pediatrics and Pediatric Endocrinology and Diabetes, Eastern Maine Medical Center, Bangor, Maine
■ *Diabetes Mellitus*

Ashima Madan, MD
Associate Professor of Pediatrics (Neonatology), Department of Pediatrics, Stanford University School of Medicine, Stanford, California; Lucile Salter Packard Children's Hospital at Stanford, Palo Alto, California
■ *Jaundice*

Anthony J. Mancini, MD
Associate Professor, Department of Pediatrics and Dermatology, Northwestern University Feinberg School of Medicine; Attending Physician, Department of Pediatrics, Children's Memorial Hospital, Chicago, Illinois
■ *Disorders of the Cutaneous Blood Vessels*

Catherine S. Mao, MD
Assistant Professor, Department of Pediatrics, Division of Pediatric Endocrinology, Harbor-UCLA Medical Center;

Data and Safety Monitor, General Clinical Research Center, Harbor-UCLA Research and Education Institute, Torrance, California
■ *Glucose and Electrolyte Disorders* ■ *Genital Disorders in Preadolescent Boys* ■ *Genital Disorders in Preadolescent Girls*

John S. March, MD, MPH
Professor and Chair, Division of Child and Adolescent Psychiatry, Department of Psychiatry and Behavioral Sciences, Duke University Medical Center, Durham, North Carolina
■ *Anxiety Disorders in Children and Adolescents*

Bruce J. Masek, PhD
Associate Professor of Psychiatry, Department of Psychiatry, Harvard Medical School; Director, Child and Adolescent Psychiatry, Department of Psychiatry, Massachusetts General Hospital, Boston, Massachusetts
■ *Obsessive-Compulsive Disorder: Cognitive-Behavioral and Psychopharmacologic Treatments*

Thornton B. A. Mason II, MD, PhD
Assistant Professor, Department of Neurology and Pediatrics, University of Pennsylvania; Attending Neurologist, Division of Neurology, The Children's Hospital of Philadelphia, Philadelphia, Pennsylvania
■ *Sleep Problems and Disorders*

Steven C. Matson, MD
Clinical Professor of Pediatrics, Department of Pediatrics, University of Wisconsin Medical School, Madison, Wisconsin; Senior Physician, Norris Health Center, University of Wisconsin, Milwaukee, Wisconsin
■ *Adolescents and Sexually Transmitted Diseases*

Doreen Matsui, MD, FRCPC
Associate Professor, Department of Pediatrics, University of Western Ontario; Department of Pediatrics, Children's Hospital of Western Ontario, London, Ontario, Canada
■ *Adherence*

Jeanne McAllister, RN, BSN, MS, MHA
Research Associate and Instructor in Pediatrics, Department of Pediatrics, Dartmouth-Hitchcock Medical Center/Dartmouth Medical School; Co-director, Center for Medical Home Improvement, Hood Center for Children and Families, Children's Hospital at Dartmouth-Hitchcock Medical Center, Lebanon, New Hampshire
■ *School Issues in Children with Chronic Illness*

Paul T. McEnery, MD
Professor of Pediatrics, University of Cincinnati College of Medicine; Professor of Pediatrics, Division of Nephrology and Hypertension, Cincinnati Children's Hospital Medical Center, Cincinnati, Ohio
■ *Long-term Management of Renal Disorders* ■ *Hypertension*

Terrence McGraw, MD, FAAP
Associate Professor, Department of Anesthesiology and Pediatrics, Oregon Health & Science University; Associate

Director, Pediatric Pain Management Center, Doernbecher Children's Hospital, Portland, Oregon
■ *Analgesics/Pain Medications/Sedation*

Gwen McIntosh, MD, MPH
Assistant Professor, Department of Pediatrics, University of Wisconsin; University of Wisconsin Children's Hospital, Department of Pediatrics, Madison, Wisconsin
■ *Adolescents and Violence*

Henry Milczuk, MD
Assistant Professor, Departments of Otolaryngology and Pediatrics, Oregon Health & Science University, Portland, Oregon
■ *Disorders of the Neck and Salivary Glands* ■ *Disorders of the Larynx and Trachea*

J. Ross Milley, MD, PhD
Director, Division of Neonatology, Department of Pediatrics, University of Utah School of Medicine; Staff, University of Utah Medical Center, Department of Pediatrics, University Hospital; Staff, Department of Pediatrics, Primary Children's Medical Center, Salt Lake City, Utah
■ *Disorders of Calcium Metabolism* ■ *Disorders of the Thyroid*

Jodi A. Mindell, PhD
Professor, Deparment of Psychology, Saint Joseph's University; Associate Director, Sleep Disorders Center, The Children's Hospital of Philadelphia, Philadelphia, Pennsylvania
■ *Sleep Problems and Disorders*

Mark M. Mitsnefes, MD, MS
Assistant Professor, Department of Pediatrics, Division of Nephrology and Hypertension, Cincinnati Children's Hospital Medical Center and University of Cincinnati, College of Medicine, Cincinnati, Ohio
■ *Hypertension*

Thomas Mock, PhD, FCACB
Clinical Assistant Professor, Department of Pathology and Laboratory Medicine, University of British Columbia; Clinical Biochemist, Department of Pathology and Laboratory Medicine, Children's and Women's Health Centre of British Columbia, Vancouver, British Columbia
■ *Laboratory Testing of Infants and Children*

Julie Mohr, MSPH, PhD
Assistant Professor, Department of Medicine, University of Chicago, Chicago, Illinois
■ *Improving Preventive Services for Children*

Rona Molodow, MD, JD
Associate Clinical Professor, Department of Pediatrics, University of California, Los Angeles, California; Department of Pediatrics, Olive View–UCLA Medical Center, Sylmar, California
■ *Approach to the Agitated Patient*

Richard A. Molteni, MD
Clinical Professor and Associate Dean, Department of Pediatrics, University of Washington School of Medicine; Vice President Medical Director, Children's Hospital and Regional Medical Center, Seattle, Washington
■ *The Ill Newborn: Early Identification and Stabilization*

Susan L. Mortweet, PhD
Assistant Professor, Department of Pediatrics, University of Missouri–Kansas City School of Medicine; Licensed Psychologist, Section of Developmental and Behavioral Sciences, Children's Mercy Hospital, Kansas City, Missouri
■ *Soiling Problems (Encopresis)* ■ *Day/Nighttime Wetting Problems (Enuresis)*

William Walker Motley III, MD, MS
Assistant Professor, Department of Ophthalmology, University of Cincinnati; Assistant Professor, Department of Ophthalmology, Cincinnati Children's Hospital Medical Center, Cincinnati, Ohio
■ *Care of the Blind Child*

William Mow, MD
Clinical Pediatric Gastroenterologist, Kaiser Permanente Medical Group, Hayward, California
■ *Disorders of the Intestine* ■ *Disorders of the Pancreas*

Charles Myer, MD
Professor, Department of Otolaryngology—Head and Neck Surgery, University of Cincinnati; Division of Pediatric Otolaryngology, Cincinnati Children's Hospital Medical Center, Cincinnati, Ohio
■ *Disorders of the Nose and Sinuses*

Jennifer M. Neal, MA
Graduate Student, Department of Psychology, The University of North Carolina, Greensboro, North Carolina
■ *Principles of Child Development and Developmental Assessment*

Robert Needlman, MD
Adjunct Associate Professor of Pediatrics, Department of Pediatrics, Case Western Reserve University School of Medicine; Attending Physician, Department of Pediatrics, MetroHealth Medical Center, Cleveland, Ohio; Vice President for Developmental and Behavioral Pediatrics, The Dr. Spock Company, Menlo Park, California
■ *Literacy*

John M. Neff, MD
Professor, Department of Pediatrics, University of Washington School of Medicine; Director, Center for Children with Special Needs, Children's Hospital and Regional Medical Center, Seattle, Washington
■ *Financial Issues and Other Resources*

Eliot Nelson, MD
Professor of Pediatrics, Department of Pediatrics, University of Vermont College of Medicine; Attending Physician, Department of Pediatrics, Vermont Children's

Hospital at Fletcher Allen Health Care, Burlington, Vermont
- *Injury Prevention*

Peter A. Nigrovic, MD
Fellow, Harvard Medical School; Fellow in Rheumatology, Division of Immunology, Children's Hospital of Boston; Fellow in Rheumatology, Division of Rheumatology, Immunology, and Allergy, Brigham and Women's Hospital, Boston, Massachusetts
- *Anti-inflammatory and Immunomodulatory Therapy*

Julie Noble, MD
Clinical Professor of Pediatrics, Department of Pediatrics, University of California, Los Angeles, California; Director of Community Health Plan, Director Low-Risk Nursery, Department of Pediatrics, Harbor-UCLA Medical Center, Torrance, California
- *Approach to the Febrile Patient* ▪ *Approach to the Ill-Appearing Child*

Laura Noonan, MD
Clinical Associate Professor, Department of Pediatrics, The University of North Carolina, Chapel Hill, North Carolina; General Pediatric Faculty, Department of Pediatrics, Carolinas Medical Center, Charlotte, North Carolina
- *Improving Preventive Services for Children*

Richard E. Nordgren, MD
Professor of Pediatrics and Medicine (Neurology), Department of Pediatrics, Dartmouth Medical School, Hanover, New Hampshire; Professor of Pediatrics and Medicine (Neurology), Department of Pediatrics, Mary Hitchcock Medical Center, Lebanon, New Hampshire
- *Myopathies and Neuropathies*

Chuck Norlin, MD
Associate Professor, Department of Pediatrics, University of Utah; Member, Medical Staff, Department of Medicine, Primary Children's Medical Center; Assistant Medical Director for Pediatrics, Department of Pediatrics, University of Utah Hospitals and Clinics, Salt Lake City, Utah
- *Pediatric Cardiac Transplantation*

Chad K. Oh, MD
Clinical Associate Professor, Department of Pediatrics, The David Geffen School of Medicine at UCLA, Los Angeles, California; Chief, Allergy and Immunology, Department of Pediatrics, Harbor-UCLA Medical Center, Torrance, California
- *Anaphylaxis* ▪ *Food and Drug Allergies* ▪ *Serum Sickness* ▪ *Insect Allergies*

Chris L. Ohlemeyer, MD
Associate Professor, Department of Pediatrics, Saint Louis University; Director, Adolescent Medicine, Cardinal Glennon Children's Hospital, St. Louis, Missouri
- *Menstrual Disorders*

Robin Ohls, MD
Associate Professor of Pediatrics, Department of Pediatrics/Neonatology, University of New Mexico; Attending Neonatologist, University of New Mexico Children's Hospital, Albuquerque, New Mexico
- *Anemia in the Neonatal Period*

Ardis L. Olson, MD
Associate Professor of Pediatrics, Dartmouth Medical School, Hanover, New Hampshire; Attending Pediatrician, Department of Pediatrics, Dartmouth-Hitchcock Medical Center, Lebanon, New Hampshire
- *Competencies Needed in Caring for Children with Chronic Conditions* ▪ *Communication with Families and Specialists* ▪ *The Primary Care Medical Home for Children with Special Health Care Needs* ▪ *Neurodegenerative Diseases*

Lucy M. Osborn, MD, MSPH, FAAP
Professor Emeritus, Department of Pediatrics, University of Utah Medical School, Salt Lake City, Utah
- *Well Child Care: A Strategic Approach* ▪ *Parasitic Infections*

Lee M. Pachter, DO
Professor of Pediatrics and Anthropology, Head, Division of General Pediatrics, University of Connecticut School of Medicine, Farmington, Connecticut; Department of Pediatrics, Saint Francis Hospital and Medical Center, Hartford, Connecticut
- *The Effects of Culture on Child Health*

Jan E. Paisley, MD
Neonatologist, Department of Pediatrics, University of Colorado Health Science Center; Neonatologist, Department of Neonatology, The Children's Hospital, Denver, Colorado; Medical Director of the Special Care Nursery, Department of Pediatrics, Poudre Valley Hospital, Fort Collins, Colorado
- *Long-term Care of the Child with Bronchopulmonary Dysplasia*

Frederick B. Palmer, MD
Shainberg Professor of Pediatrics, Department of Pediatrics, University of Tennessee Health Science Center; Director, Boling Center for Developmental Disabilities, University of Tennessee Health Science Center, Memphis, Tennessee
- *Mental Retardation*

Murray H. Passo, MD
Professor of Clinical Pediatrics, Department of Pediatrics, Division of Rheumatology, University of Cincinnati School of Medicine; Clinical Director, Division of Rheumatology, Cincinnati Children's Hospital Medical Center, Cincinnati, Ohio
- *General Approach to the Child with Suspected Rheumatologic Disease* ▪ *Juvenile Rheumatoid Arthritis* ▪ *Systemic Lupus Erythematosus and Juvenile Dermatomyositis* ▪ *Fibromyalgia and Other Idiopathic Pain Syndromes*

Kevin Patrick, MD, MS
Professor, Department of Family and Preventive
Medicine, University of California, San Diego; Editor
in Chief, *American Journal of Preventive Medicine*,
University of California at San Diego, La Jolla,
California
■ *Promoting Physical Activity*

Howard A. Pearson, MD
Professor of Pediatrics, Emeritus, Department of
Pediatrics, Yale University School of Medicine; Attending
Physician, Department of Pediatrics, Yale–New Haven
Hospital, New Haven, Connecticut
■ *Chronic Anemia*

William E. Pelham, Jr., PhD
Professor, Department of Psychology, Pediatrics, and
Psychiatry, University at Buffalo; Director, Center for
Children and Families, University at Buffalo, Buffalo,
New York
■ *Behavior Modification* ■ *Mental Health Interventions:
Evidence-Based Approaches*

Eliana Perrin, MD, MPH
Assistant Professor, Division of Community Pediatrics,
Department of Pediatrics, The University of North
Carolina, Chapel Hill, North Carolina
■ *Promoting Healthy Nutrition*

James C. Perry, MD
Chief, Section of Cardiology, Department of Pediatrics,
Yale University School of Medicine, New Haven,
Connecticut
■ *Chronic Rhythm Disorders*

Mario C. Petersen, MD
Associate Professor of Pediatrics, Department of
Pediatrics, University of Tennessee Health Science Center;
Head, Health Administration, Boling Center for
Developmental Disabilities, Memphis, Tennessee
■ *Mental Retardation*

Amy J. N. Plumb, MD
Associate Professor, Department of Pediatrics, University
of Wisconsin; University of Wisconsin Children's Hospital,
Madison, Wisconsin
■ *Risk and Resilience*

Diane Puccetti, MD
Associate Professor, Department of Pediatric Hematology/
Oncology, University of Wisconsin; Associate Professor,
Department of Pediatric Hematology/Oncology,
University of Wisconsin Children's Hospital, Madison,
Wisconsin
■ *Brain Tumors*

Ken Purdy, MD
Fellow, Pediatric Infectious Diseases, Department of
Pediatrics, David Geffen School of Medicine at UCLA,
Los Angeles, California; Department of Pediatrics,
Harbor-UCLA Medical Center; UCLA Center for Vaccine

Research, Research and Education Institute (REI),
Torrance, California
■ *Infectious Disorders of the Heart* ■ *Tuberculosis*

Bonnie Rachman, MD
Assistant Professor of Pediatrics, UCLA School of
Medicine, Los Angeles, California; Harbor-UCLA Medical
Center, Department of Pediatric Critical Care; Director,
Pediatric Critical Care Transport Team, Torrance, California
■ *Shock* ■ *Status Asthmaticus*

Susan Ralston, PharmD
Assistant Professor, University of Cincinnati, College of
Pharmacy, Cincinnati, Ohio
■ *Principles of Pharmacotherapy*

R. Lor Randall, MD, FACS
Director, Sarcoma Services; Chief, SARC Laboratory;
Assistant Professor, Department of Orthopedics,
Huntsman Cancer Institute at the University of Utah;
Assistant Professor, Division of Pediatric Orthopedics,
Primary Children's Medical Center; Tumor Consultant,
Department of Orthopedics, Shriners Hospital
Intermountain; Attending Physician, Department of
Orthopedics, LDS Hospital, Salt Lake City, Utah
■ *Nonmalignant Bone Growths*

Peter D. Rappo, MD, FAAP
Assistant Clinical Professor, Department of Pediatrics,
Harvard University School of Medicine, Boston,
Massachusetts; Brockton Hospital, Department of
Pediatrics, Brockton, Massachusetts; Children's Hospital,
Department of Pediatrics, Boston, Massachusetts
■ *Principles of Office-Based Practice*

William V. Raszka, Jr., MD
Associate Professor, Department of Pediatrics, University
of Vermont College of Medicine; Attending Physician,
Department of Pediatric Infectious Disease, Vermont
Children's Hospital, Burlington, Vermont
■ *Principles of Microbiology* ■ *Antimicrobials*

Nasser Redjal, MD, FAAP
Associate Professor, Department of Pediatrics, Harbor-
UCLA Medical Center, Torrance, California
■ *Seasonal Allergies* ■ *Asthma*

Michael Regalado, MD
Associate Professor of Clinical Pediatrics, Department of
Pediatrics, UCLA School of Medicine; Director,
Developmental and Behavioral Pediatrics, Department of
Pediatrics, Cedars-Sinai Medical Center; Adjunct
Associate Professor, Center for Healthy Children,
Families, and Communities, UCLA School of Public
Health, Los Angeles, California
■ *Developmental and Behavioral Surveillance and
Promotion of Parenting Skills*

Kirk Reichard, MD, FACS
Clinical Assistant Professor, Department of Surgery,
Johns Hopkins School of Medicine; Attending Pediatric

Surgeon, Sinai Hospital; Attending Pediatric Surgeon, Greater Baltimore Medical Center, Baltimore, Maryland
■ *Disorders of the Gastrointestinal Tract and Liver*

Jeffrey J. Ridgeway, MD
Acting Instructor, Department of Obstetrics and Gynecology, University of Washington, Seattle, Washington
■ *Standards for Routine Prenatal Care* ■ *Prenatal Factors Affecting the Newborn* ■ *Labor Management*

David S. Rosen, MD, MPH
Clinical Associate Professor, Department of Pediatrics, University of Michigan Medical School; Chief, Section of Teenage and Young Adult Health, Department of Pediatrics, University of Michigan Health System, Ann Arbor, Michigan
■ *Eating Disorders and Disordered Eating in Adolescents*

Paul Rosen, MD
Assistant Professor, Department of Pediatrics, University of Pittsburgh School of Medicine; Clinical Director, Department of Rheumatology, Children's Hospital of Pittsburgh; Children's Hospital Medical Center, Pittsburgh, Pennsylvania
■ *General Approach to the Child with Suspected Rheumatologic Disesase* ■ *Juvenile Rheumatoid Arthritis* ■ *Systemic Lupus Erythematosus and Juvenile Dermatomyositis* ■ *Fibromyalgia and Other Idiopathic Pain Syndromes*

Adam A. Rosenberg, MD
Professor of Pediatrics, Department of Pediatrics, University of Colorado School of Medicine; Director of Nurseries, University of Colorado Hospital, Denver, Colorado
■ *Long-term Care of the Child with Bronchopulmonary Dysplasia* ■ *Birth Injury and Asphyxia*

Donna A. Rosenberg, MD
Assistant Professor, Department of Pediatrics, University of Colorado Health Sciences Center, Denver, Colorado
■ *Munchausen Syndrome by Proxy*

Patti Rosquist, MD
Assistant Professor of Pediatrics, Department of Pediatrics, University of Colorado School of Medicine, Child Protection Team, The Children's Hospital Pediatrician, Denver, Colorado; Pediatrician, Department of Pediatrics, Longmont Clinic PC, Longmont, Colorado
■ *Physical Abuse and Sexual Abuse*

Lainie Friedman Ross, MD, PhD
Assistant Professor, Department of Pediatrics, University of Chicago; University of Chicago Children's Hospital, Department of Pediatrics; Assistant Director, MacLean Center for Clinical Medical Ethics, University of Chicago, Chicago, Illinois
■ *Ethical and Legal Issues in Pediatrics*

Wilma C. Rossi, MD
Clinical Associate, Department of Pediatrics, University of Pennsylvania; Attending Physician, Department of Pediatrics, The Children's Hospital of Philadelphia, Philadelphia, Pennsylvania
■ *Principles of Growth and Maturation*

Lisa A. Ruble, PhD
Assistant Professor and Director, Systematic Treatment of Autism and Related Disorders Program, Weisskopf Center for the Evaluation of Children, Department of Pediatrics, University of Louisville Health Sciences Center, Louisville, Kentucky
■ *Autism Spectrum Disorders*

Richard M. Ruddy, MD
Professor of Clinical Pediatrics, Department of Pediatrics, University of Cincinnati College of Medicine; Director, Division of Emergency Medicine, Cincinnati Children's Hospital Medical Center, Cincinnati, Ohio
■ *Injuries and Trauma*

Howard M. Saal, MD
Professor of Clinical Pediatrics, Department of Pediatrics, University of Cincinnati College of Medicine; Head, Clinical Genetics, Division of Human Genetics, Cincinnati Children's Hospital Medical Center, Cincinnati, Ohio
■ *Genetic Screening in Pediatrics*

Olle Jane Z. Sahler, MD
Professor of Pediatrics, Psychiatry, Medical Humanities, and Oncology, Department of Pediatrics, University of Rochester School of Medicine and Dentistry; Attending Physician, Departments of Hematology/Oncology and Adolescent Medicine, Golisano Children's Hospital at Strong, Rochester, New York; Medical Director, Integrated Complementary Medicine Program, Thompson Health, Inc., Canandaigua, New York
■ *Care of the Fatally Ill Child* ■ *Bereaved Children*

Karen L. Salekin, PhD
Assistant Professor, Department of Psychology, University of Alabama, Tuscaloosa, Alabama
■ *Aggressive/Oppositional Behaviors (Oppositional Defiant and Conduct Disorders)*

Susan K. Santos, MD
Assistant Professor, Department of Pediatrics, Case Western Reserve University; Ambulatory Pediatric Faculty, Department of Pediatrics, MetroHealth Medical Center, Cleveland, Ohio
■ *Obtaining Information: Parent and Child Interviewing and Rating Scales*

James D. Sargent, MD
Professor, Department of Pediatrics, Dartmouth Medical School; Hospital Staff, Department of Pediatrics, Mary Hitchcock Memorial Hospital; Director, Cancer Risk Behaviors Group, Norris Cotton Cancer Center, Lebanon, New Hampshire
■ *Smoking Cessation Counseling*

Neil Schechter, MD
Professor and Head, Division of Developmental and
Behavioral Pediatrics, Department of Pediatrics,
University of Connecticut School of Medicine,
Farmington, Connecticut; Director, Pain Relief Program,
Connecticut Children's Medical Center; Director, Section
of Developmental and Behavioral Pediatrics, Department
of Pediatrics, St. Francis Hospital and Medical Center,
Hartford, Connecticut
■ *Pain Management in Chronic Disease*

Daniel V. Schidlow, MD
Professor and Chairman, Department of Pediatrics, Drexel
University College of Medicine; Chief Medical and
Academic Officer, Attending Pulmonologist, Department
of Pediatrics, St. Christopher's Hospital for Children,
Philadelphia, Pennsylvania
■ *Bronchoscopy* ■ *Pulmonary Function Tests* ■ *Outpatient
Asthma Management*

David J. Schonfeld, MD
Associate Professor of Pediatrics and Child Study, Head,
Subsection of Developmental-Behavioral Pediatrics,
Department of Pediatrics, Yale University School of
Medicine; Yale–New Haven Hospital, New Haven,
Connecticut
■ *Normal Variations: Personality and Temperament*
■ *Helping Children Deal with Terrorism*

Jeffrey Schwimmer, MD
Assistant Professor of Pediatrics, Department of
Pediatrics, University of California at San Diego; Director,
Weight and Wellness Center, Division of Gastroenterology,
Hepatology, and Nutrition, Children's Hospital and
Health Center, San Diego, California
■ *Approach to the Child with Abdominal Pain*

Robert D. Sege, MD, PhD
Associate Professor, Department of Pediatrics, Tufts
University School of Medicine; Director, Pediatric
Adolescent Health Research Center, The Floating Hospital
for Children; New England Medical Center; Core Faculty,
Harvard Youth Violence Prevention Center, Harvard
School of Public Health, Boston, Massachusetts
■ *Violence Prevention*

James S. Seidel, MD, PhD*
Chief, Division of General and Emergency Pediatrics,
Department of Pediatrics, UCLA School of Medicine;
Chief, Division of General and Emergency Pediatrics,
Department of Pediatrics, Harbor-UCLA Medical Center,
Torrance, California
■ *Out-of-Hospital Emergency Care* ■ *Resuscitation and
Basic Life Support*

Darlene Sekerak, PT, PhD
Director and Professor, Division of Physical Therapy,
Department of Allied Health Sciences, School of

Medicine, The University of North Carolina, Chapel Hill,
North Carolina
■ *Physical Therapy*

Ann K. Seltman, MD
Resident in General Surgery, Department of Surgery,
Oregon Health & Science University, Portland,
Oregon
■ *General Surgical Interventions and Techniques*

Judith Shaw, RN, MPH
Research Assistant Professor of Pediatrics, Department of
Pediatrics, College of Medicine, University of Vermont;
Director, Vermont Child Health Improvement Program,
Department of Pediatrics, University of Vermont,
Burlington, Vermont
■ *Injury Prevention*

Terri L. Shelton, PhD
Director, Center for the Study of Social Issues, Professor
of Psychology, Center for the Study of Social Issues,
The University of North Carolina, Greensboro,
North Carolina
■ *Principles of Child Development and Developmental
Assessment*

Robert Siegel, MD
Adjunct Associate Professor of Clinical Pediatrics, Division
of General and Community Pediatrics, Cincinnati
Children's Hospital Medical Center, Cincinnati, Ohio;
Medical Director, Northern Kentucky Children's
Advocacy Center, St. Luke Hospitals, Fort Thomas,
Kentucky
■ *Domestic Violence: A Pediatric Perspective*

Monica Sifuentes, MD
Associate Professor of Clinical Pediatrics, Department of
Pediatrics, David Geffen School of Medicine at UCLA,
Los Angeles, California; Program Director and Vice Chair
for Education, Department of Pediatrics, Harbor-UCLA
Medical Center, Torrance, California
■ *Disorders of the Ear* ■ *Approach to the Deaf or Hard of
Hearing Child*

Mark L. Silen, MD, MBA
Professor of Surgery and Pediatrics, Departments of
Surgery and Pediatrics, Oregon Health & Science
University; Surgeon in Chief, Doernbecher Children's
Hospital, Portland, Oregon
■ *General Surgical Interventions and Techniques*

Alan B. Silken, MD
Assistant Clinical Professor of Pediatrics, Department
of Pediatrics, Tufts University School of Medicine,
Boston, Massachusetts; Director of Pediatric Neurology,
Department of Pediatrics, Newton-Wellesley Hospital,
Newton, Massachusetts; Clinical Associate in
Pediatrics and Neurology, Department of Pediatrics and
Neurology, Massachusetts General Hospital, Boston,
Massachusetts
■ *Long-term Management of Seizure Disorders*

* Deceased.

Thomas J. Silva, MD
Medical Director CATCH Program, Department of Pediatrics, East Boston Neighborhood Health Center, East Boston, Massachusetts
■ *Home Health Care* ■ *Technology-Dependent Therapies*

Ari Silver-Isenstadt, MD, MSEd
Pediatric Hospitalist, Department of Pediatrics, Franklin Square Hospital, Baltimore, Maryland
■ *Child Neglect: The Inadequate Promotion of Children's Health and Development*

Jeffrey M. Simmons, MD
Chief Resident, Department of Pediatrics, Cincinnati Children's Hospital Medical Center, Cincinnati, Ohio
■ *Signs and Symptoms Tables, CD-ROM*

Andrew Sirotnak, MD, FAAP
Associate Professor, Department of Pediatrics, University of Colorado School of Medicine; Director, Kempe Child Protection Team, The Children's Hospital, Denver, Colorado
■ *Physical Abuse and Sexual Abuse*

Dory P. Sisson, MA
Graduate Research Associate, Department of Psychiatry, The Ohio State University, Columbus, Ohio
■ *Sadness and Depressive Disorders*

David Skripka, MD
Assistant Professor (CHS) of Psychiatry, Department of Psychiatry, University of Wisconsin; Director, Child and Adolescent Psychiatry, Consultation-Liaison Service, University of Wisconsin Hospitals and Clinics; Attending Psychiatrist, Department of Child Psychiatry, Meriter Hospital, Madison, Wisconsin
■ *Suicide and Suicide Prevention*

John T. Smith, MD
Professor, Department of Orthopedics, University of Utah School of Medicine; Professor/Attending Surgeon, Department of Orthopedics, Primary Children's Medical Center, Salt Lake City, Utah
■ *Disorders of the Neck and Spine*

Mark S. Smith, MD
Professor, Department of Pediatrics, University of Washington; Chief, Adolescent Medicine Section, Division of General Pediatrics, University of Washington; Chief, Adolescent Services, Children's Hospital and Regional Medical Center, Seattle, Washington
■ *Chronic Fatigue Syndrome*

Charles J. Smithers, MD
General Surgery Resident, Department of Surgery, Oregon Health & Science University, Portland, Oregon
■ *General Surgical Interventions and Techniques*

Brent Snow, MD
Professor of Surgery (Urology), Department of Surgery, University of Utah; Chairman of Pediatric Urology,

Department of Surgery, Primary Children's Medical Center, Salt Lake City, Utah
■ *Chronic Genitourinary Tract Disorders*

Charles H. Song, MD
Associate Clinical Professor, Department of Pediatrics, Harbor-UCLA Medical Center; Active Staff, Department of Pediatrics, Harbor-UCLA, Torrance, California; Associate Clinical Professor, Department of Pediatrics, King Drew Medical Center, Los Angeles, California
■ *Urticaria and Angiodema*

Mary Allen Staat, MD, MPH
Associate Professor of Clinical Pediatrics, Department of Pediatrics, University of Cincinnati, College of Medicine; Director, International Adoption Center, Division of Infectious Diseases, Cincinnati Children's Hospital Medical Center, Cincinnati, Ohio
■ *Adoption*

Terry Stancin, PhD
Professor of Pediatrics and Psychiatry, Department of Pediatrics, Case Western Reserve University School of Medicine; Head, Pediatric Psychology, Department of Pediatrics, MetroHealth Medical Center, Cleveland, Ohio
■ *Obtaining Information: Parent and Child Interviewing and Rating Scales*

Martin T. Stein, MD
Professor of Pediatrics, Department of Pediatrics, University of California at San Diego; Director of Developmental and Behavioral Pediatrics, Department of Pediatrics, Children's Hospital San Diego, San Diego, California
■ *The Pediatric Clinical Interview*

Robert D. Steiner, MD
Associate Professor and Head, Division of Metabolism, Department of Pediatrics and Molecular and Medical Genetics, Oregon Health & Science University; Doernbecher Children's Hospital, Portland, Oregon
■ *Lysosomal Storage Disorders* ■ *Diagnosis and Treatment of Children with Suspected Metabolic Disease*

Peter M. Stevens, MD
Professor of Orthopedics, University of Utah, Salt Lake City, Utah
■ *Chronic Disorders of the Bones and Joints*

David K. Stevenson, MD
Harold K. Faber Professor of Pediatrics, Senior Associate Dean of Academic Affairs, Department of Pediatrics, Stanford University School of Medicine; Director, Charles B. and Ann L. Johnson Center for Pregnancy and Newborn Services, Chief, Division of Neonatal and Developmental Medicine, Department of Pediatrics, Stanford University School of Medicine, Stanford, California
■ *Jaundice*

Nava Stoffman, MD

Clinical Fellow, Department of Pediatrics, Harvard Medical School; Fellow in Adolescent Medicine, Division of Adolescent/Young Adult Medicine, Children's Hospital Boston, Boston, Massachusetts
- *Contraceptive Methods and Counseling*

Wendy L. Stone, PhD

Professor, Department of Pediatrics, Vanderbilt University Medical Center, Nashville, Tennessee
- *Autism Spectrum Disorders*

Alan K. Stotts, MD

Assistant Professor, Department of Orthopedic Surgery, University of Utah; Pediatric Orthopedic Surgeon, Department of Orthopedic Surgery, Primary Children's Medical Center, Salt Lake City, Utah
- *Disorders of the Hip*

C. Frederic Strife, MD

Professor of Pediatrics, University of Cincinnati College of Medicine; Professor of Pediatrics, Division of Nephrology and Hypertension, Cincinnati Children's Hospital Medical Center, Cincinnati, Ohio
- *Long-term Management of Renal Disorder*

Michael C. Struck, MD

Assistant Professor, Department of Ophthalmology and Visual Sciences, University of Wisconsin, Madison, Wisconsin; Physician, Department of Ophthalmology, Mercy Medical Center, Janesville, Wisconsin; Physician, Department of Ophthalmology, Meriter Hospital, Madison, Wisconsin
- *Disorders of the Eye* ▪ *Approach to the Child with Visual Impairment* ▪ *Care of the Blind Child*

Robert P. Sundel, MD

Associate Professor of Pediatrics, Harvard Medical School; Division of Pediatric Rheumatology, Immunity, and Allergy, Brigham and Women's Hospital, Boston, Massachusetts
- *Anti-inflammatory and Immunomodulatory Therapy*

Jordan Symons, MD

Assistant Professor of Pediatrics, Department of Pediatrics, University of Washington School of Medicine; Attending Nephrologist, Division of Nephrology, Children's Hospital and Regional Medical Center, Seattle, Washington
- *Disorders of the Genitourinary System in the Newborn*

Wendy Y. Tcheng, MD

Clinical Instructor, Department of Pediatric Hematology-Oncology, University of California at Los Angeles; Clinical Instructor, Department of Pediatric Hematology-Oncology, UCLA Medical Center, Los Angeles, California
- *Platelet Disorders* ▪ *Bleeding Disorders and Coagulopathies*

Elizabeth Thilo, MD

Associate Professor of Pediatrics, Section of Neonatology, University of Colorado School of Medicine; Neonatologist, Department of Neonatology, The Children's Hospital, Denver, Colorado
- *Routine Care of the Full-Term Newborn*

Eva Thomas, MD, PhD, FRCP(C)

Clinical Professor, Department of Pathology, University of British Columbia; Director, Microbiology, Virology, and Infection Control, Department of Pathology, BC Children's Hospital, Vancouver, British Columbia, Canada
- *Laboratory Testing of Infants and Children*

Gregory Thomas, MD

Assistant Professor, Department of Pediatrics, Oregon Health & Science University; Director, Oregon Hemophilia Treatment Center, Oregon Health & Science University, Portland, Oregon
- *Long-term Care of Children with Hemophilia*

Sara L. Thompson, MD, MPH

Assistant Professor of Pediatrics, Department of Pediatrics, University of California, Los Angeles, California; Department of Pediatrics, Harbor-UCLA Medical Center, Torrance, California
- *Fractures, Sprains, and Dislocations* ▪ *Nutritional Disorders*

Thomas F. Tonniges, MD, FAAP

Adjunct Professor (Clinician), Department of Pediatrics, University of Nebraska Medical Center, Omaha, Nebraska; Director, Department of Community Pediatrics, American Academy of Pediatrics, Elk Grove Village, Illinois
- *Influences of Community on Child Health and Well-being*

Ronald Turker, MD

Associate Professor, Department of Orthopedics and Rehabilitation, Oregon Health & Science University; Staff Surgeon, Shriners Hospital for Children, Portland, Oregon
- *Splinting and Casting*

Hilary Vallance MD, FRCPC, FCCMG

Clinical Associate Professor, Department of Pathology and Laboratory Medicine, University of British Columbia; Director, Biochemical Genetics Laboratory, Pathology and Laboratory Medicine, Children's and Women's Health Centre of British Columbia; Director, Newborn Screening Program of British Columbia, Department of Pathology, Children's and Women's Health Centre of British Columbia, Vancouver, British Columbia, Canada
- *Laboratory Testing of Infants and Children*

Sheryll L. Vanderhooft, MD

Associate Professor, Department of Dermatology, University of Utah School of Medicine; Director, Pediatric Dermatology Clinic, Primary Children's Medical Center; Adjunct Professor, Department of Pediatrics, University of Utah School of Medicine, Salt Lake City, Utah
- *Approach to Dermatologic Disease and Eczematoid Eruptions* ▪ *Papulosquamous Disorders* ▪ *Disorders of the Sebaceous and Sweat Glands* ▪ *Disorders of the Hair and*

Nails ■ *Vesiculobullous Disorders* ■ *Disorders of Pigmentation* ■ *Cutaneous Tumors* ■ *Dermatologic Manifestations of Systemic Disease* ■ *Acne*

René G. VanDeVoorde, MD
Chief Resident, Department of Pediatrics, Cincinnati Children's Hospital Medical Center, Cincinnati, Ohio
■ *Signs and Symptoms Tables, CD-ROM*

Dennis Vane, MD, MBA
Professor and Chairman, Division of Pediatric Surgery, Department of Surgery, University of Vermont; Vice Chairman, Clinical Affairs, Department of Surgery, Division of Pediatric Surgery, Fletcher Allen Health Care, Burlington, Vermont
■ *Burn Care* ■ *Circumcision*

Laurie Varlotta, MD
Associate Professor of Pediatrics, Drexel University College of Medicine; Director, Cystic Fibrosis Center, Section of Pulmonology, St. Christopher's Hospital for Children, Philadelphia, Pennsylvania
■ *Pulmonary Function Tests*

Anne Marie Vovakis, MD
Pediatric Nurse Practitioner, Department of Pediatrics, Community Medical Alliance, Boston, Massachusetts
■ *Home Health Care* ■ *Technology-Dependent Therapies*

Louis Wadsworth, MB, ChB, FRCP(C), FRCPath
Clinical Professor, Department of Pathology, University of British Columbia; Associate Director, Department of Pathology and Laboratory Medicine, Children's and Women's Health Centre of British Columbia; Program Director, Department of Hemopathology, Children's and Women's Health Centre of British Columbia, Vancouver, British Columbia, Canada
■ *Laboratory Testing of Infants and Children*

Lars M. Wagner, MD
Assistant Professor of Pediatrics, Division of Pediatric Hematology/Oncology, Primary Children's Medical Center, Salt Lake City, Utah
■ *Solid Tumors of Infancy and Childhood*

Linn Wakeford, MS, OTR/L
Assistant Professor, Division of Occupational Science, The University of North Carolina at Chapel Hill; Occupational Therapist, Family and Child Care Program, Frank Porter Graham Child Development Institute, Chapel Hill, North Carolina
■ *Occupational Therapy*

Cassandra Walcott, MD
Instructor in Pediatrics, Department of Pediatrics, Harvard Medical School, Boston, Massachusetts; Attending in Pediatrics, Department of Pediatrics, Caritas Good Samaritan, Brockton, Massachusetts; Instructor in Medicine, Department of Pediatrics, Boston Children's Hospital, Boston, Massachusetts
■ *Principles of Integrative Pediatrics*

Craig R. Warden, MD, MPH
Chief, Pediatric Emergency Services/Associate Professor, Department of Emergency Medicine, Oregon Health & Science University, Portland, Oregon
■ *Wound Care and Suturing* ■ *Incision and Drainage/Needle Aspiration of Cutaneous Abscesses*

G. Scott Waterman, MD
Associate Professor of Psychiatry, Director of Medical Student Education in Psychiatry, Department of Psychiatry, University of Vermont College of Medicine; Attending in Psychiatry, Director of Psychopharmacology, Psychiatry Service, Fletcher Allen Health Care, Burlington, Vermont
■ *Psychotropic Agents*

Melissa Weddle, MD, MPH
Assistant Professor, Department of Pediatrics and Adolescent Medicine, University of Wisconsin–Madison Medical School; Assistant Professor, Department of Pediatrics and Adolescent Medicine, University of Wisconsin Hospital and Clinics, Madison, Wisconsin
■ *History and Physical Examination* ■ *Health Maintenance in Adolescents*

Robert D. White, MD
Adjunct Faculty, Department of Psychology, University of Notre Dame, Notre Dame, Indiana; Director, Regional Newborn Program, Memorial Hospital, South Bend, Indiana; Clinical Assistant Professor of Pediatrics, Indiana University School of Medicine, Indianapolis, Indiana
■ *Special Issues in the Care of the Ill Premature Infant*
■ *Continuing Care of the Growing Premature Infant*

Natasha Wiebe, BMath, MMath
Research Associate, Department of Pediatrics, University of Alberta, Edmonton, Alberta, Canada
■ *Principles of Clinical Epidemiology*

D. Pauline Williams, MPA, RD, CD
Assistant Professor, Extension, Utah State University, Logan, Utah
■ *Principles of Nutrition* ■ *Nutrition in Children with Chronic Diseases*

Paul H. Wise, MD, MPH
Professor of Pediatrics and Public Health, Department of Pediatrics, Boston University School of Medicine; Director, Social and Health Policy Research, Department of Pediatrics, Boston Medical Center; Vice Chief, Division of Social Medicine and Health Inequalities, Department of Medicine, Brigham and Women's Hospital; Associate in Medicine, Department of Medicine, Children's Hospital, Boston, Massachusetts
■ *Effects of Poverty*

Michael T. Witkovsky, MD, PhD
Associate Professor, Department of Psychology and Pediatrics, University of Wisconsin at Madison; Training Director, Child and Adolescent Psychiatric Services,

University of Wisconsin Hospital; Medical Director, Child and Adolescent Psychiatric Services, Morton Hospital, Madison, Wisconsin
■ *Suicide and Suicide Prevention*

Mark Wolraich, MD
CMRI/Shaun Walters Professor of Pediatrics, Department of Pediatrics, University of Oklahoma Health Sciences Center; Department of Pediatrics, Oklahoma University Children's Hospital, Oklahoma City, Oklahoma
■ *Attention and Hyperactivity Problems and Attention Deficit Hyperactivity Disorder*

Emily J. Wong, MD
Harbor-UCLA Medical Center, Department of Pediatrics, Pediatric Infectious Disease, Torrance, California; Southern California Permanente Medical Group, Department of Pediatrics, Panorama City, California
■ *Exanthems*

Kimberly A. Worley, MD
Developmental and Behavioral Pediatric Fellow, Vanderbilt University Medical Center, Nashville, Tennessee
■ *Attention and Hyperactivity Problems and Attention Deficit Hyperactivity Disorder*

Stavra A. Xanthakos
Pediatric Gastroenterology Fellow, Department of Pediatric Gastroenterology, Hepatology and Nutrition, Cincinnati Children's Hospital Medical Center, Cincinnati, Ohio
■ *Pancreatic Disorders*

Scott Yeager, MD
Associate Professor, Department of Pediatrics, University of Vermont School of Medicine; Chief, Department of Pediatric Cardiology, Fletcher Allen Health Care, Burlington, Vermont; Associate Professor, Department of Pediatrics, Dartmouth-Hitchcock Medical Center, Lebanon, New Hampshire
■ *Long-term Medical Management of Children with Heart Disease* ■ *Electrocardiography, Echocardiography, and Cardiac Catheterization*

Sylvia Yeh, MD
Assistant Clinical Professor, Department of Pediatrics, David F. Geffen School of Medicine at UCLA, Los Angeles, California; Assistant Clinical Professor, Department of Pediatrics, Division of Pediatric Infectious Diseases, Harbor-UCLA Medical Center, Torrance, California
■ *Infections of the Bones and Joints* ■ *Approach to the Child with Recurrent Infection* ■ *Mycotic Infections*

Kelly D. Young, MD, MS
Assistant Clinical Professor of Pediatrics, Department of Pediatrics, University of California at Los Angeles, David Geffen School of Medicine, Los Angeles, California; Pediatric Emergency Medicine Faculty, Department of Emergency Medicine, Harbor-UCLA Medical Center, Torrance, California
■ *Poisoning and Drug Overdose*

Paul C. Young, MD
Professor, Department of Pediatrics, University of Utah School of Medicine, Salt Lake City, Utah
■ *Long-term Medical Management of Children with Heart Disease*

Kian-Ti Yu, MD
Associate Professor, Department of Pediatrics, Harbor-UCLA Medical Center, Los Angeles, California; Pediatric Neurologist, Departments of Pediatrics and Neurology, Kaiser Permanente Medical Group, Fontana, California
■ *Status Epilepticus* ■ *Approach to the Child with Seizures* ■ *Approach to the Child with Headache*

Kenneth M. Zangwill, MD
Associate Professor of Medicine, UCLA School of Medicine, Los Angeles, California; Department of Pediatrics, Division of Pediatric Infectious Diseases, Harbor-UCLA Medical Center, Torrance, California
■ *Infections of the Bones and Joints* ■ *Approach to the Child with Recurrent Infection*

Nataliya Zelikovsky, PhD
Assistant Professor, Department of Pediatrics, University of Pennsylvania School of Medicine; Pediatric Psychologist, Department of Nephrology, The Children's Hospital of Philadelphia, Philadelphia, Pennsylvania
■ *Adaptation in Childhood Chronic Illness: Risk and Protective Factors*

Lonnie Zeltzer, MD
Professor of Pediatrics, Anesthesiology, Psychiatry, and Biobehavioral Sciences, Department of Pediatrics, Anesthesiology, Psychiatry, and Biobehavioral Sciences, David Geffen School of Medicine at UCLA; Director, Pediatric Pain Program, Department of Pediatrics, UCLA Mattel Children's Hospital, Los Angeles, California
■ *Chronic Functional Pain/Somatic Complaints and Associated Disability*

Barry Zuckerman, MD
Professor and Chairman, Department of Pediatrics, Boston University School of Medicine; Chief, Department of Pediatrics, Boston Medical Center, Boston, Massachusetts
■ *Literacy*

FOREWORD

Given that hundreds of new texts are published each year, anyone who contemplates publishing a new medical book would be wise to ensure that it fills a special niche. This text, directed toward generalists who care for children, clearly meets that criterion. Most textbooks of pediatrics are authored by subspecialists with a disease focus, who write about diseases that are rarely seen in general practice. Although these texts fill an important role, they are not geared toward the majority of practitioners: the generalists. The goal of this book is to help generalists who practice in the community and in academic centers to deliver effective care to children and to serve those who teach children's health care.

The editors and I use the term *general pediatrics* to define the work that health care providers in the community do every day. This work involves not only a great deal of preventive, developmental, and behavioral pediatrics, but also diagnosis and management of common diseases. In addition, it includes team care for children with less-common diseases, provided by subspecialists, social workers, psychologists, and the school system. Currently, most practitioners report that one quarter to one third of all patients treated in office practice are seen for complaints that involve mental health and/or social issues. This text, unlike others, includes comprehensive coverage of both subjects.

Few books have fulfilled the complex role of this text in as clear a manner. It is one of the rare textbooks that discuss when to refer and how to co-manage children with complex chronic diseases. Rather than offer an exhaustive review of diseases, the editors—all nationally recognized leaders in academic general pediatrics—have made a concerted effort to present data in a manner that is easy to access and pertinent to the generalist. The accompanying CD-ROM includes additional content, including videos, medical procedures, audio of heart murmurs, color photographs of dermatologic conditions, and supplemental scientific data.

This text is an important resource for pediatric practitioners, residents, and students who seek to provide effective care for children in the community.

Robert J. Haggerty, MD
Professor and Chair, Emeritus
University of Rochester
School of Medicine and Dentistry

PREFACE

The practice of pediatric health care has changed dramatically in recent decades. Pediatric providers are expected not only to prevent, diagnose, and treat medical and developmental/behavioral conditions, but also to organize and provide complex care for increasing numbers of patients with chronic conditions. Moreover, this care must be delivered with an understanding of the capacities and limitations of family, community, and health care systems. Mental health concerns, child advocacy issues, new and rapidly changing technologies, complementary care, and complex health care systems present special challenges that even recently trained providers may not be adequately prepared to address.

Much of the practical information essential to the delivery of appropriate care is not available in textbooks. Even answers to relatively straightforward questions, such as which imaging study is appropriate in a given clinical situation or how to immunize a patient with hemophilia, are often hard to find. Consequently, when we, as pediatric educators, were approached by Mosby about creating a new, innovative, full-color general pediatrics textbook, the possibilities inspired us.

Our goal in the creation and organization of this text has been to provide practical information in an easily accessible, learner-friendly format. By reflecting how patients present to the health care system, the text is organized to help generalists provide optimal care. Each of the text sections is color coded for easy access. Section 1, Fundamentals, provides basic information common to a wide variety of medical conditions and practice issues. Section 2, Health Promotion and Disease Prevention, provides both the theoretical basis for and systematic methods of delivering preventive interventions. Sections 3 through 6 discuss clinical care, from general medical care (including emergent care), to chronic care, to the special care required by neonates and adolescents. Because pediatric generalists are increasingly called on to provide care for patients dealing with mental health and social issues, these subjects are covered separately in Sections 7 and 8. Section 9, Diagnostics and Therapeutics, provides not only detailed descriptions of diagnostic tests and procedures, but also a comprehensive discussion of therapeutic interventions, from pharmacotherapy and procedural medicine to rehabilitation medicine and complementary health care. Section 10, available on the CD-ROM, includes signs and symptoms tables that cluster symptoms, provide diagnostic possibilities and helpful clues, and refer the reader to key chapters in the text.

Several special features highlight important educational and clinical considerations. Each of the clinical chapters begins with a Role of the Generalist box. Depending on the medical condition, from emergencies to chronic illnesses, the pediatric generalist may be expected to provide compre-

hensive care, diagnose and triage a patient, or refer patients to specialists and then co-manage the conditions. Each Role of the Generalist box reflects the chapter author's view of the level of care that the generalist should provide and presents the educational objectives of the chapter. Also featured are "indications for referral"—when, how, and to whom to refer. Red Flag boxes list signs and symptoms for medical conditions that require urgent attention. The chronic medical care section includes recommendations for health maintenance that are specific to each condition; practical procedural information, such as how to store insulin; discussions of acute care for patients with chronic conditions; and information about co-management issues, such as coordinating care with specialists and instructing parents where to direct emergency and nonemergency calls.

Because the text is designed to present information necessary for the generalist to diagnose illnesses and manage patients with the most common conditions, when illnesses—particularly those that are unusual or rare—are not discussed comprehensively in the text, the reader is referred to textbooks, review articles, and websites in the Suggested Readings section at the end of each chapter. In addition, Mini-index of Related Topics boxes, which color code chapter listings by section, eliminate unnecessary redundancy by facilitating cross-referencing within the text. Fundamentals common to many disease entities, for example, are provided in Section 1 and are extensively cross-referenced throughout the chapters. Also listed are additional resources on the CD-ROM that complement or expand on topics in a chapter.

The inclusion of a CD-ROM has enabled us to offer content that is largely unavailable in general pediatric textbooks. In addition to the signs and symptoms tables, the CD-ROM contains videos of clinical conditions (such as seizures) and medical procedures, audio of heart murmurs, color atlases of dermatologic conditions, basic science supplements, discussion of controversial therapies, and descriptions of less-common medical conditions. All tables, boxes, and illustrations for each chapter are provided in a PowerPoint format that can be downloaded for instructional purposes.

We thank Developmental Editor Marla Sussman and the staff at Elsevier. Without them, we would not have been able to create this unique text.

We hope that this book will help meet the needs of all those who dedicate their efforts to the care of children.

Lucy M. Osborn, MD, MSPH, FAAP
Thomas G. DeWitt, MD, FAAP
Lewis R. First, MD, MS, FAAP
Joseph A. Zenel, MD, FAAP

CONTENTS

SECTION 4   CHRONIC MEDICAL CARE

SECTION 5   NEWBORN CARE

SECTION 6   ADOLESCENT CARE

SECTION 7   MENTAL HEALTH CARE

SECTION 8   SOCIAL ASPECTS OF CARE

SECTION 9   DIAGNOSTICS AND THERAPEUTICS

CD-ROM CONTENTS

Electronic image and table collection from the book, all in downloadable format

Video and audio clips as cross-referenced from the book

Supplemental materials

Signs and Symptoms Tables

Thomas G. DeWitt, Lucy M. Osborn, Jeffrey M. Simmons, and René G. VanDeVoorde III

- Abdominal Distention
- Abdominal Mass
- Abdominal Pain
- Alopecia
- Ambiguous Genitalia
- Amenorrhea
- Anemia
- Anorexia
- Antisocial Behavior
- Anuria/Oliguria
- Anxious Behavior
- Apnea
- Bruising
- Chest Pain
- Coma
- Constipation/Obstipation
- Cough, Acute
- Cough, Chronic/Recurrent
- Cyanosis
- Delirium/Agitation
- Depression
- Developmental Delay/Mental Retardation
- Diarrhea, Acute
- Diarrhea, Chronic
- Dizziness/Vertigo
- Dysmenorrhea
- Dysmorphism/Genetic Syndromes
- Dysphagia
- Dyspnea
- Dysuria
- Edema, Focal
- Edema, Generalized
- Encopresis
- Epistaxis

- Failure to Thrive
- Fatigue
- Fever, Acute
- Fever, Immunocompromised Patient
- Fever, Newborn
- Fever, Periodic
- Fever, Persistent
- Headache
- Hearing Loss
- Heart Murmur
- Hematemesis, General
- Hematemesis, Newborn
- Hematochezia and Melena
- Hematuria
- Hemoptysis
- Hepatomegaly
- Hepatosplenomegaly
- Hirsutism
- Hoarseness
- Hyperactivity/Poor Attention
- Hyperhidrosis
- Hypertension
- Hypertrichosis
- Hypotonia/Muscle Weakness
- Irregular Heart Beat/Palpitations
- Jaundice
- Jittery Infant
- Lethargy
- Limp
- Lymphadenopathy
- Menorrhagia
- Nocturia/Enuresis
- Obesity
- Odor of Body or Body Fluids

- Pain, Back
- Pain, Bone
- Pain, Ear/Otaglia
- Pain, Eye
- Pain, Joint
- Pain, Testicular
- Petechiae/Purpura
- Polyuria
- Precocious Puberty
- Pruritus
- Pubertal Delay
- Rash (refer to Chapters 69–79)
- Red Eye
- Respiratory Distress
- Rhinorrhea
- School Problems
- Scrotal Swelling
- Seizures
- Shock
- Short Stature
- Sleep Disturbance
- Sore Throat
- Splenomegaly
- Stridor
- Syncope
- Tall Stature
- Thrombocytosis
- Tics/Involuntary Movements
- Vaginal Bleeding
- Vaginal Discharge/Vaginitis
- Vomiting
- Weight Loss
- Wheezing

1

The Pediatric Clinical Interview

Martin T. Stein

The clinical interview is an opportunity beyond the collection of factual data. It defines the *therapeutic relationship* between the clinician and patient. When the relationship is viewed as an "alliance" among the child, parent, and clinician, the importance of the development of trust and rapport among the participants should be seen as a crucial factor. There is a direct relationship between the strength of a therapeutic alliance and a parent's or child's understanding of a diagnosis, their adherence to therapeutic interventions, and overall quality of care. Communication skills that enhance a therapeutic alliance focus on enhancing self-esteem; asking nonjudgmental questions; discovering the family's agenda, value system, and resources; and making practical and concrete recommendations (Table 1-1).

Table 1-1. Communication Skills in Pediatrician-Family Interactions

Goal	Example
Boost self-esteem and enhance sense of confidence and competence	"You're doing a great job."
Consider the patient and family as partners in problem solving	"How can I help you deal with the problem?"
Be open-ended	"Tell me about Billy."
Be nonjudgmental	"In this situation, anyone would get impatient."
Respect the family's agenda and timetable	"What concerns you the most about Cathy at this time?"
Explore the family's value system	"Have you discussed this problem with anyone else (e.g., your priest)?"
Use family's own resources and approaches	"Tell me what you've tried up to now. What seemed to work best?"
Make advice finite, practical, and concrete	"Do you think you could listen to him cry for about 10 minutes before going to pick him up?"
Allow yourself time to enjoy the patient as a person	"What is your favorite time at school?"
Make "contract" explicit	"How would you like to spend the time we have left before the end of our appointment?"
Don't underrate your own therapeutic potential	"This must be a really tough time for you; your next appointment is in 2 weeks, but please call me on Wednesday and let me know how things are going."

From American Academy of Pediatrics: Guidelines for Health Supervision III. Elk Grove Village, Ill, American Academy of Pediatrics, 1997 (revised 2002), p 6. Copyright © 1997 American Academy of Pediatrics. Used with permission.

CLINICAL ENCOUNTER: PLANNING AND ORCHESTRATING

The agenda for a pediatric clinical encounter has two potential sources—the clinician and the parent. The traditional pediatric interview implies the presence of a clinician's agenda (e.g., to establish a chief complaint and a history of the presenting problem or, in the case of a health supervision visit, to assess developmental skills, nutrition, and environmental safety). Simultaneously, for every pediatric clinical encounter, the parent's agenda is a crucial part of the interview. It is not uncommon for the parent's main agenda or concerns to be ignored or minimized. This situation may occur during a visit with a focus on an acute symptom, a follow-up visit for a chronic condition, and a health supervision visit. In a study of acute pediatric visits, following the history of the concern that initiated the visit, parents were asked, "What are you concerned about?" One third of the parents expressed a fear not verbalized initially about a more serious condition that could not be anticipated from the ostensible reason for the visit. A "hidden agenda" was apparent only after probing the family's main concern.

An assessment of the parent's agenda for a health supervision visit is equally important. It should be established early in the visit. A useful approach is "What are your main concerns about your child?" or "I want to be sure that we cover the things that concern you most about your child. Can you tell me them at this time?" This strategy is especially helpful for a health supervision visit in that it sets the priorities at the beginning of the visit, while sending the message that the parent's concerns are important and will be addressed. Some clinicians prefer previsit standardized forms that request parental concerns while waiting to see the clinician. The American Academy of Pediatrics published previsit forms in *Guidelines for Health Supervision III*. The forms are available for six developmental ages in a parent and a child format. In addition to asking about a parent's agenda, developmental and behavioral milestones are included on each form.

INTERACTIVE PROCESS

Clinicians who recognize the pediatric *clinical interview as an interactive process* gain more useful information for the time spent. Astute observations of parent-child interactions during an interview provide an opportunity to assess developmental skills of the child, parenting skills, and family interactions. These visual and auditory clues are usually spontaneous and often occur when least suspected. They typically do not occur in response to a specific question. They may represent a "teachable moment" in two senses of the term—an unexpected opportunity to provide information or direction to a parent (teach the parent) or an observation stored in the clinician's database for future use (teach the clinician).

During a clinical interview, children may provide important information through the use of emerging language skills. In a busy clinic setting, it is common for a clinician to see the parent as the only source of information. However, children are a rich source of medical, social, and developmental information. Most children between 2 and 3 years old have sufficient expressive and receptive language skills to communicate some symptoms and concerns to the clinician.

To ensure a child-directed interview, it is useful to direct the first set of questions to the child rather than the parent, as follows: "Why did your mom bring you to the doctor today?" or "It seems to me that you're not feeling well today. Tell me what's bothering or hurting you." In the case of a health supervision visit with a school-age child, the following approach can be used: "You are here today so that I can check on your health, to find out how your body is working and to talk about school, sports, and other activities and about your family. I am interested in knowing what you would like to talk about or what questions you might have for me." Beginning an interview with a question or comment directed to the child informs the child immediately that he or she is the patient and frequently instructs the parent in communication skills based on a broader understanding of the child's developmental achievement.

Age-appropriate words, play, and social interactions of the clinician encourage the child's participation in the interview. Direct and immediate eye contact usually engages the interest of a 4-month-old infant but may initiate fear or withdrawal in a toddler. A quick assessment of a child's temperament often guides effective communication. The availability and use of age-appropriate toys and drawing materials in the examination room may enhance the interview by engaging the child's interest and (when the clinician needs time with the parent) distracting the child.

NONVERBAL COMMUNICATION

Information derived from nonverbal observations is as important as verbal or written information. It is often the foundation for a diagnosis or observations that guide effective counseling. *Verbal information* refers to the data that patients tell clinicians about themselves, the core of the traditional medical history. *Nonverbal information* refers to observations clinicians make about the style, timing, emotive ambiance, and flow of the interview and even about what is not said. Facial expressions, posture, movements of the extremities, and the quality and tone of speech are examples of important observations that frequently provide clues to crucial aspects of a child's life and family environment. Clinicians often neglect this source of important

information, making their data gathering less efficient and less accurate.

Making use of nonverbal clinical observations requires practice, but the payoff is worth the time to learn to be an effective observer. Examples of nonverbal communication and potential clinical use are listed in Box 1-1.

USING THE CLINICAL SETTING TO OPTIMIZE THE INTERVIEW

The word *interview* is derived from two words—*between* and *seeing*. It implies that the process is a shared communication of thoughts that may be influenced by the physical space between a clinician and patient. Specific characteristics of the interview environment that may mediate the effectiveness and quality of a medical encounter are listed in Box 1-2.

Box 1-1. Examples of Nonverbal Communication and Potential Clinical Use

- Encouraging self-help skills (e.g., undressing and climbing onto the examination table) shows a parent's recognition of a child's developmental level of achievement.
- Nonverbal forms of restraint or discipline often occur during a visit to the pediatrician. Careful observations may be the only clue to a parent's discipline style.
- When a clinician's attention is focused on a child's behavior during an interview with a parent, important observations about motor, social, and language development can be made. Delays and accelerations in developmental milestones may be observed at this time.
- Observing sadness or fatigue in a parent may be a clue to depression, sleep deprivation, marital conflict, or other psychosocial stress. This nonverbal observation should lead to further evaluation.

Box 1-2. Characteristics of the Interview Environment That May Mediate the Effectiveness and Quality of a Medical Encounter

- The clinician and parent should be positioned at the same level to ensure eye contact and to prevent subservient positioning effect.
- The decision to conduct the interview in a sitting or standing position changes with the type of visit.
- For a new patient or a new problem that requires an extensive history, sitting down with the parent and child encourages greater information exchange and allows the clinician to pay more attention to nonverbal cues.
- For an established patient with an acute illness, the history may be taken while the parent and clinician are standing.
- A young child who is ill may remain in the arms of the parent.
- The placement of chairs in an examination room and the proximity of clinician and patient influence the style and content of the interview.
- A desk between the clinician and parent and child can be a barrier to optimal communication.
- Picking up a chair and moving it closer to a parent may facilitate the exchange of information; the act itself may enhance a therapeutic relationship.

COMMUNICATING WITH CHILDREN

"I think you should ask the patient what's wrong with him or her, not the parent. The parent is not sick. The kid is sick. He knows more of himself than anyone else understands."

This revealing statement, written by a school-age child, was discovered on a chair in the waiting room at the end of a clinic day. It is a reminder that pediatric patients seek an active engagement in the clinical encounter. When interviewing children who have achieved interactive language skills (beginning at about 3 to 4 years old), the clinician can speak directly to the child—asking questions and listening carefully. A useful communication tool in pediatric practice is the recognition that receptive language development is usually ahead of expressive language. A 2-year-old may understand 300 words, but expression may be limited to 50 to 100 words. Active participation of the child in the interview is an opportunity to assess language development and auditory functioning. It provides children with an experience of participating actively in the visit, which may encourage a sense of responsibility and participation in personal health and medical care. It also models for parents the role of listening to and showing respect for the opinions of children. The *TEACHER* mnemonic is a useful technique to enhance the quality of communications with children and their parents during pediatric visits (Table 1-2). This mnemonic is a guide to conduct the interview with the child and parent in a parallel fashion, engaging responses from each source interactively as opportunities surface.

Unexpected opportunities that lead to an understanding of the parent-child relationship occur when a pediatrician is sensitive to verbal and nonverbal cues and his or her own emotional experiences during a clinical encounter. In addition, the interview may provide insight into the important relationship between the child, parent, and clinician. These events, characterized as "critical incidents," require clinical vigilance. They may be fleeting and awkward, as shown in Case Study 1-1.

Table 1-2. TEACHER—a Method for Enhancing Communication with Pediatric Patients and Their Parents

T	Trust	Build trust and rapport with the child by asking nonthreatening questions not related to illness
E	Elicit	Elicit information from parent and child regarding parental fears and concerns and the child's understanding of the reason for the visit
A	Agenda	Set an agenda early in the visit to help ensure that the parents' concerns are addressed
C	Control	Help the child feel control over the visit (e.g., knowing what will and will not happen), to help decrease fear and increase cooperation
H	Health plan	Establish a health plan with the child and parent to meet the child's needs and limitations
E	Explain	Explain the health plan to the child in a way he or she can understand
R	Rehearse	Have the child rehearse the health plan as a way of assessing understanding; reinforce the child's jobs related to health care; explore any potential problems in the plan with the child and parent

From Bernzweig J, Pantell R, Lewis CC: Talking with children. In Parker S, Zuckerman B (eds): Behavioral and Developmental Pediatrics. New York, Little, Brown, 1995, p 7.

CASE STUDY 1-1

A TEACHABLE MOMENT

Jake, who has been a healthy child, arrives for his 18-month health supervision visit. As you enter the examination room, you observe Jake playing on the floor with a plastic toy with several movable parts. He appears engaged and intent on mastering the toy. You also notice that his fine motor skills are mature for his age as you observe Jake drawing a picture.

Jake appears not to notice you when you enter. Shortly after you begin to gather information from his mother, Jake's activity level and focus change dramatically. He starts hitting the toy, screams "bad, bad," and throws the toy into a wall. He starts to cry, resists his mother's attempt to hold him and provide reassuring words, and hits her with his hand several times. His mother begins to cry and says, "He was such a good baby. In the last few months, he's a different child—selfish, angry, and always throwing a tantrum."

You are faced with several options at this point:
1. Quickly perform a physical examination, check the growth chart, and order immunizations (and a blood lead level and hematocrit if appropriate).
2. Talk to Jake's mother about tantrums and the need for discipline. Provide a handout on toddler development and discipline.
3. Attempt to engage Jake with words and a toy (e.g., sit down on the floor and play with the toy; say something like, "Gee, this is a great toy. I can make the door open so the boy can go inside."). Alternatively, address Jake and say, "It's real hard to come to the doctor!" or "You are real upset at the doctor's office." Follow these words with silence and wait patiently for Jake's response.

The first option brings closure to the office visit but does not address Jake's behavior. The second option shows recognition of a problem while expanding the mother's knowledge about toddler behaviors and approaches to discipline. The third option illustrates immediate recognition of a "teachable moment."

You choose to role model an age-appropriate response to a tantrum through action and language. Engaging the child formulates the scene to the child's reality. Your language is direct and brief; you try to mirror the child's experience (i.e., feelings) with a few words and wait for a response. This technique, known as *active listening*, encourages Jake's mother to learn that she can interact with her son at these difficult moments by feeding back to him the feelings he is experiencing. It can be followed by the information exchange illustrated in the second option.

STRUCTURING THE INTERVIEW

The structure of a pediatric interview ensures the content and style of a clinical encounter and provides a framework for controlled digressions. The format of an interview should be neither too rigid nor too loose. There should always be an opportunity to inquire about issues and make observations that may not be apparent at the start of the interview.

In the case of an initial visit of a new patient, an *introduction* by name in a concerned, friendly, and empathic manner establishes a caring atmosphere. Impressions formed at the beginning of a visit encourage rapport and the formation of a therapeutic alliance. Eye contact with the parent emphasizes concern and interest in the child. An extended hand and a warm smile assist in the development of a new medical relationship.

Establishing the agenda for the visit is often useful at the start. For an acute illness visit, it may be a single symptom or a series of symptoms. In the case of a health supervision visit, the clinician may state his or her goals for the visit (e.g., developmental assessment, growth monitoring, nutritional and safety counseling); this should be followed by an invitation to the parent to express his or her goals or agenda for the visit, as follows: "What areas of your child's health would you like to discuss during this visit?" This approach early in the visit ensures that the parent or adolescent has an opportunity to state his or her agenda for the visit. It allows the clinician an opportunity to structure the visit in a format that includes that agenda.

The *content* of a pediatric interview (what parents and children tell the clinician) depends on the nature of the visit. The *process* that guides the style and tone of the interview (and the quality of the information obtained by the clinician) is something that each clinician develops with practice and self-assessment. Content is generated by the patient; process is interactive and a shared responsibility between the clinician and the patient. Often referred to as the "art of medicine," the process of an interview may include specific methods to construct an effective interview. The following communication tools can make the best use of limited time to allow parents and children "to tell their story" with clarity and appropriate detail.

Open-ended questions generate spontaneous, more elaborate, and more revealing responses. Examples in pediatric practice include the following: "How is your baby doing?" "What's new with the baby's development?" "Tell me about pain in your tummy." "The nurse tells me that you have a sore throat; tell me more about it." Open-ended questions allow parents and children to bring up problems of greatest concern to them. They acknowledge the parents' responsibility in establishing priorities in the interview. They give parents the message that their agenda is important. In contrast, *closed-ended questions* (e.g., "How long has he been coughing? When did it start? Is it more frequent during the day or evening? Does he bring up mucus or phlegm with the cough? Has he had a fever?") are important to establish the details of a history.

As a general rule, it is best to begin a medical history with an open-ended question followed by closed-ended questions that fill in the gaps. Closed-ended questions not only provide concrete data, but also shift control of the interview to the interviewer. Used too early in an interview, they may limit the quality of information. Another advantage of early open-ended questions is that they encourage parents and children to reveal their *explanatory model* of an illness, a symptom, or a behavior. The explanatory model reflects a culturally dependent perspective of an illness or symptom that the family brings to a medical encounter. When a pediatrician suspects that the explanatory model is based on a different set of assumptions, a series of focused questions yields information useful in the diagnosis or treatment or both. Box 1-3 lists questions that elaborate on the explanatory model and health beliefs that may have a cultural dimension.

Box 1-3. Explanatory Model and a Cross-Cultural Medical Interview: Questions for a Health-Beliefs History

1. What would you call this problem?
2. Why do you think your child has developed it?
3. What do you think caused it?
4. Why do you think it started when it did?
5. What do you think is happening inside the body?
6. What are the symptoms that make you know your child has this illness?
7. What are you most worried about with this illness?
8. What problems does this illness cause your child?
9. How do you treat it?
10. Is the treatment helpful?
11. What will happen if this problem is not treated?
12. What do you expect from the treatments?

From Pachter LM: Practicing culturally sensitive pediatrics. Contemp Pediatr 1997;14:139. Copyright 1997 Thomson Medical Economics. All rights reserved. Reprinted with permission.

When emotionally difficult issues are discussed, the use of *pauses and silent periods* is extremely beneficial. A silent period allows the patient time to collect thoughts and to express feelings. It carries with it the message that the clinician cares enough about the patient to take the time to listen to his or her deepest concerns about the child and family. The time and effort needed to learn to use pauses and silent periods effectively are worthwhile.

When a parent or child makes an important statement, the clinician may repeat or interpret the phrase or sentence. *Repetition of important phrases* emphasizes the significance of what has just been said and encourages elaboration and clarification. The clinician might then say, "Tell me more," followed by a pause. This technique encourages further exploration, clarification, or modification by the parent or child.

Active listening refers to the process of giving undivided attention to what a person is saying through words and body language. It requires, above all, the ability to concentrate intensely on the interview. The parent and child should feel as though they have the clinician's undivided attention, that they are the most important people to the clinician at that moment in time. The assumption underlying active listening is that the patient will provide significant information spontaneously, verbally or nonverbally, if given an opportunity.

Active listening makes use of open-ended questions, pauses, silent moments, and repetition of important phrases. Physical characteristics of the clinician that support active listening include good eye contact, leaning forward toward the parent or child at a timely moment, limited movement of hands and feet, and appropriate facial expressions. Active listening encourages an empathic interview, decreases parent and child anxieties, increases trust in the clinician, and encourages greater parent and child participation in the interview process (Box 1-4).

Primary pediatric care is based on the development of a long-term relationship with families. When continuity of health care is provided in this framework, a special relationship develops between the caregiver and the patient. In pediatric practice, parents usually have respect and admiration for their child's physician; it is the foundation for a trusting, long-term relationship. This relationship is the most powerful tool in effecting change for the child. It is also one of the rewards of primary care. At the same time, and to various degrees, as a result of this close and special relationship, a parent may respond to the pediatrician as someone who is identified symbolically and psychologically with another important person in his or her own life, past or present. For some parents, the symbolic attachment may be a father or a mother; for others, it may be an uncle or other important person in their lives.

The *transference* phenomenon may surface only at times of deep emotional expression, such as overwhelming joy, relief, and admiration for the clinician after a successful therapeutic intervention. It also may be the unconscious source of hostility directed toward the clinician by the parent of a child with a chronic, functionally disabling illness. An appreciation of parental reactions mediated by transference may assist the clinician in providing more appropriate and helpful responses during medical interviews and in understanding some aspects of the interaction. In addition, at other times, this appreciation allows for an understanding of strong personal feelings experienced by the clinician. With this insight, one does not get rid of transference in an interaction but acknowledges it, uses it for the healthy energy it provides, and keeps in check the less helpful aspects of its presence. Monitoring of one's own emotional response allows one to be aware of this phenomenon and to use it to advantage.

Pediatricians develop effective communication skills through practice and self-reflection on their perceived effectiveness (Box 1-5). Medical school and residency training is only a start. Learning to communicate therapeutically and effectively is a lifelong process. Experience with children and families, coupled with insights from one's own adult developmental path, promote competent interviewing skills.

CULTURALLY EFFECTIVE INTERVIEWS

Although most of the general principles of effective medical interviewing discussed in this chapter are applicable when there are cultural differences between a clinician and patient, culturally derived differences may pervade the encounter at many levels. Pachter defined culturally sensitive pediatrics as "care (that) respects the beliefs, attitudes, and cultural life-styles of patients. It acknowledges that concepts of health and illness are influenced by patients, ethnic values, religious beliefs, linguistic considerations, and cultural orientation." A culturally competent pediatric clinician discovers ways to blend ethnomedical interpretations of a child's illness, developmental skills, and behaviors with a biomedical understanding. Culture does not dictate the beliefs and behaviors of a child or parent in a specific way, however, but rather acts implicitly to guide a patient's decisions.

An effective medical interview between a clinician and family from a different culture is enhanced by the clinician's knowledge about the family's cultural beliefs and practices. For example, in the provision of health care, it may be important for the pediatrician to be familiar with such cross-cultural beliefs as limitation of direct and sustained eye contact in some Asian cultures; *mal de ojo*, the "evil eye" belief, found in many Latino cultures, where symptoms are perceived as arising from feelings of malevolence or jealousy; and the use of physical punishment for disruptive behaviors in children practiced by many parents in some cultures. Focused questions about health beliefs provide insights into family and cultural values (see Box 1-3). Even the act of requesting the information encourages partnerships in problem solving between clinicians, parents, and children.

Pediatricians use a model for cultural competency that focuses on three principles: awareness, assessment, and negotiation. It provides a framework for working with children and families from a culture different from the provider's background. The first step is to become *aware* of commonly held beliefs and practices specific to the family. Colleagues (including all members of the health care team), patients, and the medical anthropology literature are the usual sources of information. The National Center for Cultural Competence is a helpful resource for information on cultural competence (http://gucchd.georgetown.edu/nccc/). An example of the importance of awareness is a knowledge of the collective cultural values of Latino families: *simpatía* (kindness), *personalismo* (formal friendliness), *respeto* (respect), *familismo* (collective loyalty to the extended family), and *fatalismo* (fatalism).

The *assessment* starts with the assumption that not every family in a particular culture practices commonly held beliefs from that culture. Asking about a belief in a manner that is respectful while showing prior experience may lead to a question such as "Some parents have told me about a problem called ____; are you aware of this problem, and does it affect your child?" When a particular cultural belief related to health or illness is discovered, it should be respected. To protect against illness from the "evil eye" (*mal de ojo*), some Latino families have children wear an *azabache* (a seedlike charm) on a necklace or bracelet. The therapeutic alliance is enhanced when the clinician acknowledges the charm as a form of protection.

The *negotiation* stage is an opportunity to incorporate knowledge of cultural beliefs into education about a condition and clinical recommendations. In most situations in pediatrics, a safe, culturally derived treatment can be combined with an intervention from Western medicine. Making use of the fundamental principles of effective interviewing assists the pediatrician in successful negotiations with families from different cultures.

SUGGESTED READINGS

American Academy of Pediatrics: Guidelines for Health Supervision III. Elk Grove Village, Ill, American Academy of Pediatrics, 1997 (revised 2002).

Coleman WL: Family-Focused Behavioral Pediatrics. Philadelphia, Lippincott Williams & Wilkins, 2001.

Dixon SD, Stein MT: Encounters with Children: Pediatric Behavior and Development, 3rd ed. St. Louis, Mosby, 2000.

Lipkin ML Jr, Putnam SM, Lazare A: The Medical Interview—Clinical Care, Education, and Research. New York, Springer-Verlag, 1995.

Pachter LM: Working with Patients' Health Beliefs and Behaviors: The Awareness-Assessment-Negotiation Model in Clinical Care—Child Health in the Multicultural Environment. Report of the Thirty-first Roundtable on Critical Approaches to Common Pediatric Problems. Columbus, Ohio, Abbott Laboratories, 2000, pp 36–43.

SECTION 1   FUNDAMENTALS

2

Physical Examination: Skills and Terminology, Normal Variations, and Implications of Deviations from Normal

Paula Algranati

GOALS OF THE PHYSICAL EXAMINATION

Amid enormous diagnostic and therapeutic advances, the clinical encounter endures as the cornerstone of clinical medicine. Along with history taking, a careful, comfortable, and accurate physical examination answers fundamental clinical questions. The clinical encounter usually is sufficient to distinguish between normal and abnormal. Laying hands on children and adolescents enhances rapport, satisfies parental and patient expectations, provides information, and conveys reassurance. This chapter outlines the knowledge, attitudes, and skills necessary to determine what to examine, how to proceed, and how to determine the significance of findings for physical examinations in children and adolescents.

The importance of developmental stage is most unique to pediatrics. Attending to the patient's stages of affective, cognitive, and physical development alerts the clinician to predictable challenges, such as fears, resistance to examination, and stage-related variations of normal findings. Beginning each examination with strategies to overcome these barriers enhances cooperation and improves clinical decision making.

PLANNING THE PHYSICAL EXAMINATION

The clinician must determine which body parts to examine and which areas require the closest scrutiny. Health maintenance visits should include a comprehensive examination, a stage-related focus, and attention to individual concerns related to recent or chronic illness. The patient's age and developmental stage should guide the focus to systems that are affected most commonly by pathology, are most rapidly changing, or are most crucial to the developing child. For problem visits and hospitalized patients, the content varies substantially, depending on the acuity of the illness and the specificity of the complaint. When complaints are vague or generalized, a comprehensive approach should be refined with stage-related knowledge about disease incidence and prevalence and expected normal findings.

Obtaining and tracking objective data are essential. Determining which other measurements to obtain (e.g., vital signs, body measurements, developmental milestones, vision and hearing acuity) should be individualized to the age and stage of the patient and the purpose of the examination. Length/height and body weight are measured routinely at all health maintenance visits. The rationale for routinely measuring blood pressure beginning at age 3 years is based on incidence and prevalence data for essential hypertension and the probability that patients will be able to cooperate for measurement. Head circumference is measured routinely only during infancy, the period of maximal brain growth. Individual concerns should guide decisions about examination content for health maintenance visits and for problem-based ambulatory and hospital encounters. Measurement of blood pressure, although not routine for full-term newborns, should be performed when there is concern about a heart murmur or diminished femoral pulses and coarctation of the aorta.

APPROACH TO THE EXAMINATION

Orchestrating the examination requires attending to the physical space and its occupants. The clinician should arrange the chairs to enhance interactions and include all the participants whenever possible. A child's fears should be addressed by ensuring proximity of the child to the parent and initially distancing the child from the clinician. Attention to physical space and the patient (e.g., drawing curtains, closing doors, and using gowns and drapes) respects the concerns of older children and adolescents about physical modesty and privacy. Other decisions about positioning the participants, such as whether to examine a child on the table or in a parent's lap or whether to examine an older child with or without a parent in the room, should reflect developmental stage and individual concerns.

The sequence of examination maneuvers depends on the planned content, whether focused or comprehensive. Attending to proper sequencing and framing verbal and physical interaction effectively comfort the patient and the parent, enhance cooperation, improve efficiency, and enhance accuracy. The patient's level of understanding and ability to cooperate reflect age and developmental stage, health status, innate temperament, and previous experiences.

The clinician should carefully think out framing verbal interactions (e.g., modulating the volume, content, and tone of speech; determining whom to address) and physical interactions (e.g., making eye contact; maintaining physical distance from the patient; deciding whether to stand, sit, or kneel; modulating touch; offering distractions). All aspects of the examiner's interactions must be modulated to diminish predictable fears, such as stranger or separation anxiety. The clinician may need to avoid direct eye contact, speak softly, keep his or her distance, and sit rather than stand when entering the examination area. Speaking directly to a school-age child about activities and interests (versus asking the parent for this information) can enhance cooperation while providing useful information. The examiner should seek to familiarize the child gradually with himself or herself, the equipment (e.g., allow the patient to touch/play with the reflex hammer), and the procedures (e.g., demonstrate on the parent first).

When mechanics have been learned, the physical examination can usually be performed in 10 minutes or less. Expanding the focus beyond information gathering opens a wealth of opportunities for information gathering and developing rapport. Laying hands on distinguishes clinicians from other types of providers and satisfies parental and patient expectations. Powerful nonverbal messages can convey reassurance, empathy, validation, or even disapproval. The opportunity to establish or enhance rapport with pediatric patients includes family members. Enlisting parents as facilitators fosters relationships with them. History taking can be blended seamlessly with performing the physical examination. "Teachable moments" arise, including modeling behaviors to parents and calling attention to a child's activity to highlight a strength or achievement. The examination provides opportunities to correct misconceptions, foster positive health behaviors, defuse concerns, and reassure about normality. When the child receives verbal and nonverbal messages of the clinician's respect, self-esteem is enhanced as well.

BASIC EXAMINATION TECHNIQUES AND INSTRUMENTS

Inspection, palpation, percussion, and auscultation are fundamental elements of examinations that effectively and accurately assess relevant systems. Although the techniques themselves do not differ dramatically from techniques used on adults, the extent to which each is included reflects the patient's age and the purpose of the examination. For infants, children, and adolescents, the traditional view of inspection should be expanded to the broader concept of observation, the pediatric clinician's most powerful examination technique. Observation may replace an alternative technique that because of age-related issues may be less effective (e.g., counting the pulsations over the anterior fontanelle in a sleeping infant versus using a stethoscope to obtain heart rate after the infant awakens and begins to cry) or may be used to obtain data that are otherwise inaccessible (e.g., assessing developmental milestones in a toddler who will not "perform" for the clinician but will "play" with a parent). Watching and listening also provide data about the child's temperament and the quality of the parent-child relationship. The specific applications of palpation, percussion, and auscultation are

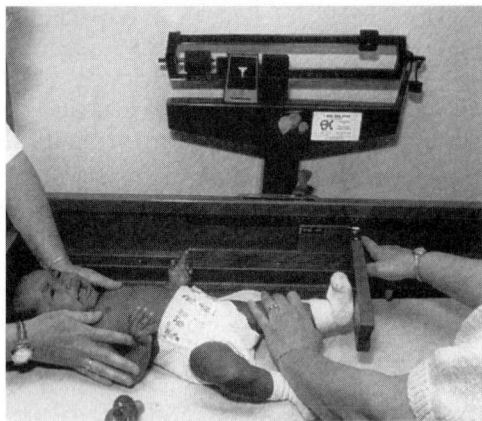

Figure 2-1. Measurement of supine length. (From Algranati PS: The Pediatric Patient: An Approach to History and Physical Examination. Baltimore, Williams & Wilkins, 1992.)

mentioned in the age-related discussions that follow. Younger and more vulnerable patients (e.g., acutely ill) benefit from an approach that minimizes invasiveness and maximizes gentleness (e.g., warm hands, warmed instruments) and graduated familiarity (e.g., introduce the patient to the instrument and technique as gradually as possible).

Examination instruments should fit the patient's age and size and the purpose of the procedure. A stethoscope with a pediatric-sized bell and diaphragm is appropriate for infants and young children. The otoscope head should be fitted with a speculum small enough to fit the ear canal yet achieve an adequate seal. Some instruments, such as an insufflator attached to an otoscope, are used more often in children than in adults.

MEASUREMENTS

Length and Height

Supine length is measured in children until age 2 to 3 years, when standing height is more appropriate. Accurate measurement of length requires placing the supine infant, legs extended, on a flat, hard table with either the top of the head or soles of the feet resting firmly up against a flat,

stationary surface angled perpendicular to the table (Fig. 2-1). A second perpendicular board is brought toward the infant's opposite end until resistance is encountered. The distance between the two boards is recorded as the supine length. Standing height is measured in children with shoes off, legs together, weight evenly distributed on both feet, standing straight, eyes directed forward, and the top of the head parallel to the floor. A straight bar parallel to the floor and perpendicular to the wall or vertical ruler is lowered until it is positioned across the crown of the head. The value for height is recorded at the point that the horizontal bar touches the vertical ruler on the wall or on the scale.

There are several pitfalls in measuring children. Because newborns frequently are flexed obligatorily at hips, knees, and elbows, the clinician should extend the limbs gently as far as possible. The correct gender-specific growth chart must be chosen when recording length/height for a toddler. Values for children ages 2 to 3 years may be recorded on either the infant charts labeled "birth to 36 months," which correspond to supine length, or the charts labeled "2 to 20 years," which correspond to standing height. See the CD-ROM for age- and gender-specific growth charts. A variety of special growth charts for children with specific health issues are available (e.g., children with Down syndrome, children with constitutional growth delay, premature infants).

Weight

Infants and young toddlers are weighed lying or sitting on a scale. Children able to cooperate may stand on an upright scale. Accurate weights require that patients wear as little clothing as possible. Values are plotted on standardized age-appropriate and gender-appropriate growth charts.

Head Circumference

Head circumference is measured routinely in infants during health supervision visits and in older children with special concerns, such as developmental delay, neurologic problems, or genetic problems. The tape should be stretched across the forehead just above the eyebrows, around to the back of the head at the level of the occipital protuberance (Fig. 2-2). The tape should be adjusted to obtain the maximal occipital-

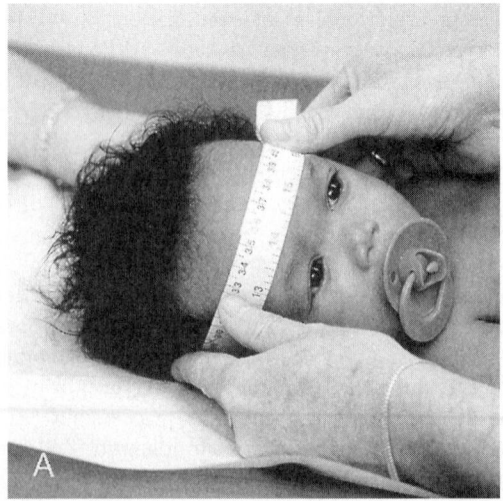
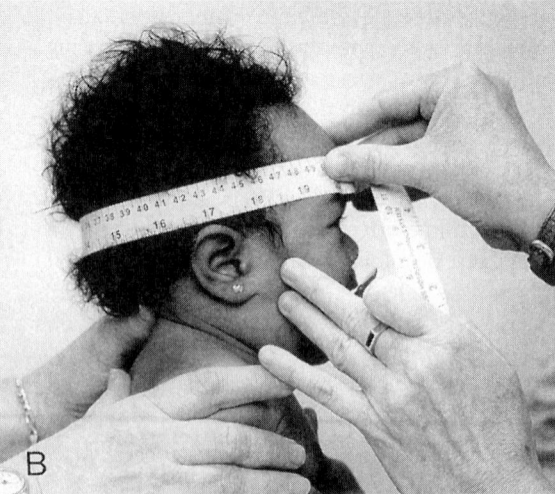

Figure 2-2. Measurement of head circumference. **A**, Anteriorly the tape is positioned over the smooth area of the frontal bone just above the eyes. **B**, Posteriorly the tape is positioned at the level of the occipital protuberance. (From Algranati PS: The Pediatric Patient: An Approach to History and Physical Examination. Baltimore, Williams & Wilkins, 1992.)

frontal circumference. Values are plotted for the patient's age on standard gender-appropriate charts. (See the CD-ROM.)

Weight for Length and Body Mass Index for Age

When accurate measurements are obtained, length/stature and weight can be used to screen for overweight and underweight children. Length/stature, weight, weight-for-length, and body mass index (BMI) should be plotted on appropriate charts (available from the National Center for Health Statistics and National Center for Chronic Disease Prevention and Health Promotion at http://www.cdc.gov/ growthcharts). For children younger than age 2 years, plotting weight versus length on a gender-appropriate chart supplies a percentile that is used to identify overweight children (Fig. 2-3). For children older than age 2 years, weight and stature are used to calculate BMI (Box 2-1). The calculated BMI value is plotted on the gender-specific chart at the patient's age (Fig. 2-4). Weight for length and BMI for age greater than 95% indicate that the patient is overweight. BMI for age greater than the 85th percentile and less than the 95th percentile indicates risk of becoming overweight. BMI for age and weight for length less than the 5th percentile indicate the patient is underweight. Although BMI does not measure body fat directly, it may be used as a proxy for body fat measurement and correlates with clinical risk factors for hyperlipidemia.

A wealth of information can be accumulated by observing and measuring many parts of the body. Questions regarding body proportions (e.g., upper segment versus lower segment ratio, arm span, philtrum length) or appearance and timing of features (e.g., number and placement of hair whorls on the head, expected time period for closure of the anterior fontanelle) can be answered by consultation of relevant reference material containing standards for norms and ranges of normal.

VITAL SIGNS

Heart Rate

Heart rate is measured by auscultation of the heart, palpation of a peripheral pulse, or observation of pulsations of a young infant's patent anterior fontanelle. Normal heart rates gradually diminish from infancy to childhood. Heart rates vary with activity level, body temperature, stress, and illness (Table 2-1).

Respiratory Rate

Respiratory rate is measured by auscultation of the chest or by observing the rise and fall of the chest wall. An accurate rate is obtained when the patient is calm. Normal respiratory rates diminish from infancy to childhood (Table 2-2).

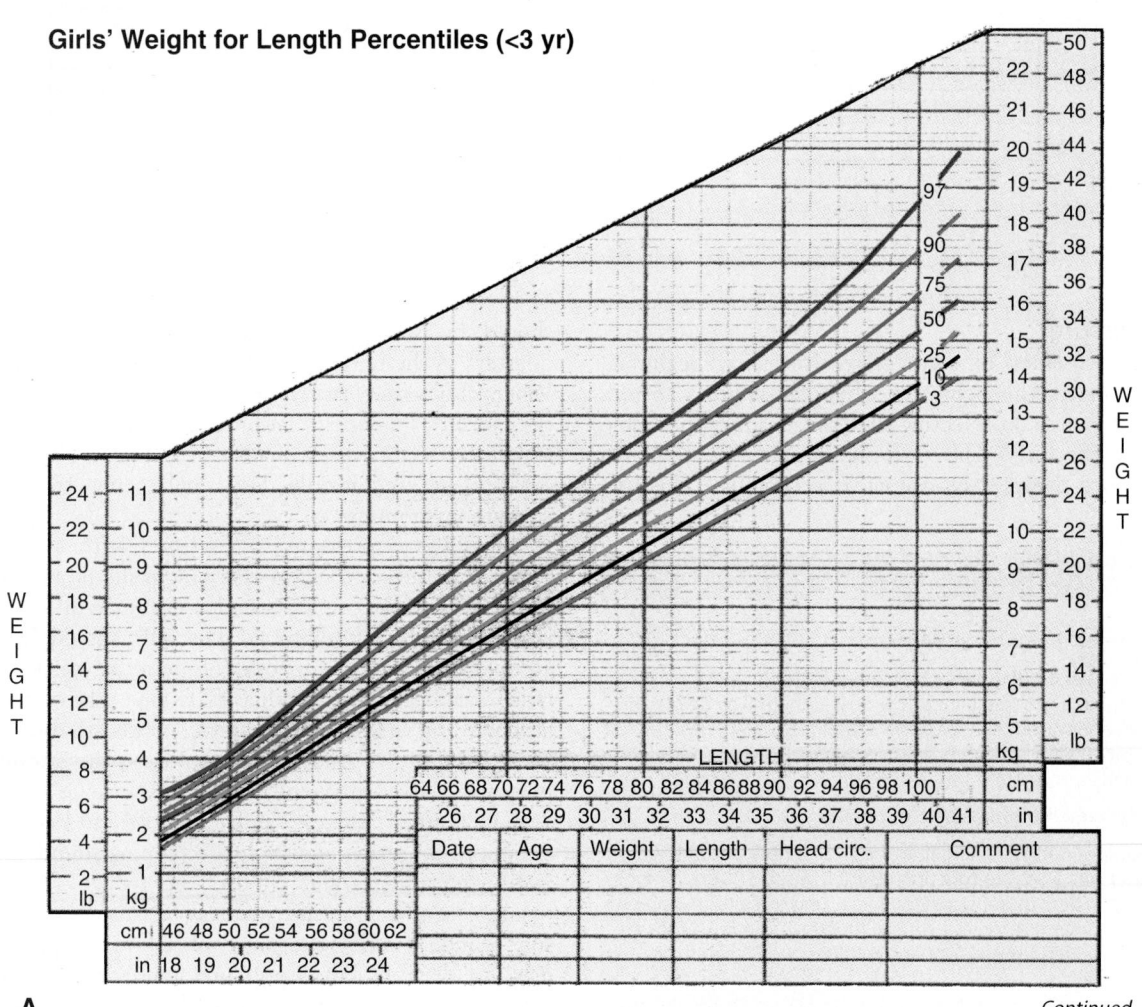

A

Continued

Figure 2-3, Gender-specific weight for length percentiles for age younger than 2 years (**A,** girls; **B,** boys). (Redrawn from the National Center for Health Statistics and National Center for Chronic Disease Prevention and Health Promotion: 2000. Available at: http://www.cdc.gov/growthcharts.)

Boys' Weight for Length Percentiles (<3 yr)

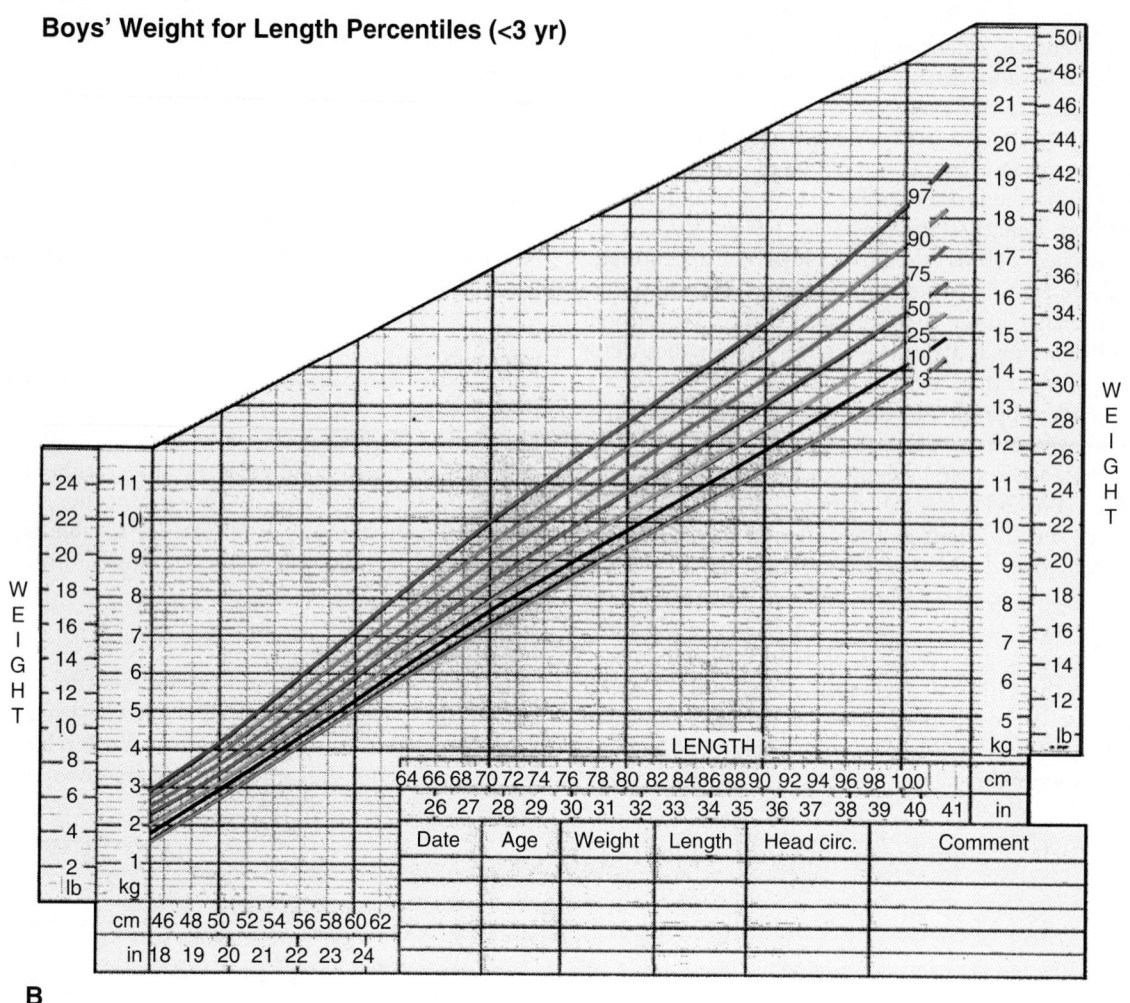

B

Figure 2-3 cont'd.

Blood Pressure

For routine screening, blood pressure is measured beginning at age 3 years in the right arm while the child is seated. Accuracy depends on selecting the correct inner inflatable bladder of the cuff. The cuff should encircle the arm circumference completely; overlap is acceptable. The cuff should be wide enough to cover approximately three quarters of the upper arm (Fig. 2-5; see also Chapter 174). When choosing between two sizes, the larger size should be selected. Underestimation of accurate blood pressure is less likely than overestimation. Electronic blood pressure devices are technically less challenging than mercury sphygmomanometers.

When blood pressure is measured with a device that requires a stethoscope, the diaphragm should be positioned over the brachial artery at the lower border of the cuff just above the antecubital fossa. The cuff should be inflated approximately 20 mm above the point at which the radial pulse disappears. With gradual deflation of the cuff, the value at which the first audible tapping sounds are discerned, K1 (first Korotkoff sound), corresponds to the systolic blood pressure. With continuing deflation, the value at which the tapping sounds become muffled is K4, and with further deflation, the value at which the tapping sounds disappear is K5. For infants and children up to age 12 years, the point of muffling, or K4, is used for diastolic blood pressure standards. K5, the point of sound disappearance, is used for diastolic blood pressure standards for adolescents age 13 years and older. Normal blood pressures gradually rise with age. Data for current blood pressure norms were obtained using mercury sphygmomanometers; fu-

---

Box 2-1. Calculation of Body Mass Index

Metric System: Weight (kg)/Height m²

Calculation: [weight (kg) / height (m) / height (m)]
If calculator has a square function, divide weight (kg) by height (m) squared, and round to 1 decimal place.
If calculator does not have a square function, divide weight by height twice, and round to 1 decimal place.

English System: Weight (lb)/Height (inches²) × 703

Calculation: [weight (lb) / height (inches) / height (inches)] × 703
If calculator has a square function, divided weight (lb) by height (inches) squared, multiply by 703, and round to 1 decimal place.
If calculator does not have a square function, divide weight by height twice, multiply by 703, and round to 1 decimal place.

From Centers for Disease Control Website: Using the BMI-for-age growth charts: 6. Calculating BMI using the metric system/English system. Available at: http://www.cdc.gov/growthcharts.

ture studies will likely use electronic devices and generate revised norms (see Tables 174-1 and 174-2 and the CD-ROM).

Temperature

Rectal measurement of temperature is the method used most widely for infants. Electronic ear canal probes are especially suited for use in young children. At around age 5 years, children are able to hold an oral thermometer under the tongue. Normal body temperature varies with age, activity, and time of day. There is approximately 1° of difference between normal temperature for infants and adolescents, with infants having a higher temperature. Because of a normal diurnal variation, body temperature is highest in the early evening and lowest in the early morning, with the difference being 2° or 3°. Rectal temperatures are approximately 1° higher than oral temperatures. The normal range of temperatures is approximately 36.9°C (97.5°F) to 38.0°C (100.4°F).

INCORPORATING DEVELOPMENTAL ASSESSMENT

Developmental monitoring, a longitudinal, multifaceted process, is incorporated routinely into all health supervision visits from newborns through adolescents. The purpose

Girls' BMI Percentiles

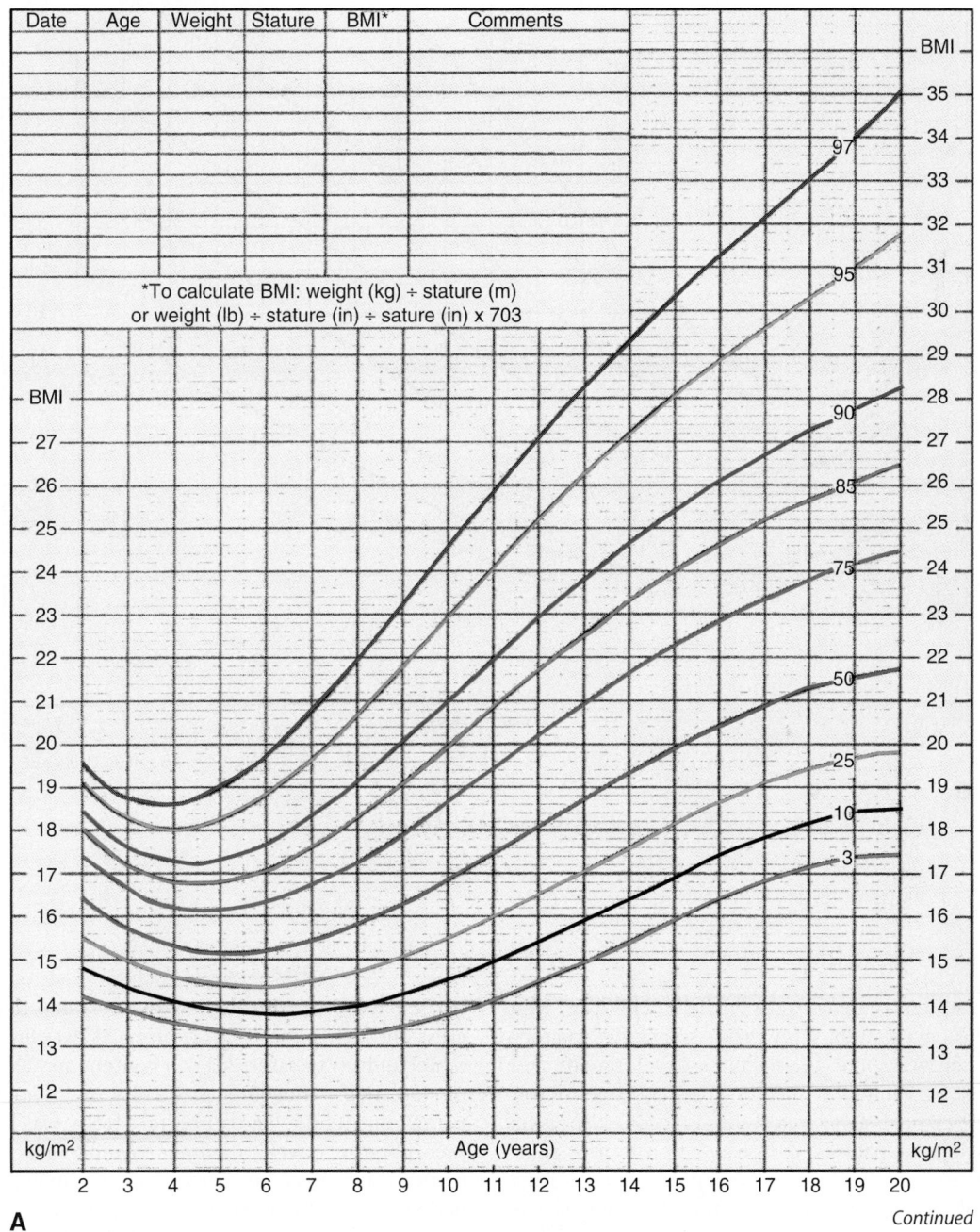

Continued

A

Figure 2-4. Gender-specific body mass index percentiles for age older than 2 years (**A,** girls; **B,** boys). Redrawn form the National Center for Health Statistics and National Center for Chronic Disease Prevention and Health Promotion: 2000. Available at: http://www.cdc.gov/growthcharts.)

Boys' BMI Percentiles

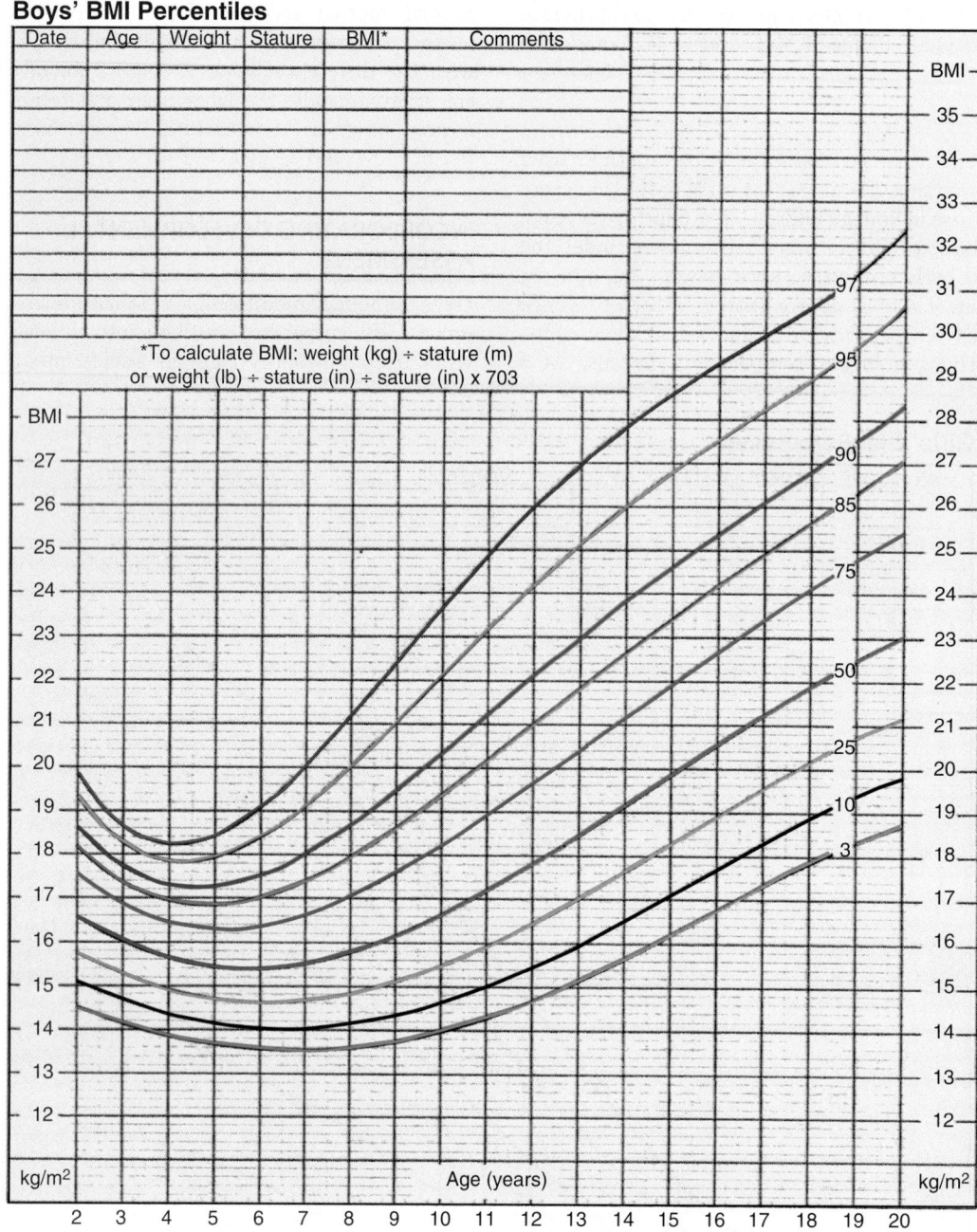

*To calculate BMI: weight (kg) ÷ stature (m)
or weight (lb) ÷ sature (in) ÷ sature (in) x 703

Figure 2-4 cont'd.

of developmental screening is to identify children who require further evaluation. The process includes history taking from parents about their child's development and their concerns. Screening for specific gross and fine motor, language, and personal/social milestones is accomplished via specific questions to parents and observation by the clinician with the use of a valid and reliable instrument. Casual observation of developmental milestones by clinicians is notoriously inaccurate. For school-age children and adolescents, developmental monitoring explores school functioning, speech and language abilities, physical activities/sports

participation, relationships with peers and family, and progress through puberty. The physical examination provides opportunities to assess speech content and clarity, dexterity of fine motor movements, quality of interaction between parent and child, and pubertal status via Tanner staging. Incorporating developmental screening into physical examinations also may be a necessary component when evaluating a specific concern. Incorporation of information regarding the patient's abilities helps the clinician predict responses and use strategies that enhance compliance or cooperation.

Table 2-1. Average Heart Rates in Children at Rest

Age	Average Rate (beats/min)	Two Standard Deviations
Birth	140	50
≤1 mo	130	45
1–6 mo	130	45
6–12 mo	115	40
1–2 yr	110	40
2–4 yr	105	35
6–10 yr	95	30
10–14 yr	85	30
14–18 yr	82	25

From Lowery GH: Growth and Development of Children, 8th ed. Chicago, Year Book, 1986, p 246.

VISION AND HEARING

Vision

Unless there are special concerns, visual acuity is assessed subjectively until approximately age 3 years. Observation by the clinician, assessing age-related abilities to fix, follow, and reach for objects, always is accompanied by querying parents whether they believe the child has normal vision. Objective screening for distance visual acuity begins at age 3 years. For children able to read letters or numbers (usually age ≥ 6 years old), the method used most widely is a Snellen wall chart with lines of letters or numbers of progressively diminishing size placed 10 ft away from the patient. For children ages 3 to 5 years, a similar process uses easier symbols, such as a Tumbling E or HOTV letters. Vision is assessed in each eye separately, with the opposite eye open but vision occluded (Table 2-3).

Hearing

Screening newborns for congenital hearing loss is accomplished using evoked otoacoustic emissions and auditory brainstem response, either alone or in combination. In the United States, the American Academy of Pediatrics supports a goal of universal hearing screening of all newborns. Beyond this age period, unless there are special concerns, hearing is assessed subjectively until approximately age 4 to 5 years, when children can cooperate for objective screening. Subjective screening is accomplished via a combination of clinician observation, assessment of age-related abilities to alert to and follow a novel sound, and history from parents. Because speech delay may indicate an underlying hearing deficit, monitoring speech development for content and clarity also is important. When the child is

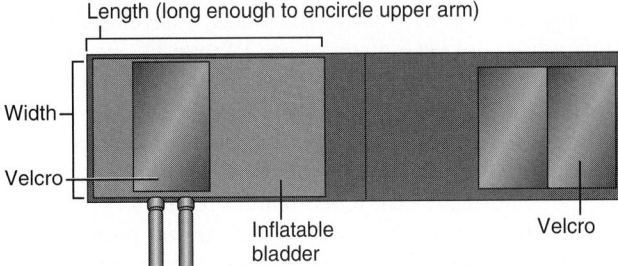

Figure 2-5. Position of blood pressure cuff on upper arm, covering approximately three fourths of arm between shoulder and elbow. (Redrawn from Algranati PS: The Pediatric Patient: An Approach to History and Physical Examination. Baltimore, Williams & Wilkins, 1992.)

able to cooperate, objective screening is performed using pure-tone audiometry. The child should respond to sounds of 1000 Hz or 2000 Hz at 20 dB and sounds of 4000 Hz at 25 dB.

DETERMINING THE SIGNIFICANCE OF FINDINGS

Evaluating the significance of findings requires knowledge of what is normal. The challenge of determining "normal" in the face of rapid development may be daunting. Interpreting physical examination data is accomplished within contexts via a series of comparisons. A fundamental level of comparison using cross-sectional data offers the opportunity to compare the patient's finding at one point in time with norms and ranges of normal for large groups of peers of the same age and gender. The patient's rate of progress can be compared with that of a reference group. Using weight and height as examples, the clinician can determine whether the child is growing at a rate that is appropriate, slower than normal, or faster than normal. Another appropriate comparison group is family members. What may seem to be an abnormality may be a benign family trait, although caution is advisable because family traits may be inherited abnormalities expressed in multiple individuals.

Equally important are comparisons that use the patient's own data over time within the context of his or her other

Table 2-2. Normal Respiratory Rates in Children

Age	Respirations/min
Newborn	30–75
6–12 mo	22–31
1–2 yr	17–23
2–4 yr	16–25
4–10 yr	13–23
10–14 yr	13–19

From Cloutier MM: Pulmonary diseases. In Dworkin PH (ed): Pediatrics. Baltimore, John Wiley & Sons, 1987, p 266. This material used by permission of John Wiley & Sons, Inc.

Table 2-3. Criteria for Referral for Ophthalmologic Evaluation: Vision Screening Guidelines*

Function	Referral Criteria
Distance visual acuity age 3–5 yr	<4 of 6 correct on 20-ft line with either eye tested at 10 ft monocularly (i.e., <10/20 or 20/40) *or* 2-line difference between eyes, even within the passing range (i.e., 10/12.5 and 10/20 or 20/25 and 20/40)
Distance visual acuity ages ≥6 yr	<4 of 6 correct on 15-ft line with either eye tested at 10 ft monocularly (i.e., <10/15 or 20/30) *or* 2-line difference between eyes, even within the passing range (i.e., 10/10 and 10/15 or 20/20 and 20/30)

*See also Table 68-2.

From Committee on Practice and Ambulatory Medicine, Section on Ophthalmology, American Academy of Pediatrics: Eye examination and vision screening in infants, children and young adults by pediatricians. Pediatrics 2003;(April):902–907. Used with permission of the American Academy of Pediatrics.

findings. An example using gross motor development is a child who is not yet walking at age 14 months. Evaluation is different for a child who stood and cruised on time than for a child whose previous motor milestones were delayed and different for a child whose strength, tone, and deep tendon reflexes are normal compared with a child with hypertonicity and abnormally brisk deep tendon reflexes.

Identifying variations of normal is as important as identifying normal. Subtleties are challenging. Many physical attributes and developmental milestones evolve gradually and progressively. Infancy, childhood, and adolescence are noted for frequent occurrences of "fits and starts." Individuals often experience unique and not always predictable periods of accelerations and plateaus or may display different rates of development for different attributes. Contextual and longitudinal perspectives are useful.

NEWBORN EXAMINATION

Box 2-2 lists the areas of concentration for a newborn examination. Box 2-3 presents the sequence of the examination.

Approach to the Examination

The newborn's physical and cognitive immaturities are factors that simultaneously hinder and facilitate the examination process. Observations and maneuvers can be performed and repeated at relative leisure without much resistance from the patient. Because of the limitations inherent in this early period of sensorimotor development, the clinician must rely almost exclusively on touch to enhance cooperation. Maneuvers are executed passively, without active assistance from the infant. Observation is crucial for the newborn. Equipment requirements are minimal and include a stethoscope, rubber glove, tongue depressor, tape measure, light source, and ophthalmoscope. The ophthalmoscope should be kept nearby, preferably with the light turned on.

The sequence of the newborn examination is influenced primarily by the newborn's state and state-to-state variations. Examination always begins with observations to form a global first impression about general state of development (e.g., term versus premature, well grown versus undernourished), obvious anomalies or asymmetries, overall coloring, ease and rate of respiration, and unusual noises or activities. If extremities are visible, the degree of flexion or extension is noted, and fingers and toes are counted and inspected for webbing (syndactyly) and abnormal curvatures (clinodactyly). Each component of the evaluation requires vigilance for congenital anomalies, birth

---

Box 2-2. Newborn Examination: Areas of Concentration

1. Congenital anomalies
2. Birth injuries
3. Acute neonatal illnesses
4. Determination of gestational age and appropriateness of size for gestational age

Adapted from Algranati PS: Effect of developmental status on the approach to physical examination. Pediatr Clin North Am 1998;45:2–3.

Box 2-3. Sequence of Newborn Examination

1. General observations
2. Eye examination/red reflex (whenever infant is calm/eyes open)
3. Auscultation of anterior chest
4. Palpation of abdomen (defer palpation of kidneys)
5. Palpation of femoral and upper extremity pulses
6. Head-to-toe examination of anterior body, including palpation of kidneys (defer Ortolani/Barlow maneuvers)
7. Head-to-toe examination of posterior body
8. Remaining neurologic assessments
9. Ortolani/Barlow maneuvers
10. Moro reflex

---

trauma, and newborn illnesses. If the infant is quiet, the examiner should proceed with auscultation of the anterior chest. For this initial auscultation, the warmed diaphragm of the stethoscope should be slipped under the blanket and shirt onto the chest with the most minimal disruption of overlying fabrics. Auscultation of the chest should be followed with gentle palpation of the abdomen for masses and organomegaly (defer palpation of the kidneys until the infant is fully undressed), then palpation of the femoral and upper extremity pulses. Palpation of the abdomen and pulses can be accomplished without undressing the infant further except to release the fastenings on the sides of the diaper. Gentle, warm touch and gradual motions minimize disturbance of sleep. Gradually increasing pressure of the fingertips, the clinician next examines for splenic enlargement (a tip is normal), locates the liver edge (may be 1 to 2 cm down from the costal margin in the midclavicular line), and palpates for masses. Some clinicians choose to auscultate for the presence of bowel sounds, but percussion of the abdomen is not routine. If the infant begins to stir, insertion of a pacifier or gloved finger to initiate sucking may maintain a calm or sleeping state and relax abdominal musculature.

The femoral pulses should feel strong, equally full, and coincident in timing with upper extremity pulses. The examination continues with head-to-toe inspection and palpation of the anterior body, deferring hip abduction until later. If the infant has remained calm, the clinician may want to examine the eyes at this time. Dimming the room lights or speaking softly to the infant may stimulate the eyes to open. Alternatively, when an examiner's hand is placed underneath the back of the head and gently raises the head off of the mattress, the eyelids should open reflexively. This maneuver allows inspection of the eyes and assessment of red reflexes, blink to light, and pupillary response to light. In dark-skinned infants, a normal red reflex is often much paler and lighter in color than in white infants. The eyes are inspected for shape, symmetry, and size (globes, palpebral fissures); presence of individual, intact structures (e.g., irises present without gaps or colobomas); spacing and positioning (e.g., eyes are not too close together or too far apart; angle of the palpebral fissures is either horizontal or consistent with the infant's racial origin) (Fig. 2-6); clarity (e.g., corneas are clear, not cloudy); and color (e.g., sclerae are white, grayish white, or bluish white). Attention next is directed to inspection and palpation of the head (for

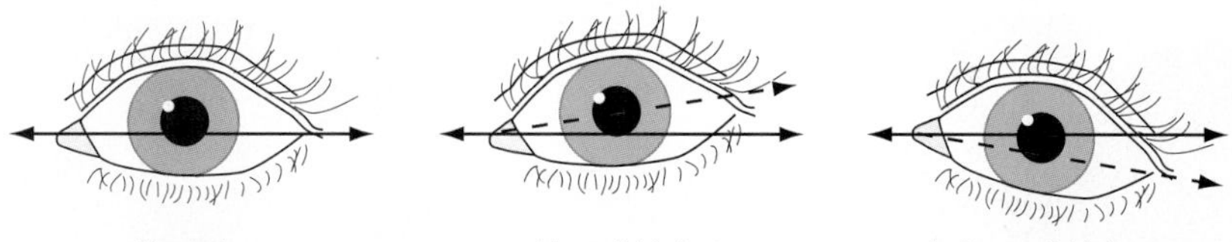

Normal	Mongoloid slant	Antimongoloid slant

Figure 2-6. Determining the angle of the palpebral fissure. (Redrawn from DeMeyer W: Technique of the Neurologic Examination: A Programmed Text, 3rd ed. New York, McGraw-Hill, 1980, p 3.)

overall shape and bulges, their location, and whether or not they are confined by or cross suture lines) (Fig. 2-7), hair (color, texture, amount, presence of unusual hair whorls), cranial sutures (overriding or widely separated) (Fig. 2-8), fontanelles (size, shape, bulging or sunken), and face (overall appearance and spatial relationships of features). Nose and ears are inspected for shape, size, placement (e.g., ears are not low set or posteriorly rotated) (Fig. 2-9), presence of abnormal pits or tags, and patency (nares, ear canals).

Otoscopic examination of the tympanic membrane is unnecessary in a healthy newborn because of the extreme unlikelihood of middle ear disease and presence of residual amniotic fluid in the external canal. Inspection of the mucosa, tongue, palate, uvula, and oral pharynx may require the use of a tongue depressor and an external light source. If the infant is crying, the clinician should peek quickly inside the mouth and observe muscles of facial expression for symmetry of movement. Inspection of the palate must be accompanied by palpation for a submucosal cleft. A gloved finger placed inside the mouth also can be used to elicit gag and sucking reflexes. The blanket and undershirt should be removed to evaluate the neck,

clavicles, anterior chest, and upper extremities. The skin is inspected for birthmarks, rashes, and jaundice. Crying also can allow observation of upper extremity movements. The extremities should have complete and normal movements. Erb's palsy and Klumpke's paralysis of upper extremities are sequelae of brachial plexus injury. Full visualization of the thyroid gland region can be accomplished only when the neck is hyperextended. The clavicles are palpated along their full lengths searching for crepitus, a sign of an underlying fracture. With the infant's chest fully exposed, auscultation of anterior lung fields can be completed. The posterior lung fields are auscultated by rolling the infant onto his or her side.

The diaper is opened anteriorly, and inspection of the abdomen is completed (e.g., sunken versus distended, presence of umbilical hernia or diastasis recti abdomini). The caudal progression continues with kidney palpation, evaluation of the external genitalia, and inspection of anterior lower extremities. To palpate the kidneys using a bimanual approach, the examiner places one hand with palm facing up underneath the infant's back just above the iliac crest (Fig. 2-10). The fingertips of the opposite hand palpate down toward the back beginning medially and progressing laterally until the kidney is located as a soft, firm mass approximately 2 cm in width and 4 cm in length, between the examiner's two hands. Because maneuvers to examine the hip are disturbing to the infant and can inter-

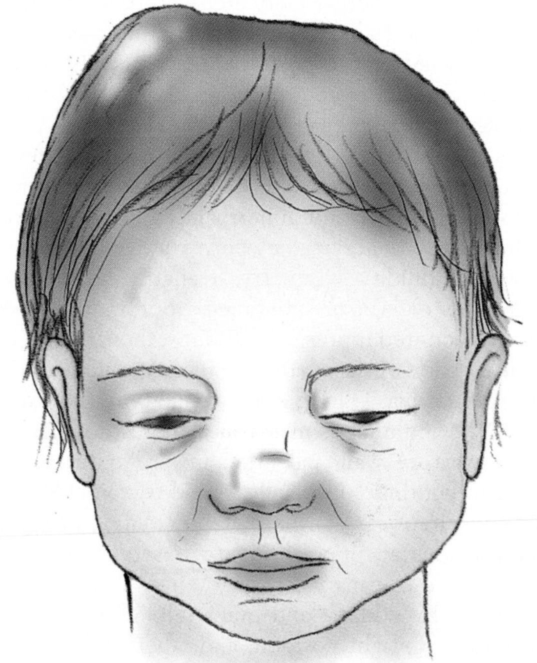

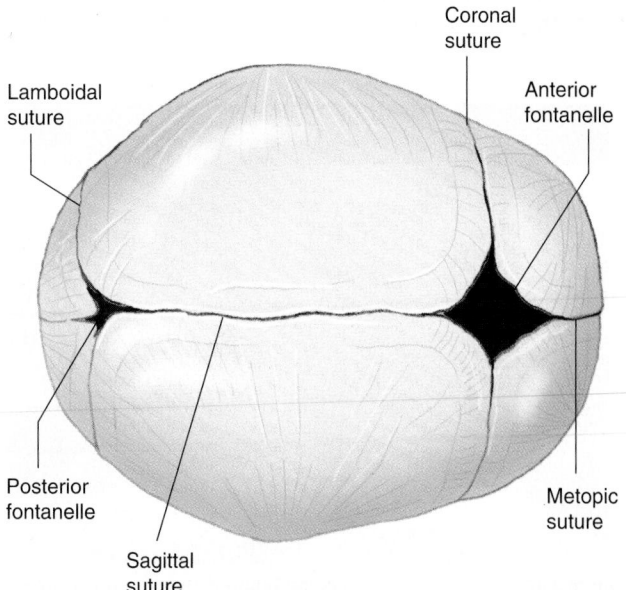

Figure 2-7. Cephalhematoma. It does not cross the suture line. (Redrawn from Algranati PS: The Pediatric Patient: An Approach to History and Physical Examination. Baltimore, Williams & Wilkins, 1992.)

Figure 2-8. Cranial sutures and fontanelles. (Redrawn from Willms JL, Lewis J [eds]: Introduction to Clinical Medicine. Baltimore, Williams & Wilkins, 1991, p 138.)

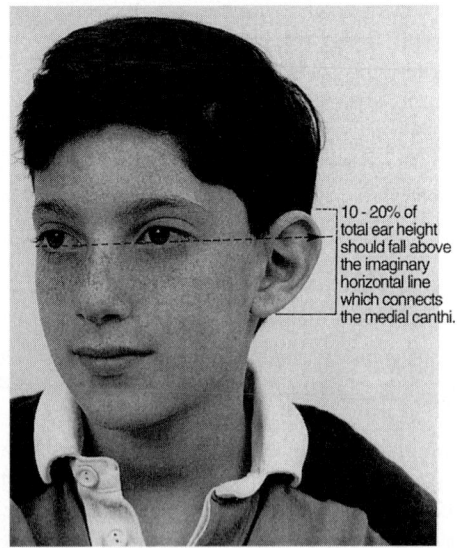

Figure 2-9. Determining low-set ears. (From Algranati PS: The Pediatric Patient: An Approach to History and Physical Examination. Baltimore, Williams & Wilkins, 1992.)

fere with accomplishing some of the remaining maneuvers, deferring hip abduction/adduction until the end of the examination is suggested. To inspect the female genitalia fully, the thighs must be flexed, abducted, and externally rotated (Fig. 2-11). After applying gentle traction to the labia, the inspection proceeds from superior to inferior visualizing in sequence the clitoris, urethra, vagina, and anus; the clinician should note that each structure is present, distinct, and appropriate in size. For male newborns, the penis is assessed for size, absence of curvature, and location of the urethral meatus (ruling out hypospadius or epispadius). The foreskin should never be retracted forcefully. Viewing the tip of the glans and urethal opening is sufficient. The scrotum is inspected and palpated for testicles (size and texture), mass, or fluid. If a testicle in not located inside the scrotum, the length of the inguinal canal is palpated. If the testicle is palpated in the inguinal canal, the clinician should attempt to milk it down into the scrotum to distinguish between a retractile and an undescended

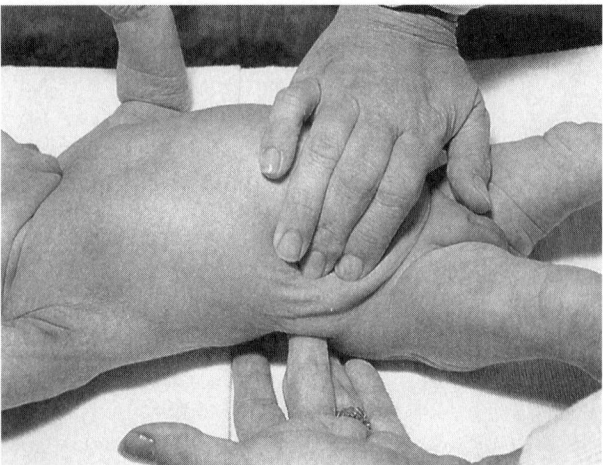

Figure 2-10. Bimanual palpation of the kidney in the newborn. (From Algranati PS: The Pediatric Patient: An Approach to History and Physical Examination. Baltimore, Williams & Wilkins, 1992.)

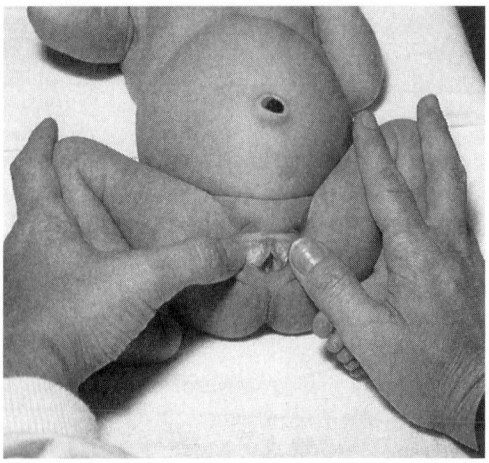

Figure 2-11. Position to inspect female genitalia in the newborn or young infant. (From Algranati PS: The Pediatric Patient: An Approach to History and Physical Examination. Baltimore, Williams & Wilkins, 1992.)

testis. A penlight or otoscope light applied directly to the scrotal surface helps assess whether a full-appearing scrotum is filled with fluid (i.e., hydrocele) or solid tissue (i.e., hernia).

After examination of the genitalia, the clinician continues caudad along the lower extremities, ending with inspection of the feet for joint flexibility and angulation and to determine that the forefoot is straight in line with the hindfoot. Before replacing the diaper, the infant is placed in the prone position. The examination continues with a head-to-toe inspection and palpation of the posterior body from the back of the head, along the length of the spine (for bony abnormalities, curvatures, dimples, pits, and overlying masses) to the buttocks, lower extremities, and feet. The eyes and hands should linger on any areas of potential abnormality to distinguish between findings such as a benign dimple in the coccygeal/gluteal cleft area compared with one in the sacral area (which may represent an occult spinal dysraphism). After the posterior inspection is concluded, the diaper and undershirt are repositioned, and the infant is consoled.

Throughout the course of the examination, the newborn's state-to-state variations can provide useful information. Cry is assessed for vigor and abnormalities in pitch and tone. Simultaneously the crying newborn's active movements are observed for fluidity, symmetry, strength, and the presence of jitteriness or lack of spontaneity. Self-induced beats of clonus are counted if present. With forethought and adaptation, other parts of the examination can continue in the face of vigorous crying. During kidney palpation, the examining hand on the abdomen is maintained in position. At the end of an expiratory wail, palpation inward onto the kidney begins and continues cyclically, timed to coincide with the infant's inspirations. The predictable voiding of the crying infant provides an opportunity to observe the force and direction of the urinary stream. When a crying infant is consoled with cuddling and quiet talk, the infant can be tilted into an upright position, and when the crying stops, the eyes open reflexively and can be examined again. It also may be possible to engage the infant in visual fixation. An assessment of doll's eye motions can be performed to assess range of motion of extraocular muscles and conjugate eye movements. While the infant is still in the clinician's arms, the examination concludes with a variety of neurologic and neurodevelopmental assessments. Play can elicit place and step, reflex grasp, and root reflexes, and tone can be assessed during ventral suspension observing for "slip through."

The last two components of the newborn examination can be performed regardless of whether the infant is calm or crying. The clinician places the infant back into the supine position and executes the Ortolani and Barlow maneuvers. The Ortolani maneuver is executed to uncover a dislocated hip, and the Barlow maneuver is executed to determine whether a hip is dislocatable (Box 2-4, Fig. 2-12, and the CD-ROM video). If a Moro reflex has not been observed, this reflex is elicited as well. Primitive reflexes (i.e., Moro reflex) primarily serve as general sensors for the integrity of the neuraxis. Their elicitation also supplies data about the status of muscle groups, nerves, and the skeletal system. Despite the dependence on observation and passive maneuvers, a relatively complete neurologic assessment of the newborn can be accomplished.

A formal assessment of gestational age is usually unnecessary for a full-term, normal-sized newborn. Formal assessment of gestational age and a determination of appropriateness of size (weight, length, and head circumference) for gestational age is appropriate for infants who appear to be premature or whose dimensions are suspiciously smaller or greater than average. (See Chapter 195.)

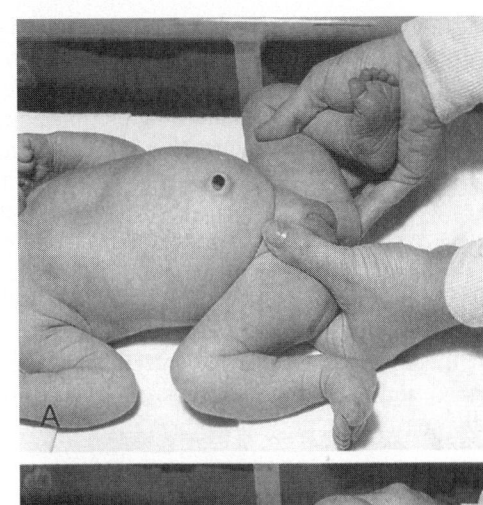

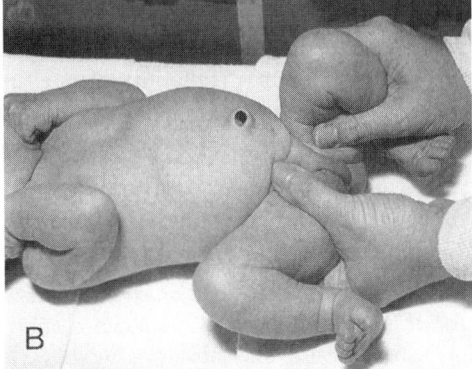

Figure 2-12. Ortolani **(A)** and Barlow **(B)** maneuvers. (From Algranati PS: The Pediatric Patient: An Approach to History and Physical Examination. Baltimore, Williams & Wilkins, 1992.)

Box 2-4. Ortolani and Barlow Maneuvers*

To Examine the Left Hip

Stabilize the infant's right hip by placing your left thumb onto the symphysis pubis and the fingers of your left hand underneath the right buttock.

To Perform the Ortolani Maneuver on the Left Hip

Using your right hand, bring the infant's left hip into 90 degrees of flexion and the knee into full flexion. The infant's posterior thigh should be resting on top of your fingertips and the lower leg/foot against your palm. Use your thumb to encircle the anterior tibia and rest it against the anterolateral thigh just distal to the inguinal fold. Your second and third fingers should rest on the posterolateral thigh over the greater trochanter.

Gently abduct the left thigh and simultaneously press the fingers resting on the posterolateral thigh upward toward the ceiling. In normal children, this maneuver is executed seamlessly or with a soft click that usually emanates from the knees.

A dislocated hip is felt to reduce or move anteriorly back into the acetabulum with a tangible or audible "clunk."

To Perform the Barlow Maneuver on the Left Hip

With your right hand maintaining the same positions on the left lower extremity (the hip and knee maintained in flexion), gently adduct the thigh and simultaneously press your thumb onto the anterolateral thigh downward toward the floor. In normal children, this maneuver is executed seamlessly or with a soft click that usually emanates from the knees.

A dislocatable hip is felt to dislocate or move posteriorly out of the acetabulum with a tangible or audible "clunk."†

*See also Figure 52-1.
†After reversing hands, repeat the Ortolani and Barlow maneuvers on the right hip.

Significance of Findings

Repetitive observation of the newborn over the 24- to 48-hour stay in the newborn nursery provides an opportunity to determine whether findings are transient or more permanent. Asymmetry of facial muscles or extremity movements can be ascertained as the patient frequently cooperates by crying, calming, yawning, and sleeping within the space of a few minutes. Most heart murmurs audible in healthy newborns disappear between 24 and 48 hours of life as a result of changing cardiovascular flow dynamics. These are soft, blowing systolic ejection murmurs usually heard at the upper left sternal border. The other benign heart murmur in the newborn, peripheral pulmonic stenosis, disappears by approximately age 3 months. This murmur is relatively quiet, short, blowing, and midsystolic and is heard with equal intensity on both sides of the anterior chest and is particularly prominent in the right axillae.

The newborn shows a wide variety of physical characteristics that are transitory, caused by physical immaturity, birth events, or maternal prenatal influences. Normal features of neonatal respiratory function are obligate nasal breathing and periodic breathing, which is not associated with deleterious consequences and resolves. The skin color varies as a result of peripheral vasculature instability, evidenced by acrocyanosis, mottling, and perioral cyanosis. These normal color changes must be distinguished from central cyanosis. Minor trauma from labor and delivery produces swellings, bruises, and molding that resolve spontaneously. The presenting part, usually the head, takes the brunt of the trauma (i.e., molding, caput succedaneum, cephalhematoma) (see Fig. 2-7). The interpretation of the significance of these findings should include differentiation from more significant trauma (e.g., cephalhematoma versus hematoma with underlying depressed skull fracture) and from congenital disorders unrelated to birth trauma (e.g., overriding sutures associated with molding at birth versus craniosynostosis). Common and benign findings also result from in utero transfer of maternal hormones to the infant, including breast swelling, secretion of a milky discharge (i.e., physiologic galactorrhea in male and female newborns), and vaginal discharge or bleeding. These conditions resolve during the first weeks of life, as hormone levels fall.

INFANT EXAMINATION

Box 2-5 lists areas of concentration for the infant examination. Areas of concentration relate to transitions in body size, physical development, and cognitive and affective capabilities.

Approach to the Examination

An infant younger than 6 months old is usually much easier to examine than an infant who is approaching 1 year old. The young infant can be examined on the examination table or the parent's lap following a sequence similar to that described for newborns. Minor obstacles and new challenges are presented by the emerging temperament and displays of varying moods. Brief but necessary interludes to feed, pacify, cuddle, or change a diaper usually suffice. Other simple maneuvers for distraction include gentle repetitive body movements (e.g., rocking) and interesting sounds (e.g., clicking noise made close to the ear as the speculum is introduced into the canal). Physically uncomfortable or intrusive maneuvers, especially examinations of the pharynx, tympanic membrane, and hips, should be deferred to the end of the examination sequence. Before development of attachment-related anxieties, infants generally enjoy being "put through their paces."

A few components of the examination merit special mention. Because of the unique orientation of the ear canal during infancy, to visualize the tympanic membrane, the pinna must be pulled down and posterior while advancing the speculum into the canal. The speculum should be long and narrow (size 2.5 mm or 3 mm). A tube attached

---

Box 2-6. Cover Test for Ocular Alignment*

This test is performed when an infant (starting around age 3 months) has the ability to fix on a object positioned approximately 10 ft away. Test one eye at a time.

1. Occlude vision of one eye. If the infant or child strongly objects to having vision occluded from one eye, referral is indicated.
2. Hold an attractive object up for the child to fix on.
3. Remove the occlusion, and observe for movement of the recently uncovered eye. An eye without ocular misalignment does not move. If the recently uncovered eye displays movement, referral is indicated. If the eye moves inward, suspect esotropia. If the eye moves outward, suspect exotropia.

*See also Figure 68-1.

---

to a rubber bulb should be connected to the otoscope (pneumatic otoscope) so that movement of the tympanic membrane can be assessed with insufflation. Evaluation for strabismus should be routine, observing for symmetric placement on the corneas of a reflection from an external light source (corneal light reflex) and by the cover test (Box 2-6). Special attention must be paid to survey for congenital anomalies and abnormalities. The eyes are inspected repeatedly for presence of complete and symmetric red reflexes, and the corneas are inspected for clarity, symmetry, and absence of bulging (i.e., congenital glaucoma). In examining for hip dysplasia, after the first several months of life, the Ortolani and Barlow maneuvers no longer are appropriate because movement of a dislocated hip in and out of the acetabulum becomes increasingly difficult. The best physical examination finding for a dislocated hip in an infant older than age 3 months is limited hip abduction. In a supine infant, the hips should be abducted while the legs are maintained at 90 degrees of flexion. The knees should touch or nearly touch the table, and the extent of abduction should be symmetric. Neurologic examination should include assessment of primitive reflexes (Table 2-4). Failure to extinguish a primitive reflex in a timely manner may indicate cerebral palsy.

For the infant age 6 months to 1 year, with the emergence of stranger and separation anxieties, approach and sequencing must become increasingly flexible, spontaneous, and responsive. Acquainting the patient with the examiner is accomplished best through a process of gradual escalation of the extent of verbal, audible, visual, and physical contact.

Box 2-5. Infant Examination: Areas of Concentration

1. Growth
2. Motor development
3. Language development
4. Affective development:
   Visibility of temperament
   Successful attachment
   Emergence of autonomy and independence
5. ≤6 months: Continued surveillance:
   Latent congenital anomalies
   Delayed sequelae of newborn problems

Adapted from Algranati PS: Effect of developmental status on the approach to physical examination. Pediatr Clin North Am 1998;45:6–7.

Table 2-4. Timing of Primitive Reflexes

Reflex	Present	Disappears
Moro	At birth (term)	6 mo
Suck	At birth	6–8 mo
Root	At birth	6–8 mo
Place and step	At birth	1–2 mo
Tonic neck	Birth–2 mo	6–7 mo
Reflex grasp	At birth	2–3 mo
Lateral prop	4–5 mo	Does not disappear
Parachute	8–9 mo	Does not disappear

From Algranati PS: Pediatric examination. In Willms JL, Schneiderman H, Algranati PS (eds): Physical Diagnosis: Bedside Evaluation of Diagnosis and Function. Baltimore, Williams & Wilkins, 1994, p 665.

For the extremely fearful infant, the examiner begins by sitting as far away as possible, avoiding eye contact, speaking softly, and moving slowly, with gradual progression toward closer contact. Instruments may be introduced casually by making them available for inspection and manipulation (e.g., place them on an accessible surface or hand something to the infant while looking at and talking with a parent). Distraction capitalizes on the infant's preoccupation with object manipulation and interest in novel sounds. To respect an infant's separation anxiety, he or she should be allowed to remain close to the parent and vice versa. The parent can stand at the clinician's side next to the examination table or hold the infant for the duration of the examination.

Observation continues to supply a great deal of information in the assessment of this age group. Infants are observed for general level of activity, overall mood, responsiveness to parental handling, and objective evidence that the infant has achieved various developmental milestones. Infants display gross motor function by attempting to roll over on the table or sitting without support in the parent's lap. Manipulation or hand transference of a pacifier or otoscope bulb supplies information about fine motor development. The infant who smiles and squeals gleefully at his or her parent but cries warily at the clinician's approach confirms that he or she has vision and offers data about muscles of facial expression, verbal development, and attachment. The infant who fixes, follows, and reaches out for an object held aloft in various directions provides evidence that extraocular muscle function, upper extremity symmetry, strength, and coordination are normal.

For a fearful infant, the choice of sequence for the hands-on portion of the examination should reflect an appreciation for stranger anxiety. Touching can be demystified by proceeding from least intrusive to most intrusive (e.g., touch first, and use invasive instruments such as the otoscope last; palpate distally before palpating centrally; use to-and-fro motions before more sustained ones).

Changing the planned sequence in midstream can enhance data collection. If the infant is sleeping, the stethoscope diaphragm should be warmed rapidly and heart and lung auscultation completed before the infant wakens. Posterior lung fields can be auscultated quickly if the infant is being held in burping position. If the infant begins to cry during auscultation of the lungs, the stethoscope should be left in place because inspiration can be evaluated adequately anyway; evaluation of expiration is deferred until the infant is calmer. With the infant still in burping position, the clinician can walk around the parent and face the infant to inspect the eyes, assess pupillary response and red reflex, and complete a cover test for strabismus. Before moving away, the cranium, sutures, and fontanelles may be palpated. The posterior fontanelle closes shortly after birth (or by 1 to 2 months of age); closure of the anterior fontanelle is less uniform, but it typically closes between 6 and 18 months (≤2 years old). Infants perceive some examination maneuvers as play. By holding onto the infant's hands and drawing the infant from supine to sitting, the extent of head lag and truncal tone are observed. Then, grasping the infant under the axillae and assisting him or her to stand, the clinician can assess the support of weight on feet and

overall tone. Finally the clinician should support the infant horizontally and move him or her through the air like an airplane to assess tone.

Examination of an ill infant presents many challenges. The most essential determination is severity of illness. Many formal scales have been developed that assess the degree of alertness or ease of arousal, state-to-state variation, quality and pitch of cry, skin color, responsiveness to social overtures, and hydration status. History complements physical examination. For the infant, assessment of hydration includes looking for tears with crying, assessing the moisture of mucous membranes, inspecting the contour of a patent anterior fontanelle (the infant must be upright), assessing abdominal skin turgor (also used as a measure of nutrition), and assessing capillary refill time. To assess skin turgor, a small portion of the abdominal skin and subcutaneous tissues is pulled up slightly and then quickly released. Normally the skin springs back quickly. To assess capillary refill time, the infant's fingertip is compressed briefly between the examiner's thumb and index finger until it blanches. The capillary refill time is normal if skin regains normal color within 2 seconds.

Significance of Findings

The enormous rate of developmental change within this age period is helpful and confounding for the clinician. The significance of findings is affected profoundly by the wide range of normal rates of growth, progress toward ambulation and conversation, and acquisition of capacity for thought. Developmental progress early in life occurs in fits and starts, adding further difficulty to decisions based on one-time observations. Caution and latitude should be exercised before concluding that a worrisome finding requires investigation or intervention. The patient's findings also must be evaluated in comparison with peers, norms, and members of the infant's family and with respect to the infant's current condition and previous progress. Input of parent opinions and concerns is essential.

Several age-related physical findings merit specific mention because of the importance of their correct interpretation. Infants younger than age 4 months commonly display intermittent periods of discordant eye movement (e.g., the eyes appear to cross) without evidence of underlying pathology. Further evaluation is indicated for fixed limitation in extraocular movement in any direction or if discordance of movements continues beyond the first 4 to 6 months of life. Pseudostrabismus is an apparent dysfunction in eye muscle coordination without true pathology. Children with pseudostrabismus frequently have epicanthal folds that create the illusion of true strabismus. Symmetry of corneal light reflex and the cover test are normal. Another important age-related finding that can be misinterpreted is presence of nuchal rigidity. Until the infant approaches age 1 year and head control is fully established, the degree of resistance to passive neck flexion is not a sensitive indicator of meningeal irritation.

With infants, several physical problems require close scrutiny and an expedient response by the clinician because of their potential for profound long-term disability if not diagnosed and treated. To recognize these problems, the examiner must be familiar with age-related norms and

21

routinely gather input from parents. Specific issues of this type are visual acuity and hearing ability, eye muscle coordination, vocalization, and attachment behaviors. Assessment most appropriately begins with careful history taking and physical examination, after which supplemental testing may be necessary. Even when diagnoses are irreversible (e.g., blindness), prompt clinical identification often profoundly affects the infant's long-term adaptive potential. Early diagnosis of treatable conditions (e.g., strabismus, glaucoma, developmental dysplasia of the hip) is essential to optimize outcome.

TODDLER EXAMINATION

Box 2-7 lists areas of concentration for the toddler examination. Areas of concentration relate to refinement of emerging verbal and motor skills.

Approach to the Examination

Toddlers' wide variations in activity levels and degrees of cooperation present the greatest examination challenges within the entire pediatric age group. Regardless of whether a toddler is highly mobile and curious or shy, cautious, and slow to warm up, the clinician's appearance at the doorway often initiates displays of heightened stranger anxiety. Predictably the toddler suddenly backs away from the doorway and clings to the nearest parent. Even as an active, inquisitive toddler races around the examination room, opportunities for data collection are present. Findings that may be assessed during this rapid-fire display include skin, gait, gross motor skills, strength, coordination, speech content and clarity during parental interaction, vision, fine motor skills during play with toys, hearing in response to parental directives, and evidence for the emergence of the preoperational stage of cognitive development (e.g., pretend play). Even the very young toddler may be enticed to come closer to participate in a game of hide-and-seek or "on-and-off" with a penlight or beeper.

The intensity of the toddler's parental attachment highlights the importance of using parents to assist the clinician. Parents provide a lap that replaces the examination table as a safe haven and base of operations and an extra pair of hands that facilitate positioning the child for examination. Additional duties may include removal or replacement of clothing, modeling as a patient (e.g., "First we'll tap mommy's knee; then we'll tap yours"), modeling as a clinician (e.g., "Watch mommy tap my knee; then we'll tap yours"), offering words of comfort, setting verbal limits, or providing physical restraint.

Box 2-7. Toddler Examination: Areas of Concentration

1. Speech clarity and content
2. Gait and appearance of lower extremities
3. Hearing and middle ear status
4. Vision and strabismus screening
5. Affective development: autonomy and independence

Adapted from Algranati PS: Effect of developmental status on the approach to physical examination. Pediatr Clin North Am 1998;45:10.

During history taking and physical examination, patient and parent display their reciprocal attachment. Children negotiate autonomy and independence issues (e.g., "No," "Me do it," "Give me that"). The clinician can observe parental management (e.g., "Stop that," "Give me that"), the "goodness of fit" between the child's behaviors and abilities, and parents' expectations. Content (i.e., what the parent says, what the child says) and process (e.g., intonation, inflection) of interactions should be assessed.

The sequence of the lap examination is governed by the philosophy of gradual familiarization. Light touch in the periphery of the body precedes firmer touch and examination of central body regions, followed by instrumentation and intrusion. The patient's temperament, the patient's fears, the purpose of the examination, and the patient's current health status dictate the exact sequence and specific choice of maneuvers.

Even a young toddler appreciates opportunities to exercise control during the encounter. Many parts of the examination (e.g., inspection and palpation of the head, face, and neck; chest auscultation; abdominal palpation; male genital examination) may be conducted even when the toddler insists on standing rather than sitting in the parent's lap. A toddler might prefer to straddle the parent's knees sideways rather than face the clinician directly. This position allows auscultation of the anterior and posterior chest walls without repositioning the patient and allows the toddler to see the parent and the clinician. It also diminishes the time the toddler is breathing directly into the clinician's face. The clinician can auscultate the lungs while compressing the chest between hands placed anteriorly and posteriorly and can uncover subtle degrees of bronchospasm during the expiratory phase of respiration. Use of a tongue depressor may be avoided if the child is willing to "pant like a doggy" or to allow the examiner to "count teeth." Offering a series of tongue depressors, one at a time, can succeed as brief diversions, as each stick is accepted, inspected, and manipulated. This distraction also may be useful for genital examinations. A female toddler, in the safe haven of a lap, may allow a parent to spread her legs, affording the opportunity for quick genital inspection.

Evaluating the middle ear is invariably a stumbling block in toddlers. Saving otoscopic evaluation for the examination's conclusion delays but does not eliminate the inevitable unpleasantness. The middle ear examination is accomplished most successfully with the toddler sitting on a parent's lap (Fig. 2-13). Visualizing the external canal as the speculum is introduced helps avoid scraping the side of the canal, a common cause of pain during the examination. Many toddlers can be distracted by clicking noises long enough for otoscopy to be completed. Pneumatic otoscopy should be performed to determine the degree of mobility of the tympanic membrane. The pharynx may be visualized with the toddler restrained similarly to that described for the tympanic membrane examination. The parent need only switch his or her hand that previously rested against the side of the toddler's head to the toddler's forehead, bracing the toddler's head against the parent's chest. The clinician is free to hold the light source in one hand and a tongue depressor in the other.

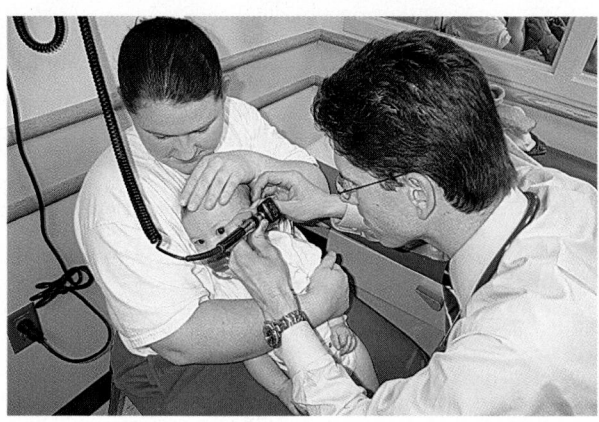

Figure 2-13. Middle ear examination with the child in parent's lap. The child is seated directly facing the examiner, with his or her legs restrained between the parent's knees. The parent encircles the child's trunk and arms with one arm, bracing the upper body against his or her own chest. With the other hand, the parent rotates the child's head to one side and holds it against the parent's upper chest. The clinician uses one hand to manipulate the pinna and the other hand to introduce the speculum into the canal, while holding the inverted shaft of the otoscope between the thumb and the forefinger and bracing the side of the hand against the child's head. (From Algranati PS: The Pediatric Patient: An Approach to History and Physical Examination. Baltimore, Williams & Wilkins, 1992.)

If the parent is unwilling or unable to provide adequate restraint or if a large amount of cerumen interferes with visualization of the tympanic membrane, the toddler should be transferred to the examination table. Assistance from a willing parent or office assistant minimizes the time of discomfort. The importance of firm restraint and efficient manipulation cannot be overemphasized. The clinician should explain the importance of the procedure, predict what will occur, and secure all necessary implements (e.g., curette) before beginning. These preparations facilitate accuracy and minimize the time of discomfort. Insufficient restraint exacerbates the potential for injury and prolongs discomfort. As soon as both tympanic membranes have been visualized, the toddler may be picked up and comforted. The pharynx can be observed quickly if the examiner switches positions with the parent. Now standing at the toddler's head, the parent is directed to lift the toddler's arms up over the head and brace each arm against the sides of the head. Positioned at the caudal end, the examiner now leans over the toddler, restraining the knees with his or her trunk, and holds the light in one hand and the tongue depressor in the other.

If gait has not yet been observed adequately and the toddler is unwilling to walk spontaneously, the clinician restrains the toddler briefly, allowing sufficient time for the parent to move to the opposite side of the room. When the toddler is allowed to escape, he or she flees quickly back to the security waiting across the room. This brief period of walking or running usually is enough to observe gait and assess for in-toeing or out-toeing (see also Chapter 51).

By age 3 to 4 years, toddlers are much more able to cooperate with an examination. Lingering fears frequently can be mitigated when conversation includes familiar subjects of interest and procedures allow for a feeling of empowerment (e.g., "Show me which ear to look in first," "Rub the stethoscope, and tell me when it's warm enough for you"). Many patients in this age group agree to sit alone on the examination table, follow directions from the clinician, and even enjoy the experience of the encounter.

In the older toddler, a head-to-toe examination sequence usually is accepted. Many toddlers have an innocent heart murmur. When careful auscultation is combined with history taking, data generally are sufficient for a clinical diagnosis of this benign entity. An innocent murmur is defined as one associated with no underlying heart disease or abnormal heart sounds. Except for a venous hum, an innocent murmur is always systolic, begins after S_1 (never coincident with S_1), is relatively quiet (not louder than a grade 3) and soft (never grating or harsh), and frequently varies with changes in the child's position (Table 2-5).

Formal neurologic examination at this age may include maneuvers that require active patient participation (e.g., "Smile and show me your teeth," "Squeeze my fingers," "Squat down like a frog and jump up really fast"). Advancing cognitive abilities in this age group frequently enable the patient to supply clinically useful information (e.g., in response to "Show me where it hurts" or "What did you eat for breakfast?") and to receive information about prevention and treatment (e.g., "Always wear your bike helmet" or "Drink this pink medicine"). The experienced practitioner is careful to avoid overdirecting the cooperative preschooler. During chest auscultation, listening without prior directives (e.g., "Take a big breath") avoids the young-ster's natural tendency to help by holding his or her breath or breathing noisily. Similarly, during abdominal palpation, some children cooperate by tensing up or holding their breath, particularly those who are ticklish. Distraction can be facilitated by guessing what was eaten for lunch while pressing onto the abdomen. Alternatively the cooperative toddler can assist by placing his or her hand either on top of or underneath the examiner's hand and complying with the request "You push in on your tummy instead of me, and I'll just leave my hand there while you do it for me" (Fig. 2-14).

Significance of Findings

The toddler examination sequence illustrates the wealth of opportunities for interpretation provided by the toddler's response to the examination. In addition to assessing affective development throughout the entire age period, an evaluation of the older toddler's achievement of independence serves a hidden and valued incidental purpose. There is a boost in self-confidence for the toddler who is congratulated for a "job well done!"

New skills usually are performed awkwardly or unsteadily, particularly with gross motor development (e.g., cruising, walking) and fine motor development (e.g., manipulation of spoon, cup). The awkwardness of newly acquired skills is an additional factor to consider when interpreting findings related to development. Normal speech patterns for this age group frequently create concerns about clarity and fluency. Disfluencies (e.g., articulation errors and letter substitutions) are by nature benign and self-limited. A good rule of thumb for clarity is that the percentage of speech intelligible by adults who are not the toddler's parents are 50% for a 2-year-old, 75% for a 3-year-old, and 100% for a 4-year-old.

Most older toddlers can cooperate for the physical examination. If a high degree of active resistance is encountered,

Table 2-5. Innocent Heart Murmurs in Childhood*

Murmur	Usual Age When First Audible	Description
Peripheral pulmonic stenosis	Newborn	Short/midsytolic/blowing Equally loud on right and left sides of anterior chest Also heard in axillae and back; often prominent in right axillae
Still's murmur	Toddler	Systolic ejection/vibratory Loudest midway between lower left sternal border and apex Increases in intensity in supine position
Venous hum	Toddler	Continuous/throughout systole and diastole Loudest at right clavicular area and may be heard at left infraclavicular area Murmur may be obliterated or modified by turning the patient's head away from the side of the murmur and by compressing the internal jugular vein on the side of the murmur Disappears in the supine position
Carotid bruit	Toddler	Systolic ejection Heard over the carotids Diminishes progressively with auscultation toward the aortic and pulmonic areas
Pulmonary flow	School-age child	Systolic ejection Loudest at the upper left sternal border, especially when recumbent May disappear completely when patient sits up

*See also Chapter 56 and CD-ROM.

From Algranati PS: Pediatric examination. In Willms JL, Schneiderman H, Algranati PS (eds): Physical Diagnosis: Bedside Evaluation of Diagnosis and Function. Baltimore, Williams & Wilkins, 1994, p 680.

the cause of this behavior should be pursued. The differential diagnosis includes cognitive delay, emotional immaturity, extremes of temperament style, inappropriate parental limit setting (e.g., absence of rules at home), reasonable fears based on previous medical experiences (e.g., frequent painful medical encounters in the past), reasonable fears based on nonmedical experiences (e.g., physical or sexual abuse history), and reasonable fears of exacerbation of existing pain (e.g., the toddler with severe otitis externa who knows that manipulation of the pinna will be painful). If ignored, the clinician may lose the opportunity to alter the toddler's response to subsequent medical experiences. In the worst-case scenario, a window of opportunity to explore potential life-threatening issues (e.g., physical or sexual abuse) may be missed as well.

Parents of toddlers frequently have questions about gait and body habitus. The gait of a new walker is wide-based, with toes frequently pointing outward. The base narrows with increasing confidence and agility. The stance of toddlers younger than age 2 is usually mildly bowlegged and evolves into a small degree of knock-kneed until school age. Toe walking is a common phenomenon and is usually transient and without pathologic significance. Careful neuromuscular and skeletal examinations are usually sufficient to rule out the more pathologic implications of toe walking (e.g., tight heel cords, cerebral palsy, tethered cord). Flatfoot is another common concern. Fat pads, an age-related phenomenon, obscure the longitudinal arch of the foot and create the illusion that the arch is absent. When walking is firmly established, parents may be concerned about in-toeing or out-toeing, most of which improves with advancing age. In toddlers and school-age children, the most common causes for in-toeing are internal tibial torsion and increased femoral anteversion. In-toeing of 30 degrees or more deviation from the forward line of progression is considered pathologic. Mild degrees of out-toeing are less frequent than in-toeing. During evaluation of lower extremities, the upright, scantily clad toddler provides the opportunity to assess body habitus. The typical pot belly and sway back result from continued laxity in abdominal muscle tone and a small degree of lumbar lordosis, both of which resolve as the thoracic cage elongates during the next several years.

SCHOOL-AGE CHILD EXAMINATION

Box 2-8 lists areas of concentration for the school-age child examination. Areas of concentration relate to individual concerns that are often troubling but relatively benign.

Approach to the Examination

The school-age child's willingness to cooperate and the unlikelihood of unexpected major discoveries allow a complete head-to-toe examination to be accomplished easily and quickly. Because resistance is unusual, its cause should be pursued. The enhanced cooperation in this age group affords the opportunity for more sophisticated information

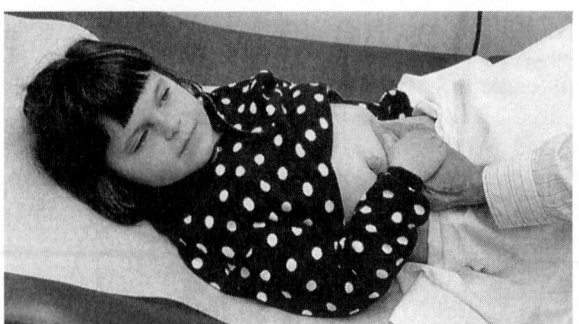

Figure 2-14. Maneuver to relax the abdomen in a child. Ask the patient to "help do the pushing." (From Algranati PS: The Pediatric Patient: An Approach to History and Physical Examination. Baltimore, Williams & Wilkins, 1992.)

> **Box 2-8.** *School-Age Child Examination: Areas of Concentration*
>
> 1. Common minor infections (e.g., respiratory, skin)
> 2. Aches and pains (e.g., headaches, stomachaches)
> 3. Allergic disorders (including asthma)
> 4. Dentition and dental development
> 5. Slow, steady growth
> 6. Scoliosis screening
> 7. *Older school-age child:* Signs of puberty
>
> Adapted from Algranati PS: Effect of developmental status on the approach to physical examination. Pediatr Clin North Am 1998;45:10.

gathering, simultaneous with performance of the relatively rote maneuvers of a standard examination. The ability to use logic and see the viewpoints of others develops with the emergence of the concrete operations stage of cognitive development (at approximately age 8).

To explore affective and cognitive functioning, the practitioner usually can engage the patient in discussions about home life, leisure pursuits, friendships, and school. Beginning with casual, innocuous, open-ended questions about familiar topics and following with requests for more specific, objective data, significant insight into functioning may be gained. "How's school going?" and "What's your most favorite or least favorite thing about school?" should be followed by "How did you do on your last report card?" or "What grades did you get in math and English?" "Do you have a friend whom you consider to be your best friend?" and "What's his or her name?" may be followed by, "What's the most favorite thing you like to do with him or her?" and "Do you do that right after school?" This style of interview can provide data regarding physical functioning. A child who reveals that he or she and a friend attend an after-school soccer program 3 days a week is implying the probability of an acceptable level of physical fitness and an age-appropriate level of peer interaction.

With physical concerns, the clinician similarly can capitalize on the patient's willingness and capacity to supply history. As the examination proceeds, the interview should continue. Exploration of symptoms should be accompanied by inquiries regarding their effect on daily functioning. A 5- or 6-year-old child may not be able to describe the quality of pain in the head or abdomen but can report needing to put his or her head down on the desk instead of going out to recess. School-age children can supply helpful history about allergies or asthma, such as the effect of symptoms on sleep or gym participation. School-age children can cooperate with the examination, including ophthalmoscopy. Another challenge with children at the younger end of this age group is a preoccupation with fear of painful procedures. When appropriate, a statement such as "No shots or needles today" may provide much needed reassurance.

At some point during the school-age years, patients begin to display physical modesty, which should be anticipated, acknowledged, and respected. Offering an examination gown to cover underwear and using a drape when appropriate conveys respect, enhances the child's sense of control during the encounter, and increases cooperation and willingness to be open. Previewing and explaining maneuvers and offering choices also acknowledge the patient's maturing cognitive capacities.

Breast and genitalia examinations are performed with substantial respect and modesty with explanations before and during the examination. Explanations and conclusions should be adjusted to the patient's educational level and emotional maturity. Reassurance about the normalcy of findings (including progression of puberty and demystification of physiologic variations of normal) is important. Assumptions that emerging physical maturity equals cognitive maturity and the use of jargon should be avoided. The Tanner system of staging pubertal development is incorporated routinely into complete examinations as soon as signs of puberty are evident. In older school-age girls and boys, breast examination and inspection of the external genitalia should be performed to assess possible acquired pathology and confirmation of normal anatomy.

School-age children show increased cognitive and social abilities, greater coordination and fluidity in gross motor skills, and greater complexity and dexterity in fine motor skills, increasing their capacity to perform the more advanced features of the neurologic examination. Ability to perform rapid alternating movements (e.g., finger to nose, finger to finger) is only one of the many new additions that the clinician can include in the neurologic examination.

Questions directed toward common symptoms or problems should accompany the examination of related body systems (e.g., tinea, acne, mild anterior knee pain in the older school-age child, upper respiratory allergies). The clinician may be inclined to overlook and underestimate the significance of some of these conditions because they are common and relatively benign. The complete examination also should investigate for stage-related problems that are usually asymptomatic (e.g., pectus excavatum/carinatum, scoliosis, kyphosis, lordosis, mild degrees of deterioration in visual acuity, dental caries or malalignments, inadequate flexibility with respect to sports readiness) (Box 2-9). Particular attention should be paid to evaluation of growth rate and body habitus. Dysfunction (e.g., anorexia in the older school-age child and obesity in the entire spectrum of this age group) is common. The prevalence of these problems mandates that regardless of the stated purpose of the encounter, the patient should be required to disrobe (e.g., wear a gown over underwear) whenever a complete physical examination is performed.

Significance of Findings

Interpretation of findings is influenced heavily by comparison with age-related norms, particularly with the lymphoid and neurologic systems. In the school-age child, the period of physiologic lymphoid hypertrophy often peaks in a child who has frequent, but normal number of minor upper respiratory infections, manifesting as large tonsils or enlarged lymph nodes. Tonsil size generally is graded on a numerical scale, such as 1 to 4, with 1/4 signifying relatively invisible or the presence of only a small amount of lymphoid tissue behind the anterior tonsillar pillars, and 4/4 signifying kissing tonsils or tonsils that meet in the midline of the pharynx. Tonsillar hypertrophy is usually benign and self-limited and does not require intervention unless airway obstruction or sleep apnea is a

Box 2-9. Screening Examination for Scoliosis, Kyphosis, and Lordosis*

1. The patient's shirt or gown is removed, and the patient is requested to "stand straight and tall," with feet together, hands at sides, and looking straight ahead.
2. Standing behind the patient, inspect and palpate the spine (looking for curvatures, feeling for prominences or areas of tenderness), and then sequentially inspect, moving caudally, the shoulders, scapulae, ribs and paraspinal musculature, hips, and buttocks (for symmetry of height and prominence).
3. The patient is instructed to bend over from the waist, keeping knees straight, head hanging down, hands dangling at sides (or clasped together in front). The spine and lateral structures are reinspected as above.
4. Moving to the side of the patient, a cross-table lateral view of the back reveals any asymmetries in height or prominence of paired structures.
5. The patient is instructed to return to the upright position so that inspection for kyphosis and lordosis is completed.
6. If kyphosis or lordosis is noted, the patient again is instructed to bend over; with this maneuver, mild kyphosis appears as a smooth small curve, and mild lordosis disappears.

*See also Figures 53-1 and 53-6.

Table 2-6. When to Be Concerned Regarding Disorders of Puberty

Disorder of Puberty	Age and Gender
Early puberty with breast development and/or pubic hair in girls	<6 yr for African-American girls <7 yr for white girls and other ethnicities
Early puberty with pubic hair and/or testicular enlargement in boys	<9 yr
Delayed puberty if there is no evidence for thelarche (breast development) in girls	>13 yr
Delayed puberty if there is no evidence for menarche (menstrual flow) in girls	>15–16 yr in girls or within 5 yr of thelarche
Delayed puberty if there is no evidence for gonadarche (testicular enlargement) in boys	>14 yr

concern. Lymph nodes that are palpable in the anterior cervical regions and are small (<1 to 2 cm in greatest dimension), mobile, and neither rock hard nor inflamed are common and almost always benign. Small shotty nodes frequently are palpated in the occiput, axillae, or groin. Lymph nodes that are larger in size, rapidly enlarging, fixed to surrounding tissues, or located low in the posterior cervical chain or anywhere in the supraclavicular regions may be pathologic and must be investigated.

Significance of neurodevelopmental findings especially depends on comparisons with age-related norms. In the school-age child, the neurodevelopmental assessment may reveal the presence of soft signs that imply a degree of neuromaturational immaturity. Soft signs are overflow movements or postures that are exhibited while the child performs a gross motor or fine motor task. Minor movements are considered normal in a child who recently has developed the capacity to perform an age-appropriate task but should disappear as the child matures. For example, a 10-year-old should demonstrate easily rapid alternating finger movements of one hand. Simultaneous mirror movements of the opposite hand in a child of this age is a "soft sign." Other examples of soft signs for school-age children are substantial mouth or tongue movements while the child is writing and dystonic posturing of arms or hands while walking on the heels. Some studies suggest a relationship to learning disabilities, whereas others dispute their significance.

Bruising and nosebleeds are common in school-age children. Normal bruising is concentrated on the anterior surfaces of the lower aspects of the lower extremities and is bilateral. History and physical examination almost always can distinguish benign bruises from bruises caused by trauma or hematologic or vascular pathology. Nosebleeds usually result from drying of mucous membranes or digital trauma (picking the nose). History and careful physical examination usually suffice to identify a benign cause.

In assessing puberty, the clinician must use data regarding puberty, its timing, and normal progression (see Chapters 4 and 151). These data can confirm normal progression and assist in predictions of upcoming events. Patients can be reassured about variations of normal (e.g., "It may seem a bit early to you, but I can assure you that this is within the range of normal"). If true precociousness is suspected, these data are useful for early identification and decision making about further investigation. Table 2-6 summarizes when the clinician should be concerned about a disorder of puberty. In girls, an emergency visit to evaluate a tender, often unilateral breast lump almost always results in the happy diagnosis of the normal onset of puberty. The intrinsic connection between the appearance of secondary sexual characteristics and growth also is useful for evaluating concerns regarding growth. For normal boys in particular, reminding the patient and family that the male growth spurt does not usually begin until genital Tanner stage 3 or peak until genital Tanner stage 4 may ameliorate concerns about short stature.

Additional Resources, CD-ROM

Heart murmurs	Audio 56-1 to 56-8
Bibliography	

SUGGESTED READINGS

Algranati PS: Effect of developmental status on the approach to physical examination. Pediatr Clin North Am 1998;45:1–23.

Algranati PS: The Pediatric Patient: An Approach to History and Physical Examination. Baltimore, Williams & Wilkins, 1992.

Barness LA, Cooper DS (eds): Handbook of Pediatric Physical Diagnosis. Baltimore, Lippincott Williams & Wilkins, 1998.

Committee on Psychosocial Aspects of Child and Family Health, American Academy of Pediatrics Committee on Psychosocial Aspects of Child and Family Health: Guidelines for Health Supervision III. Elk Grove Village, Ill, American Academy of Pediatrics, 1997.

National Center for Health Statistics and National Center for Chronic Disease Prevention and Health Promotion: 2000. Available at: http://www.cdc.gov/growthcharts.

Zitelli BJ, Davis HW (eds): Atlas of Pediatric Physical Diagnosis, 3rd ed. St. Louis, Mosby, Wolfe, 1997.

3 Principles of Dysmorphology

Kenneth Lyons Jones and Marilyn C. Jones

The word *dysmorphology* is derived from Latin *dys*—meaning "faulty"—and Greek *morphōsis*—meaning "formation." The term refers to the study of aberrations of form or birth defects. Birth defects may have a variety of causes, including genetic and environmental factors. For most birth defects, however, the specific cause is not yet identified. The goal of the dysmorphologist is to try to determine etiology and pathogenesis because it is from the establishment of a diagnosis that information regarding prognosis and recurrence risk is forthcoming. This chapter outlines the general approach used to establish a diagnosis. This approach is predicated on the fact that 90% of diagnoses are based on a careful history, a comprehensive physical examination, and knowledge of the general cause of birth defects. Although testing is available for many of the genetic conditions that are associated with birth defects, a strong clinical suspicion is necessary to direct appropriate diagnostic testing because most such tests are not part of available clinical panels.

A rational approach to the infant with birth defects is presented in Figures 3-1 through 3-4. This approach is based on the concept that the nature of the structural defects represents a clue to the time of onset, mechanism of injury, and possible etiology of the problem, all of which determine the necessary evaluation. This approach permits a systematic narrowing of the diagnostic possibilities so that one of the basic compendiums on dysmorphology can be used to make a specific diagnosis. Parents of an infant with a birth defect have little interest in the full array of diagnoses. Without the knowledge that has been accumulated from experience with other children who have the same diagnosis, it is impossible to provide appropriate prognosis and recurrence risk counseling, the information about which parents of infants with birth defects are most concerned.

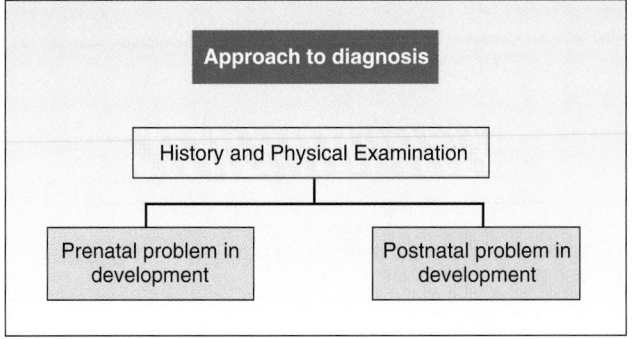

Figure 3-1. Approach to diagnosis: history and physical examination.

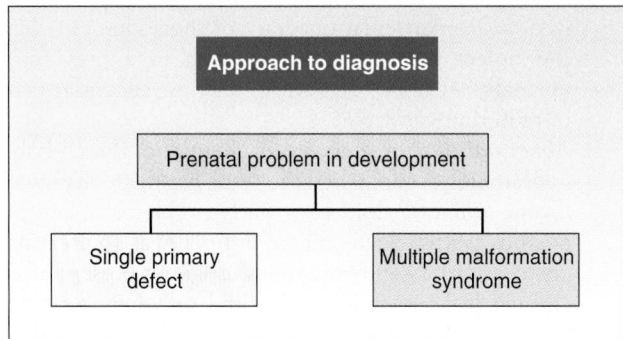

Figure 3-2. Approach to diagnosis: prenatal problem in development.

PRENATAL-ONSET VERSUS POSTNATAL-ONSET PROBLEMS IN STRUCTURAL DEVELOPMENT

Distinction between a problem in structural development with prenatal onset versus postnatal onset is determined by a directed history and detailed physical examination (see Fig. 3-1). From the standpoint of this chapter, *prenatal onset* designates structural abnormalities that are present at birth, and *postnatal onset* designates structures that have previously developed and differentiated normally. Although it is recognized that the genetic alteration responsible for many of the disorders included under postnatal-onset structural defects is present at the time of conception, the structural manifestations of that genetic alteration do not become obvious until postnatal life.

From an etiologic standpoint, prenatal-onset problems in development are the consequence of genetic or chromosomal alterations or are the result of factors unique to the pregnancy, such as environmental agents (teratogens), abnormalities of placentation, or mechanical constraint. Although the structural defects and neurologic abnormalities are present at birth, most prenatal-onset problems remain static or improve postnatally without evidence of neurologic deterioration. By contrast, postnatal-onset problems in development usually result in deterioration in structure or function that previously has been normal. Deterioration may reflect postnatal accumulation of a toxic metabolic product (as in phenylketonuria), progressive storage of a metabolite (as in Hurler syndrome), or ongoing infection (as in deafness from cytomegalovirus). Children with postnatal problems usually seem to have thrived in utero. The structural and functional consequences of the problem do not become obvious until after the newborn period.

27

The following alterations of pregnancy can be helpful in determining that an infant's structural defects are of prenatal onset:

1. *Alterations in gestational timing*—prematurity or postmaturity.
2. *Alterations in onset or nature of fetal activity.* Fetal activity usually is felt by the mother by the 18th week of gestation. Delayed onset and decreased intensity of fetal activity are associated with certain birth defects, such as meningomyelocele, different forms of arthrogryposis, and chromosomal abnormalities associated with defects in brain development (e.g., trisomy 18 syndrome). In addition, fetal movement may be localized to one particular quadrant of the abdomen when the defect represents deformation in a previously normally formed structure and is secondary to intrauterine constraint.
3. *Abnormalities in amount of amniotic fluid.* Polyhydramnios occurs when the fetus has difficulty swallowing amniotic fluid (e.g., early problems in central nervous system development or upper gastrointestinal obstruction). Oligohydramnios usually is present after chronic leakage of amniotic fluid or whenever fetal urinary excretion is decreased (e.g., renal agenesis, infantile polycystic kidney disease, or urethral obstruction).

Alterations noted at delivery associated with prenatal onset of developmental problems are as follows:

1. *Increased incidence of breech presentation.* Although breech presentation occurs in 3.1% of normal deliveries at 40 weeks' gestation, it occurs much more frequently in some disorders that adversely affect the form or function of the fetus. Defects of form include structural abnormalities, such as hydrocephalus, which would be less compatible with the vertex position because of the large head, and joint dislocations, which may limit the capacity of the fetus to alter its position. Defects of function include some conditions associated with neuromuscular dysfunction (e.g., trisomy 18 syndrome).
2. *Prenatal-onset growth deficiency.* Many of the known chromosomal, genetic, and teratogenic causes of birth defects and birth defects for which there is an unknown etiology are associated with intrauterine growth retardation.
3. *Difficulty with neonatal adaptation.* Infants with prenatal-onset structural defects frequently have problems with neonatal respiratory adaptation, probably secondary to malformations of brain structure. In these cases, one always should be cautious when attributing mental retardation to a perinatal insult. Mental retardation in such patients is more likely the result of a prenatal-onset problem in brain development.

SINGLE PRIMARY DEFECT VERSUS MULTIPLE MALFORMATION SYNDROME

Structural defects of prenatal onset can be separated into defects that represent a single primary defect in development and defects that represent a multiple malformation syndrome (see Fig. 3-2). In most cases of a single primary defect, the defect involves only a single structure, and the infant is otherwise completely normal. The seven most common single primary defects in development are congenital hip dislocation, talipes equinovarus, cleft lip with or without cleft palate, cleft palate alone, cardiac septal defects, pyloric stenosis, and defects in neural tube closure. In most cases, the etiology is unknown, and counseling as to recurrence risk is difficult. Many of the more common single primary defects are explained, however, on the basis of multifactorial inheritance, which carries a recurrence risk of 2% to 5% for the next child of unaffected parents with one affected child. The multifactorial threshold model was developed to explain the empirical 2% to 5% risk for recurrence in siblings for common single primary defects. Although this figure remains the basis for recurrence risk counseling, the model may not be completely accurate. As the genetic basis for common malformations is elucidated, genetic heterogeneity becomes apparent. For some defects, a few major genes rather than many genes may determine genetic susceptibility. For others, a monogenetic etiology may be apparent.

The extent to which multifactorial inheritance contributes to the etiology of some of the less common single defects in development is unclear. The fact that single primary defects are etiologically heterogeneous implies that some have an environmental cause and others result from dominantly or recessively inherited single altered genes. Craniosynostosis secondary to in utero constraint is an example of the former, whereas postaxial polydactyly is an example of the latter. Before multifactorial risk figures are used for counseling when a single primary defect is recognized, references should be consulted to determine whether other risk figures are available.

In contrast to the concept of the single primary defect in development, the designation *multiple malformation syndrome* is used when several observed structural defects all have the same unknown or presumed etiology (Fig. 3-3). The defects usually include many anatomically unrelated errors in morphogenesis. Multiple malformation syndromes are caused by chromosomal abnormalities, by teratogens, and by single gene defects inherited in mendelian patterns. Risks of recurrence range from zero, in cases that represent fresh gene mutations or are caused by teratogens, to 100%, in the case of a child with Down syndrome in which the mother is a balanced 21/21 translocation carrier.

Single Primary Defects in Development

Single primary defects can be subcategorized based on developmental pathogenesis into malformation, deformation, disruption, and dysplasia (Fig. 3-4). From a practical

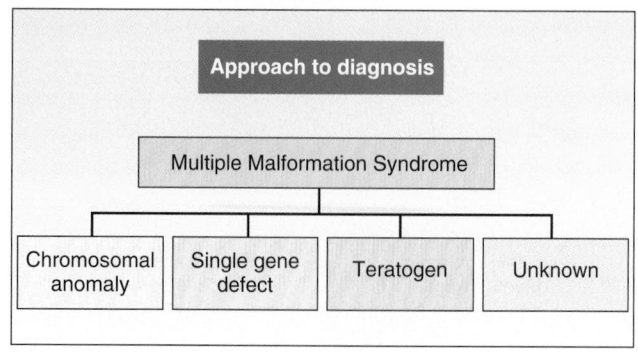

Figure 3-3. Approach to diagnosis: multiple malformation syndrome.

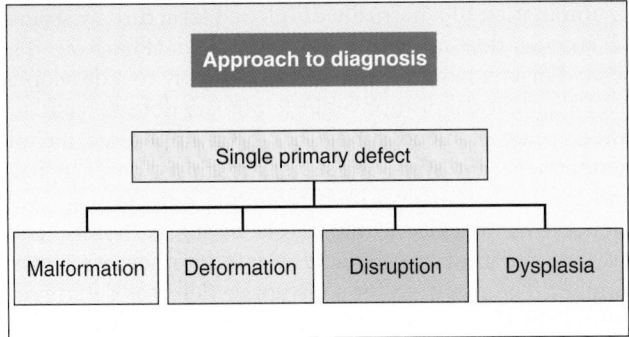

Figure 3-4. Approach to diagnosis: single primary defect.

standpoint, the purpose of making this distinction relates to prognosis.

Malformation

A malformation is a primary structural defect arising from a localized error in morphogenesis (e.g., meningomyelocele) (Fig. 3-5). For most children with a localized malformation, the prognosis is excellent after surgical correction. When neither dominant nor recessive inheritance is established, multifactorial recurrence risk factors (2% to 5%) apply to unaffected parents.

Deformation

A deformation is an alteration in shape or structure of a part that has differentiated normally (e.g., talipes equinovarus). Most deformations involve the musculoskeletal system and probably are caused by intrauterine molding. The pressure producing such molding may be intrinsic, the result of neuromuscular imbalance within the fetus, or extrinsic, secondary to fetal crowding. In either case, the impaired ability of the fetus to kick results in decreased fetal movement, an important factor in development of the normal musculoskeletal system, particularly with respect to normal joint development.

Intrinsically derived positional deformation of prenatal onset occurs in disorders involving muscle degeneration, such as Steinert disease (myotonic dystrophy), and disorders involving motor neurons, such as Werdnig-Hoffmann disease. Early defects in development of the central nervous system

are more common causes of positional deformations and should be considered seriously whenever a structural defect is thought to be intrinsically derived.

Fetal crowding, the most common cause of an extrinsically derived deformation of prenatal onset, is usually due to a decreased volume of amniotic fluid, a situation that occurs normally during the later weeks of gestation, when the fetus is undergoing extremely rapid growth. It also occurs abnormally, however, with oligohydramnios secondary to either decreased fetal urinary output or chronic leakage of amniotic fluid. Other factors associated with extrinsically derived deformation defects include breech presentation (Fig. 3-6), primigravidity, a large fetus, presence of more than one fetus, a malformed uterus, and presence of a uterine tumor. Most extrinsically derived deformations have an excellent prognosis and a low risk for recurrence. Although prognosis can be poor and recurrence risk increased with intrinsically derived defects, the physical examination often provides clues that can be helpful regarding this distinction.

Skin appears to grow passively in response to the shape and increasing size of the underlying structures. Movement produces a relative redundancy in the skin overlying the joint, allowing unrestricted mobility. Lack of movement from early in gestation is associated with pterygia or webbing of the skin surrounding the affected joint. In addition, the skin is taut and lacks the normal wrinkles and creases that are a function of movement. Smooth, stretched, wrinkle-free skin with pterygia over major joints is most common in association with an intrinsically derived deformation. In contrast, pressure applied to skin causes hypertrophy and overgrowth of the structure. Ear cartilage responds to pressure in a similar fashion. Marked redundancy of the skin and large flattened ears are characteristics of extrinsically derived deformation.

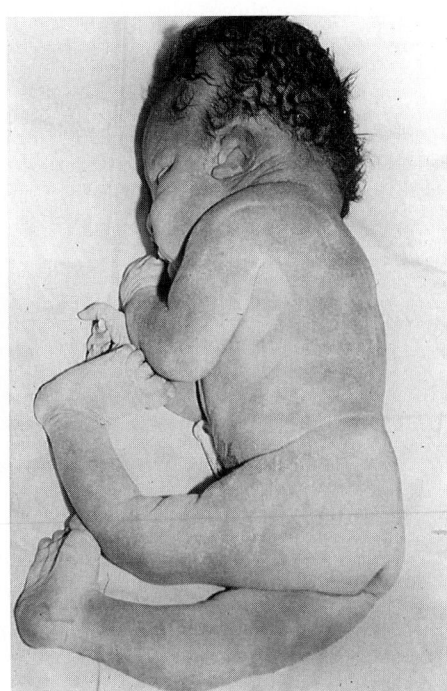

Figure 3-6. Newborn male with deformation defects secondary to breech presentation.

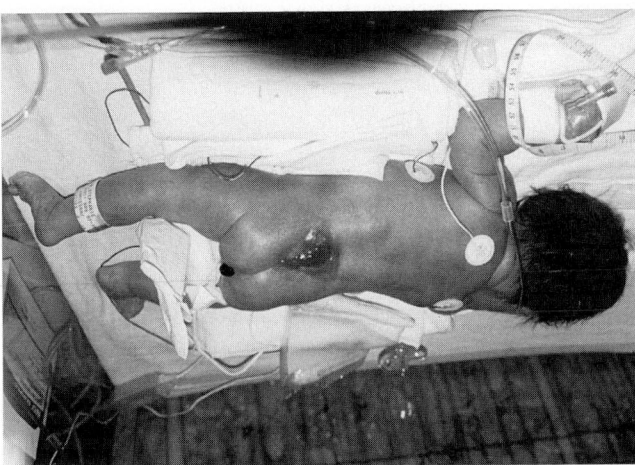

Figure 3-5. Newborn with meningomyelocele.

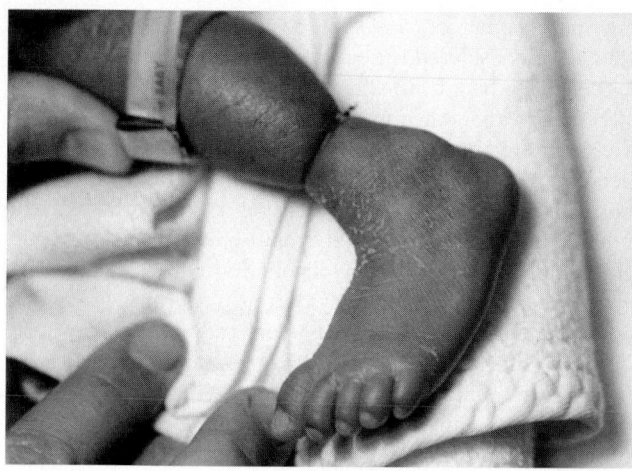

Figure 3-7. Ring constriction of lower leg caused by amniotic band.

Palmar and interphalangeal crease patterns form at about 9 weeks' postconception and reflect the planes of flexion of hand structure. In the absence of hand movement, creases do not develop. Lack of palmar crease patterns implies lack of movement before 9 weeks of gestation and is associated most commonly with intrinsically derived deformation. Crowding from extrinsic sources usually does not become significant until long after crease patterns are formed. Because the factors that produce intrinsically derived deformation defects often involve programming problems affecting overall movement, the structural defects that result tend to be symmetric in distribution. In contrast, extrinsically applied constraint can be localized, resulting in marked asymmetry of limb involvement. Although lack of amniotic fluid is a cause of deformation, polyhydramnios may be seen in association with deformation if the cause is an intrinsically derived abnormality that limits the infant's ability to swallow and ability to move. Deformations in conjunction with polyhydramnios are always intrinsically derived.

Disruption

The term *disruption* is used for a structural defect resulting from destruction of a previously normally formed part. At least two basic mechanisms are known to produce disruption. One involves entanglement followed by tearing apart

or amputation of a normally developed structure by strands of amnion floating within amniotic fluid (Fig. 3-7). The second involves interruption of blood supply to a developing part. Examples of disruptive single primary defects for which interruption of blood supply has been implicated include nonduodenal intestinal atresia, gastroschisis, porencephaly, and terminal transverse limb reduction defects (Fig. 3-8). Genetic factors play a minor role in the pathogenesis of disruptions; most are sporadic events in otherwise normal families. The prognosis for a disruptive defect is determined entirely by the extent and location of the tissue loss. A child with a limb amputation has an excellent prognosis for normal function, whereas a child with porencephaly does not.

Dysplasia

The term *dysplasia* refers to an abnormal organization of cells and the structural consequences. Localized dysplasias usually are single primary defects in development (e.g., hemangiomas). Generalized dysplasias, such as connective tissue disorders, usually present as multiple malformation syndromes in that a wide variety of structures are involved because of the widespread distribution of the dysplastic tissue. The process of dysplasia seems to involve deregulation of growth; most dysplasias change over time. Capillary hemangiomas become involuted, and bathing trunk nevi carry a risk for malignant transformation. Knowledge of the natural history of a lesion is crucial in the long-term follow-up of children with localized dysplasias.

Sequence

Sequence refers to a pattern of multiple anomalies that occurs when a single primary defect in early morphogenesis leads in a cascading fashion to secondary and tertiary errors in morphogenesis. When evaluating an infant with multiple structural anomalies, it is important to make a distinction between a sequence and a multiple malformation syndrome. In the former, recurrence risk for the multiple anomalies depends entirely on recurrence risk for the single primary defect in morphogenesis. The terms *malformation sequence*, *deformation sequence*, and *disruption sequence* are used to describe only the initiating error in morphogenesis of a sequence if it is known. For example, the Robin malformation sequence is a pattern of multiple anomalies, all of

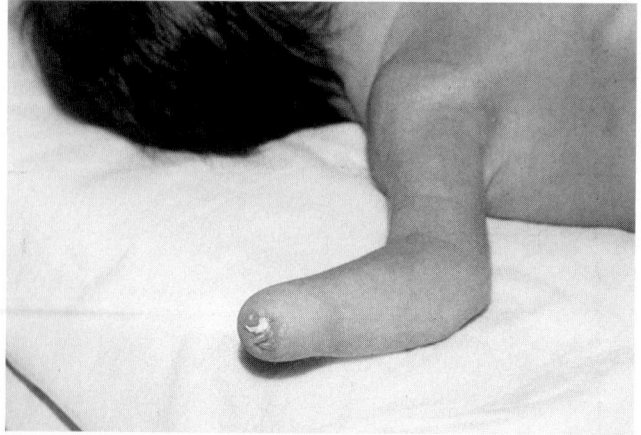

A

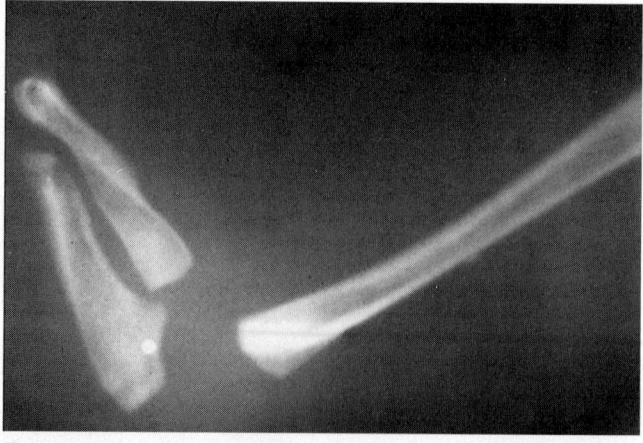

B

Figure 3-8. Transverse limb reduction defect (**A**) with corresponding x-ray (**B**).

which are produced by a single prenatal-onset defect in development, mandibular hypoplasia. Because the tongue is relatively large for the oral cavity, it drops back (glossoptosis), blocking closure of the posterior palatal shelves and causing a U-shaped cleft palate. Recognizing that all the observed defects are due to a single localized error permits recurrence risk counseling based on the single defect. It is important to recognize, however, that a sequence can occur by itself or as part of a multiple malformation syndrome. Stickler syndrome, an autosomal dominant genetically determined disorder, should be considered in any neonate with the Robin malformation sequence, particularly in those with a family history of cleft palate and in patients with dominantly inherited myopia, retinal detachment, or spondyloepiphyseal dysplasia.

Multiple Malformation Syndrome

Multiple malformation syndrome refers to a situation in which one or more developmental anomalies of two or more systems has occurred. As shown in Figure 3-3, multiple malformation syndromes can be caused by chromosomal and genetic abnormalities and by teratogens.

A karyotype should be performed in all infants with multiple malformation syndromes in which the etiology is unknown. For disorders that are due to single mutant genes (dominant or X-linked in males) or to pairs of mutant genes (autosomal recessive), the correct diagnosis depends on clinical recognition because in most cases there is no laboratory test to confirm the diagnosis. A family history of a similarly affected individual is extremely helpful. In many patients with multiple malformation syndromes of genetic etiology, the occurrence is sporadic, however, and represents fresh gene mutations. In such situations, all family members are normal, and the diagnosis depends entirely on the evaluation of the patient's phenotype. Because fresh gene mutations are associated with older paternal age, and chromosomal abnormalities are associated with older maternal age, parental ages should be documented in all cases. In addition, the presence or absence of consanguinity should be determined because of its association with some autosomal recessive disorders. A careful history of drug intake and chemical exposure also should be obtained.

Associations

The term *association* refers to a nonrandom association of malformations for which it has not been determined whether the pattern is a sequence or a syndrome. One important clinical example is the *VATER* association, which includes *V*ertebral defects, *A*nal atresia, *T*racheo*E*sophageal fistula with atresia, *R*adial upper limb hypoplasia, and *R*enal defects. Single umbilical artery and cardiac and genital anomalies also are seen in this association. These defects are likely to occur together in almost any combination of two or more and usually represent a sporadic occurrence in an otherwise normal family. The purpose of an association is to alert the clinician to search for other defects when one feature of the association is present.

Lastly, for infants with multiple malformation syndromes in whom a diagnosis has not been established and chromosomes are normal, recurrence risk is either 0% or 25%. Prognosis is based on clinical progression of the phenotype.

SUGGESTED READING

Jones KL: Smith's Recognizable Patterns of Human Malformations, 5th ed. Philadelphia, WB Saunders, 1997.

SECTION 1   FUNDAMENTALS

4 Principles of Growth and Maturation

Craig A. Alter and Wilma C. Rossi

NORMAL GROWTH

The growth of a child involves an increase in height coupled with changes in shape and body composition. By definition, *height (stature)* refers to a measurement at a single time point, and *growth (growth rate or velocity)* refers to the change in height over time. Evaluation of a child with a suspected growth disorder requires understanding normal growth at various phases of life.

Growth is maximal in utero and during infancy. In utero, with a healthy placenta and pregnancy, the fetus grows 50 cm in 9 months. During the first year of life, the growth rate can reach 25 cm/yr. After the first year, there is a marked deceleration to 5 to 7 cm/yr with a further decline just before puberty. During puberty, peak growth reaches 6 to 10 cm/yr in girls and 7 to 12 cm/yr in boys. Some children develop rapidly and have a brief, intense growth spurt, whereas others have a slower but sustained growth rate. The latter may result in more total growth. In girls, not only does puberty begin more than 1 year earlier than in boys, but the growth velocity peaks at an earlier pubertal stage. Girls reach peak growth velocity at Tanner stage 3, whereas boys peak at Tanner stage 4 (Tanner stages are discussed later in the section on sexual maturation). Pubertal growth accounts for about 15% of adult height. Postmenarche girls grow about 3% of their adult height, which is about 2 to 3 inches.

GROWTH CURVE ANALYSIS

Assessment of a child's growth is important as a key measure of well-being. Most chronic diseases affect the growth rate. The efficacy of the treatment of many chronic diseases can be monitored, in part, by analyzing the corresponding growth curves.

Standard growth curves should be plotted in all children, regardless of their health. By definition, the 50th percentile for height at a given age is the height at which 50% of children are taller and 50% are shorter. Until more recently, the 5th percentile was the lowest one shown on the most commonly used growth curves, but newer curves now highlight heights from the 3rd through 97th percentiles. The "reverse side" of most growth curves typically contain information about weight relative to a given height. Newer curves use body mass index (BMI) for age (see Chapter 2 for examples of BMI charts). These curves identify not only the underweight and overweight child, but also how the body composition is changing over time. Because the growth curves designed by the National Center for Health Statistics and National Center for Chronic Disease Prevention and Health Promotion are based on population cross-sectional data, the pattern of growth at puberty is not seen. Many children during puberty show an initial phase of decreased growth, then an acceleration followed by a slowdown before the completion of growth (Fig. 4-1). Growth charts are available online or can be ordered (http://www.cdc.gov/growthcharts).

The infant growth curves (0 to 36 months) are designed for length, whereas the curves for 2- to 20-year-olds apply to standing height. A 2-year-old infant who is standing should be plotted on the 2- to 20-year-old growth curve. Measurement of infant lengths is difficult and depends on equipment and technique. Using the typical disposable examination paper to mark off length is notoriously inaccurate. Devices that can "lock in" the length are ideal. For standing height, a stadiometer is preferred. In children with a known chronic disease or with extremes of height, measurement should be repeated to ensure accuracy. We recommend plotting parental heights on the growth charts as an indication of the family norm. Growth curves are available for children with Down syndrome, Turner syndrome, achondroplasia, and certain other genetic conditions.

FACTORS THAT INFLUENCE LINEAR GROWTH

The genetics of growth are complex. Many candidate genes are being studied. The *SHOX* (short stature homeobox) gene is located on the short arm of the X chromosome and

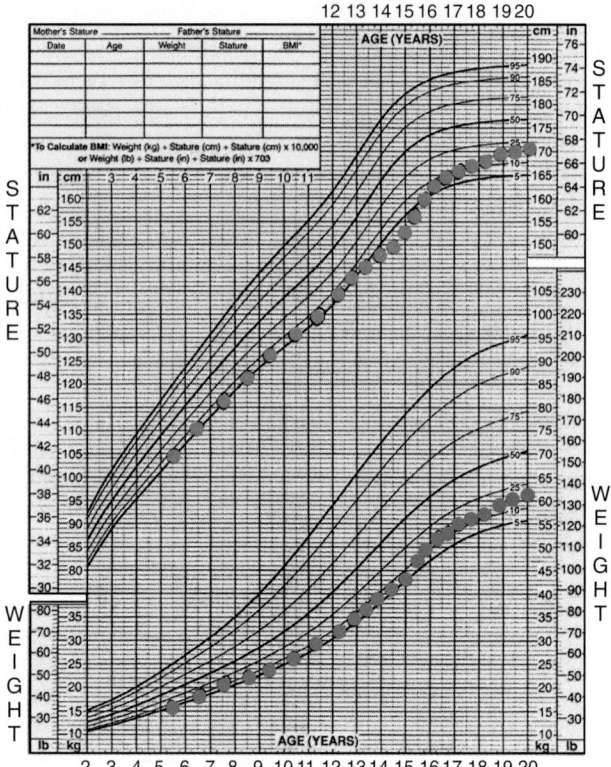

2 to 20 years: Boys
Stature-for-age and Weight-for-age percentiles

Figure 4-1. Growth curve showing peripubertal growth deceleration followed by growth spurt. (Modified from The National Center for Health Statistics and National Center for Chronic Disease Prevention and Health Promotion [2000] and the Children's Hospital of Philadelphia.)

is being studied to determine its significance in normal short children and in girls with Turner syndrome. The predicted adult heights of children in the family are usually within 10 cm of the midparental height. To compare a child's growth with the parents' heights, the parents' heights first are averaged. Then if the child is a boy, 6.5 cm is added, and if the child is a girl, 6.5 cm is subtracted from the midparental height to determine the "target height." In addition to genetic influences on height, the timing of growth and puberty tends to run in families. The age of parental maturation should be recorded. Most mothers recall the approximate age of menarche. Fathers tend to recall the timing of puberty only if they had a delayed growth spurt.

Adequate calories and nutrition are necessary for normal growth. Poor growth in infancy frequently is due to inadequate intake or to malabsorption. Families frequently ask if a better diet would increase the child's growth. If the weight for height is normal, increasing the calorie intake would not improve the growth. Certain vitamins or minerals, such as zinc, may play a role in growth. Through mechanisms not well understood, social interactions influence growth. Children exposed to an unstable environment may show periods of poor growth. Hormonal influences on growth have been well studied. Thyroid hormone is even more vital in growth than is growth hormone (GH). Deficiency of either hormone leads to an increase in weight relative to height. Adrenal insufficiency leads to a decrease in weight. Glucocorticoid excess (Cushing syndrome) leads to poor growth and rapid weight gain. The effect of puberty on growth is complex, with sex steroids being responsible for a rapid growth spurt and for epiphyseal fusion and subsequent cessation of growth. It is of note that estrogen is responsible for the epiphyseal fusion even in males. Boys have peak growth velocity at a later stage of puberty than girls. Because girls start puberty 1 year or more before boys, girls show peak growth rate about 2 years earlier.

SHORT STATURE AND POOR GROWTH

Evaluation of growth should be performed if the growth rate is low (>2 standard deviations below the mean for age) or if the child is unexpectedly short for the family. If the child's current height extended at the same percentile until adult height falls more than 10 cm below the target height, an evaluation is warranted. Causes of *short stature with a normal growth velocity* include familial short stature and constitutional delay of growth and development. In children with constitutional delay, there is a fall in height velocity in infancy or early childhood followed by a normal growth rate. Delayed dentition is typical. Family history frequently reveals a parent or relative with a similar growth pattern. The bone age is delayed, and the height plotted at the bone age rather than the chronologic age typically is at a percentile consistent with the percentile of the target height. Most growth charts do not take into account race or ethnic background. The mean adult height and weight of Asian adults is significantly less than that of white and African-American adults in North America.

Causes of *short stature with a low growth velocity* are numerous because of the multitude of factors that influence growth. Many genetic syndromes are accompanied by short stature and poor growth. Although the physiology behind poor growth is poorly understood, it has been studied in detail in Turner syndrome. The growth in girls with Turner syndrome is diminished in utero, leading to a low birth weight. Short stature is present throughout childhood, but the growth rate diminishes further after age 7 years. (See the CD-ROM for more information on Turner syndrome.)

Chromosomal patterns for girls with Turner syndrome are heterogeneous. Classic Turner syndrome occurs when there is loss of an X chromosome (45,XO); however, an equal number of cases are due to either a mosaic or a isochromosome defect. Mosaic patterns occur when some of the cells are 45,XO, but others are 46,XX. Isochromosome defects refer to the chromosome pattern in which all cells contain the same chromosome pattern, but only a piece of an X chromosome is missing. The part of the X chromosome responsible for the short stature is located on the short arm of the X chromosome and may contain the *SHOX* gene.

Noonan syndrome, sometimes referred to as *male Turner syndrome,* occurs in males and females. The karyotype is normal, but facial features are similar to the features in Turner syndrome. The heart lesions tend to be right-sided, such as pulmonic stenosis. Pubertal development may be delayed.

Children with Down syndrome also are short, although the degree of short stature may be variable and affected by family heights. Growth is poor even in infancy. Children with Down syndrome are at risk for autoimmune disorders, such as chronic lymphocytic thyroiditis (Hashimoto thyroiditis) and type 1 diabetes mellitus. The thyroid function of children with Down syndrome should be assessed annually beginning at 1 year of age to avoid clinical hypothyroidism, which could have a further impact on their growth.

Poor nutrition leading to a decrease in growth velocity can occur at any age but is most common in infancy. Parents often are frustrated by the lack of appetite of their child; however, if the weight for height is normal, poor caloric intake is not likely to be the cause of decreased growth. If the weight for height is decreased, even without severe malnutrition, nutritional status must be evaluated fully. In infancy, poor growth requires a careful nutritional assessment. Inadequate parental feeding technique, poor ability of the infant to feed, food intolerance, or malabsorption must be considered in poorly growing infants.

Infants who have a history of intrauterine growth retardation (IUGR) frequently show catch-up growth by age 2 to 3 years. Approximately 15% continue to exhibit short stature and poor growth velocity later in life, however. Infants who have IUGR early in pregnancy (symmetric IUGR) are more likely to have poor catch-up growth.

Many chronic diseases decrease growth, especially if nutrition is adversely affected. Gastrointestinal disorders, such as celiac disease (see Chapter 138) and inflammatory bowel disease (see Chapter 139), frequently are associated with poor growth and short stature. Anorexia or abdominal pain in a child beyond infancy who has poor growth, even without short stature, may be due to inflammatory bowel disease. Eating disorders also should be considered in older children with poor weight gain.

Chronic renal insufficiency is associated with profound growth failure. Chronic acidosis, poor nutrition, and retention of toxins are factors that can lead to a decreased growth rate. Renal tubular acidosis also may lead to decreased growth but without an elevation in creatinine.

Children with asthma, chronic respiratory disease such as bronchopulmonary dysplasia, and cystic fibrosis need to be followed carefully for growth failure. Steroid therapy for these conditions may have a greater impact on growth than that of hypoxia. Oral glucocorticoids can have a profound negative influence on growth. Typically, weight increases while growth rate decreases. The growth-suppressive effect of oral steroids may last many months beyond the discontinuation of the medication. Although inhaled steroids infrequently affect growth, more cases of growth suppression may emerge.

It is unlikely that the diagnosis of other chronic diseases, such as immunologic disorders, would be made from a workup for short stature. Monitoring the growth may assist in judging the effectiveness of the treatment, however.

Skeletal dysplasia can affect all bones, predominantly long bones, or just specific parts of bones. Many skeletal dysplasias have autosomal recessive inheritance. The most common form, achrondroplasia, is an autosomal dominant disorder, however, linked to the short arm of chromosome 4 (4p16.3), although 80% to 90% of cases represent new mutations. Because the long bones are predominantly stunted, the upper-to-lower body segment ratio is increased, and the arm span is decreased. Normal upper-to-lower body segment ratio is approximately 1.7 at birth, decreases to 1.1 by age 8 years, and is just above 1.0 at puberty. Although achrondroplasia is likely to be recognized early because there is such marked disproportion and short stature, hypochrondroplasia, a milder form of skeletal dysplasia, may be discovered only by noting that the legs are more affected than the upper body. Because there is no serum test to diagnose the many causes of skeletal dysplasia, diagnoses must be made based on observation of body proportions and a skeletal survey. The skeletal survey is a comprehensive series of radiographs of the long bones and vertebrae.

Psychosocial or deprivation dwarfism is a fascinating and poorly understood cause of poor growth and short stature. These children, although not calorie deprived (normal weight for their height), grow poorly (Fig. 4-2). Although the precise etiology of the poor growth is not understood, many factors are likely to be responsible, possibly including GH deficiency. Growth returns to normal when these children are placed in a nurturing environment.

Hormone abnormalities are not frequent causes of short stature. They commonly lead to increased weight for height, in contrast to the poor growth and poor weight gain seen in gastrointestinal disease. Hypothyroidism can lead to profound growth retardation (Fig. 4-3). Many patients with chronic lymphocytic (Hashimoto) thyroiditis present with a diffuse goiter and mild or no symptoms of hypothyroidism. Children who present with marked growth

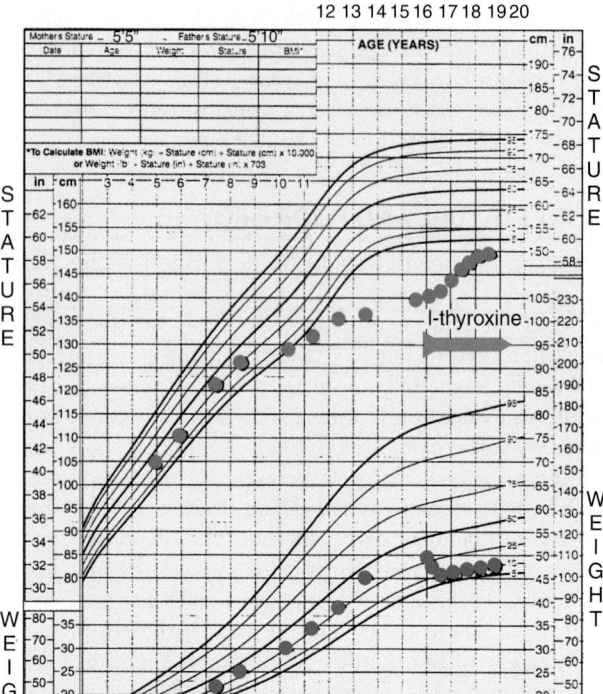

Figure 4-3. Growth chart of a girl with hypothyroidism leading to poor growth and results of treatment. (Modified from The National Center for Health Statistics and National Center for Chronic Disease Prevention and Health Promotion [2000] and the Children's Hospital of Philadelphia.)

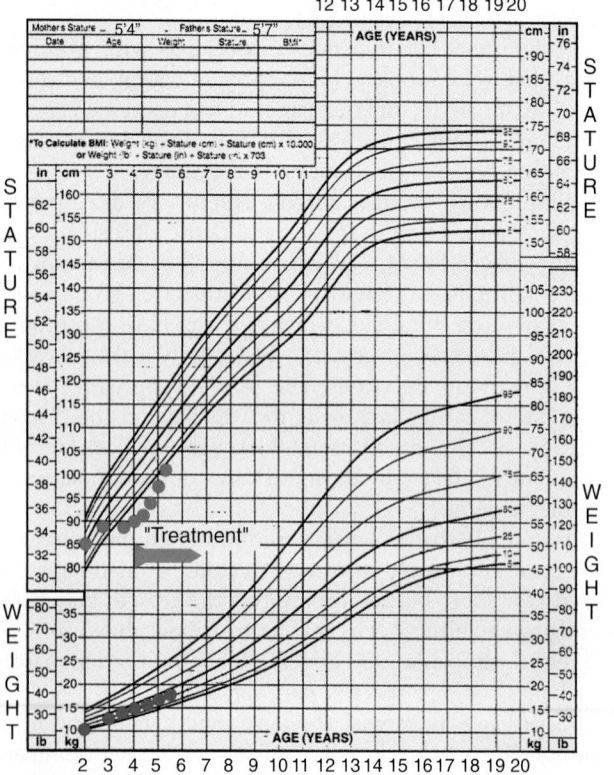

Figure 4-2. Growth curve for a girl with growth failure caused by psychosocial deprivation. (Modified from The National Center for Health Statistics and National Center for Chronic Disease Prevention and Health Promotion [2000] and the Children's Hospital of Philadelphia.)

failure frequently have no goiter because the lymphocytic destruction of the thyroid is so aggressive. With glucocorticoid excess, the growth velocity is poor while weight gain is rapid.

GH deficiency leads to variable degrees of poor growth. GH is a polypeptide synthesized by the anterior pituitary that causes the liver to release insulin-like growth factor I (IGF-I, formerly somatomedin C). Many of the anabolic effects of GH are thought to be due to IGF-I. IGF-I circulates free and in association with several binding proteins. IGF-binding protein 3 (IGF-BP3) is a marker for GH adequacy because GH induces its formation. GH deficiency may be idiopathic (72% of cases), congenital, or due to diseases of the central nervous system (CNS), head trauma, or neoplasia. Risk factors for GH deficiency include any midline defect, such as absent corpus callosum, cleft lip or palate, congenital heart disease, or underdevelopment of the optic nerve (septo-optic dysplasia). Radiation treatment to the pituitary or hypothalamus frequently results in GH deficiency, especially when doses exceed 2400 cGy. Any newborn with severe hypoglycemia, especially a boy with a small phallus, must be evaluated for hypopituitarism.

Poor growth without short stature may occur in any condition if the condition is of recent onset. Head trauma or a marked exacerbation of a chronic disease may lead to deceleration of growth and decrease in height percentiles that may be noted before actual short stature is present.

DIAGNOSING THE CAUSE OF SHORT STATURE OR POOR GROWTH

Diagnosing the cause of short stature and poor growth begins with a detailed history. History focuses on searching for signs of chronic disease, such as those mentioned in the previous section. The quality of the child's appetite, presence of abdominal pain, abnormal stools, and weight gain or loss screen for disorders of the gastrointestinal tract. Changes in psychosocial environment, such as foster care, need to be ascertained. Headaches and visual complaints or abnormal gait may signify CNS pathology and GH deficiency. Other CNS risk factors include head trauma, history of meningitis, or prior treatment of a brain tumor. Any long-term use of medication needs to be documented, especially if the medication includes steroids. Birth history searches for evidence of IUGR.

Details about the family heights should include not only the heights and percentiles of the immediate family members, but also the timing of their growth and pubertal development. Any history of delayed puberty should be documented, as should the existence of any extremely short family members (men <5 ft, 5 inches, and women <5 ft, 0 inches). The midparental height is calculated as previously described.

Analysis of the prior growth on a growth curve is essential in formulating a differential diagnosis of short stature or poor growth. A short period of poor growth must be assessed for possible measurement or plotting errors. Any concerns from the history should be correlated to the time of diminished growth. Analysis of the weight for height or the BMI curve is essential because gastrointestinal disorders tend to lead to a decrease in the weight relative to the height, whereas endocrinologic causes tend to lead to an increase (Fig. 4-4). The weight itself may not be low or high, however, and only the change in weight for height may be remarkable. Most growth curves have on the reverse side either the weight-for-height curve or the BMI-versus-chronologic age curve.

Stature that is below the third percentile but with a normal growth rate ("growth parallel to the curve") suggests familial short stature or constitutional delay. A pathologic process is suggested by a decline in growth percentiles.

Determination of the bone age helps to differentiate genetic short stature from constitutional delay. The bone age is determined by a radiograph of the left hand and wrist and compared with same-sex standards. In genetic short stature, the bone age is close to the chronologic age. In constitutional delay, the bone age is delayed. In addition, height plotted at the bone age, as opposed to the chronologic age, should be closest to the percentile of the midparental height. When the bone age indicates that the epiphyses are fused, there is no longer any potential for further linear growth. Adolescents with diminished growth rates who are at the end of their natural growth have fused or almost fused epiphyses.

Physical examination in the evaluation of short stature first focuses on the general well-being of the child. Stigmata of genetic syndromes are sought, especially the features of Turner syndrome in girls. Clinodactyly and a history of IUGR suggest Russell-Silver syndrome. Other skeletal abnormalities or abnormal body proportions suggest bony

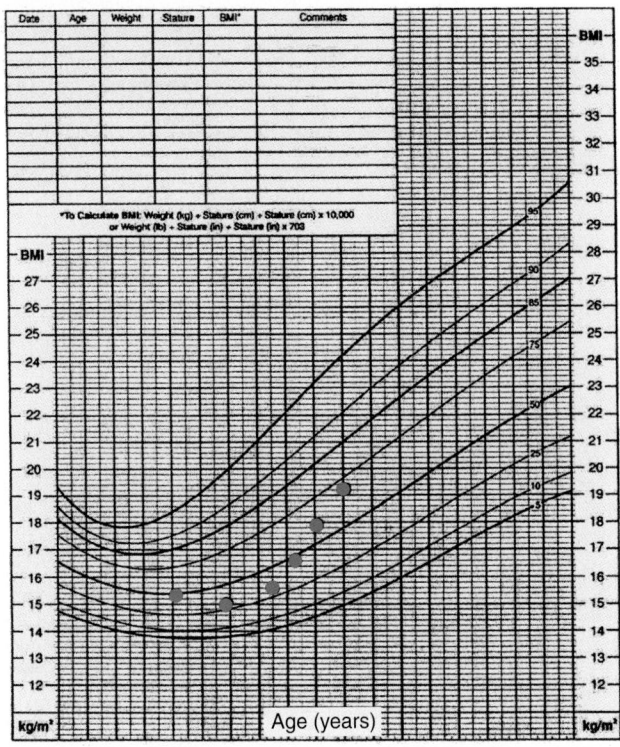

Figure 4-4. Body mass index versus age curve for a boy with growth hormone deficiency. (Modified from The National Center for Health Statistics and National Center for Chronic Disease Prevention and Health Promotion [2000] and the Children's Hospital of Philadelphia.)

dysplasia or rickets. Abnormal proportions are confirmed by calculating the upper body-to-lower body segment ratios. A high upper body-to-lower body segment ratio suggests short legs compared with the torso, which is found in several forms of skeletal dysplasia. Midline defects are risk factors for hypothalamic/pituitary disease. The thyroid should be evaluated for size and consistency. Puberty should be staged as discussed in a later section of this chapter.

Depending on the results of the history and physical examination, laboratory evaluation may not be necessary or may include tests listed in Figure 4-5, such as complete blood count, sedimentation rate, thyroid-stimulating hormone (TSH), growth factors, chemistry panel, tissue transglutaminase, antiendomysial and antigliadin antibodies, chromosomes, and urinalysis. A sedimentation rate may signal inflammatory bowel disease or another systemic disorder. Thyroid-stimulating hormone is the best screen for primary hypothyroidism. The growth factors are a screening test for GH deficiency. Growth factors include IGF-I and IGF-BP3. In children younger than age 6, it is difficult to distinguish normal from low IGF-I levels. Tissue transglutaminase antibody is a useful screening test for celiac disease. Chromosome analysis is performed in girls to search for forms of Turner syndrome; however, abnormal results are found occasionally in boys. Genetic tests are likely to increase over the next decade in the workup of short stature. Radiologic evaluation should include a bone age x-ray. A skeletal survey

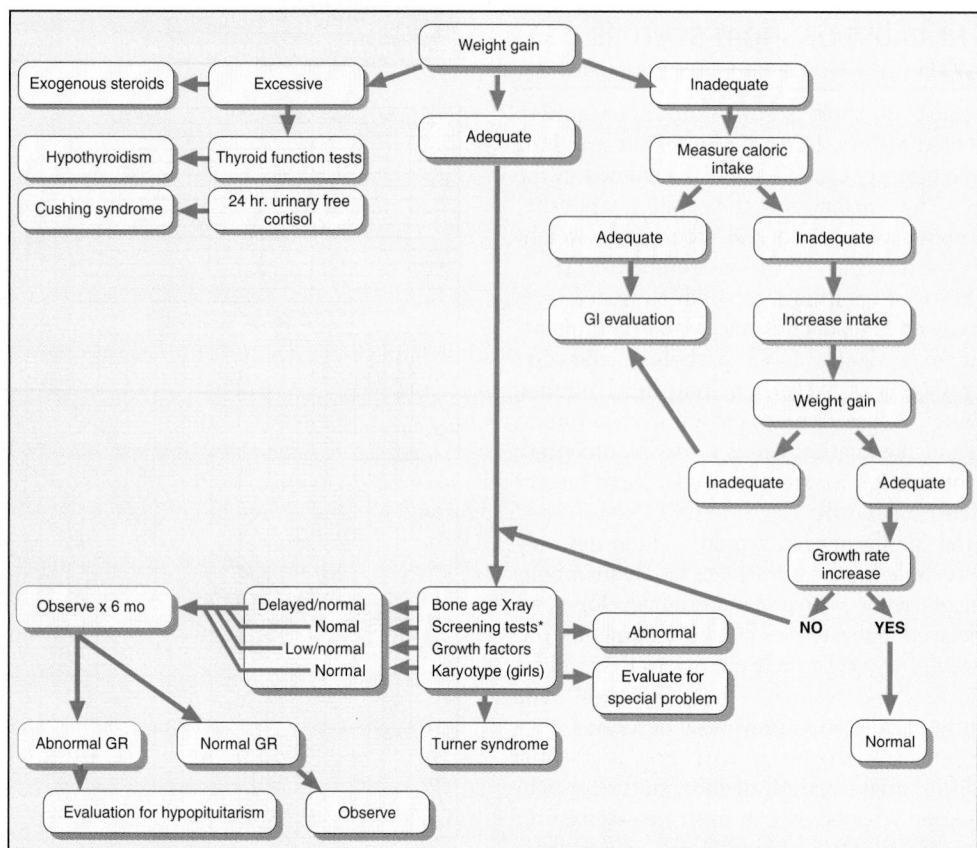

Figure 4-5. Diagnostic evaluation of growth failure. GI, gastrointestinal; GR, growth rate.

is performed only if skeletal dysplasia is a consideration, such as with extreme short stature or abnormal body proportions.

If the growth velocity is poor without explanation for an observation period of at least 6 months, referral to a pediatric endocrinologist should be considered. Referral may be contemplated if the short stature is extreme or when the projected adult height (from current percentiles) falls more than 12 cm (5 in) below the target height. A pediatric endocrinologist may do additional investigations, such as GH provocative testing. Random GH measurements are typically low and do not distinguish normal children from children with GH deficiency. Standard GH testing consists of two separate tests in which pharmacologic stimuli are given followed by multiple GH measurements. If all the GH levels on both tests are less than 10 ng/mL, the child is considered to have GH deficiency. Magnetic resonance imaging with contrast of the pituitary may reveal the cause of the GH deficiency. In approximately three quarters of cases, the etiology of the GH deficiency is idiopathic.

TREATMENT OF SHORT STATURE

If poor growth is due to a chronic disease, treatment of the chronic disease often results in catch-up growth. An exception is when the treatment is the cause of the poor growth, such as when glucocorticoids are used. Treatment of hypothyroidism usually results in rapid growth acceleration with a concomitant weight loss (see Fig. 4-4).

The current Food and Drug Administration–approved indications for treating a child with human GH are listed in Box 4-1. IUGR patients without catch-up growth by age 3 years and children with severe idiopathic short stature (growth 2.25 standard deviations below mean) have recently been added. There are ongoing studies on the usage of human GH in other conditions, including inflammatory bowel disease (IBD) and cystic fibrosis.

SEXUAL MATURATION

Puberty is defined as the period of time whereby a child's body undergoes changes in preparation for adult sexuality. Although sexual maturation often is viewed as starting in adolescence, changes begin in utero.

At 5 weeks' gestation, male and female gonads are indistinguishable. By 10 weeks' gestation, the gonads are histologically distinct. The male gonad produces testosterone and müllerian-inhibiting substance. Müllerian-inhibiting substance inhibits development of the uterus and internal vagina, whereas the androgens allow for penile development. Initially,

---

Box 4-1. FDA-Approved Indications for Human Growth Hormone Treatment in a Child with Poor Growth

- Growth hormone deficiency
- Turner syndrome
- Chronic renal insufficiency before transplantation
- Prader-Willi syndrome
- Intrauterine growth retardation
- Severe idiopathic growth stature

FDA, Food and Drug Administration.

Table 4-1. Pubertal Staging

Pubic Hair Tanner Stage (Males and Females)

1	Prepubertal, no pubic hair
2	Sparse, straight, lightly pigmented hair primarily over the base of the penis or on the labia
3	Darker, coarse, curly hair with spread onto the mons pubis
4	Similar to adult distribution but less
5	Adult distribution with spread to medial thigh

Breast Tanner Stage (Females)

1	Prepubertal, no ductile tissue palpable
2	Breast bud with minimal areolar breast
3	Breast tissue present outside of the areola
4	Areolae raised above the breast to form a second breast mound
5	Adult contour

Genital Tanner Stage (Males)

1	Prepubertal testes, scrotum, and penis
2	Testes and scrotum begin to enlarge with darkening of scrotal skin
3	Penis enlarges in length and diameter; testes and scrotum continue to enlarge, and scrotum becomes increasingly pigmented
4	Further enlargement of penis, testes, and scrotum and increased pigmentation of the scrotum
5	Adult genitalia

Adapted from Marshall WA, Tanner JM: Variations in pattern of pubertal changes in girls. Arch Dis Child 1969;44:291.

human chorionic gonadotropin, structurally similar to luteinizing hormone (LH), accounts for gonadal stimulation in both sexes. By midgestation, the maturing pituitary begins to secrete LH and follicle-stimulating hormone (FSH), resulting in continued gonadal stimulation. At birth, girls have testosterone levels less than 40 ng/dL, whereas boys average levels of 200 ng/dL—levels not reached again until puberty. Newborn boys and girls show evidence of chronic exposure to a different hormone environment.

After a few months of life, infants show minimal gonadal hormone production. Estrogen and testosterone secretion are extremely low. Simultaneously the pituitary and hypothalamus undergo changes so that the pituitary discontinues its release of LH and FSH; this characterizes the prepubertal years. The physiology behind the quiescence of the pituitary is poorly understood.

Within a year before the onset of clinical puberty, the hypothalamus begins to release gonadotropin-releasing hormone (GnRH) in a pulsatile manner to stimulate the pituitary. The pituitary responds to the pulsatile GnRH secretion by release of the gonadotropins, LH and FSH. Continuous stimulation of the pituitary with GnRH, as occurs pharmacologically with leuprolide, results in a paradoxically marked decrease in LH and FSH secretion.

In boys, LH stimulation causes the testicles to enlarge and testosterone output to increase. FSH is responsible for development of sperm production. In girls, gonado-tropin stimulation of the ovary results in production of androgens and estrogens. Estrogen is responsible for breast development. Gonadal and adrenal production of androgens accounts for pubic hair formation and acne, lowering of the voice, axillary hair, and body odor. LH and FSH control the production of gonadal androgens; the control of the adrenal production of androgens is poorly understood.

Clinical findings are described by Tanner stages (Table 4-1). In girls, breast and pubic hair development occurs at about the same time. In a study of more than 17,000 girls seen in primary care offices, the age of breast and pubic hair development was earlier than in previously established normative data (Table 4-2). Menarche occurred at a mean age of 12.18 years in African-American girls compared with 12.88 years in white girls. African-American girls began developing breast and pubic hair about 1 year before white girls, with menses beginning 0.7 year earlier.

Gonadarche or testicular enlargement in boys occurs at a mean age of 11.8 years with pubic hair noticeable at a mean age of 12.2 years. Precocious puberty in boys usually is defined as having either pubic hair or testicular enlargement before age 9 years. In contrast to girls with precocious puberty, who rarely have a significant pathologic cause, in about half of boys with precocious puberty, an intracranial process is found, making a detailed workup mandatory.

There are several normal variants of puberty that pose concerns to families. At birth, breast enlargement in

Table 4-2. Prevalence of Breast and Pubic Hair Development in White and African-American Girls 5 to 10 Years Old

	Age Range (yr)				
	5.00–5.99	6.00–6.99	7.00–7.99	8.00–8.99	9.00–9.99
Prevalence of breast development at Tanner stage 2 or greater (%)					
White	1.6	2.9	5.0	10.5	32.1
African-American	2.4	6.4	15.4	37.8	62.6
Prevalence of pubic hair development at Tanner stage 2 or greater (%)					
White	0.4	1.4	2.8	7.7	20.0
African-American	3.4	9.5	17.7	34.3	62.6

Adapted from Herman-Giddens MEP, Slora EJ, Wasserman RC, et al: Secondary sexual characteristics and menses in young girls seen in office practice: A study from the Pediatric Research in Office Settings Network. Pediatrics 1997;99:505–512. Copyright 1997. Reproduced with permission from *Pediatrics*.

boys and girls is common because of maternal estrogens. Occasionally, galactorrhea or a bloody vaginal discharge is found. Neither galactorrhea nor bloody discharge requires investigation, unless it persists beyond the first few months of life. Between age 1 and 3 years, girls may develop mild breast enlargement, a phenomenon termed *benign premature thelarche*. The breast tissue may be asymmetric and is more noticeable in a thin child. The cause of the breast enlargement is poorly understood. Although environmental factors are cited frequently, its lack of appearance in boys suggests endogenous estrogen secretion. The stimulant and source of the estrogen are unknown, however. Estradiol levels in girls with premature thelarche typically are undetectable by conventional assays. There is speculation that by using newer ultrasensitive assays low but supernormal estrogen levels may be found. Benign premature thelarche does not result in acceleration of growth or an advancement of the bone age. Breast development after age 3 years in a girl must be evaluated for potential sexual precocity.

Premature adrenarche refers to the development of pubic hair in girls younger than age 7 to 8 years or in boys younger than age 9 years in the absence of gonadarche. Essentially, premature adrenarche refers to pubic hair in girls without signs of breast development and in boys without enlargement of the testicles. As stated previously, pubic hair is found in 9.5% of African-American girls at age 7 years. Early adrenarche is common in children with obesity. It must be differentiated from other causes of early pubic hair development, such as central precocious puberty, congenital adrenal hyperplasia, ovarian cysts or tumors, adrenal tumors, and familial testotoxicosis (boys). Workup of a child with signs of early puberty is discussed later.

Central precocious puberty (CPP) refers to the process in which the gonads are actively secreting sex hormones as a result of stimulation by the pituitary gonadotropins LH and FSH. CPP in girls is most often idiopathic. The younger the girl at presentation, the more likely that a pathologic cause will be found. Signs of CPP in girls include rapid growth rate, breast development (estrogen effect), and usually pubic or axillary hair development (androgen effect). Bone age is advanced as is the dental age. CPP must be differentiated from premature adrenarche coupled with premature thelarche, from premature adrenarche and obesity but no true ductile breast development, and from early puberty due to ovarian cysts or tumor. Vaginal bleeding without significant breast development may occur as a result of an estrogen-secreting ovarian cyst or tumor, although it is usually due to vaginal trauma or foreign body and not a hormonal abnormality. Magnetic resonance imaging of the brain with contrast enhancement of girls with CPP is usually normal or shows a benign hamartoma (cells capable of producing gonadotropins but occurring in an atypical location). Risk factors for a pathologic cause of CPP include any CNS lesion, cerebral palsy, and history of head trauma or CNS infections. The presence of café-au-lait spots with irregular borders on the skin or the co-existence of bone cysts suggests McCune-Albright syndrome, a disorder that leads to multiple cysts, including in the ovary, and hyperfunctioning of endocrine glands.

Evaluation of a child with signs of early pubertal development involves searching for any CNS risk factors and determining the pace of the pubertal development. A growth curve that has a marked acceleration accompanied by a markedly advanced bone age implies more aggressive pubertal development. If the bone age is less than 1 year advanced, the patient is not likely to have significant hormone abnormalities. If the bone age is more than 1 year advanced, further evaluation is indicated. To screen for CPP in a girl with signs of breast and pubic hair development, serum levels of estradiol, testosterone, LH, and FSH are measured. Ultrasensitive assays of LH or FSH, measured by immunochemiluminescent assay, often detect increases in the gonadotropins in cases in which levels are undetectable by standard assay methods. Depending on the severity of the clinical findings, endocrinologists may perform GnRH (gonadotropin-releasing hormone) stimulation of the pituitary. If the GnRH stimulation shows evidence of CPP (rise in LH to the pubertal range), magnetic resonance imaging of the pituitary/hypothalamus should be performed. If the GnRH stimulation result is age appropriate (i.e., no rise in LH), ultrasound of the ovaries, uterus, and adrenal is indicated to locate the source of the pubertal hormones.

In boys younger than age 9 years, the workup of precocious puberty depends on the presence or absence of testicular enlargement. If the testes are enlarged (>4 mL volume or 2.5 cm length), and the GnRH stimulation test confirms CPP, magnetic resonance imaging of the brain is necessary. If the GnRH stimulation test does not confirm CPP, testotoxicosis must be considered. This is a familial disorder that is characterized by autonomous function of the testes that causes suppression of the hypothalamic-pituitary axis. McCune-Albright syndrome also can produce testicular enlargement and autonomous function. Testicular tumors must be considered when there is unilateral testicular enlargement. In boys with evidence of adrenarche but prepubertal size testes, the workup is similar to that of a girl with adrenarche but no breast development. The evaluation of a child with precocious puberty is diagrammed in Figure 4-6.

Treatment of precocious puberty depends on the etiology and must be individualized and discussed with the family. Some causes can be cured with surgical intervention (e.g., sex steroid–secreting tumors). In idiopathic CPP, the age of the child, the pace of the pubertal progression, the child's ability to cope with looking older, and the predicted height all play a role. Predicted heights are based on the current height and bone age and determined from published tables. If the puberty progresses rapidly, the bone age will continue to advance, and the predicted height may decrease.

Treatment of CPP involves pharmacologic suppression of pituitary gonadotropin secretion. Leuprolide acetate is the treatment of choice for CPP. This long-acting GnRH analogue results in the down-regulation of the GnRH receptors and halts LH and FSH release. Treatment is by intramuscular injection every 28 days, but administration may be more frequent if the response is poor. Daily injections or nasal preparations also are available but may be less effective because of poor compliance with daily therapies. In girls with early pubic hair caused by congenital

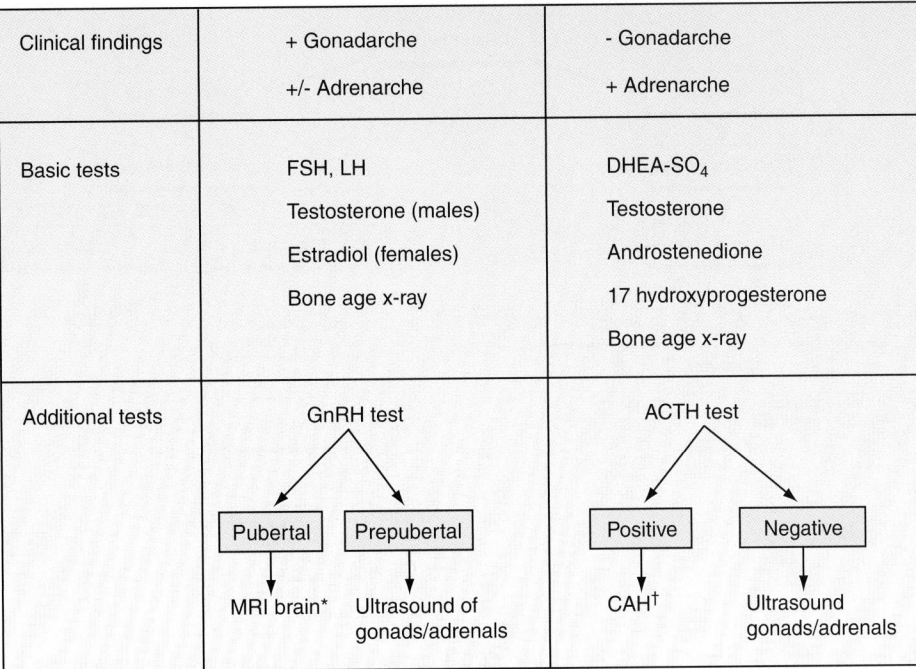

Clinical findings	+ Gonadarche +/- Adrenarche	- Gonadarche + Adrenarche
Basic tests	FSH, LH Testosterone (males) Estradiol (females) Bone age x-ray	DHEA-SO$_4$ Testosterone Androstenedione 17 hydroxyprogesterone Bone age x-ray
Additional tests	GnRH test Pubertal → MRI brain* Prepubertal → Ultrasound of gonads/adrenals	ACTH test Positive → CAH† Negative → Ultrasound gonads/adrenals

Figure 4-6. Diagnostic evaluation of precocious puberty. *Magnetic resonance imaging (MRI) of the brain should be considered early in a boy with gonadarche because there is a significant risk of central nervous system lesions as the etiology. †Adrenocorticotropic hormone (ACTH) test that results in a specific pattern of steroids that indicates a form of congenital adrenal hyperplasia (CAH).

adrenal hyperplasia, treatment with glucocorticoids must be weighed against the risk of adrenal suppression.

DELAYED PUBERTY

Delayed puberty is defined as the absence of physical changes of sexual development at a chronologic age 2 standard deviations after the mean age of onset of puberty. Evaluation is indicated in girls without breast buds by age 13 or menarche by age 15 or in boys without testicular enlargement by age 14.

Delayed puberty in boys or girls can be due to delayed activation of the hypothalamic-pituitary axis or gonadal failure (primary hypogonadism). Gonadal failure is less common than central or hypogonadotropic hypogonadism. The hallmark of primary hypogonadism is delayed puberty with elevated gonadotropins, LH, and FSH. FSH levels greater than 20 mIU/mL are diagnostic of gonadal dysfunction in both sexes.

Central hypogonadism or hypogonadotropic hypogonadism is most commonly due to constitutional delay of growth and maturation and tends to be familial. Systemic chronic diseases that affect growth usually also lead to delayed maturation. Intense exercise, anorexia, and disorders of the CNS all lead to hypogonadotropic hypogonadism. Kallmann syndrome, a disorder linked to Xp22.3, is characterized by anosmia and hypogonadotropic hypogonadism. Although it is more common in boys, it can occur in girls. The causes of hypogonadotropic hypogonadism are listed in Table 4-3. In children with iron overload, such as that secondary to treatment of chronic anemia, delayed puberty can be due to pituitary and gonadal infiltration of iron.

EVALUATION OF THE CHILD WITH DELAYED MATURATION

History focuses on any signs of chronic disease, anorexia, and prior exposure to known agents toxic to either the brain or the gonads. The child should be questioned on his or her sense of smell. A detailed neurologic and ophthalmologic history screens for brain tumors or lesions that may affect the hypothalamus or pituitary. Growth curve analysis is essential. A child who always has grown below the expected percentile of the family probably has constitutional delay of growth and maturation. Conversely a child who has grown well until the expected age of puberty suggests isolated delayed puberty, such as with Kallmann syndrome.

Table 4-3. Causes of Hypogonadism

Hypergonadotropic
Autoimmune destruction
Genetic defects (e.g., Turner syndrome)
Drug-induced (e.g., alkylating agents)
Radiation-induced
Congenital (e.g., in utero testicular torsion)
Metabolic diseases
Infectious (e.g., mumps orchitis)
Idiopathic

Hypogonadotropic
Constitutional delay
Systemic chronic diseases
Anorexia
Iron overload
Kallmann syndrome (anosmia)
Central nervous system lesions
Isolated LH/FSH deficiency
Panhypopituitarism

LH/FSH, luteinizing hormone/follicle-stimulating hormone.

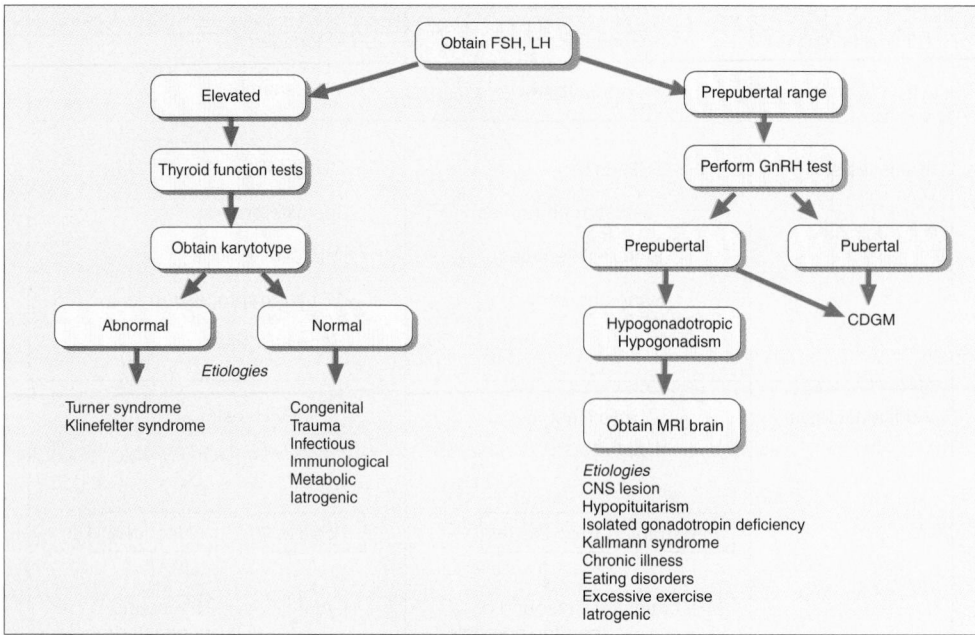

Figure 4-7. Laboratory evaluation of the child with delayed maturation. CDGM, constitutional delay of growth and maturation; CNS, central nervous system; FSH, follicle-stimulating hormone; GnRH, gonadotropin-releasing hormone; LH, luteinizing hormone; MRI, magnetic resonance imaging.

Physical examination gives additional clues to the specific diagnosis. Assessment of pubertal stage in girls involves not only examining breast and pubic hair stages, but also looking for other signs, such as growth acceleration, acne, and hirsutism. Tanner stages are summarized in Table 4-1. Subtle stigmata of Turner syndrome, such as widely spaced breasts, must be sought. In boys, abnormal testicles suggest primary testicular problems. In Klinefelter syndrome, or 47,XXY, boys typically are able to develop pubic hair, even up to Tanner stage 4, but the testicles remain small. Gynecomastia is frequent, and intelligence is low normal. It is essential in the examination of adolescent boys not only to inspect the appearance of pubic hair, but also to palpate the testicles for size and texture. Laboratory evaluation of the child with delayed maturation is shown in Figure 4-7.

Treatment of delayed puberty depends on the psychological assessment of the child; the prognosis of puberty occurring spontaneously; and any other concerns, such as decreased bone density. In boys with constitutional delay of growth and maturation, it is difficult to be certain when puberty will begin, even with detailed assessment of pituitary gonadotropin secretion. Short-term treatment with low-dose androgens sometimes is used to jump-start puberty, without adversely affecting the adult height. Treatment with estrogen in girls with permanent forms of hypogonadism is successful in promoting breast development and increasing bone density.

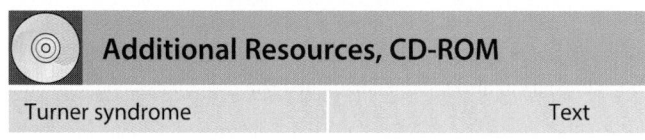

Additional Resources, CD-ROM

Turner syndrome	Text

SUGGESTED READINGS

Herman-Giddens MEP, Slora EJ, Wasserman RC, et al: Secondary sexual characteristics and menses in young girls seen in office practice: A study from the Pediatric Research in Office Settings Network. Pediatrics 1997;99:505–512.

Herman-Giddens MEP, Wang L, Koch G: Secondary sexual characteristics in boys: Estimates from the National Health and Nutrition Examination Survey III, 1988–1994. Arch Pediatr Adolesc Med 2001;155:1022–1028.

Kaplowitz PB, Oberfield SE, and The Drug and Therapeutics and Executive Committees of the Lawson Wilkins Pediatric Endocrine Society: Reexamination of the age limit for defining when puberty is precocious in girls in the United States: Implications for evaluation and treatment. Pediatrics 1999;104:936–941.

Lee PA: Central precocious puberty: An overview of diagnosis, treatment, and outcome. Endocrinol Metab Clin North Am 1999;28:901–918.

MacGillivray MH: The basics for the diagnosis and management of short stature: A pediatric endocrinologist's approach. Pediatr Ann 2000;29:570–575.

Parmert MR, Boepple PA: Variation in the timing of puberty: Clinical spectrum and genetic investigation. J Clin Endocrinol Metab 2001;86:2364–2368.

Saenger P, Albertsson Wikland K, Conway GS, et al: Recommendations for the diagnosis and management of Turner syndrome. J Clin Endocrinol Metab 2001;86:3061–3069.

5 Principles of Child Development and Developmental Assessment

Terri L. Shelton, Tracy R. Dobbins, and Jennifer M. Neal

The practice of pediatrics has changed considerably since the mid-20th century. One of the clearest examples of this is the ever-increasing role that pediatric health care providers play in enhancing the child's development in all areas, not just health. When concerned about their child's development, parents are most likely to turn to the pediatrician for advice. Knowing a child's developmental milestones is key to being able to give this advice. Having the additional working knowledge of the major developmental theories and screening and assessment measures can enhance greatly the provider's ability to anticipate difficulties and assist families in making decisions regarding referrals, interpretation of test findings, and interventions that are needed when development does not proceed as expected. This chapter presents currently held theories of cognition, language, motor, and behavior development and includes an overview of the major screening and assessment tools in these areas and how to choose a quality assessment instrument.

THEORIES OF CHILD DEVELOPMENT AND DEVELOPMENTAL MILESTONES

Numerous theories have been proposed to account for developmental processes. A *theory* generally is defined as a group of logically related statements (e.g., ideas, rules) used to explain past events and to predict future occurrences. A theory has *explanatory* and *predictive* functions. Theories of development vary in their comprehensiveness. Some theories address general principles of development, but most, especially more recent theories, focus on a specific area of development. Some theories conceptualize development as occurring in a series of stages marked by qualitative shifts over time. Others see development as evidenced by increased capacity or quantitative changes. The theories described in this chapter generally are regarded as having strong explanatory and predictive characteristics with solid empirical support.

Gesell's Maturational Theory of Development

Gesell believed that development progressed through an orderly sequence that was determined by heredity and biologic maturation and altered only somewhat by experience. In contrast to other theorists, he did not propose a formal set of stages, but rather five basic principles of development thought to be characteristic of every child's growth pattern. Although Gesell intended these principles to be applicable to all areas of development, his theory is most useful in understanding motor development in early childhood.

Gesell's *principle of developmental direction* states that development proceeds in a systematic direction as a function of preprogrammed genetic mechanisms. The prenatal development of the embryo and other aspects of physical and motor development follow two patterns. In the first pattern, *cephalocaudal*, development proceeds from the head down. Arm buds appear before leg buds in the embryo, and the infant shows voluntary motor control of the head and shoulders before control of the lower limbs. In the second pattern, *proximodistal*, development proceeds from the middle of the organism (near) to the periphery (far). In embryonic development, the spinal cord develops before the arm buds. In early motor development, the infant gains control over moving the entire arm before finer control of the individual fingers. These patterns are evident in the evolution of the motor developmental milestones summarized in Tables 5-1 and 5-2.

The *principle of reciprocal interweaving* is based on the physiologic principle of reciprocal innervations in which the complementary inhibition and excitation of different muscles result in efficient movement. This principle is illustrated in the development of walking. Walking is viewed as series of alternations between flexor (bending) and extensor (extending) dominance of arms and legs in coordination. Although flexor and extensor movements can be seen as contradictory, they result in integration and progression to a greater level of mature movement. Similar to the principle

Table 5-1. Motor Milestones in Infancy*

Motor Milestone	25% (mo)	50% (mo)	75% (mo)	90% (mo)
Lifts head up	1.3	2.2	2.6	3.2
Rolls over	2.3	2.8	3.8	4.7
Sits without support	4.8	5.5	6.5	7.8
Pulls self to stand	6.0	7.6	9.5	10.0
Walks holding onto furniture	7.3	9.2	10.2	12.7
Walks well	11.3	12.1	13.3	14.3
Walks up steps	14.0	17.0	21.0	22.0
Kicks ball forward	15.0	20.0	22.3	24.0

*The percentages indicate the approximate percentage of children who achieve the milestone by the age listed.

Table 5-2. Fine and Gross Motor Milestones in Early Childhood

2 yr	2.5 yr	3 yr	3.5 yr	4 yr	4.5 yr	5 yr
Gross Motor Skills						
Walks up and down stairs alone, one step per tread	Can walk on tiptoe	Runs well but stumbles occasionally	Runs smoothly with acceleration and deceleration	Balances on one foot for 4–8 sec	Hops on nondominant foot	Two-hand catch (may not catch ball
Can walk backward	Balances for 1 sec on one foot	Can use hands and feet simultaneously	Skillful in balancing on toes, can run on tiptoes	Skips on one foot	Leaps over objects 10 inches high	May bounce ball in place, catches each bounce
Can throw a ball overhand	Jumps with both feet in place	Can throw a ball without losing balance	Briefly hops on one foot	Goes down stairs with alternating feet (may need help)	Hops forward three hops, maintains balance	May be able to hit a swinging ball
Kicks large ball forward	Helps dress and undress	Jumps from bottom step Alternates forward foot going up stairs Rides tricycle	Catches bounced ball		Can turn somersault Dresses self except for tying shoes	Skips rope
Fine Motor Skills						
Can use some mechanical toys	Copies a crude circle	May be able to unbutton some front buttons	May be able to copy a crude square	Copies square (vertical lines usually longer)	May copy a recognizable triangle	Can button and unbutton well
	Can imitate vertical and horizontal lines	Can copy a circle		May button front buttons		
		May be able to use scissors				

of reciprocal interweaving is the *principle of self-regulatory fluctuation*. According to this principle, development goes through alternating periods of stability and instability. A distinct sequence of stages occurs that allows the organism to function while accommodating growth.

The one exception to the principle of reciprocal interweaving is the *principle of functional asymmetry*. This principle states that behaviors often go through a period of asymmetric development in the process of achieving maturity later on. An example is the asymmetric tonic neck reflex evident in early infancy. This reflex results in the infant's head turning in the direction of the outstretched hand, while the other hand bends in a type of fencer's pose. Gesell proposed that this reflex serves as the precursor of later symmetric reaching. This principle also is thought to lay the groundwork for psychomotor handedness and actions such as throwing a ball.

The *principle of individuating maturation* refers to the fact that certain prerequisite physiologic structures must be present for other development or learning to occur. It is important for an infant to have a certain degree of trunk stability for walking to occur. Providing practice in moving the legs in a stepping fashion does not facilitate walking if the necessary physiologic development is absent. This aspect was perhaps the most influential of Gesell's contribution. Although practice can accelerate the acquisition of refined motor skills, such as playing a musical instrument, or be extremely important when development has been disrupted, research tends to support Gesell's contention that biologic characteristics rather than experience are most important in the development of basic motor skills.

Principles of Cognitive Development

Views of cognitive development, as with other developmental areas, often vary along a continuum ranging from qualitative change at one end to quantitative at the other. Perhaps the best-known theory of cognitive development that illustrates the qualitative approach is that proposed by the Swiss theoretician Piaget, who stressed the active role that children take in adapting to their environment. By understanding this fact, pediatricians can help parents to enhance their child's development by providing opportunities for learning. Piaget proposed that development occurs through three mechanisms: (1) direct learning, (2) social transmission, and (3) maturation.

As the name indicates, *direct learning* is when a person actively participates and interprets new experiences. According to Piaget, children develop schemata, which are mental structures that provide a model for how to interact with the world. These schemata are adapted through the two processes of assimilation and accommodation. Assimilation occurs when someone attempts to understand new information based on existing schemata. A child may refer to a horse as "dog" because the child has a schema that says furry animals with four legs are dogs. Accommodation occurs when an existing schema must be changed to fit new information, such as when a child begins to understand that not all furry four-legged animals are dogs and uses the correct term when he or she sees a horse. The realization that schemata are inadequate and must be altered creates a state of cognitive discomfort known as *disequilibrium*. Children shift from assimilation to accommodation and back again as schemata are altered in an effort to restore equilibrium. This process is known as *equilibration*.

Piaget, similar to other theorists such as Bandura, believed that learning could occur not only through direct means, but also through *social transmission*, through observation and social contact. Disequilibration and the resulting drive to alter existing schemata can occur when the child observes or is told information that cannot be incorporated easily into existing schemata. The process is still an active one, but the child does not have to experience the event directly for learning to occur.

Piaget also recognized that development can occur through *physical maturation*. He acknowledged, although not to the same degree as Gesell, that certain biologic changes occur in neurologic and physical structures in the child that are separate from any particular experiences. These physical changes (e.g., increased myelination) make possible some of the changes in schemata (e.g., increased complexity) that occur over time.

Perhaps the best-known aspect of Piaget's theory was that there are qualitative changes in the child's thinking as he or she gets older. Older children not only have acquired more information and abilities than younger children, but they also use fundamentally different strategies to organize their thinking. As illustrated later, this means that not only do children process less information than do adults, but they also process it in qualitatively different ways that sometimes can lead to confusion and frustration on the part of children and their families. These qualitative differences also are true for children who are experiencing delays in cognitive development. Children with delays in cognitive development think in ways that are qualitatively different from their same-aged peers. Knowledge of these stages not only can help pediatricians identify possible delays in development, but also can help them support parents in setting appropriate expectations and structuring activities throughout the child's life.

Piaget described four stages of cognitive development: (1) the sensorimotor stage, (2) the preoperational stage, (3) the concrete operational stage, and (4) the formal operational stage. He proposed that these stages followed the same invariant sequence for all individuals. Although Piaget indicated the age ranges within which each stage generally occurs, the ages listed are approximate because the ages at which children proceed through the stages vary (Table 5-3).

Sensorimotor Development (Birth to 2 Years)

The first stage begins with the simple reflexes of the neonate and ends at approximately 2 years of age with the onset of symbolic thought representing early language. During this stage, the child's interactions with the environment are on an action level and involve sensory and motor movements. Major advancements during this stage include the acquisition of object permanence, discovering cause-and-effect and means-ends relationships, and, as mentioned, the onset of symbolic thought. Within this stage of development, Piaget noted six substages of qualitatively different developmental behaviors that are summarized in Table 5-3.

Preoperational Stage (2 to 7 Years)

During the preoperational stage, children are concerned with trying to make sense of their world. In doing so, they make some classic errors in thinking primarily because of the inflexibility with which they apply the rules and their limited ability to take the perspective of others. Preschoolers are not being selfish or purposely stubborn when this occurs but merely are reflecting what is an advance in their thinking. Knowledge of these characteristic patterns can help pediatricians guide parents in supporting their preschooler in their development. The main characteristics of preoperational thought are rigidity, egocentrism, semilogical reasoning, and limited social cognition.

Table 5-3. Piaget's Stages of Cognitive Development

Age	Stage	Description
Birth–2 yr	Sensorimotor	Infants understand and organize the world through sensory information and motor activity; object permanence develops
Birth–1 mo	Early reflexes substage	Reliance on and refinement of inborn reflexes; infants do not organize sensory information
1–4 mo	Primary circular reactions substage	Infants repeat enjoyable chance behaviors centering around their own bodies; begin to modify reflexes to new experiences and organize sensory information
4–8 mo	Secondary circular reactions substage	Infants repeat interesting actions on the outside world; intentional but haphazard action; begin to imitate behaviors; early object permanence
8–12 mo	Coordination of secondary circular reactions substage	Infants coordinate earlier behaviors into goal-directed behaviors; anticipation of events; early sense of time; developing object permanence (search for object in first hiding place even when they see it moved)
12–18 mo	Tertiary circular reactions substage	Children intentionally vary actions to experience the result; active overt exploration of novel objects; trial-and-error problem solving; will not search in novel place for a hidden object; imitate unfamiliar behaviors
18–24 mo	Mental combinations substage	Mental representation develops; symbolic thought to solve problems without action; deferred imitation; pretend play; full object permanence (ability to locate an object moved while out of view)
2–7 yr	Preoperational	Children use symbolic representation for events, places, and people; worldview is egocentric; language and pretend play develop
7–11 yr	Concrete operational	Children can solve logical problems about concrete physical subjects; conservation and hierarchical thinking develop
11–adulthood	Formal operational	Adolescents can reason logically about abstract topics, hypothetical problems, and possible outcomes of a situation

This rigidity is illustrated by the child's attempt to apply cognitive rules inflexibly as illustrated by what Piaget called *centration*. Centration is the tendency to focus on only one salient feature to the exclusion of other features, even when this leads to illogical conclusions. A classic example of this is when a preschooler complains that another child was given more juice because the child's glass is taller. The preschooler is unable to take into account that the glass also is thinner than the preschooler's glass. Because of centration, the preschooler focuses only on the dimension of height and ignores the dimension of width. One could try to convince the preschooler that the amount is the same, but it is much easier just to give children of this age the same-size glass. Another example of this rigidity is that preschoolers lack the concept of *constancy*. They do not realize that an object can change its appearance without changing its basic nature or identity. Children act as if a Halloween mask actually changes the identity of the person wearing it. This may explain why a child becomes upset if a parent changes a hairstyle or shaves a beard. In the child's mind, the parent actually may have changed.

Another characteristic of this age is *egocentrism*, or the tendency to view the world entirely in terms of the child's (or ego's) point of view. When talking on the phone, the preoperational child may nod or shake his or her head in answer to questions, not considering that the person on the other end of the phone cannot see the response. Piaget also thought that egocentrism was reflected in the speech and moral judgments of preschoolers. Children of this age tend to engage in "collective monologues" rather than true dialogues when they play together. With respect to moral judgments, the child judges the wrongness of an act according to external variables, such as how much damaged occurred. The child is unable to consider factors such as the person's intent or motivation. Without knowing this fact, a parent might assume when a child is being punished that he or she is uncaring or without remorse, when in fact the response merely reflects children's characteristic way of thinking.

Another characteristic of this stage is semilogical reasoning. This reasoning is reflected in what Piaget termed *transductive thinking and animism*. In transductive thinking, rather than using inductive (from the specific to the general) or deductive (from the general to the specific) thinking, the child reasons from the specific to the specific. That is, events that occur at the same time are thought to be causally related. For example, a child may assume that she caused her brother's illness because earlier that day she and her brother had fought and she had wished for something bad to happen to him. *Animism* is reflected by the child's tendency to attribute human characteristics and actions to inanimate objects (e.g., "The sidewalk made me fall").

Concrete Operational Period (7 to 12 Years)
During the concrete operational period, the child develops a set of cognitive skills or *operations* that involve the use of symbols to represent concrete objects. In Piaget's terms, operations are internalized mental actions that fit into a logical system. Children in this stage become capable of combining, separating, ordering, and transforming objects in their minds. The preschooler's thinking is characterized by egocentrism and inflexibility, whereas the school-age child's thinking is characterized by flexibility and an increased awareness of the world. Because of these new skills, children are able to benefit from language and math instruction in elementary school.

This flexibility of thought is illustrated by *decentration* and *reversibility*. Children now are capable of focusing on more than one aspect at a time. They also are able to reverse operations mentally. In contrast to preschool children, children in this age also understand that an object's *identity* remains unchanged despite physical changes as long as nothing has been added or subtracted. With the advent of decentration comes declining egocentrism. The child now is more aware of another's perspective. Children can communicate more effectively about objects a listener cannot see and are better able to adjust their speech to the needs of the listener. Children can think about how others perceive them (social perspective taking).

In addition to all the advances in reasoning that come with decentration, children in the concrete operational period have a better understanding of temporal and spatial relations. They also are less likely to use transductive reasoning and are better able to reason about the causality of events. Another way their logical reasoning is reflected is in their ability to create categories and logically classify objects. This ability often is reflected in children's growing interest in acquiring collections (e.g., baseball cards, rocks, dolls).

Formal Operational Period (12 Years to Adult)
Although children in concrete operations show great advances, their thinking still is limited to the here and now, the "concrete." With the advent of the formal operational period, the individual is able to think abstractly and to engage in hypothetical/deductive reasoning (e.g., given a premise, the individual logically can deduce the conclusion). The adolescent/adult is able to think in terms of *what may be* rather than being limited to *what is*. This ability allows the individual to consider many different solutions to a problem before acting on any one. This stage of thought influences previous conceptions of events and issues. On reaching the formal operational stage, the adolescent begins to adopt a physiologically based conception of illness, including an understanding of personal control over the onset and severity of illness.

Early in this stage, the adolescent shows a renewed egocentrism. This type of egocentrism is reflected in the self-consciousness and self-criticism that are characteristic of early adolescence. As time goes on, the older adolescent and young adult take into account how others judge them, how they judge the judgment processes of others, and how all this corresponds to social categories in the culture. These newly mastered "operations" are applied to larger issues. Adolescents and adults are able to think about politics and law in terms of abstract principles and are capable of seeing the beneficial, rather than just the punitive, side of laws.

Neo-Piagetian Theories
In reaction to research that called into question some of Piaget's assumptions (e.g., overestimating the abilities of adolescents and underestimating the abilities of young

children), a new set of cognitive theories has been developed. Often referred to as *neo-piagetian*, these theories emphasize the development of *specific* cognitive strategies and concepts rather than a generalized progression of increasingly complex mental operations applicable to any cognitive or logical problem. Case's theory proposes that there are eight domains of knowledge, each with its own central cognitive structure: number, spatial relationships, social relationships, logical analysis, language, musical ability, motor ability, and intrapersonal understanding. Throughout development, these structures undergo major transformations (i.e., qualitative changes) and increase in capacity (i.e., quantitative changes). Cognitive development is viewed as an increase in mental space or the number of schemata a child can use at once. Young children have specific and focused schemata, such as how to throw a ball or color with a crayon. As the children practice these skills, they become more adept and efficient, making available some mental space to use for new information or more challenging problems. Neurologic maturation also creates mental space. Schemata coordinate with one another to create higher order cognitive structures capable of more complex activities leading to abstract thought.

Language Development

Although Piaget's theory addressed some aspects of language development (e.g., collective monologues), it did not illuminate the major milestones of language development or specify why and how certain aspects of language develop. Linguists have attempted to account for the manner in which children accomplish the four major tasks of early language learning: (1) Children must learn the sound patterns of language, or *phonology*. (2) They must learn words and their meanings, or the *semantics* of language. (3) They must learn the morphologic rules, or *syntax* of the language, organizing words into phrases and sentences. (4) They must learn to use words in a practical or meaningful way, or the *pragmatics* of language.

Phonology and Speech Sounds

Early on, the infant must gain control over the speech apparatus—the mouth, lip, tongue, and vocal cords. Certain sounds, such as front vowels (*ah, eh, uh*) and glottal sounds (*k, l, g, h*), are mastered first. Others, such as *m, n, t,* and *b*, come later in the first year, with some consonant blends not being mastered until the end of early childhood. Infants also must learn the basic phonemes or speech sounds of their native language. Development in this area follows a general progression for most infants across all cultures, although the individual's facility with the specific speech sounds of his or her native language begin to be evident fairly early in infancy.

By early childhood, most preschoolers have mastered most of the major sounds involved in speech. Some consonant clusters continue to be difficult, however, until 7 years or so. Many 4-year-olds have difficulty with *v* and *z*. Blends or consonant clusters also are difficult ("spaghetti" as "ghepetti"). Other blends, such as *str* and *th*, are not mastered until the end of preschool and the beginning of elementary school. Some of the clusters may be mastered at the beginning of words first, with clear articulation of clusters in word endings coming later. Children who have fine or gross motor difficulties also may have difficulty in the motor aspects of language acquisition.

Words and Semantics

At around 1 year of age, most children begin saying their first words. First words are usually familiar people, body parts, animals, clothing, and several forms of negation (e.g., "no"). Comprehension precedes production. A 1-year-old may use 10 words but can understand five times that number. These single words often are used as *holophrases*. A holophrase is the use of a single word or sound to convey a complete thought. So "no" can mean a simple "no," or it can mean "No, that's mine." A nonverbal use of semantics is seen around 14 months. Infants begin to use gestures with true communicative intent. They may accompany the words with gestures that elaborate on meaning. From 18 to 24 months, first sentences are evident. Children know approximately 50 words at 18 months and about 200 by 24 months and begin to combine them into two-word sentences.

During the preschool years, there is a virtual explosion in vocabulary development. Children learn two to four new words daily. By around age 6, they use 8000 to 14,000 words. Not only the number of words, but also the variety of forms increases. Children use not only nouns, but also "w" words (e.g., *what, where, who, when, why*) and prepositions. *In* generally appears before *on*, which appears before *under*. The child's changing vocabulary reflects cognitive advances in spatial relations. Words such as *yesterday* and *tomorrow* become more prominent.

Syntax

By the time an infant becomes a toddler, he or she has begun to learn the grammatical structures of the native language. This advance reflects not only the growing social nature of language, but also the child's increasing understanding of how words are organized into phrases and sentences; this includes an increasing understanding and use of past tense verbs, possession, pronouns, and some contractions. These two-word sentences are composed of not only nouns and verbs, but also adjectives and a few articles and prepositions. These two-word sentences often are referred to as *telegraphic speech* because of the similarity to a telegram, in which only essential words are used.

In preschool, children are learning and applying the rules of language. They show an increased flexibility in verbal skills (just as in motor skills), which is reflected in their improving skills in communication. This improvement is evident in their learning of the morphology or rules of language. They show an understanding of plurals, possessives, appropriate endings on verbs, prepositions, and the various forms of "to be." Although there are advances, preschoolers tend to overapply the rules of language, which is termed *overregularization*, in much the same way as they overgeneralize cognitive rules (see earlier). The plural of *tooth* becomes "tooths," and the past tense of *run* becomes "runned." By the end of preschool age, children begin to learn not only the rule, but also the exceptions to the rule. The average length of the sentences (often termed the *mean length utterance*) also increases. Two-word sentences are replaced by three- and four-word sentences during middle preschool and six- to eight-word sentences by age 6.

Pragmatics

With the beginning of early childhood, children show great advances in the pragmatics of communication. They improve their ability to talk about things that aren't physically present. Preschoolers have some difficulty with *referential communication*, which involves describing something for someone else. Although their speech still may be egocentric, contrary to Piaget's initial views, preschoolers show an increased sensitivity to the listener and may adjust their speech to the age of the listener. Preschoolers have been observed to use "motherese" or child-directed speech (e.g., simpler words, shorter sentences, higher pitched voices) with infants and to use more polite and formal forms with adults. Some views of language development propose that egocentric speech may be more a reflection of a lack of the necessary language skills to rephrase communication rather than a true "egocentric" lack of interest in doing so.

A progression from private speech to social speech also is evident during the preschool years. *Private speech* is defined as speech that is not intended to communicate to a listener but rather seems to help children gain control over their actions. *Social speech*, as the name implies, is intended to communicate with others. Both forms are evident in preschool, and both are important. Private speech continues to represent 20% to 60% of children's verbalizations; 2- and 3-year-olds often are observed engaging in *monologues* or talking to themselves. This speech seems to serve various purposes, such as wish fulfillment, problem solving, or describing one's actions. In middle preschool, one observes with increasing frequency *collective monologues*, which are often evident during parallel and associative play in which the content may be common across preschoolers, but there is less interactive purpose. In contrast, social speech becomes more evident later in preschool.

The progression of language highlights continuities across cultures and culture-specific findings, highlighting the age-old nature-versus-nurture question. Knowledge of the major developmental milestones across these four areas (Table 5-4) and awareness of warning signs for possible delay (Table 5-5) are essential in monitoring and supporting the child's development. Similar to the theories of cognitive development, the major theories of language development emphasize different factors, with some theories highlighting environment, other theories highlighting biology, and more recent theories highlighting an interactionist approach (Table 5-6).

Learning Theories

Learning theories emphasize the role of the environment. Language develops in the same way as any other skills or behavior. Language is acquired through classic conditioning, operant conditioning, or imitation. In classic conditioning, following Pavlov's theory, the assumption is that if a word is paired reliably with an object (e.g., the mother says "bottle" every time she presents the toddler with the bottle), the child begins to understand that the word *bottle* represents the three-dimensional object. Although this

Table 5-4. Major Language Milestones

Age	Description of Milestone
Birth	*Crying*—infants cry to express discomfort; parents rely on the context to interpret intent; however, cries do have differential characteristics. A cry of pain is distinguished by high intensity. A fussy/hungry cry is low and gradually builds
2 mo	*Cooing*—infants begin to make sounds to express pleasure and contentment. This is referred to as cooing because of the absence of consonants and the predominance of the /u/ sound
6 mo	*Babbling*—consonant and vowel combinations are evident (e.g., "bababa")
6–12 mo	*Imitation*—infants accidentally imitate sounds that are heard and sounds they emit. They may engage in turn taking with their caregivers. This imitation is an important advancement for later language development and for social interaction
9–12 mo	*Expressive babbling*—often referred to as *jargon* or *patterned speech*, this patterned speech sounds much like adult speech in the sounds chosen and intonation. The speech lacks true semantic importance but expresses a feeling or a purpose
12 mo	*First words, holophrases*—first words often are linked to the infant's direct experience or actions or objects that can move or change or to communicate change in condition or quality. Infants use single words to communicate entire thoughts
18–24 mo	Vocabulary spurt using ≤300 words by age 2 and understanding ≤900; 2-word sentences consisting of noun-verb combinations
24 mo	Correct responses to indirect requests; increasing length of sentences (2–4 words); can point to object or picture when named by someone else; understand names of familiar objects, body parts, and people
30 mo	Modification of speech to take listener into account; need for clarity recognized; speech increasingly relevant to others' remarks; beginnings of true social conversation; early awareness of grammatical categories
3 yr	Use of 300–500 words; increased attention to communication; seek ways to clarify and correct misunderstandings; pronunciation and grammar sharply improve; speech with children the same age expands dramatically; use of language as instrument of control increases
4 yr	Knowledge of the fundamentals of conversation; the child is able to shift speech according to listener's knowledge; literal definitions are no longer a guide to meaning; collaborative suggestions have become common; disputes can be resolved with words; children speak well enough for strangers to understand most of the time; start to use "s" on verbs to show present tense; rapid increase in grammatical complexity over early childhood; overgeneralization of grammatical rules
5 yr	Good control of the elements of conversation; use past, present, and future tenses accurately, recall and can repeat a sentence of 8 words; talk in complex sentences that often run together
6–8 yr	Use 8000–14,000 words; use greater variety of words to express more complex meaning; more precise pronunciation, sentence structure, and word use; increased attention span for listening; can relate experiences in greater detail and in a logical way
Middle childhood	Understanding of passive forms; acquisition of written language
Adolescence	Acquisition of specialized language functions

Table 5-5. Warning Signs of a Potential Language/Communication Delay

Age	Characteristics
<12 mo	Limited verbal expression; little variability in the sounds produced; limited verbal imitation; limited interest in gesturing or any verbal sounds to communicate needs
12–18 mo	At 12 mo, infant doesn't use gestures such as waving or shaking head; doesn't say "mama" or dada" ; isn't using at least a couple of consonants. At 15 mo, doesn't understand and respond to words like "no" and "bye-bye"; isn't using at least 1–3 words. At 16 mo, doesn't point to body parts when asked. At 18 mo, isn't saying at least 6–10 words
19–24 mo	At 19–20 mo, child doesn't point out things of interest, such as bird, truck, plane. At 20 mo, isn't making at least 6 consonant sounds. At 21 mo, doesn't respond to simple directions or play pretend with toys imitating routines. At 24 mo, doesn't imitate actions or words of others; can't point to named pictures in a book; doesn't put 2 words together; doesn't know function of common household objects
25–36 mo	At 26 mo, child doesn't use any 2-word simple sentences. At 30 mo, can't name at least three body parts and can't be understood by anyone in the child's family. At 32 mo, has difficulty singing fragments of nursery rhymes. At 36 mo, doesn't ask questions; can't be understood by strangers at least half the time; is unable to articulate initial consonants (e.g., says "ow" instead of "cow"); is unable to name most common household objects
3–4 yr	At 3 yr, child can't speak in short phrases; is unable to understand short instructions; has no interest in interacting with other children. At 3.5 yr, consistently fails to add final consonant to words (e.g., says "do" instead of "dog"). At 4 yr, has difficulty producing a sound or word often accompanied by facial grimacing; isn't almost fully understandable

approach explains how children come to understand language, it does not account for how they learn to produce the sounds of language.

Operant conditioning has had more support in explaining speech production. Children are thought to emit a variety of sounds. In much the same way as Skinner described the acquisition of other behavior, language is thought to occur through reinforcement (e.g., parental attention, praise) or lack thereof (e.g., ignoring, lack of attention). As a result, certain sounds are emitted more frequently and are shaped and combined into words that have meaning within the child's language. Support for this theory can be found in language studies that show that infants across cultures emit similar sounds. Over the course of the first 2 years of life, certain sounds gain prominence and others disappear such that children begin to produce the language of their culture.

Although they are not a primary explanation for language development, social learning explanations (e.g., Bandura) also have been proposed to help explain a child's acquisition of language. Social learning theory differs from other behavioral perspectives in that it places special importance on internal mediational processes of the person in interaction with the social context. As such, learning is not restricted to trial-and-error and conditioning experience but can be expanded to include social aspects, such as

vicarious reinforcement, imitation, and observational learning. Interactions with the environment are reciprocally determined; that is, the outcome of a situation depends on the person, his or her behavior, and the environment. All three interact to produce learning.

According to social cognitive learning theory, children learn and develop their behavior through the process of modeling. They observe the behavior of a model, often a parent, other significant adult, or peer, and learn from that situation. The mechanism of this learning is through a process of observing the model, remembering the behavior exhibited, abstracting a rule from the experience, and performing the behavior for themselves. It is not necessary for the model to be reinforced for the observer to learn from his or her behavior. Imitation is another way in which children learn, with imitative behaviors of children often reinforced by parents or siblings. Although Bandura's theory and other social learning theories have been helpful in understanding behavior in general, this approach has been less helpful in understanding the totality of language development.

Nativist Explanations

Historically the most prominent nativist language theorist is Chomsky. Chomsky noted that the virtual explosion of language, particularly in early childhood, proceeds at a pace that could not be accounted for by classic or operant conditioning. In addition, there is considerable evidence that children produce a vast array of sentences that they have never heard before. Chomsky believed that although environmental factors play a role, the ability to acquire language is biologically based. He believed that there were specific inborn or biologic structures for processing language, which he referred to as *language acquisition devices*. Language acquisition devices are likened to a genetic code that matures as the child matures and interacts with the environment. This maturation enables the child to acquire and use more complex linguistic structures.

Interactionist Theories

Although the learning and the nativist theories explain aspects of language development, many developmental researchers highlighted the need for more of an inter-

Table 5-6. Major Theories of Language Acquisition

Theory	Primary Influence on Development
Learning	The environment is the primary influence with acquisition the result of reinforcement, imitation, and conditioning primarily by adults
Nativist	Heredity and biology play a major role; children are born ready to learn language and no special training is needed
Interactionist (cognitive)	Language is acquired through the interaction of social and biologic factors. Similar to cognitive development, assimilation and accommodation are involved
Interactionist (cultural context)	Language is acquired through the interaction of social and biologic factors but is mediated by culture

actionist approach. There are as many differences among these theorists, however, as there are between the learning and nativist theorists. What they do share is an appreciation of biologic structures and maturation and cultural experience and interaction.

One example of this approach that illustrates how development can be interpreted within the cultural context is the work by Bruner and colleagues. Bruner used the term *language acquisition support system* to describe the process of language acquisition. He recognized a certain amount of preprogramming related to biologic mechanisms, including the child's innate predisposition to tune into human speech and to babble. Bruner also identified the role of cultural factors, however, whereby the social environment is organized to incorporate the child (probably through learning mechanisms) as a member of an already existing language-using group. Children acquire the syntax and grammatical structures of their particular culture but do not have to be reinforced or to imitate all language to acquire these structures.

Similar to Bruner, Vygotsky highlighted the role of culture in language development. Vygotsky theorized that children's experience of language and their earliest verbalizations are social with communicative intent. He disagreed with Piaget's view that egocentric speech served no function. Rather Vygotsky believed that egocentric or private speech is derived from social speech. This inner speech influences behavior, with thought and language interconnected. Language and thought develop independently from birth through 2 years. At around age 2, there seem to be more interconnections between these two functions. Language becomes intellectual, and thinking becomes verbal. This process is mediated by the child's cultural experiences, with social reality being converted into the thoughts of the individual.

Emotional and Behavioral Development

A comprehensive review of all the theories of emotional and behavioral development is beyond the scope of this chapter. Because pediatricians are consulted more often about behavioral concerns than mental health professionals, however, some review of the major theories would be helpful in anticipating and identifying areas of difficulty, in helping families to set appropriate expectations for typically developing children and children with delays, and in helping families to enhance their child's development in these areas. For the purpose of this chapter, emotional and behavioral development theories can be categorized as addressing the development of the self, the development of parent-child relationships, and the development of relationships with friends.

Development of the Self

The rapid changes that occur in the child's cognitive, motor, language, and behavioral repertoire interact and form the framework for the child's developing sense of self. Some theories focus on the challenges that a child faces in developing an independent identity. Others focus on the specific aspects of the self that may have greater importance at certain ages. One of the best known theories in this area is that of Erikson.

Erikson's Psychosocial Theory

The ideas of Erikson have their basis in Freud's psychosexual theory and share features such as the crucial influence of emotions and relationships and a maturational order of stages. Healthy development of the self is defined as successful individuation, in which the individual is neither overly dependent on others nor overly disconnected from others. This individuation results from the satisfactory resolution of a "crisis" that varies depending on the age of the child (Table 5-7). Similar to most stage theorists, Erikson believed that there are qualitative changes in the development of the self over time. A satisfactory resolution requires the balancing of a positive characteristic (e.g., trust), which should be predominant, and a related negative characteristic (e.g., mistrust), which is also healthy to some degree. If the outcome is successful, a particular strength or virtue emerges, but regardless of the outcome, the individual moves on to the other stages without fixation. As is evident in the description of the stages, the child's experience with parents, family, or other caregivers plays an important role in determining the outcome of the stage. Three interrelated areas of life affect this course of

Table 5-7. Erikson's Psychosocial Stages and Developmental Issues

Age	Psychosocial Stage	Description (Virtue)
Birth–1 yr	Trust versus mistrust	Responsive caregiving gives infants a sense of trust in others and self and that the world is a good place—*hope*
1–3 yr	Autonomy versus shame and doubt	Children become more self-sufficient and want independence; reasonable freedom of choice leads to autonomy—*will*
3–6 yr	Initiative versus guilt	Pretend play and acceptance of responsibilities help to foster a sense of direction; children must balance this with the demands of parents—*purpose*
6–12 yr	Industry versus inferiority	Children learn to cooperate with peers and master academic tasks; competency and productivity are important—*skill*
12–18 yr	Identity versus role confusion	Adolescents strive to develop a coherent and lasting personal identity—*fidelity*
Young adulthood	Intimacy versus isolation	Young adults work to achieve intimate relationships and commitments to other people. Individuals who have not formed a strong sense of self may have difficulty—*love*
Adulthood	Generativity versus stagnation	The focus is on child rearing and work productivity to contribute to the next generation—*care*
Late adulthood	Ego integrity versus despair	Older adults attempt to reflect on their lives and feel satisfied with their successes and failures—*wisdom*

development: (1) the person's innate strengths and weaknesses; (2) the person's unique experiences, such as family life and resolution of developmental crises; and (3) the specific cultural, social, and historical circumstances surrounding the person's life.

Development of Self-Concept

Children refer to their appearance, their activities, their relations to others, and their psychological characteristics when they describe themselves. According to Harter and others who studied the development of self-concept, however, the relative weight of these characteristics changes over time, largely reflecting children's growing cognitive and language abilities. As would be expected given the concrete thinking style of younger children, they tend to describe themselves primarily in terms of the activities they engage in and to some extent their physical characteristics. As they enter into school, children describe themselves in terms of either their cognitive, physical, and social competence or a global notion of self-worth; this represents a type of *categorical* classification. The child's self-concept is largely descriptive.

As children enter into middle childhood, and their thinking allows for more complicated comparisons, the child's self-concept becomes more based in *comparative assessments*. Building on the earlier basic physical descriptions (e.g., "I am tall"), the self-concept is based on how the child measures up to others (e.g., "I am taller than my friends"). Often at this point, children who do not see themselves as "measuring up" may experience some distress; this is one of the reasons that the middle school period is such an important and often stressful transition.

In adolescence, these comparisons take on greater *interpersonal implications* (e.g., "My friends like having me on their team because I am tall"). Again reflecting the child's growing cognitive abilities, descriptions of the self shift from relatively concrete attributes to more inclusive, psychological variables (e.g., "I am a good listener"). In the healthy development of the self, the adolescent's concept of the self should reflect an increased variety of attributes used in self-description. Adolescents include not only athletic, scholastic, and job competence, but also social acceptance, romantic appeal, and conduct in their descriptions. They also tailor their descriptions of themselves to the particular context, representing what Harter described as *multiple selves*.

Gender-Role Identity

The changing view of the self is also reflected in one aspect of the self—the child's concept of gender roles. At the beginning of preschool, a child can identify whether he or she is a boy or a girl (*gender identity*) in largely descriptive terms. It is not until the end of preschool, however, with the advance of the cognitive ability of constancy, that children understand that gender remains constant regardless of the outward appearance (*gender constancy*). Children also begin to learn which behaviors accompany which gender, or knowledge of *gender roles*, with most children acquiring a gender role concept by about age 4 or 5.

Many theoretical explanations exist for this process (Table 5-8). Freud believed that it was the result of the resolution of the Oedipus or Electra complex. In striving to be like the same-gender parent after the resolution of the complex, children acquire not only the behaviors of their parents, but also their attitudes and values. Learning theorists and cognitive theorists hypothesize that gender roles are learned through the same process as other developmental milestones. Learning theorists say gender-role learning is due to direct reinforcement of particular behaviors and activities and modeling of "gender-appropriate" behavior by adults and others in the child's environment. Cognitive theorists see gender-role learning as one example of the child's schemata. Bem's gender schema theory combines these last two. This theory says that children form a concept of gender as a basic schema, but the particular meaning of gender for that child is based on social learning theory. None of these theories addresses the possible role that biologic mechanisms play in establishing gender. Bem's theory may be the most flexible, however, in accommodating the various influences.

Attachment and Development of the Relationship with Primary Caregivers

One of the important aspects of a child's emotional and behavioral development is the child's relationship with his or her parents, family, and other primary caregivers. One of the most influential theories in this area is that of attachment. Largely based on research examining the mother-child relationship, the quality of the attachment with a primary caregiver forms the basis of the child's growing "working model." This working model becomes an important foundation for peer relationships and later

Table 5-8. Four Perspectives on Gender Identification

Theory	Major Theorist	Key Process	Explanation
Psychoanalytic	Freud	Emotional	Gender identification occurs at the resolution of the Oedipus (boys) and Electra (girls) complexes when child identifies with same-sex parent
Social-learning	Kagan	Learning	Identification is a result of observing and imitating models and being reinforced for gender-appropriate behavior
Cognitive-developmental	Kohlberg	Cognitive	When a child learns he is a boy or she is a girl, the child actively sorts information by gender into what boys do and what girls do and acts accordingly
Gender-schema	Bem	Cognitive/social learning	Child organizes information about what is considered appropriate for a boy or a girl on the basis of what a particular culture dictates and behaves accordingly. Child sorts by gender because the culture dictates that gender is an important schema

adult relationships and is crucial in the development of the self.

Attachment theory was initiated by Bowlby as an evolution of Lorenz and Tinbergen's ethological theory. According to Bowlby, mother and child are prewired to respond in fixed ways to each other within the sensitive period of the first few years of life. Bowlby's research was extended by Ainsworth and others and illuminated the key factors in the development of an active, reciprocal, and affectionate relationship.

Ainsworth defined a secure attachment as an enduring affectionate tie between parent and child that is characterized by seeking contact with the object of attachment by proximity or communication. In a securely attached relationship, the mother is a "secure base" from which the child is able to explore his or her surroundings without distress, checking back with her either physically or visually for the reassurance to continue. Over the course of her research, Ainsworth defined different patterns of attachment, which she assessed in the "strange situation," a series of interactions with a stranger including separations and reunions with the child's mother (Table 5-9).

Mothers of *securely attached* children are sensitive to the needs of their children, are consistent, and are responsive to the signals that their children give. Securely attached children cry less, explore more using their parent as a secure base, are more compliant, and have higher self-esteem. Although bothered when separated from their primary caregiver, securely attached children are happy to be reunited and are consoled easily. These children also are more cooperative when playing with peers, are more readily accepting of peers, experience fewer psychological disorders, perform better in school, and are more flexible under stress. Although most children are securely attached, others are not.

One type of insecure attachment is exemplified by children who are *ambivalently attached*. These children are extremely distressed by separation; are difficult to console; and on reunion, approach the mother for comfort and resist her attempt to do so by crying, kicking, and avoiding being held. They seem to be torn in two directions: They seek contact and love from their mother, but at the same time they seem frightened by it because they fight her so much. The mothers of ambivalently attached children are less responsive and sensitive to their children than mothers of securely attached children, characterized by chaotic or inept caretaking, and are generally out of synch with their children. These mothers are often anxious in their parenting role and may have unpredictable lifestyles that lead to the anxiety that these children experience. Beyond infancy and toddlerhood, these children often are described as clingy, demanding, or anxious; show less initiation and response to social interaction; and often are victims of bullies.

Another type of insecure attachment is exemplified by *avoidant* behavior in a child. These children do not appear upset during separations and avoid seeking out their mothers for support on reunion. They react in the same way to their mother and a stranger, but they react more negatively toward the mother on reunion. These children often have endured long separation, abuse, or neglect. Mothers of avoidant children sometimes are openly rejecting of their children. For a variety of reasons (e.g., their own psychological challenges), these mothers have difficulty responding to their children's needs in a loving and contingent way. This difficulty triggers a cycle between mother and child as the child's needs are not met and he or she becomes more demanding. As a result, the mother becomes more irritated and overwhelmed. This lack of emotional and physical availability results in the avoidant type of attachment. In later childhood, these children are more likely to become aggressive and to be described as angry and are often isolated and disliked by their peers. As a result, they often have low self-esteem.

A fourth pattern of attachment has been added by Main and has been termed *disorganized/disoriented*. In the classic strange situation assessment, these children look happy on reunion but almost dazed or confused, as if to say, "I want to be held, but I am not sure that I will be held." They brighten on reunion but do not make direct eye contact. It is thought that the mothers of these children may be giving mixed messages that result in non-contingent caregiving. These children are thought to be most at risk because in contrast to the other patterns, there

Table 5-9. Patterns of Attachment

	Exploratory Behavior before Separation	Behavior during Separation	Reunion Behavior	Behavior with Stranger
Secure	Explores room, shares play with mother, friendly toward stranger, uses mother as a secure base	Might cry, is subdued at first but usually recovers and resumes play	If separation caused distress, contact with mother ends the distress, greets her warmly and initiates play	Somewhat friendly, may play with stranger after initial distress has subsided
Ambivalent	Has difficulty separating from mother to explore toys, wary of novel situations and people, maintains proximity with mother and avoids stranger	Highly distressed, hysterical crying that does not subside	Seeks comfort then rejects it, may be passive or fail to greet mother on her return, continues to cry or be fussy	Does not play with stranger, wary
Avoidant	Easily separates to explore toys, does not play with mother, shows little preference for mother over stranger	Does not show distress, continues play and interaction with stranger	Ignores mother, turns away or moves away from her	No avoidance of stranger

is not enough predictability in the parent-child relationship to develop an organized view of the relationship. This pattern has been identified in mother-infant pairs in which the mother may have some serious psychiatric difficulties (e.g., chronic, severe depression) or substance abuse.

Development of Friendships and Play
Healthy peer development and play are influenced by the child's growing physical, cognitive, and language skills and the quality of the parent-child relationship. In many theories, there is a developmental progression in the quality of peer relations and the type of play. Selman's theory of friendships closely mirrors Piaget's ideas of declining egocentrism. Children's reasoning in perspective taking and friendships is thought to begin as an egocentric, unco-ordinated understanding whereby friends are chosen by physical accessibility and then later by whether they share the same interest or do what the child wants them to do, reflecting the young child's egocentrism. With a growing understanding of another's perspective, friendships become based more on cooperation and compromise. Finally, with adolescence and adulthood, friendships are characterized by an appreciation and tolerance for the other person's need to establish relations with other people while maintaining an intimate and supportive relationship.

Similar progressions have been noted in the quality of the child's play. Parten's conceptualization, which was presented more than seven decades ago, highlights the progression from more nonsocial play during early preschool to parallel play to cooperative play in which children share an organized goal—to make something, play a formal game, or dramatize a situation. The advances in the child's language skill also make this shift possible.

Changes in the cognitive content of play also are evident. Rubin and colleagues, similar to Piaget, identified a developmental progression, in which 1- and 2-year-olds are most likely to engage in *functional play*, also called *sensorimotor play*. This type of play is defined as simple,

repetitive motor movements with or without objects. In the preschool years, children spend more of their time in *constructive play*, in which the goal is to create or construct something. Around the same time, children also increasingly engage in *make-believe play*, in which children act out everyday and imaginary roles, such as playing house or acting out scenes on television. Finally, in middle childhood (6 to 11 years old), children become more interested in *games with rules*.

Summary of Important Developmental Milestones
Although the theories of typical child development represent an important conceptual framework for identifying at-risk development, they typically focus on only one developmental domain. In reality, developmental domains are integrated, and development in one affects the other, as illustrated in the discussion of play and friendships. Another way of looking at development is to summarize the important developmental milestones within each major developmental period and to examine the important shifts that occur. This concept of biopsychosocial shifts originated with Emde and colleagues. These shifts represent periods of development in which relatively new forms of behavior emerge. These shifts are thought to be the result of changes that not only occur in the child's basic biologic makeup, but also are reflected in the child's behavior, which interacts with the child's larger social environment. The major shifts are summarized in Table 5-10. Although some of these shifts need additional empirical support, this approach provides a mechanism for organizing development across various domains.

DEVELOPMENTAL ASSESSMENT
As mentioned at the beginning of this chapter, pediatric health care providers are in key positions to monitor the development of a child and often are the first to address

Table 5-10. Biosocial-Behavioral Shifts

Developmental Period	Shift Point	Characteristics of the Shift
Prenatal	**Conception**	**Genetic material from both parents combines**
		Formation of basic organs
Early infancy (birth–2.5 yr)	**Birth**	**Transition to life outside the womb**
		Interaction with the larger environment
Middle infancy (2.5–9 mo)	**2.5 mo**	**Brain connections increase; social smiling**
		Increased memory and sensorimotor abilities
	7–9 mo	**Development of attachment; stranger and separation wariness; object permanence; beginning of goal-directed behavior**
Late infancy (9–30 mo)		Development of symbolic thought; development of new sense of self
Early childhood (2.5–6 yr)	**End of infancy (24–30 mo)**	**Development of grammatical language**
		Uneven levels of development in various areas; use of cognitive rules to explain world but cognitive rigidity and egocentrism resulting in cognitive errors; development of sex-role identity; increase in sociodramatic play; increasing interest in peers
	5–7 yr	**Gradual responsibility for tasks outside of adult supervision; application of skills; formal schooling**
Middle childhood (6–12 yr)		Increased cognitive abilities, including memory capacity and processing efficiency
	11–12 yr	**Sexual maturation**
Adolescence (12–19 yr)		Capacity for biologic reproduction; achievement of formal operations in some areas; formation of identity; increased individuation from parents

Adapted from Cole M, Cole SR: Development of Children. New York, WH Freeman, 1993.

concerns about developmental progress. The previously discussed principles and theories of development provide benchmarks of typical development and a framework for understanding typical and atypical development. Without tools to evaluate a child's progress in meeting the various developmental challenges, however, these theories may not be as helpful as they could be in enhancing a child's development. Developmental assessment provides one mechanism for operationalizing these principles of development.

In its broadest definition, assessment should be a flexible, collaborative decision-making process in which parents and professionals work together to learn about the child and reach consensus about the changing developmental, education, medical, and mental health service strengths and needs of the child. Assessment has many functions. It can help determine if a child is in need of or is eligible for services by defining the child's functioning and diagnostic characteristics. For children with an identified concern or diagnosis, assessment provides answers to important questions about program planning and intervention. For children already receiving services or for children who may be at risk, assessment can document or evaluate progress, lead to important adaptations in interventions, and provide an important way to monitor development. Assessment can take many forms (e.g., rating scales, observation, screening, full assessment batteries) and focus on various domains (e.g., cognitive, communication, personal/ social).

Since the 1990s, there has been an increase in the number of measures available to monitor child development. Most measures focus on infancy and early childhood, largely in response to the research that highlights the importance of early intervention for children with developmental risks. Many measures focus on multiple areas of development and provide a quick but reliable means of identifying children in need of more thorough or detailed evaluation. Determining which tool to use or evaluating the validity of results in a testing report from another professional can be a daunting task, but several parent and professional organizations have provided guidelines (i.e., American Academy of Pediatrics [AAP], American Psychological Association, Division for Early Childhood, Families and Advocates Partnership for Education, National Association for the Education of Young Children, National Early Childhood Technical Assistance Center, Zero to Three). Table 5-11 lists the currently available measures for assessment; these are discussed in more detail subsequently.

RECOMMENDATIONS FOR BEST PRACTICE IN ASSESSMENT

Any approach to monitoring or evaluating development must map onto the major components of the Individuals with Disabilities Education Act Amendments of 1997 (IDEA). Under Part C (neonate through 2 years old) and Part B (preschool age until kindergarten), IDEA affords young children with documented delay or in some cases developmental risk a variety of developmental services. First, the approach must provide a mechanism for eliciting

parental input and supporting the collaboration between the child's family and the pediatrician and other professionals. Not only is this input a requirement of the legislation in the development of the child's Individualized Family Service Plan (for children <3 years old) and the Individualized Educational Plan (for children >3 years old), but also, more important, research has shown the importance of parental input. Parents are the experts about their child. Although in the past, many professionals were skeptical of the validity of parental report, more recent studies have shown that parental report is predictive of developmental delay, sometimes more so than professional input because of the broader context in which the parents are able to view the child. As such, the reading level of the measure, its face validity, the degree to which it is culturally sensitive, and whether it is available in multiple languages become important considerations when choosing an approach for eliciting information from parents.

Second, pediatric clinicians should be familiar with the specific way in which their state interprets IDEA, including definitions of developmental delay (percent or amount of standard deviation required, type of instrument required); whether informed clinical opinion is acceptable and, if so, how it must be documented; whether children at environmental risk are eligible; how multiple risk factors are considered; and the frequency with which assessments should be administered. Current summaries of state requirements are available from the National Early Childhood Technical Assistance Center (http://www.nectac.org/idea/ idea.asp). As recommended by the AAP guidelines on "Developmental Surveillance and Screening of Infants and Young Children (RE0062)," best practice calls for pediatric clinicians to maintain links with other community resources, such as early intervention programs or schools, and to coordinate their screening and monitoring with the tracking and intervention services in their specific community.

Other considerations include assessing not only the child's difficulties, but also the child's strengths, abilities, and competencies and the context in which development occurs. Pediatricians should augment good clinical judgment with more standardized instruments. To have any confidence in the results, the measure should have good psychometric qualities. That is, the measure should be reliable (e.g., it should yield similar results regardless of the assessor/reporter) and valid (e.g., it should be highly correlated with future assessments or other markers of development) with estimates ideally in the 0.80s. The measure also should have good normative data based on a large, representative standardization sample that is relatively current and reflective of the children likely to be assessed with the particular measure. In addition, the manual should have clear and standardized instructions regarding administration and scoring.

Some standards relate specifically to screening measures. As stated by the AAP, clinicians must "develop a strategy to provide periodic screening in the context of office-based primary care" and must maintain and update their "knowledge about developmental issues, risk factors, [and] screening techniques." Of particular importance is the degree to which the screening measure accurately identifies

Table 5-11. Selected Developmental and Behavioral Screening and Assessment Tools

Instrument	Age Range	Administration Time, Informant, Reading Level, Translations	Domains Measured
Screening Instruments			
Ages and Stages Questionnaires (ASQ)	4 mo–5 yr	10–20 min if administered by interview; 2–3 min to score	Communication, gross motor, fine motor, problem solving, personal-social
AGS Early Screening Profiles	2–6 yr, 11 mo	15–40 min of direct testing/caregiver questionnaires	Cognitive-language, motor, self-help-social
Bayley Infant Neurodevelopmental Screen	3–24 mo	10–15 min; 10–13 directly elicited items	Neurologic, receptive, expressive functions, processing, mental activity
Denver Developmental Screening II	Birth–6 yr	10–20 min	Cognitive, motor, language, adaptive
Developmental Indicators for the Assessment of Learning (DIAL-III); Speed DIAL	3–6 yr, 11 mo	Screener administered by professionals in 15 min; Spanish version available	Motor, language, concepts, total, self-help, social, Speed DIAL
Temperament and Atypical Behavior Scale	11–71 mo	5-min parent-completed screener (see below for description)	Temperament and self-regulation behavioral indicators (e.g., activity, self-stimulatory)
Broad-Based Developmental/Achievement Assessments			
Assessment, Evaluation, and Programming System for Infants and Children (AEPS)	Birth–6 yr (covering development from birth–3 yr)	1 hr; interventionists; teachers; caregivers; compatible with curriculum guide for IFSP/IEP planning	Fine motor, gross motor, cognitive, adaptive, social-communication, social
Battelle Developmental Inventory	Birth–8 yr	10–30 min for screener; 1–2 hr for full battery	Personal-social, adaptive, motor, communication, cognitive
Bayley Scales of Infant Development (BSID-II)	1–42 mo	30–60 min; professionally administered	Mental, motor, and 30 behavior ratings
Child Development Inventories (CDI)	3 mo–6 yr	30–50 min completed by parents; 7th–8th grade reading level	Social, self-help, gross motor, fine motor, expressive language, language comprehension, letters, numbers, general development
Developmental Indicators for the Assessment of Learning (DIAL-III)	3–6 yr, 11 mo	Administered by professionals, 30 min	Motor, language, concepts, total, self-help, social, Speed DIAL
Infant-Toddler and Family Instrument	6–36 mo	45–60 min each for Caregiver Interview and Developmental Map, completed by family service providers	Fine motor, gross motor, social and emotional, language, coping, self-help
Parents' Evaluations of Developmental Status (PEDS)	Birth–8 yr	5 min completed by parent; 4th–5th grade reading level; available in Spanish	Global-cognitive, expressive language and articulation, receptive language, fine motor, gross motor, behavior, social-emotional, self-help, schools
Assessments for Specific Areas of Development			
ASEBA (Achenbach System of Empirically-Based Assessment)	1.5–18 yr	15–20 min; parent, teacher/caregiver, child report versions; available in Spanish	Total problems score, externalizing and internalizing composite, subscales (e.g., depression, aggression), competence
Behavior Assessment System for Children (BASC)	2.5–18 yr	10–20 min/30 min for child report; parent, teacher/other, child report versions; audiotaped version for low-level readers; available in Spanish	Behavior symptom index; externalizing and internalizing composites, subscales (e.g., depression, hyperactivity); adaptive skills
Temperament and Atypical Behavior Scale	11–71 mo	30 min total; parents and professionals complete; professionals score	Temperament and self-regulation behavioral indicators (e.g., activity, self-stimulatory)

children who truly need referral or further assessment *(sensitivity)* and children who are developing normally and not in need of expensive and limited assessment and intervention services *(specificity)*. These values should be in the 70% to 80% range because otherwise the measure is not doing much more than chance identification. The relative importance of overidentifying versus underidentifying children varies depending on the reason for the screening. The choice of a screening instrument always must be made in light of the referral question and the particular characteristics of the pediatrician's practice. This and other psychometric information should be readily available in the administration manual. Another important factor in selecting a screening measure is the degree to which it is

useful in the particular setting. The measure should be brief, inexpensive, and easily incorporated into an office visit. A detailed overview of screening and assessment instruments is beyond the scope of this chapter; however, a brief review of some of the major developmental assessment instruments is provided here.

Developmental Surveillance and Screening

Of all the roles in assessment, the pediatric clinician is most likely to have a direct role in the surveillance and monitoring of a child's development. In an AAP survey, 96% of pediatricians who responded indicated that they screen for developmental risk. As defined by Dworkin, developmental surveillance is a flexible, continuous process whereby knowledgeable professionals perform skilled observations of children during the provision of health care. The components of developmental surveillance include eliciting and attending to parental concerns, obtaining a relevant developmental history, making accurate and informative observations of children, and sharing opinions and concerns with other relevant professionals. First introduced in Great Britain, the rationale for surveillance is based on the limited psychometric characteristics of many of the widely used developmental screening instruments (e.g., Denver Developmental Screening Test II [DDST-II]) and the prohibitive amount of time these instruments require. Although informed clinical judgment can have its limitations, the clinician can monitor a child's development by making frequent observations during well-child visits and comparing the child's development with two to three items expected for the age of the child in each of the four major areas of development (gross motor, fine motor, speech, and personal-social) (see Tables 5-1, 5-2, 5-4, 5-5, and 5-9). The accuracy of this monitoring can be increased greatly, however, when it is augmented by parental report on checklists that can be completed before the visit or in the waiting room (e.g., Ages and Stages Questionnaire [ASQ]).

The degree to which parental report on checklists occurs may be limited in current practice. In the survey cited previously, 7 out of 10 pediatricians indicated that they use clinical assessment without a screening instrument or checklist. Pediatricians who do use a checklist typically use one completed by themselves or a staff member; 62% of pediatricians responded that they never use checklists completed by parents.

Pediatric clinicians may want to consider conducting screenings as well. Defined as a "brief assessment procedure designed to identify children who should receive more intensive diagnosis or assessment," screening measures can be completed by multiple informants (e.g., day care providers, parents, pediatric staff). Although many of the original screening measures had limited psychometric qualities and standardization samples, interest in early childhood assessment has resulted in several options that can be used to identify children at high risk for atypical development who need more in-depth evaluation. Although slightly more negative about the feasibility of surveillance and screening, Dobrez and colleagues provided a good review of cost-benefit analysis of some major developmental and behavior screens. As would be expected, costs are lowest for parent-administered developmental screens and highest for lengthy screens administered by professionals. The AAP Policy Statement on surveillance and screening of infants and young children provides an excellent summary of recommendations for both of these approaches.

The *DDST-II* is perhaps the best known of these monitoring instruments. In a survey, 34% of pediatricians reported that their clinical assessment always is guided by the DDST-II, with 40% responding that their assessment sometimes is guided by this tool. The DDST-II can be used for children from birth to 6 years old to monitor development in four areas: personal-social, fine motor-adaptive, language, and gross motor. The revision was to have addressed some of the limitations of the original test

and does to some degree. Problematic items were deleted or revised. New items were created, particularly in the language area. The items in DDST-II are scored in much the same way as the earlier version with "pass," "fail," "no opportunity," and "refusal." The DDST-II was restandardized on a larger, more ethnically diverse sample, although the sample was exclusively from Colorado. Some psychometric characteristics are quite strong (e.g., interrater reliability 99.7%), but others, such as its concurrent validity, are not addressed. The sensitivity and specificity are less than the 70% to 80% recommended guideline by the AAP. The lack of parental input and the time involved (approximately 20 minutes) render the DDST-II a less than optimal choice for detecting potential delays in young children.

The *ASQ*, the second edition of which was developed by Squires and colleagues, avoids some of the pitfalls inherent in the DDST-II. The ASQ provides a quick (10 to 30 minutes) way to identify children ages 4 through 60 months who may have potential developmental problems. Information is obtained on the child's communication, gross motor, fine motor, problem-solving, and personal-social skills through parental report and takes about 3 minutes for scoring. The ASQ can be used in 2-month intervals from 4 to 24 months, 3-month intervals from 24 to 36 months, and 6-month intervals from 36 to 60 months. There are screening cutoffs, and the manual provides information on the instrument's strong psychometric characteristics, adequate standardization sample, and cautions in using developmental cutoffs. The fact that the ASQ can be used for children 5 years of age is particularly helpful in covering the important transition between early intervention and early childhood services without changing measures. It also can be mailed to parents and completed before a pediatric visit or sent in periodically without needing a visit if development is proceeding typically. The ASQ is available in English and Spanish (Arabic and French pending) and requires only a fourth-grade to fifth-grade reading level. It is one of the measures specifically mentioned in the AAP Policy Statement and directly addresses the need for parental input and speed. The ASQ can be incorporated easily into regular pediatric visits.

Another measure mentioned as an option for surveillance purposes is the *Child Development Inventory (CDI)*. As with the ASQ, the CDI is completed by parents or caregivers for children ages 15 months to 6 years. There are three separate instruments, each with 60 yes/no items. The wide age range, the importance of parental input, and its broad coverage of eight developmental areas (social, self-help, gross motor, fine motor, expressive language, language comprehension, letters, and numbers) make the CDI an attractive option for monitoring. Although the 1992 version of the CDI represents an improvement over the earlier Minnesota Child Development Inventory in some areas, the major problem with the earlier version still remains and that relates to the standardization sample. The normative sample still is based on a small number of primarily white children from Minneapolis. Although the items have face validity and adequate psychometric characteristics, the significantly limited normative sample severely limits the utility of this measure.

Another measure that elicits parental input about their child's development is the *Parents' Evaluation of Developmental Status (PEDS)*. Appropriate for children from birth through 8 years of age, the PEDS is a prescreening measure consisting of 10 items that can be administered to parents in written or interview form. Areas assessed include global-cognitive, expressive language and articulation, receptive language, fine motor, gross motor, behavior, social-emotional, self-help, schools, and other, with one item for each area. An advantage of the PEDS is its brevity (2 to 5 minutes). Parents answer "yes," "no," or "a little," with the result being to refer for diagnostic testing, screen or refer for screening, provide brief counseling, or monitor progress at the next office visit. More information is needed about reliability and validity of the PEDS. The PEDS provides a quick, inexpensive way for parents to articulate initial concerns, however, in a broad variety of developmental domains. Other advantages are that it is available in Spanish and is written at a fourth- to fifth-grade reading level.

Several measures are available that must be administered by professionals. There are two versions of the *Early Screening Inventory–Revised (ESI-R)*: ESI-P is used for children ages 3 to 4.5 years, and the ESI-K is used for children 4.5 to 6 years; both yield an assessment of visual motor-adaptive, language and cognition, and gross motor areas. The *Developmental Indicators for the Assessment of Learning (third edition)* is designed to help identify potential difficulties for preschool children entering school for children ages 3 years, 0 months, to 6 years, 11 months. The *AGS Early Screening Profiles* examines development across the preschool period in children ages 2 years, 0 months, to 6 years, 11 months. These measures are described in more detail in the CD-ROM.

Broad-Based Developmental and Achievement Assessment

When a child is identified as being at risk through screening, additional assessment should occur. The goal here is a more in-depth analysis of the child's strengths and needs to determine if a delay or disability is present and to determine whether or not intervention is needed. According to the AAP, although a pediatric clinician is not likely to be involved in this level of assessment, he or she needs to be familiar with the measures to assist families in interpreting findings and in determining the need for referral. Measures used for this purpose are more time intensive and should be norm or criterion referenced based on a broad, representative sample that is similar to the demographic characteristics (e.g., age, ethnicity) of the child being tested. As with screening instruments, developmental assessments should have strong psychometric qualities as well.

Measures not only vary in terms of the developmental area that they assess, but also may vary depending on whether they are norm-referenced or criterion-referenced. A *norm-referenced* test compares a child's performance with that of similar students who have taken the same test. These norms can include a variety of scores, including standard scores (e.g., IQ scores in which the mean is 100 and the standard deviation is 15), percentile rankings (e.g., average = 50th percentile), or T scores (e.g., average T score = 50). In contrast, *criterion-referenced* tests measure a child's performance with respect to a well-defined domain, such as reading. Instead of obtaining scores that compare the child with other children, these tests provide information on the child's performance relative to the test items. Typically, these tests help to answer questions regarding the degree to which a child has mastered a certain level of knowledge, and they often are helpful in generating recommendations for intervention because they can be repeated frequently.

As with the screening tools, a plethora of developmental assessments exist that tap broad developmental domains. For young children age 1 month to 3.5 years, the *Bayley Scales for Infant Development (second edition) (BSID-II)* is a mainstay of many infant/toddler assessments. The BSID-II is norm referenced and includes a motor scale, which focuses on the control and skill used in body movements; a mental scale, which taps cognitive abilities; and a behavior rating scale, which assesses behavioral concerns, such as the lack of attention.

The *Battelle Developmental Inventory (BDI)* can be used for children from birth to 8.5 years of age and provides information on the child's development in five domains: personal-social, adaptive, motor, communication, and cognitive. The BDI can yield 30 profile scores within these domains. A unique option of the BDI is that the items may be administered using a structured testing format, through observation, or through parent-teacher interviews. Administration of the full battery can take 1 to 2 hours; there is a comparable screening test that takes 10 to 30 minutes. Psychometric qualities are good, as is the standardization sample providing a good basis for normative comparisons, although there are reports that the BDI overestimates preschoolers who are delayed. Raw scores can be translated into percentiles and standard scores and age-equivalent and grade-equivalent scores. A developmental quotient also can be obtained.

The *Infant-Toddler Developmental Assessment (IDA)* also is designed to improve the early identification of children who may need monitoring or intervention services. The IDA is appropriate for assessing development in young children from birth to 3 years and is conducted by teams of at least two developmental professionals. The IDA consists of six phases (referral and preinterview data gathering; initial parent interview; health review; developmental observation and assessment; integration and synthesis; and share findings, completion, and report) that provide information on the child's gross motor development, fine motor development, relationship to inanimate objects (cognitive), language communication, self-help, relationship to persons, emotions and feeling states (affect), and coping. There are some gaps in psychometric data as reported in the manual, although what is reported in terms of internal reliability is adequate. Because the IDA requires so much time and relies primarily on two professionals who are trained in the instrument, it may be less helpful for screening and monitoring that would be more typical of pediatric practice.

Some common norm-referenced assessments that tap achievement in varied domains are the *Weschler Individual Achievement Tests* and the recently revised *Woodcock-Johnson Psychoeducational Battery–III*. The Woodcock-Johnson provides a normed set of tests for measuring general intellectual ability, specific cognitive abilities, scholastic aptitude, oral language, and academic achievement in individuals age 2 to 90.

A good option for a criterion-referenced instrument to examine achievement is the Brigance Inventories. There are several inventories, but the *Brigance Inventory of Early Development–Revised* is the most recent version. Appropriate for children from birth to 7 years, the Brigance taps skills in reading, writing, and mathematics.

Specific Areas of Development

There are many options for the assessment of *cognitive development*. The reader is directed to Sattler's work for a thorough discussion and review of the instruments available. In addition to the BSID-II described earlier for young children, perhaps the best known are the Wechsler scales, which provide a mechanism for assessing intellectual abilities from preschool (Wechsler Preschool and Primary Scale of Intelligence–third edition) to childhood (Wechsler Intelligence Scale for Children [fourth edition]) through adulthood (Wechsler Adult Intelligence Scale–third edition). An overall cognitive index can be obtained from the Woodcock-Johnson as well. For infants, the BSID-II provides an evaluation of the infant's overall cognitive development and some information on motor, language, and behavior from age 1 to 42 months.

For early *language development*, the *Receptive Expressive Emergent Language Scale–2* provides information about expressive, receptive, and combined language abilities for children from birth through 3 years old. A similar measure, the *Test of Language Development–Primary (third edition)* can be used from age 4 years through 8 years, 11 months, and yields six composites of language development. For older children, measures such as the *Clinical Evaluation of Language Fundamentals–3* provide norm-referenced scores on receptive and expressive language, morphology, syntax, semantics, and memory for individuals age 6 through 21 years. The Clinical Evaluation of Language Fundamentals–3, similar to many of the more recently revised developmental assessments, has a Spanish version available.

For assessing *behavior,* there are broad-band measures that provide normative data on a child's behavior across many areas. The most frequently used measures are the *Behavior Assessment System for Children (BASC)* and the *Achenbach System of Empirically-Derived Assessment (ASEBA)*. The BASC is a multimethod, multiinformant, and multidimensional assessment system designed to assess maladaptive and adaptive behaviors for children age 2.5 through 18 years. The BASC has three core instruments: the Teacher Rating Scales, the Parent Rating Scales, and the Self-Report of Personality (ages 8 to 11 and ages 12 to 18). Similar to the BASC, the ASEBA includes parent, teacher, and self-report versions. There are three rating scales for parents. Perhaps the best known is the 118-item CBCL for parents of children ages 4 to 18 (CBCL/4–18). The CBCL/4–18 yields T scores and percentiles for internalizing, externalizing, and total problem scales and eight cross-informant areas: aggressive behavior, anxious/depressed, attention problems, delinquent behavior, social problems, somatic complaints, thought problems, and withdrawn. An additional 20 items provide estimates of specific competencies with regard to child

activities, social relationships, and school performance, along with a total competence score.

All rating scales within the ASEBA use a similar response format in which the respondent indicates the degree to which a particular behavior is true on a 3-point scale (*not true, sometimes true, very or often true)*. Depending on which scale is being used, the time frames may differ, ranging from the past 6 months for parental and self-report to the past 2 months for teacher report and parental report on the Caregiver-Teacher Report Form (C-TRF/1½–5). Similar to the BASC, a direct observation form is available. Unique to the ASEBA is the availability of a semistructured interview for children and adolescents. (See the CD-ROM for more information on the BASC and ASEBA.)

Summary

For more information on choosing and interpreting measures, the reader is directed to several sources. First, if one has access to electronic databases, the *Mental Measurements Yearbook* provides a comprehensive compendium of major developmental assessments, including the purpose of the test, domains measured, age ranges, time to administer, publisher and cost, psychometric qualities, and usually two reviews of the quality of the instrument. Most test publishers (e.g., Psychological Corporation, American Guidance Service, PRO-ED, Riverside Publishing) provide comprehensive websites where information can be obtained on the latest versions of developmental assessments as well as purchasing information. Several excellent books on assessment and assessment measures are listed in the Suggested Readings.

Screening and evaluation is not an end in and of itself but is tied ultimately to enhancing the child's development. A key part of the process is the pediatric clinician's ability to partner with families not only in eliciting information from parents, but also in communicating information about the findings and available services. As noted in the AAP Policy Statement and in federal legislation, parental observations are invaluable, and the previous skepticism about their lack of validity has not been supported. More importantly, if the child does have difficulty, it is imperative that the child's family and professionals form a partnership to ensure that the child develops to his or her fullest potential. The developmental assessment can provide a firm foundation for this partnership or can make it almost impossible for trust and collaboration to develop. A resource published by the nonprofit organization, Zero to Three, entitled *New Visions: A Parent's Guide to Understanding Developmental Assessment*, can be helpful for families and for professionals. The resource contains guidelines to help parents know what to look for in a good assessment and what to avoid. A summary of the guidelines can be obtained from the organization's website (www.zerotothree.org).

◉ Additional Resources, CD-ROM

Screening tools administered by professionals	Text
Bibliography	

SUGGESTED READINGS

American Academy of Pediatrics: Developmental surveillance and screening of infants and youngchildren (RE0062). Pediatrics 2001;108:192–196.

Anastopoulos AD, Shelton TL: Assessing Attention-Deficit/Hyperactivity Disorder. New York, Plenum/Kluwer, 2001.

Aylward GP: Practitioner's Guide to Developmental and Psychological Testing. New York, Plenum/Kluwer, 1994.

Dobrez DG, Lo Sasso AT, Holl J, et al: Estimating the cost of developmental services provided in general pediatric practice. Pediatrics 2001; 108:913–922.

Sattler JM: Assessment of Children: Behavioral and Clinical Applications. San Diego, Jerome M. Sattler Publisher, 2001.

Sattler JM: Assessment of Children: Cognitive Applications, 4th ed. San Diego, Jerome M. Sattler Publisher, 2001.

Simeonsson RJ, Rosenthal SL: Psychological and Developmental Assessment. New York, Guilford Press, 2001.

Zero to Three, New Visions: A parent's guide to understanding developmental assessment. Available at: www.zerotothree.org.

SECTION 1   FUNDAMENTALS

6 Principles of Decision Making

Olakunle B. Akintemi

Decision making is an essential part of the practice of medicine. Physicians make hundreds of decisions daily. Examples of decisions include whether to order a complete blood count and blood culture in a febrile child, whether to obtain a chest radiograph in a febrile child with cough, when to seek consultation or referral to a specialist, whether to prescribe an antimicrobial to a child with probable sinusitis, and whether a heart murmur is innocent or not.

Decision making involves a complex interaction between the physician, patient, biomedical knowledge, scientific evidence, and sociocultural factors (Fig. 6-1). Medical decisions generally are made under conditions of uncertainty and risk. Clinical data (subjective and objective symptoms, physical signs) and paraclinical data (laboratory tests) often are imperfect. There may be uncertainty in defining a disease, making a diagnosis, selecting a treatment or procedure, observing outcomes of treatment, or identifying

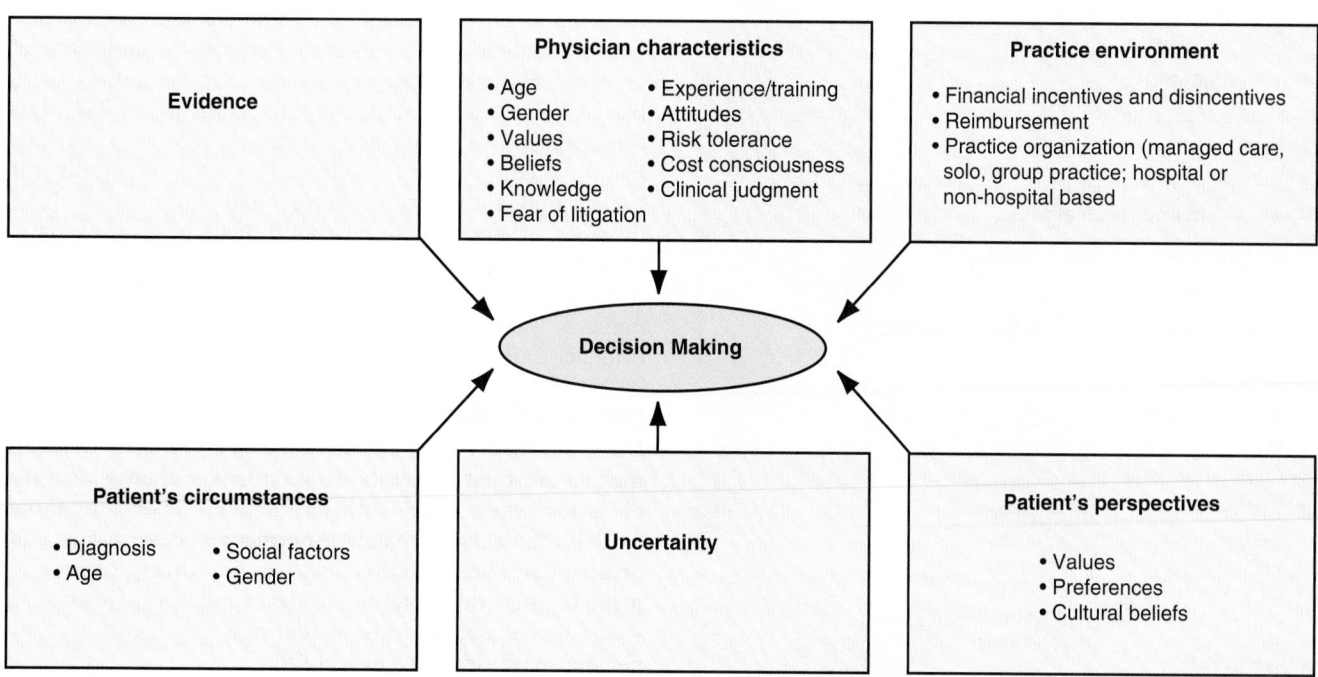

Figure 6-1. Factors influencing decision making. (Redrawn from Gifford DR, Mittman BS, Vickery BG: Diagnostic reasoning in neurology. Neurol Clin 1996;14:223–238.)

the effects of a treatment. Uncertainty is said to be the "hallmark" of clinical decision making.

A decision is a conscious, voluntary choice between alternatives to achieve goals. In medicine, the major goal of decision making is to achieve the best outcome for patients. Clinical decisions should be made after a consideration of the evidence; the benefits, risks, and cost of the alternatives; and the patient's values and preferences.

DECISION-MAKING STRATEGIES

Despite the importance of decision making in everyday practice, little is known about how physicians make decisions. Physicians make decisions based on their own experience, values, goals, and morals. A clinical decision has two distinct components—technical judgments and value judgments. Technical judgments focus on such questions as what the diagnosis is, whether to treat or to test, and how to treat. Value judgments refer to the tradeoff between positive and negative consequences of alternative management decisions.

Box 6-1 lists the strategies used in clinical decision making. *Analytic method* usually involves formal analysis and can range from problem-solving methods, such as the hypothetico-deductive, exhaustive, and arborization methods, to decision analysis. It is a slow, conscious, consistent, and accurate method of thinking that involves several steps. The first steps are to define the decision problem, specify objectives, and identify the alternative courses of action and all possible beneficial and adverse outcomes. After

identifying all the options and possible outcomes, the next step is to evaluate the benefits and harms of the alternative management strategies and choose the "best" alternative.

Although the analytic approach is rational, physicians generally do not make decisions in this manner. In reality, most clinical decisions are made intuitively by pattern recognition ("I have seen this before"), heuristics (rules of thumb), and value judgments. Other key aspects of intuitive decision making are similarity recognition (recognition of similarities and differences between past and current situations), commonsense understanding, skilled know-how, sense of salience, and deliberative rationality. *Intuitive thinking* is automatic; involves rapid, unconscious data processing; and may be highly accurate in one situation and erroneous in another (variable accuracy). It allows the physician to use past experiences and knowledge base to make decisions. Heuristics (discussed later) may be specialty dependent or personal and idiosyncratic. Although the process of formation of heuristics is poorly understood, pathophysiologic reasoning, personal experience, published research, and opinion of experts each plays a role.

The two main factors influencing the type of decision method used (analytic or intuitive) are the nature of the problem and the experience of the physician. An expert pediatric clinician in a busy office practice probably uses the intuitive method frequently. In contrast, an academic physician discussing a case in a grand rounds or clinicopathologic conference probably would use analytic and intuitive methods. Although conceptually discrete, both methods often work together, and neither is inherently superior to the other.

Physicians also may defer to experts, in the form of consultation with colleagues, local and national experts and opinion leaders, journal review articles, textbooks, clinical practice guidelines and pathways, and computerized clinical decision support systems. Expert sources of information are quick, cheap, valuable, and easy to use. Expert opinions from colleagues or local and national experts provide wisdom gained from clinical experience and clinical "pearls." However, expert opinion may be out of date, biased, and not evidence-based medicine (EBM) but "eminence-based medicine." Textbooks are easy to use, readily accessible, and moderately useful, especially for background information. Foreground information (i.e., diagnosis, therapy, and outcome) may be out of date, biased, and not evidence based. Finally, physicians may defer to and share decisions with patients and integrate patients' values and preferences with the best available evidence and clinical expertise.

Decision Theory

Decision theory is a formal theory of rational decision making designed to help a decision maker choose a course of action when faced with alternatives. There are three models of decision making—normative, descriptive, and prescriptive. The *normative model* is the theory of how to make the best decisions under ideal conditions. *Descriptive model* or behavioral decision theory is the theory of how persons make decisions in real life.

Prescriptive model is the theory of how one should make decisions to improve the quality of decisions. Application of

---

Box 6-1. Decision-Making Strategies

Analytic Method

- Hypothetico-deductive method
- Exhaustive method
- Algorithm
- Decision analysis

Intuitive Method

- Pattern recognition
- Heuristics
- Value judgment

Analytic and Intuitive Methods

- Evidence-based decision making

Defer to Experts

- Expert opinion ("eminence-based medicine")
- Colleagues
- Local experts
- National experts
- Opinion leaders
- Consultation/referral
- Textbooks
- Review articles
- Clinical practice guidelines
- Clinical pathways
- Computerized clinical decision support systems

Defer to Patients

- Shared decision

decision theory to improving physician decision making is discussed in the last section of this chapter. Neither the normative nor the descriptive theory is particularly useful in describing how physicians make most decisions. An expanded description of both normative and descriptive theories can be found on the CD-ROM.

Clinical Reasoning

Clinical decision making is a component and an outcome of the process of clinical reasoning. Clinical reasoning is enhanced by experience, knowledge, and the context in which the reasoning is occurring. The various contexts of clinical reasoning are the personal context of the patient (cultural, psychosocial values, beliefs, expectations), complexity and unique context of the clinical problem, clinical setting (inpatient, outpatient, intensive care unit), wider health care environment, personal and professional framework of the physician, and knowledge explosion (ability to manage complex and changing information). Physicians use one or more of the following strategies in medical problem solving and diagnostic clinical reasoning: pattern recognition, arborization, exhaustion, and hypothetico-deductive method.

1. *Pattern recognition* (recognition by gestalt): This is the immediate recognition that a patient's presentation is similar to one previously learned. It is a reflexive process that is acquired by clinical experience and is difficult to teach to the novice. Triggers of pattern recognition are visual, auditory, olfactory, gustatory, and tactile. Examples of visual stimuli include a herald patch (pityriasis rosea), erythema chronicum migrans (Lyme disease), and axillary freckling (neurofibromatosis). Auditory stimuli are less common; examples include stridor (upper airway obstruction), "hot potato voice" (peritonsillar abscess), and staccato cough (pertussis, *Chlamydia trachomatis* pneumonia).
2. *Arborization* (multiple branching): This involves flow charts and algorithms. An algorithm is a predetermined sequence of steps for solving problems or making decisions. Algorithms formalize the diagnostic process, present an organized and logical approach to solving clinical problems, outline which diagnostic tests to obtain, and present how the results of the tests affect subsequent management. Flow charts are printed aids that guide the clinician through a series of yes and no answers until the end point is reached. This method is applicable to evaluation of rare disorders or when diagnosis is delegated to nonphysicians.
3. *Exhaustion:* This strategy is a two-stage process—first, collecting all data conceivably relevant to the case (regardless of probability) and, second, searching through the data for the diagnosis. It is a tedious, inefficient, and time-intensive approach of the novice and seldom is used by experienced physicians. It also commonly is used in tertiary and quaternary care hospitals for evaluation of unusual diseases or unusual presentations of illness or when multiple diseases exist in a patient.
4. *Hypothetico-deductive method:* Elstein and colleagues found that physicians (experienced and novice) solve diagnostic problems by generating a limited number of hypotheses (three to five) early during clinical

encounters. Clinical maneuvers follow with additional clinical and paraclinical data to exclude any incorrect hypothesis or confirm the potential working diagnosis/hypothesis. This is the most commonly used and most effective method of clinical problem solving and is discussed fully in the section on diagnostic reasoning. Factors affecting problem-solving strategies are physician experience, case acuity, and case difficulty. Case difficulty is determined by the knowledge, experience, and practice patterns (primary care or subspecialty) of the physician. Experienced physicians use the hypothetico-deductive strategy for difficult or unfamiliar cases and pattern recognition for easy or familiar cases within their subspecialties. Also, hypothetico-deductive, exhaustion, and pattern recognition may be used in a clinicopathologic conference. Life-threatening situations requiring immediate action may be unsuitable for exhaustion or hypthetico-deductive strategies.

As stated earlier, clinical decisions are classified as either diagnostic or therapeutic. The term *diagnosis* has two different meanings in clinical medicine. First, it is the process of identifying a patient's disorder. Second, it is the outcome of the diagnostic process, which is to provide a "diagnostic label." The objectives of diagnosis are to classify the patient's condition; provide an explanation for the symptoms, signs, and clinical data; arrive at a prognosis for the patient; and select a course of action.

DIAGNOSTIC REASONING

Diagnostic reasoning is an integral part of decision making. It is a rational process, which involves logical thinking and pattern recognition. Kassirer and Kopelman proposed three basic reasoning methods used in diagnostic reasoning: (1) pathophysiologic (causal), (2) pattern recognition (categorical), and (3) probabilistic. Although conceptually discrete, these methods are complementary, they are used simultaneously, and none is inherently superior to others. In the diagnostic process, the physician makes a series of inferences about the nature of the patient's condition until a "working diagnosis" is identified with some alternatives. The essential steps in the diagnostic process are problem framing and forming the initial concept, hypothesis generation (triggering), hypothesis testing and refinement, and hypothesis verification.

Framing the Problem and Forming the Initial Concept

Early in a clinical encounter, verbal and nonverbal information (cues) is analyzed to form an initial concept about a patient's problems. The initial concept triggers ideas (initial hypothesis) from memory by pattern recognition.

Hypothesis Generation

As stated earlier, hypotheses are generated early in a clinical encounter (usually from a set of cues, such as patient's age, sex, race, appearance, and presenting complaints). Given the limited capacity of short-term memory, the number of hypotheses generated commonly is four to seven. Factors important in the generation of hypotheses are disease prevalence, heuristics (rules of thumb, certain principles, maxims, and axioms; see the CD-ROM), and the seriousness of the patient's condition.

Hypothesis Testing and Refinement

After hypotheses are generated, the next step in the diagnostic process is hypothesis-driven questioning and data gathering to test and refine these hypotheses (hypothesis evaluation and refinement). Diagnostic hypotheses form a context or framework for information gathering and hypothesis evaluation. The goals of this step are to identify likely diagnostic hypotheses, to disprove unlikely hypotheses, to differentiate among existing hypotheses, and to find diagnostic hypotheses that satisfactorily explain all available clinical data. Hypothesis refinement is a sequential iterative process of data and information gathering.

As information is gathered, some initial hypotheses are refined, revised, and made more specific; hypotheses are added; and others are dropped. Confirmation (to enhance likely hypothesis), elimination (to reduce an unlikely hypothesis), discrimination (to distinguish between two or more hypotheses), and exploration are some of the strategies used for hypothesis testing.

Differential diagnosis is the process of considering the possible causes of a patient's complaints and clinical findings (and their relative likelihoods) before making a working diagnosis. When considering a patient's differential diagnosis, one could generate a *possibilistic differential* (listing and testing all known causes simultaneously). Experienced physicians use a combination, however, of *probabilistic approach* (considering first the disorders that are more likely), *prognostic approach* (more serious if missed), and *pragmatic approach* (more responsive to treatment). The best explanation for the patient's clinical problem is termed the *leading hypothesis* or *working diagnosis*. *Active alternatives* are diagnoses that may be considered because they are likely, serious, and treatable. *Other hypotheses* are diagnoses that are not likely, serious, or treatable enough to be considered at the initial workup but are not yet excluded. *Excluded hypotheses* are diagnoses that have been rejected.

Hypothesis refinement (which may occur concurrently with hypothesis testing) may involve the use of diagnostic tests to confirm a working diagnosis and exclude the active alternatives. A specific test with a high likelihood ratio (LR) for a positive result may be chosen to confirm the working diagnosis.

Hypothesis Verification (Confirmation)

According to Kassirer and Kopelman, hypothesis verification for coherency, adequacy, and parsimony is the final step in the diagnostic process. One or more hypotheses are accepted as sufficiently valid to permit further action (e.g., observation, testing, therapy). Guidelines for hypothesis verification have been published by the Evidence-Based Medicine Working Group (Box 6-2).

PROBALISTIC MEDICAL REASONING

A 100% certainty in diagnosis is unattainable. According to Kassirer, "Our task is not to attain certainty but to reduce the level of uncertainty enough to make therapeutic decisions." Physicians often describe their belief of the likelihood of a disease by words such as *likely, unlikely, doubtful, consistent with,* or *cannot be excluded.* These words have different interpretations to different individuals, complicating communication among physicians. *Probabilistic medical reasoning* is a useful approach for dealing with uncertainties in many clinical decisions. Probability is a numerical measure of the chance or likelihood of an event. It is measured on a scale from 0 to 1. The probability that an event is certain to occur is 1; the probability that an event is certain not to occur is 0. The probability that a circumcised male infant younger than 2 years of age with fever has a urinary tract infection is between 0.002 and 0.004 or 0.2% and 0.4%.

Odds, an alternative way of expressing probability, are the ratio of the likelihood of an event occurring compared with the likelihood of an event not occurring:

$$\text{Odds} = \frac{P}{1 - P}$$

In this equation, P is the probability that an event will occur. This equation also permits the probability to be calculated if the odds are known:

$$P = \frac{\text{odds}}{1 - \text{odds}}$$

Probability may be objective (frequency based) or subjective (subjective belief of the likelihood of an event). The latter method is used more often in medicine.

Box 6-2. Explicit Tests for Verifying Patient's Diagnosis

Adequacy
- Does this diagnostic hypothesis adequately explain all the patient's clinical findings?
- If not, does the hypothesis explain the patient's important findings?

Coherence
- Does the diagnostic hypothesis fit the pathophysiologic state observed or inferred in this patient?
- Is this hypothesis pathophysiologically coherent?

Primacy
- Does this diagnostic hypothesis provide the best fit to the pattern of the patient's illness?
- Is there a hypothesis that fits the patient's illness better?

Parsimony
- Is this diagnostic hypothesis the simplest explanation of this patient's illness?
- Is there a hypothesis that is simpler?

Robustness
- Is this diagnostic hypothesis robust to attempt to falsify it?
- Has the hypothesis escaped disproof?

Prediction
- Does this diagnostic hypothesis best predict the subsequent course of the patient's illness?
- Is there a hypothesis that predicts the patient's course better?

Adapted from Richardson WS, Wilson MC, Williams JW, et al: Users' guides to the medical literature XXIV: How to use an article on the clinical manifestations of disease. JAMA 2000;284:869–875. Copyright © 2000 American Medical Association. All rights reserved. Reproduced by permission.

Prior Probability or Pretest Probability or Prevalence

During hypothesis testing and refinement, a physician may estimate the probability of a particular disease. The estimated probability, made before diagnostic testing and further information are available, is termed *prior probability* or *pretest probability*. As noted previously, the prior probability or prevalence of urinary tract infection in circumcised male infants is 0.002; the prevalence is 0.2%. Sources of information for estimating pretest probability are (1) personal experience with remembered cases, (2) population prevalence data from the medical literature, (3) published research, (4) practice databases, (5) special attributes or characteristics of the patient, and (6) clinical prediction or decision rules.

Clinical prediction rules, developed from multivariable analysis, are defined by the Evidence-Based Medicine Working Group as "clinical tools that quantify the individual contributions that various components of the history, physical examination, and basic laboratory tests make toward the diagnosis, prognosis, or likely response to treatment in an individual patient." Examples of clinical decision rules include rules developed to identify streptococcal sore throat, urinary tract infection, prognosis of children admitted to pediatric intensive care units (PRISM score), and indications for obtaining radiographs after ankle trauma (Ottawa rules). Guidelines on how to use articles about clinical decision rules have been published by the Evidence-Based Medicine Working Group and Evidence-Based Medicine in Critical Care Group (Box 6-3).

Diagnostic Tests

After estimating pretest (prior) probabilities, the next step in the diagnostic process may be diagnostic testing. Diagnostic tests are used to revise the pretest probabilities of a patient having a particular condition. Testing is necessary if it alters the diagnosis, alters the management, or provides prognostic information. Before a test is ordered, it is important to understand how to measure its accuracy, determine if it is normal or abnormal, and how to interpret the results (see Chapter 7).

LR, derived from prior (pretest) odds, is one of the methods of revising prior probability. The LR expresses the odds that the test result occurs in a patient with a target disorder compared with the odds that the test result occurs in a patient without the target disorder. The LR for a positive test (LR+) is calculated as sensitivity/(1 − specificity), and the LR for a negative test (LR−) is calculated as (1 − sensitivity)/specificity. The LR is a measure of accuracy of a diagnostic test, is less likely to change with prevalence of the disorder (i.e., more robust than sensitivity and specificity), and can be used to calculate the posttest probability.

When the LR has been determined, the posttest probability can be calculated. The Evidence-Based Medicine Working Group has proposed guidelines for the interpretation of LRs (see Table 7-1).

Bayes' Theorem

Derived from conditional probability, Bayes' theorem is a quantitative method for calculating posttest probability using the pretest probability, sensitivity, and specificity of a test. Bayes' theorem is a method used to adjust the prior probability when new information (e.g., a diagnostic test) is available.

Because of complex and awkward calculations involved in Bayes' theorem, the odds-LR form is more convenient and easier to use. The odds-LR form is expressed by the simple relationship between pretest odds and posttest odds:

$$\text{Posttest odds} = \text{pretest odds} \times \text{LR}$$

The posttest probability can be calculated indirectly from the odds ratio form of Bayes' theorem or directly from Fagan's nomogram (see Fig. 7-3).

Threshold Model of Decision Making

When faced with a decision about testing and treating, a physician has three choices—do nothing (i.e., no testing or treatment), order the test and treat on the basis of the result, or treat without testing. The following factors should be considered in deciding whether to order diagnostic tests: (1) the prior (pretest) probability of the disease; (2) the accuracy or performance characteristics, availability, and cost of the test; (3) the seriousness of the disease; (4) the benefits and harms of treatment; and (5) whether the results will change management. The decision-threshold approach, developed by Pauker and Kassirer, is a decision-making model that incorporates these factors (Fig. 6-2).

The *test threshold* is the probability above which one tests and below which one withholds treatment and testing. If the pretest probability of a disease is below the test threshold, no testing is done and no treatment is administered. If the probability is above the test threshold but below the treatment threshold, tests are performed until the posttest probability either rises above the treatment threshold or falls below the test threshold.

The *treatment threshold* is the probability at which the physician is "sure enough" of a diagnosis to begin treatment.

Box 6-3. Using Articles Describing Clinical Prediction Tools

Are the Results Valid?

1. Was a representative group of patients completely followed up?
2. Were all potential predictors included?
3. Did the investigators test the independent contribution of each predictor variable?
4. Were outcomes independent of predictors?

What Are the Results?

1. What is the prediction tool?
2. How well does it categorize patients into different levels of risk?
3. How confident are you in the estimates of risk?

Can You Apply the Prediction Tool in Your Patient Care?

1. Does the tool maintain its prediction power in a new sample of patients?
2. Are your patients similar to the patients used to develop and test the tool?
3. Would the tool improve your clinical decisions?

Adapted from Randolph AG, Guyatt GH, Calvin JE, et al: Understanding articles describing clinical prediction rules. Crit Care Med 1998;26:1603–1612.

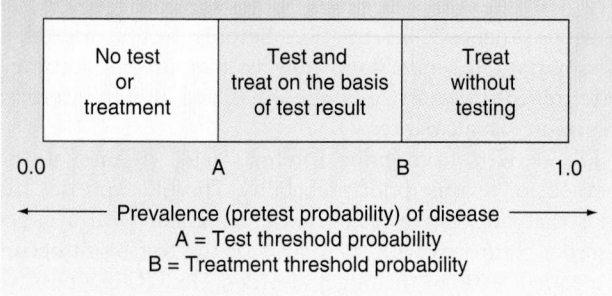

Figure 6-2. Test and treatment thresholds.

Below the treatment threshold, treatment is withheld; above the treatment threshold, treatment is administered. The optimal treatment threshold depends on the harm of treating patients without the disease and the benefits of treating patients with the disease. If the benefit of treatment is small and the harm of treatment is high (e.g., chemotherapy for a rare malignancy), the treatment threshold is high. If the benefit of treatment is high and the harm of treatment is low (e.g., prescribing an antibiotic for a febrile child with sickle cell anemia), the treatment threshold is low.

The *threshold probabilities* may be determined intuitively from the benefit-to-risk ratio or analytically (decision analysis). When harm caused by missing a diagnosis is great, a low test threshold should be chosen before the diagnosis is excluded. When there is harm associated with diagnosis (e.g., possible malignancy), however, a high treatment threshold should be chosen before beginning treatment or accepting the diagnosis.

PUTTING IT ALL TOGETHER

At the end of the diagnostic process, the physician must decide whether to initiate treatment, test, or withhold treatment. Sox recommended the steps in Box 6-4 to assist decision making. The steps are applied to a clinical case (Case Study 6-1) as follows:

1. Determine the treatment-threshold probability of occult bacteremia.
2. Estimate the pretest probability of occult bacteremia.
3. Determine whether a test result (total white blood cell count) could change the decision to treat for occult bacteremia.

First, the physician sets a treatment-threshold probability (e.g., 0.05). If the pretest probability of occult bacteremia is less than 0.05, the physician withholds treatment (i.e., parenteral antibiotic), but he or she treats if the pretest probability is greater than 0.05. A decision to treat when the pretest probability is at the threshold probability means that the physician is willing to treat 19 children without occult bacteremia to be sure of treating 1 child with occult bacteremia.

The pretest probability of occult bacteremia in the post–Hib vaccine era from the medical literature is estimated to be about 0.02 (pretest odds of 0.02). Because the pretest probability is lower than the treatment threshold probability, no diagnostic test (white blood cell count) is

---

Box 6-4. Steps in Decision Making

Step 1

Determine the treatment threshold probability of disease. This may be done intuitively or analytically (decision analysis). Below the threshold, withhold treatment; above the threshold, treat.

Step 2

Determine the pretest probability of disease. If the pretest probability is below the treatment threshold, withhold treatment. If the pretest probability is above the treatment threshold, treat.

Step 3

Determine whether testing would change your decision to treat the patient. A test should be done only if the posttest probability after a positive test is above the treatment threshold.

From Sox HC, Blatt MA, Higgins MC, et al: Medical Decision Making. Boston, Butterworths-Heidemann, 1988, pp 243–244.

---

done unless it could raise the probability of occult bacteremia to greater than 0.05 (treatment threshold).

To determine if testing could affect the decision to treat for occult bacteremia, the physician must decide if the result would increase the probability of bacteremia to greater than 0.05. In Case Study 6-1, the total white blood cell count is 20,900/mm^3 with 60% neutrophils. From a review of the medical literature, the LR for white blood cell count greater than 20,000/mm^3 is 6.0. Using Fagan's nomogram, the posttest probability of bacteremia given a white blood cell count of 20,900/mm^3 is about 0.11. The odds ratio form of Bayes' theorem also can be used to calculate the posttest probability of bacteremia given a white blood cell count of 20,900/mm^3:

$$\text{Posttest odds} = \text{Pretest odds} \times \text{LR}: 0.02 \times 6.0 = 0.12$$
Convert the odds to probability:

$$\text{Probability} = \frac{\text{odds}}{1 + \text{odds}} = \frac{0.12}{1 + 0.12}$$

Because the posttest probability of 0.11 is higher than the treatment threshold (0.05), treatment is the correct decision for this case.

CASE STUDY 6-1

CLINICAL CASE EXAMPLE

A 23-month-old, previously healthy, circumcised male infant has a 2-day history of fever. He has a rectal temperature of 39.0°C (102.2°F). There are no ill contacts; he does not attend day care. His parents are unsure if he is fully immunized. He is non–toxic appearing and has no apparent source for the fever. You are concerned that this infant may have occult bacteremia. You obtain a complete blood count and a blood culture. His total white blood cell count is 20,900/mm^3 with 60% neutrophils. You decide to treat him with an antipyretic and an intramuscular injection of ceftriaxone. Follow-up is arranged for the next day.

THERAPEUTIC DECISION MAKING

As indicated earlier, hypothesis verification is the final step in the diagnostic process, in which one hypothesis (i.e., the working diagnosis) is accepted as sufficiently valid to permit further action (i.e., therapy and prognostication). Working diagnoses are highly likely and parsimonious; they are coherent and explain all the major findings in the patient. Also, they produce valid predictions of the subsequent course of the patient's illness. Considerable diagnostic uncertainty may remain, however, at the end of the diagnostic process. Despite this uncertainty, a prognostic and therapeutic decision must be made.

Therapeutic decisions include initiating therapy (e.g., antibiotic for probable otitis media), referring to a subspecialist, arranging for a consultation, and providing patient education and counseling. Additional therapeutic decisions include transfer to a tertiary children's hospital, transfer to a pediatric intensive care unit, admission or discharge from the hospital, performance of therapeutic procedures (i.e., endoscopy for removal of an esophageal foreign body), and adjustment of medications and determination of drug levels. Although the transition from diagnosis to treatment is automatic in patients with life-threatening diseases, a deliberate, systematic, and thoughtful approach is necessary in other clinical situations. The goal of this approach is to select and tailor the right treatment for the right patient and to maximize the benefits of treatment.

According to the above-described threshold model, the decision to treat is determined by the prior probability of the disease and the calculated thresholds. The test and treatment thresholds are determined by weighing the risks (harm) and benefits (improvement) of treatment and the risks, accuracy, and costs of testing.

Some therapeutic decisions are relatively simple and straightforward, whereas others may be complex and difficult. In some cases, information from the medical literature is incomplete, invalid, or not directly relevant, increasing uncertainty. Decisions must be made, however, despite some degree of uncertainty. Therapeutic decision making is a choice of action to achieve some goals (i.e., improvement of well-being, relief of symptoms). All courses of action involve harms (risk) and benefits (improvement).

Therapeutic decision making involves choosing an action (i.e., therapy) after weighing the risks and benefits of the alternatives. There are two major components of any decision: (1) specifying the alternative actions and (2) determining the possible outcomes of each alternative action. *Decision analysis* is a formal method of making explicit the alternatives being considered and the tradeoff between risks and benefits.

Decision Analysis

Decision analysis, derived from operations research, game theory, economics, and applied mathematics, is the application of probability and utility theory to specific decisions. It is a quantitative approach for assessing the relative value of different decision options. *Decision analysis* is defined as an explicit, quantitative, and systematic approach to decision making during uncertainty. It can be applied to decisions affecting individual patients, groups of patients,

---

Box 6-5. User's Guide for Clinical Decision Analysis

Are the Results Valid?

- Were all important therapeutic alternatives (including no treatment) and outcomes included?
- Are the probabilities of the outcome valid and credible?
- Are the utilities of the outcomes valid and credible?
- Was the robustness of the conclusions tested?

Are the Valid Results Important?

- Did one course of action lead to clinically important gains?
- Was the same course of action preferred despite clinically sensible changes in probabilities and utilities?

Are the Valid Important Results Applicable to My Patients?

- Do the probabilities in this clinical decision analysis apply to my patient?
- Can my patient state his or her utilities in a stable, usable form?

Adapted from Sackett DL, Straus SE, Richardson WS, et al: Evidence-Based Medicine: How to Practice and Teach EBM. Edinburgh, Churchill Livingstone, 2000.

---

and health care policy. It also is the first step in cost-effectiveness analysis.

There are six steps in decision analysis: (1) The problem is defined. (2) The problem is structured, and a decision tree is created. (3) Probabilities are assigned to events at the chance nodes. (4) Values (utilities) are assigned to outcomes. (5) The expected utility of each chance node is calculated, and the alternative with the highest expected utility is chosen. (6) Sensitivity analysis is performed to test the validity and "robustness" of the analysis over a range of possible outcomes. An expanded description of each of these steps can be found on the CD-ROM.

A comprehensive discussion on how to perform decision analysis, influence diagrams, belief networks, Markov process (modeling future events), Monte Carlo simulation, and other decision models is beyond the scope of this discussion. Readers interested in further information about decision analysis and modeling should see the excellent tutorials by Detsky and colleagues and other textbooks. Guides for assessing the validity and applicability of clinical decision analysis have been published by Sackett and colleagues and modified by Gross (Boxes 6-5 and 6-6).

Decision analysis is a formal method of using the best available evidence to answer clinical questions quantitatively. Decision analysis allows the patient's values and preferences to be factored into medical decisions. Because it explicitly integrates the best available evidence, clinical expertise, and patient's values and preferences, decision analysis should be considered complementary to EBM.

EVIDENCE-BASED MEDICINE AND EVIDENCE-BASED DECISION MAKING

EBM is defined by Sackett as "the conscientious, explicit, and judicious use of current best evidence from clinical care research in the management of individual patients." In essence, EBM is the integration of the best research evidence with clinical expertise and patient values (expectations,

Box 6-7. Five Steps in the Practice of Evidence-Based Medicine

1. Formulate a clear clinical question about a problem.
2. Search for the best available evidence with which to answer the questions.
3. Critically appraise the evidence for its validity and applicability.
4. Integrate the evidence with clinical expertise, common sense, and patient values, and apply the results to your practice.
5. Evaluate your performance and the impact of the process on clinical practice.

preferences, concerns) (Fig. 6-3). *Current best evidence* means clinically and patient-centered research (meta-analysis, systematic review, and randomized-controlled trials). Box 6-7 lists the five steps in the practice of EBM.

Formulating a Clinical Question

The first step in the EBM approach is to ask well-built clinical questions that are answerable, searchable, and relevant to patients' problems. A well-built clinical question has four components (PICO [Box 6-8]). When a clinical question has been formulated, the next step is to find answers by searching for the best available evidence (information).

Finding the Evidence

Information seeking is an essential component of the practice of EBM; it is imperative that physicians acquire the skills to search the medical literature. The principles involved in retrieval of evidence are focusing the ques-

tion, constructing the search strategy, and filtering the literature.

Methodologic filters (clinical filters, hedges, evidence-based quality filters) are search strategies designed to retrieve high-quality articles from the medical literature for the purpose of answering patients' questions or making informed clinical decisions. Although effective in locating good evidence, filters do not retrieve all articles on a specific topic.

Filters may be downloaded from several websites. The PubMed version of MEDLINE contains a specific filter option called Clinical Queries. Filters developed at McMaster University in Canada have been published, and evidence-based filters for the OVID version of MEDLINE have been developed.

Sensitivity or recall is the likelihood of retrieving relevant articles. Specificity is the likelihood of excluding irrelevant articles. Searching the literature involves trade-offs between sensitivity (recall) and specificity (precision) of the search.

The goal of a search is to retrieve enough information and to avoid retrieving too much, too little, and insufficient relevance. Readers interested in further information about literature search for current best evidence should see the book by McKinnon entitled *PDQ-Evidence-Based Principles and Practice* and other excellent tutorials available on the World Wide Web.

Sources of Evidence

Sources of evidence include primary research, evidence-based guidelines, systematic reviews, evidence-based textbooks, bibliographic databases, evidence-based (secondary) journals, and Web-based online services (Internet). (See the CD-ROM for examples.)

Figures 6-4 and 6-5 depict a hierarchy of study designs and "synthesized" or preprocessed evidence to guide decision making.

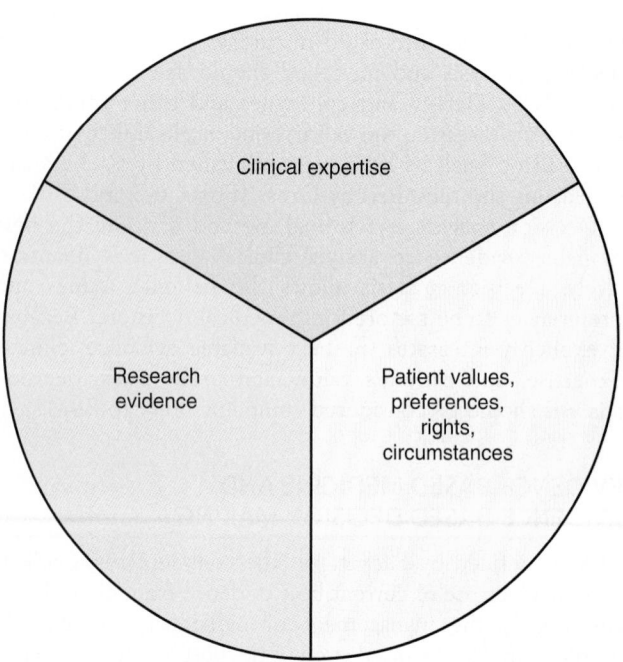

Figure 6-3. Evidence-based medicine.

Box 6-8. Four Components of a Well-Built Clinical Question

1. **P**atient and/or problem
2. **I**ntervention (exposure, diagnostic test, treatment, prognostic factor)
3. **C**omparison intervention (if necessary)
4. **O**utcome(s) of interest

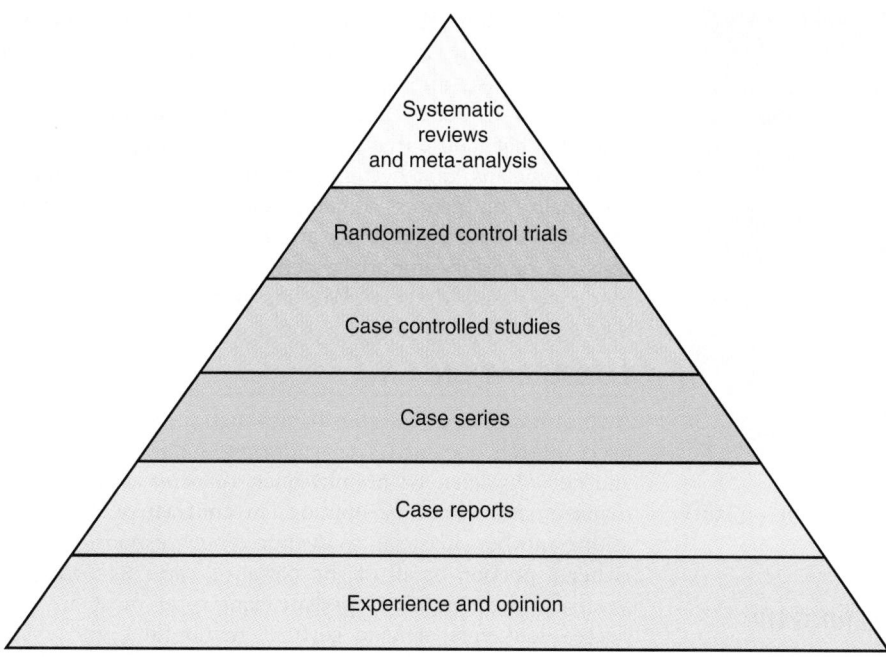

Figure 6-4. Hierarchy of evidence ("evidence pyramid").

Appraising the Evidence Critically

After retrieving the evidence, the next step is to appraise the evidence critically for its validity (strength of evidence), impact (how big is the effect), and applicability. Guidelines and worksheets have been developed to assist physicians in evaluating the validity of evidence about diagnostic tests, therapy, prognosis, clinical decision analysis, and clinical guidelines (see Chapter 7 and Richardson et al. 1999).

Applying the Evidence to Decision Making

When the evidence has been appraised, the next step is to apply it to decision making. This step involves integrating the evidence with clinical expertise and knowledge of patient values. Strategies for incorporating the patient's values

are the "paternalistic" approach (the physician decides what is best for the patient), informed choice approach (physician defers the decision to the patient), and shared decision approach (joint decision). Shared decision making may involve the use of decision aids. A systematic review suggested that decision aids improve patient knowledge, reduce decisional conflict, and stimulate patients to be more active in decision making without increasing their anxiety. Evidence of treatment effectiveness is necessary but not sufficient for management decision making and patient care. Management decision making requires making a value or preference judgment about the tradeoff between risks and benefits of the intervention. In addition to clinical expertise (scientific knowledge and clinical skills), communication skills, compassion, ethical sensitivity, and a

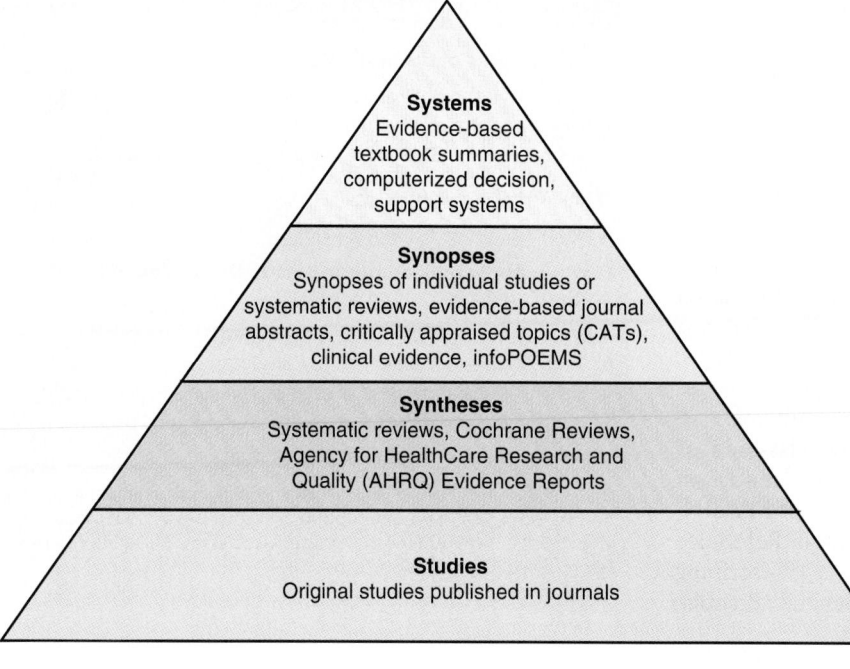

Figure 6-5. Hierarchy of preprocessed evidence. (Redrawn from Haynes RB: Of Studies, syntheses, synopses, and systems: The "4S" evolution of services for finding current best evidence. ACP J Club 2001;134:A11–A13.)

humane attitude are required for delivery of high-quality patient care.

EVIDENCE-BASED MEDICINE AND KEEPING UP WITH MEDICAL LITERATURE

Physicians are challenged to keep up-to-date with the vast medical literature. Keeping up-to-date was referred to by Sackett and colleagues as the "key to continued clinical effectiveness." It involves learning new and old information and filtering out irrelevant and outdated information. Some useful strategies for staying current are listed in Box 6-9.

COMPUTER-ASSISTED DECISION-SUPPORT SYSTEMS

Computer-assisted decision-support systems are computer applications designed to aid clinical diagnostic and therapeutic decision making. The three types of decision-support systems are (1) information-management tools, (2) attention-focusing tools, and (3) tools for providing patient-specific recommendations (management information systems).

Information management tools (health care information systems and information retrieval systems) provide clinical data and general medical knowledge without advice on how to apply the information. Information retrieval systems include electronic textbooks, bibliographic databases, full-text journals, multimedia documents, and digital libraries.

Attention-focusing tools monitor data, flag abnormal results, alert providers about drug interactions, and generate alerts or reminders. Management information systems are "formalized computer information systems that can integrate data from various sources to provide the information necessary for management decision making." The programs may be clinical algorithms, pattern recognition systems, bayesian statistics, symbolic reasoning or "expert systems" based on decision theory, and decision-analytic systems.

Management information systems can be classified as rule-based (model-driven) expert systems or data-driven systems. Rule-based expert systems include MYCIN, ONCOCIN, ILIAD, Internist/Quick Medical Reference (QMR), MEDITEL, Dxplain, PRODIGY (Prescribing Rationally with Decision support in General Practice

study), Problem Knowledge couplers, DiagnosisPro, and PEM-DxP. Only a few of these expert systems have knowledge bases appropriate to pediatric patients, however.

There is evidence from limited trials in some clinical settings that computer-assisted decision-support systems help physicians "do a better job caring for patients," improve the quality of "process of care," and assist clinical decision making. A user's guide to articles describing computer-assisted decision-support systems was published by the Evidence-Based Medicine Working Group (Box 6-10).

CONSULTATION

A consultation is not a referral, although the terms often are used interchangeably. A *consultation* is defined as asking another physician or nonphysician to offer diagnostic or management advice or opinion. In contrast, a *referral* is asking another physician to assume direct responsibility for either a portion or all of the patient's care. According to a survey, the conditions pediatricians refer most are suspected leukemia, suicide gesture, hemophilia, and cystic fibrosis. Orthopedics, dermatology, allergy, cardiology, neurology, and surgery are the six areas of subspecialty referrals most frequently requested by pediatric practitioners. Some of the criteria or reasons for consultation are shown in Box 6-11.

Consultations may be formal or informal. With formal consultations, the consultant reviews records, elicits history, examines the patient, and formally documents recommendations or advice. In contrast, with informal consultations, the consultant may neither review the patient's records nor examine the patient and does not document recommendations. Informal (curbside) consultations are potentially useful when information being sought is not available in textbooks and when verification of information from other sources is desired. They also are useful to clarify specific questions or in emergencies when immediate answers are

From Serwint J, Seidel HM: Communication: the key to effective consultation. Contemp Pediatr 1999;16:138–152.

Box 6-11. Possible Reasons for Consultation

1. Uncertainty in diagnosis, management, and therapy
2. Desire to confirm diagnosis
3. Need for specific "technical skills" required for diagnosis, management, and therapy
4. Desire to reassure patient, family, and physician
5. Need for assistance in long-term follow-up and management of chronic illness

Box 6-13. Consultation Principles

For the Primary Care Physician

- Maintain direct, ongoing communication.
- Ask clear, specific questions.
- Respect all members of the health care team.
- Discourage curbside consultations; they often are based on inadequate information.
- Establish a relationship with consultants.
- Orchestrate care and remain involved with the patient.

For the Consultant

- Be precise and prompt in providing information.
- If circumstances permit, talk to the referring physician first, before talking to the family.
- Provide a detailed report that answers the referring physician's questions.
- Be wary of curbside consultations.

required. Curbside consultations are free, are efficient, may reduce the need for formal consultations, and may offer an additional method for keeping up-to-date. Curbside consultations are not reimbursed, however, and the advice, possibly based on incomplete or inaccurate data, may be erroneous or biased.

The Judicial Council of the American Medical Association has identified nine ethical principles of consultation (Box 6-12). Good communication between the primary care physician, subspecialist, parents, nurses, and other staff is a prerequisite to effective consultation. When asking for a consultation, it is important for the pediatric clinician requesting the consultation to state the question precisely; focus on the needs of the family; be aware of patient's, family's, and his or her own uncertainty; and be responsible for coordinating information and maintaining communication. These and other principles adapted and modified from the "Ten Commandments of Effective Consultation" by Goodman are listed in Box 6-13.

ERRORS IN DECISION MAKING

Several cognitive errors (heuristics and biases) have been described in diagnostic and therapeutic decision making. Heuristics are mental shortcuts or rules of thumb commonly used in decision making; biases are faulty beliefs

Box 6-12. Nine Ethical Principles of Consultation

1. One physician should be in charge of the patient's care.
2. The attending physician has overall responsibility for the patient's care.
3. The consultant should not assume primary care of the patient without consent of the referring patient.
4. The consultation should be done punctually.
5. Discussions during consultations should be with the referring physician and only with the patient by prior consent of the referring physician.
6. Conflicts of opinion should be resolved by a second consultation or withdrawal of the consultant; however, the consultant has the right to give his or her opinion in the presence of the referring physician.
7. Consultations are indicated on "request" in doubtful or difficult cases or when they enhance the quality of medical care.
8. Consultations are primarily for the patient's benefit.
9. A case summary should be sent to the consulting physician, unless a verbal description of the case already has been given.

that affect decision making. As earlier stated, the three heuristics used in decision making are representativeness, availability, and adjustments from an anchor. Although economical and effective, they may lead to systematic errors. Cognitive biases include hindsight, ego, confirmation ("pseudo-diagnosticity," acquiring redundant information), omission, value-induced (anticipated regret), and outcome bias. A comprehensive review of decision biases, cognitive errors, and debiasing techniques is beyond the scope of this chapter. Interested readers should see the Suggested Readings.

PREVENTION OF DECISION-MAKING ERRORS AND IMPROVING CLINICAL DECISION MAKING

Key steps in the prevention or avoidance of cognitive errors are increasing physicians' awareness of possible errors in their thinking; education in formal reasoning, hypothetico-deductive method, scientific logic, probabilistic reasoning, decision theory, and EBM; and acquisition of clinical experience. Clinical decision making may be improved by using computers to support decision making and by identifying, preventing, and correcting decision-making errors.

SUMMARY

Decision making is an integral part of the practice of medicine. Physicians make innumerable decisions (autonomously or jointly with patients) that affect the care of their patients. After obtaining a history and performing a physical examination, the physician must decide on a diagnosis, whether to test, whether to treat or wait, and how to treat. Clinical decisions are characterized by uncertainty. They involve integration of personal experience, pathophysiologic reasoning with evidence from medical literature, and patients' values. Although the analytic method of decision making is logical and rational, it seldom is used. Most decisions are made by an intuitive process of pattern recognition, which is stored in the subconscious; by value judgments; and by applying shortcuts or rules of thumb (heuristics).

⊚ **Additional Resources, CD-ROM**	
Decision theory	Text
Heuristics	Text
Defining the problem: Steps in decision analysis	Text, figure
Examples of Sources of Evidence	Text
Bibliography	

SUGGESTED READINGS

Bergus GR, Cantor SB (eds): Medical decision making. Prim Care 1995;22:167–398.
Chapman GB, Sonnenberg FA (eds): Decision Making in Health Care: Therapy, Psychology, and Applications. New York, Cambridge University Press, 2000.
Detsky AS, Naglie G, Krahn MD, et al: Primer on decision analysis. Med Decis Making 1997;17:123–230.
Gifford DR, Mittman BS, Vickery BG: Diagnostic reasoning in neurology. Neurol Clin 1996;14:223–238.
Hunink M, Glasziou P (eds): Decision Making in Health and Medicine: Integrating Evidence and Values. Cambridge, Cambridge University Press, 2001.
Owens DK, Sox HC: Medical decision making: Probabilistic medical reasoning. In Shortliffe EH, Perreault LE, Wiederhold G, Fagan LM (eds): Medical Informatics, 2nd ed. New York, Springer-Verlag, 2001, pp 76–131.
Richardson WS, Wilson MC, Guyatt GH, et al: Users' guides to the medical literature XV: How to use an article about disease probability for differential diagnosis. JAMA 1999;281:1214–1219.

SECTION 1   FUNDAMENTALS

7 Principles of Clinical Epidemiology

Terry P. Klassen, Lisa Hartling, and Natasha Wiebe

Evidence-based child health care includes solving clinical problems using principles of epidemiology. Epidemiologic principles provide tools to assess the quality of evidence in the medical literature and to determine the risks and benefits of different patient management strategies. *Quality of evidence* refers to the certainty (i.e., reliability) of a study's conclusions and how likely the study is to be free from bias (i.e., validity). Clinical expertise is necessary to interpret the evidence at the level of individual patient care and to apply the evidence in the context of the values and experiences of individual children and their families.

FORMULATING THE QUESTION

The starting point for an evidence-based approach to decision making is to frame a clear, answerable question regarding a clinical dilemma (see Chapter 6). A concise question helps focus the search for evidence, assists in evaluating the relevance of studies, and ultimately yields clearer answers. There are three key components to a well-designed clinical question: (1) patient population, (2) exposure (e.g., to one or more interventions or diagnostic tests), and (3) one or more specific outcomes of interest. An example of a question about a diagnostic test is this: In febrile children with suspected urinary tract infection (*patient population*), what is the accuracy of the urine dipstick (*exposure*) in diagnosing a urinary tract infection (*outcome*)? An example of a question about a treatment

problem is this: Among children with croup (*patient population*), what is the effectiveness of glucocorticoids (*exposure*) for improving their clinical score (*outcome*)?

Having formulated a question, the next step is to identify the domain it falls into (e.g., therapy, diagnosis, prognosis, or etiology/harm). After this step, one can search for the relevant evidence and critically appraise it to determine the degree of benefit and risk related to the available options. This chapter provides an overview of tools to assess the quality of the evidence and presents various measures used to quantify the degree of benefit or risk. These tools are central to the practice of evidence-based child health. The readers are urged to consult the list of references on the CD-ROM for more in-depth reading and for original descriptions of the concepts reviewed in this chapter.

ASSESSING THE EVIDENCE

Validity

The strength of the evidence for clinical decision making depends on the validity of the study's findings. *Validity* refers to whether the results represent the true relationship between the exposure (e.g., glucocorticoids) and the outcome (e.g., croup score). There are two types of validity: Internal validity refers to whether the results represent the truth within the population under study; external validity refers to the generalizability or applicability of the results beyond the study population.

Internal Validity

Internal validity is compromised when there are systematic errors in some facet of the design or conduct of a study (bias) or when a factor other than the exposure under study is causing or distorting the relationship between the exposure and outcome (confounding).

Bias

Systematic errors, or bias, distort the estimate of the association between exposure and outcome, resulting in either an overestimate or an underestimate of the true association. While many different biases have been catalogued, they generally fall into two broad categories—selection and information (observation). *Selection bias* is a distortion in the estimate of the association between exposure and outcome resulting from systematic differences in the groups being compared. In a trial of corticosteroid use among patients with croup, bias could occur if sicker patients were assigned to the placebo arm, and it was assumed that the use of steroids accounted for the difference in outcome between the groups rather than patient selection. *Information, or observation, bias* is a misrepresentation of the association arising from systematic measurement error or misclassification of subjects on factors that are associated with exposure and outcome. Information bias would exist if the interpretation of urine dipsticks in febrile patients was systematically different depending on the patients' clinical presentation; if the physician wanted to start antibiotics because the patient looked sicker, he or she may be more likely to interpret the test as being positive.

Confounding

Confounding exists when the association between the exposure and outcome is explained or distorted by another extraneous factor. The confounding factor is associated independently with the exposure and the outcome and is not found in the causal pathway between exposure and outcome. Confounding can be controlled for in a study either at the design stage (e.g., with randomization) or during the analysis (e.g., through mathematical modeling).

In an observational analysis, pacifier use in infants was associated with early weaning. It is possible that the association is confounded by other differences between the groups who use and do not use pacifiers. Hypothetically speaking, mothers with lower levels of education may be more likely to use pacifiers to calm their infants and may be more likely to wean early (Fig. 7-1). Level of education would be acting as a confounder. When the relationship was evaluated within a randomized controlled trial (RCT), no significant association was found between pacifier use and early weaning. In this instance, other explanatory variables, such as level of education, would have been controlled for by balancing the groups through the randomization process.

External Validity

External validity, or generalizability of the study results, depends on internal validity. If the internal validity is compromised, generalizability beyond the study population should not be attempted. If the results are internally valid, informed judgment is needed to apply research findings to real-life clinical scenarios. This judgment includes com-

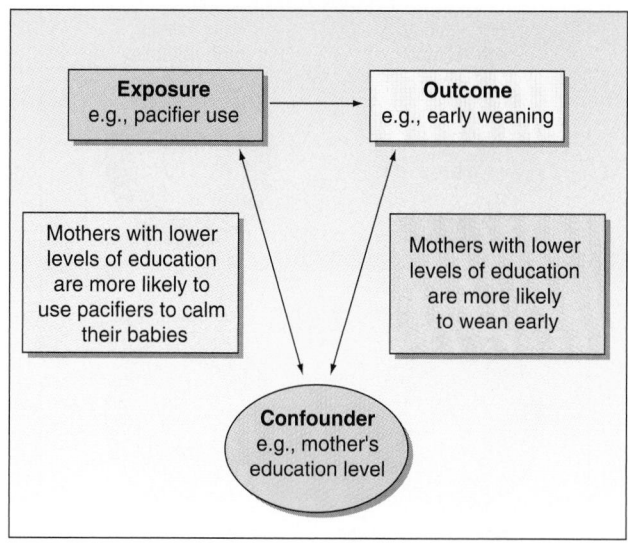

Figure 7-1. Diagrammatic representation of confounding.

paring the study population with an individual's practice in terms of demographic descriptors, severity of the disease, other comorbid conditions, and the treatment setting (e.g., hospital, emergency department, outpatient clinic).

Reliability

Reliability refers to the reproducibility of a measurement. It is compromised by random error in measuring exposures or outcomes. When evaluating the results of a study, reliability is a crucial concept because one wants to be assured that the results are due to the intervention under study and not due to inconsistencies in measuring or assessing the patient's clinical condition.

Intrarater reliability is the extent to which the same observer would measure the same value on the same patient within a time when the patient's condition would remain stable. In a population of stable asthmatic patients, the same observer may use a quality-of-life score on these patients 1 week apart. The intrarater reliability, or the extent to which the same raters' scores are similar, can be measured. *Interrater reliability* refers to the extent to which two or more independent observers measure the same value on the same patient at the same time. In a croup study, the Westley croup score for 17 patients was graded independently by two observers, and then agreement between the observers' scores was measured.

Validity and reliability act independently. For example, results can be valid without being reliable, or they can be reliable without being valid. Figure 7-2 is a diagrammatic representation of validity and reliability.

DIAGNOSIS

A major task of clinical pediatrics is to establish with some degree of certainty whether a given patient has a disease or condition. The patient's status is important to know if there is a treatment available that can improve the patient's condition when it is diagnosed or if a positive test would help predict the patient's future outcome. Evidence regarding the accuracy of a diagnostic test can be found in a valid comparative study involving patients who may have the condition of interest or a meta-analysis of such studies. Case

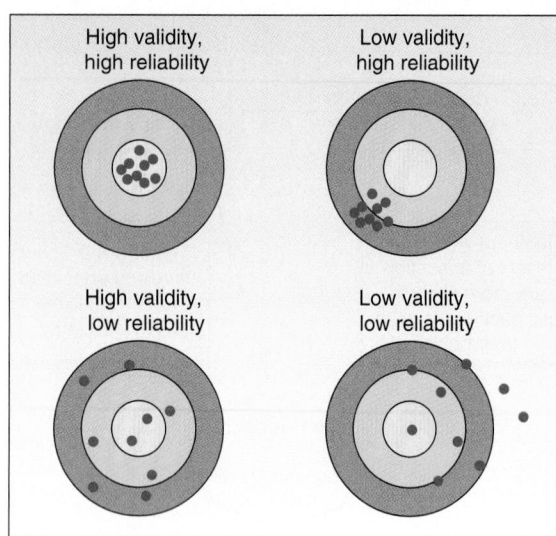

Figure 7-2. Diagrammatic representation of validity and reliability.

Study 7-1A is a hypothetical case that is used to illustrate some of the following concepts.

Sources of Bias

When reviewing the evidence on diagnostic tests, the reader must be alert to potential sources of systematic error that may affect the validity of the results. Although many potential sources of bias exist, the following discussion focuses on the methodologic weaknesses that have been shown, through empirical research, to be associated with exaggerated estimates of the accuracy of diagnostic tests.

Spectrum Bias

Diagnostic tests are used to identify the presence or absence of a condition; this is easiest to do when the distinction is clear, for example, between patients who are severely ill and persons who are healthy. In practice, a diagnostic test is most useful, however, if it can distinguish between the presence and absence of a condition in which the distinction is more ambiguous, for example, among patients who are mildly or moderately ill. The second example is more representative of most clinical situations, in which clinicians encounter patients anywhere along a continuum of disease severity.

It is important that the evaluation of a diagnostic test be done in a context similar to the clinical practice in which the test would be used. Empirical evidence has shown that the accuracy of a diagnostic test can be overestimated by 300% when the test is evaluated among patients known to be

CASE STUDY 7-1A

DIAGNOSTIC TEST

A 2-year-old girl presents to your office with a fever of 40°C and no obvious focus. You obtain a catheter urine sample, and the dipstick shows 3+ for leukocytes. How likely is it that this child has a urinary tract infection? Should you initiate treatment with antibiotics?

affected by the condition and healthy individuals versus a patient sample representing a real clinical scenario.

Differential Verification

To evaluate the accuracy of a diagnostic test, the results of the test under study are compared with the results of a reference, or gold, standard. The results of the reference standard are considered to represent the true diagnosis. The reference standard may be a definitive procedure, such as biopsy or surgery, or it may involve long-term follow-up to track the evolution of the patient's condition over time.

In situations in which the reference standard is highly invasive or costly, researchers may not subject all patients to the procedure. Positive results from the diagnostic test may be verified using the reference standard, whereas negative results are verified with another test that may be less accurate. Differential verification can result in either an overestimate or an underestimate of the accuracy of the test under study; the extent and direction of the bias depends on the relative quality of the tests being used.

Blinding

In the context of an evaluation of a diagnostic test, *blinding*, or masking, refers to keeping the person interpreting test results unaware of the results of the reference standard, or vice versa. Knowledge of the results of one test may influence the interpretation of the other, particularly if the test results are ambiguous or open to subjective assessment. In making a diagnosis of Kawasaki disease, if the clinician knows the patient has a high toxic neutrophil count, he or she may be more likely to detect the positive clinical signs consistent with the disease. Failure to blind test interpreters has been linked to a modest overestimate of the accuracy of a diagnostic test.

Reporting

The quality of reporting may be a marker for methodologic weaknesses in study design. Inadequate descriptions of the test and the study population are associated with an overestimate of the accuracy of a diagnostic test. Conversely an inadequate description of the reference standard is associated with an underestimate of the test's accuracy. When assessing studies of diagnostic tests, readers should be cautious of the findings if there is not a clear, sufficient description of the study population, the test being evaluated, or the reference standard. To date, there are no guidelines for what represents a sufficient description. One guiding principle is that methods should be reported in enough detail so that the reader could replicate the study.

Interpretation of Results

The previously described concepts are applied to the sample case in Case Study 7-1B. The next step of interest is the evaluation of the diagnostic accuracy of a test (i.e., the ability of the test to determine correctly the presence or absence of the condition). This evaluation is done by comparing test results with results obtained using a reference standard. The following discussion describes many measures commonly used to quantify the accuracy of a diagnostic test. The formulas and sample calculations are provided in CD-ROM Box 7-1. The Centre for Evidence-Based Medicine at Mount

Sinai Hospital has developed a web-based evidence-based medicine calculator that can be downloaded to a palm device (http://www.cebm.utoronto.ca/).

Pretest Probability

Pretest probability, or prevalence, is the proportion of individuals in a population with the condition of interest. The pretest probability of a condition can vary across different populations or clinical settings. Pretest probabilities can be ascertained through previous clinical experience, research studies, administrative databases, or surveillance systems. Clinical expertise is required to determine an individual patient's pretest probability of a condition, taking into account such factors as the patient's age, sex, presenting signs and symptoms, and concurrent conditions.

Posttest Probability

The posttest probability of having the target condition after a positive test result (*positive predictive value*) is the number of patients with the condition of interest who have a positive test divided by all patients with a positive test. Conversely, the posttest probability of not having the target condition after a negative test result (*negative predictive value*) is the number of patients without the condition of interest who have a negative test divided by all patients with a negative test. (See Sackett et al. 1991.)

Likelihood Ratios

The likelihood ratio (LR) for having the outcome of interest is a ratio of the likelihood that people with the outcome have positive results to the likelihood that people without the outcome have positive results. The LR for not having the target outcome also can be calculated.

An LR of 1 indicates that the pretest and posttest probabilities are exactly the same. A test with an LR close to 1 is not useful as it provides no additional information. An LR greater than 1 represents an increased probability that the patient has the condition of interest; as the LR increases, the probability that the patient has the condition increases and we are more confident in assigning a positive diagnosis. An LR of less than 1 represents a decreased probability that the patient has the condition of interest; as the LR decreases, the probability that the patient has the condition decreases and we are more confident in ruling out the diagnosis. Guidelines for assessing the magnitude of an LR are presented in Table 7-1. CD-ROM Table 7-2 presents LRs for some common pediatric conditions.

Integration of Pretest Probability, Posttest Probability, and Likelihood Ratios

Posttest probability, or the probability that the patient has the outcome, can be derived in many ways. As shown in CD-ROM Box 7-1, it can be calculated from a 2×2 table. It also can be determined using LRs and the pretest probability. This involves changing the pretest probability to an odds, then calculating the posttest odds of a positive test, and converting the posttest odds back to a probability.

An easier, more practical method is to determine the posttest probability using Fagan's nomogram for interpreting diagnostic test results (Fig. 7-3). Nomograms can be used when test results are positive (using LRs for having the outcome of interest) and negative test results are negative (using LRs for not having the outcome of interest).

LRs are useful when a series of tests is used to reach a diagnosis. Each concurrent test can increase or decrease the probability of ruling in or ruling out the disease. The pretest probability is modified by each preceding test before the ensuing test is performed.

Sensitivity

Some studies present results in terms of sensitivity and specificity. *Sensitivity* is the proportion of people with the condition of interest who are identified as having the condition by the diagnostic test. It is a measure of the probability of correctly identifying an individual with the target condition. A negative result from a highly sensitive test will rule out the condition; thus, the false negative rate will be low.

Table 7-1. Guidelines for Interpreting Likelihood Ratios

Likelihood	Ratios	Interpretation
<0.1	>10	Large, often conclusive changes from pretest to posttest probability
0.1–0.2	5–10	Moderate shifts in pretest to posttest probability
0.5–0.2	2–5	Small (but sometimes important) changes in probability
0.5–1	1–2	Small (and rarely important) changes in probability

From Jaeschke R, Guyatt G, Sackett DL: Users' guides to the medical literature: III. How to use an article about a diagnostic test: B. What are the results and will they help me in caring for my patients? JAMA 1994;271:703-707. Copyright 1994 American Medical Association. All rights reserved. Reproduced by permission.

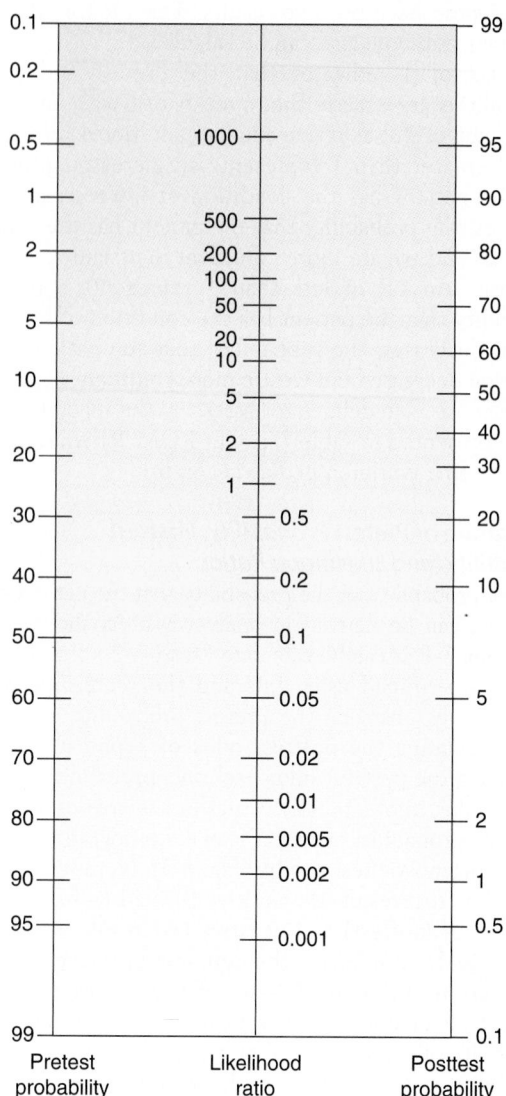

Figure 7-3. Fagan's nomogram for interpreting diagnostic test results. The left-hand column shows a range of pretest probabilities, the middle column shows likelihood ratios, and the right-hand column shows posttest probabilities. The nomogram works as follows: Anchor a straight edge to the pretest probability, shift the straight edge to pass through the appropriate likelihood ratio, and the posttest probability lies where it crosses the posttest probability axis. (Adapted from Fagan TJ: Nomogram for Bayes theorem [Letter]. N Engl J Med 1975;293:257.)

Specificity

Specificity is the proportion of people without the condition of interest who are identified as such by the test. It is a measure of the probability of correctly identifying an individual without the target condition. A positive result from a highly specific test will rule in the condition; thus, the false positive rate will be low.

Receiver-Operating Characteristics Curves

A receiver-operating characteristics (ROC) curve is a plot of sensitivity (true-positive rate) against the complement of specificity (1 – specificity; false-positive rate). Sensitivity and specificity can be calculated using different thresholds for a positive test (e.g., large, moderate, small, trace, or negative dipstick results). Changing the thresholds alters the specificity and sensitivity; either the specificity increases and the sensitivity decreases, or vice versa. Sometimes it is

more important to rule out a diagnosis (e.g., when the costs or risks of treating a patient who does not have the condition are high), and sometimes it is more important to rule in a diagnosis (e.g., when the costs or risks of potentially missing the condition in a patient are high). ROC curves give the clinician the opportunity to compare visually the diagnostic accuracy of different test thresholds.

An ROC curve is created when these sensitivity and specificity complement pairs are joined. The position of the curve gives a sense of how the diagnostic test performs (Fig. 7-4). A curve that comes close to the upper left-hand corner (perfect sensitivity and specificity) represents a better diagnostic test. Poor tests (i.e., tests that provide no additional information) have lines along the diagonal. Most tests are not perfect; there are always some patients with the disease who test negative and some patients without the disease who test positive with similar, middle-of-the-road test results. As a result, there is always some tradeoff between sensitivity and specificity.

We can also use an ROC curve to evaluate the relative accuracy of different tests; this can be done by comparing the area under the curve for each test. The larger the area under the curve (i.e., the closer the curve comes to the upper left-hand corner), the better the test.

In systematic reviews, or meta-analyses, of diagnostic tests, we can use ROC curves to exhibit and compare the results from different studies. The sensitivity and specificity complement pairs from each study are plotted in the ROC space. This plot gives the reader a visual impression of the variability surrounding the sensitivity and specificity complement pairs.

Interrater Reliability

Reliability, as discussed earlier, refers to the reproducibility of test results. Test results often are open to some degree of subjective interpretation. Readers like to know

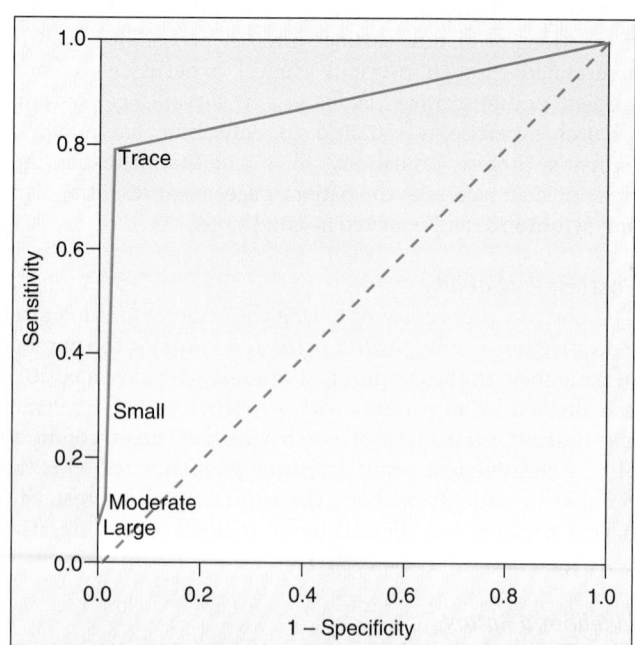

Figure 7-4. Receiver-operating characteristics curve of urine dipstick test for detecting urinary tract infections at different test thresholds (trace, small, moderate, large).

whether similar results would be obtained if the study were repeated. A high-quality diagnostic study assesses the interrater reliability before the actual study is performed. Multiple raters assess the same test results, and agreement between the raters is measured. Measures of agreement also account for the proportion of agreement that arises by chance alone. When writing an examination with true-or-false questions, by chance alone 50% of the questions should be correct. κ statistics and intraclass correlation coefficients are examples of agreement measures.

TREATMENT

Evidence from empirical research is necessary to make informed decisions regarding therapeutic options for patient care. The highest quality evidence about a therapeutic intervention is a systematic review (or meta-analysis) of RCTs or a single RCT. In some cases, there may be no meta-analyses or RCTs on a specific topic. Figure 7-5 presents different types of studies in descending order of design strength. Weaker study designs have more potential for bias, and the results of such studies should be interpreted and applied with caution (Fig. 7-6).

The study evaluating the effectiveness of pacifier use on duration of breast-feeding illustrated the difference in findings between randomized and observational study designs. The researchers conducted an RCT in which the intervention group was asked to avoid using pacifiers to calm their infants. Because mothers in both groups did use pacifiers (although fewer in the intervention group), this allowed the researchers to evaluate the results as if they had done an observational study. In the RCT analysis, the intervention had no effect on decreasing the risk of early weaning, whereas in the observational analysis, pacifier use showed a strong association with early weaning. According to this study, pacifier use is associated with early weaning, but it does not cause early weaning.

Case Study 7-2A is a hypothetical case that is used to illustrate the concepts described in the following sections.

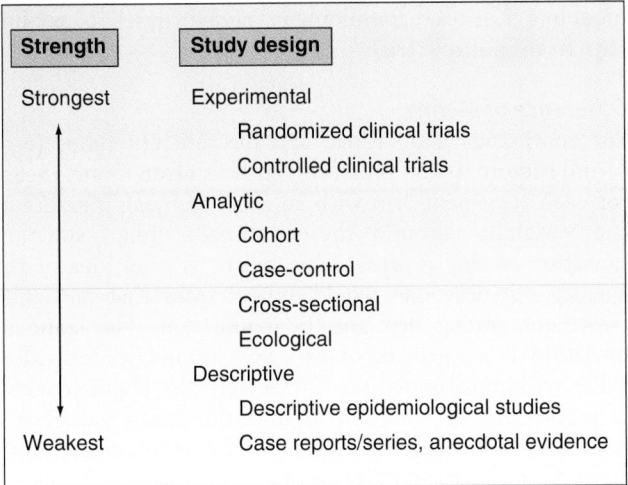

Figure 7-5. Overview of study designs.

Sources of Bias

Although systematic reviews and RCTs represent the best available evidence regarding therapeutic options, they are still open to bias. See the CD-ROM for a discussion that presents methodologic issues of RCTs and systematic reviews that empirical research has found to be associated with bias. Case Study 7-2B and Case Study 7-2C apply these concepts to the case in Case Study 7-2A.

Interpretation of Results

After the aforementioned methodologic issues have been applied to the evidence in the case (Case Study 7-2B and Case Study 7-2C), several factors need to be considered when interpreting and applying the results of a study. The first is the magnitude of the effect, the second is the precision of the estimate, and the third is the clinical (versus the statistical) importance of the findings.

Magnitude of the Effect

In clinical trials, patients most often are followed over a period of time to determine the frequency with which they experience the outcomes of interest. Then comparisons are made with respect to the frequency of the outcomes within each group. The outcomes may be dichotomous (i.e., the event occurred or did not occur), categorical (i.e., classified into two or more categories), ordinal (i.e., graded along a scale), discrete (i.e., integer values, such as blood pressure), or continuous (i.e., possible values range from negative infinity to positive infinity). Numerous measures can be used to summarize these effects, and the measures used depend on the type of outcome. The following discussion presents some of the more common statistical measures reported in the medical literature and used in the practice of evidence-based child health. The formulas and sample calculations are presented in CD-ROM Boxes 7-2 and 7-3.

Risk Difference

The risk difference (absolute risk reduction, attributable risk reduction, or absolute risk difference) is the difference between the proportion of patients with the outcome in the treatment group and the proportion of patients with the outcome in the control group. If a study found that 30% (0.30) of the control group had the outcome, but only 25% (0.25) of patients receiving treatment, the risk difference would be 5% (0.05).

Number Needed to Treat

The number needed to treat is the reciprocal of the risk difference (i.e., 1/risk difference). It provides the number of patients who would need to be treated with the intervention to produce a desired outcome or avoid an undesired outcome in one patient.

Relative Risk

The relative risk (or risk ratio) is the risk of outcome among patients receiving the new treatment, relative to the risk of outcome among controls. This risk is expressed as the proportion of patients with the outcome in the treatment group relative to the proportion of patients with the outcome in the control group.

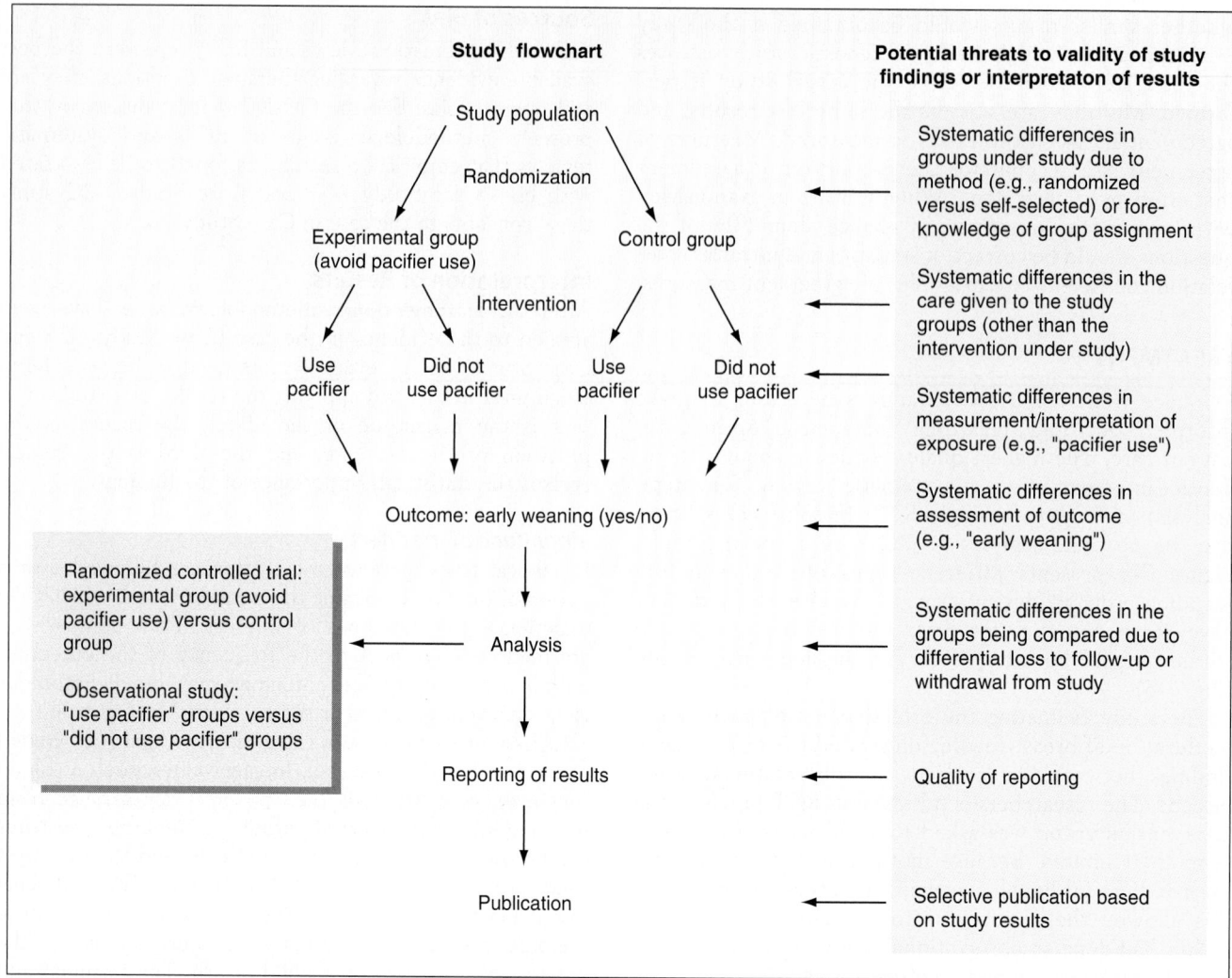

Study flowchart

Study population

Randomization

Experimental group
(avoid pacifier use)   Control group

Intervention

Use
pacifier   Did not
use pacifier   Use
pacifier   Did not
use pacifier

Outcome: early weaning (yes/no)

Randomized controlled trial:
experimental group (avoid
pacifier use) versus control
group

Observational study:
"use pacifier" groups versus
"did not use pacifier" groups

Analysis

Reporting of results

Publication

**Potential threats to validity of study
findings or interpretaton of results**

Systematic differences in
groups under study due to
method (e.g., randomized
versus self-selected) or fore-
knowledge of group assignment

Systematic differences in the
care given to the study
groups (other than the
intervention under study)

Systematic differences in
measurement/interpretation of
exposure (e.g., "pacifier use")

Systematic differences in
assessment of outcome
(e.g., "early weaning")

Systematic differences in the
groups being compared due to
differential loss to follow-up or
withdrawal from study

Quality of reporting

Selective publication based
on study results

Figure 7-6. Study design and sources of bias. (Data from Kramer MS, Barr RG, Dagenais S, et al: Pacifier use, early weaning, and cry/fuss behavior: A randomized controlled trial. JAMA 2001:286:322–326.)

Relative Risk Reduction

The relative risk reduction is the complement of relative risk. It is the difference in the proportion of patients with the outcome in the control and treatment groups (risk difference) divided by the proportion of patients with the outcome in the control group. A 20% relative risk reduction indicates that the risk of outcome was 20% less in the treatment group compared to the control group. A more effective therapy will yield a larger relative risk reduction. Although this measure is used commonly in the medical literature, it can give an exaggerated impression of the degree of benefit.

CASE STUDY 7-2A

TREATMENT

A 2-year-old boy presents to the emergency department with symptoms consistent with croup. You have heard that there is increasing evidence to support the use of glucocorticoids in the treatment of outpatients with croup. You are unsure, however, as to which glucocorticoid to use and whether one glucocorticoid is more effective than another.

Odds Ratio

The odds ratio is the ratio of the odds of the outcome in the treatment group to the odds of the outcome in the control group. The odds ratio can be used as an estimate of the relative risk in retrospective studies and in prospective studies if the outcome is rare. The odds ratio also is used often because it is more suitable for mathematical modeling. It is used commonly in meta-analyses for pooling data from multiple trials.

Difference of Means

For continuous and ordinal and discrete outcomes (e.g., serum sodium, blood pressure), authors often report means for each treatment arm with an accompanying measure of the variability around these estimates (e.g., standard deviation, standard error). The means give an idea of the average outcome one would expect from that particular treatment among that specific population. The standard deviation is a measure of variation around an individual value within a population. Conversely the standard error is a measure of variation around the mean value of a population. The standard deviation of a population is much larger than the standard error of a population. To illustrate, it is much easier to predict the average weight of 2-year-

CASE STUDY 7-2B

EVALUATING THE EVIDENCE (RANDOMIZED CONTROLLED TRIAL)

Through a search of the Cochrane Library's Cochrane Controlled Trials Register (CCTR), you have identified a randomized controlled trial comparing the efficacy of different glucocorticoids for outpatients with croup. (Klassen TP, Craig WR, Moher D, et al: Nebulized budesonide and oral dexamethasone for treatment of croup: A randomized controlled trial. JAMA 1998;279:1629–1632.)

Synopsis

The trial randomly allocated 198 children (ages 3 months to 5 years) to three treatment groups: budesonide, dexamethasone, and budesonide plus dexamethasone. The study found that there was no statistically significant difference between groups in the mean change in croup score from baseline to the final study assessment. The authors concluded that oral dexamethasone is the preferred intervention because of its ease of administration, lower cost, and more widespread availability.

Sources of Bias

Randomization: Patients were randomized to treatment groups using computer-generated random numbers.

Allocation concealment: The randomization list was kept in the central pharmacy until the end of the study.

Double-blinding: The appearance and administration of the trial drugs and the placebos are described in detail. Study personnel, the participants, and their parents were asked to guess which intervention the patient had received. Their guesses as to which drug the patients received were no better than by chance alone, suggesting that the masking was successful.

Withdrawals and losses to follow-up: Only one patient was lost to follow-up. The primary analysis was based on an intention-to-treat principle.

---

olds (measure of variation: standard error), than to predict the weight of any individual 2-year-old, sight unseen (measure of variation: standard deviation).

The difference in means between the groups gives an idea of the relative benefit one treatment would confer over the other. The difference in means often is reported with an accompanying standard error (around the difference in means); this gives an idea of how reliable the estimate is. However, confidence intervals (CIs), which are calculated from the standard errors, are more useful (see the subsequent section on precision of the estimate).

Researchers often go one step further and test for whether there is a difference between the means. Statistical testing is used to quantify the degree to which chance may account for the observed results. A measure that often is reported from tests of statistical significance is the P value, the probability of obtaining such a result if there is no relationship between the exposure and outcome. When evaluating two treatments, the researcher formulates a null hypothesis and an alternative hypothesis. The null hypothesis may be that treatment A is no more effective than treatment B, whereas the alternative hypoth-

esis may be that there is a significant difference in the relative effectiveness of treatments A and B. The authors decide a priori on a threshold P value with which to accept or reject the null hypothesis. The P value is conventionally 0.05, although 0.01 and 0.10 also commonly are used. If the P value is smaller than the prespecified threshold (e.g., 0.05), the researcher can conclude that there is a statistically significant difference between the treatment groups and reject the null hypothesis. If the P value is greater than 0.05, the null hypothesis is not rejected, and the researcher concludes that there is not a statistically significant difference in outcome between the treatment groups. CIs currently are favored in the medical literature because the P value does not take into account the size of the observed effect: A large study with a small difference in treatment effect could have the same P value as a small study that demonstrates a large difference.

Effect Size

Effect sizes also measure the difference between two populations. Effect sizes are used frequently in meta-analyses and in studies in which results are compared across

CASE STUDY 7-2C

EVALUATING THE EVIDENCE (SYSTEMATIC REVIEW)

Through a search of the Cochrane Database of Systematic Reviews (CDSR), you have identified a systematic review examining the effect of glucocorticoids for children with croup. (Ausejo M, Saenz A, Pham B, et al: Glucocorticoids for croup. Cochrane Review. In The Cochrane Library, Issue 1. Oxford, Update Software, 2001.)

Synopsis

A meta-analysis of 24 relevant randomized controlled trials was conducted. It was found that nebulized budesonide or dexamethasone, given either orally or intramuscularly, is effective in treating croup. The authors concluded that an oral dose of dexamethasone would be preferred because of its safety and efficacy.

Sources of Bias

Publication bias: The authors assessed for publication bias using quantitative methods and visually through funnel plots (Fig. 7-7). They identified a marked publication bias and the possibility that small studies with statistically negative results were not published.

Searching for the literature: The methods of searching for the identification of studies are presented in detail. The authors searched the CCTR, MEDLINE, and EMBASE; the search strategy is documented. Primary authors of the published trials were contacted to identify additional studies.

Language bias: Studies written in any language were eligible for inclusion.

Quality of evidence: Quality of the component studies was assessed based on the Jadad scale, allocation concealment, and source of funding. Two investigators independently assessed quality, and interrater agreement was measured by the intraclass correlation. Differences were resolved by consensus.

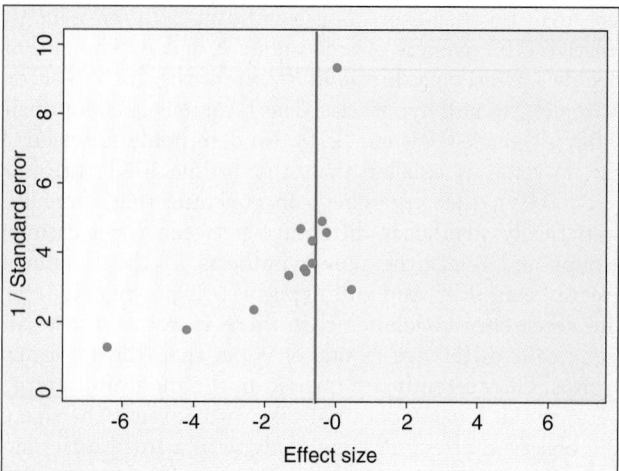

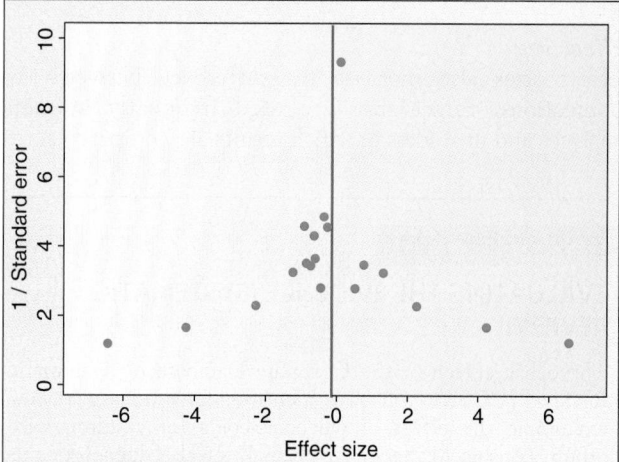

Figure 7-7. Funnel plots. The first plot is taken from a systematic review on glucocorticoids for croup. The plot is asymmetric, which may indicate publication bias. The second plot is a simulated plot adding in missing studies; the plot symmetry now indicates no publication bias. The solid line indicates the true treatment effect; the line moves slightly toward the null in the symmetric (no publication bias) plot. (Adapted from Ausejo M, Saenz A, Pham B, et al: Glucocorticoids for croup. Cochrane Review. In The Cochrane Library, Issue 1. Oxford, Update Software, 2001. This material used by permission of John Wiley & Sons, Inc.)

different scales and populations. An effect size is the difference in means divided by the pooled standard deviation (the standard deviation from the control group also may be used).

Effect sizes are in units of standard deviation. An effect size of 0.5 means the treatments differ by half of a standard deviation. An effect size of 0.2 is considered small; 0.5, moderate; and 0.8, large. How would one compare results from a Westley croup score (a 17-point scale) used in one trial with a 12-point croup score used in another trial? Units of standard deviation supply a common basis for comparison and provide fractional differences of a "natural" range of the outcomes. Effect sizes allow meta-analysts to combine outcomes using different scales.

Precision of the Estimate
The aforementioned measures give single estimates of the association between exposure and outcome, referred to as *point estimates*. Precision refers to the extent of variation

in point estimates that measure the same outcome. CIs often are calculated to assess the precision of a point estimate. These intervals give a certain degree of assurance that the "true" value is contained within. The usual measure is a 95% CI, although other ranges (e.g., 90% or 99% CIs) also are measured. Technically speaking, if a study is repeated many times and 95% CIs are calculated from each, one would expect 95% of these CIs to contain the "true" value. The true estimate is less likely to lie toward the limits of the CI; it will likely lie beyond the CI 5% of the time. This feature of the 95% CI is similar to the concept of $P < 0.05$ level of statistical significance. Generally the larger the CI, the less precise the estimate, whereas the smaller the CI, the more precise the estimate.

The principal factor affecting the precision of the results is sample size. If a therapy was evaluated among 10 randomly chosen patients in a population, the results might not represent the true outcome because of chance. If the therapy was evaluated among 1000 randomly chosen patients, there would be less variability in the estimate, and a more valid conclusion would likely be drawn.

In general, the smaller the sample size, the more variability there will be in the estimate and the less likely the results are to reflect the truth. Conversely the larger the sample, the less variability, and the more precise the estimate. Through a priori sample size calculations, researchers can assess how large a sample they need to find a statistically significant difference if the difference does exist. If a study does not find statistically significant results or if the study has only a fixed number of subjects to work with, researchers can do calculations to determine the study's potential (or power) to detect a statistically significant difference if the difference truly exists. If the power is low (e.g., <80%), it is still possible that a difference might have been detected if the sample size had been larger. Small studies with significant differences also should be suspect because chance plays a part in spuriously strong results.

Statistical versus Clinical Significance
When is a statistically significant difference meaningful? Or, how large a difference between the treatment groups do clinicians need before choosing to treat patients differently? This is called the *minimal clinically important difference* and is chosen based on clinical grounds. Clinical judgment is required to evaluate the results and potential risks and benefits to apply the results to individual patient practice. In the previously cited croup trial, a difference of 1 in the Westley croup score was considered to be a clinically important difference to detect.

CONCLUSION
The principle of evidence-based medicine is to integrate valid evidence, sound clinical judgment, and individual patient circumstances to make appropriate and well-informed decisions regarding patient care. Epidemiologic principles can assist the reader in assessing the validity of studies found in the medical literature and interpreting the results. Table 7-2 presents a glossary of all the terms

Table 7-2. Glossary of Terms*

Term	Definition	Alternate Terms (AT)/Comments
Allocation concealment	Preventing the patients and the investigators in an RCT from knowing to which group the patient will be assigned	Inadequate allocation concealment can lead to an overestimate of the treatment effect if patients with a better prognosis are assigned to the intervention group
Bias	Any systematic error that can distort the estimate of the association between exposure (or treatment) and the outcome of interest	AT: *Systematic error.* Bias can lead to either an overestimate or underestimate of the treatment effect
Blinding	Preventing study participants and personnel from knowing which treatment the patient is receiving	AT: *Masking*
Cochrane Collaboration	International organization aimed at helping people make well-informed decisions about health by preparing, maintaining, and promoting the accessibility of systematic reviews of the effects of health care interventions (http://www.cochrane.org)	
Cochrane Controlled Trials Register (CCTR)	Database of references to RCTs and CCTs in health care	
Cochrane Database of Systematic Reviews (CDSR)	Database of currently available systematic reviews produced by the Cochrane Collaboration	Database is updated quarterly
Cochrane Library (CLIB)	Collection of databases including the CDSR, CCTR, Database of Abstracts of Reviews of Effectiveness (DARE), and Cochrane Review Methodology Database	The Cochrane Library is published on the CD-ROM and is available on the Internet. It is updated quarterly
Confidence interval	Interval estimate of the "true" effect	AT: *Confidence limit*
Confounding	Factor other than the exposure under study is causing or distorting the relationship between exposure and outcome. The confounding factor is independently associated with the exposure and the outcome variables	
Controlled clinical trial (CCT)	Study that compares different treatment groups, but in contrast to an RCT does not randomly allocate the patients to the study groups	All RCTs are CCTs, but not all CCTs are RCTs
Difference of means	Difference in the mean treatment effect between the groups being compared	Difference of means provides an idea of the relative benefit one treatment would confer over the other
Differential verification	Systematic error that arises if the clinician's decision to carry out the reference standard is influenced by the results of the test being studied	Differential verification can result in either an overestimate or an underestimate of the accuracy of a diagnostic test
Double-blind	Study participants and persons assessing patient outcome in an RCT are unaware of which treatment the participants are receiving	Lack of double-blinding can result in an overestimate of treatment effectiveness
Effect size	Difference between two means of a population in a common standard deviation unit	AT: *Standardized mean difference*
External validity	Generalizability of study findings beyond the study population	
Funnel plot	Visual plot of each study's effect size against some measure of its variance (e.g., precision). In the absence of bias, the plot should look like a symmetric inverted funnel	Commonly used to detect publication bias in systematic reviews. Funnel plot asymmetry can result from various other biases and by chance
Heterogeneity	Differences between studies. Differences in the estimated treatment effects, study designs, patient populations, interventions, and outcome measures	Statistical tests for heterogeneity are used to assess whether the observed variability in study results is greater than that expected to occur by chance
Hypothesis testing	Empirically testing a tentative assumption. A researcher proposes, a priori, a null hypothesis (i.e., no difference between treatment groups) and an alternate hypothesis (i.e., there is a difference between treatments, or one treatment is better than another) and quantitatively tests for a difference	
Information bias	Distortion in the estimate of effect arising from measurement error or misclassification of subjects on factors associated with exposure and outcome	AT: *Observation bias.* Information bias can result in an overestimate or underestimate of treatment effectiveness
Intention-to-treat (ITT) protocol	All patients are accounted for at the end of the study, included in the analysis, and analyzed in the groups to which they were initially randomized, regardless of patient compliance or changes in protocol	An ITT protocol can be used to minimize selection bias arising from patient loss to follow-up or withdrawal from the study
Internal validity	Extent to which results represent the truth within the population under study	
Interrater reliability	Extent to which two independent observers measure the same value on the same patient at the same time	
Intrarater reliability	Extent to which the same observer measures the same value on the same patient within a time when the patient's condition would remain stable	
Language bias	Systematic error in results arising from the systematic exclusion of studies reported in languages other than English	

* Many of the definitions contained in this table are taken from the Clarke M, Oxman AD (eds): Cochrane Reviewers' Handbook 4.1 [updated June 2000]. In Review Manager (RevMan) [Computer program]. Version 4.1. Oxford, The Cochrane Collaboration, 2000; available at: www.cochrane.dk/cochrane/handbook/hbookCOCHRANE_REVIEWERS_HANDBOOK_GLOS.htm. Please note that this glossary is currently undergoing revision.

Table 7-2. Glossary of Terms—cont'd

Term	Definition	Alternate Terms (AT)/Comments
Likelihood ratio (LR) for a positive/negative test	Ratio of the likelihood that people with the outcome have positive/negative results to the likelihood that people without the outcome have positive/negative results	
Meta-analysis	Statistical combination of two or more studies to produce a single estimate of the effect of the treatment being evaluated	
Minimal clinically important difference (MCID)	Smallest difference in patient outcome that would result in a change in patient management	
Number needed to treat (NNT)	Number of patients who would need to be treated with the intervention to avoid or eliminate the outcome in one patient	
Odds ratio (OR)	Ratio of the odds of the outcome in the treatment group to the odds of the outcome in the control group	
Posttest probability	Number of patients with the target condition who have a positive (or negative) test divided by all patients with a positive (or negative) test	AT: *Positive predictive value* (posttest probability of having the target condition) or *negative predictive value* (posttest probability of not having the target condition)
Power	Probability of a study to detect a statistically significant difference if the difference truly exists	
Precision	Likelihood of random errors in the results of a study	
Pretest probability	Proportion of individuals in a population with the condition of interest	AT: *Prevalence*
Publication bias	Selective publication of studies based on the nature and direction of the study's findings	Studies are more likely to be published if they have positive results or if the treatment effect is large
P value	Probability of obtaining the observed result if there is no relationship between the exposure and outcome	
Quasirandomized trial	Trial that uses methods of allocating patients to study groups that are not truly random (e.g., alternation, case record number, health care number)	
Randomization	Process of allocating patients to treatment groups in a random fashion	Examples of appropriate methods of randomization include using tables of random numbers or computer-generated lists
Randomized clinical trial (RCT)	Experiment in which eligible patients are randomly allocated to two or more treatment groups	An RCT represents the highest quality of evidence for a therapeutic intervention
Receiver-operating characteristics (ROC) curve	Plot of sensitivity (true-positive rate) against the complement of specificity, 1 − specificity (false-positive rate)	An ROC curve shows the strength of a diagnostic test for a given test threshold
Reference standard	Test that is considered to represent the true state or condition being evaluated	AT: *Gold standard*
Relative risk (RR)	Risk of outcome among patients receiving the new treatment, relative to the risk of outcome among controls	AT: *Risk ratio*
Relative risk reduction (RRR)	Difference in rates of outcome between the control and treatment groups, divided by the rate of outcome in the control group	
Reliability	Reproducibility of a measurement	
Risk difference	Difference between the proportion of patients with the outcome in the treatment group and the proportion of patients with the outcome in the control group	AT: *Absolute risk reduction, attributable risk reduction, absolute risk difference*
Selection bias	Distortion in the estimate of the treatment effect resulting from systematic differences in the groups being compared	Selection bias can result in an underestimate or overestimate of treatment effectiveness
Sensitivity	Proportion of people with the condition of interest who are identified as having the condition by the diagnostic test	
Single-blind	Study participants are unaware of the treatment they are receiving	
Specificity	Proportion of people without the condition of interest who are identified as such by the diagnostic test	
Spectrum bias	Systematic error resulting from the assessment of the accuracy of a diagnostic test among a group of patients that is not representative of patients for whom the test would be used in practice	Spectrum bias can result in an overestimate of the accuracy of a diagnostic test
Systematic review	Review in which there is a comprehensive search for relevant studies on a specific topic, and the studies identified are appraised and synthesized according to predetermined and explicit methods	
Triple-blind	Study participants, persons assessing patient outcome, and the data analysts are unaware of which treatment the participants are receiving	
Validity	Extent to which study results represent the true relationship between exposure and outcome	

and principles discussed in this chapter. Many guidelines are available to assist readers when considering different types of studies (see Suggested Readings and CD-ROM references).

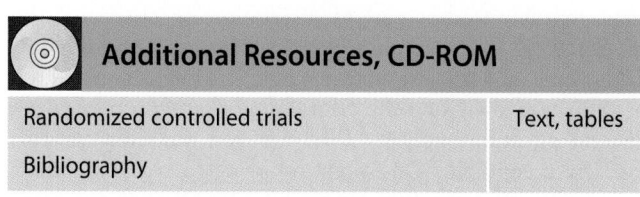

Additional Resources, CD-ROM

Randomized controlled trials	Text, tables
Bibliography	

SUGGESTED READINGS

Egger M, Smith GD, Altman D (eds): Systematic Reviews in Health Care: Meta-analysis in Context, 2nd ed. London, BMJ Books, 2001.

Guyatt G, Rennie D (eds): Evidence-Based Medicine Working Group. Users' Guides to the Medical Literature: A Manual for Evidence-Based Clinical Practice. Chicago, AMA Press, 2002.

Hennekens CH, Buring JE: Epidemiology in Medicine. Boston, Little, Brown and Company, 1987.

Laupacis A, Sackett DL, Roberts RS: An assessment of clinically useful measures of the consequences of treatment. N Engl J Med 1988;318:1728–1733.

Lijmer JG, Mol BW, Heisterkamps, et al: Empirical evidence of design-related bias in studies of diagnostic tests. JAMA 1999; 282(11):1061–1066.

Sackett DL, Haynes RG, Guyatt GH, Tugwell P: Clinical Epidemiology: A Basic Science for Clinical Medicine, 2nd ed. Boston, Little, Brown, 1991.

SECTION 1   FUNDAMENTALS

8 Principles of Office-Based Practice

Peter D. Rappo

"GOOD OLD DAYS" OF PRACTICE

As primary care practice has evolved over the last several decades, the only opinion that seems to be constant is that "things were better before." Returning to the premanaged care (in fact, to the preinsurance) era in pediatric primary care is instructive. The February 1961 issue of *Pediatric Clinics of North America* was entitled "Office Practice and Procedures." The issue was devoted primarily to clinical entities likely to be encountered by the pediatrician in practice. Information regarding billing statements is notable for the lack of any discussion about accounting, accounts receivable, collection practices, and, most important, insurance. The implication of this issue was that billing statements go to, and payment is received from, the parent of the patient. Office-based services frequently were not covered under parental insurance plans, which either excluded children from care or reimbursed only for in-hospital services. Even as fee-for-service models gradually evolved into coverage under indemnity-based insurers, children's services were covered on a sporadic basis. Pediatricians often held their fees at unrealistically low levels because of their knowledge that families were paying for services on an out-of-pocket basis and used higher paying plans to cost shift.

The problem with indemnity insurance was that there were essentially no controls on insurers, hospitals, or providers in terms of charges or expenses incurred. As health insurance increasingly was perceived as a right rather than a privilege, payment for insurance was shifted from employee to employer with minimal or no employee contribution. Indemnity insurers would calculate their loss ratios at the end of the year and then add a 10% to 15% rate increase to the following year's premium. As complaints multiplied about the increasingly chaotic fee-for-service environment, demand for managed care came from payers, whether governmental or private sector. *Managed care* is a system for providing health care services within a defined network of health care providers who are charged with the responsibility of managing the process of access, referral, and hospital services, while providing high-quality care in a cost-effective manner. More appropriately, because hospitals, health care systems, and providers render care, the term should be *managed costs*. A further refinement of this evolving system is capitation, in which a provider entity—whether hospital system, independent practice association, physician group, or individual practitioner—receives a set monthly global payment for managing part or total care of an individual patient. Capitation is a reimbursement mechanism, not a care system. The advantage to the insurer is that set costs for a panel of patients over a 1-year period can be budgeted for on a prospective basis. Intuitively the benefit is less obvious for the physician provider. Understanding historical costs for a panel of patients, understanding tools related to risk assessment and risk adjustment to better calculate appropriate capitation, and assessing adequately stop loss reinsurance needs for individual high-cost cases are skills not usually possessed by pediatric clinicians. The collection and interpretation of data become crucial in this evolving environment, yet most existing information systems are unable to quantify and evaluate these data in an objective way.

The good news is that pediatric health care providers still engender enormous loyalty among their patients, and they are highly desired by health plans as providers. From an actuarial point of view, they tend to attract younger families in the process of having children who traditionally are "preferred risks." Several studies have shown that adults tend to use a health plan that includes their children's provider. The case manager concept is valued by health maintenance organizations, and it is a concept that primary care providers not only are comfortable with, but also have long promoted. Despite their relative desirability as health care providers, the era of "hang out your shingle, and the patients will come" is over. Pediatric health care providers not only need to be caring, compassionate professionals who provide coordinated and comprehensive care for their patients, but they also need to do so in a practice environment that understands the challenges and rigors of medical administration in the 21st century.

PERSONNEL ISSUES IN PRACTICE—"HIRE WELL OR MANAGE HARD"

In an article by Roby on "Office Equipment and Supplies" in the February 1961 issue of *Pediatric Clinics of North America*, the following statement occurs: "Adequate space must be allocated to the receptionist and the bookkeeper in order for them to work efficiently." That is the only statement regarding office personnel in the entire issue on office practice and procedures. Conspicuously absent is a discussion of the role of nursing personnel because procedures such as measurements of height and weight, measurements of blood pressure and pulse, and administration of immunizations and laboratory tests were performed by the pediatrician. Also remarkable is the lack of discussion around issues related to employee policy, job interviewing, workplace administration, and provision of salary and benefits. In an era when the "single-shingle" physician ran his (or her) own office, there was a strong paternalistic aura in which the physician would "take care of his employees."

Times have changed. Although the physician-employer needs to create a positive, fulfilling, and meaningful workplace environment for his or her professional coworkers, more structure and regulatory demands exist that shape how this workplace environment is fashioned.

HIRING OF PERSONNEL

Practices tend to view recruiting, interviewing, and training of employees as an ongoing hassle that is either best avoided or dealt with in a perfunctory manner to fill a real, or perceived, need. In an ideal world, an office should hire the best-qualified applicant for a position, whether it be receptionist, coding and billing expert, nurse, medical assistant, midlevel practitioner, office manager, or new physician. The filling of a position in a hurried or careless manner is a costly mistake because a marginal candidate frequently becomes a marginal employee. Fundamental to the process is a current job description that carefully details the roles and responsibilities of the prospective employee. Screening of applicants' resumés is a crucial step, with careful attention being placed on gaps in an individual's employment history. The physician should be particularly leery of a resumé that lists many job experiences in a short time frame. Although such a resumé may reflect an individual with a broad range of experience, it usually suggests an employee with poor qualifications, wanderlust, interpersonal problems, or a lack of loyalty.

Applicants who pass initial resumé screening should receive a personal interview. Employment law has many safeguards as part of the interview process regarding how interview questions may be asked. The prospective employer needs to be aware that inappropriately asked questions may be used as part of discrimination charges if the interviewee is not subsequently offered employment. Questions such as "Are you married?" "How old are you?" or "Do you own or rent your home?" are prohibited. A general question such as "Why are you qualified for this job?" is acceptable. Questions referring to religion, ethnicity, and family structure are prohibited. Queries regarding difficulties working on weekends may disclose religious preferences, and questions regarding languages spoken and the ethnic groups that a practice sees are acceptable areas for review with a potential employee. Although it is unacceptable to ask if an employee has ever been arrested or convicted of a felony, questions related to the ability of an employee to be bonded ("All of our employees are bonded. Will that be a problem for you?") are acceptable. It is unacceptable to ask an employee about plans to marry or have children, but it is acceptable to ask an interviewee his or her career plans for the next several years. If an employee's job description requires that specific tasks, such as transcription, work with computer programs, or bookkeeping, be performed, skills tests are acceptable. References should be checked, and the reviewer should listen not only to what is said about the candidate from a positive and a negative perspective, but also to what is not said and what the reference refuses to say.

SALARY AND BENEFITS

Salary and benefits for employees in a physician's office are the largest single overhead item on the balance sheet. According to 1999 data from the National Association of Health Care Consultants, pediatric practices on average spend 23% of their revenue on this item and because of the labor-intensive nature of their practice have a full-time equivalent-to-pediatrician ratio of 3.65. Practice managers need to consult with their community colleagues to determine "fair market" salary ranges for all classes of professional employees. Although minimal wage standards are set at the state and federal level, practices in a competitive environment have to exceed or meet community standards for payment. Typical benefits include health insurance, liability insurance, life insurance, short-term disability insurance, pension and profit-sharing plan, and pay for holiday and vacation time. The increased cost of health insurance has caused some practices to move toward increased cost sharing of premiums by employees or to move to a "cafeteria-style" program in which the individual employee can determine which parts of the benefit structure he or she wishes to opt in or out of. Regulatory issues around pension plans can be particularly daunting for small practices, and an external administrator is crucial to ensure a prudent mix of investments for plan members so that a physician trustee would not be charged with an improper plan that did not satisfy his or her fiduciary responsibility to employees. Under the 1996 Health Insurance Portability and Accountability Act (HIPAA), employees changing jobs are able to do so without jeopardizing their health insurance coverage. Federal statutes require that the practice issue a departing employee a certificate notifying him or her of the opportunity to continue insurance coverage. Failure to do so carries a penalty of $100 per employee per non-notified day.

All states require workers' compensation insurance. Employees need to be classified correctly so that their insurance relativity and premium can be evaluated properly. Because compensation premiums can be high, it may be prudent for a practice to self-insure for a higher deductible or extended number of days before the workers' compensation policy is activated. Creating a safe work environment in which the risk of injury is reduced should be a fundamental part of an office's commitment to employees. Workers in the medical environment need to be trained in areas involving prevention of needle-stick injury, blood-borne pathogen standards, proper disposal of medical wastes, understanding of hazardous substance safety, and prevention of potentially infectious transmission of disease.

A wide range of state and federal laws and acts have an impact on the practice workplace. There are jurisdictional triggers for certain of these acts depending on the number of employees in the workplace. Practices that have 50 or more employees, including physicians, are subject to the Family Medical Leave Act; practices with 15 employees are subject to the Americans with Disabilities Act (ADA); and practices with 20 or more employees are subject to the Age Discrimination in Employment Act. Particular emphasis should be placed on issues related to avoidance of sexual harassment in the workplace. The U.S. Supreme Court has held that any employee who experiences a hostile work environment as a result of a supervisor's actions can recover against the employer, even if the employee did not suffer any tangible job consequences. The high court deems training programs and policies around issues of sexual harassment as a major priority.

Personnel records need to be maintained on all employees in a practice. Courts in several jurisdictions have ruled that it is inappropriate to maintain a "separate file" with information about a worker that is sensitive or inflammatory. Because a practice may be exposed to charges around discrimination, and such information can be requested by an attorney after an employee is discharged, personnel records need to be complete and adequately reflect the job experience of the employee in question.

BILLING, CODING, AND REIMBURSEMENT

The movement toward managed care was demanded neither by patients nor caretakers, but by individuals who were historically responsible for payment of health insurance premiums—employers. As health insurance gained traction in the United States, beginning in the 1940s, it was perceived as an entitlement and an obligation as a workplace benefit. The traditional model, indemnity coverage, allowed physicians to set their own fee schedules, without regulatory controls, and allowed insurers to create a usual and customary fee schedule, which would pay a maximum allowable of charges. Because there was no regulation of

inflationary costs under this model, insurers were allowed to levy double-digit premium increases on a yearly basis. This situation, coupled with the escalating costs of health care technology and advances, created a crisis in the 1980s, when health insurance costs were perceived as being out of control. Managed care, or more appropriately, managed cost, was a mechanism to decrease (it was hoped) expenditures, while maintaining quality of care through emphasis on prevention, establishment of best-practice guidelines, and the concept of a primary care physician as a "gatekeeper" to limit inappropriate access to specialty care and facilitate necessary specialty referrals. Although the promise of managed cost was compelling, the results have been mixed at best in terms of performance and success. Most problematic for the primary care community has been the concept of capitation. On a per-member, per-month basis, a gatekeeper physician receives a set budgeted amount for managing all the expenditures of a patient in his or her care. Although the concept of capitation was a sensible approach for a health insurer, because it allowed the health maintenance organization to budget appropriately and shift risk to the provider, it was less compelling in itself for physicians. Physicians not only needed high-quality data to determine their practice's performance against its budget; they also needed to understand concepts of risk assessment, risk adjustment, and stop loss reinsurance to prevent catastrophic losses from the appropriate care of seriously ill patients.

Because most physicians are unable to contract directly with health maintenance organizations as a risk-bearing entity, they frequently join with other colleagues in a variety of "alphabet soup" organizations to receive insurance contracts. Existing models include physician hospital organizations (PHO), independent practice associations (IPA), and preferred provider organizations (PPO). Under these models, the physician bills the contracting health plan for services as a pass-through via the contracting entity. The existing system of describing medical procedures and diagnoses has evolved as medical care has grown increasingly more complex. In 1966, the American Medical Association created the first edition of what then was described as *Current Procedural Terminology (CPT)*. The CPT system has become the standard medical reference for coding and describing medical encounters and procedures with patients. CPT is the first part of the Center for Medicare and Medicaid Services' (CMS) (formally the Health Care Financing Administration) global system, Common Procedure Coding System. Part One, or CPT, uses medical nomenclature to describe physician services. Part Two are so-called national-level codes for nonphysician services, supplies, and medications. Part Three describes local area codes created by regional insurance intermediaries. Part One codes are five-digit numerics, whereas Parts Two and Three are five-digit alphanumerics. The current CPT system, CPT-4, was created in 1977 with yearly updates since then. The most fundamental change regarding CPT occurred in 1991, when Medicare published a national fee schedule based on a Resource-Based Relative Value Scale, which allotted a uniquely calculated value, translatable via a multiplier conversion factor into a uniform fee, eliminating the usual and customary model. Each CPT code has a relative value that consists of three components: physician work (50%), practice costs (45%), and malpractice costs (5%). When these aggregate values are multiplied by a conversion factor (different for medical versus surgical specialties) and by a geographic adjustment, owing to increased costs in urban practice areas, a fee is produced. Beginning with the 1992 version of CPT-4, office visits were described as *evaluation and management visits*. This change in nomenclature was intended to represent fairly the cognitive contribution that traditionally had been underrepresented in prior versions of CPT.

A complete discussion of CPT coding principles is beyond the scope of this chapter. The reader is referred to the American Medical Association's yearly updated publication of *CPT* or the American Academy of Pediatrics' (AAP) text entitled *Coding for Pediatrics*. There are, however, some guiding principles that should be of use to the practitioner. The 10 basic principles of use for CPT and 8 associated rules are listed in Boxes 8-1 and 8-2.

Two other topics deserve special consideration: (1) the care of children with behavioral and mental health diagnoses and (2) the care of children with special health care needs. In 1996, the AAP, in conjunction with a broad representation from the pediatric, mental health, and medical communities, published the *Diagnostic and Statistical Manual for Primary Care, Pediatric Edition (DSM-PC)*. This book was a response to the need for a developmentally based coding manual compatible with the American Psychiatric Association's *Diagnostic and Statistical Manual of Mental Disorders, Fourth Edition*. Although this manual allows the pediatric community to speak in common terms with the mental health community, infrastructure barriers still exist around coding and reimbursement for this subgroup of patients. Health maintenance organizations frequently "carve out" behavioral and mental health services from existing risk pools for medical care and subcapitate all such services to a mental health provider network. Many diagnoses, such as attention-deficit hyperactivity disorder, enuresis, encopresis, autism, depression, and anxiety, are listed in both manuals. The primary care pediatrician who

---

Box 8-2. Helpful Current Procedural Terminology (CPT) Rules

1. A new patient is an individual who has not received services from the physician in the last 3 years.
2. Any patients seen as part of a cross-coverage arrangement are not new patients to the covering physician.
3. Time can be used as a determining factor for coding in the case of counseling or coordination of care services.
4. Although telephone codes exist in the CPT system, they usually are not reimbursed.
5. Traditionally primary care physicians cannot do "consultations" on their own patients unless requested by another physician, and a report is generated to the requesting physician. This is important because the Relative Value Units for consultations are usually twice that for comparable office visits.
6. Physicians should make careful use of the existing codes for well-child and adolescent care when performing preventive services.
7. There needs to be linkage between CPT and International Classification of Diseases (ICD)–9 diagnoses, and the support for medical necessity of services should be apparent from the use of the codes (e.g., performing a throat culture [procedural code] for a patient with a diagnosis of otitis media is a demonstration of nonlinkage and inappropriate billing).
8. Use surgical procedural codes when performing services such as laceration repair, wart removals, or reduction of a subluxed radial head because such utilization not only describes the service performed better, but also has a higher relative value.

---

cares for these patients on an ongoing basis must be willing to advocate for their needs individually and through professional advocacy organizations to ensure that patients receive appropriate care in the most appropriate setting and that providers receive appropriate reimbursement for the services rendered.

Children with special health care needs represent 10% to 30% of the U.S. child population. Three million children have illnesses of sufficient severity and chronicity that their activities of daily living are altered. Because the care of these children requires increased time, knowledge, and dedication, it is incumbent that the pediatric health care provider understand the universe of coding opportunities to appropriately capture the added effort necessary to care for this special patient population. Capitation or carve-out methodologies for this patient group should be accepted only if the care provider has an adequate data system to track utilization and expenditures on an ongoing basis.

Although children with special health care needs present unique reimbursement and office-based service challenges, the care of these children should be an integral part of the role and duty of the well-trained pediatric primary care provider. Their care serves as an opportunity for pediatric providers to distinguish themselves as individuals who are capable of caring for the needs of all children regardless of their disabilities and adopting the principles of the Medical Home as espoused by the AAP. The Medical Home is not a physical structure but is the commitment of providing health care services to all children in a high-quality and cost-effective manner. Physicians, in concert with other care providers and parents, act to identify and facilitate access for medically necessary services for their patients. The AAP posits that all children should have a medical home environment that is accessible, family-centered, continuous, com-

---

Box 8-1. Ten Basic Principles of Use for Current Procedural Terminology (CPT)

1. Select the appropriate CPT code and the diagnosis (International Classification of Diseases [ICD]) code for each patient encounter.
2. Document patient services to support the selected codes.
3. Use separate codes for separate encounters, acknowledging that approximately 20 to 30 CPT codes account for 90% of pediatric visits.
4. Create a separate fee for each code, based on some iteration of work value.
5. Use a modifier code to explain the change when altering fees or standard procedure.
6. Fees should reflect the work performed, not the reimbursement received.
7. Understand local variations and expectations for coding.
8. Inquire about change in reimbursement for a given code.
9. Review codes and fees on at least a yearly basis.
10. Use a superbill as a routing tool to assist staff in knowing what codes to use.

prehensive, coordinated, compassionate, and culturally competent. The AAP also supplies practitioners with many resources, including a Medical Home checklist for assessing health plans to determine the adequacy of coverage for children with special health care needs. This and other similar resources can be accessed at www.aap. org/advocacy/medhome/resourcesmedhomechecklist.htm.

REGULATORY AND COMPLIANCE ISSUES AFFECTING THE OFFICE-BASED PRACTICE

The term *compliance* is defined as the act of yielding or acquiescing to a demand or proposal. In medical practice parlance, compliance is the generic term that refers to the voluntary, but necessary process of satisfying many governmental or health plan–related programs that have a direct impact on patient care. Some programs, such as the ADA, apply across the entire social and workplace arena, whereas others, such as the Clinical Laboratory Improvement Amendments (CLIA), are focused primarily on the medical office. Although a comprehensive review of the full range of compliance programs is beyond the scope of this chapter, entities that have the greatest potential impact on pediatric health care providers are reviewed and are listed in Box 8-3.

The ADA stresses that individuals with disabilities should have equal opportunity to the benefits and programs offered to nondisabled individuals. The Act's provisions apply to all employers with 15 or more employees, inclusive of physicians. Discrimination is forbidden through the hiring process, the nonprovision of reasonable accommodations to the employee, and the denial of opportunity for advancement. Reasonable accommodations include making existing facilities accessible to the handicapped and allowing job restructuring or modification of work schedules to assist the disabled. Although hearing-impaired individuals (employees and patients) are entitled to telecommunication or translator assistance as result of their disability, there is no requirement for translator services for non–English-speaking patients as part of the ADA.

The Emergency Medical Treatment and Active Labor Act (EMTALA) originally was promulgated to prohibit hospitals and providers from refusing care to patients because of lack of insurance or inability to pay. It requires a medical facility to perform a screening examination on a patient arriving at the facility to determine whether or not a medical emergency exists. Even if an emergency does not exist, the lack of such a screening examination and referral to a primary care pediatric clinician's office for care would constitute a violation of the EMTALA statutes. The other piece of the statute that is relevant to pediatricians involves

transfer of acutely ill patients to a tertiary care facility. The referring hospital must receive authorization from the tertiary institution to initiate the transfer, and if the emergency department physician deems the assistance of a local pediatrician is necessary to stabilize the child before transfer, the pediatrician's presence is required.

The CLIA of the CMS is a series of regulations of laboratory investigations in medical practice. It defines levels of licensure for physician's offices involving testing procedures as follows: (1) waived: so simple that they do not require regulation, (2) essentially waived: involving microscopy as part of the physician's usual practice, (3) moderately complex: involving more sophisticated testing that requires the performance of standards and controls, and (4) highly complex: usually done in a hospital or reference laboratory setting. High accreditation costs and the reality of declining physician reimbursement for laboratory procedures have curtailed the use of the in-office laboratory.

The Needlestick Safety and Prevention Act (Public Law 106–430) is an expansion of the Exposure to Bloodborne Pathogen Standard (29 CFR 1910.1030) first promulgated in December 1991. The original standard requires a thorough understanding of potential for transmission of infection, the production of an exposure control plan, the implementation of engineering and work practice controls with the provision of personal protective equipment, the provision of hepatitis B vaccination at no charge to employees, and postexposure follow-up of vaccinated employees. The statute also requires that employees be retrained on an annual basis regarding the statute and that new hires are trained on entering a practice. The newer legislation around needle-stick prevention will require a plan for preventing needle-stick injuries, a log to document injuries when they occur, a plan for adequately treating and monitoring employees when the injury occurs, and a process to allow nonmanagerial employees to be involved in the process of testing and selecting safety sharps designed to reduce workplace accidents.

Because the U.S. government is a major payer for health care services under its obligations to the Medicare, Medicaid, and Civilian Health and Medical Program of Uniformed Services military care system, there is increasing concern regarding inappropriate payment, system waste, and outright fraud and abuse. It is incumbent on the physician community not only to understand how to bill and code appropriately, but also to have an office compliance plan regarding procedures for dealing with even the appearance of impropriety. All compliance plans for the pediatric office should include the elements listed in Box 8-4.

Resources available about compliance issues include the Office of the Inspector General's website at www.dhhs.gov/oig and www.osha.org. Although compliance programs are potentially costly and burdensome, their implications for improving patient outcomes and the success of a pediatric practice should not be minimized or ignored.

ADMINISTRATIVE DATA COLLECTION

Management of Pediatric Practice, Second Edition, was published by the AAP in 1991 as a tool to assist the pediatric practitioner in coping with the demands of administrating a

---

Box 8-3. Important Compliance and Regulatory Issues

1. Americans with Disabilities Act (ADA)
2. Emergency Medical Treatment and Active Labor Act (EMTALA)
3. Clinical Laboratory Improvement Act (CLIA)
4. Needlestick Safety and Prevention Act (Public Law 106-430)
5. False Claims Act of 1860
6. Health Insurance Probability and Accountability Act (HIPAA)

Box 8-4. Key Elements of Office Compliance Plans

1. Written standards of conduct defining fraud and abuse, coding, and appropriate relationships with other vendors or entities should be established.
2. A chief compliance officer should be appointed who is empowered to investigate and act on charges of improper conduct.
3. Regular training programs regarding compliance should be conducted for all employees.
4. A system should be in place whereby the compliance officer can receive complaints while guaranteeing anonymity to the complainant.
5. The compliance officer should be able to respond effectively to complaints and to discipline employees who violate the guidelines.
6. Audits should be used to monitor adherence to the plan.
7. Systemic issues should be identified that would interfere with continued implementation with the plan.

Box 8-6. Office Procedures for Health Insurance Portability and Accountability Act (HIPAA) Compliance

1. Designate a privacy officer (practice manager, physician, coder) who is responsible for developing and implementing an information security policy.
2. Develop policies that define how a practice safeguards the safety, security, integrity, confidentiality, and transmission of information as written, electronic, or verbal information.
3. Educate staff regarding the practice's expectations around safeguarding patient data.
4. Develop and enforce sanctions for individuals who violate a practice's policy around information handling.
5. Insure that other "business partners" with whom the practice deals are committed to a similar philosophy when handling patient information.
6. Develop a policy statement that reminds patients of their rights and responsibilities in the handling of their clinical information.
7. Establish best-practice benchmarks to reward and encourage staff around ongoing implementation and continuation of appropriate data management.

private practice. Under the section on choosing a computer system is a discussion of issues regarding data security as envisioned in the early 1990s. Lacking from this review is any discussion of data transmission and security when clinical and administrative information leaves a practice. Clinicians tend to view clinical information as being unique to each patient, and they are committed to safeguarding each patient's individual privacy and confidentiality. The number of individuals in a physician's office who have access to patient data, coupled with the potential for misdirection of such data to outside agencies, both appropriately and inappropriately, has raised increasing concerns regarding patients' needs for safeguarding confidential information. The HIPAA was passed by Congress in 1996 in an effort to remedy some of the perceived challenges regarding the handling of patient information. The four major privacy areas covered by the HIPAA are listed in Box 8-5.

Physicians had to be aware of and comply with the HIPAA as of April 15, 2003. It is the law (Public Law 104–91), and compliance is required. There are civil and financial penalties for noncompliance, and disclosures regard-

ing the inappropriate transmission of medical data in a public forum would have enormous negative impact for a practice.

To implement the HIPAA, the initial actions relate less to software or vendor solutions and more to practice administrative actions. Box 8-6 lists practice activities to facilitate complying with the HIPAA. Available resources about HIPAA implementation include state medical societies and state and national professional organizations (AAP and American Academy of Family Practitioners). Virtual resources include the main HIPAA page of the CMS website, which provides information about requirements imposed on practice groups, at www.cms.hhs.gov/hipaa/hipaa2/default.asp, or the Department of Health and Human Services website on HIPAA administrative simplification at www.hhs.gov/ocr/hipaa/.

COMPUTER HARDWARE, SOFTWARE, AND APPLICATION SERVICE PROVIDERS

Because of the ever-expanding need for data and its analysis, physicians in practice with inadequate administrative information will be severely hindered in their financial decision making and will likely be unable to survive in an ever-evolving practice environment. One cannot manage that which one cannot measure. Physicians need to deploy computer-based systems increasingly in their offices for clinical and administrative functions. Although changing technologies make it difficult—in fact impossible—to recommend one system over another, the practitioner should be guided by the following precepts. When choosing office-based hardware (i.e., the computer system), it is reasonable to ask the questions listed in Box 8-7 before purchase. Whatever system a practice chooses, there are three issues that are fundamental to a system's success: reliability, speed, and future expandability.

Although many computer users view the purchase of hardware as their most significant decision, the decision about which software system to deploy has greater and more far-reaching implications for the practice. Clinical and practice management systems often are designed for the

Box 8-5. Four Major Privacy Areas Covered by Health Insurance Portability and Accountability Act (HIPAA)

1. *Security and privacy:* HIPAA mandates that there be safeguards for patients regarding the disclosure of personal health information. Privacy legislation demands that there be appropriate levels of security and audit opportunity when data have been transmitted.
2. *Transactions:* HIPAA mandates that all electronic health care transactions, including but not limited to submission of claims, status of claims, enrollment status in a health plan, referral to another health care provider, eligibility status, and payment status, have specific standards used as part of claims processing.
3. *Identifiers:* HIPAA mandates that there be standard identifiers for patients, health plans, employers, and health care providers.
4. *Coding:* HIPAA mandates that there be standard coding for procedures (likely Current Procedural Terminology [CPT], as opposed to area-only codes), and International Classification of Diseases (ICD)–10 (under development), instead of ICD-9 for diagnosis coding.

1. How reliable is the manufacturer of the system?
2. Should I choose a brand name product, or should I choose a "PC clone"?
3. What is the support system for the product I am considering?
4. What are the cost of the system and the cost of support?
5. Is this hardware system adequate to meet my practice's professional needs?
6. Is the system expandable to meet my practice's growth, or will it be outdated within a few years?
7. Is this hardware system designed for the "industrial strength use" that is represented by a pediatric office?
8. Can multiple users interact with the system without slowing it down?
9. What is the storage capability and capacity of the system?
10. Do memory-intensive jobs, such as running billing statements, significantly slow down the system?

Box 8-9. Information and Configuration Vital for a Successful Electronic Medical Record System

1. *Data representation:* (a) growth data showing graphic display of growth patterns; (b) patient identifier to deal with name changes; (c) identification of pediatric-specific terminology; (d) age-based normal ranges for vital signs
2. *Data processing:* (a) prescription tools that allow for the appropriate calculation of doses of pediatric medications; (b) vaccine tracking; (c) reporting capability for forms to match existing formats (i.e., school forms)
3. *System design:* (a) privacy issues, including adolescent confidentiality, guardianship, and genetic information; (b) data entry tools that work efficiently in busy pediatric offices; (c) linkage to existing registry systems to improve pediatric communication

entire medical universe and have pediatric-specific components "stuck on" in an attempt to make them appear "pediatric friendly." Fundamental questions that need to be asked regarding software purchase are listed in Box 8-8.

The AAP issued a new policy statement on "Special Requirements for Electronic Medical Record Systems in Pediatrics" in August 2001. This document discusses requirements that software vendors should consider when developing information systems for pediatric patients. In the opinion of the Committee on Medical Informatics, the information and configuration listed in Box 8-9 was thought to be not only significant, but also vital for a successful electronic medical record system.

Box 8-8. Key Questions to Ask before Buying Computer Software

1. Does the software package understand primary care medicine in general and pediatrics in particular?
2. Does the software address the needs of my practice?
3. Does the software have a scheduling module for patient visits that differentiates between well and sick office visits and time differentials for acute and long-term care?
4. Can immunizations be tracked by the system?
5. Can reminders to patients regarding upcoming appointments be tracked by the system?
6. Does the billing software reduce the likelihood of errors, adequately track pending payments and receivables, and increase the frequency of clean claims via a rules engine or interface with an insurer?
7. Can the system generate detailed practice management reports that would allow me to gauge how my practice is performing in an increasingly cost-sensitive environment?
8. Can the software calculate capitated versus fee-for-service profiles to determine the profitability of a plan and the desirability of continuing as a provider for a health plan as a measure of return and investment?
9. Can the software generate lists of patients by diagnosis to determine need for recurrent services (e.g., influenza vaccination)?
10. What are the mechanism and cost for updates of the software system?

The latest innovation in software management is the introduction of *application service providers (ASPs)*. In this model, the software application for a practice is provided via an Internet connection on a subscription basis by a software vendor. The advantages relate to ease of use by a practice, lower start-up costs than simply buying a software package, reduced support needs because the updates are handled virtually by the software vendor, and the assumption of responsibility for security maintenance and upgrades and correction of flawed data being assumed by the vendor. The ability for a practice to customize the features that they desire through this application is an advantage. As with every opportunity, however, there are many potential disadvantages to be considered. Because data are not stored by a practice's server and are not under direct control, is the information regarding a patient's medical situation secure? Would the ASP attempt to share the aggregate or individual data with other vendors or interested third parties (e.g., health care systems, pharmaceutical companies)? Who owns the data? If the clinician terminates the relationship with the ASP and moves to another vendor, might the clinician be barred from receiving or using his or her own patients' information?

The well-informed clinician requires more than a sound basis and grounding in the art and science of medicine to succeed in the information age. The clinician should use all available resources from colleagues, professional societies, and independent consultants when making decisions regarding the deployment of office information systems for a practice.

PEDIATRIC CARE OFFICE OF THE FUTURE

Office-based pediatric care is facing many administrative, compliance, and clinical challenges. The era of hanging a shingle announcing the existence of one's practice in a community, financial institutions waiting in line to offer loans to the fledgling practitioner, and instant patient acceptance is over. The emphasis on preventive services and treatment of acute illness, although important and fiscally profitable, has underestimated the needs of children with special health care needs and chronic illness. Because these patient populations are difficult to care for, require greater clinical expertise on the part of the practitioner, and have not been reimbursed adequately by the existing health care system, it is vital that the health care system of the future be structured to ensure that all children, regardless of their disability, be provided with a medical home in their community. Evolving technology should facilitate the care and administrative portion of practice for the entire patient community.

What will a pediatric care office encounter look like in the foreseeable future? Just as surgeons have time parameters that involve activity at the previsit, visit, and postvisit levels for each surgical procedure, a similar process is useful to envision the process for a patient when seeking health care from a provider. At the previsit, it is likely that a patient appointment will be booked either using advanced telephony or via secure Internet messaging to the provider's office and with confirmation via a similar secure link. A reminder regarding the date of the visit will be similarly generated, and necessary preparatory forms will be forwarded to the patient. Anticipatory guidance questionnaires will be available to the patient for completion and submitted to the pediatric health care provider for review before the child's well-child visit. Issues around insurance enrollment and eligibility will be checked before the patient's arrival at the office, eliminating the inevitable bottleneck at the check-in window.

At the time of the visit itself, appropriate patient materials can be generated in anticipation of the perceived reason for the encounter. Clinicians will be able to refer the patient to their individual website to access office policies, procedures, administrative information, and clinical information. Messaging tools such as electronic communication, request for prescription refills, referrals, data forms for school and camp examinations, and immunization data as part of the practice's vaccine data tracking system also will be available. Data entry will be facilitated by bar coding technology and practice documentation templates that reflect a provider's personal practice habits and customary activities. Although some practitioners will converse with patients while entering clinical information into the practice's electronic medical system, most providers will enter data using a combination personal digital assistant/telephone device that will allow for data entered with a stylus, via bar coding, or with the use of dictation linked to a workstation via a local area network. The physician also will enter adminis-

trative data, such as CPT and ICD-10 codes, at the point of care and at the close of the patient encounter. These data will be received by the office information system before the patient checks out of the office, the information will be evaluated by the practice's eligibility claims system, the clean claim will be submitted with appropriate HIPAA encryption to the patient's insurance provider, and the transaction will result in a payment to the physician's practice checking account by the next business day.

The administrative data collected by such a system will engender reports that will allow the practitioner to analyze effectively the cost-effectiveness and appropriateness of participation in individual health care plans. After the visit, data in the system will be used to forward more information to patients regarding their diagnoses and updates around their treatment of conditions as new information becomes available. Providers will receive information at the point of care using their handheld devices and will use a variety of benchmarking tools, drug interaction information, and formulary information to improve the quality of care.

Although traditional practice marketing has involved word of mouth from satisfied patients and banner ads in telephone books, these traditional methods are unlikely to be adequate in the future for increasingly competitive practice environments. The use of a practice's individual website as its connection to the external environment will serve many functions, of which outreach and marketing is one.

No practice system, set of rules, or consultant's advice will correct a practice that is disorganized, disinterested, or slothful. The practitioners' role is to do what they traditionally have done well in the past—to be caring, compassionate, competent, and concerned caretakers for children. The office environment and administrative systems are present to ensure the completion and the comprehensiveness of such a care environment.

SUGGESTED READINGS

American Academy of Pediatrics: The Diagnostic and Statistical Manual for Primary Care (DSM-PC) Child and Adolescent Version. Elk Grove Village, Ill, American Academy of Pediatrics, 1996.

American Academy of Pediatrics: Special requirements for electronic medical record systems in pediatrics. Pediatrics 2001;108:513–515.

HIPAA regulations. Available at: www.hhs.gov/ocr/hipaa/.

Medical Home. Available at: www.aap.org/advocacy/medhome/resourcesmedhomechecklist.htm.

9 Principles of Human Genetics

Michael J. Bamshad

CORE PRINCIPLES

Biologists of the 19th century defined the study of heredity (i.e., *genetics*) as the science of variation and its causes, including the mechanisms by which traits are transferred from one generation to the next. In the 21st century, this remains as apt a definition of genetics as ever, although the scope of genetics has broadened substantially. Today, *human genetics* is the branch of science focused on the study of human variation, whereas *medical genetics* is the science of disease-causing variation. *Clinical genetics* is the branch of medicine that pertains to the care of individuals and families with medical conditions that result from disease-causing variation. Clinical genetics includes the study of inheritance of diseases in families, the identification of genes causing disease, the analysis of the mechanisms by which genes cause disease, clinical diagnosis of genetic conditions, genetic testing, and gene therapy. Consequently, medical genetics remains closely allied with laboratory-based research. Medical genetics also includes *genetic counseling*, which involves communicating information about diagnoses, occurrence/recurrence risks, and psychosocial issues to patients and their families.

Many facets of medical genetics (e.g., cancer genetics, biochemical genetics) are covered in other chapters of this book. Nevertheless, the conceptual basis of human genetics is broadly applicable to each of these topics. More important is the burgeoning realization, however, that human genetic variation underlies, in part, the variability observed in the susceptibility and natural history of most, if not all, pediatric conditions. It will become increasingly important for generalists to understand the principles of human genetics and to be able to apply this knowledge to their day-to-day practice. In addition, there are several key terms (Box 9-1) that are important to know when considering issues in medical genetics.

Traditionally, genetic disorders have been classified broadly into several major groups based on their etiology: chromosome disorders, single-gene disorders, multifactorial disorders, and disorders with nontraditional mechanisms of expression and inheritance. Chromosome disorders are conditions that result from abnormalities of chromosome number (i.e., aneuploidy) or structure (e.g., rearrangements). These conditions represent only a small fraction of the total burden of genetic disease. Disorders in which mutation in a single gene is necessary and sufficient to cause disease are called *monogenic conditions* or *single-gene disorders*. These disorders can be transmitted from parent to offspring in autosomal dominant, autosomal recessive, or X-linked patterns

---

Box 9-1. Glossary of Terms Commonly Used in Genetics

Allele—conventional abbreviation for *allelomorph*. Refers to the different forms that the DNA sequence of a gene may have in a population

Consanguinity—the mating of related individuals

Genotype—an individual's allelic constitution at a locus

Haplotype—the allelic constitution of multiple loci on a single chromosome

Incest—the mating of closely related individuals, usually first-degree relatives (e.g., father and daughter or two sibs)

Locus—the location of a gene on a chromosome (*plural, loci*)

Phenotype—the physical, physiologic, and behavioral characteristics of an individual that are produced by the interaction of genes and environment

Polygenic—traits that are caused by more than several different genes

---

and sometimes are called *mendelian* conditions. Single-gene disorders also can be produced by new mutations in a single individual that are appearing for the first time in a family; the mutation has arisen de novo in the affected family member.

Most birth defects and pediatric conditions are not caused by alterations of a single gene or chromosome (Table 9-1). Instead, they are influenced by different combinations of alleles at various loci. Traits in which variation is caused by the effects of many different genes are called *polygenic*. If the variation of a polygenic trait also is affected by nongenetic factors (e.g., environmental variables), the terms *multifactorial* and *complex* often are used to describe the trait. In contrast to single-gene disorders, multifactorial traits are not transmitted in mendelian patterns. Variation in susceptibility or resistance to many pediatric conditions is likely the consequence of multifactorial traits.

Table 9-1. Approximate Prevalence of Genetic Disease in the General Population

Type of Genetic Disease	Lifetime Prevalence per 1000
Autosomal dominant	3–9.5
Autosomal recessive	2–2.5
X-linked	0.5–2
Chromosome disorders*	6–9
Congenital malformation	20–50
Total	31.5–73

*The upper limit of this range is obtained when newer chromosome banding techniques are used.

Use of the Terms Congenital, Hereditary, and Familial

The terms *congenital, hereditary, genetic,* and *familial* are not synonymous. Conditions that are present at birth are referred to as *congenital conditions,* whether or not they are caused by genes. Prenatal infection with parvovirus, clubfeet caused by oligohydramnios, and trisomy 18 (Edwards' syndrome) all are congenital conditions. None of these conditions is usually hereditary or familial, however.

The term *hereditary* defines conditions that can be transmitted genetically from parent to offspring. All hereditary conditions are genetic conditions, but not all genetic conditions are hereditary. Cystic fibrosis is a hereditary genetic condition, whereas Down syndrome is a genetic condition that usually is not hereditary.

Conditions that seem to cluster within families frequently are called *familial conditions.* This includes familial clusters of "nongenetic" conditions (e.g., rotaviral or streptococcal infections) and genetic conditions (e.g., cystic fibrosis). Although all hereditary conditions can be familial (i.e., a parent can have more than one affected child), not all genetic conditions are familial. Turner's syndrome is a genetic condition that is usually neither hereditary nor familial. Distinguishing which term most appropriately defines a condition facilitates diagnosis, management, and counseling of families about the risk of recurrence of a condition.

Penetrance

The probability that an individual who possesses a disease-related genotype (see Box 9-1) exhibits the disease phenotype is called *penetrance.* When this probability is less than one, the disease is said to exhibit reduced (or incomplete) penetrance. Penetrance levels usually are estimated by examining a large number of families and determining what proportion of the obligate carriers (i.e., individuals who have an affected parent and an affected child and must be carriers of the altered gene) or obligate homozygotes (in the case of autosomal recessive disorders) develops the disease phenotype. Retinoblastoma is a good example of a genetic condition in which reduced penetrance is observed. Family studies have shown that approximately 10% of obligate carriers of an inherited mutation in the retinoblastoma susceptibility gene do not develop retinoblastoma. The penetrance of the condition is approximately 90%.

Variable Expressivity

Individuals with the same genetic condition or even the same genotype can have substantially different phenotypes; this is called *variable expressivity.* Within the same kindred, one sibling with neurofibromatosis type 1 (NF1) may have café-au-lait spots, axillary freckling, and sphenoid wing dysplasia, whereas another sibling with NF1 may have café-au-lait spots, a plexiform neurofibroma, and pseudarthrosis of the tibia. Although each sibling has the same genotype, the expression of the NF1 phenotype is different between them. Variable expressivity often is confused with reduced penetrance. The absence of a disease phenotype in an obligate carrier (i.e., reduced penetrance) is not considered variable expression of the condition. Compilation of the phenotypic findings of many individuals with the same genetic condition defines the phenotypic spectrum of a disorder. Not every affected individual has each of these findings.

Variable expressivity may be explained by the influence of other genes (i.e., modifying genes), environmental factors (e.g., earlier palliative intervention), or random variation. Variable expressivity among families sometimes is due to the presence of different genotypes (i.e., different mutations in the same gene). When variable expression of a disease phenotype is caused by a variety of different genotypes (i.e., alleles) at the same locus, it is said to exhibit allelic heterogeneity. In some cases, the variable expressivity is so extreme that more than one disease phenotype (i.e., distinctly different conditions with different natural histories and outcomes) is produced by different alleles (Fig. 9-1). In some genes, the same mutation can cause different syndromes in different families. A missense mutation in *fibroblast growth factor receptor 2 (FGFR2)* can cause either of two different craniosynostosis syndromes (i.e., Pfeiffer syndrome or Crouzon's disease).

Sometimes, different alleles are associated with a subset of specific traits within the phenotypic spectrum of a single condition or are associated with varying degrees of disease severity. Pancreatic insufficiency in patients with cystic fibrosis is found more commonly if they have at least one allele that is the common 3-bp deletion (ΔF508) in *cystic fibrosis transmembrane regulator (CFTR).* A potentially powerful strategy for providing affected individuals and their families with better anticipatory guidance is to estimate the correlation between genotypes and specific phenotypic characteristics (the so-called genotype-phenotype correlation).

In contrast, for some genetic conditions, the same phenotype can be produced by mutations in more than one gene. Tuberous sclerosis, an autosomal dominant disorder characterized by seizures, hypopigmented macules, multiple hamartomas, and variable mental retardation, can be caused by mutations in genes located on either chromosome 9 or chromosome 16. Mutations in more than 20 different genes have been associated with hearing loss. Conditions that can be caused by mutations in more than one gene are said to exhibit locus heterogeneity.

Pleiotropy

Genes that have more than one discernible effect on a phenotype are said to have *pleiotropic* effects. A good example of a gene that has pleiotropic effects is *fibrillin-1 (FBN1),* which is mutated in individuals with Marfan syndrome. *FBN1* encodes a protein that is a major component of extracellular microfibrils that form connective tissue in eyes, vascular tissue, and the musculoskeletal system. Mutations in *FBN1* result in abnormalities such as dislocation of the lens, aortic dilation, and tall stature. Other examples of pleiotropic genetic conditions include cystic fibrosis (characterized by abnormalities of the lungs, pancreas, and sweat glands) and osteogenesis imperfecta, in which the bones, teeth, and sclerae are affected. Pleiotropy can be caused by genes whose products play similar roles in different tissues and organs.

Pleiotropy also can be caused by genes whose protein products play varied roles in different developmental programs. Campomelic dysplasia is caused by mutations in

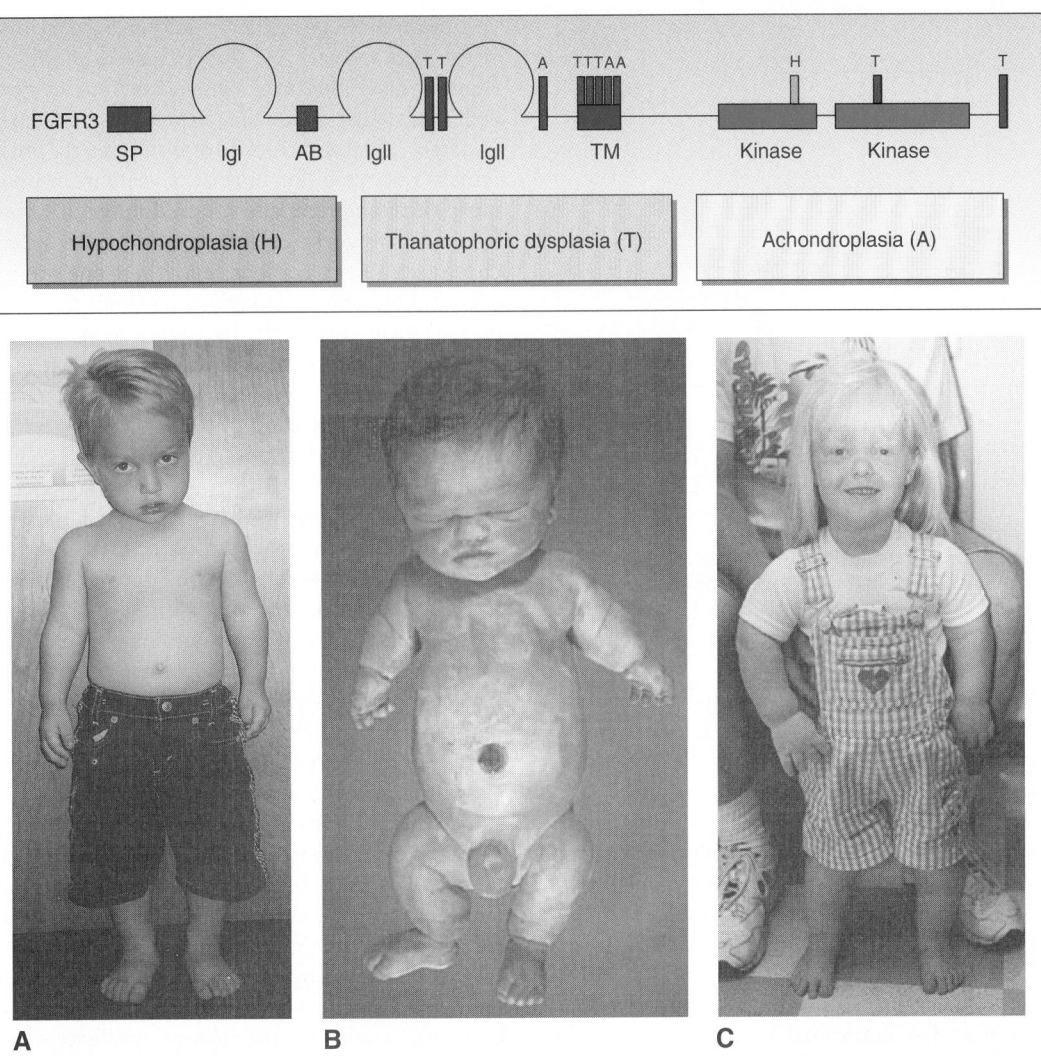

Figure 9-1. Schematic drawing of fibroblast growth factor 3 receptor (FGFR3) protein. Important functional domains of FGFR3 include a signal peptide (SP), three immunoglobulin-like (Ig) domains, an acid box (AB), a transmembrane (TM) domain, and a split tyrosine kinase (TK) domain. The locations of point mutations causing achondroplasia (A; purple), hypochondroplasia (H; yellow), and thanatophoric dysplasia (T; red) are indicated. Photographs of children with mutations in FGFR3. **A,** A boy with hypochondroplasia. He has mildly short limbs relative to his trunk. **B,** An infant with thanatophoric dysplasia, the most common of the so-called lethal skeletal dysplasias. He has markedly shortened limbs and a narrow thoracic cage. **C,** A girl with achondroplasia. She has short limbs relative to the length of her trunk resulting in redundant skin folds in the arms and legs, a prominent forehead, and a depressed nasal root. (Redrawn from Webster MK, Donoghue DJ: FGFR3 activation in skeletal disorders: Too much of a good thing. Trends Genet 1997;13:178–182. Reproduced with permission from Elsevier.)

a gene named *SRY-related HMG-BOX 9 (SOX9)*, which plays an important regulatory role in skeletal development and sexual differentiation. Individuals with campomelic dysplasia have a skeletal dysplasia that sometimes is accompanied by sex reversal.

MECHANISMS OF INHERITANCE

Autosomal Dominant Disorders

For autosomal dominant conditions, the presence of only one copy of an altered allele of a locus is sufficient to produce a disease phenotype. Genetic disorders that are inherited in an autosomal dominant pattern are the most common single-gene disorders described in humans (see Table 9-1). However, individually, each autosomal dominant disorder is relatively uncommon. Most affected offspring are produced from the mating of an affected parent and an unaffected parent, or they are the result of a

de novo mutation. A parent affected with an autosomal dominant disorder can transmit either the normal or the altered allele to his or her offspring. Each of these events has a probability of 0.5. On average, half of the children are heterozygous for the altered allele and express the disease, whereas half are homozygous for a normal allele. Matings between two individuals affected by the same autosomal dominant disorder are rare.

Brachydactyly type A-1 is characterized by shortened or missing middle phalanges of the digits and is caused by mutations in a gene encoding Indian hedgehog (a secreted signaling molecule similar to sonic hedgehog [mutations in which cause holoprosencephaly]). Brachydactyly type A-1 was described in 1903, and it is the first recorded example of a human developmental defect segregating in an autosomal dominant pattern. An idealized pedigree for this condition (Fig. 9-2) illustrates several important characteristics of autosomal dominant inheritance. First,

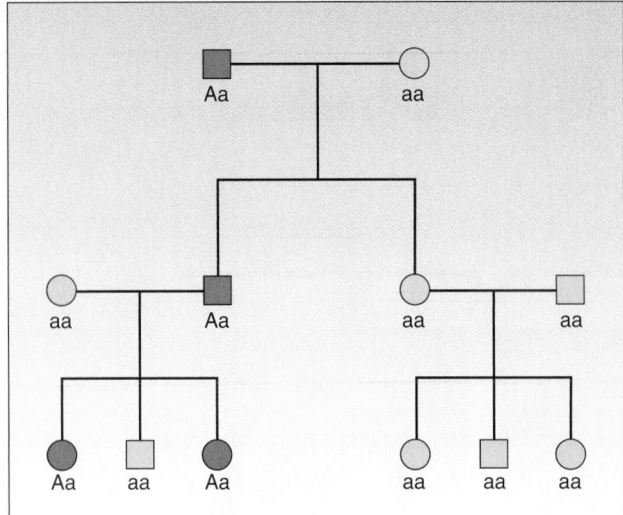

Figure 9-2. Pedigree showing the inheritance pattern of brachydactyly type A-1, an autosomal dominant disorder. Affected individuals are represented by shading. (Redrawn from Jorde LB, Carey JC, Bamshad MJ, White RL: Medical Genetics, 3rd ed. Philadelphia, Mosby, 2003, p 65.)

the two sexes exhibit the trait in roughly equal proportions, and males and females are equally likely to transmit the trait. Second, no generation is skipped. Every individual with brachydactyly type A-1 has an affected parent. Third, father-to-son transmission is observed. Although father-to-son transmission is not required to establish autosomal dominant inheritance, its presence excludes some other modes of inheritance (e.g., X-linked and mitochondrial). Last, an affected individual transmits the trait to half of his or her offspring, on average (Table 9-2).

De novo mutations are an important cause of autosomal dominant conditions. For autosomal dominant conditions that are lethal in prereproductive life (e.g., thanatophoric dysplasia, the most common lethal skeletal dysplasia), de novo mutations are the most common cause of the disorder. For some autosomal dominant conditions (e.g., achondroplasia, Marfan syndrome, Apert's syndrome), the age of the father and the likelihood of transmitting a new mutation to his offspring are positively correlated. Virtually all mutations in *FGFR2* that cause Apert's syndrome arise on the paternal

chromosome. The higher mutation rate in males seems to be caused in part by the increased number of chromosome replications in male versus female germ-producing cells (cells that produce sperm or eggs). Female germ cells undergo 23 chromosome replications to produce all of a female's oocytes. In contrast, sperm are produced continuously throughout a male's reproductive lifetime. At 15 years of age, male germ cells have undergone approximately 35 chromosome replications, and then one stem cell division occurs about every 16 days, or 23 times per year. At 30 years of age, male germ cells have undergone an average of 380 chromosome replications. Each replication provides an opportunity for mutations to occur. Not all genes exhibit an increased mutation rate in males, and only a small paternal age effect is observed for some types of mutations (e.g., deletions).

Sometimes, clearly unaffected parents have more than one child affected with an autosomal dominant disorder. Studies have shown that one of the parents in such families has two or more different cell lines in their germ cells with at least one cell line containing a mutated allele. This phenomenon is called *germline mosaicism*. Germline mosaicism seems to be more common for some disorders (e.g., osteogenesis imperfecta).

Two or more cell lines also can be found in the somatic cells of an individual (somatic mosaicism). Individuals with somatic mosaicism may have all the same characteristics found in affected individuals, exhibit abnormalities limited to only tissues containing the mutant cell line, or appear unaffected. For some genetic conditions, all affected individuals have somatic mosaicism. McCune-Albright syndrome is characterized by polyostotic fibrous dysplasia; hyperpigmented patches of the skin; and endocrinologic abnormalities, such as precocious puberty, thyrotoxicosis, pituitary gigantism, and Cushing's syndrome. It is caused by somatic mutations in *guanine nucleotide-binding protein* and *α-stimulating activity polypeptide 1 (GNAS1)*, which result in the constitutive activation of hormone-sensitive adenylate cyclase. Germline activating mutations *(GNAS1)*, however, result in embryonic lethality.

Autosomal Recessive Disorders

For autosomal recessive conditions, the presence of two copies of an altered allele of a locus is required to produce a disease phenotype. Genetic disorders that are inherited in an autosomal recessive pattern are less common than autosomal dominant disorders in most populations. Heterozygous carriers for recessive conditions are much more common than affected homozygotes. The parents of individuals affected with autosomal recessive conditions are usually heterozygous carriers.

Sickle cell disease is an autosomal recessive trait that is caused by a missense mutation (a mutation that results in an amino acid substitution) in the gene encoding β-globin, resulting in the production of an abnormal hemoglobin molecule (i.e., HbS). Exposure of HbS to a low oxygen tension results in a conformational change in erythrocytes (i.e., sickle shape) and ultimately obstruction of the microvasculature and premature destruction of red blood cells. Painful sickling crises, anemia, poor growth, and immunologic abnormalities result.

Table 9-2. Comparison of the Major Attributes of Autosomal Dominant and Autosomal Recessive Inheritance Patterns

Attribute	Autosomal Dominant	Autosomal Recessive
Usual recurrence risk	50%	25%
Transmission pattern	Vertical; disease phenotype seen in generation after generation	Horizontal; disease phenotype seen in multiple siblings, but usually no earlier generations affected
Sex ratio	Equal number of affected males and females (usually)	Equal number of affected males and females (usually)
Other	Father-son transmission of disease gene is possible	Consanguinity is seen sometimes, especially for rare recessive diseases

An idealized pedigree for sickle cell disease (Fig. 9-3) illustrates several important characteristics of autosomal recessive inheritance (see Table 9-2). First, autosomal recessive disorders usually are observed in one or more siblings but are not usually found in other generations. Second, similar to autosomal dominant conditions, males and females are affected in equal proportions, and males and females are equally likely to transmit the disease-causing mutation. Third, on average, about 25% of the offspring of two heterozygous carriers are affected. Last, consanguinity is observed more often in pedigrees of autosomal recessive disorders compared with pedigrees of autosomal dominant conditions.

The prevalence of sickle cell disease is approximately 1/400 in African Americans. This prevalence is much higher than in Northern Europeans but not as high as the prevalence in some sub-Saharan African populations. Knowledge of the prevalence of a condition facilitates estimation of its carrier frequency (i.e., individuals who carry one copy of a recessive disease allele and are unaffected). This information is important because it can be used to predict allele and genotype frequencies for disorders transmitted in mendelian patterns.

The Hardy-Weinberg law states that for a single locus in a randomly mating population (random mating also is called *panmixia*), the frequencies of genotypes within the population can be predicted on the basis of the allele frequencies. Suppose that at a locus with two alleles, the frequency, p, of an allele, A, is 0.70. Then 70% of the sperm and egg cells in a population have this allele. Because the sum of allele frequencies at a locus must equal 1, the frequency, q, of the other allele, a, is equal to $1 - p = 1.0 - 0.7 = 0.3$. Under panmixia, the probability that a sperm carrying allele A unites with an egg carrying allele A is $p \times p = p^2$ or $0.7 \times 0.7 = 0.49$

(multiplication rule). This is the probability of producing a homozygous offspring with the AA genotype. The probability of producing a homozygous offspring with the aa genotype is $q \times q = q^2$ or $0.3 \times 0.3 = 0.09$.

Heterozygous offspring can be produced two different ways. A sperm carrying allele A can unite with an egg carrying allele a, or a sperm carrying allele a can unite with an egg carrying allele A. The frequency with which either of these events occurs is equal to the product of the gene frequencies, $p \times q$. Because clinicians want to know the overall probability of both events, they use the addition rule, adding the probabilities to obtain a heterozygote frequency of $pq + pq = 2pq$. Overall, the genotype frequencies of a two-allele locus are equal to $p^2 + 2pq + q^2 = 1$. This relationship indicates that the gene frequency (q) for alleles causing sickle cell disease is equal to $(q^2)^{1/2}$ or $(1/400)^{1/2}$ or $1/20$. The frequency of normal alleles, p, is $(399/400)^{1/2}$ or approximately 1. The frequency of heterozygotes ($2pq$) is equal to $2(1)(1/20) = 1/10$. The frequency of heterozygous carriers is approximately 40 times higher than the frequency of affected individuals.

The probabilities of two carriers producing children with two normal alleles (homozygous normal), a normal allele and a disease-causing allele (heterozygous carriers), or two disease-causing alleles (homozygous affected) are 0.25, 0.5, and 0.25. On average, one quarter of the children produced by heterozygous carriers are affected with an autosomal recessive condition. If a child is known not to be affected, the likelihood that he or she is a carrier is 2 of 3 (i.e., likelihood of being a heterozygous carrier [0.5]/likelihood of being a heterozygous carrier (0.5) + likelihood of being a homozygous normal (0.25)).

X-Linked Disorders

Genes that are located on the X or Y chromosome are called *sex-linked genes*. The Y chromosome has relatively few genes and is the smallest of the human chromosomes (approximately 70 megabases [Mb]). One important gene on the Y chromosome is called the *sex-determining region Y (SRY)* gene. Mutations of *SRY* can result in XY individuals with normal external female genitalia and gonadal dysgenesis (i.e., abnormal formation of the gonads). This mutation is an uncommon cause of abnormalities of sexual differentiation in humans.

The X chromosome is almost twice as large (approximately 160 Mb) as the Y chromosome and contains thousands of genes that play a variety of roles during development and adult life. Many well-known pediatric genetic conditions are caused by alterations of X-linked genes, including hemophilia A and B, Duchenne's and Becker's muscular dystrophy, red-green color blindness, ocular albinism with neurosensory hearing loss, anhidrotic ectodermal dysplasia, and ornithine carbamoyltransferase deficiency. Additionally, more than 60 different phenotypes associated with mental retardation (e.g., fragile X syndrome) have been mapped to the X chromosome, although genes have been cloned for only a few of these conditions.

Females have two copies of the X chromosome, whereas males have only one copy of an X chromosome. The quantity of product encoded by most X-linked genes does not differ between males and females, however. The equalization of

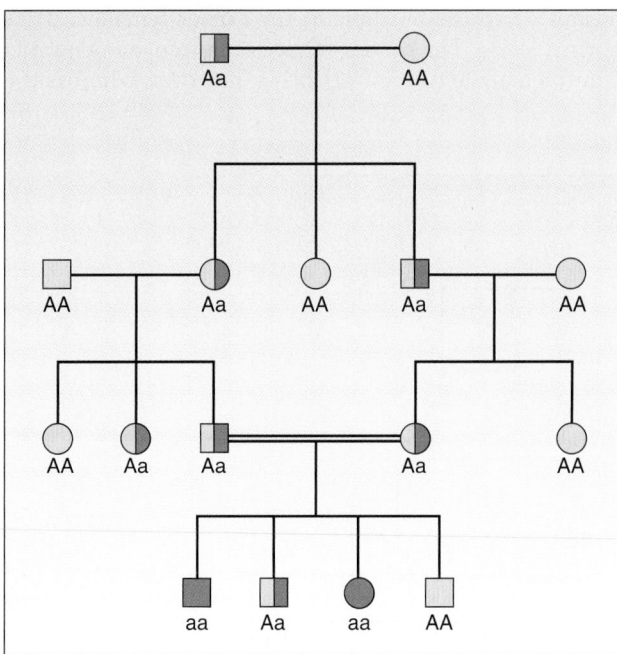

Figure 9-3. Pedigree showing the inheritance pattern of sickle cell disease, an autosomal recessive disease. Consanguinity in this pedigree is denoted by a double bar connecting the parents of the affected individuals. (Redrawn from Jorde LB, Carey JC, Bamshad MJ, White RL: Medical Genetics, 3rd ed. Philadelphia, Mosby, 2003, p 67.)

X-linked gene products is called *dosage compensation* and is produced by the inactivation of one of the X chromosomes early in female embryonic development. This inactivation process is random, so the maternally and paternally derived X chromosomes each are inactive in about half of the embryo's cells. When an X chromosome is inactivated, the same X chromosome remains inactivated in all descendants of the cell. All normal females have at least two populations of cells (somatic mosaicism), one containing a paternally derived active X chromosome and the other containing a maternally derived active X chromosome. This is clearly evident if the maternally and paternally derived X chromosomes produce different products. The retina of women who are carriers for X-linked ocular albinism show alternating patches of pigmented and nonpigmented cells corresponding to cells in which the disease-bearing X chromosome (pigmented) or the normal X chromosome (nonpigmented) have been inactivated.

Inactivation of the X chromosome occurs approximately 2 weeks after fertilization. Inactivation begins in a region of the X chromosome called the *inactivation center* and subsequently spreads along the chromosome. The X inactivation center contains at least one gene required for inactivation, *XIST*. *XIST* is transcribed only from the inactive X chromosome, but its messenger RNA (mRNA) never leaves the nucleus and is not translated into protein. The mRNA product of *XIST* appears to coat the portions of the X chromosome that subsequently are inactivated. Maintenance of inactivation seems to depend on methylation of CG dinucleotides that commonly are found in the 5′ (upstream) regions of genes. Inactivation of the X chromosome is incomplete, and genes in several regions continue to be transcribed from the inactivated X chromosome. Some of these genes have transcribed homologues on the Y chromosome; dosage compensation is maintained by their activation on both X chromosomes in females. Others do not have Y chromosome homologues and may contribute to gender differences.

The inheritance patterns of X-linked conditions differ substantially from the inheritance patterns of autosomal disorders. Females can be homozygous for a disease allele at a given locus, heterozygous for a disease allele and a normal allele, or homozygous for a normal allele at a locus. Because males have only one X chromosome, they are considered hemizygous (hemi = half) for an allele at a locus on the X chromosome. If a male inherits the altered allele for a recessive disorder, he is affected with the condition because the Y chromosome does not carry a normal allele that might compensate for the effects of the disease gene. In contrast, X-linked dominant disorders can cause the disease condition in males and females because the presence of only one copy of an altered allele is sufficient for disease expression. Only a few X-linked dominant conditions are known to exist, and these are rare.

For X-linked recessive disorders, the frequency of the disease condition in males is equal to the gene frequency, q. All males with the altered gene have the disease condition. Because females need two copies of the altered allele to manifest the condition, the frequency of the disease condition is q^2. Duchenne's muscular dystrophy has a prevalence of approximately 1/3500 males ($q = 0.0003$). It is expected that affected females will be observed in q^2 ($q^2 = 0.00000009$) or 1/12,250,000 individuals. This shows that X-linked recessive disorders are found much more frequently in males than females.

A pedigree for red-green color blindness (Fig. 9-4) illustrates some of the important characteristics of X-linked recessive conditions. First, only females are able transmit the disorder to their sons; there is no male-to-male transmission for X-linked recessive conditions. Second, sibships containing only carrier females (unaffected) and unaffected males appear as "skipped generations." In these generations, the X chromosome transmitted to the brothers of the carrier females carries a normal allele. The carrier females can transmit a normal or mutated allele to their offspring, however, whereas the

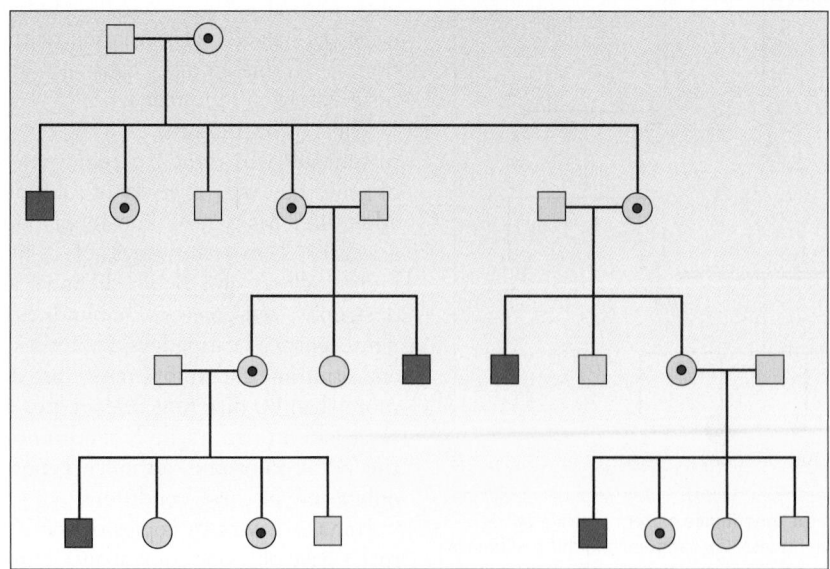

Figure 9-4. Pedigree showing the inheritance of an X-linked recessive trait. Solid symbols represent affected individuals, and dotted symbols represent heterozygous carriers. (Redrawn from Jorde LB, Carey JC, Bamshad MJ, White RL: Medical Genetics, 3rd ed. Philadelphia, Mosby, 2003, p 95.)

males can transmit only a normal allele to their daughters. An affected father transmits the disease allele to all of his daughters, who transmit it to half of their sons on average.

Some female "carriers" of X-linked recessive disorders manifest some or all of the characteristics of the condition. There are at least three mechanisms by which this can happen. First, because inactivation of the X chromosome is a random process within each cell, sometimes a much higher proportion of X chromosomes bearing a normal allele are inactivated than X chromosomes carrying a disease allele. These affected carrier females are called *manifesting heterozygotes*. For many disorders, manifesting heterozygotes have a more "mild" form of the condition compared with affected males. Approximately 5% of women carrying an allele for hemophilia A have factor VIII levels low enough to exhibit a mild form of the disease. Second, some women have only a single X chromosome (i.e., Turner's syndrome) and subsequently manifest X-linked recessive conditions for which they otherwise would have been carriers. X chromosomes with deletions sometimes are preferentially inactivated so that women who carry a mutated allele on the X chromosome without a deletion manifest disease. Last, chromosomal aberrations, such as rearrangements involving the X chromosome and an autosome, also can result in affected females. X:autosome rearrangements involving the mutation-containing X chromosome cause disease in females because the normal X chromosome is preferentially inactivated to avoid inactivating the autosome attached to the other X chromosome. These events are relatively rare.

NONTRADITIONAL MECHANISMS OF DISEASE

Anticipation

Some genetic conditions seem to display an earlier age of onset or more severe expression in the more recent generations of a pedigree. This phenomenon is called *genetic anticipation*. Some investigators had proposed that anticipation was an artifact of better observation and diagnostic tools that now are available to clinicians (e.g., a disorder previously diagnosed at age 60 now might be diagnosed at age 40). In the 1990s, it was shown that for some disorders, anticipation has a biologic basis.

One of the best examples of anticipation comes from studies of myotonic dystrophy, the most common muscular dystrophy that affects adults. Myotonic dystrophy is characterized by progressive deterioration of skeletal muscle, cardiomyopathy, testicular atrophy, and cataracts. It is caused by mutations in a gene (i.e., *DMPK*) on chromosome 19 that encodes a protein kinase or mutations in a gene (i.e., *ZNF9*) on chromosome 3 that encodes a RNA-binding protein. When caused by mutations in *ZNF9*, myotonic dystrophy seems to have a milder course.

Analysis of *DMPK* has shown that myotonic dystrophy is caused by the expansion of a CTG repeat in the 3' untranslated region of the gene (i.e., a region transcribed into mRNA but not translated into protein). Unaffected individuals have 5 to 30 copies of the repeat, mildly affected individuals may have 50 to 100 copies of the repeat, and severely affected individuals may have 100 to more than

several thousand repeats. The number of repeats is positively correlated with the severity of the disease. The number of repeats often increases with succeeding generations. As a consequence, succeeding generations have more severe disease compared with preceding generations of a pedigree (Fig. 9-5). This is strong evidence of genetic anticipation.

Imprinting

Some single-gene conditions are caused by mechanisms that are transmitted in patterns that are distinct from those of autosomal and sex-linked conditions. Many of these conditions are relatively uncommon. Nevertheless, these nontraditional mechanisms of disease often explain observations that are otherwise inconsistent with the current state of knowledge of genetic disorders. The expression of most traits is independent of the parent of origin of the causative allele. This is not always true, however. One of the most striking examples to date is caused by a deletion of 2 to 4 Mb of chromosome 15. When this deletion is inherited from the father, the offspring is born with Prader-Willi syndrome. This disorder is characterized by severe neonatal hypotonia, obesity, hypogonadism, small hands and feet, and an unusual behavioral profile including mental retardation (Fig. 9-6). In contrast, when the same deletion is inherited from the mother, the offspring manifests Angelman's syndrome. Individuals with Angelman's syndrome appear normal at birth but subsequently develop

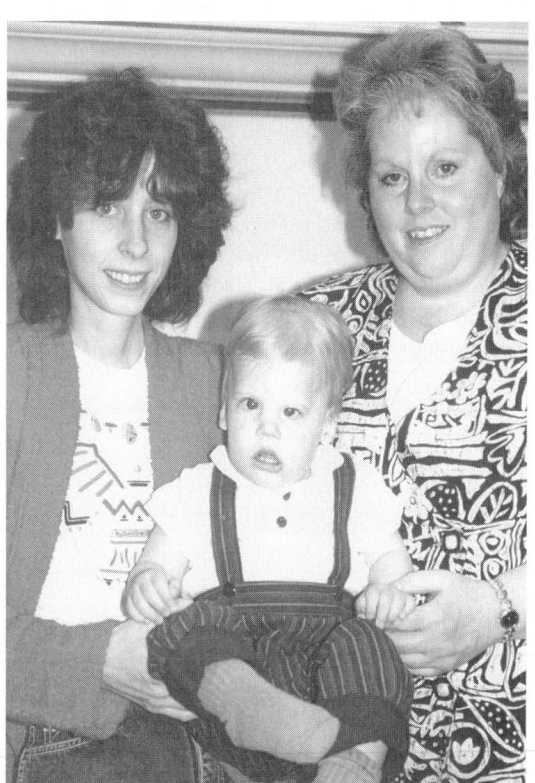

Figure 9-5. A three-generation family affected with myotonic dystrophy. The grandmother *(right)* is only slightly affected, but the mother *(left)* has a characteristic narrow face and limited facial expression. The infant is more severely affected and has the facial features of children with neonatal-onset myotonic dystrophy, including an open, triangle-shaped mouth. As expected of conditions exhibiting genetic anticipation, the degree of severity increases in each generation. (From Jorde LB, Carey JC, Bamshad MJ, White RL: Medical Genetics, 3rd ed. Philadelphia, Mosby, 2003, p 80.)

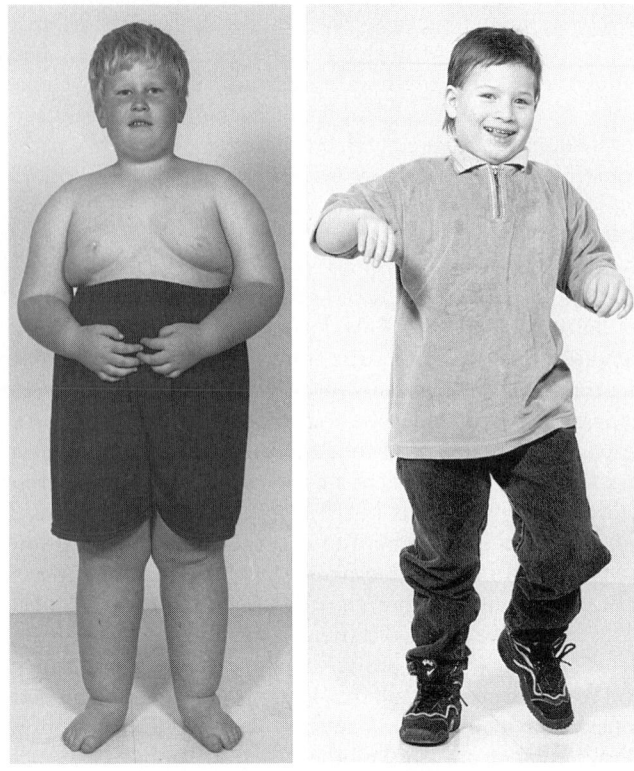

A   **B**

Figure 9-6. The effect of imprinting on chromosome 15 deletions. **A,** Inheritance of the deletion from the father produces Prader-Willi syndrome (note the inverted V-shaped upper lip, small hands, and truncal obesity). **B,** Inheritance of the deletion from the mother produces Angelman's syndrome (note the characteristic posture). (From Jorde LB, Carey JC, Bamshad MJ, White RL: Medical Genetics, 3rd ed. Philadelphia, Mosby, 2003, p 78.)

seizures, mental retardation, ataxia, and a characteristic posture (see Fig. 9-6).

Within the 2- to 4-Mb region of chromosome 15 that is deleted in these patients lie several genes that are transcriptionally active on the chromosome inherited from either the mother or the father, but not both chromosomes (i.e., they are active on only one chromosome). If these genes

are deleted, the result is a complete loss of the encoded product and a disease condition. If all of the paternally active genes are lost, the offspring has Prader-Willi syndrome (Fig. 9-7). Angelman's syndrome results from the deletion of a maternally active gene called *ubiquitin-protein ligase E3A (UBE3A)* that is involved in the degradation of proteins within the brain. The differential activation of genes contingent on whether they are maternally or paternally transmitted is called *genomic imprinting*.

Approximately 70% of cases of Angelman's syndrome or Prader-Willi syndrome are caused by chromosome deletions. Several additional mechanisms may cause these disorders, however. One of these is the inheritance of both copies of a chromosome, in part of or the whole chromosome, from only one parent. This is called *uniparental disomy*. If both copies of the maternal chromosome 15 are inherited, the resulting offspring lacks the paternally active genes and develops Prader-Willi syndrome. Conversely, uniparental disomy of paternal chromosome 15 causes Angelman's syndrome. Uniparental disomy also has been found to be responsible for some cases of Beckwith-Wiedemann syndrome. It results from two active copies of a gene called *insulin-like growth factor receptor 2* when there should be only one. Uniparental disomy has been reported for most human chromosomes, although the overall clinical significance of this finding is not yet clear.

Other cases that have been difficult to explain until more recently include the expression of autosomal recessive conditions (e.g., cystic fibrosis) in the offspring of matings between a carrier parent (i.e., heterozygous for a disease allele and a normal allele) and an unaffected parent homozygous for two normal alleles. Using molecular markers that identify each of the four parental chromosomes specifically, it was found that both copies of the chromosome bearing a disease allele were identical and inherited from the heterozygous parent. A child received two copies of the same chromosome from one parent. This is called *uniparental isodisomy*. The proportion of genetic conditions caused by this type of abnormality is unknown but likely to be low.

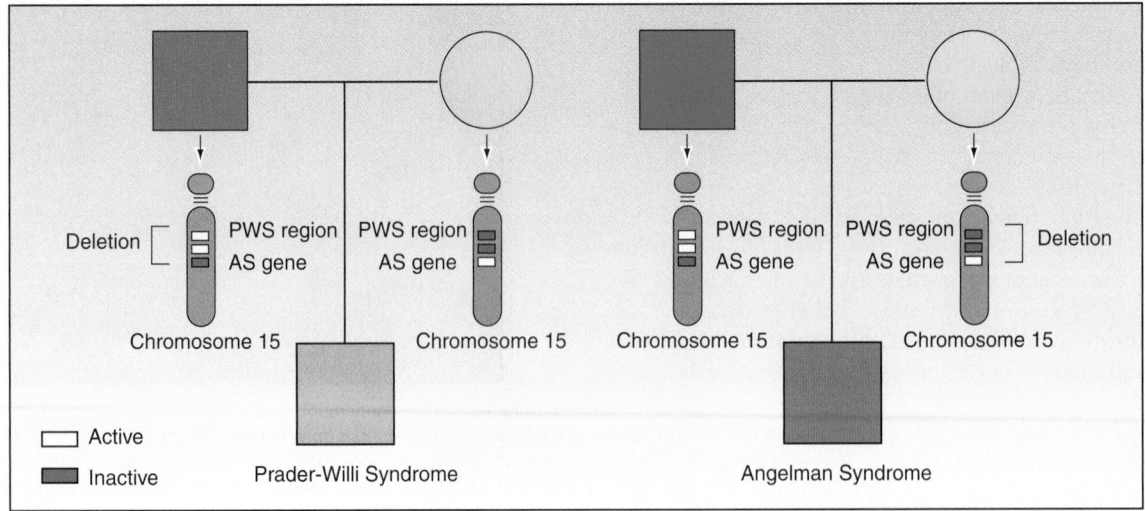

Figure 9-7. Pedigrees illustrate the inheritance pattern of the deletion of chromosome 15 that causes Prader-Willi syndrome or Angelman's syndrome depending on the parental origin of the deletion and the activation status of genes in the deleted interval. (Redrawn from Jorde LB, Carey JC, Bamshad MJ, White RL: Medical Genetics, 3rd ed. Philadelphia, Mosby, 2003, p 80.)

Mitochondrial Inheritance

Most genetic conditions are caused by abnormalities of the nuclear genome. Nevertheless, a growing number of conditions are caused by defects of the only genetic material existing outside of the nucleus, that of the mitochondrion. In contrast to the nuclear genome, which is diploid (two copies of each gene), the mitochondrial genome contains only one copy of each gene and is haploid. Because of the unique properties of the mitochondrion, these disorders exhibit a characteristic pattern of inheritance and wide phenotypic variability.

Each of the 100 to 100,000 mitochondria within a cell contains at least several copies of a 16,569-bp genome in the mitochondrial matrix, and each mitochondrial DNA (mtDNA) molecule is typically identical. The state in which all copies of mtDNA are identical is called *homoplasmy*. The mtDNA molecule encodes 13 polypeptides that are components of the oxidative phosphorylation (OXPHOS) system (another approximately 90 components are encoded by the nuclear genome), 2 ribosomal RNAs, and 22 transfer RNAs. Replication and transcription of mtDNA occur within the mitochondrion and are facilitated by nuclear-encoded proteins. In humans, mitochondria in the midpiece of the sperm may enter the egg, but the mtDNA from the sperm rarely, if ever, persists in the embryo. All of the mitochondria of the offspring are descendants of those located within the cytoplasm of the egg, and the inheritance of mtDNA is exclusively maternal.

Because there is more than one copy of mtDNA within each mitochondrion, a new mutation in an mtDNA molecule results in the emergence of two different mtDNA populations within a mitochondrion. The state of having two or more different populations of mtDNA molecules is called *heteroplasmy*. As cells divide and the mitochondria proliferate, the proportion of mutant mtDNA molecules within a cell and the proportion of cells in a tissue/organ containing mitochondria with mutant mtDNA molecules change. Mutant mtDNA diminish the efficiency of OXPHOS metabolism and cause cells to die and tissues/organs to deteriorate prematurely. A threshold of mutant mtDNA molecules within a mitochondrion must be exceeded before a biochemical defect disrupts the normal function of the OXPHOS system. The larger the proportion of mutant mtDNA molecules within a cell or tissue, the higher the likelihood of expressing a disease phenotype or the greater the severity of disease.

Mitochondrial disorders can be caused by mutations in nuclear genes or mtDNA. In general, mutations in the mtDNA molecule are either rearrangements (i.e., deletions and duplications) or point mutations (i.e., missense or nonsense mutations [a nonsense mutation is a nucleotide substitution that results in the replacement of an amino acid codon with a stop codon]). Many conditions caused by mtDNA mutations present with nonspecific neurologic findings, such as coma, seizures, and ataxia (Table 9-3). In the neonatal period, mitochondrial disorders commonly present with metabolic encephalopathy, cardiac or hepatic failure, or lactic acidemia. Although uncommon, mitochondrial disorders account for a substantial percentage of cerebrovascular accidents in children. Most mitochondrial disorders are uncommon, but mtDNA mutations also contribute to common disorders, such as deafness and diabetes mellitus. Mitochondrial mutations also have been implicated in the process of aging. It is unclear, however, whether these mutations are a cause or a consequence of the aging process.

Table 9-3. Mitochondrial Diseases Associated with Mitochrondrial DNA Mutations

Condition	Inheritance	Mutations
Mitochondrial encephalopathy, lactic acidosis, stroke (MELAS)	Maternal	tRNA
Mitochondrial encephalopathy, ragged red fibers (MERRF)	Maternal	tRNA
Neuropathy, ataxia, retinitis pigmentosa (NARP)	Maternal	ATPase
Maternally inherited Leigh's syndrome (MILS)	Maternal	ATPase
Leber's hereditary optic neuropathy (LHON)	Maternal	ND1, ND4, ND6
Kearns-Sayre syndrome (KSS)	Sporadic	Deletion
Pearson's syndrome	Sporadic	Deletion
Isolated myopathy	Both	tRNA

MECHANISMS OF MUTATION

The identification and characterization of a gene causing or influencing a condition is often the initial step in understanding the molecular pathogenesis of a disorder. Further insight often is gained by understanding the mechanism by which mutations disturb the function of a cell. Most mutations result in either a gain of function or a loss of function of the encoded product.

A disease allele occasionally results in a protein product with a novel function compared with the normal product. More commonly, a disease allele causes the overexpression of its product or expression of its product at an inappropriate time or place. Both of these types of mutations are called *gain-of-function mutations* and commonly result in conditions transmitted in a dominant pattern. Huntington's disease, a late-onset condition characterized by progressive neurologic deterioration, is caused by a gain-of-function mutation.

Some gain-of-function mutations extend the normal function of a gene. Mutations in *fibroblast growth factor receptor 3 (FGFR3)* result in the uncontrolled activation of the receptor leading to enhanced inhibition of the growth of long bones (e.g., the femur). Mutations in different regions of the gene result in varying levels of activation, and the level of activation is positively correlated with the severity of the phenotype. Depending on the location of the mutation, mutations in *FGFR3* can produce hypochondroplasia, achondroplasia, or thanatophoric dysplasia (see Fig. 9-1). This is also a good example of genotype-phenotype correlation in which the location of the mutation is associated with the altered activity level of the protein and the severity of the phenotype.

Some mutations result in the loss of 50% of the encoded product, while 50% of the product remains available (encoded by the normal allele). Often, but not exclusively, these loss-of-function mutations are observed in recessive conditions (e.g., galactosemia, Hurler's syndrome). The availability of 50% of the encoded product is often enough to prevent disease so that carriers for most recessive disorders are asymptomatic. In some cases, 50% of the encoded product is not sufficient, however, to prevent disease (i.e., haploinsufficiency). Loss-of-function mutations also can result in dominant disorders. A deletion of the gene encoding the extracellular matrix protein, elastin, results in diminished incorporation of elastin into the wall of large arteries, producing supravalvular aortic stenosis.

Another type of loss-of-function mutation results when the encoded product produced by one allele not only is nonfunctional, but also interferes with the activity of the normal product produced by the other allele in a heterozygote; this is called a *dominant negative mutation*. This type of mutation usually is observed in genes that encode proteins that are components of multimeric (containing two or more protein subunits) proteins. Mutations in one of the collagen genes *(COL1A1)* can impair the binding of collagen subunits into its normal trimeric complex, resulting in osteogenesis imperfecta.

In the 1990s, a novel type of mutation produced by an expansion of a repeated nucleotide motif was found to cause a variety of genetic conditions. Most commonly, these disorders are associated with an expansion of a trinucleotide repeat (e.g., CAG, CTG). These repeats can be located within a gene or in the 5' or 3' untranslated portions of a gene. One of the most notable of the genetic conditions caused by an expansion of a trinucleotide repeat is fragile X syndrome, the most common cause of inherited mental retardation in males (Fig. 9-8).

Fragile X syndrome is an X-linked dominant condition with 80% penetrance in males and 30% penetrance in females. It is caused by the expansion of a CGG repeat in the 5' untranslated region of a gene called *FMR1*. In unaffected men, there are typically 6 to 50 CGG repeats. Males who carry the disease allele but do not have fragile X syndrome are called *transmitting males*. An intermediate number of repeats (i.e., 50 to 230), or "premutation," is found in transmitting males and their daughters. When these female offspring transmit the gene to their offspring, the premutation sometimes expands to a full mutation ranging up to several thousand repeats. Men with full mutations have no *FMR1* mRNA in their cells, indicating that transcription of *FMR1* has been silenced. Premutations tend to become larger in successive generations, and larger premutations are more prone to expansion to a full mutation. These expansions do not occur when a male transmits the premutation. Males with a premutation cannot transmit the disease to their daughters, and grandsons and great-grandsons of normal transmitting males are more likely to be affected with fragile X syndrome.

Expansions of trinucleotide repeats also are associated with various progressive neurodegenerative disorders, including some of the spinocerebellar ataxias, Huntington's disease, and myotonic dystrophy. As discussed previously, some of these trinucleotide repeat expansions also are associated with genetic anticipation.

POPULATION VARIATION, CONSANGUINITY, AND INBREEDING

The prevalence of many genetic disorders varies extensively among human populations. The prevalence of cystic fibrosis varies from 1/313 in the Hutterites of Alberta, Canada, to 1/90,000 in Asians, a difference of nearly 300-fold. Although mutation is ultimately the source of all variation in the genome, different mutation rates among populations is not a sufficient explanation for the wide variation in prevalence rates of genetic conditions. These varied prevalence rates are the imprints left by evolutionary forces other than mutation (i.e., natural selection, genetic drift, gene flow) on disease-related variation in human populations. Explaining these patterns of disease-related genetic variation is important because it facilitates understanding the etiology and pathogenesis of genetic conditions. Estimating disease-related genetic variation depends on understanding the distribution of total (i.e., normal + disease-related) genetic variation. Since the 1990s, a variety

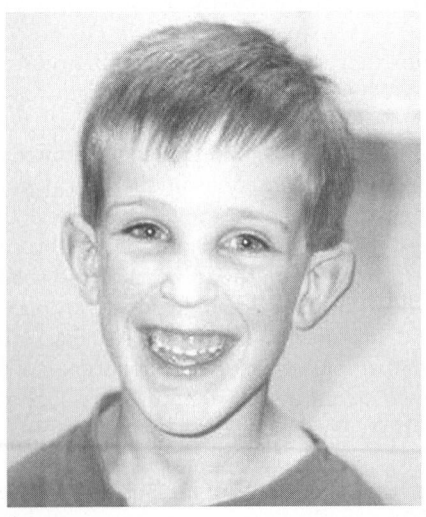 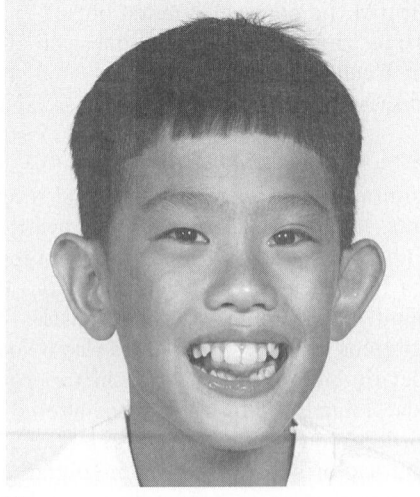 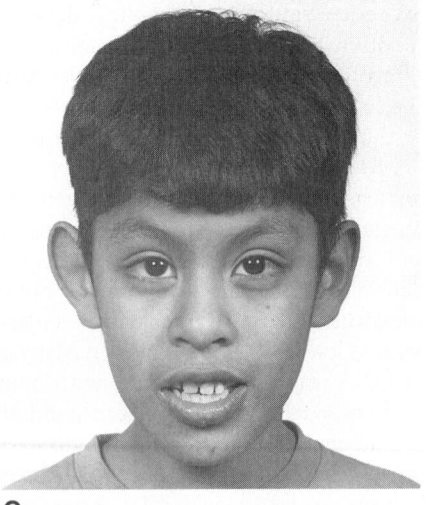

A   B   C

Figure 9-8. Boys with fragile X syndrome. Note the long faces, prominent jaws, and large ears and the similar characteristics of children from different ethnic groups: white **(A)**, Asian **(B)**, and Hispanic **(C)**. (From Jorde LB, Carey JC, Bamshad MJ, White RL: Medical Genetics, 3rd ed. Philadelphia, Mosby, 2003, p 99.)

of new molecular and statistical tools for estimating genetic variation have been applied widely to human populations to explain further the genetic basis of various medical conditions and traits, resulting in new insights about how evolutionary forces have shaped disease-related genetic variation in contemporary populations.

Genetic drift refers to the random fluctuations in gene frequencies that occur from generation to generation as a result of sampling a limited number of gametes. As the size of the population decreases, the degree of fluctuation increases. Genes that are rare in large populations may be common in small populations or vice versa. Genetic drift can be caused by a substantial reduction in the size of a population (i.e., a population bottleneck) or the separation of a subset of a larger population (founder effect). According to well-maintained historical records, the Old Order Amish in Lancaster County, Pennsylvania, were established by approximately 50 couples. Nearly half of all the reported cases of Ellis–van Creveld syndrome (an autosomal recessive skeletal dysplasia characterized by short stature, polydactyly, and cardiac defects) have been identified in the Amish population. The gene for Ellis–van Creveld syndrome was identified, but its function remains unknown. The relatively small founding population of the Amish and their custom of marrying only within their relatively isolated community (i.e., endogamy) have resulted in a high carrier frequency of the disease-causing allele of Ellis–van Creveld syndrome.

Natural selection alters the frequency of a trait (e.g., disease condition) contingent on the relative fitness of the genotype (or the success of a phenotype) in a given environmental context. Fitness reflects the ability of a genotype to survive and reproduce. As a consequence, the expectation is that phenotypes with a high fitness have been positively selected, whereas phenotypes with a low fitness have been negatively selected. Each individual's genotype is different (with the exception of monozygotic twins), however, and the lives of individuals with identical genotypes at a single locus differ. Many genes have pleiotropic effects on the phenotype. It is difficult to assign fitness to a particular genotype or phenotype.

Nevertheless, some genotypes in human populations seem to have been affected by natural selection and illustrate the relationship between natural selection, genotypes, and phenotypes. The best-known example is the effect that natural selection has had on the frequency of HbS genotypes in sub-Saharan Africa, where heterozygotes are more resistant to infection with falciparum malaria than normal homozygotes. Individuals who are homozygotes for the sickle cell mutation are much more likely to die early. There is selection for the heterozygotes and selection against the homozygotes. The result is that the sickle cell gene persists at a relatively high frequency, mainly in heterozygotes.

More recently, certain genotypes of CC *chemokine receptor 5 (CCR5)*, one of the cell surface receptors used by human immunodeficiency virus type 1 (HIV-1) to enter certain T cells and macrophages, seem to have been affected by natural selection. Individuals who are homozygous for a 32-bp deletion in *CCR5* are relatively resistant to infection with HIV-1. This polymorphism seems to have arisen relatively recently, and it has achieved a high frequency only in some European populations. This situation has led to the hypothesis that this polymorphism was positively selected in Europeans, although the selective force that was responsible remains to be identified.

Consanguinity is defined as the mating of related individuals. Although consanguinity is relatively rare in Western populations, it is common in many populations of the world. Mating between first cousins occurs in 20% to 50% of marriages in many countries of the Middle East, and uncle-niece and first-cousin marriages are common in South India. Consanguinity increases the chances that both members of a mating couple will carry the same disease allele. Consanguineous matings are more likely to produce offspring affected with autosomal recessive disorders. If the disease-causing allele shared by the couple is extremely rare in the general population, and two carriers are unlikely ever to mate with one another, the only children reported with the disease may be the offspring of consanguineous matings. The corollary of this observation is that the presentation of a child with a rare autosomal recessive disorder increases the likelihood that the mating couple share a disease allele via a common ancestor.

Many studies have shown that mortality rates among the offspring of first-cousin marriages are substantially higher than in the general population. The prevalence of genetic disease is approximately twice as high among the offspring of first-cousin marriages. Few data exist about the mating of first-degree relatives (i.e., incestuous matings), although the prevalence of mental retardation, short stature, and major congenital anomalies is higher.

MULTIFACTORIAL DISORDERS

Single-gene disorders, such as cystic fibrosis and sickle cell disease, account for a relatively small proportion of the total disease burden in the pediatric population. A much larger proportion consists of conditions that are thought to arise from the interaction of multiple genetic and environmental factors, so-called multifactorial traits. These include most cases of neural tube defects, structural heart defects, isolated cleft lip/palate, autism, and type 1 diabetes. Although these conditions are either present or absent in an individual, many quantitative traits (e.g., height, blood pressure) exhibit a normal distribution in human populations. The risk of developing a multifactorial condition is modeled by a liability distribution with a bell-shaped curve. An individual with enough liability factors to place him or her over a liability threshold will be affected with the condition.

In some cases, the threshold may be higher in one sex than in the other. Pyloric stenosis is a classic example of a multifactorial disease that seems to follow a sex-specific threshold model. It affects approximately 1 in 1000 females and approximately 1 in 200 males. The liability threshold seems to be higher for females than for males (Fig. 9-9). Accordingly, affected females should possess more liability factors than should affected males. Having more risk factors, affected females would be more likely to produce affected offspring. The recurrence risk is considerably higher for the offspring of affected females than for the offspring of affected males.

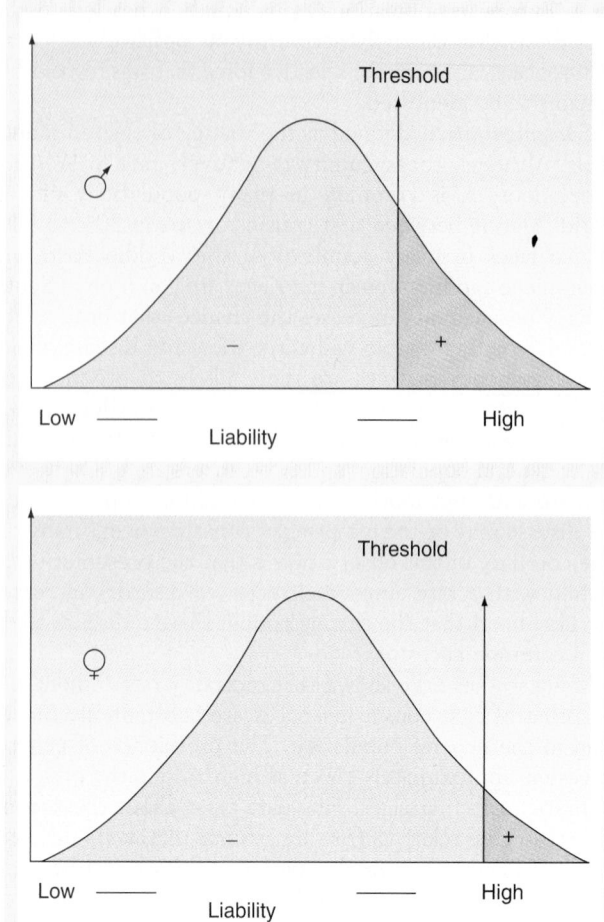

Figure 9-9. A liability distribution for a multifactorial disease in a population. To be affected with the disease, an individual must exceed the threshold on the liability distribution. This figure shows two thresholds, a lower one for males and a higher one for females (as in pyloric stenosis). (Modified from Jorde LB, Carey JC, Bamshad MJ, White RL: Medical Genetics, 3rd ed. Philadelphia, Mosby, 2003, p 241.)

Hirschsprung's disease is a malformation that results from an absence of intrinsic ganglion cells in the myenteric and submucosal plexus of the colon. Analysis of families in which Hirschsprung's disease was segregating in a mendelian pattern led to the isolation of several genes that cause Hirschsprung's disease, including *RET*, the *endothelin B receptor*, and the gene encoding its ligand, *EDN3*. Subsequently, sib pairs from families in which the Hirschsprung's disease genes seemed to be segregating like a complex trait were found to share alleles at these three loci more than 80% of the time. It seems that each allele increased the susceptibility to Hirschsprung's disease, and for most sib pairs, the combination of all disease-causing alleles at three loci led to the development of Hirschsprung's disease.

Recurrence Risks for Multifactorial Diseases

Recurrence risks for single-gene diseases are known with considerable certainty (e.g., 50% for an autosomal dominant disease). This certainty reflects the fact that the genetic mechanism and mode of inheritance are fairly well understood. In contrast, the number of genetic and environmental factors is unknown for nearly all multifactorial disorders. For these diseases, empirical recurrence risks

(i.e., risks based on direct observation) are estimated by identifying a population of affected individuals, then tabulating the proportion of their relatives who are affected by the same disease. Suppose that 1000 siblings of individuals affected with a congenital heart defect have been identified. If 50 of these siblings also are affected with a heart defect, the empirical recurrence risk is 5%. Because risk factors may vary between populations, the empirical recurrence also can vary from one population to another. Empirical risk factors are population-specific.

Patterns of recurrence risks for multifactorial disorders differ in several important ways from the patterns observed for single-gene disorders. First, the recurrence risk increases as the number of affected individuals in a family increases. The sibling recurrence risk for a ventricular septal defect is approximately 3% if one sibling is affected. If two siblings are affected in the same family, the recurrence risk increases to 10%. In contrast, recurrence risks for single-gene disorders remain the same regardless of the number of affected individuals in the family. Second, the recurrence risk is higher if the affected individual is a member of the less commonly affected sex. An affected individual who is a member of the less commonly affected sex is thought to lie farther toward the tail of the liability distribution, as discussed for pyloric stenosis. Relatives of this individual have a higher recurrence risk. Third, the recurrence risk tends to increase if the affected individual is more severely affected. More severe expression of a multifactorial disease is thought to be found in families with a greater number of risk factors. This situation should result in higher recurrence risk for relatives of the proband. The recurrence risk for relatives of an individual with bilateral cleft lip/palate is higher than that for relatives of an individual with a unilateral cleft. Fourth, the recurrence risk decreases rapidly as the degree of relationship decreases between the proband and his or her relatives. For single-gene disorders, the recurrence risk decreases by half for each successive degree of relationship (e.g., for an autosomal dominant disease, the recurrence risk is 50% for siblings, 25% for uncle-niece or grandparent-grandchild relationships, 12.5% for first cousins, and so on). The more rapid decrease seen for multifactorial disorders reflects the fact that many genetic and environmental factors typically must combine to cause the trait, and these are unlikely to be present in less closely related family members. Last, the recurrence risk for a multifactorial disorder is correlated with the prevalence of the disease in a population. In contrast, for single-gene disorders, the recurrence risk is largely independent of prevalence.

APPLICATION TO PEDIATRIC PRACTICE

The most substantial impact of genetic variation on pediatric disease is likely to be the consequence of identifying the effects of genetic variants on the pathogenesis and outcome of multifactorial traits (e.g., drug responses) and conditions previously considered to be influenced largely by the environment (e.g., infections). Some of these genetic variants have been known for decades (e.g., inherited deficiency of plasma cholinesterase and prolonged muscle relaxation with suxamethonium or FY*O Duffy allele homozygotes resistant to infection with vivax malaria). These variants are transmitted in simple mendelian patterns, whereas most drug-response and disease phenotypes are not. Using data from the Human Genome Project, newly developed analytical methods, and high-throughput screening methods, such as micro-arrays, many of the genetic variants influencing complex drug-response and disease phenotypes rapidly are becoming known.

It is becoming increasingly clear that the toxicity and treatment efficacy of various medications depend in part on heritable differences in the metabolism, disposition, and targets of drugs. The study of how an individual's genetic constitution affects his or her response to medications is called *pharmacogenetics*. Inherited differences in drug metabolism tend to be monogenic traits, whereas the overall pharmacologic effects of drugs are complex traits. Both types of genetic variants can explain observations made by the generalist pediatrician. In some children, sulfonamide-induced hypersensitivity reactions are caused by diminished acetylation activity caused by polymorphisms in the gene encoding N-acetyltransferase. Likewise, the effectiveness of inhaled β-adrenergic agonists in individuals with asthma is determined in part by polymorphisms in the gene encoding the β-adrenergic receptor. Polymorphisms in drug-metabolizing enzymes also have a major effect on the toxicity and efficacy of medications used to treat acute lymphoblastic leukemia, and, more importantly, individualizing drug dosages for children with acute lymphoblastic leukemia can improve their clinical outcome.

Susceptibility to infection and the outcome of infection with many common pathogens depend in part on host genetic variants. This situation is not surprising given that the barriers through which pathogens enter the human body and the nature and degree of the immunologic response to a pathogen are influenced by the genetic constitution of the host. Polymorphisms in the regulatory region of CCR5 have been associated with varying HIV-1 disease susceptibility and progression, including the risk of vertical transmission in children exposed perinatally to HIV-1. Polymorphisms in the gene encoding the receptor for the Fc fragment of IgG have been associated with an increased risk for pneumococcal pneumonia, and the risk of acquiring tuberculosis seems to be influenced by at least several genes. Given the complexity of host defenses and the countermeasures of pathogens, it would be a formidable task to determine which polymorphisms have the greatest effect on disease phenotypes.

Genetic polymorphisms also have been associated with diseases of unknown etiology and complex inheritance patterns. Polymorphisms in a gene called *CARDIS* have been associated with an increased susceptibility for Crohn's disease, and at least six additional loci have been associated with inflammatory bowel disease. These discoveries have provided new insights about the pathogenesis of inflammatory bowel disease. Understanding the molecular and cellular mechanism by which these polymorphisms predispose the host to Crohn's disease may facilitate the development of new therapeutic interventions.

Ultimately, knowledge of the genetic basis of the simple and complex conditions that are encountered commonly by pediatricians would enable the development of improved diagnostics (e.g., comprehensive newborn screening tests) and foster a better understanding of the natural history of these disorders. This understanding would enhance the ability of the pediatric clinician to provide improved anticipatory guidance and health care supervision, placing an even greater emphasis on preventive care. In the future, newborns may be tested to determine who among them is likely to be at higher risk for developing attention-deficit hyperactivity disorder, recurrent otitis media, acute lymphoblastic leukemia, or asthma. The health care of a child at risk for one or more of these conditions subsequently could be adapted to minimize their chances for developing the disease-related phenotype. This is analogous to the existing screening programs for phenylketonuria or galactosemia. When a child does develop an illness, however, the pediatric health care provider also would be able to organize an individually tailored therapeutic plan that is more likely to be successful and less likely to cause adverse effects.

SUGGESTED READINGS

Crow JF: The origins, patterns and implications of human spontaneous mutation. Nat Genet Rev 2000;1:40–47.

Jorde LB, Carey JC, Bamshad MJ, White RL: Medical Genetics, 3rd ed Philadelphia, Mosby, 2003.

Rimoin DL, Connor JM, Pyeritz RE (eds): Emery and Rimoin's Principles and Practice of Medical Genetics, 3rd ed. New York, Churchill Livingstone, 1997.

Scriver CR, Sly WS, Childs B, et al (eds): The Metabolic and Molecular Bases of Inherited Disease, 8th ed. New York, McGraw-Hill, 2000.

Strachan T, Read AP: Human Molecular Genetics, 2nd ed. New York, Wiley-Liss, 1999.

Table 10-2. Lymphocyte Surface Markers

CD Number	Cell Lineage	Comment
CD3	T cells	Part of TCR/CD3 complex
CD4	T cells	Helper T cells; binds to HLA class II
CD8	T cells and NK cells	Cytotoxic T cells; binds to HLA class I
CD10	Early B cells	Common ALL antigen
CD11a	Leukocytes	Adhesion molecule; with CD18 binds to ICAM-1, ICAM-2, and ICAM-3
CD11b, c	NK, granulocytes, macrophages	Adhesion molecule; with CD18 binds to C3bi
CD16	NK, granulocytes, macrophages	Fc receptor for IgG (FcγRIII)
CD19	B cells	Mature B cells
CD34	Precursor cells	Used to estimate stem cell number
CD45RO	Leukocytes	Denotes the memory T cell
CD45RA	Leukocytes	Denotes the naive T cell
CD56	NK	Used with CD16 to measure NK cells
CD69	Activated lymphocytes and macrophages	Measures activation; used as early test of lymphocyte response to stimulus

Phenotypes Used to Define Major Lymphocyte Subsets*

Immature T cell (thymocyte)
  CD3+CD4+CD8+
Mature T cells (peripheral blood or lymphoid tissue)
  CD3+CD4+CD8-RA+—recent émigré of the thymus; naive helper T cell (i.e., never antigen stimulated)
  CD3+CD4+CD8-RO+—memory helper T cell
  CD3+CD4-CD8+RA+—naive cytotoxic T cell
  CD3+CD4-CD8+RO+—memory cytotoxic T cell
Mature B cells
  CD19+
NK cells
  CD16+CD56+
Approximate percentage distribution of major subsets
  CD3+CD4+—50%
  CD3+CD8+—25%
  CD19+—20%
  CD16+CD56+—5%

*Use of multiple surface markers simultaneously is more precise. Percentages vary slightly with age; see Conley ME, Stiehm ER: Immunodeficiency disorders: General considerations. In Stiehm ER (ed): Immunologic Disorders in Infants and Children, 4th ed. Philadelphia, WB Saunders, 1996, p 217, for details.
ALL, acute lymphocytic leukemia; HLA, human leukocyte antigen; ICAM, intracellular adhesion molecule; NK, natural killer; TCR, T-cell receptor.

surface markers, CD4 and CD8. CD4-bearing T cells react with class II MHC molecules, and CD8 T cells react with class I MHC molecules. In the early stages of development, the primitive T cell bears CD4 and CD8 on its surface (double-positive cells), and the T-cell receptor (TCR) is present only in a primitive form. Only the cells that can combine with the host's transplantation antigens, which are displayed on the thymus stromal cells, are selected for further growth and development—a positive selection step. The cells that fail this first cut (95% of the precursors) die.

With further differentiation, a mature TCR is expressed, and either CD4 or CD8 is down-regulated so that only single positive TCR-bearing lymphocytes remain. The positively selected self-recognizing cells bind to the stromal cells with varying degrees of affinity. The cells that bind tightly are potentially organ destructive (too "antiself") and are eliminated—a negative selection process. Only the survivors of these initial screenings proceed through the remainder of the differentiation process and leave the thymus as mature cells, passing through the walls of medullary venules into the peripheral circulation. Circulating T cells exit from the blood via high cuboidal endothelial cells lining the venules of the paracortical areas of the lymph nodes and Peyer's patches. After a period of residence in lymph nodes, lymphocytes enter the lymphatic system via the afferent channel and travel to the thoracic duct, from which they reenter the peripheral circulation.

All antigen-recognizing receptors of the immune system have the same basic two-chain structure (Fig. 10-1). Each chain consists of a variable region, which contacts the antigenic site and is different for each lymphocyte clone that can respond, and a constant region, which is the same for all receptors, regardless of the antigen specificity. TCRs achieve their ability to combine with countless numbers of antigens through the process of gene rearrangements that generate the different variable regions. Instead of each combining site being coded by a single gene, the receptor combining sites are the results of the combination of noncontiguous blocks of DNA, known as the V (variable), D (diversity), and J (joining) segments. Selections from V, D, and J regions ultimately are combined to a constant β gene to form the β chain, whereas only V and J segments are joined to the constant region of the α chain. Each of the V, D, or J regions contains several small segments, one of which is used randomly to form the final receptor polypeptide chain. This random combination provides in the neighborhood of 10^{18} different possibilities for the combining site.

About 5% of the peripheral T cells have a TCR composed of γ and δ chains rather than α and β chains. In contrast to the α/β T cells, the γ/δ T cells can combine with antigen not complexed with MHC products. Their importance in the immune response is unknown at this time.

The antigen encounter is an external signal that notifies the T cell to initiate the remaining events of the immune response.

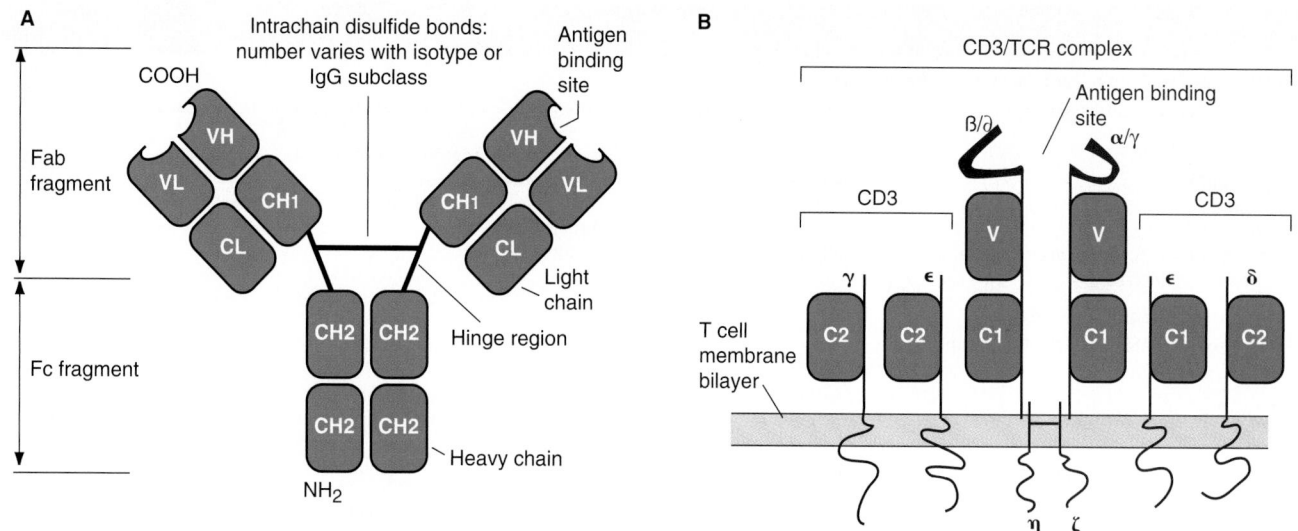

Figure 10-1. Basic immunoglobulin and T-cell receptor (TCR) structures. **A,** Immunoglobulins are composed of units consisting of two identical heavy-chain/light-chain pairs. Each chain is composed of domains that represent similar (but not identical) arrangements of approximately 110 amino acids, stabilized by disulfide bonds. Constant domains are the same for each molecule of a given isotype. The specificity for antigens is provided by the variable domains, which are different for each individual antibody. Binding occurs in the Fab fragments; amplification of the binding response (e.g., complement fixation) is accomplished by the Fc fragment, which also controls the biologic behavior (e.g., placental passage), characteristic of each isotype. **B,** The TCR also consists of two polypeptide chains (α and β) with constant and variable domains. As with immunoglobulins, antigen binding is provided by variable domains on each chain. The TCR signal must be internally transduced to initiate the T-cell response, but as can be seen, the TCR receptor chains have virtually no cytoplasmic tails. The TCR requires the complexed CD3 chains to accomplish signal transduction. The ηζ heterodimer shown is found in about 20% of the T cells; most (80%) use a ηη homodimer. The TCR also requires CD3 to be expressed on the T-cell surface. Not shown are important coreceptors that are necessary to strengthen the engagement of the T cell to the antigen-presenting cell (APC) to permit effective antigen presentation. These include CD4 and CD8, which are integral parts of the T-cell/APC interaction. The antigen to which the TCR reacts must be presented as a part of a major histocompatibility complex (MHC)/peptide complex, and CD4 or CD8 binds directly to the MHC molecule, CD4 with class II MHC and CD8 with class I MHC. C, constant domain; COOH, carboxyl terminus; Fab, antigen-binding fragment; Fc, crystallizable fragment; NH2, amino terminus; V, variable domain; α, β, the chains of the TCR; γ, δ, ε, ζ, η, the chains of CD3; C1, C2, domains of TCR and CD3 showing homology with respective immunoglobulin constant domains.

The external message must be transduced internally to produce synthesis and secretion of new proteins. The TCR lacks the intracytoplasmic extensions to accomplish signal transduction. To be functional, the TCR must be coexpressed with CD3 molecules that accomplish internal signaling. The CD3 complex is composed of five chains (γ, δ, ε, ζ, η), which embrace the short cytoplasmic tails of the TCR (see Fig. 10-1).

T cells show the capacity for long life (years), and most of the T cells in adults were differentiated well before adolescence. Because of their long-lived attributes, individuals can survive with normal T-cell function even after total thymectomy in early life. These individuals would not fare well if they had a catastrophic loss of T cells (e.g., lethal radiation or ablation for bone marrow transplantation) and were required to recreate the T-cell repertoire completely. The thymus normally involutes with age. It previously was believed that there was virtually no thymic output in adult life, but on sufficient demand, thymuses from adult patients can produce some new T lymphocytes, although the capacity is not equal to that of a young child or adolescent.

T cells accomplish their objectives through the secretion of chemicals called *cytokines*, which stimulate proliferation and promote intercellular and intracellular interactions. The cytokines important in the immune processes are termed *interleukins* (Table 10-3). Different responses are used to control different types of infectious agents. All of these final effector functions are initiated by peptides derived from proteins of the infecting agent that have been degraded in the target cell. Antigen fragments that are degraded in cytoplasmic vesicles subsequently are expressed on the cell surface complexed to MHC class II. They combine with CD4+ T cells, of which there are two subtypes, thymus helper 1 (TH1) and thymus helper 2 (TH2), classified according to the cytokine profile that they release on activation. TH1 cells secrete interferon-γ, tumor necrosis factor, CD40 ligand, granulocyte colony-stimulating factor, and Fas ligand—all of which activate macrophages. This activation results in enhanced macrophage killing and a major inflammatory response leading to granuloma formation; this would be the principal way in which T cells would combat mycobacterial or lepromatous infections. TH2 cells secrete primarily IL (interleukin)-4, IL-5, and CD40 ligand, which have their primary action on B cells, promoting antibody formation. Cytotoxic T cells (CD8+) react with MHC class I complexed peptides, which result from degraded bacterial or viral products expressed on target cell surfaces. On engagement, they release perforin, granzymes, and Fas ligand, which result in the death of the target cell by lysis or a DNA-dissolving process termed *apoptosis*. Apoptosis, or programmed cell death, is an important means of controlling virally infected cells. Apoptosis is marked by DNA fragmentation; not only nuclear DNA, but also viral DNA is susceptible. When a virally infected cell is killed by apoptotic mechanisms, the virus also is destroyed so that a shower of infectious virus cannot follow cell lysis, as would occur in cells destroyed by antibody-complement lytic mechanisms.

Table 10-3. Cytokines*

Cytokines Involved in Natural Immune Responses

Type I IFNs (IFN-α and IFN-β)	Inhibit viral replication, inhibit cell proliferation, activate NK cells, up-regulate class I MHC molecule expression
TNF-α	Mediates host response to gram-negative bacteria and other infectious agents
IL-1α and IL-β	Mediate host inflammatory response to infectious agents
IL-1Rα	Natural antagonist of IL-1; blocks signals delivered by IL-1
IL-6	Mediates and regulates inflammatory responses
Chemokines (IL-8, monocyte chemotactic protein-1; RANTES)	Mediate leukocyte chemotaxis and activation

Lymphocyte Regulatory Cytokines

Immunostimulatory or Growth-Promoting

IL-1	Costimulates activation of T cells
IL-2	Growth factor for T, B, and NK cells; activates effector cells
IL-4	T- and B-cell growth factor; stimulates IgE production; up-regulates classes I and II MHC molecule and FcRεII expression on macrophages; expansion of TH2 subset
IL-5	B-cell growth and activation; differentiation of eosinophils (?)
IL-6	Growth factor for B cells; activates T cells
IL-7	Stromal cell factor; growth factor for precursor B and T cells
IL-10	Growth and differentiation factor for B cells
IL-9	Growth factor for T cells
IL-12	Expansion of TH1 subset; activates B cells, NK cells, and monocytes
IL-13	Growth and differentiating factor for B cells; stimulates IgE production; up-regulates classes I and II MHC molecule and FcRεII expression on macrophages
TNF-β	Stimulates effector cell function
IFN-γ	Activates macrophages, NK cells; up-regulates classes I and II MHC molecule expression; inhibits IL-4- or IL-13-induced IgE production

Immunosuppressive

IL-1Rα	Regulates IL-1 activities
TGF-β	Antagonizes lymphocyte responses
IL-10	Inhibits activities of TH1 cells

Hematopoiesis-Regulating

GM-CSF, G-CSF, M-CSF	Colony-stimulating factors
Erythropoietin	Differentiation of erythroid precursors
IL-3, SCF, c-kit receptor	Regulate stem cell development
IL-4	Mast cell development
IL-5	Eosinophil differentiation and proliferation
IL-6	Differentiation of megakaryocytes, hematopoietic precursors

Proinflammatory

IL-1, TNF-α, IL-6	Participate in the acute-phase response and synergize to mediate inflammation, shock, and death

Anti-Inflammatory

IL-4	Reduces endotoxin-induced TNF and IL-1 production
IL-6	Inhibits TNF production
IL-10	Suppresses lymphocyte functions and down-regulates production of proinflammatory cytokines
IL-13	Down-regulates functions of macrophages; suppresses production of proinflammatory cytokines
TGF-β	Has immunosuppressive effects, inhibits IL-1 and TNF gene expression
IL-1Rα	Competes with the binding of IL-1 to its cell surface receptors and blocks IL-1 effects
TNFsR	Soluble TNF receptors; block interaction of TNF with target cell

*See Rosen FS, Wedgwood RJ, Eibl M, et al: Primary immunodeficiency diseases: Report of a WHO Scientific Group. Clin Exp Immunol 1997;109(Suppl):1–28, for more listings and information.

G-CSF, granulocyte colony-stimulating factor; GM-CSF, granulocyte-monocyte colony-stimulating factor; IFN, interferon; IL, interleukin; M-CSF, macrophage colony-stimulating factor; MHC, major histocompatibility complex; NK, natural killer; RANTES, regulated on activation, T-cell expressed and secreted; SCF, stem cell factor; TGF, transforming growth factor; TH1, thymus helper 1; TH2, thymus helper 2; TNF, tumor necrosis factor.

Modified in part from Buckley RH: The child with suspected immune deficiency. In Behrman RE, Kliegman RM, Jenson HB (eds): Nelson Textbook of Pediatrics, 16th ed. Philadelphia, WB Saunders, 2000, p 592.

B Cells

B cells pass through a complex series of stages before their development into antibody-producing plasma cells, occurring within the same time frame as the developing T-cell population. B-cell differentiation occurs in the fetal liver and later the bone marrow, inductive microenvironments where lymphoid progenitor cells undergo commitment to B-cell lineage.

Because the surface immunoglobulin receptor is the unique characteristic of a B cell, commitment of a stem cell to the B-cell lineage is marked by rearrangement of the immunoglobulin heavy-chain and light-chain genes. This rearrangement occurs in an orderly sequential manner, with heavy-chain gene rearrangement occurring first. These early B

cells, called *pro-B cells*, progress to the large pre-B-cell stage, which is marked by a surface receptor containing a μ-chain and a light-chain surrogate. After this receptor is triggered by an as yet unknown ligand, the large pre-B cells proliferate and give rise to a resting population of small pre-B cells, in which the light-chain genes now begin to rearrange. At this stage, IgM is found only in the cytoplasm. After productive rearrangement of the light-chain genes, a normal IgM receptor can be expressed on the surface, defining the immature B-cell stage. At this point, antigen encounters lead to deletion of the immature B cells, providing an important mechanism of creating self-tolerance. Subsequently, alternative heavy-chain splicing produces IgM and IgD, which are displayed simultaneously on the surface of what is now the mature B cell. The cell is now ready to leave the bone marrow and populate the organized collection of B cells around the body—the spleen, lymph nodes, and various tissues, such as Peyer's patches of the intestine. There, B cells encounter antigen to begin the process of acquired B-cell immunity.

The stromal cells of the bone marrow are especially adapted to promote the differentiation of B-cell progenitors. Similarly, stromal cells of the peripheral lymphoid tissues are adapted to promote antigen responsiveness and B-cell proliferation.

Activation of the B cell by antigen is accomplished by binding to the antigen receptor, the surface immunoglobulin found on each B cell, which denotes the specificity and the immunoglobulin class that is secreted. In contrast to T cells, complexing of the antigen epitope to MHC class I or class II is not required for activation. The antigen structure must be such as to cross-link the receptors (e.g., the repeating epitopes of polysaccharide coats of bacteria) to effect signal transduction; alternatively, antigens within the B-cell receptor can be presented to helper T cells, which then activate B-cell signaling. Interactions with T cells are facilitated by expression of CD40, which reacts with the T-cell CD40 ligand (CD40L or gp39), and CD80 and CD86, which interact with the T-cell molecules, CD28 and CTLA. CD40 binding with CD40L also induces class switching so that the B-cell response subsequently can include IgG, IgA, and IgE synthesis and secretion. The sequence of antibody response is IgM initially, followed by IgG, IgA, and possibly IgE, after class switching of the initial responding clone.

The signals received on the surface of the B cell are transduced internally to activate a series of cytosolic protein tyrosine kinases, initiating the cascade of events that leads to DNA binding and subsequently gene expression, immunoglobulin synthesis, and immunoglobulin secretion. For sufficient antibody to be produced to control an infection effectively, the number of B cells must be increased; this is accomplished by interactions with helper T cells, follicular dendritic cells, and macrophages, which produce the necessary growth factors. The final step in B-cell differentiation is the plasma cell. The progression from activated B lymphocyte is marked by a gradual loss of MHC class II and surface immunoglobulin molecules, along with conversion from synthesis of membrane-type to secretory immunoglobulin molecules with their hydrophilic tails. Plasma cells rarely divide and usually live for only a few days.

Some members of the activated B-cell clone do not undergo terminal plasma cell differentiation. These long-lived cells serve as memory B cells, which are triggered relatively easily by antigen on re-exposures, accounting for the anamnestic or recall antigen response, which is faster and greater in magnitude than seen with the initial encounter with antigen. The recall response also primarily involves IgG-secreting clones.

Immunoglobulins

There are five major types of immunoglobulins, termed *isotypes*: *IgM, IgG, IgA, IgE,* and *IgD*. Each has characteristics that allow the humoral immune system to operate most efficiently in different environmental conditions throughout the body and at different stages of the pathogen/host encounter. Normal serum levels vary with age (Table 10-4).

Immunoglobulins show a common structure, consisting of heavy-chain and light-chain pairs (see Fig. 10-1). The light chains have a molecular weight of 25 kd, and the heavy chains range from 50 to 60 kd. Two different light-chain classes, κ and λ, are used by all of the different isotypes. Approximately 60% of the molecules use κ, and 40% use λ. No functional differences are imposed on the molecules by either light chain. The heavy chains, through their constant regions, control the unique physiologic characteristics of the immunoglobulin molecules, such as half-life, complement fixation ability, placental passage, and polymer formation. IgM occurs naturally as a pentamer, and some IgA molecules are dimeric; polymerization is facilitated by a small polypeptide, the J chain (Fig. 10-2).

The antigen-combining site of the immunoglobulin is formed by the heavy chains and the light chains, by the variable regions formed by VDJ recombination as described previously for the TCR. The variable region is the same for all isotypes derived from the parent clone, giving rise to the same antigen specificity for IgM, IgD, IgG, IgA, and IgE derivatives. The different physiologic characteristics are conferred by the heavy-chain constant genes, which are designated by the Greek letter counterpart of the isotype name (i.e., μ, δ, γ, α, and ε) to which the variable genes are spliced.

The properties and characteristics of the different isotypes are shown in Table 10-5. Briefly, *IgM* can be considered a first line of defense. Its large size promotes binding early in the stage of antigen encounter before antibodies of higher affinity have a chance to develop, and its potent complement-activating characteristics enhance phagocytosis and complement-mediated lysis. IgG has a long half-life and can traverse the placenta. It is suited for more permanent immunity and is appropriate for passive transfer to the infant to provide protection during the early months of postnatal life.

IgA is adapted for pathogen control in the mucous secretions of the respiratory and gastrointestinal tracts, where its weak opsonic and complement-activating properties are irrelevant because these sites are lacking in phagocytes and complement. In secretions, IgA exists mostly as a dimer consisting of two units joined by a small, 15-kd polypeptide, the J chain. Secretory IgA is synthesized by plasma cells in the lamina propria of the respiratory and gastrointestinal tracts and transported through the luminal epithelium via the attachment of a 60-kd secretory component (see Fig. 10-2).

Table 10-4. Serum Immunoglobulin Levels by Age of Subject*

Age	IgG	IgM	IgA
Newborn	1031 ± 200	11 ± 5	2 ± 3
1–3 mo	430 ± 119	30 ± 11	21 ± 13
4–6 mo	427 ± 186	43 ± 17	28 ± 18
7–12 mo	661 ± 219	54 ± 23	37 ± 18
13–24 mo	762 ± 209	58 ± 23	50 ± 24
25–36 mo	892 ± 183	61 ± 19	71 ± 37
3–5 yr	929 ± 228	56 ± 18	93 ± 27
6–8 yr	923 ± 256	65 ± 25	124 ± 45
9–11 yr	1124 ± 235	79 ± 33	131 ± 60
12–16 yr	946 ± 124	59 ± 20	148 ± 63
>16 yr	1158 ± 305	99 ± 27	200 ± 61

*Values are in mg/dL ± 1 standard deviation.

Modified from Conley ME, Stiehm ER: Immunodeficiency disorders: General considerations. In Stiehm ER (ed): Immunologic Disorders in Infants and Children, 4th ed. Philadelphia, WB Saunders, 1996, p 216.

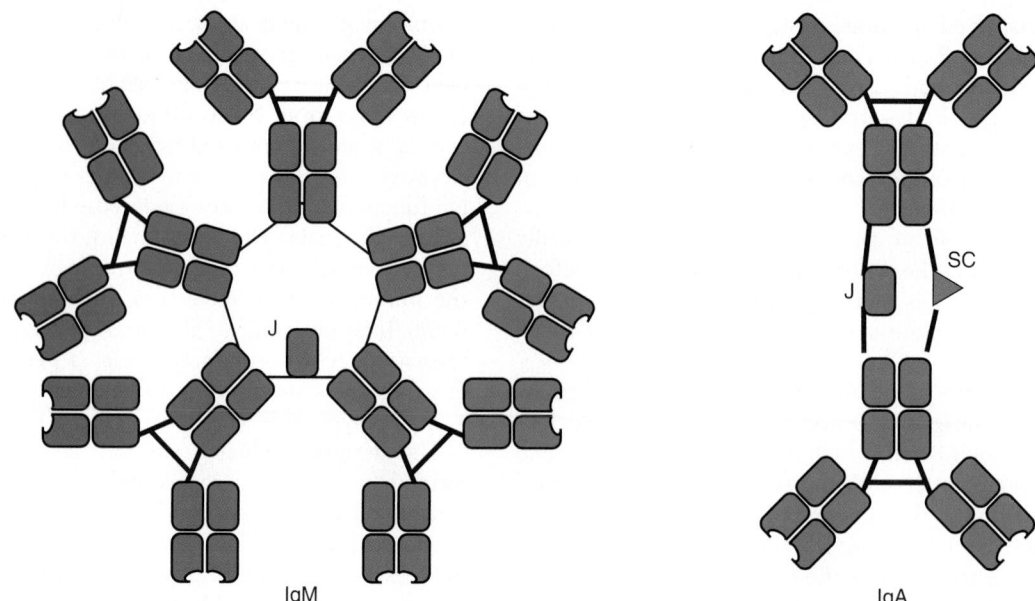

Figure 10-2. Polymeric forms of immunoglobulins. IgM is composed of five of the basic structures shown in Figure 10-1A. Polymeric forms are stabilized by J chain. Polymeric IgA is primarily a dimer. Secretory IgA, found primarily in respiratory and gastrointestinal tract secretions, contains, in addition to J chain, a fragment, secretory component (SC), produced by epithelial cells and bound to dimeric IgA to facilitate its passage into the lumen of the secretory organ.

Two subclasses of IgA, IgA1 and IgA2, are recognized. Normal serum IgA is about 90% IgA1 and 10% IgA2. In secretions, the amounts of IgA2 and IgA1 are almost equal.

IgE is bound to the surface of mast cells that secrete potent chemical mediators effective in the control of parasites. When IgE antibodies are triggered by airborne antigens, the mediator release can cause severe respiratory responses, such as bronchial constriction, and asthma results. Other allergic manifestations, such as diarrhea, anaphylaxis, urticaria, and swollen eyes, are mediated by IgE. Standards of hygiene maintained today make parasitic infestation uncommon, and the protection afforded by the IgE system usually is not needed. Nature has preserved a costly protective mechanism that is seldom, if ever, required to maintain health.

IgD is secreted primarily as a membrane protein and is involved in the differentiation of B cells. Cross-linking of the IgD molecules has a profound effect on the subsequent ability of a B cell to form antibody. IgD may play an important role in B-cell tolerization, although the specifics of its functions are unknown.

IgG also can be divided into four different *subclasses*, based on slight differences in amino acid sequence (see Table 10-5). The subclasses differ in their antigen responses and ability to activate complement, but their full impact on immune protection remains a controversial issue.

Neonatal and Infant Antibody Production

In human fetuses, the proportions of splenic lymphocytes bearing surface IgM, IgG, IgA, and IgD reach adult values by the beginning of the third trimester. Antibody synthesis in utero can be detected after the 20th week of gestation, particularly in response to intrauterine infection. Antibodies synthesized by the human fetus are mainly IgM and, to a lesser extent, IgA, although IgG synthesis in utero also has been detected under special circumstances. In the latter stages of pregnancy, however, most circulating antibodies in the fetus are obtained by transfer of maternal IgG via the placenta. The full-term human newborn infant has a serum IgG concentration slightly higher than the maternal level. Virtually no maternal IgA and IgM cross the placenta; cord blood contains less than 1% of IgA and about 10% of IgM found in maternal serum.

Maternal IgG is catabolized slowly, with a half-life of 1 month; by the third month of life, 87% of maternal IgG has been degraded. The loss of maternal IgG is replaced by the infant, but the rate of synthesis cannot maintain the serum levels at the birth values. The serum levels gradually fall, and in term infants, a nadir of approximately 400 mg/dL is reached between 3 and 4 months. Most of the maternal immunoglobulin is transferred to the infant in the last trimester, and premature infants have a lower level at

Table 10-5. Properties of Immunoglobulins

Property	IgG				IgA	IgM	IgD	IgE
	IgG1	IgG2	IgG3	IgG4				
Molecular weight ($\times 10^{-3}$ kd)	150	150	150	150	150–350	150–900	190	190
Present in secretions					++	±		
Crosses placenta	+	±	+	+	–	–	–	–
Fixes complement	++	+	++	–	–	+++	–	–
Binds to mast cells	–	–	–	+	–	–	–	++
Binds to macrophages	++	+	++	±		–		

birth and lower nadirs (60 to 104 mg/dL). Studies that tested the ability of intravenous IgG to prevent nosocomial or late-onset infections have failed to show clear-cut benefit for premature infants.

There is a hierarchy of response of the B cell to various antigens. The major clinical consequence is that the ability to make antibodies to polysaccharide antigens is delayed to relatively late in infancy. Immunization results first in the formation of IgM antibody responses, with a relatively slow progression to IgG antibody production. IgG responses are increased on recall stimulation. IgA antibody responses are more sluggish. This response pattern is reflected by the sequential acquisition of adult levels of serum immunoglobulins: IgM at 1 year, IgG at 5 to 7 years, and IgA at 10 to 14 years.

Natural Killer Cells

Some of the thymus-derived cells bear a CD8 marker but lack a TCR. They are termed *natural killer cells* because they can attack cells without prior sensitization. In vitro, natural killer cells have shown activity against tumor cells and virally infected targets. They bear the surface markers CD56 and CD16. Their role in host defense is unclear because only a few cases of absolute deficiency of natural killer cells have been reported, some with symptoms and some without. Natural killer cells seem to play a role in the early control of viral infections, particularly herpesvirus, keeping the infection under control until the immune response can accomplish elimination of the agent. There is little evidence to support natural killing as an important mechanism of tumor control.

Genes

The complexity of the interactions involved in the development and responses of the immune system involves many gene products. Mutation of a single gene can result in a primary immunodeficiency disorder. Extraordinary progress has been made in mapping of the human genome, including regions related to the immune system. To date, more than 60 genes have been described, and the first successful gene replacement has been accomplished for a disorder called *severe combined immunodeficiency disease* (Table 10-6). Because the competent immune response depends on differentiation, antigen recognition, signal transduction, proliferation, and synthesis/secretion, there are countless steps at which the process can be interrupted. The number of different immunodeficiency diseases is high (95 recognized to date), representing a formidable challenge to gene therapy.

Complement System

To contain a rapidly multiplying infectious agent effectively, the immune system needs to have a killing capacity. The antibodies produced by the B cells work in concert with the complement system to accomplish this end. In addition, complement further aids in the control of infection by promoting an inflammatory response.

The complement system consists of at least 20 serum protein components and many membrane bound proteins. A major function of the complement system is to control pathogens by lysis, which is accomplished by a group of 11 proteins, each activating another in a sequential manner, creating a biologic cascade. Other constituents of the system act as modulating influences, and others serve as cell surface receptors to focus the complement attack. These components interact in a delicately orchestrated manner, resulting in lysis of cells, phagocytosis of organisms, and local inflammation.

Activation of the complement system follows two pathways—classic or alternative. The classic route is initiated by antigen-antibody complexes and requires previous experience with the antigen to develop immunity. The alternative pathway is invoked by certain surfaces (e.g., microbial cell walls). Because specific antibody is not required, the alternative pathway is part of the innate host defenses that can be used early in life before immunization.

The classic components are denoted by the capital letter C and a number from *1* to *9* that refers to the order of their discovery, not their sequence in the cascade. The classic activation sequence nearly follows the discovery sequence except that C4 is activated before C2 (i.e., C1, C4, C2, C3, C5, C6, C7, C8, C9). The alternative pathway bypasses the initial components (C1, C4, and C2) and enters the cascade by activating C3. Thereafter, the two mechanisms follow the same pathway activating C5 through C9, leading to the formation of the macromolecular attack complex that inserts into cell membranes, resulting in lytic destruction of the target (usually a bacterium) (Fig. 10-3).

Activation of a component involves proteolytic cleavage resulting in a large fragment, designated *b* (e.g., C3b), which binds to the surface of the target and initiates cleavage of the next component of the cascade. Cleavage also generates small peptides, denoted *a*, which can induce inflammation. The early components of the alternative pathway are denoted by the capital letters *B* and *D*, and their cleavage products are denoted by *b* and *a*.

Antibody bound to antigen initiates the classic pathway as conformational changes of the antibody caused by antigen binding expose complement binding sites in the Fc portion of the immunoglobulin. IgM and all IgG subclasses except IgG4 activate complement. IgA, IgD, and IgE do not. IgM is particularly efficient, and only one molecule is required for activation, whereas two or more closely approximated molecules of IgG are necessary. Enzymatic cleavage of components C1 through C2 produces the classic pathway C3 convertase enzyme, and similarly cleavage of analogous alternative pathway early components yields the alternative pathway C3 convertase (see Fig. 10-3 for details).

C3b bound to target surfaces facilitates their interaction with cells bearing C3b receptors to enlist phagocytosis as a mode of pathogen control. Concurrently, C5 is cleaved, yielding C5b that aggregates with the later components, C6 through C9, to produce the membrane attack complex (C5b6789) that lyses the target. C5 cleavage also yields C5a, a potent anaphylatoxin and chemoattractant, causing a local inflammatory response to augment eradication of the inciting pathogen. Bound C3b also initiates activation of the entire cascade through the alternative pathway components B, D, and P, creating a positive feedback loop that greatly amplifies the magnitude of the response.

Table 10-6. Genes Involved in Primary Immunodeficiency Disease*

Disorder	Gene	Locus	Defect	Inheritance
Mostly Characterized by Defects in Antibody Production				
X-linked agammaglobulinemia (XLA)	BTK	Xq21.3	Defective B-cell development due to Bruton's tyrosine kinase deficiency	X
X-linked immunodeficiency with increased IgM (hyper-IgM syndrome)	CD40L	Xq26.3-q27.1	Deficiency of CD40 ligand without which T cells cannot effect isotype switching. T-cell deficiency also is present	X
Autosomal recessive hyper-IgM (HIGM2)	AICDA	12p13	Defect in activation-induced cytidine deaminase (AICDA); enzyme needed for isotype switching	AR
Major T-cell deficiency				
DiGeorge anomaly	DGCR	22q11.2, 10p	Monosomy at these loci lead to inadequate neural crest contribution to pharyngeal pouch derivatives with heart, facial, parathyroid, and thymus defects	AD
Interferon γ receptor deficiency	IFNGR1/2	6q23-24, 21q22.1	Mechanism unclear; increased susceptibility to mycobacteria and autoimmune endocrinopathy seen	AR
IL-12 p40 deficiency	IL12B	19p13.1	Interleukin receptor defect predisposes to mycobacterial infection	AR
Defects Involve T- and B-Cell Lines				
X-linked severe combined immunodeficiency disease (SCID)	IL2RG	Xq13.1	Normal cell growth and development prevented by defective γ chain of IL-2 receptor. B cells are present in this variety of SCID, but remain immature	X
JAK3 deficiency	Jak3	19p13.1	Janus-associated kinase3 (JAK3) is necessary for hematopoietic cell differentiation. Immature B cells are seen in this SCID variant also	AR
RAG1 deficiency	RAG1	11p13	Recombinase activating gene necessary in T/B cell differentiation to yield broadly diverse repertoire of antigen-responding cells. T and B cells are absent	AR
RAG2 deficiency	RAG2	11p13	Similar to RAG1 deficiency	AR
ADA deficiency	ADA	20q13.11	Failure to metabolize adenosine appropriately leads to accumulation of toxic metabolites, which poison lymphocytes	AR
PNP deficiency	PNP	14q13	Similar to ADA defect. Nucleoside phosphorylase metabolism is impaired. Toxic accumulations do not affect the B-cell lineage as much, however	AR
ZAP 70 deficiency	ZAP70	2q12	Defective tyrosine kinase signaling from CD3/TCR complex leads to poor T-cell lineage development. CD4+ T cells are present; CD8+ T cells are absent	AR
Affected Cell Lineages Not Clearly Defined				
Wiskott-Aldrich syndrome (WAS)	WASP	Xp11.22	The cytoskeletal protein, WASP, is altered, affecting platelet function and antigen processing	X
Ataxia-telangiectasia	ATM	11q22.3	Defects in cell cycle checkpoints lead to altered differentiation and cancer susceptibility	AR
X-linked lymphoproliferative syndrome	LYP	Xq24-q25	Inability to control Epstein-Barr virus infection leads to lymphoproliferation, aplastic anemia, and hypogammaglobulinemia	X
Defects Involving Phagocytes				
Leukocyte adhesion deficiency 1 (LAD1)	ITGB2	21q22.3	Surface receptor defect leads to poor adhesion	AR
Chronic granulomatous disease (CGD)	CYBB	Xp21.1	Cytochrome oxidase defect results in failure to produce oxidative products of the respiratory burst important in bactericidal killing	X
Autosomal recessive CGD	CYBA, NFC1, NFC2	16q24, 7q11.23, 1q25	Same as X-linked form	AR

*See Ochs H, Smith CIE, Puck JM (eds): Primary Immunodeficiency Diseases: A Molecular and Genetic Approach. New York, Oxford University Press, 1999, for additional listings. AR, autosomal recessive inheritance; X, X-linked inheritance.

Adapted from Rosen FS, Wedgwood RJ, Eibl M, et al: Primary immunodeficiency diseases: Report of a WHO Scientific Group. Clin Exp Immunol 1997;109(Suppl):15.

The extraordinary potency of the complement system is required to keep in check the powerful agents that can infect humans. Its ultimate activity must be controlled itself to prevent excessive systemic toxicity. In part, the system's effects are limited by the labile nature of the components that results in a relatively short biologic half-life. In addition, specific inhibitor proteins limit the intensity of the complement reactions. One of the most important of these is the C1 esterase inhibitor that dissociates the macromolecular complex of C1q, C1r, and C1s, which constitutes C1. Absence of C1 esterase inhibitor results in hereditary angioedema, a potentially fatal disorder, which exemplifies in a dramatic way the problems resulting from inadequate control of complement activation. Other important

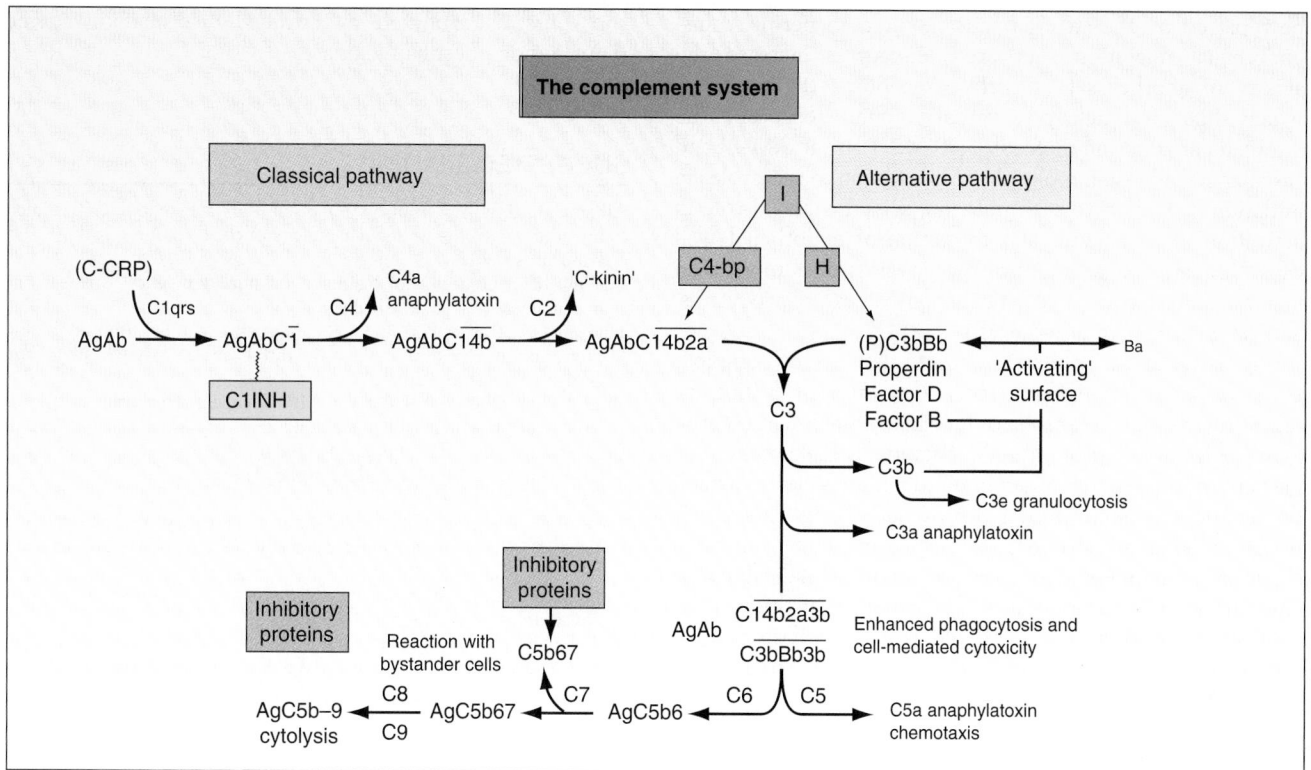

Figure 10-3. The complement cascade. Classic pathway activation is initiated by antigen-antibody (AgAb) interactions that activate the components in the sequence as shown beginning in the upper left-hand corner. As components are activated (shown by the bars over the numbers), the cleavage products initiate inflammatory activities or sequentially activate the later components in the sequence. Alternative pathway activation, shown beginning on the right, is independent of C1, C4, and C2. Both pathways can activate C3 and thereafter use the same pathway to yield cytolysis. This end point of the cascade occurs on activation of the remaining complement components from C5 to C9, yielding the membrane attack complex. Control of the cascade is maintained by inhibitory proteins (shown in boxes) that act at the sites shown by the wiggly lines. C3b can use the components of the alternative pathway in a positive feedback loop to amplify greatly the classic pathway–initiated reaction without the need of further AgAb complex formation. (Redrawn from Johnston RB Jr: The complement system. In Behrman RE, Kliegman RM, Jenson HB [eds]: Nelson Textbook of Pediatrics, 16th ed. Philadelphia, WB Saunders, 2000, p 629.)

regulators of the classic pathway include C4 binding protein and factor I, which interrupt C4/C2 interactions and promote C4b destruction.

The alternative pathway represents a way to activate the complement cascade without a preliminary antigen-antibody binding reaction. In this way, the inflammatory response generated by the complement system can be invoked in the nonimmunized individual. As such, the alternative pathway represents an innate protective mechanism.

The complement system genes are found on many different chromosomes. The genes for C2, C4, and factor B are located on chromosome 6 as part of the MHC, which, as described previously, plays a central role in the control of immune responses. Certain MHC allele patterns are associated with autoimmune diseases, suggesting a linkage of complement loci with important genetic determinants of autoimmunity. Other genes involved in the complement system are found on chromosome 1 (regulator of complement activation cluster, C1q), chromosome 11 (C1-INH), chromosome 12 (C1r, C1s), and chromosome 19 (C3).

Phagocytic System
The phagocytic cell system comprises neutrophils and monocytes/macrophages. The primary function of the phagocytic system is engulfment and killing of microbial organisms. The reticuloendothelial system, especially the spleen, also plays a

vital role in filtering pathogenic organisms from the blood. Phagocytosis is enhanced greatly by opsonization of the organisms with antibody and complement.

To accomplish their tasks, phagocytes must migrate to the area of need, engulf pathogens, and generate an inflammatory response. Vital to these functions are adherence and phagocytosis. In a manner analogous to T cells and B cells, surface receptors play important roles in initiating signaling events that activate the phagocyte for its protective roles. CR3, the complement receptor 3, consisting of an α_2 (CD11b) and a β_2 (CD18) subunit, is required for adherence and phagocytosis, whereas tumor necrosis factor receptors control inflammation.

Because the phagocytes are patrolling the body by circulating in the vasculature, to respond to areas of local need, they first must egress from the blood vessels through the capillary walls. Chemokines serve as chemoattractants and control shape change, granule release, and respiratory burst. CXC chemokines are effective for neutrophils, whereas CC chemokines are effective for monocytes, eosinophils, basophils, and lymphocytes.

A first step in initiating leukocyte extravascular emigration is slowing of rapidly flowing cells of the circulation. This phenomenon is called *rolling* and depends on surface molecules known as *selectins*, expressed on leukocytes and on endothelial cells. These relatively weak initial adhesions must be replaced by the strong bonds required to permit trans-endothelial migration. Activated leukocytes increase the avidity of another set of surface receptors, the integrins, which then bind tightly to vascular counterreceptors, the intercellular adhesion molecules (ICAM-1 and ICAM-2) and vascular cell adhesion molecule-1. In addition to their roles in initiation of leukocyte accumulation, selectins play a role in activation of leukocytes and formation of endothelial wall gaps. Similarly, engagement of the integrins does more than increase adhesiveness; cytokine responsiveness, phagocytosis, and gene expression are affected.

On arrival at the inflammatory site, leukocytes complete their response by phagocytosis and internal killing of organisms. Surface receptors for IgG and complement component C3 facilitate opsonization of bacteria by leukocytes. The particles are ingested as membrane bound vesicles to which the leukocyte granules fuse and subsequently discharge their lethal contents. In addition, the respiratory burst generates superoxide anion, hydrogen peroxide, hydroxyl radical, hypochlorous acid, and chloramines. The products of the respiratory burst are important in the control of catalase-positive organisms (e.g., *Serratia* and *Klebsiella* species). The respiratory burst is catalyzed by reduced nicotinamide adenine dinucleotide phosphate oxidase.

SUGGESTED READINGS

Alberts B, Bray D, Johnson A, et al (eds): Essential Cell Biology: Introduction to the Molecular Biology of the Cell. New York, Garland Publishers, 1997.
Conley ME: Genetics of primary immunodeficiency diseases. Rev Immunogenet 2000;2:231–242.
Janeway CA, Travers P, Walport M, Shlomchik M (eds): Immunobiology: The Immune System in Health and Disease, 5th ed. New York, Garland Publishing, 2001.
Krause K-H, Clark RA, Wymann MP: European workshop on the cell biology of phagocytes. J Leukoc Biol 1997;61:1–5.
Ochs H, Smith CIE, Puck JM (eds): Primary Immunodeficiency Diseases: A Molecular and Genetic Approach. New York, Oxford University Press, 1999.
Rosen FS, Wedgwood RJ, Eibl M, et al: Primary immunodeficiency diseases: Report of a WHO Scientific Group. Clin Exp Immunol 1997;109(Suppl):1–28.
Stiehm ER (ed): Immunologic Disorders in Infants and Children. Philadelphia, WB Saunders, 1996.
Wei J, Shaw LM, Mercurio AM: Integrin signaling in leukocytes: Lessons from the $\alpha_6\beta_1$ integrin. J Leukoc Biol 1997;61:397–407.

11 Principles of Metabolism

Nancy D. Leslie

The inborn errors of metabolism (IEOM) involve disruption of genes coding for proteins important in the intermediary metabolism of the cell. Most of these proteins are enzymes or transporters, and their function is to facilitate chemical conversion in pathways of synthesis, degradation, detoxification, or energy use. Transport function facilitates routing of the substrates to the appropriate cell or compartment for subsequent use or conversion. The traditional view is that a well-adapted organism possesses a large excess of catalytic potential at each step—hence the general rule that most inborn errors are recessive, that is, a single unaffected gene is sufficient to provide an adequate metabolic capacity in the heterozygote, but mutations in both copies (or in the only existing copy in the case of X-linked recessive conditions) result in significant deficiency and lead to phenotypic expression of the disease. Although this general rule is still relevant, exceptions do occur, and several examples are described in detail in this chapter.

A fundamental principle in intermediary metabolism is the "one gene–one enzyme" rule. The work of Beadle and Tatum using mutant yeast elegantly showed the application of this principle in a simple system. By irradiating (and mutating) yeast and growing mass cultures from single colonies, it was shown that such strains had distinct growth requirements when grown in a nutritionally incomplete medium. Nutrients essential for growth of one strain were found to be unnecessary for other strains. The different strains were able to supply required nutrients for each other, a phenomenon called *complementation*. The explanation for these phenomena was that each strain contained a mutation in one gene coding for one enzyme and that the remaining pathways were intact. The different collections of strains illustrated a series of defects in a metabolic pathway. Beadle and Tatum received the Nobel Prize in Physiology or Medicine in 1958 for this work.

Since the 1960s, numerous exceptions to the one gene–one enzyme rule have been documented, and it now is considered more appropriate to use the term *one gene–one polypeptide*. It is evident that some polypeptide subunits multitask; that is, they provide common subunits to enzymes with diverse catalytic activities. In such a situation, a mutation in the gene coding for the common subunit could produce catalytic defects in all of the assembled enzymes, even though only one mutant gene and its defective polypeptide gene product proved to be the underlying explanation. Other mechanisms for one gene affecting multiple catalytic activities are common protector proteins and common post-translational modifications (Fig. 11-1). These distinctions have practical implications in gene discovery, diagnosis, prognosis, and therapy.

The answer to the question of how much catalytic impairment is important is stated formally as the *threshold hypothesis*. This hypothesis states that a given level of substrate flux is necessary to prevent disease manifestations or, the converse, to facilitate normal metabolism. The level required depends on the requirement for production of a needed product or disposal of an upstream substrate, and the level at which pathology occurs may differ among cells, during development, or under conditions of environmental or contributory genetic stress. Perhaps the easiest way to think about this concept is to consider the consequences of construction on a major highway. Reduction of the number of available lanes or the allowable speed would curtail throughput, but still may be sufficient to get every car through that needs to pass. During peak traffic hours, such throughput would not be sufficient, however, and gridlock may occur. Should planned construction or an unplanned accident completely block the remaining lanes, no passage would occur, and the alternate routes also are likely to be flooded with extra cars.

Because metabolism is constitutive and adaptive, interruption or impairment of required pathways would be ex-pected to produce serious consequences on the cell and eventually the organism. If a pathway is constitutive and impairment nearly complete, these consequences would be expected to present early in development, perhaps during embryogenesis, and result in significant changes in cell functioning. A pathway that functions in a more adaptive manner might be called into play only when environmental stress requires it, or when disruption of other pathways amplifies its importance. The threshold hypothesis again can be invoked.

The consequences of disruption depend on what it is that perturbs the cell. Is the problem the lack of a needed product (product deficiency) or intoxication by an upstream substrate (substrate intoxication)? Necessary cofactors may be present in physiologic concentrations, which prove insufficient for an enzyme with a defective cofactor binding site. Stored product or abnormal enzyme may produce architectural distortions to cells and organs. The design of effective treatment strategies depends on the specifics of the problem. An important corollary is whether the effect of a disruption is specific to an individual cell or if the disease affects neighboring cells or distant organs. Therapy depends on the answer. Although there are many more disorders than there are clear answers to these questions, examples can be given for each type of dysfunction. Box 11-1 lists these common terms and concepts in metabolic disease.

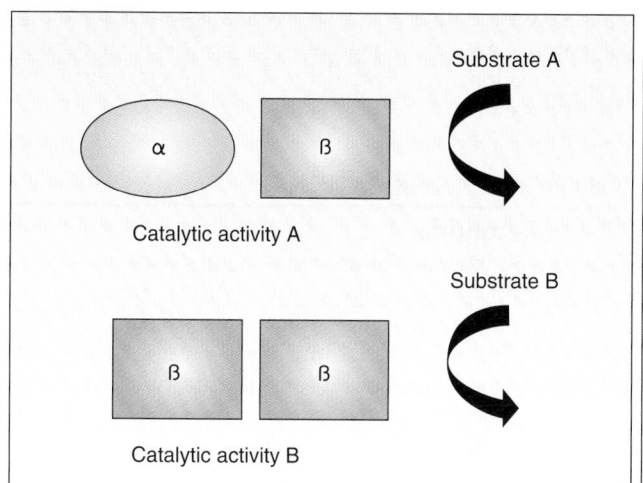

A

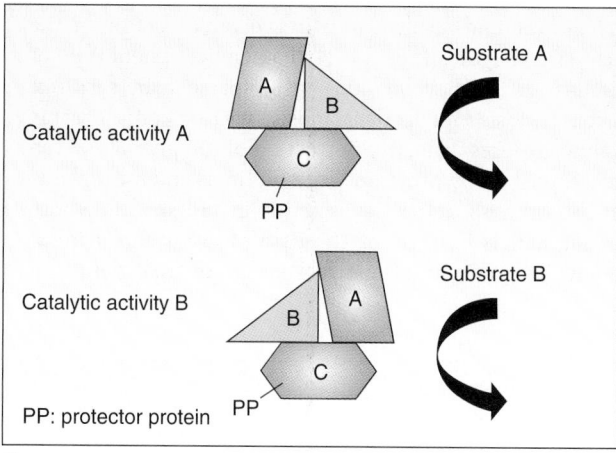

B

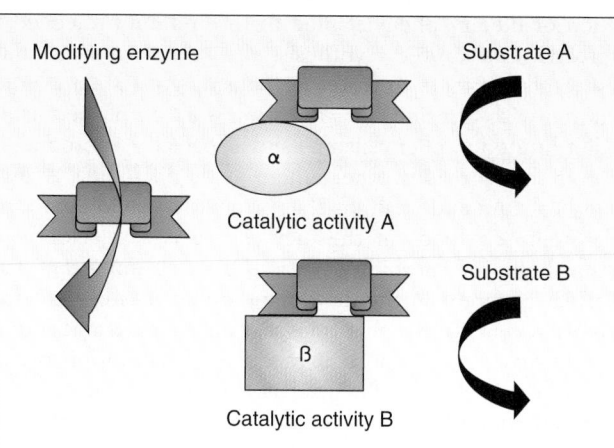

C

Figure 11-1. Exceptions to the one gene–one enzyme rule. **A,** Common units. In a heterodimeric protein, the subunits commonly are encoded by distinct genes. In the example shown, a defect in the gene encoding the a subunit would impair catalytic activity *A*, whereas a defect in the gene encoding the β subunit would impair activity *A* and *B*. **B,** A common protector protein PP stabilizes catalytic units *A* and *B*. A mutation in the gene encoding PP results in defective activities for both catalytic units. **C,** Several enzymes require activation by a common modifying enzyme. The genes and proteins for the catalytic units are intact but catalytically inactive.

Box 11-1. Common Terms and Concepts in Metabolic Disease

Product deficiency—lack of a needed product for function

Substrate intoxication—intoxication by accumulation of an upstream substrate

Cofactor dependency—disruption of the cofactor binding site by the mutation, causing poor catalytic activity at physiologic cofactor concentrations

Distortion of cell structure—substrates accumulate within organelles leading to distortion or death of cell

Cell autonomy—disruption of function within the cell expressing the gene defect

Organ-specific morbidity—the effect of a metabolic defect on specific target organs

Inborn errors of morphogenesis—endogenously produced compounds interfere with specific steps in embryogenesis

PRODUCT DEFICIENCY

Biotinidase Deficiency

Biotin is a cofactor necessary for proper activation of carboxylase enzymes. Most dietary biotin is protein bound and must be liberated for proper use. Biotin residues already present in the body are covalently attached to their cognate enzymes and must be cleaved for recycling. Biotinidase is a specific enzyme that accomplishes both of these functions. If this enzyme is deficient because of mutation in the biotinidase gene, patients become functionally biotin deficient, and the end result is impaired catalytic action of the carboxylase enzymes (Fig. 11-2). The clinical phenotype of biotinidase deficiency includes rash, sparse hair, seizures, and ketoacidosis and lactic acidosis, with specific organic acid abnormalities. Effective correction of the phenotype can be accomplished by providing free biotin as an oral replacement. Biotinidase deficiency often is included in newborn screening panels because of the ease of detection in mass screening programs and the effectiveness of treatment.

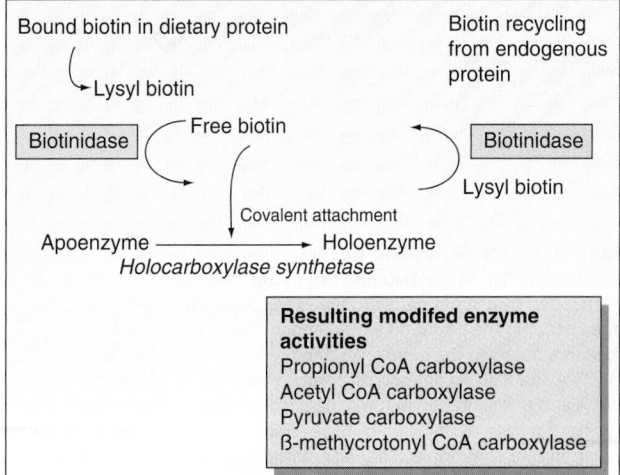

Figure 11-2. The biotinidase pathway. The enzyme biotinidase allows release of free biotin from ingested protein and recycling of biotin moieties from endogenous sources. Lack of sufficient free biotin results in impaired activation of the biotin-dependent carboxylases. The problem can be bypassed by providing readily absorbed free biotin.

Glucose-6-Phosphatase Deficiency

Circulating glucose is crucial to the fuel economy of humans. As creatures adapted to periodic meals with a long overnight fast, humans require storage of alimentary glucose and its retrieval during times of relative fasting. The formation of glycogen allows storage of glucose moieties in carbohydrate form, and the synthesis and degradation of glycogen is tightly regulated. In addition, several amino acids may be converted to glucose through the process of gluconeogenesis. The intracellular end product of glycogenolysis and gluconeogenesis is glucose-6-phosphate, which must be cleaved before free glucose can be exported from the cell for use in other tissues. Glycogen storage disease type Ia (glucose-6-phosphatase deficiency or von Gierke disease) results when all processes are intact up to the cleavage and export of glucose. The end result is significant hypoglycemia, which activates compensatory endocrine and metabolic systems. The clinical morbidity of glycogen storage disease type I is related to the hypoglycemia and the activation of these systems, which results in lactic acidemia, hypertriglyceridemia, hyperuricemia, fatty liver, and renal dysfunction. Effective treatment of this condition involves frequent daytime feedings, with continuous overnight glucose infusion through a nasogastric tube. In older infants, children, and adults, uncooked cornstarch can be substituted because it provides a source of "controlled-release" glucose over 4 hours. This treatment program requires considerable effort and compulsiveness on the part of parents and older patients but has been successful in improving longevity and decreasing chronic morbidity in these patients.

SUBSTRATE INTOXICATION

Phenylketonuria

The classic example of a condition mediated by substrate intoxication is phenylketonuria (PKU) resulting from phenylalanine hydroxylase deficiency. In this condition, phenylalanine, an essential amino acid present in all protein-containing foods, cannot be converted to tyrosine. Tyrosine itself is important, but the failure of phenylalanine throughput through the phenylalanine degradative pathway results in increased phenylalanine levels in plasma and tissues and in morbidity to the developing brain. Successful treatment requires a three-pronged nutritional approach: (1) restriction of dietary phenylalanine to the minimum needed for growth and protein synthesis, (2) provision of all unrestricted nutrients to foster anabolism, and (3) supplementation with tyrosine. This nutrition is accomplished using a diet limited in phenylalanine and a special purpose medical food that provides other amino acids, including tyrosine, and calcium and vitamins that ordinarily would come from protein-rich foods in the diet. There is a developmental threshold for morbidity, with the most important toxic effect apparent in the developing brain. It is evident from more recent studies that transport of phenylalanine into the brain may be an important modifier of natural history and therapeutic efficacy. Phenylalanine is an example of a transported metabolite: Conversion to tyrosine occurs in the liver, but the target organ is the brain. Theoretically, interruption of the transport process at any point might augment a therapeutic effect, and novel therapies that modify this process are in development.

Cofactor Dependency

Effective cooperation between enzyme and cofactor requires adequate binding of cofactor to protein. When a mutation disrupts the cofactor binding site, the enzyme may have poor catalytic activity at physiologic cofactor concentrations. Improving the concentration of the cofactor may allow sufficient reconstitution of catalytic activity to reverse the abnormal phenotype. These conditions occur for biotin in holocarboxylase synthetase deficiency, for cobalamin in certain forms of methylmalonic acidemia, for pyridoxine in some forms of homocystinuria, and for thiamine in some forms of maple syrup urine disease.

Distortion of Cell Structure

In the numerous lysosomal storage diseases, substrates accumulate within lysosomal organelles because of defective import or catalysis of lysosomal hydrolases. The result of this accumulation may be distortion or death of various cell types, with the resultant phenotype depending on the target tissue and rate of accumulation and the chemical identity of the stored substrate.

Cell Autonomy

Cell autonomy refers to disruption of function within the cell expressing the gene defect. Wiskott-Aldrich syndrome and X-linked severe combined immunodeficiency syndrome are conditions expressed almost exclusively in males. In female carriers for these mutant genes, it would be expected that random X-inactivation would result in two populations of lymphocytes—those inactivating the mutant gene (and functionally normal) and those inactivating the wild-type gene (functionally deficient). Circulating lymphocytes in these females all are functionally normal, suggesting that inactivation of the wild-type gene confers a selective disadvantage to these cells, and they fail to mature. This process must occur as a cell-autonomous process—neighboring normal lymphocyte progenitors cannot rescue the defective cells. In X-linked conditions in which cell autonomy does not occur (e.g., the urea cycle enzyme ornithine transcarbamoylase), the final phenotype, hyperammonemia, depends on the number of cells in which the wild-type genes retain activation. Both populations of cells remain because the toxic metabolites diffuse between cells, in the liver, where the wild-type cells actively contribute to their proper metabolism, and in the brain, where metabolites diffuse in from the extracellular spaces and produce morbidity. Intuitively, one would think that macromolecular defects, such as mucopolysaccharidoses, would exhibit cell autonomy, whereas some small organic acids would not. In fact, the lysosomal enzymes that hydrolyze mucopolysaccharides can be internalized and cross-correct neighboring cells, whereas small molecules, such as the highly reactive compounds that accumulate in hepatorenal tyrosinemia, tend to remain within the cell.

Organ-Specific Morbidity

The effect of a metabolic defect may occur in distant and specific target organs. α_1-Antitrypsin (α_1AT) deficiency results when a mutation in the gene for this plasma protein results in impaired secretion of the protein from the hepatocytes in which it is synthesized and deficient action of the protein in binding to neutrophil elastase in the plasma. The result of this deficiency is emphysema and in some cases liver disease. Both of these examples of organ-specific pathology show threshold effect. Lung damage is accelerated by smoking and inflammatory challenge to the limited amount of α_1AT present so that development of emphysema occurs at younger ages in smokers than in nonsmokers. For the liver lesion, accumulation of aggregated mutant protein occurs in hepatocytes as a result of an imbalance between synthesis (which is increased by stress as an acute-phase reactant), aggregation (which is increased by fever), and normal degradative processes. Although wild-type α_1AT protein may aggregate in settings of extreme imbalance, the mutant protein may produce enough aggregation to be implicated as a direct cause of liver disease, which in some cases may require liver transplantation. Although lung disease may be delayed by environmental controls (avoidance of smoking) or treated by infusion of wild-type α_1AT protein, the liver disease can be treated only by organ replacement. When a normal liver is in place secreting wild-type protein, progression of lung disease may be halted as well.

Inborn Errors of Morphogenesis

For small, easily diffusable metabolites, the placenta may protect the fetus from accumulation or deficiency by providing an equilibrium with maternal metabolic capabilities. In some cases, the mother functions as "gene therapy" for an affected fetus and vice versa. A few IEOM involve pathways important in tissue differentiation and organogenesis, however. Just as an ingested teratogen may interfere permanently with fetal development, so may an endogenously produced compound interfere with specific steps in embryogenesis, leading to fetal malformation (Table 11-1).

Smith-Lemli-Opitz syndrome first was described in 1964 as a malformation syndrome accompanied by mental retardation. Specific anomalies include polydactyly (extra digits), cleft palate and other craniofacial abnormalities, and defective virilization in males. The autosomal recessive inheritance pattern was recognized long before elucidation of the pathophysiology. In 1993, it was discovered that patients with Smith-Lemli-Opitz syndrome have markedly elevated levels of 7-dehydrocholesterol in their blood. Patients with Smith-Lemli-Opitz syndrome have mutations in the gene for 3-β-hydroxysterol-Δ7-reductase (*DHCR*). The elucidation of the biochemistry and genetics of this condition allowed recognition of less severely affected infants without malformations. The mechanism for fetal malformations is thought to be defective signaling through hedgehog proteins important in fetal morphogenesis.

FETAL-MATERNAL INTERACTIONS

In most circumstances in which small molecules pass readily through the placenta, the mother protects the fetus from the consequences of enzyme deficiency. In two scenarios, the fetal-maternal interaction is more complex. Phenylalanine embryopathy occurs when a mother with poorly treated PKU accumulates excess phenylalanine in

Table 11-1. Inborn Errors of Morphogenesis

Condition	Biochemical Effect	Enzyme (Gene)	Consequences	Mechanism
Steroid 5α-reductase deficiency	Defective conversion of testosterone to dihydrotestosterone	5α-reductase 2 (SRD5A2)	Undervirilization of external genitalia, normal wolffian structures	Product deficiency
Zellweger syndrome	Defects in peroxisomal biogenesis. Multiple peroxisomal enzyme disorders, including metabolism of very-long-chain fatty acids and bile acids	Multiple PEX genes, PEX 1 most common	Neuronal migration disorder, facial dysmorphism, renal cysts, variable hepatic, adrenal, skeletal, and eye involvement	Uncertain
Pyruvate dehydrogenase	Defective conversion of pyruvate to acetyl CoA, for entry into Krebs cycle. Lactic acidosis	Pyruvate dehydrogenase, often E1a subunit (PDHA1)	Facial dysmorphism similar to fetal alcohol syndrome, absent corpus callosum	Energy deficiency (?)
Glutaric acidemia type II	Defective transfer of electrons from fatty acid oxidation into the respiratory chain, accumulation of fatty acid metabolites as acylcarnitines or acylglycines	Electron transfer flavoprotein (ETF) or ETF dehydrogenase	Multicystic dysplastic kidneys, neuronal migration abnormalities	Toxic versus energy deficiency (?)

her plasma, and the fetus is exposed to excessive amounts of phenylalanine. The toxic effects of this situation include congenital cardiac malformations, dysmorphic facies, intrauterine growth retardation, microcephaly, and mental retardation. The infant does not have PKU and does not require dietary restriction after birth, but the consequences of the mother's poor control during pregnancy are permanent. The opposite scenario occurs with long-chain 3-hydroxyacyl coenzyme A dehydrogenase deficiency, in which an affected homozygous fetus may produce toxic compounds that cross the placenta, resulting in acute fatty liver of pregnancy in the heterozygous mother. This condition does not occur in all pregnancies affected by long-chain 3-hydroxyacyl coenzyme A dehydrogenase deficiency, but similar cases have been reported from pregnancies affected by other fatty acid oxidation defects, making a common mechanism likely.

PEDIATRIC PRINCIPLES

Age of Ascertainment as a Clue to Disease Process—Impact of Threshold and Gene/Environment Interactions

It is a common misconception that *inborn* implies the appearance of a phenotype at birth. Nothing could be further from the truth. Garrod, regarded by many as the founder of the study of inborn errors, wrote his scholarly discourse on alkaptonuria, the study of which was facilitated by the long survival and relatively benign phenotype of this condition until midadulthood. Clinical and biochemical phenotypes may have vastly different ages of onset and different thresholds of reversibility.

In conditions with a variety of levels of impairment within the same genetic locus (an example of allelic heterogeneity), the general rule is that the more severe the catalytic impairment, the more likely there is to be an early phenotypic onset. In vitro assessment of catalytic function may not tell the full story about the adequacy of pathway flux, because test tube assays usually are run at ideal conditions of pH, temperature, and substrate concentrations.

Deficiency of arylsulfatase A, a lysosomal enzyme, leads to the disease metachromatic leukodystrophy, a neurogenerative disorder. Assay of arylsulfatase activity in circulating lymphocytes reveals low catalytic capacity toward artificial substrate in affected patients. Similar results are obtained in a patient who possesses a "pseudodeficiency" allele, although the difference between true deficiency and pseudodeficiency can be discerned by more elaborate testing. When a condition presents at a later age or has more apparent catalytic activity, intuitively the prognosis should be better because the body should have either catalytic reserve or a favorable compensatory ability in other genes. Late-presenting conditions still can be fatal, perhaps because an inborn error is less likely to be considered, diagnosed, and treated in an individual who has been healthy for years. The natural history of partial enzyme defects and late presentations provides guidance for development of therapy, in that ideal therapies should be sufficient to prevent even late-presenting phenotypes. Examples of IEOM presenting in adulthood are listed in Table 11-2.

Modification of Phenotype by Other Genes or Environmental Factors
Modifier Genes

Manifestations of significant inborn errors usually result in similar biochemical phenotype, and individuals with similar defects share major clinical features. Even siblings who share the same genotype at the mutant gene may differ, however, in severity and range of clinical features. One explanation is that the entire remainder of the genome has the potential to modify threshold and clinical expression. Only identical twins and inbred mice share their entire genetic makeup with affected siblings, and mice have become the species of choice for rigorous testing of hypotheses regarding modifier genes. Many examples of phenotype modification have been shown by breeding experiments in mice, but few actual genes have been identified. Few genetic diseases present in invariant fashion, but remarkably few human modifier genes have been identified, although correlation with mouse studies has facilitated the identification

Table 11-2. Inborn Errors Presenting in Adulthood

Disorder	Enzyme (Gene)	Presenting Feature	Inheritance
McArdle disease	Muscle phosphorylase (*PYGm*)	Muscle cramps with exercise	AR
Adrenomyeloneuropathy	Adrenoleukodystrophy protein (*ALDP*)	Spasticity, adrenal insufficiency	XL (D)
Metachromatic leukodystrophy	Arylsulfatase A (*ASA*)	Dementia, ataxia	AR
MERRF	tRNA lys	Myoclonic epilepsy, deafness, myopathy	mtDNA
Gaucher disease	β-Glucosidase (*GBA*)	Splenomegaly	AR
Refsum disease	Phytanoyl CoA hydroxylase (*PHYH*)	Ichthyosis, ataxia, peripheral neuropathy	AR
Fabry disease	α-Galactosidase (*AGAL*)	Painful neuropathy, renal failure	XL (D)
Ornithine transcarbamylase deficiency	OTC (*OTC*)	Hyperammonemic encephalopathy	XL (D)
Wilson disease	Wilson ATPase (*ATP7b*)	Liver failure	AR
Acute intermittent porphyria	PBG deaminase (*PBGD*)	Acute abdominal pain	AD

AD, autosomal dominant; AR, autosomal recessive; MERRF, myoclonus epilepsy with ragged red fibers; mtDNA, mitochondrial DNA; XL (D), X-linked (dominant).

of several such candidate genes. It is likely that the search for genetic modifiers will become increasingly important in the prediction of risk and the design of new therapies.

Environmental Influences

The effect of environmental stress or adaptation as a means of phenotype modification already has been discussed as a modifier of threshold (smoking and α_1AT) or as a treatment strategy (dietary treatment of PKU or glycogen storage disease type I). Other examples of environmental influences on disease expression are listed in Table 11-3. Conversely, the effect of genetic factors on drug metabolism (efficacy and toxicity) is of increasing interest in drug development (pharmacogenomics). Some of these metabolic factors represent single-gene changes in intermediary metabolism, and others are more complex, involving subtle changes in multiple interacting genes.

Extracting a Basis for Suspicion

The most difficult step in diagnosing an inborn error of metabolism is realizing that such an entity belongs in the differential diagnosis. Sorting out which inborn error is present is a secondary concern because many have overlapping presentations, although a reasonable attempt to categorize and limit the number of entities under consideration improves efficiency. A few clues may help increase clinical suspicion.

Family History

Because most IEOM are recessive, and families tend to be small, a benign family history is rarely reassuring, but a positive family history can narrow and focus the search substantially. Specific queries should include ethnic background, possible consanguinity, and family history of unexplained neonatal death or mental retardation. Inquiring about consanguinity requires some cultural sensitivity. It sometimes is helpful to follow the questions about ethnic background ("Where would you say your ancestors came from?") with extended questions about kinship ("Have you ever been told that your families were related in some way?"). There are significant areas of consanguinity (e.g., incest) in which the information may be disclosed only in a private and trusting setting.

A general family history seeks to uncover general information about risk factors (e.g., diabetes, heart disease, asthma). Although these risk factors are important in the genetic family history, more specific and directed questioning may be necessary to elicit a history of mental retardation, especially in individuals with mild or moderate impairment. Inquiries about sudden or unexpected infant death are important, but more subtle findings in older children or adults also may provide clues. An adult with decreased stamina may have subtle myopathic symptoms or cardiomyopathy. When the patient is male, an extended query about the maternal side of the family may unmask a suspicion for X-linked disease. Diseases inherited through the mitochondrial genome are unusual in pediatrics, and the family histories in these families often are difficult to interpret because of the wide variety of possible symptoms, severities, and ages of onset.

Subtle symptoms often are ignored when they present in isolation but may take on new significance when they occur in clusters or in the face of new evidence of deterioration. These symptoms may include difficulty feeding, unusually severe symptoms with routine illnesses, or subtle delays in meeting milestones. When trying to pin down a history of regression, photographs or videotapes can be helpful. Documentation of poor weight gain or linear growth is very useful.

Physical Examination

In about two thirds of IEOM diagnoses, multiple systems are affected, but abnormalities in the nervous system occur in almost half. Specific attention to tone, alterations in mental status (which may be episodic), and developmental milestones may provide clues. Specific skeletal, ophthalmologic, and skin findings and enlargement of liver, spleen, or kidneys may be helpful in pointing to specific entities. See Table 11-4 for examples.

Table 11-3. Environmental Influences

Condition	Trigger	Effect
X-linked lymphoproliferative disease	Epstein-Barr virus	Lymphoproliferative phenotype
Acute intermittent porphyria	Barbiturates	Neurologic crisis
Galactosemia	Galactose ingestion	Acute neonatal illness
MCAD deficiency	Intercurrent illness	Reye-like syndrome

MCAD, medium-chain acyl-CoA dehydrogenase.

Table 11-4. History and Physical Examination Findings

Ascertainment	Clinical Findings	OMIM Entries*	Prototype Disease	Diagnostic Approach
History	Failure of appropriate growth	138		
	Seizures	215		
	Loss of psychomotor skills	22	Tay-Sachs disease	Lysosomal enzyme studies
	Recurrent somnolence/coma	18	Urea cycle disorders	Serum amino acids, urine orotic acid
General	Abnormal sexual differentiation	11	Smith-Lemli-Opitz syndrome	7-Dehydrocholesterol
	Arachnodactyly	12	Homocystinuria	Serum amino acids
	Hepatosplenomegaly	28	Lysosomal storage disorders	Lysosomal enzyme studies
	Kinky hair	2	Menkes syndrome	Copper studies
	Alopecia	35	Biotinidase deficiency	Serum biotinidase
	Angiokeratoma	7	Lysosomal storage disorders	Lysosomal enzyme studies
	Peau d'orange skin	0	Mucopolysaccharidosis type II	Urine GAG, lysosomal enzyme studies
	Ichthyosis	35	Sjögren-Larsson syndrome	Fatty aldehyde dehydrogenase in fibroblasts
	Coarse features	57	Lysosomal storage disorders	Lysosomal enzyme studies
Neurologic	Ataxia	132		
	Hypotonia	161		
Ophthalmologic	Cataracts	72	Lowe syndrome	Clinical
	Ophthalmoplegia	18	Kearns-Sayre syndrome	Mitochondrial DNA deletion
	Corneal clouding	20	Mucopolysaccharidosis type I	Urine GAG, lysosomal enzyme studies
	Retinopathy	41		
Audiologic	Deafness	129		
Laboratory	Metabolic acidosis	19	Organic acidurias	Urine organic acids, serum amino acids
	Lactic acidosis	12	Organic acidurias and primary lactic acidoses	Urine organic acids, serum amino acids
	Hyperuricemia	7	Lesch-Nyhan syndrome	HPRT activity in cells
	Hypouricemia	2	Molybdenum cofactor deficiency	5-Sulfocysteine in urine or blood
	Hyperammonemia	20	Urea cycle disorders	Serum amino acids, urine orotic acid
	Hypocholesterolemia	3	Smith-Lemli-Opitz syndrome	7-Dehydrocholesterol
Radiology	Dysostosis multiplex	20	Mucopolysaccharidoses	Urine GAG, lysosomal enzyme studies
	Stippled epiphyses	2	Chondrodysplasia punctata	Peroxisomal studies

*Online Mendelian Inheritance in Man database.
GAG, glycosaminoglycan; HPRT, hypoxanthine-guanine phosphoribosyltransferase.

The diagnostic utility of unusual odors is overrated, since most IEOM do not have unusual odors, and the plethora of perfumes in infant products makes their detection difficult. A few key findings may be helpful if present. The abnormal odor of maple syrup urine disease (characterized as a maple syrup, curry, or fenugreek odor) is best appreciated in cerumen. Urine odor is best characterized if collected in a bag or specimen cup, not a perfumed diaper, and the odor may be intensified if the container is capped for a few minutes, then opened briefly. Odors are not specific for IEOM, however. For unknown reasons, parent perception of unusual maple syrup odor in normal toddlers has increased in recent years and does not seem to be associated with any known biochemical pathology. An acquired body odor in a toddler may persist for months as a result of foreign bodies in the nose; in many cases, the odor is perceived in sweat or body fluids. (See the CD-ROM Odor table in the Signs and Symptoms tables.)

Often the suspicion is derived from the gestalt felt by an experienced clinician that the condition of the infant is not well explained by the history and physical findings or risk factors (e.g, apparent respiratory distress [hyperpnea] in a 24-hour-old term infant, extreme lethargy in a toddler with vomiting after only a few hours of illness, apparent "sepsis" with no risk factors or source, failure to respond to intervention as expected). Because these clinical paradoxes also are observed in situations of accidental ingestion or child abuse, it should be no surprise that one may be mistaken for the other.

Diagnostic Pathways

When a suspicion for IEOM is present, an appropriate diagnostic evaluation must be designed. The word designed is used deliberately—*there is no such thing as a complete metabolic evaluation*—and the order and urgency of tests depend on the condition of the patient, availability of testing, and access to urgent and specific treatment. Overnight express shipping has made regional reference laboratories accessible to every clinician, but sometimes it is necessary to send the patient, not the specimen. Hyperammonemic coma in a newborn is a metabolic emergency and requires urgent hemodialysis and drug therapy that is currently investigational. Other conditions may require referral to a distant center for therapy but are much less emergent (e.g., enzyme therapies for lysosomal storage disease). No matter what disposition is chosen for the patient, it is crucial to communicate the clinical scenario to the reference laboratory. Many reference laboratories, even those that handle thousands of specimens every year, provide telephone guidance to physician clients. Often the most cost-effective way to handle a diagnostic evaluation is to collect plasma and urine acutely, then get help in deciding which assays to order.

Initial Testing

The laboratory studies listed in Box 11-2 do not represent a minimum or universal initial laboratory battery; they are listed to suggest the clues that "routine" laboratory studies

Box 11-2. Suggested Laboratory Studies for Initial Metabolic Workup

Complete blood count with differential—some acute organic acid disorders present with pancytopenia. Lysosomal inclusions may be detected in peripheral leukocytes. Evidence of hemolytic anemia may be present. Abnormal red blood cell indices may provide evidence of megaloblastic anemia.

Urine dipstick—presence of ketones, reducing substances, and pH. Part of the urine should be saved in the freezer for further studies. Dipstick-positive ketones are unusual in normal newborns but may be physiologic in a toddler or older child with prolonged vomiting.

Electrolytes, blood urea nitrogen, and creatinine—look for evidence of low bicarbonate. Anion gap acidosis may signify a disorder of organic acid metabolism, whereas non–anion gap acidosis may indicate renal tubule dysfunction. A low blood urea nitrogen level may indicate low protein intake and adequate renal function, but also may be a clue to depressed urea cycle function. A rare disorder of creatine synthesis may be suspected by observation of very low (<0.1 mg/dL) serum creatinine levels.

Blood gas—is there a primary metabolic acidosis? Is there evidence of a primary respiratory alkalosis—a big clue to hyperammonemia? Blood gases and electrolytes complement each other; neither tells the whole story alone.

Plasma ammonia—specify a free-flowing stick, placed on ice, and transported to the laboratory quickly. Ammonia determinations are most useful in a patient with acute symptoms. They do not tell much in the patient running around the waiting room today who had lethargy yesterday. Ammonia determinations are notorious for artifactual elevations, but a finding of plasma ammonia increased more than threefold in the face of an ill patient should prompt immediate concern.

Blood glucose—most helpful in the acute setting before initiation of intravenous glucose. If hypoglycemia is documented, saving the remainder of the "critical" sample for specific diagnostic testing can be invaluable.

Assessment of liver function—elevated transaminases indicate leaky hepatocytes, but estimates of synthetic function may be more useful (prothrombin time, partial thromboplastin time, albumin). Certain metabolic liver diseases (e.g., hepatorenal tyrosinemia) are well known for destroying liver function, but by the time the patient is evaluated, the transaminases are normal. Elevation of unconjugated or conjugated bilirubin also may provide clues.

Lactic acid—combined lactate and pyruvate assays often are used to calculate diagnostic ratios. They often are not emergently available, however. Many automated chemistry analyzers can provide rapid, accurate assessment of lactic acid levels, which are of use in acutely ill patients.

Creatine phosphokinase—some fatty acid oxidation disorders or other disruptions of energy metabolism produce a mild or severe rhabdomyolysis.

Uric acid—may be increased in certain types of glycogen storage disease and in some fatty acid oxidation disorders and primary errors of purine metabolism. A low uric acid level may increase clinical suspicion for molybdenum cofactor deficiency, a severe condition associated with hypotonia and intractable seizures.

may provide. None of the listed studies provides specific diagnosis of any given IEOM. Even findings such as extreme hyperammonemia or lactic acidemia, although evidence of deranged metabolism, are not specific for IEOM because acquired causes for these derangements occur. These findings may be added, however, to the clues already gathered in the history and physical examination to formulate a differential diagnosis. They also provide needed information for initiation of therapy while gathering more information.

Specific Metabolic Studies

Small Molecules

Small molecules are diffusable components of body fluids, such as plasma or urine. They include organic acids, amino acids, sugars, and some fatty acid derivatives. Because most of these assays identify a spectrum of analytes, they often are used screening tests (Box 11-3).

Serum or Plasma Amino Acids. A range of amino acids can be identified and quantified using automated amino acid instruments. These dedicated instruments are a standard feature of biochemical genetic reference laboratories and use high-performance liquid chromatography–based technology with triketohydrindene hydrate (Ninhydrin) detection. (Other methodology exists: Single amino acids, such as phenylalanine, can be quantitated using enzyme-based spectrophotometric or fluorometric methods.) High-throughput newborn screening laboratories analyze many amino acids using tandem mass spectrometry. A report generally lists the amino acids present in order of elution from the column and should give reference ranges adjusted to age. Expert interpretation is important for diagnostic studies. In many cases, the pattern of findings provides clues to the diagnosis, and many physiologic or pathologic conditions can alter the pattern without yielding diagnostic findings. For this reason, it is important not to make mountains out of molehills; for example, elevated tyrosine levels are common in acute liver disease of many causes, but this does not equate to a diagnosis of hereditary tyrosinemia. Similarly, mild elevations of branch-chain amino acids are seen commonly in starvation. In a few situations, serum amino acids are virtually diagnostic as a stand-alone test. Citrulline levels of 2000 µmol/L or more are diagnostic of the urea cycle disorder argininosuccinate synthetase deficiency (citrullinemia), highly elevated methionine with increased free homocysteine is diagnostic for cystathionine β-synthase deficiency (a form of homocystinuria), and serum phenylalanine levels that are more than three to four times the upper limit of normal in an otherwise benign chromatogram are diagnostic for PKU. Refinements in these diagnoses, affecting treatment or prognosis, may require additional testing with DNA analysis or enzyme assay.

Cerebrospinal Fluid Amino Acids. From an IEOM standpoint, the most clinically useful information in the cerebrospinal fluid is measurement of glycine for diagnosis of nonketotic hyperglycinemia. Contamination with blood

Box 11-3. Screening Tests for Small Molecules

- Serum or plasma amino acids
- Cerebrospinal fluid amino acids
- Urine amino acids
- Urine organic acids
- Urinary sugar analysis
- Carnitine/acylcarnitine analysis
- Plasma long-chain fatty acids

or plasma invalidates the analysis because plasma glycine levels are 20-fold higher than normal cerebrospinal fluid glycine. Calculation of the glycine index from cerebrospinal fluid and plasma may help clarify ambiguous situations.

Urine Amino Acids. Urinary excretion of amino acids is subject to modification by tubular reabsorption, and measurement often is confounded by non–amino acid substances that react with triketohydrindene hydrate and obscure parts of the chromatogram (e.g., antibiotics such as ampicillin coelute with phenylalanine). For these reasons, quantitation of amino acids in serum or plasma is far more informative than similar analysis of urine except in situations in which renal tubular function is the issue (e.g., cystinuria).

Urine Organic Acids. The biggest difficulty with tests for urine organic acids is that nobody can remember which body fluid should be sent for which assay. Additionally confusing is the fact that all amino acids are organic by definition, but most organic acids are not amino acids (although they might be derived from them). Having said that, the analysis of urine for abnormal organic acids is an excellent first step toward characterizing suspected IEOM producing anion gap acidosis and in many other nonacute situations. The analysis of urine is preferred for several reasons. First, urine usually is available in greater quantities than serum, especially from young infants. Second, it is a simpler matrix and does not need protein removal as part of sample processing. Third, the kidney does a great job of excreting organic anions and removing water, which amplifies the findings. An acute urine sample almost always is more informative than one obtained several days later, and it is rarely necessary to collect a specimen over 24 hours. Plasma, vitreous humor, ascites fluid, and other body fluids collected at autopsy also can be analyzed. If plasma is the only specimen available, because of anuria or an infant already is deceased, analysis of plasma is worth trying, but most laboratories send back the result with the caveat that plasma organic acid analysis alone is not highly informative. Most organic acid analyses are characterized by gas chromatography, with peak identification by mass spectrometry. It is a pattern that should be interpreted, and that interpretation is most useful if clinical data (suspected diagnoses, medications, feeding history) are provided. Organic acid analysis frequently is confounded by drug and dietary metabolites, and some analytes are present in such small quantities that screening analysis is insufficient for their detection and measurement when a diagnosis is highly suspect. As with amino acid analysis, small changes may not indicate disease. Small amounts of methylmalonic acid may be physiologic or nutritional in origin, whereas massive amounts are found in the pathologic enzyme deficiencies.

Urinary Sugar Analysis. Small amounts of lactose, sucrose, and fructose commonly are found in normal specimens. Sugar analysis may be a helpful adjunct when "reducing sugars" are found in a specimen, but they are not specific. Disaccharides, such as sucrose and lactose, may be found when the intestinal brush border is disrupted, but may reflect only the sugar content of the gut, not a specific disaccharidase deficiency.

Carnitine Analysis. Plasma free and total carnitine identifies primary and secondary deficiencies of free carnitine and frequently identifies lower levels of carnitine in ill patients, most of whom do not have specific genetic conditions. An acylcarnitine profile quantitates the different fatty acid and organic acid conjugates of carnitine. Although urine acylcarnitine analysis was used several years ago, most laboratories have converted to the analysis of plasma or dried blood spots. The usual instrumentation is tandem mass spectrometry, and the expense of this instrumentation limits the number of reference laboratories offering this analysis. Acylcarnitine analysis is used primarily for the detection of abnormalities of fatty acid oxidation, although certain organic acid disorders can be detected as well. (Stable isotope analysis of acyl-glycines is another technique that provides good sensitivity and specificity in the diagnosis of fatty acid oxidation disorders.) This analysis is being used increasingly for expanded newborn screening because the same instrument can be used to screen for fatty acid oxidation disorders, several organic acid disorders, and various amino acid disorders, including PKU.

Very-Long-Chain Fatty Acids. Very-long-chain fatty acids in plasma are analyzed in a few expert reference laboratories. The primary use is detection of disorders of peroxisomal metabolism.

Large Molecules

Large molecules include enzymes, proteins, glycosaminoglycans (GAG), and DNA.

Glycosaminoglycans in Urine. Chondroitin sulfate is a normal constituent of human urine, but excretion of abnormal amounts and patterns of such compounds as heparan sulfate, dermatan sulfate, and keratan sulfate may provide evidence of abnormal lysosomal metabolism of mucopolysaccharides. The spot tests used for widespread screening for these disorders have problems with sensitivity and specificity, and further characterization of GAG excretion by quantitative dye binding and component analysis by electrophoresis or chromatography may provide additional clues to diagnosis, but these tests are rarely sufficient for diagnosis of patients with suspected mucopolysaccharide disorders. An additional caveat is that many lysosomal storage disorders are not mucopolysaccharidoses and are not associated with increased GAG excretion, and such analysis provides no information in diagnosis of these patients except a false sense of security.

Enzyme Analysis. Enzyme analysis is specific. Depending on the tissue distribution, the sample required may be erythrocytes (galactose-1-phosphate uridyltransferase for diagnosis of galactosemia), plasma (hexosaminidase A for Tay-Sachs disease), white cells (α-L-iduronidase for mucopolysaccharidosis type I or Hurler disease), fibroblasts (various enzymes implicated in methylmalonic aciduria), muscle (enzymes of the respiratory chain), or liver (phenylalanine hydroxylase for phenylketonuria or PKU). Some enzyme analyses can be done inexpensively (hexosaminidase A or galactose-1-phosphate uridyltransferase), whereas others are expensive because of the length of time it takes to do the assay or the substrates needed. In contrast to enzymes such as alkaline phosphatase, in which high-throughput automated assays are in use in most hospital laboratories, many of the diagnostic assays ordered for diagnosis of IEOM are done by hand and on individual patient samples accompanied by many controls. For these reasons, enzyme diagnosis is considered unnecessary for conditions such as PKU, in which the sensitivity and specificity of serum amino acid testing is good enough that an expensive and invasive liver biopsy becomes unnecessary. At the opposite end of the spectrum, testing for galactosemia often is done by enzyme screening in dried blood spots, and confirmatory testing in red blood cell hemolysates is the gold standard for diagnosis of this condition. In many other cases, a diagnosis can be made without enzyme confirmation, but access to therapy or clinical trials, important information about prognosis, and information needed for reproductive decision making weigh heavily in favor of an enzyme diagnosis.

Evidence of Protein Modification. α_1AT PI typing has been used for characterization of various mutant forms of these serum proteins. Transferrin isofocusing is an increasingly used test to screen for the various congenital disorders of glycosylation (formerly carbohydrate-deficient glycoprotein) syndromes. As the new field of proteomics characterizes the great diversity in protein modification, it is likely that tests in this category will become more useful.

DNA. DNA analysis is the most specific of all genetics tests, and even "complete" gene sequencing cannot find every mutation. The appeal of DNA analysis is that it is noninvasive, it provides black-and-white yes/no answers when it is informative, and it provides access to information about genes expressed in tissue sanctuaries in which no enzyme or body fluid assay ever would be of practical value. Cost and availability are significant factors, however. Frequently used assays, such as characterization of multiple mutations in cystic fibrosis, are readily available at competitive costs. Other assays, which require extensive gene sequencing, may be available, but only at costs exceeding $2000. Still others are available only through research protocols, and the results of the testing may not be provided to the patients or families. DNA testing now is being used in some situations to save the cost and risk of invasive testing (e.g., liver biopsy for glycogen storage disease type Ia).

Future Metabolic Testing

The transcriptome is the collection of expressed genes in a tissue under certain conditions. It is already possible to assess the up-regulation or down-regulation of thousands of genes using microarray technology. These tools could be used to probe just what is altering cell function and perhaps to guide the progress of therapy. Mutation "profiling" using "chip" technology is under development to design the "perfect" drug combination for patients with chronic illness, and it is increasingly likely that high-throughput mutation screening will replace body fluid or enzyme analysis for common conditions.

Application
Formulating a Differential Diagnosis

The rarest of IEOM never may be encountered by subspecialists, much less the generalist. The more common entities (e.g., cystic fibrosis) probably would be diagnosed a few times in the lifetime of a busy practice. The situations from which these patients come are encountered commonly, however. Sorting out which child needs urgent referral, routine referral, or perhaps watchful waiting are decisions

that need to be made, sometimes in the nursery, sometimes over the telephone, and sometimes in the office. Having a framework of approaches aids in this triage, definitely saves money, and may save a life.

Screening for Inborn Errors of Metabolism
Newborn Screening

The purpose of universal newborn screening for metabolic, genetic, and endocrine disorders is to identify conditions for which early diagnosis and intervention would have a significant impact on outcome and for which the cost and yield of such screening are reasonable based on the anticipated benefit. It is a significant mistake to rely on a normal newborn screen to rule out clinically suspected disease. As a public health measure, universal newborn screenings for PKU and congenital hypothyroidism have been an unqualified success in reducing morbidity from these two common conditions. Newborn screening programs are in rapid flux, with the advent of tandem mass spectrometry as an analytic tool. This technology allows screening for many more entities without significant increases in analytic cost. The cost/benefit analysis of screening for many of the more uncommon conditions is mostly theoretical and merits rigorous examination as more programs expand.

Category-Based Screening

Category-based screening refers to relatively low-yield testing of individuals with common problems (e.g., mental retardation). Mental retardation refers to substantial limitation in present functioning, including significantly subaverage intellectual function, concurrent with related limitations in two or more adaptive skill areas. The pathogenesis encompasses perhaps thousands of different entities. Genetic evaluation of individuals and families with mental retardation seeks to achieve a specific diagnosis or some understanding of the likely cause and pathogenesis. Initial estimates suggested that a diagnosis or cause could be established for 40% to 60% of patients with mental retardation, but more recent surveys are far less optimistic, despite a better armamentarium of diagnostic tools. Should mental retardation alone justify a search for an IEOM? An American College of Medical Genetics (ACMG) Consensus Conference suggested that focused testing should be considered if mental retardation is associated with suggestive clinical or laboratory findings and that such evaluation should consider selectively a variety of screening or specific tests. To evaluate the utility of the ACMG approach, the database Online Mendelian Inheritance in Man (OMIM) was searched for the combination of mental retardation and the additional findings listed in the ACMG statement. The number of genetic entities (*not* the relative frequency of affected persons) is listed in Table 11-4. As can be seen, nonspecific findings such as hypotonia do little to limit the list of diagnostic entities. Other findings, such as arachnodactyly, are quite specific. The most important point to be made is that routine "metabolic screening," mainly small molecule screens, do not facilitate further evaluation of most of the clinical problems. Two clinic-based studies confirm that the yield for metabolic evaluation is low and that unselective screening was as likely to produce falsely reassuring or false-positive results

12   Principles of Microbiology

William V. Raszka, Jr.

Traditionally and simplistically, microbes are described as invaders of the human cell and immune system. In reality, a complex interplay exists between the human host and the microbial world. This chapter outlines the characteristics of major infectious agents, explores host defense mechanisms, and reviews the basics of microbial identification.

In general, the six major groups of infectious agents that cause disease in humans are bacteria, protozoa, fungi, helminths, viruses, and prions. Ever since Leeuwenhoek first described animalis in 1676, characterizing the microbial world has been difficult. Two-compartment, three-compartment, and five-compartment models have been proposed to describe the living world. The first generalization was to distinguish between prokaryotes and eukaryotes. Eukaryotes, which include fungi, protozoa, plants, and animals, contain a nucleus and a cytoplasm that has organelles. Prokaryotes, which consist of bacteria, contain neither. The five-kingdom model places bacteria in the Monera kingdom, protozoa in the Protista kingdom, and fungi in its own kingdom. Taxonomists now use sequencing information from bacterial 16S and 23S rRNA to establish the phylogeny of bacteria. Most physicians have little need to know the taxonomy except to recognize that the shift from using morphologic characteristics to using genetic analysis on which to base taxonomy has led to the renaming of many bacteria. Some organisms even have switched kingdoms. *Pneumocystis* is now classified as a fungus rather than as a protozoan. Where to classify the viruses and the prions is confusing because they cannot live or replicate independently and they are considered separately from animals.

STRUCTURE

Bacteria

Most clinical microbiology laboratories describe bacteria, probably the dominant life form on Earth, by specific morphologic and biochemical reactions. The most common morphologic characteristics used to describe bacteria are the shape and the type of cell wall. Bacteria are round (coccus [plural cocci]), rod-shaped (bacillus [plural bacilli]), or spiraled (spirillum [plural spirilla]). Bacteria may appear singly or in pairs, chains, and clusters (Fig. 12-1). The components of the cell wall and the mechanism of bacteria division govern how bacteria appear. Streptococci appear in pairs and chains as binary fission occurs in a single plane.

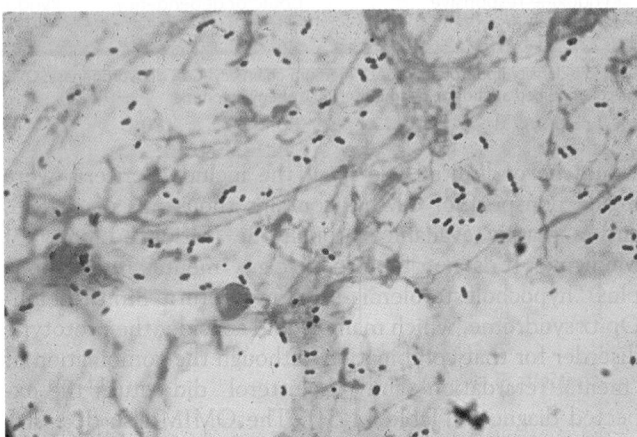

Figure 12-1. Gram stain of sputum showing bacteria arranged in pairs and short chains.

Staphylococci appear in a cluster configuration because binary fission occurs in multiple planes.

The bacterial cell wall is a complex, multilayered structure external to the cell membrane that provides structural stability and a barrier to the external environment. The principal component is peptidoglycan, a mesh of polysaccharide chains cross-linked by short peptides. Bacteria with a single inner membrane and thick cell walls interspersed with teichoic acids and coated with proteins tend to retain the crystal violet/iodine complex of Gram stain and appear blue, or gram-positive, under the microscope. Most gram-positive bacteria are linked closely phylogenetically. Bacteria that retain only the safranin counterstain of Gram stain appear pink, or gram-negative, under the microscope. These bacteria possess a thin cell wall that is external to an inner membrane and linked by lipoproteins to a lipopolysaccharide-containing outer membrane. The outer membrane contains many surface and transmembrane proteins that act to sample the external world and selectively allow passage of certain molecules. Gram-negative organisms are not related closely phylogenetically. Bacteria, such as *Rickettsiae*, *Chlamydia*, and *Mycobacterium*, with alternative cell wall structures stain poorly or not at all with Gram stain. Mycobacteria have a lipid-rich cell wall that can be stained with alternative agents and resist decolorization after acid treatment. This is the basis of the acid-fast stains, such as the Ziehl-Neelsen stain. Mycoplasmas are the smallest free-living organisms and contain no cell wall.

Bacteria contain several other external structures. Some bacteria, termed *encapsulated bacteria*, produce a viscous polysaccharide or protein coat that surrounds the cell wall. This slime layer, also called a *glycocalyx* or *capsule*, is important because it helps resist phagocytosis by neutrophils and macrophages. *Streptococcus pneumoniae, Neisseria meningitidis,* and *Haemophilus influenzae* type b all have a capsule. Many gram-negative bacteria and spirochetes possess flagella. Flagella are slender, wavy, proteinaceous appendages not usually seen under light microscopy used to propel the bacteria. Pili or fimbriae are slender, short, straighter proteinaceous appendages that bacteria use to adhere to cells and inert substances. Flagella and pili are antigenic.

The internal structures of bacteria differ from those of human cells in that they have no nucleus or organelles. Similar to all other living things, bacteria contain DNA. The bacterial DNA may be located on the chromosome or in a plasmid. Plasmids are small, circular bodies of double-stranded DNA. The extra genetic material found in plasmids may code for toxins, surface factors, and antimicrobial resistance genes. Bacteria easily may share and disseminate plasmid-mediated antimicrobial resistance genes, such as those that code for β-lactamase. Similar to human cells, bacteria contain ribosomes. The bacterial ribosome has a size of 70S, however, whereas the human ribosome is 80S in size. Antibiotics that inhibit protein synthesis exploit this difference.

Some bacteria, such as *Bacillus* and *Clostridium*, have the capacity to form spores (sporulate) when conditions are not optimal for survival. Spores are metabolically inactive cells heavily protected by layers of modified peptidoglycan. Spores can survive under inhospitable conditions, including boiling. Under favorable conditions, a spore can become a metabolically active, dividing cell. Although spores themselves do not cause disease, the products released after becoming active, such as the toxin of *Clostridium tetani*, are important causes of human disease. Table 12-1 lists medically important toxin-mediated diseases.

Although most bacteria are able to live independently, the rickettsiae and chlamydiae cannot. These organisms are small bacteria that can grow only within higher living cells. Rickettsiae and chlamydiae are bacteria because they contain DNA, ribosomes, and cell walls similar to bacteria, and they divide similar to bacteria. Chlamydiae, the size of large viruses, complete a unique developmental cycle within cells.

Protozoa

Protozoa are large single-celled eukaryotes. Most lack cell walls but undertake complex physiologic activities, including ingesting food and locomotion. The protozoa are subdivided into four phyla based on their means of locomotion. The amebae are simple, free-living forms constantly changing their shape that move by projecting and retracting protoplasm. The active form of the amebae is the trophozoite. Some amebae are able to encyst, meaning that they change into an inactive, resting form that is able to survive adverse environmental conditions. *Entamoeba histolytica* is one of the few amebae of significant medical importance. The Ciliophora have a fixed oval shape and more complex internal structures than amebae, and they move through fluids by constant beating of cilia. Few Ciliophora cause human disease. All members of the Zoomastigina or flagellates possess flagella used to propel the organisms through fluids. *Trichomonas* and *Giardia* are intestinal flagellates. *Trichomonas* causes genital mucosal disease in men and women. *Giardia* has a trophozoite and cyst stage and inhabits the proximal small intestine. Neither *Trichomonas* nor *Giardia* causes invasive disease. The hemoflagellates, such as *Trypanosoma* and *Leishmania*, enter the bloodstream after an insect bite. These organisms often have a complex life cycle that occurs in the insect and vertebrate host. Finally the Apicomplexa, such as *Plasmodium*, have no external means of locomotion but may show a gliding motion. They usually have a complex life cycle of asexual and sexual reproduction in different hosts. Table 12-2 lists several medically important protozoa and the common sites of infection.

Fungi

Fungi are complex eukaryotes with distinctive, thick cell walls. Although previously thought to be plants, fungi cell walls contain chitin, and they do not synthesize nutrients through photosynthesis. The fungal kingdom is divided into four kingdoms based on many different morphologic features of the fungus and the type of sexual reproduction. The terminology is confusing to even seasoned mycologists. Most clinicians group fungi into yeasts and molds. Yeasts are usually thick-walled unicellular organisms, which often reproduce by "budding" daughter cells. Molds consist of long chains of filamentous, branching cells containing cytoplasms and nuclei, called *hyphae*. Hyphae may be interrupted by

Table 12-1. Examples of Organisms that Release Medically Important Exotoxins and the Site of Toxin Action

Organism	Disease	Site of Action
Bacillus anthracis	Anthrax	Macrophage
Bacillus cereus	Food poisoning	Enterocyte
Clostridium botulinum	Botulism	Presynaptic nerve ending
Clostridium difficile	Pseudomembranous colitis	Enterocyte
Clostridium tetani	Tetanus	Inhibitory synapses
Corynebacterium diphtheriae	Diphtheria	Respiratory mucosa
Escherichia coli	Hemolytic-uremic syndrome	Endothelium
Staphylococcus aureus	Food poisoning	Enterocyte
S. aureus	Toxic shock	T lymphocytes
Streptococcus pyogenes	Scarlet fever	Epidermis
S. pyogenes	Toxic shock	T lymphocytes
Vibrio cholerae	Cholera	Enterocyte

Table 12-5. Representative Examples of Different Types of Transmission*

Horizontal Transmission

Airborne
- Mycobacterium tuberculosis
- Rubeola
- Varicella-zoster virus

Droplet
- Bordetella pertussis
- Neisseria meningitidis
- Streptococcus pneumoniae
- Streptococcus pyogenes pharyngitis
- Influenza
- RSV
- Many viral infections of childhood

Contact

DIRECT
- Methicillin-resistant Staphylococcus aureus
- S. pyogenes
- RSV
- Hepatitis B virus
- HSV
- Varicella-zoster virus
- Most viral infections of childhood

INDIRECT
- Clostridium difficile
- Methicillin-resistant S. aureus
- RSV
- HSV

Vertical Transmission

IN UTERO
- Treponema pallidum
- Toxoplasma gondii
- Cytomegalovirus
- HIV

PERINATAL
- Group B streptococcus
- Chlamydia trachomatis
- Neisseria gonococcus
- Cytomegalovirus
- HSV
- HIV

POSTNATAL (BREAST-FEEDING)
- HIV
- HTLV

Common Source
- Bacillus cereus
- Salmonella enteritidis
- Staphylococcal food poisoning

Vector-Borne
- Borrelia burgdorferi
- Plasmodium
- Dengue

*Horizontal transmission occurs between individuals in a population. Common source transmission is usually from a shared food or water source. Vector-borne transmission involves an animal vector to transmit the infectious agent.
HIV, human immunodeficiency virus; HSV, herpes simplex virus; HTLV, human T-lymphotropic virus; RSV, respiratory syncytial virus.

in immunocompromised hosts as *opportunistic* pathogens. For similar reasons, physicians and microbiology technologists should avoid or exercise caution in using the term *contaminant* to describe an organism isolated from a sterile site. Almost all bacteria can cause human disease under appropriate conditions. The health care team has to decide if the isolated organism is clinically relevant or not.

Bacterial Pathogenesis

Host factors that affect microbial virulence include the competency of the host immune system, concurrent or previous infectious insults, nutritional status, physiologic changes, and anatomy. Defects in any aspect of the host defense system can lead to generalized or specific susceptibility to infectious agents. Patients with acquired immunodeficiency syndrome (AIDS) are at risk for fungal,

mycobacterial, viral, parasitic, and bacterial superinfections. Individuals with terminal complement deficiency are at increased risk for invasive *N. meningitidis* infections. Previous infection may alter the host anatomy or host protective factors. Patients with influenza often develop bacterial superinfections after the viral and host immune-mediated destruction of pulmonary mucosa and clearance mechanisms. *S. pneumoniae* infection is more common after a viral illness presumably because the viral infection induces cells to express a platelet-activating factor. The pneumococcus binds to this site to gain access to the host's internal environment. Normal physiologic processes or perturbations of normal physiologic processes may alter the likelihood or severity of an infectious process. Pregnant women may develop devastating hepatitis E or varicella-zoster virus infections, whereas similarly aged nonpregnant women merely experience an unpleasant illness. *Pseudomonas aeruginosa* is a distinctly uncommon cause of pneumonia in healthy children. *P. aeruginosa* eventually infects virtually all patients with cystic fibrosis, however. The nutritional status of the host plays an important role in the virulence of an organism, as evidenced by the frequency of severe measles infections in malnourished individuals. The epidermis and mucosa are important barriers to microorganisms. Before the advent of topical antimicrobial therapy, sepsis was a common complication of severe burns. Bacteria that rarely cause disease coat most human mucosal surfaces. Human interventions, such as antibiotic consumption, significantly change this "normal" flora. This situation can lead to the development of altered resident flora and a greater likelihood of colonization and infection with multiply resistant organisms that are not usually resident on mucosal surfaces.

The intensity of the interaction between an infectious agent and the host may contribute to the virulence of that agent. *Infectivity* refers to the likelihood that an inoculum of an infectious agent will produce disease. *Vibrio cholerae*, although capable of producing severe human disease, is a high-inoculum disease. This means that a human being is unlikely to develop symptomatic cholera, unless he or she ingests a large number of organisms (i.e., 10^7 to 10^9 bacteria). *Shigella dysenteriae* is a low-inoculum organism: Ingestion of only 10^2 organisms reliably produces human disease.

Table 12-6. Examples of Diseases Associated with Arthropod Vectors

Vector	Organism	Disease
Body louse	Rickettsia prowazekii	Epidemic typhus
	Borrelia recurrentis	Relapsing fever
Fleas	Yersinia pestis	Bubonic plague
	Rickettsia typhi	Endemic typhus
Mites	Rickettsia akari	Rickettsialpox
		Scrub typhus
Mosquitoes	Wuchereria bancrofti	Filariasis
	Plasmodium	Malaria
		Dengue
		Yellow fever
Ticks	Ehrlichia	Ehrlichiosis
	Borrelia burgdorferi	Lyme disease
	Rickettsia rickettsii	Rocky Mountain spotted fever
	Francisella tularensis	Tularemia

Myriad factors govern the virulence of specific bacteria. The factors that allow bacteria to attach, replicate, damage, and disseminate themselves or products affect how virulent an organism is. Some members of a species are more virulent than closely related organisms. These more virulent organisms often contain islands of foreign genetic material that confer greater virulence over nonpathogenic strains. This genetic material often allows the organism to bind more effectively to sites or escape immune destruction.

Expression of virulence factors changes with changing environments. Bacteria are particularly adept at monitoring their environment and responding to changes in that environment. This regulation is crucial to the success of bacteria. A bacterium is likely to encounter remarkably different environments and growth conditions as it passes from the external environment to its preferred ecologic niche. Each of these environments may require specific bacterial responses to survive. Needless production of unnecessary virulence factors imposes a huge metabolic burden and a survival disadvantage. Bacteria have developed sophisticated environmental surveillance mechanisms that can trigger differential gene expression. Bacteria use many different methods to respond to an astonishing number of environmental factors, including pH, temperature, oxygen tension, iron or calcium concentration, and bacterial density. Sensor proteins embedded in the cytoplasmic membrane detect environmental stimuli and transmit signals to a response regulator protein. A conformational change in the regulator protein amplifies transcription of target genes within a regulon. Other sensor molecules act as repressor molecules that turn off gene expression after an environmental signal. Constant monitoring with positive and negative feedback on gene expression allows bacteria to exploit the environment most effectively at the lowest metabolic cost.

A crucial initial step in the pathogenesis of a bacterial infection is the attachment or adherence of the infectious agent to a particular site in the host. This step determines the cell and organ tropism of the bacterium. Other processes regulated by adherence or attachment include cell-microbe communication and internalization of the infectious agent. Most infectious agents, including bacteria, have developed specialized attachment sites. In bacteria, these sites are called *adhesins*. Adhesins and their targets, cell receptors, are composed primarily of carbohydrates, proteins, or combinations of both. Bacterial adhesins are diverse and include pili and cell membrane surface proteins. The expression of many adhesins is under positive and negative feedback control and may change under different environmental conditions. Bacteria may rely on more than one adhesin for attachment. The specific attachment systems allow organisms to exploit specific ecologic niches. Some clones of *Escherichia coli* have specific pili that allow binding to specific receptors found on urogenital mucosa. *E. coli* lacking these pili infrequently cause urinary tract infections. Other organisms exploit changes in cellular receptors. Some gram-negative bacteria release toxins or other products while in direct contact with a cell. The cell takes up the bacterial products and expresses them on the cell surface. The bacteria now can bind to the newly expressed cell surface marker and gain entry into the cell.

When established at the ecologic site, bacteria must compete with each other and host cells for nutrients. Because iron is often an essential nutrient, bacteria have developed sophisticated systems to obtain iron from the host or the environment. These mechanisms include secretion of chelating agents, such as siderophores, to remove iron from host proteins; direct uptake of complexed iron; and secretion of enzymes that release iron from heme. Expression of these processes usually is under control of a regulatory signal.

The ability of many bacteria to secrete enzymes, or exotoxins, is linked closely to their virulence. Many different types of exotoxins exist. Some exotoxins consist of a binding and transmembrane delivery domain linked with the moiety that affects cellular metabolism. Cholera toxin is a classic example of such an exotoxin. Other exotoxins are directly lytic or toxic to cells. These often form pores in the membranes of eukaryotic cells leading to cell death. The clinical consequences of exotoxin secretion are myriad (see Table 12-1). Streptolysin, secreted by *Streptococcus pyogenes*, cleaves tissue planes. The toxins elaborated by *Clostridium tetani* and *Clostridium botulinum* bind to specific neurotransmitter sites with subsequent tetany or flaccid paralysis. Superantigens, such as those elaborated by staphylococcal or streptococci involved in toxic shock syndromes, are toxins that nonspecifically stimulate large clones of T cells. Because 2% to 20% of all T cells are activated at one time, overstimulation of the immune system results, often with catastrophic consequences.

Endotoxins are not secreted by bacteria but are components of the bacterial cell wall. Lipid A, a component of the gram-negative wall, acts as a toxin with stimulation of a brisk immune response and the clinical findings of septic shock. Gram-positive bacteria also contain cell wall components that may act as endotoxins.

When the organism has established a presence in a specific niche of the human host, it needs to escape detection or destruction by host defense mechanisms. Many strategies to escape immune surveillance and destruction have evolved. Some bacteria elaborate capsules. The capsules may be composed of polysaccharides or polypeptides. Polysaccharide capsules are poorly immunogenic and block deposition of complement. The virulence effect of the capsule is dramatic. *Haemophilus influenzae* type b, a major cause of meningitis, sepsis, and pneumonia worldwide, has a polysaccharide capsule. *Nontypable Haemophilus*, so named because it contains no capsule, infrequently causes invasive disease in immunocompetent individuals. Polypeptide capsules, such as those elaborated by virulent *Bacillus anthracis*, prevent phagocytosis. Other organisms, such as *N. gonorrhoeae*, routinely change the external surface markers so that they can go unrecognized. Still others coat themselves with human-derived proteins, such as fibronectin, to escape immune surveillance.

Many organisms subvert or redirect host biologic processes to survive intracellularly. The advantage of intracellular adaptation is that the infectious agent can escape phagocyte cells, complement, and antibody. Some organisms live in the cytoplasm, but many others live in endosomes or phagosomes. Bacteria adapted for intracellular life must develop systems to escape destruction by lysosomes.

They inhibit, disrupt, or alter phagosome-lysosome fusion or adapt to low-pH environments. Intracellular bacteria pathogens are diverse and include *Rickettsia*, *Salmonella*, *Legionella pneumophila*, and *Listeria monocytogenes*.

Viral Pathogenesis

As with bacteria, the virulence of a virus depends on host and viral characteristics. Host factors include age, anatomy, genetics, nutrition, and, most importantly, the status of the cellular immune system. Viral factors include size, the presence of an envelope, and capsid structures.

Viral replication includes attachment, internalization, exposure of the genome, translocation of the genome to the site of replication, replication of the genome and viral proteins, assembly, and egress of the new virion from the cell. The virus must subvert host cellular machinery to complete these tasks. Budding virions may acquire their envelope from cell membranes. Viral replication is efficient, leading to the production of thousands of progeny virus within 6 to 8 hours for some viruses and 1 to several days for others. Typically, viral replication leads to lysis and death of the host cell. If the progeny virus escapes from the basolateral membrane, as with HIV, the virus becomes locally invasive with ultimate systemic spread. If the virus escapes from the apical or luminal surface of a cell, as with most respiratory viruses, spread is usually cell-to-cell.

As with bacteria, viruses have developed proteins that bind to specific cell receptor sites. Specific sequences on the gp120 envelope protein mediate attachment to the $CD4^+$ receptor on mature T lymphocytes and other cells. Viruses do not monitor the environment and respond to those changes as bacteria do. Viral replication allows for substantial genetic variation, however. Viruses with segmented RNA genomes, such as influenza, through genetic reassortment may express new or different surface antigens frequently. Influenza virus expressing different surface antigens (antigenic shift) may result in pandemics of severe influenza disease because preexisting immunity would not help protect against the new strain. Other viruses, particularly retroviruses, tolerate high mutation rates from inexact reverse transcription processes. This tolerance leads to swarms of a virus, such as HIV, expressing slightly different antigens. The clinical consequence may be the emergence of HIV virions resistant to antiretroviral agents or unaffected by circulating anti-HIV antibody. The rapid emergence of such viral genetic diversity makes the development of effective vaccines extremely difficult.

The consequence of naturally occurring viral infection may be complete or partial immunity, latency, or malignancy. Hepatitis A virus infection leads to durable protection against subsequent infection. Respiratory syncytial virus infection leads to protection against severe disease but not subsequent infection. Herpes DNA viruses develop latency and may lead to local or disseminated disease after reactivation. Viruses that contain DNA or a reverse transcription step from RNA to DNA usually cause chronic infection. Chronic infection develops because viral-mediated, double-stranded DNA may incorporate in host DNA. The consequence of such integration may include neoplasia, as can occur after hepatitis B and Epstein-Barr virus infections.

Protozoa and Helminthic Pathogenesis

Protozoal and helminthic infections lead to human disease through a variety of mechanisms. Some organisms cause disease through mechanical obstruction, such as occurs with large intestinal *Ascaris* worm burdens. The physical movement or migration of the organism through tissues may cause disease such as pulmonary or muscle disease that occurs with *Paragonimus* and *Trichinella* infections. Some organisms or their products are directly toxic to cells. Hookworms use teeth or cutting plates to fasten onto the mucosa or submucosa and then release anticoagulants, resulting in intestinal bleeding and, over time, anemia. Many gastrointestinal helminths compete with the host for nutrients. Significant *Taenia* or *Diphyllobothrium latum* can lead to malnutrition and anemia. The host immune response to the protozoan or helminth frequently causes disease. The inflammation that accompanies the immune response is responsible for the morbidity associated with ocular *Toxoplasma* disease. Many of these macroscopic organisms are remarkably adept at avoiding protective host immune responses. Some organisms accomplish this by routinely changing surface antigens. Few protozoal or helminth infections lead to any protection against subsequent infection.

Fungal Pathogenesis

Fungal pathogenesis depends heavily on host factors. Although occasionally healthy individuals may develop fungal disease, such as histoplasmosis meningitis or coccidioidomycosis, most fungal infections occur in immunocompromised individuals or individuals who have altered flora. Fungi and bacteria colonize mucosal surfaces and compete with each other for ecologic niches. *Candida* may contain a transmembrane protein integrin analogue. The *Candida* species that most frequently express this receptor are those most frequently isolated in human infections. Antibiotic administration may suppress the endogenous bacterial flora, allowing fungal organisms to proliferate. Fungal organisms are able to colonize organic and inorganic surfaces heavily. Immunosuppression, catheter placement, or nutrient-rich hyperalimentation fluids all allow invasion of deeper tissues.

Prion Pathogenesis

Little is known about the exact pathogenic mechanisms of prions. Heat, freezing, and irradiation do not affect prions. One hypothesis is that prion protein may lower the activation constant for conformation changes in host-derived prion protein located in the brain. Prion disease, called *transmissible spongiform encephalopathies*, may be secondary to the accumulation of these proteins.

Host Defense Mechanisms

Humans always have lived in conjunction with the microbial world and have developed sophisticated defense mechanisms. Host defense mechanisms may be nonspecific (innate) or specific (adaptive). Nonspecific host factors that decrease the likelihood of acquiring an infectious disease include the normal microbial flora, epithelial and mucosal barriers, anatomic considerations, peristalsis, excretory secretions, phagocytes, complement, and acute-phase reactants. Nonspecific defense mechanisms by definition are not organism specific, do not involve immunologic memory, and do not improve over time. Specific or adaptive immune mechanisms include cellular immune responses, such as antibody production by B cells. Adaptive immune responses are organism specific, trigger immunologic memory, and improve with subsequent exposures. See Chapter 10 for a more complete description of these mechanisms.

Role of Normal Flora

Many different bacteria and fungi colonize the epithelial and mucosal surfaces of humans. These organisms rarely cause disease, unless the host is immunocompromised. This collection of organisms, the normal flora, contributes to the health of the host in several ways. The normal flora protects against invasion by exogenous organisms. The mechanism of this protection involves competition for nutrients and host receptors for colonization and production of extracellular products that may be toxic to other organisms. Particular environments, host physiologic changes, hygiene, diet, and exposure to antibiotics all alter the normal flora. Patients hospitalized or housed in long-term care facilities are colonized with markedly different bacteria than peers in the general community. Antibiotics, particularly indiscriminate antibiotic use, have a profound effect on microbial flora. Antibiotics suppress the normal flora, allowing easier colonization by antibiotic-resistant organisms that potentially are more virulent. Finally, the constant exposure of the host to microorganisms and their products may prime the immune system, allowing a greater, more specific immune response to more virulent organisms.

ROLE OF THE MICROBIOLOGY LABORATORY

The clinical microbiology laboratory assists the physician in recovering and identifying infectious agents from clinical specimens. Several steps are involved in making the correct microbiologic diagnosis, including appropriate sampling, specimen processing, direct or indirect visualization, culture, confirmation, and susceptibility testing.

Specimen Collection

Specimen collection is the initial step in the process. The clinician first must decide what is the likely site of infection based on the history, physical examination, and previously obtained laboratory information. Knowledge of the likely site of infection determines what type of fluid or tissue specimen is sent to the laboratory to confirm or disprove the hypothesis. A few general rules apply. First, surface cultures obtained by swabbing are useful only for diagnosing specific mucosal infections at that site. They are not useful for establishing the cause of infection at a distant or deep site. Resident flora heavily contaminate mucosal surfaces, so the laboratory must know which organisms are sought so that appropriate culture techniques are used. Mucosal cultures are useful for identifying *S. pyogenes* in the pharynx; *B. pertussis* in the nasopharynx; *N. gonorrhoeae* in the urethra or cervix; and organisms that infect the gastrointestinal mucosa, such as *Salmonella* and *Shigella*.

Specimens from normally sterile sites should be obtained using clean or sterile technique to minimize the likelihood of false-positive cultures. Cleaning and disinfection of the skin before attempting to draw a blood culture at that site is crucial.

The volume of material sent to the laboratory for analysis helps determine the likelihood that an infectious agent is identified. Cotton-tipped swabs contain little clinical material and make inferior specimens. They should be used only when biopsy, aspiration, or curettage cannot be accomplished. Although blood culture systems now are quite sensitive, placing 3 to 5 mL in a blood culture vial is more likely to give a reliable result than a 100-μL sample. Similarly the clinician should aspirate a sufficient volume of purulent material from an abscess.

The higher the quality of the specimen, the more reliable is the information gained from that specimen. A sputum specimen sent for culture should contain polymorphonuclear leukocyte neutrophils (PMNs) and alveolar macrophages. Studies have shown that without evidence of these types of cells, the specimen is mostly saliva and unlikely to give useful information. Similarly, growth of bacteria in urine from specimens heavily contaminated with squamous cells should be viewed cautiously. Finally, selection of appropriate transport material is important. Fastidious or unusual organisms may require specialized transport media to support their growth.

Optimally, physicians should be in communication with technologists in the microbiology laboratory. Technologists know a great deal about specimen collection, transport, appropriate media, and ways to maximize organism recovery. Failure to communicate, whether verbally or in writing, with the microbiology staff may obscure the correct microbiologic diagnosis. Not all laboratories routinely test stool samples for *E. coli* O157. A physician caring for a child with crampy abdominal pain and bloody stools needs to notify the laboratory that *E. coli* O157 is a suspected pathogen so that a stool sample can be inoculated onto the correct medium. Similarly, laboratories look only for *S. pyogenes* on otherwise unlabeled pharyngeal swab specimens. If the clinician suspected *N. gonorrhoeae* or *Arcanobacterium haemolyticum,* unless he or she notified the laboratory, the laboratory would not culture the specimen on appropriate media and would report only on the presence of *S. pyogenes*. Laboratories develop protocols to guide technologists in the absence of clinical data, but physicians routinely should inform the laboratory of the specimen site, time of collection, and organisms suspected.

Appropriate communication with the microbiology laboratory can facilitate patient care. Although physicians often consider microbiology results as a yes or a no phenomenon, decisions in the laboratory are guided by clinical findings. In many patients, a culture of cerebrospinal fluid or blood growing coagulase-negative staphylococcus would be considered a contaminant with no further evaluation warranted. In an immunocompromised patient or a patient with a ventriculoperitoneal shunt, however, isolation of coagulase-negative staphylococci would be cause for concern. Under such conditions, the laboratory is more likely to confirm the identification and perform susceptibility testing.

Specimen Transport

Often the importance of specimen transport is unrecognized. Urine left standing at room temperature for several hours does not reflect accurately the clinical situation found

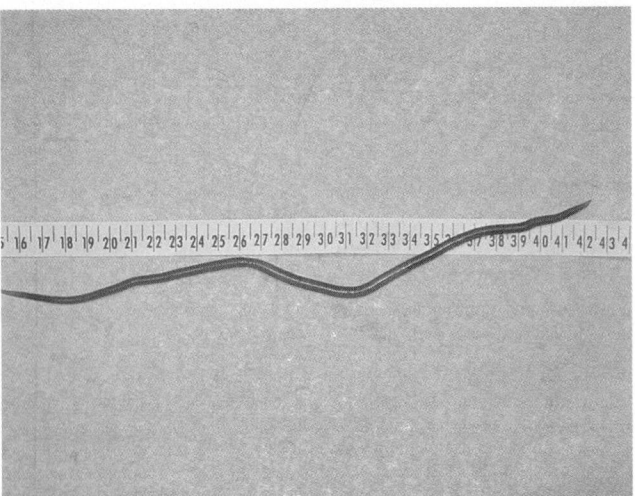

Figure 12-2. This helminth was removed from a child's rectum. Note the large size, cylindrical shape, and symmetrically tapered ends. These characteristics allow for easy identification as an adult *Ascaris lumbricoides*.

in the bladder. Some specimens require maintenance of cold temperatures. Failure to transport these specimens on ice may lead to false-negative or false-positive laboratory results. Operating room personnel should not send specimens obtained at surgery to the microbiology laboratory in preservatives. No cultures can be obtained from specimens fixed in formaldehyde.

A few general rules apply to specimen transport. When the clinician is in doubt about how to collect or transport a specimen, he or she should call the laboratory for assistance. Sealed anaerobic transport media usually support the growth of most organisms, including aerobic organisms, until the laboratory processes the specimen. Clinical samples obtained in the operating room can be placed in a sterile urine collection cup for transport to the laboratory. If material is aspirated into a syringe, the needle should be removed and the syringe sealed before sending the syringe to the laboratory. Finally, timely transport allows earlier processing by the laboratory.

IDENTIFICATION OF MICROORGANISMS

Direct Visualization

Occasionally, only inspection is necessary to identify the infecting organism. Only helminths are large enough to be visualized without diagnostic aids (Fig. 12-2). More commonly, clinicians and laboratory technologists use stains, amplification techniques, and culture media to identify an infectious agent accurately.

Direct microscopic examination of clinical specimens is a powerful tool for the rapid diagnosis of infectious processes. Several different staining and visualization techniques provide contrast between the microbial agents and the background. Staining, such as done with Gram stain, involves four steps. First, a stain is applied that binds to the target. The second step fixes the stain at the target. A decolorizing agent removes unfixed stain. Finally, a counterstain provides contrast or fixes to background material. Examination of the slide reveals the presence and number of potentially pathogenic organisms, the relative contamination by resident flora, the degree of inflammation, and the staining characteristics and morphologic features of the organisms. Staining techniques are used to identify bacteria, fungi, protozoa, and helminths. The number and type of organisms in the specimen and the skill of the microscopist limit the sensitivity and specificity of staining procedure.

The most common staining technique is Gram stain, which uses crystal violet as the primary stain and safranin as the counterstain of bacterial cell walls. Gram-negative bacteria, host cells, and exudate all stain the pink color of the counterstain (Fig. 12-3*A*). The color and morphology of certain visualized bacteria may suggest the likely organism (see Fig. 12-3*B*). Gram stain also allows identification of certain yeasts, such as *Candida* and *Cryptococcus*. Acridine orange stain is a fluorochrome stain that intercalates into nucleic acid. When viewed under ultraviolet light, bacteria and yeast appear orange-red, whereas leukocytes appear pale green. Acridine orange staining is more sensitive than Gram staining because it can detect 10^4 bacteria in a specimen compared with 10^5 bacteria for Gram staining, but it does not give the same morphologic and differential staining information.

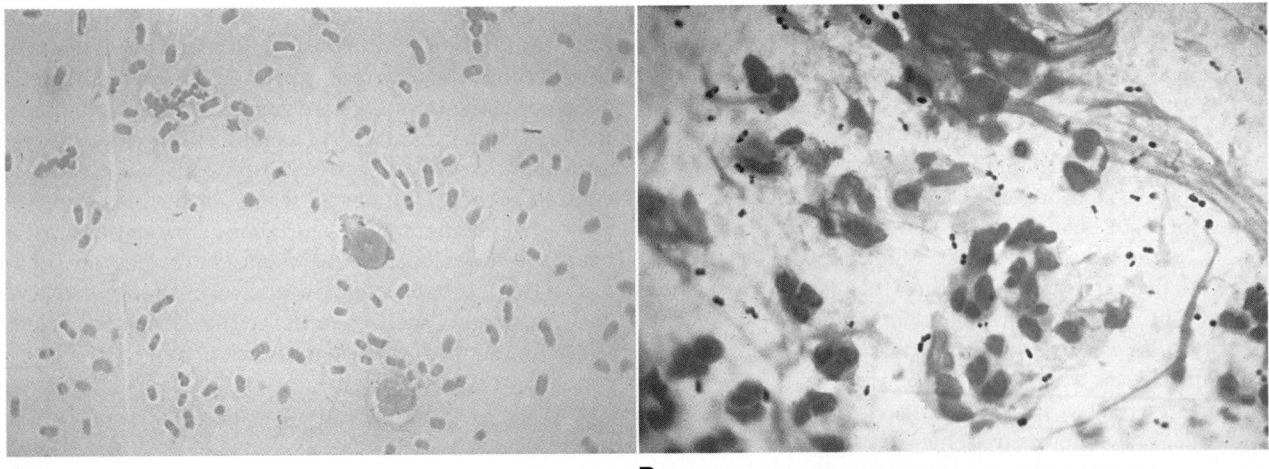

A   **B**

Figure 12-3. A, Gram stain showing a plethora of gram-negative bacilli *(Klebsiella)*. **B,** Gram stain from a clinical specimen showing the typical gram-positive diplococci of *Streptococcus pneumoniae*.

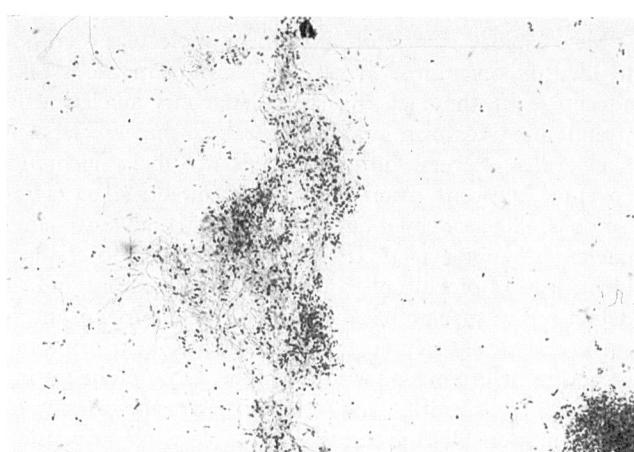

Figure 12-4. A modified Kinyoun stain from a culture. This specimen grew *Nocardia asteroides*.

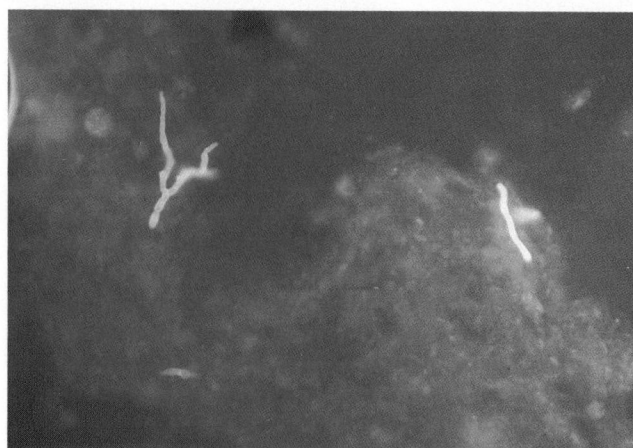

Figure 12-6. Calcofluor stain showing *Aspergillus fumigatus*.

Acid-fast stains take advantage of the fact that the lipid-rich envelope of mycobacteria resists acid decolorization. In Ziehl-Neelsen and Kinyoun stains, carbol fuchsin is the primary stain, whereas methylene blue is usually the counterstain. Mycobacteria appear as pink-red bacilli against a blue-green background. Some organisms, such as *Nocardia*, are only partially acid-fast (Fig. 12-4). An auramine-rhodamine fluorochrome stain, in which the organisms appear bright yellow or orange, is more sensitive than traditional stains (Fig. 12-5). Acid-fast stains also show the oocysts of *Cryptosporidium*, *Isospora*, and *Cyclospora* in diarrheal stools.

Many fungal stains are available. The most commonly used technique consists of examining tissue or wet mounts in 10% potassium hydroxide stained with the fluorescent reagent calcofluor white. Calcofluor white stains all fungal elements causing them to fluoresce (Fig. 12-6). Other stains include Giemsa (excellent for identification of *Histoplasma*), periodic acid–Schiff (PAS), Papanicolaou, hematoxylin-eosin, and India ink. Most laboratories infrequently use an India ink preparation to identify fungi because of its low sensitivity. Specialized stains used to identify fungi, including *Pneumocystis*, in clinical specimens include Gomori's methenamine silver stain and toluidine blue.

Stool specimens often are examined for presence of protozoa and helminths. Lugol's iodine solution applied to wet stool mounts facilitates identification of cysts. Saline wet preparations and Wheatley trichrome, methylene blue, or iron hematoxylin stains facilitate identification of trophozoites. Special stains are used to identify organisms in tissues. Giemsa is the preferred stain of blood smears and is useful for the detection of *Plasmodium*, *Leishmania*, trypanosomes, and microfilaria. Wright's or Wright-Giemsa stains may be used, however, for initial detection and Giemsa stains for defining characteristics of *Plasmodium* (Fig. 12-7).

Direct immunofluorescent stains consist of fluorescent labeled antibodies to specific microbial antigens. These preparations identify many different infectious agents, including *Bordetella*, *Legionella*, *Giardia*, *Cryptosporidium*, varicella-zoster virus, and herpes simplex virus (Figs. 12-8 and 12-9). Direct fluorescent antibody tests have variable sensitivity and specificity. Culture techniques are still preferable to diagnose *Bordetella*.

Direct, Rapid Tests for Infectious Agents

Several techniques identify infectious agents or their products in clinical specimens without the need for microscopy; these tests include latex agglutination, enzyme immunoassays, DNA hybridization, and polymerase chain reaction. In latex agglutination test kits, antiserum to specific antigen is absorbed onto latex beads. When antigen to which the

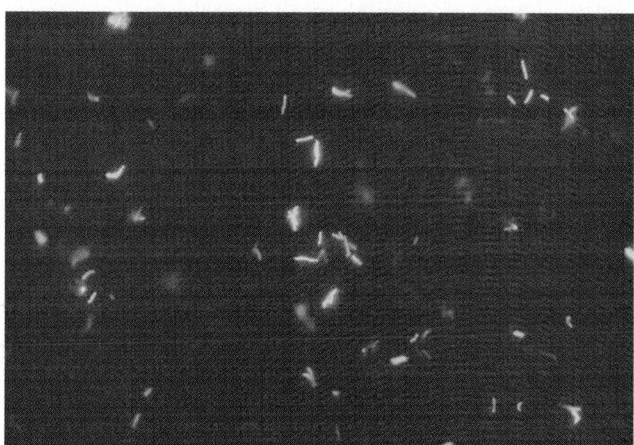

Figure 12-5. Mycobacteria detected by auramine staining. This specimen grew *Mycobacterium tuberculosis*.

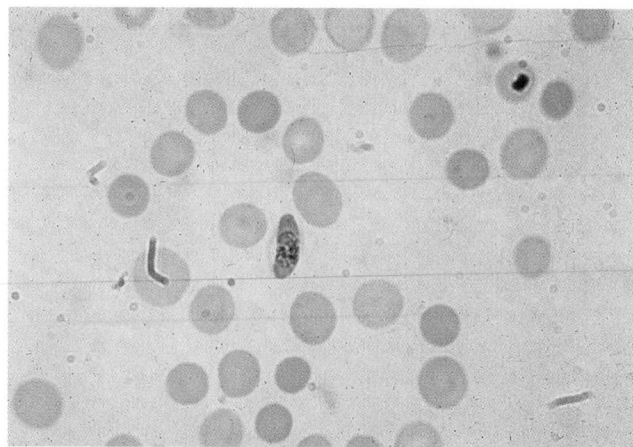

Figure 12-7. Giemsa stain of thin-preparation blood smear showing the gametocyte of *Plasmodium falciparum*.

Figure 12-8. *Legionella pneumophila* detected in sputum by direct fluorescent antibody testing.

antiserum is directed is added to the latex particles, visible agglutination of latex particles occurs. Commercially available latex agglutination test kits detect *H. influenzae* type b, *S. pneumoniae*, *N. meningitidis*, and group B streptococcus in cerebrospinal fluid. The sensitivity and specificity of latex agglutination testing of cerebrospinal fluid preclude routine use unless the patient is receiving antibiotics at the time of the lumbar puncture. The most common application of latex agglutination is to detect pharyngeal *S. pyogenes* rapidly.

Enzyme-linked immunosorbent assays (ELISA) are used to detect many different organisms. Enzyme immunoassays consist of antibody to an antigen of interest that has been absorbed to solid media. The clinical specimen, possibly containing the antigen of interest, is placed in direct contact with the bound antibody. In direct enzyme-linked immunosorbent assays, after washing, an enzyme-labeled antibody is applied. Indirect enzyme-linked assays add nonhuman animal antibodies followed by enzyme-linked antibody to the animal globulin. Enzyme-linked immunosorbent assays are inexpensive, sensitive, and easy to do. Laboratories routinely use them to detect antigens associated with *Clostridium difficile*, rotavirus, *Giardia*, cryptosporidia, microsporidia, and *C. trachomatis*.

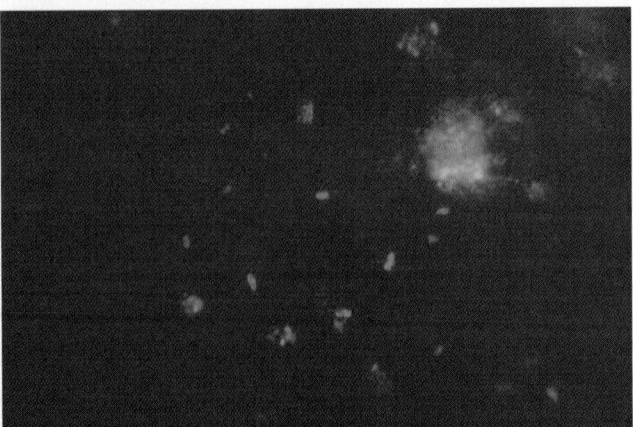

Figure 12-9. *Giardia lamblia* detected in stool by direct fluorescent antibody testing.

Microbiology laboratories use many molecular methods to identify organisms. Probe hybridization methods take advantage of the fact that complementary nucleic acid strands bind to form a stable hybrid. Probes are labeled nucleotides. Several different types of labels, including enzymes, antigens, chemiluminescent moieties, or radioisotopes, allow for easier direct detection of double-stranded nucleic acid molecules. These assays are used to confirm identification of cultures grown in the laboratory and to detect organisms in clinical samples. The material of interest is chemically treated to release nucleic acid from any organisms before mixing with the probe. DNA probe testing is sensitive, specific, and relatively straightforward to perform. Most DNA probe assays take place in a suspension in a single test tube. In situ hybridization occurs as a solid phase. DNA probes detect *N. gonorrhoeae*, *C. trachomatis*, and *M. tuberculosis* in clinical specimens.

Nucleic acid amplification and signal amplification methods are used to detect the nucleic acid of organisms. Oligonucleotide primers complementary to target sequences are incubated with clinical material that has been treated to free the nucleic acid. Hybridization occurs if complementary sequences exist. A temperature-stable polymerase extends the oligonucleotide primers to make two copies per DNA molecule of target sequence. Repetition generates an exponential number of copies. Nucleic acid amplification may amplify the target or the probe. Polymerase chain reaction (PCR) amplifies that target, whereas ligase chain reaction amplifies the probe. Branched DNA is unique in that the signal rather than the target or the probe is amplified. Currently, nucleic amplification is used most commonly to detect and quantitate HIV and hepatitis C in the blood and to detect enterovirus and herpes simplex in the cerebrospinal fluid (Box 12-1).

Culture Techniques

Growing the organism of interest in the laboratory is usually the most sensitive and specific means of recovering microorganisms from clinical specimens. Although most bacteria grow on standard media under standard conditions, some require specialized media, oxygen concentrations, or temperatures to support their growth. The laboratory must know which organisms are of major interest to ensure that media selection and environmental conditions are optimal to support the growth of all possible etiologic agents (Table 12-7). *B. pertussis* is not isolated on the usual culture

---

Box 12-1. Organisms for Which Commercial Amplification Assays Exist

- Chlamydia trachomatis
- Cytomegalovirus (plasma)
- Hepatitis B virus
- Hepatitis C virus
- Human immunodeficiency virus type 1
- Human papillomavirus
- Mycobacterium tuberculosis
- Neisseria gonorrhoeae
- Herpes simplex virus
- Enteroviruses

media that laboratories use for respiratory secretions. Nasopharyngeal secretions need to be inoculated directly onto specialized media plates (most often Regan-Lowe with and without vancomycin) that support the growth of *Bordetella* and inhibit the growth of other respiratory flora to reliably identify this organism.

The microbiology laboratory primarily uses solid or liquid media to cultivate bacteria. Solid and liquid media have unique advantages and disadvantages. Solid media are useful for small-volume inoculations. Solid media are less sensitive than liquid media except for recovering anaerobes, but they allow for discrimination among a variety of bacteria in a mixed infection, facilitate early identification based on typical colony morphologic characteristics, easily identify laboratory contaminants, and facilitate subculturing. Liquid media are useful for a larger inoculum of material and support the growth of bacteria found in small numbers. One problem with broth is that overgrowth of rapidly growing bacteria suppresses slower growing organisms. In general, liquid media systems work best when a single pathogen is expected in small numbers from a specimen. Solid media are best when a mixed population of bacteria is likely. Blood routinely is inoculated into liquid media. A fluid from normally sterile sites, such as the cerebrospinal fluid, often is inoculated into liquid media and solid media. Specimens from nonsterile sites, including urine, generally are inoculated onto solid agar media only.

Specimens obtained from sterile sites are inoculated onto nonselective media and several types of media. In this way, all potential pathogens may grow. Blood, cerebrospinal fluid, and joint fluid routinely are inoculated onto nonselective media. Specimens obtained from sites in which any number of pathogenic organisms may be found are inoculated onto differential media. Differential media contain supplements that allow for the growth and identification of organisms possessing specific metabolic characteristics. Stool contains many different bacteria and many *E. coli*. Stool specimens inoculated onto McConckey-sorbitol media allow the growth of *E. coli*. Although most *E. coli* can use sorbitol as a carbohydrate, most strains of *E. coli* O157 cannot. A pink zone surrounds most colonies of *E. coli*, whereas the zone around *E. coli* O157 is clear.

Clinical samples from heavily colonized sites are inoculated onto selective media. Selective media contain supplements that either enhance the growth of the suspected pathogen or inhibit the growth of the resident flora. Selective media are used to support the selective growth of respiratory and gastrointestinal pathogens, such as *B. pertussis*, *Salmonella*, *Shigella*, and *Campylobacter*.

When bacteria grow on solid media or in liquid media, the next task is to identify the organism. The appearance of the colonies on specific solid media may make presumptive diagnosis possible. In almost all situations, a colony from solid media or a drop of fluid from liquid media is stained with Gram stain to identify the staining characteristics and morphology of the bacteria. Characteristic patterns may yield a presumptive diagnosis. The laboratory reports only presumptive results based on strict algorithms. Physicians must keep in mind that morphologic results can give only *presumptive* results that may be confirmed or refuted by more specific testing. Additionally the physician should use the clinical information at hand to help identify the organism. Other rapid tests are available to identify quickly bacteria grown on solid media. Most laboratories test grampositive cocci appearing as clusters for evidence of coagulase to help distinguish between coagulase-negative staphylococci and *S. aureus*.

Automated systems using biochemical reactions in microtiter wells now permit identification of most organisms grown in pure culture in less than 24 hours. This methodology compares the growth pattern of the isolated organism in different chemicals with the pattern of known bacteria. If the concordance between the organism of interest and the reference pattern is greater than 95%, the laboratory reports the identification of the organism. If the concordance is less than 95% with any known pattern, the laboratory repeats the procedure or tries to reisolate the organism to minimize the likelihood of contamination.

Culturing fungi is similar to culturing bacteria in that selective and nonselective media are used. Blood may be inoculated into automated blood culture systems primarily designed to detect bacteria because many now support the growth of *Candida*. More often, the lysis/centrifugation system or a broth/agar method is employed. Although fungal blood culture systems continue to improve, all current systems have weaknesses. A presumptive diagnosis can be made based on the morphology of yeasts seen after staining

Table 12-7. Most Common Identified Bacteria in Children with Suspected Bacteremia, Sepsis, or Meningitis (A) and Pneumonia (B) by Age Group*

Age Group	Expected Bacterial Pathogens	Less Common Bacterial Pathogens
A		
0–1 mo	Group B streptococcus	*Staphylococcus aureus*
	Coliforms (*Escherichia coli*)	*Streptococcus pneumoniae*
	Listeria monocytogenes	*Neisseria meningitidis*
1–3 mo	Group B streptococcus	*S. aureus*
	Coliforms (*E. coli*)	
	Listeria monocytogenes	
	S. pneumoniae	
	N. meningitidis	
3 mo–18 yr	*S. pneumoniae*	*S. aureus*
	N. meningitidis	Group A streptococcus
B		
0–1 mo	Group B streptococcus	*S. aureus*
	Coliforms (*E. coli*)	
	L. monocytogenes	
1–3 mo	*Chlamydia trachomatis*	*S. aureus*
	S. pneumoniae	*Pneumocystis*
		Bordetella pertussis
3 mo–18 yr	*S. pneumoniae*	*S. aureus*
	Chlamydia pneumoniae	Group A streptococcus
	Mycoplasma pneumoniae	*Legionella pneumophila*

*The frequency and relative proportion of an organism may be influenced by changes in practice or immunization schedules. The widespread use of intrapartum antibiotic prophylaxis has diminished markedly the likelihood that a neonate will develop early-onset group B streptococcal sepsis. The conjugated *Haemophilus influenzae* type B vaccine makes isolation of this previously common organism rare in the United States today. Licensure of the conjugated pneumococcal vaccine is likely to lead to many fewer episodes of invasive *S. pneumoniae* disease. Knowledge of the most common bacterial agents causing pneumonia in pediatric patients is complicated by the paucity of data. Charts listing common pathogens need to be interpreted in light of current and local practices, immunization schedules, and local epidemiology.

with Gram stain and other stains or colony morphology on solid media. Molds are identified by their characteristic hyphae or conidia.

Viral culture techniques differ from culture techniques for bacteria and fungi because the media for viral culture are cells. Viruses cannot replicate in a cell-free environment. Clinical specimens are inoculated into cell lines that support the growth of the most likely pathogens from the particular clinical site. It is vital that the physician tell the laboratory which viruses are most likely, of most importance, or of most concern so that the correct cell lines can be inoculated. Some clinical specimens (i.e., blood) are toxic to cell lines and may limit the utility or yield of viral cultures from that site. Occasionally, endogenous cell line viruses may inhibit the growth of the virus of interest. After inoculation onto the appropriate cells, the cells are observed by light microscopy for any cytopathic effect.

When a cytopathic effect is seen, a presumptive identification may be made based on the speed of appearance of the cytopathic effect, the cell lines involved, and the appearance of the cells. Monoclonal antibodies or genome detection is used to make a definitive identification.

SUGGESTED READINGS

Murray PR (ed): Manual of Clinical Microbiology, 8th ed. Washington, DC, American Society of Microbiology Press, 2003.
Nissen MD, Sloots TP: Rapid diagnosis in pediatric infectious diseases: The past, the present and the future. Pediatr Infect Dis J 2002;21(6):605–612.
Root RK (ed): Clinical Infectious Diseases: A Practical Approach. New York, Oxford University Press, 1999.
Subramanian G, Mural R, Hoffman SL, et al: Microbial disease in humans: A genomic perspective. Mol Diagn 2001;6:243–252
Versalovic J, Lupski JR: Molecular detection and genotyping of pathogens: More accurate and rapid answers. Trends Microbiol 2002; 10(10 Suppl):S15–S21.

SECTION 1   FUNDAMENTALS

13 Principles of Pathophysiology

Robert Englander

Understanding pathophysiology forms the basis for a rational approach to therapeutic interventions. Too often, health care practitioners remember the "what to do," but not the "why to do it." This approach has several important caveats: (1) Continued elucidation of physiologic mechanisms may change the approach to treatments of diseases, rendering old practices obsolete. (2) Newer therapies that address more specifically the underlying pathophysiology continue to be developed, leaving behind clinicians practicing without a firm grasp of the pathophysiology. (3) Teaching the next generation of pediatricians demands a knowledge of pathophysiology. (4) Continued scientific thought and exploration are based on an underlying foundation in the principles of pathophysiology. Cases Studies 13-1 through 13-4 illustrate the importance of determining the pathophysiology. The four cases, respectively, describe the pathophysiology underlying the systemic inflammatory response syndrome (SIRS) in meningococcemia, the pathophysiology underlying the lungs in a patient with pneumonia and respiratory failure, the pathophysiology underlying the brain and intracranial vault in a patient with traumatic brain injury (TBI), and the pathophysiology underlying the immune system in a patient with severe combined immunodeficiency (SCID) syndrome secondary to adenosine deaminase (ADA) deficiency. The cases illustrate pathophysiology at the level of the organism as a whole (see Case Study 13-1), the individual organ level (see Case Study 13-2), the cel-

lular level (see Case Study 13-3), and the molecular level (see Case Study 13-4). For each case, discussion starts with the patient presentation, followed by identification of the pathophysiology, and discussion of the therapeutic plan in relation to the pathophysiology.

CASE STUDY 13-1: MENINGOCOCCEMIA

Identify the Pathophysiology
Introduction of *Neisseria meningitidis* into the bloodstream results in a systemic inflammatory cascade that wreaks havoc on the host. The two interrelated pathophysiologic processes that accompany fulminant meningococcal sepsis are *shock* and *disseminated intravascular coagulation (DIC)*. These two processes have common causal pathways and synergy in the resultant multiple organ system dysfunction that develops. An understanding of the intricate pathophysiology of *SIRS* provides the knowledge necessary for a rational approach to therapy and a glimpse into future directions for therapeutic intervention.

Shock and the Role of Meningococcal Endotoxin (Lipopolysaccharide)
The nature of shock in meningococcemia is distributive and cardiogenic. The intravascular volume is depleted as a result of capillary leak. In addition, circulating cytokines result in inappropriate vasodilation and depressed vascular tone and

MENINGOCOCCEMIA

A 10-year-old boy presents with meningococcemia. He has a 24-hour history of fever, increasing lethargy, and a rapidly progressive petechial rash. He has had no urine output in 12 hours. His vital signs are as follows: temperature, 103°F; heart rate, 140 beats/min; blood pressure, 70/30 mm Hg; and respiratory rate, 40 breaths/min with obvious hyperpnea. On physical examination, the patient is lethargic but arousable. His skin examination reveals a diffuse petechial rash that is becoming purpuric in the groin region. His capillary refill time is 4 to 5 seconds.

Laboratory data include the following: (1) complete blood count, with hemoglobin, 10 g/dL; hematocrit, 30%; white blood cell count, 2700/mm³ with 25 segmented neutrophils, 40 bands, 20 lymphocytes, 12 monocytes, 2 eosinophils, and 1 basophil; and platelet count, 43,000/µL; (2) prothrombin time, partial thromboplastin time, and fibrin degradation products, all elevated; (3) marked anion gap metabolic acidosis; (4) liver enzymes elevated (800s); and (5) blood urea nitrogen and creatinine, elevated.

act as negative inotropes with a direct myocardial depressant effect. The main activator of these derangements is meningococcal endotoxin. This toxin is a lipopolysaccharide (LPS) contained in the bacterial outer cell wall. The amount of endotoxemia produced correlates directly with the mortality rate.

Lipopolysaccharide and Cytokines

LPS in the bloodstream initially results in the release of a host of proinflammatory mediators called *cytokines*. Cytokines are synthesized and released by macrophages, monocytes, and endothelial cells and act locally on a variety of cells to signal information to adjacent cells. The two cytokines implicated as most important in meningococcemia are tumor necrosis factor (TNF)–α and interleukin (IL)-1β. These mediators have direct and indirect effects that contribute to shock. They act directly by inducing the production of the potent vasodilators, nitric oxide and prostaglandins. The prostaglandins also have a direct negative inotropic effect on the heart. TNF-α and IL-1β also affect distributive shock indirectly by inducing other cytokines and by activating neutrophils and leukocytes, which then may release potent proinflammatory cytokines that contribute to vasodilation and endothelial cell damage. These two potent mediators also enhance the adherence of polymorphonuclear leukocytes and monocytes to endothelial cells, contributing directly to capillary damage and leaking. TNF itself may have a direct negative inotropic effect on the heart. Although these two cytokines have focal roles in SIRS of meningococcemia, they are by no means the whole story. This point has been underscored by unsuccessful clinical trials using monoclonal antibodies against TNF-α or IL-1β in sepsis syndromes.

Not all cytokines are detrimental to the host in SIRS. Some have anti-inflammatory activity (e.g., IL-1 receptor antagonist, soluble TNF receptors). In addition, some cytokines may be protective in meningococcal sepsis. Carroll and colleagues found an inverse correlation between the chemokine *regulated on activation, normal T-cell expressed and secreted* (RANTES) and (1) death from meningococcal disease and (2) incidence of septic shock in meningococcal disease.

Lipopolysaccharide and the Complement System

LPS also activates the *complement system*. This system plays a key role in host defenses against bacteria, by stimulating bacterial lysis, enhancing phagocytosis by monocytes or polymorphonuclear neutrophils, and neutralizing endotoxin. In addition, the complement system is involved in regulation of other immunologic functions, control of coagulation and fibrinolysis pathways, and maintenance of vascular permeability and tone. Adequate complement is essential to the host defense against meningococcus specifically, and deficiency results in a significant increase in the risk of invasive meningococcal disease. When invasive disease occurs, however, it is characterized by excessive complement activation by LPS. The results include direct vascular injury and capillary leak, exacerbating the distributive shock.

Disseminated Intravascular Coagulation and Lipopolysaccharide

DIC is characterized by microvascular coagulation and bleeding diatheses. In meningococcal sepsis, LPS and TNF-α induce the expression of tissue factor by monocytes, macrophages, and endothelial cells. Tissue factor activates factor VII, initiating the extrinsic clotting pathway and resulting in the formation of microvascular thrombi. The proinflammatory mediator kallikrein also activates factor XII, setting the intrinsic clotting cascade in motion. Factor XII stimulates the release of bradykinin, complement, plasmin, and elastase, mitigating inflammation, fibrinolysis, tissue damage, and clot formation. In addition to the activation of the clotting cascade, meningococcal sepsis is associated with a significant decrease in the natural levels of circulating anticoagulants, particularly antithrombin III, protein S, and protein C. Clot formation is accelerated, and clot breakdown is depressed. Although microvascular thrombi result in end organ damage diffusely, the skin and adrenals seem to be particularly prone, with resultant purpura fulminans or adrenal hemorrhage and hypoadrenalism.

End Result of Shock and Disseminated Intravascular Coagulation

Shock results in inadequate delivery of substrate to tissues owing to inadequate cardiac output, further depressing function in all organ systems. Delivery of oxygen (DO_2) to tissues is represented by the following equation:

$$DO_2 = C.O. \times CaO_2$$

where C.O. is cardiac output, and CaO_2 is arterial concentration of oxygen.

The patient in Case Study 13-1 is hypotensive from the above-described vasodilatory and myocardial depressant effects of LPS. In addition, he has evidence of diffuse hypoperfusion and anaerobic respiration with a marked anion gap acidosis. Measurement of the lactic acid level would reveal significant elevation. In addition to the hypoperfusion, the patient's DIC has resulted in end organ microvascular thrombi. The two processes, shock and DIC, work synergistically to increase end organ dysfunction or failure or both. Direct organ dysfunction is evident in both of the kidneys from the elevated blood urea nitrogen and creatinine and in the bone marrow from the depressed white blood cell count and thrombocytopenia. The liver enzyme elevation is also evidence of end organ hypoperfusion. An overall schematic for the effects of LPS on proinflammatory mediators, complement, and DIC with the resultant tissue injury and organ dysfunction is presented in Figure 13-1.

Pathophysiology-Based Interventions

After attention to the "ABCs" (airway, breathing, and circulation), the most important aspect of care for the patient in Case Study 13-1 is the initiation of appropriate antibiotic therapy. Initial concerns that antibiotic treatment early in the disease result in a "showering" of LPS and worsening shock and DIC have not been borne out by experimental data. Antibiotics should be given immediately any time the diagnosis of meningococcemia is entertained.

Along with antibiotics, the focus must be on replenishing the circulating volume and providing adequate cardiac output to re-establish substrate delivery to vital organs. Isotonic crystalloid (normal saline or lactated Ringer's solution) is an adequate volume expander; 60 to 120 mL/kg may be necessary. Some clinicians support the use of fresh frozen plasma as a volume expander and to treat the bleeding dyscrasia. Conversely, fresh frozen plasma may be reserved only for patients with established significant elevations in the prothrombin time.

When the intravascular volume has been repleted, treatment with cardiotonic medications may be required for patients with a low systemic vascular resistance and persistent hypotension. Dopamine generally is the initial drug of choice and works to increase myocardial contractility by direct interactions with the β_1-receptors of the sympathetic nervous system in the heart. If dopamine fails to improve the blood pressure, norepinephrine may be added. The latter is a mixed α-adrenergic and β-adrenergic stimulating agent, with more potent α-adrenergic properties, resulting in potent vasoconstriction and an increase in the systemic vascular resistance. The potential danger with norepinephrine is the possibility of exacerbating end organ ischemia; it should be reserved for patients with significant hypotension and decreased systemic vascular resistance despite treatment with volume and dopamine. Limited success with the use of angiotensin in patients with hypotension refractory to norepinephrine treatment was reported in a case series. With aggressive and early therapy, shock generally can be reversed and end organ damage limited.

Treatments directed at interfering with the inflammatory cascade or complement activation to date have focused on monoclonal antibodies to individual agents within these systems (e.g., antibody to TNF-α or IL-1β). Although animal studies had been promising, their human counterparts have not shown benefit. A randomized controlled trial of monoclonal antibody to TNF-α in adults with severe sepsis was halted by the data-monitoring group because of increased risk in the treated group. The current hypothesis is that interference in a single pathway of this complex pathophysiologic process is simply not enough to reverse the associated shock and DIC. An alternate explanation is that these treatments are successful in animal models only when given concurrently with the endotoxin or bacterial loads, but lose their efficacy when the host has been exposed to LPS for even a brief period (minutes to a few hours).

One controversial treatment is the use of glucocorticoids. This treatment is recommended for patients with associated meningococcal meningitis if it can be given within 4 hours of antibiotics. In addition, systemic steroids have been recommended in refractory hypotension on the assumption of adrenal hemorrhages being present. Randomized controlled trials of systemic steroids in overwhelming sepsis of any kind have not proved the treatment to be beneficial, however, for prevention of either morbidity or mortality.

Future Treatments

Further elucidation of host factors that are protective and even genetic factors that play a role in morbidity or mortality from meningococcal disease should provide opportunities for investigation of novel therapies. The finding that levels of the chemokine RANTES are related inversely to outcome suggest the possibility of future investigations into RANTES as a therapy for meningococcal sepsis. This option may be subject to the same pitfalls, however, as prior trials that have targeted one aspect of the inflammatory cascade.

More likely is the development of combination therapies to block each of the pathways detrimental to the host, from proinflammatory mediators to complement activation to the coagulation pathways. Only through further efforts at elucidating the complicated pathophysiology of this ever-present bacterium, and the havoc it wreaks on the entire host, can clinicians hope to improve the current 10% to 30% mortality associated with meningococcemia.

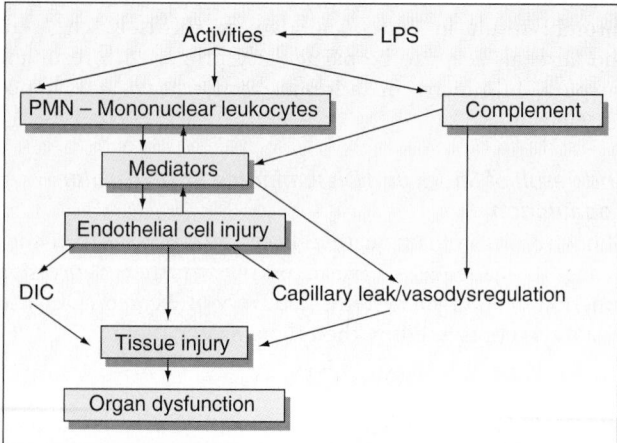

Figure 13-1. Pathophysiology of meningococcal sepsis. DIC, disseminated intravascular coagulation; LPS, lipopolysaccharide; PMN, polymorphonuclear neutrophil. (Redrawn from De Kleijn ED, Hazelzet JA, Kornelisse RF, De Groot R: Pathophysiology of meningococcal sepsis in children. Eur J Pediatr 1998;157:869–880.)

CASE STUDY 13-2: PNEUMONIA AND RESPIRATORY FAILURE

Identify the Pathophysiology

The patient in Case Study 13-2 presented with the classic findings of pneumonia resulting in respiratory failure. Specifically, despite an increase in her work of breathing, she was unable to exchange oxygen and carbon dioxide adequately. In addition, the patient developed a metabolic acidosis that exacerbated her respiratory acidosis. Her problems seemed to have started with an infection in the lungs, likely bacterial in nature given the lobar consolidation. The clinician's first goal is to understand the pathophysiology of the patient's hypoxemia, hypercarbia, and metabolic acidosis.

Hypoxemia

Hypoxemia is defined as an abnormally low P_{O_2} in arterial blood. Only four pathophysiologic processes result in hypoxemia: hypoventilation, diffusion alterations, ventilation-perfusion (V/Q) mismatch, and shunt. In the patient in Case 13-2, all four causes may be contributing to the hypoxemia.

Hypoventilation

The alveolus has a fixed partial pressure of gases that it can accommodate, represented by this *alveolar gas equation:*

$$P_{AO_2} = P_{IO_2} - P_{ACO_2}/RQ$$

where P_{AO_2} is the partial pressure of oxygen in the alveolus, P_{IO_2} is the partial pressure of oxygen in inspired air, P_{ACO_2} is the partial pressure of carbon dioxide in the alveolus, and RQ is the respiratory quotient. P_{IO_2} is defined as the O_2 fraction of inspired air (0.21) multiplied by barometric pressure (P_B) adjusted for water vapor pressure (P_{H_2O}): $P_{IO_2} = 0.21 (P_B - P_{H_2O})$. One can see from this equation that the P_{AO_2} varies inversely with the P_{ACO_2}. The patient's hypercarbia is one direct cause of hypoxemia. If it is assumed the patient is at sea level and has a normal RQ of 0.8, her P_{AO_2} would become

$$P_{AO_2} = 0.21 (760 - 47) - 60/0.8 = 75 \text{ mm Hg}$$

If the patient had a normal P_{ACO_2} of 40 mm Hg, her P_{AO_2} would have been

---

CASE STUDY 13-2

PNEUMONIA AND RESPIRATORY FAILURE

A 4-year-old girl presents to the emergency department with a 1-week history of upper respiratory tract symptoms, 3 days of high fever, and respiratory distress for several hours. On presentation to the emergency department, she is febrile (temperature 103°F), tachycardic (heart rate 140 beats/min), tachypneic (respiratory rate 44 breaths/min), and cyanotic in room air with an oxygen saturation by pulse oximetry of 77%.

Her blood gas values are as follows: pH, 7.04; P_{ACO_2}, 60 mm Hg; P_{aO_2}, 48 mm Hg; and bicarbonate, 16 mEq/L. Hemoglobin is 8.0 g/dL. Electrolyte concentrations reveal an anion gap of 24.

Chest x-ray reveals complete opacification of the right hemithorax with mediastinal shift to the left.

$$P_{AO_2} = 0.21 (760 - 47) - 40/0.8 = 100 \text{ mm Hg}$$

The patient's hypoventilation has resulted in a decrease in her P_{AO_2} (and her maximal P_{aO_2}) from 100 mm Hg to 75 mm Hg. Her measured P_{aO_2} was only 48 mm Hg, however. The other three causes of hypoxemia must be responsible for the further decrease in her P_{aO_2} from 75 to 48 mm Hg.

Diffusion Alterations

Fick's law states that the volume of a gas diffusing through a tissue is directly proportional to the area over which it diffuses and inversely proportional to the tissue thickness:

$$V_{gas} = A/T \times D \times (P_1 - P_2)$$

where *A* is the area of the diffusion sheet, *T* is the thickness of the diffusion sheet, *D* is the diffusion coefficient of the gas, and $P_1 - P_2$ is the pressure gradient across the sheet. If one were to look at the area of consolidated lung under a microscope, one would see many alveoli partially filled with exudate and an interstitium with a neutrophilic infiltration. The thickness of the gas exchange surface in these alveoli has increased dramatically, resulting in diffusion alterations that contribute to hypoxemia.

Ventilation-Perfusion Mismatch

Two potential causes of V/Q mismatch can be identified in this patient. Some alveoli, as noted previously, are partially filled with exudates, minimizing ventilation of those alveolar units. These alveoli may have slightly decreased or even normal perfusion. These alveolar units have decreased V/Q ratios and contribute to the patient's hypoxemia. The gas leaving the alveolar capillary in an alveolus with a dramatically decreased V/Q ratio has P_{aO_2} and P_{aCO_2} values that approach mixed venous blood—a P_{aO_2} of 40 mm Hg and a P_{aCO_2} of 47 mm Hg.

Other alveoli, particularly those adjacent to collapsed alveoli, may be hyperexpanded because of the interdependence of alveolar units. These alveoli may have a decrease in perfusion owing to increased alveolar pressure essentially collapsing the surrounding capillary, resulting in an increased V/Q ratio. Capillary units from alveoli with an increased V/Q ratio have P_{aO_2} and P_{aCO_2} values that approach atmospheric gas. These units *do not* contribute to the patient's hypoxemia.

Shunt

Alveoli that are perfused but completely unventilated (V/Q ratio of 0) give rise to intrapulmonary shunt. These alveolar units are abundant in the consolidated portion of lung, generally as a result of either collapse or being filled with exudate. Capillary units from alveoli with shunt have P_{aO_2} and P_{aCO_2} values equal to the mixed venous sample.

Hypercarbia

Hypercarbia also has several potential pathophysiologic etiologies: V/Q mismatch, shunt, increased carbon dioxide production, and depression of central chemoreceptors.

Ventilation-Perfusion Mismatch

Although the gradient from mixed venous to arterial blood is considerably less for carbon dioxide than for oxygen, areas with low V/Q ratios still have a higher than normal P_{CO_2}, closer to that of mixed venous blood. As the $PaCO_2$ rises, the alveoli become increasingly inefficient at removing carbon dioxide, however, resulting in increasingly larger contributions from alveoli with low V/Q ratios to the hypercarbia.

Shunt

As noted earlier, capillary units from alveoli with shunt have PO_2 and PCO_2 values equal to the mixed venous sample, contributing to hypercarbia.

Increased Carbon Dioxide Production

Fever and increased work of breathing in this patient result in a significant increase in the production of carbon dioxide. Alveolar ventilation, $PaCO_2$, and carbon dioxide production are related by the following equation:

$$VA = VCO_2/PaCO_2 \cong 863 \text{ mm Hg}$$

where VA is the alveolar minute ventilation, and VCO_2 is the production of carbon dioxide per minute. The patient in Case Study 13-2 with significant lung disease is unable to increase alveolar ventilation despite increases in carbon dioxide production, and the $PaCO_2$ increases.

Depression of Central Chemoreceptors

The respiratory cycle is under the control predominantly of central nervous system chemoreceptors in the ventral medulla. These receptors respond with exquisite sensitivity to changes in the local partial pressure of carbon dioxide. Under normal conditions, increases in the $PaCO_2$ in the ventral medulla result in stimulation of respiration and increase in the minute ventilation, with a commensurate decrease in the $PaCO_2$. When the $PaCO_2$ increases to levels greater than 60 to 70 mm Hg, however, the carbon dioxide has narcoleptic properties, resulting in a paradoxical decrease in the respiratory drive and further increases in the $PaCO_2$.

Metabolic Acidosis

In addition to respiratory acidosis, the patient in Case Study 13-2 has an anion gap metabolic acidosis. The unmeasured anion is lactic acid. This patient is set up for lactic acidosis, the result of anaerobic metabolism, which occurs with inadequate oxygen delivery to tissues, adequate delivery but inability to use oxygen delivered, or deficiencies in the aerobic metabolic pathway. The patient has two major reasons to have inadequate oxygen delivery to tissues—anemia and hemoglobin desaturation. A significant lactic acidosis can explain her anion gap.

The delivery of oxygen to tissues is represented by the following equation:

$$DO_2 = C.O. \times CaO_2$$

where DO_2 is the delivery of oxygen to tissues in mL/min; CaO_2 is the arterial content of oxygen in mL oxygen/dL blood; and C.O. is the cardiac output in L/min. The CaO_2 is the sum of the oxygen bound to hemoglobin and the oxygen dissolved in blood. It is defined by the following equation:

$$CaO_2 = (1.34 \cong Hb \cong \text{saturation}/100) + PaO_2 \cong 0.003$$

where 1.34 is the mL of oxygen that combines with 1 g of hemoglobin, *Hb* is the hemoglobin concentration in g/dL blood, *saturation* is the percent of hemoglobin saturated

with oxygen, and *0.003* is a constant with units mL oxygen/dL blood/mm Hg. The first part of the equation represents the oxygen content that is bound to hemoglobin, and the second part represents dissolved oxygen. As can be seen, the bound portion is responsible for more than 98% of the total oxygen content under normal conditions (saturation 97%, hemoglobin 12 to 14 g/dL, and PaO_2 100 mm Hg). The patient has a moderate anemia and a severe desaturation of hemoglobin, resulting in an arterial oxygen content less than half normal. Further complicating the picture is the fact that at the same time the patient has a significant *decrease in arterial content of oxygen*, she has an *increased demand for oxygen* because of fever, increased work of breathing, and infection. She has developed a lactic acidosis from inadequate delivery of substrate to supply her hypermetabolic tissues.

Pathophysiology-Based Interventions

The clinician must recognize that this patient has respiratory failure—an inability to exchange gases in the lung to meet the body's demands. The first intervention would be to intubate the trachea and provide positive pressure mechanical ventilation with 100% O_2. This intervention alone should have dramatic effects on all three of the pathophysiologic processes addressed—hypoxemia, hypercarbia, and metabolic acidosis.

Intubation and mechanical ventilation result in the following changes:

1. *Decrease in V/Q mismatching.* This occurs via expansion of partially ventilated, perfused alveoli increasing the V/Q ratio toward 1.
2. *Decrease in shunt.* Shunt is decreased by "recruitment" of nonventilated but perfused alveoli, again increasing the V/Q ratio toward 1.
3. *Improvement in diffusion.* This is accomplished by increased clearance of lymphatic and alveolar fluid, decreasing the tissue thickness across which the oxygen must diffuse (see Fick's law).
4. *Improvement in alveolar oxygenation.* Improvement occurs by providing 100% oxygen and by improving the ventilation (a decrease in the $PaCO_2$ increases the alveolar PO_2; see the alveolar gas equation).
5. *Decrease in or elimination of work of breathing.* The "work" of the respiratory system can be transferred partially or completely to the mechanical ventilator, resulting in decreased oxygen demand and decreased carbon dioxide production.
6. *Normalization of the $PaCO_2$.* This is done through proper manipulation of the ventilator (the details of mechanical ventilation are beyond the scope of this chapter).

In addition to positive-pressure ventilation, the clinician can provide several other interventions aimed ultimately at reversing the hypoxemia, hypercarbia, and metabolic acidosis. The first priority is to treat the underlying pneumonia by providing appropriate antibiotic treatment. Second, oxygen delivery can be maximized by improving oxygen content and cardiac output. Improving oxygen content can be accomplished by improving oxygen saturation as outlined previously and by transfusion of packed red blood cells. Finally, the delivery of oxygen to tissues can be improved by maximizing cardiac output, by providing adequate filling volumes and inotropic support as needed. Only through understanding the pathophysiologic processes occurring in the lungs of this patient with pneumonia and respiratory failure can the clinician focus treatment on reversal of those processes and restoration of normal physiologic function of the lungs.

CASE STUDY 13-3: TRAUMATIC BRAIN INJURY

Identify the Pathophysiology

The pathophysiology of TBI is an area of intensive investigation. With TBI, *primary injury* to neurons results in cell death and edema in the parenchyma. Primary injury is irreversible and not a source for investigation or treatment. The only treatment is prevention, and pediatric clinicians have been involved in creating and disseminating injury prevention programs for decades. Despite these efforts, head trauma remains a leading cause of morbidity and mortality in the pediatric population. An understanding of the pathophysiology and treatment of TBI is mandatory for any practitioner involved in the care of children.

After a primary neuronal injury, edema or intracranial hemorrhage increases the intracranial volume and may result in *intracranial hypertension*. Intracranial hypertension affects the *cerebral perfusion pressure (CPP)*. *Cerebral blood flow (CBF)* and *autoregulation* alterations also may contribute to the pathophysiology of TBI. Finally, several pathophysiologic processes are initiated after the primary injury resulting in further neuronal injury, called *secondary brain injury*. The following sections address the pathophysiology of intracranial hypertension and its effect on CPP, the determinants of CBF, and the pathophysiologic processes of secondary brain injury to allow an understanding of the current and potential future treatments for the patient in Case Study 13-3.

Intracranial Hypertension and Cerebral Perfusion Pressure

Primary neuronal injury results in parenchymal edema. The intracranial vault has a fixed volume consisting of brain, cerebrospinal fluid (CSF), and blood; this edema fluid must

---

CASE STUDY 13-3

TRAUMATIC BRAIN INJURY

A 2-year-old boy is unrestrained in a car seat during a motor vehicle accident. He is thrown against the window. He is unconscious at the scene and on arrival to the emergency department. His initial Glasgow Coma Scale score is 5 (no verbal response, no eye opening, and abnormal flexion to stimuli). His initial blood pressure is 150/90 mm Hg, his heart rate is 54 beats/min, and his respirations are agonal. After stabilizing the airway by endotracheal intubation and mechanical ventilation, a head computed tomography scan is ordered, which reveals a nondisplaced temporal bone fracture and a contracoup brain contusion with significant edema but no hemorrhage. An increase in the intracranial pressure is suspected.

---

displace an identical volume of cerebral blood or CSF to maintain intracranial pressure (ICP). The most readily displaced content in the intracranial vault is CSF. Under normal circumstances, the ICP is constant as a result of adjustments in CSF or CBF or both to maintain a constant intracranial volume. As a result of significant primary injury, an intracranial bleed or mass, or secondary injury, the brain's compensatory mechanisms may be overcome, resulting in *intracranial hypertension*. The compliance of the intracranial vault is such that at a critical point on the pressure-volume curve, any small further volume increase results in a logarithmic increase in the ICP.

When CSF and venous blood have been displaced maximally, small increases in any of the components of the intracranial vault result in a significant increase in the ICP. Increased ICP has a deleterious effect on the injured brain by exacerbating ischemia through reduction in the CPP. The perfusion pressure in any organ is the pressure gradient from arterial to venous circulation. In the brain, the perfusion pressure is represented by the difference between the mean arterial pressure and the central venous pressure or the ICP, whichever is higher. In TBI, the ICP becomes the determining factor for the CPP. Moderate intracranial hypertension can decrease the CPP significantly and exacerbate secondary brain injury.

In the most severe intracranial hypertension, ICP can exceed the mean arterial pressure. This condition is heralded by the presence of Cushing's triad. This triad consists of hypertension, bradycardia, and irregular respirations and results from the herniation of the cerebellar tonsils into the spinal column. Cushing's triad is an emergency requiring immediate measures to decrease the contents of the intracranial vault to allow room for the tonsils to return to their normal anatomic location. This critical situation was suggested by the case study patient's presentation in the emergency department.

Determinants of Cerebral Blood Flow

The brain has a high metabolic rate that requires a constant supply of nutrients such as oxygen and glucose. CBF is autoregulated to maintain constancy despite wide variations in systemic blood pressure. Physiologically, autoregulation results in vasodilation in arterial hypotension and vasoconstriction in arterial hypertension. CBF remains constant at mean arterial pressures between approximately 50 and 150 mm Hg in adults. Other factors also influence the CBF and merit close attention when caring for a patient with TBI. CBF is maintained at a range of oxygen partial pressures; however, when the oxygen tension falls below a critical level (around 50 mm Hg), CBF increases dramatically in an effort to maintain oxygen delivery. Conversely, $PaCO_2$ varies directly with CBF: As $PaCO_2$ increases, CBF increases, and as $PaCO_2$ decreases, as from hyperventilation, CBF decreases. Hyperventilation may result in worsening of ischemia, whereas hypoventilation may result in hyperemia and exacerbation of intracranial hypertension. The relationships between mean arterial pressure, $PaCO_2$, and PaO_2 with CBF are depicted in Figure 13-2. CBF also is coupled tightly to the metabolic rate of the brain. Efforts to control CBF include avoiding hypermetabolic states (e.g., fever) in the TBI patient.

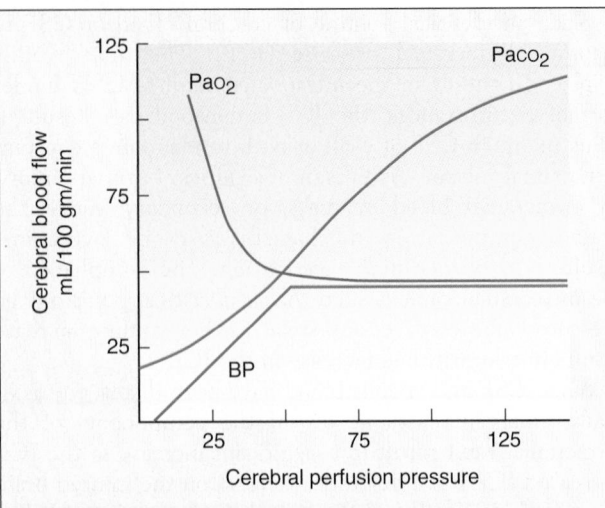

Figure 13-2. Influence of $PaCO_2$, PaO_2, and blood pressure on cerebral blood flow and cerebral perfusion pressure. (Redrawn from Poss WB, Brockmeyer DL, Clay B, et al: Pathophysiology and management of the intracranial vault. In Rogers MC [ed]: Textbook of Pediatric Critical Care. Baltimore, Williams & Wilkins, 1996, pp 645–665.)

Secondary Brain Injury

Understanding the mechanisms of secondary brain injury has formed the basis for numerous investigative efforts. Many pathophysiologic processes have been elucidated that contribute to secondary brain swelling, including ischemia, excitotoxicity, programmed cell death, axonal injury, and inflammation and regeneration. Each of these mechanisms merits some discussion because therapies designed to reverse them serve as the major focus for the future in preventing secondary brain injury. Figure 13-3 is a simple schematic representation of the pathophysiology of secondary brain injury.

Posttraumatic ischemia is a major contributor to secondary brain injury and to overall outcome. Early focus on hyperemia leading to increased brain swelling and ischemia has been altered to a focus on early hypoperfusion as the key factor in pediatric TBI ischemia. CBF is lowest in the first 24 hours after TBI in children. This ischemia from

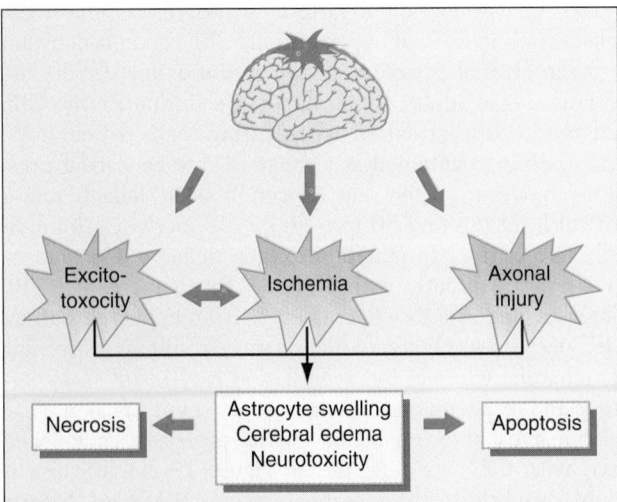

Figure 13-3. Schematic representation of the sequence of events leading to secondary brain injury.

hypoperfusion can be exacerbated severely by systemic hypotension or hypoxemia or both. The causes of this early hypoperfusion have begun to be elucidated, and several cellular and molecular biologic processes are thought to contribute. Decreased vasodilatory responses to nitric oxide, cyclic guanosine monophosphate, cyclic adenosine monophosphate, and prostanoids all have been shown in animal models of TBI. TBI also may result in the release of supranormal levels of the vasoconstricting peptide endothelin-1. Early focus for the patient in Case Study 13-3 needs to be on minimizing ongoing tissue ischemia.

Excitotoxicity

Excitotoxicity refers to the neuronal toxicity that results from inappropriately large amounts of excitatory amino acids (EAAs), especially glutamate and aspartate, after TBI. Excitotoxicity occurs in two phases. Immediately after injury, EAA-induced, sodium-dependent neuronal swelling occurs. A delayed response results in EAA-activated calcium channel overstimulation, with resultant pathophysiologic increases in intracellular calcium. This delayed event is often the harbinger of cell death. Another potential focus for this patient is on minimizing EAA action after TBI.

Programmed Cell Death and Apoptosis

After TBI, some neurons die as a result of a process called *programmed cell death*. This process is physiologic in embryos and in cells in tissues that turn over; in TBI, however, it becomes pathophysiologic. Triggering the programmed cell death process results in intranucleosomal endonucleases fragmenting DNA and dismantling cytoskeletal and nuclear structural proteins. The end result of this process is a distinct cell morphology called *apoptosis*. Programmed cell death occurs in stages and provides potential therapeutic targets at each stage.

Traumatic Axonal Injury

Traumatic axonal injury is an important pathophysiologic process in children because they are in a period of developmental axonal connectivity. Initial shearing results in axonal injury; however, adult animal studies have suggested that traumatic axonal injury is predominantly a delayed process termed *secondary axotomy*. The sequence of secondary axotomy is in the process of being elucidated. Theories have included focal ion flux, calcium dysregulation, and mitochondrial and cytoskeletal dysfunction as the triggering agents for axonal swelling and disruption of normal axonal transport functions. Although early attempts to prevent or decrease traumatic axonal injury were not successful, strategies have suggested that traumatic axonal injury may be another pathophysiologic process in the child with TBI amenable to therapeutic intervention.

Inflammation and Regeneration

An acute inflammatory reaction has been documented after TBI in numerous animal and human studies. This inflammatory process seems to be detrimental and may play a role in secondary brain swelling. One component of this reaction is neutrophil accumulation at the site of focal trauma. Neutrophil accumulation seems to have less of a

Table 13-1. Acute Inflammatory Markers in the Cerebrospinal Fluid of Pediatric Traumatic Brain Injury Patients

CSF Marker	Results	Reference
IL-6	↑↑ (60-fold)	Bell et al, 1997
IL-10	↑, associated with age <4 yr and mortality	Bell et al, 1997
IL-8	↑↑, associated with abuse and mortality	Whalen et al, 2000
Adhesion molecules (P-selectin, E-selectin, ICAM-1)	↑, similar to levels in meningitis	Whalen et al, 1998

CSF, cerebrospinal fluid; ICAM-1, intercellular adhesion molecule 1; IL, interleukin.

role in global TBI. The hypothesis is that local tissue necrosis is necessary to produce neutrophil influx. Proinflammatory cytokines, chemokines, and adhesion molecules have been shown to be elevated in the CSF of children with focal and diffuse injury. Perhaps the largest experience with investigation of these inflammatory agents in pediatric TBI comes from the CSF Bank in Pittsburgh. A summary of their findings of acute inflammatory mediators is presented in Table 13-1.

In addition to the acute inflammatory response, a subacute inflammatory process has been documented in TBI. This inflammatory response may be related to axonal regeneration, however. Current investigation is focused on further elucidation of the detrimental and beneficial effects of inflammation in an effort to elucidate further therapies that maximize benefit while minimizing risk.

Summary of the Pathophysiology of Traumatic Brain Injury

The potential pathophysiologic processes resulting in the poor neurologic condition of the patient in Case Study 13-3 have been enumerated. On the global level, cerebral swelling resulted in increased ICP, decreasing the patient's CPP and increasing secondary injury through ischemia. In addition, the patient likely had varying degrees of local hypoperfusion, excitotoxicity, apoptosis, axonal injury, and inflammation. Following is a rational and pathophysiologically based approach to the treatment of this patient with TBI.

Treatment

General Management

Endotracheal intubation and mechanical ventilation were imperative in this unconscious patient with evidence of Cushing's triad. In general, intubation should be initiated in any patient with a Glasgow Coma Scale score less than 8 because this indicates an inability to protect the airway. The patient's initial Glasgow Coma Scale score was 5. The Glasgow Coma Scale has been used in adults to predict outcome from TBI. Its predictive value in children is less

clear, although it is helpful as an estimator of severity of injury. The components of the Glasgow Coma Scale score for children are outlined in Table 13-2.

Further general management includes establishing intravenous access to maintain circulating blood volume and fully exposing the child to address any other potential injuries from the motor vehicle accident. In addition, the clinician needs to be sure to *avoid the five Hs—hyperthermia, hypotension, hypoxemia, hypoglycemia,* and *hypoventilation.* From the previous discussion of the pathophysiology of TBI, one can recognize the logic behind avoiding the five *H*s. Hyperthermia increases the metabolic rate of the brain, which has two detrimental effects: (1) increasing the metabolic rate of the brain has a direct correlation with increasing CBF, potentially exacerbating intracranial hypertension and worsening secondary brain injury through ischemia, and (2) increasing metabolic demand in hypoperfusion after TBI increases the demand/supply mismatch of substrates, increasing the likelihood of further cell death. Hypotension needs to be avoided to minimize secondary damage from hypoperfusion and to maximize the CPP. Hypoxemia and hypoglycemia result in inadequate delivery of substrate to the neurons, further increasing the likelihood of cell death. Hypoventilation should be avoided because $PaCO_2$ is noted to correlate directly with CBF, and increases in $PaCO_2$ exacerbate intracranial hypertension. Previous standard treatment included hyperventilation designed to lessen CBF. More recent animal and human adult studies suggest, however, that significant hyperventilation (to $PaCO_2$ in the 25 mm Hg range) is associated with worse outcomes.

Managing Intracranial Hypertension and Maintaining Cerebral Perfusion Pressure

Having established the airway, ensured adequate ventilation, and provided adequate volume to maintain circulating blood volume, while always attentive to avoiding the five *H*s, the clinician now must control the ICP. The goal of ICP control is to maximize the CPP and minimize secondary ischemic damage. The first step in controlling ICP is the placement of an ICP monitoring device. Without an ICP

Table 13-2. Glasgow Coma Scale Score for Children

Eye Opening	Score	Verbal Response	Score	Motor Response	Score
Spontaneous	4	Oriented	5	Responds to commands	6
To speech	3	Confused	4	Localizes to pain	5
To pain	2	Inappropriate words	3	Withdraws to pain	4
None	1	Incomprehensible sounds	2	Abnormal flexion to pain	3
		None	1	Abnormal extension to pain	2
				None	1

monitor, CPP cannot be calculated. The preferred instrument is an intraventricular catheter. This device allows measurement of ICP and concomitant drainage of ICP. This latter function provides compensation for increasing brain edema by decreasing the total intracranial volume, trying to avoid the critical volume at which ICP increases logarithmically.

In addition, as the discussion of the pathophysiology of intracranial hypertension would indicate, any measures that decrease volume in the intracranial vault should lead to a decrease in the ICP. These measures can be as simple as elevating the head of the bed to maximize venous drainage. More complex treatments, such as osmotic therapy with mannitol, have been used with moderate success in the treatment of adult TBI patients with intracranial hypertension. Intermittent doses rather than continuous infusion have been shown to have increased efficacy, although the reasons for this are not clear. Hypertonic saline also has been used with some success at controlling ICP and maintaining CPP in children with TBI. Osmolar therapy works through a rheologic mechanism—improving CBF at the same blood volume.

Barbiturates provide another pathophysiologically based therapy designed to decrease brain ischemia (inadequate substrate supply for the demand) by decreasing the brain's metabolic rate. Pentobarbital is the most frequently employed barbiturate. In addition to decreasing the metabolic rate, pentobarbital also inhibits free radical damage and improves coupling of CBF and metabolism. Induced hypothermia also has been used to decrease brain metabolism. Promising animal studies in the 1980s and 1990s were shadowed by a more recent randomized clinical trial in adults that showed no advantage to hypothermia as an intervention strategy.

Other strategies to control ICP and maintain CPP include controlled hypertension and, as an extreme measure in uncontrollable intracranial hypertension, decompression craniectomy. The latter method showed significant improvement in neurologic outcome in a randomized controlled trial in children with refractory intracranial hypertension resulting from TBI.

Preventing Secondary Brain Injury at the Cellular and Molecular Level

All of the above-described methods are designed to maintain a normal ICP and normal CPP to minimize global secondary brain injury. Understanding the pathophysiologic processes of secondary brain injury at the cellular and molecular level has allowed scientists and clinicians to begin to try to target individual pathways of secondary injury. To date, translation from the bench to the bedside has met with extremely limited success. The complexity of cellular and molecular responses, coupled with their frequent dual purposes, has made targeting strategies like walking a fine line between benefit and risk. Targeting inflammation provides an excellent example. The acute inflammatory response is detrimental, associated with increased edema and worse outcomes. In contrast, the subacute inflammatory response may be integral to regeneration of axons. Developing therapeutic strategies that target the former without ablating the latter will be the key to future endeavors.

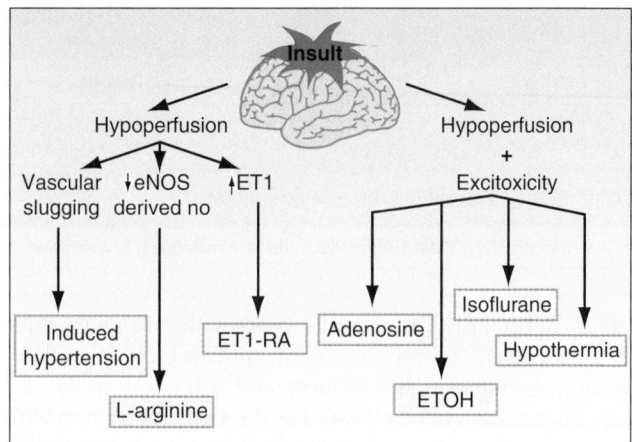

Figure 13-4. Putative strategies targeting excitotoxicity and hypoperfusion that may have field or emergency department application in the acute phase after traumatic brain injury. eNOS, endothelial nitric oxide synthase; ET1, endothelin-1; ETOH, ethyl alcohol; NO, nitric oxide. (Redrawn from Kochanek PM, Clark RSB, Ruppel RA, et al: Cerebral resuscitation after traumatic brain injury and cardiopulmonary arrest in infants and children in the new millennium. Pediatr Clin North Am 2001;48:661–681.)

Designing and testing agents that decrease early hypoperfusion and excitotoxicity also have been areas of intensive investigation. Figure 13-4 provides a graphic display of some of the putative strategies targeting specific aspects of secondary brain injury.

The next decade promises to be an exciting time in cerebral resuscitation research, as clinicians continue to apply knowledge of pathophysiology to the care of children with TBI. One can imagine a future child similar to the patient in Case Study 13-3 who, on arrival to the emergency department, has an intraventricular catheter placed and a cocktail of an EAA antagonist, anti-inflammatory agent, provasodilatory agent, and regenerative agent infused directly into the ventricle. The new intraventricular catheter also will be capable of dialyzing off the accumulated EAAs and proinflammatory mediators of the acute phase, rendering the patient awake, alert, and ready for discharge after a brief hospital stay. The TBI story would be a classic example of how expanding knowledge of pathophysiology through vigorous scientific exploration in the laboratory translates into ever-improving care at the bedside.

CASE STUDY 13-4: SEVERE COMBINED IMMUNODEFICIENCY SYNDROME

Identify the Pathophysiology

SCID syndrome represents a heterogeneous group of disorders characterized by severe impairment of humoral and cellular immunity. Patients present in early infancy with recurrent viral, fungal, and parasitic infections; failure to thrive; chronic bronchiolitis; and diarrhea. At the cellular level, the disease is characterized by an absolute lymphopenia. T cells that are present are dysfunctional, and patients have panhypogammaglobulinemia (except for passive immunity with maternal IgG). The number of B, T, and natural killer lymphocytes varies with the genetic cause of the SCID syndrome. In patients with ADA deficiency, all lymphocyte lines are severely depleted; however, natural

CASE STUDY 13-4

SEVERE COMBINED IMMUNODEFICIENCY SYNDROME

A 3-month-old girl has a history of refractory oral thrush and monilial diaper rash, chronic diarrhea, failure to thrive, and a chronic cough. Physical examination reveals oral thrush on the buccal mucosa, tongue, and palate and a severe monilial diaper rash. Her weight is in the 5th percentile and height is in the 50th percentile (she was in the 50th percentile for weight and height at birth). She has expiratory wheezes and nasal congestion. There is concern about her immune function, and after telephone consultation with an immunologist, the patient is begun on trimethoprim-sulfamethoxasole for prophylactic coverage of *Pneumocystis carinii* pneumonia. A chest x-ray reveals hyperinflation with perihilar infiltrates and no evidence of a thymus. An appointment is made with the immunologist the following day.

By the history, the immunologist is concerned about the possibility of severe combined immunodeficiency syndrome and admits the patient to the hospital. Complete blood count, antibody studies, T-cell and B-cell subset studies, and lymphocyte function studies (looking for responsiveness to mitogens and antigens) are done. A respiratory viral antigen panel is done, which is positive for parainfluenza type 3.

The immunologic workup reveals an absolute lymphopenia (total lymphocyte count <500/μL), delayed cutaneous anergy, and no lymphocytic proliferative response to mitogens or antigens. All lymphocyte cell lines (T cells, B cells, and natural killer cells) are depleted. The patient has panhypogammaglobulinemia. As a result of this evaluation, the immunologist makes the diagnosis of severe combined immunodeficiency syndrome and tests adenosine deaminase level. The results reveal severe adenosine deaminase deficiency.

Table 13-3. Classification of Severe Combined Immunodeficiency

Syndrome	T Cells	B Cells	NK Cells	Inheritance
ADA deficiency	–	–	–	AR
RAG 1, 2 deficiency	–	–	–	AR
TCR + BCR recombination gene deficiency	–	–	+	AR
CγC deficiency	–	+	–	XL
JAK3 deficiency	–	+	–	AR
IL-7Rα deficiency	–	+	+	AR
Omenn's syndrome	+	+	+	AR
MHC II deficiency	CD8+	+	+	AR

ADA, adenosine deaminase; BCR, B-cell receptors; CγC, interleukin-2 receptor common γ chain; IL7-Rα, interleukin-7 receptor α chain; JAK3, Janus-associated kinase 3; MHC, major histocompatability complex; NK, natural killer; RAG, recombination activating genes; TCR, T-cell receptors.

Adapted from Gennery AR, Cant AJ: Diagnosis of severe combined immunodeficiency. J Clin Pathol 2001;54:191–195.

deoxyadenosine, and 2'-O-methyladenosine, all of which are directly and indirectly toxic to lymphocytes. The result, as noted previously, is profound deficiency in cellular and humoral immunity.

Pathophysiology-Based Interventions

The identification of the genetic defect and resultant enzyme deficiency has resulted in several options for treatment in this previously uniformly fatal disease. All of the treatments have as their ultimate goal the creation of immunocompetent cells that express ADA.

Bone Marrow Transplantation

The efficacy of bone marrow transplantation for the treatment of SCID syndrome first was shown in 1968. Transplants have been efficacious regardless of the cause of SCID syndrome. HLA-identical sibling hematopoietic stem cells transplanted into children with ADA-deficient SCID syndrome result in ADA expression in lymphocytes and reconstitution of adequate humoral and cellular immunity. In addition, because of the lack of T-cell function in the recipient, rejection is not a complication. These patients require neither pretransplantation chemotherapy for T-cell ablation nor posttransplant prophylaxis for graft-versus-host disease.

Patients without HLA-identical sibling donors have been transplanted successfully using haploidentical hematopoietic stem cells from one of their parents. To avoid lethal graft-versus-host disease, however, the stem cells from these donors must be depleted of T cells before transplant. The results have been impressive. Stem cell transplant survival may be 96% if performed in the first 3.5 months of life. Stem cell transplantation has become the gold standard of therapy for patients with SCID syndrome. Despite the significant improvement in survival compared with uniform fatality before transplant, the mortality associated with haploidentical hematopoietic stem cell transplantation remains moderate at approximately 20% to 25%. Elucidation of the genetic defects responsible for many SCID syndrome patients makes this syndrome ideal in many ways for gene therapy research, particularly as an alternative for patients without an HLA-matched stem cell donor.

killer activity remains intact. The clinical result is an inability to combat common and opportunistic infections. Viral pneumonitis (particularly with parainfluenza B) and infection with *Pneumocystis carinii* are among the most common presenting infections. Without treatment, SCID syndrome is fatal in infancy or early childhood.

In the 1990s, there was an explosion of information elucidating many of the genetic defects and mutations that result in SCID syndrome. Table 13-3 lists some of the specific disorders that have been shown to result in SCID syndrome. All of the SCID syndromes have as their hallmark the absence of mature T cells. The individual disorders are delineated further by the presence or absence of B and natural killer cells and by their inheritance patterns.

The patient in Case Study 13-4 was identified as having an ADA deficiency. ADA deficiency–related SCID syndrome accounts for approximately 15% of patients with this immunodeficiency syndrome and half of the patients with an autosomal recessive inheritance pattern. ADA is an enzyme in the adenine nucleotide metabolic pathway (purine salvage pathway) and is crucial for the deamination of adenosine and deoxyadenosine and the formation of inosine and deoxyinosine. The enzyme is ubiquitous in the tissues and sera of all mammalian species. ADA deficiency results in an excessive accumulation of adenosine, 2'-

Gene Therapy for Adenosine Deaminase–Deficient Severe Combined Immunodeficiency Syndrome

Gene therapy for ADA deficiency first was attempted in the 1980s. Using a retroviral vector, the gene was incorporated successfully into circulating T lymphocytes with significant improvement in humoral and cellular immunity. The major problem with this therapy was the short half-life of the ADA-expressing peripheral T lymphocytes. Although the goal of gene therapy is the expression of ADA by hematopoietic stem cells, the vectors used until more recently have not been successful. Patients treated with this therapy have required frequent infusion of the gene-carrying retrovirus to maintain immunocompetency.

More recent breakthroughs have occurred in gene therapy of another type of SCID syndrome—SCID-X1 disease. This form of SCID syndrome is inherited as an X-linked condition and is caused by γc-cytokine receptor deficiency that leads to an early block in T and natural killer lymphocyte differentiation. In 2000, Cavazzana-Calvo and coworkers reported successful gene therapy in two patients with γc-cytokine receptor deficiency, resulting in incorporation of the gene in hematopoietic stem cells and restoration of immunocompetency. They also used a retroviral vector for the gene but were able to obtain gene expression from the hematopoietic stem cells.

Given the successes of gene therapy in the X1 form of SCID syndrome, further successes in patients with defined genetic causes of SCID syndrome are not far behind. Preliminary data from Europe (unpublished) suggest that successful transplantation of the ADA gene into hematopoietic stem cells has occurred in at least one patient, using a vector similar to that used by Cavazzana-Calvo and coworkers.

In the 1980s, SCID syndrome was a uniformly fatal diagnosis. As the pathophysiology of this heterogeneous set of diseases has been elucidated, SCID syndrome has become eminently treatable in most patients. The near future is likely to bring the further elucidation of genetic causes of currently unclear SCID syndrome diagnoses and the improved technology for targeting SCID syndrome at the genetic level.

CONCLUSION

The four cases studies presented in this chapter have illustrated the spectrum of pathophysiology, from the system as a whole, to an individual organ system, to individual cells and their molecular functions, and finally to the level of the single gene. In each case, elucidation of the pathophysiologic processes allows the clinician to target therapy to reverse these processes and restore normal physiologic function. In addition, scientific advancement in the understanding of the fundamentals of pathophysiology in many cases has allowed the transition from bench to bedside in treatment of diseases.

Although the material presented in this chapter is hardly even the "tip of the iceberg" of all of pediatric pathophysiology, the reader should be left with an appreciation for the importance of understanding the principles of pathophysiology in the approach to any patient. Only through such an understanding can the clinician develop a rational treatment plan, and the scientist plan directions for future research.

Additional Resources, CD-ROM

Bibliography

SUGGESTED READINGS

Fischer A, Hacein-Bey S, Le Deist F, et al: Gene therapy of severe combined immunodeficiencies. Immunol Rev 2000;178:13–20.

Kochanek PM, Clark RSB, Ruppel RA, et al: Biochemical, cellular, and molecular mechanisms in the evolution of secondary damage after traumatic brain injury in infants and children: Lessons learned from the bedside. Pediatr Crit Care Med 2000;1:4–19.

Van Deuren M, Brandtzaeg P, Van Der Meer JWM: Update on meningococcal disease with emphasis on pathogenesis and clinical management. Clin Microbiol Rev 2000;13:144–166.

West JB: Pulmonary Physiology and Pathophysiology: An Integrated, Case-Based Approach. Baltimore, Lippincott Williams and Wilkins, 2001.

14 Principles of Nutrition

D. Pauline Williams and Nedra K. Christensen

Nutrition is vital to adequate growth and good health. Assessment and education regarding the normal nutritional requirements of healthy children should be part of the overall pediatric health plan. In addition, increased or decreased needs for specific illnesses should be considered. Careful nutritional assessment, including anthropometrics, clinical examination, dietary history, and biochemical data (if indicated), is needed to ensure adequate growth and good health.

Protein-energy malnutrition is classified as marasmus or kwashiorkor. *Marasmus* results from a calorie deficit over a long time. Wasting of fat and muscle occurs. Body weight and body fat are decreased. Serum proteins, albumin and transferrin, are decreased slightly or within normal limits. *Kwashiorkor* is a result of protein deficiency and has a rapid onset, often precipitated by stress, such as an infection. Body weight and body fat are decreased. Albumin and transferrin levels and immune function are severely depressed. *Marasmic kwashiorkor* is a combined form of protein-energy malnutrition that occurs when stress is superimposed on a chronically starved patient.

Obesity, an excess accumulation of adipose tissue, also can be considered a form of malnutrition or improper nutrition. According to the National Health and Nutrition Examination Survey and the Centers for Disease Control and Prevention, the number of overweight children and teens has nearly doubled since the 1980s.

FUNDAMENTALS

Nutrition for the premature infant must consider the physiologic immaturity that renders them susceptible to malnutrition, anemia, glucose instability, decreased gastric motility, necrotizing enterocolitis, patent ductus arteriosus, respiratory distress syndrome, uncoordinated suck and swallow, hypocalcemia, fat malabsorption, heat loss, and infection. Nutritional intervention is important to optimize growth and development. *Parenteral nutrition* often is indicated in the first few days of life to allow for adaptation to the extrauterine environment before enteral feedings are begun. When parenteral nutrition is indicated, it should be initiated in the first 24 hours of life to promote energy intake, glucose homeostasis, and nitrogen balance and to prevent fatty acid deficiency. The American Academy of Pediatrics (AAP) Committee on Nutrition recommends 80 to 90 kcal/kg/day, delivered as 0.5 to 3.0 g/kg/day of fat and 2.7 to 3.8 g/kg/day of protein and glucose/dextrose at a maximum delivery of 5 to 12 mg/kg/min. Glucose/dextrose delivery

is expressed as a maximum infusion rate (mg/kg/min) to avoid hyperglycemia, phlebitis, lipogenesis, overfeeding, and cholestasis. In addition to the maximum infusion rate, the concentration of dextrose depends on the venous site. Peripheral sites should be limited to 10% to 12.5% dextrose, and central sites should be limited to 30% dextrose solutions. Vitamin, mineral, and electrolyte requirements for premature infants are extensive and may be found in texts listed in the Suggested Readings. Vitamin and mineral requirements for pediatric patients on parenteral nutrition are listed in Table 14-1. Managing *fluid needs* of premature

Table 14-1. Nutrient Needs for Parenterally Fed Pediatric Patients*

Nutrient	Amount
Vitamin A	700/2300 µg/IU
Vitamin D	10/400 µg/IU
Vitamin E	7 mg
Vitamin K	200 µg
Ascorbic acid	80 mg
Thiamine	1.2 mg
Riboflavin	1.4 mg
Pyridoxine	1.0 mg
Niacin	17 mg
Calcium	5 mg
Pantathenate	5 mg
Biotin	20 µg
Folate	140 µg
Vitamin B$_{12}$	1.0 µg
Iodide	1.0 µg/kg/day
Sodium	2–4 mEq/kg/day
Potassium	2–4 mEq/kg/day
Chloride	2–3 mEq/kg/day
Calcium	0.5–3.0 mEq/kg/day
Phosphorus	0.5–2.0 µmol/kg/day
Magnesium†	0.25–0.5 mEq/kg/day
Acetate	Balance PN
Zinc	100–300 µg/kg/day
Copper	20 µg/kg/day
Chromium	0.14–0.2 µg/kg/day
Manganese	2–10 µg/kg/day
Iron	0.1 µg/kg/day
Selenium	3 µg/kg/day, maximum 40 µg/day
Molybdenum	0.25 µg/kg/day

*Suggested dosing for vitamins provided in 5-mL pediatric multivitamin infusion (Amour Pharmaceuticals, Kankakee, IL). Give 30% to infants weighing <1 kg, 65% to infants 1–3 kg, and 100% (5 mL) to infants and children >3 kg to 11 years of age.
†Sulfate is provided with magnesium.
PN, parenteral nutrition.

infants must be individualized based on the patient's medical condition. Insensible fluid losses are high because premature skin offers little protection from evaporative losses. Radiant warmers and phototherapy used in intensive care units exacerbate this loss.

Enteral nutrition can be started when the infant has become clinically stable. Minimal amounts of feedings (trophic feedings) are suggested to give nourishment to the gut, but these do not provide a major source of nutrition. Trophic feedings minimize the chance of necrotizing enterocolitis. The AAP Committee on Nutrition recommends the premature infant receive 105 to 130 kcal/kg/day—3 to 4 g/kg/day of protein, 10.8 to 16.8 g/kg/day of carbohydrate, and 2.0 to 3.5 g/kg/day of fat—for enteral feeding. See the Suggested Readings for details on vitamin, mineral, and electrolyte recommendations.

Premature infants weighing less than 2 kg should be fed with *premature infant formulas or fortified breast milk.* The increased need for protein, sodium, phosphorus, and calcium can be met with premature infant formulas or with human milk fortifiers added to the breast milk. Breast milk fortifiers are formulated to achieve 24 kcal/oz, when one pack of fortifier is added to 25 mL of breast milk. Premature formulas are recommended until the infant is placed on a transitional formula. Transitional formulas can be started when the infant reaches 1.8 kg and should continue until the infant weighs 4 kg or more. Transitional formulas contain more protein, sodium, calcium, and phosphorus than term infant formulas, but less than premature infant formulas. Premature infant formulas and human milk fortifiers require a prescription, whereas transitional formulas do not.

Iron recommendations for premature infants are 2 to 4 mg/day when full-volume feedings have begun. This recommendation can be achieved by consumption of at least 120 kcal/kg of iron-fortified premature infant formula or

Table 14-3. Dietary Reference Intake Values for Protein for Males and Females

Age	EAR* (g/kg/day) Males	EAR* (g/kg/day) Females	RDA† (g/kg/day)	AI‡ (g/kg/day)
0–6 mo				1.52
7–12 mo	1.1	1.1	1.5	
1–3 yr	0.88	0.88	1.1	
4–8 yr	0.76	0.76	0.95	
9–13 yr	0.76	0.76	0.95	
14–18 yr	0.73	0.71	0.85	

*EAR, estimated average requirement. The intake meets the nutrient needs of half the individuals in a group.

†RDA, recommended dietary allowance. The intake meets the nutrient need of almost all (97–98%) individuals in a group.

‡AI, adequate intake. The observed average or experimentally determined intake by a defined population or subgroup that appears to sustain a defined nutritional status, such as growth rate, normal circulating nutrient values, or other functional indicators of health. The AI is used if sufficient scientific evidence is not available to derive an EAR. For healthy infants receiving human milk, the AI is the mean intake. The AI is not equivalent to an RDA.

Adapted from RDAs and DRIs (Recommended Dietary Allowances and Dietary Reference Intakes). Washington, DC, National Academy Press, 1989–2002. Reports available at: www.nap.edu. Copyright 1989–2002 by the National Academy of Sciences. Reprinted courtesy of the National Academy Press, Washington, DC.

giving a supplement to infants receiving human milk plus fortifier (human milk fortifier does not contain iron).

Nutrition during infancy provides for future health, growth, and development. An infant's growth rate is rapid, yet the ability to digest and metabolize nutrients is not developed fully. Early nutrition must meet nutrient needs while still being suited to the physiologic immaturity of the digestive system. Tables 14-2 and 14-3 present energy and protein needs for infants, Table 14-4 shows fluid needs, and Table 14-5 lists dietary reference intakes (DRIs) for nutrients.

Breast-feeding is the preferred method of providing infant nutrition. Advantages of breast-feeding include nutritional, immunologic, and psychological benefits. Colostrum, the first milk produced, has anti-infective characteristics and is high in fat-soluble vitamins, minerals, and electrolytes. Within 2 weeks, mature milk is produced. Under normal breast-feeding conditions, no additional water, food, vitamins, or minerals are needed. At 4 to 6 months of age, solid foods can be added (Table 14-6). The AAP recommends that vitamin K1 be given to all newborns as a single, intramuscular dose of 0.5 to 1 mg.

Breast milk is easily digestible and has a low renal solute load. The low protein content is adequate, without producing a high nitrogen load on the maturing kidneys. Breast milk contains essential fatty acids, saturated fatty acids, medium-chain triglycerides, and cholesterol. Docosahexaenoic acid, a long-chain fatty acid found in breast milk,

Table 14-2. Energy Needs in Pediatric Patients

Age	Estimated Energy Range Males (kcal/day): Sedentary Physical Activity Level to Active Physical Activity Level	Estimated Energy Range Females (kcal/day): Sedentary Physical Activity Level to Active Physical Activity Level
0–6 mo	570	520
7–12 mo	743	676
3 yr	1162–1485	1080–1395
4 yr	1215–1566	1133–1475
5 yr	1275–1658	1189–1557
6 yr	1328–1742	1247–1642
7 yr	1393–1840	1298–1719
8 yr	1453–1931	1360–1810
9 yr	1530–2043	1415–1890
10 yr	1601–2149	1470–1972
11 yr	1691–2279	1538–2071
12 yr	1798–2428	1617–2183
13 yr	1935–2618	1684–2281
14 yr	2090–2829	1718–2334
15 yr	2223–3013	1731–2362
16 yr	2320–3152	1729–2368
17 yr	2366–3226	1710–2353
18 yr	2383–3263	1690–2336

Adapted from RDAs and DRIs (Recommended Dietary Allowances and Dietary Reference Intakes). Washington, DC, National Academy Press, 1989–2002. Reports available at: www.nap.edu. Copyright 1989–2002 by the National Academy of Sciences. Reprinted courtesy of the National Academy Press, Washington, DC.

Table 14-4. Fluid Requirements for Pediatric Patients*

Age	Fluid Requirement
0–12 mo	150–180 mL/kg/day
> 1 yr	1.5 mL/kcal/day

*Fluid increases are needed for increased body temperature, increased environmental temperature (50–100% fluid increase), and increased physical activity (4 oz of fluid every 15 min of activity).

promotes development of the central nervous system. Breast-feeding has been associated with fewer gastrointestinal and respiratory illnesses and decreased episodes of otitis media. In addition to immunologic and nutritional benefits, breast-feeding is convenient, is economical, and enhances maternal-infant bonding. Lactating mothers should be provided with adequate education and support to encourage breast-feeding for at least the first 12 months.

Infant formulas can be used when breast-feeding is not practical or desired. Formulas provide adequate calories, fat, vitamins, and minerals, but they lack the anti-infective and other protective properties of breast milk. A variety of formulas are available. *Cow milk or standard formulas* are modified to reduce protein and mineral content, reducing the renal solute load. Standard formulas are widely used and available. *Soy-based formulas* can be used when an infant has an intolerance or allergy to cow milk–based formulas. If an infant is allergic or sensitive to the intact proteins in cow milk–based or soy-based formulas, a *hypoallergenic formula* is appropriate. Casein and whey hydrolysate formulas are hypoallergenic, but not nonallergenic; a few cases of reactions have occurred with these formulas. Older infants taking solid foods can be advanced to *follow-up formulas*, which are higher in protein and carbohydrate and lower in fat than standard formulas. No advantage to follow-up formulas compared with standard formulas has been established.

Breast-fed infants and infants fed adequate amounts of formula do not require *vitamin and mineral supplementation* during the first 6 months of life, with the exception of vitamin D. During the second 6 months of life, there are some situations in which nutrient supplementation may be needed. *Vitamin D* supplementation, according to the DRIs in Table 14-5, is recommended if exposure to sunlight is limited. The AAP recommends addition of *iron-fortified foods* after 6 months and continuing to 12 months of age or longer. Addition of iron-fortified cereals usually meets the DRI for infants. The American Dietetic Association recommends *fluoride supplementation* of 0.25 mg/day if the water supply is less than 0.3 ppm.

For infants who are not breast-fed, formulas are available in ready-to-feed, liquid concentrate, and powder forms. Care should be taken to mix formulas properly, according to the package directions. Most infant formulas have a dilution of 20 kcal/oz; however, formulas vary, and package directions should be followed. Failure to gain adequate height and weight may be an indication of improper formula preparation. Overdiluting formulas or giving water in place of formula may lead to water intoxication and poor growth. Concentrating the formula to greater than 30 kcal/oz produces a high renal solute load and may lead to renal failure and circulatory problems.

The AAP recommends that *whole cow milk and low-iron formulas not be used during the first year of life*. According to the AAP, the only acceptable alternative to breast milk during the first 6 to 12 months is iron-fortified formula, with appropriate solid foods added starting at 4 to 6 months.

Nursing bottle mouth, or baby bottle tooth decay, is the decay of the upper and sometimes the lower posterior teeth. The most common cause is extended exposure to sugary liquids, such as formulas, milk, juice, or soda. The practice of putting an infant to bed with a bottle is the major cause of this dental condition. When bottles are given at bedtime or during naps, the sweet liquid pools around the teeth creating a perfect environment for bacterial plaque. Education is the key to preventing nursing bottle mouth. Parents should be educated to feed infants when they are awake and avoid putting infants to bed with a bottle.

By 4 to 6 months, infants generally are ready to have *solid food* introduced in their diet. Table 14-6 shows when to add solid foods to the infant's diet. Initially the amounts offered should be small, with "seconds" if desired. As a first solid food, iron-fortified infant cereal, such as rice cereal, should be used, mixed with breast milk or formula. At 6 months, pureed single fruits or vegetables and fruit juices can be added. Foods can be commercially or home prepared without added salt or sugar. New foods should be added one at a time, allowing 1 week between the introduction of new foods to assess for signs of intolerance and allow time for the infant to acquire a taste for the new food. At 8 months, strained meats can be added. By 10 months, infants have a more developed biting movement and can use their fingers to feed themselves. "Finger foods" can be added at this time. Formula or breast-feeding can be decreased as more solid foods are added. Refusing new foods or textures is common; infants should be offered a variety of foods as their tastes change and grow.

The American Dietetic Association recommends avoiding early introduction of the following *common allergens:* egg whites, cow milk, citrus, wheat, chocolate, fish, shellfish, tree nuts, and nut butters (e.g., peanut butter). Adding these foods before 12 to 18 months of age may lead to allergic reactions in susceptible infants.

Energy needs of *children* vary with growth rate, physical activity, and body size. The recommended dietary allowances shown in Table 14-2 provide average energy allowances based on age and weight. These allowances can be adjusted individually to account for variable growth rates and activity. Adequate protein intake in children is needed for optimal growth. Protein needs decrease as the growth rate slows with age. Table 14-3 lists protein needs by age and weight. The DRIs for vitamins and minerals (see Table 14-5) can be met by following the recommendations of the Food Guide Pyramid for young children (www.cnpp. usda.gov/KidsPyra/). Education encouraging an increased intake of fruits, vegetables, and grains, while emphasizing low-fat choices, should be part of a child's well-care plan.

Parents often have *feeding concerns* with young children, worrying about the adequacy of the diet. Children have periods when they refuse to eat certain foods or eat only one particular food. These periods often are referred to as "food jags" and are normal behavior during the toddler and preschool years. Physicians can educate parents to use the following tips to work through these periods:

1. Offer small portion sizes of foods; a rule of thumb is 1 tablespoon of each food for every year of age (more according to the child's appetite).
2. Schedule meals and snacks at regular times.
3. Try to avoid letting the child get too hungry or tired before mealtime.
4. Create a pleasant atmosphere during feeding times.

children with a chronic disease. The integrity of the skin, lips, tongue, gums, eyes, and teeth are indications of nutritional status. Posture, skeletal development, and blood pressure are additional parameters that should be checked at each clinic visit to determine changes over time. Identifying changes could signal early nutritional intervention and prevent any long-term problems.

Diet assessment often is conducted by using one of three methods. The *24-hour dietary recall* method evaluates the diet from the previous 24 hours or the diet of a typical 24-hour period. A food frequency questionnaire uses a list of foods grouped by categories and asks the participant to list frequency and portion sizes of foods consumed. A *food diary* relies on the participant to write down the foods and amounts for an agreed-on time frame. Nutrient computer analysis programs are available to make the nutrient analysis more accurate and detailed. Individualized diet counseling occurs to improve nutrient intake from the evaluation of the diet assessment record. Counseling for improvement is received better when it is given in practical and easy-to-implement terms.

MANAGEMENT

Patients with an *eating disorder* (anorexia or bulimia) can have protein-energy malnutrition with depleted adipose and somatic protein stores. Complications from severe caloric restriction can result in hypercarotenemia, mitral valve prolapse, cardiomyopathy, congestive heart failure, delayed gastric emptying, decreased small bowel motility, constipation, bone marrow hypoplasia, anemia, osteopenia, fluid and electrolyte imbalance, and pubertal delay. Abnormalities in pancreatic enzymes can be useful in determining a pattern of binging or purging. An eating disorder, rather than pancreatic disease, is suspected when serum amylase is elevated and serum lipase is normal. Improper cholesterol metabolism has been associated with deficiencies and excesses of copper and zinc. Caution should be used in treating high cholesterol with a fat-restricted diet in the patient with an eating disorder. High cholesterol and serum amylase can be an indicator of a binge/purge eating disorder, and a fat-restricted diet may aggravate the eating disorder.

The goal for improving nutritional status for children with an *eating disorder* is to maintain growth and muscle mass. Management is achieved best with a multidisciplinary team (physician, dietitian, psychotherapist) to treat the medical, nutritional, and psychological problems these patients have. Adequate treatment settings and frequency of treatment sessions vary. Nutritional rehabilitation must begin early in treatment because psychotherapy has limited effectiveness if malnutrition and cognitive function have not been corrected. After nutritional rehabilitation has begun, psychotherapy and nutritional counseling can be coordinated for treatment.

The goal for children with *food allergies* is to prevent severe reactions and maintain adequate growth and development. Diagnosis includes obtaining a reaction history along with a 2-week food record, immunologic testing, and evaluation of diet manipulation. Diet manipulation includes food challenges, in which a suspected food is eliminated from the diet and then reintroduced to determine if the food causes symptoms or reactions. Common food allergies are listed in Box 14-2. In some children, avoidance of the food allergen while the intestinal mucosa and secretory immune system mature can result in outgrowing of the hypersensitivity. Nut, fish, and shellfish allergies are not likely to be outgrown. The therapeutic diet for the pediatric patient with food allergies should be appropriate for age and eliminate the offending food allergens. Referral to a registered dietitian is helpful, especially if the child requires the elimination of two or more foods.

Appropriately planned vegetarian diets can be healthful and nutritionally adequate. The goal for the vegetarian pediatric patient is to consume adequate amounts of all nutrients and maintain adequate growth and development. Lacto-ovovegetarians avoid meat, poultry, and fish; lacto-vegetarians avoid meat, poultry, fish, and eggs; vegans avoid meat, poultry, fish, eggs, and dairy products; and fruitarians avoid all food groups except fruits, nuts, and seeds. A diet history is essential to clarify which foods are avoided and which foods are acceptable. The clinician can suggest appropriate substitutes to meet nutrient needs.

Nutrition concerns for children on a vegetarian diet include energy, protein, iron, vitamin B_{12}, calcium, vitamin D, and zinc intake. Sufficient *energy* can be consumed by adding plant-based fats, such as avocados, olives, nuts, and seeds, to the diet. Plant *proteins* can provide adequate amounts of essential amino acids. Complementary proteins, such as beans and rice, do not need to be consumed at the same time but should be consumed over the course of the day. Dietary protein sources for vegetarians include breast milk, formula, beans, legumes, nuts, tofu, dairy products, eggs, and soy products. Risk for *iron deficiency anemia* is common in vegetarian and nonvegetarian children. Plant foods contain only nonheme iron, which is not absorbed as efficiently as heme iron. Consuming foods high in vitamin C at the same meal can enhance nonheme iron absorption. Dietary iron sources for the vegetarian include breast milk, fortified formula, fortified cereal and grain products, legumes, green leafy vegetables, eggs, soy products, and blackstrap molasses. Plant products are unreliable sources of *vitamin B_{12}*; however, some cereal products and soy milks are fortified with vitamin B_{12}. Supplementation or addition of fortified foods is advised for vegetarians who avoid or limit all animal foods. Individuals following a lacto-ovovegetarian diet generally consume adequate *calcium*, whereas other vegetarian diets may not meet calcium needs. Good sources of calcium for the vegetarian include dairy products, fortified soy milk and orange juice,

---

Box 14-2. Common Food Allergens

- Milk
- Soy
- Eggs (more often white than yolk)
- Nuts (particularly peanuts)
- Fish
- Citrus
- Chocolate
- Wheat
- Corn

calcium-precipitated tofu, and dark green leafy vegetables. Children regularly exposed to sunlight seem to have no dietary requirement for *vitamin D*. Children with limited exposure to sunlight should consume vitamin D–fortified foods, such as cow milk, soy milk, and cereals, or use vitamin D supplements. *Zinc* intake in vegetarian and nonvegetarian diets is similar. Zinc from plant products has a low bioavailability; it is difficult to determine if vegetarians are meeting zinc needs. Vegetarians should consume good sources of zinc, such as legumes, hard cheeses, whole grains, wheat germ, fortified cereals, nuts, tofu, and miso.

Complementary medicine and alternative therapies are popular in the United States. In 1997, 60 million Americans stated that they had used herbs in the previous year, yet 70% did not reveal their herbal use to their physicians or pharmacists. The extent of use of herbal medicines by children is not well known, but it is reasonable to assume that children of herbal and alternative medicines users consume more herbal medicines than children of non–alternative medicine users. Questions that the health care provider can ask patients about complementary medicine to obtain an accurate medical history and to determine an appropriate treatment program are listed in Box 14-3. Chapter 307 discusses complementary health care issues more extensively.

Childhood obesity is increasing at an alarming rate. Overweight generally is defined as equal to greater than 85th percentile of body mass index or 110% of standard weight for height and age, and obesity is defined as equal to greater than 95th percentile body mass index or 120% of standard weight. Referral to a registered dietitian for education on diet modification can benefit the patient and family greatly. Chapter 20 addresses the nutritional and functional issues of obesity more fully.

Box 14-3. Step-by-Step Strategy for the Health Care Provider to Discuss Complementary and Alternative Therapies

1. Ask the patient to identify the principal symptoms and to maintain a symptom diary.
2. Discuss the patient's preferences and expectations.
3. Review issues of safety and efficacy. Natural substances are not inherently safe (snake venom is natural, but deadly). Examples of potentially toxic herbs are sassafras, chaparral, and germander.
4. Provide key questions to be used with a licensed provider during the initial consultation.

   Is therapy based on clinical experience? Can you talk to a previous patient? What techniques or supplements would be included in the therapy? Are there potential side effects?

   How many visits are required? What is the cost per session? What is the anticipated total cost? Is third-party reimbursement available?

   Is the provider willing to communicate findings, plans, and follow-up with the primary care provider?
5. Schedule a follow-up visit in 4–8 weeks to address the response to questions, potential risks for toxicity, and any recommendations that conflict with conventional therapy.

Adapted from Eisenberg DM: Advising patients who seek alternative medical therapies. Ann Intern Med 1997;127:61–69.

Box 14-4. Nutritional Resources

- Registered dietitians
- School lunch and breakfast programs
- Food stamps
- Food banks
- Headstart
- Women, Infants, and Children (WIC)
- Expanded Food and Nutrition Education Program (EFNEP)

Sports nutrition has been acknowledged as an aid in improving performance, making young athletes vulnerable to nutrition misinformation. Adequate fluid intake and prevention of dehydration is crucial because children and adolescents compared to adults sweat less (absolute and per sweat gland), experience greater heat production with less ability to transfer heat from the muscles to the skin, and have a greater body surface area leading to excessive heat gain. Obtaining advice from physicians before starting an exercise program is recommended for children and adolescents with bulimia, congenital heart disease, diabetes mellitus, gastroenteritis, fever, or obesity because of their increased risk of developing heat-related illness. Insufficient fluid intake may occur in persons with anorexia nervosa, cystic fibrosis, mental retardation, or kidney disease, also leading to increased incidence of heat-related illness. These children and adolescents should be encouraged to participate in sports, but should be monitored closely.

The recommended distribution of calories for children and adolescents participating in sports is 55% from carbohydrate, 15% to 20% from protein, and 25% to 30% from fat. Supplements promoted to increase muscle mass and to improve performance should be used with caution or avoided.

Guidelines for *nutrition in chronic diseases* vary with each disease state. Consulting with a dietitian with expertise in pediatric nutrition is advisable because of the intricacies involved with each disease. See Chapter 130 for a brief review and starting point to initiate a diet for a child with a chronic disease.

Various nutritional resources are available and can be helpful in providing proper nutritional care of the pediatric patient. Box 14-4 lists some nutritional resources for patient referral.

OUTCOME

Quality nutritional care depends on identifying patients at nutritional risk and implementing appropriate nutritional care plans that are adapted to the specific needs of each child. Normal growth and appropriate feeding behaviors are desired outcomes of effective nutritional screening, assessment, intervention, referral, and follow-up.

FOLLOW-UP

Follow-up nutritional care depends on age, existence of chronic disease, and existence of feeding problems. Recommendations for the timing of follow-up visits vary. The infant who is not gaining weight and is at home should

15 Disease Screening and Surveillance

Wendy Lane

ROLE OF THE GENERALIST

1   Understand the principles and purposes of screening procedures.

2   Know the epidemiology and sequelae of common pediatric screening issues, including elevated lead levels, iron deficiency, tuberculosis, hypertension, vision, and hearing.

3   Know the screening recommendations for these common pediatric conditions.

4   Appreciate the evidence of the effectiveness of screening for these conditions.

5   Know how to implement condition-specific screening in practice.

Screening refers to the application of a test to detect the presence of disease in a person who is currently asymptomatic. The term *test* could refer to a blood test, imaging procedure, screening questionnaire, or physical examination. The purpose of screening is not simply to detect disease, but also to provide treatment that would reduce or eliminate the sequelae of that condition. When screening is conducted, it should be considered as not only the application of a test, but also the events that follow, including additional evaluation and decision making. Box 15-1 lists the criteria for implementation of a screening program.

Cost-effectiveness should be considered when deciding whether and whom to screen and which screening tests to perform given limited time and resources. Costs to be considered include costs of intervention and side effects; savings from avoided illness and disability; and nonmedical costs, such as transportation. Effectiveness may be measured in years of life saved or days of illness avoided.

This chapter addresses screening for specific conditions in pediatric practice, including elevated lead levels, anemia, tuberculosis, hypertension, vision, and hearing. Screening for these conditions has been recommended by authorities such as the American Academy of Pediatrics (AAP), Bright Futures, and the U.S. Preventive Services Task Force Guide to Clinical Preventive Services. Screening practices for which there is little supporting evidence, such as routine urinalysis, are not covered. Screening for hypercholesterolemia remains controversial and has not proved to be

cost-effective. A description of screening for hypercholesterolemia is included on the CD-ROM. Screening for newborns (see Chapters 11 and 21), for adolescents (see Chapter 218), and for obesity in children (see Chapter 20) are covered elsewhere in this book.

The extent to which each topic in this chapter meets the aforementioned screening criteria varies, and the strength of the recommendation for screening also varies. Screening for tuberculosis and hypertension are strongly recommended because evidence is available that meets most of the screening criteria listed in Box 15-1. In contrast, the recommendation for hypercholesterolemia screening is more equivocal because fewer screening criteria are met.

Each screening topic includes a discussion of the epidemiology and sequelae of the condition, available screening measures, evidence of the effectiveness of screening, screening recommendations, and implementation of screening in practice. Public policy considerations are included for some of the more controversial topics. Additional references are included on the CD-ROM.

SCREENING FOR ELEVATED LEAD LEVELS

Epidemiology and Sequelae of Lead Poisoning

Lead poisoning is one of the most common diseases of environmental origin among children in the United States today. Children younger than 5 years old are at particular risk because of their developing nervous systems, increased hand-to-mouth activities, and increased ability to absorb lead. Nearly 4.4% of children between the ages of 1 and 5 years, or 890,000 children in the United States, have blood lead levels at or above the current recommended cutoff level of 10 µg/dL. More recently, levels less than 10 µg/dL have been shown to have negative behavioral and cognitive effects, suggesting that an even larger number of children may be affected. Minority, urban, and low-income children are at disproportionate risk for elevated lead levels.

Major sources of lead exposure to children include lead-based paint and lead-containing dust, soil, and water. Children also may be exposed to lead contained in ceramics, lead-soldered cans, folk remedies, or cosmetics. Leaded gasoline previously was a major source of exposure in the United States. Acutely, lead has been shown to affect significantly the renal, neurologic, gastrointestinal, and hematopoietic systems, causing anemia, colic, nephropathy, encephalopathy, and death. Chronic, low-level exposure formula and cereal, it remains the most common cause of anemia and nutritional deficiency among children. The Third National Health and Nutrition Examination Survey (NHANES III) conducted between 1988 and 1994 found that 9% of infants 12 to 36 months old in the United States had iron deficiency, and 3% also had iron deficiency anemia; this corresponds to 700,000 children in the United States with iron deficiency and 240,000 children with iron deficiency anemia. Rates of iron deficiency are increased among African Americans, Native Americans, Alaskan Natives, immigrants, and children living in poverty.

Anemia is defined by the presence of a hemoglobin level below the fifth percentile for age (see Chapter 92). Iron deficiency represents a range of disorders, from depletion of iron stores to iron deficiency anemia. Although iron depletion does not cause physiologic impairment, this condition means that there are no iron stores to mobilize if the body develops increased iron needs. In contrast, iron deficiency anemia has been associated with developmental delay and behavioral disturbances in infants and preschool children. Iron deficiency anemia places children at increased risk for lead poisoning because anemia increases the ability of the gastrointestinal tract to absorb lead. Iron deficiency anemia also has been associated with conditions that affect child development, such as low birth weight, poor nutritional status, poverty, and elevated lead levels.

Children younger than 24 months old are at highest risk for iron deficiency because of rapid growth during this period. Full-term infants generally have iron stores at birth that last until 4 to 6 months of age. Iron deficiency anemia often does not become apparent until about age 9 months. Premature infants deplete their iron stores much earlier, usually by 2 to 3 months. Early introduction of whole cow milk increases the risk of iron deficiency anemia for many reasons. Cow milk does not contain significant amounts of iron and may replace other foods with higher iron content, particularly if a child drinks more than 24 oz/day after the first year of life. Whole cow milk may cause occult gastrointestinal bleeding in young children. Adolescence also is a period of risk for iron deficiency anemia in girls. Rapid growth, menstruation, and poor diet all may contribute to this risk.

Screening Measures

Hemoglobin concentration and hematocrit are the primary measures used to identify iron deficiency anemia because they are inexpensive, rapid, and easy to perform. Both of these measures determine the amount of functional body iron and are late indicators of iron deficiency. Sensitivity and specificity of hemoglobin measures vary significantly depending on the population, reference standard, and cut-point used. Reports of sensitivity have ranged from 8% to 90%, and specificity has ranged from 65% to 99%. Although capillary sampling may be easier than venous blood draws, results are less reliable. In particular, "milking" of the finger can cause hemolysis and contaminate the blood with tissue fluid leading to false low measurements. Abnormal capillary samples should be confirmed with venous blood testing.

As the prevalence of iron deficiency anemia has declined, so has the positive predictive value of an abnormal hemoglobin or hematocrit measurement. Data from the NHANES III study indicate that only one third of children

aged 1 to 5 and women of childbearing age who were anemic (hemoglobin <5th percentile) were also iron deficient. Other tests, such as *serum ferritin*, *free erythrocyte protoporphyrin*, and *transferrin saturation*, may be more accurate for the detection of iron deficiency, but are poor screening tests for iron deficiency anemia because of higher cost and less ease of use. These tests are described on the CD-ROM.

A therapeutic trial may provide the most convincing evidence of iron deficiency anemia. In the presence of a hemoglobin value of less than 10th percentile for age, a hemoglobin increase of 1.0 g/dL or more after 1 month of elemental iron, 3 mg/kg/day, is considered diagnostic of iron deficiency anemia.

Evidence of Effectiveness

Although clinical trials have shown that iron supplementation can correct iron deficiency anemia in infants and children, most also have provided mixed results as to whether iron supplementation improves clinical outcomes.

Screening Recommendations

Given the declining rates of iron deficiency anemia in the United States and the declining positive predictive value of screening tests, targeted screening currently is recommended by most groups, especially for children at high risk. Defined high-risk children include infants living in poverty, African Americans, Alaskan Natives, immigrants from developing countries, preterm and low-birth-weight infants, and infants whose primary intake is unfortified cow milk. The CDC has provided the most extensive recommendations for targeted screening (Box 15-3). The AAP and Bright Futures continue to recommend universal screening. Both authorities recommend measuring hemoglobin or hematocrit once during infancy for all children and once during adolescence for all teenagers.

Implementing Screening in Practice

Practitioners who see primarily high-risk patients (e.g., practitioners working in public health departments or underserved areas) should consider universal screening of infants for anemia. In other settings, practitioners should develop targeted screening policies based on the extensive CDC recommendations. Initial screening should be by hemoglobin or hematocrit, followed by repeat measurement to confirm abnormal values. See Chapter 92 for additional information regarding diagnosis and treatment.

SCREENING FOR TUBERCULOSIS

Epidemiology and Sequelae of Tuberculosis

Tuberculosis (TB) is one of the leading causes of death from infection worldwide. In 1996, the World Health Organization estimated that there were 8 million new cases of TB each year and 3 million deaths from the disease. Although 90% of cases occur in the developing world, about 15 million Americans are infected, accounting for 4% to 6% of the U.S. population. Risk factors for TB infection in the United States include emigration from a high-risk country, low socioeconomic status, travel to high-risk areas, human immunodeficiency virus (HIV) infection and other causes of immunodeficiency, drug use, homelessness, history of incarceration, and employment in a health care facility. Pediatric populations at highest risk for TB include foreign-born, Hispanic, and African-American children. Foreign-born children account for nearly 25% of pediatric TB infections in the United States.

Transmission of *Mycobacterium tuberculosis*, the causative organism of TB, is primarily respiratory, via inhalation of droplet nuclei that are coughed into the air by a person with contagious pulmonary TB. Several hours of contact generally are required for transmission. The most common source of exposure is household contacts. Even with active pulmonary TB, children younger than 12 years old usually are not contagious because they are infected with low numbers of organisms, and their cough is not forceful enough to expel infectious droplet nuclei. The diagnosis of latent TB infection or active disease in a child is considered a sentinel event representing recent transmission of *M. tuberculosis* within the community. The most common presentation of children with active TB is chronic cough and fever, although young children may present with failure to thrive or fever of unknown origin.

Screening Measures

Tuberculin skin testing (TST) is the standard means for identifying persons with TB infection. The Mantoux test is the recommended skin test. It contains 5 tuberculin units of purified protein derivative (PPD) and is administered intradermally. Detection of a delayed hypersensitivity reaction within 48 to 72 hours of administration is required for a positive test. False-positive results may occur more frequently in areas with a high prevalence of atypical mycobacteria, cross-reactions may lead to false-positive results, and false-positive results may occur among children who have received bacille Calmette-Guérin (BCG) vaccination (although these reactions are usually <10 mm). False-positive results also occur with improper reading (measuring erythema instead of induration), hypersensitivity to PPD components, or cellulitis. False-negative results can be seen in anergic patients, newborns, and infants younger than 3 months old, and false-negative results can occur with improper injection technique. False-negative results also may occur if the test is performed before the development of tuberculin reactivity. This reactivity generally appears 2 to 12 weeks after initial infection. The definition of a positive TST also varies according to a child's risk factors. A summary of definitions by risk factor is provided in Box 15-4.

Risk assessment questionnaires may be used to identify children with risk factors for TB who should have a TST performed. One questionnaire by Ozuah had a sensitivity of 85%, specificity of 86%, negative predictive value of 99.8%, and positive predictive value of 5.4% in a population with a prevalence of 5.8% positive TSTs. The questionnaire included questions about close contact with a person with an active case of TB, birth in or travel to an endemic region, close contact with high-risk adults, and HIV infection. Multiple puncture tests, such as tine and Mono-Vacc Test, currently are not recommended for TB screening because they have poor specificity and sensitivity compared with the Mantoux test. (See CD-ROM Chapter 17.)

Evidence of Screening Effectiveness

Detection of persons with latent TB infection (i.e., positive TST with no physical findings of disease) allows treatment of latent TB (usually with isoniazid) to prevent an individual from developing active TB. Prevention of active TB also is desirable from a societal perspective because it prevents further transmission of the organism and spread of disease. Effectiveness of latent TB treatment with isoniazid is limited by many factors. First, treatment for at least 6 months (9 months in children) generally is required, and patients may remain adherent to such a prolonged course of therapy. Second, not all organisms are susceptible to isoniazid, and persons with resistant strains do not receive adequate prophylaxis. In addition, there is a small risk of isoniazid-induced hepatitis, although the risk is much higher in adults.

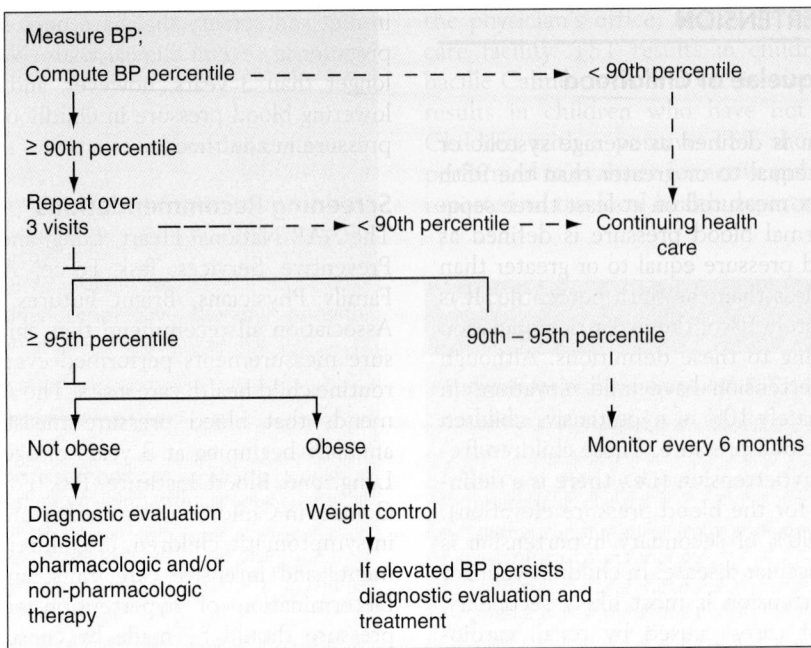

Figure 15-1. Algorithm for identifying children with elevated blood pressure (BP). (Redrawn from Task Force on Blood Pressure Control in Children: Report of the second task force on blood pressure control in children. Pediatrics 1987;79:1–25.)

visual pathways are believed to be malleable until about age 6 years. Failure to detect and treat amblyopia and its causes in early childhood may lead to permanent visual loss. This visual loss may interfere with educational and vocational opportunities and affect self-esteem. Amblyopia also is a risk factor for loss of vision in the unaffected eye. It is unclear whether there are any significant adverse effects in failing to detect refractive errors before they become symptomatic.

Accuracy of Screening Tests

Vision screening of children younger than 3 years old is problematic for many reasons, including inaccuracy of screening tests, time required for testing, and problems with cooperation. Photoscreening devices have been developed, including binocular photoscreening, in which patterns of eye reflections suggest refractive errors, strabismus, and cataracts, and monocular photoscreening, which screens only for refractive error. Owing to a wide range of sensitivities (37% to 88%) and specificities (40% to 94%), these photoscreening devices have not been recommended yet for routine use in the primary care setting.

In 3- to 5-year-old children, screening for amblyopia and strabismus may include inspection (presence of red reflex, symmetry of corneal light reflex), cover testing, visual acuity testing, and stereotesting. Visual acuity tests include Snellen letters, Snellen numbers, Tumbling E, HOTV, and various picture tests. The sensitivity of the Snellen letter test is approximately 25% to 37%. The random dot E stereo test is a common test for stereoacuity. It has an estimated sensitivity of 54% to 64% and specificity of 87% to 90% in detecting amblyopia and strabismus. Combining tests may increase sensitivity and specificity. Combined corneal light reflex symmetry, acuity testing, and stereotesting has a sensitivity of 84% and specificity of 65%. Eliminating one of the three tests raised specificity at the expense of sensi-

tivity. A study of photoscreening in children 3 months old to 8 years old (mean age >4 years old) found a sensitivity of 91% and a specificity of 74%. Visual testing in school-age children is primarily for acuity and frequently is performed in school. False-positive rates may be 30% or more.

Evidence of Effectiveness

Few data are available to assess the effectiveness of primary prevention of amblyopia. The best outcomes seem to be in children with the shortest duration of strabismus and early (<4 months) surgical treatment.

Secondary prevention involves the treatment of amblyopia before permanent visual deficits occur. Because no trials have been performed comparing treatment with no treatment, the effectiveness of treatment must be inferred from animal models, cross-sectional studies, and cohort studies. These studies provide fair evidence that early treatment does improve clinical outcomes, but as with primary prevention, success is more likely with earlier treatment. For school-age children, in whom screening is primarily for visual acuity not associated with amblyopia, secondary prevention is achieved by spectacle correction.

Few studies have assessed potential harms of screening and treatment for amblyopia or decreased visual acuity. Although eye patching may decrease visual acuity, this change is usually temporary. There is some concern that early treatment of visual impairment may interfere with the normalization of refractive errors, or emmetropization, that occurs during normal development.

Screening Recommendations

Several organizations have provided recommendations for vision screening in infants. The AAP recommends that all infants be examined by age 6 months for fixation preference, alignment, and presence of any eye disease. Subjective assessment is recommended at all routine preventive health visits until age 3 years, when objective assessment should begin. Specific screening maneuvers are presented in Table 15-2.

In 1999, an expert panel convened by the Maternal and Child Health Bureau released a task force report on preschool vision screening. The panel noted that adequate data on the validity and effectiveness of current screening programs were lacking and recommended that additional research be conducted. Until this research was available, they provided interim recommendations for vision screening in preschoolers (Table 15-3).

Many recommendations have been made for screening of children beyond the preschool years (see Table 15-2). The AAP and Bright Futures recommend objective visual acuity testing at 5, 10, 12, 15, and 18 years, with subjective testing at all other visits. The American Academy of Ophthalmology and American Association for Pediatric Ophthalmology and Strabismus recommend screening at routine school checks and for symptomatic children. The American Optometric Association recommends an optometric examination every 2 years.

Implementing Screening in Practice

Subjective assessment of visual problems should be performed on all infants and young children during routine child health visits. Recommended screening maneuvers (see Table 15-2) should be incorporated into clinicians' routine physical examination procedures. Objective visual assessment should begin in the preschool years at approximately age 3 to 4 years. If a child's lack of cooperation prevents

objective assessment at 3 years of age, rescreening should be attempted within 6 months. For older children, objective screening should be performed at the intervals noted earlier, with subjective screening at all other routine child health visits. Practitioners should have available materials to perform visual acuity and stereotesting, and procedures should be put in place to ensure that all children in need of objective screening have it performed, including children who may have missed previous opportunities for screening.

SCREENING FOR HEARING IMPAIRMENT

Epidemiology and Sequelae of Hearing Impairment in Children

Estimates of the prevalence of congenital hearing loss range from approximately 1 in 900 to 2500 live births, when hearing loss is defined as moderate, severe, or profound (at least 40 dB of loss). Approximately one to two thirds of these children have moderate bilateral hearing loss, whereas the rest have severe or profound hearing loss. The risk for hearing impairment may be 10 to 20 times greater for children who have required admission to a neonatal intensive care unit. Other risk factors for congenital hearing loss include congenital syndromes associated with hearing loss (e.g., Waardenburg's syndrome, Usher's syndrome), family history of hereditary childhood sensorineural hearing loss, congenital infections such as bacterial meningitis or TORCH (toxoplasmosis, other [congenital syphilis and viruses], rubella, cytomegalovirus, and herpes simplex virus) infections, and craniofacial anomalies. Approximately 50% to 75% of children with congenital hearing loss have an

Table 15-2. Recommended Ages and Methods for Pediatric Eye Evaluation Screening

Recommended Age	Method	Indications for Referral to an Ophthalmologist
Newborn–3 mo	Red reflex	Abnormal or asymmetric
	Inspection	Structural abnormality
3–6 mo (approximately)	Fix and follow	Failure to fix and follow in a cooperative infant
	Red reflex	Abnormal or asymmetric
	Inspection	Structural abnormality
6–12 mo and until child is able to cooperate for verbal visual acuity	Fix and follow with each eye	Failure to fix and follow
	Alternate occlusion	Failure to object equally to covering each eye
	Corneal light reflex	Asymmetric
	Red reflex	Abnormal or asymmetric
	Inspection	Structural abnormality
3 yr (approximately)	Visual acuity* (monocular)	20/50 or worse, or 2 lines of difference between the eyes
	Corneal light reflex/cover-uncover	Asymmetric/ocular refixation movements
	Red reflex	Abnormal or asymmetric
	Inspection	Structural abnormality
5 yr (approximately)	Visual acuity* (monocular)	20/40 or worse, or 2 lines of difference between the eyes
	Corneal light reflex/cover-uncover	Asymmetric/ocular refixation movements
	Red reflex	Abnormal or asymmetric
	Inspection	Structural abnormality
Every 1–2 yr after age 5	Visual acuity* (monocular)	20/30 or worse, or 2 lines of difference between the eyes
	Corneal light reflex/cover-uncover	Asymmetric/ocular refixation movements
	Red reflex	Abnormal or asymmetric
	Inspection	Structural abnormality

Note. These recommendations are based on panel consensus. Although a child may be retested if screening is inconclusive or unsatisfactory, undue delays should be avoided; if inconclusive on retesting, referral for a comprehensive pediatric medical eye evaluation is indicated.
Note. Use of medication for pupillary dilation facilitates evaluation of the red reflex. For infants, a combined weak solution of phenylephrine hydrochloride and cyclopentolate (Cyclomydril [Alcon, Ft. Worth, TX]) is associated with fewer side effects. (Isenberg S, Everett S, Parelhoff E: A comparison of mydriatic eye drops in low-weight infants. Ophthalmology 1984;91:278–279.)
*Figures, letters, "tumbling E" or optotypes, LEA symbols (Precision Vision, Inc., La Salle, IL), vision testing machines.

Table 15-3. Recommendations for Vision Screening, Age 36 to 59 Months

Function to Be Evaluated	Type of Test	Specific Test	Recommended Testing Procedures	Passing Criteria
Monocular distance acuity	Linear acuity	HOTV, Lea symbols, Tumbling E	Test distance = 10 ft (3 m)	Child must identify or match 4 of 5 optotypes on the critical line with each eye tested monocularly
	Isolated optotypes with surround bars*	HOTV cards with surround bars	Pretest (performed binocularly): test child's ability to perform test by having child identify or match each of the 4 optotypes on a line that is expected to be suprathreshold ($\geq$20/100). Child must identify successfully each of the 4 optotypes Test procedure (performed monocularly): Test child's ability to identify or match optotypes on the line used in the pretest. To proceed, child must identify or match 4 of 5 optotypes on the line used in the pretest line. Then test child's ability to identify or match optotypes on the critical line. Repeat test procedure with the other eye	Critical lines: 20/40 at 36–47 mo, 20/30 at 48–59 mo
Stereopsis	Random dot stereogram	Random Dot E	Test distance = 40 cm All testing, including pretesting, should be performed binocularly with the polarized glasses on Pretest: Test child's ability to perform test by having child identify the location of the three-dimensional E on 4 of 5 trials (E on left or right; above or below) Test procedure: Test child's ability to identify the location of the stereo E. Tester should use 5 presentations, varying location in a nonsystematic manner	Child must locate stereo E on 4 of 5 presentations

*Isolated optotypes without surround bars should not be used because they overestimate acuity in individuals with amblyopia.

From Hartmann EE, Dobson V, Hainline L, et al: Preschool vision screening: Summary of a task force report. Pediatrics 2000;106:1105–1112.

identifiable risk factor. Hearing loss in childhood has been associated with delays in speech and language acquisition, decreased cognitive ability, and problems with school achievement and employment later in life.

Chronic and recurrent otitis media with associated middle ear effusion may be associated with conductive hearing loss in infants and school-age children. The prevalence of otitis media in children younger than age 9 years is approximately 12%. Approximately 5% to 7% of children 5 to 8 years old may have a 25-dB hearing loss, which is transient and most often caused by otitis media with effusion (OME). Although correlation between OME and language delay in toddlers has been suggested, no studies have examined long-term language outcomes in children with OME.

Less common causes of hearing loss in childhood include ototoxic drug exposure, trauma, meningitis, Meniere's disease, and noise exposure. Data from the NHANES III study identified noise-induced hearing loss as a significant problem among 6- to 19-year-olds, with 12.5% having noise-induced hearing threshold shifts in one or both ears. Genetic and syndromic causes of hearing loss may be expressed during infancy but often do not become apparent until childhood or early adulthood.

Accuracy of Screening Tests

Screening for hearing impairment in newborns and infants requires electrophysiologic testing, usually by auditory brainstem response (ABR) or otoacoustic emissions (OAE). ABR measures the electrophysiologic response of the brainstem to auditory signals. ABR can detect damage to the cochlea, the auditory nerve, and auditory pathways in the brainstem. OAE primarily assesses the integrity of the cochlea and includes transient evoked tests generated in response to wide-band clicks and distortion product tests generated in response to tones.

The accuracy of newborn screening programs depends on the tests used (ABR, OAE, or both) and the criteria for defining screening failure. Sensitivity and specificity are enhanced by combining the tests and depend on the degree of hearing loss. There is a low positive predictive value in mild hearing loss, leading to many false-positive results, and a high positive predictive value in severe hearing loss.

ABR and OAE testing are limited by many factors. Both require that the infant be quiet or sleeping during the testing. Middle ear effusion or debris can lead to false-positive OAE tests. Both tests require some degree of training to achieve proficiency. Neither test is able to identify central hearing deficits that may be caused by conditions such as congenital cytomegalovirus infection or birth hypoxia. Finally, both tests require confirmation by a gold standard test. The accepted gold standard, visual reinforcement audiometry, cannot be performed until about 8 to 9 months of age. Intermediate diagnostic standards, such as a diagnostic ABR and otolaryngologic examination, must be substituted to confirm hearing loss during the first 6 months of life.

Screening for hearing impairment in school-age children usually is conducted using pure-tone (conventional) audiometry. Testing involves providing 20-dB tones at 500, 1000, 2000, and 4000 Hz in each ear and requires the cooperation of the child and a quiet environment. Sensitivity and specificity of conventional audiometry in school-age children is high (80% to 90%).

Testing for middle ear dysfunction may be performed in the primary care provider's office using tympanometry. This procedure also requires patient cooperation, however, and a good seal within the ear canal. Sensitivity and specificity of tympanometry vary significantly (60% to >90%) depending on the gold standard comparison, such as middle ear effusion or hearing loss.

Evidence of Effectiveness

It is fairly well documented that newborn hearing screening strategies can lead to earlier detection of hearing loss. There also is evidence that early diagnosis and treatment of hearing impairment can lead to improvements in language and cognitive development, although no prospective controlled studies have been completed, and family involvement seems to affect outcomes to a greater degree than early diagnosis. Treatment of hearing loss identified in the

newborn period may include amplification (use of hearing aids), cochlear implants, and speech and language therapy.

There is little evidence regarding the effectiveness of screening for hearing impairment in preschool and school-age children, with most hearing impairment in these groups caused by OME. In adults, unrecognized noise-induced hearing impairment is common among persons at high risk. Given that the NHANES III study found a 12.5% prevalence of noise-induced hearing loss in 6- to 19-year-olds, screening might be effective at identifying and treating this type of hearing loss. In OME and noise-induced hearing loss, there is little evidence documenting effectiveness of screening asymptomatic children.

Public Policy Considerations

Although the evidence for newborn screening is generally positive, some debate still exists as to the utility of screening infants without risk factors for hearing impairment. Critics of universal screening provide many arguments for limiting newborn screening to high-risk infants, including a high false-positive rate, a false sense of security created by a negative test, and parental anxiety surrounding the screening process. The increased cost of a two-stage OAE/ABR screening to identify more cases also has been considered.

Screening Recommendations

The Joint Committee on Infant Hearing has determined that there is adequate evidence to endorse universal newborn hearing screening. The Joint Committee on Infant Hearing policy does not specify whether to use OAE, ABR, or both. Some organizations believe that there continues to

---

Box 15-6. High-Risk Criteria for Hearing Loss in Children by Age Group

Neonates
- An illness or condition requiring a stay in the neonatal intensive care unit of at least 48 hours
- Stigmata or other findings associated with a syndrome that includes sensorineural or conductive hearing loss
- Family history of hereditary childhood sensorineural hearing loss
- Craniofacial anomalies, including abnormalities of the pinna and ear canal
- In utero infection, such as cytomegalovirus, herpes, toxoplasmosis, or rubella

Infants and Children ≥1 Month Old
- Parental, caregiver, or health care provider concerns regarding hearing, speech, language, or developmental delay
- Family history of hereditary childhood hearing loss
- Stigmata or other findings associated with a syndrome that includes a sensorineural or conductive hearing loss or eustachian tube dysfunction

- Postnatal infections associated with sensorineural hearing loss, including bacterial meningitis
- In utero infections such as cytomegalovirus, herpes, rubella, syphilis, and toxoplasmosis
- Neonatal indicators, such as hyperbilirubinemia at a serum level requiring exchange transfusion, persistent pulmonary hypertension of the newborn associated with mechanical ventilation, and conditions requiring the use of extracorporeal membrane oxygenation
- Syndromes associated with progressive hearing loss, such as neurofibromatosis, osteopetrosis, and Usher's syndrome
- Neurodegenerative disorders, such as Hunter's syndrome, or sensorimotor neuropathies, such as Friedreich's ataxia and Charcot-Marie-Tooth syndrome
- Head trauma associated with loss of consciousness or skull fracture
- Recurrent or persistent otitis media with effusion for at least 3 months

Adapted from Green M, Palfrey JS (eds): Appendix D: Hearing screening. In Bright Futures: Guidelines for Health Supervision of Infants, Children, and Adolescents, 2nd ed. Arlington, Va, National Center for Education in Maternal and Child Health, 2000, pp 304–306; and Joint Committee on Infant Hearing year 2000 position statement. Am J Audiol 2000;9:9–29. Copyright by the American Speech-Language-Hearing Association. Reprinted with permission.

be insufficient evidence to recommend for or against universal newborn hearing screening. For children ages 7 months through 3 years, audiologic screening is recommended for all who have not received newborn screening and any child at risk for hearing loss (Box 15-6). The AAP recommends objective screening beginning at 4 years old, with screening repeated at 5, 6, 8, 10, 12, 15, and 18 years of age. Bright Futures concurs with these recommendations and recommends additional screening if a child has any of the risk factors listed in Box 15-6.

Implementing Hearing Screening in Practice

More than 30 states now have required the implementation of universal newborn hearing screening programs by law. For infants who have not been screened, practitioners should refer either high-risk patients or all patients for audiologic evaluation, depending on their own interpretation of the evidence for and against universal screening.

For older infants and young children, referrals for audiologic screening should be made based on the presence of listed risk factors. Although good evidence supporting screening of asymptomatic older children does not yet exist, several authorities recommend screening, and it has been incorporated routinely into pediatric practice and into school-based programs. Practitioners should consider performing pure-tone audiologic screening in school-age children, with audiologic referral for screening failure.

Additional Resources, CD-ROM

Additional screening tests for iron deficiency	Text
Measurement of hypertension by sphygmomanometry	Text
Screening for hypercholesterolemia	Text, figures
Bibliography	

Mini-index of Related Topics

SUGGESTED READINGS

American Academy of Pediatrics Committee on Practice and Ambulatory Medicine: Recommendations for preventive periodic health care. Pediatrics 2000;105:645–646. Available at: www.aap.org/policy/re9939.html.

Canadian Task Force on the Periodic Health Examination: Canadian Guide to Clinical Preventive Health Care. Ottawa, Health Canada, 1994. Available at: http://www.ctfphc.org.

Green M, Palfrey JS (eds): Bright Futures: Guidelines for Health Supervision of Infants, Children, and Adolescents, 2nd ed. Arlington, Va, National Center for Education in Maternal and Child Health, 2000.

Joint Committee on Infant Hearing: Year 2000 Position Statement: Principles and guidelines for early hearing detection and intervention programs. 2000. Available at: www.aap.org/policy/jcihyr2000.pdf.

U.S. Preventive Services Task Force: Guide to Clinical Preventive Services, 2nd ed. Baltimore, Williams & Wilkins, 1996. Available at: www.ahrq.gov/clinic/uspstfix.htm.

U.S. Public Health Service: Put Prevention into Practice: Clinician's Handbook of Preventive Services, 2nd ed. McLean, Va, International Medical Publishing, 1998. Available at: www.ahrq.gov/clinic/ppipix.htm.

16 Well-Child Care: A Strategic Approach

Lucy M. Osborn

ROLE OF THE GENERALIST

1   Help parents and children understand the importance of and be partners in adherence to disease prevention and health promotion activities.

2   Ensure that all children receive appropriate health promotion and disease prevention care.

3   Perform appropriate screening, follow-up, and intervention for preventable threats to health.

4   Perform age-appropriate health promotion interventions.

5   Perform age-appropriate disease prevention interventions.

6   Select formats for well-child care that are most likely to be effective for the targeted population.

Box 16-1. Goals of Well-Child Care

1. Establish an effective clinician-patient-family relationship.
2. Help parents and children value health promotion and disease prevention.
3. Perform appropriate screening and surveillance.
4. Perform age-appropriate health promotion interventions.
5. Perform age-appropriate disease prevention interventions.

Well-child care is the foundation of the practice of pediatrics. Pediatrics evolved as a specialty from concerns about rising infant mortality that occurred during the industrial revolution when women joined the workforce. Infants were weaned early and placed on bottled milk, which, without refrigeration, rapidly became overgrown with bacteria. In the 1880s and 1890s 250 infants per 1000 died from diarrheal diseases. Milk stations were established to provide uncontaminated milk. Preventive care and health promotion rapidly followed, as providers at milk stations became concerned with infants' growth, development, and general health.

Box 16-1 lists the goals of well-child care. The importance of the social aspects of the well-child visit often is underappreciated. The establishment of an effective clinician-patient relationship is crucial to providing effective medical care and empowering the family to be active participants in that care. Trust between the parent and the physician is essential to obtaining accurate information from patients and families, to patient and family education, and to adherence to recommendations. The well-child visit is the best opportunity that clinicians have to form therapeutic alliances with families. During sick visits, families are likely to be stressed, worried, and focused on a problem. Families uniformly respond positively to the interest shown by the primary care provider in the child's health and development, in the family and its functioning, and in the child's overall environment. Well-child visits should be an enjoyable experience, with the family and the clinician collaboratively focused on common positive goals for helping children attain physical and emotional health. The clinical activities of each visit include disease screening, surveillance, and preventive interventions, such as immunization. Health promotion depends on good, interactive parent and patient education that emphasizes the crucial role that family and patient input has in fostering effective preventive activity.

Concepts essential to delivering effective well-child care are listed in Box 16-2. Continuity of care over an extended period is optimal for successful health maintenance. Teaching the concepts of prevention and the specific content recommended for each visit is time-consuming and difficult. A series of visits with the same physician or nurse practitioner allows development of a trusting relationship and effective patient education. Each visit should have a focus, balancing patient and parent agendas with anticipatory guidance. Patients with complex medical or psychosocial problems often do not receive adequate preventive care. So much

---

Box 16-2. Guidelines for Making Well-Child Care Effective

1. Establish continuity of care over an extended period.
2. Have realistic goals and objectives for each well-child visit.
3. Orient well-child care to the culture of the patient/population being served.
4. Use principles of adult education when presenting information to parents.
5. Customize each visit to the patient and family's needs.
6. Ensure that all patients, particularly children with chronic illness and children "at risk," receive well-child care.
7. Ensure that well-child visits are used for health promotion and disease prevention. When problems are found through screening and surveillance, continue well-child care and schedule a follow-up visit to address other issues.

time and attention is spent addressing problems that other health promotion and disease prevention activities are lost in the shuffle. Another common mistake made during well-child visits is using the visit to address specific behavioral or medical problems that become apparent during screening or surveillance. Issues such as unusual difficulties with toilet training or a positive lead screen need to be addressed in follow-up visits. Occasionally a problem is so urgent that the preventive visit must be put aside. In that case, the patient should be rescheduled.

Even among children born to low-risk, functional families, only a minority receives preventive care according to the recommended schedule of visits. Health maintenance should not be considered optional. Practitioners need to do everything within their power to encourage children and families to attend well-child visits. Appointment reminders for patients and a tickler file of overdue visits for the health care provider are excellent methods of increasing adherence to recommended preventive activities.

ELEMENTS OF WELL-CHILD CARE

Screening

Screening for physical, emotional, and social issues that affect the well-being of children is essential to health maintenance. The process of screening needs to be considered carefully, and the processes for effective screening need to be followed. Disease screening and surveillance is discussed in Chapter 15, and developmental and behavioral surveillance are discussed in Chapter 25. Box 16-3 lists important principles of screening. The timing of screening and the screening methods must be considered. Laboratory testing is only one method of screening. Physical screening procedures include measuring and recording growth parameters, vital signs, hearing and vision testing, and physical examination. Screening for family functioning and behavioral issues can be accomplished either by standardized assessment tools, such as the Child Behavioral Checklist, or by interview and observation. The procedures selected need to be compatible with the patient population, the practice environment, and the style of the practitioner. Methods for ensuring that screening results are interpreted accurately and followed up are essential. Positive screens should not be addressed during the well-child visit. Screening tests are not diagnostic. They simply indicate the presence of factors that place a patient at high risk to have or develop a disease. Positive screens should be explained to the family during the visit and a specific appointment made for actual testing or evaluation. Office procedures for ensuring adequate follow-up for evaluation and treatment of diagnosed conditions must be developed.

Risk assessment is also a screening activity. Assessment can be accomplished in the same manner as screening, with standardized tools or through the interview process. Chapters 23 and 24 provide detailed risk screening information for families and children, and Chapters 221, 234, and 235 are more specific to adolescents. Children at highest risk in terms of educational, community, or psychosocial risk should be reappointed for evaluation or referred or triaged to an appropriate resource or agency. Office procedures ensuring that patients not be lost and that they actually receive needed procedures are essential.

Health Promotion

Health promotion enhances the long-term life experience of children and families. Parents may be more willing to change their health behaviors for their child's benefit than they are for themselves. If the harmful effects of secondary tobacco exposure are explained to parents, they may stop smoking. Practitioners also should explain to parents the importance of role modeling. Because children learn best by example, they learn the health behaviors of their parents. Effective health promotion can occur only within the context of the family system with the family as an active participant in the process. The American Academy of Pediatrics' *Guidelines for Health Supervision III* is an excellent resource that describes activities and time frames for visits in which these activities are most likely to be effective. Immunization, promoting physical activity, promoting healthy nutrition, injury and violence prevention, and promotion of parenting skills are discussed in detail in other chapters in this section.

Family and Social Relations

One of the most essential elements of the well-child visit is formation of a trusting, interactive relationship with the child and the family. Through this relationship, the practitioner has access to information about the child's home environment that is unavailable to others. The long-term health of a child depends most on the quality of the physical, emotional, educational, and spiritual environment of the home. Practitioners too often are hesitant to ask the questions that reveal this essential information. During a well-child visit, if a trusting relationship has been established in which the parents understand that the practitioner is vested in the well-being of the child, parents generally welcome an opportunity to discuss concerns about marital relationships, substance use, siblings, violence, and economic stresses. Practitioners may be hesitant to open such discussions because they do not have "answers." The establishment of a relationship in which the views and attitudes, including cultural, of the patient and family are elicited and genuinely valued is essential to its effectiveness. The principles of screening for disease are the same in screening for family and social risk factors. The practitioner should respond to indications of detrimental family and social relationships with either a prompt reappointment for further evaluation or a referral to an appropriate resource for assistance.

Box 16-3. Principles for Effective Screening

1. The condition must have an asymptomatic state.
2. There is an effective, acceptable treatment for the condition that can prevent the disease, delay its onset, or improve the long-term outcome.
3. The risks and benefits of screening and treatment have been established.
4. The costs of screening and treatment are acceptable.
5. Patients are informed regarding the screening procedures.
6. A screening test with acceptable sensitivity, specificity, and predictive value must be available.

Anticipatory Guidance

Anticipatory guidance is one of the most valuable services that a pediatric health care practitioner can provide. Armed with knowledge of normal growth, development, and behavior, particularly in a culturally sensitive context, the practitioner can help families anticipate what to expect in the coming months. Knowing that a particular behavior or change in growth or developmental variation is normal alleviates anxiety. Raising children is a stressful responsibility that can be overwhelming to many parents. Concerns and anxiety interfere with parents' ability to enjoy their children. Teaching a parent to watch for subtle developmental milestones can help them have the same delight when they see their children achieve them as parents do with a baby's first step. Anticipation of issues such as night awakening and arming families with resources to address the issues in manners that can avoid long-term problems help parents feel confident. Through anticipatory guidance, the practitioner can build parental self-esteem and promote positive parenting skills.

Anticipatory guidance also must be planned carefully into the visit. The nature of anticipatory guidance means that parents will not ask questions about the issues that need to be covered. They are unaware of what to anticipate. Care must be taken to ensure that there is enough time during the visit to cover these crucial issues. Excellent materials regarding anticipatory guidance are available in the texts listed in the Suggested Readings at the end of this chapter.

PROCESS OF WELL-CHILD VISITS

Well-child care begins with the environment of the office. Because education of patients and families is the essence of the well-child visit, considerable thought needs to be given to creating an optimal teaching environment. Every effort must be made to make all aspects of the visit enjoyable and productive. Waiting areas should be designed to be as comfortable as possible. Carefully selected books and toys or interactive computer games can make waiting time educational for children and less stressful for parents. Culturally appropriate educational brochures and questionnaires regarding development or other aspects of child health allow productive use of this time and can make the actual visit more efficient. Although subsequent illness from exposure to communicable diseases during a well-child visit is unusual, parents understandably are concerned about bringing their healthy child to a physician's office. Separate waiting areas for well and sick children are optimal. If separate areas are not possible, scheduling well children for a specific portion of the day may be helpful.

Scheduling of patients should be done in a realistic manner, to minimize waiting times. For optimal care, families should be requested to schedule well visits for one child at a time and, if possible, bring only the child who is being seen. These requests communicate the importance of preventive care for each individual and allow the child to receive the full attention of the parent and the provider.

The family's initial contact during a health supervision visit is with office staff. Patient check-in and nursing procedures—such as measuring and graphing height, weight, and head circumference; measuring blood pressure; and

screening vision—offer an opportunity for staff to form personal relationships with patients. Families are more confident calling about a sick child if they know and trust the staff who answer the telephone. Often parents and children share information with staff that they are hesitant to share with a physician. Office staff, as an integral part of the health care team, should receive training regarding health education and "teachable moments" during their patient contact time.

Every effort should be made to minimize waiting time in examination rooms. Families who have had to entertain an active child and felt the need to contain the child's activities for more than 10 to 15 minutes are likely to be stressed and irritable. Although patients seldom complain to the physician, their frame of mind needs to be positive, open, and receptive for education to be effective.

The interview with the family and observation of the parent-child interaction by the practitioner is the most essential portion of the visit. During this communication, the basis of the provider-patient relationship is formed. While communicating with the family, the provider has an excellent opportunity not only to ascertain family values, cultural issues, and relationships, but also to observe the relationships between the parents and the child and any other family members who may be present during the visit. The interview consists of social interactions, historical data obtained for screening and surveillance, health promotion, and anticipatory guidance. Practitioners should educate themselves and develop resources for parents regarding common parenting issues, such as discipline, sleep, toilet training, and school. In a diverse population, these resources also should include an appreciation for the cultural considerations of these issues. Care should be taken during the interview to ensure that all essential aspects are covered. If the interview elicits a concern about specific issues, the practitioner must evaluate the situation and use the visit to address the problem and reschedule the well-child visit, schedule the patient for a follow-up visit for evaluation, or refer the family to an appropriate resource.

Physical examination is a screening procedure. Meticulous examination over the first 6 months of life is essential to detect congenital abnormalities. After 6 months of age, unless a parent expresses a specific concern, abnormalities on general examination are unusual. Practitioners must take care not to become lackadaisical and should be certain to focus their attention on the portions of the examination that may become abnormal over time. Box 16-4 lists some examples of considerations for focusing the general screening physical examination.

In closing the visit, the practitioner should review the findings, ensure that the parents will learn the results of any screening tests that are pending, make any referrals that are needed, and inform the family when to come for the next health maintenance visit.

METHODS OF DELIVERING WELL-CHILD CARE

Preventive care for children now often is fragmented. Because many families do not have third-party coverage for the cost of prevention or immunizations, they may receive their illness care from private practitioners or emergency

CASE STUDY 17-2

PREVENTIVE CARE AT A 13-PROVIDER MULTISPECIALTY GROUP

Conscientious Crosstown Primary Care is a 13-provider multispecialty group practice that decided to review their delivery of pediatric preventive care. In this practice, clinicians had established office-wide protocols for well-child visits. They used a standard health maintenance record. They held monthly meetings involving providers and staff. After a sample chart review of 2-year-old patient charts, they found that 80% were up-to-date on immunizations, 12% had had tuberculosis screening, 70% had been screened for anemia, and 60% had had anemia screening. A review of a sample of charts of 4-year-old patients revealed that 40% had had vision screening and 25% had had blood pressure screening. These results were discussed at the monthly practice meeting, and a decision was made to improve the delivery of preventive services.

wanted to increase efficiency by distributing the work among staff, allowing clinicians to be more focused and enabling parents' needs to be addressed more directly. This section offers some practical strategies for accomplishing these goals.

Assess Practice Performance

The first step in improving care is assessing the practice's performance. This assessment can be done through a simple chart review of a sample of 10 to 30 charts. Having data helps clinicians and staff identify opportunities for improvement, creates motivation and "buy-in" for the need for change, and provides a baseline measure that can be followed over time to determine if changes are resulting in improved care. For a simple chart review form that can be customized, see CD-ROM Box 17-1.

Create a Team to Guide the Improvement Activities

After reviewing baseline performance data, it is helpful to create a small team of physicians and staff who are committed to improving preventive care in the office. An improvement team that is motivated, is willing to try out new ideas, and can gather ideas from the rest of the practice should be chosen. The ideal team consists of a clinician, a nursing staff member, and a front office staff or administrative team member.

Keeping the improvement team small with about three to four members makes the group more effective. It also is important that the group commit to regular meetings, at least monthly or semimonthly, to review performance, plan tests of new approaches, and reflect on what has and has not been successful. Scheduling the meetings during the lunch break can increase success; alternative scheduling options include before or after office hours. It may be helpful to designate one member of the team as a "prevention coordinator," who takes responsibility for communicating and spreading the preventive services improvement strategies within the office when they have been tested adequately.

Box 17-1. Evidence-Based Strategies to Improve Preventive Care

1. Presence of a coordinator for office-based preventive services
2. Office-wide guidelines for preventive services
3. Structured assessment of patient preventive service needs at every visit
4. Methods to prompt clinicians
5. Plans for counseling
   Organized patient education materials
   Appropriately trained staff
6. Methods to promote patient communication
7. Tracking of population and follow-up
8. Regular performance monitoring and feedback

Understand Current Practice Approaches to Prevention

Prevention typically involves many strategies (Box 17-1). These strategies may be carried out differently in different offices. Some practices find it helpful to use a flow chart to identify the specific activities that take place during the office encounter. A flow chart allows the working group to identify areas of duplication and omission and can prompt discussions to delineate staff roles. Barriers that affect the practice's delivery of preventive services may arise. Some barriers may be easily amenable to change (e.g., patient flow), whereas others may be less so (e.g., lack of insurance) and may require changes outside the practice (e.g., stronger links with local social services and Medicaid agencies).

NEXT STEPS

After assessing practice performance and understanding current office processes and systems, the team should consider what tools and strategies could be tested to see if they result in improved care in the practice. Tools such as simplified guidelines, flow sheets, and educational materials can help clinicians translate processes into practice. Table 17-1 illustrates how tools can be linked to specific processes.

GUIDELINES

Almost all pediatric health care providers have a routine schedule of well-child visits and preventive services they provide. There can be variation among clinicians within a practice regarding the timing of and priority assigned to particular clinical services for patients. In many office practices, clinicians may not have come to an agreement about

Table 17-1. Office Processes and Tools to Support Them

Process	Tool
Identifying service needs	Preventive service summary sheet
Prompting provider	Chart Post-Its
Educating patients	Patient activation cards
Documenting services	Flow sheet
Following up	Tracking system
Monitoring effectiveness	Periodic chart reviews

practice-wide preventive service guidelines. One physician in a practice may conduct detailed injury prevention assessment, whereas others do not. Physicians also may have their own schedule of when to deliver certain preventive services. It is appropriate and important to vary care to meet families' needs. Unplanned variation of services within a practice can cause patient needs and risks to be overlooked, however, and opportunities and "teachable moments" for counseling to be missed. Lack of agreement about which services to perform and when to provide them also makes it difficult to enable staff to assist in care delivery. In addition, variation among clinicians can confuse staff and parents. One way of improving care is to establish practice guidelines, a recommended set of services whose priority and timing are used throughout the entire office. Practice guidelines are designed with the "average" patient in mind to ensure that services are not forgotten and have many benefits (Box 17-2). Practice guidelines are not a prescription to follow rigidly. It is important to have enough flexibility in a practice guideline to allow clinicians to tailor guidelines to each patient's needs.

Discussing and prioritizing practice guidelines enables the practice to simplify the care process for clinicians, nurses, and administrative staff. It is normal for clinicians to have a range of opinions about what clinical topics are most important. Guidelines identify *minimum* expectations that facilitate the consistent delivery of high-quality care to the entire patient population and build in an appropriate amount of flexibility that enables clinicians to tailor interventions for individual patients. Clinicians can convene a process that builds practice agreement on several key guidelines (e.g., age at screening for anemia). When some agreement has been achieved, practices can train ancillary clinical staff to assist in preventive services delivery and reduce missed opportunities.

The most reliable strategy for ensuring that guidelines are used consistently is to embed prompts and reminders in charting tools, such as preventive services prompting sheets (flow sheets), health maintenance records, and physical examination forms (see CD-ROM Box 17-2 for samples). Using these tools can open the door to others taking part in important anticipatory guidance issues, such as problem-focused counseling or assessment of patient concerns.

Box 17-2. Benefits of Practice Guidelines

1. Guidelines are associated with significant improvements in the quality of care.
2. Guidelines remind clinicians and staff about key services in the process of tailoring care to individual patient needs.
3. Guidelines ease the distribution of routine work among members of the practice.
4. Guidelines clarify the timing and priorities for particular services, making it easier and faster for everyone in the office to participate in care.
5. Guidelines define staff training priorities for clear, consistent, practice-wide approaches and roles in care delivery.
6. Guidelines make it easier to develop systems to support care for routine patients and to plan for caring for subgroups of patients with more complex problems.

PREVENTIVE SERVICE SCREENING AND PROMPTING

A routine system to screen charts and prompt clinicians about needed services at every visit is effective in improving the delivery of preventive services. These systems can be even more powerful when applied to well-child and acute care visits, encouraging providers to make every visit an opportunity for preventive care.

Given the numerous recommendations regarding preventive care, it is not surprising that clinicians may not remember what is indicated at each visit despite the establishment of practice-wide guidelines. Guidelines are more likely to be followed if they are embedded in an individualized preventive services summary (a paper or computerized summary of what services have been provided). This tool allows the clinician or the clinician's administrative staff to tell at a glance whether the child is missing any age-appropriate immunizations or other preventive care services.

Prompting the provider can be done in many ways. A preventive services summary sheet can allow all office staff, including the administrative team, to screen charts quickly to identify whether a child is missing a preventive service. Helpful reminders, such as Post-It notes affixed to the front of the chart or a quick note in the record, can alert clinicians that a preventive service is needed. Such a sheet can be referenced at non–well-child visits (e.g., acute or chronic illness visits) to identify needed care and avoid missed opportunities.

Some practices place age-appropriate prompts within health maintenance chart records that are used at well-child visits. Although this approach has the advantage facilitating documentation, it does not facilitate review of preventive services needs at all visits. These tools can be customized, however, to help divide responsibilities between nursing and physician staff (see CD-ROM Box 17-2).

Another approach process for assessing risk is to use structured assessment tools that are given to parents to complete. Nurses could be asked to administer structured assessments to parents, such as the Parents Evaluation of Developmental Status, before the clinician examines the patient. Parent risk assessment tools also can be created for other environmental risk factors (e.g., lead screening). Tools for lead, tuberculosis, and fluoride risk assessment are included in CD-ROM Box 17-3. Risk assessments are designed to identify high-risk patients, limiting unnecessary tests and adding to increased efficiency (see Chapter 15).

Strategies that divide responsibilities among office staff can free up valuable clinician time, while helping to engage all office staff in patient care. These types of strategies are easier to implement when practice guidelines are in place and commonly shared among clinicians. Practices that use flow sheets have experienced 10% to 20% increases in rates of preventive services. An electronic medical record that prompts the provider is an example of a more "high-tech" approach to undertaking this same concept. Compiling chart tools that capture all the services on the practice guideline can be daunting. A practice should start small, perhaps with a single tool, such as a flow sheet, or with a single age group.

EDUCATING PATIENTS

Educational materials work best when they address specific parental concerns (see Chapter 25). Another type of tool, sometimes called *patient activation materials*, educate parents about what will occur during the visit and prompt parents to ask questions they may have about the child's health or development. These materials, commonly handed out while parents are waiting, encourage parents to discuss concerns with the clinician and prompt parents to remember and ask questions. (An example is included in CD-ROM Box 17-4.) Studies have shown that the use of these materials can focus the encounter to ensure parents' concerns are addressed and satisfaction increased. The Parents Evaluation of Developmental Status assessment tool discussed in Chapter 25 provides some of these benefits. These materials should inform parents about what to expect at a given visit and review normal growth and development and age-appropriate health and safety topics.

COMMUNITY AND EDUCATIONAL RESOURCES

Linking families with appropriate community and educational resources is an important part of clinical practice. Taking full advantage of the resources in the community may enable the clinician to provide a wider range of services to patients. Many communities have agencies and organizations that can extend the reach of the primary care physician by supporting extended counseling, offering extensive follow-up for more complex patients, and providing targeted services for routine patients. A practice is most effective when it identifies the needs and strengths of the individual child and family, works within its own limitations, and maximizes community supports to address the wide range of issues patients face. Box 17-3 lists several key changes that practices can make that would result in more effective links with their community.

Creating effective partnerships with the community is an ongoing, evolving process. It can be daunting to identify all the community resources that the practice might want to refer patients to and to set up systems to support coordination with those resources. Lack of time, knowledge, and staff resources are among the challenges that may limit practices' use of community resources to their full potential. To avoid having the task seem insurmountable, practices can focus initially on one or two services patients need most frequently and one or two strategies for linking to those services. Learning as much as possible about community resources for those services can lead to good systems for working with the organizations that provide relevant services and translates into knowledge that a practice can use in the future.

DOCUMENTING SERVICES

Practices should use practical and efficient methods for documenting services. A flow sheet can document services and prompt staff about needed services. In addition to noting the services indicated, listing the appropriate age at the time of the indicated service makes the flow sheet a more useful reference tool (see the example in CD-ROM Box 17-2).

FOLLOWING UP

Tracking

Flow sheets in individual charts support improved delivery of preventive services to individual children when they come in for services. Some children most in need of services may not be brought in for care, however. A tracking process to identify children who "fall through the cracks" can allow a practice to be proactive at the population level, by identifying children who may be in need of services but have not come in for care.

A tracking system helps identify children who have been cared for in the practice and are behind on needed services. The first step in developing a tracking system is to determine which criteria will be used to identify children who are behind in care. Two suggested criteria are age and missed well-child visit. One can begin by generating a list of all children followed in the practice born in a particular month. Many practice information systems contain tracking features (e.g., age or missed well-child checkup). When providers have selected a tracking criterion, they can pull the charts of these patients and identify children in need of preventive services.

Even in a busy practice that sees 60 newborn infants each month, intervention is likely to be needed for only approximately 20 patients each month. Using *age* criteria, a practice may choose to focus its efforts on children 20 months old so that families can be contacted and children brought in by 24 months of age to become "up-to-date." Alternatively, one could employ a *visit measure* and use a missed 18-month-old well-child visit as a proxy for being delinquent.

Tracking systems can be either "low-tech" (e.g., an index card "tickler" file) or "high-tech" (e.g., an electronic medical record or immunization registry). Practices can use their information systems to generate the names of patients behind on services. Public agencies also may be able to provide data from statewide registries.

Box 17-3. Practice Changes That Can Result in Improved Links with the Community

- Identifying an individual or team who is responsible for coordinating with your community; this is an appropriate role for the prevention coordinator
- Determining the most frequent community resource referrals for the practice patient population
- Determining the resources in the community that may meet the needs of the patient population
- Identifying specific people at appropriate agencies that can provide the practice with information and support patients who are referred there
- Creating a listing of relevant community resources and agencies and making it available to patients and staff
- Developing simple systems to track patient care among agencies and the practice (e.g., noncarbon referral forms, obtaining eligibility criteria from agencies)

Performance Monitoring and Feedback

Monitoring rates of care over time can help offices focus their practice's efforts to improve progress when attempting improvements. Discussing results with the practice team can help reinforce practice goals. In addition, using objective measures of care directs attention to *what* the problem is rather than *who* the problem is. The practice may want to post measures publicly in the office so that staff can see and understand the link between process changes and improved outcomes. When an office system is implemented, practice teams can monitor progress by using internal chart reviews.

PUTTING PREVENTION INTO PRACTICE IN THE OFFICE: MODEL FOR IMPROVEMENT

After reviewing performance assessment and the various tools and change strategies discussed previously, the practice improvement team is ready to adapt specific strategies to the office. The Model for Improvement provides guidance and focus for implementing change in office practice. It helps identify an aim, measure, and change strategies by asking the three questions in Table 17-2. These questions are followed by the use of *small-scale, rapid* cycles of testing to evaluate changes in systems and processes. These tests are referred to as P-D-S-A *(Plan-Do-Study-Act)* cycles. P-D-S-A cycles guide improvement teams through a systematic analysis and improvement process (Fig. 17-1).

Determine the Aim

A clear aim or goal provides a target for the practice improvement team and the entire practice. Effective aim statements are clear and specific and set "stretch" goals (quantitative targets that are a real reach). An example is "we want to achieve preventive service rates of 90% for immunizations and screening for lead, tuberculosis, anemia, and visual acuity."

Use Simple Measures: How to Know if Change Is an Improvement

Measuring for improvement is different than other types of performance measurement that often reflect judgment. The Model for Improvement encourages practices to establish realistic goals with a stretch component, making the goals obtainable, but enough of a reach to be challenging. Process measures, which track incremental improvements, are an effective way to measure progress on these goals (Case Study 17-3).

Identifying, Planning, and Testing a Change

The clinician should review the strategies discussed earlier to determine which are best suited to *his or her* practice for improving preventive service delivery. The clinician

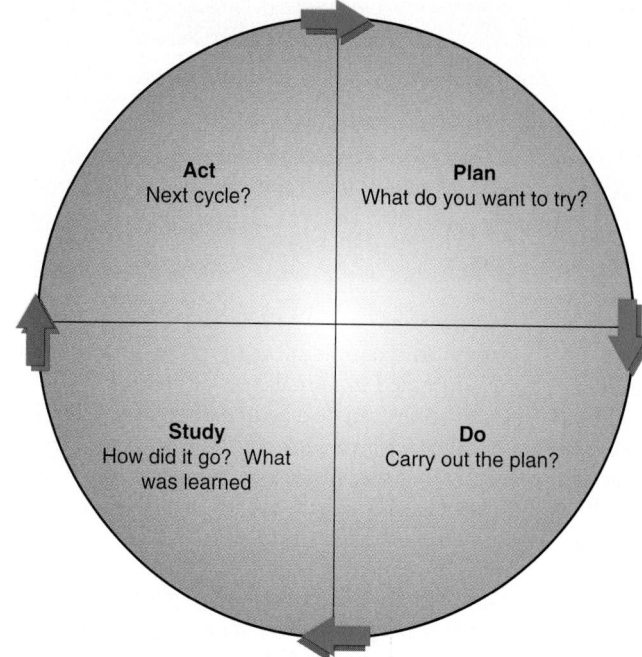

Figure 17-1. The P-D-S-A (Plan-Do-Study-Act) cycle for process improvement.

should test selected changes on a small scale, review measures, make adjustments, and measure again. The cycle is repeated until the clinician is satisfied that the results are really an improvement (Box 17-4). When planning to test a change, the clinician should specify the "who, what, where, and when" so that all project staff know their roles clearly.

CASE STUDY 17-3

MONITORING THE EFFECTIVENESS OF VISION SCREENING: USING A SMALL CYCLE TO MEASURE AND TEST CHANGE

Guidelines recommend vision screening for children beginning at 3 years of age to ensure effective identification and treatment to prevent amblyopia. Most practices do not implement vision screening routinely, however, until the prekindergarten physical examination, assuming that children younger than 5 years old would have difficulty cooperating with the screening instructions and tasks.

The physicians at Boice-Willis Pediatrics Clinic in Rocky Mount, North Carolina, wanted to implement vision screening for 3-year-olds, but the nurses who performed the screening thought this would be difficult, if not impossible. The lead physician was able to convince the nurses to try screening 3-year-olds and 4-year-olds for 2 days and keep track of the results. He employed a successful strategy for implementing improvement in the practice setting: using a small test of change to allow the staff to assess the change. A simple tracking sheet was placed next to the eye chart. The nurses found that 75% of 3.5-year-olds could be screened successfully. These encouraging data enabled the practice to increase their efforts at vision screening and improve significantly their delivery of this important service. Because of this effort, the lead physician was able to motivate the other physicians and clinician support staff to adopt vision screening in younger children.

Table 17-2.	Key Questions for Improvement Model
Aim	What are we trying to accomplish?
Measure	How will we know that a change is an improvement?
Change	What changes can we make that will result in improvement?

Box 17-4. Strategies for Small-Scale Tests

1. Test the change on a small group of volunteers before introducing it to others (e.g., members of the team who developed the change).
2. Test the change side-by-side with the existing care system.
3. Think small (e.g., conduct the test in with *one* physician, with *one* patient).
4. Conduct the test over a short period.

Box 17-6. Rationale for Small-Scale Testing

- It can help increase the belief that a specific change would result in improvement.
- It can provide opportunities for "failures" without affecting performance.
- It can help document how much improvement can be expected from a change.
- It can help those involved learn how to adapt the change to specific conditions (e.g., winter flu season, office emergencies).
- It can help in the evaluation of costs and side effects of a change.
- It can help minimize resistance on implementation.

Box 17-5 presents an example of the type of simple issue that should be addressed in a small test of change.

Identifying staff roles can be a source of great tension for the practice because *everyone usually* feels as if they have enough work to do and cannot take on *one more* task. Trying small cycles of change, for a half-day or day, allows staff to "try on" a role and determine its effect. In addition, as documented in the vision screening example in Case Study 17-3, showing an improved outcome from a change can be a great motivator for staff members as they take on new roles.

Running test cycles before full implementation offers a safe way to try something new and make modifications, while minimizing resource use and impact on the entire practice. The working group should develop the office system in a step-by-step process for the reasons noted in Box 17-6, with many of these efforts occurring simultaneously.

In addition to improving preventive services, practices should try to increase efficiency by distributing the work among staff. These changes would not help the practice or families if they increase the time the child is in office or if there is more work for clinicians. Multiple testing of ideas may be necessary before a new process is effective and practical.

Implementing

When a tool or strategy is found to be useful, the improvement team needs to determine how to implement and spread this change throughout the office. If a practice decides to implement a flow sheet, it must determine *how* to do so. The working group could decide to implement this new form on newborns only or on all well-child visits as each child comes in, or the working group could pull *all* charts and backfill these forms. Careful planning fosters successful implementation. A practice must plan for appropriate training and communication when implementing the change.

Using the strategies outlined in this chapter, the two practices described in Case Studies 17-1 and 17-2 em-

barked on a 9-month effort to improve the delivery of preventive services in their offices. Hardworking Pediatric Associates and Conscientious Crosstown Primary Care developed office systems for preventive care and improved significantly their rates of preventive service delivery. The practices chose different tools and strategies, adapting approaches to fit their staff and organizations. Conscientious Crosstown Primary Care accomplished this work more quickly because their office had more organizational processes already in place (e.g., established office protocols, office-wide use of standardized health maintenance record, and monthly staff meetings). Although Hardworking Pediatric Associates took longer to implement systems, the clinicians and staff were pleased with the improvements they made and knew they were giving more thorough care.

Additional Resources, CD-ROM

Assessment of practice performance	Text, assessment tool
Assuring delivery of preventive services	Text, preventive services prompt tool
Maintaining preventive services records	Text, children's health care improvement form
Risk assessment	Text, risk assessment questionnaire
Patient education	Text, patient activation form

Mini-index of Related Topics

Box 17-5. Using a Small Test of Change: Post-It Notes

Post-It notes can be used when reviewing a patient's chart as a way to remind the provider that services are needed. Small tests of such a change, involving three or four patients, can be used to refine the tool to meet practice needs and define staff roles and responsibilities. A key question is "Who should be responsible for reviewing a chart to determine whether services are needed and for flagging the chart with the Post-It note?" Possible choices are the clerical person pulling the chart before the visit, the front-desk person on duty when the child arrives, the nurse who checks in the patient, or the clinician who examines the patient. The answer varies depending on the practice and patient flow. Small tests of change can help answer this question.

SUGGESTED READINGS

Bordley WC, Margolis, PA, Stuart J, et al: Improving preventive service delivery through office systems. Pediatrics 2001;108(3):e41.

Langley GJ, Nolan KM, Norman CL, et al: The Improvement Guide. New York, Jossey-Bass, 1996.

Leininger L, Finn L, Dickey L, et al: An office system for organizing preventive services: A report by the American Cancer Society

Advisory Group on Preventive Health Care Reminder Systems. Arch Fam Med 1996;5:108–115.

Szilagyi PG, Bordley W, Vann JC, et al: Effect of patient reminder/recall interventions on immunization rates. JAMA 2000;284:1820–1827.

U.S. Preventive Services Task Force: Guide to Clinical Preventive Services, 2nd ed. Alexandria, Va, International Medical Publishing, 1996.

SECTION 2 HEALTH PROMOTION AND DISEASE PREVENTION

18 Immunizations: A Systems Approach

Alan Kohrt and Lois Kohrt

ROLE OF THE GENERALIST

1 Involve all clinicians and staff in the practice's immunization efforts, including education, dialogue, and quality improvement.

2 Know the current vaccine types and schedules, and provide all recommended vaccines at the appropriate time as a component of preventive care in the medical home.

3 Know and follow valid and invalid contraindications for vaccine administration, and ensure that the practice staff is using appropriate technique in vaccine storage and administration.

4 Assess the practice's immunization rates and quality assurance procedures on a regular basis to ensure 90% immunization completion.

5 Provide education for and address concerns of parents in regard to vaccines, vaccine safety, and refusal, and provide the appropriate vaccine information sheets and educational resources.

6 Understand the legal implications and documentation requirements of vaccine administration and vaccine refusal.

7 Ensure participation in governmental vaccine compensation programs and proper coding and billing to receive appropriate reimbursement for vaccination of all children

hepatitis B, measles, mumps, rubella, and *Haemophilus influenzae* type B. During the last half of the 20th century, the United States had almost a 100% decrease in the number of cases of 10 vaccine-preventable diseases (96% to 98% for pertussis and tetanus and 99% to 100% for the other 8 diseases) (Table 18-1). Primary pediatric practice has been a crucial component in this successful public health effort.

Today primary care settings provide 75% to 85% of childhood vaccines; this is a significant increase since the 1990s, in part because of the Vaccine for Children (VFC) program. The VFC program and Medicaid expansion (Children's Health Insurance Program [CHIP]) have enabled more children to receive immunizations. Although

Table 18-1. Impact of Vaccines in the 20th Century

Disease	20th Century Annual Morbidity	2001 Provisional Total	% Decrease
Smallpox	48,164	0	100
Diphtheria	175,885	2	100
Pertussis	147,271	5396	96.3
Tetanus	1314	27	97.9
Polio (paralytic)	16,316	0	100
Measles	503,282	108	100
Mumps	152,209	231	99.8
Rubella	47,745	19	100
Congenital rubella	823	2	99.8
Haemophilus influenzae (<5 yr)	20,000 (est.)	183	99.1

From CDC: Impact of vaccines universally recommended for children—United States, 1900–1998. MMWR Morb Mortal Wkly Rep 1999;48:243–248; CDC: Provisional cases of selected notifiable diseases preventable by vaccination, United States, weeks ending December 29, 2001, and December 30, 2000 (52nd week). MMWR Morb Mortal Wkly Rep 2002;50:1174-1175.

Protecting children from vaccine-preventable diseases by providing immunizations is a major component of pediatric care. The United States has been successful in immunizing greater than 98% of school-age children, and three out of four preschool children (age 18 to 35 months) are fully immunized against diphtheria, tetanus, pertussis, polio, the opportunity to protect more children has increased, the schedule, "catch-up" schedule, and immunization rules continue to become more complicated. The 2004 vaccination schedule recommends vaccines for 11 different diseases requiring 23 injections from birth to school entry. Some children also are immunized for hepatitis A, and influenza vaccine is recommended for infants 6 to 24 months old. Participation in the VFC program requires that practices have at least two different vaccine suppliers and that storage, handling, and documentation are increased. The Vaccine Injury Compensation Program has added additional education and documentation requirements to the practice, including vaccine information statements (VIS). Finally, increasing numbers of parents have questioned the need for recommended vaccines (although the primary care physician is still the most trusted source of vaccine information for families).

A primary care practice's immunization rates often are used as a measure of the overall quality of care provided by the practice. Managed care organizations and other third-party payers, Medicaid and Early and Periodic Screening, Diagnostic, and Treatment (EPSDT), VFC, and others measure the practice's immunization rates and assess if the practice is meeting quality standards for storage, handling, and delivery of vaccines. The expanded public health role for the primary care practice team, continuous government program requirements, external assessment of immunizations, and increased demands of the complex schedule also require that every practice maintain quality immunization systems to ensure that every child is immunized safely with effective vaccines. Providing vaccines in the primary care setting requires a significant investment of time and resources by the entire practice.

GENERAL PRINCIPLES OF IMMUNIZATION

Types of Vaccines

There are two types of vaccines—live attenuated vaccines and inactivated vaccines. Both types of vaccines stimulate the immune system to produce antigen-specific humoral (antibody) immunity, and live attenuated vaccines produce cellular immunity (see Chapter 10). Having the natural disease or receiving the vaccination produces *active immunity* that lasts for years; receiving live vaccines produces immunity that often lasts for life. The ability of the body to develop active immunity is affected by the presence of maternal antibody; nature and dose of antigen; route of administration; and host factors, such as age, nutritional status, and coexisting disease. *Passive immunity* occurs when preformed antibodies are given to the child. Passive immunization is temporary and includes combined and disease-specific immunoglobulins (i.e., for varicella, hepatitis B, and respiratory syncytial virus).

Live attenuated vaccines are modified viruses (e.g., mump, measles, rubella [MMR]; varicella) that can replicate in the body. Inactivated vaccines include inactivated whole viruses (e.g., inactivated poliomyelitis vaccine [IPV], influenza, hepatitis A), inactivated whole bacteria (e.g., typhoid, cholera), bacterial subunits (e.g., hepatitis B, acellular pertussis), toxoids (e.g., diphtheria-tetanus [DT] or tetanus-diphtheria [Td]), unconjugated polysaccharides

(e.g., meningococcal vaccine, pneumococcal polysaccharide vaccine [PPV]), and polysaccharide conjugates (*Haemophilus influenzae* type b [Hib], PPV). Inactivated vaccines generally require several doses to produce an adequate immune response, and antibody titers usually decrease over time.

Immunization Schedule

Recommended Schedule

Figure 18-1 shows the 2004 recommended immunization schedule. This schedule is approved by the American Academy of Pediatrics (AAP), the American Academy of Family Physicians (AAFP), and the Advisory Committee on Immunization Practices (ACIP). The schedule is updated annually and can be found at the following websites: www.aap.org/family/parents/immunize.htm#pdf (AAP), www.aafp.org/exam/rep-520.html (AAFP), or www.cdc.gov/nip (Centers for Disease Control and Prevention [CDC]). With the advent of new combination vaccines, determining how to implement the schedule within the primary care practice demands close attention to what works and what is scientifically appropriate. Studies have shown that many clinicians have difficulty in designing catch-up schedules when children fall behind. The recommendations for age-appropriate catch-up schedules are presented in sections A and B of Table 18-2.

Timing and Spacing of Vaccines

According to the General Recommendations on Immunization from the ACIP, vaccines are recommended for members of the youngest age group at risk for developing the disease for whom efficacy and safety have been shown. The number of doses of a vaccine required to develop adequate and persisting antibody response is determined by the type of vaccine and the age and immune status of the child. Some vaccines, such as DT and Td, require periodic reinforcement or booster doses. Others, such as attenuated live virus vaccines, stimulate cell-mediated immunity and neutralizing antibodies, and the second dose is not a booster, but is given to ensure that the 5% to 10% of recipients who did not respond initially now will develop immunity.

All vaccines can be given simultaneously and produce adequate levels of immunity. Vaccines should not be mixed together in the same syringe, however, unless they are licensed to be mixed by the U.S. Food and Drug Administration. As with other vaccines, MMR and varicella vaccine can be given simultaneously; however, if a child has received an MMR or varicella vaccine previously, the child should not receive another live attenuated vaccine (MMR, varicella, yellow fever) for 1 month. If the child has received immune globulin for any reason, the primary care team needs to wait 3 to 11 months depending on the blood product given before immunizing with MMR or varicella vaccines. This waiting period is not necessary when the child receives palivizumab (Synagis) for respiratory syncytial virus. If MMR and varicella vaccines are given 14 or more days before the receipt of the blood product, the vaccine should be effective.

All vaccines should not be given before the recommended minimum age and should not be given any closer

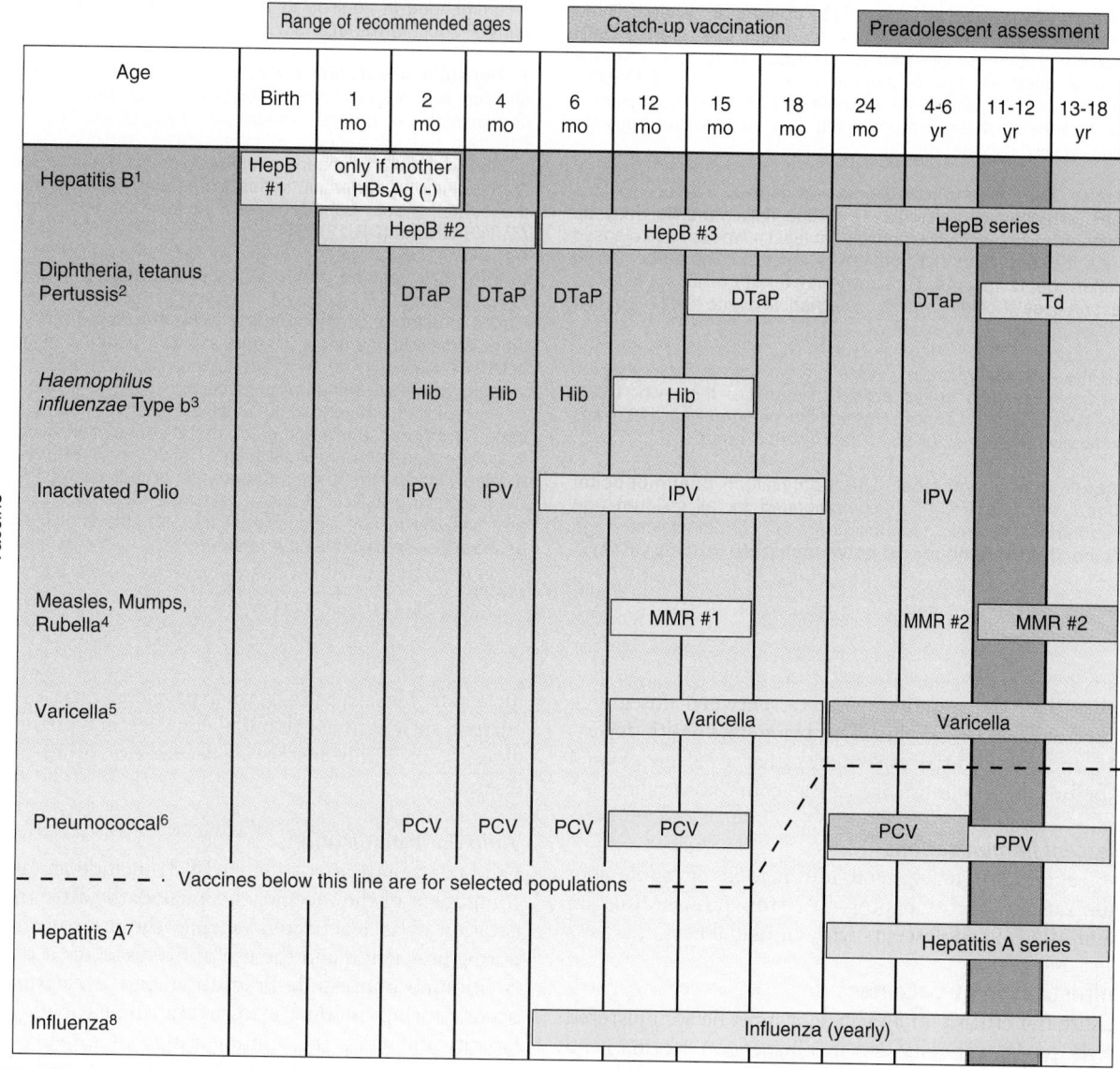

Age	Birth	1 mo	2 mo	4 mo	6 mo	12 mo	15 mo	18 mo	24 mo	4-6 yr	11-12 yr	13-18 yr
Range of recommended ages												
Catch-up vaccination												
Preadolescent assessment												
Hepatitis B[1]	HepB #1	only if mother HBsAg (-)										
		HepB #2			HepB #3				HepB series			
Diphtheria, tetanus Pertussis[2]		DTaP	DTaP	DTaP		DTaP			DTaP	Td		
Haemophilus influenzae Type b[3]		Hib	Hib	Hib	Hib							
Inactivated Polio		IPV	IPV		IPV				IPV			
Measles, Mumps, Rubella[4]						MMR #1				MMR #2	MMR #2	
Varicella[5]						Varicella			Varicella			
Pneumococcal[6]		PCV	PCV	PCV	PCV				PCV	PPV		
Hepatitis A[7]									Hepatitis A series			
Influenza[8]						Influenza (yearly)						

– – – Vaccines below this line are for selected populations – – –

Figure 18-1. Recommended immunization schedule for 2004. This schedule indicates the recommended ages for routine administration of currently licensed childhood vaccines, as of December 1, 2002, for children through age 18 years. Any dose not given at the recommended age should be given at any subsequent visit when indicated and feasible. ▓▓ Indicates age groups that warrant special effort to administer those vaccines not previously given. Additional vaccines may be licensed and recommended during the year. Licensed combination vaccines may be used whenever any components of the combination are indicated and the vaccine's other components are not contraindicated. Providers should consult the manufacturers' package inserts for detailed recommendations. For additional information about vaccines, including precautions and contraindications for immunization and vaccine shortages, visit the National Immunization Program website at www.cdc.gov/nip or call the National Immunization Information Hotline at 800-232-2522 (English) or 800-232-0233 (Spanish). (Approved by the Advisory Committee on Immunization Practices [www.cdc.gov/nip/acip], the American Academy of Pediatrics [www.aap.org], and the American Academy of Family Physicians [www.aafp.org].)

1. Hepatitis B vaccine (HepB). All infants should receive the first dose of hepatitis B vaccine soon after birth and before hospital discharge; the first dose may also be given by age 2 months if the infant's mother is HBsAg-negative. Only monovalent HepB can be used for the birth dose. Monovalent or combination vaccine containing HepB may be used to complete the series. Four doses of vaccine may be administered when a birth dose is given. The second dose should be given at least 4 weeks after the first dose, except for combination vaccines which cannot be administered before age 6 weeks. The third dose should be given at least 16 weeks after the first dose and at least 8 weeks after the second dose. The last dose in the vaccination series (third or fourth dose) should not be administered before age 6 months.

Infants born to HBsAg-positive mothers should receive HepB and 0.5 mL Hepatitis B Immune Globulin (HBIG) within 12 hours of birth at separate sites. The second dose is recommended at age 1–2 months. The last dose in the vaccination series should not be administered before age 6 months. These infants should be tested for HBsAg and anti-HBs at 9–15 months of age.

Infants born to mothers whose HBsAg status is unknown should receive the first dose of the HepB series within 12 hours of birth. Maternal blood should be drawn as soon as possible to determine the mother's HBsAg status; if the HBsAg test is positive, the infant should receive HBIG as soon as possible (no later than age 1 week). The second dose is recommended at age 1–2 months. The last dose in the vaccination series should not be administered before age 6 months.

2. Diphtheria and tetanus toxoids and acellular pertussis vaccine (DTaP). The fourth dose of DTaP may be administered as early as age 12 months, provided 6 months have elapsed since the third dose and the child is unlikely to return at age 15–18 months. **Tetanus and diphtheria toxoids (Td)** is recommended at age 11–12 years if at least 5 years have elapsed since the last dose of tetanus and diphtheria toxoid-containing vaccine. Subsequent routine Td boosters are recommended every 10 years.

Continued

3. *Haemophilus influenzae* **type b (Hib) conjugate vaccine.** Three Hib conjugate vaccines are licensed for infant use. If PRP-OMP (PedvaxHIB or ComVax [Merck]) is administered at ages 2 and 4 months, a dose at age 6 months is not required. DTaP/Hib combination products should not be used for primary immunization in infants at ages 2, 4, or 6 months but can be used as boosters following any Hib vaccine.

4. **Measles, mumps, and rubella vaccine (MMR).** The second dose of MMR is recommended routinely at age 4–6 years but may be administered during any visit, provided at least 4 weeks have elapsed since the first dose and that both doses are administered beginning at or after age 12 months. Those who have not previously received the second dose should complete the schedule by the 11–12-year-old visit.

5. **Varicella vaccine.** Varicella vaccine is recommended at any visit at or after age 12 months for susceptible children, i.e., those who lack a reliable history of chickenpox. Susceptible persons age ≥13 years should receive two doses, given at least 4 weeks apart.

6. **Pneumococcal vaccine.** The heptavalent **pneumococcal conjugate vaccine (PCV)** is recommended for all children age 2–23 months. It is also recommended for certain children age 24–59 months. **Pneumococcal polysaccharide vaccine (PPV)** is recommended in addition to PCV for certain high-risk groups. See *MMWR* 2000;49(RR-9);1–38.

7. **Hepatitis A vaccine.** Hepatitis A vaccine is recommended for children and adolescents in selected states and regions and for certain high-risk groups; consult your local public health authority. Children and adolescents in these states, regions, and high-risk groups who have not been immunized against hepatitis A can begin the hepatitis A vaccination series during any visit. The two doses in the series should be administred at least 6 months apart. See *MMWR* 1999;48(RR-12);1–37.

8. **Influenza vaccine.** Influenza vaccine is recommended annually for children age ≥6 months with certain risk factors (including but not limited to asthma, cardiac disease, sickle cell disease, HIV, diabetes, and household members of persons in groups at high risk; see *MMWR* 2002;51(RR-3);1–31), and can be administered to all others wishing to obtain immunity. In addition, healthy children age 6–23 months are recommended to receive influenza vaccine if feasible because children in this age group are at substantially increased risk for influenza-related hospitalizations. Children age ≥12 years should receive vaccine in a dosage appropriate for their age (0.25 mL if age 6–35 months or 0.5 mL if age ≥3 years). Children age ≤8 years who are receiving influenza vaccine for the first time should receive two doses separated by at least 4 weeks.

Figure 18-1 cont'd.

together than the minimum interval between doses (see section B of Table 18-2). The CDC, many state health departments, and school districts recognize that a vaccine given 4 days before the minimum age can be counted as valid.

Adolescent Immunizations

See Chapter 218 for general information on adolescent immunizations and Chapter 222 for information on immunizations in adolescents with chronic illness.

Administration of Vaccines

To ensure the efficacy of a vaccine, it must be administered properly. MMR, varicella, and meningococcal vaccine need to be administered subcutaneously, whereas diphtheria-tetanus-pertussis (DTaP), DT, Td, Hib, hepatitis A, hepatitis B, influenza, and pneumococcal conjugate vaccine (PCV7) are intramuscular injections. Pneumococcal, 23 valent (PPV23), and IPV can be given either intramuscularly or subcutaneously. Several of these vaccines (hepatitis B, pneumococcal conjugate, Hib, DTaP, and IPV) are administered intramuscularly at the 2-, 4-, and 6-month visits in the anterolateral thigh, which means two intramuscular injections in each leg. A reasonable approach is to separate the two vaccines most likely to cause local reactions (DTaP and PCVs) into different legs. Hepatitis B and Hib vaccines can be given separately in either leg or as a single Comvax injection. Multiple injections given in the same extremity should be separated by a minimum of 1 inch. The gauge and size of the needle used vary depending on the age of the child and the method of vaccination (see CD-ROM Fig. 18-1).

Valid and Invalid Contraindications to Vaccination

Invalid Contraindications

Among the most common invalid contraindications (Box 18-1) are diarrhea, minor upper respiratory tract infection with or without fever (including otitis media), mild-to-moderate local reactions to a previous dose of vaccine, current antimicrobial therapy, convalescent phase of acute illness, and family history of seizures or other neurologic diseases.

Valid Contraindications

Valid contraindications (Table 18-3) include an allergy to a component of the vaccine, encephalopathy after the administration of an inactivated vaccine, the use of live vaccines during pregnancy, and the use of live vaccines if the patient is immunosuppressed. Precaution and evaluation should occur during moderate-to-severe illness and encephalopathy following the administration of a live vaccine. If encephalopathy occurred within 7 days of pertussis vaccination, further pertussis immunization is contraindicated. If MMR is given sooner than the recommended minimum interval, the recipient should be tested for immunity, or the dose should be repeated after the appropriate interval. If the person to be vaccinated has a history of previous seizures or has an evolving neurologic condition, immunization should be deferred until the condition has stabilized and been assessed and a treatment regimen has been established. A history of egg allergy, a possible concern in yellow fever and influenza vaccines, merits further consideration and is discussed on the CD-ROM (see under Egg Allergies).

Barriers to Immunization

Even with the success of vaccines, there still are more than 1 million children in the 19- to 35-month age group who are not fully immunized. The major barriers to complete immunization of children are related to *access*, practice *systems*, and the *knowledge* of parents and practice teams. The greatest barriers for families are socioeconomic factors, especially poverty. Although the VFC program has helped address the cost, many families living in metropolitan areas and especially families living in poverty still are more likely

Table 18-2. Catch-up Schedule

A. For Children Ages 4 Months through 6 Years

Dose 1 (Minimum Age)	Minimum Interval between Doses			
	Dose 1 to Dose 2	Dose 2 to Dose 3	Dose 3 to Dose 4	Dose 4 to Dose 5
DTaP (6 wk)	4 wk	4 wk	6 mo	6 mo[1]
IPV (6 wk)	4 wk	4 wk	4 wk[2]	
HepB[3] (birth)	4 wk	8 wk (and 16 wk after first dose)		
MMR (12 mo)	4 wk[4]			
Varicella (12 mo)				
Hib[5] (6 wk)	4 wk: if 1st dose given at age <12 mo; 8 wk (as final dose): if 1st dose given at age 12–14 mo; No further doses needed: if first dose given at age ≥15 mo	4 wk[6]: if current age <12 mo; 8 wk (as final dose)[6]: if current age ≥12 mo and 2nd dose given at age <15 mo; No further doses needed: if previous dose given at age >15 mo	8 wk (as final dose): this dose necessary only for children age 12 mo–5yr who received 3 doses before age 12 mo	
PCV[7] (6 wk)	4 wk: if 1st dose given at age <12 mo and current age <24 mo; 8 wk (as final dose): if 1st dose given at age >12 mo or current age 24–59 mo; No further doses needed: for healthy children if 1st dose given at age ≥24 mo	4 wk: if current age <12 mo; 8 wk (as final dose): if current age >12 mo; No further doses needed: for healthy children if previous dose given at age ≥24 mo	8 wk (as final dose): this dose necessary only for children age 12 mo–5 yr who received 3 doses before age 12 mo	

B. For Children Ages 7 through 18 Years

Dose 1 to Dose 2	Minimum Interval between Doses	
	Dose 2 to Dose 3	Dose 3 to Booster Dose
Td: 4 wk	Td: 6 mo	Td[8]: 6 mo: if 1st dose given at age <12 mo and current age <11 yr; 5 yr: if 1st dose given at age ≥12 mo and 3rd dose given at age <7 yr and current age ≥11 yr; 10 yr: if 3rd dose given at age ≥7 yr
IPV[9]: 4 wk	IPV[9]: 4 wk	IPV[9]
HepB: 4 wk	HepB: 8 wk (and 16 wk after first dose)	
MMR: 4 wk		
Varicella[10]: 4 wk		

[1]DTaP: The fifth dose is not necessary if the fourth dose was given after the 4th birthday.

[2]IPV: For children who received an all-IPV or all-OPV series, a fourth dose is not necessary if third dose was given at age ≥4 yr. If OPV and IPV were given as part of a series, a total of four doses should be given, regardless of the child's current age.

[3]HepB: All children and adolescents who have not been immunized against hepatitis B should begin the hepatitis B vaccination series during any visit. Providers should make special efforts to immunize children who were born in, or whose parents were born in, areas of the world where hepatitis B virus infection is moderately or highly endemic.

[4]MMR: The second dose of MMR is recommended routinely at age 4–6 yr, but may be given earlier if desired.

[5]Hib: Vaccine is not generally recommended for children age ≥5 yr.

[6]Hib: If current age <12 mo and the first 2 doses were PRP-OMP (PedvaxHIB or ComVax), the third (and final) dose should be given at age 12–15 mo and at least 8 wk after the second dose.

[7]PCV: Vaccine is not generally recommended for children age ≥5 yr.

[8]Td: For children age 7–10 yr, the interval between the third and booster dose is determined by the age when the first dose was given. For adolescents age 11–18 yr, the interval is determined by the age when the third dose was given.

[9]IPV: Vaccine generally is not recommended for persons age ≥18 yr.

[10]Varicella: Given 2-dose series to all susceptible adolescents age ≥13 yr.

Note: Reporting adverse reactions: Report adverse reactions to vaccines through the fedreal Vaccine Adverse Event Reporting System. For information on reporting reactions following vaccines, visit www.vaers.org or call the 24-hour national toll-free information line (800) 822-7967.

Disease reporting: Report suspected cases of vaccine-preventable diseases to state or local health department.

For additional information about vaccines, including precautions and contraindications for immunization and vaccine shortages, visit the National Immunization Program website at www.cdc.gov/nip or call the National Immunization Information Hotline at 800-232-2522 (English) or 800-232-0233 (Spanish).

to have incomplete immunization levels compared with their suburban counterparts. Some children who are eligible for VFC are referred to public health clinics, fragmenting care and possibly delaying immunizations. Other parental/family barriers include low educational level, large family size, minority race, and young parental age. Parental lack

of knowledge may cause the late start of vaccines or lead to assumptions that a child is up-to-date when he or she is not. Clinicians and their practice teams may have knowledge gaps about recall/reminder systems, how to provide catch-up immunizations for children who are not up-to-date, restructuring and implementing schedules

Box 18-1. Invalid Contraindications to Vaccinations

- Mild illness
- Antibiotic therapy
- Disease exposure or convalescence
- Pregnancy in the household
- Breast-feeding
- Premature birth
- Allergies to products not in vaccine
- Family history unrelated to immunosuppression
- Need for tuberculosis skin testing
- Need for multiple vaccines

around a new vaccine, or the proper storage and administration of vaccines. Finally, there are still many "missed opportunities" to vaccinate.

Strategies to Improve Immunizations

Several practice-based interventions have been evaluated and shown to improve immunization rates. Interventions pertinent to the practice settings that were found to be effective and strongly recommended include *access strategies*, such as reducing the cost of vaccines to families (through VFC), and *practice systems*, including assessment and feedback for vaccine providers about immunization practices, patient reminder/recall systems, and provider reminder systems. Two other interventions were possibly effective and strongly recommended: *expanding access* in health care settings as part of a multicomponent intervention and *multicomponent interventions that include education*. Both of these interventions were listed as possibly effective because the actual effect of expanding access and education could not be separated from the other interventions implemented at the same time. Standing orders for immunizations also were effective for adults, but there was insufficient evidence in children.

The Standards for Child and Adolescent Immunization Practices (Box 18-2) were developed by the National Vaccine Advisory Committee and the Ad Hoc Working Group for the Development of Standards for Pediatric Immunization Practices. These standards address many of the barriers and focus on access, systems, and knowledge with specific subsections addressing access, assessment, communication, proper storage, handling, documentation, and implementation strategies.

Box 18-2. Standards for Child and Adolescent Immunization Practices

Availability of Vaccines

1. Vaccination services are readily available.
2. Vaccinations are coordinated with other health care services and provided in a medical home, when possible.
3. Barriers to vaccination are identified and minimized.
4. Patient costs are minimized.

Assessment of Vaccination Status

5. Health care professionals review the vaccination and health status of patients at every encounter to determine which vaccines are indicated.
6. Health care professionals assess for and follow only medically accepted contraindications.

Effective Communication about Vaccine Benefits and Risks

7. Parents/guardians and patients are educated about the benefits and risks of vaccination in a culturally appropriate manner and in easy-to-understand language.

Proper Storage, Administration, and Documentation of Vaccinations

8. Health care professionals follow appropriate procedures for vaccine storage and handling.
9. Up-to-date, written vaccination protocols are accessible at all locations where vaccines are administered.
10. Persons who administer vaccines and staff who manage or support vaccine administration are knowledgeable and receive ongoing education.
11. Health care professionals simultaneously administer as many indicated vaccine doses as possible.
12. Vaccination records for patients are accurate, complete, and easily accessible.
13. Health care professionals report adverse events after vaccination promptly and accurately to the Vaccine Adverse Event Reporting System and are aware of a separate program, the National Vaccine Injury Compensation Program.
14. All personnel who have contact with patients are vaccinated appropriately.

Implementation of Strategies to Improve Vaccination Coverage

15. Systems are used to remind parents/guardians, patients, and health care professionals when vaccinations are due and to recall patients for vaccines that are overdue.
16. Office-based or clinic-based patient record reviews and vaccination coverage assessments are performed annually.
17. Health care professionals practice community-based approaches.

DEVELOPING PRACTICE SYSTEMS FOR IMMUNIZATION

The key to a successful immunization practice begins with an aware, educated practice team using well-defined practice systems (see Chapter 17 for further discussion) designed to capture opportunities to immunize. These systems need to be refined continuously by an assessment process that periodically reviews their successes and identifies areas where improvement is needed. The following components are important to develop and maintain these systems in practice: (1) an immunization leader, (2) an

Table 18-3. Valid Contraindications and Precautions

Condition	Live	Inactivated
Allergy to component	C	C
Encephalopathy	Evaluate	C
Pregnancy	C	V
Immunosuppression	C	V
Moderate-to-severe illness	P	P
Recent blood products	P	V

C, contraindicated; P, precaution; V, vaccinate if indicated.

immunization action team, (3) regularly scheduled meeting times, and (4) written policies and procedures. Talking with parents and families about their concerns and building stronger partnerships with them also is crucial. Linking to city, county, state, or health system immunization registries is valuable for assessment, identification, reminder, and recall of children who need immunizations and other preventive services. Practices serving underserved populations, especially children in the inner cities, need to collaborate with the local health department and other community agencies and associations to ensure that children and families choose and use a medical home.

The efficiency and effectiveness of the practice depend on how well clinicians and staff operate as a team. Practice performance is enhanced when the entire staff is well informed and educated, uses appropriate skills, and has well-developed systems with written policies that use the core processes of preventive care and procedures that encourage effective communication. The practice needs to identify an immunization leader, who may or may not be a clinician, and an immunization action or work team consisting of three to four members representing physician, nursing, and practice management and billing or front office staff. Initially the leader and team need to meet on a regular and frequent basis. After policies have been developed or reviewed and rewritten, the meetings can be on a more ad hoc basis. Policies and procedures with assigned responsibilities need to be developed with regard to obtaining records; schedules; valid and invalid contraindications; protocols for nurse and medical assistant education; immunization documentation and record keeping; ordering and inventory; storage and handling; and VIS, Vaccine Adverse Event Reporting System forms, parent refusal forms, and many others (see CD-ROM Box 18-1). The practice action team should take information back to the rest of the staff at "all-staff" meetings or at physician, nursing, or clerical staff meetings. Having an educational session for the entire staff facilitated by a member of the practice or an outside group, such as the state AAP/AAFP chapter, Department of Health, VFC program, or academic medical center, may be helpful. (Contact Pennsylvania Chapter, EPIC-Immunization Education Program, at www.paaap.org or CDC, National Immunization Program, Education, Information, and Partnership Branch, to learn about practice focused educational programs.) Focusing on the diseases vaccines prevent and initiating a dialogue on practice policies also may help because many physicians, nurses, and other staff members have never seen these diseases. To facilitate following the recommendations from the Standards for Child and Adolescent Immunization Practices (see Box 18-2), the practice team can use the acronym *ASK* (Box 18-3).

Attitude

Practices often overestimate their immunization rates, and few believe they need to use recall and reminder systems. Providing practice specific data about these issues may help modify the practice's attitudes about the need for improvement in these areas. The process for obtaining these data is outlined in the next section.

Box 18-3. ASK Acronym for Immunization Standards

A is for Attitude/Assessment (and Feedback)/Access.
S is for Skills/Systems/Strategies.
K is for Knowledge.
Remember to *ASK* for immunization records at every visit and to *ASK* if the child is up-to-date at every visit.

Assessment (and Feedback)

The first step in improving a practice's performance is to determine the current performance. Each practice needs to assess (1) each chart to ensure the child is up-to-date and that the record is clear and easily accessed; (2) the practice immunization rates; (3) written policies and procedures; (4) whether the VIS was discussed, distributed, and documented; (5) the practice's storage and handling procedures; and (6) billing and reimbursement for all immunizations given.

The first practice immunization assessment should be focused on rates of immunization coverage. In a successful immunization process, a practice has some form of ongoing assessment to ensure that their immunization rates remain high and that they are not missing opportunities to immunize. The assessment can be completed as a Clinic Assessment Software Application (CASA) evaluation (available from the CDC at www.cdc.gov/nip/casa/Default.htm). CASA is a component of the VFC quality assessment program (known as the VFC/AFIX [Assessment, Feedback, Incentive, and eXchange of information] program) and is a menu-driven relational database developed as an immunization assessment tool. The program generates a report on the practice immunization rates and missed opportunities. State, county, or city departments of health, including the VFC program and others, may be available to complete a CASA evaluation in the office.

Managed care organizations and integrated delivery systems may conduct their own immunization audits through chart reviews or a Health Plan Employer Data and Information Set (HEDIS) assessment. HEDIS is a set of standardized performance measures that include immunization assessment (more information can be found at www.ncqa.org/pages/policy/hedis/hedis.htm).

Doing the assessment is only the first step; the whole practice also needs to receive feedback about how well they are doing and what steps they can take to improve. Using the information from the evaluations is key to improving the immunization delivery system. Several studies have documented the value of using the assessment and feedback, and the CDC has included it as a major component of the VFC-AFIX program.

Access

To ensure that families have access to vaccines, it is important for the practice to participate in the VFC program. The VFC program provides approximately 35% of childhood vaccines for infants and children in the United States. In the practice the VFC program provides vaccines for uninsured families, State CHIP and Medicaid enrolled families, and Native American and Alaskan Native families (for more information, see the VFC website at www.cdc.gov/nip/vfc).

Skills
Communication
Many parents today question the value of immunizations. The clinician and the entire practice team need to be able to communicate clearly the advantages and the risks of vaccine administration. The eight cardinal rules of vaccine risk communication are listed in Box 18-4.

Vaccine Administration
Ongoing staff education and competency checks ensure that vaccines are administered appropriately (see earlier section on administration of vaccines). Using a checklist of skills during this evaluation is helpful. A videotape is available from the California Health Department that can be used to educate and demonstrate proper vaccine administration technique.

Systems and Strategies
Assessing the Patient
To assess what immunizations the pediatric patient needs, the patient's immunization record should be checked at every visit. The record should be in the chart, but parents also should be encouraged to bring the child's immunization record to each visit and have it checked by the staff. The practice also needs to ensure that immunization records are updated before the patient leaves the practice.

Obtaining Records
Participating in an immunization registry will improve record availability. If no registry is available, developing a systematic process to obtain old records is a worthwhile investment of time for an often difficult process. At the time an appointment is scheduled, the parent should be told that vaccine records are needed to evaluate whether or not the child is up-to-date. Posting a reminder in a visible spot reminds the person scheduling the appointment to ask for these records. If possible, the records should arrive in the office before the patient's appointment. Otherwise the parent should be asked at the time of the reminder phone call to bring the records to the appointment. If the parent does not have the records, he or she should contact their previous provider to have the records faxed to the office

before the visit. If the parent still arrives without the records, the office can offer the use of a phone to allow the parent to call and have the records faxed. Members of the staff need to educate parents about the importance of these records before the first visit and on an ongoing basis.

Immunization Passport
Using an immunization "passport" provides parents with a small portable record of their child's immunizations. The parent presents the passport and the staff updates it each time a new vaccine is given. Then the parent has a small permanent record that can be used each time immunization information is requested. This passport shifts the responsibility to the parent and frees up the practice staff time.

Missed Opportunities
A *missed opportunity* as defined by the CDC occurs when a child in need of immunization seeks health care but either receives no immunizations or does not receive all the needed immunizations. By reviewing the child's record and determining if he or she is able to receive immunizations, the practice can avoid missed opportunities to immunize during mild acute illness, follow-up, and chronic illness visits.

Prompting the Clinician
Primary care practices are busy, and it is easy to overlook that a child needed an immunization, especially when it is a non–preventive care visit. Prompting systems to improve preventive care and decrease missed opportunities have been shown to be effective. These in-practice prompts include the immunization passport, posting the recommended schedule, posters in waiting and examination rooms that inform parents of the value and need for vaccines, front desk scripted messages and visual reminders for scheduling staff, and chart flags (see Chapter 17). Computerized encounter forms and electronic medical records and registries also can help to remind the entire staff that the child is not up-to-date. There also are billing software vendors who may have the capability of printing these statements in the header on the encounter form.

Parent-Practice Partnership
The parent-practice partnership is crucial to the immunization process in gaining the family's confidence; providing meaningful education; and ensuring that appointments are kept, immunizations are not missed, and decision making is fully informed. Taking a few minutes and helping the family identify their concerns is important in gaining their trust. Box 18-5 lists common parental questions that should be anticipated and addressed. Physicians and staff who strongly encourage and support vaccination tend to have higher immunization rates in their practices. VIS are a source of information for families and must be handed out as noted subsequently.

Documentation
Documentation of immunizations is a crucial component of the medical record. The use of a vaccine administration record is helpful in remembering the items required to be documented in the chart. These forms are available from many sources, including the AAP, the Immunization Action

> **Box 18-4.** Eight Cardinal Rules of Vaccine Risk Communication
> 1. Involve the parents.
> 2. Listen nonjudgmentally. Avoid arguing, acknowledge fears, and identify specific issues.
> 3. Be respectful of parents' need to protect their child.
> 4. Layer information given; target the response and recommendation.
> 5. Be honest, and answer questions.
> 6. Be empathetic and reassure.
> 7. Speak clearly and simply.
> 8. Check for understanding.

Coalition, and the CDC. The medical record must include the patient's name, date of birth, date and office address where the vaccine was administered, site of administration and initials of administrator, manufacturer name and lot number, and expiration date of the vial. Pertinent valid contraindications and past side effects from immunization should be documented. Additionally, the Vaccine Compensation Act of the Vaccine Injury Compensation Program requires that a VIS (available through the CDC) be provided to the parent/patient along with the date it was given and the date of publication recorded in the medical record for every immunization given. If a parent refuses a vaccine, this should be recorded in the medical chart, and a refusal-to-consent form (see CD-ROM Box 18-2) should be obtained and kept with the record. There are other written records in which vaccines need to be recorded (Box 18-6).

Reminder/Recall

Perhaps the most helpful system that can be implemented by a practice is a reminder/recall system. Studies to assess the effectiveness of these systems found that a properly implemented system showed significant improvement in kept appointments. Reminder/recall systems also are helpful during times of vaccine shortages.

The reminder component of such a system usually consists of mail or telephone messages to remind parents or guardians of vaccination due dates for their children. Reminder messages can improve parents' awareness that vaccinations are due and the importance of keeping appointments, increasing the up-to-date status of children. Reminders also increase the efficiency of the practice by reducing the number of "no show" appointments. The recall component consists of mail or telephone messages to decrease vaccination dropout rates and reduce the time children remain at risk for vaccine-preventable diseases. These systems can range from simple manual tickler systems to fully automated computer-based systems, auto dialers, or registry based programs. The system is set up to

indicate the date that the next vaccine is due, providing a retrievable list of patients to be contacted. The recall can be a phone call, postcard, computer-generated letter, or other mechanism that prompts the patient to schedule an appointment for the vaccine.

Knowledge

Equally important to increasing the awareness and focus on immunizations is providing education and timely information to all members of the staff. The first step in educating everyone is to ensure that the physicians and other providers are kept up-to-date on vaccine issues. There are many resources available to pediatricians and family practitioners to help them stay current. Some of these resources are listed in the Suggested Readings of this chapter. Various websites include the CDC, AAP, National Network for Immunization Information, and Immunization Action Coalition. Sharing this information often occurs through one or two individuals but may not reach everyone who needs to know. To avoid this situation, the practice should consider having an "immunization spark" who is responsible for communicating pertinent information in a timely manner to *all* members of the staff, including nonclinical staff. This information should be reinforced through written communication and distributed and discussed at regular staff meetings. For example, knowledge of a vaccine shortage should be communicated not only to the clinical staff, but also to individuals who are scheduling appointments. If an appointment must be delayed until the vaccine is available, the patient should be kept on a list or placed in a system to be recalled when the vaccine is received. The front desk staff should be familiar with vaccine schedules and recommendations so that they can flag a chart that a vaccine may be due at that visit. CD-ROM Box 18-4 provides questions and answers to common staff questions about immunizations, including half doses.

Other Key Immunization Systems
Medicolegal Issues
There may be legal implications of not providing immunizations to patient and staff. Clinicians may be open to a lawsuit if there is a missed opportunity to immunize and the patient develops a vaccine-preventable disease. There are several instances in which a physician was sued successfully for failure to immunize. If a parent refuses a vaccine, the physician must be certain there is a refusal-to-vaccinate form (see CD-ROM Box 18-2) mentioned previously in the patient's chart. Often a parent who is asked to sign a refusal-to-immunize consent form rethinks the decision and has the child vaccinated. Another area of medical liability may be with the practice staff and their potential exposure to preventable diseases. The ACIP recommends that health care workers be immunized against hepatitis B, influenza, measles, mumps, rubella, and varicella.

Reportable Events
All significant reactions to immunizations are a reportable event and must be reported using the Vaccine Adverse Event Reporting System form from the CDC (to contact the CDC for information or reporting, call 1-800-822-

Box 18-7. Reportable Adverse Immunization Events

- Anaphylaxis within 24 hours
- Encephalopathy within 7 days
- Collapse within 7 days
- Residual seizure disorder
- Complications or sequelae of adverse event
- Events described as contraindications in the manufacturer's insert following DTaP, MMR, IPV, and OPV
- Adverse events, such as paralytic poliomyelitis after OPV

7967). Reportable events include, but are not limited to, the events listed in Box 18-7.

Inventory

To ensure that an adequate supply of vaccine is available, a system to inventory and reorder at appropriate intervals must be developed. The practice should record the lot number and total number of doses received in its immunization log. The log is numbered and marked when the reorder spot is hit. Having a schedule or system that establishes that this log is monitored on a daily basis ensures that vaccines are ordered in a timely manner. Clear lines of responsibility need to be delineated to ensure that the appropriate staff person is notified when the reorder mark is reached.

Storage and Handling

Protecting children from vaccine-preventable diseases requires that each dose of vaccine is effective. This requires a system to ensure that vaccine is stored at the appropriate temperature and expired vaccine is discarded. Each practice needs to have vaccine storage and handling policies and procedures (see CD-ROM Box 18-3). Most vaccines must be kept at a specified temperature to ensure the efficacy of the product. It is important to develop a system (see the CD-ROM) to monitor the refrigerator and freezer temperatures on a daily basis.

Reimbursement

The economics of vaccine administration and reimbursement can be important to a practice. Missed billings can result in a 30% loss of revenue. (See the CD-ROM for additional information about key reimbursement processes, including generating appropriate bills, bulk purchases, explanation of benefits review, and billing for nurse visits for immunizations.)

CONCLUSION

Immunizations have great value not only in preventing disease, but also in increasing adherence to preventive care schedules. Children who are up-to-date for immunization are more likely to receive other preventive health care ser-

vices. Successful immunization programs require the development of a strong delivery system within the practice that uses all members of the staff, who are kept well informed and reminded frequently of the importance of the service the practice is providing to children and to society as a whole.

Additional Resources, CD-ROM

Immunization in children with egg allergies	Text
Storage and handling of immunizations	Text
Reimbursement	Text
Immunization policies and procedures with assigned responsibilities for the primary care office	Text
Refusal-to-vaccinate form	Table
Checklist for safe vaccine handling and storage	Table
Common questions and answers about immunizations	Text
How to administer intramuscular (IM) and subcutaneous (SC) injections	Figures

Mini-index of Related Topics   CH.

SUGGESTED READINGS

American Academy of Pediatrics, Childhood Immunization Support Program: Compendium of Immunization Resources and Organizations. Elk Grove Village, Ill, American Academy of Pediatrics, 2002.

American Academy of Pediatrics, Committee on Infectious Diseases: Red Book, 26th ed. Elk Grove Village, Ill, American Academy of Pediatrics, 2003.

Atkinson W, Wolfe S, Humiston S, Nelson R: Epidemiology and Prevention of Vaccine Preventable Diseases, 7th ed. Atlanta, Center for Disease Control and Prevention, 2002.

Humiston S (ed): Pediatric Immunization Update. Pediatr Ann 2001;30:6.

Lutwick LI, Rubin LG (eds): Childhood Immunizations 2000. Pediatr Clin North Am 2000;47(2).

Offit P, Bell L: Vaccines: What You Should Know, 3rd ed. Hoboken, NJ, John Wiley & Sons, 2003.

19 Promoting Physical Activity

Kevin Patrick

ROLE OF THE GENERALIST

1   Understand the importance of physical activity to optimal growth, development, and physical and mental health status.

2   Understand the definitions and use of terms related to physical activity.

3   Know national guidelines for physical activity in youth.

4   Counsel pediatric patients to improve their levels of physical activity and reduce levels of sedentary behaviors.

5   Address basic issues of physical activity for children with selected special health needs.

6   Understand how to work with family, school, and community resources to promote physical activity.

It is becoming increasingly evident that engaging in regular physical activity has positive health benefits for individuals of all ages. It is also highly probable that optimal levels of childhood physical activity yield health benefits in adulthood. Physical activity can reduce or eliminate risk factors for chronic disease, such as cardiovascular and musculoskeletal disorders and obesity. There is evidence that children and adolescents who are physically active are more likely to become active adults. Pediatricians have an opportunity to emphasize the importance of physical activity to the overall health of their patients, and evidence suggests that many pediatric patients and their families appreciate the opportunity to discuss this subject with their physician.

DEFINITIONS, EPIDEMIOLOGY, BENEFITS, AND DETERMINANTS OF PHYSICAL ACTIVITY

Several terms commonly are used to describe issues related to physical activity. Physical activity describes movement of the large skeletal muscles and involves meaningful energy expenditure. Typically, physical activity is explained in terms of *duration* (amount of time spent), *intensity* (rate of energy expenditure per unit of time), and *frequency* (how often it occurs during a specified time, such as a week). Types of physical activity are outlined in Table 19-1.

The term *exercise* often is used interchangeably with physical activity, but it is used most correctly when it applies to structured and planned activities, rather than the often-spontaneous behaviors associated with physical activity. Additionally, exercise usually is meant to produce or maintain gains in *physical fitness*. Important types of exercise include *calisthenics* (muscle fitness exercises that involve working the muscles at a higher level than they ordinarily would work [e.g., push-ups and abdominal curl-ups]) and *flexibility and stretching* (activities designed to stretch muscles and tendons to increase range of motion [e.g., hamstring stretching]).

Fitness is characterized as having two dimensions: *physical fitness*, the ability to perform a range of physical activity successfully without undue effort or risk of injury, and *health-related fitness*, considered to be the physiologic state of well-being associated with increased levels physical activity, in which risk factors for chronic disease are reduced; activities of daily living are performed in a vigorous fashion; and cardiorespiratory endurance, flexibility, and muscle strength are optimized.

An increasingly important issue for children and adolescents is *sedentary behaviors*, such as watching television and playing computer games. Because some of the determinants of sedentary behaviors are different from the determinants for physical activity, from an intervention perspective, it is important to view sedentary behaviors as a distinct class of behaviors and not just as the absence of physical activity.

Epidemiology of Physical Activity, Sedentary Behavior, and Fitness-Related Indicators

The "good news" is that young children are by nature normally physically active. The "bad news" is that most evidence suggests that this level of activity declines as children approach adolescence and that this decline continues into early adulthood. This decline is paralleled by an increase in sedentary behavior that often begins at an early age and contributes to a 100% increase in obesity in children in the United States since 1980. There is little definitive epidemiologic data on these behaviors in young children. For adolescents, data from the 1999 Youth Risk Behavior Surveillance System indicate that more than one in three high school students do not participate regularly in vigorous physical activity. From 1977 to 1995, walking and bicycling by children age 5 to 15 decreased 40%. Children age 2 to 18 spend an average of 4 hours a day watching television, playing video games, or using other forms of electronic media, with nearly one fifth spending 5 or more hours a day engaged in such activities.

The prevalence of inactivity varies by gender, age, ethnicity, and geographic region. Generally, girls become less

Table 19-1. Types of Physical Activity

Type	Definition	Examples
Aerobic	Light-to-moderate activity that requires more oxygen than sedentary activity; promotes cardiovascular fitness and other health benefits	Swimming, running, jump rope, volleyball, soccer
Anaerobic	Intense physical activity that is short in duration; requires metabolism of energy sources to create oxygen; energy sources replenished after short bouts of activity	Sprinting, maximal performance running, swimming, or biking
Lifestyle	Accomplished during normal daily activities; usually light-to-moderate intensity	Walking to/from school, climbing stairs, household chores
Play	Fun activities that usually are unstructured and self-selected	Hiking, surfing or skimboarding, playing catch
Sports	Physical activity that is organized and usually competitive; can be solo, dual, or team	Tumbling/gymnastics, "against the clock" races, tennis, soccer, baseball, basketball
Weight bearing	Activity that uses muscles to move body weight or additional weight against gravity	Jumping rope, running, weight training

active than boys as they age. Physical inactivity occurs disproportionately among individuals who are not well educated and individuals less socially or economically advantaged.

Benefits of Physical Activity

The strength of evidence varies with respect to the immediate and long-term health benefits of physical activity for infants, children, and adolescents. More evidence exists for benefits for older children and adolescents than it does for infants and younger children.

Cardiovascular Health and Related Risk Factors

Physical activity reduces systolic and diastolic *blood pressure* in hypertensive adolescents. Also, cross-sectional studies suggest that, on average, blood pressure is lower among physically active youth than their more sedentary counterparts. There is little information, however, on whether regular physical activity reduces the incidence of hypertension in apparently healthy children or adolescents.

The beneficial effect of physical activity on *lipids* in otherwise healthy children and adolescents is unclear. Cross-sectional studies indicate that active versus inactive children and adolescents have better lipid profiles, but controlled prospective trials are less convincing. There is evidence from controlled studies that lipid profiles in obese children improve with regular physical activity.

A lack of long-term prospective studies limits the amount of direct evidence that increasing the amount of physical activity, and decreasing the amount of sedentary behavior, in childhood reduces the incidence or severity of cardiovascular disease when individuals age. Evidence from autopsy studies of youth dying from other causes indicates the presence of the precursors of adult chronic cardiovascular disease, such as fatty streaking of the coronary arteries. These observations, combined with substantial evidence from several studies that coronary artery disease risk factors, such as obesity, abnormal lipids, and hypertension, track over time from adolescence into adulthood, suggest a strong benefit for optimizing these behaviors.

Obesity is an important risk factor for cardiovascular disease that can be prevented and reduced in severity by increasing physical activity and reducing sedentary behaviors. Successful interventions that address energy balance in these individuals also include modifications in dietary intake (see Chapter 20) and family or behavioral interventions. One advantage to promoting physical activity in

overweight and obese children and adolescents is that the concomitant need to reduce food intake is lessened, an important issue for children in their growing years.

Non–insulin-dependent, or type 2, *diabetes mellitus* is related closely to obesity and is a well-known cardiovascular disease risk factor. Differences have been shown between sedentary and physically active children with respect to glucose tolerance and insulin sensitivity, and developing and maintaining appropriate and consistent levels of physical activity increasingly is recognized as essential in the management of diabetes.

Cardiorespiratory fitness is also a function of adequate and regular amounts of physical activity. Improvements in cardiorespiratory fitness enable children and adolescents to participate more comfortably in a variety of recreational activities.

Bone Health

Evidence from short-term studies showed that increasing weight-bearing physical activity has positive effects—apparently independent of calcium intake—on *bone mass* gains in children and adolescents. This finding is important given that approximately 90% of adult bone mass is created by the end of adolescence, with the most rapid period of bone acquisition being late childhood and early adolescence. Current thinking is that peak bone mass is an important determinant of the ultimate risk for osteoporosis and that a stronger skeleton early in life may reduce this risk. Genetic factors determine a large part of overall skeletal health, but evaluations of young adults who were physically active during childhood showed greater amounts of bone mineral content than among their inactive counterparts. During adolescence, physical activity, hormone status, and nutritional issues interact in as yet not completely understood ways to influence optimal growth and development of bones.

Mental and Social Health

An increasing amount of evidence indicates that regular physical activity improves measures of mental and social well-being in children and adolescents. Improvements have been shown in self-esteem, anxiety and self-perceived notions of stress, and depression. Although there is no definitive evidence yet about whether increased levels of physical activity protect against the development of selected mental health disorders, limited evidence in adults suggests this is the case. Overweight and obesity in their own right are related to lower levels of self-esteem, negative self-image, and lower perceived acceptance by peers.

The social and school-related benefits of physical activity can be substantial. There is good evidence that youth participating in interscholastic sports are less likely to be regular smokers or use drugs. The social contact involved in many types of physical activity and sports generally is regarded as a determinant of overall well-being. Although other factors may come in to play, young people involved in sports and health-related physical activity programs are more likely to stay in school and perform better academically. Finally, there is evidence that girls involved in such activities are less likely to become pregnant than girls who are sedentary.

Tracking of Physical Activity Behaviors into Adulthood

One of the benefits of developing appropriate approaches to physical activity and sedentary behaviors during childhood is that these become important preconditions for such behaviors when individuals reach adulthood. Just as with selected risk factors, convincing evidence exists about the tracking of physical activity behaviors from childhood through adolescence into adulthood. Early and healthy experiences with activity also may establish the psychological and cognitive processes required to develop and maintain physically active adulthoods.

Determinants of Physical Activity in Youth

Many factors, often called *determinants*, influence whether or not children and adolescents are physically active. These determinants can be classified into four main categories: *physiologic, psychological, social*, and *environmental* (Table 19-2). It is important for clinicians to understand these factors, especially the factors that can be modified to enable or encourage appropriate levels of physical activity. If interventions to promote physical activity in children and

Table 19-2. Important Determinants of Physical Activity
Physiologic
Age
Sex
Genetic factors
Fitness
Weight status
Psychological
Self-efficacy
Enjoyment of physical activity
Problem-solving skills to overcome barriers
Perceived competence
Attitudes and knowledge
Motivation
Social
Family encouragement and assistance
Peer support
Socioeconomic status
Environmental
Availability of school and community programs
Media influences
Availability of safe areas for walking, biking
Climate/seasonal factors

Box 19-1. Familial and Social Factors That Promote Physical Activity in Children and Youth
■ Parental support of physical activity for children and adolescents
■ Parental participation in transporting children and adolescents to locations where physical activity occurs
■ Parental guidelines that limit sedentary behavior such as television and computer game use
■ Physically active peers, siblings, and role models

adolescents are to be successful, they must involve efforts to change one or more of these modifiable factors.

Physiologic factors include age and sex of the child, with general observations that levels of physical activity decline with age and that at any given age girls are less active than boys. Additional factors in this area include how physically fit a child is and whether or not the child is normal weight, overweight, or obese. Children who are overweight or lack adequate levels of fitness usually enjoy physical activity less and tend toward sedentary lifestyles.

Important psychological factors related to physical activity include how much a child enjoys being active and the child's level of confidence and self-efficacy in performing many of the skills associated with individual or group activities and sports. A child who is confident that he or she can play soccer about as well as other children the same age is more likely to enjoy doing so. This resulting self-efficacy usually derives from a combination of previous experiences in which the child had the ability to master the skills involved in soccer and self-awareness of his or her capabilities. Other psychological factors include how confident children are that they can address perceived barriers to becoming active, such as finding enough time or convincing a friend to join them and how motivated they are to become active. Familial and social factors that promote physical activity are listed in Box 19-1.

The importance of environmental factors that support physical activity in children and adolescents is being recognized increasingly. These factors range from the adequacy of school and community recreation facilities to the skills of teachers and coaches in promoting physical activity. Additional factors include general environmental characteristics, such as safety of the neighborhood, weather, and season of the year.

GUIDELINES FOR PHYSICAL ACTIVITY

How much physical activity is needed by children and adolescents to produce healthful benefits in childhood and throughout life? As with many issues in public health, there is no single recommendation endorsed by all parties in this regard. In the 1990s it was recommended that adolescents engage in physical activity daily, or nearly daily, as part of games, play, recreation, and sports and that at least three times a week adolescents engage in at least 20 minutes of moderate-to-vigorous physical activity (a threshold defined as brisk-to-fast walking). The 1996 Surgeon General's report on physical activity and health summarized the consensus at that time that people of all ages should engage

Box 19-2. Healthy People 2010 Physical Activity and Fitness Objectives for Children and Adolescents

- Increase the proportion of adolescents who engage in moderate physical activity for at least 30 minutes on 5 or more of the previous 7 days.
- Increase the proportion of adolescents who engage in vigorous physical activity that promotes cardiorespiratory fitness 3 or more days per week for 20 or more minutes per occasion.
- Increase the proportion of children and adolescents who view television 2 or fewer hours per day.
- Increase the proportion of trips made by walking.
- Increase the proportion of trips made by bicycling.
- Increase the proportion of U.S. public and private schools that require daily physical education for all students.
- Increase the proportion of adolescents who participate in daily physical education.
- Increase the proportion of adolescents who spend at least 50% of school physical education class time being physically active.
- Increase the proportion of U.S. public and private schools that provide access to their physical activity spaces and facilities for all persons outside of normal school hours (i.e., before and after the school day, on weekends, and during summer and other vacations).
- Increase the proportion of middle, junior high, and senior high schools that provide comprehensive school health education to prevent health problems in the following areas: unintentional injury; violence; suicide; tobacco use and addiction; alcohol or other drug use; unintended pregnancy, HIV/AIDS, and STD infection; unhealthy dietary patterns; inadequate physical activity; and environmental health.

HIV/AIDS, human immunodeficiency virus/acquired immunodeficiency syndrome; STD, sexually transmitted disease.
Modified from U.S. Department of Health and Human Services: Healthy People 2010: Understanding and Improving Health. Washington, DC, U.S. Department of Health and Human Services, Government Printing Office, 2000.

in 30 minutes of moderate activity (equivalent to brisk walking) on most, and preferably all, days of the week. Children's Lifetime Physical Activity Model recommendations include (1) short bouts of a variety of types of moderate and vigorous activity during the day, (2) encouragement of lifestyle activities such as walking and biking, (3) motor skill development, (4) learning behavioral skills that support lifelong physical activity, and (5) tailored activities as appropriate for higher achieving children and adolescents. More recently, the developers of this model issued recommendations that call for 60 minutes of physical activity a day for children.

Additional information on guidelines for physical activity–related factors in childhood and adolescence may be found in *Healthy People 2010*, the set of national objectives for health promotion and disease prevention. Box 19-2 summarizes the most relevant objectives.

CLINICIAN'S ROLE IN PROMOTING PHYSICAL ACTIVITY

Clinicians can contribute in many ways to encourage appropriate levels of physical activity for their patients. This encouragement can include efforts with the children themselves, with their families, and with partners in local schools and communities. Although some strategies are suggested

here for working with children and adolescents themselves, to date, there is little evidence about what works best with respect to clinically based assessment, counseling, and intervention for physical activity in children.

The concept of *determinants of physical activity* among children and adolescents was introduced earlier. Some determinants, such as age, sex, and genetic makeup, are not modifiable. Others, such as self-efficacy, barrier reduction and problem solving skills, knowledge about benefits, parental influences, and social support, can be addressed by the clinician. Which determinants the clinician addresses depends on the developmental stage of the child; the child's level of understanding of selected concepts; family, peer, and socioeconomic factors; and other issues known to the clinician through his or her contact with the patient and family. Efforts to modify some of the determinants of physical activity or sedentary behaviors can be rewarded with subtle but sometimes important changes that can lead to better outcomes.

An example of an approach based on contemporary behavioral theory is the Patient-Centered Assessment and Counseling for Exercise (PACE) program. The basis for this program consists of two of the most well-accepted theories in health behavior change—the social cognitive theory and the transtheoretical model. A useful summary of these and other theories that can be applied to health promotion is available at http://oc.nci.nih.gov/services/Theory_at_glance/HOME.html. Preliminary research using a version of PACE with adolescents age 11 to 17 showed that it is acceptable among the adolescents and their parents. Further work evaluating the efficacy of the PACE program in a controlled trial is under way. The physical activity counseling approaches shown in Box 19-3, adapted from PACE research, provide some examples of the use of this approach at different stages of change.

Given the ever-present demands on time and attention span for busy clinicians, addressing physical activity routinely with all patients can be a challenge. This challenge can be compounded as children progress in developmental stages through middle childhood and adolescence, when health guidance is needed in many areas ranging from injury prevention to sexuality to advice on drug and alcohol use. Given the importance of this issue, however, clinicians are encouraged to find creative strategies to cover the topic, if only briefly. There is evidence from studies among adolescents that patients like it when their physician brings up the issue of physical activity and exercise and discusses it in the context of the patient's medical history. Until more definitive evidence is developed about the precise clinical interventions most likely to change physical activity and sedentary behavior, clinicians are encouraged at least to model healthy behaviors themselves, to involve parents in the process of discussing enhanced physical activity for their children, and to refer their patients as appropriate to local resources that are likely to support and encourage healthy and active lifestyles.

Beyond intervening in clinical settings, clinicians can provide valuable guidance and support to school and community programs that foster appropriate levels of physical activity among youth. These programs may be receptive to input ranging from how to provide medical

Box 19-3. Strategies for Counseling Adolescents about Physical Activity

Goal: Encourage the Adolescent to Participate in Physical Activity

1. Identify the benefits of physical activity.

   Rationale: Adolescents may not be aware of the benefits of physical activity.

   Counseling statement: "Elena, being physically active is one of the most important things you can do to stay healthy, both physically and mentally. It also can help you build strong bones and feel energetic."

2. Recommend that the adolescent consider beginning some type of physical activity.

   Rationale: Evidence suggests that a physician's recommendations to exercise are taken seriously by adolescents.

   Counseling statement: "Lauren, your weight is a little above the recommended range for someone your age and height. If you were to begin something as simple as brisk walking for 30 minutes each day, I bet you'd feel a lot better, and you'd see your weight come into line with what it should be."

Goal: Help the Adolescent Develop a Plan to Participate in Physical Activity

1. Help the adolescent identify the benefits of physical activity.

   Rationale: Adolescents are more likely to participate in physical activity if they believe they will receive something in return. The health professional needs to help adolescents identify what they will gain by becoming physically active.

   Counseling statement: "Hilary, why are you interested in becoming physically active now? What do you hope to gain by participating in physical activity?"

2. Help the adolescent choose appropriate physical activities.

   Rationale: Adolescents are more likely to participate in physical activity if they are involved in planning the activities and participate in ones they enjoy. The health care professional needs to provide guidance on the duration, intensity, and frequency of activities.

   Counseling statement: "Beth, what types of physical activities do you enjoy? Are there any you have enjoyed in the past? If so, which ones? How much activity do you think you can handle right now?"

3. Help the adolescent identify barriers to physical activity.

   Rationale: Adolescents may face barriers that prevent them from participating in physical activity. Identifying these barriers is the first step toward overcoming them.

   Counseling statement: "What's keeping you from participating in physical activity (e.g., fear, embarrassment, lack of time or transportation)? If you've participated in physical activity before, why did you quit? What would help you participate in physical activity now?"

Goal: Encourage the Adolescent to Participate Regularly in Physical Activity

1. Praise the adolescent for being physically active.

   Rationale: Praising adolescents for participating in physical activity increases the likelihood that they will participate in physical activity on a regular basis.

   Counseling statement: "Susan, I am pleased that you are playing tennis regularly. I think you are doing great, and I'm behind you all the way."

2. Help the adolescent remain physically active.

   Rationale: Most people can become physically active for a short time. Maintaining physical activity is more difficult, however. The health care professional needs to help adolescents identify strategies to help them remain physically active.

   Counseling statement: "Gabriel, your physical activity plan is going well. What will help you keep this up?"

3. Help the adolescent identify social support.

   Rationale: Social support (e.g., encouragement from friends and family, participation in physical activity with others) is crucial for helping adolescents remain physically active.

   Counseling statement: "Lisa, is anyone helping you to stay physically active? You may want to ask your parents to help you. Also, it may be helpful to participate in physical activity with your family and friends."

Adapted from Patrick K, Spear B, Holt K, Sofka D (eds): Bright Futures in Practice: Physical Activity. Arlington, Va, National Center for Education in Maternal and Child Health, 2001. Used with permission from the National Center for Education in Maternal and Child Health and Georgetown University.

---

backup for interscholastic sports activities to how to develop community support to ensure the availability of playgrounds at nights and on weekends. Clinicians interested in assisting are encouraged to communicate with local school officials and representatives in the YMCA, YWCA, boys' and girls' clubs, and other organizations to explore opportunities for input and participation. Physicians, as highly credible sources of health information, have the potential to help shape community opinion about how to promote physical activity in children and adolescents (Table 19-3).

Physical Activity Issues for Special Populations

Unique issues often surface when clinicians promote physical activity with some children, including children with chronic disease, children with disabilities, and girls. Anticipating and addressing these issues can lead to more successful interventions to optimize levels of activity.

Chronic Disease

Children with chronic diseases, such as asthma or diabetes, may have the misconception that they "can't do" physical activity or that substantial limitations must be placed on what they can do. In the case of asthma, physical activity can be a trigger of exercise-induced asthma in children who previously have been diagnosed and in children who may have only a history of allergic rhinitis. When children who have asthma or who are prone to developing exercise-induced asthma are educated about how to anticipate triggers of asthma and, if appropriate, adjust the timing or dose of their medications, this helps them gain the confidence necessary to engage in many types of physical activities, including highly competitive ones (see Chapter 115).

A similar situation exists with respect to type 1 and type 2 diabetes mellitus. Regular and sufficient levels of physical activity are essential for the management of these condi-

Table 19-3. Clinician-Based Strategies to Promote Physical Activity and Reduce Sedentary Behavior

Waiting Room and Office Environment

Put up posters or photos of active children of all ages and different abilities (e.g., not just skilled athletes) in waiting and examination rooms

Have some visual aids that encourage children and adolescents to spend less time watching TV or playing computer games

Make flyers available that promote school and community programs for a wide variety of physical activity programs (e.g., dance, gymnastics, hiking)

Reception and Nursing Staff

To prompt discussion, develop a brief questionnaire about physical activity and sedentary behaviors and give it to children and parents before seeing the physician

Offer assistance for referral to school and community programs that support regular physical activity

Clinical Encounter

Ask parents and children about physical activity issues; be clear about the value you place on this for a child's health

Help the child or adolescent problem solve to overcome barriers and address other determinants

Community and School Groups

Become familiar with local school resources for physical activity

If possible, meet with school nurse or coaching staff to discuss policies and procedures for children with chronic illness (e.g., asthma, diabetes) and physical activity

Offer to participate with school and community health and safety personnel as they review playground and neighborhood safety issues

Work with community and other groups to ensure that a variety of recreational activities are available to children of all ages and athletic abilities

---

tions: Physical activity can (1) help maintain and increase muscle mass, (2) improve energy balance and body weight, (3) improve blood lipid levels, and (4) improve insulin sensitivity and overall glucose control. One of the most important things clinicians can do with children with diabetes is to counsel them and their families with the goal of obtaining a high level of self-confidence and self-efficacy for participation in regular physical activity (see Chapter 155).

Children with Disabilities and Special Needs

Disabilities in children and adolescents vary from minor conditions that are unlikely to raise the need for highly tailored physical activity recommendations to multiple physical or psychological conditions for which special activity programs are required. Overall the approach for these children should be the same as with all children—physical activity is good and should be promoted because of its beneficial effects on general health, functional status, and psychological health. Clinicians working with children with disabilities need to be aware of the physiologic and psychological limitations imposed by any disability, be it cystic fibrosis, cerebral palsy, cardiac disorders, or Down syndrome. Each condition has its own set of risks for injury or psychological outcomes associated with individual or group activities. The basic needs to be derived from physical activity still obtain for these children, however, including improved muscle strength and flexibility, weight control and energy balance, cardiovascular fitness, and multiple psychological benefits related to self-esteem and the socialization

often involved in physical activity. Taking the time with these children and their physical therapists to work through these issues and achieve higher levels of success can be one of the most rewarding activities clinicians can undertake.

Girls and Physical Activity

In an era when girls and women increasingly are portrayed in the media in sports such as soccer, gymnastics, softball, and swimming, it is important not to become complacent and assume that this is the case for all girls. Evidence still suggests that girls, as they progress through childhood into adolescence, become less physically active than their male counterparts. Also, in many locations, the opportunities for girls to participate in organized sports activities may be fewer in number or of lower quality than for boys. Developmental issues associated with puberty can lead many girls to become overly focused on body image and other issues that can conflict with developing and maintaining optimal physical activity behaviors.

Sufficient levels of activity can improve self-esteem, reduce the likelihood of school dropout, improve bone and cardiovascular health, and decrease the risk of obesity and unintended pregnancy in girls. The central challenge for clinicians caring for girls is to be supportive of the development of appropriate motor skills and physical activity participation at each growth stage. Addressing issues of self-confidence; providing accurate information on the relationships between physical activity, menstruation, weight, and nutritional behaviors; and, if requested, linking girls to community physical activity programs geared to their needs are all essential (see Box 19-3).

◎ **Additional Resources, CD-ROM**

Bibliography

Mini-index of Related Topics   CH.

SUGGESTED READINGS

Centers for Disease Control and Prevention: Guidelines for school and community programs to promote lifelong physical activity among young people. MMWR Morb Mortal Wkly Rep 1997;46(RR-6):1–36.

Patrick K, Spear B, Holt K, Sofka D (eds): Bright Futures in Practice: Physical Activity. Arlington, Va, National Center for Education in Maternal and Child Health, 2001.

U.S. Department of Health and Human Services: Physical Activity and Health: A Report of the Surgeon General. U.S. Department of Health and Human Services, Centers for Disease Control and Prevention, 1996.

20 Promoting Healthy Nutrition

Alice Ammerman, Eliana Perrin, and Kori Flower

ROLE OF THE GENERALIST

1   Be familiar with the frequency and consequences of overnutrition and undernutrition.

2   Understand how to use body mass index percentiles to classify children as "at risk" or "overweight."

3   Understand the three A's model for nutritional counseling.

4   Understand how to do a brief office dietary assessment.

5   Know how to help families access community resources to assist in nutritional assessment and counseling.

CORE PRINCIPLES

This chapter focuses primarily on the role of nutrition in the problem of obesity and on practical intervention strategies that build on the nutrition fundamentals presented in Chapter 14. Although this chapter explicitly addresses the nutritional challenges faced in obesity prevention, similar challenges to promoting a healthy diet exist for other clinical problems, including management of iron deficiency anemia, failure to thrive, food allergies, and chronic illness. The tools and solutions described in this chapter apply to a variety of nutrition-related problems in the pediatrics office. Recognizing that physical activity, in addition to appropriate nutrition, is important in obesity prevention, suggestions have been included here for initial assessment and counseling on the role of physical activity in obesity prevention. A more complete and detailed approach to physical activity is presented in Chapter 19.

Today pediatric health care providers more commonly are faced with the consequences of overnutrition rather than undernutrition. Increasing numbers of children are overweight at an early age, and clinical sequelae, such as type 2 diabetes, asthma, hypertension, hyperlipidemia, sleep apnea, and orthopedic stress injury, are presenting more frequently and earlier to the primary care practitioner. The challenge of preventing and treating childhood obesity is a daunting task for parents and health care providers. The complex relationship between environmental, familial, and genetic factors warrants a comprehensive and innovative approach to clinical care and counseling in an era when pediatric visits are becoming shorter rather than longer, with limited support for preventive care. With carefully targeted assessment and counseling, early intervention, and a willingness to think outside the clinic walls, however, pediatric health care providers are in an excellent position to help combat this alarming epidemic.

BACKGROUND

Statistics reveal an alarming increase in the prevalence of childhood obesity. Compared with the 1970s, when only 5% of U.S. children were overweight or obese, currently 10% to 15% are overweight, and another 14% are at risk for overweight. The prevalence of obesity continues to escalate, particularly in preschool and ethnic minority children. According to national data from the National Health and Nutrition Examination Survey, the prevalence of overweight among non-Hispanic African-American and Mexican-American children is nearly twice as high as in white children. Although type 2 diabetes previously was virtually unknown among pediatric populations, its incidence has increased dramatically, and it accounts for 8% to 45% of new diabetes diagnoses. Rapid increases have occurred in many other obesity-related disorders, such as hypertension, dyslipidemia, hepatic steatosis, sleep apnea, pseudotumor cerebri, polycystic ovary disease, and musculoskeletal problems. In addition to the multitude of physiologic problems associated with obesity, negative effects on psychological and social well-being are increasingly well documented. Studies show that children consistently picked overweight children last as potential. The overall quality of life of obese children is low compared with normal-weight children, with obese children having a health-related quality of life similar to that of children with cancer. The economic burden associated with childhood obesity also is being recognized. Annual childhood obesity-associated hospital costs increased from $35 million to $127 million between 1979 and 1997.

Although parents and physicians previously considered an infant's chubbiness as a temporary state soon to be outgrown, increasing evidence points to early childhood obesity as a risk factor for later childhood and adult obesity. Non–breast-fed infants who gain weight rapidly in the first year of life are more likely to become overweight by age 7. Children, especially adolescents, who are overweight are likely to remain overweight into adulthood. Having an overweight parent doubles the risk that an overweight child will become an overweight adult.

Although genetics play an important role, poor dietary habits, physical inactivity beginning at an early age, and decreased breast-feeding are thought to be major factors in the surging obesity epidemic. A strong body of evidence suggests that breast-fed infants are less likely to become obese than their bottle-fed counterparts. Childhood obesity has been associated with increased soft drink and juice consumption and a greater number of hours spent in front of the television. As serving sizes of fast food, restaurant entrees, and snack items have increased, so has the weight of children. Fewer children walk to school, and when at school they have less time for physical education classes and free play at recess. Fast food is available nearly everywhere, including the school cafeteria, and schools are making difficult decisions to accept much-needed funding from soft drink companies in exchange for exclusive contracts for high-calorie beverages. Children and their parents now face an environment that poses daily challenges to wise decision making regarding food and physical activity.

MODEL FOR TREATMENT AND PREVENTION

Given the above-described challenges, how can a pediatric health care provider hope to counteract the pervasive influences favoring poor dietary habits and weight gain among children? This chapter provides a conceptual framework (Fig. 20-1) to guide improved dietary practices within a challenging environment. The model and accompanying practical suggestions are intended to serve as a guide for implementing this framework in a busy office setting.

The conceptual framework in Figure 20-1 illustrates the relative influence of environmental factors on a child's dietary behaviors, directly and mediated through parents. The width of the arrow shaft implies the strength of the influences. This model encourages pediatricians to consider their role in influencing *environmental factors* in addition to their more direct *individual responsibilities* for the care of children and their families. Because the *food environment* exerts considerable influence on dietary behaviors of parents and children, pediatric clinicians are encouraged to target this area for change. This chapter offers specific and feasible interventions to effect change in children's nutrition at individual and environmental levels.

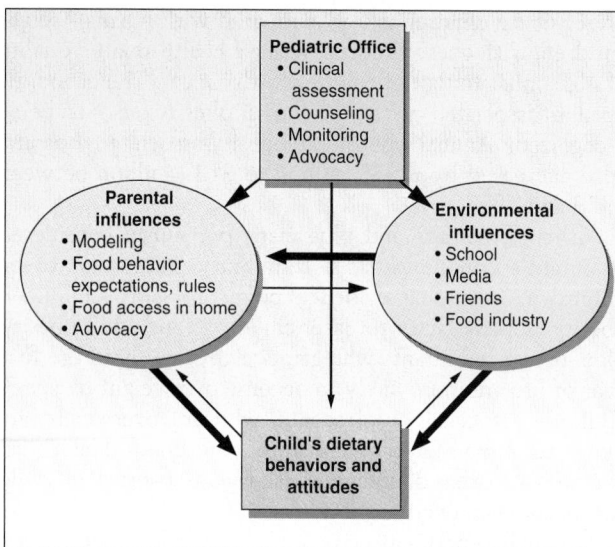

Figure 20-1. A conceptual framework to guide improved dietary practices within a challenging environment.

PROMOTING INDIVIDUAL DIETARY BEHAVIOR CHANGE: UNDERSTANDING STAGES OF CHANGE AND PUTTING THE THREE A'S INTO ACTION

To change behavior effectively, information about a healthy diet must be accompanied by problem-solving skills, motivation to change, goal setting, and reinforcement. Many behavior change theories have been used in research and clinical settings. This chapter distills some key concepts from many theories so that they can be applied in a busy office practice. These strategies are described as part of simplified versions of the stages of change theory and the five A's counseling framework that have been recommended for use by physicians in smoking cessation counseling.

Stages of Change and the Five A's Made Easy

The stages of change theory (sometimes called *stages of readiness to change* or the *transtheoretical model*) helps the provider "triage" the patient and family into those who are (1) *not ready* to tackle lifestyle change in an effort to achieve and maintain a healthy weight, (2) *ready* to make changes but unsure how to accomplish this, and (3) already *trying* to make changes but having difficulty or beginning to backslide. The stages of change theory can be simplified to these three main components (Table 20-1). In determining the stage of readiness to change, the provider can be more efficient by (1) not spending time on those patients who have no intention of changing, (2) not alienating the patient or wasting time by exhorting the patient to change when the patient already has decided to change or is in the process of trying, and (3) focusing on counseling strategies more appropriate to the specific stage of the patient. Table 20-1 presents a specific example of how this can be applied to counseling about diet and healthy weight.

The five A's have been used to guide physician counseling for smoking cessation and other behaviors (see Chapter 22). The five A's have been collapsed into three to make them easier to remember and follow: *assess, advise,* and *assist* (Table 20-2). These three A's offer a framework for counseling that begins with *assessing* the situation by asking about diet and physical activity behaviors, asking about current weight status, and agreeing on a course of action. This assessment is followed by counseling or *advising* by the health care provider, along with suggesting specific strategies and materials to help accomplish the change. Finally, the provider assists by referring for additional counseling or arranges for and schedules a follow-up appointment to monitor progress. Table 20-3 provides specific examples of how this approach can be used in obesity prevention and treatment in combination with some of the tools presented in this chapter.

Assessing the Problem
Assessment of Weight Status by Body Mass Index
In May 2000, the Centers for Disease Control and Prevention (CDC) published and recommended a new set of growth charts after the endorsement of body mass index (BMI) for diagnosis of overweight children and adolescents by two expert committees. The new growth charts and instructions for use can be accessed at http://www.cdc.gov/

Table 20-1. Stages of Readiness to Change (Modified)

Question to Ask of Child and Parents
Are you ready and willing to make some changes in the way you eat to improve your health and maintain a healthy weight?

Patient/Family Response	Stage of Change	Action
"Why go to all the trouble?"	Not ready	Discuss the reasons for concern: the possible consequences of excess weight and a poor diet. If overweight, discuss the BMI plot. Suggest that family consider this further and ask again at the next visit
"Yes, but where do we start?"	Ready	Reinforce family's willingness to make the effort and begin *ask, advise, arrange* sequence to help them get started. Use the checklist to focus on some specific areas of change
"We're trying, but struggling."	Trying	Congratulate family on positive efforts to date and use *ask, advise, arrange* approach to identify trouble spots and help with problem solving. Determine whether referral for additional help would be acceptable/useful

BMI, body mass index.

growthcharts/. Key features of the new growth charts are inclusion of graphs for age-specific and gender-specific BMI percentiles for children age 2 to 20 years (see Chapter 2). BMI levels between the 85th and 95th percentiles indicate children at risk, and levels equal to or greater than the 95th percentile indicate children who are overweight. Office settings can enhance providers' treatment practices by ensuring that the calculation of BMI is accomplished easily. Offices can adopt use of World Wide Web–based calculation programs, such as that created by the CDC (http://www.cdc.gov/nccdphp/dnpa/growthcharts/bmi_tools.htm), or begin calculating BMI percentiles using handheld personal data assistants through programs such as STAT growth charts that allow rapid calculation of BMI percentile for age. Offices also should ensure that updated CDC gender-specific and age-specific graphs to track BMI are readily available to providers. Office staff can help to support proper assessment of weight status by accurately recording heights and weights and incorporating calculation and plotting of BMI into triage.

Use of BMI percentiles to classify children as "at risk" or "overweight" is a helpful first step in assessment and treatment of weight problems. After classifying a child as at risk or overweight, pediatric health care providers can use an algorithm to evaluate health risks and recommendations associated with obesity, such as the one outlined in the Expert Committee Recommendations (see Suggested Readings). BMI percentiles are useful for continuing to follow children's weight status as they grow after dietary and lifestyle changes have been recommended. Because the

Table 20-2. Three A's of Nutritional Counseling

Counseling Element	Components of Counseling
Assess	*Ask* the child and family about Their readiness to change *If ready to make changes, proceed; if not, discuss the reasons for concern, and ask about level of interest again later* Child and family eating habits—use the checklist Parenting strategies regarding establishing norms and controlling food access Identify one or two key problem areas from the checklist and *agree* on goals to achieve before the next visit
Advise	Use information gained from the checklist to *advise* the child and family regarding changes in diet and physical activity Use suggestions in Table 20-5 regarding parenting strategies
Assist	*Assist* the family by providing relevant educational/motivational materials If feasible and available, *arrange* for the child to see a nutritionist or health educator for further assistance *Arrange* a follow-up strategy to monitor progress toward achieving goals

Table 20-3. Obesity Prevention and Treatment: Streamlined Implementation

Office Activity	Prevention Activity and Intervention
Check-in	Receptionist asks parents to complete the healthy eating and activity checklist—include with chart or ask parent/child to bring to examination room
Vital sign check	Nurse records height and weight, calculates BMI, and plots on the graph While weighing and measuring, nurse asks and records in chart What do you usually eat for snacks? What's your favorite thing to do in your free time?
During physical examination	For children age 2–10, ask while palpating abdomen "What do I feel in here—an apple? French fries? Carrots? A hamburger? I'm looking for an apple or some carrots." For children at BMI ≥85th percentile, assess health risks associated with being overweight
During counseling time	Review BMI graph with parent/child and discuss health concerns if weight trends >85th percentile and particularly 95th percentile for age Review Food and Activity checklist and encourage parents/child to move toward having all of the "yes" boxes checked
Completing encounter form	Attached to the encounter form, include a list of educational materials available in the practice. Check off relevant materials based on counseling interaction
Check-out	Receptionist pulls educational materials checked on encounter form and gives to patient when exiting, saying "The doctor would like it if you could review these carefully before your next visit."

BMI, body mass index.

CDC's BMI charts that show percentiles of BMI by age and gender do not start until age 2 and because height assessments tend to be less accurate in the first 2 years, assessment of weight alone probably is adequate to observe concerning trends in infants and toddlers up to age 2.

Assessment of Diet

For young children, dietary behavior and parental influences are closely intertwined. The older a child is, the more important it is to assess the degree to which the child controls his or her own food purchases and consumption. Table 20-4 presents quick diet assessment strategies during an office visit. More detailed and validated dietary assessments are available; however, these generally are lengthy and require software for nutrient analysis. Alternatively the quick screening questions in Table 20-4 highlight evidence-based assessment of selected dietary practices and can help start the counseling conversation. In addition to assessing a child's dietary habits, it is important to assess household practices relevant to the "food environment" at home, such as food availability and the degree to which parents regulate snack intake.

Advising

Good counseling skills are useful in many aspects of clinical practice, but they are particularly important in helping patients and families achieve lifestyle changes. When a health care provider and family have identified and *agreed* on an identified dietary problem area, the health care provider is in a good position to *advise* the family on how to make the desired change and *assist* them in reaching their goals.

Discussing Weight Status

Many pediatric health care providers are reluctant to advise or counsel about weight for fear of embarrassing the child or offending the parent. Others may worry about stimu-

lating an eating disorder. Although worry is understandable, there is currently no evidence to suggest that healthy weight counseling from a health care provider contributes to the development of eating disorders. Some evidence suggests that parents often fail to recognize the fact that their child is overweight and the degree to which this is associated with negative health outcomes. A 30-second dialogue with parents using the BMI chart to make an objective assessment of weight status can set the stage for further discussion of health risks and diet and activity changes. A sample dialogue is provided in Box 20-1 for explaining BMI charting to parents.

Discussing Diet and Physical Activity Assessment Results

Pediatric practices should consider implementing assessments of diet and physical activity at one or more points in the clinical encounter, as illustrated in Table 20-3. These assessments (1) alert the patient and parents that the health care provider is concerned about these issues, (2) help identify some habits and practices that may be problematic, and (3) start a conversation about lifestyle habits that can help maintain a healthy weight and healthy eating attitudes.

Table 20-4. Food and Activity Checklist

	No	Yes
Child eats at least 5 servings of fruit or vegetables most days*	☐	☐
Child eats ≤2 meals or snacks from a fast-food restaurant each week	☐	☐
Child drinks ≤1 soft drink a day (includes sports drinks, fruit drinks, sweet tea, lemonade, and "Koolaid"-type drinks)	☐	☐
All milk consumed is either 1% or skim	☐	☐
Snack chips are eaten ≤3 times a week	☐	☐
Candy, cookies, and other sweets are eaten ≤3 times a week	☐	☐
Most of the time, tempting unhealthy foods are not brought into the house	☐	☐
Children <10 years old are required to ask parents before helping themselves to snacks at home	☐	☐
Child is involved with some sort of regular sport or physical activity	☐	☐
TV and video watching is limited to a weekly average of ≤2 hours a day as recommended by the AAP	☐	☐
Child spends as much time playing outdoors on weekends as playing computer games or watching TV	☐	☐

*A serving is a small piece of fruit or a half cup. You can count one 8-oz serving of 100% juice a day.
AAP, American Academy of Pediatrics.

Box 20-1. Using Body Mass Index Graph to Counsel on Obesity Risk: An Example

The nurse has used a BMI graph to plot Sally's weight compared with her height so that we can see if this is a healthy weight for her.

If BMI Is >95th Percentile

With Secondary Health Problems (e.g., Hypertension)

"Sally's weight for height falls above the 95th percentile line, which means that she is heavier than is healthy for her. Sally's weight may be partly responsible for her high blood pressure as well. It is important that we start working on ways to help her 'grow into her weight over time' and ultimately maintain a healthy weight as a way to help control her blood pressure and prevent her from developing other serious health problems. Let's take a look at the checklist you completed in the waiting room."

Without Secondary Health Problems

"This is something that is important for us to start working on right away so that we can prevent Sally from developing some of the health problems that can develop in children at this weight. Let's take a look at the checklist you completed in the waiting room."

If BMI Is 85–95th Percentile

"It looks like Sally's weight for height falls between the 85th and 95th percentiles, which means that she is at risk for becoming overweight. We would like to help her so that her weight trends toward a healthier range. The good news is that we're starting early enough to prevent some serious health problems associated with being overweight. Let's take a look at the checklist you completed in the waiting room."

If BMI Is <85th Percentile (Tailored to the Degree to Which the BMI Falls Near the 85th Percentile Line)

"It looks like Sally's weight is below the 85th percentile so that her weight is currently appropriate for her height. Still, it is important that she maintain a healthy diet and physical activity habits to prevent weight gain later on. Take this checklist home and talk about how to make changes so your family can answer 'yes' to each of the questions."

BMI, body mass index.

The Food and Activity Checklist (see Table 20-4) can be scanned for "no" answers, and the child and parent can be encouraged to change behaviors so that next time they visit they are able to answer more of the questions with "yes."

Counseling Parents and Children about Dietary Change

For infants, counseling is largely anticipatory. When there is contact with the mother before delivery (through an older sibling or at a prenatal visit), she should be encouraged to breast-feed. A new mother who is breast-feeding should be encouraged to continue for 1 year as advised by the American Academy of Pediatrics, supplementing with solids beginning at 6 months. The potential to help prevent obesity can be a strong incentive to help a mother overcome challenges related to breast-feeding. During early visits with infants, parents should be reminded not to introduce solids too early and to avoid feeding excessive amounts of formula, milk, or sweetened beverages as a means to pacify the infant. Mothers who are breast-feeding should be encouraged to recognize true hunger cues versus need for alternative forms of soothing and, after the infant stage, to learn to feed by hunger rather than the clock. Families who are bottle-feeding also should be encouraged to learn about hunger cues and not to worry about finishing bottles or a prescribed number of ounces unless otherwise directed by their physician.

As children grow older, parents face an uphill battle in promoting healthy nutrition. Time is increasingly limited, meaning that fewer parents cook, and there is increased reliance on fast food and convenience items. Healthy meal choices are viewed as more time-consuming and more expensive. Many parents face their own struggles with weight control and unhealthy dietary practices, making it difficult for them to serve as role models for their children. Offices can provide lists of healthy, easy snack and meal ideas to guide healthy food choices. The CD-ROM includes a list of website sources of healthy food ideas that can be used to create individualized handouts for pediatric practices; and Table 20-5 lists parenting strategies to promote healthy nutrition.

Food plays an important role in the sociocultural lives of families, and these influences may or may not be positive in terms of healthy eating. On the positive side, the role of nutrition in good health has been highly publicized, and many parents have a sincere interest in promoting healthier eating habits among their children. Pediatric health care providers can play a crucial role in identifying and nurturing this parental interest, while respecting cultural traditions. Pediatricians can inquire about families' food preparation habits and culinary traditions. Ideas for healthful eating can take into account and draw on families' differing ethnic and cultural traditions.

Assisting: Referral to Community Resources
Dietary Counseling

When families have identified a target for dietary change, community resources can be important in supporting and facilitating change, and clinicians have an important role in linking families to these resources. Intensive individual or group dietary counseling may maximize families' chances of succeeding with dietary change. A systematic evidence

Table 20-5. Parenting Strategies to Promote Healthy Nutrition

Strategy	Application
Parents control the food environment; children control the spoon	If there is no ice cream in the house, there can be no arguments about how much a child can eat. Parents choose what foods to buy and serve for meals; children decide how much to eat
Negotiation	Seconds on favorite foods after firsts on vegetables
	Snack bars in the lunch box if the fruit is consumed, too (not traded)
	If the child does not like the dinner vegetable, raw carrots can be substituted
	Healthier dessert options (fruit juice popsicles versus cookies, candy, ice cream)
Household rules (parents have to follow them, too)	For every hour of TV/video time, there must be 1 hour of outdoor/active play time
	No eating in front of the TV
	No eating in bedrooms
	Ask a parent before getting a snack
	Serve a snack portion and put the bag/container away
	Water is the beverage of choice for quenching thirst
	Juices and sweetened beverages in moderation or diluted
	Half of Halloween candy is donated to charity
Be prepared	Carry healthy food options in the car to resist the demand to stop and buy a snack. Plan ahead when you know you'll be in the car much of the day—bring a cooler with fresh fruit and chilled water; keep a box of Cheerios or crackers in the trunk at all times
Special occasions	Slowly change the norm so that celebrations can be health-promoting
	On birthdays, cook the child's favorite meal, including favorite fruit and vegetable
	Plan birthday parties to include roller skating, swimming, or other fun physical activities. Serve lower fat options, such as sherbet and cake with limited frosting
	Do other parents a favor—give out party bags that include small trinkets and health food rather than candy
	Be matter-of-fact about going out for ice cream or buying candy—every now and then is fine; do not create a "forbidden fruit" phenomenon

review and accompanying recommendations from the U.S. Preventive Services Task Force concluded that patients who are identified as high risk and receive more intensive counseling through referral are more likely to make positive dietary changes. Potential referral resources include local health departments, outpatient hospital clinics, and nutritionists in private practice, and clinicians are encouraged to become familiar with locally available resources. Sometimes private practice nutritionists are willing to come to clinics to see patients, and this can facilitate reimbursement for their services. Seeking out nutritionists with interest and experience with children is especially helpful. Clinicians can maximize the usefulness of referral services by seeking feedback from nutrition referrals and reinforcing these counseling efforts with the patients. Reimbursement for nutrition referral services must be considered. A limited reimbursement for referral generally is available for children who have diagnostic codes that include "obesity" or "overweight" diagnoses.

Community Resources

Historically, there has been a gap between primary care clinical services and community resources that can support lifestyle change for chronic disease prevention. For parents and children with limited income, the Cooperative Extension Service and the Expanded Food and Nutrition Programs in many communities provide classes and in some cases in-home counseling. Health Department nutritionists sometimes are able to take referrals, and the Women, Infants, and Children program provides a source of nutrition education in addition to the clinical services and food supplements.

Perhaps the greatest challenge is to identify community programs and then develop systems to help patients access them. This is an excellent job for a temporary student intern or for a staff person during quieter times of the clinical year. Phone calls and websites can help establish a resource list to share with families. Health Departments may have compiled such a list already that can be adapted and modified. The Parks and Recreation Department and Cooperative Extension can be contacted and asked to have the practice office added to their mailing lists to make materials available to patients.

ENVIRONMENTAL INFLUENCES ON OBESITY

Few health care providers have the time to take on the challenge of reducing the "obesigenic" nature of the environment in which children are being raised. At the same time, chipping away at larger environmental problems one step at a time can yield positive results and provide psychological benefit to the practitioner, who otherwise might think that addressing the individual needs of obese children is a fruitless effort. There are many ways to take small steps to make a positive contribution.

Create a Supportive Office Environment

The clinician needs to ensure that the office or clinic does not perpetuate the obesigenic environment by selling candy or soda through vending machines or snack bars. In so doing, however, the clinician must avoid perpetuating media distortions of overly thin body image. Instead, it should be ensured that offices maintain a policy of promoting a healthy body image and healthy lifestyle choices. The physician can offer stickers or small toys rather than candy to reward children and have educational pamphlets and posters available that promote a social norm of good nutrition and physical activity. Anything that can be done by staff in the office informally to communicate healthy eating and physical activity helps reinforce this message over time.

Support Community Efforts

Many communities are beginning efforts to improve nutrition and physical activity opportunities for children, particularly through the schools. These activities include efforts to ban soft drink sales at school and encourage fundraising campaigns that promote healthier food or nonfood items. A letter of support to the school board from a health professional can have a lot of influence, particularly if supported with comments about the increasing numbers of obese children seen in practice. If existing community recreation resources are not well suited to the needs of overweight children, a phone call to the Parks and Recreation office could be beneficial. Many community programs are anxious to work more closely with physicians but do not know where to start. By sending patients to the directors of these programs urging modifications to meet the needs of the patients, both parties benefit.

Some communities have begun monitoring the problem of childhood overweight at the community level, to make the problem easier to visualize and to help track progress. Implementing BMI monitoring within the school system is one way for a community to track the problem of childhood overweight. Heights, weights, and calculated BMIs can be recorded annually on all schoolchildren, through either physical education classes or the school nurse. Pediatric health care providers can support this effort by ensuring that measurements are done properly and data interpreted correctly. When collected consistently across time and with sensitivity to the issues of body weight and self-esteem, these data can be a powerful catalyst for individual and community-level action.

Work through Professional Organizations to Promote Change

The pediatrician can look for opportunities within professional organizations to combine efforts with others who are working to improve policies related to improving diet and physical activity for children. These policies might include such things as restricting advertising to children, improving the school lunch program, and increasing physical activity time in schools.

SUMMARY

Obesity threatens the health of increasing numbers of children, and prevention of obesity constitutes one of the greatest nutritional challenges faced by clinicians today. Clinicians are likely to have the most influence on children's diet and activity when they intervene at multiple levels, working toward dietary change in the pediatric office and simultaneously in the community. By concentrating efforts on the broader "environmental" factors that determine children's diets as well as individual and family behaviors, clinicians are likely to achieve maximum success and satisfaction at guiding children toward healthier weights.

 Additional Resources, CD-ROM

Websites for ideas for healthy snacks and meals

Mini-index of Related Topics   CH.

SUGGESTED READINGS

Barlow SE, Dietz WH: Obesity evaluation and treatment: Expert Committee Recommendations. The Maternal and Child Health Bureau, Health Resources and Services Administration and the Department of Health and Human Services. Pediatrics 1998;102: E29.

Dietz WH: Health consequences of obesity in youth: Childhood predictors of adult disease. Pediatrics 1998;101(3 Pt 2):518–525.

Ogden CL, Flegal KM, Carroll MD, et al: Prevalence and trends in overweight among US children and adolescents, 1999–2000. JAMA 2002;288:1728–1732.

Robinson TN: Television viewing and childhood obesity. Pediatr Clin North Am 2001;48:1017–1025.

SECTION 2   HEALTH PROMOTION AND DISEASE PREVENTION

21 Genetic Screening in Pediatrics

Howard M. Saal

ROLE OF THE GENERALIST

1   Understand the importance of screening as an integral component of well-child care.

2   Know what factors make screening an effective tool in disease prevention.

3   Understand when screening for a condition should be universal and when it should be based on risk factors.

4   Know the best time for screening based on a child's age and risk factors.

5   Know the best screening tests for specific conditions.

6   Understand how to manage abnormal screening results.

At the time of birth, 3% to 5% of newborns are recognized to have a medically significant birth defect. By age 1 year, approximately 7% of infants have a recognized birth defect. Single-gene disorders, chromosome anomalies, and multifactorial disorders are responsible for 20% of hospital admissions. Nongenetic developmental disorders, including teratogen disorders and associations, account for another 14% of hospital admissions. These disorders are the leading causes of infant death, accounting for 25% of all infant deaths. It is important not only to identify but to understand the genetic and related etiologic issues regarding specific birth defects. With this understanding, it is possible to offer optimal management for the patient, appropriate genetic counseling to the patient and family, and identify appropriate support resources for the patient and family. There are genetic issues related to all aspects of health and illness. Screening for genetic disorders already is performed on almost every newborn infant. With the success of the Human Genome Project, many more common and rare disorders are likely to be identified as having some degree of genetic predisposition. Because of this likelihood, it is important to integrate genetic information into the patient health care database and to understand how to identify when more genetic information is needed and when and how to use genetic testing for diagnosis and identifying predisposition for morbid conditions.

FAMILY HISTORY

Genetic disorders may be identified at any time during one's lifetime. Most clinicians are more familiar with conditions that are seen congenitally and in early childhood, such as Down syndrome, spina bifida, sickle cell disease, cystic fibrosis, deafness, cleft lip, and cleft palate. These conditions comprise only a small proportion of all birth defects, however. It should not be the goal of the pediatric health care provider to become an expert in identifying all extremely rare disorders. The clinician must be comfortable in recognizing when a patient has a possible genetic disorder and be able to identify a consultant who could assist with diagnostic evaluation and, in many cases, management. The key to optimal management of genetic disorders and birth defects is early diagnosis. For many genetic conditions, early diagnosis often depends on knowledge of predisposition; this is the basis of prenatal screening and newborn screening.

One of the most helpful tools for identifying familial predisposition to hereditary disorders is the family history. The object is to obtain at least a three-generation family history and preferably four generations. It is most important to identify health-related issues in more closely related individuals, especially parents, siblings, aunts, uncles, and grandparents. Health and medical information about more distantly related individuals may be helpful, especially when there are suspicions of autosomal dominant disorders or in the case of consanguinity with suspected rare conditions. When drawing a pedigree, males are signified by squares, and females are signified by circles. An arrow is used to designate the proband. The pedigree is extremely useful for identifying inheritance patterns. If a condition is autosomal recessive, affected individuals usually are seen in only one generation (Fig. 21-1). When a condition is autosomal dominant, one would expect to see affected individuals in two or more generations and male-to-male transmission (Fig. 21-2) because this would exclude the possibility of an X-linked dominant trait. X-linked recessive disorders affect only males; one would expect to see only males affected with unaffected female carriers (Fig. 21-3). Often in X-linked recessive disorders, the condition may appear to "skip" generations. Multifactorial disorders, such as cleft lip, cleft palate, neural tube defects, and diabetes, may affect individuals more randomly in some families and may appear to skip generations; in fact, however, the predisposing genes are inherited from generation to generation.

In addition to identifying specific disorders in a pedigree, it is important to note additional conditions. A strong family history of infertility may indicate a chromosome translocation, uterine anomalies, or other genetic disorders, such as testicular feminization. A family history of birth defects, especially if all are similar, may indicate genetic disorders, especially single-gene disorders or chromosome disorders, particularly if there is a pattern of anomalies seen in affected individuals. Chromosome anomalies are seen in approximately 8 in 1000 live births (Fig. 21-4). Recurrent pregnancy loss often is associated with familial chromo-

some translocations (Fig. 21-5). Familial translocations can lead to live-born children with multiple malformations. When the family history is positive for multiple individuals with developmental delays and mental retardation, further evaluation is indicated to identify the etiology. When completing a pedigree, it is helpful to identify the racial and ethnic background of an individual. Because of selection factors and population migration and cultural factors, many morbid genetic disorders are common in certain populations (Table 21-1). One advantage to having knowledge of population-related risks is that targeted population screening for specific disorders can be offered to at-risk populations. Carrier testing is available for many conditions, including Tay-Sachs disease, Gaucher disease, cystic fibrosis, sickle cell disease, and the thalassemias.

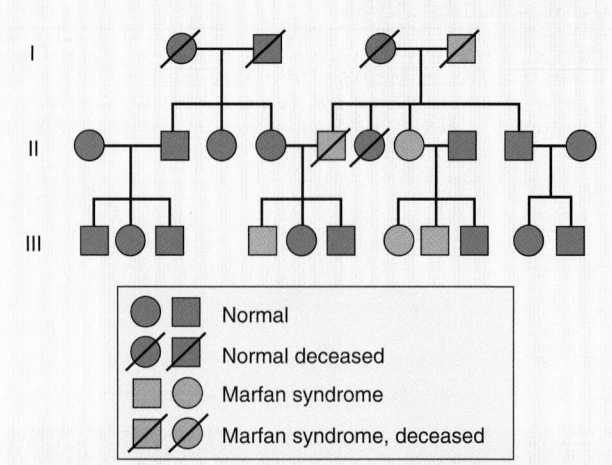

Figure 21-2. Pedigree for a family with an autosomal dominant disorder, Marfan syndrome. There is male-to-male transmission of the gene for this condition in successive generations.

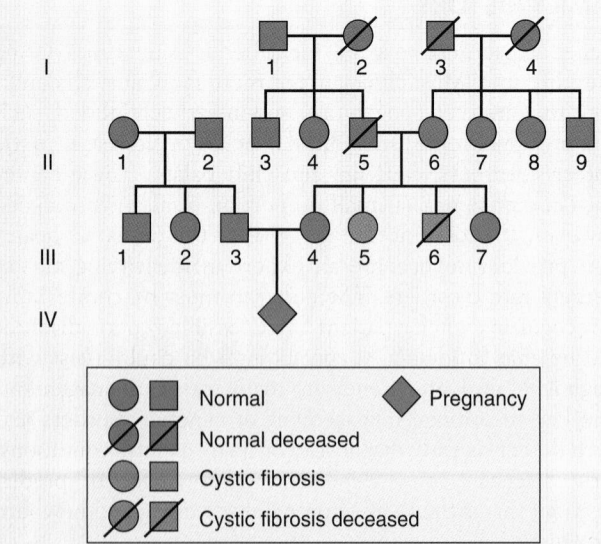

Figure 21-1. Four-generation pedigree for a family with cystic fibrosis. Siblings are affected only in one generation for this autosomal recessive disorder.

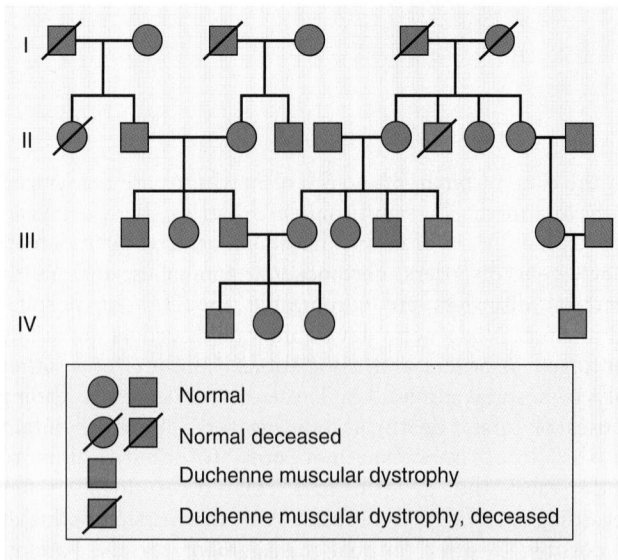

Figure 21-3. Pedigree for a family with an X-linked recessive disorder, Duchenne's muscular dystrophy. Only males are affected, and unaffected females are carriers of the gene for this disorder.

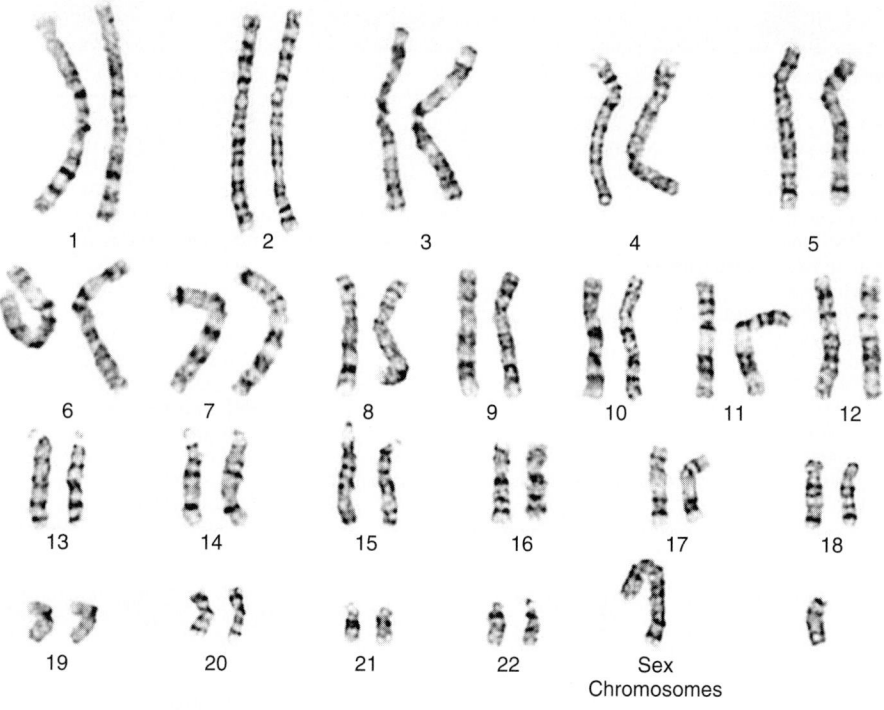

Figure 21-4. 46,XY karyotype consistent with normal male chromosomes. There are 23 pairs of chromosomes.

GENETIC INFORMATION AND THE PRENATAL VISIT

The initial pediatrics visit may be a prenatal visit. The same baseline information is helpful with the entry of any new patient (and family) into a practice. The important thing to remember in genetics, as highlighted by the family history, is that although each individual patient is important, patients still are members of a family unit. The identification of genetic or related conditions in any patient has important implications for the entire family, not only with regard to the psychosocial issues of family interactions, but also with regard to identifying other family members at risk for or predisposed to having identified genetic conditions.

Baseline information, which should be obtained for any new patient and family, should include a comprehensive family history, as outlined earlier. For the new patient, it is helpful to have the basic information of gestational length and birth complications and information regarding the

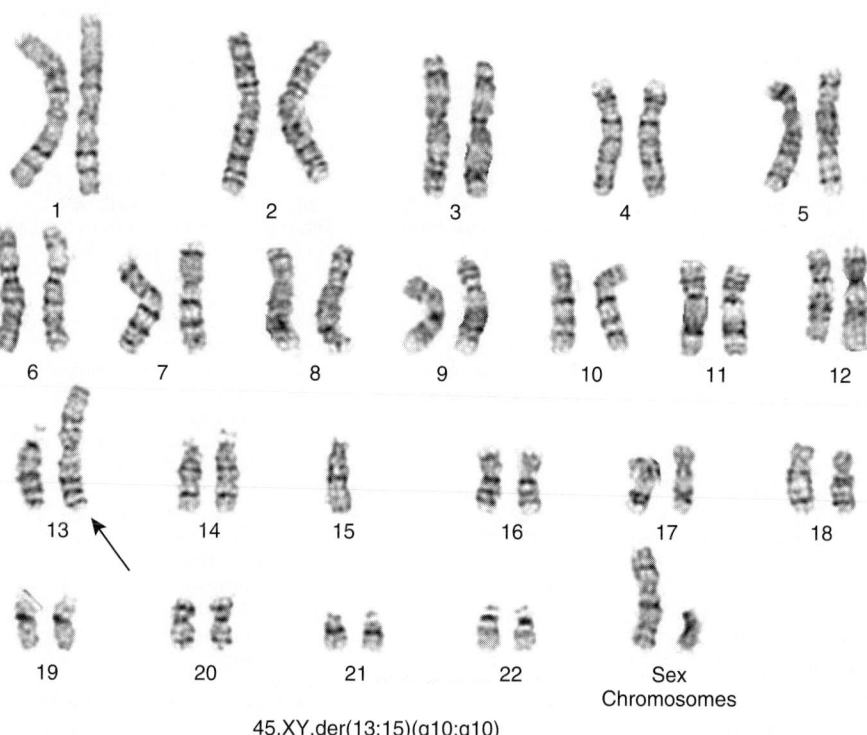

Figure 21-5. Balanced chromosome translocation with translocation of chromosome 15 to chromosome 13. There is no gain or loss of genetic material, but this male is at risk to have a child with an unbalanced karyotype, either trisomy 13 or trisomy 15 (a lethal disorder).

45,XY,der(13:15)(q10;q10)

Table 21-1. Common Racial and Ethnic Genetic Risk Factors

Racial or Ethnic Group	Genetic Disorder	Inheritance
African American	Sickle cell disease	Autosomal recessive
	Glucose-6-phosphate dehydrogenase deficiency	X-linked recessive
Ashkenazi Jewish	Tay-Sachs disease	Autosomal recessive
	Canavan disease	Autosomal recessive
	Bloom syndrome	Autosomal recessive
	Gaucher disease	Autosomal recessive
	Niemann-Pick disease type A	Autosomal recessive
	Cystic fibrosis	Autosomal recessive
	Breast/ovarian cancer (*BRCA1/BRCA2*)	Autosomal dominant
	Familial dysautonomia	Autosomal recessive
Mediterranean (Italian, Greek)	β-Thalassemia	Autosomal recessive
	Glucose-6-phosphate dehydrogenase deficiency	X-linked recessive
French Canadian	Tyrosinemia	Autosomal recessive
	Tay-Sachs disease	Autosomal recessive
Southeast Asian	α-Thalassemia	Autosomal recessive
Inuit	Congenital adrenal hyperplasia (21-hydroxylase deficiency)	Autosomal recessive
Northern European	Cystic fibrosis	Autosomal recessive

pregnancy. Prenatal history also should focus on teratogens, maternal illnesses, and exposures (Table 21-2). For example, women with diabetes during pregnancy have a twofold to threefold increased risk for having an infant with birth defects. In addition to history of medication exposure, knowledge of other exposures may have implications for fetal outcome. Such exposures include alcohol use during pregnancy, especially if excessive or if associated with binge drinking. Cigarette smoking during pregnancy is known to affect fetal growth.

Fetal radiation exposure rarely is teratogenic because the radiation doses of routine dental or chest x-rays are too low to cause any significant fetal anomalies. Exposure to other radiation sources can be teratogenic, however. This exposure would include radioactive iodine (iodine-131) and radiation therapy.

If there is a prenatal visit (or if the family of an established patient is pregnant), it is helpful to know results of any prenatal testing. Abnormal fetal sonograms usually require follow-up evaluation after delivery. Fetal growth retardation or abnormalities in the amount of amniotic fluid may indicate fetal malformations of the urinary tract or gastrointestinal system or malformations of the placenta. Amniocentesis may be performed for indications of maternal age, fetal anomalies, or family history of a chromosome or other genetic disorder. Knowledge of abnormal results of prenatal testing allows for a smoother transition from prenatal to postnatal management. This knowledge permits the pediatric clinician to be aware of any possible medical management issues for the patient, and, equally important, it allows the clinician to be involved in the support structure of the family.

The pediatric clinician can play a role in the prevention of birth defects. Encouraging the mothers of patients to take folic acid before becoming pregnant can have an effect on the risk for having an infant with a neural tube defect (spina bifida and anencephaly). Some data indicate that folic acid and possibly other B vitamins may reduce risk for other birth defects, such as cleft lip, cleft palate, and certain congenital cardiovascular malformations. Women who have had an infant with a neural tube defect should take folic acid daily before conception because neurulation

Table 21-2. Maternal Factors That Predispose to Birth Defects

Maternal Factors	Associated Birth Defects
Maternal diabetes	Vertebral anomalies, caudal regression, renal anomalies, congenital heart defects, brain anomalies
Phenylketonuria	Brain anomalies, microcephaly, ear anomalies, congenital heart defects
Maternal seizure disorder	Anomalies related to anticonvulsant medication
Myasthenia gravis	Hypotonia, weakness, poor suck
Maternal hyperthyroidism (Graves disease)	Fetal thyrotoxicosis, growth retardation, craniosynostosis, advanced bone age
Uterine anomalies (e.g., bicornuate uterus, septate uterus)	Breech positioning, clubfeet, congenital hip dysplasia, deformations
Infections	
Rubella	Microcephaly, cataracts, deafness, congenital heart defects
Cytomegalovirus	Microcephaly, intracerebral calcifications, retinal anomalies, intrauterine growth retardation, congenital hepatitis
Toxoplasmosis	Intracerebral calcifications, chorioretinitis, hydrocephalus
Parvovirus	Fetal hydrops
Medications	
Isotretinoin	Microcephaly, ear anomalies (including anotia), congenital heart defects
Diphenylhydantoin	Fetal hydantoin syndrome, cleft palate, cleft lip, nail hypoplasia, short stature, microcephaly
Valproic acid	Neural tube defects, facial dysmorphism, developmental delays
Carbamazepine	Neural tube defects
Angiotensin-converting enzyme inhibitors	Renal dysplasia, skull ossification defects
Warfarin	Calcific stippling of joints (chondrodysplasia punctata), nasal hypoplasia, facial dysmorphism
Drugs and toxic substances	
Alcohol	Intrauterine growth retardation, mental retardation, microcephaly, congenital heart defects
Tobacco	Intrauterine growth retardation
Cocaine	Vascular disruptions, porencephalic cysts, prune-belly syndrome, renal anomalies
Toluene (paint or glue sniffing)	Intrauterine growth retardation, microcephaly, mental retardation

is completed by the sixth week of gestation, and many women are not aware of pregnancy before this time.

Conversely, birth defects may be prevented if certain common supplements can be avoided. Women who take high amounts of vitamin A during pregnancy are at risk for having an infant with birth defects. The recommended daily allowance for vitamin A is 5000 IU. Women who take greater than 20,000 IU daily run a significantly increased risk for spontaneous abortion and birth defects, especially central nervous system anomalies.

NEWBORNS AND INFANTS

Most infants with birth defects are recognized easily at birth or soon after. In some cases, the birth defects are anticipated because of prenatal diagnosis. Many infants are born with birth defects such as metabolic disorders that do not become evident for weeks or years after birth, however. Although many metabolic disorders are identified by newborn screening, not all are. Many metabolic disorders are not identified until the infant presents with persistent vomiting, lethargy, or coma, and early identification is imperative to prevent serious morbidity or death.

Most structural anomalies have a genetic, teratogenic, or developmental cause. Most isolated structural defects, such as cleft lip, cleft palate, congenital heart defect, clubfoot, and neural tube defect, have a multifactorial etiology. Many infants are born with more than one congenital anomaly. In these cases, it is necessary to evaluate for a single underlying cause for all of the anomalies. In infants born with multiple anomalies, it is important to search for an underlying cause if any of the factors listed in Box 21-1 are present.

Abnormal birth weight, length, and head circumference often are associated with underlying syndromes or genetic disorders. Fetal causes of intrauterine growth retardation include chromosome anomaly (e.g., Down syndrome, trisomy 13, trisomy 18), congenital infections (e.g., cytomegalovirus, rubella, toxoplasmosis), Russell-Silver syndrome, Bloom syndrome, and Fanconi anemia. Microcephaly usually is associated with fetal causes for growth retardation and is

> **Box 21-1.** Factors Indicating a Need for Further Workup in Children Born with Multiple Anomalies
>
> 1. There are two or more major anomalies.
> 2. The anomalies are known to have a genetic etiology (e.g., polycystic kidneys, multiple fractures indicative of osteogenesis imperfecta).
> 3. The anomalies are known to be associated with a specific syndrome or genetic disorder (e.g., Pierre Robin sequence and cleft palate in Stickler syndrome, interrupted aortic arch and thymus hypoplasia in velocardiofacial syndrome).
> 4. The anomalies are rare (e.g., split hand and split foot, Dandy-Walker malformation, lissencephaly).
> 5. There is a family history of multiple malformations, known chromosome anomaly, or recurrent pregnancy loss.
> 6. There are known exposures to teratogenic agents during pregnancy.

associated with a more guarded prognosis for developmental outcome. Being large for gestational age (macrosomia) may be as likely to be associated with a genetic condition as being small for gestational age. The condition most commonly associated with being large for gestational age is maternal diabetes. A less common but still significant cause of macrosomia is Beckwith-Wiedemann syndrome (see the CD-ROM).

By age 1 year, the risk for having a medically significant birth defect is about 7%. Many infants with neuromuscular disorders or developmental disabilities may not be identified at birth, but because of feeding difficulties or motor delays they may be recognized after discharge from the hospital. Because there is not single cause for hypotonia, the prognosis depends on the specific diagnosis and what is known about the natural history of that condition (Table 21-3).

TODDLERS AND PRESCHOOL CHILDREN

Most structural anomalies should be recognized in infancy. Many genetic conditions do not come to attention, however, because the children initially may not have any

Table 21-3. Common Genetic Causes of Infantile Hypotonia

Disorder	Etiology	Genetics
Down syndrome	Sporadic; infrequently familial translocation	Meiotic nondisjunction; robertsonian chromosome translocation
Prader-Willi syndrome	Genetic—deletion or maternal uniparental disomy	Deletion of chromosome 15q11–q13 or maternal uniparental disomy chromosomome 15
Angelman syndrome	Genetic—deletion or maternal uniparental disomy; rarely a mutation of UBE3A gene	Deletion of chromosome 15q11–q13 or paternal uniparental disomy chromosome 15
Spinal muscular atrophy type II	Autosomal recessive	Chromosome 5q11.2–q13.3
Myotonic dystrophy	Autosomal dominant	Chromosome 19q13.2–q13.3; trinucleotide (CTG) repeat expansion of 50–>2000 copies
Achondroplasia	Autosomal dominant	Fibroblast growth factor receptor-3; most cases new mutations
Trisomy 13	Sporadic; infrequently familial translocation	Meiotic nondisjunction; robertsonian chromosome translocation
Peroxisome disorders—Zellweger syndrome, adrenoleukodystrophy, Refsum disease, others	Autosomal recessive, X-linked recessive	Genetic heterogeneity, multiple gene loci identified
Neurofibromatosis type 1	Autosomal dominant	Chromosome 17q11.2
Congenital muscular dystrophies	Most autosomal recessive	Genetic heterogeneity; multiple gene loci

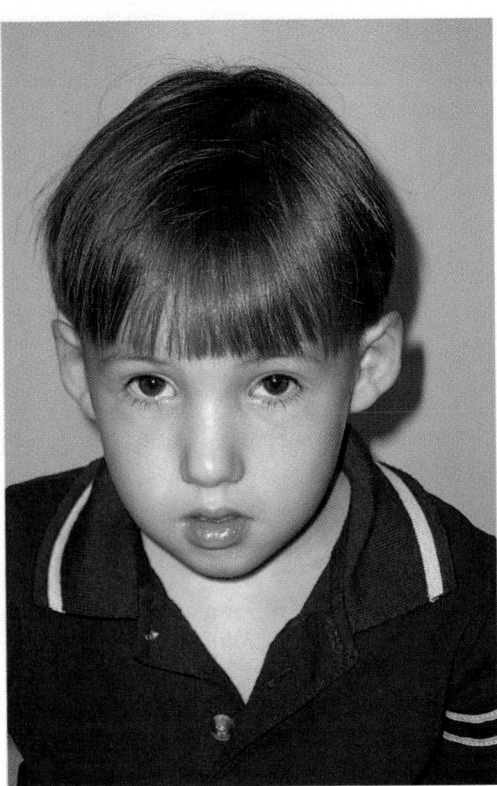

Figure 21-6. A boy with velocardiofacial syndrome caused by an interstitial deletion of chromosome 22. Note the small mouth, mildly dysplastic ears, broad nasal tip, and prominent nasal bridge.

unusual features or outward signs of an underlying disorder and are identified on the basis of developmental delays. Motor delays often are associated with hypotonia and late sitting and walking. These delays may indicate a chromosomal disorder or a neuromuscular disorder, such as Duchenne muscular dystrophy. Other conditions often associated with hypotonia and late motor milestones, such as Noonan syndrome or neurofibromatosis, have a central nervous system cause of hypotonia. Many conditions associated with abnormal central nervous system development often have associated cognitive delays as well.

Children with speech and language delays often are not identified until 2 or 3 years of age. The most common cause of speech and language delay is hearing loss. Severe-to-profound sensorineural hearing loss occurs in 1 in 1000 infants and 2 in 1000 children become deaf in early childhood. If there is a family history of deafness, especially in first-degree or second-degree relatives, a child should have a hearing evaluation done as early as possible. Early diagnosis of deafness leads to early amplification and early institution of speech therapy and a better prognosis for language development. Approximately 50% of cases of isolated deafness have a genetic cause, and of these, 80% are autosomal recessive, and 20% are autosomal dominant. Approximately 50% of cases of autosomal recessive deafness are caused by mutations of the connexin 26 gene. Genetic mutation analysis is available for this form of hereditary deafness.

Speech and language delay in the presence of normal hearing carries with it a more guarded prognosis. When speech and language delay is associated with feeding difficulties, the underlying cause may be oral motor hypotonia

or oral motor apraxia. Speech articulation defects are common, but certain types of speech problems may indicate a more serious underlying disorder. Children with hypernasal speech usually have velopharyngeal dysfunction. This condition is related most often to being born with a cleft palate. In the absence of cleft palate, other causes must be identified, including structural anomalies of the palate, especially submucous cleft palate. The conditions most commonly associated with submucous cleft palate are Stickler syndrome and velocardiofacial syndrome (deletion of chromosome 22). The most common clinical finding seen with submucous cleft palate is a bifid uvula. Velocardiofacial syndrome (Fig. 21-6) is the most common cause of velopharyngeal dysfunction (see Chapter 157). Velocardiofacial syndrome is diagnosed by confirming a deletion of chromosome 22, usually with fluorescence in situ hybridization (FISH) (Fig. 21-7).Some rare disorders are diagnosed during early childhood because of progressive physical changes or developmental degeneration. The best examples of these conditions are the mucopolysaccharidoses, especially Hunter syndrome and Hurler syndrome. (See Chapter 149 and the CD-ROM.)

SCHOOL-AGE CHILDREN

By middle childhood, almost all major genetic disorders should be evident. Most issues that present usually are related to growth disorders and learning and developmental disorders. Growth disorders usually have presented before the start of school; however, some rare skeletal dysplasias may become evident only at a later age. This is true of some forms of spondyloepiphyseal dysplasias. Spondyloepiphyseal dysplasia tarda is an X-linked disorder with onset of short stature between age 5 and 10 years. The diagnosis is made with a skeletal radiograph survey. Some girls with Turner syndrome may not be identified until short stature becomes evident or their growth velocity begins to plateau. In girls with proportionate short stature, it is important to rule out Turner syndrome with a chromosome study.

Developmental disabilities may not be recognized until a child starts school. Some conditions are diagnosed because of school problems. Neurofibromatosis type 1 is a common autosomal dominant genetic condition associated with café au lait spots (Fig. 21-8), neurofibromas, axillary and inguinal freckling, and Lisch nodules of the iris (see Chapter 15). Although neurofibromatosis type 1 is an autosomal dominant condition, 50% of cases arise as a result of a new mutation.

Some children with sex chromosome anomalies may be identified during later childhood because of school and learning difficulties. Klinefelter syndrome is a common condition in males, often associated with mental retardation, gynecomastia, and small testes. Many men are diagnosed with this condition when they are evaluated for infertility. Girls with school and learning problems also may have a sex chromosome anomaly, a 47,XXX karyotype often called the *triple X syndrome*. Fragile X syndrome may be a cause of school problems, but most affected boys should be recognized in early childhood, especially if there is a family history of males with mental retardation. Female

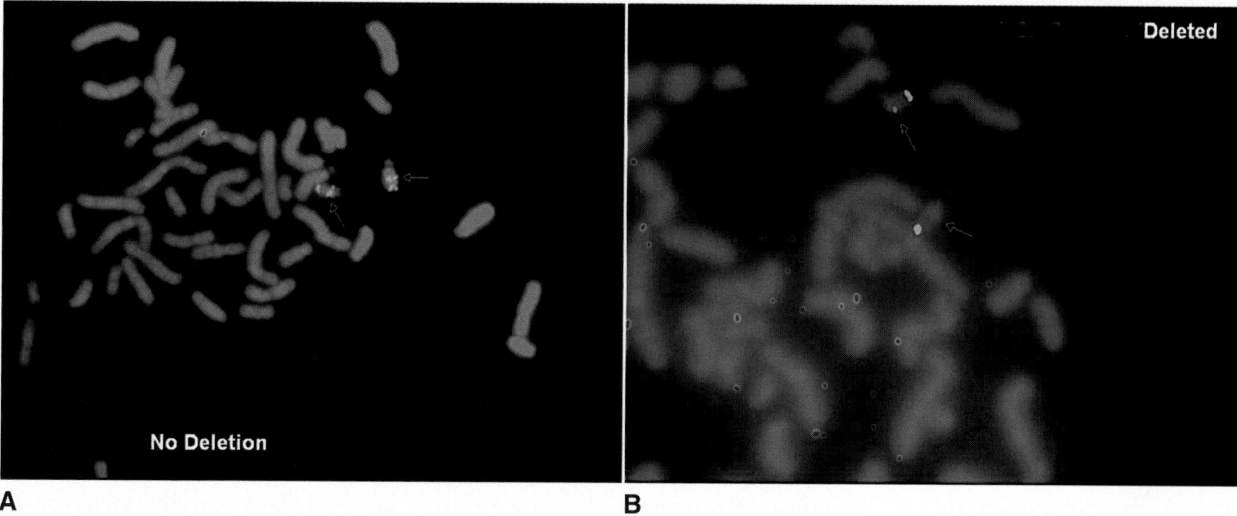

Figure 21-7. A, A normal fluorescence in situ hybridization study for deletion 22. **B,** A deletion of chromosome 22, with the lower arrow pointing to the deleted chromosome. Normal chromosome 22 should have two areas of hybridization, one for the chromosome 22 probe and one for the velocardiofacial region. The abnormal chromosome in B hybridizes only with the chromosome 22 probe but not the velocardiofacial probe because there is a deletion of this segment.

carriers of the fragile X gene are at risk also to have learning disabilities and mental retardation. In all patients presenting with developmental disabilities, the evaluation should include a chromosome study and a fragile X molecular study. A further description of all these syndromes can be found in Chapter 157.

ADOLESCENTS

When genetic conditions present in adolescence, they usually present as functional issues. Occasionally, growth delay is noted, but most cases are identified long before the teen years. During adolescence, issues related to genetic disorders present related to puberty and rapid growth. Many girls with Turner syndrome are identified because of pri-

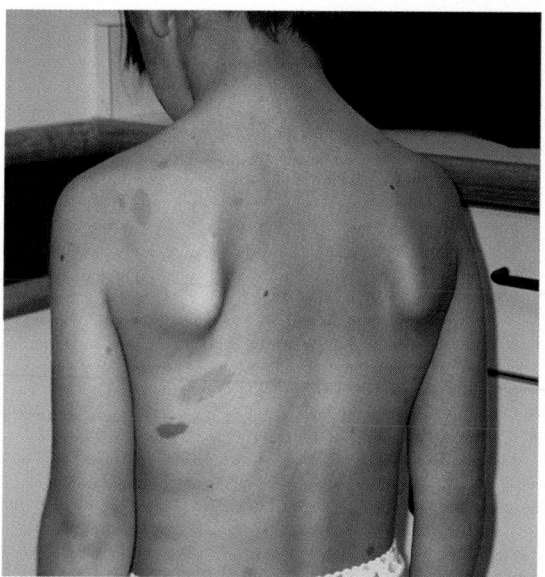

Figure 21-8. A girl with neurofibromatosis type 1. Notice she has at least eight café au lait spots.

mary amenorrhea. Chromosome studies are indicated in all girls who present with short stature and primary amenorrhea. There are many rare causes of primary amenorrhea in females, including androgen insensitivity syndrome. In this disorder, the karyotype is 46,XY. There is a mutation of the androgen receptor gene on the X chromosome (Xq11–q12). Individuals with this disorder are born with testes, but because of the abnormal androgen receptor, the penis and scrotum do not develop. These individuals are phenotypically females. They have testes and no uterus or adnexa and a blind-ending vagina. Stature and breast development are usually normal; however, most individuals have minimal axillary and pubic hair. Early identification of this disorder is important because of the risk for developing a gonadoblastoma in the intra-abdominal testes. Many girls with this disorder present with inguinal hernias in infancy. Klinefelter syndrome is another disorder often diagnosed during adolescence. During adolescence, this condition may present with gynecomastia or small testes.

Because of rapid growth during adolescence, other medical problems may become evident. Although most cases of scoliosis seem to be idiopathic, the diagnosis of scoliosis in a child who is tall and thin may indicate an underlying connective tissue disorder. The best-known condition is Marfan syndrome (see the CD-ROM). Another group of connective tissue disorders are the Ehlers-Danlos syndromes (EDS). EDS are a group of disorders associated with large and small joint hypermobility, skin hyperextensibility and fragility, and in some forms vascular and bowel fragility. This is a heterogeneous group of disorders, most of which are inherited in an autosomal dominant manner (see the CD-ROM).

ADDITIONAL CONSIDERATIONS

Many medical conditions that have a genetic predisposition may present at any time of life; this is especially true of the hereditary cancer predisposition syndromes (Table 21-4).

Colorectal cancer is one example. Several genes predispose to colorectal cancers. The best known is the adenomatous polyposis coli (*APC*) gene, which causes familial adenomatous polyposis. This autosomal dominant disorder, although rare, has a high penetrance, and almost all untreated individuals develop colorectal cancers by age 40. All first-degree relatives of individuals with familial adenomatous polyposis should be tested for this condition. *APC* mutation carriers also are at risk to develop hepatoblastoma. The risk for hepatoblastoma is 1% until age 4 years. Patients need to be followed with serial abdominal sonograms and α-fetoprotein levels (at least every 3 months until age 4 years).

Li-Fraumeni syndrome is an autosomal dominant disorder that is caused by a mutation of the *TP53* gene on chromosome 17p13 and can cause a wide range of adult-onset and childhood-onset tumors, including soft tissue sarcoma, breast cancer, leukemia, osteosarcoma, melanoma, colorectal cancer, pancreatic cancer, cancer of the adrenal cortex, and brain cancer. Multiple primary tumors can occur, and childhood cancers are common. Although genetic testing is possible and in some cases helpful, no effective screening exists for many of the cancers except breast cancer and colon cancer. Some controversy exists regarding testing children at risk for this genetic disorder in the absence of effective screening protocols.

Other hereditary cancer syndromes exist, most of which are not associated with childhood cancers. The best-known syndrome is hereditary breast and ovarian cancer. Women with a mutation of either the *BRCA1* gene (chromosome 17q21) or the *BRCA2* gene (chromosome 13q12.3) have a 50% to 80% lifetime risk for developing breast cancer and a 40% lifetime risk for developing ovarian cancer. These cancers do not occur in children. In families known to have a mutation for the *BRCA1* or *BRCA2* gene, testing is not offered to individuals younger than age 18 years because they are not able to give informed consent for testing. It is reasonable for a clinical geneticist, genetic counselor, or other health care professional to discuss issues related to hereditary breast and ovarian cancer with young adults before they reach age 18, but testing should be withheld in most circumstances until it is possible to obtain informed consent. Similar guidelines are followed for other autosomal dominant adult-onset disorders, including Huntington disease.

Multiple endocrine neoplasia type II is an autosomal dominant disorder that is caused by a mutation of the *RET* proto-oncogene. A mutation of this gene predisposes to medullary thyroid carcinoma, pheochromocytoma, and pituitary adenomas. Mutations of the *RET* proto-oncogene also have been associated with familial Hirschsprung disease. In families with medullary thyroid carcinoma, the risk for having a *RET* mutation is about 25%. In families identified with a *RET* mutation, children should be tested because the risk for medullary thyroid carcinoma is significant, and it is recommended that children with mutations have thyroidectomies at age 5 years.

WHEN TO REFER TO A CLINICAL GENETICIST

Although many pediatric clinicians believe they can diagnose and manage many genetic disorders, there are numerous instances in which the knowledge and experience of a clinical geneticist would be instrumental in this process, especially for the conditions listed in Table 21-4. The geneticist is more likely to be aware of new diagnostic tests and current therapies for uncommon and rare disorders. In addition, many genetic disorders and classes of disorders are managed best in a multidisciplinary setting, which usually includes genetics services. These services include craniofacial and cleft palate clinics, neurofibromatosis clinics, myelomeningocele clinics, and muscular dystrophy clinics.

Usually, when a child is diagnosed with a genetic disorder, the family has many questions regarding treatment, prognosis, recurrence risks, and prenatal diagnostic testing. The clinical geneticist has training and expertise not only

Table 21-4. Genetic Conditions Predisoposing to Malignancies

Genetic Condition	Common Neoplasias	Genetics
Familial adenomatous polyposis	Colorectal cancers, duodenal adenocarcinoma	Autosomal dominant; APC gene mapping to 5q21–q22
Hereditary nonpolyposis colorectal carcinoma	Colorectal cancers; endometrial carcinoma; uterine leiomyosarcoma; bladder transitional cell carcinoma; gastric, biliary, and renal cell carcinoma; hepatoblastoma	Autosomal dominant; at least 13 gene loci identified
Li-Fraumeni syndrome	Multiple tumor sites, including childhood tumors, rhabdomyosarcoma, breast cancer, osteosarcoma, leukemia, adrenocortical carcinoma, lymphomas, melanoma, lung adenocarcinoma, pancreatic carcinaoma, brain tumors	Autosomal dominant; p53 gene maps to 17p13.1
Hereditary breast/ovarian cancer*	Breast cancer, ovarian cancer, prostate cancer, pancreatic cancer, melanoma (BRCA2)	Autosomal dominant; BRCA1 gene maps to 17q21; BRCA2 gene maps to 13q12.3
Multiple endocrine neoplasia type II	Pheochromocytoma, medullary thyroid carcinoma, parathyroid adenoma	Autosomal dominant; RET proto-oncogene maps to 10q11.2
Beckwith-Wiedemann syndrome	Wilms' tumor, hepatoblastoma, adrenal carcinoma, gonadoblastoma	Sporadic, some cases autosomal dominant; maps to 11p15.5
Retinoblastoma	Retinoblastoma, osteogenic sarcoma, pinealoma, Ewing's sarcoma, lymphoma, and leukemia	Sporadic and autosomal dominant; Rb1 gene maps to 13q14.1–q14.2

*Adult-onset tumors only.

in the diagnosis of genetic disorders, but also in genetic counseling for recurrence, available options for prenatal diagnosis, and psychosocial counseling of the family with identification of appropriate support services.

As more is learned about all human disorders, it is becoming clearer that most are modified at least in some manner by an individual's genetic background. An understanding of a patient's genetic background along with a keen eye toward early identification of genetic conditions can lead to improved health care and earlier interventions. The changes and new information that are brought about by the Human Genome Project and ever-changing technology will challenge all health care professionals to remain vigilant.

Additional Resources, CD-ROM

Beckwith-Wiedemann syndrome	Text
Hutner, Hurler, and Hurler-Scheie syndrome	Text
Marfan syndrome	Text
Ehlers-Danlos syndromes	Text
Bibliography	

SUGGESTED READINGS

Cassidy S, Allanson J: Management of Genetic Syndromes. New York, John Wiley & Sons, 2001.
Information for genetic professionals. Available at: www.kumc.edu/gec/geneinfo.html.
Jones K: Smith's Recognizable Patterns of Human Malformation, 5th ed. Philadelphia, WB Saunders, 1997.
Nussbaum R, MacInnes R, Willard H: Thompson and Thompson's Genetics in Medicine, 6th ed. Philadelphia, WB Saunders, 2001.
Rimoin D, O'Connor J, Pyeritz R, Korf B: Emery and Rimoin's Principles and Practice of Medical Genetics, 4th ed. New York, Churchill Livingstone, 2002.

SECTION 2   HEALTH PROMOTION AND DISEASE PREVENTION

22 Smoking Cessation Counseling

James D. Sargent

ROLE OF THE GENERALIST

1 Know the epidemiology of adolescent tobacco use.
2 Understand and recognize the social influences that are risk factors for initiation of tobacco use.
3 Recognize the risk factors for becoming a regular smoker.
4 Assess tobacco use in children and families.
5 Apply strategies for preventing tobacco use in pediatric practice.

CORE PRINCIPLES

Overview

Addressing tobacco use in a patient is similar to addressing lead poisoning; the problem cannot be solved within the confines of the office. In addition to motivating and assisting the patient in the office setting, practitioners must consider family and community factors that contribute to the problem. Practitioners can encourage family members to quit smoking and teach parents to socialize their children against smoking. They can direct smokers to community resources that address smoking. They can pressure local retailers to reduce the display of storefront tobacco advertising. They can educate local government officials about the health implications of local ordinances restricting smoking in workplaces and restaurants. They can lobby state legislatures to increase taxes on tobacco. The benefit to health of these activities is greater than in almost any other area of prevention.

Disease Burden
Mortality

The effect of smoking on mortality is well understood as a result of multiple prospective studies conducted in the United States and other countries. Smoking is the largest preventable cause of mortality in adults, causing greater than 90% of lung cancers. Smoking is a major factor in the development of chronic obstructive pulmonary disease. A less appreciated fact is that smoking is responsible for 60% of coronary heart disease mortality occurring in middle-aged men and women. Heart disease, not lung cancer, constitutes the largest category of smoking-related mortality.

In children, the major concern is environmental tobacco smoke (ETS) exposure, which is associated with higher mortality. Postnatal ETS exposure is an independent cause of sudden infant death syndrome and has been linked to increased risk for meningococcal disease. The well-described prenatal smoking effect on birth weight is small in magnitude, but could contribute to some excess mortality, especially among very-low-birth-weight infants.

Morbidity

Children are especially sensitive to the respiratory effects of ETS exposure. ETS exposure produces a variety of acute effects involving the upper and lower respiratory tract, increasing the risk of pneumonia, acute otitis media, and chronic middle ear effusion. There is compelling evidence that ETS is a risk factor for new cases of asthma and increasing the severity of disease in children with established asthma. There also is evidence that ETS exposure affects lung growth and development as measured by small decrements in pulmonary function tests, which may persist into adulthood.

Smoking has effects on lung function, cardiovascular disease, and physical fitness. Smoking not only reduces the rate of lung growth, but also accelerates the natural decline of lung function with age, resulting ultimately in the development of chronic obstructive pulmonary disease in many lifetime smokers. As a result, teen smokers already have a higher frequency of abnormalities in small airway function compared with nonsmokers, with a higher rate of respiratory symptoms, including cough, phlegm production, wheezing, and dyspnea. Smoking also has been associated with higher levels of atherosclerosis found in adolescents who died of violent causes. Finally, smoking compromises performance and endurance in young people. The short-term consequences of *smokeless tobacco* use are leukoplakia and gum recession. Leukoplakia consists of a white patch or plaque on the gum that cannot be scraped off. This precancerous condition was present in 49% of adolescent smokeless tobacco users in one study. Gum recession is associated with long-term (>1 year) use among adolescents.

Social Influence and Addiction Models of Smoking

Adults smoke primarily because they are addicted to nicotine. This pattern of smoking is different from the pattern typically seen in adolescent experimenters. Addicted smoking is characterized by (1) smoking half a pack or more daily (the greater the number of cigarettes smoked per day, the more nicotine addicted the smoker is), (2) feeling the greatest need to smoke first thing in the morning (when blood nicotine levels are at their lowest), (3) craving a cigarette periodically as blood nicotine levels decrease below a certain level, and (4) feeling immediate relief of the craving soon after lighting up (because nicotine is free-based, so it enters the central nervous system within seconds of the first inhalation). Social influences also motivate adult smoking (e.g., a woman who quits during pregnancy is more likely to relapse if her spouse smokes), but they are, for the most part, secondary influences.

Although some work suggests that nicotine dependence might begin early in the course of initiating the smoking habit, the prevailing opinion is that social influences are the primary motivating force behind adolescent experimental smoking. Longitudinal studies suggest that adolescent smoking is an opportunistic behavior, and teenagers are capable of smoking intensively at a party one night and not smoking again for a long period without facing major withdrawal symptoms typical of addicted smokers. The intermittent smoking pattern is different from the adult pattern of smoking. In addition, the strongest predictors of initiation and maintenance of smoking during adolescence are social factors, including friend smoking, community smoking, exposure to tobacco advertising, exposure to other media containing smoking, and parental permissiveness toward smoking. These influences are best integrated into a social-cognitive learning model in which adolescents are influenced by the actions and attitudes expressed by role models they see in their immediate environment.

Adolescents move on to daily smoking over a 2- to 3-year period. By the time they are smoking half a pack per day or more, they are behaving more like nicotine addition is a factor (craving when abstinent, smoking on getting up in the morning). These half-pack-per-day smokers account for less than 20% of regular (30-day) adolescent smokers.

PEDIATRIC PRINCIPLES

Epidemiology of Adolescent Tobacco Use

Tobacco use is ascertained in adolescent populations by self-report. On anonymous surveys, adolescents report tobacco use accurately and reliably. Two primary measures are implemented to ascertain adolescent tobacco use: ever tried ("Have you ever smoked or puffed on a cigarette?") and 30-day use ("Have you smoked a cigarette in the past 30 days?"). Table 22-1 presents the rates of smoking cigarettes, smoking cigars, and using smokeless tobacco by grade, gender, and race. In addition to the information in Table 22-1, 30-day usage rates for cigarettes increased approximately 5% to 10% during the 1990s, but these rates have declined since the mid- to late 1990s. The proportion of high school seniors smoking half a pack per day or more declined from 14.3% in 1997 to 11.3% in 2000. Cigar use has not been ascertained over time in adolescents, so trend data are not available. Although spit tobacco use is more prevalent in the South and in rural versus urban areas, its use declined among adolescents during the 1990s.

Why Children and Adolescents Smoke

Understanding risk factors for smoking in adolescents can help clinicians identify high-risk adolescents for more intensive counseling or other interventions. As mentioned earlier, the most important risk factor is having friends who smoke. Other factors, such as personality characteristics of the adolescent and attitudes toward smoking, are important in determining risk of initiating smoking. In addition, some risk factors are relatively more important for young versus

Table 22-1. Smoking Rates

Tobacco Product	Tobacco Use Categories	
	Ever Tried	*30-Day Use*
Cigarettes*		
8th graders	40%	14.6%
12th graders		
Overall	63%	23.9%
White		37.9%
Black		14.3%
Hispanic		27.7%
Cigars†		
Middle school		6.1%
High school		
Overall		15.4%
Male		20.4%
Female		10.2%
White		16.1%
Black		15.1%
Hispanic		11.7%
Spit Tobacco†		
8th graders	13.0%	4.2%
12th graders		
Overall	23.0%	7.6%
Male		14.4%
Female		1.3%
White		10.5%
Black		3.8%
Hispanic		1.5%

*Monitoring of the Future Survey, 2000.
†National Youth Tobacco Survey, 1999.

older children. Parent smoking frequently is cited as a social influence on adolescents. Parent smoking is important, however, only to the extent that it strongly predicts early onset of smoking (before age 11). Risk factors are discussed by order of importance, with social influence factors first, then characteristics of the child.

Social Influences

Friends

Friend smoking is considered the most important influence of adolescent smoking and is one of the areas of widest investigation. Children become increasingly peer-oriented as they approach the end of elementary school. Adolescent never-smokers whose friends smoke are about twice as likely to initiate smoking during the following year. Friend smoking also is associated with continuation of smoking among adolescent experimenters.

Parents

Parent Smoking. Parents who smoke model the behavior for their children. This modeling, along with the greater accessibility to tobacco in the home, makes the children more likely to initiate smoking during the elementary school years. The effect of parent smoking on adolescents is weaker. Adolescents may report being disgusted with their parent's smoking and uncomfortable when forced to be with the smoker in confined spaces for long periods (e.g., car rides).

Parenting Style. In contrast to parent smoking, certain parenting practices have a moderately strong association with maintaining never-smoker status during adolescence.

The parenting characteristics associated with reduced rates of smoking include authoritative parenting (combination of supportiveness and behavioral control) and monitoring (keeping track of where the adolescent spends his or her time and with whom he or she associates). Authoritative parenting is a concept developed during the 1960s. Authoritative parents are responsive to their children and able to set limits. They validate their children's opinions and listen to their concerns. At the same time, they have no difficulty making demands and setting expectations. Monitoring probably influences adolescent smoking by modulating the influence of peer smoking.

Specific Antismoking Messages. Parents whose children perceive a strong antismoking parental attitude are less likely to start smoking. The ability to project this attitude means that the parent not only values keeping the child tobacco-free, but also believes that he or she can intervene effectively to prevent it. African-American parents tend to be strongly antitobacco and to communicate this to their children. White parents also are disturbed when their children smoke, but they tend to believe that there is nothing they can do about the behavior.

Media

Smoking is a stylized behavior. Adult smoking is ritualized, varying little from cigarette to cigarette. Adult smoking is habitual; adults light up and smoke without conscious awareness of what they are doing. Adolescent smokers tend to be experimenters, conscious of everything they do, from lighting the cigarette to offering a cigarette to others. Their smoking is not consistent; they try out things they see others do, especially in the media.

Tobacco Marketing. Tobacco companies use marketing to accomplish two main objectives. The first is to brand their product, to associate it with a series of images or ideas in order to distinguish it from or link it to other brands. The second is to discount the price through two-for-one promotions or through value-added promotions, such as clothing.

The Master Settlement Agreement (MSA) was an agreement reached in 1998 between the tobacco companies and attorney generals from each of the 50 states. The MSA eliminated some types of tobacco advertising (e.g., billboard advertising). This change did not lead to a decline in advertising expenditures, however. Instead, tobacco companies diverted their advertising dollars into areas allowed by the agreement. In 1999, tobacco marketing expenditures rose 22% to a record $8.24 billion, and by 2000, it approached $10 billion. This marketing includes media such as magazines, storefront advertising, product displays, and promotions.

Magazines. In 2000, magazine advertisements for youth brands of cigarettes reached more than 80% of young people in the United States an average of 17 times each. Tobacco magazine ads associate the product with fun times (Newport), relaxation (Parliament), and sexuality (Kool). One of the most successful advertising campaigns of all time has been the Marlboro Man campaign, associating the brand with the toughness and independence of the American cowboy for more than 40 years. The Marlboro man has changed little since he was introduced in the 1960s and can be seen in almost every country worldwide.

Billboards and Storefront Advertising. The MSA eliminated billboards but did not affect storefront advertising. Tobacco companies rent counter space from retailers for promotional setups. This arrangement accounts for substantial revenues for small retail stores and serves to convey visual images and product promotions to customers. It also explains why storeowners typically line up with the tobacco industry against higher tobacco taxes and other antitobacco legislation.

Tobacco Company Promotions. Adolescents spend a lot of time thinking about the clothes they wear because clothing is an important part of their identity. It makes sense, then, that dressing them in clothing that bears a tobacco logo might influence their image of themselves and their subsequent smoking behavior. Tobacco promotional items are articles of clothing such as t-shirts and backpacks or smoking paraphernalia that display the brand logo. These items were distributed during the 1990s through value-added coupons and could be ordered through catalogues available at retailers. Depending on the region, 20% to 40% of adolescents owned tobacco promotional items during this period. Even for never-smokers, ownership of a promotional item proved to be a strong predictor of the initiation of smoking, almost as strong as friend smoking. Acquisition of an item increases the risk of trying out smoking, and losing the item decreases the risk. Although the MSA restricts distribution of tobacco promotional items by mail, they can be found at road races, such as NASCAR events. A survey of Northern New England adolescents in 1999 showed that approximately 20% of young adolescents owned tobacco promotional items.

Another form of promotion is discounting. Adolescent smoking is correlated to tobacco price. From a tobacco control perspective, the main point of increasing tobacco taxes at the state level is that it causes some people to quit smoking and others to refrain from starting in the first place. Tobacco companies are aware of this and undercut state tax increases by offering discounts. This action cuts profits, but tobacco is so profitable that significant discounts can be offered without eliminating the profit margin.

Movies and Television. Compared with magazine advertising, the modeling of smoking on screen is a powerful visual input. It is happening in real time, and children are able to assimilate the demonstrated stylistic elements of tobacco use. Tobacco use also is modeled by a larger-than-life hero, the screen star. Although tobacco use always has been depicted prominently in movies, until relatively recently, little tobacco use was depicted on television.

The average adolescent watches two to three movies per week. How much tobacco use is seen depends on the type of movie. The median numbers of tobacco occurrences by movie rating are as follows: G, 2; PG, 4; PG-13, 4; and R, 8. The adolescent who watches three R-rated movies per week sees smoking depicted by a movie star about 24 times. Tobacco brands are depicted in one third of movies, and actors endorse brands while lighting up about 10% of the time. When the movie is distributed internationally, these brand appearances result in worldwide promotion for the tobacco company.

The question of whether exposure affects behavior is just beginning to be examined. Cross-sectional studies have established that adolescents who prefer stars who smoke are more likely to be smokers themselves and that adolescent never-smokers who prefer stars who smoke are more likely to have favorable attitudes toward smoking. Cross-sectional and longitudinal studies have shown a strong and independent association between direct measures of exposure to tobacco use in movies and adolescent smoking. Finally, one study showed that adolescents whose parents restrict access to R-rated movies have lower rates of tobacco and alcohol use.

Characteristics of the Child

Some adolescents have personality characteristics that make them more apt to experiment. Others have interests that make them more likely to find themselves in situations where peers smoke. This section describes characteristics associated with initiating smoking.

Sensation Seeking. Sensation seeking refers to the tendency to seek out novel, exciting experiences. It is related to the concept of risk taking. Some children are by nature cautious, whereas others are more willing to take risks and try new things. Sensation seekers are more likely to try many risky activities, from physical risks (jumping a bike or skateboard) to experimentation with tobacco or other drugs.

Rebelliousness. Rebellious adolescents are more likely to question authority. To the extent that adolescent tobacco use is restricted by authority figures, smoking could consolidate the identity for a rebellious teen. Rebelliousness is an independent predictor of teen smoking. It is a common misconception that most teens are rebellious and that this factor explains why they engage in risky behaviors. Most teens score low on rebelliousness scales.

Poor School Performance. Teens who perform poorly in school are more likely to become smokers. Poor school performers tend to be teens who are alienated from the mainstream and who are less involved in academic and extracurricular activities and therefore have additional free time. They are less likely to be engaged in sports (a protective factor) and are much more likely eventually to drop out of school. School dropouts have high smoking rates.

Attitudes That Predict Smoking. Attitudinal susceptibility to smoking is a measure of intentions, resistance to peer offers, and measures of the teen's perception of the utility of smoking and is a powerful predictor of initiation. Teens who cannot rule out smoking in the next 6 months or if offered a cigarette by a friend are twice as likely to start smoking. Having the view that there is something to be gained from smoking, termed *positive utilities*, is also a predictor of the behavior. This type of attitude is assessed by questions such as "Do you think you might enjoy smoking?" Finally, viewing smoking as normative is linked with the behavior. Many adolescents think that most of their peers smoke. This is not surprising; smoking is highly visible, and nonsmokers are, for the most part, silent about their nonsmoking status. One component of successful school-based social influence programs has involved teaching adolescents that most of their peers do not smoke.

Community Environment

Communities where smoking is restricted have lower rates of adult and teen smoking. Community smoking restrictions make it harder to find a place to smoke and place a greater burden on the smoker, increasing the relative value of cessation. In addition, community smoking restrictions limit the visibility of smoking to impressionable teens. California, which has some of the most stringent environmental smoking bans in its cities and towns, has rates of adult and teen smoking 5% to 7% lower than the rest of the United States. The passing of local ordinances restricting smoking in public places is a keystone of the tobacco control movement.

Preventing Tobacco Use in Pediatric Practice
Smoking Cessation Counseling

The *Guide to Clinical Preventive Services* is an established reference source for clinicians needing evidence-based recommendations on preventive services. This source gives clinical interventions to promote smoking cessation an "A" recommendation, meaning there is good evidence to support this activity; there are few counseling activities that receive an "A" rating. Multiple randomized clinical trials show that smoking cessation counseling increases the chances of quitting. Brief advice exerts a small effect (1% to 2%) on the quit rate; a much larger effect is seen when the advice is coupled with follow-up and pharmacotherapy (12% to 15%). One of the biggest disappointments with smoking cessation counseling is that most physicians overlook it, despite almost 100 randomized clinical trials showing efficacy of this clinical activity, and despite evidence that physicians are extremely effective in prompting change in their patients. To help address this issue and facilitate tobacco prevention and counseling in the office, it is important to set up a systematic approach. Table 22-2 provides an overview of such a systematic approach and its elements. There are four steps to cessation counseling, embodied in the four A's—ask, advise, assist, and arrange.

Ask about Family Smoking

Clinicians do not address tobacco use unless they are prompted to do so. The pediatric office system should include routine inquiry about family smoking. This inquiry

Table 22-2. Supporting Tobacco Cessation in the Office

Ask about Smoking in Families

Incorporate smoking into vital signs assessment to prompt clinician to ask.

Designate someone in the office (typically the person who prepares patient) to fill out vital signs stamp.

Know key questions for assessing smoking status, quit history, and gauging motivation to quit.

Advise Smokers to Quit

Tailor motivational statement according to patient's level of interest in quitting.

For those not considering quitting: "I really want you to think about quitting smoking."

For those considering quitting: "I'm really pleased you are planning to quit smoking."

Assist and Arrange

Designate an office person to be a tobacco cessation support. This person's job is to know about community cessation counseling resources, be able to assist a parent in choosing the best resource for his or her needs, facilitate the referral, and do telephone follow-up.

Refer tobacco users interested in quitting to community or World Wide Web resources.

can be accomplished by incorporating assessment of parent smoking into the process of taking vital signs at every visit.

The clinician needs to know how to take a smoking history. Table 22-3 includes a series of questions that evaluate how much the patient smokes and whether he or she is interested in cessation. Table 22-3 has been modified to serve as a standardized history form. The key elements of the assessment are to establish how much the patient smokes, how long the patient has been smoking, the patient's level of addiction, and the patient's interest in quitting and to explore potential barriers to quitting.

Advise

Brief Advice. Brief advice involves giving a motivating message tailored to the patient's intentions. The motivational message should be clear, strong, and personalized. For patients not considering quitting in the next 6 months, the goal is to nudge them in the direction of considering quitting with a message something like "I really want you to think about quitting smoking. This is the most important thing you can do for your health and the health of your family, especially as smoking makes your daughter's asthma worse." The advice also can be tailored to address a perceived barrier to quitting: "I really want you to think about how you could structure your workday to avoid being around smokers during breaks." Alternatively, emphasis can be on a perceived benefit: "You will save $30 a week by quitting."

Motivational Interviewing. Some pediatricians may want to go beyond brief advice in their approach to motivating behavior change in patients. Motivational interviewing is a widely used approach, but it takes much more time than the brief advice intervention. Motivational interviewing is a "directive, client-centered counseling style for eliciting behavior change by helping clients to explore and resolve ambivalence." The principles of motivational interviewing apply to adult and adolescent smokers and to other behavior change issues. Adolescents may be motivated to quit for many reasons. Some want to quit because of sports or because they perceive an impact on their health. Some are forced into cessation by their parents or school officials. Regardless of the reason, the discussion begins by assessing motivators and barriers to quitting. Table 22-4 summarizes the three steps in a motivational counseling strategy that focuses on decisional balance. The first step is to clarify issues by having the patient list factors that work for continuing smoking and factors that work for quitting. There are several indirect ways to lower resistance and several direct lines of inquiry designed to increase motivation.

Assist

Brief Advice. In the case of a patient or parent who wants to quit, the physician's role is to facilitate the process. For clinicians who desire to limit their involvement to brief advice, someone in the office should be familiar with community cessation resources. This makes it easy to arrange for assistance. The physician's message for individuals considering cessation is something like "I'm really happy you are considering giving up smoking. Let's get Sandy to help you think about where you can get some help. I really think you should consider using the patch or the gum this time." The office cessation expert can engage

Table 22-3. Assessment Questions for Adolescent Smoking

Key Assessment Factors	Question
Smoking Experience	
Ever tried	"Have you ever tried smoking (or smokeless tobacco)?"
30-day use	"Have you smoked (or used smokeless tobacco) in the past 30 days?"
Daily use	"How many packs (or cans) per day do you smoke (chew)?"
Cost	"How much do you spend on cigarettes (or cigars, chew) each week?"
Never-Smokers	
Susceptibility*	
Intentions	"Do you think you might try smoking in the coming year?"
Resistance to peer offers	"Do you think you would smoke if a friend offered?"
Positive utilities	"Do you think you might enjoy smoking?"
Peer smoking	"Do any of your friends smoke?"
Smokers	
Level of addiction: Hooked on Nicotine Checklist	1. Have you ever tried to quit, but couldn't?
	2. Do you smoke now because it is really hard to quit?
	3. Have you ever felt like you were addicted to tobacco?
	4. Do you ever have strong cravings for tobacco?
	5. Have you ever felt like you really needed a cigarette?
	6. Is it hard to keep from smoking in places where you are not supposed to, like school or work?
	When you try to stop smoking (or, when you have not used tobacco for a while),
	7. Do you find it hard to concentrate because you couldn't smoke?
	8. Do you feel more irritable because you couldn't smoke?
	9. Do you feel a strong need or urge to smoke?
	10. Do you feel nervous, restless, or anxious because you couldn't smoke?
Quit history	"Have you ever tried quitting?"
	"What is the longest time you remained abstinent?"
	"What caused your relapse?"
	"Have you ever tried aids, like nicotine replacement or Zyban (the pill)?"
Interest in quitting†	"Do you think you might try quitting in the next 6 months?"
	"Do you think you might try quitting in the next month?"
Motivational factors	Evaluate resistance
	"Let's list all of your reasons for not quitting." (e.g., nerves)
	"Can you think of barriers to your quitting?" (e.g., all my coworkers smoke)
	Evaluate motivation
	"Let's list all of your reasons for quitting." (e.g., it costs a lot)

*Must answer "definitely not" to all three questions to be considered not susceptible.
†"No" to the first question means the individual is in the precontemplative stage. "Yes" to the first and second questions means the individual is contemplating quitting. Those actively planning quitting are in the preparation phase, and those actually quitting are in the action or maintenance phase.

the patient in cessation counseling or determine where best to refer the patient for more intensive counseling (see CD-ROM Tables 22-1 and 22-2 for Internet resources and state-specific tobacco quit-line information).

Cessation Counseling. The basics of cessation counseling are listed in Table 22-5 and include helping patients with a quitting plan that includes setting a quitting date, preparing them for quitting, discussing pharmacologic assistance, and giving key advice on successful smoking cessation. The physician should discuss pharmacologic aids to quitting because many smokers have only a rudimentary knowledge about this. There have been few randomized trials to define the role of pharmacotherapy as an aid to cessation in adolescents. The published results are disappointing for nicotine replacement therapy and not recommended for most adolescents. For addicted adolescents, a better choice is bupropion, marketed as Zyban for smoking cessation. For more information on pharmacologic aids, see the article by Hughes and colleagues.

Arrange for Follow-up

One important element of cessation assistance is to arrange for follow-up. The most difficult period of abstinence is the first 6 weeks. During this time, the individual is coping with physiologic craving for nicotine and having to work through the behavioral elements of avoiding tobacco use. The clinician should follow up 2 weeks after the quit date and every month thereafter for one to three visits. During the follow-up visits, the clinician should engage the patient in a discussion of relapses that includes the following questions: How many? How often? What prompted them? How can you avoid them in the future? For clinicians not wanting to spend face-to-face clinical time doing this kind of counseling, ancillary personnel can be trained to do follow-up by telephone.

Counseling to Prevent Smoking

The *Guide to Clinical Preventive Services* also gives an "A" rating to including antitobacco messages in health promotion counseling of children and adolescents, but states that there is no study that evaluates the effectiveness of clinical counseling to prevent the initiation of tobacco use. It follows that rather than spending large amounts of time engaging in direct counseling, the clinician should develop materials to give to parents at each visit. The materials should be dispensed with brief advice and should be designed to prompt a discussion between the parent and the child (e.g., around expectations regarding tobacco

Table 22-4. Motivational Interviewing

Tasks	Questions or Examples
Clarify Issues	
Assess willingness to quit	"Are you thinking about quitting in the next 6 months?"
Assess decisional balance	"Let's see how the pros and cons of quitting balance out for you."
Motivation	
Assess benefits of smoking	"Let's list the things you like about smoking."
Assess negative aspects of quitting	"Are there some things you would be worried about if you quit?"
Resistance	
Assess negative aspects of smoking	"Are you having some concerns about your smoking?"
Assess benefits of quitting	"Can you think of some advantages to quitting?"
Scale importance	"I want you to rate the importance of your reasons to continue smoking on a scale of 1–10, 10 being very important and 1 being not important at all." (Repeat for reasons to quit)
Lower Resistance: Indirect Inquiry	
Use simple reflection	"Smoking relieves your nerves?"
Probe priorities	"If you look over all your reasons to smoke, which one do you think is the most important?"
Use double-sided reflection	"On one hand, you tell me smoking helps you relax. On the other hand, you tell me your smoking makes you concerned about your son's asthma."
Explore the future	"I want you to think about how your health has changed in the past 5 years and extend that into the future. What do you think your health will be like 5 years from now?"
Acknowledge ambivalence	"Everybody has mixed feelings about continuing to smoke. When you think about all your reasons for smoking and reasons for quitting at once, does this change the way you think about quitting?"
Emphasize personal choice	"In the end, it's your decision whether you want to quit or continue smoking."
Increase Motivation: Direct Intervention	
Substitute benefits	"I'm wondering if there are some other ways you could find to help yourself relax."
Bring the future to the present	"At the last visit you mentioned some things that could affect your health in the future. What if one of those things happened sooner, like this week; do you think that would change how you think about your smoking?"
Clarify values	"I hope you don't mind me making a point of this, but I was wondering if you could think about what's more important to you—the relaxation smoking brings to you versus your son's asthma?"
Use discrepancies	"You're saying one thing but doing another."
Use differences in motivational reasons	"I'm seeing how important it is to you to protect your son's health, and I'm wondering what it would take for you to use that same motivation to protect your own health by not smoking."
Reframe issues	"You say smoking helps you relax, but you know that sense of relaxation is really just a sign of nicotine addiction. When you haven't had a cigarette for a while, you feel edgy because you get a craving for nicotine. Did you ever think that smoking might be adding to your stress by making you edgy?"
Arrange Follow-up	
At follow-up, reassess resistance and motivation	Telephone follow-up is a cost-effective way to follow-up on a patient's quit status.

Table 22-5. Basics of Cessation Counseling

Action	Strategies for Implementation
Help patient with a quit plan	Set a quit date—ideally within 2 wk.
	Make preparations for quitting.
	Inform family, friends, and coworkers and request understanding and support.
	Remove cigarettes from your environment. Before quitting, avoid smoking in places where you spend a lot of time (e.g., home, car).
	Review previous quit attempts. What helped you? What led to relapse?
	Anticipate challenges to planned quit attempt, particularly during the first few weeks (when most relapse occurs). Anticipate nicotine withdrawal symptoms (irritability, moody, increased stress, cravings).
	Strategize coping mechanisms.
Encourage pharmacologic assistance	For adults: encourage the use of nicotine patch or nicotine gum for smoking cessation.
	For adults and for selected adolescents: encourage the use of bupropion.
Give key advice on successful quitting	Abstinence—total abstinence is essential; the best predictor of relapse to regular smoking is taking even a single puff of a cigarette.
	Alcohol—drinking alcohol is highly associated with relapse. Those who stop smoking should review their alcohol use and consider limiting/abstaining from alcohol during the first 2 mo of abstinence.
	Other smokers in household—the presence of other smokers in the household, particularly a spouse, is associated with lower quitting success. Patients should consider quitting with their significant others and/or developing specific plans to stay quit in a household where others smoke.
Provide supplementary materials	Sources—these include federal agencies; nonprofit agencies; drug companies that market cessation aids; or local/state health departments.
	Location—materials must be readily available in the clinic.

Adapted from Treating Tobacco Use and Dependence—Clinical Practice Guideline, USDHHS, Washington DC, June 2000. Available at: www.surgeongeneral.gov/tobacco/clinpak.html.

use) or to motivate a behavior change (e.g., to motivate a parent to get rid of tobacco promotional items around the house).

CD-ROM Tables 22-3, 22-4, and 22-5 list developmentally appropriate tobacco prevention strategies, interventions that address factors that contribute to adolescent smoking, and prevention activities with regard to tobacco control in the community. The tables are designed to help the practitioner link concepts described in this chapter to practical clinical approaches. In addition, CD-ROM Tables 22-1 and 22-2 list tobacco control resources on the Internet and state-specific tobacco quit-line contact information.

Additional Resources, CD-ROM

Tobacco control resources on the Internet	Table
State-specific tobacco quit-line contact information	Table
Developmentally appropriate tobacco prevention strategies	Table
Interventions that address factors that contribute to adolescent smoking	Table
Prevention activities for tobacco control in the community	Table

Mini-index of Related Topics   CH.

SUGGESTED READINGS

Botelho R: Beyond Advice: 1. Becoming a Motivational Practitioner. Rochester, NY, Motivate Healthy Habits, 2002.

Botelho R: Beyond Advice: 2. Developing Motivational Skills. Rochester, NY, Motivate Healthy Habits, 2002.

Fiore MC, Bailey WC, Cohen SJ, et al: Treating Tobacco Use and Dependence. Clinical Practice Guideline. Rockville, Md, U.S. Department of Health and Human Services, Public Health Service, 2000.

Hughes JR, Goldstein MG, Hurt RD, Shiffman S: Recent advances in the pharmacotherapy of smoking. JAMA 1999;281:72–76.

Lynch BS, Bonnie RJ: Growing Up Tobacco Free: Preventing Nicotine Addiction in Children and Youths. Committee on Preventing Nicotine Addiction in Children and Youths, Division of Biobehavioral Sciences and Mental Disorders, Institute of Medicine. Washington, DC, National Academy Press, 1994.

National Cancer Institute: Smoking and Tobacco Control Monograph 10. Health Effects of Exposure to Environmental Tobacco Smoke. National Institutes of Health, 1999. Available at: http://rex.nci.nih.gov/NCI_MONOGRAPHS/MONO10/MONO10.HTM.

U.S. Department of Health and Human Services Preventing Tobacco Use Among Young People: A Report of the Surgeon General. Atlanta, Ga: U.S. Department of Health and Human Services, Public Health Service, Centers for Disease Control and Prevention, National Center for Chronic Disease Prevention and Health Promotion, Office on Smoking and Health, 1994.

23 Injury Prevention

Judith Shaw and Eliot Nelson

ROLE OF THE GENERALIST

1 Understand and apply knowledge of the epidemiology and impact of unintentional injuries in children and adolescents.

2 Understand and apply the principles of injury prevention, including the role of host, agent, and environment.

3 Use developmentally appropriate and age-appropriate interventions in scheduled office-based counseling and teachable moments.

4 Use effective communication techniques for injury prevention counseling.

5 Use community partnerships and resources to enhance office-based prevention activities.

Injuries are the leading cause of death and disability in children and adolescents. Counseling parents about how to prevent injuries is an important component of care provided by the primary care provider. By understanding the risk of injury and the associated prevention strategies, pediatricians can work with parents to impart knowledge and create a safer environment for children.

The pediatric health care provider is in a unique position to offer guidance to parents about safety and to promote injury prevention more broadly in the community. The American Academy of Pediatrics Committee on Practice and Ambulatory Management and Bright Futures recommend that primary care providers counsel families and children on injury prevention. Every interaction between the health care provider and parents is an opportunity for imparting information about maintaining a safe environment in which the child can grow, learn, and thrive. Clinicians can use a variety of strategies to provide anticipatory guidance, including using a schedule for injury prevention counseling, taking advantage of teachable moments, and reinforcing positive behaviors.

The scope of injury prevention is enormous because injury is a leading public health problem in the United States. Although this chapter focuses primarily on clinical counseling as a tool for injury prevention, clinicians should recognize that community-based programs, legislative initiatives, and engineering advances often have surpassed individual clinical educational interventions in reducing the toll of injury in society. Understanding this fact can help pedi-

atric health care providers to support advocacy and other efforts to complement their own anticipatory guidance.

EPIDEMIOLOGY

Injury has become increasingly prominent as a childhood health problem in the United States over the last century, primarily because other causes of morbidity and mortality (e.g., infectious diseases) have decreased dramatically as a result of improvements in public sanitation, nutrition, and advances in medical care. Although injury death rates overall have declined more slowly than death rates from other causes, some areas of injury death rates have declined substantially. This decline reflects the potential for having an impact on injury with appropriate public health measures.

This chapter focuses on *unintentional injuries* in children and adolescents, as opposed to *intentional injuries*. The latter include assault, homicide, and suicide. Pediatric death rates in these categories have been virtually unique in showing increases in recent decades in the United States. Most pediatric homicide and suicide deaths occur in mid- to late adolescence, and 60% to 70% of these deaths are firearm deaths. Although the prevention of intentional injuries is complex, many of the successful approaches to prevention of unintentional injury discussed in this chapter (e.g., safe storage of firearms) show promise for reducing the risk of intentional injury as well. Violence prevention (see Chapter 24) and issues of adolescent injury prevention, including suicide (see Chapters 219, 233, and 235), are discussed elsewhere in this book.

In the United States in 2000, almost 12,500 children and adolescents 0 to 19 years old died of unintentional injuries. Of the total of 26,000 pediatric deaths after age 1 year, slightly less than half (44.5%) resulted from unintentional injury. Among teenagers, unintentional injury accounted for nearly 50% of all deaths. Overall injury death rates show a bimodal age distribution, with high rates in early childhood and higher rates in late adolescence. Almost 54% of all pediatric unintentional injury deaths occur in adolescents 15 to 19 years old. Boys have significantly higher injury rates than girls in virtually all injury categories and at all ages. Table 23-1 shows death rates for selected major categories of injuries by pediatric age groups. Pediatric clinicians should consider the leading causes of injury death for children at various ages in guiding their anticipatory guidance. The Centers for Disease Control and Prevention's WISQARS website from the National Center for Injury Prevention and

Table 23-1. Unintentional Injury Deaths and Death Rates* by Type of Injury and Age Group, United States, 2000

Type of Injury	Age Group				
	0–1, No. Deaths (Rate)	1–4, No. Deaths (Rate)	5–9, No. Deaths (Rate)	10–14, No. Deaths (Rate)	15–19, No. Deaths (Rate)
All Unintentional Injury	881 (22.90)	1826 (12.05)	1391 (7.03)	1588 (7.98)	6755 (33.97)
Selected Injury Categories					
Motor vehicle occupant†	152 (3.95)	388 (2.56)	490 (2.47)	630 (3.16)	4565 (22.95)
Pedestrian	16 (0.41)	269 (1.78)	222 (1.12)	199 (1.00)	332 (1.67)
Pedal cyclist	0 (0)	4 (0.02)	57 (0.29)	107 (0.54)	59 (0.30)
Drowning	75 (1.95)	493 (3.25)	201 (1.02)	174 (0.87)	371 (1.87)
Falls	8 (0.20)	36 (0.24)	16 (0.08)	21 (0.11)	99 (0.50)
Residential fire/flame	35 (0.91)	277 (1.83)	171 (0.86)	78 (0.39)	72 (0.36)
Firearm	1 (0.02)	18 (0.11)	18 (0.09)	49 (0.25)	107 (0.54)
Suffocation/choking	526 (13.67)	151 (1.00)	45 (0.23)	72 (0.36)	70 (0.35)
Poisoning	14 (0.36)	32 (0.21)	17 (0.08)	28 (0.14)	351 (1.77)

*Rates are per 100,000 persons.
†Counts and figures for motor vehicle occupant deaths include a prorated portion of motor vehicle traffic deaths that are coded as "unspecified." Most such deaths are believed to be "occupant" deaths, not specified as such simply due to coding challenges posed by police reports. A small portion of "unspecified" deaths are believed to be motorcyclist deaths instead of motor vehicle occupant deaths.

From Centers for Disease Control and Prevention: National Center for Injury Prevention and Control. Available at: http://www.cdc.gov/ncipc/.

Control provides state-by-state data on injury mortality, which can help clinicians to tailor their approaches to injury prevention for their patient populations.

Injury causes a huge amount of costly morbidity. Experts estimate that for every injury death, there are approximately 20 injuries serious enough to require hospital admission and 200 to 300 injuries that require some form of medical care. Falls and poisoning are major examples of injuries that rarely are fatal but that nonetheless result in high hospitalization rates and enormous costs.

The injury categories shown in Table 23-1 may obscure the importance of certain injury problems, such as head injuries, which overlap many of the categories shown. Even more important to prevention efforts, the categories do not reveal the contribution of certain "root causes" of injury mortality and morbidity, such as alcohol and drug use or poverty. Addressing these root causes, which is beyond the scope of this chapter, can be expected to have an impact on childhood injury.

PRINCIPLES OF INJURY PREVENTION

Ever since the seminal work of Haddon beginning in the 1960s, experts increasingly have recognized that effective prevention of injuries involves a *multidisciplinary approach* focused on the interrelated triad of the *host*, *agent*, and *environment*. Appropriate supervision of children and adolescents should address developmental and behavioral vulnerabilities of the child (*host*) at all ages. Although supervision is always important, modifications of *agents* and the *environment* often are more likely to reduce injury risks. Safe cribs, child-proof caps on medication, safe playgrounds, child car seats, bicycle paths, pool fences with self-latching gates, trigger locks or lock-boxes for guns, and smoke detectors all offer better ways of protecting children than supervision alone or simply teaching to "be careful." Protective measures that work *passively* (i.e., without requiring *active* or repetitive steps by child or parent) often are most effective.

OFFICE COUNSELING FOR INJURY PREVENTION

The pediatric health care provider is in a unique position to offer guidance to parents about safety and to promote injury prevention in the office and more broadly in the community. Education for injury prevention in the health supervision setting has long been considered valuable. The breadth of injury risk coupled with limited time during visits presents a challenge, however, regarding what to counsel, when, and to what extent. An even more important caveat is that *there is not strong evidence for the effectiveness of counseling alone to prevent injuries*. Clinicians cannot assume that increasing parental knowledge by itself is sufficient to produce changes in *behavior* that are key to reducing risk.

The previous statement does not preclude counseling efforts. Rather, effective anticipatory guidance in the office should seek to help parents identify developmentally based risks of injury for their children, then to identify specific ways of modifying agents or the environment to reduce the risks of these injuries. Studies show that the effectiveness of office education can be enhanced by coupling information with specific suggestions and with the provision of devices themselves or with the provision of help in obtaining them (e.g., discount coupons). Counseling can reinforce the use of legally mandated devices, such as car seats, smoke detectors, bicycle helmets, or pool fences in communities where such laws exist. Regular counseling can convey a clear and consistent message to parents that injuries occur in predictable patterns, that they can be prevented with reasonable measures, and that health care providers view injury prevention efforts as crucial to good health maintenance. Office-based counseling can occur through a predesigned scheduled format, through "teachable moments" that present themselves in a variety of ways in office encounters, and through use of reinforcing strategies.

Guidelines for Injury Prevention Counseling in Health Supervision Visits

- Consider the *developmental level* of the child.
- *Gather information* from caregivers about what they see as risks and what steps they already may have taken to reduce injury risks.
- Give *positive reinforcement* where appropriate.
- Help caregivers *focus on one or a few of the most serious injury risks* for children at this age.
- Give *hopeful* message that there are reasonable ways proven to prevent serious injuries.
- Provide *specific* suggestions on how to reduce risks of particular injuries.
- *Acknowledge costs* and potential inconvenience of injury-prevention steps.
- *Allow caregivers time* to consider suggestions, and *follow-up* by the next visit to address difficulties in taking steps to reduce injury risks.

SCHEDULED COUNSELING FOR INJURY PREVENTION

Counseling of parents or caregivers to reduce injury risk should respect individual differences in home and community environments and should recognize the efforts that most already have made to protect their children. Studies suggest that parents want information but are unlikely to be receptive if they are merely "told what to do." A good general approach for injury prevention counseling in health supervision visits is outlined in Box 23-1.

As mentioned previously, the breadth of injury risk coupled with limited time during a health supervision visit presents a challenge regarding what to counsel, when, and to what extent. The information communicated should be culturally relevant so that parents can understand what is being said and should take into consideration the child and family's particular environment and situation. Families residing in farm communities have different risks and different needs compared with families living in cities. Children relying on public transportation rather than an automobile present differing risks. Knowing basic risk factors and associated injury prevention strategies for each of the age groups allows the clinician to target the counseling to the environment and situation to meet the needs of the family and child.

The American Academy of Pediatrics provides recommendations for injury prevention counseling based on age and injury topic area. The American Academy of Pediatrics supplemental materials and tools for counseling, The Injury Prevention Program, offer surveys to assess for risk and parent educational handouts to complement the counseling provided. Table 23-2 lists age-appropriate and developmentally appropriate injury prevention counseling.

TEACHABLE MOMENTS

Teachable moments are situations that present as opportunities for counseling families or children. Used as an adjunct to a counseling schedule, teachable moments can be used to impart new information or reinforce previous counseling.

All encounters with children and families provide opportunities for instructing about safety. Injury prevention counseling should not be limited to well-child visits; it can occur during acute care visits, phone calls, and other encounters when teachable moments arise (Box 23-2).

REINFORCING STRATEGIES

In addition to following a counseling schedule or taking advantage of teachable moments, injury prevention counseling can be done to reinforce safe behaviors. With this approach, information is offered in recognition of a safe practice or behavior. Rather than providing new information, an existing safe behavior is recognized, and new or supporting information is shared.

A child properly restrained in a child safety seat while waiting in the examination room is an opportunity to recognize and support child safety seat use. A simple comment such as, "I see you have placed Lily in a child safety seat, and that the straps are snug and that you have no padding between her and the seat," recognizes what the parent has done to create a safe environment for the child. This comment acknowledges the safety behavior while offering information on snug straps and the importance of no additional padding between the child and the safety seat. Depending on the need of the family at the time of the visit, additional information can be offered at this time, such as placement of the seat in the car, transitioning to a larger seat, or even the use of a tether strap. This approach recognizes the effort the parent has made in creating a safe environment for the child and reinforces this positive behavior.

BEYOND OFFICE-BASED COUNSELING: COMMUNITY INVOLVEMENT AND ADVOCACY

Because they are respected for their special knowledge and their natural interest in promoting child health, pediatric clinicians are in a unique position to further injury prevention efforts at the community, state, and national levels. Working in partnership with other interested community leaders, including educators, health department workers, recreation department officials, and other government and business leaders, clinicians can offer appropriate perspective regarding children's developmental capabilities. They can help ensure that injury prevention programs are respectful of scientific evidence of effectiveness and take leading roles in campaigns to promote specific safety strategies, such as bicycle helmet use, as exemplified by the pioneering Seattle Bicycle Helmet Campaign begun in the 1980s. These partnerships also can help facilitate the development of community safety check programs and hotlines that can serve as ready resources for families and organizers of child and adolescent activities.

Legislative initiatives can lead to implementation of safe product design and usage and can add crucial incentive for people and communities to modify environments or change behavior, in situations in which knowledge alone might have been insufficient to effect such changes. The federal Poison-Prevention Packaging Act of 1970 is a prime example of such legislation; laws mandating the use of child safety seats in cars and of smoke detectors in homes have

Table 23-2. Age-Appropriate and Developmentally Appropriate Injury Prevention Counseling

Topic	Sample Specific Advice or Strategy	Topic	Sample Specific Advice or Strategy
For 0–1 yr		Firearms	Store securely.
Motor vehicle occupant	Use rear-facing car seat until at least 1 yr and 20 lb.		Ask parents of playmates about firearm presence and safe storage.
	Never place car seat in front of an active airbag.	Fires and burns	Review previous sections.
Fires and burns	Use smoke detectors.		Do not allow loose clothing around kitchen flame.
	Keep hot water temperature <120°F.		Establish home escape plan and drill.
Poisonings	Keep National Poison Prevention hotline available: 1-800-222-1222.	**For 10–14 yr**	
Suffocation	Beware of small toys and foods such as raisins, grapes, popcorn, firm vegetable or fruit pieces.	Motor vehicle occupant	Place in rear seat until at least age 13.
			Use seatbelts for every ride.
	Review first-aid for choking.		Never ride in pickup truck bed.
Falls	Do not use mobile infant walkers.	Bicycle	Helmet use is mandatory.
	Use stairway gates.		Traffic laws apply to bicyclists.
	Install window bars.	Firearms	Store safely.
			Enroll child in hunter safety course if applicable.
For 1–4 yr			Review guidelines to remove guns from homes (e.g., risk factors for violence or suicide).
Motor vehicle occupant	Check appropriate car seat or booster seat.		
	Place child in rear seat/out of airbag path.	Drowning	Review boating safety guidelines; use flotation devices.
Pedestrian	Supervise play in fenced yards or parks.		
Drowning	Review constant bathtub supervision.		Review diving risks in pools and natural bodies of water.
	Pool fences should be 4-sided enclosures with a self-latching gate.	Sports injuries	Use protective equipment.
	Keep buckets empty, toilet lids closed.		Review concussion guidelines.
Fires and burns	See previous section.	**For 15–19 yr**	
	Remove access to lighters and matches.	Motor vehicle occupant	Support graduated driver licensing.
Firearms	Store securely.		Review strategies to avoid riding with alcohol- or substance-using driver.
Kitchen safety check	Review choking foods (see previous section).		Use seatbelts.
	Remove access to knives/sharp objects.		Turn off and put away cellular phone while driving.
	Keep a fire extinguisher on hand.	Firearms	See previous section.
For 5–9 yr			Never trust that a gun is unloaded.
Motor vehicle occupant	Use a booster seat until child is 57 inches tall.	Drowning	Review hazards of natural bodies of water (diving, hypothermia, changing currents).
	Place child in rear seat.		Review boating risks.
Pedestrian	Prohibit independent street crossing until 8 yr.	Poisonings	Consider potential unintentional medication overdose.
	Ensure fenced play.		
Bicycle safety	Helmet use is mandatory.		
Drowning	Provide swim lessons.		
	Use pool fences (see previous section).		

Box 23-2. Teachable Moments for Injury Prevention Counseling

1. When writing a prescription or handing out a sample medication, instruct parents of young children about the importance of storing medications in a high, locked cabinet.
2. When washing your hands in the sink, discuss with the parent the importance of checking the hot water temperature in their residence.
3. When placing an infant on the examination table, discuss never leaving an infant unattended on a high surface.
4. When an active toddler is climbing around the examination room, discuss the risk of falls (e.g., windows, stairs, or playground falls).
5. A parent bringing a hot beverage into the examination room provides an opportunity to discuss the risk of scald burns.
6. Visits around a holiday provide the opportunity to discuss the injury risks associated with that holiday (e.g., fireworks on Fourth of July).
7. Any injury-related visit provides an opening for discussing strategies for prevention.

been credited with major reductions in injury morbidity and mortality from leading injury killers. Pediatric clinicians can reinforce the value of such laws in individual and group discussions. They also can support advocacy efforts to enact new and better laws and can offer valuable assistance in education of the public and of legislators. Although such efforts can be time-consuming, they offer the ultimate potential for greater impact in injury prevention than might be achievable through office-based efforts alone.

Mini-index of Related Topics

SUGGESTED READINGS

American Academy of Pediatrics: Injury Prevention and Control for Children and Youth. Elk Grove Village, Ill, American Academy of Pediatrics, 1997. Available at: http://www.aap.org.

American Academy of Pediatrics: The Injury Prevention Program (TIPP) and a Guide to Safety Counseling in Office Practice. Elk Grove Village, Ill, American Academy of Pediatrics. Available at: http://www.aap.org.

American Academy of Pediatrics: Physician's Resource Guide for Bicycle Safety Education. Elk Grove Village, Ill, American Academy of Pediatrics, 1994. Available at: http://www.aap.org.

Behrman R (ed): Unintentional Injuries in Childhood. The Future of Children. The David and Lucile Packard Foundation. Spring/Summer 2000;10(1).

Centers for Disease Control and Prevention: National Center for Injury Prevention and Control. Available at: http://www.cdc.gov/ncipc/.

Christoffel T, Gallagher SS: Injury Prevention and Public Health: Practical Knowledge, Skills, and Strategies. Gaithersburg, Md, Aspen Publishers, 1999.

National SAFE KIDS Campaign: Washington, DC, National SAFE KIDS Campaign. Available at: www.safekids.org.

U.S. Consumer Product Safety Commission: Washington, DC, U.S. Consumer Product Safety Commission. Available at: www.cpsc.org.

SECTION 2   HEALTH PROMOTION AND DISEASE PREVENTION

24   Violence Prevention

Robert D. Sege

ROLE OF THE GENERALIST

1   Understand the key elements of primary prevention of violence.
2   Convey general messages on violence prevention to all parents.
3   Screen for risks and resilience.
4   Obtain a violence history.
5   Prevent reinjury.
6   Make appropriate referrals.
7   Understand the process of mobilizing community resources.

Violence is one of the leading causes of death and serious injury for children in the United States. Gunshot injuries claim more lives of children and adolescents than do all natural causes combined. As a result of many studies in the 1980s and 1990s that delineated certain risk and resilience factors, there is a new understanding of the role physicians can take in preventing youth violence.

Several key observations underlie the approach to violence prevention presented here. First, most violence results from conflicts between people who know each other well. Children who solve their problems violently are likely to get hurt. Children can be encouraged to solve their conflicts nonviolently and taught specific, age-appropriate skills. Second, children learn about violence through social learning—exposure to violence at home, on television, or in the community increases the risk for subsequent violence. Modeling and teaching nonviolent problem-solving skills is key. Finally, the presence of handguns greatly increases the risks for serious injury from violence.

In general, there are two forms of violence prevention activities in the physician's office. First, anticipatory guidance offers the opportunity to teach parents and children effective techniques for minimizing the risk of violence. Second, the treatment of children injured in a fight offers a "teachable moment"—the opportunity to intervene with children at a high risk for violence. Clinicians have opportunities for both types of activities.

This chapter first discusses anticipatory guidance, or primary prevention of violence-related injury, with general messages for parents and a review of screening tools that identify risk and resilience factors. Next, techniques used for taking a violence history are introduced, better connecting injured patients and their families with community resources and other referral sources to facilitate prevention of future reinjury.

ANTICIPATORY GUIDANCE: PROMOTING PROSOCIAL LEARNING

Health care providers caring for children usually understand the basics of good parenting. This section addresses specific topics that are particularly germane to the risk of subsequent violence. Many successful practices use ancillary personnel—nurses, aides, and receptionists—and materials—printed handouts, posters, and cards—to help reinforce important messages. Key concepts in teaching parenting skills are listed in Box 24-1.

Box 24-1. Key Concepts in Teaching Parenting Skills

- Be supportive—parents are trying to do what is best for their child.
- Address the parent's concerns—these can be elicited with a question from you.
- Be practical—teach specific skills and techniques.
- Place the behavioral issues in the context of the child's cognitive and emotional development.

Toddlers

At about age 18 months, toddlers begin to develop more autonomy and have a much greater need to explore and to separate from their parents and other caregivers. The verbal skills and physical abilities of toddlers lag behind this newfound need for independence. One result is frustration at this inability to communicate, which occasionally results in tantrums. When toddlers climb furniture, refuse to eat some foods, run around a lot, and generally lack good common sense, parents are left feeling frustrated and frazzled. At this point, two things happen: many parents use corporal punishment, and many have difficulty setting limits of any sort. Both of these responses to the toddler's need for autonomy—lax parenting style and corporal punishment—have been linked to subsequent aggressive or violent behavior.

One key to positive parenting at this stage is to understand that the child still craves parental attention and approval. Perhaps the easiest and most powerful technique to teach parents is the use of positive reinforcement. The clinician should remind parents of the struggle their child is going through and ask them to "catch the child being good." Parents can say, "I love it when you do that" or "What a good big brother you are!" In general, parents should be advised to avoid the temptation of ignoring a well-behaved child and paying attention only when the child is doing something unsafe or undesired. The clinician needs to teach parents to pay attention for the behavior they *want* to see.

Time-out is a natural outgrowth of this approach. When a child misbehaves, the parent or caregiver stops the behavior and ritualistically ignores the child for a brief period, as a consequence of the misbehavior. The key components of a time-out for misbehavior are listed in Box 24-2.

School-Age Children

As children move to the more structured environment of school, the potential for conflict between children becomes much more pronounced. Playground fights begin, and the

Box 24-2. Key Elements of Time-Out

- Time-out needs to be immediate.
- Child needs to know *why* the time-out was given (e.g., "No hitting. Time-out.").
- Time-out needs to be brief (corresponding to the brief attention span of the young child).
- Do not talk with the child during the time-out, even to discuss the misbehavior.

nearly universal phenomenon of bullying appears. These are different phenomena, and a careful history easily brings out the distinctions.

Playground Fighting

Fighting by children generally begins in the later elementary school years. For the pediatric health care provider, the approach is fairly straightforward. The health care provider elicits a story of how the fighting-related injury occurred. The health care provider explores with the child if there would have been a way to resolve the conflict without fighting. It should be emphasized to the patient and the parents that times have changed, and the best protection is to learn how to avoid fighting, rather than being able to win. Children who fight frequently should be referred for further counseling.

Bullying

Bullying is characterized by repeated acts of violence or intimidation by a stronger child inflicted on a weaker one. Bullies often lead a small pack of hangers-on, who reinforce the bullying behavior, while the victims often are socially isolated. Among boys, bullying usually involves physical aggression. Bullying among girls typically manifests as social isolation and teasing.

Bullying occurs at all socioeconomic levels and in ethnically and socioeconomically homogeneous and heterogeneous environments. Prevention of bullying has been the focus of large-scale intervention efforts, and proven anti-bullying programs are available to school administrators.

Victims of Bullies

Often, victims of bullies present directly. A parent may say, "My child is being picked on at school." Bullying also needs to be considered for children who present with school phobia, depression, or a sudden worsening of school performance. Violence of one sort or another often explains the inattentiveness at school of children who do not have a previous history of attentional problems.

It is important to know where and when the bullying occurs. Because the behavior seldom happens in the classroom, parents should be advised to seek the assistance of the school principal or guidance counselor. The clinician must ensure that the victim knows that it is the bully who has the problem—it is not due to any physical or behavioral feature of the victim. The child should be encouraged to make friends either at school or in another social environment. The mastery of a sport, music, or other pursuit may make a child less likely to be victimized or at least more psychologically resilient.

Children Who Are Bullies

Most often, bullies escape direct attention and punishment for bullying at school. When these children do receive the attention of the school administration, however, it is imperative that the school, the physician, and the parents work together to help resolve the bullying behavior. Long-term studies have shown that without intervention, elementary-school bullies are less likely to complete their education, marry (or form other stable intimate relationships), or hold down jobs as adults.

Bullies often are described by their parents as difficult children. The first step is to help the parents establish and enforce simple household routines and rules. Whenever possible, family therapy or parent education programs should be instituted to help with this process. In encouraging this approach, the practitioner should expect some resistance from the child and family. Bullies seldom see the problems in their behavior, and their families often concur. Nevertheless, with support from the schools, simple but effective behavior management programs can be instituted and are likely to benefit the child.

Adolescents

The emphasis on avoiding physical fighting continues through adolescence. There are two new components, however: dating violence prevention and a more conceptual discussion of nonviolent problem solving. The clinician should consider having these conversations with adolescents alone, with the parents excused from the examination room.

Dating Violence Prevention

Although most dating violence involves male aggressors and female victims, the clinician needs to be aware that this is not always the situation and use open-ended questions to elicit a history. All teens need to receive a consistent message that violence is not an acceptable part of dating relationships, and that nothing either partner does, including drinking, using drugs, or infidelity, excuses this type of behavior. Screening for dating violence is discussed in Chapter 235.

Gay, Lesbian, Bisexual, and Transgender Adolescents

Gay, lesbian, bisexual, and transgender adolescents experience violence at rates far higher than the general population. Clinicians and their staffs who care for adolescents cannot assume that all patients are heterosexual. Clinicians should consider including information concerning hotlines or support groups for gay, lesbian, bisexual, and transgender patients along with other materials focused on adolescents and their parents (see Chapter 255).

SCREENING FOR RISK

Other than taking a direct violence history and responding to clinical manifestations of violence, screening for certain overriding risks deserves serious attention. Screening for violence risk is done best in the context of overall anticipatory guidance. Environmental risks for violence—domestic violence, media exposure, and the presence of firearms in the home—may be assessed periodically. Because violence-related injury is related to other risky adolescent behavior, violence history should be a core component of the assessment of risk in adolescent patients.

Television and Media Exposure

Exposure to television violence begins near birth and constitutes the best-studied and most ubiquitous risk for violence in modern society. With an average of 12 to 14 violent acts per hour, children's television is by far the most violent genre of television programming. The average American child, who watches more than 4 hours of television per day, sees greater than 10,000 acts of violence per year. Because television does not require reading—or even words—to make its impression, the violence on television affects preliterate and even preverbal children. Hundreds of studies conducted over decades have established that exposure to media violence increases the risk of subsequent violence. Although other forms of violent entertainment have not been studied in as much detail, it is likely that violent interactive games and movies are similarly unhealthy. Box 24-3 lists possible approaches to reducing television viewing, especially viewing violence.

Domestic Violence

Children exposed to domestic violence experience many direct and indirect effects. Child abuse, depression, posttraumatic stress disorder, and behavioral problems all are associated with domestic violence. In addition, young children exposed to domestic violence are more likely to experience violence themselves later in life, either as a victim or as a perpetrator. (See Chapter 266.)

Beginning with the prenatal visit, the clinician should ask about domestic violence. Some practices place small cards with domestic violence hotline numbers in the rest rooms. The clinician must have access to skilled domestic violence counselors or social workers to help parents who are the victims of violence. The clinician needs to be alert to the possibility of child abuse in families with domestic violence. If child abuse reporting is necessary, the clinician must be certain to discuss the mother's safety with the child protective service caseworker.

Firearms in the Home

The safest home for a child is one without guns. Although many people bring handguns into the home because they fear a criminal intruder, the handgun is much more likely to be used on a friend or family member, often with tragic consequences. The presence of a gun in the home dramatically increases the risk of homicide and suicide and escalates the consequence of childhood aggression. Research has shown that gun safety programs designed to

---

Box 24-3. Counseling Strategies Regarding Television Viewing

- Consider having no TV in your office waiting room, or if there is one, tune into public TV or selected videos. Post a notice: "This TV set shows only nonviolent programming."
- Remind parents that the American Academy of Pediatrics recommends no more than 2 hours per day of total screen time, including TV, videos, and video games.
- Help parents brainstorm other activities for their children, and let them know that the boredom resulting from TV restriction seldom lasts more than 2 weeks.
- Advise parents and grandparents not to place a TV set in the child's bedroom.
- Let parents know that parents who watch TV with their children and discuss with their children the violent messages that they have just seen reduce the risks associated with TV exposure.
- Support TV tune-out weeks and media literacy programs in the schools.
- Discuss the association of excessive TV viewing with obesity and poor school performance.

Box 24-4. Gun Safety Preventive Approaches

- Obtain posters or other information concerning the risks of handgun ownership.
- Ask parents directly if there is a gun in the home.
- Suggest that parents inquire about whether there are handguns in other homes where their children visit.
- In areas of the United States with a high prevalence of handgun ownership, consider distributing gunlocks.

teach young children not to touch guns are not effective. For teenagers, the risks of either serious violence-related injury or completed suicide attempts dramatically increase in homes with guns. Box 24-4 lists preventive approaches for health care providers with regard to gun safety.

Adolescent Violence History

Because of the potential serious consequences of violence, health care providers should consider taking a specific violence history from adolescent patients. See Chapter 235 for further discussion of this issue, including screening tools.

APPROACH TO THE INJURED CHILD

Children and adolescents who have been injured in a fight or by any other violent act face a higher risk for another injury. When health care providers are aware of this risk factor, they can use this occasion to help reduce the risk of another injury. Health care providers can take a history of the incident (Box 24-5), institute crisis intervention if needed, and implement a long-term risk reduction strategy. Successful risk reduction strategies often involve collaborations between physicians, nurses, social workers, community-based organizations, the patient, and the patient's family. The medical record should contain a summary of the cause of injury, who reported the history, and a physical description of the injury received.

Intervention

Generally, injuries treated in the primary care setting are minor and unlikely to lead to long-term disability. The most serious long-term sequela to these injuries may be future injuries. The clinician should talk with the patient about how the fight started, not how it ended. Rather than ask who won the fight, the clinician should ask how the fight might have been avoided. The clinician should inform the patient that although this injury is minor, it is nevertheless worrisome because young people who get in a lot of fights have a higher risk of getting severely injured. Because risk factors cluster, it also is appropriate to ask about other risk factors, especially school success and illicit drug use.

Box 24-5. History of Injury Incident

- "How did you get hurt?"
- "Did you know the other person(s) involved?"
- "Were any weapons involved?"
- "What are your plans when you leave?"
- "Do you have a safe place to go to?"

Implementation of intervention requires forethought. Risk assessment and intervention planning may be spread out between the initial injury visit and subsequent follow-up visits. The assistance of a social worker to gather risk information and to plan an intervention can be exceedingly helpful. Studies suggest that the highest chance of long-term risk reduction occurs when the patient is connected with community-based programs, ranging from mentoring (e.g., Big Brother/Big Sister programs) to after-school basketball. When all staff members are aware of the high risk of reinjury, the patient and the family receive a consistent message about the serious risks of future violence-related injuries that these young patients face.

OTHER CLINICAL PRESENTATIONS

The issue of violence is common enough in the United States that it also needs to be considered in the differential diagnosis of many other chief complaints.

School Dysfunction

Health care providers often assess children who have difficulty in school. Children who experience abuse, threats, intimidation, or physical or sexual harassment often have difficulty focusing on their schoolwork. Hallmarks of school dysfunction caused by violence (or other psychosocial issues) include reluctance to go to school and a relatively sudden or dramatic change in school performance or attendance. Occasionally, patients are reluctant to discuss these issues; however, many willingly volunteer information when asked. The health care provider should consider asking the patient either open-ended questions (e.g., "Why don't you like to go to school? What is the worst thing about school this year?") or more directed questions (e.g., "Does anyone bother you at school? Do you feel safe going to school?"). Further assessment of school dysfunction is best postponed until after any violence or intimidation is addressed.

Other Risk Behaviors

A related concern is that adolescents who are doing poorly at school or who drop out of school—for any reason—are at higher risk for violence-related injury. Many of these young people would benefit from a more complete psychosocial risk assessment and intervention. School failure is one of many coexisting risk factors or risky behaviors that characterize some adolescents. The same group of adolescents simultaneously may abuse alcohol or other drugs, engage in unsafe sexual practices, drop out of school, and get involved in fights. Interventions focused on a particular risky behavior provide an opportunity to screen for and address other high-risk activities.

MOBILIZING COMMUNITY RESOURCES

School Programs

Throughout the 1990s, many school curricula designed to teach conflict resolution or otherwise reduce interpersonal violence were developed and tested throughout the United States. Many of these programs showed modest success in reducing violence-related attitudes and beliefs and, in some cases, seemed to reduce the number of physical altercations observed in school playgrounds. The Centers for Disease Control and Prevention has reviewed many of these programs. Box 24-6 lists common features in these successful programs.

Several programs beyond classroom activities are also effective. Peer mediation offers middle school and high school students an opportunity to resolve conflicts without fighting or losing face and has been shown to be successful not only in the school, but also in the surrounding communities. Well-run after-school programs have the potential to engage young people positively from 3:00 to 6:00 P.M., when risky behaviors often occur. Finally, because students who drop out of school are at the highest risk, programs that seek to reduce dropout rates also may decrease the overall incidence of youth violence.

Other types of school-based programs do not seem to offer significant positive results. Some programs attempt to shock or scare young people by exposing them to the consequences of violence or delinquency, by introducing them to prison or emergency department environments. When used by themselves, these programs have not been shown to work. In all likelihood, the highest risk young people already are well aware of the consequences of violence—often through either personal experience or the experience of a close friend or family member. Many high-risk adolescents join gangs or arm themselves in the mistaken belief that these actions offer improved safety and security. On the contrary, successful programs teach students to learn to channel this fear into prosocial behavior that is likely to reduce their personal risk.

More recently, several computer programs and other screening tools have been offered to help administrators identify adolescents at risk of violence. In general, these tools are borrowed from criminal justice or inpatient psychiatry tools and have not been validated adequately in the general population. There is a great deal of concern that their widespread use would stigmatize some children unfairly without any significant improvement in overall safety.

> **Box 24-6.** Elements of Successful Violence Reduction School Intervention Programs
>
> - Students are engaged actively in creating safe school communities.
> - Role-playing, drama, or other types of activities allow students to rehearse what they would do in situations of conflict.
> - Teachers and administrators model nonviolent conflict resolution.

Mental Health

As mentioned earlier, violence-related issues may be the presenting symptoms of more complex mental health issues. Physician's offices serving children should have resource lists available of counseling centers, social workers, and psychologists who can assist children in trouble. In the case of adolescents, follow-up often is necessary to ensure that the referral appointment is kept.

Community-Based Organizations

Many community-based organizations offer services to children and adolescents ranging from sports to drug treatment. The success in reducing youth violence in many U.S. cities has come from successfully integrating the energy and social competence of these organizations into comprehensive violence prevention strategies. Health care providers serving children may want to find out about these organizations and the services they offer. Many physicians have found more active involvement, often as advisors or advocates, to be particularly rewarding.

SUGGESTED READINGS

Thornton T, Craft C, Dahlberg L, et al: Best Practices of Youth Violence Prevention: A Sourcebook for Community Action. Atlanta, Centers for Disease Control and Prevention, National Center for Injury Prevention and Control, 2000.
Youthwork Links and Ideas: Youth Issues. Available at: www.AAP.org/VIPP.

25 Developmental and Behavioral Surveillance and Promotion of Parenting Skills

Michael Regalado and Neal Halfon

ROLE OF THE GENERALIST

1 Employ a surveillance strategy toward child development and behavior.

2 Elicit and examine parents' concerns about development and behavior.

3 Monitor developmental progress.

4 Evaluate the psychosocial environment and family context.

5 Evaluate child behavior.

6 Evaluate parents' knowledge, skills, and resource needs.

7 Manage common behavioral problems and concerns.

8 Refer to appropriate diagnostic, intervention, or service agency.

9 Monitor and coordinate child, parent, and family service needs.

BACKGROUND

This chapter provides an overview of primary care health supervision activities addressing child development and behavior during the first 5 years of life. This overview considers current guidelines for health supervision, research evidence for the effectiveness of services, and practical constraints in offering recommendations. This chapter provides a general discussion of strategies that have been shown to work and offers some guidelines for organizing health supervision for the individual child and family.

A major challenge for practitioners is to organize health supervision activities into an effective health care strategy. Health supervision guidelines enumerate a comprehensive list of activities to perform at recommended health visits. Few data exist, however, to guide the clinician in determining health visit priorities and selecting specific services (i.e., defining the content of the health visit for the individual child and family). How clinicians address child development during the health visit varies as much as individual children vary in their developmental profiles and clinical

histories and as much as parents vary in their needs and concerns relevant to child rearing.

Despite a long tradition in pediatrics, preventive health care addressing child development has not been particularly effective. Three quarters of children with disabilities are identified after school entry and are more likely to be identified by a nonmedical professional; half of parents or more do not receive basic information about child rearing or developmental topics from their physicians; and identification rates of important, treatable psychosocial risk factors are unacceptably low. Reasons for these deficiencies are not clear. Little effort has been directed toward understanding how the process of health care delivery can support better the development of children.

A significant gap exists between what we know about supporting the development of children and what characterizes the standard of care in pediatrics. Over the past several decades, the role of experience in shaping child development has become evident. *Experience for young children is mediated through social relationships with their caregivers.* From an ecologic perspective, these relationships are influenced by community social structures and by social and economic policy. Health supervision activities intended to promote and support child development must understand and work with the child's social relationships, especially the parent-child relationship, and these activities must include knowledge of the community context and relevant health and social policy.

DEVELOPMENTAL SURVEILLANCE: ROLE OF THE GENERALIST

The health supervision role of primary care providers has been conceptualized in terms of *developmental surveillance* and *anticipatory guidance. Developmental surveillance* emphasizes eliciting and evaluating parents' concerns, monitoring developmental progress, and performing skilled observations in a continuous manner. *Anticipatory guidance* refers to the teaching role of pediatricians and work with families to adopt preventive health practices. A surveillance approach to addressing child development and behavior replaces the more narrowly focused concept of developmental screening, although selective use of a developmental screening test is still an important observation that a clinician may make. The requisite skills to perform developmental surveillance effectively include sound knowledge of child development and of community resources, strong communication and observational skills, and a commitment to providing this kind of support for children and families.

There are at least two other considerations relevant to a surveillance approach to care. First, as in any clinical activity, a theoretical model should guide appraisals and interventions. In the case of health supervision promoting optimal child development, this model should address the significance of the parent-child relationship. Primary care approaches to child development have directed little attention to matters beyond monitoring developmental milestones and providing information or universal prescriptions for a few topical issues. The most significant advancements in this field have been in understanding of the role that experience plays in brain development and the importance of the parent-child relationship to that experience. These are matters that are largely social and emotional, with much effort from parents toward helping infants and children learn to regulate their behavior (i.e., their states of consciousness, emotional responses, attention, and communicative bids) so that cognitive and social experiences are optimized. Health care providers must have a solid understanding of the psychology of the parent-child relationship if health supervision is to be effective. The second issue to address is the scope of clinical care. Important considerations are identification of specific clinical outcomes that providers should strive to achieve, boundaries and relationships between health care and other community service providers, and strategies that are feasible and reimbursable. These are important considerations now that a multidisciplinary expertise has evolved around early childhood care enabling a continuum of care between the health care provider and other community providers.

Evidence

The evidence for primary care activities addressing child development was summarized in a review of the literature. This review was organized around a typology of recommended activities (Table 25-1) from the two major guidelines for pediatric health supervision published by the American Academy of Pediatrics and the Bright Futures Project. Briefly the major findings of the review are as follows:

1. Structured assessments provide valid means for eliciting and appraising parents' needs and concerns, examining the psychosocial environment, understanding child temperament, and monitoring developmental progress.
2. Effective physician teaching should address ways to optimize the parent-child social relationship by emphasizing emotionally and cognitively stimulating social interaction and by considering the child's individuality to facilitate child-rearing approaches.
3. Primary care counseling interventions for common behavioral concerns are efficacious.
4. Care coordination linking the primary care office to developmental services and providers in the community has not received adequate attention.

Assessment Activities

A structured approach to eliciting and assessing parents' concerns about their children's development and behavior has two important effects. First, communication between physician and parent around concerns about behavior and development is improved. For a variety of reasons, most concerns about behavior and development are raised infrequently or addressed inadequately at the health visit. A structured form or questionnaire that raises these issues with parents sends the message that they are appropriate topics for discussion with the physician. Second, the nature and number of parents' concerns are associated with different probabilities of having true developmental problems. Knowledge of these associations provides physicians with valuable information to focus discussion more efficiently at the health visit and to make clinical decisions around the management of developmental concerns.

Other assessments have been developed to identify problems in the psychosocial environment (e.g., maternal depression, domestic violence, substance abuse, housing instability, histories of child abuse), to examine the quality of the home environment to nurture developmental progress, and to examine the quality of social interaction between parent and child. Assessments of temperament help parents understand their child's behavior and are useful in adapting child-rearing strategies. Behavior checklists provide means for identifying significant behavior problems.

Education

A variety of educational activities intended to promote optimal development were identified. Several studies have shown that physicians' teaching efforts can be effective in promoting healthy development regarding many child-rearing topics and concerns (Box 25-1). Effective physician teaching emphasizes parental warmth in social interaction with children, consistency in caregiving approaches, and an appreciation of children's individuality or behavioral style when incorporated into discussions about soothing fussy infants (or infant colic), sleep habits, book-sharing activities, or discipline approaches. General discussions about child development ("what to expect") are not likely to be effective. A potentially valuable approach is temperament-based anticipatory guidance, in which temperament assessments are linked to specific parenting advice to match different profiles. Group well-child care is an alternative format for the health visit that seems to promote discussion of personal issues, parenting, and child behavior concerns in low-risk populations.

Intervention

Physicians are consulted about the management of a variety of behavioral concerns. Infant crying behavior and sleep disturbances are common clinical concerns during the first 5 years. In both cases, counseling parents seems effective in providing guidance for calming fussy infants or in managing night waking and bedtime settling difficulties. The effectiveness of handouts or medication in the management of sleep problems is unclear. Although many other behavior concerns present to pediatric health care providers (biting, temper tantrums, and other forms of aggressive behavior),

Table 25-1. Developmental Services Typology

Service	Timing*			Source
	Prenatal	**Perinatal**	**Postnatal**	
Assessment				
Parental concerns				
Parental concerns assessment				APP, BF
Developmental screening				
Developmental history				
Developmental screening test			1, 3	AAP, BF
Psychosocial risk screening				
Psychosocial history			1, 2, 3	
Psychosocial risk assessment	2	2		AAP, BF
Stress management interview				
Home environment screening			1, 2, 3	AAP, BF
Parent-child relationship				AAP, BF
Parent-child interaction observation				AAP, BF
Behavior concerns		1, 2, 3		AAP, BF
Child behavior problems assessment			1, 2, 3	
Temperament assessment			1, 2, 3	AAP, BF
Education				
Anticipatory guidance				
Optimizing parent-child interaction		1, 2, 3	1, 2, 3	AAP, BF
Temperament-based counseling				
Sleep habits counseling				AAP, BF
Promoting children's learning				
Discipline practices counseling				
Parent education/support groups				
Developmental behavioral brochures		1, 2, 3	1, 2, 3	
Audiovisual materials			1, 2, 3	
Parenting classes/training				
Group well-child care				
Intervention				
Problem-focused intervention				
Office counseling				AAP, BF
Telephone advice line				
Home visitation	2	1, 2, 3	1, 2, 3	BF
Care coordination				
Office care coordinator			1, 2, 3	
Developmental passport/journal			1, 2, 3	
Subspecialist/program referrals			1, 2, 3	
Developmental services resource manual		1, 2, 3	1, 2, 3	
Office tracking system			1, 2, 3	AAP, BF

*Suggested timing of services based on risk status: [1]biological; [2]psychosocial; [3]multiple.
AAP, American Academy of Pediatrics; BF, Bright Futures.

Sources: American Academy of Pediatrics: Guidelines for Health Supervision, 3rd ed. Elk Grove Village, Ill, American Academy of Pediatrics, 1997; Green M, Palfrey JS (eds) Bright Futures, Guidelines for Health Supervision of Infants, Children, and Adolescents, 2nd ed. Arlington, Va, National Center for Education in Maternal and Child Health, 2000. From Regalado M, Halfon N: Primary Care Services: Promoting Optimal Child Development from Birth to Three Years. UCLA Schools of Medicine and Public Health, The Commonwealth Fund, September 2002.

the literature is limited regarding the effectiveness of pediatric recommendations or management in these other areas.

Care Coordination

The management of developmental and behavioral concerns frequently requires other services and the participation of other providers outside the pediatric office. Ideally,

Box 25-1. Areas of Demonstrated Effectiveness of Physician Teaching

- Social interaction with infants
- Temperament
- Healthy sleep habits
- Ways to promote learning
- Use of discipline

practitioners should develop plans for the types of concerns that they can address in the office or refer to the community, which would include services mandated by the Individuals with Disabilities Education Act (IDEA), Title V services for children with special health care needs, early intervention programs (e.g., Head Start and Early Head Start), mental health services, programs/groups for parents, and social services.

The issue of care coordination raises many questions, particularly regarding feasibility, time and labor costs, and boundary issues with other professionals (e.g., developmental-behavioral pediatrics, psychology, and psychiatry). When a developmental problem is suspected, a referral is required to confirm a diagnosis and arrange for appropriate services if indicated. Although a workforce of specialist providers and services can be mobilized, the fragmentation of care that is created frequently leaves families on their own to navigate the system. The process is often stressful for families who are coping with the news or uncertainty of having a child with a disability at the same time. Health care providers can play a crucial role in providing stability, continuity, advocacy, and support through this process by having procedures in place to help parents navigate the various systems.

Applying a Theoretical Framework to Developmental Health Supervision

Effective health supervision should work with and within the rules or code of the parent-child social relationship. A model for understanding clinical issues relevant to the parent-child relationship is needed to guide clinical care. This is a crucial point because the current model that drives clinical care is the disease model, and most developmental issues and concerns are not diseases. Instead, developmental and behavioral concerns organize around a theme of *normative change and adaptation*. Most clinical issues and concerns are not unique to either the child or the parent but pertain to both in a unique relationship. To illustrate this idea, consider the toddler who is having difficulty settling to sleep. A disease model approach would target either the child or the parent, frequently the child, by prescribing a sedative at bedtime or suggesting a child-focused behavioral strategy, such as extinction (letting the child "cry it out"). If the difficulty includes setting appropriate limits to the child's behavior, this is likely to be unsuccessful. Ironically, for developmental matters, a disease model approach is akin to treating the symptoms and not the disease. A "relationship-based" approach would consider the child's contribution in terms of temperament, relevant developmental issues (e.g., autonomy versus dependency), and medical history; the parent's beliefs and practices; contextual factors (e.g., work-related stress); and the history that defines their relationship.

One potential model for this task that avoids the pitfalls of the traditional medical approach examines developmental issues as a framework for understanding adaptation from the perspective of the parent-child relationship. In this model (Table 25-2), development is not viewed in terms of milestones or stages as we typically consider it. Instead the focus is on how well or effectively the parent-child relationship adapts to developmental change in terms of behavioral self-regulation as it moves from *dyadic* (relying heavily on the parent's supportive presence) to *self-*regulation (guided by the child's own cognitive appraisals and internalized standards).

Physiologic Regulation (0 to 3 Months)

During the first 3 months, caregiving is organized around achieving regulation of the infant's physiologic processes. The parent's social interactions and routines assist the infant in regulating activities of feeding, sleeping, and elimination. Caregiving routines that are responsive, contingent, and predictable lead to familiarity on the infant's part and a sense of efficacy in the parent in meeting the infant's needs. Much of parents' efforts are directed at helping the infant maintain stable behavioral states of sleep and wakefulness. As these states become better organized, they prepare the infant for later sustained social interaction and learning.

Reciprocal Dyadic Interaction (4 to 6 Months)

The second 3 months are a period of harmonious and reciprocal social interaction between parent and infant with social exchanges that occur in caregiving activities (e.g., feeding, dressing, diapering, bathing). The parent guides and helps the infant to remain attentive in social interaction, which is important to remaining attentive for optimal learning.

Formation of Attachment (7 to 12 Months)

The second half of the first year is organized around the formation of attachment between infant and parent. During this period, the infant is capable of intentional and goal-directed behavior, while the parent is available to respond when needed. The infant now takes the initiative in social interaction.

Exploration and Mastery (13 to 18 Months)

The infant's exploration and experimentation toward mastery of the environment highlight the next 6-month period. The parent provides a "secure base" for the infant's activity. If the parent consistently provides emotional feedback, the infant explores actively.

Individuation (19 to 30 Months)

The ensuing year is highlighted by individuation (i.e., the emergence of an autonomous, aware self). Parents must set reasonable limits to their children's behavior in a manner that encourages exploration for the sake of learning, while creating a safe environment and teaching acceptable social behavior. The challenge is to set limits and maintain the child's positive sense of self.

Management of Impulses, Gender Role Identification, and Peer Relations (31 to 60 Months)

The preschool period is highlighted by the emergence of self-control. Children develop greater inhibitory capacities (e.g., fewer tantrums) and show internalized standards for behavior (e.g., greater compliance to caregiver). They identify with adult role models whose behavior they emulate.

This developmental framework highlights key themes and issues for the parent-child relationship in a manner that is particularly well suited to health supervision. Anticipatory guidance organized by these developmental issues

Table 25-2. Developmental Model for Parent-Child Relationship

Age (mo)	Developmental Issue	Caregiver's Role
0–3	Physiologic regulation	Smooth, harmonious caregiving routines
4–6	Management of tension	Sensitive, cooperative interaction
7–12	Forming an effective attachment	Responsive availability
13–18	Exploration and mastery	Secure base
19–30	Individuation (autonomy)	Firm support
31–60	Management of impulses, sex-role identification peer relations	Clear roles, values; flexible self-control

Adapted from Stroufe LA, Cooper R, Dehart G: Child Development: Its Nature and Course, 3rd ed, McGraw-Hill, 1996.

highlights the social and emotional aspects in the development of self-regulation, providing a conceptual basis for many topical priorities outlined in pediatric health supervision guidelines (e.g., sleep habits, discipline, and temper tantrums).

Defining the Scope of Pediatric Health Supervision

Several decisions must be made in determining the content of health supervision addressing child development. The scope of clinical care recommended by current health supervision guidelines is defined broadly by the four categories of assessment, education, intervention, and care coordination (see Table 25-1). From these categories, a long and comprehensive list of service choices is generated. Priorities must be set for each family, and some individualization of services has to occur to best meet families' needs around these developmental issues. Determining the content of service provision also requires that health care providers identify their own limitations and individual practice goals for providing developmental care. Developmental services are a high priority for many practitioners. Other practitioners may want to limit their office activity in providing developmental services if they have a high volume of patients and limited office resources. This desire should not limit services to families, provided that there is access to other community resources and providers. If a parent desires discussion about discipline approaches that is more than a practice can provide, the practice may wish to establish a referral link to parenting groups or classes.

DEVELOPMENTAL ACTIVITIES FOR PRIMARY CARE HEALTH SUPERVISION

Assessment at the Health Visit

Assessment at the health visit differs from other assessments of children's development. The term *assessment* is used to refer to the use of skilled observations or validated measures to obtain information about the child and family for monitoring the child's developmental progress and providing assistance to the parent and family to nurture and support their efforts. As much as possible, child assessment should characterize the child's maturational progress and social and emotional capacities to engage the environment. Parents' concerns, needs, and beliefs are important to elicit and understand so that they can be addressed specifically to promote competence and confidence in that role. The environment should be assessed, not only in terms of risks and protective factors that impede or support the child's development, but also in terms of the adaptations made to the child's transactions with the environment.

Structured versus Unstructured Assessments

The clinical interview should provide most of this information if conducted skillfully and if the physician-parent relationship encourages communication around child development concerns. Several tools are available, however, that may increase the accuracy and efficiency of assessment. Theoretical advantages with structured approaches include greater accuracy in identifying problems and consistency in facilitating the discussion of important developmental

topics. Disadvantages include increased administrative work and concerns about legal and ethical issues that may arise with gathering and charting sensitive information. There is the risk of relying too heavily on instruments and using them as a substitute for good communication practices and skilled observations and concerns about how these instruments will be interpreted. Common misapplications of developmental screening tools include incomplete or inappropriate administration and making diagnostic interpretations of the results. The assessments reviewed in the literature for use in pediatric settings *are not diagnostic tools* and should be viewed as adjuncts intended to increase the efficiency and effectiveness of care.

Structured assessments combined with the clinical interview and office observations should help the clinician to make decisions about whether to provide information (anticipatory guidance), help parents with problematic concerns in the office, recommend further assessments, or refer to other specialists for diagnostic assistance and intervention. At the same time, these assessments should help the clinician to comment on aspects of the child's development and parenting that are progressing well and to encourage practices that are adaptive. The following discussion examines specific instruments, their indications for use, and recommendations for incorporating them into an assessment strategy for the office. Table 25-3 presents a suggested timetable for structured and unstructured (clinical interview) assessment of development and behavior issues in primary care.

Eliciting and Evaluating Parents' Concerns

Checklists of common concerns or topics for discussion at the health visit have been developed to elicit concerns about development (e.g., checklists provided by the American Academy of Pediatrics or Bright Futures). A modification of this approach, the Parents' Evaluation of Developmental Status (PEDS), is a 10-item, validated questionnaire that elicits parents' concerns about development and behavior and provides an appraisal of a child's risk for having significant developmental problems. The PEDS elicits parents' concerns about global/cognitive, gross motor, fine motor, expressive language, receptive language, behavior, social, self-help, and learning skills. In addition to evaluating risk for developmental problems, the PEDS helps the physician identify topics of importance to the parent for discussion. It can be administered and scored in less than 5 minutes and classifies concerns in terms of their associated probabilities with developmental problems. A "significant concern" is associated with an increased probability of having a developmental problem. Two or more significant concerns are elicited in 11% of parents, 70% of whom have children with undetected developmental problems. This risk is sufficiently high to refer the child for a diagnostic assessment if the parent agrees. One significant concern is elicited in 23% of parents, 29% of whom have children with undetected developmental problems. This risk is moderate and should be verified by confirmatory screening. Twenty percent of parents have "nonsignificant" concerns about behavior, of whom 7% have undetected developmental problems. The behavior problems of these children should be appraised in some manner, with a

Table 25-3. Suggested Timetable for Assessment of Development and Behavior Issues in Primary Care

Age (mo)	Routine Structured Assessments			Clinical Interview	
	Parent Concerns	Psychosocial Assessment	Other Assessments (Optional)	Behavior/Developmental Progress	Parenting
0–2 wk		Demographic risk Psychosocial risk	CLNBAS	* *	Newborn care Soothing strategies Feeding/sleep
2		Psychosocial risk		*	Psychosocial stress Routines Feeding/sleep
4	PEDS	Psychosocial risk	ASQ	*	Psychosocial stress Routines Feeding/sleep
6	PEDS	Home environment	ASQ	*	Psychosocial stress Discipline Sleep Routines
9	PEDS		ASQ	*	Psychosocial stress Feeding/sleep Dsicipline Book sharing
12	PEDS	Psychosocial risk	ASQ	*	Psychosocial stress Toilet training
15	PEDS		ASQ	*	Psychosocial stress Discipline Toilet training Book sharing
18	PEDS	Home environment Psychosocial risk	ASQ	*	Psychosocial stress Feeding/sleep Discipline Toilet training
24	PEDS		ASQ	*	Psychosocial stress Sleep Discipline Toilet training Book sharing
36	PEDS	Home environment Psychosocial risk	ASQ PSC	*	Psychosocial stress Book sharing Psychosocial stress
48	PEDS	Home environment Psychosocial risk	START ASQ PSC	*	Book sharing Psychosocial stress
60	PEDS	Home environment Psychosocial risk	START ASQ PSC	*	Book sharing Psychosocial stress

ASQ, Ages and Stages Questionnaire; CLNBAS, Clinical Newborn Behavior Assessment Scales; PEDS, Parents' Evaluation of Developmental Status; PSC, Pediatric Symptom Checklist; START, Simultaneous Techniques for Acuity and Readiness Testing.

validated behavioral assessment (see later) if indicated, to determine if the behavior problem is of sufficient concern to warrant a referral. If not, counseling in the area of concern and continued monitoring are warranted. Of parents, 43% have no concerns, and of these, 5% have undetected developmental problems. Routine monitoring and anticipatory guidance is indicated. This process is depicted in Figure 25-1.

Monitoring Developmental Progress

Another approach to identify children who may have developmental problems is the Simultaneous Technique for Acuity and Readiness Testing (START). START uses observations of the preschool child's behavior in the office to screen for developmental and visual acuity problems. The simplicity, accuracy, and efficiency of the PEDS and START make them highly useful adjuncts to clinical care that can be integrated easily into office protocols. They are reliable instruments, require no special training, and can be

administered by ancillary staff without infringing on the clinical interview.

The use of developmentally timed questionnaires that query parents about current developmental function is a third option for monitoring developmental progress. The Ages and Stages Questionnaire monitoring system links parent-reported developmental achievements with the health visit. This system requires more organization in providing the questionnaires to parents in advance of the visit, scoring the forms, and managing the extra paperwork. Its accuracy and supplemental materials (e.g., intervention activities and adaptations for home visits) counterbalance those drawbacks.

Developmental Screening

The Committee on Children with Disabilities recommends that pediatricians use periodic screening to detect developmental delays as early as possible. There are technical reasons to discourage mass screening approaches for devel-

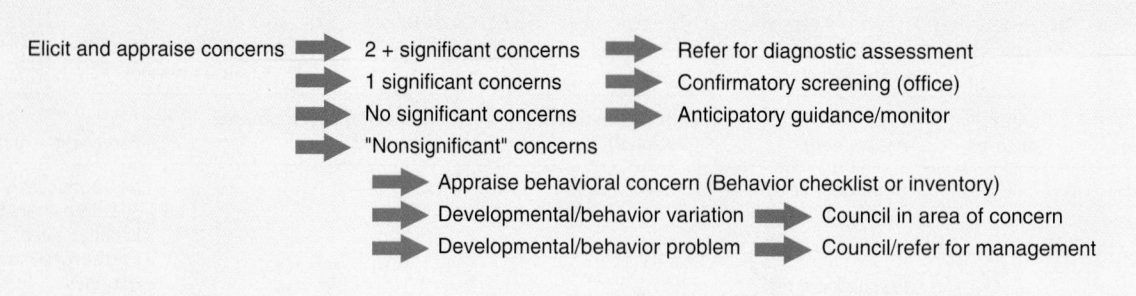

Figure 25-1. Developmental surveillance assessment strategy using the Parents' Evaluation of Developmental Status.

opmental problems, not the least of which is a relatively low accuracy of most screening tools (a sensitivity or specificity of 0.80 is considered "acceptable" for developmental screening tests). The advancements in assessment noted earlier allow for other options, however. The accuracy of the PEDS for identifying children with true developmental problems is comparable to that of lengthier tools (Table 25-4) and probably is increased when confirmatory screening is done with other validated tools for children identified as having a moderate risk. Another consideration in administering screening tests is that the type and timing of screening are associated with accuracy for predicting later school problems. Tests of adaptive and neurologic function at 9 months, 2 years, and 3 years may yield better predictions of later school problems. These two considerations suggest the selective use of developmental screening tools for moderate-risk cases and special populations (e.g., high-risk infants).

Psychosocial Assessment

Assessment of the psychosocial environment has received relatively little attention despite its importance as a factor in child development. Three types of approaches have been evaluated: (1) identification of psychosocial risk factors to parenting, (2) examination of the home environment, and (3) observations of parent-child interaction. The Family Psychosocial Screening Questionnaire seems to improve the identification of important psychosocial risk factors, including maternal depression, parent substance abuse, domestic violence, housing instability, and parental history of abuse as a child. Most of these risk factors can be addressed by social or mental health services. We suggest assessments at birth, 4 months, 9 months, and 18 months (important developmental transitions when environmental stress may be heightened and risk factor screening may be more meaningful to parents), then annually. There are no

clear guidelines for using this instrument, however. The Home Screening Questionnaire (HSQ) examines the quality of the home environment to identify families who may need assistance in supporting their child's development from birth to 6 years. Without any empirical guidelines for using these assessments, we have staggered the HSQ with other psychosocial assessments beginning at 6 months so that anticipatory guidance targeting parent-child activities and early learning (e.g., book sharing) might be addressed. Finally, direct assessments of the parent-child relationship are limited, although measures such as the HSQ provide some insight into this. The Pediatric Review of Children's Environmental Support and Stimulation (PROCESS) combines a 24-item questionnaire that addresses the organization and quality of the child's environment with a 20-item inventory rating observations of parent-child interaction during the office visit. This system has not been widely disseminated, and it is unclear how much expertise is required to administer and interpret this approach. Table 25-5 lists age-specific psychosocial assessment tools.

Behavioral Assessments

Two approaches to assessment of child behavior are available. Both approaches seek to characterize the behavioral individuality of the child to enable caregiving choices that are most responsive to the child's needs. The Clinical Newborn Behavioral Assessment Scale consists of 18 behavioral and reflex items, designed to examine the newborn's physiologic, motor, state, and social capacities over the first 2 months of life. This scale provides a profile intended to promote parents' understanding of their infant's behavior. Temperament questionnaires provide similar information for older children. Temperament questionnaires query parents about typical behavior in a variety of contexts and allow a description of the child's behavioral individuality in terms of different temperamental characteristics (e.g., activity, emotionality). These questionnaires are lengthy and must be used selectively as indicated clinically.

Table 25-4. Selected Development Screening Tests for Confirmatory Screening or High-Risk Groups

Test	Sensitivity/Specificity
Parents' Evaluation of Developmental Status (4–72 mo)	0.79/0.72
Ages and Sages (4–60 mo)	0.72/0.86
Brigance Screens (0–90 mo)	NA
Child Development Inventory (0–72 mo)	0.65/0.67
Early Language Milestone Scales–2 (0–36 mo)	0.91/0.84

NA, not available.

Table 25-5. Selected Psychosocial Assessment Tools

Test	Age Range (yr)
Pediatric Symptom Checklist	4–15
Eyberg Child Behavior Inventory	2–11
Child Behavior Checklists	18 mo–5 yr
Home Screening Questionnaire	0–3; 0–6
Family Psychosocial Screening Questionnaire	Not specified

Physicians can inquire about the child's temperament most of the time with open-ended questions by asking parents to describe their child's personality and how they are managing as parents. Because pediatricians have limited expertise in the evaluation of behavior concerns, determining when a clinically significant behavior problem exists can be a challenge. When this question arises, problem-oriented questionnaires, such as the Pediatric Symptom Checklist, the Eyberg Scales, and the Child Behavior Checklist, provide useful adjuncts (see the references on the CD-ROM).

Education Activities at the Health Visit

Several aspects of anticipatory guidance have been evaluated and shown to be efficacious in narrow contexts, including advice to soothe fussy infants, to help infants sleep better, to discipline effectively, and to promote learning. Incorporating anticipatory guidance about these activities into practice requires more than adding them to the health visit agenda for two reasons. First, there is not sufficient time to address each topic. Decisions must be made regarding what to discuss. Second, the important factor in effectiveness of physician teaching seems to be how well the physician addresses issues relevant to the parent-child relationship. Counseling that does not consider parent-child developmental issues is unlikely to have more than superficial relevance to many families. Eliciting parents' concerns about development and behavior frequently identifies a specific topic of discussion of interest and concern to the parent that can be addressed at the health visit. At the same time, the developmental framework outlined by Sroufe is useful to organize anticipatory guidance around important developmental topics from the perspective of the parent-child relationship.

Infant Crying and Colic

The first 3 months of life is a particularly valuable period for educating parents. Several studies have shown the effectiveness of educating parents about their infant's behavioral capacities in terms of the quality of later parent-infant interaction and parental knowledge and confidence. In general, parents can be guided in responding to their infants in ways that promote self-soothing and stable states of sleep and wakefulness. Beginning in the early newborn period, parents should have some understanding about infant sleep and waking behavior. Neurobehavioral assessment is a particularly effective way to show the infant's self-regulatory capabilities. With an understanding of these capabilities, the parent can know how to help the infant maintain longer states of sleep and wakefulness over time. At the 2-week visit, parents should be encouraged to feed their infants whenever they awaken. Around the end of the first month, feedings can be postponed slightly for a little social interaction with the infant to encourage maintenance of an alert state and stretching out the feeding interval slowly to 3 to 4 hours during the day.

Individual differences in physiologic regulation may make self-regulation more difficult for some infants. Excessive crying is a common behavioral concern that is brought to physicians at this time. Infants who cry excessively and who are labeled "colicky" seem to differ from other infants in that they are more difficult to soothe once they have begun

to cry. That is, they cry as often as other infants do but for longer periods. Conceivably, caregiving challenges with fussy infants could be mitigated in several ways. Neurobehavioral assessment may identify infants who are more difficult to soothe. Psychosocial assessment could identify families more likely to have difficulty providing support or environmental adaptations to cope with a challenging infant. Interventions that minimize environmental stimulation have been most effective in the management of infant colic. One of the difficulties for physicians is that challenges related to excessive crying occur between the 2-week and 2-month scheduled visits. Having this information before that time allows for focused, specific teaching.

Sleep Habits

Counseling about sleep habits builds on the counseling activities of the first 3 months. At the 4-month visit, parents should be encouraged to institute a sleep routine that supports infant self-soothing—placing the infant into bed while still awake and allowing the infant an opportunity to fall asleep on his or her own. Anticipatory guidance at this time coupled with a handout is effective in encouraging this bedtime routine and minimizing night waking at 9 months. The 4-month visit also is a good time to discuss co-sleeping, which many parents prefer for a variety of reasons. Address the pros and cons of this practice in a nonjudgmental way, particularly the difficult issue of transitioning the child out of the family bed later on, and support the parents' decision. Between 7 and 9 months, night waking may occur again, perhaps because of the excitement of other developmental achievements that make it difficult for infants to settle back to sleep. Although parents may feel compelled to intervene, the infant probably will return to sleep if he or she has self-soothing strategies and has practiced settling without parental help in the past. Sticking to a bedtime ritual that facilitates self-soothing is important.

Discipline

Physicians are encouraged to begin discussions about approaches to discipline with parents at the 9-month health visit. The American Academy of Pediatrics policy statement, "Guidance for Effective Discipline," cites three components to effective discipline as noted in Box 25-2.

It is easy to take for granted the first component of the committee's policy statement (i.e., the importance of a positive and supportive learning environment). Most attention has focused on the use of corporal punishment. The quality of the learning environment reflects the quality of the parent-child relationship, however. Parental warmth, affection, and consistency are important in promoting infant self-regulation, secure attachment, exploration, and learning. These qualities also indicate the extent to which parents are emotionally available and able to convey affective meaning to their child around issues of discipline. Sensitive and responsive caregiving helps the infant organize behaviorally at a physiologic level. With the emotional basis for optimal communication in place, teaching from the parent's perspective and learning from the infant's perspective is facilitated. Although conflict is inevitable, its impact and frequency are mitigated when the parent and child communicate effectively.

Although physicians are advised to begin discipline counseling around 9 months, a small percentage of parents will have spanked their infants by this time. Counseling parents to avoid hitting their children is crucial because any corporal punishment is associated with an increased risk of later depression, suicide, aggression, violence, low self-esteem, and negative effects on learning. These risks increase as the level and duration of corporal punishment increase. All parents should be aware of these risks and should be helped to learn other approaches. Parents who report depressive symptoms on psychosocial screening and who express ambivalence, a lack of confidence that they can meet their infants needs, high levels frustration, or aggravation with parenting should receive closer attention and help with child rearing. Although the number of parents who believe that corporal punishment is necessary has declined to about 55% since 1968, the number of parents of toddlers who spank remains high at about 90%; this suggests that many more parents are open to discussions about alternative discipline practices.

Promoting Cognitive Development

Anticipatory guidance promoting children's learning through book-sharing activities seems particularly promising as an educational strategy. Pediatric programs such as Reach Out and Read increase parents' reading activities with their children and promote children's language development. Parents are less likely to read to their infants than to their toddlers, however, finding it difficult and not particularly rewarding. Helping parents to understand their infant's behavior and to interact with them in affectively positive ways that promote sustained states of attention increases the likelihood that cognitively stimulating activities such as book sharing will be positive emotional experiences.

Toilet Training

Helping parents prepare for independent toileting typically occurs in the second year. As with discipline, a strained parent-child relationship is likely to result in difficulty with this activity. Important aspects of facilitating toilet training include discussing with parents their plans for toilet training their child and identifying the child's and parent's readiness. Child readiness issues are listed in Box 25-3. Parent considerations include discussing perceptions and expectations.

Summary of Education Activities

Effective educational approaches to promoting child development share the common characteristic of working to promote a positive and harmonious social relationship

---

Box 25-2. Three Essential Components for Effective Discipline

1. Positive and supportive learning environment
2. Proactive strategy for teaching and strengthening of desired behaviors
3. Reactive strategy for decreasing or eliminating undesired or ineffective behaviors

---

Box 25-3. Child Considerations for Readiness for Toilet Training

- Signs of bladder physiologic maturity (voiding large amounts, remaining dry for several hours, awareness of need to void)
- Motor development (capable walking and sitting)
- Cognitive development (receptive language skills and communicative intent)
- Social skills (dressing/undressing, imitation)
- Temperament

---

between parent and child; this is done most efficiently when a developmental perspective to that relationship is taken. This approach also has the theoretical advantage of enabling selective teaching strategies based on a clearer understanding of the individual needs of each parent and child. Details about the content of developmental anticipatory guidance that were omitted from this discussion can be found in other sources (e.g., NC Center for Children's Healthcare Improvement).

CARE COORDINATION

The coordination of patient care around developmental and behavioral concerns is an important aspect of health supervision. There are no data to inform this aspect of care. It makes intuitive sense, however, that a practice is most effective when it coordinates developmental services from the office with available community supports (see Fig. 25-1). Individual practices should identify what services are priorities to address from the office. Next the practice should examine the community network of complementary diagnostic, educational, and therapeutic services that are available. A systematic approach to linking practices with community resources has been developed by the National Initiative for Children's Healthcare Quality. Steps include (1) determining the needs of the practice population, (2) identifying information about community programs and resources of the practice, (3) assigning a practice community coordinator, (4) selecting a strategy and developing a system for linking with the community, and (5) monitoring the system when in place.

Important resources for developmental and behavioral concerns include early intervention and special education programs (e.g., IDEA), Title V programs (e.g., for children with special health care needs), home visiting programs (e.g., Early Head Start), nutrition counseling programs (e.g., Women, Infants, and Children), preschool programs (e.g., Head Start), parent support services, mental health providers, and social service agencies. Knowing the range of services provided by various subspecialists, including psychologists, developmental and behavioral pediatricians, child psychiatrists, and social workers, also is important.

Many communities and practices have developed approaches to addressing developmental concerns in primary care and systems for coordinating services. The Denver General Hospital and Clinics system and the Healthy Steps for Young Children Program are examples. (See Fig. 25-2 and the text on the CD-ROM for further discussion of these examples.)

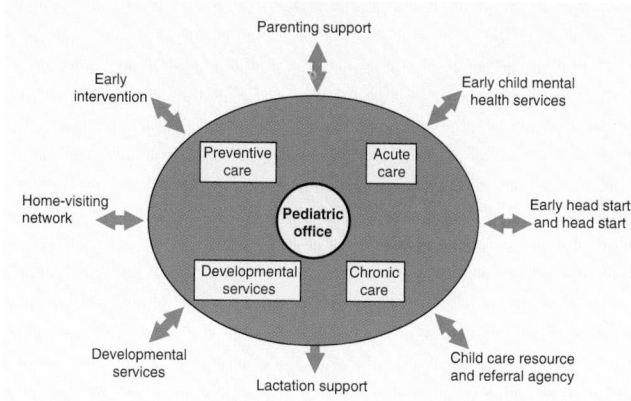

Figure 25-2. Service organization for early child development and parenting.

Mini-index of Related Topics

SUMMARY

This chapter addressed primary care approaches to developmental and behavioral concerns. The concept of developmental surveillance and information from a review of the literature was used to guide strategies for delivering this type of care. Although the literature provides support for the concept of developmental surveillance and the efficacy of many primary care developmental services, no strategies have been proposed for putting a long list of recommended health supervision activities into a feasible, effective model of care. Evidence in this area also highlights the importance of efforts intended to optimize the parent-child relationship. As such, a conceptual model was presented in which understanding developmental issues pertinent to the parent-child relationship was helpful in guiding clinical decisions and care provision. Efforts to prioritize and set appropriate limits to service delivery are needed to create a feasible model of care. Finally, four categories of developmental services were identified with recommendations for *assessment*, a developmental approach to the parent-child relationship relevant to patient *education* and office *intervention*, and considerations for *coordinating care* around developmental concerns.

Additional Resources, CD-ROM

The Denver system	Text, figure
Healthy steps	Text, box, figure
Bibliography	

SUGGESTED READINGS

Achenbach TM, Rescorla LA: Manual for the ASEBA Preschool Forms and Profiles. Burlington, Vt, University of Vermont, Research Center for Children, Youth, and Families, 2000.

American Academy of Pediatrics: Guidelines for Health Supervision, 3rd ed. Elk Grove Village, Ill, American Academy of Pediatrics, 1997.

Brazelton TB: Touchpoints: Your Child's Emotional and Behavioral Development. Reading, Mass, Perseus Books, 1992.

Bricker D, Squires J: Ages and Stages Questionnaires (ASQ): A Parent-Completed Child-Monitoring System. Baltimore, Paul H. Brookes Publishing, 1999.

Committee on Children with Disabilities: Developmental surveillance and screening of young infants and children. Pediatrics 2001; 108:192–196.

Committee on Psychosocial Aspects of Child and Family Health: Guidance for effective discipline. Pediatrics 1998;101:723–728.

Frankenburg WK, Coons CE: Home screening questionnaire: Its validity in assessing home environments. J Pediatr 1986;108:624–626.

Glascoe FP: Parents' concerns about children's development: Pre-screening technique or screening test? Pediatrics 1997;99:522–528.

Green M, Palfrey JS (eds): Bright Futures: Guidelines for Health Supervision of Infants, Children, and Adolescents, 2nd ed. Arlington, Va, National Center for Education in Maternal and Child Health, 2000.

Kemper KJ, Kelleher KJ: Family psychosocial screening: Instruments and techniques. Ambulatory Child Health 1996;4:325–339.

National Initiative for Children's Healthcare Quality: A Practical Guide to Implementing Office Systems for Anticipatory Guidance. 2002. Available at: www.nichq.org/resources/PracticalGuide/030602.pdf.

Regalado M, Halfon N: Primary care services promoting optimal child development from birth to age 3 years: A review of the literature. Arch Pediatr Adolesc Med 2001;155:1311–1322.

Sturner RA, Funk SG, Green JA: Simultaneous Technique for Acuity and Readiness Testing (START): Further concurrent validation of an aid for developmental surveillance. Pediatrics 1994;93:82–88.

SECTION

GENERAL MEDICAL CARE

3

26   Out-of-Hospital Emergency Care

James S. Seidel

ROLE OF THE GENERALIST

1. Prepare outpatient clinics and offices to respond to emergencies.
2. Equip and supply offices for emergency situations.
3. Prepare office staff to respond to emergency situations.
4. Know how and when to access emergency medical service (EMS).
5. Assist local EMS agencies to develop EMS for children within the EMS system.

Box 26-1. Key Components of Emergency Medical Services

- Personnel
- Training
- Communication
- Transportation
- Medical facilities
- Critical care units
- Public safety agencies
- Access to care
- Patient transfer
- Coordinated patient record keeping
- Public information and education
- Review and evaluation
- Disaster linkage
- Mutual aid

The primary care provider is an integral part of the health care delivery system in the community. Out-of-hospital care includes emergency care rendered in offices, in schools, by lifeguards, by emergency medical technicians (EMTs), and by paramedics. To ensure the best possible outcomes, pediatricians must be prepared to respond to emergencies and know how and when to access the emergency medical services (EMS) system. As advocates for the children in the community, pediatricians should assist local EMS agencies in the development of EMS for children (EMSC) within the EMS system.

EMERGENCY MEDICAL SERVICES SYSTEMS

The organization of EMS systems varies throughout the United States. Some communities rely on volunteer EMTs and ambulance drivers that serve all of the EMS needs of a community. Other agencies have combinations of volunteer and paid staff. In some communities, out-of-hospital care is provided by the fire department, whereas in others it is contracted to another public service agency or a private company. The essential components of an EMS system are listed in Box 26-1. The types of EMS providers vary widely. There are four levels of providers:

1. *First responders* are individuals who may be volunteers or professionals from law enforcement units, fire departments, park services (i.e., park rangers), or other public service agencies. They can provide extrication, basic airway support and cardiopulmonary resuscitation, hemorrhage control, and first aid. These individuals usually are the first on the scene and stabilize the patient until EMS arrives.
2. *Basic emergency medical technicians* can provide basic life support and operate an automated external defi-

brillator. In some EMS systems, they also can use an EpiPen (automatic intramuscular injection device to administer epinephrine), give inhaled β-agonists, and administer sublingual nitroglycerin.
3. *Intermediate emergency medical technicians* can start intravenous lines and give certain medications under medical control.
4. *Paramedics* are trained in assessment and emergency stabilization of medical and traumatic illness. They can deliver advanced cardiac life support and administer certain medications for specific conditions. They operate under medical control that may be direct via a radio or indirect by written protocols.

In some systems, emergency nurses and physicians give direct medical control to EMTs and paramedics in the field by radio. They operate under standardized protocols and direct the EMS providers to deliver specific care and destination.

The goal of EMS is to "get the right patient, to the right place, in the shortest amount of time"; this is particularly important for children, who often require specific expertise to care for illness or injury. EMSC is a component of the EMS system that attends to the special needs of children. Ideally an EMSC component provides a seamless system of care from problem identification through out-of-hospital care, to transport to the emergency department (ED) and admission to specialized care and rehabilitation. The care should be integrated with the medical home and be family centered.

EMERGENCY MEDICAL SERVICES AND THE PRIMARY CARE PEDIATRICIAN

Pediatricians should be knowledgeable about the EMS system in their community. Not all ambulances are equipped and supplied for pediatric emergencies. The pediatrician can help the EMS agency by becoming a consultant and ensuring that the minimal ambulance equipment and supplies suggested by the Federal EMSC program are available (Boxes 26-2 and 26-3).

The pediatric protocols that guide field care usually are determined by the local EMS agency. Pediatricians can be involved in EMSC by reviewing these protocols and serving on field treatment committees. There are two types of medical direction. In some systems, all advanced life support runs are directed on-line by medical contact via radio with a physician or nurse at a base hospital. The dialogue between medical control and the paramedics determines the field treatment and destination of the patient. In other

---

Box 26-2. Basic Life Support Ambulance Pediatric Supplies and Equipment

Essential

- Oropharyngeal airways—infant, child, and adult (00–5)
- Self-inflating resuscitation bag—child and adult[1]
- Masks for bag-valve-mask device—infant, child, and adult[2]
- Oxygen masks—infant, child, and adult
- Nonrebreathing mask—pediatric and adult
- Stethoscope
- Backboard
- Cervical immobilization device[3]
- Blood pressure cuff—infant, child, and adult
- Portable suction unit with a regulator
- Suction catheters—tonsil tip and 6 Fr to 14 Fr
- Extremity splints—pediatric
- Bulb syringe
- Obstetric pack
- Thermal blanket[4]
- Water-soluble lubricant

Desirable

- Infant car seat[5]
- Nasopharyngeal airways (18 Fr to 34 Fr or 4.5 mm to 8.5 mm)[6]
- Glasgow Coma Scale reference
- Pediatric trauma score reference
- Small stuffed toy

---

[1]A self-inflating resuscitation bag should be self-refilling, should have an oxygen reservoir, and should not have a pop-off valve. A child bag has a reservoir of 450 mL, whereas an adult bag has a reservoir of at least 1000 mL.

[2]A neonatal mask may be necessary for rescue units that may deliver a premature infant in the field.

[3]Many types of cervical immobilization devices are available, including wedges and collars. The type of device used depends on local preference and policies and procedures. Whatever device is chosen should be stocked in a variety of sizes to fit infants, children, adolescents, and adults. The use of sandbags to meet this requirement is discouraged because they may cause injury if a patient has to be turned.

[4]A thermal blanket may help minimize heat loss. Hypothermia complicates many illnesses and injuries, particularly in infants and young children. The type of material used depends on local preference, protocols, and procedures but may include Mylar, standard blankets, or aluminum foil for small infants.

[5]Infants should be restrained in ambulances. Car seats may be used for medical emergencies or in trauma when the infant already is restrained in a seat and not critically injured. Traumatically injured infants should be restrained on a gurney if they are not already in a seat. Many types of seats are available to meet this guideline. A more recently developed seat is collapsible and easy to store. The type of seat that is procured is determined by local preference, policy, and procedure.

[6]A nasopharyngeal airway may be useful when the upper airway compromises respiration and an oral airway cannot be secured. Providers must be trained in its use and know the contraindications for insertion of this device.

Box 26-3. Advanced Life Support Equipment and Supplies

All advanced life support ambulances should carry everything on the basic life support list (see Box 26-2) plus the following:

Essential

- Transport monitor
- Defibrillator with adult and pediatric paddles[1]
- Monitoring electrodes—pediatric
- Laryngoscope—straight blades (0–2) and curved blades (2–4)
- Endotracheal tube stylets—pediatric and adult
- Endotracheal tubes—uncuffed (2.5–6.0) and cuffed (6.0–8.0)
- Magill forceps—pediatric and adult
- Nasogastric tubes—8 Fr to 16 Fr[2]
- Nebulizer
- Intravenous catheters—16-gauge to 24-gauge
- Intraosseous needles
- Length/weight–based drug dose chart or tape[3]
- Needles—20-gauge to 25-gauge
- Resuscitation drugs and intravenous fluids that meet the local standard of practice

Desirable

- Blood glucose analysis system[4]
- Carbon dioxide detection device (disposable)

---

[1]A defibrillator should be able to deliver 5 to 360 J. The addition of pediatric paddles may give the responding unit enhanced capabilities, but is not essential for units that rarely use this equipment. The defibrillator may be equipped with only adult paddles/pads or pediatric paddles and adult paddles/pads. Units carrying only adult paddles/pads should ensure that providers are trained in the proper use of adult paddles in infants and children. When the defibrillator cannot deliver a low dose of joules for infants, shock should be applied at the lowest possible energy level.

[2]Nasogastric tubes may be useful when the transport time is greater than 30 minutes in patients who have abdominal distention that may impede respiration.

[3]One example of a commercially available item that correlates length with weight to generate accurate drug doses and equipment needed for resuscitation is the Broselow Tape. Other length/weight tapes or charts may be substituted for this device.

[4]Many emergency medical services systems estimate blood glucose in the field. The accuracy of a blood glucose test is influenced by many factors, such as the shelf life of the particular strip used, how the blood sample was obtained, and the education of the providers performing the skill. Quality improvement is an important component of any laboratory analysis and should be applied to this field procedure. Universal precautions always must be followed when handling blood.

---

systems, all field treatment is guided by off-line written protocols that are followed by the out-of-hospital providers. Radio contact is made only in certain circumstances.

Patient destination policies are particularly important for pediatric patients. Most systems transport patients to the nearest appropriate ED. This destination is important for patients needing immediate resuscitation, but it may not be appropriate for some pediatric patients who need a higher level care than can be given at the local ED. Bypassing of EDs for children can be achieved only if the appropriate facility is within a 15- to 20-minute transport time; if this cannot be accomplished, secondary transport needs to be arranged. Pediatricians serving on-call for ED consultation should be involved in the assessment and transfer of children requiring higher levels of care in a neonatal or pediatric intensive care unit. In rural areas, secondary transport usually is required and may be done by land or air transportation. The distance to the receiving hospital, the weather, and the condition of the patient dictate the type of transport used. There are different configurations for EMSC in rural and urban areas.

Office emergencies are common. The average pediatrician has two emergencies in the office weekly, for which office staff and the office must be prepared. Staff should have protocols on how to access emergency assistance through 9-1-1 or another emergency phone number. The pediatrician also should be aware of the capabilities of the local ED to manage pediatric emergencies. If there is more than one ED in the area, the one with the best capabilities for children should be recommended. The Federal EMSC program has a recommended list of minimal ED equipment and supplies (Box 26-4).

All office staff should be trained in basic life support. Physicians and nurses should have training in pediatric

---

Box 26-4. Emergency Department Essential Equipment and Supplies

Essential

Monitoring
- Cardiorespiratory monitor with strip recorder
- Defibrillator (0–400 J capability) with paddles—pediatric and adult (4.5 cm and 8 cm)
- Monitor electrodes—pediatric and adult
- Pulse oximeter with sensors—newborn through adult
- Thermometer/rectal probe[1]
- Sphygmomanometer
- Doppler blood pressure device
- Blood pressure cuffs—neonatal, infant, child, adult, and thigh
- Method to monitor endotracheal tube placement[2]

Vascular Access
- Butterfly needles—19-gauge to 25-gauge
- Catheter-over-needle devices—14-gauge to 24-gauge
- Infusion device[3]
- Tubing for infusion device
- Intraosseous needles—16-gauge and 18-gauge[4]
- Arm boards—infant, child, and adult
- Intravenous fluid/blood warmer[5]
- Umbilical vein catheters—3.5 Fr and 5 Fr[6]
- Seldinger technique vascular access kit catheters—3 Fr, 4 Fr, and 5 Fr

Airway Management
- Clear oxygen masks—preterm, infant, child, and adult
- Nonrebreathing masks—infant, child, and adult
- Oral airways—00–5
- Nasopharyngeal airways—12 Fr to 30 Fr
- Bag-valve-mask resuscitator, self-inflating—450-mL and 1000-mL
- Nasal cannulae—infant, child, and adult
- Endotracheal tubes—uncuffed (2.5–8.5) and cuffed (5.5–9.0)
- Stylets—pediatric and adult
- Laryngoscope handle—pediatric and adult
- Laryngoscope blades—curved (2 and 3) and straight (0–3)
- Magill forceps—pediatric and adult

- Nasogastric tubes—6 Fr to 14 Fr
- Suction catheters—flexible (5 Fr to 16 Fr) and Yankauer suction tip
- Chest tubes—8 Fr to 40 Fr
- Tracheostomy tubes—00–6[7]

Resuscitation Medications
- Medication chart
- Tape or other system to ensure ready access to information on proper per-kilogram doses for resuscitation drugs and equipment sizes[8]

Miscellaneous
- Infant and standard scales
- Infant formula and oral rehydrating solutions
- Heating source[9]
- Towel rolls/blanket rolls or equivalent
- Pediatric restraining devices
- Resuscitation board
- Sterile linen[10]

Specialized Pediatric Trays
- Tube thoracotomy with water seal drainage capability
- Lumbar puncture—spinal needles 20-gauge, 22-gauge, and 25-gauge
- Urinary catheterization with pediatric Foley catheters—5 Fr to 16 Fr
- Obstetric pack
- Newborn kit—umbilical cannulation supplies and meconium aspirator
- Venous cutdown
- Surgical airway kit[11]

Fracture Management
- Cervical immobilization equipment—child to adult[12]
- Extremity splints
- Femur splints—child and adult

Desirable
- Medical photography equipment

---

[1]Suitable for hypothermic and hyperthermic measurements with temperature capability of 25–44°C.
[2]May be satisfied by a disposable end-tidal carbon dioxide detector, bulb, or feeding tube methods for endotracheal tube placement.
[3]To regulate rate and volume.
[4]May be satisfied by standard bone marrow aspiration needles, 13-gauge or 15-gauge.
[5]Available within the hospital.
[6]Available within the hospital.
[7]Ensure availability of pediatric sizes within the hospital.
[8]System for estimating medication doses and supplies may use the length-based method with color codes or other predetermined weight (kg)/dose method.
[9]May be met by infrared lamps or overhead warmer.
[10]Available within hospital for burn care.
[11]May include any of the following items: tracheostomy tray, cricothyrotomy tray.
[12]Many types of cervical immobilization devices are available, including wedges and collars. The type of device chosen depends on local preference and policies and procedures. Whatever device is chosen should be stocked in sizes to fit infants, children, adolescents, and adults. The use of sandbags to meet this requirement is discouraged because they may cause injury if the patient has to be turned.

Note. The equipment and supplies in this box represent a minimum list. An emergency department may choose to modify this list to meet the acuity level of the patient population. Emergency departments that see a high volume of ill and injured pediatric patients may need additional items not on this list. When purchasing equipment and supplies, consideration should be given to the growing problem of latex sensitization of patients and health care workers. The use of hypoallergenic materials for routine and special pediatric procedures is encouraged.

advanced life support. This training enables health care providers to recognize a child in respiratory failure or shock, perform crucial interventions, and transfer to the appropriate level of inpatient care. Courses in basic life support are available through the American Heart Association and the Red Cross. The pediatric advanced life support course is available through the American Heart Association. Having mock codes in which the entire office staff participates in the exercise periodically also helps prepare the office for emergencies.

Pediatric offices should have an emergency bag or cart that contains a length-based weight tape (see Fig. 27-7), resuscitation drugs and fluids, and equipment and supplies (Table 26-1). This bag should be checked periodically, and

all staff should know where it is kept. All offices should have an oxygen source. Office preparation is key to having a good outcome when emergencies are encountered.

Children with special health care needs should have the American Academy of Pediatrics/American College of Emergency Physicians emergency information sheet updated regularly by the pediatrician. It also may be helpful for local EMS providers and EDs to have a copy of the emergency information sheet.

CONCLUSION

Pediatricians and the medical home should be integrated into the local EMS system. Emergencies occur in the field, at school, at recreational sites, and in the office. Pediatricians need to become educated about the local EMS system, how to access emergency care, which EDs are prepared to care for children, and the location of the nearest institution with a neonatal intensive care unit or pediatric intensive care unit. Pediatricians need to know what pediatric equipment and supplies are available in local ambulances. Pediatricians need to educate the office staff in basic life support and pediatric advanced life support and have the office emergency-ready by having equipment and supplies available.

Table 26-1. Office Emergency Equipment and Supplies

	Priority
Airway	
Oxygen and delivery system	E
Bag-valve-mask (450 mL and 1000 mL)	E
Clear oxygen masks, breather and nonrebreather, with reservoirs (infant, child, adult)	E
Suction device, tonsil tip, bulb syringe	E
Peak flowmeter	E
Nebulizer (or metered-dose inhaler with spacer/mask)	E
Oral airways (00–5)	E
Nasal airways (12 Fr to 30 Fr)	S
Magill forceps (pediatric, adult)	S
Suction catheters (5 Fr to 14 Fr)	S
Nasogastric tubes (6 Fr to 14 Fr)	S
Pulse oximeter	S
Laryngoscope handle (pediatric, adult) with extra batteries, bulbs	S
Laryngoscope blades (straight, 0–4; curved, 2–3)	S
Endotracheal tubes (uncuffed, 2.5–5.5; cuffed, 6.0–8.0)	S
Stylets (pediatric, adult)	S
Fluid Management	
Butterfly needles (19-gauge to 25-gauge)	S
Catheter-over-needle device (14-gauge to 24-gauge)	S
Arm boards, tape, tourniquet	S
Intraosseous needles (16-gauge, 18-gauge)	S
Intravenous tubing, microdrip	S
Miscellaneous Equipment and Supplies	
Color-coded tape or preprinted drug doses	E
Cardiac arrest board/backboard	E
Sphygmomanometer (infant, child, adult, thigh cuffs)	E
Splints, sterile dressings	E
Spot glucose test	S
Stiff neck collars (small/large)	S
Length-based weight tape	E

E, essential; S, strongly suggested.

Mini-index of Related Topics CH.

SUGGESTED READINGS

Emergency Medical Services for Children National Task Force on Children with Special Health Care Needs: EMS for children: Recommendations for coordination of care for children with special health care needs. Ann Emerg Med 1997;30:274–280.

Seidel JS, Chair, Committee on Ambulance Equipment, NERA: Guidelines for pediatric equipment and supplies for BLS and ALS ambulances. Ann Emerg Med 1996;28:699–710.

Seidel JS, Knapp J (eds): Preparing the Office, Hospital and Community for Childhood Emergencies: Organizing Systems of Care. Elk Grove Village, Ill, American Academy of Pediatrics, 2000.

27

Resuscitation and Basic Life Support

James S. Seidel

The "chain of survival" for pediatric patients describes the crucial links of primary prevention, early cardiopulmonary resuscitation (CPR), early activation of emergency medical services, early and effective basic life support (BLS) and advanced life support, and postresuscitation stabilization and definitive pediatric critical care. Except for cases of sudden infant death syndrome, cardiopulmonary arrest in children is rarely a sudden event. It generally is secondary to respiratory or circulatory failure. Early recognition and intervention can prevent poor outcomes, which are seen most often in pediatric asystolic cardiopulmonary arrest. Outcomes in children also can be improved if there is immediate bystander CPR and appropriate, early defibrillation. If the child is pulseless and apneic on arrival in the emergency department, survival rate is poor. When CPR is initiated in the out-of-hospital setting, the survival rate is 26% compared with an overall survival rate of 8.4%.

BASIC LIFE SUPPORT

BLS is the support of the airway, breathing, and circulation (ABCs). All health care providers and office staff should have training in BLS. For the lay public, checking for a pulse no longer is suggested when a child is found unconscious. Immediate airway support is indicated using mouth-to-mouth rescue breathing, mouth-to-nose rescue breathing, or a manual resuscitation device (bag-valve-mask device). Health care providers first should look, listen, and feel for breath and begin rescue breathing followed by a pulse check. The pulse is palpated best in the brachial or femoral areas. All health care providers should be trained in bag-mask ventilation. When a patient is found unresponsive, the health care provider should use the following sequence: assessment, ventilation, oxygenation, perfusion, ventilation and oxygenation, foreign body removal, chest compression, and use of automated external defibrillators.

Assessment

The patient is assessed for vital functions (i.e., for ventilation, oxygenation, and perfusion). First health care provider determines if the patient's ventilation is effective.

Ventilation

The health care provider should perform the following actions:

1. Observe for ventilatory effort, increased work of breathing, and signs of respiratory distress
2. Assess tidal volume by observation of chest excursion in older children and abdominal excursions in infants
3. Listen to breath sounds in the axillae bilaterally, then at the base and apex of the lungs

Sounds produced during respiration are caused by turbulence across a narrowed airway and may include gurgling, stridor, snoring, and grunting. Grunting is an indication of partial closure of the glottis during end expiration and is a sign of lower airway disease. Increased work of breathing may be evident by observation of nasal flaring, retractions, and use of accessory muscles.

Oxygenation

The health care provider assesses oxygenation by observing the color of the skin, the nail beds, and the mucous membranes. Signs of peripheral cyanosis include perioral and extremity cyanosis. The tongue and mucous membranes are blue in central cyanosis, a sign of a serious problem with oxygenation. The brain is sensitive to poor oxygenation, and an altered level of consciousness may accompany hypoxia. The child may be lethargic, combative, or unresponsive.

Perfusion

The health care provider should use the following procedures to determine the adequacy of the child's perfusion:

1. Palpation of the pulses peripherally and centrally
2. Assessment of skin temperature and moisture
3. Assessment of capillary refill
4. Measurement of blood pressure
5. Auscultation of the heart
6. Assessment of the mental status

Cardiac rhythm can vary greatly, particularly in young children. Vital signs are age specific, and anxious, ill, or injured patients may have rapid heart rates (Table 27-1). The initial rhythm is assessed with the "quick look" paddles. Bradycardia is an ominous sign that may indicate impending circulatory failure. Bradycardia is precipitated most often by hypoxia or acidosis or both. The status of the patient is assessed along with the rhythm. Ventricular rhythm disturbances may be more common in children than previously suspected. The clinician must remember: *Treat the patient, not the rhythm.*

The clinician continually monitors all patients and reassesses frequently, particularly after any intervention. Pulse oximetry should be used, if available, to assess oxygenation. As mentioned previously, it no longer is recommended that laypersons do a pulse check. A layperson should observe for signs of life, such as respirations and movement. When health care providers take over BLS from a layperson, a pulse check should be performed.

Ventilation and Oxygenation

Airway obstruction in children often is due to posterior placement of the tongue and relaxation of the muscles of the pharynx. The health care provider should use the following procedures to relieve this obstruction:

1. Open the airway with the head-tilt/chin-lift maneuver.
2. If trauma is suspected, avoid manipulation of the neck, and open the airway by using the jaw thrust. An additional rescuer should ensure that the cervical spine is secure during the procedure.
3. If there is adequate ventilation and no evidence or history of trauma, allow the patient to assume a position of comfort, and provide oxygen as tolerated.
4. If there is no spontaneous breathing, begin rescue breathing, while maintaining the patient's airway with the chin lift or jaw thrust.
5. Use mouth-to-nose breathing to provide rescue breathing for infants and mouth-to-mouth breathing for older children. Mouth-to-mask ventilation, using a mask with a one-way valve, is recommended whenever possible for rescue breathing.
6. Initiate ventilation with the use of a manual resuscitator (bag-mask ventilation) and 100% oxygen as soon as possible. A bag with a minimum reservoir of 450 mL should be used even for small infants. If only one pediatric bag is to be purchased, a 750-mL bag is recommended and can be used in all pediatric patients.

The procedure for bag-valve-mask ventilation is as follows. Masks should be transparent and have a small dead

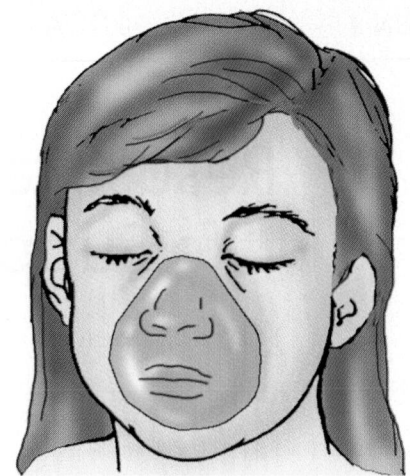

Figure 27-1. Proper mask placement. (Adapted from American Heart Association: Textbook of Pediatric Advanced Life Support. Dallas, Tex, American Heart Association, 1990. Copyright American Heart Association.)

space. A clear mask allows visualization of any emesis. The facemask should be the smallest size that completely covers the nose and mouth and does not compress the eyes (Figs. 27-1 and 27-2). A mask of the correct size is needed to ensure a good seal. Many mask sizes should be available.

Preparation
The health care provider should prepare as follows:

1. Select the correct mask size.
2. Select the correct bag size.
3. Attach an oxygen source to the bag.

Procedure
The health care provider should proceed as follows:

1. Open the airway, using the head-tilt/chin-lift or jaw-thrust technique.

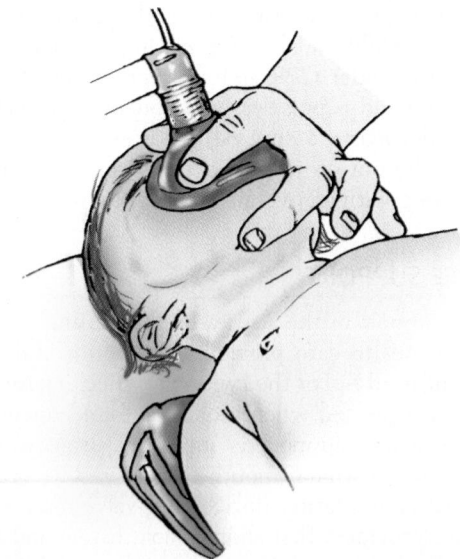

Figure 27-2. One-handed mask grip. (Adapted from American Heart Association: Textbook of Pediatric Advanced Life Support. Dallas, Tex, American Heart Association, 1990. Copyright American Heart Association.)

Table 27-1. Vital Signs by Age

Age	Respiration (breaths/min)	Pulse (beats/min)	Blood Pressure (Systolic) (mm Hg)
Newborn	30–60	100–160	50–70
1–6 wk	30–60	100–160	70–95
6 mo	25–40	90–120	80–100
1 yr	20–30	90–120	80–100
3 yr	20–30	80–120	30–110
6 yr	18–25	70–110	80–110
10 yr	15–20	60–90	90–120

2. Place the patient's head in a neutral position (sniffing position).
3. Insert an oropharyngeal or nasopharyngeal airway, as appropriate.
4. Secure the mask to the patient's face, using a one-handed grip (Fig. 27-3).
5. Push the mask down with gentle pressure to create a seal.
6. Use the last two or three fingers to support the mandible. Place the thumb and first two fingers over the mask to seal the mask to the face.
7. Ensure that the mask is not covering any part of the eyes.
8. Use a one-handed head-tilt/chin-lift maneuver.
9. Squeeze the bag with one hand, maintaining the mask seal with the other.
10. Choose the correct ventilation rate: infant, 30 breaths/min; child, 20 breaths/min.
11. Provide an exhalation time of 1 to 1.5 seconds.
12. Recite the following mnemonic slowly, to ensure adequate time for exhalation: "Squeeze, release, release."
13. Assess the effectiveness of ventilation by means of the following: (a) observation of the chest rise and (b) auscultation of the breath sounds over the lung fields; begin with listening in the axillae.

The most effective method for ventilation and oxygenation using a manual resuscitator can be accomplished by using the two-rescuer, two-handed technique. One rescuer maintains the seal of the mask and head position, while the other operates the bag device.

Complications

When a manual resuscitator is used, there is always a risk of gastric distention, which can compromise lung expansion and increase the risk of vomiting. Pneumothorax can occur with excessive pressures.

The clinician observes the chest excursions and listens for breath sounds during rescue breathing and ventilation with

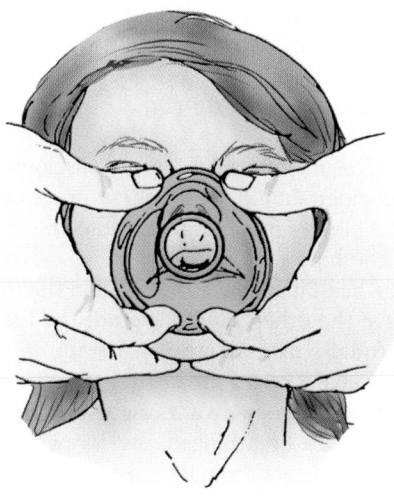

Figure 27-3. Two-hand mask grip. (Adapted from American Heart Association: Textbook of Pediatric Advanced Life Support. Dallas, Tex, American Heart Association, 1990. Copyright American Heart Association.)

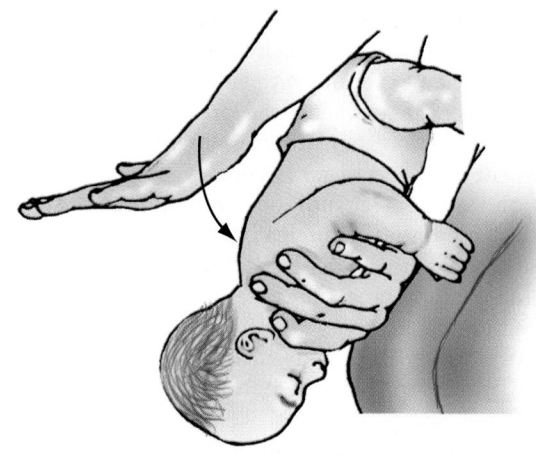

Figure 27-4. Back blows to dislodge a foreign body. (Adapted from American Heart Association: Textbook of Pediatric Advanced Life Support. Dallas, Tex, American Heart Association, 1990. Copyright American Heart Association.)

a bag-valve-mask. Improper opening of the airway is the most frequent cause of airway obstruction in an unconscious patient. If ventilation is difficult or ineffective or both, the clinician repositions the airway. If ventilation continues to be difficult, the clinician should consider the presence of a foreign body and initiate intervention for foreign body removal.

Foreign Body Removal

More than 90% of the deaths from foreign bodies are in children younger than 5 years of age. Prehospital care providers must be experienced in the maneuvers to remove foreign material from the airway. Commonly ingested objects include food such as hot dogs, balloons, and small toy parts. The prehospital care provider should consider removal of a foreign body from the airway, when the event has been witnessed, if there are persistent signs of complete airway obstruction that cannot be cleared with repositioning the airway or if there is the sudden onset of respiratory distress associated with coughing, gagging, or stridor. If the patient has no respiratory distress and can cough or speak, foreign body removal can be deferred until arrival at the hospital. Maneuvers that are suggested to remove a foreign body from the airway include back blows, chest thrusts, and abdominal thrusts, depending on the age of the child.

Removal of a Foreign Body from an Infant

To clear a foreign body from an infant less than 1 year of age, the health care provider should follow these procedures:

1. Hold the infant with the abdomen resting your forearm, with the head in a dependent position and your forearm resting on your thigh. Support the infant's head by holding the jaw.
2. Deliver five blows, using the heel of the hand, to the middle of the back between the shoulder blades (Fig. 27-4).
3. After delivering the back blows, gently turn the infant by sandwiching the body between two hands, ensuring that one hand still supports the head and jaw.
4. If the foreign body has not been expelled, execute five chest compressions, using two fingers on the lower third

of the sternum (one fingerbreadth below the nipple line). Chest thrusts are delivered at a rate of approximately one per second with enough force to create an artificial cough to dislodge the foreign object (Fig. 27-5).

5. Remove the foreign material if observed in the mouth. Do not use blind finger sweeps.
6. If the airway remains obstructed, repeat steps 1 through 6 until the foreign body is expelled.

If the infant becomes unconscious, the health care provider should follow these procedures:

1. Position the airway.
2. Look for a foreign body in the mouth and pharynx and, if observed, remove it.
3. Attempt rescue breathing.
4. If rescue breathing is unsuccessful, reposition the airway and reattempt ventilation.
5. If ventilation is unsuccessful, give five back blows and five chest thrusts.
6. Look for a foreign body in the mouth and pharynx and, if present, remove it.
7. If ventilation continues to be impaired, initiate advanced airway management.

Removal of a Foreign Body from a Conscious Child

To remove a foreign body from a conscious child, the health care provider should follow these procedures:

1. Stand behind the child and place the arms under the axillae of the child, encircling the body (Fig. 27-6).
2. Make a fist with your hand and place the thumb side of the fist against the child's abdomen in the midline just above the navel. Avoid placing the hands near the xiphoid process, which is at the lower end of the sternum.
3. Grasp the fist with the other hand, and give a series of upward thrusts.
4. Each thrust should be a separate, distinct movement avoiding the upper part of the abdomen. Pressure

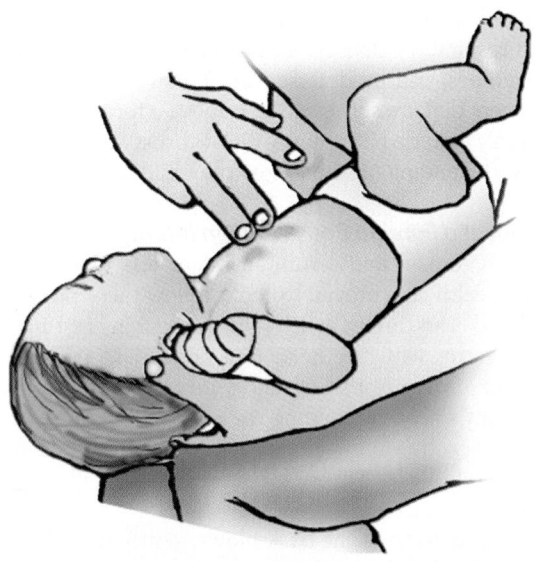

Figure 27-5. Chest thrusts to dislodge a foreign body. (Adapted from American Heart Association: Textbook of Pediatric Advanced Life Support. Dallas, Tex, American Heart Association, 1990. Copyright American Heart Association.)

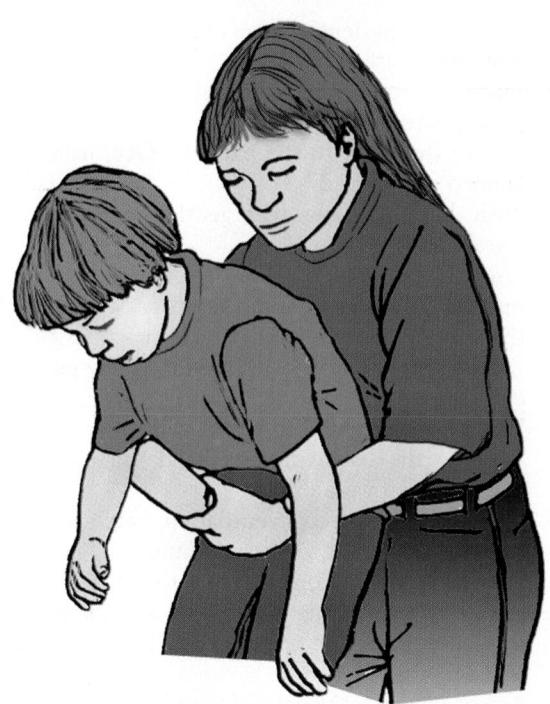

Figure 27-6. Abdominal thrust technique for conscious foreign body removal. (Adapted from American Heart Association: Textbook of Pediatric Advanced Life Support. Dallas, Tex, American Heart Association, 1990. Copyright American Heart Association.)

applied to this area may cause damage to the internal organs.

5. Continue the sequence of five abdominal thrusts until the foreign body has been dislodged or the child loses consciousness.

If there is loss of consciousness, the health care provider should follow these procedures:

1. Open the airway and look in the mouth and pharynx for a foreign body. If present, remove it.
2. Perform rescue breathing. Position the airway in a neutral position.
3. If the child's level of consciousness does not improve, follow the procedures for removal of a foreign body from an unconscious child listed next.

Removal of a Foreign Body from an Unconscious Child

To remove a foreign body from an unconscious child, the health care provider should follow these procedures:

1. Place the child supine, and straddle the child at the level of the hips.
2. Place one hand just above the navel in the midline and then place the other hand on top of the fist.
3. Give a quick upward thrust to the abdomen. If necessary, give a series of thrusts.
4. Remove the foreign body if it can be seen in the mouth.
5. Perform rescue breathing if the foreign body is not removed by the abdominal thrusts.
6. If unsuccessful, begin CPR.

Blind finger sweeps are not recommended because they may push the foreign material into the airway. If the foreign body is in the upper airway (mouth or pharynx), the clinician may attempt to remove the material with pediatric Magill forceps.

Chest Compression
If signs of circulation are absent or the heart rate is less than 60 beats/min and the child shows signs of poor perfusion, the health care provider should initiate chest compression.

Infant
The two-thumb hand encircling technique is now the preferred method for chest compressions in an infant. The health care provider places two thumbs in the midline just below the nipple line and encircles the chest with the hands. The lateral walls of the chest should not be compressed with the hands. Chest compressions are delivered on the sternum with the two thumbs. If the infant is too large for this technique, the two-finger method should be used. The health care provider places two or three fingers one fingerbreadth below the intermammary line. The sternum is compressed to a relative depth of approximately one third to one half the anterior-posterior diameter of the chest at a rate of at least 100 times per minute. In newborns, one third of the diameter of the chest is compressed. Adequate compressions should generate a pulse.

Child
The health care provider places the heel of the hand one fingerbreadth above the intersection of the ribs and sternum. The sternum is compressed to a relative depth of approximately one third to one half the anterior-posterior diameter of the chest at a rate of 100 times per minute. For all patients, the health care provider should ensure that each compression and relaxation phase is of equal length and that the fingers or hand is not removed from the chest during the relaxation phase of chest compressions. Compressions and ventilation should be coordinated in a 5:1 ratio. In children older than 8 years of age, the ratio is 15 compressions to 2 ventilations.

Use of Automated External Defibrillators
The use of automated external defibrillators is now recommended in children older than 8 years of age who are in cardiopulmonary arrest. Collapse in this age group is associated with ventricular rhythm disturbances, which can be treated successfully with electrical shocks to convert the rhythm. These devices cannot be used in younger children because the minimum voltage dispensed might damage the myocardium of a small child permanently. If the child is in standing water, the health care provider should remove the child from the water, dry the child, and apply the pads of the automated external defibrillator. The health care provider should not use an automated external defibrillator over an implanted defibrillator/pacemaker and should not place the pads over transdermal medication patches.

PEDIATRIC ADVANCED LIFE SUPPORT
Pediatric advanced life support involves advanced airway management, obtaining vascular access, the use of drugs for cardiopulmonary arrest and rhythm disturbances, and postresuscitation care.

Advanced Airway Management
Endotracheal intubation is the best way to manage the airway during cardiopulmonary arrest. Only an experienced provider should perform endotracheal intubation. The indications for endotracheal intubation include the following:

1. Need for assisted ventilation to maintain effective alveolar gas exchange
2. Inadequate central nervous system control of ventilation resulting in apnea or inadequate respiratory effort
3. Excessive work of breathing leading to fatigue
4. Lack of airway protective reflexes
5. Airway obstruction
6. Control of the airway during procedures or for diagnostic studies

The endotracheal tube (ETT) size is estimated by matching the diameter of the ETT to the width of the nail of the fifth finger. Alternatively, the following formula can be used:

$$4 + \text{(the patient's age)}/4$$

A tape that correlates weight with length and gives fairly precise sizes of supplies, including ETT sizes, and appropriate drug doses is commercially available (Broselow Tape, Vital Signs Corporation) (Fig. 27-7). One ETT size larger and one ETT size smaller than the one estimated always should be immediately available (Table 27-2). A straight Miller laryngoscope blade is generally used for pediatric intubation. Cricoid pressure (the Sellick maneuver) during intubation may help visualize the airway and prevent regurgitation of stomach contents. A tonsil tipped suction device and an appropriate-sized suction catheter should be readily available during intubation. If cervical spine trauma is a concern, an assistant should maintain in-line stabilization during the intubation; traction or movement of the neck should be avoided. Tube placement is verified by clinical examination: The health care provider listens for equal breath sounds in the axillae and observes a good chest rise with ventilation. A chest radiograph or direct visualization through a laryngoscope confirms proper ETT placement.

End-tidal carbon dioxide monitoring using a disposable colorimetric device may be used for confirmation of ETT placement. The color should change from purple to yellow with ventilation. A yellow color change during resuscitation means there is carbon dioxide production, a purple color means there is no carbon dioxide production, and a tan color means the clinician needs to consider whether there is a problem with the tube or equipment. Good color change during CPR confirms proper tube placement. A negative test may indicate a misplaced tube or poor perfusion.

Fluid Administration
If shock and circulatory collapse are the primary cause of cardiopulmonary arrest, the health care provider should rapidly infuse an initial volume expansion of 20 mL/kg of isotonic crystalloid. The type of fluid used—lactated Ringer's solution or normal saline—depends on institutional preference (see Chapters 28 and 42).

Rhythm Disturbances
The rhythms commonly seen in pediatric patients can be divided into three categories: slow, fast, and nonperfusing or collapse rhythms. The health care provider needs to

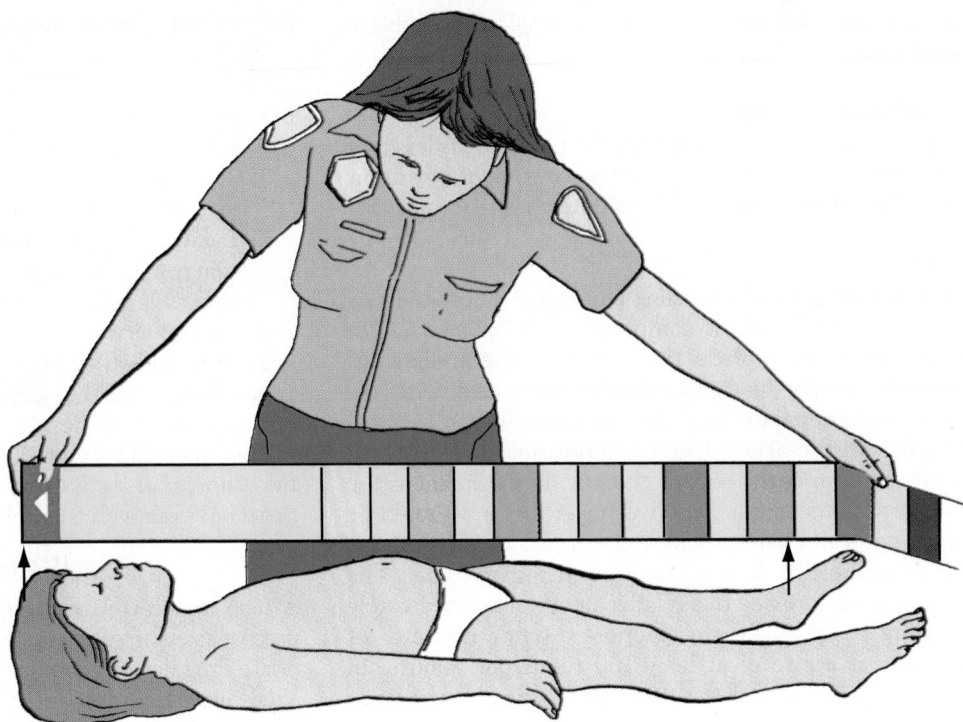

Figure 27-7. Use of the Broselow weight/length–based tape.

determine the configuration of the cardiac rhythm. Unstable or collapse rhythms need to be treated. Treatment of acute rhythm disturbances is discussed in Chapter 59 and on the CD-ROM.

Collapse Rhythms
Asystole

Asystole is treated with ventilation, oxygenation, and chest compression. Vascular access should be achieved rapidly by means of a peripheral vein or intraosseous routes. Until vascular access is achieved, drugs may be given through the ETT, including lidocaine, epinephrine, atropine, and naloxone. The drug may be instilled directly into the ETT and followed by a flush of 2 mL of saline. The exact doses of drugs for ETT instillation have not been determined;

however, high-dose epinephrine should be used: 0.1 mg/kg (0.1 mL/kg of a 1:1000 solution). When vascular access has been established, epinephrine, 0.01 mg/kg (0.1 mL/kg of a 1:10,000 solution) intravenously or intraosseously, is given every 3 to 5 minutes.

Pulseless Ventricular Tachycardia and Ventricular Fibrillation

Pulseless ventricular tachycardia and ventricular fibrillation are seen most commonly in patients with submersion injuries, in patients who have had cardiac surgery, and in patients with congenital heart disease. These rhythms are more common than previously thought and may be seen in the field. The complexes are fast, wide, and irregular (Fig. 27-8). The clinician should perform CPR on any patient with a nonperfusing ventricular rhythm and immediately defibrillate with 2 J/kg for the first energy dose and 4 J/kg for all subsequent doses. The patient is assessed after each countercurrent shock for the rhythm and a pulse. If there is no return to spontaneous circulation after the first three defibrillation cycles, the clinician should give epinephrine at the standard dose intravenously or intraosseously (0.1 mL/kg of a 1:10,000 solution) and defibrillate again. If pulseless ventricular tachycardia and ventricular fibrillation continues after repeated shocks, the clinician should give amiodarone, 5 mg/kg by rapid bolus, followed by another defibrillation attempt. Amiodarone does not terminate ventricular fibrillation but can prevent recurrence after defibrillation. If a pulse returns, give lidocaine, 1 mg/kg; this may be repeated as necessary for a total dose of 3 mg/kg. Bretylium no longer is recommended because of the lack of evidence of effectiveness and the significant risk of hypotension. Lidocaine also no longer is considered a first-line drug for shock-resistant ventricular tachycardia and ventricular fibrillation but may be

Table 27-2. Guidelines for Endotracheal Tube and Suction Catheter Sizes

Age	Weight (kg)	ETT Size (mm)*	Suction Catheter Size (Fr)
Premature infant	<1000 g	2.5	5
	1–2	3.0	6–8
Newborn	2–3	3.0–3.5	6–8
Newborn–1 mo	3–4	3.5–4.0	8
1–6 mo	4–8	3.5–4.5	8–10
6–12 mo	6–12	4.0–4.5	8–10
18 mo	10–12	4.0–4.5	8–10
3 yr	12–16	4.5–5.0	10
6 yr	18–25	5.0	10
8 yr	22–32	5.5–6.0	10
10 yr	25–40	5.5–6.0	10
12 yr	40–50	6.0–6.5	10
15 yr	48–70	6.5–8.0	10–14

*Tubes 2.5-6.0 uncuffed.
EET, endotracheal tube.

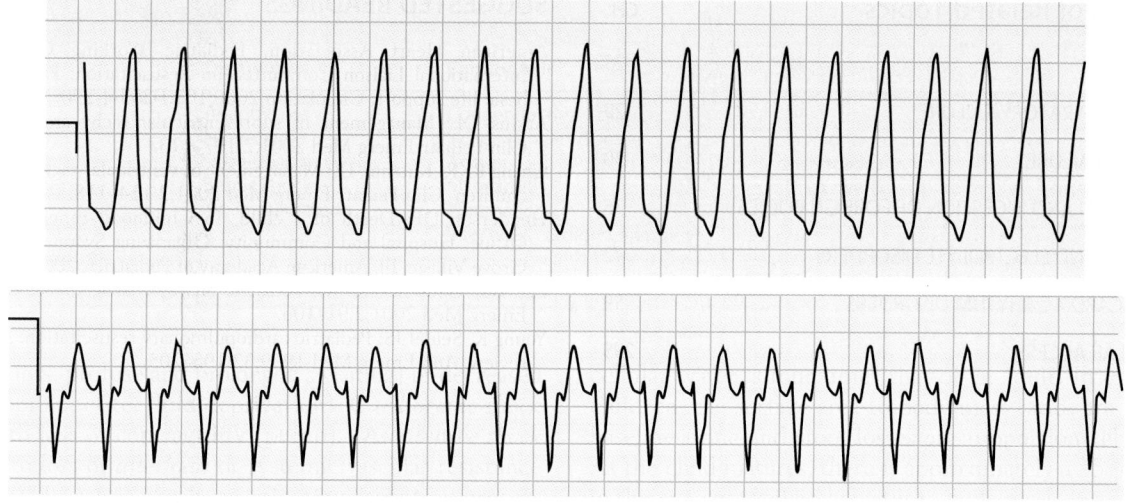

Figure 27-8. Electrocardiogram of ventricular tachyarrhythmia. (Courtesy of T. Knilans, MD, Cincinnati Children's Hospital Medical Center.)

considered in this setting. High-dose epinephrine also can be considered.

Pulseless Electrical Activity

Pulseless electrical activity is by definition electrical activity of the heart that does not generate a perfusing pulse. The complexes may be slow or fast but generally are wide and of lower voltage than normal. This rhythm is seen most commonly with trauma. When a clinician sees pulseless electrical activity, he or she should think of the following treatable causes, the four *t*s and the four *h*s: tension pneumothorax, pericardial *t*amponade, pulmonary *t*hromboembolus, *t*oxins, *h*ypovolemia, *h*ypoxia, *h*ypothermia, and *h*ypokalemia. These rhythms may be reversed to normal activity with a pulse when the underlying cause is treated.

The clinician should assess the patient carefully and perform appropriate maneuvers.

Postresuscitation Care

Careful attention should be directed toward continuous monitoring and stabilization. The health care provider should assess the ABCs frequently. The health care provider should ensure the patient is kept normothermic and is not hypoglycemic. All pediatric patients who have had a cardiopulmonary arrest with return to spontaneous circulation should be cared for in a pediatric intensive care unit. Transport to a tertiary care facility should be arranged whenever possible to avoid secondary complications.

Medications

Table 27-3 lists resuscitation medications.

Parental Presence for Cardiopulmonary Resuscitation

Many studies have shown that parents prefer to be in the room during CPR. Although this situation may cause great anxiety for the medical staff, parents do not get in the way and do not become a burden if there is a protocol in place and they are "chaperoned" during the CPR. Most family members who have been present during CPR state that even if the patient does not survive, they feel that being in the room helped them and the patient cope with the situation. It also made subsequent grieving easier, knowing what occurred. Contrary to common fears, having family members present does not generate more liability claims.

Table 27-3. Drugs for Resuscitation

Drug	Dosage	Quantity/Other
Epinephrine	Asystole—0.01 mg/kg IV/IO Tracheal—0.1 mg /kg	mL/kg 1:10,000 0.1 mL/kg 1:1000 Repeat every 3–5 min Consider high dose: 0.1–0.2 mg/kg
Atropine	0.02 mg/kg IV/IO/IT	Minimum 0.2 mg
Glucose	0.5–1.0 g/kg IV/IO	1–2 mL/kg D50W or 2–4 mL/kg D25W or 5–10 mL/kg D10W
Sodium bicarbonate	1 mEq/kg IV/IO	1 mL/kg
Lidocaine	1 mg/kg IV/IO	
Calcium chloride	20 mg/kg IV/IO	
Amiodarone	5 mg/kg IV/IO	Infuse over 20–60 min
Adenosine	0.1 mg/kg IV	Maximum 12 mg
Naloxone	<5 yr or 20 kg: 0.1 mg/kg >5 yr: 2 mg IV/IO/IT	
Defibrillation	2 J/kg 4 J/kg on repeat	

D10W, D25W, D50W, 10%, 25%, 50% dextrose in water; IO, intraosseous; IT, intratracheal; IV, intravenous.

Modified from American Heart Association and American Academy of Pediatrics: PALS Provider Manual. Dallas, Tex, American Heart Association, 2002.

Additional Resources, CD-ROM

Vascular access	Text, figures
Rhythm disturbances	Text, figures

Table 28-4. Adrenergic Drugs

Drug	Dose Range (µg/kg/min)	Receptors	Use	Risk
Dopamine	2–20	α, β, dopamine	Renal effects, early inotropy needs, septic shock	Peripheral vasoconstriction
Dobutamine	3–20	β_1 primarily	Contractility	Tachycardia, vasodilation
Epinephrine	0.01–2	β > α, but both	Contractility vasoconstriction (higher doses)	Tachycardia, vasodilation
Milrinone	0.3–0.7	Phosphodiesterase inhibitor	Inotropy, vasodilation	Tachycardia, vasodilation

deficit signifying tissue hypoperfusion, decreased mixed venous oxygen saturation on venous blood gas, and electrolyte abnormalities related to the cause of shock.

In hypovolemic shock, findings on the physical examination include dry mucous membranes, absent tears, decreased urine output, poor perfusion, delayed capillary refill, diminished peripheral pulses, and poor color. Diagnostic studies in hypovolemic shock include increased blood urea nitrogen and, to a lesser extent, increased creatinine; small cardiac silhouette on chest x-ray; and low central venous pressure. Pertinent history with cardiogenic shock includes congenital heart disease, recent cardiac surgery, other diseases associated with cardiac problems (e.g., Duchenne's muscular dystrophy), and recent viral infection. The physical examination may reveal a heart murmur, especially with new, extra heart sounds, such as a gallop and a friction rub. Diagnostic studies may reveal a large cardiac silhouette or pulmonary edema on chest x-ray, increased troponin if an infection is present, and elevated central venous pressure. In distributive shock, the history may include a recent allergic exposure (beesting, peanuts, other agent with prior history of severe reaction) or traumatic or surgical spinal cord injury. The physical examination reveals bounding pulses, well-perfused skin, and low blood pressure requiring large volumes of fluid. Clues in the history for septic shock include immune suppression, fever, and exposure to infectious agents. Pertinent findings on physical examination include initially bounding pulses, fever, and poor perfusion. Laboratory values include high or low white blood cell count and coagulopathy.

MANAGEMENT

Management always starts with the ABCs (airway, breathing, and circulation). The need to establish an airway varies depending on the cause of shock. Patients may need intubation or other respiratory support, particularly to help manage a prolonged metabolic acidosis. Oxygen therapy should be instituted even though oxygen saturation may be normal.

After securing the airway and ensuring that ventilation is adequate, volume should be administered. Preload (volume) replacement must be made with isotonic and usually iso-oncotic fluids. Normal saline is the preferred solution because of its wide availability. The initial volume must be at least 20 mL/kg; in most cases of early shock, it takes more volume than this to correct deficits. There is no need to be hesitant initially with fluids. For later fluid resuscitation, losses should be replaced with the specific isotonic/iso-oncotic fluid that is needed, such as packed red blood cells for hemorrhage or fresh frozen plasma; 5% albumin also is appropriate. Fluid should be given through the largest bore intravenous line obtainable, but any intravenous line would work. An intraosseous line also can be used. A central line is another option if it is available. Patients who are not responsive to 60 mL/kg over 30 to 45 minutes have refractory shock, and the next intervention may include boluses using 5% albumin or pressors or both.

Special situations warrant consideration. In hypernatremic dehydration, the initial resuscitation is identical to that for isonatremic dehydration. The fluid deficit should be replaced slowly over 48 hours. Although there are controversial issues in the treatment of hypernatremic dehydration, several principles are agreed on: the need for careful, frequent monitoring of serum sodium and osmolarity; the need to decrease serum sodium slowly (1 mEq/hr); and the need to monitor the patient closely for changes in mental status or the occurrence of seizures. Complications before therapy include the risk for intracerebral thrombosis from dehydration or hemorrhage from rupture of the bridging vessels of the subarachnoid and subdural spaces when the central nervous system volume contracts. Patients are at risk for cerebral edema during the resuscitation and rehydration phase as the extracellular fluid osmolarity decreases and fluid is shifted intracellularly.

Hyponatremic dehydration is another special situation that requires close treatment and monitoring. The initial resuscitation is the same as for isotonic dehydration except

Table 28-5. Vasoconstrictive Agents

Drug	Dose Range (µg/kg/min)	Receptor Activity	Use	Risk
Dopamine	2–20	α, β, dopamine	Renal effects, early inotropy needs, septic shock	Peripheral vasoconstriction
Epinephrine	0.01–2	β > α	Anaphylaxis, cardiogenic shock	Ischemia, hypertension
Norepinephrine	0.05–1	α > β	Severe vasodilation, hypotension	Acidosis from poor perfusion, ischemic injury
Phenylephrine	0.1–0.5	α selective	Severe hypotension, tetralogy of Fallot spells	Acidosis, ischemic injury

Table 28-6. Vasodilator Agents

Drug	Dose Range (µg/kg/min)	Site of Action	Use	Risk
Nitroprusside	0.3–7	Arteries > veins	Afterload reduction	Cyanide toxicity, hypotension
Nitroglycerin	0.5–5	Venodilation and dilation of coronary arteries	Preload and afterload reduction, coronary vasospasm	Hypotension, methemoglobinemia

if children are having seizures or are unresponsive to normal saline boluses. For these patients, 3% normal saline is given in 5 mL/kg boluses until the seizure stops. Each bolus should increase the plasma sodium by 5 mEq/L. The specifics of the rate of correction and the sodium concentration of the replacement fluid often are debated, but close monitoring and slow correction is the usual choice. Central pontine myelinosis is at least a theoretical complication associated with the rapid correction of hyponatremia.

After fluid resuscitation is addressed, cardiac contractility should be assessed. In theory, the stronger the contraction, the greater the pulse pressure and the potential for pumping greater amounts of fluid. The main pathway of action is through adrenergic receptors. There are two types of adrenergic receptors: α and β. α receptors are found in the peripheral vasculature. Stimulation of these receptors causes vasoconstriction. There are two types of β receptors: β_1 and β_2. β_1 receptors are found in the myocardium and when stimulated improve inotropy and chronotropy. β_2 receptors are found in the lungs and peripheral vasculature. When stimulated, they cause smooth muscle relaxation, vasodilation, and bronchodilation. Table 28-4 lists adrenergic drugs and their actions.

Afterload and systemic vascular resistance also can be changed. *Systemic vascular resistance* refers to vascular tone, whereas *afterload* refers to the force against which the heart must pump. This force includes stenotic valves or other outflow obstructions and vascular tone. In some ways,

systemic vascular resistance and vascular tone can counteract each other. Decreases in afterload decrease the amount of work against which the heart must pump. As a result, cardiac output increases, as does blood pressure. Commonly, afterload is decreased by inducing vasodilation, and blood pressure decreases. Table 28-5 lists doses of vasoconstrictive agents, their use, and their risks. Table 28-6 lists vasodilator agents. Table 28-7 provides a summary of treatment of shock.

OUTCOME

Shock is an evolving process that is a symptom of other clinical conditions. Children in shock are critically ill and at risk for progression to multiorgan failure and death. Prognosis depends on how early shock is recognized and treated and on the underlying cause. Prompt, appropriate therapy has a significant and positive impact on morbidity and mortality.

FOLLOW-UP

Follow-up depends on the underlying cause of the patient's dehydration and shock and on any morbidity associated with treatment. Follow-up is needed with the patient's regular pediatrician and any subspecialists who may manage additional problems the patient may have.

Table 28-7. Treatment Summary

Hypovolemic shock—a preload issue	Volume, volume, volume
Cardiogenic shock—a contractility issue	Volume first, because increasing the preload can get the heart to a better point on the Frank-Starling curve. Early use of inotropic agents to improve contractility; dobutamine is usual first choice. Only after blood pressure is stabilized and patient is fluid resuscitated, consider vasodilator agents to reduce afterlod
Distributive shock—a systemic vascular resistance issue	First give volume to fill the tank. Consider vasoconstrictive agents to increase vascular tone. Dopamine usually is first choice except in anaphylaxis, when epinephrine is first choice
Septic shock—a combination of the three	Volume first, then frequently vasoconstrictive agents. Dopamine usually is used first

SUGGESTED READINGS

Centers for Disease Control and Prevention: The management of acute diarrhea in children: Oral rehydration, maintenance and nutritional therapy. MMWR Morb Mortal Wkly Rep 1992;41:1–20.

Holliday M: The evolution of therapy for dehydration: Should deficit therapy still be taught? Pediatrics 1996;98:171–177.

Tobin JR, Wetzel RC: Shock and multi-organ system failure. In Rogers MC (ed): Textbook of Pediatric Intensive Care, 3rd ed. Baltimore, Williams & Wilkins, 1996, pp 584–588.

29

Acute Respiratory Failure

Harold N. Amer

ROLE OF THE GENERALIST

1 Recognize children at risk for respiratory failure.

2 Determine immediate management strategies by assignment of patients with respiratory disorders into a physiologic category of stable, respiratory distress, or respiratory failure.

3 Institute immediate, effective, simple measures to stabilize patients with respiratory failure.

4 Refer patients to appropriate specialist or tertiary care center for assistance with diagnosis and management.

DEFINITION

The condition of *respiratory failure* is aligned closely with the concept of pulmonary gas exchange, and the condition of *respiratory distress* is aligned closely with the concept of work of breathing. *Pulmonary gas exchange* refers to the molecular movement of oxygen (O_2) and carbon dioxide (CO_2) between the alveolar airspace and the juxta-alveolar capillary blood. All of this movement is passive, driven by gradients between the alveolar and capillary gas concentrations (expressed quantitatively as the partial pressures P_{O_2} and P_{CO_2}). *The clinical condition of respiratory failure is a reflection of the pathophysiologic condition of inadequate pulmonary exchange of O_2 or CO_2 or both.*

Work of breathing refers to the effort that a patient expends inhaling and exhaling to supply fresh gas to the alveoli for the conduct of pulmonary gas exchange. The effort required under normal physiologic conditions is minimal, but under pathologic conditions this effort can increase

dramatically. *The clinical condition of respiratory distress is predominantly a reflection of the pathophysiologic condition of increased work of breathing.*

Pulmonary gas exchange and work of breathing are related to one another, but they are distinctly different. One may have increased work of breathing with or without adequate pulmonary gas exchange. Alternatively, one may have inadequate pulmonary gas exchange with or without increased work of breathing. Based on these concepts, all patients with respiratory illness can be categorized into one of three physiologic states: (1) in respiratory distress, (2) in respiratory failure, or (3) in neither respiratory distress nor respiratory failure (i.e., physiologically stable). Arterial blood gas values that are typical of each of these states are presented in Table 29-1.

FUNDAMENTALS

The causes of respiratory failure can be grouped into five disease categories (Table 29-2):

1. *Upper airway obstruction:* Examples are croup and epiglottitis.
2. *Restrictive lung disease:* Examples are pneumonia and atelectasis.
3. *Obstructive lung disease:* Examples are asthma and bronchiolitis.
4. *Pulmonary vascular diseases:* One example is pulmonary hypertension. These conditions share the common element of depriving a ventilated alveolus of proximate blood flow, creating "wasted ventilation." These diseases are unusual. Management is complex, and immediate referral for tertiary care is usually necessary.

Table 29-1. Physiologic Categories of Respiratory Status

Category	Stable	Respiratory Distress	Respiratory Failure
Arterial blood gases	Pa_{O_2} >60 mm Hg on room air Pa_{CO_2} <45 mm Hg, pH >7.35	Pa_{O_2} >60 mm Hg on Fi_{O_2} = 60% Pa_{CO_2} <45 mm Hg, pH >7.30	Pa_{O_2} <60 mm Hg on Fi_{O_2} = 60% Pa_{CO_2} >55 mm Hg, pH <7.30

Physical examination	Normal work of breathing
	Normal gas exchange
		Increased work of breathing
		  Tachypnea
		  Nasal flaring
		  Diaphoresis
		  Retractions
		  ↑ Accessory muscle use
		  Grunting
		  Head bobbing
			Impaired gas exchange
			  Bradypnea
			  Diminished chest excursions
			  Diminished breath sounds
			  Cyanosis
			  Altered mental status

Table 29-2. Disease Categories

	Upper Airway Obstruction	Restrictive Lung Disease	Obstructive Lung Disease	Pulmonary Vascular Disease	Neuromuscular Disease
Dominant Pathology	Difficulty inhaling	Alveolar collapse (derecruitment)	Difficulty exhaling	Wasted ventilation (dead space)	Difficulty inhaling and alveolar collapse
Typical Diseases	Croup Epiglottitis Laryngomalacia Tonsil/adenoid hypertrophy Foreign-body aspiration	Atelectasis Pneumonia Chest wall deformity Abdominal distention Congestive heart failure ARDS	Asthma Bronchiolitis Bronchopulmonary dysplasia Bronchomalacia Cystic fibrosis	Pulmonary emboli Sepsis Pulmonary hypertension Zone I–II mechanical ventilation	Postictal state Intoxication Head and cervical spine trauma Guillain-Barré syndrome Infant botulism Meningoencephalitis Exhaustion
Prevalence	Common	Common	Common	Uncommon	Common
Management Complexity	++	++	+	++++	+++
Specific Therapy	Aerosolized epinephrine Corticosteroids Intubation	Diuresis Inotropes Mechanical ventilation	Aerosolized albuterol Corticosteroids	Hyperoxygenation Hyperventilation Inhaled Nitric Oxide	Intoxication antidotes Intubation Mechanical ventilation

5. *Neuromuscular diseases:* These conditions can have elements of upper airway obstruction (as a result of loss of airway protective reflexes) and restrictive lung disease (as a result of atelectasis). Many neuromuscular diseases associated with altered respiratory drive or respiratory muscle weakness are included in this category. Any condition among the preceding four categories of lung disease that progresses to a point of physical exhaustion also is classified in this category. Some of these conditions resolve spontaneously, such as the postictal state. Patients in this category have little or no "reserve." The severity of the physiologic compromise may be subtle because patients often do not manifest increased work of breathing. Patients in this category are at the highest risk for sudden respiratory arrest.

DIAGNOSIS

Most health care providers can identify the common physical findings of respiratory distress and failure. Most health care providers are not accustomed, however, to subcategorizing these findings in a physiologically meaningful way. The goal of the focused physical assessment is to categorize the patient into one of three physiologic states—stable, respiratory distress, or respiratory failure. The pediatric advanced life support methodology as taught by the American Heart Association uses this paradigm.

Findings that indicate increased work of breathing include tachypnea, grunting, retracting, accessory muscle use, head bobbing, nasal flaring, and diaphoresis. These findings identify the patient as having respiratory distress. A child with a neuromuscular etiology may have minimal evidence of increased work of breathing. These children often manifest respiratory "failure" with little or no sign of "distress." The examination for respiratory failure seeks out evidence of inadequate gas exchange. The crucial findings on physical examination are those indicating reduced minute ventilation, cyanosis, and altered mental status.

Minute ventilation is the arithmetic product of respiratory rate and tidal volume. An abnormally slow respiratory rate almost always indicates decreased minute ventilation because compensation would require the conduct of supranormal tidal volumes, which is virtually never seen. More commonly, patients present with tachypnea. In these cases, diminished chest excursions on visual assessment or diminished breath sounds on auscultatory assessment may indicate decreased minute ventilation. Findings consistent with decreased minute ventilation, as a result of either inadequate respiratory rate or tidal volume, suggest the presence of hypercarbia.

Central cyanosis, evidenced by duskiness of the lips and tongue, indicates hypoxemia. Occasionally a hypoxemic child is not cyanotic, as with severe anemia, when desaturated hemoglobin levels are insufficient to cause changes in color. Some children experience vasoconstriction with hypoxemia and appear pallid rather than cyanotic.

Altered mental status can be the result of either hypercarbia or hypoxemia, usually of a severe degree, and is a particularly ominous finding in the context of respiratory illness. A common clinical pitfall is to be relieved when a crying, agitated child becomes peaceful. This change may reflect an improvement to a mental status of comfort or a deterioration to obtundation. A thorough assessment is essential to clarify which of these alternatives is most likely.

A more detailed discussion of the physiology of gas exchange and work of breathing is presented on the CD-ROM but is not necessary to discuss the management of respiratory distress and failure. Based on the assignment of the patient to a physiologic category (stable, in respiratory distress, or in respiratory failure), subsequent management strategies are determined.

MANAGEMENT
General Approach
The management strategies appropriate to the patient's physiologic state are outlined in Table 29-3. All children with complaints suggesting a respiratory disease at some point require a specific diagnosis to deliver appropriate, disease-specific therapy. For a child who is judged to be

Table 29-3. Management

Stable	Respiratory Distress	Respiratory Failure
Disease-specific evaluation	Remain with parent	Evaluate and secure airway
Disease-specific therapy	Position of comfort	Humidified oxygen
Re-evaluate for physiologic deterioration	Humidified oxygen	Ineffectual ventilation → BVM ventilation
	Suctioning as needed	Marginal ventilation → Optimize patient position; aerosolized medications
	Pulse oximetry	Pulse oximetry
	NPO	NPO
		Cardiac monitoring
		Intravenous access

BVM, bag-valve-mask; NPO, nothing per mouth.

physiologically stable (based on the focused physical examination described earlier), disease-specific actions may proceed immediately.

For a child who is judged to be in respiratory distress but not in failure, some simple nonspecific interventions should be undertaken first. By definition, all children in respiratory distress have normal mental status. Allowing them to remain with a parent is appropriate and may be therapeutic because emotional distress often worsens respiratory distress. If airway secretions seem to be causing distress, gentle suctioning is indicated. Provision of supplemental oxygen is technically simple but not always well tolerated. If tolerance is a problem, altering the delivery device or involving the parent (or the child) in applying the device can help. Humidification should be added as soon as possible to avoid drying secretions. Oral intake should be suspended until it is clear the patient is improving and intubation will not be necessary. Oxygen saturation should be monitored with pulse oximetry if available.

For a child who is judged to be in respiratory failure, diagnostic considerations are secondary. Immediate aggressive resuscitation becomes the primary concern. The airway should be evaluated and cleared if necessary. Oxygen should be administered in maximal concentrations. If spontaneous ventilation appears to be nil, artificial ventilation should be provided with bag and mask. If spontaneous ventilation appears to be marginal or bag/mask ventilation is met with resistance, patient positioning should be optimized, and appropriate aerosolized medications should be administered. In addition to pulse oximetry, cardiac monitoring should be performed and intravenous access obtained whenever possible.

Repeated physical assessment is the primary means of determining the progress of the patient. Ancillary diagnostic studies, such as chest x-rays, blood gases, end-tidal CO_2 monitoring (discussed on the CD-ROM), and other laboratory studies, may be conducted as appropriate, but it is paramount that diagnostic studies must *not* delay resuscitation when the physical examination indicates respiratory failure.

Airway: Specific Skills, Equipment, and Interventions

The most common reason for obstruction of the airway is posterior displacement of the tongue. The typical patient with altered mental status, lying in the supine position, often requires assistance clearing the tongue from the posterior pharynx. Two hand skill maneuvers, the head tilt/chin lift and the jaw thrust, may be used for this purpose. These airway management techniques are shown in Figures 29-1 through 29-5. It also may be helpful to place neck/shoulder padding behind the patient to compensate for the head/body disproportion that tends to force infants and small children into a position of neck flexion. If clearance of the tongue from the airway is especially problematic in an unconscious patient, use of an oropharyngeal airway may resolve the problem.

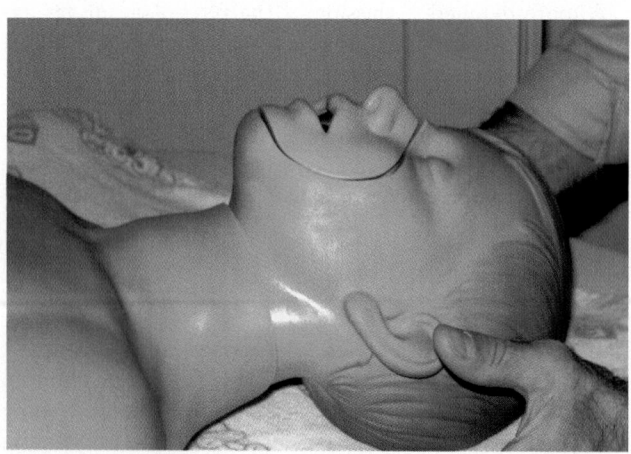

Figure 29-1. Patient in neutral position.

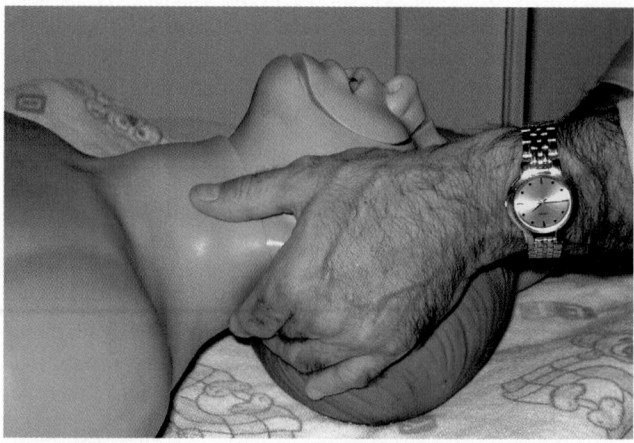

Figure 29-2. Head tilt, viewed from left side. The left hand lifts to provide a fulcrum for tilting the head.

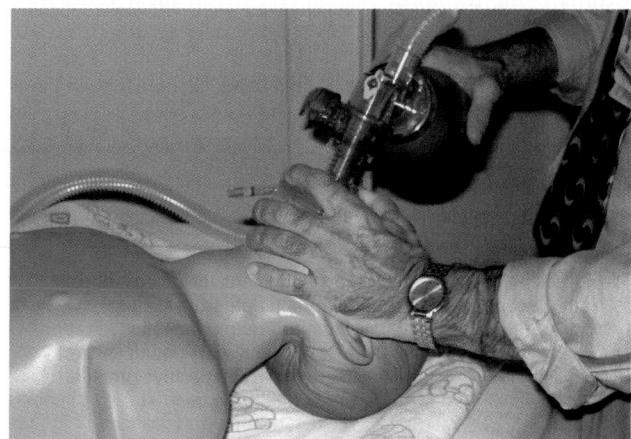

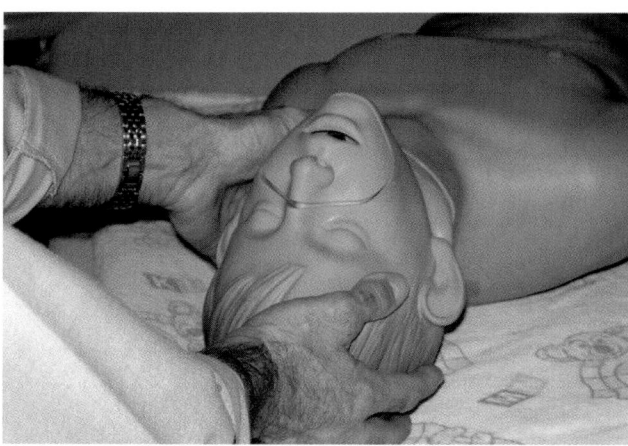

Figure 29-3. Head tilt, viewed from head of the bed. The right hand maintains the head in an extended position.

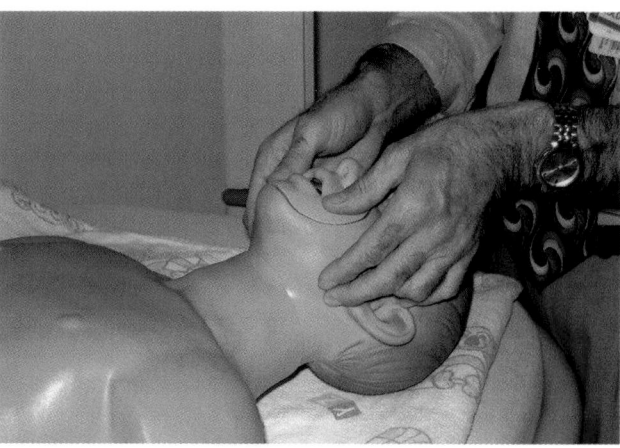

Figure 29-5. Jaw thrust. Fingertips lift toward the ceiling.

Secretions exacerbate airway obstruction. Rigid, large-bore suctioning devices, such as the Yankauer catheter, should be used for suctioning the oropharynx. Soft catheters or aspirating bulbs can be used for suctioning the nose and nasopharynx. Because young infants are obligate nose breathers, relatively small secretion volumes may cause severe obstruction.

If a foreign-body obstruction is suspected, choosing the best intervention depends on the setting. If an individual skilled in airway management is immediately available, visualization by direct laryngoscopy may be preferred. In most circumstances, however, the Heimlich maneuver achieves the most expeditious result. Infants and small children should have compression applied over the sternum rather than the epigastrium to avoid injury to abdominal organs.

Breathing: Specific Skills, Equipment, and Interventions

When the airway is cleared, several simple interventions may benefit a spontaneously breathing child further. Infants and children are extremely diaphragm-dependent for ventilation and oxygenation. Upright positioning relieves pressure on the underside of the diaphragm by displacing abdominal contents. Deflation of a distended stomach with a nasogastric tube has a similar effect.

Many children present with findings characteristic of asthma or croup for which aerosolized albuterol or epinephrine is indicated. There is little reason to insist on definitive diagnoses early in the resuscitation of acute respiratory failure. Administration of albuterol to any patient with wheezing or racemic or L-epinephrine to any patient with stridor is recommended when respiratory distress or failure is present.

For a patient who requires positive-pressure ventilation, immediate endotracheal intubation usually is *not* necessary. Bag-valve-mask (BVM) ventilation is sufficient to stabilize most children with respiratory failure until an individual with intubating skills is available. A caveat to this statement relates to the ability to achieve good BVM ventilation in the face of a partially obstructed airway or lungs with poor compliance. In either case, relatively high airway pressures may be needed, and the ability to maintain a tight facemask seal is paramount. This seal is achieved best by combining the jaw-thrust airway maneuver with facemask application using the thumbs and thenar eminences. This hand skill is far easier to learn and retain than that of endotracheal intubation. A second resuscitator must compress the insufflating bag. BVM techniques are shown in Figures 29-6 and 29-7.

Table 29-4 lists hand skills and equipment that are essential for complete initial stabilization of a child with respi-

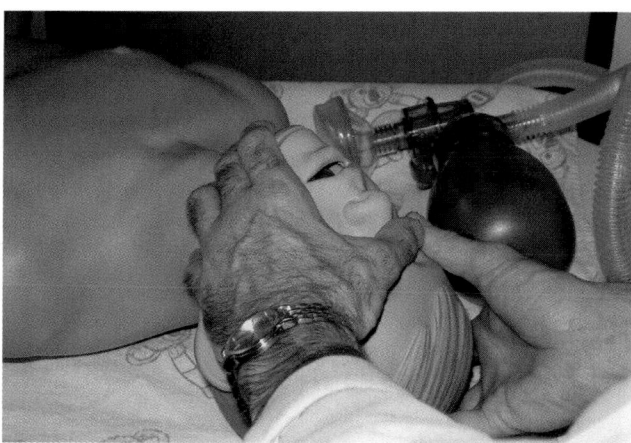

Figure 29-4. Head tilt with chin lift. The left hand moves to the chin and lifts.

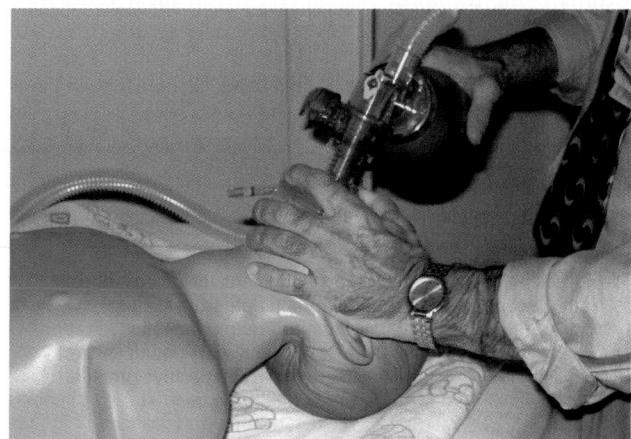

Figure 29-6. Head-tilt/chin-lift maneuver with bag-valve-mask ventilation.

30 Cardiac Failure

Barry G. Baylen

DEFINITION

Extraordinary advances in basic science and related clinical developments have led to better understanding of underlying pathophysiologic processes and management of heart failure in ill newborns, infants, and children. Early definitions of *heart failure* characterized the condition solely as a failure of "pump function." More recent studies have shown that the heart and peripheral circulation are a complexly integrated system controlled by the endocrine, paracrine, and neuroautonomic systems and a host of circulating vasoactive substances, local autoregulatory controls, and cellular controls. Current definitions go beyond consideration of the disordered heart, defining heart failure as a maladaptation or exhaustion of the "peripheral" systems and the compensatory mechanisms required to maintain metabolic homeostasis and organ function. Therapeutic strategies have shifted away from primarily influencing variables related to pump function. The use of positive inotropic agents may be detrimental to myocardial oxygen demands, increase the risk of dysrhythmia, and have a negative impact on elements of contraction. Therapy that acts to enhance the physiology of the peripheral circulation and affect systemic metabolic requirements favorably is key in the management of heart failure.

Application of these concepts to pediatric patients requires consideration of the unique interaction of congenital and acquired cardiac disorders and fundamental developmental processes. Pediatric patients with congenital heart disease present a host of clinical situations associated with "maldistribution" of cardiac output. A shunt into the pulmonary circulation away from the systemic circulation (left-to-right) may be associated with "adequate" pump performance and ventricular output but maldistribution of cardiac output (away from the body). In some conditions, systemic flow is normal, but recirculation of poorly oxygenated venous blood into the systemic (body) circulation (right-to-left shunt) leads to reduced oxygen delivery (the product of cardiac output and oxygen content). Inflow or outflow obstruction of a cardiac chamber may lead to quantitatively reduced systemic blood flow. Frank myocardial dysfunction secondary to constriction, infection, infiltration, cardiomyopathy (muscle disorder), or arrhythmias may lead to inadequate oxygen delivery to vital organs.

A definition of heart failure in children must take into account the variable metabolic requirements ("demands") of newborns compared with infants and young children. Development and related nutritional and growth requirements must be considered in defining "inadequate" oxygen delivery. Metabolic demands are relatively high in newborns during the first months after birth. From the perspective of the Frank-Starling principles, the "matching" of pump performance or cardiac output to venous return is irrelevant in the forms of congenital heart disease associated with abnormal venous connections to the atrial or ventricular chambers.

FUNDAMENTALS

The pathophysiology of heart failure has been described as a disorder of myocardial and ventricular pump function leading to a decrease in cardiac output and inadequate oxygen delivery to meet systemic metabolic needs. The classic determinants of heart function and early measures to improve ventricular function were focused on four variables: heart rate, preload, afterload, and contractility of the ventricle. According to the Frank-Starling relationship, cardiac pump performance (represented by ventricular output) is related directly to increased venous return up to a maximum value (Fig. 30-1). Depression of muscle contraction may lead to a decrease in output at any filling pressure or volume (sometimes referred to as *preload*). A significantly diminished cardiac output at normal or low filling volume may occur secondary to decreased contractility, fluid losses, or diuretics, leading to clinical "fatigue." When severe ventricular dysfunction ensues, low cardiac output is associated with increased residual ventricular diastolic filling volume/pressure leading to left atrial and pulmonary venous hypertension; extravasation of interstitial and alveolar fluid; and respiratory symptoms, such as tachypnea, coughing, wheezing, and sleeplessness (symptoms of pulmonary edema). Primary involvement of the right ventricle, pulmonary hypertension, or impaired right ventricular filling caused by compression by a distended left ventricular chamber leads to systemic "passive" venous congestion, including congestion of the liver and gastrointestinal tract, and signs of fluid retention, a constellation of symptoms and findings termed *congestive heart failure.* Strategies directed at improving the magnitude and force of contraction (inotropic agents) and achieving optimal preload or fluid status (diuretics) produce temporary clinical improvement but often are ineffective and potentially deleterious in chronic heart failure.

More recently the importance of peripheral neural, endocrine, and paracrine circulatory adjustments has become central to the understanding of pathophysiology and management of heart failure (Fig. 30-2). Low cardiac output leads to "compensatory" circulatory adjustments, such as stimulation of baroreceptors; secretion of renin-angiotensin-aldosterone, atrial natriuretic peptide, and catecholamines; and release of other vasoactive agents, such as endothelin, prostaglandins, and nitric oxide. These adjustments lead to increased total body fluid and sodium retention, generalized vasoconstriction (increased afterload), and redistribution of blood flow to central organs. The clinical correlates of these disturbances include diaphoresis, cool extremities, diminished skin perfusion, organ congestion, edema, and oliguria. The impaired ventricle of the developing heart is particularly vulnerable to increased vascular impedance or resistance (often termed *afterload*). Current therapeutic strategies are directed at establishing peripheral circulatory and neuroendocrine homeostasis using vasodilating (afterload-reducing) agents, hormonal antagonists (angiotensin "blockade," aldosterone antagonists), and β-blocking agents.

Because of the variable structural nature of congenital heart disease and evolving developmental and metabolic factors, the previously described pathophysiologic processes do not explain sufficiently the nature of heart failure

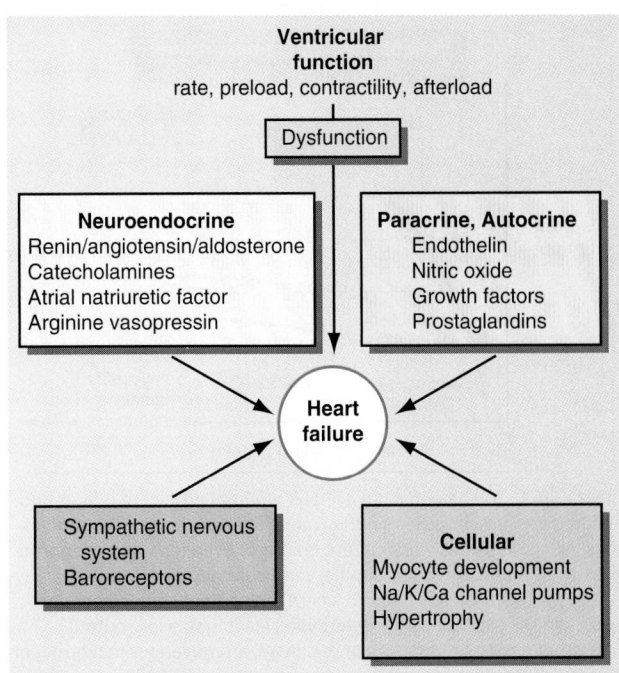

Figure 30-2. Pathophysiology of heart failure. The integrated circulatory system consists of integrated mechanisms maintaining circulatory homeostasis. Variables influencing cardiac pump function interact with a host of peripheral circulatory and neuroendocrine feedback systems. Exaggeration of exhaustion of these systems leads to heart failure.

in children. The neonatal and infant myocardium, when compared with that of older children and adults, is relatively deficient in myocytes. Incomplete sympathetic enervation renders the heart more dependent on circulating catecholamines. Electromechanical properties related to immature cell membrane and calcium uptake release, mechanisms that regulate myocyte contraction and relaxation, and differences in metabolic processes and contractile proteins lead to relatively less ventricular pumping capacity in the newborn and infant heart. Because newborns and young infants have increased systemic metabolic requirements, the heart functions closer to its capacity during the first months after birth, leading to relatively less pump "reserve." This reduced reserve leads to the young heart being less capable of responding to the abnormal loading forces on the myocardium associated with congenital heart disease.

The infant heart may be more adapted to conditions of hypoxia. The paradigm of "pump failure" and low cardiac output may not apply to many common forms of congenital heart disease in which the primary disorder is abnormal blood flow distribution (left-to-right shunt) or decreased oxygen delivery (right-to-left shunt, cyanotic heart disease [Fig. 30-3]). Ventricular dysfunction and a low output state may manifest suddenly at "end stage," however, with mixed shunting lesions, obstructive lesions (aortic stenosis and coarctation of the aorta), or acquired heart disease.

CONDITIONS COMMONLY ASSOCIATED WITH HEART FAILURE

The most common group of congenital heart lesions presenting as heart failure in infants and older children are lesions associated with left-to-right shunt, defined anatomi-

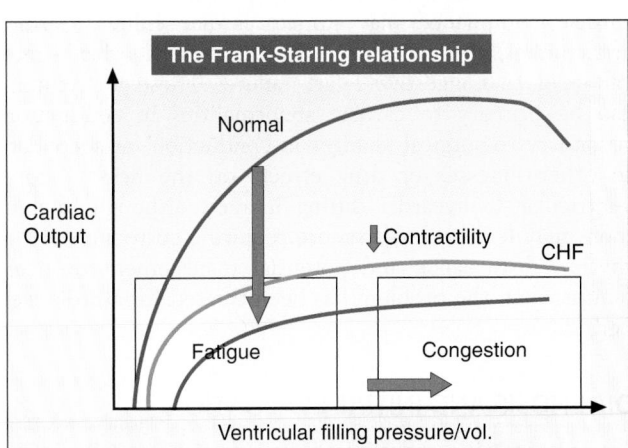

Figure 30-1. The Frank-Starling relationship. Ventricular output corresponds to ventricular filling volume or pressure. A decrease in contractility at any filling volume is associated with a decrease in cardiac output. A cardiac output insufficient to meet metabolic needs at any filling pressure *(lower curve/left)* is associated with fatigue at rest or "exercise." As contraction deteriorates, increased ventricular residual volumes lead to congestive symptoms (congestive heart failure).

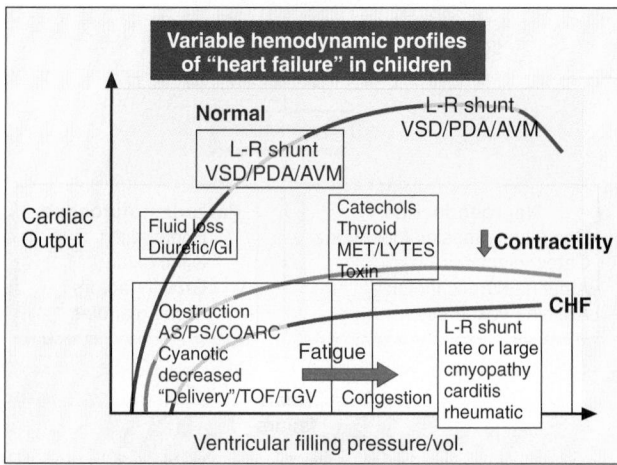

Figure 30-3. The hemodynamic (Frank-Starling) profiles of infants and children are superimposed on the Frank-Starling function. The profiles may vary considerably for different lesions or even for a single lesion as the condition evolves. For example, ventricular septal defect (VSD) may present with a relatively high left ventricular output state *(upper right)*, and eventually function may deteriorate, leading to a low-output "congestive state." AS, aortic stenosis; AVM, arteriovenous malformation; COARC, coarctation of aorta; GI, gastrointestinal; MET/LYTES, metabolic/electrolytes; PDA, patent ductus arteriosus; PS, pulmonary stenosis; TGV, transposition of the great vessels; TOF, tetralogy of Fallot.

cally as flow from the left to right heart chambers or vessels. These include ventricular septal defect and patent ductus arteriosus. When the pulmonary vascular resistance decreases from its intrauterine level and the hemoglobin decreases in the first 2 and 3 months of life, blood is shunted from the systemic high-pressure ventricle or aorta into the lower resistance pulmonary circulation. If the communication is large, the "steal" of flow away from the systemic circulation and the lower hemoglobin level lead to a fall of tissue/organ oxygen delivery, increased pulmonary blood flow, and altered mechanical properties of the lung. Increased pulmonary flow leads to excessive blood return to the left ventricle. Increased volume load and filling pressure cause pulmonary congestion. Although total left ventricular output often is increased initially, actual systemic flow and oxygen delivery may be reduced. Eventually, left ventricular function may be compromised, further reducing systemic flow. Other large systemic (cerebral/hepatic) arteriovenous fistulae, an unusual cause of heart failure in infants, may mimic patent ductus arteriosus.

Atrial septal defects are associated with increased right heart volume and pulmonary flow but only rarely cause clinical symptoms and usually are diagnosed later secondary to detection of the associated heart murmurs. A special form of combined atrial and ventricular septal defect (atrioventricular septal defect or endocardial cushion defect) associated with mitral insufficiency, common in children with trisomy 21, often presents with heart failure during the first weeks after birth. Obstructive lesions of the left and right ventricular outflow (aortic and pulmonary valve stenosis, coarctation of the aorta) generally do not present with heart failure with moderate obstruction. The most severe forms may present with cyanosis, low cardiac output, heart failure, or shocklike syndrome in the neonatal

period. Anomalous origin of the left coronary artery may present as a "near-miss" sudden death or myocardial infarction and a low cardiac output or shock syndrome at approximately 2 to 3 months of age.

Cyanotic congenital heart conditions are structural disorders that produce a right-to-left shunt by recirculation of systemic venous blood with reduced oxyhemoglobin saturation into the systemic (whole-body) arterial circulation. Usually this recirculation involves flow from the right heart or pulmonary circulation to the left heart or aorta. The degree of cyanosis is related in part to the amount of admixture of returning fully saturated pulmonary venous blood. In conditions associated with decreased pulmonary blood flow, the patient is severely cyanotic. Patients with increased pulmonary flow may be relatively "acyanotic" because the returning saturated blood from the lungs "dilutes" the poorly saturated systemic venous return. These conditions are classified for clinical and diagnostic purposes as conditions associated with decreased pulmonary blood flow and conditions with increased pulmonary flow (Table 30-1). Commonly, right heart obstructive lesions, such as tricuspid atresia, critical pulmonary valve stenosis or atresia, and tetralogy of Fallot (TOF), are associated with decreased pulmonary flow. Conditions associated with increased pulmonary flow include transposition of the great vessels (TGV), total anomalous pulmonary venous connection with obstructed veins (TAPVC), and hypoplastic left heart syndrome (HLHS).

A host of acquired heart conditions may lead to ventricular dysfunction and low cardiac output heart failure in newborns, infants, and older children. These conditions may be categorized as infectious (i.e., viral and bacterial myocarditis, toxic septicemia, bacterial endocarditis); metabolic (i.e., cardiomyopathy or generalized metabolic nutritional or electrolyte disturbances); rheumatic and other autoimmune or collagen vascular diseases; Kawasaki disease (a nonspecific vasculitis associated with coronary and myocardial involvement); and infiltrative disorders, occasionally including neoplasia. Infiltrative disorders may produce "diastolic dysfunction," in which restriction of cardiac compliance may impair cardiac filling. Cardiac arrhythmias, either from too slow a rate or too fast a rate, can lead to congestive heart failure. These arrhythmias can be primary to cardiac abnormalities in conduction, secondary to surgical changes in conduction, or secondary to other illnesses or drug effects on the heart. Supraventricular tachycardia during infancy, although uncommon, may lead to heart failure requiring correction of the rhythm disturbance and potential management of heart failure when the problem has been treated for a prolonged period.

DIAGNOSIS AND INITIAL EVALUATION

The presentation and clinical findings of heart failure vary with condition and age (summarized in Fig. 30-4). Heart failure in the neonate is discussed in Chapter 203. In older infants and children, the manifestation of clinical signs and symptoms of failure are related to the degree of cardiac reserve available. Heart failure may be difficult to identify in young infants because clinical signs of failure can be

Table 30-1. Differential Diagnosis of Neonatal Cyanotic Congenital Heart Diseases

Sign/Symptom	Decreased Pulmonary Blood Flow* ECG (QRS) Axis				Increased Pulmonary Blood Flow* ECG Ventricular Forces		
	<0°† Tricuspid Atresia	0–90° Critical PS PA/IVS	90–150° TOF	>150° Complex CHD with PS or PA	Normal d-TGA	Abnormal TAPVC	HLHS
Systolic murmur	0 or long	0 or long	Short	0 or long	0	0	0 or long
Pulses	N or ↓	N or ↓	N or ↑	N	N	0–+	0–+
S₂	Single	Single	Single	Single	Single	± split†	Single
Hepatomegaly	+	+	0	0	0	+++↑	+++↑
CXR findings	CM (↑ RA)	CM (↑ RA)	"Boot"† Right arch	CM	"Egg shape"	No CM Edema†	CM Edema†
Other ECG	LVH, RAE, ↓ RV	RAE, ↑ RV	RVH	RVH	N (RVH)†	RAE, RVH	RVH, LV
Po₂ (mmHg)	30–60	30–60	30–60	30–60	<30	<30	30–90†

*Chest radiograph.
†Important differential feature.
+ = present; 0 = absent; ↓ = decreased; ↑ = increased.
CHD, congenital heart disease; CM, cardiomegaly; CXR, chest radiograph; d-TGA, d-transposition of great arteries; ECG, electrocardiogram; HLHS, hypoplastic left heart syndrome; IVS, intact ventricular septum; LVH, left ventricular hypertrophy; N, normal; PA, pulmonary atresia; Po₂, arterial oxygen tension; PS, pulmonary stenosis; RAE, right atrial enlargement; RV, right ventricle shadow; RVH, right ventricular hypertrophy; TAPVC, total anomalous pulmonary venous connection (obstructed); TOF, tetralogy of Fallot.

nonspecific in this age group. Cardinal signs include feeding difficulty, failure to thrive, diaphoresis, irritability, and weak cry. Respiratory symptoms may be subtle and include chronic pulmonary symptoms, such as tachypnea, cough, wheeze, or cyanotic episodes (particularly in TOF). Feeding history should be detailed because infants with heart failure are likely to take less volume per feeding. They may feed more frequently, but spend less time at the breast or taking from the bottle. Infants may become diaphoretic and tachypneic during feeding. Older children with heart failure manifest with symptoms of reduced activity. They present more frequently with findings of a specific acquired condition (e.g., rheumatic heart disease) and early or late findings of decompensation, such as fatigue, shortness of breath, exercise intolerance, pulmonary symptoms, and fluid retention (see Fig. 30-3). Fatigue in older children may be manifested in changes in age-specific activities, such as riding a bicycle or participation in physical education classes. History should include queries designed to

determine the condition causing the heart failure (see Chapters 59, 60, and 203).

Although in current practice the physical examination often assumes a backseat to echocardiography, correct diagnosis of cardiac defects frequently can be straightforward. Physical examination should begin with vital signs (respiratory rate, heart rate, blood pressure, differential leg-arm blood pressures, weight); assessment of perfusion (capillary refill time, strength of pulses, pallor); and an evaluation of the general appearance of the child, including general signs of systemic congestion, such as periorbital edema. Oxygen saturation, when available, should be obtained. Major and minor malformations should be noted, particularly malformations that indicate syndromes associated with cardiac lesions, such as trisomy 21. Color and level of respiratory distress are crucial. Commonly, right heart obstructive lesions in the newborn, such as tricuspid atresia, critical pulmonary valve stenosis or atresia, and TOF, are associated with decreased pulmonary flow. These

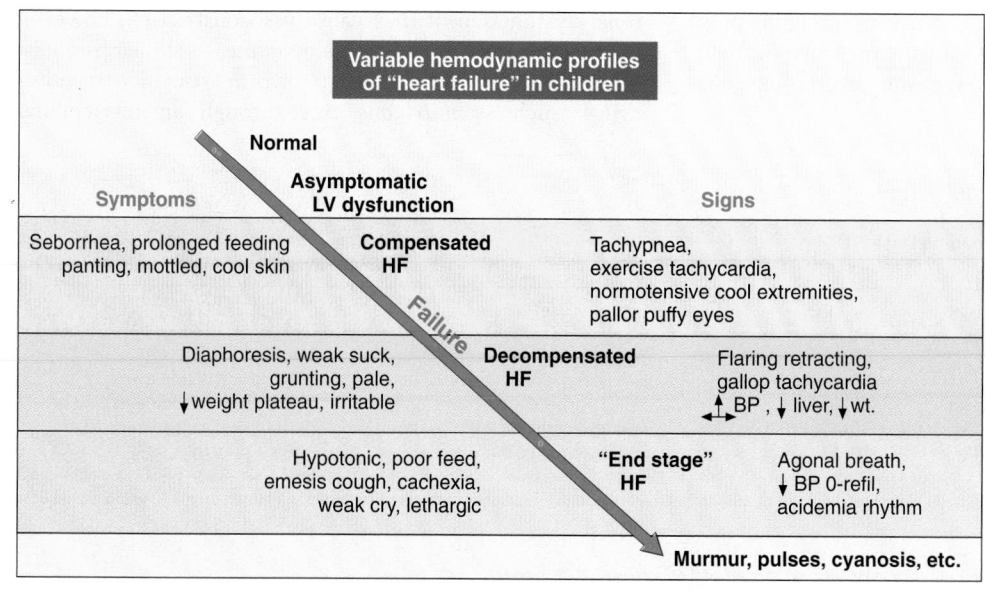

Figure 30-4. Symptoms and signs of heart failure (HF) in children vary with condition, age, and stage (early or late). This illustration of evolving signs and symptoms of HF in newborns, infants, and children indicates how these are associated with advancing clinical HF. BP, blood pressure; LV, left ventricular.

lesions generally present with central or whole-body cyanosis during the first days after birth, when the ductus arteriosus begins to constrict. Conditions associated with increased pulmonary flow include TGV, TAPVC, and HLHS. TGV and TAPVC present with severe cyanosis and pulmonary congestion soon after birth, whereas HLHS presents with a pulseless shocklike picture or "gray infant" when the ductus arteriosus constricts from 2 to 3 days up to 2 to 3 weeks of age.

Respiratory effort should be noted, including ease of respiration, use of accessory muscles to breathe, intercostal and subcostal retractions, and flaring of the alae nasi. In general, newborns with critical right heart obstructions and decreased pulmonary blood flow have tachycardia and short, shallow/effortless respirations ("happy" tachypnea). Newborns with increased pulmonary flow associated with pulmonary congestion have labored grunting, retractions (supracostal, infracostal, and intercostal), and overexpansion of the chest. Auscultation of the lungs may reveal wheezing in infants and basilar crackles in older children.

Examination of the heart may reveal a wide variety of physical findings, including active precordium; loud, "busy" heart sounds; and gallop rhythm, although, importantly, a heart murmur may be absent in newborns with certain structural lesions (TGV, pulmonary or aortic valve atresias, TAPVC, HLHS). Heart sounds and murmurs should be characterized carefully (see Chapter 56). The finding in patent ductus arteriosus is a continuous murmur associated with bounding pulses; the finding in a ventricular septal defect is harsh systolic murmur with normal pulses; the findings in an atrial septal defect are soft systolic and diastolic murmurs with "fixed split" second sound. Murmurs or rubs or both can be heard in children with rheumatic carditis or other infectious or inflammatory causes of heart failure. In most cases of myocarditis, because cardiac output is reduced, murmurs frequently are not appreciated. Other associated findings on physical examination include hepatomegaly, edema, and signs of associated diseases (i.e., swollen red joints in rheumatic fever, erythema of the oral and pharyngeal mucosa with Kawasaki disease).

Indicated laboratory investigations include chest x-ray and electrocardiography. Echocardiography is useful in assessing ventricular function. In addition to screening pulse oximetry, it is important to assess for the presence of metabolic acidosis and the degree of systemic arterial oxygenation with arterial blood gas.

MANAGEMENT

Management of newborns with heart failure is discussed in Chapter 203. Heart failure in older infants and young children generally is associated with congenital or acquired conditions, often of gradual onset and occasionally of chronic duration. In these situations, management assumes a more conventional therapeutic approach, with initiation of inotropes and diuretics and often the use of vasodilators or inodilators. After initial stabilization and institution of therapy as appropriate, consultation with a pediatric cardiologist should be obtained promptly. The cardiologist can provide invaluable assistance on-line via computer/Internet or telephone assistance to the on-site echocardiography technician and can make recommendations to the generalist regarding urgent medical management and preparation for transport to a tertiary center. Therapies or diagnostic procedures that increase stress and oxygen demand should be avoided when treating heart failure, particularly in young infants or any child with distress.

Drug therapy is indicated to improve cardiac contractility and function. *Digoxin* improves myocardial function by augmenting the rate and force of contraction. In addition, digoxin's vagotonic effects slow cardiac rate, and its baroreceptor inhibition reduces the vascular resistance or afterload. Many schemes of "digitalization" are available depending on acuity varying from ½, ¼, and ¼ of the total dose orally or intravenously in 12 to 24 hours. Suggested schedules and doses are listed in Table 30-2. Total digitalizing dose and maintenance doses are given in micrograms per kilograms per 24 hours. Intravenous doses are generally 20% less than oral doses, and recommended doses vary by age. Digoxin toxicity includes vomiting, diarrhea, bradycardia, and atrial or ventricular arrhythmias. Digoxin levels may be of value in monitoring some infants, particularly infants with shock or renal dysfunction. Patients with low cardiac output, impaired perfusion, and a preshock or shocklike state need more intensive rapid-onset inotropic pharmacologic management and usually require β-agonists. *Dopamine* improves contractility and force of contraction and in low "renal" doses (<5 µg/kg/min) has renal vasodilating effects. With higher doses or in the presence of renal dysfunction, it may cause vasoconstriction, however, increasing ventricular work. *Dobutamine* has similar β-agonist effects with lower vasoconstrictor properties. Postreceptor drugs, such as *milrinone*, act through an intracellular

Table 30-2. Digitalization regimens*

Age and Weight	Loading Dose (TDD) (Give ½, ¼, ¼ of total every 8 hr)		Maintenance	
	IV/IM	PO	IV/IM	PO
Premature	15 µg/kg	20 µg/kg	3–4 µg/kg; divide every 12 hr	5 µg/kg; divide every 12 hr
Full-term	20 µg/kg	30 µg/kg	6–8 µg/kg; divide every 12 hr	8–10 µg/kg; divide every 12 hr
<2 yr	30–40 µg/kg	30 µg/kg	7.5–9 µg/kg; divide every 12 hr	10–12 µg/kg; divide every 12 hr
2–10 yr	20–30 µg/kg	30–40 µg/kg	6–8 µg/kg; divide every 12 hr	8–10 µg/kg; divide every 12 hr
>10 yr, <100 kg	8–12 µg/kg	10–15 µg/kg	2–3 µg/kg; give daily	2.5–5 µg/kg; give daily

*Loading dose (total digitalizing dose [TDD], give ½, ¼, ¼ of total every 8 hr. Obtain electrocardiogram 6 hr after dose to assess for toxicity. Maintenance: <10 yr old, divide dose twice daily; >10 yr old give dose daily.
IM, intramuscular; IV, intravenous; PO, oral.

Adapted from Siberry GK, Iannone R (eds): The Harriet Lane Handbook, 15th ed. St. Louis, Mosby, 2000, p 692.

mechanism inhibiting phosphodiesterase and increasing intracellular cyclic adenosine monophosphate; the latter leads to greater contractility and has beneficial vasodilating (afterload-reducing) effects.

Diuresis reduces systemic congestion and body edema and improves the fluid and sodium imbalance characteristic of patients with advanced heart failure. Respiratory mechanics, such as compliance and airway resistance, and gas exchange are improved. Heart function is moved to a more favorable position on the Frank-Starling curve (see Fig. 30-1). When acute management is required, preferred treatment is intravenous administration of a loop diuretic that dramatically increases sodium and water excretion. The usual *furosemide* dose is 1 mg/kg every 6 to 12 hours until objective signs of improvement are observed (diuresis, weight loss, reduced respirations, and reduced hepatomegaly). Because associated hypercalciuria may lead to microtubular nephrolithiasis, conservative oral dosing (1 to 2 mg/kg/24 hr) is preferred for chronic diuresis or change of drug to a tubular diuretic, such as hydrochlorothiazide.

Aldosterone antagonists improve outcome of chronic heart failure. Primary and secondary (to the stimulus of diuretics) hyperaldosteronism can interfere with the efficacy of conventional diuretics. Aldosterone antagonists, such as *aldactone*, augment diuresis, have a potassium-sparing effect, and may influence favorable myocardial remodeling.

Afterload-reducing agents, to reduce the cardiac pump working against extra pressure, such as angiotensin-converting enzyme inhibitors, reduce afterload and improve ventricular performance by inhibiting conversion of angiotensin 1 to angiotensin 2 (a vasoconstrictor). They are particularly useful in the immature heart and in various congenital heart conditions associated with left-to-right shunt. Reduction of systemic vascular resistance using angiotensin-converting enzyme inhibitors is associated with decreased left-to-right shunt and decreased volume overload of the left ventricle. Currently, short-acting (e.g., *captopril*) and long-acting (e.g., *lisinopril*) oral agents are available. Side effects include hyperkalemia, hypotension, and chronic cough. These drugs generally are contra-indicated in primary renal dysfunction.

Nutritional requirements of children with heart failure are increased. Infants with large left-to-right shunts may require 130 kcal/kg. Caloric augmentation of standard infant formula by altered dilution or caloric additives to 24 to 27 kcal/oz and adding small amounts of supplemental lipids may be useful. Attention must be directed at maintenance of normal fluid and electrolyte requirements and electrolyte balance. Occasionally, nasogastric or parenteral feeding is required in cachectic infants or to achieve positive metabolic balance before stressful operative procedures.

The homeostatic role of the peripheral circulation and its controlling factors has assumed prime importance in the management of heart failure in children. Heart failure is a complex combination of ventricular dysfunction and disordered peripheral regulation or exhaustion of compensatory homeostatic circulatory mechanisms. Future directions for management include β-blockade, which seems to up-regulate myocardial β receptors, improving contractility. Other strategies are leukotriene inhibitors, anti–tumor necrosis factors, growth factors, and even agents that may influence myocardial remodeling favorably.

OUTCOMES AND LONG-TERM FOLLOW-UP

Medical and surgical management of heart failure in congenital heart disease has improved viability and long-term outcomes for newborns with serious congenital heart disease. Arterial switch correction for TGA and most other common congenital heart lesions has approached a 96% success rate. In most other common lesions, the variable most closely associated with mortality and morbidity is delayed diagnosis and medical management. The optimal approach when technically and anatomically feasible is "complete open heart repair" (i.e., for TOF, truncus arteriosus, pulmonary valve stenosis, or TAPVC). The availability of bedside extracorporeal membrane oxygenators and the use of the inhaled pulmonary vasodilator, nitric oxide, have improved postoperative management and survival for the most serious immediate postoperative complications, ventricular dysfunction and pulmonary hypertension. Many defects cannot be repaired primarily and require "palliation," such as aorta-to-pulmonary shunt or pulmonary artery banding and subsequent complete repair. Many so-called corrective procedures may have considerable residual structural or functional limitations, however, requiring additional medical and surgical management, and in some conditions, "repair" may constitute solely a "bridge" for ultimate cardiac transplantation. The long-term results and management of cardiac transplantation have improved with more effective means of immunosuppression.

The medical management of acute-onset heart failure, including arrhythmia control, currently is highly effective, and in patients with acquired heart disease, many conditions can be managed successfully for extended periods. When indicated, these patients are better candidates for surgical repair, such as valve replacement or even cardiac transplantation. The evolving discipline of interventional cardiac catheterization currently eliminates surgical treatment of many congenital valve stenoses, patent ductus arteriosus, and atrial septal defects, and arrhythmia management often can be achieved by radiofrequency ablation.

The ongoing long-term management of children with congenital and acquired heart diseases requires close collaboration between the pediatric generalist and subspecialist and a thorough understanding of the specific illness, medications, and adverse affects in the unique setting of the developing child and family unit. Ultimately the goal of the family, specialist, and generalist is optimal physical rehabilitation and neurodevelopmental outcome. Studies indicate the relationship of preexisting neurologic disorder/deficit, timing of repair, effectiveness of medical management, and type and duration of cardiopulmonary bypass as important variables influencing ultimate neurologic outcome. Ultimately, favorable functional and neurodevelopmental outcomes require expert medical assessment, coordination with physiotherapy, and communication with the school system. These challenges are managed best by the general pediatrician who can follow, evaluate, and manage ongoing medical issues and ensure the best neurodevelopmental

Table 31-1. Children's Coma Scale

	Points
Ocular Response	
Pursuit	4
Extraocular muscles intact Pupils reactive	3
Extraocular muscles impaired	1
Pupils fixed	2
Extraocular muscles paralyzed	1
Pupils fixed	
Verbal Response	
Cries	3
Spontaneous respirations	2
Apneic	1
Motor Response	
Flexes and Extends	4
Withdraws from pain	3
Hypertonic	2
Flaccid	1

with a sinus thrombosis, from increased jugular venous pressure, or from increases in the arterial volume related to hypercarbia.

Increases in ICP become critical when perfusion pressure is compromised, which first occurs when ICP is about 70 mm Hg less than the mean arterial pressure. Perfusion is compromised dangerously when ICP approaches 40 to 50 mm Hg less than the mean arterial pressure. When the pressure of the intracranial components overtakes the arterial blood pressure, creating inadequate tissue perfusion, irreversible tissue damage occurs. Decreased perfusion produces swollen damaged tissue, exacerbating the pressure-volume problem in a "snowballing" fashion.

Acute changes in pressure in an intracranial compartment may produce a pressure gradient and precipitate a brain herniation syndrome. An ominous heralding sign of transtentorial herniation of the uncus of the temporal lobe is full pupillary dilation and loss of the light reflex caused by entrapment of cranial nerve III. Herniation often produces vascular compromise of other tissues by compression of the posterior cerebral artery, causing further tissue necrosis, edema, and pressure increases that produce irreversible brainstem damage. Posterior fossa pressure may result in a pressure cone downward through the foramen magnum leading to apnea and death. *A marginally compensated pressure gradient may be decompensated by an ill-advised lumbar puncture.*

Symptoms of increased ICP include loss of appetite, nausea, vomiting, headache, and lethargy. More prolonged increased ICP may produce decreased visual acuity. Findings on examination include inattention, decreased arousability, papilledema, up-gaze paresis, hypertonia, positive Babinski reflexes, and impaired gait. Decreased pulse rate and increased blood pressure may occur as a sign of worsening ICP. The child also may have history and focal signs compatible with an intracranial mass or may have a mass lesion, cerebral edema, or enlarged ventricles on an imaging study. An infant with increased ICP may show reluctance to feed, irritability, scalp vein distention, full fontanelle, spreading of sutures with abnormal skull percussion, increasing head

size, and "sunsetting" of the eyes as a result of failure of up-gaze. Papilledema is rare in infants.

DIAGNOSIS

The extent and severity of the encephalopathy and its etiology must be diagnosed. The neurologic examination establishes the extent and severity of CNS involvement. The direction and rate of progression of the acute encephalopathy can be determined by careful, serial examinations. The causes of encephalopathy are diagnosed from the history, clinical setting (age of the patient, other diagnoses or conditions, and where and when the encephalopathy began), and laboratory investigations. Pertinent history includes behavioral changes and the events leading to them; drug or toxic exposures (medicine cabinet inspections may be necessary); recent or concurrent fever, infection, and infectious exposures; systemic illness; and previous personal or family history of encephalopathy, epilepsy, or migraine. Physical examination may provide clues, such as evidence of trauma, skin lesions, presence of a ventricular shunt, or meningeal signs.

When the history and clinical setting point to a specific diagnosis, appropriate laboratory investigations should be undertaken. Otherwise, studies should be obtained in a stepwise fashion (Box 31-3). First, complete blood counts, electrolytes, glucose, blood urea nitrogen, liver function tests including an ammonia level, serum osmolality, and anticonvulsant levels if the patient has taken them and urine for analysis and toxicology screen should be requested. If there is fever, blood and urine cultures also should be obtained. Next, a computed tomography (CT) scan of the head should be done. If there is evidence of unexplained trauma, a dilated ophthalmologic examination, a skeletal survey, and a radionuclide bone scan should be done to look for evidence of abuse. If studies are nondiagnostic, a lumbar

Box 31-3. Laboratory Investigations for Acute Encephalopathy

- Complete blood count, coagulopathy screen
- Electrolytes, blood urea nitrogen, creatinine
- Glucose, calcium, phosphate
- Serum osmolality
- Liver function tests
- Anticonvulsant levels
- Arterial blood gas
- Urinalysis, urine organic acids
- Serum lactate/pyruvate, ammonia, amino acids
- Cultures
- Chest x-ray
- Electrocardiogram
- Electroencephalogram
- Evoked potentials
- Computed tomography scan
- Magnetic resonance imaging
- Head ultrasound (neonate)
- Cerebrospinal fluid examination
- Toxicology screen
- Skeletal survey

puncture with manometry should be done looking for signs of infection, subarachnoid hemorrhage, or increased ICP. Calcium, phosphate, and thyroid function tests help establish parathyroid and thyroid disorders, although these conditions are rare. Blood gases and pH are useful when the cause is respiratory or metabolic. If blood gases or chest sounds are abnormal, an electrocardiogram and chest x-ray should be requested. If there is metabolic acidosis or an anion gap, serum lactate, serum free and esterified carnitine, urine organic acids, and urine and plasma amino acids should be obtained.

The electroencephalogram (EEG) assesses the degree of encephalopathy as revealed by the frequency of background rhythms and can indicate specific abnormalities, such as periodic lateralized epileptiform discharges in a temporal lobe in herpes encephalitis, triphasic waves in hepatic encephalopathy, or focal slowing in ischemic cortex. Magnetic resonance imaging (MRI) using diffusion mapping techniques discerns infarcted tissue early after an hypoxic-ischemic insult and detects demyelinated or edematous white matter and mass lesions more readily than CT. Angiography is needed to diagnose a clot or other source of hemorrhage if there is evidence of a clinical stroke or early decreased diffusion signal or a hypodense lesion in a vascular distribution on MRI. MRI also readily delineates the findings of hypertensive encephalopathy. Coagulation studies should be added if there is evidence of a stroke, hemorrhagic diathesis, or coagulopathy. An echocardiogram is useful when an embolic stroke from a cardiac source is likely.

Hypoxic-ischemic injuries usually are suspected from the history or clinical setting. Box 31-4 lists frequent causes of hypoxemic-ischemic encephalopathy in children. If the hypoxic-ischemic insult is severe enough, other organs also are affected, although the CNS may be the most sensitive. Acute tubular necrosis in the kidneys, liver function abnormalities, and cardiac enzyme elevations may accompany CNS failure. The CNS injury may evolve through stages, including an initial partial recovery after cardiorespiratory restoration, then a worsening after the first few hours as cytotoxic cerebral edema progresses, damaging or causing dysfunction in tissue that survived the initial insult.

Infections, trauma, and seizures are common causes of acute encephalopathy in children. Intracranial infections include meningitis, encephalitis, and focal inflammations, which can produce widespread CNS involvement through generalized cytokine responses. Acute disseminated post-

Table 31-2. Closed Head Trauma

Injury	Findings
Concussion, a clinical syndrome	Immediate and transient impairment of neurologic function. Findings may include alteration of consciousness, amnesia, or disturbance of vision or equilibrium
Cerebral contusion, bruising of the brain parenchyma	Focal signs and symptoms at site of injury (coup) or on the side opposite the injury (contracoup)
Subdural hematoma, bleeding between the dura and brain parenchyma from a tear of an artery or bridging vein	Loss of consciousness, signs of increased intracranial pressure
Epidural hematoma, rapidly accumulating blood between dura and cranium	Loss of consciousness, severe headache. Biphasic course of impaired consciousness followed by lucid period, then abrupt evolution to impaired consciousness is less frequent in children than in adults

infectious encephalomyelitis is a rare cause and presumably involves a dysimmune mechanism. "Patchy" or diffuse white matter involvement associated with mildly inflammatory CSF parameters (e.g., CSF white blood cells <25 mm^3) is the most common presentation. Accidental trauma in an older ambulatory child and nonaccidental trauma in an infant also are common causes of encephalopathy. Table 31-2 lists types of head trauma and their findings. Nonaccidental trauma must be considered when the history does not correspond with the severity of the injuries to the CNS (see Chapter 269). Seizures may be symptomatic of either a separate acute brain process or an idiopathic disorder producing only the ictal state intermittently. Findings that suggest a seizure include rhythmic, clonic movements or lightning, myoclonic jerks; rapid or variable changes of tone or posturing distinct from decerebrate posturing; abrupt or fluctuating changes of autonomic function (e.g., heart rate, blood pressure, pupillary size); saliva production without swallowing; and history of prior seizures. Sometimes only direct EEG monitoring or the immediate response to a therapeutic anticonvulsant dose can establish ongoing seizure activity as the cause of the change in level of responsiveness.

Ingestions of toxic substances commonly cause childhood encephalopathy. Box 31-5 lists specific signs and symptoms that accompany encephalopathy from toxin exposures. Features that indicate the encephalopathy may be caused by a metabolic disorder are listed in Box 31-6. The pattern of organic acids and amino acids present on a screen may help suggest a possible diagnosis. Urea cycle disorders generally do not produce acidosis. An abnormal level of citrulline or the presence of orotic acid helps establish these diagnoses. Some organic acidurias also have hyperammonemia. Some disorders may require muscle biopsy tissue to assay for specific defects (see Chapter 146).

Box 31-7 lists causes of recurrent acute encephalopathies. Complicated or confusional migraine sometimes presents a diagnostic challenge. If a child is confused and the headache symptom cannot be elicited, the diagnosis becomes one of exclusion. The possibility of a space-occupying lesion should be eliminated by imaging studies

Box 31-4. Frequent Causes of Hypoxic-Ischemic Encephalopathy

- Submersion accident
- Strangulation
- Trauma with severe hemorrhage
- Septic shock
- Smoke inhalation
- Aspiration of foreign body
- Ingestion of a central nervous system depressant
- Acute epiglottitis with airway obstruction
- Cardiac failure
- Apparent life-threatening event

compromised, and the flattened diaphragm is forced to contract with shortened muscle fibers.

Patients who have had previous life-threatening attacks or were admitted to the hospital in the past year are most at risk for mortality. Fatal cases occur in patients who have a psychological disorder or depression or who lack parental or medical support systems. African-American urban boys younger than 15 years old have a 50% higher mortality rate than girls of the same age. Other contributing causes include inappropriate use of sedatives and complications of asthma medications. In many cases, morbidity and mortality are related to the cerebral anoxia occurring before hospital admission or barotrauma during mechanical ventilation. The two most common modes of death from asthma are hypoxic cardiac arrest and pneumothorax. Most deaths from asthma seem to occur in newly diagnosed or mildly affected asthmatic children who experience a sudden, severe bronchospastic attack resulting in cardiac arrest and children with an established diagnosis who are steroid-dependent and who have poor asthma control, often with histories of previous ventilatory failure. Few in-hospital deaths occur, suggesting that aggressive pharmacotherapy and judicious use of positive-pressure ventilation of severe asthmatics results in favorable outcomes.

DIAGNOSIS

Clinical evaluation of a patient with asthma and deteriorating gas exchange or progressive dyspnea must be completed quickly. As complete a history as possible should define the degree of underlying pulmonary disease, potential inciting events, and response to treatment; prior history of wheezing; what maintenance medications the child takes; compliance; time of last aerosol; previous office, clinic, or emergency department visits; previous hospitalizations; intubations; last steroid course; when this exacerbation began; precipitating factors; other nonasthma medications; and general medical history. The differential diagnosis of status asthmaticus is listed in Box 32-1.

The physical examination of the lung fields should define the degree of airflow obstruction and assess respiratory

---

Box 32-1. Differential Diagnosis of Respiratory Distress

- Pneumothorax
- Endobronchial lesion
- Pulmonary edema, cardiogenic or noncardiogenic
- Foreign body
- Enlarged lymph nodes from infection or tumor
- Anaphylaxis
- Bronchiolitis
- Cystic fibrosis
- Aspergillosis
- Congenital anomalies
  - Laryngotracheomalacia
  - Vocal cord paralysis
  - Tracheal or bronchial stenosis
  - Gastroesophageal reflux
  - Vascular ring
- Toxic fume exposure

---

reserve. The presence or absence of wheezes on lung examination can be an important indicator of the degree of airflow obstruction and the potential for respiratory failure. Wheezes can be a sign of improving pulmonary function for a patient with severe bronchospasm who previously had such low expiratory flow that no wheezes were audible. Breath sounds should be symmetric. Some asymmetry may be heard with asthma alone as a result of mucous plugging and atelectasis. Unilateral increased wheezing may indicate a foreign body. Significant unilaterally decreased breath sounds may be caused by pneumothorax or pneumonia. Use of accessory muscles (abdominal paradoxical breathing, sternocleidomastoid use, nasal flaring, intercostals retraction) correlates with the severity of airflow obstruction. Wheezing is a less sensitive indicator of the degree of obstruction present.

Pulsus paradoxus is the difference in systolic blood pressure between the pressure at which an observer first hears faint pulse sounds and the pressure at which all sounds are heard. It is measured best with a sphygmomanometer and a stethoscope. Pulsus paradoxus of 10 to 15 mm Hg indicates the effect that air trapping is having on cardiac output and correlates well with moderate-to-severe disease. The presence of crepitus in the neck or chest wall signifies air leak and significant obstruction. If evaluation of the patient's mental status reveals any confusion or obtundation, significant hypercapnia or hypoxemia should be considered; if present, this necessitates immediate action.

Laboratory evaluation includes a white blood cell count to evaluate the likelihood of infection and tests to assess gas exchange. Most often an arterial blood gas evaluation is necessary to document the degree of hypoxemia, response to supplemental oxygen, and degree of hypoventilation or hyperventilation. Clinicians must be prepared to act on the information obtained from blood gases and should make judgments regarding the need for blood gases and immediate intervention based on clinical information (e.g., worsening of or improvement in clinical condition). The degree of hypoxemia is extremely variable and does not correlate with the overall severity of airway constriction. The presence of a metabolic acidosis accompanied by an anion gap suggests inadequate oxygen delivery from either impaired cardiac output or hypoxemia. Acidosis may be caused by the combined effects of hypoxemia, myocardial compromise, increased work of breathing, and oxygen demand of the respiratory muscles. Capillary blood gases are adequate for evaluating PCO_2 after good perfusion of the site has been ensured. In older children and adults, serial monitoring of peak expiratory flow may provide a useful guide to clinical response to therapy. A chest x-ray can document pulmonary infiltrates and potential infection, lung disruption, and evidence of atelectasis. Segmental atelectasis commonly is present in children with acute asthma. The presence of multiple infiltrates indicates an infectious component.

Criteria for admission to the pediatric intensive care unit are not absolute. The most important consideration is to admit the patient who continues to deteriorate despite aggressive therapy. Some clinical indications for pediatric intensive care unit admission are the use of accessory muscles, pulsus paradoxus greater than 12 mm Hg, diaphoresis, inability to recline, hypercapnia, peak expiratory flow rate less than 40% predicted, disturbed consciousness, previous history of respiratory failure, drug toxicity, metabolic acidosis, respiratory treatments greater than every hour, inability to provide adequate staffing on general wards, and respiratory arrest and the need for mechanical ventilation.

MANAGEMENT

Principles for managing status asthmaticus are listed in Box 32-2. The first essential step in management is to improve oxygen delivery. High-flow oxygen should be administered immediately and continued until hypoxemia has resolved. Hypoxemia, often the cause of morbidity and mortality from asthma, may produce pulmonary hypertension, bronchoconstriction, and decreased oxygen delivery in the face of increased myocardial oxygen consumption. Because hypoxemia most commonly is due to V/Q mismatching, it usually is reversed with supplemental oxygen, which improves systemic oxygen delivery and minimizes hypoxia caused by β_2-agonist–enhanced pulmonary vasodilation to low ventilated alveolar units. The benefit of improved oxygen delivery is much greater than any theoretical risk of oxygen-induced respiratory depression. Hypoxemia may produce pulmonary hypertension, bronchoconstriction, and decreased oxygen delivery in the face of increased myocardial oxygen consumption.

Inhaled β_2-agonists are the drugs of choice in the treatment of the smooth muscle–mediated component of acute asthma. Albuterol and metaproterenol are used most frequently because their onset of action is rapid and side effects are rare. Albuterol may have some advantage over metaproterenol because of its slightly longer duration of action and greater β_2 selectivity resulting in less cardiac stimulation. Because dose response and duration of activity of these agents can be decreased by limitations of airflow caused by bronchoconstriction, impaired delivery secondary to airway inflammation and edema, and altered patient cooperation and breathing patterns, larger and more frequent dosing often is required in the treatment of status asthmaticus. Continuous therapy with β-agonists can be an effective method of delivering bronchodilators because it does not require cooperation or coordination of inspiratory effort and can be administered without waking the patient.

The ventilator circuitry, ventilator settings, and site of administration within the ventilator circuit influence delivery of inhaled β-agonists to the intubated patient. Other factors that affect delivery are presence of infection, thoracic volume alterations, fluid overload, and other drug interactions. Therapeutic regimens must be tailored to the individual patient. Generally, supranormal doses should be administered and then adjusted according to clinical and physiologic parameters. The comparative efficacy of inhalations of metered-dose inhalers varies. Intubated patients generally require higher doses than spontaneously breathing patients to achieve the desired physiologic effects. The use of intravenous bronchodilators in severely ill intubated children with asthma has never been evaluated.

Nebulized albuterol delivers the drug locally to β-receptors in the lung, achieving therapeutic effects with fewer side effects than systemically administered β_2-adrenergic agents. Hemodynamic effects of β_2-agonists include tachycardia, dysrhythmias, hypertension, possible myocardial ischemia, skeletal muscle tremor, and central nervous system stimulation. Metabolic side effects include hyperglycemia, hypokalemia, rhabdomyolysis, lactic acidosis, and hypophosphatemia.

Anticholinergics, such as ipratropium bromide and glycopyrrolate, tend to produce less bronchodilation than β-agonists. Onset of action may be slower, but duration of action is prolonged; peak onset of action occurs after 2 hours but lasts 6 hours. Absorption of inhaled anticholinergics from the airways is limited and does not seem to impair mucociliary clearance. Because ipratropium bromide seems to augment the bronchodilating effects of β-agonists, combining inhaled anticholinergics with β_2-agonists may yield enhanced and prolonged bronchodilation. A 30% reduction in hospital admission has been observed in patients treated with multiple doses.

Corticosteroids have a dual action: the early facilitation of β_2-agonist bronchodilation followed by a later anti-inflammatory role. They should be initiated immediately because the clinical response occurs 6 to 8 hours after administration. Maximal effect is obtained after 6 to 12 hours. Corticosteroids decrease mucus production, mediator release, and the late response (cellular) inflammatory process. They also increase the affinity of β-adrenergic receptors and reverse the increased capillary permeability seen in exacerbations. Side effects include hyperglycemia and hypertension.

Intravenous terbutaline has replaced isoproterenol almost entirely for use in particularly severe asthmatics. It is used widely in treating moderate-to-severe asthma exacerbations when frequent or continuous aerosols have been ineffective or if initial presentation is especially severe. Terbutaline is easily titrated and has a short half-life with an onset of action of less than 5 minutes and peak effects occurring by 90 to 120 minutes. Side effects include tachycardia, lowering of diastolic blood pressure, hyperglycemia, hypokalemia, and worsening hypoxia caused by increased V/Q mismatching and rhabdomyolysis. Heart rate must be monitored closely for tachycardia and electrocardiogram ST interval changes. Occasionally creatine phosphokinase levels are impressively elevated, particularly the MM fraction. The implication of increased creatine phosphokinase levels without electrocardiogram changes is unclear. Terbutaline increases lipolysis, gluconeogenesis, and glycogenolysis, resulting in an increase in insulin levels, blood glucose, and lactate and a decrease in serum potassium. As the patient improves, terbutaline is weaned before albuterol.

Box 32-2. Management Principles in Treating Status Asthmaticus

- Improve gas exchange, particularly ensuring adequacy of oxygenation
- Relieve bronchospasm
- Treat cause
- Therapy directed toward decreasing airway inflammation
- The key to successful management is early, aggressive medical management and appropriate use of mechanical ventilation

If aggressive medical therapy is unsuccessful, mechanical ventilation is the next step. Arterial blood gas is not always a good indication of the need for mechanical ventilation. Clinical criteria for intubation and ventilation are listed in Box 32-3. Although hypercapnia in acute severe asthma is worrisome, most patients do not require mechanical ventilation. The only absolute indication for ventilatory support occurs in patients who present in cardiac arrest.

Mechanical ventilation can rest the inspiratory muscles, provide adequate gas exchange, and decrease dynamic hyperinflation until the severe airway obstruction can be reversed. Limiting minute ventilation using an appropriately low but adequate tidal volume and respiratory rate decreases hyperinflation. Adequate gas exchange should be achieved with the lowest peak inspiratory pressure and lowest expiratory lung volume, avoiding intrinsic peak end-expiratory pressure. Regular, frequent suctioning of the endotracheal tube must be performed to prevent mucous plugging.

Although no ventilation method has been proved to be superior in status asthmaticus in children, volume-controlled mode usually is employed. This method guarantees reproducible tidal volume despite variations of airways resistance, but the consequent uses of pressure must be limited. In the pressure control mode, variation in resistance induces variations of tidal volume. No matter which mode of ventilation is used, ventilation must be monitored continuously. Parameters include inspiration and expiration, oxygen saturation, capnography, and arterial blood gases. Use of positive end-expiratory pressure is controversial. In most cases, none should be applied to reduce the risk of auto–positive end-expiratory pressure, compromised venous return, and decreased cardiac output.

Permissive hypercapnia is a ventilatory strategy used to minimize barotrauma. Ventilation is maintained at the lowest level, allowing a relatively high $PaCO_2$ if oxygenation remains adequate and pH remains greater than 7.20. Risks of permissive hypercapnia include worsening of preexisting intracranial hypertension (cerebral vasodilation and edema), myocardial depression, and pulmonary vasoconstriction.

The complications of mechanical ventilation include pneumothorax, pneumomediastinum, pneumoperitoneum, and interstitial emphysema. After intubation, the patient may have hypotension as a result of hyperinflation, hypovolemia, and sedation. Treatment consists of a rapid fluid bolus and modification of the ventilator settings. Other complications include tissue hypoxia, arrhythmias, edema, mucous plugs, atelectasis, and nosocomial infections including pneumonia and sinusitis.

In refractory cases, general inhalational anesthesia has been advocated for sedation and to decrease airway resistance in patients with persistent severe asthma. Halothane, enflurane, and isoflurance effectively have lowered airway resistance and improved gas exchange. Response is expected within the first hour of therapy. In most cases, the anesthetic gases can be discontinued within 12 hours. Patients may develop hypotension from inhalational anesthetics because of peripheral vasodilation and decreased venous return as a result of high intrathoracic pressures. Hypotension is controllable by temporarily lowering the concentration of the agent while providing volume expansion.

Supportive care for a patient with status asthmaticus includes the judicious use of antibiotics and fluid management. Approximately 10% of asthmatic children undergoing an acute exacerbation have a bacterial infection. Antibiotics should be given only to patients with clinical, biologic, or radiographic signs of bacterial infections, such as otitis, sinusitis, or pneumonia. Some children with status asthmaticus may present with mild-to-moderate dehydration as a result of increased metabolism, increased respiratory fluid losses, vomiting, and decreased fluid intake.

Controversial therapies in the treatment of status asthmaticus include the use of methylxanthines, sodium bicarbonate ($NaHCO_3$), magnesium sulfate, and ketamine. Use of methylxanthines, magnesium sulfate, and ketamine is discussed on the CD-ROM. Infusion of $NaHCO_3$ has been proposed in two main clinical situations: (1) for the partial correction of severe metabolic acidosis in a spontaneously breathing child who has responded well to bronchodilators but with persistent dyspnea and hyperventilation and (2) during mechanical ventilation with persistent hypercapnia to maintain pH greater than 7.3. The optimal pH threshold during $NaHCO_3$ infusion is not clear. The side effects of metabolic acidosis include myocardial depression; decreased effectiveness of β-agonists; and stimulation of ineffective, rapid, shallow ventilation. $NaHCO_3$ may lower intracellular and cerebrospinal fluid pH, lower serum potassium, and increase the affinity of hemoglobin for oxygen.

OUTCOME

Outcome of status asthmaticus depends on the condition of the patient on arrival to the hospital. If the patient arrives in full arrest, outcome is dismal from anoxic damage to the brain and other organs. In-hospital deaths are rare.

FOLLOW-UP

Patients who are hospitalized with severe status asthmaticus should be referred to a specialist with experience in dealing with asthma. These patients are at high risk for further morbidity and mortality. All patients should continue to be followed by their pediatrician. Appropriate

Box 32-3. Criteria for Intubation and Mechanical Ventilation

1. Respiratory muscle fatigue, obvious exhaustion, disappearance of pulsus paradoxus
2. Decrease of thoracic amplitude during respiratory movements
3. Diminution of air entry into the lungs: quiet chest, absence of audible wheezes
4. Pulsus paradoxus >20–40 mm Hg
5. Deterioration of mental status (lethargy, agitation, confusion, coma)
6. Diaphoresis in recumbent position
7. Respiratory or cardiac arrest
8. Failure of maximal pharmacologic therapy
9. Cyanosis and hypoxemia (PaO_2 <60 mm Hg) unrelieved by oxygen
10. $PaCO_2$ >50 mm Hg and increasing >5 mm Hg/hr

long-term therapy is the mainstay in preventing further exacerbations. Families must be educated on the management of asthma and the importance of long-term medications even in the face of a well-appearing child.

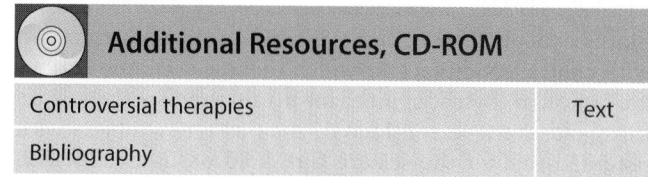

Additional Resources, CD-ROM

Controversial therapies	Text
Bibliography	

SUGGESTED READINGS

American Thoracic Society: Chronic bronchitis, asthma, and pulmonary emphysema. Am Rev Respir Dis 1962;85:762–768.
Bulloch B, Ruddy RM: Asthma update: Managing asthma in the pediatric emergency department. Pediatr Emerg Med Rep 1998;3:39–50.
Cohen NH, Eigen H, Shaughnessy TE: Status asthmaticus. Crit Care Clin 1997;13:459–476.
DeNicola LK, Monem GF, Gayle MO, Kissoon N: Treatment of critical status asthmaticus in children. Pediatr Clin North Am 1994;41:1293–1323.
Kulick RM, Ruddy RM: Allergic emergencies. In Fleisher GR, Ludwig S (eds): Textbook of Pediatric Emergency Medicine, 3rd ed. Baltimore, Williams & Wilkins, 1993, pp 858–867.

SECTION 3   GENERAL MEDICAL CARE: *Emergent Medical Care*

33 Status Epilepticus

Kian-Ti Yu

ROLE OF THE GENERALIST

1 Recognize and classify the different clinical manifestations of status epilepticus.

2 Apply the appropriate general resuscitative and supportive measures and specific pharmacologic therapies in the management of status epilepticus.

3 Refer to a specialist for the management of refractory status epilepticus.

4 Ensure follow-up evaluation in the treatment of status epilepticus.

DEFINITION

Status epilepticus is a common neurologic emergency. Status epilepticus may be life-threatening to the patient and a challenge to the treating physician. It is estimated that 3% to 16% of all patients with epileptic seizures develop status epilepticus at some point in their lives. In some patients, it may be the presentation of the initial seizure disorder.

The cardinal feature of status epilepticus is continuous or repeating seizures that occur so rapidly that the patient does not recover consciousness between them. Status epilepticus has various forms of clinical presentations. *Convulsive status epilepticus* involves motor activity and includes tonic-clonic status and myoclonic status. Complex partial status epilepticus and absence status epilepticus are classified as *nonconvulsive status epilepticus*. There is impairment of consciousness with varying other symptoms, depending on the seizure type. *Focal status epilepticus* involves continuous focal clonic movements. *Psychogenic status epilepticus* involves continuous factitious "seizures"—voluntary movements, in the absence of an abnormal brain discharge.

Tonic-clonic status epilepticus typically has been defined as repetitive generalized tonic-clonic seizures lasting 30 minutes or longer or seizures without full return of consciousness between episodes. The stereotyped nature of the motor activity in *generalized tonic-clonic seizures* makes them relatively easy to diagnose. Typically the seizures consist of five clinical phases (Table 33-1): flexion, extension, tremor, clonic, and postictal. Consciousness is lost during the flexion phase. Apnea may occur during the extension phase, possibly caused by a central effect combined

Table 33-1. Five Clinical Phases of Tonic-Clonic Seizures

Phase	Description
Flexion phase	Brief, usually begins with the eyes opening, ocular globes rotating upward, mouth held rigidly half open, flexion of arms and legs. Consciousness lost during this phase
Extension phase	Begins with extension of back and neck, mouth forcibly closed resulting in tongue biting, apnea may occur, extension of the arms and legs
Tremor phase	Tonic rigidity replaced by a fine tremor that increases in amplitde and decreases in frequency as the clonic phase is entered
Clonic phase	Muscle relaxation is interspersed with tonic contractions. Alternating increase and decrease in muscle tone result in rhythmic jerks, which decrease in frequency as the seizure continues
Postictal phase	Patient is flaccid and unconscious, slowly resolves through stages of consciousness, although some may progress into sleep without awakening

with sustained contraction of the respiratory muscles. The tongue may be bitten in either the extension or the clonic phase. Between the last clonic jerk and the immediate postictal phase, the bladder sphincter relaxes, and incontinence may result. During the immediate postictal period, the patient remains unconscious and flaccid; as the postictal phase continues, the patient may awaken slowly by passing through successive stages of coma, stupor, confusional states, and drowsiness. Some patients progress directly into sleep without awakening.

Myoclonic status epilepticus is seen commonly among comatose patients after asphyxia or cardiac arrest. Other causes include drug intoxication, toxic exposure to pesticides, renal or hepatic failure, and end-stage neurodegenerative disorders. With *complex partial status epilepticus*, consciousness is impaired, with a blank stare, rambling speech, or mute presentation. A waxing and waning state alternating between agitation and obtundation is characteristic. Inappropriate laughing or crying may occur. Hallucinations also may occur, and a complete amnesia for the attacks is characteristic.

Absence status epilepticus is characterized by evenly sustained impairment of consciousness or intellectual dysfunction, facial twitching or eye blinking, staring, and occasional motor automatisms. Many patients have spontaneous or reactive automatisms and can perform activities of daily living, such as eating, drinking, and dressing. Because there is reduction of vigilance, however, unintentional injuries usually occur in the process of carrying out daily activities. *Focal status epilepticus* involves continuous clonic movements of one or two extremities, which the patient is unable to control. A hemiparesis that may last for days can result if the condition is treated in an untimely fashion. The disorder often is related to an acute hemispheric lesion, such as hemorrhage or metastasis.

Psychogenic seizures may occur comparatively frequently in patients with proven seizure disorder. Several clinical features help distinguish psychogenic status epilepticus. Jerking movements are out of phase and asynchronous, with forward thrusting of the pelvis. Screaming during the jerking movements, dilated but reactive pupils, intact gag reflex, and absence of tongue biting are other prominent features. Between jerking movements, some patients may speak brief sentences indicating major distress.

EVALUATION

Status epilepticus may occur de novo or may be associated with clinical conditions for which therapeutic interventions are indicated. Potential mechanisms that reduce the seizure threshold must be considered, such as a new illness with potential to alter the seizure threshold or, in a child with seizure disorder, the onset of symptoms that reduces the seizure threshold or who does not have a therapeutic level of anticonvulsant to match the seizure threshold risk currently. Evaluation includes determining the type of status epilepticus and the underlying cause. Common causes of status epilepticus include (1) rapid discontinuation of barbiturates and benzodiazepines, (2) change in antiepileptic drugs or bioavailability, (3) hypoxic-ischemic encephalopathy, (4) central nervous system infections (bacterial meningitis/viral encephalitis), (5) stroke, (6) intracranial tumor or metastasis, (7) head trauma, (8) drug or alcohol abuse, (9) hypoglycemia, and (10) hyponatremia.

MANAGEMENT

The goals in the management of status epilepticus, specifically the generalized tonic-clonic status, are simple: Stop seizure activity as quickly as possible, protect neurons from seizure-induced damage, and allow for full recovery from the episode. Physiologic changes that occur in late status epilepticus can produce systemic complications and place neurons in jeopardy of permanent damage or death (Table 33-2). The longer status epilepticus persists, the more likely neurons are to be damaged by exposure of N-methyl-D-aspartate receptors to the excitatory amino acid neurotransmitter glutamate.

The management of status epilepticus can be divided into general measures and specific pharmacotherapy. General measures include immediate emergency cardiovascular and pulmonary support; fluid and electrolyte management, especially immediate management of hypoglycemia; and evaluation and correction of physiologic abnormalities that

Table 33-2. Physiologic Changes in Generalized Convulsive Status Epilepticus

Transient or Early (0–30 min)	Late (after 30 min)
Arterial hypertension	Arterial hypotension
Cerebrovenous pressure raised	Cerebrovenous pressure raised or normal
Arterial P_{O_2} low or normal	Arterial P_{O_2} low or normal
Arterial P_{CO_2} high	Arterial P_{CO_2} or high
cvP_{O_2} (low or high)	cvP_{O_2} normal or low
cvP_{CO_2} high	cvP_{CO_2} normal (or high)
Cerebral blood flow increased	Cerebral blood flow increased, normal, or decreased
Hyperglycemia	Normoglycemia, hypoglycemia
Hyperkalemia	Hyperkalemia
Lactic acidosis	Hyperthermia (secondary)

cvP_{CO_2}, cerebrovenous partial pressure of carbon dioxide; cvP_{O_2}, cerebrovenous partial pressure of oxygen; P_{CO_2}, partial pressure of carbon dioxide; P_{O_2}, partial pressure of oxygen.

may occur as a consequence of the episode of status epilepticus or may be causing the seizure.

Successful management of status epilepticus is contingent on the use of drugs with the characteristics listed in Box 33-1. New formulations of drugs relevant to the treatment of status epilepticus include diazepam rectal gel, fosphenytoin, and intravenous valproate. Table 33-3 is a suggested protocol for the treatment of status epilepticus in children. If status epilepticus persists despite adequate initial pharmacotherapy or in complex cases in which adverse side effects are to be expected, the generalist may wish to call for the assistance of specialists.

Administration of *diazepam rectal gel (Diastat)* may be preferred when intravenous access is difficult or impossible. In addition, the rectal route offers the advantage of treating status epilepticus in the prehospital setting. The high lipid solubility of diazepam solutions permits rapid absorption and penetration into the central nervous system. Rectal diazepam has been shown to cause electroencephalogram changes consisting of fast activity that appears 1 to 9 minutes after administration. Diastat is a gel that contains diazepam provided in a prefilled, unit-dose, rectal delivery system, available in 2.5-, 5-, and 10-mg dosage strengths in pediatric preparations.

Fosphenytoin is a water-soluble phosphate ester prodrug of phenytoin. It is converted rapidly and completely to phenytoin after parenteral administration with little intrinsic pharmacologic activity before conversion. Organ and blood phosphatases cleave phenytoin from the prodrug. The conversion half-life is 8 to 15 minutes. Fosphenytoin has a pH of 8.6 to 9.0, may be admixed with many standard intravenous solutions, and is stable at room temperature for several months. In contrast, *phenytoin* has a pH of 12, is not to be diluted, and should be administered only with normal saline. Phlebitis and other serious cutaneous side effects

Table 33-3. Timetable for Treatment of Status Epilepticus* (Generalized Tonic-Clonic)

Minutes	Action
0–5	1. Confirm diagnosis observing active seizure while placing patient in safe position in office or emergency department 2. Position head and airway, assess oxygenation and ventilation; initiate supplemental oxygen by nasal cannula or simple mask or bag-valve-mask when respiratory assistance is needed. Obtain suction with rigid suction catheter (Yankauer) to clear airway as necessary. Prepare for endotrachea intubation for persistent respiratory insufficiency 3. Obtain and record vital signs, establish ECG monitoring, and evaluate oxygenation with pulse oximetry: continue to observe; treat any abnormalities 4. Obatin IV access, keep open with 0.9% saline 5. Obtain rapid glucose measure. Obtain venous blood for glucose, serum chemistries, hematology, toxicology, and serum anti–epileptic drug levels as indicated 6. If hypoglycemic or if blood glucose measurement is not available, give glucose in children, 2 mL/kg of 25% glucose (in young infants, consider use of 5 mL/kg of 10% glucose) 7. Ascertain pertinent historical and current therapy from parent/provider
6–9†	1. Administer lorazepam, 0.1 mg/kg IV at 2 mg/min up to 4 mg total 2. For difficult IV access, administer rectal diazepam, 0.5 mg/kg for ages <6 yr, 0.3 mg/kg for age 6–11 yr, and 0.2 mg/kg for ages ≥12 yr 3. Reassess ABCs, especially oxygenation, ventilation, and perfusion 4. Repeat dose as above if no response in 5 min
10–20	1. Administer fosphenytoin (or phenytoin) at 20 mg/kg phenytoin equivalents at maximum of 6 mg phenytoin equivalents/min. Phenytoin at 1 mg/kg/min (IV fluid must be 0.9% saline as phenytoin crystallizes in D5W solution) *or* Administer valproate (Depacon) IV, 25 mg/kg at a rate of 3 mg/kg/min 2. Reassess respiratory status and monitor blood pressure and ECG during infusion
20–60	1. If seizure continues for >15–20 min after 20 mg/kg of phenytoin or fosphenytoin, give additional phenytoin or fosphenytoin at 5 mg/kg until a maximum of 30 mg/kg 2. If seizure persists, give valproate IV as above *or* If the second-line drug use was valproate IV and seizure persists, give 20 mg/kg of phenytoin or fosphenytoin as above *or* Administer phenobarbital, 20 mg/kg IV at rate of 2 mg/kg/min (maximum 100 mg/min) Assisted ventilation usually required 3. If status persists 20 min after previous therapy, administer midazolam as a loading dose of 0.2 mg/kg slow IV bolus, followed by 0.05–0.3 mg/kg/hr. Adjust maintenance dose to stop seizure based on EEG monitoring. The primary end point for therapy is suppression of EEG spikes 4. Expect apnea, particularly if the patient has received benzodiazepines. Assist ventilation; intubation is required, patient requires a monitored PICU bed
>60	Pentobarbital or other general anesthetics may be added for the refractory status; vasopressors often required

*Use this timetable for a seizure that starts within medical care. Because more commonly the seizure has begun before arrival, it is safe to assume a minimum of 10 minutes (if initial time is not available).

†Early treatment is the goal, particularly when simple seizures in childhood often stop spontaneously in <5 min. The goal is to administer therapy early, particularly when the seizure may have been unwitnessed or begun before "starting the clock."

ABCs, airways, breathing, circulation; D5W, 5% dextrose in water; ECG, electrocardiogram; EEG, electroencephalogram; IV, intravenous; PICU, pediatric intensive care unit.

linked to intravenous administration of phenytoin do not occur with fosphenytoin. Although fosphenytoin can be administered intramuscularly, drugs ideally should not be given intramuscularly in status epilepticus because absorption is slow and may be erratic. The maximal recommended infusion rates of fosphenytoin (150 mg phenytoin equivalents [PE]/min or 3 mg PE/kg/min) are three times the maximum rate for phenytoin, allowing administration of a 20 mg PE/kg loading dose of fosphenytoin in less than 10 minutes.

The antiepileptic drugs available for parenteral use are phenobarbital, fosphenytoin, phenytoin, diazepam, lorazepam, and intravenous valproate (Depacon). Phenobarbital undergoes less rapid penetration of the blood-brain barrier, and peak brain concentrations are achieved 15 to 20 minutes after peak serum concentrations. This medication also is associated with sedation and respiratory depression. Phenytoin is much less sedating than phenobarbital and is not associated with respiratory depression. Its use is accompanied, however, by the risk of injection site complications in view of its high alkalinity; hypotension and cardiac arrhythmia can occur secondary to its propylene glycol content when infused too rapidly. The recommendation is to infuse at no greater than 1 mg/kg/min. Fosphenytoin, being soluble in aqueous solutions, circumvents the adverse effects of phenytoin, but still has limited value in the treatment of myoclonic, atonic, and absence seizures.

Valproate offers treatment for a broad spectrum of seizure types, and the new intravenous form facilitates administration of loading doses in the treatment of status epilepticus. The ideal loading dose for achieving a target concentration of 100 to 150 µg/mL is 25 mg/kg of intravenous valproate. The rate of infusion for status epilepticus in pediatric patients may be 3 mg/kg/min. Valproate is tolerated best when infused intravenously at a minimal dilution of 1:1 with 5% dextrose in water, normal saline, or lactated Ringer's solution.

Treatment of complex partial status epilepticus should be aggressive. Animal studies indicate that electrical status may produce neuronal damage even when the animal is paralyzed and systemic homeostasis is maintained. Memory disturbances may result from complex partial status epilepticus even if patients do not have any changes involving their vital signs during the prolonged seizures. Intravenous lorazepam or rectal diazepam may be used as the first-line drug, with intravenous phenytoin, fosphenytoin, or valproate as second-line drugs.

Aggressive treatment also is recommended in absence status epilepticus. Although many children can perform activities of daily living, such as eating, drinking, and dressing, they are prone to unintentional injury because of sustained impairment of consciousness. The initial therapy for *absence status epilepticus* is usually intravenous lorazepam or rectal diazepam. If the initial therapy fails to halt the seizures, intravenous valproate should be administered.

FOLLOW-UP EVALUATION AND TREATMENT

When status epilepticus has been treated successfully, the etiologic and precipitating factors of the episode should be determined. If the patient is a known epileptic, it is important to note the serum antiepileptic drug level before

---

Box 33-2. Calculations for Appropriate Dose for Mini-Load

Formula: $D = Vd \times (C1 - C0)$

where D = dose; Vd = volume of distribution; C1 = the desired concentration; and C0 = the starting concentration.

For a drug with a Vd of 1 L/kg, a loading dose in mg/kg is equal to the desired increase in serum concentration in mg/L. A close approximation for clinical purposes is to give a mini-loading dose of 1 mg/kg for each 1 mg/L desired increase in serum concentration.

---

the administration of any drugs to treat status epilepticus. If the serum level was low, a review of potential causes—inadequate dosing, change in bioavailability, and possible noncompliance—should be reviewed with the patient, and appropriate measures should be taken. If the serum level was high, the decision of adding a second drug to control seizures should be made with potential alteration of the first medication.

When status epilepticus occurs in the absence of a history of a seizure disorder, it is necessary to determine whether this is a first presentation of chronic epilepsy or a complication of a severe systemic or central nervous system disorder. Evaluation and treatment should be directed at the cause, whether it is the specific epileptic syndrome or the specific illness that caused the status epilepticus.

Administration of a partial loading dose of a drug after status epilepticus has been treated successfully may be necessary to increase the steady-state concentration of the drug. This situation is most common when phenytoin is used to protect against recurrence of status epilepticus. Calculations for the appropriate dose for such a "mini-load" are listed in Box 33-2. Using the formula, an example of a mini-loading dose is as follows: A patient is found to have a phenytoin serum concentration of 12 mg/L and the desired maintenance concentration of phenytoin concentration is 20 mg/L; the mini-loading dose required to achieve this concentration is 8 mg/kg.

Mini-index of Related Topics   CH.

SUGGESTED READINGS

Holmes GL: Diagnosis and Management of Seizures in Children. Philadelphia, WB Saunders, 1987.

Treiman DM: Treatment of status epilepticus. In Engel J, Pedley TA (eds): Epilepsy: A Comprehensive Textbook. Philadelphia, Lippincott-Raven, 1997.

Wheless JW, Venkataraman V: New formulation of drugs in epilepsy. Exp Opin Pharmacother 1999;1:49–60.

Willmore JL: Epilepsy emergencies. Neurology 1998;51(Suppl 4):S34–S38.

Working Group on Status Epilepticus: Treatment of convulsive status epilepticus. JAMA 1993;270:854–859.

34 Injuries and Trauma

Richard M. Ruddy

ROLE OF THE GENERALIST

1 Differentiate high-risk injury from less serious injury.
2 Initiate care of the injured child.
3 Recognize injuries that need evaluation and treatment by a trauma specialist.
4 Understand the role of the pediatrician at a trauma center or community emergency department or hospital.
5 Triage care of injured children appropriately.

Table 34-1. Epidemiology of Death from Injury in Children (1998)

	<1 yr	1–4 yr	5–14 yr	All
Deaths	976	1714	2936	5626
Motor vehicle	147	654	1766	2567
Drowning	68	458	333	859
Burn	50	225	252	527
Firearm	15	70	253	338
Fall	23	32	66	121
Poisoning	15	31	50	96
Homicide*	332	415	326	1073

*Not cause but intentional.

Data from National Vital Statistics Report 2003;52(3). Available at: www.cdc.gov/nchs/data/nvsr52/nvsr52_03.pdf.

Trauma is the leading cause of death in children older than 1 year of age and one of the most frequent causes of hospitalization, chronic disability, missed school, and activities. Increased resources are required to address the public health issues of trauma, including trauma primary prevention and efficient and appropriate treatment (secondary prevention). Primary care practitioners should be able to differentiate high-risk injuries from less serious injuries. Generalists should initiate care and recognize injuries that need to be evaluated by a trauma specialist who can provide specific care to the child. Community physicians should understand the role of the pediatrician at a trauma center and the responsibility of a pediatrician at a community emergency department (ED) or hospital. Key in the office practice of pediatricians is to understand the risks to children of inappropriate triage and underreferral for specialized trauma care when it is needed.

FUNDAMENTALS: MECHANISMS OF INJURY

Trauma is differentiated into two broad categories—blunt and penetrating. *Blunt trauma* is more common, responsible for 85% to 90% of injuries to children. Classic examples are motor vehicle crash in which riders are injured or a pedestrian is struck by a moving object. Although blunt trauma is often serious and can cause long-term disability or death, it is usually "nonoperative." Operative blunt injury most often involves significant long bone fractures, but also can be seen with head trauma and serious chest or abdominal injury. *Penetrating trauma* can result from a knife or other sharp object or a gunshot causing injury from the bullet traversing vital structures. In adolescent boys, particularly in inner-city environments, the highest risk of death is from gunshot wounds or motor vehicle crash.

These situations commonly require rapid exploration or an operation to define and treat the injuries. In penetrating injury, the external examination may be benign, even with serious injury.

Other types of trauma include drowning and burns, the second and third leading causes of injury deaths in many age groups and regions. The major issue in drowning or submersion is the degree of resulting asphyxia. Incidence of drowning injuries/deaths has two peaks—the first in early childhood and the second in adolescence. Adolescent drowning frequently is associated with alcohol or drug use. Burns cause tissue injury to varying depths from flame, scald, or chemical agents. Although the rate of burn deaths has decreased since the 1990s, many burns still can be prevented through the proper use of smoke detectors and the maintenance of safe home environments. Survivors of significant burns can have systemic toxicity, significant end organ failure, and skin scarring with its subsequent negative psychosocial impact.

Table 34-1 lists the causes of injury deaths in children from the National Center for Health Statistics. Injuries still are the leading cause of deaths in childhood after the first year of life. Older adolescents are at high risk of death from motor vehicle crash, firearm injury, and suicide.

ASSESSMENT OF INJURY

All providers who care for children need to understand the emergency medical services within their community to comprehend their role in the management of injuries (see Chapter 26). The pyramid of emergency medical care described in Chapter 26 shows the potential access for care with them. Risk of ventricular fibrillation/arrest is higher. Internal burns not seen on the surface may lead to tissue, muscle, or bone necrosis, requiring surgical care or fasciotomy. Prevention of all of these injuries requires anticipatory guidance at each developmental stage—toddlers for home electrical cord risks and older children and adolescents (and the whole family) for thunderstorm safety and risk of high-energy electrical injury.

HYPOTHERMIA AND HYPERTHERMIA

Cold and heat exposures in children are important causes of significant morbidity and occasional deaths. Risk is increased significantly with chronically ill and very young children who may have impaired internal temperature control, in families with low socioeconomic status who are homeless or destitute, and in dysfunctional families when impaired guardians do not protect children adequately from environmental exposures.

Hypothermia most often is a problem with extended outdoor exposure when an unprotected, exposed extremity—hand, foot, nose, ear, or face—is exposed to extreme cold. Wet gloves, socks, or clothing further enhances the lowering of temperature and potential damage. *Frostnip* is the mildest local form of hypothermia, with pain, pallor, and numbness of the body part. It is rapidly reversible in almost all children. *Frostbite* is local freezing of tissue and can be categorized similar to burns by the degree of injury. Depending on the degree and duration of exposure, injuries range from superficial skin "burn" causing blistering to subcutaneous and muscle/bone necrosis. Treatment is removal from the cold environment, removal of wet clothing, and covering with warm blankets. Warm drinks are encouraged. The frostbitten body part should be rewarmed externally with warm water (40°C [104°F]) for 20 to 30 minutes to enhance circulation.

Systemic hypothermia is defined as the lowering of the core body temperature a minimum of 2°C (3.8°F) from the normal body temperature. Initial response of a normal child includes reflex vasoconstriction to spare the central circulation and involuntary shivering to raise the temperature. Continued lowering of core temperature further impairs homeostasis, leading to neurologic symptoms, cardiac dysrhythmias, and other end organ dysfunction. Cardiac arrest may follow ventricular fibrillation as the temperature decreases to less than 24°C (75.2°F) to 10°C (64.4°F). Children with "apparent" death from primary cold exposure may be resuscitated, but resuscitation of cardiac arrest rarely is successful in children who present as hypothermic but for whom the cause of arrest is not primary cold exposure. Hypothermia may be a sign of other serious problems, such as sepsis, hypothyroidism, or drug exposure.

Treatment of primary hypothermia includes accurate ascertainment of the core temperature and early control of ventilation to improve oxygenation and to maintain normocapnia. Mild-to-moderate hypothermia (temperature >32°C [89.6°F]) may require only passive external rewarming using dry, insulated materials and a warm environment. Because rewarming leads to peripheral vasodilation, fluid resuscitation may be needed. When the temperature is less than 32°C (89.6°F), rewarming may require warmed intra-

venous fluids, external warmed blankets or warmed bags, or warmed humidified oxygen. Immersion rewarming in a 40°C (104°F) bath is difficult. Regional centers are prepared for active rewarming regimens that may use gastrointestinal irrigation, peritoneal dialysis, thoracic lavage, and, rarely, cardiopulmonary bypass.

Hyperthermia, the elevation of body temperature secondary to environmental heat stress with subsequent inability to maintain homeostasis and secondary organ injury and potential death, most often occurs in extreme exposure (infants left in locked automobiles in the summer) or when heat exposure is subacute with inadequate fluid and electrolyte repletion. Infants are at higher risk because of their inability to ask for assistance and their higher body surface area to body size. Exertional heatstroke occasionally affects older children or adolescents, although the classic examples are military recruits who are overworked. Risk can be increased during early morning exercise from extreme physiologic stress the previous day. Risk also is increased in children with chronic conditions that affect sweating or temperature control. Drug overdoses, malignant hyperthermia, and neuroleptic syndromes are important secondary causes of hyperthermia that are life-threatening if not recognized and appropriately treated.

Heat cramps occur often in heat exhaustion, either in isolation or as part of more symptoms, and generally respond to salt solutions. They can occur with excessive hydration with water and subsequent hyponatremia. *Heat syncope* is a manifestation of intravascular volume depletion and requires oral or intravenous fluid resuscitation, depending on the degree of symptoms. Heat syncope must be distinguished from the more familiar vasovagal syncope. Heat exhaustion usually is more subacute, manifesting over several days with salt and water depletion. Heat exhaustion is differentiated from heatstroke by maintenance of body temperature at less than 39.4°C (103°F) to 40.0°C (104°F).

Management of *heat exhaustion* is oral and intravenous hydration and reduction of elevated temperatures to normal. Rehydration may be accomplished over 36 hours, provided that the environmental cause of the problem has been removed. Cooling may be accomplished by application of wet, cool towels, fanning, ice bags, or immersion in ice water. Prevention includes personal awareness of exposures; acclimatization; hydration with appropriate beverages; and conditioning with particular attention to infants, toddlers, and adolescents in early conditioning.

Management of *heatstroke* requires emergency management of the airway in all unconscious patients, establishment of intravenous access, and administration of a 20 mL/kg intravenous bolus of normal saline. Cooling measures should be initiated immediately with ice-water immersion. Core cooling techniques may be necessary in rare circumstances with the help of consultants. Prognosis may be good in 90% but is more guarded in patients with temperatures greater than 41°C (105.8°F) at presentation.

BITES AND ENVENOMATION

Animal bites are a common acute injury in children; dog bites account for more than 80% of mammalian bites. Important issues are cosmetic outcome of the injury; acute infection at the site; and risk of late infectious complications, such as tetanus or rabies. Wounds suffered from animal bites need to be managed to maximize cosmetic outcome. For most children, facial lacerations warrant primary closure after copious exploration, irrigation, and preparation. Although dog bites carry only a 2% to 3% rate of infection, most often with *Staphylococcus aureus*, but also with *Pasteurella multocida* in 15% to 20% of infections, antibiotic prophylaxis for dog bites is routine, particularly when the wound is closed. Wounds with a puncture entry where organisms from the animal's oropharynx may be deposited deep in the wound are more risky to close and a higher risk for infection. Antibiotic treatment should be considered for all wounds in which treatment has been delayed, all human and cat bites, and all wounds in children with underlying immune disorders. High-risk wounds often are treated with amoxicillin-clavulanic acid with erythromycin an alternative for penicillin-allergic patients. Cat bites, which tend to be puncture wounds, carry a higher risk of infection with *P. multocida*.

Closure of simple wounds may not require special skills, whereas a complex wound usually requires general or plastic surgical intervention to obtain the best cosmetic and functional outcomes. In making recommendations to a family, it is best to consider the known skills of local physicians rather than to refer to a specific credentialed group.

If the epidermis has been penetrated or disrupted, tetanus immunization status and risk of other delayed complications, particularly rabies, must be investigated. Although the risk of rabies is low, prophylaxis is safe now when it is indicated. The history of the type and health of the animal should be obtained. The greatest risk is from wild carnivores and bats. The risk of rabies from domesticated dogs or cats does not warrant immunization, unless the animal's health deteriorates over the next 2 weeks or the animal is not known or found. Prophylaxis should be considered in bat incidents even with scratches or abrasions. Dosing includes rabies immune globulin, 20 IU/kg, at day 1 and vaccine (human diploid cell rabies vaccine), 1 mL intramuscularly, at days 0, 3, 7, 14, and 28.

SUMMARY

The management of minor and severe trauma in children requires the efforts of a strong multidisciplinary team in the community. Although prevention efforts are crucial, when the child has an injury, care needs to be delivered from the initial transport to the incorporation back to the community (Fig. 34-2). Organization and use of regional resources is key to this success.

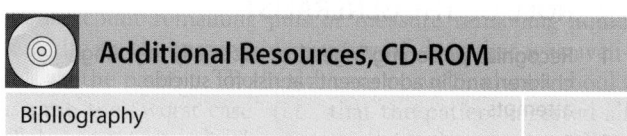

Additional Resources, CD-ROM

Bibliography

Mini-index of Related Topics

SUGGESTED READINGS

Auerbach PS: Wilderness Medicine: Management of Wilderness and Environmental Emergencies, 3rd ed. St. Louis, Mosby, 1995.

Cantor RM, Leaming JM: Evaluation and management of pediatric major trauma. Emerg Clin North Am 1998;16:229–257.

Committee on Trauma: Advanced Trauma Life Support for Doctors. Chicago, American College of Surgeons, 1997.

Jaffe D, Wesson D: Emergency management of blunt trauma in children. N Engl J Med 1991;324:1477–1482.

Moore E (ed) and the Committee on Trauma: Early Care of the Injured Patient. Toronto, BC Decker, 1990.

Ziegler MM, Gonzalez JA: Major trauma. From Fleisher GR, Ludwig S (eds): Textbook of Pediatric Emergency Medicine, 4th ed. Philadelphia, Lippincott Williams & Wilkins, 1999.

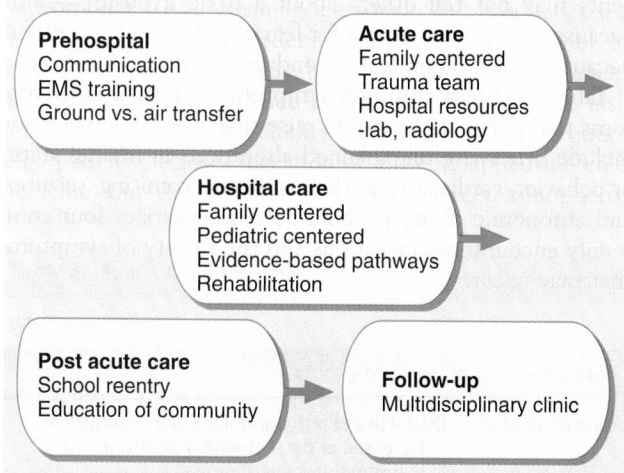

Figure 34-2. Continuum of care. EMS, emergency medical services.

Table 35-5. Toxidromes

Toxin	Symptoms	Treatment
Narcotics	Respiratory depression, miosis, altered mental status or coma	Naloxone
Organophosphates, cholinergics	*SLUDGE* mnemonic: *s*alivation, *l*acrimation, *u*rination, *d*iarrhea, *g*astrointestinal cramping, *e*mesis. Also bronchorrhea, bronchospasm	Atropine, pralidoxime
Tricyclic antidepressants	Seizures, prolonged QRS, altered level of consciousness, dysrhythmias	Sodium bicarbonate
Anticholinergic	Flushing ("red as a beet") Dry skin and mucous membranes ("dry as a bone") Hyperthermia ("hot as a hare") Delirium ("mad as a hatter") Mydriasis, tachycardia, urinary retention	Supportive care
Sympathomimetic	Mydriasis, anxiety, tachycardia, hypertension, hyperthermia, diaphoresis	Quiet environment and benzodiazepines

information. The anion gap is calculated as [Na] – ([Cl] + [HCO₃]) and is normally 8 to 12 mEq/L. An elevated anion gap indicates metabolic acidosis. Differential diagnosis can be remembered using the *MUDPILES* mnemonic: *m*ethanol ingestion, *u*remia, *d*iabetic ketoacidosis, *p*araldehyde or *p*henformin ingestion, *i*ron or *i*soniazid ingestion, *l*actic acidosis, *e*thylene glycol or *e*thanol ingestion, *s*alicylate or *s*olvent (e.g., toluene) ingestion. The osmolar gap is the difference between the measured serum osmolarity and the osmolarity calculated as 2[Na] + [glucose]/18 + [blood urea nitrogen]/2.8 and is normally less than 10 mOsm. An elevated osmolar gap is seen with ingestion of the alcohols (ethanol, methanol, ethylene glycol, and isopropyl alcohol).

Table 35-6. Laboratory and Diagnostic Tests

Routine Laboratory
Specific drug levels as indicated
Acetaminophen, salicylate, ethanol levels
Serum chemistries, calculated anion gap
Serum osmolarity, calculated osmolar gap
Rapid bedside glucose test
Urine pregnancy test in childbearing-age female

Laboratory, if Indicated
Arterial blood gas
Urinalysis

Diagnostic Studies, if Indicated
Electrocardiogram
Chest radiography
Plain abdominal radiography for radiopaque tablets
Endoscopy

Arterial blood gas analysis is indicated if acidosis, hypoxemia, or abnormal hemoglobins (carboxyhemoglobin or methemoglobin) are suspected. Because hypoglycemia is common to many ingestions, a rapid bedside glucose test should be done on all patients. If rhabdomyolysis is suspected or associated with the toxic exposure, urinalysis should be performed. All girls of childbearing age should have a urine pregnancy test.

Other diagnostic studies include pulse oximetry and cardiorespiratory monitoring for all poisoning patients, an electrocardiogram if cardiac toxicity is suspected or abnormalities (including tachycardia) are noted on physical examination, and imaging studies. Specific imaging studies may be indicated for certain ingestions, such as a chest radiograph in hydrocarbon ingestion to assess for aspiration and pulmonary toxicity. A plain abdominal radiograph (kidney, ureter, and bladder film) may identify certain radiopaque substances, as recalled by the mnemonic *CHIPETS*: *c*hloral hydrate, *h*eavy metals, *i*ron, *p*henothiazines, *e*nteric-coated medications, *t*ricyclic antidepressants, and *s*low-release medications. An abdominal radiograph is primarily useful in iron ingestions to determine whether significant amounts of drug are present or remain after gastric decontamination procedures. Other diagnostic studies may be indicated for a specific toxin (e.g., endoscopy after ingestion of caustic acids or alkalis).

Table 35-7 lists thresholds for probable toxicity and expected severity of poisoning by serum levels for acetaminophen, iron, and alcohols. In acetaminophen ingestion, the Rumack nomogram is used to plot a 4-hour postingestion level for determining the severity of expected toxicity. Baseline liver function tests also should be checked. Ingestions of iron at a dose of 20 mg/kg or less are unlikely to produce symptoms. A plain abdominal radiograph may show radiopaque tablets. If tablets are present, attempts should be made to remove them through gastric decontamination and, in extreme cases, endoscopy or even surgery to prevent further absorption. Repeat iron levels should be performed at 4 to 6 hours and 8 to 12 hours postingestion to rule out bezoar formation or ingestion of a

Table 35-7. Toxicity: Threshold Dose and Expected Toxicity by Serum Level

Ingestant	Ingested Dose for Probable Toxicity	Expected Toxic by Serum Levels
Acetaminophen	Child: 140 μg/kg, toxicity likely Adolescent: 6g, toxicity likely	4-hr level: 150–200 μg/mL, possible toxicity >200 μg/mL, probable toxicity
Iron	<20 mg/kg, symptoms unlikely 40 mg/kg serious toxicity >60 mg/kg, potentially lethal	450–500 μg/dL, toxicity likely 800–1000 μg/dL, severe toxicity
Ethanol	3–5 g/kg, toxicity likely	100 mg/dL, significant toxicity
Isopropyl alcohol	2–3 g/kg	50 mg/dL, toxicity likely
Methanol and ethylene glycol	1–2 mL/kg	20 mg/dL, toxicity likely

sustained-release product. Ingestion of alcohols may be suspected by the presence of an anion gap acidosis and an osmolar gap. The Breathalyzer may offer a rapid assessment of ethanol ingestion.

The threshold for toxicity in tricyclic antidepressants is low; moderate-to-severe symptoms can occur with doses of 10 to 20 mg/kg. Levels may be available for some tricyclic antidepressants, but results usually are not immediately available and may be difficult to interpret. Diagnosis is by clinical suspicion. An electrocardiogram should be performed to assess cardiac toxicity, including initial sinus tachycardia; prolonged QRS interval; prolonged P-R interval; prolonged Q-T interval; and in severe toxicity, progression to potentially life-threatening wide-complex tachycardia.

MANAGEMENT

Management strategies are specific to the toxin and the symptoms of the patient. Initial management must focus on the basic ABCs (airway, breathing, circulation) of resuscitation. General management of poisoning includes decontamination methods if indicated, specific antidotes if available, and close observation and supportive care. Details of toxic exposures by the ophthalmic and dermal routes are not discussed in this chapter, but general management includes copious irrigation with water or normal saline. Exposures to acids should *not* be treated by attempted neutralization with bases, and vice versa.

Several methods of decontamination exist (Table 35-8). Syrup of ipecac and gastric lavage theoretically decrease absorption by removing residual toxin in the stomach. Toxicologists no longer recommend their use because studies have shown these techniques to be relatively ineffective, particularly as the time since ingestion increases, and they may interfere with the use of activated charcoal. Complications include aspiration and esophageal trauma. Some toxicologists recommend use only if they can be applied within 30 minutes of ingestion of a liquid or 1 hour of ingestion of solids. The American Academy of Pediatrics no longer recommends ipecac as a home treatment strategy. Neither induction of vomiting nor lavage should be used in patients with hydrocarbon or caustic acid or alkali ingestions. Care should be taken in patients with altered mental status who may not be able to protect their airway from aspiration.

Activated charcoal is the mainstay of therapy for most ingestions. Charcoal binds toxins, preventing their absorption; the charcoal-toxin complex is then eliminated. The optimal dose of charcoal is 10 times the amount of toxin ingested. Because the exact amount of toxin ingested is often unknown, charcoal usually is administered at doses of 1 to 2 g/kg. The amount of charcoal given is limited only by what the patient is able to tolerate. The mnemonic *PHAILS* may be used to recall the few substances not bound to charcoal: *p*esticides; *h*ydrocarbons; *a*cids, *a*lkalis, and *a*lcohols; *i*ron; *l*ithium; and *s*olvents.

Charcoal may be mixed with soda or juice to enhance voluntary administration. Because charcoal has an unappetizing black color, placement in a cup with an opaque lid and administration through a straw may be helpful. A charcoal product is available for home use. If the patient

refuses charcoal, it may be administered through a nasogastric tube. Care must be taken with patients at risk for aspiration (young children, children with altered mental status) because it can result in serious pneumonitis. Endotracheal intubation to protect the airway may be required before charcoal administration in these patients. Correct placement of the nasogastric tube in the gastrointestinal tract should be verified before administration.

Cathartics (e.g., magnesium citrate, magnesium sulfate) have been mixed with charcoal to decrease transit time, enhance elimination, and counteract the constipating effects of charcoal. No significant benefit of cathartic use has been shown. Adverse effects, including dehydration and electrolyte disturbances, may occur, especially in young children. Cathartics are not recommended, but if used, they should never be given in repeated doses.

Multiple-dose charcoal, less commonly used and often referred to as *gastrointestinal dialysis*, involves repeated administration of activated charcoal every 4 hours. This method may promote diffusion of the drug back into the gastrointestinal tract with binding to the charcoal. Cathartics should not be given with charcoal in repeated doses. Multiple-dose charcoal may be useful for phenobarbital, theophylline, and carbamazepine overdoses. It is not recommended for overdoses of drugs that cause ileus, such as tricyclic antidepressants.

Whole-bowel irrigation uses solutions prescribed to clean out the gastrointestinal tract in preparation for colon

Table 35-8. Summary of Gastric Decontamination Techniques

Technique	Dose	Contraindications
Syrup of ipecac	6 mo–1yr: 10 mL (use with caution) 1–12 yr: 15 mL >12 yr: 30 mL Follow with 8 oz water	ALOC Caustics: acids and alkalis Hydrocarbons Expected ALOC (tricyclic antidepressants)
Gastric lavage	15 mL/kg aliquots normal saline to maximum of 400 mL until lavage is clear (may be several liters)	ALOC with unprotected airway Caustics: acids and alkalis Hydrocarbons Expected ALOC >1 hr since ingestion
Activated charcoal	1–2 g/kg *or* <6 yr: 25–50 g >6 yr: 50–100 g	ALOC with unprotected airway Absent bowel sounds, bowel obstruction Substance not bound by charcoal
Cathartics	Magnesium citrate, 4 mL/kg 70% Sorbitol, 1 g/kg	Repeated doses can cause dehydration or electrolyte imbalances
Whole-bowel irrigation	Toddler and preschool age: 500 mL/hr Adolescent and adult: 1–2 L/hr Continue until rectal effluent is clear	Bowel obstruction, ileus, perforation, hemorrhage ALOC with unprotected airway

ALOC, altered level of consciousness.

surgery (e.g., GoLYTELY). It may be indicated for slow-release medications, tablets that dissolve slowly and may cause concretions (e.g., iron), and ingestions in which charcoal is not effective. Administration by nasogastric tube usually is required to accomplish a rate of 500 mL/hr in young children and 1 to 2 L/hr in older children and adolescents. The end point is clear rectal effluent. Contraindications include bowel obstruction, ileus, gastrointestinal perforation, hemorrhage, and altered mental status with an unprotected airway.

Hemodialysis may be used for severe ingestions of ethylene glycol, methanol, phenobarbital, lithium, salicylate, or theophylline. Charcoal hemoperfusion involves passing blood through a charcoal cartridge instead of a dialysis machine and may be used for severe theophylline poisoning.

Urinary alkalinization via administration of sodium bicarbonate intravenously can enhance elimination of weak acids. The toxin is kept in its ionic state, preventing reabsorption in the renal tubule. This method is used primarily in severe salicylate and phenobarbital poisonings.

Antidotes are available for only a few ingestions (Table 35-9). Naloxone may reverse rapidly respiratory depression from narcotic overdose. *N*-acetyl cysteine (NAC), if administered in time, prevents severe liver toxicity in acetaminophen ingestion. Bicarbonate administration may ameliorate the cardiac toxicity of tricyclic antidepressants. Digoxin immune Fab (Digibind) is used to bind digoxin, and deferoxamine is used to chelate iron.

Referral and consultation depends on the specific substance ingested and the resources available. The regional poison center should be contacted for recommendations regarding management, disposition, and length of observation time required for asymptomatic patients. Symptomatic patients and patients who require a long observation period to rule out toxic effects should be admitted to the hospital. Severely toxic patients require management in an intensive care unit (ICU). A toxicologist should be consulted on such patients if one is available. Otherwise the poison center can be used for follow-up and recommendations.

Table 35-9. Common Antidotes

Toxin	Antidote
Acetaminophen	*N*-Acetyl cysteine
Anticoagulants (warfarin-like)	Vitamin K
Anticholinergics	Physostigmine
Benzodiazepines	Flumazenil
β-blockers	Glucagon
Calcium channel blockers	Calcium, glucagon
Carbamate pesticides	Atropine
Carbon monoxide	Oxygen
Cyanide	Cyanide antidote kit
Digoxin	Digibind
Ethylene glycol	Ethanol
Iron	Deferoxamine
Isoniazid	Pyridoxine
Lead	Dimercaprol, EDTA, DMSA
Mercury	Dimercaprol, DMSA
Methanol	Ethanol, fomepizole
Methemoglobinemia	Methylene blue
Narcotics	Naloxone
Organophosphate pesticides	Atropine, pralidoxime
Tricyclic antidepressants	Sodium bicarbonate

DMSA, dimercaptosuccinic acid; EDTA, ethylenediaminetetraacetic acid

Management of acetaminophen overdose involves the antidote NAC. NAC acts as a substitute for glutathione, which normally binds the toxic metabolite of acetaminophen, but is overwhelmed in an overdose. An initial dose of 140 mg/kg orally, followed by 70 mg/kg every 4 hours for 17 doses, is the traditional protocol. In other countries, NAC may be delivered intravenously. Activated charcoal is not used if it would interfere with NAC administration. Any vomiting should be treated aggressively with antiemetics to avoid interference with NAC. Patients with potentially toxic ingestions must be observed in the ICU. Patients with severe toxicity not prevented by NAC may require transfer to a liver transplant center.

Deferoxamine is given to chelate iron in potentially serious overdoses, at a rate of 10 to 15 mg/kg/hr intravenously. Activated charcoal is not effective for binding iron. Gastric lavage may be used early after ingestion or if radiopaque tablets are still visible on plain abdominal radiographs. Presence of concretions or bezoars may require whole-bowel irrigation, endoscopy, and, in rare cases, surgical removal. Dialysis is used to remove the deferoxamine-iron complex if renal failure occurs. Patients with potentially serious ingestions or undergoing chelation therapy should be admitted to the ICU.

Treatment of alcohol poisoning is primarily supportive and includes airway management/protection; fluid administration; and treatment of significant acidosis, hypocalcemia, and hypoglycemia with bicarbonate, calcium, and dextrose administration. Activated charcoal is not useful for alcohols. Gastric lavage is not recommended in a patient with significant altered mental status unless the airway is protected. Ethanol has been used as an antidote for severe methanol and ethylene glycol poisonings. Fomepizole is a new antidote available for methanol overdose and is preferred over ethanol administration. Dialysis may be required for life-threatening overdoses, severe acidosis, renal failure, and methanol overdose causing visual symptoms not reversed by fomepizole.

Treatment of tricyclic antidepressant poisoning includes supportive care, close monitoring, activated charcoal, and sodium bicarbonate for cardiac toxicity. ABCs should be assessed and stabilized immediately, and the patient should be placed on a cardiorespiratory monitor. Cardiac toxicity may be treated with sodium bicarbonate, 1 to 2 mEq/kg intravenously initially, then continuous infusion to maintain a serum pH of 7.45 to 7.55. Tricyclic antidepressants block the fast sodium channel, and sodium bicarbonate administration counteracts this effect. Lidocaine, 1 mg/kg slow intravenous bolus, then continuous infusion at 20 to 50 µg/kg/min, may be used for wide-complex tachyarrhythmias. Seizures should be treated with benzodiazepines. Hypotension should be treated with fluid boluses; Trendelenburg positioning; sodium bicarbonate; and, if needed, pressors, such as norepinephrine and low-dose dopamine. Because of the low threshold for toxicity, all patients with tricyclic antidepressant ingestion warrant admission to an ICU.

Anticipatory guidance and parental education are important in prevention (Box 35-1). Management of a less serious accidental ingestion provides an excellent opportunity for parental education. Emphasis should be placed on safe storage of toxic substances and access to the regional poison

Box 35-1. Education Points for Anticipatory Guidance

Safe Storage

1. Keep potential toxins out of reach of children. Lock cabinets storing toxic substances.
2. Never store substances in unmarked containers, especially containers that typically hold beverages (e.g., old soda bottles or cups).
3. Advise visitors (e.g., grandparents) to store medications out of reach of children.
4. Dispose of unneeded toxic substances and unused or outdated medications.

Education

1. Discuss safety issues with children as developmentally appropriate (e.g., not ingesting unknown substances).
2. Do not refer to medication as "candy" to entice young children to take it.
3. Discuss risks in depressed adolescents; advise parents to keep toxins out of reach of potentially suicidal family members.

Poison Center

1. Keep the regional poison center and local emergency department or pediatrician's telephone numbers readily available. Many poison centers provide stickers for household telephones.

Therapy

1. Consider advising parents to have activated charcoal in the home.
2. Parents should administer activated charcoal *only* if instructed by the poison center staff or medical staff.

---

center phone number. Parents should be reminded that potential toxins include not only prescription medications, but also over-the-counter medications, vitamins, herbal preparations, alternative medications, household products, toxic plants, gardening and hobby chemicals, and kitchen items such as alcohol or oil of wintergreen.

OUTCOME AND FOLLOW-UP

Prognosis depends on the specific toxin but is generally good. Most ingestions are not serious, and fatalities are rare. Advances in education of the public, poison center use, and child-safe packaging have reduced fatalities further. Prognosis is more likely to be poor in intentional ingestions if the patient does not disclose ingestion or delays disclosure. The severity of poisoning is distinct from the seriousness of suicidal intention. Patients may have been quite serious about committing suicide, yet taken an inconsequential amount of drug or a drug that is relatively safe in overdose. In contrast, patients hoping to make a suicidal gesture unwittingly may expose themselves to a potentially fatal ingestion. Follow-up involves repeated anticipatory guidance and psychiatric consultation for intentional ingestions.

Mini-index of Related Topics

SUGGESTED READINGS

American Academy of Pediatrics, Committee on Injury and Poison Prevention: Handbook of Common Poisonings in Children, 3rd ed. Elk Grove Village, Ill, American Academy of Pediatrics, 1994.

Erickson JB: Toxicology: Ingestions and smoke inhalation. In Gausche-Hill M, Fuchs S, Yamamoto L (eds): APLS: The Pediatric Emergency Medicine Resource. Boston, Jones and Bartlett, 2004, pp 234–267.

Perry H, Shannon H: Poisoning. Pediatr Ann 1996;25:19–29.

Tenenbein M: Poisoning. In Barkin RM (ed): Pediatric Emergency Medicine Concepts and Clinical Practice. St. Louis, Mosby-Year Book, 1997, pp 527–534.

Tenenbein M, Cohen S, Sitar DS: Efficacy of ipecac-induced emesis, orogastric lavage and activated charcoal for acute drug overdose. Ann Emerg Med 1987;16:838–841.

36 Aspiration and Ingestion of Foreign Bodies

Jane Knapp

ROLE OF THE GENERALIST

1 Manage basic life support competently for a choking child.

2 Diagnose aspirated foreign body in a timely and accurate manner.

3 Recognize the pitfalls related to the diagnosis of aspirated or ingested foreign bodies.

4 Manage aspirated and ingested foreign bodies appropriately.

5 Refer to a specialist when assistance is needed with foreign body removal.

6 Provide follow-up for children who have aspirated or ingested foreign bodies.

7 Provide anticipatory guidance for parents in the prevention of choking and esophageal foreign bodies.

8 Advocate for regulations to decrease or eliminate choking hazards from toys.

ASPIRATED FOREIGN BODIES

Of cases of foreign-body aspiration, 70% occur in children younger than 2 years of age. Choking accounts for many preventable childhood deaths. The National Safety Council reported that in 1995, 5% of all unintentional deaths in children younger than age 4 years were due to mechanical suffocation, with 65% of the deaths occurring in children younger than 2 years old. Behavioral and developmental factors account for the increased risk of foreign-body aspiration in young children. Newly gained mobility as young children learn to crawl, walk, and climb allows greater exploration of their environment with their hands and mouth. Younger children also are more likely to cry or run with objects in their mouths. Until approximately 2 years of age, children do not have the molar teeth necessary to chew hard foods adequately. Children with neuromuscular disorders who have difficulties coordinating swallowing or with poorly protected airways also are at high risk for foreign-body aspiration

Food items are the most commonly aspirated substance, particularly peanuts, popcorn, and hot dogs. Nonfood items such as balloons, pieces from toys, and other small household objects also present a high risk for aspiration.

Diagnosis and Management

Aspirated foreign bodies produce either partial or complete obstruction of the airway. A partial or incomplete obstruction is differentiated quickly from complete obstruction by the patient's ability to cough or phonate. Complete airway obstruction results in inability to phonate or cough. The presentation of a child with an aspirated foreign body varies from subtle to dramatic and life-threatening. The variation in presentation is related to the degree of obstruction, location of the foreign body in the airway, nature of the foreign body, and length of time to presentation.

Laryngotracheal locations are most likely to lead to complete airway obstruction. Conforming objects such as balloons and round or cylindrical objects such as hot dogs or marbles have been implicated most frequently in deaths. Latex balloons, including examination gloves blown up as balloons, are the most frequent nonfood objects causing death. Deaths from balloon aspiration also are noteworthy because they account for a significantly higher proportion of choking deaths among children 3 years old and older than among children younger than 3 years.

Early diagnosis of an aspirated foreign body prevents serious complications and is associated with a better outcome. Box 36-1 lists signs and symptoms that should cause clinicians to consider foreign-body aspiration. A history of a gagging, choking, or coughing episode is classic and should not be disregarded, even if the child is symptom-free at presentation. A recent or past history of a gagging, coughing, or choking episode should be sought actively in all young children who present with a first-time episode of wheezing;

Box 36-1. Signs and Symptoms of Aspirated Foreign Body

1. Inability to cough or phonate—indicates complete airway obstruction and requires emergency intervention
2. History of a gagging, coughing, or choking episode in young children
3. First episode of wheezing, particularly without family history of reactive airway disease
4. Unexplained or chronic cough or hoarseness
5. Repeated or persistent pneumonia

who have an unexplained or chronic cough or hoarseness; or who have repeated or persistent pneumonia, unexplained fevers, or dysphagia. Food aspirations can be subtle when presenting symptoms involve complications such as pneumonia. Although careful history taking is vital to the diagnosis of aspirated foreign body, some events are unwitnessed or unreported by preverbal children. Foreign-body aspiration should remain in the differential even when history is unavailable or lacking. Family history of asthma or reactive airway disease is important in assessing for the likelihood of reactive airway disease in a child who presents with a first wheezing episode.

The most serious sequela of foreign-body aspiration is complete airway obstruction. To be prepared for such an event, the generalist periodically must update personal basic and advanced life support skills in the management of a choking infant and child.

Figure 36-1 shows the utility of a lateral neck x-ray in diagnosing a radiopaque upper airway foreign body that is causing symptoms of partial obstruction. Aspirated radiopaque foreign bodies are readily identified on chest x-ray. Inspiration/expiration chest x-rays are positive in a high percentage of instances of radiolucent foreign-body bronchial aspirations into a bronchus and are not difficult to interpret (Fig. 36-2). Inspiration and expiration views of the chest are compared. Typically on the inspiration view, both lungs appear well inflated. When a foreign body is present, the expiration film shows hyperaeration on the involved side from air trapping. A drawback is that inspiration and expiration views require expertise and timing on the part of the technologist and a degree of cooperation from the patient. In situations in which these views are impossible to obtain, lateral decubitus radiographs are an alternative method for showing air trapping. On a decubitus view, a lung with trapped air does not allow the expected downward shift of the mediastinum to the dependent side (Fig. 36-3). The uninvolved side, when dependent, allows

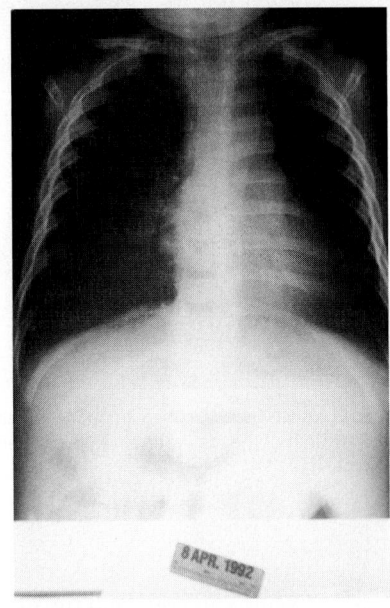

A

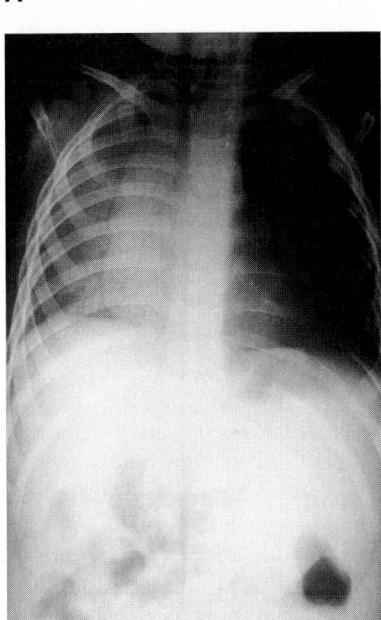

B

Figure 36-2. Inspiration (A) and expiration (B) chest x-rays in a patient with a radiolucent foreign body. Note air trapping on involved left side.

compression of the lung and a resulting downward shift of the mediastinum. Other chest x-ray findings that are consistent with the diagnosis of foreign-body aspiration and should raise concerns when present in children younger than 2 years old are atelectasis, infiltrates, emphysema, and pneumomediastinum. Fluoroscopy can be used to study respiratory excursion of the diaphragm as another method for detecting trapped air. There is decreased diaphragmatic movement on the involved side.

Bronchoscopy also can be used diagnostically, especially in confusing cases or when a delayed presentation is suspected. Direct bronchoscopy by an experienced consultant is the gold standard for foreign-body removal and is successful in most cases. The specialist consulted to perform the

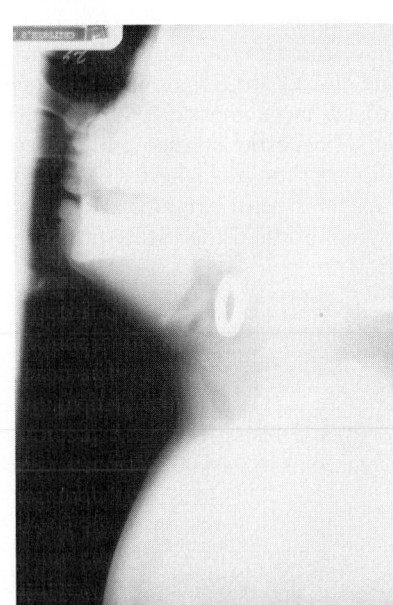

Figure 36-1. Lateral neck x-ray shows a radiopaque upper airway foreign body.

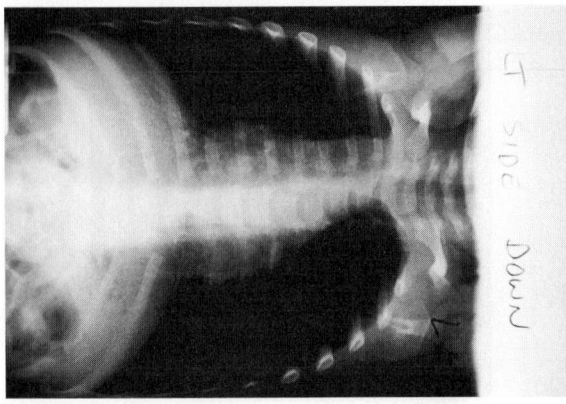

Figure 36-3. Decubitus view with trapped air on the left and absence of expected downward shift of the mediastinum when the left side is dependent.

procedure (e.g., surgeon; ear, nose, and throat specialist; or pulmonologist) depends on local resources. There is some controversy among endoscopists over whether flexible or rigid bronchoscopy is most appropriate for foreign-body removal. Flexible bronchoscopy has the advantage of a greater peripheral range, allowing diagnosis of foreign bodies missed when the rigid bronchoscope is used. Flexible bronchoscopy can be done with intravenous sedation and topical anesthesia. Rigid bronchoscopy requires general anesthesia. Flexible bronchoscopy has less superior optics, is more likely to occlude airways, and affords a smaller working space that technically can hinder or defeat foreign-body removal.

Outcome

With either a flexible or a rigid instrument, procedure-related morbidity for bronchoscopy is low, on the order of 2% to 3%. The complication rate is related to the length of time the foreign body has been in the tracheobronchial system. Foreign bodies removed less than 12 hours after aspiration have the fewest complications. The major complications are pneumothorax, perforation, hemorrhage, and cardiac arrest. Mortality is 0% to 1.6%. In the rare instance when bronchoscopy is unsuccessful, thoracotomy is indicated.

Prevention

Because choking deaths are preventable, the generalist has an important role in providing anticipatory guidance to parents and in advocacy. TIPP (The Injury Prevention Program of the American Academy of Pediatrics) assists pediatricians in injury prevention counseling. Given the advice and encouragement of their pediatrician, parents can be motivated to protect their children from injuries such as choking and to learn basic life support for use should a choking emergency occur.

Generalists have an advocacy role through their support of regulations governing the design of toys and toy parts and the identification of toy hazards. Generalists should have an understanding of the purpose and use of the small parts test fixture, sometimes called a *choke tube*. The small parts test fixture is a cylinder of defined measurements used to test objects for use by young children. An object that easily passes through the tube is considered a potential choking hazard. A cardboard tube from toilet paper can substitute as a simple, readily available choke tube for parents. *Finally, the generalist has a role in prevention by not using latex gloves as a substitute for toys or balloons at office visits.*

INGESTED FOREIGN BODIES

The peak incidence for ingested foreign bodies is between 6 months and 3 years of age. Esophageal foreign bodies present the greatest risk for impaction in the gastrointestinal (GI) tract and subsequent need for removal. The most common sites of esophageal impaction are the thoracic inlet, the aortic knob, or the gastroesophageal junction. Lodged esophageal foreign bodies are most common in children younger than 10 years old, mentally disabled children, and children with esophageal abnormalities. Children with strictures from previous surgery, ingestion of caustic agents, or other injuries are at higher risk for retained esophageal foreign body at the point of the stricture.

Diagnosis and Management

Ingestion of a foreign body should be suspected with a history of a choking, gagging, or coughing episode followed by symptoms of increased salivation, drooling, dysphagia, chest pain, or vomiting (Box 36-2). Cough, tachypnea, wheeze, and stridor unresponsive to pharmacologic therapy can occur secondary to compression of the trachea by the foreign body or overflow of food or secretions into the larynx from the site of obstruction. Unwitnessed ingestions may present as unexplained crying or irritability, new-onset feeding problems, or unexplained vomiting without other attendant illness. Bloody vomiting can be present if laceration or injury has occurred. Fever, bleeding, or respiratory difficulties occur with delayed presentation or perforation. When ingestion of a foreign body has been witnessed or is suspected, the primary decisions for the generalist concern the need for diagnostic studies and a choice of conservative management versus referral for endoscopic or surgical removal (Table 36-1). Given that most objects pass without problems, a conservative approach with observation at home is reasonable. Diagnostic studies and interventions can be confined to children at highest risk for complications. The most important considerations in this regard are the presence of symptoms and the nature of the foreign body.

Box 36-2. Signs and Symptoms of Ingested Foreign Body

1. History of choking, gagging, or coughing episode followed by symptoms of salivation, drooling, dysphagia, chest pain, or vomiting
2. Cough, tachypnea, wheeze, or stridor unresponsive to pharmacologic therapy
3. Unexplained crying or irritability
4. New-onset feeding problems
5. Unexplained vomiting
6. Bloody vomiting

Table 36-1. Indications for Diagnostic Studies or Intervention

Object	Diagnostic Testing	Indications for Removal
Disk battery	X-ray neck, chest, and abdomen	Emergent removal when in esophagus
Sharp, pointed, or elongated objects	X-ray of neck, chest, and abdomen	Older children: diameter >5 cm, thickness >2 cm, length >10 cm Infants and young children: diameter >3 cm, length >20 mm
Coins	Controversial, see text. Micromedex Health Care Series* recommendations: x-rays for diagnostic localization in children ≥2 yr old if size of penny or greater; x-rays for all children <2 yr old	Children with esophageal strictures, esophageal impaction

*Micromedex Health Series. Available at: http://micromedex.hcn.net.au.

Disk batteries, sharp or elongated objects, and coins are the objects that raise the most concerns. Disk batteries can leak alkaline contents, causing serious mucosal burns when they are lodged in the esophagus or fail to progress through the GI tract. Sharp or elongated objects account for one third of the perforations associated with foreign-body ingestion. Coin ingestions are common but controversial with respect to management.

When ingestion of a disk battery is suspected, the child should have x-rays of the neck, chest, and abdomen to determine the location of the battery in the GI tract. This knowledge helps to determine management. Emergent endoscopic removal is recommended in a symptomatic patient or when the battery is located in the esophagus. If the battery is beyond the esophagus, the patient may be observed at home with instructions for the parents to watch for vomiting, tarry or bloody stools, fever, abdominal pain, or decreased appetite. Repeat radiographs are recommended to assess the progress of the battery through the GI tract. If the patient has not had the documented passage of the battery in 1 week, a follow-up radiograph is prudent. Referral for endoscopic removal is indicated in symptomatic patients, when there is evidence of a corroding battery, or when the battery stops progressing through the GI tract. Regional poison control centers are excellent sources of advice for management of disk button battery ingestions. Alternatively, the National Button Battery Ingestion Hotline may be reached at (202) 625-3333 for treatment advice.

Management decisions regarding sharp, pointed, or elongated ingested foreign bodies are challenging because there are no definite established guidelines. Objects such as chicken bones or fish bones, long straight pins, razor blades, open safety pins, and toothpicks have been identified as unusually high risk. In general, in an older child or adolescent, oval objects greater than 5 cm in diameter or 2 cm in thickness can lodge in the stomach. Thin objects greater

than 10 cm in length are more likely to fail to negotiate the duodenum and should be considered for removal. In infants and young children, the dimension is 3 cm or longer than 20 mm. Referral for possible endoscopic removal is indicated for high-risk objects or objects that exceed the dimensions noted.

The necessity for x-rays with all coin ingestions is controversial. The controversy surrounds the risk for esophageal injury when coins are lodged in the esophagus but the child is asymptomatic. Clinicians who favor x-rays for all children who have a history of a coin ingestion believe that this is a simple way to determine an esophageal location and prevent complications with early removal. Clinicians who favor observation believe that children who are asymptomatic and can tolerate oral fluids are at low risk for esophageal impaction and that the radiation and added expense of x-rays are unwarranted.

The individual generalist's management of coin ingestions may best be guided largely by personal experience and the relationship with the family. A reasonable conservative approach would be to follow the recommendations of the Micromedex Healthcare Series. These recommendations suggest diagnostic localization in asymptomatic children 2 years old or older who swallow objects the size of a penny or greater in diameter and localization for all swallowed foreign bodies in children younger than 2 years old.

When x-rays are used as an aid to diagnosis or localization, a foreign-body series should be ordered. This series consists of views of the anteroposterior and lateral neck, chest, and abdomen, allowing for full visualization of the GI tract. When a radiopaque object is present, the foreign-body series discriminates an esophageal from a tracheal or distal GI location. A barium swallow can be used to show evidence of a radiolucent foreign body lodged in the esophagus. Handheld metal detectors have been found to be useful in discriminating between an esophageal or gastric location for coins and potentially eliminating the need for x-rays.

Alternatively, endoscopy can be used for diagnosis and subsequent removal of the foreign body. Endoscopy offers the additional advantage of direct inspection of the esophagus, allowing identification of esophageal injury or other unsuspected foreign bodies. Esophageal bougienage is a safe and effective method used to push an ingested coin from the esophagus to the stomach. Criteria for bougienage include an acutely ingested single coin radiographically localized to the esophagus in a child with no previous history of an esophageal disease process or surgery. Fluoroscopic Foley catheter removal also is safe and effective for removing coins in children without underlying esophageal lesions and a short duration of impaction. In a comparison of the endoscopy, bougienage, and Foley catheter methods, all were found to have high success and low complication rates. The complications that occurred were usually minor. Endoscopy was the most expensive of the three methods studied, with costs fourfold higher than those of Foley catheter or bougienage.

Bezoars are an accumulation of foreign material found in the stomach or intestine that are classified on the basis of composition. Common examples are trichobezoars, which are composed of hair; phytobezoars, which are composed of plant material; and lactobezoars, which are composed of the high casein or calcium content of some formulas for premature infants. Other nondigestible substances, such as plastic, also can form bezoars when ingested in quantity.

Bezoars can become large and cause symptoms of gastric outlet obstruction. Patients may complain of abdominal pain and distention. Symptoms can include vomiting, anorexia, and weight loss. On physical examination, a firm mass may be palpable in the left upper quadrant. Abdominal plain films suggest the presence of a mass that can be confirmed by barium, ultrasound, or endoscopic examination. Lactobezoars can be treated conservatively with hydration and withholding of feedings. Other bezoars can be removed with endoscopy. If endoscopy is impractical or unsuccessful, surgical removal is needed.

Outcome

Esophageal foreign bodies that are retained over a length of time can cause erosion through mucosal tissue with resulting mediastinal inflammation and infection. Once in the stomach, 95% of all objects pass without difficulty. Of ingested foreign bodies, 10% to 20% require endoscopic removal, and 1% require surgery. Perforation of the GI tract is estimated to be less than 1% and tends to occur in areas of physiologic sphincters, congenital malformations, or previous bowel surgery.

SUMMARY

Foreign-body aspiration or ingestion is common in children, especially children younger than 2 years of age. The generalist's responsibility is to diagnose an aspiration or ingestion and make an appropriate referral. Follow-up is dictated by the clinical situation and presence and severity of complications. The generalist also has an important role in anticipatory guidance in the prevention of choking and in advocacy.

Additional Resources, CD-ROM

Bibliography	Text

Mini-index of Related Topics

SUGGESTED READINGS

Biehler JL, Tuggle D, Stacy T: Use of the transmitter-receiver metal detector in the evaluation of pediatric coin ingestions. Pediatr Emerg Care 1993;9:208–210.

Bonadio WA, Jona JZ, Glicklich M, Cohen R: Esophageal bougienage technique for coin ingestion in children. J Pediatr Surg 1988;23:917–918.

Byrne WJ: Foreign bodies, bezoars, and caustic ingestion. Gastrointest Endosc Clin North Am 1994;4:99–119.

Rimell FL, Thome A, Stool S, et al: Characteristics of objects that cause choking in children. JAMA 1995;274:1763–1766.

Schmidt H, Manegold BC: Foreign body aspiration in children. Surg Endosc 2000;14:644–648.

37

Approach to the Febrile Patient

Julie Noble

ROLE OF THE GENERALIST

1 Distinguish hyperthermia from fever.
2 Document temperature accurately, and understand the pathophysiology of fever.
3 Recognize the significance of fever in various age categories and have a logical approach to its evaluation.
4 Use signs, symptoms, and selected laboratory tests to identify the underlying cause of fever.
5 Have a treatment plan for fever.
6 Have a treatment plan for the etiology of fever.
7 Recognize the need for specialist referral for treatment of infections or immunologic causes of fever.

Fever is an elevation of body temperature resulting from a physiologic response to an insult to the body's inflammatory defense system. It may be a symptom of a range of stimuli, from a self-limited viral infection to a serious bacterial infection or an immunologic response to a systemic process. As a symptom of illness, fever is responsible for 10% to 30% of all pediatric office and emergency department visits. Because fever is such a frequent chief complaint, a logical approach to its assessment is essential for a practicing clinician.

Fever must be differentiated from hyperthermia, an elevation of body temperature resulting from thermoregulatory failure. Environmental heat, overproduction of heat, or a reduced ability to dissipate heat by vasodilation or sweating can cause hyperthermia. Severe hyperthermia can occur when a child is left in a closed car on a hot day. In contrast to fever, hyperthermia can cause temperature elevation to a pathologic level, causing tissue injury or death.

Normal body temperature has a diurnal pattern referred to as a *circadian rhythm* with a nadir of 36°C in the early morning to a peak of 37.5°C in the afternoon. The most commonly accepted minimum temperature defining a fever is 38°C (100.4°F) rectally. Many techniques are available to measure body temperature. Ear, skin, and axillary measurements may underestimate a fever. The most accurate measurement is obtained by rectal thermometry. If a child is older than 36 to 48 months of age, an oral temperature is acceptable and may be preferable secondary to patient comfort. Tactile temperature is not a reliable indication of

true fever; if a child is younger than 2 years and fever is greater than 38.9°C, however, it may be a reliable historical finding.

In evaluating fever in a pediatric patient, the age of the patient is essential because it determines the immunologic competence of the child, influences the physician's ability to assess the child, determines which infectious etiologies are likely, and guides management. The incidence of fever in infants younger than 3 months old is low, but these infants generally are regarded as immunocompromised hosts. They are at risk for perinatally acquired infection, have greater difficulty in localizing infection, and are more difficult to assess clinically because of neurodevelopmental immaturity. An aggressive approach to diagnosis and treatment is recommended in this age group.

Children 3 months to 3 years old frequently present with fever because they are exposed to numerous infectious agents for the first time. Although clinical assessment is easier and more reliable, even febrile children in this age category who are not toxic appearing are at risk for bacteremia and subsequent serious bacterial infection, including sepsis, meningitis, septic arthritis, osteomyelitis, and pneumonia. After 3 years of age, children are at minimal risk for bacteremia. Serious bacterial infection usually is apparent on examination, and evaluation is directed by the appearance of the child.

Duration of the fever is essential to its evaluation. A fever that has persisted for more than 7 to 10 days is considered to be *prolonged*. A fever of this duration without a known cause is called *fever of unknown origin (FUO)*. For prolonged fever and FUO, an in-depth evaluation must be done.

FUNDAMENTALS

The febrile response is generated when an insult to the body causes monocytes, neutrophils, and macrophages to release cytokines, interleukin-1 and interleukin-6, and tumor necrosis factor. These endogenous pyrogens travel to the preoptic nucleus of the anterior hypothalamus and stimulate vascular endothelial cells to produce prostaglandin E_2; this raises the set-point of thermoregulation to a higher temperature. The autonomic nervous system responds by generating heat through shivering and vasoconstriction, elevating body temperature (Fig. 37-1). Body temperature seldom exceeds 41.1°C (106°F).

With hyperthermia, the hypothalamic set-point remains normal, but body temperature rises secondary to the in-

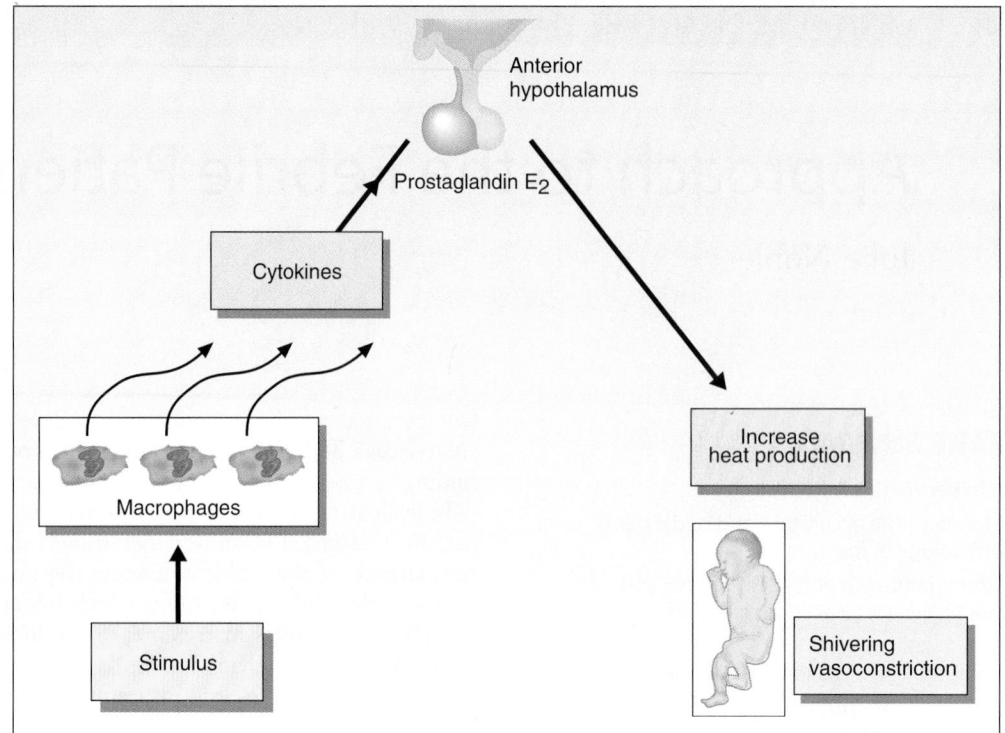

Figure 37-1. Fever results from generation of shivering and vasoconstriction, responses to the autonomic nervous system.

ability to dissipate heat or the body's overproduction of heat. An example occurs in the overproduction of heat with exercise in a hot environment producing heatstroke. In contrast to fever, temperature elevation from hyperthermia may exceed 107°F and cause neuronal damage.

The most common etiology for fever in any age group is an infectious agent. Viral disease is the most frequent offender, and most of these infections are self-limited. If a cause is not identified after a complete history and physical examination, the urinary tract should be evaluated as a source.

Infants younger than 3 months of age may present with fever or may be hypothermic in response to an infection. Infants are at risk for community-acquired infections and maternally derived pathogens (Table 37-1). *Listeria monocytogenes*, group B β-hemolytic streptococci, gram-negative organisms, and enterococci all are possible pathogens in the neonatal period. Infants also are at greater risk of non-localization of infection and developing sepsis and meningitis. They show decreased opsonin, macrophage, and neutrophil activity.

In children 3 months to 3 years old, community-acquired infections are the most common causes of fever (see Table 37-1). Generally a complete history and physical examination reveal a source. Of patients, 20% have no source of infection identified after a complete examination. Of this 20%, 3% of children have unsuspected bacteremia, making them at risk for serious bacterial disease (Box 37-1). Children younger than 2 have poor immunoglobulin G antibody response to encapsulated bacteria. *Streptococcus pneumoniae* is the predominant organism in bacteremia, although the prevalence of this pathogen should decrease after the routine administration of conjugated pneumococcal vaccine. *Neisseria meningitidis, Salmonella*, group A

streptococci, *Escherichia coli, Haemophilus influenzae*, and *Staphylococcus aureus* also are found. With the widespread use of *H. influenzae* conjugate vaccine, this pathogen is now rarely seen in immunized children.

Children older than 3 years of age have a significantly lower risk for bacteremia. They localize infections better and acquire community-related infections with their exposures in school and social settings.

In evaluating prolonged FUO, infection still is the most common etiology and is seen in 50% of cases. Bacterial and viral causes are seen. Epstein-Barr virus is a frequent culprit. Collagen vascular disease, neoplasms, and inflammatory disorders also are major categories of disease causing prolonged FUO (Table 37-2). Most patients with prolonged FUO more commonly have unusual presentations of common disease rather than unusual diseases.

Table 37-1. Etiologies of Fever

Maternally Derived Infection (Infants <3 mo)	Community-Acquired Infection
Bacterial	Bacterial
Group B β-hemolytic streptococci	*Streptococcus pneumoniae*
Listeria monocytogenes	Group A streptococci
Gram-negative organisms	*Staphylococcus aureus*
Enterococci	*Salmonella*
Chlamydia	*Haemophilus influenzae* type b
	Neisseria meningitidis
Viral	Viral
Herpesvirus	Respiratory syncytial virus
	Rotavirus
	Rhinovirus
	Influenza
	Parainfluenza
	Coxsackievirus

DIAGNOSIS

The major diagnostic goal in evaluating children with fever is to differentiate a child with serious disease from a child with a minor acute illness (see Box 37-1). The second goal is identification of the etiologic agent responsible for the fever. Most conditions causing fever in children can be diagnosed by a thorough history and physical examination. The relevant history includes past medical history, recent ill contacts, day care attendance, immunization history, current medications, and community epidemics. If the patient is an infant, the birth history and history of any maternal illnesses should be included. The fever pattern can be helpful. With malaria, a relapsing fever pattern is typical. The height of the fever correlates with an increased proba-

Table 37-2. Etiologies of Fever of Unknown Origin

Infectious Diseases
Viral
Epstein-Barr virus
Cytomegalovirus
HIV
Hepatitis
Bacterial
Brucellosis
Cat-scratch disease
Tularemia
Rickettsial disease
Other Infectious Agents
Lyme disease
Tuberculosis
Histoplasmosis
Malaria
Toxoplasmosis
Leptospirosis

Collagen Vascular Disease
Henoch-Schönlein purpura
Juvenile rheumatoid arthritis
SLE
Rheumatic fever

Malignancy
Leukemia
Lymphoma
Neuroblastoma

Miscellaneous
Drug fever
Inflammatory bowel disease
Kawasaki's disease
Sarcoidosis

HIV, human immunodeficiency virus; SLE, systemic lupus erythematosus.

bility of a serious bacterial infection. A history of the child's ability to play, or lack thereof, can denote the seriousness of the infection. This aspect can be difficult to assess in young infants whose behavioral skills are less well developed. Children with urinary tract infection typically are playful, although their fever can be high. Symptoms localizing an infectious process, such as nasal congestion, cough, ear pain, eye discharge, sore throat, inability to swallow, rash, vomiting, diarrhea, abdominal pain, dysuria, and seizures, should be evaluated.

The physical examination should preferably be done with the patient unclothed to maximize the ability to observe perfusion, rash, respiratory effort, and joint mobility. A complete set of vital signs is essential. If an afebrile patient has a history of documented fever at home, it should be considered the same as office documentation. Ascertainment of home use of antipyretics is important. Elevated respiratory rate and increased respiratory effort have long been thought to indicate pulmonary infection, but according to more recent information, pulse oximetry less than 95% is a better predictor of pulmonary infection than respiratory rate. Tachypnea may reflect a metabolic acidosis with respiratory compensation.

The clinical appearance of a child can be helpful in assessing the severity of disease but does not predict the etiology. Criteria have been developed to assess toxicity in a child (see Chapter 38). Playfulness, eye contact, peripheral perfusion, and respiratory effort are all components to assess the level of toxicity. A cooperative patient facilitates the physical examination. Cooperation can be fostered by keeping a young child in the mother's arms or by lowering the fever before the examination. The examination should be performed in an order that is least upsetting to the child. Examining the ears and throat last may postpone crying to the end. The skin should be examined thoroughly for lesions and rashes. Petechiae raise concern for sepsis, specifically from *N. meningitidis*. The examination should concentrate on identifying the source of the fever.

When a diagnosis is not readily apparent after a complete history and physical examination, as occurs in about 20% of cases, the child has fever without a source. There is a risk for occult bacteremia if the child is younger than 3 years of age. Factors correlated with occult bacteremia include the child's appearance (toxic appearing or not), height of fever (temperature ≥39°C [>102.2°F]), and white blood cell (WBC) count (≥15,000/mm^3).

In neonates 1 to 28 days old, accepted practice is a complete septic evaluation with blood culture, complete blood count, urinalysis and culture, and lumbar puncture. A chest x-ray should be performed if there are clinical indications of pulmonary infection. Stool culture is indicated if there is a history of diarrhea. If an infant is 1 to 3 months old and is toxic appearing, the same evaluation is necessary. If an infant is not toxic appearing and meets low-risk criteria, the physician has the option of evaluation with blood, urine, and cerebrospinal fluid cultures or blood and urine cultures only and outpatient management. Low-risk criteria include a previously healthy term infant, no focal bacterial infection on examination, WBC count less than 15,000/mm^3, less than 1500 bands/mm^3, negative urinalysis, cerebrospinal fluid less than 8 WBCs/mm^3, and negative Gram stain (Fig. 37-2).

If the child is 3 months to 3 years of age, the patient's appearance and the height of the fever dictate the treatment plan. If the child is toxic appearing, a complete septic workup is indicated. If the child is not toxic appearing and the temperature is less than 39°C (<102.2°F), no diagnostic tests are necessary. If the temperature is equal to or greater than 39°C (≥102.2°F), a urinalysis and complete blood count should be ordered with a blood culture sent if the WBC count is equal to or greater than 15,000/mm^3 (or absolute neutrophil count ≥10,000/mm^3) (Fig. 37-3).

With the decrease in *H. influenzae* type B disease, secondary to widespread vaccination usage, the incidence of bacteremia and subsequent invasive disease from this organism has decreased greatly. Routine administration of the new conjugate pneumococcal vaccine (seven serogroups) should decrease cases of pneumococcal bacteremia by 90%. In the future, evaluations for bacteremia no longer will be productive enough to justify the expense and patient discomfort.

In evaluating a child older than 3 years of age for fever, laboratory evaluation should be directed at symptoms or physical findings. A urinalysis should be considered routinely, if there are no physical findings. Laboratory evaluation for occult bacteremia is not necessary.

In evaluating a child with a prolonged fever, presence of fever should be confirmed. The physical examination always should be repeated completely over the course of the illness. New findings on repeated examination are reported in 25% of cases. An assessment of growth parameters is essential because serious systemic disease usually affects growth. Laboratory tests may be necessary to aid in diagnosis. If the child has localized symptoms or physical findings, laboratory tests should be ordered accordingly. If there are no specific findings, the laboratory workup should be a progression of reasonable tests, beginning with complete blood count; urinalysis; erythrocyte sedimentation rate;

Non-toxic-appearing
28–90 days and
"low-risk" (defined below)

No

Admit to hospital

Blood culture
Urine cultue
Lumbar puncture
Parental antibiotics
Chest radiograph*

Yes

Outpatient Management

Option 1
Blood culture
Urine culture
Lumbar puncture
Ceftriaxone 50 mg/kg intravenously or intramuscularly
Re-evaluation within 24 hr

Option 2
Blood culture
Urine culture
Re-evaluation within 24 hr

*Chest radiograph if signs of pneumonia: respiratory distress, abnormal breath sounds, tachypnea, pulse oximetry <95%

Follow-up of low-risk infants treated as outpatients with positive culture results:

Blood culture positive (pathogen): Admit for sepsis evaluation and parenteral antibiotic therapy pending results

Urine culture positive (pathogen): Persistent fever. Admit for sepsis evaluation and parenteral anitbiotic therapy Results. Outpatient antibiotics if afebrile and well

Low-risk criteria for febrile infants:

Clinical criteria:
- Previously healthy, term infant with uncomplicated nursery stay
- Nontoxic clinical appearance
- No focal bacterial infection on examinaton (except otitis media)

Laboratory criteria:
- WBC count 5000–15,000/mm^3, <1500 band/mm^3, or band/neutrophil ratio <0.2
- Negative Gram stain of unspun urine (preferred), or negative urine leukocyte esterase and nitrite, or <5 WBCs/hpf
- When diarrhea present: <5 WBCs/hpf in stool
- CSF: <8 WBCs/mm^3 and negative Gram stain (option 1 only)

Figure 37-2. Algorithm for the management of a previously healthy infant (birth to ≤3 months old) with fever without a source with a temperature of equal to or greater than 38.0°C (≥100.4°F). CSF, cerebrospinal fluid; hpf, high-power field; WBCs, white blood cells. (Adapted from Baraff LJ: Management of fever without source in infants and children. Ann Emerg Med 2000;36:602–614. Reprinted with permission of American College of Emergency Physicians.)

Child appears toxic

Yes	No
Admit to hospital **Sepsis workup** **Parenteral antibiotics** **Yes**	**Temperature ≥ 39.0°C** **No** 1. No diagnostic or antibiotics 2. Acetaminophen 15 mg/kg/dose q4h or ibuprofen 10 mg/kg/dose q6h for fever 3. Return if fever persists >48 hours or if condition deteriorates

1a. Urine leukocyte esterase (LE) and nitrite or urinalysis and urine culture:
   All male ≤6 months and uncircumcised males 6–12 months
   All females <12 months
   If urine screening test is positive: Outpatient antibiotics (oral third-generation cephalosporin)
1b. Urine LE and nitrite or urinalysis and hold urine culture
   Circumcised males 6–12 months and all females 12–24 months
   If urine screening test positive: Send urine culture and outpatient (oral third-generation cephalosporin)
2. For infants and children who have not received the conjugate *S. pneumoniae* vaccine:
   Temperature ≥39.5°C: Obtain WBC count (or ANC) and hold blood culture
   If WBC count ≥15,000 (or ANC ≥10,000 mm^3):
           Send blood culture
           Cetriaxone 50 mg/kg up to 1 g

3. Chest radiograph: If SaO$_2$ <95%, respiratory distress, tachypnea, rales, or temperature ≥39.5°C and WBC count ≥20,000 mm^3 (see below)
4. Acetaminophen: 15 mg/kg/dose q4h or ibuprofen 10 mg/kg/dose q6h for fever
5. Return if fever persists >48 hours or condition deteriorates

Follow-up of low-risk children treated as outpatients with positive culture results:

Blood culture positive (pathogen): Admit if febrile or ill-appearing
                                   Outpatient antibiotics if afebrile and well

Urine culture positive (pathogen): Admit if febrile or ill-appearing
                                   Outpatient antibiotics if afebrile as well

Figure 37-3. Algorithm for the management of a previously healthy child (3 months to 3 years old) with fever without a source. ANC, absolute neutrophil count; LE, leukocyte esterase; WBC, white blood cell. (Adapted from Baraff LJ: Management of fever without source in infants and children. Ann Emerg Med 2000;36:602–614. Reprinted with permission of American College of Emergency Physicians.)

C-reactive protein; cultures of blood, urine, and stool; purified protein derivative; and chest x-ray. Liver and kidney function studies also should be considered. If the initial studies are negative, antinuclear antibody, rheumatoid factor, antistreptolysin O, and Epstein-Barr virus titer can be helpful. Additional studies include an upper gastrointestinal series looking for inflammatory bowel disease and a bone marrow aspirate to evaluate for leukemia, metastatic disease, or infection. A gallium scan or bone scan might be considered, but "a shotgun approach" is frequently unproductive and has low yield.

When a child is diagnosed with a specific infection, it is important to consider whether this is a recurrent infection. If the child has a pattern of repeated infections, he or she may have an underlying immunodeficiency syndrome. Failure to thrive would support this diagnostic impression. A laboratory evaluation with complete blood count, chest

x-ray, quantitative immunoglobulins, and skin tests to assess T-cell function should be ordered (see Chapter 116).

MANAGEMENT

Goals for managing febrile children are listed in Box 37-2. Toxic-appearing febrile children without a diagnosis should be admitted to the hospital for antibiotic therapy. In managing the febrile child who is not toxic appearing, the most important variable, as with diagnosis, is the age of the child. All neonates younger than 28 days of age who present with documented fever should be hospitalized for intravenous antibiotic treatment pending culture results. Antibiotics should provide coverage for gram-negative pathogens. Treatment with ampicillin, 100 to 200 mg/kg/24 hr intravenously every 6 hours, and gentamicin, 6 to 7.5 mg/kg/24 hr intravenously every 8 hours, or cefotaxime,

100 to 200 mg/kg/24 hr intravenously every 6 hours, would be acceptable.

In managing an infant 1 to 3 months old, hospitalization is necessary if the infant is toxic appearing. If the infant meets low-risk criteria, he or she can be managed as an outpatient (see Fig. 37-1). The "low-risk" infant should have a septic evaluation and receive ceftriaxone, 50 mg/kg intramuscularly or intravenously. Alternatively, blood and urine cultures alone may be obtained with no treatment. Both groups of infants need re-evaluation in 24 hours. If the blood or the urine culture is positive and the infant is febrile, admission is necessary.

Children 3 months to 3 years old who are not toxic appearing are still at risk for occult bacteremia. If they have an identified source of infection, they should be treated with the appropriate antibiotic and evaluated if fever persists or symptoms worsen. If the temperature is less than 39°C (<102.2°F), these children can be managed with acetaminophen or ibuprofen and re-evaluated if the fever persists for more than 48 hours. If the fever is equal to or greater than 39°C (≥ 102.2°F) and the urine screen is positive or WBC count greater than or equal to 15,000/mm^3, appropriate urine and blood cultures should be sent. A child with a positive urine culture can be treated by oral antibiotics if the child is not vomiting; suspected bacteremia should be treated with ceftriaxone, 50 mg/kg intramuscularly (≤1 g dose) (see Fig. 37-3).

Older children are managed by treatment specific to the identified etiology of fever. Antibiotic or antiviral treatment should be directed to the most likely pathogen. If the child's course is atypical, fever is persistent, the infection is unusual, or the condition deteriorates, consultation with an infectious disease specialist is appropriate. In managing prolonged FUO, accurate documentation of the fever is important. Hospitalization may be necessary to assess fever pattern and to facilitate a diagnostic evaluation. Consultation with specialists in hematology-oncology, infectious disease, or immunology may be helpful depending on the initial evaluation and laboratory results.

Treatment of fever itself is a controversial issue. Hyperthermia should be managed by physical cooling to lower body temperature, but fever may have an important role in immune function in fighting infection. Fever enhances neutrophil migration, promotes T-cell proliferation, and increases the release of interferon. Suppression of fever has been shown to prolong the course of infection with rhinovirus and varicella. The presence of fever sets off a parental alarm, however. It has been reported that 91% of caregivers believed fever could cause harmful effects, and 85% believed that fever could be dangerous for the child. Educating parents regarding these misconceptions is an important part of the management of fever. Fever in response to an insult seems to be physiologically controlled to remain within benign limits as long as hydration is maintained.

Antipyretic therapy is designed to lower the hypothalamic set-point by decreasing cyclooxygenase activity, preventing the synthesis of prostaglandin. It is not effective for treatment of hyperthermia. Treatment with antipyretics decreases the metabolic demands of fever, including increased oxygen consumption and heart rate. Antipyretics also improve patient comfort and confer a feeling of well-being. Either acetaminophen, 10 to 15 mg/kg/dose orally or per rectum every 4 hours to a maximum of 4 g/24 hr, or ibuprofen, 5 to 10 mg/kg/dose orally every 6 to 8 hours to a maximum of 40 mg/kg/24 hr, may be prescribed. Tepid water sponging alone does not decrease body temperature significantly. It may increase the rate at which the temperature decreases when used with an antipyretic, but also may increase shivering and patient discomfort. Some believe that side effects of sponging outweigh the benefit. Alcohol sponging should never be used because acute poisoning has been documented.

Febrile seizures occur in 2% to 4% of children younger than age 5 with fever. These seizures generally are benign, and there is no proof that antipyretic treatment is effective in preventing febrile seizures. If febrile seizures are recurrent, anticonvulsant therapy can be considered. Fever also may lower the threshold for seizures in children with a seizure disorder. A seizure disorder should be considered if seizures are atypical or recurrent. An evaluation with an electroencephalogram and neurologic consultation should be considered.

OUTCOME

Fever is a symptom of an underlying disease process. It generally is a self-limited and benign symptom with no sequelae. The disease process causing the fever may have significant sequelae if not treated in a timely fashion or if the disease process is serious. Infections in infants are more likely to have complications. Late diagnosis always increases complications. In untreated occult bacteremia, the complication rate is 4% to 20% depending on the organism. If fever persists despite antibiotic treatment for a bacterial focus, the child should be evaluated for a complication. Examples of complications to consider include a subdural effusion during treatment for meningitis or a concurrent viral infection, such as mononucleosis, during therapy for streptococcal pharyngitis. With prolonged FUO, 40% of patients have a serious disorder with lasting sequelae. Early identification is important for optimal outcome.

FOLLOW-UP

Follow-up evaluations are essential in febrile children; it is essential to ensure that the disease is responding to treatment. A telephone call may be sufficient. If symptoms are resolved, an office visit may not be necessary. If infants are treated as outpatients and meet criteria for bacteremia, an office visit for re-evaluation is required in 24 hours. With certain foci of infection, such as pneumonia or cellulitis in an older child who is stable for outpatient therapy, a return visit in 24 hours is important. If the child is improving on treatment, an evaluation at the end of treatment should be scheduled. If the child with fever is followed closely for resolution, the rate of complications and missed diagnoses is minimal.

Additional Resources, CD-ROM

Bibliography

SUGGESTED READINGS

Baker MD: Evaluation and management of infants with fever. Pediatr Clin North Am 1999;46:1061–1072.
Baraff LJ: Management of fever without source in infants and children. Ann Emerg Med 2001;36:602–614.
Crocetti M, Moghbeli N, Servant J: Fever phobia revisited: Have parental misconceptions about fever changed in 20 years? Pediatrics 2001;107:1241–1246.
Kupperman N: Occult bacteremia in young febrile children. Pediatr Clin North Am 1999;46:1073–1109.
McCarthy PL: Fever. Pediatr Rev 1998;19:401–407.

SECTION 3   GENERAL MEDICAL CARE: *Emergent Medical Care*

38 Approach to the Ill-Appearing Child

Julie Noble

ROLE OF THE GENERALIST

1 Distinguish an ill-appearing from a well-appearing child.

2 Use a logical approach to determine the pathophysiologic cause of the child's appearance.

3 Differentiate an acutely ill child from a chronically ill child, and understand the different approaches to determine cause.

4 Stabilize an acutely ill child rapidly, and determine further management.

5 Recognize the need for critical care or specialist referral.

6 Prevent morbidity and mortality by early recognition and treatment.

7 Educate parents and office staff to recognize signs of serious illness in children.

When a child of any age presents to a medical setting—office, community clinic, urgent care clinic, or emergency department—the first important assessment is whether the child appears ill. A rapid ascertainment of this parameter facilitates evaluation and stabilization of the patient.

The clinical judgment of a child as ill or well often takes years of experience and observation of children to perfect. A practitioner develops a "gestalt," an impression comprising clinical evidence obtained through history, physical examination, and observation of the child. An ill-appearing child has objective findings that suggest compromise of bodily functions. Astute clinicians also recognize that a child can have significant illness and not appear ill. Experience and knowledge of age-specific behavioral activities improve a clinician's ability to determine the level of illness of an individual patient. The assessment of an infant frequently is more difficult than the assessment of an older child who has better developed behavioral and communication skills.

A chronically ill-appearing child exhibits different clinical findings than an acutely ill-appearing child. In an acutely ill-appearing child, the level of severity of illness frequently is referred to as *toxicity*. This term originally referred to a patient who displayed signs of being poisoned or exhibited effects from toxins of infectious agents. *Toxic* now denotes an ill-appearing child who appears to be at risk for having a clinically severe illness. If febrile, an ill-appearing child is more likely to have an infectious disease. Prompt, logical evaluation of an ill-appearing child is essential to ensure early treatment and prevent morbidity and mortality in the child with serious illness.

Table 38-1. Severity Index Scoring System

Variable	Point Value		
	0	1	2
Respiratory effort	Labored or absent	Some distress	No distress
Color	Cyanotic	Pale, mottled, flushed	Normal
Activity	Delirium, stupor, coma	Lethargy	Normal
Temperature	<97.4°F or >104°F	101.1–104°F	97.4–101°F
Play	Refuses to play	Decreased	Normal

From Nelson KG: An index of severity for acute pediatric illness. Am J Public Health 1980;70:804–807. Copyright © 1980, American Public Health Association. Used with permission.

FUNDAMENTALS

The determination of ill appearance is based on observation of signs and symptoms that indicate either acute or chronic pathophysiology. This observation includes determination of cardiorespiratory status, activity level and behaviors, mental status, and growth and nutritional parameters. Respiratory status should be noted for breathing pattern, hyperventilation, respiratory distress, stridor, hypoventilation, and wheezing. Skin is observed for color; cyanosis; pallor; and evidence of rash, bruises, or poor perfusion, which can present as a *mottled* appearance. An ill-appearing child may exhibit decreased muscle tone and activity that may represent fatigue.

Mental status is evaluated for level of alertness, responsiveness to environment, and evidence of lethargy. The child's behavior is an important component of the clinician's assessment of a child as ill appearing. Behavior is evaluated by eye contact, social smile, interest in toys, and ability to play. These parameters may be unreliable if the child is influenced by pain, hunger, stranger anxiety, or situational anxiety. The child must be as comfortable as possible for the clinician to make valid observations. Knowledge of and experience with age-specific behaviors are essential to evaluation of behavior in children.

A chronically ill-appearing child may exhibit some of the previously mentioned findings, including fatigue. The child frequently has a decreased ability to play and decreased interest in interacting with the environment. Growth may be affected, and there may be evidence of malnutrition. Skin should be evaluated for bruises and rashes. Abdominal distention may be present.

In an effort to quantify and define symptoms consistent with an acutely ill-appearing child, several scoring systems have been developed for assessing level of illness and triaging patients for care. Table 38-1 presents an index of objective criteria to rate the severity of illness of children. The scoring system, used for triage, selected the following five variables as the best predictors of severity of illness: (1) respiratory effort, (2) color, (3) activity, (4) temperature, and (5) play. The variables are rated on a 0-to-2 scoring system, with 2 being normal for that parameter. A well-appearing child would receive a score of 10; a moderately ill–appearing child would receive a score of 8 to 9; and a very ill–appearing child would receive a score of 7. This index can be used as a triage tool in assessing toxicity. The tool has a predictive accuracy for nonsevere illness of 98.7% with a 1.3% false-negative rate. In predicting significant illness, the index is 84.2% accurate.

Table 38-2 (the Yale Observation Scale) lists criteria used specifically for evaluating febrile ill-appearing children 3 years old or younger. The variables are playfulness, alertness, consolability, motor ability, eating, color, respiration, and hydration. Playfulness is identified as a key variable.

Table 38-2. Yale Observation Scale

Observation Variable	Normal (1)	Moderate Impairment (3)	Severe Impairment (5)
Quality of cry	Strong with normal tone or contents and not crying	Whimpering or sobbing	Weak or moaning or high-pitched
Reaction to parent stimulation	Cries briefly, then stops or content	Cries on and off	Continual cry or hardly responds
State variation	If awake, stays awake, or if asleep and stimulated, wakes up quickly	Eyes close briefly when awake or awakes with prolonged stimulation	Fall to sleep or cannot be aroused
Color	Pink	Pale extremities or acrocyanosis	Pale or cyanotic or mottled or ashen
Hydration	Skin normal, eyes normal, and mucous membranes moist	Skin and eyes normal and mouth slightly dry	Skin doughy or tented and dry mucous membranes or sunken eyes
Response (talk, smile) or social overtures	Smiles or becomes alert	Brief smile or becomes alert briefly	No smile, anxious, dull, expressionless, or cannot be alerted

From McCarthy PL, Sharpe MR, Spiesel SZ, et al: Observation scales to identify serious illness in febrile children. Pediatrics 1982;70:802–809. Copyright 1982. Reproduced with permission from *Pediatrics*.

Box 38-1. The Young Infant Observation Scale

Affect

- Smiling or not irritable (1)
- Irritable, consolable (3)
- Irritable, not consolable (5)

Respiratory Status/Effort

- No impairment, vigorous (1)
- Mild-to-moderate compromise (tachypnea, retractions, grunting) (3)
- Respiratory distress or inadequate effort (apnea, respiratory failure) (5)

Peripheral Perfusion

- Pink, warm extremities (1)
- Mottled, cool extremities (3)
- Pale, shock (5)

Data from Bonadio WA, Hennes H, Smith D, et al: Reliability of observation variable in distinguishing infectious outcome of febrile young infants. Pediatr Infect Dis J 1993;12:111–114.

Box 38-2. Diagnostic Goals and Challenges for Evaluating an Ill-Appearing Child

1. Prompt recognition of an ill-appearing child
2. Rapid evaluation of a child who appears acutely ill
3. Determine underlying pathologic process causing physiologic compromise
4. Determine appropriate diagnostic tests

This scale uses quality of cry, reaction to parent stimulation, state variation, color, hydration, and response to social overtures as the significant observation variables. The total score ranges from 6 to 30, with a higher score indicating a more ill-appearing child. If the Yale Observation Scale score is less than or equal to 10, the rate of serious illness is 2.7%. If the total Yale Observation Scale score is greater than 16, the rate of serious illness is 92.3%. The scale is not helpful in predicting bacteremia but may be helpful in assessing a nonfebrile ill-appearing child.

Box 38-1 shows the Young Infant Observation Scale. In this scale, young infants are rated for three variables: (1) affect, (2) respiratory status and effort, and (3) peripheral perfusion. Scores range from 3 to 15. A normal infant would receive a score of 3, and a severely ill child would receive a score of 15. A score greater than 7 has a sensitivity of 75% and specificity of 75% for predicting serious bacterial disease. When using this rating scale, an infant can appear normal and have significant disease.

Any of the aforementioned scoring scales can be used as an adjunct to assist a physician in determining the level of illness of a child. These scales are more appropriate in evaluating an acutely ill-appearing child versus a chronically ill-appearing child.

DIAGNOSIS

A child can be identified as appearing ill by office staff, the health care provider, or parents. The assessment of trained and experienced professionals is more accurate than that of parents. Parents can overestimate the severity of illness, usually secondary to parental anxiety or experience with previous childhood illness. Overestimation of severity of illness by parents is not related to socioeconomic status.

A patient observed to be ill appearing requires a prompt evaluation by the health care provider. Box 38-2 lists the diagnostic goals and challenges for an ill-appearing child. Complete vital signs, including temperature, respiratory rate, heart rate, blood pressure, and pulse oximetry, should

be obtained. A complete physical examination of the patient without clothing should be performed. If the child is acutely ill appearing and febrile, infectious diagnoses, such as sepsis, meningitis, pneumonia, and encephalitis, should be considered. If the patient is stable, antipyretic treatment may improve the child's clinical appearance because fever itself can make a child appear "toxic."

In evaluating all ill-appearing children, the organ system most compromised should be identified by thorough evaluation of the history and physical examination findings. Signs of respiratory distress suggest airway, pulmonary, or cardiac problems. Hyperventilation can be seen with metabolic acidosis secondary to hyperglycemia, lactic acidosis, or metabolic disorders. Poor perfusion may indicate sepsis, vascular collapse, anaphylaxis, dehydration, or cardiovascular shock. Irritability or lethargy and change in mental status and behavioral activities may indicate central nervous system infection, toxin ingestion, nonaccidental trauma, metabolic error, central nervous system hemorrhage, or hypoperfusion. If the parental history cannot account for the severity of the child's illness, an unobserved ingestion or nonaccidental trauma should be suspected.

A chronically ill-appearing child, if febrile, may have an infectious, autoimmune, or neoplastic process. If the child is nonfebrile, malnutrition, starvation, child abuse, or anorexia nervosa should be considered. A chronically ill-appearing child with or without fever could present later with inflammatory bowel disease or malignancy (Table 38-3).

In evaluating an acutely ill-appearing child, initial diagnostic tests include a complete blood count, urinalysis, blood glucose, and electrolytes. If respiratory distress is apparent, a chest x-ray and blood gas analysis are indicated. If the child is febrile, a blood culture and urine culture should be ordered. Also the child should be assessed for the need for a lumbar puncture for cerebrospinal fluid analysis and culture. If there is a change in mental status, a toxicology screen, blood ammonia, and computed tomography scan of the head should be obtained. Further diagnostic workup should be guided by the specific findings in the history and physical examination. Determining the etiology of the child's clinical compromise is essential to further treatment and management.

MANAGEMENT

Management goals are listed in Box 38-3. The management of an ill-appearing child should be optimal to prevent a catastrophic event. Parents should be educated to recognize signs of serious illness so that a child can be identified early. Office staff should be educated to perform effective triage. Recognition of a child with clinical compromise of an organ

Table 38-3. Differential Diagnosis of an Ill-Appearing Child

	Chapter
Acutely Ill Child	
Shock	
Cardiogenic	28
Hypovolemic	42
Toxin-induced	35
Respiratory	
Aspiration	36
Asthma	32
Epiglottitis	111
Croup	111
Pneumothorax	113
Asphyxia	110
Infection	
Sepsis	117
Pneumonia	113
Meningitis	108
Encephalitis	108
Ingestion	35
Nonaccidental trauma	269
Cardiac	
Failure	30
Arrhythmia	59
Metabolic	
Inborn error of metabolism	146
Electrolyte abnormality	42
Diabetes mellitus	155
Adrenal insufficiency	154
Anaphylaxis	43
Acute abdominal event	81
Intracranial	
Increased pressure	31
Hemorrhage	34
Child with Chronic Illness	
Infection	
HIV	171
Chronic or recurrent infection	116
Malnutrition	
Inflammatory bowel disease	139
Nutritional	86
Malabsorption	138
Anorexia nervosa	232 and 254
Chronic child neglect	268
Neoplastic	162
	163
	164
	165
Renal failure	173
Hepatic failure	90
Chronic toxin exposure	
Lead poisoning	109

HIV, human immunodeficiency virus.

system should prompt immediate intervention for evaluation and stabilization. Venous access should be obtained, and resuscitation should ensue, if indicated by respiratory, cardiac, or volume compromise. Diagnostic evaluation to identify the cause of the compromise can proceed when the child is stable. When the etiology is identified, therapy directed at that diagnosis can begin. Specialist consultants are helpful if the diagnosis is complicated or the etiology is unusual. If the child requires intensive care management, transport to a pediatric intensive care unit is essential. Many ill-appearing children require hospitalization for therapy, and many chronically ill-appearing children may require hospitalization for diagnostic evaluation.

Box 38-3. Management Goals for an Ill-Appearing Child

1. Effective triage to facilitate rapid identification of an ill-appearing child
2. Appropriate resuscitation as indicated
3. Stabilization and therapy for identified cause of compromise
4. Use of consultants when indicated for an identified condition
5. Parental and staff education for early identification of severe illness
6. Prevention of a catastrophic event

OUTCOME

The outcome for an ill-appearing child depends on two parameters. The first parameter is early recognition of a serious disease process. Treatment is more effective for any disease process if begun early. If meningitis is detected early, the sequelae of neurologic deficits are reduced. With malignancy, the earlier the disease is diagnosed, the more likely the process will remit with treatment. The second parameter is the severity of the disease process. If a child appears ill as a result of influenza, his or her outcome is much better than that of an ill-appearing child diagnosed with sepsis. Accurate diagnosis is essential to treatment and prognosis.

Outcome can be improved with educational efforts for parents, triage staff, and physicians aimed at early recognition of an ill-appearing child. Improving resuscitation skills and physician education for current therapies should be ongoing in any practice setting.

Mini-index of Related Topics

	CH.
RESUSCITATION AND BASIC LIFE SUPPORT	27
SHOCK	28
ACUTE RESPIRATORY FAILURE	29
CARDIAC FAILURE	30
CENTRAL NERVOUS SYSTEM FAILURE	31
APPROACH TO THE FEBRILE PATIENT	37
THE ILL NEWBORN: EARLY IDENTIFICATION AND STABILIZATION	195

*See also Table 38-3.

SUGGESTED READINGS

Bonadio WA: The history and physical assessments of the febrile infant. Pediatr Clin North Am 1998;45:65–77.

McCarthy PL, Jekel JF, Stashwick CA, et al: Further definition of history and observation variables in assessing febrile children. Pediatrics 1981;67:687–693.

McCarthy PL, Liem RM, Baron MA, et al: Predictive value of abnormal physical examination findings in ill-appearing and well-appearing febrile children. Pediatrics 1985;70:167–171.

McCarthy PL, Sznajderman S, Lustman K, et al: Mothers' clinical judgment: A randomized trial of the Acute Illness Observation Scales. J Pediatr 1990;116:200–206.

Mower WR, Sacks C, Nicklin EL, Baraff LJ: Pulse oximetry as a fifth pediatric vital sign. Pediatrics 1997;99:681–686.

39

Approach to the Agitated Patient

Rona Molodow

ROLE OF THE GENERALIST

1   Differentiate the causes of agitation in infants and children.
2   Assess an agitated child systematically.
3   Manage agitation based on the underlying etiology.
4   Determine which patients can be managed by the general practitioner and which patients require referral.

DEFINITION

Agitation commonly is accepted as a state of increased arousal, with signs and symptoms including anxiety, irritability, restlessness, tremulousness, and frank psychosis or delirium. This chapter focuses on children in whom agitation is the primary or predominant presenting complaint. An age-based approach is useful for the differential diagnosis, recognizing that there is overlap between groups.

FUNDAMENTALS

As diverse as the signs and symptoms constituting agitation may be, the differential diagnosis is perhaps even broader. Causes include pain, anxiety, cardiopulmonary disorders, toxic ingestion and intoxication, and metabolic and endocrine disturbances. In assessing an agitated child, the practitioner must consider the age of the patient, associated complaints, the onset and duration of symptoms, previous episodes, the setting of presentation, and exactly what is considered "agitation." The generalist must differentiate "normal agitation," seen in many children as a result of fear or anxiety, from agitation that suggests an underlying pathologic condition. An infant who appears agitated in the course of a well-child visit likely has a different cause than an agitated adolescent brought to the emergency department by police. Although management varies with the underlying cause, the first principle in caring for agitated patients is offering a calm environment while providing appropriate supportive care.

DIAGNOSIS AND MANAGEMENT

Although some causes of agitation cross all age groups (Table 39-1), others are highly age specific (Table 39-2), allowing for the practitioner to assess agitation by age of the

Table 39-1. Differential Diagnosis of Agitation*

Infection
  Septicemia
  Meningoencephalitis
Neurologic
  Seizures (temporal lobe epilepsy)
  Confusional migraine
  Intracranial injury
Psychiatric disorders
  Anxiety disorders
  Oppositional-defiant disorder
  Posttraumatic stress disorder
Hypoxia
Obstructive sleep apnea
Metabolic/endocrine disease
  Hypoglycemia
  Hyponatremia
  Hypomagnesemia
  Hypocalcemia
  Hyperthyroidism

*Diagnoses common to all age groups.

affected child. Precise symptoms also vary with age. In neonates, agitation may be manifested by little more than crying and fussiness, with symptoms such as restlessness and anxiety becoming more obvious with increasing age.

In all age groups, the evaluation starts with a complete history of the present illness, focusing on related symptoms and on events that may have triggered the episode. It must be determined whether onset was acute or insidious and whether symptoms are chronic or intermittent. Any interventions and their success or failure should be noted, as should a history of similar episodes in the past. General health status, including previous illnesses and drugs (prescription or otherwise), must be assessed, and in infants and neonates, prenatal and peripartum history should be explored. A psychosocial history also is crucial, focusing on the child's usual level of functioning. The physical examination begins with observation of the child's general status: Is the child calm or agitated at the time of the examination; does the child appear well or ill? Next, the examiner must look for signs that may point toward systemic disease. Vital signs, including pulse oximetry, are crucial. Is the child hypoxic; is the child tachycardic or hypertensive? A thorough physical examination should follow. The neurologic examination is particularly important: Does the child react to the examiner? Does he or she behave age appropriately? Is the child confused or delirious? Can he or she move all extremities? Are the child's pupils small or large, and are they responsive? The examination

Table 39-2. Differential Diagnosis of Agitation by Age

Neonate	Infant	Toddler/Preschooler	School-Age Child	Adolescent
Normal crying	Teething	"Terrible twos"	Developmental disorders*	Intoxication withdrawal
Colic	Stranger awareness	Toxic ingestion	Autism spectrum disorders	Alcohol
Occult head trauma	Occult head trauma	Sympathomimetics	Pervasive developmental	Barbiturates
Withdrawal from maternal	Cardiac disease	Anticholinergics	delay	Opioids
drug use		Salicylates	Specific developmental	Psychiatric disease†
Cardiac disease		Sleep disorders	disabilities	Schizophrenia
Supraventricular		Night terrors	Psychiatric disorders*	Bipolar disorder
trachycardia			Attention-deficit hyperactivity	
Anomalous coronary			disorder	
arteries				
Congestive heart failure				

*May be seen in younger and older children.
†May be seen in younger children.

does not end here. A systematic examination of the undressed child reveals associated signs and clues to possible etiologies for the agitation. As with many medical complaints with a broad differential diagnosis, the question of what laboratory data to collect depends on information from the history and physical examination.

Infants

Crying and irritability are common medical complaints during the neonatal period. Although some authors disagree about its existence as a distinct entity, reports of "colic" have been recorded in medical literature since at least the 18th century. Early descriptions still are used today to define colic, such as the "rule of three" (excessive crying for 3 hours a day, 3 days a week, for 3 weeks). Illingworth vividly depicted the affected infant: "violent screaming attacks in the evening … his face flushes, his brow furrows, and then he draws his legs up, clenches his fist, and emits piercing, high pitched screams."

"Colicky" and "noncolicky" infants cry most during evening hours, with episodes peaking at about 6 weeks and declining thereafter until 4 months of age. Although multiple researchers have attempted to delineate risk factors for colic, no consistent features have been identified. Management efforts typically include comforting measures, such as swaddling and gentle rocking, and some authorities tout the use of hydrolyzed casein formula. Reassurance is vital. Crying invariably decreases in frequency and intensity with age, although more recent studies suggest that colicky infants tend to be more fussy and aggressive as children.

Other disorders also may present with crying in early infancy, and duration of symptoms is an important differentiating feature. Gastroesophageal reflux may be present with symptoms similar to colic but often is associated with other symptoms, such as vomiting or poor weight gain. Acute pain also may be responsible for agitation, but may be difficult to identify in infants. A thorough examination, including a fluorescent eye examination to detect a corneal abrasion, may reveal the cause of the pain. Hair tourniquets, unrecognized fractures, and otitis media frequently are implicated and may be identified via a systematic assessment. Infections such as bacteremia, urinary tract infection, and meningoencephalitis may present with cry-

ing or irritability. Fever and an ill appearance usually are noted.

The possibility of drug withdrawal after in utero exposure also must be explored. Signs and symptoms of withdrawal may include irritability, restlessness, crying, and poor feeding. The abstinence syndrome is defined best in narcotic exposure, in which symptoms peak at 3 to 14 days of life and may persist 4 to 6 months. Although not as pronounced as with opiates, withdrawal also is described in neonates exposed to marijuana and cocaine. The maternal and prenatal history are essential in evaluating the irritable neonate or infant. Urine drug screening may provide confirmatory evidence.

A frequent occult cause of agitation in infants is intracranial injury, especially that associated with abusive head trauma. In a study of "missed cases" of abusive head trauma, in two thirds of missed cases the infants were described as "irritable" at the time of their first health care encounter. Frequent misdiagnoses included viral gastroenteritis, influenza, accidental head injury, possible sepsis, otitis media, and reflux. The possibility of head trauma should be considered in an infant who presents with agitation with or without symptoms such as vomiting or fever. Associated findings may include cutaneous bruises, fractures, and retinal hemorrhages.

Tachyarrhythmias during infancy also may present with irritability and fussiness. Supraventricular tachycardia is the most common pediatric tachyarrhythmia. If circulation is not compromised, a rapid heart rate may be the sole physical sign, and if the arrhythmia is intermittent, the tachycardia may go undetected. In such cases, the practitioner may elicit a history of discrete episodes, manifested by sudden onset and resolution of irritability. If the tachycardia is prolonged, the child may present in florid heart failure. An electrocardiogram or, if no signs are evident on presentation, a Holter monitor confirms the diagnosis and differentiates forms of tachyarrhythmia. Other cardiac disorders that may masquerade as agitation include anomalous coronary arteries and congestive heart failure, although in such cases irritability is rarely an isolated symptom. After immediate stabilization, referral to a pediatric cardiologist is mandatory.

Teething is a universal experience. Different studies present conflicting results about whether symptoms such as irritability, wakefulness, and ear rubbing are associated significantly with teething. Temperature greater than 102°F (38.9°C), decreased appetite for liquids, cough, and rash not linked to teething suggest, however, an easy distinction between systemic illness and teething.

Toddlers and Children

When children are ambulatory, they are at risk for other disturbances, such as ingestions. Children younger than 6 years old account for more than 50% of emergency department visits for accidental ingestions. Agitation is reported with many different medications, including anticholinergics, sympathomimetics (albuterol and over-the-counter preparations containing epinephrine and pseudoephedrine), hypoglycemic agents, and, rarely, thyroid hormones. The practitioner must be alert not only to medications used by children, their parents, and grandparents, but also to other substances to which they might have access, such as heavy metals, plants, and illicit drugs. The presence of other specific physical findings, such as dilated pupils, hyperventilation, and diaphoresis (sympathomimetics), or dry mouth, urinary retention, and respiratory depression (anticholinergics), suggests an ingestion and the potential agent. Precise management depends on the material consumed, but standard care includes toxicology screening, administration of charcoal as indicated, and supportive measures.

"Night terrors" may account for a history of nocturnal agitation and crying in toddlers and preschoolers. Affected children generally appear well in the practitioner's office, but parents describe episodes in which children awaken, scream or cry, and are inconsolable for 30 minutes before falling back to sleep. Care should be taken to explain night terrors as a normal developmental variant, likely to resolve by middle childhood. Because episodes are more likely to occur with stress or fatigue, attempts should be made to investigate and relieve these factors.

Hypoxia is a serious and potentially lethal cause of restlessness and irritability, particularly if unrecognized and managed with sedation. Agitation generally improves when hypoxia is corrected, but the ease of correction depends on the etiology and duration. In contrast to an adult, in whom daytime sleepiness predominates, recurrent hypoxia and sleep disruption may combine to result in agitation and hyperactivity in children of any age with obstructive sleep apnea.

Children with psychiatric and behavioral disorders, such as attention deficit hyperactivity disorder, oppositional-defiant disorder, anxiety disorder, and bipolar disorder, may manifest increased levels of activity, especially in the school setting. Similarly, autistic or developmentally delayed children and hearing-impaired or aphasic students may become agitated in unfamiliar settings. The diagnosis of these conditions is usually not problematic, although management may require psychiatric, behavioral, or pharmacologic interventions.

Adolescents

Ingestions, common in toddlers and preschoolers, again surface as a culprit for agitation in adolescents. In adolescents, the ingestion itself is rarely accidental, however.

Sympathomimetic drugs of abuse are especially common. These include amphetamines, phencyclidine, and cocaine. Ecstasy (3,4-methylenedioxymethamphetamine) is an amphetamine analogue, whereas "herbal ecstasy" contains ephedrine. In contrast, an adolescent who chronically abuses substances such as alcohol, barbiturates, or narcotics may show agitation not as a result of intoxication but secondary to withdrawal. The examination may reveal signs consistent with a toxidrome, and toxicologic testing can provide confirmatory evidence. Management of intoxication and withdrawal requires a calm environment, with appropriate monitoring and supportive measures. A thorough evaluation for possible substance abuse is necessary, and enrollment in a treatment program may be indicated.

Although the agitation of intoxication is generally acute, more insidious development of symptoms may be a clue to serious psychiatric disease. Schizophrenia, bipolar, obsessive-compulsive, and anxiety disorders and depression may present with agitation. Early recognition is often difficult, secondary to the gradual onset of symptoms and the reluctance of practitioners to label patients as mentally ill, with time from onset of symptoms to diagnosis often exceeding 1 year in this age group. As always, making the diagnosis depends on a systematic history and physical examination, centering on onset of symptoms and premorbid condition. Although orientation, memory, and intellectual functioning may be impaired in an intoxicated child, they generally remain intact in patients with psychiatric disease. On physical assessment, altered level of consciousness and abnormal vital signs may be observed in an intoxicated or systemically ill adolescent but not in a youngster with psychiatric illness. Nonetheless, mental illness and substance abuse may coexist as an adolescent attempts "self-medication," also contributing to the difficulty in prompt recognition of psychiatric disorders. Even if psychiatric illness is suspected, toxicology screening is warranted in most situations.

Additional medical illnesses that may present with agitation include temporal lobe epilepsy and hyperthyroidism. Patients with hyperthyroidism have additional symptoms, such as increased appetite without weight gain, palpitations, and dyspnea. A child with hyperthyroidism may exhibit tremor; mild-to-moderate exophthalmos; smoothed, flushed skin with diaphoresis; and tachycardia. Temporal lobe seizures may manifest with bizarre or agitated behavior. Amnesia following an episode suggests seizure activity.

OUTCOME

Sometimes agitation can signify a normal developmental variant and at other times it can be evidence of a medical emergency. The key is recognizing that agitation is a symptom, not a disease in itself. The differential diagnosis is broad, and management requires determining the underlying cause via a thorough assessment, which must include attention to age, surrounding circumstances and associated complaints, premorbid status, and physical signs. Collection of laboratory data should be based on this information.

SUGGESTED READINGS

Illingworth RS: "Three months" colic. Arch Dis Child 1954;29:165–174.

Jenny C, Hymel KP, Ritzen A, et al: Analysis of missed cases of abusive head trauma. JAMA 1999;281:621–626.

Macknin ML, Piedmonte M, Jacobs J, Skibinski C: Symptoms associated with infant teething: A prospective study. Pediatrics 2000;105:747–752.

Oberklaid F: Persistent crying in infancy: A persistent clinical conundrum. J Pediatr Child Health 2000;36:297–298.

Thiedke CC: Sleep disorders and sleep problems in childhood. Am Fam Physician 2001;63:277–283.

SECTION 3   GENERAL MEDICAL CARE: *Emergent Medical Care*

40 Hypertensive Crisis

Sudhir K. Anand

ROLE OF THE GENERALIST

1. Recognize hypertensive crisis.
2. Distinguish hypertensive emergency from hypertensive urgency.
3. Institute appropriate emergency treatment.
4. Diagnose etiology of hypertensive crisis.
5. Refer to appropriate specialists for assistance in diagnosis and management when needed.

DEFINITION

Hypertensive crisis implies profound hypertension requiring prompt therapy to prevent permanent sequelae. Hypertensive crisis usually is subdivided into hypertensive emergencies and hypertensive urgencies. *Hypertensive emergency* is an acute symptomatic clinical state in which uncontrolled hypertension is associated with acute end organ damage and requires immediate, carefully monitored therapy to reduce blood pressure (BP) to prevent further organ damage. Hypertensive urgency is defined as a significant elevation in BP without evidence of end organ damage. In hypertensive urgency, reduction of BP may occur over a few to 48 hours, usually with oral agents in an ambulatory setting. Both of these conditions are uncommon in children who were previously healthy; they usually occur in children with pre-existing renal disease or other known causes of hypertension.

NORMAL BLOOD PRESSURE, HYPERTENSION, AND HYPERTENSIVE CRISIS

Systolic and diastolic BP in children gradually increase from the newborn period through adolescence; age-appropriate norms should be used to classify a given BP reading as normal or hypertensive (see CD-ROM Tables 174-1 and 174-2). A BP reading of 136/85 mm Hg may be regarded as normal in a 17-year-old, but it would be regarded as severe hypertension in a 6-month-old and require immediate attention.

Based on the Report of the Second Task Force on Blood Pressure Control in Children in 1987 and an update of this report in 1996, BP readings persistently greater than the

95th percentile adjusted for patient age and height are regarded as hypertension, whereas readings greater than the 99th percentile are termed *severe hypertension*. Hypertensive crisis is characterized by markedly increased BP (>99th percentile) usually in association with end organ damage.

CLINICAL PRESENTATION

Children with mild hypertension are usually asymptomatic. Children with hypertensive crisis present with one or more of the symptoms and signs listed in Box 40-1. The child may have central nervous system symptoms and signs, including headache, vomiting, altered mental state, seizures, and paralysis. Cardiovascular symptoms and signs include tachycardia, tachypnea, enlarged liver, or frank heart failure. Urine output may be diminished, and renal failure may be present. Visual changes may be present; an examination of the fundus may show vascular changes with exudates and papilledema. Symptoms and signs of the primary disorder that led to the crisis are superimposed on the aforementioned findings (e.g., hematuria in a patient with acute glomerulonephritis).

ETIOLOGY

Disorders that cause hypertension also can lead to hypertensive crisis (Table 40-1). Hypertensive crisis can be caused by a wide variety of conditions but most often is secondary to renal disorders. In some patients, the disease is acute in onset, whereas in others hypertension is chronic (although its preexistence may not have been known), with an abrupt increase in BP. The etiology of hypertension varies with the age of the child.

PATHOPHYSIOLOGY

The development of hypertensive crisis is based on sudden change in the rate of BP increase and not an arbitrary number. Because of adaptive changes in blood vessels, patients with chronic hypertension often are asymptomatic, even with markedly increased BPs. These patients are less likely to develop crisis with acute changes in BP. Children with previously normal BP can develop hypertensive crisis at considerably lower BPs (e.g., 145/95 mm Hg) in acute glomerulonephritis.

The pathogenesis of hypertensive crisis and accompanying end organ damage is incompletely understood. Plasma and/or tissue levels of vasoconstricting agents (e.g., angiotensin II, norepinephrine, and endothelin I) increase, and vasodila-

Table 40-1. Etiology of Hypertensive Emergencies

System	Etiologies
Renal	Renal parenchymal diseases: scarred or dysplastic kidney(s)
	Glomerulonephritis: acute or chronic
	Hemolytic uremic syndrome
	Blood transfusion in chronic renal failure patient
	Renal transplant rejection
	Vascular disease: renal artery stenosis, thrombosis
	Vasculitis: systemic lupus erythematosus, polyarteritis
	Renin-secreting tumor
Endocrine	Neuroblastoma/ganglioneuroblastoma
	Pheochromocytoma
	Cushing's disease
	High-dose steroid treatment
	Riley-Day syndrome
Cardiovascular	Coarctation of the aorta
Pregnancy related	Preeclampsia, eclampsia
CNS disorders	Gullain-Barré syndrome
	Head injury
	CNS hemorrhage
	Brain tumor
Drugs	Cocaine, amphetamines
	Phencyclidine
	Cyclosporine
	Erythropoietin
	Sudden antihypertensive withdrawal
Unknown	Essential hypertension

CNS, central nervous system.

tors (e.g., nitric oxide and prostacyclin) decrease. These changes result in increased vascular resistance, severe vasoconstriction, fibrinoid necrosis, and endothelial damage in small arterioles, especially in the kidneys, brain, retina, and myocardium. The endothelial damage leads to platelet and fibrin deposition and may lead to partial or complete occlusion of the vessel. Ensuing ischemia triggers further release of vasoconstrictive substances, resulting in a vicious cycle of vasoconstriction, intimal damage, and ischemia.

Hypertensive encephalopathy occurs in association with diffuse or focal cerebral edema from endothelial damage, disruption of the blood-brain barrier, and a failure of cerebral blood flow autoregulation. Clinically, hypertensive encephalopathy is characterized by one or more of the following symptoms (Box 40-2): headache, lethargy, confusion, nausea, vomiting, visual disturbances (including blindness), or focal or generalized weakness or seizures. Hypertensive retinopathy and papilledema usually are present. If encephalopathy is not treated adequately, cerebral hemorrhage, coma, and death can ensue.

Box 40-1. Signs and Symptoms of Hypertensive Crisis

- *Central nervous system:* headache, vomiting, altered mental state, seizures, paralysis
- *Cardiovascular:* tachycardia, tachypnea, enlarged liver, frank heart failure
- *Renal:* diminished urine output, renal failure
- *Ophthalmologic:* visual changes, fundus with vascular changes, exudates, papilledema

---

Box 40-2. Signs and Symptoms of Hypertensive Encephalopathy

- Headache, lethargy, confusion
- Nausea, vomiting
- Visual disturbances (including blindness)
- Focal or generalized weakness or seizures
- Hypertensive retinopathy and papilledema usually present

CLINICAL EVALUATION AND LABORATORY WORKUP

Based on the previously described clinical presentation, a directed evaluation should be performed to determine any underlying etiology, preexisting hypertension, or other disorders; the extent of neurologic dysfunction, retinopathy, congestive heart failure, and renal failure; and whether the patient requires emergent or urgent treatment. Upper and lower extremity BPs should be measured. An electrocardiogram, urinalysis, complete blood count, serum creatinine, blood urea nitrogen, electrolyte measurements, and chest x-ray should be obtained.

Depending on the extent of end organ damage described earlier, laboratory findings may show hemolytic anemia with fragmented red blood cells and thrombocytopenia, proteinuria and microhematuria, increase in blood urea nitrogen and serum creatinine, hypokalemia (hyperkalemia with severe renal damage), and increase in lactate dehydrogenase and liver enzymes. Electrocardiogram may show ST changes and evidence of myocardial isehemia. Chest x-ray may show pulmonary edema. The presence of these findings distinguishes hypertensive emergency from urgency.

MANAGEMENT

Hypertensive emergency should be distinguished from hypertensive urgency by the criteria discussed earlier. Hypertensive emergency is managed best in an intensive care unit. An intra-arterial catheter should be placed for continuous BP monitoring. While such measures are being instituted, therapy should be initiated in the emergency department with close monitoring of vital signs and BP.

The immediate goal of therapy in a hypertensive emergency is a prompt, but gradual reduction of BP. A reasonable goal, based on the experience in adults, is to reduce mean arterial pressure by 20% to 25% (but not <100 mm Hg diastolic) over 15 minutes to 2 hours. BP reductions to normal or hypotensive levels should be avoided to avoid end organ ischemia or infarction and worsening of function. Children generally seem to tolerate BP reductions better than adults.

If during the management of hypertensive encephalopathy, neurologic function deteriorates, antihypertensive therapy should be stopped, and BP should be allowed to

increase. When neurologic function stabilizes, BP should be reduced more slowly. Hypertension often is present in patients with subarachnoid or cerebral hemorrhage, stroke, central nervous system tumors, status epilepticus, vasculitis, and encephalitis. In these conditions, antihypertensive therapy usually is withheld, unless the BP is extremely elevated, because the higher pressure enables better cerebral perfusion, and BP decreases may induce ischemia.

Hypertensive urgencies usually are managed with oral medications. As in hypertensive emergencies, the aim is to lower mean BP by 20% to 25% (but not <90 to 100 mm Hg diastolic), but not to decrease BP precipitously to hypotensive levels. Patients should be observed in the emergency department for at least 6 hours after the initial therapy to monitor for adverse effects and orthostatic hypotension before being discharged home on continuing oral drugs and appropriate follow-up.

DRUG THERAPY

A variety of drugs are available for treatment of hypertensive emergencies. Gradated doses of parenteral drugs are preferred over oral drugs. The etiology (if known) and the nature of the end organ damage help determine which particular drug is most suitable. Table 40-2 lists the usual drugs used in the management of children with hypertensive emergencies along with doses, onset, duration of action, and adverse effects. Initiate with the lowest dose and titrate until the desired effect is obtained. Intravenous sodium nitroprusside, a potent vasodilator, is safe and effective in most situations. Its onset is almost immediate, and discontinuation leads to return to previous BP within 1 or 2 minutes. Although sodium nitroprusside helps achieve precise BP control, continuous infusion and monitoring is required, making it usually unsuitable for immediate use in the emergency department. When desired BP control is achieved for a few hours, oral therapy should be started and intravenous nitroprusside gradually tapered. Prolonged use of nitroprusside may lead to thiocyanate toxicity. In aortic dissection caused by severe hypertension, nitroprusside should be used along with β-blockade (aortic dissection is rare, however, in pediatric patients).

Other drugs that are suitable in most hypertensive emergencies are intravenous labetalol and the calcium channel blocker, nicardipine. Labetalol has α- and β-blocking action

Table 40-2. Parenteral Medications Used in Hypertensive Emergencies

Drug	Dose	Onset	Duration	Adverse Effects
Sodium nitroprusside	0.25–10 µg/kg/min	Immediate	1–2 min	Hypotension, nausea, vomiting, cyanate toxicity especially in renal failure
Labetalol	Bolus: 0.2 mg/kg (max: 20 mg/dose) Infusion: 15–50 µg/kg/min	5–10 min	2–6 hr	Hypotension, nausea, vomiting, heart block, bronchospasm
Nicardipine	Bolus: 30 µg/kg Infusion: 0.5–5.0 µg/kg/min	5–10 min	2–4 hr	Reflex tachycardia, flushing
Hydralazine	0.1–0.25 mg/kg over 30 min every 4 hr	10 min	2–6 hr	Reflex tachycardia, headache, nausea
Fenoldopam	Infusion: 0.1–0.3 µg/kg/min	5–10 min	10–15 min	Hypotension, headache
Enalaprilat	5–10 µg/kg bolus	15 min	4–6 hr	Hypotension, renal failure
Diazoxide	1 mg/kg/dose, can repeat every 10 min to maximum 6 mg/kg	1–5 min	6–12 hr	Hypotension, tachycardia, nausea, vomiting, hyperglycemia, may exacerbate myocardial ischemia, aortic dissection
Phentolamine	0.05–0.1 mg/kg/dose every 1–2 hr	1–2 min	3–5 hr	Reflex tachycardia, headache, hypotension

Table 40-3. Oral Medications Used in Hypertensive Urgencies

Drug	Dose	Onset	Duration	Adverse Effects
Nifedipine	0.25–0.5 mg/kg/dose Maximum 10 mg/dose	5–10 min (sublingual) 10–20 min (oral)	3–6 hr	Headache, dizziness, flushing, hypotension
Enalapril	10–50 µg/kg/dose	10–30 min	12–24 hr	Hypotension, tachycardia, headache, cough, use caution in renal disorders
Clonidine	5–10 µg/kg/dose	30–60 min	8–12 hr	Sedation, dry mouth
Hydralazine	0.25–1.0 mg/kg/dose	30–60 min	4–6 hr	Headache, tachycardia

but primarily works through β-adrenergic blockade, which leads to a reduction in cardiac output. It also has a mild peripheral vasodilator action through β$_2$-agonist activity in the peripheral vasculature. Excessive hypotension is uncommon. Labetalol may be used in the emergency department without an intra-arterial line and has an added advantage in that when desired BP control has been obtained it can be changed gradually to oral therapy. Disadvantages are that it is less effective than nitroprusside or nicardipine, and it occasionally may cause bronchospasm.

Intravenous nicardipine is a calcium channel blocker that primarily dilates peripheral arteries. It has a rapid onset of action and lasts 2 to 4 hours. BP control is gradual, and excessive hypotension is uncommon. Nicardipine also may be used in the emergency department. Fenoldopam, a dopamine agonist, is a newer agent found to be effective in hypertensive emergencies in adults. Experience in children so far is limited. Hydralazine is used primarily in the management of hypertensive emergency associated with preeclampsia or eclampsia and sometimes in acute glomerulonephritis.

Angiotensin-converting enzyme inhibitors usually are not used in acute hypertensive emergencies, especially in patients with renal disorders. These drugs further reduce the already compromised renal circulation and function and sometimes precipitate acute renal failure. They sometimes are useful in refractory patients in whom sodium nitroprusside or other drugs need to be discontinued because of toxicity. Phentolamine, a potent α-adrenergic blocker, is used primarily for patients in whom catecholamine-secreting tumors are suspected or known. Diazoxide was used commonly for hypertensive emergencies, but because of frequent hypotension and other complications, it is no longer a drug of choice.

Hypertensive urgencies can be treated with the drugs listed in Table 40-3. Patients should be treated in the emergency department and observed for a minimum of 6 hours. They should be monitored carefully for adverse effects and orthostatic hypotension, and appropriate follow-up should be ensured before discharge on continuing oral drugs.

Additional Resources, CD-ROM

Blood pressure levels for the 90th and 95th percentiles of blood pressure for boys ages 1 to 17 years by percentiles of height	Table 174-1
Blood pressure levels for the 90th and 95th percentiles of blood pressure for girls ages 1 to 17 years by percentiles of height	Table 174-2

Mini-index of Related Topics

SUGGESTED READINGS

Calhoun DA, Oparil S: Treatment of hypertensive crisis. N Engl J Med 1990;323:1177–1183.

Groshong TD: Hypertensive emergencies in the pediatric intensive care unit patient. In Tobias JD (ed): Pediatric Critical Care: The Essentials. Armonk, NY, Futura Publishing, 1999, pp 377–387.

Update on the Taskforce (1987) on High Blood Pressure in Children and Adolescents: A working group from the National High Blood Pressure Education Program. Pediatrics 1996;98:649–658.

Vaughan CJ, Delanty N: Hypertensive emergencies. Lancet 2000; 354:411.

required. When the insulin infusion is stopped, subcutaneous insulin is given 30 minutes before the infusion is terminated. The usual initial dose is 0.25 U/kg subcutaneously of regular insulin.

If the previously mentioned steps are followed, most patients correct their acidosis with fluids and insulin alone. Bicarbonate therapy poses some problems and may produce lactic acidosis, may worsen hypokalemia, and may worsen cerebral acidosis. For these reasons, bicarbonate therapy is limited to the situations listed in Box 42-5.

DKA has many manifestations, and some children with mild DKA (pH >7.25, bicarbonate 15 mEq/L) may be managed in an emergency department or hospital short stay unit. Some children have severe metabolic derangements and require intensive care expertise. Patients at highest risk are infants younger than 1 year of age, patients with alterations in mental status, and patients with hypernatremia or hypokalemia on initial laboratory determination. The management of DKA can be intense, and attention to detail is necessary. The resources of the hospital and personnel delivering the care are important determinations of when to refer the patient to a tertiary care setting or for specialty management. Cerebral edema may present with alterations in mental status a few hours after treatment is initiated. For all patients with diabetes mellitus, comanagement with an endocrine specialist is helpful for ongoing care.

In a child with profound dehydration, intravenous fluid should be administered on an emergent basis, even before a complete evaluation of the patient is undertaken. In less urgent situations, before administration of fluids, the patient should be evaluated clinically and the type and quantity of fluids calculated. In isonatremic dehydration, the net loss of isotonic fluid from the body produces clinical manifestations resulting predominantly from plasma volume depletion. In this situation, isotonic solutions are indicated for the immediate restoration of ECF volume because movement of sodium from intracellular spaces is gradual and complete only with full restoration of intracellular potassium levels, a process that may take several days.

Relatively greater losses of sodium than of water produce hyponatremic dehydration. Treatment of hyponatremic dehydration is similar to that for isonatremic dehydration except that the extra losses of sodium should be taken into account when calculating electrolyte administration. Administering the extra sodium needed to replace losses can be spread over 12 to 24 hours so that gradual correction of the hyponatremia is accomplished as the volume is expanded. Serum sodium concentrations should not be elevated abruptly by administering hypertonic saline solutions, unless symptoms such as seizures appear. Hyponatremia with difficult to control seizures, rare in the face of hyponatremic dehydration, presents in water intoxication or with SIADH. Use of 3% solution of sodium chloride (0.5 mEq/mL) to raise the sodium to 125 mEq/L is the initial treatment. An infusion of 12 mL/kg over 60 minutes raises the serum sodium by 10 mEq. Lower the rate if the seizure stops during the infusion.

Fluid therapy for hypernatremic dehydration can be difficult because severe hyperosmolality may result in cerebral damage with widespread cerebral hemorrhages, thromboses, and subdural effusions. Even in the absence of obvious pathologic lesions, patients with severe hypernatremia are vulnerable to seizures. Frequently, seizures occur during treatment as the serum sodium is returning to normal. During dehydration, in response to increased plasma osmolality, water shifts out of cerebral cells. To prevent cellular dehydration, neurons make specialized idiogenic osmoles, however, such as taurine, myo-inositol, glutamine, and glycerophosphorylcholine. With a rapid decrease in ECF osmolality as a result of changes in serum sodium and, occasionally, a decrease in the concentration of other osmotically active substances, such as glucose, there may be excess movement of water into cerebral cells during rehydration, with the subsequent development of cerebral edema. In some patients, this edema may be irreversible and lethal. This situation may occur during an overly vigorous correction of hypernatremia or with the use of initial rapid intravenous hydrating solutions that are not isotonic. The incidence of these complications may be reduced by correcting dehydration and hypernatremia slowly over several days. Therapy is adjusted to return the serum sodium levels toward normal by not more than 10 mEq/L/24 hr.

Because the sodium deficit in hypernatremic dehydration is relatively small and the ECF volume relatively well maintained, the amounts of sodium and water to be administered in this phase of treatment are lower than those in hyponatremic or isonatremic dehydration. A suitable regimen is a 5% dextrose solution containing 25 mEq/L of sodium as a combination of the bicarbonate and chloride. Others have suggested 40 mEq/L of sodium and 40 mEq/L of potassium. Fluids with even higher sodium concentrations have been proposed. Although these fluids result in excess sodium administration to the patient, they may protect against abrupt falls in serum sodium. Most studies indicate that the composition of the rehydration solution is less important than careful adherence to a slow and gradual restoration of the deficit over 48 to 72 hours, which is associated with a slow return of serum sodium values to normal. If seizures occur, they often can be controlled by anticonvulsants; intravenous administration of 3 to 5 mL/kg of a 3% sodium chloride solution; or measures to reduce increased intracranial pressure, such as mannitol or hyperventilation.

Treatment of hypernatremic dehydration with large amounts of water, with or without salt, frequently results in expansion of the ECF volume before there is any notable excretion of chloride or correction of the acidosis. As a consequence, edema and occasionally cardiac failure may develop. Hypocalcemia occasionally occurs during treatment of hypernatremic dehydration and may require intravenous administration of calcium. Another complication is renal tubular injury with azotemia and loss of concentrating ability.

Although hypernatremic dehydration can be treated successfully, management is difficult, and seizures frequently occur, even with the best-designed regimens. It is important to emphasize prevention of neurologic sequelae. The complications of hypernatremic dehydration, especially cerebral edema, often are not the result of hypernatremia per se but of inappropriate and aggressive rehydration.

Problems with potassium require careful attention to cardiovascular status, and an ECG should be obtained and continuous cardiac monitoring provided whenever an increased or decreased potassium level exists. Referral for intensive care may be necessary when ECG changes occur, but treatment should be initiated quickly without delays for transport. The management of hyperkalemia requires a multifaceted approach to remove potassium from the body; to enhance the shift of potassium intracellularly; and, if arrhythmias are present, to reverse the cellular membrane effects of potassium. Calcium acts on the cell membrane and is used when arrhythmias or ECG changes are present. Calcium gluconate 10% (100 mg/kg) is given intravenously over 5 minutes. The effects are rapid, and if they are not present in 5 to 10 minutes, the dose can be repeated. The duration of action is brief, only 30 to 60 minutes, and it does not lower the potassium level, so additional treatment must be given along with calcium. Continuous ECG monitoring is important, and the infusion should be stopped if the patient's heart rate is less than 100 beats/min. Insulin works to transfer potassium intracellularly and is given with glucose. An insulin dose of 0.1 U/kg intravenously is accompanied by 0.5 to 1 g/kg of glucose and is given slowly over 30 minutes. An effect is produced in 30 minutes and lasts 4 to 6 hours. The dose may be repeated, and glucose levels should be followed carefully. Alkalinization also shifts potassium intracellularly, and sodium bicarbonate, 1 to 2 mEq/kg intravenously over 5 to 10 minutes, produces a rapid effect (5 to 10 minutes), which lasts 2 hours. It can be repeated if there is no effect in 15 minutes. Finally, sodium polystyrene sulfonate is a cation exchange resin that promotes gastrointestinal elimination of potassium. Potassium levels are reduced 1 mEq/L for each 1 g/kg of resin. The resin is given orally or as a retention enema at a dose of 0.5 to 1 g/kg. The enema must be retained 30 minutes, and for both routes the resin is mixed with sorbitol to enhance elimination. Doses can be repeated every 6 hours, and a decrease in potassium concentration is expected in 4 to 6 hours. Mild hyperkalemia that is asymptomatic may respond to use of the resin alone, without intravenous therapy. Because the resin is not totally specific, potassium, magnesium, and calcium levels must be followed frequently. If unsuccessful, the patient may need hemodialysis and referral for that procedure.

Hypokalemia is best treated slowly and orally, when the patient is known to be urinating. This approach avoids possible hyperkalemia resulting from potassium replacement. If the patient is alkalotic, the potassium value should be corrected upward 0.6 mEq/L for each 0.1 unit change in pH. Correction of the alkalosis may correct the potassium level without any additional potassium. If the patient is dehydrated, it is necessary to provide a volume bolus of normal saline to stop renal losses of potassium. When administering potassium replacement, potassium chloride should be used for patients who are alkalotic, potassium citrate or potassium gluconate should be given orally, and potassium acetate should be given intravenously for patients who are acidotic. Oral doses are 1 to 4 mEq/kg/day given two to four times daily; in periodic paralysis, the dose is 2 to 6 mEq/kg/day. Replacement occurs over 2 to 3 days. If the patient is symptomatic, or if the potassium level is less than 3 mEq/L, admission and intravenous potassium replacement may be necessary. A concentration of 40 mEq/L may be used peripherally and 80 mEq/L in central lines with replacement rates of 0.2 to 0.3 mEq/kg/hr for most cases, up to 1 mEq/kg/hr for life-threatening arrhythmias. Continuous ECG monitoring is necessary for higher infusion rates, and frequent monitoring of potassium concentration should be performed whenever intravenous potassium replacement is given.

OUTCOME

The outcome of glucose and electrolyte disorders depends on the severity of the disorder and the underlying cause of the derangement. Permanent neurologic injury can result from disorders of glucose and sodium and in some cases may be fatal. Seizures can be a manifestation of hypoglycemia, hyponatremia, and hypernatremia. Potassium disorders can cause life-threatening arrhythmias. The paralysis of hypokalemia can produce respiratory failure, but usually the muscles of respiration are spared.

FOLLOW-UP

Recommendations for long-term follow-up of children with glucose and electrolyte disorders depend on whether the child has a chronic illness that produced the metabolic derangement or whether the metabolic abnormality was due to a transient illness or event. All children with diabetes mellitus require ongoing care by the primary care provider and a specialist (see Chapter 155). Most children with transient illnesses or events producing a disorder of glucose, sodium, or potassium homeostasis can be followed by the primary care provider, perhaps with initial consultation with a specialist at the time of hospital admission or treatment. Children with chronic problems usually are comanaged with a specialist. Ongoing developmental assessments and early intervention are important, particularly for patients with serious derangements in infancy and patients with neurologic presentations of their illnesses.

Additional Resources, CD-ROM

Hypoglycemia Ketotic and nonketotic hypoglycemia Hyperinsulinism Special considerations in infancy Special considerations in childhood Uncommon causes of hypoglycemia Treatment of hypoglycemia Diagnostic workup	Text, tables, figure
Hyperglycemia Stress response Drugs Diagnostic evaluation Acute treatment	Text, tables
Hyponatremia SIADH Cerebral salt wasting syndrome	Text
Hypernatremia Diabetes Insipidus	Text
Bibliography	

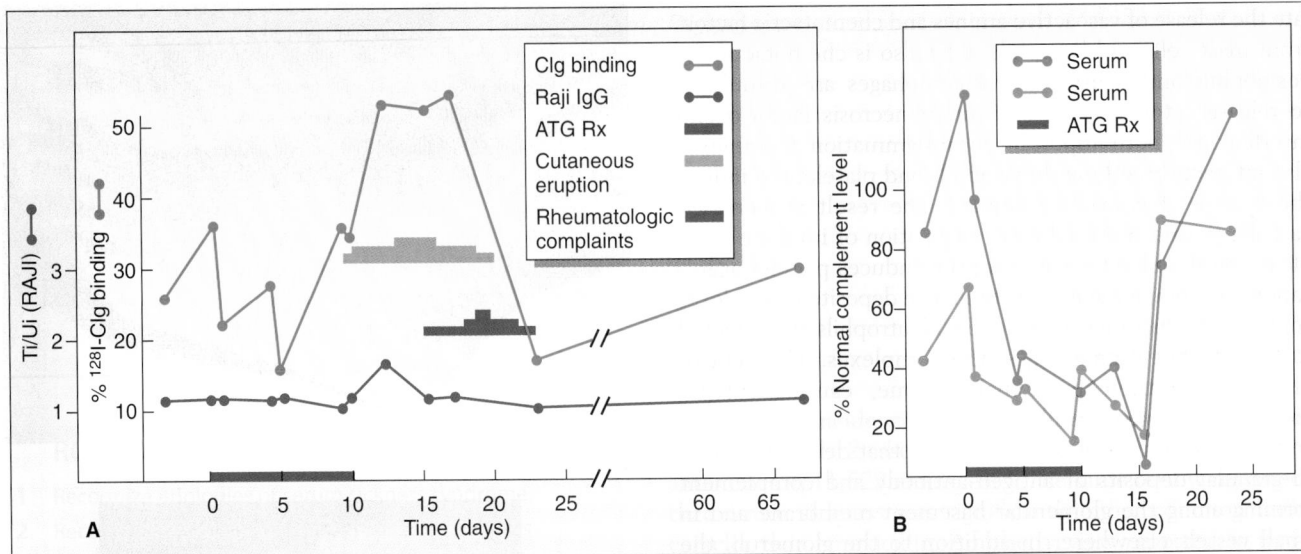

Figure 45-2. Circulating immune complex levels were maximally elevated at the time of cutaneous eruptions and arthralgias **(A)**, and serum complement C3 and C4 levels declined during serum sickness **(B)** in a representative patient with serum sickness after treatment with antithymocyte globulin (ATG). CIg, intracytoplasmic immunoglobulin. (From Lawley TJ, Bielory L, Gascon P, et al: A prospective clinical and immunologic analysis of patients with serum sickness. N Engl J Med 1984;311:1407–1413. Copyright 1984 Massachusetts Medical Society. All rights reserved. Used with permission.)

A febrile response after a skin eruption may make one suspect an infection or other conditions. Polyarthralgias and fever may be mistaken for rheumatic fever. Fever, joint pains, and adenopathy may suggest infectious mononucleosis. The history of antecedent foreign protein or nonprotein drug administration with accompanying immune complex elevation is an important clue suggesting a serum sickness syndrome. This condition is self-limited, and if symptoms persist for more than 1 month, the diagnosis must be reconsidered.

Laboratory Findings

Initial leukocytosis is followed by leukopenia, neutropenia, and thrombocytopenia. Peripheral eosinophilia may be present. There is a marked decrease in serum C3 and C4 that generally parallels the increase noted in immune complex levels (Fig. 45-2). Immune deposits on skin lesion biopsy specimens may show IgM, IgE, IgA, and C3. A polyclonal gammopathy with free light chains in the serum or transient monoclonal IgG proteins has been reported. Circulating immune complexes may be positive.

TREATMENT

When the diagnosis has been established, the offending agent should be discontinued, and symptomatic management should be initiated. Intense itching associated with urticaria can be treated as urticaria from any other cause with the use of oral antihistamines. In severe cases, glucocorticoids may be helpful in controlling symptoms. Corticosteroids may need to be administered and tapered over 10 to 14 days. Aspirin may be useful for fever, arthralgia, and myalgia.

OUTCOME

The prognosis for serum sickness syndrome is excellent. Complete recovery, even from the severe form, occurs. The syndrome may recur, however, with re-exposure to the same antigens with worse reactions than during the original episode. In most cases, the offending antigen can be identified and avoided.

Mini-index of Related Topics   CH.

SUGGESTED READINGS

Erffmeyer JE: Serum sickness. Ann Allergy 1986;56:105–110.
Heckbert SR, Stryker WS, Coltin KL, et al: Serum sickness in children after antibiotic exposure: Estimates of occurrence and morbidity in a health maintenance organization population. Am J Epidemiol 1990;132:336–342.
Lawley TJ, Bielory L, Gascon P, et al: A prospective clinical and immunologic analysis of patients with serum sickness. N Engl J Med 1984;311:1407–1413.
Naguwa SM, Nelson BL: Human serum sickness. Clin Rev Allergy 1985;3:117–126.
Platt R, Dreis MW, Kennedy DL, et al: Serum sickness like reactions to amoxicillin, cefaclor, cephalexin and trimethoprim-sulfamethoxazole. J Infect Dis 1988;158:474–476.

46 Urticaria and Angioedema

Charles H. Song

ROLE OF THE GENERALIST

1 Distinguish isolated urticaria from manifestations of a systemic illness.
2 Formulate a systemic diagnostic approach to identify etiology.
3 Formulate treatment plan.
4 Follow the progression of symptoms and adjust the treatment.
5 Refer refractory and difficult cases to a specialist for assistance with diagnosis and management.

DEFINITION

Urticaria is characterized by the appearance of circumscribed areas of skin elevation accompanied by erythema and pruritus. Microscopic examination of biopsy specimens shows dilation of small venules and capillaries in the superficial dermis. *Angioedema* is manifested by diffuse swelling of the skin areas and is associated with a burning sensation rather than pruritus. Microscopic findings, although similar to urticaria, are distinguished by involvement of the deeper dermal layer and subcutaneous tissue. Urticaria may occur on any part of the body, whereas angioedema more commonly involves the vascular areas, such as tongue, lips, genitalia, and extremities.

Although urticaria is a common condition with a cumulative prevalence rate of 15% to 25% of the general population, the precise incidence in children is unknown. Urticaria usually resolves spontaneously after a few days or in response to elimination of the causative agents. The symptoms may last for months or years, however. The condition is defined as chronic when symptoms persist longer than 6 weeks.

FUNDAMENTALS

Skin tissue is a target for immunologic and nonimmunologic reactions. Immunologically, these tissues are home to circulating leukocytes and to residential cells, including mast cells. Mast cells play a central role in the development of urticaria. In chronic urticaria, inflammatory leukocytes assume a more significant role.

In allergic type I hypersensitivity urticaria (as in reactions to drugs or foods), mast cells are activated by IgE. Activated mast cells produce histamine and other mediators, such as prostaglandins and leukotrienes, causing the skin reaction of urticaria: vasodilation (erythema), increased vascular permeability (edema), and axon reflex (flare and erythema). Inflammatory cells that accumulate in the skin during the late phase of allergic reactions produce their own mediators, which may be responsible for the protracted release of histamine in an IgE-independent manner.

The second pathway leading to urticaria formation involves complement products. In immune complex diseases (type II) such as systemic lupus erythematosus, activated complement products (C3a, C5a) are responsible for the mast cell activation.

The third pathway involves kinin-generating systems. In either type I or type III hypersensitivity diseases, increased vascular permeability induces activation of the plasma kinin-forming pathways. Increased kinin production causes further vascular permeability, resulting in tissue edema. Angioedema also may occur in a mast cell–independent manner by means of other kinin-releasing mechanisms, as seen in hereditary angioedema.

Urticaria can be produced by nonimmunologic activation of mast cells. Many drugs, including opioids and antibiotics, are direct stimulants of mast cells. Neuropeptides from autonomic nerve endings also can activate cells directly.

DIAGNOSIS

Acute urticaria occurs more commonly in atopic children and may be associated with infection and ingestion of drugs or foods. In chronic urticaria, the process of identifying an etiology is more difficult and frustrating. Data in adults indicate identification of an etiology in less than 10% to 15% of cases, although the rate may be higher in children. In the absence of clinical clues, screening laboratory tests (Table 46-1) are in order, although the yield generally is low. A systematic approach to evaluation is described in Figure 46-1 and Tables 46-2 and 46-3.

Some forms of urticaria are associated with unique physical appearances. Papular or pustular urticaria in exposed skin areas suggests insect bites or scabies. Pinpoint wheals suggest cholinergic urticaria or rarely aquagenic (induced by exposure to water) urticaria. *Cholinergic urticaria* (5% of all urticaria) occurs most commonly in individuals 10 to 30 years old and is induced by conditions that increase the core body temperature (e.g., exercise, hot shower, and anxiety). Lesions tend to appear first in the neck and upper chest and later spread to the rest of the body. These characteristic

Table 46-1. Screening Laboratory Tests

Laboratory Tests	Associated Diseases
CBC with ESR	Eosinophilia: allergy and parasites ↑ESR > infections, immune complex diseases
UA	Urobilinogen in hepatitis, blood, or protein in some vasculitis
LFT	↑ in viral hepatitis
TFT, thyroid antibodies	TFT ↑ or ↓ in autoimmune thyroid diseases, antithyroglobulin, or antimicrosomal antibodies in thyroiditis and some euthyroid patients

CBC, complete blood count; ESR, erythrocyte sedimentation rate; LFT, liver function test; TFT, thyroid function test; UA, urinalysis.

Table 46-2. Diagnostic Evaluation

History	Associated Diseases
Temporal relationship to drugs, foods, and contactants	Adverse reactions to penicillin, fish, latex
Travel history	Hepatitis, parasites
History of physical exposure	Physical urticaria (cold, heat, pressure, vibratory, aquagenic, solar)
Induced by exercise	Cholinergic, exercise-induced urticaria and anaphylaxis
History of trauma	Hereditary angioedema
Systemic illness	Viral/bacterial/mycoplasmal infections, vasculitis including systemic lupus erythematosus and serum sickness, Henoch-Schönlein purpura
Family history	Hereditary angioedema, amyloidosis with deafness and urticaria, C3b inactivator deficiency
Physical Examination	
Size of urticaria	Cholinergic, cold-cholinergic, aquagenic, insect bites, scabies
Exposed areas	Physical urticaria (cold, dermatographism, solar, pressure, vibratory, aquagenic)
Angioedema	Hereditary angioedema, acquired angioedema associated with malignancy, drug, or contactant
Dependent area	Vasculitis
Involves palms and soles	Vasculitis
Thyroid enlargement	Thyroiditis

wheals can be reproduced by methacholine challenge test (intradermal injection of 0.01 mg of methacholine in 0.1 mL of saline) in one third of affected patients.

Location of lesions can be a helpful clue. Lesions appear at the sites where contactants or physical stimuli (physical urticaria) are applied. *Dermatographism*, the most common form of physical urticaria, affects 2% to 5% of the population and may appear in association with other forms of urticaria. The diagnosis can be confirmed by stroking the skin with a narrow object. In a small fraction of these patients, the condition is severe enough to warrant treatment.

Cold urticaria accounts for approximately 3% of cases of chronic urticaria. Its presentation varies depending on whether it is the acquired or familial form. *Acquired cold urticaria* is the more common of the two forms. The cause of primary acquired cold urticaria is unknown, although studies implicate an autoimmune process. In the rare instance of secondary acquired cold urticaria, urticaria is induced by the presence of cryoglobulins or cold agglutinins associated with malignancies and autoimmune disorders. Cold drinks may cause lesions on the lips, tongue, and throat. Swimming in cold water can induce anaphylactic shock. The diagnosis is confirmed by placing an ice cube on the forearm for 4 minutes and watching for the appearance of lesions over the next 10 minutes. *Familial cold urticaria* is differentiated from the acquired variety by the presence of a positive family history (autosomal dominant inheritance), lesions characterized by burning erythematous papules rather than large wheals or edema, and a negative ice cube test. Two forms of familial cold urticaria have been identified: an immediate form with symptoms developing 30 minutes to 3 hours after cold exposure and a rare delayed form with onset after 9 to 18 hours.

Pressure urticaria commonly is associated with chronic idiopathic urticaria presenting as deep, localized, and painful swelling 3 to 6 hours after sustained pressure to the skin for at least 2 minutes. Typically the soles, palms, buttocks, and skin beneath the belt are affected.

In addition to size and location, other physical attributes of lesions, such as duration and color, are helpful diagnostic clues. In contrast to the waxing and waning nature of urticarial lesions in general, lesions associated with vasculitis, such as erythema multiforme and systemic lupus erythematosus, tend to persist for longer than 24 hours and may not blanch with pressure. Although the lesions of urticaria and vasculitis can appear annular with central clearing, the

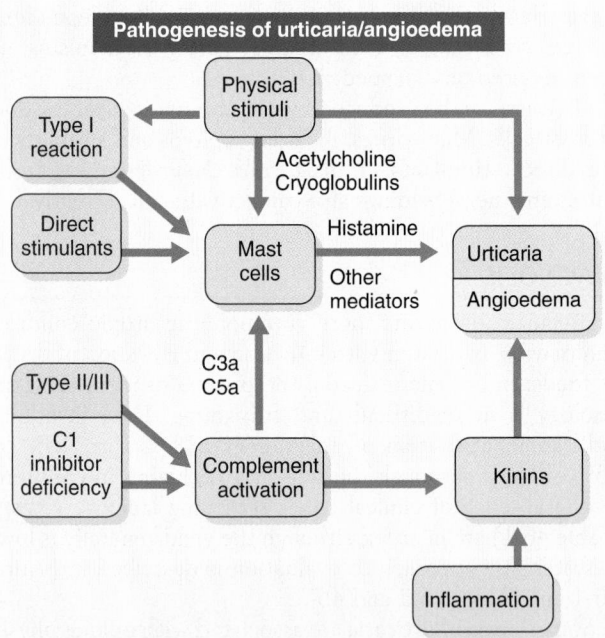

Figure 46-1. Mast cells are activated by various mechanisms: type I hypersensitivity (IgE mediated), type III hypersensitivity (immune complex mediated via C3a, C5a), or direct stimulation (e.g., by opioids, radiocontrast media, chemokines). Mediators from activated mast cells produce urticaria and angioedema. Some physical stimuli (e.g., dermatographism, sunlight) may operate through type I hypersensitivity. In cholinergic urticaria, acetylcholine from the nerve endings may activate mast cells. Deficiency in C1 inhibitor results in increased vasoactive kinin levels leading to angioedema, bypassing mast cell activation pathways.

Table 46-3. Diagnostic Tests for Specific Urticaria and Angioendema

Suspected Etiology	Mechanism	Tests
Food/drug/contactant reaction	Type I (II, III)	Elimination and challenge of offending agents, skin tests, RAST (e.g., fish, latex)
Infection	? (II, III)	HSV, EBV titers, mycoplasma titers, LFT, stool for ova and parasites
Physical urticarias	Type 1 in some, but unknown most cases	
Dermatographism		Stroking the skin with a blunt narrow object
Cholinergic		Methacholine test, exercise test
Heat		Positive local heat test with negative exercise test
Cold		Ice cube test
Aquagenic		Apply water at body temperature
Pressure		Apply sustained pressure (wheals last >24 hr)
Solar		Apply light at certain wavelengths
Vibratory		Apply vibration
Vasculitis	Type III	CBC, ESR, CH_{50}, C4, TFT, skin biopsy
Hereditary angioedema	Complement activation	CH_{50}, C3, C4, Cl inhibitor level and functional assay
Acquired angioedema	Complement activation	CH_{50}, C1q
Urticaria pigmentosa	Mast cell tumor	Skin biopsy, bone marrow biopsy, 24-hr urine collection for mediators

CBC, complete blood count; CH_{50}, 50% hemolyzing dose of complement; EBV, Epstein-Barr virus; ESR, erythrocyte sedimentation rate; HSV, herpes simplex virus; LFT, liver function test; RAST, radioallergosorbent test; TFT, thyroid function test.

latter have a dark cyanotic central area and tend to involve the palms and soles. Lesions in *urticaria pigmentosa* are associated with typical small yellow-tan to red-brown macules or papules. Urticaria pigmentosa is the most common manifestation of indolent systemic mastocytosis in children and adults.

Urticaria may be a manifestation of other systemic diseases, including malignancy, thyroiditis, and infections. In chronic urticaria, thyroid antibodies are detected in not only patients with autoimmune thyroiditis, but also patients without thyroid diseases. Their causal relationship to the pathogenesis of urticaria is unclear. Hepatitis viruses A, B, and C and hemolytic streptococci also are associated with acute urticaria.

Despite intensive searching, the etiology reportedly is elusive in more than 80% of chronic urticaria cases. Lately in a significant portion of these cases of so-called chronic idiopathic urticaria in adults, autoantibodies (IgG) directed to the α-chain of the high-affinity IgE receptor (Fc receptor I) or IgE have been found. These antibodies have been shown to induce urticarial lesions when injected into the human skin.

Angioedema coexists in half of urticaria cases. Isolated angioedema indicates other diagnoses, however, such as hereditary angioedema or acquired angioedema. *Hereditary*

angioedma, the best-known entity, is rare, representing only 1% of all cases of angioedema. It is inherited as an autosomal dominant trait and results from C1 inhibitor deficiency. C1 inhibitor inactivates various components of the immune/hematologic system, including coagulation, kinin, and complement systems. Uncontrolled activation of these pathways leads to the formation of bradykinin and C2 kinin, which induce edema formation. Angioedema frequently involves the face, lips, scrotum, and extremities; usually is secondary to minor trauma or stress; and generally subsides within a few days. Involvement of the larynx, if left untreated, may lead to asphyxiation in half of patients. Bowel wall edema may cause acute abdominal pain indistinguishable from surgical emergencies. Family history is an important clue. Other genetic causes of angioedema are listed in Table 46-3.

MANAGEMENT

Figure 46-2 outlines management of urticaria. If a specific diagnosis is made, appropriate treatment should be instituted, such as avoidance of the offending drug in drug-induced urticaria or cold objects or environments in cold urticaria. When a thorough search does not yield a cause,

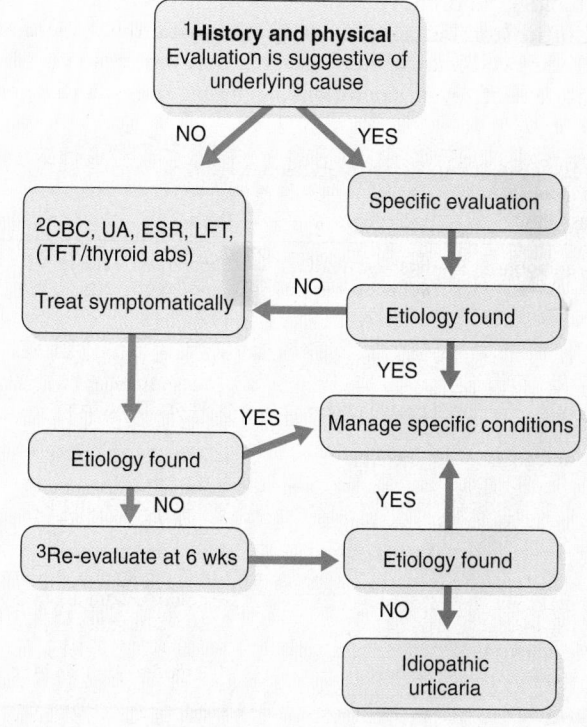

Figure 46-2. When the initial history and physical examination *(1)* yield a specific diagnosis, such as cholinergic urticaria or food allergy, the condition should be managed accordingly. When the history and physical examination yield no result, screening laboratory tests *(2)* should be done, and symptomatic treatment should be started. If the screening laboratory tests indicate a specific diagnosis, such as thyroiditis or hepatitis, the condition should be managed accordingly. If no cause is found, the evaluation is repeated in 6 weeks *(3)*. If still no diagnosis is obtained, management should be as for idiopathic urticaria. abs, antithyroid antibodies; CBC, complete blood count; ESR, erythrocyte sedimentation rate; LFT, liver function test; TFT, thyroid function test; UA, urinalysis.

symptomatic treatment needs to be initiated. Patients should be informed of the results of diagnostic evaluation and reassured about the prognosis, which is good in most instances. Reassurance is especially important in managing chronic urticaria, because anxiety and frustration contribute to the disease process. If the symptoms worsen or do not improve despite standard therapy, the patient should be referred to an allergist/immunologist or a dermatologist.

Table 46-4 lists pharmacologic agents used in the treatment of urticaria. Antihistamines remain the drugs of choice for control of urticaria. First-generation and second-generation antihistamines are equally effective in controlling the symptoms and signs of the disease. Although first-generation antihistamines, especially hydroxyzine, are effective, their use sometimes is limited by undesirable side effects, including somnolence, sedation, and paradoxical hyperactivity, particularly in young children. Although the sedative effect tends to lessen with time, a practical approach is to use these drugs at bedtime in combination with daytime use of second-generation antihistamines. If one antihistamine is not effective, it is advisable to try another, because individuals' response to individual agents may vary. Addition of H_2 antagonists is controversial but may be tried in recalcitrant cases. Doxepin, a tricyclic agent with H_1 and H_2 antagonist properties, is effective in adults, especially adults with increased anxiety, and may be tried with older children.

Corticosteroids can provide symptomatic relief. Because of their well-known side effects, they are reserved for treatment of severe conditions, including unresponsiveness to antihistamines, acute exacerbations, serum sickness, vasculitis, and delayed pressure urticaria. If used, corticosteroids should be tapered to low-dose, alternate-day therapy as soon as possible.

OUTCOME AND FOLLOW-UP

Most cases of urticaria are caused by benign conditions and resolve spontaneously or with avoidance of causative agents or events. Urticaria may be associated, however, with potentially life-threatening systemic illnesses, such as anaphylaxis and serum sickness. With these two disorders, the outcome depends on the nature of the systemic illness.

Physical urticarias, including acquired cold urticaria, solar urticaria, and cholinergic urticaria, tend to resolve after a few to several years. Even in idiopathic urticaria, the prognosis is good. In a review of chronic urticaria in 94 children, the median age of onset was 6 years, and the median duration of urticaria was 16 months.

Although prognosis is good in general, it is important to follow the patient closely. In rare instances, urticaria may be the earliest manifestation of certain systemic illnesses, such as hepatitis or malignancy. Inadequate control of symptoms and exacerbations requires adjustment of the dosage, schedule, or type of drugs. Optimal management of the disease requires more than controlling symptoms; it requires improving the quality of life. To achieve this outcome, the clinician has to pay close attention to subjective and objective details of the disease process.

Table 46-4. Drug Therapy Guidelines

Category	Medication	Dose
H_1 antagonist	Hydroxyzine HCl	2 mg/kg qd ÷ 6–8 hr
	Diphenhydramine	5 mg/kg qd ÷ 6 hr
H_1 antagonist, nonsedating	Cetirizine	½–5 yr: 2.5 mg qd; >5 yr: 5–10 mg qd
	Loratodine	3–5 yr: 5–10 mg qd; >5 yr: 10 mg qd
	Fexofenadine	6–11 yr: 30 mg bid; >11 yr: 60 mg bid
H_2 antagonist	Cimetidine	Infants: 10–20 mg/kg qd ÷ 6–12 hr; Children: 20–40 mg/kg qd ÷ 6 hr
	Ranitidine	Infants and children: 4–5 mg/kg qd ÷ 8–12 hr
Tricyclic ($H_1 + H_2$ antagonist)	Doxepin	For older children: 10–25 mg qhs
Steroids	Prednisone	1–2 mg/kg qd ÷ 12–24 hr
	Methylprednisolone	0.5–1.7 mg/kg qd ÷ 6–12 hr

Bid, two times a day; qd, every day; qhs, at hour of sleep; ÷, divided by.

Mini-index of Related Topics

SUGGESTED READINGS

Greaves M: Chronic urticaria. J Allergy Clin Immunol 2000; 105:664–672.
Kaplan AP: Urticaria and angioedema. In Middleton E, Reed CE, Ellis EF, et al (eds): Allergy, Principles and Practice, 5th ed. St. Louis, Mosby, 1998, pp 1104–1122.
Wander AA, Bernstein IL, Goodman DL, et al: The diagnosis and management of urticaria: A practice parameter. Ann Allergy Immunol 2000;85:525–544.
Zacharisen MC: Pediatric urticaria and angioedema. Immunol Allergy Clin North Am 1999;19:363–382.

47 Seasonal Allergies

Nasser Redjal

DEFINITION

Most allergic diseases, such as asthma, allergic rhinitis, allergic conjunctivitis, and atopic dermatitis, are multifactorial. They result from a combination of hereditary and environmental factors. Some are perennial, some are seasonal, and others are perennial with seasonal exacerbation. Multiple factors have been identified that predispose patients to develop allergic diseases. Abnormal sensitivity (atopy) is mediated by IgE. Atopy tends to occur in families with a history of asthma, allergic rhinitis, and atopic dermatitis. Atopy occurs in about 20% to 30% of the general population; 10% to 15% of all children are atopic. Allergic rhinitis is one of the most common types of allergy.

Rhinitis is diagnosed based on symptoms that last for at least 1 hour per day on most days. Clinical features of rhinitis include sneezing, nasal blockage, nasal irritation, and itchiness. Etiologic factors, such as exposure to cigarette smoke and allergens (most commonly pollens, house dust mites, and pets), contribute to these symptoms. In some cases of rhinitis, an etiologic factor cannot be identified.

FUNDAMENTALS

Functions of the Nose

The nose is a conduit for airflow. Anatomically the nasal cavity has a narrow, irregular shape, promoting turbulent airflow that serves a protective function. Harmful inhaled particles are impacted in the nasal cavity and do not enter the bronchial tree. The impacted foreign particles become trapped in the nose, moved into the pharynx by means of ciliary transport, and swallowed.

The "nasal cycle" leads to alternating congestion and decongestion of the right and left nasal cavities. The duration of one cycle may vary from 50 minutes to 4 hours. Filtration conditioning and humidification of inspired air begins in the vibrissae, which are the hairs that grow in the nasal vestibule and are able to filter airborne particles larger than 15 μm in diameter. The mucus effectively filters and removes almost all particles greater than 5 μm in diameter. The nose partially filters some gases, such as ozone and sulfur dioxide. Inspired air is warmed and humidified from an ambient air temperature of 20°C to 31°C in the pharynx and 35°C in the trachea. As the air is warmed, it also is fully humidified.

Nasal protective reflexes are sneezing, diving reflex, reflex stimulation, and nasonasal secretory reflex. Cholinergic reflex stimulation is involved in most of these reflexes because they are inhibitable by parasympathetic blockade.

The sense of smell may be affected if there is an obstruction impeding airflow into the olfactory area causing hyposmia or anosmia. An obstruction may be nasal congestion, nasal polyp, mucosal inflammation, or other structural abnormalities.

Allergic Rhinitis

Allergic rhinitis is a constellation of symptoms that occur on exposure to specific antigens. Symptoms result from immunologic responses that may cause specific nasal conditions and may lead to complications such as sinusitis, recurrent otitis, and nasal polyps. Allergic rhinitis may be seasonal or perennial depending on when the allergen is present in the environment. Offending allergens in seasonal allergic rhinitis are most likely aeroallergens, such as pollens, fungal spores, and outdoor insect particles. Patients with perennial allergic rhinitis are sensitive to indoor allergens, such as dust mites, animal dander, cockroaches, and indoor fungi.

Allergic rhinitis has a large genetic component. When both parents have a family history of allergic rhinitis or asthma, a child has a 70% chance of developing either of the conditions; the chance is only 50% if only one parent is affected. The response to an antigen is under the control of autosomal dominant immune response genes that appear to be linked to major histocompatibility loci. The mode of inheritance has yet to be established.

Approximately 10% of the general population has allergic rhinitis. Allergic rhinitis gradually increases in prevalence from less than 1% in infancy, to 5% in childhood (ages 5 to 9 years old), 10% in adolescence, and 15% in late adolescence. Allergic rhinitis decreases in adulthood. A strong inverse relationship of allergic rhinitis with family size has been noted, with first-born children being at greatest risk. The relative risk for developing rhinitis doubles for children living in damp houses and having parents who smoke. Modern energy-efficient "tight" buildings encourage the growth of house dust mites and molds from the higher humidity and warmth and increase the exposure to potential allergens. Environmental pollution and occupational agents contribute to allergic sensitization, perhaps accounting for the increase in the occurrence of allergic rhinitis in many industrialized countries since the 1980s.

PATHOPHYSIOLOGY

In an atopic individual, sensitivity is observed after inhalation of a specific antigen. The mechanism of allergy requires the soluble antigen to pass through the nasal mucosa and react with IgE fixed onto mast cells. The specificity of this response presumably is provided by $CD_4^+Th_2$ phenotype T cells, which possess the correct antigen specificity and the ability to produce appropriate cytokines. The cytokines, such as interleukin-4, produced on activation of mast cells stimulate B-cell differentiation into IgE-producing plasma cells. Allergen-specific IgE antibodies bind to receptors on mast cells, basophils, monocytes, eosinophils, lymphocytes, and platelets.

Mast cells degranulate, releasing multiple inflammatory mediators (histamine, N-α-tosyl-l-arginine methyl ester, leukotrienes, prostaglandins, and kinins) that stimulate the nasal end organs, producing itching, sneezing, rhinorrhea, and congestion. After the early reaction in some individuals, symptoms spontaneously recur 3 to 11 hours after the initial challenge. The cellular influx in the late phase includes eosinophils, neutrophils, basophils, mononuclear cells, and the recruitment of the Th_2 phenotype T cell–producing cytokines that induce IgE production and recruitment of basophils and eosinophils. Mast cell degranulation underlies the release of histamine in the early response, and basophil influx seems to explain histamine release in the late response. The priming response induces greater symptoms and response to an equivalent mediator release. The dose of allergen required to elicit a response may be reduced by 100 times when challenges are repeated within 24 hours.

SYMPTOM PRESENTATION

Clinical aspects of allergic rhinitis may be divided into three forms. Seasonal allergic rhinitis occurs in temperate climates where allergenic pollens and fungal spores are airborne during circumscribed times of the year. In many areas of the United States, pollen is released from trees in early spring, grasses in later spring, and ragweed in early fall. Perennial allergic rhinitis is classically associated with exposure to indoor allergens, such as dust mites. Patients who have allergies to indoor and outdoor allergens have perennial rhinitis with seasonal exacerbation. Episodic allergic rhinitis is an almost immediate onset of acute allergic rhinitis on exposure to allergens. An example is a cat-sensitive person visiting a home with a cat.

Typical symptoms of seasonal allergic rhinitis, often following allergen exposure, include itchiness, clear watery discharge, congestion, paroxysmal sneezing, and nasal blockage. Some patients complain of conjunctival symptoms of itching and an increase in tearing or an itchy throat

and soft palate. Recurrent epistaxis, pain over the sinuses, headache, postnasal discharge, hoarseness, and dry cough may accompany allergic rhinitis. The dominant symptoms may differ, however, from one patient to another.

PHYSICAL EXAMINATION

Several facial features are associated with allergic rhinitis. Allergic shiners are infraorbital dark circles related to venous plexus engorgement probably secondary to mucosal edema of the nose and sinuses. Dennie's sign (also called *Morgan's line*), a wrinkle just beneath the lower eyelids, is present from early infancy and is associated with atopic dermatitis and allergic rhinitis. Allergic gape or adenoid facies is secondary to chronic mouth breathing during the first several years of life that results in a characteristic pattern of maldevelopment of facial bones causing a high arched palate, flat maxilla, and angulated mandible yielding a recessed chin and dental malocclusion. The "allergic salute" involves using palms of the hand in an upward thrust of the nares to relieve itching and open the nasal airway. A transversal nasal crease is a hypopigmented or hyperpigmented groove at the junction of the tip of the nose and the more rigid nasal bridge that develops after 2 years of constant upward rubbing of the nose. This groove should be differentiated from a familial transverse nasal groove that is inherited as a dominant trait, a groove that is not obliterated by downward pressure on the tip of the nose. Geographic tongue is characterized by sharply outlined white patches on the tongue and is seen in some patients with allergic rhinitis.

Postnasal discharge and hypertrophic lymphoid follicles in oropharynx often can be seen in patients with allergic rhinitis. Associated disorders that can occur as complications of allergic rhinitis, such as serous otitis media and sinusitis, also should be noted as part of the routine examination.

DIAGNOSIS

Table 47-1 summarizes the differential diagnoses for allergic rhinitis. A careful history and physical examination are essential to diagnose allergic rhinitis. The history begins with determining the onset of disease, the duration of symptoms, a relationship with seasons, and the amount and characteristics of secretions (purulent versus clear). The clinician watches for clinical signs of other types of rhinitis or complications of rhinitis, such as sinusitis, postnasal drip, halitosis, snoring, coughing, and morning sore throat. A complete ear, nose, and throat examination with special attention for a sinus infection is essential. After examination of the external nares, a nasal speculum should be used to examine the anterior third of the nasal cavity. The size and color of the turbinates and mucous membrane and the color and amount of nasal secretion should be noted. Pooling of secretions under the inferior turbinate is seen with immotile cilia syndrome or with total nasal obstruction. Unilateral signs, particularly purulent drainage, should raise suspicion for foreign bodies. Diagnosis and differentiation of allergic rhinitis can be confirmed by laboratory tests and diagnostic studies.

Table 47-1. Differential Diagnosis of Allergic Rhinitis

	Allergic Rhinitis	Nonallergic Rhinitis with Eosinophilia Syndrome	Vasomotor Rhinitis
Occurrence	Seasonal Perennial Perennial with seasonal exacerbation	Perennial	Perennial
Age	Most <20	Mostly adult	Mostly adult
Family history of allergy	Positive	Mostly negative	Negative
Sex	Male, female	Male, female	Mostly female
Symptoms			
Itchy nose	Common	Rare	Rare
Sneezing	Common	Rare	Rare
Allergic salute	Positive	Negative	Mostly negative
Nasal discharge	Watery profuse	Mucoid profuse	Watery profuse
Allergic conjunctivitis	Often present	Absent	Absent
Nasal eosinophilia	Common	Very common	Negative
Allergic skin tests and in vitro tests	Always positive	Negative	Negative
Therapeutic effects			
Corticosteroids (topical and systemic)	Excellent	Excellent	Rarely helpful
Antihistamines	Beneficial	Helpful	Rarely helpful
Decongestants	Helpful	Some help	Some help
Cromolyn	Helpful	Limited help	Limited help
Ipratropium	Limited	Limited	Helpful
Immunotherapy	Good	None	None

Laboratory Tests

Nasal cytology samples of superficial nasal mucosal cells can be obtained by a small bulb syringe, by blowing the nose directly onto wax paper or cellophane, or by scraping the surface of the inferior turbinate with a plastic curette. The specimen is transferred to a glass slide and stained with Wright stain, and the types of cells are counted. Predominance of neutrophils suggests an infectious etiology. Presence of clumps of eosinophils or eosinophils that constitute more than 10% of the total white blood cells indicates a probable allergic cause. Seasonal exposure to an allergen and the total eosinophil density on nasal smear are strongly correlated. Total serum IgE, measured by enzyme-linked immunosorbent assay test, is elevated 2 standard deviations above healthy control values in 60% of patients with asthma or allergic rhinitis. Eosinophilia on a peripheral blood count suggests allergy. A moderate eosinophilia greater than 10% can be present, especially during the offending pollen season, but marked allergic symptoms can occur in its absence.

Offending allergens can be determined by in vitro methods of measuring specific IgE antibodies (e.g., radioallergosorbent, fluoroallergosorbent, or multiple allergosorbent test) against a large number of allergens. Disadvantages include reduced sensitivity compared with intradermal skin tests, lack of immediately available results, limited allergen selection, and increased expense. Advantages are no risk to the patient, lack of dependence on skin reactivity, and stability of the antigens in the solid phase state. These tests are indicated in patients who have histories of anaphylactic sensitivities, poor skin reactivity, and positive dermatographia and who are taking antihistamines.

Diagnostic Studies

Fiberoptic rhinoscopy is used to diagnose structural abnormalities that may present with rhinitis. In patients with allergic rhinitis, endoscopy reveals watery nasal secretions and swollen mucosa.

Allergy skin testing should be carried out when there are no other obvious reasons for the nasal symptom. Epicutaneous testing (puncture or prick) remains the most useful method of establishing specific causative allergens. Epicutaneous skin testing is less helpful before 3 years of age because skin reactivity is reduced in young children. In these young patients, intradermal test of household inhalant allergens can yield positive reactions. Intradermal tests can verify suspicious positive or negative epicutaneous tests.

Intradermal tests are not useful for diagnosing food allergies. They often give false-positive results and have been associated with fatalities resulting from systemic anaphylaxis. Food elimination and challenge can be helpful. If the patient's history suggests a food allergy, a skin-prick test or in vitro test may help prove the food allergy. Diagnoses of food allergy depend on the elimination of the suspected food, however, and the subsequent challenge that results in the production of clinical symptoms.

When skin testing is negative, nasal provocative tests may be helpful. Direct application of the specific allergen to the nasal mucosa provokes symptoms of rhinitis, such as nasal discharge, sneezing, and itchiness. Provocative testing is time-consuming, because only one antigen can be tested at a time and can provoke a systemic reaction.

COMPLICATIONS

Sinusitis is common in patients with rhinitis from obstruction of the sinus ostia. Nasal polyps may occur. They appear as shiny gray or white gelatinous masses originating from the ostia of the maxillary or ethmoid sinuses or from the surface of the middle turbinate. Nasal polyps are rare in children with allergic rhinitis and if present raise concern about cystic fibrosis. Severe generalized reactions to aspirin and nonsteroidal anti-inflammatory drugs can occur in patients with the classic triad of aspirin intolerance, asthma, and nasal polyp. Nasal obstructions cause disturbances in taste and olfaction. Chronic mouth breathing affects the growth of the mandible and maxilla, causing facial abnormalities such as retrognathic maxilla, crossbite, high arched palate, and adenoid facies. These cosmetic changes mandate aggressive interventions for children before they reach full growth. Nasal obstructions can cause snoring and sleep apnea. Obstruction of the eustachian tube predisposes to otitis media. Activation of nasal reflexes secondary to a nasal obstruction causes bronchospasms and increases asthma symptoms.

TREATMENT

The most important element in treatment is educating the patient and the parents regarding the disease. Successful therapy of allergic rhinitis involves three general considerations:

1. Identification and avoidance of specific allergens and contributing factors
2. Pharmacologic management to reduce and to prevent symptoms
3. Immunotherapy to alter the patient's response to the allergen

When feasible, avoidance of the allergen is the best therapy for allergic rhinitis. Elimination of animal dander by removing feather pillows or a pet from the house may provide significant relief. Avoidance of more ubiquitous allergens, such as dust, molds, and pollens, is much more difficult. Measures to control house dust mites should be concentrated within the patient's bedroom and should include the use of airtight mattress and box spring covers and the removal of dust collectors, such as stuffed toys, bookshelves, drapery, and carpet underpads wherever possible. Thorough weekly cleaning and vacuuming can reduce house dust. Air conditioning is especially helpful for a pollen-sensitive patient because the house can be isolated effectively during summer months.

Several pharmacologic agents are available for the treatment of rhinitis. A combination of drugs with different effects, such as antihistamines and decongestants, can be more beneficial than either drug used alone.

Antihistamines, the most used agents in the treatment of allergic rhinitis, show greatest efficacy in the relief of sneezing, itching, and rhinorrhea. Best results are shown when given before exposure to known allergens. During symptomatic periods, regular daily administration rather than intermittent use should be employed. H_1 antagonists are competitive inhibitors of histamine. They bind to the H_1 receptor and are classified as first-generation and second-generation antihistamines. First-generation drugs pass through the blood-brain barrier and can produce somnolence, impair psychomotor performance, interfere with learning, and decrease work productivity. Second-generation drugs penetrate poorly into the brain and are much less likely to have adverse effects on the central nervous system. Because antihistamines do not block the actions of other mediators, they cannot control symptoms of allergic rhinitis completely. First-generation antihistamines have pharmacologic anticholinergic activity that can control rhinorrhea and sneezing but also can produce side effects, such as blurred vision, difficulty urinating, and dry mouth. Other side effects

are nervousness, insomnia, excitation, somnolence, dizziness, lack of coordination, palpitations, headaches, anorexia, nausea, vomiting, constipation, and tinnitus. Most of these symptoms subside after a few days of therapy. Other side effects of antihistamines are delayed reaction time and inability to concentrate, without the patient being aware of any impairment. The patient may be at risk if driving or operating machinery. Second-generation nonsedating antihistamines, such as loratadine, desloratadine, fexofenadine, and astemizole, do not cause drowsiness and do not produce anticholinergic side effects.

Topical and systemic decongestants are α-adrenergic receptor stimulants controlling vasoconstriction of mucosal vessels. Topical application has fewer side effects compared with oral administration, although large doses administered intranasally may cause the same side effects seen with oral decongestants. Use of decongestants should be limited to a few days to avoid rebound congestion and rhinitis medicamentosa. Oral decongestants may be used alone or in combination with antihistamines. Some patients experience side effects such as tachycardia, insomnia, nervousness, irritability, headache, high blood pressure, and gastrointestinal symptoms.

Oral corticosteroids are more effective and rapid in controlling symptoms than topical corticosteroids. Oral corticosteroids should be considered only if other conventional treatments have failed. A short course of therapy of 7 to 10 days should be applied. Topical corticosteroids are indicated for seasonal allergic rhinitis and chronic rhinitis. Intranasal corticosteroids are safe and effective when used on a daily basis for periods of time during the allergy season. Topical corticosteroids, such as beclometasone, fluticasone, triamcinolone, flunisolide, budesonide, and mometasone, are highly potent and safe. Topical dexamethasone is absorbed in its active form and can cause systemic side effects. Its use should be limited to 6 weeks.

Cromolyn sodium inhibits mediator release by stabilizing mast cell membrane and decreasing the activation of eosinophils, neutrophils, and monocytes. It is effective in allergic rhinitis but not in nonallergic rhinitis.

Anticholinergics are effective in treating rhinorrhea associated with allergic and nonallergic rhinitis, "skier's" or "jogger's" nose, gustatory rhinitis, and upper respiratory infection. Ipratropium bromide does not pass through the blood-brain barrier, works topically without systemic side effects, and is available in two concentrations of 0.03% and 0.06% administered intranasally.

Immunotherapy should be considered when systematic drug therapy and avoidance techniques cannot control symptoms. Immunotherapy has been shown to be effective in treating allergic rhinitis related to allergens such as pollens, house dust mites, and animal dander, providing clinical improvement in more than 80% of patients with pollen-induced allergic rhinitis. Immunologic responses are due to allergen-specific blocking antibody (IgG), increased allergen-specific suppressor T cells, decreased lymphocyte-cytokine response to allergen, and decreased basophil histamine release in response to an allergen. Treatment involves using increasing doses of allergic extracts in the buildup phase and then maintenance treatment of stable amounts of extract for 3 to 5 years.

OUTCOME

Seasonal allergies are chronic conditions. Early diagnosis and aggressive treatment minimize serious complications, such as sinusitis, otitis media, disturbance of taste and smell, nasal polyps, sleep apnea and sleep disturbance, activation of nasal-bronchial reflexes, and disturbances of facial growth and development (that is, increased length of face, high arched palate, and crossbite). Referral to an allergist or to an otolaryngologist is warranted if the patient does not respond to conventional treatment. Specific studies, such as allergy skin testing, or surgical procedures, such as adenoidectomy, tympanostomy tube placement, sinus surgery, or polypectomy, may be indicated in some cases.

Additional Resources, CD-ROM

Nasal anatomy and physiology	Text, figure

SUGGESTED READINGS

Howard MD: Allergic and non-allergic rhinitis. In Middleton E Jr, Reed CE, Ellis EF, et al (eds): Allergy Principles and Practice. St. Louis, Mosby, 1998, pp 1005–1016.

Lasley MV, Shapiro GG: Testing for allergy. Pediatr Rev 2000;21:30–43.

Lieberman P: Rhinitis. In Lieberman P, Anderson IA (eds): Allergic Diseases, Diagnosis, and Treatment. Totowa, NJ, Humana Press, 1997, pp 131–149.

Lierl MB: Allergy of the upper respiratory tract. In Lawlor GJ Jr, Fischer TJ, Adelman DC (eds): Manual of Allergy and Immunology. Boston, Little, Brown, 1995, pp 94–103.

Nimmagada SR, Evans III R: Allergy: Etiology and epidemiology. Pediatr Rev 1999;20:111–115.

SECTION 3   GENERAL MEDICAL CARE: *Allergic Disorders*

48 Insect Allergies

Barbara K. Ariue and Chad K. Oh

ROLE OF THE GENERALIST

1 Recognize the stinging insect.
2 Diagnose insect allergy.
3 Recognize the various classes of reactions.
4 Treat insect allergy.
5 Refer to an allergy specialist when appropriate.
6 Educate patients on avoiding insect stings and preventing life-threatening reactions.

DEFINITION

Insect allergy refers to a hypersensitivity reaction from a small group of stinging insects of the *Hymenoptera* order. The clinically important families of this order are the Apidae, Vespidae, and Formicidae. The relevant winged insects are members of two insect families: the *apid* family (consisting of honeybees, Africanized bees, and bumble-

bees) and the *vespid* family (consisting of yellow jackets, hornets, and wasps). Fire ants and harvester ants are part of the nonwinged *formicid* family.

Although most children experience only mild swelling and redness at the site of an insect sting, some have a more severe reaction. The exact incidence of insect allergy is not known, but it is estimated to be 0.3% to 3% of the general population. Children are more likely to come across stinging insects and to have allergic reactions than adults. An estimated 40 to 50 people die each year from insect sting allergy in the United States.

FUNDAMENTALS

The well-recognized American honeybee (Fig. 48-1) originated in Asia, evolved in Europe, and was imported to the United States for domestication. These temperate bees usually sting in defense of their disturbed colony. The honeybee stings with two barbed lancets thrust into the skin and then anchored by the barbs. The stinger with the connected venom sac remains in the skin as the bee flies

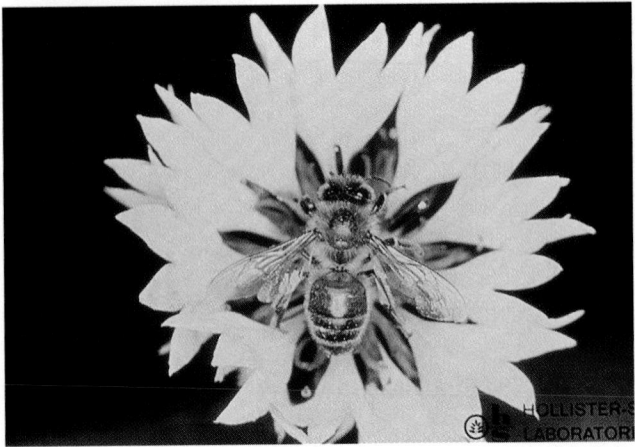

Figure 48-1. American honeybee. (Courtesy of Hollister Stier Laboratories.)

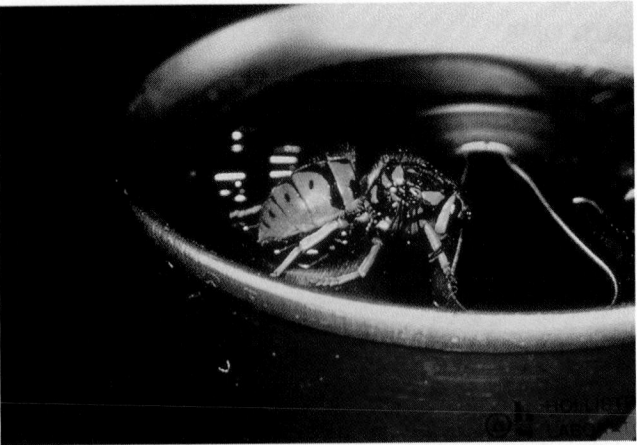

Figure 48-3. Yellow jacket. (Courtesy of Hollister Stier Laboratories.)

away to die. Although intimidating in appearance, the bumblebee (Fig. 48-2) is docile. Its stinger is not barbed, so it may sting more than once. Bumblebee stings usually are not associated with systemic allergic reactions.

African honeybees initially were brought to Brazil in 1956. The hybrid Africanized bee since has spread northward through South America, Central America, Mexico, and the United States. Africanized bees sting on the slightest disturbance of their nest, sending out thousands of bees, which can result in a massive attack of hundreds to thousands of stings.

The sting of the yellow jacket (in the vespid family) (Fig. 48-3) is a common cause of insect allergy. Yellow jackets build their nests on the ground and often are found scavenging for foods in trash, predominantly in the late summer and early fall. Hornets (Fig. 48-4) also are aggressive. They are similar in appearance to yellow jackets but have a larger black area between the eyes and mandible. Hornets build nests in trees and shrubs, so attacks usually occur as people garden. The paper wasp (Fig. 48-5) generally is not as aggressive as the other vespids. Its nests can be found in protected areas under the edges of buildings.

Imported fire ants from South American countries are found predominantly along the Gulf Coast states in the southeastern United States. When their nest mound is disturbed, fire ants may sting multiple times, producing sterile pustules at the sting sites. Harvester ants inhabit the

southern and western United States. Their stings rarely cause anaphylaxis.

Insect venom consists of mainly peptides and enzymes. Vasoactive amines, such as histamine, serotonin, dopamine, and norepinephrine, are nonallergenic components. The enzymes phospholipase A and hyaluronidase cause most of the allergic reactions. Phospholipase A cleaves membrane phospholipids with resultant smooth muscle contraction, mast cell degranulation, and increased capillary permeability. Hyaluronidase increases the action of other venom components. Another major allergen in the honeybee is mellitin, which can hemolyze erythrocytes and leukocytes.

The pharmacologic properties of the venom and the insect sting commonly result in a *local reaction* of redness, swelling, and pain at the sting site. This is a self-limited process, which lasts less than 24 hours. *Large local* reactions have more extensive areas of swelling and redness greater than 10 cm. This reaction is continuous with the sting site, peaks in 1 to 3 days, and may last 7 days. *Systemic reactions* are a generalized non–life-threatening event that usually is limited to the skin with urticaria and angioedema (Fig. 48-6). *Anaphylaxis* is the most severe, life-threatening, IgE-mediated reaction. In addition to cutaneous symptoms, there usually is respiratory compromise with laryngeal edema and wheezing and cardiovascular symptoms of hypotension and circulatory collapse.

Large local reactions are IgE mediated with 84% of children showing a positive skin test to venom. Large local,

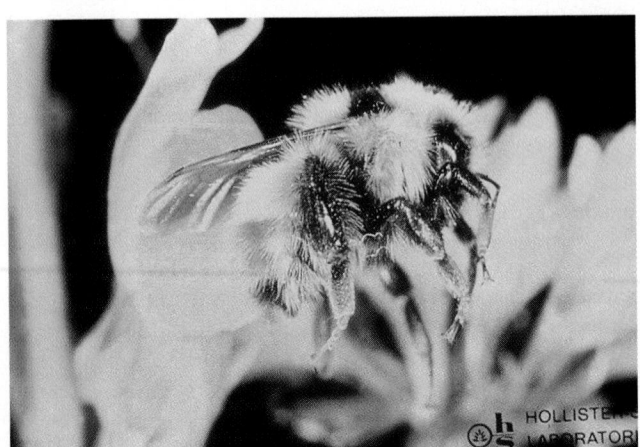

Figure 48-2. Bumblebee. (Courtesy of Hollister Stier Laboratories.)

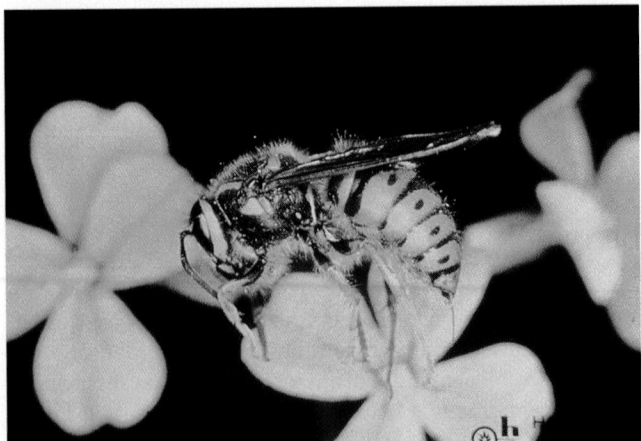

Figure 48-4. Hornet. (Courtesy of Hollister Stier Laboratories.)

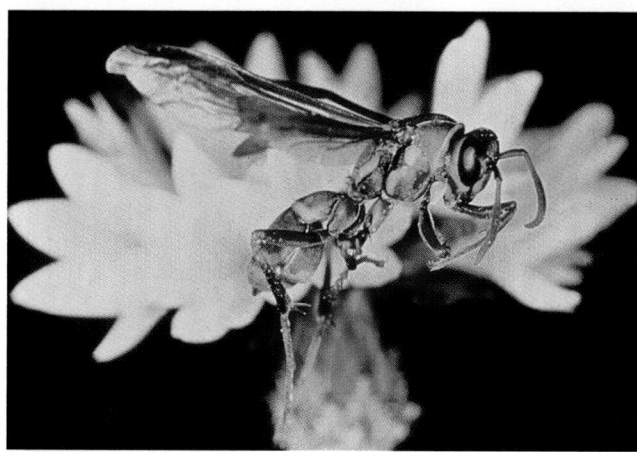

Figure 48-5. Yellow wasp. (Courtesy of Hollister Stier Laboratories.)

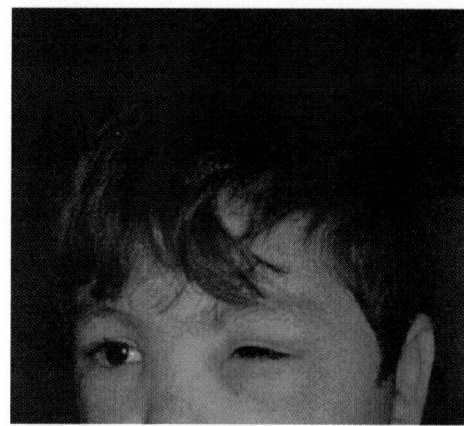

Figure 48-6. Child after insect attack. (From Franca FOS, Benvenuti LA, Fan HW, et al: Severe and fatal mass attacks by "killer" bees (Africanized honey bees—*Apis mellifera scutellata*) in Brazil: Clinicopathological studies with measurement of serum venom concentrations. Quart Journ Med 1994;87:269–282. Reproduced by permission of Oxford University Press.)

systemic, and anaphylactic reactions are IgE-mediated Gell and Coombs type I hypersensitivity to insect venom (Table 48-1). Venom components interact with IgE antibodies bound to mast cells with subsequent release of histamine and other pharmacologically active mediators. Anaphylactoid reactions are clinically similar to anaphylaxis but are non–IgE mediated and may be seen after a massive attack of Africanized bees. Hundreds to thousands of stings may result in a direct toxic effect of the vasoactive amines from the insect venom.

In addition to immediate reactions after insect stings, delayed reactions have been reported in children. Most delayed reactions that occur within 72 hours of an insect sting are primarily urticaria. Seven to 14 days after an insect sting, some patients develop a serum sickness–type reaction with joint swelling, urticaria, and arthralgia. All patients with a serum sickness–type reaction seem to have venom-specific IgE in the serum, whereas only 25% have venom-specific IgG. Serum sickness is a Gell and Coombs type III hypersensitivity reaction (see Table 48-1). This reaction develops when excess antigen combines with circulating IgG to form antigen-antibody immune complexes that cannot be cleared and are deposited into tissue. The complement system is activated with inflammation and tissue damage.

DIAGNOSIS

A well-taken clinical history helps in identification of the stinging insect. Important information to gather includes a physical description of the insect, location of the stinging event, nest location, evidence of aggressive behavior in the insect, and presence of embedded stinger in the patient. In addition, the time between the stinging event and patient's

symptoms and a description of the symptoms clarify the classification of the reaction.

In children with signs and symptoms remote from the sting site, skin testing with insect venom is indicated and is a sensitive method of detecting venom-specific IgE. Venom extracts are commercially available for honeybee, yellow jacket, wasp, yellow hornet, and white-faced hornet. Testing for imported fire ants is accomplished with whole-body extracts. Patients may be evaluated accurately for winged venom-specific IgE within 1 week of a systemic reaction. Prick tests at a concentration of 1 µg/mL are placed initially. If prick tests are negative, intradermal tests from 1 ng/mL to 1 µg/mL are performed. Venom concentrations at 1 µg/mL may produce a false-positive skin test as a result of an irritant effect.

Venom-specific IgE also may be detected with in vitro immunoassays, such as the radioallergosorbent test. Radioallergosorbent test is considered to be less sensitive with a 15% false-negative rate. However, one report drew attention to a subset of patients who are skin test negative but later experience a systemic reaction. These patients have a variable low sensitivity to skin tests, may be initially positive by radioallergosorbent test, and may have venom-specific IgE detected by either test in 3 to 6 months.

MANAGEMENT

Most reactions to insect stings are mild and require only analgesia and cold compresses to the sting site (Box 48-1). A stinger embedded in the skin may be removed carefully

Table 48-1. Hypersensitivity Type Reactions

Hypersensitivity Type	Immune Mediator	Mechanism	Examples
Type I	IgE	Mast cell mediator release	Anaphylaxis, allergic reactions
Type II	IgG/IgM	Complement-mediated lysis	Autoimmune hemolytic anemia
		Cytotoxic action against cell surface	Pemphigus, myasthenia gravis
Type III	IgG/IgM immune complexes	Complement activation	Serum sickness, arthus reaction
		Recruitment of neutrophils/macrophages	
Type IV	T cell	Macrophage-activated cytotoxicity	Contact dermatitis, tuberculin reaction
		Lymphokine activation of macrophage	Leprosy granuloma

| Box 48-1. | Immediate Therapy |

Local Treatment

1. Remove sting by scraping with sharp object, avoiding squeezing.
2. Apply cold compress.
3. Apply steroid cream.
4. Apply calamine lotion.

Systemic and Anaphylactic

1. Secure airway.
2. Administer 100% oxygen.
3. Place on cardiorespiratory monitoring devices.
4. Administer epinephrine (1:1000) 0.01 mL/kg subcutaneously.
5. Give antihistamine: Diphenhydramine, 1–2 mg/kg orally.
6. Give H_2 receptor blockade.
7. Consider corticosteroids.

| Box 48-2. | Indications for Referral to an Allergist |

1. Systemic reaction to insect sting
2. Anaphylactic reaction and insect is thought to be the cause
3. Toxic reaction to insect sting

0.01 to 0.1 μg and continues with a buildup phase of increasing incremental doses to a maintenance dose of 100 μg. This maintenance dose is given every 4 to 8 weeks for 3 to 5 years. Immunotherapy is a well-tolerated and effective treatment for children. In one study of children, immunotherapy was associated with a 5% risk of anaphylaxis, which is similar to other pollen immunotherapy regimens. Children subjected to in-hospital sting challenges after 15 weeks of immunotherapy showed a 97% protection rate.

OUTCOME

The outcome and follow-up of insect stings depend on the severity of the reaction. Most mild reactions are self-limited. Systemic reactions require intervention and referral. Children with large local reactions to insect stings initially show an elevated venom-specific IgE that declines over 3 to 5 years. Repeat stings result in a systemic reaction in 2% of children with large local reactions. The natural history of untreated insect sting anaphylaxis in children reveals a 30% risk of recurrence into adulthood. Children with systemic reactions and the presence of venom-specific IgE require venom immunotherapy and close follow-up. Children treated with venom-specific immunotherapy have a decrease in skin test sensitivity with less than 5% risk of future anaphylaxis after stopping treatment.

by scraping with a sharp object. It is important to avoid squeezing. Large local reactions are treated with the aforementioned measures plus oral antihistamines. Corticosteroids may be considered in severe cases.

Immediate therapy for systemic reactions to insect stings is similar to the general treatment of anaphylaxis. The medication of choice is epinephrine (1:1000), 0.01 mL/kg, given intramuscularly or subcutaneously. The dose may be repeated in 10 to 15 minutes and then given every 4 hours until the reaction is controlled. The pharmacologic properties of epinephrine include vasoconstriction, bronchodilation, positive inotropic and chronotropic effects on the myocardium, and inhibition of histamine release. H_1 receptor antagonists also help to block histamine, one of the major mediators of anaphylaxis. Corticosteroids may help alleviate late-phase reactions. Additional treatment may incorporate nebulized albuterol for bronchospasm and intravenous fluids and vasopressors for hypotension.

Preventive management begins with patient education regarding insect avoidance and prevention of anaphylaxis. Children should wear protective covering of shoes, hat, long pants, and long-sleeved shirts when playing outdoors and gloves when helping in the garden. Insect attractants, such as floral and pastel clothing, perfumes, and scented cosmetics, should be avoided. Caution should be taken in areas where children are likely to encounter stinging insects, such as flower fields, picnics, and trash sites. Children with insect allergy should wear an identification alert bracelet or necklace at all times. Physicians can prescribe emergency epinephrine kits and instruct patients and parents on the proper use and indications of self-administered epinephrine.

Referral to an allergy specialist is indicated for children with a systemic, anaphylactic, and serum sickness–type reaction to insect stings (Box 48-2). If venom-specific IgE can be shown, the child is a candidate for venom-specific immunotherapy. In children with exclusively dermal manifestations, immunotherapy is not indicated. The dosing schedule of immunotherapy begins with an initial dose of

Mini-index of Related Topics   CH.

SUGGESTED READINGS

Ariue B: Multiple bee stings in a child. Pediatrics 1994;94:111–115.

Kemp SF, deShazo RD, Moffitt JE, et al: Expanding habitat of the imported fire ant: A public health concern. J Allergy Clin Immunol 2000;105:683–691.

Resiman RE: Allergy to stinging insects. In Patterson R, Grammer LC, Greenberger PA (eds): Allergic Diseases: Diagnosis and Management, 5th ed. Philadelphia, Lippincott Williams & Wilkins, 1997, pp 253–264.

Schuberth KC, Lichtenstein LM, Kagey-Sobotka A, et al: Epidemiologic study of insect allergy in children: II. Effect of accidental stings in allergic children. J Pediatr 1983;102:361–365.

Yunginger JW: Insect allergy. In Middleton E, Reed CE, Ellis EF, et al (eds): Allergy, Principle and Practice, 4th ed. St. Louis, Mosby-Year Book, 1993, pp 1511–1520.

49 Sports Medicine

Paul Fu, Jr.

ROLE OF THE GENERALIST

1 Educate young athletes on safe sports participation and injury prevention before, during, and after sports activities.

2 Identify, manage, and treat basic sports injuries.

3 Diagnose and refer appropriately severe, complex, or chronic sports injuries to a specialist.

4 Assist with rehabilitation and return to participation for injured athletes.

An estimated 35 million children, adolescents, and young adults 6 to 21 years old participate in some form of sports activities through clubs, leagues, or schools. Participation can benefit children by influencing the development of self-image and independence, fostering confidence, promoting leadership skills, enhancing peer socialization, and developing physical and psychological strength. These benefits accrue from focusing on the positive experiences and attainable goals of sports activities.

Injuries related to sports participation can cause significant morbidity if not recognized and managed appropriately. Sports for children are relatively safe. Because of the greater forces involved, however, sports for adolescents—especially collision/contact sports, such as football and ice hockey—have significantly greater risk for participants.

DEFINITIONS

Most sports-related injuries are due to either acute soft tissue trauma or overuse. A *significant injury* is one that results in a decreased level of participation. *Acute soft tissue injuries* include concussions, contusions, sprains, strains, and ligament disruptions, all of which may result from forceful impacts or from sudden changes in directional motion. Table 49-1 defines and classifies acute soft tissue injuries.

Overuse injuries result from repetitive stresses that overload the muscle-tendon unit and lead to microtrauma, causing localized inflammation, edema, and pain with or without motion. Risk factors for overuse are listed in Box 49-1. Overuse injuries may be prevented by providing adequate flexibility and strength training; using gradual increases in training to reach a desired level or performance; and having sufficient warm-up, stretching, and cooldown periods. Pain in grade I overuse injuries occurs only during activity. With grade II overuse injuries, pain persists through

Table 49-1. Definition and Classification of Acute Soft Tissue Injuries

Sprain	Any injury to a ligament or joint capsule
Grade I	Mild sprain. Involves microcirculation or limited ligamentous disruption only. Minimal swelling, tenderness, no loss of joint stability, no loss of function
Grade II	Moderate sprain. Involves partial ligamentous disruption. Moderate swelling, tenderness, pain. Limitation in range of motion and slight loss of stability
Grade III	Severe sprain. Complete ligamentous disruption. Severe swelling, tenderness, pain. Total loss of range of motion and joint stability
Strain	Any injury to a tendon or muscle-tendon attachment
Grade I	Mild strain. Involves microcirculation or limited muscle or tendon fiber disruption only. Minimal swelling, tenderness, no significant weakness
Grade II	Moderate strain. Involves partial muscle or tendon disruption. Moderate swelling, tenderness, pain. Moderate weakness
Grade III	Severe strain. Complete rupture of muscle or tendon. Severe swelling, tenderness, pain. Severe weakness
Dislocation	Complete displacement of bony elements within joint
Subluxation	Partial displacement of joint surfaces

activity and the immediate postactivity period. Pain associated with grade III overuse injuries is continuous.

Treatment usually involves rest from activity. *Relative rest* is a decrease in intensity and duration of activities that exacerbate injury from previous levels. *Complete rest* involves a complete cessation of activity to facilitate the healing process.

Preparticipation Sports Physical Examination

A good preparticipation sports physical examination is a key component in the management of the health of a young athlete. The physician should reassure the participant that

Box 49-1. Risk Factors for Overuse Injuries

- Changes in exercise regimens (intensity, frequency, or duration)
- Level of activity
- Prior injury
- Level of conditioning
- Existing anatomic abnormalities
- Inadequate equipment (e.g., shoes or protective gear)
- Poor biomechanics

the goal is not to disqualify, but to modify, participation where appropriate. A thorough family history of sudden death and other familial risk factors, such as hypertrophic cardiomyopathy, prolonged Q-T syndrome, or aortic rupture associated with Marfan syndrome, is crucial. A review of the athlete's history should include any past injuries and syncopal episodes.

A sports physical examination can be performed rapidly during a routine office physical examination (Table 49-2). Abnormal findings should be assessed for relevance to the particular sport in which the athlete wishes to participate.

Injury Evaluation

A thorough history and physical examination guide the diagnosis of a sports injury. History should include the type of sport that was being played; the specific action in which the injury occurred (acute) or the type of activity that produces the complaint (overuse); actions that alleviate the complaint; actions that exacerbate the complaint; a general description of the complaint itself, such as pain intensity, quality, duration, radiation, weakness, and joint stability; and any treatment or medication that has been used.

On physical examination, the clinician should look specifically at limb symmetry, anatomic abnormalities or deformities, swelling or contusions, muscle wasting, and tenderness to palpation. Any detectable masses should be assessed for size and whether bony or soft tissue in nature. Pulses should be checked distally, and capillary refill time should be noted. Sensory impairment should be assessed. Joint range of motion testing should be performed last to avoid involuntary guarding or apprehension from causing pain. Voluntary (active) and involuntary (passive) range of motion should be performed and the joint assessed as too lax or too rigid. Strength also should be assessed, although testing should never exceed comfortable limits or elicit significant pain. Further testing may be indicated depending on the type and location of the injury.

Team Physician

Although an orthopedic specialist may serve as a team physician, true orthopedic emergencies are uncommon, and a general pediatrician with knowledge of sports injuries can fill the role and counsel patients about proper conditioning and training. Because involvement of a team physician can vary, the pediatrician should clarify his or her role when volunteering.

A team physician has two broad roles. The first is that of educator, working with the coaching and training staff and student athletes to develop exercise and competition regimens that are designed to prevent injury. These programs include progressive workout routines that increase in intensity, frequency, or duration no more than 10% per week and modified depending on the individual and the level of competition.

The second role is to assist with the management of acute and overuse injuries. Certified athletic trainers are valuable assistants. Attendance at sporting events, planning the response to injury, and initial treatment of acute on-field injuries are responsibilities of a team physician.

ACUTE MANAGEMENT OF SPORTS INJURIES

The team physician should use a playbook to help manage on-field injuries. Information about the appropriate responses to a catastrophic injury and assignment of roles to specific individuals should be included (e.g., who should respond on the field, what their roles are, who will activate the emergency medical services response, whether there is a standby ambulance, how the immobilized player will be removed from the field of play).

Most on-field injuries are not catastrophic. The first role of the team physician as responder is to maintain leadership and calm. The second role is to begin the injury evaluation. Evaluation should begin with the assessment of the ABCs (airway, breathing, circulation), consciousness, and any injury or anatomic deformity. The goal of on-field triage is to determine whether the injured player requires immediate transport to a receiving facility for further management and evaluation or merely assistance off the field of play for further evaluation. Players with critical injuries should be immobilized and transported directly to a waiting ambulance or emergency medical services response vehicle. Movement should be minimized. Players rendered unconscious and who are initially unresponsive in a contact sport should have the cervical spine immobilized and the body logrolled for evaluation of any spinal process or body fracture through palpation of the entire spine. After inspection, the athlete should be placed on a backboard for stabilization and transport to a receiving facility.

Table 49-2. 90-Second Sports Physical

Instruction to Patient	What is Screened
"Stand up straight and face me."	Acromioclavicular joints, symmetry of extremities
"Look up, down, left, right, and shrug your shoulders."	Cervical spine range of motion
"Shrug your shoulders again [against resistance]."	Trapezius strength
"Let your arms hang at your sides, then slowly bring them up fully outstretched to reach up above your head."	Shoulder range of motion
"Let your arms down again. Raise your elbows at your side like wings."	Deltoid strength
"Reach your arms straight out in front of you. Flex and extend your elbows."	Elbow range of motion
"Let your arms down again. Flex your elbows so that your hands reach straight out. Turn your wrists in and out."	Wrist range of motion (pronation/supination)
"Show me your hands. Spread your fingers out (resist spreading). Make a fist and squeeze."	Hand/finger range of motion and strength
"Lift your right leg up, bent at the knee. Now lift the other leg."	Leg symmetry, knee or ankle effusion
"Squat like a duck, and walk four steps away from me."	Hip, knee, and ankle range of motion
"Stand up again. Keep your knees as straight as you can, and try to touch your toes. Straighten slowly."	Shoulder symmetry, scoliosis, hip range of motion, hamstring tightness
"Stand up on your tiptoes."	Calf symmetry, leg strength

Adapted from Garrich JG: Sports medicine. Pediatr Clin North Am 1977;24:737–747.

If the athlete is conscious, he or she should be asked to identify the source of pain. If the player is conscious and able to ambulate, he or she should be assisted off the field. If he or she is unclear or unable to ambulate because of pain or medical contraindication, transport off the field should be arranged. Immediate swelling, body tenderness, any deformity, limitations in range of motion, or limb or joint instability indicates that assistance should be provided in moving the athlete off the field of play.

Off the field, the examination should be repeated with the player in the position most suited for a thorough examination of injury; this may require movement into the clubhouse or training room. Off-field evaluation of non-critical injuries should include visual inspection and palpation and assessment of range of motion and joint and limb stability. Stability of joints is best examined immediately, before the onset of edema, inflammation, hemorrhage, or guarding. Minor injuries in which function and strength are not impaired should not prevent a return to play and may be treated with protective taping or bracing. Protective taping or bracing is inadequate treatment for significant injuries.

Heat injuries are relevant in hot and cold climates but are more prominent when the heat index is higher than the ambient temperature. Temperatures at the playing field may be higher than ambient air temperature, especially with artificial surfaces. Players who are obese, who are in poor physical condition, who have preexisting dehydration, who have a poor tolerability to heat, or who participate with full-body uniforms or layers of protective gear are at higher risk.

Heat cramps are painful contractions of muscles that tend to be due to dehydration and overexertion (not electrolyte imbalances). Treatment is rest, massage and stretching, and lots of fluid (sports rehydration drinks or cold water). Players may return to play when adequately hydrated. *Heat syncope (hypotensive syncope)* occurs after a sudden stop to prolonged physical activity when decreased peripheral vascular resistance leads to venous pooling and exacerbates hypotension caused by dehydration. Treatment involves sitting or lying down and significant fluid intake. Athletes should be forbidden from resuming participation. *Heat exhaustion* is more severe and indicates a significant hypovolemia. Athletes may appear pale, with poor peripheral circulation, central nervous system symptoms (dizziness, visual disturbances, syncope), and elevated core body temperature. Significant nausea and vomiting also may result and prevent oral hydration. Hydration should be aggressive and should include intravenous 0.5 normal saline for all patients with central nervous system manifestations. Affected players should not return to play, all other players should be evaluated for heat exhaustion, and coaches should be advised to cut the practice short. *Heatstroke* represents imminent vascular collapse, and central nervous system symptoms such as delirium, convulsions, and loss of consciousness should be considered medical emergencies requiring immediate transport to the nearest emergency department for admission and monitoring for possible multiorgan system failure. Core body temperatures may be greater than 41°C (106°F). Treatment while awaiting transport should include ice packs and intravenous 0.5

normal saline. Coaches should end practice immediately. Prevention includes the ready availability of fluids at all practices and no "penalty" or perceived weakness for water breaks. Daily weigh-ins should be used with restrictions for athletes with greater than 3% day-to-day weight loss, practices should be modified on hot days (no contact, no pads), and, most important, coaching staff should be vigilant for signs of early heat exhaustion.

SPORTS NUTRITION

Advocating proper nutrition for athletes goes beyond the food pyramid. Athletes in training, especially athletes in weight-sensitive competitive sports, such as football, wrestling, or gymnastics, often feel pressured to gain or lose weight while maintaining optimal conditioning for strength and flexibility. Expensive, over-the-counter nutritional supplements are obtained easily from stores or through the Internet and are increasingly popular among student athletes. Although some of these supplements are relatively benign, it may be difficult to determine the true active ingredients for any given supplement. Name clues may help; for example, supplements ending in *-one*, *-ione*, or *-ane* are likely to contain a steroid or steroid derivative. At the collegiate level, deterrents to steroid use include random drug urine screening, and severe penalties for use or abuse of a long list of banned substances that range from suspension to complete loss of eligibility and scholarships to school sanctions.

There is no universal screening in high school sports, and, though many high schools have zero-tolerance drug policies, there are no fixed penalties and sanctions. In competitive sports whose players are recruited heavily by colleges, students may feel pressure to bulk up to perform at a higher level. Pediatricians should ask patients routinely about the use of nutritional supplements during the Home, Education, Activities, Drugs, Sexuality, Suicide/Depression (HEADSS) assessment. Providing accurate information about supplements also is important. Amino acid supplements have not consistently been shown to help with strength or weight gain and may cause increased diarrhea and abdominal pain as a result of increased osmotic load. Nutritional supplements used to lose weight also may contain banned substances and may affect overall conditioning and stamina adversely.

Weight gain also is required by some sports. Pediatricians should promote gain in lean body mass (muscle) over fat mass. Many adolescent and young adult athletes mistakenly equate increased protein intake with increased weight gain potential. The American diet is rich in protein; total caloric intake may need to be increased, and this is accomplished best through complex carbohydrates. Dietary intake should be reviewed in collaboration with a registered dietitian.

Wrestlers, gymnasts, figure skaters, distance runners, or any athlete with weight classes to meet, a low center of balance to maintain, or less weight to carry for long periods may be concerned with weight loss. Questions should screen for eating disorders. Just as weight gain is accomplished best by increasing caloric intake above the level of caloric expenditure, weight loss is achieved best by increasing caloric expenditure above the level of caloric intake. The ideal rate of loss is no more than 1 to 2 lb (0.5 to 1 kg) per week, with less loss for smaller athletes. Aggressive weight loss may result in ketosis, loss of lean body mass (muscle), dehydration, and electrolyte disturbances.

Game day nutrition also is important for sports such as football, ice hockey, field hockey, basketball, and soccer. A meal consisting of complex carbohydrates should be consumed 2 to 3 hours before the game, allowing sufficient time for digestion. High-sugar snacks (power bars, candy, high-sugar sodas) should be avoided immediately before the game because of the possibility of rebound hypoglycemia during the contest. During the competition, most fluid loss is through sweating and can be replenished with cold water. Sports drinks that contain electrolytes are probably necessary only for prolonged physical exertion. Athletes should be reminded that thirst is not a timely indicator of hydration status and that they should hydrate constantly between shifts or plays. After the competition, hydration continues to be important to replenish body volume. High-fat foods require longer digestive periods and may result in postprandial drowsiness as a result of gastrointestinal tract shunting. As with pregame dining, complex carbohydrates are sources of energy replacement after the game.

SPORTS INJURIES

Head and Neck Injuries

Head and neck injuries have potential for catastrophic sequelae. They occur most frequently in collision or contact sports (football and ice hockey) and typically are acute injuries.

A *concussion* ("ding," "seeing stars") is a transient loss of consciousness or significant impairment of cognitive function after closed head injury. The most sensitive test is an evaluation of recent memory, such as the ability to recall home address or scripted plays. Players who fail the memory test or who have loss of consciousness should be withdrawn from participation and observed closely. Postconcussive headaches may persist for hours to days and are a contraindication for future play. Rehabilitation should be gradual. Players should be banned permanently from returning to participation after the third episode of concussive head injury. Players reluctant to accept this restriction should be reminded that even elite professional athletes retire as a consequence of repeated concussive episodes.

Frequent headaches, difficulty concentrating and focusing on tasks, irritability, decreased academic performance, and persistent loss of some cognitive function are symptoms of *postconcussive syndrome*. A computed tomography scan is indicated to look for intracranial hemorrhage.

Brachial plexus injuries ("stingers," "burners") result from hyperextension or lateral flexion of the neck that stretches the brachial plexus. Pain radiates unilaterally and is sharp and burning in quality. Grade I brachial plexus injuries are brief, lasting seconds to days, and resolve completely without residual pain or weakness. Players may return to play when there is no residual weakness. Grade II injuries persist for weeks to months. Grade III injuries are diagnosed after more than 1 year of persistent symptoms and preclude return to play. Bilateral pain or cervical spine tenderness should be managed with cervical spine immobilization and immediate imaging to rule out spinal cord injury or traumatic disk herniation. Patients without radiographic findings should be followed up 1 to 2 days after injury to assess for posttraumatic edema.

Back and Spine Injuries

During adolescence and early adulthood, back and spine injuries are likely to be due to overuse, mechanical strain, developmental abnormality, or a combination of factors. Symptoms may persist for weeks to months. The evaluation of back or spine pain in a child athlete also should include a consideration of infectious or malignant etiologies. Football and gymnastics are the two sports with the highest incidence of back injuries.

Strains are the most common cause of back and spine injuries and usually are due to overuse in adolescents and young adults. Typical presentation includes back pain, loss of flexibility, loss of rotational range, and loss of strength. Muscle relaxants rarely are required for severe cramping and spasm. *Intervertebral disk injuries* usually are the result of repeated spinal loading (as with weightlifting and football). Lower back pain is the presenting concern. Sciatica is uncommon in young athletes. Magnetic resonance imaging frequently is needed to confirm the diagnosis. Successful rehabilitation for sprains and disk injuries includes sufficient rest to begin healing, ice and nonsteroidal anti-inflammatory drugs (NSAIDs) for inflammation, and a progressive stretching and strengthening back exercise program. *Spondylolysis* (unilateral or bilateral stress fracture of the pars interarticularis of the lower lumbar spine in an adolescent athlete), spondylolisthesis (slippage of a superior vertebra on a lower vertebra associated with bilateral spondylolysis), and Scheuermann's epiphysitis (associated with kyphosis and wedge vertebrae) are other injuries that may be related to sports participation.

Upper Extremity Injuries

Injuries to the shoulder, arm, and hand are frequent reasons for visits to the pediatrician. Acute injuries to the shoulder joint are not uncommon, because the joint is not intrinsically stable and is vulnerable to sudden and traumatic dislocation. These injuries include glenohumeral dislocation or subluxation, acromioclavicular joint dislocation or subluxation, and sternoclavicular joint dislocation or subluxation. Table 49-3 lists acute shoulder injuries and their treatment.

Overuse injuries of the upper extremity occur from repetitive stresses, and most may be rehabilitated with ice to decrease inflammation, relative rest to allow recovery and healing of microtrauma, NSAIDs for pain and inflammation control, and a well-designed stretching and strengthening rehabilitation program started after the resolution of pain and continued throughout resumption of sports activities.

Rotator cuff impingement syndrome (tennis shoulder) often presents as pain with either full flexion or partial flexion with internal rotation of the humerus that worsens progressively during an overhand throwing workout. Tenderness is greatest over the greater tuberosity, where the supraspinatus tendon is attached. Successful rehabilitation also requires total upper body conditioning to maintain

Table 49-3. Acute Shoulder Soft Tissue Injuries

Location of Injury	Symptoms/Signs	Treatment
Glenohumeral joint	Usually anterior dislocation; painful; results from forced abduction, lateral rotation, and hyperextension	Immobilization; reduction; stretching and strengthening exercises
AC joint		
Grade I	No palpable defect; mild pain; no disruption of ligaments	Rest; NSAIDs; stretching and strengthening; protective equipment
Grade II	Subluxation palpable; moderate-to-severe pain; AC ligament disrupted, trapezoid and conoid ligaments partially disrupted	
Grade III	AC joint elevated; very painful; all ligaments disrupted	
Sternoclavicular joint	Less common; painful; localized swelling; anterior or posterior dislocation	Immediate traction and reduction; figure-of-eight appliance or sling; stretching and strengthening; protective equipment

AC, acromioclavicular; NSAIDs, nonsteroidal anti-inflammatory drugs.

correct throwing biomechanics. Steroid injections may be used for accompanying bursitis. Surgery rarely is employed.

Thoracic outlet syndrome is a clinical diagnosis that consists of vague, intermittent, and variable shoulder and arm pain caused by compression of structures running through the thoracic outlet. It is rare in childhood but can be seen in later adolescent years. A positive Adson test is diagnostic. Radiographic studies are recommended to rule out anatomic abnormalities. Initial treatment should involve stretching. Failure to improve should prompt referral.

The elbow is at particular risk for overuse injuries. *Flexor-pronator tendinitis* occurs with progressive inflammation of the medial structures in the elbow from persistent microtrauma. This condition also is called *little leaguer's elbow*, owing to the repetitive rotational stress from learning how to throw a curveball or slider. Pain can be elicited over the pronator teres and medial epicondyle, and forearm pronation and wrist flexion are resisted. Ulnar nerve inflammation and dysfunction may be present. Radiographic studies should rule out medial physis fractures. Rehabilitation should include correction of throwing biomechanics.

Panner's disease (osteochondrosis of humeral capitellum) is the likely diagnosis for acute onset of medial elbow pain while throwing in an athlete younger than 11 years old. Radiographic studies show the fragmentation of the capitellum ossific nucleus with minimal deformity of the capitellum itself. A more gradual development of sharp elbow pain with or without locking of the elbow is found in *osteochondritis dissecans*. Radiographs and computed tomography scans looking for avascular necrosis may be required for diagnosis. Standard overuse rehabilitation usually is adequate for both injuries. Failure to resolve pain in a timely fashion should prompt referral.

Flexion contractures result from repetitive hyperextension with subsequent anterior joint capsule fibrosis. Athletes may be asymptomatic initially. Contractures less than 30 degrees should be treated with relative rest and stretching and strengthening exercises. Contractures greater than 30 degrees should be treated with complete rest and targeted active and assisted range-of-motion rehabilitation.

Olecranon bursitis is a painful inflammation caused by intrabursal bleeding from traumatic impact. Rest and joint compression until symptoms resolve constitute adequate therapy, but significant swelling may require needle aspiration. There is a low risk for permanent disability.

Unusual in older adolescents, *lateral epicondylitis (tennis elbow)* manifests with lateral epicondyle point tenderness and pain secondary to extensor overuse from activities in which a firm grip is maintained continuously (like holding onto uneven bars or a racquet). It may be precipitated by a change in equipment or biomechanics. Swelling and loss of range of motion are atypical. Standard rehabilitation is adequate. Elite athletes may require steroid injections.

Wrist sprains are the most common wrist injury and are noted by pain with palpation and motion of affected ligaments. Wrist fractures should be excluded by radiographs. Treatment with a neutral-position wrist splint, ice, and NSAIDs usually is adequate. Return to play is possible with resolution of pain with motion.

Ligamentous disruption of the wrist is rare but may occur with forceful wrist dorsiflexion. Scaphoid-lunate ligaments are affected most commonly. This condition requires referral to an orthopedic specialist. *Triangular fibrocartilage tears* occur with forceful simultaneous wrist dorsiflexion and pronation, presenting with ulnar surface pain that worsens with forearm rotation and radioulnar compression. Magnetic resonance imaging usually is required to confirm the suspected diagnosis. Orthopedic referral is recommended for patients who do not respond to conservative therapy. Stress fractures of the distal radial physis, navicular or hamate fractures in the wrist, and intra-articular and extra-articular hand fractures also may occur from either acute trauma or overuse.

"Jammed" fingers, the most common finger injury, result from hyperextension of the proximal interphalangeal (PIP) or distal interphalangeal (DIP) joints. Symptoms are moderate swelling and pain with range-of-motion limitation. Radiographs should be obtained for injuries to an athlete's dominant hand. In-line traction and reduction of dorsal displacements may be attempted if no neurovascular compromise or angular malalignment is present, followed by buddy splinting and range-of-motion exercises to minimize fibrosis. Return to participation depends on the ability to protect the injury. Volar displacements should be referred.

Skier's thumb occurs when there is a fall onto the outstretched hand causing a sudden radial extension of the thumb. A complete tear requires orthopedic intervention, especially in the dominant hand. *Jersey finger* is the avulsion of the flexor digitorum profundus tendon and results in the inability to flex the DIP joint. Surgical intervention is necessary for reattachment.

Mallet finger is the disruption of the terminal extensor mechanism and occurs with severe or forced flexion of the

DIP joint and avulsion of the extensor tendon. *Boutonnière deformity* is caused by rupture of the central slip of the extensor tendon over the PIP joint. The result is a 15- to 30-degree flexion of the PIP joint with swelling and point tenderness and a hyperextended DIP joint. Continuous full-extension PIP joint splinting for 6 to 8 weeks is required for mallet finger and boutonnière deformities. Referral is advised because avulsion may require surgery.

Lower Extremity Injuries

Proper conditioning of the school-age athlete is important. Warm-ups, stretching, postactivity cooldowns, and progressive programs of strength and skills acquisition are crucial in the prevention of all sports injuries but are especially important for the prevention of lower extremity ailments.

Medial tibial stress syndrome (shin splints) occurs in runners and jumpers and is marked by pain along the distal posteromedial border of the tibia, where there is inflammation of the periosteum. Shin splints worsen with progressive exercise, improve with rest, and often are related to overtraining or sudden changes from short distance to long distance running. Rest, ice, and NSAIDs are used until the athlete is asymptomatic. Recurrence is reduced with rehabilitation involving frequent calf/heel cord stretches and ankle plantar flexion exercises and lower extremity strengthening. Orthotics may be necessary to correct pronation.

Stress fractures manifest by well-localized tenderness over the proximal half of the tibia or fibula and result from constant, repetitive trauma, such as long distance running over hard surfaces. Fractures may be small areas of periosteal reaction without cortical defect, so oblique radiographs are recommended to make the diagnosis. Technetium bone scans also are helpful. Complete rest is recommended for 6 to 8 weeks.

Compartment syndrome is associated with running microtrauma. This syndrome is characterized by a period of exercise lasting 10 minutes, followed by progressively worsening achy, tight, pounding pain that can persist for hours after activity. There may be some numbness or tingling in the feet. Athletes with suspected compartment syndrome should be referred to orthopedists for definitive management.

Avulsion fractures typically occur over the anterior superior iliac spine and are heralded by the acute onset of severe pain and sudden loss of function after an episode of strenuous activity. Treatment involves a regimen of stretching and strengthening. *Stress fractures of the femur* may occur in distance runners as a result of constant foot pounding on hard surfaces and presents as an aching, vague thigh pain. Radiographic confirmation may require oblique views or technetium bone scans. Casting should be done to prevent bony displacement. A progressive strengthening program is essential.

Iliac apophysitis also occurs in adolescent long distance or cross-country runners. Palpation over the iliac crest elicits significant pain. Radiographs should exclude avulsion fractures. Return to activity usually occurs within 4 to 6 weeks after rest and pain resolution. *Iliac crest contusions* ("hip pointer") are painful periosteal hematomas caused by trauma, usually at the anterior superior iliac crest. Ice, rest, and padding are indicated. Athletes may return to participation when there is full strength and range of motion without limp. No long-term disability occurs with either injury.

Traumatic impact to the upper portion of the lower extremity can result in a *quadriceps contusion*. Moderate-to-severe pain on knee flexion is present. Play should be restricted immediately after injury. Treatment involves stopping acute bleeding with ice, pressure, and elevation. Severe injuries carry a high risk for myositis ossificans. After rehabilitation, return to play may occur when there is no pain and equal strength.

Knee injuries are common in athletes of all sporting activities, presenting as chronic and acute complaints. *Tibial tuberosity apophysitis* (Osgood-Schlatter disease) is the most common cause of knee pain in a skeletally immature athlete. Repetitive avulsion stresses manifest as variable tenderness over the tibial tubercle and local soft tissue swelling. Jumping, squatting, or kneeling activities can exacerbate the usually unilateral pain, although 20% to 30% of patients have bilateral involvement. Radiographs are indicated with atypical presentation or to rule out malignancy. Symptoms resolve when the proximal tibial epiphysis closes (age 14 to 16 years), so symptomatic treatment is adequate. Immobilization should be minimized.

Patellofemoral stress syndrome (chondromalacia, peripatellar pain syndrome), one of the most common sports medicine complaints, presents with an anterior and circumferential, chronic, dull, and aching pain. Pain is exacerbated by climbing stairs, prolonged sitting, or patellar trauma. It occurs commonly in athletes who run frequently and can persist over the entire career of the athlete. Painful isometric quadriceps contraction is considered diagnostic. Examination also may produce clicking or popping sounds with knee movement and pain with patellar compression. *Chondromalacia patella* has a similar clinical picture but has pathologic softening or erosion of patellar articular cartilage on radiographs, which also are indicated to rule out malignancy or fracture after nonresponse to treatment. Treatment for both conditions involves relative rest and rehabilitation with progressive stretching and strengthening of the hamstrings and quadriceps. Hyperpronation, femoral anteversion, and external tibial torsion may require modification of future activity or the use of orthotic devices.

Patellar tendinitis is a chronic anterior knee pain that occurs with running and jumping and is more common in older adolescents. The pain is not disabling but may lead to poor flexibility of quadriceps and hamstrings. Treatment involves complete rest for 6 to 8 weeks and subsequent rehabilitation. Recurrences are common. Surgical débridement may be required for pain after more than 12 months of complete rest. *Sinding-Larsen-Johannson syndrome* is patellar tendinitis in a preteen athlete. Pain and tenderness occur over the inferior pole of the patella. Radiographs show an ossicle adjacent to the inferior pole. This condition is self-limited, usually resolving with skeletal maturation of the athlete. An abnormal *patellar tilt* is caused by chronic increased loading on the lateral facet of the patella causing pain with patellar motion. Management is relative rest, stretching and strengthening, and patellar stabilization. *Patellar dislocation and subluxation* may occur with sudden trauma and is the second leading cause of hemarthrosis.

Iliotibial band friction syndrome is the most common cause of lateral knee pain in runners and occurs when a taut iliotibial band (from running on banked roads) is irritated by constant friction across the lateral femoral epicondyle, causing a dull, achy pain without swelling or weakness. Orthotic heel wedges may be necessary after rest and rehabilitation to correct biomechanics.

Prepatellar bursitis (turf knee) usually results from a sharp blow directly on the patella that causes a prepatellar bursal contusion, intrabursal bleeding, and anterior swelling and ballotable fluid over the patella. Knee flexion is painful but is relieved by ice and compression. Aspiration rarely is indicated. Recurrence is common, especially when playing on artificial surfaces. Return to participation requires full range of knee motion and symmetric strength. Minimal-to-mild pain is not a contraindication to return to play.

Peripatellar contusions may result from a sharp blow to soft tissue around the patella or from forced knee flexion with contracted quadriceps. The development of large hematomas is common and prompts slower rehabilitation. Often, compression is necessary to stop the bleeding. Rehabilitation should be slow and avoid unnecessary knee flexion.

Acute knee ligament injuries are uncommon in younger athletes but increase in frequency during adolescence with a higher incidence in sports that require rapid leg planting and shifts in direction (e.g., soccer, volleyball, basketball) or contact sports (e.g., football).

The *medial collateral ligament* sprain is the most common knee injury in contact sports and usually occurs through a direct blow to the lateral aspect of the planted leg. Moderate-to-severe injury causes immediate excruciating pain and loss of active motion. The *lateral collateral ligament* sprain is uncommon at all ages and occurs with excess force placed on the medial aspect of the planted leg. Significant knee laxity suggests involvement of other ligaments and posterior capsule injury. Complete rest and immobilization for 2 to 3 days is indicated for both injuries, followed by assisted ambulation and gradual rehabilitation. Orthopedists should be consulted because surgery may be necessary. A normal, painless examination is required for return to participation.

Anterior cruciate ligament sprains are the most common ligamentous knee injury across all age groups. Complete disruption presents with the classic "pop" sensation and is exquisitely painful, precluding activity. Swelling worsens over several hours, and a hemarthrosis can result. Many younger patients do well with nonoperative management, but orthopedic consultation is recommended for all anterior cruciate ligament injuries. *Posterior cruciate ligament* sprains are uncommon and unusual in patients with open growth plates. Although pain is sharp, the knee is usually stable. Management is nonoperative with surgical reconstruction for failed rehabilitation only in elite athletes. Radiographs are recommended.

Immediate and significant swelling of the knee joint after acute trauma suggests a *meniscal injury*. Most meniscal injuries have an insidious onset, however, and present with limping, decreased knee range of motion, and synovitis. Magnetic resonance imaging assists in diagnosis. Referral is necessary because treatment is surgical.

Ankle sprains are the most common acute injury to the lower extremity, but serious injury to ankle ligaments is uncommon in younger children because the force required to produce ligamentous injury in young adults or older teens usually causes fractures in patients with open physes. The usual mechanism of injury is plantar flexion and inversion (twisting) that leads to lateral ligament disruption. Pain is immediate, and there is often swelling from bleeding. Tenderness anterior and inferior to the lateral malleolus is more suggestive of soft tissue injury than ligamentous damage. The Ottawa ankle rules were developed for adults but are applicable for older adolescents as well. The Ottawa ankle rules state that radiographic studies are required only if the patient has pain located near the malleoli, is unable to bear weight, or has bony point tenderness. Sprains may be treated with relative rest, ice, compression, elevation, and progressive stretching and strengthening. Athletes may return to full participation when there is no pain with lateral movement. Ankle taping or other orthotic devices that enhance ankle stability may be helpful for future exercise. Surgery is indicated only for elite athletes who require absolute ankle stability.

Older adolescents and young adults participating in running, dancing, or jumping sports may develop microtears leading to *Achilles tendinitis*. Pain over the posterior aspect of the heel is worsened by exercise. Associated swelling is minimal, and the tendinitis usually is self-limited. Symptoms resolve by the closure of the apophysis. Rest and stretching and strengthening of the gastrocnemius and soleus muscles, heel lifts or cups, and well-cushioned athletic shoes are usually adequate. When the heel is nontender, the athlete can return to training.

◎ Additional Resources, CD-ROM	
Sports injuries	Text, table
Spondylolisthesis	
Spondylolysis	
Scheuermann's epiphisitis	
Glenohumeral dislocation or subluxation	
Acromioclavicular (AC) joint dislocation or subluxation	
Sternoclavicular (SC) joint dislocation or subluxation	
Stress fractures of the wrist	
Intra-articular and extra-articular hand fractures	
Patellar dislocation and subluxation	
Sever's disease (calcaneal apophysis)	
Iselin's disease	
Jones fracture	
Plantar fasciitis	

SUGGESTED READINGS

American Academy of Pediatrics, Committee on Sports Medicine and Fitness: Climatic heat stress and the exercising child. Pediatrics 2000;106:158–159.

American Academy of Pediatrics, Committee on Sports Medicine and Fitness and Committee on School Health: Organized sports for children and preadolescents. Pediatrics 2001;107:1459–1462.

Bernhardt DT, Landry GL: Sports injuries in young athletes. Adv Pediatr 1995;42:465–500.

Herring SA, Nilson KL: Introduction to overuse injuries. Clin Sports Med 1987;6:225–239.

Landry GL: Sports injuries in childhood. Pediatr Ann 1992;21:165–168.

Loosli AR, Benson J: Nutritional intake in adolescent athletes. Pediatr Clin North Am 1990;37:1143–1152.

SECTION 3 GENERAL MEDICAL CARE: *Musculoskeletal Disorders*

50 Fractures, Sprains, and Dislocations

Sara L. Thompson

ROLE OF THE GENERALIST

1 Recognize developmental and physiologic changes that predispose children to different patterns of musculoskeletal injury.

2 Diagnose a sprain, fracture, or dislocation by medical history, physical examination, and radiographic evaluation.

3 Recognize fractures and dislocations requiring emergent specialty care.

4 Refer for orthopedic specialty care when assistance is needed for medical management and follow-up of sprains, fractures, and dislocations.

5 Treat sprains and dislocations that do not require orthopedic specialty care.

6 Recognize injuries resulting from nonaccidental trauma.

7 Address safety issues that may prevent the occurrence of future injuries.

DEFINITIONS

Musculoskeletal trauma accounts for 10% to 25% of childhood injuries and, depending on a child's level of musculoskeletal maturation, may result in a bone fracture, ligament sprain, or joint dislocation. A *fracture* is a disruption of the bony cortex or periosteum or both and may occur at either a macroscopic or a microscopic level. By age 16, 42% of boys and 27% of girls have sustained a fracture. *Ligamentous sprains* are due to overstretching and partial tearing of a ligament and, although uncommon in children, are seen more frequently than musculotendonous strains. Sprains are most common in children before the growth spurt and in adolescents after closure of the physis. *Joint dislocations* are uncommon pediatric injuries and occur when there is complete separation of the bones that normally oppose each other within a joint. *Joint subluxation* is incomplete separation with partial contact of the bones of the joint.

Fracture patterns are described according to the anatomic location, the fracture configuration, the relationship of the fragments to one another, and the relationship of the fragments to the overlying tissue. The anatomic location on the bone may be the diaphysis, metaphysis, epiphysis, or physis. The configurations include plastic deformation, buckle (torus) fracture, greenstick fracture, and complete fracture (Fig. 50-1). *Plastic deformation*, bending of a bone past its point of elastic recoil with persistent deformity, most commonly occurs in the ulna or fibula in association with a fracture of the paired bone (radius or tibia). A *buckle (torus) fracture*, frequent in young children with more porous bone, is due to compression of the bone, most commonly at the diaphyseal/metaphyseal junction. This fracture most commonly occurs at the distal radius. In a *greenstick fracture*, one portion of the periosteum and cortex remains intact along the fracture line. The intact portion undergoes plastic deformation and does not recoil to its anatomic position. This fracture is common in the diaphysis or metaphysis of the bone and occurs in young children with

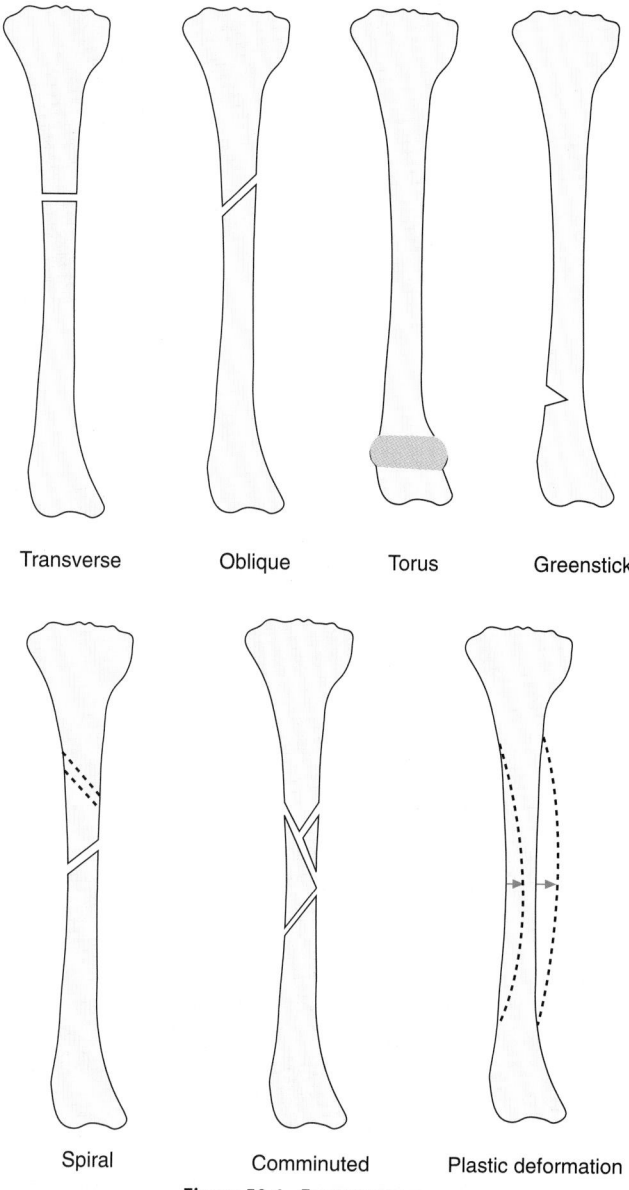

Transverse   Oblique   Torus   Greenstick

Spiral   Comminuted   Plastic deformation

Figure 50-1. Fracture types.

more porous bone. A *complete fracture* propagates through the entire bone and may be described as *transverse* (at a right angle to the longitudinal axis of the bone), *oblique* (at an angle to the longitudinal axis of the bone), *spiral* (an oblique fracture line that encircles the shaft of the bone), or *comminuted* (fracture site in multiple fragments).

Fractures that involve the growth plate, or physis, of a bone are described according to the Salter-Harris classification system, based on whether the fracture involves the physis, the metaphysis, or the epiphysis (Fig. 50-2). Because the physis changes throughout childhood, patterns of physeal fractures change with age. Type I Salter-Harris fractures occur more commonly in younger children. As the epiphysis ossifies with age, type II through IV Salter-Harris fractures increase in frequency.

The relationship of bone fragments to one another may be angulated, overriding, or bayonet. *Angulation* is the presence of an angle between the fragments, *overriding fragments* are fragments that are displaced and adjacent without cortical contact, and *bayonet fragments* are mini-

mally displaced with cortical contact. The relationship of fracture fragments to surrounding soft tissue defines whether a fracture is open or closed. An *open fracture* breaks the overlying skin, increasing risk for subsequent infection. A closed fracture has intact skin over the fracture.

Stress fractures, small breaks in the bony cortex caused by repetitive stress or minor trauma, occur at a microscopic level and are not uniformly visible on radiographs. *Pathologic fractures* occur in bone with abnormal structure from infection, tumor, abnormal metabolism, or hereditary disease. The abnormal structure predisposes the bone to fracturing with relatively minor trauma.

FUNDAMENTALS

Musculoskeletal injury patterns in children differ with age as a result of anatomic differences in bone composition. Children have more porous and plastic bone from a greater number of vascular channels and lower levels of mineralization, making their bones more prone to fracture than bones of adults. Children's bones can respond to forces by buckling and bending, resulting in a greater propensity for greenstick fractures, torus fractures, and plastic bone deformation. Ligamentous strength around a child's joint is greater than the strength of the physis. A child is less likely to sustain a dislocation, subluxation, sprain, or strain with a traumatic force to the joint and is more likely to sustain an apophyseal avulsion, epiphyseal displacement, or physeal injury. The periosteum of the pediatric diaphysis and metaphysis is thick and may remain intact even in the presence of a fracture, decreasing the prevalence of fracture displacement.

The presence of the physis, or growth plate, is unique to pediatric bone. Injuries to this area account for 15% of all children's skeletal injuries. This region of the bone contains a high ratio of cellular components (chondrocytes) to matrix and is more vulnerable to fracture than other areas with a higher proportion of matrix. Local joint anatomy also affects the likelihood of physeal injury. Because ligamentous strength is greater than physeal strength, a ligamentous insertion on the metaphysis of a bone protects the physis from injury, but insertion on the epiphysis leaves it vulnerable. Physeal injuries are most common at times of rapid growth, particularly during the growth spurt of puberty.

When a fracture does occur, a child's bone heals more rapidly and has greater capacity to remodel poorly united or angulated fragments than adult bone. Rapid healing is attributed to high levels of osteogenic activity and greater vascularity. The mechanism by which remodeling occurs is unknown. The greatest remodeling is seen with fractures close to the growth plate and with bone angulation in the plane of the extremity's movement. Remodeling occurs as long as longitudinal bone growth is taking place. Type I and II Salter-Harris fractures have the greatest potential for remodeling.

DIAGNOSIS

The diagnosis of a sprain, fracture, or dislocation is determined by the medical history, physical examination, and radiographic findings. The mechanism of injury (e.g., con-

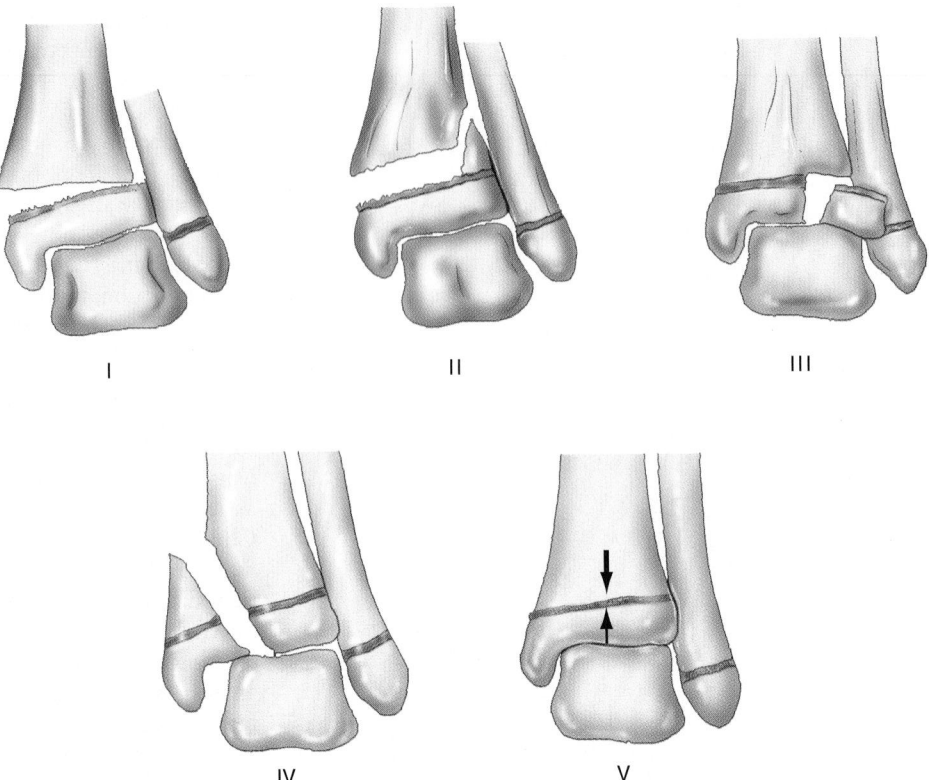

Figure 50-2. Salter-Harris fractures: I, pure separation through physis; II, metaphyseal spike; III, separation through physis and vertically through epiphysis; IV, fracture through metaphysis, through physis, and vertically through epiphysis; V, pure compression injury. (Adapted from Green NE, Swiontkowski MF: Skeletal Trauma in Children, 2nd ed. Philadelphia, WB Saunders, 1998, p 22.)

tact during sports, a fall or twisting motion) helps to create the differential diagnosis of suspected injuries. Weakness, paresthesias, pallor, and disproportionate pain indicate the presence of neurovascular compromise or a compartment syndrome. The general physical examination of musculoskeletal injury includes inspection, palpation, range of motion, and testing for neurovascular sufficiency.

The radiographic evaluation of musculoskeletal injuries may include x-rays, nucleotide bone scans, computed tomography, or magnetic resonance imaging. Anteroposterior and lateral radiographs are standard views for evaluation of bone, although an oblique view may be helpful if the injury involves a joint, such as the shoulder, hip, or knee (Table 50-1). In cases of suspected long bone injury, the joints on either side of the injury should be included on the radiographs. Comparison views of the unaffected extremity also may provide valuable information if findings from the initial x-rays may be developmental variations and not traumatic findings. Not all fractures are visible on x-ray. Type I Salter-Harris fractures often are diagnosed by clinical findings alone. If subtle fractures are not radiographically visible, they may be diagnosed with a nucleotide bone scan. Repeat x-rays in 10 to 14 days may show callus or periosteal reaction. Computed tomography and magnetic resonance imaging are used to evaluate suspected growth plate injury.

Examination of the upper extremity begins with the shoulder. Shoulder injuries typically involve either the humerus or the clavicle. Any visible deformity, pain to palpation, or limitation of shoulder movement warrants radiographic evaluation. Clavicle fractures commonly are sustained during the birth process, in short falls, and with direct trauma to the shoulder. Distal clavicle fractures are the most common and may result from mechanisms that

cause acromioclavicular sprains and separations in adolescents and adults. Clavicle fractures, acromioclavicular ligament sprains, and acromioclavicular joint separations all result in pain with arm and neck movement and localized tenderness. The fracture itself may be palpable. Proximal humerus fractures, which account for less than 1% of pediatric fractures, may be difficult to differentiate from clavicle fractures. They commonly are due to a fall on an outstretched, externally rotated arm.

Table 50-1. Radiographic Views for Assessment of Musculoskeletal Injury

Location	Standard Radiographic Views	Additional Radiographic Views
Clavicle	AP	
Shoulder	AP (internal or external rotation); axillary or Y-view	
Elbow	AP; lateral	
Arm/forearm	AP; lateral	
Hand/wrist	PA; lateral; oblique	Scaphoid view (for scaphoid bone)
Pelvis/hip	AP; frog-leg lateral	
Leg	AP; lateral	
Knee	AP; lateral	Internal and external oblique views (for femoral condyles, tibial tuberosities, medial and lateral patella); sunrise view (for patella)
Ankle	AP; lateral; mortise view*	
Foot	AP; lateral; oblique	

*Mortise view provides a true AP view of the ankle.
AP, anteroposterior.

Although uncommon, glenohumeral (shoulder) dislocations may be seen in adolescents, particularly athletes, and usually are due to a fall on an outstretched, extended arm. Of pediatric shoulder dislocations, 95% are anterior. Posterior dislocations are associated with congenital joint instability. With anterior dislocations, the deltoid appears flattened; the acromion is prominent; and the humeral head is anterior, inferior, and medial to the glenoid. The arm is held in external rotation and slightly abducted. With posterior dislocations, the arm is internally rotated and adducted. Because shoulder dislocations are associated with brachial plexus and vascular injuries, a complete neurovascular examination is essential.

Examination of the arm includes palpation of the biceps, brachialis, and triceps muscles, along with finger and wrist flexors and extensors. The humeral, radial, and ulnar shafts should be palpated, as should the ulnar head and styloid process, radial head and styloid process, lateral humeral condyle, medial humeral epicondyle, and olecranon. The child should be asked to flex and extend the elbow and wrist and to supinate and pronate the forearm. Any localized pain or swelling or limited elbow motion is an indication for radiographic evaluation.

Humeral shaft fractures account for 2% of pediatric fractures, whereas radial and ulnar fractures account for 30% to 50%. Forearm fractures are classified into three categories: fracture-dislocations, midshaft fractures, and distal fractures. Fracture-dislocations include the Monteggia and Galeazzi injury patterns. Supracondylar fractures account for 60% of fractures and are most common in children 3 to 10 years old. Supracondylar fractures are due to a fall on an outstretched arm and result in localized distal humeral tenderness and an inability to flex the elbow; 15% have associated nerve injury. Vascular injury is less common. Lateral condyle fractures, the second most common elbow fractures, result from a varus force on a supinated arm and typically are type IV Salter-Harris injuries that present with localized lateral tenderness. Early diagnosis is important because there is a high rate of nonunion during the healing process. Medial epicondyle fractures account for 5% to 10% of elbow injuries and typically occur in children 9 to 14 years old. These fractures are due to a valgus stress on an extended arm, present with localized medial tenderness, and commonly are associated with elbow dislocations.

The elbow is the most commonly dislocated joint in childhood. Dislocations account for 5% of all elbow injuries and are particularly common in children older than age 8. Dislocations commonly occur from a fall on an outstretched arm and may be associated with medial condyle, coronoid process, or radial neck fractures. The forearm may appear visibly shortened, the olecranon may be prominent, and the elbow may be held in flexion. A thorough neurologic assessment for ulnar nerve palsy is essential.

Radial head subluxation is most common in children 1 to 3 years old and is due to abrupt traction on a pronated arm. The affected arm is slightly flexed, pronated, and held close to the body. Radiographic evaluation is unnecessary, unless arm movement is not restored after several attempts at reduction or bony tenderness is present.

Examination of the hand should note any swelling or bony deformities, and palpation should include the carpal bones, metacarpals, and phalanges. Particular attention should be paid to the anatomic snuffbox region (the scaphoid bone). Range of motion should include finger flexion and extension and opposition of the thumb. Neurologic evaluation should include sensation in the radial, median, and ulnar nerve distributions. Hand fractures are common pediatric fractures and typically are due to crush injuries in young children and sports-related injuries in adolescents. Phalangeal neck fractures and intercondylar (involving the joint) fractures are at risk of malunion and avascular necrosis, and prompt diagnosis is important.

Evaluation of the lower extremity includes palpation of the long bones and individual joint examination. The hip should be evaluated for flexion/extension, internal/external rotation, and abduction/adduction. Any evaluation for knee pain should include an examination of the hip, assessment of gait, inspection for an effusion or soft tissue swelling, and tracking of the patella with knee flexion/extension. The medial and lateral collateral ligaments, patella, patellar tendon, tibial tubercle, and areas of the femoral and tibial growth plates should be palpated (Fig. 50-3). Palpation of the ankle and foot should include the distal fibula and lateral malleolus; distal tibia and medial malleolus; tibial and fibular physes; all tarsals, metatarsals, and phalanges; and medial and lateral ankle ligaments (Fig. 50-4). Refusal to bear weight, bony tenderness, soft tissue swelling, and the presence of an effusion are indications for radiographic evaluation.

Tibial and fibular fractures are the most common fractures of the lower extremity. Injuries of the proximal and distal ends may result in nonspecific knee and ankle findings, such as decreased range of motion and effusions. Such injuries include avulsion of the tibial tubercle (and associated patellar ligament injury), avulsion of the tibial spine (with anterior cruciate ligament injury), and proximal or distal tibial epiphyseal fractures. Proximal epiphyseal injury is associated with popliteal artery damage and requires a thorough examination for vascular sufficiency. Nondisplaced spiral tibial fractures in children 1 to 4 years old may be noted after minor trauma or a history of leg twisting. These fractures, in the absence of other concerning findings, are termed *toddler* or *CAST* (childhood accidental spiral tibial) fractures and do not indicate child abuse.

Although less common, ligamentous knee injuries do occur. Sprains of the medial and lateral collateral ligaments should be suspected with tenderness over the medial or lateral physes or over the ligaments themselves. Ligamentous laxity may or may not be present. These injuries may be associated with femoral, tibial, and fibular avulsion fractures.

The ankle joint is stabilized by the anterior talofibular ligament (ATFL), posterior talofibular ligament, calcaneofibular ligament, and deltoid ligament (see Fig. 50-4). Because the medial ligaments of the ankle are stronger than the lateral ligaments, the ankle is more susceptible to inversion injury than eversion injury. When eversion injuries occur, they generally are more serious and are likely to include a fracture. Because of the epiphyseal insertions of the ligaments, ankle fractures have a higher likelihood of epiphyseal or physeal involvement and subsequent growth abnormalities.

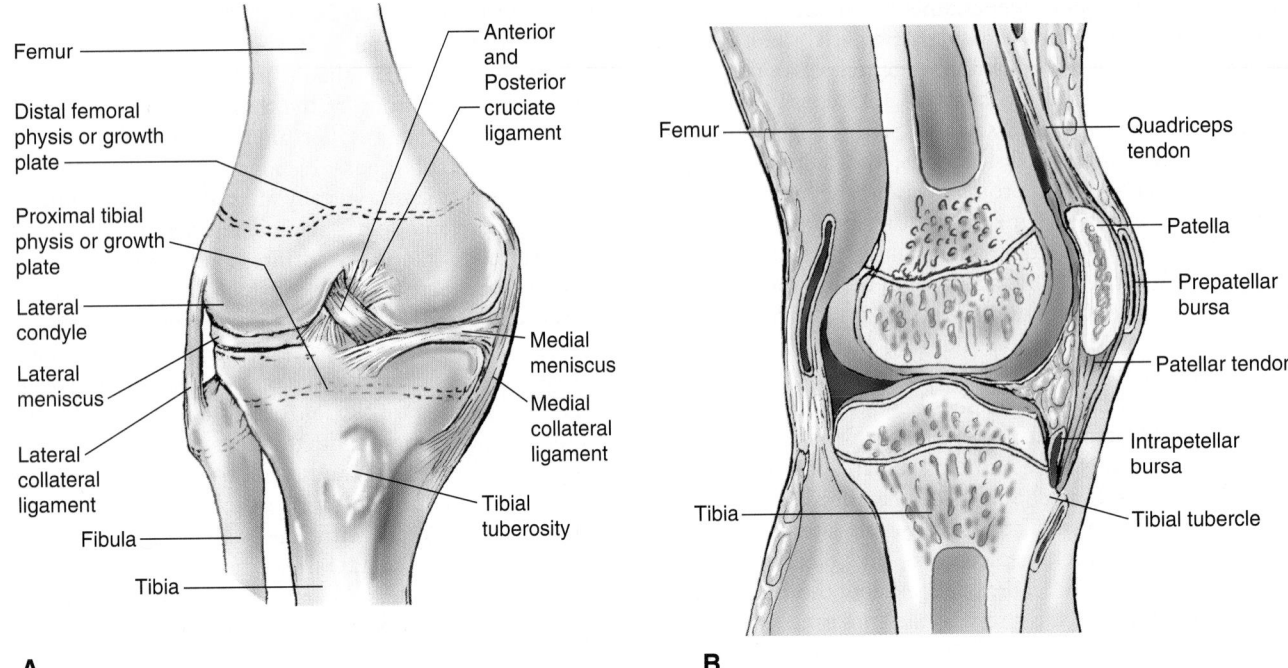

Figure 50-3. Knee anatomy. **A,** Anterior view (patella removed). **B,** Sagittal section. (Adapted from Fleisher GR, Ludwig S, Henretig FM, et al: Textbook of Pediatric Emergency Medicine, 4th ed. Philadelphia, Lippincott Williams & Wilkins, 1999, p 340.)

Ankle sprains are one of the most common sports-related and activity-related injuries and most frequently involve the ATFL. In children with open physes, ankle ligaments are stronger than the physes, however, and ankle sprains are less common. Ankle sprains are associated with localized tenderness over the injured ligament, swelling, and ecchymosis. Ligament stability can be assessed with the anterior drawer test. The ankle is placed at 90 degrees, the tibia is held firm, and the foot is drawn forward. ATFL instability is indicated by 3 to 5 mm of talar movement. The talar tilt test also may indicate ATFL and calcaneofibular ligament instability. The ankle is inverted, and the degree of talar tilt during this inversion is compared with the unaffected side. A difference of 10 degrees of tilt is significant. Rarely the tibiofibular syndesmosis may be sprained in association with a deltoid ligament injury. In these cases, tenderness may be elicited by squeezing the tibia and fibula.

Ankle sprains are graded according to the severity of ligamentous injury and the resulting clinical manifestations (Table 50-2). Because ankle sprains may be associated with avulsion fractures of the fibula, malleolus, talus, or base of the fifth metatarsal, any moderate-to-severe sprain first must be considered to be a possible fracture requiring radiographic evaluation. Clinical algorithms, such as the Ottawa rules, have been developed for the evaluation of ankle injuries in adults. No similar algorithm has been validated for children.

MANAGEMENT

General management principles for musculoskeletal injury include the minimization of edema (RICE [rest, ice, compression, elevation]), immobilization, analgesia, and recognition of conditions requiring orthopedic referral. Analgesia often is addressed inadequately. The resulting pain and

muscle contraction counteracts efforts at reducing fractures and dislocations. Analgesia and sedation requirements may be beyond the resources available in a pediatrician's office and require referral to an emergency department or short-stay observation unit.

The most emergent conditions requiring orthopedic consultation are neurovascular compromise, compartment syndrome, open fractures, and open dislocations. Additional conditions requiring immediate referral are structurally significant fractures; obvious limb deformities; and fractures that are shortened, are angulated, are rotated, are intra-articular, involve the growth plate, or are at statistically high risk of neurovascular compromise. Appropriate reduction must be obtained in these cases to minimize the risk of neurovascular damage and subsequent growth abnormalities. Hospitalization may be indicated for fractures at high risk of neurovascular compromise after reduction and immobilization.

Immobilization of musculoskeletal injuries minimizes the risk of further injury, protects neurovascular integrity, and reduces pain. Primary care providers should place a splint on the injury before orthopedic referral. Fractures should be splinted in the extremity's position of function. Splinting should include the joints above and below the fracture. Dislocations should be splinted to include the bones above and below the affected joint. The area should be well padded, with particular attention to areas of bony prominence, and the splint should not be wrapped tightly (to avoid a compartment syndrome). Immobilizers purchased in standard adult sizes usually do not fit children and should not be used. Common splint configurations include long arm and long leg splints, short arm and short leg posterior splints, thumb spica, and sugar-tong and double sugar-tong splints (Table 50-3). Medial or lateral splints tend to have greater longevity in children than posterior

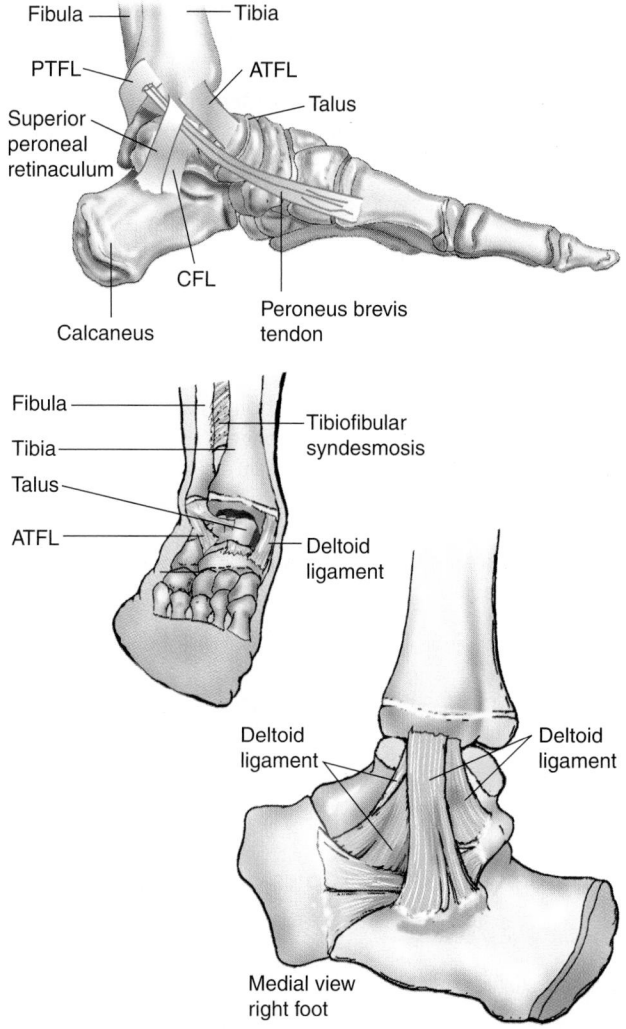

Fibula — Tibia

PTFL — ATFL

Talus

Superior peroneal retinaculum

CFL

Calcaneus

Peroneus brevis tendon

Fibula

Tibia

Talus

ATFL

Tibiofibular syndesmosis

Deltoid ligament

Deltoid ligament

Deltoid ligament

Medial view right foot

Figure 50-4. Ankle anatomy. ATFL, anterior talofibular ligament; CFL, calcaneofibular ligament; PTFL, posterior talofibular ligament. (Adapted from Fleisher GR, Ludwig S, Henretig FM, et al: Textbook of Pediatric Emergency Medicine, 4th ed. Philadelphia, Lippincott Williams & Wilkins, 1999, p 325.)

splints. Splints also should be placed well up the arm or leg and to the full length of the hand or foot to obtain adequate stabilization of a fracture in an active child.

Most dislocations require orthopedic referral. Treatment requires adequate pain control and muscle relaxation, and for these reasons referral to an emergency department or treatment unit may be necessary. Postreduction treatment of dislocations includes rest, ice, immobilization for several weeks, and orthopedic follow-up.

Table 50-2. Classification Guidelines for Ankle Sprains

Grade I	Mild sprain. Involves stretching and minimal interstitial tearing of the ligament. Minimal swelling, tenderness, or loss of function
Grade II	Moderate sprain. Involves partial ligamentous disruption. Moderate swelling and loss of function, diffuse tenderness, difficulty with weight bearing
Grade III	Severe sprain. Complete ligamentous disruption. Extensive swelling and joint instability, marked tenderness, inability to bear weight

CHAPTER 50 Fractures, Sprains, and Dislocations

Table 50-3. Splinting Techniques and Indications

Splint Type	Indication
Long leg splint	Knee immobilization (knee positioned in extension)
	Distal femur, proximal and midshaft tibia/fibula fractures (knee positioned in flexion)
Short leg posterior splint	Distal leg, foot, and ankle fractures
Sling and swathe	Upper extremity injuries between sternoclavicular joint and elbow
Long arm splint	Forearm and distal radius fractures
Posterior arm splint	Elbow and forearm injuries
	Wrist injuries requiring no forearm rotation or elbow flexion
Sugar-tong splint	Humerus, forearm, elbow, and wrist injuries
Ulnar gutter splint	Nondisplaced fractures of fourth and fifth fingers
Thumb spica splint	Thumb injuries and scaphoid fractures

The subluxed radial head can be reduced safely without orthopedic consultation by one of two methods. In the first method, the patient's hand is taken as if to shake it, the affected elbow is held with the thumb of the physician's other hand over the radial head, and in one fluid motion the arm is supinated and the elbow is flexed. In the second method, the elbow is held firmly while the wrist is hyper-pronated. With both methods, another reduction should be attempted if there is no return of arm function within 15 minutes. Radiographs should be obtained after two to three unsuccessful reduction attempts.

Treatment of sprains depends on the degree of ligamentous laxity and disruption and length of time since the injury. For grade I to II ankle sprains, treatment in the first 48 hours includes RICE. Pain and inflammation may be treated with nonsteroidal anti-inflammatory drugs, and crutches should be used if there is pain with weight bearing. Two to 5 days after the injury, range of motion and weight bearing should increase gradually, and the RICE protocol should be used after activity. After 5 days, range of motion and weight bearing should continue to increase as tolerated. Grade III ankle sprains, eversion ankle injuries, and any uncertain diagnoses require orthopedic referral.

A final aspect of managing musculoskeletal injury is the recognition of pathologic and inflicted injuries. Pathologic fractures occur in bone with abnormal structure and often are detected as fractures in uncommon locations, with uncommon configurations, or are due to a minimal degree of trauma. Additional clinical findings and radiographically visible osteopenia may help to determine subsequent laboratory workup and referrals.

Inflicted trauma often is detected if a traumatic injury is not consistent with the history provided or the developmental ability of the child, if the injury is known to have a high association with physical abuse, or if the child has additional physical findings that indicate abuse (Table 50-4). If inflicted trauma is suspected in a child 0 to 2 years of age, a radiographic skeletal survey should be obtained to evaluate for the presence of additional fractures. Between age 3 and 5 years, the skeletal survey should be obtained in highly suspicious cases. These may include cases with at least one suspicious injury or focal bony tenderness

363

Table 50-4. Specificity of Skeletal Fracture Characteristics as an Indication of Child Abuse (in the Absence of a History of Significant Accidental Trauma)

High specificity	Metaphyseal fracture
	Rib fracture
	Sternal fracture
	Scapular fracture
	Spinous process fracture
Moderate specificity	Multiple fracture locations or ages
	Hand fracture
	Foot fracture
	Complex skull fracture
	Vertebral body fracture
Low specificity	Diaphyseal fracture
	Clavicle fracture
	Linear skull fracture

on examination. When physical abuse is suspected, it is appropriate to notify local child protective services and law enforcement immediately.

OUTCOME

Fractures in children heal more rapidly and the bones have a greater ability to remodel than in adults because of the higher vascularity and osteogenic activity in the bones of children. These processes may be impaired by the loss of cellular components that facilitate healing (e.g., with an open fracture) or the loss of blood supply (e.g., with severe soft tissue injury).

Two complications of fractures in children—limb overgrowth and growth plate arrest—are unique to the child's growing skeleton. Bone overgrowth may occur after long bone fractures, and although the exact mechanism is unknown, it has been attributed to the increased vascularity and periosteal damage at the fracture site. Bone overgrowth is seen most commonly after femoral fractures in children 3 to 9 years old, but also may be seen with other fractures. It results in limb-length discrepancy that requires orthopedic referral.

Growth plate arrest can result from a fracture of the physis and may lead to limb-length discrepancy. The arrest may be partial or complete, peripheral or central. Peripheral arrest may lead to an angular deformity and the limb-length discrepancy. This complication may be diagnosed several months to years after the injury and is seen most often after type IV and V Salter-Harris fractures.

Open fractures heal more slowly than closed fractures and are at risk for infection, especially in children older than age 12 years. The risk of infection is minimized with prompt surgical irrigation and débridement.

Sprains and dislocations in children may recur. Risk can be decreased with muscle-strengthening exercises to stabilize the affected joint. Shoulder dislocations in children younger than age 10 almost universally recur. Radial head subluxations recur in one quarter to one third of patients.

FOLLOW-UP

Children who have sustained long bone fractures need to be monitored for limb-length discrepancy, and an orthopedic referral is indicated if this complication develops. Parents and caretakers also should receive anticipatory guidance regarding the circumstances of the trauma and should be educated regarding safety equipment in an effort to avoid future injuries.

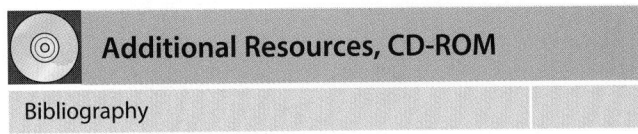

Additional Resources, CD-ROM

Bibliography

Mini-index of Related Topics

	CH.
SPORTS MEDICINE	49
PHYSICAL ABUSE AND SEXUAL ABUSE	269
SPLINTING AND CASTING	299

SUGGESTED READINGS

Della-Giustina K, Della-Giustina DA: Emergency department evaluation and treatment of pediatric orthopedic injuries. Emerg Med Clin North Am 1999;17:895–922.

Huurman WW, Ginsburg GM: Musculoskeletal injury in children. Pediatr Rev 1997;18:429–440.

Lyon RM, Street CC: Pediatric sports injuries: When to refer or x-ray. Pediatr Clin North Am 1998;45:221–243.

Sports Shorts. Available at: http://www.aap.org/family/sportsshort.htm.

Shaw DC, Heckman JD: Principles and techniques of splinting musculocutaneous injuries. Emerg Med Clin North Am 1984; 2:391–407.

51 Disorders of the Lower Extremities

Geeta Grover

ROLE OF THE GENERALIST

1 Recognize rotational and angular problems, and diagnose the most common causes.

2 Perform a detailed physical examination, including assessment of gait, rotational profile, and neurologic and musculoskeletal function.

3 Provide appropriate education and reassurance to parents regarding most of the conditions that produce rotational deformities and physiologic bowlegs and knock-knees.

4 Refer to a specialist when a pathologic condition is suspected or when the course of a rotational or angular deformity deviates from the normal developmental sequence.

5 Prevent long-term sequelae from pathologic conditions by accurate diagnoses and timely referral to a specialist when appropriate.

Rotational and angular deformities of the lower extremities occur frequently in infants and young children. Although most of these problems generally do not require any treatment and only rarely lead to physical limitations, they are a common cause of parental concern. Most rotational problems and physiologic angular deformities, such as bowlegs and knock-knees, can be managed adequately by the primary care physician. Pathologic cases of bowlegs and knock-knees are uncommon. Congenital clubfoot, which generally is a pathologic condition, has been included in the discussion of rotational problems because it often is confused with conditions of the feet that produce in-toeing.

FUNDAMENTALS

Rotational problems, such as in-toeing and out-toeing, are deformities in the transverse plane of the body, occurring when a bone rotates either internally or externally along its long axis. Rotational problems that fall within the normal range are referred to as *version*. Tibial version is the angular difference between the axis of the knee and the transmalleolar axis. Femoral version is the angular difference between the transcervical and transcondylar axes. The normal tibia is laterally rotated, and the normal femur is anteverted. Torsion is abnormal limb rotation 2 standard deviations from the mean and is described as a *deformity*.

Angular deformities, such as bowlegs and knock-knees, are deformities in the frontal plane. In bowleg deformity, the legs distal to the knees are angled toward the midline of the body. The legs are tilted away from the midline in knock-knee deformity (Fig. 51-1). Knee angle variations that fall within the normal or physiologic range are referred to as *bowlegs* and *knock-knees*. Knee angle variations that fall outside the normal range are referred to as *genu varum* for bowlegs and *genu valgum* for knock-knees.

ROTATIONAL PROBLEMS

The causes of in-toeing and out-toeing may be classified according to a child's age at presentation and anatomic location of the problem (Table 51-1). The normal developmental sequence of torsional problems follows a predictable course based on a child's age. Metatarsus adductus may be first noticed at birth or during early infancy and generally resolves by the first birthday. The newborn lateral (external) rotation contracture of the hips produces out-toeing during the latter part of the first year. In-toeing secondary to tibial torsion presents between 12 and 24 months and resolves by 3 to 4 years. Medial femoral torsion generally presents between 3 and 5 years of age, when the congenital lateral rotation contracture of the hips has resolved completely.

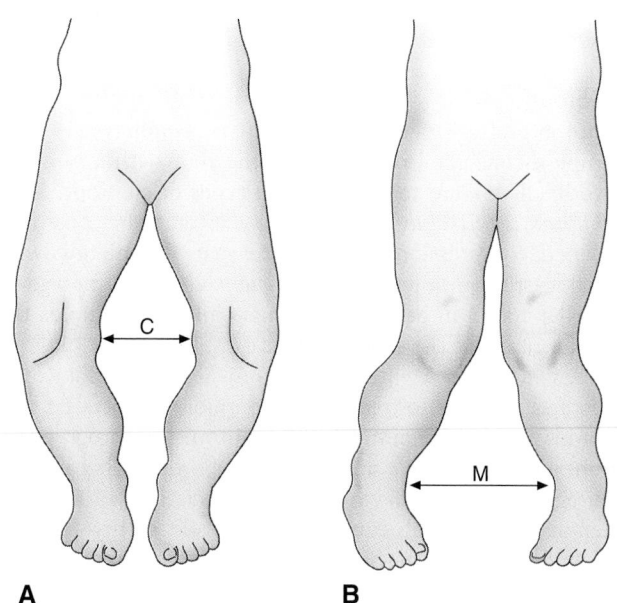

A   **B**

Figure 51-1. Comparison of bowleg deformity **(A)** with knock-knee deformity **(B)**. C, intercondular distance; M, intermalleolar distance.

Table 51-1. Age of Presentation and Location of Lower Limb Rotational Problems

Problem	Location	Age at Presentation	Description
In-Toeing			
Searching toe	Toe	Infancy	Big toe points medially
Clubfoot	Foot	Birth	Pathologic deformity
Metatarsus adductus	Foot	Birth/infancy	Forefoot angles toward midline
Metatarsus varus	Foot	Birth/infancy	Forefoot angles to midline and is inverted
Medial tibial torsion	Tibia	Toddler (12–24 mo)	Tibia rotated internally
Medial femoral torsion	Femur	Early childhood (3–5 yr)	Hip condition; entire leg internally rotated
Out-Toeing			
Physiologic out-toeing	Hips	Infancy	Feet turn outward with weight bearing
Lateral tibial torsion	Tibia	Childhood	Tibia rotated externally

Femoral torsion resolves slowly and may persist into adulthood.

Metatarsus adductus, medial tibial torsion, and newborn lateral rotation contracture of the hips all are related to intrauterine positioning. Sleeping in the prone position with the legs internally rotated may perpetuate internal tibial torsion or metatarsus adductus. A familial pattern of torsional abnormalities is noted frequently, with parents having the same rotational deformity (e.g., medial femoral torsion) as their children.

In the normal developmental sequence, internal (medial) rotation of the lower limb brings the big toe to the midline during the early intrauterine period. External (lateral) rotation occurs throughout the remainder of the intrauterine period, infancy, and childhood. Alterations in this normal lateral rotational process caused by either genetic or environmental factors (e.g., intrauterine molding) may lead to torsional problems.

In-Toeing

Searching Toe

The searching or adducted great toe is a dynamic deformity resulting from the relative overpull of the abductor hallucis muscle pulling the toe toward the midline during the stance phase of gait. In contrast to the other causes of in-toeing, which are structural and present at rest, this condition is observed only when the child is weight bearing.

Clubfoot

Clubfoot, also referred to as *talipes equinovarus*, is a complex congenital deformity of the foot with a range in severity. There are four recognized types of clubfoot. *Mild (deformational) clubfoot*, caused by intrauterine postural-induced compression, generally resolves completely with serial casting. *Idiopathic* or *classic clubfoot*, a polygenic disorder found in otherwise normal children, occupies the middle range of the severity spectrum. *Syndromic clubfoot* is seen in children with other anomalies and tends to be rigid and resistant to treatment. Commonly associated syndromes include amniotic band syndrome, arthrogryposis, prune-belly syndrome, and Möbius' syndrome. *Acquired or neurogenic clubfoot* may be seen in association with myelomeningocele, spinal tumors, poliomyelitis, myopathies, cerebral palsy, Guillain-Barré syndrome, or diastematomyelia.

Clubfoot occurs in about 1 in 1000 live births, has a male-to-female ratio of 2:1, and is bilateral in about 50% of cases. The diagnosis is made at birth based on the presence of forefoot varus, heel varus, and ankle equinus (Fig. 51-2). In severe clubfoot, the deformity is rigid, and the forefoot cannot be brought into a neutral position by passive abduction. In mild cases, the forefoot can be brought toward the midline with gentle pressure. Mild clubfoot may be confused with severe metatarsus varus or metatarsus adductus. The equinus component of clubfoot clearly differentiates it from these other two conditions.

The pathology of clubfoot includes abnormalities of cartilage and bone. The talus is most deformed, and the tarsal bones are hypoplastic. The bones are misaligned at the joints. Other notable changes include ligamentous thickening and muscle hypoplasia. These pathologic changes result in a generalized shortening of the leg on the affected side with hypoplasia of the calf muscles and a shortening of the foot.

Metatarsus Adductus and Metatarsus Varus

Metatarsus adductus and metatarsus varus are foot deformities, characterized by a medial deviation of the forefoot. Some authors do not differentiate between the two conditions and instead prefer to describe metatarsus adductus as a spectrum of foot deformities of varying degrees. Both conditions can be bilateral or unilateral. The incidence of metatarsus adductus and metatarsus varus is about 1 to 2 per 1000 live births, with metatarsus varus constituting 10% of cases in the spectrum of deformities. Because these conditions are thought to be secondary to intrauterine crowding, infants with these foot deformities should be examined for other molding disorders, such as neck torticollis and hip dysplasia (seen in 2% to 10% of cases).

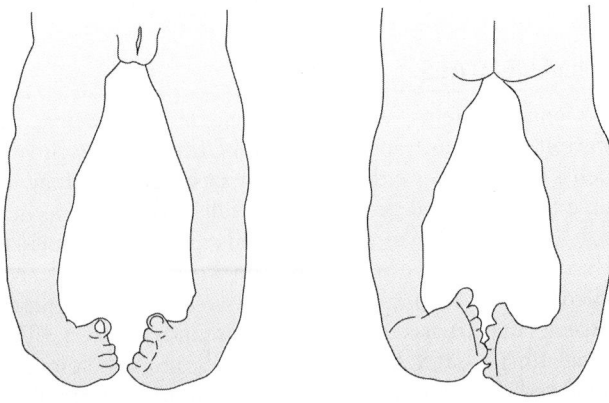

Figure 51-2. Clubfoot deformity.

Metatarsus adductus is a functional deformity in which the forefoot is adducted with respect to the hindfoot (Fig. 51-3*A*). The forefoot can be brought into a neutral position either by gently straightening it or by stroking the lateral border of the foot. In metatarsus varus, the forefoot is inverted and adducted with respect to the hindfoot (Fig. 51-3*B*). It is a bony abnormality caused by the subluxation of the tarsometatarsal joint with adduction of the metatarsals. Metatarsus varus is a fixed deformity, and the foot cannot be brought into the neutral position. On examination, the medial border of the foot is concave, there is convexity of the lateral border, and there is a prominence of the base of the fifth metatarsal. A deep crease may be noted along the plantar surface of the tarsometatarsal joints. Severe forms of metatarsus varus can be differentiated from clubfoot by normal dorsiflexion of the ankle.

Medial Tibial Torsion

Medial tibial torsion, a molding disorder secondary to intrauterine crowding, generally is first noticed by parents when children begin to walk. This condition, which is often bilateral, is the primary cause of in-toeing during the second year of life. Observation of gait reveals that as the child walks, the feet turn inward, but the knees point straight. The site of the rotational deformity can be isolated to the lower leg, if the feet are normal and no metatarsus adductus or metatarsus varus is present.

Medial Femoral Torsion

Medial femoral torsion usually is first evident at about 3 to 4 years of age, is most severe between 4 and 6 years of age, and then gradually resolves. This condition may have been present at birth, but generally is not noted until age 3 to 4 years because it has been masked by the lateral rotatory forces of infancy. Medial femoral torsion is the primary cause of in-toeing during early childhood. Children with this condition stand with the knees medially rotated ("kissing patella") and can sit in the W position with both legs behind them (Fig. 51-4). The knees and the feet appear to turn inward when children stand or walk.

Femoral anteversion describes the forward placement of the femoral head with respect to the femoral shaft. In adults, the normal angle of anteversion is about 10 to 15 degrees. In some children, muscle balance or familial tendencies lead to a wider angle than normal (femoral antetorsion). Conceptually, when a child with this condition lies on his or her back, the torsion causes the femoral head to protrude instead of lie flat within the acetabulum. The presence of medial femoral torsion causes the entire leg distal to the hip joint to turn inward when the femoral head articulates normally with the acetabulum.

Out-Toeing
Physiologic Out-Toeing of Infancy

Physiologic out-toeing of infancy classically is seen during the second half of the first year of life in infants who are learning to walk. Both feet appear to turn outward when the child is held in a standing position. This condition is believed to be secondary to a lateral rotation contracture about the hips as a result of intrauterine positioning. Sleeping in the prone, frog-leg position, which does not allow for stretching of the external rotators of the hips, may perpetuate this condition.

Lateral Tibial Torsion

Out-toeing that presents in children who are 3 to 5 years old may be due to lateral tibial torsion. Approximately 5 degrees of out-toeing is normal after age 3 years. Because the tibia normally rotates laterally with time, this condition may become more severe with age. Malalignment between the knee and the direction of gait may produce knee pain.

Angular Deformities

The most common angular deformities of the lower extremities, bowlegs and knock-knees, are generally variations of normal that resolve with time. As the angular alignment at the knees changes with age, relative bowing of the legs normally progresses to knock-knees and eventually straight legs. Appreciation of the normal developmental sequence of angular deformities and knowledge of pathologic causes of genu varum and genu valgum allow the primary care physician to identify pathologic cases in a timely manner and initiate prompt treatment (Table 51-2).

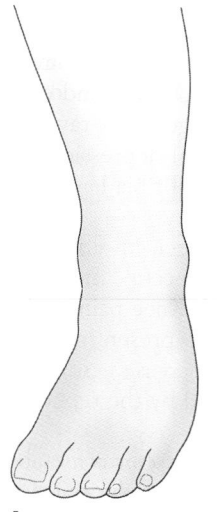
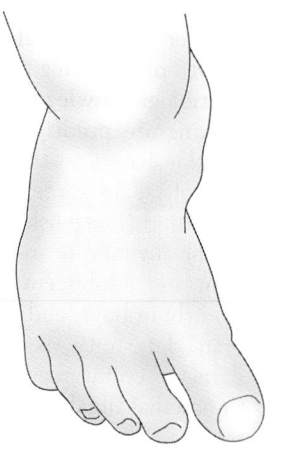
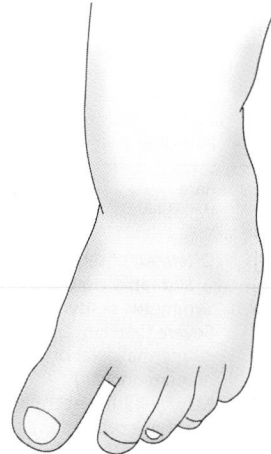

Figure 51-3. A, Metatarsus adductus. **B,** Metatarsus varus.

A   **B**

52 Disorders of the Hip

Alan K. Stotts

ROLE OF THE GENERALIST

1   Be proficient in the examination of the child's hip.
2   Recognize and diagnose instability of the child's hip.
3   Diagnose and treat transient synovitis of the hip.
4   Evaluate and diagnose a child with a painful hip.
5   Recognize and diagnose Legg-Calvé-Perthes disease.
6   Recognize and diagnose slipped capital femoral epiphysis.
7   Refer for specialist care when assistance is needed for diagnosis, treatment, or management of hip disorders in children.

The child's hip is a frequent source of concern for the physician and the patient or family. The term *hip* usually refers to the proximal femur, the acetabulum, and the articulation, or joint, between the bones. Because the development of the hip is crucial to the long-term functioning of the joint, every effort should be made to diagnose pathologic conditions early and institute appropriate care. Although genetics and certain medical conditions of the patient can affect the hip, normal development of the femoral head and acetabulum depends on the presence of a well-reduced joint such that the acetabulum can shape itself around the spherical head. One of the most distinguishing features of the hip in a child is the growth potential of the hip to shape itself in response to this articulation. The growth plates that allow this adaptive change also can be the source of problems in the hip through growth arrest or slippage with injury to the plates. The circulation of blood to the femoral head in an immature patient differs from that of an adult and is susceptible to disruption at the level of the growth plate. Disruption of the blood supply results in osseous necrosis of the head. With care in diagnosis and management, many of the long-term problems of the hip can be avoided.

DEVELOPMENTAL DYSPLASIA OF THE HIP

Previously called *congenital dysplasia of the hip*, the term *developmental dysplasia of the hip* (DDH) now is preferred to acknowledge that the condition is not consistently present at birth and may present later in life. *Teratologic* hip problems—those associated with a disorder that affects the musculoskeletal system, such as arthrogryposis—are difficult to treat.

DDH represents a broad spectrum of pathology in the hip ranging from subtle bony changes seen on x-ray to instability of the joint and even complete dislocation. Approximately 1% of all children have some degree of instability on newborn examination. The cause of DDH is multifactorial. Box 52-1 lists risk factors for developing DDH. Incidence varies with ethnic background, with Native Americans and Lapps having the highest incidence (25 to 50 per 1000 births) and African and Chinese populations having a much lower incidence. Postnatal care is a contributor because populations that swaddle children with the legs together and the hips extended place the hips into potentially unstable positions. The higher incidence in females is believed to be due to muscle and ligamentous relaxation from hormonal stimulation. Risk from breech presentation is secondary to the extreme flexion position adopted by the joint. Approximately 20% of DDH cases have a history of breech presentation. Factors such as oligohydramnios decrease fetal movements and cause "packing disorders," giving rise to common associations between DDH and torticollis and metatarsus adductus. The presence of either of these latter two disorders should raise concern about DDH.

Diagnosis

Screening all infants for hip instability on newborn physical examination is essential. Accurate examination requires that the infant be relaxed. Use of a bottle-feeding or pacifier during examination may help. The child's diaper should be opened to allow inspection of the skin and a comparison of the skinfolds present in either thigh. Asymmetry in the number of creases between the sides may indicate a shortened thigh with dislocation of the hip, which would

---

Box 52-1. Risk Factors for Developmental Dysplasia of the Hip

- Breech presentation
- Female gender
- Primigravid mother
- Positive family history
- Ethnicity (especially Native American or Lapp)
- Oligohydramnios
- Lower limb malformation
- Concomitant disorders (e.g., arthrogryposis)

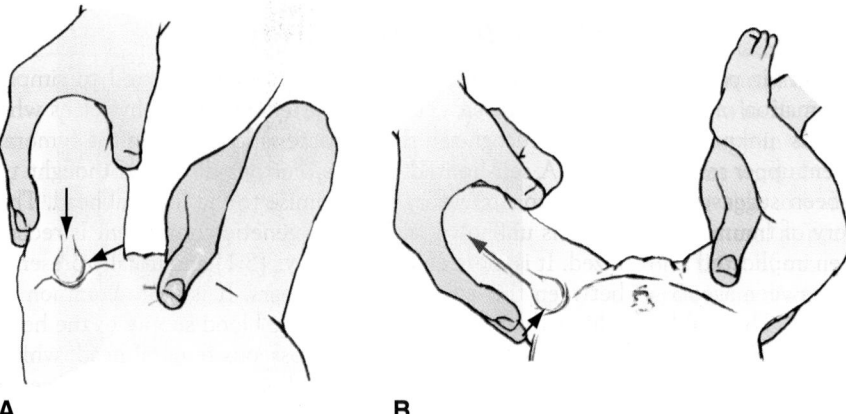

A   **B**

Figure 52-1. Barlow and Ortolani maneuvers. **A,** Barlow maneuver. With the left hand stabilizing the child's buttocks and pelvis, the right hand is used to examine the left hip by gently holding the child's flexed left knee and adducting the thigh with the hip flexed to 90 degrees, while gently pushing posteriorly along the thigh. **B,** Ortolani maneuver. The thumb rests on the medial aspect of the thigh, and the long finger is positioned laterally over the greater trochanter. The thigh is abducted gently as slight traction is placed on the thigh, and the examiner uses the long finger to press and lift the trochanter medially toward the acetabulum.

result in additional skinfolds on the affected side. This finding is not consistent and should serve only to alert the examiner to the possibility of underlying problems. The thighs are held gently and the hips are flexed to 90 degrees to note any difference in length between them, looking again for shortening on one side (a positive Galeazzi sign). The thighs are abducted at the same time, and the abduction should be symmetric. Normally an infant has wide abduction with the hips flexed. A restriction of abduction, especially in an older child, may be the clearest sign of a hip dislocation that is fixed in the dislocated position such that it no longer feels unstable.

Two specific maneuvers, the Barlow and the Ortolani maneuvers, for instability testing should be performed. Figure 52-1A illustrates the Barlow maneuver, which is an attempt to subluxate or dislocate the hip. The examiner feels the hip shift out of the acetabulum if the hip is unstable. It may be easier to feel the shift if the examiner extends his or her middle finger along the thigh and rests the tip at the level of the greater trochanter. There is commonly a "click" present in the newborn examination that represents soft tissue passing over a bony prominence, such as the greater trochanter, or bony movement at the knee and is not indicative of hip pathology. This click is to be distinguished from the true feeling of the bones moving past one another, which has been described as a "clunk."

The second test, the Ortolani maneuver, is an attempt to relocate a dislocated hip. The examiner's hand position changes only subtly (see Fig. 52-1B). The examiner is feeling for the shift of the hip as the femoral head is relocated, which would indicate a dislocated hip that is reducible. Commonly, when a positive test is felt for the first time, the examiner is surprised by the lack of force on the child's thigh required to produce the shift. The feeling of both of these maneuvers is quite characteristic when the hip does shift, and clinicians who perform newborn examinations are encouraged to seek out "positive" examinations to learn this.

Plain radiographs are unreliable in a newborn because of the lack of ossified bone. Ultrasonography performed by an experienced person frequently is helpful for patients whose examinations are unclear or to define hip anatomy more clearly. The sonographer also can perform the Ortolani and Barlow maneuvers while directly observing the hip joint in real time. Anteroposterior x-ray of the pelvis should be obtained in infants older than 3 to 4 months with a suspected pathologic condition. Film measurements may be helpful in evaluating the hips in the infant (Fig. 52-2).

Management

Infants with an abnormal physical examination or imaging studies should be referred to a pediatric orthopedist for follow-up and management. Common treatment of instability in infants includes use of the Pavlik harness, which attempts to hold the hip in a reduced position while the tissues tighten around the joint. Occasionally the joint must be reduced manually under an anesthetic and then the infant is casted. Surgery may be employed for hips that are difficult to reduce or are too unstable to be held in a cast. The development of the hip is monitored with growth, and additional procedures, such as osteotomies, are performed, if needed, to optimize outcome by maintaining reduction of the hip so that the femur and acetabulum can develop together. Long-term follow-up of children who have been treated is essential to ensure that the joint forms normally. Early detection and initiation of treatment for children with hip disorders improves the possible outcome.

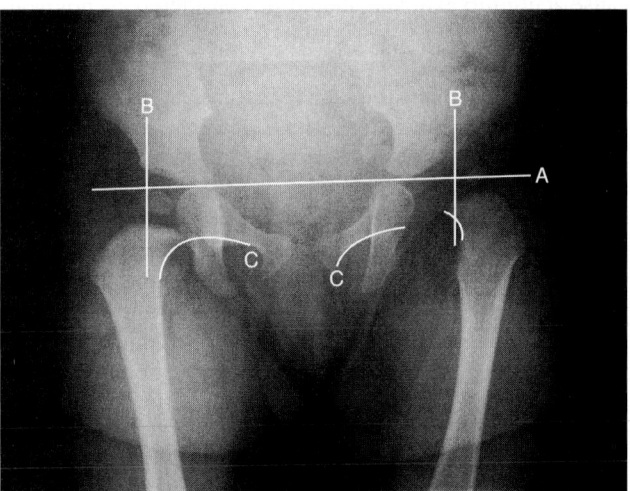

Figure 52-2. Left hip dislocation seen on x-ray compared with normal right side. The femoral head is smaller on the left. The head lies above the horizontal line (A) drawn between the triradiate cartilages and lateral to the vertical line (B) drawn from the lateral aspect of the acetabulum. The curvilinear line (C) around the inferior pubis should be continuous with the inferior neck of the femur as it is on the right.

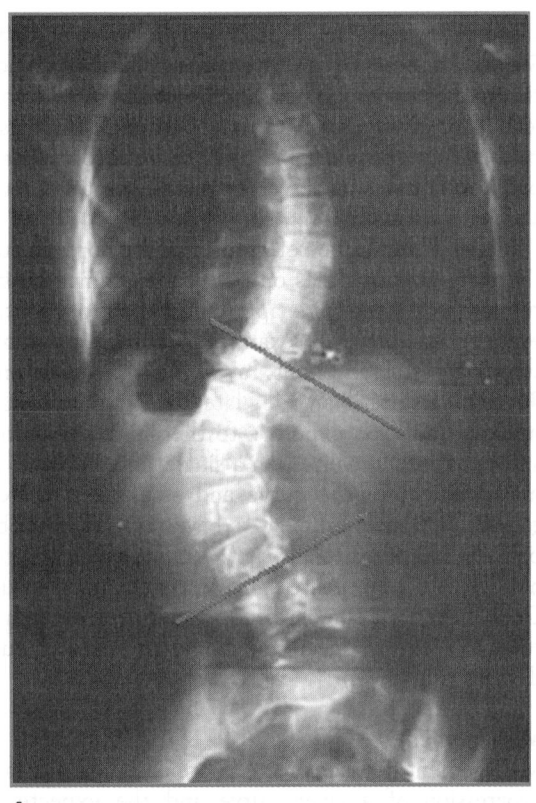

A

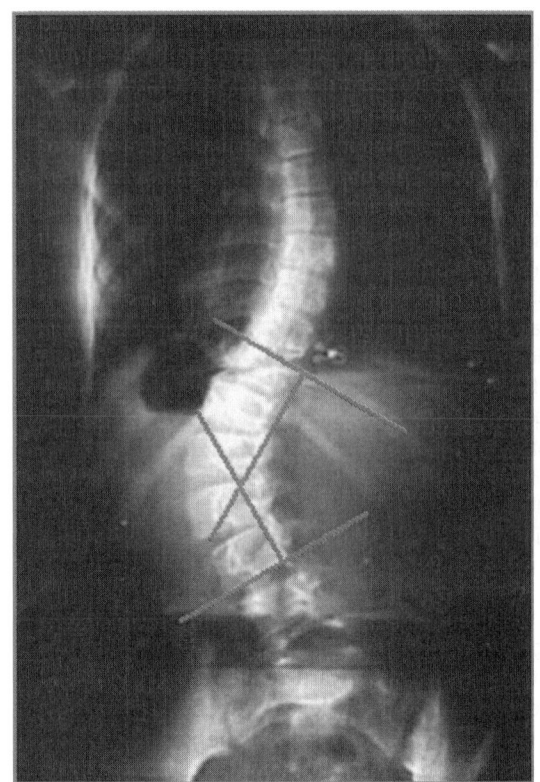

B

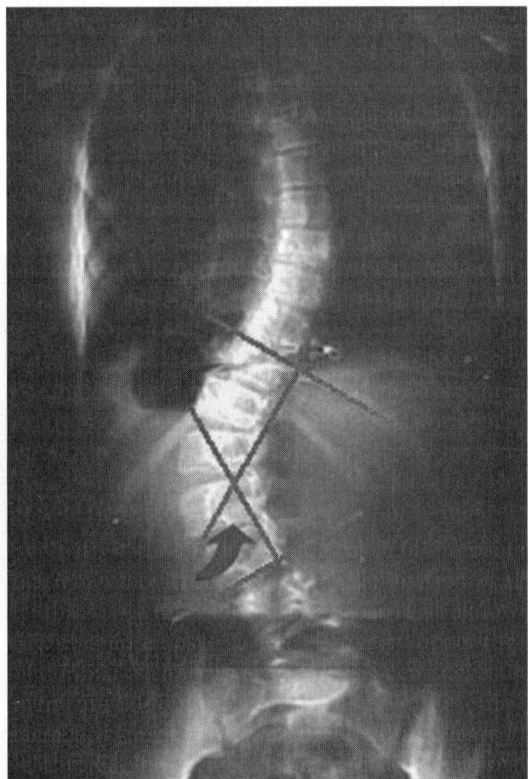

C

Figure 53-2. A–C, Cobb method of measuring scoliosis.

presenting before menses, thoracic curves, and female gender. A rapidly progressing curve can change 1 to 2 degrees per month during the adolescent growth spurt. Curves of less than 30 degrees at the completion of growth are unlikely to progress during adulthood and are not associated with back pain or physical deformity. Curves greater than 50 degrees at skeletal maturity tend to progress in adulthood at a rate of 1 to 2 degrees per year. Curves greater than 80 degrees often are painful later in life and have adverse effects on pulmonary and cardiac function.

Observation, bracing, and surgery are three accepted methods of treating scoliosis. Observation is appropriate for curves less than 20 degrees before the end of growth or for curves less than 50 degrees after skeletal maturity. Bracing is a means to stop curve progression and is indicated for curves between 20 and 40 degrees when there is still growth remaining. A brace cannot "correct" the curve; however, by preventing further progression of the curve, it is possible to alter the natural history of a given curve and avoid the need for surgery. Studies indicate that bracing is effective at stopping curve progression in 70% to 80% of curves during growth.

Surgery is indicated for curves greater than 40 to 50 degrees, in which progression after skeletal maturity is expected. The goal of surgery is to prevent further progression of the curve, preserve a physiologic balance to the spine, and improve the cosmetic appearance of the back. Modern surgical techniques allow the surgeon to obtain significant correction of the curve (Fig. 53-3).

Idiopathic scoliosis also has infantile and juvenile forms. Infantile idiopathic scoliosis presents before age 3, is rare, but can be aggressive in terms of severity and progression. All children with infantile scoliosis require a complete evaluation, with attention focused on detecting associated anomalies of the spine and spinal cord and cardiac and genitourinary anomalies. All children with spinal deformities should be referred to a specialist with expertise in pediatric spinal deformity for this evaluation. Many children with infantile scoliosis require either bracing or surgery.

The diagnosis of juvenile idiopathic scoliosis is made when curves present between the ages of 3 and 10 years. The cause is unknown, but the prognosis is poor because these children have a tremendous amount of growth remaining. The management principles are similar to those for AIS.

Congenital Scoliosis

Congenital scoliosis is defined as a curvature of the spine that results from malformations of the vertebral elements. The elements of the spinal cord and vertebral structures develop in unison between 3 and 6 weeks of gestation. Given the complexity of embryologic development, it is miraculous that congenital vertebral malformations are relatively rare. Congenital vertebral anomalies commonly are associated with malformations of other structures that are developing concurrently, such as the genitourinary tract, heart, cervical spine, and spinal cord. The overall incidence of associated anomalies has been reported to be 61%. Malformations of the spinal cord also are common and should be sought if there is any suggestion of spinal dysraphism (dimples, hairy patches, pain, or spasticity in the lower extremities).

Evaluation of a child with suspected congenital scoliosis begins with a thorough search for associated congenital anomalies. Anteroposterior and lateral radiographs of the entire spine confirm the diagnosis of congenital scoliosis. Radiographs allow for classification of the type and severity of the congenital vertebral malformations and provide a basis for long-term prognosis and prediction of progression of the deformity. Renal ultrasound is recommended as part of the routine screening assessment if congenital scoliosis has been confirmed. Magnetic resonance imaging of the spinal cord may be indicated if spinal dysraphism is suspected or if there is unexplained rapid progression of the curve.

Congenital scoliosis can be classified into three groups: failure of formation, failure of segmentation, and a combination of these defects. The most common failure of formation is a hemivertebra. Hemivertebrae produce a growth imbalance in the spine and result in secondary curvature. Failures of segmentation include block vertebra and unilateral bars, which produce a growth tether of the spine. Finally, when these conditions occur in combination, such as a hemivertebra on one side and a bar on the other, curves can progress in an aggressive manner.

Treatment of congenital scoliosis is based on the prediction of the potential abnormal growth associated with a particular pattern of malformation. An isolated hemivertebra in the midportion of the spine has a low potential for significant progression with growth, whereas a hemivertebra with a contralateral bar progresses aggressively at an early age. Each pattern of malformation is unique, and the treatment plan should be based on the risk of curve progression during growth.

Treatment options in congenital scoliosis include observation, bracing, and surgery. The goals of treatment are to allow the child to reach the end of growth with a reasonably straight, balanced spine and to preserve as much trunk height as possible. For younger children, chest cavity growth and development that allows for increase in lung size increasingly is recognized as an important consideration in the overall treatment plan. The outcome of a short but straight spine is questioned in the current management of congenital scoliosis. Newer techniques and hardware are being developed that allow for gradual correction of the curvature without early spinal fusion.

Observation is appropriate for small curves and balanced patterns of malformations. Bracing rarely is valuable in congenital scoliosis. Bracing secondary curves that result from the congenital malformation sometimes is useful, but primary congenital curves do not respond to bracing. The role of surgery is to attempt to maintain spinal balance, while preserving as much trunk height as possible during growth. Surgical procedures must be individualized and should be attempted only by surgeons with experience in the management of congenital spinal deformities.

Neuromuscular Scoliosis

The term *neuromuscular scoliosis* is used to describe curvature of the spine in children with any disorder of the neurologic system. Common categories include cerebral palsy, spina bifida, muscular dystrophies, and traumatic injury to the spine. Most affected children have truncal

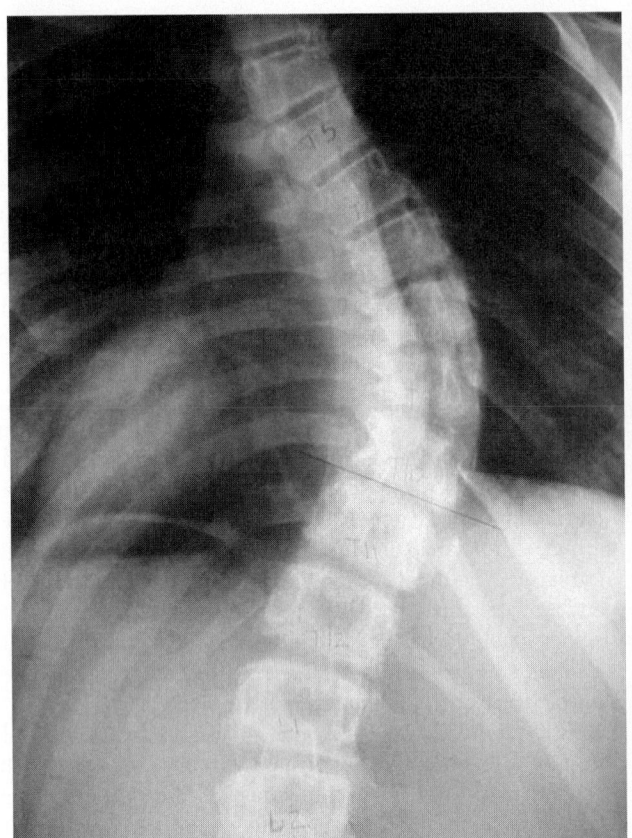

A

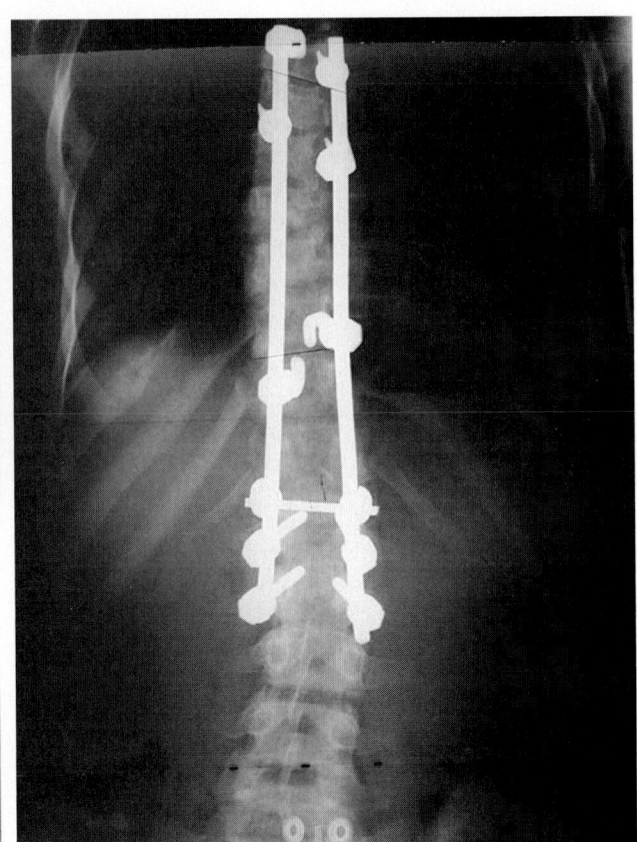

B

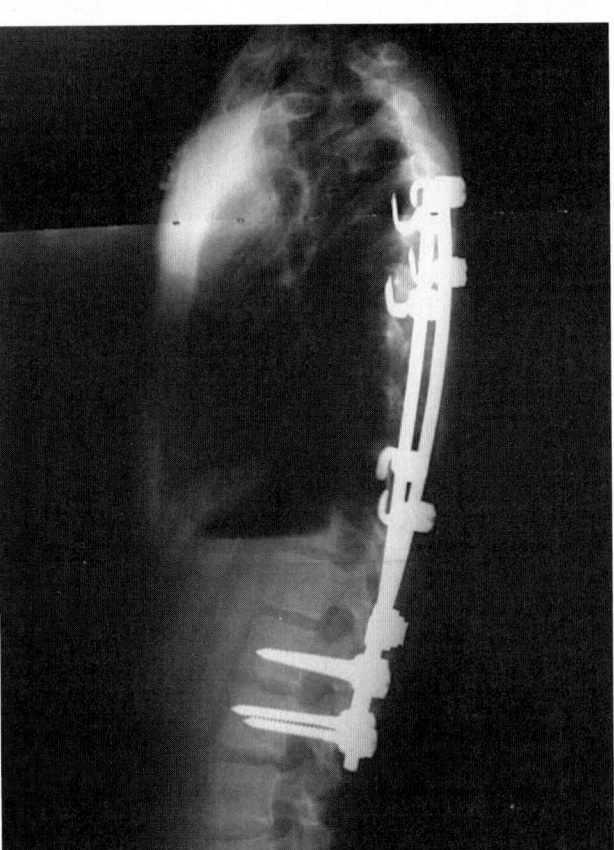

C

Figure 53-3. **A–C,** Surgical correction of adolescent idiopathic scoliosis.

weakness. As they grow and the truncal weakness increases, the spine progressively collapses, producing a long, c-type curve. These curves progress, with the rate of progression accelerating during growth. For children confined to a wheelchair, progressive curves may affect the child's ability to sit comfortably, affecting the quality of life and function.

The treatment of neuromuscular scoliosis must be individualized. Bracing may provide support for the trunk in the seated position, but usually does not stop progression of the curve over time. Seating modifications, such as inserts into wheelchairs, may help with positioning the child, but also do not correct the scoliosis. Alternative therapies, such as insertion of an intrathecal baclofen pump, produce a reduction in spasticity but do not affect the long-term progression of scoliosis. Injection of botulinum toxin (Botox) into the paraspinal musculature temporarily reduces the tone in these muscles but has no proven long-term efficacy in the treatment of neuromuscular curves.

A fundamental question to be addressed by the family and physician is whether preservation of functional seating posture by invasive surgery would maintain or improve the child's quality of life and function. For children with cognitive or visual/sensory impairment, these decisions are particularly difficult because the children may not understand the surgery and the pain accompanying the procedure.

KYPHOSIS

Kyphosis is a curvature of the spine when viewed from the side or sagittal plane that is normal in the thoracic spine when the kyphosis is between 20 and 50 degrees. Kyphosis greater than 50 degrees is abnormal and may present as "poor posture." Parents are concerned that despite their persistent reminders, their child will not stand up straight.

Evaluation of kyphosis begins by viewing the child from the side. There are no clear visual clues that distinguish normal from abnormal kyphosis. The clinician's intuition is usually the best indicator for when the amount of kyphosis is abnormal. The kyphosis may be accentuated with forward bending. The patient should be examined carefully for concomitant scoliosis and other spinal anomalies. If excessive kyphosis is suspected, x-rays are required to measure the degree of kyphosis. The x-ray should be taken in the standing position and should include posteroanterior and lateral views using a single 36-inch cassette to allow for accurate measurement of the degree of kyphosis and the sagittal balance.

The two most common forms of kyphosis encountered in adolescents are Scheuermann's kyphosis and postural roundback. Scheuermann's kyphosis, most commonly found in adolescent boys, is characterized by a short, sharp kyphosis in the midthoracic spine and may be associated with aching back pain (Fig. 53-4). Kyphosis tends to be rigid on clinical examination. Radiographic criteria to establish a diagnosis of Scheuermann's kyphosis are a curve greater than 50 degrees, irregularity of the vertebral end plates, and wedging of three consecutive vertebrae of greater than 5 degrees. The curves occur over a short number of vertebral segments and are typically in the thoracic spine. A mild degree of scoliosis is common in adolescents with Scheuermann's kyphosis.

Postural roundback is characterized by a smooth, flexible kyphosis and is not typically associated with pain. The curve is corrected easily by asking the child to stand up straight. Radiographically the criteria for the diagnosis of postural roundback are kyphosis greater than 50 degrees, but *without* vertebral end plate irregularity and wedging. These curves tend to be mild in severity and extend over a longer number of vertebral segments compared with Scheuermann's kyphosis.

Treatment decisions regarding kyphosis are based on the expected natural history, the degree of deformity, the risk of progression during and after growth, and the severity of symptoms associated with the kyphosis. Treatment options for kyphosis include observation, bracing, and surgery.

Kyphosis of less than 50 degrees requires no treatment. If there is significant growth remaining or persistent back pain, kyphosis of 50 to 75 degrees may be managed in a brace. Kyphosis bracing is technically difficult. The brace must be custom made to fit the child properly and requires a three-point bend to achieve correction of the curve while wearing the brace. In contrast to scoliosis bracing, kyphosis bracing may produce sustainable correction of the curve if worn consistently during growth.

Surgery is reserved for curves greater than 75 degrees, when there is concern that there will be gradual progression after the completion of growth or if there is progressive loss of bone mass in late adult life. Surgical treatment consists of a correction of the deformity using spinal instrumentation and fusion of the involved portion of the spine to prevent progression later in life.

BACK PAIN IN CHILDREN AND YOUNG ADULTS

Back pain is much less common in children and young adults than in adults older than age 25. Approximately one in five children has back pain at some point during their childhood and early adult years. The causes of back pain in children are different from the causes in adults. Nearly 50% of children who see a physician for back pain have a medically definable cause of the pain. In contrast, most adults have more general disorders, such as back strain or overuse syndrome. Accordingly, significant back pain in children and young adults requires a careful, systematic evaluation by a physician.

The common causes of back pain in children tend to be age specific. In children younger than 10 years old, infections of the intervertebral disks and abnormal growths or tumors in the spine are the most common causes of pain. In children older than age 10, a developmental abnormality in the bones of the lower lumbar spine, such as spondylolysis or spondylolisthesis, can cause low back pain, whereas Scheuermann's disease is a likely cause of back pain in a child who has kyphosis. In addition, nonmusculoskeletal problems, such as renal disease, peptic ulcer disease, and pancreatitis, can present with back pain.

Every child with back pain requires a careful and complete evaluation. The evaluation begins with a thorough medical history and physical examination. Significant back pain should be evaluated further with an x-ray of the spine. If the diagnosis remains unclear, technetium bone scan, computed tomography scan, and magnetic resonance

CRP are most useful as tools to follow a child's response to therapy. Continued elevation of either ESR or CRP often indicates a complicated course. Blood cultures should be obtained and are positive in 30% to 40% of cases of septic arthritis and 35% to 75% of osteomyelitis.

Etiologic diagnosis usually is obtained with bone biopsy (osteomyelitis) or arthrocentesis (septic arthritis). Arthrocentesis often is required to diagnose septic arthritis definitively. Synovial fluid should be cultured and examined for white blood cell count and differential, glucose and protein concentration, pH and Gram stain. A white blood cell count of 25,000 to 250,000 cells/mL (with a polymorphonuclear cell predominance of around 90%) and a low synovial-to-serum glucose ratio usually are found. Synovial fluid cultures are positive in about 50% to 60% of cases with septic arthritis.

Radiologic examinations often are helpful in confirming the diagnosis of septic arthritis or osteomyelitis. In osteomyelitis, the earliest findings (within 5 to 7 days) may be deep soft tissue swelling or loss of an adjacent fat pad. More pronounced radiographic changes of osteomyelitis typically do not appear until at least 7 to 14 days from the onset of symptoms. These changes may include lytic lesions, periosteal elevation, new bone formation, or osteoporosis. When plain radiographs do not clarify the diagnosis, ultrasonography or a technetium bone scan can be helpful. Ultrasonography is less expensive, it is most often readily accessible, and it can be performed as a bedside procedure. Ultrasound findings suggesting osteomyelitis are (1) a thickening of the periosteum with hypoechoic areas superficial and deep to it, creating a "sandwich" appearance; (2) subperiosteal elevation greater than 2 mm indicating subperiosteal pus; and (3) swelling of overlying tissues occasionally with altered echogenicity. These changes often can be appreciated 24 hours after the onset of symptoms. Ultrasonography is useful in distinguishing infection from vaso-occlusive disease in children with sickle cell disease. Ultrasonography is limited, however, because its accuracy is operator dependent. A standard technetium bone scan follows intravenous administration of the radionucleotide that preferentially is taken up by osteoclasts in the bone marrow. In the first minutes after administration, increased blood flow can be detected. Two to 5 hours later, areas of increased ("hot spot") or decreased ("cold spot") bone uptake are seen with osteomyelitis in greater than 90% of cases. This test may be positive at presentation, in contrast to plain radiographs.

Computed tomography and magnetic resonance imaging (MRI) increasingly have been used to diagnose osteomyelitis. MRI probably is most useful in delineating the extent of infection when cellulitis cannot be differentiated clinically from osteomyelitis or septic arthritis. MRI often is helpful in the context of infection after a traumatic injury, when the extent of disease is unclear. Computed tomography scans are better than MRI in detecting sequestra and showing intraosseous gas in cases of complicated osteomyelitis.

Findings on plain radiographs in septic arthritis include joint space widening, soft tissue swelling with obliteration of normal fat planes, and effusion of the joint. Ultrasonography is most useful in excluding septic arthritis when fluid in the joint space cannot be shown. Bone scan can help to delineate septic arthritis from osteomyelitis or determine the exact location of bone or joint involvement when it is unclear. Uptake is increased in the area surrounding the joint during the vascular phase, but the bone is spared on delayed images.

Osteomyelitis and septic arthritis are different in newborns. Early signs and symptoms may be subtle. Neonates may have no localized findings and simply may be irritable with minimal or no fever. Decreased use or an asymmetric positioning of the involved extremity may be noted. Differentiation between septic arthritis and osteomyelitis is difficult in this age group. Neonates with osteomyelitis may have rapid extension of the infection and present with generalized symptoms (e.g., fever, irritability, and possible toxic appearance) with significant involvement of the bone. Surrounding structures may be swollen, red, and tender to palpation with severe limitation in movement (pseudoparalysis). In contrast to older children, neonates are more likely to have more than one bone or joint involved. Bone scan in this age group is insensitive but informative if positive.

In all age groups, the differential diagnosis of acute localized bone pain includes osteomyelitis, septic arthritis, trauma, cellulitis, toxic synovitis, reactive arthritis, malignancy, collagen vascular disease, acute rheumatic disease, thrombophlebitis, and bone infarction. Other specific conditions also must be considered depending on the age of the patient and the location of the involved joint. In the case of the hip, Legg-Calvé-Perthes disease, slipped capital femoral ephiphysis, psoas abscess, diskitis, and vertebral osteomyelitis should be excluded.

Toxic synovitis is a transient inflammation of a joint and is the most common cause of hip pain in children. It typically affects children 4 to 10 years old and is twice as common in boys. Most children with toxic synovitis report an antecedent upper respiratory tract infection and present with leg pain and limp with limitation on internal rotation of the hip. Most children have a modestly elevated temperature, white blood cell count, and ESR and a normal plain film, but some may show a small effusion. If septic arthritis cannot be excluded, a joint aspirate for synovial fluid examination and Gram stain and culture is imperative. Toxic synovitis is a self-limiting condition, and children typically recover without sequelae within a few days.

Reactive arthritis is inflammation at one or more joints that is distant from the site of infection and occurs 1 to 3 weeks after the inciting infection. Reactive arthritis has been associated with previous gastrointestinal infections (*Salmonella, Shigella, Campylobacter,* or *Yersinia*), sexually transmitted infections, and group A streptococcal infections. Synovial fluid examination may be similar to septic arthritis, but cultures are sterile. Therapy is primarily supportive. If the precipitating infection has not been treated adequately, appropriate antimicrobial therapy should be initiated targeting the inciting infection.

MANAGEMENT

The therapeutic goal in the management of children with osteomyelitis and septic arthritis is to prevent the development of long-term sequelae. Treatment should be initiated quickly, always includes antibiotics, and may require a drainage procedure. Reasonable attempts to obtain cultures from the blood and at the site of infection should be pursued (fluoroscopically or sonographically guided arthrocentesis). Empirical antibiotic therapy should be begun when the clinical findings are clear.

Management of children with uncomplicated skeletal infections may involve collaboration between the pediatrician, orthopedic surgeon, and infectious disease specialist. Management of children with complicated disease always should include subspecialty input. Empirical antibiotics should be initiated as soon as possible. The choice of antibiotic agent should be based on the most likely etiologic organisms. Table 54-4 lists examples of initial antibiotic choices. In acute hematogenous osteomyelitis in otherwise healthy children, most frequently the etiologic agent is S. aureus. For osteomyelitis, surgical intervention usually is needed only in instances of a course complicated by persistent fevers despite appropriate antibiotics, persistent pain, radiologic evidence of involucrum or sequestrum formation, or persistently elevated markers of inflammation (ESR or CRP). Septic arthritis involving the hip is a surgical emergency. Early drainage often is needed to minimize potential compromise of the vascular supply to the femoral head. The need for and method of surgical intervention of infections that involve other skeletal areas are variable. Arthrocentesis may be necessary to evaluate synovial fluid to differentiate between septic arthritis and toxic synovitis. In septic arthritis, some surgeons defer open drainage of a joint by performing daily aspirations. If fluid persists in the joint space after 4 to 5 days, open drainage must be considered.

Duration of antimicrobial therapy needs to be tailored individually, based on the patient's clinical history, site and extent of infection, response to prior therapy, etiologic organism (when known), age, and social support systems. Skeletal infections traditionally have been treated with a prolonged course of antibiotics. Most physicians initiate therapy with intravenous antibiotics. S. aureus osteomyelitis typically requires at least 3 weeks of antibiotic therapy to minimize the risk of recurrent or chronic infection. A combination of intravenous and oral therapy may be considered, but compliance with therapy and follow-up must be ensured. Oral therapy typically requires higher than standard dosing to achieve sufficient antibiotic levels in the bone. In the neonate, prolonged intravenous antimicrobial therapy is the rule. In this instance, care should be managed by the primary care provider with specialty consultation.

OUTCOME

Although most children recover without significant sequelae if appropriately managed, it may take several months to years before sequelae are recognized clinically. The complication rate or frequency of long-term sequelae after hematogenous osteomyelitis is approximately 4% to 10%. Complications may be due to inadequate therapy or the disease process itself and include persistent (chronic) infection, sequestrum formation (dead bone), involucrum, relapse of infection, limb-length discrepancy, gait abnormalities, and scoliosis. Certain clinical features and laboratory findings early in the course of osteomyelitis may predict an increased risk of complications, including persistent fever, swelling and erythema, and pain or restriction of mobility for more than 7 to 10 days; the need for more than one surgical drainage procedure; involvement of more than one focus; sepsis; and persistently elevated CRP after 5 to 7 days of therapy.

FOLLOW-UP

Besides routine pediatric care, patients with a history of osteomyelitis and septic arthritis should be followed closely for gait abnormalities and possible leg-length discrepancy. Any potential problems should be referred to a pediatric orthopedic specialist. As previously mentioned, sequelae may take years to develop, and families should be informed of the potential need for long-term evaluations.

Mini-index of Related Topics

SUGGESTED READINGS

Krogstad P: Osteomyelitis and septic arthritis. In Feigin RD, Cherry JD, Demmler GJ, Kaplan SL (eds): Textbook of Pediatric Infectious Diseases, 5th ed. Philadelphia, WB Saunders, 2004, pp 713–736.

Maxson S, Darville T: Acute hematogenous long-bone osteomyelitis. Semin Pediatr Infect Dis 1997;8:220–233.

Trujillo M, Nelson JD: Suppurative and reactive arthritis in children. Semin Pediatr Infect Dis 1997;8:242–249.

Table 54-4. Suggested Empirical Antibiotic Choices for Osteomyelitis

Patient Factors	Empirical Choices*
Neonate	Nafcillin/oxacillin + gentamicin
Child, normal host	Nafcillin/oxacillin or cefazolin
Child with sickle cell disease	Nafcillin/oxacillin + cefotaxime
Child on chemotherapy	Nafcillin/oxacillin + ceftazidime

*If methicillin-resistant Staphylococcus aureus is suspected, vancomycin, clindamycin, or trimethoprim/sulfamethoxazole should be considered.

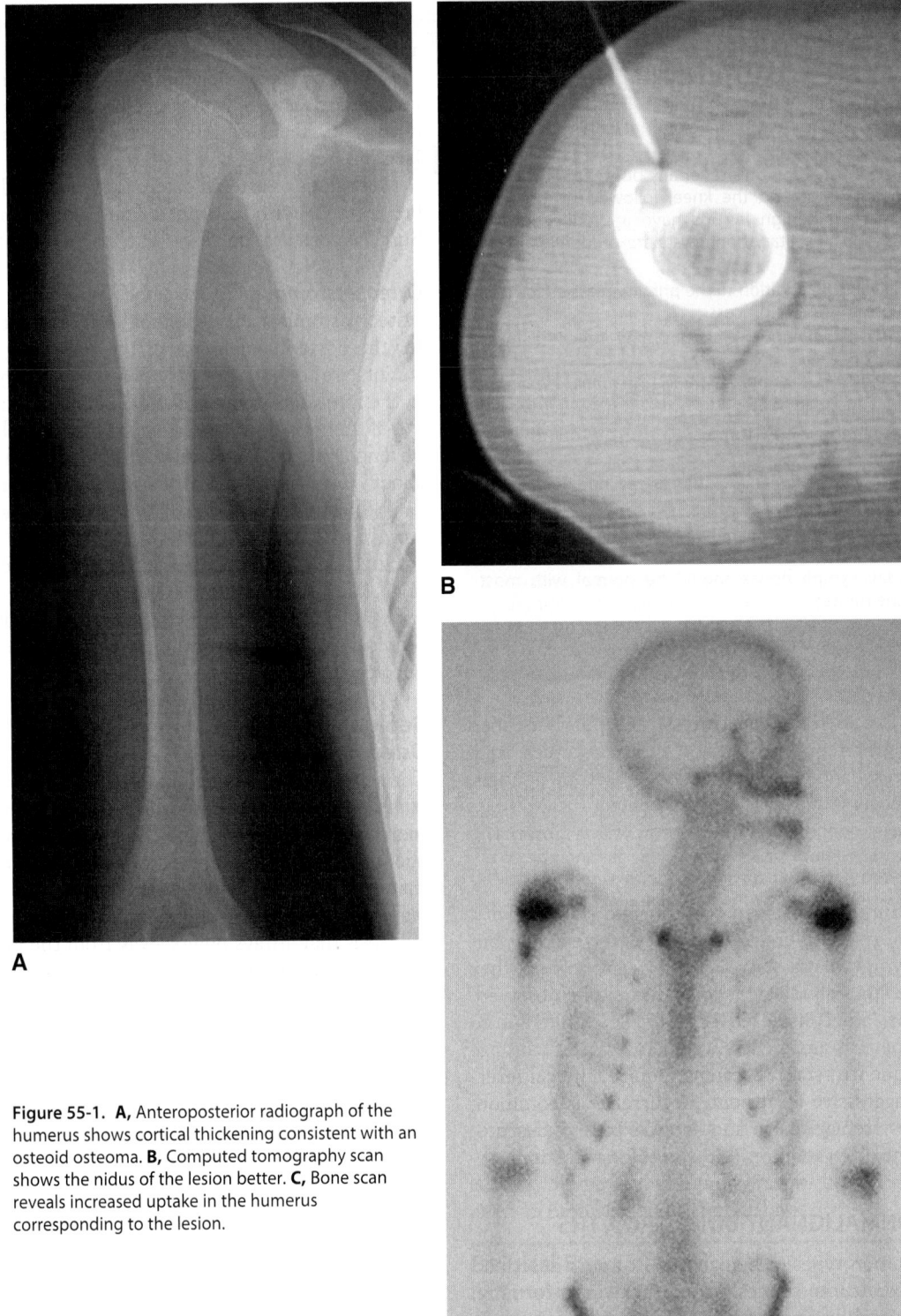

Figure 55-1. A, Anteroposterior radiograph of the humerus shows cortical thickening consistent with an osteoid osteoma. **B,** Computed tomography scan shows the nidus of the lesion better. **C,** Bone scan reveals increased uptake in the humerus corresponding to the lesion.

cases, the lesion may be palpable and irritating. Surgical removal is appropriate only to treat symptoms, *not* as a prophylaxis for chondrosarcomatous degeneration. In multiple hereditary exostoses, symptomatic lesions are surgically removed as needed. In adults, a previously quiescent lesion that begins to enlarge should be removed.

Enchondroma

Enchondroma is a relatively common, centrally located cartilage tumor; 50% are found in the small tubular bones of the hands and feet. These tumors develop as hamartomatous processes in growing bones. Because they are frequently asymptomatic, enchondromas may not be detected

Table 55-1. Histologic and Radiographic Features of Nonmalignant Bone Growths

Tumor	Histologic Features	Radiographic Features
Osteoid-Forming Tumors		
Osteoid osteoma	Nidus aggressive, but benign woven bone formation, large numbers of osteoblasts and osteoclasts in vascular stroma. No lymphocytes or plasma cells	Central lytic nidus, measures 1 cm, extensive reactive sclerosis, creating fusiform bulge
Osteoblastoma	Identical to osteoid osteoma with excessive osteoblastic activity, osteoid formation. Numerous giant cells in a vascular stroma	Nidus >1 cm, more lytic and destructive than osteoid osteoma, less sclerotic reactive bone at periphery. May have appearance of aneurysmal bone cyst
Chondroid-Forming Tumors		
Osteochondroma	Cartilage cap similar in appearance to physeal plate with maturation via enchondral ossification; bony base contiguous with hematopoietic or fatty marrow	Pedunculated or sessile projection in continuity with medullary canal; well demarcated
Enchondroma	Hypocellular with uniform chondrocytes with no atypia in bland cartilage stroma	Geographic lysis with sharp margination and central calcification. In hand, cortex thinned out with slight dilation. In long bone, lesion central with minimal erosion or dilation
Chondroblastoma	Stromal cells polyhedral, associated with streaks of calcification giving "chicken wire" appearance, chondroid metaplasia essential to diagnosis	Lytic tumor with sharp sclerotic margin, stippled or flocculated calcification in chondroid portion

until adulthood. The lesion may be discovered in association with a pathologic fracture or as an incidental finding on a routine radiographic examination.

Radiographic features of enchondromas are shown in Figure 55-4 and described in Table 55-1. An enchondroma of the large long bones is centrally located with minimal evidence of cortical erosion or dilation. Enchondromas are either stage 1 or 2 lesions.

Multiple enchondromatosis, or *Ollier's disease,* is a rare nonfamilial dysplasia typically confined to half of the body. Extensive involvement of the metaphyseal areas can result in bowing and shortening of the long bones. The cortical thinning and epiphyseal involvement in Ollier's disease are seen rarely in a solitary enchondroma. In patients with *Maffucci's syndrome,* enchondromatosis is seen in association with multiple soft tissue hemangiomas.

Fewer than 5% of large solitary enchondromas of the large bones convert to a low-grade chondrosarcoma during adulthood, whereas solitary enchondromas of the hand rarely become malignant. Because secondary chondrosarcoma in Ollier's disease occurs in 20% to 30% of cases, and the incidence is even higher in Maffucci's syndrome, any patient with either of these conditions should be evaluated by an orthopedic oncologist.

Treatment of an asymptomatic patient with a solitary enchondroma of the hand or foot is unnecessary. If the patient has a pathologic fracture, it is best to allow the fracture to heal and remove the lesion surgically at a later date if necessary.

Chondroblastoma

Chondroblastoma is a benign cartilage-forming tumor seen almost exclusively in the epiphysis or apophysis (Fig. 55-5). Most arise after age 10 years. Boys are affected more often than girls. The most common location is the proximal humeral epiphysis, followed by the distal femoral and proximal tibial epiphyseal areas. Because of its proximity to a joint, chondroblastoma can present with a symptomatic joint effusion. Histologic and radiographic features are

described in Table 55-1. Most chondroblastomas are stage 2 lesions, but some can be stage 3 lesions.

Although the chondroblastoma is considered benign, and spontaneous conversion of chondroblastoma to a malignant tumor is extremely rare, it has been reported to metastasize to the lung on rare occasions. Nevertheless, chondroblastoma carries an excellent prognosis. Treatment for chondroblastoma consists of surgical management by an orthopedic oncologist.

Benign Fibrous Tumors of Bone
Fibrous Cortical Defect

Fibrous cortical defects or cortical desmoids are small hamartomatous fibromas seen almost exclusively in the metaphyseal areas of the lower extremities of growing children. They can be multiple, are usually asymptomatic, and are found in 25% of normal children at 5 years of age. Bone remodeling tends to cause lesions to disappear before skeletal maturity. If excessive stress is placed across the lesions, they can become symptomatic. The radiographic appearance is so characteristic of this entity that a biopsy usually is not necessary. Lesions may cause increased activity on bone scan. These are stage 1 lesions and generally can be observed.

Nonossifying Fibroma

The nonossifying fibroma is considered a larger form of the fibrous cortical defect. Lesions typically are seen in the lower extremity. Because of its size, a nonossifying fibroma may persist into adult life. Pathologic fractures may occur if the lesion approaches 50% of the diameter of the bone. The fracture healing process may facilitate resolution of the lesion. Fracture prophylaxis should be considered for large lesions only. Nonossifying fibromas are stage 1 lesions. Fibrous cortical defects and nonossifying fibromas do not require biopsy because their radiographic appearance is so characteristic (Fig. 55-6).

Nonossifying fibromas may be multiple lesions that take on the appearance of fibrous dysplasia and can be associated

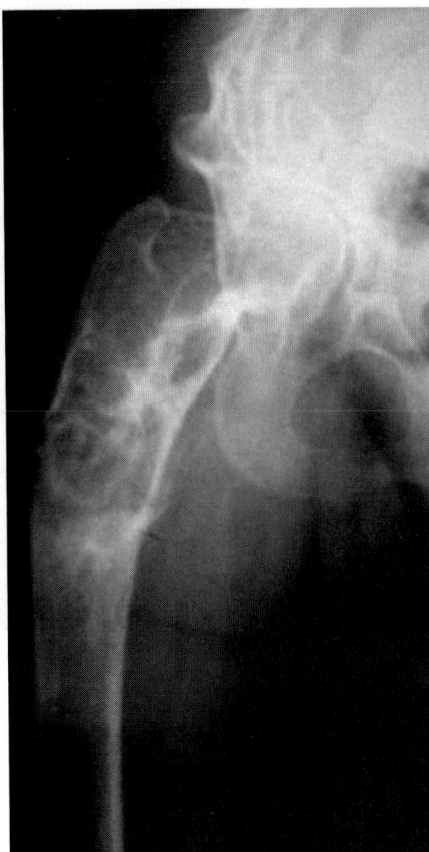

Figure 55-7. Polyostotic fibrous dysplasia.

nates has been shown to be beneficial in some cases. Irradiation is contraindicated because it may lead to irradiation-induced sarcoma at a later date.

Cystic Lesions of Bone
Solitary Bone Cyst

Solitary bone cyst is a common pseudotumor of bone and is the most frequent cause of pathologic fractures in children. The bone cyst typically affects patients 5 to 15 years old and occurs more often in boys than in girls. It is found in the proximal humerus in 50% of cases and in the upper femur in 25%. Patients are asymptomatic until a pathologic fracture occurs. Fractures seem to arise from the central metaphyseal side of an epiphyseal or apophyseal growth plate. The cystic process continues to grow away from the physis. When it remains in contact with the physis, it is termed *active*. When it separates, it is termed *inactive*.

Histologic and radiologic findings are described in Table 55-1. Figure 55-8 depicts a solitary bone cyst. Because the periosteal covering of a cyst is normal, pathologic fractures heal normally and, in most cases, do not require surgery. The cyst usually persists after fracture union and requires further treatment.

Solitary bone cysts generally are considered stage 1 lesions. Occasionally, they may be stage 2. Currently, treatment is a function of location. In weight-bearing bones, lesions should be treated aggressively. Initial management usually involves aspiration/injection with either bone marrow or corticosteroid. Results are best in patients 5 to

15 years old, when macrophage activity is greatest in the cyst lining.

Aneurysmal Bone Cyst

Aneurysmal bone cyst is a hemorrhagic expansile lesion. Of aneurysmal bone cysts, 75% occur in patients 10 to 20 years old; they are more common in girls. The femur is the most frequently affected site, followed by the tibia, pelvis, and spine. In the spine, two thirds of aneurysmal bone cysts arise from posterior elements.

Radiographic and histologic features are described in Table 55-1. Initially, aneurysmal bone cysts can appear on radiographs as an aggressive osteolytic lesion with cortical attenuation that may mimic a malignant process, such as Ewing's sarcoma or hemorrhagic osteosarcoma (Fig. 55-9).

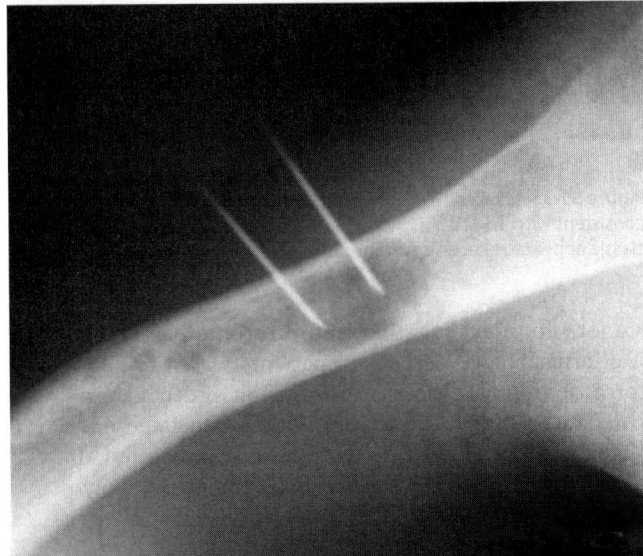

A

B

Figure 55-8. A, Solitary bone cyst before injection. **B,** After injection of radiocontrast material to reveal the cavitary nature.

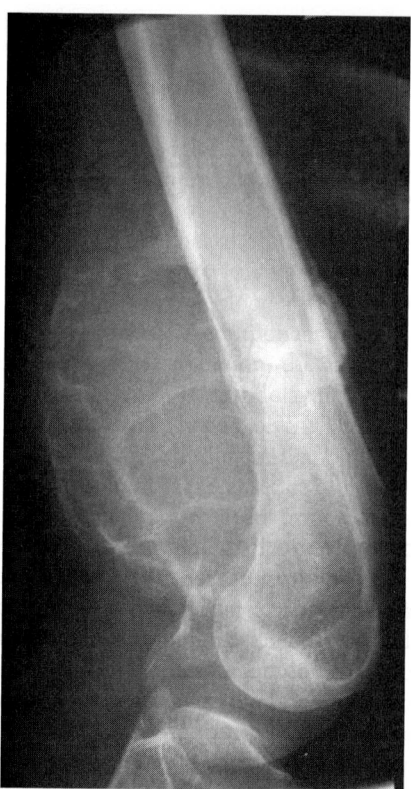

Figure 55-9. Lateral radiograph of the distal femur shows the aggressive appearance of an aneurysmal bone cyst.

Aneurysmal bone cyst is either a stage 2 or a stage 3 lesion and is frequently symptomatic.

If an aneurysmal cyst is left untreated, it may involute spontaneously, developing a heavy shell of reactive bone at the periphery. This involutional process can be hastened by surgical manipulation. Another option for treating extremely large lesions is repeated embolization to reduce the rate of hemorrhagic expansion.

Hemangioma

Hemangioma of bone is a hamartomatous process that occurs more frequently in girls than in boys and is seen most commonly in vertebral bodies. It is found only rarely in the diaphysis of long bone. Hemangiomas of bone can be associated with hemangiomas of soft tissue. Spinal lesions usually are discovered as an incidental radiographic finding and show a characteristic vertically oriented honeycombed or moth-eaten appearance. Rarely a lesion can cause cord compression that may require immediate surgical consultation.

Mini-index of Related Topics

SUGGESTED READINGS

Dorfman HD, Czerniak B: Bone Tumors. St. Louis, Mosby, 1998.

Huvos AG: Bone Tumors: Diagnosis, Treatment, and Prognosis, 2nd ed. Philadelphia, WB Saunders, 1991.

Johnston JO, Randall RL: Tumors in orthopedics. In Skinner HB (ed): Current Diagnosis and Treatment in Orthopedics, 2nd ed. New York, Lange Medical Books/McGraw-Hill, 2000, pp 247–325.

Scarborough MT, Moreau G: Benign cartilage tumors. Orthop Clin North Am 1996;27:583–589.

Schmale GA, Conrad EU, Raskind WH: The natural history of hereditary multiple exostoses. J Bone Joint Surg Am 1994;76(7):986–992.

PATHOLOGIC MURMURS

Pathologic Systolic Ejection Murmurs

Pathologic systolic ejection murmurs are due to either obstruction of flow across one of the outflow tracts or a "relative stenosis" secondary to a large left-to-right shunt causing an increased ejection volume across a normal-sized RV outflow tract.

Left Ventricular Outflow Tract Stenosis

Pathologic systolic ejection murmurs resulting from turbulence from LV outflow tract obstruction can be caused by stenosis in the subvalvar, valvar, or supravalvar areas. *Subvalvar aortic stenosis*, which can be caused either by a discrete membrane or by asymmetric septal hypertrophy from hypertrophic cardiomyopathy, causes a soft or harsh systolic ejection murmur that usually is loudest at the left mid-sternal border with radiation to the apex and right upper sternal border. The dynamic obstruction resulting from hypertrophic cardiomyopathy causes the murmur to increase on changing from a lying to standing position, which produces a decrease in preload and afterload, decreasing the diameter of the LV outflow tract and increasing the obstruction. Because of the thickened ventricular muscle, hypertrophic cardiomyopathy causes diastolic dysfunction and commonly is associated with a gallop.

The murmur of *valvar aortic stenosis*, a common congenital heart defect, usually is harsh and loudest at the right upper sternal border with radiation to the carotid arteries and commonly to the apex. An ejection click frequently can be appreciated immediately before the murmur of valvar aortic stenosis. The intensity of the aortic component of S_2 frequently is decreased in valvar and subvalvar aortic stenosis of a moderate or severe degree.

Supravalvar aortic stenosis, a rare condition seen mainly with Williams syndrome, produces a murmur that is similar to valvar aortic stenosis except that the aortic component of S_2 is loud from the increased pressure above the aortic valve, and an ejection click is absent. Reversed or "paradoxical" splitting of S_2 is rare and heard only in severe LV outflow tract obstruction at any level. Decreased peripheral pulses can be noted in any moderate-to-severe obstruction of LV ejection.

Aortic coarctation gives rise to a systolic ejection "murmur" caused by turbulent flow across an obstruction into the proximal descending thoracic aorta. The precordial murmur usually is loudest at the mid- to upper left sternal border, radiating to the left back between the spine and scapula. A difference between the pulses and systolic blood pressures of the upper and lower extremities is present with a significant aortic coarctation. At a minimum, the blood pressure should be checked in the right arm and leg of every patient with a murmur or hypertension. The systolic pressure in the leg should not be significantly lower than the pressure in the arm.

Right Ventricular Outflow Tract Stenosis

Pathologic systolic ejection murmurs resulting from turbulence from RV outflow tract obstruction also can be caused by stenosis in the subvalvar, valvar, or supravalvar areas. In all of these conditions, the murmur is louder with inspiration, and the area of maximal intensity is the left upper or midsternal border with radiation to the axillae or back or both. If the stenosis is more than mild, splitting of S_2 is constant.

Subvalvar pulmonary stenosis, rarely caused by a discrete membrane, usually is due to dynamic obstruction from infundibular hypertrophy and, as in the case of tetralogy of Fallot, malalignment of the infundibular septum. The murmur of *valvar pulmonary stenosis*, a relatively common congenital heart defect, usually is harsh, with an ejection click at the beginning of the murmur. The intensity of the pulmonic component of S_2 frequently is decreased in moderate-to-severe valvar or subvalvar pulmonary stenosis.

Supravalvar pulmonary stenosis, a narrowing of the main pulmonary artery, is a rare condition seen mainly with the postrubella syndrome or Noonan's syndrome. Pathologic *branch pulmonary stenosis* also is rare as an isolated condition; however, it is a common problem in patients with other congenital cardiac abnormalities with decreased pulmonary blood flow, such as tetralogy of Fallot. Both of these types of pulmonary arterial obstruction produce a murmur that is similar to valvar pulmonary stenosis except that the pulmonic component of S_2 is loud from the increased pressure above the valve, an ejection click is absent, and the radiation to the axillae and back is particularly loud.

Atrial Septal Defects and Anomalous Pulmonary Venous Return

A moderate-to-large, left-to-right shunt at the level of the atria or vena cava causes enough increase in the RV stroke volume to create a "relative stenosis" across the infundibulum and pulmonary valve and produce a systolic ejection murmur similar to pulmonary stenosis. This murmur usually is soft or blowing, loudest at the mid- to upper left sternal border, with constant splitting of S_2. If the atrial septal defect shunt is large, S_2 splitting is wide and fixed, without any respiratory fluctuation in the interval between the two components. Frequently a mid-diastolic rumble can be heard.

Regurgitant Systolic Murmurs

Either AV valve regurgitation or a ventricular septal defect is the cause of a regurgitant systolic murmur.

Mitral Regurgitation

The systolic murmur of mitral regurgitation is loudest at the cardiac apex and usually radiates to the left axilla. When the regurgitation is due to *mitral valve prolapse*, the murmur extends from mid- to late systole, increasing in intensity with standing up and decreasing in intensity and duration with squatting or lying down. In mitral valve prolapse, usually, but not always, a midsystolic click just precedes the murmur. The systolic murmur of mitral regurgitation without mitral valve prolapse is holosystolic.

Tricuspid Regurgitation

The murmur of tricuspid regurgitation, which is rare in pediatric patients, is holosystolic, loudest at the lower left sternal border, and increases in intensity with inspiration. If the regurgitation is severe, prominent jugular venous pulsations may be visible in older children, or a pulsatile liver might be palpated.

Ventricular Septal Defect

The regurgitant systolic murmur of a ventricular septal defect usually is loudest at the left lower or midsternal border with diffuse radiation proportional to the loudness. A tiny defect, or rarely a ventricular septal defect associated with severe pulmonary hypertension, causes a murmur from early to midsystole because flow across the defect is minimal in late systole. Larger defects without severe pulmonary hypertension produce a holosystolic murmur.

Early Diastolic Murmurs

Regurgitation of either semilunar valve can produce a murmur that begins at S_2 and decrescendos in early diastole. The quality of these murmurs usually is soft. If the semilunar valve insufficiency is severe, a gallop generally is present.

Aortic Insufficiency

The early diastolic murmur of aortic valve regurgitation is loudest at the left midsternal border and radiates to the cardiac apex. The intensity of the murmur may increase with leaning forward while sitting or with squatting. With severe aortic insufficiency, the peripheral pulses are increased, the pulse pressure is widened, and the diastolic blood pressure may be below normal.

Pulmonic Insufficiency

The early diastolic murmur associated with pulmonic insufficiency also ordinarily is loudest at the left midsternal border, but radiates down to the left lower sternal border and not to the apex. The intensity of this murmur usually increases with inspiration.

Mid-diastolic or Mid-to-Late Diastolic Murmurs

Mid-diastolic and mid-to-late diastolic murmurs result from turbulent flow across one of the AV valves. LV diastolic murmurs are heard best with the patient in the left lateral decubitus position.

Mid-diastolic Rumble

Increased flow across a normal-sized AV valve can cause a prolonged low-frequency, rumbling sound following an S_3 gallop. When this sound occurs in the left ventricle, it is loudest at the apex, and when it occurs in the right ventricle, it is loudest at the lower left sternal border. An LV rumble can occur with a large left-to-right shunt from a ventricular septal defect or a patent ductus arteriosus or with severe mitral regurgitation. An RV rumble can be heard with a large atrial septal defect left-to-right shunt or with severe tricuspid regurgitation.

Mitral Stenosis

The murmur of mitral stenosis is soft or rumbling in quality, is loudest at the apex, may be associated with a loud S_1, or may be preceded immediately by a mid-diastolic "opening snap." If severe, the murmur can extend from mid- into late diastole.

Tricuspid Stenosis

The murmur of tricuspid stenosis is similar to that of mitral stenosis except that it is loudest at the left lower sternal border, may increase in intensity with inspiration, and may cause prominent A waves in the jugular venous pulsations seen in older children.

Continuous Murmurs

Pathologic continuous murmurs are caused by either aortopulmonary or arteriovenous shunts.

Patent Ductus Arteriosus or Surgical Aortopulmonary Shunt

The "continuous" murmurs of patent ductus arteriosus or surgical aortopulmonary shunt peak at S_2 and if from a large shunt can be associated with increased peripheral pulses, a wide pulse pressure, and a low diastolic blood pressure. The murmur of a patent ductus arteriosus usually is loudest at the upper left sternal border. If severe pulmonary hypertension from high pulmonary vascular resistance is present, the murmur of any aortopulmonary shunt decreases in intensity and in duration, sometimes becoming only systolic without extension into diastole.

Arteriovenous Malformations

The "continuous" murmur of an arteriovenous fistula peaks in systole. A pulmonary arteriovenous malformation murmur may increase in intensity with inspiration. Thoracic arteriovenous malformations of either the systemic or the pulmonary circulations are heard best over the ipsilateral chest, commonly including the axilla.

INDICATIONS FOR REFERRAL

Patients with a benign murmur are normal and should be treated as such. They should be followed routinely by their primary care physician, but they do not require any limitations of physical activity or any other precautions. If after a careful cardiovascular history and physical examination the primary care specialist has any doubt that the murmur is innocent, the patient should be referred to a pediatric cardiologist for further evaluation. A 12-lead electrocardiogram is indicated when making a referral to a cardiologist, but a chest radiograph is not necessary. The generalist should not order an echocardiogram. Echocardiograms in children are performed best under the guidance of a pediatric cardiologist who already has examined the patient. Most children referred for evaluation of a murmur do not require an echocardiogram after examination by a pediatric cardiologist.

FOLLOW-UP

Patients with an innocent murmur are normal and do not require follow-up beyond routine well-child surveillance visits. The fact that an innocent murmur is a normal finding should be stressed to the parents because most parents initially assume that the mere presence of a murmur is abnormal. Almost all forms of congenital heart defects except for secundum atrial septal defect or mild mitral valve prolapse without any regurgitation should receive presenting symptom in patients with mediastinal tumors. Collagen vascular disease resulting in pleurodynia and pleural effusion is an uncommon cause of chest pain.

Cardiac chest pain from ischemia is rare in children but can be life-threatening. Causes of coronary insufficiency include prior surgery for congenital heart disease, coronary artery atresia (or stenosis), other congenital coronary anomalies, coronary abnormalities caused by Kawasaki disease, hypertrophic cardiomyopathy, familial hypercholesterolemia with premature coronary atherosclerosis, and use of cocaine. Structural heart disease, such as aortic stenosis and mitral valve prolapse, also may present with chest pain. Pericarditis and myocarditis from viral, bacterial, or other causes sometimes present with chest pain. Pericarditis from bacterial (e.g., *Staphylococcus*, *Streptococcus*) and viral pathogens may cause pericardial effusion, friction rubs, and pain. Myocarditis, mostly viral (e.g., coxsackievirus, adenovirus), often presents with chest pain, ventricular arrhythmia, ventricular dysfunction, tachycardia, and tachypnea. Young children often report palpitation, particularly sustained tachyarrhythmias, as chest pain. Prolonged episodes of otherwise benign tachycardia also can lead to ischemia and may cause chest pain. Life-threatening ventricular tachycardia can present as isolated chest pain. Dissecting aortic aneurysm is rare in children but should be considered in children with Marfan syndrome.

DIAGNOSIS

In most cases, the cause of chest pain can be identified by a thorough history and physical examination. Selective use of laboratory tests is helpful in some cases to determine the cause of chest pain. Box 57-2 summarizes the clinical evaluation of a child with chest pain by history, physical examination, and selective laboratory tests.

The age of the patient is an important consideration in determining the cause of the pain. Organic causes of pain are more common in younger children, whereas psychogenic pains are seen frequently in adolescents, especially girls. The characteristics (sharp, dull, burning), onset (sudden or gradual), duration, frequency, location, and severity of the pain are helpful clues. Whether the pain is associated with meals, activity or physical exertion, breathing or coughing, and position (supine or upright) and whether the symptom disrupts the child's activity should be determined. Previous history of cardiac or pulmonary disease, surgery, Kawasaki disease, and trauma should be explored carefully. Family history of hypercholesterolemia, hypertrophic cardiomyopathy, arrhythmia, or sudden death raises the index of suspicion for cardiac etiology.

In conjunction with a thorough history, careful physical examination is likely to reveal the cause of pain. Children with abnormal vital signs or apparent distress should be evaluated and managed immediately. Poor weight and height suggest the presence of a significant chronic illness. The chest should be inspected and palpated for bruises or rashes, chest wall deformity, presence of a mass, or tenderness. Finding bruises or rib fractures suggests trauma. In such cases, physical abuse should be considered, especially in younger children. Palpation may elicit tenderness of

---

Box 57-2. Clinical Evaluation of Chest Pain

History

1. Characteristics (sharp, dull, burning), onset (sudden or gradual), duration, frequency, location, and severity of the pain
2. Association of the pain with meals, activity or physical exertion, breathing or coughing, position (supine or upright), and whether the symptom disrupts the child's activity
3. Previous history of cardiac or pulmonary disease, surgery, Kawasaki disease, and trauma
4. Family history of hypercholesterolemia, hypertrophic cardiomyopathy, arrhythmia, and sudden death

Physical Examination

1. Vital signs or apparent distress
2. Weight and height plotted on growth chart
3. Inspection of the chest for skin bruises or rashes, chest wall deformity, and presence of a mass or swelling
4. Palpation for tenderness of specific muscles, tendons, joints, or bone
5. Signs suggesting pulmonary disease, including cyanosis, wheezing, intercostal retraction, decreased lung sounds, and asymmetric chest expansion
6. Cardiac auscultation for heart sounds (muffled or not), murmurs, friction rubs, clicks, and gallop

Laboratory Tests

1. *Chest x-ray*—fractures, pneumothorax or pneumomediastinum, pleural effusion, cardiomegaly, pulmonary edema, infiltrates, atelectasis, consolidation
2. *12-Lead electrocardiogram*—arrhythmia, preexcitation, prolonged Q-T interval, ST-segment changes, abnormal Q waves, diffuse low voltages
3. *Blood tests*—complete blood count, cardiac enzymes, erythrocyte sedimentation rate
4. Urine toxicology screen
5. Echocardiogram
6. Exercise stress test

---

specific muscles, tendons, or joints, suggesting a musculoskeletal origin of the pain. Tietze's syndrome is characterized by fusiform shape swelling at the sternoclavicular or chondrosternal junction and commonly is diagnosed by inspection and palpation of the chest wall.

Cyanosis may be a sign of underlying cardiac or pulmonary disease. Wheezing and intercostal retraction are signs of reactive airway disease or asthma. Decreased lung sounds on auscultation suggest pneumothorax, consolidation of the lung, pneumonia, atelectasis, or pleural effusion. In the process of cardiac auscultation, attention should be paid to the heart sounds and murmurs. Muffled heart sounds or friction rubs suggest the presence of pericarditis or pericardial effusion. Heart murmurs and ejection clicks may signify congenital heart disease. A gallop rhythm is associated with heart failure, which may be the presenting feature of myocarditis.

If the history and physical examination suggest chest trauma or when cardiac or pulmonary causes are suspected, a chest x-ray should be considered. In inspecting the x-ray, attention should be paid to fractures, pneumothorax or pneumomediastinum, pleural effusion, cardiomegaly, pulmonary edema, infiltrates, atelectasis, and consolidation.

An electrocardiogram should be performed in children with suspected arrhythmias, a history of heart disease, or significant cardiac physical findings. Findings of a short P-R interval, wide QRS, and a delta wave on electrocardiogram are diagnostic of Wolff-Parkinson-White syndrome and suggest intermittent supraventricular tachycardia as the cause of chest pain. Premature ventricular contractions are seen frequently in children with myocarditis. In pericarditis, diffuse low voltages may be seen in the precordial leads when there is significant pericardial effusion. ST-segment changes and abnormal Q waves may be seen in patients with myocardial ischemia or infarct. Finally, a prolonged Q-T interval suggests the need to explore further the possibility of the long Q-T syndrome, especially in patients with a significant family history of cardiac problems.

Blood tests may provide useful information in acute chest pain. Cardiac enzymes such as creatinine kinase with MB fraction and troponin T level may be elevated in myocardial ischemia or infarct, although these conditions are rare in children. Abnormal white blood cell counts and elevated erythrocyte sedimentation rate are seen in infection, malignancy, collagen vascular disease, and postpericardiotomy syndrome. Urine toxicology screen should be considered in adolescents when cocaine or other illicit drug use is suspected. An echocardiogram is indicated in children with history of heart disease, suspected myocarditis, pericarditis, or structural heart disease (e.g., aortic stenosis, coronary artery anomaly, and hypertrophic cardiomyopathy). The echocardiogram may show structural heart disease or abnormal segmental ventricular wall motion if myocardial ischemia or infarct in patients with structurally normal hearts is present. An exercise stress test using a treadmill or cycle ergometer is helpful in patients older than age 4 years to evaluate exercise-induced chest pain. Ischemia during exercise, as evidenced by ST-segment elevation, suggests coronary insufficiency. For patients who achieve maximal exercise as measured by heart rate or oxygen consumption or who experience chest pain during the test, the lack of ST-segment changes is reassuring and suggests that cardiac ischemia is not the cause of chest pain. Other conditions that may be diagnosed by stress testing include exercise-induced asthma and arrhythmias.

MANAGEMENT

Treatments for chest pain depend on the underlying causes. In children with musculoskeletal, psychogenic, or idiopathic chest pain, it is important to reassure the patient and family that the chest pain is not of cardiac origin and will not result in a heart attack or other life-threatening event. Musculoskeletal pain generally responds to nonsteroidal anti-inflammatory drugs. Patients with significant, prolonged musculoskeletal pain can be given a 2- to 3-week course of nonsteroidal anti-inflammatory medication. If reflux is suspected, a trial treatment can be diagnostic and therapeutic.

If cardiac chest pain is suggested by initial evaluation, a pediatric cardiologist should be consulted. An echocardiogram either excludes or establishes the diagnosis of structural cardiac abnormalities, such as valve stenosis or ventricular dysfunction. In children with suspected coronary ischemia, cardiac catheterization with coronary angiogram is used to evaluate coronary anomalies, aneurysms, atresia, or stenosis. Coronary vasodilators, such as sublingual nitroglycerin, the mainstay of treatment for adults with chest pain caused by coronary disease, rarely are indicated in children. In some cases, hospitalization may be necessary for patients with severe distress, abnormal vital signs, or significant cardiac or pulmonary conditions, such as pneumothorax, myocarditis, and ventricular arrhythmias.

FOLLOW-UP

Because chest pain in children may be present for months to years, and initial evaluation may not be conclusive, appropriate follow-up is needed. Clues as to the cause of chest pain first may appear at follow-up visits. If no significant cardiac or pulmonary etiology is found, it seldom is necessary to restrict activities of children with chest pain. During follow-up visits, the primary care physician should ensure that children with complaints of chest pain are not restricted by their parents or teachers. Parents and children should be encouraged to return to normal activity with the resumption of the customary lifestyle for the family and patient when cardiopulmonary etiologies have been excluded.

OUTCOMES

The outcomes of children with chest pain generally are good unless significant cardiopulmonary, hematologic, or oncologic disease is involved. Many children with musculoskeletal or idiopathic pains continue to have intermittent symptoms for years. Psychogenic causes of chest pain and excessive anxiety on the part of the parent or child should not be ignored. When simple reassurance does not relieve the anxiety, short-term counseling may be indicated, especially for families who have visited multiple pediatricians and pediatric subspecialists. In most cases of pediatric chest pain, the general pediatrician can provide a great service to the family and the child by a thorough evaluation and simple reassurance.

Mini-index of Related Topics

SUGGESTED READINGS

Driscoll DJ, Glicklick LB, Gallen WJ: Chest pain in children: A prospective study. Pediatrics 1976;57:648–651.
Fyfe MD: Chest pain in pediatric patients presenting to a cardiac clinic. Clin Pediatr 1984;23:321–340.
Selbst SM: Evaluation of chest pain in children. Pediatr Rev 1986;8:56–62.

Selbst SM, Ruddy RM, Clark BJ: Pediatric chest pain: A prospective study. Pediatrics 1988;823:319–323.
Wiens L, Sabath R, Ewing L, et al: Chest pain in otherwise healthy children and adolescents is frequently caused by exercise-induced asthma. Pediatrics 1992;90:350–353.

58 Approach to the Child with Syncope

Ruey-Kang R. Chang and Thomas S. Klitzner

ROLE OF THE GENERALIST

1 Distinguish syncope from seizure, dizziness, vertigo, and presyncope.

2 Distinguish cardiac from noncardiac syncope.

3 Perform a basic evaluation of a child with cardiac syncope.

4 Refer a child to a cardiologist or neurologist as indicated.

5 Implement emergency management of syncope.

6 Follow-up children with syncope.

DEFINITION

Syncope, a common, often benign problem in children, is a sudden loss of consciousness and postural tone resulting from transient cerebral underperfusion with spontaneous recovery. Syncope in children may cause significant anxiety at home or at school. Although syncope can occur in children of all ages, it is more common in adolescents. The age-adjusted incidence is higher for girls (166/100,000) than boys (93/100,000). Although syncope accounts for only 0.125% of pediatric emergency department visits, 15% of children report at least one syncopal episode.

Children with syncope complain of a variety of symptoms, including lightheadedness, dizziness, blacking out, and visual changes. The pediatrician must differentiate between fainting episodes and other conditions, such as dizziness, vertigo, presyncope, and seizures. In general, dizziness, vertigo, and presyncope are not associated with loss of consciousness, the hallmark of true syncope. Dizziness is a frequently reported prodrome of syncope and must be distinguished from *vertigo*, a feeling of "spinning" resulting from vestibular dysfunction. In contrast to patients with true syncope, patients with presyncope usually report the feeling of "about to pass out" but do not lose consciousness.

ETIOLOGY

The causes of syncope in children can be defined broadly as neurally mediated, cardiogenic, and miscellaneous (Table 58-1). Because certain forms of cardiogenic syncope may lead to fatal outcomes, syncope of cardiac etiology must be diagnosed. Cardiac causes of syncope are characterized by inadequate cardiac output and decreased cerebral perfusion, which may be the result of obstruction of systemic outflow, myocardial dysfunction, or arrhythmia. Children with aortic valve stenosis, subvalvar stenosis, and hypertrophic cardiomyopathy with dynamic subaortic obstruction frequently present with syncope during exercise. Cardiac rhythm disturbances causing syncope include bradycardia (sick sinus syndrome, complete heart block) and tachycardia (supraventricular or ventricular). Common causes of arrhythmia in children with structurally normal hearts include preexcitation syndrome, long Q-T syndrome, and congenital heart block. Children with supraventricular tachycardia usually tolerate the arrhythmia well and rarely present with syncope. Ventricular tachycardia may be tolerated for a short time or may cause syncope at the onset of tachycardia. Arrhythmias may occur before or after surgical repair in children with congenital heart disease. Myocardial dysfunction from acute myocarditis, cardiomyopathy, coronary artery anomaly (e.g., an anomalous coronary artery that courses between the great arteries), and pulmonary hypertension also may cause inadequate cerebral perfusion, especially during exercise, and lead to syncope. Only 3% of

Table 58-1. Cardiac and Noncardiac Causes of Syncope in Children

Mechanism	Disorder
Neurally mediated	Vasovagal (neurocardiogenic)
	Situational—micturition, hair grooming, coughing
	Hypervagal
	Neurologic disorder—seizures, migraine, space-occupying lesions (tumor, vascular malformation), familial dysautonomia
Cardiac	LVOT obstruction—aortic stenosis, subaortic stenosis, hypertrophic cardiomyopathy
	Arrhythmia—ventricular tachycardia, supraventricular tachycardia, sinus node dysfunction, heart block, long Q-T syndrome
	Others—coronary artery anomaly, pulmonary hypertension, acute myocarditis, dilated cardiomyopathy
Miscellaneous	Orthostatic (hypovolemia)—dehydration, anemia, blood loss
	Metabolic—hypoglycemia, electrolyte imbalance
	Medications or toxins—carbon monoxide, sedatives, antihypertensives
	Respiratory—breath-holding spells, hyperventilation
	Psychiatric disorders—hysteria, conversion disorder, depression, panic attack
	Idiopathic
	Malingering

all syncopal episodes occur during exercise; however, exercise-induced syncope raises the index of suspicion for cardiac etiology.

Neurally mediated syncope includes vasovagal, situational (reflex), and neurologic disorders. Vasovagal syncope, also called *vasodepressor syncope, neurocardiogenic syncope,* and *common fainting,* is the most common cause of syncope in children and adolescents, accounting for 50% to 75% of all cases. Vasovagal syncope usually occurs after prolonged standing; after a sudden change of postural position; during emotional distress; with sudden unexpected pain or fear; or with the introduction of an unpleasant sight, sound, or smell. Vasovagal episodes typically last a few seconds to minutes and involve complex, poorly understood pathophysiologic mechanisms. The commonly used model is the Bezold-Jarisch reflex. This reflex is initiated by excessive venous pooling, decreased left ventricular filling, and increased sympathetic output that lead to increased myocardial contractility. The mechanoreceptor of the left ventricle detects the change and transmits the signal to the medulla. Sympathetic withdrawal and increased vagal activity result, causing hypotension, bradycardia, decreased cerebral perfusion, and loss of consciousness. Reflex syncope episodes commonly occur in conjunction with micturition, defecation, cough, hair grooming, stretching, swallowing, or noxious and emotional stimuli. The cause of reflex syncope episodes is thought to be a sudden increase in vagal tone resulting from a reflexive response to a physiologic or environmental stimulus. Although true neurologic disorders (seizures and migraine variants) may not present with typical syncopal episodes, they need to be considered in the differential diagnosis, especially for younger children.

Miscellaneous causes of syncope include anemia, hypovolemia, hypoglycemia, electrolyte imbalance, use of medications (antihypertensive and antidepressant agents), and toxin inhalation or ingestion. Syncope also is seen as the result of neurally mediated respiratory problems, either breath-holding spells (in infants and toddlers) or hyperventilation (in older children and adolescents). Psychiatric disorders (e.g., hysteria, conversion disorder, and malingering) also should be considered when evaluating syncope in pediatric patients.

DIAGNOSIS

Box 58-1 outlines the clinical evaluation of syncope. When a child with syncope who has or has not regained consciousness arrives in the emergency department, general assessment should begin with the ABCs (airway, breathing, and circulation). Vital signs, including orthostatic blood pressure and pulse oximetry, should be obtained immediately on arrival to the emergency department. After initial assessment and stabilization, a detailed history and thorough physical examination are likely to establish the cause of syncope and determine the patient's risk of future injury or sudden death. Selective use of laboratory tests may be helpful in some patients.

History should be obtained from the patient, parents, and any witnesses of the syncopal episode. The onset, prodrome, associated symptoms (e.g., chest pain, nausea, palpitations), duration of unconsciousness, association with exercise, predisposing factors (e.g., prolonged standing, noxious stimuli, hyperventilation, or breath-holding), use of medication, exposure to drugs or toxins, and frequency of syncope should be explored carefully. Neurally mediated syncope usually occurs with sudden, unexpected pain or fear or an unpleasant sight, sound, or smell or after prolonged standing. Reflex or situational syncope occurs in certain specific situations, such as micturition, swallowing, coughing, and defecation. Orthostatic hypotension occurs within minutes after changing from a recumbent or sitting position to an upright posture. If syncope occurs during exercise; is associated with chest pain, palpitations, previous cardiac disease or with a family history of sudden death; or is not associated with a history of prodrome, suspicion for cardiac syncope is increased. Syncope associated with abnormal movements, such as tonic or clonic activity, suggests seizures. The possibility that seizures are a result of prolonged cerebral underperfusion from other causes must be explored carefully.

Past medical history of heart disease; cardiac surgery; trauma; and neurologic, psychiatric, and metabolic disorders should be investigated. A family history of syncope, arrhythmia, sudden or early death, seizure, migraine, and deafness is relevant and should be considered carefully.

Physical Examination

A complete physical examination, including thorough cardiac and neurologic evaluations, should be performed. A decrease in systolic blood pressure from baseline by 30 mm Hg when changing from supine to upright position is considered orthostatic hypotension. This is a useful test to identify hypovolemia (from dehydration, blood loss, or other causes) and patients with abnormal vagal reflex

59 Acute Cardiac Rhythm Disorders

James J. Joyce and Barry G. Baylen

ROLE OF THE GENERALIST

1   Distinguish normal variant cardiac rhythms from dysrhythmias.

2   Diagnose the type of dysrhythmia and search for an underlying cause.

3   Treat the dysrhythmia as indicated and maintain hemodynamic stability.

4   Treat any underlying cardiac or noncardiac disorder.

5   Refer to a pediatric cardiologist when indicated.

6   Ensure appropriate long-term follow-up of patients with chronic dysrhythmias or with a risk of recurrent dysrhythmia.

A cardiac rhythm disorder, or dysrhythmia, is an abnormality in the rate, regularity, or sequence of cardiac activation. This chapter discusses the recognition and short-term therapy of acute cardiac dysrhythmias at the time of initial presentation. Subsequent to initial stabilization, patients with a significant cardiac dysrhythmia should be referred to a pediatric cardiologist for follow-up (see Chapter 135). Immediate telephone consultation with a pediatric cardiologist during the initial stabilization can be extremely helpful. Failure to treat a life-threatening dysrhythmia quickly can result in tragedy; however, inappropriate or overly aggressive therapy can be just as dangerous.

FUNDAMENTALS

Basic Electrocardiogram Terminology

An electrocardiogram (ECG) is a graphic record of the total cardiac electrical current (see also Chapter 276). The scalar ECG is an inexpensive and widely used clinical tool that is acquired easily and is the mainstay in the differential diagnosis of a cardiac dysrhythmia. Although computer interpretations of ECGs are readily available, the clinician's role as final interpreter must not be diminished, especially because computerized interpretations often are erroneous. Figure 59-1 shows a typical example of a sinus rhythm ECG waveform.

Common Benign Rhythm Disorders, Including Isolated Prematurities

Normal sinus rhythm is identified on the ECG by a regular rhythm, a normal P-wave axis (0 to 90 degrees, positive or isoelectric P-wave deflections in leads I and aVF), and a normal P-QRS-T sequence. Minor cardiac rhythm disturbances, which are benign and do not require any specific therapy, are seen frequently. *Sinus arrhythmia*, a regularly irregular sinus rhythm that varies with respiration, is extremely common in pediatric patients. A normal variant that is much less common is *low right atrial rhythm*, which closely resembles sinus rhythm except for an abnormal P-wave axis (negative P-wave deflection in aVF). The *junctional escape rhythm* (regular narrow QRS rhythm without associated P waves), which is rarer, also can be normal if the rate is adequate. Normal variant rhythms generally are seen on ECG during periods of rest, especially deep sleep, when the heart rate is slower. If the average heart rate is sufficient, no specific therapy is needed (see Table 2-2).

Sinus bradycardia, a sinus rate lower than established lower limits of normal for age, is especially common in athletic children and adolescents. Specific therapy is necessary only when signs and symptoms of decreased cardiac output are present. Causes of marked sinus bradycardia include vagal stimulation, hypoxemia, drug effect, hypothermia, increased intracranial pressure, and hypothyroidism.

Sinus tachycardia is a sinus rhythm with a rate greater than normal for age, which in children is usually a normal physiologic response to a precipitating factor, such as exertion, anxiety, pain, and fear. Other more significant causes include fever, anemia, hypovolemia, hypoglycemia,

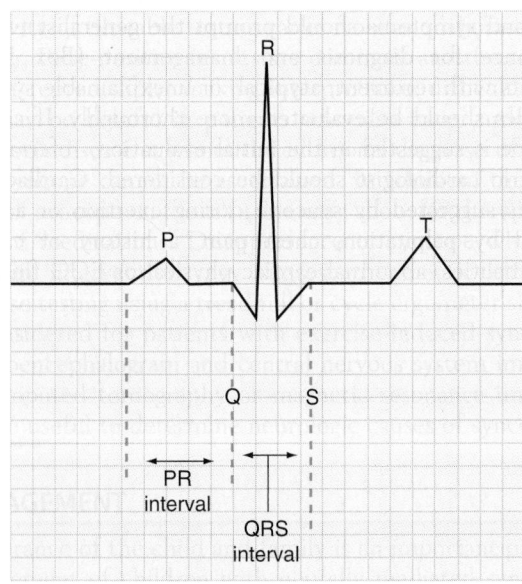

Figure 59-1. Electrocardiogram terminology and sinus rhythm.

hypoxemia, hypercapnia, hyperthyroidism, drug effect, and heart failure. Treatment should be aimed at the underlying cause. Attempts to decrease the heart rate directly by medication are inappropriate except during the early phase of therapy for hyperthyroidism.

Premature atrial complexes are typically benign, especially if they are isolated and unifocal, and should not cause great concern unless there are other symptoms or signs of heart disease. These rhythms are especially common during the first few days of life.

Isolated, unifocal *premature ventricular complexes* are generally benign. Premature ventricular complexes are almost certainly benign if there is no evidence of underlying heart disease, and the premature ventricular complexes disappear with exercise. When there is an associated cardiac or extracardiac disorder, treatment should be directed initially at the underlying disease. The presence of ventricular couplets, two ventricular premature complexes in a row, greatly increases the risk of ventricular tachycardia.

GENERAL PRINCIPLES OF THERAPY

In the treatment of a cardiac dysrhythmia, prime consideration should be given to the clinical setting and the natural history of the rhythm disorder. Antiarrhythmic drug therapy should be initiated with some knowledge of the most likely underlying mechanism responsible for the dysrhythmia. Tachycardic rhythm disturbances caused by enhanced automaticity often must be treated differently from tachydysrhythmias caused by reentry. *Direct current*

cardioversion is effective only in the reentry type of tachydysrhythmias.

Cardiac dysrhythmias may occur without underlying structural heart disease. A thorough evaluation for primary cardiac disease should be undertaken quickly, however. Examples include congenital heart defects, myocarditis, Kawasaki disease, Lyme disease, rheumatic heart disease, cardiac trauma, myocardial tumors, and dilated or hypertrophic cardiomyopathy. Extracardiac disorders also can cause rhythm disturbances, especially drug side effects, electrolyte imbalance, hypoglycemia, acidosis, and hypoxia.

With rare exception, antiarrhythmic drug therapy should be initiated with a single agent. Simultaneous administration of multiple drugs can make it impossible to determine which medication is responsible for the desired effect and, more important, which drug is the cause of any undesirable side effect that might occur. Combination drug therapy should be considered only when one antiarrhythmic drug given in an adequate dose fails to control, or only partially controls, a dysrhythmia. Amiodarone and procainamide should *not* be administered together because both prolong the Q-T interval and can produce ventricular arrhythmias. Pediatric antiarrhythmic drug dosage ranges are listed in Table 59-1.

The other important determinant of initial therapy is hemodynamic instability in the patient, manifested by hypotension; altered consciousness; prolonged capillary refill time; and signs of heart failure, such as a loud gallop, hyperdynamic precordial impulse, basilar crackles, tachypnea, jugular venous distention, edema, and hepatomegaly.

Table 59-1. Pediatric Antiarrhythmic Drug Dosages

Drug	Route	Dose	Frequency
Adenosine	IV bolus	0.1 mg/kg initial bolus (maximum first dose 6 mg; maximum second dose 12 mg)	May repeat in 2–4 min at 0.2 mg/kg
Amiodarone	IV load	5 mg/kg rapid bolus if pulseless, otherwise over 20–30 min (maximum 15 mg/kg/day, not to exceed 2 g/day)	May repeat once
	IV maintenance	7 µg/kg/min	Continuous infusion
Atenolol	PO	1–2 mg/kg	Once daily
Atropine	IV bolus	0.02 mg/kg (minimum bolus 0.1 mg; maximum bolus 1 mg; maximum total 2 mg)	May repeat once in 3–5 min
Digoxin	PO load	Total loading dose: 20 µg/kg preterm infant, 30 µg/kg term infant, 40 µg/kg young child, 30 µg/kg older child	Total loading dose divided into 3 doses over first 24 hr
	PO maintenance	2.5–5 µg/kg	Every 12 hr
	IV load and maintence	75% of PO doses	As above
Diltiazem	IV load	0.1–0.2 mg/kg over 2 min	15 min later may give second loading dose at 0.2–0.35 mg/kg
	IV maintenance	1–3 µg/kg/min (maximum 10 mg/hr)	Continuous infusion
Epinephrine	IV bolus	0.01 mg/kg (1:10,000 = 0.1 mL/kg; maximum 1 mg/dose)	Every 3–5 min
	Endotracheal	0.1 mg/kg (1:1000; 0.1 mL/kg)	Every 3–5 min
Esmolol	IV load	0.5 mg/kg over 1 min	May repeat every 4 min
	IV infusion	50–200 µg/kg/min	Continuous infusion
Lidocaine	IV load	1 mg/kg bolus	May repeat once or twice at 5–15 min intervals
	IV infusion	20–50 µg/kg/min (maximum 4 mg/min)	Continuous infusion
Magnesium sulfate	IV bolus	25–50 mg/kg over 30–60 min (maximum dose 2 g)	May repeat if serum magnesium level low
Procainamide	IV load	7–15 mg/kg over 30–60 min	
	IV infusion	30–60 µg/kg/min	Continuous infusion
Propranolol	PO	0.5–1 mg/kg	Every 6 hr

IV, intravenous; PO, oral.

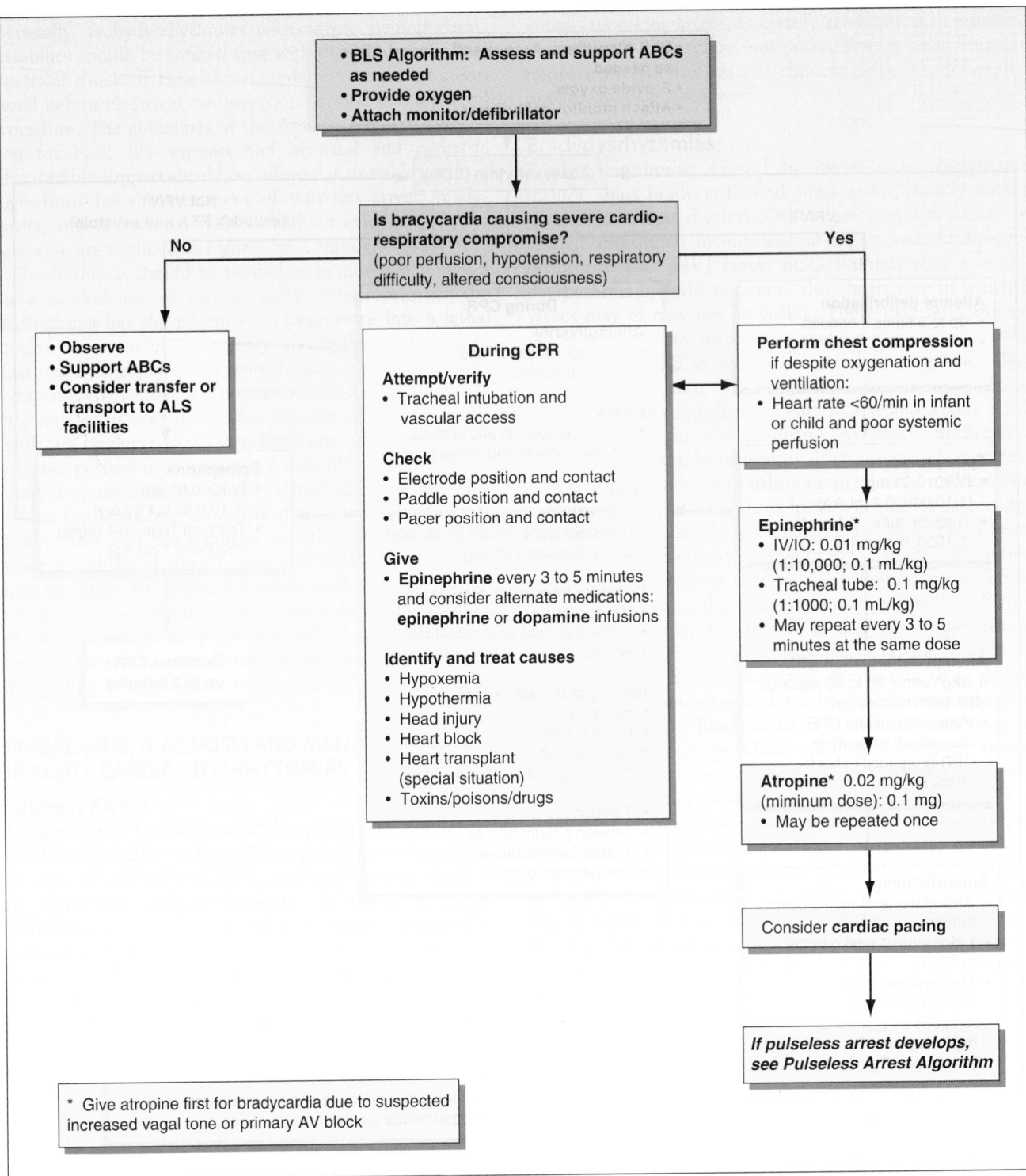

Figure 59-3. Bradycardia algorithm. ABCs, airway, breathing, circulation; ALS, advanced life support; AV, atrioventricular; BLS, basic life support; CPR, cardiopulmonary resuscitation; IO, intraosseous; IV, intravenous. (Modified from American Heart Association: Circulation, vol. 102, no. 8, pt. 10. Philadelphia, Lippincott, Williams & Wilkins, 2000.)

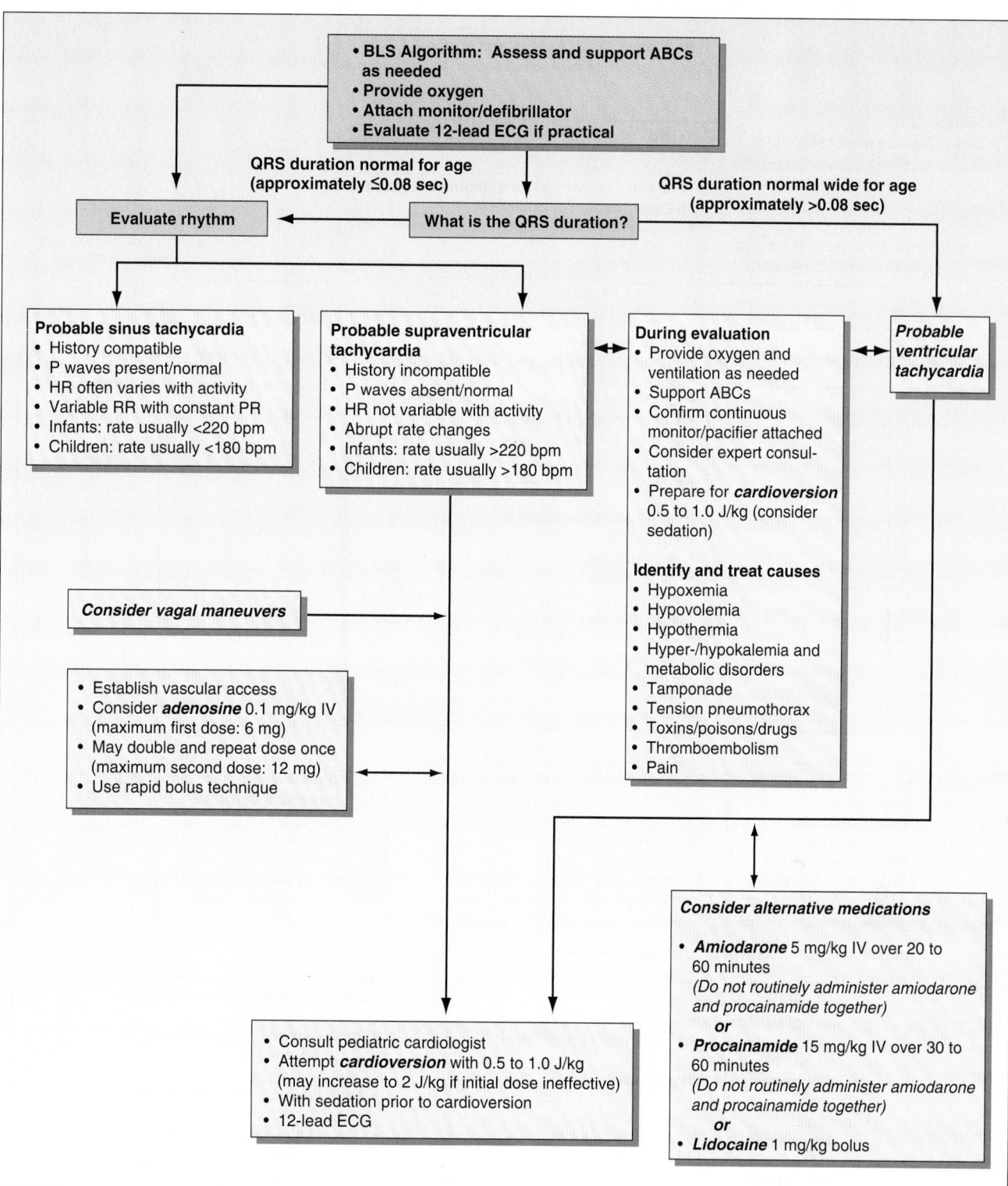

Figure 59-4. Tachycardia algorithm for infants and children with rapid rhythm and adequate perfusion. ABCs, airway, breathing, circulation; BLS, basic life support; ECG, electrocardiogram; HR, heart rate; IV, intravenous. (Modified from American Heart Association: Circulation, vol. 102, no. 8, pt. 10. Philadelphia, Lippincott, Williams & Wilkins, 2000.)

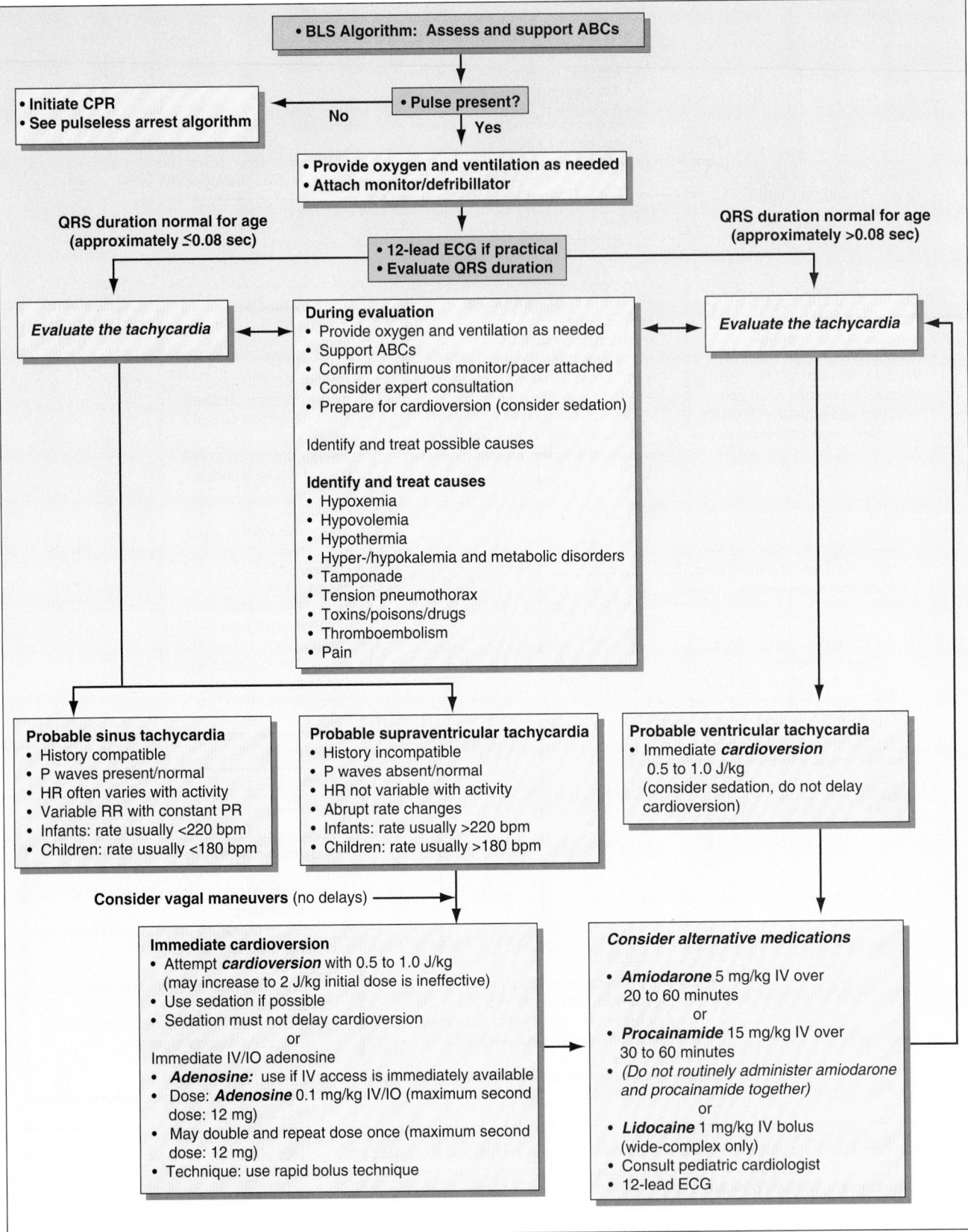

Figure 59-5. Tachycardia algorithm for infants and children with rapid rhythm and evidence of poor perfusion. ABCs, airway, breathing, circulation; BLS, basic life support; CPR, cardiopulmonary resuscitation; ECG, electrocardiogram; HR, heart rate; IO, intraosseous; IV, intravenous. (Modified from American Heart Association: Circulation, vol. 102, no. 8, pt. 10. Philadelphia, Lippincott, Williams & Wilkins, 2000.)

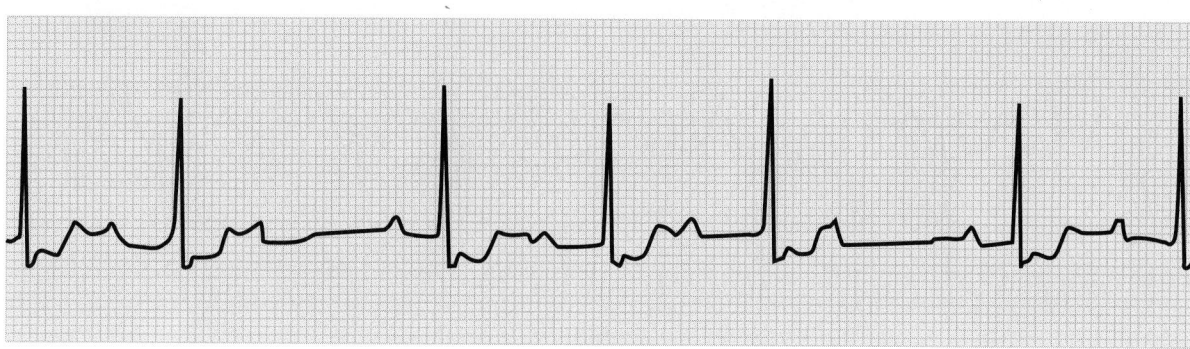

Figure 59-6. Wenckebach second-degree heart block.

and a maximum single dose of 0.5 mg for a child or 1 mg for an adolescent; the dose can be repeated in 3 to 5 minutes to a maximal total dose of 1 mg for a child or 2 mg for an adolescent.

If bradycardia responds only transiently to initial drug therapy with bolus epinephrine or atropine, despite adequate ventilation and oxygenation, a continuous infusion of epinephrine or dopamine should be considered. In patients with bradycardia unresponsive to medical therapy, emergency transcutaneous pacing should be attempted. The negative electrode should be placed over the anterior chest near the apex of the heart, and the positive electrode should be placed behind the heart on the back. Pacemaker output requires adjustment to ensure that each pacemaker electrical impulse results in a ventricular depolarization and contraction. Because of large pacing artifacts with transcutaneous pacing, determination of whether ventricular depolarization is taking place is difficult without palpating for a pulse.

Tachydysrhythmias

Supraventricular tachycardia (SVT) is a rapid regular rhythm, which is generally paroxysmal and produced in most cases by a reentry mechanism involving the AV node and an accessory AV pathway, called *AV reentry tachycardia* (Fig. 59-8). This accessory pathway usually is concealed from lack of antegrade conduction, but in some patients it is manifest during sinus rhythm, with antegrade conduction causing preexcitation of the ventricle and the ECG delta wave of Wolff-Parkinson-White syndrome. Fewer pediatric patients have SVT caused by AV nodal reentry tachycardia by virtue of dual nodal pathways. Although SVT usually is well tolerated for a short time in

most patients, it can lead to cardiovascular collapse, especially in small infants. The heart rates during SVT vary with age. In infants, SVT typically is faster than 220 beats/min and often faster than 240 beats/min. In children, SVT characteristically is faster than 180 beats/min. During SVT, there is almost no beat-to-beat variation, and the heart rate does not vary with activity, in contrast to sinus tachycardia. Onset and termination of SVT is usually abrupt, whereas with sinus tachycardia the heart rate accelerates and decelerates more gradually. The rhythm is usually regular, and distinct P waves may not be seen. If P waves can be identified in SVT, the P-wave axis is typically abnormal. In most cases, the QRS duration is normal. SVT with aberrant conduction causing a wide QRS is rare in infants and children, but when present may be difficult to distinguish from ventricular tachycardia. Because either SVT or ventricular tachycardia can cause hemodynamic instability, assumptions about the mechanism should not be based on the hemodynamic status of the patient. In most cases, wide-complex tachycardias should be treated as if they are ventricular tachycardia (see Fig. 59-4).

If a patient with SVT is hemodynamically stable, vagal maneuvers, such as an ice-cold object applied to the face, a gag reflex, or a Valsalva maneuver, can be attempted first. Crushed ice mixed with water in a plastic bag or glove is most effective in infants and young children, but care must be used to avoid obstructing ventilation when applying to the face. Regardless of which maneuver is attempted, the ECG must be monitored continuously during and shortly after the maneuver. Adenosine, which causes a temporary block of conduction through the AV node, interrupting the reentry circuit, is the initial drug of choice for treatment of SVT without hemodynamic compromise. The initial

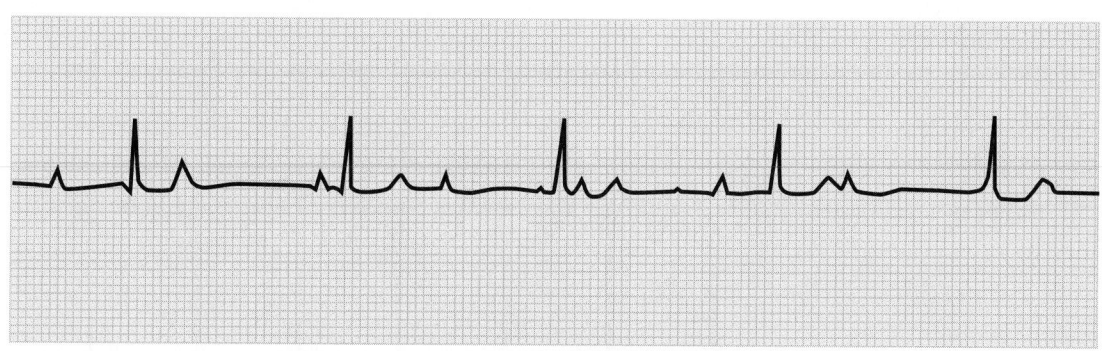

Figure 59-7. Third-degree heart block.

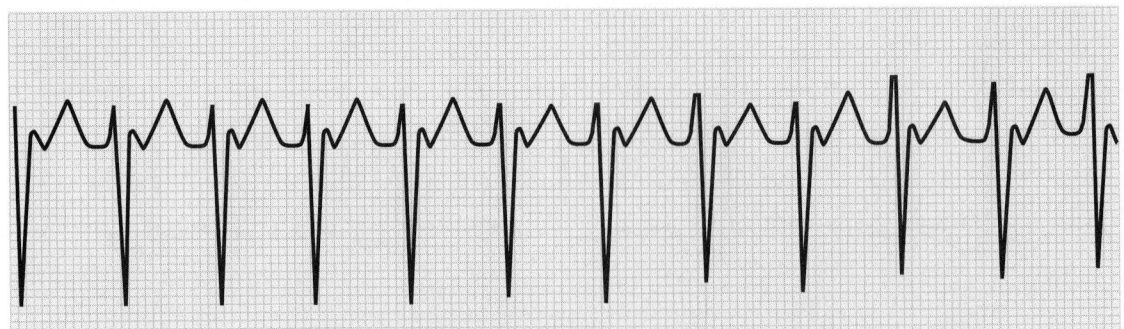

Figure 59-8. Atrioventricular reentry tachycardia.

dose, which should be given in a rapid bolus intravenously, is 0.1 mg/kg followed immediately by a rapid bolus of a few milliliters of normal saline. A continuous ECG should be recorded during bolus infusion. If there is no effect, the dosage should be doubled and repeated. The adenosine dose should not exceed 0.25 mg/kg or 12 mg. Side effects, such as flushing, dyspnea, chest pain, or irritability, occur frequently but along with the concomitant bradycardia, usually resolve completely within 1 minute. *Calcium channel blockers, particularly verapamil, should not* be used to treat SVT in infants, children with congestive heart failure, children receiving β-adrenergic blocking drugs, or anyone with Wolff-Parkinson-White syndrome because profound hypotension and cardiac arrest have been reported in these situations. Procainamide or amiodarone can be used in infants and children with hemodynamically stable SVT.

If a patient with SVT is hemodynamically unstable (see Fig. 59-5), DC cardioversion should be attempted initially at 0.5 J/kg; it can be increased to 2 J/kg if necessary. The synchronizer circuit must be activated first, and the discharge button must be pressed and held until the countershock is delivered. If vascular access is already available, adenosine may be tried quickly before electrical cardioversion, but cardioversion should not be delayed if an intravenous line is not already in place in an unstable patient.

An unusual type of reentry SVT, which is difficult to treat and highly recurrent, is permanent junctional reciprocating tachycardia. This diagnosis should be considered in a patient with SVT that responds only briefly to adenosine or DC cardioversion and then quickly recurs. Rarely, SVT is not due to a reentry mechanism, but rather is due to enhanced automaticity, which does not respond at all to adenosine or DC cardioversion. Ectopic atrial tachycardia and junctional ectopic tachycardia are automatic tachy-

dysrhythmias, which generally are chronic and almost incessant, typically accelerating and decelerating gradually on initiation and termination. A pediatric cardiologist should be consulted for therapy of these unusual types of SVT, which are difficult to control and commonly cause congestive heart failure if prolonged.

Atrial flutter, recognized by the sawtooth flutter waves of atrial activation as shown in Figure 59-9, is a regular rapid atrial rhythm, commonly with 2:1 AV conduction. With variable AV conduction, the ventricular response is irregular. *Atrial fibrillation* is identified by a chaotic rapid atrial rate with changing fibrillation waves associated with an irregularly irregular, less rapid ventricular response. With atrial flutter and atrial fibrillation, if the patient is hemodynamically stable, medical therapy can be attempted. Adenosine is unlikely to convert either of these atrial dysrhythmias because their reentry pathways do not involve the AV node. Typically, medical therapy can start with a β-blocker, such as esmolol, propranolol, or atenolol, to slow the ventricular rate. Calcium channel blockers, especially diltiazem, also can be used to slow the ventricular response, but only if there are no contraindications as mentioned earlier for patients with SVT. If myocardial function seems to be depressed, and there is no evidence of Wolff-Parkinson-White syndrome preexcitation, digoxin is preferred. In patients with congestive heart failure and preexcitation, amiodarone is recommended. After acute control of the ventricular rate in atrial flutter or atrial fibrillation, pharmacologic or electrical cardioversion of the atrial dysrhythmia can be attempted under the direction of a cardiologist. Atrial fibrillation and, to a lesser extent, atrial flutter are associated with a risk of atrial thrombus formation when present for more than 2 days. Because transesophageal echocardiography and anticoagulation may be indicated before cardioversion in such circumstances, a cardiology

Figure 59-9. Atrial flutter.

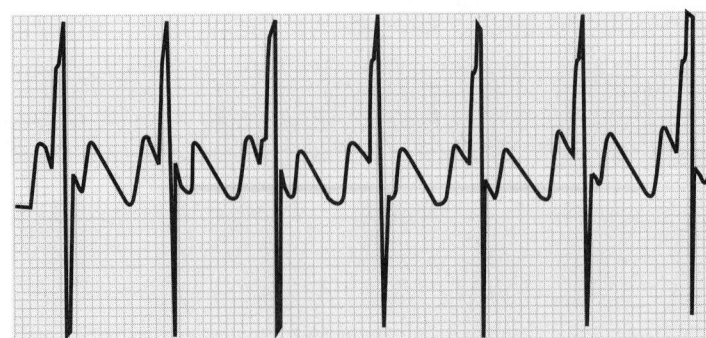

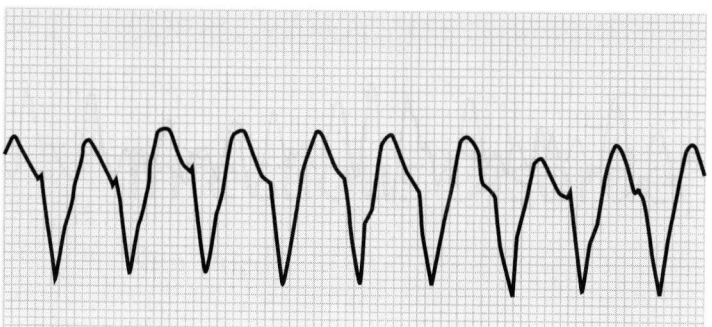

Figure 59-10. Ventricular tachycardia.

consultation should precede elective cardioversion in these cases. Synchronized electrical cardioversion is the treatment of choice for atrial fibrillation or atrial flutter with evidence of hemodynamic instability. The initial DC cardioversion dose is 0.5 J/kg, which can be increased to 2 J/kg.

Ventricular tachycardia is recognized by a regular, uniform pattern wide QRS complex tachycardia with no associated P waves (Fig. 59-10). About 10% of pediatric cardiac arrest patients have pulseless ventricular tachycardia or ventricular fibrillation. Ventricular tachycardia without a pulse should be treated the same as ventricular fibrillation, beginning with an unsynchronized DC electrical shock (see Fig. 59-2). In a patient with sustained ventricular tachycardia and a pulse but who is hemodynamically unstable, DC cardioversion beginning with 1 to 2 J/kg should be performed immediately (see Fig. 59-5). When sustained ventricular tachycardia presents in a hemodynamically stable patient, who is alert with good distal pulses, intravenous lidocaine, procainamide, or amiodarone can be tried first in consultation with a cardiologist. If such an antiarrhythmic drug is ineffective, DC cardioversion with sedation, starting at 1 J/kg, is a reasonable alternative. After stabilization, a careful search should be undertaken for an underlying myocardial disease, unless there is an obvious noncardiac cause, such as severe potassium imbalance or drug toxicity.

Rarely, ventricular tachycardia can be polymorphic with a variable QRS configuration. Typically, this rhythm is associated with underlying Q-T prolongation and produces a twisting pattern called *torsades de pointes* (Fig. 59-11). In such cases, antiarrhythmic medications that may prolong the Q-T interval, such as procainamide and amiodarone, must be avoided. If torsades de pointes is suspected, 25 mg/kg of magnesium sulfate should be given by slow intravenous bolus over 10 to 20 minutes. If the patient is hemodynamically unstable, DC cardioversion should be

administered quickly. Because recurrence is common, a cardiologist should be consulted as soon as possible.

Ventricular fibrillation is a pulseless rhythm with a rapid chaotic wide-complex pattern on the ECG (Fig. 59-12). The emergency therapy for this rhythm is outlined in Figure 59-2. Adult-sized paddles should be used for defibrillation shocks if the patient's chest size permits complete contact. The larger paddle size lowers the transthoracic impedance, resulting in a higher current flow facilitating defibrillation. A cardiologist should evaluate thoroughly survivors of cardiac arrest without an obvious transient cause, such as a drug overdose.

INDICATIONS FOR REFERRAL

When the patient's rhythm and cardiopulmonary status are stable, the clinician should perform a rapid secondary survey and monitor temperature closely. The clinician should consider obtaining any indicated laboratory studies, such as serum glucose, electrolytes, hematocrit, or arterial blood gas. If the patient has the potential to become unstable again, he or she should be transferred expeditiously to an appropriate medical facility. As mentioned earlier, after initial stabilization, a pediatric cardiologist should evaluate most pediatric patients who have had a significant dysrhythmia.

FOLLOW-UP

Children with minor acute cardiac rhythm disturbances that have a transient, easily treatable cause do not require more than routine well-child follow-up. A pediatric cardiologist should evaluate all other dysrhythmia patients, however, even after the acute dysrhythmia has resolved. Appropriate cardiac follow-up and precautions are outlined by the cardiology consultant. Tests that are used frequently

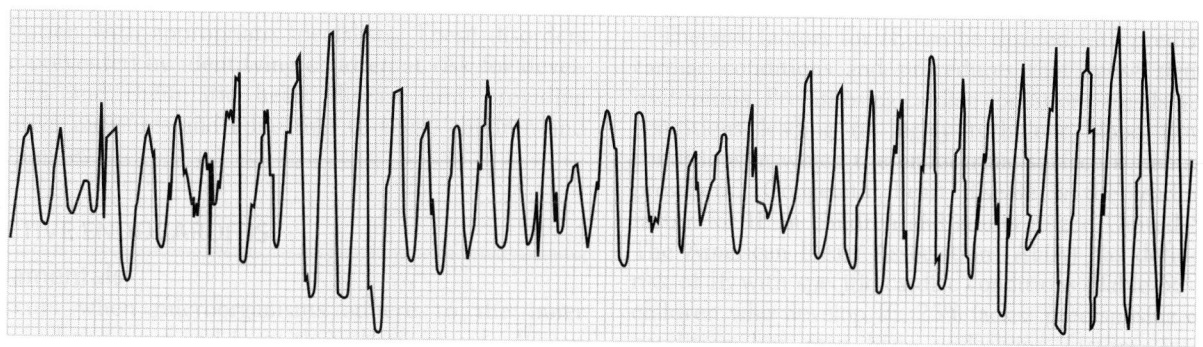

Figure 59-11. Torsades de pointes (polymorphic ventricular tachycardia caused by Q-T prolongation).

associated with a poor medical prognosis. Surgery often is indicated for ruptured chordae tendineae or papillary muscles, refractory heart block, abscesses, and postoperative endocarditis occurring less than 8 weeks after cardiac surgery.

Outcome

Before the availability of anti-infective therapy, IE was universally fatal. Today, mortality among children with IE has been reduced to less than 10%. Recurrent endocarditis is common among children who undergo surgery before infected vegetations are sterilized, but urgent and lifesaving procedures should not be deferred solely because of the likelihood of recurrent infection.

Follow-up and Prevention

Many cases of pediatric IE can be prevented by the use of appropriate antimicrobial prophylaxis. Antimicrobial prophylaxis for IE is thought to work by preventing the adherence of bacteria to sterile vegetations rather than killing them in the bloodstream. Antimicrobial prophylaxis for IE differs from that of rheumatic fever in that it is episodic.

Endocarditis prophylaxis is indicated for a specific procedure only if a patient is known to have a high- to moderate-risk cardiac lesion and if the procedure induces significant bacteremia. Specific prophylaxis regimens depend on the site of the procedure. Dental, oral, respiratory tract, and esophageal prophylaxis regimens are shown in Table 60-2. Different prophylaxis regimens, usually consisting of two doses, are used for genitourinary and gastrointestinal tract procedures. These regimens are listed in the American Academy of Pediatrics' *Red Book*, which is updated regularly to reflect current AHA recommendations.

Table 60-2. Prophylactic Regimens for Dental, Oral, Respiratory Tract, or Esophageal Procedures

Situation	Agent	Regimen*
Standard general prophylaxis	Amoxicillin	Adults, 2 g; children, 50 mg/kg orally 1 hr before procedure
Unable to take oral medications	Ampicillin	Adults, 2 g IM or IV; children, 50 mg/kg IM or IV within 30 min before procedure
Allergic to penicillin	Clindamycin *or*	Adults, 600 mg; children, 20 mg/kg orally 1 hr before procedure
	Cephalexin† or cefadroxil† *or*	Adults, 2 g; children, 50 mg/kg orally 1 hr before procedure
	Azithromycin or clarithromycin	Adults, 500 mg; children, 15 mg/kg orally 1 hr before procedure
Allergic to penicillin and unable to take oral medications	Clindamycin *or*	Adults, 600 mg; children, 20 mg/kg IV within 30 min before procedure
	Cefazolin†	Adults, 1 g; children, 25 mg/kg IM or IV within 30 min before procedure

*Total children's dose should not exceed adult dose.
†Cephalosporins should not be used in individuals with immediate-type hypersensitivity reaction (urticaria, angioendema, or anaphylaxis) to penicillins.
IM, intramuscularly; IV, intravenously.

Children with high- to moderate-risk cardiac conditions or their parents should be given an AHA wallet card that lists up-to-date prophylaxis regimens. Patients and their families should be instructed to inform other health care providers about their risk for IE and to show health care providers their prophylaxis cards as needed.

INFECTIOUS MYOCARDITIS

Fundamentals

Myocarditis comprises a diverse group of infectious and noninfectious disorders that lead to inflammation of the myocardium. Noninfectious causes of myocarditis include autoimmune disorders (rheumatic fever, lupus erythematosus, KD, dermatomyositis, scleroderma, and sarcoidosis), substance abuse (alcohol, cocaine), medications (doxorubicin, cyclophosphamide, phenothiazines), toxins (lead, mercury), genetic disorders (familial dilated cardiomyopathies, spinocerebellar ataxia, Duchenne's muscular dystrophy, myotonic dystrophy), and endocrinologic or metabolic disorders (thyrotoxicosis, hypothyroidism, hypocalcemia, hypophosphatemia). With the exceptions of KD and rheumatic myocarditis, noninfectious myocarditis occurs primarily among adults and older children.

Infectious myocarditis is relevant to the general pediatric provider as an important cause of sudden death and has been documented in 28% of children and adolescents who have died sudden cardiac deaths. Although the incidence of infectious myocarditis is not known precisely, it is most common among neonates. It is one of the causes of sudden infant death syndrome.

Innumerable infectious agents can cause myocarditis. Viruses are the most common and include group B coxsackieviruses, echoviruses, and other enteroviruses; adenoviruses; cytomegalovirus and Epstein-Barr virus; human immunodeficiency virus (HIV) type 1; and influenzaviruses. Bacterial causes include group A streptococci, *S. aureus*, salmonella, *Neisseria meningitidis*, *Mycoplasma pneumoniae*, *Rickettsia rickettsiae*, *Brucella melitensis*, *Mycobacterium tuberculosis*, and *Borrelia burgdorferi*. Myocarditis is the leading cause of death from toxin-producing *Corynebacterium diphtheriae* and remains common in countries where children are not immunized routinely. A parasite, *Trypanosoma cruzi* (the agent of Chagas' disease), is the predominant cause of myocarditis in South America, where it infects 18 million individuals. Chagas' myocarditis is unusual in that it tends to manifest years after primary infection, although it may present acutely and initially involves the right ventricle. Other parasitic causes include *Toxoplasma gondii*, *Trichinella spiralis*, and the agents of African trypanosomiasis. Fungal myocarditis is rare and typically affects severely immunocompromised adults. Reported fungal causes include *Cryptococcus neoformans*, *Candida*, and *Aspergillus*.

Diagnosis

Most cases of infectious myocarditis are subclinical. Symptomatic cases often have an insidious presentation. A high index of suspicion is required to make the diagnosis. Rarely, infectious myocarditis is fulminant, but even then, disease may be mistaken for bacterial sepsis, adult respiratory distress syndrome, or toxic shock because of concomitant multiorgan failure.

Initial symptoms are vague and may be limited to fatigue and malaise. Fever, pharyngitis, rhinorrhea, and cough may precede viral myocarditis, but these symptoms generally are absent or forgotten by the time clinical cardiac disease is apparent. Parents may note pallor, irritability, and difficulty feeding in young infants.

The most common and often sole sign is tachycardia, which is frequently out of proportion to the height of fever. Later findings include diminished arterial pulses, pulsus alternans, a hypoactive precordium on palpation, and ventricular gallops, reflecting dilated cardiomyopathy; tachypnea, dyspnea, and bibasilar rales; and, rarely, hepatomegaly, reflecting left-sided or bilateral cardiac failure. In young infants, a sepsis-like syndrome may occur, with lethargy, cutaneous mottling, cool extremities, and, rarely, frank circulatory collapse.

Electrocardiograms may be normal during the early stages, but supraventricular tachycardia, ventricular extrasystoles, or signs of ischemia, including ST-segment elevations or T-wave changes (inversions, biphasic patterns, or notching), may be observed. Diffuse low voltages, which are QRS complexes less than 0.5 mV (5 mm in height on a standard tracing), are less common. Chest radiographs are initially normal, but may show cardiomegaly or pulmonary edema with disease progression. Cardiac enzymes, including the MB fraction of creatine kinase (CK-MB) and troponins T or P, can be elevated in later disease, but these are nonspecific because other causes of myocardial necrosis, including infarction and noninfectious myocarditis, can lead to similar elevations.

Echocardiography has become the most useful diagnostic modality, and serial studies are indispensable for managing severe cases. Early echocardiographic findings include regional myocardial edema and focal and intermittent wall motion abnormalities. Later findings include dilation of the left or both ventricles, persistent wall motion abnormalities, and decreased ventricular systolic function.

Endomyocardial biopsy is the most specific diagnostic test. Isolation of the causative agent from the myocardium or detection of its specific proteins or nucleic acids within myocardial tissue provides a definitive diagnosis. Complications from the procedure occur in 6% of adult cases and include perforation, tamponade, and death. Biopsy is performed only when the benefit of knowing the diagnosis outweighs the risks of the procedure. Isolation of a suspected infectious agent from a commonly infected body site (e.g., enteroviruses from the stool or adenoviruses from the throat) provides circumstantial evidence of causality if the agent has been shown to cause myocarditis.

Management

Patients with signs of early, dilated cardiomyopathy should be hospitalized in an intensive care unit, and infectious disease and cardiology specialists should be consulted. Treatment of infectious myocarditis is directed against the specific infectious agent when feasible. Ganciclovir has been used successfully to treat cytomegalovirus myocarditis, but data for other antivirals are lacking. Supportive care is the usual mainstay of care. Strict bed rest and attentive cardiac monitoring are essential, and oxygen is provided as needed. Dopamine and dobutamine are used most commonly to improve cardiac output. Phosphodiesterase inhibitors such as milrinone have afterload-reducing and inotropic effects and may improve ventricular relaxation. Antiarrhythmic medications, if needed, should be used cautiously in patients with depressed left ventricular function or failure because all can depress left ventricular function further, precipitating or worsening heart failure. Amiodarone and lidocaine cause the least added impairment of left ventricular function. There is no consensus regarding use of corticosteroids, cellular immunosuppressants (azathioprine, cyclosporine, and others), and intravenous immunoglobulins (IVIG) as adjunctive therapies.

Outcome

Death from congestive heart failure or sudden death from dysrhythmias occurs in one third of children who develop acute dilated cardiomyopathy, usually within 1 or 2 years after onset of disease. Survival with residual cardiac dysfunction occurs in one third, and one third have a full recovery. Prognosis among neonates with coxsackievirus B or adenovirus myocarditis is dismal. Fulminant infectious myocarditis has the highest mortality, but survivors have relatively few long-term sequelae. Less than half of children who develop chronic dilated cardiomyopathy progress to have end-stage cardiomyopathy requiring cardiac transplantation.

Follow-up and Prevention

Children with chronic myocardial dysfunction and immunocompromised children, including children with HIV disease and transplants, generally require long-term subspecialty care. Agents to manage chronic congestive heart failure occasionally are needed. β-Blockers or pacemakers are effective in preventing sudden death from dysrhythmias. Generalist pediatricians continue to provide the most effective protection against diphtheritic myocarditis by immunizing their patients.

INFECTIOUS PERICARDITIS

Pericarditis of any etiology is rare, particularly among children (see the CD-ROM). Most clinically significant pericarditis affects adults, is chronic, and represents a complication of prior pericardial inflammation. Noninfectious causes of pericarditis include rheumatic fever, systemic lupus erythematosus, chronic uremia, cardiac or mediastinal malignancy, mediastinal radiation therapy, and hypersensitivity reactions to various medications. Most infectious pericarditis in children is viral, acute, mild, and self-limited. Viral pericarditis often is due to the same viruses that cause myocarditis: coxsackieviruses and echoviruses, adenoviruses, herpesviruses (including herpes simplex, cytomegalovirus, and varicella-zoster virus), and influenzaviruses. Enteroviruses and adenoviruses may cause myocarditis and pericarditis simultaneously in infants, in whom mortality is high.

Fever is the most common symptom of infectious pericarditis, affecting more than half of patients. Chest pain can be significant and often is aggravated by lying in the supine

61

Disorders of the Ear

Monica Sifuentes

ROLE OF THE GENERALIST

1   Distinguish otitis externa from otitis media.

2   Recognize complications associated with otitis media.

3   Treat infections of the external and middle ear appropriately.

4   Diagnose masses of the middle ear.

5   Recognize traumatic abnormalities of the tympanic membrane.

6   Consult otolaryngologist as needed for assistance with medical and surgical management.

7   Prevent long-term sequelae associated with untreated disorders of the ear, including sensorineural hearing loss.

8   Provide appropriate follow-up for children who have recurrent otitis media, hearing loss, and traumatic perforations of the tympanic membrane.

DEFINITION

Disorders of the ear in pediatric patients include infections of the middle ear, infections of the external ear canal, congenital and acquired masses, and complications related to blunt or direct head trauma. Early and correct recognition of these conditions is essential.

Otitis media (OM) is an acute or chronic inflammation of the middle ear. Acute OM (AOM) is an acute infection of the middle ear with middle ear effusion (MEE) by otoscopic examination. The tympanic membrane (TM) often is red, bulging, and opaque. AOM usually is manifested by ear pain or tugging or rubbing of the ear. Fever and irritability may be present. OM with effusion (OME) is a painless collection of fluid in the middle ear without any signs of acute inflammation or infection. Most cases evolve from AOM, but a preceding infection is not necessary.

Recurrent AOM is defined as three new episodes of AOM within 6 months or four episodes within 1 year. Resolution of the infection should be documented between each episode of AOM, but this may be difficult if OME develops. Chronic OM is the presence of MEE for more than 3 months. Recurrent and chronic disease can occur simultaneously because the presence of one condition often predisposes to the other.

Complications of OM can be divided into intratemporal and intracranial causes (Table 61-1). Children differ from

adults in that complications are more likely to occur from AOM than chronic ear disease and often are the result of delayed treatment. Hearing loss, the most prevalent complication, can be conductive, sensorineural, or mixed. The magnitude of the conductive hearing loss ranges from 15 to 40 dB and seems to result from the quantity, rather than the quality, of fluid in the middle ear. This type of hearing loss disappears when the MEE resolves. Infectious or inflammatory mediators in the middle ear or in the labyrinth can cause sensorineural hearing loss.

Children with AOM usually have fluid present in the mastoid air cells because of the direct connection with the middle ear (Fig. 61-1). Mastoiditis, an inflammatory process that accompanies OM, develops when there is destruction of bone or formation of a subperiosteal abscess within the cavity. Early in its course, mastoiditis may resolve spontaneously. When the infection persists for more than 1 week, inflammatory granulation tissue forms, and a series of changes occurs within the cavity, resulting in either acute or chronic mastoiditis. Acute mastoiditis is subdivided into pathologic stages depending on the progression of the disease within the mastoid air cells. Chronic mastoiditis almost always is associated with chronic suppurative OM, a chronic (≥2 months) drainage from the middle ear and the mastoid through either a perforation of the TM or a tympanostomy tube.

The most common suppurative intracranial complication of OM and mastoiditis is bacterial meningitis, although its incidence has decreased dramatically since the advent of antibiotic therapy for acute infections and routine immunization against *Haemophilus influenzae* type B. Other

Table 61-1. Complications and Sequelae of Acute Otitis Media

Intratemporal	Intracranial
Chronic suppurative otitis media	Bacterial meningitis
	Extradural abscess
Perforation of the tympanic membrane	Subdural empyema
	Lateral sinus thrombosis
Hearing loss (conductive and sensorineural)	Brain abscess
	Otitic hydrocephalus
Cholesteatoma	
Mastoiditis	
Petrositis	
Facial nerve paralysis	
Labyrinthitis	
Osteomyelitis of the temporal bone	
Bezold's abscess	

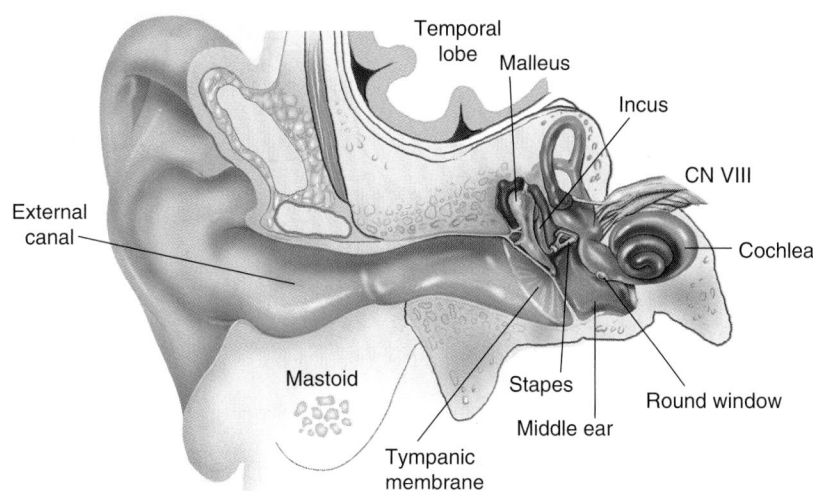

Figure 61-1. External, middle, and inner ear anatomy. (Modified from Bluestone CD, Klein JO: Otitis in Infants and Children. Philadelphia, WB Saunders, 1988.)

intracranial complications, such as subdural empyema and brain abscess, occur rarely in developed countries and are associated more often with other chronic diseases, such as sinusitis, rather than AOM.

Otitis externa (OE) refers to inflammation and infection of the external ear canal or the auricle. It is commonly known as *swimmer's ear*, an acute diffuse inflammation of the external auditory epithelium extending from the pinna all the way to the TM. Although inflammation of the TM also may occur, it usually can be differentiated from AOM by pneumatic otoscopy.

Perforations of the TM may be temporary or permanent depending on whether they are associated with AOM, a chronic infection, a surgical procedure, or trauma. Permanent perforations are classified as central or marginal. In central perforations, the fibrous annulus is unaffected, and the TM circumscribes the entire intact ring. Marginal perforations involve the fibrous annulus, and the defect is seen posteriorly on the TM. Abnormal growth of squamous epithelium into the middle ear as a result of destruction of the margin of the TM may lead to formation of a secondary cholesteatoma.

The most common ear mass in children is a cholesteatoma, a histologically benign lesion in the middle ear, mastoid space, or petrous bone containing keratinizing squamous epithelium. Occasionally a cholesteatoma may be found in the external auditory canal. Congenital, or primary, cholesteatoma is defined as the presence of squamous epithelium medial to an intact TM without a significant past history of AOM or eustachian tube dysfunction. Acquired, or secondary, cholesteatoma occurs more commonly as a complication of chronic OM. Cholesteatomas are locally invasive and can destroy important structures, such as the ossicles, cochlea, or semicircular canals.

FUNDAMENTALS

Figure 61-1 illustrates the normal anatomy of the ear and the relationship of the external, middle, and inner ear to one another. The location of the eustachian tube acts as a conduit connecting the middle ear to the nasopharynx. The development of OM in children is the direct result of

abnormal function of this tube. Anatomic features, such as its length and position relative to the posterior nasopharyngeal wall, contribute to increased frequency of OM. The eustachian tube in young infants is shorter and more horizontal than in older children (Fig. 61-2).

The eustachian tube has three major physiologic functions: (1) ventilation of the middle ear, (2) drainage of middle ear fluid, and (3) protection of the middle ear from nasopharyngeal secretions. These functions occur via active dilation of the tube by contraction of the tensor veli palatini

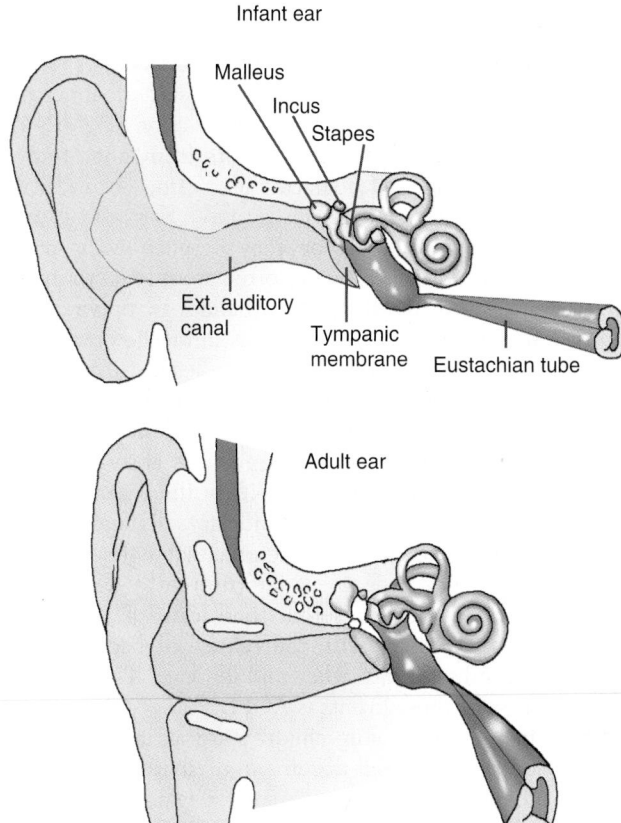

Figure 61-2. Adult and infant eustachian tube. (Modified from Bluestone CD, Klein JO: Pediatric Otolaryngology. Philadelphia, WB Saunders, 1996.)

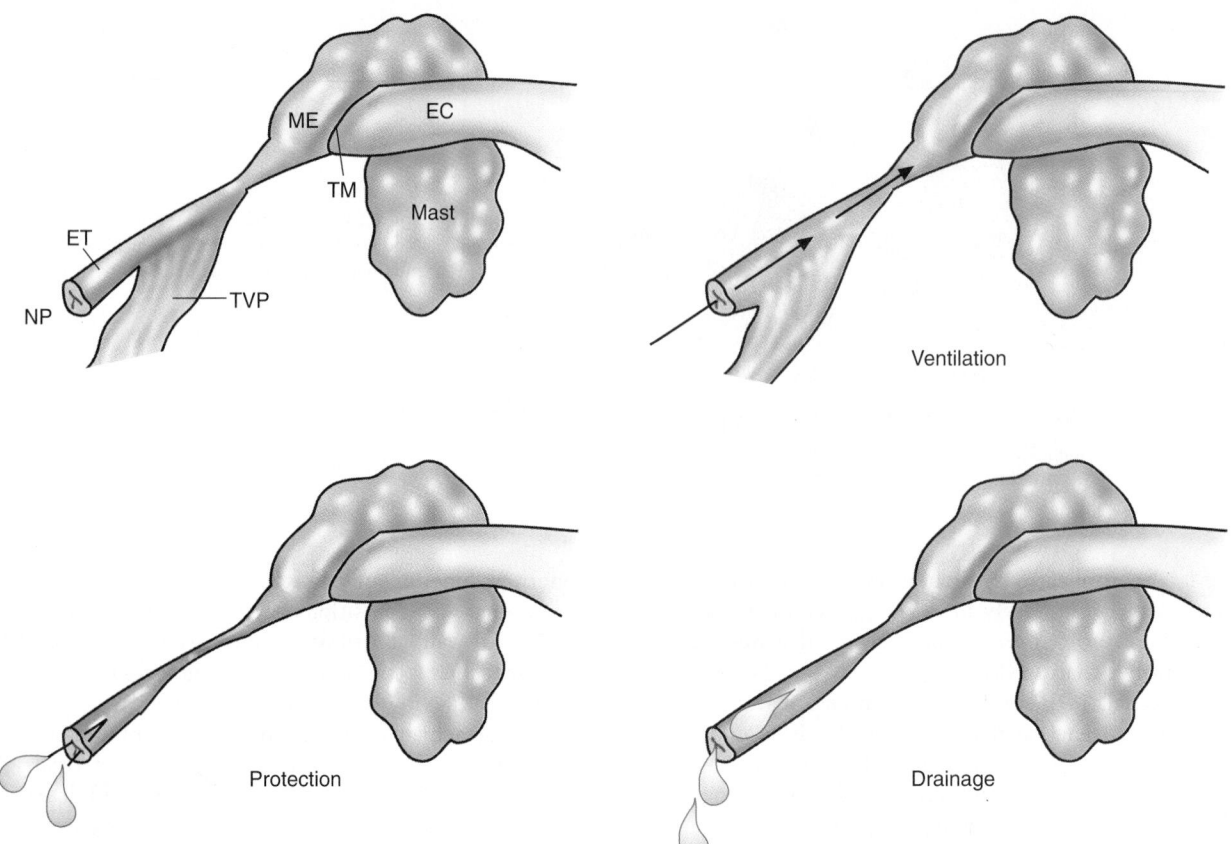

Figure 61-3. Functions of the eustachian tube. EC, external canal; ET, eustachian tube; ME, middle ear; NP, nasopharynx; TM, tympanic membrane; TVP, tensor veli palatini. (Modified from Bluestone CD, Klein JO: Otitis Media in Infants and Children. Philadelphia, WB Saunders, 1988.)

muscle (Fig. 61-3). Normal function of this muscle is essential in preventing MEE and acute infections.

Eustachian tube dysfunction is the result of abnormal patulence of the tube, mechanical obstruction (Fig. 61-4), or both. Functional obstruction results from poor tensor veli palatini function. Mechanical obstruction occurs from either an extrinsic or an intrinsic cause. Extrinsic causes include enlarged adenoids or the presence of a naso-pharyngeal tumor. Intrinsic causes often are related to injury or inflammation of distal tubal epithelium by upper respiratory infections with viruses such as influenza or respiratory syncytial virus. Epithelial damage leads to increased mucus secretion and cellular debris, which then obstructs the lumen. If the eustachian tube is occluded, negative middle ear pressure develops as oxygen is absorbed from this space. Transudative serous capillary fluid accumulates in the middle ear and the mastoid air cells and can be infected with nasopharyngeal bacteria that enter through the eustachian tube as it opens intermittently. Replication of the bacteria within the serous fluid leads to a series of inflammatory processes with the release of bacterial and host cell products into the middle ear. The clinical manifestation of these events is AOM.

Some infants and young children are at increased risk for developing OM. Well-documented environmental risk factors include passive tobacco smoke exposure, lack of breast-feeding, bottle-propping, poor socioeconomic status, and day care attendance. Children with craniofacial anomalies or congenital or acquired immunodeficiency syndromes have a higher incidence of OM and recurrent disease, as do

certain ethnic groups, including whites, Alaskan Eskimos, and Native Americans.

The peak incidence of AOM occurs during the first 2 years of life, particularly between 6 and 12 months of age. Another peak occurs after the time of school entry. In temperate areas of the world, most infections occur during the fall, winter, and early spring, seasons when most viral upper respiratory infections occur in young children. Recurrent disease after age 5 years should prompt a more extensive evaluation to exclude other predisposing factors, such as allergies or an underlying immunologic condition.

Streptococcus pneumoniae, nontypable *H. influenzae*, and *Moraxella catarrhalis* account for approximately 85% of acute infections. Gram-negative enteric bacilli account for about one fifth of middle ear effusions in infants younger than 6 weeks old. Other, less common bacteria reported to cause AOM include group A, C, and G streptococci; *Staphylococcus aureus; Streptococcus epidermidis;* and mixed flora. The role of viral pathogens has become much more apparent with more sensitive laboratory detection methods. Common virus isolates from middle ear fluid in acute infections include respiratory syncytial virus, influenza A and B, rhinovirus, adenovirus, coronavirus, and parainfluenza (types 1, 2, and 3). Some studies report that 25% of middle ear effusions are "sterile." Approximately 70% of isolates from chronic MEE yield bacterial growth. In MEE *Pseudomonas aeruginosa* and coagulase-negative staphylococci play a prominent role.

Mastoiditis is an extension of the acute inflammatory process of OM. At birth, the mastoid air cell system com-

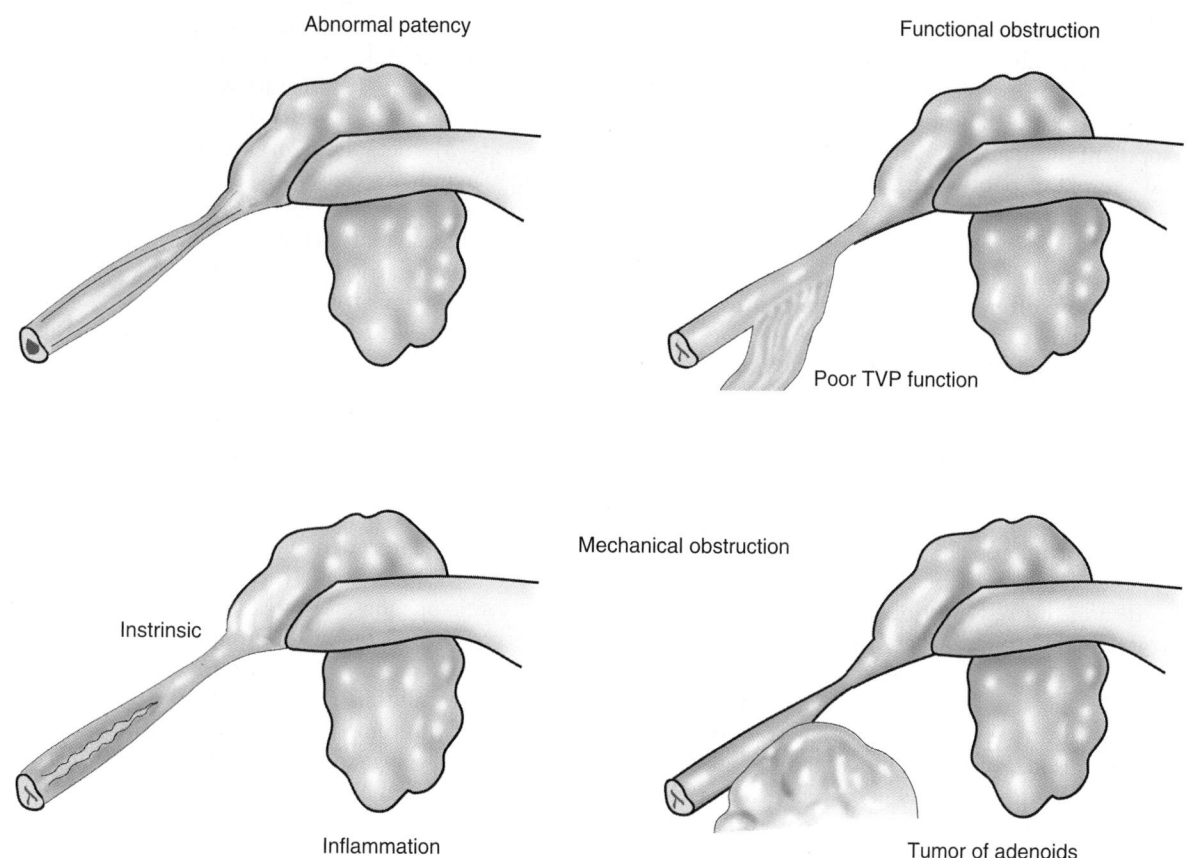

Abnormal patency

Functional obstruction

Poor TVP function

Instrinsic

Mechanical obstruction

Inflammation

Tumor of adenoids

Figure 61-4. Eustachian tube dysfunction. TVP, tensor veli palatini muscle. (Modified from Bluestone CD, Klein JO: Otitis Media in Infants and Children. Philadelphia, WB Saunders, 1988.)

prises a single cell, the antrum, which is connected to the middle ear by a small channel called the *aditus ad antrum*. Pneumatization of the mastoid bone begins soon after birth and continues throughout life. By age 2, this process is usually extensive. All mastoid air cells end up interconnected with the antrum, which sometimes is referred to as the bottleneck when an acute infection cannot drain from the mastoid into the middle ear.

Clinically significant disease develops when an infection within the mastoid cavity spreads to the periosteum covering the mastoid process. With further progression, the bony trabeculae that separate the mastoid air cells are destroyed, resulting in a mastoid empyema. Invasion of adjacent structures leads to formation of a soft tissue, subperiosteal abscess, or chronic mastoiditis. Rarely, further extension into the petrous portion of the temporal bone may occur, resulting in petrositis. A classic triad of retrobulbar pain, persistent otorrhea, and ipsilateral abducens nerve palsy (Gradenigo's syndrome) is seen in patients with this complication. Infection also can spread to the labyrinth and facial nerve or into the intracranial cavity causing more serious morbidity and mortality. Acute mastoiditis occurs most commonly as a complication of chronic suppurative OM but can develop after an acute infection. Acute TM perforation and the presence of a cholesteatoma are predisposing factors.

Currently the incidence of mastoiditis is reportedly less than 0.1%. The incidence may change with recommendations to use oral antibiotics only in children with unequivocal acute infections of the middle ear. Countries in which

acute OM is observed initially, rather than treated with antimicrobials, do not have a higher incidence of mastoiditis. Most cases of acute mastoiditis are caused by the same organisms that cause AOM. Other pathogens include *Streptococcus pyogenes* and *S. aureus*. In subacute or chronic cases, *S. aureus* and gram-negative enteric bacilli, such as *Escherichia coli*, *Proteus*, and *P. aeruginosa*, are common isolates from persistent and indolent infections.

The external ear consists of the pinna and the external auditory canal, which consists of a lateral cartilaginous portion (approximately one third of the canal) and a medial osseous portion. Before development of the osseous portion during infancy, the external auditory meatus is predominantly cartilaginous. The squamous epithelium is thicker over the lateral cartilaginous portion of the canal compared with the osseous portion from subcutaneous tissue containing hair follicles and sebaceous and ceruminous glands. The sebaceous glands, located superficially in the dermis, secrete an oily substance called *sebum*, whereas the apocrine (ceruminous) glands secrete a milky opaque fatty fluid. Cerumen is a mixture of these two secretions and desquamated epithelial cells. Its purpose is to form a protective acidic lipid layer that limits pathogenic bacterial overgrowth and inhibits maceration from water or sweat.

OE develops from alterations in the pH of the external auditory canal, local trauma, or secondary maceration of the skin. High humidity, increased environmental temperature, and water contamination increase the pH of the canal and subsequent risk for acute OE. Moisture in the canal raises the pH and removes the protective lipid layer of the skin, leading to edema and maceration of the epithelial lining. Excessive sweating, absence of cerumen, hearing aid irritation or improper fit, earplug usage, and the insertion of a foreign body to scratch the ear canal also can play a role in the development of infection. Water that has high bacterial counts and the pH of pool water play an important role in OE rather than the number of bacteria in the water. Hot tubs, whirlpools, and pressurized ear irrigation are other sources of water contamination.

OE is seen most often in the summer months in temperate climates and year round in warmer areas. Most cases are unilateral, with mild-to-moderate diffuse inflammation. Rarely, in severe cases, infection may extend to the surrounding soft tissue and lymph nodes. The organisms primarily responsible for acute OE are *P. aeruginosa* and *S. aureus*. Other organisms include *S. epidermidis, Proteus, Enterobacter, Klebsiella*, and streptococci. Many acute infections are polymicrobial, with aerobic and anaerobic bacteria. Acute otomycosis (fungal OE) accounts for 10% of cases of OE and is caused most often by *Aspergillus niger*.

Acute tympanic perforations are secondary to trauma or AOM. Certain racial groups may experience perforations with AOM at a higher rate than the general population. Spontaneous eardrum perforation has been reported with almost every episode of AOM in Eskimos and Native Americans. Chronic perforations occur under a variety of circumstances, including (1) when an acute perforation fails to heal after an episode of AOM, (2) after spontaneous extrusion (or removal) of a tympanostomy tube, (3) after long-standing atelectasis of the TM, and (4) when an acute traumatic perforation fails to close. Small chronic perforations, regardless of their location, have little impact on hearing in the absence of other abnormalities. Large perforations can be associated with a 20- to 30-dB conductive hearing deficit.

Traumatic perforations of the TM occur from rapid changes in ambient pressure that occur with certain sports, such as diving, water-skiing, and surfing, or with activities such as flying in an unpressurized airplane. Blunt trauma with child abuse (e.g., the slap of an open hand against a child's ear by an angry parent) can rupture the TM. TM lacerations may occur by the accidental or intentional placement of a foreign body, such as a cotton-tip applicator or hairpin, into the external auditory canal. Some injuries are severe enough to damage the ossicular chain or cause a perilymphatic fluid leak or fistula.

Congenital cholesteatoma is an asymptomatic keratotic white mass located behind an intact membrane in a patient with no significant history of recurrent middle ear disease or previous ear surgery. Although the origin of the lesion is not well understood, it is presumably present since birth. The most widely accepted theory is that congenital cholesteatoma results from a persistent epidermoid formation in the developing middle ear that, under normal circumstances, disappears after 33 weeks' gestation. The most common age of diagnosis is 4 years, but this also can range from infancy to adolescence. Boys are affected more commonly than girls in a ratio of 3:1.

Most acquired cholesteatomas occur as a complication of chronic OM and arise as a focal area of retraction of the TM. Three main theories exist to explain their patho-genesis: (1) implantation and invasion of squamous epithelium into the middle ear secondary to ear surgery or temporal bone fracture, (2) migration and invasion of squamous epithelium through a perforation of or retraction of the TM, and (3) metaplasia of low cuboidal epithelium of middle ear mucosa caused by infection. Regardless of the etiology, certain children are at increased risk for the development of secondary cholesteatoma, including children with cleft palate, trisomy 21, and aural atresia or stenosis. In the case of aural atresia, occult lesions can develop in the remnant of the external auditory canal or in the middle ear cleft.

DIAGNOSIS

In the verbal child, the diagnosis of AOM is usually straight-forward, with the patient complaining of ear pain (otalgia), fever, and an antecedent upper respiratory infection. The affected TM appears markedly erythematous or injected and often is opaque and thickened, obscuring visualization of the bones (ossicles) in the middle ear. The TM is "full" or bulging. An air-fluid level also may be seen.

Preverbal children and infants are a greater diagnostic challenge. Symptoms often are nonspecific, such as irritability, poor sleeping, and decreased appetite. Unaccustomed ear tugging or rubbing can be seen, but is inconsistently predictive. The cartilaginous external ear canal of an infant can be tortuous, making visualization of the TM difficult. Accurate assessment of the color and opacity of the TM is particularly hard in an apprehensive, febrile, crying toddler, sometimes requiring the use of additional diagnostic procedures, such as tympanometry.

Tympanometry is an objective test that measures the mobility, or compliance, of the TM and the middle ear. It does not evaluate hearing but is sensitive in detecting MEE. Compliance is measured via a probe tone presented to the sealed canal. Compliance is reported as high (≥ 0.5 mL), intermediate (<0.5 mL but >0.2 mL), or low (≤ 0.2 mL). A tympanogram also measures middle ear pressure, which is categorized as normal, negative, or positive and represented as a curve, or peak, on a graph (reported in mm H_2O). A peak between -100 mm H_2O and $+50$ mm H_2O is normal. A peak less than -100 mm H_2O signifies high negative pressure, and a peak at greater than $+50$ mm H_2O is consistent with high positive pressure. A sharp tympanometric peak suggests a low likelihood of MEE; a rounded one suggests a greater likelihood of fluid. A flat one is highly suggestive of MEE. Tympanometry alone cannot distinguish between an acute infection of the middle ear and an uninflamed effusion (OME). The highly compliant cartilaginous walls of the external canal of infants younger than 6 months old can expand when air pressure is increased in the canal in this age group and result in a falsely normal reading.

All examinations of the middle ear should include a determination of the mobility of the TM via pneumatic otoscopy. Normal mobility is shown when positive pressure is applied in the external auditory canal and the TM moves rapidly inward (away from the examiner). When the bulb is released, negative pressure is created, and the TM moves outward (toward the examiner). Mobility of the TM is reduced greatly by fluid or pus in the middle ear.

Tympanocentesis, needle aspiration of the middle air space, is a diagnostic and therapeutic procedure. It may be indicated to determine the causative organism of a middle ear effusion in infants younger than 6 weeks old, children who are immunocompromised, or children who are toxic or have signs of invasive bacterial disease. Presence of suppurative complications also may warrant this procedure. Tympanocentesis may be indicated if the diagnosis of AOM is unclear or if the patient is not improving after appropriate therapy. Potential complications include chronic perforation of the TM, facial nerve paralysis, dislocation of the incudostapedial joint, and bleeding from an exposed jugular bulb. The risks and benefits must be weighed carefully when considering the procedure.

Myringotomy is an incision into the TM to drain middle ear fluid acutely and usually is preceded by tympanocentesis. Indications for myringotomy include treatment for complications of purulent OM, such as mastoiditis, labyrinthitis, or facial nerve paralysis. Severe otalgia may be relieved by myringotomy.

Most cases of OME are identified when children return for follow-up after a recent AOM. OME also may be an incidental finding. Residual fluid in the middle ear may represent incomplete resolution of the acute infection or the natural course of an uncomplicated treated infection. Distinguishing between these two entities can be particularly challenging (Table 61-2). Figure 61-5 shows the persistence of MEE after a diagnosis of AOM. Approximately 40% of children continue to have an effusion at 4 weeks, 20% at 8 weeks, and 10% at 12 weeks. Frequently these patients are asymptomatic (e.g., no fever, normal hearing), but occasionally children continue to complain of unilateral hearing loss.

The TM of OME is retracted (as indicated by a prominent short process of the malleus) with minimal or no signs of inflammation. Pneumatic otoscopy reveals diminished-to-absent mobility of the TM. In equivocal cases, tympanometry can be a useful adjunct. The positive predictive value of an abnormal or flat tympanogram is 49% to 99%, which means that half the number of ears with abnormal tests may have OME. A normal tympanogram more accurately predicts absence of an effusion.

The development of an intratemporal complication of acute or chronic ear disease should be suspected by clinical signs and symptoms. Acute mastoiditis usually presents with fever and postauricular swelling, erythema, and tenderness

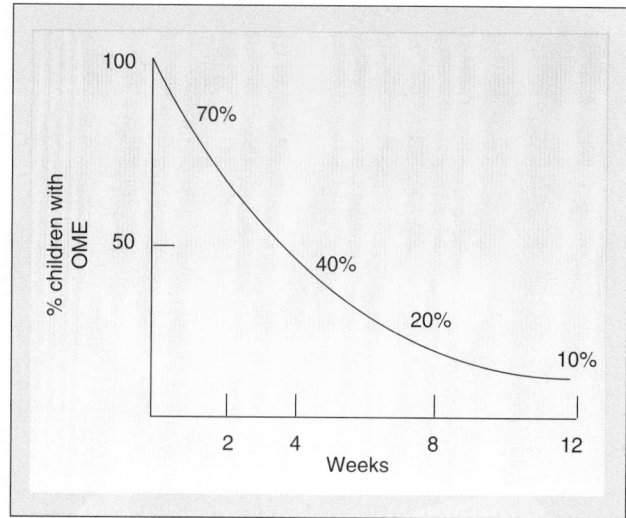

Figure 61-5. Persistence of middle ear fluid after onset of acute otitis media. OME, otitis media with effusion. (Modified from Teele DW, Klein JO, Rosner BA: Epidemiology of otitis media in children. Ann Otol Rhinol Laryngol 1980; 89:5.)

to palpation. Common symptoms associated with AOM also may be present, such as otalgia and hearing loss. The pinna is displaced downward and outward, with swelling or sagging of the posterosuperior canal wall (Fig. 61-6). Acute otorrhea may be seen as the result of a perforation in the TM. The canal is filled with purulent material and debris. Visualization of the TM can be difficult, but it is important to differentiate between AOM with a spontaneous perforation and mastoiditis. In such cases, assistance from an otolaryngologist may be needed. Rarely a postauricular fistula may develop from the mastoid area, or a fluctuant subperiosteal abscess may be palpated in the same region. Children who have persistent retroauricular pain and a history of recurrent OM may not have other signs of an acute infection but may have clinically significant disease.

The diagnosis of acute and chronic mastoiditis is confirmed by computed tomography of the temporal bone. Even in the absence of fluid in the middle ear by otoscopy, any haziness, distortion, or destruction of the bony trabeculae in the mastoid cavity by computed tomography indicates the presence of mastoiditis. These findings should prompt the generalist to seek consultation from an otolaryngologist for assistance in the evaluation and treatment of this condition, especially because a surgical procedure may be indicated. Other indications for consultation include a history of recurrent or chronic OM, especially if the condition is bilateral, and a concern that the child's hearing, speech, or language development is abnormal.

The presence of otorrhea or blood in the external canal suggests the possibility of an acute perforation of the TM or chronic suppurative OM with or without cholesteatoma. The challenge for the clinician is to distinguish these two entities from simple OE. Specific features of the history and physical examination associated with each condition are summarized in Table 61-3.

Patients with acute OE complain of pruritus, the acute onset of unilateral ear pain that is worsened by applying pressure to the tragus or with movement of the pinna, and sometimes a sense of aural stuffiness or fullness. Significant

Table 61-2. Clinical Characteristics of Acute Otitis Media (AOM) and Otitis Media with Effusion (OME)

Signs and symptoms	AOM	OME
Upper respiratory infection	+	+/–
Otalgia, irritability	+	–
Fever	+	–
Otorrhea	+	–
Hearing impairment	+/–	+ (usually)
Middle ear effusion	+	+
Opaque TM	+	– (air-fluid level)
Bulging TM	+	–
Retracted TM	–	+/–
Decreased mobility of TM	+	+

TM, tympanic membrane.

β-lactamase–producing *H. influenzae* and resistant strains of *S. pneumoniae*. Antibiotics currently recommended for second-line therapy are those that are effective against these organisms while achieving adequate concentrations in the middle ear. High-dose amoxicillin-clavulanate (90 mg/kg/day of amoxicillin component, with 6.4 mg/kg/day of clavulanate in two divided doses) and many of the oral cephalosporins (cefuroxime axetil, cefpodoxime, and cefdinir) are second-line therapies. According to a Centers for Disease Control and Prevention working group on drug-resistant *S. pneumoniae*, clindamycin might be effective against pneumococci that are resistant to β-lactam antibiotics. A 3-day course of ceftriaxone (50 mg/kg/day), either intravenously or intramuscularly, can be used in children vomiting or in other clinical situations that preclude administration of oral antibiotics. A substantial number of pneumococcal isolates are resistant to erythromycin. Therefore, erythromycin-sulfisoxazole is not optimal second-line therapy for AOM. The use of trimethoprim-sulfamethoxazole as an alternative agent is controversial because pneumococcal surveillance studies indicate that approximately 25% of isolates are resistant.

Failure of second-line therapy is an indication for tympanocentesis to confirm the diagnosis of OM and to obtain a specimen for culture. Before this procedure, patient compliance must be ascertained. If good compliance can be confirmed, the infection is most likely due to a resistant strain of pneumococci. The role of intramuscular ceftriaxone in this setting has been investigated and is advocated by most experts. Others recommend referral to an otolaryngologist, however, in the case of recurrent disease for placement of tympanostomy tubes. Adenoidectomy is reserved for children older than 4 years of age who need tympanostomy tubes a second time.

Children with acute inflammation of the middle ear may benefit from symptomatic therapy to reduce pain. Oral acetaminophen and ibuprofen are acceptable analgesics for most cases of mild-to-moderate pain. Topical anesthetics include benzocaine formulations (Auralgan and Americaine). Some families may use home remedies for the treatment of ear discomfort, such as placing a clove of garlic or warm olive oil in the external auditory canal. The role of antihistamines and decongestants in the treatment of acute infections has not been well supported. Although these medications may improve symptoms associated with a viral upper respiratory tract infection, studies have not shown that they eradicate middle ear fluid any faster. Corticosteroids also have no role in the treatment of AOM, although their use remains controversial for long-standing MEE.

Longitudinal studies of OME show that most effusions resolve spontaneously within 3 months. Specific recommendations have been developed for young children age 1 through 3 years who are otherwise healthy (e.g., with no craniofacial or neurologic abnormalities or sensory deficits). Highlights from a U.S. consensus panel in 1994 include a short period of observation for most children, a hearing evaluation if the effusion is bilateral and present for more than 3 months, control of environmental risk factors such as exposure to tobacco smoke, and antimicrobial therapy for the few children whose effusions persist. Because most middle ear effusions resolve without treatment, the general

pediatrician should reexamine the asymptomatic child 6 weeks from initial diagnosis with pneumatic otoscopy. If the effusion persists at follow-up, its presence should be confirmed by tympanometry, followed by oral antibiotic therapy for 10 days. For young children that continue to have OME 3 months after the initial diagnosis, a hearing evaluation should be performed and a referral made for possible myringotomy with tympanostomy tube placement, especially if the patient is found to have a hearing deficit. Steroid medications, antihistamine/decongestant therapy, and adenoidectomy with or without tonsillectomy are not recommended for the treatment of OME in otherwise healthy children 1 through 3 years old. The reader is referred to the practice guideline published by the American Academy of Pediatrics for further details regarding the management of OME in young children. Adenoidectomy has been shown to be of value in children older than 4 years of age with bilateral effusion.

Antimicrobial prophylaxis should be reserved for patients with a history of recurrent OM and administered during the months when upper respiratory infections are the most prevalent. Current treatment options are a single daily dose of amoxicillin, 20 mg/kg, and sulfisoxazole, 75 mg/kg/day divided in two doses. Children who continue to have episodes of AOM despite medical prophylaxis should be referred to an otolaryngologist for further evaluation and consideration for tympanostomy tube placement. The administration of prophylactic antibiotics for the prevention of MEE is not advisable because of bacterial resistance.

Parental education and the administration of specific immunizations can play a major role in the prevention of AOM. As a part of anticipatory guidance, the generalist always should review the role of passive tobacco smoke exposure, bottle-feeding instead of breast-feeding, and pacifier use in the development of AOM. Additional interventions include providing the influenza vaccine for children who are particularly susceptible to an acute infection during the winter months and administering the heptavalent conjugate pneumococcal vaccine routinely at well-child visits. Data report that the pneumococcal vaccine reduces the incidence of AOM by 6% to 8%.

The management of acute mastoiditis may be medical or surgical, depending on the extent of bony destruction. Mastoiditis is an indication for referral to an otolaryngologist. For uncomplicated mastoiditis, intravenous antibiotic therapy is the mainstay of treatment. A myringotomy also may be necessary to decompress the middle ear and is important to provide a specimen for culture and sensitivity. If there is evidence of significant destruction of the bone or no improvement while on intravenous medication, a mastoidectomy is indicated. The goal is to clean out and drain the mastoid air cell system into the middle ear. In addition, a tympanostomy tube is inserted to allow further drainage and ventilation of the middle ear.

Mild-to-moderate OE can be managed by the general pediatrician with the primary goals of therapy aimed at controlling the inflammation and infection. Although difficult and occasionally painful for the patient, the ear canal should be cleansed gently of the debris from the entire length of the external auditory canal. This cleansing may be accomplished by gentle irrigation with warmed saline or 2.5% acetic acid solution. Gentle suctioning adequately clears the canal. Most cases also require the instillation of ototopical drops into the ear canal or onto a wick if there is significant edema. Classes of ototopical medications include steroids, acidifying agents, antiseptics (alcohol), and antibiotics. Many of the most commonly used products contain polymyxin B or E, neomycin, and hydrocortisone. The usual dosage schedule is three to four times a day for 7 to 10 days. If a wick is placed, it should be removed within 24 to 72 hours. Newer fluoroquinolone topical antibiotics contain ciprofloxacin/hydrocortisone and ofloxacin. Patients who do not respond well to initial treatment should be switched to drops containing ciprofloxacin or tobramycin. Otomycosis requires treatment with antifungal drops, such as clotrimazole.

Swimming should be prohibited during the course of treatment. Further episodes of OE can be prevented through the use of earplugs while swimming. Other recommendations include the use of acidic solutions in the ear canal after exposure to water, drying the ear with a hair dryer set on low heat from 1 foot away for 60 seconds, and avoiding manipulation of the ear canal with cotton swabs and other objects to avoid irritation and maceration of the skin. Cases of OE that are persistent or recurrent warrant a culture of the ear discharge and the assistance of a specialist to evaluate the child for cholesteatoma or another undiagnosed condition.

Traumatic perforations of the TM should be managed in consultation with an otolaryngologist. Although small perforations often heal spontaneously within a few weeks after the injury, larger perforations may persist. Consultation with a specialist is essential to evaluate the extent of the defect, any associated complications such as involvement of the ossicular chain, and the timing of any surgical procedures.

The management of cholesteatoma is surgical and requires the expertise of a pediatric otolaryngologist. The goals of surgery are twofold: (1) to eradicate the squamous epithelium from the middle ear, mastoid, or both and (2) to preserve or restore hearing. The initial surgical procedure is aimed at direct removal of the squamous epithelium. Removal is done either through the ear canal or by a postauricular approach, depending on the size of the external auditory canal and location of the lesion. Commonly, with acquired cholesteatoma, mastoidectomy also is necessary to remove the entire lesion. Other surgical procedures may include ossicular chain reconstruction. Hearing aids often are necessary for children who are awaiting elective surgery and have significant bilateral hearing loss or who are not candidates for ossicular chain reconstruction.

OUTCOME

Children with uncomplicated AOM generally have a favorable outcome depending on their age at diagnosis, frequency of infections, and length of time for fluid in the middle ear to resolve. Severe adverse sequelae of treated OM are rare. The most common adverse outcomes include hearing impairment, speech delay, and significant TM perforation.

Various studies indicate that recurrent disease or prolonged MEE in young infants may affect hearing and normal speech and language development. Referral to a pediatric otolaryngologist for tympanostomy tube placement is essential for children with severe-to-profound hearing loss or children with abnormal speech development. Other children should be evaluated on a case-by-case basis to assess whether medical prophylaxis (antibiotics) should be initiated before the referral. For children who require a second placement of tympanostomy tubes, adenoidectomy without a tonsillectomy has been shown to be an effective additional procedure to prevent recurrent disease.

The outcome of intracranial complications of AOM, such as meningitis, is variable, ranging from full recovery with no long-term sequelae, to mild hearing loss with minimal associated neurologic deficits, to recurrent seizures, to developmental delay. Reported mortality rates in severely affected children range from 0% to 20%. The outcome of intratemporal complications depends on the particular condition being considered. Mastoiditis usually has a favorable outcome if the infection is controlled acutely.

The outcome of TM perforation depends on the size and location of the defect and any associated complications. Most lesions heal spontaneously, however. After an uncomplicated TM perforation, a mild conductive hearing loss may be observed on audiometric testing. Destruction of the margin of the TM may lead to additional complications, such as secondary cholesteatoma formation.

In children, cholesteatoma is thought to be an aggressive disease that, if not discovered early, may have a poor outcome. Because extensive disease usually is found at the time of surgery and there are higher rates of residual and recurrent disease after surgery, the outcome is variable.

FOLLOW-UP

General recommendations for follow-up of AOM are based on several factors, the most important being the amount of time for the accompanying MEE to resolve. Because approximately 80% of effusions resolve by 8 weeks after the acute infection, most practice guidelines recommend reexamination of the TM within 6 to 8 weeks of the initial diagnosis. Audiologic testing usually is reserved for children with a history of recurrent OM, chronic MEE, or suspected speech delay. An evaluation by a speech therapist is warranted for abnormal language development, especially during the first 4 years of life.

A child diagnosed and treated for mastoiditis should continue to be screened for further episodes of OM in consultation with an otolaryngologist. Children with traumatic perforations should be screened initially for a hearing deficit and then followed until complete resolution of the defect has been documented. All children with cholesteatoma should continue to be followed by a subspecialist so that recurrent lesions can be prevented and controlled.

 Additional Resources, CD-ROM

Bibliography

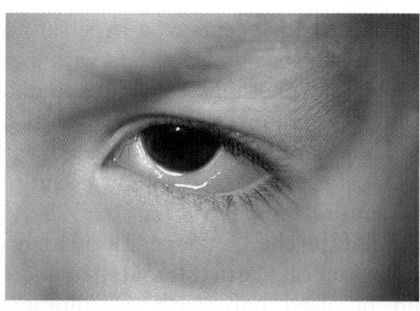

A

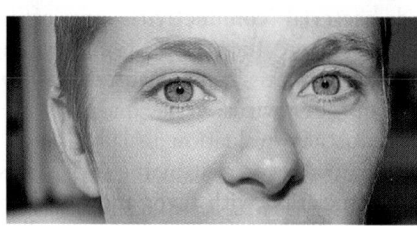

B

Figure 62-7. A, Conjunctival injection (prominent blood vessels) edema of the conjunctiva and fine wrinkles on the eyelid are markers of chronic rubbing. **B,** Repeated rubbing of the itchy nose as a result of allergic rhinitis has produced a horizontal crease on the nose. (From Chaudhry B, Harvey D: Mosby's Color Atlas and Text of Pediatrics and Child Health. St. Louis, Mosby, 2001.)

inflammation of the cornea. The corneal keratitis may last for weeks or months and often significantly reduces vision. Epidemic keratoconjunctivitis is highly contagious, and strict isolation is mandatory. Patients with pharyngo-conjunctival fever and epidemic keratoconjunctivitis should be referred to the ophthalmologist; treatment is supportive but often involves topical steroids and may have a prolonged course. *Herpetic conjunctivitis* is associated with "dendritic" keratitis and is a leading cause of infectious vision loss in the United States (Fig. 62-8). It usually is caused by herpes simplex virus type 1, is recurrent, and has a predilection for mucous membranes. The lesions on the skin are vesicular, but lesions on the conjunctiva and cornea are ulcerative (Fig. 62-9). In the immunocompromised host and neonate, the lesions are ulcerative. Eye infection is almost always unilateral. Prevention of advancement of the

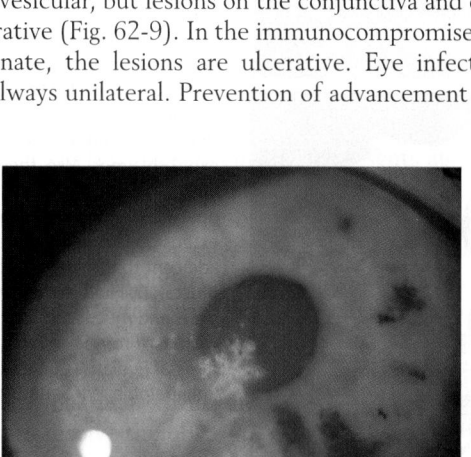

Figure 62-8. Herpes simplex keratitis. Infection of the corneal epithelium with herpes simplex virus produces a pattern of fluorescein staining that resembles a neuronal dendrite. Conjunctival injection typically is present. (From Zitelli BJ, Davis HW: Atlas of Pediatric Physical Diagnosis. St. Louis, Mosby, 1997.)

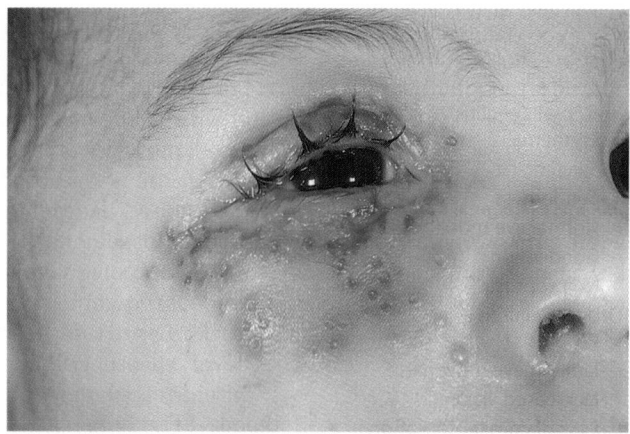

Figure 62-9. Herpes keratoconjunctivitis. Primary infection by herpes simplex in a 9-month-old infant. Multiple vesicles were present that quickly progressed to pustular and scab formations. The cornea was not involved. Herpes simplex virus type 1 (HSV-1) was cultured from the vesicle (ocular infections usually are caused by HSV-1 except in newborns, in whom HSV-2 predominates). (From Shah BR, Laude TA: Atlas of Pediatric Clinical Diagnosis. Philadelphia, WB Saunders, 2000.)

ocular infection to corneal stromal disease is paramount. This advancement may be hastened with inappropriate use of topical steroids. Ophthalmology referral is essential if herpes is suspected. Treatment of the acute ocular infection is with topical trifluorothymidine. Current recommendations for recurrent ocular herpes simplex virus infection include prolonged suppression with oral acyclovir.

Hordeolum and Chalazion

Meibomian glands are the sebaceous glands at the eyelid margin. Infection of the glands can result in formation of a hordeolum (Fig. 62-10). Blockage of the orifice of the gland by desquamation, inflammation, or infection leads to stagnation of the lipids and secondary internal inflammation of the glands. The resulting chalazion (Fig. 62-11) is usually a sterile inflammatory process, but may be secondarily infected and present more acutely. Treatment of hordeolum and chalazion includes hot packs, lid hygiene (tearless soap scrubs), massage, topical antibiotics, and occasionally oral antibiotics. Occasionally, referral for surgical drainage may be required.

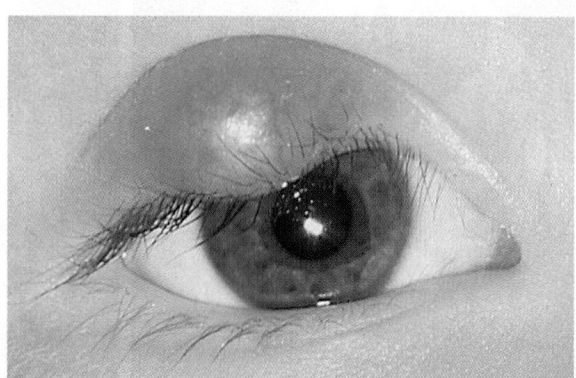

Figure 62-10. Acute hordeolum of the eyelid (pointing externally) with swelling, induration, and purulent contents. (From Zitelli BJ, Davis HW: Atlas of Pediatric Physical Diagnosis. St. Louis, Mosby, 1997.)

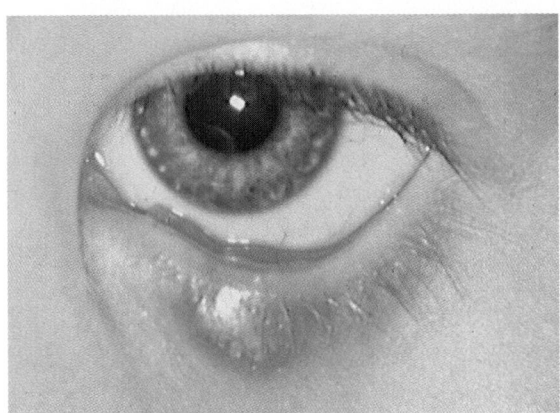

Figure 62-11. Chalazion, a painless lid mass pointing externally or internally. (From Zitelli BJ, Davis HW: Atlas of Pediatric Physical Diagnosis. St. Louis, Mosby, 1997.)

Immune-Mediated Disease

An inflamed red eye may be the sign of an internal inflammatory process affecting the uveal layer of the eye. Clinically, high-power magnification is used to identify cells and flare circulating in the anterior chamber; additionally, white blood cells can deposit on the inner layer of the cornea and are called *keratic precipitates*. This type of iritis may be painful, and affected children are photosensitive. Iritis in association with juvenile rheumatoid arthritis is often asymptomatic and can lead to serious complications, especially if not properly identified. The mainstay of treatment is topical steroids, at times on an hourly basis. Steroids may be injected periocularly in recalcitrant cases; oral steroids have little proven benefit. Topical mydriatics also are used to limit internal scarring of the pupil and cataract formation. The differential diagnosis for sterile inflamed red eye includes uveitis, Stevens-Johnson syndrome, Kawasaki disease, toxic epidermal necrolysis, atopic conjunctivitis, and episcleritis.

Disorders of the Anterior Segment

Corneal leukoma, or literally *white cornea*, has several important etiologies (Fig. 62-12). Congenital glaucoma, corneal dystrophy, anterior chamber dysgenesis syndromes, sclerocornea, birth trauma, and infections all can compromise the corneal integrity and result in permanent damage to the ocular surface. Treatment is directed at the underlying etiology.

Aniridia is a heritable condition caused by a PAX-6 gene mutation. The gene is located on chromosome 11, next to the gene for Wilms' tumor. Because nonfamilial or "sporadic" aniridia can be associated with deletion of the Wilms' tumor gene, patients with nonfamilial aniridia should be evaluated for this condition. Most aniridics are missing all iris tissues except for a peripheral stump. They present with congenital nystagmus, reduced vision, and hypoplastic macula and are at high risk for development of glaucoma. *Coloboma* is a congenital malformation caused by incomplete fusion of the apposing margins of the embryonic fissure. There is a resulting gap of tissue inferiorly. Iris colobomas result from a full-thickness loss of iris tissue, resulting in a keyhole-shaped pupil. As a rule, eyes with isolated iris colobomas are normal size and have normal sight. Colobomas may be associated with other congenital anomalies (CHARGE association—*c*oloboma, *h*eart disease, *a*tresia choanae, *r*etarded growth and developmental or central nervous system anomalies, *g*enital anomalies or hypogonadism, and *e*ar anomalies or deafness).

Congenital *glaucoma* is a rare but aggressive condition involving elevation of the intraocular pressures. Classic symptoms include epiphora, photophobia, and blepharospasm. Continued elevated pressure leads to buphthalmos (enlarged eye) and clouded cornea (Fig. 62-13). Treatment as a rule is surgical lowering of the intraocular pressure.

Cataracts

Congenital cataracts pose a serious threat to normal visual development. Early visual rehabilitation, before 8 to 12 weeks of age, is crucial for restoring the developing visual system. Although congenital cataracts are familial in origin, early detection of an abnormal red reflex by the primary care provider is the only reliable screening mechanism for providing timely and appropriate treatment (Fig. 62-14). Unilateral congenital cataracts are the most devastating to the visual system. Posterior hyperplastic primary vitreous and posterior lenticonus are the most frequent causes.

Developmental cataracts are a challenge to detect and manage. These cataracts are believed to develop between 2 and 10 years of age as a result of mild defects that do not reduce optical clarity during the critical neonatal period. With time, the opacity increases, resulting in a clinically significant cataract. Differentiating these conditions can be difficult; however, prognosis is significantly better than in the undiagnosed unilateral congenital cataract. Results after treatment for childhood cataracts have improved steadily since the 1990s; optical rehabilitation with contact lenses and patching and diligent follow-up are the crucial determining factors in successful visual recovery.

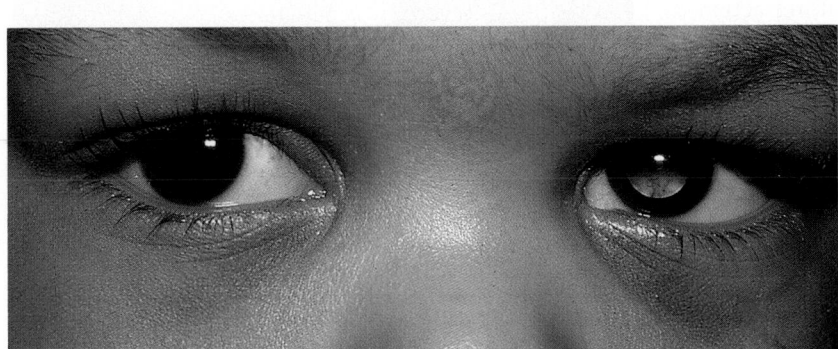

Figure 62-12. Leukocoria. The patient's left eye has a white papillary reflex produced by reflection of light from a retinoblastoma. Leukocoria is the most common presenting sign (60%) of retinoblastoma. (From Zitelli BJ, Davis HW: Atlas of Pediatric Physical Diagnosis. St. Louis, Mosby, 1997.)

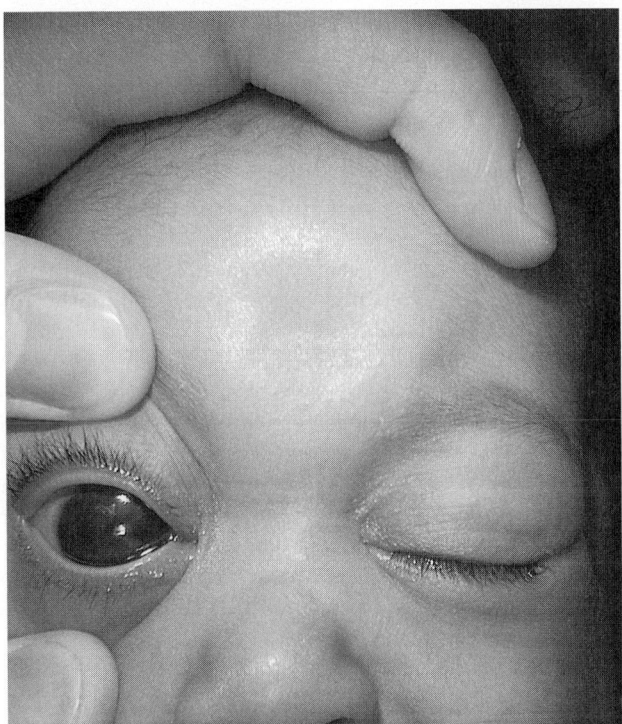

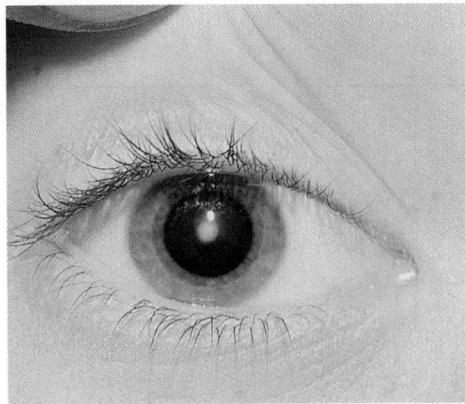

Figure 62-14. Anterior polar cataract. This type of lens opacity is a developmental abnormality that in most cases remains stable and rarely affects vision. (From Zitelli BJ, Davis HW: Atlas of Pediatric Physical Diagnosis. St. Louis, Mosby, 1997.)

Figure 62-13. Infantile glaucoma with megalocornea (hardly any sclera can be seen) in a 3-month-old infant. In a patient with unilateral eye involvement, which allows comparison with the normal eye, the diagnosis of megalocornea is made easily. Diagnosis often is delayed in patients with bilateral involvement. Diagnosis is especially difficult in the absence of corneal cloudiness or when bilateral corneal enlargement is symmetric. (From Shah BR, Laude TA: Atlas of Pediatric Clinical Diagnosis. Philadelphia, WB Saunders, 2000.)

rhages, vitreous hemorrhages, chorioretinal scars, optic atrophy, retinoschisis (splitting of the retinal layers), and retinal ischemia are all found in a child who has been physically abused. Retinoschisis and retinal folds in association with hemorrhages are pathognomonic for traumatic insult in a child abuse victim. Other much less frequent causes of retinal hemorrhages include diabetes, leukemia, thrombocytopenia, retinal infection (human immunodeficiency virus, cytomegalovirus, septic emboli), vein occlusion, and hemorrhage associated with disk edema.

Hereditary Retinal Dystrophy

The definitive retinal dystrophy is retinitis pigmentosa, in which a defect in the rhodopsin gene causes a slowly progressive deterioration in function of the retinal photoreceptors. Pigment deposition in the fundus, optic disk pallor, and retinal vessel attenuation are the hallmark signs of retinitis pigmentosa. Many other types of retinal dystro-

Lens ectopia and subluxation occasionally are the first diagnostic signs of a systemic condition. Most commonly, lens subluxation is seen in Marfan syndrome, but it also is seen in Weill-Marchesani syndrome, homocystinuria, and hyperlysinemia. Some cases are idiopathic.

Retinal Disorders

Pigmentary abnormalities of the retina, including albinism, nevi, and blue sclera, can affect visual functioning significantly. Albinism can involve only the eye (ocular albinism) or the entire integumentary system (oculocutaneous albinism). Either condition has profound detrimental effects on visual development and processing. The eye findings include nystagmus, hypopigmented (blue) irides, iris transillumination, and retinal hypopigmentation. The vision deficit is proportional to the degree of pigment loss and nystagmus. Treatment involves optimal refraction, darkly tinted spectacles, and treatment of secondary strabismus. Nevus of Ota is a congenital melanosis of the periocular skin and uveal tract of the eye that occurs unilaterally. There is a low rate of malignant transformation to melanoma, for which routine surveillance is warranted. Blue sclera may be associated with Ehlers-Danlos syndrome, osteogenesis imperfecta, and high myopia. Regular eye examinations are indicated.

Vitreous and retinal hemorrhage strongly suggests child abuse (Fig. 62-15). Hemorrhages are multiple and may be unilateral or bilateral. Retinal hemorrhages, preretinal hemor-

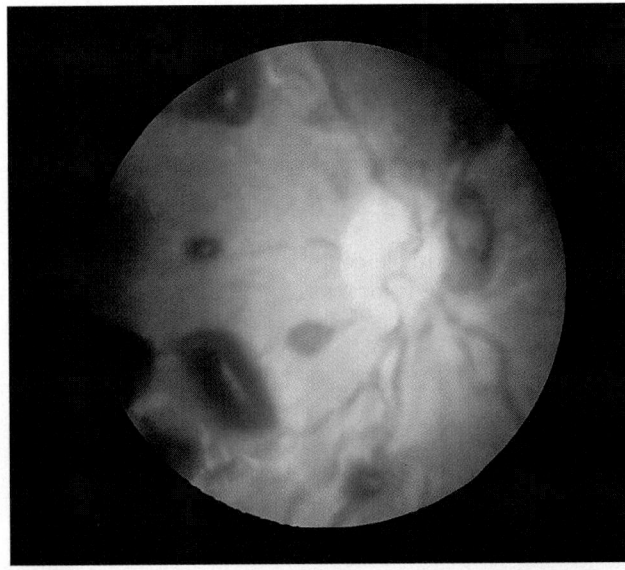

Figure 62-15. Multiple retinal hemorrhages are seen on funduscopic examination of this infant, who was a victim of "shaken baby" syndrome. Subdural hematoma and multiple metaphyseal "shake" fractures are typical associated findings. (Courtesy of Dr. Stephen Ludwig, Children's Hospital of Philadelphia.)

phy exist, presenting in early childhood through adolescence. Some of the other, more common dystrophies include Stargardt's disease, Best's dystrophy, X-linked retinoschisis, congenital stationary night blindness, cone dystrophy, mitochondrial dystrophy, and Usher's syndrome. Advances in genetic testing have improved understanding of how these conditions affect retinal functioning. Directed treatments are being developed.

Disorders of Optic Nerves

Any discussion of congenital anomalies of the optic nerve must include septo-optic dysplasia, or de Morsier's syndrome. Hypoplasia of either one or both optic nerves is seen frequently in association with absence of the septum pellucidum, pituitary hypoplasia, and central nervous system abnormalities. Visual functioning may range from "normal" 20/20 vision to complete blindness. Nystagmus often is present and the presenting symptom in secondary strabismus and ocular torticollis. Evaluation of endocrine function is appropriate.

Papilledema and pseudopapilledema are often emergent reasons for referral to a pediatric ophthalmologist and can cause considerable distress among patients, their families, and general health care providers. Papilledema is the swelling and elevation of the optic nerve head as a direct result of elevated intracranial pressure and by definition is bilateral. Pseudopapilledema is the blurring of disk margins, with the appearance of swelling without elevated pressures. Papillitis or optic neuritis is swelling of the disk caused by inflammation; it is unrelated to the intracranial pressure and usually is unilateral. The signs of true papilledema are elevation of the disk (best seen stereoscopically), blurring of the margins with obscuration of the retinal vessels as they cross the disk, loss of the central cup and absence of spontaneous venous pulsations, engorgement of the retinal veins, and splinter hemorrhages at or near the disk margin. Papilledema usually is associated with normal 20/20 visual acuity, an enlarged blind spot on visual field testing, and reversible peripheral visual field loss. Occasionally, papilledema may cause ischemic optic neuropathy and permanent visual loss. In contrast, papillitis often is associated with dramatic vision deficit in the range of 20/200 to light perception.

Tumors

Tumors of the eye, orbit, and periocular region are considered best in terms of benign and malignant. Common benign tumors include dermoid, lipodermoid, plexiform neurofibroma, hemangioma, and lymphangioma. Dermoid tumors are choristomas that typically are located along the lateral aspect of the brow. These are present at birth but often grow and become obvious in the first year of life. Progressive slow growth is characteristic, and rupture of the capsule surrounding the dermoid can result in an intense inflammatory response that simulates cellulitis. Removal is recommended. In contrast, lipodermoids usually are associated closely with the globe and orbital structures. They most often are visible laterally as pinkish, fleshy tissue on the surface of the eye. Removal is not indicated in most cases because the adipose tissue "wraps" around the globe, and removal results in scarring and limited motility of the eye. Hemangiomas are hamartomas and can occur anywhere in the body. When the tumor involves the orbit or lids, progressive growth can lead to loss of visual function and deprivational amblyopia. If the visual axis is uninvolved, treatment is conservative observation. If vision is threatened, treatment, including corticosteroids, is required. Steroids can be given orally (1 mg/kg/day) or intralesionally.

Malignant tumors of the orbit and eye include rhabdomyosarcoma, optic nerve glioma, and retinoblastoma. Rhabdomyosarcoma presents rapidly as painful proptosis in childhood (age 5 years) through adolescence. Although these tumors are aggressive, if they are limited to the orbit at the time of presentation, survival is dramatically improved. Any acquired proptosis should be evaluated with orbital CT scan and emergent ophthalmology consultation. Optic nerve glioma is often seen in association with neurofibromatosis type 1, but also can be seen in isolation. The tumor may involve the orbital or intracranial portion of the nerve or chiasm. Vision loss is seen in association with local compressive effects, and treatment is reserved for cases in which growth is causing progressive damage to the visual fields. Retinoblastoma is often seen first by the parents or an astute clinician who notes leukocoria; urgent ophthalmic referral should be requested. Peak incidence is at age 3, and the tumor may present as uveitis, strabismus, cataract, intraocular hemorrhage, or glaucoma. Evaluation includes CT scan of the orbit, possible ocular ultrasound, and careful dilated examination of both eyes. The genetics of retinoblastoma are well characterized. The possible inheritance of the cancer should be discussed with the parents after certain diagnosis is made.

Orbital pseudotumor is an inflammatory orbital condition that is neither a benign nor a malignant tumor, but it results in a painful and recurrent inflammatory proptosis of the orbit. Recurrence of the condition can lead to fibrotic ocular restriction and loss of motility. The condition responds to steroids, which may require prolonged taper over months.

Mini-index of Related Topics

SUGGESTED READINGS

Wright KW: Pediatric Ophthalmology for Pediatricians. Philadelphia, Lippincott Williams & Wilkins, 1998.
Wu G, Lampert R (eds): Ophthalmology for Primary Care. Philadelphia, WB Saunders, 1997.

63 Disorders of the Nose and Sinuses

Debora W. Goebel and Charles Myer

A myriad of disorders may affect the pediatric sinonasal tract, including congenital, inflammatory, neoplastic, traumatic, iatrogenic, and metabolic etiologies. Because of the obligatory nasal respiration of newborns and young infants up to several months of age, the importance of proper, timely diagnosis and treatment of pediatric sinonasal pathology cannot be overemphasized. Several theories have been postulated regarding this obligate nasal respiration. First, the infant larynx is situated relatively cephalad in the neck, resulting in close apposition of the soft palate to the tongue and epiglottis. Also, a patent rigid nasal airway aids during suckling and feeding and provides safety in infants, who spend a large amount of time supine and sleeping. Although bilateral complete obstruction invariably produces respiratory distress with associated intermittent cyanosis, apnea, and failure to thrive, even unilateral obstruction may cause airway distress and difficulty with feeding. The degree and duration of obligate nasal breathing may vary with the infant; infants with more advanced neurologic development and maturity may adapt to oral respiration more rapidly.

CHRONIC NASAL AIRWAY OBSTRUCTION

Unrecognized chronic nasal airway obstruction may lead to anatomic and physiologic changes in the growing infant and child. Chronic mouth breathing with secondary abnormal tongue positioning may result in anomalies in craniofacial development. The altered dental arch leads to the "long face syndrome," or adenoid facies, characterized by vertical excess in the lower third of the face, lip incompetence, and a high-arched palate. Controversy exists regarding the cause-and-effect relationship between nasal airway obstruction and aberrant craniofacial development.

The most worrisome complication is the cardiopulmonary physiology alterations that may be seen with obstructive sleep apnea secondary to nasal airway obstruction. Obstructive sleep apnea may manifest as enuresis, daytime hypersomnolence, decreased mental and physical performance, and, occasionally, hyperactivity and behavioral problems. A history of snoring almost invariably is present. Associated hypoxia may lead to alveolar hypoventilation and pulmonary hypertension and ultimately to cor pulmonale. Another phenomenon possibly associated with nasal obstruction is the hypothalamus-mediated nasopulmonary reflex, through which increased nasal resistance produces heightened pulmonary resistance and decreased compliance with alveolar hypoventilation. The end result is a clinical picture similar to that described for obstructive sleep apnea.

History

A thorough history is paramount in assessing sinonasal disorders in pediatric patients. Associated symptoms, such as nasal discharge, snoring, stertor, or cyanosis, should be sought. In an infant, bilateral nasal airway obstruction may manifest as respiratory distress relieved with crying and warrants urgent airway management. The infant's ability to feed should be assessed. The parent should be questioned regarding day care, a family history of atopy, and any maternal history of medications taken during the pregnancy. Narcotics, antihypertensives, β-blockers, and antidepressants are known causes of neonatal nasal obstruction.

Examination

The overall condition of the infant or child should be evaluated, noting stridor, stertor, retractions, and abnormalities of oxygen saturation. Any change in airway symptoms associated with crying should be assessed. A thorough head and neck examination includes assessment for any abnormalities that may account for nasal airway obstruction. Craniofacial anomalies such as those seen in Crouzon disease or Pfeiffer syndrome should be sought, and stigmata of Down syndrome similarly should be identified because midface and nasopharynx abnormalities may predispose to nasal airway obstruction in these disorders. Allergy or adenoid hypertrophy may manifest as adenoid facies, as described earlier, and the allergic patient also may have allergic "shiners," a transverse nasal crease, a broadened nose, and perioral or nasal pallor.

The external nasal examination may reveal anatomic abnormalities or a mass. Rhinoscopy and nasopharyngoscopy allow assessment of the nasal septum, lateral nasal walls, and nasal airway. Any mass lesions should be identified. In neonates, nasal airway patency may be assessed by passage of a soft suction catheter (5 Fr to 6 Fr) to at least a length of 32 mm; this rules out choanal atresia. Prompt otolaryngologic consultation is warranted for any confirmed or suspected nasal abnormality, especially in cases with associated respiratory distress. Flexible fiberoptic nasopharyngoscopy is a valuable tool in the otolaryngologist's armamentarium for diagnosis of intranasal or nasopharyngeal abnormalities.

CONGENITAL NASAL AIRWAY OBSTRUCTION

Box 63-1 lists effects of pediatric nasal airway obstruction. Box 63-2 lists congenital causes of pediatric nasal airway obstruction. Syndromic or nonsyndromic craniofacial abnormalities may cause nasal obstruction as a result of altered midfacial anatomy. Congenital nasal anomalies also may arise secondary to aberrant embryologic development of the sinonasal tract itself. Arrhinia, polyrrhinia, and proboscis lateralis are extreme and rare congenital nasal anomalies.

Choanal atresia, noted in 1 in 5000 to 8000 births, is the most common congenital anomaly. From a pathophysiologic standpoint, failure of buccopharyngeal membrane breakdown during embryogenesis or persistence of intranasal epithelial cell rests produces this entity (Fig. 63-1). Bony atresia occurs more commonly than the membranous form, and unilateral cases are twice as common as bilateral cases. Girls are affected twice as often as boys. In many choanal atresia patients, other anomalies exist, such as coloboma, heart disease, retarded neurologic development, genital hypoplasia, and ear abnormalities, which together are characterized as *CHARGE* association (Box 63-3).

Examination of an infant with suspected choanal atresia should include passage of a 5 Fr to 6 Fr gauge suction catheter through each nasal cavity; successful passage excludes atresia (Box 63-4). If suspicion remains high, prompt otolaryngologic consultation with nasal endoscopy is warranted. Helpful imaging studies include computed tomography (CT) performed in the axial planes parallel to the hard palate and the nasal airway (Fig. 63-2).

Bilateral choanal atresia is an airway emergency in infants (see Chapter 191). Temporizing management options include a taped-in oropharyngeal airway, a McGovern nipple, and orotracheal intubation along with nasogastric feeding. Definitive surgical intervention is pursued preferably via the transnasal route, given the potential for altered midfacial growth patterns, presumably caused by disruption of

---

Box 63-1. Effects of Pediatric Nasal Airway Obstruction

- Changes in craniofacial growth and development
- Obstructive sleep apnea
- Nasopulmonary reflex
- Pulmonary hypertension
- Cor pulmonale

Box 63-2. Causes of Congenital Nasal Airway Obstruction

- *Maternal medications*—narcotics, antihypertensives, β-blockers, antidepressants
- Craniofacial anomalies
- Arrhinia
- Polyrrhinia
- Proboscis lateralis
- Choanal atresia
- Choanal stenosis
- Pyriform aperture stenosis
- Dacrocystocele
- *Midline nasal masses*—dermoid cyst, glioma, encephalocele
- *Other cystic lesions*—dentigerous, nasoalveolar, mucus retention cysts

---

the palatal mucoperichondrium. Long-term stenting is required postoperatively (Fig. 63-3).

In contrast to bilateral atresia, diagnosis of unilateral choanal atresia frequently is delayed and may not cause respiratory distress. Surgical management is the same as for the bilateral form but is not urgent. Choanal stenosis may not become symptomatic until the child acquires a respiratory tract infection. If stenosis is severe, it may be obvious and mimic choanal atresia. CT differentiates the two entities. Selected stenosis cases may be managed conservatively with topical steroid or saline drops or both.

Pyriform aperture stenosis occurs uncommonly and is secondary to overgrowth of the medial maxillae and causes anterior nasal obstruction. Examination reveals shelflike projections laterally into the vestibule, and CT confirms the diagnosis. Symptomatic cases require surgery by a sublabial approach with drilling of the excess bone. Stents are left in place postoperatively.

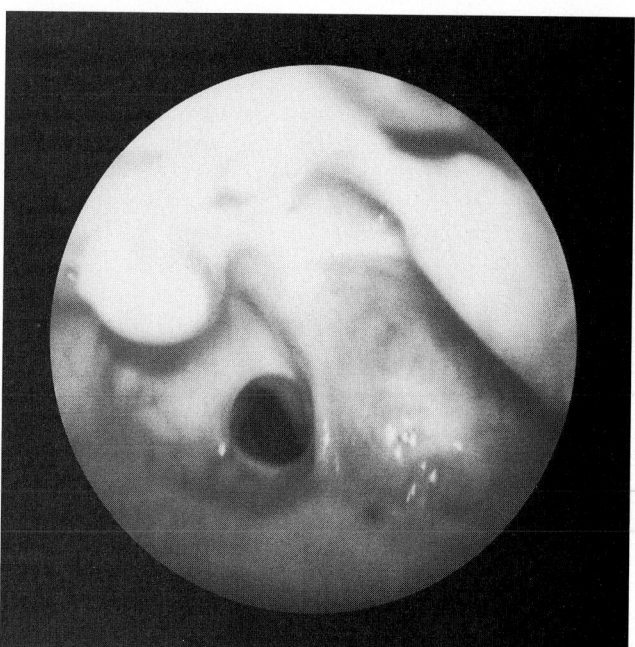

Figure 63-1. Endoscopic view of unilateral choanal atresia and contralateral choanal stenosis from nasopharynx.

Box 63-3. CHARGE Association

- Coloboma
- Heart disease
- Atresia choanae
- Retarded neurologic development
- Genital hypoplasia
- Ear anomalies

Box 63-4. Workup for Suspected Choanal Atresia

1. Transnasal passage of 5 Fr to 6 Fr catheter
2. Ear, nose, and throat consultation/flexible fiberoptic naso-pharyngoscopy
3. Axial computed tomography

Various congenital cysts may manifest in the nasal cavity. Dacryocystocele, or nasolacrimal duct cyst, presents within the first weeks of life and appears as a unilateral or bilateral anterior nasal swelling arising from the inferior meatus with medial displacement of the inferior turbinate. CT or magnetic resonance imaging should be done to confirm the diagnosis and evaluate for intracranial extent in the case of dermoid cyst, glioma, or encephalocele. Management of dacrocystocele consists of intranasal marsupialization; ophthalmologic consultation for concomitant nasolacrimal duct stenting is recommended (see Chapter 62). Other cystic lesions include nasoalveolar, dentigerous, and mucus retention cysts.

Congenital midline nasal masses include dermoid cysts, gliomas, and encephaloceles (Fig. 63-4). Dermoids contain ectomesodermal elements and are connected to the nasal dorsum skin by a fistulous tract. Half may extend deep to the nasal bones, and 25% show intracranial extension. Gliomas represent extradural glial tissue and most commonly occur extranasally, although some present wholly intranasally or with intranasal and extranasal components. Of gliomas, 15% maintain a connection to the subarachnoid space in the form of a fibrous stalk but with no continuity to the cerebrospinal fluid. Herniation of cerebral contents into the nasal cavity may manifest as a meningocele, meningoencephalocele, or encephalocele, depending on the contents of the herniation. CT scan is crucial to evaluate the skull base and to assess for any continuity of the lesion with the intracranial space. Biopsy is contraindicated until such a connection is ruled out. In questionable or confirmed cases of intracranial extension, neurosurgical consultation is mandated. Treatment is surgical.

OTHER CONDITIONS

Inflammatory

Inflammatory conditions represent the most common etiology of pediatric nasal obstruction (Box 63-5). Rhinitis of infancy denotes mucosal edema with airway obstruction and may be due to a multitude of conditions, such as meconium aspiration, chlamydial infections, gastroesophageal reflux, and idiopathic vasomotor rhinitis. Chlamydial infection may manifest with fiery red erythema of the nasal mucous membranes. Purulent secretions, if present, should be cultured, especially for chlamydia, and local measures, such as saline or decongestant nasal drops, may be instituted, although decongestant medications should be administered with caution in neonates. In some cases, topical or systemic steroids may be warranted. Although emphasis is placed on ruling out an infectious etiology of nasal obstruction, irritative rhinitis secondary to gastroesophageal reflux with nasopharyngeal regurgitation or primary nasal regurgitation of oral feedings must be considered.

Acute viral infection (the common cold) is the most common etiology of pediatric nasal obstruction and rhinorrhea. Responsible viruses include rhinovirus, adenovirus, myxoviruses (influenza, parainfluenza, and respiratory syncytial virus), and coxsackievirus A and B. The prodromal phase of other viral illnesses may involve nasal obstruction and rhinorrhea; these conditions include mumps, measles, infectious mononucleosis, and poliomyelitis.

Bacterial infection often results secondarily from preexisting viral, allergic, or vasomotor rhinitis; prolongation of the vasomotor reaction leads to obstruction and mucostasis.

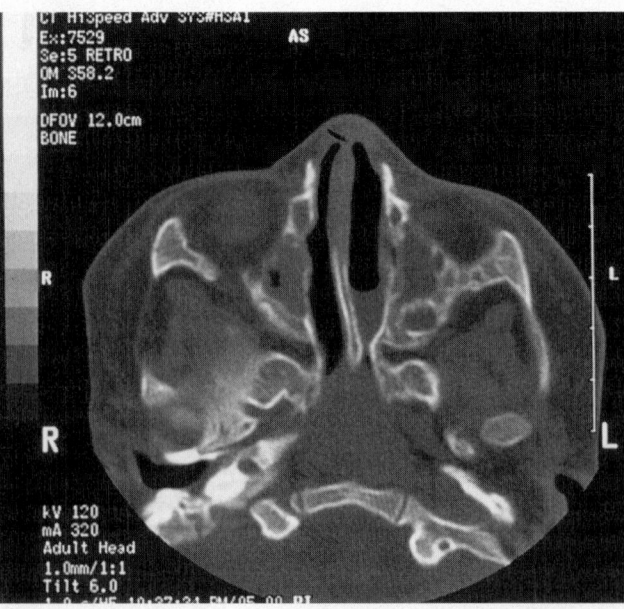

Figure 63-2. Axial computed tomography scan through the level of the nasal cavity and nasopharynx. Unilateral bony choanal atresia with air-fluid level is on the left.

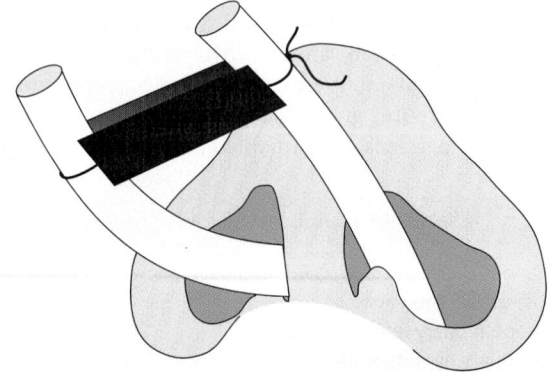

Figure 63-3. Soft bilateral nasal stents with anterior strut that protects the alar rims and columella.

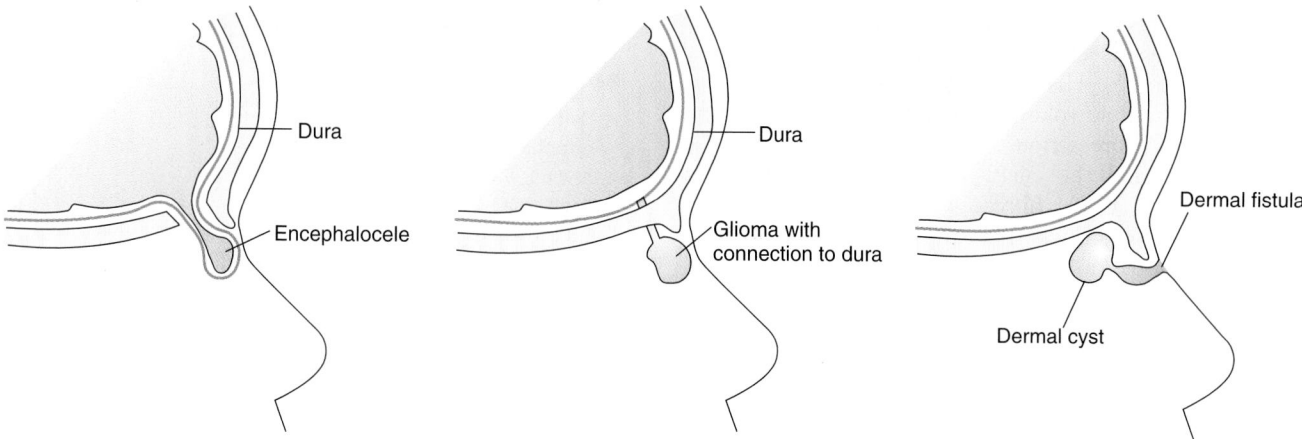

Figure 63-4. Differentiation of midline nasal mass anatomic features: encephalocele (left), glioma (middle), and dermoid cyst (right).

Seven percent of all upper respiratory infections become complicated by acute bacterial sinusitis. Common offending organisms include *Streptococcus pneumoniae, Haemophilus influenzae,* and *Moraxella catarrhalis.* In cases of chronic rhinosinusitis, anaerobic organisms, *Staphylococcus* species, and *Pseudomonas* species become more prevalent as the oxygen tension decreases within the obstructed sinuses. With the increase in inflammatory exudate seen with bacterial infection, rhinorrhea becomes more purulent. Acute bacterial sinusitis is characterized by upper respiratory infection symptoms persisting for more than 10 days without improvement. This appropriate historical information coupled with confirmation of mucosal edema and purulence aid in establishing the diagnosis. Routine radiologic imaging generally has low specificity and is not recommended routinely. CT is indicated, however, in the case of suspected orbital or intracranial complications associated with acute sinusitis. Additionally, confirmation of chronic sinusitis as a diagnosis may warrant CT after appropriate aggressive medical management. A diagnosis of recurrent or chronic sinusitis should alert the physician to the possibility of an immunodeficiency disorder.

Antibiotic therapy of acute sinusitis involves use of the most narrow-spectrum agent active against the most likely pathogens, taking into account the local bacterial resistance patterns and the child's risk factors for harboring a resistant strain of *S. pneumoniae.* These risk factors include day care attendance, antibiotic administration within the preceding 30 days, age younger than 2 years, and exposure to tobacco smoke (Box 63-6). Supplemental symptomatic therapy in the form of systemic or topical decongestants and antihistamines has not been shown to result in a significant decrease in severity, frequency, and time to resolution of upper respiratory infection symptoms.

Rare inflammatory conditions include tuberculosis, diphtheria, and syphilis. Syphilis, caused by *Treponema pallidum,* may be congenital or acquired; in the congenital form, early involvement manifests with thin watery discharge that becomes mucopurulent in addition to nasal obstruction, both of which result in noisy breathing or "snuffles." Obstruction and purulent sanguineous discharge secondary to gummatous involvement accompany the later stage of congenital syphilis. Sinonasal fungal infection must be included in the differential diagnosis of sinonasal symptoms, especially in immunocompromised and debilitated patients. *Mucor* species and *Aspergillus* are the most common pathogens, and diagnosis is confirmed by culture or biopsy.

Allergy may play a role in nasal obstruction and rhinorrhea. The Gell and Coombs type I anaphylactic IgE-mediated reaction results ultimately in an intense vasomotor reaction with increased capillary permeability and vasodilation from mast cell degranulation. Watery rhinorrhea, obstruction, sneezing, and pruritus are hallmark signs of allergic rhinitis. The turbinate mucosa may appear pale or bluish, and the classic adenoid facies may be apparent in a slightly older child. A family history of atopy may be elicited, and a history of chronic eczema, middle ear effusion, or sinusitis may accompany the rhinitis. Drops containing saline, decongestant, or steroid may be instituted, and antihistamine therapy may be appropriate if copious secretions dominate as the main factor in the obstruction.

Box 63-5. Inflammatory Conditions

- *Rhinitis of infancy*—meconium aspiration, chlamydial infection, gastroesophageal reflux
- *Viral rhinitis/sinusitis*—rhinovirus, adenovirus, myxovirus (influenza, parainfluenza, respiratory syncytial virus), coxsackie A and B, mumps, measles, poliomyelitis
- *Bacterial rhinitis/sinusitis*—*Streptococcus pneumoniae, Haemophilus influenzae, Moraxella catarrhalis,* anaerobic species, *Staphylococcus aureus, Pseudomonas*
- Tuberculosis
- Syphilis
- Fungal rhinitis/sinusitis
- Allergic rhinitis
- Adenoid hypertrophy

Box 63-6. Risk Factors for Bacterial Resistance

- Day care attendance
- Age <2 years
- Antibiotic use within previous 30 days
- Tobacco smoke exposure

Chronic allergy may lead to polyp formation secondary to the chronic hypersecretion and hyperplasia of the nasal mucosa (Fig. 63-5). Histologically, there is an increase in the intracellular fluid volume. Sinonasal polyps also may be a harbinger of more serious conditions, however, such as cystic fibrosis and the ciliary dyskinesia syndromes. As mentioned later, cystic fibrosis may manifest as chronic sinusitis with foul, thick rhinorrhea and nasal polyposis. Primary ciliary dyskinesia (immotile cilia syndrome) manifests as chronic rhinitis/sinusitis, nasal polyposis, chronic otitis media, and chronic bronchitis; a diagnosis of situs inversus in addition to this clinical picture represents Kartagener syndrome.

Adenoidal hypertrophy is a fairly common cause of nasal obstruction and rhinorrhea. Adenoid tissue is minimal in size at birth and increases over 1 to 2 years; the adenoids then generally recede at puberty. Part of Waldeyer's ring, this tissue plays a role in the immune system because the adenoid pad is in constant contact with antigens in inspired air and nasal secretions (see Chapter 64). The nasal obstruction resulting from adenoid hypertrophy with or without tonsillar hypertrophy may lead to obstructive sleep apnea and, eventually, alveolar hypoventilation with resultant increased pulmonary vascular resistance and cor pulmonale.

Neoplastic

Although rare, a myriad of neoplasms may arise within the sinonasal tract; lesions include those of ectodermal, mesodermal, neurogenic, or odontogenic origin (Box 63-7). Nasal obstruction, rhinorrhea, and epistaxis compose a triad of symptoms associated with sinonasal tumors, although tumors arising from the sinuses or nasopharynx may remain asymptomatic until extension into the nasal cavity occurs.

Hemangioma and lymphangioma are the most common benign lesions and usually arise from the nasal vestibule or external nasal skin. Juvenile nasopharyngeal angiofibroma is a distinct entity specific to adolescent boys, with symptoms generally manifesting around age 14 years. This lesion is

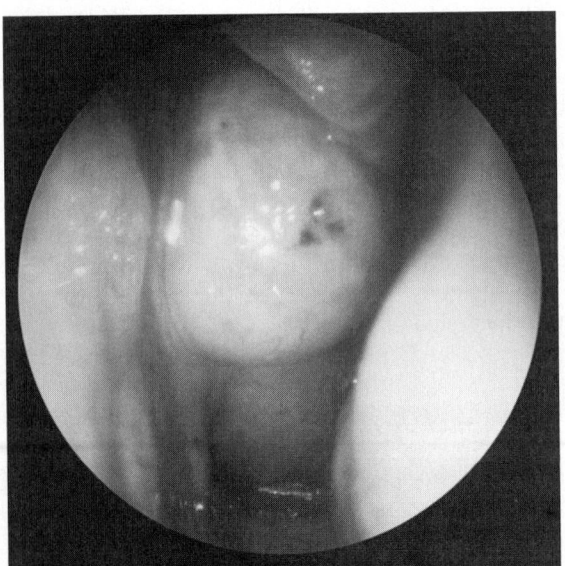

Figure 63-5. Nasal polyposis, endoscopic view.

Box 63-7. Sinonasal Neoplasms

Benign

- Hemangioma
- Lymphangioma
- Juvenile angiofibroma
- Papilloma
- Fibro-osseous lesions
- Neurogenic lesions (schwannoma, neurofibroma)
- Aneurysmal bone cyst
- Teratoma

Malignant

- Rhabdomyosarcoma
- Nasopharyngeal carcinoma
- Olfactory neuroblastoma
- Lymphoma

---

highly vascular and arises from the posterolateral aspect of the nasal cavity superiorly. Unilateral nasal obstruction becomes bilateral over time with extension across the midline posteriorly, and epistaxis is invariably present. Given the propensity for hemorrhage, biopsy of any lesion suspicious for juvenile nasopharyngeal angiofibroma should be performed in the operating room with ample packing supplies available. Other less common tumors include papillomas, fibro-osseous lesions, schwannomas, aneurysmal bone cysts, and teratomas, which are congenital neoplasms.

Rhabdomyosarcoma is the most common tumor of the pediatric sinonasal tract. Nasopharyngeal carcinoma presents with nasal symptoms as growth continues beyond the site of origin in the nasopharynx. Olfactory neuroblastoma is another uncommon tumor that arises from the olfactory mucosa superiorly within the nasal vault; generally, this tumor remains clinically silent until it reaches a large size. Hematopoietic system tumors, such as lymphoma, are rare and may arise primarily within the sinonasal tract or metastasize from distant sites.

Traumatic

Traumatic causes of pediatric nasal airway obstruction are listed in Box 63-8. Nasal trauma resulting in septal deviation may affect newborns. Of neonates, 70% may show subtle nasal septal abnormalities on examination, whereas 1% experience significant deflection of the septum. Nasal septal trauma may be noted in infants delivered by either vaginal or cesarean delivery; etiologies include various intrauterine forces depending on head presentation. These forces flatten the nasal tip and deflect the septum. Additionally, traumatic vaginal delivery, especially in the occipitoposterior position or with associated forceps use, may lead to septal deflection.

Box 63-8. Trauma as a Cause of Pediatric Nasal Airway Obstruction

- Nasal septal deflection
- Septal hematoma/abscess
- Foreign body

Management of neonatal septal deviation depends on the severity of the injury. In most infants, the deformity resolves on its own, usually within the first year of life. If there is displacement from the maxillary crest vomerine groove accompanied by external deformity and airway compromise, observation alone is not adequate. Instead, closed reduction is warranted; special neonatal septal manipulation forceps or small elevators may be employed.

Septal hematoma is a possible sequela from nasal trauma and is considered an otolaryngologic emergency (Fig. 63-6). Disruption of septal vessels with an intact mucoperichondrium results in a hematoma; devitalization of the septal cartilage secondary to ischemia may lead to necrosis within 48 hours and eventually cause saddle nose deformity. The mucoperichondrium in pediatric patients is thicker and more elastic than that of adults; this entity is seen more commonly in children. Associated symptoms include intermittent epistaxis and nasal obstruction. It may take several days for the hematoma to become clinically apparent. Drainage in a timely manner is the standard of care. Occasionally the hematoma is complicated further by abscess formation; urgent drainage is mandatory. Systemic antibiotic therapy should be instituted in all cases of septal hematoma.

Foreign bodies of the nasal cavity cause internal nasal trauma, which in some cases is quite serious. Toddlers, younger children with older siblings, and children with neurologic deficits or psychiatric issues are the most likely to present with a nasal foreign body. The object or material generally causes an intense vasomotor reaction with congestion and rhinorrhea, usually fetid. In any case of unilateral nasal obstruction with foul discharge, a retained foreign body must be sought. Disk batteries in particular pose an emergency, and prompt extrication prevents or diminishes the mucosal and cartilaginous damage seen with leakage of the battery's chemical contents. If suspicion is high yet identification of a battery proves difficult, an x-ray in the lateral plane may be obtained; a radiopaque bilaminar object is virtually diagnostic of a disk battery (Fig. 63-7). Unilateral

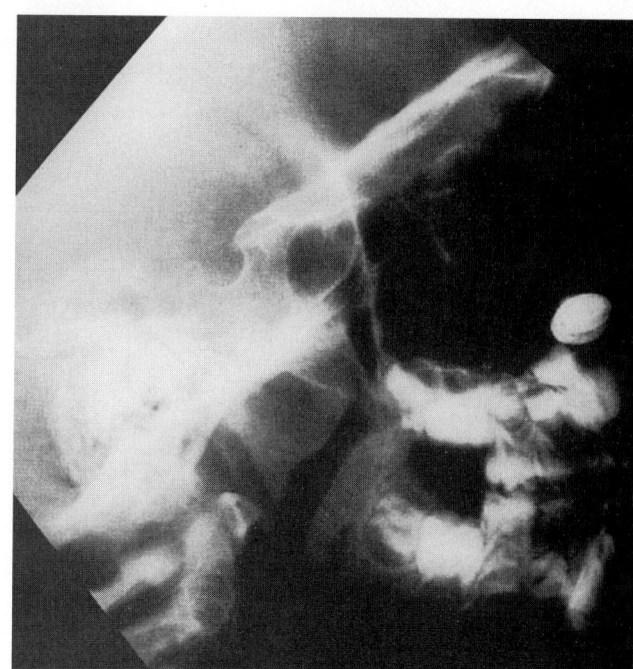

Figure 63-7. Plain radiograph of radiopaque foreign body in the nasal cavity, most consistent with a disk battery. Note bilaminar appearance.

purulent rhinorrhea almost always is associated with a nasal foreign body or unilateral choanal atresia.

Nasal decongestion should precede any attempt at removal of a nasal foreign body, and topical anesthetic may be considered. Suction aids in identification of the object, whereas alligator forceps or a blunt right-angle hook may be used for foreign-body removal. Otolaryngologic consultation should be considered. In the face of many prior unsuccessful attempts, controlled removal under a brief general anesthetic is warranted. In every case of nasal foreign body, bilateral nasal examination should be performed.

Metabolic

Certain endocrinologic and metabolic factors may intensify the vasomotor reaction. Endogenous and exogenous hormones may potentiate nasal mucosa edema and secretion; estrogen is one example. Deficiencies of calcium and magnesium may modify the mucosal basement membrane permeability with resultant congestion; low levels of ionic calcium are seen in the hypothyroid state. Chronic nasal infection may stem from aberrant carbohydrate metabolism caused by disruption of the system by which nasal mucosal cells release antibodies.

Cystic fibrosis leads to nasal obstruction and production of viscid mucus. The secretions show pronounced adhesiveness and an altered water-binding capacity related to increased calcium concentrations. The stasis resulting from congestion and tenacious secretions leads to chronic secondary infection in 90% of patients with cystic fibrosis; frequently isolated pathogens include *S. aureus*, *Pseudomonas*, *Streptococcus viridans*, *H. influenzae*, and *M. catarrhalis*. Nasal polyposis is also a prominent feature. Chronic nasal obstruction, thick, foul rhinorrhea, and polyps should heighten suspicion for cystic fibrosis, and appropriate diagnostic measures should be undertaken.

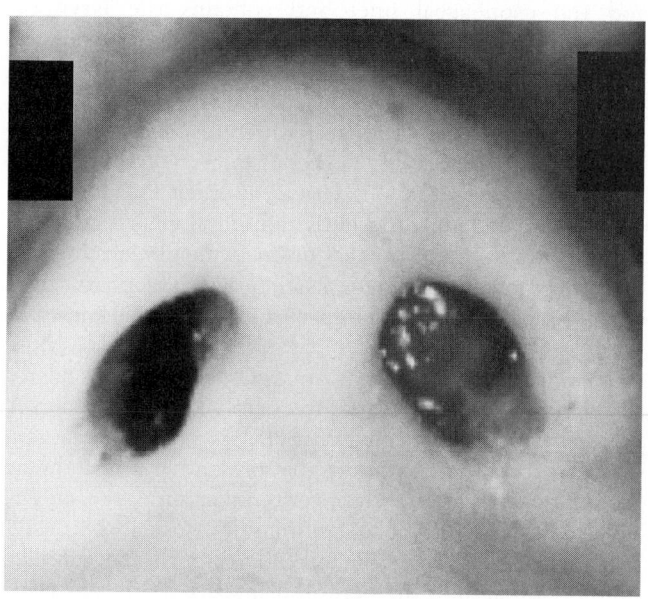

Figure 63-6. Left-sided septal hematoma.

SUGGESTED READINGS

Coates HL: Nasal obstruction in infancy. In Cotton RT, Myer CM (eds): Practical Pediatric Otolaryngology. Philadelphia, Lippincott-Raven, 1999, pp 449–468.

Hepler KM, Woodson GE, Kearns DB: Respiratory distress in the neonate: Sequela of a congenital dacryocystocele. Arch Otolaryngol Head Neck Surg 1995;121:1423–1425.

Magit AE: Tumors of the nose, paranasal sinuses, and nasopharynx. In Bluestone CD, Stool SE, Kenna MA (eds): Pediatric Otolaryngology, 3rd ed. Philadelphia, WB Saunders, 1996, pp 893–904.

Saluke A, Bird S, Cottongim T: Evidence based clinical practice guideline for children with acute sinusitis. Health Policy and Clinical Effectiveness Program, Children's Hospital Medical Center, Cincinnati, Ohio, 2001.

Settipane GA, Klein DE, Settipane RJ: Nasal polyps: State of the art. Rhinol suppl 1991; 11:33–36.

SECTION 3   GENERAL MEDICAL CARE: *Disorders of the Head and Neck*

64 Disorders of the Pharynx

Stanley H. Inkelis

ROLE OF THE GENERALIST

1   Differentiate between infectious and noninfectious disorders of the pharynx.

2   Distinguish between viral and bacterial causes of pharyngeal disorders based on clinical presentation.

3   Recognize the physical findings diagnostic of infectious disorders of the pharynx.

4   Treat infectious and noninfectious disorders of the pharynx based on the etiology of the disorder.

5   Educate parents about the judicious use of antibiotics only for bacterial infections of the pharynx.

6   Diagnose obstructive sleep apnea disorders, and determine the underlying pathophysiologic process.

7   Refer children with anatomic or surgical disorders of the pharynx to an otolaryngologist for consultation and management.

DEFINITION

Pharyngeal disorders, particularly sore throat, are among the most common diseases seen by the generalist. These disorders may occur in any of the three parts of the pharynx—nasopharynx, oropharynx, or hypopharynx—extending from the base of the skull to the esophagus (Fig. 64-1). The nasopharynx is the upper portion of the pharynx, above the palate, containing the adenoids (pharyngeal tonsils) and the eustachian tubes. The part of the pharynx from the palate to the tip of the epiglottis containing the palatine tonsils is the oropharynx. The most inferior part of the pharynx, the hypopharynx, is located between the tip of the epiglottis and the esophageal inlet and contains the laryngeal structures. Most pharyngeal disorders seen by the generalist involve the oropharynx, which is the main focus of this chapter. Craniofacial anomalies, eustachian tube dysfunction, abnormalities of laryngeal structures, and swallowing difficulties are discussed in other chapters.

The most frequent pharyngeal disorder in children is pharyngitis (including tonsillitis and tonsillopharyngitis), an inflammatory illness of the mucous membranes of the throat, commonly known as a *sore throat*. Nasopharyngitis, when nasal symptoms accompany a sore throat, is known as an *upper respiratory infection* (i.e., the common cold). Most often, pharyngitis is due to a virus, but bacteria, particularly *Streptococcus pyogenes*, more frequently known as group A β-hemolytic streptococcus (GABHS), is a common cause.

Several bacterial conditions that present with sore throat require immediate attention. Peritonsillar abscess, a suppurative complication of bacterial tonsillitis, usually is caused by GABHS. The infection extends through the tonsillar fibrous capsule into the peritonsillar space. A retropharyngeal abscess is an infection of the retropharyngeal space,

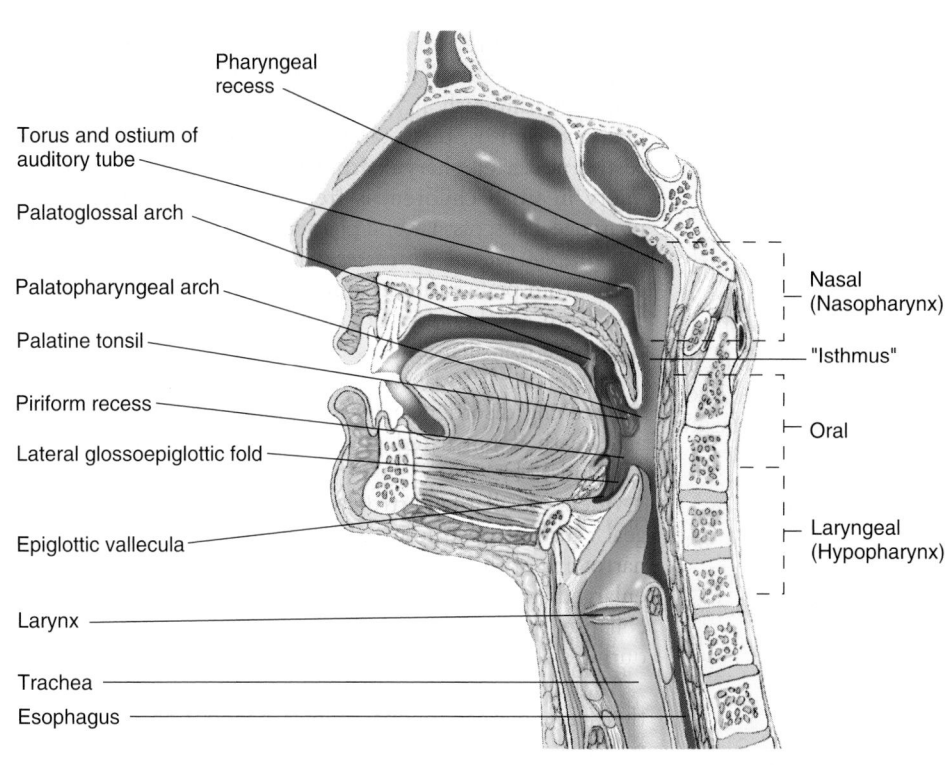

Pharyngeal recess

Torus and ostium of auditory tube

Palatoglossal arch

Palatopharyngeal arch

Palatine tonsil

Piriform recess

Lateral glossoepiglottic fold

Epiglottic vallecula

Larynx

Trachea

Esophagus

Nasal (Nasopharynx)

"Isthmus"

Oral

Laryngeal (Hypopharynx)

Figure 64-1. Pharyngeal anatomy.

between the prevertebral fascia of the cervical vertebrae and the posterior pharyngeal wall. A lateral pharyngeal abscess (parapharyngeal abscess) is an infection of the lateral pharyngeal space that is contiguous with the retropharyngeal space. In addition to GABHS, *Staphylococcus aureus* and oropharyngeal anaerobic organisms may be involved. Epiglottitis (supraglottitis), a bacterial infection of the epiglottis, aryepiglottic folds, arytenoid soft tissue, and uvula, most commonly was caused by *Haemophilus influenzae* type b before the *H. influenzae* type b vaccine. Thermal epiglottitis may occur from hot foods or liquids or from smoking freebase cocaine. Laryngotracheobronchitis, or croup, a viral infection of the upper airway, has a similar clinical presentation to epiglottitis.

Physiologic adenotonsillar hyperplasia refers to the fact that tonsils and adenoids are normally larger in children than in adults. Without symptoms of infection or obstruction, adenotonsillar size has no medical significance. Adenotonsillar hypertrophy may occur acutely with infection or may be chronic, resulting in pathologically enlarged tonsils that cause obstruction of airflow and result in an obstructive sleep disorder. Obstructive sleep apnea or obstructive sleep apnea syndrome has a prevalence of approximately 2% and occurs most commonly in children 2 to 5 years old (see the CD-ROM and Chapters 63 and 251).

Pharyngeal tumors in children are uncommon. Benign tumors of the oropharynx and hypopharynx include juvenile nasopharyngeal angiofibroma, hamartomas, hemangiomas, and neurofibromas. The most common malignant tumors of this region are lymphoma and rhabdomyosarcoma.

Trauma to the pharynx, most often from foreign objects, such as pencils, sticks, or toys, may cause injuries such as contusions, lacerations, and penetration of the pharyngeal structures. Burns and caustics also may cause trauma to the pharynx.

FUNDAMENTALS

Sore throat accounts for approximately 5% of all pediatric visits, is less common in children younger than 1 year old, and peaks between 5 and 8 years of age. Viral pharyngitis occurs most commonly in the summer and fall. Bacterial pharyngitis occurs most frequently in the winter and spring and is uncommon in children younger than 3 years old. Approximately 15% of cases of pharyngitis in school-age children are caused by GABHS.

Typically, viral pharyngitis follows inhalation of airborne droplets or self-inoculation of organisms into the nasal mucosa or conjunctiva and viral invasion of the respiratory epithelium. Pain results from the effect of inflammatory mediators on vascular permeability and on pain nerve endings. Bacterial organisms, in particular GABHS, directly invade the mucous membranes. Streptolysin O and hyaluronidase, enzymes produced by GABHS, facilitate the local spread of infection.

Viruses are the most common cause of nasopharyngitis and pharyngitis in children (Table 64-1). Rhinovirus typically is associated with upper respiratory symptoms, such as cough and rhinorrhea. Adenovirus often causes an exudative pharyngitis, usually in children younger than 3 years old. Parainfluenza virus, respiratory syncytial virus, and influenza virus cause sore throat and croup. Coxsackievirus and echovirus (enteroviruses) are the usual cause of herpangina, sore throat that may be associated with high fever, irritability, and refusal to eat or drink leading to dehydration. Enteroviral infections are most common in the late spring, summer, and early fall. Epstein-Barr virus (EBV) usually is associated with tonsillar exudate and is often difficult to distinguish from GABHS infection.

The most common cause of bacterial pharyngitis in children (usually >3 years old) is GABHS. Other bacteria that

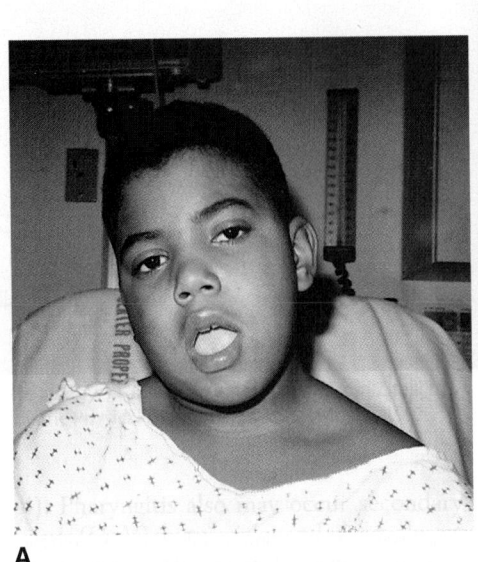

A

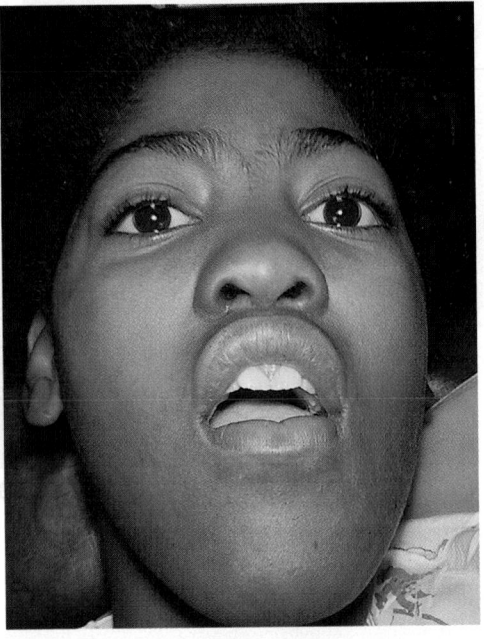

B

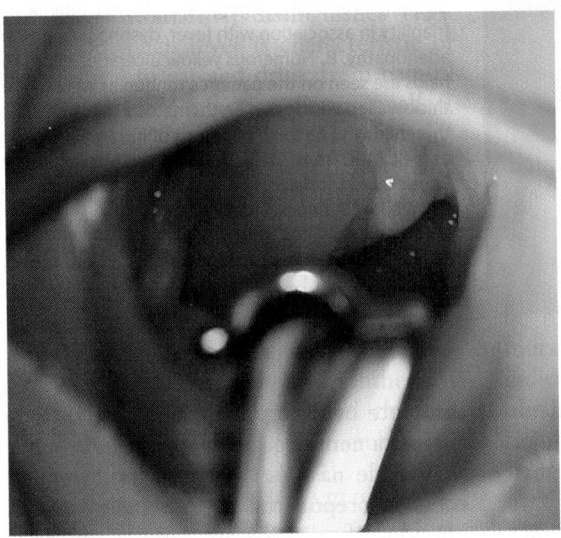

C

Figure 64-6. Peritonsillar abscess. **A,** This patient exhibits the torticollis often seen with a peritonsillar abscess in an effort to minimize pressure on the adjacent, inflamed tonsillar node. **B,** Sympathetic inflammation of the pterygoid muscles causes trismus, limiting the patient's ability to open the mouth. **C,** This photograph, taken in the operating room, shows an intensely inflamed soft palatal mass that obscures the tonsil and bulges forward and toward the midline, deviating the uvula. (From Zitelli BJ, Davis HW: Atlas of Pediatric Physical Diagnosis. St. Louis, Mosby, 1997.)

lymphoma. Lymphoma also should be considered in children with rapid bilateral tonsillar enlargement.

Symptoms of pharyngeal and laryngeal injury include dysphagia, odynophagia, and dysphonia. Crepitance in the neck may be present. Respiratory distress and stridor suggest airway obstruction and may require endotracheal intubation. Vascular injury should be considered with trauma to the posterior pharyngeal wall, persistent bleeding, or an enlarging hematoma. Parents should be asked to provide any suspected penetrating object to be examined for pieces that may have been broken off and been retained in the area of injury. With caustic ingestions, the type of product, the brand name, and quantity ingested should be determined. Drooling and refusal to eat or drink are common symptoms of caustic oropharyngeal burns. Physical examination should note the extent of injury and involvement of surrounding structures so that the appropriate imaging studies may be obtained and appropriate consultants notified.

Laboratory tests and imaging studies are often helpful in the diagnosis of pharyngeal disorders. Throat culture is the most reliable test for confirming the diagnosis of bacterial pharyngitis, particularly GABHS. The large number of children who are streptococcal carriers (15% to 20%) causes a high rate of false-positive throat cultures. The false-negative rate is approximately 10%. The throat culture is the gold standard by which other tests are judged. The greatest disadvantage of throat cultures is that results are not final for 1 to 2 days. Although rapid streptococcal antigen detection tests provide immediate results and are reliable when they are positive (approximately 95% specificity), they are less reliable when negative (approximately 80% to 90% sensitive). Because newer optical immunoassay and chemoluminescent DNA rapid streptococcal antigen tests are as sensitive as throat cultures, confirmatory culture no longer is recommended routinely (see the CD-ROM).

Determination of the precise cause of viral pharyngitis is rarely necessary. In unusual instances, when there is a

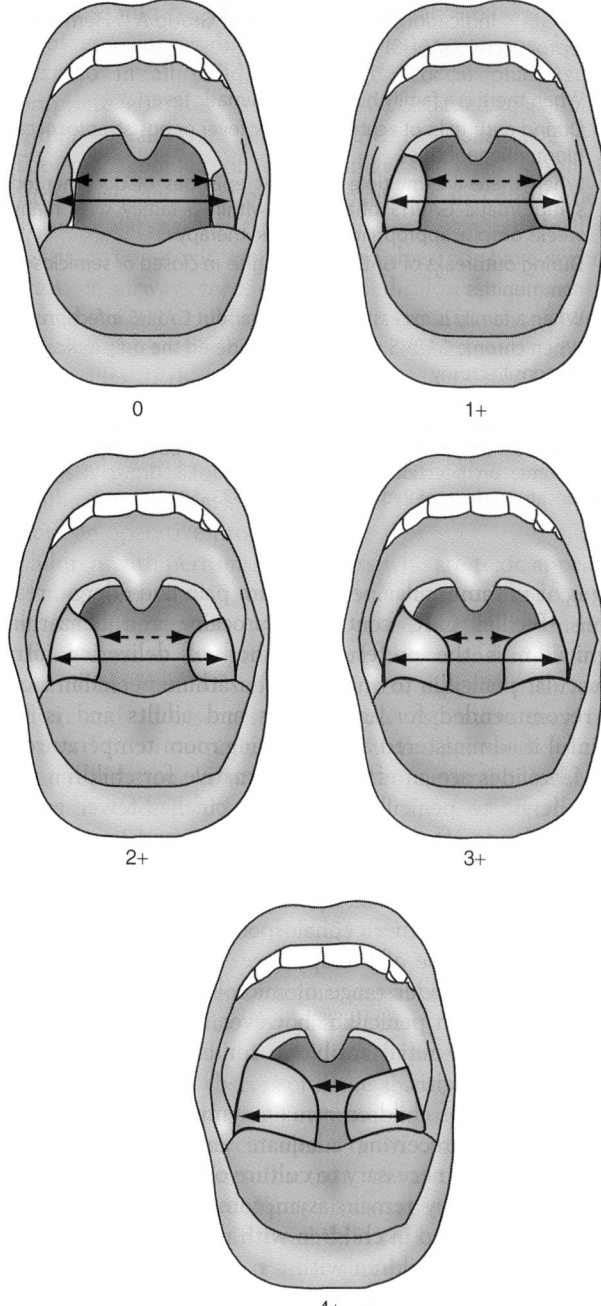

0   1+

2+   3+

4+

Figure 64-7. Tonsillar grading classification. Grundfast KM: The Pediatric Clinics of North America, vol 36, number 6. WB Saunders, Philadelphia, December 1989.

Imaging studies are particularly useful for the diagnosis of deep infections of the pharyngeal space. Lateral soft tissue radiographs of the neck are helpful in patients suspected of having a retropharyngeal abscess and may be used as a screening study. If the lateral neck film suggests a retropharyngeal abscess or if there is a high degree of clinical suspicion for this diagnosis, computed tomography (CT) scan with contrast enhancement from the base of the cranium to the upper mediastinum usually is recommended for better delineation of the abscess and surrounding tissue. A CT scan also should be obtained if there is suspicion of a lateral pharyngeal abscess. Peritonsillar abscess is usually a clinical diagnosis, but in cases in which the diagnosis is not clear, CT scan is beneficial. The information obtained by CT is comparable to that of magnetic resonance imaging, and CT generally is more readily available and is less costly. Ultrasound examination of the head and neck for deep infection has not been shown to be as good an imaging study as CT. Chest radiographs or CT may be helpful if there is concern of extension of the infection into the mediastinum.

Epiglottitis usually can be diagnosed clinically. In cases in which there is suspicion of epiglottitis but the diagnosis is unlikely, a lateral neck x-ray may be helpful. A portable x-ray in the emergency department is preferable to sending the patient to radiology because of the potential of respiratory compromise.

All of these studies should be performed with the immediate availability of oxygen, bag-valve-mask ventilation, and endotracheal intubation. A physician should be present who is capable of performing endotracheal intubation if the patient has significant airway compromise during the study.

Children with adenotonsillar hypertrophy and obstructive sleep apnea disorders often are diagnosed clinically and do not need further diagnostic studies. In some cases, polysomnography, also known as a *sleep study*, is useful in confirming the diagnosis of obstructive sleep apnea, particularly when the history is unclear or when surgery may be more complex and of higher risk, such as in children with craniofacial anomalies.

Pharyngeal foreign bodies and subcutaneous air from trauma sometimes may be seen on lateral neck or chest x-ray. CT scan with contrast enhancement is the best imaging study for delineating laryngeal trauma. The extent of tumors of the pharynx is determined best with CT or magnetic resonance imaging.

MANAGEMENT

The management of pharyngeal disorders is varied and depends on the etiology. Pharyngitis usually is viral in origin and may be treated symptomatically with analgesics, such as acetaminophen or ibuprofen, to relieve pain of pharyngitis and promote oral hydration. Parents should be instructed about monitoring fluid intake and the signs of dehydration. An older child may derive some relief from gargling with warm salt water or sucking on hard candy or mentholated throat lozenges.

If the pharyngitis is bacterial in origin, antibiotic treatment is indicated. GABHS is treated with penicillin. Evidence suggests that antibiotic treatment provides more rapid relief of symptoms, shortens the course of illness, and prevents suppurative complications and rheumatic fever.

treatable systemic infection, such as encephalitis caused by HSV, viral throat cultures and acute and convalescent titers may be helpful. Infectious mononucleosis is diagnosed best with a heterophil agglutination test, particularly in children older than 4 years of age and later in the course of illness. A white blood cell count with a predominance of lymphocytes or greater than 10% atypical lymphocytes supports the diagnosis of infectious mononucleosis.

Gonorrheal pharyngitis may be diagnosed by a positive culture on a Thayer-Martin plate. Tularemia may be diagnosed with a serum agglutination test, and confirmatory diagnosis of diphtheria may be made by culture of the pseudomembrane or by fluorescent antibody technique.

airway is secured, pulmonary edema is the most common complication, occurring in about 9% of patients in one study. Extraepiglottic complications, such as pneumonia and cervical adenitis, occur commonly, whereas meningitis is rare. Adverse outcome, including hypoxic central nervous system injury and mortality, almost always can be prevented with early establishment of an airway.

The outcome for benign pharyngeal tumors is usually excellent. The outcome of juvenile nasopharyngeal angiofibromas is generally good if complete surgical removal is successful. Most complications are related to the inability to remove the tumor completely because of anatomic locations or to the surgery itself. Complications of malignant tumors usually relate to the anatomic structures involved and to the surgery. The outcome in children with pharyngeal malignant tumors depends on the type of tumor and its associated morbidity and mortality.

Accidental trauma to the pharynx usually is minor, and the outcome is excellent. Adverse outcomes may occur owing to complications associated with the injury if the trauma is to the lateral soft palate, peritonsillar area, or posterior pharynx. These areas are near vital structures, such as the carotid artery, which can become contused with potential subsequent thrombosis. Edema or hematomas from trauma may lead to respiratory compromise. Penetrating trauma from guns or knives often is associated with a bad outcome. The outcome from burns or chemicals is related to the extent of the trauma.

Most children with obstructive sleep disorders with adenotonsillar hypertrophy undergo successful adenotonsillectomy. Bleeding is the most concerning complication. Severe pain and persistent vomiting also may occur with an associated decrease in oral fluid intake and subsequent dehydration. Snoring and apnea sometimes continue after adenotonsillectomy. Other surgical and nonsurgical forms of therapy are beneficial to many patients with persistent symptoms. Tracheostomy rarely is needed for the child who is not responsive to other forms of treatment.

FOLLOW-UP

Children with viral pharyngitis and bacterial pharyngitis rarely need follow-up because these are self-limited diseases. If EBV is the cause of the pharyngitis, good anticipatory guidance regarding airway obstruction should be provided. If a child with EBV pharyngitis has evidence of early airway obstruction or is hospitalized for airway obstruction, close follow-up should be arranged. Children with recurrent bacterial tonsillitis should return for follow-up. Parents should be instructed to return for follow-up if, after 48 hours of antibiotic treatment, the child continues to have severe pain, difficulty swallowing, drooling, or a fever equal to or greater than 38.3°C.

The child treated for a deep neck abscess, epiglottitis, or penetrating trauma should be followed by an otolaryngologist in conjunction with a generalist. Children with minor trauma to the pharynx can be followed as needed. Children with burns or chemical injuries should be followed according to the severity of the injury by the generalist and an otolaryngologist or gastroenterologist or both. Pharyngeal tumors should be followed by an otolaryngologist. If the tumor is malignant, an oncologist also should be involved in follow-up care.

Complete resolution of symptoms is typical in patients with obstructive sleep apnea after adenotonsillectomy. If symptoms persist, postoperative polysomnography should be obtained. Postoperative sleep studies also should be obtained in children with severe preoperative obstructive sleep apnea and in children with craniofacial anomalies or neurologic deficit. These high-risk patients are more likely to have recurrences and require more frequent and longer term follow-up.

Additional Resources, CD-ROM

Tests for diagnosis of group A β-hemolytic streptococcus	Text
Epiglottitis and croup	Text
Obstructive sleep apnea	Text
Bibliography	

Mini-index of Related Topics

SUGGESTED READINGS

Attia M, Zaoutis T, Eppes S, et al: Multivariate predictive models for group A beta-hemolytic streptococcal pharyngitis in children. Acad Emerg Med 1999;6:8–13.

Berkowitz RG, Makadevan M: Unilateral tonsillar enlargement and tonsillar lymphoma in children. Ann Otol Rhinol Laryngol 1999;108:876–879.

Bower CM, Gungor AG: Pediatric obstructive sleep apnea syndrome. Otolaryngol Clin North Am 2000;33:49–75.

Herzon FS, Nicklaus P: Pediatric peritonsillar abscess: Management guidelines. Curr Probl Pediatr 1996;26:270–278.

Nicklaus PJ, Kelley PE: Management of deep neck infection. Pediatr Clin North Am 1996;43:1277–1296.

65 Disorders of the Neck and Salivary Glands

Henry Milczuk

DEFINITIONS

Of structures contained within the head and neck, lymph nodes account for most problems in children. *Benign lymphadenopathy*, increased size of lymph nodes, is not associated with other symptoms and usually results from nonspecific inflammation. Cervical lymph nodes greater than 1.5 cm in size (larger than the average adult fingertip) are considered enlarged. *Lymphadenitis* is invasion of microorganisms into the cervical lymph nodes. An acute cervical lymphadenitis develops over a few days with other signs and symptoms of infection. Other microbes cause a granulomatous reaction and chronic inflammation of the lymph nodes. *Chronic lymphadenitis* may have few symptoms other than slow growth of the mass in the neck over weeks. Granulomatous lymphadenitis occasionally may suppurate or lead to overlying skin changes and skin necrosis. The challenge for the generalist is differentiating benign but persistent lymphadenopathy from conditions that merit further evaluation and treatment.

Many types of *congenital masses* may occur because of the complex embryology of the head and neck. A congenital neck mass is not always found at birth. Location of congenital neck masses reflects their embryologic origin and migratory pattern during structural development. Remnants from the branchial apparatus and the thyroid anlage contain secretory epithelium that can form a cystic mass. Vascular malformations are named by the primary vascular component: lymphatic malformation (cystic hygroma, lymphangioma), venous malformation, or arteriovenous malformation. Hemangiomas contain proliferating and hyperplastic endothelium that may enlarge or encroach on adjacent areas during the first year of life. Traumatic passage through the birth canal or forceps delivery can injure the sternocleidomastoid

(SCM) muscle, causing fibrosis and a firm mass within the muscle that has been given various names, including congenital muscular torticollis (CMT), fibromatosis colli, SCM tumor of infancy, and pseudotumor. CMT may not be related to birth trauma or another apparent etiology.

Neoplasms in the head and neck region are rare, but the generalist should remain suspicious of an atypical head and neck mass. The most common head and neck malignant tumor in children is lymphoma, which is usually nodal. Hodgkin's disease also can affect cervical lymph nodes. The most common malignant soft tissue tumor in the head and neck region is rhabdomyosarcoma. Rarely, cervical neuroblastoma arises from the cervical autonomic plexus.

There are two sets of major salivary glands—the parotid and submandibular glands—and minor salivary glands throughout the mouth and pharynx, including the sublingual glands. All salivary glands contain secretory glandular structures with ducts that conduct the saliva to the oral cavity (or pharynx). Lymph nodes can be found within the salivary glands, especially the parotid gland. The major salivary glands and their associated lymph nodes may become infected, the ducts can become obstructed, or, rarely, these structures may become involved with a neoplastic process.

FUNDAMENTALS

The neck is rich in lymphatic vessels and lymph nodes. More than 25% of all lymph nodes are above the clavicles (Fig. 65-1). Nodes generally are not palpable during the newborn period. Cervical lymph nodes frequently are stimulated and enlarge over time from numerous upper respiratory tract infections. The cervical lymph nodes may remain enlarged after the acute infection resolves. *Benign cervical lymphadenopathy* is common with lymph nodes anterior to the SCM muscle. The jugulogastric lymph nodes, found near the angle of the mandible, drain the pharynx and tonsillar regions and commonly are enlarged. Benign lymphadenopathy is not associated with other symptoms, such as pain, redness, or fevers. *Generalized lymphadenopathy*, affecting other lymph nodes such as the axillary or inguinal regions, also can involve the neck. Typically a systemic disease, such as an autoimmune disorder, viral illness (e.g., Epstein-Barr virus), or serum sickness, may be the cause.

Acute lymphadenitis develops when microorganisms directly invade the cervical lymph nodes. Affected lymph nodes are tender and erythematous, and the patient may normal position, is indicated by mobility of the tooth and usually means that the periodontal ligament has been damaged or lacerated, affecting the teeth's neurovascular supply. Displaced teeth also suggest the possibility of fracture of the root or the supporting alveolar bone. Intrusion occurs when a tooth is driven into the socket, damaging the periodontal ligament and fracturing the alveolar socket. Avulsion refers to loss of the tooth from the alveolus. If possible, avulsed permanent teeth should be replaced in the socket as soon as possible. Fractures through the enamel (Ellis class I) have no dentin, or pulp is visible at the fracture site. Fractures through the dentin (Ellis class II) are characterized by exposure of yellow dentin at the fracture site. Dentin fractures are sensitive to changes in temperature and touch. Tubules running from the dentin to pulp can transmit infection toward the pulp, especially in children younger than age 12 who have thinner dentin. In fractures through the pulp (Ellis class III), bleeding comes from the fracture site. Children with class III fractures may have constant pain or, paradoxically, little pain if the neurovascular bundle has been disrupted completely. Root fractures lie below the alveolar ridge and require radiographic evaluation for diagnosis and are suggested by unusual mobility or sensitivity to percussion. Alveolar fractures also require radiographic diagnosis and may be accompanied by other dental injuries, soft tissue swelling and tenderness, step-offs, or changes in occlusion. A tooth also may be missing after trauma. It should not be assumed that the tooth was lost at the injury scene; radiographic evaluation may be necessary to assess whether the missing tooth may have been aspirated; swallowed; or intruded into the socket, nasopharynx, or sinus cavity.

MANAGEMENT

Although most definitive management of dental disorders is done by dentists, primary care providers play an important role in early identification of dental pathology and in facilitating prompt referrals. Generalists also can take advantage of a teachable moment to emphasize the importance of prevention after dental pathology is discovered or dental injury has occurred.

If access to dental care is limited, primary care providers can intervene actively when early carious lesions or white spots are identified. Application of fluoride varnish to the teeth can help to remineralize and reverse early lesions. Counseling on diet and oral hygiene is important. When a child has more advanced caries, prompt referral to a dentist is indicated. Pulpal involvement and abscess formation may result if a carious lesion is ignored. If dental care is not immediately available, antibiotics and analgesics may alleviate symptoms temporarily; however, more definitive treatment (root canal or extraction) is necessary to remove the source of infection and prevent recurrence of symptoms and further complications.

Children with persistent gingivitis or with risk factors for periodontal disease should be identified and referred in the early stages of disease. In the early stages, gingivitis can be reversed through the institution of regular brushing and flossing to remove plaque, but signs such as gingival swelling,

bleeding, the presence of plaque and purulent debris, and regression of the gum line indicate the need for prompt dental referral.

Irrigation and analgesics usually are the first steps in caring for a dental injury. Tetanus prophylaxis should be considered for children with avulsion, laceration, or intrusion injuries. The timing of dental referral after dental injury depends on the type of injury. With more extensive or complex injuries, early consultation with a dental specialist should occur. In certain circumstances, antibiotics may be indicated. Radiographic evaluation is often necessary to determine if the alveolus or other bones are fractured.

Children with central concussion injuries and Ellis class I fractures (involving only the enamel) can be seen at the next available dental appointment. Children who have sustained a dental concussion may have tenderness when pressure is applied to the tooth. Treatment is a soft diet and analgesics. Sharp edges from an enamel fracture can be filed down to prevent soft tissue injury.

Children with class II fractures and intrusion injuries should be seen by a dentist within 1 to 2 days. Young children with class II fractures should be seen by a dentist within 12 hours because thinner dentin allows spread of infection to the pulp to occur more quickly. While waiting for the appointment, the child can be treated with soft diet and analgesics. Although intruded teeth may be allowed to re-erupt, many of these teeth ultimately show pulpal deterioration and require root canal therapy.

Class III fractures, root fractures, avulsions, and luxations require prompt dental care. Alveolar fractures and more complex facial fractures require immediate consultation, usually with an oral surgeon. In an otherwise stable and alert child, an avulsed permanent tooth can be rinsed in tap water or saline and, holding the tooth by the crown (avoiding the root to prevent damage to the periodontal ligament fibers), manually reimplanted in the socket. The child can hold the tooth in place either with his or her finger or by biting onto a gauze pad. The child should be seen urgently by a dentist. Primary teeth should not be reimplanted because doing so risks damaging the underlying developing permanent dentition. The shorter the time between tooth loss and replacement into the socket, the greater the chance for retaining tooth viability. If the tooth cannot be replaced immediately into the socket, it should stored in saline or cold milk or held in the child's buccal vestibule (only if the child is alert and cooperative) until definitive care is rendered. Commercially available tooth-preserving systems also can be used. Water is not a desirable transport medium because its low osmolality can lead to cellular damage. Other liquids, such as juice or bleach, should not be used.

Care of traumatized primary teeth is different. Damage to the primary teeth may affect the developing permanent teeth located in close proximity to the primary teeth roots. Priority should be placed on maintenance of permanent teeth. Avulsed primary dentition should not be replaced because doing so may damage the developing permanent teeth. Children with luxated or intruded primary teeth should be referred for same-day dental care. If there is risk of tooth aspiration or if a dentist is not immediately available, primary care providers can remove loose primary teeth (the provider should not attempt to remove intruded teeth). Dentists may allow an intruded tooth to re-erupt before extracting it, but primary teeth intrusions require close follow-up to prevent complications. Dentoalveolar fractures involving the primary dentition are less common than luxation injuries in young children because the alveolus in young children is more porous and vascularized, providing elasticity with a blow. If a primary tooth fractures and the pulp is involved, a same-day visit is needed because of risk of infection through the exposed pulp. Children with uncomplicated primary tooth fractures should be seen by a dentist within a few days.

PREVENTION

Prevention of dental disorders and promotion of good oral health are the responsibility of the primary physician. In 2003, the American Academy of Pediatrics issued a recommendation that pediatricians and other pediatric health care providers begin regular oral health anticipatory guidance and risk assessment before their patients are 6 months old. Protection against all decay is theoretically possible. Important preventive practices include regular home oral hygiene; access to routine dental care; sound dietary practices, including avoiding frequent or prolonged exposure to fermentable carbohydrates, especially sucrose; regular use of fluorides; and sealant application. Community water fluoridation provides an effective, inexpensive, and important source of fluoride. Regular use of toothpaste provides another good means of fluoride delivery. Children at high risk for dental decay may need additional sources of fluoride. Sealants placed on the pit and fissure surfaces of the permanent molars can defend against caries in these surfaces. Children should be seen by a dentist for evaluation for sealant placement within 6 to 12 months of eruption of their first permanent molars. Prevention of periodontal disease also should begin during childhood with development of a regular home oral hygiene regimen. Tooth brushing can begin with first tooth eruption. By age 7 years, most children have developed sufficient fine motor skills to begin flossing their teeth. Brushing and flossing facilitate removal of plaque.

Certain types of malocclusion are preventable. Because caries and trauma can lead to premature tooth loss and subsequent loss of spacing and overcrowding, prevention minimizes the need for orthodontic treatment. Prolonged digit sucking (after about age 4 years) may cause malocclusion. The most common types of malocclusion associated with digit sucking are anterior open bite (posterior teeth come together, but there is an opening between the maxillary and mandibular anterior teeth), overjet, maxillary protrusion, posterior crossbite, and retrusion of the mandible (Fig. 66-10).

Generalists can play an important role in the prevention of all injuries, including dental injuries. Use of restraint systems appropriate for a child's age and size while riding in the car minimizes the risk of craniofacial injuries. Dental injuries during sports such as soccer, football, baseball, hockey, skateboarding, and scooter and bicycle riding are common in older children. Mouth guards provide effective protection

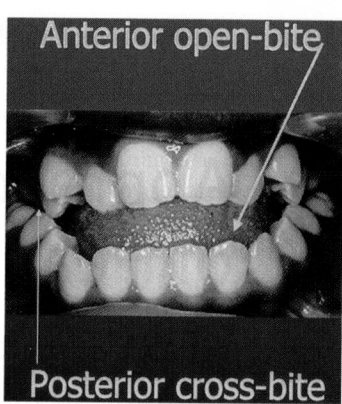

Figure 66-10. Anterior open bite and posterior crossbite.

against orofacial trauma. Custom-made, self-adapted (so-called "boil and bite"), and stock mouth guards are available.

OUTCOMES

Many dental disorders are preventable. Early identification and prompt referral can prevent complications. In the past, edentulism in adulthood resulting from decay and periodontitis was common. Fluoride use and proper preventive oral health have reduced this condition. Prompt referral also is necessary to prevent serious complications from certain types of dental injuries. Even in the best hands, some permanent teeth cannot be saved after extensive injury. In these cases, dental implants or dentures may be possible.

FOLLOW-UP

Good oral health and preventive oral hygiene must begin in early childhood. Children should have their first visit with a dental professional by age 1 year for those at high risk for dental decay and by 3 years for others. Physicians can function as advocates for their patients by facilitating dental referrals and following up to ensure a dental visit has occurred.

Mini-index of Related Topics   CH.

SUGGESTED READINGS

Holt R, Roberts G, Scully C: ABC of oral health: Oral health and disease. BMJ 2000;320:1652–1655.

McTigue DJ: Diagnosis and management of dental injuries in children. Pediatr Clin North Am 2000;47:1067–1084.

Oral Health in America: A Report of the Surgeon General. Rockville, Md, National Institute of Dental and Craniofacial Research, National Institutes of Health, U.S. Department of Health and Human Services, 2000.

Recommendations for using fluoride to prevent and control dental caries in the United States. MMWR Morb Mortal Wkly Rep 2001;RR-14:1–42.

Vig KW, Fields HW: Facial growth and management of orthodontic problems. Pediatr Clin North Am 2000;47:1085–1123.

strabismus beyond this age is abnormal, requiring referral to a pediatric ophthalmologist.

Incomitant strabismic deviations often require a more extensive evaluation with the involvement of multiple pediatric specialists. Parents may not recognize the strabismus and frequently complain of abnormal "eye movement" or abnormal head posture. The causes include the developmental abnormalities Duane's syndrome, Möbius' syndrome, Brown's syndrome, and ocular fibrosis syndrome or nerve palsies of the third, fourth, or sixth cranial nerves.

Duane's syndrome is an absence of the abducens nerve nucleus that results in aberrant innervation of the lateral rectus muscle from branches of the third cranial nerve. There is a deficiency of abduction, with cocontraction of the lateral and medial rectus muscles on attempted adduction. This cocontraction results in globe retraction with attempted adduction, narrowing of the palpebral fissures in adduction, and widening of the palpebral fissures on attempted abduction. Compensatory head posturing is variable, but it most often results in the affected eye turned slightly in adduction with a head turn toward the affected side. Of affected individuals, 10% have an associated hearing loss. Although surgery is usually unnecessary, patients should be referred to a pediatric ophthalmologist.

Möbius' syndrome of congenital facial diplegia (cranial nerve VII) and failure of abduction (cranial nerve VI) may be associated with multiple cranial nerve involvement. Möbius' syndrome can be unilateral or bilateral and variably is associated with horizontal gaze palsy and third, fifth, and eighth cranial nerve paresis. Multiple systemic findings have been described in association, a few of which include tongue hypoplasia, agenesis or dysgenesis of limbs, Poland's anomaly (absent pectoralis major and minor), dental anomalies, and brain malformations.

Brown's syndrome is inability to elevate the affected eye in the adducted field. It is caused by a restriction of the superior oblique tendon as it traverses the trochlea. The restricted superior oblique is unable to extend fully, and the eye is unable to elevate. Brown's syndrome is sporadic, isolated, and relatively more common than other causes of incomitant strabismus. Surgery rarely is required; amblyopia and secondary strabismus occur. Referral to a pediatric ophthalmologist is appropriate.

Congenital fibrosis of the ocular muscles is an autosomal dominant disorder with high penetrance. One or multiple muscles of one or both eyes may be involved. The involved muscles are fibrotic and smaller than normal on computed tomography scan of the orbits. The presentation is variable depending on the muscle involved, but ptosis and amblyopia are common associations. Surgery is often, but not always, required.

Oculomotor (cranial nerve III), trochlear (cranial nerve IV), and abducens (cranial nerve VI) nerve palsies have characteristic associated deficits in ocular muscle function. A full history is important, including history of recent illness, viral infection, trauma, headaches, fever, medications, and general health status. Oculomotor palsies are associated with ptosis, exotropia, and hypotropia of the affected eye. The pupil is usually dilated but can present constricted in a congenital palsy. Fourth nerve palsy is usually either congenital or traumatic. The child may present years after the initial insult. Presenting symptoms often include ocular torticollis with a head tilting to the contralateral side. Occasionally, an older child complains of vertical double vision. Fourth nerve palsies are the most common of the three cranial nerve palsies affecting the ocular muscles. Sixth nerve palsies present with an acute esotropia, abduction deficit, head turn toward the affected side, and self-occlusion (squint) of the affected eye. Neuroimaging is required because sixth nerve palsy may be the presenting sign of increased intracranial pressure or neoplasm.

Nystagmus

Nystagmus involves the oscillation of the eye in a rhythmic manner. Nystagmus in children can be classified as *sensory* (secondary to a visual deficit), *motor* (benign idiopathic), and neurologic or neuromuscular nystagmus. Most nystagmus is of the benign or sensory type, and the presenting signs, features, and timing usually can eliminate a sinister cause of nystagmus without unnecessary neuroimaging. History is a key component in the evaluation. Congenital motor nystagmus is often present before 3 months of age and sometimes is present at birth; congenital motor nystagmus is associated with an autosomal dominant transmission. The further evaluation of nystagmus is determined by the child's visual development and physical examination. Visual evoked cortical potential recordings often can determine the visual acuity. In the setting of normal visual development and normal ocular examination (clear visual media, normal funduscopic examination, absence of albinotic features), the next step in the evaluation of nystagmus is eye movement recordings and electroretinography. Eye movement recordings are characteristic in the benign "motor" type of nystagmus and are diagnostic. Electroretinography is essential in establishing the diagnosis of cone dystrophy, rod dystrophy, or ocular albinism, among others, in sensory nystagmus with normal ocular examination. Neurologic nystagmus includes acquired nystagmus after 6 months of age, vertical nystagmus, gaze-evoked nystagmus, seesaw nystagmus, and vestibular nystagmus (nystagmus associated with oscillopsia or vertigo) and requires neuroimaging, including computed tomography or magnetic resonance imaging. Vertical nystagmus always should be evaluated for the possibility of pharmacologic causes or intracranial disorders. A final important category is nystagmus in association with head oscillations. *Spasmus nutans* is a self-limiting, benign triad of pendular nystagmus, head nodding, and ocular torticollis. The head nodding behavior and the nystagmus are usually horizontal. Various theories of head nodding to suppress or compensate for the nystagmus have been proposed. The condition resolves completely by 5 years of age, leaving no permanent vision impairment.

Nystagmus may be associated with significant vision loss as with congenital optic nerve hypoplasia or cortical visual impairment; however, most nystagmus is associated with relatively normal visual function. Most nystagmus is of the benign congenital type, which can be diagnosed on the basis of clinical findings and has no significant comorbid central nervous system pathology.

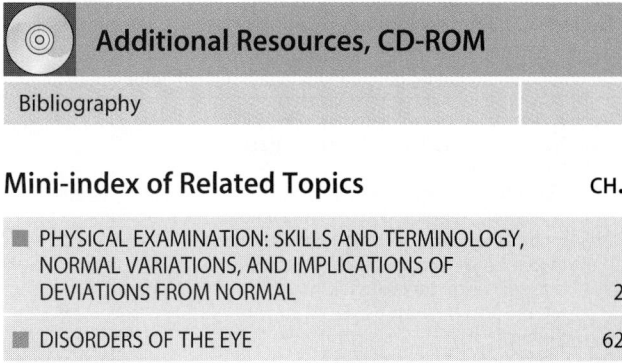

Additional Resources, CD-ROM

Bibliography

Mini-index of Related Topics

SUGGESTED READINGS

Campbell LR, Charney E: Factors associated with delay in diagnosis of childhood amblyopia. Pediatrics 1991;87:178–185.

Friendly DS: Amblyopia: Definition, classification, diagnosis, and management considerations for pediatricians, family physicians, and general practitioners. Pediatr Clin North Am 1987;34:1389–1401.

Paysse EA, Williams GC, Coats DK, Williams EA: Detection of red reflex asymmetry by pediatric residents using the Bruckner reflex versus the MTI photoscreener. Pediatrics 2001;108:E74.

Simon JW, Kaw P: Vision screening performed by the pediatrician. Pediatr Ann 2001;30:446–452.

Stager DR, Birch EE, Weakley DR: Amblyopia and the pediatrician. Pediatr Ann 1990;19:301–315.

SECTION 3   GENERAL MEDICAL CARE: *Disorders of the Skin*

69

Approach to Dermatologic Disease and Eczematoid Eruptions

Mark Herron, Christopher M. Hull, and Sheryll L. Vanderhooft

ROLE OF THE GENERALIST

1 Develop a systematic, appropriate general approach to examination of the skin.

2 Identify primary and secondary cutaneous lesions.

3 Define the configuration and distribution of a cutaneous disorder.

4 Identify the key elements of the dermatologic history.

5 Understand the basic laboratory studies that are helpful in the evaluation of a patient with a cutaneous disorder.

6 Recognize the clinical features of atopic dermatitis.

7 Know the diagnostic criteria of atopic dermatitis.

8 Educate patients and parents about the chronic nature, triggering factors, and long-term management of atopic dermatitis.

9 Recognize that successful management of atopic dermatitis requires a multimodal approach.

10 Understand the differential diagnosis of diaper dermatitis.

11 Diagnose and manage pompholyx.

12 Be aware of less common eczematous eruptions, including lichen simplex chronicus, lichen striatus, intertriginous dermatitis, frictional lichenoid dermatitis, and nummular dermatitis.

13 Recognize common causes of contact dermatitis.

14 Understand the different potencies, side effects, and appropriate uses of topical steroids.

FUNDAMENTALS

Although the skin is examined easily, the diagnosis of skin disorders often eludes generalist clinicians. There are hundreds of cutaneous diseases, and the morphology of any given disease may vary considerably. Skin lesions evolve over time so that the appearance of lesions varies depending on the stage of evolution in which they are encountered. The classic approach in medicine is to allow the history to guide the examination and further diagnostic evaluation. In dermatology, the morphology of the skin lesions is of prime importance, and historical information is supplementary. For a reasonable differential diagnosis of a dermatologic disorder to be formulated, a systematic approach to examination of the skin is absolutely essential.

General Approach to Examination of the Skin

As with any aspect of pediatrics, preparation is essential for the best possible examination. Without good lighting, the color of a skin lesion may be distorted. Natural light or artificial light that closely resembles natural light is preferable. Tangential lighting helps in the identification of mild elevations and depressions in the skin. Magnification using a hand lens enhances the surface characteristics of skin lesions and is helpful in the evaluation of subtle lesions.

The child's general appearance is an important consideration. Fever and irritability accompany viral exanthems; drug eruptions; and systemic diseases with dermatologic manifestations, such as acute juvenile rheumatoid arthritis or systemic lupus erythematosus. Cachexia and wasting are

Table 69-1. Regional Anatomy of the Skin

Face
  Forehead, glabella, eyes, conjunctivae, medial and lateral canthi, malar surface, nasolabial folds, nasal root, ala nasi, columella, philtrum, vermilion border, oral mucosa
Scalp
  Frontal, temporal, parietal, vertex, occipital, posterior auricular
Ears
  Helix, antihelix, tragus, antitragus, external auditory canal, lobe
Chest
  Axillary folds, inframammary creases, presternal area
Abdomen
  Umbilicus
Back
Arms
  Flexor and extensor surfaces
Hands
  Ulnar and radial aspects, palmar and dorsal surfaces, MCP, PIP, DIP joint surfaces
Legs
  Flexor and extensor surfaces
Feet
  Interdigital web spaces, plantar and dorsal aspects
Nails
  Nail plate, nail bed, proximal and lateral nail folds, lunula, cuticle

DIP, distal interphalangeal; MCP, metacarpophalangeal; PIP, proximal interphalangeal.

Table 69-2. Primary Lesions—Definitions and Examples

Term	Example
Macule: flat lesion, <1 cm diameter, consisting of change in the surface color; the surface itself is normal	Freckle
Patch: flat lesion, >1 cm diameter	Café au lait spot
Papule: palpable, raised lesion, <1 cm diameter	Insect bite
Plaque: palpable, raised lesion, >1 cm diameter, often formed by a coalescence of papules	Psoriasis
Nodule: raised lesion that extends into the dermis or subcutaneous tissue, <2 cm diameter	Lipoma
Tumor: large, deep, solid lesion, >2 cm diameter	Deep hemangioma
Wheal: white-to-pink or pale red elevated evanescent lesion caused by local, superficial, transient edema in the skin	Urticaria
Vesicle: fluid-filled lesion, <1 cm diameter (small blister)	Varicella zoster
Bulla: fluid-filled lesion, >1 cm diameter (large blister)	Bullous impetigo
Pustule: vesicle with purulent contents	Folliculitis
Telangiectasia: permanent dilation of superficial vessels of the skin	Spider veins
Petechiae: deposit of blood in the skin, <0.5 cm	Meningococcemia
Purpura: deposit of blood in the skin, >0.5 cm diameter	Purpura fulminans

signs of chronic systemic disease. Obesity may accompany specific skin disorders, such as acanthosis nigricans. Characteristic facies and structural malformations provide helpful clues in the diagnosis of genetic syndromes.

The entire skin surface should be examined, including the hair, nails, and mucous membranes (Table 69-1). The skin color should be noted, as should the degree of moisture, texture, and mobility. Dryness of the skin may result from excessive bathing; a dry climate; or a systemic condition, such as hypothyroidism. Excessive oiliness often is present in acne vulgaris. Roughness may represent chronic atopic dermatitis or hypothyroidism. Loss of mobility of the skin is seen in scleroderma. Hair distribution, density, color, and texture also need to be noted. Nails should be observed for color, thickness, and uniformity.

Primary and Secondary Lesions

Accurate description of cutaneous lesions is the key to dermatologic diagnosis. An understanding of dermatologic terminology is essential in establishing the correct diagnosis and subsequent management of skin disorders. *Primary lesions* are the most representative, but not necessarily the earliest or the most visible, lesions produced by a cutaneous disorder (Table 69-2). Identifying the newest, most representative lesions aids the formulation of a differential diagnosis. Lesions that have been altered or traumatized by scratching (secondary changes) can be misleading. *Secondary lesions* represent evolutionary changes that occur during the course of a cutaneous disorder or as the result of scratching (Table 69-3).

Color

Color in the skin is determined primarily by melanin content, thickness of the skin, carotene, and blood flow. Lesions that are red usually are inflammatory or related to vascular proliferation or increased cutaneous blood flow. Brown

lesions often are secondary to abnormal pigment production or deposition in the skin. White lesions typically represent partial or complete loss of normal pigment. Yellow or orange lesions usually contain lipid or sebum. Flesh-colored lesions usually are associated with thickening of the epidermis.

Table 69-3. Secondary Lesions—Definitions and Examples

Term	Example
Scale: accumulation of "dead skin" from the outermost layer of the epidermis; thin flake of exfoliated epidermis	Psoriasis
Crust: dried residue of serum, blood, pus, or exudates; "scab"	Impetigo
Erosion: focal loss of epidermis, leaving a shallow opening in the skin; usually heals without scarring	Eczema
Ulcer: an open and significantly depressed wound, resulting from total loss of the epidermis, part or all of the dermis, and underlying subcutaneous tissue. Ulcers heal with scarring	Pyoderma gangrenosum
Excoriation: linear or oval erosion caused by scratching of the skin	Atopic dermatitis
Fissure: linear crack of the skin, extending into the dermis, resulting from marked drying and long-standing inflammation of the skin	Chronic hand or foot dermatitis
Lichenification: thickening of the skin secondary to chronic rubbing or scratching, characterized by accentuation of the normal skin lines	Atopic dermatitis
Atrophy: thinning of or a depression in the skin, often with a shiny or translucent surface	Lichen sclerosus
Scar: permanent fibrotic change in the skin after damage to the dermis	Burn

Configuration

Configuration refers to the general shape of the lesion. Many cutaneous diseases are defined by their configuration (Table 69-4). The border of a lesion can be poorly defined, with the area of abnormal skin merging into normal skin, such as in eczema. Lesions with well-circumscribed borders show a clear separation between normal and abnormal skin, as in psoriasis.

Location and Distribution

Determination of the anatomic *location* and *distribution* of lesions is a key element of the skin examination (Table 69-5). Distribution of cutaneous lesions is determined by the areas of involvement. Areas of sparing may be just as significant in formulating a differential diagnosis. When an eruption develops in a photodistribution, the face, posterior neck, "V" of the chest, and dorsal aspect of the hands and forearms typically are affected, whereas the areas behind the ears, under the chin, and under the eyebrows usually are spared. Symmetric lesions usually have an endogenous etiology, such as atopic dermatitis, psoriasis, or a drug eruption. Asymmetric lesions are more likely to be due to an external cause, such as contact dermatitis. Many diseases have a characteristic anatomic distribution. Acne vulgaris typically affects the face, chest, and back. Psoriasis most often affects the extensor surfaces of the knees and elbows, whereas atopic dermatitis affects primarily the flexor surfaces.

History

Questioning the parent and child before, during, and after the skin examination provides insight regarding the nature of the skin disease. Discussion can ascertain whether the skin disorder has provoked anxiety or emotional upset in the parent or child. Focused questioning based on the physical findings provides data to formulate a differential diagnosis. Specific questions regarding the disorder are crucial. Past medical and surgical history, history of medication use and allergies, and family and social history also are important to consider.

When Did This Start? Where on the Body Did It Begin? Where Did It Spread?

The most important aspect of the history is to have the patient or parent clearly indicate where the problem exists. The parent should focus on when and where the problem began. Lesions that have been present for a long time should be distinguished from lesions that have been present for only a few days or weeks.

How Long Do the Lesions Last? How Do They Evolve?

Duration and evolution of the lesions are crucial when evaluating cutaneous lesions, especially eruptions. The lesions of urticaria and erythema multiforme can look alike. A history of migratory lesions, in which lesions come and go within a 24-hour period, suggests urticaria. Erythema multiforme is a fixed eruption that can take weeks to resolve. Herpes simplex infections last approximately 7 to 10 days. Lesions evolve from vesicles on an erythematous base to crusts. Recurrent lesions tend to arise at the same anatomic site.

Does It Itch? Is It Painful?

Pruritus is a common complaint associated with skin disorders. It is a symptom, not a diagnosis. Appropriate assessment of pruritus provides insight, however, into the level of distress the skin disorder is causing the child. The presence of pruritus also may determine the course of treatment because patients appreciate symptomatic relief even if a skin disorder is self-limited and benign. Pruritus without

Table 69-4. Configuration—Definitions and Examples

Term	Examples
Annular: ring-shaped lesions with an active margin and relative central clearing	Tinea corporis, nummular dermatitis, granuloma annulare
Arcuate: lesions with an arclike shape	Erythema multiforme, urticaria
Confluent: small lesions that run together to form larger areas of involvement	Drug eruption, viral exanthem
Dermatomal: follows a dermatome	Herpes zoster
Discrete: individual lesions that tend to remain separated from others	Melanocytic nevus
Grouped: lesions that cluster close together	Herpes simplex, insect bites
Guttate: droplike lesions	Guttate psoriasis
Iris: lesions with concentric rings (target lesions)	Erythema multiforme
Linear: forms a line or band of involvement	Excoriations, plant contact dermatitis, linear epidermal nevus
Morbilliform: measles-like	Drug eruption, viral exanthem
Polycyclic: oval lesions containing more than one ring	Urticaria
Reticulated: netlike pattern	Cutis marmorata, livedo reticularis
Serpiginous: snakelike pattern	Cutaneous larva migrans

Table 69-5. Distribution—Definitions and Examples

Term	Examples
Localized	Contact dermatitis
Generalized	Drug eruption, viral exanthem
Migratory	Urticaria
Sun-exposed (photodistribution): face, ears, posterior neck, "V" of the chest, dorsal aspect of the hands and forearms	Photosensitizing drugs, collagen vascular disease
Intertriginous (body folds): anterior neck, axillae, inframammary, groin	Candidiasis, erythrasma
Acral (hands and feet)	Erythema multiforme, Rocky Mountain spotted fever
Palmar/plantar	Dyshidrotic eczema
Scalp, genital (seborrheic)	Seborrheic dermatitis, psoriasis
Flexor (especially antecubital and popliteal fossae, flexural folds of the wrists and ankles)	Atopic dermatitis
Extensor (especially elbows and knees)	Psoriasis
Follicular	Folliculitis, keratosis pilaris
Periorificial	Perioral dermatitis contact dermatitis, zinc deficiency
Mucosal (mouth, eyes, genitals, perirectal)	Herpes simplex, syphilis, warts

primary lesions may be caused by an underlying systemic disorder, such as lymphoma, renal insufficiency, diabetes, or hepatitis. Pain may be associated with infectious skin disorders, such as furuncles, carbuncles, cellulitis, and viral infections. The pain may be boring, burning, shooting, or throbbing.

Has Treatment Been Attempted? What Makes It Better or Worse?

Most patients have tried some form of topical preparation to treat a skin problem before seeing a physician. The physician needs to be persistent when questioning the parent about use of topical and systemic medications and the response to treatment. Many parents do not consider over-the-counter products or herbal remedies important when providing a medication history. They also may not know what they have used. Providing examples of over-the-counter medications may help in obtaining a medication history. Many over-the-counter topical preparations (e.g., anesthetics, antibiotics, and antihistamines) contain ingredients that may exacerbate the primary skin problem by causing a contact allergy or irritation of the skin. When an eczematous eruption worsens with topical therapy, a superimposed contact allergic dermatitis must be considered. Whether the topical agents used were ointments or creams needs to be established. An ingredient in the base, not the active ingredient, may be causing the problem. Eliciting a history of adverse reactions to topical and systemic medications is crucial. Drug reactions are common. They can present with a wide variety of morphologies and may simulate systemic illness. Drug eruption should be considered in the differential diagnosis for almost any skin disease.

Does Anyone Else in the Family Have a Skin Problem? Is It the Same as the Patient's?

Family history may be helpful in the formulation of a diagnosis. A child with chronic eczema is more likely to be diagnosed with atopic dermatitis if there is a positive family history of eczema, asthma, allergies, or hay fever. Information about similar skin problems in household contacts is also important from an environmental standpoint. Tinea capitis often is transmitted among family members through grooming with a common brush or comb. Scabies often is present in more than one member in a household at any given time. In the case of a patient with insect bite reaction, family contacts generally do not have similar problems since typically only one individual in a family is the object of arthropod assaults.

Exposure History

Exposure history is particularly useful when evaluating dermatitis. Information about hobbies, chemical exposure, exposure to animals, and exposure to ill individuals can be helpful in determining a cause for the eruption.

Laboratory Evaluation
Mycology

If a lesion is red and scaly, cutaneous fungal infection should be considered, and a potassium hydroxide preparation should be done. Scale from the border of the lesion is removed with a no. 15 scalpel blade, the scale is placed on a glass slide, and a coverslip is placed over the scales. Potassium hydroxide is added to the edge of the coverslip and is drawn under it by capillary action. Flame heating the slide allows the scales to dissolve quickly. The slide should be examined under a light microscope. Dermatophytes are identified as branched hyphae crossing cell walls. The white exudate of *Candida albicans* shows interwoven pseudo-hyphae and yeast forms on a potassium hydroxide preparation. Scales can be sent in a Petri dish or sterile urine cup to the microbiology laboratory for fungal culture. Fungal cultures should be obtained to confirm the diagnosis whenever the use of systemic antifungal medication is considered. It may take 4 weeks to obtain the final result.

Bacteriology and Virology

Swabs taken from vesicles, pustules, erosions, or ulcerations may be cultured for bacteria or viruses. Crusts should be removed and the underlying exudate swabbed. Standard bacterial cultures with antibiotic sensitivities are recommended for all patients with primary or secondary skin infection to rule out resistant organisms. Viral cultures require a special transport medium.

Skin Biopsy

A skin biopsy may be required to make the diagnosis in patients with lesions or eruptions that cannot be identified by morphologic pattern alone. These patients should be referred to a dermatologist.

ECZEMATOUS ERUPTIONS

Eczematous eruptions are a diverse and common group of inflammatory skin conditions whose cardinal features are pruritus and cutaneous reactivity. The term *eczema* (meaning to boil over) has been used for years by the public and by many physicians to refer generally to the pediatric form of atopic dermatitis. *Eczema* (or dermatitis) is a descriptive term (not a specific disease) that should be reserved for describing a complex of symptoms that includes itching, burning, redness, papules, vesicles, and crusting in its acute phases and thickened plaques with accentuated skin markings *(lichenification)* and scaling in its chronic phases. Eczematous lesions are found in skin diseases other than atopic dermatitis, such as allergic and irritant contact dermatitis, seborrheic dermatitis, and diaper dermatitis. Eczema is better thought of as a reaction pattern to many different stimuli and should be used to classify a group of disorders that have similar clinical and histologic characteristics.

Atopic Dermatitis
Definition

Atopic dermatitis (atopic eczema, infantile eczema) is a chronic, relapsing inflammatory eczematous disorder characterized by severe pruritus and cutaneous inflammation.

Fundamentals

The prevalence of atopic dermatitis is rising, having increased severalfold since the 1980s. It is one of the most common skin disorders seen in infants and children, affecting approximately 10% to 15% of the pediatric population. Most children who develop atopic dermatitis manifest the disease during early childhood. Approximately 35% to 60% of children who develop atopic dermatitis develop the disease by 1 year of age, and most other cases arise by 5 years of age. Although most children improve over time, approximately 60% of patients continue to have skin problems ranging from dryness, to sensitive skin, to continuing dermatitis.

The pathogenesis of atopic dermatitis is not fully understood; it seems to be multifactorial, with contributions from genetic and environmental factors. Atopic dermatitis appears primarily in individuals who show IgE-mediated skin reactions and who have a propensity for developing other allergic (atopic) conditions, such as asthma, allergies, or hay fever. Of children with atopic dermatitis, 30% to 50% go on to have asthma or hay fever. Atopic dermatitis seems to have a familial basis; risk is increased for a child to develop atopic conditions if one or both parents are affected. If one parent is atopic, at least half of the children develop allergic symptoms during childhood. In cases in which both parents have atopic dermatitis, approximately 80% of the children also have the disease. Among monozygotic twins, 85% are affected if the other twin has atopic dermatitis. An inheritance pattern for atopic dermatitis has not been identified. Genetic susceptibility to asthma has been linked to several chromosomes, but there is no association yet identified with atopic dermatitis.

The role of allergens, especially foods, in the pathogenesis of atopic dermatitis is controversial. Approximately 10% to 20% of patients with atopic dermatitis have clinically relevant food hypersensitivity. Of patients with atopic dermatitis, 50% to 85% have one or more positive prick tests or positive radioallergosorbent tests (RAST) to food allergens, but only 25% to 30% of patients with positive skin tests react with oral food challenge. The most common food allergens are eggs, peanuts, milk, fish, soy, and wheat. These account for greater than two thirds of clinically relevant food allergies in atopic individuals. Even if an allergen is detected with formal allergy testing, removing it from the patient's diet does not necessarily lead to improvement of the condition of the skin. Routine testing for food allergies is not recommended. Allergy testing may be helpful in a child with difficult-to-manage atopic dermatitis.

Diagnosis

Atopic dermatitis is divided into three stages: (1) infantile atopic dermatitis, 2 months to 2 years of age; (2) childhood atopic dermatitis, 2 to 10 years of age; and (3) adolescent and adult atopic dermatitis. Atopic dermatitis undergoes an evolution from the characteristic acute inflammatory eczematous dermatitis of childhood to a chronic lichenified dermatitis in older patients. The sites of predilection of cutaneous involvement vary with age. Infants tend to have diffuse involvement, including the face and scalp (Figs. 69-1 and 69-2). There is a predilection for the extensor surfaces (elbows, knees) during the crawling stage (Fig. 69-3). The diaper area usually is spared. Toddlers and older children tend to have involvement of the flexor surfaces (antecubital and popliteal fossae, neck, wrists, ankles) (Figs. 69-4 and 69-5) and hand and foot dermatitis. Adolescents and adults also have involvement of flexor surfaces, hands, and feet,

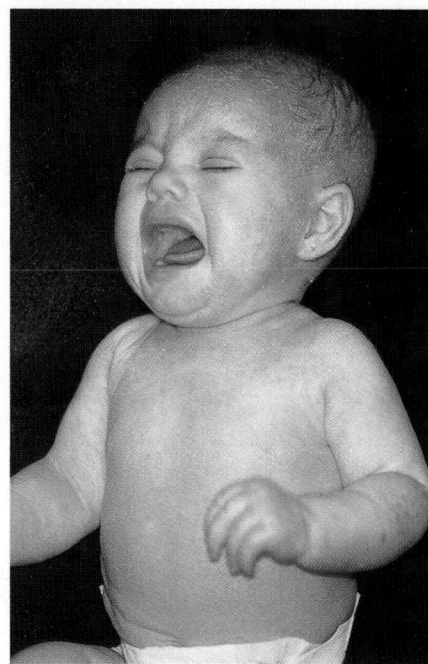

Figure 69-1. Infant with atopic dermatitis, displaying diffuse body, face, and scalp involvement.

but the lesions tend to be more chronic and lichenified (Figs. 69-6 and 69-7). The hallmark at all ages is pruritus. The itching often precedes the onset of skin lesions. Atopic dermatitis has been referred to as the "itch that rashes." Several secondary changes occur in the skin because of the persistent inflammation and altered immune responsiveness and chronic scratching, including lichenification, xerosis, excoriation, weeping, and secondary infections (Fig. 69-8).

A set of major and minor diagnostic criteria has been defined to establish guidelines for making a diagnosis of atopic dermatitis (Box 69-1). These criteria have been modified to assess atopic dermatitis in infancy (Box 69-2). CD-ROM Figures 69-9 through 69-17 depict many of the minor features often encountered in individuals with atopic dermatitis.

The diagnosis of atopic dermatitis usually is straightforward, although other inflammatory skin conditions can resemble atopic dermatitis. The major and minor diagnostic

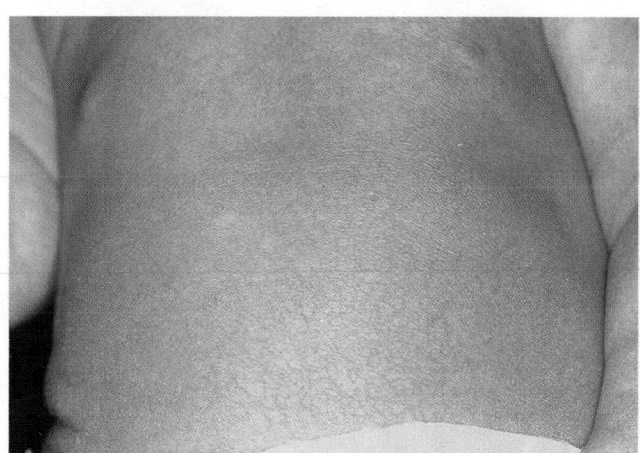

Figure 69-2. Close-up of abdomen of the infant shown in Figure 69-1 shows erythematous patches with scale.

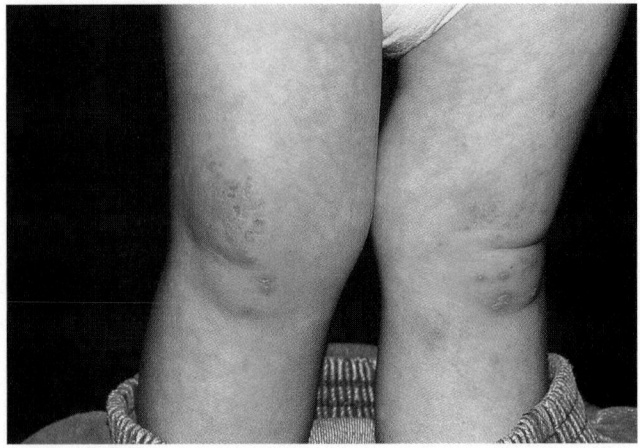

Figure 69-3. Eczema involving the extensor surfaces of the knees in an atopic child secondary to crawling.

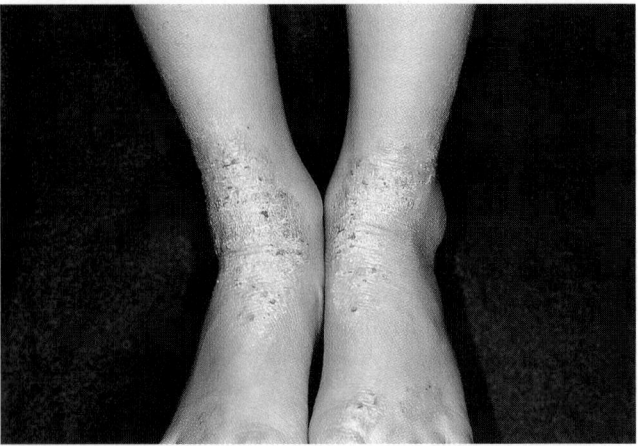

Figure 69-5. Same child shown in Figure 69-4, showing erythematous scaly excoriated plaques of the flexor aspect of the ankles.

criteria are useful in differentiating atopic dermatitis from other eczematous eruptions, including seborrheic dermatitis, contact dermatitis, nummular dermatitis, psoriasis, and scabies. Seborrheic dermatitis tends to have a characteristic greasy yellow scale, involves intertriginous areas, and has minimal associated pruritus. Contact dermatitis can mimic any form of dermatitis. It tends to be more localized than atopic dermatitis; geographic configurations of the lesions that conform to external contact points with the skin can help differentiate it from atopic dermatitis. Nummular dermatitis can be recognized by the characteristic coin-shaped lesions with an annular configuration; often the lesions have peripheral erosions and crusts. Psoriasis can be differentiated from atopic dermatitis by the well-demarcated red plaques, silvery or micaceous scale, predilection for extensor surfaces, and associated nail involvement. Scabies can mimic closely atopic dermatitis in infants and young children; the eczematous eruption of scabies in this

setting can be generalized, with involvement of the face, scalp, and body (Fig. 69-9). The palms and soles of infested infants typically show vesicles and pustules. Sites of predilection in older children, adolescents, and adults include the axillae and genital areas, locations that typically are spared in atopic dermatitis. The diagnosis of scabies can be confirmed by identification of a primary lesion (the pathognomonic burrow or a linear papulovesicle) (Fig. 69-10) or finding a mite, eggs, or feces (scybala) on microscopic examination of skin scrapings. Other conditions to include in the differential diagnosis of atopic dermatitis include metabolic disorders, nutritional deficiencies, and immunologic abnormalities (see Chapter 79).

Management

There is no cure for atopic dermatitis. The first and most important principle of successful management is education. Parents and patients need to be counseled about the chronic nature of the disease, the general principles of long-term therapy, and strategies to prevent and modulate trigger factors. The approach to treatment of atopic dermatitis is multimodal (Box 69-3). Management is directed at preventing pruritus, inflammation, and secondary infections. Therapy depends on anti-inflammatory agents, lubrication of the skin, antipruritics, and antimicrobial agents when

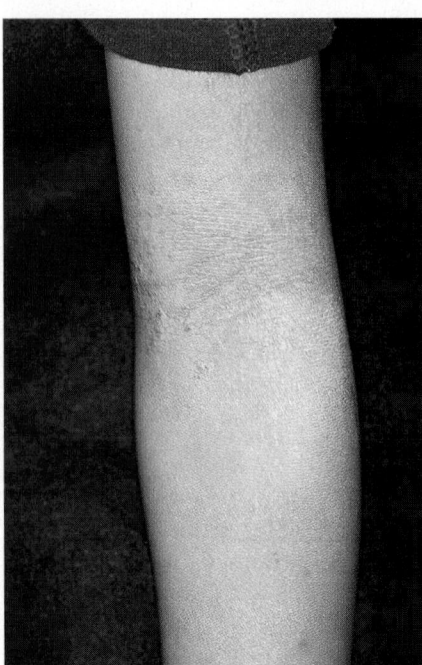

Figure 69-4. Child with atopic dermatitis, demonstrating a slightly erythematous lichenified excoriated plaque within the antecubital fossa.

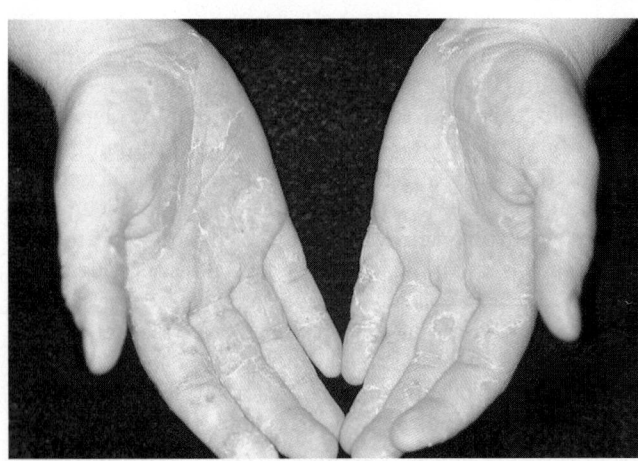

Figure 69-6. Chronic hand dermatitis in an atopic teenager.

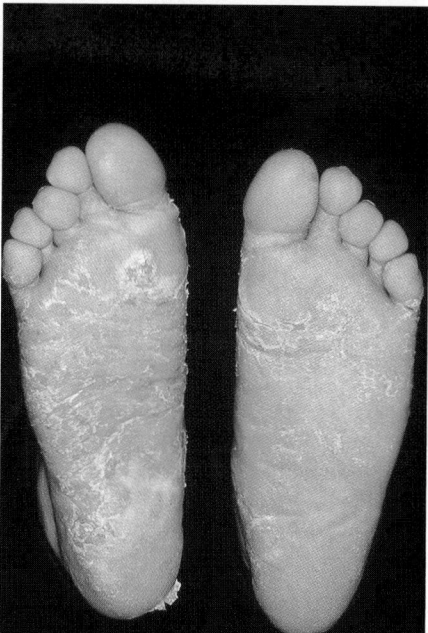

Figure 69-7. Foot dermatitis in the same teenager shown in Figure 69-6.

indicated. Patients need to learn how to avoid trigger factors, such as skin irritants, overheating, emotional stress, and known allergens. This education is crucial to help patients and parents manage this chronic and often frustrating disease.

Topical corticosteroids have been the mainstay of therapy for atopic dermatitis for decades because of their anti-inflammatory, antipruritic, and vasoconstrictive properties. Generally a midpotency to high-potency topical steroid is required to control acute inflammation in older children, adolescents, and adults (Table 69-6); infants typically do

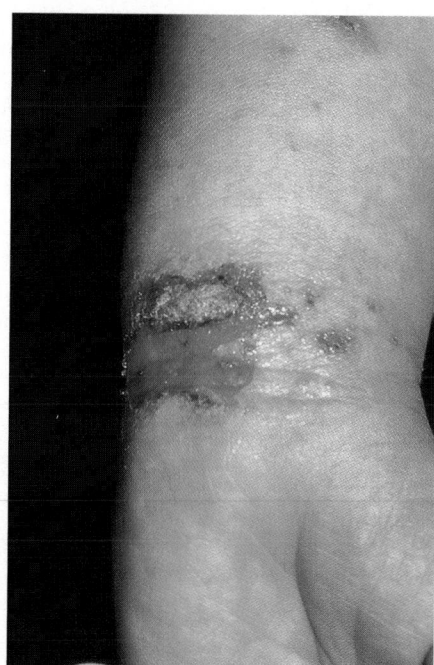

Figure 69-8. Secondarily infected, lichenified excoriated plaque on the flexor aspect of the wrist in an atopic toddler.

Box 69-1. Major and Minor Diagnostic Criteria of Atopic Dermatitis

Major Criteria

Must have three of the following:

- Pruritus
- Typical morphology and distribution
- Chronic or chronically relapsing dermatitis
- Personal or family history of atopy

Minor Features

Must have three of the following:

- Generalized
  - Xerosis
  - Ichthyosis, keratosis pilaris, or hyperlinear palms
  - Pityriasis alba
  - Perifollicular accentuation
  - White dermatographism
  - Susceptibility to skin infections, including *Staphylococcus aureus*, herpes simplex, *Candida*, and molluscum contagiosum
- Localized
  - Facial pallor or erythema
  - Scalp dermatitis
  - Cheilitis
  - Periauricular fissures
  - Anterior neck fold involvement
  - Hand/foot dermatitis
  - Nipple dermatitis
- Orbital/ocular
  - Dennie's lines/Morgan's fold (linear tranverse fold below edge of lower eyelid)
  - Orbital darkening
  - Conjunctivitis
  - Keratoconus
  - Anterior subcapsular cataracts
- Symptomatic
  - Early age of onset
  - Itch when sweating
  - Intolerance to wool and lipid solvents
  - Food intolerance
  - Course influenced by environmental/emotional factors
- Laboratory
  - Elevated serum IgE
  - Immediate (type I) skin test reactivity

Adapted from Hanifin JM, Rajka G: Diagnostic features of atopic dermatitis. Acta Derm Venereol Suppl 1980;92:40–47.

well with low-potency topical steroids. After control has been achieved, the strength of the topical steroid can be tapered, or the use of the original topical steroid may be tapered over a few weeks. Topical steroids should be applied twice daily; application after bathing helps increase efficacy. Ointments provide the best barrier protection and emollient action and in general for a given topical steroid molecule are more potent than cream, gel, or lotion formulations (Box 69-4). Use of ointment formulations is recommended for most patients with atopic dermatitis except in humid environments or in patients who tend to trap heat and do worse with more occlusive ointments.

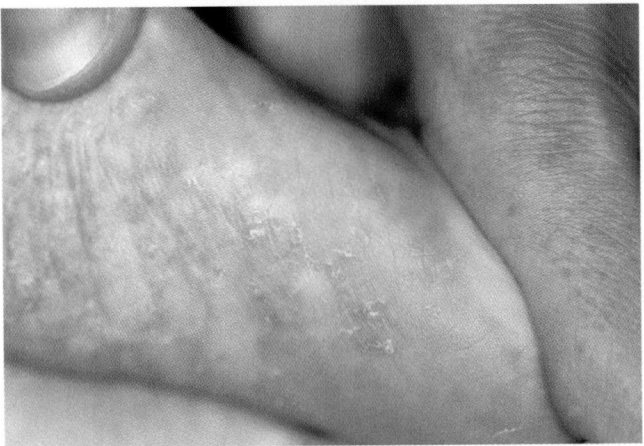

Figure 69-10. Scabietic burrows on the soles of the foot in a toddler.

Two topical nonsteroidal immunomodulators (tacrolimus 0.03% and 0.1% ointment, pimecrolimus 1% cream) have been designed specifically for the treatment of atopic dermatitis and have been shown to be safe and effective nonsteroidal topical alternatives. These agents have a similar efficacy profile as midpotency topical steroids but lack the adverse effects of cutaneous atrophy, steroid-induced acne, telangiectasias, and striae. They should be applied twice daily and are safe to use on the face, groin, and intertriginous areas.

The most common factor that exacerbates atopic dermatitis is the tendency toward dry skin. Lubricants should be applied to the skin at least twice daily, if not more often. Emollients should be applied over slightly moist skin to seal in moisture; application immediately after bathing is recommended. Oil-based products (ointments and heavy creams) are better emollients than water-based ones (light creams and lotions), but water-based products are more cosmetically acceptable. Ointments and creams such as petrolatum, Aquaphor, Cetaphil, and Eucerin are preferred. Products with fragrance are discouraged. Alpha hydroxy acid–containing moisturizers, such as Lac-Hydrin 12% cream or lotion or Eucerin Plus cream or lotion, are needed in patients with concomitant keratosis pilaris and ichthyosis; these products sting when applied if there are open areas on the skin and must be used with care.

The control of pruritus is important but often difficult to achieve. Systemic antihistamines are commonly used, but their efficacy is questionable. Sedating antihistamines can be useful at night to help patients sleep and to control nighttime itching. When tolerance to one antihistamine develops, another sedating antihistamine should be selected; these may be used on a rotating basis to maintain the soporific effect. Nonsedating oral antihistamines can be beneficial to some individuals with atopic dermatitis for daytime use. Topical lotions or sprays containing pramoxine (e.g., Aveeno anti-itch lotion) or menthol and camphor (e.g., Sarna anti-itch lotion) or menthol alone (e.g., Eucerin anti-itch spray) also can be useful adjunctive agents to help control itching. Topical diphenhydramine can cause allergic contact dermatitis and should be avoided. Doxepin cream is helpful to break the itch-scratch cycle and is marketed for use four times daily for 8 days at a time. Wet soaks or compresses using dilute potassium permanganate solution (1:8000) or aluminum acetate solution (Burow solution) can provide symptomatic relief for acute, weeping, oozing, or crusted lesions.

Recognition and control of secondary infections is key to the successful management of atopic dermatitis. Individuals with atopic dermatitis have an impaired skin barrier, and their skin is colonized and infected easily with *Staphylococcus aureus* and *Streptococcus*. Infected areas are typically excoriated and have golden crusts and at times weeping. Mupirocin cream or ointment can be used for localized secondary infections on a twice-daily basis until the open areas have healed. More widespread involvement requires systemic antibiotic therapy directed at *S. aureus* and *Streptococcus*, often for a 2-week course or longer. Skin cultures should be obtained in patients who do not respond,

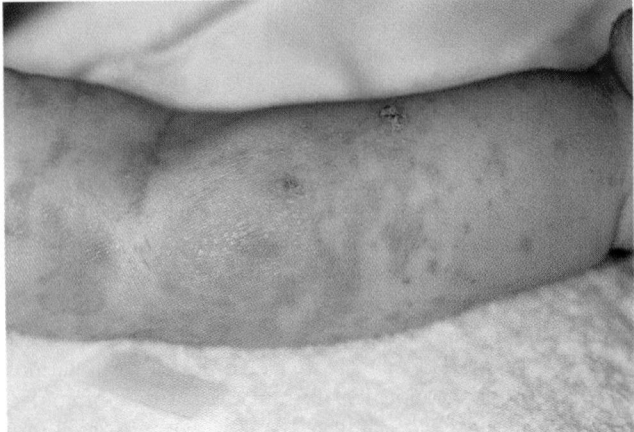

Figure 69-9. Infant with an eczematous excoriated patch on the upper extremity.

to rule out resistant organisms (i.e., methicillin-resistant *S. aureus*). Secondary infection of the skin with herpes simplex may be widespread (eczema herpeticum) and requires systemic antiviral medications (e.g., acyclovir). Inpatient management may be required for toxic-appearing children to administer intravenous fluid hydration and intravenous acyclovir. Secondary fungal infection with *Candida* or dermatophyte organisms can be treated with topical antifungal agents, although systemic treatment may be indicated in some patients. Given their decreased skin barrier function, atopic children also are prone to widespread molluscum contagiosum; the viral infection spreads readily as the child scratches at the lesions and autoinoculates other areas.

Avoidance of irritants to the skin is helpful for most atopic individuals. Although some patients can tolerate daily baths, most patients should limit bathing to a few times a week. Mild cleansers (e.g., Cetaphil, Aquanil, Dove, Purpose, Basis, Oil of Olay) should be used sparingly, and children should not be allowed to sit in sudsy water. Addition of oils to the bath water is helpful for some; many benefit from addition of coal tar solution to the bath water, which decreases inflammation and pruritus. When the child exits the bath, the skin should be patted dry, not rubbed; topical medications should be applied to inflamed areas and lubricants should be applied to the remaining areas. Fragrance-free, dye-free powder or liquid detergent should be used for the laundry; the clothes should be double

Table 69-6. Potency Ranking of Selected Topical Corticosteroids

Class	Generic Name	Trade Name	Concentration	Formulation
I	Betamethasone dipropionate (augmented)	Diprolene	0.05%	O, G, L
	Clobetasol propionate	Temovate	0.05%	C, O, G, S
		Cormax	0.05%	C, O, S
		Clobevate	0.05%	G
		Olux	0.05%	Foam
	Diflorasone diacetate	Psorcon	0.05%	O
	Halobetasol propionate	Ultravate	0.05%	C, O
II	Amcinonide	Cyclocort	0.1%	O
	Betamethasone dipropionate	Diprolene AF	0.05%	C
	Betamethasone dipropionate	Diprosone	0.05%	O
	Desoximetasone	Topicort	0.25%	C, O
		Topicort	0.05%	G
	Diflorasone diacetate	Psorcon	0.05%	C
		Psorcon E	0.05%	O
	Fluocinonide	Lidex	0.05%	C, O, G, S
	Halcinonide	Halog	0.1%	C
	Mometasone furoate	Elocon	0.1%	O
	Triamcinolone acetonide	Aristocort	0.5%	O
III	Amcinonide	Cyclocort	0.1%	C, L
	Betamethasone dipropionate	Diprosone	0.05%	C
	Betamethasone valerate	Valisone*	0.1%	O
	Desoximetasone	Topicort LP	0.05%	C
	Diflorasone diacetate	Psorcon E	0.05%	C
	Fluocinonide	Lidex E	0.05%	C
	Fluticasone propionate	Cutivate	0.005%	O
	Halcinonide	Halog	0.1%	O, S
	Triamcinolone acetonide	Aristocort	0.5%	C
IV	Betamethasone valerate	Luxiq	0.12%	Foam
	Fluocinolone acetonide	Synalar	0.025%	O
	Flurandrenolide	Cordran	0.05%	O
	Hydrocortisone valerate	Westcort	0.2%	O
	Mometasone furoate	Elocon	0.1%	C, L
	Triamcinolone acetonide	Aristocort	0.1%	C, O
		Kenalog	0.1%	C
V	Betamethasone dipropionate	Diprosone	0.05%	L
	Betamethasone valerate	Valisone*	0.1%	C
	Fluocinolone acetonide	Synalar	0.025%	C
	Flurandrenolide	Cordran	0.05%	C, L
	Fluticasone propionate	Cutivate	0.05%	C
	Hydrocortisone butyrate	Locoid	0.1%	C, O, S
	Hydrocortisone valerate	Westcort	0.2%	C
	Prednicarbate	Dermatop	0.1%	C
	Triamcinolone acetonide	Kenalog	0.1%	L
VI	Alclometasone dipropionate	Aclovate	0.05%	C, O
	Betamethasone valerate	Valisone*	0.1%	L
	Desonide	DesOwen	0.05%	C, O, L
		Tridesilon	0.05%	C
	Fluocinolone acetonide	Synalar	0.01%	C, S
	Triamcinolone acetonide	Aristocort	0.025%	C
VII	Hydrocortisone	Hytone	1%, 2.5%	C, O, L

*Valisone no longer is available in the United States; betamethasone valerate is available generically.
C, cream; G, gel; L, lotion; O, ointment; S, solution.

rinsed, and fabric softeners should be avoided. Use of 100% cotton clothing and bedding is recommended. Avoidance of wool and synthetic fibers is important. The child's room should be kept cool. Use of a humidifier may be helpful.

Systemic corticosteroids should be reserved for extensive, severe atopic dermatitis that is refractory to other treatment measures. Corticosteroids have no role in the daily management of chronic disease because of the many potential side effects. Patients with severe, widespread, difficult-to-control disease should be referred to a dermatologist who may use more aggressive therapy, such as ultraviolet light, methotrexate, cyclosporine, azathioprine, or mycophenolate mofetil.

Diaper Dermatitis
Definition
Diaper dermatitis (diaper rash, nappy rash) refers to inflammation that involves the skin of infants and children in the area covered by diapers. This condition is one of the most common cutaneous disorders of infancy, affecting an estimated 7% to 35% of infants at any given time. The highest prevalence of diaper dermatitis occurs between ages 9 and 12 months. Diaper dermatitis is not a specific clinical entity, but rather a geographic diagnosis; it represents a family of inflammatory disorders that occur in the anogenital region. The differential diagnosis of eruptions involving the diaper area is outlined in Box 69-5.

Fundamentals
The pathogenesis of diaper dermatitis is usually multifactorial. The most common factors associated with diaper dermatitis include increased skin wetness, increased frictional forces, contact irritation from urine and feces, and secondary bacterial and candidal colonization and infection. Increased skin wetness compromises the physical barrier of the skin and leads to a greater susceptibility to frictional breakdown in areas of rubbing, such as the inner thighs, inguinal creases, and lower abdomen.

Diagnosis
The most common cause of rash in the diaper area is irritant dermatitis (Fig. 69-11). Irritation of the skin occurs after contact with urine, feces, harsh soaps, detergents, and topical medications. Irritant contact dermatitis tends to affect the convex surface of the buttocks, genitals, lower abdomen, and proximal thighs, with sparing of the inguinal folds. The skin is erythematous with a glazed appearance. Because of the moisture in the diaper area, scaling is usually minimal.

Allergic contact dermatitis is an unusual cause of diaper dermatitis. The most common offending agents are topical medications, including antibiotics, and detergents. Although commercially available disposable diapers have a low allergenicity, some infants become sensitized to the elastic in the waist and leg bands. Allergic contact dermatitis in the diaper area presents as diffuse erythema, edema, papules, and occasionally vesicles and scale, usually sparing the intertriginous areas. The diagnosis often is made by clinical suspicion. Allergy patch testing rarely is required in infants.

Seborrheic dermatitis occasionally presents in the diaper area. It is easy to recognize when the characteristic well-

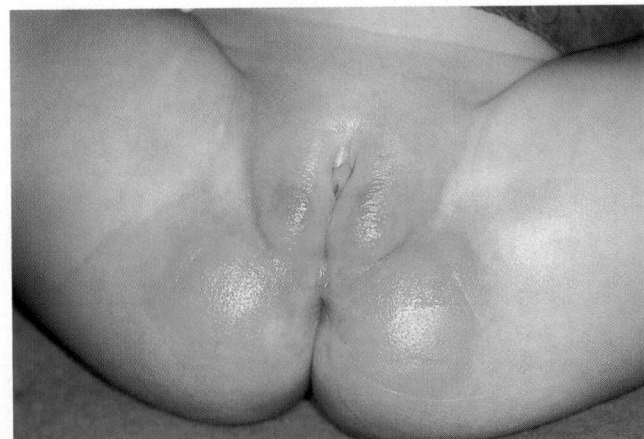

Figure 69-11. Irritant contact dermatitis of the diaper area (photograph taken after application of A & D ointment.)

circumscribed erythematous patches with yellow greasy scale are present in the diaper area; involvement of more commonly affected sites, such as the scalp (cradle cap), face, postauricular areas, and neck, provides a clue to the diagnosis. Lesions of seborrheic dermatitis are usually asymptomatic, although mild pruritus may be present on occasion.

Psoriasis of the diaper area (see Fig. 70-9) can mimic seborrheic dermatitis. The characteristic silvery scale is usually absent because of the moisture and maceration of the diaper area. Identification of more typical features of psoriasis on examination of the skin leads to the correct diagnosis.

Candidiasis is an important disorder to consider when evaluating a patient with diaper dermatitis. It may present as a primary process or represent a secondary infection of a persistent dermatitis. *Candida* may be introduced into the diaper area from the upper gastrointestinal tract (oral thrush) or lower gastrointestinal tract, or transmission can occur from a caregiver's hands. Candidiasis is common after treatment with systemic antibiotics. Clinically, *Candida* diaper dermatitis presents as coalescence of erythematous papules involving the buttocks, scrotum or labia majora, inguinal folds, inner thighs, and lower abdomen with satellite erythematous papules and pustules (Figs. 69-12 and 69-13). A fine white scale sometimes is present. The diagnosis can be confirmed by microscopic examination of potassium hydroxide–treated skin scrapings from the leading edge of the eruption or a satellite pustule; this reveals budding hyphae and pseudohyphae.

Perianal streptococcal infection often is overlooked as a cause of diaper dermatitis. It is characterized by a persistent, bright red, often pruritic or tender perianal eruption that is sharply demarcated from the normal surrounding skin. The diagnosis is confirmed with bacterial culture taken from a swab of the perianal area. Although it responds well to systemic antibiotic therapy, 40% of children experience recurrences.

Tinea cruris ("jock itch"), caused by dermatophyte infection, is an unusual cause of rash in the diaper area in infants; it is seen most commonly in adolescents and adults. The eruption tends to be more reddish brown in color compared

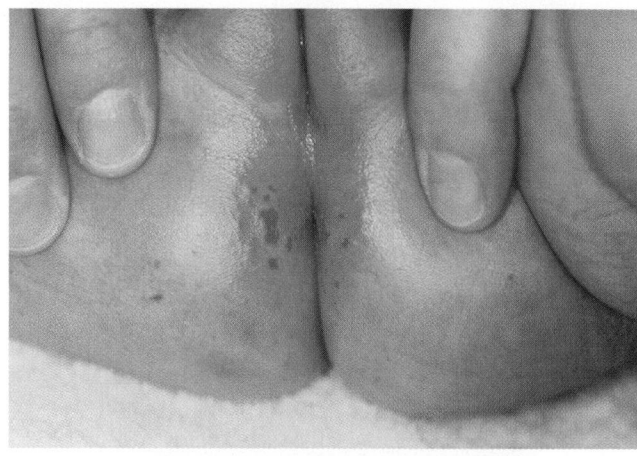

Figure 69-13. Perianal candidiasis in an infant.

with irritant or allergic contact dermatitis or candidiasis; in addition, tinea cruris tends to spare the scrotum and labia, whereas dermatitis and candidiasis often involve these areas. The diagnosis can be confirmed by microscopic examination of potassium hydroxide–treated skin scrapings from the leading edge of the eruption; this reveals branching hyphae.

Chronic and recurring eruptions in the diaper area are encountered commonly in metabolic disorders, nutritional deficiencies, and immunologic abnormalities. These are discussed in Chapter 79.

Letterer-Siwe disease is a rare and severe histiocytosis that can present with an eruption in the diaper area. It occurs almost exclusively in infants and young children, usually before age 3 years. Cutaneous involvement is found in most cases and usually presents with an eruption resembling seborrheic dermatitis, characterized by scaling erythematous papules involving the scalp, axillae, and diaper area (Figs. 69-14 and 69-15). Petechiae, purpuric papules, and occasionally vesicles are also present. Systemic features include fever, anemia, thrombocytopenia, hepatosplenomegaly, and lymphadenopathy. A skin biopsy confirms the diagnosis.

Management

The treatment of diaper dermatitis to some extent depends on the exact cause of the eruption. In many instances, however, therapy is the same regardless of the underlying

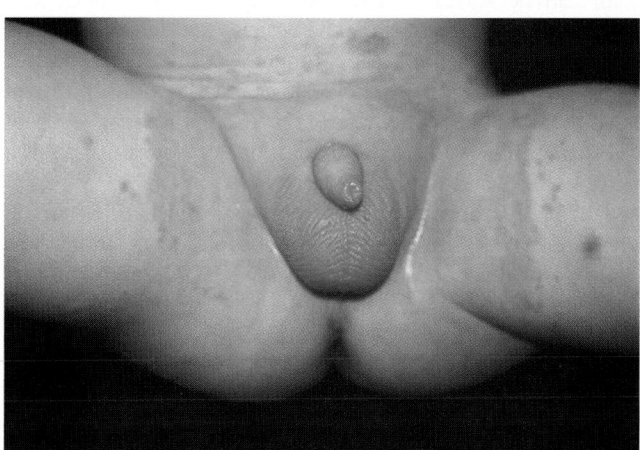

Figure 69-12. Candida diaper dermatitis with coalescence of erythematous papules involving the buttocks, scrotum, inguinal folds, inner thighs, and lower abdomen, with satellite erythematous papules. (Courtesy of the Department of Dermatology, University of Utah, Salt Lake City, Utah.)

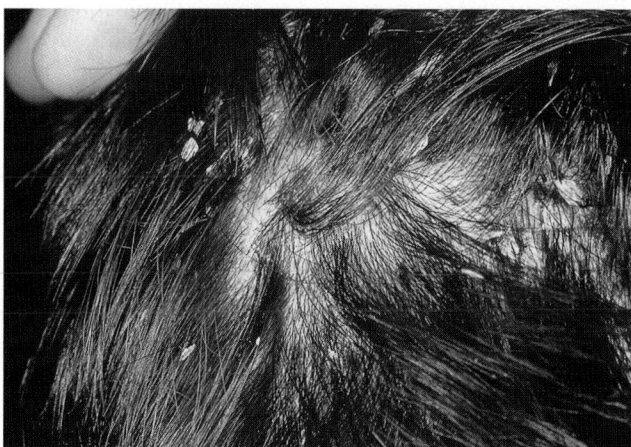

Figure 69-14. Scalp of an infant with Letterer-Siwe disease, showing thick, yellow scales adherent to the hairs.

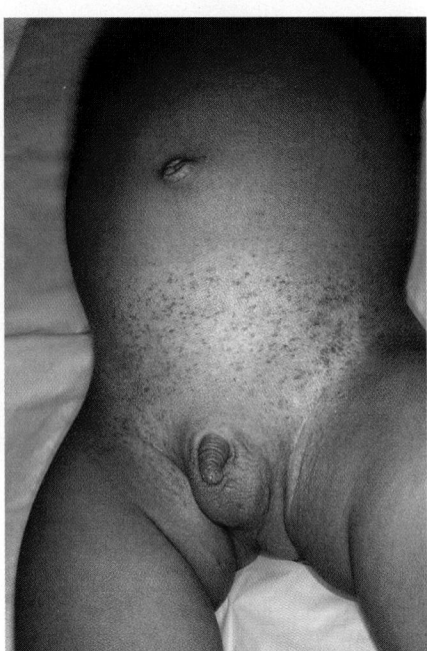

Figure 69-15. Same infant as in Figure 69-14, showing petechiae and purpuric papules on the lower abdomen and diaper area; this child also had hepatosplenomegaly.

problem. Prevention of irritation and secondary infection are the primary goals of treatment. Diapers should be changed frequently and the area cleansed with water or a mild cleanser. The use of absorbent disposable diapers has been shown to be superior to reusable cloth diapers for preventing diaper dermatitis. Exposure of the diaper area to air is an additional measure that may help prevent the development of dermatitis. Barrier agents (ointments, creams, powders) help protect the skin from irritants and moisture. The most commonly used agents are petrolatum and zinc oxide. Dusting powders, such as cornstarch and talcum powder, can be used to reduce moisture and frictional irritation. Sucralfate has been useful in some difficult cases of diaper dermatitis; this is a pastelike substance that provides a physical barrier and the ability to bind bile salts and positively charged proteins. Barrier agents should be applied after each diaper change.

Diaper dermatitis that does not respond to barrier protection alone requires addition of topical medications. Topical corticosteroids are used to treat inflammation; only low-potency nonfluorinated topical steroids, such as hydrocortisone or desonide, should be used. Combination topical steroid/antifungal creams (e.g., Lotrisone cream) contain high-potency fluorinated corticosteroids and should be avoided in the diaper area. Secondarily infected dermatitis should be treated with topical antibiotics or antifungal agents. Mild bacterial infections can be treated with topical mupirocin ointment, whereas more severe cases require systemic therapy directed at *S. aureus* and *Streptococcus*. Cutaneous candidiasis usually can be treated with topical antifungal agents, such as nystatin, clotrimazole, or econazole; occasionally, systemic antifungal therapy is required. Most patients with diaper dermatitis benefit from combination therapy with a topical antifungal or antibacterial cream, a low-potency topical steroid ointment, and a barrier ointment, applied in layers at each diaper change until the

eruption has resolved. Rashes that do not respond to treatment may require skin biopsy for further evaluation.

Seborrheic Dermatitis
Seborrheic dermatitis is discussed in detail in Chapter 70.

Intertriginous Dermatitis
Intertriginous dermatitis (intertrigo) is a superficial inflammatory dermatitis that occurs within skin folds. As a result of recurrent rubbing, heat, and trapping of moisture, the skin becomes erythematous and macerated. Secondary infection with bacteria and *Candida* is common. Intertriginous dermatitis occurs most commonly during hot and humid weather and in obese individuals. Commonly affected areas include the inframammary creases; neck; axillae; finger webs; antecubital fossae; umbilicus; and inguinal, perineal, and intergluteal creases. The primary intervention is elimination of the macerated skin. Apposing skin surfaces can be separated with gauze or wet compresses. Drying or dusting powders, such as cornstarch and talcum powder, can be used to decrease skin wetness. Low-potency nonfluorinated topical steroids can be used on a limited basis for inflammatory lesions. Secondarily infected areas should be treated with topical antibiotics or antifungal agents.

Periorificial Dermatitis (Perioral Dermatitis)
Periorificial dermatitis is discussed in Chapter 71.

Lichen Simplex Chronicus
Lichen simplex chronicus is unusual in infants and children and is identified more commonly in adolescents and adults, with the highest prevalence in adults 30 to 50 years old (Fig. 69-16). This condition is discussed on the CD-ROM.

Pompholyx (Dyshidrotic Eczema)
Pompholyx (dyshidrotic eczema) is a chronic form of vesicular dermatitis affecting the palms and soles. Pompholyx derives from the term *cheiropompholyx*, which means "hand and bubble" in Greek. The disease is characterized by recurrent episodes of vesicles affecting the palms, soles, and lateral aspect of the fingers and toes. Pruritus and burning pain can be severe and occasionally may be experienced before the vesicles appear. The vesicles are deep seated and have a tapioca-like appearance without surrounding erythema. Occasionally the vesicles may become confluent and form bullae. The blisters typically resolve without rupturing, followed by desquamation. Episodes usually last 3 to 4 weeks and tend to recur.

Pompholyx occurs equally in boys and girls. It occurs at any age but is most common in adolescents and young adults and develops more commonly in warmer climates and during spring and summer months. The etiology of pompholyx is unknown. The original hypothesis of sweat gland dysfunction is incorrect, and the term *pompholyx* (not *dyshidrotic eczema*) is preferred. There is no abnormality of the sweat ducts, and hyperhidrosis is usually not present. Atopy may predispose patients to pompholyx because 50% of affected individuals have atopic dermatitis. Emotional stress and exogenous factors, such as seasonal changes, hot or cold temperatures, humidity, nickel sensitivity, and dermatophyte infections, may trigger or exacerbate episodes.

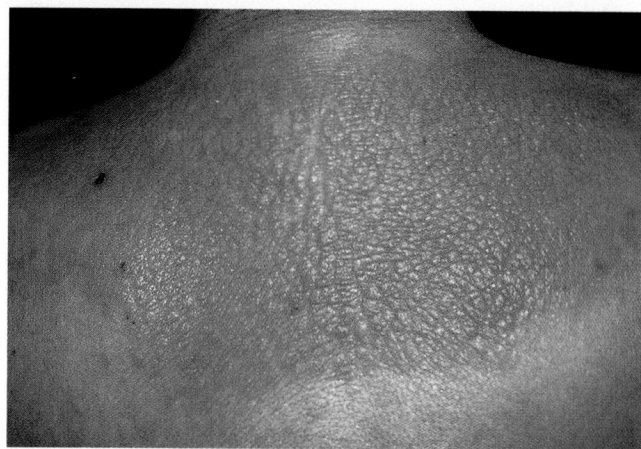

Figure 69-16. Lichen simplex chronicus. (Courtesy of the Department of Dermatology, University of Utah, Salt Lake City, Utah.)

The differential diagnosis of pompholyx includes allergic contact dermatitis, irritant dermatitis, pustular psoriasis, and superficial fungal infections. Dermatophyte infections are usually unilateral, and microscopic examination of potassium hydroxide–treated skin scrapings or fungal culture can exclude this diagnosis. Distinguishing pompholyx from contact or irritant dermatitis can be difficult and may require allergy patch testing. The typical scaling plaques and nail changes can help differentiate pustular psoriasis from pompholyx.

Treatment can be difficult and frustrating. Wet soaks or compresses using dilute potassium permanganate solution (1:8000) or aluminum acetate solution (Burow solution) can provide symptomatic relief. Treatment with high-potency topical steroids may hasten resolution of lesions and decrease the associated pruritus and burning. Secondary bacterial infection is common. If infection is suspected, cultures should be taken, and the patient should be treated with systemic antibiotics directed at *S. aureus* and *Streptococcus*. Refractory and severe cases warrant referral to a dermatologist and may require treatment with ultraviolet light, cyclosporine, methotrexate, or other systemic immunosuppressive medications.

Lichen Striatus

Lichen striatus is a self-limited, linear dermatitis of uncertain etiology that develops primarily in children. Girls outnumber boys by at least 2 to 1, and it generally affects children between ages 5 and 10 years. Infants and adults also can be affected. Lichen striatus is characterized by the sudden eruption of a narrow, linear band of small, slightly scaly, flat-topped, pink or flesh-colored papules (Fig. 69-17). Lesions tend to occur on a proximal extremity, but the face and trunk are affected occasionally. Bilateral or multiple bands are seen rarely. Lichen striatus generally resolves spontaneously within 3 to 12 months and may leave a linear streak of postinflammatory hypopigmentation that also eventually disappears in most cases.

The diagnosis usually is straightforward when a linear band of dermatitis is identified in a child. The differential diagnosis includes linear lichen planus, linear psoriasis, tinea corporis, verruca plana, linear epidermal nevus, and inflammatory linear verrucous epidermal nevus. In some instances, a skin biopsy may be necessary to exclude other linear eruptions.

In general, no treatment is required. Parents should be reassured of the favorable prognosis and notified of the expected spontaneous resolution. Topical steroids and emollients, especially those containing alpha hydroxy acids (e.g., Lac-Hydrin 12% cream or lotion or Eucerin Plus cream or lotion) can be used to treat associated dryness and pruritus. These medications may hasten resolution of the lesions.

Frictional Lichenoid Dermatitis
Definition
Frictional lichenoid dermatitis (also termed *summertime pityriasis of the elbows and knees, Sutton summer prurigo,* or *summer lichenoid dermatitis*) is a dermatosis of the elbows and knees seen primarily in children. The typical age of onset is 4 to 12 years, and it affects boys more commonly than girls (ratio 3:1).

Fundamentals
Frictional lichenoid dermatitis appears during spring and early summer, when outdoor activities and minor frictional trauma are common, and often spontaneously remits in the autumn. The lesions are characterized by small, flat-topped papules involving areas subjected to trauma and friction, such as the elbows, knees, and dorsal aspect of the hands (Fig. 69-18). Hypopigmentation and pruritus are variably present.

Diagnosis
The differential diagnosis of frictional lichenoid dermatitis includes atopic dermatitis, psoriasis, lichen simplex chronicus, and Gianotti-Crosti syndrome. The appearance of a self-limited dermatitis in the summertime involving areas of chronic friction and trauma usually makes the diagnosis

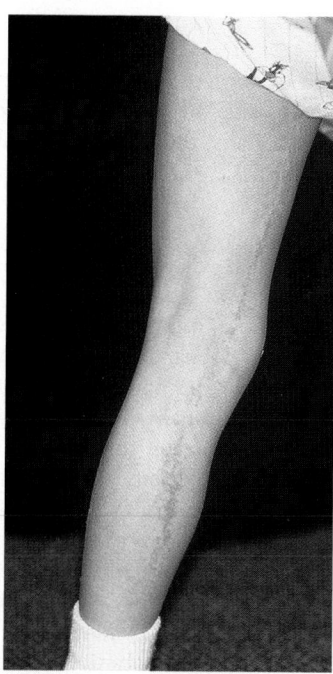

Figure 69-17. Narrow, linear band of flat-topped pink papules on the lower extremity of a young girl with lichen striatus.

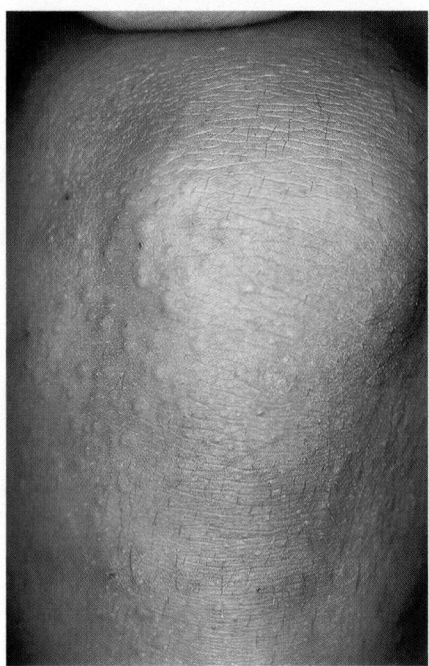

Figure 69-18. Flat-topped, flesh colored papules on the knee of a preteen girl with frictional lichenoid dermatitis.

straightforward. Psoriasis commonly involves the elbows and knees, similar to frictional lichenoid dermatitis, but larger plaques with prominent scaling usually are found in psoriasis. Additionally, patients with psoriasis may have evidence of nail disease, such as pitting and separation of the nail plate (onycholysis); scalp disease; or arthritis. Lichen simplex chronicus generally presents as a solitary plaque, and the patient usually gives a history of chronic scratching and rubbing. When the diagnosis is in question, or the patient fails to respond to appropriate therapy, a skin biopsy may be required.

Management

Treatment should be directed at limiting frictional trauma to the affected areas and the use of topical corticosteroids and emollients, especially those containing alpha hydroxy acids (e.g. Lac-Hydrin 12% cream or lotion or Eucerin Plus cream or lotion).

Nummular Dermatitis
Definition

Nummular dermatitis (nummular or discoid eczema) is defined by its clinical appearance as coin-shaped lesions. The lesions of nummular dermatitis appear in a distinctive manner. They begin as small vesicles and papules that enlarge by peripheral extension to form the characteristic erythematous coin-shaped lesions with peripheral erosions and crusts. Central clearing may be present, at times leading to a configuration that resembles tinea corporis (Fig. 69-19). In the acute phase, small papules and vesicles with edema, exudation, and formation of crusts are present. With time, lesions change and become more scaly, hyperpigmented, and lichenified. Excoriations are often present. Pruritus is variable; it can be severe and lead to significant emotional stress and difficulty sleeping.

Nummular dermatitis generally affects the extensor surfaces of the arms and legs. Involvement of the dorsal aspect of the hands and trunk is variably present, and involvement of the face and scalp is unusual. Nummular dermatitis is rare in children. It occurs most commonly in adults and more frequently in men. The peak age of onset is 55 to 65 years.

Fundamentals

The cause of this disease is unknown. It is exacerbated by local factors, including excessive bathing and irritants such as wool and harsh soaps. Nummular dermatitis is seen more frequently in individuals with dry skin and during winter months. Exacerbations may occur after secondary infection with staphylococci. Nummular dermatitis seems to be a distinct disease entity from atopic dermatitis. There are no associations with other atopic diseases, such as asthma and hay fever, and serum IgE levels are normal.

Diagnosis

The differential diagnosis of nummular dermatitis includes allergic contact dermatitis, atopic dermatitis, superficial fungal infections, and psoriasis. Microscopic examination of potassium hydroxide–treated scale scraped from the lesion fails to reveal fungal elements in nummular dermatitis and excludes the diagnosis of tinea corporis (Fig. 69-20). A contact allergen should be suspected when a patient fails to respond to appropriate therapy. Atopic dermatitis usually is associated with a personal or family history of eczema, allergies, hay fever, or asthma.

Management

Treatment consists of use of midpotency to high-potency topical steroids. Liberal lubrication of the skin and avoidance of irritants while bathing and doing the laundry are

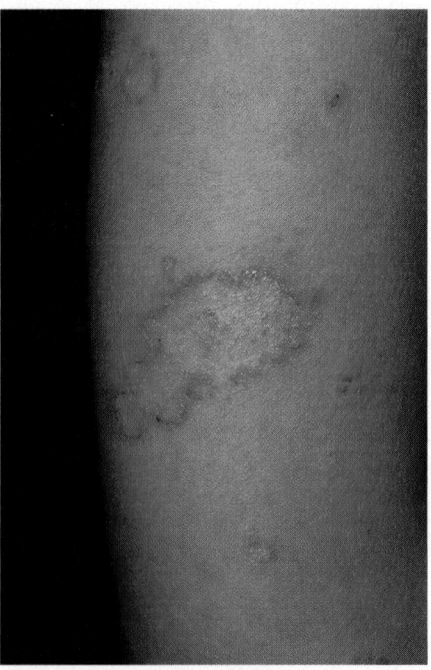

Figure 69-19. Teenage boy with nummular dermatitis. The central lesion is large and polycyclic; the peripheral lesions are more coin-shaped. All of these lesions show central clearing and peripheral erosions and crusts.

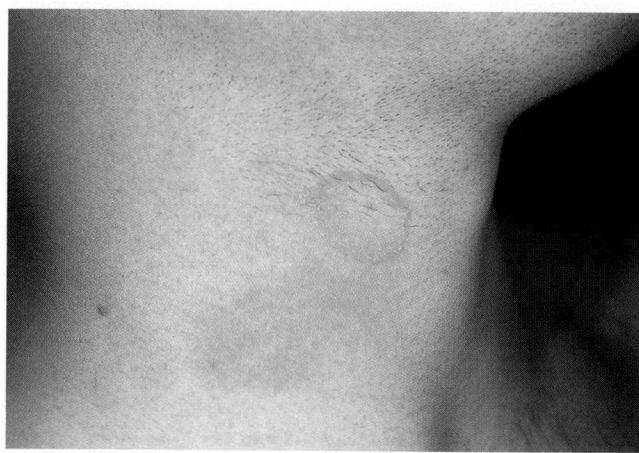

Figure 69-20. Tinea corporis on the neck of a young man. (Courtesy of the Department of Dermatology, University of Utah, Salt Lake City, Utah.)

important long-term changes that affected individuals should make. Oral antihistamines may help control pruritus. If secondary infection is suspected, treatment with an oral antistaphylococcal antibiotic is indicated.

Juvenile Plantar Dermatosis

Juvenile plantar dermatosis ("sweaty sock syndrome") is a common form of irritant dermatitis that develops primarily in children. It is characterized by a smooth, glazed-appearing, erythematous scaly eruption affecting the weight-bearing surfaces of the feet, sparing the interdigital spaces (Fig. 69-21). Patients usually complain of pain and burning of the feet, rather than pruritus, because of fissuring of the skin. The cause of this disorder is unclear, but it likely develops as a result of hyperhidrosis and rapid drying, resulting in chapping and fissuring of the skin. This disorder is associated with hyperhidrosis and generally presents in children with a tendency to atopy. Treatment consists of application of topical steroids and emollients, wearing white cotton socks that are changed frequently, and control of hyperhidrosis with topical aluminum chloride (e.g., Drysol).

Contact Dermatitis
Definition
Contact dermatitis is an inflammatory eczematous eruption caused by contact of substances with the skin. There are two forms of contact dermatitis: irritant and allergic. Irritant contact dermatitis is a nonimmunologic inflammatory reaction to a substance that occurs in nearly all persons exposed to it. Allergic contact dermatitis is an allergic or immunologic acquired sensitivity to a substance that occurs in a subset of patients previously exposed to the allergen.

Fundamentals
Development of irritant contact dermatitis requires no previous exposure to an irritating substance; the reaction may occur within minutes or hours after exposure. The primary factors that can influence the severity of the reaction include the condition of the skin at the time of exposure, strength or concentration of the irritant, location of contact, skin moisture, and occlusion or trapping of the irritant on the skin. Common agents that cause an irritant contact dermatitis in infants and children include alkalis, such as soaps, detergents, and bleaches; acids; antiseptics; certain foods; saliva; urine; and feces. The common locations for irritant contact dermatitis in children include the lips (lip licking, pacifier use), face, hands, and diaper area (Fig. 69-22). Clinically, irritant contact dermatitis presents as erythematous patches and plaques with scaling and occasionally blister formation. Treatment consists of avoiding the irritating substance; application of barrier protectants, such as zinc oxide ointment or petrolatum; and limited use of low-potency to midpotency topical steroids.

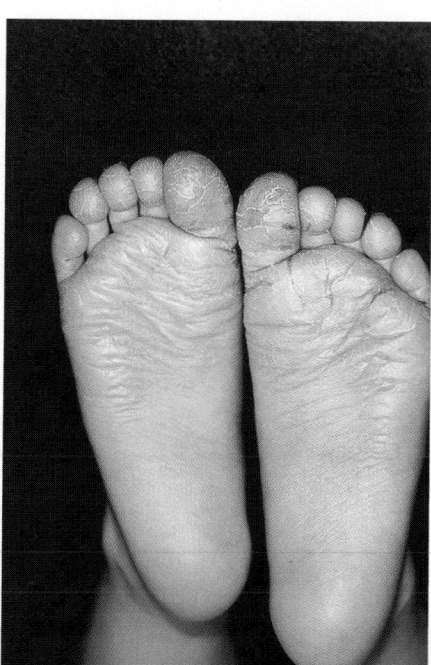

Figure 69-21. Boy with juvenile plantar dermatosis. The forefoot is smooth and glazed appearing. Fissures, erythema, and scale are present on the toes.

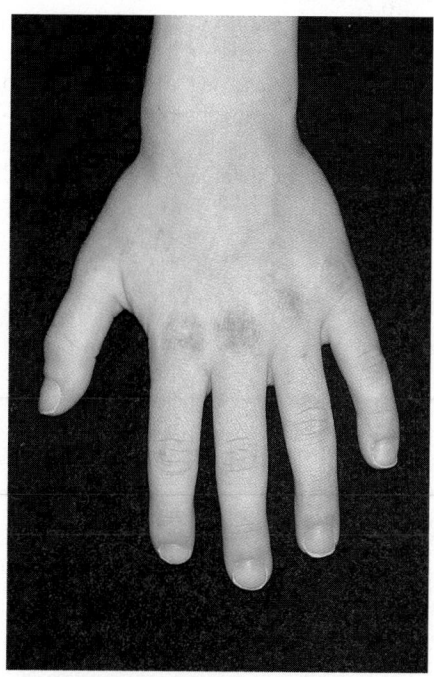

Figure 69-22. Irritant contact dermatitis.

Allergic contact dermatitis develops after exposure of previously sensitized skin to certain allergens. The incidence of allergic contact dermatitis in infants and children is unknown, but it occurs less commonly than in adults because of a diminished reactivity of children's skin to certain allergens and less opportunity of exposure to allergens often encountered in the occupational setting. Despite the decreased reactivity to contact allergens in childhood, allergic contact dermatitis may represent 20% of all cases of dermatitis in children.

Allergic contact dermatitis is caused by an immunologic type IV delayed hypersensitivity response. The initial phase is termed *sensitization*. This phase develops after penetration of an antigen into the skin. The antigen is processed by Langerhans cells in the skin and presented to T lymphocytes. The T lymphocytes undergo clonal expansion bearing specific receptors for the antigen then enter the circulation. During the sensitization phase, no reaction on the skin develops. Subsequent exposure to the antigen on the skin leads to the elicitation phase. Previously sensitized, clonal T lymphocytes interact with the antigen, proliferate, and release inflammatory mediators. When an area has been exposed to an allergen, repeated contact results in an allergic inflammatory response with subsequent dermatitis. Allergic contact dermatitis generally develops within 24 to 48 hours after exposure to the allergen. If untreated, the dermatitis can persist for weeks to months.

Many allergens can result in allergic contact dermatitis. Box 69-6 lists the most common causes of allergic contact dermatitis in the United States. The diagnosis of allergic contact dermatitis is made by recognizing the characteristic appearance and distribution of the eruption, identifying potential allergens by history, and using allergy patch testing. Clinically, allergic contact dermatitis presents as a pruritic eczematous eruption usually localized to the site of allergen contact. Patients with allergic contact dermatitis may experience widespread involvement, however, with erythematous pruritic papules distant from the site of contact (autoeczematization or id reaction). Potent allergens, such as poison ivy, oak, or sumac, produce intensely inflammatory lesions consisting of erythema, induration, oozing, crusting, and occasionally blisters (Fig. 69-23). Less potent allergens produce a subacute eruption consisting of erythema, scaling, and thickening of the skin. Blisters are unusual in subacute reactions. The distribution of the reac-

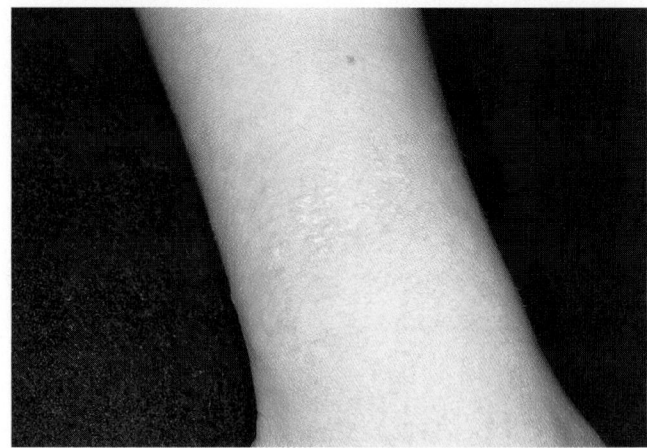

Figure 69-23. Prominent vesiculation and mild erythema on the forearm of a girl with allergic contact dermatitis.

tion can help distinguish allergic contact dermatitis from other forms of dermatitis. Allergic contact dermatitis tends to produce unusual shapes and often is localized to one skin area. A linear eruption strongly suggests allergic contact dermatitis. The distribution of the dermatitis may help identify the cause of allergic contact dermatitis. Dermatitis on the face may represent allergic contact dermatitis to foods or preservatives in cosmetics, chewing gum, hair spray, or shampoo. Dermatitis localized to the feet may result from allergy to rubber products in shoes and elastic stockings. Dermatitis in the V distribution of the neck, periumbilical area (Fig. 69-24), or earlobes suggests nickel allergy from necklaces, pants snaps, or earrings.

Diagnosis

In most cases, an allergen can be identified from the history and physical examination. In cases in which the allergen cannot be recognized and allergic contact der-

---

Box 69-6. Most Common Causes of Allergic Contact Dermatitis in the United States

- *Toxicodendron* (poison ivy, oak, and sumac)
- Nickel
- Neomycin
- Fragrance
- Thimerosal (preservative)
- Balsam of Peru (fragrance)
- Formaldehyde (preservative)
- Bacitracin
- Quaternium-15
- Rubber compounds

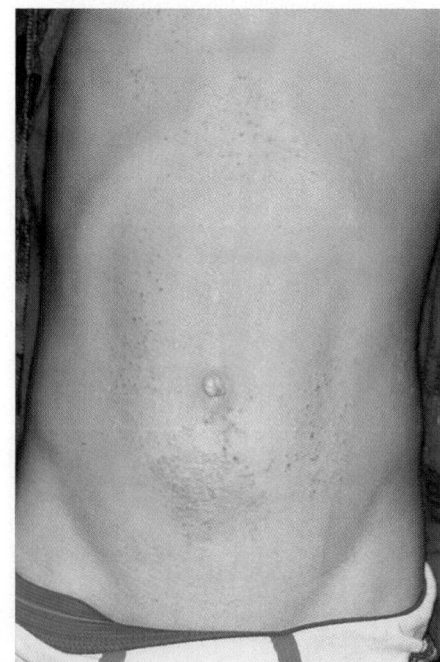

Figure 69-24. Allergic contact dermatitis secondary to nickel contained in the metal snap on the pants of a young boy.

matitis is suspected, the patient should be referred to a dermatologist for allergy patch testing. Patch testing is a safe and reliable method that involves placement of different allergens on the skin and assessment of the tested area for evidence of dermatitis. Patch testing is unreliable in children who are younger than 1 year of age and often is difficult to interpret in children who are younger than 8 years of age. Nevertheless, patch testing is a valuable tool in making the diagnosis of allergic contact dermatitis and in the identification of specific allergens. Patch testing involves the application of numerous diluted allergens to the skin. The allergens are placed in special metal (Finn) chambers and are taped to the upper back. The patch tests are removed 48 hours later and the sites are examined; the sites are reexamined at 4 to 5 days. Positive reactions consist of erythematous papules, edema, and vesicles.

Management

The best treatment for allergic contact dermatitis is recognition and avoidance of exposure to the specific allergen. Patients need to be educated about the allergen and instructed about specific products containing it. Most patch test clinics provide written educational handouts about the allergen and potential sources of exposure. Prevention is the most important means of avoiding recurrences of allergic contact dermatitis. Low-potency to high-potency topical steroids should be used for the treatment of acute lesions, depending on the body area affected. Systemic steroids are required for severe or widespread reactions.

Additional Resources, CD-ROM

Lichen simplex chronicus	Text, figure
Color atlas	Figures
Minor features of eczema	Figures
Bibliography	

Mini-index of Related Topics CH.

SUGGESTED READINGS

Guenst BJ: Common pediatric foot dermatoses. J Pediatr Health Care 1999;13:68–71.

Habif TP: Clinical Dermatology: A Color Guide to Diagnosis and Therapy, 3rd ed. St. Louis, Mosby-Year Book, 1996.

Habif TP, Campbell JL, Quitadama M: Skin Disease: Diagnosis and Treatment. St. Louis, Mosby, 2000.

Hauber K, Rose C, Brocker EB, Hamm H: Lichen striatus: Clinical features and follow-up in 12 patients. Eur J Dermatol 2000; 10:536–539.

Kazaks EL, Lane AT: Diaper dermatitis. Pediatr Clin North Am 2000; 47:909–919.

Ong PY, Leung DY: Atopic dermatitis. Clin Allergy Immunol 2002; 16:355–379.

Weston WL, Bruckner A: Allergic contact dermatitis. Pediatr Clin North Am 2000;47:897–907.

70 Papulosquamous Disorders

Mark Herron and Sheryll L. Vanderhooft

ROLE OF THE GENERALIST

1   Recognize pityriasis rosea and distinguish it from secondary syphilis.

2   Manage seborrheic dermatitis.

3   Identify the specific presentations of psoriasis, including psoriasis of infancy, plaque-type psoriasis, guttate psoriasis, pustular psoriasis, and erythrodermic psoriasis.

4   Recognize the significance of exfoliative erythroderma.

5   Refer children with psoriasis that is refractory to conventional therapy to a dermatologist for ongoing management.

6   Recognize the emotional effects of psoriasis on children.

7   Recognize less common papulosquamous disorders, such as pityriasis rubra pilaris and lichen planus, and provide appropriate treatment and triage.

8   Recognize Gianotti-Crosti syndrome, and provide appropriate treatment and triage.

9   Understand that children with lymphomatoid papulosis are at risk for lymphoma and require close long-term follow-up.

FUNDAMENTALS

Papulosquamous disorders are a diverse group of inflammatory skin conditions characterized by raised (papular) and scaling (squamous) lesions. The papules coalesce into plaques that have well-demarcated borders, a feature that helps distinguish a papulosquamous disorder from an eczematous process, the lesions of which typically have ill-defined margins.

PITYRIASIS ROSEA

Pityriasis rosea is a self-limited inflammatory disorder that affects primarily adolescents and young adults. Its etiology is unknown. Its seasonal clustering (fall, winter, and spring) and the association with a prodrome of headache, malaise, and pharyngitis in some affected individuals suggest a viral cause. Attempts to isolate an infectious agent have been disappointing, however. Pityriasis rosea begins with a single oval, pink–to–brownish red patch with raised borders and peripheral scale (the "herald patch") (Fig. 70-1). After 1 to 2 weeks, a generalized eruption arises on the trunk, extremities, and neck, consisting of smaller, oval, salmon-colored scaly papules with a collarette of scale distributed along the relaxed skin tension lines (Fig. 70-2), giving the distribution of the eruption the appearance of a Christmas tree. The trunk is involved most frequently. Sun-exposed skin (e.g., the face, hands, and feet) usually is spared. An atypical form of pityriasis rosea presents with an inverse distribution, with lesions on the face, axillae, groin, upper and lower extremities, and hands and feet. Some children may present with lesions that are purpuric (Fig. 70-3). The eruption usually resolves within 6 to 12 weeks.

The differential diagnosis of pityriasis rosea includes guttate psoriasis, secondary syphilis, nummular dermatitis, seborrheic dermatitis, tinea corporis, tinea versicolor, viral exanthem, and drug eruption. The herald patch of pityriasis rosea may be mistaken for tinea corporis; a potassium hydroxide preparation of the scales fails to reveal fungal elements in pityriasis rosea. A potassium hydroxide preparation can help the clinician distinguish tinea versicolor from pityriasis rosea. In sexually active adolescents and young adults with a widespread papulosquamous eruption,

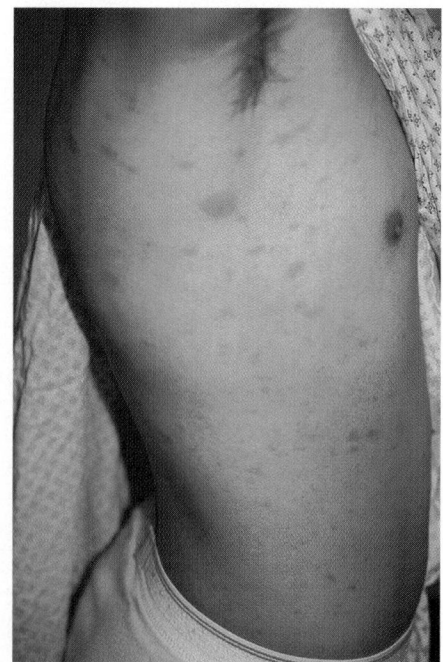

Figure 70-1. Pityriasis rosea in a young man, with a herald patch below the axilla. (Courtesy of Department of Dermatology, University of Utah School of Medicine, Salt Lake City, Utah.)

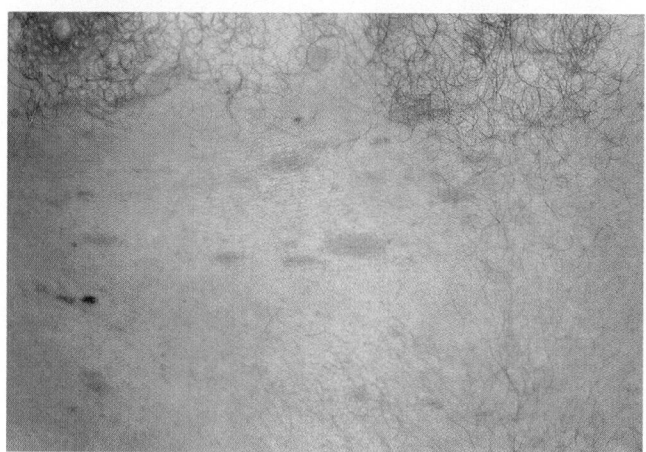

Figure 70-2. Pityriasis rosea with oval, salmon-colored, scaly papules distributed along the relaxed skin tension lines.

SECONDARY SYPHILIS

Similar to pityriasis rosea, secondary syphilis favors the trunk and presents with multiple scaling, reddish brown macules and papules along the relaxed skin tension lines. The palms and soles often are involved, a clinical feature that can help distinguish secondary syphilis from pityriasis rosea. Secondary syphilis usually presents 6 to 8 weeks after the appearance of the primary chancre, which is still present in approximately one third of individuals with secondary syphilis. History of a preceding mucosal (genital or oral) ulceration points toward syphilis and away from pityriasis rosea. Generalized lymphadenopathy, fever, malaise, headache, and anorexia are more prominent in secondary syphilis. Serologic tests are always positive at the time of the cutaneous eruption of secondary syphilis and confirm the diagnosis. Treatment of secondary syphilis is with intramuscular injections of benzathine penicillin G. In penicillin-allergic patients, either oral erythromycin or doxycycline may be used.

secondary syphilis is a concern. Further evaluation should include examination of the oral mucosa and genitals for ulcerative lesions and a serologic test for syphilis. In some instances, a skin biopsy may be necessary to make a definitive diagnosis, especially if the herald patch is absent or if presentation of the disorder is atypical.

In general, no treatment is required for pityriasis rosea. Antipruritic lotions containing pramoxine (e.g., Aveeno anti-itch lotion) or menthol and camphor (Sarna anti-itch lotion) can decrease pruritus; oral antihistamines may be beneficial as well. Topical steroid therapy is indicated for patients with moderate pruritus but may not hasten resolution of the lesions. Ultraviolet light therapy (ultraviolet B [UVB]) or sunlight exposure may be employed for patients with more severe pruritus and can hasten resolution of the lesions. Erythromycin given orally for 2 weeks also may lead to more rapid resolution of the eruption.

SEBORRHEIC DERMATITIS

Seborrheic dermatitis is a common chronic cutaneous disorder marked by redness and scaling of areas of densest concentration of the sebaceous glands (scalp, eyebrows, eyelids, nasal creases, ears, upper chest, and body folds). It presents as a spectrum of severity, ranging from fine flaking to coarse yellow scaling, with or without underlying pink-to-erythematous skin, to large erythematous plaques with loose, moist, yellow greasy scales (Figs. 70-4 and 70-5). The differential diagnosis includes psoriasis, atopic dermatitis, contact dermatitis, tinea capitis, tinea versicolor, and pityriasis rosea.

The infantile form of seborrheic dermatitis occurs as yellow waxy adherent scales over the fontanelle and vertex of the scalp (cradle cap), typically between the 2nd and 10th weeks of life. It also may present as well-demarcated erythematous patches in the diaper area (napkin dermatitis), which may spread to intertriginous areas, such as the axillae and neck. Seborrheic dermatitis in infants usually clears by 8 to 12 months of age and typically recurs during puberty. Therapy of seborrheic dermatitis is usually a long-

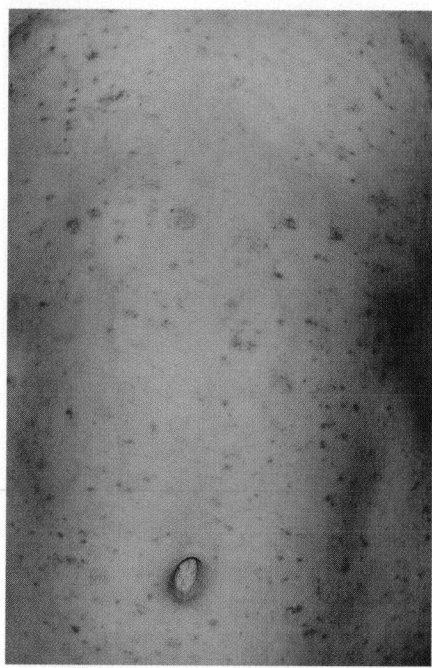

Figure 70-3. Purpuric variant of pityriasis rosea in a young boy.

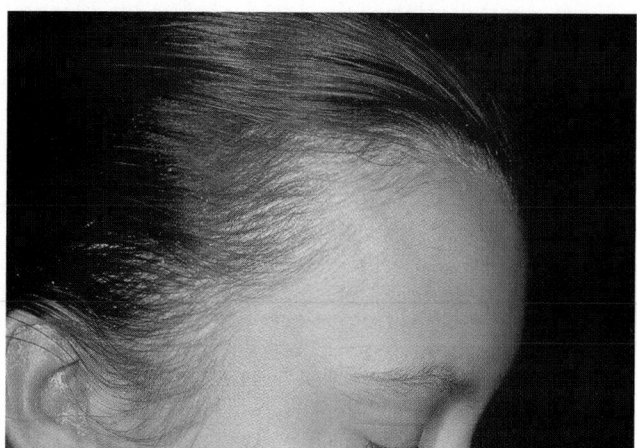

Figure 70-4. Seborrheic dermatitis characterized by dense, fine flaking of the scalp in a teenage girl with atopic dermatitis.

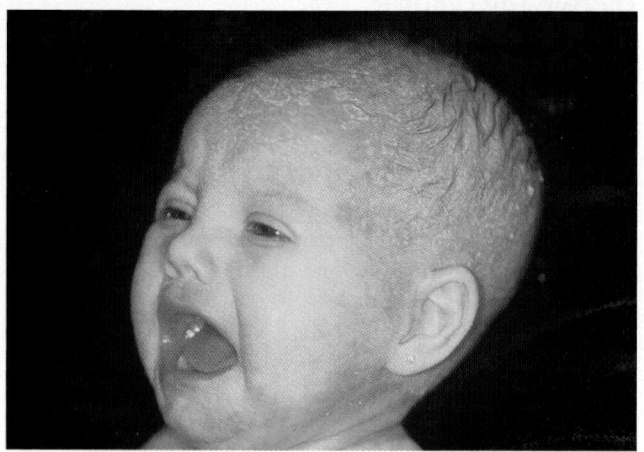

Figure 70-5. Severe seborrheic dermatitis in an infant with atopic dermatitis.

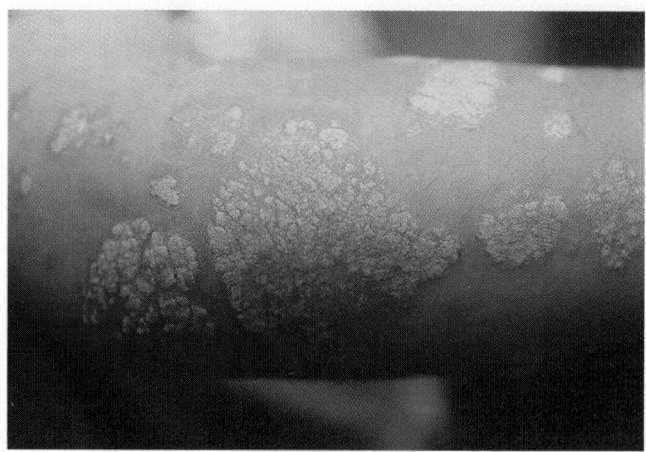

Figure 70-6. Psoriasis on the arm of a teenage girl.

term commitment because of its chronic and recurring nature. Medicated shampoos containing salicylic acid, selenium sulfide, tar, or zinc are useful in minimizing the scale and may be required on a maintenance basis. It is important to counsel parents and patients about proper use of the shampoo, which consists of allowing the shampoo to be in contact with the scalp for 5 to 10 minutes before rinsing out the lather. Daily shampooing is recommended to get the scaling under control and then is done a few times a week to keep the seborrhea under control. Ketoconazole-containing shampoo (or cream for the skin) also is effective in suppressing seborrheic dermatitis, probably by reducing *Pityrosporum ovale* organisms on the skin, which may contribute to seborrheic dermatitis in some individuals. Topical corticosteroids lessen the inflammatory component of seborrheic dermatitis and are useful for patients who do not respond to medicated shampoo alone. Corticosteroids may be used in solution or foam form for application to the scalp or in cream form for the skin.

PSORIASIS

Psoriasis is an autosomal dominant inherited disorder that requires interplay of genetic and environmental factors for complete clinical expression. It affects 1% to 3% of the general population. More than one third of psoriasis patients report developing the disorder before age 20 years. Although psoriasis affects men and women in equal numbers, childhood psoriasis is more common in girls, with a female-to-male ratio of 2:1. It is uncommon for psoriasis to present during the first 2 years of life; congenital psoriasis has been reported rarely in the literature. The most frequently observed variant of psoriasis during childhood is the plaque type, followed by the guttate form and juvenile psoriatic arthritis. Pustular psoriasis and erythrodermic psoriasis are rare forms of the disease, but can be seen during childhood from infancy to adolescence.

Plaque-type psoriasis presents as erythematous papules with a silvery white scale that enlarge and coalesce into thick, red, scaling, well-demarcated plaques (Fig. 70-6). There is a predilection for the extensor surfaces of the elbows and knees and the lumbosacral area, although the plaques may be scattered diffusely on the extremities, torso

(especially within and around the umbilicus), and face. When the top layer of scale is removed from the lesions, punctate bleeding occurs (Auspitz sign). The scalp frequently is involved with thick, erythematous plaques with silvery scale (Fig. 70-7), often with involvement of the frontal hairline extending onto the forehead and in the posterior auricular areas. "Pinking" of the intergluteal folds is common, characterized by mild erythema but no scale given the moistness of the area. The palms and soles frequently are involved (Fig. 70-8). Nail involvement occurs in more than half of cases. Pitting of the nail plate, separation of the plate from the nail bed (onycholysis) (see CD-ROM Fig. 72-26), focal brown discoloration of the nail (oil spot changes), and nail thickening with subungual debris may occur in association with psoriasis.

Psoriasis spreads in areas of trauma to the skin (Koebner phenomenon) a response that may be induced by excoriations, lacerations, abrasions, surgical incisions, sunburns,

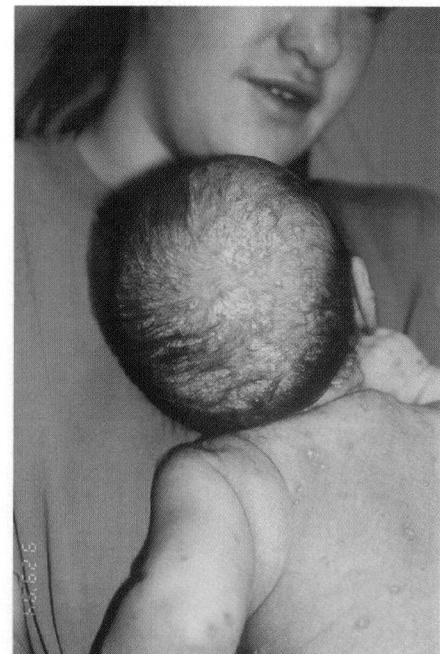

Figure 70-7. Prominent scalp involvement in a 6-week-old boy with psoriasis.

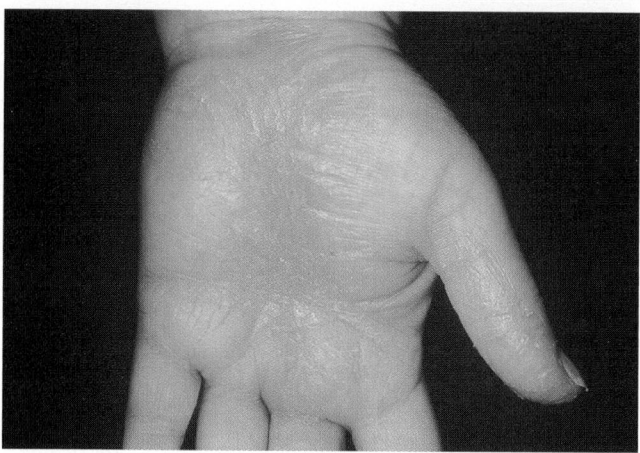

Figure 70-8. Psoriasis of the palm in a middle-aged woman. (Courtesy of Department of Dermatology, University of Utah School of Medicine, Salt Lake City, Utah.)

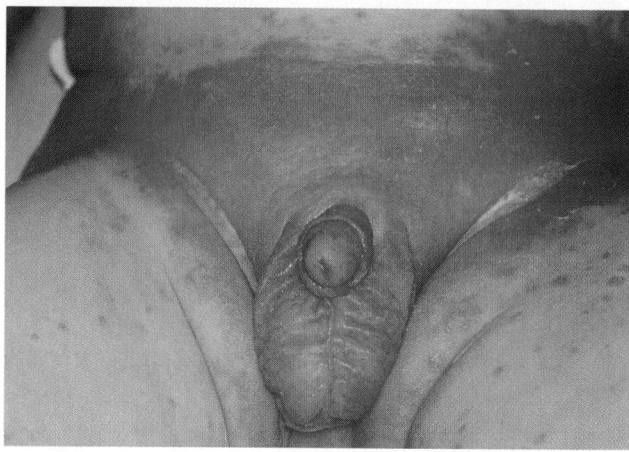

Figure 70-9. Involvement of the diaper area in a toddler with guttate psoriasis.

insect bites, or pressure. Koebner phenomenon is not unique to psoriasis and is shared by many other cutaneous disorders (Box 70-1). The diaper area usually is involved in infants with psoriasis (Fig. 70-9), most likely secondary to constant maceration of the involved site. The inverse form of plaque-type psoriasis presents with lesions in a flexural distribution, involving the axillae, groin, central chest, and umbilical area, with or without involvement of more typical sites of predilection. The differential diagnosis of plaque-type psoriasis includes pityriasis rosea, seborrheic dermatitis, nummular dermatitis, pityriasis rubra pilaris (PRP), and lichen planus.

Guttate ("droplike") psoriasis presents with generalized small, red, silvery scaling papules (Fig. 70-10). Despite the diffuse involvement, accentuation over the trunk and the proximal extremities often is seen. This variant of psoriasis most commonly occurs in children and young adults, often appearing 1 to 3 weeks after an upper respiratory tract infection, and may be the initial presentation of psoriasis in genetically susceptible individuals. Guttate psoriasis has been associated closely with preceding streptococcal pharyngitis or tonsillitis. Perianal streptococcal infection also has been reported with acute guttate psoriasis. Other viral and bacterial infections may precipitate guttate psoriasis. Management of acute guttate psoriasis includes systemic antibiotics, typically directed at streptococcal infections. Acute guttate psoriasis responds well to treatment, but the psoriasis often recurs with the more typical plaque-type morphology. Guttate psoriasis may be confused with

pityriasis rosea, secondary syphilis, a morbilliform viral exanthem, or drug eruption.

Pustular psoriasis seldom is seen in children. The localized form, known as *pustulosis palmaris et plantaris*, is restricted to the palms and soles; a variant known as *acrodermatitis continua* typically is restricted to the fingers (Fig. 70-11). Localized psoriasis presents with deep-seated pustules that heal with crusting and peeling. It may be confused with bullous tinea pedis, impetigo, and contact dermatitis. The differential diagnosis also includes Reiter's disease, characterized by the triad of urethritis, arthritis, and nonbacterial conjunctivitis; these patients can develop palmoplantar pustules that become hyperkeratotic and scaly when they dry (keratoderma blennorrhagicum).

Generalized pustular psoriasis is a severe form of psoriasis. It presents with the explosive onset of widespread sterile pustules and erythematous, scaly papules. The pustules may coalesce to form "lakes of pus" (Fig. 70-12). When the pustules dry, coarse scales form, and subsequently sheets of skin peel off; this may lead to exfoliative erythroderma (see description later). Noncutaneous features of pustular psoriasis include fever, chills, malaise, and arthralgias. Elevated white blood cell count, elevated erythrocyte sedimentation rate, hypoalbuminemia, and hypocalcemia may be associated with generalized pustular psoriasis. When

Box 70-1. Disorders That Show Koebner Phenomenon (Isomorphic Response)

- Allergic contact dermatitis
- Bullous pemphigoid
- Psoriasis
- Lichen planus
- Lichen nitidus
- Molluscum contagiosum
- Verruca vulgaris
- Vitiligo

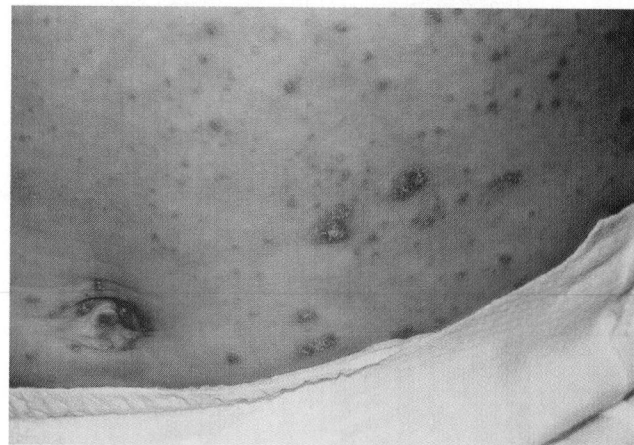

Figure 70-10. Guttate psoriasis of the abdomen in the same toddler depicted in Figure 70-9.

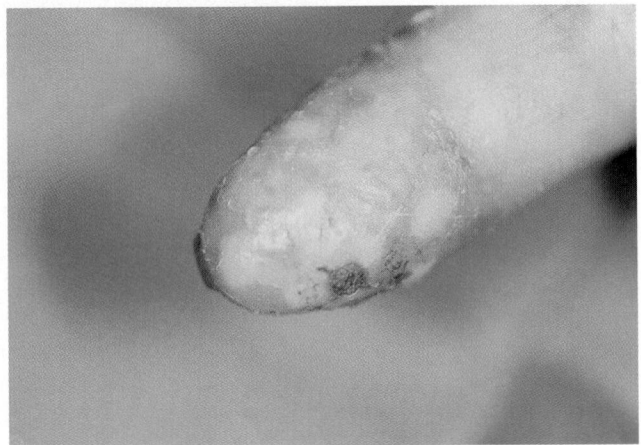

Figure 70-11. Localized psoriasis (acrodermatitis continua) of the index finger in a middle-aged woman.

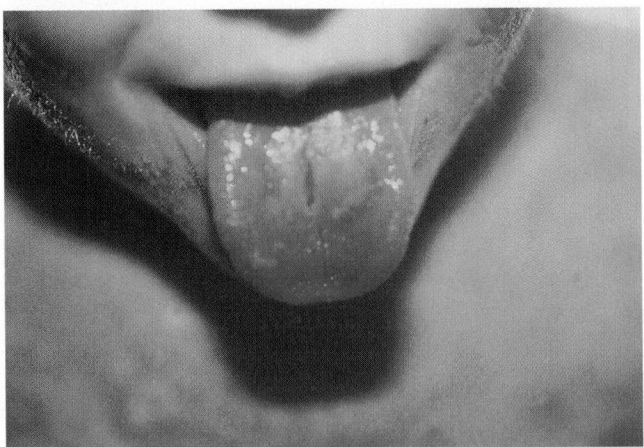

Figure 70-13. Geographic tongue in the same boy depicted in Figure 70-12.

generalized pustular psoriasis occurs in infancy, it is difficult to control. Mucous membrane involvement (geographic tongue) is much more common in pustular psoriasis than in plaque-type psoriasis (Fig. 70-13). Pustular psoriasis may arise after cessation of systemic steroid therapy in a patient with plaque-type psoriasis. It also can be precipitated by acute infection, pregnancy, hypocalcemia, emotional stress, and exposure to certain medications, including antimalarials, β-blockers, lithium, sulfonamides, nonsteroidal anti-inflammatory drugs, progesterone, and iodides. The differential diagnosis of generalized pustular psoriasis includes cutaneous candidiasis; subcorneal pustular dermatosis of Sneddon and Wilkinson; and acute generalized exanthematous pustulosis, a pustular form of drug eruption.

Erythrodermic (exfoliative) psoriasis is the most severe form of the disorder. It occurs in a small percentage of adults with psoriasis and rarely in children. It presents with widespread erythema and massive exfoliation involving almost the entire cutaneous surface. It is abrupt in onset and often is associated with pruritus and burning sensation. It may involve the scalp and result in alopecia. Noncutaneous features include fever, chills, malaise, tachycardia, pedal edema, lymphadenopathy, and hepatomegaly. Patients with erythroderma have difficulty regulating their body temperature and are at risk for high-output cardiac failure. Erythrodermic psoriasis generally occurs as a complication of chronic psoriasis and may be triggered by sunburn (from natural sunlight or as a complication of ultraviolet light therapy), severe emotional stress, excessive alcohol consumption, or systemic viral or bacterial infection; it is rarely the initial presentation of psoriasis. Erythroderma also can arise as a complication of other cutaneous disorders (Fig. 70-14; Box 70-2). Evaluation of a patient who presents with erythroderma includes obtaining skin biopsy speci-

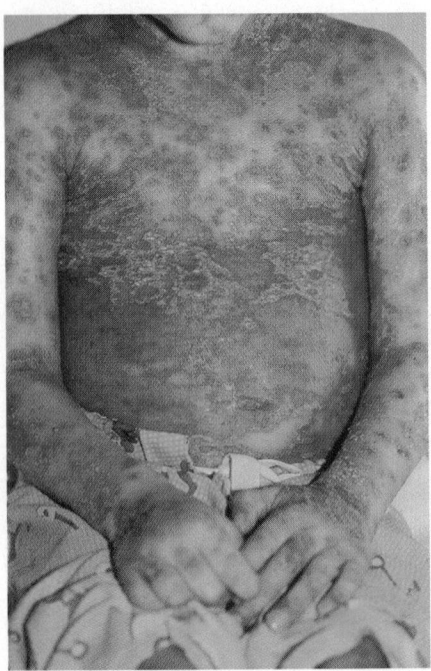

Figure 70-12. "Lakes of pus" on the upper abdomen in a young boy with extensive pustular psoriasis.

Figure 70-14. Erythroderma in a teenage girl with severe atopic dermatitis.

mens in an attempt to identify the underlying cutaneous disorder.

Treatment objectives in childhood psoriasis are to normalize the appearance of the skin as much as possible, to afford physical relief, and to employ treatments that do not endanger the health or the future development of the child. Topical therapeutic modalities include corticosteroids, coal tar preparations, anthralin, calcipotriene (Dovonex), and retinoids (tazarotene [Tazorac]). These preparations may be used as monotherapy or in combinations. It is not unusual for a patient to stop responding to a particular topical medication after a period of time (tachyphylaxis); *rotational therapy* is advocated for most patients for this reason. Intralesional corticosteroid injections are useful for plaques that are recalcitrant to topical therapy. For scalp psoriasis, medicated shampoos (as outlined earlier in the section on Seborrheic Dermatitis); topical corticosteroid solutions, gels, or foams; and calcipotriene solution are used to decrease inflammation and scaling.

When psoriasis is widespread, topical therapy becomes more difficult to use successfully. Systemic corticosteroids should not be used in psoriasis because of the risk of severe rebound or the induction of pustular psoriasis when the steroids are discontinued. Other options include natural sunlight exposure, phototherapy using UVB or photochemotherapy with psoralen (taken orally or applied topically) plus ultraviolet A light (PUVA), oral retinoids, and systemic immunosuppressive medications. UVB and PUVA treatments are associated with an increased risk of skin cancer and are best avoided in children. Oral retinoids, methotrexate, and cyclosporine are used in severe cases unresponsive to other treatment modalities, such as recalcitrant psoriasis with arthritis, and in crisis situations, such as generalized pustular or erythrodermic psoriasis. All of these medications have significant potential toxicities, and laboratory monitoring on a regular basis is required. Management of a child with severe psoriasis employing any of these medications is best left to the dermatologist. Patients with generalized pustular or erythrodermic psoriasis often require hospitalization and treatment with topical steroids under occlusion, conservation of body heat, intravenous fluid replacement, and at times phototherapy or administration of systemic therapies.

It is important to emphasize to parents and patients the chronic and recurring nature of childhood psoriasis. Most

cases of childhood psoriasis continue into adult life and are marked by remissions and exacerbations. The course is variable and unpredictable, but overall most patients have chronic localized involvement. Parents should understand that the severity of psoriasis can be lessened, and the potential for remission is possible with ongoing treatment. Children and adolescents have a difficult time accepting psoriasis because they see themselves as disfigured and unattractive. Adolescents need strong emotional support. Exacerbations of psoriasis occur at times of emotional stress. Participation in stress management workshops is recommended as a way for parents and children to learn to cope with the physical and psychological aspects of the disorder. Although trauma to the skin may induce psoriasis, restriction of activities may stigmatize the child further and is unwarranted. An excellent resource for patients and their families is the National Psoriasis Foundation (6600 SW 92nd Avenue, Suite 300, Portland, OR 97223-7195, 800-723-9166, www.psoriasis.org).

PITYRIASIS RUBRA PILARIS

PRP is an uncommon papulosquamous disorder that typically is acquired, although a familial autosomal dominant form also exists. Of affected individuals, 40% develop the disorder during childhood. The classic juvenile form of PRP typically begins during the first few years of life and is the presentation for one fourth of the pediatric cases. It is clinically identical to the classic adult form, characterized by perifollicular erythema that expands into large salmon-colored plaques with fine scale and a nutmeg grater texture, distributed on the torso and extremities (Figs. 70-15 and 70-16). "Islands of sparing" represent normal areas of skin surrounded by and sharply demarcated from involved skin. The face and scalp may be diffusely erythematous with fine

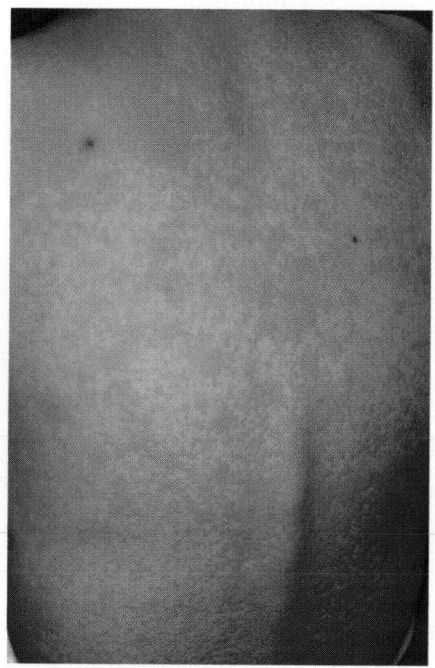

Figure 70-15. Pityriasis rubra pilaris in a young boy. (Courtesy of Department of Dermatology, University of Utah School of Medicine, Salt Lake City, Utah.)

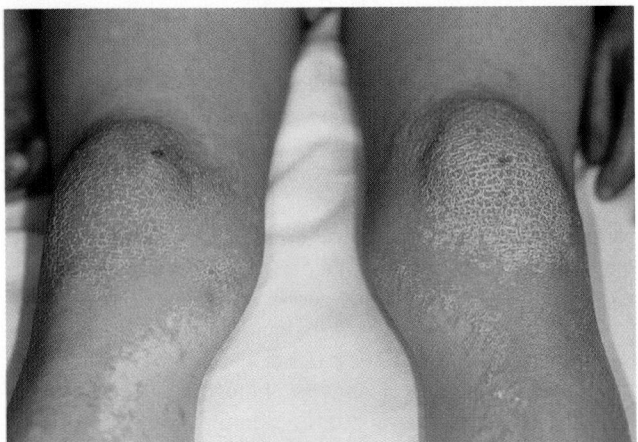

Figure 70-16. Lower extremities of the same boy depicted in Figure 70-15. (Courtesy of Department of Dermatology, University of Utah School of Medicine, Salt Lake City, Utah.)

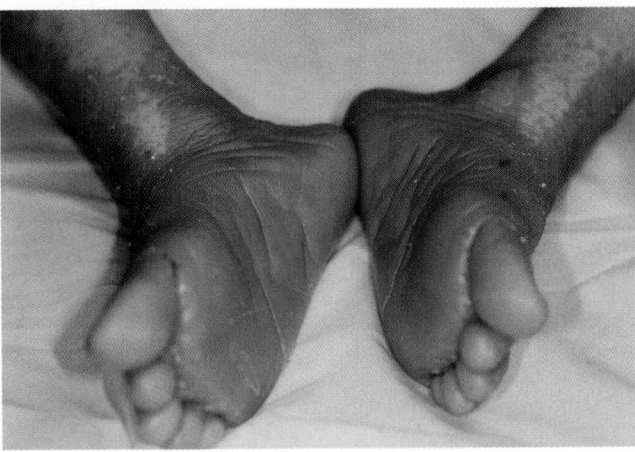

Figure 70-18. Soles of the same boy depicted in Figures 70-15, 70-16, and 70-17. (Courtesy of Department of Dermatology, University of Utah School of Medicine, Salt Lake City, Utah.)

scale. Follicular keratotic papules arise on the dorsal aspect of the hands and are pathognomonic for this disorder. The palms and soles become thickened and exhibit an orange hue (Figs. 70-17 and 70-18); painful fissuring of the palms and soles is common. The nails often are thickened with subungual debris, and the nail plates may become opaque. A waxy texture may develop on the face, with subsequent development of ectropion. Pruritus may or may not be a significant feature. PRP can progress to an exfoliative erythroderma, with associated fevers, chills, and malaise. Although this form of PRP may follow a protracted course, spontaneous remissions occur in 50% of affected individuals within 2 to 3 years after onset.

The circumscribed juvenile form of PRP accounts for approximately 60% of pediatric cases. It usually presents in prepubertal children and is characterized by salmon-colored scaly plaques on the elbows, knees, and other bony prominences. This form of PRP tends to follow a protracted course, persisting into adulthood. The atypical juvenile form of PRP is the least common presentation in children. It typically begins during the first few years of life and persists throughout life; familial cases of PRP tend to fit into this category.

Mild forms of PRP may be managed successfully with topical medications. Topical corticosteroids can decrease the erythema and pruritus but may not alter the course of PRP. Keratolytic agents, including salicylic acid, lactic acid, urea, and topical retinoids, are useful adjuncts, although burning and irritation often limit their use. Topical calcipotriene has been reported to be beneficial in some patients. Systemic corticosteroids are generally ineffective in the treatment of PRP. When PRP is either persistent or disabling, systemic therapy is indicated. Systemic retinoids can be effective in the management of PRP. Systemic retinoids may be associated with serious toxicity, however, and serum fasting lipid profiles and liver function tests must be monitored. Methotrexate also is effective in severe cases of PRP; given its potential for toxicity, it must be used with caution in children.

LICHEN PLANUS

Lichen planus is a pruritic eruption that is not commonly encountered in children. It is characterized by flat-topped, violaceous polygonal papules that typically are clustered and may coalesce into plaques (Fig. 70-19). Lacy white lines, called *Wickham's striae*, may be appreciated when the lesions are moistened and magnified with a hand lens. Sites of predilection include the flexural aspect of the wrists and ankles, forearms, overlying the shins, the inner aspect of the knees and thighs, and genitals. Lichen planus is associated with the Koebner phenomenon, with new lesions arising at sites of injury to the skin and the presence of lesions arranged in a linear configuration.

Mucosal involvement is seen in approximately one third of children with lichen planus. White papules form a lacy reticulated pattern on the buccal mucosa or the gingiva; the palate, tongue, and lips also may be involved. Oral lichen planus has the potential to become erosive and painful and may interfere with proper intake of nutrients. Lichen planus also may involve the scalp and may cause a scarring alopecia, but this complication is rarely encountered in children. Nail changes are seen in approximately 10% of individuals with lichen planus and include brittleness, thinning, roughness, and longitudinal ridging of the nail plates;

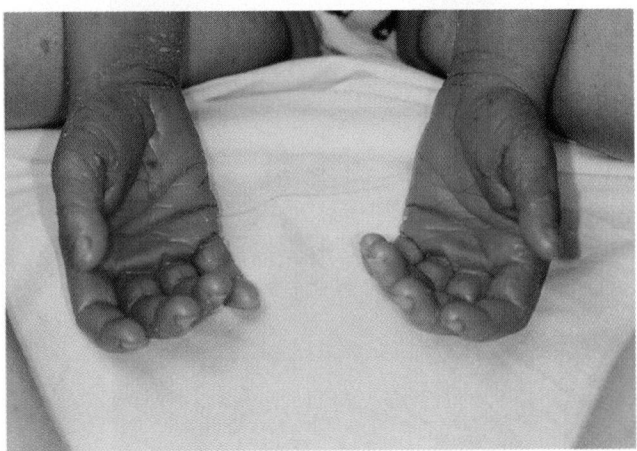

Figure 70-17. Palms of the same boy depicted in Figures 70-15 and 70-16. (Courtesy of Department of Dermatology, University of Utah School of Medicine, Salt Lake City, Utah.)

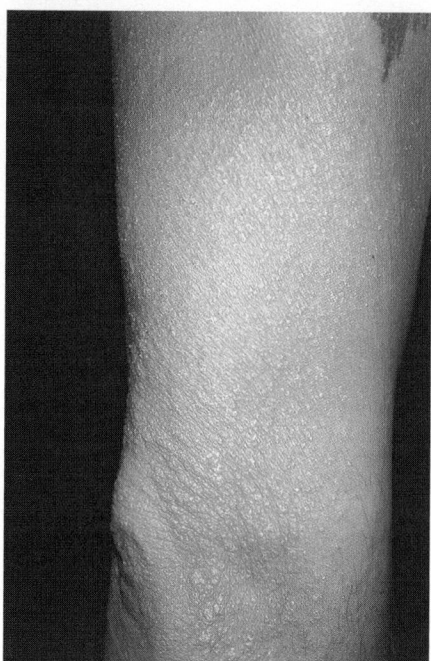

Figure 70-19. Arm of a man showing the *P*s of lichen planus: planar (flat-topped), pruritic, purple, polygonal papules. (Courtesy of Department of Dermatology, University of Utah School of Medicine, Salt Lake City, Utah.)

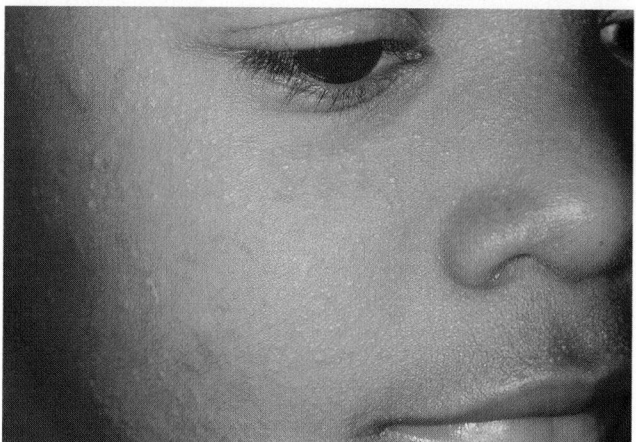

Figure 70-20. Lichen nitidus on the face of a young boy.

ptyergium formation and complete and permanent loss of the nail may occur. Trachyonychia (20 nail dystrophy) may represent an early form of lichen planus in some children, with the nail changes preceding the onset of cutaneous lesions (see CD-ROM Fig. 72-22 and the discussion in CD-ROM Chapter 72).

Topical corticosteroids are the mainstay of treatment for lichen planus. Intralesional steroid injections are helpful for thick lesions that do not respond to topical steroids. Intralesional steroid therapy also can be effective in treating nail lichen planus, with the maximal effect seen in 2 months. Systemic corticosteroids are of benefit in patients with widespread lesions that prove to be unresponsive to topical corticosteroids. When the lesions of lichen planus resolve, often prominent postinflammatory hyperpigmentation remains and may take several months to fade. One quarter of patients with lichen planus may expect a recurrence; recurrences also are responsive to corticosteroid therapy. For refractory cases of lichen planus, systemic dapsone therapy or PUVA may be employed. Patients with mucosal involvement may be treated with an elixir formulation of topical steroid. Topical anesthetics, such as viscous lidocaine, are helpful for patients with painful oral erosions and ulcerations.

LICHEN NITIDUS

Lichen nitidus is a chronic, yet usually asymptomatic, self-limited papulosquamous disorder that most often is encountered in preschool and school-age children. It is characterized by pinpoint flesh-colored, flat-topped shiny papules arranged in clusters typically on the torso, genitals, and extremities (Fig. 70-20). Lichen nitidus exhibits the Koebner phenomenon, with new lesions arising at sites of trauma; lesions frequently are present in a linear config-

uration. Lichen nitidus can be distinguished clinically from keratosis pilaris, which is a common chronic disorder characterized by follicular rough, flesh-colored papules with a collarette of erythema that typically arise on the cheeks, upper outer arms, thighs, and buttocks (Fig. 70-21). Reassurance is central to the treatment of lichen nitidus. Topical corticosteroids and keratolytics may be of some benefit.

GIANOTTI-CROSTI SYNDROME

Gianotti-Crosti syndrome (papular acrodermatitis of childhood) is a self-limited process that presents with the abrupt onset of flat-topped, dome-shaped succulent erythematous papules localized to the malar areas of the face, upper and lower extremities, palms, soles, and buttocks (Figs. 70-22 and 70-23). The trunk often is spared. The

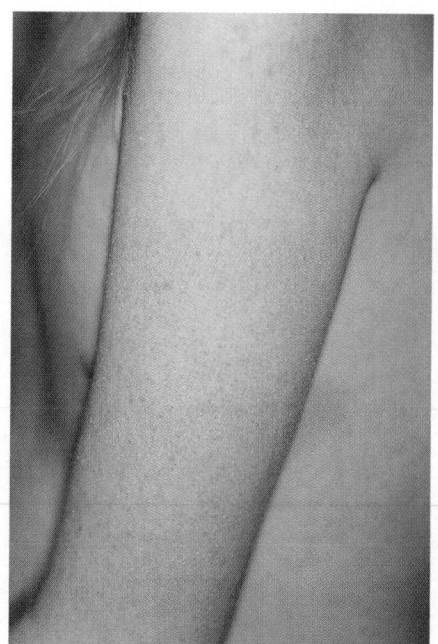

Figure 70-21. Extensive keratosis pilaris on the upper arm of a young girl.

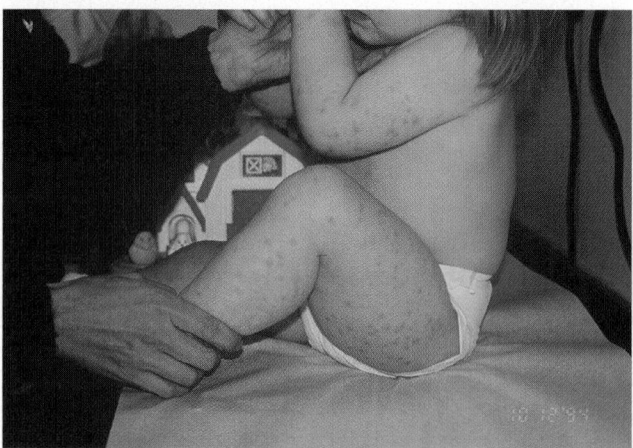

Figure 70-22. Gianotti-Crosti syndrome in a toddler.

lesions are usually asymptomatic, although children with diffuse involvement may have severe pruritus. The mean age of onset is 2 years old. Symptoms of an upper respiratory tract infection may precede the cutaneous eruption. The eruption may be accompanied by low-grade fever, malaise, lymphadenopathy, hepatomegaly, and elevated liver transaminases.

Gianotti-Crosti syndrome originally was reported in association with hepatitis B infection. It subsequently has been reported in association with a wide variety of infectious agents and administration of immunizations (Box 70-3) and likely represents a specific reaction pattern to a nonspecific infectious process. The lesions of Gianotti-Crosti syndrome typically resolve within 3 weeks, although it may take several weeks to clear completely in some children. Treatment with topical corticosteroids may or may not decrease the erythema associated with the lesions, and such treatment is unlikely to hasten resolution of the eruption. Topical antipruritics and systemic antihistamines are indicated if there is associated pruritus.

PITYRIASIS LICHENOIDES

Pityriasis lichenoides is a cutaneous disorder of unknown etiology. It arises in an acute form, known as *pityriasis lichenoides et varioliformis acuta (PLEVA)* or *Mucha-* *Habermann disease*, and a chronic form, *pityriasis lichenoides chronica (PLC)*. PLEVA primarily affects children and young adults, whereas PLC is more common in adolescents and young adults; clinical and histopathologic overlap between these two forms often is encountered in children.

PLEVA is a polymorphous eruption characterized by reddish brown, scaly macules and papules that arise in crops and evolve into vesicular, necrotic, and sometimes purpuric lesions (Fig. 70-24). Because there are typically numerous lesions at various stages of evolution, PLEVA often is mistaken for varicella. PLEVA has a generalized distribution, but lesions tend to be more concentrated on the trunk and flexor surfaces of the proximal extremities. Patients are usually asymptomatic, and there is minimal pruritus associated with the lesions. There is, however, a severe variant of PLEVA that presents with fever, malaise, ulceronecrotic lesions, and elevated C-reactive protein or erythrocyte sedimentation rate. The ulceronecrotic lesions may predispose the patient to cutaneous superinfection and bacteremia. The more deeply ulcerated lesions heal with scarring; transient postinflammatory hyperpigmentation or hypopigmentation may be seen. PLEVA typically persists for several weeks to several months and then spontaneously resolves, although some individuals may experience recurrences that continue for a few years.

PLC may arise de novo or evolve from PLEVA. It is characterized by reddish brown, firm papules with adherent scales that are thicker in the center than at the edges of the lesions (Fig. 70-25). As the papules recede over several weeks, the scale separates from the surface, revealing postinflammatory hyperpigmented or hypopigmented macules. The macules fade after several months; the lesions heal

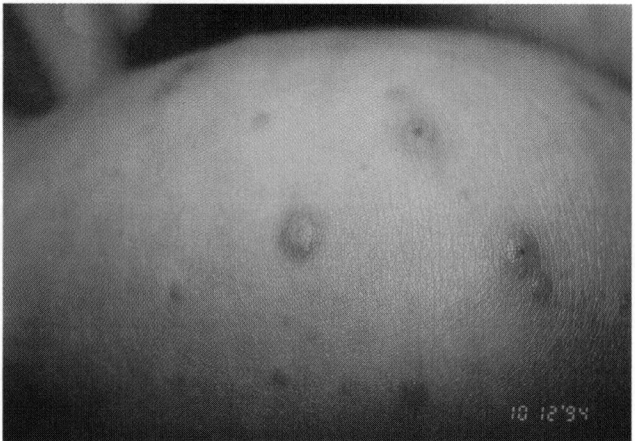

Figure 70-23. Close-up of succulent papules on the knee of the same girl depicted in Figure 70-22.

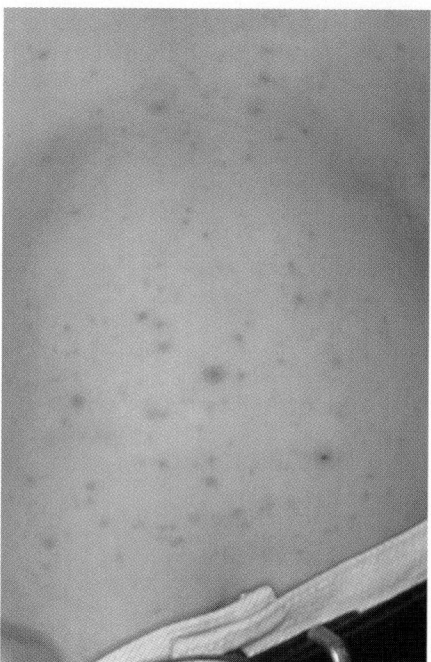

Figure 70-24. Pityriasis lichenoides et varioliformis acuta on the abdomen of a young girl.

without scarring. PLC tends to follow a more protracted course than PLEVA, with lesions recurring for 6 months to several years.

The differential diagnosis of PLEVA includes varicella, insect bite reaction, scabies, impetigo, and vasculitis. PLC may be confused with Gianotti-Crosti syndrome, papular eczema, pityriasis rosea, secondary syphilis, guttate psoriasis, and lichen planus. A skin biopsy often is needed to make a definitive diagnosis.

Pityriasis lichenoides has a tendency to wax and wane in severity. In the acute stages, it is not uncommon for the patient to experience exacerbations and remissions, lasting several months at a time, with eventual clearing. Although there are no data to support an infectious etiology for pityriasis lichenoides, a several-week course of oral erythromycin (40 mg/kg/day) is often beneficial for young children with PLEVA; adolescents and adults may be treated with oral tetracycline in high doses (2 g/day). Midpotency topical corticosteroids applied twice daily may decrease the

inflammatory component of PLEVA, but they may have no effect on the overall course of the eruption; PLC tends to be less responsive to topical corticosteroid therapy. Most patients respond favorably to natural sunlight used with topical coal tar preparations or UVB therapy in a dermatologist's office or a tanning salon. Methotrexate and PUVA therapy are reserved for treatment of children with more severe, ulceronecrotic cases of PLEVA or adults with prolonged debilitating cases of PLC.

Reports in the literature suggest that pityriasis lichenoides may be part of the spectrum of cutaneous T-cell lymphoma. Although most of the individuals with malignant transformation are adults, there are a few reports of children with chronic pityriasis lichenoides evolving into cutaneous T-cell lymphoma after several years. Individuals with pityriasis lichenoides that proves to be unremitting and individuals who develop atypical lesions should have biopsies performed to look for malignant transformation.

LYMPHOMATOID PAPULOSIS

Lymphomatoid papulosis is a recurrent, self-healing, papulonecrotic eruption that histologically resembles lymphoma. It is considered by some to be a variant of pityriasis lichenoides, a pseudolymphoma, or a low-grade form of cutaneous T-cell lymphoma. It is rarely encountered in children. Of patients with lymphomatoid papulosis, 10% to 20%, usually adults, have or are diagnosed later with a lymphoma, such as cutaneous T-cell lymphoma, Hodgkin's disease, or non-Hodgkin's lymphoma. Lymphomatoid papulosis is characterized by mildly pruritic, reddish brown papules with a smooth surface that become scaly and develop hemorrhagic necrotic crusted centers (Fig. 70-26). Ulcerated nodules may form in some cases (Fig. 70-27). The lesions arise in crops and are localized to the trunk and proximal extremities. The papules and nodules evolve over

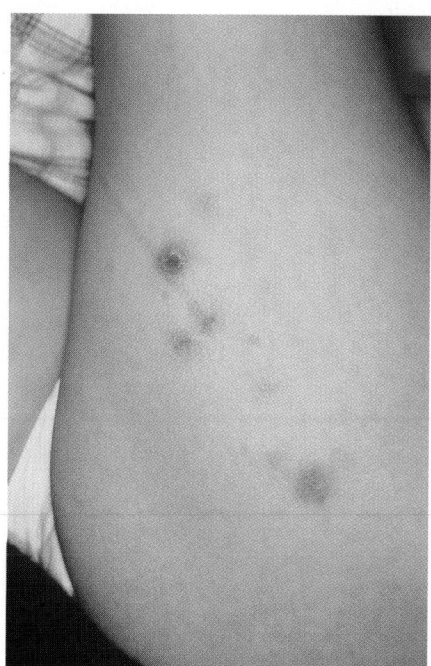

Figure 70-26. Lymphomatoid papulosis on the posterior thigh of a young girl.

Figure 70-25. Pityriasis lichenoides chronica on the back of a young girl.

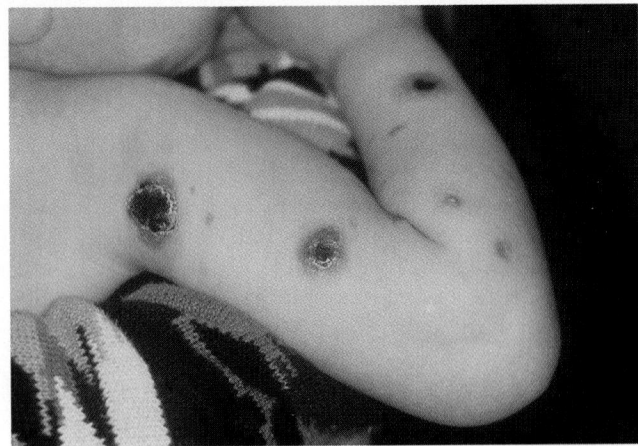

Figure 70-27. Ulcerated nodules in a young boy with lymphomatoid papulosis.

several weeks and eventually involute, leaving behind post-inflammatory hyperpigmentation, hypopigmentation, and scars. Lymphomatoid papulosis may follow a protracted course, with new crops of lesions arising over several years. The differential diagnosis of lymphomatoid papulosis in childhood includes insect bite reaction, pityriasis lichenoides, pseudolymphoma, primary cutaneous Hodgkin's disease, and large cell anaplastic lymphoma.

Midpotency topical corticosteroids and systemic antibiotics (erythromycin or tetracycline) have been used with variable success in lymphomatoid papulosis. Pulsed application of ultrapotent topical corticosteroids has been more efficacious. Although the risk is small, childhood-onset lymphomatoid papulosis may be a harbinger of lymphoma. Careful ongoing surveillance of children with lymphomatoid papulosis is imperative.

Additional Resources, CD-ROM

Color atlas	Figures
Bibliography	

Mini-index of Related Topics

	CH.
◼ DISORDERS OF THE HAIR AND NAILS	72
◼ VESICULOBULLOUS DISORDERS	73
◼ INFECTIOUS DISEASES IN THE NEONATE	209
◼ ADOLESCENTS AND SEXUALLY TRANSMITTED DISEASES	224

SUGGESTED READINGS

Hartley AH: Pityriasis rosea. Pediatr Rev 1999;20:266–269.
Leman J, Burden D: Psoriasis in children: A guide to its diagnosis and management. Paediatr Drugs 2001;3:673–680.
Nelson JS, Stone MS: Update on selected viral exanthems. Curr Opin Pediatr 2000;12:359–364.
Sharma R, Maheshwari V: Childhood lichen planus: A report of fifty cases. Pediatr Dermatol 1999;16:345–348.
Vanderhooft SL, Francis JS, Holbrook KA, et al: Familial pityriasis rubra pilaris. Arch Dermatol 1995;131:448–453.

71

Disorders of the Sebaceous and Sweat Glands

Mark Herron and Sheryll L. Vanderhooft

ROLE OF THE GENERALIST

1   Identify age-specific presentations of acne in a newborn, infant, preadolescent, and adolescent.

2   Recognize when evaluation for an underlying endocrinologic abnormality is indicated in a patient with acne.

3   Refer to a dermatologist for treatment of severe, nodulocystic, scarring acne or acne that is refractory to conventional treatment.

4   Recognize acne variants, including periorificial dermatitis, drug-induced acne, and acne keloidalis nuchae.

5   Recognize hidradenitis suppurativa and Fox-Fordyce disease as apocrine disorders.

6   Recognize and manage disorders of the eccrine sweat glands, including miliaria, hyperhidrosis, and palmoplantar eccrine hidradenitis.

FUNDAMENTALS

Pilosebaceous units consist of sebaceous glands in association with a hair follicle (Fig. 71-1). They are found everywhere on the body except the palms and the soles. Sebaceous glands develop early in embryogenesis at 3 months, from a bulge in the hair follicle. The sebaceous glands are well differentiated alongside the hair follicles at 4 months' gestation. Pilosebaceous units become active at birth as a reaction to maternal hormones. Sebaceous glands, large in newborn infants, diminish in size early in childhood and are quiescent during most of childhood. Sebaceous glands begin to enlarge at 10 or 12 years of age, become active during adolescence, and continue to grow until adulthood.

Apocrine sweat units, generally confined to the axillae, areolae, and anogenital region, are connected to the opening of the hair follicle, rather than the skin surface. Apocrine glands form from the upper portion of the hair follicle beginning in the fourth month of gestation and coinciding with new hair formation. Although immature apocrine sweat glands are found covering the entire surface of the fetus, they regress as the fetus reaches term.

Eccrine sweat units are found virtually all over the human body but are most abundant on the palms, soles, forehead,

and axillae. The germinative eccrine units develop on the palms and soles in the fourth month of gestation, appear over the axillae early in the fifth month, and develop over the entire body later in the fifth month. Differentiation of the secretory units continues until term. At 9 months' gestation, the eccrine glands morphologically resemble eccrine glands in adults. Eccrine glands of the palms and soles are functional at birth; the sweat glands of the rest of the skin become functional within months. Heat is the primary stimulus that causes the eccrine sweat glands to produce sweat; mental and gustatory stimuli also affect sweat production. Eccrine sweating is controlled by the sympathetic nervous system.

Acne is an inflammatory disease of the pilosebaceous unit that is characterized clinically by comedones (blackheads and whiteheads) (Fig. 71-2), inflammatory papules, pustules, nodules, and cysts. Acne affects 17 million people in the

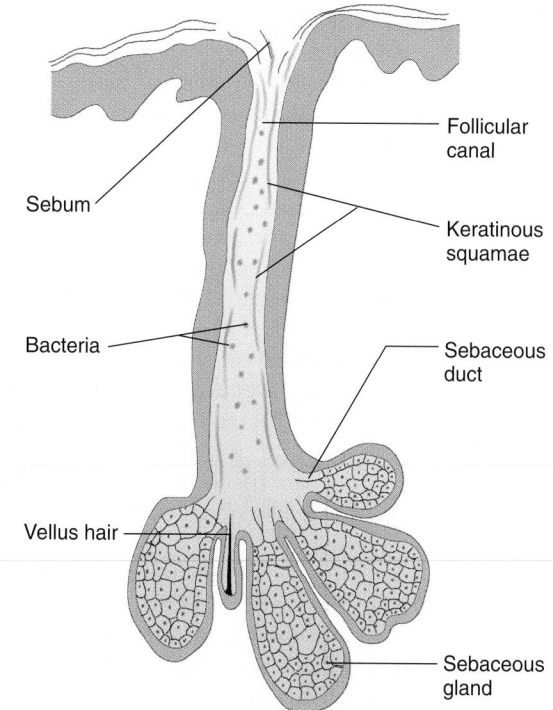

Figure 71-1. The pilosebaceous unit. (Adapted from Leyden JJ: New understandings of the pathogenesis of acne. J Am Acad Dermatol 1995;32:S15.)

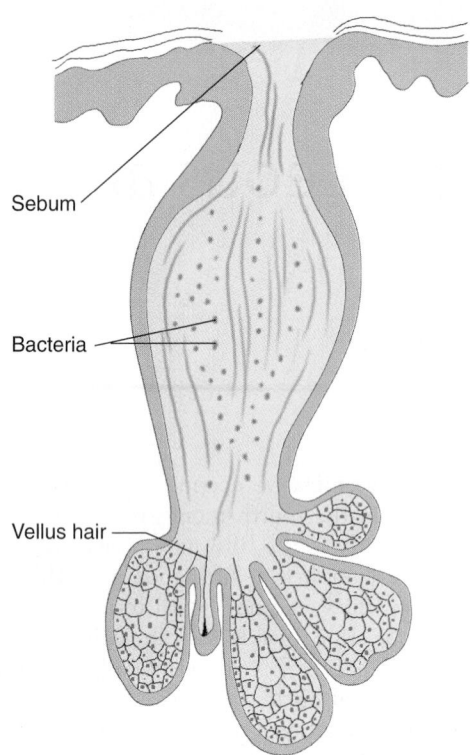

Figure 71-2. Microcomedone. (Adapted from Leyden JJ: New understandings of the pathogenesis of acne. J Am Acad Dermatol 1995;32:S19.)

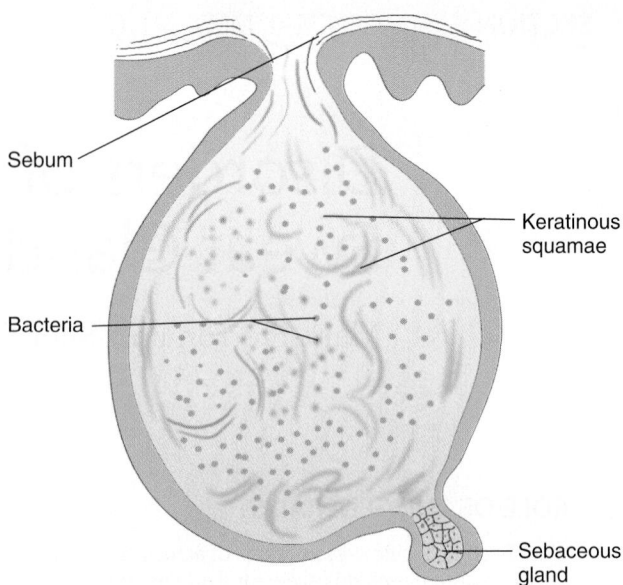

Figure 71-3. Closed comedone. (Adapted from Leyden JJ: New understandings of the pathogenesis of acne. J Am Acad Dermatol 1995;32:S19.)

United States and is the most common skin condition treated by physicians. It affects 80% of people 10 to 30 years old. Acne in adolescence is discussed in Chapter 223. Noninflammatory acne is characterized by open and closed comedones. If the opening of the follicle is tight, a *closed comedone* (whitehead) is produced (Fig. 71-3). These are small white papules beneath the skin surface. Closed comedones have no surrounding erythema. *Open comedones* (blackheads) are keratin-filled follicles with a dilated opening (Fig. 71-4). The blackness of the tip of the open comedone results from the presence of melanin, not dirt. Inflammatory acne is characterized by erythematous papules, pustules, nodules, and cysts. The most severe form is nodular disease that has undergone suppuration. Scarring occurs in adolescents who have nodular acne; however, any inflammatory lesion may produce scarring.

Hidradenitis suppurativa is a chronic suppurative scarring disorder of the apocrine sweat glands. Occlusion of the apocrine duct is the inciting event. Keratin plugs form and dilate the ducts. Secondary bacterial infection and abscess formation with subsequent rupture promote the extension of the process to deeper tissue. *Fox-Fordyce disease* (apocrine miliaria) is caused by obstruction and rupture of the apocrine ducts, leading to apocrine sweat retention.

Miliaria is caused by sweat retention resulting from obstruction of the eccrine sweat ducts. Excessive hydration of the stratum corneum secondary to prolonged exposure to perspiration leads to maceration and keratinous plugging of the sweat ducts; disruption of the ducts allows the eccrine sweat to escape into the skin below the level of the obstruction, causing miliaria. The incidence of miliaria is highest during the first few weeks of life, when the eccrine

ducts are not completely developed. Aerobic bacteria increase in number as a result of hydration of the epidermis and may play a role in the obstruction of the eccrine ducts. *Hyperhidrosis* refers to excessive eccrine sweat production. *Palmoplantar eccrine hidradenitis* is an inflammatory condition affecting the eccrine sweat glands.

ACNE

Neonatal Acne

Neonatal acne occurs as a response to maternal hormonal stimulation of pilosebaceous glands that have not yet involuted into the childhood state of inactivity. It is seen in 20% of newborns, with a slightly higher incidence in boys. It is characterized by superficial inflammatory papules, pustules, and closed comedones that usually are confined to the cheeks but also may arise on the chin and forehead

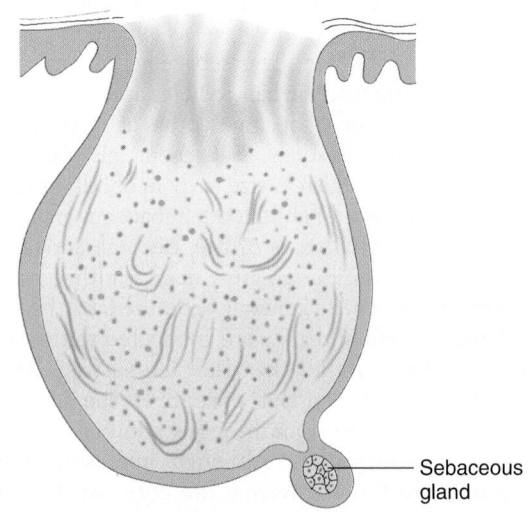

Figure 71-4. Open comedone. (Adapted from Leyden JJ: New understandings of the pathogenesis of acne. J Am Acad Dermatol 1995;32:S19.)

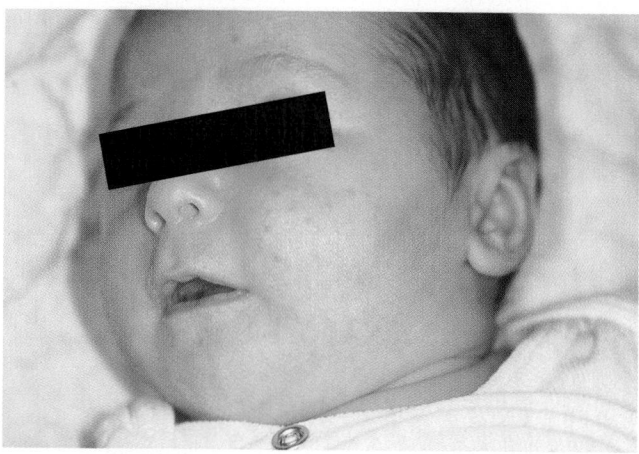

Figure 71-5. Neonatal acne. (Courtesy of Department of Dermatology, University of Utah, Salt Lake City, Utah.)

(Fig. 71-5). The closed comedones can be distinguished from milia, which appear as 1- to 2-mm pearly white or yellow papules, most commonly located on the nose, although they also may be seen on the forehead, cheeks, and chin. Milia develop from retention of keratin and sebum within the pilosebaceous apparatus of the newborn. They usually last 3 to 4 weeks, although they may persist for months. Neonatal acne and milia require no therapy. Picking and squeezing the lesions should be discouraged because this may cause scarring. Gentle cleansing with a mild soap is all that is necessary; scrubbing should be avoided.

Infantile Acne

Infantile acne presents at 3 to 6 months of age, with a higher incidence in boys. It is due to precocious secretion of androgens by the gonads. Numerous comedones may progress to inflammatory papules and pustules (Fig. 71-6). Rarely, nodules and scar formation accompany infantile acne. Infantile acne may resolve in the second or third year, although persistence into the teens may occur. In contrast to neonatal acne, infantile acne is associated with a family history of moderate-to-severe acne, and infants with the disorder are at higher risk to develop moderate-to-severe acne during adolescence. A complete physical examination is indicated to evaluate the possibility of an underlying

endocrine disorder, with special attention paid to height and weight, which are increased in precocious puberty. The scrotum should be evaluated for hyperpigmentation, and the abdomen should be palpated carefully for masses. Laboratory screening should include adrenocorticotropic hormone (ACTH), 17-hydroxyprogesterone, dehydro-epiandrosterone sulfate, and androstenedione levels. If the ACTH is elevated, magnetic resonance imaging of the brain should be obtained to evaluate the pituitary gland. If the ACTH is normal or low and any of the other laboratory tests are high, magnetic resonance imaging of the abdomen should be obtained to evaluate the adrenal glands. An infant with acne should be approached in a fashion similar to a teenager with acne vulgaris (see Chapter 223), with combination therapy using topical comedolytic agents and topical or oral antibiotics. In cases of severe cystic scarring in infantile acne, treatment with oral isotretinoin may be required.

Prepubertal Acne

Prepubertal acne is primarily comedonal with a midfacial predilection. It is correlated more with pubertal stage than with age. Comedonal acne arises during Tanner stage I and is seen in 100% of children at Tanner stage IV. Inflammatory acne is not seen during Tanner stage I but is seen in 50% of children at Tanner stage IV. Prepubertal acne is common and should not prompt an evaluation for an underlying endocrine disorder. Comedonal acne may be seen in 5-year-olds. Acne usually begins 1 to 2 years before the onset of puberty.

Acne Vulgaris

Acne vulgaris during the teen years arises on the face, upper neck, chest, and back, where the pilosebaceous units are densely concentrated. The diagnosis and management of acne vulgaris are discussed in Chapter 223.

Cystic acne is the most severe form of acne vulgaris. The predominant lesions are deep-seated nodules that suppurate and resolve with prominent scarring. *Acne conglobata* is an unremitting suppurative form of acne seen primarily in men 18 to 30 years old. Cysts and abscesses develop interconnecting sinus tracts that burrow underneath the skin surface. These cysts are localized to the forehead, cheeks, and anterior neck. The result is prominent scarring, often with keloid formation. A rare syndrome of synovitis, acne, pustulosis, hyperostosis, and osteitis, or *SAPHO syndrome*, is associated with a variety of inflammatory skin conditions. SAPHO syndrome is characterized by chronic recurrent multifocal osteomyelitis, osteoarticular inflammation, and severe acne. Other cutaneous features include palmoplantar pustulosis, nonpalmoplantar pustulosis, and psoriasis. This disorder affects children and young adults, particularly men.

PERIORIFICIAL DERMATITIS

Periorificial dermatitis is a chronic condition seen most commonly in young and middle-aged women, but it can be seen in infants and prepubertal children. Periorificial dermatitis is characterized by erythematous pinpoint papules, sometimes with overlying scale, and pustules confined to the perioral, perinasal, and periorbital areas

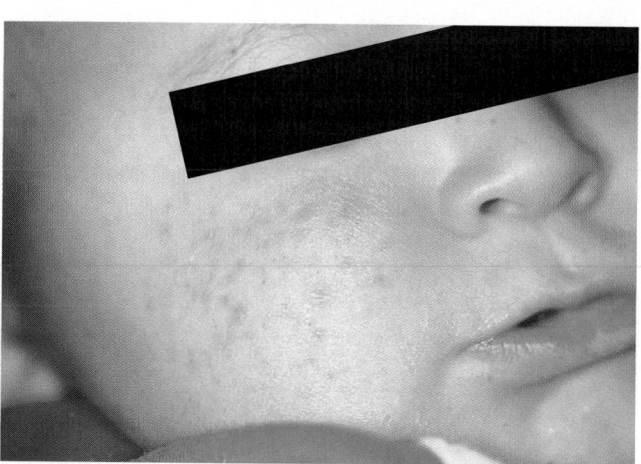

Figure 71-6. Infantile acne.

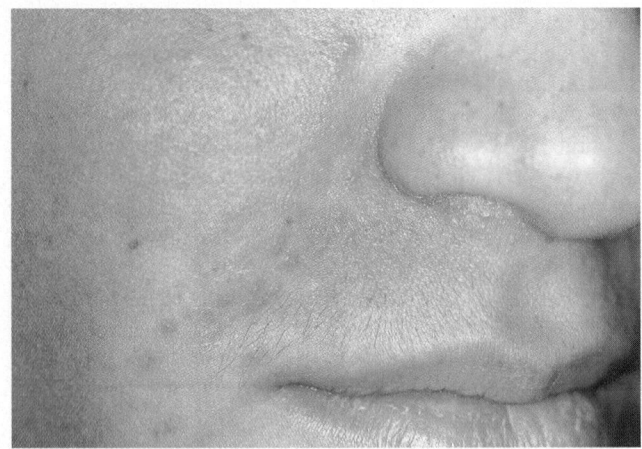

Figure 71-7. Periorificial dermatitis in a teenage boy.

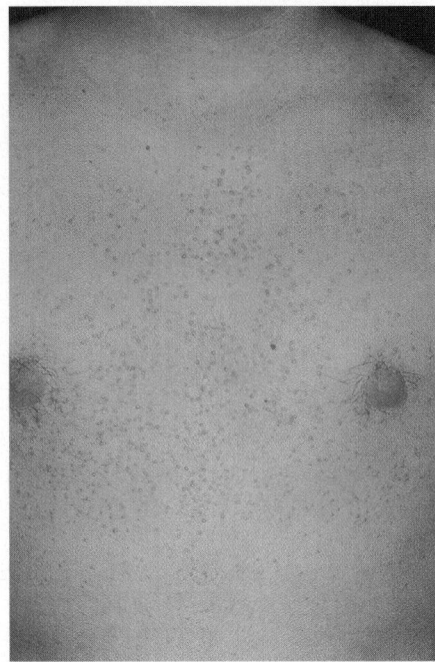

Figure 71-8. Steroid folliculitis in a patient with dermatomyositis.

with a clear zone around the vermilion border of the lips (Fig. 71-7). Patients may describe burning and stinging; pruritus is uncommon. The dermatitis tends to wax and wane for months. It may arise as a primary entity or may follow treatment of facial dermatitis with potent fluorinated topical corticosteroids. It also has been linked to fluoride in toothpaste. Treatment includes topical metronidazole, topical erythromycin, and oral erythromycin in more extensive or refractory cases; oral tetracycline may be used in older children and teenagers. In many cases, an initial worsening of the eruption may occur with initiation of treatment. The patient should be made aware of this complication. In cases of long-term topical steroid abuse, the dermatitis worsens when the topical steroids are withdrawn, and a low-dose topical steroid, such as hydrocortisone 1% cream, may be employed for a short course. Periorificial dermatitis can be chronic and recurring.

DRUG-INDUCED ACNEIFORM ERUPTIONS

Drugs may induce a folliculitis that resembles acne but differs from true acne because of the absence of comedones. Systemic corticosteroids employed as immunosuppressive therapy are notorious for producing this type of eruption, particularly when the doses are tapered. The eruption presents as monomorphous erythematous papules and pustules, located predominantly on the chest, back, upper arms, and neck (Fig. 71-8). Iodides found in vitamin and mineral supplements cause follicular pustules on the face and upper chest; bromides used to treat myoclonic epilepsy cause the same type of eruption. Isoniazid can cause an acneiform eruption characterized by reddish brown follicular papules that begin on the face and spread to the trunk. Treatment consists of avoiding the offending drug if possible and use of topical or oral antibiotics.

ACNE KELOIDALIS

Acne keloidalis, a chronic folliculitis and perifolliculitis predisposed to the nape of the neck (Fig. 71-9), is seen most frequently in postpubertal African-American male patients. Because comedones are absent, this is an acneiform eruption rather than true acne. The chronic folliculitis leads to keloid formation over the affected area. Treatment

includes topical and systemic antibiotics and intralesional corticosteroids.

HIDRADENITIS SUPPURATIVA

Hidradenitis suppurativa is characterized by tender erythematous papules, cysts, and nodules arising in apocrine sweat gland–bearing skin in the axillary, anogenital, and breast regions (Fig. 71-10). Fluctuant cysts rupture and cause suppuration and sinus tract and scar formation. The disorder typically presents at puberty, affects girls more commonly than boys, and is worsened by obesity. Weight loss may improve the condition. Hidradenitis can be controlled but not cured by medication. Intralesional steroids reduce the inflammation and pain of the nodules and cysts. Oral antibiotic therapy should be directed by culture of purulent lesions and draining sinus tracts, which often consists of long-term use of tetracycline, minocycline, or sulfa drugs. Isotretinoin may be useful, but recurrences are frequent after discontinuation. Early referral to a general

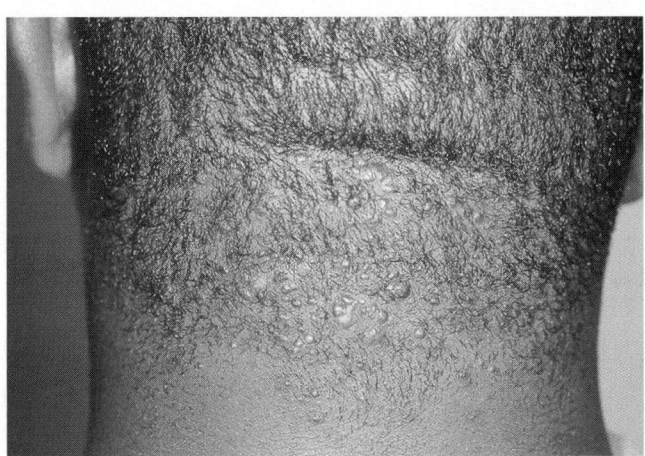

Figure 71-9. Acne keloidalis nuchae.

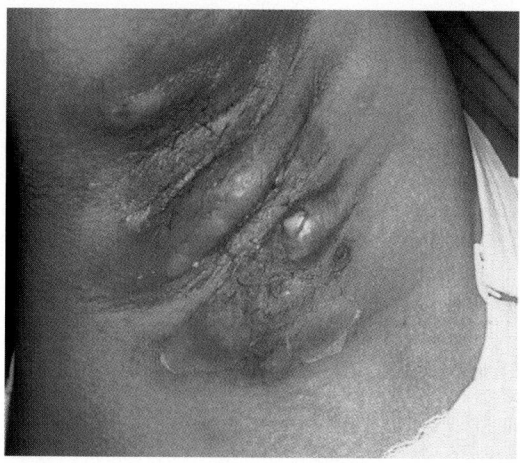

Figure 71-10. Hidradenitis suppurativa. (From Kaminer MS, Gilchrest BA: The many faces of acne. J Am Acad Dermatol 1995;32:S9. Courtesy of Richard B. Odom, MD, San Francisco, California.)

or plastic surgeon for surgical removal of the affected areas followed by skin grafts should be considered for patients who do not respond to medical management.

MILIARIA

Fox-Fordyce disease (apocrine miliaria), a chronic pruritic papular eruption affecting the axillae, periareolar and intermammary regions, and groin, most commonly affects adolescent girls and young women. The follicular papules are small, smooth, and flesh colored. Patients should be advised of the chronicity of this disorder and the possible need for long-term therapy. Keratolytic agents and topical antibiotics (e.g., clindamycin) have been used to treat patients with recalcitrant disease. High-dose estrogen oral contraceptives, estrogen creams, and testosterone creams have been reported to be beneficial in some women.

Miliaria crystallina is caused by a superficial obstruction of the eccrine sweat ducts. The lesions appear in crops within days of exposure to a hot environment. It affects approximately 5% of infants, with a peak incidence at 1 week of age, and presents with pinpoint asymptomatic vesicles arising in crops, typically localized to the head, neck, axillae, and areas on the trunk covered by clothing

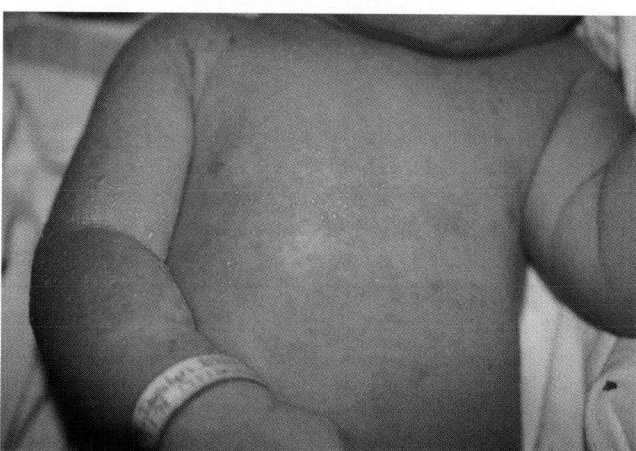

Figure 71-11. Miliaria crystallina in a newborn whose mother had a fever before delivery.

(Fig. 71-11). The vesicles rupture easily and resolve spontaneously with superficial desquamation.

Miliaria rubra ("prickly heat"), the most frequently encountered variant of miliaria, is characterized by pruritic erythematous papules and papulovesicles. It can be differentiated from folliculitis by the lack of hairs arising from the center of the lesions, which most commonly are found on the neck, upper torso, axillae, and groin. Lesions resolve spontaneously within days.

Miliaria profunda, the most severe form of miliaria, is caused by deep obstruction of the eccrine sweat ducts and is seen almost exclusively in tropical climates. It is characterized by firm white papules on the trunk and extremities and may resemble gooseflesh, although the lesions are not follicular. Management involves prevention of sweating by limiting exposure to excessive heat and humidity, taking cool baths, and wearing light and loose-fitting clothing. Topical anhydrous lanolin may prevent blockage of the sweat ducts and has been reported to dramatically improve some patients who are prone to miliaria. The pruritus of miliaria rubra may be treated with antipruritic lotions containing camphor and menthol (e.g., Sarna anti-itch lotion) or a topical anesthetic, such as 1% pramoxine (e.g., Aveeno anti-itch lotion).

HYPERHIDROSIS

Hyperhidrosis, characterized by excessive sweating of the palms, soles, and axillae, may have autosomal dominant inheritance. It typically begins during childhood or at puberty and persists throughout life. Hyperhidrosis of the axillae and palms can be a socially disturbing condition. Occlusive sneakers, boots, and shoes enhance hyperhidrosis of the soles of the feet. Fissuring and cracking arise from the repetitive cycles of wetting and drying. Hyperhidrosis may contribute to tinea pedis and contact dermatitis. Prevention of hyperhidrosis can be accomplished with the use of absorbent powders (e.g., ZeaSorb), avoidance of occlusive footwear, frequent changes of the socks, and applications of light emollients to prevent drying. Aluminum chloride hexahydrate 20% solution (Drysol) blocks the sweat pores and can reduce sweating when applied nightly for 1 week. With the reduction of sweating, the patient can maintain the response with less frequent applications. When no response is seen, the solution may be applied under occlusion with plastic wrap for several consecutive nights until sweating is reduced. A patient with axillary hyperhidrosis should wear light-colored clothing made of natural and absorbent fabric, avoid high-buttoned collars, use talcum powder or cornstarch, and shave the axillae if appropriate.

Dermatologists may treat patients with hyperhidrosis using iontophoresis, low-voltage electric current held against the skin of the palms and soles while immersed in an electrolyte solution. Iontophoresis is difficult to apply in axillary hyperhidrosis and impossible to use in diffuse hyperhidrosis. *Botulinum* toxin injections have been used for axillary hyperhidrosis, with the decrease in sweating lasting approximately 6 to 12 months. Excision of the axillary sweat glands may be considered in severe axillary hyperhidrosis. Sympathectomy to interrupt nerves that trigger the sweat glands is an option for severe facial, palmar, and axillary hyperhidrosis refractory to medical management.

PALMOPLANTAR ECCRINE HIDRADENITIS

Palmoplantar eccrine hidradenitis is characterized by the sudden onset of tender erythematous papules, plaques, and nodules on the plantar surfaces of the feet (Fig. 71-12) and,

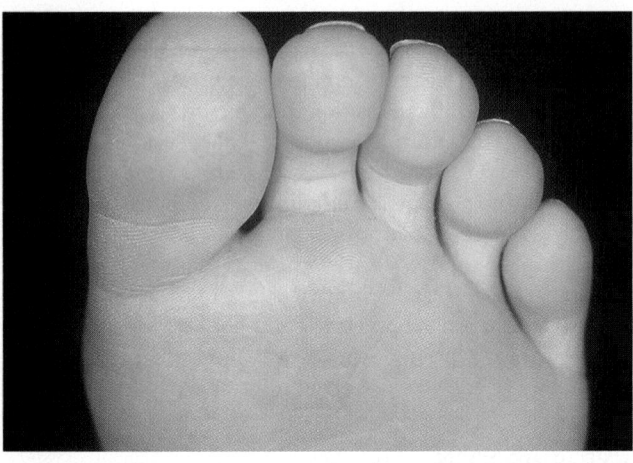

Figure 71-12. Palmoplantar eccrine hidradenitis.

less commonly, the palmar surfaces of the hands. The cause is unknown, although mechanical or thermal trauma leading to rupture of the palmoplantar eccrine glands has been suggested as a potential cause. The disorder presents most commonly during the autumn and the spring. Most children have self-limited lesions, with resolution in 1 to 3 weeks, but recurrences are seen in some patients. The pain associated with the lesions may limit ambulation. Nonsteroidal anti-inflammatory drugs may be beneficial.

Mini-index of Related Topics	CH.
■ DISORDERS OF PUBERTAL DEVELOPMENT	151
■ ACNE	223

SUGGESTED READINGS

Landau M, Metzker A, Gat A, et al: Palmoplantar eccrine hidradenitis: Three new cases and review. Pediatr Dermatol 1998;15:97–102.
Lucky AW: A review of infantile and pediatric acne. Dermatology 1998;196:95–97.
Manders SM, Lucky AW: Perioral dermatitis in childhood. J Am Acad Dermatol 1992;27:688–692.
Simon M, Cremer H, von den Driesch P: Idiopathic recurrent palmoplantar hidradenitis in children: Report of 22 cases. Arch Dermatol 1998;134:76–79.

SECTION 3   GENERAL MEDICAL CARE: *Disorders of the Skin*

72 Disorders of the Hair and Nails

Mark Herron and Sheryll L. Vanderhooft

ROLE OF THE GENERALIST

1 Recognize normal hair growth cycle.
2 Identify different patterns of hair loss.
3 Formulate a differential diagnosis, and initiate appropriate laboratory investigation.
4 Differentiate between hypertrichosis and hirsutism.
5 Recognize normal anatomy and development of the nail unit.
6 Recognize nail disorders that signify underlying systemic illness.
7 Refer to dermatologist for assistance in evaluation or management when needed.

DISORDERS OF HAIR

Fundamentals

In the human fetus, buds of follicular cells appear in the epidermis at 8 weeks of gestation. These buds differentiate to form hair follicles. Hair growth begins between 8 and 12 weeks of gestation. *Lanugo hairs* are fine, soft, and poorly pigmented and are present during the fetal and neonatal periods. They appear over the entire cutaneous surface of the fetus. In utero, lanugo hairs are shed during the last few weeks of gestation. Premature infants frequently are covered diffusely with lanugo hairs. *Vellus hairs* are fine and lightly pigmented. They are present on the arms and face of children and the faces of women. *Terminal hairs* are mature, thick, dark hairs on the scalp, eyebrows, eyelashes, axillae, and groin.

The hair growth cycle is characterized by three distinct phases (Fig. 72-1). During the *anagen phase*, the hairs are actively growing. This phase lasts 2 to 6 years (average 3 years). The length of the anagen phase determines how long the hairs grow. Scalp hair has a long anagen phase; eyebrows and eyelashes have a short anagen phase. The *catagen phase* is a short period of 10 to 14 days during which the follicle undergoes partial regression. The *telogen phase* is a resting period that lasts 3 to 4 months; all activity ceases, and the follicle rests. At the end of the telogen phase, new hair growth is initiated. The new growing anagen hairs push out the old telogen hairs that have remained in the follicles. The telogen hairs that are shed are called *club hairs* because they have a solid white node at the proximal end (Fig. 72-2). This white node represents a lack of pigment.

The average human scalp contains approximately 100,000 hairs. In the healthy scalp, 85% of the hair is actively growing, 5% is in a state of involution, and 10% is in the resting phase. Each day, 50 to 100 hairs are shed and replaced. The average growth rate of a terminal hair is 0.3 to 0.4 mm/day, which is equivalent to on average 2.5 mm/week or 10 mm/month.

Terminal hairs begin growing actively at birth. Within the first few days of life, there is a physiologic conversion from the anagen phase to the telogen phase. This conversion leads to shedding of a large portion of the newborn scalp hair within the first 4 months of life. Telogen shedding of a newborn may occur suddenly or gradually and typically is generalized over the scalp. Replacement of the first terminal hairs is complete by the first 6 months of life. Frequently the neonate has a hairline of terminal hairs that extends along the forehead to the temples and the lateral margins of the eyebrows. These terminal hairs convert to vellus hairs during the first year of life.

Diagnosis

When evaluating a child with hair loss, it is helpful to know whether the process is congenital or acquired. The physician needs to determine whether the hair loss was gradual or sudden in onset; the hair density usually is reduced by 50% before thinning is apparent. A history of preceding physical or psychological stress (e.g., illness with high fever, surgical procedures, hospitalizations, trauma, move to a new home, birth of a sibling, divorce of parents, death of a family member) may indicate a temporary upset in the hair growth cycle. The presence of systemic disease may point to an underlying cause for the hair loss (e.g., thyroid disease). Medications the child has taken should be studied thoroughly for their association with alopecia. A family history of hair loss is significant.

During the examination, the pattern of hair loss needs to be identified because this leads to formulation of a differ-

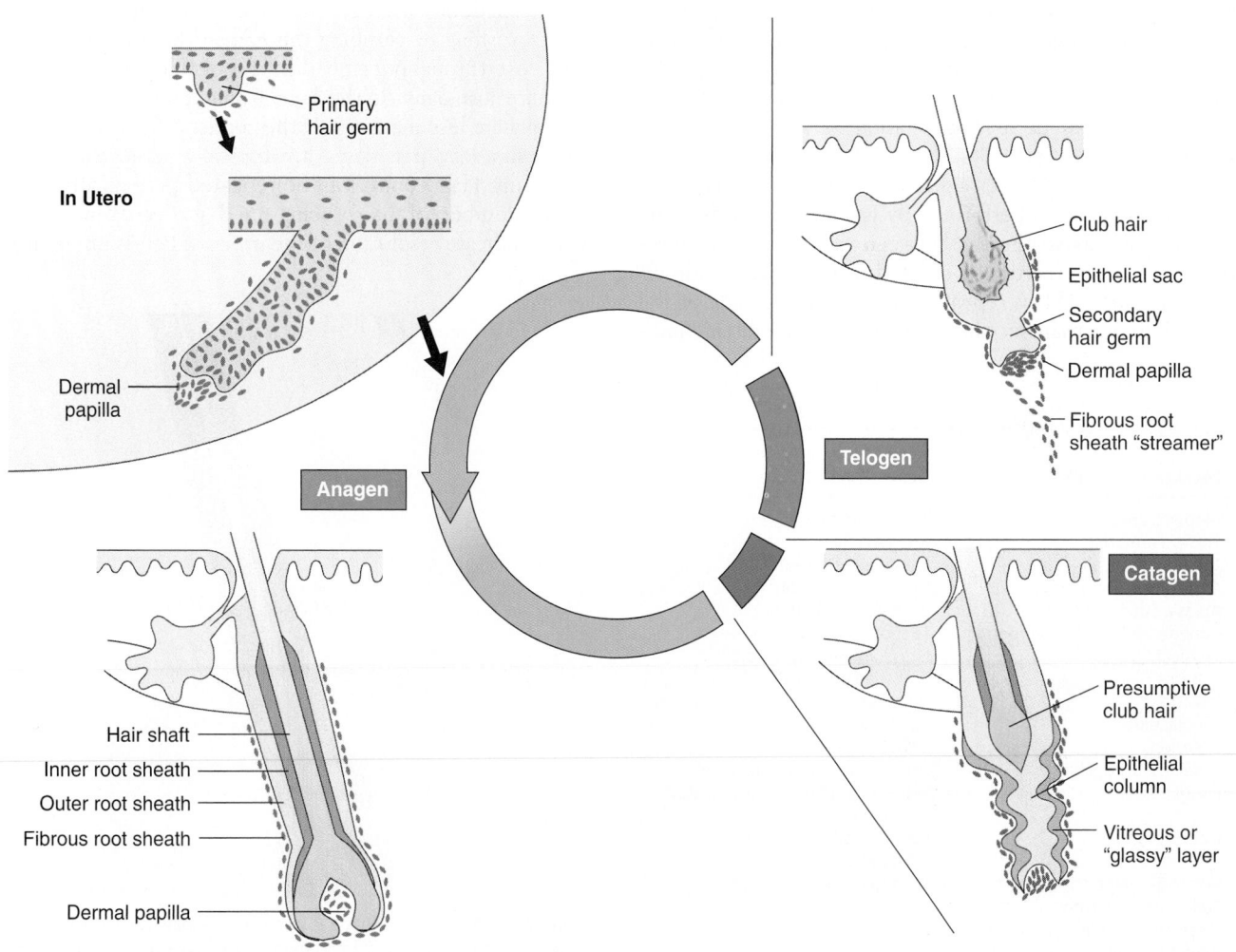

Figure 72-1. Normal hair growth cycle. (From Sperling LC: Hair anatomy for the clinician. J Am Acad Dermatol 1991;25:4.)

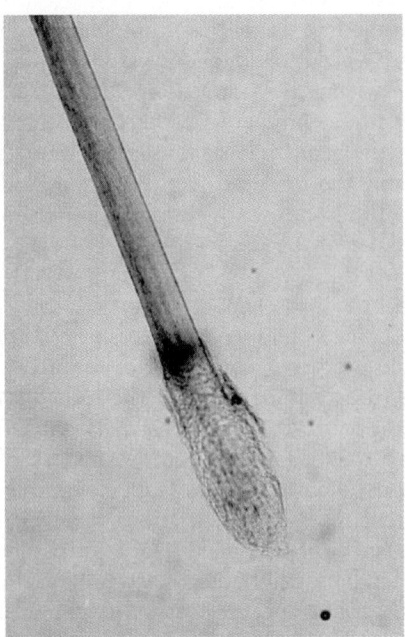

Figure 72-2. Shed telogen hair with a club-shaped bulb. (From Sperling LC: Evaluation of hair loss. Curr Prob Dermatol 1996;8:104.)

Table 72-2. Scarring versus Nonscarring Alopecia

Scarring	Nonscarring
Aplasia cutis congenita	Telogen effluvium
Kerion	Anagen effluvium
Chemical or thermal injury	Metabolic disorders or nutritional deficiencies
Traction alopecia (chronic)	Alopecia areata
Trichotillomania (chronic)	Androgenetic alopecia
Lupus	Traction alopecia
Lichen planopilaris	Trichotillomania
Keratosis pilaris atrophicans	Congenital triangular alopecia
Folliculitis decalvans	Loose anagen syndrome
Dissecting cellulitis of the scalp	Hair shaft abnormalities
Acne keloidalis	Hereditary hypotrichosis
	Secondary syphilis

ential diagnosis. The hair loss should be described as localized or generalized (Table 72-1) and scarring or nonscarring (Table 72-2), and associated scale and erythema should be noted, which could indicate an inflammatory or infectious process. The physician needs to determine whether the hair loss is from the roots or secondary to hair breakage; the latter can result from trauma to the hair, can result from infection, or can be a manifestation of a structural hair abnormality.

Several diagnostic tests aid in the evaluation of hair loss. The *hair pull test* is performed by grasping about 50 hairs on the scalp above the ear between the thumb and forefinger. Constant traction is exerted as the fingers slide up the hair shafts. This is repeated on the opposite side of the scalp. If more than six club hairs are extracted, this indi-

cates the presence of telogen effluvium. The *hair pluck test* is a more painful technique. Approximately 50 hairs are grasped firmly using a hemostat with rubber-covered tips to extract the hairs, which are placed between two glass slides and examined under a microscope *(trichogram)*. The telogen hairs have bulbs that are small, round, and without pigment (see Fig. 72-2). The anagen hairs have bulbs that are pigmented and elongated (Fig. 72-3). The hairs also can be evaluated for abnormalities along the hair shafts that could indicate a hair shaft malformation (Fig. 72-4).

Hair counts are an exhaustive way to evaluate the degree of hair shedding. The patient collects hairs in a plastic bag when brushing or combing the hair in the morning and all hairs lost throughout the day, if possible. Normally 100 hairs are lost daily. If the hair is shampooed daily, counts typically are less than 100. If the counts reflect greater than 100 hairs lost per day, this typically indicates telogen effluvium. Hair counts can be repeated periodically to see if the number of hairs being shed is decreasing, which would indicate resolution of the process. Potassium hydrox-

Table 72-1. Localized versus Generalized Hair Loss

Localized Hair Loss	Generalized Hair Loss
Alopecia areata	Telogen effluvium
Trichotillomania	Anagen effluvium
Traction alopecia	Metabolic disorder
Androgenetic alopecia	Nutritional deficiency
Aplasia cutis congenita	Alopecia areata (severe)
Congenital triangular alopecia	Trichotillomania (severe)
Physical trauma	Loose anagen syndrome
Burns	Hair shaft abnomalities
Infection	Hereditary hypotrichosis
Folliculitis	Lupus (severe)
Kerion	Lichen planus (severe)
Secondary syphilis	Folliculitis decalvans (severe)
Lupus	Dissecting cellulitis of the scalp (severe)
Lichen planus	Keratosis pilaris atrophicans (severe)
Keratosis pilaris atrophicans	Secondary syphilis
Folliculitis decalvans	
Dissecting cellulitis of the scalp	
Acne keloidalis	

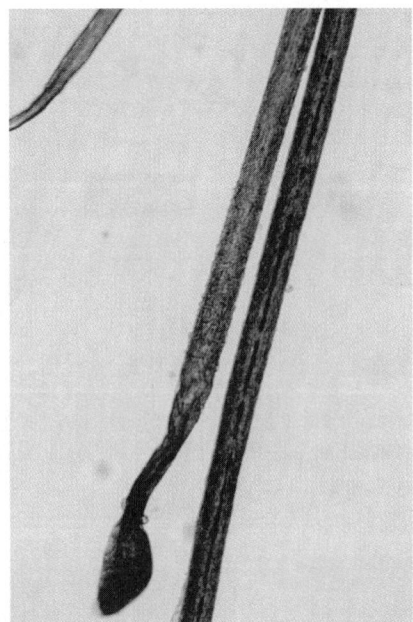

Figure 72-3. Anagen hair that has lost its root sheaths as an artifact of plucking. (From Sperling LC: Evaluation of hair loss. Curr Prob Dermatol 1996;8:105.)

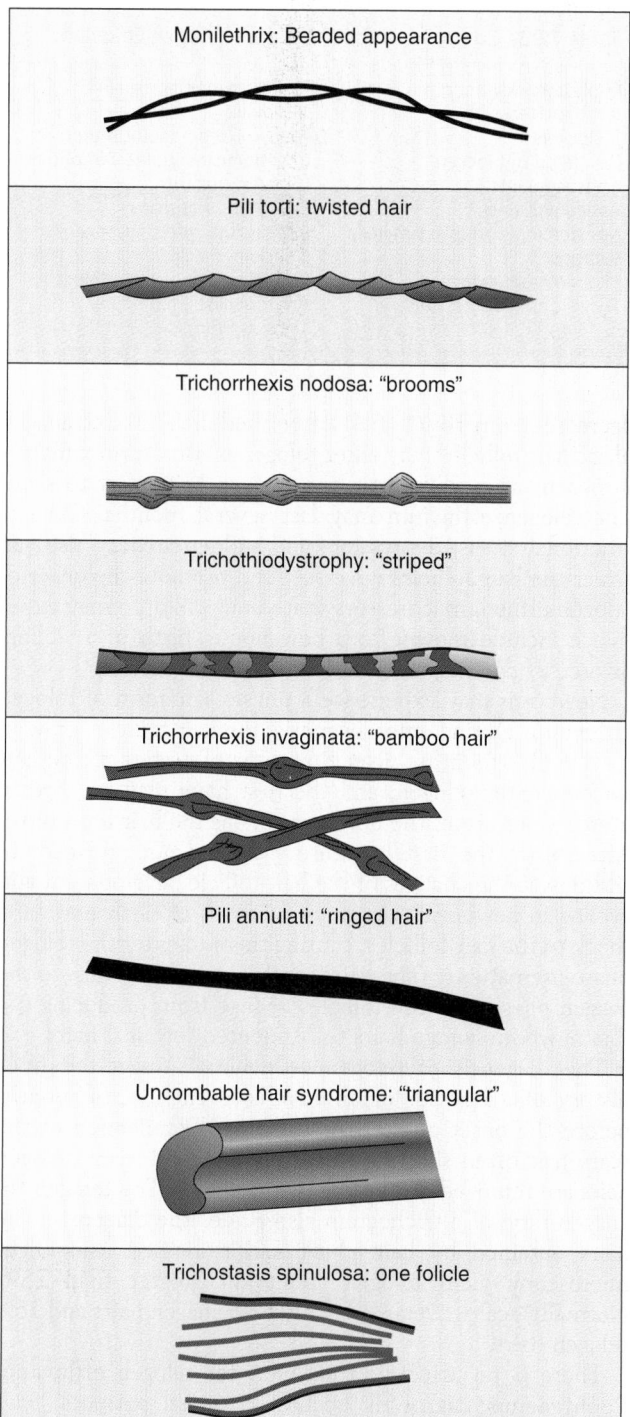

Monilethrix: Beaded appearance

Pili torti: twisted hair

Trichorrhexis nodosa: "brooms"

Trichothiodystrophy: "striped"

Trichorrhexis invaginata: "bamboo hair"

Pili annulati: "ringed hair"

Uncombable hair syndrome: "triangular"

Trichostasis spinulosa: one follicle

Figure 72-4. Schematic diagram of various hair shaft abnormalities.

ide examination and fungal culture of scales and hairs are used to diagnose fungal infections. Scalp biopsy may be indicated when the diagnosis is still in question. Determinations of thyroid function and the status of iron stores may be indicated; obtaining hormone levels is appropriate when virilization is suspected.

Congenital Hair Loss

Aplasia cutis congenita (congenital absence of skin) is a congenital anomaly present at birth in which there is localized absence of the epidermis, the dermis, and at times the subcutaneous fat. Although it typically arises on the

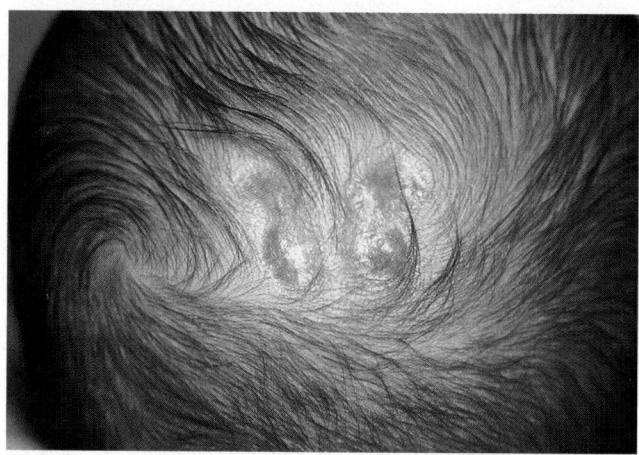

Figure 72-5. Aplasia cutis congenita in a newborn. Note open, eroded areas.

vertex of the scalp, it can be found anywhere on the scalp and body. This condition presents with an eroded area usually measuring a few centimeters in diameter (Fig. 72-5) that heals rapidly with a scar. Hair follicles are absent, so the affected area remains hairless (Fig. 72-6). Aplasia cutis congenita usually is seen as an isolated, sporadic defect, but it can be inherited as an autosomal dominantly. It has been linked to exposure to methimazole during pregnancy. Aplasia cutis congenita can be associated with other developmental anomalies, including limb reduction defects, myelomeningocele, spinal dysraphism, cranial stenosis, omphalocele, gastroschisis, and gastrointestinal atresia. It also may be part of a malformation syndrome, such as trisomy 13, 4p- syndrome, oculocerebrocutaneous syndrome, and focal dermal hypoplasia. Most lesions require no intervention. Extensive lesions can be closed surgically. Cosmetically, scars can be excised completely, or normal hair follicles can be transplanted to the affected area.

Congenital triangular alopecia is characterized by localized nonscarring alopecia over the frontotemporal portion of the scalp in a triangular configuration, with the wide end of the triangle facing inferiorly and anteriorly and the tip of the triangle pointing superiorly and posteriorly. This condition is discussed and shown on the CD-ROM (see CD-ROM Fig. 72-7).

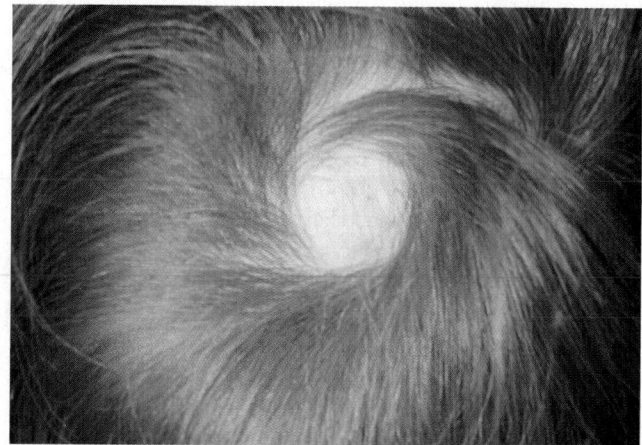

Figure 72-6. Aplasia cutis congenita in an older child. The affected area has healed with scarring alopecia.

Loose anagen syndrome is characterized by anagen hairs loosely anchored in the hair follicles. These hairs may be pulled from the scalp effortlessly. It usually is diagnosed between ages 2 and 5 years, when patients present with the complaint that "the hair does not grow" or that the child has "never needed a haircut." Affected children typically are blond girls with sparse, short, fine hair that is pulled out easily with brushing. Extensive alopecia of the posterior scalp may arise from rubbing on the pillow while sleeping, leaving the frontal scalp relatively less affected. Eyebrows and eyelashes are normal. With light microsopy, anagen hairs can be seen to lack an inner and outer root sheath. Loose anagen syndrome tends to improve with age. There is no effective treatment.

Structural abnormalities of the hair shafts can lead to unusual-appearing hair, with or without increased fragility. A variety of hair shaft abnormalities are distinguished by the morphology of the hair shafts as seen with light microscopy (see Fig. 72-4). These may present as isolated anomalies or may be part of a syndrome. There is no specific treatment for these disorders. Reduction of mechanical and chemical trauma to the hair helps minimize breakage in conditions that are associated with hair fragility. Uncommon hair shaft abnormalities, including monilethrix (beaded hair), pili torti (twisted hair), trichorrhexis nodosa, trichothiodystrophy, trichorrhexis invaginata, pili annulati, pili trianguli et canaliculi (uncombable hair syndrome, "spun glass hair"), wooly hair, trichostasis spinulosa, and trichorrhexis nodosa, are discussed on the CD-ROM.

Hereditary hypotrichosis (Marie Unna syndrome) is an autosomal dominant condition characterized by sparse or absent scalp hair, eyebrows, and eyelashes. Normal hair may be present during the neonatal period, but it is replaced during early childhood with coarse and twisted hairs. During puberty, the alopecia progresses, and the hairs become sparse. There is no known treatment.

Acquired Hair Loss

Telogen effluvium, the most common form of alopecia in children, is characterized by shedding of several hundred hairs a day globally over the scalp, leading to diffuse thinning of the hair. The normal phase of hair growth is terminated prematurely by a physical or psychological stressor so that a larger proportion of hairs than usual enter the resting phase of the hair cycle. A few months later, when the new anagen hairs begin to grow in the follicles, the old telogen hairs are shed. Telogen effluvium usually develops slowly over several months. The severity of the alopecia is related to the duration and severity of the stressor that altered the hair cycle. Recovery and return to normal hair density are slow and can take many months.

Physical stressors that can cause telogen effluvium include febrile illnesses, surgical shock, crash diets, injury, and exposure to certain medications (Table 72-3); discontinuation of estrogen-dominant oral contraceptives also can lead to telogen effluvium. High body temperatures stress the dividing cells of the hair follicles. Acute blood loss starves the hair follicles of nutrients, forcing the follicles into reduced activity. Postpartum alopecia is a common form of telogen effluvium. During the late stage of pregnancy, the percentage of hair follicles in the telogen phase

Table 72-3. Common Drugs That Cause Telogen Effluvium

Cholesterol-lowering drugs	Clofibrate, gemfibrozil
Antihypertensives	Diazoxide
β-Blockers	Atenolol, propranolol, metoprolol
Histamine H$_2$ blockers	Cimetidine, ranitidine, famotidine
Anticoagulants	Heparin, warfarin
Anticonvulsants	Phenytoin, valproate
Nonsteroidal anti-inflammatory drugs	Aspirin, ibuprofen, naproxen, indomethacin
Vitamin A derivatives	Retinoids, retinol, isotretinoin
Tricyclic antidepressants	Amitriptyline, imipramine, doxepin

decreases from 10% to 5%. After childbirth, 60% of anagen phase hair follicles may enter telogen phase. Approximately 3 months after childbirth, the telogen hairs start to shed. The telogen effluvium may last several months. Chronic emotional stress, depression, and sudden anxiety also can affect the hair follicles adversely and promote the onset of telogen effluvium. Stressors that young children may experience include moving to a new home, birth of a sibling, divorce of parents, and death of a family member.

Newborns may experience a physiologic form of telogen effluvium. During embryogenesis, the hair follicles grow in a cycle of 8 months. After 8 months of gestation, the hair follicles enter telogen, and the first hairs may be shed in utero. More often, the newborn retains the hair until birth. After birth, the first hairs are shed and not replaced. In addition to the changes of the hair follicle development and cycling in newborns, the physical stress of birth may be a shock to the hair follicles, causing them to enter the telogen phase prematurely. The hair follicles gradually return to the anagen phase, and the follicles change from producing the fine newborn lanugo hairs to pigmented terminal hairs.

The diagnosis of telogen effluvium is suggested by a history of a stressor or an adverse event 2 to 4 months before the onset of the hair thinning. Examination of the scalp hair often shows diffuse thinning, and many telogen hairs are removed during the hair pull test. The telogen-to-anagen ratio of a trichogram also guides the diagnosis. The hairs obtained by hair pluck and examined using light microscopy yield telogen counts of greater than 25%. Normally, scalps average roughly 85% anagen hairs and 15% telogen hairs.

There is no effective treatment for telogen effluvium. Spontaneous regrowth occurs in most patients. Full recovery usually is expected. If prolonged illness with high fevers completely destroys the follicles, hair regrowth may be partial. Patients should avoid excessive manipulation of the hair with shampooing, combing, and brushing until new hair growth begins. Minoxidil solution promotes telogen hair follicles to enter the active anagen growth phase and may be used to treat telogen effluvium in children. Parents can perform hair counts at home periodically to see if the number of hairs being shed is decreasing over time.

Anagen effluvium results from the inhibition of cell division in anagen hair follicles, leading to a sudden cessation of hair growth. The hair roots become tapered, and the hair shafts constrict. The tapered hair root tips and thinner hair shafts are shed intact, but the hair follicles do not enter the resting telogen phase as they do in telogen effluvium (Table

Table 72-4. Comparison of Telogen Effluvium and Anagen Effluvium

	Telogen Effluvium	Anagen Effluvium
Onset of shedding from inciting event	2–4 mo	1–4 wk
Degree of hair loss	20–50%	90%
Characteristics of shed hairs	Normal club hair with white bulb	Anagen hair with pigmented bulb
Hair shaft appearance	Normal	Narrowed and fractured

72-4). Because on average 85% to 90% of the hairs on the scalp are in the anagen phase at any given time, anagen effluvium can result in a severe diffuse alopecia. It develops rapidly over 1 to 4 weeks after the triggering event. When conditions become more favorable, the onset of regrowth is as sudden as the initial loss. Patients with 10% of hair remaining after an insult should be considered to have anagen effluvium.

Extensive anagen effluvium is seen most often in people undergoing chemotherapy for cancer treatment. Folic acid antagonists, purine antagonists, alkylating agents, and natural alkaloids are common agents that cause anagen hair loss (Table 72-5). Anagen effluvium has been described with excessive radiation exposure to the scalp. Toxicity from lead, boric acid, mercury, thallium, arsenic, and bismuth can cause anagen effluvium. The extent of anagen effluvium depends on the agent; severe toxicity may lead to profound hair loss. Anagen effluvium may be reversed by discontinuation of the offending agent. Minoxidil solution has been used to reduce the extent of anagen effluvium caused by chemotherapeutic drugs.

Metabolic and nutritional deficiencies may lead to diffuse hair thinning, typically by inducing telogen effluvium. Hypothyroidism is associated with diffuse hair thinning. Crash dieting over a long time can alter the hair cycle. The follicular cells have a high degree of metabolic activity. With crash dieting, the hair follicles have a limited source of energy, vitamins, and minerals. Hair thinning begins several months after the diet begins and persists for several months after diet completion. In malabsorption states, the prolonged deficiency of essential fatty acids can lead to diffuse alopecia. The hairs become dry and change color. Treatment consists of topical or oral safflower oil (linoleic acid). Deficiencies of iron and zinc also are associated with diffuse hair thinning. Vegetarians are particularly susceptible to zinc deficiency. Chelated zinc in supplement form is easy to absorb and has considerably fewer gastrointestinal side effects compared with inorganic zinc sulfate. Because

Table 72-5. Drugs That Induce Anagen Effluvium

Alkylating agents	Cyclophosphamide, nitrogen mustard, chlorambucil, thiotepa
Antimetabolic agents	Methotrexate, 5-fluorouracil, 6-mercaptopurine
Cytostatic agents	Colchicine, actinomycin D, vinblastine, vincristine, cytosine, doxorubicin, arabinoside
Vitamin A derivatives	Retinoids, retinol, isotretinoin
Other drugs	Bleomycin, cytarabine, thioguanine

copper and vitamin C aid absorption and use of iron, deficiency of these minerals may indirectly cause hair thinning.

Alopecia areata, an autoimmune disorder with a prevalence of 1:1000, can occur at any age. Incidence is increased in Down syndrome. Familial predisposition is seen in 10% to 20% of cases, occurring with thyroid disease, pernicious anemia, diabetes, adrenal disease, vitiligo, and atopy. Alopecia areata is characterized by the sudden onset of localized well-circumscribed patches of hair loss. In children, patches may have an irregular border with scattered long hairs within the areas of hair loss. The scalp skin is soft and almost devoid of hair (Fig. 72-7). Rarely, early lesions may show edema and erythema. Older patches of alopecia may have depigmented hair shafts within them. Eyebrows and eyelashes may be involved. In 10% to 20% of children, the fingernails may have rows of pits, proximal separation with subsequent shedding (onychomadesis), or longitudinal ridging (Fig. 72-8). Nail dystrophy may progress to roughness of the entire nail surface (trachyonychia) or opacification. Opaque white nails are seen with complete loss of the scalp hair (alopecia totalis).

The diagnosis of alopecia areata usually is made on clinical examination. Hairs that are removed along the periphery of the patch of alopecia may show tapering of the shaft to an attenuated bulb, giving them the appearance of an exclamation point. Alopecia areata can be differentiated from trichotillomania by the bizarrely shaped patches of alopecia with broken hairs seen with trichotillomania. Tinea capitis differs from alopecia areata in the scaling of the scalp, with or without erythema. If the diagnosis is in question, a scalp biopsy may be performed. Children with alopecia areata should be screened for associated thyroid disease, anemia, or latent diabetes.

The course of alopecia areata is unpredictable. Most children have complete regrowth of the hair within 1 year, regardless of whether treatment is attempted. One third

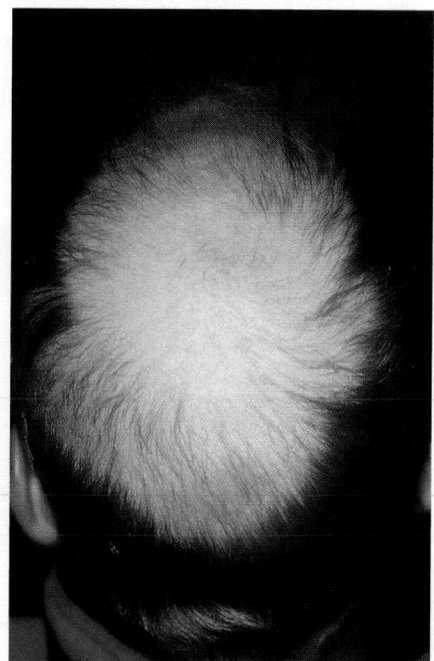

Figure 72-7. Extensive alopecia areata on the top of the scalp in a prepubertal boy.

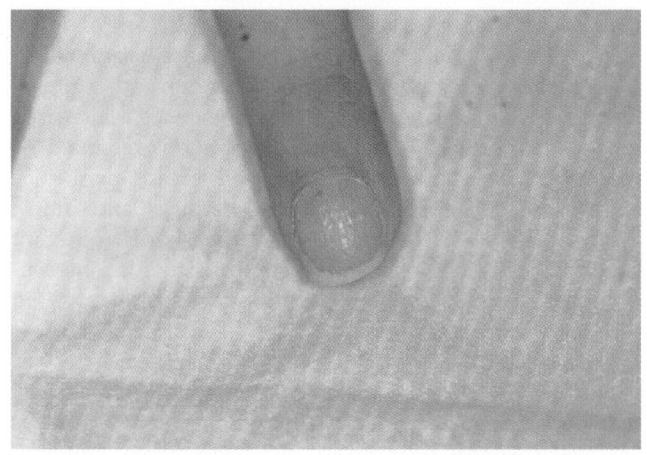

Figure 72-8. Pitting of the nail in a boy with alopecia areata.

of patients experience recurrent hair loss. The pattern of hair loss can be diffuse, and progression can be rapid. Approximately 5% to 10% of patients develop alopecia totalis, which tends to develop gradually and is seen more frequently in children than in adults. Prognosis is poor with young age at onset or if the patient develops alopecia universalis, or complete loss of all body hair. Prognosis for hair growth is poor with hair loss in the ophiasis distribution (along the occipital portion of the scalp extending anteriorly above the ears bilaterally [Fig. 72-9]).

Initial treatment with topical or intralesional steroids is of greatest benefit early in the course of the disease and in patients with less than 75% hair loss. Topical steroids frequently affect hair regrowth within 4 to 6 weeks. Intralesional injections of corticosteroids can be used every 4 to 6 weeks. For severe and refractory alopecia areata, prednisone, 1 to 2 mg/kg/day, may be given for 4 to 6 weeks, followed by tapering to alternate-day therapy and discontinuation over the following 6 weeks. High-dose pulse corticosteroids have been used successfully in the treatment of severe alopecia areata. Short-term and long-term side effects should be explained in detail to parents before initiation of systemic corticosteroids; hairs that regrow during systemic steroid therapy may be lost when the steroids are discontinued. Cyclosporine also has been used in cases of severe alopecia areata. Psoralens and ultra-

violet A treatments are another option, although many treatments are required to induce hair regrowth, and light treatments increase the lifelong risk of skin cancer. Dermatologists have used dinitrochlorobenzene, diphencyprone, and squaric acid dibutyl ester topically to produce a mild allergic contact dermatitis; these chemicals typically are applied weekly to induce and maintain contact sensitization. Anthralin may be used in a similar fashion to produce an irritant dermatitis. Topical minoxidil has modest success in one third of patients. Although there is no specific treatment for the nail dystrophy, resolution of the alopecia areata may be associated with normalization of the appearance of the nails. The National Alopecia Areata Foundation (710 C Street, Suite 11, San Rafael, CA 94901, 415-456-4644, www.alopeciaareata.com) is an excellent source of support for affected individuals and their families.

Androgenetic alopecia is a polygenically inherited disorder. Androgen-sensitive follicles arise on the top of the scalp. Androgen-independent follicles arise on the sides and the posterior portion. Terminal hairs in the androgen-sensitive areas may be replaced by miniaturized vellus hairs secondary to the influence of circulating androgens. Severity of alopecia is related to age of onset; it is more severe when it arises during childhood.

Uniform recession of the frontal hairline is seen in 96% of boys and 80% of girls during adolescence; it is not characteristic of androgenetic alopecia and does not portend baldness. The earliest stage of male pattern alopecia is characterized by hair loss on the frontoparietal portion of the scalp, with a triangular pattern of hair loss bilaterally, and may occur during adolescence or in early adulthood, causing stress and emotional disturbance. Male pattern hair loss progresses slowly. By the time a man with male pattern hair loss reaches his 30s or 40s, balding on the top of the scalp is evident. Androgenetic alopecia tends to be less noticeable in a genetically predisposed woman. The frontal hairline is unaffected. The hair tends to thin slowly after puberty, and the hair part widens. Androgenetic alopecia that accompanies hirsutism, acne, and menstrual irregularity in a female patient should be evaluated with free testosterone, dehydroepiandrosterone, and testosterone binding globulin levels to evaluate for an underlying endocrine abnormality. Genetic disorders associated with early-onset androgenetic alopecia include Ehlers-Danlos syndrome and trisomy 21 (Down syndrome).

Topical minoxidil solution produces acceptable hair growth in approximately 30% of patients. The solution must be applied to a dry scalp twice a day. Hair growth becomes evident within 4 to 12 months of continuous use. One third of patients grow hair that is long enough to be cut or combed. Minoxidil may halt the progression of androgenetic alopecia. If successful, the therapy must be continued throughout the patient's life. Young individuals with frontal recession of less than 5 years respond favorably to topical minoxidil. Adverse effects are irritation from the vehicles of the solution and contact allergy to minoxidil. Cutaneous adverse effects include erythema, pruritus, and dermatitis. Because minoxidil may exacerbate sun-exposure damage, sunburn should be avoided while using minoxidil. Oral finasteride, another treatment option, is best reserved for men with androgenetic alopecia.

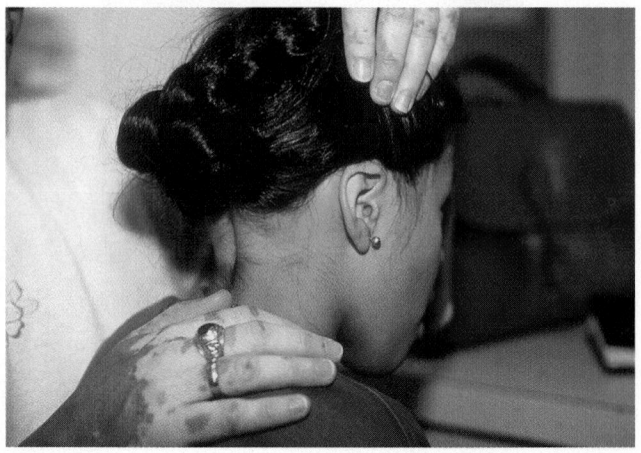

Figure 72-9. Ophiasis distribution of hair loss in a girl with alopecia areata. Her mother's hands show vitiligo.

Trauma-Related Alopecias

Traction alopecia is hair loss resulting from cosmetic practices, such as braiding; wearing pony tails; use of tight hair rollers, barrettes, or elastics; hair straightening; and use of hot combs. Peripheral scalp hair loss occurs with hair worn in a tight ponytail. Hair loss around the margins of the scalp and on the frontal scalp occurs in patients who use hair rollers. Hot comb alopecia occurs with hair straightening and occurs on the vertex and the marginal areas of the scalp.

After the traumatic cause has ceased, new hair growth may take 3 months. Chronic traction can lead to fibrosis around the hair follicles, irreversible scarring, and permanent hair loss. Treatment is hair transplantation.

Trichotillomania, alopecia from the habit of hair pulling or twisting, begins as an irregular area of partial hair loss, most commonly in the frontoparietal region. It is seen most commonly in children between 4 and 10 years old. The patient either consciously or subconsciously plucks, twirls, or rubs the hair-bearing areas, resulting in breakage of hair shafts. Commonly, neither the patient nor the parents fail to notice the habit, which can be associated with thumb sucking and nail biting in young children. It usually is performed at bedtime before the child falls asleep as a comfort technique and can be a response to emotional stress. Trichotillomania may be triggered by hospitalization, difficulties at school, severe sibling rivalry, or disturbed parent-child relationship. Association of trichotillomania with obsessive-compulsive disorder increases with age.

The hallmark of trichotillomania is an irregular outline and short, stublike broken hairs. The patches of hair loss have reduced hair density, but are never completely bald. Approximately 70% of cases involve the scalp, 50% involve eyebrows or eyelashes or both, 30% involve pubic hair, 20% involve body hair, and 10% involve facial hair. Hairs are broken, shortened, and vary in length. When the diagnosis is in question, a biopsy specimen of the most recently involved area shows traumatic damage of the hairs in the follicles.

Direct confrontation and accusation are rarely helpful because patients frequently deny pulling the hairs. Although trichotillomania is associated with some psychological disorders, fewer than 5% of patients with the disorder have severe emotional problems. Parents need to be accepting and supportive rather than judgmental. Patients should be given the opportunity to discuss their stressors. The prognosis is generally good, and with behavioral modification, many children outgrow the habit. Patients with obsessive-compulsive disorder benefit from treatment with fluoxetine and clomipramine. Since 1991, a support network has been in place for individuals affected with trichotillomania (Trichotillomania Learning Center, 1215 Mission Street, Suite 2, Santa Cruz, CA 95060).

Infection-Related Alopecias

Tinea capitis is a fungal infection of the scalp caused by a dermatophyte. Dermatophytes chiefly infect children between ages 4 and 7 years. The incidence in school-age children can reach 12%. The risk of infection seems to be higher in urban areas and in African Americans. In urban schools with high rates of infection, 15% of children may be asymptomatic carriers. Boys are five times more likely to

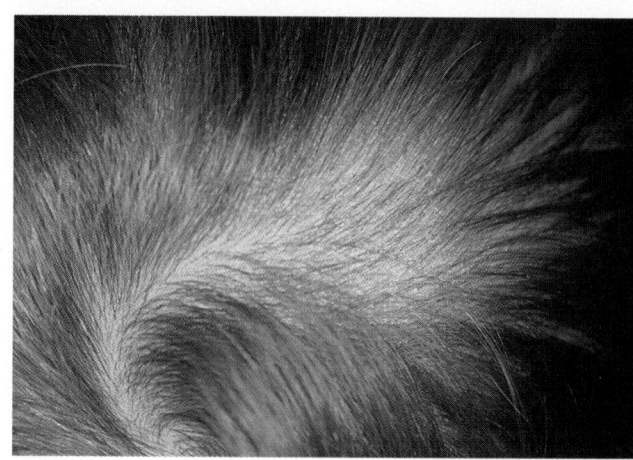

Figure 72-10. Tinea capitis presenting with a scaly patch and minimal hair loss.

be affected than girls. Approximately 95% of tinea capitis infections in the United States are caused by *Trichophyton tonsurans*, an organism that can live for prolonged periods on combs, hats, and toys. Transmission often occurs in families from shared use of grooming instruments. Asymptomatic carriage provides a route for transmission, infection, and reinfection.

Tinea capitis is characterized by scaly, round-to-oval patches of partial alopecia with broken hairs that typically measure 1 to 5 cm in diameter (Figs. 72-10 through 72-12). Lesions may be erythematous, and the active borders may be slightly elevated. The broken hairs may resemble black dots ("black dot ringworm"). Secondary bacterial infection may be present. Children with tinea capitis often have posterior cervical lymphadenopathy. A kerion is a painful, inflamed, boggy plaque on the scalp that often is surrounded by pustules and vesicles. A kerion represents an intense allergic and inflammatory response to *Microsporum canis*, *Trichophyton verrucosum*, and *T. tonsurans*. When the inflammatory response is severe, healing is prolonged, and scarring is irreversible.

The diagnosis of tinea capitis is made by demonstration of fungal elements on a potassium hydroxide preparation from scales and hairs. Potassium hydroxide preparations may be negative because the fungus often is situated deeply

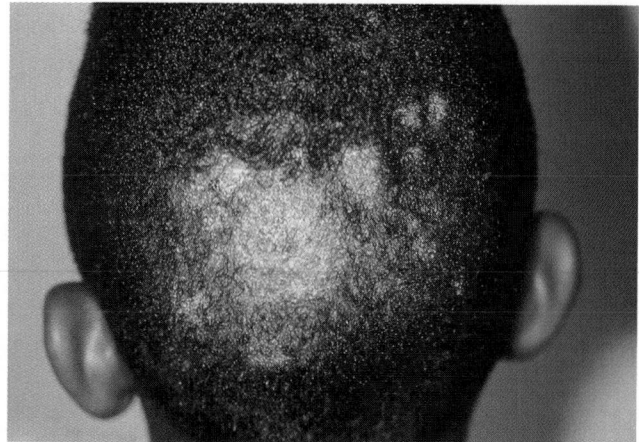

Figure 72-11. Tinea capitis with extensive hair loss and pustule formation (secondary staphylococcal infection).

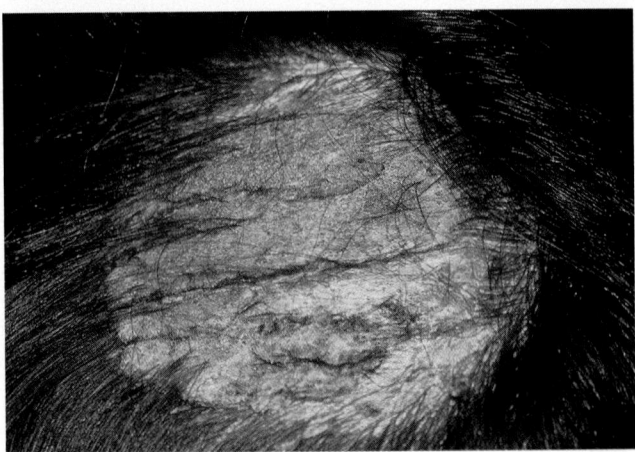

Figure 72-12. Tinea capitis with thick, adherent scale.

in the hair follicles. Fungal cultures of affected hairs and scales help confirm the diagnosis in these cases. The hairs are plucked using a hemostat, and scales are scraped with a scalpel blade; alternatively a sterile cotton swab or sterile toothbrush may be used to collect samples for culture in a less traumatic manner. The specimens may be collected directly on Sabouraud's glucose agar or submitted to the microbiology laboratory in a Petri dish to be placed on agar. Growth and identification of the fungal organism occur within 5 to 14 days but may take 4 weeks. Wood's lamp illumination usually is not helpful because the most common causative organism, *T. tonsurans*, does not fluoresce; *M. canis* does fluoresce.

Treatment of tinea capitis requires systemic antifungal medication (Table 72-6). Topical antifungals do not cure tinea capitis because they do not reach the hair bulb. Griseofulvin has a long track record of safety and is approved by the U.S. Food and Drug Administration for the treatment of tinea capitis in children. Griseofulvin enters skin, hair, and nails, where it exerts a fungistatic effect.

Treatment duration is 6 to 12 weeks and should continue for 2 weeks beyond clinical resolution. Griseofulvin is best taken with a fatty food, such as milk or ice cream, which aids in absorption. Griseofulvin is well tolerated by children; potential side effects include hypersensitivity (morbilliform eruptions or urticaria), photosensitivity, gastrointestinal upset, headaches, and reversible leukopenia. Rare complications include aplastic anemia and precipitation of acute porphyria. Griseofulvin is teratogenic and embryotoxic. Drugs that interact with griseofulvin are listed in Table 72-7.

Fluconazole, itraconazole, and terbinafine are systemic antifungals that seem to be safe and efficacious in the treatment of fungal infections of the scalp in children, although they are not approved by the Food and Drug Administration for this indication. They have a high affinity for keratin. These medications have long half-lives and persist in the skin for several weeks after cessation of therapy. Studies of itraconazole indicate the drug is retained in keratin for 4 weeks after discontinuation of treatment. Steady clinical improvement and mycologic cure have been shown even after discontinuation of itraconazole therapy. Efficacy of itraconazole is 70% to 100% after 2 to 4 weeks of therapy for *Trichophyton* and *Microsporum*. Fluconazole and itraconazole are fungistatic and impair the synthesis of the fungal cell wall. Fluconazole is water soluble and can be taken without food. Itraconazole is absorbed best when taken with food. Side effects include headache, diarrhea, and papular eruptions. Because itraconazole can contribute to congestive heart failure, history or signs of cardiac disease are contraindications for its use. Terbinafine, an allylamine, selectively inhibits an early step of fungal cell membrane sterol synthesis causing accumulation of squalene, which is cytotoxic to fungus. Terbinafine has a 93% cure rate for tinea capitis and 90% cure rate for other dermatophyte infections in children. Terbinafine therapy for 4 weeks is as efficacious as 8 weeks of griseofulvin in the treatment of tinea capitis.

Regardless of which oral antifungal medication is used, a selenium sulfide–containing shampoo should be used to decrease shedding of fungal spores from the infected scalp. Family members should be evaluated for asymptomatic carriage to prevent reinfection. If the fungal culture identifies an organism of animal source (e.g., *M. canis*), household pets should be evaluated by a veterinarian.

Syphilitic alopecia consists of patchy alopecia with the papulosquamous lesions of secondary syphilis (diffuse,

Table 72-6. Systemic Antifungal Treatment Options for Tinea Capitis

Antifungal	Dosage
Griseofulvin	Microsized (125 mg/5 mL): 20 mg/kg/day for 6–12 wk
	Ultramicrosized (tablets): 10–15 mg/kg/day for 6–12 wk
Fluconazole (liquid or tablet)	Option 1: 6 mg/kg/day for 20 days
	Option 2: 6 mg/kg/day for 14 days, with an extra week of treatment 2 wk later if clinically indicated when the patient is evaluated 4 wk after beginning therapy
	Option 3: 5 mg/kg/day for 30 days
	Option 4: 8 mg/kg once a week for 4–8 wk
Itraconazole (100 mg capsules)	<10 kg: 5 mg/kg/day for 4 wk
	10–20 kg: 1 capsule every other day for 4 wk
	21–30 kg: 1 capsule daily for 4 wk
	31–50 kg: 1 capsule/day alternating with 2 capsules/day for 4 wk
	>50 kg: 2 capsules daily for 4 wk
Terbinafine (250-mg tablets)	<20 kg: 62.5 mg daily for 4 wk
	20–40 kg: 125 mg daily for 4 wk
	>40 kg: 250 mg daily for 4 wk

Table 72-7. Systemic Antifungal Medications and Drug Interactions

Griseofulvin: barbiturates, warfarin, cyclosporine, oral contraceptives, rifampin
Fluconazole: astemizole, calcium channel blockers, carbamazepine, cisapride, cyclosporine, diazepam, digoxin, lovastatin, midazolam, phenobarbital, phenytoin, protease inhibitors, quinidine, rifampin, simvastatin, terfenadine, triazolam
Itraconazole: astemizole, cisapride, cyclosporine, hydrochlorothiazide, oral hypoglycemic agents, phenytoin, rifampin, terfenadine, theophylline, warfarin
Terbinafine: cimetidine, cyclosporine, rifampin, theophylline

brownish red macules and papules, including the palms and soles). The alopecia commonly is described as "moth-eaten," but also may arise as diffuse thinning of the scalp hair. Erythema, scaling, and induration are absent. Serologic tests for syphilis confirm the diagnosis when patchy or diffuse alopecia is unexplained and there is a high index of suspicion.

Scarring Alopecias

Scarring alopecias, including discoid lupus on the scalp, lichen planopilaris, keratosis pilaris atrophicans (see CD-ROM Figs. 72-14 and 72-15), folliculitis decalvans (see CD-ROM Fig. 72-16), dissecting cellulitis of the scalp, and acne keloidalis, are described and discussed on the CD-ROM.

Hypertrichosis and Hirsutism

Hypertrichosis is a pattern of excessive hair growth that is not androgen dependent. It may be localized or generalized and congenital or acquired. Hypertrichosis occurs without any evidence of masculinization or menstrual abnormality and is best described as an excessive amount of hair in a normal location on the body compared with individuals of the same sex, age, and ethnic background (Fig. 72-13). Drugs that cause hypertrichosis include phenytoin, minoxidil, cyclosporine, corticosteroids, diazoxide, streptomycin, interferon, and acetazolamide. Transplant patients treated with cyclosporine commonly develop either generalized hypertrichosis or hypertrichosis limited to the forearms. Acquired hypertrichosis lanuginosa is the development of fine, long, unpigmented hairs in association with malignancy.

Hirsutism refers to excessive growth of hair in a woman or child in an androgen-dependent pattern (upper lip, chin, sideburn areas, neck, anterior chest, breasts, abdomen, upper inner thighs, and legs). Fine vellus hairs are transformed to visible, thickened terminal hairs as a result of androgenic stimuli. Idiopathic hirsutism usually begins around puberty and is genetically determined, often related to ethnicity. Hirsutism also is a sign of polycystic ovarian disease. For only a few female patients, hirsutism signals a serious medical problem, such as an ovarian tumor, an adrenal tumor, congenital adrenal hyperplasia, or Cushing's syndrome. Signs of virilization accompany hirsutism in these disorders, including acne and increased sebum production, clitoral hypertrophy, decreased breast size, deepening of the voice, increased muscle mass, heightened libido, and irregular or absent menses. Hormonal screening tests, including dehydroepiandrosterone sulfate, prolactin, and total free testosterone, are helpful in diagnosing girls with pathologic hirsutism. Tests that help define the disease process include 17α-hydroxyprogesterone, serum 11-deoxycortisol, follicle-stimulating hormone, luteinizing hormone, 24-hour urinary cortisol concentrations, and dexamethasone suppression test.

Even when hypertrichosis and hirsutism are not associated with an underlying medical condition, excess hair growth is considered to be cosmetically undesirable by many girls and women. Treatment is hair removal by plucking, wax epilation, electrolysis, or laser.

Pigmentary Changes of the Hair

The spontaneous appearance of green discoloration of the hair in light-haired children may occur as a result of copper used as an algae retardant in swimming pools. In such cases, the use of a copper-based algicide should be discontinued. Copper-induced discoloration can be treated with topical application of a chelating agent containing ethylenediamine tetraacetic acid. Premature graying of the hair is caused by a reduction in the activity of melanocytes within the follicles. Graying may be an early sign of pernicious anemia or thyrotoxicosis, and it is seen in vitiligo, alopecia areata, and tuberous sclerosis. Premature graying also is a feature of progeria, Werner's syndrome, Rothmund-Thomson syndrome, poliosis, Waardenburg's syndrome, and Vogt-Koyanagi syndrome.

DISORDERS OF THE NAILS

Fundamentals

The nail matrix is present at 10 weeks of gestation. The nail plate grows out of the nail matrix and becomes keratinized at 15 weeks of gestation. The nail plate is well formed at birth. The nail plate is thin in childhood and is attached to the nail bed by protein fibers. The nail plate is relatively transparent in childhood. The nail matrix lies under the proximal nail fold (Fig. 72-14). The cuticle is an outgrowth of the proximal nail fold. The lunula is the white crescent at the proximal aspect of the nail. The nail plate distal to the lunula looks pink because of the vascularity of the underlying nail bed.

Fingernails grow at a rate of approximately 1 cm every 3 months. Nail growth is faster on the fingers than the toes. Nail growth is faster on the larger fingers, on the right hand, in the summer, during the daytime, and in association with nail biting or nail trauma.

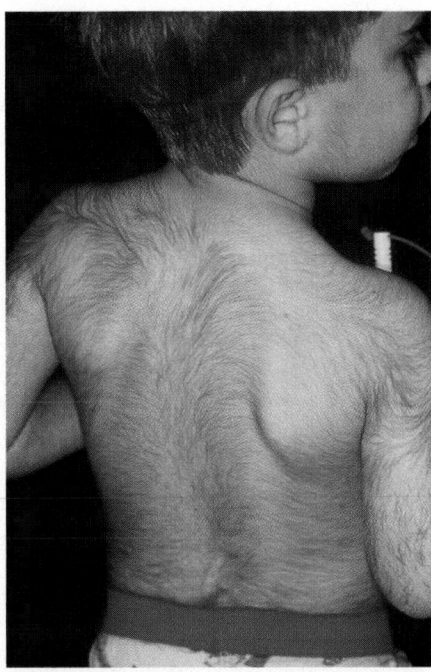

Figure 72-13. Young boy with gingival fibromatosis and hypertrichosis, an autosomal dominant condition.

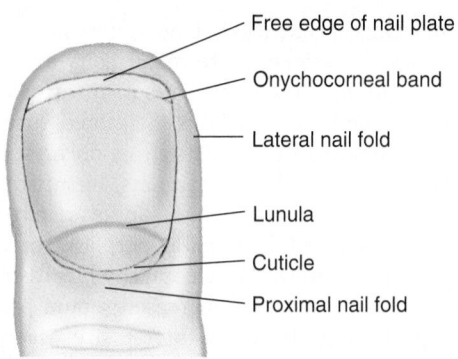

- Free edge of nail plate
- Onychocorneal band
- Lateral nail fold
- Lunula
- Cuticle
- Proximal nail fold

Figure 72-14. Surface anatomy of the nail. (From Lowry M, Rich P: The nail apparatus: A guide for basic and clinical science. Curr Prob Dermatol 1999;11:169.)

Congenital Nail Disorders

Congenital nail disorders, which are rare, are discussed on the CD-ROM, including median nail dystrophy (see CD-ROM Fig. 72-19), congenital malalignment of the great toenails (see CD-ROM Fig. 72-20), nail-patella syndrome, and pachyonychia congenita (see CD-ROM Fig. 72-21).

Acquired Nail Disorders

Several acquired disorders of the nails are discussed on the CD-ROM, including trachyonychia ("twenty nail dystrophy"; see CD-ROM Fig. 72-22), familial clubbing of the nails, Beau's lines (see CD-ROM Fig. 72-24), onychomadesis (see CD-ROM Fig. 72-25), onycholysis (see CD-ROM Fig. 72-26), leukonychia (see CD-ROM Fig. 72-27), chromonychia, and koilonychia.

Although *clubbing of the nails* may be familial or idiopathic, it is seen most commonly in association with hypoxic disorders. Clubbed nails show an increase of the angle between the nail plate and the phalanx to 180 degrees or greater (Fig. 72-15). As clubbing progresses, the normal depression found at the proximal nail fold is lost. In late clubbing, the nail plate becomes visibly enlarged and is spongy when palpated. Pulmonary diseases that cause chronic clubbing include cystic fibrosis, emphysema, bronchiectasis, and tuberculosis. Cyanotic congenital heart disease, subacute bacterial endocarditis, cirrhosis, obstructive liver disease, ulcerative colitis, and thyrotoxicosis all cause clubbing. Nail clubbing has been described as a sign of human immunodeficiency virus infection in infected children presenting with acute pneumonia.

Splinter hemorrhages are extravasations of blood from vessels into the nail bed. Because the blood attaches to the underside of the nail plate, splinter hemorrhages grow out with the nail. The splinter hemorrhage appears stationary if the blood attaches to the nail bed. Trauma to the nails is the most common cause of splinter hemorrhages. Simultaneous appearance of splinter hemorrhages in several nails should prompt consideration of a systemic etiology, including endocarditis, cystic fibrosis, diabetes, peritoneal dialysis, cirrhosis, hepatitis, hypertension, leukemia, hereditary hemorrhagic telangiectasia, rheumatoid arthritis, systemic lupus erythematosus, thyrotoxicosis, and vasculitis. Splinter hemorrhages also may occur in primary dermatologic conditions, such as eczema and psoriasis.

Habit-tic dystrophy is caused by chronic rubbing or picking of the nail cuticle of a digit on the hand by another digit on the same hand, most commonly the thumbnail, caused by rubbing with the index finger. The nail has a longitudinal depression or split down the center with numerous horizontal ridges extending outward. As opposed to median nail dystrophy, the configuration of the dystrophy in habit-tic deformity has the appearance of an upright Christmas tree. Treatment consists of discontinuing the habit.

Subungual hematomas of the nail bed are common and related to trauma. Loss of the nail plate is likely when more than 25% of the nail bed is affected. Severe hematomas may lead to nail bed injury and deformity of the nail. Evacuation of the hematoma decreases the pain. Puncturing the nail plate with a sterile, heated, and pointed instrument provides immediate relief.

Subungual exostoses are fibrous nodules that arise on the distal phalanx of a finger or toe just under the free edge of the nail plate (Fig. 72-16). These bony tumors cause the distal edge of the nail plate to lift up and detach from the nail bed. These lesions may result from trauma and often are mistaken for subungual warts. The great toes are affected most commonly. A plain radiograph is diagnos-

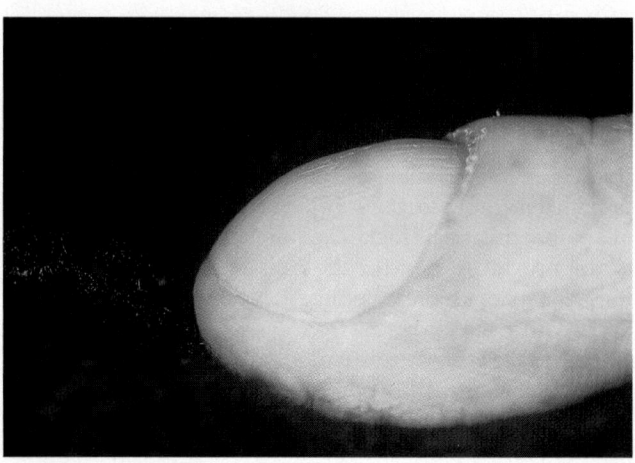

Figure 72-15. Familial clubbing in an adult.

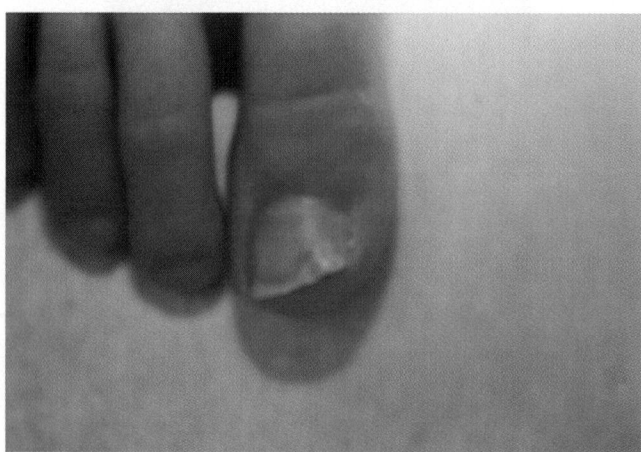

Figure 72-16. Subungual exostosis.

tic. When the diagnosis is made, the patient should be referred to an orthopedic surgeon for definitive surgical management.

Ingrown toenails result from the lateral edge of the nail plate penetrating into the soft tissue of the lateral nail fold, causing erythema, swelling, and pain of the affected soft tissue. The great toenails are affected most commonly. Ingrown toenails usually are related to improper clipping of the toenail or poorly fitting shoes. Ingrown toenails also may be seen as a transient phenomenon of newborns, which typically resolves spontaneously during the first year of life. Preventive measures include allowing the nail to grow out beyond the distal aspect of the lateral nailfolds, careful nail trimming, and wearing properly fitting shoes. When ingrown nails are a chronic problem, surgical removal of the lateral portion of the nail plate and destruction of the lateral aspect of the nail matrix prevent regrowth of the problematic portion of the nail.

Infection-Related Nail Dystrophies

Acute *paronychia* presents as erythema, swelling, and pain of the nail folds and can have purulent drainage and is caused most commonly by *Staphylococcus aureus*, *Streptococcus*, or *Pseudomonas* (which can cause green color of the nail folds and the drainage).

Chronic paronychia typically is caused by *Candida albicans*. Acute and chronic paronychias may lead to osteomyelitis. Incision and drainage provides immediate relief of the discomfort and evacuates the infection. The drainage should be cultured to guide appropriate systemic antimicrobial therapy. Warm compressive soaks and pain control are important adjunctive treatments. Sterile chronic paronychia can be seen in primary cutaneous disorders, such as eczema or psoriasis, and are treated with topical or intralesional steroids.

Onychomycosis is a chronic fungal infection of the nails caused by dermatophytes, most commonly *Trichophyton rubrum*, *Trichophyton mentagrophytes*, and *Epidermophyton floccosum*. Onychomycosis is unusual without a primary dermatophyte infection of the skin, typically occurring in association with tinea pedis or tinea manus. Toenails are involved more often than fingernails. *Candida* also causes onychomycosis (Fig. 72-17). Maceration of the nails and

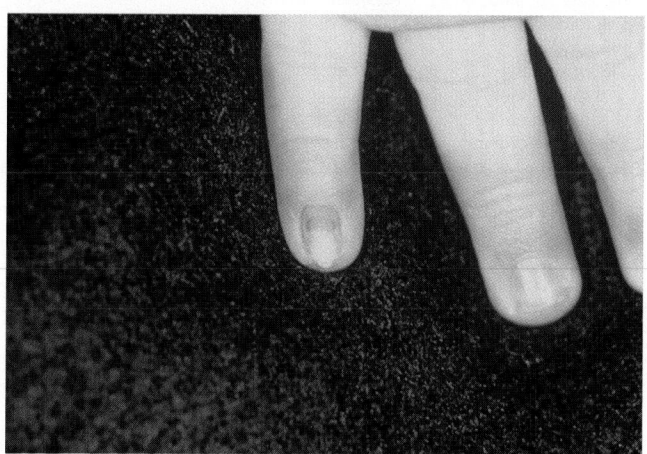

Figure 72-17. *Candida albicans* onychomycosis in an infant.

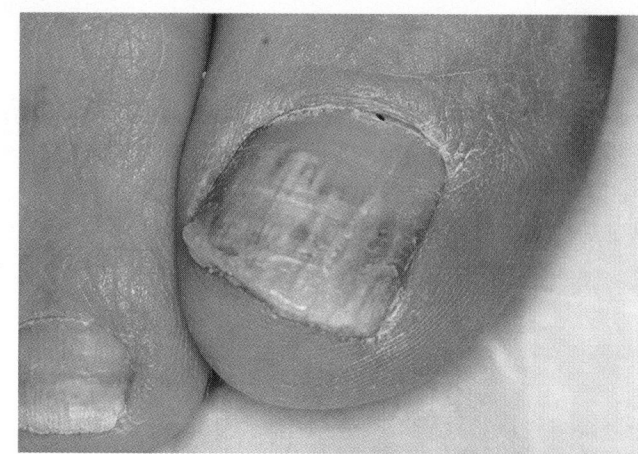

Figure 72-18. Distal subungual onychomycosis that has progressed proximally to involve most of the affected nail plates. (Courtesy of Department of Dermatology, University of Utah, Salt Lake City, Utah.)

nail folds from thumb or finger sucking provides a portal of entry for *Candida* into the nail plate.

Distal subungual onychomycosis is the most common presentation of dermatophytic nail infection. Infection begins at the distal and lateral free edges of the nail with white, yellow, or brown discoloration of the nail plate. Subungual debris collects as the nail becomes discolored, thickened, and friable (Fig. 72-18). Because onychomycosis is uncommon in children, it is imperative to distinguish it from nonfungal nail dystrophies, especially dystrophies seen in association with eczema, psoriasis, and lichen planus. Accurate diagnosis depends on the presence of fungal organisms on a potassium hydroxide preparation or identification of the fungus by culture. Scrapings of the nail surface frequently do not show fungal organisms; samples for potassium hydroxide preparation and fungal culture must be taken from subungual debris and fragments of the nail plate. When onychomycosis is suspected clinically and the potassium hydroxide preparation and fungal cultures are negative, a nail clipping sent for histopathologic examination can be diagnostic with a sensitivity of 85%.

Treatment of onychomycosis requires long-term, systemic therapy. Topical antifungal therapy may be employed if only a few nails are involved, and they are chemically or surgically avulsed before treatment; superficial white onychomycosis (Fig. 72-19) also may be managed with topical therapy. Options for systemic treatment of onychomycosis are outlined in Table 72-8. Parents should be advised that prolonged oral therapy may not achieve a complete cure, and there is a risk of recurrence. Griseofulvin and terbinafine cannot be used to treat *Candida* because it is not sensitive to these medications.

Nail Dystrophy of Atopic Dermatitis, Psoriasis, and Lichen Planus

Children with atopic dermatitis may have enough inflammation of the distal digits to cause inflammation in the nail matrices. The nails may develop irregular pits, ridges, roughened surfaces, or thickening (Fig. 72-20). At times, the surfaces of the nails are smooth and shiny from chronic scratching and rubbing of the nails against the skin.

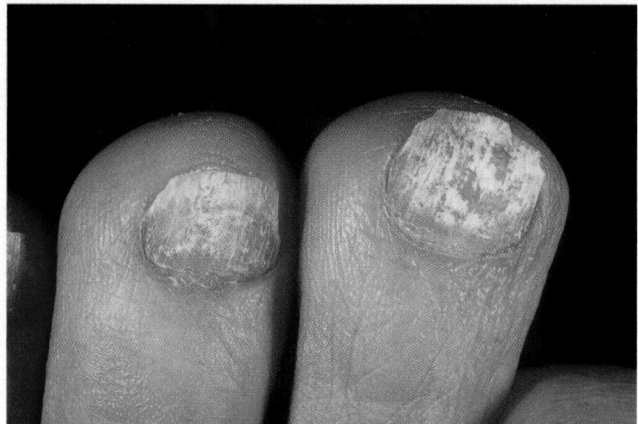

Figure 72-19. Superficial white onychomycosis. (Courtesy of Department of Dermatology, University of Utah, Salt Lake City, Utah.)

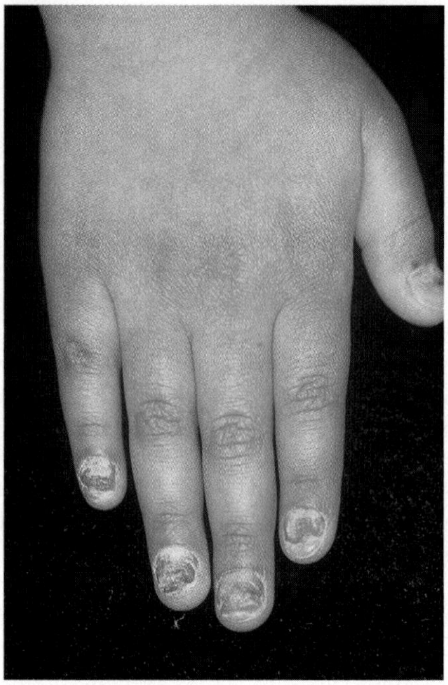

Figure 72-20. Nail dystrophy in a patient with atopic dermatitis.

Nails are involved in most patients with psoriasis. Psoriatic nail dystrophy may be mistaken for onychomycosis. Onycholysis (see CD-ROM Fig. 72-26), punched-out depressions or pits, and subungual hyperkeratosis are changes associated with psoriasis. Subungual hyperkeratosis of the nails represents the proliferative state of psoriasis. Psoriasis should be considered in children with nail pits, although they also can result from trauma and are seen in alopecia areata. Psoriatic patients with nail involvement are prone to have arthritis.

Nail dystrophy occurs in 10% of patients with lichen planus. The nails are brittle and ridged, and complete shedding and subungual hyperkeratosis may occur. Trachyonychia has been described as the presenting feature of lichen planus. The proximal portion of the nail may fold onto the nail bed and obliterate the nail plate. This pterygium formation is a characteristic of the severe effect that lichen planus may have on the nails.

Discoloration of the Nails

Table 72-9 lists diagnostic considerations when nails are discolored.

Table 72-8. Systemic Antifungal Treatment Options for Onychomycosis

Medication	Dosage
Griseofulvin—fingernails for 6 mo, toenails for 12 mo	Microsized (125 mg/5 mL): 20 mg/kg/day Ultramicrosized (tablets): 10–15 mg/kg/day
Fluconazole (liquid or tablet), intermittent therapy—fingernails for 12 wk, toenails for 26 wk	3–6 mg/kg, one dose per wk
Itraconazole (100-mg capsules), pulse therapy—fingernails, 2 pulses; toenails, 3 pulses	10–20 kg: ½ capsule every other day for a 1-wk pulse per mo 21–30 kg: 1 capsule daily for a 1-wk pulse per mo 31–40 kg: 1 capsule/day alternating with 2 capsules/day for a 1-wk pulse per mo 41–50 kg: 2 capsules daily for a 1-wk pulse per mo >50 kg: 2 capsules twice daily for a 1-wk pulse per mo
Terbinafine (250-mg tablets)—fingernails for 6 wk; toenails for 12 wk	<20 kg: 62.5 mg daily 20–40 kg: 125 mg daily >40 kg: 250 mg daily

Table 72-9. Diagnostic Considerations of Nail Discoloration

Systemic Drugs	Systemic Disease	Nail Infections
Tetacycline: brown, red	Melanoma: gray-black	*Pseudomonas*: green
Minocycline: blue-gray	Lymphedema: yellow	Bacteria: yellow
Chloroquine: blue-brown	Bronchiectasis: yellow	Fungal: white, yellow, brown, black
Cyclophosphamide: black	Wilson's disease: blue lunulae	
Melphalan, bleomycin, and daunorubicin: brown	Addison's disease: brown	
Zidovudine: hyperpigmented longitudinal streaks	Ochronosis: gray-blue	
Phenytoin: brown	Argyria: blue	
Fluoride: brown bands	Diabetes: yellow	
	Anemia: pallor	
	Carbon monoxide poisoning: cherry red	
	Cardiac failure: red lunulae	
	Cushing's syndrome: black	
	Cyanotic disease: blue	
	Hyperbilirubinemia: brown	
	Hyperthyroidism: brown	

Additional Resources, CD-ROM

Color atlas	Figures
Congenital triangular alopecia	Text, figure

Structural abnormalities of the hair shaft:
  Monilethrix (beaded hair)
  Trichorhexis nodosa
  Trichothiodystropy
  Trichorrhexis invaginata
  Pili trianguli et canaliculi (uncombable hair syndrome, "spun glass" hair)
  Wooly hair
  Trichostasis spinolosa
  Trichorrhexis nodosa
	Text

Scarring alopecias:
Discoid lupus on the scalp
  Lichen planopilaris
  Keratosis pilaris atrophicans
  Folliculitis decalvans
  Dissecting cellulitis of the scalp
  Acne keloidalis
	
	Text
	Text
	Text, figures
	Text, figure
	Text
	Text

Congenital disorders of the nails:
  Median nail dystrophy
  Congenital malalignment of the great toenails
  Nail-patella syndrome
  Pachyonychia congenita
	
	Text, figure
	Text, figure
	
	Text
	Text, figure

Rare acquired disorders of the nails:
  Trachyonychia ("twenty nail dystrophy")
  Beau's lines
  Onchomadesis
  Onycholysis
  Leukonychia
  Chromonychia
  Koilonychia
	
	Text, figure
	
	Text, figure
	Text, figure
	Text, figure
	Text, figure
	Text

Mini-index of Related Topics   CH.

	CH.
■ APPROACH TO DERMATOLOGIC DISEASE AND ECZEMATOID ERUPTIONS	69
■ ANTIMICROBIALS	284

SUGGESTED READINGS

Gupta AK, Chang P, Del Rosso JQ, et al: Onychomycosis in children: Prevalence and management. Pediatr Dermatol 1998;15:464–471.

Gupta AK, Hofstader SLR, Adam P, Summerbell RC: Tinea capitis: An overview with emphasis on management. Pediatr Dermatol 1999;16:171–189.

Madani S, Shapiro J: Alopecia areata update. J Am Acad Dermatol 2000;42:549–566.

Olsen EA: Hair disorders. In Harper J, Oranje A, Prose N (eds): Textbook of Pediatric Dermatology. Oxford, Blackwell Science, 2000, pp 1463–1490.

Scher RK, Daniel CR: Nails: Therapy, Diagnosis, Surgery, 2nd ed. Philadelphia, WB Saunders, 1997.

73 Vesiculobullous Disorders

Clive M. Liu and Sheryll L. Vanderhooft

ROLE OF THE GENERALIST

1. Understand the structure of the skin, and recognize the clinical appearance of blisters at different levels.
2. Recognize the major categories of blistering disorders.
3. Use a logical diagnostic approach to a child with a blistering disorder.
4. Implement a basic approach to treatment of various blistering disorders.

FUNDAMENTALS

Blisters arise from a pathologic process that causes a split or separation within the skin. *Vesicles* are small, well-defined blisters less than 1 cm in diameter. *Bullae* are blisters that are greater than 1 cm in size. The normal structure of the skin is shown in Figure 73-1. The epidermis and dermis are joined by the basement membrane zone. Within the basement membrane zone are attachment complexes that play a role in maintaining the integrity of the skin (Fig. 73-2). Disruption of these attachment complexes forms blisters.

Blistering disorders may be categorized based on the level in the skin in which the separation or cleavage occurs (Table 73-1). *Subcorneal blisters* are caused by cleavage just below the stratum corneum, resulting in shallow flaccid bullae. Because these fragile blisters rupture easily with minimal trauma, they often are not seen on clinical evaluation, but rather present as erosions. The split in *intraepidermal blisters* occurs anywhere within the epidermis and presents with flaccid bullae. These bullae extend laterally with the application of pressure, a phenomenon known as the *Asboe-Hansen sign*. The deepest blisters at the dermal-epidermal junction are called *subepidermal blisters*. These bullae are tense and do not enlarge when manipulated. The *Nikolsky sign* refers to blistering of uninvolved skin after rubbing.

DIAGNOSIS

Bullous disorders are divided into several etiologic categories: infectious disorders, reaction to an external process, photosensitivity disorders, hypersensitivity reactions,

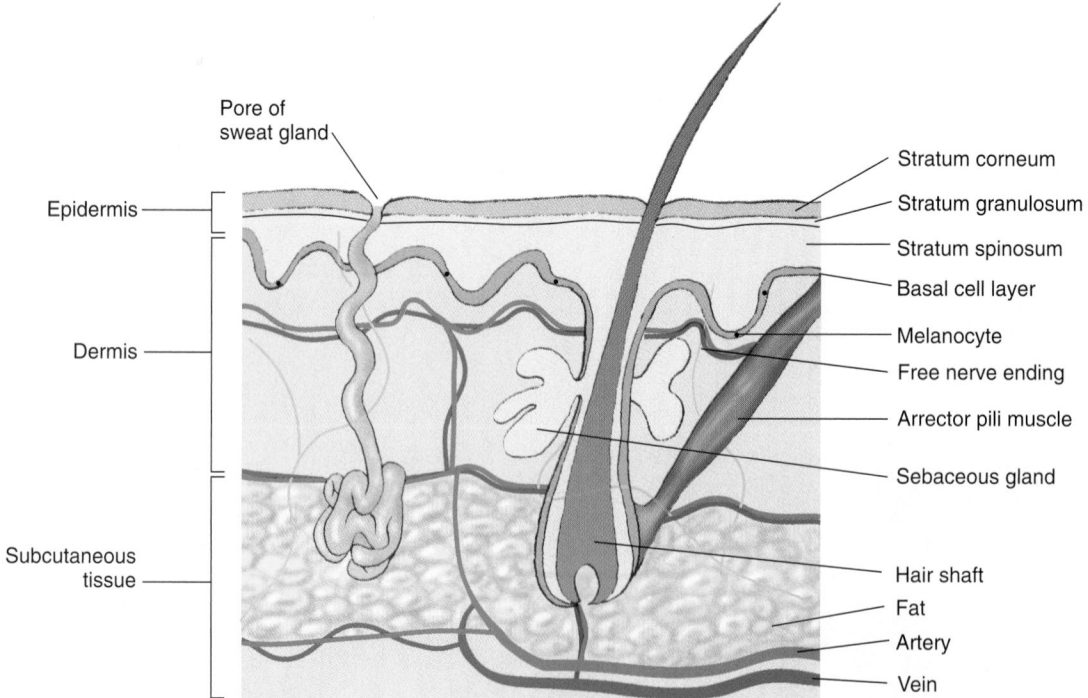

Epidermis

Dermis

Subcutaneous tissue

Pore of sweat gland

Stratum corneum
Stratum granulosum
Stratum spinosum
Basal cell layer
Melanocyte
Free nerve ending
Arrector pili muscle
Sebaceous gland

Hair shaft
Fat
Artery
Vein

Figure 73-1. Cross section of normal skin. (Adapted from Zitelli BJ, Davis HW [eds]: Atlas of Pediatric Physical Diagnosis. St. Louis, Mosby, 1997, p 212.)

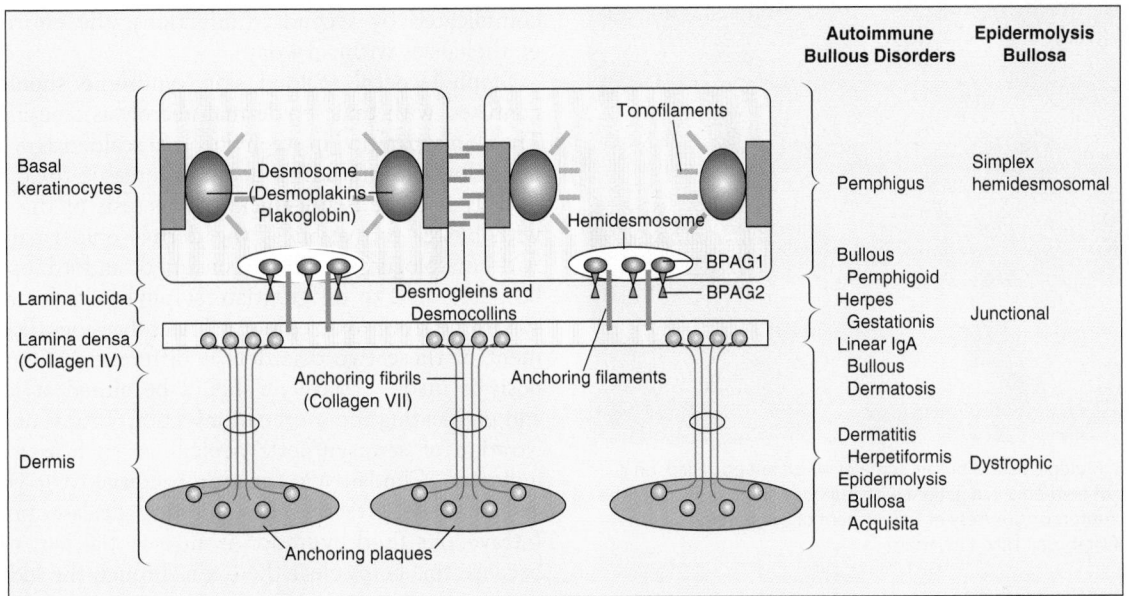

Figure 73-2. Structures comprising the basement membrane zone of the skin. The level in the skin at which separation occurs in mechanobullous disorders and autoimmune bullous disorders is noted. (Adapted from Bowen AR, Zone JJ: Bullous diseases. In Callen JP, Jorizzo JL, Bolognia JL, et al [eds]: Dermatological Signs of Internal Disease, 3rd ed. Philadelphia, Saunders/Elsevier, 2003, p 81.)

congenital mechanobullous disorders, autoimmune mediated blistering diseases, and other disorders in which blisters are encountered. Given that there are numerous infectious causes of cutaneous blistering, the first step in evaluating a vesiculobullous disease is to rule out an infectious cause.

Table 73-1. Infectious, Inflammatory, and Mechanical Causes of Blistering Arising in Different Levels of the Skin

Level of Skin	Disorder
Subcorneal blisters	Bullous impetigo
	Staphylococcal scalded skin syndrome
	Candidiasis
	Bullous tinea pedis
	Pustular psoriasis
	Subcorneal pustular dermatosis
	Friction blisters
Intraepidermal blisters	Herpes simplex
	Varicella zoster/herpes zoster
	Hand-foot-mouth disease
	Contact dermatitis (allergic and irritant)
	Phototoxic/photodrug eruption
	Pemphigus foliaceus
	Pemphigus vulgaris
	Intraepidermal IgA pemphigus
	Thermal or chemical burns
	Epidermolysis bullosa simplex
Subepidermal blisters	Insect bites
	Bullous mastocytosis
	Coma blisters
	Erythema multiforme
	Stevens-Johnson syndrome
	Toxic epidermal necrolysis
	Bullous pemphigoid
	Cicatricial pemphigoid
	Herpes gestationis
	Epidermolysis bullosa aquisita
	Bullous lupus erythematosus
	Dermatitis herpetiformis
	Linear IgA bullous disease
	Epidermolysis bullosa-junctional and dystrophic

Gram stains, bacterial cultures, Tzanck smears, and viral cultures of blister contents are key diagnostic tests. Viral serologies also may be helpful. Potassium hydroxide preparations can show hyphae in fungal infections, although fungal culture may be required for a definitive diagnosis. Skin biopsies are indicated if an infectious workup is unrevealing.

INFECTIOUS DISEASES

Several infectious diseases that are associated with cutaneous blisters are discussed in Chapters 76 and 77, including herpes simplex virus, varicella zoster virus, and candidiasis.

Bullous Impetigo

Bullous impetigo is a superficial skin infection that is a blistering variant of impetigo contagiosa, caused by group 2 *Staphylococcus aureus*, phage type 71. These organisms produce an exfoliatoxin that directly disrupts the cell adhesion molecules in the epidermis by binding to desmoglein 1. Bullous impetigo is seen most often in children, especially infants, and can involve any aspect of the cutaneous surface. Patients present initially with macular erythema that progresses into large, multiple flaccid bullae, many of which become filled with purulent material (Fig. 73-3). These blisters rupture easily, leaving behind a characteristic annular circinate scale with a honey-colored crust. Constitutional symptoms, including fever, weakness, and diarrhea, also may occur.

Bullous impetigo is treated with systemic antibiotics. First-generation cephalosporins and penicillinase-resistant penicillins remain the standard therapy. Given the increased prevalence of resistant organisms, however, a culture should be performed. If a resistant organism is encountered, sensitivities should guide the choice of an antibiotic.

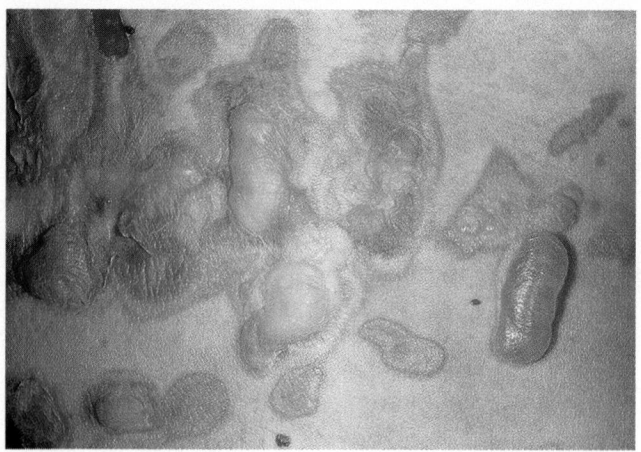

Figure 73-3. Multiple flaccid bullae, some of which are pus-filled, on a background of erythema in a patient with bullous impetigo. Some of the bullae have ruptured. (Courtesy of Department of Dermatology, University of Utah, Salt Lake City, Utah.)

Staphylococcal Scalded Skin Syndrome

Staphylococcal scalded skin syndrome, also called *Ritter's disease*, is a generalized exfoliative dermatosis also caused by toxin-producing group 2 *S. aureus*, phage type 71. Although the pathology is similar to that of bullous impetigo, the actual site of the staphylococcal infection is often remote from the involved skin. The toxin, released into the systemic circulation, is deposited in the skin, where it binds with desmoglein 1, resulting in a generalized exfoliative eruption. Because the toxin is cleared through the kidneys, staphylococcal scalded skin syndrome typically affects infants and young children with immature kidneys and elderly and debilitated individuals with poor renal function. Patients present with fever and malaise along with a rapidly progressing tender macular erythema. Initially the erythema involves the face, neck, and intertriginous areas, but eventually generalizes to involve the total body surface area with sparing of the palms, soles, and mucous membranes (Fig. 73-4). The Nikolsky sign is positive. Over the ensuing few days, the skin develops a fine wrinkly crust and scale, which is removed easily with gentle manipulation. Unless

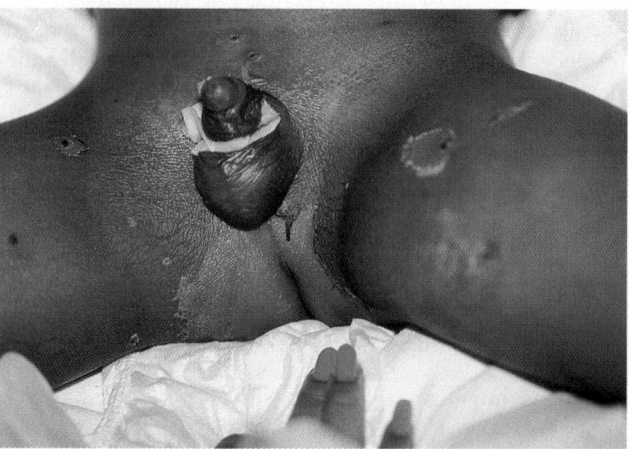

Figure 73-4. Child with staphylococcal scalded skin syndrome presenting with blisters and exfoliation in the diaper area. The source of the staphylococcal infection was a secondary infection of varicella zoster lesions at a distant site.

complicated by secondary infections, the entire skin re-epithelializes within 14 days.

Staphylococcal scalded skin syndrome should not be confused with toxic epidermal necrolysis (see Fig. 79-13). The skin separation in staphylococcal scalded skin syndrome lies below the stratum corneum, whereas in toxic epidermal necrolysis there is full-thickness necrosis of the epidermis with blister formation at the dermal-epidermal junction. A dermatologist should be consulted, and a biopsy should be performed to differentiate staphylococcal scalded skin syndrome from toxic epidermal necrolysis because management of these two disorders is different. When the diagnosis is made, treatment should be aimed at identifying and eradicating the source of infection. Intravenous administration of semisynthetic penicillins, such as nafcillin, is indicated. Clindamycin can stop bacterial toxin production and may be effective in inhibiting disease progression. Intravenous fluid hydration is an essential part of therapy because this helps clear the toxin through the kidneys.

Blistering Distal Dactylitis

Blistering distal dactylitis is a bullous disease caused primarily by β-hemolytic streptococci and at times by *S. aureus*. It most commonly affects children and presents with tender tense bullae with surrounding erythema localized to the pads of the fingers or toes (Fig. 73-5). Some affected individuals have accompanying fever. The differential diagnosis includes bullous impetigo, herpetic whitlow, and friction blisters. Bacterial cultures help make the correct diagnosis. The lesions resolve rapidly after drainage of the blisters and systemic administration of penicillin, penicillinase-resistant penicillins, or first-generation cephalosporins.

Hand-Foot-and-Mouth Disease

Hand-foot-and-mouth disease is a viral disorder often attributed to coxsackievirus, but it also can be caused by other enteroviruses. Symptoms usually begin with fever and

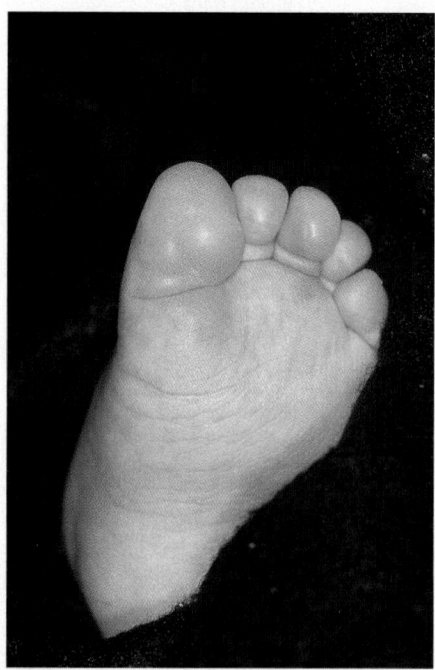

Figure 73-5. Child with blistering distal dactylitis on the toes.

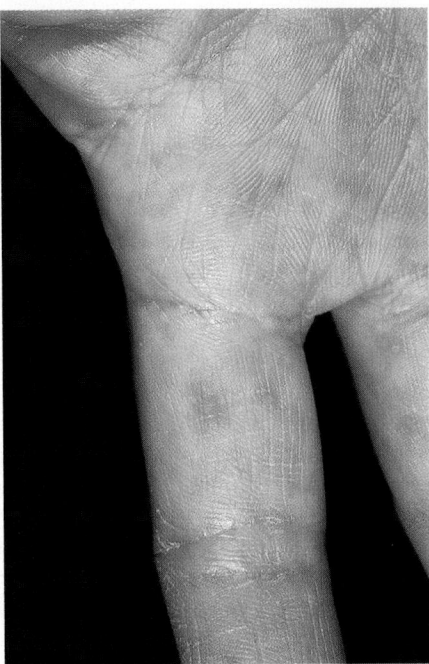

Figure 73-6. Palmar aspect of the fingers of a young adult with hand-foot-and-mouth disease.

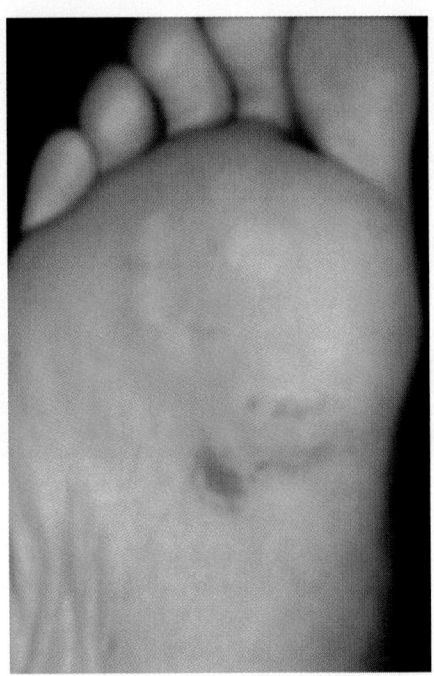

Figure 73-8. Child with bullous tinea pedis. A potassium hydroxide preparation of the blister fluid showed branched hyphae.

soreness of the oral mucosa. As the disease progresses, small vesicles with surrounding erythema develop on the buccal mucosa, tongue, gingiva, and palate. Tender vesicles also involve the palms and soles and have a tendency to follow skin lines (Figs. 73-6 and 73-7); lesions also may arise on buttocks, knees, and ankles. Lesions usually resolve in 1 week, and no intervention other than supportive care is necessary.

Bullous Tinea

Tinea is a superficial fungal infection caused by a dermatophyte organism. It is a common dermatologic ailment that is known by many names (e.g., *ringworm*, *athlete's foot*, *jock itch*). Classically the lesions present with annular erythematous patches with raised margins and scale. At times, a vigorous inflammatory response that results in blister formation may be seen. These reactions most commonly occur on the palms and soles (Fig. 73-8) and are associated with significant pain and pruritus. A potassium hydroxide preparation of scales from the leading edge of the lesion or from vesicle fluid should be performed. When fungal elements have been confirmed, topical antifungal therapy should be administered; at times, oral antifungal medication is required to induce an adequate remission.

REACTION TO EXTERNAL PROCESSES

Arthropod Assaults

Insect bites from mosquitos, fleas, or scabies induce an immediate hypersensitivity reaction by introducing sensitizing components from their saliva into the skin. Often erythema and pruritus are the only presenting sign and symptom. Some individuals may develop a vigorous inflammatory response, however, with severe edema and blister formation (Fig. 73-9). Lesions tend to be distributed in areas not covered by clothing. Oral antihistamines and topical steroids can provide symptomatic relief.

Scabies

Scabies is discussed in Chapter 69 in the differential diagnosis of atopic dermatitis and in Chapter 76. Typically, scabies presents as an eczematous eruption with a predilection for involvement of the axillae and genital areas in older children, adolescents, and adults. In infants, the eruption

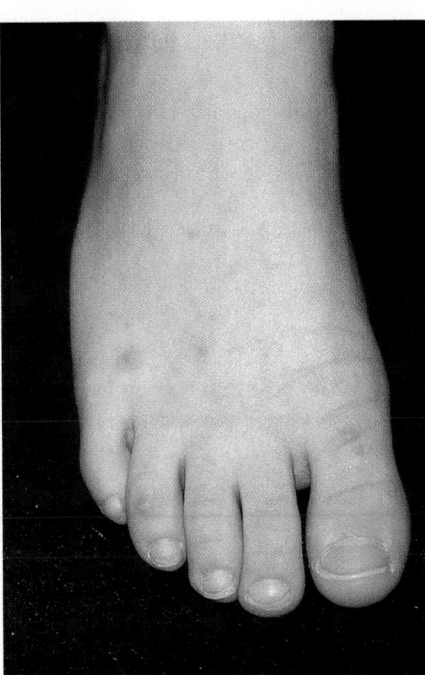

Figure 73-7. Child with hand-foot-and-mouth disease, with vesicles on the top of the foot.

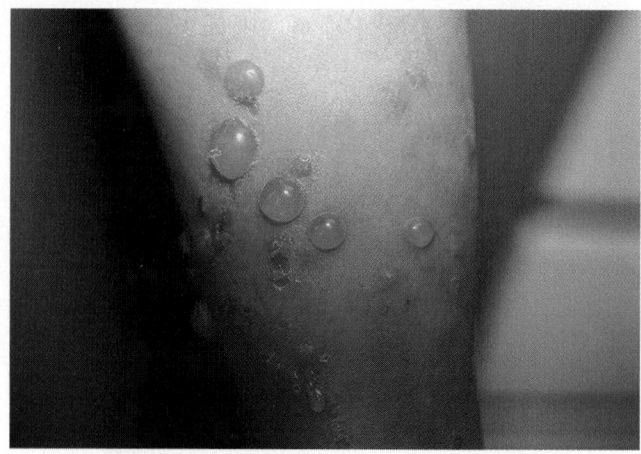

Figure 73-9. Child with bullous insect bite reaction on the leg.

can be generalized, with involvement of the face, scalp, and body; vesicles and pustules on the palms and soles are common.

Contact Dermatitis

Contact dermatitis is discussed in detail in Chapter 69. In some instances, the reaction can be severe, and blister formation can occur.

PHOTOSENSITIVITY DISORDERS

Polymorphous Light Eruption

Polymorphous light eruption is a phototoxic delayed hypersensitivity response to ultraviolet light of unknown etiology. It is extremely common in Native Americans, suggesting a possible genetic factor in some individuals. It is characterized by erythematous papules, urticarial plaques, and vesicles distributed in sun-exposed areas, typically the face, arms, and "V" of the chest (Fig. 73-10). Pruritus is variable

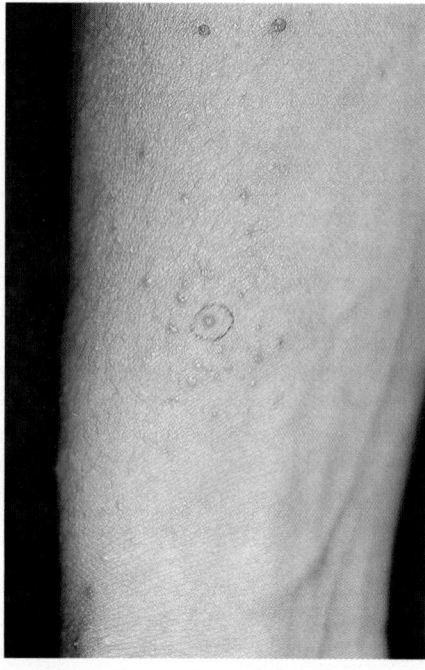

Figure 73-10. Adolescent with polymorphous light eruption on the forearm characterized by erythematous papules and vesicles.

and may be completely absent or quite intense. The lesions typically resolve over 1 to 2 weeks but recur with subsequent sun exposure. Polymorphous light eruption typically presents during childhood and in young or middle-aged adults. It usually flares during early spring, but with subsequent sun exposure, the skin "hardens," and the eruption flares less and less as summer wears on. Although the diagnosis is suggested by clinical presentation, skin biopsy often is performed to confirm the diagnosis and to distinguish it from other photosensitivity disorders, including lupus erythematosus.

Polymorphous light eruption is managed best with sun avoidance and protection, including broad-spectrum ultraviolet A protective sunscreens. Topical and systemic steroids can ameliorate the pruritus of an intense flare of the disease. Oral psoralen combined with ultraviolet A light therapy (PUVA) may be initiated during the early spring to accelerate the "hardening" process, although the risk for skin cancer in later life makes this a less attractive treatment option in children. Beta carotene may be beneficial to some patients. For severely affected individuals, oral administration of antimalarial agents may be considered; because of the potential for ocular complications, use of oral antimalarials should be restricted to short intermittent courses.

Hydroa Aestivale and Vacciniforme

Hydroa aestivale (summer prurigo of Hutchinson) is a blistering disorder that primarily affects children, with summertime recurrences. It is seen in boys twice as often as it is in girls. Some authors consider it a variant of polymorphous light eruption. The term *hydroa vacciniforme* refers to more severe cases in which scarring occurs. Hydroa aestivale is a delayed phototoxic reaction that presents as pruritic edematous papules and vesicles on sun-exposed surfaces that arise within hours or days of ultraviolet light exposure (Figs. 73-11 and 73-12). The lesions can develop central necrosis and heal with varioliform scars. Recurrence of the eruption with subsequent sun exposure is typical. Most patients experience spontaneous resolution by the teen years. The differential diagnosis of hydroa aestivale includes polymorphous light eruption and porphyrias (e.g., erythropoietic protoporphyria, porphyria cutanea tarda, pseudoporphyria) (Fig. 73-13). Treatment of hydroa aestivale is similar to that of polymorphous light eruption, with the exception of PUVA treatments.

HYPERSENSITIVITY REACTIONS

Erythema multiforme, Stevens-Johnson syndrome, and toxic epidermal necrolysis are discussed in Chapter 79.

MECHANOBULLOUS DISORDERS

Epidermolysis Bullosa

Epidermolysis bullosa is a family of rare inherited disorders characterized by absence or dysfunction of protein components comprising the attachment structures of the basal layer of the epidermis, the basement membrane zone, and the papillary dermis. They share the common feature of spontaneous blister formation from mechanical injury to

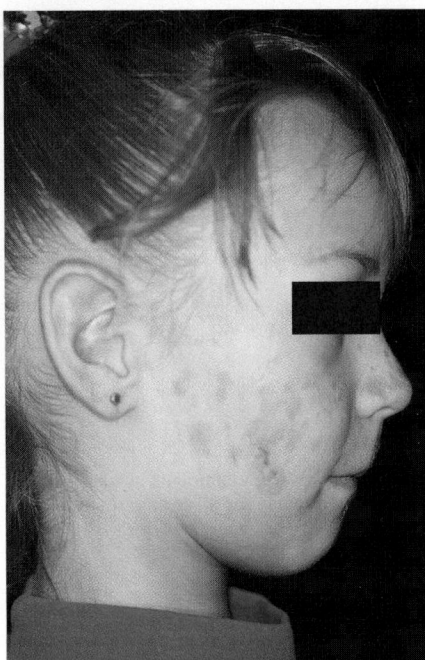

Figure 73-11. Young girl with hydroa vacciniforme, with scarring on the face.

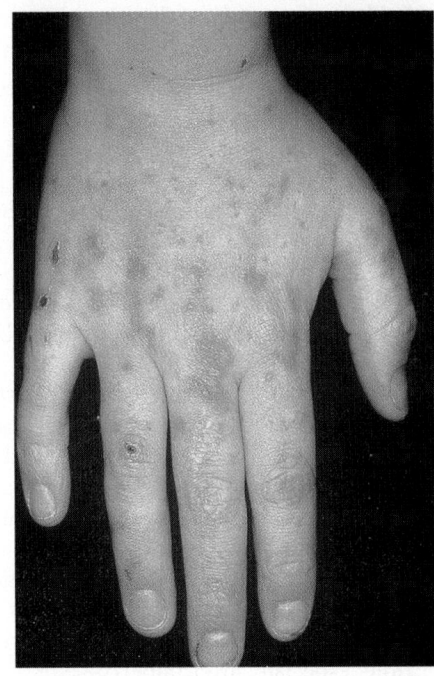

Figure 73-13. Child with short-bowel syndrome with pseudoporphyria secondary to a nonsteroidal anti-inflammatory drug. Note the erosions on the dorsal aspect of the hand, which are identical to lesions seen in porphyria cutanea tarda.

the skin. As depicted in Figure 73-2, there are numerous structural components within the epidermis and dermis that maintain the integrity of the skin. A heterogeneous group of 20 phenotypes of epidermolysis bullosa have been described and categorized based on the level of blister formation within the skin. With the advent of new molecular genetic techniques, the exact molecular defects of these disorders have been elucidated. Epidermolysis bullosa now is categorized into four main groups: simplex, hemidesmosomal, junctional, and dystrophic (Table 73-2).

Epidermolysis Bullosa Simplex

Epidermolysis bullosa simplex, a group of autosomal dominant disorders, is the most common form of epidermolysis bullosa, with approximately 50,000 cases in the United States. The defect lies with the congenital absence or dysfunction of keratins 5 and 14. Keratins are intracellular intermediate filaments that maintain the cytoskeletal structure of keratinocytes. Keratins 5 and 14 are found only within the basal cells of the epidermis. The defective keratins result in cell fragility that leads to blister formation after trauma to the skin. Because the cleavage of the blister is intraepidermal, scarring typically does not occur. There are three main clinical phenotypes of epidermolysis bullosa simplex.

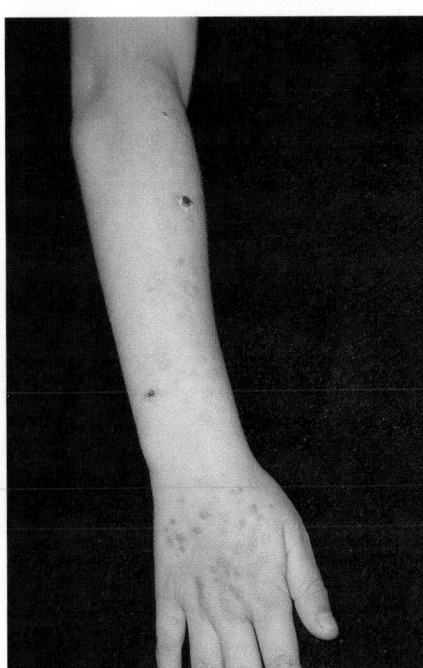

Figure 73-12. Forearm and hand of the girl shown in Figure 73-11.

Table 73-2. Categorization of the Main Types of Epidermolysis Bullosa

Epidermolysis bullosa simplex	Localized (Weber-Cockayne)
	Generalized (Koebner)
	Herpetiformis (Dowling-Meara)
Epidermolysis bullosa, hemidesmosomal	Epidermolysis bullosa with late-onset muscular dystrophy
	Generalized atrophic benign epidermolysis bullosa
	Epidermolysis bullosa with congenital pyloric atresia
Epidermolysis bullos, junctional	Herlitz
	Non-Herlitz
Epidermolysis bullosa dystrophica	Dominant (Cockayne-Touraine, Pasini)
	Recessive (Hallopeau-Siemens)

Localized Epidermolysis Bullosa Simplex (Weber-Cockayne)

Localized epidermolysis bullosa simplex presents with localized blistering. Blister formation usually requires a relatively high level of physical injury and tends to occur in areas subjected to repeated trauma, such as the hands and feet (Fig. 73-14). Lesions can start in infancy, but usually begin later in life as the child learns to crawl and walk. Hyperhidrosis and thickening of the palms and soles are common. Symptoms are exacerbated by warm weather, but most affected people do not find this disease debilitating.

Generalized Epidermolysis Bullosa Simplex (Koebner)

Generalized epidermolysis bullosa simplex is characterized by generalized blister formation, milia, and mucosal erosions. Symptoms usually begin at birth and progress as the child learns to ambulate. Vigorous suckling may lead to mild oral erosions, but scarring and atrophy do not occur. Symptoms are worst during the summer months and improve as the temperatures cool. In general, patients with the Koebner variant of epidermolysis bullosa improve with the passage of time, especially after puberty.

Epidermolysis Bullosa Simplex Herpetiformis (Dowling-Meara)

Epidermolysis bullosa simplex herpetiformis is the most severe form of simplex disease. Infants develop widespread bullae formation with a characteristic grouped herpetic configuration (Figs. 73-15 and 73-16). These often heal with the development of milia, but no scarring. Prominent blistering can be seen on the palms and soles, resulting in thickening of the skin. Many patients have oral mucosal erosions with esophagitis and nail dystrophy. The Dowling-Meara variant of epidermolysis bullosa simplex has significant morbidity and mortality, with many infants dying

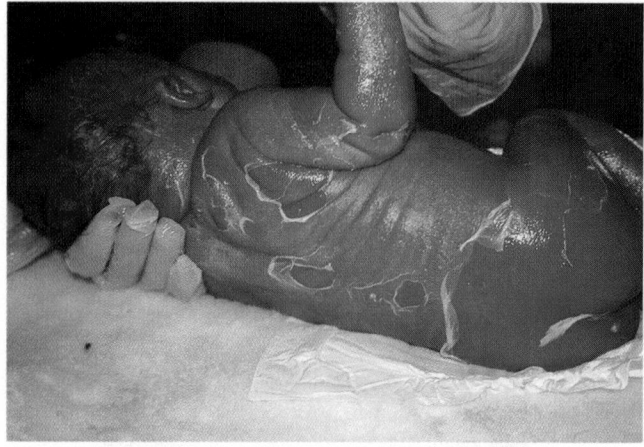

Figure 73-15. Newborn with epidermolysis bullosa simplex herpetiformis (Dowling-Meara), showing diffuse erythema of the skin and extensive erosions.

within the first few months of life. Similar to the Koebner variant, patients with the Dowling-Meara variant tend to blister less over time (Fig. 73-17). In contrast to other forms of epidermolysis bullosa, patients with the Dowling-Meara type tend to have less blister formation with heat exposure.

Hemidesmosomal Epidermolysis Bullosa

Hemidesmosomal epidermolysis bullosa is a new category of epidermolysis bullosa. Initially, these phenotypically distinct disorders were combined in the simplex or junctional forms of epidermolysis bullosa. With recent molecular genetic analysis, however, it has become clear that these disorders represent a distinct class of epidermolysis bullosa. In contrast to epidermolysis bullosa simplex, the defect in hemidesmosomal epidermolysis bullosa resides in abnormalities in the hemidesmosomal complexes at the dermal-epidermal junction. These attachment structures, in contrast to desmosomes, bind the keratinocytes to the underlying substrates in the dermis. Currently, there are three recognized variants of hemidesmosomal epidermolysis bullosa.

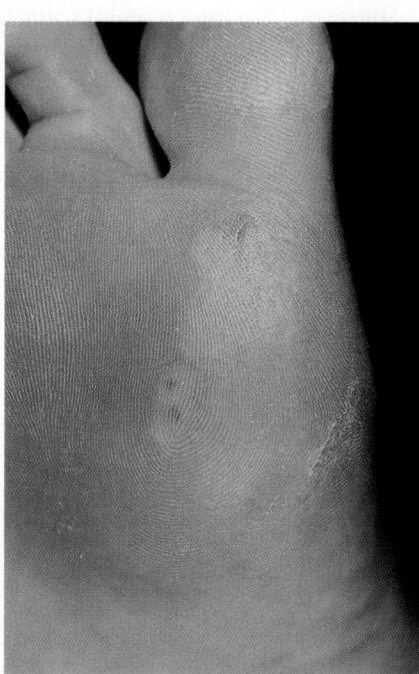

Figure 73-14. Deep-seated blisters on the foot of a young main with localized epidermolysis bullosa simplex (Weber-Cockayne). (Courtesy of Department of Dermatology, University of Utah, Salt Lake City, Utah.)

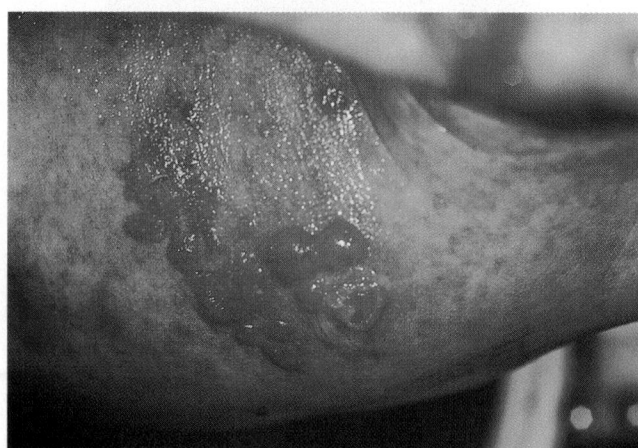

Figure 73-16. Same infant shown in Figure 73-15, with development of herpetiform bullae on the chest 6 days later. The diffuse erythema of the skin has diminished.

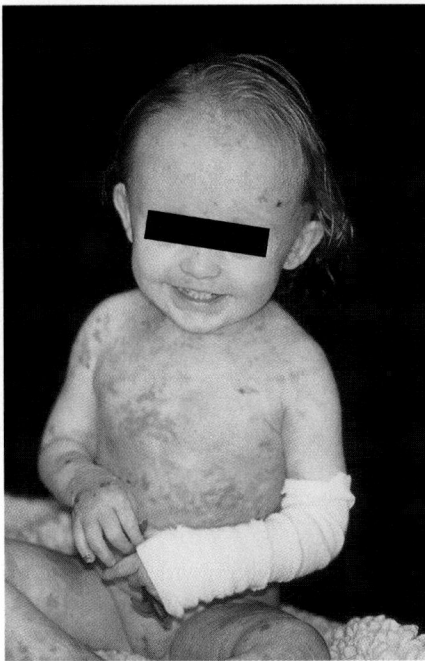

Figure 73-17. Same infant shown in Figures 73-15 and 73-16, now at 21 months of age. Although her skin continues to blister, her disease is much less severe compared with the neonatal period.

Epidermolysis Bullosa with Late-Onset Muscular Dystrophy

Epidermolysis bullosa with late-onset muscular dystrophy is a rare autosomal recessive disorder characterized by widespread blistering at birth with scarring, milia formation, and nail abnormalities. Muscular dystrophy with progressive weakness and wasting occurs later in life. The defect lies in the abnormal synthesis of plectin, a large intracellular adhesion molecule expressed in the basal keratinocytes and in the hemidesmosomes of sarcolemma of muscles.

Generalized Atrophic Benign Epidermolysis Bullosa

Generalized atrophic benign epidermolysis bullosa is an autosomal recessive disorder that presents at birth with generalized bullae that heal with atrophy. Many affected individuals have nail dystrophy, tooth enamel defects with caries and subsequent loss of teeth, and scarring alopecia of the scalp along with mucosal erosions. Although the disease process can be severe, most patients survive into adulthood. The defect lies in the dysfunction of type 17 collagen, a 180-kd transmembrane component of the hemidesmosomal complex.

Epidermolysis Bullosa with Congenital Pyloric Atresia

Epidermolysis bullosa with congenital pyloric atresia is an autosomal recessive disorder characterized by severe widespread bullae, oral mucosal erosions, and pyloric atresia at birth. Some patients also develop urethral strictures requiring surgical intervention. Most neonates die from the skin disease even with repair of the pyloric atresia. If the infant survives the neonatal period, however, the blistering tends to improve over time. The defect is due to an abnormal $\alpha_6\beta_4$ integrin, a hemidesmosomal transmembrane protein.

Junctional Epidermolysis Bullosa

Junctional epidermolysis bullosa, a recessively inherited disorder, is a mechanobullous disorder characterized by a split at the lamina lucida of the basement membrane zone. There is a wide spectrum of clinical severity, ranging from a mild localized (non-Herlitz) variant to a more severe generalized (Herlitz) type. On the mild end of the spectrum, neonates present with bullae on the extremities with nail and hair abnormalities, but otherwise limited systemic concerns. The more severe Herlitz type tends to present with generalized bullae; most infants do not survive because sepsis and sloughing of the respiratory mucosa leading to obstruction are major contributors to mortality. Tooth, laryngeal, pulmonary, gastrointestinal, and genitourinary abnormalities all can be seen. In infants who survive, growth retardation and anemia may be prominent. The defect lies in the mutation of laminin 5, a component of the anchoring filaments, found on three different genes. The clinical severity is determined by the degree of functionality of the abnormal laminin 5.

Dystrophic Epidermolysis Bullosa

Dystrophic epidermolysis bullosa is a scarring form of epidermolysis bullosa that has been mapped to a defect on chromosome 3, which encodes type VII collagen, the anchoring fibril protein. Because the blistering arises in the sublamina densa, lesions heal with significant scarring. Currently the dystrophic forms of epidermolysis bullosa are separated into dominantly and recessively inherited types. The dominant dystrophic type is characterized by relatively limited disease compared with its recessively inherited counterpart. This spectrum of severity of disease is related to the functionality of type VII collagen.

Dominant dystrophic epidermolysis bullosa can present with localized or more generalized bullous eruptions. The localized variant, known as *Cockayne-Touraine*, tends to have lesions limited to the extremities that heal with milia and hypertrophic scarring (Figs. 73-18 and 73-19). Some affected individuals can present at birth, whereas milder cases may not be diagnosed until later in life. In the *Pasini* variant, blistering tends to be more widespread; in addition, patients typically develop small hypopigmented, ivory-colored papules on the trunk, called *albopapuloid lesions*. In

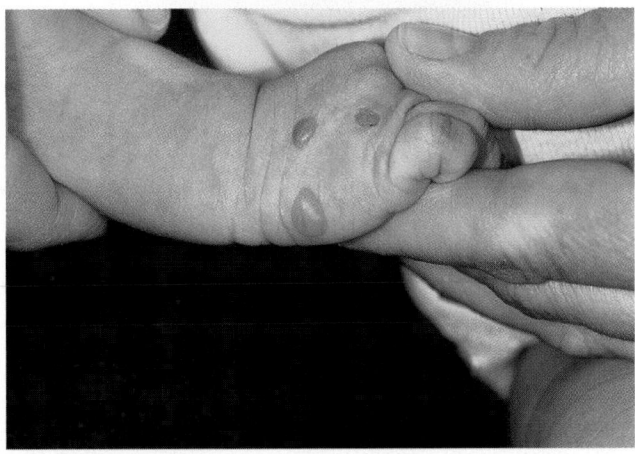

Figure 73-18. Bullae on the hand of an infant with dominant dystrophic epidermolysis bullosa localized variant (Cockayne-Touraine).

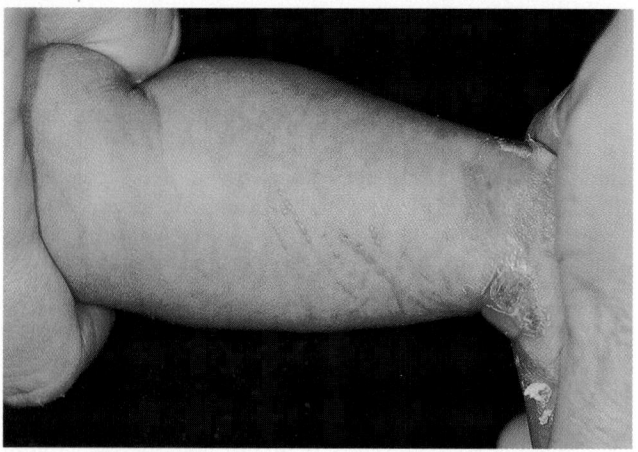

Figure 73-19. Same infant shown in Figure 73-18. Note the linear array of vesicles on the lower leg caused by scratches from toenails on the infant's contralateral foot.

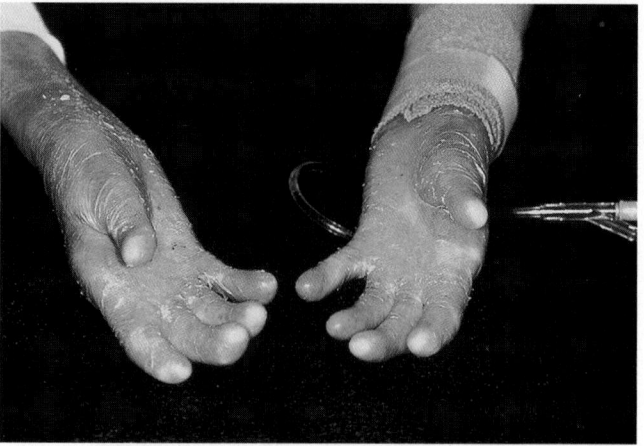

Figure 73-21. Same girl shown in Figure 73-20.

dominant dystrophic epidermolysis bullosa, the nails are often dystrophic or completely absent, but teeth and mucosal abnormalities are more limited.

Recessive dystrophic epidermolysis bullosa (Hallopeau-Siemens) is the most debilitating form of epidermolysis bullosa. It is characterized at birth by widespread blister formation that heals with atrophic scars and milia. The nails are often dystrophic. Mucosal erosions are extensive with involvement of the oral, ocular, esophageal, and genital mucosa. Scarring leads to hoarseness, strictures, and esophageal and anal stenosis. Dental caries is common, arising as a result of poor oral hygiene. Digital fusion and "mitten deformities" of the hands and feet develop from repeated episodes of blistering (Figs. 73-20 and 73-21). Given the chronic hyperplastic nature of the skin, many patients develop squamous cell carcinomas that can be aggressive and must be treated accordingly. Affected individuals are at risk for poor nutrition, growth retardation, and anemia. Most die in young adult life, with chronic infection and mucosal malignancy major contributors to mortality.

When evaluating a newborn with a blistering disorder, an infectious cause needs to be ruled out first. Table 73-3 outlines the diagnostic considerations in this setting. In general, after an infectious cause has been ruled out, the neonate should be referred to a dermatologist for a skin biopsy for routine histologic examination. When the diagnosis of epidermolysis bullosa is seriously considered, electron microscopy or immunofluorescent mapping of the skin can be helpful. If necessary, DNA analysis may be performed at available referral centers.

Management of epidermolysis bullosa depends on severity. In most cases of epidermolysis bullosa simplex, gentle wound care with whirlpool, topical antibiotics, and moisturization is sufficient. Blisters should not be removed, but instead decompressed with a sterile needle to prevent their extension. An effort should be made to avoid trauma to the skin; most patients tend to tolerate a cool environment better. In severe cases, especially recessive dystrophic epidermolysis bullosa, a multidisciplinary management approach is required. A dentist should be consulted for adequate oral hygiene. An occupational therapist can help delay the onset of mitten deformities, but ultimately surgical intervention

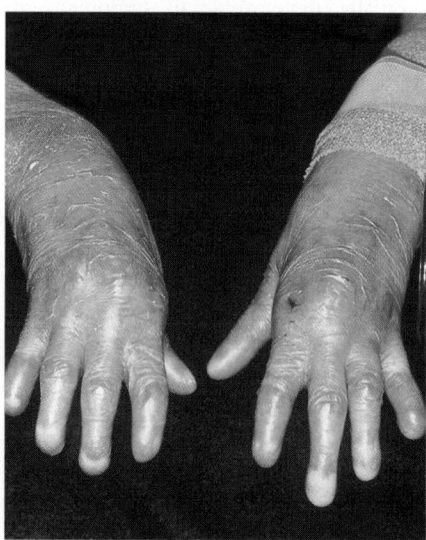

Figure 73-20. Mitten deformities of the hands in a teenage girl with recessive dystrophic epidermolysis bullosa (Hallopeau-Siemens).

Table 73-3. Diagnostic Considerations in the Evaluation of the Newborn with Blisters

Infection	Bullous impetigo
	Staphylococcal scalded skin syndrome
	Candidiasis
	Herpes simplex
	Varciella infection
	Congenital syphilis
	Scabies
Inflammation	Miliaria
	Erythema toxicum neonatorum
	Transient neonatal pustular melanosis
	Transient cephalic neonatal pustulosis
	Mastocytosis
	Sucking blisters
	Contact dermatitis
	Toxic epidermal necrolysis
Genodermatoses	Bullous congenital ichthyosiform erythroderma
	Ectodermal dysplasia
	Incontinentia pigmenti
	Epidermolysis bullosa

may be needed. It is important that these patients have an adequate nutritional intake. Referral to appropriate specialists should be guided by the symptoms the patient develops (e.g., esophageal strictures, squamous cell carcinomas). Ultimately, management is based on preventing trauma to the skin, treating secondary infections of the skin, and minimizing potential complications of cutaneous and non-cutaneous structures. The Dystrophic Epidermolysis Bullosa Research Association (DEBRA) is an excellent support group available to patients with all forms of epidermolysis bullosa and can be contacted via their website at http://www.debra.org.

OTHER HEREDITARY OR CONGENITAL DISORDERS

Incontinentia pigmenti typically presents with blisters and pustules at the time of birth. This condition is discussed in Chapter 74. Aplasia cutis congenita may present with bullae, rather than open erosions, at birth; this is discussed in Chapter 72. Other disorders that may present with blistering at birth include bullous congenital ichthyosiform erythroderma, an autosomal dominant type of ichthyosis, and some types of ectodermal dysplasias.

AUTOIMMUNE BLISTERING DISORDERS

Autoimmune blistering disorders are a group of diseases that result from the deposition of immunoglobulins against normal structural and adhesive components of the skin, with subsequent induction of inflammation and blister formation. It remains unclear what initiates the immune system to produce these autoantibodies. Historically, immunobullous diseases were categorized based on phenotypic features of each disorder. With the advent of immunofluorescent techniques in the 1960s, it was discovered that most autoimmune blistering disorders could be categorized based on characteristic immunofluorescent patterns. These features include the type of antibody involved and the level of distribution in the skin (Table 73-4).

Differentiating autoimmune bullous disorders from other blistering diseases can be difficult on a clinical basis. When evaluating a child with a blistering disorder, a workup to rule out an infectious process should be undertaken first. Skin biopsy specimens are essential to make the diagnosis of an immunobullous disorder. Biopsy specimens for routine histology are obtained from involved skin. Biopsy specimens for immunofluorescence studies are obtained from perilesional skin, about 5 mm from the edge of a blister; the specimen should be sent to the laboratory in Michel's medium or on a saline-soaked gauze and refrigerated until processing is undertaken.

Pemphigus

Pemphigus is a bullous disorder that presents most often in adults in their 40s to 60s. Although rarely encountered in children, there is a variant of neonatal pemphigus that results from the transient transfer of immunoglobulins from affected mothers.

Pemphigus vulgaris is the most severe form and is characterized by flaccid blisters on normal-appearing skin or on an erythematous base involving the scalp, neck, axillae, or groin (Fig. 73-22). These bullae form above the basal layer of the epidermis and rupture easily, resulting in painful bloody erosions that enlarge with minor trauma. The Nikolsky sign is present. Oral lesions are common and often precede the onset of the cutaneous eruption (Fig. 73-23). Erosions can extend from the lips to the pharynx, larynx, and esophagus and can affect oral intake significantly. The mucosa of the eyes and genital and anal areas also may be involved. *Pemphigus vegetans* is a rare variant of pemphigus vulgaris characterized by verrucous plaques surrounded by pustules that develop from open areas along the body folds, the groin, and the face. Because bullae may not be encountered, pemphigus vegetans should be considered in the differential diagnosis of any chronic papillomatous process of unknown etiology.

Pemphigus foliaceus is a superficial, less severe variant of pemphigus in which the split occurs more superficially in the skin, within or just beneath the granular layer of

Table 73-4. Autoimmune Bullous Disorders

Name	Level of Blister Formation	Direct Immunofluorescence Pattern	Autoantigens
Intraepidermal IgG			
Pemphigus vulgaris	Suprabasal	IgG and C3 between keratinocytes	Desmoglein 3 (and 1)
Pemphigus foliaceus	In or below granular layer	IgG and C3 between keratinocytes	Desmoglein 1
Intraepidermal IgA			
IgA pemphigus	Subcorneal pustules	IgA between keratinocytes	Desmocollin 1
	Intraepidermal vesicles	IgA between keratinocytes	Desmoglein 1 and 3
Subepidermal IgG			
Bullous pemphigoid	Subepidermal	Linear IgG and C3 at the BMZ	BPAg 1, BPAg 2
Cicatricial pemphigoid	Subepidermal	Linear IgG and C3 at the BMZ	BPAg 1, BPAg 2, laminin V, β_4-integrin, type VII collagen, 45 kd keratin
Herpes gestationis	Subepidermal	Linear C3 at the BMZ	BPAg 2
Epidermolysis bullosa acquisita	Subepidermal	Linear IgG and C3 at the BMZ	Type VII collagen
Subepidermal IgA			
Dermatitis herpetiformis	Subepidermal	Granular IgA in the dermal papillae	Epidermal tissue transglutaminase
Linear IgA bullous dermatosis	Subepidermal	Linear IgA at the BMZ	BPAg 2, type VII collagen

BMZ, basement membrane zone.

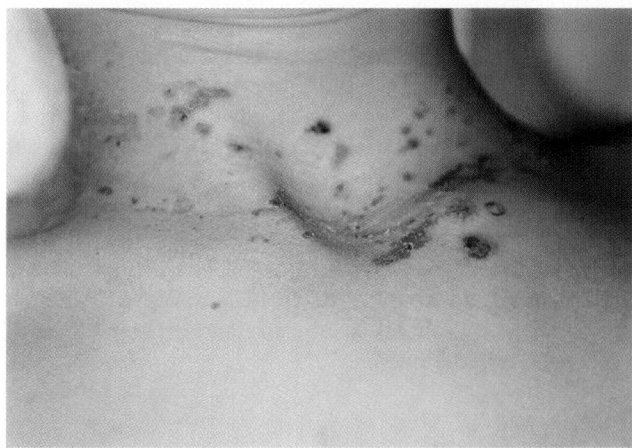

Figure 73-22. Erosions on the neck of a young boy with pemphigus vulgaris.

the epidermis. Although also uncommon in children, there seems to be a higher prevalence compared with pemphigus vulgaris. Lesions begin as small flaccid bullae that rupture easily, leaving behind shallow crusted erosions that often have an eczematous or exfoliative appearance (Fig. 73-24). The scalp, face, chest, and back are most commonly involved. In contrast to pemphigus vulgaris, oral lesions are rarely encountered in pemphigus foliaceus. There is an endemic form of the disease in Brazil, called *fogo selvagem*.

IgA pemphigus presents with pustules and vesicles involving primarily the axillae and groin (Fig. 73-25). Oral mucosal involvement is rare. Two histologic patterns are recognized, the subcorneal pustular type and the intraepidermal type. As opposed to the other variants of pemphigus, IgA pemphigus is distinguished by IgA deposition in the skin, rather than IgG.

Topical and systemic steroids remain the initial therapy for pemphigus. Steroid-sparing agents, such as azathioprine, methotrexate, cyclophosphamide, mycophenolate mofetil, and intramuscular gold, can be used as single agents or in combination therapy in more severe cases. Plasmapheresis and intravenous immunoglobulin may be helpful in recalcitrant patients. Dapsone is the treatment of choice for IgA pemphigus.

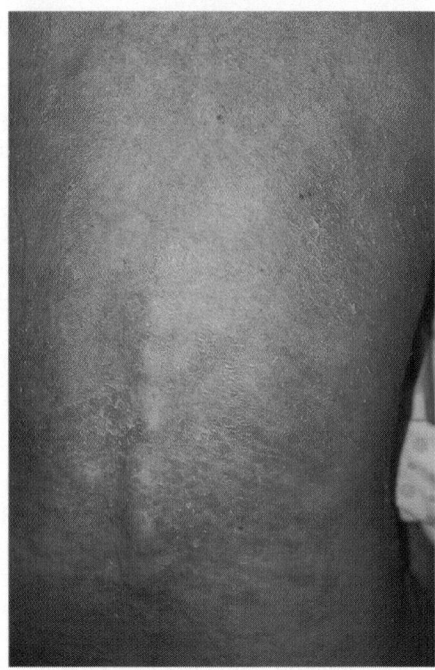

Figure 73-24. Pemphigus foliaceus in a middle-aged woman. (Courtesy of Department of Dermatology, University of Utah, Salt Lake City, Utah.)

Bullous Pemphigoid and Cicatricial Pemphigoid

Bullous pemphigoid is a relatively common autoimmune bullous disorder that predominantly affects the elderly and is rarely found in children. Bullous pemphigoid begins as large tense bullae on either normal-appearing skin or an erythematous base (Fig. 73-26). Cicatricial pemphigoid represents a unique and scarring subset of pemphigoid. Most cases are seen in middle-aged to elderly individuals, with rare cases reported during childhood. Bullous pemphigoid and cicatricial pemphigoid are discussed on the CD-ROM.

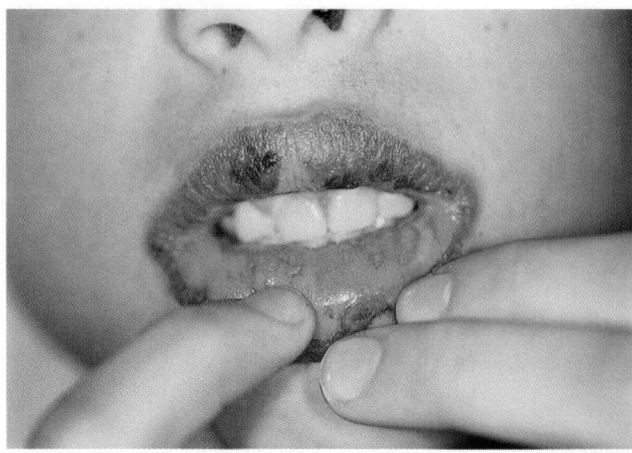

Figure 73-23. Oral mucosal involvement of the child shown in Figure 73-22 with pemphigus vulgaris.

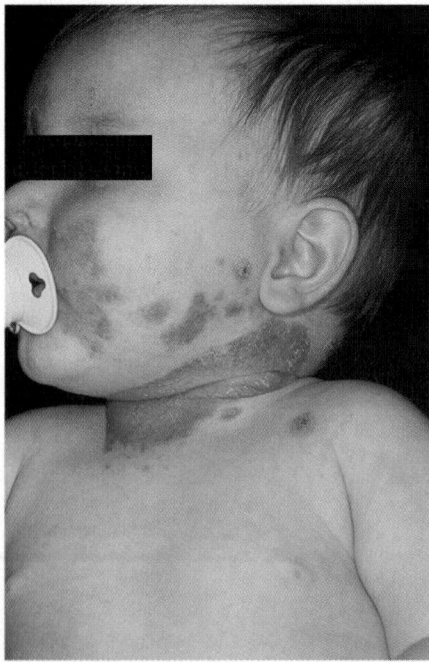

Figure 73-25. Subcorneal pustular type of IgA pemphigus in an infant, characterized by large erosions studded with pustules at the margins.

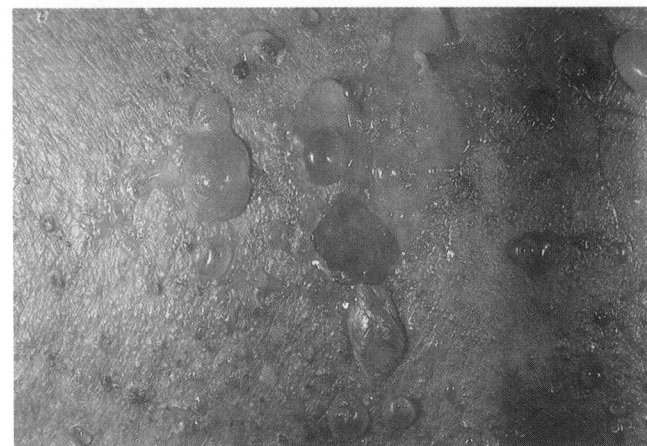

Figure 73-26. Tense bullae on erythematous skin in an elderly man with bullous pemphigoid. (Courtesy of Department of Dermatology, University of Utah, Salt Lake City, Utah.)

Herpes Gestationis

Herpes gestationis is a relatively uncommon immunobullous dermatosis of pregnancy with histologic features similar to bullous pemphigoid (Fig. 73-27). Herpes gestationis is discussed on the CD-ROM.

Epidermolysis Bullosa Acquisita

Epidermolysis bullosa acquisita is an uncommon acquired blistering disorder that is encountered most commonly in adults and is characterized by trauma-induced blisters on the extensor surfaces, especially on the hands, that heal slowly with scarring. Formation of milia at sites of prior involvement is typical. Epidermolysis bullosa acquisita is discussed on the CD-ROM.

Dermatitis Herpetiformis

Dermatitis herpetiformis, also known as *Duhring's disease,* is a chronic recurring blistering disorder that can arise at any age, but generally is seen in adults. Most affected children develop cutaneous lesions after age 5 and continue to have the disorder into adulthood. Childhood dermatitis herpetiformis is clinically and histologically identical to the adult form.

Dermatitis herpetiformis classically presents with extremely pruritic papules and vesicles on the elbows, knees, upper back, and buttocks (Fig. 73-28). The distribution is surprisingly symmetric. The vesicles develop in small grouped configurations, with a "herpetiform" morphology. Given the pruritic nature of this disease, erosions are encountered more often on physical examination than intact vesicles. Other less common areas of involvement include the palms, soles, and face. Oral and ocular lesions are rare.

An interesting aspect of dermatitis herpetiformis is its association with gluten-sensitive enteropathy. Most patients have little if any complaints of abdominal discomfort and diarrhea, as commonly seen in celiac sprue. Endoscopic evaluation often reveals varying degrees of intestinal villous atrophy, however, histologically identical to celiac disease. In addition, patients with dermatitis herpetiformis have exacerbations of the skin disease by the presence of gluten in their diet. It has been shown that the autoantigen in dermatitis herpetiformis is epidermal tissue transglutaminase. Affected individuals develop highly adherent antibodies against epidermal transglutaminase when challenged with gluten. This immune complex is deposited in the skin.

When dermatitis herpetiformis is suspected, a dermatologist should be consulted. Direct immunofluorescence in most cases is diagnostic. Antiendomysial antibodies are found in the blood of about 85% of patients with dermatitis herpetiformis and should be evaluated in conjunction with immunofluorescence studies of the skin.

Dapsone, a sulfone, is the most effective treatment for dermatitis herpetiformis. There are severe side effects, however, that must be monitored closely. Hematologic abnormalities include anemia, methemoglobinemia, leukopenia, and rarely agranulocytosis. Although hemolysis occurs in all patients, a severe form of hemolytic anemia is seen in patients with glucose-6-phosphate dehydrogenase deficiency. Other less frequent side effects include abnormal liver function tests and peripheral neuropathy. Before initiation of therapy, baseline complete blood count, liver functions, and glucose 6-phosphate dehydrogenase should be checked. A complete blood count should be monitored weekly for 4 weeks, then monthly for 6 months, then every 6 months

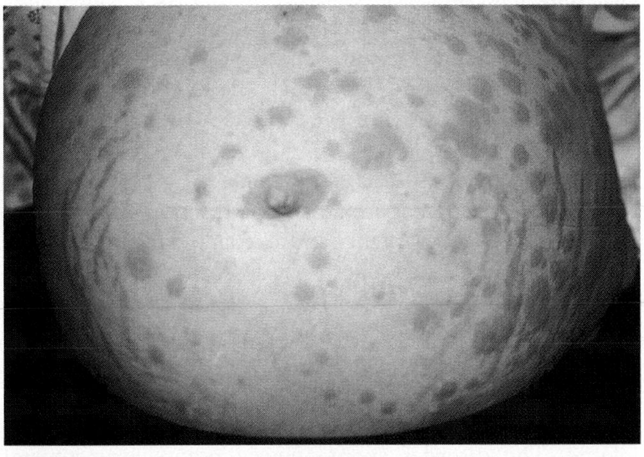

Figure 73-27. Urticarial papules and plaques on the abdomen of a pregnant woman with herpes gestationis. (Courtesy of Department of Dermatology, University of Utah, Salt Lake City, Utah.)

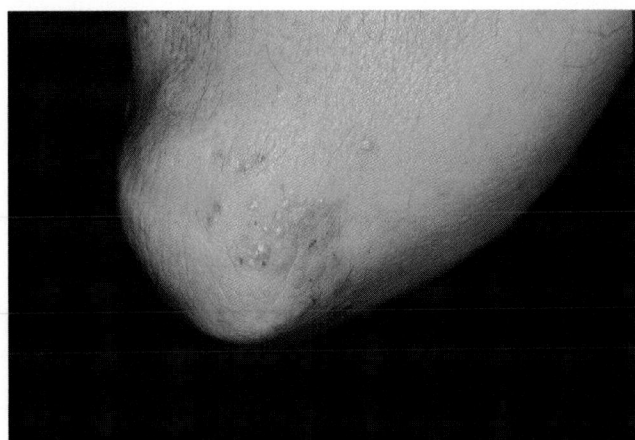

Figure 73-28. Grouped erythematous papules, vesicles, and erosions on the elbow of a man with dermatitis herpetiformis. (Courtesy of Department of Dermatology, University of Utah, Salt Lake City, Utah.)

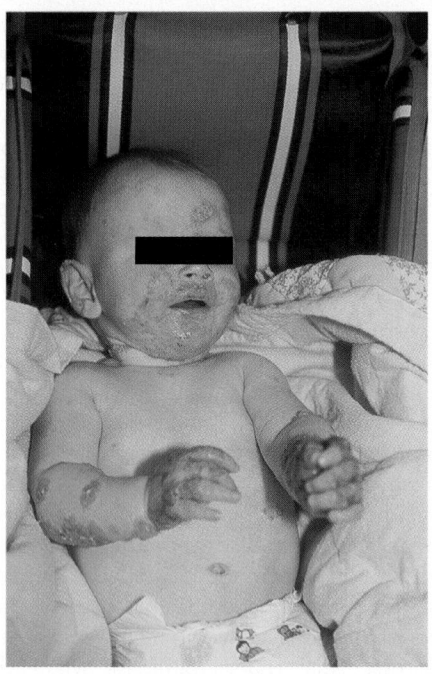

Figure 73-29. Infant with chronic bullous disease of childhood.

thereafter. Liver functions should be monitored every 2 weeks for 4 months, then every 3 to 6 months thereafter.

Sulfapyridine, another sulfur-based medication, had long been used for dermatitis herpetiformis before the discovery of dapsone. Currently, it is available only from the manufacturer directly and is used most often in patients with refractory disease or who are intolerant of dapsone therapy. The side-effect profile is similar to dapsone, as is blood monitoring.

Because of the association with gluten sensitivity, a gluten-free diet can generate a long-term remission for patients with dermatitis herpetiformis. Gluten is found in wheat, rye, and barley flour (corn has no gluten). This diet can be difficult to adhere to, especially given the predominance of wheat products in the food supply. Consultation with a nutritionist can be invaluable in maintaining strict adherence. After 5 to 12 months of gluten avoidance, complete remission with discontinuation of systemic therapy often can be maintained.

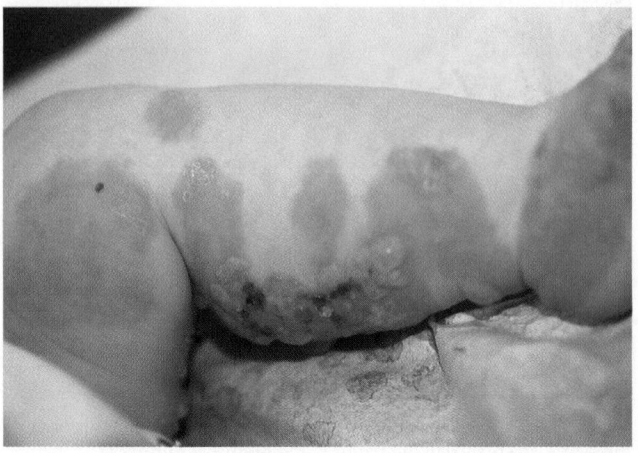

Figure 73-30. Same infant shown in Figure 73-29.

Linear IgA Bullous Disease

Linear IgA bullous disease (chronic bullous disease of childhood) is a distinct clinical entity that shares with dermatitis herpetiformis IgA deposition in the skin, but similar to bullous pemphigoid, the pattern of deposition is a linear band along the dermal-epidermal junction. Children usually are affected within the first 10 years of life, and although most cases remit within 3 years, some patients continue to be affected into adulthood. Clinically, patients can present predominantly with vesicles resembling dermatitis herpetiformis or large tense bullae as seen in bullous pemphigoid. Many develop an interesting annular or "crown of jewels" configuration, in which new bullae develop at the periphery of an erythematous patch with older lesions (Figs. 73-29 and 73-30). There is no characteristic area of predilection, as seen in dermatitis herpetiformis, and any part of the skin may be involved. Oral mucosal erosions are seen in about 60% of patients, and pruritus can be variable. In contrast to dermatitis herpetiformis, there is rarely an association with gluten sensitivity.

The treatment of linear IgA bullous disease is similar to that of dermatitis herpetiformis. Dapsone and sulfapyridine are effective in maintaining a disease-free remission in most affected individuals. For more limited involvement of the skin, ultrapotent topical steroids can be considered, but should be used cautiously because of concerns of cutaneous atrophy and systemic absorption in young children. A trial of gluten avoidance is not recommended routinely, given the rare association with gluten sensitivity, unless celiac disease is documented.

OTHER BULLOUS DISORDERS

Acropustulosis of Infancy

Acropustulosis of infancy arises typically between birth and age 2 years and has a predilection for black infants. It is characterized by recurrent crops of intensely pruritic papules, vesicles, and pustules on the palms and soles, waxing and waning every few weeks (Fig. 73-31). It is four times more common in boys than in girls. Some cases arise after a scabies infestation. The differential diagnosis includes ongoing scabies infestation, dyshidrotic eczema, pustular psoriasis, impetigo, and subcorneal pustular dermatosis/IgA pemphigus. Topical steroids are relatively ineffective at controlling the pruritus; oral antihistamines are helpful. Oral therapy with erythromycin or sulfa-based antibiotics may be of benefit. Dapsone, 2 mg/kg/day, can be helpful to keep the lesions under control until they spontaneously remit.

Eosinophilic Pustular Dermatosis

Eosinophilic pustular dermatosis is a disorder of unknown etiology that affects infants and is characterized by recurrent crops of pustules on the scalp, palms, soles, and at times torso (Figs. 73-32 and 73-33). Some consider it to be a longer lasting variant of erythema toxicum neonatorum. It is distinct from eosinophilic folliculitis, often associated with human immunodeficiency virus infection in adults. Male infants are affected nearly five times as often as female infants. The disorder spontaneously remits after several months or a few years. The differential diagnosis includes acropustulosis of infancy and scabies. Treatment with

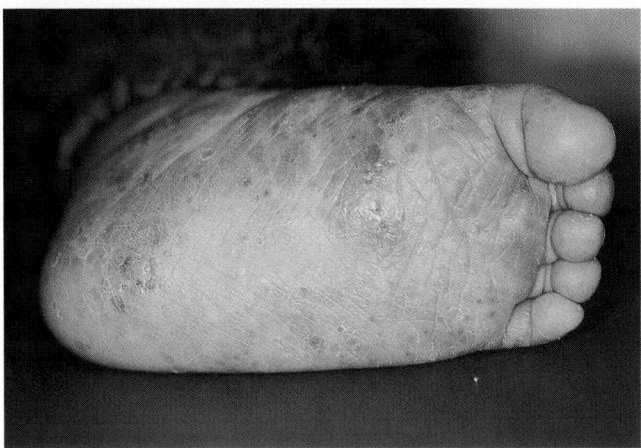

Figure 73-31. Papules, vesicles, and erosions on the sole of the foot of an infant with acropustulosis of infancy.

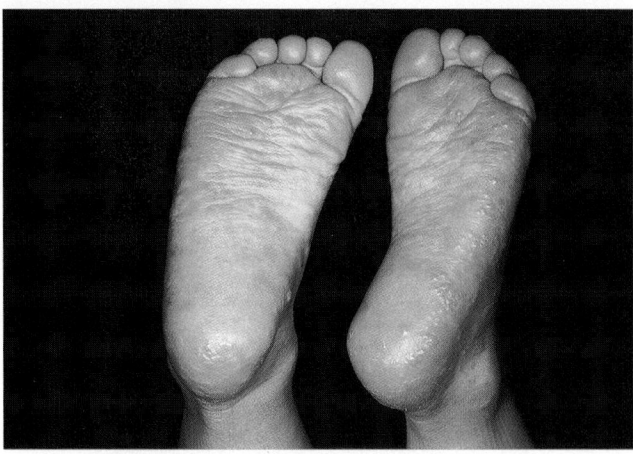

Figure 73-33. Vesicles on the soles of the feet in another infant with eosinophilic pustular dermatosis.

topical steroids is beneficial in some, and oral erythromycin given for a few months may be associated with remission.

Pompholyx

Pompholyx is discussed in Chapter 69.

Cutaneous Mastocytosis

Cutaneous mastocytosis is a heterogeneous group of disorders characterized by the accumulation of mast cells within the dermis. It may be seen from birth to adulthood. There are five main types of mastocytosis: (1) solitary mastocytosis, (2) urticaria pigmentosa, (3) diffuse cutaneous mastocytosis, (4) telangiectasia macularis eruptiva perstans, and (5) systemic mastocytosis. The most common types seen in pediatric patients are solitary mastocytosis and urticaria pigmentosa. Bullous variants may be seen with both of these forms of mastocytosis in children.

Solitary mastocytomas present as isolated, yellowish brown papules, plaques, or nodules, most often located on

the extremities, neck, and trunk (see Fig. 78-17). Although most cases are solitary, multiple lesions are not uncommon. Lesions typically present at birth or during early infancy. The clinical diagnosis is suggested by the presence of localized erythema, edema, or urticaria after vigorous stroking (Darier's sign); this phenomenon results from the mechanical release of histamine from the mast cells. Vesicles or bullae can arise during a vigorous histamine response. Treatment is symptomatic. Topical and intralesional steroids can be effective in controlling pruritus and thinning of the lesions. Most mastocytomas become less reactive after several years and typically resolve by puberty.

Urticaria pigmentosa is characterized by numerous red-brown macules or papules that over time become hyperpigmented (see Fig. 78-18). It arises predominantly in children, but can be seen in adults. Darier's sign is usually positive. Lesions can affect any cutaneous surface and usually are found on the trunk, face, scalp, and extremities. As with solitary mastocytomas, a vigorous histamine response induced by mechanical stimulation (e.g., rubbing the skin or hot baths) or spontaneous degranulation of mast cells caused by certain medications (Box 73-1) or foods (e.g., spicy foods, cheese, alcohol) can result in blister formation (Fig. 73-34).

In children, urticaria pigmentosa is essentially a cutaneous disorder with complete resolution seen by adolescence in most cases. Onset of urticaria pigmentosa during adolescence or adulthood has a higher risk of associated

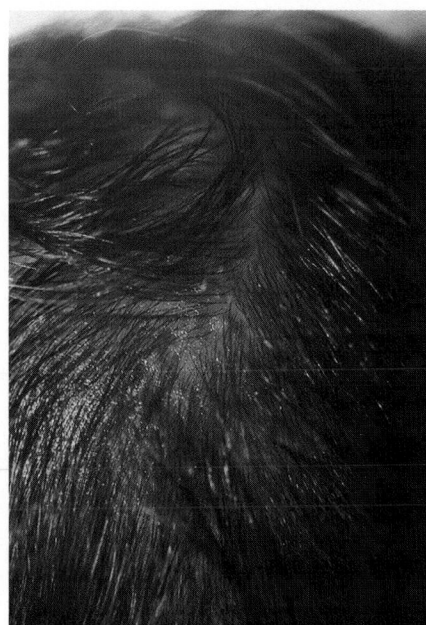

Figure 73-32. A crop of pustules on the scalp of an infant with eosinophilic pustular dermatosis.

Box 73-1. Medications That Spontaneously Degranulate Mast Cells and Should Be Avoided in Patients with Urticaria Pigmentosa

- Aspirin
- Opiate narcotics
- Procaine
- Polymyxin B
- Radiographic contrast dyes
- Scopolamine
- Tubocurarine
- Gallamine
- Decamethonium
- Pancuronium

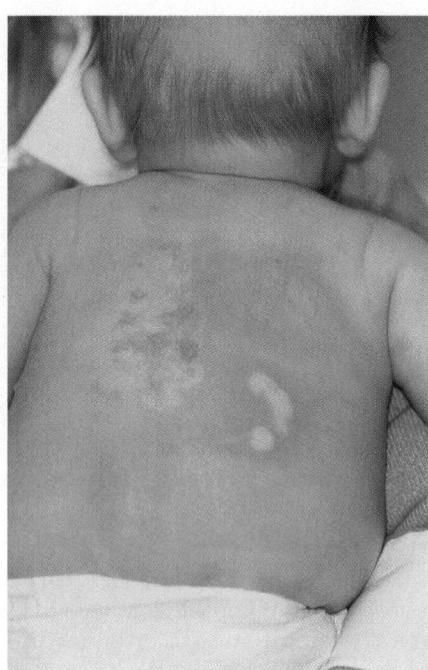

Figure 73-34. Infant with bullous mastocytosis.

systemic disease, however, and a workup for liver, spleen, and bone marrow involvement should be considered. Urticaria pigmentosa in most cases can be controlled with topical steroids, oral antihistamines (H_1 and H_2 blockers), and oral administration of mast cell stabilizers (e.g., cromolyn or ketotifen). In refractory cases, PUVA can be considered, but must be weighed against the potential consequences of future development of skin cancer.

Additional Resources, CD-ROM

Color atlas	Figures
Bullous pemphigoid	Text, figure
Cicatricial pemphigoid	Text
Herpes gestationis	Text, figure
Epidermolysis bullosa acquisita	Text
Bibliography	

Mini-index of Related Topics   CH.

SUGGESTED READINGS

Bowen AR, Zone JJ: Bullous diseases. In Callen JP, Jorizzo JL, Bolognia JL, et al (eds): Dermatological Signs of Internal Disease, 3rd ed. Philadelphia, WB Saunders, 2003, pp 81–93.

Fesq H, Ring J, Abeck D: Management of polymorphous light eruption: Clinical course, pathogenesis, diagnosis and intervention. Am J Clin Dermatol 2003;4:399–406.

Heide R, Tank B, Oranje AP: Mastocytosis in childhood. Pediatr Dermatol 2002;19:375–381.

Patel GK, Finlay AY: Staphylococcal scalded skin syndrome: Diagnosis and management. Am J Clin Dermatol 2003;4:165–175.

Weston WL, Morelli JG, Huff JC: Misdiagnosis, treatments, and outcomes in the immunobullous diseases in children. Pediatr Dermatol 1997;14:264–272.

74 Disorders of Pigmentation

Mark Herron and Sheryll L. Vanderhooft

ROLE OF THE GENERALIST

1   Know the congenital and acquired causes of pigmentary abnormalities.

2   Identify when a pigmentary abnormality may be associated with an underlying disorder.

3   Distinguish hypopigmentation from depigmentation.

4   Recognize pigmentary changes along the lines of Blaschko and their possible genetic implications.

5   Counsel parents of patients with pigmentary abnormalities about appropriate photoprotection.

6   Refer to a specialist when the etiology of a pigmentary abnormality is unclear.

FUNDAMENTALS

Melanin is a brown-to-black pigment in the skin that serves to protect it from the acute and chronic damage of ultraviolet (UV) radiation. Melanin is responsible for the pigmentation of hair and skin. Melanin is synthesized in the melanocytes found along the basal layer of the epidermis. The melanocytes travel from the neural crest to the epidermis during embryogenesis. Tyrosine in the melanocytes is converted by tyrosinase to dihydroxyphenylalanine (DOPA), which eventually is converted to melanin. Melanocytes transfer the melanin via their dendritic processes to the keratinocytes, where the melanin is dispersed in the cytoplasm. Normal pigmentation of the skin is influenced by the amount, type, and location of melanin; by the degree of dermal vascularity; by the presence of carotene; and by the thickness of the stratum corneum of the epidermis. The intensity of pigmentation depends on the size and number of melanosomes in the melanocytes and the keratinocytes.

Hyperpigmentation refers to an excess of color within the skin. The term *hypopigmentation* is used to describe diminished color within the skin; this may result from reduction in the number of melanocytes or abnormally low melanin production. *Depigmentation* refers to complete loss of pigment in the skin. The loss of pigment usually is considered to be a loss of melanin, although other pigments, such as iron and carotene, also may be absent. The distinction between hypopigmentation and depigmentation is seen best with the use of Wood's lamp (365 nm). This distinction is important in fair-skinned children and most white infants because of their light skin color. Hypopigmented lesions appear dull white under Wood's lamp illumination, whereas depigmented lesions appear starkly bright white. A Wood's lamp examination also is useful in the evaluation of hyperpigmented lesions and helps determine the location of the excess pigment. When the long-wavelength UV light shows enhanced contrast between the abnormally hyperpigmented skin and the normal surrounding skin, the excess melanin is located in the epidermis. Examples of lesions with excess epidermal pigmentation that accentuate with Wood's lamp include freckles, lentigines, café au lait spots, and melanocytic nevi. When the UV light does not show enhancement between the hyperpigmented lesion and the normal-appearing skin, the excess melanin is present within the dermis. Dermal pigmentation occurs in disorders such as postinflammatory hyperpigmentation and deposition of drug metabolites in the skin. A skin biopsy also can be performed to identify the location and type of pigment deposition within the skin.

Many cutaneous disorders are characterized by lesions that follow the *lines of Blaschko*, which form arcs on the chest, S shapes on the abdomen, and V shapes on the posterior midline (Fig. 74-1). These lines should not be confused with dermatomes. They represent embryonic migration planes and are clinically evident only when adjacent populations of cells are genetically distinct, usually caused by chromosomal mosaicism. *Chromosomal mosaicism* occurs in the presence of two or more genetically distinct cell populations in an individual derived from a single zygote. The mosaicism affects single genes, groups of genes, or entire chromosomes. Mosaicism arises from a postzygotic chromosomal nondisjunction during mitosis or a somatic mutation during embryogenesis. Many of the pigmentary anomalies following the lines of Blaschko represent a cutaneous manifestation of chromosomal mosaicism. This includes the hyperpigmented streaks and swirls found in incontinentia pigmenti and linear and whorled nevoid hypermelanosis and the hypopigmented streaks and swirls of hypomelanosis of Ito. Serum karyotype is recommended in patients with pigmentary changes along the lines of Blaschko when structural malformations or developmental delay is present; if the serum karyotype is normal, karyotyping from fibroblasts obtained from skin biopsy specimens of normally and abnormally pigmented skin is recommended.

DIAGNOSIS

When approaching a child with a pigmentary abnormality, it is helpful to know whether the pigmentary change is congenital or acquired and whether it follows a certain

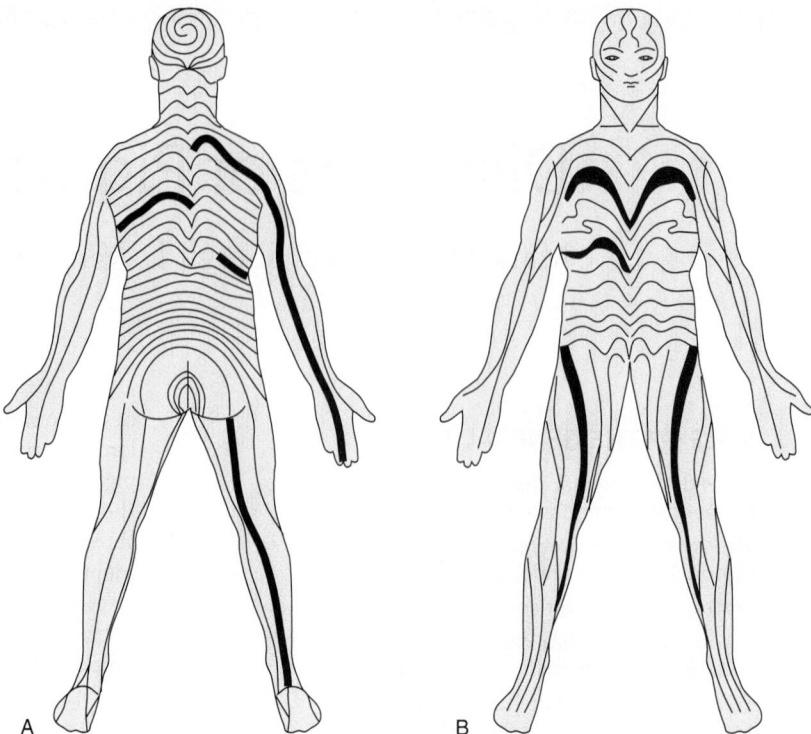

Figure 74-1. A and **B,** Lines of Blaschko. (Adapted from Bolognia JL, Orlow SJ, Glick SA: Lines of Blaschko. J Am Acad Dermatol 1994;31:159–190.)

A   B

pattern (e.g., following the lines of Blaschko, unilateral, or bilateral and symmetric). Congenital and acquired pigmentary disorders are outlined in Tables 74-1 and 74-2.

DISORDERS OF HYPERPIGMENTATION

Freckles (Ephelides)

Freckles are small, light brown macules occurring exclusively on sun-exposed areas, especially the nose, rest of the face, shoulders, and upper back (Fig. 74-2). They develop during early childhood and fade in adulthood. They are seen most commonly in children with fair skin, especially children with red or blonde hair. Freckles become darker and more conspicuous in response to UV light exposure and fade when there is less exposure. Histologically, freckles are characterized by an increase in melanin pigmentation of the basal layer of the epidermis without an increase in the number of melanocytes. Freckles are not associated with an underlying systemic disorder, although excessive freckling in infancy may be a sign of congenital photosensitivity, such as xeroderma pigmentosum. The best management for

freckles is avoidance of sun exposure and regular application of sunscreen with a high sun protection factor. This not only leads to less prominence of the freckles, but also protects the child from the acute and chronic hazards of sunlight exposure, such as sunburn, photoaging, and skin cancer.

Lentigines

Lentigines are brown-to-black macules that are distinguished from freckles by their darker color, scattered distribution, tendency to have an irregular configuration, and lack of darkening with sun exposure (Fig. 74-3). They may arise during childhood and are encountered commonly in older adults. Lentigines histologically show an increased number of melanocytes within the basal layer of the epidermis and increased melanization of the basal keratinocytes. The presence of congenital or multiple lentigines in a child should raise the suspicion about an underlying lentiginous syndrome, as outlined subsequently.

Peutz-Jeghers Syndrome

Peutz-Jeghers syndrome is an autosomal dominant disorder characterized by lentigines of the lips, buccal mucosa, tongue, palate, face, digits, palms, and soles (Fig. 74-4). The

Table 74-1. Congenital and Acquired Causes of Hyperpigmentation

Congenital	Acquired
Lentigines	Freckles
Peutz-Jeghers syndrome	Lentigines
Multiple lentigines syndrome	Café au lait spots
Café au lait spots	Nevus of Ota
Mongolian spots	Postinflammatory hyperpigmentation
Nevus of Ota	Metabolic disorders
Nevus of Ito	Drug induced
Incontinentia pigmenti	Heavy metal exposure
Linear and whorled nevoid hypermelanosis	

Table 74-2. Congenital and Acquired Causes of Hypopigmentation

Congenital	Acquired
Achromic nevus	Ash-leaf macules
Nevus anemicus	Postinflammatory hypopigmentation
Ash-leaf macules	Pityriasis alba
Hypomelanosis of Ito	Tinea versicolor
Albinism	Vitiligo
Piebaldism	
Waardenburg's syndrome	

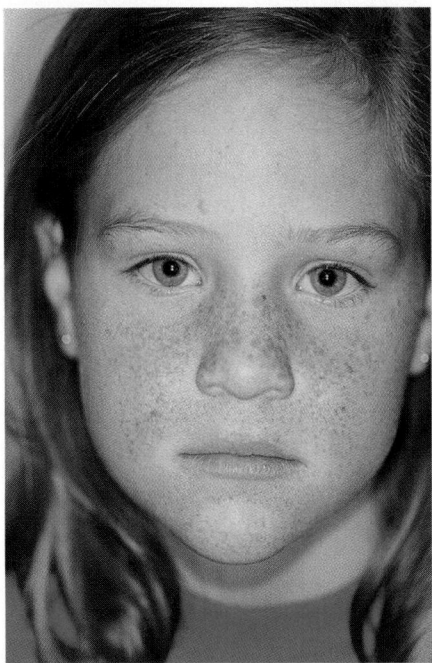

Figure 74-2. Freckles on the face of a young child.

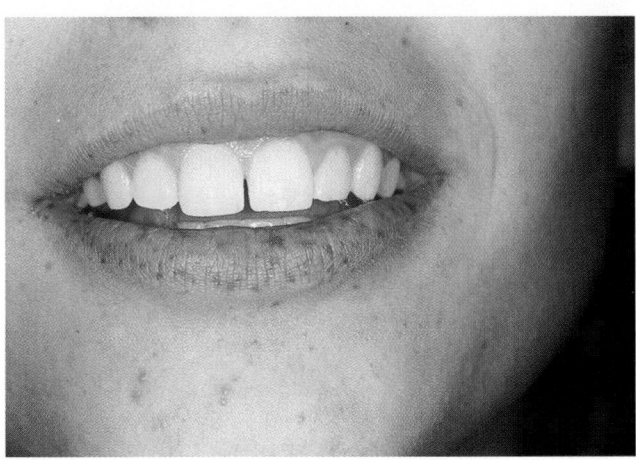

Figure 74-4. Lentigines on the lips in a teenage girl with Peutz-Jeghers syndrome.

lentigines are present at birth or arise during the first few years of life. The lentigines on the lips and skin may fade after puberty, but those on the oral mucosa usually persist. Hamartomatous polyps in the gastrointestinal tract are the other main feature of Peutz-Jeghers syndrome. Multiple hamartomatous polyps arise in any region of the gastrointestinal tract, but are particularly common in the small intestine. The hamartomas may cause abdominal pain, gastrointestinal bleeding, anemia, obstruction, and intussusception. Malignant degeneration of the polyps is uncommon, but this potential complication warrants close surveillance of patients with Peutz-Jeghers syndrome by a gastroenterologist. There is an increased frequency of breast, ovarian, uterine, cervical, testicular, and pancreatic cancers in affected patients, typically arising at relatively young ages. Patients must be followed carefully for these potential complications. The pigmented macules on the lips are cosmetically bothersome to some patients and may be lightened with laser treatment.

Café au Lait Spots

Café au lait spots are well-delineated macules and patches with the tan–to–light brown color of "coffee with milk." They may be congenital or acquired. As an isolated finding, they are relatively common; 10% to 20% of the general population has one or a few café au lait spots. Individuals with multiple café au lait spots are at risk of having an underlying disorder (Box 74-1). Treatment of café au lait spots is medically unnecessary and variably successful; bleaching agents are ineffective, and laser treatment may lead to only transient lightening.

Neurofibromatosis

Neurofibromatosis is an autosomal dominant disorder with an incidence of 40 per 100,000 live births. An estimated 50% of cases represent new mutations. There are eight different subtypes, with type 1 accounting for at least 85% of cases. Neurofibromatosis 1 is characterized by multiple café au lait spots (Fig. 74-5), neurofibromas, and central nervous system and skeletal anomalies. Multiple café au lait spots are present in 90% of patients with neurofibromatosis 1; the presence of six or more café au lait spots having a diameter larger than 5 mm in prepubertal children and larger than 15 mm in adults suggests this disorder. The café au lait spots may be present at birth, with their number and size increasing during childhood. Smaller café au lait spots in the axillary and inguinal areas (axillary and inguinal freckling, also known as *Crowe's sign*) are seen in 20% of cases. The diagnosis of neurofibromatosis 1 may be difficult to make in prepubertal children who do not have sufficient numbers of café au lait spots and lack other diagnostic features of the disorder (Box 74-2); these children need to

Figure 74-3. Lentigines on the back of a woman with a history of extensive sun exposure.

Box 74-1. Disorders with Multiple Café au Lait Spots
▪ Neurofibromatosis ▪ McCune-Albright syndrome ▪ Tuberous sclerosis ▪ Proteus syndrome ▪ Familial café au lait spots ▪ Watson syndrome ▪ Fanconi's anemia

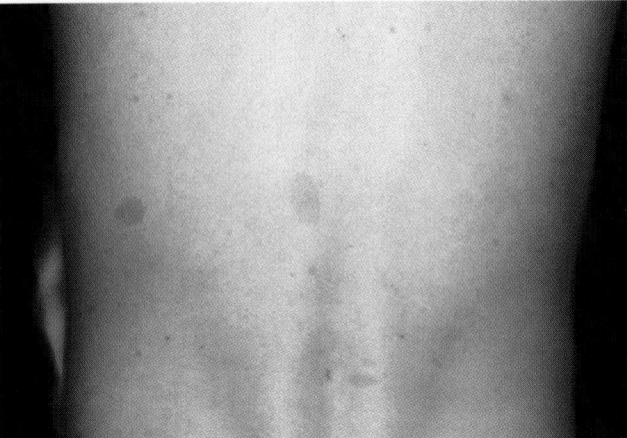

Figure 74-5. Multiple café au lait spots in a child with neurofibromatosis type I.

be followed closely over time because eventually many meet criteria for the diagnosis. Neurofibromatosis is discussed in detail in Chapter 157.

When an infant or young child with a large or giant café au lait spot is encountered (Fig. 74-6), it is often difficult to discern whether the patient has neurofibromatosis 1, segmental neurofibromatosis, or McCune-Albright syndrome (see discussion later) or is an otherwise healthy child without a predisposition to any of the previously mentioned disorders. Although the large café au lait spots of McCune-Albright syndrome tend to respect the midline and have more jagged edges compared with the giant café au lait spots of neurofibromatosis, these features are not sufficient to distinguish neurofibromatosis from McCune-Albright syndrome. Children with giant café au lait spots also must be followed carefully over time.

McCune-Albright Syndrome

McCune-Albright syndrome consists of café au lait spots, polyostotic fibrous dysplasia of long bones, and endocrine dysfunction, especially precocious puberty in girls and hyperthyroidism. Café au lait spots may be present at birth and tend to be large, unilateral, and segmental, stopping abruptly at the midline. The borders of the café au lait spots are jagged and likened to "the coast of Maine," as opposed

---

Box 74-2. Criteria for the Diagnosis of Neurofibromatosis 1*

- Six or more café au lait spots >5 mm in greatest diameter in prepubertal children and >1.5 cm in postpubertal adolescents and adults
- Two or more neurofibromas of any type or one plexiform neurofibroma
- Multiple freckles (Crowe's sign) in axillary or inguinal areas
- Osseous lesion, such as sphenoid dysplasia or thinning of the long bone cortex, with or without pseudarthrosis
- Optic glioma
- Two or more iris hamartomas (Lisch nodules) on slit-lamp examination
- First-degree relative with neurofibromatosis 1

*Must meet two or more criteria to make a diagnosis of neurofibromatosis 1.

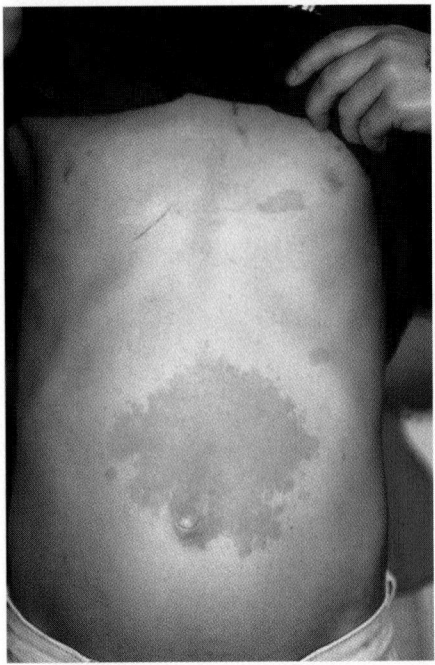

Figure 74-6. Giant café au lait spot on the abdomen in the same child in Figure 74-5.

to the café au lait spots in neurofibromatosis that have smooth borders similar to "the coast of California." Patients with McCune-Albright syndrome can have recurrent fractures, bowing of the limbs, and limb-length discrepancies. Evaluation of the bones corresponding to the segmental café au lait spots may reveal bone lucencies. When the diagnosis of McCune-Albright syndrome is confirmed, the patient should be referred to an orthopedist and endocrinologist.

Dermal Melanosis

Dermal melanosis refers to deposition of melanin in the dermis. The pigment may be present in dermal melanocytes, in macrophages, or in the extracellular portion of the dermis. Because of scattering of short wavelength light, the lesions of dermal melanosis have increased blue light reflectance and display a deep blue or slate-gray discoloration (Fig. 74-7).

Mongolian Spots

Mongolian spots present at birth as blue-gray patches, typically on the lumbosacral area; the buttocks; and at times the lower extremities, back, and shoulders. They are seen in most African-American, Native American, Asian, and Hispanic infants; only 10% of white infants are born with mongolian spots. Mongolian spots have collections of spindle-shaped melanocytes deep in the dermis, likely resulting from arrest of migration of the melanocytes from the neural crest to the epidermis. Mongolian spots tend to fade during the first decade of life, although some may persist into adulthood. These lesions have no malignant potential.

Nevus of Ota (Nevus Fuscoceruleus Ophthalmomaxillaris)

Nevus of Ota is a congenital or acquired unilateral slate-gray to blue-brown patch, often intermingled with speckling of smaller darker macules, arising in the distribution

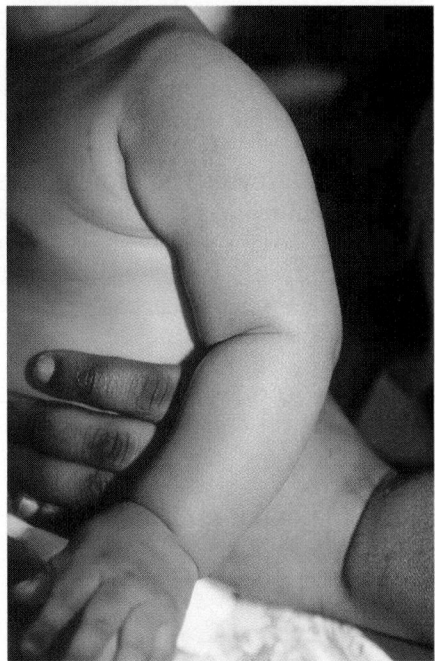

Figure 74-7. Dermal melanosis on the arm of an infant.

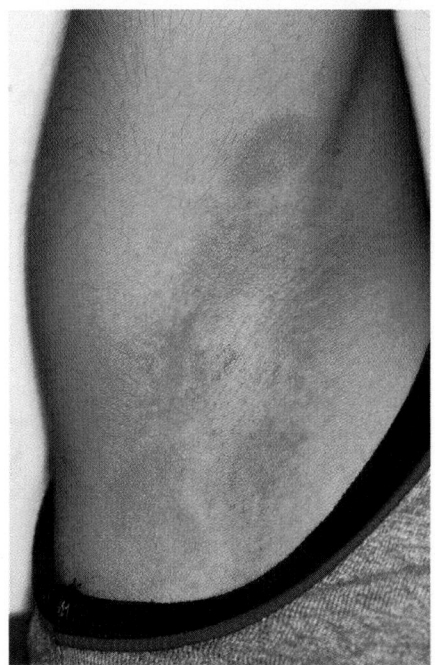

Figure 74-9. Postinflammatory hyperpigmentation of the axilla in a teenage girl after contact dermatitis caused by her deodorant.

of the first and second divisions of the trigeminal nerve (Fig. 74-8). It may involve the periorbital, temporal, malar, and frontal areas of the face. Pigmentation often is noted on the ipsilateral sclera. Occasionally, nevus of Ota is bilateral. It occurs commonly in Asians and African Americans; it rarely occurs in whites. There may be a female predilection. Melanin-producing melanocytes and melanin-laden macrophages are found in the reticular dermis in the nevus of Ota. Although a rare occurrence, intraocular melanoma, leptomeningeal melanosis, and leptomeningeal melanoma have been reported in association with nevus of Ota. Patients should be examined periodically by an ophthalmologist for signs of early intraocular melanoma. The pigmentation of the nevus of Ota generally persists, although some may fade over time. Repeated cryosurgery has been reported to help fade the pigmentation. Laser surgery has been effective in treatment of nevus of Ota.

Nevus of Ito (Nevus Fuscoceruleus Acromiodeltoideus)

Nevus of Ito has the same clinical features as nevus of Ota, but it occurs on the scapula, deltoid region of the shoulder, side of the neck, or supraclavicular area.

Postinflammatory Hyperpigmentation

Postinflammatory hyperpigmentation is one of the most common causes of hyperpigmentation. It results from increased melanin production after inflammation in the skin. It is most common in darker skinned individuals. A history of previous inflammation in the involved area is a clue to the diagnosis (Fig. 74-9). The hyperpigmentation may resolve after several months; if there is retention of melanin in dermal melanophages, it may persist indefinitely. Treatment of postinflammatory hyperpigmentation consists of sun avoidance or bleaching agents containing hydroquinone. If the hyperpigmentation is caused by a recurrent inflammatory condition, adding topical steroid therapy minimizes the occurrence of new areas of pigmentary change.

Incontinentia Pigmenti (Bloch-Sulzberger Syndrome)

Incontinentia pigmenti is an X-linked dominant disorder that is usually fatal in utero to hemizygous male fetuses. It is characterized by four distinct phases of cutaneous involvement, although all four phases may occur simultaneously; in addition, patients may present at birth during any phase, having already gone through the earlier cutaneous changes in utero. The first phase features grouped vesicles and bullae on an erythematous base distributed in a swirly pattern on the trunk and extremities along the lines of Blaschko (Fig. 74-10). Blistering may be present for several weeks or months. The second phase is characterized by verrucous papules found in the same distribution as the blisters. As the verrucous lesions resolve, they are replaced

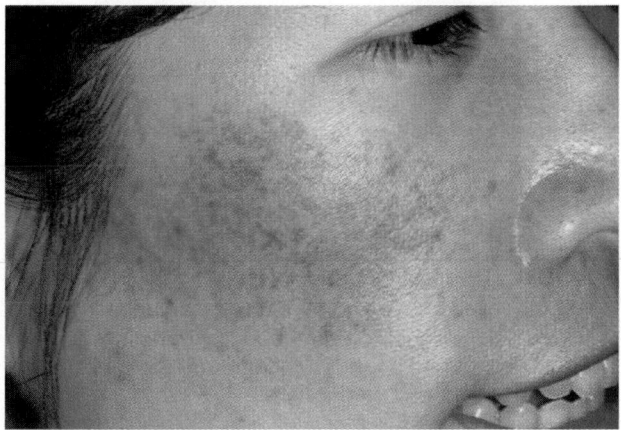

Figure 74-8. Nevus of Ota. (From Salmon JK, Frieden IJ: Congenital and genetic disorders of hyperpigmentation. Curr Prob Dermatol 1995;7:185.)

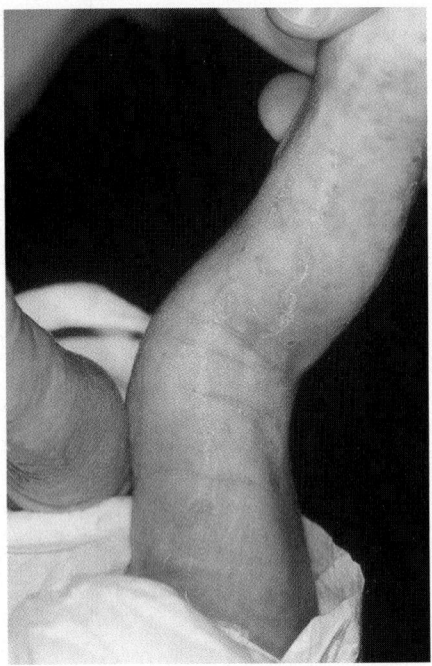

Figure 74-10. Incontinentia pigmenti, first phase.

by blue-gray–to–brown swirly patches following the lines of Blaschko (third phase) (Fig. 74-11). The hyperpigmentation fades and is replaced with subtle hypopigmentation and slight cutaneous atrophy that may persist into adulthood (fourth phase). Most affected girls have no serious sequelae. Associated abnormalities include scarring alopecia, abnormal dentition (peg-shaped teeth, oligodontia, hypodontia, microdontia, delayed eruption of the teeth), ocular abnormalities (retinal vascular proliferation, colobomas, strabismus, cataracts, optic atrophy, retrolental mass), central nervous system abnormalities (mental retardation, seizures,

spastic diplegia, hemiplegia, quadriplegia), and cardiac and skeletal malformations. Girls with incontinentia pigmenti should be followed by a pediatric ophthalmologist and dentist. Appropriate genetic counseling is required.

Linear and Whorled Nevoid Hypermelanosis

Linear and whorled nevoid hypermelanosis presents at birth or in the first years of life as swirly hyperpigmentation along the lines of Blaschko that is not preceded by inflammation (Fig. 74-12). Although it is a phenotype for chromosomal mosaicism, most patients have no associated extracutaneous anomalies. It may become less noticeable over time. Linear and whorled nevoid hypermelanosis may be difficult to distinguish clinically from the third phase of incontinentia pigmenti; skin biopsy can be helpful.

Diffuse Hyperpigmentation Caused by Metabolic Disorders

Metabolic disorders associated with hyperpigmentation are outlined in Table 74-3.

Exogenous Causes of Hyperpigmentation

Long-term use of various medications (Table 74-4) may be associated with deposition of pigment in the skin; this may or may not resolve on cessation of the medication. Patients taking minocycline on a prolonged basis for the treatment of acne may develop blue-gray macules within acne scars, on the buccal mucosa, or anywhere else on the cutaneous surface (Fig. 74-13); this represents deposition of metabolites of minocycline in the skin and typically resolves when the drug is discontinued. Exposure to heavy metals, such as silver, gold, and mercury, can cause a similar-appearing, blue-gray discoloration of the skin. Carotenemia is an orange discoloration of the skin that results from ingestion of excessive carotene sources, such as carrots, squash, pump-

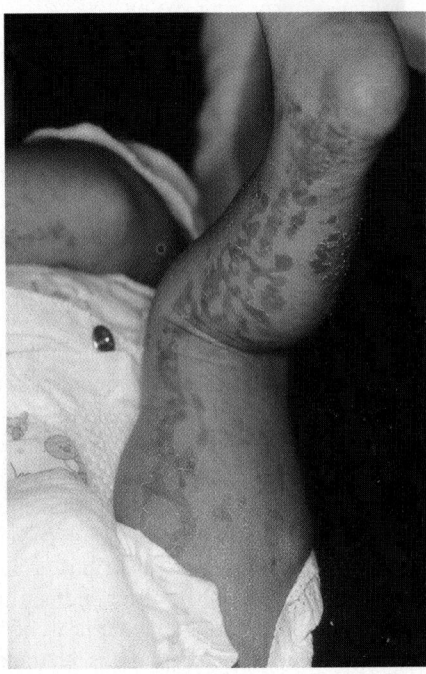

Figure 74-11. Incontinentia pigmenti, evolving from second phase to third phase.

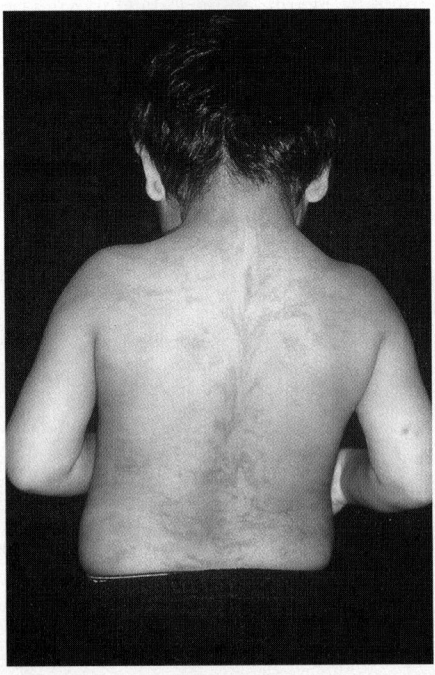

Figure 74-12. Nevoid hypermelanosis in a boy with chromosomal mosaicism (karyotype from fibroblasts of hyperpigmented skin showed 47,XY, whereas normally pigmented skin was 46,XY).

Table 74-3. Diffuse Hyperpigmentation from Metabolic Disorders

Disorder	Color	Distribution
Hepatobiliary disease	Bronze	Generalized; accentuation of freckles, hyperpigmentation of nipples
Hemochromatosis	Gray; bronze	Generalized; pronounced on the face, forearms, body folds, and genitocrural area
Adrenal insufficiency (Addison's disease)	Brown-black	Generalized; pronounced in sun-exposed areas, axillae, palmar and plantar creases, nipples, genitals, conjunctivae, and oral mucosa. Darkening of nevi and hair may be seen
Cushing's syndrome	Brown	Generalized; may have a pattern of accentuation similar to that of adrenal insufficiency
Hyperthyroidism	Brown	Generalized
Hyperpituitarism	Brown	Generalized; may have a pattern of accentuation similar to that of adrenal insufficiency
Ochronosis (alkaptonuria)	Blue-brown; blue-black	Nose, malar areas, sclerae, ears, axillae, genitals, and nail beds

kins, sweet potatoes, peaches, and apricots. Carotenemia is seen most commonly in infants and children. Carotenemia can be differentiated from jaundice by the presence of high serum carotene levels and normal serum bilirubin.

DISORDERS OF HYPOPIGMENTATION

Achromic Nevus (Nevus Depigmentosus)
Achromic nevus is a macule or patch of hypopigmentation seen in approximately 5% of whites. It is present at birth or in early childhood and grows in proportion to the growth of

Table 74-4. Medications Most Commonly Associated with Pigment Deposition in the Skin

Antibiotics
  Doxycycline, minocycline, ofloxacin, sparfloxacin, tetracycline
Anticonvulsants
  Carbamazepine, phenytoin, tiagabine, topiramate
Antifungals
  Amphotericin B, griseofulvin, ketoconazole
Antimalarials
  Chloroquine, hydroxychloroquine, pyrimethamine, quinacrine
Antimycobacterials
  Isoniazid, rifabutin, rifapentine
Antipsychotics and tranquilizers
  Chlorpromazine, fluphenazine, haloperidol, loxapine, mesoridazine, molindone, perphenazine, prochlorperazine, promethazine, risperidone, thioridazine, thiothixene, trifluoperazine
Antiretrovirals
  Indinavir, zidovudine
Antivirals
  Cidofovir, foscarnet, ganciclovir
Cardiac and antihypertensive medications
  Amiodarone, betaxolol, bisoprolol, captopril, carteolol, labetalol, lidocaine, metoprolol, minoxidil, nisoldipine, quinidine, spironolactone, timolol
Chemotherapeutic agents
  Bleomycin, busulfan, carmustine, cisplatin, cyclophosphamide, dactinomycin, daunorubicin, doxorubicin, etoposide, fluorouracil, ifosfamide, mercaptopurine, methotrexate, mitomycin, mitotane, procarbazine, thiotepa, vinorelbine
Immunomodulators
  Azathioprine, clofazimine, corticosteroids, dapsone, hydroxyurea, leflunomide, sulfasalazine
Hormonal agents
  Estrogens, leuprolide, oral contraceptives, toremifene
Parkinson's disease medications
  Carbidopa, donepezil, methyldopa, ropinirole, tolcapone
Serotonin reuptake inhibitors
  Citalopram, fluoxetine, fluvoxamine, olanzapine, paroxetine
Tricyclic antidepressants
  Amitriptyline, clomipramine, desipramine, imipramine

the child. Achromic nevus usually is located on the trunk or extremities and may have the configuration of an ash-leaf macule of tuberous sclerosis (Fig. 74-14) or may appear as irregular bands or streaks of hypopigmentation that resemble "splashed paint." No treatment is available. Lesions may be camouflaged with cosmetic cover-ups.

Nevus Anemicus
Nevus anemicus, an oval or round, pale or mottled patch with irregular edges, appears at birth or in early childhood. Its blanched appearance is secondary to a focal developmental anomaly of increased vascular tone. Because it is not an abnormality of pigmentation, Wood's lamp illumination does not accentuate the lesion. Rubbing the nevus anemicus causes redness of the surrounding normal skin, but the lesion itself stays blanched. No treatment is available. Lesions may be camouflaged with cosmetic cover-ups.

Hypomelanotic Macules (Ash-Leaf Macules)
Hypopigmented macules and patches are seen in nearly 90% of individuals with tuberous sclerosis, an autosomal dominant condition with variable penetrance characterized by the triad of seizures, adenoma sebaceum, and mental retardation. The incidence of tuberous sclerosis is estimated at 5 to 7 per 100,000 live births. Most cases are attributed to a spontaneous gene mutation. Hypopigmented macules and patches constitute the earliest cutaneous sign of tuberous sclerosis; they may be present at birth or appear with

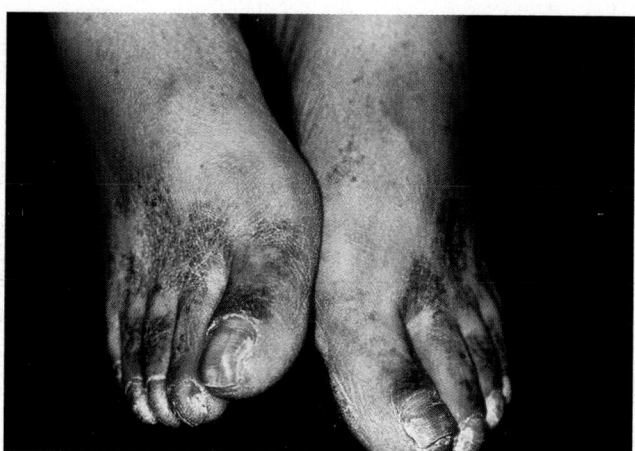

Figure 74-13. Blue-gray discoloration of the skin in a young man overdosed with minocycline for acne.

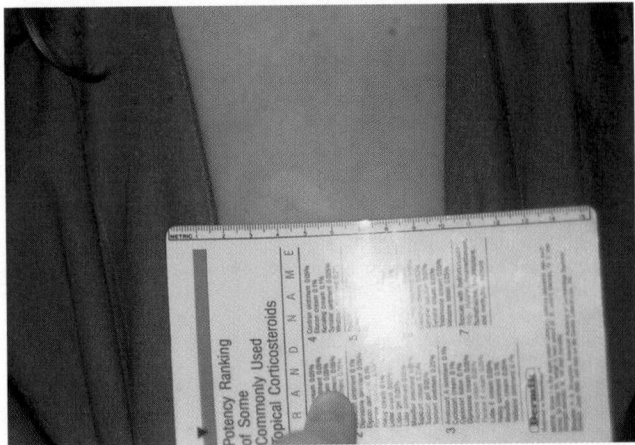

Figure 74-14. Achromic nevus on the abdomen of a young girl that has the configuration of an ash-leaf macule.

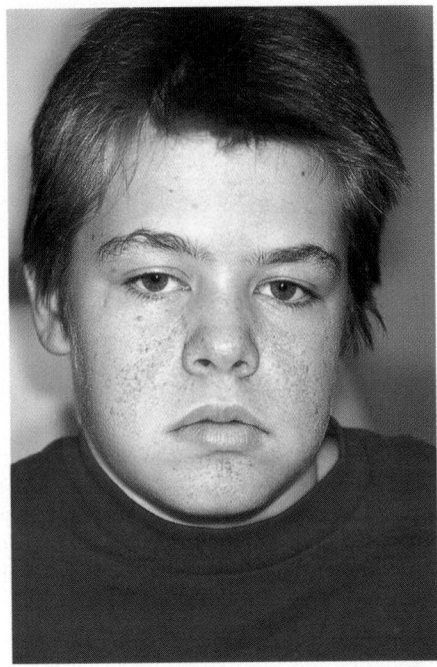

Figure 74-15. Adenoma sebaceum (angiofibromas) on the face of a teenage boy with tuberous sclerosis.

increasing numbers during the first few years of life. The hypopigmented macules and patches are asymmetrically distributed and are found most commonly over the trunk, buttocks, and extremities; facial involvement is rare. The lesions typically are greater than 1 cm in diameter with a lancet-shaped configuration, resembling an ash leaf. Multiple clustered hypopigmented macules with the appearance of "confetti" also may be seen. Hypopigmented lesions range in number from several to hundreds. Some may be subtle and are best found with Wood's lamp examination.

Additional cutaneous features of tuberous sclerosis include adenoma sebaceum, periungual fibromas, shagreen patches, and café au lait spots. Adenoma sebaceum are angiofibromas that typically present as erythematous, smooth papules involving the nasolabial folds, cheeks, and chin in a symmetric distribution (Fig. 74-15). They are found in 70% to 90% of patients with tuberous sclerosis older than age 5 years. Periungual fibromas (Koenen's tumors) are pink–to–flesh-colored papules ranging in size from 1 mm to 1 cm that arise from the toenail bed or less commonly from the fingernail bed. They can be located in the lateral nail groove, under the nail plate, or along the proximal nail groove (Fig. 74-16). They usually appear at puberty and are present in about 20% of cases of tuberous sclerosis. Shagreen patches (connective tissue nevi) are flesh-colored or yellowish brown–to–pink, pebbly firm plaques that usually are found on the forehead or lumbosacral area. They vary in size from a few millimeters to 10 or more centimeters. Shagreen patches rarely are found in infancy and become more common after puberty. Café au lait spots may occur in 10% to 20% of patients with tuberous sclerosis. Café au lait spots are not included as a diagnostic sign of this disorder, however.

Other types of cutaneous fibromas may arise in patients with tuberous sclerosis. These include (1) large, asymmetric fibromas of the face and scalp; (2) soft, pedunculated growths on the neck, trunk, or extremities (molluscum fibrosum pendulum); (3) grouped, firm papules of the neck, trunk, and extremities; and (4) pedunculated or sessile nodules of the buccal or gingival mucosa. Noncutaneous features of tuberous sclerosis include hamartomas of the cerebral cortex ("tubers"), focal or generalized seizures, mental retardation, retinal and optic nerve gliomas, renal angiomyolipomas and cysts, cardiac rhabdomyomas, and pulmonary leiomyomatosis.

When a normally developing child without a history of seizures or a family history of tuberous sclerosis presents with a single or a few hypopigmented macules, the most likely diagnosis is achromic nevus. These children should undergo Wood's lamp examination of the entire cutaneous surface, however, to exclude the presence of other, more subtle areas of hypopigmentation. Complete skin examination should focus on ruling out the presence of other cutaneous features of tuberous sclerosis. Indirect ophthalmoscopy also can be considered to rule out retinal gliomas.

Postinflammatory Hypopigmentation

Postinflammatory hypopigmentation is most noticeable in darkly pigmented individuals. It represents a temporary decrease in skin pigmentation after inflammation associated with disorders such as eczema, psoriasis, pityriais rosea,

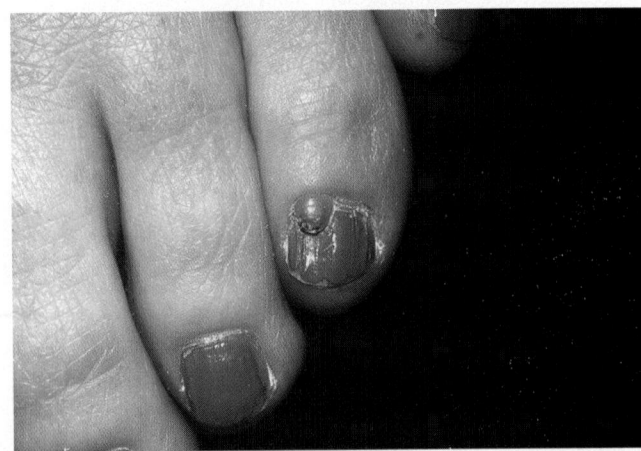

Figure 74-16. Periungual fibroma in a woman with tuberous sclerosis.

bullous diseases, and tinea corporis (Fig. 74-17). The decrease in pigmentation may be secondary to temporary disruption of melanin transfer to keratinocytes injured by the inflammatory process. The diagnosis of postinflammatory hypopigmentation is confirmed by a history of preceding eruption in the hypopigmented areas. Postinflammatory hypopigmentation resolves spontaneously after several months. Because tanning of the normally pigmented skin enhances the contrast between the normal and hypopigmented areas, protection from sun exposure is indicated.

Pityriasis Alba

Pityriasis alba, a low-grade dermatitis, presents as rough, scaly hypopigmented patches, most commonly located on the cheeks of school-age children (Fig. 74-18). It is more prominent in darkly pigmented individuals and is encountered frequently in individuals with atopic diathesis. Pityriasis alba can be distinguished from postinflammatory hypopigmentation by the rough, scaly texture. It is treated with low-potency topical steroids. When the roughness and scale resolve, the normal pigmentation returns, but this may take several months. Sun protection is advised.

Tinea Versicolor

Tinea versicolor, most common in adolescents and young adults, is caused by overgrowth of a normal inhabitant of the skin, *Pityrosporum* yeast. It usually presents as slightly scaly, hypopigmented macules and patches; however, the color of the lesions can range from pink to tan. Tinea versicolor typically is located on the upper trunk and upper arms in a "capelike" distribution (Fig. 74-19), although involvement of the neck and face also can be seen. Because involved areas fail to tan, they become more prominent after sun exposure. Light microscopy of a potassium hydroxide preparation of the scales reveals short hyphae and spores in clusters ("spaghetti and meatballs"). Treatment of

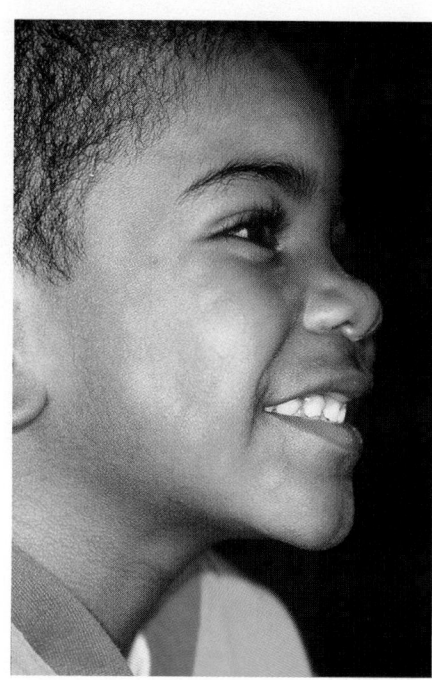

Figure 74-18. Pityriasis alba on the cheek of an African-American boy.

tinea versicolor is with selenium sulfide 2.5% lotion, used as an overnight application weekly for 1 month, then monthly for several months to prevent recurrence. The hypopigmented areas resolve after several months.

Hypomelanosis of Ito (Incontinentia Pigmenti Achromians)

Hypomelanosis of Ito is characterized by hypopigmented patches and swirls along the lines of Blaschko (Fig. 74-20). It may be present at birth or develop early in childhood. It represents a phenotype rather than a distinct disorder and

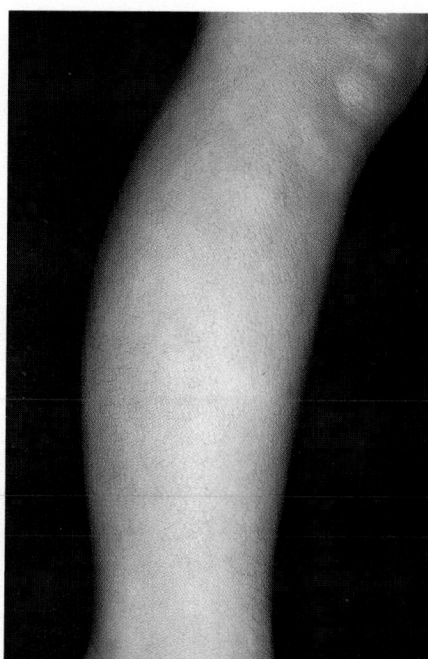

Figure 74-17. Postinflammatory hypopigmentation in a Hispanic boy with atopic dermatitis.

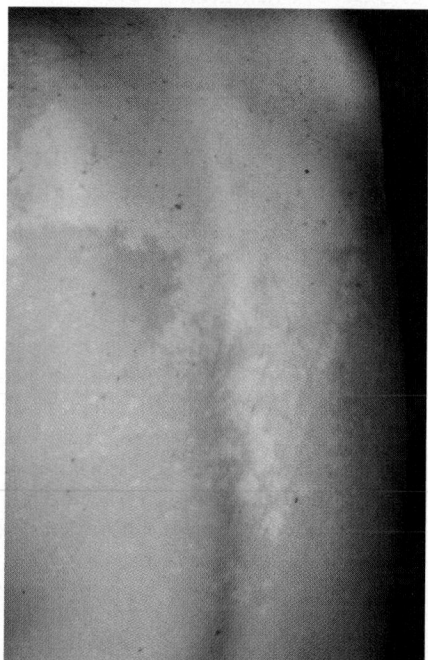

Figure 74-19. Tinea versicolor on the back of a young man. (Courtesy of Department of Dermatology, University of Utah, Salt Lake City, Utah.)

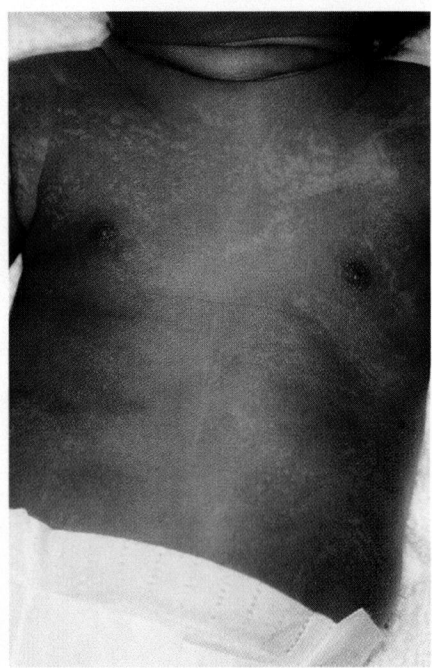

Figure 74-20. Hypomelanosis of Ito in a female infant with Turner's syndrome (45,X).

can be seen in association with a wide variety of associated anomalies, including mental retardation, seizures, and structural brain malformations. Chromosomal mosaicism has been found in 50% of affected children. Karyotyping of the serum, and, if that is normal, of fibroblasts from biopsy specimens taken from hypopigmented and normally pigmented skin, should be performed in a child with hypomelanosis of Ito if development is abnormal or if the child has seizures or structural malformations. No treatment is available for the hypopigmentation, which may fade with age.

DISORDERS OF DEPIGMENTATION

Vitiligo

Vitiligo, a pigmentary disorder caused by the idiopathic loss of melanocytes, affects approximately 1% of the general population. It presents with partially to completely depigmented ivory-white macules and patches and may arise in areas of trauma (Koebner phenomenon). Vitiligo may develop at any age, although its usual onset is between 5 and 30 years of age. Half of affected individuals develop vitiligo before age 20, and 25% develop it before age 10. Girls are more commonly affected than boys. The relative risk of developing vitiligo for first-degree relatives of an affected individual is 10-fold higher than the general population risk. Approximately 25% of vitiligo patients have a positive family history. Studies have linked vitiligo with HLA-DR4. Vitiligo can be seen in association with a wide variety of autoimmune disorders, including hyperthyroidism, hypothyroidism, adrenal insufficiency, diabetes, pernicious anemia, myasthenia gravis, and alopecia areata.

The generalized form of vitiligo is the most common presentation. The depigmented macules and patches arise in a bilaterally symmetric distribution, with a predilection for periorificial areas (eyelids, nostrils, mouth, umbilicus, genitals, anal area), the dorsum of the hands and feet, neck,

torso, and extremities, especially over bony prominences. Generalized vitiligo may progress slowly over years, although spontaneous repigmentation is common. Vitiligo rarely progresses to complete depigmentation of the skin. In some individuals, vitiligo may remain localized, affecting less than 20% of the body surface.

The segmental form of vitiligo, encountered more frequently in children than in adults, is characterized by a patch of vitiligo expanding over a particular segment of the skin, such as the upper arm or thigh (Fig. 74-21). Although segmental vitiligo may follow the path of a particular cutaneous nerve, its distribution is not dermatomal and usually does not cross the midline.

Spontaneous repigmentation can occur but tends to be incomplete. Partial repigmentation typically occurs on sun-exposed skin. Repigmentation occurs when melanocytes from the hair follicles migrate to the depigmented skin and repopulate the epidermis. Repigmentation often appears first as round perifollicular brown macules. When the hairs within the patches of vitiligo lack pigment, the follicular reservoir of melanocytes is absent, and prognosis for repigmentation is poorer (Fig. 74-22).

For dark-skinned individuals, vitiligo can be disfiguring because of the stark contrast between the depigmented and normally pigmented skin. Aggressive treatment should be instituted as early as possible to prevent further spreading of the vitiligo. Response to treatment is variable. Early institution of treatment with topical steroids is warranted for children. Moderate-potency to ultrapotent topical steroids need to be used. Patients need to be re-evaluated every few months for the development of cutaneous atrophy.

UV light treatment is an option for patients with extensive generalized vitiligo. Narrow-band UVB treatment has been shown to be effective in pediatric patients. Topical photochemotherapy with sunlight or a handheld home

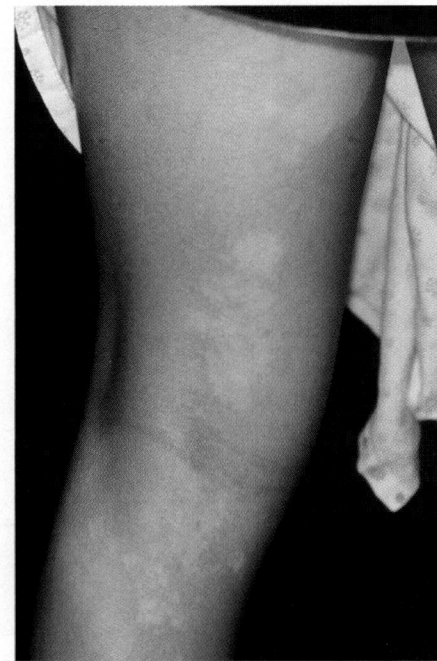

Figure 74-21. Segmental vitiligo on the upper thigh of a girl.

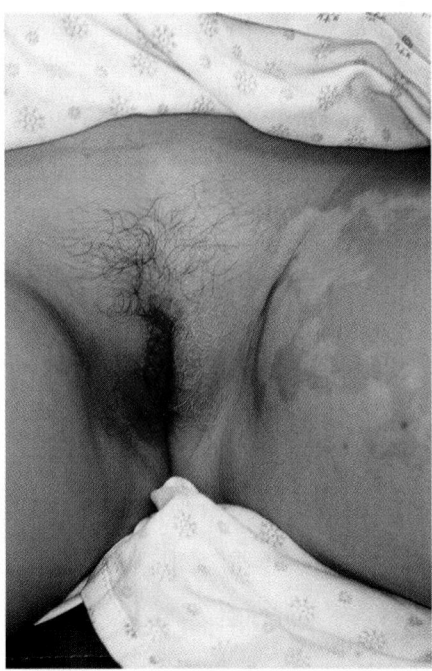

Figure 74-22. Same girl as in Figure 74-21. Note the depigmented hairs on the left side of the genital area overlying the patch of vitiligo.

UVA light and trioxsalen cream also can be considered, although extreme caution must be taken to avoid sunburning. Systemic psoralen photochemotherapy (PUVA) administered in a dermatologist's office has more side effects and should be reserved for individuals with extensive involvement. PUVA therapy is not recommended for children younger than 12 years old. Side effects of PUVA include nausea and vomiting, pruritus, hypertrichosis, premature aging of the skin, skin cancer, and cataracts. PUVA and narrow-band UVB treatments require highly motivated parents and children. The treatment is time-consuming and often requires 100 to 200 treatments for a response. The patient must travel to the physician's office for treatment two to three times a week for 1 year.

Patients with vitiligo should be counseled that the affected areas lack photoprotection and that extra precautions need to be taken to avoid sunburns. Depigmented skin is also at higher risk for photoaging and skin cancers. Sun avoidance, protective clothing, and liberal use of sunscreens are essential, not only to protect the vitiliginous skin, but also to prevent tanning of the normally pigmented skin that enhances the contrast between the normal and abnormal skin. Cosmetic camouflage is an option for all vitiligo patients and is especially useful for patients who do not want to risk the side effects of treatment or for whom treatment was unsuccessful. The National Vitiligo Foundation (611 South Fleishel Avenue, Tyler, TX 75701, (903) 531-0074, www.vitiligofoundation.org) is a superb support group.

Oculocutaneous Albinism

The albinisms are a group of autosomal recessive disorders characterized by absent or reduced pigment production despite the presence of normal numbers and structure of melanocytes. Several different gene defects can cause a reduction in melanin pigment biosynthesis. The molecular analysis of these gene defects has become integral in delineating the different types of albinism and has provided an explanation for overlap of the phenotypes. Oculocutaneous albinism is characterized by absent or reduced pigment in the skin, hair, and eyes. The skin has a pink-white–to–cream color, and the hair has a cream-to-yellow color. The irides are translucent, and there is a prominent red reflex. Optic track misrouting, foveal hypoplasia, greatly impaired visual acuity, nystagmus, and photophobia usually are present. These patients are prone to premature aging of the skin, actinic keratoses, squamous cell carcinoma, and basal cell carcinoma. Sun protection is vital to diminish these complications. Patients with oculocutaneous albinism should undergo regular skin cancer screening. Early referral to an ophthalmologist is helpful. The National Organization for Albinism and Hypopigmentation (NOAH) (P.O. Box 959, East Hampstead, NH 03826-0959, (800) 473-2310, www.albinism.org) is the support group for patients with albinism.

Piebaldism (Partial Albinism)

Piebaldism is an autosomal dominant disorder characterized by a congenital white lock of hair above the forehead ("white forelock") and circumscribed areas of depigmentation on the face, neck, anterior trunk, and midextremities (Figs. 74-23 and 74-24). There may be islands of normal pigmentation within the depigmented patches. The depigmentation is stable and results from failure of melanocytes to migrate from the neural crest into the epidermis during embryogenesis. Although most individuals with piebaldism are healthy, there is an association with deafness, heterochromia irides, facial dysmorphism, ataxia, mental retardation, and Hirschsprung's disease. Overall, children with piebaldism seem to cope better with the pigmentary disorder than children who acquire vitiligo. Sun protection is an important part of their lifestyle. Camouflage in the form of hair dye and cosmetic cover-ups may be helpful.

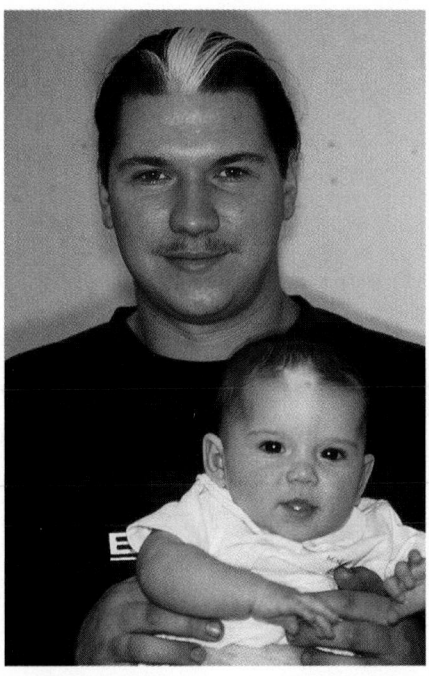

Figure 74-23. A father and his infant daughter with piebaldism, showing prominent white forelocks.

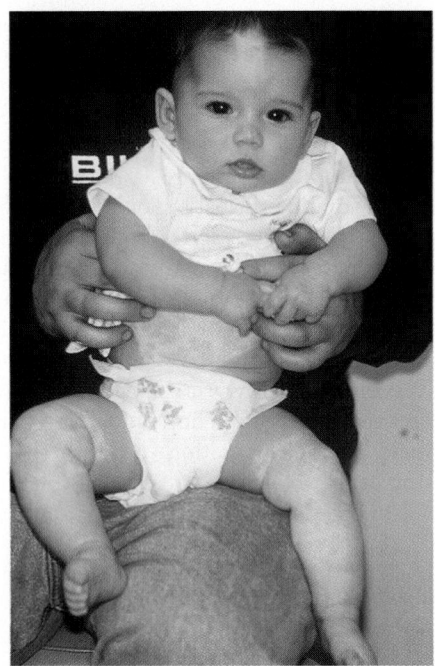

Figure 74-24. Infant shown in Figure 74-23, showing widespread depigmented patches.

Waardenburg's Syndrome

Waardenburg's syndrome is a rare autosomal dominant disorder characterized by depigmented macules, white forelock, heterochromia irides, lateral displacement of the medial canthi (dystopia cantharum), broad nasal root, and congenital sensorineural deafness. The depigmented macules

---

Box 74-3. Sun Protection Guidelines

1. Minimize the exposure to ultraviolet radiation, especially between 10:00 A.M. and 4:00 P.M., when the chance of developing sunburn is greatest. Sit in the shade whenever possible.
2. Wear protective clothing. Hats with a 4-inch brim all around are best because they protect the neck, eyes, and scalp. Wide-brimmed hats, sunglasses, long-sleeved shirts, and pants are the mainstays.
3. Use sunscreen whenever outdoors. This is particularly important when on sand, snow, and water and at high elevations.
4. Sunscreens should be applied about 20 minutes before going outdoors. Sunscreens should be reapplied often, about every 2 hours or after swimming.
5. Rely on hats, clothing, and shading rather than sunscreens.
6. Use sunscreens with a sun protective factor greater than 30. This includes lip balm with sunscreen in it.

---

are totally devoid of melanocytes. The white forelock may disappear over time as the depigmented hairs are replaced with normally pigmented ones. Hirschsprung's disease may be seen in some patients with Waardenburg's syndrome. The features of Waardenburg's syndrome result from a defect in neural crest cell migration. All patients with Waardenburg's syndrome need a thorough audiology evaluation. Sun protection is important for individuals with depigmented macules in exposed areas.

Photoprotection Strategies

Photoprotection for patients with disorders of pigmentation are outlined in Box 74-3.

Additional Resources, CD-ROM

Color atlas	Figures
Rare disorders of hyperpigmentation:	
LEOPARD syndrome	Text
Centrofacial lentiginosis	Text
NAME syndrome	Text
LAMB syndrome	Text
Carney complex	Text
Bibliography	

Mini-index of Related Topics CH.

SUGGESTED READINGS

Hann SK, Nordlund JJ: Vitiligo: A Comprehensive Monograph on the Basic and Clinical Science. Oxford, Blackwell Science, 2000, pp 35–70.
Landau M, Krafchik BR: The diagnostic value of café-au-lait macules. J Am Acad Dermatol 1999;40:877–890.
Loomis CA: Linear hypopigmentation and hyperpigmentation, including mosaicism. Semin Cutan Med Surg 1997;16:44–53.
Sybert VP: Genetic Skin Disorders. New York, Oxford University Press,1997, pp 262–334.
Vanderhooft SL, Francis JS, Pagon RA, et al: Prevalence of hypopigmented macules in a healthy population. J Pediatr 1996;129:355–361.

75

Disorders of Cutaneous Blood Vessels

Anthony J. Mancini

ROLE OF THE GENERALIST

1 Classify disorders of cutaneous blood vessels.
2 Distinguish proliferative vascular tumors from vascular malformations.
3 Recognize possible syndromes and complications associated with cutaneous vascular disorders.
4 Treat and manage patients with disorders of the cutaneous blood vessels.
5 Refer patients to specialists when necessary for assistance with diagnostic or therapeutic considerations.

FUNDAMENTALS

Disorders of cutaneous blood vessels are classified on the basis of the clinical manifestations of the lesions, the natural history (Fig. 75-1), and the histopathologic characteristics. Based on this classification, cutaneous vascular anomalies can be divided into proliferative tumors *(hemangiomas)* and nonproliferative malformations *(vascular malformations)*.

Hemangiomas are the most common soft tissue tumor of infancy. These tumors are characterized by a period of rapid postnatal growth (proliferating phase) and slow spontaneous regression (involuting phase). Lesions may be superficial in the skin (previously referred to as *strawberry hemangioma*) or reside in the deeper dermis and

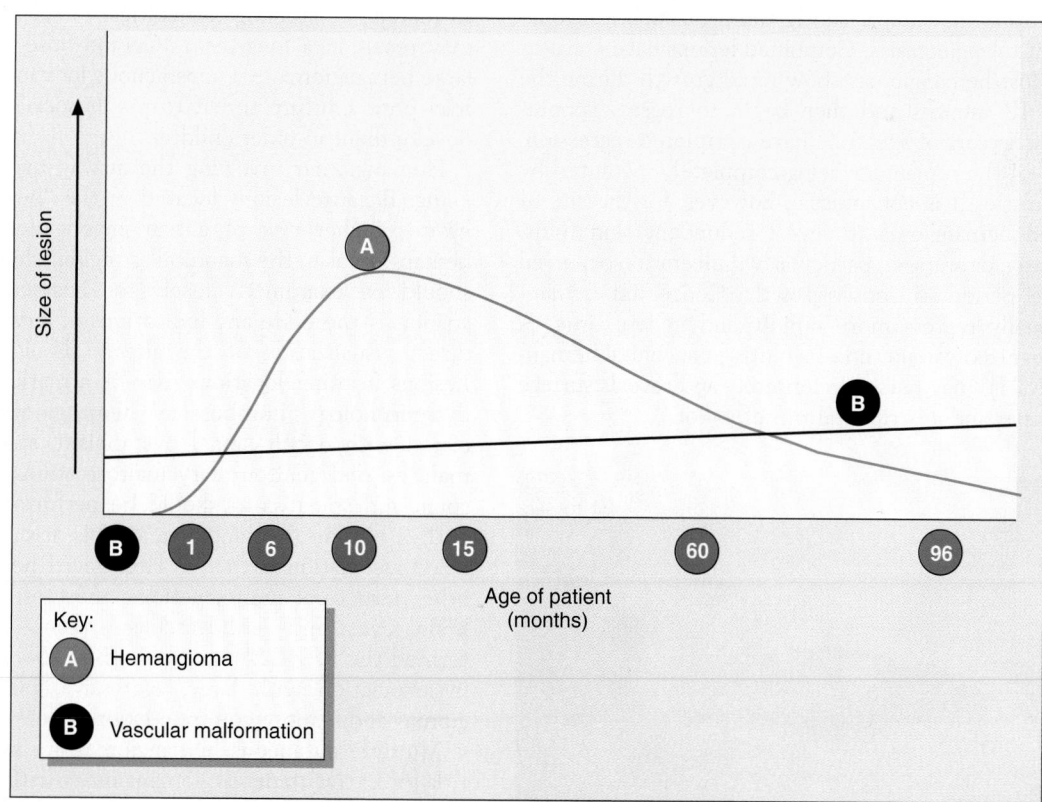

Figure 75-1. Natural history of vascular malformations and hemangiomas. For *hemangioma,* note growth, plateau, and involution phases; rates shown are average, with exact length of each phase varying among patients; some may present at birth, with more rapid involution phase. For *vascular malformation,* note mild increase in size with time, commensurate with growth of the patient.

subcutaneous tissues (previously referred to as *cavernous hemangioma*).

Vascular malformations are developmental errors of vascular morphogenesis and by definition are present at birth. They are composed of dysmorphic channels lined by flat endothelium, without evidence of proliferative cellular turnover, although they may increase in size proportionate with the child's overall growth because of progressive ectasia of the existing vessels. Vascular malformations are divided into slow-flow lesions (venous, capillary, and lymphatic malformations) and fast-flow lesions (arterial malformations, arteriovenous malformations [AVMs], and arteriovenous fistulae).

DIAGNOSIS

Hemangiomas occur in 10% of children 1 year old or younger. Girls are three times more likely than boys to have a hemangioma, and their incidence is higher in premature infants, with more than 20% of infants weighing less than 1000 g affected. Typically, lesions first become evident around 2 weeks of age, although congenital hemangioma is a well-recognized variant. The initial appearance is usually that of a flat red or blue patch or an area of telangiectasias, and the head and neck are the most common sites of involvement. Ulceration occasionally may be the initial sign of a hemangioma. Although usually solitary, multiple lesions may occur in 20% of affected infants.

Superficial hemangiomas are bright red with a surface that may resemble a strawberry (Fig. 75-2). Deep lesions present as soft subcutaneous tumors and may have normal-appearing overlying skin or subtle findings, such as a blue hue or faint telangiectasias. Combined lesions have features of both. Most hemangiomas show rapid growth during the first 8 to 12 months and then begin to regress spontaneously. By 5 years of age, 50% have completed regression, with most of the remainder being completely involuted by 10 years of age. It is not unusual, however, for the site of a regressed hemangioma to reveal redundant skin folds, telangiectasia, or scarring, particularly if ulceration occurred during the period of active growth. Congenital hemangiomas usually regress more rapidly and in less time. A newly recognized variant, non-involuting congenital hemangioma (NICH), may persist indefinitely and reveals surface telangiectasias and a peripheral rim of pallor.

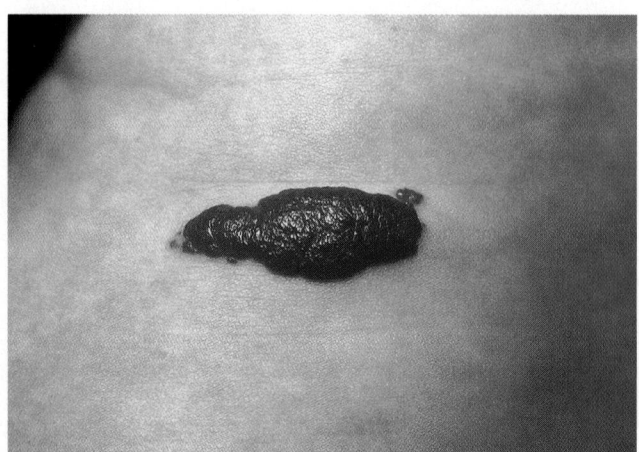

Figure 75-2. Superficial hemangioma.

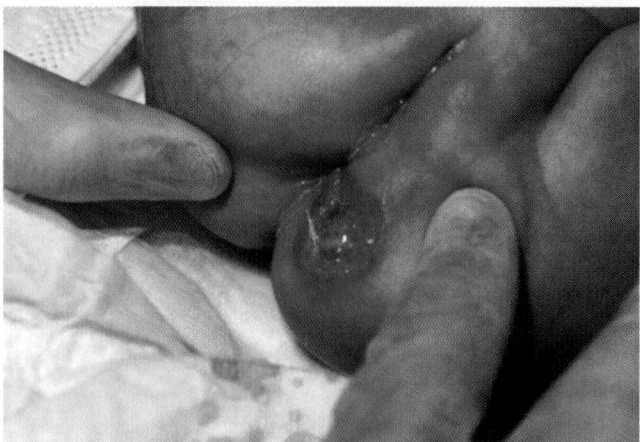

Figure 75-3. Ulcerated perianal hemangioma.

Although most hemangiomas follow a benign course, some progress to skin breakdown, functional compromise, cosmetic deformity, and occasionally systemic symptoms related to internal involvement. Ulceration is a common complication in rapidly proliferating lesions. It is accompanied by pain, irritability, and feeding intolerance in younger infants. When lesions become secondarily infected, permanent scarring nearly always results. Lesions in the diaper region are the most frequent to ulcerate.

Hemangiomas in certain locations tend to be problematic. Eyelid lesions may pose a risk to vision by causing light deprivation amblyopia or astigmatism. Ear involvement may obstruct the external auditory canal. Lesions on the lips or perianal area may ulcerate (Fig. 75-3) and often contribute to feeding or stooling difficulties. Nasal tip hemangiomas may result in a long-term "Cyrano nose" deformity. Any large hemangioma in a conspicuous location (e.g., the face) may pose a future threat to psychosocial and self-esteem development in older children.

Hemangiomas involving the airway may be life-threatening. Because lesions located in the "beard" distribution have a higher risk of airway involvement, infants with hemangiomas in the mandibular region, chin, or upper neck should be examined closely for hoarseness or biphasic stridor. If there are any indications of airway involvement, direct visualization of the airway should be performed. Lesions in other locations may be a marker for associated dysmorphology. Lumbosacral hemangiomas can be associated with occult spinal dysraphism, spinal cord abnormalities, and genitourinary malformations. Imaging of the spine and spinal cord should be performed in all infants with a midline hemangioma in this area. Another recognized association is that of large facial hemangiomas with other structural malformations, most often involving the brain, eyes, and cardiovascular system. This association, termed the *PHACES syndrome* (Box 75-1), usually is seen in association with large, aggressive, plaquelike hemangiomas and is more common in girls.

Multiple cutaneous hemangiomas are associated with a risk for extracutaneous hemangiomas with their complications. *Diffuse neonatal hemangiomatosis* describes infants with multiple cutaneous and visceral lesions. Internal lesions, especially those in the liver, may be associated with high-output congestive heart failure and anemia. Other organ systems that may be involved include the gastrointestinal tract, lungs, central nervous system, and eyes. Any infant with multiple cutaneous hemangiomas (Fig. 75-4) should be followed closely, with consideration given to screening abdominal ultrasonography (Box 75-2). Hepatic lesions may occur in the presence of only a few or no cutaneous hemangiomas. *Benign neonatal hemangiomatosis* describes infants with multiple cutaneous lesions without internal involvement.

Kasabach-Merritt phenomenon is the association of an enlarging vascular lesion with coagulopathy and thrombocytopenia. This phenomenon is not seen with classic hemangioma, but rather has been shown to be associated with other vascular tumors, most commonly kaposiform hemangioendothelioma or tufted angioma. Patients present with an enlarging, firm, dusky violaceous tumor associated with a consumptive coagulopathy, profound thrombocytopenia, and hemolytic anemia. Because this process requires aggressive therapy and has a high mortality rate, prompt recognition and referral are essential.

Pyogenic granuloma, or lobular capillary hemangioma, is a common acquired benign vascular tumor in children. These lesions are common on the face and the extremities and usually present as a solitary, red, dome-shaped papule with a moist, friable surface (Fig. 75-5). A collarette may be present around the base of the lesion, and the parent often reports bleeding. Lesions occasionally occur on the oral mucosa, although this presentation is most common in gravid women.

Vascular malformations can be divided into lesions that resolve spontaneously and lesions that do not. The most common vascular malformation, the *salmon patch* (also called *nevus simplex*) falls into the former category and occurs in 40% of newborns. These faint pink patches most commonly are located on the glabella ("angel's kiss") (Fig. 75-6), the occipital scalp and posterior neck ("stork bite"), and occasionally the nose and superior eyelids. Facial lesions tend to fade completely by 1 year of age, although they may reappear during episodes of crying or exertion. Posterior scalp and neck lesions may take several years to fade.

Port-wine stain (PWS) refers to a darker red, congenital vascular malformation that does not spontaneously involute. It occurs in 0.5% of newborns and is composed of mature dermal capillaries. PWSs are most common on the face but may occur anywhere on the skin surface. Location and associated findings are important in the evaluation of the patient with a PWS because there are several potential syndrome associations with these lesions (Table 75-1). *Sturge-Weber syndrome*, the most commonly associated syndrome, consists of the triad of facial PWS, leptomeningeal angiomatosis, and glaucoma. The vascular malformation in this disorder involves the ophthalmic division (V1) of the trigeminal nerve (Fig. 75-7), although involvement of other ipsilateral branches or bilateral involvement may be present. Common neurologic symptoms include seizures and mental retardation. Sturge-Weber syndrome occurs in 6% to 8% of patients with facial PWSs that involve the forehead or upper eyelid. The risk of central nervous system or eye involvement is higher with bilateral trigeminal involvement, upper and lower eyelid involvement, and ipsilateral involvement of all three branches of the trigeminal nerve. *Klippel-Trenaunay syndrome* refers to the constellation of PWS; venous varicosity; and bone and soft tissue hypertrophy of an extremity, usually a leg (Fig. 75-8).

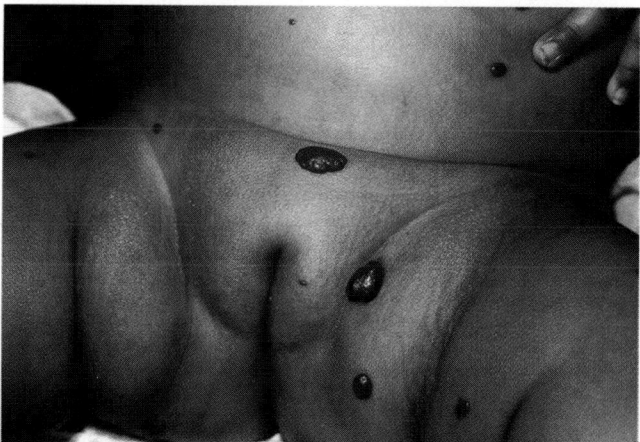

Figure 75-4. Neonatal hemangiomatosis.

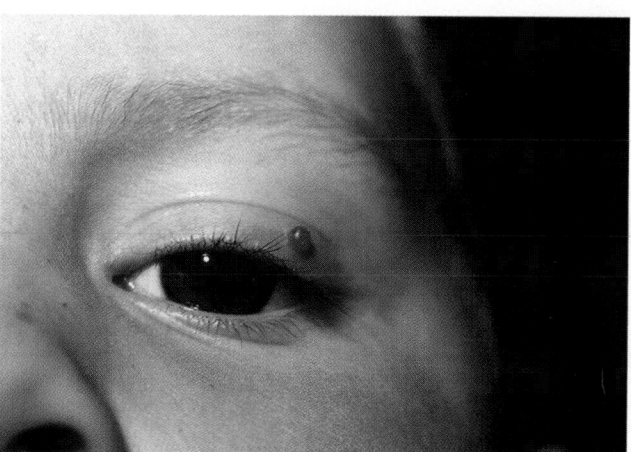

Figure 75-5. Pyogenic granuloma.

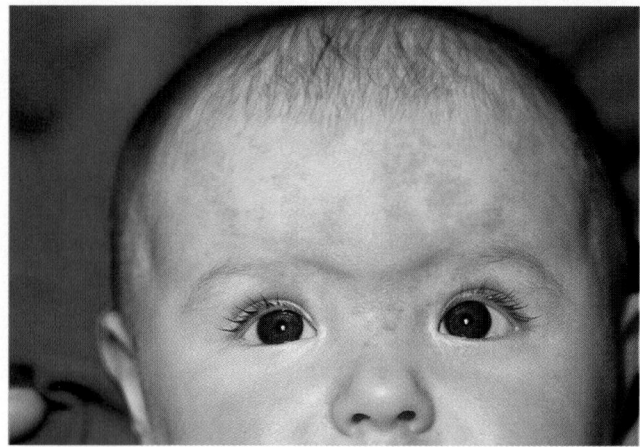

Figure 75-6. Glabellar salmon patch. Note also superior eyelid involvement.

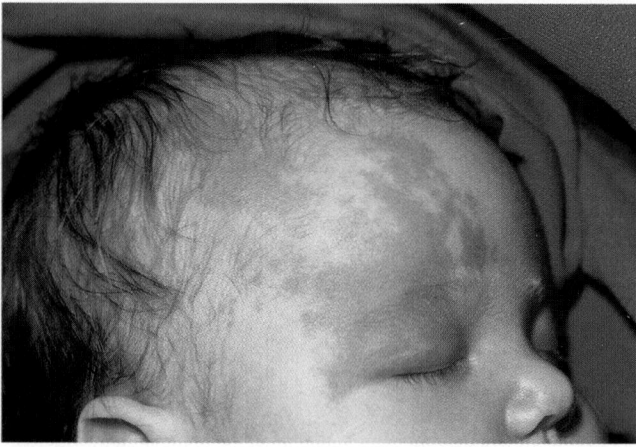

Figure 75-7. Port wine stain in V1 distribution.

Venous malformation, another type of vascular malformation, presents as a blue or purple nodule. These malformations may occur singly or in groups and sporadically or in association with syndromes. *Blue rubber bleb nevus syndrome* is the association of multiple venous malformations in the skin and gastrointestinal tract and less commonly other organ systems. *Maffucci syndrome* consists of multiple venous malformations with enchondromas, which result in marked bony and soft tissue deformities. The enchondromas in this condition carry a risk of malignant transformation into chondrosarcoma.

Telangiectases are permanently dilated small blood vessels in the skin that may or may not blanch with pressure. Telangiectases occur sporadically and in association with some disease states. Prolonged use of topical corticosteroids may result in telangiectases. *Spider angioma* is the most common form of telangiectasia and presents as a central vascular papule (arteriole) with radiating fine telangiectatic vessels around the periphery. Spider angioma may occur sporadically (most common in children) or in association with pregnancy or liver disease. *Unilateral nevoid telangiectasia* presents with multiple telangiectases on the face, neck, chest, and arms in a unilateral distribution. Although affected individuals usually are otherwise healthy, pregnancy and liver disease may be predisposing factors.

Hereditary hemorrhagic telangiectasia (HHT), or *Osler-Weber-Rendu syndrome*, is an autosomal dominant disorder that results in mucocutaneous telangiectases and visceral AVMs, most notably in the lungs, brain, spine, liver, and gastrointestinal tract. Telangiectases in this disorder are distributed most commonly on the lips, fingers, and nose and in the oral cavity. Patients frequently have a history of recurrent epistaxis and may have clinical manifestations referable to hemorrhage or shunting in other affected organs.

Cutis marmorata telangiectatica congenita (CMTC) is a rare disorder that presents at birth with exaggerated cutis marmorata–like mottling of the skin (Fig. 75-9) that does not disappear with rewarming. The reticulated, blue-violet vascular lesions of CMTC may be generalized or localized; may reveal skin and subcutis atrophy; and may be associated with body asymmetry and limb discrepancy, most commonly hypoplasia, of the affected extremity. The pathogenesis and exact nature of the vascular anomaly are poorly understood. Associated defects include ocular and neurologic abnormalities, although most patients have a benign course with gradual fading of the cutaneous lesions. Because exaggerated physiologic cutis marmorata may occur in Down syndrome and de Lange's syndrome, these entities should be considered in the differential diagnosis of CMTC.

Table 75-1. Port Wine Stain–Associated Syndromes

Syndrome Name	Port Wine Stain Characteristics	Associations
Sturge-Weber	Ophthalmic (V1) branch trigeminal nerve	Leptomeningeal angiomas, glaucoma, seizures, DD, MR
Klippel-Trenaunay	Extremity, usually leg	Venous varicosity, bone and soft tissue hypertrophy; Parkes-Weber variant with underlying AVMs
Cobb	Dermatomal distribution on trunk or extremity	AVM in corresponding spinal cord metamere
Wyburn-Mason	Telangiectatic; periocular	Ipsilateral AVM of retina and brain
Proteus	Common, but also venous or lymphatic malformations	Connective tissue nevus, epidermal nevus, overgrowth (bone and fat), hyperostoses
Phakomatosis pigmentovascularis	Associated with verrucous nevus, mongolian spots, nevus spilus, nevus anemicus	May have associated abnormalities (eye, CNS, skeletal)

AVM, arteriovenous malformation; CNS, central nervous system; DD, developmental delay; MR, mental retardation.

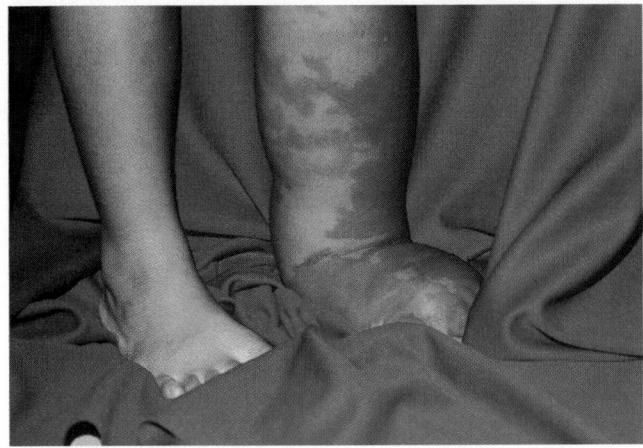

Figure 75-8. Port wine stain, varicosities, and limb hypertrophy in Klippel-Trenaunay syndrome.

Table 75-2. Medical Therapies for Hemangiomas

Therapy	Comments
Topical antibiotic cream/ointment, nonstick wound dressing	For eroded or ulcerated lesions; Ace or Coban wrap useful for extremities
Oral antibiotics	If secondary infection (crusting, exudate) present
Acetaminophen or acetaminophen with codeine	Occasionally indicated for pain
Intralesional corticosteroids	Triamcinolone, maximum dose 3–5 mg/kg; caution with periocular lesions (retinal artery occlusion)
Oral corticosteroids	Mainstay of therapy; prednisone or prednisolone, 2–4 mg/kg/day; gradual taper over months; avoid live vaccinations while on therapy
Interferon alfa-2a, -2b	1–3 million U/m²/day, subcutaneous injection; fever and irritability common; spastic diplegia in 20%

MANAGEMENT

Although most hemangiomas are uncomplicated and spontaneously involute without incident, certain clinical situations may require therapeutic intervention, including (1) rapidly growing or ulcerative lesions, (2) lesions with life-threatening or potentially functional consequences (e.g., periocular lesions at risk for resulting in astigmatism), and (3) lesions likely to result in significant disfigurement or psychosocial distress for the patient. Any complicated hemangioma or lesion that seems to warrant therapy should be referred to a physician or center with experience in the management of these patients.

In uncomplicated cases, an approach of "active nonintervention" has been advocated, using parental education and reassurance, anticipatory guidance, psychosocial support, and frequent patient follow-up. Medical therapies for hemangiomas (Table 75-2) include symptomatic care, corticosteroids, and interferon alfa. Pulsed dye laser therapy usually is restricted to superficial, early hemangiomas given its limited depth of penetration, although it is helpful in ulcerated lesions for hemostasis and pain control. Lastly, surgical intervention may be an appropriate consideration in some cases, including pedunculated lesions that are likely to result in fibrofatty residua and life-threatening or deforming lesions in which pharmacologic therapy is deemed ineffective or intolerable. Many factors must be weighed when surgical intervention for a hemangioma is being considered.

Treatment of Kasabach-Merritt phenomenon is difficult at best. Therapies aimed at reversing the thrombocytopenia and inhibiting the disseminated intravascular coagulopathy may be necessary. Reported treatments include corticosteroids, interferon alfa, aspirin, heparin, dipyridamole, ε-aminocaproic acid, cyclophosphamide, embolization, and surgical excision.

Pyogenic granuloma usually is treated easily with shave excision followed by electrocautery, which assists in hemostasis and in the prevention of recurrence. Pulsed dye laser therapy may be useful for smaller lesions.

PWSs are treated most successfully with the flashlamp-pumped pulsed dye laser. This laser has high specificity and safety and adheres to the principle of "selective photothermolysis," with thermal injury largely confined to the targeted blood vessels in the malformation and minimal damage to surrounding tissues. Although significant improvement may occur, complete clearing is less common, and multiple treatments are usually necessary. PWSs involving the central face are less responsive to pulsed dye laser therapy. Cosmetically significant telangiectases also may be treated with the pulsed dye laser or alternatively with electrofulguration.

A multidisciplinary approach is vital in caring for patients with PWS-associated (or other vascular malformation–associated) syndromes. The specialties most often involved include pediatrics, dermatology, ophthalmology, orthopedic surgery, neurology, neurosurgery, interventional radiology,

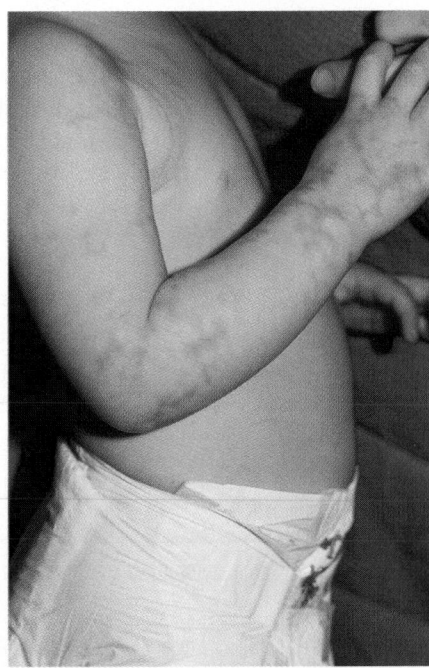

Figure 75-9. Cutis marmorata telangiectatica congenita.

surgery, and genetics. Physical and occupational therapy, referral to national associations, use of support groups, and adequate psychological and social support all are important considerations. Patients with Klippel-Trenaunay syndrome may benefit from the use of compressive garments for the affected extremity and may require referral to a national odd-shoe exchange program.

Most of the morbidity associated with HHT is due to hemorrhage from the vascular lesions, and therapy needs to be tailored to the individual patient and sites of involvement. Presymptomatic screening for pulmonary and cerebral AVMs should be considered in patients with known HHT or a family history of the disease. Treatment options for affected individuals include the administration of antifibrinolytic agents, hormonal therapy, and DDAVP and surgical excision of the AVM when feasible. Red blood cell transfusions may be necessary. In addition, HHT-associated recurrent epistaxis may be treated with embolization or septal dermoplasty, and transcatheter embolization is useful in treating pulmonary AVMs. Genetic counseling is vital, and prenatal and molecular diagnosis is possible.

Patients with CMTC rarely require therapy. A careful clinical evaluation with special attention to associated orthopedic, ophthalmologic, or neurologic complications is warranted.

OUTCOME

The outcome for patients with hemangiomas, vascular malformations, or associated syndromes depends on the extent of organ involvement and related complications. Most patients with uncomplicated hemangiomas have an excellent prognosis and do well. Psychosocial concerns and emotional well-being are the greatest concerns for disfiguring facial hemangiomas. Adverse effects include parental reactions of disbelief, fear, and mourning; poor parent-child interaction; and lack of acceptance of the child by the extended family. Attention to these potential concerns is vital for the clinician caring for these patients.

The prognosis for infants with diffuse neonatal hemangiomatosis depends most on the extent of visceral involvement, especially the liver. These high-flow lesions increase the potential morbidity, with the mortality rate approaching 40% to 80%. Despite the multiple therapies reported for Kasabach-Merritt phenomenon, the mortality rate remains high (20% to 30%).

The outcome for patients with Sturge-Weber syndrome is variable. Poor prognostic indicators include cortical changes in the first months of life, early onset of seizures, and poorly controlled seizures. Distributions of PWS that seem to correlate with a higher seizure risk include bilateral involvement and involvement of all three (V1, V2, and V3) divisions of the trigeminal nerve. Developmental delay, emotional and behavioral difficulties, and poor intellectual functioning also seem to be correlated to early onset and severity of seizure activity.

Most patients with Klippel-Trenaunay syndrome do well with appropriate education, support, and encouragement. Complications include leg-length discrepancy, which may require orthopedic intervention when greater than 2 cm,

Box 75-3. Follow-up for Patients with Complex Lesions or Syndromes

1. Appropriate well-child care, with attention to immunizations and normal parameters of growth and development
2. Psychological support for patients, parents, and families affected by vascular disorders
3. Referral to national organizations and use of appropriate support groups as indicated
4. Consideration of delayed surgical intervention for select patients with complicated hemangiomas
5. Appropriate ongoing orthopedic follow-up for patients with lesions or syndromes predisposing to asymmetric overgrowth or undergrowth

although differences in limb girth alone are more common. Thrombosis, infection, bleeding, coagulopathy, and pulmonary embolism are uncommon complications.

The natural history of HHT is heterogeneous and may be due in part to genotype/phenotype correlation; pulmonary AVM seems more common in kindreds with an *endoglin* mutation as opposed to kindreds with a mutation in the *ALK-1* gene. In general, 20% of patients with HHT have pulmonary AVMs, and 5% to 10% develop cerebral AVMs.

Most patients with CMTC do quite well, with gradual fading of the skin lesions over time. Morbidity usually is related to the extent of extracutaneous involvement, especially neurologic, orthopedic, and any deeper vascular lesions. Eye involvement seems to be a greater risk in patients with periocular skin involvement with the vascular malformation.

FOLLOW-UP

Multidisciplinary or specialty follow-up is indicated for patients with hemangioma-related or vascular malformation–related syndromes or complex vascular lesions. The frequency of evaluation is best left to the individual specialty service(s) and depends on extent of involvement and severity of disease. For some disorders, specific multispecialty clinics are coordinated, primarily at larger tertiary care institutions, and usually meet with high patient and parent acceptance. Box 75-3 lists recommendations for patients with complex lesions or related syndromes.

Additional Resources, CD-ROM

Color atlas	Figures
Bibliography	

Mini-index of Related Topics CH.

SUGGESTED READINGS

Drolet BA, Esterly NB, Frieden IJ: Hemangiomas in children. N Engl J Med 1999;341:173–181.

Enjolras O, Mulliken JB: Vascular tumors and vascular malformations (new issues). Adv Dermatol 1998;13:375–423.

Frieden IJ, Eichenfield LF, Esterly NB, et al: Guidelines of care for hemangiomas of infancy. J Am Acad Dermatol 1997;37:631–637.

Mulliken JB, Glowacki J: Hemangiomas and vascular malformations in infants and children: A classification based on endothelial characteristics. Plast Reconstr Surg 1982;69:412–420.

Shovlin CL, Guttmacher AE, Buscarini E, et al: Diagnostic criteria for hereditary hemorrhagic telangiectasia (Rendu-Osler-Weber syndrome). Am J Med Genet 2000;91:66–67.

SECTION 3   GENERAL MEDICAL CARE: *Disorders of the Skin*

76 Infections of the Skin

Rekha Krishnankutty

ROLE OF THE GENERALIST

1   Recognize various types of skin infections, and use appropriate diagnostic tools to determine the responsible pathogen and the extent of disease.

2   Treat infections of the skin with appropriate medical therapy, and recognize the need for drainage procedures in certain types of infections.

3   Choose appropriate topical, oral, or parenteral antibiotic therapy to treat skin infections.

4   Distinguish patients with potentially serious and life-threatening illnesses from patients who can be treated as an outpatient, and quickly refer ill-appearing patients for inpatient care.

5   Establish adequate follow-up when treating patients in the outpatient setting, ensuring proper response to therapy.

Infections of the skin can be caused by a variety of agents and may manifest in different ways. Proper diagnosis and treatment of skin infections are important to prevent progression and transmission to others. This chapter discusses common bacterial, fungal, viral, and parasitic infections of the skin.

BACTERIAL SKIN AND SOFT TISSUE INFECTIONS

Bacterial infections of the skin are common during childhood. Children are especially prone to breaching the protective skin barrier through superficial cuts, abrasions, insect bites, or burns of the skin; they are at high risk for inoculation, replication, and development of infection by bacteria on the skin surface. Normal skin flora, such as coagulase-negative staphylococci, rarely cause infection and may be protective against more pathogenic bacteria. Organisms that colonize the skin after being introduced from the environment, most commonly group A β-hemolytic streptococci (GABHS) and *Staphylococcus aureus*, are more likely to cause infection. These organisms can inhabit the nasopharynx or the skin, especially under conditions of warm climate, humidity, poor hygiene, and crowded living conditions. Prior antibiotic use also can alter the normal skin flora and predispose to infection.

Any preexisting skin condition that weakens the skin barrier, such as dermatitis, chickenpox, or tinea, predisposes to bacterial colonization and infection, with potential for rapid spread. An immunosuppressed state may prevent the body from adequately combating skin infection after inoculation and may lead to more serious complications.

Presentation
Impetigo and Ecthyma
Impetigo typically is described as multiple "honey-crusted" lesions, most commonly on the face, nares, and extremities of preschool-age children (Fig. 76-1). There is superficial bacterial invasion of the upper epidermis, which usually is breached after minor skin trauma or an insect bite. Several days later, small vesicles or pustules form and then unroof and crust over. Regional lymphadenopathy is common. *S. aureus* is more frequently a pathogen than GABHS. Impetigo can be pruritic, stimulating scratching of the lesions and promoting spread to adjacent skin and transmission to others. *Bullous impetigo* is caused by *S. aureus* and is more common in the intertriginous areas, such as the axillae and diaper area, of infants and younger children. Blisters form, and when the blister breaks, rim desquamation surrounds the moist, shallow skin erosion. The lesions are thought to be a localized form of staphylococcal scalded skin syndrome.

Ecthyma also involves a break in the epidermal barrier with subsequent bacterial inoculation, but in contrast to impetigo, ecthyma involves the entire epidermis. It may

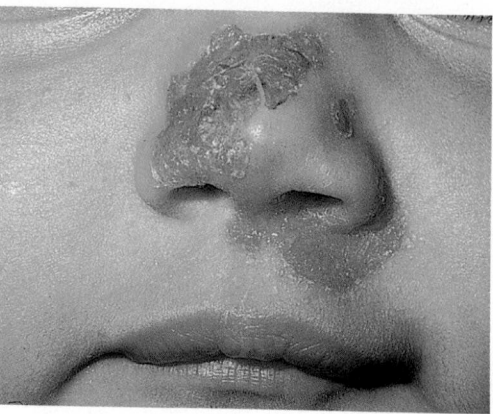

Figure 76-1. Impetigo. (From Weston WL, Lane AT, Morelli JG: Color Textbook of Pediatric Dermatology, 3rd ed. St. Louis, Mosby, 2002, p 45.)

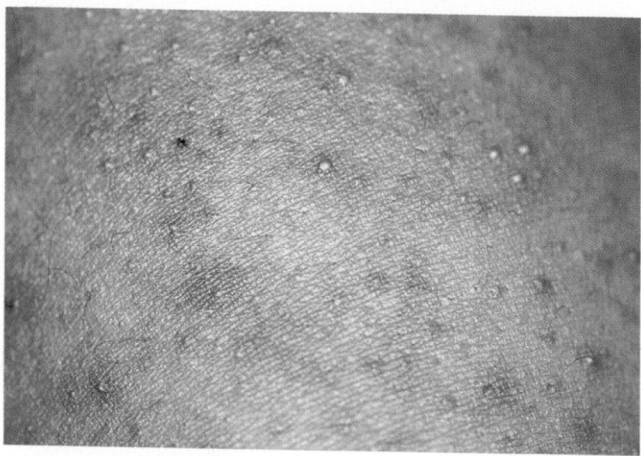

Figure 76-3. Folliculitis. (Courtesy of Sheryll L. Vanderhooft, MD, University of Utah Medical Center.)

begin similarly to impetigo, but the lesions later develop thick, dry, dark, adherent crust with surrounding erythema and induration (Fig. 76-2). Lesions are painful, and pus often can be expressed with direct pressure on the crust. Predisposing factors include tropical climate; undernutrition; poor hygiene; and presence of pruritic lesions, such as insect bites or scabies. The lesions of *ecthyma gangrenosum* are hemorrhagic papules, pustules, and bullae with necrosis. This disease is associated with *Pseudomonas aeruginosa* sepsis and occurs in patients with underlying immunosuppression.

The differential diagnosis of impetigo and ecthyma includes other skin diseases that also may manifest with

crusted or bullous lesions, such as dermatitis; viral infections, such as herpes and varicella; scabies; burns; or other immunobullous diseases. Bacterial culture of expressed purulent material should confirm the diagnosis.

Folliculitis, Furunculosis, and Skin Abscesses

Folliculitis is infection of the hair follicle. Manifestations vary with the location of inflammation within the follicle. *Superficial folliculitis* results from occlusion of the follicular opening and invasion of the follicular wall by bacteria, usually by normal skin flora. Inflammation of the mouth of the hair follicle develops and appears as crops of small 1- to 2-mm pustules on an erythematous base (Fig. 76-3); impetigo also may be present. *Deep folliculitis*, or *furunculosis*, involves inflammation of the base of the follicle and the adjacent deep dermis and presents as deeper set, painful erythematous nodules (Fig. 76-4). Multiple furuncles can coalesce to become a soft and fluctuant mass, or *abscess*; they also may develop into interconnecting dermal and subcutaneous abscesses, called *carbuncles*, which are more likely to be associated with fever, chills, and malaise.

Prolonged moisture and occlusion of the follicles predispose to the development of these infections; areas

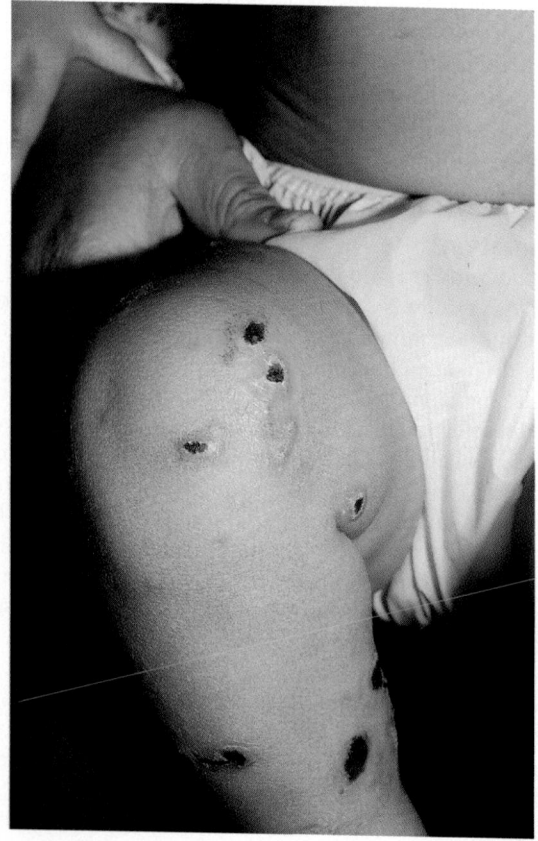

Figure 76-2. Ecthyma. (Courtesy of Stanley Inkelis, MD, Department of Pediatrics, Harbor–UCLA Medical Center.)

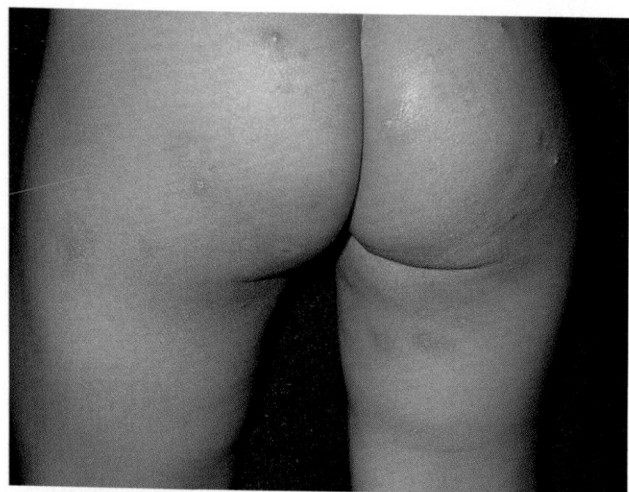

Figure 76-4. Furunculosis. (Courtesy of Stanley Inkelis, MD, Department of Pediatrics, Harbor–UCLA Medical Center.)

such as the axilla, buttocks, and inner thighs, especially with tight clothing, are common locations. *S. aureus* typically is cultured from these lesions, but gram-negative bacteria also can be found; submersion in *Pseudomonas*-contaminated water, as in poorly chlorinated hot tubs and pools, predisposes children to so-called hot tub folliculitis. Patients with recurrent furuncles may be carriers or may be in contact with carriers of *S. aureus* in the nostrils, axilla, or groin. The differential diagnosis of bacterial folliculitis includes acne and folliculitis from chemical contact or fungal skin infections.

Paronychia

Periungual abscess, or paronychia, is an abscess that develops superficially in the tissue surrounding the fingernail or toenail; it also can occur under the cuticle (Fig. 76-5). Predisposing factors include anything that causes trauma to the tissue, such as nail biting, chewing or clipping cuticle or hangnails, and finger sucking. Ingrown nails, which occur as a result of improperly cut nails, predispose to paronychia by growing into the nail fold and lacerating the tissue. Patients experience tenderness, erythema, and swelling at the nail fold, which subsequently develops an abscess. If treatment is delayed, the abscess can burrow underneath the base of the nail, leading to an onychia, or subungual abscess. *S. aureus* is the usual pathogen, although anaerobic bacteria also may be present.

Perianal Streptococcal Dermatitis

Perianal streptococcal dermatitis is also known as *perianal dermatitis*, *perianal cellulitis*, and *perianal streptococcal cellulitis* (Fig. 76-6). It presents as superficial, well-circumscribed, and often tender perianal erythema, most commonly in children between ages 6 months and 10 years. Edema, purulent discharge, and perianal fissures may be present, but patients typically are afebrile. The vulvovaginal and penile areas may be involved. Symptoms may include perianal pruritus and painful defecation with blood-tinged stools and constipation. GABHS is often responsible, and many patients may have concomitant pharyngitis with positive pharyngeal cultures for the organism. The infection may spread among household contacts, especially when

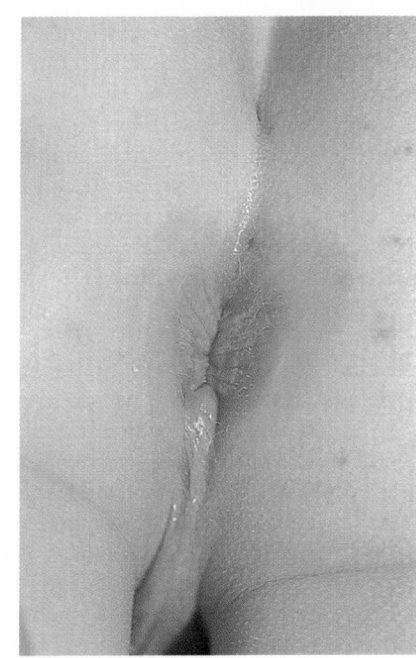

Figure 76-6. Perianal streptococcal cellulitis. (From Weston WL, Lane AT, Morelli JG: Color Textbook of Pediatric Dermatology, 3rd ed. St. Louis, Mosby, 2002, p 47.)

bath water is shared. The differential diagnosis of perianal streptococcal dermatitis includes psoriasis, candidiasis, seborrheic dermatitis, pinworms, sexual abuse, and inflammatory bowel disease.

Cellulitis

Cellulitis is bacterial infection and inflammation of the subcutaneous fat underlying the skin; it may extend to the layer of the deep dermis (Fig. 76-7). This infection is found most commonly on the face and extremities, and it commonly is introduced after a local trauma to the skin. Cellulitis also can be of hematogenous origin or can extend upward from a deeper infection, such as a dental abscess, osteomyelitis, or lymphangitis. Cellulitis is characterized by tenderness, erythema, induration, and sometimes warmth of the overlying skin. The borders of the swelling and erythema are indistinct. Regional lymphadenopathy and systemic symptoms, such as fever, chills, malaise, and

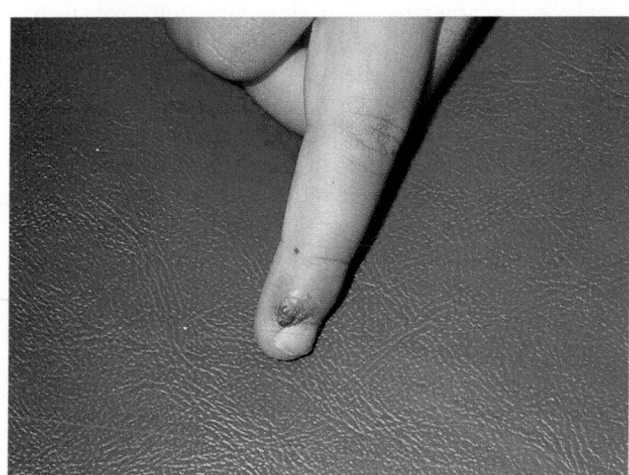

Figure 76-5. Paronychia. (Courtesy of Stanley Inkelis, MD, Department of Pediatrics, Harbor–UCLA Medical Center.)

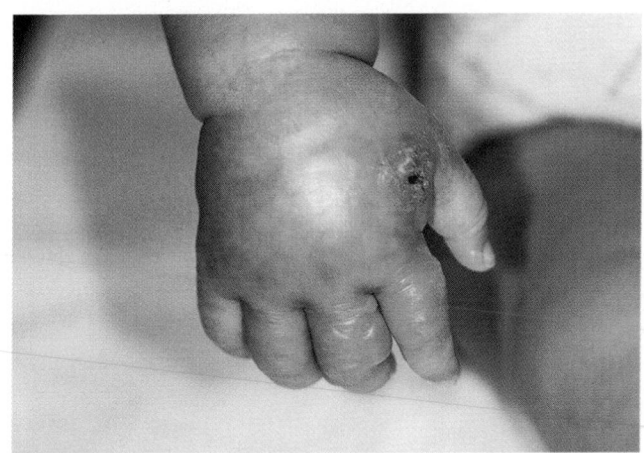

Figure 76-7. Cellulitis. (Courtesy of Sheryll L. Vanderhooft, MD, University of Utah Medical Center.)

headache, may be found; these symptoms are more common with hematogenous origin of infection or spread from deeper structures.

Skin lesions resulting from insect bites or stings, giant urticaria, pressure erythema, or early-stage contact dermatitis may mimic cellulitis, but in contrast to cellulitis, these are nontender lesions. Fracture or septic joint may have associated overlying redness or swelling and also should be considered in the differential diagnosis.

Erysipelas

Erysipelas is an infection by GABHS of the dermis and superficial lymphatic system, which occurs in a localized fashion (Fig. 76-8). There is a prodrome of fever and chills, sometimes with headache, nausea, and vomiting. The patient develops a painful, well-demarcated, raised red or pink macular lesion, sometimes with red lymphatic streaks advancing toward the nearest regional lymph nodes. The skin is edematous, is exquisitely hot and tender to palpation, and may have a peau d'orange quality on close inspection. Erysipelas can occur on any part of the skin, but the face is the most common area of involvement. This infection usually results from inoculation of a break in the skin by organisms carried in the upper respiratory tract of the affected patient, but some cases are thought to have spread hematogenously. There is risk of bacteremia and metastatic spread of infection, especially in infants.

Necrotizing Fasciitis

Necrotizing fasciitis also has been called *streptococcal gangrene*, *necrotizing erysipelas*, *synergistic cellulitis* or *gangrene*, and more recently *flesh-eating bacteria* or *killer strep* disease. It is a severe necrotizing infection of the soft tissue, which can begin as cellulitis and progress to involve deeper structures; bacteria invade through the dermis and subcutaneous tissue to the deep fascial sheaths and sometimes the underlying muscle. Pathogens include GABHS, *S. aureus*, *P. aeruginosa*, *Escherichia coli*, and mixed organisms. The infection spreads rapidly, causing edema and compromise of blood flow in fascial compartments, leading to infarction of skin and soft tissue. Patients with compromised immune systems and diabetes are at higher risk, especially if they have preexisting skin and soft tissue infections, deep surgical or traumatic wounds, history of injec-

tions, or any break in the protective skin barrier. Newborns with omphalitis, or infection of the periumbilical skin, are at high risk for necrotizing fasciitis.

Symptoms of necrotizing fasciitis initially are similar to the symptoms of cellulitis; however, in patients with necrotizing fasciitis, systemic symptoms are more prominent, and the lesions may progress over hours. Compared with cellulitis, necrotizing fasciitis is exquisitely painful even early in the course of disease. The induration and edema are present in deeper structures, and the affected area may be unusually firm in consistency. If the edema involves the skin, lesions may resemble erysipelas. Necrotizing fasciitis changes in color from red or purple to grayish blue, and bullae may appear; later, central necrosis leads to formation of a black eschar. Sensation is decreased as a result of destruction of the cutaneous nerves that travel through the fascia and subcutaneous tissue. If anaerobic bacteria are involved, there may be crepitance of the skin or subcutaneous emphysema on x-ray.

As the skin and soft tissue lesions worsen, systemic symptoms also progress. In addition to fever, patients can develop signs and symptoms of shock, including poor perfusion with generalized pallor and mottling and altered level of consciousness with obtundation and grunting respirations. Necrotizing fasciitis may lead to death if not adequately treated.

Diagnosis

The diagnosis of most infections of the skin is clinical, based on the history, signs and symptoms, and physical examination findings. The classic recognizable features of each disease process, as described previously, allow the initiation of therapy based on clinical diagnosis alone. Tools such as Gram stain and cultures may be helpful in confirming the responsible organism and may indicate the need to modify current treatment.

Infections of the skin that involve abscesses, vesicles, bullae, or any other lesions from which material can be obtained should be cultured by draining or unroofing the lesions. The lesions of cellulitis and erysipelas can be cultured via tissue aspirate; after injection into the lesion of nonbacteriostatic saline, high-pressure suction is applied with a large syringe. Wound infections also can be cultured to help direct therapy. Any skin infection that is not responding to therapy should be cultured to modify therapy properly. Cultures of the nasopharynx and throat of patients who have serious or recurrent skin infections may show colonization by a particular organism, such as GABHS or methicillin-resistant *S. aureus*, and may indicate prophylaxis to prevent future infections.

In patients with skin infections who have systemic signs or symptoms, such as fever, blood cultures may show bacteremia, either as a complication of or as the origin of the infection. Blood cultures are necessary in patients with suspected serious infections, such as erysipelas or necrotizing fasciitis, or in any ill-appearing child.

Imaging techniques may help to assess the extent of disease in infections that are located or suspected to have spread from deeper structures. Magnetic resonance imaging is a useful tool in determining the extent of involvement in necrotizing fasciitis.

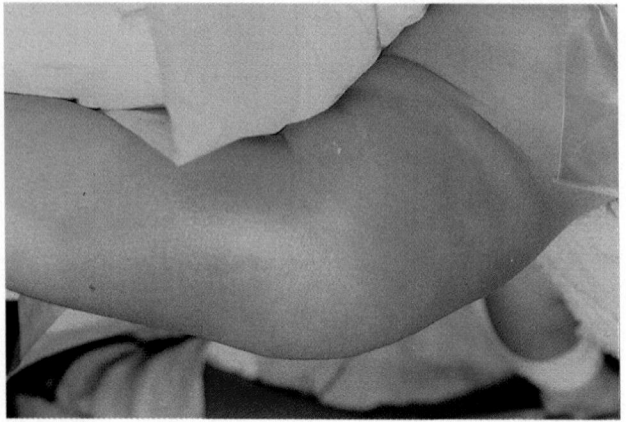

Figure 76-8. Erysipelas. (Courtesy of Stanley Inkelis, MD, Department of Pediatrics, Harbor–UCLA Medical Center.)

Management

Management of children with bacterial skin infections varies depending on the type of lesions, extent of disease, accompanying signs and symptoms, and overall appearance of the child. Antibiotics alone can be used for most simple bacterial skin infections, but infections involving collections of purulent material, such as abscesses and paronychia, require drainage for adequate treatment. A child who has fever or other systemic signs of infection or who has failed outpatient treatment may require admission to the hospital and intravenous antibiotic therapy. Any child who appears ill with signs or symptoms of shock should be taken immediately to an emergency department.

Skin infections caused by GABHS and *S. aureus* often present similarly, and initial empirical antibiotic therapy should cover both types of bacteria (see Chapter 284). If cultures are performed, therapy should be tailored based on identification and sensitivity of the responsible organism. Oral antibiotic choices should include penicillinase-resistant β-lactam drugs, such as cloxacillin and dicloxacillin, or first-generation or second-generation cephalosporins, such as cephalexin. The intravenous forms of these drugs, including nafcillin, oxacillin, and cefazolin, should be administered in patients with more severe infections. Macrolide antibiotics are an option for patients with penicillin allergy, but they should not be used as first-line therapy, owing to concerns about emerging bacterial resistance to these drugs. The topical antibiotic mupirocin is used to treat mild skin infections, but other topical antibiotics, such as bacitracin and neomycin, should be used only to prevent infection after minor skin trauma.

Without treatment, *impetigo* resolves spontaneously over several weeks, but antibiotic therapy is important in reducing transmission to others. Mild cases of impetigo may be treated with mupirocin ointment for a 7- to 10-day course. Seven days of oral antibiotics should be prescribed if the lesions are extensive or if household contacts also have lesions. If the lesions are on the face, the nares may be the reservoir for the offending bacteria, and systemic therapy is indicated. Patients with recurrent impetigo who are nasal carriers of *S. aureus* may benefit from nasal mupirocin therapy. Adequate treatment of *ecthyma* requires oral antibiotics. Impetigo and ecthyma are contagious lesions that should be treated with at least 24 hours of antibiotics before children are allowed to return to school.

Folliculitis usually is treated with mupirocin, but patients also may benefit from antibacterial soaps, such as chlorhexidine. If the lesions are severe, oral antibiotics are indicated. Hot tub folliculitis resolves spontaneously over 7 to 10 days without therapy, if the water is adequately chlorinated and frequently changed. Skin *abscesses* and deep *furuncles* should be drained and treated with oral antibiotics, but *carbuncles* are treated best with intravenous antibiotics, owing to the higher risk of secondary bacteremia. Lesions that extend into deeper soft tissue may need surgical incision and drainage, in addition to intravenous antibiotic therapy. A child with chronic recurrent furunculosis may be a carrier of *S. aureus* in the nares and may benefit from a 5-day course of mupirocin nasal ointment or long-term antibiotic therapy.

Treatment of *paronychia* is aimed at drainage of the superficial abscess (see Chapter 298). Drainage may be achieved via incision, with subsequent soaks in clean, warm water. Topical antibiotics in an occlusive dressing applied for 5 days also has been found to soften the skin enough to allow spontaneous drainage and subsequent resolution of the infection. Oral antibiotics should be considered if the lesion does not respond to these treatments or if there is more severe skin or soft tissue involvement. If a paronychia is related to an ingrown toenail, the nail may need to be removed partially or fully from the nail bed to prevent recurrence.

Perianal streptococcal dermatitis can be treated with a 10-day course of oral penicillin V or intramuscular benzathine penicillin. Mupirocin alone also has been successful.

In a nontoxic patient, mild-to-moderate *cellulitis* may be treated with oral antibiotics for 7 to 10 days. Moderate-to-severe cellulitis and *erysipelas* should be treated in a hospital with intravenous antibiotics.

Treatment of *necrotizing fasciitis* requires prompt surgical débridement with aggressive fluid resuscitation and intravenous antibiotic therapy. Ultimately, skin grafts may be indicated, depending on the extent of skin lost.

Outcome

In the immunocompetent host, most bacterial infections of the skin resolve with adequate antibiotic therapy and drainage of any abscesses, with the potential to leave scars. If left untreated, however, infections such as ecthyma, cellulitis, erysipelas, and abscesses may lead to serious illness. The mortality rate of necrotizing fasciitis can be high (70%), especially when diagnosis is delayed or débridement is inadequate.

Follow-up

Patients being treated in the clinic with antibiotics for mild-to-moderate skin infections should be seen again by a physician in 1 to 2 days for follow-up to ensure that current therapy is adequate. If patients continue to experience recurrent skin infections, further testing, such as nasopharyngeal cultures and immune workup, should be considered. Good hygiene should be strongly encouraged because it can help to prevent the further spread of many of these lesions.

FUNGAL SKIN INFECTIONS

Fungal infections of the skin occur via invasion and proliferation of dermatophytes or yeasts in the outer layer of the epidermis, causing an inflammatory response. The most common predisposing factor is contact with infected persons or pets, but warm and humid conditions also contribute to these infections. Dermatophyte infections are called *tinea*, or *ringworm*. *Candida* and *Pityrosporum* are the most common causes of yeast infections of the skin.

Presentation

Tinea Corporis

Tinea corporis, also known as *ringworm*, is a superficial infection of the skin that causes erythematous, pruritic, and scaly lesions that often have an annular shape (Fig. 76-9; see also Chapter 74). The outer circumference of each lesion consists of papules and microvesicles that burst and scale; as

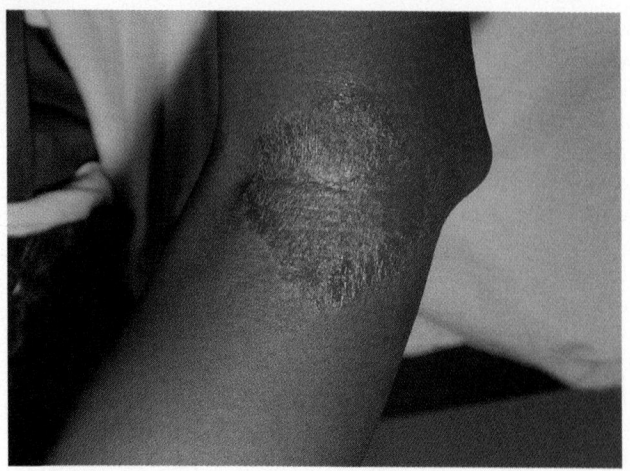

Figure 76-9. Tinea corporis. (Courtesy of Stanley Inkelis, MD, Department of Pediatrics, Harbor–UCLA Medical Center.)

this active portion of the ring-shaped lesion grows outwardly, the inner portion of the lesion begins to resolve, leading to central clearing. Tinea corporis may begin as a single lesion, which can grow to 5 cm in diameter, but the lesions often spread to other areas of the skin via autoinoculation from the primary patch. Tinea incognita is a lesion with less distinct borders and less scaling, due to erroneous treatment with topical steroids.

The inflammatory nature of the lesions may lead the clinician to confuse them with atopic dermatitis, especially if they do not have the characteristic ring-shaped appearance. Tinea can be differentiated from atopic dermatitis by its contagious nature, asymmetric distribution, and central clearing of the lesions. The herald patch of pityriasis rosea also may be mistaken for tinea corporis but is distinguishable by its central scaling.

Tinea Pedis

Also known widely as *athlete's foot*, tinea pedis is a fungal infection of the feet that is most common among adolescents. Predisposing factors include contaminated floors (shower, bathroom, gym, and locker room) and the warmth and moisture associated with prolonged wearing of shoes. The infection affects especially the web spaces in between the toes, but it can spread to the dorsum and sole of the foot. Patients experience burning and itching of the affected areas, which are characterized by scaling and cracking and sometimes maceration and vesiculopustular lesions.

Contact dermatitis of the feet, which is often an allergic reaction to some component of the shoes, spares the web spaces and can be distinguished from tinea pedis. Other skin conditions, such as atopic dermatitis, scabies, juvenile plantar dermatosis, and dyshidrotic eczema, also may mimic tinea pedis.

Tinea Versicolor

Tinea versicolor is another superficial fungal infection of the skin, caused by *Pityrosporum*, also called *Malassezia furfur* (Fig. 76-10; see also Chapter 74). It can occur in all age groups but is more common in adolescents and young adults. Tinea versicolor appears as multiple, small, oval-shaped lesions with fine scale that sometimes occur on the

face but more frequently affect the upper chest, back, and proximal arms. Lesions may be hypopigmented, especially over tanned areas of skin; however, in non–sun-exposed areas, lesions are hyperpigmented with tan or reddish color. Tinea versicolor is usually asymptomatic but may be associated with mild pruritus. Lesions display orange fluorescence on Wood's lamp examination.

Pityriasis alba, vitiligo, and postinflammatory hypopigmentation can mimic tinea versicolor, but these lesions lack scale. In contrast to tinea versicolor, vitiligo does not show residual pigmentation in affected areas. Postinflammatory hypopigmentation has an associated history of prior skin involvement.

Candidal Diaper Dermatitis

Candidal diaper dermatitis, a common skin infection in infants and toddlers, presents as a bright red rash with distinct and raised borders and satellite lesions in the intertriginous parts of the diaper area (see Figs. 69-13 and 69-14). It is caused by *Candida albicans*, and predisposing factors to infection include oral thrush and recent antibiotic therapy, in addition to prolonged warmth and moisture of the skin. It frequently is diagnosed after the rash fails to respond to the usual moisture-barrier creams and ointments.

Diagnostic Tools

The diagnosis of fungal skin infections is often clinical but can be confirmed with potassium hydroxide preparation and microscopic examination of skin scrapings of the active portion of a lesion. The presence of long, septate, branching rods of uniform width, called *hyphae*, indicates dermatophytic infection. Budding yeasts and pseudohyphae are typical of *Candida*. *Pityrosporum* has a characteristic "spaghetti-and-meatballs" appearance under the microscope, indicating hyphal and yeast forms.

Treatment

Topical antifungal creams applied twice a day for 3 to 4 weeks are usually sufficient to treat superficial dermatophytic skin infections. These creams include the imidazoles (miconazole, clotrimazole, econazole, ketoconazole, naftifine, and tolnaftate). Allylamines such as terbinafine and

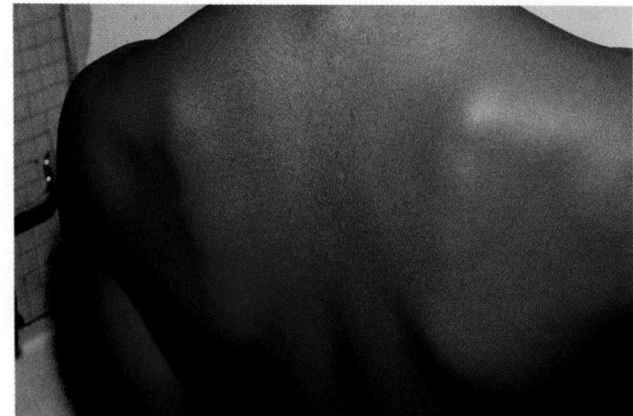

Figure 76-10. Tinea versicolor. (Courtesy of Stanley Inkelis, MD, Department of Pediatrics, Harbor–UCLA Medical Center.)

butenafine, are generally more expensive than imidazoles, but their shorter course of treatment may improve patient compliance and effectiveness.

For tinea pedis, topical antifungal creams, sprays, or powders may be used. It also is necessary to reduce moisture of the foot in as many ways as possible, including careful drying after bathing, wearing cotton socks, and wearing shoes that provide maximal aeration, such as sandals. A positive response to therapy should be seen within 2 weeks of starting therapy.

Tinea versicolor may respond to topical desquamating agents, such as selenium sulfide lotion or shampoo, for 10 minutes per day for 2 weeks. Ketoconazole shampoo is effective over a 3-day course, but is not approved by the U.S. Food and Drug Administration for tinea versicolor. Well-localized lesions can be treated with antifungal creams. There is a high risk of recurrence, and patients should be counseled that lesions might remain hypopigmented for months, even after adequate therapy.

The usual treatment of choice for candidal diaper dermatitis is topical nystatin, but other antifungal creams also are effective. There is evidence that mupirocin also eradicates *Candida* and is more effective for wound healing than nystatin. The perineal area should be kept as dry as possible, with frequent diaper changes. Response to therapy should be seen within 5 to 7 days, and treatment failures usually are due to poor compliance.

Systemic therapy has more risk of side effects, but it may be required to treat extensive lesions. For dermatophytic infections, griseofulvin is approved by the U.S. Food and Drug Administration. Itraconazole, fluconazole, and terbinafine also are effective.

VIRAL SKIN INFECTIONS

Herpes Simplex Infections

Also called *human herpesvirus 1* and *2*, herpes simplex virus (HSV) types 1 and 2 usually infect the skin and mucous membranes. These viruses cause primary infection and then enter a latent stage during which they reside in local sensory nerve ganglia. Reactivation of the virus, with subsequent recurrent infection, can occur at any time and may be related to a variety of precipitating factors, including fever, sun exposure, trauma, emotional or physical stress, and menses. Regardless of the location, HSV infections present as grouped vesicles on an erythematous base. HSV is spread via contact with human secretions, often by viral shedding from an asymptomatic person. HSV type 1 is the more common pathogen, and HSV type 2 typically is associated with genital infections.

Primary skin infections occur after a break in the skin barrier, with subsequent viral inoculation via contact with people who have shedding herpetic lesions. Primary skin lesions are painful, thick-walled vesicles on an erythematous base, which may become pustular and then coalesce and burst, leading to thick crusting (Fig. 76-11; see also Chapter 209). These infections most often occur on the lips and fingers *(herpetic whitlow)* but occasionally may be found over the periorbital areas, with increased risk of *herpetic keratoconjunctivitis.*

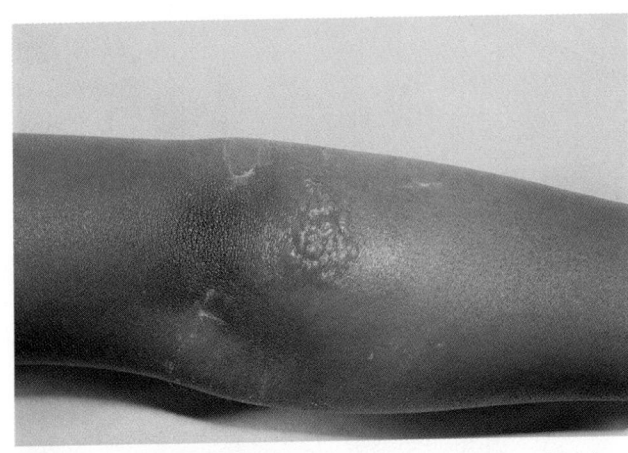

Figure 76-11. Herpes simplex infection of the skin. (Courtesy of Stanley Inkelis, MD, Department of Pediatrics, Harbor–UCLA Medical Center.)

HSV infection in immunocompromised patients can lead to disseminated disease with central nervous system involvement and even death. These patients include neonates, patients with genetic immune deficiencies, patients on immunosuppressive drugs, and patients with severe malnutrition. *Kaposi varicelliform eruption*, also called *eczema herpeticum*, is a severe form of HSV skin infection, found in patients with underlying chronic dermatitis or in burn victims. This disease may mimic varicella infection, with high fever, irritability, and local discomfort, but there is a high risk of disseminated infection and death, depending on the extent of involvement.

Recurrent HSV infections usually are well localized to the area of the previous primary infection, most commonly on the perioral region, and may occur secondary to the previously mentioned triggers. Recurrent lesions appear after a prodrome of burning, stinging, or itching at the involved site. These lesions are smaller than primary lesions, with thin-walled vesicles filled with serous fluid and some crusting. Fever and systemic symptoms are not present during recurrences.

HSV type 2 is the predominant cause of genital herpes, which is transmitted through sexual contact. As with other herpes infections, recurrent genital herpes may involve a prodrome of pain and is contagious to others. Neonates may acquire HSV type 2 via passage through the birth canal.

Herpes infections may be diagnosed clinically, but if the diagnosis is uncertain, Tzanck smear of the scrapings of a vesicle base can be performed to look for multinucleated giant cells. A lesion also can be unroofed and swabbed for viral culture, with results in 24 to 48 hours.

Treatment for herpes simplex usually is not indicated for localized infections, but systemic acyclovir started within 72 hours of onset has been useful in treating moderate-to-severe herpes infections. Herpes infections in patients with compromised immune function, as discussed earlier, should be admitted to the hospital, monitored closely, and treated with intravenous acyclovir. Systemic therapy usually is not indicated for recurrent herpes unless it is severe; oral acyclovir prophylaxis does not fully prevent recurrences, but it may help to reduce the frequency of outbreaks. Patients and their families should be educated regarding

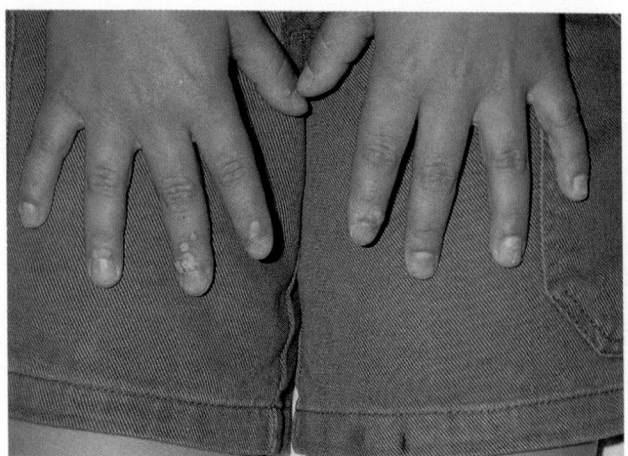

Figure 76-12. Common warts, or verruca vulgaris. (Courtesy of Stanley Inkelis, MD, Department of Pediatrics, Harbor–UCLA Medical Center.)

the contagious nature of HSV infection and potential precipitating factors for recurrences.

Warts

Certain viruses can produce warts, which are benign tumors of the skin. A break in the skin barrier allows inoculation of human papillomavirus (HPV), with subsequent infection of the epithelium, proliferation of keratinocytes, and formation of warts. HPV is spread by human contact, sometimes from mother to newborn infant. Common warts, or *verruca vulgaris*, are dry, rough, skin-colored papules found most commonly on the hands and frequently are periungual in children who bite or pick at their nails (Fig. 76-12). Flat warts, or *verruca plana*, are mildly hyperpigmented flat lesions typically found on the face and extremities and are spread by scratching. *Plantar warts* may be transmitted through contaminated floor surfaces and can be symptomatic because the wart may extend much farther below the visible skin surface, causing pain during walking. True *condylomata acuminata*, or genital warts, should arouse suspicion of sexual abuse in children, but verruca vulgaris also can present in the genital area, especially in toddlers. Most warts are asymptomatic and self-limited, resolving over approximately 1 to 2 years, and if they are widespread and persistent, immune deficiency should be considered. Diagnosis is clinical, and therapy of warts most commonly includes cryotherapy and salicylic acid, but duct tape also has been studied as a method of treatment. Recurrence rates for all types of therapy are high, and multiple treatments often are necessary.

INFESTATIONS

Scabies

Acarus scabiei is a mite that burrows under the skin to cause the highly contagious infestation called *scabies*. It commonly presents with extremely pruritic erythematous papules in the webs of fingers and toes, but also appears in the groin, buttocks, axillae, arms, or trunk of children; infants and toddlers also may have lesions on the head, neck, palms, and soles and all aspects of the foot. The burrows of the mites often are visible as scaly linear papules;

this finding is pathognomonic for scabies (Fig. 76-13). The mite is transmitted by direct contact from already infested humans and is clinically apparent approximately 4 to 6 weeks after contact. The red and intensely pruritic lesions are thought to represent a hypersensitivity reaction to the mites and their eggs and feces. Complications of scabies include excoriation, secondary bacterial infections, and the development of an eczema-like condition.

Scabies usually is diagnosed clinically, but scrapings of a skin burrow can be examined under the microscope to look for evidence of mites. Under low power, mites are visible as eight-legged arachnids, the eggs are approximately one half the size of a mite with a smooth ovular shape, and the feces appear as clusters of reddish brown pellets.

Permethrin 5% cream is the treatment of choice for scabies. All members of the household must be treated, and all clothing and linens must be washed thoroughly to eradicate the mites from the house. Secondary to the hypersensitivity reaction, symptoms may persist for 7 to 10 days after the mites are killed. If necessary, topical steroids and oral antipruritic agents may be used.

Helminths (Parasitic Worms)

Cutaneous larva migrans, also known as *creeping eruption*, is caused most commonly by *Ancylostoma braziliense*, a hookworm of cats and dogs. The ova are found in the soil or sand of the southern United States shoreline, South and Central America, the Caribbean, Africa, and the Far East. The hatched larvae penetrate and migrate through the skin of the soles of the feet and occasionally the arms and legs. They migrate approximately 1 to 2 cm per day, causing characteristic pruritic serpiginous lesions. The larva cannot be removed manually from the skin; treatment is topical thiabendazole for 5 to 7 days. The lesions of cutaneous larva migrans are not contagious, and one treatment is usually curative.

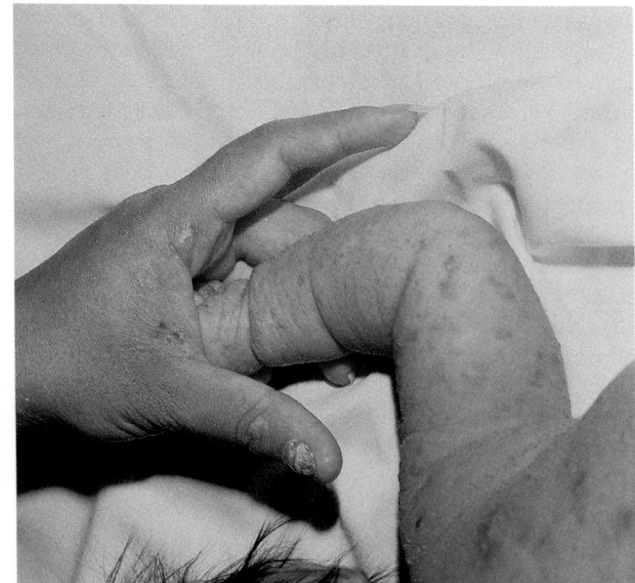

Figure 76-13. Scabies infestation in a mother and infant. (Courtesy of Stanley Inkelis, MD, Department of Pediatrics, Harbor–UCLA Medical Center.)

SUGGESTED READINGS

Mancini AJ: Bacterial skin infections in children: The common and not so common. Pediatr Ann 2000;29:26–35.

Vander Straten M, Tyring SK: Mucocutaneous manifestations of viral diseases in children. Clin Dermatol 2002;20:67–73.

Weston WL, Lane AT, Morelli JG: Color Textbook of Pediatric Dermatology, 3rd ed. St. Louis, Mosby, 2002.

Zitelli BJ, Davis HW: Atlas of Pediatric Physical Diagnosis, 4th ed. Philadelphia, Mosby, 2002.

Zuber TJ, Baddam K: Superficial fungal infection of the skin: Where and how it appears help determine therapy. Postgrad Med 2001;109:117–132.

SECTION 3 GENERAL MEDICAL CARE: *Disorders of the Skin*

77 Exanthems

Emily J. Wong

ROLE OF THE GENERALIST

1 Distinguish viral exanthems from serious bacterial or rickettsial infections and from allergic reactions.
2 Recognize and differentiate the clinical manifestations of common viral exanthems.
3 Diagnose the specific viral etiology when possible.
4 Provide supportive or definitive therapy.
5 Recognize common complications and high-risk individuals.
6 Prevent disease through immunization.

DEFINITIONS

An *exanthem* is any eruption on the surface of the skin, usually temporary, and an *enanthem* is an eruption on a mucosal surface. Although exanthems and enanthems have a wide range of infectious and noninfectious causes, most are due to viruses. A pediatric *common viral exanthem* is a rash with an established viral etiology that has been recognized to occur frequently and consistently in children.

Historically the common viral exanthems were numbered from one to six, but this system has become outdated. Although the first (measles), third (rubella), fifth (erythema infectiosum), and sixth (roseola infantum) diseases are due to viruses, the second (scarlet fever) and fourth (Filatov-Dukes disease) are not. There also are newer viral exanthems that have been recognized. Rather than use the old numbering system, this chapter discusses the exanthems according to the likelihood that they would be encountered by the clinician.

The appearance of the exanthems can be typical or variable with a combination of elements. A *macule* is a discoloration of the skin without elevation. A *papule* is a small, circumscribed, superficial elevation of the skin. A *vesicle* is a small, circumscribed epidermal elevation usually less than 5 mm that contains clear fluid (see Chapter 69).

Clinical diagnosis of the exanthems can be augmented by laboratory testing. Some viruses responsible for exanthems can be grown in *culture* using specific media. Various assays of *serology* measure the level of IgG or IgM antibodies to the infectious agent in the serum. An *acute* serum specimen obtained at the onset of illness and a *convalescent* specimen obtained 3 to 4 weeks later can show a serologic response by an elevated or rising antibody titer. *Indirect* and *direct immunofluorescence assays* use fluorescein-labeled antibodies to detect viral antigens in a tissue sample or scraping. *Polymerase chain reaction* amplifies the viral DNA so that its presence can be detected.

Some common viral exanthems can be prevented by *immunization*. Administration of an attenuated (less virulent) form of the virus causes a child's immune system to recognize and attack the virus if encountered later on.

FUNDAMENTALS

Viral exanthems have a variety of clinical manifestations and can be difficult to recognize. It is important to distinguish exanthems from other infectious agents or from noninfectious causes. The differential diagnosis should include bacterial sepsis, toxic shock syndrome, rickettsial diseases, Kawasaki disease, Stevens-Johnson syndrome, autoimmune diseases, rheumatic diseases, and other etiologies. It is particularly crucial that emergently life-threatening and potentially treatable diseases, such as meningococcemia, Rocky Mountain spotted fever, and toxic shock syndrome, are considered.

A knowledge of the epidemiology of these viruses is important for diagnosis. Viruses have a predilection for certain age groups and often attack in a geographic location at a particular time of year. In addition to an individual child's exposure to ill contacts, it is helpful to be aware of local outbreaks. Table 77-1 summarizes the epidemiology and presentation of viruses that commonly present with exanthems.

Certain exanthems have been identified with individual viruses, such as measles, rubella, and varicella. Some exanthems are caused by a family of viruses, however, which can be difficult to distinguish from each other. Examples of this are human herpesvirus (HHV) 6 and HHV 7, which cause roseola infantum, and the enteroviruses, which cause hand-foot-and-mouth disease and a variety of exanthems and enanthems. In such cases, it is usually more important for the clinician to recognize the family of viruses causing the exanthem, rather than the individual virus.

Most healthy children recover from most viral exanthem infections, although occasionally there are complications. Immunocompromised children are at high risk, however, for severe or life-threatening infections from these viruses. Any infected neonate or child with an immune deficiency, with human immunodeficiency virus infection, or receiving immunosuppressive therapy (e.g., chemotherapy or prolonged corticosteroid therapy) should be monitored carefully and given maximal therapy.

Because the common viral exanthems are so prevalent and can cause severe disease, prevention of infection is an important goal. Vaccines have resulted in a significantly decreased morbidity and mortality for measles, rubella, and varicella. Appropriate isolation measures also can decrease the spread of infection.

PRESENTATION AND DIAGNOSIS

Enterovirus is a large family of more than 30 viruses, including echovirus and coxsackievirus. These viruses are more common in the late summer and early fall, and they are spread by the fecal-oral route. After an incubation period of 3 to 7 days, the clinical manifestations are varied, with an exanthem more often in younger children and

Table 77-1. Epidemiology and Presentation of Common Viral Exanthems

Exanthem and Viral Etiology	Epidemiology	Signs and Symptoms

Enteroviral rash, hand-foot-and-mouth disease
  Coxsackievirus
  Echovirus
  Other enterovirus
	Young children
	Late summer–early fall
	Fecal-oral route
		Variable—erythematous maculopapular rash, vesicles, oral ulcers
		Fever, URI symptoms, vomiting, diarrhea
		Aseptic meningitis

Roseola infantum (exanthem subitum)
  HHV 6
  HHV 7
  Adenovirus
  Parainfluenza
	6 mo–3 yr
	Respiratory secretions
		High fever 3–5 days
		Pink macules and papules after defervescence
		Cough, coryza, headache, abdominal pain
		Febrile seizures

Erythema infectiosum (fifth disease) Parvovirus B19	5–15 yr Late winter–early spring Respiratory secretions	Bright red facial erythema, lacy reticular truncal rash, recrudescence Polyarthropathy Aplastic anemia
Chickenpox Varicella-zoster virus	School-age children, unvaccinated adolescents Late winter–early spring Aerosolized respiratory droplets	Crops of erythematous papules, vesicles, crusts, and scabs Fever, malaise
Measles Rubeola virus	Unvaccinated children Winter–spring Respiratory droplets	Morbilliform—confluent, erythematous macules, papules Koplik's spots Fever, cough, coryza, conjunctivitis
German measles Rubella virus	Unimmunized adolescents and adults Spring Respiratory droplets	Discrete pink maculopapules Lymphadenopathy, arthralgias

HHV, human herpesvirus; URI, upper respiratory infection.

central nervous system symptoms more often in older children. A diffuse erythematous maculopapular rash occurs, sometimes appearing morbilliform, scarlatiniform, vesicular, petechial, or urticarial (Fig. 77-1). Fever, upper respiratory symptoms, vomiting, or diarrhea commonly accompanies the rash. Aseptic meningitis causing headache, nausea, or vomiting also can be associated. A well-known syndrome is hand-foot-and-mouth disease, caused by coxsackievirus (Fig. 77-2). Large vesicles progressing to ulcers are present on the buccal mucosa, tongue, palate, anterior tonsillar pillars, and uvula. Vesicles also appear on the dorsal hands and feet, palms and soles, and groin area and occasionally in a diffuse distribution.

Although usually mild, enteroviruses can cause severe disseminated disease in neonates or children with agammaglobulinemia. Rarely, enteroviral infections also can cause myocarditis, pericarditis, parotitis, hepatitis, pancreatitis, or encephalitis. Diagnosis is made by viral culture of the oropharynx, stool, or rectum. If the child has meningitis, the virus can be detected in cerebrospinal fluid by polymerase chain reaction. Because there are so many serotypes, it is not practical to obtain serology except to detect a particular serotype (e.g., in an outbreak situation).

Roseola infantum (exanthem subitum) is associated most commonly with HHV 6, but also can be caused by HHV 7, adenovirus, or parainfluenza (Fig. 77-3). Most children are infected in the first 2 years, predominantly between age 6 and 12 months, and there is no apparent seasonality. The virus most likely is shed in respiratory secretions and has an incubation period of 5 to 15 days. Initially a child has a high fever for 3 to 5 days without other symptoms. At the time of defervescence, the exanthem appears as small pink macules or maculopapules that last for hours up to 2 days. The rash can be accompanied by an enanthem of pink elevations on the uvula and soft palate or by cough, coryza, headache, or abdominal pain. Because of the high fever in the initial phase, roseola has been associated with febrile

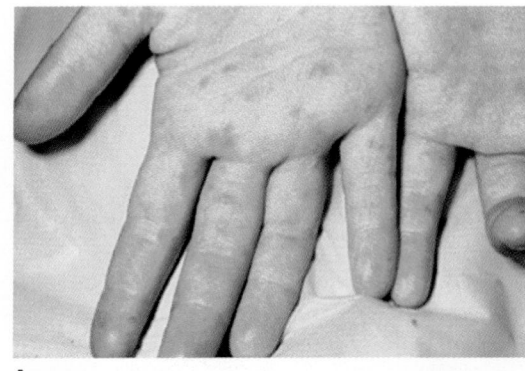

A

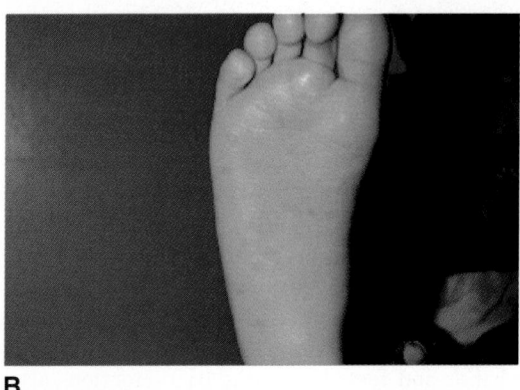

B

Figure 77-2. Hand-foot-and-mouth disease is characterized by vesiculopustular lesions on the hands and fingers, feet, and buttocks and in the oropharynx; it commonly is caused by infection with coxsackievirus A16. **A,** Characteristic lesions on hands. **B,** Lesions on foot. (From Mandell GL, Wilfert CM [eds]: Atlas of Infectious Diseases, Vol XI. Pediatric Infectious Diseases. Philadelphia, Churchill Livingstone, 1998, p 6.8.)

seizures in infants. Diagnosis usually is made by the clinical presentation. Roseola serology is performed at reference laboratories and is not widely available.

Parvovirus B19, also known as *Erythrovirus B19*, is the cause of *erythema infectiosum* (fifth disease) (Fig. 77-4). In the late winter and early spring, this infection is spread by respiratory secretions among children age 5 to 15 years. The incubation period of 4 to 14 days is followed by a nonspecific prodrome of mild fever, malaise, myalgia, headache, coryza, and sore throat. Subsequently the exanthem appears in three stages. First is a rapid onset of facial erythema: A bright red macular rash occurs on the cheeks with

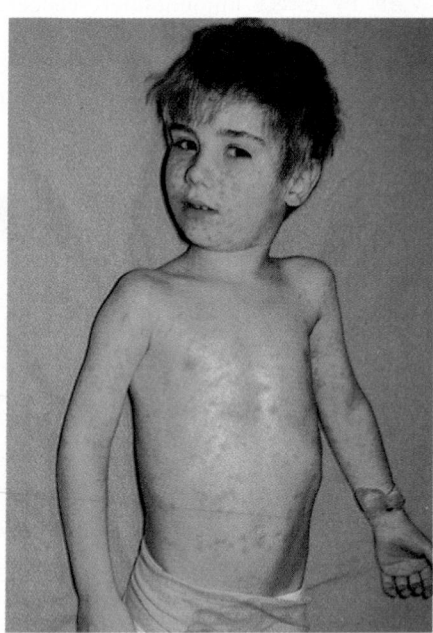

Figure 77-1. A discrete maculopapular rash caused by echovirus. (From Hart CA, Broadhead RL: Color Atlas of Pediatric Infectious Diseases. St. Louis, Mosby, 1992, p 148.)

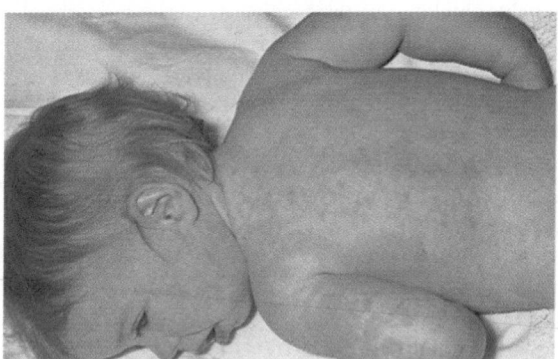

Figure 77-3. A child with roseola infantum. The delicate erythematous rash is visible over the face and trunk. (From Hart CA, Broadhead RL: Color Atlas of Pediatric Infectious Diseases. St. Louis, Mosby, 1992, p 143.)

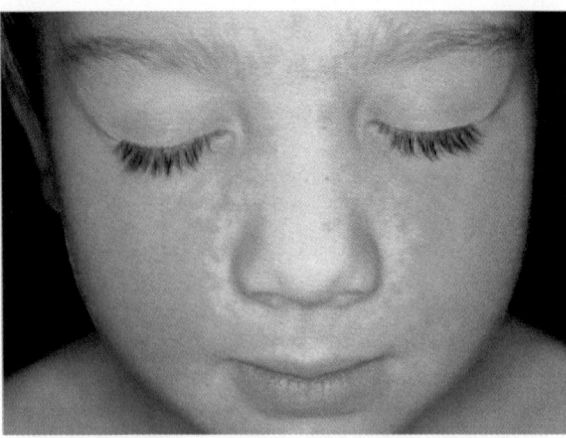

Figure 77-4. Erythema infectiosum. The rash gives the child the characteristic slapped cheek appearance. (From Hart CA, Broadhead RL: Color Atlas of Pediatric Infectious Diseases. St. Louis, Mosby, 1992, p 142.)

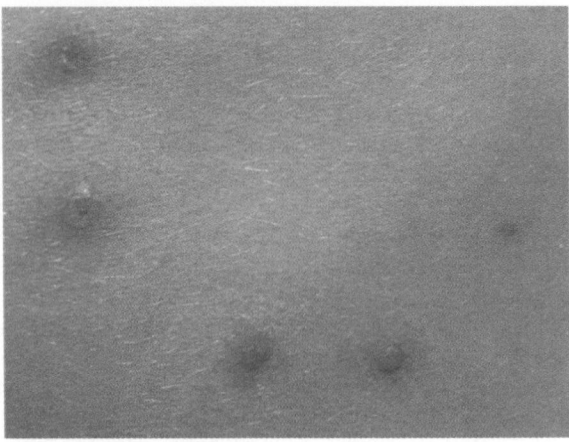

Figure 77-5. Varicella showing all of the stages of evolution of the rash. (From Hart CA, Broadhead RL: Color Atlas of Pediatric Infectious Diseases. St. Louis, Mosby, 1992, p 140.)

circumoral sparing, causing a "slapped cheeks" appearance. Next the trunk and extremities develop an erythematous maculopapular rash that becomes lacy and reticular. Finally the rash fades but can have episodes of recrudescence over 1 to 3 weeks. Adolescents and adults often have an associated symmetric polyarthropathy involving the small joints of the hands and feet. Parvovirus B19 infections also have been reported to cause encephalitis, neurologic symptoms, myocarditis, vasculitis, hepatitis, and a papular-purpuric gloves-and-socks syndrome.

Because parvovirus B19 is cytotoxic to erythroblasts, there is an acute self-limited cessation of red blood cell production. Children with a hemolytic anemia (e.g., sickle cell disease, spherocytosis, or thalassemia) are at high risk for a transient aplastic crisis. These children are usually viremic and remain infectious throughout the infection. Immunocompromised patients may develop a chronic infection with persistent red blood cell aplasia. If a woman acquires parvovirus B19 infection during pregnancy, there is a risk of transplacental transmission resulting in fetal hydrops. Diagnosis of parvovirus B19 infection is made on a clinical basis and by serology.

Chickenpox caused by *varicella-zoster virus* (VZV) used to be one of the most commonly encountered exanthems by pediatricians (Figs. 77-5 and 77-6). Since licensure of the vaccine, the incidence of disease has decreased significantly, especially in areas of widespread vaccine use. Previously, chickenpox predominantly affected school-age children, but now it may be seen more often in adolescents and adults. Varicella occurs in the late winter and early spring and is transmitted by aerosolized respiratory droplets or by direct contact with a lesion. After exposure, the incubation period is 10 to 21 days. Systemic symptoms of low-grade fever and malaise are accompanied by the onset of red macules, which develop into papules and then crops of small vesicles surrounded by 1 to 2 mm of erythema. The lesions, which are pruritic, eventually crust and form scabs. Appearing first on the face, scalp, and trunk, the rash spreads peripherally to the extremities and is distinctive for the concurrent presence of lesions at different stages. The mucous membranes can be involved with ulcers on the conjunctiva, pharynx, tonsils, palate, and genital area.

It has been shown that chickenpox is associated with invasive group A β-hemolytic streptococcus. As a result of the significant disruption of the skin barrier, children may develop bacteremia, cellulitis, myositis, or necrotizing fasciitis secondary to group A β-hemolytic streptococcus. Immunocompromised children are at high risk for severe life-threatening VZV disease. They can develop pneumonia, encephalitis, hepatitis, or dissemination to other organs.

VZV establishes latency in the dorsal nerve root during primary infection. Reactivation of the virus results in shingles or varicella zoster (Fig. 77-7). Vesicles appear in the distribution of the nerve root. Patients can present with pain along the dermatome, before onset of the rash. Usually there are no systemic symptoms. Pain can persist after the infection has resolved (postherpetic neuralgia).

Diagnosis of chickenpox and herpes zoster usually can be made on a clinical basis. For confirmation, an intact vesicle may be unroofed, and a scraping of the surface may be tested for VZV by direct immunofluorescence assay or culture or both. Although commonly used in the past, a Tzanck preparation is not specific for VZV, and the study can be positive as a result of infection with other members of the herpesvirus family.

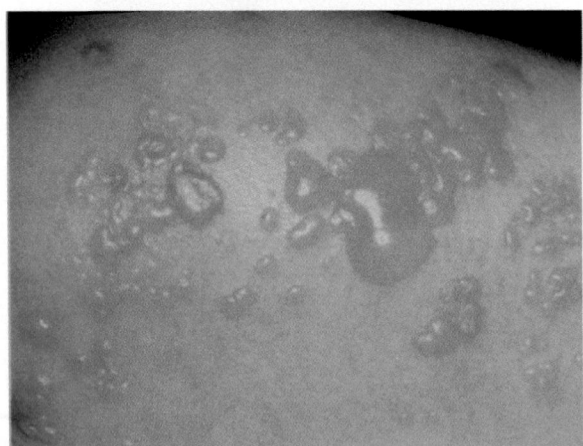

Figure 77-6. The typical "teardrop" varicella papules and developing pustules with umbilication. (From Hart CA, Broadhead RL: Color Atlas of Pediatric Infectious Diseases. St. Louis, Mosby, 1992, p 141.)

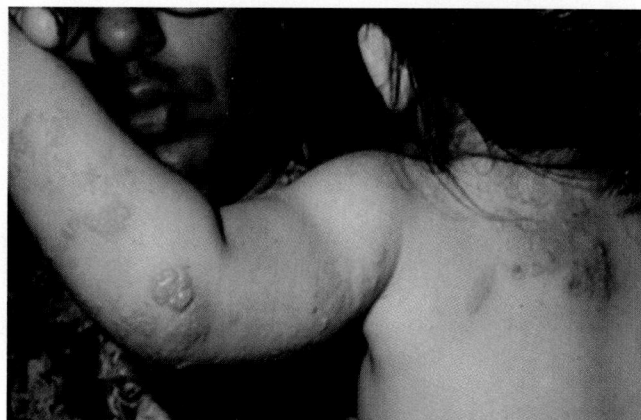

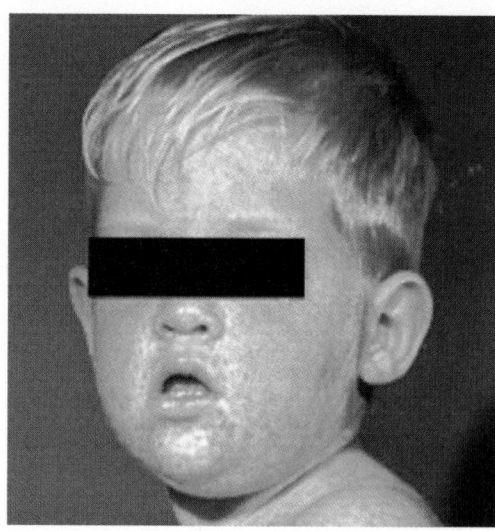

Figure 77-7. Herpes zoster rash. Varicella-zoster virus reactivation from latency causes a localized, unilateral, pruritic vesicular rash involving the dermatomal distribution of one or more adjacent sensory nerves. The rash often is preceded by several days of pain, and acute pain and hypersensitivity accompany the rash. The vesicles coalesce into larger, fluid-filled lesions as the infection progresses. Scattered cutaneous lesions outside the primary dermatome are observed occasionally. (From Mandell GL, Wilfert CM [eds]: Atlas of Infectious Diseases, Vol XI. Pediatric Infectious Diseases. Philadelphia, Churchill Livingstone, 1998, p 5.11.)

Figure 77-9. Early measles exanthem, day 3. This young boy displays the classic form of the early measles exanthematous phase, with conjunctivitis, coryza, and an initially discrete maculopapular rash beginning on the face and spreading to the trunk and extremities. The rash begins to coalesce in a cephalocaudal direction as seen in this child. (From Mandell GL, Wilfert CM [eds]: Atlas of Infectious Diseases, Vol XI. Pediatric Infectious Diseases. Philadelphia, Churchill Livingstone, 1998, p 1.3. Courtesy of Centers for Disease Control.)

Traditionally known as the "first" exanthem, *measles* infection has decreased dramatically since the widespread use of measles vaccine. There have been epidemics in the United States, however, among unvaccinated urban children. Occurring in the winter and spring, the measles virus is spread by respiratory droplets and has a 10-day incubation period. A prodrome of fever, cough, coryza, conjunctivitis, and malaise lasts 3 to 4 days, accompanied by an enanthem known as *Koplik's spots* (Fig. 77-8). Multiple 1- to 2-mm white or blue-gray punctate spots on an erythematous base appear on the buccal and labial mucosa. The typical "morbilliform" exanthem is an erythematous maculopapular rash that becomes confluent, beginning on the forehead and upper neck and spreading to the trunk and

extremities over 3 days (Figs. 77-9 and 77-10). As the rash resolves, other symptoms disappear as well, although measles can be complicated by otitis media, diarrhea, pneumonia, myocarditis, postinfectious encephalitis, or subacute sclerosing panencephalitis (Table 77-2).

Modified measles is a milder form of illness that occurs in children with partial immunity (from transplacentally acquired maternal antibodies, receipt of intravenous immunoglobulin, or vaccine failure). After a shorter prodrome, a less severe exanthem similar to other viral exanthems appears with or without confluence or Koplik's spots. Atypical measles occurs in individuals who received the killed measles vaccine from 1963 to 1967. If infected with measles, these individuals develop an abrupt onset of fever, headache, and myalgias for 3 days, followed by an erythematous papular, vesicular, or petechial exanthem spreading from the extremities to the head. A segmental

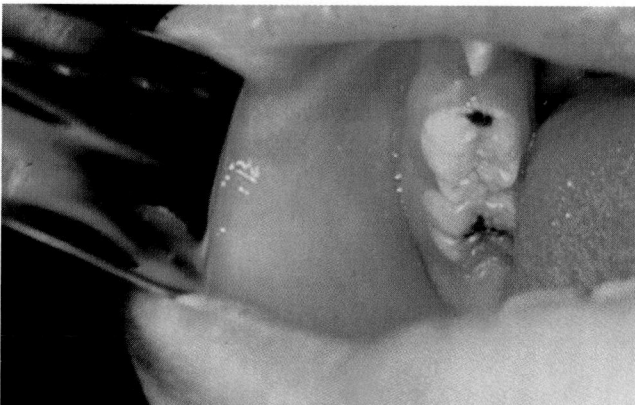

Figure 77-8. Koplik's spots. The enanthem of measles infection is manifested primarily by erythematous oral mucosa and by Koplik's spots, which are white, macular, 1-mm lesions that appear on the buccal mucosa usually opposite the premolars. These lesions eventually may coalesce and spread throughout the buccal mucosa, including the hard palate. Koplik's spots precede the development of the classic measles exanthem by 2 to 3 days and may be fleeting, usually lasting only 12 to 72 hours. (From Mandell GL, Wilfert CM [eds]: Atlas of Infectious Diseases, Vol XI. Pediatric Infectious Diseases. Philadelphia, Churchill Livingstone, 1998, p 1.3. Courtesy of Centers for Disease Control and Prevention.)

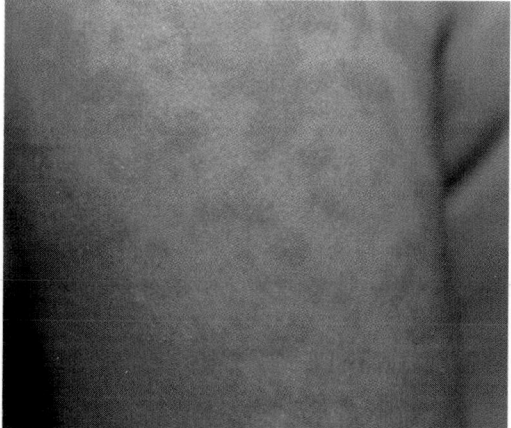

Figure 77-10. Close-up of the maculopapular measles rash. (From Hart CA, Broadhead RL: Color Atlas of Pediatric Infectious Diseases. St. Louis, Mosby, 1992, p 136.)

Table 77-2. Complications of Measles

System	Complication
Respiratory	Croup
	Otitis media
	Sinusitis
	Pneumonitis
	Superinfection with bacterial pneumonia
	Giant cell pneumonia
	Reactivation of tuberculosis
Cardiovascular	Myocarditis
Central nervous system	Seizures
	Encephalitis
	Subacute sclerosing panencephalitis
Hematologic	Idiopathic thrombocytopenic purpura
	Hemorrhagic measles

nodular pneumonia with effusion is common and can be severe. Measles infections can be diagnosed clinically and with serology.

Another previously common but now rare viral exanthem is *rubella*, known as *German measles*. Because of the efficacy of the vaccine, rubella is now more common in unimmunized adolescents or adults. It usually occurs in sporadic outbreaks in the spring and is spread by respiratory droplets. After a long incubation period of 15 to 21 days, the infected person experiences a prodrome of fever, headache, malaise, eye pain, cough, and sore throat. The exanthem, beginning centrally on the face and trunk and extending to the extremities, is a discrete pink maculopapular rash that is less confluent than measles (Fig. 77-11). *Forschheimer spots* refers to the enanthem of pinpoint pink petechiae and macules on the soft palate. When adolescents or adults are infected with rubella, they are likely to have lymphadenopathy (suboccipital or postauricular) (Fig. 77-12) and arthralgias or arthritis. Unimmunized pregnant women who acquire infection are at risk for having an infant with congenital rubella. Serology is useful for augmenting the clinical diagnosis.

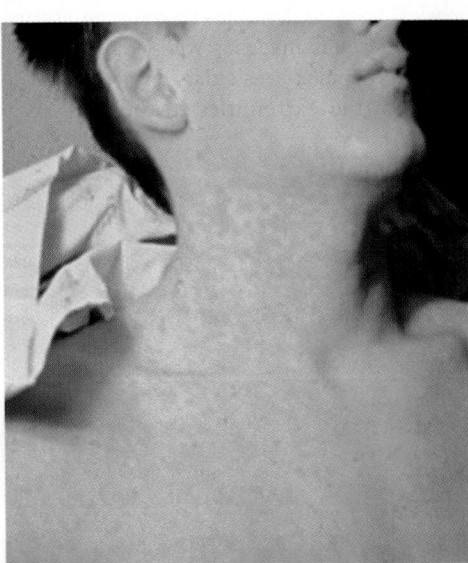

Figure 77-11. Rash of acquired rubella. The rash of acquired rubella is usually maculopapular, which may coalesce eventually. The rash is usually mild. (From Mandell GL, Wilfert CM [eds]: Atlas of Infectious Diseases, Vol XI. Pediatric Infectious Diseases. Philadelphia, Churchill Livingstone, 1998, p 1.11.)

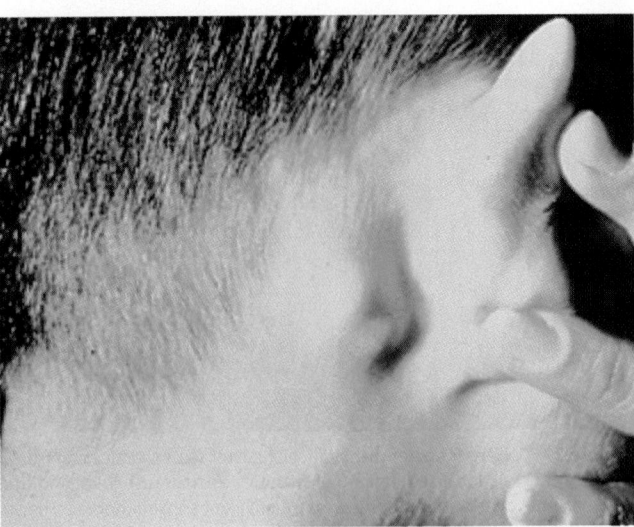

Figure 77-12. Posterior auricular adenopathy associated with acquired rubella. Posterior auricular adenopathy is associated most frequently with acquired rubella infection. (From Mandell GL, Wilfert CM [eds]: Atlas of Infectious Diseases, Vol XI. Pediatric Infectious Diseases. Philadelphia, Churchill Livingstone, 1998, p 1.11.)

Other viral infections in childhood commonly can involve an exanthem. *Adenovirus* causes a variable maculopapular, morbilliform, or petechial rash associated with fever, upper respiratory symptoms, and conjunctivitis. It can be diagnosed by viral culture or serology. *Epstein-Barr virus* by itself can cause a maculopapular, petechial, urticarial, or erythema multiforme–like rash (Fig. 77-13). If treated with an antibiotic, such as amoxicillin or ampicillin, a patient with Epstein-Barr virus infection may develop an erythematous, morbilliform, coalescent rash on the entire body. *Gianotti-Crosti syndrome*, also called *papulovesicular acrolocated syndrome*, is an erythematous, polymorphous, pruritic rash associated with fever, malaise, and hepatosplenomegaly. It has many different viral etiologies, including hepatitis B virus, enterovirus, Epstein-Barr virus, cytomegalovirus, parainfluenza, and hepatitis A virus (see Chapter 70).

MANAGEMENT

Therapy for the viral exanthems is predominantly supportive. Management of fever is important, particularly with roseola, to decrease the likelihood of febrile seizures and to

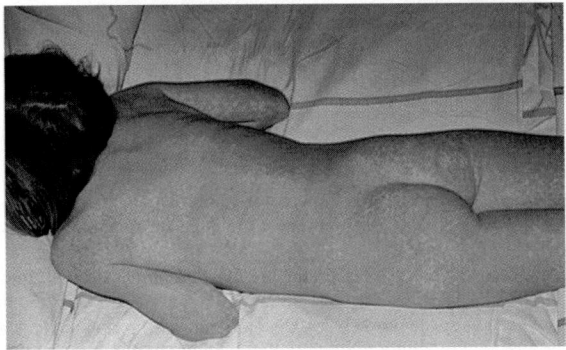

Figure 77-13. A typical discrete maculopapular rash on a child with infectious mononucleosis. (From Hart CA, Broadhead RL: Color Atlas of Pediatric Infectious Diseases. St. Louis, Mosby, 1992, p 146.)

ensure the comfort of the child. Acetaminophen, ibuprofen, and cool baths may be used, but salicylates should be avoided because of the risk of Reye's syndrome. If there are open skin lesions, such as with chickenpox, it is important to keep the skin clean and dry to prevent secondary bacterial infections with group A β-hemolytic streptococcus, staphylococcus, or other skin flora. As with other viral infections, it is important for the child to have sufficient hydration and rest.

Children infected with VZV who are at risk for moderate-to-severe disease (adolescents, children with chronic skin or pulmonary disease, children receiving long-term salicylate or steroid therapy, and immunocompromised children) should receive acyclovir therapy. Immunocompetent children can be treated with oral acyclovir, 80 mg/kg/day (maximum 3200 mg/day) in four divided doses for 5 days. Immunocompromised children should receive intravenous acyclovir, 1500 mg/m^2/day (30 mg/kg/day for infants) in three divided doses for 7 to 10 days. After exposure to VZV, an immunocompromised child should receive VZV immunoglobulin prophylaxis within 96 hours, preferably as soon as possible. The only specific antiviral therapy for enterovirus is pleconaril, which is being evaluated for the treatment of enteroviral infection in immunocompromised children and children with aseptic meningitis. Currently, there are no indications for use of pleconaril in a healthy child with a routine viral exanthem.

Adjunctive therapies can be beneficial in specific circumstances. Vitamin A deficiency is associated with severe measles infections. Any measles-infected child from a community with vitamin A deficiency or a mortality from measles that is greater than 1% or who is hospitalized with measles between 6 months and 2 years of age should receive vitamin A therapy. The dose is 200,000 IU orally for children 1 year old and older and 100,000 IU for infants 6 to 12 months old. Immunocompromised children who develop chronic or severe infections from enterovirus or parvovirus may benefit from intravenous immunoglobulin. In addition, parvovirus-infected children with aplastic crisis may require blood transfusion.

Any severe case of a viral exanthem, particularly if the child is immunocompromised or develops complications, should be referred to an infectious disease specialist. Intensive care may be required if the infection disseminates to the lungs, liver, central nervous system, or other organs or if there is hematologic or cardiovascular compromise (e.g., disseminated intravascular coagulation or shock). Pregnant patients who acquire a viral exanthem should be counseled regarding the risk of congenital infection.

OUTCOME

Most healthy immunocompetent children have a good outcome without sequelae after a viral exanthem infection. Complications can occur on rare occasions, however. A child who develops a secondary bacterial infection causing sepsis or necrotizing fasciitis may experience organ damage or loss of a necrotic appendage. Viral meningitis or encephalitis may result in neurologic sequelae. These outcomes are unusual in a normal child, but immunocompromised hosts have a higher likelihood of having an adverse outcome.

FOLLOW-UP

If a healthy child resolves his or her viral exanthem, there is no specific follow-up required. A child who has a seizure, meningitis, or encephalitis should have a careful examination to detect any neurologic sequelae. After a severe course of infection or complications, a child may need monitoring for any loss of organ function. Any pregnant patient at risk for congenital infection should have close prenatal monitoring, particularly for signs of malformations or fetal hydrops.

PREVENTION

The lack of specific antiviral therapy emphasizes the importance of immunization in the prevention of disease. Measles, rubella, and varicella vaccines all are available as live attenuated virus vaccines and have resulted in significant declines in incidence, morbidity, and mortality from these diseases. Special circumstances surrounding immunocompromised children or children who have received immunoglobulin therapy should be observed.

Isolation precautions should be used for infected hospitalized patients and for infected household contacts of immunocompromised children to prevent the spread of infection. VZV and measles virus require airborne respiratory isolation, whereas rubella parvovirus and possibly HHV 6 require respiratory droplet isolation. Only children in the early (pre-exanthem) stage of parvovirus or immunocompromised children with prolonged parvovirus infection are contagious. Contact isolation is needed for enterovirus, particularly when handling an infant's diapers.

Additional Resources, CD-ROM

Color atlas	Figures

SUGGESTED READING

Pickering LK (ed): Red Book: 2003 Report of the Committee on Infectious Diseases, 26th ed. Elk Grove Village, Ill, American Academy of Pediatrics, 2003.

78 Cutaneous Tumors

Mark Herron and Sheryll L. Vanderhooft

Virtually all children have many benign growths on their skin. Parents who ask the clinician to look at a growth usually are concerned that the lesion may be cancerous or precancerous. The ability to differentiate a benign or self-limited process from a serious or malignant one is a skill that comes with experience. Many papules and nodules that arise in children have characteristic clinical features that allow a diagnosis to be made without the aid of histologic or radiographic evaluation. Other lesions may be nonspecific in appearance and require a skin biopsy for diagnosis. In some situations, obtaining an imaging study is desirable before a biopsy is performed. Lesions along the midline of the face, scalp, and back frequently have connections to the brain or spinal cord, and care must be taken to avoid biopsy of any midline lesion until such a communication is ruled out by computed tomography or magnetic resonance imaging (MRI).

Features of a cutaneous neoplasm that heighten concern about malignancy are listed in Box 78-1 and include onset during the neonatal period, rapid or progressive growth,

---

Box 78-1. Features Associated with Malignancy

- Onset during neonatal period
- Rapid or progressive growth
- Skin ulceration
- Fixation to or location deep to the fascia
- Firm mass >3 cm in diameter
- Blue skin nodules

---

skin ulceration, fixation to or location deep to the fascia, and a firm mass greater than 3 cm in diameter. Blue skin nodules should raise the concern about malignancy, including leukemia cutis, lymphoma cutis, and neuroblastoma. In the absence of any of these findings, 99% of lesions prove to be benign. Presence of some of these findings need not always prompt a biopsy. Hemangiomas typically arise during the neonatal period, grow rapidly, and may ulcerate, but they are benign vascular tumors that are self-limited and eventually involute.

Nevus is a circumscribed abnormality of any cell type. Accurate description of a nevus requires specification of the particular cell type (e.g., melanocytic nevus, epidermal nevus, sebaceous nevus, vascular nevus). The most common, but technically incorrect, use of the term *nevus* is to equate it with a mole. A *hamartoma* is a tumor arising from misplaced embryonal cells. It is characterized by an abnormal arrangement of normal tissue elements. The defect in its arrangement stems from faulty embryogenesis.

FUNDAMENTALS

The anatomy of normal skin is illustrated in Figure 73-1. Neoplasms may arise from any of these normal structures. Epidermal nevi arise from keratinocytes, melanocytic nevi arise from melanocytes, dermatofibromas arise from dermal collagen, angiofibromas arise from dermal fibroblasts and blood vessels, pilomatricomas arise from hair follicles, nevus sebaceus arises from sebaceous glands, smooth muscle hamartomas arise from arrector pili muscles, and lipomas arise from subcutaneous fat.

DIAGNOSIS

Cutaneous tumors can be diagnosed best by categorization by their color and texture. Although there may be some variability in the color of a tumor, Table 78-1 outlines the most typical colors at presentation of commonly encountered cutaneous tumors in children. Table 78-2 categorizes cutaneous tumors by their texture.

FLESH-COLORED LESIONS

Epidermoid Cysts

Epidermoid cysts arise from occluded pilosebaceous units or from traumatic implantation of epidermal cells into the dermis. They often erroneously are referred to as *sebaceous cysts*. They grow slowly as keratin accumulates within them

Table 78-1. Differential Diagnosis of Cutaneous Tumors by Color

Color	Lesion
Flesh-colored	Epidermoid cyst
	Dermoid cyst
	Lipoma
	Connective tissue nevus
	Smooth muscle hamartoma
	Verruca vulgaris
	Molluscum contagiosum
	Trichoepithelioma
	Syringoma
	Cylindroma
	Neurofibroma
	Recurring digital fibroma
	Subungual exostosis
	Basal cell carcinoma
Yellow	Epidermoid cyst
	Sebaceous nevus
	Juvenile xanthogranuloma
	Pilomatricoma
	Calcinosis cutis
	Osteoma cutis
	Nevus lipomatosus
Red	Hemangioma
	Pyogenic granuloma
	Tufted angioma
	Angiokeratoma
	Pilomatricoma
	Spitz nevus
	Keloid/hypertrophic scar
	Angiofibroma
	Hematoma
Blue	Cavernous hemangioma
	Lymphangioma
	Philomatricoma
	Blue nevus
	Extramedullary hematopoiesis
	Leukemia cutis
	Lymphoma cutis
	Neuroblastoma
	Infantile myofibromatosis
Reddish brown	Mastocytoma
	Juvenile xanthogranuloma
	Spitz nevus
	Granuloma annulare
	Dermatofibroma
	Dermatofibrosarcoma protuberans
	Infantile myofibromatosis
	Leukemia cutis
	Lymphoma cutis
Brown	Epidermal nevus
	Becker's nevus
	Smooth muscle hamartoma
	Neurofibroma
	Melanocytic nevus
	Speckled lentiginous nevus
	Malignant melanoma

Table 78-2. Differential Diagnosis of Cutaneous Tumors by Texture

Texture	Lesion
Hard	Pilomatricoma
	Calcinosis cutis
	Osteoma cutis
	Subungual exostosis
Firm	Dermatofibroma
	Dermoid cyst
	Keloid
	Trichoepithelioma
	Angiofibroma
	Syringoma
	Juvenile xanthogranuloma
	Subcutaneous granuloma annulare
	Leukemia cutis
	Lymphoma cutis
	Neuroblastoma
Soft	Neurofibroma
	Lipoma
	Connective tissue nevus
Cystic	Epidermoid cyst
	Dermoid cyst

necessary to prevent recurrence. If the cyst ruptures when it is being removed, care must be taken to irrigate all of the keratin out of the wound to prevent formation of a foreign-body granuloma. Oral antibiotic therapy is indicated if an epidermoid cyst becomes inflamed or infected.

Dermoid Cysts

Most dermoid cysts are noted at birth. They arise primarily along lines of embryonic fusion as firm, partially mobile subcutaneous nodules. They grow slowly to a few centimeters in diameter. They contain keratin; some also may contain hair, bone, tooth, or nerve tissue. They are located most commonly along the lateral third of the eyebrow, forehead, scalp, and anterior and lateral aspects of the neck. Definitive treatment is surgical removal. Radiographic imaging with computed tomography or MRI is recommended for dermoid cysts arising near the medial canthus of the eye, along the nose, or along suture lines of the skull because they may have an intracranial extension. If an intracranial connection is identified, the child should be referred to a neurosurgeon.

and present as elevated, round, flesh-colored or yellow papules or nodules (Fig. 78-1), often with a discernible overlying punctum. When they rupture, the keratin released has a cheesy consistency, often with a sour odor. Although epidermoid cysts typically appear after puberty, they are not unusual in young children. They arise most commonly on the face, scalp, neck, back, and scrotum. Management consists of incision and drainage of the keratinous contents followed by extraction of the cyst lining through the incision or incisional or excisional removal of the intact cyst. Removal of the entire epidermal lining of the cyst is

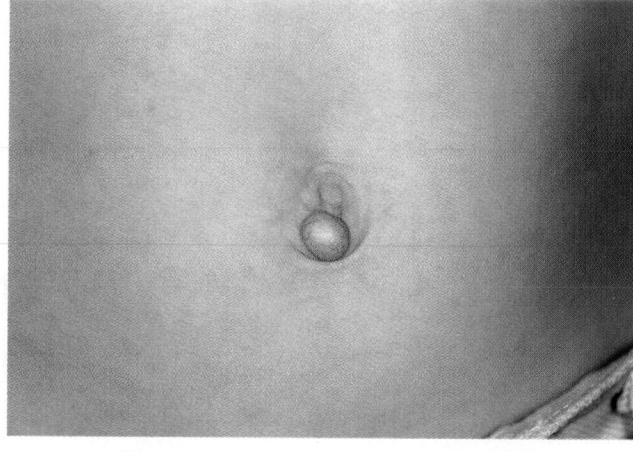

Figure 78-1. Epidermoid cyst of the umbilicus.

Lipomas

Lipomas are soft, mobile, and nontender subcutaneous nodules with a lobular and rubbery texture. They arise from subcutaneous fat anywhere on the body, but are found most commonly on the neck, shoulders, back, and abdomen. Lipomas may be left untreated, unless they become uncomfortable, are growing, or are cosmetically unacceptable. Surgical excision typically is curative. Malignant degeneration is rare in lesions smaller than 10 cm in diameter.

Connective Tissue Nevus

Connective tissue nevi are localized hamartomas of dermal collagen and elastic tissue. They appear early in childhood or in adulthood. They present as firm, flesh-colored, sometimes pebbly plaques distributed on the abdomen, back, buttocks, arms, or thighs (Fig. 78-2). Connective tissue nevi may be familial or seen as part of a genodermatosis. The "shagreen patch" of tuberous sclerosis is a connective tissue nevus. Connective tissue nevi also are seen in the Buschke-Ollendorff syndrome, characterized by osteopoikilosis, a hereditary dysplasia of the long bones, pelvis, hands, and feet. Biopsy of a connective tissue nevus is performed when the diagnosis of the lesion is in question. These nevi require no specific treatment, but children with connective tissue nevi should be evaluated for the possible association of tuberous sclerosis or Buschke-Ollendorff syndrome.

Smooth Muscle Hamartomas

Smooth muscle hamartomas are congenital proliferations of smooth muscle within the dermis, typically arrector pili muscles, which may not be noted until later in childhood or adulthood (see CD-ROM Fig. 78-3).

Verruca Vulgaris (Wart)

Warts are a common skin infection caused by human papillomavirus. The virus is spread by skin-to-skin contact. The virus induces epidermal proliferation, causing rough-surfaced papules and plaques, often with superficial thrombosed capillaries, commonly referred to by the layperson as "seeds" (see Fig. 78-3). When present on the hands, the surface may be dome shaped from wear and tear. On the soles of the feet, warts may invaginate from repetitive pressure of walking and standing. On the face, they

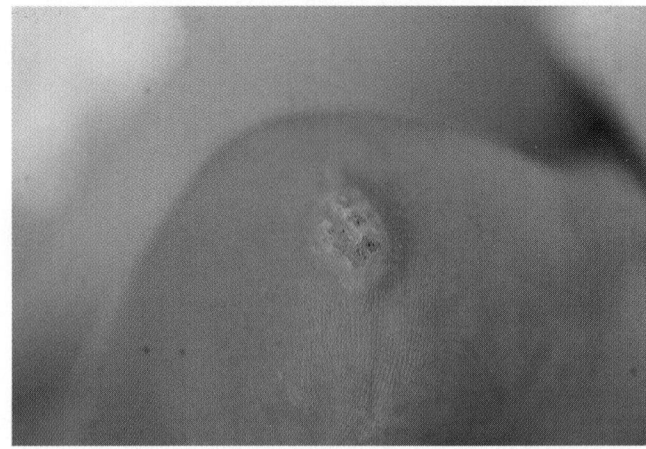

Figure 78-3. Verruca on the heel with superficial thrombosed capillaries.

may grow as filiform projections or flat-topped papules (flat warts) (Fig. 78-4). Warts spontaneously resolve. On average, 75% of warts in children resolve without treatment within 3 years. Treatment should be no worse than the cutaneous viral infection itself. Too often, traumatic treatments are used because patients or their parents want to "just get rid of" the warts. No treatment is guaranteed to eradicate warts successfully.

The most important management principle in treatment of warts is provision of guidance and education and avoidance of treatments that can cause scarring. The treatment method should be based on the extent of the lesions, age of the child, and willingness of the child to participate in treatment. Treatment options include salicylic acid liquid or pads used on a daily basis for several months, liquid nitrogen cryotherapy every few weeks, cantharidin blistering every few weeks, topical formaldehyde or glutaraldehyde, bleomycin injections, curettage with electrodessication, carbon dioxide or yellow pulsed-dye laser surgery, tretinoin cream for facial flat warts, and podophyllum resin for mucosal warts. Oral cimetidine, although advocated by some, has been ineffective in placebo-controlled trials. Imiquimod cream, which is approved by the U.S. Food and Drug Administration only for treatment of genital warts in adults, is gaining favor.

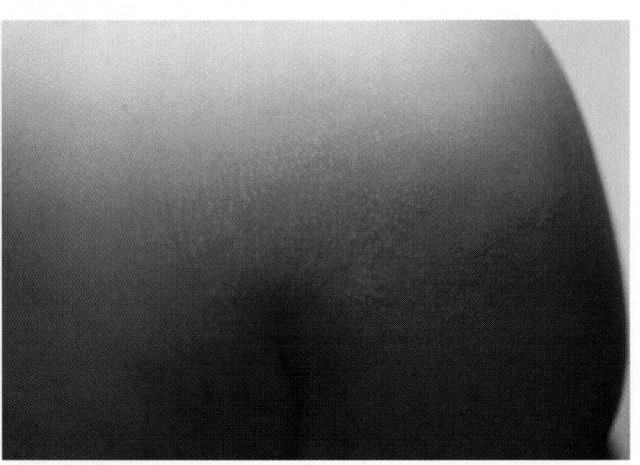

Figure 78-2. Connective tissue nevus on the shoulder.

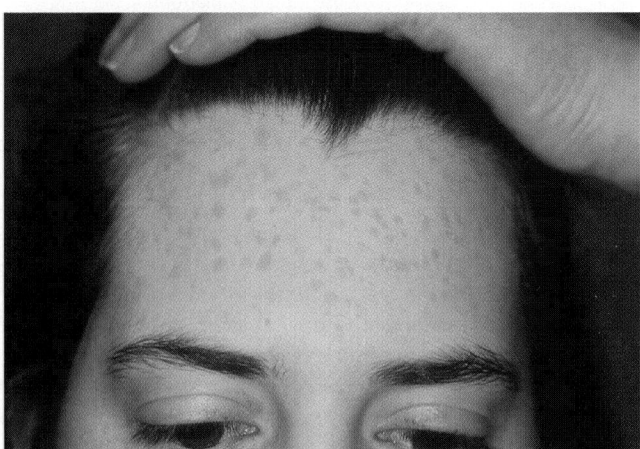

Figure 78-4. Flat warts on the forehead.

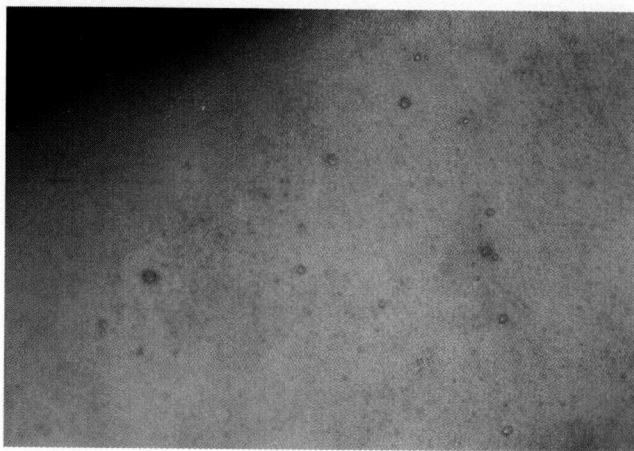

Figure 78-5. Molluscum contagiosum with secondary irritant dermatitis.

Molluscum Contagiosum

Molluscum contagiosum is caused by a poxvirus that spreads by skin-to-skin contact and presents as crops of flesh-colored to pink papules with central umbilication (Fig. 78-5). The face, trunk, extremities, and genitalia commonly are involved. Molluscum spontaneously resolves in 6 months to 2 years. As old papules involute, new crops often form. Involvement is more widespread in children with atopic dermatitis from decreased skin barrier function and autoinoculation of the virus from scratching. More widespread involvement also is seen in patients with immunodeficiencies or immunosuppression from cancer chemotherapy or organ transplantation. Education and avoidance of potentially traumatic treatments are the most important aspects of managing molluscum. Treatment should be individualized for the patient's age, extent of the lesions, and desire for treatment. No intervention while awaiting the host immune response is reasonable. Treatment does not speed the host immune response. A pinpoint depressed scar may remain after spontaneous resolution; destructive treatments do not increase risk of scarring. Treatment options include liquid nitrogen cryotherapy every few weeks, cantharidin blistering every few weeks, curettage, and tretinoin cream for a few months. Imiquimod cream, approved by the Food and Drug Administration only for treatment of genital warts in adults, has been shown to be safe and effective in the treatment of molluscum in pilot studies.

Trichoepithelioma

Trichoepitheliomas may mimic molluscum contagiosum. They are benign cutaneous tumors of hair follicle origin, present as solitary or multiple small, flesh-colored translucent papules, typically on the central portion of the face. Some have overlying telangiectasias and can be mistaken for a basal cell carcinoma. Multiple trichoepitheliomas occur in an autosomal dominant pattern, with lesions arising during childhood or at puberty. Solitary lesions typically are removed by punch biopsy for histologic evaluation. Treatment options for multiple lesions include surgical removal, curettage with electrodesiccation, cryosurgery, and dermabrasion.

Syringomas

Syringomas are benign, small, flesh-colored translucent papules occurring primarily on the lower eyelids derived from eccrine sweat glands. Syringomas appear in early adolescence, usually as multiple lesions, with a greater incidence in girls than boys. Syringomas are seen in 37% of children with Down syndrome. Treatment consists of destruction by electrodesiccation, cryosurgery, carbon dioxide laser ablation, or surgical excision.

Cylindroma

Cylindroma is discussed on the CD-ROM.

Neurofibromas

Neurofibromas are benign neoplasms of nerve tissue that may appear as solitary lesions in otherwise healthy individuals or as multiple lesions in association with neurofibromatosis (Fig. 78-6). They appear initially in early childhood or adolescence as smooth, polypoid, soft, flesh-colored tumors. As they enlarge, neurofibromas become pink, blue, or brown. They gradually increase in size and, in patients with neurofibromatosis, in number. Neurofibromas occur anywhere on the cutaneous surface, but palms and soles tend to be spared. When moderate digital pressure is applied to the surface of a small neurofibroma, it may invaginate into the dermis, which is referred to as "buttonholing." Surgical excision is performed on tumors that are disfiguring; tumors that interfere with function; and tumors that are subject to irritation, trauma, or infection.

Recurring Digital Fibroma

Recurring digital fibroma is discussed on the CD-ROM (see CD-ROM Fig. 78-8).

Subungual Exostoses

Subungual exostoses are discussed on the CD-ROM (see CD-ROM Fig. 78-9).

Basal Cell Carcinomas

Basal cell carcinomas present as flesh-colored–to–erythematous papules with pearly surfaces, rolled borders, and overlying telangiectasias. Although basal cell carcinomas typically are seen in adults with a history of extensive sun exposure, particularly those with fair complexions, they can occur in childhood and must be considered when evaluating a growing skin lesion or an ulcerated lesion that shows no evidence of healing (see also CD-ROM Fig. 78-10).

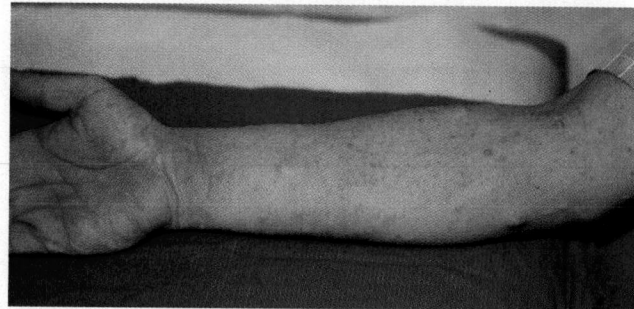

Figure 78-6. Multiple neurofibromas in an individual with neurofibromatosis.

YELLOW LESIONS

Nevus Sebaceus of Jadassohn

The nevus sebaceus is composed of collections of normal sebaceous glands. It presents at birth as a solitary, well-circumscribed, round or oval, hairless, yellowish orange plaque, often with a lobular texture (Fig. 78-7). The predominant sites of involvement are the scalp, face, and neck. The nevus sebaceus grows in proportion to the child's growth. With the onset of puberty, the sebaceous glands within the nevus sebaceus become functional, and the plaque thickens and may develop wartlike projections and a greasy appearance. Secondary neoplasias arise in 10% to 15% of these lesions, typically in adulthood, and most commonly are benign tumors of epidermal appendage origin. Malignant degeneration (basal cell carcinoma, squamous cell carcinoma) is uncommon, with more recent literature estimating a less than 1% risk. Changes of the nevus sebaceus that should prompt consideration of a biopsy include friability, focal nodularity, and rapid enlargement. Periodic evaluation for changes of the nevus sebaceus during infancy, early childhood, and into adulthood is recommended. Large lesions may be associated with ophthalmologic, nervous system, skeletal, and visceral abnormalities, commonly referred to as the *nevus sebaceus syndrome*. Management includes biopsy of any changing area or full-thickness excision if the lesion is bothersome. Prophylactic excision before puberty no longer is routinely recommended.

Juvenile Xanthogranuloma

Juvenile xanthogranulomas are non-Langerhans histiocytic dermal proliferations that present as dome-shaped papules with a yellow-orange or reddish brown color (Fig. 78-8). They are distributed most commonly on the head, neck, upper trunk, or proximal extremities. The lesions may be solitary or multiple. They appear at birth or within the first year of life. Children with multiple juvenile xanthogranulomas on the face should be evaluated by an ophthalmologist to rule out intraocular involvement. When lesions in the iris or the epibulbar region are left untreated, there is a risk of glaucoma or intraocular hemorrhage. Juvenile xanthogranu-

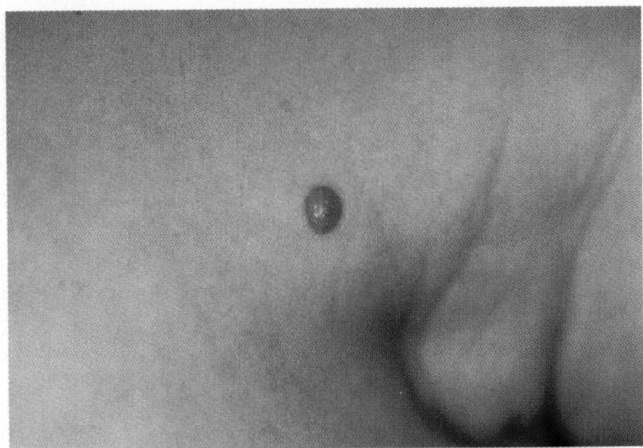

Figure 78-8. Juvenile xanthogranuloma near the axilla in an infant.

lomas may involve the lung, pericardium, liver, spleen, central nervous system, and testes. Children with neurofibromatosis and juvenile xanthogranulomas are at risk for developing leukemia. The clinical differential diagnosis of a juvenile xanthogranuloma includes Spitz nevus, mastocytoma, Letterer-Siwe disease, and xanthoma. Individual lesions undergo spontaneous involution over a few years and do not require removal unless they are causing functional compromise.

Pilomatricoma (Calcifying Epithelioma of Malherbe)

Pilomatricoma (calcifying epithelioma of Malherbe) is discussed on the CD-ROM (see CD-ROM Fig. 78-13).

Calcinosis Cutis

Cutaneous calcification arises secondary to trauma or in association with metabolic diseases (e.g., parathyroid neoplasms, hypervitaminosis D, renal disease) and connective tissue diseases (e.g., CREST [calcinosis, Raynaud phenomenon, esophageal involvement, sclerodactyly, and telangiectasia] syndrome, dermatomyositis). Calcinosis cutis may be a focal process or it may be more widespread. The condition presents as hard nodules with chalky material within them (Fig. 78-9). The clinical differential diagnosis includes osteoma cutis. The treatment of choice is surgical removal.

Nevus Lipomatosus

Nevus lipomatosus is a congenital hamartoma of mature fat cells in which fatty tissue is found high within the dermal layer of the skin. It appears as a soft, flesh-colored–to–yellow fatty plaque (Fig. 78-10). The lumbosacral region, buttocks, and proximal lower extremities are common locations. These lesions are asymptomatic and have no malignant potential. If a nevus lipomatosus becomes disfiguring, it may be surgically excised.

RED LESIONS

Vascular tumors, such as hemangiomas, pyogenic granulomas, and tufted angiomas, are discussed in Chapter 75.

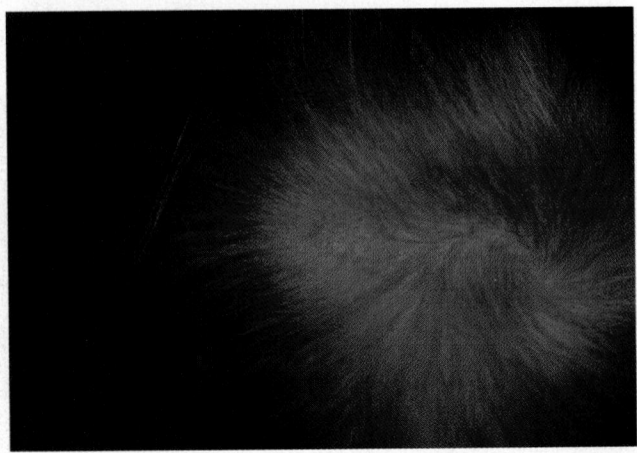

Figure 78-7. Nevus sebaceus on the scalp of an infant.

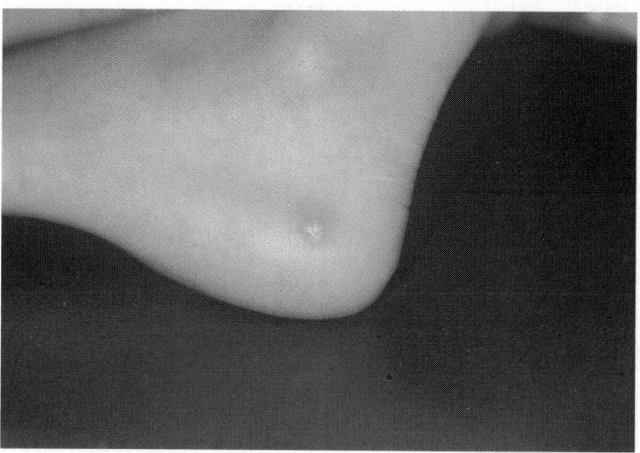

Figure 78-9. Calcinosis cutis on the heel of a child who sustained multiple heel sticks in the neonatal intensive care unit ("heel-stick nodule").

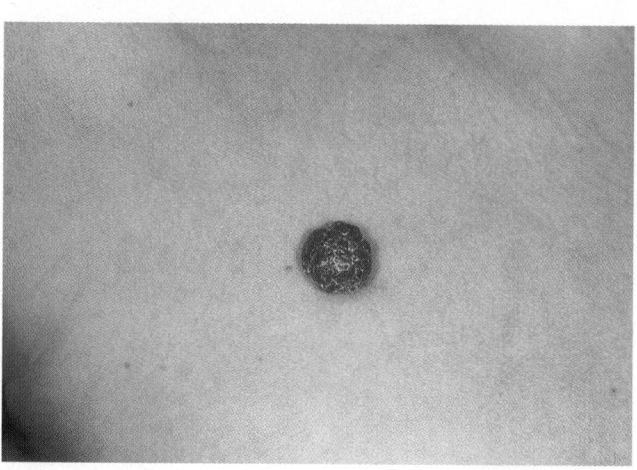

Figure 78-11. Spitz nevus.

Spitz Nevus

The Spitz nevus is a melanocytic tumor that is unique to children and adolescents. The most common clinical presentation is a smooth, dome-shaped papule that may be pink or reddish brown with telangiectasias on the surface (Fig. 78-11). They are located most commonly on the face and are usually solitary. Spitz nevi may grow rapidly and change colors, features that may raise concern about melanoma. The clinical differential diagnosis includes intradermal melanocytic nevus, hemangioma, pyogenic granuloma, juvenile xanthogranuloma, dermatofibroma, mastocytoma, and amelanotic melanoma. The histology of a Spitz nevus shows moderate atypia and may be confused with melanoma. Conservative but total surgical excision is recommended.

Hypertrophic Scar/Keloid

Hypertrophic scar/keloid is an exaggerated connective tissue response to dermal injury. They are thick, firm, pink-to-red plaques (Fig. 78-12). The hypertrophic scar usually flattens and fades to a white shiny discoloration. Keloids may appear long after the original injury and may continue to enlarge. They do not resolve spontaneously. Management consists of potent topical steroid massage, intralesional steroid injections, and topical silicone gel. Surgical revision of a keloid must be done with care because recurrences are common.

Angiofibromas

Angiofibromas are small, pink, dome-shaped papules that may be solitary or multiple and are distributed symmetrically on the nasolabial folds, cheeks, and chin (Fig. 78-13). Because the "adenoma sebaceum" of tuberous sclerosis are angiofibromas, presence of multiple angiofibromas should raise concern regarding this diagnosis. Multiple facial angiofibromas also may be seen with multiple endocrine neoplasia syndrome type I. Although angiofibromas may arise in early childhood, they typically do not present until puberty. Over time, they may evolve into verrucous or polypoid growths. Treatment includes cryosurgery with liquid nitrogen, curettage with electrodessication, dermabrasion, and laser ablation.

Hematomas

A hematoma is a collection of blood that has extravasated into the dermis or underlying soft tissue that presents as reddish blue tender nodules. Hematomas may become firmer over time if they calcify and take months to reabsorb.

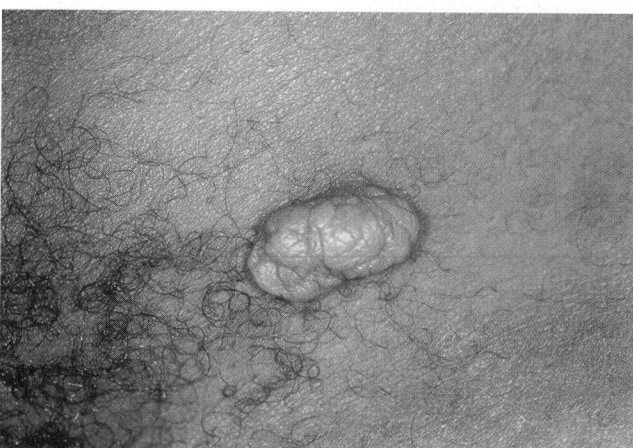

Figure 78-10. Nevus lipomatosus in the groin area of a teenage boy.

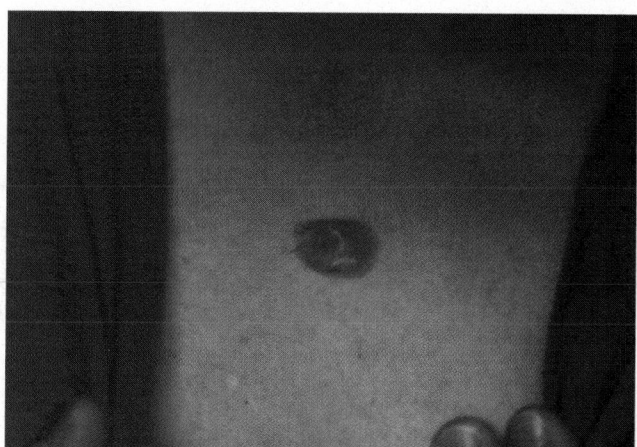

Figure 78-12. Keloid on the upper chest of a child that arose from a chickenpox lesion.

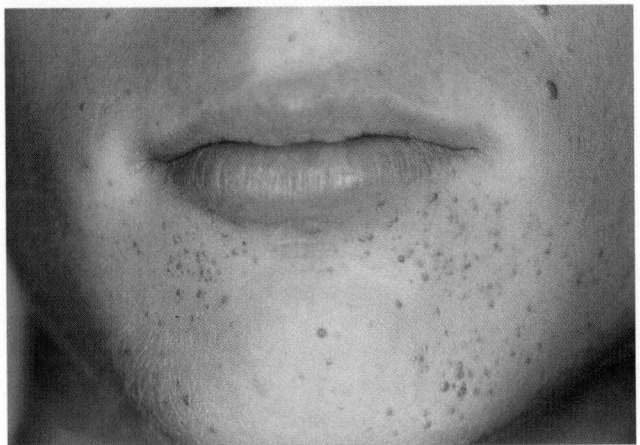

Figure 78-13. Angiofibromas in a teenage boy with tuberous sclerosis.

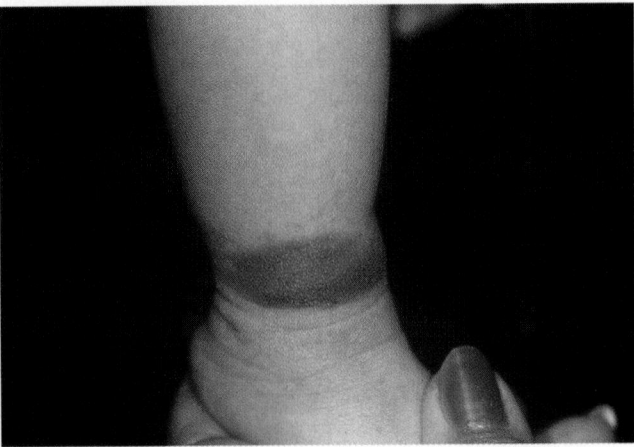

Figure 78-15. Congenital blue nevus on the ankle.

BLUE LESIONS

Blue Nevi

Blue nevi derive their color from elongated spindle-shaped melanocytes distributed among the collagen fibers deep in the dermis. The blue nevus typically presents as a small, dome-shaped papule most often located on the dorsa of the hands and feet (Fig. 78-14). Congenital blue nevi present as blue patches or plaques that may be several centimeters in diameter (Fig. 78-15). The differential diagnosis of a blue nevus includes Spitz nevus, graphite traumatic tattoo, and malignant melanoma. Melanoma may arise in a blue nevus. Biopsy is necessary to make the diagnosis and exclude malignancy.

Extramedullary Hematopoiesis

Extramedullary hematopoiesis presents at birth or within the first 24 hours of life with blue macules and infiltrative papules distributed over the scalp, face, neck, torso, and extremities, giving the neonate the appearance of a "blueberry muffin." Lesions occur when hematopoiesis takes place in the dermis secondary to severe hemolytic anemia or bone marrow infiltration with an infectious or malignant process. Lesions typically resolve in several weeks. Associated conditions include congenital infections (rubella, toxoplasmosis, and cytomegalic inclusion disease), neuroblastoma, congenital leukemia, erythroblastosis fetalis, and twin

transfusion syndrome. The differential diagnosis includes leukemia cutis and neuroblastoma. Skin biopsy is necessary to differentiate between extramedullary hematopoiesis and a malignant process.

Leukemia Cutis

Cutaneous lesions of leukemia appear as discrete, firm, bluish purple or reddish brown papules and nodules. Lesions with a green hue (known as granulocytic sarcomas or chloromas) can arise at the same time as acute granulocytic leukemia, and their presence may be noted for 1 year or more before leukemia is diagnosed. Congenital leukemia presents with firm, blue, red, or purple nodules in a generalized distribution (Fig. 78-16), and the cutaneous lesions may precede the other manifestations of the leukemia by months. The natural history of congenital leukemia does not seem to be altered by the presence of leukemia cutis. Biopsy is necessary to confirm the diagnosis.

Lymphoma Cutis

Cutaneous lesions of Hodgkin's lymphoma are seen in 8% of affected patients and typically are seen as a late manifestation. They may appear as bluish purple, pink, or reddish brown papules and nodules that may coalesce to form large tumors and plaques. These lesions are localized to the upper trunk, neck, and scalp. Cutaneous lesions of non-Hodgkin's lymphoma are bluish purple to dusky red

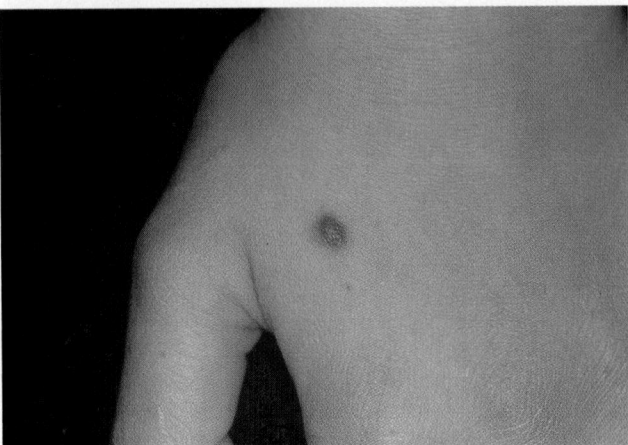

Figure 78-14. Acquired blue nevus on the hand.

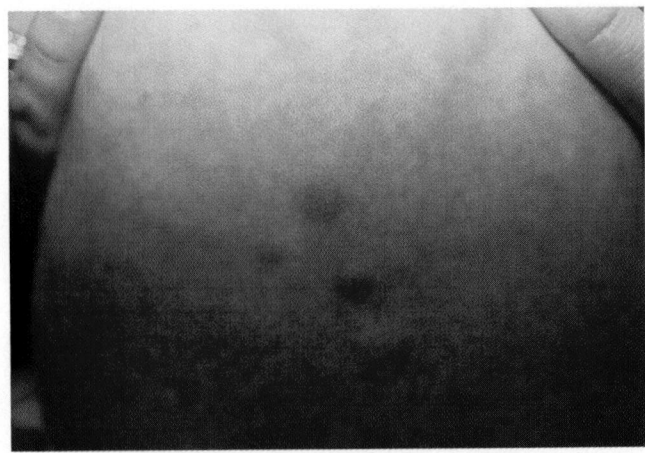

Figure 78-16. Congenital leukemia.

or brown nodules arranged in an annular or arciform configuration. Biopsy is necessary to confirm the diagnosis.

Neuroblastoma

Neuroblastoma is a tumor that arises from the primitive neural crest cells that form the adrenal medulla and sympathetic nervous system. It typically presents in newborns or in young children with an abdominal mass. Skin metastases are firm, blue-gray nodules that blanch and develop a surrounding halo of erythema within minutes of being palpated, stroked, or rubbed secondary to release of catecholamines. Biopsy is necessary to confirm the diagnosis.

REDDISH BROWN LESIONS

Mastocytoma

Mastocytomas are benign collections of mast cells in the dermis. They may be solitary or multiple; when multiple, they are referred to as *urticaria pigmentosa*. Mastocytomas usually arise during the first 2 years of life. Solitary mastocytomas present as reddish brown papules, sometimes with a yellow hue, plaques, or nodules (Fig. 78-17). They occur most frequently on the arms, wrists, neck, and trunk. Urticaria pigmentosa is characterized by yellow-red or reddish brown papules and plaques that may be distributed diffusely over the cutaneous surface. Gentle stroking or rubbing of the mastocytoma causes the mast cells to release histamine, which produces an urticarial response, called *Darier's sign* (Fig. 78-18). Blisters may form when the lesions are rubbed vigorously. Pruritus is an associated symptom of histamine release. Solitary mastocytomas become less reactive over time and typically resolve within several years. When urticaria pigmentosa presents before age 10 years, the prognosis is excellent, and the disease tends to resolve by puberty. Urticaria pigmentosa that presents during adolescence or adulthood has a higher risk of associated systemic involvement, including mastocytomas of the bones, liver, spleen, intestines, and lymph nodes and a risk of developing mast cell leukemia. Patients with systemic involvement may have flushing attacks, episodes of hypotension, headaches, tachycardia, and diarrhea. Systemic involvement, if severe, can be life-threatening. Although the risk of systemic involvement is low in childhood-onset urticaria pigmentosa, it is reasonable to

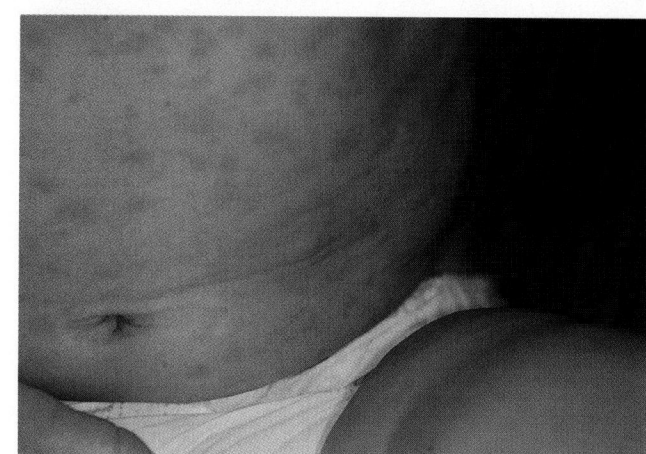

Figure 78-18. Urticaria pigmentosa showing a positive Darier's sign on the right lower abdomen.

obtain a complete blood count in affected children and to monitor for the aforementioned symptoms. Parents must be counseled to avoid triggers that induce mast cell degranulation, including aspirin, opioid narcotics, radiographic contrast dyes, polymyxin B, tubocurarine, scopolamine, gallamine, decamethonium, pancuronium, alcohol ingestion, and spicy foods and cheeses. In addition, children with urticaria pigmentosa should avoid physical stimuli that cause mast cell degranulation, such as hot baths, skin friction, and cold stress. Treatment is largely symptomatic. Potent topical steroids with or without occlusion may be used on extremely reactive mastocytomas. Oral antihistamines usually control pruritus, flushing, and blistering; they may be administered during episodes of flaring in children with mild-to-moderate symptoms or given "around the clock" in children with more pronounced symptoms. At times, H_2 blockers are used in addition to H_1 blockers to control the symptoms. Oral cromolyn may be used in more severely symptomatic children. Psoralens and ultraviolet A (PUVA) is helpful for children with extensive symptomatic urticaria pigmentosa complicated by frequent episodes of blistering (bullous mastocytosis). Problematic solitary mastocytomas may be surgically excised, but given that these lesions spontaneously resolve, this decision must not be made lightly. Parents of children with urticaria pigmentosa should be reassured and counseled that the disease ordinarily disappears with minimal sequelae.

Granuloma Annulare

Although granuloma annulare is an idiopathic inflammatory rather than a neoplastic process involving the dermal collagen, the firmness of the lesions often raises concern about malignancy. It presents most commonly in children and young adults as localized, firm aggregates of flesh-colored or reddish brown papules that coalesce into annular plaques, often with central clearing (Fig. 78-19). There is a subcutaneous variant that presents as firm lobular nodules that can raise concern about malignancy; subcutaneous granuloma annulare histologically mimics a rheumatoid nodule ("pseudorheumatoid nodule"). Granuloma annulare most commonly arises on the dorsal aspect of the hands and feet. It is usually asymptomatic, but lesions on the feet can become tender if they rub on the shoes. The disseminated

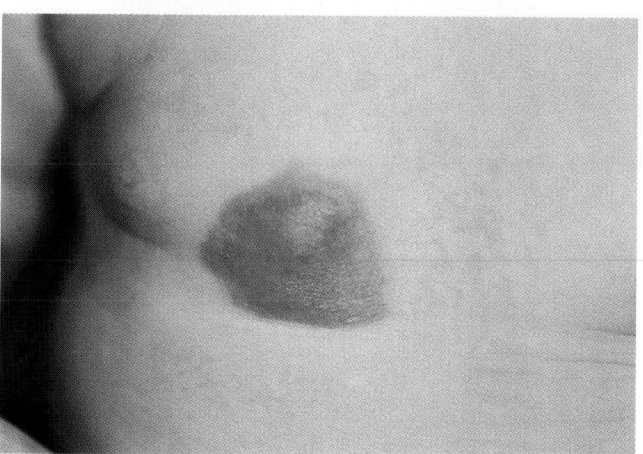

Figure 78-17. Solitary mastocytoma.

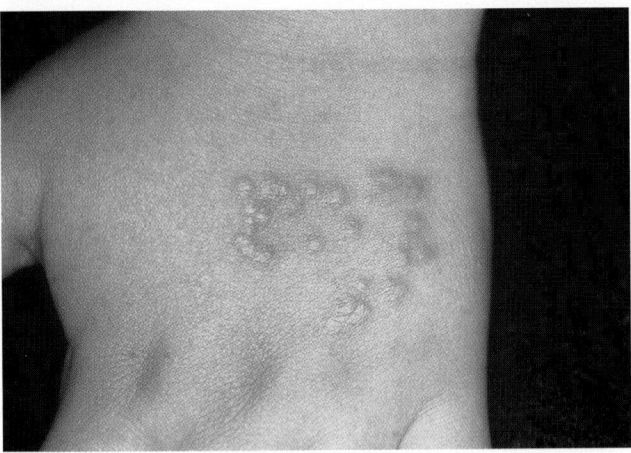

Figure 78-19. Granuloma annulare characterized by coalescing firm papules in an annular configuration with central clearing.

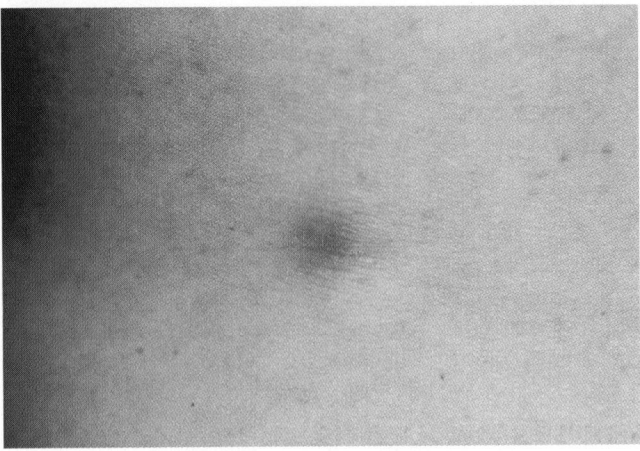

Figure 78-21. Dermatofibroma.

form of granuloma annulare, characterized by numerous small, reddish brown papules diffusely distributed on the torso and at times the extremities, is rare in children. Granuloma annulare may be seen in association with diabetes mellitus, arising either before the diagnosis of diabetes is made or afterward, although this is rare in children. Because of its annular configuration with central clearing, granuloma annulare often is misdiagnosed as tinea corporis; granuloma annulare lacks the overlying scale that is seen in a cutaneous fungal infection (Fig. 78-20). Spontaneous resolution occurs within several years in most patients. Reassurance is an important aspect of management, and expectant observation is a reasonable approach. Symptomatic lesions may be treated with topical or intralesional steroids, which are variably successful. Disseminated granuloma annulare may be treated with potassium iodide (SSKI), systemic steroids, chloroquine, niacin, dapsone, or PUVA.

Dermatofibromas

Dermatofibromas are benign neoplasms of dermal connective tissue that may vary tremendously in their appearance. Some dermatofibromas present as small, firm, reddish brown, sclerotic papules that exhibit dimpling of the overlying skin when they are squeezed (Fig. 78-21). Others

present as dome-shaped pink, red, or reddish brown tumors (Fig. 78-22). Dermatofibromas are freely movable over the subcutaneous fat. They may grow slowly and then remain stable in size for years. They are found most commonly on the anterior surface of the lower extremities. No intervention is required unless the lesion is progressively growing, in which case a biopsy should be performed to rule out dermatofibrosarcoma protuberans or another type of fibrous tumor.

Dermatofibrosarcoma Protuberans

Dermatofibrosarcoma protuberans is discussed on the CD-ROM.

Infantile Myofibromatosis

Infantile myofibromatosis is discussed on the CD-ROM (see CD-ROM Fig. 78-28).

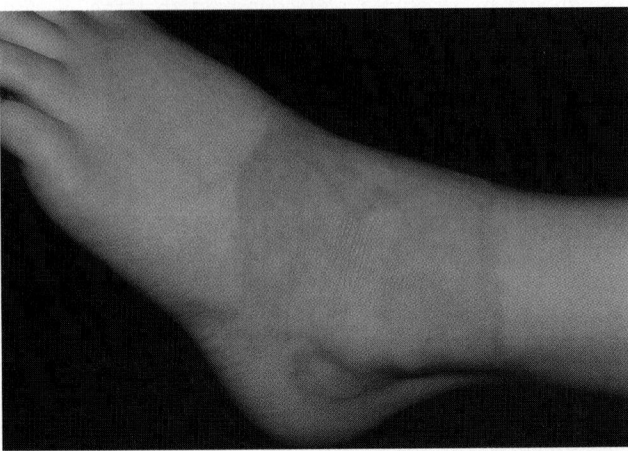

Figure 78-20. Large plaque of granuloma annulare. There is no overlying scale, but lesions with this morphology often are mistaken for tinea corporis.

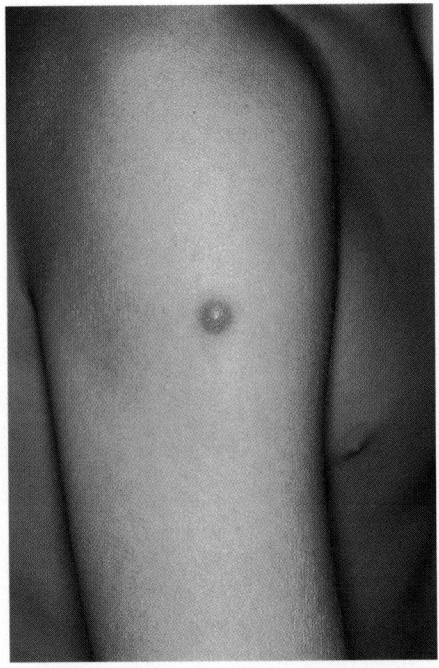

Figure 78-22. Dermatofibroma.

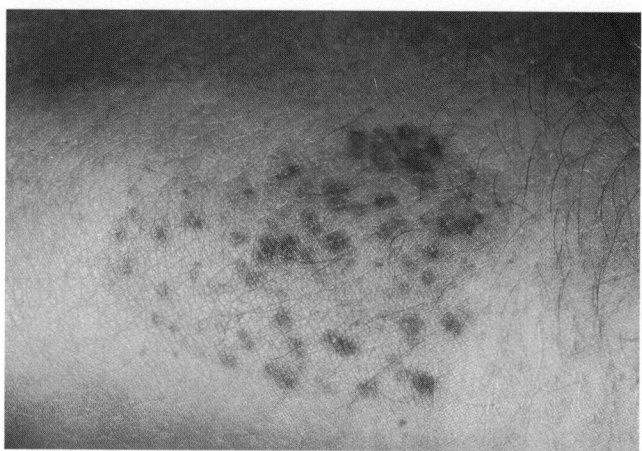

Figure 78-23. Epidermal nevi.

BROWN LESIONS

Epidermal Nevi

Epidermal nevi are epidermal neoplasms that present as yellowish brown, velvety, granular, or warty plaques (Fig. 78-23). They may occur as single or multiple lesions and typically have a linear or whorled configuration, following the lines of Blaschko (Fig. 78-24; see also Chapter 74). Epidermal nevi may be present at birth, but they most often appear during early childhood and evolve until puberty. They may arise anywhere on the cutaneous surface and may involve the oral mucosa and ocular conjunctiva. Malignant degeneration (e.g., basal cell or squamous cell carcinoma) of epidermal nevi is rare. Epidermal nevi may be generalized (nevus unius lateris, systematized epidermal nevus) and associated with abnormalities of the skeletal, central nervous, and cardiovascular systems, commonly referred to as the *epidermal nevus syndrome*. This syndrome does not represent a distinct entity, but rather is a family of disorders that share extensive epidermal nevi and associated structural malformations. Skeletal abnormalities include vertebral defects, hemihypertrophy, short limbs, phocomelia, and kyphoscoliosis. Central nervous system involvement includes brain tumors, hydrocephaly, mental retardation, and seizures. Cardiovascular abnormalities include patent ductus arteriosus and coarctation and hypoplasia of the aorta. Ocular abnormalities and increased susceptibility to visceral malignant tumors also have been reported in association with extensive epidermal nevi. Patients with large epidermal nevi should have an extensive history taken and physical examination performed with particular emphasis on development and structure of the musculoskeletal, central nervous, and cardiovascular systems and the eyes.

A subset of epidermal nevi represents somatic mutations for the same keratin gene abnormality that causes bullous congenital ichthyosiform erythroderma, a severe autosomal dominantly inherited ichthyosis. This subset of epidermal nevi displays the same histologic finding as is seen in patients with bullous congenital ichthyosiform erythroderma—epidermolytic hyperkeratosis. Individuals with large epidermal nevi should have a biopsy of the nevus performed before they are of childbearing potential to identify whether or not their nevus shows epidermolytic hyperkeratosis; if so, appropriate genetic counseling is required because the individual may carry the keratin gene mutation in the gonads and theoretically can have offspring with bullous congenital ichthyosiform erythroderma.

Inflammatory linear verrucous epidermal nevi are another variant of epidermal nevi. These are erythematous, slightly verrucous linear pruritic plaques (Fig. 78-25) that may be misdiagnosed as psoriasis, chronic eczema, or lichen striatus. Topical or intralesional steroids give temporary relief from the inflammation.

Management of epidermal nevi is difficult. Topical keratolytics, such as ammonium lactate cream, urea cream, tretinoin cream, and 5-fluorouracil cream, can help smooth the epidermal nevi but need to be used long term to maintain the effect. Cryosurgery, curettage, dermabrasion, and carbon dioxide laser resurfacing have been performed; however, recurrences or scarring is common with these treatments. Full-thickness surgical excision is curative for a

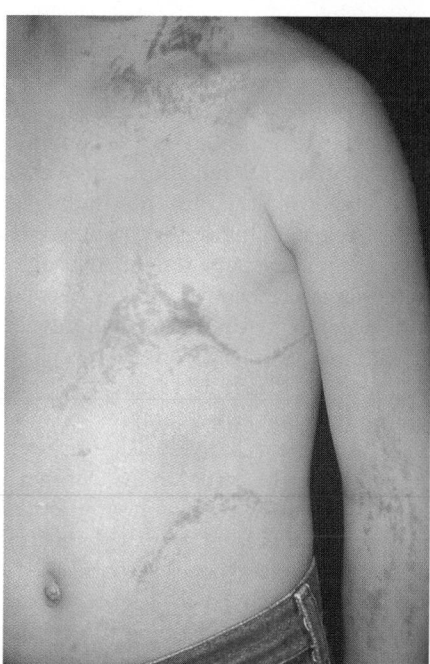

Figure 78-24. Extensive epidermal nevus showing linear and whorled pattern following the lines of Blaschko.

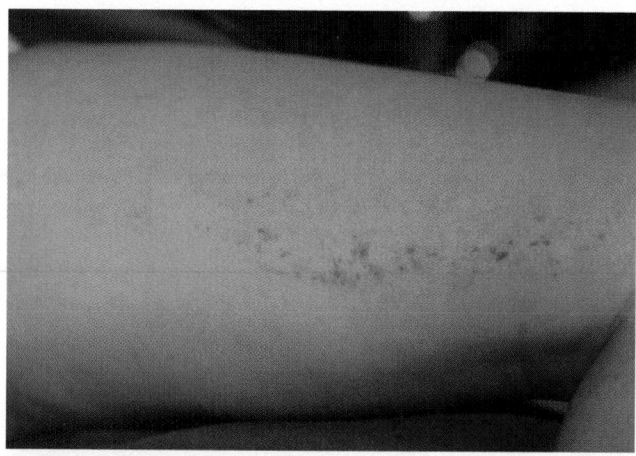

Figure 78-25. Inflammatory linear verrucous epidermal nevus on the inner thigh.

completely developed epidermal nevus. Surgical planning must take into account the size and location of the nevus and the age of the patient because excision of a lesion that has not evolved completely may lead to recurrence. Surgical excision should be delayed if possible until the lesion is fully evolved, which typically occurs at puberty.

Becker's Nevus

Becker's nevus is discussed on the CD-ROM (see CD-ROM Fig. 78-32).

Congenital Melanocytic Nevus

Congenital melanocytic nevi are benign tumors of melanocytes that present at or shortly after birth. They may be light or dark brown with stippling of the pigmentation, macular or papular, and with or without overlying hypertrichosis. They may appear on the face, scalp, torso, and extremities. They grow in proportion to the child's growth and typically darken, thicken, and become hypertrichotic as the child matures. Small congenital melanocytic nevi measure less than 2 cm in largest diameter (Fig. 78-26). Intermediate-sized congenital melanocytic nevi measure 2 to 20 cm in largest diameter. Giant congenital melanocytic nevi measure greater than 20 cm in largest diameter (Fig. 78-27). A lesion that is small during the newborn period may qualify as an intermediate-sized lesion later in life. Infants with congenital melanocytic nevi measuring 9 cm on the head and 6 cm on the body will have giant nevi by the time they become adults. The main reason to be as precise as possible in classifying congenital melanocytic nevi as to size is that the risk of developing malignant melanoma within a given congenital melanocytic nevus is relative to the size of the lesion and probably is reflective of total melanocyte burden.

Small congenital melanocytic nevi are seen in about 1% of the general population. They have an estimated lifetime risk of developing melanoma within them of approximately 2% to 4%. Statistically, these melanomas are most likely to arise at or after puberty. On a statistical basis, prophylactic excision of small congenital melanocytic nevi may be deferred until puberty, as long as there are no worrisome changes arising in the lesion that could indicate malignant degeneration. Surgical removal is not mandatory, as long as the parents, and the child when mature, are capable of

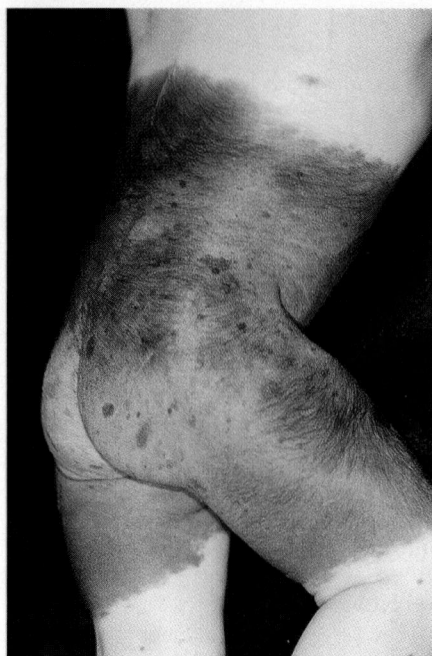

Figure 78-27. Giant congenital melanocytic nevus (bathing trunk nevus).

performing regular inspection of the nevus. Excision is strongly recommended, however, for lesions in locations that are difficult to follow (e.g., scalp, back, genital area) or lesions that are atypical appearing, in which early detection of melanoma would be difficult. Parents should examine the nevus on a monthly basis. Evaluation by a dermatologist is essential if there are questions about the appearance of the lesion.

Giant congenital melanocytic nevi have an estimated lifetime risk of developing melanoma within them of approximately 5% to 10%. Greater than 60% of the melanomas arise before puberty, and 25% arise before 2 years of age. Melanoma within a giant nevus may arise in utero (congenital melanoma). The prognosis of melanomas arising in giant nevi tends to be poor secondary to early and widespread metastasis. Another potential complication of a giant congenital melanocytic nevus is neurocutaneous melanosis, in which melanocytes are located in the leptomeninges. At risk for neurocutaneous melanosis are children with "garment" nevi involving the posterior midline areas of the back, head, or neck and children with numerous congenital nevi but no predominant large lesion. Although some children with leptomeningeal involvement remain asymptomatic, most become symptomatic before age 2 years, manifesting with macrocephaly from hydrocephalus, seizures, papilledema, headaches, paresis, cranial nerve palsies, developmental delay, and spinal cord compression. The prognosis is poor in symptomatic individuals; even benign leptomeningeal lesions can be structurally damaging and clinically malignant. More than 50% of symptomatic patients die within 3 years of presentation with neurologic manifestations; 70% die before age 10 years. Leptomeningeal melanoma has been reported in 40% to 64% of symptomatic patients. Diagnosis is made with MRI with gadolinium contrast enhancement (although a normal scan does not rule out neurocutaneous melanosis) or with cerebrospinal fluid cytology.

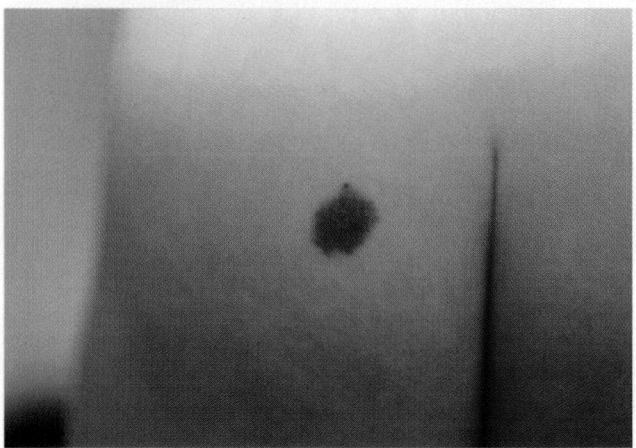

Figure 78-26. Small congenital melanocytic nevus on the buttock.

Parents should be counseled about the potential for malignancy of giant congenital melanocytic nevi and the risk for neurocutaneous melanosis. Regular inspection of the giant nevus is advised and may be aided with serial photographs. Surveillance skin biopsy specimens may need to be obtained from time to time to rule out the possibility of development of melanoma. Whether or not to proceed with surgical removal is an individual decision; complete removal often is not possible, and the risk of melanoma cannot be reduced to zero for patients whose parents desire surgical intervention. For parents and patients interested in surgical removal, excision and grafting or excision combined with tissue expansion should be started as early as possible. Patients with symptomatic neurocutaneous melanosis probably should not be subjected to multiple cutaneous surgical procedures because of their poor prognosis.

Intermediate-sized congenital melanocytic nevi are the least studied subgroup of congenital melanocytic nevi. These lesions have an estimated lifetime risk of developing melanoma within them of approximately 4%. Recommendations as to how to approach these lesions typically depend on where in the 2- to 20-cm size spectrum individual lesions lie.

Acquired Melanocytic Nevus

Acquired melanocytic nevi are benign neoplasias of melanocytes. They typically appear as brown macules after the first 6 to 12 months of life. The size and number of acquired nevi increase during childhood, and the lesions may thicken, especially during puberty. The number of new acquired nevi typically peaks during a person's 20s and 30s. Thereafter, acquired nevi may lose their pigment, become more fleshy and taglike, and slowly regress. Most acquired nevi may be left alone. It is important for individuals to perform skin self-examinations on a monthly basis to become familiar with the characteristics of their nevi such that if there is a change, medical attention can be sought promptly. Features that can indicate malignant degeneration include loss of symmetry, irregularity of the borders, change of color (especially red, blue, gray, white, or black), rapid growth, or itching or bleeding. Any of these changes in an adult warrants a biopsy; some of these changes may be seen as part of the natural evolution of an acquired nevus in a child and must be evaluated on an individual basis.

Atypical Melanocytic Nevus

Atypical melanocytic nevi are acquired nevi that appear irregular in their configuration, pigmentation, or size. These nevi present as macules or papules with variegated color, including tan, brown, pink, or black (Fig. 78-28). They have a fuzzy or irregular border and may be greater than 6 mm in diameter. Atypical melanocytic nevi frequently occur in prepubertal children and adolescents and likely represent growing nevi in growing individuals. These nevi may occur in the absence of a personal or family history of melanoma, but when present in this setting, an atypical melanocytic nevus may represent a precursor to melanoma. These patients should perform skin self-examinations every month, and family members should be enlisted to aid in examination of areas that are difficult for the patient to inspect. These patients also should have complete skin examina-

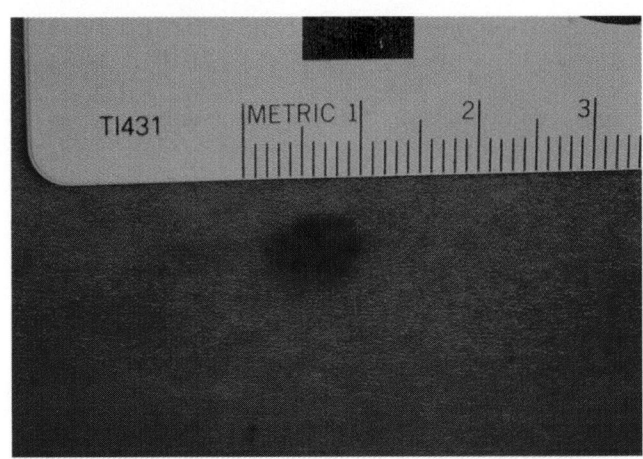

Figure 78-28. Atypical melanocytic nevus in a teenage girl.

tions, including the scalp, genital area, and between the fingers and toes, performed by a dermatologist on a semi-annual basis. Patients with numerous atypical melanocytic nevi often benefit from systematic photography and "mole mapping" because clinical photographs can be invaluable for detecting changing lesions or new lesions over time.

Halo Nevus

A halo nevus is a melanocytic nevus that develops a rim of depigmentation around it (Fig. 78-29). This phenomenon is thought to arise as a result of immunologic destruction of the melanocytic nevus. Acquired and congenital melanocytic nevi may be affected. Halo nevi typically are benign in children. The appearance of a halo nevus in a child should trigger a careful examination for associated features, however, including atypical melanocytic nevi and vitiligo, the latter of which may be seen in 30% of individuals with halo nevi. Although malignant melanoma is rare in children, melanoma may develop a halo of depigmentation around it,

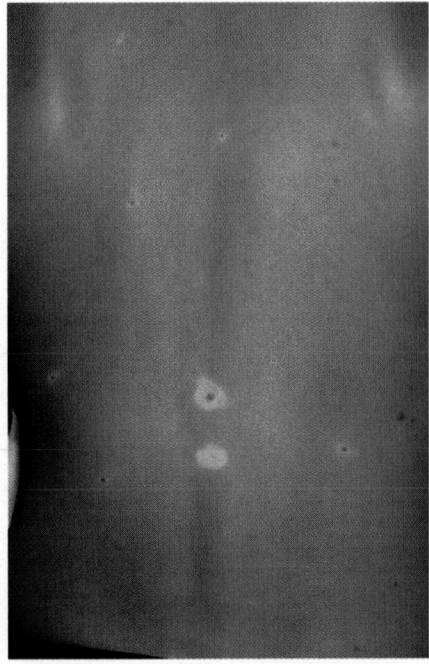

Figure 78-29. Multiple halo nevi on the back of a teenage boy.

and halo nevi may develop in patients with a melanoma at a distant site.

Speckled Lentiginous Nevus (Nevus Spilus)

Speckled lentiginous nevi are benign neoplasms of melanocytes that appear as tan patches with darker brown macules or papules studding the surface. These lesions may be congenital or acquired and are seen in 2% of the general population. Although melanoma may arise in a speckled lentiginous nevus, the risk is lower compared with a congenital melanocytic nevus of the same size because the melanocyte density of a speckled lentiginous nevus is lower. These lesions typically are observed and biopsy is performed if there are changing areas, although lesions in children are expected to develop additional darker flecks of pigment within them over time. Surgical excision can be considered.

Malignant Melanoma

Malignant melanoma, a neoplasm of melanocytes, appears as an unevenly pigmented brown or black macule, papule, or nodule (Fig. 78-30). Melanomas may have shades of red, blue, gray, or white. They affect both sexes equally, arising most frequently on the head and trunk of men and on the arms and legs of women. The lifetime risk of developing malignant melanoma in the U.S. white population is 1 in 76. Approximately 2% of melanomas occur in individuals younger than 20 years old, with 0.3% to 0.5% of melanomas occurring in prepubertal children. Stage for stage, the prognosis of melanoma in childhood is similar to that of adults. Overall outcome is worse in children, however, because the stage at presentation is more advanced secondary to delay in diagnosis. The overall 5-year survival in children with melanoma is 33%. Risk factors for melanoma in descending order include xeroderma pigmentosum, familial atypical mole and melanoma syndrome, increased number of acquired melanocytic nevi, atypical melanocytic nevi, giant congenital melanocytic nevus, previous melanoma, immunosuppression, melanoma in a first-degree relative, excessive sun exposure, and sun sensitivity. Approximately 50% of melanomas arise in a preexisting melanocytic nevus.

Immediate referral for biopsy is imperative for any lesion with features suggesting malignant transformation of a melanocytic nevus (Box 78-2). Differential diagnosis includes Spitz nevus, traumatized nevus, blue nevus, atypi-

Box 78-2. Signs and Symptoms of Malignant Transformation of a Melanocytic Nevus

- Loss of symmetry
- Irregularity of borders
- Change of color
- Rapid growth
- Itching or bleeding

cal melanocytic nevus, pyogenic granuloma, hemangioma, and angiokeratoma.

Parents and children should be educated on the dangers of sun exposure and counseled regarding photoprotection techniques. Regular avoidance of sun exposure should be advocated. Children should avoid playing outside in the sun during peak-intensity hours of the day—typically 10:00 A.M. until 4:00 P.M. When children are outside, they should wear long-sleeved shirts and long pants constructed from a tightly woven fabric. They also should wear a wide-brimmed hat and seek shade when possible. Avid use of sunscreen with protection against ultraviolet B and A rays should be encouraged. Although sunscreen should be reapplied every few hours, especially after exposure to water, parents must be warned that sunscreen use does not imply unlimited protected time in the sun. Sunscreen should be considered the last line of defense against sun exposure.

MIDLINE LESIONS

Thyroglossal Duct and Branchial Cleft Cysts

Thyroglossal duct cysts are embryonic remnants that present as flesh-colored or red papules that sometimes drain and are located over the midline of the anterior aspect of the neck near the hyoid bone (Fig. 78-31; see also Chapter 65). Branchial cleft cysts arise from a defect in the embryonic development of the branchial arches (see also Chapter 65). They present as small cystic papules or larger masses laterally displaced on the side of the neck.

Nasal Gliomas

Nasal gliomas are composed of ectopic neural tissue and typically present at or after birth as firm, reddish blue swellings over the nasal root. They may have an intracranial

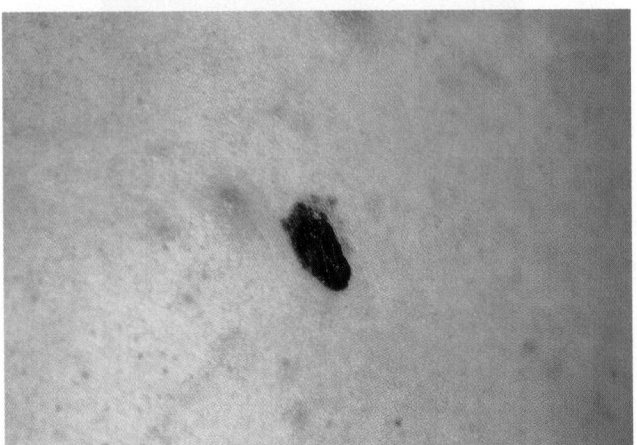

Figure 78-30. Malignant melanoma.

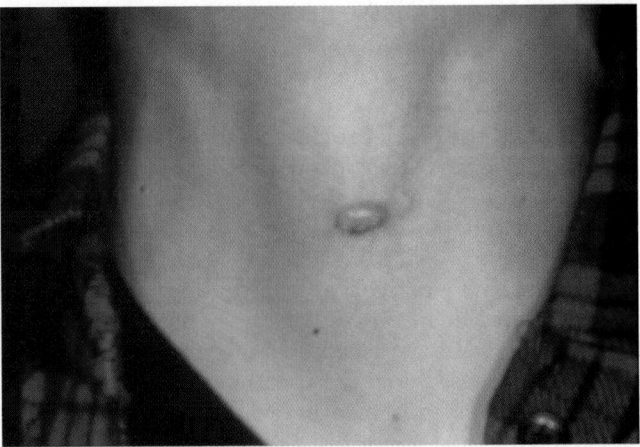

Figure 78-31. Thyroglossal duct cyst in a teenage boy.

connection and typically do not enlarge with crying, as would be expected with an encephalocele. They may extend into the nasal passage or oropharynx. The differential diagnosis includes encephalocele, hemangioma, nasal dermoid cyst, lacrimal duct cyst, neuroblastoma, or rhabdomyosarcoma. MRI delineates any soft tissue invasion. Children with nasal gliomas need to be referred to a neurosurgeon for surgical removal.

Encephaloceles

Encephaloceles arise anywhere along the midline of the upper face and scalp (see CD-ROM Fig. 78-40; see also Chapter 176). *Meningocele* is a herniation of the neural tube without ectopic brain tissue (see Chapter 177).

Meningeal Hamartomas

Meningeal harmartomas, rests of meningeal tissue outside the calvaria, present as firm, flesh-colored or pink subcutaneous nodules on the scalp or forehead. Some may overlie a port wine stain, and they may have an associated dark tuft of hair surrounding them ("hair collar sign") (see CD-ROM Fig. 78-41). When these lesions present along the midline or over sutures of the skull, an imaging study is indicated to assess whether a connection to the central nervous system exists. Surgical excision is curative.

⊚ **Additional Resources, CD-ROM**	
Color atlas	Figures
Unusual lesions:	
Flesh-colored lesions	
Smooth muscle hamartoma	Text, figure
Cylindroma	Text
Recurring digital fibroma	Text, figure
Subungual exostoses	Text, figure
Basal cell carcinoma	Text, figure
Yellow lesions	
Pilomatricoma (calcifying epithelioma of Malherbe)	Text, figure
Osteoma cutis	Text
Reddish brown lesions	
Dermatofibrosarcoma protuberans	Text
Infantile myofibromatosis	Text, figure
Brown lesions	
Becker's nevus	Text, figure

SUGGESTED READINGS

Ceballos PI, Ruiz-Maldonado R, Mihm MC Jr: Melanoma in children. N Engl J Med 1995;332:656–662.

Paller AS, Pensler JM, Tomita T: Nasal midline masses in infants and children: Dermoids, encephaloceles, and gliomas. Arch Dermatol 1991;127:362–366.

Wagner A: Lumps and bumps in childhood. Curr Probl Dermatol 1996;8:137–188.

Williams ML, Pennella R: Melanoma, melanocytic nevi, and other melanoma risk factors in children. J Pediatr 1994;124:833–845.

79 Dermatologic Manifestations of Systemic Disease

Mark Herron and Sheryll L. Vanderhooft

ROLE OF THE GENERALIST

1 Recognize cutaneous conditions associated with underlying systemic illness.

2 Evaluate patients to determine associated medical conditions.

3 Refer to appropriate specialist when needed for assistance in diagnosis or management.

Although many disorders of the skin are local primary abnormalities, skin lesions may be secondary to a systemic process. Skin manifestations may be part of a syndrome that involves other organ systems or may be associated with other conditions in which the causal relationship between the systemic condition and the skin disorder are poorly understood. Finally, skin lesions may be one of the more obvious signs of multisystem processes, such as infection or inflammation.

ACANTHOSIS NIGRICANS

Acanthosis nigricans is characterized by thickened brown plaques, often with a velvety or verrucous texture, found on the nape and sides of the neck, on the axillae, on the groin, below the breasts, and on the abdomen (Fig. 79-1). The neck is the site most commonly affected in children. Other areas that may be involved include the knuckles, antecubital and popliteal fossae, genitalia, thighs, face (particularly the perioral area), and oral mucosa. Although acanthosis nigricans can be present at birth or develop during childhood, it most often arises during puberty or in adulthood. It is a clinical marker of insulin resistance that is seen in association with a variety of endocrinopathies, obesity, medications, and malignancy and as a feature of several syndromes (Boxes 79-1 and 79-2). The presence of acanthosis nigricans in some of these disorders and syndromes cannot be explained by insulin resistance, however, and the etiology of acanthosis nigricans in these instances is unclear. Acanthosis nigricans may be noted before, concomitant with, or after the onset of an endocrinopathy or internal malignancy. In some cases, there is a familial autosomal dominant component. Acanthosis nigricans is more common in populations with darker skin pigmentation; the prevalence is highest in African Americans, Native Americans, and Hispanics.

The presence of acanthosis nigricans in a child should prompt a search for an underlying endocrinopathy. Screening tests for diabetes include fasting glucose and glycosylated hemoglobin. When screening for insulin resistance, a fasting plasma insulin level should be obtained; it is abnormally elevated in individuals with insulin resistance. Malignancy coinciding with acanthosis nigricans is rare in children; it usually is seen in middle-aged and older adults.

Correction of hyperinsulinemia often leads to improvement of the appearance of acanthosis nigricans. When it is associated with obesity, acanthosis nigricans may regress with weight loss. Topical keratolytics, such as 10% urea, lactic acid (e.g., Lac-Hydrin 12% lotion), topical retinoids (e.g., Retin-A cream), and salicylic acid, are beneficial and may reduce the thickness and brown discoloration of the plaques.

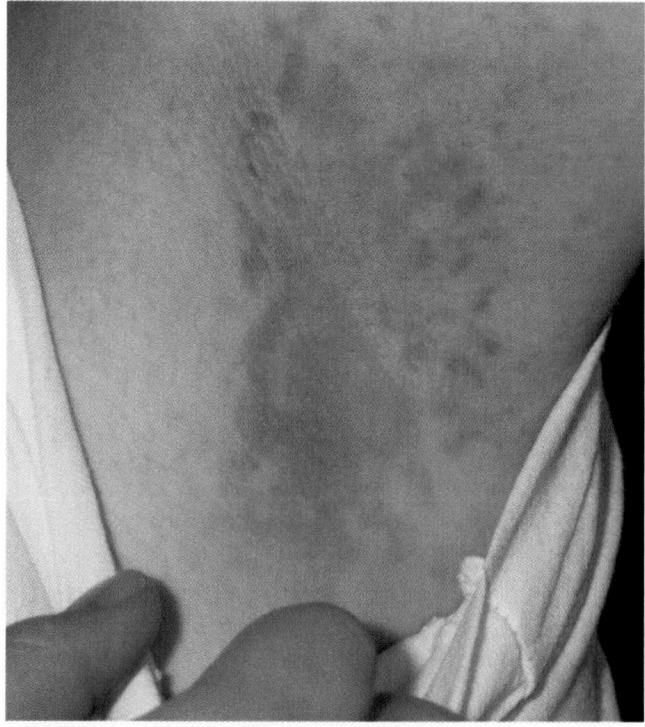

Figure 79-1. Acanthosis nigricans in the axilla of a teenage girl with recent weight gain, which resolved after weight loss.

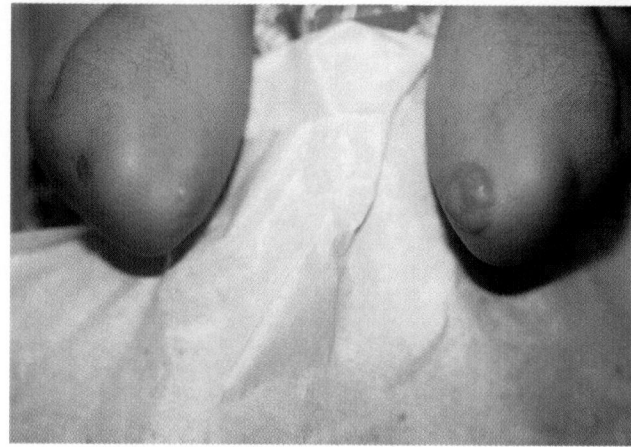

Figure 79-2. Tuberous xanthomas on the elbows of a pubertal girl with normal serum lipids.

NECROBIOSIS LIPOIDICA DIABETICORUM

The initial lesion of necrobiosis lipoidica diabeticorum is a well-circumscribed erythematous papule. The lesion progresses to a depressed, atrophic, yellow-red–to–brown plaque; the periphery of the lesion is erythematous and raised (see CD-ROM Fig. 79-2). The presence of necrobiosis lipoidica diabeticorum in any child should prompt evaluation for underlying diabetes. This condition and its implications are discussed on the CD-ROM.

XANTHOMAS

Xanthomas are lipid-filled, yellow papules and nodules that may be found anywhere on the cutaneous surface and arise most commonly as a result of abnormal lipid metabolism. *Plane xanthomas* are yellow macules or papules that typically arise on the upper eyelids (xanthelasma) during middle age, although they also may be seen elsewhere on the face, sides of the neck, upper torso, elbows, and knees; they are rare in children and adolescents. Approximately two thirds

of individuals with plane xanthomas have normal lipid levels, but they can be the first manifestation of hyperlipoproteinemia type II. When seen in a child, plane xanthomas also may indicate underlying diabetes, Hand-Schüller-Christian disease, myeloma, or liver disease.

Eruptive xanthomas occur as crops of small yellow-orange papules on an erythematous base on the buttocks, shoulders, and extensor surfaces of the extremities. The lesions frequently are pruritic. Eruptive xanthomas are associated with hypertriglyceridemia, particularly in patients with diabetes, hypothyroidism, nephrotic syndrome, or hyperlipoproteinemia types I, III, IV, and V.

Tendinous xanthomas present as flesh-colored or yellow, mobile, nontender subcutaneous nodules attached to the extensor tendons of the elbows, knees, heels, hands, and feet. They appear almost exclusively in patients with hypertriglyceridemia and hypercholesterolemia caused by hyperlipoproteinemia types II and III.

Tuberous xanthomas are large, flesh-colored or yellowish red nodules or tumors arising on the palms, elbows, knees, hands, and buttocks (Fig. 79-2); they are not attached to underlying structures, as are tendinous xanthomas. They are seen in patients with hypertriglyceridemia, either acquired or as part of hyperlipoproteinemia types II, III, and IV.

Evaluating for diabetes and a primary hyperlipidemia is essential in individuals with xanthomas. Fasting glucose and glycosylated hemoglobin are the best screening tests for diabetes. Fasting triglycerides and cholesterol effectively screen for an abnormality of lipid metabolism. Often the treatment of the underlying hyperlipidemia results in resolution of the xanthomas. Diet, exercise, and drug therapy all are essential components of treating hyperlipidemia.

DERMATITIS

Dermatitis, a common disorder in infants and young children, is usually atopic. Other common causes are contact irritant dermatitis, contact allergic dermatitis, and seborrheic dermatitis. Because dermatitis can be a manifestation of other conditions, consideration also must be given to the possibility of an underlying metabolic, nutritional, or immunologic abnormality. This is particularly important when evaluating a neonate with erythroderma or extensive

Table 79-1. Metabolic Disorders Associated with Neonatal Erythroderma or Infantile Dermatitis

Disorder	Features	Enzyme Deficiency
Biotin deficiency—neonatal (multiple carboxylase deficiency)	Seborrheic dermatitis Alopecia Ketoacidosis Dehydration Coma Death	Holocarboxylase synthetase
Biotin deficiency—infantile (multiple carboxylase deficiency)	Seborrheic or erosive dermatitis Alopecia Developmental delay Hypotonia Ataxia Seizures Hearing loss Keratoconjunctivitis Blepharitis	Biotinidase
Hartnup disease	Photosensitivity Pellagra-like lesions (eczematous eruption with hyperpigmentation on the face, neck, hands, and legs) Chronic diarrhea Failure to thrive Short stature Brittle hair Developmental delay Cerebellar ataxia Nystagmus	Transport abnormality of tryptophan, which is a precursor of nicotinic acid (niacin); clinically, Hartnup disease resembles niacin deficiency (pellagra)
Iminopeptiduria	Dermatitis Abnormal connective tissue Leg ulcers	Prolidase
Phenylketonuria	Photosensitivity Dermatitis Hypopigmentation Scleroderma-like skin changes Developmental delay Seizures Microcephaly Short stature	Phenylalanine hydroxylase
Propionic acidemia	Dermatitis Ketoacidosis Neutropenia Thrombocytopenia Osteoporosis Developmental delay Seizures	Propionyl-CoA carboxylase
Methylmalonic acidemia	Dermatitis Cutaneous candidiasis Ketoacidosis Neutropenia Thrombocytopenia Osteoporosis Growth retardation	Methylmalonyl-CoA mutase
Maple syrup urine disease	Dermatitis Maple syrup odor of skin, hair, or urine Feeding difficulty Irregular respirations Severe hypoglycemia Seizures Death	Branched-chain ketoacid decarboxylase

seborrheic dermatitis and in infants with dermatitis that is refractory to treatment, especially in conjunction with failure to thrive, developmental delay, or alopecia. Table 79-1 outlines the *metabolic disorders* associated with neonatal erythroderma or infantile dermatitis.

Nutritional deficiencies associated with neonatal erythroderma or infantile dermatitis are listed in Box 79-3. Acrodermatitis enteropathica and essential fatty acid deficiency may present with an erosive dermatitis involving the perioral area and diaper area. The dermatitis of biotin deficiency, whether acquired or from a metabolic defect, can

have a similar appearance. Acquired biotin deficiency arises in individuals who consume an unbalanced diet containing excessive raw egg whites. Biotin binds to avidin found in egg whites, resulting in malabsorption of biotin from the intestinal tract. Patients with pancreatic tumors that secrete glucagon can develop a periorificial and intertriginous erosive dermatitis that resembles acrodermatitis enteropathica, known as *necrolytic migratory erythema*. It is rare in children.

Acrodermatitis enteropathica is an autosomal recessive disorder in which there is an abnormality of zinc-binding

> **Box 79-3.** Nutritional Deficiencies Associated with Dermatitis in Infants
>
> - Acrodermatitis enteropathica—abnormal zinc-binding ligands
> - Protein-calorie malnutrition
> - Essential fatty acid deficiency—linoleic and linolenic acids
> - Malabsorption
> - Acquired deficiencies
>   - Zinc
>   - Biotin
>   - Niacin
>   - Riboflavin (vitamin B_2)
>   - Pyridoxine (vitamin B_6)

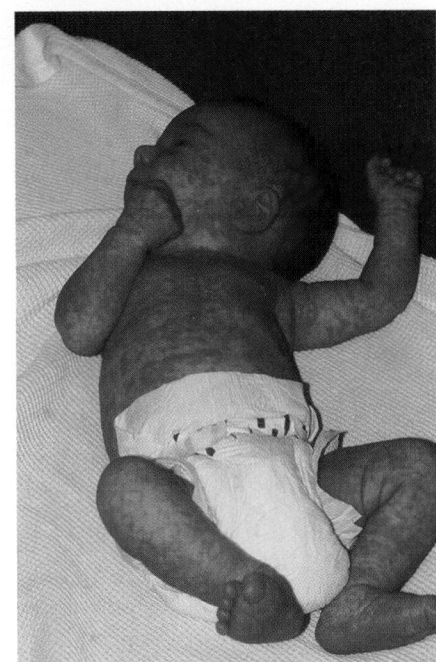

Figure 79-4. Extensive dermatitis in an infant with acrodermatitis enteropathica.

ligands, leading to zinc deficiency. The binding ligands transport zinc into the epithelial cells. Because zinc is exceptionally well absorbed from breast milk, infants with acrodermatitis enteropathica typically do not show features of the disorder until after being weaned from the breast. Infants with acrodermatitis enteropathica also show acral erythema and paronychia, nail dystrophy, glossitis, stomatitis, and secondary *Candida* and *Staphylococcus* infections of the skin (Figs. 79-3 and 79-4). Alopecia of the scalp, eyelashes, and eyebrows is prominent. Diarrhea and failure to thrive simultaneously develop with the cutaneous eruptions in zinc deficiency. Neurologic abnormalities in acrodermatitis enteropathica include progressive ataxia, irritability, and lethargy. Incomplete expression of these skin findings may be confused with perioral dermatitis, hand dermatitis, candidiasis, and pustular psoriasis. Other causes of zinc deficiency are listed in Box 79-4.

Measurement of plasma zinc is diagnostic, provided that the sample is not hemolyzed or contaminated; particular care needs to be taken to ensure that test tubes used to collect the blood specimen and measurement equipment are free of zinc. Serum zinc levels, levels of zinc metalloenzymes (e.g., alkaline phosphatase), and urinary excretion of zinc are abnormally low in patients with zinc deficiency. Lowered zinc levels in the plasma may occur in the absence of true zinc deficiency. Levels fall nonspecifically in the acute phases of cardiac, hepatic, renal, pulmonary, neurologic, infectious, and malignant disorders. Urinary excretion of zinc is decreased only as a result of zinc deficiency.

Deficiency of zinc can be corrected easily with oral supplementation of elemental zinc, 0.5 mg/kg/day. Response to therapy is dramatic. Skin lesions, diarrhea, and behavioral abnormalities reverse within days to weeks. Hair growth and growth of the infant normalize over the course of months.

Immunologic abnormalities associated with dermatitis are listed in Box 79-5. These disorders are associated with recurrent cutaneous and systemic infections and chronic dermatitis. Markedly elevated serum IgE levels (10 to 100 times normal) are found in *hyperimmunoglobulin E syndrome*. Severe combined immune deficiency is characterized by deficiency of T-lymphocyte and B-lymphocyte function. Wiskott-Aldrich syndrome is an X-linked recessive disorder characterized by thrombocytopenia and platelet dysfunction. *Leiner phenotype* is a term used to represent a heterogeneous group of diseases with common clinical features, including erythroderma; failure to thrive; diarrhea; and decreased C3, C4, and C5 levels. Some cases of "Leiner's disease" have been reclassified later as Netherton's syndrome (ichthyosis linearis circumflexa and trichorrhexis invaginata), Omenn's syndrome (familial

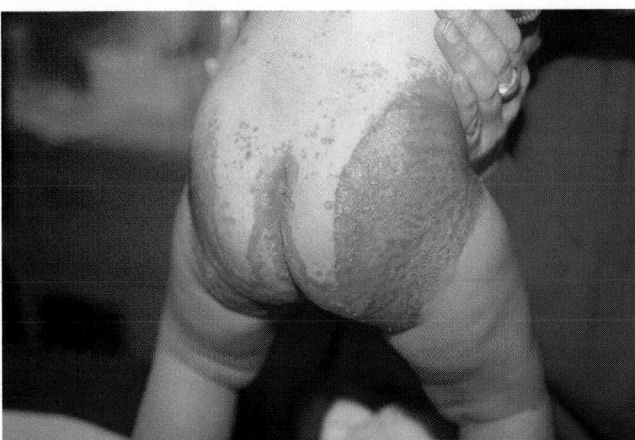

Figure 79-3. Erosive dermatitis of the diaper area in an infant with acrodermatitis enteropathica.

> **Box 79-4.** Causes of Zinc Deficiency
>
> - Acrodermatitis enteropathica
> - Dietary deficiency
>   - Zinc-deficient vegetarian diet
>   - Alcoholism
>   - Long-term total parenteral nutrition with inadequate zinc supplementation
> - Malabsorption
>   - Cystic fibrosis
>   - Intestinal bypass
>   - Crohn's disease
>   - Prolonged diarrhea

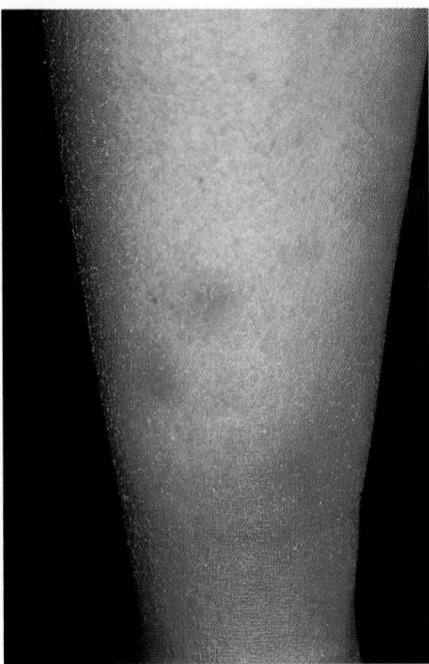

Figure 79-5. Erythema nodosum on the shin of a girl with ulcerative colitis.

reticuloendotheliosis with eosinophilia), and severe combined immune deficiency with graft-versus-host disease.

ERYTHEMA NODOSUM

Erythema nodosum is an inflammatory disease involving the subcutaneous fat. It is seen most often in the fall and spring and is three times more common in girls than in boys. The lesions appear as crops of red painful subcutaneous nodules, most often located on the extensor surfaces of the lower extremities (Fig. 79-5), often accompanied by fever and malaise. Joint complaints, ranging from arthralgias to oligoarthritis and migratory polyarthritis, occur in most patients. Articular symptoms may antedate the skin lesions. The duration of erythema nodosum is usually 3 to 6 weeks. Protracted courses of 18 weeks and recurrences have been reported in association with non-Hodgkin's and Hodgkin's lymphomas. Recurrences otherwise are seen in 10% of affected patients. Disorders associated with erythema nodosum are listed in Table 79-2.

Leading causes of erythema nodosum in children are viral upper respiratory tract infections, streptococcal infections (especially pharyngitis), primary tuberculosis, and chronic inflammatory conditions. In many cases, the cause is not determined. Initial evaluation should include a throat culture, complete blood count, erythrocyte sedimentation rate, antistreptolysin-O titer, chest radiograph, and tuberculosis skin test. Other laboratory studies should be based on the history and physical examination. Any identified underlying disorder should be treated and symptomatic treatment provided, including bed rest, leg elevation, and nonsteroidal anti-inflammatory medication. Oral potassium iodide or colchicine is beneficial to some patients. Systemic or intralesional corticosteroids can hasten the recovery.

Table 79-2. Disorders Associated with Erythema Nodosum

Infections	Inflammatory Disorders	Malignancies	Medications	Other

Bacterial infections
  Streptococcal (especially upper
    respiratory tract)*
  Primary tuberculosis*
  Mycobacterium marinum
  Leprosy
  Salmonella gastroenteritis*
  Yersinia
  Tularemia
  Mycoplasma
  Chlamydia (including cat-scratch disease)
Fungal infections
  Coccidioidomycosis
  Histoplasmosis
  North American blastomycosis
  Trichophyton superficial cutaneous
    infections
Protozoal infections
  Leishmaniasis
Viral infections
  Epstein-Barr virus
  Hepatitis B virus
	Crohn's disease*
	Ulcerative colitis
	Behçet's syndrome
	Sarcoidosis*
		Leukemia
		Lymphoma
			Phenytoin
			Sulfonamides
			Oral contraceptives
			Bromides
				Pregnancy

*Most common in children.

PYODERMA GANGRENOSUM

Pyoderma gangrenosum is a severe inflammatory ulcerative disease. Inflammatory bowel disease is the single most commonly associated disorder with pyoderma gangrenosum. When seen in association with inflammatory bowel disease, the activity of pyoderma gangrenosum parallels the activity of the bowel disease. Other diseases associated with pyoderma gangrenosum are listed in Box 79-6. In 27% of cases of pyoderma gangrenosum in children, no underlying disorder can be identified. Pyoderma gangrenosum is characterized by rapidly expanding ulcers with a purulent base and violaceous undermined borders (Fig. 79-6). The most common site of involvement is the lower extremity. It may involve peristomal and incision sites, extremities, chest, back, abdomen, head, and neck (Fig. 79-7).

The diagnosis of pyoderma gangrenosum is one of exclusion. Biopsies often are required to rule out other causes of ulceration. Management of pyoderma gangrenosum revolves around topical care of the ulcers, immunosuppressive therapy, and treatment of the underlying disorder. Topical therapy is directed toward débridement of the ulcers

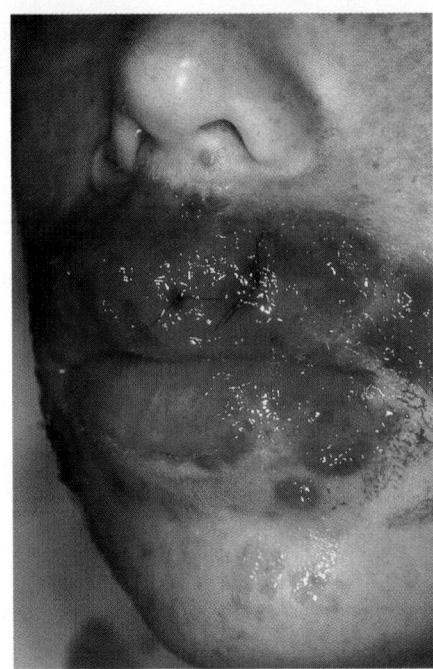

Figure 79-7. Pyoderma gangrenosum of the perioral area in a teenage boy with Crohn's disease.

with wet dressings and whirlpool baths. Débridement is followed by topical or intralesional corticosteroids, topical cromolyn, or topical tacrolimus. Although some patients have been managed successfully with local measures alone, most patients with pyoderma gangrenosum require systemic immunosuppression, including systemic steroids, cyclosporine, or azathioprine

SWEET'S SYNDROME (ACUTE FEBRILE NEUTROPHILIC DERMATOSIS)

Sweet's syndrome is a hypersensitivity response, rarely seen in children, characterized by painful, indurated, red–to–plum-colored papules, plaques, and nodules distributed asymmetrically on the face, neck, and limbs (see CD-ROM Fig. 79-9). Disorders associated with Sweet's syndrome are listed in Box 79-7. This disorder is discussed on the CD-ROM.

LEUKOCYTOCLASTIC VASCULITIS

Leukocytoclastic vasculitis is a descriptive term for a small vessel vasculitis. The cutaneous findings are nonpalpable petechial macules and patches and palpable purpuric

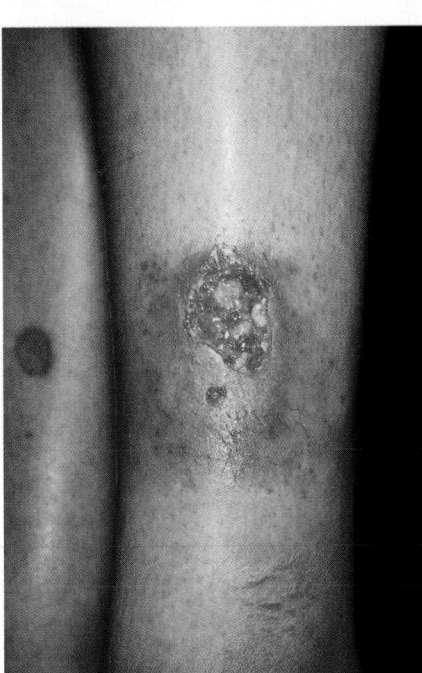

Figure 79-6. Pyoderma gangrenosum. (Courtesy of the Department of Dermatology, University of Utah, Salt Lake City, Utah.)

papules coalescing into plaques (see CD-ROM Fig. 79-10). The disorders and medications most frequently associated with leukocytoclastic vasculitis are outlined in Box 79-8. This disorder is described on the CD-ROM.

HENOCH-SCHÖNLEIN PURPURA

Henoch-Schönlein purpura, the most common form of vasculitis encountered in children and young adults, is a specific subtype of leukocytoclastic vasculitis that is characterized by IgA antibody deposition in cutaneous blood vessel walls and renal mesangium. Cutaneous lesions consist of crops of erythematous macules and papules that become purpuric and resolve with hyperpigmentation over several days, after which new crops may arise, giving the eruption a polymorphous appearance (Fig. 79-8). Lesions are distributed most commonly on the lower extremities, although they also may be present at sites of pressure, including the buttocks and elbows. In children younger than 3 years old, edema of the hands, feet, periorbital area, and scrotum may be seen. Other hallmark features are arthritis, abdominal pain, and hematuria.

This hypersensitivity vasculitis results in localized or widespread vascular damage. Although the etiology is unknown, it is clear that IgA antibodies play a crucial role. Serum IgA levels and IgA-containing circulating immune complexes are increased. Bacterial and viral infections often are implicated as the trigger of Henoch-Schönlein purpura.

Although the condition generally is benign and self-limiting, one third of patients have recurrence of symptoms, and many have complications in the acute phase, most commonly gastrointestinal bleeding and glomerulo-

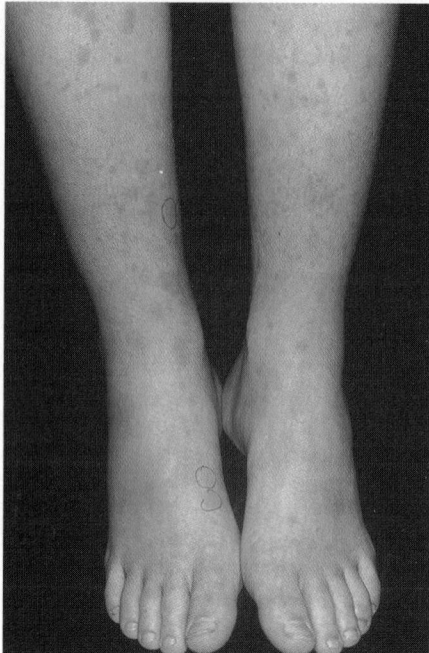

Figure 79-8. Henoch-Schönlein purpura.

nephritis. Hypertension is a common feature of Henoch-Schönlein purpura acute nephritis. Approximately 5% of children with nephritis progress to end-stage renal disease. Severe gastrointestinal vasculitis and kidney disease account for mortality in 3% of affected children. Other less common complications include pulmonary hemorrhage, cerebral vasculitis, pericarditis, and myocardial necrosis. Acute scrotal purpura, swelling, and pain occur in 20% of boys. Scrotal involvement improves with systemic corticosteroid therapy.

Treatment of patients with Henoch-Schönlein purpura is primarily symptomatic. The joint pain and edematous, purpuric cutaneous lesions may improve with analgesics and nonsteroidal anti-inflammatory drugs. Although the use of systemic steroids may not alter the course of Henoch-Schönlein purpura, patients tend to feel better with such therapy. Early treatment with high-dose corticosteroids combined with oral cyclophosphamide or azathioprine reduces proteinuria, may halt progression to chronic renal insufficiency, and improves outcome.

URTICARIAL VASCULITIS

Urticarial vasculitis, a rare condition that clinically resembles urticaria but actually is a leukocytoclastic vasculitis, is characterized by erythematous edematous papules and wheals that usually are generalized and frequently are accompanied by a stinging or burning sensation (see CD-ROM Figs. 79-12 and 79-13). This condition is discussed fully on the CD-ROM.

CUTANEOUS DRUG REACTIONS

Cutaneous drug reactions commonly are encountered by primary care providers. Reactions to drugs may assume a variety of morphologies. A given drug can cause different types of reactions in different patients and even in the same patient. Most drug reactions are benign in nature and self-

---

Box 79-8. Disorders and Medications Most Frequently Associated with Leukocytoclastic Vasculitis

Medications

- Nonsteroidal anti-inflammatory drugs
- Penicillins
- Phenytoin
- Sulfonamides
- Tetracyclines

Infection

- Upper respiratory tract (especially streptococcal)
- Viral hepatitis
- Influenza
- Rocky Mountain spotted fever
- Meningococcemia
- Gonococcemia
- Mononucleosis
- Human immunodeficiency virus infection

Collagen Vascular Disease

- Juvenile rheumatoid arthritis
- Systemic lupus erythematosus

Inflammatory Bowel Disease

Cystic Fibrosis

Cryoglobulinemia

Malignancy

limited. Exanthematous (morbilliform) eruptions and urticaria constitute the most common expression of drug sensitivity. Although discomfort from pruritus often is present with these types of drug reactions, there are no long-term sequelae associated with them. Severe drug reactions, such as vasculitis, Stevens-Johnson syndrome, and toxic epidermal necrolysis, are serious and have great morbidity and risk for mortality.

Essential to the management of any drug reaction is the identification and the elimination of the offending medication. When attempting to determine if a patient's eruption is secondary to a medication, and in the case of the patient taking many medications which medication could be the culprit, several historical factors must be weighed. The interval between the introduction of a medication and the onset of the eruption must be determined. Allergic drug reactions usually begin within 7 to 20 days after the initiation of a new medication. If a patient previously was sensitized to the medication, a drug reaction can occur within 2 days. All medications that the patient has taken during the 3 weeks before the onset of the eruption must be considered. This includes all prescription and over-the-counter medications, topical agents, vitamins, and herbal and homeopathic remedies. Medications taken by nursing mothers often are excreted in the breast milk and become a source of drug exposure for the nursing infant. Drugs ingested by the mother during pregnancy may account for a cutaneous eruption in a newborn. History of past medication exposure also is important; multiple courses of drug therapy and prolonged administration of a drug can cause allergic sensitization. Some drugs are more likely to cause reactions than others. The Boston Collaborative Drug Surveillance Program has published rates of drug reactions for the most commonly used medications, and using these statistics, it is possible to look at a patient's medication list and determine which ones are the most likely to cause a drug reaction. It also is helpful to note whether there is improvement after the suspect drug is withdrawn; some drug eruptions may continue to worsen for several days after the offending drug has been discontinued, and clearing of lesions may take 2 weeks. If the patient is rechallenged with the suspect drug and there is no reaction on readministration, it was unlikely to have been the cause of the prior eruption.

Minor drug reactions resolve slowly when the offending agent is discontinued. For mild eruptions with no severe signs or symptoms, no further medical evaluation is necessary when the causative agent has been identified. Persistent pruritus may be controlled with oral antihistamines. Emollients and moisturizing lotions are beneficial during the late desquamative phase. Topical steroids may be combined with oral antihistamines. Complications are uncommon with mild eruptions.

Avoidance of the identified drug is absolutely necessary in severe drug reactions. In the case of minor morbilliform eruptions, if there are no alternatives to the culprit medication, it is possible to administer it in the future and "treat through the rash" symptomatically. A list of the patient's drug allergies and emergency identification wristbands or cards should be used to prevent future exposure and reactions. Parents should be counseled regarding cross-reactivity with other medications. Common cross-reactivities include penicillins with cephalosporins, phenytoin with phenobarbital and carbamazepine, and sulfonamides with other sulfa-containing drugs (see also Chapter 44).

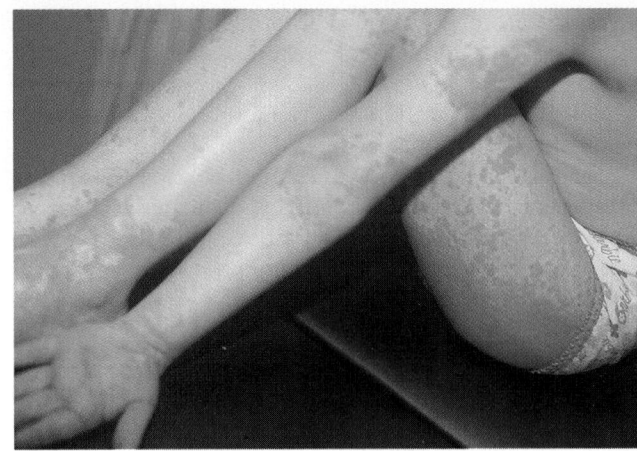

Figure 79-9. Erythema multiforme.

ERYTHEMA MULTIFORME

Erythema multiforme is characterized by fixed annular red macules, papules, plaques, and urticarial wheals symmetrically distributed on the torso, extensor surfaces of the arms and legs, tops of the hands and feet, and palms and soles (Fig. 79-9); there may be progression to the neck and face. Target lesions are the hallmark finding, characterized by an erythematous ring with a dusky violaceous center; these typically are seen on the palms and soles (Fig. 79-10). At times, bullae form, typically at the sites of target lesions. The lesions have a burning sensation but are not typically pruritic. Mucous membrane involvement is either absent or limited to one surface; gingival lesions are rare in erythema multiforme.

An acute hypersensitivity reaction to herpes simplex virus is the cause of erythema multiforme in most affected children. Other infectious agents that have been well documented as precipitating factors for erythema multiforme include orf virus, Epstein-Barr virus, and histoplasmosis. Many other infectious agents, including *Mycoplasma pneumoniae* and varicella-zoster virus, and medications and immunizations have been implicated as triggers of erythema multiforme. Some patients with herpes simplex

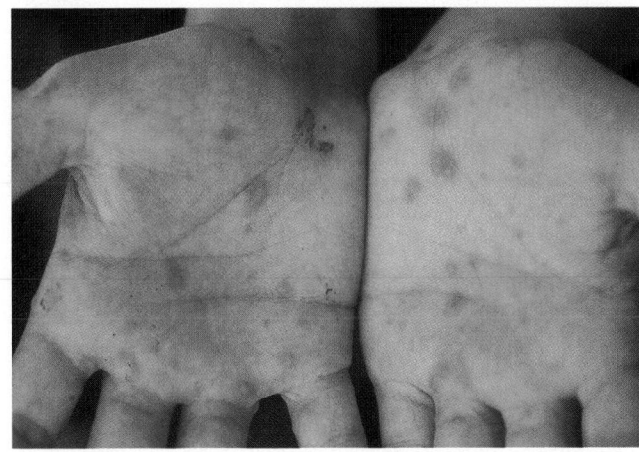

Figure 79-10. Target lesions on the palms in a patient with erythema multiforme.

virus–associated erythema multiforme have recurrences of erythema multiforme with recurrences of the herpes simplex infection. Often the cause of erythema multiforme is not determined. Erythema multiforme occurs most commonly in the spring and fall.

Clinical and laboratory evaluation of erythema multiforme is directed toward identifying the underlying trigger. Mild cases of erythema multiforme require only symptomatic treatment with oral antihistamines, topical antipruritics, and topical steroids. Analgesics and cold compresses also are beneficial. Use of systemic steroids is controversial, but if used early in the presentation, they may ameliorate the reaction. If the patient is developing Stevens-Johnson syndrome, systemic steroids may increase the risk of secondary infection and delay wound healing. Patients with herpes-induced erythema multiforme benefit from oral acyclovir therapy. Prophylactic acyclovir is effective in decreasing the frequency and severity of recurrent erythema multiforme associated with recurrent herpes. Erythema multiforme is self-limited and has minimal morbidity. The cutaneous lesions resolve without sequelae in 2 to 4 weeks.

STEVENS-JOHNSON SYNDROME (ERYTHEMA MULTIFORME MAJOR)

Stevens-Johnson syndrome is a mucocutaneous hypersensitivity reaction considered by some to be a severe form of erythema multiforme, hence the term *erythema multiforme major*. Others argue that Stevens-Johnson syndrome is distinct from erythema multiforme because it is more often a reaction to medications than to an infectious agent. Factors that may precipitate Stevens-Johnson syndrome are listed in Box 79-9. Patients typically show a prodrome of fever, malaise, headaches, cough, coryza, sore throat, vomiting, diarrhea, myalgia, and arthralgias 1 week before the onset of the eruption. The lesions are similar to what is seen in erythema multiforme, although target lesions may be less prominent; however, there is more extensive cutaneous involvement than with erythema multiforme, and bullae may be widespread but cover less than 20% of the body surface area (Fig. 79-11). Two or more mucous membranes are involved. Bullae, mucosal erosions, edema, and hemor-

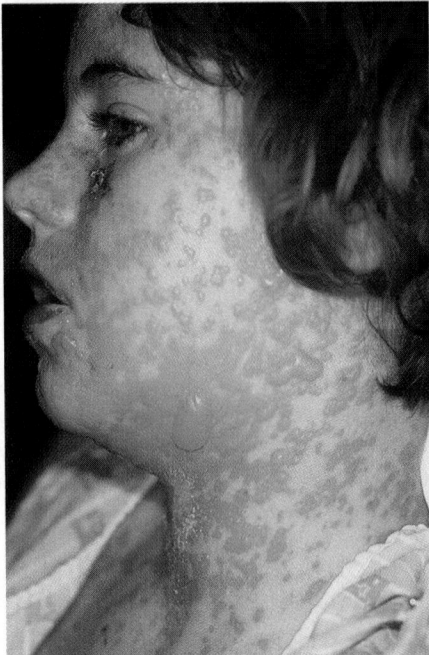

Figure 79-11. Stevens-Johnson syndrome with bulla formation in a girl taking cefaclor (Ceclor).

rhagic crusts appear on the mucous membranes of the eyes, nose, lips, genitalia, and anus (Fig. 79-12). Gingival lesions are more prevalent in Stevens-Johnson syndrome than in erythema multiforme. Involvement of the mucous membranes may precede the skin lesions and is debilitating. Oral pain is severe and limits the patient's ability to eat, drink, and open the mouth. Ocular involvement occurs in most patients with Stevens-Johnson syndrome. Ocular complications include corneal ulceration, corneal opacities, anterior uveitis, symblepharon formation, and blindness. Stevens-Johnson syndrome carries significant morbidity, including secondary infections, fluid and electrolyte imbalances, and multiorgan involvement, and has a mortality rate of 5% to 15%.

Laboratory evaluation is important in assessing the extent of systemic involvement of the hypersensitivity reaction in Stevens-Johnson syndrome. Often a complete blood count reveals a mild leukocytosis and anemia. Marked elevation of the white blood cell count indicates an underlying infection. Electrolytes and renal function are the best screens for

---

Box 79-9. Most Commonly Implicated Factors in Stevens-Johnson Syndrome and Toxic Epidermal Necrolysis

Medications
- Nonsteroidal anti-inflammatory drugs
- Sulfonamides
- Anticonvulsants
- Penicillins
- Tetracyclines

Infection
- *Mycoplasma pneumoniae*
- Herpes simplex virus
- Other viral, bacterial, and deep fungal infections
- Syphilis
- *Mycobacterium tuberculosis*
- Bacille Calmette-Guérin (BCG) immunization

Radiation Therapy

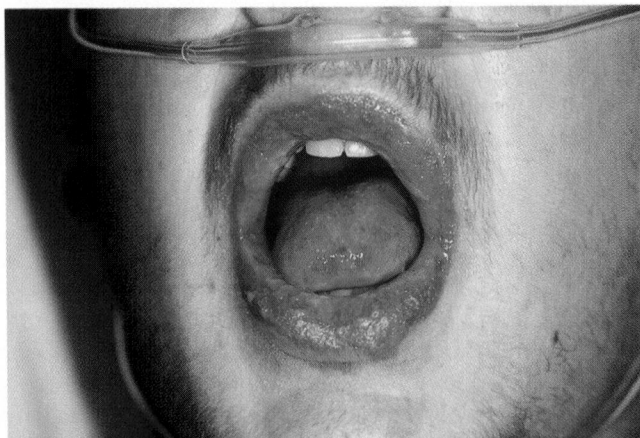

Figure 79-12. Oral mucosal involvement in Stevens-Johnson syndrome.

dehydration and renal involvement. Cultures should be collected if an infection is suspected.

Stevens-Johnson syndrome runs a protracted and severe course. Prompt withdrawal of any medications should be a priority when blisters and erosions appear in a patient suspected of having a drug eruption. Patients with Stevens-Johnson syndrome warrant hospitalization for supportive care, including intravenous fluids and hyperalimentation. The empirical use of systemic antibiotics is not recommended; when there is clinical evidence of secondary infection, antibiotics are directed against the causative organism. Meticulous skin care by nursing staff improves the outcome of the patient. Nonadherent dressings, such as Vaseline gauze, are best for covering and protecting the eroded areas. Oral care consists of gentle débridement of crusts and topical anesthetic mouthwashes, such as a mixture of equal proportions of magnesia and alumina, diphenhydramine, and viscous lidocaine. Oral antihistamines and topical antipruritics may ease pruritus. Ophthalmologic consultation is mandatory. Stevens-Johnson syndrome may require 6 weeks to resolve. Scarring is more common on mucosal than cutaneous surfaces.

TOXIC EPIDERMAL NECROLYSIS

Toxic epidermal necrolysis is a life-threatening hypersensitivity reaction that presents with generalized erythema, diffuse bulla formation (covering >20% of the body surface area), and exfoliation of the epidermis, leaving the dermis exposed (Fig. 79-13). A prodrome of fever, malaise, and upper respiratory symptoms often precedes the cutaneous sloughing. The initial manifestation is the appearance of an erythematous confluent morbilliform eruption associated with pain. Rapid exfoliation of the skin at the dermal-epidermal junction results in peeling of large sheets of necrotic epidermis. Photophobia, conjunctival edema, and ulceration with crusting are common ocular findings that begin shortly after the appearance of the skin lesions. Painful inflammation and blistering of the oropharynx limit oral intake.

Toxic epidermal necrolysis is usually a reaction to systemic medications and should be considered drug-induced necrosis of the skin. The other precipitating factors are outlined in Box 79-9; toxic epidermal necrolysis has been reported with the combined use of natural medications, vitamins, and minerals.

Complications of toxic epidermal necrolysis include dehydration, leukopenia, bacterial infections, and septicemia (most commonly secondary to *Pseudomonas aeruginosa*, *Staphylococcus aureus*, gram-negative bacteria, and disseminated *Candida albicans*), gastrointestinal hemorrhage, and renal insufficiency. Involvement of the bronchial epithelium is suggested when the patient has dyspnea, bronchial hypersecretion, and hypoxemia in the face of a normal chest radiograph. Bronchial injury in toxic epidermal necrolysis portends a poor prognosis and is associated with a high risk of mortality. Bronchopneumonia results in respiratory failure, which may require ventilatory support. Glomerulonephritis is a common complication observed in toxic epidermal necrolysis. Disseminated intravascular coagulation is encountered frequently. Urethral involvement may produce urinary retention and secondary urinary tract infec-

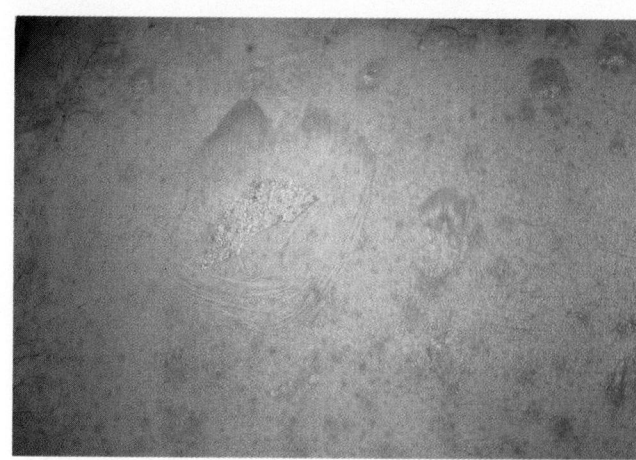

Figure 79-13. Toxic epidermal necrolysis, showing wrinkling of the epidermis that has sheared off the dermis and adjacent erosions with exposed dermis. (Courtesy of the Department of Dermatology, University of Utah, Salt Lake City, Utah.)

tion. Esophageal and vaginal stenosis may occur. Ocular involvement includes symblepharon, entropion, ectropion, trichiasis, and corneal opacities, all of which may lead to blindness. These major complications contribute to the mortality rate of approximately 15% to 40%. When toxic epidermal necrolysis presents in early infancy (<6 months old), it carries an extremely poor prognosis and is almost uniformly fatal.

Initial evaluation of a patient with toxic epidermal necrolysis should include a complete blood count to evaluate for leukopenia, metabolic profile to monitor renal and electrolyte abnormalities, and urinalysis to monitor for hematuria and proteinuria. Cultures should be taken based on the history and signs of infection. Skin biopsy specimens should be obtained as soon as possible to confirm the diagnosis.

Children with toxic epidermal necrolysis are critically ill, have large areas of skin loss, and require specialized skin care. Prompt intervention includes withdrawal of drugs suspected as causative agents, admission to a tertiary burn center, volume replacement and hyperalimentation, removal of devitalized tissue, and application of biologic dressings. Meticulous wound care and close monitoring for secondary infection are required. Prophylactic antibiotics and empirical use of systemic steroids have no proven benefit; systemic steroids may delay wound healing and increase the risk of secondary infection. Early plasmapheresis and administration of intravenous immunoglobulin have halted progression of this severe reaction in some patients. As is true for Stevens-Johnson syndrome, ophthalmologic consultation is mandatory. Adequate analgesia is important in the management of this painful condition.

Additional Resources, CD-ROM

Color atlas	Figures
Unusual conditions:	
Necrobiosis lipoidica diabeticorum	Text, figures
Sweet's syndrome	Text, figure
Leukocytoclastic vasculitis	Text, figure
Urticarial vasculitis	Text, figures

SUGGESTED READINGS

Saulsbury FT: Henoch-Schonlein purpura. Curr Opin Rheumatol 2001;13:35–40.

Vanderhooft SL: Is the rash a drug reaction? Contemp Pediatr 1998;15:118–137.

Weston W: Erythema multiforme, Stevens-Johnson syndrome and toxic epidermal necrolysis. In Harper J, Oranje A, Prose N (eds): Textbook of Pediatric Dermatology. Oxford, Blackwell Science, 2000, pp 628–636.

SECTION 3 GENERAL MEDICAL CARE: *Gastrointestinal and Nutritional Disorders*

80 Approach to the Child with Difficulty Swallowing

Janet K. Harnsberger

ROLE OF THE GENERALIST

1 Recognize the symptoms of dysphagia in each of the pediatric age groups.

2 Identify a likely etiology for the swallowing difficulty.

3 Recognize associated complications of the various causes of dysphagia.

4 Use a detailed history to guide appropriate diagnostics, treatment, and referral.

The impairment of swallowing, *dysphagia*, is a problem seen in all pediatric age groups. Swallowing disorders are common; 7% of the U.S. population complains of dysphagia at some point in their lives. Because the physiology of the movement of food and liquids from the mouth to the stomach is complex, many different problems can interrupt the normal processes of swallowing.

The mechanics of swallowing can be considered in three stages. The initiation of a swallow, the *oral stage*, is under voluntary control. It encompasses the choice and enjoyment of foods, mastication, and the propulsion of a bolus into the pharynx. The *pharyngeal stage* of swallowing, under reflexive regulation through the medulla, is a swift coordinated movement, which allows transit of the bolus, protection of the airway, and opening of the upper esophagus. The final *esophageal stage* of swallowing begins with pharyngeal contraction. The longitudinal esophageal muscles shorten, while the circular esophageal muscles contract in series, creating peristalsis. The primary esophageal peristalsis is initiated in response to the oral act of swallowing. Secondary peristalsis occurs with luminal distention in the esophagus to clear any undigested material or refluxate that is present after the primary peristaltic wave. The relaxation of the lower esophageal sphincter, in reality occurring almost simultaneously with the opening of the upper esophagus, should allow for the movement of the ingestate completely into the stomach.

FUNDAMENTALS

Structural dysphagia occurs if there is a fixed narrowing or an anatomic malformation that inhibits the passage of food and liquids from mouth to stomach. Conditions that alter oral skills and esophageal motility cause *functional dysphagia* (Table 80-1).

Table 80-1. Functional Dysphagia in Pediatric Patients

Oropharyngeal Dysphagia	Esophageal Dysphagia
Inflammatory	**Inflammatory**
Stomatitis	Esophagitis from acid reflux,
Pharyngitis	infection (CMV, thrush, herpes),
Corrosive ingestion	allergy/eosinophilia, corrosive,
Metabolic: thyroid disease,	"pill" induced
diabetes mellitus	Barrett esophagus
Toxic: rabies, tetanus, lead	Crohn disease
poisoning, botulism	Epidermolysis bullosis
Neurogenic	**Generalized Neuromuscular Diseases**
CNS malformations: Chiari,	Myasthenia: maternal/congenital,
syringobulbia	acquired
Stroke, CNS stroke/tumor/trauma	Prematurity
Oculopharyngeal dystrophy	Cerebral and bulbar palsy
Myopathies	Muscular and myotonic
	dystrophy
	Guillain-Barré syndrome
	Familial dysautonomia
Psychogenic	**Rheumatologic Disorders**
Globus	Dermatomyositis/polymyositis
Food aversion	Scleroderma
Miscellaneous	**Isolated Esophageal Neuromuscular Disorders**
Medications that decrease saliva	Nonspecific motility disorders of
production	the esophagus
	Diffuse esophageal spasm
	Achalasia
	Cricopharyngeal
	Lower esophageal sphincter
	Pseudoachalasia

CMV, cytomegalovirus; CNS, central nervous system.

Most children with dysphagia present with complaints of difficulty swallowing, but in newborns and patients with neuromuscular disorders, a careful history may reveal that dysphagia is at the root of a variety of presenting symptoms, such as wheezing, drooling, and failure to gain weight. A guided patient interview should elicit information concerning the age of onset, whether the dysphagia is acute or indolent in development, and the anatomic location of the swallowing difficulty. It is important to determine the degree of swallowing difficulty (i.e., for liquids, solids, hot foods, or cold drinks). Dysphagia may be progressive or intermittent and may be associated with pain on swallowing (odynophagia).

The most common causes of swallowing difficulty vary with age. *Obstructive anatomic abnormalities* of esophageal development present at birth with a history of maternal polyhydramnios. The newborn has a scaphoid abdomen and inability to handle oral secretions. In the toddler and early school-age years, *caustic and foreign-body ingestions* are common causes of acute-onset dysphagia. Older school-age children and adolescents are more likely to have swallowing difficulty as sequelae of *gastroesophageal reflux*. Neuromuscular diseases may present with dysphagia in all age groups, from the earliest signs of cerebral palsy to myotonic diseases of older children. Behavioral dysphagia (temperamental swallowing refusal), perhaps with its teleologic roots in protection from nonfoods and contaminated food, is a functional pediatric problem that is more challenging to manage than the anatomic and motility

abnormalities of the esophagus. *Acute onset of the inability to handle oral secretions indicates that a severe obstruction needs emergency evaluation and intervention.*

A careful history and direct observation of swallowing help locate the likely site and cause of the underlying disorder. *Oropharyngeal* abnormalities are most likely with symptoms of choking, gurgling, coughing, cyanosis, and nasal regurgitation during the initiation of a swallow. There may be accompanying symptoms of voice abnormalities, dysarthria, recurrent pharyngitis, and aspiration when dysphagia is secondary to a supraesophageal etiology. *Esophageal dysphagia* presents most commonly with a sensation of food or liquid "sticking" in the mid- or low substernal area. Rumination and heartburn in the patient's history help to differentiate esophagitis from esophageal stricture.

PRESENTATION AND INITIAL EVALUATION

Table 80-1 lists functional causes of swallowing difficulty, and Table 80-2 lists structural abnormalities that result in swallowing difficulty. A newborn presenting with intolerance of initial feedings and trouble handling oral secretions should have supplemental oxygen, the head of the bed elevated, and an oropharyngeal tube placed gently for suction. A chest x-ray and consultation with the radiologist are needed emergently to evaluate for esophageal atresia, web, duplication, tracheoesophageal fistula, and diaphragmatic hernia. The physical examination should include careful evaluation for choanal atresia, cleft palate, and anomalies associated with congenital syndromes.

Beyond the early newborn period, an infant with a swallowing disorder presents with a wide array of overt and covert symptoms. Gagging, choking, and coughing are recognized easily as dysphagia. More subtle swallowing problems may present with drooling, hoarseness, refusal to eat and drink, posturing during feedings, wheezing, pneumonias, and rumination. A toddler with dysphagia may show any of these symptoms seen in infancy and intolerance to textured foods and oral food hoarding. A communicative child or adolescent easily describes difficulty initiating a swallow or in passing the bolus from pharynx to stomach. A child or teenager who is observed to have prolonged chewing or

Table 80-2. Structural Abnormalities Causing Dysphagia in Pediatric Patients

Oropharyngeal	Esophageal
Choanal atresia	Esophageal stenosis: congenital,
Macroglossia	inflammatory, cicatricial
Cleft lip and palate/submucous	Esophageal atresia/web/ring
cleft	(including Schatzkis)
Laryngeal, pharyngeal, and	Tracheoesophageal fistula
retropharyngeal abscess/	Esophageal diverticula/
neoplasm	duplication
Foreign body/hematoma	Foreign body
Micrognathia	Ectopic tracheobronchial rest
Thyromegaly	Paraesophageal hernia
Lymphadenopathy	Diaphragmatic hernia
Tonsillar hyperhypertrophy	Anomalies of the great vessels
Scarring from tracheostomy/	Thoracic tumors/abscess/
surgery	adenopathy
Zenker diverticulum	

guzzling of liquids during meals should be evaluated for esophageal abnormality.

DIAGNOSIS

Oropharyngeal Dysphagia

Anatomic abnormalities causing *oropharyngeal dysphagia* include clefts of the soft and hard palate, pharyngeal abscesses and hematoma, laryngeal scarring secondary to tracheotomy or other neck surgery, and tumors. These conditions usually are identified readily from the history, physical examination, direct laryngoscopy, and computed tomography of the head and neck. *Functional oropharyngeal dysphagia* is caused by neurologic disease, infection, foreign-body retention, and temperament. Neuromuscular diseases that lead to functional oropharyngeal dysphagia are more common than the anatomic etiologies. Symptoms typically are associated with other neurologic deficits. The dysphagia marks a potentially severe risk for life-threatening aspiration and malnutrition. Bulbar palsy, cerebral palsy, stroke, muscular dystrophy, myasthenia, myotonia, Chiari malformations, and brainstem lesions all may present early in life as swallowing difficulty. A guided barium swallow study done with thick and thin barium liquids and barium-impregnated solids can identify the degree of dysphagia and aspiration risk in patients with functional dysphagia. A more isolated neuromuscular condition, cricopharyngeal incoordination, is currently a subject for study and categorization in pediatric intestinal motility centers. *Infectious causes* of oropharyngeal dysphagia include thrush, herpetic stomatitis, and pharyngitis. A pharyngeal foreign body often presents with remarkable halitosis. *Behavioral oral dysphagia* is diagnosed readily by the history of hoarding and spitting only foods that are disliked. A compassionate approach to the parent and child in the setting of behavioral dysphagia is an important step in developing a therapeutic plan.

Esophageal Dysphagia

Anatomic abnormalities leading to *esophageal dysphagia* are caused by intrinsic and extrinsic obstruction of the esophagus. The congenital anomalies of esophageal formation are listed in Table 80-2. If the anomaly creates a low-grade obstruction, such as seen in H-type tracheoesophageal fistula, diverticulum, duplication, and congenital stenosis, special studies may be needed for diagnosis. The H-type fistula may be shown only by barium esophagography done with the patient in a head-down position or by bronchoscopy. Esophageal stenosis can occur as a congenital anomaly (Fig. 80-1) or can result from inflammatory sequelae of ingestions, impactions, infection, and radiation or chemotherapy. Stenosis may have a normal caliber on ingestion of liquid barium but may impede the passage of a 13-mm barium tablet. Duplications and diverticula not shown with esophagography may require computed tomography to be seen.

There are multiple *inflammatory* causes of *esophageal dysphagia*. The most common in all age groups is esophagitis secondary to gastroesophageal reflux disease. Many pediatric patients with extensive esophageal inflammation do not have esophodynia or heartburn associated with dysphagia. Some cases of *eosinophilic esophagitis* have been

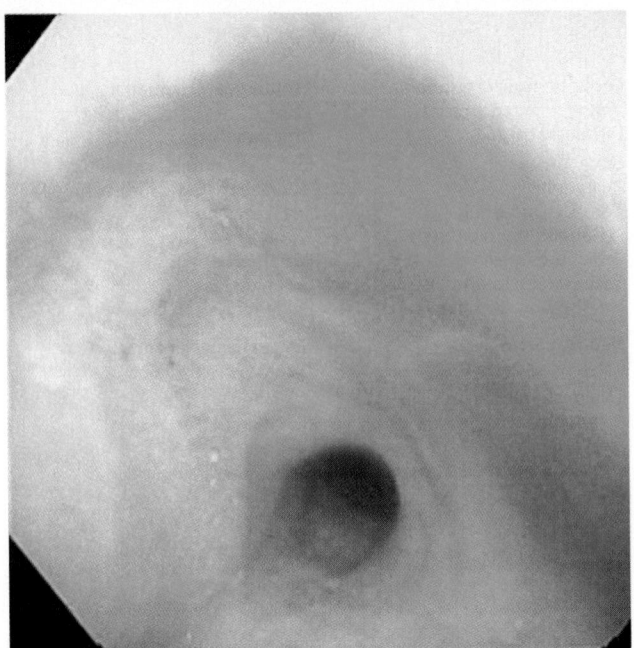

Figure 80-1. Recurrent esophageal stenosis after tracheoesophageal fistula repair.

shown to respond to a hypoallergenic diet and steroid treatment, leading researchers to conclude an *allergic* etiology is present in a subset of esophagitis patients. Crohn disease and connective tissue diseases also can present with esophageal inflammation. *Infectious esophagitis* can be seen in immunocompromised and immunocompetent children and teenagers. With the advent and use of potent broad-spectrum antibiotics, thrush esophagitis (Fig. 80-2) is becoming more common. The prolonged use of gastric acid–suppressant medications also may contribute to persistence of esophageal infections. In addition to *Candida*, cytomegalovirus and herpesvirus can infect the esophageal

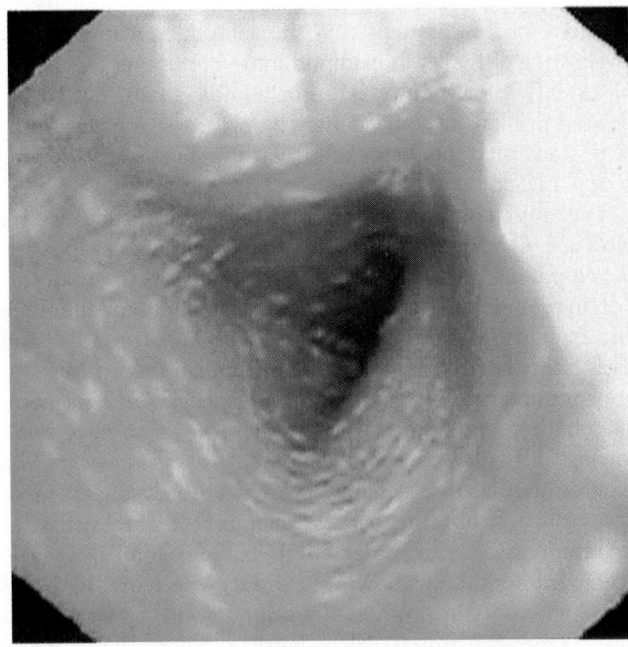

Figure 80-2. Thrush esophagitis in an immunocompetent infant.

mucosa; anti-infective therapy and supportive therapy including hydration and pain management are necessary.

The acute onset of intense substernal pain and dysphagia should suggest traumatic esophagitis as a differential diagnosis. Caustic ingestion carries with it the added concerns of esophageal perforation, stricture, and systemic poisoning. "Pill" esophagitis occurs when a medication is not taken with sufficient water to allow passage into the stomach. Direct pressure from a large capsule and erosion from the medication itself can cause deep ulceration (Fig. 80-3). Pill esophagitis seems to be most common in teenagers taking acne or nonsteroidal anti-inflammatory drugs at bedtime. A careful history often is needed to discover the initial pill ingestion; expectant treatment with liquid pain relievers and fluid nutrition leads to resolution of symptoms within 7 to 10 days.

Medications that impair saliva production also can cause *functional* esophageal dysphagia. Antihistamines, tricyclics, and anticholinergics need to be discontinued if they are interfering with swallowing function. Endoscopy and biopsy of the esophagus is the diagnostic study to determine the nature and extent of esophageal inflammation and to tailor an appropriate treatment plan.

Other *functional esophageal disorders causing dysphagia* can be localized or systemic in origin. Primary esophageal motility disorders cause intermittent dysphagia to liquids and solids. The diagnosis of these disorders may be suggested by history and barium swallow study, but referral for esophageal manometry is needed to confirm the dysmotility. The symptoms of *spastic esophageal motility* disorders are intermittent and usually brought out with hot or cold liquids. There often is chest pain—hence the term *nutcracker esophagus*—associated with the dysphagia. *Globus*, the sensation of something sticking in or blocking the upper esophagus without any demonstrable lesion, suggests an underlying trigger of anxiety. *Achalasia* of the esophagus is diagnosed by two hallmarks: a lack of relaxation in the lower esophageal sphincter and a loss of peristalsis in the lower two thirds of the esophagus. Transport of liquids and solids is progressively impaired as the

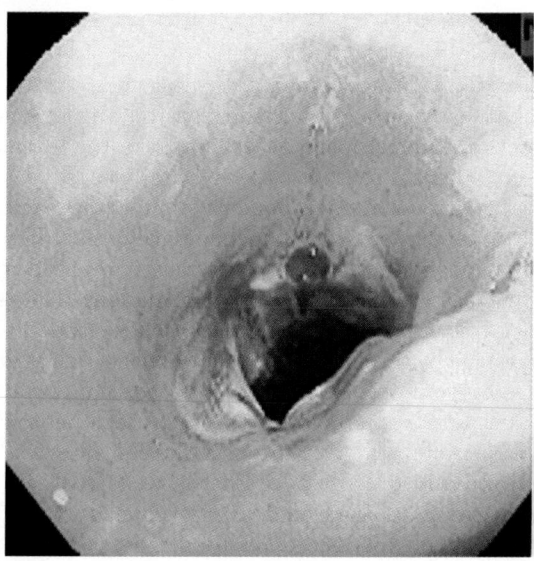

Figure 80-3. Pill esophagitis from a tetracycline capsule in a teenage boy.

Table 80-3. Syndromic Achalasia

Syndrome	Features
Allgrove syndrome	Alacrima, ACTH insensitivity with sensorineural neuropathy, achalasia
Anderson-Fabry disease	Paresthesias, angiokeratomas in skin and mucous membranes, hydrohyphosis, corneal and lenticular opacities, achalasia
Rozychi syndrome	Deafness, vitiligo, muscle weakness, short stature, cricopharyngeal dysphagia from Chiari malformation
McKusick syndrome	Microcephaly, motor neuropathy, dysautonomia, adrenal leukodystrophy, achalasia

achalasia becomes more advanced. Patients give a history of "filling up," literally, with meals. A chest x-ray in a patient with achalasia can show an air-fluid level in the upper esophagus and the shadow of a markedly widened esophageal diameter. Multiple pediatric syndromes include achalasia as a part of their spectrum of symptoms (Table 80-3). As noted earlier, multiple lesions and diseases of the central nervous system also lead to swallowing disorders.

TREATMENT

Therapy for swallowing disorders is directed at the underlying cause. Surgical correction of congenital anomalies, extrinsic obstructions, and inflammatory masses usually is curative. Endoscopic removal of foreign objects and dilation of strictures can allow for either permanent or transient improvement in dysphagia. Repeated dilation in the setting of recurring stricture or spastic esophageal motility disorders sometimes is necessary to treat periodic symptoms. The identification of infection, allergy, or acid irritation leads to effective definitive therapy with diet or medication. Therapy for functional disorders of motility usually is only palliative.

An experienced gastroenterologist should treat achalasia. Therapies available for achalasia include pneumatic dilation of the lower esophageal sphincter, injection of the sphincter with botulinum toxin, surgical myotomy, calcium channel blockers, and nitrates. Other primary disorders of esophageal motility are amenable to treatment by the primary care provider. There are programs available through pediatric physical therapy and speech therapy departments to help patients with swallowing safety and efficiency. Physical therapists and speech therapists can augment swallowing enjoyment and technique and help determine the best food texture, feeding tools, and positioning for effective deglutition. If nutritional sufficiency cannot be attained by oral feedings, nasogastric or gastrostomy tube feedings must be instituted. Pharmacologic therapy with metoclopramide, bethanechol, or hyoscyamine may help many patients with esophageal motility symptoms. Psychotherapy, play therapy, and biofeedback treatment programs are useful for patients with behavioral and anxiety-related dysphagia. *To minimize the risk of esophageal injury, the primary care practitioner should include advice about safe storage of caustic agents and effective pill-swallowing techniques in regular well-child care visits.*

OUTCOME

The outcome of therapy for dysphagia is linked to the successful treatment of the underlying disorder. Esophagitis from acid reflux, allergy, or infection can be expected to resolve with appropriate medication, diet, or surgical intervention. Ancillary health care support from physical therapists and speech therapists can be effective in the development of feeding programs for patients debilitated from neurologic, functional, and emotional conditions. When malnutrition or oropharyngeal aspiration risk is significant, enteric feeds can be used permanently or as a transitional treatment for maintenance of health and growth.

FOLLOW-UP

Effective and comfortable swallowing, important for the maintenance of nutrition, is also one of the vital elements in the enjoyment of life. The identification of the nature and extent of dysphagia allows for a treatment program to be developed that promotes good health and general well-being. Follow-up of the patient should include regular weights, an assessment of long-term swallowing tolerance, and maintenance of appropriate therapies.

SUGGESTED READINGS

Khan S, Orenstein SR, Di Lorenzo C, et al: Eosinophilic esophagitis: Strictures, impactions, dysphagia. Gastroenterology 2000;532:A66.

Rosario JA, Medow MS, Halata MS, et al: Nonspecific esophageal motility disorders in children without gastroesophageal reflux. J Pediatr Gastroenterol Nutr 1999;28:480–485.

Wyllie R, Kay M: Pediatric therapeutic endoscopy: Strictures of the upper gastrointestinal tract and achalasia. Practical Gastroenterol 1997;9–18.

SECTION 3   GENERAL MEDICAL CARE: *Gastrointestinal and Nutritional Disorders*

81

Approach to the Child with Abdominal Pain

Jeffrey Schwimmer and Silvia Buratti

ROLE OF THE GENERALIST

1. Establish a logical, stepwise approach to a child with abdominal pain.
2. Diagnose medical and surgical emergencies.
3. Recognize warning signs of serious disease.
4. Treat the underlying process causing the abdominal pain.
5. Recognize the typical features of functional abdominal pain, and establish an adequate management (education, diet, empirical therapy).
6. Refer the patient to an appropriate specialist when expert assistance is needed for diagnosis or therapeutic management or procedures.
7. Ensure appropriate follow-up and re-evaluate the diagnosis over time, especially if new signs and symptoms occur.

Abdominal pain is a common presenting complaint in children and adolescents. An understanding of the neuroanatomic basis of abdominal pain is essential in the diagnostic process. Different sensory pathways are involved. *Visceral pain* is experienced when noxious stimuli (mechanical or chemical) affect nociceptors in abdominal organs. This pain usually is poorly localized and generally is referred to the periumbilical, epigastric, or suprapubic midline. The pain is described as dull, achy, crampy, or colicky and often is accompanied by secondary autonomic effects, such as sweating, nausea, vomiting, and pallor. *Somatoparietal pain* travels the somatosensory pathways from the parietal peritoneum, abdominal wall, or retroperitoneal skeletal muscles. This pain usually is described as sharp, well localized, and intense, and it is aggravated by movement or coughing. *Referred pain* is experienced in areas remote to the affected organ. This pain is the result of the convergence of visceral afferent neurons with somatic afferent neurons from different anatomic regions at the same spinal segment. The classic example is abdominal pain as initial presentation of pneumonia.

Abdominal pain is classified as acute or chronic. Acute abdominal pain occurs suddenly without any previous history, is considered an emergency, and should be evaluated promptly. Chronic abdominal pain relates to symptoms continuing for 3 or more months and often is referred to as *recurrent abdominal pain*.

ACUTE ABDOMINAL PAIN

Acute abdominal pain is defined as abdominal pain of recent onset that triggers an urgent need for prompt diagnosis and active treatment. Although most children have self-limiting conditions, the challenge for the primary care provider is to identify rapidly conditions that are potentially life-threatening and either treat the underlying condition or refer the patient to an appropriate specialist.

Diagnostic Approach
History
A detailed history is essential in the evaluation of a child with abdominal pain. The age of the child (Table 81-1), the onset (Table 81-2), and site and radiation of the pain (Table 81-3) are helpful in the diagnostic process. The sequence and timing of symptom progression may reveal the extension of the inflammatory process from the viscus to parietal peritoneum (as in appendicitis). Relationship with food, bowel movement, stress, medications, and movement is helpful (e.g., fatty meals trigger biliary colic). Constitutional symptoms (fever, weight loss, anorexia, joint pain), vomiting (bilious, feculent, hematemesis), altered bowel pattern, hematochezia, melena, urinary symptoms, menstrual irregularities, vaginal bleeding or discharge, coughing, and chest pain should be considered.

A detailed past medical history should investigate any prior episode of abdominal pain, trauma or abdominal surgery, exposure to toxic agents or infections (endemic area, travel), medications (antibiotics, steroids, immunosuppressants), and menstrual and sexual history in an adolescent. Pain in the context of chronic disease (renal/liver disease, immune deficiency, sickle cell disease, diabetes mellitus, choledocholithiasis) is likely to be related to the primary condition. The family history may reveal important information (inflammatory bowel disease, peptic ulcer disease, biliary disease, sickle cell disease, porphyria, hereditary angioedema).

Table 81-1. Principal Causes of Acute Abdominal Pain Classified by Age

Infancy	Colic, intussusception, volvulus, incarcerated hernia, perforation, Hirschsprung's disease
Childhood	Gastroenteritis, appendicitis, pancreatitis, urinary tract infection, pneumonia, peptic ulcer disease, Henoch-Schönlein purpura, hemolytic uremic syndrome
Adolescence	Inflammatory bowel disease, peptic ulcer disease, biliary disease, pelvic inflammatory disease, dysmenorrhea, pregnancy, testicular/ovarian torsion

Table 81-2. Characteristics of Abdominal Pain at Onset

Sudden	Perforation, intussusception, torsion, ruptured ectopic pregnancy
Gradual	Inflammatory process (appendicitis, pancreatitis, cholecystitis)
Intermittent	From muscular viscus (intestine, biliary tree, pancreatic duct, uterus, fallopian tube)
Severe constant	Inflammatory bowel disease, sickle cell anemia

Physical Examination
A careful systemic examination determines the degree of illness and uncovers helpful clues for the diagnostic and decision-making process. *General appearance* may reveal typical features of peritoneal irritation (lying quiet), colicky pain (moaning, rocking back and forth), retroperitoneal inflammation (leaning forward), shock (lethargy), or sepsis (toxic state).

The *vital signs* can provide several clues. Fever is usually present during any inflammatory process. Hypertension is possible in Henoch-Schönlein purpura and in hemolytic uremic syndrome. Hypotension or shock is a warning sign of rupture (ruptured ectopic pregnancy). Tachycardia is the response to hypovolemia in intra-abdominal hemorrhage, sepsis, and shock. A patient with peritonitis or pneumonia is tachypneic. Kussmaul's respirations are a typical feature of ketoacidosis.

During the *abdominal examination*, observation can reveal distention, visible peristaltic waves, hernia, or evidence of trauma or previous surgery. Auscultation is helpful in detecting hyperperistalsis, typical of intestinal obstruction or gastroenteritis; hypoactive or absent bowel sounds may be associated with peritonitis. Gentle palpation of the abdomen reveals organ size and the presence of masses, tenderness, rigidity, guarding, and rebound tenderness. Percussion may detect tympany as a result of excessive abdominal gas, whether intraluminal (as in intestinal obstruction) or extraluminal (as in perforation). Rectal examination is indicated in all cases of acute abdominal pain.

Genital and pelvic examination is necessary to exclude conditions such as inguinal hernia, cryptorchidism (or a high-riding testicle), and testicular torsion in boys and vaginal atresia and imperforate hymen in girls. *Skin* should be inspected carefully for rash, petechiae, purpura, jaundice, or other lesions (e.g., erythema nodosum, pyoderma gangrenosum). *Chest examination* may reveal findings suggesting pneumonia. Box 81-1 lists "red flags" from the history or physical examination that should alert the physician to the possibility of urgent or serious medical or surgical conditions.

Table 81-3. Location of Pain and Structures Involved

Epigastric	Esophagus, stomach, duodenum, biliary tree, pancreas
Periumbilical	Small bowel, proximal colon
Hypogastric	Distal colon, bladder, ovary, fallopian tubes
Left upper quadrant	Pancreas, diaphragm
Right upper quadrant	Liver, gallbladder, diaphragm
Shoulder	Diaphragm
Back	Pancreas, peritoneum, sacrum, spine
Right scapula	Gallbladder

Laboratory Workup

All patients with acute abdominal pain should have a complete blood count with differential, serum electrolytes, glucose, creatinine, and urinalysis. Amylase, lipase, and liver function tests should be ordered in patients with upper abdominal pain. A peripheral smear may be diagnostic of hemolytic uremic syndrome or sickle cell disease. *A pregnancy test always should be performed in any postmenarcheal female patient before any radiologic study.* Cultures of cervical and vaginal smears may be helpful if pelvic examination is performed.

Imaging

Plain abdominal films in supine and upright or left lateral decubitus positions may show air-fluid levels, free air, bowel obstruction, calcifications, foreign bodies, or masses. Abdominal ultrasound may be helpful when abdominal films are equivocal or to evaluate liver, gallbladder, pancreas, kidneys, uterus, and adnexa. A computed tomography scan is indicated for patients with abdominal trauma or masses. In patients with respiratory symptoms, a chest x-ray may reveal lower lobe pneumonia. In patients with acute pain in the scrotum, a testicular blood flow scan is diagnostic.

Diagnosis and Management of Acute Appendicits

Acute appendicitis is the most common childhood condition requiring emergency abdominal surgery. Clinical signs and symptoms depend on the stage of the disease at the time of examination. The triad of classic signs and symptoms is abdominal pain, vomiting, and fever.

During the initial phase, the *pain* is periumbilical. As inflammation progresses to involve the serosa, the pain migrates to the point of peritoneal irritation, usually the right lower quadrant. If the appendix is retrocecal, the pain can be lateral or posterior or may mimic signs of septic arthritis. If the appendix perforates, the pain may remit for a brief period and then it becomes generalized. *Emesis* may follow the onset of pain. Anorexia is a much more common symptom, however. *Fever* usually is low grade, unless the appendix has perforated. The onset of pain before vomiting is an important feature in distinguishing appendicitis from infectious enteritis.

Physical Examination

The child may move hesitantly, with a hunched-over posture. If the abdomen is distended on inspection, perforation or obstruction should be suspected. Bowel sounds may be normal or hyperactive in the early stages of the disease and hypoactive as the process progresses to perforation. Palpation should be performed carefully and gently, with examination of the right lower quadrant reserved until rapport with the child has been established. Testing for rebound tenderness and rectal examination should be performed at the end of the examination. If the history and physical examination are convincing, rectal examination can be omitted, but it can be useful in younger children and in adolescent girls.

Laboratory Findings

The diagnosis of appendicitis depends on the clinical examination. A complete blood count and urinalysis may be helpful. Laboratory studies are most useful for excluding other diagnoses. Imaging studies may be helpful if the clinical diagnosis is in doubt.

Treatment

Referral to a surgeon should be made as soon as the generalist has a high suspicion of the diagnosis. Treatment is removal of the appendix. If the appendix has perforated, fluid resuscitation and broad-spectrum antibiotics that cover commonly encountered abdominal organisms *(Bacteroides, Escherichia coli, Klebsiella, and Pseudomonas)* should be instituted (see Chapter 284). Nasogastric suction may be needed if the patient has significant vomiting or abdominal distention.

Diagnosis and Management of Other Causes of Acute Abdominal Pain

If the abdominal pain is severe and a definitive diagnosis cannot be made, the child should be hospitalized for further workup or observation. In the setting of emergency medical care, the management of a child with severe abdominal pain involves basic life support: monitoring of vital signs for early recognition of shock; assessment and management of airways, breathing, and circulation; and establishing intravenous access. The child should not be allowed to take anything by mouth until a diagnosis can be made.

Consultation
Surgeon

In the event of any uncertainty in the diagnosis or when an acute surgical abdomen is suspected, a pediatric surgeon should be consulted immediately. The surgeon often is involved when invasive diagnostic investigations are required (peritoneal lavage, laparoscopy, or exploratory laparotomy).

Gastroenterologist

In some cases, the recognition of typical patterns of abdominal diseases is difficult because one third of patients exhibit significantly atypical features. In these cases and in cases of uncommon gastrointestinal conditions presenting with abdominal pain, a pediatric gastroenterologist should be involved early in diagnosis and management.

CHRONIC ABDOMINAL PAIN

Chronic recurrent abdominal pain is a common clinical problem encountered by primary care physicians. A survey of middle school and high school students revealed that

13% to 17% have weekly abdominal pain, which affected activity in 21%. *Recurrent abdominal pain* is defined as intermittent abdominal pain in children between the ages of 4 and 16 years that persists for more than 3 months and affects normal activity. Classification of recurrent abdominal pain includes five categories: anatomic, infectious, noninfectious inflammatory, biochemical, or functional. A structural or biochemical cause is identified in only 10% of cases; functional abdominal pain (FAP) is the most common cause of recurrent abdominal pain. FAP is a complex neurobiologic disorder. Several studies have shown that patients with FAP have a decreased threshold for perception of abdominal pain; the visceral hyperalgesia may be due to a dysregulation in any part of the pain routes (viscera, extrinsic primary afferent tracts, or central nervous system). Psychological, developmental, and psychosocial factors influence the clinical expression of pain.

Clinical Presentations

Table 81-4 lists Rome II criteria for symptom-based diagnosis of FAP. Children with FAP may exhibit three different clinical presentations. *Isolated paroxysmal pain* refers to FAP that presents as clustering of pain episodes, lasting several weeks or months, during which pain may occur daily. The pain is periumbilical or midepigastric (90%), and radiation is rare. It is more frequently constant than colicky and has no temporal relationship with meals, exercise, or bowel movements. The pain can be variable in nature and severity. It can be associated with symptoms such as nausea, headache, pallor, and dizziness.

Dyspepsia typically is localized to the epigastrium. This presentation may include pain, discomfort, bloating, early satiety, nausea, or vomiting. Other symptoms are heartburn, oral regurgitation, excessive hiccups, and flatulence. There is often a temporal relationship with meal ingestion.

When FAP is *associated with altered bowel pattern (irritable bowel syndrome)*, the symptoms suggest colonic dysfunction and include change in frequency or consistency of the stool, bloating, sense of incomplete evacuation, urgency, straining, pain relieved by defecation, and passage of mucus per rectum. The character of pain is similar to that described for isolated paroxysmal abdominal pain, and dyspeptic symptoms may be present.

Despite the heterogeneous clinical presentations, children with FAP share historical features that are extremely characteristic, as follows:

1. *Physical or psychosocial stress factors.* Physical stress (acute or chronic illness) or psychological stress (abuse, death or separation, school problems, recent geographic moves, financial or health problems in the family) often is reported at the onset of symptoms. Patients with FAP often show signs of internalizing behavior, coping deficits, and social anxiety.
2. *Illness behavior.* Illness behavior includes how symptoms are perceived, evaluated, and acted on. The pain behavior evokes a characteristic reinforcement response from parents, who excuse children from normal life activities and tolerate misbehavior; from school personnel, who send home the child when pain is present; and from physicians, who continue diagnostic testing and empirical medical therapies.
3. *Family history.* Family history may be positive for gastrointestinal disorders (irritable bowel syndrome, peptic ulcer disease), migraine headache, or maternal depression or anxiety.

Diagnostic Approach

Criteria for the diagnosis of FAP include a characteristic history, normal physical examination (except for abdominal pressure tenderness), and negative results of screening laboratory studies, if performed. FAP is not a diagnosis of exclusion; the diagnosis can be made in a positive fashion when the described criteria are identified. Further diagnostic evaluation should be driven by an index of suspicion based on pertinent indicators obtained from history and physical examination.

Key Elements of History

The characteristics of pain should be investigated carefully (chronicity, frequency, severity, character, location, radiation, worsening or relieving factors, associated signs and symptoms, influence on normal activity). Review of systems is often helpful in the differential diagnosis. History of constitutional symptoms and weight loss is particularly important; menstrual and sexual history is mandatory in adolescents. Medication use and past medical history (infections, surgery) also are necessary. Risk factors for parasitic or bacterial infections should be considered. Dietary history may iden-

Table 81-4. Rome II Criteria: Diagnosis of Functional Gastrointestinal Disorders*

Functional Abdominal Pain	Functional Dyspepsia	Irritable Bowel Syndrome
Continuous abdominal pain in a school-age child or adolescent *and*	Persistent or recurrent pain or discomfort centered in the upper abdomen (above the umbilicus) *and*	Abdominal pain or discomfort with at least two of the following: relief with defecation, onset associated with a change in frequency of stool, onset associated with a change in form (appearance) of stool
No or only occasional relationship of pain with eating, menses, or defecation *and*	No evidence (including EGD) that organic disease is likely to explain the symptoms *and*	There are no structural or metabolic abnormalities to explain the symptoms
The pain is not feigned *and*	No evidence that dyspepsia is relieved exclusively by defecation or associated with the onset of a change in stool frequency or stool form	Associated symptoms: abnormal stool frequency (<3 times per week or >3 times per day), stools alternate between hard and loose, straining, urgency, passing mucus, bloating, and abdominal distention
The patient has insufficient criteria for other functional gastrointestinal disorders that can explain the pain	Ulcer-like: pain is the predominant symptom dysmotility-like: fullness, early satiety, and nausea are the predominant symptoms	

*Abdominal pain of at least 12 weeks' duration in the preceding 12 months.
EGD, esophagogastroduodenoscopy

tify nutritional factors in irritable bowel syndrome (fiber intake, sugars). Family history should focus on the presence of gastrointestinal disorders, migraine headaches, and other risk factors (e.g., Middle Eastern ancestors for familial Mediterranean fever). Different psychosocial factors should be investigated, including family structure (maternal depression, overprotectiveness), recent stressful life events, coping style (internalizing behavior), and illness behavior phenomena (e.g., school absenteeism).

Key Elements of Physical Examination

Physical examination is crucial to localize the pain, identify abdominal masses, evaluate the liver and spleen, inspect the perinanal area, and perform a rectal examination with Hemoccult test. A systemic examination for extra-abdominal manifestations of the underlying disease may narrow the differential diagnosis (skin rashes, mucosal ulcerations, joint swelling). Evaluation of growth parameters is essential.

Screening Laboratory Tests

A limited initial screen may include complete blood cell count with differential, erythrocyte sedimentation rate, chemistry profile, urinalysis, and stool studies for enteric bacterial pathogens and parasites. Patients with chronic diarrhea and history of antibiotic therapy should be evaluated for *Clostridium difficile* toxin. Box 81-2 lists red flags that should raise concern that the cause of the abdominal pain is organic and that further investigation is warranted.

Targeted Testing

If signs of malabsorption are identified (diarrhea, bloating), lactose breath hydrogen test should be considered. Abdominal ultrasound is indicated for patients with signs of hepatic, biliary, pancreatic, or renal disease. Upper gastrointestinal series and small bowel follow-through help to evaluate malrotation and Crohn's disease. Esophagogastroduodenoscopy and colonoscopy are used increasingly in clinical practice to evaluate recurrent abdominal pain, especially when signs of nonfunctional disorders are present (see Chapter 273).

Management of Functional Abdominal Pain

FAP is a multidimensional illness that encompasses functional, psychological, cognitive, and social factors. All factors have to be addressed to improve symptoms and prevent social dysfunction. The primary outcome is resumption of a normal lifestyle.

Education

The first step is to create a sympathetic supportive relationship with the patient and family. Parents need to understand that significant pathology has been ruled out and that this problem is common among children. The pain is real, but it can be exacerbated by emotional factors that must be identified and minimized. Lifestyle must be normalized regardless of pain, and illness behavior must be reversed.

Dietary Modification

Foods that may act as provocative stimuli, including high-sorbitol and high-fructose products (candies, fruit juices), carbonated beverages, and dietary starches, should be avoided. If dyspeptic symptoms are present, nonsteroidal anti-inflammatory drugs, caffeine, spicy foods, and fatty foods must be avoided. Small frequent meals may be helpful in preventing early satiety. A high-fiber diet or fiber supplements often are useful to decrease frequency and severity of pain, even if constipation is not evident.

Empirical Therapy

If the above-described measures fail, pharmacologic treatment should be considered and targeted at major symptoms. The role of antidepressants (desipramine, imipramine, amitriptyline) in the management of visceral hypersensitivity has been shown. Relatively low doses are used (0.2 to 0.4 mg/kg or 10 mg before bed and advance toward 25 mg daily). Amitriptyline is recommended in patients with difficulty sleeping or with diarrheal component; imipramine is recommended if constipation is predominant. A trial of antacids or H_2 receptor antagonists for patients with dyspeptic symptoms is reasonable. For the treatment of abdominal pain, anticholinergic medications (dicyclomine hydrochloride, hyoscyamine sulfate) are used frequently. When diarrhea is the predominant symptom of irritable bowel syndrome, antidiarrheal agents (e.g., loperamide) or a bile salt–binding agent (e.g., cholestyramine) seem to be effective.

Referral
Gastroenterologist

A specialist should be involved in the case of failure to respond to appropriate treatment or prompt recurrence of symptoms after stopping medications, when atypical clinical features require a second opinion, for evaluation of less common disorders, or when invasive or specialist diagnostic investigations are considered essential.

Esophagogastroduodenoscopy often is used after failure of empirical therapy to evaluate the presence of mucosal pathology such as acid-related disease, infection *(Helicobacter pylori)*, eosinophilic esophagitis or gastroenteritis, food allergy, or inflammatory bowel disease. Hematemesis, persistent vomiting, dysphagia, odynophagia, intractable pain, and weight loss should prompt endocopic evaluation. Colonoscopy always should be considered in the presence of bleeding or when inflammatory bowel disease is suspected.

Box 81-2. Red Flags: Warning Signs That Should Raise Concern About Nonfunctional Disease and Lead to Further Investigations

- Age <5 years
- Constitutional symptoms (fever, weight loss, growth delay, joint pain, rash)
- Pain awakening patient from sleep
- Pain localized away from umbilicus
- Radiation of pain to back, shoulder, or lower extremities
- Hematochezia (occult blood in stool) or steatorrhea
- Emesis, especially if bilious or blood stained
- Perianal disease (skin tags, fissures, fistulae)
- Family history of significant gastrointestinal disease (e.g., inflammatory bowel disease, peptic ulcer disease)

Psychologist/Psychiatrist

If psychological triggers play a significant role in the onset and perpetuation of symptoms, individual or family counseling may be necessary. Stress reduction techniques (muscular relaxation, biofeedback) help to reduce pain and improve function. Referral to a pediatric psychiatrist or psychologist is indicated if symptoms suggest a psychiatric disorder (anxiety, depression, extreme internalizing behavior).

Gynecologist/Obstetrician

In an adolescent girl, if menstrual dysfunction, pelvic inflammatory disease, or pregnancy is suspected, she should be referred to a specialist.

Outcome

Long-term studies indicate that pain resolves in 30% to 50% of patients within 2 to 6 weeks after diagnosis, suggesting that reassurance, education, and environmental modification are effective. Of patients, 30% to 50% experience pain and 70% develop other chronic complaints (headaches, backaches, menstrual irregularities) as adults. FAP has been suggested as a potential precursor of irritable bowel syndrome in adolescents and young adults.

Additional Resources, CD-ROM

Bibliography

SUGGESTED READINGS

Boyle JT, Hamel-Lambert J: Biopsychological issues in functional abdominal pain. Pediatr Ann 2001;30:32–40.

Hyams JS, Hyman PE: Recurrent abdominal pain and the psychosocial model of medical practice. J Pediatr 1998;133:473–478.

Milla PJ: Irritable bowel syndrome in childhood. Gastroenterology 2001;120:287–290.

Silen W: Cope's Early Diagnosis of the Acute Abdomen. New York, Oxford University Press, 1991.

Young GP: Abdominal catastrophes. Emerg Med Clin North Am 1989;7:699–719.

SECTION 3   GENERAL MEDICAL CARE: *Gastrointestinal and Nutritional Disorders*

82

Approach to the Child with Diarrhea

Mary Ann Limbos

ROLE OF THE GENERALIST

1 Differentiate acute from chronic diarrhea.
2 Diagnose the etiology of diarrhea.
3 Determine the degree of dehydration.
4 Initiate appropriate fluid and dietary therapy.
5 Use appropriate adjunctive therapy in acute diarrhea.
6 Treat acute bacterial gastroenteritis appropriately with antibiotics.
7 Refer patients to specialists as needed for assistance in diagnosis and management.

FUNDAMENTALS

An estimated 4 million children worldwide die from diarrhea and dehydration each year, and many more have malnutrition and delayed growth. In the United States, diarrhea accounts for 20% of acute medical visits for children younger than 2 years of age. Although most children have mild symptoms, each year an average of 220,000 children are hospitalized in the United States, and approximately 300 die from diarrhea. Because stool volumes differ by age and the normal variation in stool number and frequency is large, diarrhea is defined as either an increase in stool frequency or a decrease in stool consistency.

The underlying pathophysiology of diarrhea can be grouped into four categories: osmotic, secretory, motility disorder, and inflammatory. In many disease states, more than one mechanism exists. *Osmotic diarrhea* occurs when malabsorption of a solute creates an osmotic load in the distal small bowel and colon, resulting in increased fluid losses. Osmotic diarrhea stops when feeding is discontinued. An example is diarrhea from excessive intake of juices by toddlers. *Secretory diarrhea* results from active secretion of water and electrolytes, primarily chloride, into the bowel lumen. Stools tend to be large volume and watery. Secretory diarrhea continues even when the patient is not being fed. Because there is no intestinal inflammation, the stool does not contain fecal leukocytes or occult blood. Causes of secretory diarrhea include (1) congenital disorders of fluid and electrolyte metabolism, such as congenital chloridorrhea; (2) mucosal disorders, such as microvillus inclusion disease; (3) tumors, such as neuroblastoma; and (4) infection with enterotoxin-producing bacteria that stimulate adenylate cyclase activity. Disorders that produce either *increased* or *decreased motility* may result in diarrhea. Increased intestinal transit time has been implicated in chronic nonspecific diarrhea, or toddler's diarrhea. Disorders associated with decreased intestinal motility, such as Hirschsprung's disease, may result in bacterial overgrowth in the small intestine, causing mucosal injury and a subsequent inflammatory diarrhea. *Inflammatory diarrheas* are usually acute illnesses with an infectious etiology and are manifested by exudation of mucus, protein, and blood into the gastrointestinal lumen and loss of fluids, electrolytes, and proteins. Noninfectious inflammatory diarrheas include inflammatory bowel disease and celiac disease. Inflammatory diarrheas often are accompanied by secretory, osmotic, and motility-induced components.

Chronic diarrhea is defined as diarrheal symptoms of 2 or more weeks' duration. The differential diagnosis of chronic diarrhea is extensive and varies greatly with the child's age at presentation (Table 82-1). The most common cause of chronic diarrhea in young infants is *cow milk protein intolerance.* Symptoms usually begin at 2 weeks to 2 months of age and include poor feeding, vomiting, diarrhea, and, occasionally, bloody stools. Other manifestations are recurrent respiratory infections, wheezing, chronic rhinitis, and eczema. In severe, protracted cases of formula intolerance, infants may have malabsorption, malnutrition, and failure to thrive. Stools may be positive for reducing substances or have a pH less than 5.5, suggesting carbohydrate malabsorption and small bowel mucosal injury. Leukocytes also may be present, which suggests colitis. Congenital transport defects, such as *congenital chloridorrhea* and *congenital glucose-galactose malabsorption,* may cause diarrhea from birth. Congenital lactase deficiency also causes diarrhea from birth, whereas sucrase isomaltase deficiency produces symptoms after introduction of sucrose into the diet. Other rare causes of chronic diarrhea in infants include microvillus inclusion disease and autoimmune enteropathy, both of which require biopsy for diagnosis. *Hirschsprung's disease* should be considered in any infant with intractable diarrhea because this disease occasionally presents as enterocolitis. *Munchausen syndrome by proxy,* in which a caregiver administers laxatives, needs

Table 82-1. Causes of Chronic Diarrhea

Infants	Toddlers	Older Children and Adolescents
Cow milk, soy protein intolerance	Chronic nonspecific diarrhea	Inflammatory bowel disease
Congenital transport defects	Protracted viral enteritis	Acquired lactase deficiency
Microvillus inclusion disease	Giardiasis	Perforated appendix
Autoimmune enteropathy	Celiac disease	Constipation with encopresis
Hirschsprung's disease	Sucrase isomaltase deficiency	
Munchausen syndrome by proxy	Tumors	
	Inflammatory bowel disease	

to be considered in an infant with unexplained chronic diarrhea.

The most common cause of chronic diarrhea in toddlers is *chronic nonspecific diarrhea,* or *toddler's diarrhea.* Symptoms of intermittent loose watery stools usually begin between 6 months and 2 years of age. The cause of this disorder is unknown. Unless these children are placed on calorie-restricted diets in an attempt to control the diarrhea, growth is unaffected. *Protracted viral gastroenteritis* begins with a viral infection, such as rotavirus. In response to the acute diarrheal illness, the child is fed a high-carbohydrate, low-fat, low-protein diet, including large amounts of hyperosmolar beverages, such as apple juice. An osmotic diarrhea results, and the mucosal injury from the viral enteritis persists. *Celiac disease,* also referred to as *celiac sprue* and *gluten-sensitive enteropathy,* results in chronic small bowel inflammation after ingestion of gluten, a protein in wheat, oats, barley, and rye. Symptoms, which begin when these foods are introduced into the diet, include chronic diarrhea, abdominal pain, poor growth, weight loss, and failure to thrive. Rare causes of chronic diarrhea in toddlers include congenital *sucrase isomaltase deficiency, secretory diarrheas from certain tumors,* and *inflammatory bowel disease.*

Inflammatory bowel disease should be considered in a school-age child with chronic diarrhea but may present simply with growth failure or fever of unknown origin. *Crohn's disease* and *ulcerative colitis* occur with similar frequency. Other symptoms include blood and mucus in the stool and crampy abdominal pain. Growth failure is common, especially in Crohn's disease. *Acquired lactase deficiency* is seen between age 3 and 5 years in children with a genetic predisposition for lactose intolerance, when lactase levels begin to drop. Symptoms include gradual development of flatulence, abdominal pain, and loose stools after ingestion of milk and milk products. A *perforated appendix* may cause diarrhea for several days or weeks from inflammation in the region of the cecum. Occasionally, patients with *constipation* present with a complaint of chronic diarrhea from fecal impaction with overflow incontinence, or encopresis, which is interpreted by caregivers as diarrhea.

Most *acute diarrhea* is caused by infection. Although most cases in children are caused by viral, bacterial, and parasitic pathogens, no specific pathogen can be identified in more than half of children with diarrheal illnesses. Worldwide, *rotavirus* causes more cases of diarrheal disease in children than any other agent. In the United States, it is the most frequently identified pathogen in children requiring hospitalization. Epidemics occur in the late fall and winter months with virtually no cases in the summer. Children between 6 and 24 months old most commonly are affected. Illness begins suddenly with fever, vomiting, and watery diarrhea. Gross or occult blood may be present in the stools. Symptoms last 2 to 8 days. In a few children, the vomiting and diarrhea may be severe enough to cause dehydration. Diarrhea resulting from *enteric adenovirus* infection is generally of longer duration than that from rotavirus and may last 2 weeks. Other viral pathogens in children include the Norwalk virus and caliciviruses. Diarrhea from the Norwalk virus is more common in older children and adults, and symptoms generally last only 24 to 48 hours. Calicivirus has been documented to cause diarrhea in children in day care centers.

Although *Salmonella* infection can have varied clinical manifestations, the most common illness associated with nontyphoidal *Salmonella* organisms is gastroenteritis. Children younger than 5 years old and adults older than 70 are at highest risk for infection. Transmission generally is through animal products, including meat, poultry, eggs, and unpasteurized milk. Fruits and vegetables can transmit the disease if contaminated by infected animals or humans. Other modes of transmission include ingestion of contaminated water; contact with infected reptiles (e.g., pet turtles); and contact with contaminated medication, dyes, or medical instruments.

Symptoms of *Shigella* can range from mild watery diarrhea with minimal or no constitutional symptoms to profuse watery diarrhea with fever, headache, and malaise. Abdominal cramping and tenderness, tenesmus, and stools containing blood or mucus or both are characteristic of large bowel disease (bacillary dysentery). Seizures sometimes can occur. Although the Shiga toxin is neurotoxic, it is now believed that the fever accompanying the *Shigella* infection causes seizures. Feces of infected humans serve as the source of infection; there is no known animal reservoir for *Shigella*. Infection also may be transmitted through ingestion of contaminated food or water, contact with a contaminated inanimate object, and anal intercourse. Flies can serve as vectors of infection by physically transporting infected feces.

Campylobacter jejuni is found in the gastrointestinal tract of domestic and wild birds and animals. Transmission occurs through ingestion of contaminated food, such as unpasteurized milk or untreated water, or by direct contact with fecal material from infected animals or persons. *Campylobacter* infection usually presents as frequent, watery stools and fever. Occasionally the diarrhea is bloody. Abdominal pain is common and may mimic appendicitis. Most patients recover without treatment in less than 1 week, although 20% of individuals have a more severe, prolonged illness.

Escherichia coli that cause diarrhea are classified into four major groups based on pathogenic mechanism of disease. Enterotoxigenic *E. coli* and enteropathogenic *E. coli*

are major causes of infantile diarrhea in underdeveloped countries; the former also is the causative organism in traveler's diarrhea. *E. coli* that causes a dysentery-like illness and enterohemorrhagic *E. coli*, which causes hemorrhagic colitis, are enteroinvasive. Enterohemorrhagic *E. coli* infection, specifically infection with *E. coli* 0157:H7, is of particular importance in the pediatric age group because of the risk of hemolytic uremic syndrome.

Infections with *Clostridium difficile* include antibiotic-associated diarrhea and pseudomembranous colitis. When antimicrobial therapy diminishes the normal intestinal flora, *C. difficile* proliferates and elaborates toxins. Penicillins, clindamycin, and cephalosporins are associated most frequently with C. *difficile* colitis, but almost every antibiotic has been implicated. *Aeromonas hydrophila* typically causes diarrheal disease in children younger than 2 years old. Symptoms range from mild watery diarrhea to bloody stools to persistent diarrhea.

Giardia lamblia is the most common intestinal parasite in the United States and is contracted through contaminated food or water or by person-to-person contact. Children present with loose watery stools, crampy abdominal pain, and weight loss secondary to malabsorption. *Entamoeba histolytica* can cause several different clinical syndromes, including noninvasive intestinal infection, intestinal amebiasis, acute fulminant colitis, ameboma, and liver abscess. More severe disease is seen in immunocompromised patients, very young patients, and patients with malnutrition. Patients with noninvasive intestinal infection may be asymptomatic or have vague gastrointestinal tract complaints, whereas patients with intestinal amebiasis generally have 1 to 3 weeks of diarrhea, often with grossly bloody stool, abdominal pain, fever, and weight loss.

DIAGNOSIS

Because the morbidity and mortality associated with diarrhea in young children stems from dehydration, the first step in evaluation is assessment of the degree of dehydration. Documentation of change in the child's weight is the most accurate method. Other clinical indicators crucial to the initial evaluation are accurate vital signs, determination of mental status—done most easily by observing the child's interaction with the environment—and a focused physical examination to identify signs of dehydration. This quick assessment should determine whether a child is dehydrated and allows classification of dehydration as mild (equivalent to a 3% to 5% loss of body weight), moderate (6% to 9% of body weight), or severe ($\geq$ 10% loss). Moderate and severe dehydration require immediate, emergent stabilization and management.

Initial assessment should be followed by a detailed history and thorough physical examination. The diarrhea first should be classified as acute or chronic, with chronic diarrhea being defined as having persisted for a minimum of 2 weeks. The stool should be characterized, including frequency, color, estimated volume, and presence of blood or mucus. In cases of acute disease, pertinent historical facts include ill contacts, recent travel, ingestion of unusual foods, day care attendance, contact with pets or other animals, and recent antibiotic use. In chronic diarrhea, the history should be guided by the age of the patient, seeking details to support or eliminate the conditions listed in Table 82-1 and described in the fundamentals section. In acute diarrhea, history of vomiting, amount of fluid intake, and types of fluids given help guide the need for laboratory evaluation and management. Nutritional data, growth data, and family history are particularly important in chronic diarrhea.

Important findings on physical examination include vital signs; mental status; fever; capillary refill time; and general appearance, including signs of malnutrition, such as presence of a potbelly or muscle wasting. Skin should be examined for color, tone, and presence of rashes. The abdomen should be examined carefully for tenderness, bowel sounds, masses, and organomegaly. Rectal examination may reveal perianal skin tags (Crohn's disease), impaction (chronic constipation), or tenderness (perforated appendix).

Most children with diarrhea do not need laboratory evaluation. Children with frequent or prolonged vomiting or who have signs of severe dehydration should have serum electrolytes measured. Diagnosis of rotavirus can be made by examining stool for rotavirus antigen (enzyme-linked immunosorbent assays) or antibodies to rotavirus particles (radioimmunoassay, latex particle agglutination, immunofluoresence, and immunoelectron microscopy.) C. *difficile* is diagnosed by detecting the toxin in the stool. Stool can be examined microscopically for blood, leukocytes, and ova and parasites. Microscopic examination for G. *lamblia* cysts may be normal in 50% of patients; examination of three specimens increases the sensitivity to 95%. Stool cultures should be obtained only if the diarrhea is bloody or if examination of a fecal smear reveals white blood cells.

Children with chronic diarrhea may need additional testing or procedures such as colonoscopy or barium enema, which require the assistance and expertise of specialists.

MANAGEMENT OF ACUTE DIARRHEA

Management of chronic diarrhea depends on the etiology of the disease and is discussed in the chapters on each specific disease entity (see Mini-index). Management of acute diarrhea generally consists of supportive care. Antimicrobial therapy is indicated only in specific conditions.

Fluid Therapy

The cornerstone of management is fluid and electrolyte replacement. For mild-to-moderate dehydration, oral rehydration therapy is the preferred method. Oral rehydration is safe, rapid, and inexpensive and has been shown to be as effective as intravenous solutions in achieving hydration. It is less invasive than intravenous therapy, can be administered at home, and costs only about 12% of a similar course of intravenous therapy. Intravenous fluid therapy is required for children with shock or severe electrolyte imbalances and for children who fail to improve on oral therapy. Intravenous fluid resuscitation is discussed in Chapter 28. Treatment of children with electrolyte disorders is discussed in Chapter 42.

The principal underlying oral rehydration is the phenomenon of coupled transport. When one glucose molecule is absorbed across the intestinal epithelium, one sodium ion travels with it in an obligatory, linked fashion (Fig. 82-1). Clinical observations have confirmed that adding glucose to

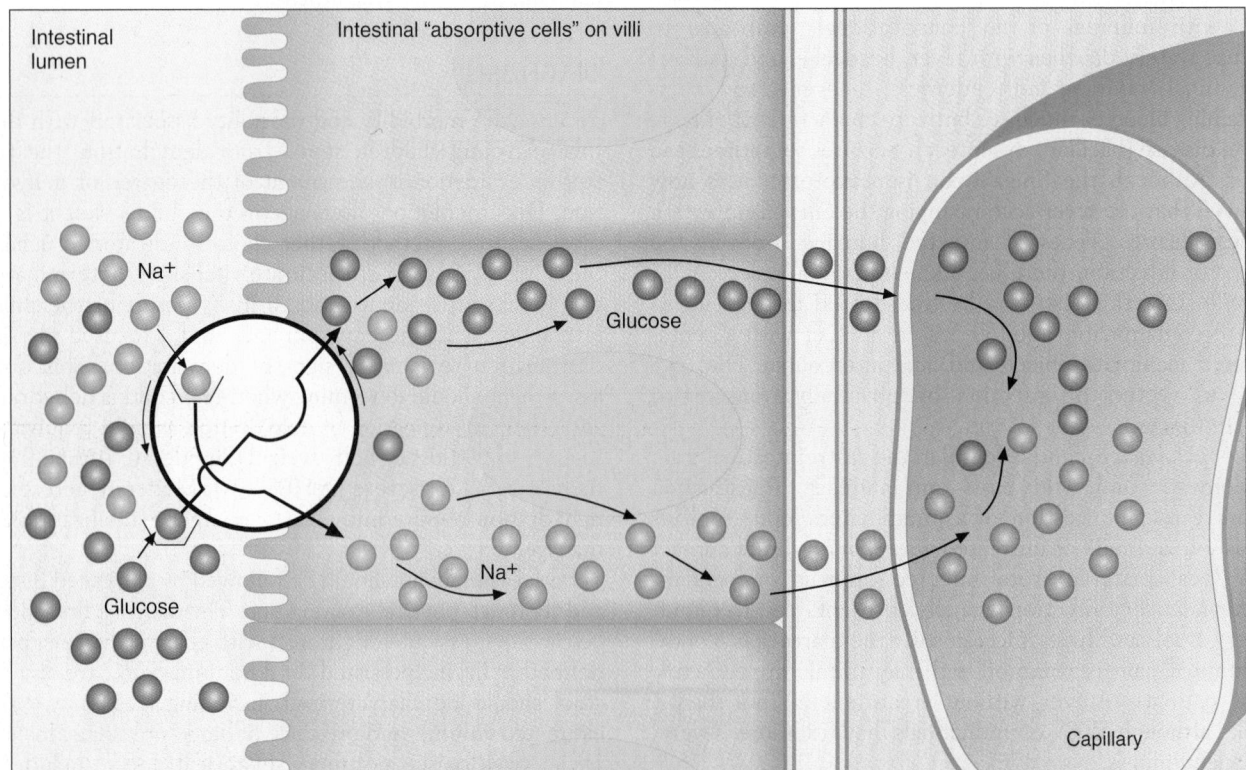

Figure 82-1. The cotransport mechanism of sodium and glucose. Every glucose ion that crosses the intestinal epithelium brings a sodium ion with it, increasing the concentration of ions in the bloodstream and pulling water out of the gut. (Redrawn with permission from Kevin A. Somerville. Copyright 1995.)

Table 82-2. Composition of Oral Rehydration Solutions and Common Clear Liquids

	Carbohydrate (g/L)	Sodium (mEq/L)	Potassium (mEq/L)	Base (mEq/L) (citrate or bicarbonate)	Osmolarity (mM/L)
Recommended					
WHO ORS	20 (glucose)	90	20	30	310
Pedialyte	25 (glucose)	45	20	30	270
Infalyte	30 (rice syrup solids)	50	25	30	200
Not Recommended					
Cola	50–150 (glucose and fructose)	2	0.1	13	550
Apple juice	100–150 (glucose and fructose)	3	20	0	700
Chicken broth	0	250	5	0	450
Gatorade	45 (glucose, fructose, and sucrose)	20	3	3	330
Tea	0	0	0	0	5

WHO ORS, World Health Organization oral rehydration solution.

sodium-containing solutions used for patients with cholera results in the net movement of sodium and fluid from the intestines into the bloodstream. Maximal uptake of water and electrolytes from the intestinal lumen occurs when the carbohydrate-to-sodium ratio is 1. Carbohydrate-to-sodium ratios of 3:1 have been shown to be safe and effective. The American Academy of Pediatrics recommends using higher sodium solutions containing 75 to 90 mEq of sodium per liter for initial rehydration. After rehydration, solutions with lower sodium concentrations (40 to 60 mEq/L) are recommended until a normal diet is re-established. Most commercially available solutions in the United States have sodium concentrations ranging from 45 to 50 mEq/L. Although these products are best used as maintenance solutions, they can be used to rehydrate children who are mildly to moderately dehydrated. Composition of oral rehydration solutions and commonly used clear liquids are presented in Table 82-2.

Glucose-based rehydration solutions do not reduce stool volume or frequency, and they do not shorten the duration of illness. Cereal-based solutions contain polymers from starches and simple proteins. Although composed of many molecules, these polymers have the same osmotic effect as a single molecule. When the polymer is hydrolyzed at the intestinal cell surface, its glucose or amino acid components

are absorbed quickly into the bloodstream, bringing sodium and water with them (Fig. 82-2). Despite the large number of molecules created by digestion of the polymer, the osmolarity of the gut is not increased because of rapid uptake by the villus cells. Studies evaluating mixtures made from rice or wheat indicate they are at least as effective for rehydration as glucose-based solutions. A meta-analysis showed that compared with glucose-based oral rehydration solutions, rice-based solutions reduced stool volume by a mean of 32% in children with cholera and by 18% in children with noncholera diarrhea. Duration of diarrhea was reduced by 8 hours in both groups. Decreasing stool volume and duration of diarrhea holds potential benefits for a child's nutritional status and may decrease the use of potentially harmful medications, such as antidiarrheal agents and antibiotics. Cereal-based and rice-based solutions are not commercially available at present and should not be confused with available solutions that derive their carbohydrate from glucose polymers purified from rice or with homemade rice water solutions that have low concentrations of glucose and glucose polymers. Many commonly used liquids, such as fruit juices, teas, sports drinks, and carbonated beverages, have low electrolyte concentrations and high concentrations of sugars (see Table 82-2). Fruit juices in particular may exacerbate diarrhea because of their

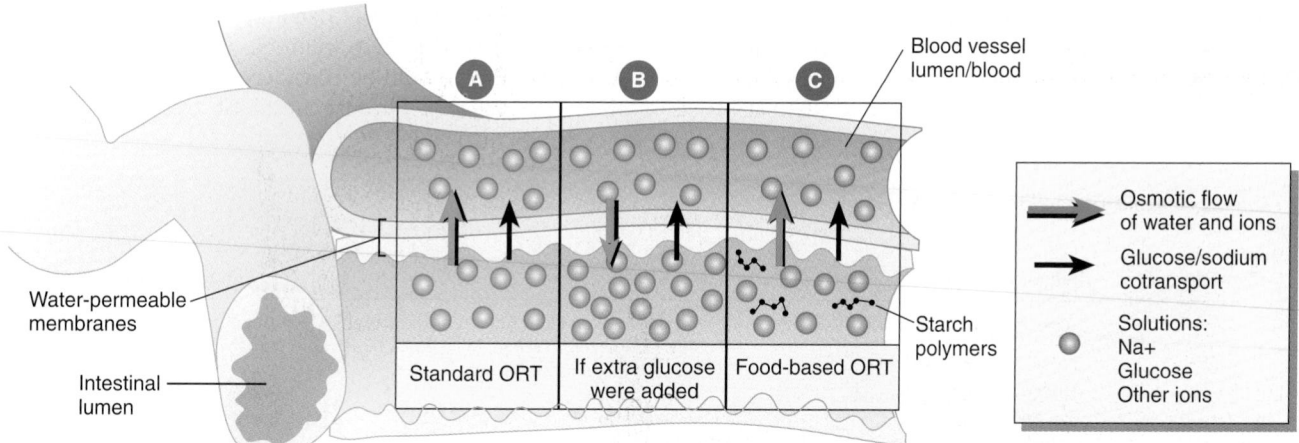

Figure 82-2. Effective rehydration depends on the composition of fluids. ORT, oral rehydration therapy. (Redrawn with permission from Kevin A. Somerville. Copyright 1995.)

high osmolarity. Parents should be discouraged from using these nonphysiologic liquids to treat children with diarrhea.

Successful oral therapy requires not only the appropriate solutions, but also a technique for ensuring that the child drinks adequate amounts. The volume required is determined by the amount of dehydration present (Table 82-3). Almost all children with vomiting and dehydration can be rehydrated orally. The key is to offer the oral rehydration solution in small quantities at short intervals. Small volumes of 5 to 10 mL can be given slowly by spoon, syringe, or medicine cup every 15 to 20 minutes. As dehydration and electrolyte imbalances are corrected, vomiting often lessens in frequency. As the vomiting decreases, larger amounts of solution can be given at longer intervals until the child can drink normally. Stool losses should be replaced with approximately 10 mL/kg of oral solution for each diarrheal stool.

Oral rehydration solution can be administered via a nasogastric tube in the emergency department in a child who refuses to drink or who has frequent vomiting. Nasogastric infusion also can be used as a temporary measure while intravenous access is being established. Nasogastric infusion is contraindicated in a child who is comatose or who may have an ileus or intestinal obstruction.

Dietary Therapy

Early refeeding with an age-appropriate diet is an important component of therapy for children with diarrhea. Even a few days of fasting results in substantial intestinal villus atrophy and a decrease in absorptive surface area. Children with no or mild dehydration should be fed throughout their illness, whereas children with moderate-to-severe dehydration should begin feeding as soon as possible after rehydration. Taking a stepwise approach from diluted to full-strength formula is unnecessary. Unrestricted diets do not worsen the course or symptoms of mild diarrhea and can decrease stool output compared with fluid therapy alone.

The use of cow milk formula during an acute diarrheal episode is controversial. Numerous clinical trials have shown that children tolerate lactose-containing diets as well as lactose-free diets if they had no or mild dehydration or if they have been rehydrated appropriately after being moderately to severely dehydrated. Although intestinal brush border damage can produce a transient lactase deficiency, most children have no clinical signs or symptoms of malabsorption and can resume breast-feeding or their regular formula safely. The few children who have worsening diarrhea when a lactose-containing formula is reintroduced can be placed on a soy-based formula temporarily. Clinical trials

on refeeding have suggested that foods low in fats and simple sugars and high in complex carbohydrates are tolerated better. These foods include breads, cereals, starches, lean meats, yogurt, fruits, and vegetables. The traditional BRAT diet of bananas, rice, applesauce, and toast, although generally well tolerated, is low in energy density, protein, and fat.

Treatment of milk protein intolerance is elimination of milk from the diet. Alternatives include soy or hydrolyzed milk protein formulas. Of infants with cow milk protein intolerance, 30% to 50% also have soy protein hypersensitivity. Most patients respond well to protein hydrolysate formulas, although occasionally amino acid formulas may be required. For toddler's diarrhea, a high-fat, low-carbohydrate diet has been found to improve symptoms by reducing osmotic load and decreasing intestinal motility. Toddler's diarrhea is a self-limiting disease and usually resolves spontaneously before age 4. Children with protracted viral gastroenteritis respond well to a diet high in protein and fat. Contrary to popular belief, lactase deficiency is usually not a significant problem, and in most cases, a lactose-free diet is unnecessary.

Adjunctive Therapies

Antimicrobial therapy for acute bacterial diarrhea is summarized in Table 82-4. Antibiotics are indicated only in specific situations because bacterial gastroenteritis generally is self-limited, and the clinical effectiveness of antibiotics has not been established clearly for some pathogens even when in vitro susceptibility is shown.

Antibiotics do not shorten the duration of disease in *Salmonella* infection and can promote asymptomatic carriage and excretion of the organism. Treatment is indicated for patients at risk for developing invasive disease, including infants less than 3 months of age and patients with malignancies, hemoglobinopathies, human immunodeficiency virus infection and other immunosuppressive conditions, chronic gastrointestinal tract disease, or severe colitis. Antibiotics are indicated for *Shigella* because they shorten the duration of symptoms and decrease excretion of the organism.

Treatment of *C. jejuni* infection usually is not necessary because symptoms are mild and resolve quickly. Organisms can be excreted for 7 weeks, however. Antibiotic therapy can decrease excretion and should be considered for children attending day care centers. Antibiotic therapy for *E. coli* diarrhea should be considered only if the diarrhea is moderately severe. Because antibiotic treatment in *E. coli*

Table 82-3. Fluid Therapy for Diarrhea

Degree of Dehydration	Rehydration Phase	Maintenance Phase	Stool Replacement
None	None. Proceed to maintenance phase	*Infants:* Breast milk or full-strength formula *Older infants and children:* Milk, foods high in complex carbohydrates	10 mL/kg ORS for each diarrheal stool
Mild (3–5%)	ORS 50 mL/kg (over 4–6 hr)	Same as above	Same as above
Moderate (6–9%)	ORS 100 mL/kg	Same as above	Same as above
Severe (≥10%)	IV fluids: 20 mL/kg of normal saline until vital signs normalize, then 100 mL/kg IV fluids or ORS	Same as above	Same as above

IV, intravenous; ORS, oral rehydration solution.

Table 82-4. Antimicrobials for Acute Bacterial Gastroenteritis in Children

Organism	Effectiveness of Antibiotics	Preferred Agent	Alternate Agent(s)	Comments
Salmonella	Not effective	Third-generation cephalosporin	TPM-SMZ, ampicillin, fluoroquinolones	Antibiotics indicated only for patients with or at risk for invasive disease; high rates of resistance in some areas to TMP-SMZ Fluoroquinolones are not recommended for children <18 years old except when potential risks are less than potential benefits
Shigella	Highly effective	Third-generation cephalosporin	Ampicillin, TMP-SMZ, azithromycin, fluoroquinolones	High rates of resistance in some areas to TMP-SMZ See previous comment regarding fluoroquinolones
Campylobacter	Effective; indicated in some circumstances	Erythromycin, azithromycin	Tetracycline	Tetracycline should not be used in children <8 years old
Enterotoxigenic *Escherichia coli*	Effective; indicated in some circumstances	TMP-SMZ		

TMP-SMZ, trimethoprim and sulfamethoxazole.

0157:H7 infections increases the risk of developing hemolytic uremic syndrome, antimicobial therapy should not be started until the stool culture confirms that the strain of *E. coli* is one that is treated appropriately with antibiotics. In infections with *C. difficile*, the diarrhea stops simply by discontinuing the offending antibiotic. Treatment with oral metronidazole is recommended if the diarrhea persists or is severe, or if the antibiotics must be continued. Metronidazole is the treatment of choice for *G. lamblia*. A 5- to 7-day course of treatment has a cure rate of 80% to 95%. If therapy fails, the course can be repeated. Metronidazole followed by a luminal amebicide is the recommended treatment for mild-to-moderate intestinal amebiasis.

Bismuth subsalicylate, an over-the-counter medication widely used for the treatment of diarrhea, has antimicrobial, antisecretory, and anti-inflammatory properties. It has been shown to be effective as prophylaxis and treatment of travelers' diarrhea. Although bismuth subsalicylate at doses of 100 to 150 mg/kg/dose has been shown to decrease stool output and duration of diarrhea significantly without adverse effects, its use cannot be recommended routinely for the treatment of diarrhea in children because of concerns about potential toxicity.

Antimotility agents, such as loperamide (Imodium) and diphenoxylate with atropine (Lomotil), are not indicated in the management of acute diarrhea in infants and young children and should be used with caution in older children. Although effective for the symptomatic relief of diarrhea, these agents have harmful and potentially fatal side effects, including sedation, respiratory depression, and ileus. Because inhibition of intestinal motility can lead to overgrowth of the infecting organism, these agents are contraindicated in children with bloody or inflammatory diarrhea.

Probiotics, such as *Lactobacillus* and *Bifidobacterium*, have been used in acute diarrhea to alter the intestinal microflora. When an episode of diarrhea diminishes the intestinal flora, production of short-chain fatty acids is reduced, and colonic absorption of water is impaired. Although oral administration of bacteria, such as *Lactobacillus*, *Bifidobacterium bifidum*, and *Streptococcus thermophilus*, has been shown to shorten the course of the diarrhea, evidence that probiotics significantly alter the course of acute diarrhea in

children still is limited, and their use is not recommended routinely.

PREVENTION

The most powerful tool for controlling diarrheal illness is prevention. Prevention includes simple interventions, such as promoting breast-feeding and encouraging good personal hygiene, particularly good hand washing. On a global scale, no intervention has had as great an impact as ensuring a safe water supply. Research is ongoing to develop safe and effective vaccines against diarrheal pathogens such as rotavirus and cholera.

SUGGESTED READINGS

American Academy of Pediatrics, Provisional Committee on Quality Improvement, Subcommittee on Gastroenteritis: Practice parameter: The management of acute gastroenteritis in young children. Pediatrics 1996;97:424–433.

Branski D, Lerner A, Lebenthal E: Chronic diarrhea and malabsorption. Pediatr Clin North Am 1996;43:307–331.

Laney DW, Cohen MD: Approach to the pediatric patient with diarrhea. Gastroenterol Clin North Am 1993;22:499–516.

83 Approach to the Child with Constipation

Mary Ann Limbos

ROLE OF THE GENERALIST

1 Diagnose constipation by history, physical examination, and ancillary tests if indicated.

2 Distinguish functional constipation from Hirschsprung disease and other organic causes.

3 Manage chronic constipation in three phases: disimpaction, maintenance, and weaning.

4 Treat functional constipation using a combination of dietary measures, pharmacologic therapies, and behavioral modification techniques.

DEFINITION

Constipation is a common pediatric complaint, accounting for nearly 5% of all outpatient visits to a primary care physician and 20% to 25% of referrals to pediatric gastroenterologists. *Constipation* is defined as delay or difficulty in defecation that is present for 2 or more weeks and that is sufficient to cause significant distress to the patient. It is characterized by the infrequent passage of hard, painful stools. The definition of constipation suggests there is a departure from the normal stooling pattern. Because of the normal variation of frequency of bowel movements at different ages of childhood, some clinicians prefer to define constipation simply as the difficult passage of large or hard stools, regardless of the frequency. Constipation is a symptom and not a diagnosis. Box 83-1 lists the differential diagnoses of nonorganic constipation. Table 83-1 lists organic causes. Most infants and children with constipation have functional, or nonorganic, constipation.

Box 83-1. Differential Diagnosis of Constipation: Nonorganic Causes of Constipation

- Coercive toilet training
- School bathroom avoidance
- Fear of toilet
- Sexual abuse
- Attention deficit disorder

Table 83-1. Differential Diagnosis of Constipation: Organic Causes of Constipation

Disease Classification	Disease Entities
Dietary	Low-fiber diet
	Dehydration
	Malnutrition
Endocrine/metabolic	Hypothyroidism
	Hypercalcemia
	Hypokalemia
	Cystic fibrosis
	Diabetes mellitus
	Gluten enteropathy
Neurologic	Congenital aganglionic megacolon (Hirschsprung disease)
	Myelomeningocele/spinal cord abnormalities
	Botulism
Anatomic malformations	Imperforate anus/anal stenosis
	Anterior ectopic anus
	Pelvic mass
Collagen vascular disease	Scleroderma
	Lupus
	Dermatomyositis
Drugs	Opiates
	Phenobarbital
	Tricyclic antidepressants
	Antacids
	Antihypertensives
	Anticholinergics
Other	Lead poisoning

FUNDAMENTALS

Pathophysiology

The colon reabsorbs fluid and electrolytes, serves as the storage organ for fecal material, and conducts feces along its length from cecum to rectum. Fecal material is emptied rapidly from the cecum and the ascending colon and then generally remains in the transverse colon for several hours. The descending colon conducts stool into the sigmoid colon, where it is stored. After ingestion of a meal, colonic contractions propagate down the sigmoid colon, which delivers stool into the rectum (gastrocolic reflex).

Defecation is controlled by the pelvic complex, consisting of two overlapping muscle sphincters that form a funnel-like structure surrounding the anus. Figure 83-1 illustrates the anatomy of the anorectum and explains the process of defecation. If defecation is not convenient or is painful, the external anal sphincter and the gluteal muscles can be

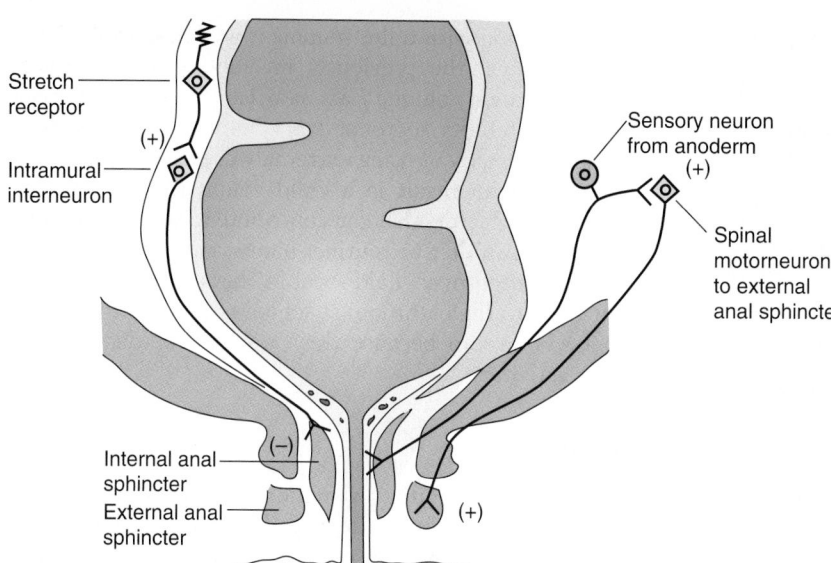

Figure 83-1. Anorectum, internal anal sphincter involuntary smooth muscle, and external sphincter voluntary skeletal muscle. Continence is maintained by resting tonic contraction of internal anal sphincter. Stretch receptors are activated when greater than 15 mL of stool enters rectum. Inhibitory neurons decrease the resting tone of the internal anal sphincter. Stool reaches the external anal sphincter, creating the urge to defecate. During defecation, squatting position straightens the anal canal, Valsalva maneuver increases intra-abdominal pressure, the external anal sphincter relaxes, and the rectum is evacuated of stool. (Adapted from Rudolph CD, Benaroch L: Hirschsprung disease. Pediatr Rev 1995;16:5–11. Copyright 1995.)

tightened voluntarily, pushing the fecal mass back into the rectal vault. The urge to defecate subsides until the rectum is distended again. Repetitive stool withholding leads to stretching of the rectum and, eventually, the lower colon, producing a reduction in muscle tone and retention of stool. The longer the stool remains in the rectum, the more water is removed, resulting in a larger and harder stool that gradually becomes impacted.

Encopresis

Unresolved constipation may lead to fecal retention, impaction, and eventually overflow incontinence. Encopresis, or the involuntary passage of stool from the anus, usually results from stool leaking or overflowing from a rectum that has been distended by retained stool. Anorectal motility studies show decreased sensitivity to distention in a chronically distended rectum, and the child is not aware of the soiling until it is nearly complete. Encopresis is three to six times more common among boys than girls and usually presents between 3 and 7 years of age. Most children have a history of chronic problems with stooling. Rarely, voluntary soiling may occur in children from anxiety or severe passive-aggressive behavior.

Hirschsprung Disease

Hirschsprung disease, or congenital aganglionic megacolon, is the most common cause of lower intestinal obstruction in neonates and must be considered in the differential diagnosis of any child with severe constipation. It is a relatively rare condition, occurring in 1 in 5000 births. The male-to-female ratio is 4:1, and there is no racial predilection. Although a clear pattern of inheritance has not been established, there seems to be a strong genetic influence. A positive family history is found in 7% of cases, whereas 21% of cases with total colonic aganglionosis have an affected family member. Several syndromes are associated with Hirschsprung disease, the most common being Down syndrome. Other associated conditions include Waardenburg syndrome, Smith-Lemli-Opitz syndrome, Laurence-Moon-Bardet-Biedl syndrome, congenital deafness, and congenital central hypoventilation (Ondine's curse).

Hirschsprung disease is characterized by the absence of intramural ganglion cells of the submucosal (Meissner's) and myenteric (Auerbach's) plexus from the distal rectum to a variable length proximally. The pathogenesis of the disease is believed to be an arrest of the migration of ganglion cell precursors from the neural crest to the distal bowel during early embryogenesis. In 75% to 80% of affected children, the aganglionic segment does not extend above the sigmoid colon. The entire colon and some small bowel may be involved in the 3% of children who have long-segment Hirschsprung disease.

The presentation of Hirschsprung disease is variable and depends on the length of colon involved. Presentation occurs before 3 months of age in more than 60% of affected individuals and by 1 year of age in 80%. Fewer than 10% of patients present after 3 years of age. Short-segment and ultra-short-segment (<5 cm) Hirschsprung disease more commonly is present at later ages. Infants with Hirschsprung disease commonly exhibit constipation, abdominal distention, vomiting, diarrhea, or failure to thrive. The classic sign to suggest Hirschsprung disease in a neonate is delayed passage of meconium. Almost all full-term infants pass their first meconium stool within 48 hours after birth. Because only 40% of infants with Hirschsprung disease have delayed passage of meconium, normal passage of meconium does not exclude the diagnosis of Hirschsprung disease. Occasionally, infants may develop bowel obstruction with perforation or enterocolitis and sepsis. These infants are ill appearing and present with sudden onset of fever; abdominal distention; and explosive, bloody diarrhea. These complications occur most often during the second or third months of life in infants with undiagnosed Hirschsprung disease and have an associated mortality of 20%. Older children with short-segment or ultra-short-segment disease may present only with constipation that is recalcitrant to medical therapy. Historical points and physical examination findings that raise suspicion for Hirschsprung disease are presented in Table 83-2 and are compared with findings that suggest functional fecal retention.

An unprepared barium enema is often the initial study in the evaluation of a child with possible Hirschsprung

Table 83-2. Comparison of Hirschsprung Disease with Functional Fecal Retention

Signs and Symptoms	Hirschsprung Disease	Functional Fecal Retention
Delayed passage of meconium	Common	Rare
Symptoms from birth	Common	Rare
Soiling	Rare	Common
Obstructive symptoms	Common	Rare
Large-caliber stools	Rare	Common
Stool-withholding behavior	Rare	Common
Stool in rectal ampulla	Rare	Common

disease. The barium enema examination may show the transition zone at the junction of the dilated, normally innervated proximal colon and the narrowed, aganglionic distal colorectal segment. This sign may be absent in the first few weeks of life, however, because the normal ganglionic bowel may not have had sufficient time to dilate with stool. In addition, the barium enema may not show a transition zone in cases of Hirschsprung disease in which the entire colon is involved or in ultra-short-segment disease. The diagnosis of Hirschsprung disease cannot be excluded by barium enema alone.

Rectal biopsy and anorectal manometry are the only two tests that can exclude the diagnosis of Hirschsprung disease reliably. Anorectal manometry evaluates the response of the internal (involuntary) anal sphincter to the inflation of a balloon in the sphincter. When the rectal balloon is inflated, normally there is a reflex relaxation of the internal anal sphincter. In Hirschsprung disease, there is no relaxation because the inhibitory reflex is absent. There may even be a paradoxical contraction of the sphincter. Anorectal manometry is particularly useful when the results of radiologic or pathologic studies are equivocal or the aganglionic segment is short. If relaxation is normal, the diagnosis of Hirschsprung disease can be excluded. If manometry results are abnormal, diagnosis should be confirmed with a biopsy.

A tissue biopsy specimen of the rectal wall showing the absence of ganglion cells in the submucosal plexus is required to make a definitive diagnosis of Hirschsprung disease. If ganglion cells are shown on suction biopsy, Hirschsprung disease can be excluded. If no ganglion cells are present, a full-thickness biopsy often is performed to obtain a better tissue sample.

Functional Constipation

Functional fecal retention, or functional constipation, with voluntary withholding of stool, is the most common cause of constipation in childhood. Functional constipation usually is initiated by the passage of a hard, painful stool or the fear of the toilet. This situation begins a cycle of events in which the child voluntarily tightens the external anal sphincter and contracts the gluteal muscles to prevent the passage of stool. With chronic stool hoarding, the stool becomes larger and harder and causes even more pain when eventually passed, perpetuating the cycle. Many events can lead to stool withholding. The association of functional fecal retention with toilet training is well described. During toilet training, the previously involuntary act of stooling must become a voluntary act associated with social expectations. Attempts to toilet train before a child is developmentally ready or using extremely coercive toilet training techniques can result in a child voluntarily holding back stool. Other factors that can contribute to stool withholding are changes in diet or routine, illness, and stressful events. Older children may "hold stool in" because they are reluctant to go to the bathroom at school or may postpone going to the bathroom because they are busy or distracted by other activities.

DIAGNOSIS

The goal in the initial evaluation of infants and children with constipation is to identify the small number of children with an organic cause for their constipation and begin appropriate care. A thorough history and physical examination and screening laboratory and radiographic investigations when indicated allow the primary care provider to differentiate functional fecal retention from organic causes of constipation; to begin treatment of functional constipation; and to refer children with an organic cause of constipation to a pediatric gastroenterologist or other specialist.

History

Evaluation of a child who presents with constipation often can be limited to a thorough history and physical examination. After determining what the family and child are considering as "constipation," a complete birth and medical history should be obtained. Important information to obtain in this history include timing of the passage of meconium; the length of time the constipation has been present; frequency, consistency, and size of the bowel movements; whether the child has painful bowel movements or abdominal pain; the presence of blood on the stool or toilet paper; and use of medications. "Red flags" in the history that could be signs of an organic disorder include fever, abdominal distention, anorexia, vomiting, or weight loss. A history of retentive posturing, infrequent stooling in the toilet, and soiling strongly suggest functional fecal retention. Although sometimes overlooked, a psychosocial history can provide important clues as to the cause of constipation. Elements of the child's psychosocial history that are important to assess include family structure, the child's interactions with peers, and the possibility of abuse.

Physical Examination

The aim of the physical examination is to identify signs of systemic disease. The physical examination should begin with documentation of height and weight and, if the information is available, a review of previous growth velocity. Areas of particular focus are the abdomen, the rectum, and the lumbosacral area. The abdominal examination should assess distention and the presence of masses. Stool may be palpable in the sigmoid and distal colon in the left lower quadrant and above the pubic symphysis. Inspection of the anal area can show fissures, ulcerations, or hemorrhoids (rare in children) and the position of the anal opening relative to the vaginal or scrotal fourchette (to assess for possible anterior ectopic anus). The anal reflex, or anal wink, is a visible contraction of the external anal sphincter in response to stroking of the perianal skin and, when present, confirms the integrity of the sensorimotor pathway that maintains continence.

A digital rectal examination to assess rectal tone and the amount and characteristic of stool in the rectal ampulla is recommended at the initial evaluation, although this may not be achievable in all patients. The child should be positioned as comfortably as possible, either on the examination table or on the parent's lap. The normal rectal ampulla is dilated slightly and may contain stool. Hard stool in a dilated rectum suggests functional constipation. One also should palpate for masses or asymmetries along the rectal wall. Finally, the lumbosacral area should be inspected for hair tufts, dimples, or vascular lesions that may signify an underlying spinal deformity.

Role of Radiographs

An abdominal radiograph is not indicated routinely in the evaluation of a child with constipation. Radiographs are indicated in a child with a good history for constipation who does not have large amounts of stool on rectal examination. Other specific cases in which a radiograph may be helpful include a child who is obese in whom an abdominal and digital rectal examination is difficult; a child who refuses a rectal examination; and a child with critical psychological factors, such as sexual abuse.

Role of Laboratory Tests

Laboratory investigations are indicated if suggested by findings of the history or physical examination or if appropriate therapy has been ineffective. These tests include thyroid function tests, serum electrolyte levels including calcium and magnesium, lead level, and celiac disease antibodies.

MANAGEMENT

Referral to a Specialist

Children who do not respond to therapy or whose management has become complex should be referred to a pediatric gastroenterologist. When an organic cause is suspected from the history, physical examination, or screening laboratory tests mentioned previously, referral to a gastroenterologist or other specialist may be appropriate (see Chapter 89).

Management of Functional Constipation

The management of children with functional constipation can be divided into three therapeutic phases: disimpaction, maintenance, and weaning (Table 83-3). The important first step before initiating therapy is to educate the child and family and to demystify constipation by explaining its possible causes. If there is associated encopresis, it is important to explain to the family and child why the soiling is occurring. Education should continue throughout the treatment process.

Phase 1: Disimpaction

The first phase of therapy requires removal of the hard fecal mass and the emptying of the rectum completely either by enemas or by oral agents. In uncontrolled clinical

Table 83-3. Treatment of Functional Constipation

Phase 1: Disimpaction (2–3 days)	Phase 2: Maintenance (3–12 mo)	Phase 3: Weaning

Enema
  Mineral oil
  Hypertonic
    phosphate
  Milk and molasses
Oral/nasogastric
  Mineral oil
  Polyethylene glycol
Manual disimpaction
  (rarely needed)
	Oral laxatives
	High-fiber diet
	Increased fluid intake
	Behavior modification
		Tapering of
		  laxative dose
		High-fiber diet
		Increased fluid
		  intake

trials, the oral route, the rectal route, and a combination of the two all have been shown to be effective for disimpaction. Although the rectal route is faster, children with functional constipation already are sensitized to pain in the anal area and may be unwilling to have any intervention per rectum. Although the oral route is less invasive, large doses of oral medications are required. It may be difficult for the child and family to adhere to the treatment regimen. The choice of treatment is best determined after discussing the options with the family and child. Phosphate soda enemas, saline enemas, or mineral oil enemas followed by a phosphate enema have been used and are effective for rectal disimpaction. Milk and molasses enemas mixed 1:1 also have been found to be effective and safe in a child without a cow milk allergy. Parents should be cautioned to allow the mixture to cool before it is inserted. *Enema preparations of soapsuds, tap water, and magnesium are not recommended because of their toxicity.* Hypernatremia and hyperphosphatemia have been reported in infants and young children after use of commercially available hypertonic phosphate (Fleet) enemas.

The recommended regimen for rectal disimpaction is a series of two to three enemas given 1 day apart. For a child who refuses an enema or fails enema therapy, disimpaction can be accomplished with large doses of mineral oil (1 oz per year of age up to 8 oz/dose given twice daily for 2 to 3 days). Some children with severe constipation may require admission for nasogastric administration of polyethylene glycol electrolyte solution. In rare cases of a large impacted mass, a pediatric gastroenterologist or surgeon must be consulted for manual disimpaction under sedation.

Phase 2: Maintenance

After successful disimpaction, maintenance therapy is begun and consists of laxatives, dietary changes, and behavioral modification. The primary goal of maintenance therapy is for the child to have one or two loose bowel movements daily. Loose stools ensure that they will not be painful, that the child will not be able to hold the stools in, and that the rectum will be emptied completely. Lactulose, milk of magnesia, and mineral oil are effective oral laxatives that are safe even for long-term use. The choice of laxative should be based on the child's preference, ease of administration, and safety. The starting dose should be adjusted to achieve the goal of one to two loose stools per day. Palatability of the medications can be increased by mixing them with various foods and beverages. Because the maintenance phase of therapy requires months of laxative use, parents may express concerns about the safety of long-term use and laxative dependence. Most of the medications used to treat constipation when given appropriately are safe for long-term use. Mineral oil should not be used in young children or children who are neurologically impaired because of the risk of lipid pneumonitis if it is aspirated.

Dietary changes that commonly are advised include increased intake of fluids and dietary fiber. A balanced diet that includes whole grains, fruits, and vegetables should be recommended rather than adherence to a strict diet.

Behavioral modification should focus on establishing regular toilet habits. Parents of young children can be taught appropriate toilet training techniques. A positive reinforcement program with a reward system can be used with older children. Using a calendar with stickers, children can record each stool that is passed in the toilet. Biofeedback also has been used successfully with older children.

Phase 3: Weaning

When the child has had months of painless, daily bowel movements, the laxative dose can be tapered gradually. One recommendation is a decrease in laxative dosage of 25% every 1 to 2 months. During this weaning period, the child must continue to have daily painless bowel movements. If the child stops having regular bowel movements or has painful bowel movements, the laxative dose should be increased to previous levels for several more weeks. Frequent office visits every 4 to 8 weeks is essential to monitor compliance and provide ongoing education and support to the family.

TREATMENT OUTCOMES

Treatment failures occur in about 20% of children with encopresis. Failure is more likely in children with a longstanding problem that has had a negative impact on their self-esteem or in children who receive a secondary gain from encopresis. A small subgroup of children with fecal soiling have what is termed *antisocial soiling, or nonretentive functional soiling*, and require psychological intervention. These children do not have a history of prior constipation, and they have no evidence of fecal retention on radiographic examination. They generally display other maladaptive behaviors. Laxative therapy in these children worsens their soiling behavior.

Mini-index of Related Topics

SUGGESTED READINGS

Abi-Hanna A, Lake AM: Constipation and encopresis in childhood. Pediatr Rev 1998;19:23–30.
Baker SS, Liptak GS, Colletti RB, et al: Constipation in infants and children: Evaluation and treatment. J Pediatr Gastroenterol Nutr 1999;29:612–626.
Parker PH (guest ed): Pediatric Constipation and Encopresis. Pediatr Ann 1999;28(5):283–290.

84

Approach to the Child with Gastrointestinal Bleeding

George Gershman

Gastrointestinal (GI) bleeding in pediatric patients is uncommon. It could be a sign of various diseases either localized to the GI tract or more generalized and systemtic. Knowledge of age-specific causes of GI bleeding, along with the details of different clinical presentations, can help with appropriate diagnostic and therapeutic actions.

DEFINITIONS

There are four ways for blood loss from the GI tract to occur: hematemesis, melena, occult bleeding, and hematochezia. *Hematemesis* is vomiting of blood that may be "fresh" and bright red or old, brown, and denatured; the latter commonly is described as "coffee-ground" emesis. Usually, hematemesis reflects bleeding from the esophagus, stomach, or proximal duodenum. Swallowing of maternal blood in neonates and epistaxis in older children should be ruled out to avoid unnecessary invasive procedures. *Melena* is liquid, black, tarry, foul-smelling stool. It suggests bleeding from the upper GI tract. Occasionally, the site of bleeding can be found in the ileum or right colon.

Occult bleeding in pediatric patients, defined as a guaiac-positive stool, is secondary to blood loss, which is often chronic. There are two ways of testing for occult bleeding: the Hemoccult test and the Hemoquant test. Hemoccult stool test is the reaction of a dye, guaiac, with peroxidase-containing substances and hydrogen peroxide. It is not specific for presence of blood (hemoglobin) in stool. False-positive results can be caused by peroxidase activity in cantaloupes, radishes, bean sprouts, cauliflower, broccoli,

grapes, red meat, and iron preparations. False-negative results of the Hemoccult stool test can occur because of prolonged colonic transient time and bacterial degradation of hemoglobin to porphyrin, which does not have peroxidase activity. An alternative assay is the Hemoquant test (SmithKline Diagnostics Inc., San Jose, California), which is specific because it fluoresces hemoglobin-derived porphyrin and is qualitative and quantitative. Disadvantages are that the test is time-consuming and requires a reference laboratory.

Hematochezia is the passage of bright red blood per rectum. As a rule, it is a sign of lower GI bleeding from the distal ileum or colon. Because hematochezia may occur with massive bleeding from the duodenum, bleeding from the upper GI tract should be ruled out first to ensure the appropriate management of an unstable patient.

GI bleeding may be acute or chronic. Acute bleeding is more dramatic. The child may be in shock even before hematesis, melena, or hematochezia becomes obvious. Chronic blood loss usually manifests with pallor, fatigue, lightheadedness, or irritability. The patient's respiratory system and hemodynamics may be stable, but if the bleeding is untreated, decompensation eventually occurs.

ASSESSMENT AND INITIAL MANAGEMENT

Initial assessment of a child with suspected GI bleeding should be focused and rapid. Four major questions (Box 84-1) must be answered promptly. Red food and medications can stain stool or vomitus. Cranberry juice, beets, candies, amoxicillin, phenytoin, and rifampin can change color of stool and vomitus to red or burgundy. Bismuth, activated charcoal, iron, spinach, blueberries, and licorice can simulate bleeding by black staining of vomitus and stool.

An appropriate history, a normal physical examination, guaiac-negative stool, and Gastroccult test (SmithKline Diagnostics Inc., San Jose, California) negative vomitus are sufficient to rule out a true bleeding episode. Hematemesis

Box 84-1. Essential Questions in the Assessment of Gastrointestinal Bleeding in Children

1. Is the bleeding real?
2. Is the patient stable?
3. Where is the source of bleeding?
4. What is the best approach to hemostasis?

and melena can be secondary to epistaxis. A quick examination of the nose and oropharynx can lead to the correct diagnosis.

A prompt examination to assess blood loss and determine the degree of shock should be done using objective criteria, such as skin color, pulse, blood pressure, capillary refill, urinary output, mental status assessment, and orthostatic maneuvers (see Chapter 28). Special attention should be focused on tachycardia, which could be the earliest sign of shock. Hypotension is an ominous finding because it usually occurs in the late phase of shock in children. Good venous access has to be established simultaneously for adequate volume resuscitation (see Chapter 295). Two large-bore peripheral intravenous lines or a central line should be placed and secured. Blood should be typed and screened. Resuscitation should be completed before any diagnostic procedure is done. If the source of bleeding is not obvious, the placement of a nasogastric tube is useful. The largest bore tolerable tube should be placed for adequate gastric lavage and decompression in an unstable patient. Room-temperature normal saline solution is an optimal fluid for this procedure. Iced saline lavage is not recommended because it may induce hypothermia, especially in infants, and can cause platelet dysfunction. A bloody or coffee-ground aspirate indicates upper GI bleeding, if swallowed blood (e.g., epistaxis) was ruled out. The absence of blood in the stomach does not exclude an upper GI bleed because the source of bleeding can be in the duodenum. The presence of coffee grounds in a gastric aspirate that promptly clears by gastric lavage suggests that bleeding has stopped. Fresh blood with or without clots that does not clear rapidly indicates ongoing bleeding from the esophagus, stomach, or duodenum.

Laboratory data that are immediately helpful include hemoglobin, mean corpuscular volume, and blood urea nitrogen. Anemia (low hemoglobin) with normal red blood cell indices indicates rapid blood loss. Elevated blood urea nitrogen in patients with acute bleeding suggests absorption

of blood in the small intestine, poor renal perfusion, or both. Low hemoglobin and low mean corpuscular volume in hemodynamically stable patients is consistent with chronic GI blood loss. Intensity and persistence of lower GI bleeding can be assessed based on characteristics of stool. Stool should be examined for presence of fresh blood, clots, streaks of blood, or guaiac-positive stool and stool output, combined with serial hemoglobin, hematocrit, and red blood cell count.

When the patient has been stabilized, the source of bleeding becomes the target question. Detailed history and physical examination help determine the cause. Jaundice, hepatomegaly, spider hemangiomas, prominent vessels of the abdominal wall, and ascites are signs of chronic liver disease and suggest portal hypertension as the possible source of bleeding. GI bleeding in an acutely ill, febrile child could be secondary to sepsis-induced ulceration of the stomach or the duodenum or a coagulopathy. Careful assessment of the perineum can reveal fissures, fistulae, or perianal induration.

DIAGNOSIS AND MANAGEMENT

Knowledge of common causes of GI bleeding in age-specific groups of children helps with the diagnostic strategy (Table 84-1).

Neonates

In the first few days of life, hematemesis or bloody stools in otherwise healthy neonates most likely are caused by swallowed maternal blood, either during delivery or during breast-feeding. In such cases, the Apt test should be performed to differentiate between maternal and infant blood. The Apt test is based on the chemical reaction of adult hemoglobin with sodium hydroxide, which leads to a color change from bright red to yellow or crusty brown. Fetal hemoglobin is resistant to hydroxylation, and blood

Table 84-1. Common Causes of Gastrointestinal Bleeding in Children

Age	Upper GI Bleeding	Lower GI Bleeding
Neonates (0–30 days)	Swallowed maternal blood Hemorrhagic disease of the newborn Stress ulcers/sepsis Hemorrhagic gastritis	Necrotizing enterocolitis Midgut volvulus Anal fissure Hirschsprung disease Vascular malformation
Infants (30 days–6 mo)	Cow milk or soy protein allergy Esophagitis Mallory-Weiss tear Portal hypertension	Anal fissure Allergic proctitis or enterocolitis Nodular lymphoid hyperplasia Intussusception
Infants and children (6 mo–6 yr)	Epistaxis Esophagitis Portal hypertension Drug-induced ulcers Gastritis	Anal fissures Intussusception Meckel diverticulum Nodular lymphoid hyperplasia Polyps Infectious colitis Hemolytic uremic syndrome Henoch-Schönlein purpura
Children and adolescents (7–18 yr)	Epistaxis Drug-induced gastropathy and ulcers Peptic ulcer Esophagitis Gastritis Portal hypertension	Infectious colitis Ulcerative colitis Crohn disease Polyps Polyposis Hemorrhoids

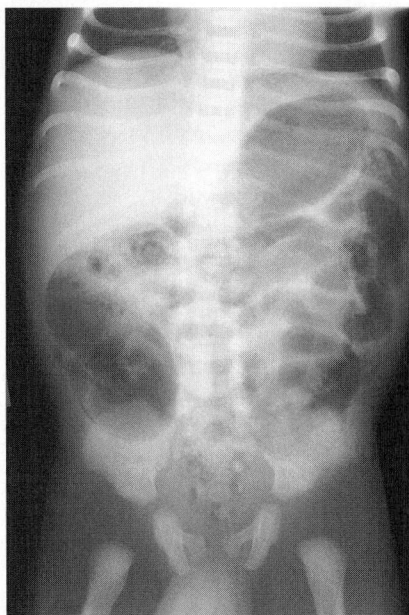

Figure 84-1. Plain film of abdomen (kidney, ureter, and bladder) in a 1-day-old infant shows distention in the cecal region and probable intramural gas to the right of the first lumbar vertebra. (Courtesy of Michael J. Diament, MD, Pediatric Radiology Department, Harbor–UCLA Medical Center.)

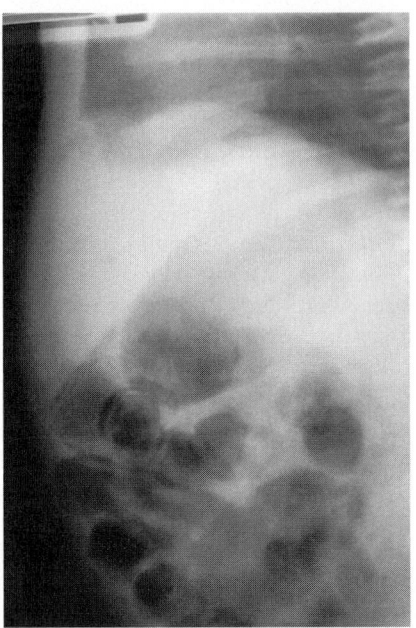

Figure 84-2. Lateral view of the abdomen obtained at the same time in the same patient as in Figure 84-1 shows definite portal venous gas. (Courtesy of Michael J. Diament, MD, Pediatric Radiology Department, Harbor–UCLA Medical Center.)

from the infant remains bright red. Anal fissures are a common cause of bleeding in neonates. A fissure is initiated by passage of a firm stool that makes a small tear along the anal canal. Hemorrhagic disease of the newborn is rare in the United States and other developed countries. Breast-feeding neonates who did not receive vitamin K are at greatest risk. Acute gastric or duodenal ulcerations should be suspected in a stressed or septic infant. GI bleeding is a common manifestation of necrotizing enterocolitis, particularly in preterm neonates. The warning signs of necrotizing enterocolitis are abdominal distention, feeding intolerance with increased gastric residuals, mild diarrhea, and stool positive for blood and reducing substances.

Plain x-rays show nonspecific distribution of bowel gas, pneumatosis intestinalis (Fig. 84-1), or gas in the portal vein (Fig. 84-2), reflecting the degree of bowel ischemia. Rare causes of GI bleeding in the first months of life include Hirschsprung enterocolitis, midgut volvulus, duplication cyst, and vascular malformation.

Infants to 6 Months of Age
One of the leading causes of GI bleeding in infants younger than 6 months old is enterocolitis from cow milk or soy protein allergy. The spectrum of symptoms includes recurrent vomiting with or without hematemesis, failure to thrive, and diarrhea with guaiac-positive stools or hematochezia. Rarely, exclusively breast-feeding infants may develop similar symptoms, secondary to the presence of antigenically intact protein from the maternal diet in breast milk. Maternal dietary protein restriction is often successful when infants have eosinophilic proctitis and less effective in infants with enterocolitis or IgE-mediated disease. Most infants with milk-related hypersensitivity intestinal disease improve within the first week of treatment with hydrolyzed protein formulas.

Intermittent rectal bleeding with streaks of frank blood mixed with normal-appearing stool could be secondary to *nodular lymphoid hyperplasia* of the colon or terminal ileum. Multiple hemispheric smooth nodules less than 5 mm, with or without halos of hyperemia, can be seen in clusters or diffusely throughout the GI tract (Fig. 84-3). It is considered to be a response of lymphoid tissue to variety of antigens (e.g., food-related or infectious [viral]). Spontaneous regression of lymphoid follicles is the rule. In addition to parental reassurance, an elimination diet for nursing mothers is a reasonable initial treatment. If food allergy is strongly considered on the basis of positive family history of eosinophilic infiltration of the lamina propria, feeding with a hydrolyzed protein formula is the next step

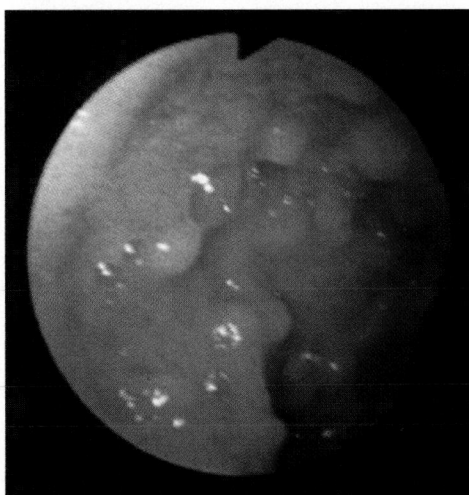

Figure 84-3. Nodular lymphoid hyperplasia in an infant with recurrent episodes of rectal bleeding. Multiple, 3- to 4-mm hemispheric nodules are seen in the terminal ileum. Similar nodules can be found in the colon or duodenum.

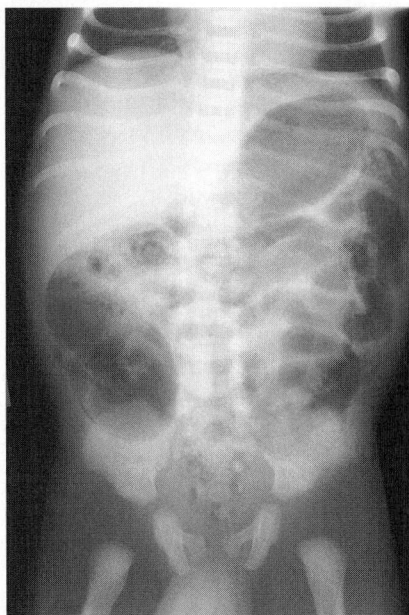

of the therapy. Corticosteroid therapy is restricted to infants with a severe form of this disease who present with significant anemia, persistent rectal bleeding, diarrhea, failure to thrive, lymphadenopathy, and intermittent intestinal obstruction. In these cases, immune deficiency has to be excluded.

Esophagitis can be the source of bleeding in infants with a history of recurrent emesis or in "slower eaters" with interrupted feeding patterns associated with crying, irritability, or arching. Patients with repaired esophageal atresia with or without tracheoesophageal fistula are at higher risk of severe reflux disease and esophagitis. Bleeding induced by esophagitis is usually recurrent and not intensive. Patients may have hematemesis with streaks of blood or small clots or guaiac-positive stool. The presence of a large amount of blood in vomitus should raise concern about portal hypertension. Esophageal varices are the most common site of bleeding in children with intrahepatic-sinusoidal and extrahepatic-presinusoidal forms of portal hypertension.

Hypertensive gastropathy has to be ruled out in children with parenchymal liver diseases. Bleeding secondary to portal vein thrombosis, as the most common cause of the extrahepatic form of portal hypertension, usually occurs in the first 3 years of life. The risk factors for the presinusoidal form of portal hypertension are omphalitis, history of umbilical vein cannulation, and dehydration. The sinusoidal form of portal hypertension can occur in children with biliary atresia, α_1-antitrypsin deficiency, congenital hepatic fibrosis, and many other types of parenchymal liver disease. In these patients, bleeding may occur at any age.

Infants and Children Younger than 7 Years of Age

Intussusception, common in the first 2 years of life, is strongly considered in infants and children with sudden onset of severe cramping abdominal pain intercepted with pain-free episodes and currant-jelly stools. Diagnosis is confirmed by air contrast (Fig. 84-4), barium enema (Fig. 84-5), or ultrasonography. A mass acting as a lead point is often present in children older than 2 years of age.

Meckel diverticulum is the most common congenital GI anomaly in children, with 1% to 4% of all infants having a

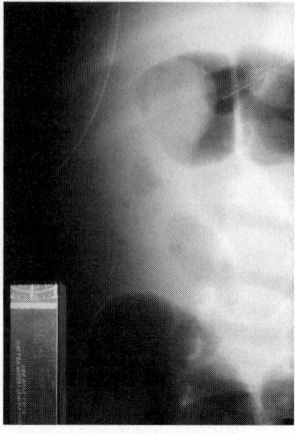

Figure 84-4. An air enema shows the intussusceptum outlined by air in the proximal transverse colon. (Courtesy of Michael J. Diament, MD, Pediatric Radiology Department, Harbor–UCLA Medical Center.)

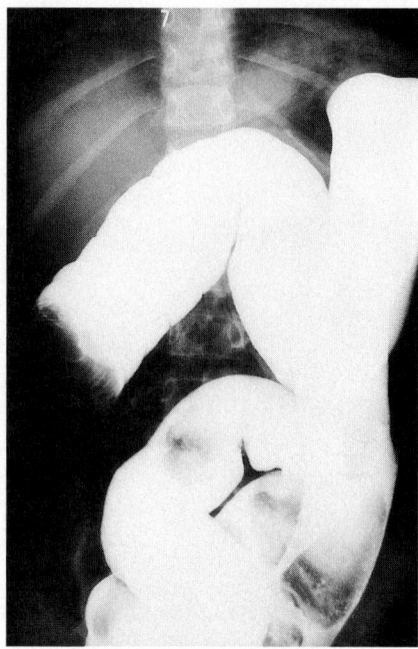

Figure 84-5. A barium enema shows the intussusceptum in the mid-transverse colon. (Courtesy of Michael J. Diament, MD, Pediatric Radiology Department, Harbor–UCLA Medical Center.)

remnant of omphalomesenteric duct. Less than 5% of children develop complications, including GI bleeding. The predominant location of the diverticulum is the 40 to 50 cm of the distal ileum. Ectopic tissue is present in 40% to 80% of symptomatic patients. Gastric mucosa is the most common type of ectopia. The cause of bleeding is peptic ulceration at the junction of the ectopic gastric mucosa and normal ileum, so-called marginal ulcer. The bleeding can be massive, but it may cease spontaneously secondary to contraction of the splanchnic vessels in response to hypovolemia. This phenomenon explains the intermittent nature of bleeding from Meckel diverticulum. Bleeding is usually painless, but sometimes it coincides with recurrent abdominal pain. The diagnostic procedure of choice is a "Meckel scan," which has sensitivity of 85% and specificity of 95% (Fig. 84-6). The scan uses technetium, which is taken up by ectopic gastric mucosa.

Juvenile polyps may occur in 1% of children, with peak incidence from 2 to 5 years of age. The common clinical presentation is recurrent painless bleeding with a small amount of blood on formed stool. Diarrhea and tenesmus can occur when the polyp is large and located in the left colon. Typical juvenile polyps are smooth, rounded, and red. Polyps less than 1 cm usually are sessile; polyps larger than 1 cm have a short or long stalk (Fig. 84-7). Juvenile polyps are composed of normal and cystically dilated crypts embedded in an abundant lamina propria. Adjacent to the large polyp mucosa has a distinctive, so-called goose-skin appearance (Fig. 84-8). Colonoscopy is indicated because of the high incidence (almost 50%) of coexisting polyps in the descending and more proximal portions of the colon. Endoscopic polypectomy is the treatment of choice. Because a single juvenile polyp is not a premalignant condition, removal of a solid juvenile polyp is curative. Surveillance colonoscopy is not indicated unless the child develops a new episode of rectal bleeding.

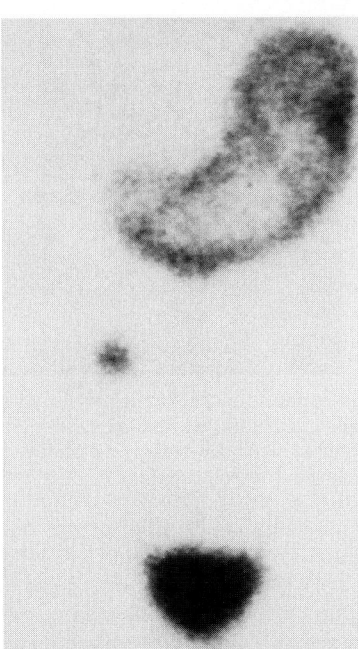

Figure 84-6. A technetium pertechnetate scan (Meckel scan) shows abnormal activity in the right lower quadrant consistent with ectopic gastric mucosa in a Meckel diverticulum. There is normal uptake in the stomach and excretion of isotope into the urinary bladder. (Courtesy of Michael J. Diament, MD, Pediatric Radiology Department, Harbor–UCLA Medical Center.)

Children with multiple juvenile polyps must be followed differently. Most children with fewer than five juvenile polyps have a clinical course similar to patients with a single juvenile polyp. Juvenile polyposis syndrome (JPS) should be strongly considered in children with five or more juvenile polyps throughout the GI tract or patients with juvenile polyps and a family history of juvenile polyposis. Children with JPS are at risk for failure to thrive, significant anemia, protein-losing enteropathy, and malignancy. As the disease progresses, the number of polyps increases to 50 to 200 or

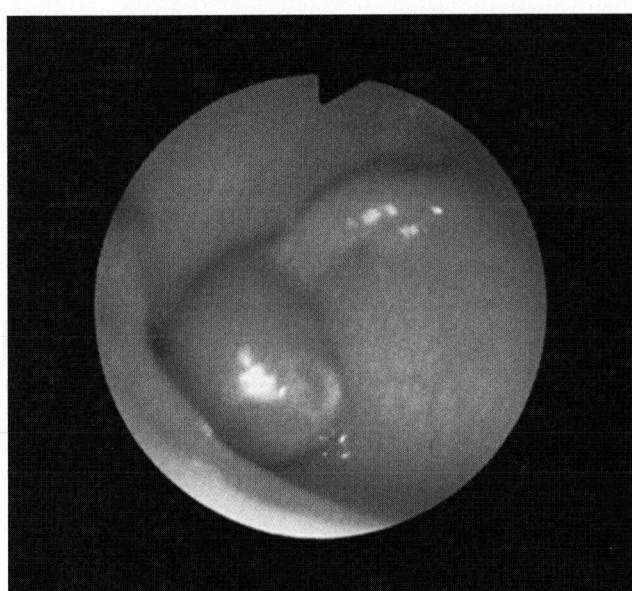

Figure 84-7. A large juvenile polyp of sigmoid colon. Exudate and small ulcerations of the head of the polyp are seen.

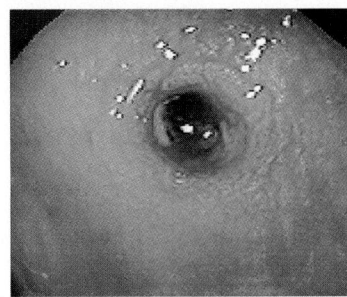

Figure 84-8. So-called goose-skin appearance of the mucosa adjacent to the amputated large colonic polyp. The presence of the clot at the base of the former polyp indicates the recent amputation manifested by bleeding.

more. Coexistence of juvenile and adenomatous polyps and juvenile polyps with adenomatous elements have been documented. Data from St. Mark's Hospital (London) showed that 18 of 87 patients with juvenile polyposis developed colorectal carcinoma at a mean age of 34 years (range 5 to 59 years). These data strongly support the opinion that JPS is a premalignant condition.

JPS is a rare disorder with familial and sporadic cases. The familial form has an autosomal dominant mode of inheritance. It usually is diagnosed before age 10. Sporadic cases of JPS have a tendency to present earlier. Associated anomalies include digital clubbing, alopecia, macrocephaly, congenital heart diseases, cleft lip or palate, genitourinary abnormalities, and mental retardation. In infants with JPS, bloody diarrhea and protein-losing enteropathy lead to severe malnutrition and failure to thrive. In generalized juvenile polyposis, polyps may be found throughout the GI tract or may be confined to the stomach. Colectomy is indicated if clearing of the polyps by colonoscopy is not possible or high-grade dysplasia is found.

Hemolytic uremic syndrome always should be suspected in infants and toddlers with bloody diarrhea, which is present in three quarters of children with epidemic hemolytic uremic syndrome. In two thirds of these children, *Escherichia coli* 0157:H7 can be isolated. The cause of bloody diarrhea in hemolytic uremic syndrome is hemorrhagic colitis from endothelial damage produced by verotoxin and Shiga toxin and submucosal hemorrhages. In HUS, tenesmus is common, and severe abdominal pain with peritoneal signs can occur. Extensive colonic "thumbprinting" is prominent on barium enema. Colitis-related symptoms last no longer than 1 week, followed by signs of hemolytic anemia and oliguria. Known GI complications of hemolytic uremic syndrome are intussusception, pancreatitis, intestinal obstruction, and small or large bowel perforation, which may occur during peritoneal dialysis.

Henoch-Schönlein purpura is most common in children younger than 7 years old. The median age is 4 years. Henoch-Schönlein purpura should be suspected in children with sudden onset of severe diffuse abdominal pain, vomiting, and hematochezia, especially after a prodromal viral illness in winter and early spring and about 1 week after purpuric-type skin lesions appeared on the buttocks or lower extremities. Rarely, GI manifestations may precede the skin rash. Severe anemia is uncommon. Purpura lesions on the small and large bowel are apparent on small bowel x-ray series or barium enema with coarsening of folds and thumbprinting. Abdominal pain and hematochezia are self-limited. Treatment with corticosteroids is controversial, but may shorten the course of GI symptoms of abdominal pain by 1 or 2 days.

Children 7 Years and Older

Drug-induced gastritis should be suspected strongly in children treated with nonsteroidal anti-inflammatory drugs (NSAIDs). This can be complicated by various degrees of bleeding. The usual clinical presentation is the sudden onset of abdominal discomfort followed by hematemesis or melena. Hemorrhage usually originates from the stomach. Two types of lesions are seen: gastropathy or acute gastric ulcers from alteration of the mucosal microcirculation and of mucosal cytoprotection related to suppression of local synthesis of prostaglandins. The incidence of NSAID-related GI bleeding is much higher in patients with *Helicobacter pylori* gastritis than without *H. pylori* gastritis. Therefore, eradication of *H. pylori* gastritis is recommended before long-term therapy with NSAIDs.

Although *peptic ulcer disease* is relatively rare in pediatric patients, it constitutes at least half of the cases of upper GI bleeding in school-age children. Most bleeding ulcers are located in the duodenal bulb. At least 80% of bleeding episodes from duodenal ulcers cease spontaneously. If the bleeding is arterial, it may recur and become life-threatening. Patients with severe bleeding from the upper GI tract present with hemodynamic instability, hematemesis with bright red blood, failure to clear gastric aspirate, and hematochezia. Urgent endoscopy is necessary as soon as the patient becomes clinically stable by volume resuscitation.

If spurting blood or a visible bleeding vessel is found, the risk of recurrent bleeding is high even after initially successful endoscopic hemostasis. These patients require careful observation and treatment with proton-pump inhibitors and antibiotics if *H. pylori* is suspected. Recurrence of bleeding most often occurs during the 3 days after the initial episode. If an ulcer has a clear base or pigmented spot, the risk of further bleeding is minimal, and therapeutic endoscopy is not indicated.

Rectal bleeding in older children and adolescents most commonly is caused by *colitis*. Infectious colitis is more common than inflammatory bowel disease (i.e., ulcerative colitis or Crohn disease). Bacterial colitis is an acute, usually self-limited disorder manifested by sudden onset of fever, tenesmus, and bloody diarrhea lasting 5 to 7 days. Chronic diarrhea (≥2 weeks) is usually associated with chronic inflammatory bowel disease. Rare causes of chronic infectious colitis are *Yersinia enterocolitica*, tuberculosis, *Entamoeba histolytica*, *Strongyloides stercoralis*, and opportunistic infections in immunocompromised patients. *Clostridium difficile* colitis should be ruled out, especially in children treated with antibiotics or hospitalized patients. Ulcerative colitis (Fig. 84-9) and Crohn disease (Fig. 84-10) have a more indolent onset but rarely present as fulminant colitis, mimicking severe bacterial *dysentery*. Differentiation between bacterial colitis and the early stage of chronic inflammatory bowel disease is always a challenge. A high index of suspicion and negative bacterial stool culture results, including *Yersinia* and other rare pathogens, should assist with early diagnosis and treatment.

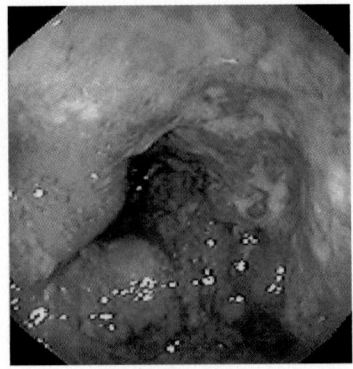

Figure 84-9. Severe diffuse erythema, edema, loss of vascular pattern and folds, multiple ulcerations, and whitish exudates are seen. The patient was diagnosed with a severe form of ulcerative colitis. The onset of disease was fulminant, resembling acute bacterial colitis.

GI polyposis is an unusual cause of GI bleeding in this age group. *Peutz-Jeghers syndrome* is a rare (1/120,000 births) autosomal dominant polyposis associated with mucocutaneous pigmentation. A family history is reported in 50% of patients. Pigmented lesions occur on the lips; the buccal mucosa; and occasionally the hands, feet, and eyelids in most cases. The most common clinical manifestations are recurrent abdominal pain, frequently associated with intussusception and anemia. Fewer than 5% of patients have cutaneous pigmentations without GI polyps. The entire GI tract may be involved with the highest frequency of polyps in the small intestine. Polyps vary from small, rounded, pink, and sessile to pedunculated large, red, and lobulated masses, which may occupy the entire intestinal lumen (Fig. 84-11). The risk of malignancy is well documented in teenagers and young adults. In addition to carcinoma of the GI tract, unusual tumors such as Sertoli cell tumor of the ovary and testicular tumor, can occur. Children with small bowel polyps larger than 1.5 cm require laparotomy with intraoperative enteroscopy. Patients with polyps 1 cm or less benefit from prophylactic endoscopic polypectomy.

Familial adenomatous polyposis is an autosomal dominant condition. It is related to a defect of the *APC* gene on chromosome 5q21. Sporadic mutation of the *APC* gene is accounted for in 20% of patients. The incidence in the general population is approximately 1 in 8000 births. There are hundreds to thousands of adenomas in the colon. The

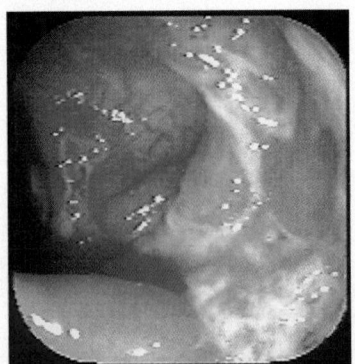

Figure 84-10. Multiple deep, longitudinal ulcers and areas with normal-appearing mucosa are typical for Crohn disease. The patient was diagnosed with Crohn disease and treated successfully with steroids and an antimetabolite agent.

polyps are usually small and sessile (Fig. 84-12). Extra-intestinal manifestations, such as osteomas of the skull, epidermoid cysts, subcutaneous fibromas, and desmoid tumors, generally are associated with Gardner syndrome. Symptoms usually do not begin until 10 years of age. Diarrhea is the earliest symptom. It may be associated with abdominal pain or hematochezia or both. Careful examination of the retina should be performed, looking for congenital hypertrophy of the retinal pigment epithelium, which is a marker for adenomatous colonic polyposis.

If these patients are untreated, the risk of developing colon cancer by age 55 years is almost 100%. Annual endoscopic surveillance is mandatory. Colectomy is the only effective therapy. In the absence of severe dysplasia, colectomy usually is performed in patients in their mid- to late teens or early 20s.

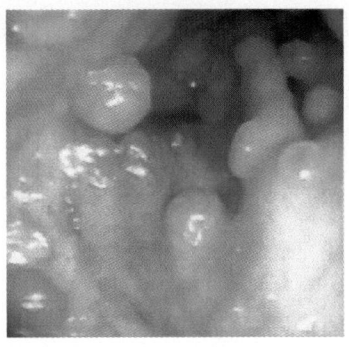

Figure 84-12. Multiple sessile adenomatous polyps in a patient with Gardner syndrome. The same patient was found with adenoma in the second portion of the duodenum, which is the second most common area of adenomatous changes and subsequent malignancy.

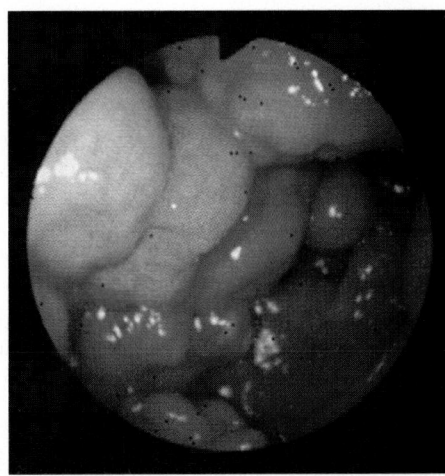

Figure 84-11. Multiple sessile hamartomas in the duodenum were found in a 16-year-old patient with Peutz-Jeghers syndrome. He also had multiple polyps throughout the gastrointestinal tract and a history of testicular tumor. The patient experienced recurrent abdominal pain secondary to chronic intussusception and chronic anemia. Exploratory laparotomy with intraoperative enteroscopy revealed multiple small and large polyps of the small intestine. One removed polyp had a focus of carcinoma in situ.

Mini-index of Related Topics

SUGGESTED READINGS

Fox VL: Gastrointestinal bleeding in infancy and childhood. Gastroenterol Clin North Am 2000;29:37–67.

Heitlinger LA, McClung HJ: Gastrointestinal hemorrhage. In Wyllie R, Hayms JS (eds): Pediatric Gastrointestinal Disease: Pathophysiology, Diagnosis, and Management, 2nd ed. Philadelphia, WB Saunders, 1999, pp 64–72.

Oldham KT, Lobe TE: Gastrointestinal hemorrhage in children: A pragmatic update. Pediatr Clin North Am 1985;32:1247–1263.

Teach SJ, Fleisher GR: Rectal bleeding in the pediatric emergency department. Ann Emerg Med 1994;23:1252–1258.

85 Ascites and Peritonitis

Linda S. Book

ROLE OF THE GENERALIST

1 Recognize the clinical features of ascites, differentiating them from other causes of abdominal distention.

2 Recognize the clinical features of chronic liver disease, the most common cause of ascites.

3 Recognize and refer patients with ascites caused by secondary peritonitis from intra-abdominal surgical conditions.

4 Refer patients with liver disease to appropriate centers and specialists.

5 Diagnose and treat spontaneous bacterial peritonitis, and decide if paracentesis can be performed accurately and safely in the local medical center.

6 Comanage the child with a chronic liver disease specialist to ensure general pediatric care (e.g., immunization) is performed.

7 Refer patients to appropriate specialists when expert assistance is needed for management or diagnosis.

DEFINITIONS

Ascites is the accumulation of fluid in the abdomen; nearly 80% of the time it is associated with chronic liver disease. The ascitic fluid typically is straw colored, containing plasma proteins and leukocytes that have extravasated into the peritoneum. *Chylous ascites* represents a lymphatic leak; it is milky and opaque owing to its high fat content. *Urinary ascites* occurs with rupture or leak anywhere in the urinary system and contains a urea content much higher than plasma. *Pseudoascites* refers to abdominal fluid compartmentalized into a cyst.

Peritonitis is inflammation or infection of the peritoneal cavity and generally is accompanied by ascites. Peritonitis may be caused by microorganisms (bacteria, viruses, or fungi), irritating chemicals (bile, pancreatic fluid, or intestinal contents), or both. *Primary peritonitis* or *spontaneous bacterial peritonitis* refers to infection without any underlying abdominal cause. It occurs frequently in patients with chronic ascites with 25% experiencing this complication. *Secondary peritonitis* refers to inflammation or infection caused by an intra-abdominal condition, such as appendicitis. Peritonitis can progress to generalized sepsis, can be life-threatening, and requires urgent medical management and sometimes surgical intervention.

The procedure for obtaining a sample of the ascitic fluid for analysis by inserting a needle or catheter through the abdominal wall into the peritoneal cavity is called *paracentesis*. Paracentesis also is performed to remove larger amounts of fluid when ascites results in so much distention that respiratory effort is compromised.

FUNDAMENTALS

Table 85-1 lists the causes of ascites. Ascites most commonly is associated with portal hypertension secondary to chronic liver disease. Chronic liver disease with cirrhosis in children is seen in biliary atresia, neonatal hepatitis, α_1-antitrypsin deficiency, autoimmune hepatitis, and metabolic disorders. The development of ascites can be the first indication of hepatic disease (see Chapter 141).

Portal hypertension also occurs with thrombosis or cavernous transformation of the portal vein. Portal vein

Table 85-1. Differential Diagnosis of Ascites

Cause of Ascites	Disorders
Portal hypertension	Portal vein thrombosis
	Cirrhosis
	Tumors
	Hepatic fibrosis
	Budd-Chiari syndrome
Hypoalbuminemia	Nephrotic syndrome
	Protein-losing enteropathy
	Malnutrition
	Hydrops fetalis
	Malabsorption syndromes
Infection	Spontaneous bacterial peritonitis
	Secondary peritonitis
	Fungal peritonitis
	Tuberculous peritonitis
	Cytomegalovirus
Chylous ascites	Traumatic
	Lymphatic obstruction
	Lymphatic abnormalities
	Cytomegalovirus
	Lymphoma
Urinary	Posterior urethral valves
	Bladder perforation
	Ureteral and urethral stenosis
Pancreatic	Pancreatitis
	Trauma
	Ruptured pseudocyst
Bile	Rupture of bile duct
	Rupture of choledochal cyst
Miscellaneous	Hypothyroidism
	Gynecologic disorders
	Ventriculoperitoneal shunts
Pseudoascites	Mesenteric cysts
	Duplication cysts

thrombosis can be a consequence of omphalitis in infancy, hypercoagulable states, and inflammatory bowel disease. Although portal vein thrombosis commonly is thought to be a complication of umbilical vein catheterization, this is actually a rare cause of portal vein thrombosis. Occlusion of hepatic veins, or Budd-Chiari syndrome, also results in portal hypertension.

The reasons for the formation of ascites in portal hypertension are complex. Increased hydrostatic portal venous pressure occurs when blood return to the heart is impeded by resistance from a firm cirrhotic liver or by occluded portal or hepatic veins. Hypoalbuminemia from decreased synthesis of albumin in a chronically diseased liver results in decreased oncotic pressure, favoring extravasation of fluid into the peritoneal cavity. Excretion and reabsorption of renal sodium by the kidney is altered, and hepatic lymph formation is increased. When extravasation into the abdominal cavity exceeds the ability of lymphatics to resorb fluid, ascites results. Ascites that develops in heart failure and constrictive pericarditis is due to an increase in hydrostatic portal venous pressure. Associated protein-losing enteropathy and decreased oncotic pressure also may contribute.

In nephrotic syndrome, ascites results from hypoalbuminemia caused by proteinuria and subsequent decreased oncotic pressure. In malabsorptive states, ascites occurs secondary to low oncotic pressure from hypoalbuminemia resulting from decreased synthesis. Malignancies, which seed the peritoneum, also cause ascites. Lymphoma may be associated with chylous ascites from lymphatic obstruction. Pancreatic ascites occurs in blunt abdominal trauma and pancreatitis. It is caused by leaking of pancreatic secretions into the abdominal cavity. Intestinal obstruction, especially in the newborn, can occur with ascites.

The newborn may present with abdominal distention owing to ascites. The volume may be great enough to impede normal ventilation and require emergency paracentesis. The most common cause is urinary ascites from a congenital anomaly. Urine extravasates into the peritoneal cavity. The urea content of the ascitic fluid is elevated many times that of plasma. Congenital lymphangiectasia or congenital infection can result in chylous ascites.

Large-volume ascites with protein levels of less than 1 g/dL is a particular risk for spontaneous bacterial peritonitis. Not only is the fluid an excellent culture medium; in addition, there is a low concentration of defense factors, such as opsonizing proteins. Infection results from translocation of bacteria from the intestinal lumen. Malnutrition, a comorbid condition in many children with ascites, increases their susceptibility to infection. Children with chronic liver disease, nephrotic syndrome, peritoneal dialysis, and ventriculoperitoneal shunts are at risk for peritonitis. Secondary peritonitis results from abdominal trauma with ruptured viscus or from an inflammatory process, such as appendicitis. Secondary peritonitis frequently is polymicrobial and anaerobic.

DIAGNOSIS

The diagnostic goals and challenges for a child with ascites are listed in Box 85-1. Evaluation begins with a careful history and physical examination. Pertinent history includes

> **Box 85-1.** Diagnostic Goals and Challenges for Assessment of Ascites and Peritonitis
>
> 1. Differentiate ascites from other causes of abdominal distention.
> 2. Recognize significant respiratory distress as a complication of ascites.
> 3. Determine or refer for subspecialty evaluation for the underlying cause of ascites.
> 4. Recognize features of chronic liver disease and cirrhosis.
> 5. Distinguish portal vein thrombosis from chronic liver disease as a cause of ascites.
> 6. Diagnose and determine the underlying cause of peritonitis.

perinatal complications, a history of esophageal varices, unexplained gastrointestinal bleeding, or iron deficiency anemia.

Physical examination shows a distended abdomen. Fullness may be appreciated in the pelvic area and the flanks. As fluid accumulates, abdominal protuberance develops. The accumulation of fluid may cause umbilical hernias, inguinal hernias, scrotal swelling, and hydroceles. When the patient's position changes from supine to lateral, percussion findings may change. This "shifting dullness" results from movement of the intra-abdominal fluid. The onset of ascites is generally gradual with fullness of the abdomen and weight gain. Onset may be sudden when the cause is peritonitis, cardiac failure, abdominal trauma, pancreatitis, or fulminant hepatic failure. The abdominal girth may become so massive that respiration is compromised, especially while supine. Not all patients with abdominal distention have ascites. Pseudoascites resulting from a cyst may have physical examination features that are identical to ascites. Other important findings on physical examination are splenomegaly, prominent veins on the anterior abdominal wall (portal hypertension), and jaundice (a variable finding in a child with liver disease). Cutaneous findings include bruising, xanthomas, and spider angiomas.

Cardinal symptoms of peritonitis are fever, abdominal tenderness often with rebound, and abdominal distention. Children with peritonitis may appear toxic and septic. Decreased appetite, lethargy, and irritability are common. When liver disease is present, deterioration in hepatic or renal function or encephalopathy may be present. Peritonitis also can occur in the absence of fever or with only low-grade intermittent fever. Symptoms may be only decreased appetite, vague abdominal discomfort, and malaise or irritability. Elective paracentesis in adults with chronic ascites revealed that 25% have positive bacterial cultures.

Laboratory evaluation of a patient with ascites begins with abdominal radiographs, which are useful in identifying obstruction or diffusely dilated and fluid-filled loops of bowel. In ascites alone, air-filled bowel rises to the anterior abdomen and is visualized in the center of the film. Abdominal ultrasound should be performed in anyone with new-onset ascites to confirm the diagnosis, exclude portal vein obstruction, evaluate for abdominal mass, evaluate renal anatomy, and identify a cyst. Ultrasound also is useful in guidance for the site of paracentesis. Abdominal

Table 85-2. Classification of Ascites and Diagnostic Tests

Classification	Ascitic WBC/mm³	Serum Albumin Gradient (g/dL)	Other
Portal hypertension			
Cirrhosis	<250 PMN	>1.1	Low serum albumin
Portal vein thrombosis			Ultrasound abnormal
Budd-Chiari			Ultrasound abnormal
Fulminant hepatic failure			Low serum albumin
Cardiac			
Heart failure	<250 PMN	<1.1	
Constrictive pericarditis	<250 PMN	<1.1	
Malignancy	>250 PMN	>1.1	Abnormal cytology
Infection	>250 PMN	<1.1 with no portal hypertension >1.1 with portal hypertension	Culture positive in 50%
Pancreatic ascites	Variable, often increased	Variable	Ascitic amylase greatly increased
Renal			
Nephrotic syndrome	<250 PMN	<1.1	
Urinary	<250 PMN	<1.1	Increased urea in fluid
Chylous ascites	>250 mononuclear	<1.1	Triglyceride >200 mg/dL

PMN, polymorphonuclear neutrophils; WBC, white blood count.

computed tomography and magnetic resonance imaging are not routinely required. A complete blood count may show a low platelet count or pancytopenia resulting from splenic sequestration if portal hypertension is present. A prolonged prothrombin time and low serum albumin indicate impaired synthetic function of the liver, which is characteristic of cirrhosis but typically is not seen in portal hypertension caused by portal vein thrombosis.

Examination of the ascitic fluid is crucial in determining the cause of ascites (Table 85-2). Patients with a known diagnosis of liver disease do not need paracentesis when ascites develops. When spontaneous bacterial peritonitis is suspected, fluid must be obtained. Patients with ascites secondary to acute abdominal trauma, obstruction, or perforation should not have paracentesis but immediate operative intervention. Most other patients with new onset of ascites should undergo diagnostic paracentesis.

Ascites should not be classified as either transudate or exudate because there are too many overlapping situations. The best method to distinguish ascites caused by portal hypertension from other forms of ascites is the serum ascites-to-albumin gradient, which is calculated by subtracting the ascitic albumin concentration from the serum albumin concentration. In portal hypertension, this value is greater than 1.1 g/dL. In most other forms of ascites, the value is less than 1.1 g/dL. This value cannot be interpreted accurately if the serum albumin is less than 1 g/dL. Ascitic fluid is normally clear and straw colored. The appearance of the fluid is cloudy or turbid when the leukocyte count is elevated. The PMN or neutrophil count determines if infection is likely. Bloody fluid, which does not clot, usually indicates abdominal trauma. Other studies that may be obtained by a specialist to evaluate a patient with ascites include computed tomography, visceral angiography, magnetic resonance angiography, lymphangiography, and endoscopic retrograde pancreatogram.

There are few contraindications to paracentesis. A distended bladder should be emptied with a Foley catheter if necessary. Caution should be taken when there are distended bowel loops. Any site with obvious cutaneous infection or inflammation should be avoided as the puncture site. Coagulopathy and thrombocytopenia are relative contraindications, but even though many patients with liver disease have coagulopathy, paracentesis can be accomplished without administration of blood products. Ultrasound is recommended to localize an appropriate puncture site for the generalist who performs the procedure infrequently. Ultrasound also is advised when there has been prior abdominal surgery or distended bowel, to avoid perforation of the bowel. Locations for paracentesis are midline 2 cm caudad to the umbilicus and 1 to 2 cm lateral and caudad to the umbilicus. Abdominal scars should be avoided. A "Z" technique is used for puncture, whereby one slides the skin 2 cm laterally while the puncture is performed. This technique results in skin puncture and peritoneal puncture occurring in different locations and reduces leaking of fluid after the procedure. Although no more painful than an injection, sedation may be necessary to ensure a cooperative patient. The equipment necessary and technique for abdominal paracentesis are listed in Table 85-3, and interpretation of laboratory findings is summarized in Table 85-2. *When chylous ascites is a consideration, the clinician should be certain the patient has ingested a high-fat meal several hours before the paracentesis so that the milky character of the fluid is prominent and triglyceride level definitive when measured.*

MANAGEMENT

Most children with ascites require referral to a specialist. The generalist must decide based on an initial evaluation what type of referral is appropriate. When peritonitis is diagnosed, surgical consultation is necessary to exclude causes of secondary peritonitis. Chronic liver disease is crucial to recognize because ascites in this context signifies serious disease, which may require liver transplantation.

Initial management of ascites resulting from portal hypertension involves modest salt restriction of 1 to 2 mEq/kg/day (Box 85-2). Spironolactone, an aldosterone inhibitor, should be started at 2 to 3 mg/kg/day three times daily. Weight loss of 300 to 800 g/day for older children or approximately 10 to 30 g/kg for infants is appropriate. Bed rest helps mobilize fluid. Hospitalization may be necessary for children with marked ascites so that electrolytes and

Table 85-3. Equipment and Technique for Performing Paracentesis

Equipment

1. Skin cleansing solution and sterile gauze
2. Sterile gloves and mask
3. Sterile drapes
4. Lidocaine (usually with epinephrine)
5. 5-mL syringe for anesthetic with 25-gauge needle
6. 20-mL syringe for diagnostic tap
7. 50-mL syringe and stopcock for fluid reduction
8. 18- to 20-gauge angiocath or needle with stylette
9. Optional 3-way stopcock and intravenous connecting tubing

Technique

1. Explain procedure and obtain consent
2. Abdominal films to exclude free air/obstruction
3. Empty bladder with Foley if necessary
4. Ultrasound to assess appropriate site
5. Position patient in horizontal decubitus position (may tilt to side of collection)
6. Prepare skin and drape with typical site 2 cm below umbilicus to avoid scars
7. Infiltrate skin with lidocaine, then direct needle perpendicular to peritoneum
8. Using "Z" technique (see text), slowly introduce angiocath or needle with frequent pause and aspiration
9. When fluid is identified, angle needle or catheter toward pelvic hollow and withdraw style
10. Withdraw fluid with 20-mL syringe. Sometimes fluid is obtained by letting drip (i.e., lumbar puncture into sterile container)
11. Collect sample in anticoagulated tube for count, albumin. Inoculate 10–20 mL fluid directly into blood culture vials. Send fluid for amylase, cytology, and triglyceride as indicated

weight loss can be monitored closely. Excessive, rapid weight loss can be associated with hypotension. Nutritional status should be monitored carefully because gastric compression from the fluid can interfere with adequate caloric consumption. Restriction of water intake is not usually necessary, but if hyponatremia is present, it needs to be addressed. Additional diuretics, such as furosemide at 0.25 to 1 mg/kg/dose two or three times daily, may be required. Hypoalbuminemia can be corrected with albumin infusion of 0.5 to 1 g/kg over 1 to 2 hours, followed by furosemide to facilitate diuresis of mobilized fluid.

For patients who do not respond to medical management, there are surgical options. Interventional radiologists can place transjugular intrahepatic percutaneous shunts, in which a venous connection is made between the jugular vein and the portal vein branches within the liver. Splenorenal and mesocaval shunts can be considered. A

Box 85-2. Management Goals for Children with Ascites and Peritonitis

1. Diagnose and treat or refer for treatment for the underlying cause.
2. Use diuretics and salt restriction as treatment modalities for ascites from portal hypertension.
3. Monitor serum electrolytes in children receiving diuretic therapy.
4. Choose appropriate antibiotics for treatment of peritonitis and refine choice after culture of the ascitic fluid.
5. Perform paracentesis or refer for paracentesis patients with marked respiratory distress.

child with uncontrolled ascites from chronic liver disease is a candidate for liver transplantation.

Spontaneous bacterial peritonitis is treated with antibiotics selected for the most likely organism. *Streptococcus pneumoniae* was the main cause of peritonitis in children with nephrotic syndrome, but gram-negative bacilli and *Staphylococcus aureus* are now as frequent. In cirrhotic children, enteric microorganisms account for more than two thirds of pathogens. *Escherichia coli* is the most frequent pathogen, followed by *Klebsiella pneumoniae*, *Streptococcus pneumoniae*, and other streptococcal organisms, including *Enterococcus*. Anaerobes are much less common. Infections usually are monomicrobial in spontaneous bacterial or primary peritonitis. Peritonitis secondary to an intra-abdominal or secondary peritonitis may be polymicrobial and anaerobic. Occasionally, *Mycobacterium tuberculosis* or fungi may cause peritonitis. Gram stains are positive in less than 10% of patients. The initial choice of antibiotic is often empirical based on the most likely pathogens. The antimicrobial regimen is modified when the results of the culture and susceptibility tests are available. Approach to appropriate antibiotic treatment is described in Chapter 284. Approximately 25% of patients have features consistent with peritonitis but negative cultures. Reasonable regimens include a third-generation cephalosporin or ampicillin and gentamicin. Broad-spectrum penicillins, such as piperacillin and tazobactam, also are acceptable. Early diagnosis and treatment produce the best survival rates. Nearly 75% of patients have septicemia with the same organism and require treatment for shock or renal insufficiency.

Chylous ascites is treated with dietary intervention. A response usually is seen with low-fat diets and when most fat is administered as medium-chain triglyceride. Intravenous albumin and gamma globulin may be necessary to replace protein losses. Chylous and malignant ascites do not respond to salt restriction or diuretics.

Massive ascites accompanied by respiratory distress requires therapeutic removal of fluid by paracentesis. If this is done, albumin should be infused intravenously at a rate of 20 mL of 5% albumin for every 100 mL of fluid removed.

OUTCOME

When ascites occurs secondary to cirrhotic liver disease in children, liver transplantation frequently is necessary within 1 to 2 years. Children should be referred to centers where pediatric transplantation is available. The generalist plays a crucial role in the preparation of children for transplantation, especially immunization before transplantation. The survival for most children after transplantation approaches 90%. Children with ascites secondary to malignancy, cardiac failure, and renal problems should be referred to appropriate specialists; their prognosis depends on the diagnosis and treatment of the underlying condition.

Although the reported mortality in adults with peritonitis is 30% to 90%, most children who receive prompt treatment survive the initial infection. Recurrence is high (50% or 60%). All patients with ascites should be educated about the signs and symptoms of peritonitis.

In portal vein thrombosis, the liver is not diseased, so in most cases transplantation is not required. Some patients develop collateral vessels that decompress portal pressure and do not require surgical intervention, whereas others are candidates for surgical shunts.

Mini-index of Related Topics

SUGGESTED READINGS

Hardy S, Kleinman RE: Cirrhosis and chronic liver failure. In Suchy FJ, Sokol RF, Balistreri WF (eds): Liver Disease in Children. Philadelphia, Lippincott Williams & Wilkins, 2001, pp 89–129.

Holcomb GW III, Gheissari A, Sharter N, et al: Chylous peritonitis in children: Case report and literature review. J Pediatr Gastroenterol Nutr 1990;10:114–116.

Larcher VF, Manolaki N, Vegnente A, et al: Spontaneous bacterial peritonitis in children with chronic liver disease: Clinical features and etiologic factors. J Pediatr 1985;106:907–912.

Levison ME, Bush LM: Peritonitis. In Mandell GL, Bennett JE, Dolin R (eds): Mandell, Douglas, and Bennett's Principles and Practice of Infectious Diseases, 5th ed. Phildelphia, Churchill Livingstone, 2000, pp 821–837.

Runyon BA: Care of the patient with ascites. N Engl J Med 1994;330:337–342.

SECTION 3   GENERAL MEDICAL CARE: *Gastrointestinal and Nutritional Disorders*

86 Nutritional Disorders

Sara L. Thompson

ROLE OF THE GENERALIST

1 Understand basal metabolic requirements for infants and children.

2 Recognize signs and symptoms of vitamin and mineral deficiencies.

3 Diagnose failure to thrive and establish its cause.

4 Diagnose obesity, establish its cause, and evaluate for comorbid states.

5 Treat obesity and failure to thrive owing to undernutrition.

6 Refer for specialty care if diagnosis is uncertain, if case is severe or refractory, or if a comorbid state exists.

7 Oversee a multidisciplinary approach to treatment.

8 Establish an ongoing relationship with the patient and family and a long-term treatment plan.

DEFINITIONS

To grow and thrive, humans rely on daily food intake to supply the energy and nutrients that are the substrate for the body's ongoing cellular processes. The calorie is the basic unit of metabolic energy that is used to quantify the energy content of food. The most commonly used unit is the *kilocalorie (kcal)*, defined as the amount of heat necessary to raise the temperature of 1 kg of water by 1°C. Calories are used to maintain body processes, such as physical activity, digestion, growth, and basal metabolism. The caloric value of a particular food is its quantitative balance of protein, carbohydrates, and fat.

Proteins are high-molecular-weight polypeptides and are a component of all body tissues. The function of each protein is dictated by the sequence of its constituent amino acids. Of the 20 amino acids that comprise the body's proteins, the body does not synthesize the nine essential amino acids. Carbohydrates are composed of carbon, hydrogen, and oxygen and function predominantly as an energy source for the body. They may be configured as monosaccharides (glucose, fructose, galactose), disaccharides (sucrose, lactose), or polysaccharides (glycogen, starch). Fats are a heterogeneous group of compounds that serve as an energy source; are present in all body tissues; and are found in plasma in the form of triglycerides, free fatty acids, lipoproteins, and phospholipids. Cholesterol often is classified as a fat, but it is a sterol with a different chemical structure.

The most common state of overnutrition is *obesity*, an excess of body fat, specifically defined as a *body mass index (BMI)* greater than the 95th percentile for age. States of undernutrition in a child are termed *failure to thrive, kwashiorkor, marasmus,* and *marasmic kwashiorkor*. The latter three terms refer to states of severe protein and calorie malnutrition.

Failure to thrive is poor growth in a child younger than 2 years and is defined in one of two ways: a child with a height or weight less than the third or fifth percentile for age or with decreased growth velocity that crosses two major percentile lines on a standard National Center for

Health Statistics growth chart. Failure to thrive has been categorized as organic (caused by a medical condition) and nonorganic (caused by psychosocial factors). Newer theories do not favor this classification, using instead a "transactional model," whereby poor growth and delayed attainment of developmental milestones are affected by poor nutrition and impaired emotional and physical nurturing. Impaired nurturing is the result of interactions among multiple factors, including family economics, social supports, child and family health status, health beliefs, and interpersonal interaction patterns (including the influence of child and caretaker temperaments).

Kwashiorkor is a state of inadequate body protein stores that may be secondary to inadequate intake or may occur after a marginal dietary intake becomes inadequate from the catabolic stress of an acute or chronic infection. *Marasmus* is a disorder of energy intake, but also may be associated with inadequate protein, vitamin, or mineral intake. *Marasmic kwashiorkor* is a clinical state of combined protein and energy undernutrition, with the clinical manifestations of each.

FUNDAMENTALS

The body requires nutrient energy intake to maintain its basal metabolic rate and digestion and to support physical activity and growth. A caloric intake of 100 kcal/kg/day (range 80 to 120 kcal/kg/day) is sufficient to maintain growth during the first year of life. After the first year, caloric needs decrease by an average of 10 kcal/kg/day per 3-year period (Table 86-1). After the onset of puberty, the proportional increase in lean body mass is greater in boys than in girls, resulting in a greater caloric requirement for basal metabolism and activity. This gender-specific difference in caloric requirement persists through adulthood.

Of a child's daily caloric intake, 15% to 20% should be from protein, 45% to 55% should be from carbohydrates, and 30% should be from fat. Because the body has no ability to store protein, it must be an ongoing part of daily nutrition. Protein requirements are difficult to categorize by age because they depend on each individual child's lean body mass and growth rate. Preterm infants have higher requirements than term neonates, and infants have higher requirements than older children. Protein sources are classified as high and low quality, depending on the essential amino acid content.

Carbohydrates are not essential because they can be synthesized from proteins and fat. Prolonged absence of carbohydrates from the daily diet results, however, in ketosis and acidosis. Fats also can be synthesized from proteins and carbohydrates, but some fatty acids are essential and must be a part of dietary intake. Because the daily requirement of essential fatty acids is low, deficiency is rare.

Vitamins and minerals are essential for tissue function and cellular metabolism, and except for vitamin D, vitamin K, and vitamin B_{12}, they must be a part of dietary intake. The recommended daily allowances of vitamins for children are based on limited data. Vitamin deficiencies are rare in the United States as a result of the popularity of over-the-counter vitamins and fortified foods. Examples of food fortification include iron-fortified infant formulas and cereals, folic acid–enriched grain products, vitamin D–fortified milk, and calcium-enriched orange juice. Calcium, magnesium, and phosphorus account for 98% of the body's minerals by weight. Trace elements are iron, zinc, copper, fluoride, iodine, selenium, manganese, chromium, cobalt, molybdenum, nickel, silicon, and vanadium.

Nutritional status can be assessed by anthropometric measurements and evaluation of dietary intake. The most common measurements are height and weight. In the assessment of nutritional status, these measurements must be evaluated in relation to each other (e.g., with weight-for-height calculations and the BMI). The most reliable and simply calculated indicator of body fatness in children and adolescents is the BMI, defined as weight (kg)/height (m^2). BMI is the recommended measure of body adiposity for routine clinical and public health use.

A child's dietary history can be documented on a 3-day diet history or a 24-hour dietary recall. The diet history is preferred because it accounts for the variability in day-to-day food intake and is not dependent on a child or parent's recall.

PRESENTATION AND INITIAL EVALUATION

The assessment of pediatric nutritional disorders includes identification of disease states contributing to a child's nutritional difficulties, acknowledgment of psychosocial and economic factors affecting nutritional intake, and recognition of disease states secondary to the child's nutritional problems. Adequate nutritional assessment is achieved best through a multidisciplinary health care team.

Obesity is the result of energy intake in excess of energy expenditure. In children, it can result from genetic or endocrine abnormalities. Between 1971 and 1991, the national prevalence of obesity increased by 66% in 6- to 11-year-old boys, 150% in 6- to 11-year-old girls, 140% in 12- to 17-year-old boys, and 22% in 12- to 17-year-old girls. All children with a BMI greater than the 95th percentile for age should have an in-depth medical assessment for the cause and complications of obesity. Children with a BMI between the 85th and 95th percentiles should be evaluated for the complications of excess body fat.

Factors contributing to the development of obesity in children include genetic predisposition, environmental and psychosocial factors, and metabolic changes. Metabolic changes may result from a change in activity level or from

Table 86-1. Daily Caloric Requirements by Age

	Age (yr)	Average Daily Energy Requirement (kcal/kg/day)
Infants	0–1	100
Children	1–3	100
	4–6	90
	7–10	70
Girls	11–14	45
	15–18	40
Boys	11–14	55
	15–18	45

From Farris RP: Pediatric nutrition guidelines. In Suskind RM, Lewinter-Suskind L (eds): Textbook of Pediatric Nutrition, 2nd ed. New York, Raven Press, 1993, pp 531–547.

Table 86-2. Conditions Associated with Childhood/Adolescent Obesity

Condition	Signs and Symptoms
Genetic	
Bardet-Biedl syndrome	Developmental delay, digital, gonadal, and retinal anomalies
Prader-Willi syndrome	Developmental delay, males with undescended testes, short stature, almond-shaped eyes, small hands and feet
Cohen's syndrome	Developmental delay, microcephaly and craniofacial anomalies, poor visual acuity, short narrow hands and feet
Turner's syndrome	Short stature, broad chest, widely spaced nipples, lymphedema, characteristic facies, low posterior hairline, webbed neck, extremity anomalies, congenital heart disease
Endocrine	
Hypothroidism	Poor linear growth, cold intolerance, edema, constipation, decreased energy level
Cushing's syndrome	Poor linear growth, violaceous striae, hirsutism, truncal obesity, buffalo hump, delayed puberty, school difficulties, hypertension
Polycystic ovary syndrome	Amenorrhea, hirsutism, acanthosis nigricans
Psychological	
Depression	Sleep and eating disturbances, behavior difficulties, anxiety, fatigue, suicidal ideation

endocrine pathophysiology. The child's past medical history, family history, and review of systems should focus on the presence of genetic, endocrine, and psychological disorders that may contribute to the development of obesity (Table 86-2).

A child's dietary and activity histories are essential in evaluating obesity. A child's diet and activity may depend on parental perceptions of appropriate food intake and activity levels. A dietary history includes who prepares the child's meals, whether television is watched during meals, who shops for the child's food, and what meals the child eats at school. This information indicates which individuals and behaviors affect the child's daily food intake. The child's 3-day diet history or 24-hour dietary recall and a dietary history for other family members provide information on the family's overall dietary habits.

An activity history includes in-school and out-of-school activities and daily time spent using a television, video machine, or computer. Other factors that affect a child's activity level are neighborhood safety, the accessibility of facilities where the child can play or participate in sports, and the presence of an adult caretaker in the home after school.

Subjective and objective data should be gathered to document when the obesity began and whether the family perceives a weight problem and nutritional disorder. Plotting prior height and weight on a growth chart indicates the trend in growth parameters over time. These objective data do not always coincide with the parental perception of when the child became obese. The child and the family should be asked about prior attempts at weight control and

methods used. Adolescents often use tobacco as a method of weight control.

Psychosocial factors that influence weight include school, economic, and family or social stressors that may result in increased caloric intake or decreased energy expenditure. Parent/child interactions also may be observed during the medical visit and may provide insight into family interpersonal behavior patterns. Children, especially adolescents, should be screened for eating disorders, body image distortions, and self-esteem problems that may have led to or been a result of the child's obesity.

Questions in the past medical history and review of systems should focus on the orthopedic, respiratory, neurologic, gastrointestinal, endocrine, and cardiovascular complications of obesity (Table 86-3). A family history of hypertension, coronary artery disease, or dyslipidemia increases the child's risk of developing these particular complications of obesity.

The physical examination of an obese child focuses on detecting any underlying medical etiologies and any complications of obesity (see Tables 86-2 and 86-3). Children who are obese from excess intake or decreased energy expenditure are typically tall, whereas children with underlying endocrine pathology are short. The heart rate may be low in hypothyroid children. Blood pressure may be elevated in Cushing's syndrome or as a complication of obesity. The laboratory evaluation of an obese child includes a fasting lipid profile (low-density lipoprotein, very-low-density lipoprotein, total cholesterol, triglyceride), fasting insulin and glucose, liver function tests, and a thyroid-stimulating hormone level. Additional laboratory or radiographic evaluation is guided by clinical judgment.

Many of the same concepts apply to the evaluation of failure-to-thrive cases. The primary care provider is most often the first to detect a problem. The National Health and Nutrition Examination Survey III (1988–1991) found

Table 86-3. Medical Complications of Obesity

Condition	Signs and Symptoms
Orthopedic	
Slipped capital femoral epiphysis	Hip or knee pain, externally rotated lower extremity, leg-length discrepancy
Blount's disease (tibia vara)	Bowed lower extremities
Neurologic	
Pseudotumor cerebri	Headache, visual changes, papilledema
Respiratory	
Sleep apnea	Snoring, daytime somnolence
Hypoventilation syndrome	Somnolence, cyanosis
Gastrointestinal	
Cholelithiasis	Abdominal pain, jaundice
Hepatic steatosis	Abdominal pain, hepatomegaly
Endocrine	
Insulin resistance/ non–insulin-dependent diabetes	Polyuria, polydipsia, acanthosis nigricans
Cardiovascular	
Hypertension Dyslipidemias	Elevated blood pressure

a 2.7% prevalence of low weight among children 2 to 5 years old. Failure to thrive has been correlated with low socioeconomic status, low level of maternal education, greater number of feeding difficulties, premature birth, low birth weight, and prolonged hospitalization after birth. A child's failure to thrive may be a marker for a family's psychosocial stressors or medical issues, such as low food security, maternal depression, homelessness, or mismatched temperaments that result in the child being labeled as "difficult." Although inadequate nutrition is the immediate cause of failure to thrive, the multiple factors that lead to malnutrition also must be addressed to treat failure to thrive adequately. Review of systems and past medical history should be used to assess physiologic conditions that could affect a child's growth status (Table 86-4).

Birth history may reveal a predisposing medical condition for the development of failure to thrive and provide insight into psychosocial issues affecting maternal-infant bonding. Birth history includes the infant's gestational age, Apgar scores, prenatal complications, birth weight and length, and exposure to drugs or infections. Infants exposed to tobacco, alcohol, or illicit drugs may have temperaments that are labeled as "difficult" and may not respond to nurturing from their caretakers. An unwanted pregnancy or a newborn's prolonged hospitalization may result in impaired maternal-child bonding.

Family history should focus on sibling medical problems, history of infant deaths, sudden infant death syndrome, or apnea (raising the level of concern for child abuse or neglect in the home). Parental height and weights should be obtained. Social history may reveal that siblings in the home may dominate caretaker time and result in a child's poor nutrition or that a new parent has inadequate parenting skills. Substance abuse by caretakers can result in poor parental judgment in feeding the child. Any history of prior child abuse reports or involvement with child protective services increases the level of concern for the child's health and well-being in the home environment. Major life events, such as marriage, divorce, loss of employment, change in custodial parent, family move to a new location, birth of a child, or parental incarceration, may affect financial stability, the availability of food, social support, and interpersonal dynamics. Availability of food, maternal anger or depression, infant fussiness, and child behavioral problems ultimately can affect a child's nutritional intake. A temporal relationship between these life events and a child's growth impairment can be seen on a growth curve over time.

Dietary history is essential in order to assess whether the child has adequate caloric intake to sustain normal growth. Inappropriate foods may be offered as a part of nontraditional dietary practices, as a result of poverty, or as a result of inadequate knowledge of appropriate feeding practices. Failure to thrive also may result from inadequate intake if the child refuses to eat, if the child has oral anomalies or dental caries, or if insufficient time is allotted for feeding. Nutrient retention may be inadequate if the child has recurrent vomiting or diarrhea. Infant intake may be estimated rapidly by approximating caloric intake as 20 kcal/oz of formula and 80 kcal/4 oz jar of baby food (baby foods range from 40 to 140 kcal/jar). Occasionally, a caretaker intentionally or unintentionally may dilute or concentrate a child's formula or food, resulting in inadequate nutrition, emesis, or diarrhea. Repeated dietary assessments over time may be necessary to obtain accurate information.

Physical examination of an infant with growth impairment includes an assessment for signs of undernutrition and for underlying medical etiologies of the growth problems. It also provides an opportunity to observe parent-child interactions. An infant or child's lack of eye contact with a parent, withdrawal, and hypertonic posturing when held all indicate an inadequate nurturing relationship with the parent. Severe undernutrition and a slowed basal metabolic rate may cause hypothermia and a low heart rate. Low blood pressure is consistent with inadequate hydration. Acute starvation results in weight that is decreased out of proportion to a child's height. Chronic undernutrition results in a low weight and height. The child's prior growth parameters must be charted to assess the timing and trends in the growth impairment, and the BMI needs to be calculated to determine the child's body fatness. A BMI less than the fifth percentile for age is consistent with a diagnosis of undernutrition. Wasting of the buttocks and buccal fat pads indicate low body fat. Generalized signs of starvation include hypotonia, muscle wasting, edema, and a protuberant abdomen. Vitamin or mineral deficiencies may result in

Table 86-4. Systemic Disorders Associated with Failure to Thrive

Symptom/System Affected	Disorders
Difficult feeding	Craniofacial anomalies (cleft lip and palate, micrognathia, genetic syndrome–associated anomalies)
	Dental caries
	Cerebral palsy
Vomiting	Gastroesophageal reflux
	Gastrointestinal tract obstruction
	Intracranial pathology (increased intracranial pressure)
Diarrhea	Infection (bacterial, parasitic)
	Celiac disease
	Cystic fibrosis
	Inflammatory bowel disease
	Chronic hepatitis or cirrhosis (multiple etiologies)
	Carbohydrate or protein intolerance
Chronic infection	HIV
	Tuberculosis
	Urinary tract infection
	Congenital infection (syphilis, CMV, rubella)
Cardiac	Congenital heart disease (associated with congestive heart failure or cyanosis)
Pulmonary	Cystic fibrosis
	Bronchopulmonary dysplasia
Renal	Chronic renal insufficiency
	Renal tubular acidosis
Endocrine	Pituitary insufficiency
	Hypothyroidism
	Growth hormone deficiency/resistance
	Rickets (in younger children)
Genetic/congenital syndromes	Chromosomal anomalies (Turner's syndrome, Down syndrome, trisomy 13, trisomy 18, DiGeorge syndrome)
	Inborn errors of metabolism
Intrauterine exposure	Fetal alcohol syndrome
	Dilantin

CMV, cytomegalovirus; HIV, human immunodeficiency virus.

hair or skin changes. Physical findings that indicate an underlying medical etiology for the growth impairment also may be present (see Table 86-4).

Laboratory evaluation establishes the cause of failure to thrive in infants and children in less than 1% of cases and should be guided by a health care provider's clinical findings in the history and physical examination. The most commonly recommended screening tests include hemoglobin level, urinalysis, lead level (in areas of high prevalence), stool culture, stool Hemoccult, and bone age. Nutritional status is monitored with serum protein markers, such as prealbumin and albumin levels. Prealbumin is preferred because its shorter half-life reflects nutritional status in the preceding several days.

Kwashiorkor, marasmus, and marasmic kwashiorkor are states of severe protein and energy malnutrition. Kwashiorkor and marasmus may be differentiated by their specific physical findings. Marasmic kwashiorkor manifests some of the findings of each. Worldwide, these conditions are associated with poverty and inadequate nutritional intake. They are less common in the United States and typically are due to a predisposing disease state, such as chronic infection or malignancy. These conditions often are associated with vitamin and mineral deficiencies.

Kwashiorkor results from inadequate protein intake and worldwide is seen most commonly in toddlers and older children who no longer are breast-fed. Many children do not become symptomatic until a marginally appropriate protein intake becomes inadequate from the catabolic stress of infection. Physical findings include irritability or apathy, skin darkening unrelated to sun exposure, sparse or coarse hair, hypotonia, edema, hepatomegaly (from fatty infiltration of the liver), and weight loss. Edema may cause the child's wasting to be difficult to observe. Late in the course of the disease, cardiomegaly or impaired renal tubular function can occur. Laboratory evaluation may show low serum albumin, prealbumin, glucose, potassium, magnesium, cholesterol, amylase, lipase, or aminotransferase levels or an anemia that is microcytic, normocytic, or macrocytic.

Marasmus is seen most commonly in younger children and results from inadequate caloric intake. Children may be hypotonic and irritable, but the most notable physical finding is extreme wasting of muscle and subcutaneous tissue.

The most common vitamin and mineral deficiencies in children are of calcium, iron, zinc, magnesium, vitamin B_6, and vitamin A (Tables 86-5 and 86-6). Young children are at the greatest risk for iron deficiency because of their rapid growth and high nutritional requirements. Full-term infants are born with iron stores that meet their growth requirements until 4 to 6 months of age, when most infants have begun cereal and solid foods that provide iron. Premature

Table 86-5. States of Vitamin Excess and Deficiency

Name	Effects of Deficiency	Effects of Excess	Dietary Sources
Vitamin A (retinol)	Night blindness, xerophthalmia, keratomalacia, poor bone growth, follicular hyperkeratosis	Hyperostosis, hepatomegaly, alopecia, increased cerebrospinal fluid pressure	Liver, egg, cheese
Biotin	Seborrheic dermatitis, anorexia, pallor, alopecia, myalgias, paresthesias	Unknown	Liver, egg yolk, soybeans, milk, meat
Vitamin B_{12} (cyanocobalamin)	Pernicious anemia	Unknown	Meat, fish, poultry, cheese, milk, eggs
Folate	Megaloblastic anemia, impaired cellular immunity, irritability, paranoia	May mask pernicious anemia in vitamin B_{12} individual	Yeast, liver, leafy green vegetables, oranges, cantaloupe
Niacin	Pellagra: dermatitis, diarrhea, dementia	Flushing, pruritus, hyperuricemia, decreased LDL and increased HDL cholesterol	Milk, eggs, poultry, meat, fish, whole grains, enriched grains
Vitamin B_6 (pyridoxine)	Irritability, depression, dermatitis, glossitis, cheilosis, peripheral neuritis; in infants: convulsions, microcytic anemia	Neuropathy, photosensitivity	Liver, meat, whole grains, legumes, potatoes
Vitamin B_2 (riboflavin)	Photophobia, cheilosis, glossitis, poor growth	Unknown	Meat, dairy products, eggs, green vegetables, whole grains, enriched grains
Vitamin B_1 (thiamine)	Beriberi: neuritis, edema, congestive heart failure, hoarseness, anorexia, aphonia	Unknown	Enriched grains, lean pork, whole grains, legumes
Vitamin C (ascorbic acid)	Scurvy: diarrhea, bleeding gums, perifollicular hemorrhage	Nephrolithiasis, nausea, abdominal pain	Papaya, citrus fruits, tomatoes, cabbage, potatoes, cantaloupe, strawberries
Vitamin D	Rickets: osteopenia, fractures	Hypercalcemia, azotemia, poor growth, vomiting, nephrocalcinosis	Fortified milk and margarine, fish, liver, egg yolk
Vitamin E	Hyporeflexia, neurologic abnormalities	Bleeding, impaired leukocyte function	Sardines, green leafy vegetables, wheat germ, whole grains, liver, egg yolk
Vitamin K	Bleeding	Hyperbilirubinemia, hemolysis	Cow milk, green leafy vegetables, pork, liver

HDL, high-density lipoprotein; LDL, low-density lipoprotein.

Adapted from Committee on Nutrition, American Academy of Pediatrics: Vitamins. In Kleinman RE (ed): Pediatric Nutrition Handbook, 4th ed. Elk Grove Village, Ill, American Academy of Pediatrics, 1998, pp 267–281.

Table 86-6. States of Mineral Excess and Deficiency

Name	Effects of Deficiency	Effects of Excess	Dietary Sources
Calcium	Rickets, poor growth, tetany	Unknown	Milk, cheese, green leafy vegetables
Chloride	Alkalosis	Unknown	Table slat, milk, meat, eggs
Chromium	Impaired glucose utilization	Unknown	Meat, cheese, whole grains, yeast
Cobalt	Unknown	Few toxic effects	Green leafy vegetables
Copper	Sideroblastic anemia, poor growth, osteoporosis, neutropenia, hypopigmentation	Few toxic effects	Shellfish, meat, legumes, whole grains
Fluoride	Dental caries	Fluorosis of teeth	Tap water, seafood
Iodine	Goiter	Few toxic effects	Table salt, seafood
Iron	Anemia	Abdominal pain, emesis, diarrhea, edema, acidosis, renal or hepatic failure	Liver, meat, egg yolk, green leafy vegetables, legumes, whole grains
Magnesium	Tetany	Few toxic effects	Whole grains, beans, legumes, green leafy vegetables
Manganese	Unknown	Few toxic effects	Nuts, whole grains, tea
Molybdenum	Unknown	Gout symptoms	Meats, grains, legumes
Phosphorus	Rickets, muscle weakness	Few toxic effects	Meat, milk, egg yolk, legumes, whole grains
Potassium	Muscle weakness, anorexia, nausea, confusion, tachycardia	Heart block	All foods
Selenium	Cardiomyopathy	Irritation of mucous membranes, pallor, irritability	Seafood, meat, whole grains
Sodium	Nausea, diarrhea, muscle cramps, dehydration	Edema	Table salt, milk, eggs
Sulfur	Unknown	Few toxic effects	Meat
Zinc	Anorexia, poor growth, delayed puberty, impaired wound healing, acrodermatitis enteropathica	Few toxic effects	Liver, meat, whole grain, cheese

Adapted from Committee on Nutrition, American Academy of Pediatrics: Trace elements. In Kleinman RE (ed): Pediatric Nutrition Handbook, 4th ed. Elk Grove Village, Ill, American Academy of Pediatrics, 1998, pp 247–266.

infants have lower body stores that are depleted by 2 to 3 months of age and have a higher growth rate than full-term infants. As a result, they require iron supplementation in addition to regular dietary intake. Risk of iron deficiency declines between 3 years of age and puberty but increases again with the adolescent growth spurt and the onset of menarche. Other children at risk for inadequate iron intake include infants greater than 6 months of age who are exclusively breast-fed and children with excessive cow milk intake. Laboratory findings of iron deficiency anemia include microcytosis, a low ferritin level, and a red blood cell distribution width greater than 17.

At least 50% of children younger than 5 years old, 65% of boys aged 12 to 19 years, and 85% of girls aged 12 to 19 years do not meet the daily recommended calcium intake. The major source of calcium for children in the United States is dairy products. Groups at particular risk for calcium deficiency include preterm infants, adolescents, vegetarians, and lactose-intolerant individuals. Diets high in sodium or phosphate and the use of steroids, diuretics, or aluminum-containing antacids all decrease total body calcium and predispose a child to osteopenia. Calcium requirements are proportional to bony storage needs and are greatest at times of rapid growth. Preterm infants experience rapid bone growth and have high needs. Adolescents have rapid growth and typically low levels of intake. Fast-food meals that are high in sodium and low in calcium and the substitution of soft drinks (with a low calcium-to-phosphorus ratio) for milk contribute to inadequate calcium intake.

Because the serum ionized calcium level is regulated closely, total body calcium stores may be low despite a normal serum level. Laboratory evaluation for calcium deficiency includes a serum calcium level, phosphorus level, parathyroid hormone, alkaline phosphatase, 25-dihydroxy-vitamin D, and 1,25-dihydroxyvitamin D. There may be radiographic evidence of osteopenia. Bone mass measurements currently are not used for the clinical evaluation of bone density in children.

MANAGEMENT

Management of nutritional disorders is most optimal when it is done through a multidisciplinary team that includes a pediatric health care provider, nutritionist, social worker, and psychologist when necessary. Intervention should be initiated as early as possible in the child's life. Because children are dependent on the family unit and adult caretakers, the treatment plan must include the child's family and primary caretakers.

The management of obesity requires multiple components. The child may need subspecialty referral for diagnosis and treatment of a medical condition causing the obesity or for evaluation of a medical complication of obesity. The child also may require referral to a specialized pediatric obesity treatment center. Criteria for such a referral include obesity in a child younger than 2 years old, the presence of severe obesity, or the presence of a medical condition with serious morbidity requiring rapid weight loss. Although there are few specialized centers to accept such referrals, they may be available to clinicians for phone consultation. Behavioral goals, weight goals, and medical goals must be set for the child and the family. Behavioral goals include changes in the child's eating and activity and changes in parenting behaviors. Medical goals include the improvement of complications, such as hypertension or insulin resistance, and weight goals include weight maintenance or weight loss (Fig. 86-1). The child and the family should be advised that behavior and weight changes are small and gradual.

Weight loss should not be attempted until a family displays an ability to maintain the child's current weight. If successful in preventing further weight gain, weight loss should not exceed 1 lb/mo. The child should be monitored for medical complications of weight loss, including cholelithiasis, slowing of linear growth, loss of lean body mass, and psychological issues, such as eating disorders, difficulties with self-esteem, frustration, unrealistic expectations, and preoccupation with weight and body image.

Needed changes in parenting behaviors include establishment of regular mealtimes and snack times, provision of only healthy food options, and use of a favorite activity or time with a caretaker as a reward instead of food. Parents must learn that they, and not the child, determine the food that is offered at mealtime and that the child determines whether or not to eat the food that is offered. Parents must act as role models during mealtimes and be consistent in their actions related to food. For an older child or adolescent, parental support is important in helping them make healthy food and activity choices.

Children and adolescents should participate in at least 30 minutes of vigorous activity on most days. The easiest way to maintain such activities is if they are part of a child's daily routine. Children may prefer different categories of activities, such as team sports, individual sports, or activities with parents or siblings. After-school organized activities, regular playtime with friends or family, walking to and from school, and household chores decrease sedentary behavior.

Children should have no more than 1 to 2 hours of television, videos, or computer time per day. Decreasing sedentary behaviors in children who are not interested in initiating physical activity ultimately can divert their interest into other, more active endeavors.

The goal of dietary management for an obese child is to establish permanent changes in eating habits that result in healthier, more balanced meals. This goal is accomplished most effectively with the help of a nutritionist. Commercial weight loss programs are not recommended because their impact on a child's growth and well-being is unknown. Children and parents must be taught to address nutritional questions, to make healthy food choices outside of the home, and to self-monitor the feeling of hunger and to eat only when hungry. Multiple methods are available to teach children and parents which foods to eat. Forbidding certain foods has not been as effective as teaching moderation in intake and by teaching a family to eliminate certain high-calorie foods slowly from the family diet. Substitution of high-calorie foods with low-calorie foods containing saccharin or aspartame, without other dietary changes, has been shown to have no significant effect on daily caloric intake because these individuals tend to consume other high-calorie foods on a daily basis.

Treatment of children with failure to thrive is a multidisciplinary effort that involves dietary, social work, occupational therapy, and medical expertise. Infants and children also may require specialist referral for evaluation of conditions causing the growth impairment. Child protective services should be notified at the discretion of the health care team in cases of failure to thrive if there is intentional withholding of food or other abusive or neglectful circumstances.

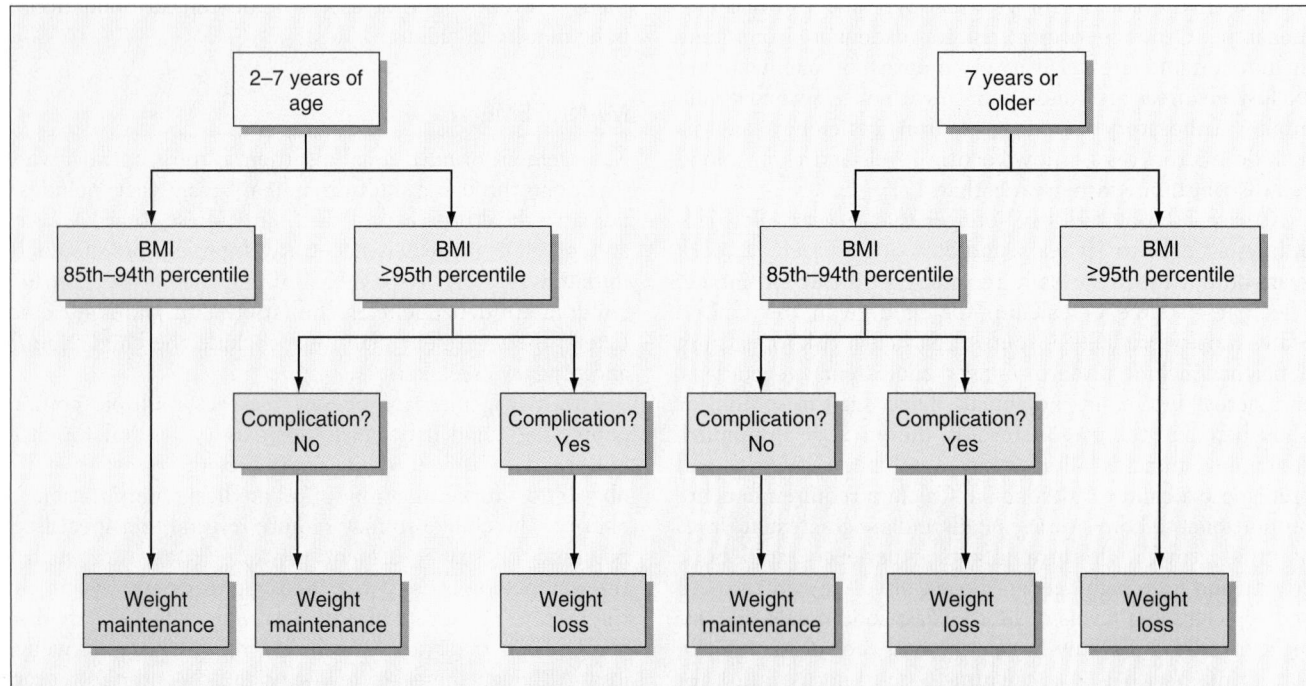

Figure 86-1. Recommended weight goals for obesity treatment. (Modified from Barlow SE, Dietz WH: Obesity evaluation and treatment: Expert committee recommendations. Pediatrics 1998;102:E29. Copyright 1998. Reproduced with permission from *Pediatrics*.)

Many cases of failure to thrive may be managed on an outpatient basis. Criteria for inpatient admission include serious malnutrition, failure to thrive that is refractory to outpatient intervention, and evidence of trauma or abuse that raises a concern for the child's safety in the home environment.

Depending on the severity of undernutrition and the primary care provider's level of expertise, initial dietary changes may be started before dietary consultation. To meet the child's needs for catch-up growth, daily caloric intake should be 1.5 to 2 times the usual daily intake by increasing the caloric density of the child's food, rather than by increasing the amount. Formula may be concentrated from 20 kcal/oz to 24 kcal/oz (Table 86-7), glucose polymers may be added as additional carbohydrates, or medium-chain triglyceride oil or corn oil may be added as a fat source. For children older than 2 years of age, breakfast shakes may be made with milk and eaten at any time of day, in addition to regular meals, to increase caloric intake. Older children also may eat high-calorie foods, such as peanut butter, cheese, cream, or margarine. Because during the period of catch-up growth, infants and children have higher protein needs than others their age, the balance of caloric intake with protein, carbohydrates, and fat requires ongoing monitoring. If a child does not gain weight on an adequate caloric intake, he or she may be admitted for monitored feeding sessions, or a nasogastric tube may be placed to facilitate feedings.

Because most cases of failure to thrive also involve issues of interpersonal interaction, mothers must be educated on recognizing infant cues for hunger and satiety and creating nurturing interactions with their infants or children. Distractions must be eliminated from mealtime. Parents must be taught appropriate feeding techniques and to avoid a pattern of force feeding. Support from public services, counseling, a visiting home nurse, or respite care also may be helpful for the family and improve the child's nutritional intake.

Children with severe protein or calorie malnutrition should be admitted to the hospital, and refeeding should be done in consultation with an expert in pediatric nutrition. The type of nutritional deficiency (protein, calorie, or vitamin/mineral), the extent of the dehydration, and presence of electrolyte imbalances all must be determined.

Although some children have an increase in total body water, most are intravascularly depleted. Electrolyte imbalances may include hypokalemia, hypomagnesemia, and hypoglycemia. Because infection is prevalent in severely malnourished infants, a screening chest x-ray and blood, urine, and stool cultures should be sent.

Refeeding is begun with special formulas, often via a nasogastric tube, with a goal to deliver approximately 175 kcal/kg/day and 4 g protein/kg/day. Vitamins and minerals also must be supplemented as needed (see Tables 86-5 and 86-6). Social work or psychological assessment of the caretakers may help to determine the factors that led to the undernutrition, and child protective services should be notified at the discretion of the health care team. For a malnourished child with developmental delay, psychological stimulation also may help in the "catch-up" of developmental abilities. Children with suspected vitamin excess or deficiency should be managed in conjunction with a pediatric nutritional specialist and with appropriate specialists who can address the complications of these disorders.

OUTCOME

Obese children have greater success with weight loss and weight maintenance if the entire family is involved in the treatment plan and supports the child's lifestyle changes. Strategies for weight maintenance have not been well studied and are not based on reliable data. The presence of obesity at progressively older ages in a child or adolescent is correlated with a higher risk of adult obesity and its associated morbidity and mortality.

The outcomes of patients with failure to thrive or severe undernutrition are best if they are treated by multidisciplinary teams and not by the primary care provider alone. The risk of permanent growth impairment (even after intervention) is greatest in patients with a younger age of onset and longer duration. Studies of patients have found a higher prevalence of intellectual, language, and motor delays and behavioral problems compared with well-nourished children. It is unclear whether these issues are the result of undernutrition, the lack of a stimulating social environment, or both.

FOLLOW-UP

Nutritional disorders, including obesity, failure to thrive, and severe vitamin or mineral deficiencies, require frequent and long-term medical follow-up. Children require monitoring for appropriate food intake, and the family benefits from ongoing support of lifestyle changes and counseling for new psychosocial stressors that may arise.

Children with a history of undernutrition are at risk for cognitive and developmental delays and behavioral difficulties, whereas children with a history of obesity are at risk for eating disorders and other psychological disorders. These children should undergo periodic developmental or psychological assessments to detect cognitive, developmental, or behavioral problems that may be long-term sequelae of the nutritional disorder.

Table 86-7. Formula: Water Ratios for Increasing Caloric Density of Infant Formulas

kcal/oz	Amount of Powder or Concentrate	Volume of Water (oz)
Powdered Formula*		
20	2 scoops	4
24	3 scoops	5
30	9 scoops	12
Liquid Concentrate†		
20	13 oz (1 can)	13
24	13 oz	8.5
30	13 oz	4

*Powdered formula = 40 cal/tbsp (= 40 cal/scoop).
†Liquid concentrate = 40 cal/oz.

Additional Resources, CD-ROM

Bibliography

Mini-index of Related Topics

SUGGESTED READINGS

Barlow SE, Dietz WH: Obesity evaluation and treatment: Expert committee recommendations. The Maternal and Child Health Bureau, Health Resources and Services Administration, and the Department of Health and Human Services. Pediatrics 1998;102:E29.

Dietz WH, Robinson TN: Use of the body mass index as a measure of overweight in children and adolescents. J Pediatr 1998;132:191–193.

Gahagan S, Holmes R: A stepwise approach to evaluation of undernutrition and failure to thrive. Pediatr Clin North Am 1998;45:169–187.

Must A, Jacques PF, Dallal GE, et al: Long-term morbidity and mortality of overweight adolescents: A follow-up of the Harvard Growth Study of 1922–1935. N Engl J Med 1992;327:1350–1355.

Story M, Neumark-Sztainer D: Promoting health eating and physical activity in adolescents. Adolesc Med 1999;10:109–123.

Strauss R: Childhood obesity. Curr Probl Pediatr 1999;29:5–29.

SECTION 3   GENERAL MEDICAL CARE: *Gastrointestinal and Nutritional Disorders*

87 Gastroesophageal Reflux

George Gershman

ROLE OF THE GENERALIST

1. Apply a consistent diagnostic approach to patients with recurrent emesis.
2. Recognize signs of significant disease.
3. Distinguish gastrointestinal reflux from gastroesophageal reflux disease (GERD).
4. Provide management of GERD for affected infants.
5. Treat the complications of GERD.
6. Refer to a pediatric gastroenterologist when assistance is needed with diagnosis or management of GERD.

FUNDAMENTALS

Definition and Epidemiology

Gastroesophageal reflux (GER) is an effortless passage of gastric contents into the esophagus. Most episodes of GER are brief and harmless and can occur 20 to 50 times per day in healthy infants, children, and adults. Most infants and children with GER have no definable anatomic, metabolic, infectious, or neurologic problems. GER can be non-regurgitant or regurgitant. *Nonregurgitant* or *silent GER* implies the movement of the gastric content into the distal or middle esophagus. *Regurgitant GER* involves the retrograde movement of gastric contents to the level of the oral pharynx and is restricted mostly to infants who manifest effortless dribbling or spitting up of swallowed breast milk or infant formula. Regurgitation at least once per day is reported in 50% of infants younger than 3 months old. Regurgitation peaks at 4 months of age, reaching 67%, and sharply decreases to 21% in infants 6 to 7 months old. Less than 5% of infants remain symptomatic by 12 months of age. Most infants with regurgitation are healthy and have normal development—the so-called *happy spitter*. Infants are more likely to regurgitate because the esophagus is shorter, they are usually recumbent, feeds are predominantly liquid, and caloric density of food is much higher compared with older children and adults. Maturation of gastric compliance, improved truncal tone, upright posture, gradually decreasing caloric density, and more solid food are responsible for the natural course of diminishing infantile reflux with age.

If recurrent emesis does not cease after 1 or 1.5 years of age, spontaneous resolution is unlikely. Data regarding prevalence of regurgitation in children 2 years and older are sparse but suggest a prevalence of GER of 2% and 8% in children 3 to 9 years old and 10 to 17 years old, respectively. The percentage of children with recurrent emesis and heartburn who have *gastroesophageal reflux disease (GERD)* is unclear.

The major difference between uncomplicated GER and GERD is the degree of associated pathologic conditions

(Box 87-1). GERD not only is a more complex disorder, but also has a more chronic and relapsing course, comparable with adult GERD. According to an Australian study of 126 infants (mean age 2 months) with GERD, less than 40% of infants with esophagitis and only three fourths of infants with failure to thrive or respiratory diseases had satisfactory response to medical treatment. One study indicates that less than 40% of symptomatic children 3 years and older were symptom-free 1 to 8 years after initial treatment.

Physiology

The esophagus conducts liquid and solid food to the stomach and prevents regurgitation of gastric contents into the airways. Coordinated contraction of the esophagus (peristalsis) and swallow-related opening of the upper esophageal sphincter (UES) and lower esophageal sphincter (LES) conducts liquid and food to the stomach. Regurgitation is prevented by a constant positive-pressure gradient between the LES and the stomach and closure of the UES between swallows. The UES consists of the cricopharyngeal muscle and a caudal portion of the inferior pharyngeal constrictor. The UES closes with stimulation of the somatic nerves and relaxes with swallowing. Inhibitory stimulation from the swallowing center in the brainstem is conducted by the vagus nerve. The UES opens right before and closes right after pharyngeal constriction. The UES pressure increases with esophageal distention and presence of acid in the esophagus. The latter phenomenon is absent in infants less than 10 weeks old. The UES pressure increases during inspiration, protecting the lungs from aspiration and excessive insufflation of the esophagus. It decreases during the first stage of sleep and diminishes to a greater extent during deep sleep.

The LES is a complex functional unit, which consists of intrinsic muscles of the distal esophagus augmented by the oblique fibers of the proximal stomach and extrinsic muscles of the crural diaphragm. The LES is relatively short (about 1 cm) at birth, growing to 4 cm in length in adults. At birth, the range of LES pressure in full-term infants is equal to adults' values and is almost twice as high in the first week of life than at 6 months. The LES is kept closed at rest, creating a constant pressure gradient toward the stomach. Small minute-to-minute fluctuations in pressure are related to LES contractions. Large fluctuations in LES pressure are linked with the activity of the migrating motor complex of the stomach and contractions of the crural

Table 87-1. Effects of Pharmacologic Agents on the Lower Esophageal Sphincter

Increases LES Pressure	Decreases LES Pressure
α-Adrenergic agonists	β-Adrenergic agonists
Bethanechol	α-Adrenergic antagonists
β-Adrenergic antagonists	Anticholinergics
Metoclopramide	Dopamine
Domperidone	Calcium channel blockers
Cisapride	Caffeine
	Nicotine
	Nitrates
	Theophylline

Adapted from Castell DO: Anatomy and physiology of the esophagus and its sphincters. In Castell DO, Richter JE, Dalton CB (eds): Esophageal Motility Testing. New York, Elsevier Biomedical, 1987, p 24.

diaphragm. LES pressure peaks before the onset of gastric contractions and increases with each inspiration. LES tone is influenced by different foods: Protein-rich food increases and fatty foods, chocolate, and coffee lower LES pressure. Table 87-1 lists the many drugs that can affect the LES. LES muscle tone is controlled by shifts of intracellular stores of calcium in smooth muscle and efferent vagal stimulation of neurons in the myenteric plexus. Swallowing-induced relaxation of the LES occurs with postganglionic transmission of nitric oxide and vasoactive intestinal peptide. Swallowing-induced relaxation of the LES is coupled with synchronous selective inhibition of the crural diaphragm.

Pathophysiology

The main mechanism of GER in normal children and adults and patients with reflux disease is transient LES relaxation. Transient LES relaxation is not mediated by swallowing. It is a long-lasting period (10 to 60 seconds) of simultaneous relaxation of the LES and the crural diaphragm. Transient LES relaxation is accompanied by inhibition of primary esophageal peristalsis and partial inhibition of esophageal body tone. Gastric distention increases the frequency of these relaxations.

Frequent and prolonged reflux can create enough contact of the esophageal mucosa and hydrochloric acid to increase regional blood flow and local tissue content of prostaglandin E2. As permeability of the mucosa to acid increases, inflammation occurs that itself may impair motility of the distal esophagus and the LES, enhancing GER and esophagitis. Involvement of the vagal nerve endings also may exacerbate LES dysfunction, promote pylorospasm, and delay gastric emptying, a common finding in children with GERD. Because esophageal, bronchial, and alveolar vagal nerve endings have the same embryonic origin, irritation of the vagal nerve endings can mediate vagovagal reactions of apnea, bradycardia, cough, laryngospasm, and bronchospasm.

DIAGNOSIS

Uncomplicated infantile GER is a clinical diagnosis that does not require confirmation by any available techniques. Diagnosis is based on a history of recurrent spitting up or emesis, normal development, and a normal physical examination. Environmental factors should be analyzed carefully, including the experience and anxiety of the mother and risk

Box 87-1. Complications Related to Gastroesophageal Reflux and Gastroesophageal Reflux Disease

- Failure to thrive
- Apnea and bradycardia
- Asthma
- Recurrent pneumonia
- Stridor
- Sandifer syndrome
- Esophagitis
- Esophageal stricture
- Barrett's esophagus

factors for GER, such as overfeeding, complications of pregnancy or delivery, infant age of onset, characteristics of the emesis, and family history of cow milk protein allergy. In most cases, this information should alert the clinician to underlying problems that can induce vomiting (Box 87-2). The volume of vomited breast milk or formula and the frequency of emesis are not indications for barium or esophageal pH study in thriving and otherwise healthy infants. "Red flags" or warning signs that require a prompt and thorough diagnostic workup of vomiting infants are listed in Box 87-3.

Complicated Gastroesophageal Reflux or Gastroesophageal Reflux Disease

The presence of acid in the esophagus explains neither the cause of symptoms nor the cause of GER. The main goal of confirmatory studies in GERD is to establish a strong association between symptoms or pathologic conditions and acid reflux.

Infants with forceful or projectile, bilious or nonbilious vomiting; cough initiated by feeding; refusal to eat; and failure to thrive should be studied first with an upper gastrointestinal (GI) series to detect anatomic abnormalities, such as malrotation, hiatal hernia, esophageal stricture, tracheoesophageal fistula, antral/duodenal web, and small bowel obstruction. In addition, barium swallow video study is an excellent tool for the diagnosis of cricopharyngeal abnormalities in pediatric patients. Upper GI series should not be used to diagnose GER. Sensitivity and specificity are low compared with esophageal pH monitoring.

Box 87-2. Disorders Associated with Vomiting in Infants and Children

- Obstruction of gastrointestinal tract
  - Pyloric stenosis
  - Malrotation with intermittent volvulus
  - Incarcerated hernia
  - Hirschsprung disease
  - Foreign body
  - Antral/duodenal web
- Acute and chronic gastrointestinal disorders
  - Gastroenteritis
  - Food allergy
  - Pancreatitis
  - Peptic ulcer disease
- Infections
  - Sepsis
  - Meningitis
  - Urinary tract infections
  - Otitis media
- Increased intracranial pressure
- Endocrine/metabolic
  - Congenital adrenal hyperplasia
  - Galactosemia
  - Hereditary fructose intolerance
  - Urea cycle defects
- Toxic
  - Lead
  - Iron
  - Medications

Box 87-3. Red Flags: Warning Signals in Vomiting Infants

- Bilious or forceful vomiting
- Hematemesis
- Hematochezia
- Failure to thrive
- Onset of emesis after 6 months of age
- Diarrhea
- Constipation
- Abdominal tenderness
- Abdominal distention
- Fever
- Lethargy
- Hepatosplenomegaly
- Bulging fontanelle
- Macrocephaly or microcephaly
- Seizures
- Down syndrome and other genetic disorders

Regurgitation of barium to the midesophagus or even into the mouth during an otherwise normal study means only that an infant or child had one or more episodes of GER. It does not provide any information regarding the reproducibility of this event or association with the patient's symptoms. Because barium is an inert substance that does not activate various receptors coordinating gastric emptying, an upper GI series cannot be used to assess gastric emptying, a common abnormality in children with GERD.

Prolonged esophageal pH monitoring is the gold standard for the diagnosis of pathologic acid reflux. The ambulatory version is well adapted to a more physiologic setting and the patient's routine environment. Changes of esophageal pH can be measured and analyzed for frequency, duration, correlation with the child's activity, position, feeding, symptoms, time, efficacy of medical therapy, and surgical correction of GER. The test can be limited by the buffering action of large amounts of neutral infant formula to the gastric acidity, which makes interpretation of the postprandial portion of the tracing difficult. The most common technique used to overcome this limitation is addition of hydrochloric acid, 0.1 N, to the formula or the substitution of apple juice for at least one regular feeding. Currently, prolonged esophageal pH monitoring is not recommended just for confirmation of clinically suspected GER. It is also indicated to (1) establish the relationship of GER with respiratory symptoms, (2) document pathologic GER before fundoplication or laryngeal surgery, and (3) assess the efficacy of medical treatment or performed surgery. In infants with frequent apnea and bradycardia, prolonged esophageal pH monitoring must be combined with a pneumogram, a synchronous recording of nasal air flow, respiratory rate, heart rate, and oxygen saturation.

Esophagogastroduodenoscopy (EGD) with target biopsy is a safe and reliable method for detection of mucosal lesions of the esophagus, stomach, and duodenum. Box 87-4 lists indications for esophagogastroduodenoscopy. It is a gold standard for diagnosis of esophagitis, Barrett's esophagus, and concomitant gastric or duodenal lesions. Pathologic GER is always present in infants and children with esophagitis, but only 50% of pediatric patients with GERD have detectable inflammation of the esophagus. An endoscopically "normal" esophagus does not rule out esophagitis in pediatric patients. A target biopsy specimen always should be obtained during endoscopy in infants and children with suspected GERD. Erosions, ulcers, and "vertical lines" are more reliable endoscopic signs of esophagitis.

A technetium-99m-radiolabeled meal is used for scintigraphic evaluation of GERD, a noninvasive test with low radiation. Scintiscan allows for the diagnosis of postprandial reflux independently from esophageal acidification, the assessment of gastric emptying, and the detection of aspiration. Disadvantages of the method are the brevity of the evaluation period and insensitivity for late postprandial reflux. Sensitivity of the test varies from center to center. In experienced hands, sensitivity may reach 60% or 70% compared with esophageal pH monitoring. To improve sensitivity, 24-hour delayed images after a single meal have been used. False-negative results can occur in patients with infrequent aspiration. Specificity of GERD scintigraphy is greater than 80%.

Therapeutic response to the treatment of GERD may be considered as a diagnostic test. Symptomatic improvement and subsequent worsening of symptoms when therapy is discontinued provide a reasonable indication of reflux-related problems. Empirical therapy should be short (2 to 3 weeks). Empirical therapy is contraindicated in infants and children with the red flags and warning signals listed in Box 87-3.

Approach to the Infant with Recurrent Vomiting

Recurrent regurgitation or emesis in infants can be divided in three broad categories: "happy spitter," GERD, and vomiting secondary to underlying disorders. Detecting vomiting from underlying disorders (see Box 87-2) should be the focus of the initial evaluation because delayed or incorrect diagnosis can lead to a catastrophic outcome.

Analysis of patient history and physical examination are the only way to decide what test, if any, should be ordered. Bilious vomiting is a red flag for small bowel obstruction and malrotation until proved otherwise. Upper GI series should be ordered without delay. Nonbilious, forceful, projectile vomiting is a warning sign of pyloric stenosis or an antral web. If ultrasound detects a normal pyloric channel, a contrast study of the stomach is the next reasonable choice. Delayed passage of meconium in full-term newborns or the presence of abdominal distention in infants with vomiting should trigger concern about Hirschsprung disease and a request for barium enema and rectal suction biopsy.

Diagnosis of esophagitis, Mallory-Weiss syndrome, cow milk protein allergy, or eosinophilic gastritis should be entertained in infants with hematemesis. Upper GI endoscopy is the best diagnostic study in these circumstances. Sudden onset of vomiting in newborns never should be assumed as simple GER, and a sepsis workup is mandatory. Infants with recurrent emesis and irritability or crying after feeding, refusal to eat, hematemesis, or chronic respiratory problems (e.g., poor response to conventional therapy for asthma) should be referred to a pediatric gastroenterologist. Parental reassurance and education regarding the difference between uncomplicated infantile reflux and GERD are sufficient for *happy spitter* patients.

Recurrent Vomiting and Poor Weight Gain

GERD is not a frequent cause of poor weight gain. Other reasons for failure to thrive should be considered first. *Is the intake of calories adequate for the infant to thrive?* Dietary history, including technique of formula preparation and frequency and volume of feeding, gives a preliminary estimation of caloric intake. *Is the infant able to take the offered volume of food?* If a problem is found (e.g., improperly prepared formula) and resolved, close follow-up determines the need for further evaluation. If weight gain is suboptimal despite the estimated adequacy of caloric intake, complete blood count; comprehensive metabolic panel; urinalysis, including ketones; review of neonatal screening tests; and upper GI series to assess anatomy should be considered. Three additional diagnostic options can be used in situations in which reasonable explanations for poor weight gain are not found: (1) empirical trial with thickened or hypoallergenic formula, prokinetics, and acid-suppressive agents; (2) upper GI endoscopy with biopsy to rule out esophagitis; and (3) hospitalization for close observation of parent-child interaction and elimination of problems related to socioeconomic status or child neglect.

Recurrent Vomiting and Irritability

Healthy infants cry for an average of 2 hours daily, although some infants may cry 6 hours a day. The intensity of the crying usually peaks at 6 weeks of age. Significant subjectivity exists in parental perception of infant fussiness, cry, or sleep pattern: What is normal for some could be unacceptable for other parents, even inside the same family. In daily practice, uncertainty in association between infants' irritability, disturbed sleep patterns, and GER leaves pediatricians and gastroenterologists with the dilemmas of lack of evidence and parental frustrations. Limited and conflicting data do not allow for conclusions regarding the degree of association between infantile colic and GER. In one study, simultaneous video recording and esophageal pH monitoring showed some linkage between grimacing and GER. In two other studies, no correlation was found between excessive crying, irritability, back arching, and pathologic acid reflux. Significant decrease of crying was found in 5 infants with esophagitis after treatment with H_2 receptor antagonists (H_2RAs) compared with 13 untreated infants without esophagitis.

In the absence of warning signs, the clinician first should determine the magnitude of the problem using a symptom diary and eliminate inadequate feeding as a reason for crying and irritability. If recurrent vomiting and irritability are confirmed, two different strategies can be offered. The first one is a 2-week trial of a hypoallergenic formula, if there is a family history of dairy product allergy or intolerance. If symptoms persist, it should be followed by a 2- to 3-week trial of acid suppression therapy. Prolonged esophageal pH monitoring to assess effectiveness of acid suppression therapy or upper GI endoscopy with a biopsy to rule out esophagitis can be performed. The second approach is more aggressive and consists of initial (baseline) esophageal pH monitoring to calculate a symptoms, index—the ratio of the reflux-associated symptoms, for example, crying episodes associated with esophageal pH below 4 divided by total number of crying episodes during the study. If these studies are normal and response to empirical therapy has not occurred, GER is not a contributing factor to the symptoms.

Approach to Children 2 Years and Older with Gastroesophageal Reflux

Recurrent Vomiting

Nonbilious, nonbloody vomiting occasionally can occur postprandially on exertion in otherwise normal children. It is unclear to what extent it is a medical or behavioral social problem. Upper GI series can exclude anatomic abnormalities. If vomiting persists, upper GI endoscopy is suggested by some experts, but the diagnostic yield is relatively low. An empirical trial with prokinetic agents is a reasonable choice. If the patient improves, long-term therapy with prokinetics is an option.

Heartburn, Chest Pain, and Dysphagia

Heartburn, chest pain, and dysphagia, the typical adult-type presenting symptoms of GERD, can be difficult to identify in small children. If a careful history and physical examination suggest an esophageal origin of the problem, a 2- to 4-week therapeutic trial with H_2RAs or proton-pump inhibitors (PPIs) is recommended for children with heartburn and chest pain. For children with dysphagia, barium esophagram is advocated to assess for abnormalities, such as strictures, vascular or Shatzki ring, or radiologic signs of achalasia. Upper GI endoscopy with biopsy is performed in all children with dysphagia and the subset of patients with heartburn or chest pain who do not improve after an initial therapeutic trial.

In children with histologically proven esophagitis, follow-up endoscopy usually is unnecessary. If the patient remains symptomatic, esophageal pH monitoring is recommended while therapy is continued to estimate the efficacy of acid suppression.

A repeat endoscopy is required for children with erosive esophagitis to assess healing. If resolution of the symptoms does not occur or mucosal defects persist despite appropriate acid suppression, esophageal pH monitoring 72 hours after discontinuation of therapy is recommended. If pH monitoring is normal, the diagnosis of reflux esophagitis is unlikely.

Gastroesophageal Reflux Disease and Airway Disorders

The esophagus and airways are derived from the embryonic foregut and share some elements of innervation and protective systems. Vagal nerve endings of the esophagus and upper and lower airways have similar embryonic origin, and the UES constricts with inspiration to prevent aspiration into the lungs and excessive insufflation of the esophagus. Congenital anomalies of the esophagus and lung, such as esophageal atresia with tracheoesophageal fistula, bronchoesophageal fistula, and pharyngeal cleft, are seen often in conjunction with each other. This relationship provides the possible underlying link between some symptoms and conditions such as cough, emesis, apnea, bradycardia, laryngospasm, bronchospasm, aspiration, and GER.

Apnea

Apnea may be triggered by GER from vagovagal reactions resulting from hypersensitivity of the vagal nerve ending of the esophagus or sudden esophageal distention. The most convincing evidence that apnea is reflux induced is when it occurs within 1 hour after feeding with the infant awake and recumbent or during some activity (e.g., diaper change soon after a meal). Apnea may or may not be associated with overt regurgitation. The spectrum of apnea secondary to GER varies. Most episodes are brief (<20 seconds) without change of color or with acrocyanosis. Spontaneous resolution of these episodes is the rule. More severe episodes are rare, such as apnea of 20 seconds or longer with change in color and muscle tone, choking, and gasping—an apparent life-threatening event (ALTE). Appropriate intervention by the caretaker is necessary and may be lifesaving. Other causes of apnea, such as tracheomalacia, seizure/central nervous system disorders, and sepsis or other infections, should be ruled out before the initiation of a GER workup. In patients with recurrent ALTE in which the role of GER is uncertain, prolonged esophageal pH monitoring with simultaneous recording of nasal air flow, respiratory and heart rates, and oxygen saturation can assess for association between ALTE and acid reflux. Medical therapy combining formula thickening, positioning, and prokinetic and acid-suppressant medications is sufficient for most patients. Surgery as a treatment option should be discussed with parents but reserved only for infants with severe ALTE secondary to GER.

Asthma

Pathologic GER has been detected frequently (25% to 75%) in infants and children with asthma undergoing esophageal pH monitoring. Although patients with asthma frequently, but not always, have regurgitant reflux, GER can contribute to the severity of asthma either by microaspiration of gastric acid triggering hypersensitivity of the airway or by vagovagal reactions after esophageal acid exposure. Prolonged and aggressive treatment of GER has been associated with significant symptomatic or clinical improvement and a reduction in the intensity of conventional therapy needed in many patients with severe and persistent asthma.

Impressive data are reported for antireflux surgery (fundoplication) in selected pediatric patients with severe persistent asthma and proven pathologic GER by esophageal pH monitoring. Aggressive 3-month empirical therapy with H_2RAs or PPIs and prokinetic agents is recommended for adults with severe asthma and suspected GER. Similar therapy is justifiable for pediatric patients with severe and persistent asthma and GERD symptoms or selected patients with nonregurgitant pathologic reflux diagnosed by esophageal pH monitoring.

Laryngeal Inflammation

Laryngeal symptoms, such as hoarseness or stridor, in children can be secondary to GER. Laryngoscopic examination often reveals airway erythema, edema, vocal cord nodules, granuloma, and cobblestoning. The sensitivity and specificity of these findings are unknown in children and adults, although even small amounts of acid in prolonged contact with the larynx from poor laryngeal acid clearance could produce epithelial damage. Currently, there is no standard approach to this cohort of patients. Diagnostically motivated empirical therapy or esophageal pH monitoring, especially before laryngeal surgery, is justifiable.

Recurrent Pneumonia

Repeated aspiration of small amounts of gastric or swallowed fluids may lead to chronic inflammation of the lungs, pulmonary fibrosis, and severe impairment of pulmonary function. Evidence supporting this association includes reported improvement in pediatric patients with recurrent pneumonia after medical or surgical therapy of GER. In otherwise normal children, other causes of recurrent pneumonia, such as defective mechanism of swallowing, laryngeal cleft, tracheoesophageal or tracheobronchial fistula, pulmonary sequestration, foreign body, cystic fibrosis, and immune deficiency, should be excluded before considering GER as a potential cause of recurrent pneumonia. If abnormal swallowing is suspected, especially in neurologically compromised children, an assessment by an experienced occupational therapist and video swallowing study can be diagnostic. Radionuclide "salivagram" is a new diagnostic test, which may help to detect aspiration after a single ingestion of technetium-99m sulfur colloid.

Esophageal pH monitoring is indicated for a subset of neurologically compromised patients with frequent and radiologically documented aspiration pneumonia to justify fundoplication. Nuclear scintigraphy is noninvasive, has low radiation exposure, and can be repeated. Sensitivity of scintigraphy is higher when 24-hour delay images are taken. If both tests are negative, but a clinical suspicion for GER is high, flexible bronchoscopy with pulmonary lavage can be done to detect lipid-laden alveolar macrophages.

TREATMENT OF GASTROESOPHAGEAL REFLUX DISEASE

The current medical therapy of GERD has three essential elements: (1) selection of the therapy to match the degree of symptoms and severity of GERD-related complications, (2) validation of empirical therapy for certain types of GERD scenarios, and (3) reassessment of the therapeutic efficacy for further treatment options and revision of the diagnosis. Initial treatment of infants and children with uncomplicated GER does not require medication, but rather usually consists of parental reassurance and lifestyle modification. Potentially beneficial environmental changes for infants are improvement in mother-infant interaction, changes of the formula, and changes in sleep position.

Changing infant formula usually is useless, unless there is a strong family history of dairy products or other food allergy or intolerance. In these circumstances, hypoallergenic casein hydrolysate–based formula is the best choice. Cessation of vomiting within the first days of a trial is a good clinical indicator for a food allergy as the cause of GER.

Formula thickening with agents such as rice cereal does decrease the frequency of regurgitation but not other symptoms of GER. Increased volume and caloric density of formula is associated with high frequency of transient LES relaxation and more frequent cough in infants. Therefore, formula thickening is indicated primarily for infants with uncomplicated GER. One or two teaspoons of rice cereal can be added to 1 oz of formula. One tablespoon of rice cereal to 1 oz of regular 20 kcal/1 oz infant formula increases caloric density to 34 kcal/oz. If formula is thickened noncommercially, the nipple should be cross-cut for adequate flow. Commercially thickened formulas have proved to be effective in Europe. Currently, some formulas with rice starch, carob flour, and locust bean gum are available in the United States.

Limited studies regarding the influence of nasogastric tube on frequency and other characteristics of GER suggest that small (6 Fr to 8 Fr) feeding tubes do not promote GER in infants and children. Nasogastric or nasojejunal tube overnight feeding has been used successfully to improve nutrition of infants with GERD.

Position during sleep is a factor known to affect the frequency of transient LES relaxation. Prone position in infants and left lateral position in adults have been associated with reduced frequency of reflux. Prone position in infants has been associated with sudden infant death syndrome (SIDS), however. Although supine position is inferior to prone position for the control of reflux, it has been associated with a substantial decline in the rate of SIDS. The supine position is recommended even for infants with GERD. The prone position can be used for infants with high risk of death from complicated GERD. Parental education regarding soft bedding as a risk factor for SIDS in infants placed prone is extremely important. Lifestyle modification should be limited to suggestions to avoid chocolate, spicy food, or other products, which may aggravate symptoms. Similarly, caffeine restrictions, smoking cessation, and drinking alcohol should be emphasized for teenagers with GERD.

Pharmacotherapy

The goal of pharmacotherapy of GERD is to increase LES tone, decrease acid production, and promote gastric emptying. Two groups of medications have been used successfully: prokinetics and acid suppressants (H₂RAs and PPIs).

Prokinetics

When cisapride was readily available, it was prescribed for infants or children who failed treatment with lifestyle modification. Cisapride is a non–dopamine receptor–blocking, noncholinergic prokinetic drug with 5-hydroxytryptamine-antagonistic properties. Cisapride has been shown to reduce GER-related symptoms and promote healing of mucosal defects in children with esophagitis. Because cisapride can affect potassium channels in the myocardium and induce prolongation of the Q-T interval, it currently is available only by limited access protocol in the United States. Other prokinetics, such as metoclopramide and bethanechol, have many side effects, including dystonic reactions, irritability, dry mouth, urinary retention, and potential to aggravate bronchospasm. The frequency of these side effects usually outweighs the efficacy. Treatment should be started with the lowest recommended therapeutic doses.

Acid Suppressors
H₂-Receptor Antagonists

H₂RAs reduce acid secretion by blocking the H₂ receptors on the parietal cells. Effectiveness of this type of medication has been proved in numerous studies in adults. H₂RAs are more effective for patients with mild-to-moderate esophagitis than severe esophagitis. Effectiveness of H₂RAs in pediatric patients has been assessed less intensively. In one randomized control study of patients with esophagitis, patients who received cimetidine had significant improvement in symptoms and histology compared with the control group. The therapeutic effect usually is achieved at doses higher than recommended by pharmaceutical companies (Table 87-2). The common problem with H₂RAs is escape from the acid suppression action within 6 weeks of treatment.

Proton-Pump Inhibitors

PPIs are the most effective acid suppressive medications. They deactivate the hydrogen/potassium pump in parietal cells. PPIs should be activated by acid in the target cells. They are most effective when given 30 minutes before a meal to archive peak plasma concentration at the time of maximal acid stimulation by food. Numerous studies show superior efficacy of PPIs compared with H₂RAs in the treatment of erosive esophagitis in adults. Symptoms often recur after discontinuation of therapy. Headache, dry mouth, and diarrhea are common side effects. Hepatitis and interstitial nephritis have been reported less frequently. Because PPIs can affect liver metabolism of some drugs, such as benzodiazepines, warfarin, phenytoin, and cyclosporine, drug interaction should be considered before PPI administration.

Currently, there is no standard pediatric recommendation for PPI treatment. Use of PPIs is appropriate in infants and children who failed standard therapy or patients with severe respiratory manifestations of GERD.

Surgical Therapy

Surgery usually is reserved for infants and children with the most severe forms of GERD who have failed medical therapy. In most patients, the indication for fundoplication is respiratory complications related to GERD. In smaller groups of pediatric patients, antireflux surgery has been performed for uncontrolled esophagitis, esophageal stricture, or Barrett's esophagitis. A laparoscopic version of Nissen or Thal fundoplication is now available and compatible in its efficacy and morbidity to the standard surgical techniques. In the largest pediatric series, success rate approached 90%. The major complications after fundoplication are breakdown of the fundoplication wrap, intrathoracic herniation of the wrap, slipping at the wrap, excessive tightness of the fundoplication, and intestinal obstruction. The reported incidence of this complication is less than 15%. Gas bloat syndrome, dysphagia, dumping syndrome, gagging, and retching are less serious but potentially debilitating complications, especially in the first few months after surgery. These symptoms tend to resolve or improve in time. In infants and young children, fundoplication is performed in combination with gastrostomy to prevent gas bloat syndrome or to initiate enteral feeding.

Table 87-2. Pharmacologic Treatment of Gastroesophageal Reflux Disease

Type of Medication	Recommended Oral Dosage	Side Effects/Precautions
H₂-receptor antagonists Cimetidine (Tagamet)	40 mg/kg/day divided tid or qid	Rash, bradycardia, dizziness
Ranitidine (Zantac)	9–12 mg/kg/day divided tid (maximum 150 mg tid)	Headache, dizziness, rash
Famotidine (Pepcid)	1–2 mg/kg/day divided bid	Headache, dizziness
Proton-pump inhibitors	1–3.5 mg/kg/day divided	Headache, diarrhea
Lansoprazole (Prevacid)	1.5–3.5 mg/kg/day divided	Headache, diarrhea
Rabeprazole (Aciphex)	Adult dose: 20 mg qd	Headache, diarrhea, abdominal pain, nausea
Prokinetic		
Cisapride (Propulsid)	0.8 mg/kg/day divided qid	Available only by limited

Bid, twice a day; qd, everyday; qid, four times a day; tid, three times a day.

Adapted from Rudolph CD: Gastroesophageal reflux. In Lifschitz CH (ed): Pediatric Gastroenterology and Nutrition in Clinical Practice. New York, Marcel Dekker, 2002, p 494.

SUGGESTED READINGS

Boyle JT: Gastroesophageal reflux in pediatric patients. Gastroenterol Clin North Am 1989;18:315–337.

Orenstein SR, Izadnia F, Khan S: Gastroesophageal reflux disease in children. Gastroenterol Clin North Am 1999;28:947–969.

Rudolph CD: Gastroesophageal reflux. In Lifschitz CH (ed): Pediatric Gastroenterology and Nutrition in Clinical Practice. New York, Marcel Dekker, 2002, pp 481–500.

Vandenplas Y: Gastroesophageal reflux in children. Scand J Gastroenterol 1995;30(Suppl 213):31–38.

SECTION 3   GENERAL MEDICAL CARE: *Gastrointestinal and Nutritional Disorders*

88 Disorders of the Stomach

Ranjan Dohil

ROLE OF THE GENERALIST

1   Identify peptic disorders.

2   Exclude conditions that mimic peptic disorders.

3   Complete a through psychosocial evaluation to determine stress factors that predispose to nonulcer dyspepsia.

4   Consider a trial of therapy with antacids or H_2 blockers (≤4 weeks), which, if successful, may assist in the diagnosis of underlying peptic disorders.

5   Refer to specialists when assistance is needed in the diagnosis and management of patients with peptic disorders.

DEFINITIONS

Peptic disorders encompass a spectrum of diseases involving the esophagus, stomach, and duodenum, ranging from the histologic evidence of inflammation *(esophagitis, gastritis, duodenitis)* to the endoscopic finding of erosions and mucosal ulceration *(peptic ulcer disease)*. Peptic disorders are diagnosed at the time of upper gastrointestinal (GI) endoscopy or from gastric and duodenal biopsy specimens taken at the time of this procedure. Diagnosis of peptic disorders is not made by clinical history or serologic or radiologic tests.

FUNDAMENTALS

Typically, gastric acid production begins immediately after birth with the gastric luminal pH decreasing to 4 or less within the first hour of life and 1 by 48 hours postpartum.

Peptic disorders may arise anytime after birth and are thought to occur with an imbalance between aggressive factors and mucosal protective mechanisms. Any disturbance in the production of mucus, which normally forms a protective layer over the gastric and duodenal epithelium, or in the secretion of bicarbonate into the mucous layer ("mucus-bicarbonate barrier") exposes the underlying cell surface to the damaging effects of acid and pepsin. Prostaglandins play an integral role in gastric mucosal protection through (1) maintenance of microvascular circulation, (2) stimulation of epithelial cell turnover, (3) inhibition of gastric acid, and (4) stimulation of bicarbonate production. Aggressive factors that provoke mucosal damage include conditions associated with increased acid and pepsin production, such as stress, drugs, and infection. The degree of imbalance between the protective and aggressive factors ultimately accounts for the spectrum of peptic diseases, ranging from gastritis and duodenitis to ulceration, with its long-term sequelae (e.g., stricture formation).

Gastritis may or may not be associated with symptoms in children. The prevalence of gastritis in children is unknown, but is likely to be far less than that seen in adults, in which the gastritis-inducing effects of caffeine, nicotine, drugs, and alcohol contribute to the disorder. Gastritis may occur as a result of a targeted insult to the stomach (e.g., *Helicobacter pylori* infection) or may arise as part of a systemic disorder, such as stress, Crohn's disease, allergy, graft-versus-host disease, and cytomegalovirus infection. Understanding the pathogenesis of gastric inflammation is crucial to successful management of a child who presents with upper GI symptoms.

Peptic ulcers are characterized as primary or secondary, with primary ulcers occurring more often in the duodenum and secondary ulcers occurring more often in the stomach.

Secondary ulcers occur more often in children than do primary ulcers, usually in association with aspirin or non-steroidal anti-inflammatory drug (NSAID) ingestion or with underlying systemic disease, such as Crohn's disease, stress, and sepsis. Primary ulcers occur with conditions that cause acid hypersecretion, such as *H. pylori* infection, Zollinger-Ellison syndrome, and short bowel syndrome. Typically, primary peptic ulcers are chronic with histologic evidence of granulation tissue and fibrosis underlying an active inflammatory infiltrate. Secondary peptic ulcers usually are more acute in onset and usually do not have histologic evidence of fibrosis. Box 88-1 lists causes of gastritis and ulceration in children.

Determination of the nature of the underlying peptic disease may not be possible simply from the child's presenting complaints. Symptoms of most peptic disorders are similar. Mild esophagitis, gastritis, and severe duodenal ulceration may present with identical pain characteristics, despite the severity of the inflammation or its underlying etiology. Although abdominal pain is the most common symptom suggesting peptic disease, peptic disorders account for only 5% of children who present with chronic abdominal pain, even to a subspeciality clinic. Because a tertiary care children's hospital with a referral population of 3 million would be expected to diagnose only six to eight new cases of primary peptic ulcer disease per year, the approach to suspected ulcer disease in children is different from that in adults.

Helicobacter pylori

H. pylori is an important cause of peptic disease in children and adults and of gastric malignancy in adults. *H. pylori* is a gram-negative, urease-producing, motile bacillus that colonizes the stomach in 50% of the world's population. The prevalence of *H. pylori* gastritis in children in the United States is age dependent, with *H. pylori* accounting for few cases of gastritis in patients younger than age 5 years, but increasing to become the most common cause of gastritis in teenagers. Risk factors for infection include low socioeconomic status with familial overcrowding, birth in a developing country, and race (blacks > Hispanics > whites).

Virtually all people infected with *H. pylori* develop chronic active gastritis. When the infection is eradicated, the gastritis resolves. *H. pylori* infection is associated with 90% of diagnosed duodenal ulcers and to a lesser degree with gastric ulceration in children. It is a cofactor in the development of gastric B-cell lymphoma arising from mucosa-associated lymphoid tissue. Although most reports of *H. pylori*–associated gastric malignancy are in adults, rare cases also have been described in children age 11 to 16 years, with subsequent cure following *H. pylori* eradication in some. Gastric adenocarcinoma also is associated with *H. pylori* infection, and although it is reported only in adults, childhood aquisition is an important risk factor in its development.

For unknown reasons, only a few *H. pylori*–infected patients develop ulcer disease or malignancy. Suggested mechanisms include the interplay between certain bacterial virulence factors, such as cytotoxins *Vac A* and *Cag A*, which are produced by some subtypes of *H. pylori*, and the host's immune response. The host's response to gastric colonization with *H. pylori* may differ not only from person to person, but also from child to adult. Typically, infected children and adults develop chronic active antral gastritis, whereas only adults may develop atrophic gastritis, a condition that predisposes to gastric adenocarcinoma (Fig. 88-1).

Many diagnostic tests for *H. pylori* are available (Box 88-2). Commercially available serologic assays for IgG levels against *H. pylori* are a satisfactory screening tool but should not be the basis for treatment. *H. pylori* IgG levels may remain elevated for years after effective eradication or resolution of the infection. Positive serology does not always imply active infection. The most accurate noninvasive method for detecting active *H. pylori* is the ^{13}C or ^{14}C urea breath test. This semiquantitative test relies on the conversion of labeled urea to ammonia and bicarbonate and then to labeled carbon dioxide within the lungs. The carbon dioxide is measured within an expiratory breath and approximates bacterial load within the stomach. Urea breath testing is an accurate and easy means of confirming effective eradication of infection. The gold standard for the diagnosis of *H. pylori* infection is endoscopy with gastric antral biopsy. The organism can be seen best histologically by using a Steiner or Giemsa stain.

Nonsteroidal Anti-inflammatory Drugs and Other Drugs

NSAIDs produce mucosal injury through local irritant and systemic effects. A single dose of aspirin may cause petechial hemorrhages in the stomach within a few hours and erosions within 24 hours. These early lesions usually are of little clinical significance and do not predict whether ulcer formation will occur. In children, lesions caused by NSAIDs are more commonly gastric than duodenal and may include hemorrhagic gastritis and ulceration. Bleeding from these

---

Box 88-1. Peptic Disorders Affecting Children

- *Helicobacter pylori* gastritis
- Stress gastropathy
- Hypersecretory states
  - Zollinger-Ellison syndrome
  - Systemic mastocytosis
  - Cystic fibrosis
  - Short bowel syndrome
  - Hyperparathyroidism
- Crohn's gastritis
- Allergic gastritis
- Eosinophilic gastritis
- Neonatal gastritis
- Traumatic gastropathy
- Aspirin and other NSAIDs
- Corrosive gastropathy
- Exercise-induced gastropathy/gastritis
- Cytomegalovirus gastritis
- Radiation gastropathy
- Graft-versus-host disease
- Henoch-Schönlein gastropathy
- Ménétrier's disease
- Gastritis with autoimmune diseases
- Other infectious gastritides

NSAIDs, nonsteroidal anti-inflammatory drugs.

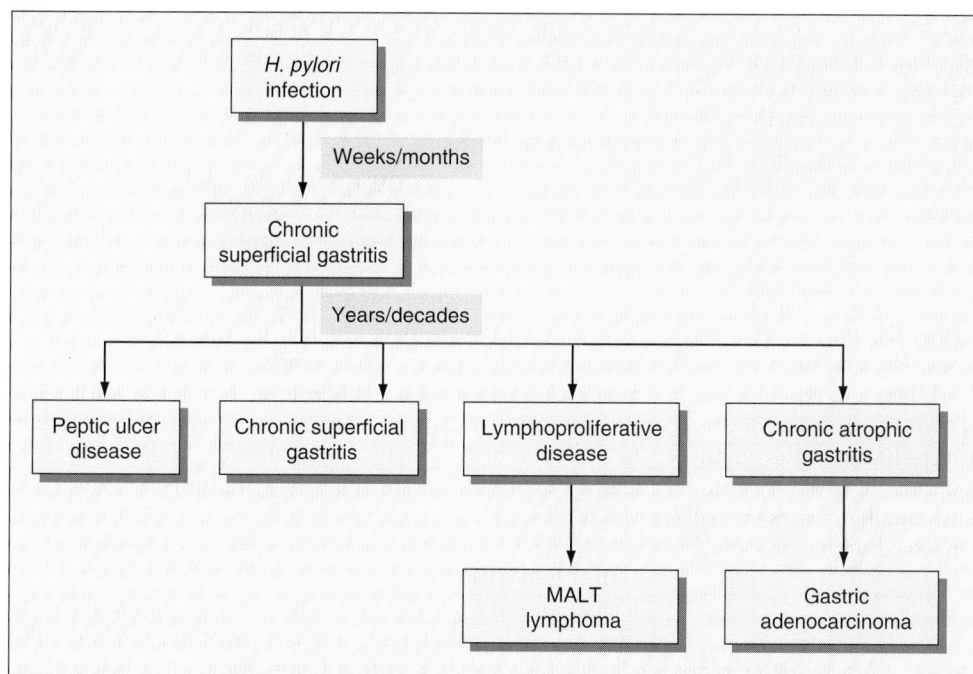

Figure 88-1. Natural history of *Helicobacter* infection.

lesions after NSAID ingestion in children has been well documented. Among children with juvenile rheumatoid arthritis who take one or more NSAIDs for more than 2 months, 75% have endoscopic evidence of gastritis, erosions, or ulcers; of these, two thirds may have anemia and abdominal pain. Other drugs implicated in the development of erosive or hemorrhagic gastropathy include valproic acid, dexamethasone, chemotherapeutic agents, alcohol, potassium chloride, and some antibiotics.

Stress Gastritis

Stress gastritis usually occurs within 24 hours of the onset of critical illness, such as shock, hypoxemia, acidosis, sepsis, burns, major surgery, multiple organ system failure, or head injury. These stressors cause reduction of gastric blood flow with subsequent mucosal ischemia and breakdown of mucosal defenses. In addition, sepsis and head trauma may be associated with acid hypersecretion. The resultant stress erosions are typically asymptomatic, are multiple, and do not perforate, but when they are symptomatic, the major symptom is overt upper GI hemorrhage. Newborns and infants seem to be more prone to perforations.

Crohn's Disease

Crohn's disease is the most common cause of granulomatous gastritis, and involvement of the stomach may occur in the absence of upper GI symptoms and sometimes even precedes the diagnostic features in the colon. Gastric involvement is relatively common, with ulceration, mucosal

swelling, and luminal narrowing occurring in 30% of children with the disease (Fig. 88-2). Symptoms similar to those of acid peptic disease and of delayed gastric emptying may occur, with hematemesis and melena occurring less frequently.

Hypersecretory States

Zollinger-Ellison syndrome is rare in children. In addition to the typical pancreatic gastrinomas, Zollinger-Ellison syndrome has been reported in children with solitary extra-pancreatic gastrinomas in stomach, liver, and kidney. Other conditions associated with acid hypersecretion include short bowel syndrome, hyperparathyroidism, systemic mastocytosis, and cystic fibrosis. Gastric acid hypersecretion is a transient phenomenon that can occur after massive small bowel resection (greater than two thirds) in infants and adults. The etiology is unclear, but the increased acid production may lead to peptic ulceration. Hypergastrinemia usually is observed and may be due to reduced levels of intestinal gastrin inhibitory factor.

Box 88-2. Tests for Suspected Ulcer Disease

- *Helicobacter pylori* serology—does not distinguish between recently treated and newly acquired infection
- ^{13}C urea breath test—detection of active *H. pylori* infection
- Upper gastrointestinal endoscopy and biopsy

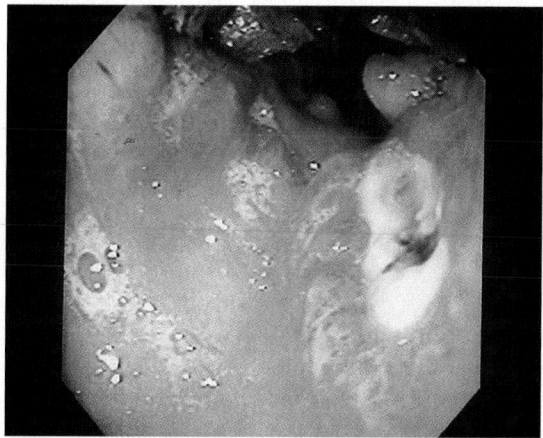

Figure 88-2. Chronic gastric ulceration in a child with Crohn's disease.

Allergic Gastritis

Allergic gastritis is the gastric component of allergic gastroenteritis and usually is associated with a specific allergen, such as cow milk or soy milk protein. Symptoms usually arise within the first 6 to 12 months of life. Gastric erosions may occur. Reintroduction of the antigen almost always is possible by 24 months of age or earlier.

Eosinophilic Gastroenteritis

Although eosinophilic gastroenteritis may share some common features with allergic gastritis, it is a chronic, severe disease, of unknown etiology, characterized by the presence of upper GI symptoms and signs and poor growth, GI bleeding, and often diarrhea. Iron deficiency anemia and hypoproteinemia with protein-losing enteropathy commonly are present. In most, but not all, patients, serum IgE is elevated, and peripheral eosinophilia is present. All layers of the gastric wall may be involved with eosinophilic infiltrate.

Traumatic Gastropathy

Traumatic gastropathy, also known as *prolapse gastropathy*, is due to forceful retching or vomiting causing trapping of the proximal stomach into the distal esophagus, resulting in vascular congestion and hemorrhages in the stomach. Mallory-Weiss tears in the gastroesophageal junction zone also may occur. Although prolapse gastropathy and tears tend to resolve quickly, they can result in significant blood loss. Suction through nasogastric tubes, ingestion of foreign bodies, and endoscopic procedures, such as diathermy, are common causes of subepithelial hemorrhages and focal erosions.

Neonatal Ulcers

A high prevalence of hemorrhagic gastropathy has been reported in sick neonates in intensive care units. These infants usually do not manifest upper GI symptoms or signs. These neonatal gastropathies are probably stress lesions but with a greater predilection to hemorrhage and perforation.

Autoimmune Disease

In children and adults with connective tissue diseases, mast cell and eosinophilic gastritides have been described. In a large group of children with insulin-dependent diabetes mellitus, 7% underwent upper GI endoscopy; 48% had evidence of erosions and ulcers, none from *H. pylori*.

Corrosive Gastropathy

The most common ingestants affecting the stomach are acids, iron, and strong alkalis; the last mentioned predominantly involve the esophagus, but occasionally involve the stomach. When gastric injury does occur, the pyloric area often is involved, with ulceration, hemorrhage, and rarely perforation.

Henoch-Schönlein Gastritis

Endoscopy seldom is required for diagnosis of Henoch-Schönlein gastritis, but it may be helpful if the diagnosis is uncertain, showing a hemorrhagic and erosive picture typical of this disorder. Although gastric mucosal biopsy specimens usually are too superficial to show typical histologic changes, they may show a vasculitis similar to that seen in the skin.

Other Infections

Rare causes of gastritis, erosions, and ulcers include *Helicobacter heilmannii*, herpes simplex, and cytomegalovirus in immunosuppressed patients; herpes zoster; influenza A; and *Mycobacterium tuberculosis* (usually associated with tuberculosis elsewhere or with immune deficiency). Fungal infections of the stomach, such as *Candida albicans*, histoplasmosis, and mucormycosis, may occur, especially in sick neonates, malnourished children, and children with burns or immune deficiencies. Acute gastric *anisakiasis* occurs in areas of high raw fish consumption. Early endoscopy allows for diagnosis and relief of symptoms by removal of the worm.

Other Gastritides

Celiac disease, hepatic cirrhosis, uremia, graft-versus-host disease, sickle cell disease, exercise, radiation, and bile reflux all may be associated with inflammation, ulcer disease, and hemorrhage.

DIAGNOSIS AND MANAGEMENT

Figure 88-3 summarizes the basic evaluation of children with persistent symptoms of upper GI disease. Symptoms of gastritis or peptic ulcer can be mimicked by nonulcer dyspepsia, constipation, esophagitis, gallbladder or liver disease, pneumonia, pancreatitis, or giardiasis (Table 88-1). Typical symptoms of peptic ulcer disease reported by adults, such as meal-exacerbated epigastric pain or discomfort and nocturnal wakening, may not always be present in children, particularly children younger than 8 to 10 years old. Young children may not be able to localize the pain to the epigastrium. They may present with anorexia and irritability with meals, nausea, early satiety, recurrent vomiting, anemia, and, to a lesser extent, weight loss. Pain that truly is localized to the epigastrium is relatively uncommon in children and always requires investigation, as does upper GI bleeding with or without pain. Most primary peptic ulcers in children occur between the ages of 8 and 17 years (mean 12 years), whereas secondary ulcer disease occurs at all ages. GI bleeding may occur with long-standing antecedent epigastric pain or other symptoms, but painless bleeding may be the only manifestation of ulcer disease; 25% of children, particularly with duodenal ulcers, have this "silent" presentation. Epigastric tenderness on examination is an unreliable sign of gastritis or ulcer disease.

The management of *H. pylori* infection is still controversial in children. This ubiquitous organism causes symptoms and ulcers in a relatively small number of infected children. The presence of *H. pylori* infection, in the absence of ulceration, does not automatically necessitate eradication therapy. The decision to test for *H. pylori* should be made only in patients in whom treatment is planned if the result is positive. Children who should be tested are those with chronic upper GI symptoms. The most accurate test is upper GI endoscopy, which not only confirms or excludes the presence of *H. pylori* infection and ulceration, but

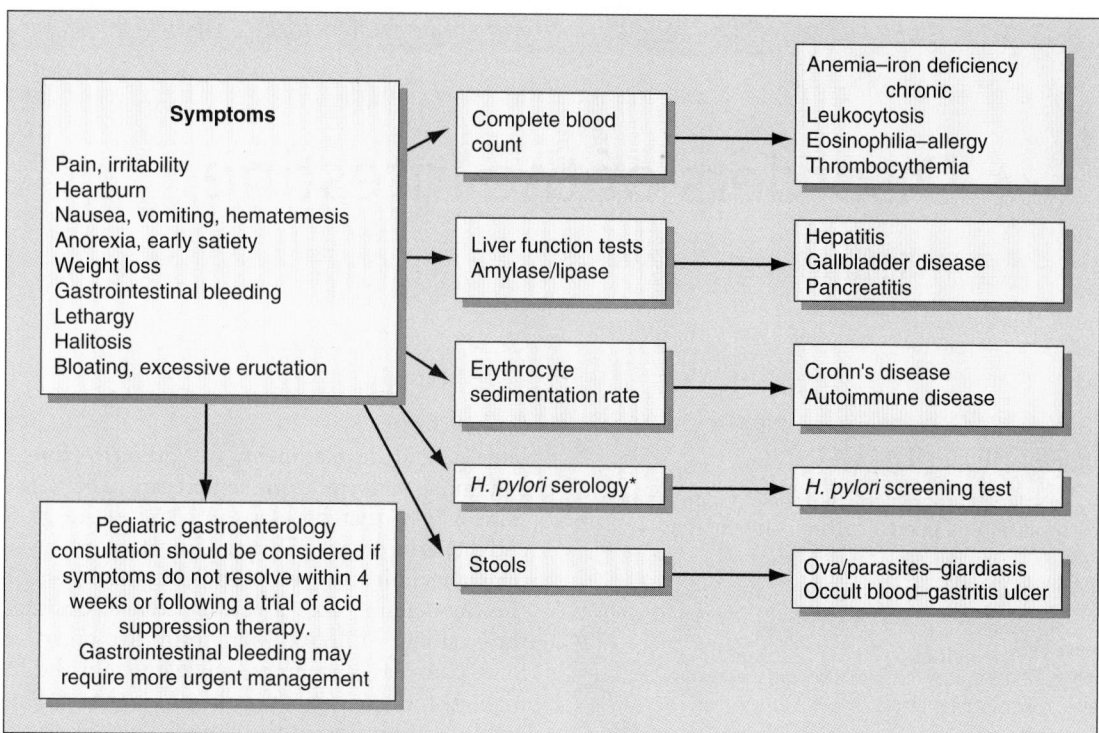

Figure 88-3. Basic evaluation of children with persistent symptoms of upper gastrointestinal disease.
*Although *Helicobacter pylori* serology is a useful screening test, its place in clinical practice is still unclear. Positive serology may represent old infection and is not an absolute indication for starting *H. pylori* eradication treatment.

also may diagnose other conditions that can cause identical symptoms, such as esophagitis, giardiasis, and eosinophilic gastritis (see Table 88-1). Screening tests, such as *H. pylori* serology, are of little value in the management of these children. Urea breath tests are valuable in confirming successful eradication of *H. pylori* infection after treatment. Upper

GI contrast studies are not useful in diagnosing ulcer disease in children.

Healing of peptic ulcers in most cases is achieved through adequate acid suppression using H_2 blockers or proton-pump inhibitors. Ulcer recurrence is prevented by effective treatment of the underlying cause. In the case of *H. pylori*, treatment of the infection is recommended with a combination of proton-pump inhibitor, clarithromycin, and either metronidazole or amoxicillin for 2 weeks. *H. pylori* eradication therapy may be offered to children who have GI symptoms even in the absence of ulcer disease, provided that other diagnoses have been excluded, and the infection is proved to be current. Other therapies for peptic ulcer disease include removal of a possible dietary allergen in allergic conditions and celiac disease and corticosteroids for eosinophilic gastritis, Crohn's disease, and autoimmune disease.

Table 88-1. Diagnostic Red Flags for Peptic Ulcer Disease and Conditions That May Mimic This Disorder

Condition	Red Flags
Peptic ulcer disease	Meal-related symptoms, nocturnal wakening, epigastric tenderness, relief with antacids
Nonulcer dyspepsia	Stress factors, symptoms may occur in clusters and be of varying severity, not typically meal related
Giardiasis	Bloating, flatulence, lactose intolerance, camping and foreign travel
Constipation	Bowel irregularities, anal fissures/tags, constipating drugs (e.g., opiates, anticholinergics, anticonvulsants)
Allergy/eosinophilic gastroenteropathy	History of allergy, diarrhea, growth delay, peripheral eosinophilia, and elevated serum IgE
Gallstones	Family history, hyperlipidemia, TPN, obesity, Crohn's disease, hemolytic anemia, cystic fibrosis, severe vomiting
Pancreatitis	Abdominal trauma, sudden onset, hyperlipidemia, drugs (e.g., corticosteroids, 6-mercaptopurine, furosemide)

TPN, total parenteral nutrition.

Mini-index of Related Topics

SUGGESTED READINGS

Dohil R, Hassall E: Peptic ulcer disease in children. Ballieres Best Pract Res Clin Gastroenterol 2000;14:53–73.

Dohil R, Hassall E, Jevon G, Dimmick J: Gastritis and gastropathy of childhood. J Pediatr Gastroenterol Nutr 1999;29:378–394.

89 Disorders of the Intestine

William Mow

ROLE OF THE GENERALIST

1   Use knowledge of embryology to understand the timing and presentations of congenital anomalies of the intestine.

2   Diagnose congenital anomalies of the intestine, and refer to appropriate surgical specialist for treatment and management.

3   Diagnose inflammatory bowel disorders, and refer to pediatric gastroenterologist.

4   Diagnose malabsorption syndromes, treat disaccharidase deficiencies with elimination diet, and refer other patients as needed for assistance in diagnosis and management.

5   Comanage patients with chronic disorders of the gastrointestinal tract with a pediatric gastroenterologist.

Embryology

During fetal development, the primitive foregut, midgut, and hindgut form from endoderm. These three regions form a tube that develops into the entire gastrointestinal and hepatic organs. During development of the foregut, which includes the esophagus, stomach, and duodenum, the duodenum takes a retroperitoneal position, fixed via the ligament of Treitz. Many primitive organs, such as the liver, pancreas, and lungs, originate from the foregut. The midgut, connected to the yolk sac via the vitelline duct with its blood supply from the superior mesenteric artery, gives rise to the jejunum, ileum, and ascending and first half of the transverse colon. During early development, each segment of the primitive gut elongates. Most of the midgut and hindgut are contained within a large umbilical herniation at around 8 weeks of gestational age, a process called *physiologic umbilical herniation* (Fig. 89-1). Normally the midgut is rotated 270 degrees around the superior mesenteric artery and vitelline duct (Fig. 89-2). By the third month, the embryo has developed enough abdominal space

FUNDAMENTALS

The small intestine and colon process food so that it can be absorbed and used. The intestinal enterocyte, found on the villi and microvilli of the small bowel, secretes and absorbs water, electrolytes, amino acids, carbohydrates, fat, bile acids, and vitamins. Digestion and absorption of chyme, a mixture of gastric fluids and mechanically digested food, is completed by pancreatic digestive enzymes and by intrinsic intestinal disaccharidases and is absorbed primarily in the jejunum. Iron is absorbed in the duodenum, and vitamin B_{12} and bile salts are absorbed in the ileum.

Carbohydrates are digested by salivary and pancreatic amylase into oligosaccharides and disaccharides that are digested by disaccharidases into monosaccharides, each with a specific transporter for absorption. Protein is digested by gastric and pancreatic peptidases into oligopeptides and absorbed into the enterocyte via specific transporters. Dietary triglycerides are digested by lingual, gastric, and pancreatic lipase into insoluble free fatty acids and monoglycerols. These attach to bile acids, forming micelles that are absorbed into enterocytes, esterified back into triglycerides, packaged into lipoproteins, and sent to the liver for processing via lacteals and the lymphatic system. Medium-chain triglycerides are absorbed directly by the enterocytes.

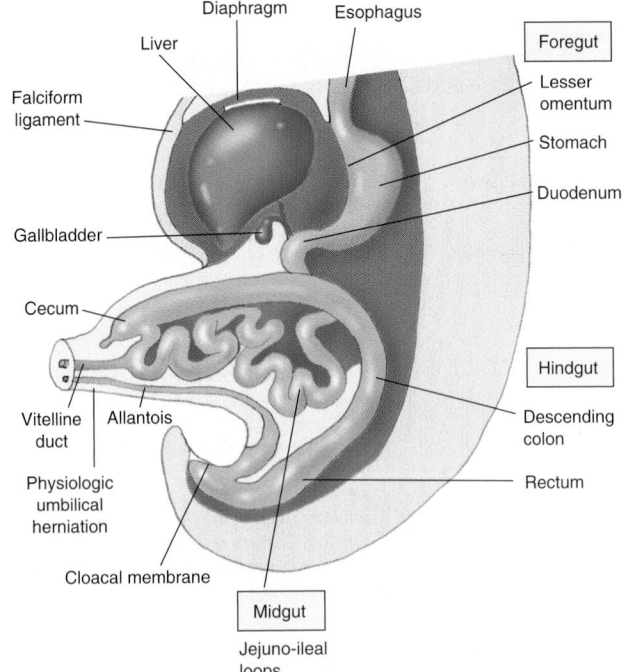

Figure 89-1. Umbilical herniation. At approximately 8 weeks, most of the midgut and hindgut are contained within a physiologic umbilical herniation.

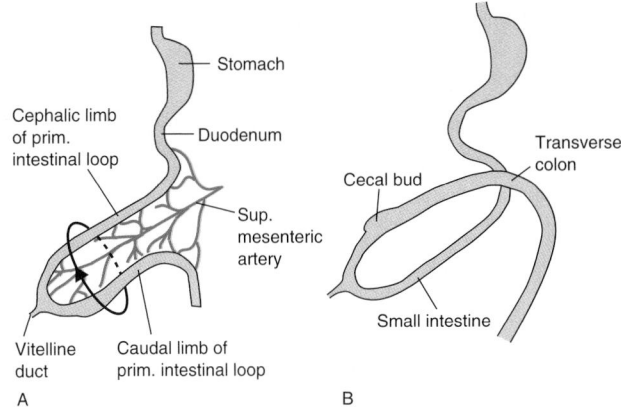

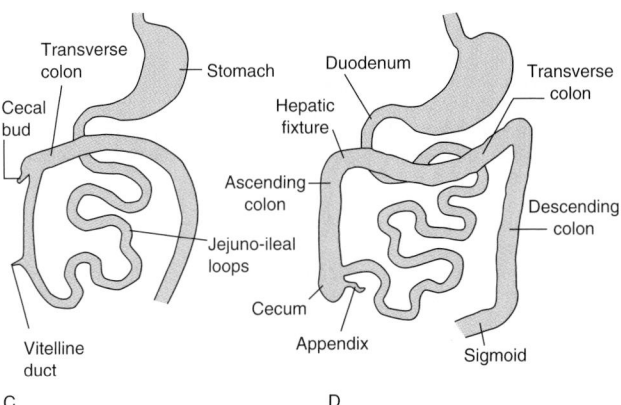

Figure 89-2. Intestinal rotation. **A,** Lateral view of the midgut before rotation. The arrow indicates counterclockwise rotation around the superior mesenteric artery. **B,** After 180 degrees counterclockwise rotation. **C,** Anterior view after 270 degrees rotation. **D,** Final position of intestines, with the cecum fixed in the right lower quadrant and the duodenum fixed by the ligament of Treitz.

for the intestine to return gradually into the peritoneal cavity. The jejunum, the first portion to enter the abdominal cavity, comes to lie in the left side of the abdomen. The ileum and colon follow so that the ileum fills the right side of the abdomen, and the cecum takes a position in the right lower quadrant. The hindgut forms the second half of the transverse colon, descending colon, sigmoid, and rectum. Its blood supply is from the inferior mesenteric artery. The cloacal membrane prevents drainage of contents of the hindgut into the amniotic fluid.

DIAGNOSIS AND MANAGEMENT OF SPECIFIC DISORDERS

Table 89-1 outlines the diagnosis and management of congenital disorders of the intestines. Table 89-2 describes the diagnosis and management of noncongenital disorders. See the mini-index and the CD-ROM for further discussion.

Meckel Diverticulum

Meckel diverticulum, a remnant of the omphalomesenteric duct found in 2% to 3% of infants, is the most common congenital gastrointestinal anomaly (Fig. 89-3). The "rule of twos" describes its location, usually approximately 2 feet proximal to the ileocecal valve, and its length, about 2 inches. Of these defects, 80% contain gastric mucosa, which can lead to ulceration of the mucosa and gastrointestinal bleeding. The most common presentation, found in about one third of patients, is intestinal obstruction, with Meckel diverticulum acting as a lead point for intussusception. Patients can present with painless rectal bleeding in the first 2 years of life. Meckel diverticulum should be considered in the differential diagnosis in any infant or toddler with bright red blood per rectum or melena. Meckel diverticulum also can mimic acute appendicitis, presenting as diverticulitis with fever, right lower quadrant tenderness, and leukocytosis. Diagnosis is made with the Meckel scan, a nuclear medicine scan that has a sensitivity of 80% to 90% and a specificity of 95%. Treatment is surgical, requiring Meckel diverticulectomy.

Malrotation and Midgut Volvulus

Malrotation, present in approximately 1 in 500 live births, is due to incomplete rotation of the gut during development and incomplete fixation of the duodenum by the ligament of Treitz and of the cecum in the right lower quadrant (Fig. 89-4). Malrotation can be asymptomatic until the midgut rotates or twists around the superior mesenteric artery causing a volvulus, a process that can lead to occlusion of the superior mesenteric artery, bowel ischemia, and symptoms of bowel obstruction. Approximately 50% of malrotations present in the first month of life, and 90% present within the first year. Patients present with bilious emesis, crying, irritability, and abdominal distention. Only 10% of patients pass blood per rectum. Malrotation is associated with other disorders, such as abdominal heterotaxia and asplenia-polysplenia syndromes. Diagnosis is made by an upper gastrointestinal series that shows the ligament of Treitz to be malpositioned and may show volvulus with the classic "corkscrew" deformity. Patients with malrotation and midgut volvulus require emergent laparotomy and Ladd procedure. The surgeon must unwind the rotated gut before the bowel becomes infarcted and is damaged beyond salvage. The surgeon must lyse the Ladd bands and rearrange the intestines so that a volvulus does not occur again. The mortality rate for this disorder is around 20%, and significant morbidity is associated with short gut syndrome after extensive bowel resections.

Intussusception

Intussusception, an invagination of the bowel within itself, typically affects children age 5 to 12 months old and is the most common cause of intestinal obstruction in patients age 3 months to 6 years. The incidence is 1 to 4 per 1000 live births with a male-to-female ratio of 4:1. Although lead point may initiate the process, often one is not found. In children, hypertrophied Peyer patches, possibly secondary to viral illnesses, often act as the lead point at which the bowel intussuscepts. The most common type of intussusception is the ileocolic intussusception, in which the ileum passes into the colon. Affected patients typically present with severe intermittent colicky abdominal pain, bilious emesis, lethargy, fever, and bloody stools. After 24 hours,

Table 89-1. Diagnosis and Management of Congenital Disorders of the Gastrointestinal Tract

Diagnosis	Presentation	Management
Gastroschisis	Newborn with abdominal wall hernia with evisceration of intestine, liver, colon	Cover the exposed viscera with saline-dampened sterile gauze and an impermeable barrier, such as plastic wrap, immediately after delivery Place a nasal or oral gastric tube for decompression Notify pediatric surgeon Manage fluids and electrolytes, with attention to possibility of severe third spacing until surgeon arrives
Omphalocele	Newborn, midline sac filled with intestinal contents at base of the umbilical cord	Note whether sac is intact If sac is ruptured, follow same procedure as for gastroschisis Notify pediatric surgeon
Intussusception	Usually infants 5–12 months old, severe intermittent colicky abdominal pain, bilious emesis, lethargy, fever, and bloody, "currant jelly" stools. After 24 hours, may present with shock	Intravenous fluids and antibiotics if shock, sepsis, or peritonitis present Admission to intensive care if patient critically ill Referral to radiologist for retrograde enema with air or barium Referral to surgeon for urgent laparotomy if noninvasive reduction fails If noninvasive reduction successful, careful follow-up for recurrence (10%) or complications
Atresia	Newborn, bilious emesis, abdominal distention, failure to pass meconium, and the "double-bubble" sign on abdominal radiograph	Stabilize patient with fluid and electrolytes Upper gastrointestinal series Referral for exploratory laparotomy
Stenosis	Newborn through childhood, can be difficult to diagnose, consider with feeding difficulties, failure to thrive, and diarrhea from bacterial overgrowth	Upper gastrointestinal series with small bowel follow through Referral to pediatric surgeon for surgical resection of affected area
Hirschsprung disease	Any age, most frequently present in infancy with history of constipation since birth, abdominal distention, obstruction, bilious emesis, and persistent need for rectal stimulation or enemas for defecation, perforation of appendix and/or cecum	Barium enema without "clean-out" Anorectal manometry Referral to surgeon for suction biopsies or open full-thickness rectal biopsies
Imperforate anus and anorectal malformations	Newborn, abnormal appearance of the genitalia, imperforate anus, or failure to pass meconium	Recognize defect Recognize associated congenital defects Abdominal and pelvic ultrasound Echocardiography in patients with complex and more proximal lesions Referral to a pediatric surgeon Identify need for colostomy Long-term follow-up for constipation, fecal incontinence, and soiling

the risk for bowel wall infarction increases, and patients can present with septic shock. The classic currant-jelly stool, seen in approximately 60% of patients, is due to venous congestion and diapedesis of red blood cells into the lumen. Intussusception always should be considered in the differential diagnosis for infants and toddlers with bloody stool, vomiting, and abdominal pain. A left upper quadrant mass can be felt in only 40% to 70% of children with intussusception.

Patients with signs of shock, peritonitis, pneumatosis intestinalis, or free air on x-ray or who appear critically ill should be stabilized with intravenous rehydration and antibiotics and admitted to the intensive care unit, and the intussusception should be surgically reduced. In stable patients in whom intussusception is suspected, diagnosis and reduction can be accomplished with retrograde enema with either air or barium, depending on whether or not there is concern for perforation and the preference of the radiologist. Radiologists successfully reduce intussusception in 75% to 80% of cases done within 48 hours of the onset and in 50% of cases done after 48 hours. The use of barium carries a 0.5% to 2.5% risk of perforation, whereas air

enema carries a 0.1% to 0.2% risk. Ten percent of patients treated by retrograde enemas have a recurrent episode of intussusception. If noninvasive reduction is not successful, urgent laparotomy is necessary to reduce the defect and avoid ischemic damage to the bowel. Intraoperatively the surgeon typically looks for a lead point, such as a Meckel diverticulum, intestinal polyp, duplication, or abdominal tumor, and often performs an appendectomy. Risk for recurrence of the intussusception after surgical reduction is 2% to 5%. Intussusception is associated with Henoch-Schönlein purpura, cystic fibrosis, Meckel diverticulum, polyposis syndromes, intestinal hemangiomas, and hemolytic uremic syndrome. Ileoileo intussusception is a more rare form. It presents with signs of small bowel obstruction and can be difficult to diagnose. Because hydrostatic reduction is not feasible, the treatment is surgical.

Intestinal Atresias and Stenoses

Atresias and stenoses are the most common defects isolated to the midgut. Atresias are defects in which the lumen is completely obstructed, whereas stenoses are defects in which a small, constricted lumen still is present. Atresias

Table 89-2. Diagnosis and Management of Noncongenital Disorders of the intestines

Diagnosis	Presentation	Management
Crohn disease	Childhood–adulthood: Chronic abdominal pain, bloody diarrhea, and weight loss, Right lower quadrant mass indicating terminal ileal inflammation. Fever, growth retardation, perirectal disease Extraintestinal manifestations: arthritis, erythema nodosum, pyoderma gangrenosum, aphthous ulcers, uveitis, iritis, hypercoagulability, nephrolithiasis, sclerosing cholangitis, chronic hepatitis, pancreatitis, and anemia	Stool cultures CBC, ESR Albumin, prealbumin Stool for WBCs Referral to a pediatric gastroenterologist if patient anemic, hypalbuminemic, or if ESR elevated
Ulcerative colitis	Childhood–adulthood: Bloody diarrhea and abdominal pain >14 days, urgency, nighttime bowel movements, tenesmus, weight loss Extraintestinal manifestations: pyoderma gangrenosum, arthritis, biliary diasese (primary sclerosing cholangitis), iritis, and uveitis.	Stool culture CBC, ESR Albumin, prealbumin, liver function tests Serum iron Stool for cells pANCA Referral to gastroenterologist for colonoscopy Long-term comanagement with gastroenterologist
Food allergies	Infancy–adulthood: Vomiting, diarrhea, malabsorption with protein-losing enteropathy, rectal bleeding, irritability, urticaria, angioedema, wheezing, and anaphylaxis	Refer to allergist for testing and evaluation
Idiopathic eosinophilic gastroenteritis	Childhood: Diarrhea, protein-losing enteropathy, growth failure, weight loss, and abdominal pain	Stool culture Stool for WBCs Serum albumin IgE CBC with differential Consultation of a pediatric gastroenterologist for endoscopic biopsy Long-term comanagement with gastroenterologist
Malabsorption	Infancy–adulthood: Diarrhea, weight loss, failure to thrive, and poor linear growth	Stool for blood, WBCs, reducing substances, *C. difficile* toxin, bacteria, and ova and parasites CBC, electrolytes, BUN, creatinine, calcium, phosphorus, albumin, and total protein Urinalysis Referral to pediatric gastroenterologist for assistance in evaluation and management
Disaccharidase deficiency	Newborn–adulthood: Watery diarrhea, cramping, abdominal pain	Elimination of disaccharide from diet
Protein-losing enteropathy	Newborn–adulthood: Diarrhea, chronic abdominal pain, and dependent edema	Serum albumin Identify cause of protein-losing enteropathy Treat underlying disorder Refer to pediatric gastroenterologist as needed for assistance in diagnosis and treatment of underlying disease
Celiac disease	Celiac crisis: malnutrition, dehydration, shock Toddlers: failure to thrive, diarrhea, abdominal pain or distention, anorexia and irritability, foul-smelling greasy stools Older children: minor abdominal complaints, short stature, delayed, puberty, anemia, and arthritis	Refer to pediatric gastroenterologist for assistance in diagnosis and long-term management Implementation of a strict gluten-free diet

BUN, blood urea nitrogen; CBC, complete blood count; ESR, erythrocyte sedimentation rate; pANCA, perinuclear antineutrophilic cytoplasmic antibody; WBC, white blood cell.

are more common than stenoses by a ratio of at least 10:1 and are discussed in Chapter 204 and on the CD-ROM.

Intestinal stenoses sometimes are difficult to diagnose. They can present similarly to atresias with bilious emesis and abdominal distention or more indolently. Often they present with feeding difficulties, failure to thrive, and diarrhea from bacterial overgrowth. The diagnosis is made by upper gastrointestinal series with small bowel follow through. Treatment usually is surgical resection of the affected area.

Hirschsprung Disease

In Hirschsprung disease, the ganglion cells of the intestine and colon are absent. The ganglion cells of the myenteric plexus of Auerbach and the submucosal plexus of Meissner are essential for autonomic control of the intestines. These nerves are involved integrally with parasympathetic control of gut motility and function. In Hirschsprung disease, neural crest cells fail to migrate from a cephalad to caudad direction along the vagus nerve and into the bowel wall. Ganglion cells play an important role in defecation. When

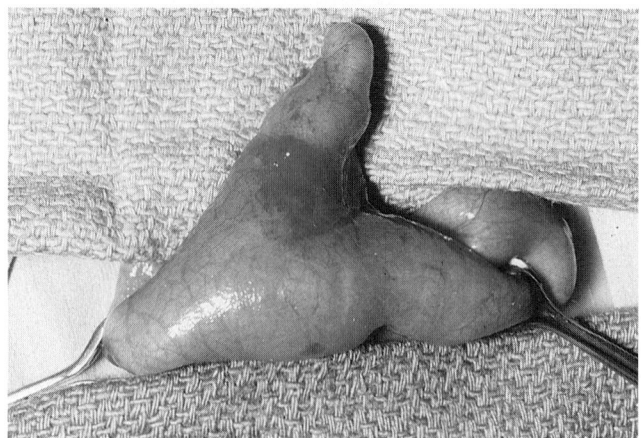

Figure 89-3. Meckel diverticulum. (From Schwartz M: Meckel's diverticulum and other omphalomesenteric duct remnants. In Wyllie R, Hyams J [eds]: Pediatric Gastrointestinal Disease, 2nd ed. Philadelphia, WB Saunders, 1999, p 485.)

the rectal vault fills with stool, ganglion cells are responsible for sending inhibitory reflexes to the involuntary internal anal sphincter. When the internal anal sphincter relaxes, the sensation to defecate is translated to the human brain because there also is voluntary contraction of the external anal sphincter to control the timing of defecation.

The incidence of Hirschsprung disease is estimated at 1 in 5000 live births with a male predominance and often a family history of the disease. Many genes have been identified in association with Hirschsprung disease. Other congenital anomalies can be seen in 30%, such as Down syndrome, Waardenburg syndrome, multiple endocrine neoplasia type IIa, and Smith-Lemli-Opitz syndrome. The longer the length of the aganglionic segment, the higher the association with other congenital anomalies and with the likelihood of another affected family member.

Affected patients can present at any age, but classically present in infancy with a history of constipation since birth, abdominal distention, obstruction, bilious emesis, and persistent need for rectal stimulation or enemas for defe-

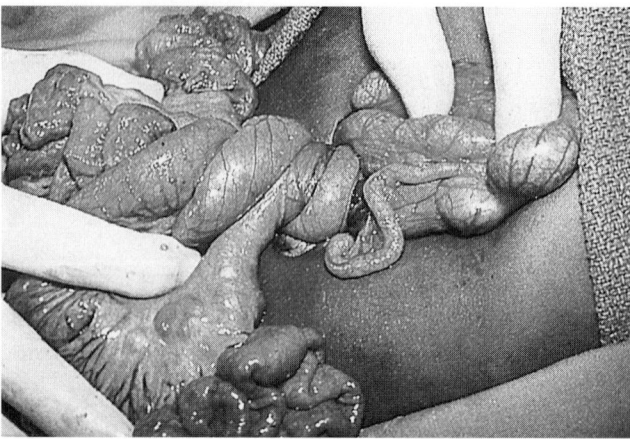

Figure 89-4. Malrotation with midgut volvulus. Vascular compression and intestinal ischemia resulting from twisting of the midgut around the superior mesenteric artery pedicle. (From Phillips JD: Abdominal surgical emergencies. In Wyllie R, Hyams J [eds]: Pediatric Gastrointestinal Disease, 2nd ed. Philadelphia, WB Saunders, 1999, p 142.)

cation. Many of these patients have a history of failing to pass meconium in the first day of life. In neonates, Hirschsprung disease can present with intestinal obstruction; any child with a history of perforation of the appendix or cecum should undergo a workup for Hirschsprung disease. In older children, Hirschsprung disease can be differentiated from functional constipation by a lack of soiling or encopresis and the presence of failure to thrive and abdominal distention with Hirschsprung disease. On physical examination, patients with functional fecal retention have a lax anal sphincter and large dilated rectum filled with stool, whereas patients with Hirschsprung disease have a tight anal sphincter with a small rectum and only a small amount of stool at the tip of the examiner's finger.

The diagnosis of Hirschsprung disease is made after anorectal manometry, barium enema, and rectal suction biopsy or open full-thickness rectal biopsy. Anorectal manometry shows a lack of an inhibitory response of the internal anal sphincter to rectal balloon dilation. The barium enema shows a small rectum and colon and a transition zone to the large, dilated proximal bowel. The rectal biopsy specimens show the absence of ganglion cells and the presence of hypertrophic nerves.

The goals of surgical treatment are removal of the aganglionic segments and creation of a new rectum. In the Soave procedure, the entire aganglionic portion of colon is removed except the rectal stump. The mucosa is stripped in the rectal stump, and the ganglionic bowel is sewn in, creating a new ganglionic rectum. Often the surgery is successful, but complications such as enterocolitis, anastomotic stenosis, constipation, and incontinence can be seen.

Before surgical resection, these patients are at increased risk for the development of enterocolitis, acute colonic perforation, and toxic megacolon. Parents should be informed that fever, severe abdominal pain, bilious emesis, rectal bleeding, and lethargy are symptoms of these serious complications of Hirschsprung disease.

Appendicitis

Acute appendicitis is a relatively common cause of acute abdominal pain. The diagnosis is based on history and physical examination, but in many cases this diagnosis is elusive. Acute appendicitis is seen most commonly in children and young adults.

Pathophysiology

The appendix is a diverticulum that comes off the cecum. In patients with normal intestinal rotation, the cecum is in the right lower quadrant. The varied clinical presentation of acute appendicitis may be related to the orientation of the cecum. Acute appendicitis is thought to be caused by obstruction of the lumen as a result of a fecalith or lymphoid tissue with inflammation and swelling of the appendix. Initial swelling of the appendix causes stimulation of T10 dermatome, which classically is experienced as periumbilical pain. As the inflammation and swelling progress, the pain is localized to the right lower quadrant from involvement of the overlying peritoneum. Perforation occurs within 36 to 48 hours, with an 80% perforation rate by 48 hours. After perforation, the body makes attempts to confine the infection, but these mechanisms often fail, and shock and sepsis can occur.

Diagnosis

The diagnosis of appendicitis is made clinically. Most patients have severe worsening of abdominal pain in the umbilical area and right lower quadrant. Many have vomiting and anorexia. Fever is common, but not universal. Pain at McBurney point, a point located two thirds the distance between the umbilicus and the anterior superior iliac spine, is characteristic. On physical examination, palpation of the right lower quadrant elicits pain. Signs of peritonitis, such as guarding and rebound tenderness, indicate possible perforation. Retroperitoneal involvement can be assessed with the psoas and obturator signs. Rectal examination may reveal tenderness in cases in which the appendix is oriented posteriorly. Infants can develop acute appendicitis, but the diagnosis is difficult because of an inability to convey characteristic symptoms. Diagnosis can be difficult in sexually active female patients because appendicitis can be confused with ovarian torsion and pelvic inflammatory disease.

Laboratory Findings

Urinalysis is essential to rule out a urinary tract infection. A white blood cell count can be helpful if elevated, but often is normal. Inflammatory markers, such as C-reactive protein, sometimes can be used to assist in the diagnosis in difficult cases.

Radiologic Findings

A radiologic workup is not necessary if the diagnosis is made clinically. If there is uncertainty, especially in infants, a computed tomography (CT) scan can be helpful. A thin-cut helical computed tomography scan with rectal contrast enhancement has good sensitivity and specificity (approximately 94%) and is much more sensitive than ultrasound. The utility of ultrasound in the diagnosis of acute appendicitis is variable, especially in young patients, obese patients, and sexually active female patients.

Differential Diagnosis

The differential diagnosis of acute appendicitis includes gastroenteritis, constipation, Crohn disease, pelvic inflammatory disease, ovarian cyst or torsion, pneumonia, mesenteric adenitis, and typhlitis. These entities are not discussed here, but are addressed in greater detail in other chapters.

Treatment

Intravenous antibiotics with broad-spectrum coverage to include *Enterococcus* and gram-negative organisms should be started in all patients with appendicitis. If perforation is suspected, anaerobic coverage should be added. Because of the natural progression of acute appendicitis to perforation, shock, and sepsis, appendectomy must be done in a timely manner. The risks of perforation typically are thought to outweigh the risks of surgery. Although open appendectomy has been the classic method of operation for many years, laparoscopic appendectomy has been useful in cases of nonperforated appendicitis; in diagnostic dilemmas, such as a sexually active female patient; or for interval appendec-

tomy. The use of laparoscopy in complicated, perforated acute appendicitis is controversial. For patients who present after perforation and abscess formation, many practitioners elect to place peritoneal drains with computed tomography or ultrasound guidance and treat acutely with intravenous antibiotics, with an interval appendectomy planned 6 to 8 weeks after the initial presentation.

Inflammatory Disorders

Ulcerative colitis and Crohn disease are discussed on the CD-ROM and in Chapter 139.

Allergic Disorders and Eosinophilic Gastroenteritis

Food allergies, cow milk protein allergy, and eosinophilic gastroenteritis seem like similar disorders, but each has a different pathogenesis. The diagnosis is often difficult to make in children. Food allergies are typically IgE-mediated hypersensitivity reactions in which there are reproducible responses to a food protein. In eosinophilic gastroenteritis, there is an idiopathic infiltration of the gut mucosa with eosinophils. Cow milk protein allergy is a common disorder in which IgE-mediated and non–IgE-mediated factors cause the clinical disease (see Chapter 44).

Although food allergies are perceived to be common in children, prospective studies indicate the prevalence of proven food allergies ranges from 1.9% to 8%. Infants younger than 1 year old are the most likely to have IgE-mediated hypersensitivity reactions, with most of these reactions to cow milk protein or soy protein. Hypersensitivity to cow milk protein, soy protein, egg, fish, peanut, and wheat account for 90% of all food allergies in children. Children with food allergies present with a myriad of symptoms associated with ingestion of the inciting allergen within minutes to less than 2 hours. These symptoms include vomiting, diarrhea, malabsorption with protein-losing enteropathy, rectal bleeding, irritability, urticaria, angioedema, wheezing, and anaphylaxis. Children with suspected food allergies should be referred to an allergist for evaluation and testing.

Idiopathic eosinophilic gastroenteritis, a chronic inflammatory condition characterized by eosinophilic infiltration of the gut, usually is accompanied by peripheral eosinophilia and can be difficult to discriminate from cow milk protein allergy. Many disorders can cause eosinophilia of the gut, including parasitic infections, vasculitis, inflammatory bowel disease, celiac disease, chronic granulomatous disease, lymphoma, malignancy, food or drug allergies, and hypereosinophilic syndrome. Patients with eosinophilic gastroenteritis typically present with diarrhea, protein-losing enteropathy, growth failure, weight loss, and abdominal pain. The initial workup should include stool culture, stool for white blood cells, serum albumin, IgE, and complete blood count with differential, followed by consultation with a pediatric gastroenterologist. Diagnosis usually is made after endoscopic biopsy evaluation showing significant eosinophilic infiltration of the gut mucosa. Sometimes eosinophilic gastroenteritis can present with gastric outlet obstruction, which mimics hypertrophic pyloric stenosis. It is important to look for an inciting food allergen by skin testing and IgE radioallergosorbent test testing. The results of these tests may direct therapy toward dietary elimination of the offending agent. Dietary therapy rarely works for eosinophilic gastroenteritis, however. Corticosteroids are the mainstay of therapy. Other agents, such as mast cell stabilizers and antihistamines, have been tried with variable results.

Malabsorption, Sucrase-Isomaltase Deficiency, Glucose-Galactose Malabsorption, and Congenital Lactase Deficiency

Digestion starts in the mouth, where salivary amylase and lipase are excreted. In addition, a carrier protein for vitamin B_{12}, named *R binder*, is secreted to aid in transport and absorption of vitamin B_{12}. In the stomach, gastric acid, lipase, pepsinogen, and intrinsic factor are secreted to aid in digestion. Intrinsic factor replaces R binder protein and takes over the role of transporting vitamin B_{12} to the terminal ileum, where it is absorbed. Gastric acid converts pepsinogen to its active form pepsin. The pancreas secretes bicarbonate for neutralization of gastric acid, lipase for fat digestion, trypsinogen for protein digestion, and amylase for carbohydrate digestion. Absorption of fats requires bile excretion by the liver. Bile aids the absorption of fats by forming micelles, which are absorbed by the intestinal enterocyte. Cholestatic disorders are known to cause fat malabsorption.

The small intestinal mucosa possesses enzymes essential for the digestion and absorption of carbohydrates. Brush border enzymes are responsible for the digestion of disaccharides and polysaccharides into monosaccharides that can be absorbed via simple diffusion, facilitated diffusion, or sodium-coupled transporters. Congenital deficiencies of lactase, sucrase-isomaltase, and maltase are exceedingly rare. Glucose-galactose malabsorption results from a defect in the transporter responsible for the absorption of glucose and galactose. Affected children have severe carbohydrate malabsorption.

Breakdown of proteins to amino acids in the small intestine is initiated by enterokinase, which activates intraluminal proteases, such as trypsinogen and procolipase. Sodium-coupled transporters undertake the absorption of amino acids. Defects in these extremely rare transporters are the cause of Hartnup disease, lysinuric protein intolerance, blue diaper syndrome, Oasthouse syndrome, and Lowe syndrome.

After digestion, fats are emulsified with bile acids to form micelles, which are absorbed into the lymphatic system and processed into chylomicrons. Proper processing of these chylomicrons requires lipoproteins. In abetalipoproteinemia, absence of or defect in these proteins causes ineffective chylomicron formation. Patients cannot process ingested fat and have systemic symptoms of acanthosis, retinal disorders, and ataxia. Treatment includes dietary restriction of triglycerides and supplementation with medium-chain triglycerides, which can be absorbed directly by enterocytes.

Severe damage to the intestinal mucosa, as seen with inflammatory bowel disease, celiac disease, and cow milk protein allergy, also can cause malabsorption by disrupting functions of the gut. Cardiac failure can cause malabsorption from bowel wall edema by inhibiting lymphatic drainage (also seen in intestinal lymphangiectasia) and slowing removal of the chylomicrons from the lymphatics. Microvillus inclusion disease and tufting disease are two other rare malabsorption defects (see Chapter 138).

Malabsorption should be suspected in patients with a history of diarrhea, weight loss, failure to thrive, and poor linear growth. A good history should ascertain the details of the patient's diarrhea, diet, energy level, time course of disease, associated symptoms, travel history, and family history. The physical findings usually coincide with the degree of malnutrition. Height, weight, and head circumference should be measured and plotted according to chronologic age. Examination of the trunk, buttocks, and extremities for fat and muscle mass may reveal the extent of malnutrition. Delayed sexual maturation is a common feature in malnourished children. Close examination of the skin, eyes, tongue, hair, and nails reveals manifestations of vitamin deficiencies. The presence of a cardiac gallop may steer the diagnosis toward congestive heart failure–induced malabsorption.

The initial workup for malabsorption includes examination of the stool for blood, white blood cells, reducing substances, C. *difficile* toxin, bacteria, and ova and parasites; blood studies, such as complete blood count, electrolytes, blood urea nitrogen, creatinine, calcium, phosphorus, albumin, and total protein; and a routine urinalysis. Patients with chronic malabsorption commonly exhibit hypoalbuminemia and anemia from iron, folate, or vitamin B_{12} deficiency, and these patients should be referred to a pediatric gastroenterologist because there are many other studies that can be done to assess for malabsorption (intestinal absorption studies, breath tests, prolonged stool fat collections).

Protein-Losing Enteropathy

Protein-losing enteropathy is characterized by disruption of tight junctions between the enterocytes, leading to leakage of proteins into the stool. Infection, inflammation, and lymphatic drainage problems are common causes of protein-losing enteropathy. The diagnosis is made by measuring α_1-antitrypsin in the stool. α_1-Antitrypsin is a serum protein, roughly the same size as albumin, that normally is not excreted into the stool and is not a component of most diets. Most patients with protein-losing enteropathy present with diarrhea, chronic abdominal pain, and dependent edema. The history must identify the cause of the protein-losing enteropathy by ascertainment of allergies, diet history, weight loss, travel history, ill contacts, and past medical history. Laboratory tests may show hypoalbuminemia.

Infections are a common cause of protein-losing enteropathy. Elevations in fecal α_1-antitrypsin level can be seen with viral gastroenteritis but should not persist for longer than 5 days. Other common infectious causes include *Giardia lamblia*, cytomegalovirus, *Helicobacter pylori*, C. *difficile*, *Clostridium perfringens*, measles, rotavirus, *Salmonella*, and *Strongyloides stercoralis*. In general, chronic infections with the aforementioned organisms are more likely to result in low albumin, whereas short-lived infections rarely cause hypoalbuminemia.

Noninfectious causes of protein-losing enteropathy include allergic enteropathies (e.g., cow milk protein allergy), inflammatory bowel disease, graft-versus-host disease, Henoch-Schönlein purpura, intestinal lymphangiectasia, systemic lupus erythematosus, juvenile rheumatoid arthritis, polyposis, reflux esophagitis, celiac disease, and malnutrition. Differentiation of this diverse differential diagnosis must begin with a thorough history and physical examination. Management is aimed at treating the underlying disorder. Depending on the primary disorder, these patients universally are followed by pediatric specialists.

Celiac Disease

Celiac disease, a genetic disorder in which patients have permanent intolerance to dietary wheat proteins, such as gliadin, leads to mucosal flattening and protein-losing enteropathy. Celiac disease tends to run in families and has a high concordance between monozygotic twins. Certain HLA markers, *DQA1* and *DQB1*, have been highly associated with celiac disease, suggesting their role in presenting gliadin fragments to T cells, activating mucosal inflammation. The prevalence of symptomatic celiac disease varies by location. Screening tests have indicated that celiac disease may be highly underdiagnosed in the United States; 8 in 2000 healthy blood donors were found to be positive for antiendomysial antibodies.

The pathogenesis of celiac disease is complex. Gliadin-driven T-cell activation may lead to mucosal inflammation. The classic pathologic feature in celiac disease is mucosal flattening, but patients can have a variety of abnormal features, such as elongated crypts, increased intraepithelial lymphocytes, and villous atrophy.

Toddlers with celiac disease present with features such as failure to thrive, diarrhea, abdominal pain or distention, anorexia, and irritability. An accurate growth chart shows growth failure starting when wheat is introduced. Stools are foul smelling, greasy, and bulky. In severe cases, children can present in "celiac crisis" with severe malnutrition, dehydration, and shock. In older children, symptoms include minor abdominal complaints, short stature, delayed puberty, anemia, and arthritis. Celiac disease is associated with dermatitis herpetiformis, autoimmune disorders, inflammatory bowel disease, Down syndrome, IgA deficiency, cystic fibrosis, and cow milk protein intolerance. These patients also have an increased risk of small bowel lymphoma when not maintained on a gluten-free diet.

The diagnosis of celiac disease should be made in conjunction with a pediatric gastroenterologist. In patients with suspicious serology results and clinical histories, upper endoscopy should be performed. Diagnosis of this disorder is based on pathologic findings, including villous atrophy.

Therapy involves implementation of a strict gluten-free diet. This diet excludes wheat, rye, and barley. The role of oats in the gluten-free diet is controversial, but oats should be excluded as well. These patients can tolerate rice-based and maize-based diets, and most do well if maintained on a gluten-free diet.

Additional Resources, CD-ROM

Omphalocele and gastroschisis	Text, figures
Atresias	Text, figure
Meconium ileus and meconium plug	Text, figure
Imperforate anus and anorectal malformations	Text
Crohn disease	Text
Ulcerative colitis	Text
Bibliography	

Mini-index of Related Topics

SUGGESTED READINGS

Branski D, Lerner A, Lebenthal E: Chronic diarrhea and malabsorption. Pediatr Clin North Am 1996;43:307–332.

Hyams JS: Crohn's disease in children. Pediatr Clin North Am 1996;43:255–277.

Kirschner BS: Ulcerative colitis in children. Pediatr Clin North Am 1996;43:235–254.

Troncone R, Greco L, Auricchio S: Gluten-sensitive enteropathy. Pediatr Clin North Am 1996;43:355–374.

90 Acute Hepatobiliary Disorders

Linda S. Book

ROLE OF THE GENERALIST

1   Recognize the clinical features of acute liver disease.

2   Identify features of chronic liver disease.

3   Recognize the clinical features of severe hepatic dysfunction, including fulminant liver failure.

4   Recognize acute and chronic cholecytitis, and refer patients for surgical treatment.

5   Initiate prophylaxis and control measures for transmission of infectious hepatitis.

6   Refer patients with severe liver hepatic dysfunction, fulminant failure, and chronic liver disease to appropriate centers and specialists.

7   Diagnose and treat uncomplicated viral hepatitis.

8   Comanage a child with chronic hepatitis B and C and liver disease occurring as a manifestation of other illnesses.

9   Refer patients to appropriate specialists when expert assistance is needed for management or diagnosis.

FUNDAMENTALS

Hepatitis means inflammation or necrosis of the liver. The most common acute liver disease is hepatitis, which usually is caused by five major hepatitis viruses, *A* through *E*. In children, the most frequent cause of acute liver disease is hepatitis A. Numerous other viruses also may infect the liver. Acute liver disease may occur in metabolic disorders, from toxic reactions to drugs or toxins, and in association with systemic disorders. *Cholecystitis*, inflammation of the gallbladder, usually occurs with gallstones *(cholelithiasis)*. Stones also may obstruct the biliary or cystic ducts.

Jaundice, fever, anorexia, vomiting, general malaise, and abdominal pain are common presenting symptoms of hepatobiliary disorders. Most cases of acute hepatitis in children younger than 6 years old have minimal symptoms and no jaundice. Approximately 70% of older children and adolescents with hepatitis have jaundice. Urine may be brown from excretion of water-soluble direct bilirubin. Stools may be light yellow or nearly white (acholic), particularly when there is biliary obstruction. Physical examination typically shows hepatomegaly with mild-to-moderate tenderness. Splenomegaly is less common and when present should raise suspicion of chronic liver disease. Other signs that indicate chronic liver disease rather than an acute process are a prominent venous pattern on the abdomen and ascites, both of which suggest portal hypertension. The triad of fever, right upper quadrant pain, and jaundice is classic for acute cholecystitis.

DIAGNOSIS AND EVALUATION

A careful history is invaluable as part of the evaluation of a child with acute hepatobiliary disease. Knowing the immunization status of a child is important because hepatitis A and B occur rarely in immunized children. Risk factors for hepatitis A include attendance in day care centers, exposure to an individual with jaundice or hepatitis, and travel to an endemic area. Hepatitis A occurs at a younger age in low socioeconomic environments and with crowded living conditions. Because hepatitis A is spread by the fecal-oral route, close personal contact is required for infection to occur, such as with a parent or individuals living in the same household. Day care centers in which there are infants in diapers and centers with large numbers of children pose a particular risk. The clinician should inquire about international travel or contact with international travelers as sources of potential exposure for hepatitis A and E. Hepatitis A also is endemic within several areas of the United States. Hepatitis E is recognized infrequently in the United States, but is endemic in areas of Asia, Africa, and South America. Hepatitis A also may be spread by food-borne or water-borne outbreaks, so inquiry about exposure to known sources in a community should be made. The time of the potential exposure also is important to consider with regard to the various incubation periods for the hepatitis viruses (Table 90-1).

A history of parenteral exposure is the major risk factor for hepatitis B and C. High-risk behaviors and hepatitis status of the mother are important historical facts in infants with acute liver disease. Sexual transmission occurs regularly with hepatitis B, less commonly with hepatitis C, and rarely with hepatitis A. Since the advent of careful screening of blood in the United States, blood transfusions seldom are associated with hepatitis B or C. Patients who require multiple transfusions and pooled blood products such as gamma globulin and clotting factors are at increased risk. Although hepatitis B is seen worldwide, the prevalence is particularly high in Southeast Asia, Africa, South America, and Eastern Europe. Adoptees from these areas should be screened.

Exposure to hepatotoxins should be determined, including use of acetaminophen, anticonvulsants, salicylates, carbon tetrachloride, and herbal remedies. Intentional or inadvertent acetaminophen overdose is one of the most

Table 90-1. Characteristics of Viral Hepatitis

	HAV	HBV	HCV	HDV	HEV
Transmission	Fecal-oral	Parenteral, sexual	Parenteral	Parenteral	Fecal-oral
Incubation (wk)	2–6	4–26	4–?	4–26	2–10
Chronic disease	No	Infants 90% <6 yr 30% Adult 1–5%	>80%	With HBV	No
Prophylaxis	Gamma globulin immunization	HBIG, gamma globulin immunization	None	None	None
Hepatic failure	<1%	<1%	Rare	Rare	Pregnant women

HAV, hepatitis A virus; HBIG, hepatitis B immunoglobulin; HBV, hepatitis B virus; HCV, hepatitis C virus; HDV, hepatitis D virus; HEV, hepatitis E virus.

common hepatotoxic exposures in children. Ingestion of toxic mushrooms can result in hepatic failure.

Acute hepatic dysfunction may be the initial presentation of children with underlying metabolic disorders. Children with an acute hepatic presentation of a metabolic disease may have a history of developmental delay, weakness, or seizures (see Chapter 146).

A history of bruising or bleeding could indicate hepatic decompensation and fulminant hepatic failure (Box 90-1). Lethargy, excessive sleeping, irritability, and disorientation are seen in fulminant failure and metabolic and toxic hepatopathy.

Severe colicky pain occurring after eating should alert the clinician to the possibility of cholecystitis. Anemia, jaundice, and family history of anemia suggest hemolysis and cholecystitis secondary to bilirubin gallstones.

Physical Examination

The physical examination aids in distinguishing acute from chronic liver disease. Jaundice can be recognized as scleral icterus ranging from a barely detectable yellow hue at bilirubin levels of 1.5 to 3 mg/dL to deep green-yellow at higher levels. The skin is noticeably pigmented at bilirubin levels greater than 6 mg/dL. When there is biliary obstruction, there may be scratch marks secondary to pruritus. Bruising usually indicates more severe hepatic dysfunction or vitamin K deficiency or both.

The level of alertness should be noted, and the clinician should distinguish an inactive, uncomfortable child from one with mild encephalopathy. Box 90-2 shows the grading of encephalopathy.

Abdominal examination typically shows hepatomegaly with mild-to-moderate tenderness to palpation. Splenomegaly is less common and when present should raise suspicion for chronic liver disease. A prominent venous pattern on the abdomen and abdominal distention from ascites indicate portal hypertension and chronic liver disease. Splenomegaly can be seen particularly in Epstein-Barr virus and cytomegalovirus infections. Skin lesions may be present

with cytomegalovirus, Epstein-Barr virus, and enteroviruses. A raised red papular rash can be seen in hepatitis B.

The triad of severe right upper quadrant pain, jaundice, and fever suggests acute cholecystitis. Pain may radiate to the right scapular or shoulder area. Pancreatitis may be present as well with radiation of pain to the lower thoracic spine.

Diagnostic Testing

The generalist should order liver enzymes in individuals suspected to have acute hepatobiliary disease, including aspartate aminotransferase (AST), alanine aminotransferase (AST), alkaline phosphatase, and gamma glutamyl transpeptidase. Bilirubin should be fractionated. The degree of elevations of these tests identifies liver injury but do not predict severity or etiology, although there is a trend toward more marked elevations with more severe disease. When abdominal pain radiates to the shoulder or back, amylase and lipase values should be determined because pancreatitis may accompany cholecystitis. Table 90-2 lists tests commonly needed in the evaluation of hepatobiliary disorders and significant characteristics of the tests.

Prothrombin time is normal in uncomplicated hepatitis. Abnormalities indicate impaired hepatic synthetic function, and marked elevations are seen in fulminant hepatic failure. The generalist should consult with a specialist for patients with elevated prothrombin times.

Blood tests for specific viral causes should be ordered based on the history (Table 90-3). An abdominal ultrasound performed while fasting is an excellent test for identification of cholecystitis with or without gallstones. Findings may include thickening of the gallbladder wall, stones, and dilation of the extrahepatic or intrahepatic bile duct.

SPECIFIC CLINICAL ENTITIES

Viral Hepatitis

Hepatitis A is an asymptomatic infection in 70% of children younger than 6 years old. In older children and adolescents, jaundice is present along with malaise, nausea, and vomit-

---

Box 90-1. Red Flags: Signs of Fulminant Hepatic Failure or Metabolic or Toxic Hepatopathy

- History of bruising and bleeding
- Lethargy
- Excessive sleeping
- Irritability
- Disorientation

Box 90-2. Grades of Hepatic Encephalopathy

0—Alert and oriented
1—Confused; fatigue
2—Drowsy; inappropriate behavior
3—Lethargic but arousable; marked confusion; slurred speech; obeys simple commands
4—Coma

ing. The peak period of infectivity is during the incubation period (average 30 days.) There is minimal shedding of virus in stool by 1 week after the onset of jaundice, at which time children may return to school or day care. Enzyme elevations and bilirubin levels return to normal values by about 2 months. A more protracted cholestatic course occurs in some patients. The disease is more severe with increasing age, when there is coinfection with hepatitis B or C, when alcoholic hepatitis is present, with immunosuppression, and when chronic liver disease is present. A posthepatitic syndrome is possible with prolonged malaise, fatigue, anorexia, and hepatic tenderness lasting weeks. Liver failure is rare, and chronic disease does not occur. Immunity after natural infection is probably lifelong. Prophylaxis for unimmunized close contacts is 85% protective if given within 2 weeks of exposure. The dose for immune globulin prophylaxis is 0.02 mL/kg intramuscularly, which affords 3 months of protection. Infants and pregnant women should receive preparations free of thimerosal. Strategies for reducing transmission of the virus, which is spread via the oral-fecal route, include washing hands after using the toilet, after changing diapers, and before food preparation and appropriate disposal of diapers and clothing contaminated with feces or bile. Swimming in water potentially contaminated by sewage should be avoided.

Hepatitis E is transmitted by the fecal-oral route often via contaminated water and less often by human contact. Its symptoms are similar to hepatitis A. There is no vaccine and no immunoprophylaxis. Chronic disease does not occur, and liver failure is rare except during pregnancy. Control measures are similar to hepatitis A.

Hepatitis B is transmitted through parenteral and sexual routes. Unimmunized close household contacts become infected 40% of the time. Postexposure prophylaxis for unimmunized individuals consists of initiation of hepatitis B immunization and hepatitis B immunoglobulin in selected cases, according to Centers for Disease Control and Prevention guidelines, which can be found in the American Academy of Pediatrics *Redbook*. The infection may be asymptomatic. Acute liver failure occurs but is uncommon. Greater than 90% of infants and 1% to 5% of older children remain chronic carriers.

Hepatitis C is transmitted primarily parenterally and less often sexually. Spread to household contacts is uncommon. The acute phase of the infection usually goes unrecognized. The risk of perinatal transmission is estimated at 10%. At least 80% of cases remain chronic with an estimated prevalence rate in the United States of 1.8%. Complications from this disease are the major cause of liver transplantation. There is no immunization or postexposure prophylaxis available.

Hepatitis D occurs only as a coinfection with hepatitis B. It is acquired parenterally. Hepatitis D may worsen the course of hepatitis B, including progression to hepatic failure.

Other viruses that cause hepatitis but have their major source of replication in organs other than the liver include coxsackievirus, influenza, echovirus, adenovirus, parvovirus, varicella, and herpesvirus. Epstein-Barr virus causes clinical hepatitis less than 25% of the time, but enzyme abnormalities are seen in 80% of cases when looked for. Splenomegaly is common. Hepatitis from cytomegalovirus occurs typically in infants and immunocompromised individuals.

Fulminant Hepatic Failure

Fulminant liver failure is an emergency, and when recognized the patient should be transferred to a facility capable of offering liver transplantation. The etiology may be viral, toxic injury, or metabolic, but often the cause is unknown. The patient has or develops encephalopathy (see Box 90-2). Marked coagulopathy is present with prolongation of the prothrombin time, and blood ammonia typically is elevated,

Table 90-3. Tests for Diagnosis of Viral Hepatitis

Virus	Test	Comments
HAV	IgM anti-HAV	Acute infection
	IgG anti-HAV	Past infection
HBV	IgM anti-HBc	Acute infection
	HBsAg	Acute and chronic infection
	HBV/DNA	Active viral replication
	HBeAg	Active viral replication
	anti-HBs IgG	Recovery or immunization
	anti-HBc IgG	Current, past, or resolved infection
HCV	anti-HCV IgG	Acute and chronic infection
	HCV RNA or PCR	Viral replication
HDV	IgM/IgG anti-HDV	Rapid conversion to IgG antibody
HEV	IgM/IgG anti-HEV	Rapid conversion to IgG antibody

HAV, hepatitis A virus; HBc, hepatitis B core; HBeAg, hepatitis B antigen; HBs, hepatitis B surface; HBsAg, hepatitis B surface antigen; HBV, hepatitis B virus; HCV, hepatitis C virus; HDV, hepatitis D virus; HEV, hepatitis E virus; PCR, polymerase chain reaction.

Table 90-2. General Tests for Evaluation of the Liver

Test	Comments
AST	>500–8000 IU in acute hepatitis. Rises before bilirubin. Values >2500 IU seen in fulminant failure. Enzyme also found in heart, muscle, brain, and blood cells
ALT	Same as AST, but enzyme found predominantly in liver and is a more specific test for liver disease
Alkaline phosphatase	Released from bile ducts and sinusoids. May be 5× normal values in hepatitis, especially cholestatic phase. Increased in biliary obstruction and chlolecystitis. Found in bone, intestine, kidney, leukocytes. Elevated during periods of bone growth
GGT	When elevated with alkaline phosphatase, confirms hepatobiliary source. Elevated in biliary tract disease. Found in cell membranes of many other tissues
Bilirubin	Total bilirubin level elevated. Direct fraction typically represents 20–30%. Higher direct bilirubin in cholestatic phase of hepatitis and in biliary disease
Albumin	Synthesized by liver with long half-life. Normal in acute liver disease. Low in chronic liver disease, malnutrition
Prothrombin time	Sensitive test of liver synthetic function. Typically normal in acute hepatitis. Rising values indicate poor prognosis; remains elevated in liver failure

ALT, alanine aminotransferase; AST, aspartate amino transferase, GGT, gamma-glutamyl transpeptidase.

distinguishing it from other causes of encephalopathy. The clinician should be aware of the special circumstance in which a patient with apparent recovery from viral hepatitis A relapses with jaundice and marked elevations of AST and ALT, followed by rapid onset of encephalopathy. A history of drug exposure, particularly acetaminophen, should be considered, with toxic screen and acetaminophen levels obtained. The symptoms of hepatic failure from acetaminophen develop 48 hours or more after the acute ingestion so that blood levels are not elevated.

Other Causes of Acute Liver Disease

Reye syndrome is a toxic encephalopathy characterized by mitochondrial dysfunction. Features are hypoglycemia and hyperammonemia. It occurs in the context of an acute infection, especially but not exclusively influenza and varicella, and there often is exposure to salicylates or other drugs. The incidence of Reye syndrome has declined dramatically in part owing to avoidance of aspirin in children and adolescents and for unknown reasons. Illnesses that resemble Reye syndrome may result from metabolic disorders such as fatty acid oxidation defects. Some patients in previous years diagnosed with Reye syndrome likely had metabolic disorders.

Acute hepatic dysfunction can occur in systemic diseases and after toxic exposures. Table 90-4 lists the systemic causes of acute hepatic dysfunction.

Cholecystitis

Cholecystitis and cholelithiasis are recognized increasingly in pediatric patients. Children with hemolytic disorders form bilirubinate stones that may predispose to obstruction and cholecystitis. Incidentally identified gallstones that are asymptomatic do not require treatment, but one needs to be aware that acute obstruction of the cystic or common bile duct with cholangitis and cholecystitis can develop in this situation. Symptoms of acute cholecystitis are right upper quadrant pain, vomiting, fever, and jaundice. Chronic cholecystitis is characterized by intermittent postprandial pain in the right upper quadrant. Cholecystitis may be associated with gallstones and some degree of biliary obstruction and bile duct dilation or may occur without gallstones, acalculous cholecystitis.

MANAGEMENT AND OUTCOME

The treatment of acute hepatitis is supportive. The patient may experience significant fatigue, and bed rest may be appropriate. Anorexia and nausea occasionally are marked, and attention needs to be directed at adequate hydration. Although the magnitude of ALT and AST elevation does not predict recovery or severity of disease in an individual case, patients with enzyme values greater than 2500 IU should be followed more carefully. Children with hepatitis A may return to school 1 week after the onset of jaundice if feeling well. The physician should verify that liver enzyme tests have normalized by 3 months for hepatitis A and by 6 months for hepatitis B. Patients who have an atypical course of hepatitis A with failure to resolve symptoms and laboratory abnormalities by 3 months should be referred. The clinician also should determine the hepatitis B surface antigen status as a reflection of chronic hepatitis B and refer children who remain positive for more than 6 months. All patients diagnosed with hepatitis C should be referred because this nearly always is a chronic disease.

The most serious complication of hepatitis is fulminant hepatic failure. Significant prolongation of the prothrombin time, acidosis, hyperammonemia, hypoglycemia, and hypoalbuminemia indicate hepatic decompensation, and consultation should be obtained. Encephalopathy is a medical emergency, and the patient requires hospitalization in a center capable of providing liver transplantation to children. When referral is prompt, survival approaches 80% with the option of liver transplantation. Conversely, mortality for patients who reach grade III encephalopathy who do not receive transplantation can approach 90%.

Individuals with features of portal hypertension and liver disease with growth failure should be referred to a pediatric liver specialist for evaluation of chronic liver disease (see Chapter 141). A child or adolescent presenting with acute

Table 90-4. Causes of Hepatic Dysfunction

General Category	Specific Causes
Infection	Sepsis
	Hepatitis
Drugs	Acetaminophen
	Amiodarone
	Aspirin
	Azathioprine
	Carbamazepine
	Chemotherapy agents
	Ecstasy (3,4-methylenedioxymethamphetamine)
	Erythromycin
	Estrogens
	Halothane
	Isoniazid
	Ketoconazole
	Penicillins
	Phenobarbital
	Phenytoin
	Propylthiouracil
	Retinoids
	Sulfonamides
	Valproic acid
Toxins	Carbon tetrachloride
	Mushrooms
Cardiac	Congenital heart disease
	Congestive heart failure
	Shock
Nutritional	Parenteral nutrition
	Obesity
	Malnutrition
Malignancy	Leukemia
	Neuroblastoma
	Bone marrow transplantation
	Lymphoma
Immunologic disorders	Inflammatory bowel disease
	Lupus erythematosus
	Autoimmune liver disease
	Juvenile rheumatoid arthritis
	Immune deficiency
Metabolic disorders	
Endocrine disorders	Diabetes
	Thyroid disorders
Hematologic	Sickle cell disease
	Hemolytic disorders

right upper quadrant pain may have either hepatitis or biliary disease, and an ultrasound evaluation is necessary to assess the gallbladder and bile ducts. When cholecystitis and biliary obstruction are identified, surgical consultation is necessary. When fever is present, antibiotics should be administered for presumed cholangitis.

Mini-index of Related Topics

SUGGESTED READINGS

American Academy of Pediatrics: Summaries of infectious diseases. In Pickering L (ed): 2000 Redbook Report of the Committee on Infectious Diseases, 25th ed. Elk Grove Village, Ill, American Academy of Pediatrics, 2000, pp 278–308.
Fagan EA, Harrison TJ: Viral Hepatitis: A Handbook for Clinicians and Scientists. Oxford, BIOS Scientific Publishers Limited, 2000.
Kelly D, Skidmore S: Hepatitis C–Z recent advances. Arch Dis Child 2002;86:330–343.
Lobe TE: Cholelithiasis and cholecystitis in children. Semin Pediatr Surg 2000;9:170–176.
Yazigi N, Balistreri WF: Acute and chronic viral hepatitis. In Suchy FJ, Sokol RF, Balistreri WF (eds): Liver Disease in Children. Philadelphia, Lippincott Williams & Wilkins, 2001, pp 365–429.

SECTION 3   GENERAL MEDICAL CARE: *Gastrointestinal and Nutritional Disorders*

91 Disorders of the Pancreas

William Mow

ROLE OF THE GENERALIST

1 Understand normal embryologic development of the pancreas.
2 Diagnose congenital anomalies of the pancreas.
3 Diagnose and manage acute pancreatitis.
4 Diagnose pancreatic insufficiency.
5 Refer to specialist for treatment.

DEFINITIONS

Disorders of the pancreas are rare in children. The *endocrine* functions of the pancreas include control of glucose homeostasis through the production of insulin and glucagon. The *exocrine* functions of this organ are important for proper digestion of fat, protein, and carbohydrates. Without a properly functioning pancreas, malabsorption of nutrients results in failure to thrive and fat-soluble vitamin deficiencies.

FUNDAMENTALS

The pancreas is formed from two buds of endoderm—one from the duodenum, the dorsal pancreatic bud, and the other from the liver bud, the ventral pancreatic bud. These two buds, which first appear around 30 days' gestation, develop into pancreatic tissue with individual ductal systems by 6 weeks' gestation (Fig. 91-1). The ventral bud drains via the duct of Wirsung through the major papilla (along with the common bile duct) into the duodenum, and the dorsal bud drains through the minor papilla via the duct of Santorini into the duodenum. At around 6 weeks' gestation, the ventral bud rotates to fuse with the dorsal bud. Abnormalities in the ductal system are relatively common, but they are usually clinically insignificant.

Pancreatic exocrine function is important for proper digestion and absorption of nutrients by the small bowel. Pancreatic secretion of bicarbonate and digestive enzymes occurs as a result of vagal nerve stimulation and the secretion of two hormones from the duodenal epithelium, secretin and cholecystokinin. Secretin release is stimulated by the presence of acid and fats in the duodenum after gastric emptying. Secretin stimulates pancreatic secretion of bicarbonate to neutralize the acid in the gastric chyme. Cholecystokinin release is stimulated by the presence of fat in the chyme and stimulates the pancreas to secrete enzymes involved in digestion of protein, fat, and carbohydrate. Trypsinogen and chymotrypsinogen are secreted by the pancreas into the duodenum, where enteropeptidases help convert them into their active forms, trypsin and chymotrypsin. These two enzymes are essential for the digestion of protein. The pancreas also secretes α-amylase, which breaks down starch and glycogen into trisaccharides

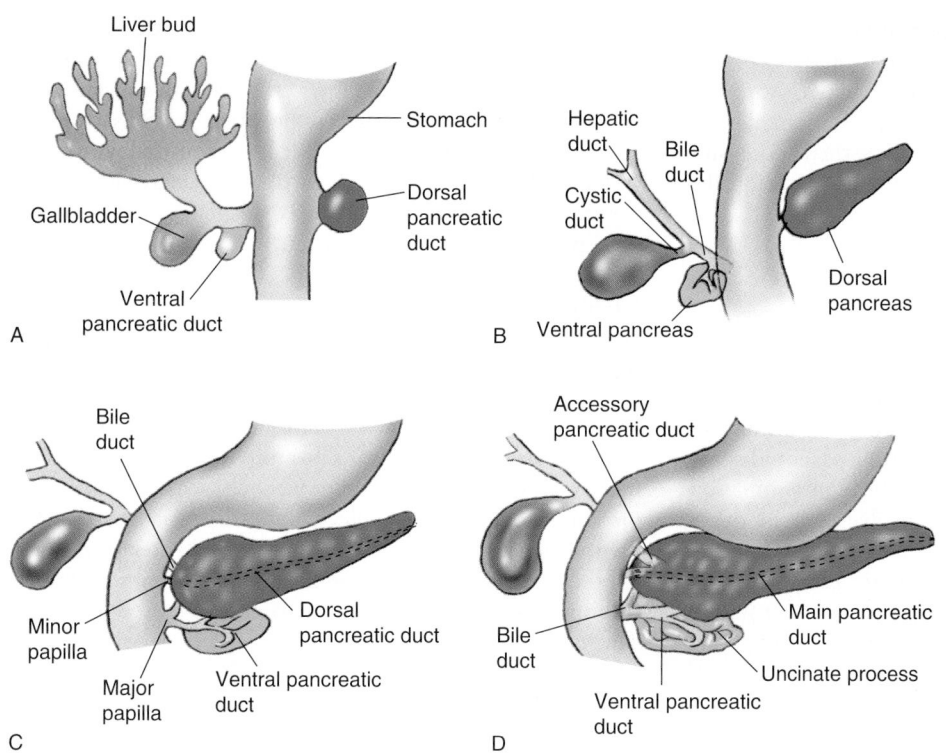

Figure 91-1. Embryologic development of the pancreas. **A,** At 4.5 weeks. **B,** At 5 weeks. The ventral pancreatic bud originates near the liver bud. **C,** At 6 weeks. The ventral pancreatic bud has migrated posteriorly and is in close contact with the dorsal pancreatic bud. **D,** Fusion of the pancreatic buds and ducts.

and disaccharides for further digestion by intestinal enzymes into absorbable sugars. Pancreatic lipase, the most important of the pancreatic enzymes, is secreted in conjunction with an activating enzyme procolipase. It breaks down triglycerides into 2-monoglycerides and free fatty acids for absorption in micelles. In addition to its exocrine functions, the pancreas is essential in glucose homeostasis. Hormone-producing cells in the pancreatic islets of Langerhans produce glucagon, insulin, somatostatin, and pancreatic polypeptide.

CONGENITAL ANOMALIES OF THE PANCREAS

Congenital malformations of the pancreas are not rare, but they are diagnosed rarely because they usually are asymptomatic. Pancreatic ductal variations are present in 10% of the population. Development of the pancreas is complex, and problems lead to congenital malformations, such as pancreatic divisum and annular pancreas.

Pancreatic divisum is a disorder in which the dorsal and ventral pancreatic buds fail to fuse, leaving two separate regions with individual drainage systems. This malformation is seen in 0.5% to 11% of the population. Its role in recurrent pancreatitis is controversial. Current evidence indicates that pancreatic divisum can be a normal variant. Pancreatic divisum is found in 15% of autopsy specimens from patients without a history of chronic pancreatitis. In some patients, this malformation is seen in conjunction with chronic-recurrent pancreatitis, failure to thrive, and chronic abdominal pain. Diagnosis is made with either endoscopic retrograde cholangiopancreatography (ERCP) or magnetic resonance cholangiopancreatography (MRCP). Patients with pancreatic divisum and recurrent pancreatitis need to be followed by a pediatric gastroenterologist and a surgeon. Treatment is good nutrition, supplemental fat-soluble vitamins, and replacement pancreatic enzymes. If

medical therapy is unsuccessful, the pancreatic drainage problem may need to be corrected surgically.

Annular pancreas is a disorder in the development of the pancreas in which the dorsal and ventral pancreatic buds fail to align properly before fusion. As the two buds fuse, they constrict the duodenum, causing some degree of intestinal obstruction (Fig. 91-2). This disorder frequently is associated with other congenital malformations, such as malrotation, duodenal web or atresia, cardiac defects, and tracheoesophageal fistula. It also is seen more commonly in patients with trisomy 21. Because many of these patients present in the first few days of life with intestinal obstruction, diagnosis usually is made at the time of surgery. Surgery involves bypass of the obstruction. Most patients with this malformation alone do well. When annular pancreas does not cause obstruction, it usually is found incidentally on an imaging study or on autopsy specimens.

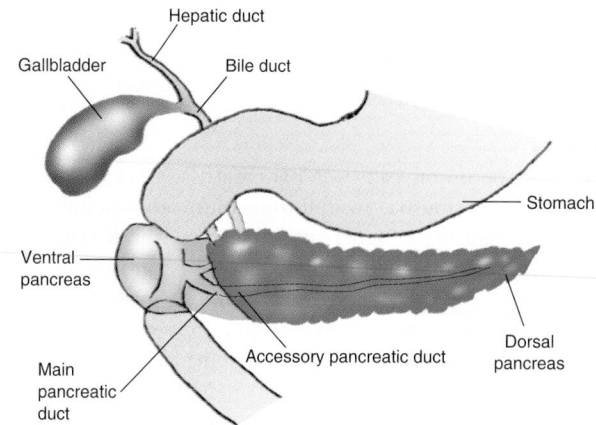

Figure 91-2. Annular pancreas. A ring around the duodenum formed by the ventral pancreas.

Ectopic pancreatic rests are benign nodules of pancreatic tissue usually found in the greater curve or antrum of the stomach. Endoscopically, these rests look like 1- to 3-cm smooth round bumps with a central umbilication. Rarely, these lesions are found on upper gastrointestinal series and are found in 1% to 2% of autopsy specimens. Occasionally, they are associated with gastric outlet obstruction.

PANCREATITIS

Pancreatitis, an uncommon disorder in children, is inflammation of the pancreas. Pancreatitis can be caused by trauma, viral infections, stones, multisystem diseases, congenital malformations to the ducts, and certain drugs. In children, the etiology of pancreatitis often is not discovered. Acute pancreatitis is described as acute inflammation of the pancreas without significant involvement of other organ systems. It can vary from mild to severe based on the degree of organ dysfunction and systemic effects of the pancreatitis. In chronic pancreatitis, there is continued inflammation, structural changes, and pancreatic exocrine and endocrine dysfunction.

Acute Pancreatitis
Pathophysiology
Although theories about the pathogenesis of acute pancreatitis have yet to be proven, they provide a foundation for understanding the disorder. The pancreas is responsible for the secretion of digestive enzymes. Usually these enzymes are secreted as proenzymes, which need to be activated by other enzymes in the duodenum. The obstruction-secretion hypothesis states that in acute pancreatitis, outflow of digestive proenzymes from the pancreas is obstructed, leading to premature activation and autodigestion of the pancreas itself. The fact that many patients with biliary stones and choledocholithiasis have associated pancreatitis supports this theory. The hypothesis is contradicted by the fact that most adult patients with chronic pancreatitis have normal sphincter of Oddi pressures and normal pressures within the duct of Wirsung. It also seems logical that direct trauma to the pancreas would lead to the release of pancreatic enzymes and edema, which could be responsible for ductal obstruction. If this process of inflammation progresses, it is likely that there will be continued edema, necrosis, and pancreatic insufficiency. Complications and systemic effects of acute pancreatitis include systemic inflammatory response syndrome, shock, sepsis, pancreatic abscess or pseudocyst, and immunosuppression.

Etiology
The most common cause of pancreatitis is accidental and nonaccidental trauma. In children, blunt abdominal blows can create significant pancreatic damage without significant external abdominal wall findings because children are relatively thin, and the pancreas lies directly over the spinal column. Stones are rare in children but can be seen in children with risk factors for cholelithiasis (e.g., family history, hemolytic disease, obesity). Multisystem disease, such as systemic lupus erythematosus, Kawasaki disease, hemolytic uremic syndrome, and inflammatory bowel disease, can be associated with the development of pancreatitis. Drugs are a common cause of pancreatitis in chronically ill children who are exposed to a large variety of medicines and chemotherapy. Viral infections can cause pancreatitis, including mumps, hepatitis A, coxsackievirus B, human immunodeficiency virus, cytomegalovirus, and varicella. Congenital anomalies of the pancreas are associated with chronic pancreatitis, although their role in susceptibility to pancreatitis is unclear.

Clinical Presentation and Diagnosis
Patients classically have severe epigastric abdominal pain that is constant and radiates to the back. In most cases, the pain continues to worsen over the first 24 to 48 hours. Patients also may have fever, vomiting, and pain with eating. In most cases, the process is self-limited, with slow improvement over the next week. In more severe cases, patients can present in shock with electrolyte disturbances, ascites, pleural effusions, and dehydration. Some degree of abdominal tenderness and distention usually is present on physical examination. Bowel sounds usually are decreased or absent. The classic findings of pancreatitis, Cullen's sign (bluish periumbilical area), and Grey Turner's sign (bluish discoloration of the flanks) are seen only in severe cases.

The diagnosis of acute pancreatitis should be suspected in any child with acute-onset abdominal pain and nonspecific symptoms, such as fever, nausea, and back or chest pain. It should be suspected in children with severe abdominal pain and vomiting during seasons not typically associated with viral gastroenteritis. Serum amylase and lipase are simple serologic tests that can be used to diagnose this disorder. Amylase can be elevated for many reasons other than pancreatitis, such as biliary disease, bowel obstruction, duodenal ulcer, parotitis, ectopic pregnancy, burns, head trauma, and acute appendicitis. An elevated amylase level should be verified with a lipase level to help confirm the diagnosis. Elevation of amylase and lipase to three times the upper limit of normal is diagnostic of pancreatitis. A pancreatic ultrasound study is recommended to assess presence of biliary stones, pancreatic pseudocysts, and pancreatic ductal dilation. Abdominal computed tomography (CT) usually is performed in cases in which the ultrasound is inconclusive or when pancreatic or extrapancreatic fluid collections are seen on ultrasound. Findings on ultrasound and CT often are initially negative for pancreatitis. These imaging studies are important to help define the anatomy and degree of damage and inflammation in the pancreas. MRCP and ERCP are reserved for chronic or severe cases.

Treatment
Most generalists can manage mild and moderate cases of acute pancreatitis. Patients require fluid and electrolyte replacement and pain management with meperidine. Morphine is contraindicated because of the possibility of sphincter of Oddi spasm. If patients have a significant amount of vomiting, a nasogastric tube should be placed for decompression. Bowel rest for a short time usually is indicated. Oral refeeding can begin when these patients express hunger, have increased bowel sounds, pass stool and rectal gas, have decreased pain, and have decreased nasogastric tube output. Reintroduction of food can begin before

serology values have normalized, but food is a major stimulus to the pancreas and can cause recurrence of symptoms.

Approximately 15% of cases of acute pancreatitis are defined as severe. These cases often are associated with systemic inflammatory response syndrome, which has a mortality of 21% in children. In these more severe cases, the aforementioned management approach also applies. These patients are more likely to have problems with hypocalcemia, anemia, hypoalbuminemia, hypoxemia, and sepsis. No medicines have been proved to be effective in acute pancreatitis. Often these patients are given acid-blocking drugs, however, such as H_2 blockers or proton-pump inhibitors. Prophylactic antibiotics are discouraged in patients who are not in shock. These patients are at great risk for complications, and serial CT scans should be followed. Surgery is indicated in cases of ductal rupture and pancreatic abscess. Pancreatic pseudocysts are rare and rarely require surgery. In severely sick patients with fever and shock, differentiation of a pseudocyst from an abscess is difficult. After resolution of a severe case of pancreatitis, an ultrasound at 2 to 4 weeks usually is recommended to evaluate for pseudocysts. Pseudocysts less than 4 cm are generally benign. Pseudocysts larger than 4 cm may require surgical or percutaneous drainage. Use of ERCP has been reported in acute pancreatitis resulting from choledocholithiasis for stone removal and sphincterotomy and in other cases for the evaluation of the pancreatic and biliary ductal systems.

Chronic Pancreatitis

Chronic pancreatitis is defined as morphologic changes in the organ and pancreatic malfunction. Chronic pancreatitis has continuing necrosis and inflammation of the pancreas causing scarring, tissue damage, and eventually organ dysfunction. In adults, the most common cause of this disorder is alcoholism. In children, the cause usually is not found. It can be caused by recurrent pancreatitis secondary to congenital anomalies or any chronic obstructive lesion of the pancreatic duct. It also is associated with pancreatic ductal damage after trauma. In some cases, there may be a need for referral to a tertiary center for pancreatic surgery. Chronic recurrent pancreatitis also is associated with hyperlipidemia, cystic fibrosis, α_1-antitrypsin deficiency, sclerosing cholangitis, and inflammatory bowel disease. Hereditary pancreatitis is a rare autosomal dominant disorder caused by a defect in the trypsinogen gene. These patients usually have chronic pancreatitis and are at increased risk for the development of pancreatic cancer.

Clinical Presentation

Many patients present with recurrent episodes of what seems to be acute pancreatitis. With each recurrence, the pancreatic exocrine and endocrine functions are damaged further, although exocrine dysfunction and malabsorption are not seen until 98% of the pancreas is lost. Diabetes also can occur.

Diagnosis

The diagnosis is suspected in patients with recurrent episodes of pancreatitis. Imaging studies can be done to show calcification of the pancreas, which confirms the diagnosis. ERCP is being used commonly to evaluate the ductal systems of these patients for congenital anomalies, ductal strictures, or other abnormalities.

Treatment

Treatment should be in conjunction with a pediatric gastroenterologist and surgeon. The mainstay of therapy revolves around pain management, pancreatic enzyme replacement, and somatostatin therapy. In cases that fail medical management, endoscopic and surgical attention may be necessary to relieve obstruction from ductal strictures. When diabetes occurs, it can be treated with insulin. These patients are at greater risk for hypoglycemia secondary to lack of glucagon excretion. These patients usually are chronically ill and require close follow-up.

EXOCRINE INSUFFICIENCY

There are several disorders of pancreatic exocrine dysfunction, the most common of which is cystic fibrosis (CF). These disorders usually present in infancy and early childhood with failure to thrive secondary to malabsorption. Some of the more common causes of exocrine pancreatic insufficiency are discussed briefly. These patients should be followed in conjunction with a pediatric gastroenterologist.

CF is the most common inherited disorder of pancreatic exocrine dysfunction. It is seen in 1 in 2500 live births in white families. At this time, more than 600 mutations of the CF transmembrane regulator (CFTR) on chromosome 7 have been described. These defects cause the pancreas to be unable to secrete its digestive enzymes. About 85% of patients with CF have some degree of exocrine pancreatic insufficiency. These patients often present in the first 2 to 4 months of life with severe malnutrition and failure to thrive. They usually have a history of malodorous, voluminous, greasy, yellow stools. As a result of the severe protein and calorie malnutrition, these patients typically are hypoalbuminemic and immunosuppressed. In addition, they may have manifestations of zinc, iron, and trace element deficiencies and fat-soluble vitamin deficiency. CF should be suspected in all children with malabsorption in infancy. The diagnosis of CF can be established with a sweat test containing greater than 60 mEq/L of sodium chloride and CF gene mutation analysis. Treatment usually is initiated at a CF treatment center and revolves around minimizing pulmonary disease and giving supplemental pancreatic enzymes.

Shwachman's syndrome is a rare disorder seen in 1 in 200,000 live births. The constellation of symptoms seen in this disorder includes exocrine pancreatic insufficiency, neutropenia, metaphyseal dysostosis, and short stature. Shwachman's syndrome has a variable presentation, but most patients initially are referred to pediatric gastroenterologists for malabsorption and failure to thrive. In addition to the aforementioned findings, patients are known to have a predilection for the development of acute myelogenous leukemia. Treatment is symptomatic and includes pancreatic enzyme supplementation. Some studies advocate the use of granulocyte colony-stimulating factor in patients with neutropenia. Studies have shown that some of these patients outgrow the disease.

Other syndromes that are associated with pancreatic insufficiency include Johanson-Blizzard syndrome and Pearson's syndrome. Both of these disorders are extremely rare. Johanson-Blizzard syndrome involves a constellation of features including hypoplastic alae nasi, short stature, dental defects, and deafness. Pearson's syndrome is a mitochondrial disorder characterized by sideroblastic anemia and exocrine pancreatic insufficiency. It is a rare disorder and is fatal.

A few known diseases involve a deficiency in the pancreatic production of lipase and colipase. As a result of these deficiencies, patients typically have severe fat malabsorption without other extrapancreatic sequelae. These disorders are diagnosed with pancreatic function tests. Patients should be followed in conjunction with a pediatric gastroenterologist.

 Additional Resources, CD-ROM

Bibliography

SUGGESTED READINGS

Cipolli M, D'Orazio C, Delmarco A, et al: Shwachman's syndrome: Pathomorphosis and long-term outcome. J Pediatr Gastroenterol Nutr 1999;29:265–272.

Kilman W, Berk R: The spectrum of radiologic features of aberrant pancreatic rests involving the stomach. Radiology 1977;123:291–296.

Lehman GA, Sherman S: Pancreatic divisum. Gastrointest Endosc Clin North Am 1995;5:145–170.

SECTION 3   GENERAL MEDICAL CARE: *Disorders of the Hematopoietic System*

92 Anemias and Other Disorders of Red Blood Cells

Karen Ann Kalinyak

ROLE OF THE GENERALIST

1 Provide dietary counseling for anemia prevention.

2 Provide screening for anemia.

3 Diagnose anemia and refer to hematologist if assistance is needed for diagnosing cause of anemia.

4 Diagnose and treat iron deficiency anemia.

5 If other nutritional anemias are suspected, refer to hematologist for assistance with diagnosis and treatment.

6 Comanage patients with chronic anemias (see Chapter 159).

DEFINITION

Anemia is a condition in which the concentration of hemoglobin or the number of red blood cells is less than normal, resulting in decreased oxygen-carrying capacity of the blood and a reduction in the oxygen available to the tissues. Table 92-1 outlines the normal values of hemoglobin and mean corpuscular volume (MCV) by age. The signs and symptoms of anemia are a result of failure to oxygenate tissues and speed of onset (gradual onset of anemia allows time for compensatory mechanisms to increase oxygenation).

Symptoms are related to the degree of anemia, occurring in the following order: (1) pallor, fatigue, increased pulse rate, tachypnea, (2) irritability, headache, dizziness, nausea, heart murmur, and finally (3) chest pain, congestive heart failure, shock, coma.

FUNDAMENTALS

Anemia is the result of diverse underlying pathophysiologic processes. Anemias can be classified either by causative (etiologic) mechanisms or by red blood cell morphology. Classification of anemias by etiology is (1) acute or chronic hemorrhage, (2) increased loss or destruction of red blood

Table 92-1. Normal Hematologic Values*

Age (years)	Hemoglobin† (g/dL)		Mean Corpuscular Volume (fL)	
	Mean Value	Lower Limit	Mean Value	Lower Limit
0.5–2.0	12.0	11.0	77	70
2–6	12.5	11.0	81	74
6–12	13.5	11.5	86	76
12–18 Adult				
Female	14.0	12.0	88	78
Male	14.5	13.0	88	78

*Note the developmental changes in hemoglobin and mean corpuscular volume.
†The mean hemoglobin concentration is about 0.5 g/dL lower in the black population.

From Dallman PR, Siimes MA: Percentile curves for haemoglobin and red cell volume in infancy and childhood. J Pediatr 1979;94:26–31.

Newborn screening to identify infants born with significant hemoglobinopathies, such as sickle cell disease or thalassemia intermedia or thalassemia major, is currently done in almost every state in the United States. Physicians are notified of abnormal results and babies are retested so that those with disease can be referred to appropriate specialty clinics. This approach allows appropriate education, counseling, and medical care to occur prior to the child's first symptom.

cells, or (3) impaired hemoglobin and red blood cell formation (Table 92-2).

Anemias that are classified morphologically are based on the values of MCV and mean corpuscular hemoglobin concentration (MCHC). In this classification schema, anemias fall into one of three general categories: (1) normocytic, normochromic anemias, in which both the MCV and the MCHC are normal, (2) microcytic hypochromic anemias, in which both the MCV and MCHC are less than normal, or (3) macrocytic anemias, in which the MCV is increased. Table 92-3 lists morphologically classified anemas.

DIAGNOSIS

The initial approach to the evaluation of the anemic child includes a detailed history, physical examination, and a minimum of laboratory studies. Historical factors of importance are outlined in Table 92-4. Significant physical findings are summarized in Table 92-5. The initial laboratory studies should include a determination of the white blood cell count, platelet count, and hemoglobin concentration and measurements of the red blood cell indices. These values are all included in the automated, electronic counter that reports the complete blood count (CBC). In addition, the red blood cell distribution width (RDW) is provided as part of the CBC. The RDW is an index of the variation in red blood cell size, and thus can be used to detect anisocytosis. The RDW reflects the ratio of the standard deviation and MCV. Table 92-6 shows the relationship of the RDW and MCV in various diseases.

The examination of the peripheral blood smear is the single most useful procedure in the initial evaluation of the patient with anemia. The blood smear should be examined first under low power to scan the cells, look at the adequacy of the cell distribution and staining, and to find the best area on the smear to examine by higher power. Signs of a poor area of the smear include loss of central pallor in the red blood cells, artifactually large spherocytes, and polygonal-shaped red blood cells. Caution must be taken never to try to interpret a poorly made smear or an inappropriate area of the smear. A classification of red blood cell hemolytic disorders based on their predominant morphology is presented in Table 92-7. Table 92-8 outlines the various red blood cell inclusions and their significance.

Table 92-2. Etiologic Classification of Anemia

Etiology	Anemic Disorder
Blood loss	Acute
	Chronic
Increased blood destruction	Intrinsic red blood cell defects
	▪ Defects of hemoglobin (hemoglobinopathies such as sickle cell anemia, thalassemia)
	▪ Defects of red blood cell membrane (hereditary spherocytosis, elliptocytosis, pyropoikilocytosis, stomatocytosis, etc.)
	▪ Defects of red blood cell metabolism
	Extracorpuscular factors
	▪ Immune-mediated (autoimmune, Rh antibodies)
	▪ Nonimmune mechanisms (infectious agents, chemical agents, physical trauma such as thermal injury, march hemoglobinuria, hemolytic-uremic syndrome, thrombocytic thrombocytopenic purpura, associated with chronic inflammatory disorder, malignancy, or other causes such as hypersplenism)
	Interaction of intracorpuscular and extracorpuscular factors
	▪ Associated with membrane defect: paroxysmal nocturnal hemaglobinuria
	▪ Hemoglobinuria
	▪ Associated with enzyme defect: favism, glucose-6-phosphate deficiency
	▪ Lead poisoning
	▪ Nutritional deficiencies
Impaired production	Nutritional deficiencies
	Suppression or inhibition of bone marrow
	▪ Infection
	▪ Drug reaction
	▪ Physical agents
	▪ Immune mechanisms
	▪ Idiopathic bone marrow failure
	Mechanical interference and replacement of bone marrow by abnormal cells
	▪ Osteopetrosis
	▪ Myelofibrosis
	▪ Malignancies (leukemia, neuroblastoma)
	Secondary relative marrow failure
	▪ Infection
	▪ Chronic inflammatory disease
	▪ Renal disease
	▪ Liver disease
	▪ Malignancy
	▪ Endocrine disorders
	Dyserythropoiesis (ineffective erythropoiesis)
	▪ Primary
	▪ Secondary

Note: Anemias that are classified *morphologically* are based on the values of mean corpuscular volume (MCV) and mean corpuscular hemoglobin concentration (MCHC). In this classification anemias fall into one of three general categories: (1) normocytic, normochromic anemias, (2) microcytic, hypochromic anemias, or (3) macrocytic anemias (see Table 92–3).

Table 92-3. Morphologic Classification of Anemia

Morphologic Type	Causes

Normocytic, normochromic anemias	With reticulocytosis
	  ■ Acute blood loss
	  ■ Hemolysis
	  ■ Splenic pooling
	Without reticulocytosis
	  ■ Primary bone marrow failure
	  ■ Secondary bone marrow failure
	  ■ Expanded plasma volume
	  ■ Chronic disease

Microcytic, hypochromic anemias	Iron deficiency Thalassemia syndromes Lead poisoning Pyridoxine-responsive anemias Copper deficiency Sideroblastic anemia
Macrocytic anemias	Folate deficiency Vitamin B_{12} deficiency Orotic aciduria Bone marrow hypoplasia Thiamine-responsive anemia Dyserythropoietic anemias Hypothyroidism Liver diseases Aplastic anemia Diamond-Blackfan syndrome

REFERRAL TO A HEMATOLOGIST

Mild anemias that are not causing medical problems for the child can be evaluated by the primary care provider. Because the most common anemia in the young child is iron deficiency, if the CBC demonstrates a microcytic picture suggestive of iron deficiency, treatment with iron may be begun. If the child does not respond despite appropriate doses of iron and appropriate dietary counseling, further studies are indicated.

Referral to a hematologist is indicated if the cause of the anemia remains uncertain, the anemia is severe, or significant hemolysis is evidenced by the blood smear and elevated bilirubin. If the anemia is also accompanied by low white blood cell counts or low platelet counts, referral to a hematologist would be appropriate to rule out a significant bone marrow disorder, such as leukemia or aplastic anemia (Box 92-1).

Infants identified by newborn screening as having a significant hemoglobinopathy, such as sickle cell disease, should be retested and referred to an appropriate clinic or hematologist.

PREVENTION

Acquired, nutritional anemias can be prevented with appropriate nutritional counseling. The iron stores of full-term infants should last 4 to 6 months without iron supplementation. Infants exclusively breast-fed after 6 months of age should be given a multivitamin with iron. Infants on iron-fortified formulas are not at risk of developing nutritional iron deficiency anemia until they are switched from the formula to cow milk. Most pediatric providers recommend keeping the child on breast milk or formula until 12 months of age before switching to cow milk. This practice has significantly decreased the incidence of iron deficiency in the child younger than 1 year of age. If, however, the older infant is switched to cow milk at 12 months of age and consumes excessive amounts of cow milk, the child can become iron deficient in a matter of months. Parents should be counseled to limit the amount of cow milk the child consumes to less than 16 oz a day, preferably from a cup, to eliminate the risk of developing nutritional iron deficiency anemia. Careful dietary history should be taken after formula is discontinued to determine if screening for iron deficiency should be done.

NUTRITIONAL ANEMIAS

Most nutritional anemias including those of iron, folate, and vitamin B_{12} deficiency, are associated with a decrease in the release of young red blood cells from the bone marrow and a decrease in the reticulocyte count. Lack of the essential nutrient restricts cell proliferation or differentiation. Although a nutritional anemia is often thought of as

Table 92-4. Historical Factors in Diagnosing Causes of Anemia

Factor	Possible Cause of Anemia
Age Newborn	Most common causes of anemia in this age group include blood loss, isoimmunization, congenital infection, congenital hemolytic anemia Hyperbilirubinemia in the newborn period may suggest presence of congenital hemolytic anemia: spherocytosis, G6PD deficiency Prematurity predisposes to early development of iron deficiency
Age 3–6 months	Congenital disorders of hemoglobin synthesis or hemoglobin structure; almost never nutritional iron deficiency in otherwise normal infant who was full term
Older infant and toddler	Nutritional iron deficiency in those switched to whole cow milk
Sex	Consider X-linked disorders in males: glucose-6-phosphate dehydrogenase (G6PD) deficiency, phosphoglycerate kinase deficiency
Race/ethnicity	Hemoglobins S and C are more common in blacks β-Thalassemia more common in people of Mediterranean background α-Thalassemia trait most common among black and yellow races G6PD deficiency observed with increased frequency among Sephardic Jews, Filipinos, Greeks, Sardinians, and Kurds
Diet	History of pica, geophagia, or pagophagia suggests presence of iron deficiency Document sources of iron, vitamin B_{12}, folic acid, and vitamin E in diet (e.g., infants fed goat milk are at risk for developing folic acid deficiency because goat milk is a poor source of folate)
Drugs	Various drugs can induce megaloblastic anemia (anticonvulsants, chemotherapy) Drug-induced aplastic anemia vs. drug-induced bone marrow suppression that is reversible upon discontinuing the drug Oxidant-induced hemolytic anemia
Infection	Hepatitis-induced aplastic anemia, infection-induced red blood cell aplasia or hemolysis
Inheritance	Family history of anemia, jaundice, gallstones, splenectomy
Diarrhea	Small bowel disease with malabsorption of folate or vitamin B_{12} Inflammatory bowel disease with blood loss

Table 92-5. Physical Findings as Clues to the Etiology of Anemia

Location	Physical Finding	Type of Anemia
Skin	Hyperpigmentation	Fanconi's aplastic anemia
	Petechiae, purpura	Autoimmune hemolytic anemia with thrombocytopenia, hemolytic-uremic syndrome, bone marrow apasia, bone marrow infiltration
	Carotenemia	Suspect iron deficiency in infants
	Jaundice	Hemolytic anemia, hepatitis, and aplastic anemia
	Cavernous hemangioma	Microangiopathic hemolytic anemia
	Ulcers on lower extremities	S and C hemoglobinopathies, thalassemia
Facies	Frontal bossing, prominence of the malar and maxillary bones	Congenital hemolytic anemias, thalassemia major, severe iron deficiency
Eyes	Microcornea	Fanconi's aplastic anemia
	Tortuosity of the conjunctival and retinal vessels	S and C hemoglobinopathies
	Microaneurysms of retinal vessels	S and C hemoglobinopathies
	Cataracts	G6PD deficiency, galactosemia with hemolytic anemia in newborn period
	Vitreous hemorrhages	S hemoglobinopathy
	Retinal hemorrhages	Chronic, severe anemia
	Edema of the eyelids	Infectious mononucleosis, exudative enteropathy with iron deficiency
	Blindness	Osteopetrosis
Mouth	Glossitis	Vitamin B_{12} deficiency, iron deficieny
	Angular stomatitis	Iron deficiency
Chest	Unilateral absence of the pectoral muscles	Poland's syndrome (increased incidence of leukemia)
	Shield chest	Diamond-Blackfan syndrome
Hands	Triphalangeal thumbs	Red blood cell apasia
	Hypoplasia of the thenar eminence	Fanconi's aplastic anemia
	Spoon nails	Iron deficiency
Spleen	Enlargement	Congenital hemolytic anemia, leukemia, lymphoma, acute infection, portal hypertension

being the result of a single nutrient, a diet lacking in one nutrient may also lack other substances, resulting in a mixed or masked deficiencies. Therefore, a careful nutritional history is important.

Iron Deficiency Anemia

Iron deficiency remains the most common cause of anemia in childhood despite improvements in diet and education. The most common factors that contribute to the development of iron deficiency in children are as follows:

1. Increased demand during times of rapid growth (expansion of the blood volume). These periods include infancy, early childhood (toddler), and adolescence.

2. Deficient intake. For example, whole cow milk has virtually no bioavailable iron, which means that none of the iron in cow milk is absorbed.

3. Blood loss (acute or chronic). This loss may be a result of excessive menstrual losses, whole cow milk sensitivity, gut changes from primary iron deficiency, gastritis or ulcer disease, bleeding diathesis, or other disorders.

4. Decreased absorption secondary to severe diarrhea or inflammatory bowel disease.

5. Prematurity. Premature infants have fewer iron stores and are at greater risk for developing iron deficiency.

Table 92-9 outlines the three stages in the development of iron deficiency anemia.

The first stage consists of depletion of storage iron (decrease in serum ferritin and bone marrow iron). The second stage consists of a decrease in transport iron and is characterized by a declining concentration of serum iron and increase in the total iron-binding capacity (TIBC). These changes result in a decrease in the transferrin saturation that is calculated from the ratio of the serum iron to the TIBC. The third stage of iron deficiency develops when the supply of transport iron decreases sufficiently to restrict hemoglobin production. This stage is characterized by an elevation of free erythrocyte protoporphyrin (FEP) and zinc protoporphyrin (ZPP) and the gradual development of detectable anemia (decreased hemoglobin) and microcytosis (decreased MCV). The decrease in MCV should be proportional to the decrease in hemoglobin. A minimal anemia caused only by iron deficiency should have a slightly decreased MCV. A profound anemia would have a very low MCV.

Nonhematologic abnormalities associated with iron deficiency include behavioral changes, impaired intellectual function, abnormal neutrophil function and cellular

Table 92-6. The Relationship of Red Blood Cell Distribution Width (RDW) and Mean Corpuscular Volume (MCV) in a Variety of Disease States

RDW	Low MCV	Normal MCV	High MCV
Normal	Heterozygous α- or β-thalassemia		Aplastic anemia
High	Iron deficiency hemoglobin H	Chronic disease	Folate deficiency
	S β-thalassemia	Liver disease	Vitamin B_{12} deficiency
		Myelotoxic chemotherapy	Immune hemolytic anemia
		Chronic lymphocytic or myelogenous leukemia	
		Mixed deficiencies	
		Sideroblastic hemoglobin SS or SC	
		Myelofibrosis	

Table 92-7. Morphologic Classification of Red Blood Cell Hemolytic Disorders

Spherocytes

Hereditary spherocytosis
ABO incompatibility in neonates
Immunohemolytic anemias with IgG- or C3-coated red blood cells*
Acute oxidant injury (hexose monophosphate shunt defects during hemolytic crisis, oxidant drugs and chemicals)
Hemolytic transfusion reactions*
Clostridium welchii septicemia
Severe burns, other red blood cell thermal injury
Spider, bee, and snake venoms
Severe hypophosphatemia
Hypersplenism†

Bizarre Poikilocytes

Red blood cell fragmentation syndromes (micro- and macroangiopathic hemolytic anemias)
Acute oxidant injury†
Hereditary elliptocytosis in neonates
Hereditary pyropoikilocytosis

Elliptocytes

Hereditary elliptocytosis
Thalassemias
(Other hypochromic-microcytic anemias)
(Megaloblastic anemias)

Stomatocytes

Hereditary stomatocytosis
Rh⁰ blood group
Stomatocytosis with cold hemolysis
(Liver disease, especially acute alcoholism)
(Mediterranean stomatocytosis)

Irreversibly Sickled Cells

Sickle cell anemia
Symptomatic sickle syndromes

Intraerythrocytic Parasites

Malaria
Babesiosis
Bartonellosis

Spiculated or Crenated Red Blood Cells

Acute hepatic necrosis (spur cell anemia)
Uremia
Red blood cell fragmentation syndromes†
Infantile pyknocytosis
Embden-Meyerhof pathway defects†
Abetalipoproteinemia
Heat stroke†
McLeod blood group
(Postsplenectomy)
(Transiently after massive transfusion of stored blood)
(Anorexia nervosa)†

Target Cells

Hemoglobins S, C, D, and E
Hereditary xerocytosis
Thalassemias
(Other hypochromic-microcytic anemias)
(Obstructive liver disease)
(Postsplenectomy)
(Lecithin: cholesterol transferase deficiency)

Prominent Basophilic Stippling

Thalassemias
Unstable hemoglobins
Lead poisoning†
Pyrimidine 5′-nucleotidase deficiency

Nonspecific or Normal Morphology

Embden-Meyerhof pathway defects
Hexose monophosphate shunt defects
Unstable hemoglobins
Paroxysmal nocturnal hemoglobinuria
Dyserythropoietic anemias
Copper toxicity (Wilson disease)
Cation permeability defects
Erythropoietic porphyria
Vitamin E deficiency
Hemolysis with infections†
Rh hemolytic disease in neonates*
Paroxysmal cold hemoglobinuria
Cold hemagglutinin disease*
Hypersplenism
Immunohemolytic anemia

Note: Nonhemolytic disorders of similar morphologic type are in parentheses.
*Usually associated with positive Coombs' test.
†Disease sometimes associated with this morphologic type.

Table 92-8. Diagnostic Significance of Red Blood Cell Inclusions

Type of Inclusion	Staining Agent	Diagnostic Significance
Basophilic stippling	Wright's stain	Represent aggregated ribosomes; may be observed in thalassemia syndromes, lead poisoning, iron deficiency syndromes accompanied by ineffective erythropoiesis and pyrimidine 5′-nucleotidase deficiency
Howell-Jolly bodies	Wright's stain	Represent nuclear remnants; observed in asplenic and hyposplenic states, pernicious anemia, dyserythropoietic anemias, and severe iron deficiency anemia
Cabot rings	Wright's stain	Appear as basophilic rings, circular, or twisted figures-of-eight; considered to be nuclear remnants or artifacts; observed in lead poisoning, pernicious anemia, and hemolytic anemias
Heinz bodies	Brilliant cresyl blue, methyl violet	Represent denatured or aggregated hemoglobin; observed in patients with thalassemia syndromes or unstable hemoglobins, following oxidant stress in patients with enzyme deficiencies of the pentose phosphate pathway, and in patients with asplenia or chronic liver disease
Siderocytes	Prussian blue counterstained with safranin O	Represent nonhemoglobin iron within erythrocytes; seen in increased numbers in periphereal circulation following splenectomy; observed in increased numbers in patients with chronic infection, aplastic anemias, or hemolytic anemias

Table 92-10. Treatment of Iron Deficiency Anemia

Age	Daily Dose
Premature infants	2–4 mg elemental Fe/kg/24 hr divided qd-bid po Maximum dose: 15 mg elemental Fe/24 hr
Children	3–6 mg elemental Fe/kg/24 hr divided qd-tid po
Adults	60 mg elemental Fe bid-qid po

immune responses, malabsorption, edema secondary to a protein-losing enteropathy, spoon-shaped nails, decreased exercise tolerance, and high-output heart failure.

Treatment includes oral iron supplementation and dietary counseling (especially important if the cause is excessive whole milk ingestion in a toddler). Table 92-10 outlines treatment. Table 92-11 lists iron preparations. The normal sequence of response is as follows:

1. 12 to 24 hours: subjective improvement is noted in mood and appetite.
2. 36 to 48 hours: marrow erythroid response occurs.
3. 48 to 72 hours: reticulocytosis occurs (peaks in 5 to 7 days).
4. Week 2: hemoglobin should increase by 0.5 to 1.0 g/day.
5. Once hemoglobin level has normalized, the iron stores are replenished.

Folic Acid (Pterolyglutamic Acid, Folate) Deficiency Anemia

The best sources of folic acid are meat, green vegetables, and cereals. Goat milk is severely deficient. Folic acid is readily absorbed in duodenum and jejunum. The liver is the main storage site and stores a sufficient quantity for only a few months.

The hematologic features of folic acid deficiency include increased MCV with macro-ovalocytes, anisocytosis, and poikilocytosis (some polychromasia and basophilic stippling can also be seen) Hypersegmentation of the neutrophils occurs early. If the deficiency is severe, there is evidence of leukopenia, large platelets, and thrombocytopenia.

The causes of folic acid deficiency are listed in Box 92-2. The diagnosis is made by the clinical history, hematologic features, and decreased serum and red blood cell folate

levels. Treatment usually requires 1 to 5 mg/day of folic acid. Reticulocytosis should be evident in 48 to 72 hours. A major caution to be considered is the exclusion of vitamin B_{12} deficiency. Folate partially corrects hematologic abnormalities while neurologic signs progress; folate can lower seizure threshold in some epileptics. Table 92-12 outlines treatment of folic acid deficiency.

Vitamin B_{12} (Cobalamin) Deficiency Anemia

Vitamin B_{12} is found in meats and dairy products (animal sources only). Vitamin B_{12} is actively absorbed in the terminal ileum and is dependent on intrinsic factor (glycoprotein secreted by gastric parietal cells). Cobalamin requires transcobalamin II for transport. The liver is the main storage site and can store sufficient amounts for about 2

Table 92-9. Stages in Development of Iron Deficiency

Stage I: loss of storage iron*
  ↓ Serum ferritin
Stage II: loss of circulating iron†
  ↓ Serum ferritin
  ↓ Serum iron/TIBC ↑
Stage III: decreased hemoglobin production‡
  ↓ Serum ferritin
  ↓ Serum iron/TIBC ↑
  ↓ Hemoglobin
  ↓ Mean corpuscular volume (MCV)
  ↑ Free erythrocyte protoporphyrin

*Stage I consists of depletion of storage iron (decrease in serum ferritin and bone marrow iron).
†Stage II consists of a decrease in transport iron and is characterized by a declining concentration of serum iron and increase in the total iron-binding capacity (TIBC).
‡Stage III is characterized by a decrease in hemoglobin production and the gradual development of anemia and microcytosis (decreased MCV). The decrease in MCV is proportional to the decrease in hemoglobin.

Table 92-11. Iron Preparations

Iron Preparation	Dose
Ferrous Sulfate (20% Elemental Fe)	
Drops (Fer-In-Sol)	75 mg (15 mg Fe)/0.6 mL (50 mL)
	125 mg (25 mg Fe)/1 mL (50 mL)
Syrup (Fer-In-Sol)	90 mg (18 mg Fe)/5 mL (5% alcohol)
Elixir (Feosol)	220 mg (44 mg Fe)/5 mL (5% alcohol)
Capsules	250 mg (50 mg Fe)
Tablets	195 mg (39 mg Fe)
	300 mg (60 mg Fe)
	324 mg (65 mg Fe)
Ferrous Gluconate (12% Elemental Fe)	
Elixir	300 mg (34 mg Fe)/5 mL (7% alcohol)
Tablets	240 mg (27 mg Fe, as Fergon)
	300 mg (34 mg Fe)
	320 mg (37 mg Fe)
	325 mg (38 mg Fe)
Sustained-release capsules	320 mg (37 mg Fe)
	435 mg (50 mg Fe)
Capsules	86 mg (10 mg Fe)
	325 mg (38 mg Fe)
	435 mg (50 mg Fe)
Ferrous Sulfate, Exsiccated/Dried (30% Elemental Iron)	
Tablets	200 mg (65 mg Fe)
Extended release tablets	160 mg (50 mg Fe)
Capsules	190 mg (60 mg Fe)
Extended release capsules	159 mg (50 mg Fe)
Polysaccharide-Iron Complex (Niferex)	
Expressed in mg elemental iron	
Tablets	50 mg
Capsules	150 mg
Elixir	100 mg/5 mL (10% alcohol)

Adapted with permission from Siberry GK, Iannone R: The Harriet Lane Handbook, 15th ed. Philadelphia, 2000 p 744.

Box 92-2. Causes of Folic Acid Deficiency

- Deficient intake (relatively exclusive carbohydrate diet, goat milk, breast-feeding from folate-deficient mother, excessively cooked food, phenylketonuric diets)
- Increased demand (rapid growth, hemolysis, pregnancy, infection)
- Decreased absorption (congenital antimetabolites such as methotrexate and sulfisoxazole trimethoprim)
- Metabolic defects (congenital, antimetabolites, liver disease)

Box 92-3. Causes of Vitamin B_{12} (Cobalamin) Deficiency

- Deficient intake (strict vegetarian diet, breast-fed infant of a mother with pernicious anemia or vitamin B_{12} defiency secondary to malnutrition)
- Decreased absorption (due to decreased intrinsic factor with congential pernicious anemia [PA], juvenile PA, gastrectomy, structurally abnormal intrinsic factor, primary intestinal disease such as Crohn's disease, transcobalamin II deficiency, congenital abnormality of vitamin B_{12} metabolism, drug use such as alcohol or colchicine)

to 4 years. The daily requirement of vitamin B_{12} is about 2 to 3 µg.

The hematologic features of deficiency are the same as noted for folic acid deficiency. Physical abnormalities include glossitis and neurologic symptoms. Causes of vitamin B_{12} deficiency are listed in Box 92-3. The diagnosis is made by the hematologic features, decreased vitamin B_{12} level, diagnostic Schilling test to distinguish if the vitamin B_{12} malabsorption is secondary to intrinsic factor deficiency, intestinal disease, or decreased transcobalamin II levels.

The treatment is 500 to 1000 µg every 1 to 2 months or more frequently if neurologic signs are present.

Anemias Caused by Other Nutritional Deficiencies

Copper deficiency can cause anemia under unusual circumstances or may be iatrogenic. Protein and calories malnutrition can also cause anemia. Vitamin E deficiency can cause hemolytic anemia with fragments, thrombocytosis, and possible edema. Deficiency seen is with prematurity, fat malabsorption, and hereditary abetalipoproteinemia. Deficiencies of vitamin A, pyridoxine, riboflavin, and vitamin C have all been associated with anemias.

Mini-index of Related Topics   CH.

Table 92-12. Treatment of Folic Acid Deficiency

Infants	Children (1–10 yr)	Adults (>11 yr)
Initial Dose (po, im, iv, sc)		
15 mcg/kg/dose; maximum dose 50 mcg/24 hr	1 mg/dose	1–3 mg/dose divided qd-tid
Maintenance (po, im, iv, sc)		
30–45 mcg/24 hr qd	0.1–0.4 mg/24 hr qd	0.5 mg/24 hr qd Pregnant/lactating women: 0.8 mg/24 hr qd

Adapted with permission from Siberry GK, Iannone R: The Harriet Lane Handbook, 15th ed. Philadelphia, 2000 p 723.

Note: Tablets: 0.4, 0.8, 1 mg; oral solution: 1 mg/mL; injection: 5 mg/mL (1.5% benzyl alcohol).

SUGGESTED READINGS

Irwin JJ, Kirchner JT: Anemia in children. Am Family Physican 2001;64(8):1379–1386.
Lillyman JS, Blanchette VS, Hann IM (eds): Pediatric Hematology, 2nd ed. New York, Churchill Livingstone, 1999.
Nathan D, Orkin S (eds): Nathan and Oski's Hematology of Infancy and Childhood, 5th ed. Vol. 1. Philadelphia, WB Saunders, 1998.

93 Presentation and Initial Evaluation of Disorders of White Blood Cells

Paul Fu, Jr.

 ROLE OF THE GENERALIST

1   Recognize normal and abnormal white blood cell (WBC) values.
2   Evaluate suspected WBC disorders appropriately.
3   Refer patients to the appropriate specialist for further evaluation of suspected WBC disorders.
4   Manage care of children with chronic WBC disorders in collaboration with the specialist.

In diagnosing and treating diseases, the pediatric generalist often orders screening laboratory studies and a quantitative measurement of the total WBC count. The WBC count is often used to determine the presence of or risk for disease. The most frequent use of the WBC count is related to infectious disorders. WBCs, also known as leukocytes, form the primary systemic defense mechanisms that fight infection and serve in a host of immunologic processes. The system is dynamic and is capable of reacting swiftly and accurately to infection, trauma, inflammation, and other noxious stimuli. WBCs can release colony-stimulating factor, which stimulates the bone marrow to increase WBC production and to release available mature cells from the marrow reserve.

Results in hand, the generalist must determine whether the findings (an elevation or depression of the WBC count or an abnormal distribution of leukocytes) represent a disease entity that may be managed by the generalist or that requires referral to a specialist.

FUNDAMENTALS

Leukocyte is a generic term applied to all WBCs. Granulocytes belong to a morphologic subclass of leukocytes with intracytoplasmic granules on microscopic examination and include neutrophils, basophils, and eosinophils. The term is often used incorrectly as a synonym for *neutrophils*.

Neutrophils are the largest and shortest-lived population of circulating WBCs. Bands (or stabs) are an immature form of circulating neutrophil. Segmented neutrophils ("segs") are the mature form. Neutrophils from undifferentiated stem cells are produced and mature over 6 days in bone marrow. Approximately 85% of available neutrophils reside within the marrow at any given point in time. After storage in marrow for 6 to 8 days, neutrophils are released to the general circulation into one of two pools: the circulating pool (approximately 5% of all available neutrophils) and the marginating pool, where they adhere to blood vessels' endothelium (approximately 10%). Cells circulate for 6 to 12 hours before migrating into tissue via diapedesis, where tissue half-life is about 2 days. Neutrophil production may be increased as a result of a variety of conditions that stimulate production of proinflammatory mediators and chemotactic factors, such as bacterial infection. Once activated, neutrophils are strongly phagocytic.

Monocytes share the same stem cell as neutrophils. After production in the marrow, monocytes circulate for 6 to 8 days before entering tissue, where they differentiate into macrophages. As macrophages, they process foreign antigens and present them to immunocompetent lymphocytes. Macrophages are also capable of phagocytosis.

Eosinophils respond chemotactically to cytokines produced by stimulated mast cells or bacteria. Eosinophil counts are increased in chronic allergic reactions and parasitic infections. Eosinophil granules contain basic proteins that are toxic to certain parasites. The life span is similar to that of neutrophils.

The phagocytic system of neutrophils, eosinophils, and monocytes and their derivatives constitutes the primary defense against bacterial and fungal infections. Disorders of phagocytes are discussed further in Chapter 169.

Basophils are the least numerous of the leukocytes. They are similar to mast cells in appearance and function but are distinct cell types. Basophils have a rich complement of IgE receptors, suggesting a role in allergic responses. When stimulated, they produce vasoactive mediators (histamine, leukotrienes, and platelet-activating factors) and chemotactic factors for neutrophils and eosinophils.

Lymphocytes are produced in a variety of lymphoid organs and are responsible for both cellular and humoral immune response. They are the second most numerous of the circulating leukocytes. Adequate levels of circulating lymphocytes are crucial to the function of the immune system.

INITIAL EVALUATION

The initial evaluation of the child with a suspected WBC dysfunction consists of a thorough history of present illness, past medical history, past family history, physical exami-

Box 93-1. Initial Evaluation of a White Blood Cell Disorder

History of Present Illness

Symptoms

Onset, duration, and recurrence of symptoms

Location, radiation, and intensity of symptoms

Past Medical History

Frequency and severity of previous disease (e.g., infection, reaction, symptoms)

Exposure to medications, toxins, and environmental agents that can cause bone marrow suppression

Family History

Other family members with frequent recurrence of symptoms or disease states

Other family members with cancer or recurrent infection

Early childhood or in utero deaths

Physical Examination

Skin (open wounds, healing, scarring)

Mucous membranes (oral, perianal)

Lymph nodes

Liver

Spleen

Laboratory Studies

Complete blood cell count

WBC differential and smear to assess morphologic appearance of cells

Blood culture if concerned with recurrent infection

---

nation, and requisite laboratory studies. Box 93-1 outlines an appropriate approach to a child with a suspected WBC disorder.

The heterogeneous origin and function of the various leukocyte cell types means that no single constellation of signs and symptoms signals or causes a clinician to suspect a WBC disorder. Likewise, the quantitative enumeration of WBCs in the basic complete blood count (CBC) is not indicative of a specific disorder. The total WBC count is useful for establishing whether the number of cells is abnormally high or low. Without additional clinical information, a WBC count cannot establish an accurate diagnosis. Because each leukocyte form has its own function, a differential WBC count (either automated or manual) is crucial with every CBC when an acute or chronic dysfunction of the immune system is being considered.

Assessment of a microscopic blood smear is a crucial part of any evaluation of WBC function. Toxic granulations (deeply basophilic granules in neutrophils) or Döhle's bodies (basophilic cytoplasmic masses) may suggest or confirm the presence of severe infection. Serial blood cell counts and blood smears may be helpful in establishing the chronicity of the complaint. Automated laboratory instruments, rather than technicians, are often used to perform routine smear evaluation. Modern hematopathologic instruments are highly sensitive and reliable and provide accurate interpretations. However, abnormal results should always be confirmed by manual differential blood cell count and microscopic evaluation.

Reference ranges may vary from laboratory to laboratory, but the normal values listed in Table 93-1 are acceptable for general use. The clinician should always use the appropriate, laboratory-specific reference range values when interpreting individual laboratory results.

DIAGNOSIS AND ASSESSMENT OF DISORDERS OF LEUKOCYTE PRODUCTION

Leukopenia is a dearth of WBCs and leukocytosis a surplus of WBCs in the circulating blood. If either condition is present, the adequacy of each WBC count component should be assessed to determine the type of WBC disorder. WBC disorders are classified by the component of the WBC population causing the increase or decrease in the total number of WBCs. Significant deficiencies or excesses of neutrophils and lymphocytes, the largest components of the WBC pool, are most likely to parallel the total WBC counts. Because monocytes, eosinophils, and basophils constitute a relatively low proportion of the total WBC pool, a deficiency or excess for each cell type can be present without concomitant leukopenia or leukocytosis. To diagnose disorders for cell types that constitute a low proportion of the total count, confirmatory diagnosis must be made by the absolute blood cell count and comparison to reference normal values. Figure 93-1 categorizes clinically significant WBC disorders.

Leukopenia

Leukopenia is defined as a total WBC count of less than 4000 cells/mm^3. Leukopenia can be caused by viral infection, overwhelming bacterial infection, and bone marrow dysfunction from a variety of triggers, including pharmaceuticals. Box 93-2 lists drugs that may induce leukopenia. These agents trigger a decrease in WBC count through marrow failure, peripheral destruction, or a shift into the storage or marginated compartments. Once a leukopenic

---

Table 93-1. Normal Values for White Blood Cells: Total and Differential Counts

Age	WBC*	Neu (%)	Lym (%)	Mono (%)	Eos (%)	Baso (%)	Neu*	Lym*	Mono*	Eos*
0–3 d	10.5–30.5	28–65	20–55	2–12	0–8	0–2	6.5–17.8	2.7–7.1	0.8–2.0	0.0–2.4
3–7 d	7.0–18.2	28–65	20–55	2–12	0–8	0–2	4.0–10.2	2.3–5.2	0.3–1.1	0.5–1.0
7–13 d	6.2–16.1	28–65	20–55	2–12	0–8	0–2	1.8–5.9	3.3–6.6	0.5–1.7	0.5–1.0
14–28 d	7.2–19.8	23–62	20–54	2–12	0–8	0–2	1.8–7.2	4.1–7.8	0.5–1.7	0.5–1.1
1 mo–1 yr	6.9–17.2	23–62	20–54	2–12	0–8	0–2	1.0–6.5	4.0–9.2	0.5–1.5	0.0–0.4
1–12 yr	4.0–12.0	29–65	24–60	2–11	1–8	0–2	1.7–7.0	1.2–6.0	0.4–1.4	0.0–0.5
>12 yr	4.0–10.0	30–75	20–40	2–12	0–8	0–2	1.7–7.0	0.8–4.0	0.1–1.0	0.0–0.5

Note: Cell counts are given in units of 1000 cells/μL (mm^3) and are estimates of 95% confidence limits. Percentages relate to total white blood cell count.
Baso, basophils; Eos, eosinophils; Lym, lymphocytes; Mono, monocytes; Neu, neutrophils; WBC, total white blood cell count.

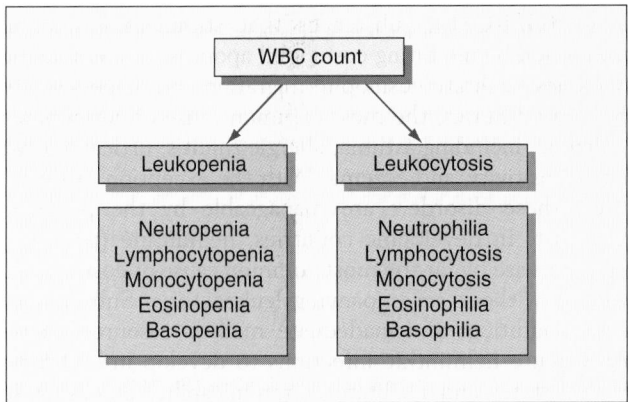

Figure 93-1. Categorization of clinically significant white blood cell (WBC) disorders.

state is recognized, the specific WBC types affected must be identified immediately.

The most common type of leukopenia is neutropenia, both because neutrophils represent the greatest proportion of WBCs and because neutrophils are active in the most common infections and immunologic processes. Neutropenic patients should be protected from interventions that may disrupt skin integrity, such as injections or rectal temperature readings, and from prolonged exposure to acutely or chronically infectious patients while the workup is in progress. The risk of infection from neutropenia is inversely proportional to the number of neutrophils present (the absolute neutrophil count, or ANC). Mild neutropenia (<1500 cells/mm^3) increases the risk for significant but localized infections of the mucous membranes and skin. Severe neutropenia (<500 cells/mm^3) may present with systemic toxicity (fever, chills, shock) as the absence of adequate numbers of neutrophils results in susceptibility for gram-negative septicemia. Chronic neutropenia may be manifested by extensive necrotic and ulcerative lesions of the mucous membranes. Disorders of the function of neutrophils are described in Chapter 169.

Transient neutropenia caused by temporary bone marrow suppression by viral or other infectious agents typically resolves spontaneously. Care while awaiting resolution of transient neutropenia is supportive. Hospitalization and broad-spectrum parenteral antibiotics that include coverage for gram-negative organisms should be considered for any neutropenic patient presenting with signs and symptoms of severe systemic infection. In the infant younger than 3 months of age, concomitant presence of clear neutropenia and infection should be considered a significant risk factor for severe illness, because the neutrophil reserves in this age

Box 93-2. Drugs That May Induce Leukopenia

Analgesics	Antithyroid drugs
Antibiotics	Arsenic-based drugs
Anticonvulsants	Barbiturates
Anti-inflammatory drugs	Cardiovascular drugs
Antimetabolites	Diuretics
Antineoplastic agents	Heavy metals

group are extremely limited. Severely hypocellular peripheral smears should prompt consideration of a bone marrow evaluation and referral to the pediatric hematologist/oncologist.

Other forms of WBC deficiencies are much less common. Lymphocytopenia may be seen with corticosteroid treatment, chemotherapy, irradiation, sex-linked agammaglobulinemia, certain lymphomas, and some chronic diseases, such as sarcoidosis, tuberculosis, human immunodeficiency virus (HIV) infection, and systemic lupus erythematosus (SLE). Unless these disorders are diagnosed relatively late in their course, lymphocytopenia may not be apparent on initial evaluation. Corticosteroids can also induce a transient monocytopenia that usually resolves within 12 hours of administration. Infections associated with endotoxemia have also been known to depress monocyte counts. Eosinophils and basophils exhibit diurnal variation, being lowest in the morning and highest in the evening. Eosinopenia and basopenia may be seen with corticosteroids, acute physiologic stress, and acute interleukin 5 (IL-5)–mediated inflammation. Basopenia may also be seen with hyperthyroidism or thyroid storm. These disorders do not typically cause catastrophic illness, and the cause is often evident without significant workup (recent steroid therapy for asthma or chemotherapy or radiation therapy). Persistent or chronic leukopenia should be referred to a pediatric hematologist or oncologist for further evaluation and management.

Leukocytosis

Leukocytosis refers to an increase of the total WBC count above normal range, usually an inflammatory response to noxious stimuli, such as infection, allergy, malignancy, or hereditary disorders. Leukocytosis is mediated by a complex network of growth factors (e.g., granulocyte colony-stimulating factor, granulocyte-monocyte colony-stimulating factor, c-Kit ligand), adhesion molecules (e.g., CD11b/CD18), and cytokines (e.g., IL-1, IL-3, IL-6, tumor necrosis factor) that act in conjunction to coordinate the production and release of cells from storage pools, the demargination of cells, and diapedesis.

Box 93-3 lists the differential diagnosis of leukocytosis. Most commonly, neutrophils and lymphocytes are markedly increased with leukocytosis. Toxic granulations or Döhle's bodies may be present on microscopic examination. In younger children, the release of immature granulocytes into circulation during acute physiologic stress may result in a leukemoid reaction in which granulocyte counts may exceed 50,000 cells/mm^3. Leukemoid reactions can be differentiated from leukemia by (1) absence of other cell line depression, (2) evidence of infection, and (3) absence of blasts on bone marrow smear. The urgency of subspecialty consultation is directly proportional to the elevation of the total WBC count. Hyperleukocytosis (>100,000 cells/mm^3) has significantly high morbidity and mortality rates from the high cell burden, regardless of underlying cause, and should prompt immediate and emergent referral to a pediatric hematologist/oncologist for evaluation and treatment of leukemia (e.g., acute myelogenous leukemia) or myeloproliferative disorder.

Leukocytosis resulting from neutrophilia commonly results from an acute infection. Slight leukocytosis may be

Table 94-3. Causes of Neonatal Thrombocytopenia

Increased Destruction
Immunologic Causes
Neonatal alloimmune thrombocytopenia (due to platelet antigen incompatibility)
Neonatal autoimmune thrombocytopenia (due to maternal ITP)
Maternal drug-induced
Drugs
Infections
Nonimmunologic Causes
Disseminated intravascular coagulation
Kasabach-Merrit syndrome
Cyanotic congenital heart disease

Decreased Production
Congenital infections
Thrombocytopenia with absent radii (TAR) syndrome
Congenital idiopathic amegakaryocytic thrombocytopenia
Fanconi's anemia
Wiskott-Aldrich syndrome
Metabolic disorders
Maternal hyperthyroidism
Osteopetrosis
Congenital leukemia

Kasabach-Merritt syndrome is thrombocytopenia in infants with giant hemangiomas. Thrombocytopenia results from platelet trapping within the hemangioma. A localized consumptive coagulopathy can occur, leading to low fibrinogen levels and elevated fibrin degradation products. Thrombocytopenia resolves as the hemangioma regresses.

Thrombocytopenia occurs frequently in children with cyanotic congenital heart disease, usually when the hematocrit is greater than 60%. Although the exact mechanism is unclear, platelet consumption may be initiated by platelet margination in the small blood vessels or by low-grade DIC. Thrombocytopenia resolves if the polycythemia is corrected by therapeutic phlebotomy or repair of the cardiac lesion.

Thrombocytopenia from Decreased Production
Table 94-4 lists the congenital and acquired causes of hypoproductive thrombocytopenia. The most common causes of thrombocytopenia from decreased production are acquired conditions that affect bone marrow function. The most frequently observed cause is bone marrow suppression secondary to drugs, such as immunosuppressants and chemotherapeutic agents, or radiation therapy. Infiltrative processes within the bone marrow, such as leukemia, neuroblastoma, myelofibrosis, osteopetrosis, and genetic storage diseases, can also cause thrombocytopenia, often in conjunction with red and white blood cell abnormalities. Thrombocytopenia can occur with acquired aplastic anemia. In this condition other cell lines are also affected.

Congenital hypoproductive thrombocytopenias are rare and may occur secondary to a viral infection, an idiopathic etiology, or as part of an inherited disorder (see Table 94-4). Thrombocytopenia with absent radii (TAR) syndrome is an autosomal recessive condition, typically recognized in the newborn period, characterized by thrombocytopenia, skeletal anomalies (most commonly radial agenesis), and renal and cardiac abnormalities. Severity of thrombocytopenia is variable. Some infants may require platelet trans-

fusions. Bone marrow examination demonstrates absent or markedly reduced megakaryocytes, which are often dysplastic. After 1 year of age, many patients experience a spontaneous increase in megakaryopoiesis.

Thrombocytopenia from Splenic Sequestration
One third of the body's platelets are normally located within the spleen, serving as a reserve pool for hemostatic stress. The number of platelets sequestered in splenomegaly is directly proportionate to spleen size. Thrombocytopenia from splenic sequestration is mild, with platelet counts ranging from 50,000 to 150,000/mm^3. Platelet counts less than 50,000/mm^3 should not be attributed to splenomegaly alone.

Thrombocytosis
The most common cause of a high platelet count is reactive thrombocytosis from an underlying inflammatory condition, such as infection, rheumatoid disease, or Kawasaki disease. The degree of thrombocytosis usually parallels the activity of the underlying disease process. Therapy to reduce platelets in patients with these conditions is not indicated because they are not at increased risk for thrombotic complications and the thrombocytosis resolves when the underlying disease process is treated. Rarely, thrombocytosis in a child may be secondary to a primary myeloproliferative disorder. Essential thrombocythemia, polycythemia vera, and chronic myelogenous leukemia, are associated with a primary megakaryocytic proliferation.

Qualitative Platelet Disorders
Acquired Disorders of Platelet Function
Acquired disorders of platelet function occur after exposure to drugs or toxins that inhibit platelet function. The most commonly observed drug effects involve inhibition of the cyclooxygenase enzyme, which is crucial in arachidonic acid metabolism. When a platelet is activated arachidonic acid is released from the platelet membrane and

Table 94-4. Thrombocytopenia Secondary to Decreased Production

Congenital Disorders
Thrombocytopenia with absent radii (TAR) syndrome
Congenital idiopathic amegakaryocytic thrombocytopenia
Bernard-Soulier disease*
May-Hegglin syndrome*
Fanconi's aplastic anemia
Wiskott-Aldrich syndrome*
X-linked thrombocytopenia
Metabolic disorders
Congenital immune deficiencies

Acquired Disorders
Aplastic anemia
Bone marrow infiltrative processes
 Malignancy
 Osteopetrosis
 Storage disorders
Drug-induced
Radiation-induced
Nutritional deficiency states

*These hereditary thrombocytopenias are also associated with abnormalities of platelet function.

metabolized through the action of cyclooxygenase to generate thromboxane A_2. Thromboxane A_2 stimulates platelet aggregation and vasoconstriction. Aspirin irreversibly inhibits cyclooxygenase, thereby affecting platelets for the duration of their life span (7 to 10 days). Because nonsteroidal anti-inflammatory agents reversibly inhibit cyclooxygenase, the antiplatelet effect lasts only as long as the active drug is circulating. Abnormalities in platelet function also occur in uremia, liver disease, and DIC.

PRESENTATION AND EVALUATION

Mucocutaneous bleeding is the hallmark for disorders of primary hemostasis such as platelet disorders and von Willebrand disease (vWD). Petechiae, purpura, ecchymoses, epistaxis, menorrhagia, gastrointestinal hemorrhage, hematuria, and excessive bleeding from injuries or surgery are all bleeding manifestations of platelet disorders and vWD. The hemarthroses and deep muscle hematomas that typically occur in patients with disorders of secondary hemostasis, such as hemophilia A or B, do not occur with platelet disorders or vWD.

Thrombocytopenia may be detected in a patient with mucocutaneous bleeding or as an incidental finding. Thrombocytopenia occurs in four clinical settings: a healthy child, a child with evidence of an underlying illness, a toxic-appearing child, and the neonate. Most etiologies of thrombocytopenia can be determined by a thorough history, physical examination, and review of a peripheral blood smear.

When evaluating a patient with a low platelet count, thrombocytopenia must first be confirmed. Platelet counts can be spuriously low from aggregation of platelets within the syringe or blood tube, platelet cold agglutinins, or platelet adherence to white blood cells (platelet satellitism). Evaluation of a peripheral blood smear shows clumps of agglutinated platelets near the periphery of the blood film or platelet satellites. Artifactual thrombocytopenia may also occur as a result of in vitro platelet agglutination secondary to ethylenediaminetetraacetic acid (EDTA)-dependent antibodies, which can be in the patient's serum. Correction of the platelet count using a different anticoagulant such as citrate confirms the diagnosis.

A healthy child who presents with the sudden onset of bruising and petechiae with isolated thrombocytopenia most likely has acute ITP. A history of a nonspecific viral illness or immunization within the previous 3 weeks is present in 50% to 80% of cases. Bleeding symptoms include petechiae, purpura, mucosal bleeding (10% to 30% of patients), and hematuria or gastrointestinal bleeding (less than 10%). Intracranial hemorrhage, a rare but devastating complication, occurs in 0.1% to 0.5% of ITP patients. At any platelet count, the risk of bleeding in ITP is much lower compared to thrombocytopenia from leukemia, aplastic anemia, or chemotherapy, because ITP patients have an excellent bone marrow reserve and the platelets in circulation are young and healthy.

The physical examination in acute ITP is significant only for mucocutaneous bleeding. Hepatosplenomegaly and lymphadenopathy are notably absent. A complete blood count (CBC) shows isolated thrombocytopenia, often less than 20,000/mm³ at diagnosis. White blood cell count, hemoglobin (unless there has been significant bleeding secondary to thrombocytopenia), and the mean corpuscular volume (MCV) are normal. The mean platelet volume (MPV) is often increased. The peripheral blood smear shows normal red and white blood cell morphology and few large platelets.

Acute ITP is diagnosed on history and clinical findings. In a patient with a history, physical examination, and laboratory findings consistent with acute ITP, a bone marrow biopsy is not indicated. If the patient is to be treated with corticosteroids, most hematologists recommend a bone marrow biopsy to rule out occult leukemia because steroid treatment can delay diagnosis and adversely affect long-term prognosis. Prothrombin time, activated partial thromboplastin time, and antiplatelet antibody assays are normal and not indicated. The bleeding time may be prolonged, depending on the degree of thrombocytopenia, but is not needed for the diagnosis of ITP.

Chronic ITP presents in two different ways. Patients can present suddenly with severe thrombocytopenia, are initially diagnosed as having acute ITP, but the thrombocytopenia persists beyond 6 months. Chronic ITP can present with an insidious onset of bruising over several months and milder thrombocytopenia. Chronic ITP is generally benign with few patients having serious bleeding complications. Except for bruising, the physical examination is normal. The CBC is remarkable only for thrombocytopenia, typically in the 40,000 to 80,000/mm³ range. Platelets on peripheral smear have normal morphology. Additional workup is warranted to rule out an underlying cause, such as an autoimmune disorder, congenital immune deficiency, or HIV infection. Antinuclear antibody test and anti-double-stranded DNA test should be done on a yearly basis, as many autoimmune conditions can present initially with ITP. Approximately 20% of patients with chronic ITP have positive results on an antinuclear antibody test. A quantitative immunoglobulin test should also be performed to rule out a congenital immune deficiency. If corticosteroids are considered for therapy or if there are abnormalities in the other blood cell lines, a bone marrow biopsy is indicated

If thrombocytopenia presents with fever, bone pain, weakness, or pallor, an underlying disease process such as leukemia or aplastic anemia should be considered. Most children with leukemia present with pallor, petechiae, hepatosplenomegaly, and lymphadenopathy. The CBC often reveals abnormal white blood cell counts, anemia, thrombocytopenia, and blasts on peripheral blood smear. Aplastic anemia may initially present with isolated thrombocytopenia before full-fledged pancytopenia develops. Other hematologic abnormalities, such as macrocytosis and mild neutropenia, may be present. A bone marrow biopsy is absolutely indicated if other blood cell lines are involved or if the presentation is atypical for classic ITP.

A toxic-appearing child with thrombocytopenia is likely to have a serious life-threatening condition such as sepsis, DIC, HUS, TTP, or liver disease. Fever, lethargy, petechiae, and hypotension can occur with sepsis and DIC. Laboratory findings typically show leukopenia or leukocytosis, anemia, thrombocytopenia, prolonged prothrombin time and partial thromboplastin time, decreased fibrinogen, and schistocytes (red blood cell fragments) on peripheral blood smear. HUS presents with recent gastroenteritis, acute renal failure, thrombocytopenia, and a microangiopathic hemolytic anemia. TTP presents with fever, acute renal failure, neurologic abnormalities, thrombocytopenia, and microangiopathic hemolytic anemia. Laboratory findings for both HUS and TTP show elevated blood urea nitrogen and creatinine, thrombocytopenia, anemia, and schistocytes on peripheral smear.

Thrombocytopenia is seen commonly in the critically ill neonate as a manifestation of a systemic disease such as sepsis, shock, birth asphyxia, or DIC. Thrombocytopenia may also be secondary to medications, congenital infections, constitutional disorders, neonatal alloimmune thrombocytopenia, or neonatal autoimmune thrombocytopenia. The presentation of neonatal alloimmune thrombocytopenia is dramatic with petechiae, purpura, and severe thrombocytopenia in an otherwise healthy-appearing infant. Bleeding symptoms can occur within minutes of birth and include petechiae, purpura, gastrointestinal bleeding, hematuria, bleeding from the umbilicus or skin puncture sites, and intracranial hemorrhage. Diagnosis is confirmed by detection of antiplatelet antibody in mother's serum, and platelet antigen typing of mother and father. A normal maternal platelet count helps differentiate this disorder from neonatal autoimmune thrombocytopenia (caused by maternal ITP). In maternal ITP, the mother's platelet count is depressed secondary to autoimmune antibodies. Maternal ITP typically causes a milder neonatal thrombocytopenia. Bleeding symptoms tend to be milder and the risk of intracranial hemorrhage is less than 1%.

Reactive thrombocytosis is usually detected as an incidental finding in a child being evaluated for an inflammatory disease process such as infections or a rheumatoid disorder. In patients with thrombocytosis secondary to a primary myeloproliferative disorder, systemic symptoms of fever, bone pain, fatigue, pallor, weight loss, and night sweats are often present. The CBC reveals abnormalities in the other cell lines. Patients are at risk for both thrombotic and hemorrhagic complications.

Qualitative platelet disorders may be detected during an evaluation of a child who presents with a chronic history of petechiae, easy bruising, epistaxis, or other mucosal bleeding. When evaluating a child for a potential qualitative platelet disorder, useful screening tests include a platelet count, bleeding time, and peripheral smear to evaluate platelet morphology. A prolonged bleeding time in a patient with a normal platelet count is suggestive of a platelet disorder. Because a prolonged bleeding time does not distinguish between the different steps in primary hemostasis, patients with vWD or collagen vascular disorders, such as Ehlers-Danlos syndrome, also have prolonged bleeding times. If a patient does not have evidence of a collagen vascular disorder and if the vWD workup is negative, patients should be referred for platelet aggregation studies that measure platelet aggregation in response to a number of different agonists (thrombin, ADP, epinephrine, collagen, and ristocetin). A number of qualitative platelet disorders have unique platelet aggregation patterns. These tests should be performed in specialized coagulation laboratories experienced in platelet aggregation studies.

Box 94-1. Indications for Referral to Hematologist-Oncologist

- Acute ITP: serious bleeding, atypical presentation, hepatosplenomegaly, lymphadenopathy, multiple cell line involvement
- All children with chronic ITP
- Infants suspected of having neonatal alloimmune thrombocytopenia
- Neonates with physical findings of a congenital platelet disorder (absent radii, limb abnormalities, giant hemangioma)
- Chronic history of mucocutaneous bleeding symptoms
- Thrombocytosis when there is evidence of myeloproliferation

Referral

Box 94-1 lists indications for referral of children with suspected platelet disorders. Although most cases of acute ITP can be diagnosed and managed by the pediatrician, a telephone consultation with a pediatric hematologist-oncologist prior to treating the patient is recommended. Children with serious bleeding or atypical presentations (hepatosplenomegaly, lymphadenopathy, or evidence of multiple cell line involvement) should be referred to a pediatric hematologist-oncologist. Children who develop the chronic form of ITP should also be evaluated by a pediatric hematologist.

Thrombocytopenia in a critically ill neonate or child is often associated with a systemic illness such as sepsis, shock, DIC, or liver disease, and consultation with a pediatric hematologist-oncologist is not necessary. Infants suspected of having neonatal alloimmune thrombocytopenia should be evaluated by a pediatric hematologist immediately because of the risks of serious hemorrhage. Neonates with physical findings suggestive of a congenital platelet disorder (absent radii, limb abnormalities, giant hemangioma) should also be evaluated by a pediatric hematologist-oncologist.

In general, children with a reactive thrombocytosis can be managed by the pediatrician. If there is evidence of an underlying myeloproliferative disorder, referral to a pediatric hematologist-oncologist is indicated.

A hematology consultation is recommended in a child with a chronic history of mucocutaneous bleeding symptoms for evaluation of a possible congenital bleeding disorder such as vWD or qualitative platelet disorder.

MANAGEMENT

Acute ITP is managed with supportive measures, patient/parent education, and pharmacologic therapies. Supportive measures include avoidance of aspirin, ibuprofen, and other antiplatelet medications; avoidance of intramuscular injections; and postponement of immunizations and allergic desensitization injections that may exacerbate the degree of thrombocytopenia. Physical activity should be limited, with specific instruction to avoid activities that may cause head injury. Children with signs of mucocutaneous bleeding should be instructed to avoid contact sports, climbing, and bicycle riding. Protective headgear has also been advocated for toddlers and young active children. Parents should be educated regarding the specific signs and symptoms of bleeding and given instructions on whom to contact and what to do in the event of an emergency. Parents should be aware that headache and vomiting are potential signs of an intracranial hemorrhage.

For uncomplicated cases of acute ITP, children can be followed on an outpatient basis. Platelet counts should be monitored regularly, often daily at the onset of disease when the thrombocytopenia is severe and intervention may be required. Subsequently, the frequency with which the platelet count is monitored depends on the severity of the thrombocytopenia, the presence of bleeding symptoms, and the rate of change in the platelet count. When the patient's symptoms have stabilized, the platelet count can be followed on a weekly and then monthly basis.

Pharmacologic treatment of acute ITP remains controversial. Most cases resolve spontaneously without intervention. The primary reason to treat this disorder is to prevent an intracranial hemorrhage; however, there are no data to confirm whether any currently available therapies actually prevent this complication. Primary drug treatments are corticosteroids, intravenous immunoglobulin (IVIG), and anti-D immunoglobulin. Although the platelet count increases more rapidly with use of these agents, whether the risk of intracranial hemorrhage is reduced remains unknown. The decision to treat must be individualized to each case, taking into consideration the child's age, bleeding symptoms, activity level, and parental anxiety level. Pharmocologic therapy is certainly indicated in a child with clinically significant mucous membrane bleeding. In the absence of significant bleeding, some hematologists treat if the platelet count is less than 10,000 to 20,000/mm^3, because most cases of intracranial hemorrhage occur in patients with platelet counts less than 20,000/mm^3. Others advocate intervening only in those patients with clinically significant bleeding symptoms.

Table 94-5 lists the common dosing regimens, side effects, advantages, and disadvantages of corticosteroids, IVIG, and anti-D immunoglobulin. Corticosteroids are believed to act by blocking the Fc receptors of macrophages in the spleen and reticuloendothelial system, allowing antibody-coated platelets to pass through without being ingested and by reducing the synthesis of antiplatelet antibodies. IVIG also acts by blocking Fc receptors of the reticuloendothelial system. Anti-D immunoglobulin, which can be used only in Rh-positive patients, acts by binding to the D antigen (Rh antigen) of red blood cells. Immune clearance of antibody-coated red blood cells results in a longer life span for antibody-coated platelets.

Patients with chronic ITP should be referred for management of the disorder, and care is coordinated between the general pediatrician and the pediatric hematologist. Most patients do not require treatment. Those with persistent bleeding symptoms may benefit from therapy to maintain a more normal lifestyle. Therapeutic options for chronic ITP include observation without therapy, regular infusions of IVIG or anti-D immunoglobulin, immunosuppressive agents, and splenectomy. Immunosuppressive agents have been studied, but data do not support their use in children. Splenectomy is successful in raising the platelet count levels that reduce bleeding symptoms in 60% to 80% of cases. Splenectomy by laparoscopy can be performed with minimal morbidity. The major risk after splenectomy is sepsis from encapsulated organisms, such as *Streptococcus pneumoniae*, *Haemophilius influenzae*, and *Neisseria meningitidis*. Because the risk of sepsis is higher in children younger than 5 years, splenectomy should be postponed if possible. Immunizations against encapsulated organisms should be performed prior to splenectomy (see Chapter 167).

All infants suspected of having neonatal alloimmune thrombocytopenia or qualitative platelet disorders should be evaluated immediately by a pediatric hematologist. Infants with alloimmune thrombocytopenia are at significant risk for intracranial hemorrhage, often necessitating initiation of therapy prior to laboratory confirmation of alloimmunization. Treatment options include transfusion of maternal washed platelets, corticosteroids, and IVIG. Transfusion with compatible platelets (maternal platelets) corrects the thrombocytopenia immediately; therefore, it

Table 94-5. Drug Treatments for Acute Idiopathic Thrombocytopenic Purpura

Features of Treatment	Corticosteroids	Intravenous Immunoglobulin	Anti-D Immunoglobulin
Dosing regimens	2–4 mg/kg/day orally for several days to weeks, followed by taper	1 g/kg/day IV for 2 days (each dose infused over 4–6 hours)	50 µg/kg IV as a single dose (infused over 3–5 minutes)

Side effects	With long-term use:
	  Growth retardation
	  Osteoporosis
	  Immunosuppression
	  Cataracts
	  Cushingoid facies
	  Fluid retention
	  Hypertension
	  Acne
	  Pseudotumor cerebri
	  Psychosis
		Headache
		Nausea/vomiting
		Fever
		Chills
		Aseptic meningitis
		Anaphylaxis in IgA-deficient patients
		Hemolytic anemia (rare)
			Fever
			Chills
			Headache
			Hemolytic anemia
			Renal failure (rare)

Advantages	Easy oral administration Inexpensive	Prompt rise in platelet count after infusion	Quick IV administration Inexpensive Well-tolerated
Disadvantages	Serious side effects with long-term use Bone marrow biopsy needed prior to steroid therapy to rule out leukemia	Long infusion time, often requiring hospitalization Expensive Side effects can be severe	Causes a drop in hemoglobin Use only in Rh-positive patients

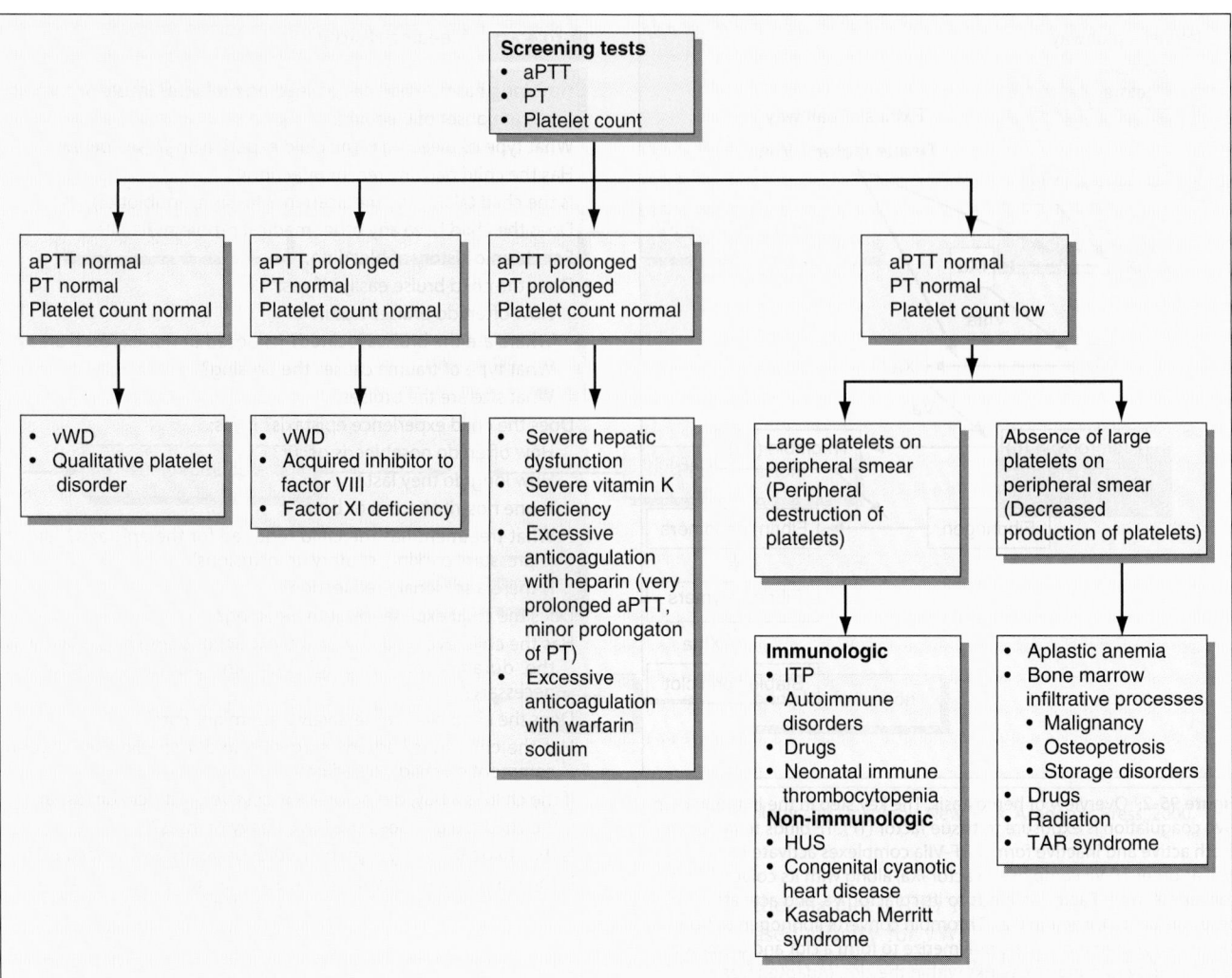

Figure 95-3. Evaluation of child with mucocutaneous bleeding and excessive bleeding during or after surgery. aPTT, activated partial thromboplastin time; PT, prothrombin time; vWD, von Willebrand disease; ITP, idiopathic (immune) thrombocytopenic purpura; HUS, hemolytic uremic syndrome; TAR, thrombocytopenia with absent radii syndrome. (Adapted from Lusher JM: Approach to the bleeding patient. In Nathan DG, Orkin SH (eds): Nathan and Oski's Hematology of Infancy and Childhood. Philadelphia, WB Saunders, 1998, p 1575.)

weight neonates. In infants, bleeding may occur after circumcision (in 30% of affected males) or with intramuscular injections such as immunizations. Oral bleeding may also occur when the teeth erupt. As the child becomes more mobile with age and starts to crawl and walk, the bleeding pattern changes. Superficial hematomas, easy bruising, oral bleeding (especially from a torn frenula), intramuscular hemorrhages, and occasional hemarthroses can occur. The ankle is the most frequent site of hemarthrosis in toddlers. As the child gets older, the knee and elbow become the most common bleeding sites. Throughout most of childhood and adulthood, intramuscular hemorrhages and hemarthroses are the major bleeding symptoms.

Intramuscular hemorrhages usually occur deep in the muscle, causing it to become swollen, hard, and painful. Patients may experience a vague feeling of pain on movement of the muscle. Bleeding within the forearm, gastrocnemius, and quadriceps can lead to compartment syndrome with resultant tissue ischemia, fibrosis, atrophy, and possible neuropathy. Fibrosis and atrophy can lead to severe muscular contractures resulting in muscle weakness. Weak muscles can then predispose to joint hemorrhage. Bleeding

into large muscles may also lead to anemia. Because large volumes of blood can be lost into the iliopsoas, it can present like an acute surgical abdomen. Pain can occur in the anterior thigh, groin, or lower abdominal region mimicking appendicitis.

Hemophilia patients who experience a hemarthrosis describe an initial tingling, warm sensation followed by increasing pain, swelling, and decreased range of motion of the affected joint. On examination, the joint is warm, swollen, and tender with limited range of motion. Older children are able to verbalize when a hemorrhage is starting prior to the onset of physical signs. In younger children, significant joint swelling and pain can occur before the hemorrhage is localized. Fussiness and refusal to use the affected extremity are often the only initial symptoms. As the child gets older, a cycle of recurrent hemorrhages into the same joint, known as the "target" joint, develops and, if not appropriately treated, can lead to long-term morbidity. Repeated bleeding into a joint irritates the synovial lining, causing proliferation and vascularization. As the synovium hypertrophies, it becomes thick and friable, predisposing the joint to more bleeds. Eventually, the cartilage erodes

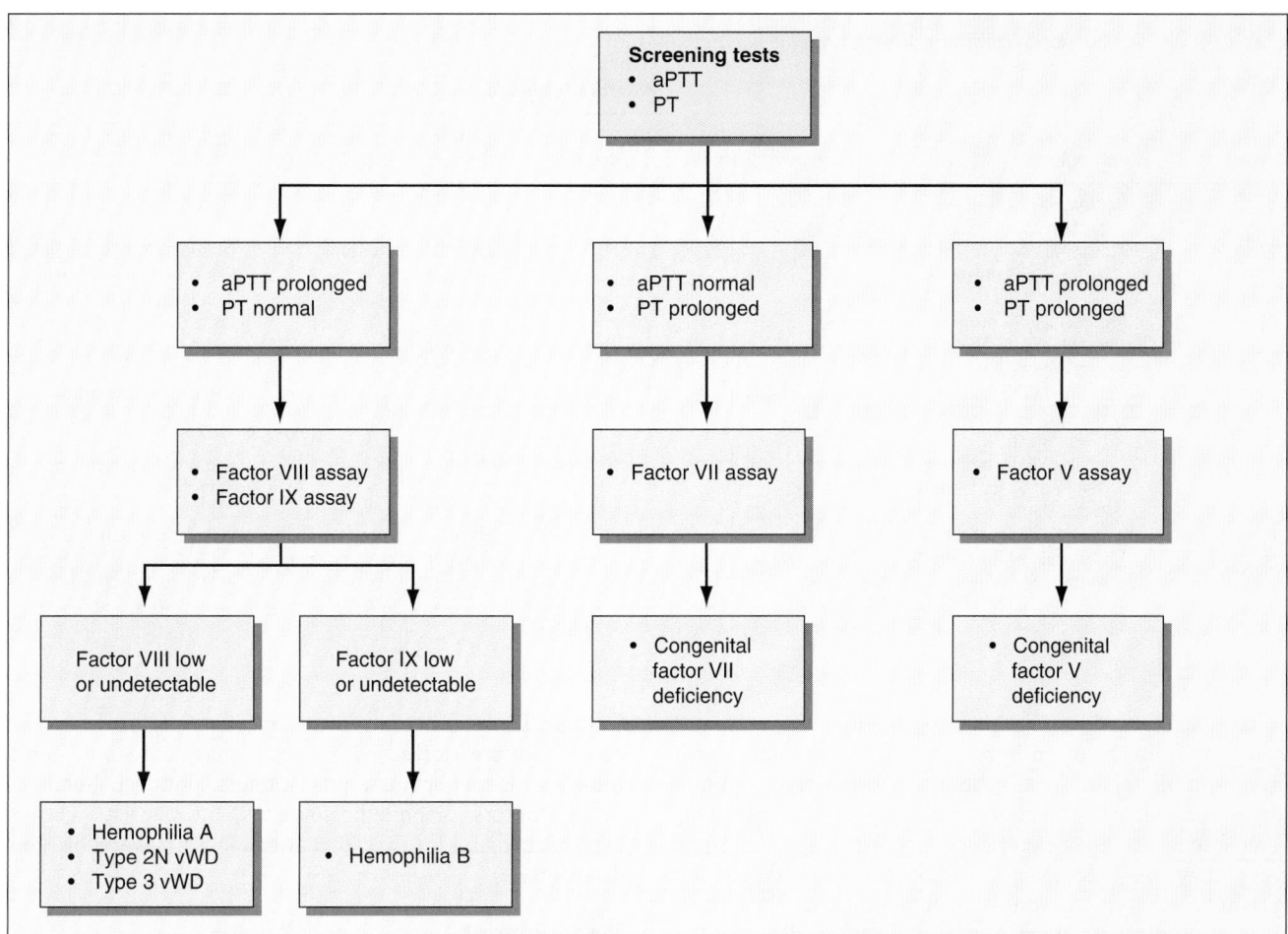

Figure 95-4. Evaluation of child with bleeding into joints/muscles and excessive bruising. aPTT, activated partial thromboplastin time; PT, prothrombin time; vWD, von Willebrand disease. (Adapted from Lusher JM: Approach to the bleeding patient. In Nathan DG, Orkin SH (eds): Nathan and Oski's Hematology of Infancy and Childhood. Philadelphia, WB Saunders, 1998, p 1575.)

and the joint space narrows, resulting in a chronic arthropathy

Hemorrhage within the central nervous system (CNS) is a potentially life-threatening complication and should be considered a medical emergency. Toddlers and young children are prone to falling and sustaining a head injury. Minor head trauma can lead to CNS bleeding, and in some cases, there is no history of trauma. Symptoms are often minimal at first. Late signs and symptoms include headache, vomiting, altered mental status, lethargy, focal neurologic changes, and seizures. Common sites of hemorrhage in patients with hemophilia are listed in Box 95-2.

When the diagnosis of hemophilia is suspected in a patient on the basis of positive family history or clinical findings, initial screening tests should include an activated PTT, PT, and platelet count. If these values are abnormal, referral to a hematologist should be considered. If the PTT is prolonged, a factor VIII assay should be obtained, and if normal, a factor IX assay should be done. If the factor VIII is abnormal, additional studies for von Willebrand disease should be performed to distinguish factor VIII deficiency from von Willebrand disease. Patients with normal factors VIII and IX assays should be screened for rarer bleeding disorders. Prenatal diagnosis in pregnant carriers can be performed during the first trimester (11 to 13 weeks) by chorionic villus sampling. Genetic diagnosis during the second trimester can be performed at 16 weeks using amniocentesis for DNA analysis and at 18 to 20 weeks using umbilical cord fetal blood sampling for analysis of factor VIII or IX activity. Factors VIII and IX do not cross the placenta; therefore, activity for both these factors can be tested from the cord blood or from a peripheral blood sample from the infant at birth. Factor IX levels are physiologically low in neonates; therefore, mild hemophilia B may be difficult to rule out at birth. All degrees of hemophilia A can be diagnosed during the newborn period.

Mucocutaneous bleeding is the classic bleeding pattern seen in von Willebrand disease. Bleeding symptoms include ecchymoses, epistaxis, menorrhagia, and posttraumatic or

Box 95-2. Sites of Hemorrhage in Hemophilia

Hemarthroses
Intramuscular hematomas
Mucocutanous bleeding
Central nervous system (intracranial or intraspinal)
Retropharyngeal
Retroperitoneal
Gastrointestinal
Genitourinary tract

709

Table 95-2. Types of von Willebrand Disease and Their Testing Patterns

Type	Pathogenesis	Laboratory Testing Profile					Therapy
		vWF Antigen	Ristocetin activity	Factor VIII	Multimers	Platelet Count	
1	Decreased levels of vWF protein	↓ to N	↓ to N	↓ to N	N	N	DDAVP
2A	Abnormal vWF protein causing loss of HMWM	↓	↓↓	N	Loss of HMWM	N	DDAVP (effective in 10%) Factor VIII concentrate with vWF
2B	Abnormal vWF protein with increased binding to platelet GPIb	↓ to N	↓ to N	N	Loss of HMWM	↓ to N	Factor VIII concentrate with vWF
2N	Abnormal vWF protein that lacks a factor VIII binding site	↓	↓	↓↓	N	N	Factor VIII concentrate with vWF
3	Absent vWF protein with resultant absent to low factor VIII	Absent	Absent	Absent	Absent	N	Factor VIII concentrate with vWF
Platelet-type	Platelet GPIb receptor has "gain of function" mutation	↓ to N	↓ to N	N	Loss of HMWM	↓ to N	Platelet transfusions

DDAVP, vasopressin; HMWM, high-molecular-weight multimers; N, normal; vWF, von Willebrand factor.

postsurgical bleeding. Patients with type 1 or 2 von Willebrand disease often have very mild symptoms, and it may go undetected until the patient undergoes minor surgery or a dental procedure and has prolonged bleeding. Female teenagers may experience menorrhagia, and in some cases they may develop an associated iron deficiency. Patients with type 3 von Willebrand disease have more frequent and severe symptoms and are often diagnosed at an earlier age. These patients can have bleeding symptoms that are similar to those seen in patients with moderate to severe hemophilia A.

Given the cost and complexities of laboratory testing for von Willebrand disease, a referral to the hematologist is appropriate when the diagnosis is suspected. A PTT may or may not be prolonged, and a normal result does not preclude the diagnosis of von Willebrand disease. The bleeding time is often used as a screening test, but it is extremely unreliable in children and can be normal in patients with known von Willebrand disease. Specific tests for von Willebrand disease include vWF antigen, ristocetin cofactor activity, vWF multimers, and factor VIII level. Characteristic results of this panel of testing can indicate the type of von Willebrand disease. Table 95-2 lists the types of von Willebrand disease and their respective testing patterns. Testing for von Willebrand disease can be challenging because vWF protein levels can vary. vWF is an acute phase reactant, and stress and trauma can transiently increase vWF levels into the normal range. Repeated testing is often required to accurately diagnose von Willebrand disease.

REFERRAL

All patients who present with a significant bleeding history should be referred to a pediatric hematologist for an evaluation. Subsequently, patients with hemophilia, severe von Willebrand disease, or rare bleeding disorder should be referred to a local Hemophilia Comprehensive Treatment

Center. These centers provide excellent multidisciplinary care. They are staffed with a team that consists of hematologists, nurses or nurse practitioners, physical therapists, social workers, orthopedic surgeons, and dentists who are experienced in the care of patients with severe bleeding disorders.

Management

Care of patients with bleeding disorders must be coordinated between the primary care provider and the hematologist. Patients and parents should always know when and whom to call. Primary care providers should know protocols for treatment of bleeding episodes and emergency treatments. Box 95-3 lists general guidelines for initial treatment of bleeding episodes in hemophilia A and B. Table 95-3 lists types of bleeding episodes and recommended treatment.

Prevention and early treatment of bleeding episodes, family education, and good well-child care are all important components of excellent hemophilia care. Parental and patient education can be provided by the local Hemophilia Comprehensive Treatment Center. Parents should be educated about hemophilia, the signs and symptoms of a bleeding episode, indications for treatment, and the appropriate action to take in the event that treatment is needed.

Box 95-3. General Guidelines for Initial Treatment of Bleeding Episodes in Hemophilia A and B

Do not delay treatment. Administer factor immediately and prior to performing radiographic or diagnostic tests.

Factor product is contained in vials with the number of units written on the label. When calculating the dose of factor, use the number of vials closest to the calculated dose. Administer the entire vial(s).

Inquire about inhibitors prior to treating.

Contact the patient's hematologist immediately.

Table 95-3. Initial Treatment of Bleeding Episodes in Hemophilia A and B*

Type of Hemorrhage	Desired Level
Major Bleeds	
Central nervous system Neck/throat (airway) Severe injury Limb-threatening muscle hematoma (compartment syndrome) Iliopsoas hemorrhage Surgery	100% for all major bleeds. Patients with major bleeds will need on-going treatment after initial therapy. Major bleeds should be referred to hemophilia center for therapy.
Minor Bleeds	
Early hemarthrosis/muscle Mucocutaneous	50–60%, may need more than one dose 30–50%, antifibrinolytic agents useful

*Factor VIII: number of units to infuse = weight (kg) × desired level (%) × 0.5. Factor IX: number of units to infuse = weight (kg) × desired level (%).

In addition, parents need to be taught how to properly store factor, reconstitute the factor, and start an intravenous infusion in their child and administer factor as needed. As the child gets older, he can be taught to start an intravenous infusion himself and self-administer the factor. By teaching parents and the patient how to administer factor at home, early treatment can be provided and the long-term morbidity associated with hemophilia may be avoided. Every child should have a Medic-Alert bracelet stating the type and severity of his hemophilia and the name and dose of his factor product.

Childhood immunizations should be administered subcutaneously according to the regular schedule. The hepatitis B series and the hepatitis A vaccine should be administered as early as possible to minimize risk of infection. Immunizations generally are well tolerated because of their small volume; however, direct pressure should be applied for at least 5 minutes to prevent excessive bleeding. Intramuscular injections should be avoided. Aspirin, ibuprofen, and other antiplatelet medications ought to be avoided as well, and prophylactic dental care should be emphasized. During infancy, padded cribs and playpens are often recommended, and during the toddler months, when the patient is crawling and learning to walk, knee pads and helmets can be helpful. As the child grows older, regular exercise to strengthen muscles and protect joints should be encouraged. Nontraumatic sports such as swimming are recommended. Contact sports and other activities that can result in head injury should be avoided. Restriction of physical activities needs to be individualized to each patient, taking into account the severity of hemophilia, bleeding history, presence of inhibitors, and the patient's lifestyle preferences and acceptance of risk.

Prompt, early treatment of bleeding episodes is key to preventing the long-term complications associated with hemophilia (see Box 95-3 and Table 95-3). Life-threatening hemorrhages such as CNS bleeding, exsanguinating hemorrhages, and bleeding around the airway require immediate replacement therapy. If a CNS hemorrhage is suspected, immediate factor replacement to 100% is necessary prior

to radiographic evaluation. After factor has been infused, a head computed tomography or magnetic resonance imaging scan can be performed to document bleeding. Depending on the severity of the bleed, treatment may be required for several days or weeks.

In 15% to 25% of patients with severe hemophilia A and in 1% to 4% of patients with severe hemophilia B, polyclonal antibodies to infused factor can develop. These antibodies, known as inhibitors, neutralize the clotting activity of infused factor and pose a major therapeutic problem. An inhibitor may be detected on a routine screening test or it may be detected because a patient suddenly fails to respond to therapy. Affected patients may be "low responders" who maintain a low titer of antibody even when exposed to repeated doses of factor. "High responders" are patients who have a true anamnestic response and develop a high-titer antibody when exposed to factor. The development of inhibitors does not appear to be related to the number of factor infusions.

When a patient with hemophilia presents with signs or symptoms of bleeding, it is important to quickly inquire about the severity of hemophilia, current factor replacement product and dose, and the presence of inhibitors. Most patients and their families are very knowledgeable about their hemophilia and treatment and can provide insight to the problem. Timely consultation with the patient's hematologist is recommended. In particular, patients with inhibitors require individualized treatment plans using special products; therefore, a call to the hematologist is recommended prior to treatment. For patients without inhibitors, treatment should not be delayed.

Treatment of hemophilia patients with inhibitors is complicated and should be performed by experts in hemophilia management. Treatment of acute bleeding depends on whether the patient has low-responding or high-responding titers. Patients with low-responding factor VIII inhibitors can usually be treated with higher doses of factor VIII concentrates. Treatment for patients with high-responding inhibitors is more difficult and includes the use of recombinant factor VIIa, continuous factor VIII infusions, porcine factor VIII concentrates, prothrombin complex concentrates, or activated prothrombin complex concentrates. Treatment of hemophilia B patients with factor IX inhibitors includes the use of factor VIIa and activated prothrombin complex concentrates. Immune tolerance programs have been developed for long-term management of patients with inhibitors.

Treatment of von Willebrand disease depends on the specific type of disease. For patients with type 1 von Willebrand disease, DDAVP is the primary treatment. DDAVP leads to the release of stored vWF from endothelial cells. The dosing for DDAVP is the same as for adjunctive therapy in patients with mild to moderate hemophilia A. For minor procedures, it can be given once prior to surgery. For major surgeries it can be given on a daily basis. Tachyphylaxis can occur with repeated dosing. Approximately 10% of type 2A patients respond to DDAVP; therefore, a therapeutic trial is worthwhile. For patients with DDAVP-unresponsive type 2A von Willebrand disease, and patients with type 2B, type 2N, or type 3 disease, infusion of plasma-derived factor VIII concentrates that contain vWF is indicated. Patients with "platelet"-type von Willebrand disease require platelet transfusions for severe bleeding episodes. For all types of von Willebrand disease, antifibrinolytics are a useful adjunct when treating nasal or oral bleeding.

Outcome

The major complications of children with hemophilia are orthopedic disability, inhibitor development, and infectious complications of therapy. Chronic arthropathy is a significant disabling complication for many patients with hemophilia. Fortunately, with the advent of home therapy, aggressive treatment regimens, and prophylactic regimens, the incidence of hemophilic arthropathy is decreasing. The reduced morbidity associated with arthroscopic synovectomy and radiosynovectomy has also improved outcome. Treatment of patients with inhibitors continues to be challenging, and in general, these patients experience more short-term and long-term complications than children without inhibitors. Immune tolerance offers the best long-term option for these patients, with an overall success rate of 60% to 80%. Unfortunately, these programs can be time-consuming, difficult to implement, and costly. The infectious risks of plasma-derived products are exceedingly low as a result of monoclonal antibody purification techniques, viral inactivation methods, and new assays that can determine viral load. The incidence of transmission of hepatitis B, hepatitis C, or human immunodeficiency virus (HIV) is negligible with these products; however, the transmission of hepatitis A and parvovirus is not prevented. With recombinant factor products, the risk of infection is almost non-existent and transmission of blood-borne or animal viruses has not been seen. As newer factor products continue to be developed, even safer and more effective products will become available.

FOLLOW-UP

Standard of care for patients with hemophilia, type III von Willebrand disease, and other rare bleeding disorders requires a multidisciplinary approach with a team of providers including the pediatrician, hematologist, nurse practitioner, social worker, physical therapist, dentist, orthopedic surgeon, and psychologist. This comprehensive approach, described in Chapter 161, reduces the short- and long-term complications of hemophilia and improves patient performance in school and in the workplace.

Mini-index of Related Topics   CH.

SUGGESTED READINGS

Bell B, Canty D, Audet M: Hemophilia: An updated review. Pediatr Rev 1995;16:290–298.

Jones P: Living with Hemophilia. New York, Oxford University Press, 1995.

Lanzkowsky P: Manual of Pediatric Hematology and Oncology. New York, Churchill Livingstone, 1995.

Lusher JM: Approach to the bleeding patient. In Nathan DG, Oski FA (eds): Hematology of Infancy and Childhood. Philadelphia, WB Saunders, 1998, pp 1574–1584.

Montgomery RR, Gill JC, Scott JP: Hemophilia and von Willebrand disease. In Nathan DG, Oski FA (eds): Hematology of Infancy and Childhood. Philadelphia, WB Saunders, 1998, pp 1631–1659.

96 Hematuria and Glomerular Disorders

Sudhir K. Anand

ROLE OF THE GENERALIST

1   Recognize the usual benign nature of asymptomatic microhematuria detected during screening of normal children versus more serious causes of hematuria.

2   Provide initial evaluation of children with hematuria with emphasis upon detailed history, especially family history.

3   Recognize indicators of significant renal disease in children with asymptomatic hematuria who need referral to a specialist.

DEFINITION

Hematuria, meaning literally blood in the urine, is common and may be visible (gross hematuria) or microscopic (microhematuria). Hematuria can develop from abnormalities anywhere along the genitourinary tract from the kidneys to the urethra. The finding of hematuria may signify a serious medical problem or may be incidental and inconsequential. Hematuria is usually identified in one of the three following manners (Box 96-1): screening in an asymptomatic child; a patient who presents with red urine, or microscopic or gross hematuria with other significant clinical or laboratory findings.

FUNDAMENTALS

Epidemiology

Gross hematuria resulting in an emergency department visit is approximately 1 to 2 per 1000 patient visits, with urinary tract infection (documented or suspected) being the cause in half of the patients. Microhematuria is usually asymptomatic and is most often detected by dipstick testing during

---

Box 96-1. Identification of Hematuria

- Dipstick test is positive for microscopic hematuria in an asymptomatic child detected by a screening urinalysis during a routine physical examination.
- Patient presents with red urine and no other symptoms.
- Patient presents with microscopic or gross hematuria and has other findings (e.g., edema, hypertension, burning urination, history of trauma) or dipstick urinalysis shows proteinuria or leukocyturia.

---

screening urinalysis at periodic physical examinations, especially before starting kindergarten or elementary school. The prevalence varies between 0.5% and 2% depending upon the age of patient and the number of samples checked per child.

Detecting Hematuria and Normal Values

Small amounts of blood (less than 1 mL/L of urine) can cause the urine to appear red. Red urine also may be secondary to other causes, such as hemoglobinuria, certain foods, food dyes, and drugs. Because dipsticks detect hemoglobin, dipsticks are positive in patients with hemoglobinuria and myoglobinuria and with hematuria. Microscopic examination of the urine must be done to verify presence of red blood cells (RBCs). The first-voided urine in the morning is the best urine sample to examine because it is concentrated. Urine should be examined within 2 hours of voiding to prevent lysis of casts.

Dipsticks are fairly sensitive in detecting the presence of hemoglobin and RBCs, but are not precise in quantifying the number of RBCs. In the United States, hematuria is usually quantified and recorded as the number of red blood cells per high-power field (RBC/HPF) in a centrifuged specimen. In children, the readings of negative and trace positive are usually regarded as normal. Presence of more than 5 RBC/HPF is considered abnormal. A highly positive dipstick reading usually signifies more than 20 RBC/HPF. In European countries, an uncentrifuged specimen is measured in a counting chamber and recorded as number of RBCs per cubic millimeter. The latter numerical values are two to three times higher than the former.

Presence of RBC casts indicates a glomerular lesion. Their absence does not exclude a glomerular disorder. Examination of fresh urine with phase contrast microscopy may distinguish glomerular from nonglomerular hematuria even in the absence of RBC casts. In glomerular hematuria RBCs appear dysmorphic and may be fragmented, have blebs, or take bizarre shapes. RBCs have normal morphology in nonglomerular hematuria. Presence of 2+ or more protein on dipstick usually suggests glomerular hematuria, but its absence does not exclude a glomerular disorder.

Hematuria Detected in Asymptomatic Normal Schoolchildren During Screening

Studies of normal schoolchildren indicate that 0.5% to 1.0% may have more than 5 RBC/HPF (or 6 RBC/mm^3) in consecutive samples. Children with isolated microscopic

Box 96-2. Indicators for Referral in Children with Asymptomatic Microscopic Hematuria

Associated proteinuria

Previous episodes of gross hematuria

Family history of renal disease, hematuria, renal failure, stones, cystic kidney, sickle cell disease, or deafness

Increased BUN or serum creatinine

Table 96-2. Etiology of Gross Hematuria in Children Seen in the Pediatric Emergency Setting

Cause	Number of Patients (%)
Documented urinary tract infection	39 (26%)
Suspected urinary tract infection	35 (23%)
Perineal irritation	16 (11%)
Meatal ulcer	11 (7%)
Trauma	10 (7%)
Recurrent hematuria	7 (5%)
Acute glomerulonephritis	6 (4%)
Stones	3 (2%)
Tumor	1 (1%)
Miscellaneous	9 (6%)
Unknown	13 (9%)
Total number of patients	150 (100%)

Modified from Ingelfinger JR, Davis AE, Grupe WE: Frequency and etiology of gross hematuria in a general pediatric setting. Pediatrics 1977; 59:557–561.

hematuria (without proteinuria) rarely have serious renal disease. Although the usefulness of screening urinalysis in detecting significant occult renal disease is questionable, the American Academy of Pediatrics recommends at least one screening urinalysis at age 4 to 6 years as a baseline test. Asymptomatic children with isolated microscopic hematuria can be followed with periodic (every 6 months) dipstick testing but need not be subjected to radiologic or invasive investigations, such as renal biopsy or cystoscopy. Normal persons following exercise and athletes following both contact and noncontact sports can develop microscopic hematuria (rarely gross hematuria) that spontaneously resolves and usually does not need investigation.

Indicators of significant renal disease in children with asymptomatic microscopic hematuria are listed in Box 96-2. Children with hematuria and these findings should be referred to a pediatric nephrologist for further evaluation.

Etiology of Hematuria

Hematuria is seen in a wide variety of renal disorders (Table 96-1). The disorders are generally divided into three groups: renal, bladder or urethral (postrenal), and systemic hemostatic disorders sometimes called prerenal disorders. The renal group is further divided into two subgroups: glomerular and nonglomerular disorders. Glomerular hematuria is characterized by the presence of one or more of the following: RBC casts, dysmorphic RBCs, more than 2+ proteinuria; but these findings are not always present. All types of glomerulonephritis have microscopic or gross hematuria.

Urinary tract infection, which may be bacterial or viral, is the most common cause of gross hematuria in children seen in the emergency department (Table 96-2). Approximately 8% to 10% of patients with blunt abdominal trauma have urinary tract injury and hematuria. Ten percent of trauma patients with hematuria also have preexisting renal disease (e.g., hydronephrosis, cystic kidneys). Children of parents with renal stones often develop hematuria associated with hypercalciuria long before they themselves develop kidney stones. Wilms' tumor is the predominant tumor leading to hematuria in children. Renal cell carcinoma and transitional cell carcinoma of the bladder are extremely uncommon in children.

EVALUATION OF HEMATURIA

The evaluation of a child with hematuria should proceed in a systematic manner starting with the history, physical examination, and then, in an algorithmic fashion, appropriate laboratory tests. History should include preceding respiratory or skin infections, and time interval between infection and hematuria; relationship of hematuria to exercise; past history of hematuria; past or recent history of edema; whether the hematuria is associated with burning urination, passage of clots, or gravel; whether the hematuria is present throughout urination or only terminal (at the end of urination); and if there is family history of hematuria,

Table 96-1. Etiology of Hematuria

Renal Causes of Hematuria

Glomerular Disease

Recurrent hematuria syndrome:

    Benign sporadic, benign familial (with or without thin glomerular basement membrane)*†

    IgA nephropathy (Berger's disease)*†

    Hereditary nephritis (Alport syndrome)*

Acute glomerulonephritis (poststreptococcal, others)*

Membranoproliferative glomerulonephritis

Schönlein-Henoch purpura†

Lupus nephritis

Hepatitis B or C associated glomerulonephritis

Anti-GBM glomerulonephritis

Hemolytic-uremic syndrome

Extraglomerular Causes

Urinary tract infection, renal tuberculosis

Sickle cell trait or disease†

Genitourinary trauma*

Hydronephrosis, polycystic kidney disease and other congenital lesions†

Idiopathic hypercalciuria and renal stones*†

Hyperuricosuria

Renal neoplasm (Wilms' tumor)*†

Interstitial nephritis

Bladder or Urethral (Postrenal) Causes of Hematuria‡

Urinary tract infection (hemorrhagic cystitis)*

Perineal irritation, meatal ulcers

Trauma to bladder or urethra*

Following catheterization of bladder

Suprapubic bladder puncture

Miscellaneous: stones, vesicoureteral reflux, posterior urethritis, urethrorrhagia, hemangioma, tumors, urethral prolapse, and fictitious hematuria

Systemic (Prerenal) Causes of Hematuria

Bleeding disorders: idiopathic thrombocytopenic purpura, hemophilia, disseminated intravascular coagulation

Clotting disorders: renal artery or vein thrombosis

*Common causes of microscopic or gross hematuria.

†Causes of recurrent hematuria.

‡Exclude menstrual period in any girl older than age 10 years.

stones, deafness, or death from renal disease. A complete physical examination should be performed with special attention to the presence of hypertension, fever, edema, rash, abdominal mass or tenderness, examination of genitalia, and if necessary, a rectal examination.

Urinalysis quantifies the magnitude of hematuria and detects the presence of RBC casts or dysmorphic RBCs, coexisting proteinuria, or leukocyturia. A urine culture should be done if clinical findings suggest urinary tract infection. African-American children should be tested for sickle cell disease unless the test has been performed previously. Immediate family members should be screened for hematuria, and if appropriate, the extended family should be investigated to determine an inheritance pattern.

Blood testing should be based on the suspected diagnosis and may include a complete blood count (including platelets), serum creatinine, blood urea nitrogen (BUN), electrolytes, C3, C4, antistreptolysin O (ASO) or anti-DNase B titer (if indicated), antinuclear antibody (ANA), hepatitis B and C. C3 is low in poststreptococcal glomerulonephritis (GN), membranoproliferative GN, and lupus nephritis. Urine calcium and creatinine as well as uric acid and creatinine ratios should be measured on a spot urine test to evaluate hypercalciuria and hyperuricosuria, respectively. Borderline positive tests should be confirmed by measuring urinary calcium or uric acid in a 24-hour collection. Depending upon the suspected diagnosis, the child may continue to be observed for 1 to 2 years or may be evaluated with renal and bladder ultrasound.

Cystoscopy is rarely indicated in the evaluation of children with hematuria. It is reserved for children who have hematuria and persistent lower urinary tract symptoms (e.g., burning urination, but with sterile urine culture and normal urinary calcium excretion). Cystoscopy is also indicated in some patients with terminal (end of urination) or initial hematuria.

Kidney biopsy is indicated in some children with recurrent hematuria if the diagnosis is uncertain and in those with persistent high-grade (>20 RBC/HPF) hematuria, proteinuria greater than 1g/24 hours, reduced kidney function, or deafness.

RECURRENT HEMATURIA

Recurrent hematuria is characterized by repeated episodes of gross hematuria, usually following an upper respiratory infection (URI) or exercise. The latent period is usually 1 or 2 days rather than the 1 to 3 weeks observed in acute poststreptococcal glomerulonephritis. During the interval, either the urine is normal or there is microscopic hematuria. Edema and hypertension are usually absent. Serum creatinine and BUN are usually normal, although occasionally they may be transiently elevated during an episode of gross hematuria or severe relapse. The disorders that may result in recurrent hematuria are listed in Tables 96-1 and 96-3 and include benign sporadic or familial hematuria with thin or normal glomerular basement membrane (GBM), Alport syndrome, IgA nephropathy, Schönlein-Henoch purpura, sickle cell trait or disease, idiopathic hypercalciuria or stones, polycystic kidneys, and Wilms' tumor.

Table 96-3. Renal Biopsy Diagnosis in Children Presenting with Recurrent Gross or Persistent Microscopic Hematuria

Finding	Schroder et al	Piqueras et al
Benign hematuria	33 (familial 23)	98
Thin GBM	23 (familial 18)	50
Normal GBM	10 (familial 5)	48
Alport syndrome	8	86
IgA nephropathy	16	78
Hilar vasculopathy		28
Miscellaneous	8	32
Total number of patients	65	322

GBM, glomerular basement membrane.

Modified from Schroder CH, Bontemps CM, Assmann KJM: Renal biopsy and family studies in 65 children with isolated hematuria. Acta Paediatr 1990; 79:630–636; and Piqueras A, White RH, Raafat F, et al: Renal biopsy diagnosis in children presenting with hematuria. Pediatr Nephrol 1998;12(5):386–391.

Benign Recurrent Hematuria (Familial/Sporadic) and Thin Glomerular Basement Membrane Disease

Over the past 10 to 20 years so called benign recurrent hematuria has emerged as one of the more common diagnoses in children with episodes of asymptomatic recurrent gross hematuria or persistent microscopic hematuria. The usual onset is in childhood or early adult life. In approximately half to two thirds of the patients, the disease is familial with autosomal dominant transmission. Other family members have hematuria, but no deafness, and only rarely progress to renal failure. Patients are usually otherwise asymptomatic, but 10% to 15% may have loin (flank) pain during the episode of hematuria. The diagnosis is suggested by family history, an autosomal dominant mode of transmission, and a benign course. The diagnosis can usually be confirmed by renal biopsy. Light microscopy may be normal or show mild mesangial increase. Immunofluorescence is negative. The hallmark of the disorder is the finding of uniformly thin GBM with thickness less than 60% of normal for age and sex (Fig. 96-1). The disorder is termed thin GBM disease or thin basement membrane nephropathy. Some families with thin GBM disease have been found to have mutations in the same genes as auto-

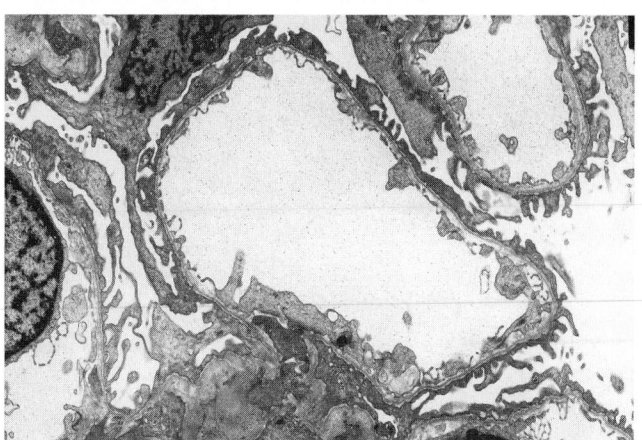

Figure 96-1. Thin glomerular basement membrane (GBM) disease: thin basement membrane nephropathy. The capillary GMBs are uniformly thin, about half the thickness of normal GBMs. (Courtesy of Dr. Arthur Cohen.)

somal recessive Alport syndrome affecting collagen IV α3 or α4 chains.

The clinical course in patients with the sporadic form of benign recurrent hematuria is similar, but family history is negative. Screening urinalysis of asymptomatic family members must be done to confirm the sporadic nature of disease in these patients.

Alport Syndrome

Alport syndrome (AS) is a genetic disorder of basement membrane type IV collagen synthesis, resulting in progressive nephropathy. In many families with AS, sensorineural hearing loss and eye lesions are also present. In 85% of families the inheritance pattern is X-linked dominant due to mutations in the gene for α5 chain of collagen IV, and in the remaining 15% inheritance is autosomal recessive due to mutation in the gene for α3 or α4 chain of collagen IV. In rare patients, transmission may be autosomal dominant. Male patients with the X-linked disorder usually present with asymptomatic microscopic or gross hematuria during the first decade of life. As the disease gradually progresses, proteinuria and hypertension may develop. During the second or third decade, male patients develop end-stage renal disease. Progressive sensorineural deafness is present in 50% to 70% patients. Initially, hearing loss is limited to high tones, but loss gradually progresses to all tones and complete deafness ensues. Macular lesions are present in 20% to 25% of patients and 5% develop lenticonus.

Most girls and women who are X-linked carriers for AS are normal or have microscopic hematuria only during the first 3 to 4 decades. Subsequently most remain asymptomatic, but some develop progressive renal disease. Autosomal recessive AS is equally severe in girls and boys, and like the X-linked disorder in boys, patients clinically present during the first decade of life and gradually progress to end-stage renal disease during the second or third decade.

Pathologic findings are variable, depending upon the stage of AS. During the first few years of life, the basement membrane may be thin, making it hard to differentiate from thin GBM disease. By the end of the first decade, most patients with AS show characteristic splitting or multilayering and wide thickening of GBM and electron-dense deposits on electron microscopy (Fig. 96-2). Light microscopy may show mesangial proliferation in the

glomeruli and foam cells in the interstitium. Immunofluorescence studies are negative except that most patients with AS (unlike normal persons) do not bind anti-GBM antibodies obtained from patients with Goodpasture syndrome. The diagnosis of AS can also be confirmed by genomic DNA analysis.

There is no definitive treatment for AS. Progression of the disease may be slowed by adequate control of blood pressure and use of angiotensin-converting enzyme (ACE) inhibitors. Most patients with AS are suitable candidates for dialysis and renal transplantation. A few patients, however, develop anti-GBM nephritis because their native kidneys lack certain collagen IV GBM antigens, which the transplanted kidney possesses.

IGA Nephropathy (Berger's Disease)

IgA nephropathy is the most common form of glomerulonephritis in the world. The prevalence is high in Asian countries along the Pacific rim and relatively low in the United States and Europe. The disease is less common in blacks. The renal biopsy is characterized by mesangial proliferation and matrix expansion under light microscopy and mesangial deposition of IgA demonstrated by immunofluorescence (Fig. 96-3). The pathologic findings are identical to those in Schönlein-Henoch purpura. The two disorders are differentiated by the clinical presentation.

Recent evidence suggest that the disease results from altered structure of IgA or altered regulation of its production. The glycosylation of IgA in the hinge region of its heavy chains is reduced, making it more prone to aggregation and deposition in the mesangium.

In children with IgA nephropathy, 80% to 90% present with asymptomatic gross or microscopic hematuria 1 to 2 days following a URI or other infection; proteinuria is mini-

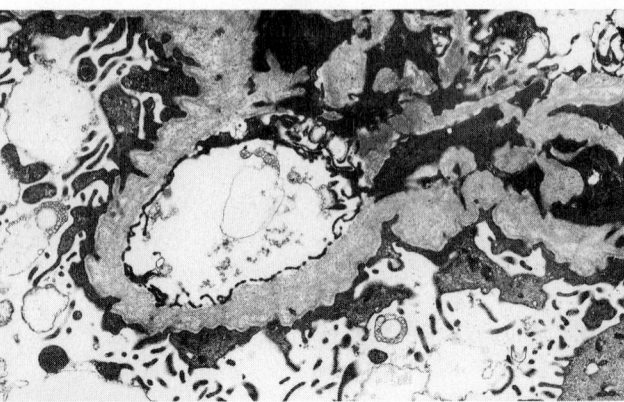

Figure 96-2. Alport syndrome. The glomerular basement membrane is thick and multilayered, with an irregular subepithelial border. (Courtesy of Dr. Arthur Cohen.)

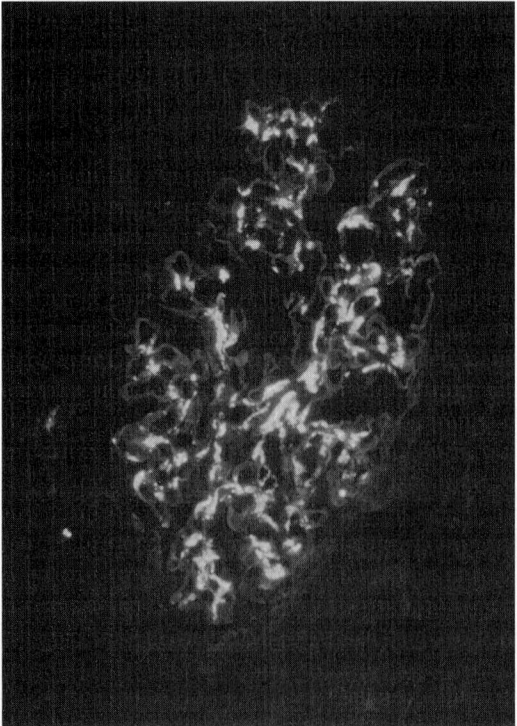

Figure 96-3. IgA nephropathy. Granular deposits of IgA are in the mesangium. (Courtesy of Dr. Arthur Cohen.)

mal and renal function is normal. The remaining 10% to 20% of children may have associated proteinuria, acute glomerulonephritis features, nephrotic syndrome, or rapidly progressive glomerulonephritis.

IgA nephropathy generally is a chronic disorder with episodes of hematuria alternating with long asymptomatic periods. Most children with the disorder recover or remain stable; however, 20% to 40% of patients develop progressive renal disease and chronic renal failure after 10 to 20 years of disease.

No therapy has been proved beneficial in controlled studies of patients with IgA nephropathy. Patients with mild IgA nephropathy without any proteinuria need no treatment. Omega-3 fish oil and ACE inhibitors seem to improve hematuria or proteinuria in some patients with moderate IgA nephropathy. Patients with heavy proteinuria or rapidly progressive IgA glomerulonephritis seem to benefit from treatment with steroids and immunosuppressive agents. IgA nephropathy may recur in a renal transplant patient.

Acute Glomerulonephritis

Acute glomerulonephritis (AGN) is clinically characterized by the sudden onset of gross hematuria, edema, hypertension, oliguria, and renal failure in a previously healthy child. In more than 90% of affected children AGN follows a streptococcal infection of the throat or skin and is called poststreptococcal AGN (PSAGN). In the remaining 10% AGN may follow other bacterial, viral, rickettsial, or protozoal infections, and the disorder is called postinfectious AGN. There is usually a latent period of 1 to 3 weeks between the infection and onset of hematuria or edema.

Epidemiology

PSAGN predominantly affects children 2 to 10 years old but can occur in any age group. During winter months PSAGN usually follows streptococcal pharyngitis or otitis media, whereas it follows streptococcal impetigo or pyoderma during the summer months. Only certain strains of streptococci, called nephritogenic strains, cause PSAGN. Most cases are sporadic, but epidemics of the disorder due to specific strains have been described.

Pathology

On light microscopy, PSAGN shows generalized diffuse proliferation and inflammation. Glomeruli appear enlarged, and have an increased number of mesangial and endothelial cells and infiltration of polymorphonuclear cells in the mesangium and capillary lumina (Fig. 96-4). In severe cases, there is proliferation of parietal epithelial cells and accumulation of macrophages in Bowman's space in the form of crescents; interstitial edema and inflammation may also be present. Immunofluorescence microscopy shows coarse deposits of C3 and IgG on the epithelial side of GBM. Electron microscopy reveals large subepithelial immune deposits.

Pathogenesis

Although, deposits of C3 and IgG in the glomerular capillaries along with decreased C3 levels in blood would suggest that PSAGN is mediated by immune complexes, the precise mechanism of renal injury in PSAGN is still uncertain. It remains unclear whether the disorder is medi-

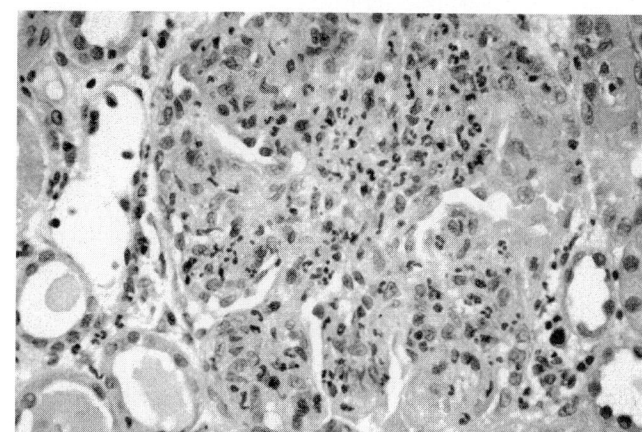

Figure 96-4. Acute poststreptococcal glomerulonephritis. The glomerulus is enlarged and markedly hypercellular with numerous leukocytes in the capillary lumen.

ated by circulating or in situ formed immune complexes, or both. The proposed nephritogenic antigens include endostreptosin and others; however, none of them has been uniformly and reproducibly shown to be present in the subepithelial immune deposits. In postinfectious AGN due to other organisms, the respective antigen usually can be demonstrated in the immune deposits.

Clinical Findings

Most children with PSAGN present with abrupt onset of tea- or coke-colored urine along with a history of mild insidious onset of edema of face or legs for a few days. Many children also have malaise, nausea, and upper abdominal pain. Hypertension is present in the majority of patients. Urinalysis shows dysmorphic RBCs or RBC casts. Mild to moderate proteinuria is usually present. Heavy (>2 g/m^2/day or 4+ protein) nephrotic range proteinuria is uncommon. Serum creatinine and BUN are increased in nearly half the patients. Mild anemia (due to hemodilution) is present in the majority of patients. Radiographs of the chest may show perihilar hyperperfusion or pulmonary edema. The ASO titer is increased in 80% of patients, and anti-DNase B titer is increased in 95%. C3 is reduced in more than 90% of patients.

Severe cases may present with congestive heart failure or hypertensive encephalopathy and seizures. Some patients develop rapidly progressive glomerulonephritis (RPGN) and have marked oliguria/anuria, markedly increased serum creatinine and BUN, and acute renal failure. These patients should be referred to a pediatric nephrologist for help with management.

Management

All patients with hypertension, decreased urine output, or increased BUN/creatinine should be hospitalized. Only the mildest asymptomatic patients may be managed as outpatients with close daily follow-up. Treatment consists of appropriate fluid and salt restriction based upon the daily urine output and presence of hypertension. Oliguria sometimes successfully responds to diuretics. Hypertension may be treated with nifedipine, labetalol, or hydralazine. Dialysis is rarely indicated in most PSAGN patients, but may be necessary in RPGN patients.

Prognosis

The great majority (>90%) of patients with PSAGN recover completely. Edema, gross hematuria, and hypertension resolve within 2 weeks. Documentation that C3 has returned to normal in PSAGN patients (usually within 6 weeks) is essential because membranoproliferative GN patients may initially present in a similar manner to PSAGN, but C3 remains chronically low. Microhematuria may persist for a few months to a couple of years. In patients with severe AGN or RPGN and acute renal failure, recovery is slower and chronic renal failure may develop.

Disorders such as benign recurrent hematuria, IgA nephropathy, and Alport syndrome are usually easy to differentiate from PSAGN (Table 96-4). Patients with membranoproliferative GN generally have heavy proteinuria. Glomerulonephritis due to systemic lupus erythematosus (SLE), Schönlein-Henoch purpura, or vasculitis may mimic PSAGN, but patients usually have other clinical or laboratory findings that help differentiate the disorders.

Hemolytic-Uremic Syndrome

Hemolytic-uremic syndrome (HUS) is characterized by microangiopathic hemolytic anemia, thrombocytopenia, and acute renal failure. Although a wide variety of disorders can lead to the same findings, typically, HUS in young chil-

dren follows acute diarrhea/colitis caused by O157:H7 strain of *Escherichia coli*, which produces Shiga-like toxin (also called verotoxin). Shiga-like toxin in some children, most likely based on genetic susceptibility, causes endothelial damage, platelet aggregation, and fibrin deposition in the kidneys, colon, brain, and sometimes in other organs, such as pancreas, heart, and muscle. The pathogenesis of HUS is not completely known, but thrombotic activity increases and fibrinolytic activity decreases in the coagulation cascade (Fig. 96-5).

Children usually present with a prodrome of diarrhea often bloody, followed 2 or 3 days later by pallor, abdominal pain, petechiae, and decreased urine output. More severe cases may present with an acute abdomen or seizures usually associated with hypertension. If the renal failure worsens, the patient may develop signs of uremia, hyperkalemia, or arrhythmias. Fluid overload and hypertension may lead to congestive heart failure.

Urinalysis (if the patient is not anuric) shows mild to moderate proteinuria along with microscopic hematuria. Anemia may be severe; hemoglobin usually varies between 5 and 10 g/dL. Platelet count is usually less than 100,000/mm^3 and the reticulocyte count is greater than 5%. The hallmark of HUS is the presence of fragmented RBCs (schistocytes, helmet and burr cells) on the smear. PT and PTT are usually normal, but recent data show that plasma concentrations of prothrombin fragments 1 and 2, tissue plasminogen activator (tPA) antigen, tPA inhibitor type 1 (PAI-1) complex, and D-dimer are increased. Serum creatinine and BUN are increased. With worsening of HUS, BUN and creatinine can become markedly elevated. Bilirubin may be increased due to excessive hemolysis.

The management of HUS is primarily directed toward meticulous care of acute renal failure (Chapter 98) including appropriate restriction of fluids and electrolytes. If renal failure is severe, early introduction of peritoneal or hemodialysis is critical. Hemoglobin should be maintained at greater than 8 g/dL using packed RBC transfusions if necessary. Platelet transfusions are rarely indicated and reserved for children with bleeding manifestations or platelet counts less than 10,000/mm^3. Adequate nutrition should be provided to prevent excessive tissue breakdown. Anticoagulation, thrombolytic therapy, plasma exchange, antiplatelet drugs, and steroids have not been proved to have any benefit in the management of patients with *E. coli* or diarrhea-associated HUS.

In familial HUS, recurrent HUS, and especially TTP, plasma exchange or infusions are helpful in the treatment. Steroids and other drugs may also be indicated.

The majority (65% to 80%) of children with diarrhea-associated acute renal failure recover normal renal function. Of the remaining patients, a few die acutely, whereas others have significant persistent renal dysfunction. Some of the latter patients may develop early or late chronic renal failure and progress to end-stage disease, requiring dialysis or transplantation.

Idiopathic Hypercalciuria

Idiopathic hypercalciuria (IH) may present as microscopic or gross hematuria and dysuria. Serum calcium level is normal in patients with IH. Family history of urinary stones

Table 96-4. Comparison of Acute Poststreptococcal Glomerulonephritis and Recurrent Hematuria Syndrome

Characteristic	Acute Poststreptococcal Glomerulonephritis	Recurrent Hematuria Syndrome
History of preceding skin or throat infection	Usually +	±
Latent period	7–21 days	1–3 days
Edema	Frequent	Usually absent
Hypertension	Frequent	Usually absent
ASO or anti-DNase B titer	Usually ↑	Normal
C3	Usually ↓	Normal
Kidney function (GFR)	Usually ↓	Normal or transiently ↓
Renal biopsy	Generalized diffuse, proliferation with exudation; Immunofluorescence: subepithelial C3 and IgG deposits	Focal segmental mesangial proliferation; Immunofluorescence IgA nephropathy shows mesangial IgA and C3; EM: benign hematuria may show thin GBM; Alport syndrome: thickened, fragmented GBM
Recurrence	Rare	Common
Prognosis	Generally good	Benign hematuria: generally good; IgA nephropathy: some have progressive disease; Alport syndrome: slow progression to renal failure

ASO, antistreptolysin O; EM, electron microscopy; GBM, glomerular basement membrane; GFR, glomerular filtration rate.

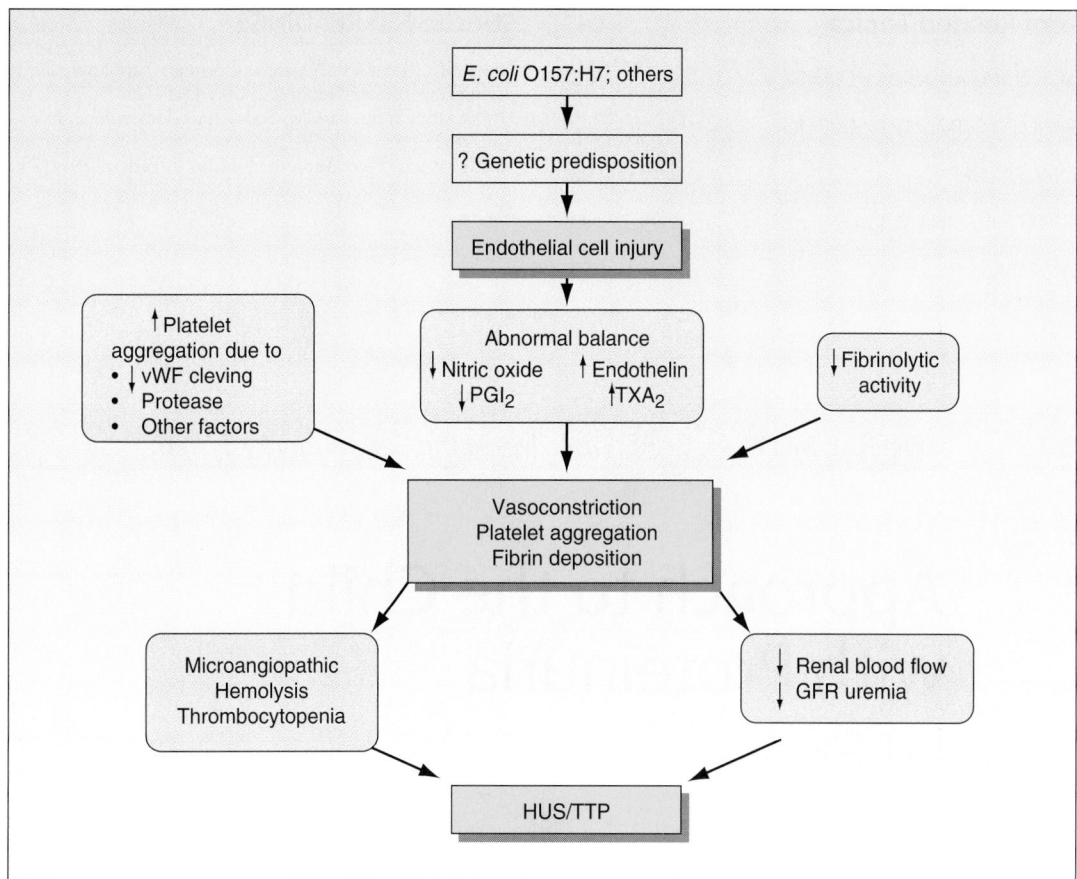

Figure 96-5. Pathogenesis of hemolytic-uremic syndrome (HUS) and thrombotic thrombocytopenic purpura (TTP). GFR, glomerular filtration rate; HUS, hemolytic-uremic syndrome; PGI$_2$, prostaglandin I$_2$; TXA$_2$, thromboxane A$_2$; vWF, von Willebrand factor.

is often positive. Children, however, develop hematuria due to IH long before actual stone(s) develop or are demonstrable by various radiologic investigations. IH may result from excessive calcium absorption (absorptive type) in the gastrointestinal (GI) tract or from a defect in renal tubular calcium reabsorption (renal leak). Although exquisite sensitivity to vitamin D has been postulated as a possible cause of excessive calcium absorption in the GI tract, the exact defects that lead to either excessive GI absorption or renal leak are unknown. Absorptive hypercalciuria and renal leak hypercalciuria are difficult to differentiate clinically. Hypercalciuria may cause hematuria by microdeposition or tubular cell injury. The precise mechanisms remain unknown. Hypercalciuria is documented by measuring either 24-hour urinary calcium excretion (normal: <4.0 mg/kg/24 hours in children >6 years old) or spot urinary

calcium and creatinine ratio (normal less than 0.22 in the first-voided urine in the morning; Table 96-5). Conditions that cause hypercalcemia may also be associated with hypercalciuria, hematuria, and renal stone(s) and must be differentiated from IH.

Hypercalciuria is treated by increasing daily fluid intake to 1.5 to 2.0 times the daily recommended allowance for weight of the patient to enable the urine volume to double. When urine specific gravity decreases to near 1.010 the likelihood of stone formation is substantially reduced. Low-sodium diet and decrease in animal protein intake also reduce the chances of stone formation. Calcium intake should be normal; decrease in calcium intake does not prevent stone formation and may lead to osteoporosis. If gross hematuria is frequent or high-grade microhematuria persists, the patient may be treated with hydrochlorothiazide at 1 mg/kg/day (25 mg max) to decrease urinary calcium excretion. Patients should be closely monitored for hypokalemia. If hypokalemia develops, it should be treated aggressively to restore normal levels. Hypokalemia tends to decrease urinary citrate excretion and increase urinary calcium ion levels and stone formation.

Table 96-5. Normal Values for Urinary Calcium-Creatinine Ratios

Age	Urine Calcium-Creatinine Ratio*
<7 months	≤0.86
7–18 months	≤0.60
19 months to 6 years	≤0.42
6 years to adult	≤0.22

*The calcium and creatinine concentrations must be in the same units (mg/dL) before the ratio can be calculated.

Modified from Sargent JD, Stukel TA, Kresel J, et al: Normal values for random urinary calcium to creatinine ratios in infancy. J Pediatr 1993;123(3):393–397.

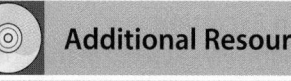

Additional Resources, CD-ROM

Bibliography

SUGGESTED READINGS

Diven SC, Travis LB: A practical primary care approach to hematuria in children. Pediatr Nephrol 2000;14:65–72.

Hricik DE, Chung-Park M, Sedor JR: Glomerulonephritis. N Engl J Med 1998;339:888–899.

Northway JD: Hematuria in children. J. Pediatr 1971;78:381–396.

SECTION 3   GENERAL MEDICAL CARE: *Disorders of the Genitourinary System*

97

Approach to the Child with Proteinuria

Sudhir K. Anand

ROLE OF THE GENERALIST

1. Recognize the transient and benign nature of proteinuria detected during screening of asymptomatic schoolchildren.

2. Recognize other transient (functional) causes of proteinuria, especially postural proteinuria.

3. Diagnose causes of proteinuria, especially nephrotic syndrome (NS).

4. Recognize when to refer patients to a pediatric nephrologist for help with management.

5. Recognize complications of NS and its treatment.

Proteinuria is a common finding detected during screening of asymptomatic children receiving routine well-child care or a medical visit for a nonrenal condition (Box 97-1). In the overwhelming majority, it is a transient and insignificant finding. Proteinuria, however, is an important marker of glomerular disease and may be the only early finding in some patients with renal disorders. Moreover, in the past 10 years most nephrologists believe that proteinuria itself induces renal damage and worsening of chronic renal diseases.

FUNDAMENTALS

Normal Daily Urine Protein Excretion

A small amount of protein is normally excreted in the urine, approximately 50 mg/day in adults and 30 mg/m²/day in children. The upper limits of normal are up to 150 mg/24

Box 97-1. Clinical Presentation of Proteinuria

Proteinuria is usually identified in one of the following clinical settings:

Dipstick test is positive for proteinuria during screening of an asymptomatic child receiving routine physical examination.

Child presents with edema and has isolated proteinuria.

Child presents with one or more of the following clinical or laboratory findings along with proteinuria: hematuria, hypertension, burning urination, tubular dysfunction, and renal failure.

---

hours in adults and 100 mg/m²/24 hours in children. About one third of this protein is albumin. The remainder is primarily Tamm-Horsfall mucoprotein, secreted by the thick ascending limb of the loop of Henle and is the main constituent of various casts. Small amounts of low-molecular-weight globulins are also normally present in the urine.

Methods of Detection of Proteinuria

The urine dipstick, a fairly sensitive test for detection of protein, primarily detects albumin, which is better for diagnosing glomerular disorders than tubular disorders in which low-molecular-weight globulins are excreted in the urine. The dipstick test may be falsely positive at the level of 1+ or 2+ in patients with gross hematuria or pyuria, or if the urine is alkaline. Sulfosalicylic acid (SSA) is the semiquantitative method used by most laboratories to measure 24-hour urine proteins. SSA is falsely positive if radiopaque dyes, oral antidiabetic agents, or some antibiotics (e.g., oxacillin) are being excreted in the urine. Both dipstick and

SSA tests are affected by urine concentration. A highly concentrated urine may show 3+ protein on a dipstick but only mild to moderate proteinuria on a 24-hour collection. By contrast, a dipstick reading of 1+ in a very dilute urine may reflect moderate proteinuria with a 24-hour collection. Proteinuria is more accurately determined by performing 24-hour or timed (4- to 8-hour) urine collections. Alternately, protein and creatinine ratio may be determined in a random sample, preferably the first morning urine specimen. The normal ratio is less than 0.2. A ratio greater than 3.0 usually indicates heavy proteinuria and NS.

In patients with diabetic nephropathy, proteinuria by a positive dipstick reading is a relatively late event, usually indicating considerable damage to glomerular capillaries. To detect early diabetic nephropathy, measurement of minute amounts of albumin (microalbuminuria) is done by radioimmunoassay. Special dipsticks are now available to detect microalbuminuria (3 to 20 mg/dL).

Proteinuria Detected during Screening of Asymptomatic Schoolchildren

The prevalence of proteinuria in healthy schoolchildren varies considerably (1% to 11%), depending upon the magnitude of the proteinuria and the number of samples tested for persistence of proteinuria. The prevalence of trace (≥ 10 mg) protein in the initial urine has been reported to be as high as 11%. Prevalence of 1+ protein is approximately 1% and 2+ protein is 0.2%. The prevalence of proteinuria appears to increase with age until puberty. Most children with proteinuria at a 2+ level or more have postural proteinuria. Identification of serious renal disease through screening is rare. Box 97-2 lists indications for referral to a pediatric nephrologist.

Postural or Orthostatic Proteinuria

Postural proteinuria primarily occurs in adolescents and young adults with onset beginning about 10 to 12 years of age. Children with this disorder excrete normal amounts of protein while supine. While lying down during the night children excrete less than 30 mg/m^2 and adults less than 50 mg during the 8 hours. While upright during the day affected children excrete 500 to 1000 mg (rarely more) protein. Proteinuria is always asymptomatic and is usually identified during a routine medical evaluation. Spot urine testing may show 1+ to 3+ protein during the day, but the first-voided urine in the morning is usually negative. Three different strategies can be used to confirm the presence of postural proteinuria. The first option requires the parents to evaluate all voided urine by a dipstick at home over a weekend for 36 to 48 hours. If all the night time or first-

---

Box 97-2. Indications for Referral to a Pediatric Nephrologist

Proteinuria greater than 1 g/day
Proteinuria with hematuria
Proteinuria with renal dysfunction, including increased serum creatinine or increased BUN
NS with frequent relapses or steroid-dependent or -resistant NS
Diagnosis not clear and patient needs renal biopsy for further evaluation

---

Box 97-3. Causes of Transient (Functional) Proteinuria

Exercise
Fever
Exposure to heat or cold
Congestive heart failure
Adrenaline (epinephrine) administration
Following abdominal operation

---

voided specimens in the morning are negative, but daytime (upright posture) urine samples are 1+ to 3+ for protein, a presumptive diagnosis of postural proteinuria can be made. The second option is to measure urine protein/creatinine ratio on first morning specimen voided immediately after waking up. The third option requires collection of two separate urine samples from 8:00 AM to 8:00 PM (the urine voided 8:00 AM at the beginning is discarded; start with an empty bladder and end with an empty bladder) and supine urine from 8:00 PM to 8:00 AM. During the night collection, the child must remain supine. If the postural nature of the proteinuria can be verified by the preceding tests and urinalysis is otherwise normal (no hematuria or leukocyturia), no further evaluation is necessary. If BUN, creatinine, and C3 are measured, they are normal.

Postural proteinuria is a benign condition. At 10-year follow-up, 50% of young adults with postural proteinuria still have proteinuria; in others the condition spontaneously resolves. At 20-year follow-up, only 17% continue to have proteinuria. Renal function remains normal. Although no long-term studies are available in children, they are believed to have equally good prognosis.

Transient Proteinuria

Transient proteinuria is found in several physiologic and nonrenal pathologic conditions (Box 97-3). The proteinuria is asymptomatic and usually registers 1+ to 2+, rarely 3+. Although the precise pathogenesis of proteinuria in these conditions is not known, it is thought to be mediated by angiotensin II or norepinephrine induced alterations in glomerular permeability.

Five percent of children with fever of 40°C (104°F) or higher have proteinuria. Some children may have mild proteinuria even with lesser increases in temperature to 38.3°C (101°F) or higher. Proteinuria disappears once fever resolves. Proteinuria may follow vigorous exercise. It usually spontaneously resolves within 48 hours.

"Benign" Persistent Proteinuria

Some asymptomatic children have persistent proteinuria, both during the day and when supine at night. They have normal renal function and no obvious renal or systemic abnormality. In the past, this condition was labeled benign persistent proteinuria because studies found no progression of proteinuria or deterioration of renal function over 5 years. Other studies with a 10-year follow-up have found deterioration of renal function or renal biopsy showed focal sclerosis. These findings suggest that persistent proteinuria may not always be a benign condition and all patients with persistent proteinuria need long-term follow-up with periodic blood pressure measurements, urinalysis, urine protein/

creatinine ratio, and blood chemistries. These children should be managed in consultation with a pediatric nephrologist because some may need a renal biopsy to ascertain renal damage and progression.

Proteinuria in Renal Disorders

Proteinuria may be present in a variety of renal disorders. In some disorders, proteinuria is minimal even though the underlying renal disease is of a serious nature. In other renal disorders, proteinuria is one of the major problems and may result in NS. Proteinuria has been generally grouped in the following three categories, based on 24-hour protein excretion:

Mild: less than 500 mg/m^2/day in children or less than 1000 mg/day in adults; spot urine test shows less than 1.0 mg protein per 1.0 mg creatinine.

Moderate: 500 to 2000 mg/m^2/day in children or 1000 to 3500 mg/day in adults; spot urine test shows 1.0 to 3.0 mg protein per 1.0 mg creatinine.

Severe: more than 2000 mg/m^2/day in children or over 3500 mg/day in adults; spot urine test shows more than 3.0 mg protein per 1.0 mg creatinine.

Table 97-1 lists various disorders that may present with mild, moderate, or severe proteinuria. This classification is somewhat arbitrary because the same disorder (e.g., diabetes mellitus) may start out with mild proteinuria and gradually progress to severe proteinuria. Most benign renal conditions tend to be asymptomatic and have mild proteinuria. Severe (heavy) proteinuria is identical to NS and may be present with disease onset or may develop gradually. Most patients with glomerulonephritis at onset have microhematuria or gross hematuria and coexisting moderate proteinuria; the level of proteinuria may sometimes overlap into nephrotic range proteinuria.

EVALUATION

Evaluation of a child with proteinuria should progress systematically starting with history, physical examination, and then, in an algorithmic fashion, appropriate laboratory studies. The history should elicit information about recent or past edema, hematuria, reduced or increased urine output, burning urination, fever, rash, headaches, and previous renal disease. Family history of edema, hematuria, renal disease, or diabetes should be sought. A complete physical examination should be performed with special attention to edema, hypertension, fever, and rash.

Urinalysis is performed to quantify the magnitude of proteinuria and detect the presence of coexisting hematuria, pyuria, casts, oval fat bodies, or other abnormalities. Urinary protein excretion is quantified either by 24-hour urine collection or by measuring urine protein/creatinine ratio. Supine and upright differential protein excretion should be determined if postural proteinuria is suspected.

Blood testing is based upon suspected diagnosis and may include measurement of serum creatinine, urea nitrogen, electrolytes, calcium, total protein, albumin, cholesterol, uric acid, C3, C4, antinuclear antibody (ANA), and hepatitis B and C. Renal ultrasound or DMSA may be necessary to rule out structural anomalies or reflux nephropathy. Renal biopsy is usually reserved for situations when the diagnosis is unclear, evaluating adolescents with NS, or diagnosis when there is associated hematuria.

NEPHROTIC SYNDROME

The hallmark of NS is heavy proteinuria (>2 g/m^2/day). Associated findings usually include hypoproteinemia (albumin <3.0 g/dL), generalized edema, and hypercholesterolemia (cholesterol >250 mg/dL). A wide variety of renal and systemic disorders can lead to NS in children. More than 90% of the children have idiopathic NS. Minimal change nephrotic syndrome (MCNS) is the most common lesion on biopsy (Table 97-2). In children with NS seen by pediatric nephrologists, the percentage who have focal sclerosis appears to be increasing.

Table 97-1. Disorders Causing Proteinuria

Type of Proteinemia	Disorder
Mild proteinuria: In most of these disorders, proteinuria is asymptomatic and usually other clinical and laboratory findings help point to the specific diagnosis.	Postural proteinuria Physiologic or nonrenal causes of transient proteinuria "Benign" persistent proteinuria Severe obesity Acute or chronic pyelonephritis/reflux nephropathy Renal tubular disorders, e.g., Fanconi syndrome, cystinosis, Dent's disease Congenial dysplastic lesions Chronic interstitial nephritis/analgesic abuse Hypokalemic, hypercalcemic and uric acid nephropathy Early diabetes nephropathy Early hypertensive nephropathy Early hereditary nephritis (Alport syndrome)
Moderate proteinuria: Many disorders included in this category have associated hematuria, which helps in the differential diagnosis.	Acute post-streptococcal glomerulonephritis Membranoproliferative glomerulonephritis Lupus and Schönlein-Henoch purpura nephritis Hereditary nephritis (Alport syndrome) Chronic (atrophic) pyelonephritis and reflux nephropathy Chronic interstitial nephritis/analgesic abuse Diabetic nephropathy Hypertensive nephropathy

Severe proteinuria (nephrotic syndrome): In all patients with severe proteinuria appropriate workup should be done to determine the cause.	Congenital or infantile nephrotic syndrome
	Idiopathic (primary) nephrotic syndrome
	  Minimal change
	  Focal glomerulosclerosis
	  Mesangial proliferation
	  Membranoproliferative glomerulonephritis
	  Membranous nephropathy
	Secondary nephrotic syndrome
	  Infection: secondary syphilis, quartan malaria, hepatitis B or C, human immunodeficiency virus
	  Metabolic: diabetes mellitus
	  Collagen vascular disease: lupus, Schönlein-Henoch purpura
	  Malignancy: lymphoma, Hodgkin's disease, and other malignancies
	  Drugs: nonsteroidal anti-inflammatory drugs, gold

Table 97-2. Renal Lesion in Idiopathic (Primary) Nephrotic Syndrome

Histopathologic Type	Children 1–16 years		Adults
	Unselected Group	Referred Group	
Minimal change	88–90%	75%	15–25%
Focal sclerosis	5%	10–12%	10–20%
Proliferative	5%	10–12%	15–30%
Membranous	1–2%	2%	35–40%

Modified from White RH, Glasgow EF, Mills RJ: Clinicopathological study of nephrotic syndrome in childhood. Lancet 1970;1:1353–1356 and others.

Epidemiology

NS is a relatively common chronic childhood disorder with an annual incidence of 2 to 5 per 100,000 children and a prevalence of 15 per 100,000 children. The peak age at onset is 2 to 6 years with a boy-to-girl ratio of 3:2. Three to 5% of children with MCNS have an affected sibling. Familial NS is similar to nonfamilial NS in its presentation, histopathologic features, steroid response, and clinical course.

Etiology and Pathogenesis

The etiology and the exact pathogenesis of MCNS are still unknown. There are no immune deposits or complement alterations in MCNS, unlike some other disorders resulting in NS, such as membranoproliferative glomerulonephritis or lupus. Factors that suggest that MCNS is an immune disorder due to T-cell abnormalities are response to steroids; higher incidence of allergy in MCNS patients; presence of vascular permeability factor; increased levels of IgM and decreased levels of IgG, suggesting impaired IgM-IgG switching; and presence of soluble immune response suppressor.

Proteinuria has been generally attributed to alterations in the glomerular basement membrane (GBM) porosity or loss of negative charge in the GBM. In MCNS, some studies show decreased GBM charge, but other studies do not confirm this. Recent studies suggest proteinuria results from damage to foot processes of the podocytes (glomerular visceral epithelial cells) or their interlinking, bridging slit membrane. Nephrin gene and its mutations causing alterations in the slit membrane were recently identified as the cause of the Finnish-type congenital NS, one of the most severe proteinuria disorders. Mutations in two other genes, which help anchor foot processes to GBM, are known to cause NS with focal glomerulosclerosis. Although the foot processes in MCNS show effacement (fusion), so far no other specific alterations in podocytes have been identified.

Edema in NS results from hypoalbuminemia and low oncotic pressure in peripheral capillaries as well as from yet incompletely defined mechanisms that promote increased sodium reabsorption and retention of water by renal tubules.

In NS increased infection with capsular organisms such as *Pneumococcus* and *Escherichia coli* results from loss of factor B or D of alternate complement pathway and reduced opsonization. Decrease in IgG levels and steroid treatment further increase chance of infection.

Clinical Presentation

Children with NS usually present with gradually worsening edema around the eyes upon awakening, or in the lower extremities during the day. With time the edema becomes generalized and ascites or plural effusion may develop. Parents may notice decrease in urinary output. Gross hematuria is absent. Most relapses and the initial episode often follow a viral upper respiratory infection. Some children may present with a more serious infection, such as peritonitis or pneumonia. Mild hypertension is present in 10% to 15% children with NS.

Laboratory Findings

Urinalysis usually shows 3+ to 4+ protein on a dipstick. Urine sediment is usually normal, but may show oval fat bodies or hyaline casts. Ten to 15% of children with MCNS have microscopic hematuria. In other types of NS microhematuria is present in 25% to 100% of affected children. Hemoglobin and hematocrit are usually normal, but may be increased in some children, with severe intravascular volume depletion from hemoconcentration. Erythrocyte sedimentation rate (ESR) is increased even though NS is not an inflammatory condition and the child may not have an accompanying infection. Increased erythrocyte sedimentation rate is caused by an increase in plasma fibrinogen values and loss of select proteins in urine that normally prevent RBC rouleaux formation.

Serum creatinine and BUN are usually normal, but may be slightly increased with intravascular volume depletion. Rarely they are markedly increased from accompanying acute renal failure. Serum total protein and albumin are decreased, albumin values in severe cases may be less than 1.0 g/dL. Serum lipids and cholesterol are markedly elevated. The greater the decrease in serum albumin, the greater the increase in cholesterol. C3 is normal in MCNS, but decreased in NS caused by membranoproliferative glomerulonephritis (MPGN) and lupus nephritis. Depending on the age of presentation and clinical findings, other laboratory tests may include tests for ANA, hepatitis B and C, venereal disease (VDRL), HIV (human immunodeficiency virus), and parvovirus antibody.

Renal biopsy is usually reserved for children who at presentation are younger than age 1 year or older than age 12 years, if the diagnosis is unclear, or if there is no response to 6 to 8 weeks of steroid treatment.

Management

The management of NS starts with education of the family regarding the chronic relapsing and remitting nature of the disease, the need for compliance with medicines and the low-salt diet, possible complications of the disease and its treatment, and keeping a record of proteinuria by using urine dipsticks at home. Polyvalent pneumococcal vaccine should be administered to all children with NS.

The mainstay of MCNS treatment is prednisone 2 mg/kg/day given as a single dose in the morning with a maximum of 60 mg/day. For the large adolescent (weighing more than 80 kg) sometimes prednisone 80 to 100 mg/day may be given. Once a patient has achieved sustained remission, meaning no proteinuria for 3 to 5 days, prednisone should be changed to same dose every other day for 8 expansion and diuresis, but its superiority over D₅ normal saline and furosemide has not been established. If oliguria persists despite the foregoing measures, ATN should be suspected and fluid administration reduced to prevent the possibility of developing fluid overload, edema, hypertension, or congestive heart failure.

Renal ultrasonography is the most useful test for differentiating between intrinsic ARF and postrenal ARF or identifying congenital anomalies and chronic renal failure. Renal ultrasound can detect the presence or absence of kidneys, enlarged or small scarred kidneys, dilated pelvocalyceal system, or distended bladder. Other investigative tests such as renal scans, spiral computed tomographic (CT) scan, voiding cystourethrography, or angiography may occasionally be necessary, but are generally not indicated in children with ARF.

Urgent renal biopsy is sometimes indicated to differentiate ATN from rapidly progressive glomerulonephritis or interstitial nephritis as the cause of ARF. The renal biopsy may be also helpful for guiding appropriate treatment and predicting more accurate prognosis.

MANAGEMENT

The initial care of patients with ARF is focused on treating and reversing the underlying cause(s) and correcting fluid and electrolyte imbalances. Prompt treatment of prerenal ARF with volume expanders and inotropic agents improves renal perfusion and may prevent development of intrinsic ARF. Nephrotoxic agents such as aminoglycoside antibiotics should be avoided in high-risk patients. If essential for treatment, they should be monitored meticulously, with frequent measurements of blood levels.

Once intrinsic renal failure from ATN is established, no current therapy can speed the recovery of renal function. The goal of management of ATN patients is maintenance of normal body homeostasis while awaiting spontaneous improvement.

Daily fluid intake is limited to replacement of insensible water loss (about 30% of daily recommended fluid intake for age), urinary losses, and fluid losses from nonrenal sources (e.g., nasogastric drainage). Overhydration should be avoided in patients with ARF because it can cause edema, congestive heart failure, hypertension, hyponatremia, encephalopathy, or seizures. Patients with ARF who already

have congestive heart failure or patients whose fluid intake cannot be restricted because of management of the primary or associated disorders should have continuous renal replacement therapy (CRRT) initiated early even though BUN and creatinine levels may not be markedly increased.

Children with anuria lose virtually no sodium or potassium unless they have vomiting, diarrhea, or nasogastric tube suction. Therefore, sodium intake is restricted to replacement of urinary losses (preferably by measuring daily urinary sodium excretion) and losses from other sites (if any).

Once ARF is suspected, potassium intake from all sources should be restricted. Severe hyperkalemia can often be avoided early in the course of the disease with strict adherence to potassium restriction. The level of serum potassium as well as ECG changes should be closely monitored. Patients with mild hyperkalemia may be treated with ion exchange resins; sodium polystyrene sulfonate (Kayexalate) may be given orally or by retention enema (1 to 2 hours retention) every 4 to 6 hours. Dialysis is more effective for treating hyperkalemia and may be warranted if serum potassium has been rising steadily over several days, especially if dialysis is also indicated for other reasons. In children with hyperkalemia at the onset, with serum potassium greater than 7.0 mEq/L or ECG showing tall peaked T waves and widened QRS complexes or arrhythmias, treatment should begin immediately with intravenous calcium gluconate, followed by insulin and glucose (Table 98-3). The role of sodium bicarbonate in treatment of hyperkalemia without acidosis is controversial, but most pediatric nephrologists continue to recommend its use. β_2-Adrenergic agonist agents, such as albuterol given by inhalation, are also effective in lowering serum potassium. Because the duration of action of these agents is limited, arrangements should also be made for initiating early dialysis.

Hypocalcemia and hyperphosphatemia are common in ARF, and small alterations in levels of calcium and phosphorus require no treatment. For serum phosphate levels greater than 8 mg/dL, phosphate binders such as calcium carbonate or sevelamer hydrochloride may be used. If serum calcium is less than 8 mg/dL, intravenous or oral calcium should be given to prevent tetany. Uric acid may also be markedly elevated, but does not need treatment in children.

Mild metabolic acidosis is common in ARF and requires no treatment. If blood pH is less than 7.2 or serum bicar-

Table 98-3. Treatment of Hyperkalemia in Acute Renal Failure

Drugs/modality	Dose	Onset	Duration	Mechanism	Remarks
1. Calcium gluconate 10% solution	0.5–1 mL/kg IV maximum 20 mL	1–2 min	30–60 min	Increases threshold potential	Give IV over 3–5 min; monitor heart rate
2. NaHCO₃	1–2 mEq/kg IV	5–10 min	1–2 hr	Intracellular shift of potassium	Give IV over 10–15 min; may cause tetany
3. Insulin and glucose	0.1–0.2 μ/kg/hr IV 25% glucose 1–3 mL/kg/hr	30–60 min	2–4 hr	Intracellular shift of potassium	Do not exceed 0.8 g glucose/kg/hr; monitor glucose qh
4. Albuterol inhalation or IV albuterol	5 mg to 20 mg by nebulizer 0.25 to 0.5 mg IV	30–60 min	2–4 hr	Intracellular shift of potassium	Dose is 2 to 8 times higher than for asthma
5. Kayexalate with 10–20% glucose or sorbitol	1 g/kg/dose Oral or enema	1–4 hr	Few hr	Removal of potassium	1–2 hr retention enema
6. Hemodialysis		30 min–1 hr	Several hr	Removal of potassium	Technical difficulties

bonate is less that 12 mEq/L, sodium bicarbonate may be administered cautiously so as not to precipitate tetany.

Adequate nutrition is important in ARF because it prevents excessive tissue breakdown. If renal failure is expected to be short in duration (3 to 4 days), most calories may be provided as carbohydrates. If ARF is expected to last longer, adequate calories in the form of carbohydrates along with daily protein intake of 1 g/kg should be provided.

Low-dose dopamine has often been recommended as a renoprotective drug in ARF; however, no clear experimental or clinical data from well-controlled studies support such a claim. Once intrinsic ARF has developed, use of continuous furosemide drip or repeated administration of high-dose furosemide in controlled studies has shown few benefits, does not improve outcome, and may cause ototoxicity. Several other drugs, such as atrial natriuretic peptides, calcium-channel blockers, ATP-MgCl$_2$, thyroxine, prostaglandin E$_1$, theophylline, insulin-like growth factors (IGF-1), antiendothelin receptor antagonists, anti-ICAM-1 antibodies, and platelet-activating factor antagonists, have been used experimentally in animals and for some of these drugs in human trials also, with variable results. In human ARF, none of these treatments has shown consistent benefit, and some have actually shown overall deterioration.

Many children with ARF can be managed by the conservative measures described here. If renal failure lasts more than 5 to 7 days or if complications develop, however, dialysis should be performed. On the other hand, critically ill children with multiorgan failure including ARF, usually require early introduction of continuous renal replacement therapy by hemofiltration or hemodiafiltration.

The usual indications for dialysis include uncontrollable hyperkalemia or acidosis, volume overload with potential for pulmonary edema or congestive heart failure, and progressive uremia with BUN greater than 120 mg/dL or creatinine greater than 6 to 8 mg/dL. The choice of peritoneal dialysis versus hemodialysis or hemofiltration is usually based upon the primary disorder, clinical condition of the child, availability of the technique, and experience of the center providing care.

CLINICAL COURSE

Nonoliguric ARF is generally associated with a shorter clinical course than oliguric ARF. The duration of oliguria in ARF may be short (1 to 2 days) or long (a few weeks). Recovery is usually first indicated by an increase in urinary output. BUN and creatinine may rise during the first few days of diuresis before beginning to return to normal. During diuresis, large quantities of sodium and potassium may be lost in the urine. Serum electrolytes should be closely monitored during this phase, and adequate replacements should be made to prevent hyponatremia or hypokalemia.

PROGNOSIS

In children with ARF, the prognosis largely depends upon the primary condition, the severity of damage to the kidneys and other organs, and physician expertise in managing ARF and critically ill children. Most children with ATN recover complete renal function usually within 4 to 6 weeks. In some children, recovery may extend over several months. Children with more severe renal damage from renal cortical necrosis or rapidly progressive glomerulonephrosis may develop residual renal impairment or chronic renal failure. Although, it has often been stated that mortality rate from ARF in adults has remained unchanged for the past several decades and continues to be in the 30% to 60% range, closer review suggests that this reflects inclusion of progressively more severely ill patients with ARF during this period. In a recent study of pediatric patients with ARF, no deaths occurred in children in whom a primary urinary tract disorder was the cause of ARF.

Mini-index of Related Topics

	CH.
▪ SHOCK	28
▪ CARDIAC FAILURE	30
▪ HYPERTENSIVE CRISIS	40
▪ GLUCOSE AND ELECTROLYTE DISORDERS	42
▪ HEMATURIA AND GLOMERULAR DISORDERS	96
▪ FLUIDS AND ELECTROLYTES	292

SUGGESTED READINGS

Anand, SK: Acute renal failure (in the newborn infant). In Taeusch HW, Ballard RA, Avery ME (eds): Diseases of the Newborn, 6th ed. Philadelphia, WB Saunders, 1991, pp 892–897.

Brady HR, Brenner BM, Clarkson MR, Lieberthal W: Acute renal failure. In Brenner BM (ed): The Kidney, 6th ed. Philadelphia, WB Saunders, 2000, pp 1201–1262.

Lameire N, Vanholder R: Pathophysiologic features and prevention of human and experimental acute tubular necrosis. Am Soc Nephrol J 2001;17:S33–39.

Sehic A, RW Chesney: Acute renal failure: Diagnosis and the therapy. Pediatr Rev 1995;16:101–106, 137–141.

Thadani R, Pascual M, Bonventre JV: Acute renal failure. N Engl J Med 1996;334:1448–1460.

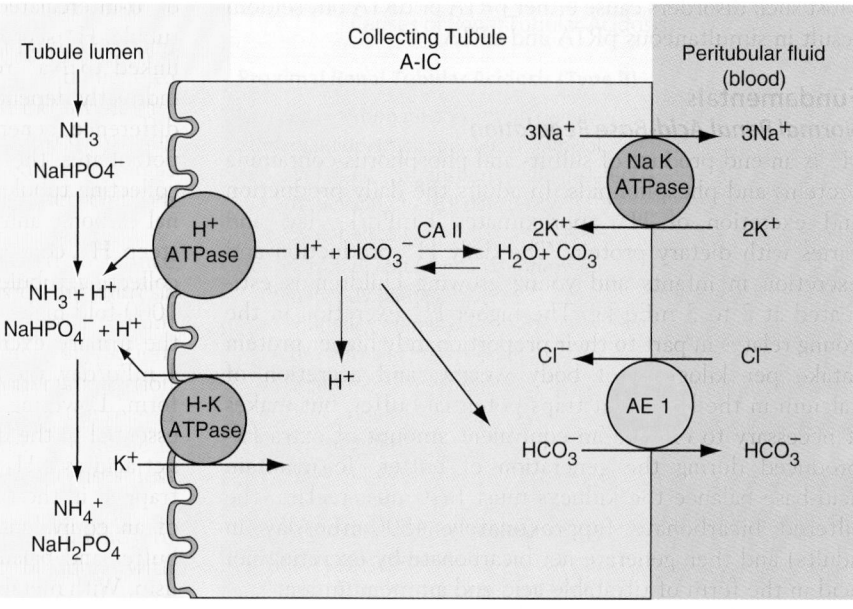

Figure 99-2. H$^+$ secretion and excretion of net acid, NH$_4$, and titratable acid in collecting tubule. (Modified from Anand SK: Renal tubular disorders. A-IC, alpha intercalated cells. In Taeusch HW, Ballard RA, Avery ME (eds): Diseases of the Newborn, 6th ed. Philadelphia, WB Saunders, 1991, pp 920–926.)

(albeit at a lower plasma HCO$_3^-$ value), because the distal tubular function is normal, the secreted H$^+$ allows urine pH to become less than 5.5. This allows excretion of NH$_4^+$ and titratable acid in sufficient amount to balance the daily metabolic production of H$^+$. The new bicarbonate threshold usually varies between 12 and 18 mEq/L.

Proximal RTA may occur as an isolated defect in the reabsorption of HCO$_3$ (at normal plasma HCO$_3^-$ values), but more commonly occurs as a component of a generalized defect in proximal tubular reabsorption including glycosuria, generalized aminoaciduria, and phosphaturia (Fanconi syndrome).

Distal (Classic) Type I Renal Tubular Acidosis

Distal RTA may occur from inability of the α-intercalated cells of collecting tubules to adequately secrete H$^+$, secondary to mutations in H$^+$-ATPase located in the luminal border or to mutations in AE1 transporter in the basolateral membrane (see Fig. 99-2) that normally allows return of HCO$_3^-$ from cell to blood. A defect in AE1 results in accumulation of HCO$_3^-$ in cells and a decrease in further secretion of H$^+$. Either of these two defects results in failure of urine pH to fall below 6.0 and leads to minimal excretion of net H$^+$ as NH$_4^+$ or titratable acid. Thus, in distal RTA even during severe metabolic acidosis (unlike proximal RTA) net H$^+$ is markedly diminished, leading to consumption of body buffer reserves in bone and gradually worsening acidosis. Hypercalciuria, hypokalemia, and hypocitraturia frequently accompany distal RTA. Nephrocalcinosis is common. Hypokalemia results from increased K$^+$ secretion in the collecting tubule that is unable to secrete H$^+$. Distal RTA may be a primary inherited disorder or may occur secondary to a number of disorders listed in Box 99-2.

Hyperkalemic, Type IV Renal Tubular Acidosis

Hyperkalemic RTA results from a decrease in sodium reabsorption in the collecting tubule or a decrease in the amount of sodium reaching the collecting tubule, both of which impair generation of a negative electrical potential difference necessary for maximal secretion of H$^+$ and K$^+$.

The ability of the collecting tubule to lower urine pH below 5.5, however, is maintained. The disorder is typically seen in children with aldosterone deficiency or reduced tubular responsiveness to aldosterone.

Diagnosis

Clinical Presentation

Inherited forms of RTA usually present during the first 18 months of life with nonspecific findings including failure to thrive, irritability, vomiting, constipation, polyuria, polydipsia, dehydration, and deep breathing from acidosis. In infants older than 9 months, rickets may be present. Other clinical findings depend upon the type of RTA and the primary disorder that led to RTA. In some patients RTA is identified during investigation of an unrelated disorder.

Evaluation

The laboratory characteristics of various types of RTA are summarized in Table 99-3. The diagnosis of RTA should be considered in any infant who presents with hyperchloremic metabolic acidosis (normal anion gap) and in whom other causes of metabolic acidosis have been excluded. The urine pH should always be interpreted in relationship to plasma bicarbonate values. A persistently alkaline urine (or pH >6.0), irrespective of the severity of metabolic acidosis, is strongly suggestive of distal RTA. Urinary citrate is reduced. In distal RTA at presentation or during induced metabolic acidosis, urinary cation gap Cl$^-$ − (Na$^+$ + K$^+$) is ≤ 0, whereas in normal persons during metabolic acidosis the cation gap is greater than 20 mEq/L because of the excretion of NH$_4^+$. Patients with proximal RTA at presentation (during metabolic acidosis) frequently have a urine pH value less than 6.0. However, when serum bicarbonate level is raised above the set threshold level by alkali therapy, the urine pH promptly becomes alkaline (even though serum bicarbonate values remain less than what is usually considered normal for age). Because most patients with proximal RTA have Fanconi syndrome, urine should be screened for aminoaciduria, phosphaturia, glycosuria, and excretion of small-molecular-weight proteins (e.g., β$_2$–microglobulin).

Table 99-3. Clinical and Laboratory Characteristics of Various Types of Renal Tubular Acidosis

Laboratory Feature	Type I (Distal, Classic)	Type II (Proximal)	Type IV (Hyperkalemic)
During acidosis (low serum bicarbonate)			
Urine pH	>6.0	<5.5	<5.5
Serum potassium	N or ↓	N or ↓	↑
Urine Cl^- – (Na^+ + K^+)	≤0	>20	?
Urinary citrate	↓	↑	?
Aminoaciduria, glycosuria	–	±	–
Titratable acid and ammonium excretion	↓	N or ↓	↓
Following therapy (normal bicarbonate)			
Fractional excretion of bicarbonate	3%–5%	>15%	1%–5%
Serum potassium	N	N or ↓	N or ↑
Urinary-blood P_{CO_2} difference	<20	>20	<20
Daily alkali treatment (mEq/kg/day)	1–4	5–20	1–4
Nephrocalcinosis	Common	Rare	Absent

N, normal.

Type IV RTA should be suspected when the patient has persistent hyperkalemia with hyperchloremic metabolic acidosis. Plasma renin and aldosterone should be measured to help determine the cause of type IV RTA.

Radiographs of long bones may show rickets both in distal and proximal RTA. In distal RTA rickets occurs from hypercalciuria and undefined mechanisms, and in Fanconi syndrome (proximal RTA) rickets are due to hypophosphatemia and alterations in vitamin D metabolism. Renal ultrasound may identify nephrocalcinosis both in distal RTA as well as in Dent's disease causing proximal RTA.

Usually these tests are sufficient to confirm the diagnosis and differentiate between various types of RTA. If the diagnosis is in doubt, patients may require bicarbonate titration studies, measurement of fractional excretion of bicarbonate and urinary/blood P_{CO_2} gradient, or measurement of urinary excretion of NH_4 and titrable acid in order to differentiate between various types of acidosis (see Table 99-3).

Treatment

The therapy for RTA is relatively simple but demands sustained compliance to maintain normal serum bicarbonate and potassium levels. Patients with severe metabolic acidosis and hypokalemia should be treated initially with intravenous therapy. Otherwise, most patients can be managed by oral therapy. Patients may be given sodium bicarbonate or sodium citrate, usually administered as Bicitra. Most patents also require supplementation with potassium citrate. Most patients with distal RTA require 2 to 3 mEq/kg/day of sodium bicarbonate or an equivalent citrate given in three or four divided doses.

Patients with proximal RTA may require 5 to 15 mEq/kg/day of sodium bicarbonate to maintain normal serum bicarbonate and pH values. Patients with Fanconi syndrome also require phosphate supplementation and treatment with calcitriol (1:25 $(OH)_2$ D_3) or some other vitamin D analog. Some patients with proximal RTA do not tolerate such high doses of bicarbonate therapy and may benefit from thiazide diuretics (hydrochlorothiazide 1 mg/kg/day). The thiazide diuretics increase proximal tubular reabsorption of bicarbonate by inducing extracellular volume contraction. Patients with type IV RTA and aldosterone deficiency usually benefit from use of a mineralocorticoid (fluorohydrocortisone). Other patients with type IV RTA require 1 to 2 mEq/kg/day of sodium bicarbonate to correct acidosis. Patients with Gordon syndrome need to be treated with thiazide diuretics.

Prognosis

Although patients with distal RTA caused by H^+-ATPase mutations have a lifelong disorder, with early recognition and adequate sustained therapy normal growth may be achieved. Bicarbonate therapy in some patients is able to prevent nephrocalcinosis, but is often ineffective in improving nephrocalcinosis that is already present. Bicarbonate therapy is ineffective in preventing or improving deafness in patients with *ATP6B1* mutation. Patients with inadequate therapy of acidosis develop growth retardation, progressive nephrocalcinosis, and ultimately renal failure.

Most infants with isolated proximal RTA usually have a transient disorder lasting a few months to a few years. Although they initially require a large amount of bicarbonate therapy, their long-term prognosis is excellent. The prognosis in patients with Fanconi syndrome depends on the cause of the syndrome. Similarly, prognosis of type IV RTA depends upon the cause of the disorder.

Mini-index of Related Topics   CH.

SUGGESTED READINGS

Chan JCM, Scheinman JI, Roth KS: Renal tubular acidosis. Pediatr Rev 2001;22:277–297.

Leung AKC, Robson WLM, Halperin ML: Polyuria in childhood. Clin Pediatr 1991;30:634–640.

Scheinman SJ, Guay-Woodford L, Thakker RV, Warnock DG: Genetic disorders of renal electrolyte transport. N Engl J Med 1999;340:1177–1187.

Soriano JR: Renal tubular acidosis: The clinical entity. J Am Soc Nephrol 2002;13:2160–2170.

Watnick T, Germino GG: Introduction to genetic renal disease. In Schrier RW (ed): Diseases of the Kidney and Urinary Tract, 7th ed. Philadelphia, Lippincott Williams & Wilkins, 2001, pp 491–519.

100 Urinary Tract Infections

Sudhir K. Anand

Urinary tract infection (UTI) is the most common genitourinary disorder affecting infants and children. These infections cause acute morbidity and occasionally result in long-term problems. UTIs may be asymptomatic or may present with urinary or systemic symptoms and are occasionally accompanied by sepsis. In most children UTIs resolve completely. In a few children, especially those with recurrent pyelonephritis, delayed or inadequate treatment, vesicoureteral reflux (VUR), or obstructive uropathy, UTIs may lead to renal scarring and sometimes are a risk factor for development of hypertension or end-stage renal failure in later childhood.

FUNDAMENTALS

Clinical Presentation

UTI is usually identified in one of the following three clinical settings:

- *Acute pyelonephritis* is a symptomatic infection of renal parenchyma and is characterized by one or more of the following clinical findings: high fever, chills, flank or abdominal pain, nausea, vomiting, dysuria (burning urination), frequency, foul-smelling urine, and costovertebral angle tenderness. Clinical findings in the newborn and young infants are nonspecific and include fever, irritability, poor weight gain (or loss), vomiting, and jaundice. In infants with sepsis, temperature instability, cyanosis, or disseminated intravascular coagulation (DIC) may occur. Chronic pyelonephritis implies scarred kidneys caused by a previous pyelonephritis usually demonstrated by a nuclear scan or an intravenous pyelogram.

- *Cystitis* implies infection localized to the bladder and is characterized clinically by dysuria, frequency, urgency or hesitancy, foul-smelling urine, and suprapubic pain or tenderness. Rarely, gross hematuria is present. Fever, if present, is low grade. Urethritis, usually from a venereal disease, in the teenager may mimic cystitis. In many young children and 10% to 20% schoolchildren, it is hard to differentiate between acute pyelonephritis and cystitis because of overlapping findings. When symptoms are overlapping, children should be regarded as having pyelonephritis and managed accordingly.

- *Asymptomatic bacteriuria* and *screening bacteriuria* are synonymous terms that refer to bacteriuria identified by dipstick or culture during screening of healthy children receiving routine physical care. Screening bacteriuria is a preferable term because some affected children, on close questioning, actually have symptoms such as perineal irritation, dysfunctional voiding, and daytime or nighttime incontinence.

Epidemiology

Symptomatic UTIs occur in approximately 0.4% to 1% of newborns and young infants. In the first 2 to 3 months of life UTI is more common in boys than girls, and about 5 to 10 times more common in uncircumcised boys than circumcised boys. After 3 to 6 months of life the incidence and prevalence of UTIs becomes higher in girls than boys and circumcision status is less significant. The prevalence of UTI is 3% to 8% among febrile infants younger than 24 months who do not have another potential source of fever on clinical evaluation. UTIs seem to be more common in white infants and children than in other races.

PATHOPHYSIOLOGY

UTI is an ascending infection in almost all children except in some newborn infants, immunocompromised hosts, and children with overwhelming systemic infection, in whom it may be blood-borne. The pathogenesis of bacteria ascending from urethra to bladder and kidney and causing UTI involves interaction between various bacterial factors and protective host defense mechanisms.

Bacterial Factors

Many microorganisms can colonize the urinary tract, but the overwhelming majority of symptomatic UTIs in children are caused by gram-negative bacteria. In immunocompromised children *Candida* or other fungi may colonize or cause invasive infection. Adenovirus 11 and occasionally other viruses cause hemorrhagic cystitis in children. *Escherichia coli* accounts for 80% to 90% of first infections. The remainder are caused by *Proteus, Klebsiella, Enterobacter,* and gram-positive cocci *Enterococcus* and *Staphylococcus saprophyticus*. *S. saprophyticus* (a coagulase-negative staphylococcus) infections are primarily seen in adolescents with UTI. *Pseudomonas* primarily causes infection in children with recurrent infections and those who have been previously treated with antibiotics or have undergone previous catheterization or other instrumentation.

Most bacteria that cause UTIs originate from the fecal flora and enter the urinary tract by an ascending route. In girls prone to UTIs, the bacteria first colonize the introitus, periurethral skin, and distal urethra before inducing infection. Factors that predispose bacteria to adhere to uroepithelium and cause infection are not well understood. Bacterial adhesion in *E. coli* is mediated by fimbriae, which are fine, hairlike projections from the bacterial cell wall. In many children with acute pyelonephritis, UTI is caused by *E. coli* with P-fimbriae, which adhere to *Gal-Gal* receptors on uroepithelium; however, in the majority of children with VUR and renal scarring, the infection is caused by *E. coli* that lack P-fimbriae.

Host Factors
Host factors that contribute to the pathogenesis of UTI include age and gender of the child, family history and genetic makeup, VUR (see Chapter 172 for discussion of vesicoureteral reflux), abnormal voiding habits leading to incomplete bladder emptying and residual urine, labial adhesions, severe constipation, and immune response to bacterial colonization and infection. In teenage girls sexual activity and pregnancy may further contribute to UTIs. The uroepithelium of school-age girls and adult women who develop recurrent UTIs binds *E. coli* more avidly than uroepithelium from nonsusceptible persons, perhaps because of higher density or type of receptors, and this predisposition is in part genetically determined. Urinary tract obstruction, neurogenic bladder dysfunction, or other anomalies contribute to development of UTIs in less than 5% of children.

EVALUATION

The evaluation of a child with UTI should proceed in a systematic manner, starting with history, physical examination, appropriate urine collection for urinalysis and urine culture, and then proceeding to other tests (Fig. 100-1). Clinical findings in the newborn and young infants are often nonspecific. Therefore, a high degree of suspicion for UTIs must be maintained and a urine culture obtained in all infants and young children with fever without an apparent source. In male infants and young boys, one should inquire about the force of the urinary stream and the presence of urinary dribbling. In older children, besides the typical clinical findings described earlier, history of previous UTIs, dysfunctional voiding, daytime or nighttime enuresis, and constipation should also be sought.

A complete physical examination should be performed with special attention to the presence of abdominal masses; costovertebral or suprapubic tenderness; genitalia for severe phimosis in boys; introital or labial redness, labial adhesions, or vulvovaginitis in girls; dribbling of urine and wet underwear. The lumbosacral area should be examined for anomalies such as hair tuft or sinus tract suggestive of spina bifida occulta. In children with constipation, a rectal examination may be indicated.

Laboratory Tests
The diagnosis of UTI is established by documenting significant bacteriuria; however, a dipstick test or complete urinalysis (Table 100-1) can be performed rapidly, and a positive result from these tests is highly suggestive of UTI in a child who presents with positive clinical findings and suggests the need for antibiotic treatment, pending culture results.

In young infants not yet 24 months old with fever in whom UTI is considered or suspected, a urine specimen for culture should always be obtained by catheterization or bladder puncture. Bag urine sample has a high contamination rate, making it unsuitable for evaluation of an acute infection. In older children who have attained bladder control, a midstream urine collection is satisfactory for urine culture. To reduce contamination of midstream urine, it is advisable to position girls facing backward on the toilet seat to help spread the labia apart during urination.

Most patients with a UTI have urine bacterial counts greater than 100,000/mL on a voided or catheterized urine sample. However, some infected children and adult women have counts of less than 1000/mL. In urine samples obtained by suprapubic puncture, growth of any organism is significant unless the organisms grown are skin contaminants. Midstream "clean catch" urine is usually considered positive if it grows 100,000/mL or more of a single organism, and counts between 10,000 and 100,000 are considered suspect and need to be reconfirmed with a second specimen. In catheterized urine samples, colony counts greater than 10,000/mL of a pathogenic organism are considered positive. Counts between 1000 and 10,000 of pure growth of a single organism are also considered positive if the patient has clinical findings or urinalysis suggestive of UTI; otherwise, the count may be considered indeterminate.

Urine dipstick, routine urinalysis, and Gram stain of the urine are rapid tests that are quite sensitive and specific in diagnosing UTI (see Table 100-1); however, the diagnosis of UTI should not be based on these tests alone. The diagnosis needs to be confirmed by urine culture. Many young infants with UTIs (20% to 50% who are less than 8 weeks old) may not manifest leukocyturia; thus, their diagnosis is substantiated only by a positive urine culture. Moreover, leukocyturia may occur in other renal disorders in the absence of UTI. The false negative rate for the nitrite test is nearly 50% in children with UTI.

Erythrocyte sedimentation rate (ESR) and C-reactive protein are increased in infants and children with high fever and findings suggestive of acute pyelonephritis. On the other hand, children with cystitis tend to have normal results. These tests, however, are nonspecific and by themselves are not very useful in deciding the need for further urinary evaluation or antibiotic treatment. Moreover, in young children, either upper or lower urinary tract infections mandate imaging studies described next.

SUGGESTED READINGS

Leppik IE: Contemporary Diagnosis and Management of the Patient with Epilepsy, 5th ed. Newton, Pa., Handbooks in Health Care, 2000.

Schacter SC, Schomer DL: The Comprehensive Evaluation and Treatment of Epilepsy: A Practical Guide. New York, Academic Press, 1997.

Shields WD: Catastrophic epilepsy in childhood. Epilepsia 2000; 41(suppl 2):S2–6.

SECTION 3 GENERAL MEDICAL CARE: *Disorders of the Nervous System*

104 Approach to the Child with Breath-Holding Spells

Kenneth Huff

ROLE OF THE GENERALIST

1 Distinguish breath holding from other paroxysmal behaviors by history.

2 Rule out less benign entities when the history is questionable.

3 Reassure parents.

Breath-holding spells are a common paroxysmal nonepileptic behavior in infants that has been recognized for centuries. Despite the frightening appearance of the spells, they are benign and self-limited in the majority of cases. Children are otherwise healthy and develop normally. Pharmacologic intervention is rarely necessary.

Two primary types of breath-holding spells have been described: (1) the more common cyanotic breath-holding spells and (2) the probable vagally mediated pallid infantile syncope. Both are circumstantially provoked and result in a brief loss of responsiveness related to cerebral anoxia but have different pathophysiologic mechanisms. The distinction of type of spell is relevant to the presentation and to prognosis for later syncope in the latter type of spell.

DEFINITION

The syndrome is defined by the behavior during an episode. Spells occur when the infant is awake. Infants undergo a relatively stereotypic sequence of events that include being emotionally upset (usually related to fear or anger) in response to a provocative happenstance (such as a minor fall or a toy being removed from them), followed by crying, with a subsequent silent attempt at expiration, color change, and often, loss of consciousness. Cyanotic breath-holding spells, the most common, are accompanied by glottis closure in expiration. After several seconds of apnea, cyanosis develops. The spell may terminate at this point, or the child may proceed to lose consciousness. The pallid spells occur after a briefer initial cry with more rapid loss of consciousness and are accompanied by a brief period of asystole. Following loss of consciousness most children are limp, although a minority have a few clonic jerks or develop rigid opisthotonic posturing before becoming atonic. Normal respiration is then resumed. Children usually regain responsiveness shortly, frequently seem tired for several minutes, but then resume normal play.

FUNDAMENTALS

The prevalence of breath-holding spells in all children ages 6 months to 6 years is 5%. Although breath-holding spells are related to developmental stage and familial tendency, their pathophysiology is not well understood. The age of onset is 6 to 12 months with only 15% beginning before 6 months. The peak frequency is at 12 to 18 months of age, and spells usually end by age 3 years, although some have continued to age 7 years. Affected children frequently have several spells a week. Boys and girls are equally affected. Thirty-four percent have a positive family history. Because there is a high incidence in proband parents and sibs, an autosomal dominant mode of transmission with variable expressivity is proposed. Affected children have a normal developmental history, no past history of neurologic or respiratory problems, and a normal neurologic examination. No single behavioral profile other than the occurrence of the paroxysms identifies children with breath-holding spells. Some breath-holding infants may have more sleep disturbances than other children. In one study monitoring a single night, breath-holding infants had less stage III sleep, more arousals and stage changes, more sweating, and more frequent and longer airway obstructions than control infants.

Cerebral anoxia is the factor ultimately responsible for the loss of consciousness observed in breath-holding spells. This occurs either from lack of oxygen intake through nonventilation combined with Valsalva maneuver and preceding hypocapnia in the cyanotic spells or from lack of cardiac output to supply the brain in the pallid spells. Children with cyanotic spells may have an underlying autonomic dysregulation as evidenced by mildly abnormal postural autonomic parameters produced by evocative tests (greater pulse increase and diastolic pressure decrease with rising from supine to standing). Valsalva maneuver and an abnormal reflexive glottis closure may also be part of this dysregulation. Voluntary breath holding has been used as a technique to assist with functional brain magnetic resonance imaging by assessing cerebral oxidative metabolism and blood oxygen level dependency functions related to changes in cerebral vessel dilation from hypercapnia. The pathogenesis of cyanotic breath-holding spells does not seem to involve an insensitivity to hypercapnia or hypoxia.

Pallid syncope is associated with vagally induced asystole during the initial stage of the spell. There may be less respiratory sinus arrhythmia related to a primary parasympathetic disturbance in children with pallid syncope compared to children with cyanotic spells or children without any spells. There may also be autonomic dysregulation with a greater decrease in mean arterial pressure and pulse rate with rising to standing. The diagnosis of pallid infantile syncope is supported by performing an ocular compression polygraph. The polygraph relies on surprise and ocular pain to provoke a spell and to produce several seconds of asystole, which is vagally mediated. Though this test illustrates a physiologic mechanism, it is rarely necessary for the diagnosis, because the historical description is sufficient. Pallid breath-holding spells may be related to preterm bradycardic spells, apparent life-threatening events, and sudden infant death syndrome through the mechanism of paroxysmal vagal overactivity.

DIAGNOSIS

Key factors in the diagnosis of breath-holding spells are an identifiable precipitating event or emotion, often accompanied by crying and a normal neurodevelopmental history and examination (Table 104-1). Information about what the child did during the spell and the child's color before and during the spell, and a family history of similar spells in infancy is useful. If the description is unclear or atypical, standard electroencephalogram (EEG), video EEG (if spells are frequent and if the standard interictal EEG is normal), electrocardiogram (ECG), or sleep studies should be considered.

Breath-holding spells are largely an infantile disorder, not occurring in the neonatal period and rarely after preschool age. In the latter group, seizures are a diagnostic consideration. Seizures are not usually accompanied by precipitating factors and may also occur at night. Seizures may be accompanied by a rapid fall and by tonic stiffening unless they are atonic seizures. Breath-holding spells rarely have opisthotonus if any stiffening occurs, and if opisthotonus or any rhythmic jerking occurs, it happens after prolonged apnea and color change. Atonic seizures do have a brief loss of tone, but occur most frequently in children with an abnormal neurologic examination, developmental delay, and an EEG with generalized polyspike discharges or rhythmic slowing interictally. Apnea has been reported as an isolated manifestation of seizures in infants, but such spells are unprovoked and accompanied by either an abnormal interictal EEG or abnormal video EEG. Seizures are known to elevate prolactin levels acutely, whereas breath-holding spells do not.

Startle disease begins in infancy, is dominantly inherited, and does not generally completely remit by school age. Attacks are provoked in response to tactile, auditory, or visual stimuli in infants, or emotional stress in older children. They may occur in sleep. Exaggerated startling is often accompanied by clonus or sometimes loss of muscle tone. Crying is absent unless the individual was truly injured by a subsequent fall caused by the startle reaction. No loss of consciousness occurs. In the minor form, there

Table 104-1. Diagnosis of Breath-Holding Spells

Feature	Breath Holding	Atonic Seizures	Startle Disease	Central Apnea	Obstructive Apnea	Gastric Reflux	Benign Vertigo	Cardiogenic Syncope	Cataplexy
Age	Infant	All	Infant	Neonate	Older child	Infant	Preschool	Older child	Adolescent
Neurodevelopment	Normal	Abnormal	Abnormal	Normal	Normal	Normal	Normal	Normal	Normal
Electroencephalogram	Normal	Abnormal	Normal	Normal	Normal	Normal	Normal	Normal	Abnormal
Family history	Yes	No	Yes	No	No	No	Yes	Some	Some
Crying	Yes	No	No	No	No	Yes	No	No	No
Loss of consciousness	Yes	Yes	No	Yes	Yes	No	No	Yes	No
Spells provoked	Yes	No	Yes	No	No	No	No	No	Yes
Sleep	No	Yes	Yes	Yes	Yes	Yes	No	Some	Yes
Follows feeding	No	No	No	No	No	Yes	No	No	No
Nystagmus	No	No	No	No	No	No	Yes	No	No
Abnormal electrocardiogram	No	No	No	No	Some	No	No	Yes	No
Tone stiff	Some	Yes	Yes	No	No	Yes	No	No	No
Aura	No	No	No	No	No	No	No	Yes	No

757

are no associated neurologic abnormalities, but in the major form, hypertonia, hyperreflexia, clonus, spasticity, and gait ataxia are found.

Central and obstructive apnea must be distinguished from breath-holding spells. Central apnea may be related to prematurity. Spells occur most often in sleep. They are not provoked by external circumstances but can be aborted by stimulated arousal. Persistent, severe sleep apnea, or "Ondine's curse," necessitates artifical ventilation during sleep. Obstructive apnea also occurs in sleep but is usually seen in older children. It is related to deficient pharyngeal muscle tone or excessive weight of tissue in the pharynx, airway, or chest wall that impairs air movement during automatic respiratory drive in sleep. Diagnosis is confirmed by overnight sleep study.

Gastroesophageal reflux, a recurrent syndrome of infancy, is accompanied by color change, hypertonicity, posturing including opisthotonus, and a startled expression on the child's face. Episodes are not stimulated by external provocative factors, and there is no more than momentary loss of responsiveness. Generally episodes follow feeding.

Benign paroxysmal vertigo also occurs in the preschool child, may have a sudden onset, and can cause the child to become pale, frightened, and drop to the floor. Episodes last longer than a few minutes. The child is not unresponsive or unconscious and exhibits nystagmoid eye movements during the spell. Children with benign paroxysmal vertigo often have a positive family history of migraine.

Cardiogenic syncope and mitral valve prolapse syndrome may mimic breath-holding spells in the older child. These conditions persist past the age of 6 years. Congenital and acquired cardiac conditions, including mitral prolapse, can produce arrhythmias or Stokes-Adams attacks as the basis for cardiogenic syncope. Generally there are no precipitating factors. The patient may experience palpitations, light-headedness, vertigo, or fading vision before the loss of consciousness, followed by momentary confusion and lethargy. A longer period of cerebral ischemia may be accompanied by convulsive symptoms. The potential for cardiogenic syncope caused by arrhythmias or prolonged QTc (corrected QT interval) syndrome is confirmed by ECG and by tilt table testing.

Cataplexy is characterized by sudden falling with loss of tone or the sensation of wobbly knees following an emotional stimulus such as surprise, anger, or laughter. Attacks last only a few seconds. It is very rare before adolescence. Consciousness and memory are completely preserved. Attacks are typical in patients with narcolepsy. There is also a relationship with paralysis experienced while entering REM (rapid eye movement) sleep. Polysomnography discloses the characteristic abnormal pattern of REM sleep at the onset of sleep.

MANAGEMENT

Management is simple reassurance regarding the benign self-limited nature of the breath-holding spells and parental support for limit setting if spells occur in the course of discipline. Education about spells reduces parental anxiety. A spell brought on by child frustration with caretaker limit setting should not be a reason to forgo the latter. Generally, pharmacologic therapy is neither effective nor necessary.

A subgroup of infants with breath-holding spells have iron deficiency anemia. Iron therapy may treat not only the anemia, but also the breath-holding spells. Pallid infantile syncope may respond to atropine sulfate, which is used on an ongoing basis if spells are frequent, or intermittently if spells are situationally predictable (such as with venipuncture).

Seizures lasting longer than 10 minutes have been known to occur following breath-holding spells. Presumably these seizures occur in individuals with a familial predisposition and a lowered seizure threshold. The temporary ischemic insult from the breath-holding spell precipitates neuronal depolarization leading to an ictal event. Such rare occurrences have been effectively aborted acutely by intravenous anticonvulsants. Prolonged seizures have been effectively prevented with oral anticonvulsants that predictably do not prevent the breath-holding spells.

OUTCOME

Although breath-holding spells may recur frequently in infancy, they generally have a good long-term prognosis and resolve by early childhood. In a prospectively studied cohort of 95 children, the peak frequency of spells occurred between 12 and 18 months. The median frequency of spells was weekly but 30% had daily spells. The oldest age at time of latest spell was 7 years, and most resolved by 4 years. In this study, hypoxic convulsions occurred in less than 15% of the subjects. Infants who have had pallid infantile syncope sometimes present later in childhood with syncopal spells, usually of the vasodepressor type.

Breath-holding spells are not generally associated with behavioral difficulties in the child. In another prospective study, children in whom breath-holding spells were identified at age 3 years showed no differences from control subjects in problems of behavior or development when studied 5 years later. However, other evidence suggests mothers of children with breath-holding spells may experience more stress and disruption of their attachment or understanding of their child compared with control mothers.

FOLLOW-UP

Follow-up should include an assessment of subsequent spells including a precise description to determine if there is any change in impressions about the nature of atypical spells. An assessment of efficacy of iron therapy should be made if such treatment was initiated. Family anxiety must be addressed along with further education and reassurance. In severely disruptive situations, referral for counseling or family therapy may be needed, but in most cases families are able to adapt over time to the benign nature of the condition.

⊙ **Additional Resources, CD-ROM**	
Breath-holding spell	Video 104-1
Bibliography	

SUGGESTED READINGS

Breningstall GN: Breath-holding spells. Pediatr Neurol 1996; 14(2):91–97.
DiMario FJ: Breath-holding spells in childhood. Am J Dis Child 1992;146(1):125–131.

DiMario FJ: Prospective study of children with cyanotic and pallid breath-holding spells. Pediatrics 2001;107(2):265–269.
Evans OB: Breath-holding spells. Pediatr Ann 1997;26(7):410–414.
Saul JP: Syncope: Etiology, management, and when to refer. J S C Med Assoc 1999;95(10):385–387.

SECTION 3   GENERAL MEDICAL CARE: *Disorders of the Nervous System*

105 Approach to the Child with Headache

Kian-Ti Yu

ROLE OF THE GENERALIST

1 Distinguish primary from secondary (organic) headaches.
2 Determine etiology of headache.
3 Provide treatment for primary headaches.
4 Refer patients with secondary headaches to appropriate specialist.
5 Refer patients with primary headaches when assistance is needed with evaluation or management.

The medical model for the evaluation of a child with headache includes a carefully obtained medical history, a general physical examination, and a thorough neurologic examination. Identification or exclusion of a serious underlying cause of the headache is of utmost importance. A differential diagnosis should be formulated based on the history and physical examination. Appropriate laboratory tests may be ordered to confirm the diagnosis or rule out serious or life-threatening causes, and treatment is initiated. Follow-up of the clinical course is necessary to ensure that the diagnosis is correct, and the treatment is appropriate.

MEDICAL HISTORY

The patient's history is the most important factor in determining the correct diagnosis. The headache first needs to be carefully characterized including onset, location and duration of pain, frequency and timing, quality of the pain, and temporal pattern. Factors that trigger or ameliorate the headache should be elicited. Patients should also be asked about family history, medication history, and other medical conditions. The first and most important distinction is differentiating organic or secondary headache from primary headache (Box 105-1).

Box 105-1. Red Flags: Signs and Symptoms of Secondary or Organic Headaches

Headache worsening in frequency and severity
Nocturnal headache, headache awakens patient from sleep
Headache worse on waking in the morning, associated with vomiting
Fixed location, occipital headache
Headache worse with Valsalva maneuvers (sneezing, coughing), recumbent position, or change in position
Rapid onset of first headache, or "worst headache of my life"
Systemic signs and symptoms (fever, weight loss)
Profound hypertension
Abnormality on neurologic examination

Headache Onset

Headaches that occur after head injury suggest postconcussive headache disorder or intracranial pathology, though migraine and cluster headaches may also be triggered by head trauma. A psychological basis is suggested by onset following stressful events such as parental separation, the death of a loved one, or moving to a different locale. Onset with exertion suggests subarachnoid hemorrhage or other serious causes as well as benign exertional headache. Migraine headaches usually begin in the first decade of life; whereas most chronic, nonprogressive headaches, especially if daily, occur during adolescence.

Location and Duration of Pain

Most children with migraine describe bifrontal or bitemporal pain. Occipital pain is strongly indicative of organic disease, specifically posterior fossa tumors. Other causes of occipital headaches are basilar artery migraine, occipital neuralgia, and craniocervical junction abnormality such as Chiari malformation. Cluster headaches are almost always unilateral pain that occurs in or around one eye, the temple, or adjacent areas. Tension headaches are usually bifrontal or bioccipital, or may have a hatband distribution. The pain from maxillary sinusitis is commonly located between the eyes, while ethmoidal and sphenoidal sinusitis causes deep midline pain behind the nose. Prolonged ocular near-fixation in a child with a latent disturbance in convergence may cause dull aching pain behind the eyes that is quickly relieved when the eyes are closed. This pain is termed eyestrain. Refractive errors in children do not cause eyestrain as presbyopia does in adults.

More than 80% of patients with brain tumor have pain on the side of the tumor. Patients with migraines may have unilateral, hemicranial pain; although the pain may have a predilection for one side, it may also change sides from attack to attack. Unvarying location of headache should alert the clinician to the possibility of brain tumor. Migraines in young children last 1 to 3 hours. Cluster headaches usually last 30 to 60 minutes. Chronic nonprogressive or tension headaches may last all day. Headaches of organic origin do not have a characteristic duration.

Frequency and Timing of Headaches

Morning headache or headaches that awaken the child from sleep are classic symptoms of the dependent edema of intracranial lesions and obstructive hydrocephalus. Pseudotumor cerebri, also known as benign intracranial hypertension, also presents with signs of increased intracranial pressure. Migraines may occur at random, with menstrual cycle, or with specific temporal patterns. Chronic nonprogressive or tension headaches may occur daily. Cluster headaches occur in a regular pattern, at similar times of the day or night.

Quality of Pain

Migraines usually begin as dull, steady aches, and may not throb until the pain becomes moderate to severe. Tension headaches are dull and bandlike. Cluster headaches are described as deep, boring, or piercing. Brain tumor headaches may resemble tension or migraine headaches. Ruptured arteriovenous malformations may present with a continuous, intense, aching, or throbbing pain.

Temporal Pattern of Headache

Headaches that began in the recent past and are rapidly becoming more severe and are associated with neurologic signs and symptoms suggest an organic process. Headaches that are intermittent and unchanging over the course of months to years are more likely to represent a primary headache condition such as migraine. Headaches that are daily or almost daily from the time patients awaken until the time they go to bed, and have been present for months to years, with no associated neurologic signs and symptoms, represent a chronic nonprogressive type of headache.

Trigger Factors

Migraines may be brought about by stress, relaxation after stress, menstruation, food (chocolate, cheese, red wine, citrus, aspartate, monosodium glutamate [MSG]), physical exercise, and weather changes. Ingesting alcohol during a cluster period may trigger the attack. Daily stress aggravates chronic nonprogressive or tension headaches. Headache from brain tumor may be intensified by exertion, postural changes, bending over, or coughing. Pain in sinusitis is exaggerated by blowing the nose or quick movements of the head, especially bending forward.

Ameliorating Factors

Lying down motionless in a dark, quiet room may relieve a migraine headache. Patients with cluster headaches need to sit upright, pace back and forth, or engage in vigorous movements to relieve the pain. Relaxation, rest, and sleep relieve tension headaches.

Associated Features

Nocturnal or morning emesis, with or without headache, suggests increased intracranial pressure and is a common symptom of tumors arising near the floor of the fourth ventricle. Persistence of symptoms between headaches, such as behavioral changes, cognitive decline, ataxia, weakness, or abnormal eye movements, raises the likelihood of a space-occupying lesion.

Family History

Approximately 50% to 60% of migraine sufferers have a parent with the disorder. Among patients with tension headaches, 40% may have another family member with similar headache. Cluster headaches rarely occur within the same family.

Past Medication History

Willful or unwitting overuse of over-the-counter analgesics and excessive use of medications containing ergots, caffeine, narcotics, barbiturates can lead to rebound or withdrawal headaches. Avoidance of medication overuse is an essential step in headache control.

Other Medical Conditions

Certain types of headaches are found more frequently with pseudotumor cerebri and intracranial tumors. Pseudotumor cerebri has been associated with metabolic disorders, infections, medications, hematologic disorders, and venous thrombosis. Intracranial tumors are found in neurofibromatosis.

PHYSICAL EXAMINATION

Tentative diagnosis made after the history should be kept in mind while performing the general physical examination. The vital signs are important. Presence of fever may indicate an infectious process. Hypertension, especially if severe or recent, may cause headache. Hyperventilation may be indicative of anxiety. The presence of café-au-lait spots or ash leaf spots may implicate a neurocutaneous syndrome and its associated central nervous system lesions such as astrocytoma. Striae suggest illicit use of steroids with concomitant hypertension. Presence of a butterfly rash over the cheeks may indicate systemic lupus erythematosus and vasculitis of the central nervous system.

Meticulous neurologic examination, the key to the diagnosis and management of headaches, begins with examination of the head. An enlarged head in a child with headaches may suggest hydrocephalus or neurofibromatosis (if the corresponding skin lesions are present). Auscultation of the cranium for an asymmetric machinery-like bruit detects an underlying vascular abnormality. Palpation of the scalp and skull should be performed. Localized areas of tenderness or fluid may indicate trauma or a skeletal defect.

Five key points in the main neurologic examination should be documented: optic disks, eye movements, pronator drift, tandem gait, and deep tendon reflexes. The presence of papilledema and inability to move the eyes in the lateral direction indicate increased intracranial pressure. Patients with posterior fossa lesions may be ataxic, may have wide-based gait, and therefore cannot perform the tandem gait. Unilateral pronator drift and depressed deep tendon reflex indicate a mass lesion on the contralateral hemisphere.

LABORATORY TESTS

The choice of laboratory tests rests on the differential diagnosis suggested by the history, physical examination, and neurologic examination. The main indication for a neuroimaging study is an abnormality on neurologic examination (Box 105-2). The electroencephalogram (EEG) is of limited value in evaluating headaches in children. If the child's headache is associated with impaired consciousness, automatisms, or abnormal movements such as clonic or myoclonic movements, an epileptic seizure may be in the differential diagnosis, in which case an EEG may be useful. It is important to recognize, however, that 10% of migraine patients have focal epileptiform discharges that are not related to headaches. A magnetic resonance arteriography should be done at the same time as the magnetic resonance imaging if the patient's headache is assessed to be secondary to a vascular event. Lumbar puncture is indicated to determine the presence of an infectious process as the cause of headache, or to measure cerebrospinal fluid (CSF) pressure if pseudotumor cerebri is suspected. Lumbar puncture should not be performed if a space-occupying cranial lesion is suspected. Psychological tests may be indicated for individuals with chronic nonprogressive or tension headaches. When school problems coexist, psychoeducational testing may also be useful.

Box 105-2. Red Flags: Indications for Neuroimaging Studies in Children with Headache

High Priority

Chronic progressive pattern
Age <3 years
Acute headache: worst headache of life, thunderclap headache
Focal neurologic symptoms
Abnormal neurologic examination
Presence of ventriculoperitoneal shunts
Presence of neurocutaneous syndrome (neurofibromatosis or tuberous sclerosis)

Moderate Priority

Headache or vomiting on awakening
Unvarying location of headache
Meningeal signs

PSEUDOTUMOR CEREBRI

Pseudotumor cerebri, also known as benign intracranial hypertension, is a clinical syndrome of increased intracranial pressure with normal cerebrospinal fluid and normal ventricular size, anatomy, and position. Table 105-1 lists the causes of pseudotumor cerebri.

Pseudotumor cerebri produces the same symptoms as increased intracranial pressure from other causes, such as brain tumor or hydrocephalus. The headache may be severe, may be worse in the morning, can awaken the patient from sleep, may be exacerbated or improved by change in position, and may worsen with Valsalva maneuvers with coughing, sneezing, or straining, or during projectile vomiting without nausea. Blurred vision or diplopia are frequent accompanying complaints. Most patients are alert and have no other constitutional symptoms.

Physical examination reveals papilledema with an enlarged blind spot. Sixth cranial nerve palsy, ataxia, and occasionally spasticity, may be found on physical examination. In infants, examination may reveal a bulging fontanelle or a resonant sound on percussion ("cracked-pot sound" or Macewen's sign). No other focal neurologic defects should be found on examination. If present, they indicate a different underlying process.

Table 105-1. Causes of Pseudotumor Cerebri

Metabolic Causes	Infections
Galactosemia	Roseola
Hypoparathyroidism	Guillain-Barré syndrome
Pseudohypoparathyroidism	Chronic otitis media
Hypophosphatasia	Mastoiditis
Addison's disease	
Obesity	**Hematologic Causes**
Menarche	Polycythemia
	Hemolytic anemia
Drugs	Iron-deficiency anemia
Corticosteroids	Winscott-Alrich syndrome
Vitamin A	
Tetracycline	**Miscellaneous Causes**
Oral contraceptives	Pregnancy
Nalidixic acid	Venous thrombosis
Nitrofurantoin	
Isotretinoin	

Diagnostic tests for pseudotumor cerebri include computed tomography (CT) or magnetic resonance imaging (MRI) scan with a lumbar tap to measure intracranial pressure.

Pseudotumor cerebri is generally a self-limiting condition. The prime goals of management are discovery and treatment of the underlying cause, relief of symptoms, and prevention of complications, which include optic atrophy and blindness.

For some patients, a single lumbar puncture may be both diagnostic and therapeutic. If symptoms recur, treatment with steroids and acetazolamide may be used. Repeated lumbar punctures are sometimes indicated.

If increased intracranial pressure persists, repeat neuro-radiologic studies are indicated to look for a slow-growing tumor. These patients should also be followed regularly by an ophthalmologist to prevent damage to the visual system. Intractable pseudotumor cerebri can damage the optic nerve. The nerve can be protected by fenestration of the optic nerve sheath or by placement of a lumbar peritoneal shunt.

HEADACHE TREATMENT

If an ominous secondary headache is suspected, consultation with a pediatric neurologist for assistance in diagnosis and management is needed. Patients should be referred promptly for any signs of increased intracranial pressure, dependent edema of intracranial lesions, or obstructive hydrocephalus. If the patient's blood pressure is highly elevated, hypertensive crisis must be considered and urgently treated.

If the diagnosis of primary headache disorder has been established, treatment may be initiated in the office setting. Confident reassurance to the patient and his family that no intracranial abnormality is present is the most helpful initial step. The treatment of migraine headache (Box 105-3) begins with simple observation and asking the patient to maintain a headache calendar, especially in those patients whose migraine attacks are short and self-limited and few and far between. If head pain and vomiting are disabling or bothersome to the patient, medication can be initiated immediately.

Medication can be given to alleviate the patient's symptoms. Non-narcotic analgesics, such as ibuprofen and acetaminophen, are valuable. The use of an antiemetic orally or rectally is quite useful in those in whom vomiting is marked and interferes with oral medication. Medications that induce sedation such as diphenhydramine are also useful, as

---

Box 105-4. Indications for Chronic Preventive Treatment

Significant headache-related disability occurs (e.g., four or more attacks per month, or if less, attacks produce disability lasting 3 or more days).
Symptomatic or abortive medications are contraindicated, produce intolerable side effects, or are ineffective.
Symptomatic or abortive medications are being overused.
Special situations exist, such as hemiplegic migraine or risk of permanent neurologic injury.

---

it is well established that sleep relieves migraine in a significant number of children.

When the use of symptomatic medication is unsuccessful or has to be used more often than twice a week, the use of abortive and prophylactic medications should be considered. Abortive medications include nonsteroidal anti-inflammatory drugs (NSAIDs), dihydroxyergotamine (DHE), and the triptans. Four triptan medications are currently available: sumatriptan, naratriptan, zolmitriptan, and rizatriptan. There is definitely a subset of children who do not respond to or who have conditions that contraindicate the use of symptomatic and or abortive medications, for which preventive treatment may be required (Box 105-4).

Preventive medications are given on a daily basis, whether or not headache is present, to reduce the frequency or severity of attacks. Patients may need to take the medication daily for 2 to 3 months before the efficacy can be noted. However, preventive treatment need not be "lifelong" because the patient can be weaned off the medication after the headaches have been under control for 6 to 12 months. Based on the U.S. Headache Consortium Guidelines, the following medications available in the United States, with proved high efficacy and mild to moderate side effects, are recommended for preventive treatment of migraine: valproate, amitriptyline, and propranolol. Divalproex sodium is presently available in the extended release tablet (Depakote ER) to make the dosing simple (once daily) for migraine prevention.

For chronic nonprogressive headaches, judicious use of valproate or amitriptyline, together with nonpharmcologic approaches such as biofeedback, relaxation training, cognitive training, counseling, and family counseling, have all been used. It is the psychologist who determines the most cost-effective method of dealing with the family.

Because cluster headaches are rare and sometimes difficult to manage, all patients suspected of having this condition should be referred to a neurologist or a headache specialist for evaluation and management.

Box 105-3. Pediatric Migraine without Aura: Diagnostic Criteria

A. At least five attacks fulfilling following items B through D
B. Headache attack lasting 30 minutes to 48 hours
C. Headache has at least two of the following qualities:
    1. Bilateral (fronto/temporal) or unilateral location
    2. Pulsating quality
    3. Moderate to severe intensity
    4. Aggravation by routine physical activity
D. During headache, at least one of the following occurs:
    1. Nausea or vomiting
    2   Photophobia or phonophobia

Mini-index of Related Topics

SUGGESTED READINGS

Fenichel GM: Clinical Pediatric Neurology: A Signs and Symptoms Approach, 2nd ed. Philadelphia, WB Saunders, 1993.

Rothner AD: The evaluation of headaches in children and adolescents. Semin Pediatr Neurol 1995;2(2):109–118.

Rothner AD: Headaches in children and adolescents: Update 2001. Semin Pediatr Neurol 2001;8(1):2–6.

Rothner AD, Linder SL, Wasiewski WW, O'Neill KM: Chronic nonprogressive headaches in children and adolescents. Semin Pediatr Neurol 2001;8(1):34–39.

Silbersten SD: Practice parameter: Evidence-based guidelines for migraine headache (an evidence-based review). Neurology 2000;55:754–763.

Silberstein SD, Lipton RB, Goadsby PJ, Smith RT: Headache in Primary Care. Oxford, UK, Medical Media, 1999.

SECTION 3   GENERAL MEDICAL CARE: *Disorders of the Nervous System*

106

Approach to the Child with Weakness or Paralysis

Kenneth Huff

ROLE OF THE GENERALIST

1. Recognize the signs and symptoms of types of acute or subacute weakness.
2. Localize the site of the lesion by examination.
3. Use appropriate laboratory tests to support the clinical impression.
4. Institute a treatment plan with the assistance of specialists' opinions.
5. Oversee and coordinate long-term care and follow-up.

Acute or subacute weakness or paralysis is an urgent problem with potentially dire implications for a child's ultimate well-being. Appropriate diagnosis and therapeutic strategies may improve the potential for full recovery. Clinicians must have knowledge and skills to act in a timely manner. Longstanding weakness also requires a diagnostic strategy but allows for a more methodical approach, and even if not cured, patients can still benefit from directed care.

The range of diagnostic possibilities for a problem of weakness is wide. The clinician can narrow this list first by localizing the level of the lesion within the child's entire nervous system, from the cerebral cortex down to the muscle. The course of illness over time, the pattern of the weakness and other findings on neurologic examination, and laboratory tests help establish a specific diagnosis.

Therapy depends on diagnosis and may be related specifically to the biochemistry or physiology of the level of the nervous system, general immune modulation, or simply supportive care.

DEFINITIONS

Weakness is defined as decreased power or movement of a muscle. The degree of weakness observed can be graded on a subjective scale (Box 106-1). More objective measurements of power can be achieved with a strain gauge, but this assessment is not usually necessary for diagnosis. Hypotonia may be the cause of weakness in an infant or child who cannot or will not cooperate voluntarily for strength testing against resistance. Hypotonia is lower than normal resistance to passive motion across a joint. Although this resistance has other components, muscle strength is a key component. The examiner can obtain clues regarding the presence, pattern, and degree of weakness by observing the child's posture in standing, sitting, or lying positions. Swayback posture in standing may indicate hip girdle or proximal weakness. Asymmetric weight bearing may indicate hemiparesis. Pointed toes in supine position may indicate an upper motor neuron lesion. Strength is best assessed in an alert child by requested or imitated actions or tasks such as walking on toes or heels, running, climbing stairs, stooping and recovering an object from the floor, getting up from a

---

Box 106-1. Assessment of Muscle Strength

Normal as assessed with resistance against the examiner
Decreased power but active movement against both gravity and resistance
Active movement only against gravity
Active movement only with gravity eliminated
A trace of muscle contraction
No muscle contraction

supine position or a chair, reaching for something high, or drawing with a crayon or pencil.

FUNDAMENTALS

Weakness can result from lesions at various points in the nervous system: in the cerebral hemispheres affecting the pyramidal system of upper motor neurons at their cortical cell bodies; along the pyramidal tracts through the hemispheres and brainstem; in the spinal cord affecting the white matter pyramidal tracts before their synapse with the anterior horn cells; in the anterior horn cells of the ventral gray of the spinal cord; in the ventral roots exiting the spinal canal; along the peripheral nerve, either myelin sheath or axon; at the neuromuscular junction; and in the muscle, affecting its ability to contract. Systemic disorders can also cause dysfunction of the central nervous system or peripheral neuromuscular apparatus. Distinction of upper motor neuron weakness from lower motor neuron and peripherally caused weakness is a useful first step in making a diagnosis.

Upper motor neuron weakness may be associated with abnormalities of other brain function such as state of alertness, attention, and cognition or with signs of increased intracranial pressure such as vomiting or irritability and a tense fontanelle in an infant. Chronic problems involving upper motor neuron weakness with signs of encephalopathy may be more difficult to discern than acute lesions, particularly if the clinician is unfamiliar with the immature and changing developmental status of the central nervous system. Signs of weakness from upper motor neuron disease are listed in Box 106-2. Spasticity may not accompany pyramidal tract lesions for some time after the insult. Dysmorphic features and malformations of other organs may suggest cerebral dysgenesis as the source of the weakness.

The neuromuscular unit includes the anterior horn cell, nerve root, peripheral nerve axon and myelin sheath, the neuromuscular junction, and the muscle (Fig. 106-1). Lesions of this unit generally occur in the absence of signs of encephalopathy, and the child may have an interested and visually attentive facial appearance. Neuromuscular lesions produce a decrease or loss of deep tendon reflexes. The pattern of weakness is generally, though not always,

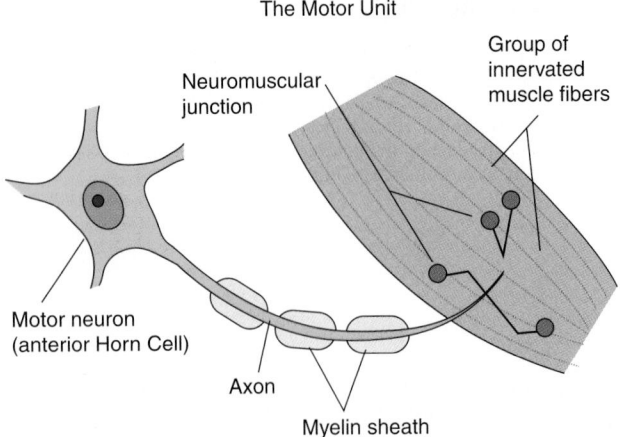

The Motor Unit

Figure 106-1. The neuromuscular unit.

symmetric in agonists and antagonists across a particular joint, and there should be no accompanying spasticity or rigidity.

Weakness or paralysis can be caused by many different types of physiologic, ultrastructural, or biochemical pathologic conditions. The frequency of neuronal action potentials in the motor neurons may change. Either upper or lower motor neurons may be necrotic or experience apoptotic death. Myelin sheaths in peripheral or central motor fibers can be temporarily or permanently lost. Chemical, immunologic, or physical changes at the neuromuscular junction can affect the synaptic efficiency. Muscle fiber structural or energy metabolism may be affected.

DIAGNOSIS

Disorders causing weakness are listed in Table 106-1 with associated signs and symptoms and diagnostic tests that are useful in making each diagnosis. Acute bilateral weakness from an upper motor neuron lesion is usually accompanied by a change in level of consciousness with lethargy, obtundation, or coma. An asymmetric or unilateral "sudden" upper motor neuron weakness may suggest either an "electric" or a "vascular" cause such as a postictal hemiparesis after an unwitnessed partial seizure or a vascular occlusion (stroke) or hemorrhage. If headache and a history of migraine are present, hemiplegic migraine should be considered after other causes have been excluded.

A weakness with a less acute onset may suggest a space-occupying lesion such as an extra-axial hemorrhage or hemispheric mass, but usually other symptoms and signs of increased intracranial pressure are present, such as lethargy, headache, vomiting, Parinaud's eye signs, and papilledema. If the weakness is bilateral but asymmetric and accompanied by cranial nerve signs or ataxia, a brainstem or cerebellar lesion, particularly a tumor, should be considered. Subacute weakness may be from a demyelinating process, such as a postinfectious disseminated encephalomyelitis or a relapse of multiple sclerosis. Both disorders have accompanying signs depending on where plaques of demyelination occur.

Chronic problems involving the cerebral hemispheres (upper motor neuron involvement) can be either progres-

---

Box 106-2. Signs of Weakness Secondary to Upper Motor Neuron Disease

General Signs

Deep tendon reflexes may be normal or increased

Babinski reflex may be dorsiflexor

Hemiparesis or upper extremity extensor weakness and lower extremity knee flexor, ankle dorsiflexor, and ankle everter weakness

Signs in Infants

Fisting of the hands

Scissoring of the extended legs on vertical suspension

Movement through postural reflexes such as the asymmetric tonic neck reflex

Table 106-1. Diagnosis of Weakness

Cause of Weakness	Associated Symptoms	Accompanying Signs	Laboratory Tests
Upper Motor Neuron			
Stroke	Sudden onset	Aphasia, visual field defect	MRI diffusion
Postictal hemiparesis	Seizure	Confusion	EEG
Extra-axial hemorrhage	Trauma	Increased sleepiness	CT
Posterior fossa tumor	Vomiting	Cranial nerve palsies	MRI
Postinfectious disseminated encephalomyelitis	Recent infection	Encephalopathy	MRI
Multiple sclerosis	Previous bouts	Visual, spinal cord	MRI
Aminoacidopathies and organic acidurias	Poor feeding, seizures	Encephalopathy	Metabolic screen
Storage disorders	Regression	Organomegaly	Lysosomal screen
Leukodystrophies	Learning problems	Decreased DTRs	VLCFA, lysosomal screen, enzyme assessment
Hypoxic-ischemic insult	Perinatal problems	Decreased alertness	EEG
Intraventricular hemorrhage	Prematurity	Respiratory distress syndrome	Head ultrasound
Periventricular leukomalacia	Ischemic insult	LE>UE	MRI
Cerebral dysgenesis	Developmental delay	Dysmorphisms	MRI
Transverse myelopathy	Bladder obstruction	Sensory level	Sensory evoked potentials
Spinal cord tumor	Back pain	Sensory loss	MRI
Spinal cord tethering	Constipation, leg weakness	Dimple, mass	MRI
Neuromuscular Unit			
Enteroviral poliomyelitis	Fever	Asymmetry	CSF cells, culture
Spinal muscular atrophy	Regression	Loss of DTRs	Gene test
Guillain-Barré syndrome	Prior illness	Ascending	Nerve conduction
Bell's palsy	Sudden onset	Hyperacusis	None
Hereditary sensory and motor neuropathy	Family history	Distal wasting	Gene test
Toxic neuropathy	Exposure	Sensory loss	NCV, EMG
Myasthenia	Fatigability	Cranial nerves	Tensilon test

CSF, cerebrospinal fluid; CT, computed tomography; DTR, deep tender reflex; EEG, electroencephalogram; LE, lower extremity; MRI, magnetic resonance imaging; NCV, nerve conduction velocity; UE, upper extremity; VLCFA, very long chain fatty acids.

sive, as in a degenerative disorder, or static. Degenerative disorders involving the central nervous system include aminoacidopathies and organic acidurias that present most commonly in the neonatal period. Storage disorders and leukodystrophies appear more commonly in the infantile and later childhood periods. Inborn errors often manifest with variants of the classic forms and may present outside their usual age of presentation. Because both peripheral and central myelin are lost in leukodystrophies, both lower motor neuron signs, including loss of reflexes, and upper motor signs and dementia are seen. A family history of other affected individuals suggests a genetic pattern and is helpful in diagnosing a degenerative cause for the progressive weakness.

Static encephalopathies with weakness usually present with delay in motor developmental milestones without loss of any skills already attained. Because the insult often occurred prenatally or perinatally, history of loss of fetal movements, complicated delivery, or prematurity are important. The pattern of disability might suggest the mechanism of the insult: quadruparesis or bilateral hemiparesis suggests an hypoxic-ischemic insult; hemiparesis, a prenatal stroke, or infarct related to an intraventricular hemorrhage in a premature infant; and diplegia with weakness greater in lower extremity than upper extremity suggests periventricular leukomalacia related to either prenatal ischemic insults in a full-term infant or postnatal ischemic insults in a premature infant.

Cerebral dysgenesis can result in a static encephalopathy and weakness. Cerebral dysgenesis includes prosencephalization abnormalities accompanied by specific facial anomalies, neuroglial precursor migration defects, rostral neural tube anomalies, and malformation at the microscopic or ultrastructural level. Although sometimes the dysgenetic insult produces microcephaly, often the brain is normal-sized but clearly functionally deficient (Down syndrome). Weakness is usually associated with cognitive deficits that become more apparent as the child grows older.

Acute bilateral weakness with loss of sphincter function and a dermatomal level below which there is loss of pain sensation suggest an acute transverse myelopathy, such as a spinal stroke. Deep tendon reflexes may be depressed initially, even below the level of the lesion. Most often the spinal infarct is in the thoracic cord producing a marked discrepancy between normal upper and flaccid lower extremity strength. A spinal cord tumor must be considered with subacute presentation of these signs accompanied by back pain. Presence of a skin hemangioma or hairy patch, a dermal sinus tract, or an intradermal lipoma in the midline sacral region in an infant suggests an occult spinal dysraphism. Spinal cord tumors and occult dysraphism may also extend into the spinal canal and produce acute infectious or compressive pathology. All these stigmata may also present with a chronic and progressive course from tethering of the spinal cord, leading to lower extremity weakness and caudal spine dysfunction.

Anterior horn cell disorders can be acute or chronically progressive. Acute flaccid weakness with loss of deep tendon reflexes, fever, and a patchy distribution may represent enteroviral poliomyelitis. Spinal muscular atrophy is a progressive disorder that produces areflexia and symmetric, proximal greater than distal, weakness and spares diaphragm, face, eye movements, and intellect.

One of the leading causes of acute generalized weakness in a fully alert child is acute postinfectious polyradiculoneuritis or Landry-Guillain-Barré syndrome. The weakness develops rapidly over a few days, usually after a mild infectious illness. Generally, symptoms begin distally in the legs and progress with loss of ambulatory ability, loss of hand and arm strength, and finally loss of ventilatory capacity. Deep tendon reflexes are lost soon after onset. Often mild sensory symptoms accompany the weakness at the outset. Autonomic symptoms, including hypertension, are relatively common. Symptoms suggesting another diagnosis include fever at the onset of weakness, asymmetry of weakness, objective pain sensory loss, persistent sphincter dysfunction, and progression of weakness beyond 2 weeks.

The pathophysiology of Landry-Guillain-Barré syndrome involves primarily a dysimmune response following which regeneration of nerve fibers or myelin sheaths must occur. Although many different infectious agents have been associated with the disorder, *Campylobacter jejuni* is the most commonly associated pathogen and has a common antigenic epitope with peripheral nerve gangliosides. A rare variant (Miller-Fisher syndrome) includes cranial nerve findings and ataxia.

Focal acute peripheral nerve weakness may occur secondary to immune dysfunction. Bell's palsy, sudden isolated cranial nerve VII weakness, has been associated with herpesvirus type 6 infection. Sudden appearance of an abducens nerve palsy, a less common problem in children, may also be related to antecedent infection or immune dysfunction.

Chronic peripheral neuropathies producing weakness in children most often result from a slowly progressive hereditary disorder, but occasionally may be related to a toxin. Hereditary sensory and motor neuropathies are classified by their electrophysiologic characteristics and inheritance pattern. Symptoms are symmetric distal weakness, lower leg first, then hand. The child may present with an awkward gait, difficulty running, and absent ankle jerks. Eventually muscle atrophy may evolve with "stork leg" deformity and loss of thenar and hypothenar bulk. Progression may occur over decades. The diagnosis may be facilitated by examining one or both parents. Cancer chemotherapy with vincristine, which disrupts axoplasmic transport, may produce a toxic neuropathy. Deep tendon reflexes are lost early, and there may be transient sensory symptoms. The severity of the weakness is dose-dependent so that long-term disability usually can be avoided.

Neuromuscular junction disorders, including childhood myasthenia, are characterized by fatigability and weakness. Although these symptoms can be general, cranial muscles are most often affected, particularly the levator palpebri, the extraocular muscles, and the jaw and palatal muscles. Patients may present with ptosis, diplopia, difficulty chewing, or nasal speech. They report needing frequent rests during physical activities such as climbing steps or walking long distances. Although myasthenia is a chronic condition, with symptoms fluctuating during the day as well as day to day, patients can present with acute severe weakness. Deep tendon reflexes are preserved but the patient has difficulty with sustained activity such as upgaze or finger tapping.

During a myasthenic crisis there may be marked generalized weakness.

Other less common neuromuscular junction disorders include infantile botulism, aminoglycoside paralysis, and tick paralysis. They produce a similar pattern of weakness as myasthenia. Infantile botulism has an insidious onset with intestinal *Clostridium* colonization leading to toxin production. The child may exhibit poor feeding, hypotonia, and constipation as well as the cranial nerve signs, and the diagnosis may be missed. Eventually weakness may progress and involve almost every muscle including pupillary constrictors and gut smooth muscle. Aminoglycoside paralysis may follow surgery or renal failure and is related to toxic serum levels. Tick paralysis toxin blocks motor terminal depolarization.

Marked neonatal weakness may be seen with congenital neuromuscular junction and muscle disorders (Figure 106-2). The weakness may be of such severity that multiple joint contractures or arthrogryposis is produced. Congenital myasthenia most often results from transplacental antibody transmission from maternal myasthenia. The infant with congenital myasthenia has fluctuating signs and symptoms of a weak cry, sucking difficulties, ptosis, and dysconjugate gaze. The neonate with congenital myotonic dystrophy has a history of polyhydramnios, has sucking problems, and may have severe generalized weakness and respiratory problems but does not demonstrate myotonia. Because the mother usually transmits the gene for congenital myotonic dystrophy, an examination of the mother can provide clues to the diagnosis. The mother may exhibit characteristic signs of frontal balding, myopathic facial appearance, and percussion or hand grasp myotonia. Rare congenital myopathies are of variable severity and result in static, slowly resolving, episodic, or progressive weakness. Many are defined only by ultrastructural features of the muscle biopsy such as nemaline rods, central cores, abnormal mitochondria, or myotubules. Others are defined by metabolic abnormalities including defects of glycogen metabolism, glycolysis, fatty

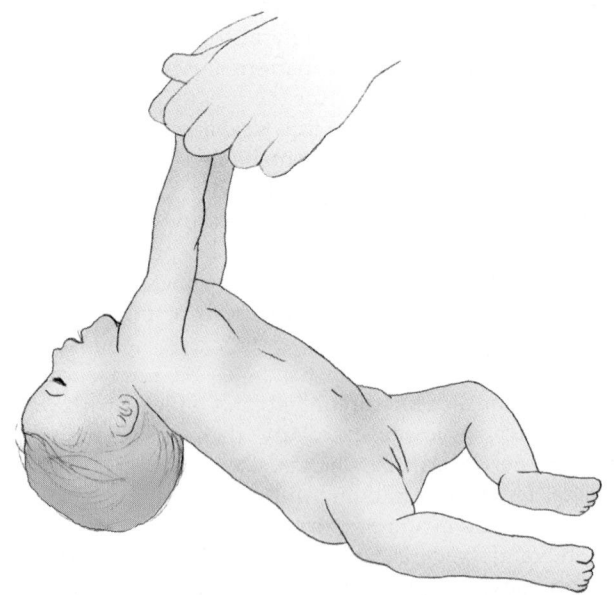

Figure 106-2. Posture of a hypotonic infant.

acid metabolism, intracellular fuel transport, amino acid metabolism, or defects producing lactic acidosis secondary to Kreb's cycle, pyruvate metabolism, or electron transport chain abnormalities. Other congenital muscle disorders with a poor prognosis are associated with eye abnormalities and migrational brain malformations.

An acute or subacute form of myopathy producing childhood weakness is myositis. The spectrum of conditions includes primary autoimmune dermatomyositis, myositis associated with systemic connective tissue disorders, and infectious myositis. The myopathic pattern of weakness involves trunk hyperlordosis, neck flexion weakness in rising from the supine position, poor shoulder girdle fixation with weight bearing and scapular winging, hip girdle extensor weakness, and Gower's sign—hands climbing up the legs in rising from prone position because of hip extensor weakness (Fig. 106-3). Muscles are generally tender. Dermatomyositis includes rash on extensor joint surfaces, periorbital skin discoloration, sometimes muscle calcinosis, and generalized discomfort.

The muscular dystrophies are disorders that present with the myopathic pattern of weakness but are chronic and progressive. The X-linked Duchenne's dystrophy is the most common. Deep tendon reflexes are depressed and the calf muscles show pseudohypertrophy. Seventy-five percent have an abnormal electrocardiogram (ECG) and most have mild intellectual impairment. Less common autosomal dominant and recessively inherited dystrophies have the same pattern of weakness but progress more slowly.

Laboratory studies should be determined by the history of progression and localizing signs on neurologic examination. Weakness associated with acute encephalopathy, signs of increased intracranial pressure, or potential intracranial surgical lesions requires an imaging study. Although calcification, hemorrhage, and mass lesions are often apparent on computed tomography (CT), ischemic insults are better seen acutely by a diffusion-weighted magnetic resonance imaging (MRI) scan. MRI is also more useful to delineate subtle malformations and the scars of periventricular leukomalacia. Electroencephalogram (EEG) is useful for assessing ischemic insults and seizures as a cause of weakness. Hematologic studies are necessary to determine the cause for acute thrombosis or spontaneous hemorrhage. Spinal cord, canal, and dysraphic lesions are best seen with MRI scan, and sensory-evoked potentials may help confirm a nonmass lesion within the cord. A cerebrospinal fluid (CSF) examination may confirm a subarachnoid hemorrhage, infection, inflammation, necrosis, or spinal block, or measure the degree of increased pressure.

Other laboratory studies are useful in confirming diagnoses within the neuromuscular unit. Nerve conduction studies can delineate a segmental demyelinative nerve block, confirm radiculopathy, or help determine an axonal versus demyelinative neuropathy. Electromyography can define muscle areas that have been denervated for at least 2 weeks, confirm electrical responses of a neuromuscular junction problem, and provide nonspecific signs consistent with a primary myopathy. An intravenous edrophonium test and serum acetylcholine receptor antibodies are useful to confirm myasthenia. A serum creatine phosphokinase

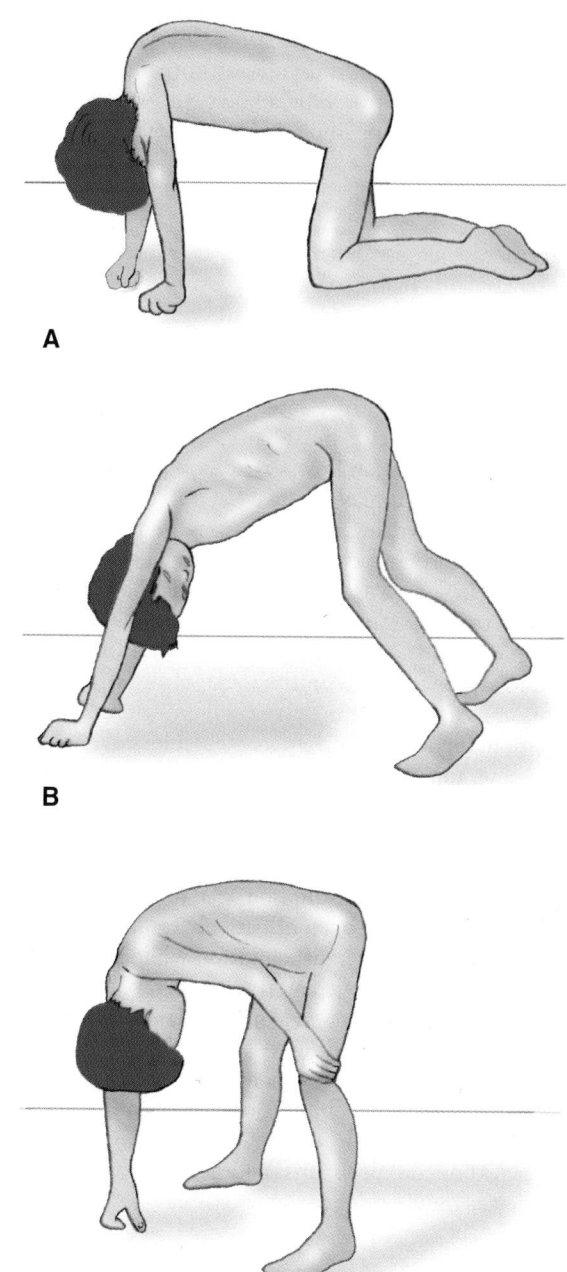

Figure 106-3. Gower's sign. The child is asked to get to a standing position from a supine position. The child will roll over and rise to kneeling **(A)**, progressively walk the hands up the legs **(B)**, and use the hands to push off the knees to a standing position **(C)**.

(CPK) is highly elevated in dystrophies and myositis, sometimes mildly elevated in nonprogressive myopathies, and occasionally mildly abnormal in neuropathies. Muscle biopsy is indicated to diagnose a dystrophy or progressive myopathy. Immunohistochemistry is helpful when a DNA study is uninformative and an ultrastructure examination is helpful for abnormal mitochondria or other areas of fiber architecture.

The diagnosis of many degenerative or progressive disorders is made by biochemical tests. Leukodystrophy tests rely on enzymatic assays or very long chain fatty acid profiles; mitochondrial disorder tests on urine organic acids, serum amino acids, and carnitine levels; and familial disorders such as spinal muscular atrophy and progressive neuropathies, as well as Duchenne's and other muscular dystrophies, rely on specific DNA mutation probes.

MANAGEMENT

Management includes both specific therapies and general supportive care (Table 106-2). Acute severe weakness management mandates addressing the respiratory problems related to the weakness. With acute neuromuscular crises (Landry-Guillain-Barré syndrome, myasthenic relapse, or muscular dystrophy with an intercurrent respiratory illness) the ventilatory capacity must be assessed and monitored with vital capacity, peak flow, or a blood gas measurement. Ventilatory support may be needed in an intensive care unit. Frequently a rising heart rate may be the only sign of ventilatory failure in a child too weak to show other signs. In addition, in some cases the airway must be protected by intubation because there is pharyngeal weakness.

Treatment of acute upper motor neuron weakness related to stroke depends on the cause of the stroke: hypertransfusion is indicated for sickle cell hemoglobinemia, anticoagulation for a chronic hypercoagulable state, or factor replacement for a clotting deficiency causing hemorrhage. Central demyelinative disorders may benefit from a brief course of steroid therapy. Mass lesion and increased intracranial pressure problems should receive neurosurgical consultation and oncologic consultation if a tumor is diagnosed. Leukodystrophies have been effectively treated but at great risk with bone marrow transplantation while several inborn errors of metabolism are treated with dietary therapies.

Patients with chronic weakness related to an upper motor neuron cause should have physical and occupational therapy. The goals of therapy include teaching strategies for overcoming functional limitations, obtaining necessary orthotics or other hardware for mobility and daily care, avoiding orthopedic problems, and achieving as much age-appropriate independence as possible. Severely weak children may also require feeding assistance, ongoing gastroenterologic care, and gastrostomy appliances to maintain adequate nutrition. Patients with a spinal cord lesion also frequently need urologic care because of sphincter/detrusor problems, risk of infection, and eventual kidney failure.

When weakness is related to immune dysfunction, immunotherapy should be instituted in a timely manner. Immunotherapy for Guillain-Barré syndrome, when delayed past 5 days after the onset of symptoms, is less efficacious. Plasmapheresis has demonstrated benefit in children and intravenous gamma globulin is beneficial in adult subject studies. Gamma globulin is easier to administer in young children because plasmapheresis requires venous access through a large-bore needle. Indications for these interventions include severe weakness early in the course, rapid progression to loss of ambulation, or impending use of artificial ventilation. Intensive care monitoring of ventilation and autonomic dysfunction is also indicated. After the nadir of weakness is reached, non-weight-bearing physical therapy can be introduced for rehabilitation. Bell's palsy should also be treated early with immune suppression. Data indicate that when treatment with prednisone is delayed 48 hours it is not effective. A dose of 2 mg/kg with rapid tapering is used. Chronic relapsing polyneuritis is also treated with immune supression measures of steroids, imuran, and plasmapheresis when necessary.

Myasthenia is generally treated with anticholinesterase medications such as pyridostigmine (Mestinon) to boost acetylcholine levels in the neuromuscular synaptic cleft. Steroids are also beneficial as nonspecific immunosuppression but have side effects that are particularly undesirable in young children. Thymectomy, which requires a thoracotomy, is beneficial in a little over 50% of children and may result in obviation of medication afterward. Plasmapheresis and intravenous gamma globulin are particularly useful in a severe crisis requiring artificial ventilation. These modalities are also effective for periodic outpatient immunosuppression. Other immunosuppressive agents such as imuran and cyclosporine are used in refractory cases.

Table 106-2. Treatment Modalities for Types of Weakness

Diagnosis	Pharmacologic	Immunologic	Other Treatment
Stroke	Thrombolytics		Hypertransfusion
Postictal hemiparesis	Anticonvulsants		
Extra-axial hemorrhage			Surgery
Posterior fossa tumor	Chemotherapy	Steroids	Surgery, radiation
Postinfectious disseminated encephalomyelitis		Steroids	
Multiple sclerosis		Interferons, copolymer	
Aminoacidopathies and organic acidurias	Cofactors		Dietary manipulation
Storage disorders and leukodystrophies			Bone marrow transplant
Intraventricular hemorrhage			Manage hydrocephalus
Spinal cord tumor	Chemotherapy	Steroids	Surgery, radiation
Spinal cord tethering			Surgery
Guillain-Barré syndrome		Plasmapheresis, IVIG	
Bell's palsy		Steroids	
Myasthenia	Anticholinesterases	Steroids, plasmapheresis, IVIG	Thymectomy
Infant botulism		Trivalent antisera	
Tick paralysis			Remove tick
Myositis		Steroids, antimetabolites	
Muscular dystrophy		Steroids	

IVIG, intravenous immunoglobulin.

Infant botulism is treated with specific antibotulinum toxin antisera and supportive therapies. Antibiotics are ineffective. Dermatomyositis is treated with medium dose prednisone (less than 1 mg/kg). When this is not effective, cytotoxic drugs or cytokine production inhibitors are used. Metabolic myopathies are still poorly understood and therapies are largely empiric. These approaches have included thiamine, riboflavin, nicotinamide, vitamin C, vitamin K, coenzyme Q_{10}, biotin, L-carnitine, succinate, and medium chain triglycerides (MCT) oil.

No curative therapies are yet available for spinal muscular atrophy or the muscular dystrophies. However, affected children and their familes benefit from information provided from the physician, protection from unproved therapies, support from paramedical and lay support groups, and hospice support when progression is at end stage. Because of an inflammatory component in dystrophic muscle, prednisone has been used in a palliative way (such as to prolong ambulation) in Duchenne's muscular dystrophy. Until a cure is found, treatment is directed toward maintaining mobility and preventing contractures through therapy, casts, braces, and surgery. Inactivity increases disability. New hardware technologies (long leg braces, electric wheelchairs, battery-powered ventilators, and noninvasive positive pressure ventilation devices) have allowed affected children to overcome previously insurmountable disabilities.

OUTCOME

The prognosis for weakness related to immune-mediated disorders is generally good. Most children with Guillain-Barré syndrome recover (77%), although it may take weeks. Only a small percentage relapse. Patients with Bell's palsy have a 70% chance of full recovery. Chronic relapsing polyneuritis also may resolve in time. Myasthenia can be controlled by oral medication in some cases. Thymectomy can lead to cure but in many cases the disease persists despite thymectomy. Dermatomyositis can be successfully treated in most cases.

The outcome for genetic progressive disorders is often poor. The course of spinal muscular atrophy depends on the allele present for the survivor motor neuron gene. Age of onset and rapidity of progression are determined by which allele is present. Type I infants have an onset before 6 months, never sit, and die by 2 years; type II have an onset before 18 months and never walk; and type III walk later but have progressive weakness into adulthood. Boys with Duchenne's muscular dystrophy almost never are able to run, begin to have difficulty walking by 2 to 5 years, are wheelchair-bound by 7 to 13 years, and finally develop ventilatory failure by their late teens. Children with a leukodystrophy who do not get a bone marrow transplant survive only a few years. On the other hand, children who have myotonic dystrophy or one of the other congenital myopathies gain strength with development and progress into adulthood, although with some degree of disability, if they survive the neonatal period.

FOLLOW-UP

Mild cases of Guillain-Barré syndrome need early and frequent follow-up until the nadir of strength in the course occurs. The frequency of follow-up for children with myasthenia and myositis is based on the severity of the disorder, its progression or regression, and the frequency of relapses. For example, patients taking steroids require at least monthly follow-up visits. Patients with degenerative disorders should be followed at a frequency of 1 to 3 months, depending on the rapidity of their course, to ascertain new disabilities. Patients with a mild static weakness need monitoring of their therapies, hardware needs, and coordination of their care at least every 6 months. Patients with more severe chronic weakness may need close follow-up to monitor for incipient respiratory failure in times of intercurrent respiratory illness.

 Additional Resources, CD-ROM

| Gower's sign | Video 106-1 |

Mini-index of Related Topics

SUGGESTED READINGS

Crawford T: Clinical evaluation of the floppy infant. 1992;21:348–354.
Dubowitz V: Muscle Disorders in Childhood, 2nd ed. Philadelphia, WB Saunders, 1995.
Fenichel G: Flaccid limb weakness in childhood. In Fenichel GN: Clinical Pediatric Neurology: A Signs and Symptoms Approach, 4th ed. Philadelphia, WB Saunders, 2001, Chap. 7, pp 171–198.
Huff K: Hypotonia. In Berkowitz C (ed): Pediatrics: A Primary Care Approach. Philadelphia, WB Saunders, 2000, pp 432–436.
Ouvrier R: Hereditary neuropathies in children: The contribution of the new genetics. Semin Pediatr Neurol 1996;3:140–151.

107 Approach to the Child with Movement Disorders

Kenneth Huff

ROLE OF THE GENERALIST

1   Characterize and define the type of movement disorder.
2   Determine any associated medical or neurologic problems.
3   Use appropriate screening laboratory tests to assist in specific diagnosis.
4   Initiate treatment for paroxysmal movement disorders.
5   Initiate treatment for comorbid learning disabilities and psychologic conditions when present.
6   Coordinate care and refer to appropriate specialists when assistance is needed with diagnosis, treatment, and comanagement.

The clinical presentation of movement disorders distinguishes them from other paroxysmal or sustained disorders of behavior. The type of movement problem and the clinical setting can localize the lesion within the nervous system and lead to laboratory tests used to specify the diagnosis. Diagnosis can also be suggested by a combination of a particular type of movement with other associated findings or symptoms.

Although most movement disorders in children are chronic, some are reversible. Reversible disorders respond to specific treatments, but chronic nonreversible disorders may be amenable to effective treatments that minimize disability. Although some treatments are based on specific diagnoses, most are based on the type of movement problem. Distinguishing different types of movement problems both narrows the specific diagnostic possibilities and assists in selecting therapies.

DEFINITION

Movement disorders are neurologic dysfunctions with either too much movement (hyperkinetic disorders) or too little movement (bradykinetic disorders) in the absence of spasticity or weakness. Parkinsonian signs such as bradykinesia are rare in children. Hyperkinetic disorders are much more common. Pyramidal lesions, characterized by weakness, spasticity, hyperreflexia, and Babinski signs, can be distinguished from movement disorders related to extrapyramidal lesions by slowness of movement, muscle

rigidity, and involuntary movements. Older children with extrapyramidal lesions can be misdiagnosed as hysterics when psychologic or behavioral disorders coincide with or antedate the extrapyramidal symptoms.

Abnormal movements can be characterized by their timing, the circumstances at occurrence, characteristics of the movement, and their distribution. Their timing can be paroxysmal or continuous, sustained or nonsustained posturing, and rhythmic or random. Movements should be specified as occurring at rest or with action, with a specific task or nonspecifically, during sleep or during waking; as being suppressible or not suppressible; and as being influenced or uninfluenced by sensory stimuli. The characteristics of the movement may be either patterned or nonpatterned, fast or slow, high or low amplitude, and forceful or weak. The distribution may be focal, segmental, multifocal, unilateral, or generalized. There may be an association with other movements, other neurologic conditions, or other medical disorders. Some movement disorders in the adolescent age group may be associated with dementia: dystonia with Wilson disease, Hallervorden-Spatz disease, and metachromatic leukodystrophy; chorea with Huntington's disease; and myoclonus with Lafora's disease, subacute sclerosing panencephalitis, and AIDS (acquired immunodeficiency syndrome) dementia complex. Table 107-1 describes types of movement disorders in children (see also the videos on the CD-ROM).

Tics are brief, abrupt nonpurposeful movements or utterances usually involving the face, neck, or arms. They may look like normal movement or behavior, but can be distinguished by their repetitive and nonvoluntary nature. Tics can be voluntarily suppressed temporarily. They can be complex or may involve a series of orchestrated simple movements. Most often they are simple recurrent behaviors that vary in frequency with other activities, emotion, or stress. There is often a sense of a buildup of the need to tic, which increases if the child attempts to suppress the movement. Once the movement is made, there is a temporary relief until the sense of the need for the next movement begins again. Box 107-1 lists different types of repetitive behaviors.

Dystonia is abnormal sustained muscle contraction at the point of highest amplitude of movement. It also frequently involves twisting and repetitive movements, or abnormal postures. The speed of contractions may be rapid when not at the point of highest amplitude of the movement.

Table 107-1. Child Movement Disorders*

Movement Disorder	Syndromes
Tics	Tourette's syndrome
	Stimulant medications
Dystonia	Torsion (dystonia musculorum deformans)
	Torticollis
	Wilson's disease
	Hallervorden-Spatz disease
	Lipidoses, metachromatic leukodystrophy, Lesch-Nyhan syndrome, aminoacidopathies
	Dopamine-responsive dystonia
Chorea	Benign
	Cerebral palsy
	Postcardiac surgery
	Sydenham's chorea
	Other encephalitides
	Huntington's chorea
	Other degenerative disorders
	Metabolic—hypocalcemia, hypothyroidism, hepatic failure
Myoclonus	Opsoclonus-myoclonus syndrome
	Juvenile myoclonic epilepsy (Janz)
	Benign myoclonus of infancy
	Hypoxic-ischemic encephalopathy
	Degenerative disorders—Lafora's disease, lipidoses, mitochondrial cytopathies, subacute sclerosing panencephalitis

*See the videos on the CD-ROM.

Contractions may have a consistent directional or postural character. Dystonia is also described by the affected body parts. It may be focal, segmental, multifocal, hemiballism, or generalized. Most commonly in children, a focal dystonia progresses over time to a generalized pattern. Dystonia usually occurs during or is aggravated by a voluntary movement or with voluntary maintenance of a posture of the limbs or body. It can vary with changes in posture or specific actions and can be improved by certain actions. For example, attempted flexion of the fingers to hold a pen may lead to flexion of additional fingers, extension of the wrist, or movements of the opposite hand. Sensory tricks can lessen the contractions, such as pressing a finger to the side of the jaw opposite the direction of a spasmodic torticollis. Dystonia often worsens with stress or fatigue, and gets better with rest, sleep, or hypnosis.

Chorea is an involuntary, irregular, rapid, and uncontrolled movement that flows from one part of the body to another at random. Limb movements are jerky or "dancing." The child appears restless and unable to sit still. Excessive movements of the legs and body make walking

Box 107-1. Repetitive Behaviors

Tics
Compulsions
Stereotypies
Perseverative behaviors
Self-injurious behaviors
Addictive behaviors
Habits
Mannerisms
Anger outbursts

appear bizarre and can produce involuntary throwing of objects or falling to the ground. Athetosis is a slower writhing or twisting movement. Choreoathetosis, the most common type of chorea in children, is a combination of flitting and writhing movements. Hemiballism is a higher amplitude throwing movement of the limb usually of greater amplitude on one side and is sometimes considered in the same class of movements as chorea and athetosis. These movements occur at rest even in the absence of voluntary movement.

Myoclonus is involuntary, sudden, rapid, brief, electric shock–like movements. They involve usually only a few related muscle groups but may cause a jerk of the upper body or the whole body and cause the child to fall. Myoclonus may be triggered by a startle, sensory stimulation, or attempts at voluntary movement. The appearance of myoclonus may also occur in young children in association with opsoclonus, conjugate chaotic dancing eye movements producing random fast amplitude saccades in all directions.

Paroxysmal dyskinesias produce dystonic posturing with choreoathetotic, dystonic, or clonic movements that are episodic and provoked. Between spells the child is completely normal in strength and coordination. The spells, which may occur many times a day, can be socially and athletically disabling and dangerous because spells can occur while crossing the street.

Stereotypies are involuntary, coordinated, patterned, repetitive, rhythmic, purposeless but sometimes seemingly purposeful or ritualistic movements, postures, or utterances. They may be made by normal children when they are bored, excited, or engrossed in an activity. The onset is usually less than 2 years of age and the pattern is usually fixed. Examples include hand or arm flapping, rocking while sitting, head banging, and slapping. Children can be unaware they are making the movements. In some cases they may be able to suppress them when made aware. They are associated with and occur more frequently in autism and global developmental delay and are labeled "self-stimulatory" behaviors in children who may have a limited repertoire of other play behaviors. Self-injurious behaviors are a type of self-stimulatory behavior and include biting the wrist or back of the hand, head hitting, head banging, and skin scratching. Perseverative behaviors, repeated complex movements often involving an object (such as twirling a string), may also be seen in autistic or retarded children.

FUNDAMENTALS

The brain localization of most involuntary movement disorders is hemispheric deep gray matter structures, including the basal ganglia and diencephalic and midbrain nuclei. The caudate nucleus and putamen have internal cholinergic connections, and connections to the substantia nigra pars reticulata and globus pallidum interna that involve inhibitory neurotransmitters (γ-aminobutyric acid, GABA) through both direct and indirect pathways, allowing for modulation of the inhibition (Fig. 107-1). These nuclei have an inhibitory influence on the thalamus that facilitates the cerebral cortex and the pyramidal upper motor neurons, the final common pathway for generating voluntary movement. The

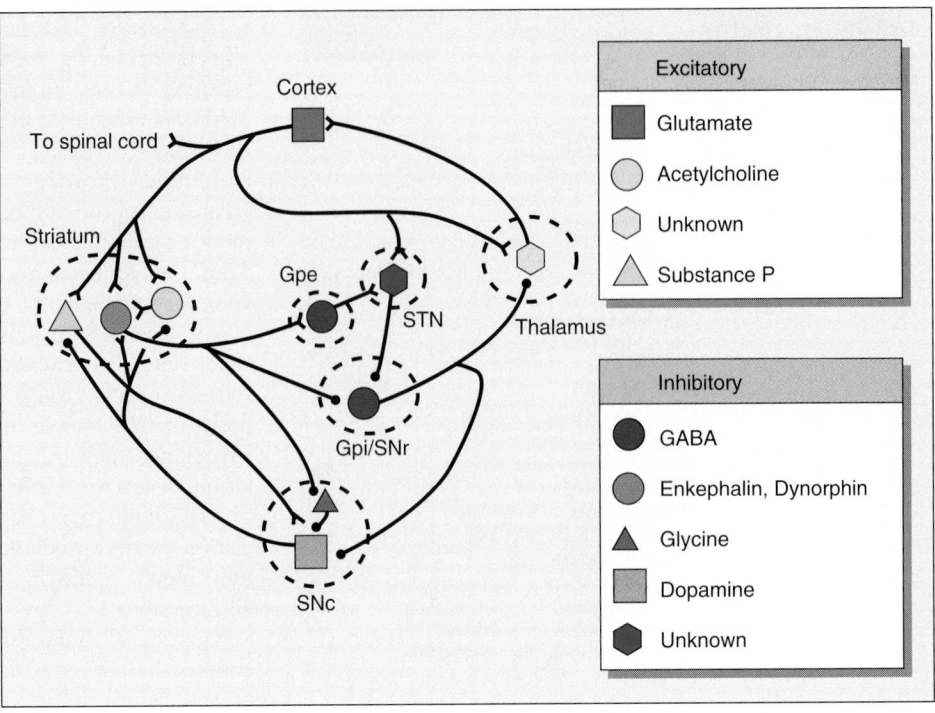

Figure 107-1. Brain nuclei and transmitters involved in movement disorders. Only selected connections are illustrated. The "striatum" includes caudate nucleus, putamen, and nucleus accumbens. Only some of the peptidergic neurons in the striatum are indicated which provides inhibitory input to both direct and indirect pathway stations. The medial pallidum or globus pallidus interna functions together with the pars reticulata of the substantia nigra in the "direct pathway" to the thalamus. The lateral palladium or globus pallidus externa functions separately from the internal portion in the "indirect pathway" to the thalamus by way of the subthalamic nucleus. The pars compacta of the substantia nigra functions separately from the pars reticulata as a separate source of inhibitory dopaminergic input back to the striatum. Gpe, globus pallidus externa; Gpi/SNr, globus pallidus interna/substantia nigra pars reticulata; SNc, substantia nigra pars compacta; STN, subthalamic nucleus.

purpose of the basal ganglia in controlling movement may be to select certain patterns and inhibit "nearby" patterns depending on the child's motivations and sensory milieu. The selected pattern is then transmitted back to the cortex and amplified to initiate movement. If this finely tuned system is damaged, errors may occur in the pattern through excessive or insufficient feedback.

Centers that control movement are easily disrupted to produce disease states. Their complex circuitry and numerous different neurotransmitters are subject to metabolic aberrations. High levels of energy are necessary to maintain membrane polarization of densely packed neuronal connections and for neurotransmitter release and postsynaptic signal transduction to ion channels. The region is vulnerable to hypoxia, vasculopathy producing local ischemia, diseases of energy substrate production (e.g., mitochondrial disorders), toxins of energy production machinery, defects in neurotransmission, and autoimmune insults.

The circuitry connecting parts of the frontal lobe cortex with the caudate and putamen are involved in the pathogenesis of tic disorders, including Tourette's syndrome. The response to different types of medications indicates the complexity of the circuitry and transmitters involved in the disorder. Family and twin studies have supported a genetic etiology for Tourette's syndrome. Linkage evidence suggests several chromosome sites of involvement. The male-to-female ratio is 3:1, implicating developmental sexually dimorphic brain circuitry or chemistry. Androgens exacerbate tics, indicating later hormonal effects as well.

Pediatric autoimmune neuropsychiatric disorder associated with streptococcus (PANDAS) is an immune-related disorder producing tics or obsessive-compulsive disorder (OCD) symptoms in prepubertal children. Symptoms are episodic with abrupt exacerbations associated with group A beta-hemolytic streptococcal infections. In addition to

tics or OCD, children may have choreic movements and hyperactivity. Some children have antineuronal antibodies and the B lymphocyte antigen D8/17 that is also seen with rheumatic fever and autism with compulsive or repetitive behaviors.

The stretch reflex may be important in disorders of tone. Alpha motor neurons stimulate muscle fibers that move the body, and gamma motor neurons adjust the sensitivity of the intrinsic spindle fibers that sense the length or velocity of the muscle's movement. Spindles send signals to the alpha motor neurons that resist external forces on the limbs. This reflex is modulated by signals from above and must be inhibited for normal voluntary movement so that an opposing contraction is not triggered. Damage to the descending tracts causes reduced inhibition and an increase of the "gain" (amplification of output over input) of the stretch reflex over time. The precise mechanism of dystonia is not well understood. Basal ganglia cells that help coordinate cortical and brainstem outflow of descending fibers to the spinal motor neurons respond abnormally to movements of more than one limb rather than a single limb, suggesting lack of precision between signals to different body parts.

Chorea results from damage to the basal ganglia, particularly of the indirect pathway, that inhibits initiation of extraneous movements. Cells in the striatum and globus pallidum are imprecisely targeted resulting in variably and randomly generated muscle signals in both agonist and antagonists, causing cocontraction of these muscle groups.

Myoclonus results from decreased inhibition in the cerebral cortex, a similar mechanism with some types of epilepsy. Startle myoclonus results from hyperexcitable brainstem circuits and decreased inhibition of spinal circuits from defective glycine receptors.

Whether paroxysmal dyskinesias are related more to epilepsies or persistent movement disorders is controversial.

Because affected children remain aware and responsive during episodes, which are precipitated by external factors, and not accompanied by ictal discharges on clinical EEG, the episodes resemble movement disorders. On the other hand, they are associated with mutations in shared specific ion channels with epileptic disorders and have been seen in the same pedigrees as infantile epilepsies. Paroxysmal kinesigenic choreoathetosis (PKC), one of the paroxysmal dyskinesias, is known to be very responsive to traditional anticonvulsants. The paroxysmal dyskinesias may be dominantly inherited with variable penetrance or sporadic.

Stereotypy is both a self-generating sensory stimulus seen in animals subjected to environments of low stimulation and a motor expression of underlying tension and anxiety that accompanies a variety of behavioral disorders.

DIAGNOSIS

Some movement disorders are suppressible or infrequent and may not be seen during the examination. The examiner should therefore observe the patient unobtrusively in the waiting room or while interviewing the parent. Asking the parent to imitate the movements or viewing a home videotape are very helpful. Articulate children can describe their sensations and observations.

Tic disorders are classified as simple transient tics, lasting less than 12 months and related to particular environmental or psychological situations; chronic tics, lasting longer than 12 months but monomorphic; and Tourette's syndrome. Box 107-2 lists the types of tics. Although Tourette's syndrome may be manifested as isolated tics, it is often a combined movement and behavior problem with a wide spectrum of expression and comorbidities. Criteria for the diagnosis of Tourette's syndrome are listed in Box 107-3.

Nonvocal tics associated with Tourette's syndrome include blinking, eyebrow raising, head shaking, grimacing, neck stretching, chin rubbing, shoulder shrugging, eye rolling, nodding, arm jerking or stretching, nose wrinkling, crotch grabbing, finger flexing, and jaw moving. Vocal tics include sniffing, grunting, spitting, throat clearing, squeaking, sucking, clicking, gulping, kissing, hiccoughing, gasping, blowing. Other common tic manifestations include syllables, irrelevant or nonsense words, pallilalia (repeating the end of one's own phrase), echolalia (repeating another's phrase), echopraxia (repeating another's movement), coprolalia

(obscene speech), copropraxia (obscene gestures), coprographia (obscene writing), other socially inappropriate words or gestures, and touching or smelling things or other people.

Diagnosis of Tourette's syndrome is often delayed. Unusual symptoms are attributed to attention-seeking or psychological problems or a normal "developmental phase." Vocal tics have been attributed to upper respiratory, sinus, or bronchial problems or allergies. Eyeblinking or other ocular tics have been erroneously considered as ophthalmologic abnormalities. The belief that tics must be severe and observable in the office is incorrect. A common mistake is to wait for coprolalia to appear before making the diagnosis. Tourette's syndrome patients have a high incidence of comorbid problems, as listed in Box 107-4. Many children with Tourette's syndrome have attention deficit disorder.

Dystonia in children can occur as a genetic disorder or can be secondary to a static insult, structural lesion, medication reaction, degenerative condition with additional manifestations, or conversion disorder. Formerly called dystonia musculorum deformans, juvenile or adolescent limb-onset dystonia has a mean age of onset of 12 years, spreads to other limbs and the trunk within 5 years, and infrequently involves cranial musculature. Inheritance may be autosomal dominant, but penetrance is only 30% of individuals at risk. Cases are usually from deletion mutations in the *DYT1* gene, which encodes for torsin A. Cell density in the pars compacta of the substantia nigra is abnormal. Another gene, *DYT5*, encodes for guanosine triphosphate (GTP) cyclohydrolase I, leading to dopamine-responsive dystonia. This disorder has a characteristic diurnal pattern for symptoms, a progressive course starting with clumsiness and then gait disturbance beginning at 1 to 12 years, and uniformly responds to treatment. Other types of genetic dystonias have been described.

Dystonia may be secondary to early static insults such as hypoxic injury, kernicterus, malformations, and strokes, although it may not manifest for several months. Occasionally head trauma, encephalitis, and brain tumors produce dystonia. Numerous degenerative disorders with

---

Box 107-3. Diagnostic Criteria for Tourette's Syndrome

Combined movement/behavior problem
Onset before 18 years, duration longer than 1 year
Multiple motor and vocal tics evolving
Waxing and waning course
Tics not explained by another condition

Box 107-2. Types of Tics

Clonic
Dystonic
Complex
Sensory
Echopraxic
Copropraxic
Coprographic
Vocalized
- Air movement sounds from pharynx
- Syllables, irrelevant words, nonsense
- Pallilalia, echolalia
- Coprolalia

Box 107-4. Tourette's Syndrome: Associated Problems

Attention deficit hyperactivity disorder
Obsessive-compulsive disorder
Behavioral and emotional problems
Learning disabilities
Impaired visual motor skills
Impaired visual motor performance
Disturbed auditory discrimination
Speech and language disorders
Sleep disorders

general loss of cognitive function and several metabolic disorders including Wilson disease may include dystonia. Several classes of medications including neuroleptics, antiemetics, and calcium-channel blockers may idiosyncratically produce acute dystonia. A tardive dystonia may also be produced by long-term use of an antipsychotic. Toxins including carbon monoxide, cyanide, methanol, and ethylene glycol are also potential etiologic agents.

Chorea may accompany a static injury (perinatal insults or postencephalitis) or may be immune-mediated, drug-induced, hereditary, or a manifestation of a metabolic disorder. Sydenham's chorea follows a group A beta-hemolytic streptococcal infection and can be associated with acute rheumatic fever. Typically it occurs in children 5 to 15 years of age and is associated with hypotonicity, clumsiness, and emotional lability. Other primary dysimmune disorders displaying chorea include lupus erythematosus, Schönlein-Henoch purpura, antiphospholipid antibody syndrome, and chorea gravidarum. Benign hereditary chorea, inherited as an autosomal dominant trait, has an early onset with delayed milestones, has some degree of cognitive impairment, and is nonprogressive with gradually less movement with age. Metabolic disorders including organic acidurias such as glutaric aciduria type I and thyrotoxicosis may also produce chorea. Cardiac patients after cardiopulmonary bypass may develop a transient chorea syndrome lasting several weeks.

Myoclonus can be classified as physiologic, epileptic, or symptomatic. There are numerous physiologic examples, which include hypnagogic jerks in stage II sleep, hiccoughs, exercise or anxiety-induced myoclonus, and benign infantile myoclonus usually occurring with feeding. Epileptic myoclonus includes juvenile myoclonic epilepsy (JME), Otohara's myoclonic epilepsy of infancy, West's syndrome of infantile spasms, and Lennox-Gastaut syndrome. Myoclonus can also be associated with metabolic, storage, or degenerative disorders including Batten's, Lafora's, or Wilson disease and the lipidoses; renal or liver failure; strokes or carbon monoxide poisoning; slow viral encephalitides such as subacute sclerosing panencephalitis (SSPE) related to a defective measles virus; or a paraneoplastic syndrome such as the opsoclonus-myoclonus association with neuroblastoma.

Paroxysmal kinesigenic choreoathetosis and paroxysmal dystonic choreoathetosis are paroxysmal dyskinesias. Paroxysmal kinesigenic choreoathetosis, the more common of the two, is characterized by episodes of sudden assumption of a dystonic posture, a bout of choreoathetosis, or both, lasting less than 5 minutes. A sudden movement or a startle precipitates these brief episodes. Paroxysmal dystonic choreoathetosis, described in several families, is characterized by a brief aura of "tugging" or "stiffness" and then dysarthric speech, dystonic flexion of upper extremities, hand clenching, and flexion or extension of legs and inversion of feet, accompanied by irregular clonic movements, choreoathetosis, or tonic spasms. These attacks can last up to 4 hours and are often precipitated by alcohol, fatigue, coffee, or stress.

Stereotypies are seen most often in mentally retarded or autistic children. Behaviors such as thumb sucking, body rocking, or head banging are classified as stereotypic when they occur after the age when they are considered to be developmentally normal. Rett's syndrome is an autistic disorder seen almost entirely in girls. Acquired finger and hand skills gradually are replaced by stereotypic hand movements including hand wringing, clenching, finger joint flexion and extension, patting, and rubbing. Additionally Rett's syndrome patients exhibit body rocking and weight shifting while standing. Patients with Asperger's syndrome, William's syndrome, and fragile X syndrome show better communication skills than patients with other autistic disorders but also frequently display stereotypies that do not necessarily involve the hands. Stereotypies are also seen in children with schizophrenia. Stereotypies are rarely seen as part of tardive syndromes in children treated chronically with dopamine receptor blocking drugs (neuroleptics). A common example of tardive dyskinesia is the orofacial-lingual-masticatory movement and examples of tardive akathisia include crossing and uncrossing of the legs, picking at clothes, or face rubbing.

Laboratory studies can assist in making a specific diagnosis for the movement disorder. Screening studies may be useful, but laboratory studies should be directed by clues from the history and examination. All patients should be evaluated for treatable etiologies (Table 107-2), such as drug side effects or intoxications, Wilson disease and metabolic cofactor deficiencies, and dopa-responsive dystonia. Screening tests include a complete blood count (CBC) with smear (looking for acanthocytes), electrolytes, blood urea nitrogen (BUN), creatinine, glucose, liver function tests, thyroid function tests, ceruloplasmin or urinary copper excretion, erythrocyte sedimentation rate (ESR) and autoimmune serologies (such as antinuclear antibody, ANA), a metabolic screen to include urine organic acids and oligosaccharides, serum amino acids and carnitine, urine high-performance liquid chromatography (HPLC) toxicologic screen, cerebrospinal fluid (CSF) examination, electroencephalogram (EEG), magnetic resonance imaging (MRI) scan, psychometric testing, and blood buffy coat electron microscopy. General invasive tests include muscle, skin, nerve, or brain biopsy. Specific CSF studies may help diagnose slow virus infections such as subacute sclerosing panencephalitis (SSPE). Functional imaging studies such as positron emission tomography (PET), single photon emission computed tomography (SPECT), or functional MRI

Table 107-2. Potentially Reversible Causes of Movement Disorders

Type of Disorder	Specific Examples
Metabolic imbalance or enzymatic/cofactor deficiency	Hyperthyroidism, some amino acidopathies (including urea cycle disorders), GTP cyclohydrolase deficiency (DYT5 gene-encoded, leads to dopamine-responsive dystonia)
Medication side effects and other intoxications	Neuroleptics, anticonvulsants, tricyclics, stimulants, anesthetics, opiates, lead, strychnine
Metal dysmetabolism	Copper (Wilson's disease)
Immune disorders	Sydenham's chorea, lupus, PANDAS
Tumors	Remote (neuroblastoma), CNS tumors
Infections	Meningoencephalitis

CNS, central nervous system; GTP, guanosine triphosphate; PANDAS, pediatric autoimmune neuropsychiatric disorder associated with streptococcus.

may assist in establishing the area of the nervous system involved. Deep brain recording is sometimes used in planning for stimulation or surgical ablative treatments. An increasing number of specific gene tests are available when the family history suggests heritability or the symptoms point to the possibility of a particular disorder.

MANAGEMENT

Patients with movement disorders generally need to be comanaged with specialists. Treatment modalities address both the movement disorder and the underlying condition. Treatments for movement disorders other than Tourette's syndrome are outlined in Table 107-3. For example, treatment may involve sodium benzoate for some urea cycle disorders; restriction diets for aminoacidopathies; copper chelation for Wilson disease; biotin, pyridoxine, vitamin B_{12}, or dopamine replacement in deficiency states; tumor removal (e.g., neuroblastoma) for paraneoplastic movement problems; antibiotics or acyclovir for an infection; immuno-suppressant therapy for dysimmune problems; and reduction or removal of offending medication or other toxic ingestion.

Direct treatment of the movement disorder may be complicated. The biochemical lesion or even the neuro-transmitter system that mediates the disorder may be undefined. The movement control circuitry is complex. The promiscuity of present medications for nonspecific receptor subtypes creates neurologic side effects. Individual response varies because of pharmacologic factors. However, a number of medications act at various sites, and a combination of rational and empiric approaches to treatment can be taken. Generally, one should start from a low dose per kilogram of body weight and titrate up to reach the minimally effective dose, thus avoiding untoward side effects.

One goal in the treatment of tics is to improve the quality of life and reduce social embarrassment. Tics may be treated with clonidine, an α-adrenergic blocker, using a transdermal patch which also can be titrated in strength. An alternative in this class of medication is guanfacine. The major tranquilizer, haloperidol, a dopamine type 2 receptor blocker, has been a longstanding effective agent for tics. Although it is occasionally effective at very low doses (0.5 mg/day), higher doses may be required, creating the risk of learning suppression and dyskinesia over the long term. Alternatives to haloperidol include pimozide, fluphenazine, and trifluroperazine. The class of atypical neuroleptics, including risperidone, olanzapine, and ziprasidone, and the benzodiazepine clonazepam have also shown some usefulness. An electrocardiogram (ECG) is recommended with initiation of many neuroleptics to determine risk related to prolonged QT_c interval. There is some anecdotal evidence for the usefulness of tetrabenazine, pergolide, calcium channel blockers, and nicotine in treating tics.

Treatment for children with Tourette's syndrome often must be multimodal to address all problematic aspects of the syndrome. Box 107-5 outlines treatments and the side effects of medications used to treat the disorder. Learning disabilities, particularly attention deficit disorder, should be managed with individualized instruction or stimulants if they do not worsen tics. Clonidine or a tricyclic antidepressant may be used if tics are worsened by stimulants. Obsessive-compulsive symptoms within Tourette's syndrome may be treated with fluoxetine or clomipramine. Children and their families often benefit from educational materials, lay support groups, and psychological counseling, especially when there are primary psychobehavioral or secondary social or emotional problems.

Oral treatments for dystonia include L-dopa, anticholinergics, and GABA agonists. In most cases, primary dystonia should be first treated with L-dopa to determine if it is a dopa-responsive dystonia as this is the most easily treated and dramatically responsive type of dystonia. Anticholinergics include trihexyphenidyl, benztropine, and the antihistamine diphenhydramine, which has anticholinergic effects. Trihexyphenidyl is effective in doses of 50 to 100 mg/day but must be started at 1 mg/day and titrated upward over 3 to 6 months to avoid side effects of chorea. Neuroleptic-induced acute idiosyncratic dystonia is treated effectively with a single dose of diphenhydramine 12.5 to 50 mg. Baclofen has also been used for chronic dystonia, starting at 5 to 10 mg twice a day and increasing by 10 to 15 mg/day at weekly intervals up to a total of 150 to 200 mg/day in older children. The limitation is sedation. Other classes of medications, including benzodiazepines, reserpine, and valproic acid, have been used with less success.

Nonoral treatments for dystonia include botulinum toxin, intrathecal baclofen, and surgery. Focal dystonias can be treated with botulinum toxin injections into specific

Table 107-3. Therapies for Movement Disorders Other Than Tourette's Syndrome

Movement Disorder	Pharmacologic Therapy	Other Treatment
Dystonia	Neuroleptic-induced—diphenhydramine, benztropine. Generalized—levodopa/carbidopa, benzodiazepines, anticholinergics, dopamine depletors, baclofen	Intramuscular botulinum toxin injection Intrathecal baclofen pump Intracranial surgery—thalamotomy, deep brain stimulation (globus pallidus)
Chorea	Immunologic—steroids, corticotropin, intravenous immunoglobulin Nonimmunologic—haloperidol, valproate, pimozide, clonazepam, fluphenazine, reserpine, baclofen	
Myoclonus	Epileptic—benzodiazepines, valproate, primidone, phenobarbital, baclofen Posthypoxic—5-hydroxytryptophan	
Paroxysmal dyskinesias	Carbamazepine, phenytoin, phenobarbital, clonazepam	
Sterotypies	Benzodiazepines, baclofen, lithium, opioid antagonists, clomipramine, other neuroleptics	Behavior modification

FUNDAMENTALS

Bacterial meningitis occurs when bacteria enter the CNS either from the bloodstream or directly from a local site. The most common initial portal of entry into the bloodstream is from an infection of either the nasopharynx or lung. Direct local spread may occur from otitis media, sinusitis, cerebral sinus thrombosis, or a structural abnormality (myelomeningocele or traumatic CSF leak). White blood cells (WBCs), mostly polymorphonuclear leukocytes (PMNs), migrate across the blood-brain barrier (brain endothelial cells and glial cells) into the areas around the brain blood vessels and eventually into the CSF. The inflammation that results from the PMN invasion causes the normally tight blood-brain barrier to leak, altering its normal function, allowing fluids and serum protein into the brain, causing brain edema. Both the PMNs and brain glial cells react to the bacterial infection by secreting inflammatory substances called cytokines, leukotrienes, prostaglandins, and platelet activating factor. These inflammatory substances further enhance inflammation, PMN migration, and intravascular coagulation cascade. The vasculitis and enhanced coagulation cause small vessel venous thromboses in the brain that further accentuate brain edema, leading to an increase in intracranial pressure. The end effect of excessive intracranial pressure, if the skull sutures are closed (after 15 to 18 months of age), is to reduce the brain blood flow, leading to poor oxygen delivery to brain tissue and brain infarcts. Reduction in brain blood flow also can occur from concomitant sepsis and the resulting systemic inflammatory response or septic shock.

In animal models of bacterial meningitis, therapeutic antibiotic administration has been shown to increase meningeal inflammation as a result of the breakup of bacteria into fragments, notably endotoxin in gram-negative bacteria and lipoteichoic acid in gram-positive bacteria. This enhanced inflammation can lead to circulatory collapse and shock or further outpouring of inflammatory substances, causing further brain edema and microvascular thromboses. Therefore, although potent antibiotics that enter in high concentrations into the CSF are required to treat bacterial meningitis, the treatment itself may increase the inflammation in the brain and lead to deleterious effects. This development is especially likely when there are large numbers of bacteria in the CSF. The dual effects of the PMNs to engulf and kill bacteria, yet also secrete proinflammatory substances that promote brain edema and vascular thromboses, has led researchers to look at means to decrease this inflammation while still allowing for antibiotic-enhanced bacterial destruction. Dexamethasone, a corticosteroid, has been shown in

animal models of both gram-positive and gram-negative bacterial meningitis to reduce indices of inflammation in the CSF and brain edema especially when administered before antibiotic treatment.

A successful animal model of viral meningitis, the leading cause of aseptic meningitis, has not been established. A mechanism similar to bacterial meningitis, involving the spread of the virus into the CNS from a respiratory tract source, is thought to occur in humans who develop viral meningitis. However, the type and severity of inflammation in this process are different. Similarly, there are few animal models of encephalitis and the large number of conditions and types of infections that are associated with encephalitis make a single animal model relevant to human disease unlikely.

The microorganisms that cause meningitis and encephalitis in children vary by age group and are different from those found in adults (Table 108-1). The recent advent of conjugate polysaccharide vaccines against *Haemophilus influenzae* type b, *Streptococcus pneumoniae*, and polysaccharide vaccines against certain types of *Neisseria meningitidis*, has changed the incidence of childhood bacterial meningitis in the United States. From 1987 to 2002, the Centers for Disease Control (CDC) reported a 99.8% reduction in cases of *H. influenzae* type b (Hib) invasive diseases, including meningitis, from 4.2 to 0.1 cases per 100,000 U.S. population less than 5 years of age. In 1995, the most common cause of bacterial meningitis over all age groups was *S. pneumoniae*, causing 1.1 cases per 100,000 population, and the next most frequent cause was *N. meningitidis*, causing 0.6 cases per 100,000 population. This order of relative incidences of types of bacterial meningitis is the same for all age groups except adolescents, neonates, and the elderly (>60 years of age). Recent use of conjugate pneumococcal vaccines in infancy should further reduce the incidence of pneumococcal meningitis in the United States, making *N. meningitidis* the most frequent cause of childhood and young adult bacterial meningitis. Neonates and young infants up to 3 months of age have a predilection for acquiring meningitis from gram-negative bacteria, group B streptococcus, and *Listeria monocytogenes*. Two thirds of adolescents with bacterial meningitis are infected with *N. meningitidis*, one third with *S. pneumoniae*, and the other third with *H. influenzae*, *Listeria monocytogenes*, and group B streptococcus. The elderly are more likely to acquire meningitis from *S. pneumoniae* and *Listeria monocytogenes*.

The etiologic agents of aseptic meningitis, encephalitis, and meningoencephalitis are listed in Table 108-2. The causes of aseptic meningitis, encephalitis, or meningoencephalitis vary by age group, immune status, season, and geographic

Table 108-1. Etiology of Bacterial Meningitis in the United States by Age Group

Pathogen	Neonate (<1 Month)	Infant/Toddler (1–23 Months)	Child/Adolescent (2–18 Years)
Streptococcus pneumoniae	5–10%	40–60%	30–40%
Neisseria meningitidis	1–2%	30–50%	50–60%
Haemophilus influenzae	1–2%	1–2%	0–8%
Group B streptococcus	40–50%	10–20%	0–3%
Listeria monocytogenes	5–10%	0–1%	0–2%
Gram-negative enteric bacteria	20–30%	0%	0%
Other	5–10%	0–2%	0%

Table 108-2. Microorganisms Associated with Aseptic Meningitis, Encephalitis, and Meningoencephalitis

Type of Pathogen	Associated CNS Disease	Susceptible Host	Route of Transmission/Vector	Geographic Distribution
Virus				
Herpes simplex, types 1, 2	Encephalitis, meningitis, meningoencephalitis	Neonate, rarely older child	Human to human	Worldwide
Cytomegalovirus	Encephalitis	Neonate and IC	Human to human	Worldwide
Epstein-Barr	Encephalitis, aseptic meningitis, myelitis	Child/adolescent and IC	Human to human	Worldwide
Varicella-zoster	Postinfectious encephalitis, aseptic meningitis, myelitis	Child or adolescent	Human to human	Worldwide
Human herpes, type 6	Encephalitis	Young infants and children	Human to human	Worldwide
Adenovirus	Encephalitis, aseptic meningitis	Child/adolescent and IC	Human to human	Worldwide
Vaccinia	Postinfectious encephalitis	Young children	Smallpox vaccine	Worldwide
Western equine encephalitis	Encephalitis, aseptic meningitis	Children	Mosquitoes/birds	West of Mississippi (U.S.)
Eastern equine encephalitis	Encephalitis, aseptic meningitis	Children	Mosquitoes/birds	Atlantic and Gulf Coast (U.S.)
Venezuelan equine encephalitis	Encephalitis, aseptic meningitis	Children	Mosquitoes/horses	Central and South America, Southwestern United States
La Crosse encephalitis	Encephalitis, aseptic meningitis	Children	Mosquitoes/birds	Northeast and Midwest (U.S.)
St. Louis	Encephalitis, aseptic meningitis	Children	Mosquitoes/birds	All areas of the U.S
West Nile encephalitis	Encephalitis, aseptic meningitis	Rare in children/adolescents	Mosquitoes/birds	Atlantic and Gulf Coast (U.S.)
Japanese B encephalitis	Encephalitis, aseptic meningitis	Common in young infants, adolescents	Mosquitoes/pigs and birds	Asia
Enteroviruses	Encephalitis, aseptic meningitis, myelitis	Common in young infants and children	Human to human (fecal-oral)	Worldwide
Measles, mumps	Meningoencephalitis, aseptic meningitis, myelitis	Children	Human to human (respiratory)	Worldwide
Influenza	Postinfectious encephalitis	Children/adolescents	Human to human (respiratory)	Worldwide
Rabies	Encephalitis, meningoencephalitis	Children/adolescents	Animal bite	Worldwide
Human immunodeficiency virus	Encephalitis	Children/adolescents	Human to human (blood)	Worldwide
Lymphocytic choriomeningitis	Encephalitis, aseptic meningitis	Children/adolescents	Rodent	Worldwide
Bacterial (Not Cultured on Routine Media)				
Rickettsia rickettsii (RMSF)	Encephalitis	Children/adolescents	Tick bite	South and Eastern United States and Western Hemisphere
Borrelia burgdorferi (Lyme disease)	Aseptic meningitis, cranial nerve palsies	Children/adolescents	Tick bite	Worldwide
Bartonella henselae (cat-scratch disease)	Encephalitis	Younger children	Scratch of cat, flea	Worldwide
Mycobacterium tuberculosis	Meningoencephalitis	Children/adolescents	Human to human (respiratory)	Worldwide
Mycoplasma pneumoniae	Aseptic meningitis, encephalitis	Children/adolescents	Human to human (respiratory)	Worldwide
Fungi				
Coccidioides immitis	Aseptic meningitis, encephalitis	Rarely in adolescents	Soil inhalation or inoculation	Southwestern United States and Central/South America
Aspergillus, Mucor, Candida	Meningoencephalitis	Immunocompromised	Soil inhalation or inoculation	Worldwide
Toxoplasma gondii	Aseptic meningitis, brain abscess	Immunocompromised, neonates	Cat to human, feces, uncooked meat	Worldwide
Taenia solium (cysticercosis)	Cysts in brain and spinal cord	Children/adolescents	Pig to human, feces	Worldwide
Acanthamoeba, Naegleria	Meningoencephalitis	Rarely in children/adolescents	Fresh water in nose or eyes	Worldwide
Plasmodium falciparum	Meningoencephalitis	Children/adolescents	Mosquito bite	Tropical/subtropical

IC, immunocompromised hosts.

location. The most common cause of these diseases are viruses. Enteroviruses are the most common cause of aseptic meningitis and produce outbreaks in the summer and autumn in temperate climates. Herpes simplex, mumps, mosquito/tick-borne arboviruses and enteroviruses account for the majority of viral agents causing encephalitis and meningoencephalitis. *Mycobacterium tuberculosis* and invasive dimorphic fungi may not grow on routine bacterial media and have to be considered in susceptible hosts when a subacute clinical presentation of aseptic meningitis occurs. However, they remain rare causes of aseptic meningitis in children. Children may develop symptoms of encephalitis

Box 108-1. Complications of Bacterial Meningitis
Subdural effusions
Cerebritis
Hearing loss
Ataxia
Neurologic motor deficits seizure disorder
Cognitive deficits
Shock
Syndrome of inappropriate secretion of antidiuretic hormone
Reactive or suppurative arthritis
Pericardial effusion
Secondary fever (steroids)
Blindness

after a respiratory viral (adenovirus, parainfluenza, or influenza virus) or *Mycoplasma pneumoniae* infection. Additionally, postimmunization neurologic symptoms of encephalopathy with evidence of immune-mediated encephalitis have occurred in children who are administered rabies, Japanese encephalitis, smallpox, typhoid, and rarely yellow fever, mumps, influenza, or live measles virus vaccines.

Despite new powerful antibiotics, steroid use, and more intensive care, many centers in the United States have not documented any change in the mortality rate from bacterial meningitis, which remains about 20% to 25%. The frequency of neurologic sequelae or death after either bacterial meningitis or encephalitis is substantial and is related to the time to initiation of effective treatment and the presence of signs and symptoms of neurologic dysfunction during hospitalization. A retrospective study of bacterial meningitis in adults found that the mortality rate was increased (7.4% versus 35.7%) if antibiotics were delayed more than 4 hours from the time of hospital admission as a result of delays in performing either a lumbar puncture or a head computed tomography (CT) scan. A few studies comparing neurologic abnormalities in children who had received prior antibiotic treatment with those who had not received prior antibiotic treatment found a higher rate in the former. This difference was thought to be due to a delay in diagnosis and treatment of children with partially treated bacterial meningitis. The complications of

bacterial meningitis are varied and are listed in Box 108-1. Prevention of these complications requires clinicians to make an early diagnosis of bacterial meningitis by performing lumbar punctures on all infants and children with signs and symptoms of meningitis, early institution of appropriate antibiotic therapy, and possible consideration of adjunctive anti-inflammatory therapy.

DIAGNOSIS

The diagnosis of meningitis or encephalitis can be difficult, especially in the neonate or young infant, whose symptoms may be nonspecific. A high index of suspicion and a low threshold for performance of a lumbar puncture are essential in diagnosing this condition.

A careful and complete history is essential. The history should include a timeline of when the symptoms started, how they progressed during the illness, and a list of medications used to treat the symptoms. History of birth, immunizations, travel/pets, previous infectious diseases, immunologic defects, and any prior episodes of CNS infections also should be obtained. The signs and symptoms of bacterial meningitis are listed in Table 108-3 and for encephalitis are listed in Box 108-2. The most specific symptoms for either meningitis or encephalitis are neurologic symptoms and include an altered level of consciousness or motor/sensory impairment. Fever may be absent, particularly in some age groups. Intractable vomiting in a systemically ill infant or child may be the hallmark of increased intracranial pressure from a CNS infection. A generalized seizure with a prior onset of fever always should raise concern of a CNS infection but by itself is too nonspecific for uniformly mandating the performance of a lumbar puncture. Benign febrile convulsions are common in otherwise healthy infants and children between the ages of 6 months to 5 years of age. They usually occur once in the first 24 hours of fever, are brief in duration (less than 5 minutes), and are symmetric without signs of system illness or neurologic dysfunction before or after the seizure. If an infant or child has a seizure associated with fever and does not fit the clinical characteristics of a typical benign febrile convulsion, a lumbar puncture, neurologic imaging, and consultation with a pediatric neurologist should be considered.

Table 108-3. Signs and Symptoms of Bacterial Meningitis According to Age

Neonates and Young Infants (0 to 3 Months of Age)	Older Infants (3–24 Months of Age)	Children and Adolescents (2 to 18 Years of Age)
Fever (40% may not have fever, but more have temperature instability)	Fever	Fever (44% may not have fever if older than 6 years)
Lethargy	Lethargy or altered level of consciousness	Lethargy, confusion, coma
Vomiting or poor feeding	Vomiting	Vomiting
Seizure	Seizure	Seizure
Irritability	Irritability	Headache and photophobia
Respiratory distress	Respiratory symptoms (in up to one third)	Respiratory symptoms (in up to one third)
Apnea		Focal neurologic signs (hemiparesis and cranial nerve palsies)
Bulging fontanelle and splitting of the coronal sutures		Papilledema (rarely)
Neck stiffness (rare and late finding, 15% at most)	Neck stiffness	Neck stiffness (~50%)
Petechiae or decreased capillary refill	Petechiae or decreased capillary refill	Kernig/Brudzinski signs +(~50%)
Jaundice in newborns		

Signs and Symptoms of Encephalitis in Children and Adolescents

Headache or irritability
Altered level of conciousness
Behavioral or personality changes
Seizures
Paralysis or cranial nerve abnormalities
Movement disorders, tremor, or abnormalities in muscle tone
Ataxia
Neck stiffness

A lumbar puncture is performed at the L3–L4 intervertebral space to obtain an opening pressure, WBC and differential counts, protein, glucose, Gram stain, and culture, which are the minimum tests required to make the diagnosis of a CNS infection. The normal CSF opening pressure varies with age and the patient's position. The normal opening pressure is 20 to 110 mm H_2O for newborn infants and less than 200 mm H_2O for children. In most cases of CNS infections, this pressure is elevated. Lumbar punctures are contraindicated in children with focal neurologic findings, focal seizures, coma, or papilledema on funduscopic examination until brain imaging with and without contrast medium rules out a space-occupying lesion or noncommunicating hydrocephalus. Brainstem herniation can occur in these conditions. Children with severe coagulation defects or compromised cardiopulmonary status also should not have a lumbar puncture performed until their clinical status is stabilized.

Depending on the likelihood of a diagnosis of encephalitis or aseptic meningitis, other cultures (i.e., viral, fungal, mycobacterial) and special stains should be requested. Additionally, molecular tests to detect the genome of viral or other unusual pathogens may be requested from CSF or blood (e.g., polymerase chain reaction of the CSF for herpes simplex virus, enterovirus, *Mycobacterium tuberculosis*). Acute and convalescent serologic tests may be required to diagnose CNS infections from *Mycoplasma pneumoniae*, respiratory viruses, and syphilis. Many of these tests are not routinely available in most hospitals, and consultation with the hospital microbiologist regarding sending the appropriate specimens to a reference laboratory may be required.

Computed tomography or magnetic resonance imaging of the head should be considered in patients with contraindications to performance of a lumbar puncture, suspected complications of bacterial meningitis, suspected brain abscesses, encephalitis, or other diseases of the CNS. The

type of imaging scan depends on the suspected pathologic process, and a consultation with a radiologist proficient in childhood neurologic disease imaging is useful.

The CSF test results assist in predicting the type of CNS infection (Table 108-4). The CSF indices and pressure help distinguish between bacterial meningitis (high CSF protein, pressure, and WBCs with predominantly PMNs; low CSF glucose), aseptic meningitis (lower CSF WBCs, predominantly mononuclear cells; normal CSF protein, glucose, and pressure), and encephalitis (lower CSF WBCs, predominantly lymphocytes; often a high CSF protein and pressure; normal CSF glucose). Because there is significant overlap of individual test results they should not be considered diagnostic of a certain CNS infection and must be considered in light of the clinical presentation and other tests.

The physical examination of an infant, child, or adolescent with a suspected CNS infection should be extensive and cover all body systems, including a careful and complete neurologic examination. Vital signs and findings of a systemic inflammatory response (respiratory distress, capillary refill, warmth and color of the extremities, quality of pulse) may alert the clinician to an impending circulatory collapse. The overall level of consciousness, using the modified Glasgow Coma Scale is helpful and is predictive of neurologic outcome (see Fig. 31-15). A complete neurologic examination should be performed, including head circumference measurement, palpation of the sutures and fontanelles, funduscopic examination, assessment of neurologic reflexes, motor strength and tone, and sensory nerve and cranial nerve assessment. Funduscopic examination is important to detect papilledema associated with brain edema and hemorrhages or retinitis associated with CNS infections. The neck should be examined for stiffness and for reflex flexion of the knees (Brudzinski's sign). To elicit Kernig's sign, the patient's knee should be flexed and then extended; a positive sign occurs when pain is elicited in the extensor muscles of the thigh. Although neck stiffness and either Kernig's or Brudzinski's sign are elicited in some children and adolescents with meningitis and meningoencephalitis, the absence of these physical signs does not eliminate these conditions. Mucous membranes and skin should be examined to detect a rash that may occur with meningococcemia, enterovirus, herpesviruses, or other infections.

The diagnosis of partially treated bacterial meningitis is often problematic. Clinicians are usually faced with a negative CSF and blood culture after prior oral or parenteral antibiotic treatment and a CSF with at least one index suggestive of bacterial meningitis (low glucose, high

Table 108-4. Laboratory Cerebrospinal Fluid Indicies in Central Nervous System Infections

Diagnostic Test	Bacterial Meningitis	Partially Treated Bacterial Meningitis	Aseptic Meningitis	Encephalitis
CSF pressure (mm H_2O)	Increased (average 300)	Increased or normal	Normal	Increased
CSF WBC count (cells/mm³)	300–50,000*	300–6000	100–500	10–2000
Predominant WBC type	PMN†	PMN	Early PMN and then MN	Lymphocytes
CSF protein (mg/dL)	High (100–500)	High	Normal	Elevated (75–200)
CSF glucose (mg/dL)	Low (<40 in 50% of cases)	Low	Normal	Normal

*Except can be <100 in meningococcal, tuberculous, early, or overwhelming infection.
†Except can be lymphocytic in tuberculosis and monocytic in *Listeria* infection.
CSF, cerebrospinal fluid; MN, mononuclear cells; PMN, polymorphonuclear leukocytes; WBC, white blood cell.

protein, high WBC with a predominance of PMNs). Owing to the significant sequelae of bacterial meningitis, children with suspected partially treated bacterial meningitis should be treated with parenteral antibiotics. Consultation with a pediatric infectious disease specialist is advised early in the management of a patient with a CNS infection unless it is clear from all clinical and laboratory information that the patient has an uncomplicated viral meningitis.

The most common pitfall in the diagnosis of a CNS infection is failure to suspect the diagnosis early in the course of the disease. Since institution of the use of conjugate *H. influenzae* type b and pneumococcal vaccines, acute bacterial meningitis is less frequently seen. Because infants younger than 6 months of age have generally not received more than two immunizations, they are still at risk for *H. influenzae* or pneumococcal meningitis. Children who have emigrated from countries in which these vaccines are not routinely given have an increased risk for these infections. Infants and neonates with meningitis rarely have a stiff neck and even in older children a stiff neck or Kernig's or Brudzinski's signs may be elicited only late in their course of bacterial meningitis. The early rash of meningococcemia may be macular, resembling a viral exanthem rather than purpuric. Neonates with herpes simplex encephalitis may present with fever, irritability, and a few or no vesicles on the skin or mucous membranes. The mother of the neonate may not recollect having had any genital vesicles. In older children and adolescents, headache, fever, and irritability may occur but are nonspecific, occurring in any viral syndrome or a migraine associated with an upper respiratory illness, making a decision regarding the need for a lumbar puncture difficult.

When the diagnosis of meningitis or encephalitis is suspected, a lumbar puncture should be performed. Even if the CSF does not show indices of inflammation, careful follow-up is important because laboratory studies may be normal early in the course of illness. If symptoms worsen, a repeat lumbar puncture is indicated. Anticipatory guidance to parents regarding what signs or symptoms to monitor should be given, along with an appointment for re-evaluation. The parents should be asked to bring their infant, child, or adolescent back for re-evaluation for the occurrence of persistent high fever, signs of toxicity, convulsions, cold and white extremities, intractable vomiting, new appearance of a rash, or the development of increased sleepiness or extreme irritability.

MANAGEMENT

The initial antibiotic treatment for suspected bacterial meningitis in children over 1 month of age is the intravenous administration of a third-generation cephalosporin (usually cefotaxime 275 to 300 mg/kg/day divided in three or four doses or ceftriaxone 100 mg/kg/day given in one or two doses) and vancomycin 60 mg/kg/day divided in four doses. This choice of antibiotics reflects the need to administer agents that target beta-lactamase-producing *H. influenzae* and penicillin- and cephalosporin-resistant *S. pneumoniae*, both of which have become increasingly common. Third-generation cephalosporins have retained their activity against both *H. influenzae* and *N. meningitidis*.

Full-term, healthy neonates with suspected bacterial meningitis may be treated initially with either intravenous ampicillin 150–200 mg/kg/day divided in three to four doses and gentamicin 5.0–7.5 mg/kg/day divided in two or three doses or ampicillin and a third-generation cephalosporin (cefotaxime 150–200 mg/kg/day divided in three or four doses or ceftazidime 150 to 200 mg/kg/day divided in three doses). Ampicillin is used to cover *Listeria monocytogenes*, group B streptococcus, and the rare case of *Enterococcus* spp. Third-generation cephalosporins or aminoglycosides are chosen to cover gram-negative bacterial pathogens. The CSF Gram stain may assist in the early determination of the likely pathogen. Neonatal gram-negative meningitis also warrants the use of two antimicrobial agents, such as a third-generation cephalosporin and an aminoglycoside. Gram-negative meningitis is particularily severe in neonates and is often difficult to treat. Coliform bacteria may possess inducible beta-lactamases that can be produced on extended treatment with single-agent cephalosporin antibiotic treatment. Aminoglycosides, although able to penetrate into the CSF during acute inflammation, may not penetrate as well after meningeal inflammation is reduced during antimicrobial therapy. Repeat lumbar punctures every 24 to 72 hours are routinely performed in gram-negative enteric bacterial meningitis and in cases of meningitis caused by resistant organisms until no growth from the CSF culture is obtained. Generally the doses of antibiotics used to treat bacterial meningitis are higher than those used to treat pneumonia or bacteremia, and in neonates doses vary with weight and postgestational age.

Generally it is recommended to treat noncomplicated *H. influenzae* or pneumococcal meningitis with intravenous antibiotics for 10 days and *N. meningitidis* meningitis for 7 to 10 days. Group B streptococcal and *Listeria monocytogenes* meningitis usually require a course of 14 to 21 days of antimicrobial therapy, and gram-negative meningitis requires 21 days minimum and often 4 to 6 weeks of intravenous antibiotic therapy. Most physicians routinely consult a pediatric infectious disease specialist when a neonate or child presents with bacterial meningitis. Careful observation and evaluation of neurologic and cardiorespiratory status in an intensive care unit is often required for the first 24 to 72 hours when the meningeal inflammation and brain swelling are most severe. Comatose or semicomatose individuals require intubation and artificial ventilation to control their airway and regulate CO_2 production that may have deleterious effects on cerebral perfusion. Children with meningitis often are dehydrated owing to vomiting and accumulation associated with sepsis and may need initial fluid and electrolyte rescuscitation. Management may include monitoring serum/urine electrolytes and osmolality for the syndrome of inappropriate antidiuretic hormone secretion and fluid restriction for the first 24 to 72 hours of hospital admission.

Dexamethasone administered intravenously in a dosage of 0.6 mg/kg/day in four divided doses for the first 2 days of antimicrobial therapy of infants and children 6 weeks of age and older should be considered in patients with suspected bacterial meningitis. Several clinical studies show a reduction in the incidence of significant hearing loss and or other neurologic sequelae in dexamethasone-treated children predominantly with *H. influenzae* meningitis. The efficacy of dexamethasone in adjunctive treatment of *S. pneumoniae* or *N. meningitidis* meningitis has not been established, and some clinicians do not recommend its use in these cases. Maximal effect of dexamethasone administration occurs when it is administered 15 to 20 minutes before or simultaneously with the first dose of antibiotic. Many experts believe that dexamethasone administration may be ineffective if administered 2 to 4 hours after the first dose of antibiotic. Dexamethasone therapy should be avoided in cases of concomitant active gastrointestinal bleeding, consumptive coagulopathy, or in herpes simplex viral CNS infections. It has been used in cases of postinfectious encephalitis caused by vaccine or respiratory viruses with some success and should be considered in all cases of tuberculous meningitis.

Prolonged fever is a common occurrence during treatment of bacterial meningitis. If adjunctive dexamethasone treatment has been given, fever recurrence is common 1 to 2 days after the steroid is discontinued. Fever alone, lasting up to 5 days after initiation of antibiotics, is not of concern. However, if the fever persists longer, if the neurologic response is slow, or if new neurologic signs or symptoms develop after treatment, then a repeat lumbar puncture and neuroimaging should be considered. Consultation with a pediatric neurologist and infectious disease specialist should also be considered if they are not already being involved. Complications that may produce persistent fever and neurologic abnormalities include subdural effusions, cerebritis, abscess formation, and ongoing antibiotic-resistant bacterial meningitis (see Box 108-1). Other causes of fever should be sought, including superficial venous thrombosis associated with antibiotic administration, reactive arthritis, another focus of infection, and antibiotic drug hypersensitivity. Generalized seizures are not uncommon in the first 24 to 48 hours and are usually easily controlled with anticonvulsant medication. Seizures that are focal, prolonged, or poorly controlled or occur after 48 hours from initiation of antibiotic treatment are reasons for concern and are associated with increased incidence of neurologic sequelae and require clinical re-evaluation by a pediatric neurologist.

Aseptic meningitis caused by viruses is usually a mild self-limited illness in children with normal immune status and requires supportive care only. Brief hospitalization is warranted for the more severely ill child, the young infant, or the child who has received prior antibiotic therapy when there is difficulty in distinguishing partially treated bacterial meningitis from viral meningitis. Older infants, children, and adolescents with typical CSF findings of viral meningitis, particularly those who present during the summer or fall months of the year, can be treated symptomatically as outpatients with close follow-up examinations.

The treatment of encephalitis depends on the likely cause. Neonates 1 to 6 weeks of age with symptoms and CSF findings consistent with encephalitis are usually treated with intravenous acyclovir 60 mg/kg/day in three or four divided doses for 3 weeks because of the likelihood and the high frequency and morbidity of herpes simplex virus encephalitis. Superficial (mouth, eye, skin lesion), urine, stool, and CSF viral cultures and CSF polymerase chain reaction tests for herpes simplex virus and enteroviruses

may be useful in determining the need for and duration of acyclovir treatment. Older infants, children, and adolescents may or may not be empirically treated with acyclovir, depending on the history, symptoms, physical examination, CSF findings, neuroimaging studies, and other test results. Other than acyclovir and anticonvulsants to control seizure activity, the management of children with encephalitis is largely supportive in nature.

OUTCOME AND FOLLOW-UP

The most prevalent neurologic sequela of bacterial meningitis is hearing loss, which occurs in 5% to 15% of cases of *H. influenzae* type b meningitis and up to 30% of cases of *S. pneumoniae* meningitis. Motor paralysis in bacterial meningitis is more common early in the course of illness (13%) and usually resolves. Persistant neurologic abnormalities are seen in about 2% of children. Children with confirmed long-term neurologic deficits are at high risk for a subsequent seizure disorder. Ataxia is seen during hospitalization in 3% but rarely persists beyond 1 to 6 months after hospitalization. Visual disturbances may be due to cranial nerve paralysis that leads to problems in accommodation but also may be secondary to optic nerve damage, as seen in the children with neurologic devastation and vegetative state after severe bacterial meningitis.

In some studies, the mortality rate from viral encephalitis is highest in infants. The rates of neurologic sequelae from encephalitis vary with the responsible microorganism but are generally more severe and more frequent than in children with bacterial meningitis. All children with CNS infections should have a hearing test performed shortly after resolution of their acute condition. The test should be repeated 1 to 3 months later if abnormal. Follow-up neurologic examinations and behavioral and developmental assessments are important to detect not only motor and cognitive deficits, but also learning difficulties, attention deficits, and behavioral problems that may not be appreciated initially. An ophthamologic examination should be performed in cases of encephalitis involving newborns or young infants to detect changes associated with congenital CNS infections and subsequent cranial nerve or retinal abnormalities related to the episode of encephalitis.

Mini-index of Related Topics

Table 110-1. Anatomic Factors That Affect Respiratory Function in Infants and Small Children

Anatomic Factor	Effect	Clinical Effects
Small midface, tongue large and close to palate	Obligate nose breathers	Distress from nasal congestion
Larynx higher in neck, epiglottis in contact with soft palate	Obstruction of oral airway	Distress from nasal or oral secretions
Laryngeal cartilage and tracheal rings less rigid	Laryngomalacia	Stridor, wheezing that worsens with agitation and increased respiratory effort
Smaller airways	Increased airway resistance	Wheezing and respiratory distress during bouts of bronchiolitis
Smaller number of alveoli, smaller size alveoli	Predisposition to alveolar collapse	Increased risk for rapid development of hypoxemia
Nonrigid chest wall	Retraction of chest wall and compression of lungs	Increased risk for airway obstruction, hypoxia, hypercarbia, respiratory failure

When approaching a child with respiratory distress, the clinician must assess the severity of the distress rapidly. Severe distress initially should be approached in an *ABC* fashion—airway, breathing, and circulation. The goal is to treat and diagnose simultaneously, preventing life-threatening hypoxia. When the patient is stable or if he or she initially has less severe distress, a more expansive evaluation can ensue safely.

FUNDAMENTALS

Developmental anatomic factors increase the risk of respiratory distress in infants and small children. Table 110-1 lists features of the respiratory tract in infants and small children that affect respiratory function compared with adults and older children. The laryngeal cartilage and the tracheal rings are less rigid in the infant, contributing to laryngomalacia and tracheomalacia. Both improve as the cartilage stiffens with age. Infants and small children have smaller airways throughout the respiratory tract. Relatively small changes in the radius of the subglottic space result in large increases in resistance to gas flow in viral croup (Fig. 110-1). Greater peripheral airway resistance causes wheezing and respiratory distress during bouts of bronchiolitis.

The increased surface tension of the smaller alveola predisposes infants to alveolar collapse. An infant is at greater risk

for rapid development of hypoxia than an older child or adult because of decreased oxygen diffusing capacity and the fact that the resting oxygen consumption is about twice that of an adult's. Because the chest wall is not rigid and the muscles are less developed and fatigue more easily, infants and young children are at increased risk of airway obstruction, hypoxia, hypercarbia, and respiratory failure.

Other nonpulmonary processes may affect a patient's breathing pattern and should be considered when evaluating a child in respiratory distress. Box 110-1 lists some nonpulmonary causes of hyperventilation. Diseases that cause a primary metabolic acidosis (e.g., diabetic ketoacidosis or sepsis with a lactic acidosis) stimulate a compensatory respiratory alkalosis. Reflexive hyperventilation lowers the arterial carbon dioxide and increases the arterial pH. Hysteria also can cause dyspnea and hyperventilation. The diagnosis can be made by history with the only laboratory abnormality being a primary respiratory alkalosis if the child is still hyperventilating.

Disorders of the brain also can alter respiratory patterns. Comatose patients with bilateral cortical dysfunction may have *Cheyne-Stokes* breathing, a pattern of increasing speed and depth of respiration followed by a gradual decrease in both that may proceed to apnea. The pattern increases and decreases in a repeating crescendo-decrescendo pattern. Comatose children with dysfunction of the brainstem may have irregular or slow breathing that requires immediate intubation and establishment of adequate ventilation. Adequate airway, breathing, and circulation must be established in all children with altered mental status and respiratory distress, followed by immediate referral to an emergency department for further evaluation.

Small changes in arterial oxygen concentration do not affect respiratory rate or effort. As the arterial oxygen level

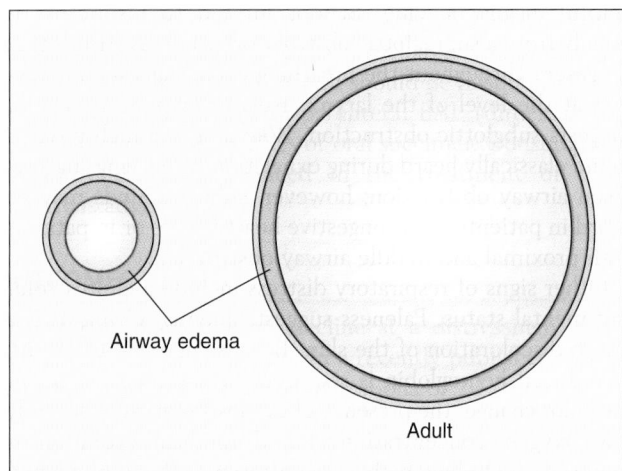

Figure 110-1. Comparison of change in airway radius owing to the same amount of airway edema in an infant and adult.

Airway edema

Adult

Box 110-1. Nonpulmonary Causes of Hyperventilation

- Metabolic acidosis (e.g., sepsis, diabetic ketoacidosis, inborn errors of metabolism)
- Congestive heart failure
- Intoxications (e.g., aspirin, iron)
- Hemoglobinopathies (e.g., carbon monoxide poisoning, methemoglobinopathies)
- Severe intracranial processes (e.g., bilateral cortical disease, pontine hyperventilation)
- Hysteria

decreases to less than 60 mm Hg and the arterial hemoglobin saturation is less than or equal to 90%, however, the chemoreceptors respond to *hypoxemia* and stimulate an increase in the minute ventilation in an attempt to increase the arterial oxygen concentration and the arterial oxygen content. Hypoxia may be primarily from heart disease, diseases of hemoglobin such as methemoglobinopathies, carbon monoxide poisoning, or pulmonary disease.

DIAGNOSIS

The first step in approaching a child with respiratory distress is to classify the process as an upper airway disorder, a lower airway disorder, or a nonpulmonary process resulting in hyperventilation, with consideration of the child's age. Upper airway disease typically presents with congestion, noisy breathing, or stridor. Table 110-2 presents causes of nasal obstruction in newborns and toddlers. Inability to breathe at birth through the nares requires establishment of an emergency airway by either intubation or placement of an oral airway. If a 5 Fr or 6 Fr suction catheter cannot be passed through the nares, the diagnosis of *choanal stenosis* or atresia is suggested and can be confirmed by a computed tomography scan of the nares. Surgical management is required.

Table 110-3 presents causes of upper airway obstruction that are below the nose. *Laryngomalacia* is the most common congenital anomaly of the larynx. Infants have a high-pitched inspiratory stridor that sometimes is relieved by placing the child prone. Crying exacerbates the stridor. Fluoroscopy or laryngoscopy can be used to confirm the diagnosis. Laryngomalacia resolves by age 1 to 2 years and usually requires only supportive care. Consultation with a specialist is appropriate for any newborn with stridor, a hoarse cry, choking with feeding, or obvious craniofacial anomalies.

Stridor in older infants and children can be divided into chronic and acute stridor. Chronic stridor usually is caused by congenital disorders and typically presents in the first year of life. Acquired causes of chronic stridor include tumors, trauma, vocal cord paresis after neck or chest surgery, and vocal cord dysfunction. Screening tests for evaluation of chronic stridor include radiographs of the chest and neck to assess airway patency and chest abnormalities. A barium swallow to assess compression by a vascular ring and fluoroscopy also may be indicated. Ultimately, laryngoscopy and bronchoscopy may be required. These patients must be referred to a pediatric pulmonologist or pediatric otolaryngologist.

Table 110-2. Patient Age and Causes of Nasal Obstruction

Age	Cause
Newborn	Choanal stenosis/atresia
	Midface hypoplasia with craniofacial syndromes
	Nasal encephalocele
	Nasal tumor—teratoma
Infant	Viral upper respiratory tract infection
	Foreign body
Toddler	Adenoid hypertrophy
	Foreign body

Table 110-3. Patient Age and Upper Airway Obstruction

Age	Cause
Newborn	Laryngomalacia
	Laryngeal web, laryngeal cyst, laryngocele, tumor
	Congenital subglottic stenosis
	Tracheoesophageal fistula
	Vascular ring
	Cystic hygroma
	Birth trauma with vocal cord paresis
	Craniofacial anomalies
Infant	Croup
	Tracheoesophageal fistula
	Vascular ring
	Foreign body
	Acquired subglottic stenosis (past history intubation)
	Airway hemangioma
	Retropharyngeal abscess
	Bacterial tracheitis
	Epiglottitis
Toddler	Croup
	Adenoid hypertrophy
	Foreign body
	Caustic ingestion
	Acquired subglottic stenosis (past history intubation)
	Retropharyngeal abscess
	Bacterial tracheitis
	Epiglottitis
Child	Spasmodic croup
	Retropharyngeal abscess
	Peritonsillar abscess
	Epiglottitis
	Bacterial tracheitis
	Trauma

The diagnosis and management of conditions that cause acute stridor are discussed in Chapter 111. The most common cause is *laryngotracheobronchitis* or croup. It primarily affects children age 6 months to 3 years. Affected children generally have low-grade fevers, and their cough is worse at night. *Bacterial tracheitis* may complicate croup. Similar to patients with croup, patients have stridor, but they typically have high fever, hoarseness, and very thick, copious secretions. Other infectious causes of stridor include epiglottitis, retropharyngeal abscess, and peritonsillar abscess. The prevalence of epiglottitis has decreased dramatically with infant vaccination for *Haemophilus influenzae*. A high fever, stridor, drooling, and hoarse voice characterize epiglottitis. The child sits in a "sniffing" position to help maintain a patent airway. Epiglottitis is a medical emergency because the child may occlude the airway acutely. A lateral neck radiograph has the characteristic "thumbprint" sign as a result of edema of the epiglottis. The child should be left in a position of comfort, and unnecessary procedures should be avoided. Intubation should be managed by an anesthesiologist with a surgeon present in case a tracheostomy is required. Neuromuscular blocking agents should be avoided because relaxation of the airway muscles may precipitate total occlusion of the larynx and preclude successful intubation. Cultures of the epiglottis and blood should be obtained, and empirical antibiotics with activity against *Staphylococcus aureus*, *H. influenzae*, *Streptococcus pyogenes*, and *Streptococcus pneumoniae* should be instituted.

Children with *retropharyngeal abscess* and *peritonsillar abscess* also present with fever, muffled voice, and drooling.

Retropharyngeal abscess is more common in children younger than 3 years old. A lateral radiograph reveals widening of the soft tissues between the air column and the cervical vertebrae. Treatment requires surgical drainage and antibiotics. Peritonsillar abscess is uncommon in young children and usually can be seen by examination of the oral cavity with a bulge between the base of the tongue and the lateral pharyngeal wall. Treatment requires antibiotics and aspiration if the child has severe respiratory distress.

Lower airway disease includes obstructive lung diseases, such as asthma or bronchiolitis, or restrictive processes, such as pneumonia or acute respiratory distress syndrome. Children with obstructive processes have an elevated respiratory rate and may have nasal flaring, wheezing, and retractions. Children with severe lower airway obstruction may not have loud wheezing because of limited air movement. Patients generally can maintain normal carbon dioxide levels by increasing their respiratory rate; hypercarbia is a relatively late sign of respiratory insufficiency. Patients with restrictive lung disease typically do not wheeze but may have crackles noted with auscultation of the chest. Tactile fremitus suggests lung consolidation or pleural effusion, whereas egophony suggests consolidation. Children with restrictive lung disease may have grunting, dyspnea, and hypoxemia. Patients who are weak or overmedicated with narcotic or sedative agents make poor respiratory effort with small and infrequent breaths leading to failure of the respiratory "pump." They experience hypoxia and hypercarbia.

Table 110-4 lists potential causes of lower airway disease in children. When assessing children with lower airway disease, the child's age, medical history, and physical examination may be all that is required. If a child has a history of asthma and started wheezing after contracting an upper respiratory tract infection but has been afebrile, a radiograph of the chest may not be necessary. For most other cases of respiratory distress, two radiographic views of the chest are generally helpful.

TREATMENT

Children with respiratory distress should be assessed and monitored. Rapid visual inspection can reveal pallor, cyanosis, or poor respiratory effort. Patients who present in extremis need immediate supplemental oxygen and establishment of an adequate airway and breathing. Respiratory rate and effort, heart rate, blood pressure, and arterial saturation should be determined and followed during assessment and therapy until they are stable. The child's voice quality and ability to phonate should be assessed. Children who are severely short of breath may be able to speak only single words.

Arterial saturation is an important and noninvasive method of monitoring arterial oxygen concentration. The relationship between hemoglobin saturation and arterial oxygen concentration is described by a sigmoidal curve (Fig. 110-2). Small decreases in oxygen concentration less than 60 mm Hg (a saturation of about 90%) result in large decreases in saturation. Because arterial saturation is related directly to the blood oxygen content, efforts to prevent decreases in oxygen concentrations less than 60 mm Hg are generally appropriate. Hyperoxia does not increase oxygen content significantly because oxygen is poorly soluble in blood at normal body temperature.

Patients should receive supplemental oxygen to maintain arterial saturations greater than 90%. Patients with cyanotic congenital heart disease should receive supplemental oxygen if they are desaturated below their usual level. If

Table 110-4. Patient Age and Lower Airway Disease

Age	Reactive Disease	Obstructive Disease	Pump Failure
Newborn	Aspiration Hyalin membrane disease Meconium aspiration Pneumonia Lung hypoplasia Diaphragmatic hernia Pulmonary edema	Congenital lobar emphysema	CNS depression Congenital myasthenia gravis
Infant	Pneumonia Pulmonary edema Aspiration Acute respiratory distress syndrome Pleural effusion Tumor Pulmonary hemorrhage	Bronchiolitis Bronchopulmonary dysplasia Reactive airway disease	Infantile botulism CNS depression Cervical spine injury
Children	Pneumonia Pulmonary edema Aspiration Acute respiratory distress syndrome Pleural effusion Pulmonary contusion Pulmonary hemorrhage Tumor Smoke inhalation Medication toxicity (antineoplastic)	Asthma Bronchitis	CNS depression Cervical spine injury Myasthenia gravis Muscular dystrophy Spinal muscular atrophy Guillain-Barré syndrome Transverse myelitis Multiple sclerosis

CNS, central nervous system.

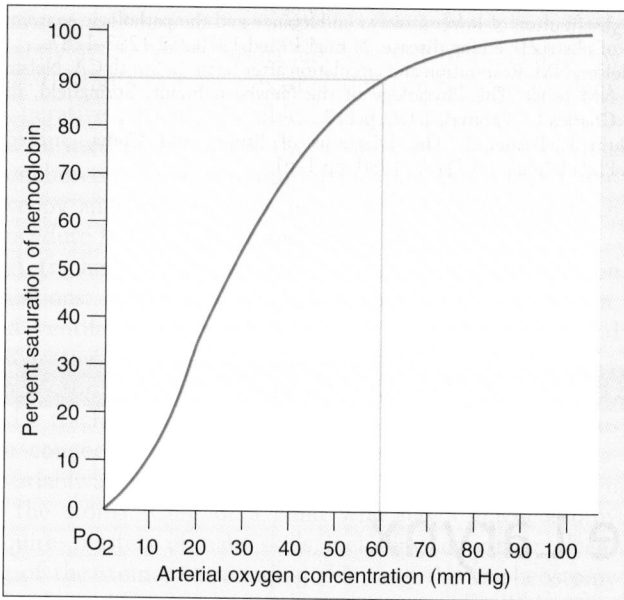

Figure 110-2. Oxyhemoglobin dissociation curve. An arterial oxygen concentration of 60 mm Hg corresponds to a saturation of 90%.

Table 110-5. Monitors, Equipment, and Medications for Intubation

Monitors

Continuous pulse oximeter
Continuous electrocardiogram
Blood pressure measurements every 2–4 min during procedure
Exhaled carbon dioxide detector

Equipment

Bag with appropriate-sized mask
Oxygen source connected to bag at 10–15 L/min
Suction catheter and wall suction
Appropriate-sized endotracheal tubes
Stylet for the endotracheal tube
Laryngoscope with appropriate-sized blades (check battery before laryngoscopy)

Medications

Sedative/amnestic medication
Neuromuscular blocking agent (succinylcholine or rapid-onset nondepolarizing agent [e.g., rocuronium])

nasal prong administration of 3 to 4 L/min of oxygen is inadequate, a mask should be used. Simple facemasks using 6 to 10 L/min of gas flow can deliver 30% to 55% oxygen, whereas nonrebreathing masks can deliver almost 100% oxygen, provided that the gas flow to the reservoir is sufficient to keep the bag distended throughout the respiratory cycle.

Accurate noninvasive methods to measure carbon dioxide levels are not currently available. Capillary blood gases for pH and capillary carbon dioxide levels can be obtained by a finger or toe stick. Inadequate ventilation generally is suspected by observation. An arterial or capillary carbon dioxide of greater than 50 to 55 mm Hg is confirmatory.

Intubation should be considered if the patient has a restrictive lung process, and saturations of equal to or greater than 90% cannot be maintained when breathing 0.6 inspired oxygen or if there is inadequate ventilation. Intubation of asthmatic children should be considered when they are hypoxic, have an altered mental status, or have rising arterial carbon dioxide levels. Modest levels of hypercapnia should be followed closely in an intensive care unit without intubation while the child receives bronchodilators and corticosteroids. Emergency intubation also should be considered in all patients with altered mental status who cannot protect their airway or who make inadequate respiratory efforts. Urgent intubation is recommended for patients with facial burns or smoke inhalation because they may have airway swelling from the burn.

Successful laryngoscopy and tracheal intubation requires careful positioning of the patient, proper equipment, and training. Meticulous patient monitoring is essential to prevent hypoxemia and hypotension during sedation for airway management. Appropriate monitors and equipment are listed in Table 110-5. Continuous pulse oximetry is mandatory, and blood pressure should be measured every 2 to 4 minutes while the child is receiving potent sedative agents to facilitate intubation. Exhaled carbon dioxide monitors

exhibit color changes when carbon dioxide is present and should be used routinely to confirm successful intubation of the trachea in addition to auscultation of the chest to confirm equal breath sounds and the presence of mist in the endotracheal tube.

The intubating provider must be competent in techniques of bag-mask ventilation, use of potent sedative and neuromuscular blocking agents, and airway techniques including rapid sequence intubation and modified rapid sequence intubation. Neck or facial trauma or anomalies that limit range of motion of the jaw or neck may complicate visualization of the larynx, and an airway expert should be consulted rapidly before administration of sedatives or neuromuscular blocking agents. Bag-mask ventilation can be lifesaving and should be used as the first method to stabilize the child in an emergency before laryngoscopy and intubation.

Mini-index of Related Topics

Table 111-1. Differential Diagnoses for Airway Lesions by Etiology

Congenial	Infectious	Tumors	Trauma
Laryngomalacia	Croup	Subglottic hemangioma	Postextubation stridor (subglottic stenosis)
Subglottic stenosis	Supraglottitis	Laryngeal	Foreign-body aspiration
Vocal cord paralysis	Bacterial tracheitis	Papillomatosis	
Tracheomalacia			
Laryngeal web			
Laryngeal cleft			

Laryngomalacia must be differentiated from other causes of inspiratory stridor during infancy (Table 111-1). Tracheomalacia may be confused with laryngomalacia. The two differ in etiology, natural history, and treatment (Table 111-2). Occasionally, tracheomalacia may present with chronic cough, with stridor heard only with careful auscultation. Tracheomalacia should be suspected if there is no response to bronchodilator therapy. Bronchoscopy should be performed with the child breathing spontaneously so that airway dynamics can be seen easily. With expiration, the intrathoracic pressure increases and collapses the trachea (see CD-ROM Video 111-2). Tracheomalacia often is associated with cardiovascular abnormalities, vascular rings, and gastroesophageal reflux. Supportive measures should be used to prevent complications, such as recurrent pneumonia. A common cause of extrinsic or secondary tracheomalacia, innominate artery compression of the trachea, has a characteristic appearance at bronchoscopy. Magnetic resonance imaging of the thorax can show other associated vascular abnormalities. If severe, the segment of tracheomalacia can be "stented" by suturing the adventitia of the aorta to the sternum, pulling the trachea anteriorly. Severe cases of tracheomalacia usually require tracheostomy to stent open the trachea and provide positive airway pressure. Mechanical ventilation support may be needed for years.

Other congenital lesions that cause upper airway obstruction and stridor include laryngeal webs, cysts, vocal cord paralysis, and subglottic stenosis. These lesions produce inspiratory or biphasic stridor unaffected by other activity, such as feeding. The infant's cry may be muffled or absent. These lesions may be seen on bedside flexible laryngoscopy. Treatment varies based on the severity of airway stenosis.

Although occasionally a small laryngeal web or cyst can be removed endoscopically, many patients require tracheostomy and subsequent open airway reconstruction. Many infants born with vocal cord "paralysis" eventually develop adequate vocal cord mobility, which has tempered the need to operate early to expand the airway in these infants. Tracheostomy may be required during early infancy if the vocal cord dysfunction creates airway obstruction.

Infections

Infectious causes of upper airway obstruction usually present with acute stridor. Supraglottitis must be differentiated from croup (Table 111-3). Supraglottitis is an acute, life-threatening infection caused by bacteria localized to the structures of the larynx above the vocal cords. The vocal cords and subglottis are spared. *H. influenzae* type b infection was responsible for most reported cases in the past. The incidence of this infection has decreased significantly since the introduction of the HiB conjugate vaccine. Other bacterial causes include group A β-hemolytic streptococcus, *Staphylococcus aureus*, and *Streptococcus pneumoniae*. The child usually presents with acute onset of high fever, stridor, dysphagia, and air hunger to the point the child is focused only on breathing.

If supraglottitis is the suspected cause of respiratory distress, the airway must be secured safely in the operating room, preferably with a pediatric anesthesiologist and otolaryngologist. The child should be kept calm, often in the parent's arms, en route to the operating room. The diagnosis is confirmed by direct laryngoscopy when a swollen, red supraglottic larynx (Fig. 111-1) is seen. The patient should be transferred to the pediatric intensive care unit

Table 111-2. Comparison between Laryngomalacia and Tracheomalacia

	Laryngomalacia	Tracheomalacia
Stridor	Inspiratory only	Biphasic or expiratory
Etiology	Weak cartilage of the larynx or inadequate neuromuscular tone of the larynx	Widened tracheal rings (primary)
		Extrinsic compression (secondary)
Symptoms in severe cases	Failure to thrive, cyanosis, or apnea	Reflex apnea ("dying spell")
Associated findings	Gastroesophageal reflux common	Chronic cough (may be "barking")
		Cardiovascular abnormalities
		Gastroesophageal reflux
Endoscopic findings	Collapse of epiglottis, arytenoids, or both on inspiration	Normal larynx
	Normal trachea	Posterior tracheal wall "fish mouth" to anterior wall
		May be short or long segment
		Bronchomalacia
Treatment	Expectant management	Aortopexy if innominate artery compression
	Supraglottoplasty in severe cases	Tracheotomy in severe cases
Natural history	Spontaneous resolution by 18 months old	Recurrent "croup" episodes
		Narrow segment less critical with growth

Table 111-3. Comparison between Supraglottitis and Croup

	Supraglottitis	Croup
Peak age	4–5 yr	1–2 yr
Quality of stridor	Wet	Loud
Fever	Often high	Usually low grade
Cough	No	Barking
Dysphagia	Yes, may be drooling	No
Dysphonia	Muffled voice	Hoarse
Toxicity	Yes	No

when the airway is secured by endotracheal intubation. The patient usually can be extubated within 24 to 48 hours when air leaks around the endotracheal tube, signifying resolution of edema. Intravenous antibiotics for about 7 days are indicated. Prognosis is excellent. Some patients with supraglottitis present with a more indolent course, especially older children. Onset of stridor is acute, but the child is not in extremis. Lateral soft tissue neck x-ray can be diagnostic (Fig. 111-2). A "thumbprint" sign indicates an inflamed epiglottis.

Croup is the most common cause of upper airway obstruction in children (see Chapter 110). Parainfluenza virus types 1 and 2 are the most common pathogens. Affected children are usually 6 months to 6 years old, with peak incidence between 1 and 2 years old (see Table 111-3). Typically, viral upper respiratory symptoms precede development of a barking cough, inspiratory stridor, and retractions. Onset may be gradual or rapid. Symptoms generally begin at night and last 2 to 7 days. If the child is not in extremis, an anteroposterior soft tissue neck film can be obtained (Fig. 111-3). The narrow, inflamed subglottic airway is seen as the "steeple sign." Treatment for mild-to-moderate croup is nebulized epinephrine or budesonide, parenteral dexamethasone (0.15 mg/kg), or both. Some children do not respond to initial outpatient treatment and need to be monitored and treated in the hospital. Most children have an uncomplicated course, but occasionally airway obstruction becomes life-threatening and requires intubation. An endotracheal tube smaller than usual should be used to avoid injury to the subglottic mucosa. The

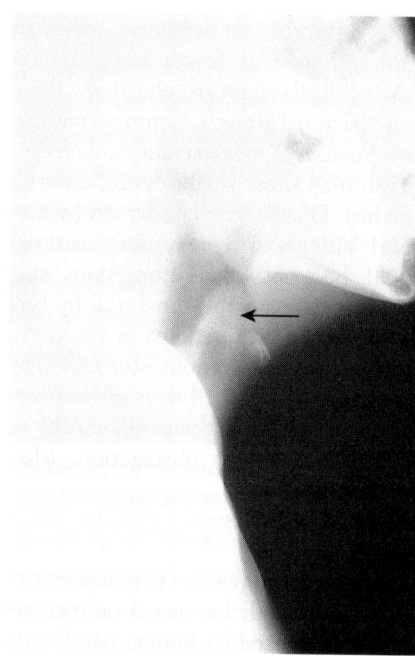

Figure 111-2. Soft tissue lateral neck radiograph of a child with supraglottitis. Note the thickened epiglottis (thumbprint sign [arrow]) indicating soft tissue edema. Anteroposterior radiograph was normal (not shown).

prognosis of croup is excellent. Recurrent croup should be evaluated with direct laryngoscopy and bronchoscopy to exclude airway stenosis when the child is well.

Bacterial tracheitis is an uncommon cause of upper airway obstruction. A viral upper respiratory tract infection often precedes the onset, which may occur in all ages of childhood. Symptoms are similar to croup with a barking cough, retractions, and inspiratory stridor. Additional symptoms include paroxysmal cough with thick sputum, hoarse-

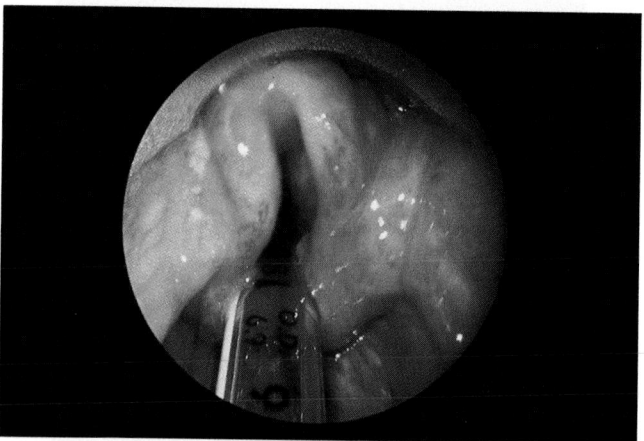

Figure 111-1. Supraglottitis resulting from *Haemophilus influenzae* type b infection in a child who had received 4 vaccines for *H. influenzae* type b. This photo was taken shortly after intubation in the operating room. Note the swollen and hemorrhagic epiglottis. There were no changes at or below the vocal cords (not seen).

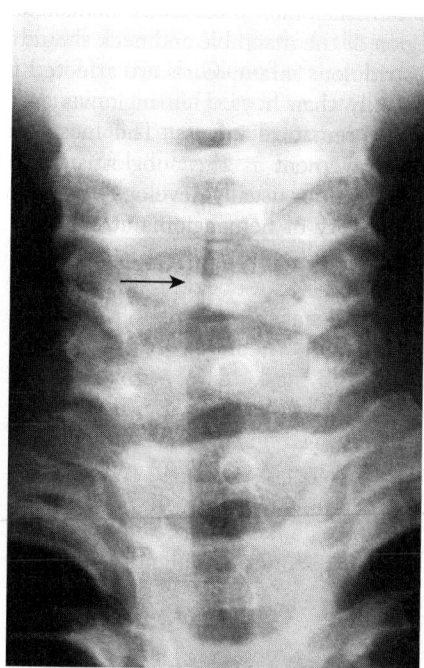

Figure 111-3. Soft tissue anteroposterior radiograph of a child with croup. Note the narrowing to a point (steeple sign [arrow]) in the subglottic airway. Lateral radiograph was normal (not shown).

Pulmonary embolism results from the breaking off and dissemination of a fibrin-platelet clot from a vascular source, usually a deep vein of an extremity. Although rare in children, the occurrence of a pulmonary embolism in a pediatric patient warrants a search for an inherited deficiency of anticoagulation system. Congenital protein C, protein S, and antithrombin III deficiencies all have been associated with pulmonary embolism in patients of all ages. Children with malignancies, central venous catheters, recent operations, obesity, nephrotic syndrome, trauma, ventriculoatrial shunts, and dehydration are at a higher risk of thromboembolic disease owing to hypercoagulable states, endothelial tissue damage, or vascular stasis. Children with systemic lupus erythematosus produce lupus anticoagulants and anticardiolipin antibodies (also found in other autoimmune diseases, certain medications, and neoplasms), a finding associated with thromboses in 25% to 50% of patients with systemic lupus erythematosus. Distal pulmonary infarction, associated with poor lung tissue oxygenation and necrosis, rarely occurs because there are multiple sources of oxygen supply to the lung that can bypass the pulmonary artery obstruction. When distal pulmonary infarction occurs, it usually is associated with hemorrhage into the airways and is manifested by the coughing up of blood (hemoptysis). A condition associated with recurrent chronic airway hemorrhage of unknown etiology is called *idiopathic pulmonary hemosiderosis.*

Disorders of lung and pleura may result in a mismatch of ventilation and perfusion of the lung. Ventilation-perfusion mismatch may occur by continued pulmonary perfusion to the atelectatic, consolidated, or fluid-filled areas of the lung or by ongoing ventilation to underperfused areas of the lung. Ventilation-perfusion mismatch is the primary means by which hypoxemia occurs. Conditions that increase lung stiffness or cause hyperinflation increase the work of breathing and may increase tissue oxygen requirement and result in hypoxemia. Infants and children with disorders of the lung and pleura have increased metabolic and hydration requirements. Chronic fluid loss in a tachypneic infant in respiratory distress needs to be replaced. This replacement may not be achieved by the oral route because of the interference of respiratory distress with oral feeding, necessitating intravenous rehydration and nutrition.

DIAGNOSIS

The precise clinical diagnosis of disorders of the lungs and pleura is often difficult to make on the basis of history and physical examination alone. Signs and symptoms of disorders overlap. Many of the disorders have respiratory distress, including tachypnea, shortness of breath, chest wall retractions, and occasionally central cyanosis when the disorder is advanced. There are several clinical caveats, however, which bear reviewing. Generally, respiratory distress caused by pleural effusions, pneumothorax, or pulmonary embolus and pulmonary infarction does not occur until a large area of the lung and pleura is affected. Chest pain that increases with deep respiration usually occurs earlier when the pleura is inflamed from pneumonia, pulmonary infarction secondary to a pulmonary embolus, or the accumulation of fluid or air in the pleural space. A

moderate-grade or high-grade fever (>38.5°C) is more likely to indicate an infectious process (e.g., pneumonia, pleural empyema, bronchiolitis) than a noninfectious process (e.g., pulmonary embolus, pulmonary edema); however, fever does not distinguish well between bacterial and nonbacterial etiologies. Viral bronchiolitis may cause a fever of 40°C and significant respiratory distress in an infant, making the distinction between bronchiolitis and bacterial pneumonia difficult. The presence of fever does not rule out noninfectious etiologies of respiratory distress because low-grade to moderate-grade fevers (≤38.5°C) are common in pulmonary embolus, atelectasis, and neoplasm.

Important history that can help differentiate disorders of the lungs and pleura from each other includes the duration and acuity of the respiratory distress and cough. The type of cough is important and may be paroxysmal in pertussis, mycoplasma, and some viral infections or sound staccato-like in *Chlamydia trachomatis* lower respiratory tract infections. Often the cough is nonproductive of sputum (dry cough), although it may be productive of sputum (type, color, blood) in some older children. Children younger than 5 to 8 years old often swallow their sputum and cannot provide this information. A prodromal upper respiratory tract infection is a common presentation of pneumonia. A sudden occurrence of acute respiratory distress, especially if there is an absence of associated fever, may make the clinician think more about foreign-body aspiration, pulmonary embolus with infarction, and pulmonary hemorrhage. A history of infectious contact in the home, in friends' homes, or day care allows clinicians to consider respiratory viruses, mycoplasma, or pertussis as the cause of lower respiratory tract infection. A history of documented recurrent pulmonary infections raises concerns about immune deficiency, tuberculosis, neoplasm, cystic fibrosis, foreign-body aspiration (especially if it is the same lobe involved), or a congenital/iatrogenic structural anomaly of the lung (e.g., bronchiectasis, tracheomalacia or bronchiomalacia, vascular ring, bronchogenic cyst, postintubation trauma). It is important to search for associated symptoms, including symptoms related to sinusitis, choking event, neurologic disorder, cardiac disorder, autoimmune disorder, weight loss, night sweats, esophageal reflux, odynophagia, or deep venous thrombosis, which may suggest a specific etiology. A careful history of any chronic recreational or medicinal drug use, smoking in adolescents, exposure to tuberculosis, previous immunizations (*H. influenzae* type b, *S. pneumoniae*, bacille Calmette-Guérin) or prior hospitalizations for respiratory distress should be elicited.

The physical examination should include vital signs, growth parameters, general appearance, and nutritional status. The presence of failure to thrive, poor nutritional status, and evidence of chronic sinusitis or otitis media should cause clinicians to consider cystic fibrosis, immune deficiency, or tuberculosis.

Of all the physical signs, the resting respiratory rate is the most sensitive means of diagnosing a disorder of the lung and pleura. The World Health Organization has developed a highly sensitive clinical algorithm based on resting respiratory rate to predict pneumonia in infants and children in developing countries who present with cough and fever. A resting respiratory rate of greater than 50 breaths/min for infants younger than 12 months old and greater than 40 breaths/min for children 12 months old and older suggests a clinical diagnosis of lower respiratory tract infections. The presence of crackles and retractions of the chest wall improves the overall sensitivity in the diagnosis of pneumonia when used in conjunction with the respiratory rate, but the specificity is poor. The specificity of the diagnosis of pneumonia is improved when a chest radiograph is evaluated.

The physical examination of the chest should include the palpation of any cervical or supraclavicular lymphadenopathy that may be due to tuberculosis or neoplasm arising in the chest. The trachea should be palpated and assessed for deviation from midline. Tracheal deviation can occur secondary to expansion of the lung on one side from air or fluid accumulation in the pleural cavity (trachea moves away from affected side) or collapse of an airway that occurs with atelectasis (trachea moves toward the affected side). The observation of general expansion of the chest, presence of chest wall retractions (supraclavicular, substernal, and intercostal) or nasal flaring may indicate respiratory distress. Young infants may make a grunting sound when they experience respiratory distress. This grunting represents an attempt to increase their airway end-expiratory pressure. Percussion of the chest when the patient is sitting upright indicates dullness in an area of consolidation from pneumonia or pleural effusion. If the affected side is hypertympanic on percussion, a pneumothorax should be considered. Auscultation of the chest may indicate decreased air entry or abnormal breath sounds on an affected side of pneumonia, pulmonary infarction, pleural effusion, or pneumothorax. Crackles are intermittent high-pitched or low-pitched sounds heard on auscultation of the chest, usually occur during inspiration, and indicate the opening or closure of small airways caused by fluid. Wheezes may be heard during the expiratory phase or continuously throughout respiration. They are high-pitched musical sounds that result from air moving through narrowed airway passages.

The overall clinical status of the infant or child is important. A child who appears toxic may have an infection. An ashen, lethargic child or a child who is irritable and inconsolable with diminished air entry on chest auscultation, even in the absence of significant respiratory distress, may be in impending respiratory failure from diaphragmatic and accessory muscle fatigue. The paradoxical rising of the abdominal wall during inspiration suggests that the child needs prompt oxygen administration and a secured airway to provide assisted ventilation (see Chapter 29).

A chest radiograph including upright anteroposterior and lateral views should be obtained in all infants and children with significant respiratory distress. Alveolar infiltrates associated with lobar consolidation and air bronchograms suggest bacterial pneumonia. Perihilar interstitial infiltrates suggest viral or mycoplasmal pneumonia, but significant overlap between radiographic presentations of bacterial or nonbacterial pneumonia exists. Bronchiolitis typically shows peribronchial thickening, interstitial infiltrates, areas of atelectasis, and general hyperinflation on chest x-ray. Pulmonary tuberculosis is often silent clinically in children younger than 7 to 10 years old and may be detected only by the presence of significant hilar or paratracheal lymphadenopathy. Hilar lymphadenopathy also can occur in dimorphic fungal infections of the lung and in pulmonary anthrax. Pulmonary anthrax is rare in North America but needs to be considered in the current era of bioterrorism threats. The chest radiograph in cases of pulmonary anthrax may show focal pneumonitis caused by hemorrhagic necrosis of lung tissue and mediastinal widening caused by hemorrhagic necrosis and rupture of the mediastinal lymph nodes. Older children and adolescents with pulmonary hemorrhage usually present with patchy areas of alveolar infiltrates that may be confused with pneumonia. Pulmonary edema usually causes fluffy alveolar infiltrates and interstitial infiltrates (owing to the engorged lymphatics) that are greatest in the dependent lobes of the lung and are seen in association with a dilated failing heart. Air bronchograms, although unusual in cases of pulmonary edema, may not be seen in all cases of pneumonia either. Further compounding the difficulties in distinguishing pulmonary edema from pneumonia is that infants and children with pulmonary edema and congestive heart failure are at increased risk of concomitant respiratory infections probably on the basis of diminished lung defense mechanisms. It is not unusual for patients placed on a ventilator for pulmonary edema also to manifest a pulmonary infection that is not distinguishable on the basis of radiologic examination alone. Clinicians should assess these patients carefully for purulent change in tracheal secretions, fixed patches of infiltrates that do not change with the use of diuretic medication, and an unexplained increase in temperature or elevation in white blood cell count.

Atelectasis is another condition that is difficult to distinguish from pneumonia and may require the assistance of a pediatric radiologist. The radiographic findings of linear infiltrates that cause the normal lobar fissure lines to deviate toward the affected area are typical for this condition. Chest plain films should be taken in inspiration and expiration if there is concern that a foreign body may have been aspirated. If present, there may be unilateral hyperinflation of the distal affected lobe in the expiratory phase because of the ball-in-valve effect of partial airway obstruction.

A minimum of 400 mL of pleural fluid is required to show obliteration of the costophrenic angle of the lung shadow on an upright chest radiograph in the older child or adolescent. The lateral decubitus view may detect only 50 mL of pleural fluid. Loculated effusions, seen often in pleural empyema, are suspected when the fluid fails to shift during the change in position from upright to decubitus. Large pleural effusions can mask an underlying contributing lobar infiltrate. Ultrasound or computed tomography (CT) of the chest may be useful in determining the state of the lung parenchyma obscured by the effusion and the thickness of the pleura or the presence of any loculations where needle aspiration would be problematic. A loculated pleural effusion secondary to an underlying pneumonia often needs to be differentiated from lung abscess for management reasons, and CT is the best radiologic means to do this. CT of the chest provides useful information to assess lung involvement in interstitial lung processes, to evaluate a suspected congenital anomaly of the lung, and as a more sensitive means to detect hilar lymphadenopathy in suspected cases of pulmonary tuberculosis in children. Consultation with a pediatric radiologist is suggested whenever the diagnosis of these uncommon disorders of the lung and pleura are considered.

In addition to the chest radiograph, other tests that should be considered routinely in infants and children with respiratory distress include pulse oximetry, complete blood count with differential, electrolytes, total serum protein/albumin, lactate dehydrogenase, liver and renal function tests, and, in certain patients with chronic respiratory disorders, a capillary or arterial blood gas to assess oxygen and carbon dioxide concentrations.

Patients with suspected bacterial pneumonia should have a blood culture obtained. Nasopharyngeal secretions for rapid identification and culture for pertussis, C. trachomatis, and respiratory viruses should be considered, especially in infants younger than 2 years old with a perihilar, patchy interstitial, or peribronchial pneumonia. Sputum Gram stain and bacterial culture should be performed whenever feasible in children older than age 5 to 8 years with presumed bacterial pneumonia. Children younger than 5 years old generally are not compliant with attempts to retrieve sputum. Even older children 5 to 10 years old may have difficulties in producing sputum, and they may be assisted in producing sputum using hypertonic saline mask inhalation. Children requiring intubation for respiratory failure and pneumonia should have the secretions from the first suction after intubation sent for, at minimum, Gram stain and routine bacterial culture. Immunocompromised children with serious respiratory compromise may require protective bronchoscopy, bronchoalveolar lavage, bronchial brushings, and bronchial biopsy for bacterial, mycologic, mycobacterial, and viral special stains and cultures to determine the etiology of the pneumonia.

In all patients with suspected tuberculosis, 5 tuberculin units of purified protein derivative (PPD) containing heat-killed tubercle bacilli antigens should be injected intracutaneously in a forearm with a tetanus or Candida control antigen. Pulmonary tuberculosis should be suspected in all children with HIV infection, chronic or recurrent pneumonia, hilar lymphadenopathy, large pleural effusions, or positive tuberculosis contact history. Infants and children with a positive PPD skin test and abnormal chest radiograph should have three early-morning gastric aspirates (or sputum samples if capable of providing) obtained for mycobacterial stains and cultures.

Pulmonary hemorrhage can be diagnosed by the finding of hemosiderin-laden alveolar macrophages on cytologic evaluation of bronchoalveolar lavage fluid specimens. Children with suspected pulmonary embolism should have a careful examination of the deep venous system using Doppler ultrasound, an electrocardiogram to look for the classic S1Q3T3 (S wave in lead I, Q wave and T wave inversion in lead III) changes indicating right heart strain, and an arterial gas to look for an abnormal P(A-a) oxygen gradient. Often these diagnostic modalities, including chest radiograph, are negative in children. Ventilation-perfusion scans look for abnormalities in lung ventilation and perfusion caused by a clot in a pulmonary vessel. They are nonin-

vasive tests, but they may not detect all cases of pulmonary embolus. A more invasive procedure, and the gold standard for the diagnosis of pulmonary embolus, is pulmonary angiography. It should be considered in patients suspected of having a pulmonary embolus whose initial workup with other noninvasive tests is negative.

MANAGEMENT

All infants and children with pneumonia do not require admission to the hospital. Consideration regarding admission includes age, clinical status, and the ability to take oral medications (Box 113-1). Most infants with bronchiolitis do well with symptomatic treatment at home. Hospitalization is required, however, for infants with significant respiratory compromise.

There are not sufficient randomized, controlled antibiotic treatment trials of children with pneumonia that have sufficient power, defined end points, and a clear distinction between bacterial and nonbacterial etiologies to determine outcomes related to antibiotic treatment choices. Treatment considerations are empirical and based largely on local antibiotic resistance patterns. Outpatient treatment of an older infant or child with presumed bacterial pneumonia may include treatment with either amoxicillin-clavulanate (40 mg/kg/day orally in three divided doses) or a second-generation cephalosporin (cefuroxime [30 mg/kg/day orally in two divided doses]). The addition or substitution of one of these antibiotics with a macrolide antibiotic, such as erythromycin (40 mg/kg/day orally divided in four doses), clarithromycin (15 mg/kg/day orally in two doses), or azithromycin (10 mg/kg/day loading dose, then 5 mg/kg/day orally), depends on the likelihood of an atypical pathogen and the prevalence of macrolide-resistant S. pneumoniae isolates in the local community. Children older than age 2 years have been shown to have significant respiratory disease caused by M. pneumoniae, and the use of one of the newer macrolides in such a child or adolescent with perihilar interstitial infiltrates is reasonable. In communities with significant erythromycin-resistant S. pneumoniae, combination therapy of either amoxicillin-clavulanate or cefuroxime plus a newer macrolide (clarithromycin or azithromycin) is recommended. Infants 3 to 24 months old being managed as outpatients are more likely to have presumed viral pneumonia and do not require antibiotic

---

Box 113-1. Factors to Consider Regarding Decision to Admit a Child with Pneumonia to the Hospital

- Age <6 months
- Toxic appearance
- Moderate-to-severe respiratory distress
- Ongoing oxygen requirement
- Dehydration
- Vomiting and unable to take oral medication
- Immunocompromised
- Previous pneumonia requiring intubation
- Failure of outpatient treatment
- Poorly compliant

treatment, unless a secondary bacterial pneumonia or bacterial infection elsewhere (e.g., otitis media, urinary tract infection) is suspected. Infants 1 to 3 months old with afebrile pneumonitis may have either pertussis or *C. trachomatis*. These infants should be treated with erythromycin (40 mg/kg/day orally in four divided doses).

All outpatient antibiotic treatment for pneumonia should be for 7 to 10 days. Generally, repeat chest radiographs are not performed unless symptoms persist because chest films take several weeks to clear despite resolution of clinical signs and symptoms. Although a single episode of pneumonia is unlikely to cause significant sequelae, multiple or recurrent episodes of pneumonia may leave a patient with some loss of lung function, pulmonary fibrosis, and chronic lung disease later in life. To minimize these sequelae, a pediatric infectious disease specialist and pulmonologist should assess infants and children with recurrent episodes of pneumonia.

Previously healthy infants and children hospitalized for pneumonia should be treated with a second-generation cephalosporin (cefuroxime sodium [150 mg/kg/day intravenously in three divided doses]) plus either erythromycin (40 mg/kg/day intravenously/orally) or one of the newer macrolides for 7 to 10 days. Neonates, debilitated patients with chronic respiratory diseases, and patients with nosocomial pneumonia may require intravenous oxacillin (or vancomycin if methicillin-resistant *S. aureus* is suspected or prevalent in the hospital or community) plus either a third-generation cephalosporin (ceftazidime) or an aminoglycoside or a uredo-penicillin/β-lactamase inhibitor combination (piperacillin-tazobactam) to cover routine respiratory bacteria, gram-negative bacteria, and *S. aureus*. Immunocompromised children may require a similar combination of antimicrobial agents plus trimethoprim and sulfamethoxazole (trimethoprim 20 mg/sulfamethoxazole 100 mg/kg/day intravenously in two divided doses) to ensure coverage against *P. carinii*. Acute aspiration usually causes chemical inflammation in the lung and is manifested as a new infiltrate that generally improves markedly within 48 hours. If there is no improvement within 48 hours or if there is persistent moderate or high fever, a secondary bacterial pneumonia should be suspected, and treatment should be initiated with the following regimen: oxacillin plus a uredo-penicillin/β-lactamase inhibitor combination (piperacillin-tazobactam), a third-generation cephalosporin (ceftazidime), or an aminoglycoside in addition to metronidazole (30 mg/kg/day intravenously in three divided doses).

Viral pneumonia and bronchiolitis in infants usually respond to symptomatic treatment. Hospitalization is reserved for patients with evidence of significant hypoxic or moderate-to-severe respiratory distress. Humidified oxygen by nasal cannula, fluid rehydration, and oral feeding as tolerated are instituted as appropriate. Parenteral or inhaled steroids or bronchodilators have not been shown conclusively to be beneficial in treating these disorders. Close outpatient follow-up to assess hydration and respiratory status of infants during the first 3 days of illness, when their disease is maximal, is recommended.

Significant atelectasis often responds to physiotherapy aimed at dislodging mucous plugs that cause segmental lobar collapse. The use of incentive inspirometry for postoperative patients reduces this condition. Patients with persistent significant atelectasis without re-expansion of one lobe lasting several weeks should be referred to a specialist, who may perform a bronchoscopic evaluation to rule out neoplasm or foreign body and to remove whatever is causing the obstruction (see Chapter 36).

Large pleural effusions should be tapped early in their course for symptomatic relief and diagnosis. The generalist may wish to refer patients for this procedure. Pleural fluid should be sent for routine biochemistry, Gram stain, routine bacterial culture, and cytopathology if neoplasm is considered (Table 113-3). When tuberculosis or pleural neoplasm is suspected, a pleural biopsy can be performed simultaneously with the pleural tap. Additionally, 10 mL of pleural fluid should be inoculated into a routine aerobic and anaerobic blood culture bottle if there has been prior antibiotic use and into a mycobacterial blood culture bottle if pulmonary tuberculosis is likely. A pleural effusion that either grows a likely pathogen or has cell or biochemical indices suggesting empyema should be drained completely by the insertion of a chest tube. Failure to drain adequately an infected pleural effusion or empyema within 1 week from diagnosis frequently leads to a thickened pleura that contains multiple loculations of infected pus that are difficult to drain. Occasionally, these patients have daily spikes of high temperature and require open thoracotomy and decortication of the pleural surface to avoid later severe pleural scarring and restrictive lung function. Parapneumonic effusions that are sterile and do not have cell or biochemical indices indicating empyema usually respond within a few days to appropriate antimicrobial therapy, resolve completely over several weeks without sequelae, and do not require chest tube insertion. Ideally a pediatric infectious disease specialist and general surgeon should be consulted in patients with a large pleural effusion.

Treatment of pneumothorax varies with its extent and its underlying cause. Treatment of air leaks in newborns is

Table 113-3. Differential Diagnosis of Pleural Effusions

Transudate	Exudate
Congestive heart failure	Empyema due to infection
Pericardial disease	Neoplasm
Cirrhosis	Hemothorax and trauma
Nephrotic syndrome	Pancreatitis
Peritoneal dialysis	Intra-abdominal abscesses
Chylothorax	Sarcoidosis
Collagen vascular diseases	Drugs: phenytoin, isoniazid, nitrofurantoin, amiodarone, antimetabolites
Parapneumonic effusion	Congenital lymphagiectasia or irradiation
Pulmonary embolus and infarction	Post–cardiac surgery (Dressler's syndrome)
Hypothyroidism	Esophageal perforation
Vitamin A intoxication	Urinary tract obstruction
Inflammatory bowel disease	Yellow nail syndrome
Pulmonary arteriovenous malformation	
Iatrogenic (catheters, ventriculoperitoneal shunts)	
Postoperative atelectasis	

discussed in Chapter 213. Children with underlying disease, such as cystic fibrosis or asthma, already may be under the care of a specialist, who should be consulted urgently should a pneumothorax occur. A small pneumothorax (occupying <5% of the hemithorax) in a patient with asthma may resolve spontaneously. Administering 100% oxygen may be helpful, hastening resolution by increasing resorption of free air. Needle aspiration usually is required for a pneumothorax that occupies 15% or more of the hemithorax. Patients on mechanical ventilation usually are treated with tube thoracostomy. Spontaneous pneumothorax and recurrent primary pneumothorax in a previously healthy child or adolescent should be referred to a specialist for evaluation. Tension pneumothorax leads to hypoxemia, impaired venous return, and shock. Emergency treatment consists of decompression by needle aspiration, followed by placement of a chest tube. A large-bore needle, with or without a three-way stopcock, should be inserted over the second or third rib anteriorly and air aspirated (see Chapter 298). Mediastinal air rarely requires treatment. Evacuation of a pneumomediastinum is indicated if it compromises cardiac output.

If a patient is suspected to have a pulmonary embolus, urgent consultation is indicated. Patients with documented pulmonary embolus should be treated with anticoagulation therapy under the direction and dosing of a pediatric hematologist. Children with massive pulmonary embolus and hemodynamic instability may require consultations by a pediatric cardiologist, pediatric intensivist, and cardiothoracic surgeon. Tissue plasminogen activator or urokinase intravenous drip may be given in a pediatric intensive care unit to dissolve the clot. Rarely, children require a surgical embolectomy by a cardiothoracic surgeon to remove the clot.

Mini-index of Related Topics

SUGGESTED READINGS

Alkrinawi S, Chernick V: Pleural infection in children. Semin Respir Infect 1996;11:148–154.

Boyer KM: Nonbacterial pneumonia. In Feigin RD, Cherry JD (eds): Textbook of Pediatric Infectious Diseases, 4th ed. Philadelphia, WB Saunders, 1998, pp 260–269.

Freeman L: Pulmonary embolism in a 13-year-old boy. Pediatr Emerg Care 1999;15:422–424.

Gruber WC: Bronchiolitis: Epidemiology, treatment and prevention. Semin Pediatr Infect Dis 1995;6:128–134.

Jadavji T, Law B, Lebel MH, et al: A practical guide for the diagnosis and treatment of pediatric pneumonia. Can Med Assoc J 1997;156: S703–S711.

114 Tuberculosis

Ken Purdy

ROLE OF THE GENERALIST

1 Know the difference between tuberculosis exposure, latent infection, and disease.

2 Obtain specimens for culture and susceptibility testing from children suspected or known to have tuberculosis disease.

3 Place contagious adolescents in appropriate isolation until they are noninfectious.

4 Use one of three combinations for initial therapy of all children with uncomplicated tuberculosis.

5 Report each child with suspected or known tuberculosis promptly to local public health departments.

6 Perform human immunodeficiency virus testing for all children and adolescents with tuberculosis.

7 Treat patients with susceptible isolates for at least 6 months.

8 Evaluate adolescents who are smear-positive after 3 months of therapy for potential nonadherence or infection with drug-resistant strains.

9 Perform tuberculin skin testing on high-risk children and adolescents.

10 Treat all persons with latent infection unless documentation of prior treatment is available.

Terms for tuberculosis in the languages of major civilizations (Sanskrit, *rajayakshma*; Greek, *phthisis*; Latin, *tabes*; and even an older English term, *consumption*) denote wasting, a classic sign of advanced disease. Tuberculosis was the leading cause of death in the United States in the 19th century and was highly prevalent in densely populated industrial cities such as New York, Boston, and Philadelphia.

During the first half of the 20th century, public health measures and significant improvements in sanitation and nutrition dramatically reduced the incidence of tuberculosis in the United States. In 1943, streptomycin became the first antimicrobial shown to be effective in treating patients with tuberculosis. Later, isoniazid (1952) and rifampin (1970) were shown to have superior sterilizing activity and fewer adverse effects; the latter have remained the most important therapeutic agents.

Despite major strides in prevention and therapy, tuberculosis remains a global menace. It is the largest single infectious cause of death in the world. More than one third of the world's population is infected with *Mycobacterium tuberculosis*. A 6-month course of combination drug therapy cures 90% to 95% of patients with pulmonary tuberculosis, even in high-prevalence countries. The 6-month course of drug therapy costs U.S. $11 per course in some nations, but it is inaccessible to more than half of the world's inhabitants. If current trends continue, between 2000 and 2020, nearly 1 billion people will be newly infected, 200 million people will develop active disease, and 35 million people will die from tuberculosis. Of these, 28 million cases of disease and at least 4 million deaths will occur among children 0 to 14 years old. The National Academy of Sciences has described tuberculosis as "the most neglected infectious disease of our time."

Tuberculosis also has re-emerged in the United States. Re-emergence began during the 1970s after rates of disease reached an all-time nadir, and federal funding of programs to prevent tuberculosis was reduced. From 1985 to 1992, as a result of a languishing public health infrastructure and acquired immunodeficiency syndrome (AIDS), the incidence of tuberculosis in the United States increased 20% overall and 35% among children. The incidence of disease has declined slowly since 1992, but the proportion of U.S. cases among persons born in high-prevalence countries is rising. The steady immigration of persons from endemic areas, the growing proportion of urban children who are homeless or live in poverty, and the alarming spread of human immunodeficiency virus (HIV-1) among young women and minorities in inner cities foreshadow that tuberculosis, including pediatric disease, will remain a public health problem for many years to come.

Elimination of tuberculosis among U.S.-born individuals within the 21st century may be feasible with currently available resources. The successful control of tuberculosis transmission and disease requires improved communication between primary care providers and local public health departments, including reporting of all suspected and known cases of tuberculosis disease, the use of targeted tuberculin skin testing (TST) to enhance the identification of latent infection and disease among high-risk persons, and adequate treatment of all cases of latent tuberculosis infection and disease. The goal of this chapter is to improve the generalist's ability to diagnose, report, and treat children with latent tuberculosis infection and uncomplicated tuberculosis disease.

FUNDAMENTALS

Tuberculosis exposure is defined as significant contact with an adult or adolescent who has contagious pulmonary or laryngeal tuberculosis. Some exposed patients become infected and subsequently develop a positive TST, but others do not. The two cannot be distinguished reliably when exposure has been recent. By definition, exposed patients never have a positive TST, symptoms or signs of disease, or laboratory or radiographic findings of disease. Children 0 to 3 years old who are exposed to tuberculosis are treated for presumed latent infection because TST may take much longer to become positive in young children, and the risk of central nervous system (CNS) or disseminated tuberculosis is especially high, particularly among infants younger than 2 years old. Individuals who are at least 5 years old do not require therapy for exposure.

Latent tuberculosis infection is manifested by a positive TST. The term *latent tuberculosis* excludes individuals with symptoms, signs, or laboratory or radiographic findings of active disease. Chest radiographs of children with latent infection often are completely normal. The presence of one or two calcified or noncalcified nodules in the lung parenchyma or a few calcified regional lymph nodes usually reflects latent infection and only rarely is a manifestation of active disease. All children and adolescents with latent tuberculosis infection are treated to prevent active disease and to limit the transmission of tuberculosis.

Tuberculosis disease is defined as the presence of symptoms, signs, or radiographic or laboratory evidence of active tuberculosis. Disease tends to occur in two chronologically distinct patterns: primary disease, which occurs within months after primary infection, and reactivation disease, which generally occurs years after primary infection, mostly among elderly adults and immunocompromised individuals. Disease in very young children is nearly always primary disease because infants and toddlers tend to lack effective cell-mediated immunity.

Several epidemiologic factors are associated reproducibly with an increased risk for developing tuberculosis. Among U.S. adults and children, these factors include coinfection with HIV, birth (or residence during childhood) in a country with a high prevalence of tuberculosis, homelessness, abnormally low body weight (usually reflecting malnutrition), and, to a lesser extent, urban residence and nonwhite race. Residence or close contact with an adolescent or adult who has any of the preceding risk factors is another proven risk factor. Non-HIV immunocompromising conditions are associated with a 10-fold to 30-fold increase in the rate of disease; these include lymphoma and other hematologic malignancies, high-dose or long-term therapy with immunosuppressive agents including corticosteroids or chemotherapeutic agents, chronic renal failure, chronic hemodialysis, and solid-organ transplantation. Very young age is associated with a twofold to fivefold increase in the probability of disease. Diabetes mellitus and other metabolic disorders are associated with a modest increase in risk. Adolescents have unique risk factors for tuberculosis, including incarceration or residence in correctional facilities and injection drug use. With the exception of health care workers, occupational exposure is uncommon. Many genetic factors, including conditions that impair the normal interaction of macrophages and T cells, also may increase susceptibility to disease.

Although primary infection may occur at any age, the incidence of disease varies tremendously among different age groups. Adults 65 years old and older account for most cases reported in the United States, but the highest incidence of disease (new cases per period of time per population) occurs among children 0 to 2 years old. Children 5 to 14 years old have the lowest overall incidence of disease.

More than 95% of tuberculosis is caused by *M. tuberculosis*, an exclusively human pathogen that is believed to have evolved from bovine tubercle bacilli. *Mycobacterium bovis*, the second most common pathogen, is the agent of bovine tuberculosis; cattle are the definitive hosts. Accidental infection of humans is an important cause of human tuberculosis in countries where cow milk is not pasteurized routinely. A third cause, *Mycobacterium africanum*, is found primarily in Africa and is rare. The three organisms are slow-growing, obligate aerobes and collectively are termed *tuberculous mycobacteria* or *tubercle bacilli*. More than 50 species of mycobacteria, several of which are pathogenic in humans, do not cause pulmonary tubercles and are referred to as *nontuberculous mycobacteria*. All tuberculous and nontuberculous mycobacteria have thick, waxlike cell walls that stain poorly with Gram stain, but well with carbol-fuchsin and fluorochrome dyes. Because they uniquely resist decolorization with acid-alcohol after primary staining, mycobacteria also are called *acid-fast bacilli* (AFB).

The primary route of transmission of tuberculosis is inhalation. More than 98% of transmission occurs when an adult or adolescent with contagious pulmonary tuberculosis coughs or sneezes or when an individual with laryngeal tuberculosis speaks loudly or sings. These four processes generate fine airborne droplets containing tubercle bacilli that are inhaled by uninfected individuals. Droplets that are smaller than 5 to 10 mm^3 can enter the small airways of the lung. A single inhaled organism is sufficient to establish infection. Before adolescence, children with pulmonary tuberculosis are seldom contagious because they cough less frequently and with less expulsive force than older individuals. Tubercle bacilli rarely are transmitted from a pregnant woman to her fetus, either hematogenously across the placenta if the mother has disseminated tuberculosis or by infected amniotic fluid if she has tuberculous endometritis. The most frequent route of transmission to infants is perinatal or postnatal inhalation of organisms from a contagious mother or household member.

Inhaled tubercle bacilli multiply and establish one to several primary foci of infection in the lung. Macrophages migrate to these foci and ingest tubercle bacilli, but virulent organisms survive and replicate intracellularly within macrophage phagolysosomes. Infected macrophages then enter the lymphatics and become concentrated in the regional lymph nodes that drain each primary focus. In the lymph nodes, macrophages process and present mycobacterial antigens to T cells, some of which become sensitized to these antigens and proliferate. Sensitized T cells enter the bloodstream and migrate to primary foci, where they release potent inflammatory cytokines, including interferon-γ, that enhance the ability of macrophages to engulf and digest organisms and necrotic cells. When enough T cells have been sensitized, they can display a delayed hypersensitivity response when a purified antigen, tuberculin, is injected into the dermis. This response consists of a local area of induration and erythema that appears within 6 to 12 hours, peaks in 2 to 7 days, and slowly subsides. Older children and adults develop delayed hypersensitivity within 2 to 12 weeks after inhalation of organisms, but young children and immunocompromised individuals may require months or may not develop a response at all (a condition called *anergy*).

Normally, cytokines produced by T cells at the primary foci induce macrophages to differentiate into epithelioid cells that encase primary foci and lead to the formation of granulomas. Latent infection results when the host effectively has walled off all primary foci. Six to 12 months after their formation, each granuloma begins to undergo caseous necrosis and calcifies within years. Untreated, tubercle bacilli within these lesions survive for decades.

Reactivation disease occurs when waning host immunity allows latent tubercle bacilli to re-establish productive lung infection or, less commonly, when new tubercle bacilli are inhaled after latent infection already is established. In both instances, previously sensitized memory T cells generate a brisk anamnestic proliferation of cytotoxic and helper T cells that migrate to the infected sites in the lung. The enormous number of T cells produces significantly more inflammation than the usual T-cell response to primary infection and can lead to the formation of cavitary lesions in the lung containing more than 1000 times the number of tubercle bacilli found in primary lung disease. Patients of any age with cavitary lung disease are highly contagious and usually have numerous AFB on sputum smears.

DIAGNOSIS

The earliest symptoms of tuberculosis—malaise, fatigue, anorexia, and night sweats—can occur with disease at any anatomic site but are nonspecific and often are missed in very young children. Cough is common among individuals with pulmonary tuberculosis and may be chronic, but it often is absent in young children. Most children with tuberculosis lack overt signs of disease, but fever and mild-to-moderate cervical, axillary, or supraclavicular adenopathy occasionally are present. Weight loss and anemia may be apparent with pulmonary or extrapulmonary disease.

All children who have been exposed to tuberculosis or who are suspected to have latent tuberculosis infection or disease should undergo skin testing. Nearly 90% of children with pulmonary tuberculosis, but less than one quarter with CNS or disseminated disease, have a positive TST. Placement and interpretation of TSTs are discussed in the section on prevention.

The most common anatomic site of tuberculosis among all ages is the lung (Table 114-1). Primary infection may be present in any lobe or lobar segment, but reactivation disease in immunocompetent persons tends to occur at the apices. Auscultation in children seldom reveals abnormalities, although rales may be present with tuberculous pneumonia. Anteroposterior and lateral chest radiographs generally reveal one or two segmental-to-lobar infiltrates

Table 114-1. Sites of Tuberculosis among U.S. Children 0 to 14 Years of Age, 1989 and 1999

Site of Disease	Reported Cases, 1989 (%)	Reported Cases, 1999 (%)
Pulmonary	1007 (76.2)*	821 (78.6)[†]
Lymphatic	228 (17.3)	160 (15.3)
Pleural	24 (1.8)	12 (1.1)
Meningeal	25 (1.9)	17 (1.6)
Bone/joint	15 (1.1)	10 (1.0)
Genitourinary	3 (0.2)	—
Peritoneal	3 (0.2)	5 (0.4)
Other	16 (1.2)	19 (1.8)
Miliary	10 (0.8)	17 (1.6)
Total	1321	1044

*Includes 10 cases of pulmonary disease with extrapulmonary or miliary disease.
[†]Includes 17 cases of pulmonary disease with extrapulmonary or miliary disease.
Data courtesy of Marisa Moore, MD, MPH; Centers for Disease Control and Prevention.

(depending on the number of primary foci) and associated hilar or mediastinal lymphadenopathy (Fig. 114-1). Radiographic evidence of tuberculosis may be absent on plain films with early pulmonary disease, particularly in children. When the diagnosis is probable (e.g., in a child with known recent exposure and suggestive symptoms), computed tomography of the chest is more likely to detect early lesions. Although hilar or mediastinal adenopathy also may be caused by malignancy, systemic autoimmune disorders, or pulmonary fungal infections including coccidioidomycosis or histoplasmosis, these findings strongly suggest tuberculosis when compatible clinical and epidemiologic findings are present.

Sites of extrapulmonary tuberculosis depend primarily on age, but also on the immune status of the patient. The most common site of extrapulmonary disease is the lymphatic system (see Table 114-1). Tuberculous lymphadenitis tends to affect the cervical nodes, but also may involve the supraclavicular or axillary nodes. Cervical lymphadenitis, known historically as *scrofula*, is most common among elementary school–age children, but can affect individuals of any age. Bilateral involvement is uncommon, and the degree of adenopathy can be impressive. In patients who delay seeking medical attention, nodes may suppurate and form fistulous tracts, in which case surgical excision expedites healing and decreases the likelihood of large, cosmetically undesirable scars. In the absence of fistulae, medical management is sufficient.

Pleural tuberculosis is the second most common extrapulmonary site and occurs primarily among older adolescents and young adults. The diagnosis is suggested when signs of a pleural effusion are present with clinical or epidemiologic findings that suggest tuberculosis, but also should be considered among all patients with pleural effusions of unclear etiology who fail to improve with conventional antimicrobial therapy. Tuberculous pleural fluid is chylous to purulent in appearance and tends to be extremely high in protein and low in glucose. AFB are observed in less than one third of stained specimens. Video-assisted thoracoscopy or open thoracotomy with decortication of diseased pleurae, combined with antimycobacterial agents, is the definitive therapy. Surgery also permits the

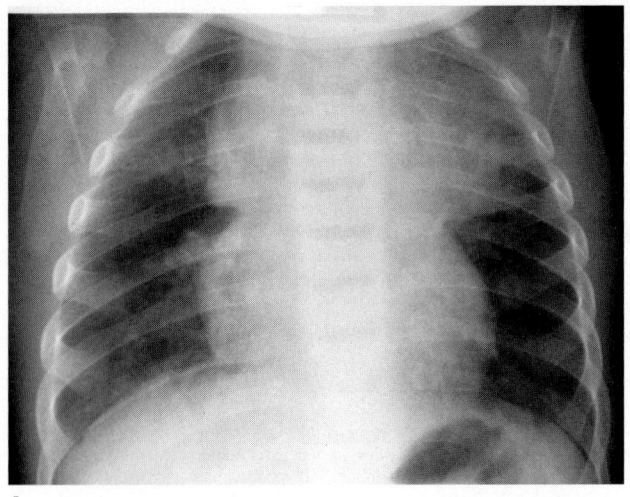

A

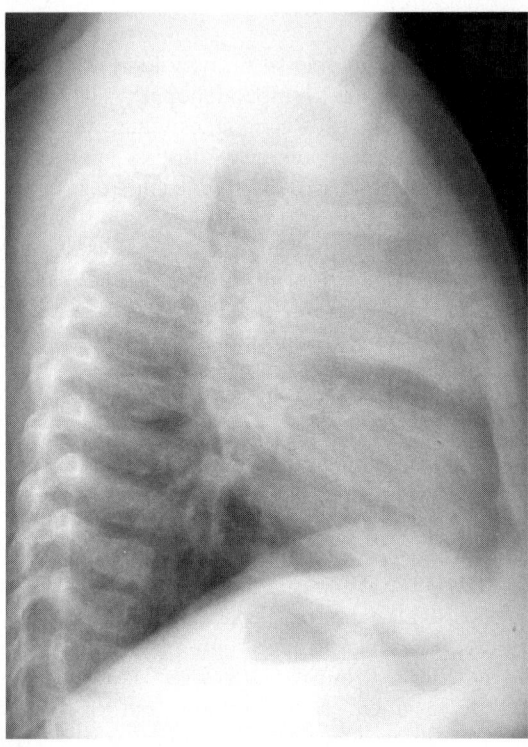

B

Figure 114-1. Anteroposterior **(A)** and lateral **(B)** chest radiographs of a 7-month-old infant with tuberculosis of the anterior segment of the left upper lobe. Chest films obtained 2 weeks earlier had been interpreted as showing a prominent left lobe of the thymus. *Mycobacterium tuberculosis* was isolated from gastric aspirate cultures. (Courtesy of Michael J. Diament, MD, and Bradley K. Ackerson, MD.)

collection of pleural tissue for culture when alternative specimens are negative or unavailable.

The CNS is the third most common extrapulmonary site of tuberculosis infection. CNS disease affects 1% to 4% of children with untreated tuberculosis. Tuberculous meningitis is the most common form and accounts for 85% to 90% of children with CNS disease. The highest incidence is among children 0 to 2 years old. Tuberculomas, masses of tubercle bacilli that resemble tumors, affect fewer than 10% of children with CNS disease, but may occur anywhere in the brain parenchyma and frequently are associated with meningitis.

Meningitis has been classified into three stages (Table 114-2). Stage I includes patients presenting with nonspecific symptoms (fever, anorexia, intermittent headache, or vomiting) and no definite signs of CNS involvement. Stage II patients have more specific signs of CNS involvement (lethargy, disorientation, meningismus, or acute cranial nerve palsies) but lack profound alteration of consciousness. Cranial nerve palsies, usually of the abducens or facial nerves, but also of the oculomotor nerve and others, are particularly suggestive of the etiology in children with clinical meningitis. Stage III patients have florid alteration of consciousness and obvious signs of increased intracranial pressure; more than half progress to coma and death. Less than one third of children with tuberculous meningitis have TSTs greater than 10 mm, and most are completely anergic. Stage I meningitis usually develops within 1 week of the onset of symptoms, and stage II develops within 2 to 3 weeks. Stage III meningitis generally occurs after the third week of illness, but it may be observed earlier in very young or immunocompromised children. Most patients with meningeal tuberculosis are not diagnosed until stages II or III because of the indolent and nonspecific nature of stage I findings.

Computed tomography of the brain with contrast enhancement is useful for diagnosing CNS tuberculosis and helps exclude critical mass effect before lumbar puncture. The use of contrast material allows detection of basilar enhancement of the meninges, a relatively specific finding, and of masses (tuberculomas or tuberculous brain abscesses). The cerebrospinal fluid of children with tuberculous meningitis tends to have fewer than 500 white blood cells/mm^3, an elevated protein, and a low glucose. The yield of cerebrospinal fluid AFB stains and culture is low (10% to 20%). Cerebrospinal fluid polymerase chain reaction of *M. tuberculosis* DNA improves the likelihood of establishing a microbiologic diagnosis, but is negative in more than half of individuals with CNS tuberculosis. Epidemiologic and clinical findings alone lead to the diagnosis of most cases.

One third to one half of children with CNS tuberculosis have permanent neurologic sequelae, including seizure disorders, hydrocephalus requiring the placement of ventriculoperitoneal shunts, or mild-to-gross cognitive impairment. Children with tuberculomas may require

Table 114-2. Stages of Tuberculosis Meningitis

Stage	Symptoms
Stage I	Nonspecific symptoms with no definite signs of CNS involvement Fever Anorexia Intermittent headache Vomiting
Stage II	CNS symptoms, but without profound alteration of consciousness Lethargy Disorientation Meningismus Acute cranial nerve palsies
Stage III	Florid alteration of consciousness and obvious signs of increased intracranial pressure

CNS, central nervous system.

surgical resection in addition to antimycobacterial therapy. The administration of corticosteroids with antimycobacterial therapy can relieve mass effect caused by tuberculomas and can be lifesaving when critical intracranial hypertension is present.

Tuberculous osteomyelitis and septic arthritis occurs among only 1% to 2% of untreated children. Osteomyelitis has a propensity for the vertebrae, particularly the inferior thoracic and superior lumbar vertebrae, and is termed *tuberculous spondylitis*. Spondylitis tends to have an indolent presentation. Patients often are diagnosed 2 to 3 months after the onset of symptoms—usually back pain and local soft tissue tenderness. Severe, deforming involvement with kyphosis is known by the eponym *Pott's disease* and represents late spondylitis. Other complications of spondylitis include paravertebral or psoas abscesses, spinal cord compression, and cord injury leading to lower extremity paresis and bowel or bladder dysfunction. Septic arthritis is rare and usually involves the knee or hip, but it may involve any joint.

The gastrointestinal system is an uncommon site of disease. Gastrointestinal tuberculosis may occur when tubercle bacilli are ingested (primary gastrointestinal disease), when infectious secretions from the lungs are swallowed (secondary gastrointestinal disease), or when tubercle bacilli infect the gastrointestinal tract hematogenously (disseminated disease). Of these three, disseminated gastrointestinal disease is most common in the United States and includes such manifestations as peritonitis, hepatitis, and pancreatitis. Primary or secondary intestinal disease usually occurs in the terminal ileum and cecum (ileocecitis), is more frequent with *M. bovis* than with *M. tuberculosis*, and has become exceedingly rare in the United States. Tuberculous ileocecitis shares numerous clinical and histologic features with Crohn's disease, for which it has been mistaken and treated with corticosteroids, leading to serious and occasionally fatal complications. Stools range from blood-tinged diarrhea to frank hematochezia, and abdominal pain and distention often are present. Untreated, ileocecitis may lead to small bowel obstruction, bowel perforation, polymicrobial peritonitis and sepsis, and death.

Genitourinary tuberculosis may involve the kidney, ureters, or reproductive tract of both sexes. It arises hematogenously, and tubercle bacilli in these organs are latent for years before disease is apparent clinically. Renal tuberculosis is rare before adulthood, and in the pediatric population it occurs primarily among adolescents. Renal involvement may be manifested by flank pain, sterile pyuria, or hematuria, but tuberculosis is seldom the cause when these findings are encountered in children.

Tuberculous pericarditis is rare in the United States, but it is an important cause of chronic constrictive pericarditis in high-prevalence countries. Biopsy and culture of pericardial tissue is the best way to make the definitive diagnosis. Nonimmunocompromised adults with tuberculous pericarditis have better outcomes when corticosteroids are added to antimycobacterial therapy for several weeks. Open drainage of pericardial effusions seems to prevent their reaccumulation and may promote more rapid healing, but data are insufficient to determine whether partial or total pericardiectomy improves outcome.

Primary or reactivation tuberculosis that is ineffectively controlled by host immune mechanisms may lead to disseminated (or miliary) tuberculosis. In disseminated tuberculosis, tubercle bacilli within the lung enter the bloodstream and may establish infection throughout the lung, liver, bone marrow, spleen, adrenal glands, CNS, musculoskeletal system, genitourinary tract, and other organs. Hematogenous lesions range in size from microscopic to a few millimeters in diameter. Their resemblance to fine seeds on gross pathology is the origin of the term *miliary tuberculosis* (Latin *milia*, "millet seeds"). Organisms that become lodged in pulmonary capillaries and arterioles produce miliary pulmonary tuberculosis, which is characterized on plain radiographs by a diffuse reticulonodular disease pattern. Disseminated disease may occur in very young children, the elderly, and immunocompromised individuals of any age; it has the highest morbidity and mortality of all forms of tuberculosis.

MANAGEMENT

In the near future, more U.S. individuals with tuberculosis are likely to be evaluated and treated by primary care providers and clinicians in managed care organizations than by specialty public health clinics. In light of this change, the Infectious Disease Society of America and the Centers for Disease Control and Prevention have published a new set of recommendations and performance indicators to help primary care clinicians improve the outcome of patients treated for latent tuberculosis infection and uncomplicated disease. This section paraphrases these guidelines as they apply to the care of children and adolescents.

Whenever possible, specimens should be collected for mycobacterial staining and culture from all children and adolescents suspected of having pulmonary tuberculosis and children who have disease at other readily accessible sites (e.g., meningeal disease). Children with pulmonary tuberculosis who are younger than 10 years old may lack a cough and rarely produce sputum. Aspiration or lavage of early morning gastric contents is an alternative method to obtain isolates from children. The yield of culture from children who have had early morning gastric aspirates collected on 3 consecutive, separate days is 50%. Gastric content collection can be performed on an outpatient basis. Treatment is more likely to succeed when the identification and susceptibilities of the patient's organism are known. Knowledge of susceptibilities also allows detection of multidrug-resistant tuberculosis, defined as isolates that are resistant to isoniazid and rifampin. Detection of these strains mandates referral of patients to specialists who are experts in treating multidrug-resistant tuberculosis because the mortality rate is 30% to 80% even when optimal therapy is provided.

Young children with tuberculosis rarely require isolation, but all children with pulmonary tuberculosis who are at least 10 years old and patients of any age with laryngeal tuberculosis or cavitary lesions should be placed in negative-pressure isolation rooms until noninfectious. All health care personnel should wear fitted particulate respirators when in contact with potentially contagious individuals. Patients can be considered noninfectious when they are receiving effective therapy, are improving clinically, and have had negative AFB stains of sputum obtained on 3 separate, consecutive days. When families already have been exposed to a contagious adolescent or child and are not at increased risk of tuberculosis (i.e., if there are no infants or immunocompromised individuals), it may be appropriate to discharge patients to home if they agree not to have contact with susceptible individuals until they have been deemed noninfectious and if compliance with medications and follow-up visits can be ensured.

Children and adolescents with confirmed or suspected tuberculosis should *begin therapy immediately* with one of the following regimens, depending on local resistance patterns: (1) isoniazid, rifampin, and pyrazinamide; (2) isoniazid, rifampin, pyrazinamide, and ethambutol; or (3) isoniazid, rifampin, pyrazinamide, and streptomycin. Regimens 2 and 3 are used in areas of the United States where 4% or more of isolates are resistant to isoniazid because strains from these areas are more likely to be resistant to more than one drug and three drugs may be inadequate to treat them effectively. Regimen 1 may be used if less than 4% of local isolates are isoniazid resistant, if a child has acquired disease recently from a person whose strain is known to be susceptible to isoniazid, or if the susceptibility of a child's isolate is known before therapy has been initiated. Characteristics of common antimycobacterial agents are summarized in Table 114-3.

All children and adolescents who are suspected or known to have tuberculosis should be reported to the local public health department. Reporting patients allows public health investigators to determine if other cases of untreated infectious tuberculosis are present in the community, to identify infected contacts and administer treatment of latent infection to appropriate candidates, to monitor patients' adherence to therapy, and to perform surveillance and analysis of local efforts to control tuberculosis. Cases that are suspected to have disease because of clinical findings or the presence of AFB in clinical specimens should be reported before culture confirmation of tubercle bacilli. Reporting within 7 days of the diagnosis of suspected or known cases allows public health workers to visit and establish continuity of care with inpatients before they are discharged from the hospital.

Children with tuberculosis should undergo HIV testing within 2 months of diagnosis. This recommendation is especially important for infants and adolescents, the two groups

Table 114-3. First-Line Drugs for the Treatment of Tuberculosis Disease in Children

Drug	Daily Dose	Twice-Weekly Dose	Adverse Effects	Recommended Monitoring	Comments
Isoniazid (oral, intravenous, or intramuscular)	Children: 10 mg/kg Adolescents: 300 mg (Maximum: 300 mg)	Children: 20–30 mg/kg Adolescents: 15 mg/kg (Maximum: 900 mg)	Peripheral neuropathy, hypersensitivity reactions, fever, hepatitis (rare)	Bilirubin and transaminase levels at baseline and monthly for children with significant hepatic disease	Overdose may precipitate seizures or death; given with pyridoxine in pregnant women and breast-feeding infants to decrease neuropathy
Rifampin (oral or intravenous)	Children: 10–20 mg/kg Adolescents: 600 mg (Maximum: 600 mg)	Children: 10–20 mg/kg Adolescents: 600 mg (Maximum: 600 mg)	Hepatitis, rash, fever, nausea and vomiting, flulike syndrome with high doses, reduced blood levels of many medications	Bilirubin and transaminase levels at baseline and monthly for children with significant hepatic disease	Commonly causes orange discoloration of urine, sweat, and tears; rifabutin is substituted in most HIV-infected patients; contraindicated during pregnancy
Pyrazinamide (oral)	Children: 20–30 mg/kg Adolescents: 1.5 g (≤50 kg), 2 g (51–74 kg), 2.5 g (≥75 kg), (Maximum: 2 g for children; 2.5 g for adolescents)	Children: 40–50 mg/kg* Adolescents: 2.5 g (≤50 kg), 3 g (51–74 kg), 3.5 g (≥75 kg) (Maximum: 3.5 kg for adolescents)	Hepatitis (particularly with twice-weekly dosing), hyperuricemia (subclinical in young persons), nausea and vomiting, anorexia, fever	Bilirubin and trasaminase levels at baseline and monthly for children with significant hepatic disease	Risk of hepatitis is increased when given with rifampin
Ethambutol (oral)	All age groups: 15–25 mg/kg (Maximum: 2.5 mg)	Children: 30–50 mg/kg* Adolescents: 50 mg/kg*	Occasional optic neuritis (uncommon with lower doses and reversible in most cases when drug is withdrawn)	Color vision testing and visual acuity at baseline and monthly while on therapy	May need to avoid in children too young to cooperate with vision testing
Streptomycin (intramuscular or intravenous)	Children: 20–40 mg/kg Adolescents: 20–40 mg/kg (Maximum: 1 g)	—	Vestibular or cochlear damage (may be irreversible), renal failure (usually reversible)	Baseline audiometry, renal function testing, and electrolytes	Warm compresses at injection site may reduce pain; seldom needed >2 mo

*A maximum twice-weekly dose has not been established.
HIV, human immunodeficiency virus.

of children at highest risk for recent infection with HIV. Successful therapy of tuberculosis in HIV-infected individuals requires treatment of both diseases. Many coinfected patients also are at risk for other infections and may benefit from chemoprophylaxis and other measures.

Children and adolescents who do not have HIV disease and who have strains of *M. tuberculosis* that are sensitive to all standard drugs are treated for 6 months. Isoniazid and rifampin are given throughout the course of therapy with pyrazinamide added during the first 2 months. Only children with drug-susceptible isolates who have miliary, meningeal, or bone or joint disease require a longer course of therapy: 12 months of isoniazid and rifampin with streptomycin and usually pyrazinamide added during the first 2 months. Among patients who cannot tolerate one drug, substitutions are permissible but should be made by a physician who is experienced in treating tuberculosis.

Patients infected with strains that are resistant to isoniazid alone are treated with 6 months of rifampin, ethambutol, and pyrazinamide. Miliary, meningeal, or bone or joint disease requires a treatment duration of 12 months with streptomycin added during the first 2 months. A longer regimen is needed to treat patients with resistance to rifampin, and expert consultation is recommended. Patients with isolates that are resistant to more than one drug should be referred to tuberculosis specialists. Patients with isolates resistant to isoniazid and rifampin require at least 18 to 24 months of treatment and should be managed by an expert in multidrug-resistant tuberculosis.

The optimal therapy for children and adolescents with HIV infection who have active tuberculosis is unknown. The American Academy of Pediatrics recommends at least 9 months of therapy for uncomplicated disease using at least three drugs: isoniazid, rifampin, and pyrazinamide. Ethambutol or streptomycin may be added during the first 2 months of therapy, and consultation with a specialist experienced in managing HIV-infected persons with tuberculosis is advisable. Additionally, HIV-infected children and adolescents in many parts of the United States are more likely to have isolates that are resistant to one or more drugs. Obtaining specimens for culture from these patients is crucial and improves the likelihood of successful treatment.

Nonadherence to antimycobacterial therapy is the primary reason for treatment failures and the development of drug-resistant strains. Directly observed therapy (DOT) has been shown repeatedly to improve the success of therapy and to prevent the emergence of drug resistance. In U.S. studies, greater than 95% of children and adolescents with tuberculosis, including children with isoniazid-resistant strains, are cured with their first round of DOT. DOT is available free of charge to all patients through local public health departments and is recommended for all children and adolescents with tuberculosis.

Adolescents and the few children who are contagious should be assessed at least monthly while on therapy to monitor their symptoms and their sputum smears and cultures. If clinical improvement is not apparent, or if smear and culture results remain positive after 3 months of therapy, treatment failure should be suspected. The most common reason for treatment failure is noncompliance with medications. Whenever nonadherence is suspected, DOT should be instituted immediately, and health departments may need to be notified for the rare situations in which detention is needed to ensure compliance with therapy. Among children already receiving DOT, drug resistance should be considered and may be de novo (primary resistance). When drug resistance is suspected, repeat culture and susceptibility testing is indicated to determine if drug resistance has been acquired since the initial isolate was obtained. Experts in the treatment of tuberculosis should be consulted to evaluate individuals with potential treatment failure. When treatment failure is suspected and noncompliance has been excluded, experts usually add two or more new agents to the current regimen.

PREVENTION

TST is the most important diagnostic test to perform in individuals suspected to have disease and is the only proven method of diagnosing latent or recent primary infection. The currently recommended technique of placing TSTs is the Mantoux method, in which 5 units of tuberculin (0.1 mL) are administered intradermally using a 27-gauge needle. Only experienced health care personnel who have been trained in the proper techniques should place and interpret TSTs. Control tests (e.g., tests using mumps or candida antigens) to assess cutaneous anergy no longer are recommended and do not contribute information about the patient's immune status that cannot be discerned by more reliable clinical or laboratory findings. The size of induration should be recorded 48 to 72 hours after placement. Erythema alone does not represent delayed hypersensitivity and should not be recorded.

Interpretation of TSTs depends on the patient's age, the patient's immune status, and the prevalence of tuberculosis in the area where he or she resides (or resided during childhood if from a high-prevalence area). Positive TST results are described in Table 114-4. False-positive TSTs can occur if an individual is infected with nontuberculous mycobacteria or if he or she has been vaccinated recently with live attenuated *M. bovis* (bacille Calmette-Guérin; see later). False-negative TSTs may be observed among infants and toddlers; immunosuppressed persons; persons with CNS or disseminated disease; and children who have received measles, mumps, and rubella (MMR) vaccine within the past 6 weeks. The effect of varicella vaccine on tuberculin reactivity is unknown. TSTs can be administered, however, with any vaccine at the same visit without affecting the result at 48 to 72 hours. All patients with positive TSTs should have their history taken, a physical examination, and a chest radiograph to exclude disease before therapy for latent infection is initiated.

The Centers for Disease Control and Prevention has recommended targeted TST. Limiting testing to individuals who are at high risk for developing tuberculosis disease and treating all who have latent infection is the most efficient way to reduce transmission of tuberculosis in the community and to limit reactivation disease. Those who are at high risk include individuals who have had recent infection and others who are at increased risk of reactivation of latent infection (i.e., immunocompromising conditions). Testing

Table 114-4. Definitions of Positive Tuberculin Skin Test Results*

Induration ≥5 mm

Children in close contact with suspected or known contagious cases of tuberculosis disease
   Children residing in households with persons who have or who recently have had contagious tuberculosis disease (if their noninfectious status was not documented before the child's exposure)
   Children residing in households where treatment of the contagious person was initiated after the child's exposure
   Children residing in households with an individual suspected to have reactivation tuberculosis
Children suspected or known to have tuberculosis disease
   Children with chest radiographs consistent with active or previously active tuberculosis
   Children with clinical evidence of tuberculosis disease†
Children receiving immunosuppressive therapy or who have immunosuppressive conditions
   Children with HIV infection
   Children receiving immunosuppressive doses of corticosteroids

Induration ≥10 mm

Children at increased risk of disseminated disease
   Children 0–3 years of age
   Children with lymphoma, Hodgkin's disease, chronic renal failure, malnutrition, or diabetes mellitus
Children with increased exposure to tuberculosis disease in their community
   Children born in high-prevalence regions of the world
   Children whose parents or guardians were born in high-prevalence regions of the world
   Children frequently exposed to high-risk adolescents or adults (e.g., adults with HIV disease, individuals with a history of recurrent injection drug use or incarceration, and homeless persons)
   Children residing in high-prevalence areas of the United States
   Children who have resided for significant periods in high-prevalence regions of the world

Induration ≥15 mm

Children ≥4 years of age without any of the preceding risk factors

*These definitions apply regardless of previous bacille Calmette-Guérin administration.
†Symptoms, signs, radiographic findings, or microbiologic evidence of active disease (see text).
HIV, human immunodeficiency virus.

From American Academy of Pediatrics: Tuberculosis. In Pickering L (ed): Red Book: 2003 Report of the Committee on Infectious Diseases, 26th ed. Elk Grove Village, Ill, American Academy of Pediatrics, 2003, p 643.

individuals who have agreed to undergo a medical evaluation if positive (including chest radiographs) and to complete 9 months of therapy with monthly outpatient evaluations is a wiser use of resources than testing all high-risk persons, including persons who may be unable to attend visits or adhere to therapy.

The only recommended regimen for children and adolescents who have latent tuberculosis infection and who have not been treated for latent infection previously is 9 months of isoniazid. Isoniazid can be administered to children daily by household members or can be given by DOT twice weekly if another individual in the same household is receiving DOT for disease. Children 0 to 3 years old who are exposed to tuberculosis also should receive isoniazid for 9 months. Some experts recommend treating HIV-infected children with isoniazid for at least 12 months. Children and adolescents without significant liver disease who receive isoniazid do not require measurement of liver enzymes because isoniazid-related hepatotoxicity is negligible in this age group. Children and adolescents with latent tuberculosis infection from a strain that is resistant only to isoniazid may receive therapy for latent infection with rifampin for a minimum of 6 months if there are no contraindications (e.g., severe liver disease, the use of medications with potentially harmful interactions, or pregnancy).

Compliance with self-administered therapy for latent tuberculosis infection is poor and occasionally is related to misconceptions concerning potential toxicities of isoniazid. Primary care providers should reassure parents of children and adolescents taking isoniazid and should assess compliance of patients receiving therapy for latent tuberculosis infection at least monthly. By doing so, primary care providers can limit effectively the spread of tuberculosis and the risk of future reactivation disease among patients.

Additional Resources, CD-ROM

Bibliography	

SUGGESTED READINGS

American Academy of Pediatrics: Tuberculosis. In Pickering LK (ed): 2000 Red Book: Report of the Committee on Infectious Diseases, 25th ed. Elk Grove Village, Ill, American Academy of Pediatrics, 2000, pp 593–613.

Geiter L (ed): Institute of Medicine (U.S.). Committee on the Elimination of Tuberculosis in the United States. Ending Neglect: the Elimination of Tuberculosis in the United States. Washington, DC, National Academy Press, 2000.

Horsburgh CR Jr, Feldman S, Ridzon R: Practice guidelines for the treatment of tuberculosis. Clin Infect Dis 2000;31:633–639.

Small PM, Fujiwara PI: Management of tuberculosis in the United States. N Engl J Med 2001;345:189–200.

Starke JR: Tuberculosis of the central nervous system in children. Semin Pediatr Neurol 1999;6:318–331.

115   Asthma

Nasser Redjal

ROLE OF THE GENERALIST

1   Detect and diagnose asthma in children with recurrent respiratory complaints.

2   Recognize conditions masquerading as asthma in young children and infants.

3   Use established guidelines to develop a treatment plan for children with asthma.

4   Treat asthma exacerbations, recognizing the severity of illness and treating patients in the correct setting.

5   Recognize and manage respiratory failure.

6   Develop reasonable and rational therapeutic outcomes for asthma therapy in coordination with the child and the family.

7   Use available therapies, recognizing their indications and potential toxicities.

8   Evaluate adherence and response to asthma therapy, and ensure appropriate follow-up.

Asthma is the most common chronic illness of childhood and is a leading cause of emergency department visits, hospital admission, and school absenteeism. About 5% to 10% of children have signs and symptoms compatible with asthma during childhood. Over the last several decades, the prevalence of asthma has shown a worldwide consistent pattern of increase estimated at 5% to 15% for the entire pediatric population. The increase varies from 40% in some areas of the United Kingdom and Australia to 3% in Indonesia, China, and India. Asthma prevalence and mortality and hospitalization are higher in blacks than in whites. Low socioeconomic status is associated with an increase in asthma prevalence and morbidity and mortality. The male-to-female ratio is 2:1 until age 10 and is equal from age 10 to 14; after puberty, asthma incidence is greater in girls and women.

DEFINITION

Asthma is a heterogeneous syndrome characterized by chronic inflammation of airways, hyperresponsiveness to a variety of stimuli, episodic bronchospasm, and airflow obstruction that is reversible either spontaneously or with treatment. In young children, the practitioner must consider all other possible causes of reactive airways disease because not all children who wheeze have asthma. Clinically, asthma is characterized by recurrent episodes of cough, chest tightness, dyspnea, prolonged expiration, wheezing, hyperinflation of the chest (air trappings), use of accessory chest muscles (retractions), and, in severe cases, cyanosis.

FUNDAMENTALS

Many factors contribute to the development of asthma. Environmental factors, including pollutants such as ozone, sulfur dioxide, and nitrogen dioxide, and particulate matter, such as diesel exhaust, have been implicated in the etiology of asthma. Numerous studies have shown a consistent relationship between high ozone exposure and emergency department visits and hospital admissions. Because visits and admissions occur on the day after exposure to ozone, the asthma exacerbation seems to be a function of airway inflammation rather than a simple reflex bronchospasm. Ozone exposure also worsens the subsequent response to allergens and intensifies the early-phase and late-phase response to allergens. Airborne particulates may contain elemental carbon, metals, organic residues (e.g., diesel exhaust), and biologic residues (e.g., endotoxin), all of which can induce proinflammatory and inflammatory changes in the airways. Diesel exhaust particles can act as an adjuvant and exacerbate symptoms in patients who already are sensitized. Endotoxin, which is prevalent in the air around farms, also can heighten the inflammatory response to allergens in patients with atopic asthma. Indoor pollutants that may be associated with asthma include fumes from unvented gas, oil, or kerosene stoves; wood burning appliances; or fireplaces and spray and strong odors.

Genetic factors also play an important role. The atopic phenotype of asthma represents the sum of multiple genotypic and environmental influences. There are at lease 50 genes that influence susceptibility to asthma and its clinical expression. Sites located on chromosomes 6p and 12q, 5q, 11q, and 16p are known to be associated with allergic diseases and encoding for major histocompatibility complex, IgE, interferon, and cytokine.

Infection, particularly respiratory infections, can play a variety of roles in asthma, influencing not only its exacerbation, but also its inception and persistence. Viral infections, such as respiratory syncytial virus, influenza virus, and rhinovirus, are the most frequent precipitants of asthma exacerbations in infancy. Because young children have smaller sized airways, they are more predisposed to have bronchial obstruction and wheezing during viral infections. Some infections, such as respiratory syncytial virus, may play roles as a risk factor for inception of asthma in some patients who are deficient in their ability to produce Th1-like cytokines and instead mount a Th2-type response, which raises the risk of developing allergy and possibly asthma. *Mycoplasma* and *Chlamydia* infections can cause wheezing and persistence of asthma; some respiratory tract infections may have the potential to prevent the development of asthma, depending on host and environmental variables and the time of life during which respiratory infections occurred.

Individuals at the extremes of age (infants and elderly) have lower levels of lung function and are more susceptible to asthma and airway hyperresponsiveness. In early life, peculiar anatomy and physiology of lung compared with adults predispose infants to obstructive airway disease, such as deficient number and size of the pores of Cohn and Lambert's canals, causing deficient collateral ventilation and development of atelectasis distal to obstructed airway. Mucous gland hyperplasia favors increased intralumial mucus production. Decreased smooth muscle in the peripheral airway results in less support and narrow airway. Decreased number of fatigue-resistant skeletal muscle fibers in the diaphragm and its horizontal insertion to the rib cage (versus oblique in adult) and highly compliant rib cage increase work of breathing in a poorly equipped diaphragm. Decreased static elastic recoil predisposes to early airway closure during tidal breathing, resulting in mismatching of ventilation and perfusion and hypoxemia.

Cigarette smoking is associated strongly with asthma, particularly maternal smoking and the development of asthma during the first year of life. Smoking during pregnancy is associated with decrease in pulmonary function at 1 month of age. Exposure of a child to tobacco smoke (second-hand or passive smoking) can be documented by cotinine level (a metabolite of nicotine). Exposure to environmental tobacco smoke contributes to the cause of asthma and the exacerbation of the disease in affected children.

Inhalant allergens, particularly indoors, play an important role. The most important allergens are house dust mite feces (Der P1 and 2), cat dander (Feld1), and cockroach saliva (Bla g2, 4, and 5). House dust mite antigen (Der P1) stimulates the response causing an increase in IgE synthesis by impairing T-cell proliferation and interferon-γ secretion. Other inhalant allergens, such as dog dander and outdoor fungus (i.e., *Alternaria*) and some pollens, also play a role in asthma.

Pathogenesis

Inflammation plays a major role in the pathogenesis of asthma. The histopathology of asthma includes denudation of airway epithelium, edema, infiltration by inflammatory cells (neutrophils, eosinophils, mast cells, lymphocytes [Th2-like cells]), collagen deposition beneath basement membrane, and smooth muscle hypertrophy. The particular role of eosinophils in asthma is suggested by their presence in sputum and their increased numbers in the circulating blood. Airways of living subjects with mild-to-moderate asthma have been studied either by bronchal biopsy specimens or bronchoalveolar lavage (BAL). BAL fluid from asthmatic subjects contains increased numbers of mast cells, eosinophils, macrophages, epithelial cells, and activated T cells. Elevated levels of histamine, prostaglandin D_2, and cysteinyl leukotrienes have been reported.

Mast cells obtained from BAL fluid of asthmatic patients release more histamine, and the eosinophils contain more major basic protein, a protein that has been shown to cause damage and shedding of airway epithelium. These alterations in the content of BAL fluid correlate with the extent of airway hyperresponsiveness to different stimuli, suggesting a causal relationship between the mediator and hyperresponsiveness in asthma. Similarly the degree of airway hyperresponsiveness correlates with the severity of the asthma. Interaction between cells and mediators leads to the development and maintenance of inflammation. In acute severe asthma, lymphocytes become activated by increasing interleukin (IL)-2 receptor class II major histocompatibility complex antigen and VLA-1 expression and generating cytokines that recruit eosinophils. Macrophages are capable of generating chemotactic factors and proinflammatory cytokines. The epithelial cells generate a range of cytokines. Myofibroblasts also contribute to inflammation, serving as a source of granulocyte-macrophage colony-stimulating factor, whereas fibroblasts serve as a source of C-kit ligand (a stromal cytokine that regulates mast cell development, differentiation, proliferation, and function). Lipid mediator plays an important role in inflammation; for instance, platelet-activating factor is a potent eosinophil chemotaxin. Leukotriene B_4 is a potent neutrophil and monocyte chemotaxin.

Interaction and cooperation between inflammatory leukocytes and vascular endothelium is basic to the pathology of asthma. Vascular endothelium has an important role in the recruitment of leukocytes to an inflammatory focus in the lung. Activation of vascular endothelium by various inflammatory stimuli causes expression of various endothelial cell adhesion molecules, such as selectin, which is involved in a wide range of cellular events. P-selectin and E-selectin recognize carbohydrate domains on the leukocyte cell membrane, facilitating recruitment of them to an inflammatory focus. Adhesion molecules expressed on leukocytes recognize counterreceptors on vascular endothelium.

Clinical Manifestations

Symptoms of asthma increase in severity as the condition persists. If untreated, a patient may present with any or all of the following: cough, shortness of breath, prolonged expiration, use of accessory muscles of respiration, wheezing, complaints of "chest tightness or congestion," hyperinflation of chest, cyanosis, exercise intolerance, tachycardia, and abdominal pain. These symptoms of asthma vary not only between individuals, but also in the same individual over time. The onset of an asthma attack may be with wheezing and dyspnea or sometimes can be insidious with coughing or a feeling of chest discomfort, without overt wheezing. The cough, which sounds tight and nonproductive early on, increases in frequency and severity, especially during pollen season or with a viral respiratory infection. When an acute attack is brought on by exposure to irritants, such as noxious fumes, cold air, exercise, or allergens, wheezing is present because of turbulent air in larger airways. Small airways are often "silent" because the airflow there is laminar rather than turbulent. When obstruction is confined to smaller airways, there may be no audible wheezing. Instead, patients complain of cough or a feeling of chest discomfort. When a patient experiences severe obstruction and extreme respiratory distress, wheezing may be absent owing to poor air movement. Wheezing may appear after bronchodilator treatment, owing to partial opening of the airway.

In severe asthma, a patient may assume a hunched-over, tripod-like seated position that makes it easier to breathe. Abdominal pain is common, especially in younger children. Vomiting also is common in younger children and may be followed by temporary relief of symptoms. During an acute asthma attack, a low-grade fever, profuse sweating, and fatigue from the hard work of breathing may be apparent. Clubbing of the fingers, even in severe asthma, is rare and suggests other chronic respiratory illness.

DIAGNOSIS AND ASSESSMENT

The history is essential in establishing a proper diagnosis and determining the appropriate therapy. In a patient with recurrent episodes of coughing and wheezing, particularly if accentuated by exercise, the diagnosis of asthma is made easily. Asthma should be suspected with a history of cough (worse at night), difficulty breathing, and chest tightness. Asthma also should be considered when symptoms occur or worsen with exercise, viral infection, airborne allergens (pollen, animal dander, house dust mites), airborne chemicals, smoke (wood, tobacco), strong emotional expression (laughing or crying hard), and menses. The 1997 National Heart, Lung and Blood Institute of the National Institutes of Health (NHLBI) expert panel guideline suggests that the medical history of a patient with asthma includes the items listed in Table 115-1.

A medical history such as that outlined in Table 115-1 helps to delineate the extent of symptoms from asthma to assess the severity of asthma and to identify possible precipitating factors. If the diagnosis is unclear on clinical grounds, specific laboratory studies must be performed to document asthma or rule out disorders that mimic it. Patients who present with a history of isolated chronic cough or wheezing that occurs only with exercise can be diagnosed by the reversibility of symptoms with bronchodilator. When necessary, this impression can be confirmed

---

Table 115-1. Signs and Symptoms of Asthma

Symptoms
Cough
Wheezing
Shortness of breath
Sputum production

Pattern of Symptoms
Perennial, seasonal, or both
Continual, episodic, or both
Onset, duration, frequency (number of days or nights, per week or month)
Diurnal variations, especially nocturnal and on awakening in early morning

Precipitating/Aggravating Factors
Viral respiratory infections
Environmental allergens, indoor (e.g., mold, house dust mite, cockroach, animal dander or secretory products) and outdoor (e.g., pollen)
Exercise
Occupational chemicals or allergens
Environmental change (e.g., moving to new home; going on vacation; and/or alterations in workplace, work processes, or materials used)
Irritants (e.g., tobacco smoke, strong odors, air pollutants, occupational chemicals, dusts and particulates, vapors, gasses, and aerosols)
Emotional expressions (e.g., fear, anger, frustration, hard crying or laughing)
Drugs (e.g., aspirin; β-blockers, including eye drops; nonsteroidal anti-inflammatory drugs; others)
Food, food additives, and preservatives (e.g., sulfite)
Change in weather, exposure to cold air
Endocrine factors (e.g., menses, pregnancy, thyroid disease)

Development of Disease and Treatment
Age of onset and diagnosis
History of early-life injury to airways (e.g., bronchopulmonary dysplasia, pneumonia, parental smoking)
Progress of disease (better or worse)
Present management and response, including plans for managing exacerbations
Need for oral corticosteroids and frequency of use
Comorbid conditions

Family History
History of asthma, allergy, sinusitis, rhinitis, or nasal polyps in close relatives

Social History
Characteristics of home, including age, location, cooling and heating system, wood-burning stove, humidifier, carpeting over concrete, presence of molds or mildew, characteristics of rooms where patient spends time (e.g., bedroom and living room with attention to bedding, floor covering, stuffed furniture)
Smoking (patient and others in home or day care)
Day care, workplace, and school characteristics that may interfere with adherence
Social support/social networks
Level of education completed
Employment (if employed, characteristics of work environment)

Profile of Typical Exacerbation
Usual prodromal signs and symptoms
Usual patterns and management (what works?)

Impact of Asthma on Patient and Family
Episodes of unscheduled care (emergency department, urgent care, hospitalization)
Life-threatening exacerbations (e.g., intubation, intensive care unit administration)
Number of days missed from school/work
Limitation of activity, especially sports and strenuous work
History of nocturnal awakening
Effect on growth, development, behavior, school or work performance, and lifestyle
Impact on family routines, activities, or dynamics
Economic impact

Assessment of Patient's and Family's Perceptions of Disease
Patient, parental, and spouse's or partner's knowledge of asthma and belief in the chronicity of asthma and in the efficacy of treatment
Patient perception and beliefs regarding use and long-term effects of medications
Ability of patient and parents, spouse, or partner to cope with disease
Level of family support and patient's and parents', spouse's, or partner's capacity to recognize severity of an exacerbation

From National Institutes of Health, National Heart, Lung, and Blood Institute. Guidelines for the Diagnosis and Management of Asthma. Expert Panel Report 2. NIH Publication No. 97-4051. Bethesda, Md, U.S. Department of Health and Human Services, 1997.

by routine pulmonary function tests or methacholine bronchoprovocation test.

Pulmonary function tests are noninvasive, objective, and cost-effective in the diagnosis and follow-up of patients with asthma (see Chapter 275). These tests can be performed in children older than age 5 years with appropriate coaching and teaching to achieve good techniques and reliable results. Depending on the severity of the asthma, a variety of abnormalities may be detected in the lung function tests. Dynamic tests of airflow, such as forced vital capacity, forced expiratory volume in 1 second (FEV_1), and maximum expiratory flow between 25% and 75% of vital capacity (FEF_{25-75}), are decreased, but total lung capacity, functional residual capacity, and residual volume are increased in symptomatic asthmatic patients. After the administration of an aerosolized bronchodilator, dynamic tests of air flow increase or return to normal. A greater than 15% improvement in FEV_1 is virtually diagnostic of asthma, but lack of improvement in FEV_1 does not preclude asthma. In severe airway inflammation, a 1- to 2-week course of oral corticosteroid may be necessary to show a reversible component to airflow obstruction.

Peak flowmeters, which measure forced peak expiratory flow (PEF), are useful in the office and at home to monitor expiratory flow rate. A 4-year-old child can be taught to use a peak flowmeter two to three times a day. A decrease in PEF predicts the onset of an exacerbation and suggests the need for early intervention using additional drug therapy. The PEF provides the clinician with an objective measurement of the degree of airway obstruction between office visits.

Exercise tolerance tests using a treadmill or a free running exercise followed by pulmonary function tests can be performed; a decrease greater than 15% in FEV_1 or 30% in FEF_{25-75} is diagnostic of exercise-induced asthma. Chemical challenge tests using methacholine or histamine are valuable in a patient with a chronic cough, normal pulmonary function tests, and an inconclusive therapeutic trial with antiasthma medications. Inhalation challenge using specific antigens may offer valuable diagnostic information regarding asthma triggers; however, in practice antigen inhalation challenge has severe limitations. These tests are potentially dangerous and should be preformed only by a specialist.

Asthmatic sputum is tenacious, rubbery, and whitish. Sputum smear, stained with eosin–methylene blue, may show numerous eosinophils and granules from disrupted white blood cells, eosinophils, and epithelial cells. The presence of greater than 5% to 10% eosinophils suggests allergic inflammatory disease. Other findings in sputum include Curschmann's spirals, which are threads of glycoprotein; Creola bodies, which are clusters of epithelial cells; and Charcot-Leyden crystals, which are derived from eosinophils. Peripheral eosinophilia usually are greater than 250 to 400 mm^3.

Allergy skin testing or serologic testing, such as radioallergosorbent testing, is indicated to identify potentially important environmental allergens (see Chapter 278). Allergens may play a significant role in asthma, and 85% of asthma patients have a positive skin test reaction to common aeroallergens. Although true positive skin tests indicate the presence of antigen-specific IgE, a positive test does not predict uniformly that exposure will create clinically significant disease. The predictive value of a positive test is enhanced if the reactivity is intense and occurs in conjunction with a positive provocative history. Total serum IgE is not as helpful as antigen-specific IgE, but it is elevated in 80% of children with allergen-induced asthma. Serum IgE levels do not have practical value in the management of asthma and are not usually indicated except in a patient with bronchopulmonary aspergillosis.

Children suspected of having asthma, especially children requiring hospitalization, should have a chest radiograph to eliminate other pathology. X-ray findings may range from normal to hyperinflation, increased bronchial marking, and atelectasis, especially during acute exacerbation. Infiltration, pneumothrax, pneumomediastinum, and pneumonia are less common.

DIFFERENTIAL DIAGNOSIS

Diagnosing asthma in children requires the exclusion of other causes of recurrent respiratory symptoms (Box 115-1). Most children with coughing and recurrent wheezing have asthma. Particularly in children younger than 3 years old, other conditions have to be eliminated. These include foreign-body aspiration; respiratory infections, especially bronchiolitis, croup, epiglottitis, tonsillitis, and tonsillar abscess; congenital heart disease causing left ventricular failure, especially with pulmonary edema; hyperventilation from anxiety attack; laryngeal dysfunction and hysterical laryngospasm (factitious asthma); pneumothorax; and pulmonary embolism (in patient with history of oral contraceptive use). Cystic fibrosis can present as a chronic obstructive pulmonary disease with cough, wheezing, recurrent infections, malabsorption, and failure to thrive.

α_1-Antitrypsin deficiency, an autosomal recessive disorder, causes liver disease and emphysema in young adulthood. Chronic upper respiratory obstruction may be caused by enlarged adenoids; hypertrophic tonsils; foreign body; tracheal tumor; endobronchial tuberculosis; carcinoid syndrome; immunodeficiency disease; hypersensitivity pneumonitis; bronchopulmonary aspergillosis; and a variety of rarer conditions, such as parasitic infections and tropical eosinophilia.

Box 115-1. Differential Diagnosis of Recurrent Cough and Wheezing in Infancy

- Recurrent respiratory tract infections
- Sinusitis with postnasal drip
- Pulmonary infection (bacterial, viral, fungal)
- Allergy and asthma
- Aspiration syndromes (gastroesophageal reflux, oropharyngeal dyscoordination, tracheoesophageal fistula)
- Foreign body
- Cystic fibrosis
- Pulmonary edema (cardiogenic or noncardiogenic)
- Toxic exposure
- Central airway anomalies (vascular ring, tracheomalacia)
- Congenital lung anomalies (bronchogenic cyst, sequestration)
- Ciliary dyskinesia

CLASSIFICATION OF ASTHMA SEVERITY

An accurate assessment of asthma severity guides the clinician toward the appropriate use of medication in the long-term management of asthma. The NHLBI expert panel classifies asthma, based on severity, as determined by careful assessment of symptom frequency during the day and at night and pulmonary function testing, into four catergories: *mild intermittent, mild persistent, moderate persistent,* and *severe persistent asthma* (Table 115-2).

Mild Intermittent Asthma

Patients experience daytime symptoms of asthma two or fewer times per week and nighttime symptoms two or fewer times per month. Symptomatic episodes are brief and resolve spontaneously or with the use of a β_2-agonist. Patients are asymptomatic and have normal pulmonary function tests between episodes; daily functioning and exercise tolerance are normal; and there are no emergency department visits or school absenteeism because of asthma. FEV_1 or PEF is equal to or greater than 80% of predicted and peak flow variability is less than or equal to 20%.

Mild Persistent Asthma

Patients experience the symptoms of asthma more than twice a week, but less than on a daily basis, and nighttime symptoms more than two times a month. Exacerbation of asthma may affect activity. The FEV_1 or PEF is usually greater than or equal to 80% of predicted, and PEF variability is 20% to 30% at most.

Moderate Persistent Asthma

Patients experience daily symptoms and asthma symptoms at night more than once weekly. Exacerbations occur more than twice a week, may last for days, and affect patient activity. The FEV_1 or PEF is reduced to between more than

60% and less than 80% of predicted, and PEF variability is more than 30%.

Severe Persistent Asthma

Patients have continuous symptoms, frequent exacerbations, and limited physical activity. Nighttime symptoms are frequent. FEV_1 or PEF, is less than or equal to 60% of predicted, and PEF variability is more than 30%.

Because asthma symptoms may be highly variable, categories may overlap. The presence of one of the features of severity is sufficient to place a patient in that category. Patients in any category may have severe exacerbations of asthma.

MANAGEMENT AND MEDICATIONS

Pharmacologic measures form the basis for the symptomatic and anti-inflammatory treatment of asthma. The choice of medications is based on the history, physical examination, pulmonary function testing, and other laboratory tests and is predicated on the severity of the asthma, as categorized according to NHLBI guidelines.

Nonpharmacologic measures aim at prevention and serve as an adjunct to drug therapy. All modalities should be assessed frequently to determine whether the goals of therapy are being achieved (Box 115-2).

Nonpharmacologic Measures
Asthma Education

Asthma education is the cornerstone of asthma management. The more patients and parents understand asthma, the better they can cope with its symptoms and comply with treatment. A partnership between the patient, family, and physicians is paramount in managing asthma. Educational topics such as pathophysiology, signs and symptoms, characteristic changes in airway triggers, and

Table 115-2. Classification of Severity of Asthma: Clinical Features before Treatment*

	Symptoms†	Nighttime Symptoms	Lung Function
Step 1: Mild Intermittent	Symptoms ≤2 times a week Asymptomatic and normal PEF between exacerbations Exacerbations brief (from a few hours to a few days); intensity may vary	≤2 times a month	FEV_1 or PEF ≥80% predicted PEF variability <30%
Step 2: Mild Persistent	Symptoms >2 times a week but <1 time a day Exacerbations may affect activity	>2 times a month	FEV_1 or PEF ≥80% predicted PEF variability 20–30%
Step 3: Moderate Persistent	Daily symptoms Daily use of inhaled short-acting β_2-agonist Exacerbations affect activity Exacerbations ≥2 times a week: may last days	>1 time a week	FEV_1 or PEF >60–<80% predicted PEF variability 20–30%
Step 4: Severe Persistent	Continual symptoms Limited physical activity Frequent exacerbations	Frequent	FEV_1 or PEF ≤60% predicted PEF variability >30%

*Patients at any level of severity can have mild, moderate, or severe exacerbations. Some patients with intermittent asthma experience life-threatening exacerbations separated by long periods of normal lung function and no symptoms.
†The presence of one of the features of severity is sufficient to place a patient in that category. An individual should be assigned to the most severe grade in which any feature occurs. The characteristics noted in this table are general and may overlap because asthma is highly variable. An individual's classification may change over time.
FEV_1, forced expiratory volume in 1 second; PEF, peak expiratory flow.

Adapted from National Institutes of Health, National Heart, Lung, and Blood Institute Guidelines for the Diagnosis and Management of Asthma. Expert Panel Report 2. NIH Publication, No. 97-4051. Bethesda, Md, U.S. Department of Health and Human Services, 1997.

Table 116-1. Anatomic and Physiologic Factors that Predispose to Recurrent Infection in Children with an Otherwise Normal Immune System

Infection Type	Selected Predisposing Abnormalities
Otitis media	Allergy
	Gastroesophageal reflux
	Cleft lip and palate
	Structural abnormalities
Sinusitis	Allergy
	Ciliary dysfunction (e.g., cystic fibrosis, Kartagener's syndrome)
Pneumonia	Gastroesophageal reflux
	Tracheoesophageal fistula
	Ciliary dysfunction (e.g., cystic fibrosis, Kartagener's syndrome)
	Pulmonary sequestration/cysts
	Tracheal/bronchial obstruction (foreign body, tracheal web, vascular ring)
Urinary tract infection	Genitourinary tract abnormalities (duplication, cysts, fistulas, obstruction)
	Posterior urethral valves
	Vesicoureteral reflux
Meningitis	Midline dermal sinus
	Occult cerebrospinal fluid leak/skull fracture
	Neuroenteric fistulae
Soft tissue infection	Paresthesia
	Lymphedema
	Skin disorders (e.g., epidermolysis bullosa, eczema)

Adapted from Buescher ES: Evaluation of the child with suspected immunodeficiency. In Long SL, Pickering LK, Prober CG (eds): Principles and Practice of Pediatric Infectious Disease New York, Churchill Livingstone, 1997.

predispose children to recurrent respiratory infections include Kartagener's syndrome and cystic fibrosis, both of which impair ciliary motility and mucus clearance.

Certain exposures may result in unusual or serious infections. For example, *Salmonella* infections (gastroenteritis, sepsis, and meningitis) in neonates and infants are frequently associated with contact with a household pet that serves as the reservoir (i.e., iguanas or turtles). Travel to developing countries or regions where specific diseases are endemic may place a child at risk of infection (tuberculosis, malaria, dysentery, histoplasmosis).

Factors that may decrease the frequency of infections include breast-feeding and handwashing. Breast-fed infants are less likely to develop acute otitis media, pneumonia, bacterial sepsis, and gastroenteritis compared to infants who are exclusively bottle-fed. Breast-feeding is also associated with a reduced duration of illness with gastroenteritis (primarily from rotavirus infections). Handwashing continues to be the most effective measure against transmission of infectious agents in all settings.

PRESENTATION AND INITIAL EVALUATION

Children with immune defects typically present with either (1) severe, deep tissue or possibly life-threatening infections, (2) recurrent or protracted infections, or (3) infections with unusual organisms. In evaluating an individual child's history of recurrent infections, certain features that provide reassurance about the child's immune status are (1) prior diagnoses are vague without clear documentation, (2) lack of any deep tissue infections, (3) the presence of normal

growth and development, and (4) general wellness as measured by overall activity and absence of complaints between infectious episodes.

Table 116-2 lists the characteristics of several immune defects and their common presentations. For example, anatomic defects may present with recurrent infections at a site contiguous to the abnormality. Defects of the urinary tract (ureteropelvic junction obstruction, vesiculoureteral reflux, or duplicating urinary system) can predispose to and often present with multiple urinary tract infections. Meningomyelocele may disrupt the skin barrier, allowing entry of organisms into the central nervous system. Children with cystic fibrosis and other disorders related to the ciliary clearance of mucus often present with recurrent and protracted infections of the ciliated respiratory tract (sinusitis and pneumonia).

Children with defects of antibody production (usually IgG or IgA deficiencies) are most susceptible to frequent bacterial infections of the sinopulmonary system. With IgA deficiencies, children are also susceptible to recurrent gastrointestinal infections owing to its relative deficiency on the mucosal surfaces. Unlike other inherited disorders of the immune systems in which infants may be quite ill at an early age, children with disorders of primarily antibody production do not usually present with symptoms until about 5 to 7 months of age, when passively transferred maternal antibody reaches its nadir. The age of presentation may be younger in prematurely born children.

Phagocytes and T cells are required for clearance of organisms that can survive intracellularly. Therefore, children with defects of these cell lines often present with infection with unusual organisms such as *Pneumocystis jiroveci* (PCP), *Mycobacterium* spp., cryptococcosis, or severe infections with viruses, most frequently of the herpesvirus family (herpes simplex virus, cytomegalovirus, Epstein-Barr, and varicella-zoster virus).

It is essential to obtain a thorough history in the evaluation of a child in whom an immune deficiency is suspected. The history should include the prenatal and perinatal history and an account of all types of illnesses and hospitalizations. Each infectious episode should be detailed, including date, duration, method of making the diagnosis, severity, treatment, and response to treatment. Clarification of the child's immunization status, growth and development patterns, medication history and compliance, and presence of underlying conditions is also necessary. Special dietary information and travel history that may indicate exposure to unusual pathogens should also be sought. A family history of unusual early deaths may provide a clue because many primary immune deficienices are inherited. A complete review of systems is also important. Failure to thrive is often seen with HIV or other T-cell disorders and may guide the clinical evaluation process. Skin disorders (such as eczema seen with Wiskott-Aldrich syndrome) or a history of neurologic problems (ataxia telangiectasia) or motor weakness (associated with recurrent aspiration pneumonia) may also provide some direction. Certain infectious presentations may suggest a specific immune defect as detailed in Table 116-3.

A complete physical examination, including documentation of the child's weight, other growth parameters, and

Table 116-2. Defects of the Immune System in Children

Affected System	Typical Presentation	Age of Onset	Disease Examples	Characteristic Presentations or Pathogens
Innate immunity				
Epithelial/mucosal barriers	Recurrent infections at the same location or anatomic system	Variable	Cystic fibrosis	Impaired pulmonary and pancreatic function
			Gastroesophageal reflux	
Complement deficiencies	Deficiency of early components associated with autoimmune disease	Variable	Lupus	Susceptible to encapsulated organisms (*Streptococcus pneumoniae*)
	Deficiency of late components associated with bacterial infections esp. *Neisseria* sp.		C9 deficiency	Typically, CH_{50} approximately 50% normal
Phagocytic	Recurrent skin infections often with abscesses	Early (<6 months of age)	Chronic granulomatous disease	Infections with catalase-producing organisms (*Staphylococcus aureus*, *Serratia* sp. fungi)
			Natural killer cells deficiency	Increases susceptibility and severity to herpesviruses
			Leukocyte adhesion deficiency	Delayed cord separation
			Chediak-Higashi syndrome	Giant leukocyte granules, partial albinism
			Cyclic neutropenia	Recurrent episodes of neutropenia with 14–28 day cycles
Adaptive immunity				
Antibody production				
Predominantly B cells	Recurrent sinopulmonary infections occasionally associated with recurrent or severe gastrointestinal infections	Delayed (after maternal antibody wanes, 5–7 months of age)	X-linked agammaglobulinemia	Bacterial infection, increased susceptibility to recurrent or severe infections with Enteroviruses
			IgA deficiencies	Sinopulmonary and gastrointestinal infections. May be associated with autoimmune disorders
			Common variable immunodeficiency	Sinopulmonary infections. Variable age onset, may present in adulthood. IgG usually <50% normal, IgA and IgM may also be reduced
Cellular defects Predominantly T cells	Failure to thrive, recurrent bacterial infections, persistent oral thrush	Early (<6 months of age)	DiGeorge anomaly	Congenital hypoparathyroidism and heart disease, abnormal facies, extent of immunodeficiency variable
	Increased susceptibility to virus (herpes); intracellular bacteria (*Mycobacterium, Listeria, Legionella*); Protozoan (PCP, Toxo, *Cryptosporidium, Giardia*); fungal (Crypto, Histo, Cocci); mucocutaneous candidiasis		HIV	Higher susceptibility to infections with PCP, mycobacteria; mucocutaneous candidiasis
Combined antibody and T cells	Features of both antibody and cellular deficiencies	Early (<6 months of age)	Severe combined immunodeficiency	Absent thymus
			Hyper IgM	Frequent bacterial infections and intracellular organisms (PCP)
			Wiskot-Aldrich syndrome	X-linked, petechiae, thrombocytopenia, eczematoid rash
			Ataxia-telangiectasia	Progressive ataxia, oculocutaneous telangiectasia, frequent sinopulmonary infection; variable endocrinopathies

Cocci, Coccidioides immitis; Crypto, Cryptococcus neoformans; Histo, Histoplasma capsulatum; PCP, Pneumocystis carinii pneumonia; Toxo, Toxoplasma gondii.

vital signs, is a key component of the evaluation. The presence of thrush or other mucosal lesions (suggestive of a T-cell or phagocytic defect), wheezing (common in children with cystic fibrosis), hepatomegaly or splenomegaly (indicative of an underlying medical condition or type of infection), eczema, telangiectasia, or albinism (suggestive of Wiskott-Aldrich, ataxia-telangiectasia, Chediak-Higashi

syndrome, respectively), or neurologic deficits (ataxia-telangiectasia) may suggest specific disorders.

Laboratory testing may be necessary when a child presents with a history of frequent infections that seems out of the range of normal. Such testing will help to confirm that a child is normal, or suggest the need for further diagnostic testing or referral. Although laboratory testing

Lyme Disease
Fundamentals

Lyme disease is caused by the spirochete *Borrelia burgdorferi*. Humans acquire infection through *Ixodes* tick bites; the animal reservoir is small mammals (especially mice) and deer. Many infections occur after bites by small, often unnoticed, nymphal ticks, usually between April and October. In the United States the majority of cases are reported from the Northeast (Massachusetts to Maryland) and the upper Midwest (especially Wisconsin and Minnesota); cases are reported in lower numbers from the West coast. Lyme disease also occurs in Canada, Europe, and Asia. Because of the evolving nature of this illness, clinicians should check with state and local health authorities for up-to-date information about their region.

Clinical Presentation

Three stages of symptomatic illness are recognized. In *early localized Lyme disease*, an annular rash, erythema chronicum migrans, gradually develops 1 to 2 weeks after and centered around a tick bite (Fig. 118-1). This slowly expands to an average of 15 cm. Although classically showing central clearing, the rash may be uniformly erythematous, or may develop a vesicular or necrotic center. The rash

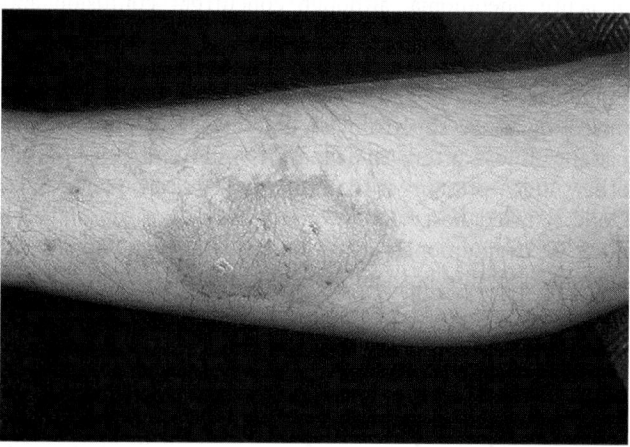

A

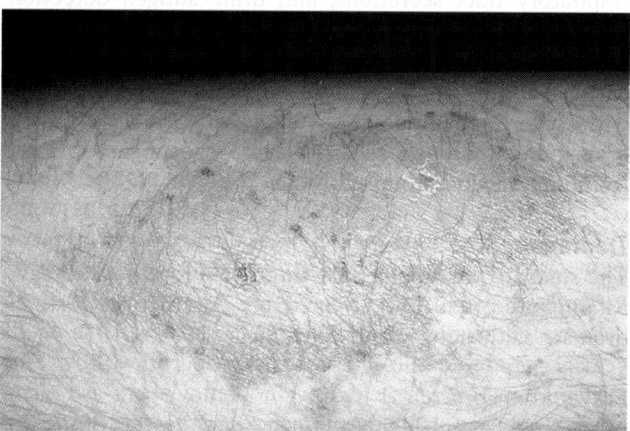

B

Figure 118-1. A-B, Erythema chronicum migrans, the annular rash of Lyme disease, after two nearby tic bites.

lasts for at least 1 to 2 weeks and will resolve spontaneously. Systemic symptoms such as fever, fatigue, and myalgia may occur at this stage.

In *early disseminated Lyme disease* (stage 2), multiple, smaller, secondary erythema chronicum migrans lesions appear at sites distant from original rash/tick bite. At this stage, systemic symptoms, conjunctivitis, aseptic meningitis, carditis (heart block), and focal neurologic involvement can occur.

Arthritis develops as the manifestation of *late disseminated Lyme disease* (stage 3) in approximately 7% of untreated children. This stage typically occurs months after the original rash appeared. Large joints, especially the knee, are most commonly involved. If untreated, joint swelling will resolve over a course of weeks, only to recur in the same or other joints. Over time, the frequency of recurrences diminishes. If treated, joint swelling resolves, but 5% to 10% may have recurrent arthritis. Late central nervous system complications are rarely reported in children.

Diagnosis

The erythema chronicum migrans rash of Lyme disease in the correct epidemiologic setting allows for clinical diagnosis of the illness. At this stage, serologic testing is likely to be negative and may remain so with successful treatment. In patients with suspected disseminated (early or late) infection, serologic testing should be obtained. Two-stage testing with screening ELISA (enzyme-labeled immunosorbent assay) and confirmatory Western blot is recommended to maximize sensitivity and specificity. PCR testing of skin biopsy and joint fluid may prove to be an useful test in the future.

Treatment

Treatment composition and duration depends on stage and location of infection. Recommendations for treatment of children are extrapolated from results in adults. Erythema chronicum migrans or early disseminated disease is treated for 21 days with amoxicillin, cefuroxime, or doxycycline (if child is older than 8 years). If there is cranial nerve involvement or arthritis, treatment is extended to 30 days. If there is carditis, meningitis, neurologic disease, or unresolved arthritis, then parenteral ceftriaxone or penicillin G is recommended for 14 to 21 days.

Outcome

Treatment for early Lyme disease is highly effective. Prolonged symptoms related to disseminated and late Lyme disease are not related to persistent infection and prolonged or repeated courses of antibiotics are not needed.

Prevention

Although vaccines have been developed, none are currently marketed in the United States. Avoidance of tick-infested area and use of long sleeved/legged clothing and insect repellent are valuable. Checking children for adherent ticks is also useful since, in general, ticks must be attached for at least 24 hours for infection to occur. Antibiotic prophylaxis after tick bite is controversial; local experts should be consulted for advice.

Nocardia Infections
Fundamentals

Nocardia species are aerobic actinomycetes from soil which grow as branched filaments in culture. Gram stain shows thin, branching forms with a beaded or weak gram-positive appearance. A modified acid-fast stain will also be positive. The most common species isolated in human disease are *N. asteroides* complex, *N. brasiliensis* and *N. pseudobrasiliensis*.

Nocardia infections are uncommon in children. The organism is found in the soil worldwide. Infection is acquired via inhalation or via contamination of the skin. Person-to-person transmission does not occur. Complicated and symptomatic infection can occur in compromised hosts, including those receiving steroids or cancer chemotherapy, as well as those with HIV infection, chronic granulomatous disease, and cystic fibrosis.

Clinical Presentation

Lung, skin, and brain are the most common sites of infection. Pulmonary disease can be acute, subacute, or chronic with cough, respiratory distress, and weight loss; chest radiographic patterns include lobar pneumonia, nodules, lung abscess, cavitation, and interstitial infiltrate. Skin manifestations include cellulitis, abscess, ulcers, and mycetoma; nodular lymphadenitis also occurs. Disseminated disease, especially brain abscess, occurs most often in immunocompromised hosts, and virtually any organ can be affected in such patients. Clinical course depends on the health of the host with more chronic illness and complications in those with more comorbidity.

Diagnosis

Specimens can be stained with Gram or modified acid-fast stains. The organism can grow on media for mycobacteria as well as conventional blood and chocolate agar if cultures are maintained for several weeks. Growth from respiratory tract secretions is complicated by overgrowth of more rapidly growing organisms. The laboratory should be aware if *Nocardia* species are suspected. *Nocardia* species should be sought in the setting of pulmonary disease and brain abscess in compromised hosts as well as in chronic unexplained pulmonary and skin disease in normal hosts.

Treatment

Trimethoprim-sulfamethoxazole or sulfonamides alone are drugs of choice. The new agent, linezolid, may develop a role in primary or salvage therapy. Duration of therapy is prolonged in all cases, especially in brain disease and in compromised hosts.

Outcome

Prognosis is guarded in compromised hosts, and nocardial infection may lead to death.

Pertussis
Fundamentals

Bordetella pertussis, a small gram-negative coccobacillus, is the major cause of whooping cough, also known as pertussis syndrome. *B. parapertussis* and *B. bronchiseptica* are less common causative agents. These bacteria are challenging to isolate and require special media for growth. *B. pertussis* has a number of virulence factors, including pertussis toxin, filamentous hemagglutinin, periactin, and tracheal cytotoxin, which are important for pathogenesis and immunity.

Pertussis is highly communicable; prior to vaccination programs in the United States, over 200,000 cases were reported each year. Transmission is via respiratory droplets, and after an incubation period of 3 to 12 days, approximately 80% of susceptible household contacts become ill. Worldwide pertussis remains an important threat, with an estimated 300,000 deaths in children per year. Currently, cases in the United States peak in the summer and fall. There is no animal reservoir; adolescents and adults serve as the source of infection because immunity wanes over time after both natural infection and immunization.

The introduction of pertussis vaccination in the 1940s led to a dramatic decline in reported cases from over 200,000 per year to less than 3000 per year by 1980. The subsequent increase in cases in the 1990s to 5000 to 8000 per year may be related to cyclicity of disease, vaccine coverage, and changes in adolescent and adult immunity. The stable incidence in children aged 6 months to 4 years suggests that the change in vaccine recommendation from DTP (diphtheria, tetanus, pertussis) to DtaP (diphtheria, tetanus, acellular pertussis) vaccine has not increased the risk for this age group. Among reported cases, children under age 1 year have the highest incidence of infection, but the greatest increase in cases has been in adolescents and adults.

Clinical Presentation

The classic pertussis syndrome is divided into three stages and the disease specifically lacks fever, rash, tachypnea, or diarrhea. The first or catarrhal stage, lasting 1 to 2 weeks is a nonspecific upper respiratory infection. The second, paroxysmal stage is heralded by development of dry cough, which evolves into prolonged coughing fits that end with a deep inspiration or "whoop" (see the video on the CD-ROM.) This stage can last from days to several weeks and coughing fits often conclude with vomiting. During the convalescent stage coughing fits become both less frequent and less severe. Infants may present with choking or apnea rather than coughing and whooping. Immunized children and adults may have a less distinctive clinical course.

Adults and adolescents with pertussis may lack the inspiratory whoop but have a prolonged duration of cough (mean 36 to 48 days) with a paroxysmal pattern. In many studies of adults, a cough of greater than 7 to 21 days' duration was attributed to pertussis in 12% to 32% of cases. Features such as emesis and choking after coughing fits may occur. Complications in older patients include sweating, syncope, rib fracture, hernia, incontinence, and back pain.

Physical examination findings are few, and usually, lower respiratory tract findings are absent. Petechiae and conjunctival hemorrhages may occur as a result of the coughing fits.

Complications of pertussis include apnea, secondary bacterial pneumonia, seizures, encephalopathy, and death. Apnea and respiratory fatigue is most common in young infants. Because pertussis usually lacks fever and lower respiratory manifestations, the development of these problems plus tachypnea and increased neutrophil count should suggest bacterial pneumonia. Persistent apnea or pneumonia may require mechanical ventilation. The high pressures generated during coughing fits may cause petechiae, pneumothorax, subcutaneous emphysema, and conjunctival, CNS, or retinal hemorrhages. CNS abnormalities may be caused by hypoxia or CNS hemorrhage associated with coughing spells. Death is usually attributed to bacterial pneumonia, but pulmonary hypertension is increasingly recognized as a factor in fatal cases.

Diagnosis

The presence of absolute lymphocytosis (15,000 to 100,000/μL) on complete blood count (CBC) with differential is an important clue to pertussis (in infants only) and is rare in other respiratory illnesses. Greater magnitude of lymphocytosis and thrombocytosis is associated with worse prognosis. Chest x-ray may be normal or show a nonspecific perihilar infiltrate. Specific diagnosis requires detection of the organism by culture or the more sensitive PCR test. Direct fluorescent antibody testing of nasopharyngeal secretions is a rapid method of diagnosis but suffers from false positive and false negative results in many laboratories. All three tests are done on nasopharyngeal secretion specimens. Serologic testing requires convalescent specimens and is not helpful in diagnosis of acute infection.

Testing should be done in all suspect cases to ensure appropriate antimicrobial therapy, monitor community activity of disease, prompt contact tracing to limit spread, and aid in prognosis.

Treatment

Treatment with 14 days of erythromycin is the standard of care, and efficacy is greatest when treatment is started early. Other macrolide agents are likely to be effective but should be considered alternatives. Although treatment does not always provide a clinical benefit to the patient, it limits further spread. Bronchodilators and corticosteroids do not have an established role in treatment. Supportive care to prevent hypoxia, dehydration, and malnutrition during prolonged illness may be needed, especially in young infants.

Outcome

Cough can persist for many weeks. Pulmonary function test abnormalities are common even in uncomplicated pertussis for 6 to 12 months, but most children eventually make complete recoveries.

Prevention and Control

Immunization for pertussis is discussed in Chapter 18. Droplet precautions (masks) are used to prevent spread to health care workers. Close contacts should be immediately treated with erythromycin regardless of immunization history or symptoms. All suspected and proved cases should be promptly reported to local health authorities. Control of pertussis in adults and adolescents using acellular pertussis vaccine is recommended in some countries and is under study in the United States.

Rickettsial Diseases

Fundamentals

Rickettsiae are small, gram-negative, coccobacilli. Because they are obligate intracellular pathogens, they cannot be grown in cell-free media. Most have arthropod vectors, including ticks, fleas, and lice. The incubation period is often about 1 week, but ranges from 2 to 14 days. The most significant of these organisms is *Rickettsia rickettsii*, which causes Rocky Mountain spotted fever (RMSF). Other diseases caused by rickettsial organisms include rickettsialpox caused by *Rickettsia akari*, murine/endemic typhus *(R. typhi)*, and epidemic typhus *(R. prowazekii)*.

Clinical Presentation

History of exposure to arthropod vectors is important when evaluating a child for possible infection. Rickettsial organisms can cause systemic capillary and small-vessel vasculitis. Common clinical features of infection include fever, rash, myalgia, headache, nausea, vomiting, photophobia, and conjunctival hyperemia. The rash of RMSF usually occurs before the sixth day of illness. Initially the rash may be erythematous and macular, but eventually it becomes maculopapular, often with petechiae. The rash begins on the extremities (wrists and ankles), spreads to the trunk, and involves the palms and the soles, but it usually spares the face. The illness can last up to 3 weeks and can be severe. Acute complications include hyponatremia, which can be profound, mild anemia, thrombocytopenia, acute respiratory distress, renal failure, and hypotension. Disseminated intravascular coagulopathy can occur with shock, leading to death. Long-term complications include paraparesis, hearing loss, peripheral neuropathy, and other neurologic dysfunction.

Diagnosis

Initial diagnosis must be made clinically. Diagnosis can be made by using rickettsial group-specific serologic tests. Testing of acute and convalescent-phase sera is recommended. Culture and isolation of the organism from tissues is restricted to research laboratories.

Treatment

Early treatment with antibiotics is essential. Patients treated within 4 days of onset of illness have significantly better outcomes than those treated later. Doxycycline is the drug of choice *for all age groups*. Even though use of tetracyclines is generally not recommended for children younger than 8 years of age, doxycycline is the drug of choice for RMSF. Less likely than tetracycline to stain teeth, the 7- to 10-day course of therapy for RMSF is too brief to cause noticeable tooth staining; it is effective against ehrlichial infections, which can mimic RMSF; and the main alternative, chloramphenicol, has serious adverse effects and is not widely available in the United States.

Supportive measures should be provided as indicated, with particular attention to fluid and electrolyte imbalances and fluid therapy.

Prevention and Control

Avoidance of tick-infested areas is the best preventive measure. Children who might be exposed to ticks should wear protective clothing that fits tightly around the wrist and ankles and use insect repellent. Ticks should be removed promptly and properly. Prophylactic antibiotics after a tick bite are not recommended.

SPIROCHETAL INFECTONS

Leptospirosis

Fundamentals

The *Leptospira* genus includes spirochetes of several species that cause human disease. These organisms are widespread in both wild and domestic animals; human infection is via direct or indirect contact with animal urine. Animals may shed the bacteria in their urine for long periods, sometimes for the life of the animal. Most human cases are acquired through contact with contaminated water in which, under favorable pH conditions, the leptospira can survive for 3 months. High-risk groups include veterinarians, slaughterhouse workers, and farmers and their families. Children are likely to become infected after contact with contaminated water through swimming, splashing, and wading.

Clinical Presentation

Most patient suffer from the "anicteric" form of leptospirosis. After an incubation period of 7 to 14 days, there is an acute onset of fever, headache and myalgia sometimes associated with gastrointestinal symptoms and conjunctival suffusion. Generally this 4- to 7-day phase of the illness, during which the organism is present in blood, CSF, and urine, is self-limited, but it can be severe. Subsequently, there can be an "immune" phase of the illness during which headache, rash, myalgia, and nuchal rigidity occur. Other complications include encephalitis, Guillain-Barré syndrome, neuropathies, nephritis, acalculus cholecystitis, and uveitis.

Approximately 10% of patients have a more severe acute illness known as "icteric" leptospirosis or Weil syndrome. In these patients, jaundice, renal failure, and occasionally cardiac failure develop during the first week of illness.

Infection of pregnant women has been reported with a high rate of abortion and congenital infection.

Diagnosis

Leptospira species can be cultured under special conditions not available in most laboratories; hence, most cases must be diagnosed retrospectively using serologic testing. Diagnosis should be pursued in cases of unexplained illness and in situations in which cases are linked to a water or animal source.

Treatment

Little prospective data support the use of specific antibiotics in leptospirosis, but animal experiments and in vitro susceptibility testing support the use of intravenous penicillin for suspected severe infection and oral amoxicillin or doxycycline (for children over 8 years) for less severe infection.

Prevention

Animal immunization is available. Children should not swim or play in potentially infected waters.

Tetanus

Fundamentals

The anaerobic, spore-forming, gram-positive bacillus, *Clostridium tetani*, causes the clinical syndrome known as tetanus by producing toxins. *Clostridium tetani* spores are ubiquitous worldwide in soil and feces but do not cause disease unless they become vegetative in tissue in the setting of injury or inoculation. Tetanospasmin, also known as tetanus toxin, is produced by growth of C. *tetani* and causes local or distant muscle spasm, depending on the amount produced and mechanism of spread. This toxin causes muscle spasm by preventing acetylcholine release from inhibitory neurons and leads to unopposed muscle contraction.

Tetanus became uncommon in the United States during the 20th century prior to the institution of routine childhood tetanus immunization in the 1940s. Since the 1960s it has become extremely rare, with only 50 to 100 cases reported per year in the United States. Worldwide, if immunization is not universal, it remains an important cause of morbidity and death in adults and children; it is a substantial pediatric problem with an estimated 270,000 neonatal deaths annually. The incubation period is usually about 1 week (range of 3 to 21 days). Introduction to the body is typically through a wound, although the wound may be minor, inapparent, or intentional (drug use). Other mechanisms of acquisition are surgery, burns, crush injury, otitis media, animal bites, abortion, and pregnancy. It is not spread from person to person.

Clinical Presentation, Course, and Complications

Four syndromes are recognized. Both localized tetanus, in which spasm is limited to the area of injury/inoculation, and cephalic tetanus, in which the cranial nerves are involved, are uncommon. Most cases in the United States are generalized tetanus in which jaw muscle spasm (trismus, lockjaw) develops first, followed by descending neck, back, and abdominal contractions. Spasms may be triggered by stimuli, can last several minutes, and can continue for weeks, even with treatment. Elevated temperature, heart rate, blood pressure, and sweating also occur. Complications include airway obstruction, apnea, fractures, hypertension, and arrhythmias. Neonatal tetanus occurs in infants of inadequately immunized mothers, often in the setting of nonsterile umbilical cord care. After a presentation of poor feeding at 1 to 2 weeks of age, generalized spasms and opisthotonus develop. Most cases are fatal, and survivors may have cognitive disability.

Diagnosis

Tetanus is a clinical diagnosis and is occasionally confirmed by growth of toxin-producing C. *tetani* from wounds. In the setting of inadequate immunization and clinical findings, a history of chronic infection, injection, or minor surgery can be sought. Important diseases to include in the differential diagnosis include meningitis, hypocalcemia, seizure, dystonic medication reactions, and strychnine poisoning. Treatment should not be delayed while awaiting microbiologic confirmation.

Treatment

Treatment of tetanus requires a multidisciplinary team in an intensive care unit to provide respiratory and nutritional support in a minimally stimulating environment. Human tetanus immune globulin is used to neutralize free toxin, wounds are debrided to remove dead tissue, and penicillin or metronidazole is given for at least 10 days to kill any remaining *C. tetani* organisms. Muscle spasms can be limited with benzodiazepines or neuromuscular blockade if necessary. α-Adrenergic and β-adrenergic blockade may be required. Surviving patients require immunization because the very potent toxin does not generate an adequate response.

Prevention and Control

Routine childhood and adult immunization eliminates the risk of tetanus. Use of tetanus toxoid (dT) and tetanus immune globulin (TIG) for wounds depends on number of previous vaccine doses received as shown in Table 118-2.

Tularemia
Fundamentals

Francisella tularensis is an aerobic gram-negative coccobacillus that can infect more than 100 animal species. Humans acquire infection through direct contact with infected animals, ingestion of game meat, or bites from insects, mostly ticks, that have fed from infected animals. Small wild mammals such as rabbits are more important reservoirs than domestic animals. Most of the 100 to 200 cases reported each year in the United States occur between June and September when tick bites are most frequent. Person-to-person transmission of tularemia does not occur.

Table 118-2. Guide to Tetanus Prophylaxis in Routine Wound Management

History of Absorbed Tetanus Toxoid (doses)	Clean, Minor Wounds		All Other Wounds*	
	Td[†]	TIG[‡]	Td[†]	TIG[‡]
<3 or unknown	Yes	No	Yes	Yes
≥3[§]	No[‖]	No	No[¶]	No

¶Td indicates adult-type diphtheria and tetanus toxoids vaccine; TIG, tetanus immune globulin (human).
*Such as, but not limited to, wounds contaminated with diet, feces, soil, and saliva; puncture wounds; avulsions; and wounds resulting from missiles, crushing, burns, and frostbite.
†For children younger than 7 years of age, diphtheria and tetanus toxoids and acellular pertussis (DTaP) vaccine is recommended; if pertussis vaccine is contraindicated, diphtheria and tetanus toxoids (DT) vaccine is given. For people 7 years of age or older, Td vaccine is recommended.
‡Equine tetanus antitoxin should be used, if available, when TIG is not available.
§If only three doses of fluid toxoid have been received, a fourth dose of toxoid, preferably an adsorbed toxoid, should be given. Although licensed, fluid tetanus toxoid rarely is used.
‖Yes if more than 10 years since last dose.
¶Yes, if more than 5 years since last dose. More frequent boosters are not needed and can accentuate adverse effects.

From American Academy of Pediatrics: Tetanus. In Pickering LK (ed): Red Book 2003: Report of the Committee on *Infectious Diseases*, 26th ed. Elk Grove Village, Ill, American Academy of Pediatrics, 2003, p 614.

Clinical Presentation

Several distinct clinical syndromes occur, but most reported cases have tender regional adenopathy with or without a distal ulcerated lesion at the site of inoculation. When the conjunctivae are infected, nodules and ulcers of this surface may occur, followed by painful preauricular adenopathy. Typhoidal tularemia resembles bacterial sepsis, has a high mortality rate in untreated cases, but unfortunately lacks the cutaneous ulcers or enlarged lymph nodes to suggest the diagnosis. Aerosol acquisition leads to pneumonic tularemia, which can be fatal. Laboratory workers have been infected by this route, which is also considered a possible method of bioterrorism. Table 118-3 lists common syndromes and symptoms and findings of infection.

Diagnosis

Culture should be done only in specialized laboratories after informing staff of the suspected diagnosis because laboratory workers are at risk of acquiring infection. Diagnosis can be confirmed retrospectively by serologic testing.

Treatment

Gentamicin, amikacin, and streptomycin are the recommended agents for treatment of all forms of tularemia. Relapses can occur, in which case imipenem or fluoroquinolones can be used. Intensive supportive care may be required.

Prevention

Avoidance of exposure to ticks and potentially infected animals will prevent infection. A live attenuated vaccine is available but is used only for laboratory workers.

Yersinia Species
Fundamentals

Yersinia species are gram-negative bacilli; the genus includes three important human pathogens: two (*Y. enterocolitica* and *Y. pseudotuberculosis*) cause diarrhea and abdominal symptoms; the third, *Y. pestis*, is the cause of plague. The typical characteristics of illness caused by the three species are presented in Table 118-4.

Table 118-3. Clinical Syndromes of Tularemia

Syndrome	Route of Acquisition	Symptoms/Findings
Glandular	Cutaneous inoculation	Tender regional adenopathy
Ulceroglandular	Cutaneous inoculation	Papule or ulcer distal to tender regional adenopathy
Oropharyngeal	Contaminated food or water	Tonsil inflammation, oral ulceration, cervical adenopathy
Typhoidal	Contaminated food or water	Gastrointestinal symptoms, hepatosplenomegaly, sepsis syndrome
Pneumonia	Inhalation or secondary to hematogenous spread from other site	Lobar pneumonia with or without effusion

Table 118-4. Typical Characteristic Features of Illness Caused by the Three Species of *Yersinia*

Feature	*Y. enterocolitica*	*Y. pseudotuberculosis*	*Y. pestis*
Reservoir	Pigs and other animals	Many animals and birds, including pets	Rabbits, prairie dogs, bobcats, squirrels, coyotes, mice, and rats
Sources of infection	Pig contact, pig intestines (chitterlings)		Rat fleas, wild animal contact, rarely person-to-person (pneumonic plague)
Clinical syndromes	Gastroenteritis, fever, bloody stool, sometimes prolonged	Mesenteric adenitis (pseudoappendix), Kawasaki disease mimic	Tender regional adenopathy followed by sepsis, bronchopneumonia with sepsis, isolated sepsis, meningitis
Complications	Intestinal perforation, mesenteric adenitis, terminal ileitis; see text for extraintestinal complications	Rarely sepsis	Disseminated intravascular coagulation, rapid death
Diagnosis	Stool culture for prolonged or bloody diarrhea, notify laboratory that *Yersina* infection is suspected	Stool culture, mesenteric node culture	Gram stain of blood, sputum, cerebrospinal fluid, or node aspirate; blood culture
Treatment	TMP/SMX, ceftriaxone, cefotaxime	Usually self-limited; susceptible to TMP-SMX, ampicillin in vitro	Streptomycin
Prevention	Careful food preparation, especially with pork	Good hygiene around animals	Rat and flea control

TMP-SMX, trimethoprim-sulfamethoxazole.

Clinical Presentations, Diagnosis, Treatment

Y. enterocolitica can also cause bacteremia after intestinal infection especially in infants and those with iron overload syndromes (hemochromatosis, repeated transfusion, oral iron supplements). After bacteremia, a variety of focal complications can develop, including granulomatous hepatitis, pancreatitis, meningitis, osteomyelitis, pyomyositis, and renal abscess.

Y. pseudotuberculosis is uncommon but causes both mesenteric adenitis, mimicking appendicitis, and a syndrome with fever, rash, and oral findings mimicking Kawasaki disease.

Plague is currently rare in the United States and largely has been limited to western state residents with wild animal contact. *Y. pestis* is considered to be a possible agent of bioterrorism, in which case it would likely be spread as an aerosol causing epidemic pneumonic plague. Because the recommended treatment, streptomycin, is unlikely to be used empirically for community-acquired pneumonia, awareness of this organism in an unexpected outbreak of pneumonia is important.

Additional Resources, CD-ROM

Pertussis	Video 118-1

Mini-index of Related Topics — CH.

SUGGESTED READINGS

Feigin RD, Cherry J, Demmler G, Spector S (eds): Textbook of Pediatric Infectious Diseases. 5th ed. Philadelphia, WB Saunders, 2003.

Long SS, Pickering LK, Prober CG (eds): Principals and Practice of Pediatric Infectious Disease. New York, Churchill Livingstone, 1997.

Pickering LK (ed): Red Book: 2003 Report of the Committee on Infectious Diseases, 26th ed. Elk Grove Village, Ill, American Academy of Pediatrics, 2003.

119 Viral Infections

Paul F. Lewis

Because this text is organized to discuss diseases as they are likely to present to the practitioner, most infectious disorders are found in chapters that cover specific organ systems. Viral illness is the most common acute disease among children. Because most viral illnesses cause symptoms referable to a specific organ system, discussion of most viruses is found in those sections of the text. This chapter discusses general issues related to viral infections and viral infections that are not discussed in chapters related to disorders of specific organs or organ systems.

FUNDAMENTALS

Viruses are commonly classified according to nucleic acid type, DNA or RNA, and whether they carry a single or double strand of genetic material. Other characteristics such as the presence of an envelope, the type of replication, and biologic properties are also used in classification. A clinically useful classification is according to mode of transmission: enteric, respiratory, sexually, or vector-borne. Viral structure and pathogenesis are discussed in Chapter 12.

CLINICAL PRESENTATION AND DIAGNOSIS

Viral illnesses can present with generalized symptoms, such as fever and malaise, or with symptoms related to the infected organ. Some viruses produce clinical syndromes that are distinct enough to be diagnosed reliably without laboratory testing. For example mumps, measles, chickenpox, parvovirus B-19 (Fifth disease), and enteroviral hand-foot-and-mouth disease have features rarely seen with other illnesses. Because most nonspecific viral illness is self-limited and few antiviral agents are available, making the diagnosis of a specific infectious agents is often unnecessary. When identification of a specific agent is desired, diagnosis can be pursued with viral culture, antigen testing, polymerase chain reaction (PCR), or serologic testing.

TREATMENT

Because few antiviral therapies are available (see Chapter 284) therapy for viral infections is generally directed toward alleviation of symptoms and physiologic support, such as fluids and electrolytes (see Chapters 42 and 292).

PREVENTION AND CONTROL

Prevention of many viral illnesses is possible through routine immunization (see Chapter 18). The spread of viral illness to other susceptible individuals can be greatly decreased by careful hygiene, especially of the hands. Good hygiene is particularly important in day care centers.

SPECIFIC VIRAL INFECTIONS

Dengue Fever
Fundamentals
Dengue fever is a common mosquito-borne flaviviral infection responsible for millions of cases of febrile illness in tropical countries. Dengue hemorrhagic shock syndrome (DHSS) is a severe complication. The only areas in the United States that are at risk for this disease are those that border Mexico.

Clinical Presentation
Dengue can present with multiple signs and symptoms, usually fever, rash, and headache, and also hepatitis, upper gastrointestinal bleeding, pneumonia, splenic rupture, and encephalopathy. DHSS results in hypotension, shock, and generalized bleeding.

Diagnosis
Diagnosis is made by culturing the virus in the blood or with reverse transcriptase polymerase chain reaction (RT-PCR).

Treatment
Treatment is supportive and consists of careful clinical monitoring and fluid resuscitation.

Outcome
Most patients with good supportive care recover within 48 hours. Fatality occurs in approximately 10% of cases.

Human Herpesvirus Type 8

Fundamentals

Human herpesvirus type 8 (HHV-8) is the most recently discovered member of the herpesvirus family.

Clinical Presentation

The spectrum of clinical disease is as yet unknown, although the virus has been associated with Kaposi sarcoma in the elderly and in those with human immunodeficiency virus (HIV) infection.

Diagnosis

Tests for detection of HHV-8 are limited to research laboratories.

Treatment

No treatment is known.

Hantavirus

Fundamentals

Hantavirus, an RNA virus in the Bunyaviridae family, is transmitted by rodents and is particularly prevalent in the four-corners area of the United States (Utah, Arizona, Colorado, and New Mexico). Sporadic cases of Hantavirus have been reported throughout the United States.

Clinical Presentation

Hantaviral infections present with three different syndromes: hemorrhagic fever with renal syndrome (HFRS), a noncardiogenic pulmonary edema, or hantaviral pulmonary syndrome (HPS). A nonspecific prodromal illness (3 to 7 days) consists of fever, chills, headache, myalgias, nausea, vomiting, diarrhea, and dizziness. Respiratory symptoms of pulmonary edema and severe hypoxemia can occur suddenly after 3 to 7 days of illness.

Diagnosis

Sin Nombre virus (SNV, causes noncardiogenic pulmonary edema) RNA can be detected by reverse transcriptase polymerase chain reaction assay (RT-PCR) of peripheral blood mononuclear cells. Hantavirus-specific immunoglobulin antibodies are present at onset of the disease and can be detected using a rapid immunoblot assay or enzyme immunoassay that is available through many state health departments and the Centers for Disease Control and Prevention (CDC).

Treatment

No specific therapy is available. Because the mortality rate from hantaviral infections is high, patients should be transferred immediately to a tertiary care facility for intense supportive therapy.

Prevention and Control

No immunization is available. Rodent populations in the home and work environment should be controlled through limiting food sources to rodents, limiting nesting sites, and using traps. Dusty or dirty areas in which rodents have been detected should be moistened with a 10% bleach solution or other disinfectant before being cleaned.

Influenza

Fundamentals

Although there are three antigenic types of influenza virus (influenza A, influenza B, and influenza C), only influenza A and B cause epidemic disease. Surface antigens are important determinants of immunity. Major changes in the surface antigens are called antigenic shifts. Minor changes are labeled antigenic drift. Antigenic shift has occurred only with influenza A. Antigenic shift is important in producing epidemics. Recent analysis demonstrates that influenza infections are responsible for nearly as many pediatric hospitalizations as respiratory syncytial virus (RSV).

Clinical Presentation

Influenza presents with sudden onset of fever, chills, headache, myalgia, malaise, and cough. Other respiratory symptoms, such as sore throat and rhinitis, appear subsequently. Other signs and symptoms include conjunctival injection, nausea and vomiting, and abdominal pain. Influenza can cause a sepsis-like illness in young children, as well as bronchitis, bronchiolitis, croup, and pneumonia. In older children, calf tenderness resulting in refusal to walk may occur after several days of illness. Influenza has also been associated with Reye syndrome and encephalopathy.

Diagnosis

During acute illness, rapid diagnostic tests of nasopharyngeal secretions and viral culture can be performed for diagnosis. Serologic testing can establish the diagnosis retrospectively.

Treatment

Although antiviral agents are available for treatment of influenza infection, only amantadine has been approved for use in children. Amantadine and rimantidine, effective only against influenza A, can result in reduction of symptoms when administered within 48 hours of onset of illness. Rimantidine is not approved for use in children 13 years old or younger. Antiviral treatment should be considered in children at increased risk for severe or complicated influenza infection, such as those with chronic pulmonary disease, or in healthy children with severe disease. Supportive treatment is important, particularly in children with underlying chronic conditions. Aspirin for treatment of fever must be avoided because of the risk of Reye syndrome. Patients should be monitored for bacterial superinfection, particularly pneumonia. For up-to-date treatment options, see www.cdc.gov/flu/professionals/antiviralpack.htm.

Prevention

Inactivated vaccines against influenza are available and should be given annually in the fall to children at high risk for complications of influenza such as those with underlying cardiac or pulmonary disease. Routine immunization of healthy children over the age of 6 months is now recommended by the American Academy of Pediatrics (AAP) to prevent infant hospitalization and decrease the adult burden of illness.

ASPERGILLOSIS

Fundamentals

Aspergillus species are ubiquitous molds, widespread in the environment in soil, plants and decomposing organic matter. Aspergillosis is usually acquired by inhalation of spores; therefore, lungs and sinuses are the most common sites of primary infection. Most cases of aspergillosis are caused by *Aspergillus fumigatus*, followed by *A. flavus*, and to a lesser extent *A. nidulans*, *A. niger*, and *A. terreus*. Neutropenia and neutrophil dysfunction are the major risk factors for invasive aspergillosis. Prolonged neutropenia is the single most important risk for aspergillosis among patients with leukemia and bone marrow transplants.

Clinical Presentation, Course, and Complications

Aspergillus species can cause three clinical syndromes: (1) colonization that results in an allergic response (allergic bronchopulmonary aspergillosis), (2) colonization of a preexisting cavity (aspergilloma), and (3) invasive aspergillosis of the bronchopulmonary system, paranasal sinuses, central nervous system (CNS), skin, bone, and heart. Allergic bronchopulmonary aspergillosis (ABPA) is a hypersensitivity disease of the lungs marked by episodic asthma-like symptoms, history of pulmonary infiltrates, and central bronchiectasis. Chest radiographs can reveal transient consolidation, unilateral or bilateral, usually in the upper lobes. ABPA can progress through the clinical stages of acute corticosteroid-responsive asthma to corticosteroid-dependent asthma to, ultimately, fibrotic end-stage lung disease.

The most common site of noninvasive colonization of preexisting cavities is in the lung (aspergilloma), but the sinuses can also be involved. In pediatrics, aspergilloma is most common in patients with cystic fibrosis. On chest radiograph, an aspergilloma can appear as a solid oval or round mass within a cavity and separated from the wall of the cavity by an airspace of varying size and shape. Aspergilloma can progress to invasive disease. Hemoptysis is a common symptom and can be the cause of death in up to 26% of patients with aspergilloma.

Invasive disease is marked by angioinvasion of the organism. With angioinvasion, thrombosis, infarction, and necrosis of surrounding lung tissue follow. The lungs are the most common site of initial infection, but the sinuses are another common site. Invasive disease is seen most often in the context of a patient with profound neutropenia (from leukemia or lymphoma with chemotherapy) or in patients with chronic granulomatous disease (CGD). In the neutropenic child, the most common presentation of invasive *Aspergillus* infection is persistent fever despite use of broad-spectrum antibiotics, frequently without any respiratory tract symptoms, although nonproductive cough may at times be present. Chest radiographs may reveal wedge-shaped, pleural-based densities and cavities, both of which are late findings, or diffuse pulmonary infiltrate. Computed tomography (CT) scan is more sensitive and may show abnormalities before they are seen on the chest radiograph. Distinctive lesions are small nodules or small pleural-based lesions surrounded by a zone of low attenuation, also known as the "halo sign." These nodules can cavitate, resulting in the "crescent sign," with a thin crescent of air near the edge of a lung nodule. In the patient with CGD, fever is often the initial symptom, with few pulmonary symptoms. Chest radiographs can reveal multiple nodular infiltrates. The course of aspergillosis in patients with CGD is more indolent, but there may be contiguous spread into the ribs or spine.

The CNS is the most common secondary site of infection and is involved in 10% to 20% of cases. *Aspergillus* infections in the CNS usually manifest as single or multiple cerebral abscesses, meningitis, epidural abscess, or subarachnoid hemorrhage.

Diagnosis

For the diagnosis of APBA, the clinical criteria described previously need to be met. Peripheral blood eosinophilia, elevated IgE levels, an immediate prick test reaction to *Aspergillus* antigen, and precipitating antibodies to *Aspergillus* antigen are also required for the diagnosis of APBA.

Definitive diagnosis of invasive aspergillosis requires both histopathologic evidence of branching, septate, nonpigmented hyphae in lung tissues and the isolation of the organism in culture. Because the hyphae of *Aspergillus* may resemble those of *Fusarium*, *Scedosporium*, and many other nonpigmented molds, histologic identification without a culture yields only a probable diagnosis. Recently a new rapid test for *Aspergillus* galactomannan antigen in blood was approved by the Food and Drug Administration (FDA). In clinical studies, the test has about 81% sensitivity and 89% specificity. The utility of this test for screening febrile neutropenic hosts compared to confirmation of diagnosis in immunosuppressed patients with a clinical syndrome suspicious for *Aspergillus* infection remains to be determined.

Treatment

The treatment of choice for invasive aspergillosis is amphotericin B in relatively high doses. Lipid formulations may be considered for children who are unable to tolerate regular amphotericin B. Itraconazole can be considered for mild to moderate cases of aspergillosis if the isolate is susceptible. However, safety and efficacy of itraconazole in children has not been established. Caspofungin and voriconazole are newer agents licensed by the FDA for treatment of aspergillosis in adults. Data on the safety and efficacy of both of these agents in children are very limited. Surgical excision of a localized lesion may be indicated.

Allergic bronchopulmonary and sinus aspergillosis are usually treated with corticosteroids. Systemic antifungal therapy in allergic aspergillosis or nonallergic colonization is not indicated.

Prevention and Control

Minimization of exposure to spores in the environment is important. Live plants and flowers should be removed from the patient's room and food items that can be contaminated with *Aspergillus* species (such as spices and nuts) should be avoided. Use of sterile laminar air flow rooms or rooms with HEPA filtration is effective but limited when patients must be transferred to other areas. Patients should not be housed in environments adjacent to or exposed to construction work, which can release mold spores. No vaccine is available, and to date, antifungal prophylaxis has not demonstrated significant efficacy.

BLASTOMYCOSIS

Fundamentals

Blastomycosis is caused by *Blastomyces dermatitidis*, a dimorphic fungus reported worldwide. In the United States, endemic areas are the southeastern and central states, and the midwestern states bordering the Great Lakes. The natural reservoir is not well known, but the organism is believed to be a soil saprophyte. Infection occurs by inhaling into the lungs fungal spores, which then may disseminate. Person-to-person transmission does not occur.

Clinical Presentation, Course, and Complications

The major clinical manifestations of blastomycosis are pulmonary, cutaneous, and disseminated disease. Primary pulmonary infection may be asymptomatic, but approximately 50% of infected children develop symptomatic illness, presenting as an acute or chronic pulmonary process. Cough, fever, malaise, and chest pain are the most common symptoms in patients with blastomycosis. Chest radiographs in children reveal extensive consolidation of involved lobes, but can also demonstrate mass effects or fibronodular patterns. Skin lesions can be pustular, ulcerative, nodular, or verrucous, with minimal inflammation, often in sun-exposed parts of the body. Disseminated disease is present in 50% to 80% of children diagnosed with blastomycosis. The most common site is the bones (long bones, ribs, and vertebrae are most common), but disease can also involve the central nervous system, abdominal viscera, kidneys, and the skin. Prior to the availability of active antifungal therapy, the mortality rate of blastomycosis was over 60%.

Diagnosis

Definitive diagnosis requires culture of *B. dermatitidis* from sputum, bronchoalveolar lavage, or tissue. Presumptive diagnosis may be made if characteristic yeasts are seen in sputum, tracheal aspirates, cerebrospinal fluid (CSF), urine, purulent material, or histopathologic specimens treated with 10% potassium hydroxide or a silver stain. Serologic assays are insensitive with high cross-reactivity with other mycoses and therefore are not useful in the clinical setting.

Treatment

For severe or life-threatening infections, amphotericin B is the treatment of choice. For less severe infections, a short course of amphotericin B followed by oral itraconazole or fluconazole may be used. Oral therapy is usually continued for 6 months for pulmonary and extrapulmonary disease and 1 year for osteomyelitis.

Prevention and Control

There is no effective preventive measure currently available.

COCCIDIOIDOMYCOSIS

Fundamentals

Coccidioidomycosis is caused by *Coccidioides immitis*, a dimorphic fungus found in soil and endemic in the Western Hemisphere between the 40°N and 40°S latitudes. In the United States, endemic areas include western Texas, northwestern Utah, New Mexico, Arizona, and California. Coccidioidomycosis is also known as "San Joaquin fever" or "valley fever." Infection arises from inhalation of fungal arthroconidia, which become airborne during windstorms or disruption of soil by construction and farming. Person-to-person transmission does not occur. Primary pulmonary infection often is self-limited, but infection can disseminate and become fatal. Age, sex, and racial features do not appear to change an individual's susceptibility to infection with *C. immitis*, but the risk of disseminated disease is increased in infants, Filipinos, Hispanics, African Americans, pregnant women, elderly, and immunosuppressed individuals.

Clinical Presentation, Course, and Complications

Primary pulmonary infection is asymptomatic or self-limited in 60% of children. In the remainder, severity of illness varies from insignificant flu-like illness (with fever, cough, myalgia, headache, and chest pain) to severe lower respiratory illness with lobar pneumonia, pleural effusion, and occasionaly pericarditis. Diffuse erythematous maculopapular rash, erythema multiforme, erythema nodosum, and arthralgias can occur and may be the only manifestation in some children.

Disseminated disease is rare (less than 1% of infected persons) but can involve the skin, bone and joints, and central nervous system (CNS). Skin manifestations include nodules or verrucous granuloma, which is characteristically located at the nasolabial fold. Chronic osteomyelitis may drain into overlying soft tissues, and radiographs will often reveal lytic lesions. Meningitis is a life-threatening manifestation of disseminated disease and is a granulomatous and suppurative basilar meningitis, frequently with parenchymal and spinal cord involvement. Meningitis may present with the primary infection or may occur many months later. Symptoms usually consist of headache, sluggishness, ataxia, and vomiting. Meningeal signs are often absent, although there may be signs of focal neurologic deficits.

Diagnosis

With primary pulmonary infection, chest radiographs are nonspecific: Bronchopenumonic infiltrates with hilar lymphadenopathy, sequential or lobar consolidation, or nodular or patchy pulmonary infiltrates are some common findings. Only 5% of infected individuals have residual findings on chest radiograph consisting of nodules, or thin-walled cavities (coin lesions) that are typically solitary and less than 6 cm. In meningitis, CSF analysis often reveals a moderate pleocytosis with mononuclear cell predominance, low glucose level, and elevated protein level.

Suspicion of infection with *C. immitis* involves obtaining a travel history if a patient does not reside or present in an endemic area. Confirmation of the diagnosis may be made by serologic test, histopathologic examination, and culture. Serologic tests available include IgM (detected by latex agglutination, enzyme immunoassay, immunodiffusion, or tube precipitin) and IgG (detected by immunodiffusion, enzyme immunoassay, or complement fixation). IgM is detectable 1 to 3 weeks after onset of symptoms and usually lasts 3 to 4 months. IgG can be useful as a prognostic indicator as transient or asymptomatic disease often have low titers, but severe disease and disseminated infection usually have high persistent titers (≥1:32). Antibodies may also be detected in CSF. Increasing titers suggest progressive disease, whereas decreasing titers suggest resolution. Low titers should be interpreted with caution in immunocompromised individuals. Histopathologic features may reveal large spherules typical of C. *immitis*. Culture of the organism from infected sites is possible but potentially hazardous to laboratory personnel. The laboratory should be made aware if coccidioidomycosis is suspected to ensure appropriate safety equipment and procedures are employed.

Treatment

Primary pulmonary infection is a self-limited illness in more than 90% of children, and therapy is not indicated in the vast majority of cases. These patients can be followed clinically and radiographically. Treatment is recommended for patients with persistent fevers for more than 1 month, severe or progressive lung disease, disseminated disease, or an underlying immunocompromising condition such as human immunodeficiency virus (HIV) infection, organ transplant, or high doses of steroids; for infants; and during pregnancy. Children from high-risk populations, such as Filipinos and African Americans (170 times and 10 times the risk of dissemination, respectively, compared to non-Hispanic whites), may also be considered for therapy.

For diffuse pneumonia, disseminated infection not including the CNS, and infection in children with immunocompromising conditions, amphotericin B is the recommended initial therapy, and may be replaced later with oral "azole" therapy including fluconazole, ketoconazole, or itraconazole. For less severe disseminated disease, itraconazole and fluconazole may be used. For CNS infection, fluconzaole is recommended. This therapy may be augmented with intrathecal administration of amphotericin B if the CNS infection is not responsive to fluconazole alone. Duration of therapy varies from months to years to lifelong, depending on site of infection and underlying host factors. Surgical débridement may be helpful in cases of osteomyelitis and cavitary pulmonary disease.

Prevention and Control

Because the organism is inhaled when spores become airborne, measures to control dust in endemic areas with excessive soil disruptance are recommended. Persons with immunocompromising conditions living or traveling in endemic areas should be advised to avoid activities in which soil can become airborne.

CRYPTOCOCCOSIS

Fundamentals

Cryptococcosis is caused by *Cryptococcus neoformans*, a monomorphic, encapsulated yeast. The organisim is found in soil enriched with bird droppings and is acquired by inhalation of the yeast into the lungs. From the lungs, the organism can then hematogenously disseminate to the CNS or the skin. Other sites of dissemination are the eye, prostate, adrenal gland, liver, heart, bone, lymph node, joint,

or kidney. Systemic infection can occur in both immunocompetent and immunocompromised persons, but most cases occur in immunocompromised patients, specifically those with cell-mediated immune defects. HIV-infected children have a lower incidence of cryptococcosis than do HIV-infected adults.

Clinical Presentation, Course, and Complications

Infection with C. *neoformans* begins with a primary pneumonia, which can be asymptomatic, mild, or severe. Primary pneumonia in immunocompetent individuals is usually asymptomatic or mild. Productive cough, pleuritic chest pain, and fever are the most common manifestations. Chest radiographs may reveal single or multiple lung nodules, mediastinal lymphadenopathy, and occasionally pleural effusion. Dissemination in the immunocompent host is rare. In the immunocompromised host, the primary pneumonia is often more severe, with a more rapid course.

Cryptococcal meningitis is the most common manifestation of disseminated disease. Fever and headache are the most common presentations. Nausea and vomiting may be seen in about one half of patients. Meningeal signs may be seen in 70% of nonimmunocompromised individuals, but only in 33% of patients with AIDS (acquired immunodeficiency syndrome). Other less frequent signs include altered mental status, focal neurologic deficits, seizures, signs of increased cranial pressure, and ataxia. Symptoms may be present for less than 1 week up to 18 months before patients present or are diagnosed with cryptococcal meningitis.

Cutaneous manifestations of cryptococcosis include ulcers, nodules, vesicles, abscesses, papules, cellulitis, acneiform plaques, purpuric lesions, and sinus tracts.

Diagnosis

In cryptococcal meningitis, the CSF may have normal to minimally eleveated leukocyte count, rarely more than 100 cells/mm^3. CSF glucose level is usually normal or minimally low. Definitive diagnosis of cryptococcosis is made by demonstrating the organism during the active infection. In CSF, urine, and sputum, the organism may be visualized with an India ink preparation. The organism can also be cultured. Antigen testing of serum or CSF is also available and useful for diagnosis.

Treatment

For meningitis or other serious cryptococcal infections, amphotericin B in combination with oral flucytosine is the treatment of choice. Lipid formulations of amphotericin B may be used instead of conventional amphotericin B if there is renal impairment. In the immunocompetent host, combination therapy is continued for 2 weeks or until CSF culture results are negative, followed by 4 weeks of amphotericin B or 10 weeks of fluconazole. Immunosuppressed patients should be treated for at least 2 weeks of combination therapy with amphotericin B and flucytosine, followed by 10 weeks of fluconazole, and then continued on suppressive doses of fluconazole for 6 to 12 months or lifelong, depending on the underlying host factors.

For less severe cryptococcal infections, fluconazole or itraconazole may be used for therapy for 6 to 12 months in nonimmunocompromised patients, or lifelong in HIV-infected children.

Prevention and Control

There are no known measures effective for preventing cryptococcal infections. There is no vaccine for C. *neoformans*.

HISTOPLASMOSIS

Fundamentals

Histoplasmosis is caused by *Histoplama capsulatum*, a dimorphic fungus encountered worldwide, and endemic in eastern and central United States, especially in Mississippi, Ohio, and the Missouri River Valley. The organism grows in moist soil with a predilection to soil enriched with bird droppings and bat guano. Spores become airborne in dry and windy weather and with activities that disturb soil. Infection is acquired by inhalation of spores.

Clinical Presentation, Course, and Complications

Clinical manifestation of infection with H. *capsulatum* varies, depending on inoculum of organism inhaled, underlying immune status, and the virulence of the strain. Approximately 95% of infections are asymptomatic. In those with symptoms, histoplasmosis may present with pulmonary, cutaneous, ocular, or disseminated disease. Acute pulmonary histoplasmosis can present with influenza-like illness with nonpleuritic chest pain, hilar adenopathy, and mild pulmonary infiltrates. Symptoms last for 2 days up to 2 weeks. Severe pulmonary disease presents with prolonged fever, fatigue, weight loss, and diffuse nodular pulmonary infiltrates and may last 10 to 21 days. Hepatosplenomegaly and erythema nodosum may be present in some cases of histoplasmosis.

Disseminated histoplasmosis occurs usually with immuno-compromised hosts and infants younger than 2 years of age. Progressive disseminated histoplasmosis is an overwhelming infection of the reticuloendothelial system by yeast forms of the organism. Prolonged fever, failure to thrive, and hepatosplenomegaly are early manifestations and can progress, if untreated, to malnutrition, diffuse adenopathy, pneumonia, mucosal ulceration, pancytopenia, disseminated intravascular coagulation, and gastrointestinal bleeding with or without involvement of the CNS.

Diagnosis

Definitive diagnosis is made by culture of H. *capsulatum* from bone marrow, blood, sputum, and tissue specimens. The organism can also be visualized with special stains of tissue, blood, bone marrow, or bronchoalveloar lavage specimen and can support the diagnosis when clinical and epidemiologic factors are consistent. Antigen detection of H. *capulatum* in serum, urine, or bronchoalveolar lavage specimens is specific. A negative test does not exclude the diagnosis, but a positive antigen test can be used to monitor the response to therapy and possibly identify relapse of infection in HIV-infected individuals.

Treatment

Because the vast majority of individuals resolve this infection without sequelae, immunocompetent children with primary pulmonary histoplasmosis do not require anti-fungal therapy in most cases. Progressive disseminated histoplasmosis in infants and acute infection in immuno-compromised children should have antifungal therapy. Immunocompetent children with pulmonary symptoms lasting more than 4 weeks, serious illness with high inoculum, and granulomatous adenitis causing functional obstruction should also receive antifungal therapy.

For disseminated disease and other serious manifestations of infection, amphotericin B is the drug of choice. For less serious disease, fluconazole and itraconazole may be used. For disseminated disease, amphotericin B should be administered for 4 to 6 weeks. Alternatively, if there is significant clinical improvement, amphotericin B may be administered for 2 to 3 weeks followed by 3 to 6 months of itraconazole. Milder disease may be treated with itraconazole for 3 months. In patients with HIV infection, lifelong suppressive therapy with itraconazole or fluconazole is required to prevent relapse.

Prevention and Control

There are no vaccines for H. *capsulatum*. During outbreaks, it is necessary to determine the common source of infection. Avoidance of soil with significant bird or bat dropping is important for immunocompromised individuals. Specific guidelines for preventing histoplasmosis for professionals involved with activities that might cause soil to be airborne are available through the National Institute for Occupational Safety and Health.

PARACOCCIDIOIDOMYCOSIS

Fundamentals

Paracoccidioidomycosis, also known as South American blastomycosis, is caused by *Paracoccidioides brasiliensis*, an imperfect, dimorphic fungi. This pathogen is limited to various Latin American countries. The reservoir and mode of transmission are unknown, but the organism is suspected to reside in soil, and there is no person-to-person spread. Most cases are in adults, and disease in children is rare.

Clinical Presentation, Course, and Complications

The clinical manifestations of paracoccidioidomycosis include acute pneumonia, chronic pneumonia, and disseminated disease. Acute pneumonia and disseminated infection occur in children but make up only 3% to 5% of para-coccidioidomycosis cases. Pneumonia, lymphadenopathy, hepatosplenomegaly, mucosal and skin ulceration, adrenal insufficiency, and cachexia can be present with disseminated disease. Chronic disease is seen primarily in adults and is marked by pulmonary lesions that progress over months to years. Symptoms may include cough, sputum production, weight loss, and dyspnea. Lymphadenopathy, hepatosplenomegaly, or skin and mucosal ulcerative lesions may occur in some patients. Chest radiograph may review dense bilateral nodular, fibrotic, and cavitary lesions, with propensity to involve the central or basilar lung fields. Over time and with healing, lesions become fibrotic in affected tissues.

Diagnosis

Anemia, elevated sedimentation rate, severe hypoalbuminemia, and hypergammaglobulinemia can be seen frequently. The diagnosis can be made by culture or by visualization of characteristic multiple-budding cells with a pilot's wheel appearance on 10% potassium hydroxide preparations of specimens. Serologic antibody detection can also be performed using complement fixation, enzyme immunoassay, and immunodiffusion methods.

Treatment

For severe cases of paracoccidioidomycosis, amphotericin B is the preferred treatement. For less severe or localized cases, itraconazole can be used. Therapy for at least 6 months is recommended to prevent relapse.

Prevention and Control

There is no known measure effective for preventing infection. No vaccination exists for *P. brasiliensis*.

SPOROTRICHOSIS

Fundamentals

Sporotrichosis is caused by *Sporothrix schenckii*, a dimorphic fungus found in soil, hay, straw, thorny plants, sphagnum moss, and decaying vegetable matter or plant debris. It is a ubiquitous organism found worldwide but is most common in tropical and subtropical regions of Central and South America. In the United States, there is a concentration in the Midwest along the Mississippi and Missouri River areas. Infection in humans usually occurs by direct inoculation of the organism into a minor wound. Activities that involve gardening, farming, and mining place an individual at risk of infection. Transmission from animals or family members with cutaneous disease has been reported, but is uncommon.

Clinical Presentation, Course, and Complications

The most common manifestation of sporotrichosis is a cutaneous infection. Pulmonary infection from inhalation of spores can occur as well as disseminated disease but are uncommon in children. Cutaneous infection initially starts with a firm, slightly tender, subcutaneous nodule at the site of inoculation. This lesion can then progress along draining lymphatic channels to form multiple nodules. These lesions enlarge and then become ulcerative and suppurative. Pulmonary sporotrichosis mimics tuberculosis with cavitary lesions often in the upper lobes.

Extracutaneous disease can affect any organ, but bones and joints are most commonly affected. Disseminated disease typically occurs by hematogenous spread from a primary skin or pulmonary infection, and can involve one or more sites (eyes, genitourinary tract, or CNS). Disseminated disease occurs primarily in immunocompromised individuals.

Although sporotrichosis may resolve spontaneously, treatment is often indicated. Cutaneous lesions usually respond well, but extracutaneous lesions are associated with a greater risk of morbidity and death and may result in some residual disability, depending on the organ system involved.

Diagnosis

The gold standard for diagnosis of sporotrichosis is culture of *S. schenckii* from tissue, wound drainage, or sputum specimens. *S. schenckii* can also be isolated from blood and suggests disseminated disease. Histopathologic tests can be performed but require special stains. Some reference laboratories offer a latex agglutination assay, but no standardized serologic test is available.

Treatment

The treatment for cutaneous sporotrichois is itraconazole for 3 to 6 months. A saturated solution of potassium iodide is an alternative therapy that is effective and is given orally until several weeks after lesions are healed. For osteoarticular disease, itraconazole is the treatment of choice. For pulmonary infections, itraconazole or amphotericin B can be used, depending on severity of illness. Surgical débridement may be necessary with cavitary lesions. For disseminated disease and infection in immunocompromised children, amphotericin B is the drug of choice.

Prevention and Control

The best measure of prevention is the wearing of protective gloves and clothing when engaging in activities associated with exposure to potential infection (gardening and farming).

Mini-index of Related Topics

SUGGESTED READINGS

Feigin RD, Cherry J, Demmler G, Spector S (eds): Textbook of Pediatric Infectious Diseases, 5th ed. Philadelphia, WB Saunders, 2003.

Long SS, Pickering LK, Prober CG (eds): Principals and Practice of Pediatric Infectious Disease. New York, Churchill Livingstone, 1997.

Pickering LK (ed): Red Book: 2003 Report of the Committee on Infectious Diseases, 26th ed. Elk Grove Village, Ill, American Academy of Pediatrics, 2003.

121 Parasitic Infection

Lucy M. Osborn

ROLE OF THE GENERALIST

1 Evaluate and diagnose children with possible parasitic infection.

2 Provide treatment of children with common parasitic infections.

3 Consult with specialists for assistance with diagnosis, treatment, or long-term management for children with less common parasitic infections.

FUNDAMENTALS

Disease from protozoal or helminthic infection occurs through a number of different pathogenic processes. Mechanical obstruction can result from large burdens of intestinal parasites, such as *Ascaris* worms. Many gastrointestinal helminths cause disease by robbing the host of nutrients, causing malnutrition. Organisms can migrate to the lungs or muscles, such as occurs with *Paragonimus* and *Trichinella* infections. Some organisms are directly toxic to cells; for example, hemolysis and subsequent anemia are caused by the erythrocytic phase of *Plasmodium* in malaria. The host's immune response causes the toxicity experienced from some parasitic infections, as in the ocular disorder from *Toxoplasma*. Because many parasitic organisms do not evoke a protective immune response, few infections with protozoa or helminths result in protection against subsequent infection.

Most infections with specific protozoa and helminths are covered on the CD-ROM (see the Additional Resources, CD-ROM box at the end of this chapter).

SPECIFIC PROTOZOAN INFECTIONS

Enterobiasis
Fundamentals
Enterobius vermicularis, a nematode known as the pinworm, is the cause of the most common helminthic infection in the United States and temperate climates. Oral-fecal transmission is the most common route, with eggs being deposited on perianal skin and then transmitted by fingers and hands to bedding, clothing, and toys.

Clinical Presentation
Infection is benign. The most common symptom is perianal pruritus. Other symptoms are vulvar and vaginal pruritus, grinding of teeth at night, and possibly enuresis. Children may also present with worms in stools or in the perianal region, seen by the parents when changing a diaper. On rare occasions, the adult may enter the urethra, causing abacterial urethritis or cystitis. In addition, pelvic granulomas may occur when the adult worm migrates to the vagina, uterus, and fallopian tubes.

Diagnosis
Adult worms may be visualized in the perianal region or the stool. Otherwise, eggs can be seen with application of a transparent tape to the perianal skin in the morning, prior to bathing.

Treatment
Table 121-1 lists treatment options for pinworms. The drugs of choice are abendazole, mebendazole, and pyrantel pamoate.

Prevention and Control
Clothes and bed linens should be washed in hot water at the time of treatment. Other family members should be treated if infected. All should practice good hygiene, with careful handwashing.

Malaria
Fundamentals
Malaria is caused by four species of parasites: *Plasmodium falciparum*, *P. vivax*, *P. ovale*, and *P. malariae*. Malaria is endemic throughout the tropical areas of the world, with a worldwide incidence of 300 million to 500 million cases per year. Transmission is through bites from *Anopheles* mosquitoes. Malaria occurs in temperate climates where *Anopheles* mosquitoes live.

Many clinical symptoms of malaria are related to the life cycle of the organism. Once *sporozoites* enter the human body, they first invade hepatic parenchymal cells. The parasites undergo asexual multiplication (schizogony) and then emerge as merozoites to invade red blood cells, causing the symptomatic phase of the disease. Parasites of the

Table 121-1. Treatment Options for Pinworms

Drug	Dosage
Abendazole	400 mg once, repeat in 2 weeks
Mebendazole	100 mg once, repeat in 2 weeks
Pyrantel pamoate	11 mg/kg base once (max. 1 g); repeat in 2 weeks

857

relapsing species of *Plasmodium* can enter a quiescent stage. Once inside the red blood cell, parasites can undergo either asexual or sexual reproduction, a necessary step for transmission of the disease. Rupture of red blood cells with release of merozoites into the bloodstream leads to fever and exacerbation of other malarial symptoms.

Clinical Presentation

Paroxysmal high fever with chills that last 10 to 12 hours is the classic presenting symptom of malaria. Timing of paroxysms is related to the infecting species. *P. malariae* has a cycle of 72 hours; the other species have paroxysms every 44 to 48 hours. Profuse sweating occurs with defervescence. Anemia and thrombocytopenia are common and hepatomegaly may be present.

Infection with the various malarial parasites can cause several clinical syndromes, which are listed in Table 121-2. Initial infection with *P. falciparum* may not present with paroxysmal fever in nonimmune individuals, but rather with fever and a flu-like illness with headache, diarrhea, vomiting, cough, malaise, myalgia, arthralgia, and abdominal pain.

Diagnosis

The most important aspect of diagnosis is considering malaria in the differential diagnosis, particularly in the United States. The diagnosis is made by identifying the organism in thick or thin blood films. The thick film allows identification of the organism that may be present in small numbers. The thin film allows specific species identification and an estimate of the level of parasitemia. If malaria is considered, but the initial tests do not identify the organism, testing should be repeated every 12 to 24 hours for 72 hours.

Treatment

Chemotherapy is based on the infecting species, the severity of the disease, immune status of the host, and the possibility of drug resistance (see Chapter 284). Patients must be carefully evaluated and observed for complications of

the disease (see Table 121-2) and provided with appropriate supportive therapy.

Outcome

Fatality from malaria occurs mostly with *P. falciparum* infections, usually from cerebral malaria. Most deaths in the United States are due to delay in the diagnosis. Relapsing disease can occur when the infecting organism is *P. vivax* or *P. ovale*.

Prevention and Control

Preventive strategies consist of control of the *Anopheles* mosquito population, treatment of infected persons, and chemoprophylaxis of travelers to endemic areas. Recommendations for chemoprophylaxis in children are identical to those for adults. The most current information regarding recommendations for travelers can be found by contacting the Centers for Disease Control at http://www.cdc.gov.

Toxoplasmosis
Fundamentals

Congenital infection with toxoplasmosis is covered in Chapter 209. Toxoplasmosis is caused by *Toxoplasma gondii*, an obligate intracellular protozoan parasite. It is the only *Toxoplasma* species that is pathogenic for humans. The distribution of *T. gondii* is worldwide, infecting most species of warm-blooded animals. Cats are the most common host to pass infection to humans. Endogenous infection can be reactivated in immunocompromised individuals.

Clinical Presentation

Toxoplasma infection acquired after birth can be asymptomatic or can cause lymphadenopathy with or without fever. Symptoms of infection are nonspecific, including fever, sore throat, malaise, and myalgia. *Toxoplasma* can also cause a mononucleosis-like illness. The disease is usually self-limited. Primary infection or reactivation of latent infection in an immunocompromised host can involve any organ, particularly the central nervous system.

Diagnosis

Diagnosis depends on serologic testing. Because tests require careful interpretation, the assistance of a specialist is often needed.

Treatment

Acquired infection often does not require treatment. When treatment is needed (e.g., for chorioretinitis or significant organ damage), the agents used are pyrimethamine and sulfadiazine. Consultation with a specialist is recommended.

Outcome

Outcome of acquired disease is usually excellent because of the benign nature and self-limiting nature of the disease in immunocompetent hosts. In those who are immunocompromised, outcome depends on the extent of organ involvement. Patients with acquired immunodeficiency syndrome (AIDS) who have toxoplasmosis encephalitis should receive lifelong suppressive therapy.

Table 121-2. Clinical Syndromes in *Plasmodium* Infections

Organism	Syndrome
P. falciparum	Cerebral malaria with neurologic symptoms
	Severe anemia
	Hypoglycemia
	Respiratory compromise, adult respiratory distress syndrome
	Renal failure
	Vascular collapse and shock
P. vivax and *P. ovale*	Hypersplenism
	Anemia
	Relapse
P. malariae	Nephrotic syndrome
	Chronic asymptomatic parasitemia

Prevention and Control

Pregnant women should avoid exposure to cat feces. Oral ingestion can be avoided by cooking meat well, washing fruits and vegetables, and careful handwashing, particularly after gardening.

SPECIFIC HELMINTHIC DISEASES

Ascaris lumbricoides Infection
Fundamentals

Ascaris lumbricoides, a nematode, is the most common cause of parasitic infection of humans. Adult worms live in the small intestine. The female worm produces large numbers of eggs that are excreted and then incubated in the soil, from which they are then transmitted to humans by ingestion of moist soil. Although the organism is best suited to warmer climates, the eggs are resistant to many environmental stressors. Infection is most common in tropical areas where human feces are used for fertilizer and in areas where sanitation is poor.

Clinical Presentation

Clinical symptoms are produced from both larval and adult migration, which occurs under stressful host conditions, such as fever or illness. Most infected individuals are asymptomatic. Larval migration is through the lungs, causing pulmonary microhemorrhages, inflammation, and exudation of fluid that results in an acute pneumonitis (Loeffler syndrome). Symptoms are fever, cough, dyspnea, wheezing and mild hemoptysis. Marked eosinophilia may occur. Symptoms of adult worms in the gastrointestinal tract include epigastric pain and diffuse abdominal pain. Acute intestinal obstruction from heavy infection occurs more frequently in children than in adults because the intestinal lumen is smaller. Worm migration can cause peritonitis and obstruction of the common bile duct. Chronic infection has been associated with malnutrition, steatorrhea, growth retardation, and impaired intellectual development.

Diagnosis

Diagnosis of the infection is established by identification of the characteristic ova in the stool. Occasionally, patients will pass adult worms from the rectum or from the nose.

Treatment

Treatment of intestinal infection without obstruction and pulmonary infection is with one dose of pyrantel pamoate or albendazole or with three doses of mebendazole. Piperazine citrate via a gastrointestinal tube can be used with intestinal obstruction, but occasionally surgery is required. Supportive therapy for intestinal obstruction should be provided, including intravenous hydration, nasogastric suctioning, and careful observation of electrolyte status.

Prevention and Control

Improved sanitation with appropriate disposal of human feces offers the most effective method of prevention.

Toxocariasis
Fundamentals

Toxocariasis is caused by two tissue nematodes that invade the deep and superficial tissues. *Toxocara canis* are common roundworms of dogs and *Toxocara cati* are found in cats. Transmission occurs when eggs from the feces of dogs or cats embryonate in soil and then are ingested by children.

Clinical Presentation

Most children who are infected are asymptomatic. Visceral larva migrans occurs most commonly in young children with a history of pica. Symptoms include fever, hepatomegaly, occasionally cough, and malaise. The disorder can be accompanied by leukocytosis, persistent eosinophilia, hypergammaglobulinemia, and anemia. Ocular invasion may occur in older children, presenting with changes in vision and strabismus. The organism causes endophthalmitis or retinal granulomas.

Diagnosis

Diagnosis is made by suspecting the disease and supportive labortoray data, such as elevated IgE and elevated eosinophil count. Specific IgG and IgM antibodies can be detected by enzyme immunoassay, but the test is not available in most clinical laboratories.

Treatment

Therapy is with mebendazole or albendazole, but does not reliably reduce symptoms. These drugs may not be effective in ocular larva migrans. Patients with ocular disease should be referred to an ophthalmologist for treatment, which may conisist of injection of corticosteroids or surgery if the granulomas have caused retinal detachment.

Prevention and Control

No effective preventive measures have been devised. Sand boxes of playgrounds should be covered after use each day to prevent defecation of cats and dogs in the sand.

Additional Resources, CD-ROM	
Cryptosporidium	Text
Cyclospora	Text
Leishmoniasis	Text
Anisakis	Text
Cysticercosis and tapeworm	Text
Enterobiasis	Text
Hookworms	Text
Schistosomiasis	Text
Trichinosis	Text
Trichuriasis	Text
Bibliography	

conditions. Effective primary care clinicians develop a knowledge base about the common educational and community issues encountered at different stages of illness and times of transition, allowing them to anticipate issues and plan strategies with families.

Children with chronic conditions often receive care from many providers. To improve outcomes for children with chronic conditions, close collaboration among the patient's providers is needed. Participating as a member of a team, contributing to without directing the process, may be a new role for some clinicians. An effective member of a health care team must understand the perspectives of other providers as well as the delivery systems in health and community settings. A broad perspective about how the clinician's efforts integrate with those of the entire team can help create effective collaboration.

SPECIAL SKILLS FOR CHRONIC ILLNESS CARE

Communication Skills

Organization and advanced communication skills are needed to monitor illness issues efficiently, implement participatory decision making, and empathetically include the child and family in the visit. Nuances in the tone of the visit, such as how well the clinician listens, play an important role in the overall effectiveness of the session (see Chapter 123).

Delivery of Structured Flexible Care

The effective clinician is proactive in providing care at several levels. Just as well-child care has predictable issues and challenges that occur at different stages, common issues and transitions exist for chronic conditions. These must be assessed and monitored in addition to the usual illness parameters and in addition to acute exacerbations and complications. Comprehensive care often requires either an extended well-child visit or a separate management visit. As children grow and the frequency of recommended health maintenance visits decreases, scheduled assessment visits increase in importance. Initiating all visits by determining families' priorities ensures flexibility in responding to their needs. During an acute care visit, the clinician may respond to unresolved needs and priorities for the near future or family priorities in planning for developmental or illness transitions. Flow sheets, which help the provider cover a wide range of issues for health maintenance, can help ensure that key issues are addressed over a number of visits. Providers can create their own flow sheets from the topics listed in Table 122-1 and from the condition-specific issues discussed in other chapters in this section.

Effective Patient Education

Two different kinds of patient education are required with chronic conditions: The practitioner must (1) explain the disease and its process and treatments clearly and (2) seek to change patient and family behaviors.

The clinician's explanation should be a dialogue in which families receive digestible amounts of information and have the opportunity to ask questions. Complex terminology, medications, and tests usually require repeated explanations and illustrations or written instructions for families to

Table 122-1. Issues to Monitor in Chronic Care
Child's Daily Life
Strengths/assets/recent accomplishments
Coping/psychosocial adjustment
Family Life
Parental stress/depression/coping
Sibling adjustment/coping
Recreational opportunities
Respite or relief time
Developmental/School/Child Care Issues
Adequacy of program/services
Appropriate social experiences
Preparing for school transition
Financial Issues
Receiving appropriate public benefits
Adequacy of insurance coverage
Patient Education
Assessment of patient education knowledge/needs
Illness management skills
Progressive independence by child/adolescent
Long-term Care Issues
Long-term prognosis/outcomes
Shifting to adult care
Vocational/work issues

review later. Even if the specialist has already provided the family with information, it is important for the generalist to check for understanding and clarify any misconceptions.

The clinician's role of changing patient and family behaviors is also crucial, because controlling the disease often involves daily treatments administered at home. Patients and their families are the primary managers of chronic diseases, guided and coached by the clinician to devise the best therapeutic regimes. Asthma research has shown that this approach of partnership to motivate families and to plan changes is effective in improving health outcomes without increasing the length of the visit. However, providing knowledge, although important in preparing patients to act, is insufficient to change health behaviors. Care is based on the theory of self-regulation in which patients develop the ability to observe themselves, make sensible judgments, feel confident, and recognize desirable outcomes. The clinician helps patients recognize areas in which their daily lives are adversely affected by disease. Together, patient, family, and clinician develop strategies to manipulate the circumstances. Through a process of self-assessment and planning, the patient and family learn which approaches work. This self-regulation requires observation, judgment, and realistic and appropriate reaction to one's efforts to manage a task. In this approach, clinicians help families or patients determine how they will proceed, given their own specific goals, the social context, and their perceptions of their own capabilities. Primary care clinicians usually have received little training in these techniques. Further information on this approach can be found in the Suggested Readings listings and in Chapter 279.

Assessment of Psychosocial Issues

With chronic conditions, interviewing and screening approaches must routinely assess common emotional and behavioral sequelae. In particular, depression in children with chronic conditions who are not acting out often goes undetected (see Chapter 247).

During clinical care, the provider typically develops a close relationship with the parents. Efforts must be directed at helping the parents and the family of the patient to receive optimal care. Family stress, level of coping, and mood must be carefully monitored. Providing complex care at home can be a chronic burden that leads to exhaustion, isolation, and discouragement. The rate of depression in mothers of children with chronic conditions can be as high as 60%. Parents who are depressed may not appear so during the visit. In these cases, depression may be detected only if the clinician is willing to inquire directly. Often parents feel guilty and inadequate, and in order to accept help they need the assistance of their child's health care professionals in understanding that these problems are common and treatable.

Provision of Community Linkages and Resources

Each community varies in the types of family support; nursing; and educational, developmental, and mental health services available for families with children. Some services are specific for children with certain impairments; others are for all families under stress. Because the community-based clinician is in a unique position to link families to these supports, knowledge of the types of services provided, eligibility, and referral mechanisms is essential. Although another staff member in the office may serve to help families in more depth, clinicians must understand the options. Personal connections to key individuals in community organizations made on a patient's behalf can be even more effective. Some providers introduce themselves and learn about programs through phone calls, others visit agencies or schools, and still others invite program representatives into the practice to meet with the entire office staff. These connections enhance communication and build the credibility needed to act as an advocate on behalf of the family or to act as an advocate for broader issues that affect large numbers of children. Key community contacts are listed in Table 122-2. Clinicians can gain expertise in community resources by gradually making these connections over a 6- to 12-month period. Effective linkages are made only through such efforts.

Resources at the state or regional level can often be accessed through nurse coordinators or social workers in disease-specific specialty care programs or the state agency responsible for services for children with special health care needs. The state agency usually receives funding from the federal Bureau of Maternal and Child Health Title V to assist children and improve services in the state. Families can provide a great deal of information resources and educational materials for unusual conditions. Many states also have active family organizations that provide advocacy and support. Family Voices, a parent organization whose focus is

Table 122-2. Key Community Agency/Organization Links That Can Enhance Effectiveness

Schools
School nurse
Special education director
Guidance counselor
Coordinator of school services for ages 3 to 5

Early Intervention Program
Services Agency for Developmentally Delayed or Mentally Retarded Children
Family support

Public Health Nursing
Parent Support Centers or Organizations
Home visiting programs

Mental Health Services
Major providers of child/youth services
Case management services

children with chronic illnesses and disabilities, has chapters in all states.

It is estimated that about one in five children has some type of significant chronic condition. About a third of these children have conditions that impact their lives daily. With continued advancements in the treatment of many previously life-limiting conditions, the primary care clinician is likely to devote increasing clinical time to the care of children with chronic conditions. Optimal care requires that clinicians evaluate their perspectives and enhance their chronic care skills. Clinicians who use this approach will find caring for patients with chronic conditions both productive and satisfying.

Mini-index of Related Topics   CH.

SUGGESTED READINGS

Clark NM, Gong M: Management of chronic disease by practitioners and patients: Are we teaching the wrong things? BMJ 2000;320:572–575.
Family Voices. Website links to chapters in all states and parental support and advocacy assistance. Available at: http://www.FamilyVoices.org.
Nickel RE, Desch LW: The Physician's Guide to Caring for Children with Disabilities and Chronic Conditions. Baltimore, Paul H. Brooks, 2000.
Wilson G, Cooley WC: Preventive Management of Children with Congenital Anomalies and Syndromes. Cambridge, Cambridge University Press, 2000.

123 Communication with Families and Specialists

Ardis L. Olson

ROLE OF THE GENERALIST

1   Develop the knowledge, attitudes, and skills necessary to communicate effectively with families with children with chronic illness.

2   Approach families using principles of family centered care.

3   Communicate with and support families during the time of initial diagnosis.

4   Use specific skills to communicate effectively with families during times of stress.

5   Discuss roles and expectations with families.

6   Recognize families' culture and beliefs and adapt care and communication accordingly.

COMMUNICATION WITH FAMILIES

The first step in communication with families is to discuss the role of the primary care provider in the ongoing care of the child. Families may be aware of their primary care provider's role in the usual well-child and acute care visits only; they may be unaware of the primary care provider's potential role in chronic illness care. Although medical and surgical specialists provide expert care for specific diseases, the relationship with the primary care provider is essential for comprehensive, long-term care of children with chronic conditions. The primary care clinician can provide support for the family, serve as an interpreter between the specialist and family, and ensure that secondary impact of the disease and its treatment is minimized. Active participation by primary care providers can ensure that care is not fragmented. Primary care providers are guides who help families navigate through complicated medical care and educational and social service systems. The provider should allow enough time during the first visit to discuss the various issues and problems associated with different chronic conditions, family preferences, and provider styles. See Table 123-1 for other important topics of discussion during the initial visit.

Primary care providers face challenges in communication in caring for children with chronic health conditions that are less likely to emerge in acute and well-child care. The involvement of multiple specialists, agencies, and systems of care can result in disjointed and erratic communication for both families and primary care clinicians. Clinician interaction with patient and family is a key component of care in chronic illnesses. Effective communication under these circumstances requires more than the good interpersonal and interviewing skills used in all patient care. Specific communication areas can be problematic in this situation.

Families are now more likely to take an active role, expressing how they want health professionals to interact with them. The child resides within a family that is ultimately responsible for care coordination and management. Well-intended clinicians may find themselves assuming that their expertise allows them to best determine the most effective approach. Yet unless family preferences and priorities are considered and understood, care is less likely to be successful. Box 123-1 presents nationally developed family centered care principles. These principles can help providers examine whether their approach acknowledges the central role that the family plays. Families of chronically ill children have determined how they would like medical services to be provided (Table 123-2). They want to be included as partners in the process of their care, they want their providers to listen carefully and elicit their concerns and priorities, and they want their clinician respond comfortably and acceptingly when strong emotions arise during the course of care. Understanding a patient's experiences and perspectives enables the clinician to develop relevant advice and guidance for specific situations.

Table 123-1. Issues to Discuss at the Onset of Care

Role of Primary Care Provider vs. Specialist

What primary care provider will deal with in visits that differs from what specialists will deal with

How often primary care provider wishes to see patient for illness monitoring and health supervision visits

Who will help the family with school and community issues

Whom to call for different types of issues

What to Do When Care Does Not Go Well

The role of primary care provider as interpreter and advocate

The primary care clinician's willingness to share with the family that his or her practice's care is not optimal

Practical Issues

Understanding tertiary care systems

The referral process

Family financial barriers to adequate care

Logistics of the primary care provider's practice

Box 123-1. Family Centered Care

Family centered care involves the following:
- Recognition that the family is the constant in the child's life
- Facilitation of parent-professional collaboration at all levels of health care
- Sharing of unbiased and complete information with the parents on an ongoing basis
- Implementation of appropriate programs and policies to support the family
- Encouragement of parent-to-parent support
- Assurance of a delivery system that is flexible, accessible, and responsive to family needs

Communication during Stressful Times

Provider communication with the family during the time surrounding the initial diagnosis is particularly important. Either the primary care clinician or specialist may convey the initial diagnosis. An example of how to impart initial bad news is provided in Chapter 158. Clinicians need to understand that their concepts of severity of any illness may not be shared by families. Those who are learning about illnesses such as asthma may have difficulty processing the information initially provided. Parents value ongoing contact with their child's primary care physician particularly when their child is hospitalized and receiving care from specialists with whom they are not familiar. Regular visits by or telephone conversations with the primary care provider showing support and concern for families are essential. The first couple of days after discharge is also a pivotal time in which a telephone call or a scheduled visit with the primary care provider is crucial. Early communication of support and participation with the specialist in the care plan are key in defining roles in ongoing care. Additional attention is crucial at other stressful times, such as exacerbation of the illness, family crises, life stage transitions, and the transfer of care to adult providers.

Communication about Roles and Expectations

With the variety of primary care roles possible with respect to different conditions, families and clinicians both benefit if the provider sets time aside to discuss the partnership among providers. Sometimes this occurs most optimally at the time of diagnosis. Sometimes it is better accomplished when the child's condition provides more of a challenge and multiple providers and care coordination become necessary. The provider should clarify his or her role in the medical and psychosocial aspects of management, the suggested frequency of visits to the primary care provider to monitor the child's progress, the primary provider's role in school or other community issues, the importance of health supervision visits, what to do and whom to call when the child becomes ill and when other issues arise. A discussion of the family's preferences and desires is important in determining the generalist's role. The older child can be included in this discussion. During life transition points or major changes in disease severity, these issues should be revisited with the family. The time spent establishing expectations in partnership with the family help avoid miscommunications, inappropriate use of specialty care, and alienation from primary care over time.

Enhancing Outpatient Communications

Families dealing with chronic conditions often need more access to the office and office staff than do families of other patients. Facilitation of communication with the clinicians or their staff is crucial. Many issues, such as prescriptions, referrals, or letters, can be handled by designating one person in the office as the family's contact for nonclinical issues. Electronic mail, practice websites, and fax technology can facilitate families' ability to share information (e.g., glucose monitoring) and to get answers to nonurgent questions. A designated phone hour for patients with chronic illnesses can ease the burden of crisis calls during patient care.

Arrangements for after-hours care are particularly important for families with a chronically ill child. During evenings and weekends families receive care from other providers in the practice or call network. Families can become frustrated when no mechanisms are in place for the clinicians to communicate key issues in the acute care of the conditions involved. Defining the practice's population of children with chronic care allows development of systematic approaches for their unique care needs. Care summaries and acute treatment protocols provided to parents, colleagues, or emergency room staff have been shown to decrease inappropriate care.

Cultural Issues

Communication with families of different cultural backgrounds, especially if they are not fluent in English, presents additional challenges. Cultural differences may also significantly alter perceptions of disease and treatment. Frustrations arise when families are not compliant with the clinician's expectations. Those in the community who work with a given population can provide cultural understanding, as can medical anthropology literature. Families may also be willing to share their cultural beliefs and values when queried respectfully. For families that do not speak English, medical interpretation services are essential. Telephone-based services are available through American Telephone and Telegraph (ATT). If the child or a family member is the only available interpreter, caution must be exercised. Family members who are emotionally involved may omit

Table 123-2. Approaches Desired by Families/Adolescents

Recognize the Patient and Family as Partners in the Care Process
Acknowledge their front-line expertise and knowledge.
Learn and accept families' values and preferences.
Reach joint decisions together whenever possible.

Recognize the Entire Child and Family, Not Just Their Illness
Discuss the child's strengths and accomplishments.
Assess and support family coping and resources.
Attend to the practical issues that limit daily quality of life.
Discuss both short-term and long-term care issues.

Listen Carefully to Families and Adolescents for the Following Purposes:
To understand their lives
To respond to their issues
To recognize when the parent is distressed

or edit unacceptable information, may have insufficient education to translate medical topics, or may avoid psychosocial issues.

COMMUNICATION WITH THE CHILD

Over time clinicians often develop a strong connection to the parents of children with chronic health conditions; they tend to focus interactions primarily on the parents, treating the child as a more passive participant. Even in routine health care, pediatricians often interact with the child on the initial visit when gathering data but not when discussing the diagnosis and treatment. Clinicians must make an active effort to include the child with a chronic condition at a level appropriate for his or her condition and developmental level. The parents of children with marked cognitive impairment state that they want the clinicians to value their children, interact with them in the visit, and comment positively about them. Many chronic illnesses require discussion of home monitoring and treatments primarily performed by the parents. As children mature, they need to be provided appropriate explanations and to become partners in decision making about their care. Illness management must be gradually shifted to adolescents to prepare them to make the transition to adult care systems and independent care. Some advice from children with chronic illnesses is provided in Table 123-2.

Concepts of body function and illness at different stages must be understood for effective communication with children and adolescents. Until about ages 5 to 7, children define illness by external events and symptoms and are illogical in how they connect them. They understand illness by its individual symptoms only. They are egocentric and construct their world by following rules. They believe that they become ill because of their specific actions and recover simply if they adhere to treatments. Early to mid-elementary school-age children begin to use logical rules and principles. They still commonly understand illnesses as contagious and external in origin, with the body playing a passive role. By 10 to 12 years of age, children start to understand illness as a more complex, multifaceted process. Children may not understand the role of the body's internal mechanisms in illness until well into the teen years. More sophisticated understanding of how personal actions can exacerbate or prevent illnesses is developmentally unlikely before adolescence.

Children's understanding of their illness and its pathophysiology can be quite varied with chronic health conditions and disabilities. For conditions such as diabetes mellitus and asthma, age-appropriate educational materials can help children achieve advanced comprehension for their age. For many conditions, however, age-appropriate educational materials are not available. The clinician must recognize that children can have superficial understanding of the words and jargon associated with their condition without any real understanding of body processes and the way that prevention or treatment works.

The level of cognitive understanding of their illness issues may influence how children with chronic conditions emotionally respond to their condition. Well into the grade school years, children with cardiac disease, diabetes, and

other conditions have been known to blame themselves and feel guilt that is based on magical notions about how their actions or behaviors are linked to the onset or progression of disease. Adolescents with chronic conditions struggle with issues of self-esteem and identity. Children whose cognitive processes have not yet matured need their clinicians to help provide them with both cognitive and emotional insights that will allow them to become meaningfully involved in the self-management of their conditions.

COMMUNICATION WITH SPECIALISTS

Although the consultation process has the potential to provide optimal medical care for a child with a chronic condition, it can also result in fragmented care and frustration for both the provider and parent. Limitations by insurers have made the process more cumbersome and sometimes have restricted access to specialists with pediatric expertise. Expectations regarding the referral must be crystal clear. Although referral forms often specify the number of visits approved, the primary care providers must clearly state the level of involvement desired. Options for the level of specialty involvement are described in Box 123-2 and must be clearly stated in the initial referral. Primary care providers should state whether they are seeking specific guidance in the diagnosis only or whether they wish the specialist to assume a portion of the patient care. Ongoing management may consist of periodic re-evaluation by the specialist, with the primary care clinician providing the majority of the management, or it may consist of all aspects of care for the chronic condition being provided by the specialist. Variations in the collaboration between primary care provider and specialists vary with different conditions, geographic constraints, and family preferences. Clarification of the desired roles by the primary care clinician and specialists opens the door for dialogue about the expected course of the illness, frequency of monitoring visits, and the responsibilities of each care provider. Families must also understand the roles that each provider will perform, and their preferences must be considered.

When referring children with chronic conditions for consultation or management, the specialist will benefit by receiving from the primary care physician the information provided in Box 123-3. Primary care clinicians can enhance communication with specialists by telling them the best times to call, letting them know whether they wish to be contacted by e-mail, and providing fax numbers. During ongoing care, specialists require a two-way communication process. When they see a patient in follow-up, they value the primary care provider's continuing input. Supplying

Box 123-2. Primary Care Referral Options
Guidance in diagnosis only
Assumption of some aspects of ongoing care of the condition by specialist
Primary care management with periodic re-evaluation and input from specialist
Handling of all aspects of care for the chronic condition by specialist

Box 123-3. Information for Specialist on Initial Referral

Primary Care Provider Concerns/Priorities

Family concerns/priorities

Clinical observations as problem has evolved

Psychosocial/family background information

Copies of Key Laboratory and Other Diagnostic Tests

Radiologic studies rather than written interpretations

Treatments and medications used and patient response

information, providing laboratory results, or posing questions by electronic mail or fax before the patient visit can improve care.

When a child receives ongoing specialty care, the specialist is a clinical resource to the primary care clinician. Specialists should communicate key issues to monitor, red flags that indicate the need for re-evaluation, and acute care and health supervision needs to the generalist provider. The chapters on specific chronic conditions later in this section provide condition-specific information to assist the generalist in comanagement. With this background, the primary care clinician can refine with the specialist individual patient-level monitoring and treatment for the individual patient.

Mini-index of Related Topics CH.

SUGGESTED READINGS

"Bandaids and Blackboards: When chronic illness or some other medical problem goes to school." Available at: http://www.faculty.fairfield.edu/fleitas/mdtips.html.

Fadiman, Anne: The Spirit Catches You and You Fall Down. New York, Noonday Press, 1997.

The Family Village. Available at: http://www.familyvillage.wisc.edu.

The National Organization for Rare Disorders. Available at: http://www.rarediseases.org.

Compassionate care ensures that families and their primary care providers have a shared stake in the outcome of care, including the successes and the failures. The appreciation that families feel for a caring physician is often expressed in terms of the small kindnesses that he or she has extended to them. Medical Homes must specialize in the pursuit of professional excellence that is wrapped more in a cloak of empathy than in a starched white coat.

Cultural competence requires an in-depth awareness of the cultural context of the community surrounding a Medical Home. Effective communication requires the development or identification of educational materials in the languages of the local community as well as plans for accessing translation services when needed. Recognition and respect for the cultural values of others requires an awareness of one's own cultural heritage and its influence on attitudes.

IMPROVING PRIMARY CARE FOR CHILDREN WITH SPECIAL HEALTH CARE NEEDS

Developing a fully functioning Medical Home is an enormous task that requires commitment and openness to thinking "out of the box" with respect to the usual processes of care. Realistically, practices must work gradually toward the Medical Home goal by progressively implementing activities that address various elements of the American Academy of Pediatrics' definition of Medical Home. Most primary care offices are so busy that large-scale change seems impossible. Practitioners must therefore adopt an incremental approach to change and engage in a systematic process to bring about improvements.

The first step is to understand the current strengths and weaknesses in a practice's care of children with special health care needs. Tools are available to assess the practice and chart a course for initial improvement ideas. The Medical Home Index and the Medical Home Family Index (www.medicalhomeimprovement.org) can help practices measure the degree to which they have achieved "medical homeness" and can identify areas for improvement. To begin systematically changing the practice, the professional and administrative leadership and provider colleagues must be supportive. Establishing a team devoted to quality improvement activities for the office's chronic illness care

can provide the structure to bring about incremental change. It is important to work with families of children with special health care needs who utilize their services. The input received from families during patient care can differ greatly from that received from families during a practice improvement effort. Families can help identify and implement changes aimed at enhancing both the child's health and the overall child and family functioning and satisfaction with care delivered.

MEDICAL HOMES AND THE FUTURE OF PRIMARY CARE

Pediatric primary care is by its very nature proactive and forward-looking. Pediatricians and other primary care providers are geared toward the anticipation of problems and the implementation of preventive measures. Most individual practitioners aspire to deliver care in keeping with the Medical Home model. The issues and challenges rest with the systems that surround well-meaning and capable professionals. The redesign of these systems requires patience and commitment, but the result can deliver care that is not only more effective and satisfactory for children and their families, but also more satisfying and rewarding for pediatric practitioners and for all those who work with them in office settings. This redesign can help to transform primary pediatric care from an increasing routine and productivity-driven series of brief encounters to a dynamic, evidence-based, and proactive community resource.

Mini-index of Related Topics

SUGGESTED READINGS

Medical Home Policy statement. Pediatrics 2002;110:184–186.
The National Medical Home Initiatives Center. Available at: http://www.medicalhomeinfo.org.

125 School Issues in Children with Chronic Illness

Jeanne McAllister

School-age children who face the challenges of living with a chronic health condition are also expected to master age-appropriate developmental skills in the areas of social development and school performance. Almost 40% of children and adolescents with chronic health conditions experience school-related problems. Preventing these problems is essential to a child's adaptation to life with a chronic health condition. Health needs and related educational implications are interrelated for these children, creating unique opportunities for pediatricians to offer support and interventions. The generalist can partner with the family on behalf of the child, and together they can develop a course of care. By establishing communication among the child, family, practice, and school, the health care provider can also help establish continuity of care.

When a generalist (1) offers guidance that prepares and supports family interactions with the educational system and (2) advocates for proactive approaches in the school environment, outcomes for the child and care-giving family are enhanced. These outcomes include optimizing student and family management of the chronic condition, improving school attendance and participation, and improving academic performance. Additionally, increased knowledge and sensitivity enable educators to help these children succeed socially and academically. Pediatric support and involvement reduce stress on families as they balance their family and work lives. Coordinated efforts help families succeed in providing a positive educational experience for their children as they address urgent and fluctuating health concerns.

National efforts by organizations such as Family Voices, Parent-to-Parent initiatives, and related projects funded by the United States Maternal and Child Health Bureau emphasize the identification of child/youth and family needs and the inclusion of these needs in the development of supportive interventions and health system design. Studies of students, families, pediatric practices, and schools have attempted to ascertain what contributes to a successful school experience for students with chronic health conditions. Factors that are necessary to enhance education, provide essential information, and improve communication are summarized in Table 125-1.

The quality of health or educational interventions depends on the development of a partnership with the child/youth and family. Assessment of children and their community and school-based needs is a stepping stone to qualitative collaboration. Assessment should include both the physical and psychosocial component. The effects of physical symptoms and treatment side effects on learning should be considered. A determination of how a child/youth is handling his or her condition and its treatment and how the care is integrated into the school environment is crucial.

Asking the right questions and being prepared for strong parental responses is an essential role for the generalist. The inquiry "How is school going?" is better phrased "What do you need from me to help school go more smoothly?" This demonstrates to parents that they can expect the health care provider's help and acknowledges the energy, skill, and hard work that go into ensuring a successful school experience for the child. For some parents this acknowledgment may be all that is needed. Others will communicate what assistance they need—a letter, a phone call, a school visit, help educating the school staff about their child's condition, or the stronger support represented by the health care provider's voice or presence.

Pediatricians have a long history of school advocacy and of interest in the integration of health and education. Without health it is difficult to learn. Without a good education it is difficult to develop the skills necessary to promote health. A fast-paced primary care office may be a difficult environment in which to foster successful family/school communication, but strategies for promoting

Table 125-1. Student, Family, and School Staff Needs and Pediatric Responses: Students with Chronic Health Conditions, Their Families, School Educators, and Implications for the Generalist Pediatrician

Students living with chronic health conditions state they want to be considered as individuals and
- Communicated with as a person, not as a disease
- Not have their condition referred to publicly in the classroom
- Be responded to sensitively by staff who demonstrate a knowledge of their condition and health regimen, not blaming everything on the condition
- Be challenged academically but flexibly considering the course of their illness or condition

Parents are looking for the school to do the following:
- Value their children and not see them as health problems
- Value the role that they, the parents, play in their child's life and in the daily care and treatment of their child's condition
- Partner with them and their child's health care provider to establish goals for school learning and social success and to provide for ongoing meaningful communication
- Be educated and sensitive to their children's needs and flexibly incorporate medical recommendations into the school environment

School professionals have expressed their lack of preparedness to educate and support students with health problems and unease around illness. Their concerns include the following:
- Insufficient planning time
- A lack of funding for appropriate programs including staff development
- Vague guidelines about program and service eligibility in school
- Role confusion around planning, coordinating, and providing health related services
- Communication gaps among parents, school, and health care providers

How the *Generalist* Can Respond
- Partner with families.
- Assess needs and help link chronic conditions and learning implications.
- Prepare the family for school offering proactive skills.
- Know school law.
- Create and share written care plans.
- Educate those who will use the care plan.
- Be a voice of advocacy in the community for the population of children with disabilities and chronic health conditions.

optimal processes for successful family communication and collaboration exist. They include (1) offering child and family support or intervention in addressing the child's school needs; (2) providing anticipatory guidance for both families and schools about the child's condition and its related school implications; and (3) developing and using office tools (care plans) that assess and document needs, articulate concerns, and stress assets of the child and family. Such tools can be shared among the family, school, and practice.

FAMILY SUPPORT: A RESULT OF THE PROVIDER'S RELATIONSHIP WITH THE FAMILY

Fundamental to offering family centered care is establishing a partnership with the child/youth and family. This relationship acknowledges the family as the central, consistent caregiver for the child. It also demonstrates respect for what the family has learned about their child and what the family accomplishes on a daily basis. Families must work to gain a sense of rhythm and balance with the health care system in caring for their children's medical needs. Then they are faced with learning "the rules" of the

community-based school system and building a rapport with the school professionals who have a significant impact on their children's daily lives. The health care provider's offer to be the families' point person, an advocate, and an additional voice for their children in the community can ease their sense of isolation in the challenges that they face. The health care provider's rapport with the family is an essential form of family support.

By modeling family centered approaches, health care providers can promote the central role of the family to school staff members. Communication with the school by phone, letter, or e-mail should reflect the fact that recommendations and interventions are created from decisions made mutually among the family and the primary care provider and specialists. Conversations with the school should always emphasize respect for families, their privacy, and their role as primary decision-makers and caregivers for their children. Goals set by the student, family, and physicians, including goals that address the necessary increase in the child/youth's own responsibility for his or her condition, should be apparent in each communication between the practice and the school. By keeping the family central to the conversation and sharing goals for the student's own self-competence, the generalist models family support and demonstrates the value of partnership with the family.

ANTICIPATORY GUIDANCE AND SCHOOL HEALTH LAW

The generalist should acquaint families with community and state services and systems that can be used together to promote optimal care for their children. Families benefit from help that prepares them for their ongoing role as the primary communicator with the school system. The generalist can advise families on taking proactive steps to help their children, such as getting in touch with specific school personnel and getting to know and helping to educate the principal, the school nurse, teachers, counselors, school psychologists, and others who interact with their children at school. Parents may need help identifying the one or two people who can best serve as the school point person. Often one point person will be the school nurse. Sometimes, however, the age of the child/youth and the availability of school nurse coverage will require the identification of another primary advocate.

Complex school laws and programs have been designed to help and protect students with special health or learning needs. The pediatrician must know and understand these laws and must share them with the families. In the 1970s, federal laws affirming the right to an equal education supported the integration into public schools of the first wave of schoolchildren with special needs, specifically those with mental and physical disabilities. Since that time advances in the medical sciences have created a second wave of schoolchildren with special needs, those with chronic medical illnesses such as asthma, diabetes, cancer, and cystic fibrosis. Their full inclusion in the school experience has not been accompanied by federal mandates to meet their health and educational needs, however. This has presented unique challenges to families, educators, and health professionals.

IDEA AND 504

The individual with disabilities education act (IDEA [public law 94-142]) and Section 504 of the Rehabilitation Act of 1973 are federal laws that help protect the rights of students with disabilities. IDEA provides federal funds to states to help provide special education and related services to eligible children. Parts A and B cover eligibility procedures and required services for children ages 3 to 21, and Part C covers services for infants and toddlers. IDEA protects students who need specialized instruction and related services because of one or more of the following disabilities: autism, deaf-blindness, deafness, developmental delay (ages 3 to 9), serious emotional disturbance, hearing impairments, mental retardation, multiple disabilities, orthopedic impairments, other health impairments (limited strength, vitality, or alertness because of chronic or acute health problems [such as heart conditions, tuberculosis, rheumatic fever, nephritis, asthma, sickle cell anemia, hemophilia, epilepsy, lead poisoning, leukemia, or diabetes] that adversely affect a child's educational performance), specific learning disabilities, speech and language impairment, traumatic brain injury, and visual impairments.

An IEP (Individual Educational Plan) is required if a child is eligible for services under IDEA. This is a written plan describing a student's ability, a student's goals, and the family's, student's, and school's collaborative plan to meet these goals. A written plan is also required if a student is eligible for services under Section 504 (Table 125-2). Section 504 of the Rehabilitation Act of 1973 prohibits discrimination against any person with a disability by any federally funded agency or school. This applies to any person who has a physical or mental impairment limiting one or more major life activities (breathing, self-care, hearing, learning, performing manual tasks, seeing, speaking, walking, or working).

A frank discussion with the family about what is needed at school and the best means of achieving these goals is most worthwhile. As with any "unfunded mandate," these laws promise more than they can deliver (or more than the school communities can deliver), and they may set up expectations that can be quickly and disappointingly dashed. It is best first to set goals in partnership with families and then to inquire of the school the most effective approach for fostering best practices in school for a student with a chronic health condition.

CARE PLANS

Simple care plans offer a centralized place for the family to pull the pieces together. Diagnosis, treatment, generalists' and specialists' names and numbers, and intervals for rechecks are important information for adults who are responsible for children with special needs. Care plans should include vital medical information but should also communicate the strengths, assets, and goals of the child and family. Families coordinate multiple, complex aspects of their children's lives; a care plan assists them in this management and supports them in their ongoing representation of the child's story.

Approaches to care plans vary, but the consensus among most providers and families is the need for simplicity. Some practices choose an existing care plan template that works well for them, whereas others opt for a simple assessment or a checklist crafted with respect to the needs of child, family, and providers. Such a checklist may include whether the practice has provided materials and resource information to the family. It also can serve as a prompt or script to help the provider inquire about school concerns and to ascertain whether support and advocacy are needed and welcomed by the family. Numerous examples of care plans are available on the World Wide Web (www.BrightFutures.org, www.medicalhomeimprovement.org) or through the American Academy of Pediatrics website (www.aap.org). It is important to select a care plan template that works well in an individual practice and meets the needs of the families. Providers should start by using only one. A more ambitious template referred to as the School-Family-Practice Information Exchange (see the CD-ROM) aims to address aggressively the need for enhanced communication among family, pediatrician, and school staff members. This combined template sets up information that the family and the pediatrician can share with the school and offers a template for the family and the school to share with the practice in return.

FINAL STRATEGIES

A pediatrician's partnership with families sets up the child, the family, and the medical practice as a team; this team can then proactively extend the hand of collaboration toward the school/community. Everyone wins. The student, the family, the school, and the practice all benefit. Numerous other pediatric activities can foster enhanced and productive partnerships with schools as well. Serving on the board of a community family organization or on the local school board or offering an educational session once or twice a year on a topic of the school's choice are examples. Meeting with school nurses, principals, or both at regular intervals for an informal lunch fosters informal collegiality. Inviting school nurses to work per diem in the provider's office during the summer or possibly to use the practice as a site for a physical assessment skill refresher can enhance future collaborations by creating opportunities for practitioners and school staff to match faces with names. These are examples of family centered approaches working to promote school performance and social development for each child with a chronic health condition. Table 125-3 provides a summary of steps for generalists to take in their effort to link families, school, and primary care pediatricians for the benefit of children and their families.

Table 125-2. School Health Laws and Requirements

Law	Focus	Application
IDEA	Specialized instruction	Individual Educational Plan (IEP)
504 (Rehabilitation Act)	Reasonable Accommodation	Individual Health Plan (IHP)

Table 126-1. Condition Parameters at a Glance

Parameter	Considerations	Risks Factors	Protective Factors
Condition variables	Type	Brain involvement	Good prognosis
	Severity	Severity inconclusive	Few observable signs
	Duration	Longer duration	No physical impairment
	Functional status	Poor functional status	
Medical treatment	Medical procedures	Past negative experience	Appropriate explanations
	Surgery	Perceived threat	Coping skill training
	Transplant	Invasive nature	Available support
Medical regimen	Frequency	Many medications	Good self-care skills
	Complexity	Several regimen components	Parental supervision
	Adherence	No parental monitoring	Simpler regimen
		Side effects	Clear instructions

hospital setting. It is crucial that health care professionals develop an open, trusting relationship with the patient and family.

Common factors of chronic illness are the complex course of treatment and the associated demands of frequent appointments, testing, procedures, and hospitalizations. Adjusting to a novel and complicated medical regimen is stressful, overwhelming, and time consuming. With time, many families are successfully able to integrate medical regimens into their daily routine. Parental monitoring of medication adherence in a supportive manner can buffer the potentially negative impact of burdensome medical regimens. A patient centered approach by practitioners can facilitate identification of nonadherence and foster a working relationship with the family (see Table 126-1).

INDIVIDUAL CHARACTERISTICS OF THE CHILD

Reports of effects of demographic variables (i.e., age, gender) and children's adjustment are variable and depend on the source of information (Table 126-2). Whereas teachers and parents report boys to have more behavior problems, girls themselves report more internalizing symptoms. Although age of the child has not proven to be significant, the child's age at diagnosis may play an important role in promoting or hindering resilience. The child's age may affect tolerance of medical stressors and development of effective coping

strategies. Younger children do not have as much experience dealing with medical events and may therefore require more time to develop effective coping strategies. Adolescents are faced with unique challenges related to peer pressures, increased risk-taking behavior, and desire for autonomy. Health care professionals (in consultation with psychosocial team) must understand the child's developmentally expected behaviors and level of understanding and make information accessible and digestible.

The depth of children's understanding and perceptions of their experiences with their surroundings seem to affect long-term adaptation to chronic illness. Perceived stress by the child may result in low self-esteem, depressive and anxious mood, and behavior problems. Similarly, negative perception of physical appearance has been related to declining mood states and low self-esteem. Positive self-concept, academic success, social competence, and positive perceptions of the mothers were associated with fewer adverse psychiatric diagnoses.

Premorbid developmental and psychiatric history of the child and family impact the course of adaptive development. Significant history includes traumatic experiences, persistent symptoms of depression or anxiety, significant familial conflict, and deaths of close family members or friends (see Table 126-2). Economic strains (e.g., cumulative effects of poverty, need for parents to work extended hours or additional jobs) exacerbate the stress of caring for a medically ill child. In the context of chronic problems and

Table 126-2. Individual Child Factors at a Glance

Parameter	Considerations	Risk Factors	Protective Factors
Demographics	Sex	Gender and age are mixed;	No consistent findings for
	Age	Reporter dependent	Demographics serving a protective role
	Age of onset	Younger age more impact	
Cognitive processes	Comprehension	Poor understanding	Age-appropriate knowledge
	Developmental	Inappropriate reactions	Behavior consistent w/age
	Perception	Perception of increased stress and lacking support	Perception of manageable stress and social support
Adjustment history	Psychological	Premorbid functioning	Minimal psychological history
	Intrapersonal	Numerous stressors	Positive social adaptation
	Interpersonal	Social difficulties	History of effective coping
Coping reactions	Coping methods	Negative thinking	Positive approach behavior
	Locus of control	Denial and avoidant style	Optimistic view of future
	Efficacy	Attribute health to others	Acceptance of diagnosis
		Feeling ineffective	Strong sense of efficacy
		Inactive in treatment	Internal locus of control

maladaptive patterns of interaction, a child's medical condition can threaten an already vulnerable situation. Social support by peers and health care professionals can buffer the impact of unfortunate histories.

A child's belief in the source of health problems and outcomes is often overlooked. Children who have an internal locus of control may be more responsible in managing their illness and have a stronger sense of competency or belief in their ability to comply with medical tasks. These children may also be at greater risk for maladjustment if their efforts do not yield positive outcomes. Children who believe in "powerful others" as the primary focus of their health can develop internalizing problems. A related concept is that of self-efficacy, the belief that one can affect the environment in a way that can result in a beneficial or self-advantageous outcome. Children who feel ineffective in managing their illness may develop emotional problems and a sense of helplessness. Children who have a strong sense of self-efficacy despite periodic disappointments may protect themselves by taking a more optimistic, goal-oriented approach to their concerns.

FAMILY AND SOCIAL SUPPORT

Understanding families is crucial in assessing risk and protective factors in childhood chronic illness. Within the child's social ecology, the family (inclusive of immediate and extended family) determines, in large part, the child's well-being. Most children cannot seek medical care without parental consent and must rely on adults to assure the necessary environment in which treatment is provided. The family coordinates complex care and assures continuity of care across time and health care and educational systems.

Literature that portrayed families as vulnerable to disintegration in the face of serious childhood illness, portending the likelihood of divorce and parental psychopathology, has been refuted. Studies show that families of chronically ill children are not generally dysfunctional, but rather are like "normal" families, albeit undergoing the severe disruption(s) associated with illness and treatment. Families are viewed as competent but stressed, different but not deficient. The most effective approach to families is therefore to normalize issues and support child and family development whenever possible while also identifying families with more severe difficulties.

What are indicators of potential family risk in childhood chronic illness? With regard to family structure, single parent homes and larger families tend to have more difficulties, often complicated by problems related to poverty and social class. The tangible resources available to families also affect well-being, particularly with the limitations associated with managed health care and nonreimbursed costs for obtaining medical and educational care for children. The family's beliefs regarding the child's illness and treatment and the family's views of the future additionally affect well-being.

One of the most important predictors of well-being is social support. Families that are socially isolated are at greater risk for long-term difficulties than those who have supportive family, friends, and communities. The family's social context includes relationships with health care teams, school personnel, and providers in the community. All are central in establishing ongoing connections to ensure a child's well-being. The ability to meet the necessary challenges in making such connections appears to be a strong predictor of well-being.

ASSESSING COMPETENCE AND RISKS

In light of the long-term nature of the care of chronically ill children, attention must be paid to continuity of care, beginning with the point of initial assessment. Ideally, multidisciplinary care includes early identification (e.g., interviews, psychosocial screeners) of the family's psychosocial risks and competencies. Table 126-3 outlines the *process* of assessment of competence and risk in families with a chronically ill child and provides suggestions for developing and maintaining relationships with families over time.

The majority of families with a chronically ill child experience periods of distress and disorganization, but rebound and stabilize in ways that promote the ongoing care of the child. Examples of "stress points" for families include diagnosis, developmental changes (e.g., parent-adolescent conflict, school graduations), relapses or onset of new medical problems, and family difficulties that tax overall coping responses (e.g., another child's behavior problem, substance abuse, marital stress, death of family members). There are also problems that are predictable and "normal" in the course of chronic illness (e.g., pain, adherence, school difficulties, and peer relationships), albeit often warranting additional psychological care.

Table 126-3 outlines general areas for questions related to psychological well-being of children with chronic illnesses and their families. Sample questions are provided, although any question should be integrated as part of conversations with the family and framed in a manner that is comfortable for patient, staff, and family. Open discussion of potentially sensitive issues early in the relationship with families helps identify the types of intervention needed at an early point when preventive interventions can be implemented.

A coordinated plan of care for chronically ill children should include psychosocial treatment goals and, ideally, psychosocial collaborators to help implement related interventions. In addition to helping patients and families, consultation with colleagues with expertise in managing psychosocial challenges acknowledges that the comprehensive care of these complex patients cannot be completed by a single health care professional. A referral for additional psychological support should be determined by indicators of problems for the child and/or family (e.g., unresolving pain, anxiety, nonadherence to a treatment protocol, suicidal ideation) or by the provider's knowledge that his or her care of the patient would be enhanced by a consultation.

Successful referral for mental health consultation may be more likely when presented in the following manner: "Like other children I treat, Johnny seems sad. The best care that we can provide includes helping Johnny with his sadness. I am an expert at treating Johnny's [asthma, diabetes, muscular dystrophy] but I am not an expert at treating sadness. I would like to ask another doctor to help *us* with this." This approach maintains the centrality and responsibility of the primary treatment team (e.g., the consultant

Table 126-3. Assessing Competence and Risk in Families of Children with Chronic Illness

Family Structure	Understand who the family considers part of the family and the roles and relationships in the family. Introduce yourself to family members who you do not know. Recognizing the diversity of family structures, be open and curious, inviting the family to share with you who is important in the care of the child. Examples: "Who is in the family [name, relationship]?" "Who lives in your home?" "I saw (a woman) here yesterday who seemed to be helping you." In connecting with family members, briefly identify family members' roles and interests, and reflect on how their family may work ("So, Johnny has many people who care for him. How does this usually work in your busy morning while preparing for school?").
Risks and Competencies	Let family members know that you will ask them some questions about how they are doing in order to identify ways to help them best. Most families respond positively to your interest in them. It may take time for a family to warm up to you or other members of the team. Asking questions in a manner that is respectful and honest is the best way to gain the trust of the patient and child. Examples: "Tell me about how Johnny is doing [prior to his diagnosis, since I last saw you, since we started the new medication]." "This protocol can be quite demanding. "How are you doing with it?"
	Your goal in asking these questions is to identify the areas associated with better or worse functioning, e.g., child behavioral problems, school difficulties, adherence concerns, conflicts among family members that impact the child's treatment, parental psychological difficulties, substance use. It is appropriate to ask directly about these issues. One might say, for example, "All families have areas in which they struggle. When a child is ill, these problems can become more difficult. I'd like to ask you about some things that families sometimes encounter. Has Johnny or anyone else in your family had behavior problems or seen a counselor, psychologist, or psychiatrist?"
Social Support	Given the importance of social support (and the risks associated with isolation), assessment of social support is essential. Examples of inquiries include the following: "I am wondering who helps you [with physical care of your children, with your questions about your child's care, when you are upset or uncertain, when you need concrete help with something at home]." If the family seems isolated, this process can help identify the need for additional resources and support. Support can be informal (family, friends) or formal (health care providers). Be attentive to how family members relate to you and to your efforts to establish relationships with them.
Family Beliefs and Expectations	The sense that families make of their children's conditions and their general and illness-related world views are heterogeneous. However, these beliefs impact relationships with health care providers, adherence to protocols, and long-term adjustment. One area of exploration relates to previous experiences with chronic illness, experiences with the health care system, and religious beliefs and/or practices that may impact on the child's care and treatment. Other areas include ways in which families relate generally to others and how they view the adversities they face: Does the family tend to be optimistic or pessimistic when misfortunes occur? Does the family believe in being active in the child's treatment, or prefer that others provide most of the information?

will help us) and normalizes the request (other children feel sad, parent and family are *not* "crazy").

INTERVENTIONS TO PROMOTE SUCCESSFUL ADAPTATION

Many effective psychological interventions are available to assist children and families with the difficulties associated with chronic childhood illness. The process of deciding what type of intervention may be helpful begins during the initial assessment. The clinician may decide to consult psychosocial professionals when the difficulties noted in the assessment (e.g., isolation, family stress, behavior problems, and concerns about pain or adherence) warrant further attention. The process of intervention begins merely by asking questions about these areas and listening to families' concerns.

The major category of interventions that have been evaluated empirically in childhood chronic illness are behavioral, or cognitive behavioral, in focus. Behavioral approaches are well known to most health care providers, although they may be difficult to implement effectively (see Chapter 302). Families and school personnel can implement behavioral approaches, providing a continuity of care essential for chronically ill children.

Cognitive behavioral approaches are widely used and effective for a range of problems experienced by chronically ill children, such as pain, adherence, illness-related symptoms, and coping with invasive procedures (see also

Chapters 128 and 279). Children with cancer, for example, face the administration of chemotherapy. They may come to believe that they will have difficulty during a clinic visit, that they are alone, or that they are disappointing their health care providers by becoming upset. Using a cognitive behavioral intervention, children may be coached to see that they are able to cope with small parts of the adversity, that they have people they can count on, and that being upset is a normal part of treatment. By changing their beliefs, children can change their behaviors (e.g., use more effective coping techniques during the clinic visit).

Given the importance of families in providing care for chronically ill children, family intervention approaches are important to consider when integrating psychological interventions (see Chapter 237). One family intervention approach is conducting behavioral and/or cognitive behavioral techniques in a family context (e.g., assuring that families participate actively in the implementation of the intervention). Another focuses on problems at a broader family systems level (e.g., how can the whole family organize to care for the child while facing many potentially disorganizing life strains?

A variety of individual, family, and environmental factors may influence a child's adjustment to chronic illness. The parameters that pose risks for youngsters with health conditions include chronicity combined with poor functional status, premorbid psychiatric history, limited financial resources, and a conflictual family environment. Patients who establish trusting and open relationships with their medical team, participate actively in their treatment, and have a strong social support network may buffer the impact of medical stressors. Clinicians are encouraged to promote families' strengths to support their trajectory toward resilience.

Mini-index of Related Topics

SUGGESTED READINGS

Bauman LJ: A patient-centered approach to adherence: Risks for nonadherence. In Drotar D (ed): Promoting Adherence to Medical Treatment in Chronic Childhood Illness: Concepts, Methods, and Interventions. Mahwah, NJ, Lawrence Erlbaum Associates, 2000, pp 71–94.

Kazak A, Rourke M, Crump T: Families and other systems in pediatric psychology. In Roberts M (ed): Handbook of Pediatric Psychology, 3rd ed. New York, Guilford, 2003, pp 159–175.

Masten AS: Ordinary magic: Resilience processes in development. Am Psychol 2001;56:227–238.

Quittner AL, DiGirolamo AM: Family adaptation to childhood disability and illness. In Ammerman RT (ed): Handbook of Pediatric Psychology and Psychiatry, Vol. 2: Disease, Injury, and Illness. Boston, Allyn and Bacon, 1998, pp 70–102.

Wallander JL, Thompson RJ: Psychosocial adjustment of children with chronic physical conditions. In Roberts MC (ed): Handbook of Pediatric Psychology, 2d ed. New York, Guilford Press, 1995, pp 124–141.

SECTION 4   CHRONIC MEDICAL CARE: *Issues in Chronic Illness*

127

Financial Issues and Other Resources

John M. Neff

ROLE OF THE GENERALIST

1. Provide a Medical Home for chronically ill children.
2. Assist families in identifying potential insurance limitations for their children.
3. Provide families with resource information concerning financial support and how to access this information.
4. Identify individuals in the private or public sector who can assist families in interacting with insurance agencies.
5. Counsel families on the need for long-term financial planning and provide estimate of long-term needs of children.
6. Assist families in addressing issues regarding transition of their children to adult care.

Approximately 13% of children have a chronic health condition and have special needs, such as medications, durable equipment, specialized treatment therapies, or home nursing care. The expenses involved in caring for these children are 2 to more than 10 times higher than for children who are healthy. Most chronic conditions are not expected and the family is not prepared, personally or financially, for the added expenses.

In the late 1980s the majority of care for children was provided through fee for service, with surprisingly little attention paid to children with chronic illnesses and their impact on the overall expenses in the children's health care system. The limits of care were defined primarily by the insured parent's benefit package, with few restrictions on the use of medical services. For uninsured children and those whose benefit package was inadequate, Medicaid, Supplemental Security Income (SSI), and the Maternal and Child Health and Crippled Children's program (Title V of the Social Security Act) provided the safety net. Eligibility or disability standards varied widely from state to state. The Federal Government, through the process of Title V block grants, gave increasing authority to the states for administration and allocation of funds for children with chronic conditions. As non-Medicaid dollars available for direct care for children with chronic conditions decreased, Medicaid became the main safety net for those with chronic conditions.

Since 1990, changes in the financing and provision of health care have had an impact on children with chronic conditions. Private insurers and state Medicaid programs developed managed care. Many employment-based insurance programs provided previously lacking insurance benefits to support children with chronic conditions, and a significant number of children had no insurance at all.

In 1996, as part of welfare reform, the link between Medicaid and welfare was severed, making enrollment/termination of Medicaid no longer automatic with receipt or loss of welfare cash assistance. In 1998, the U.S. government initiated a State Children's Health Insurance Program (SCHIP) to increase the number of children insured and to improve their benefits. The result has been that nearly all states have raised income eligibility standards for government-sponsored health insurance to at least 200% above the federally recognized poverty level. Because the Medicaid and SCHIP benefit package have been broadened to encompass most of the needs of children with chronic conditions, Medicaid and SCHIP have become the major safety nets for children, especially those with chronic health conditions. The federal government placed a greater emphasis on diagnostic rather than functional criteria, and restricted eligibility for SSI to only the most disabled, a population that represents less than 1% of all children. The role of the family's practitioner is to help the family work through this funding maze.

Although currently coverage is better and coordinated care improved, tightly managed care practices have limited some children's access to needed specialty services. Payment arrangements in some managed care programs often have not adequately reimbursed providers who care for the complex care that these children require. Benefit packages from one employer and from one state to another are inconsistent. Insurance for dental and mental health services is often quite limited.

By the year 2000, with the return to double-digit health care inflation and the SCHIP initiative, states faced the cost of increased enrollment, as well as the cost of improved benefits. Federal and state governments are reluctant to support both health insurance for all children and comprehensive benefit programs. The conflict will continue between comprehensive coverage and comprehensive benefits and between allocation of resources between children and the aging adult population, where health care inflation is the highest.

Although implementation of managed care has assured for the first time that all children will be assigned to a health plan and provider, increased financial management has placed greater responsibilities on the families and providers to be certain that these children receive adequate services.

DISTRIBUTION OF HEALTH CARE DOLLARS TO HEALTHY AND CHRONICALLY ILL CHILDREN

Distribution of health care expenses are unevenly distributed between children who have chronic illnesses and those who do not. For example, approximately 60% of children's Medicaid expenditures are for the chronically ill. For a healthy child, expenditures are primarily for physician and outpatient costs, while for children with a chronic condition, expenditures are primarily for hospitalizations, medications, equipment, and home nursing care. Because few health care plans recognize this difference in expendi-

tures, children with chronic conditions and their providers often are underfunded.

MAJOR FINANCIAL ISSUES FOR IMPROVED CARE

Benefit package: The minimum benefit package must support a wide range of services including dental, mental health, nutritional, equipment, special medications, and rehabilitation. Copayment arrangements should be based on the family's ability to pay. Total and annual limits should be sufficient so that families are not vulnerable to the loss of coverage. Commitment from both private and public insurers and agencies is required to develop uniform acceptable benefits for this population, so that moving from one plan or from one state to another will not disadvantage families. SCHIP programs should be enhanced to assure access and broad coverage.

Home/respite care: Families need specialized home and/or respite care. For families in the welfare system, there must at least be adequate specialized childcare services. If the family support system breaks down, care rapidly becomes more costly.

Risk payment system and provider reimbursement: Payment systems should provide adequate support to health plans in the form of risk adjustment payments. This methodology is available and better than systems that adjust only by age and gender. Methods should be developed and implemented to assure that funds are distributed to individual providers and practice settings, in proportion to the percentage of children with chronic problems that are seen by that practice.

CURRENT CHALLENGES TO FAMILIES

Each child with a chronic condition should have a Medical Home that provides coordination and comprehensive care, and serves as an information resource on specific conditions and available community resources. Without a Medical Home, the burden of coordination and identification of resources rests heavily on the family.

Limits of insurance: If a child has insurance, the burden to the family may be the limits of total lifetime or annual expenditures, or limits of specific benefits, such as those for mental health, dental, special nutritional needs or diets, specialized durable equipment, respite care, or home nursing care.

Out-of-pocket expenses: Out-of-pocket expenses are significant, including copays, premium sharing, payment for medications, therapies, or equipment not included in the insurance, home remodeling, specialized transportation, and other important lifestyle expenses. In 1996, of the $62 billion spent on medical care for children, $12.8 billion (20.5%) was paid out of pocket.

Employment: In a family of two employed adults, one adult often has to stop employment to take care of the child with a chronic condition. The decision on who stops work usually depends on insurance status. A single parent may have to keep working just to maintain income and insurance, creating hardship on both child and parent. One study has demonstrated that half of families caring for a chronically ill child reported spending $1000 in the preceding year; 10% reported spending in excess of $5000. Half of the parents in the labor force said that they stopped working because of their child's chronic health care, and half of those still working said they had reduced working hours to meet their child's need.

Additional medical care responsibilities: Recent trends to reduce hospitalization and institutionalization have placed more responsibilities on families for direct nonreimbursed care. Many must provide direct health care at home each week in the form of physical therapy, equipment care, dressing care, and so forth, which can require 20 or more hours each week.

Welfare: States' work requirements vary considerably. Some states grant temporary exemptions from work for parents of severely impaired children, but still expect that the parent eventually work. Some states classify as work care for a chronically ill child at home or in a community setting. If no work exceptions are allowed, the child with a chronic illness is dependent on family members, friends, or the scarce availability of qualified childcare or respite facilities. Even under the best of circumstances, the income from most welfare to work programs is insufficient to meet the needs of the child. All of these issues are magnified for a single parent.

Transition to adult care: Transition of the child with a chronic problem to adult care creates new challenges. When a child reaches adulthood, health insurance status will change and benefits may be lost. If a child moves out of the home, there will be long-term support expense, depending on the child's ability to be self-sufficient. All of these issues can be overwhelming for individual families and they should engage in long-term financial as well as health and social planning.

RECOMMENDATIONS FOR PROVIDER

Table 127-1 lists challenges to families that providers must help address. Most families are overwhelmed when they have a child with complex needs and do not know where to turn. The practitioner must guide families through their financial issues. Families need to be in direct contact with their insurance program to clarify the extent and limitation of their coverage. The practitioner can assist families in identifying potential gaps in their insurance with special attention to copays, long term limits, direct medical expenditures, special medications, and nutritional supplements. In the absence of adequate coverage, families should be directed to available local, state, and federal programs. Practitioners can encourage families to engage in long-term

Box 127-1. Information Services
■ Social Security Administration: Benefits for Children with Disabilities http://www.ssa.gov/pubs/10026.html ■ Children's Health Insurance Program: CHIP or Healthy Kids Now! http://www.insurekidsnow.gov/ ■ NeedyMeds.com http://www.needymeds.com ■ Disability Resources Monthly Guide to Disability Resources on the Internet (Financial Information) http://www.disabilityresources.org/ ■ Family Village Financial Information on the Internet http://www.familyvillage.wisc.edu/hospital/financing.html ■ Financial Planning for your Special Needs Child http://www.pueblo.gsa.gov/cic   text/children/special-child/special11.html

planning with special attention to issues related to transition to adult care. Most states have some coordinators for special needs children. Information resources are available on the Internet or through local public health departments or other community-based agencies. In large practices, one person can be identified as a consistent resource for families. Smaller practices may have to rely directly on the Internet and provide education on how to access this information. Those for whom English is not their primary language and those who are not computer literate will need direct counseling from culturally and linguistically trained individuals. Box 127-1 lists websites that provide useful information for providers and families regarding financing the cost of care for chronically ill children. Finally, practitioners should be aware of their own practice patterns, financial profiles, and costs for contract negotiation purposes.

ADVOCACY

Practitioners and families need to advocate broadly for everyone to change an imperfect health care system that has yet to embrace the financial issues of children with chronic conditions. Organizations that are already involved are the American Academy of Pediatrics, the National Association of Children's Hospitals and Related Institutions, and Family Voices.

 Additional Resources, CD-ROM

Bibliography

Table 127-1. Challenges to Families
1. Identify a Medical Home for the child for coordinated and comprehensive care. 2. Be knowledgeable about insurance coverage and potential limits for the child. 3. Make careful assessment of out-of-pocket expenses. 4. Engage in long-term financial and employment planning. 5. Initiate plans as early as possible for transition to adult care, including estate planning.

SUGGESTED READINGS

Family Voices at the Federation for Children with Special Health Care Needs, April 2000. Available at: http://www.familyvoices.org.

Ireys HT, Anderson GF, Shaffer TJ, Neff JM: Expenditures for care of children with chronic illnesses enrolled in the Washington State Medicaid Program, Fiscal Year 1993. Pediatrics 1997;100:197–204.

Light JL: Appendix II, Resource. In Light JL: Clinician's Guide to Pediatric Chronic Illness, 1st ed. New York, McGraw Hill, 2001, pp 421–440.

McCormick MC, Weinick RM, Elixhauser A, et al: Annual report on access to and utilization of health care for children and youth in the United States–2000. Ambul Pediatr 2001;1:3–15.

SECTION 4   CHRONIC MEDICAL CARE: *Issues in Chronic Illness*

128 Pain Management in Chronic Disease

Neil Schechter

ROLE OF THE GENERALIST

1   Assess pain and associated symptoms.
2   Provide pain relief, sleep hygiene, and elimination of nauseas.
3   Communicate with the family.
4   Coordinate care for children with chronic pain.
5   Encourage normal development.
6   Prevent "vulnerable child syndrome."

Over the past decade research on pain in children has been conducted at both the clinical and neurodevelopmental level. Results indicate fetuses have the anatomic and neurochemical capabilities of experiencing pain by the end of the second trimester. Research has emphasized as well the short-term and long-term consequences of inadequate pain treatment. For example, when compared to uncircumcised newborns, babies circumcised without adequate anesthesia have significant differences in response to pain at their 4 and 6 month immunizations. Children who undergo painful procedures without anesthesia report more pain associated with subsequent procedures than those who initially had adequate pain control.

Management of pain in children has improved as a result. Postoperative pain is more often treated adequately than in the past. Children with cancer now generally have adequate sedation for painful diagnostic procedures. No infant undergoes surgery without adequate anesthesia. Unfortunately, data suggest success is more limited in children with the less predictable, intermittent pain associated with chronic disease.

FUNDAMENTALS

The International Association for the Study of Pain defines pain as "an unpleasant sensory and emotional experience associated with actual or potential tissue damage or described in terms of such damage." The definition states that pain is always subjective, learned through experiences related to injury early in life. This definition implies that pain results not only from a nociceptive stimulus, but also from the individual's experience and interpretation of that stimulus. Discomfort caused by the noxious stimulus can be either magnified or dampened depending on a number of modifying factors (age of the child, sex, culture, context of meaning of the pain, temperament, and affective state). In general, younger children and girls experience more pain from a given stimulus than do older children and boys. Response to pain also varies culturally. If the pain represents possible relapse of an illness or increasing disfigurement, the same stimulus may be experienced more intensely than without those implications. Less adaptable children are more responsive to a given stimulus than those with "easier" temperamental characteristics. Anxiety and depression clearly have a role in amplifying pain.

Although the multifactorial nature of pain is well accepted, other aspects of this definition are debated, particularly the concept that pain is learned. This implies that newborns cannot experience pain. Some propose that pain perception represents an inherent quality of life that appears early in development and serves as a signaling system for tissue damage.

Pain is categorized by its time course and by its pathophysiology. Pain can be classified as acute (immediate), chronic (at least 3 months' duration), or recurrent (occurring at least monthly for at least 3 months with some disruption of daily living). Nociceptive pain that results from noxious stimulation of nociceptors may require different treatment strategies from those for neuropathic pain that stems from nerve injury. Chronic pain can be associated with illness such as cancer, sickle cell disease, HIV/AIDS, or rheumatologic diseases or may stem from a variety of syndromes with less clear origins such as fibromyalgia (see Chapter 187).

GENERAL PRINCIPLES FOR TREATMENT OF CHRONIC PAIN

Box 128-1 and Table 128-1 outline general principles that apply to all categories of chronic pain in children. These include promotion of normal development despite the difficulties the child is experiencing, adequate assessment of the pain regardless of its origin, a system-wide approach to the pain, anticipation of the pain if at all possible, and empowering the family to control the pain and avoid learned helplessness. These principles with some variation also apply to children with pain associated with a chronic illness.

Painful diagnostic and treatment procedures should be approached aggressively. For many children, painful procedures are the worst part of their illness. If inadequately treated during the initial diagnostic phases, children experience significantly more pain associated with subsequent procedures compared to those whose pain was appropriately managed. Adequate treatment may prevent development of overwhelming fear and anxiety, which can affect children's entire hospital experience and their relationship with health care providers.

Severe pain occurs intermittently during chronic disease. Whether unrelated to the disease process or the result of a flare or progression of the disease, it should be considered an emergency and treated rapidly.

Parents should be actively involved in the child's medical care. Parents are the best source of information about how a child will handle an upcoming procedure. They are far better than medical staff at discerning subtle cues that indicate the child's pain. They should be used as "coaches" during medical procedures. Parental involvement decreases both the parents' and child's anxiety, which has a clear impact on decreasing pain.

Box 128-1. Principles for Management of Chronic Pain

1. Painful diagnostic and treatment procedures should be approached aggressively and treated as an emergency.
2. Severe pain occurs intermittently during chronic disease.
3. Parents should be actively involved in the child's medical care.
4. Behavioral, cognitive, and pharmacologic strategies as well as physical strategies should be used in all children.
5. Alleviation of pain is essential to allow restorative sleep.
6. Noxious routes of administration of medication should be avoided.
7. Addiction is extraordinarily rare in children who use analgesia for legitimate medical problems.
8. The right dose of opioid is the dose that relieves the pain.

Table 128-1. Guidelines in Management of Chronic Pain

Promote normal development. While pain needs to be addressed, normative behavior needs to be reinforced so that development can proceed. Social interactions need to be maintained.
Action: Provide a forum in which pain can be discussed and minimize secondary gain from the pain.
Ongoing, adequate, meticulous assessment regardless of the origin of the pain.
Action: Create a pain problem list. Children with chronic disease may have many different types of pain and these should be assessed independently. Assessment should occur in a developmentally appropriate manner using instruments that have been generally agreed upon by those caring for the child. The child's self-report of pain should be believed. A pain diary to be filled out at home may be beneficial.
Develop a system-wide approach. Children with chronic pain generally are involved with multiple providers who may have different perspectives on the origin of the discomfort. Multiple medications that potentially interact may be used.
Action: Track all the medications that have been prescribed, their efficacy and potential interactions. The primary care physician is ideal for this critical integrative role.
Anticipate the pain. It takes far less analgesia to prevent pain than to treat it.
Action: Premedicate child before painful procedures or aggressive physical therapy, or if pain occurs at predictable times of the day.
Empower child and family to take over control of the pain so that learned helplessness can be avoided.
Action: Use or refer families so they can learn behavioral and cognitive approaches. Use of handheld medical records, self-administered analgesia, and other strategies can enable children and families to feel more control over their life circumstances.

Behavioral, cognitive, and pharmacologic strategies as well as physical strategies should be used in all children. Often pain persists and cannot be entirely eliminated pharmacologically. Cognitive strategies that involve improving coping capabilities can be extremely beneficial. When less invasive strategies are effective, the result is decreased need for medication and avoidance of unintended side effects such as sedation that have an impact on the child's quality of life.

Alleviation of pain is essential to allow restorative sleep. Pain impairs sleep in many children with chronic disease. Some types of pain such as bone pain tend to be worse at night. The child's sleep habits should be investigated and analgesics, alternative medications, or behavioral strategies should be used to allow restorative sleep at night.

Noxious routes of administration of medication should be avoided whenever possible. Intramuscular, rectal, or intranasal routes of administration are uncomfortable and serve as a disincentive for children to report pain. Oral or intravenous routes should be used if at all possible.

Addiction is extraordinarily rare in children who use analgesics for legitimate medical problems. Addiction should not be confused with dependence, a physiological condition that occurs in all individuals who take opioids for over a week. Addiction is a psychological preoccupation with the drug and the feelings and paraphernalia associated with it. Dependence is easily treated by slowly weaning the child from the medication. Addiction is extraordinarily rare in children. Concern about addiction should never constrain the appropriate use of analgesics. Concern about the possibility of parental diversion should not limit the child's access to adequate pain relief. If parents are at risk for using or selling pain medications, strategies such as having medication administered in school or by a visiting nurse or trusted guardian must be employed.

The ultimate goal of therapy, acceptable level of pain relief, should be discussed among the child, family, and staff. Realistic goals should be decided on, recognizing that complete elimination of pain may not be possible.

The traditional guidelines for analgesic usage apply to opioid naive patients. *The right dose of opioid is the dose that relieves the pain.* Children with chronic pain problems will almost always require more medication than is listed in the traditional analgesic tables for children. Increased need for analgesics should not automatically be viewed as tolerance until the disease extension has been ruled out. If a child complains of increasing discomfort despite a dose of an analgesic that had previously been adequate, a thorough search for disease extension should be undertaken before the increased pain is dismissed as tolerance to medication.

ASSESSMENT

Developmentally appropriate assessment is the cornerstone of pain treatment. Pain cannot be treated adequately if its existence is not identified and if the efficacy of treatment is not measured. Because pain is inherently a subjective experience, the individual's report of his or her discomfort has always been the standard by which pain is assessed. In adults and children over the age of 8, pain intensity is assessed by use of a visual analogue scale, typically a 10-centimeter line that is anchored by "no pain" at one end and the "most pain imaginable" on the other end. Children or adults are asked to rate their pain on that line. Because children under the age of 8 are often incapable of such complex quantitative thinking, a number of modified self-report scales have been developed for children between the ages of 3 and 8. These may use colors, cartoon faces, photographs of children experiencing pain, a pain thermometer, or poker chips or other manipulatives representing various gradations of pain. For children who are younger than 3 or who are developmentally delayed, nonspecific proxy measures of pain must be used. Behavioral markers of pain include position, crying, appetite suppression, and facial expression. Specific techniques for evaluating facial expression appear to be reliable and reproducible. Physiologic markers that correlate with pain include increased heart rate, respiratory rate, and blood pressure, and decreased oxygen saturation and vagal tone. Composite scales for neonates, infants, and older nonverbal children include the CHEOPS, CRIES, OPS, and PIPP.

While assessment of pain intensity is essential for acute pain, it is often less helpful in chronic pain situations. Children may report severe pain yet in all other ways appear to be improving. As a result, for children with continuous pain in whom disease progression is unlikely (fibromyalgia, headache, recurrent abdominal pain, reflex sympathetic dystrophy), progress should be monitored through increasing function (improved activity level, concentration, sleep, appetite, mood) and not solely by report of decreasing pain intensity. Repeated discussion about pain may in fact reinforce oversurveillance and focused attention on pain and create increased pain-related disability.

THERAPEUTICS

Treatment of pain in children with chronic illness requires multiple modalities. Pharmacologic treatment of pain is discussed on the CD-ROM and in Chapter 285.

PSYCHOLOGICAL AND BEHAVIORAL STRATEGIES

Behavioral and cognitive strategies have efficacy in the management of pain in children. These techniques can ameliorate pain during procedures and can be modified for treatment of chronic pain as well.

Preparation: Preparing children for impending procedures has clearly been demonstrated to decrease the discomfort associated with them. Preparation must be done in a developmentally appropriate manner and have two key elements: description of the procedure and a description of how it will feel. The variations in children's personalities and temperaments require individualization and limit the value of a "one size fits all" approach to preparation.

Parental presence: Parents should be involved in all aspects of their child's treatment. During procedures, parents can be taught specific techniques to help their children. This can decrease parents' sense of helplessness and comfort children by having familiar individuals working with them. Parents should be queried regarding their knowledge of the child's historic response to such situations, encouraged to accompany the child to painful procedures, and taught distraction and relaxation techniques. Parents of children with painful chronic diseases can be taught methods to help children cope, and can learn to assist children in practicing and mastering these techniques.

Distraction/hypnosis: A host of techniques have been developed to help distract children from their discomfort. These range from breathing, blowing, and counting to telling children their favorite stories or looking at a book together. Music can also be used. Children can learn meditation techniques. Hypnosis involves the more active involvement of the child in this process through the use of suggestion and fantasy. Hypnotic techniques such as the "magic glove" or "pain switch" can help a child reframe an experience and reduce pain as a result.

Increased self-control/rehearsal: Helping children increase their sense of control over the environment reduces anxiety. Allow children to have some role in the procedure such as selection of site and time of day. Patient-controlled analgesia decreases the sense of helplessness by allowing them to administer medication when they need it. The method of rehearsal has the child rehearse impending procedures on a stuffed animal or talk to other children about the procedure. Visiting the place where the procedure will occur or watching a videotape about it is helpful.

PHYSICAL APPROACHES

Physical approaches to pain reduction work primarily at the level of dorsal horn by stimulating the larger afferents that carry messages that dampen the impact of the pain. Nonnoxious stimuli such as heat, cold, massage, and vibration are used to reduce pain. Transcutaneous electrical nerve stimulation uses a specifically designed instrument to generate various patterns of electrical sensation. When an individual has pain in an isolated area such as a limb, electrodes can be placed in the appropriate location for that area and different patterns of electrical impulses can be tried to dampen the pain message. This technique provides effective relief for many localized chronic pain problems.

SPECIFIC PAIN PROBLEMS

Specific management for the pain in sickle cell disease, cancer, and HIV is found on the CD-ROM.

Procedure pain: For many children, the necessary medical procedures associated with the diagnosis and treatment of disease is the worst part of their illness. For children with chronic disease, these procedures dominate their life experience. Pain must be aggressively treated and managed during procedures, especially at the outset of an illness. If inadequate analgesia is provided initially, the cycle of dread and fear of future procedures can be hard to eradicate.

Applying general principles of pain management can minimize the pain and distress associated with procedures. The intervention should be tailored to the severity of pain associated with the procedure and the individual characteristics of the child, such as age or temperament. If the child is very young, if the parents predict the child will have a particularly difficult time, or if conscious sedation has been unsuccessful in the past, then general anesthesia should be considered at the outset. Preparation should occur in a developmentally appropriate way, ideally with involved parents who can remain with the child. Parents should be taught how to work with their child and function as coaches throughout the procedure. If procedures are performed in the hospital, they should be done in a separate treatment room so the child's room can remain a refuge from painful events. Behavioral and pharmacologic strategies should be used regardless of the severity of pain associated with the procedures.

During the procedure, local anesthetics should be used for all needle procedures. A number of topical agents and delivery systems are now available. If the pain associated with the procedure is moderate or severe, sedation should be considered and, if performed, the American Academy of Pediatrics guidelines should be followed carefully. These state clearly that there should be one individual in the room to monitor the child and another individual who is skilled in airway maintenance. Monitoring and resuscitative equipment and resuscitative drugs should be available.

Typically, conscious sedation involves the use of an opioid, often morphine or fentanyl, and a short acting benzodiazepine, typically midazolam. Chloral hydrate alone can be used for painless procedures that require immobilization. Additional agents such as propofol, nitrous oxide, and ketamine should be administered by appropriately credentialed practitioners.

To manage pain each clinician depend on personal experience and training and the specific logistics at his or her site. For painless procedures such as MRIs, high dose chloral hydrate may be all that is necessary. For mildly painful procedures, such as intravenous cannulation or venipuncture, parental presence, appropriate preparation, and local anesthetics should be considered. Distractive techniques should be used. For painful procedures, parental presence

and preparation are essential. In addition, local anesthesia should be used as well as appropriate sedation and analgesia, often fentanyl and midazolam in combination, prior to the procedure. Cognitive behavioral techniques are also of value.

Specific management for pain in sickle cell disease, cancer, and HIV is found on the CD-ROM.

SUMMARY

Although the management of pain in children has undergone remarkable changes in a short period of time, these changes have been most pronounced in predictable pain problems. Pain associated with chronic disease is often more complex and requires more vigilance to evaluate and treat.

The treatment of pain requires an understanding of its nature as well as a system of assessment by which its intensity can be gauged and interventions appropriately evaluated. Pharmacologic therapy, cognitive behavioral approaches, and physical approaches have a role with all children who have pain associated with chronic disease. Pain should be anticipated and treated in a preventive manner.

Chronic illness poses enormous burdens on children and their families. Relief of pain and suffering eliminates some of those burdens and should be viewed as an essential part of the compassionate practice of medicine.

Additional Resources, CD-ROM

| Pharmacologic treatment of pain | Text |
| Pain treatment in sickle cell disease, cancer, and HIV | Text |

Mini-index of Related Topics

SUGGESTED READINGS

Ballas S: Sickle Cell Pain: Progress in Pain Research and Management, Vol. 11. Seattle, IASP Press, 1998.
Cancer Pain Relief and Palliative Care in Children. Geneva: World Health Organization, 1998.
McGrath PJ, Finley GA: Chronic and Recurrent Pain in Children and Adolescents: Progress in Pain Research and Management, Vol. 13. Seattle, IASP Press, 1999.
Schechter N, Berde C, Yaster M: Pain in Infants, Children, and Adolescents, 2d ed. Philadelphia, Lippincott Williams and Wilkins, 2002.
Weisman SJ (ed): Pain management in children. Child Adolesc Psychiatr Clin N Am 1997;6:687–923.
Yaster M, Krane E, Kaplan R, et al: Pediatric Pain Management and Sedation Handbook. St. Louis, Mosby, 1997.

Table 130-1. Nutrient Deficiencies and Toxicities—cont'd

Nutrient	Signs of Deficiency/Low Intake	Signs of Toxicity/Excess Intake	Treatment
Iodine	Goiter; cretinism	Enlarged thyroid	*Deficiency:* utilize iodized salt in diet *Toxicity:* decrease use of iodized salt, seafood, and any supplements containing iodine
Iron	Anemia; fatigue	Liver damage; may occur with hemochromatosis	*Deficiency:* increase red meats and dark green leafy vegetables; take high iron foods with citrus fruits to increase absorption *Toxicity:* Discontinue supplement use; blood withdrawal for chronic iron overload
Magnesium	Nausea; vomiting; muscle weakness	Nausea; vomiting; low blood pressure; usually from nonfood sources	*Deficiency:* increase intake of nuts, dark green vegetables, whole grains, and dried beans *Toxicity:* discontinue supplement use
Manganese	Abnormal bone and cartilage formation; impaired glucose tolerance; poor growth	Uncommon	*Deficiency:* increase intake of nuts, whole grains, fruits, and vegetables
Phosphorus	Poor bone and teeth structure; weakness	Poor bone structure. Rare	*Deficiency:* increase intake of meat, dairy products, dried beans, and whole grains
Potassium	Lethargy; weakness; poor appetite; irregular heart rhythm	Toxicity unlikely unless associated with renal disease; irregular heart rhythm	*Deficiency:* increase intake of potatoes, tomatoes, apricots, cantaloupe, dried beans, spinach, bananas, and milk
Selenium	Muscle pain and weakness	Nausea; diarrhea; vomiting; fatigue; hair loss; fingernail loss	*Deficiency:* increase intake of seafood, organ meats, and eggs *Toxicity:* discontinue supplement use, decrease intake of selenium-containing foods
Zinc	Poor growth; prolonged wound healing; loss of appetite; decreased immune function	Decreased copper absorption; decreased immune function	*Deficiency:* increase intake of meat, seafood, milk, whole grains, and eggs *Toxicity:* discontinue supplement use
Molybdenum	Rare; may occur with prolonged TPN use	Joint inflammation	*Toxicity:* discontinue supplement use; food sources vary in content depending on soil
Fluoride	Increased dental carries; possible reduced bone density	Mottled teeth; impaired kidney, nerve, and muscle function	*Deficiency:* add fluoride supplements; check for fluoridated water sources *Toxicity:* discontinue supplement use; check for fluoridated water sources

developmental disabilities increase the metabolic rate and increase need for energy intake. See Box 130-1 for ideas on increasing intake; however, care should be taken that the foods used to increase intake do not pose other problems. An example is using a high-potassium food to increase intake in a renal patient can be damaging.

Box 130-1. Ideas for Increasing Energy and Protein Intake — "Power Packing Food"

1. Use instant breakfast and other liquid nutritional supplements.
2. Add dry powdered milk to shakes, casseroles, soups, puddings, and cereals to increase protein and calcium.
3. Add butter or liquid/soft tab margarine to vegetables, breads, and casseroles to increase calories.
4. Add pasteurized powdered egg whites (found in the baking section of the store) to shakes, soups, and mashed potatoes.
5. Take advantage "good days" — offer more food.
6. Have favorite foods and snacks easily accessible and available.
7. Try adding sweet sauces to meats to reduce the "metallic" taste often experienced with some medications. For example, use ham and pineapple, pork chops and applesauce, apricot jam and chicken.

Special Diets. Caring for a child with a chronic disease is challenging at best. For many people, diet is one of the easiest things to control. For each carefully researched and proven therapeutic diet there is one or more nonresearched and unproven diet. Some special diets, such as the ketogenic diet for seizure patients, have shown patient improvements, while other diets, such as limited sugar for attention deficit disorder, have no research backing. When working with a patient and family who want to use a special diet, ask the following questions. Will the diet harm the patient in any way? Does the diet eliminate one or more food groups and will these eliminations lead to potential nutrient deficiencies? What is the source of the diet; is the source reputable? Are there any peer-reviewed studies on this diet? Many special diets will neither harm nor help the patient physically, but there may be psychological benefits. Care should be taken with special diets so nutritional status and health are not compromised.

DIAGNOSIS

Chapter 14 has guidelines for conducting a nutritional assessment to determine nutritional status and risk for malnutrition.

MANAGEMENT

Information on specific guidelines for managing the nutritional care of the patient with a particular chronic disease is provided in tabular form on the CD-ROM. The table includes information on nutritional considerations for the specific disease, nutritional requirements, nutritional assessment, treatment and management, special effects of medications used in each disorder, pearls for nutritional management, and "red flags."

Nutritional care in oncology should focus on preventing protein-energy malnutrition (PEM) caused from too little intake. Too little intake may be due to irradiation of the head, neck, esophagus, abdomen, or pelvis or frequent courses of chemotherapy, making eating difficult and unpleasant. Nutrition should focus on increasing energy and protein intake to allow for tissue repair and to spare breakdown of lean body mass.

The goal for nutritional care in renal disease is to provide adequate nutrients for growth while minimizing the consequences of renal disease. Adjustments to protein, potassium, sodium, calcium, phosphorus, and fluid are needed.

In the pediatric patient with hyperlipidemia, the nutritional goal is to support growth while preventing the development of coronary heart disease (CHD). For the patient with congenital heart disease, calories may need to be increased to achieve good nutritional status before surgery.

Treatment of celiac disease requires avoidance of gluten in the diet. This requires meticulous reading of food labels and creativity in food preparation. Vitamin and mineral supplements as well as medications need to be scrutinized to determine if they contain modified food starch or flavoring, since a small amount of gluten is enough to trigger a reaction in the small intestine. Inflammatory bowel disease (IBD) can cause malabsorption as a result of an inflammation of the mucosa. Patients with bowel resections may malabsorb nutrients because of the shortened bowel length. An estimated 30% of children with inflammatory bowel disease develop growth failure.

In the child with HIV infection opportunistic infections and side effects of medications are intertwined with nutrient intake. Nausea, vomiting, abdominal pain, diarrhea, oral ulcers, and metallic taste may influence intake.

Medical nutrition therapy of diabetes mellitus involves intensive nutritional education incorporated into self-care management education. Comprehensive instruction leads to self-care management of the day-to-day adjustments needed for growth, insulin reactions, and dietary alterations. Insulin, diet, and exercise patterns must be individualized to the patient's lifestyle. The meal pattern must be established according to the family lifestyle and not to the insulin prescription. The insulin prescription can and should vary with growth and activity, and should be planned around the nutrient intake to achieve near normal blood glucose and normal glycosylated hemoglobin levels.

Cystic fibrosis (CF) requires extensive nutrition therapy. Children with cystic fibrosis are prone to nutritional deficiencies from decreased intake, malabsorption, and increased requirements, because of the following: (1) impaired release of pancreatic enzymes (lipase, trypsinogen, chymotrypsin, and maltase); (2) inadequate pancreatic bicarbonate secretion (thus the gastric acid entering the duodenum may lower the intestinal pH in the jejunum); lipase is denatured by a low pH; (3) excessive mucus on the intestinal wall, which impairs nutrient absorption; and (4) recurrent vomiting from coughing. Energy losses may also result from gastroesophageal reflux, steatorrhea from improper bile-salt metabolism, hepatobiliary disease, short gut as a result of resection after meconium ileus, and glucose loss from diabetes mellitus. A high-fat, high-calorie diet with vitamin and mineral supplementation is needed to prevent malnutrition.

Nutrition treatment for phenylketonuria (PKU) consists of providing a nutritionally balanced diet containing enough phenylalanine to meet the needs of a growing child without exceeding the child's capacity to metabolize phenylalanine. Untreated patients (patients on a regular diet) have mental retardation, diminished pigmentation, eczema, hypertonicity, seizures, a musty odor, and an abnormal electroencephalogram. The biochemical defect in phenylketonuria is a deficiency in the enzyme phenylalanine hydroxylase, which cannot be replaced at this time. A dietitian should work with the patient and guardian to instruct them on the types and amounts of food that can be combined with the medical formulas for a balanced diet.

Nutrition treatment for the child with cerebral palsy is very individual. Calorie needs are based on changes in weight and height and may change frequently, depending on muscle tone. Feeding difficulties such as problems with sucking, swallowing, chewing, tongue thrust, dental problems, and poor tongue and lip control may lead to poor intake.

A special diet, the ketogenic diet, has resurfaced as a treatment for seizures in patients nonresponsive to medications. Growth is stunted for the 2 to 3 years the child is on the ketogenic diet, but some catch-up growth is seen after returning to a regular diet. Specific diet modifications for ketogenic diets are found on the CD-ROM.

Management of the overweight or obese child includes goals to avoid short- and long-term health problems and encourage healthy lifestyle behaviors. The degree of diet modification and exercise frequency depends on the medical condition, age, level of obesity, psychosocial factors, and parental involvement.

Nutritional goals for the patient with anorexia nervosa (AN) or bulimia nervosa (BN) include support of growth and maturation, normalization of eating patterns, and development of self-management and control. Psychotherapy is a crucial aspect of treatment. In the severely malnourished patient, nutritional support must begin so the patient is cognitively functional during psychotherapy. Nutrition therapy should be individualized for each patient's situation. Generally, a normal diet without restrictions is recommended.

Feeding children with special needs may be stressful and often requires extra time, attention, and patience. Parents and family may often turn to nonresearched special diets for treatment. Care should be taken that these diets do not pose any harm or risk for malnutrition. For the child with a cleft palate special attention to positioning for breast- and bottle-feeding is needed. The trial and error approach for

Table 131-2. Chronic Disorders of the Bones and Joints

Skeletal Dysplasias

Abnormal growth; abnormalities in size, number, or shape of one or more bones:

1. Achondroplasias
2. Arthrogryposis
3. Osteogenesis imperfecta
4. Rickets
5. Hereditary multiple exostoses

Limb Deficiences

1. Amelia
2. Phocomelia
3. Hemimelia
4. Polydactyly
5. Syndactyly
6. Hemiatrophy
7. Hemihypertrophy

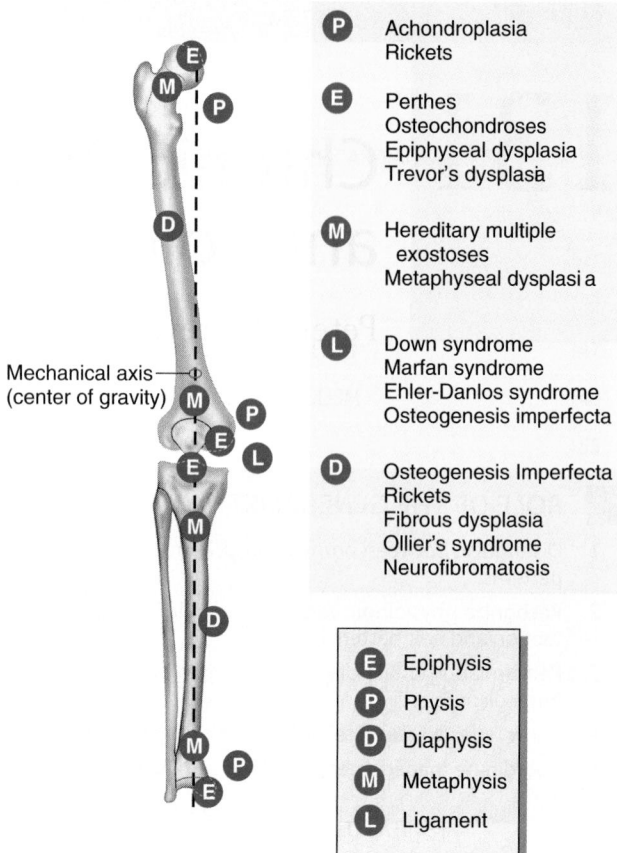

- **P** Achondroplasia
  Rickets
- **E** Perthes
  Osteochondroses
  Epiphyseal dysplasia
  Trevor's dysplasa
- **M** Hereditary multiple exostoses
  Metaphyseal dysplasi a
- **L** Down syndrome
  Marfan syndrome
  Ehler-Danlos syndrome
  Osteogenesis imperfecta
- **D** Osteogenesis Imperfecta
  Rickets
  Fibrous dysplasia
  Ollier's syndrome
  Neurofibromatosis

Mechanical axis (center of gravity)

- **E** Epiphysis
- **P** Physis
- **D** Diaphysis
- **M** Metaphysis
- **L** Ligament

Figure 131-1. Anatomy of a long bone, with indications of areas affected in various disorders.

disorders. After limb development, growth continues and is affected by the intrauterine environment. With the in-migration of muscles, and formation of joint clefts, intrauterine fetal movement plays a crucial role in limb mobility and growth. Abnormalities that constrict or compress the fetus, such as bicornuate uterus, oligohydramnios, and amniotic bands, can lead to a variety of limb deformities, joint contractures (arthrogryposis), or even autoamputation (Streeter dysplasia). Maternal exposure to toxins and teratogens (the classic example being thalidomide) may also result in gross limb deficiencies.

DIAGNOSIS

Although many disorders are evident prior to birth or at delivery, the evaluation of chronic bone disorders begins with a careful history. Family history is particularly important and should alert the clinician to various inheritable conditions, such as hereditary multiple exostoses, achondroplasia, and osteogenesis. Trauma or illness during pregnancy and exposure to drugs or toxins predispose to gestational and intrauterine problems. An abnormal uterus that restricts fetal movement raises the prospects of problems with fetal development.

Table 131-3. Four Phases of Limb Formation

Phase	Week of Gestation
1. Initiation of limb buds	4
2. Specification of limb pattern	5
3. Differentiation of tissues and shaping of limb*	5–8
4. Growth of the miniature limb to adult size†	>40

*Differentiation: With respect to the appearance and development of the skeleton, the limb structure sequence involves three processes: (1) mesenchymal condensations, (2) Y-shaped branching, forming parallel bones (radius/ulna, tibia/fibula, rays/digits), and (3) segmentation, forming joints.

†Intrauterine growth: Subsequent to limb development, growth continues in the intrauterine environment, subject to the conditions in the womb. With the inmigration of muscles, and formation of joint clefts, intrauterine fetal movement plays a critical role in limb mobility and growth. It is well recognized that anatomic factors such as bicornuate uterus, oligohydramnios, and amniotic bands may exert compressive or constrictive effects on the developing fetus, resulting in a variety of limb deformities, joint contractures (arthrogryposis), or even auto-amputation (Streeter's dysplasia). Maternal exposure to a variety of toxins and teratogens (the classic example is thalidomide) may have a deleterious effect on the formation of the skeletal structures as well, resulting in gross limb deficiencies.

Table 131-4 lists orthopedic abnormalities that are obvious on physical examination of the newborn. Certain limb malformations, such as clubfoot (talipes), tibial absence, or proximal femoral focal deficiency (PFFD), are clearly visualized by intrauterine ultrasonography and may have been diagnosed prior to birth. Problems such as polydactyly, neonatal contractures, asymmetric limb appearance or mobility are readily evident. For the osteochondral dysplasias, measurement of the crown to rump length compared to limb lengths, the head circumference, and the percentile on the growth charts may indicate disproportionate growth of the long bones compared to the flat bones.

Subtle departures from the norm may become more evident during growth and maturation. Klippel-Trenaunay-Weber syndrome is an example of an extensive hemangioma or arteriovenous malformation that causes progressive

Table 131-4. Obvious Orthopedic Anomalies Noted at Birth

Limb Anomalies (Deformed or Absent)

1. Contractures
2. Hypoplasia
3. Hyperplasia
4. Duplication
5. Focal defects

General Skeletal Anomalies (Osteochondral Dysplasias)

1. Rizomelic: proximal limbs most affected
2. Mesomelic: middle portion of limb affected
3. Acromelic: distal (hands and feet) most affected

overgrowth of the involved extremity. A missing fifth toe may be the presenting sign of postaxial hypoplasia, resulting in progressive limb length inequality, knee and ankle valgus, and instability. A dimple or hairy nevus over the lumbosacral spine may reflect spinal dysraphism, with potential spinal cord tethering during growth. Periodic assessment of motor milestones and neurologic development during childhood and growth may reveal latent problems that, although congenital, were not apparent at birth. Asymmetric limb lengths and unilateral, symptomatic, or excessive angular deformities warrant referral and further investigation. These conditions are best evaluated with full-length weight-bearing radiographs.

Sonoembryology has become a standard method of assessing intrauterine fetal development; improved technique and resolution enable the early recognition of specific orthopedic conditions affecting the appendicular and the axial skeleton. Fetal nomograms have been established to assess linear growth of the limbs after the 11th week of gestation. The femur-to-foot ratio should remain 1:1 throughout intrauterine growth. This ratio helps differentiate between intrauterine growth retardation and osteochondral dysplasias. The discovery of a limb anomaly should alert the clinician to the possibility of other problems and warrants a detailed anatomic survey of the fetus. Relative foreshortening of the limbs may be either early or late in onset. The latter may be seen in osteogenesis imperfecta and achondroplasia. This later appearance highlights the benefits of repeated and comparative ultrasonography when monitoring certain abnormalities. Fetal short limbs or polydactyly may serve as a marker for chromosomal anomalies or syndromes, prompting genetic consultation and counseling.

Following birth, a skeletal survey may be helpful in pinpointing the diagnosis and screening for related clinical problems such as hip instability, birth fractures, flat and long bone deformities, and growth disturbances. Because the ossific nucleus of the femoral head may not be visible until the age of 6 months, an ultrasound of the hips may help to differentiate between coxa vara and developmental dislocation of the hip. The orthopedic management of these two conditions differs radically, so it is important to document the true cartilaginous deformity prior to initiating treatment.

In the older ambulatory child, a full-length standing radiograph is invaluable for assessing limb length and alignment problems. The legs should be equal in length and the mechanical axis (center of gravity) should bisect the knee when a line is drawn from the center of the femoral head to the center of the ankle. The diaphysis of each long bone should be straight, and gross assessment of the bone density should be noted. The physes should be horizontal and clearly visible, unless the child is nearing maturity. The appearance of the epiphyses, metaphyses, and diaphyses is noted, along with the apparent density and overall quality of the bones. The proportion and length of the long bones, as well as the mechanical axis, are readily measured on the radiograph. In some cases, a skeletal survey, which includes the upper extremities, spine, and skull, is useful in pinpointing the specific syndrome or diagnosis. Although scanograms or teleroentgenograms are still popular, they demonstrate only a true anteroposterior (AP) view of each joint; diaphyseal deformities cannot be appreciated. Furthermore, they do not include the pelvis or foot, and they are not taken in a weight-bearing position; therefore, the effects of gravity cannot be demonstrated.

"Weight-bearing" (sitting or standing) AP and lateral radiographs of the thoracolumbar spine are useful in detecting scoliosis, kyphosis, or other vertebral anomalies, which may be an integral part of a skeletal dysplasia. Lateral flexion and extension views of the cervical spine may reveal instability patterns that are best recognized prior to surgical intervention requiring intubation; this problem is frequently encountered in children with Down syndrome and Morquio syndrome.

Computed tomography (CT) scan and magnetic resonance imaging (MRI) are reserved for specific situations requiring three-dimensional imaging or cartilage and soft tissue delineation. Recently, bone densitometry has been extended for pediatric usage. However, normative data for younger age groups are still incomplete.

MANAGEMENT

Patients with these disorders require multidisciplinary care. The primary care clinician should coordinate the care, screening for associated medical problems, and referring patients to appropriate health care providers for intervention. For obvious "birth defects," timely orthopedic referral should transpire within the first weeks of birth. Decisions must be made regarding the long-term functional prognosis and the timing of intervention via some combination of bracing, prosthetics, physical or occupational therapy, and surgery. Genetic counseling may be needed to specify the diagnosis and the likelihood of recurrence in future offspring.

Presently the pediatric orthopedist is called on to assess the child and provide the family with a long-range functional prognosis. The familiar questions ("Will he or she walk?" "Will braces or physical therapy be required?" "Will surgery be necessary?") must be anticipated and answered with objectivity and confidence.

For certain teratologic *limb deficiencies*, timely ablation and prosthetic fitting remain the standard of care and may be preferable to "high-tech" limb salvage techniques. The definitive procedure is accomplished before walking age so that the patient and family can adapt readily with minimal down time for the child. Advantages of this approach are the relative simplicity and efficacy—a single operative intervention with early rehabilitation. When specific criteria are met, limb salvage may be more appropriate; this approach may require complex and staged reconstructive surgery, including limb lengthening and joint reduction and stabilization. The family must be well informed, and realistic goals must be established before embarking on this course. Once they commit to this choice, it is difficult to give up and revert to ablation and prosthetic fitting.

Joint instability, due either to intrinsic collagen defects, deficient bone growth, or increasing angular deformity, may compromise function and cause pain. Some of the more common associated conditions seen are Down syndrome, Ehlers-Danlos syndrome, Marfan syndrome, achondroplasia, rickets, and osteogenesis imperfecta. In younger children, bracing may provide temporary reprieve from symptoms caused by flatfeet and ankle or knee instability. However, braces are supportive, not corrective; they are not a definitive solution to the problem. Adaptive physical education and restriction of certain activities (trampolines, gymnastics, contact sports) are wise precautions. Physical therapy may be helpful for strengthening muscles and adapting to activities of daily living, but it has no effect on ligamentous laxity or limb deformity. With increasing forces from growth and increased body mass, skeletal deformities may progress unless surgical correction is undertaken. This correction may require joint stabilization and correction of angular and rotational deformities in order to normalize the forces of gravity and protect the ligaments.

Diaphyseal bowing, as is often encountered in osteogenesis imperfecta, neurofibromatosis, fibrous dysplasia, and rickets, may best be managed with corrective osteotomies and intramedullary pin or rod fixation. For pathologic bone deformities, the rods may be left in place permanently, in order to reinforce the weak bone(s) and to prevent recurrent bowing or fracture. Juxta-articular (epiphyseal or metaphyseal) deformities may warrant corrective osteotomies with cross pin, staple, or plate fixation. Surgical interventions have been extended by the use of techniques for growth manipulation to correct angular deformities and limb-length discrepancies. Around the knee, staples may be applied to one (for angular correction) or both (for length correction) sides of the physis to accomplish a temporary epiphysiodesis or tether. This mechanical bracket effectively inhibits longitudinal growth while the staple(s) are present, and growth resumes upon staple removal. At the ankle a similar effect may be used to correct valgus, using a cannulated screw in the medial malleolus. These minimally invasive techniques are applicable in a wide variety of circumstances and for diverse etiologies. These procedures are performed on an outpatient basis, requiring no cast immobilization and no change in bracing or physical therapy regimens. The caretakers must understand that initially there is no perceived change in alignment; however, as the child grows, there is gradual but steady improvement. The staples and screws are removed when the alignment is neutral and the limb lengths equal. If there is rebound growth leading to recurrent deformity, the technique may be safely repeated. Although staples have been available since 1945, this procedure was reserved for teenagers. However, with further experience, modern imaging, and meticulous technique it has been successfully used in children as young as 3 years old.

Table 131-5. Spondyloepiphyseal Dysplasia Syndromes

Type	Features	Complications
Achondroplasia	Short limbs, long narrow trunk	
	Large head	
	Thoracic gibbous deformity	
	Hydrocephalus	
	Stenosis, foramen magnum	Hypotonia, failure to thrive, quadriparesis, apnea, sudden death
	Stenosis, lumbar spine	Paresthesias, numbness, claudication in the legs, loss of bowel/bladder control
	Frequent otitis, hearing loss	
	Leg bowing	
	Dental crowding	
Achondrogenesis II	Severe shortening of neck, trunk, limbs	Lethal, stillborn or death shortly after birth
	Large soft head	
	Hydrops fetalis	
	Prematurity	
Kniest dysplasia	Short trunk	Motor delay
	Short limbs	Normal intelligence
	Flat face with prominent eyes	Hearing loss
	Cleft palate	Painful joints, flexion contractures with subsequent muscle atrophy
	Club foot	
	Enlarged joints	
Multiple epiphyseal dysplasia	Short stature	Osteoarthritis
	Foreshortened limbs	
Pseudoachondroplasia	Gait abnormalities	Normal development and intelligence
	Short stature	Osteoarthritis
	Joint laxity	
Schmidt metaphyseal dysplasia	Mild short stature	Normal development and intelligence
	Bowing of legs	No extraskeletal symptoms
	Waddling gait	
Spondyloepiphyseal dysplasia congenita	Normal head and face	Normal development and intelligence
	Cleft palate	Waddling gait
	Short neck	Respiratory compromise
	Barrel chest	Spinal cord compression
	Kyphosis	Retinal detachment
	Exaggerated lordosis	Osteoarthritis
	Proximal limb shorter than hands and feet	
Stickler dysplasia (hereditary arthro-ophthalmopathy)	Cleft palate	Severe myopia
	Micrognathia (Pierre Robin syndrome)	Retinal degeneration
		Hearing loss
		Osteoarthritis

Table 131-6. Multidisciplinary Care for Medical Issues in Children with Spondyloepiphyseal Dysplasia Syndromes

Age	Medical Issue	Management/Referral
Newborn	Respiratory distress, upper airway obstruction, apnea	Neonatology, pulmonary
	Recurrence risk to parents	Genetic counseling
	Emotional support	Psychosocial counseling, parent groups
Infancy/childhood	Hydrocephalus	Follow head size closely, referral to neurology/neurosurgery if hydrocephalus suspected
	Spinal cord compression, stenosis of foramen magnum	Computed tomography scan, referral to neurology/neurosurgery
	Instability of cervical vertebrae	Orthopedics/neurosurgery
	Skeletal (kyphosis, scoliosis, lordosis, hip dysplasia)	Orthopedic surgery
	Muscular (hypotonia, contractures)	Physical therapy/occupational therapy
	Otolaryngologic (otitis media, conductive and neurosensory hearing loss)	Ear, nose, and throat; speech and hearing
	Ophthalmologic (cataracts, myopia, retinal detachment, blindness)	Ophthalmology
	Nutritional (obesity)	Nutritionist

Management of children with *skeletal dysplasias* varies with the diagnosis. Table 131-5 lists *spondyloepiphyseal dysplasia* syndromes with their findings and associated features. Table 131-6 lists medical issues with suggestions for management and referral. Many children with these syndromes will have neurosensory hearing loss, visual problems, and osteoarthritis. Surveillance for these problems with appropriate referral is important to their long term health. *Achondroplasia* is the most common chondrodysplasia. Physical abnormalities include short limbs, long narrow trunk, large head with midfacial hypoplasia, large head with prominent forehead, and thoracic gibbus deformity. Although the head is large, only a few will develop hydrocephalus. Careful monitoring of head size, compared to standards for children with achondroplasia, is essential. Stenosis of the spinal canal can occur at the foramen magnum and in the lumbar region. Stenosis of the foramen magnum can lead to central apnea and sudden death, failure to thrive, and hypotonia. At the lumbar level it can lead to paresthesias, numbness, claudication, and eventually loss of bowel and bladder control. Patients should be referred promptly if stenosis is suspected. Other common complications include hearing loss from frequent otitis, bowing of the legs, dental crowding, and obesity.

As the Human Genome project nears completion, the way we perceive, evaluate, and manage congenital bone abnormalities will change profoundly. The historic method of descriptive dysmorphology, which relies on "classic" phenotypic and radiographic features, will yield to more rational and defensible classifications based on understanding of the complex interaction of collagen genes, fibrillin genes, growth factors, and a myriad of other genetic mechanisms that govern the manufacture and maintenance of bony architecture. The evolving field of functional genomics may guide in determining the treatment of choice for future generations.

OUTCOME

Whether congenital bone problems are noted prenatally by intrauterine ultrasound or at birth, or whether they are of insidious onset, they need to be carefully assessed in light of the family history and other organ system involvement or syndromes before initiating treatment. Radiographs of the affected extremity, or of the entire skeleton, serve as a baseline for prognostication and for future comparison. Ultrasound or MRI may be useful in specific patients for visualizing structures that are not observed roentgenographically.

From the orthopedic perspective, a successful outcome could be broadly defined as the improvement in comfort, function, and lifestyle. When possible, bracing should be minimized or eliminated while independent activities of daily living are facilitated. When comparing treatment alternatives, the goal should be to accomplish a successful outcome with the least necessary cost and risk. The treatment and optimal timing of intervention are varied, and these decisions are sometimes difficult; this situation may be compounded by unfiltered information on the Internet and well-meaning advice from people who may lack perspective and expertise. Although research and new technologic wonders hold hope for the future, skeletal growth is inexorable and imparts a certain urgency to be prompt and practical. Orthopedists delight in "straightening things that are crooked." However, this goal is only one component of care; we need validated instruments that are suited for this patient population in order to measure outcomes. Objective input from primary care providers, physical and occupational therapists, orthotists, school teachers, patients, and their families is integral to decision making and to assessing the risk/cost/benefit ratios of our treatment methodologies. Information sharing among support groups and expanding databases will continue to be helpful in redefining and further refining our management skills.

Additional Resources, CD-ROM

Milestones in skeletal sonoembryology	Table
Bibliography	

Table 132-2. Differentiating Bone Formation and Bone Resorption Disorders

Laboratory Test	Bone Formation	Bone Resorption
Serum calcium	Normal or decreased	Normal
Serum phosphate	Decreased	Normal
Calcium × phosphate product	Decreased	Normal
Serum alkaline phosphatase	Increased	Normal
Serum osteocalcin	Increased	Normal
Urine calcium/creatinine	Normal	Increased
Urine phosphate/creatinine	Normal	Increased

Radiographic studies of long bones or the knees may aid in making the diagnosis of MBD (Table 132-3). The presence of fractures, radiolucent bones, and cupping, fraying, or flaring of the epiphysis are suggestive of MBD. Multiple fractures are more indicative of osteogenesis imperfecta. Dense long bones and sclerosis of the skull on x-rays are suggestive of osteopetrosis. Though bony deformities are the hallmark of advanced rickets, weight bearing can exaggerate leg deformities of other disorders. Table 132-4 lists disorders that produce leg bowing and mimic rickets.

SPECIFIC METABOLIC BONE DISEASES

Rickets is a disorder of mineralization of the bone matrix, or osteoid in growing bone. It involves both the growth plate (epiphysis) and newly formed trabecular and cortical bone. Osteomalacia also is a defect in bone matrix mineralization, but it occurs after the cessation of growth and involves only the bone and not the growth plate. The mineralization defect in rickets is mainly a bone formation problem caused by deficiencies in calcium, phosphate, or vitamin D. Low calcium phosphate concentration in the extracellular fluid surrounding rachitic cartilage and bone contributes to the undermineralization. Classification of rickets is shown in Table 132-5.

X-linked hypophosphatemic rickets (also known as familial hypophosphatemic rickets), and vitamin D–dependent rickets (VDDR), types I and II, are rare inborn errors of renal tubular function and vitamin D metabolism. Vitamin D–dependent rickets is inherited as an autosomal recessive trait. Clinical, radiographic, and biochemical features of these disorders are similar to vitamin D–deficiency rickets. However, these disorders do not respond to the usual vitamin D replacement therapy, but may respond to pharmacologic doses of vitamin D (>20,000 IU daily). These disorders differ in the circulating concentrations of 1,25-dihydroxyvitamin D, the therapeutic response to vitamin D, and obviously in their primary defect. Table 132-6 lists the different types of rickets, common laboratory findings, and the therapeutic response to vitamin D. X-linked hypophosphatemic rickets has an abnormality in the renal proximal tubule that impairs phosphate reabsorption. Vitamin D–dependent rickets, type I, has a defect in renal 25-hydroxyvitamin D 1-hydroxylase enzyme with low concentrations of 1,25-dihydroxyvitamin D, and the type II disorder has a presumed intracellular 1,25-dihydroxyvitamin D receptor defect with normal or elevated 1,25-dihydroxyvitamin D levels.

Table 132-4. Conditions That Produce Leg Bowing and Mimic Rickets

Conditions	Specific Disorders
Intrinsic diseases of bone	Achondrodysplasia
	Chondrodysplasias (metaphyseal)
	Jansen
	Schmid
	McKusick
Growth-cartilage hyperplasia	Ollier disease
Genetic mucopolysaccharides	Morquio syndrome
	Hurler syndrome
Hormonal disorders	Hypo- and hypergonadism
	Hypo- and hyperpituitarism
	Hypo- and hyperthyroidism
	Hypo- and hypercortisolism
	Parathyroid disorders
	Primary or secondary hyperparathyroidism
Nutritional deficiencies	Vitamin C deficiency (scurvy)
Localized disorders	Blount disease
	Mechanical trauma
	Radiation
	Myelodysplasias

Table 132-5. Classification of Rickets

Type of Disturbance	Specific Disorders
Calcium and phosphate	Dietary calcium deficiency
	Dietary vitamin D deficiency
	Vitamin D malabsorption
	Sunlight deficiency
	Liver disease
	Drug-related enzyme induction—anticonvulsants
	Deficiency of 25-hydroxyvitamin D$_1$ α-hydroxylase (vitamin D–dependent type 1)
	End-organ unresponsiveness to 1,25-hydroxyvitamin D$_2$ (vitamin D–dependent type II, resistant rickets)
	Renal osteodystrophy
Phosphate	Renal tubular disorder with loss of phosphorus
	Fanconi syndrome
	Hereditary hypophosphatemic rickets
	X-linked hypophosphatemic rickets
	Renal tubular acidosis
	Low phosphorus intake
	Dietary phosphorus deficiency—human milk
	Phosphorus malabsorption—antacid use, short guts
	Total parenteral alimentation

Table 132-3. X-ray Findings of Metabolic Bone Disease

Disease	Bone Mass	Fractures
Rickets	Decreased	Few
Osteoporosis	Decreased	Few
Osteogenesis imperfecta	Very decreased	Multiple
Osteopetrosis	Increased	Few

Table 132-6. Usual Laboratory Findings in Different Types of Rickets

Condition	Serum Calcium	Serum Phosphate	Serum Alkaline Phosphatase	Serum 1,25-(OH)$_2$-Vitamin D	Serum Parathyroid Hormone	Urine Amino Acids	Response to Vitamin D
Vitamin D deficiency	Dec	Dec	Inc	Normal	Inc	Inc	Good
X-linked hypophosphatemic	Normal	Dec	Inc	Normal	Normal	Normal	Fair to large doses
Vitamin D–dependent type I	Dec	Dec	Inc	Dec	Inc	Inc	Fair to large doses
Vitamin D–dependent type II	Normal	Dec	Inc	Inc	Inc or normal	Inc or normal	Poor

Dec, decrease; inc, increase.

The diagnosis of osteoporosis in children is usually made when skeletal radiographs reveal a generalized decrease in mineralized bone. During bone remodeling, bone resorption is increased in osteoporosis. However, an inherited group of disorders known as osteogenesis imperfecta usually represents defects in bone-forming cells in which mutations in one of the two gene-encoding type I procollagens produce a defective matrix. Table 132-7 shows a classification of osteoporosis.

Osteogenesis imperfecta (OI) is an inheritable congenital form of osteoporosis and is often called brittle bone disease. The pathogenesis of all types of OI centers on a qualitative or quantitative abnormality of the most abundant protein in bone, type I collagen that is produced by the osteoblasts. The clinical hallmark of OI is osteoporosis associated with recurrent fractures and skeletal deformity. However, type I collagen is also present in teeth, ligaments, skin, and sclera. Many patients with OI have dental disease caused by defective formation of dentin (dentinogenesis imperfecta) as well as abnormalities of other tissues that contain this fibrous protein. Joint hypermotility and lax skin are common in this disorder. Besides the defective collagen synthesis, OI also has increased bone resorption from increased number of osteoclasts. Table 132-8 shows classification of OI by inheritance and clinical findings.

Osteopetrosis (marble bone disease) is inherited as an autosomal dominant benign or an autosomal recessive malignant disease. The pathogenesis of this MBD is diminished or absent osteoclasts with the resultant accumulation of unresorbed bone matrix. Benign osteopetrosis is often asymptomatic but can manifest as a developmental disorder. The long bones are brittle and fractures can occur. Deafness, facial palsy, visual or auditory impairment, progressive leukoerythroblastic anemia, and osteoarthritis can be part of the presentation. The malignant form begins in infancy and presents with growth failure, nasal stuffiness from malformations of paranasal sinuses, and neurologic impairment of optic, oculomotor, and facial nerves from narrowed cranial foramina.

Management
The principles of therapy are promotion of linear growth without skeletal deformities, avoidance of drug toxicity, and genetic counseling. Table 132-9 outlines the medical approach to MBDs.

In disorders of bone formation, osteoblast activity is increased from mineral or vitamin D deficiencies but the rate of bone formation is decreased. Therapy should be aimed at correcting the deficiencies and increasing bone formation. All children with MBD should be ingesting adequate amounts of calcium (Table 132-10). Vitamin D–deficient rickets should be treated with 800 to 1600 IU of vitamin D daily. In vitamin D–dependent rickets, type I, in which the 1,25-dihydroxyvitamin D levels are low, giving 1,25-dihydroxyvitamin D (calcitriol) has promoted bone mineralization and healing.

Bone loss from increased bone resorption requires that the osteoclast activity decreases or stabilizes. Estrogen, calcitonin, and bisphosphonates have emerged as antiosteoclast agents but are of limited use in pediatric subjects. Estrogen therapy has been used in adolescents with Turner syndrome and amenorrhea. Calcitonin has been tried in subjects with OI, but bisphosphonates appear to be more beneficial.

Immobilization causes bone loss, and physical activity or exercise appears to stimulate bone mass in children and adolescents. Although the type and duration of load-bearing activity on the children's bones are unknown, routine physical activity is recommended for children with MBD.

Referral
An orthopedist and physical therapist should evaluate all children with skeletal deformities of the long bones or spine. Children on hormonal therapy should be evaluated

Table 132-7. Classification of Osteoporosis

Type of Disorder	Specific Diseases
Congenital	Osteogenesis imperfecta
Juvenile	Paget disease
Immobilization	
Endocrine	Hyperthyroidism
	Diabetes mellitus
	Hyperadrenocorticism
	Growth hormone deficiency
	Hypogonadism
Arthritic	Juvenile rheumatoid arthritis
Genetic	Turner syndrome
	Down syndrome
Metabolic	Cystic fibrosis
	Riley-Day syndrome
	Menke syndrome
	Marfan syndrome
	Ehlers-Danlos syndrome
Blood	Leukemia
	Lymphoma
	Waldenström's macroglobulinemia
	Multiple myeloma
	Heparin therapy
Malnutrition	Vitamin C deficiency
	Protein deficiency

Table 132-8. Classification of Osteogenesis Imperfecta

Type	Inheritance	Clinical Findings
Type I	AD	Bone fragility and blue sclerae, scoliosis and growth retardation, hearing loss, walks independently
Type II	AD or AR	Marked bone fragility in utero and blue sclerae, perinatal death
Type III	AD or AR	Bone fragility and growth retardation, mild blue sclerae
Type IV	AD	Osteoporosis, bone fragility and fractures with long bone deformities, normal sclerae

AD, autosomal dominant; AR, autosomal recessive.

and followed by an endocrinologist. The physical therapist may help in providing a physical exercise program and may provide developmental assistance.

A nephrologist should be consulted for all children with renal tubular disorders causing MBD. Phosphate, vitamin D and its metabolites, and calcium supplementation require close follow-up.

Hearing and eyes should be evaluated in MBD. Sensorineural hearing loss is prominent in children with OI and osteopetrosis. Infants with osteopetrosis may develop optic nerve atrophy. Blindness, corneal opacification, and glaucoma have been reported in OI.

Follow-up

Generalists should follow the child's linear growth closely. Any progressive bone deformities, delays in functional motor capabilities, or recurrent fractures require yearly monitoring and appropriate referral. Careful evaluation of progressive scoliosis greater than 50 degrees or kyphosis greater

Table 132-9. General Therapy for Metabolic Bone Disorders

Actions	Bone Formation	Bone Resorption
Bone cell effect	Osteoblast increase	Osteoclast stabilization
Target	Low bone turnover	High bone turnover
Medications	Calcium, phosphate, vitamin D	Estrogen, calcitonin, bisphosphonates

Table 132-10. Daily Calcium Requirements

Age	Calcium Requirement
Birth to 6 months	400 mg
6–12 months	600 mg
1–5 years	800 mg
6–10 years	800–1200 mg
11–24 years	1200–1500 mg

than 45 degrees should be made to avoid complications of the child's pulmonary function and neurologic loss of motor or sensory function. Generally, progressive spinal deformities decrease after puberty.

Because of the bone deformities and limited physical and developmental capabilities, the generalist should assist patients with MBD in obtaining the optimal quality of life. Daily problems of care for the family should be minimized. Special education services and nursing care should be available. Efforts should be made to reduce physical barriers in the home, school, and community.

Mini-index of Related Topics CH.

SUGGESTED READINGS

Avioli LV, Krane SM: Metabolic Bone Disease and Clinically Related Disorders. San Diego, Academic Press, 1998.

Castells S, Finberg L: Metabolic Bone Disease in Children. New York, Marcel Dekker, 1990.

DeLuca HF, Constantine A: Pediatric Diseases Related to Calcium. New York, Elsevier, 1980.

Favus MJ: Primer on the Metabolic Bone Diseases and Disorders of Mineral Metabolism. Philadelphia, Lippincott Williams & Wilkins, 1999.

Maroteaux P: Bone Diseases of Children. Philadelphia, JB Lippincott, 1979.

133 Long-term Medical Management of Children with Heart Disease

Paul C. Young and Scott Yeager

ROLE OF THE GENERALIST

1 Provide a competent and credible Medical Home for the child with heart disease.

2 Perform regular monitoring related to the child's heart disease.

3 Recognize all clinically important alterations in cardiac function.

4 Understand the appropriate dosing, actions, adverse effects, and potential drug interactions of cardiac medications.

5 Recognize the signs and symptoms of complications that may result from the child's heart disease or its treatment.

6 Recognize how heart disease affects the management of common childhood illnesses.

7 Understand the long-term history of and potential problems of both treated and untreated specific cardiac lesions.

8 Provide guidance regarding exercise and sports participation.

9 Provide appropriate prophylaxis to prevent endocarditis.

The generalist responsible for providing care for a child with heart disease will be most successful employing the model of the Medical Home that provides regular health supervision (well-child care); all standard immunizations as well as those indicated as a result of the child's heart condition (e.g., influenza); periodic evaluations for problems of health, growth, behavior, or development; and anticipatory guidance (nutrition, injury prevention, behavior, development, promotion of a healthy lifestyle). In addition, to provide the required level of comprehensive pediatric care, the generalist must make the commitment to acquire the skills, knowledge, and attitudes about the patient's heart condition to be competent in meeting the child's needs and, perhaps of equal importance, to appear credible to the family and the child's cardiologist. All too frequently, the child's primary care clinician is bypassed when the child with a heart condition is ill or when other issues arise. A primary care clinician who has developed a relationship with the family and with the child is ideally suited to

provide the long-term clinical monitoring and care relevant to both the heart condition and the child's general health and to provide all the other components of an ideal Medical Home. Clarifying with the family and the specialists that the generalist expects to and is capable of playing a primary role in the child's medical care is of utmost importance in overcoming any real or potential barriers.

The chapters on long-term management of children with cardiac conditions provide a description of the issues that confront generalists as they assume primary care responsibility for a child with an abnormal heart. Although there are many similarities in management that are independent of the specific lesion or conditions, important differences require an understanding of the particular child's anatomy, physiology, and therapy. Generalist must be certain that they have received this information in a comprehensible and pragmatic way.

MONITORING THE CHILD WITH HEART DISEASE

The initial step in providing ongoing care is to determine what parameters should be monitored and with what frequency. Creating a child-specific flow sheet (an example for a 3-year-old child who is status post Fontan procedure is shown in Table 133-1) can be a useful and efficient method of guiding the visit, recognizing changes, and communicating with the family and child and with the child's cardiologist. The generalist must communicate with the child's cardiologist to define parameters of the child's condition and identify what constitutes important changes from baseline. Following the child for the wrong issues is as much of an error as not following him for the right ones. Depending on the child's age, the *subjective data* might include the following: feeding problems, respiratory symptoms, exercise tolerance, intercurrent illnesses, hospitalizations, emergency department visits, school attendance, and oxygen needs. *Objective* data would include growth measures, vital signs, color or oxygen saturation, indicators of congestive heart failure (respiratory rate, heart rate, gallop, liver size, crackles, edema, etc.), changes in murmurs (particularly those related to shunts, conduits, valves), and rhythm changes. *Laboratory tests*, such as hemoglobin for children with low oxygen saturation or electrolytes for those on diuretics, may be indicated. The child's medications and his adherence to the prescribed schedule should be recorded.

Table 133-1. Flow Sheet for Monitoring Child with Heart Disease

Date					
Height/length					
Weight					
Blood pressure					
Pulse					
Respiratory rate					
Oxygen saturation					
Feeding/nutrition					
Activity					
Illnesses					
ED visits					
Hospitalization					
Oxygen need					
Lungs					
Rhythm					
Murmur					
Liver					
Pulses					
Digoxin					
Lasix					
Aldactone					
ASA					
Hemoglobin					
Lab results					
Problems?					
Notes					

The frequency of visits to the generalist depends on the nature of the child's problem, her age, her cardiovascular status and function, the frequency of her visits to her specialist and the time and effort required to travel to the medical center. More frequent visits should be considered early in the course of the relationship between the patient and the generalist in order to establish the generalist's role in the child's ongoing care. Although it may be possible to combine a well-child or health supervision visit with one directed toward the heart disease, it is better to schedule these appointments separately so that each issue can receive the attention it requires. Although many experienced generalists are able to comfortably "shift gears" between primary care and secondary care issues in the same visit, regular visits specifically directed toward the issues relevant to the heart disease help to focus the attention of both the physician and the family. In addition, systematic visits directed toward the child's cardiovascular status provide the essential background from which to recognize important changes. Also, health maintenance issues, particularly developmental assessment, family and school problems, and anticipatory guidance, can easily be overlooked unless preventive care visits are scheduled separately.

Recognizing Changes

When a child with heart disease displays signs or symptoms that are concerning to the parent or physician, it is important to distinguish between problems related to worsening of cardiac status, an intercurrent and unrelated problem, or a combination of the two. Sometimes an illness can increase the demands on an already compromised cardiovascular system, resulting in signs or symptoms of congestive heart failure. Alternatively, tachypnea, tachycardia, and poor feeding may be related to a minor self-limited viral illness. Like many situations in primary care that are characterized by uncertainty, the generalist has three general options to assist decision making: obtain consultation, order a test (e.g., a chest x-ray to look for cardiomegaly), or a therapeutic trial of an intervention (which may be only observation) combined with careful follow-up.

Congestive heart failure (CHF) can develop acutely or insidiously and should be looked for carefully in any child with actual or potential decreased myocardial contractility; a residual, persisting, or surgically created left-to-right shunt; or incompetence with regurgitation of the mitral or aortic valve or in situations that can result in volume overload such as intravenous fluid therapy. The clinical findings associated with CHF are listed in Box 133-1. In young infants, the effort associated with feeding from the breast or bottle may result in them having to stop to "catch their breath" and often results in sweating that can be seen on the forehead. Toddlers and older children are more likely to have decreased appetite and activity. In the context of potential air trapping associated with bronchiolitis or other pulmonary disease the liver may be displaced and appear to be enlarged; percussing the span to assess size may be helpful. Although the specificity and sensitivity of delayed capillary refill has been questioned, the examiner must consider it along with the strength of the pulses, color, and blood pressure in making an assessment of the child's perfusion. Edema is a less common manifestation of CHF in

children than in adults, but subtle changes in facial puffiness (typically more obvious to the parents) or in dependent regions (i.e., the sacral area) should be searched for.

Pulmonary hypertension can develop in children with chronic heart disease—particularly in those who have large left-to-right shunts or conditions associated with impaired pulmonary venous return, including mitral stenosis, anomalous pulmonary venous return with obstruction, or left-sided obstructive lesions such as aortic stenosis or coarctation of the aorta. Children with Down syndrome are particularly prone to develop pulmonary hypertension and may do so even after surgical repair of, for example, their endocardial cushion defect.

Symptoms, signs, electrocardiogram (ECG), and x-ray findings of pulmonary hypertension are listed in Box 133-2. Symptoms typically develop gradually, but some, such as hemoptysis, can be quite dramatic and ominous. Pulmonary hypertension can cause chest pain. A single or very narrowly split and loud second heart sound in a child in whom it was previously normal should alert the physician to the possibility of pulmonary hypertension.

When the generalist is concerned that pulmonary hypertension is present or worsening, contact and referral to the child's cardiologist should be undertaken promptly. In the primary care or community hospital setting, oxygen and ventilatory support may be initiated, but treatment for this condition is likely to be difficult and complex.

Medications are usually an important part of the treatment of children with functionally significant heart disease and should be monitored as part of the scheduled visits. It is important to verify adherence to prescribed doses and schedules (Chapter 279). Changes in the child's status may be associated with failure to give medications as prescribed. Familiarity with the appropriate doses, potential side effects, and drug interactions is essential. Some patients may be taking prescribed drugs with which the generalist is unfamiliar because they are relatively new or because experience with their use in children is limited. In the latter case, it is particularly important that the cardiologist

---

Box 133-1. Symptoms and Signs of Congestive Heart Failure

Symptoms

Tachypnea
Difficulty feeding, sweating with feeding
Decreased exercise tolerance
Irritability
Poor sleep
Poor or dusky color

Signs

Tachypnea
Crackles on lung examination
Tachycardia
Gallop rhythm
Hepatomegaly
Decreased perfusion (pulses, capillary refill, color)
Edema

X-ray

Cardiomegaly
Increased vascular markings

Box 133-2. Clinical Manifestations of Pulmonary Hypertension

Symptoms

Dyspnea and fatigue
Headache, syncope
Chest pain, hemoptysis

Signs

Cyanosis
Clubbing
Hepatomegaly, edema, other signs of right-sided heart failure
Prominent single second heart sound

Electrocardiogram

Right-axis deviation and right ventricular hypertrophy

Chest X-ray

Heart size normal unless congestive heart failure present
Prominent main pulmonary artery segment with clear lung fields

Table 133-2. Commonly Used Chronic Medications in Pediatric Cardiac Patients

Medication	Category	Approximate Maintenance Dose	Common Side Effects	Drug Interactions	Comments
Digoxin	Inotrope	5–10 µg/kg/day, 2 doses	Arrhythmias, nausea, vomiting	Diuretics	Increased potential for side effects with hypokalemia (diuretics, gastroenteritis)
Fursosemide	Loop diuretic	1–6 mg/kg/day, 2–3 doses	Hypokalemia, hyperuricemia, azotemia, rash	Digoxin	
Spironolactone	Diuretic (aldosterone antagonist, potassium-sparing)	1–3 mg/kg/day, 1–3 doses	Hyperkalemia	ACE inhibitors	Additive effect for hyperkalemia with ACE inhibitors
Captopril	ACE inhibitor	Infant: 0.5–0.6 mg/kg/day, 1–4 doses Child: 12.5 mg per dose, 1–2 times per day	Hypotension	Diuretics	
Enalapril	ACE inhibitor	0.1 mg/kg per dose, 1–2 times daily; maximum: 0.5 mg/kg/day	Hypotension	Diuretics	
Verapamil	Calcium-channel blocker	3–5 mg/kg/day, 3 times daily	Hypotension, bradycardia, cardiac depression	β-Adrenergic blockers	
Aspirin	Anticoagulant (antiplatelet)	3–5 mg/kg/day, once daily	Bleeding	Warfarin	
Warfarin	Anticoagulant	1–5 mg/day, once daily	Bleeding	Aspirin, NSAIDs	Keep INR at 2.5–3.5

ACE, angiotensin-converting enzyme; INR, international normalized ratio; NSAIDs, nonsteroidal anti-inflammatory drugs.

communicate information about the medication and its effects to the generalist. Table 133-2 lists some of the more commonly used chronic medications, their usual maintenance doses, important side effects, and potential drug interactions. Antiarrhythmic medications and transplant-related medications are discussed in Chapters 59, 135, and 136.

COMMUNICATION WITH THE CHILD'S CARDIOLOGIST

Although most generalists anticipate receiving information regarding their patient's visits to specialists, it has not been standard practice for the results of visits to generalists to be communicated back to the specialist. In the model of shared care, data collected and recorded on a flow sheet could be easily transmitted by fax or e-mail (or by "snail" mail) between the child's physicians or other providers (Chapter 123). The cardiologist may recognize a change or problem from the data that was not apparent to the generalist at the time of the visit or may be reassured that the child is doing well. This two-way flow of information also facilitates access for the generalist on those occasions when the need for urgent communication arises.

The concept of *family-centered care* is important for all children with chronic conditions or special needs, and sending copies to the parents of all communications about their child should be the general rule. Occasionally a family will need assistance in meeting the complex needs of their child; making this issue explicit and identifying the resources in the community or at the medical center that can provide assistance is much more likely to be helpful than ignoring the problem or not acknowledging that one exists.

PROBLEMS AND COMPLICATIONS

Depending on the particular condition, children with heart disease may be more likely to develop certain problems or complications when compared to children without heart disease. Because of this increased underlying prevalence, certain signs or symptoms may have an increased or more specific *positive predictive value* for the condition in question. Management may need to be altered for some relatively common problems such as upper respiratory or gastrointestinal infections based on the child's cardiac problem or its treatment.

Altered Mental Status

When a child with heart disease presents with sudden changes in neurologic status, the generalist must strongly consider the possibility of a cerebrovascular accident (CVA) or a brain abscess. Conditions that are associated with either cyanosis or right-to-left shunts predispose the child to a CVA, the former because of increased viscosity of the blood, the latter because of the risk of paradoxical emboli. Relative or mild iron deficiency in children who have a need for higher hemoglobin results in the production of microcytes. These small cells appear to be less deformable and may contribute to the risk of stroke. Younger infants with cyanosis, especially those under 1 year, are at highest risk. Febrile illnesses, especially those associated with dehydration, are frequent triggering events. Signs and symptoms can include hemiplegia or other, more focal, motor deficits, seizures, ataxia, and confusion. A *brain abscess* must be considered in any child with cardiac disease with acute neurologic changes. Fever or other signs of infection may be present, but their absence does not exclude abscess. Recent events such as dental work, surgery, or trauma that might have led to bacteremia or endocarditis may be contributory. Immediate imaging by computed tomography (CT) or magnetic resonance imaging (MRI) should be followed by other studies and consultation as indicated. Important preventive interventions are ensuring adequate iron intake for cyanotic infants, attention to appropriate prophylaxis against bacterial endocarditis, and prompt recognition and treatment of dehydration.

Fever

Although most children with heart disease do not have increased susceptibility to serious infections (children with asplenia associated with hetertotaxy syndromes *do* have an increased risk), the presence of fever deserves special consideration because of the possibility of endocarditis and the increased metabolic demands imposed by an elevated temperature. The generalist must always consider the possibility of infective endocarditis when evaluating a febrile child with heart disease. Clues from the history include a recent localized infection such as cellulitis, a urinary tract infection, and a history of recent dental work or surgery. Suggestive physical findings include a change in the murmur, splenomegaly, or petechiae. However, in most febrile children, these findings will be absent, and the generalist must maintain a high index of suspicion. Children who do not appear particularly toxic and who have a clear source for the fever on examination need only careful follow-up, but in those who do not have such a focus, blood cultures should be obtained. Starting antibiotics without a clear indication and doing so without first obtaining at least one blood culture is not advisable. The patient will be better served by careful follow-up examinations. Because of the increasing metabolic demand, fever from any cause may be poorly tolerated by children whose cardiac function is compromised, and reduction of the fever with appropriate antipyretic therapy is essential.

Respiratory Infections

Children with heart disease have the same risk for developing respiratory infections as other children, but the generalist needs to consider whether the illness has the potential to have a significant impact on the child's functioning. For children at risk for cardiac failure, the additional stress imposed by the illness can precipitate decompensation. The changes may be subtle and difficult to differentiate from those associated with the respiratory illness. A chest x-ray to evaluate heart size and for the presence of lower respiratory infection may be helpful. The generalist should be alert for signs or symptoms suggesting pneumonia in children with increased pulmonary blood flow from a left-to-right shunt because some seem to be at increased risk of developing secondary bacterial lower respiratory tract infections when they have colds. Children with increased pulmonary resistance or existing pulmonary hypertension tolerate lower respiratory tract infections poorly and their symptoms may worsen significantly. Those with single ventricle physiology, with Glenn or Fontan connection, may do particularly poorly with increased pulmonary vascular resistance as pulmonary blood flow is by a passive mechanism.

Management of viral or bacterial respiratory infections does not differ from children without heart disease, but it may be necessary to carefully monitor the respiratory status and provide additional respiratory support.

Despite a lack of proved efficacy, decongestant and other cough and cold medications are widely used by parents. Parents should be advised to avoid those that contain sympathomimetic compounds such as pseudoephedrine. Antibiotics should be given only when there is clear evidence of a bacterial infection. Effective preventive interventions include immunization against influenza and *Streptococcus pneumoniae*. The role of palivizumab in children with heart disease to prevent respiratory syncytial virus (RSV) infection is, currently, uncertain. The use of RSV immune globulin in children with cyanotic congenital heart disease has been associated with poor outcomes and is not recommended. A decision to use palivizumab in an infant who meets the criteria based on prematurity or pulmonary disease but who also has heart disease should be made in conjunction with the child's cardiologist.

Gastroenteritis and Dehydration

Gastrointestinal illnesses can complicate the care of children with heart disease in several ways: Vomiting may result in the child being unable to keep down needed medications. Diuretics may need to be adjusted if dehydration appears to be developing. Because the risk of a CVA or clotting off shunts or conduits is increased if the child develops hemoconcentration from dehydration, maintaining adequate fluid intake is crucial. In children whose cardiac reserve is limited, any illness can precipitate CHF.

In most children with viral gastroenteritis, small amounts of fluids along with their medications will be tolerated. As a rule of thumb, if the child keeps the medication down for 20 to 30 minutes, it is not necessary to repeat it. Diuretics should usually be held in a child with symptoms of dehydration such as decreased urine output, dry mucus membranes, or decreased tear production. Electrolytes should be checked in children with evidence of dehydration. Once the child is able to take oral fluids diuretics can be restarted unless the stool volume loss remains quite high or electrolyte abnormalities are present. If diuretics are held, the child must be carefully monitored for evidence of CHF. In most situations, oral administration of electrolyte-containing fluids is advisable to prevent dehydration or to rehydrate the child with mild dehydration, rather than immediate employment of intravenous fluids.

SLOW WEIGHT GAIN AND GROWTH DELAY

Frequent assessment of weight gain and growth are important in any child with heart disease, but are crucial in young infants awaiting surgery until they reach a certain age or size. Increased energy expenditure, fatigue with feeding, and the need to avoid excessive volumes of formula can all contribute to slow weight gain. Formulas with higher caloric density, such as 24, 27, or even 30 kcal per ounce, may be required. Supplementation using feeding tubes, particularly at night, may be needed. In some situations it may be necessary to utilize a gastrostomy tube to provide adequate nutrition. The generalist should be prepared to advise parents on implementing these approaches or be sufficiently familiar with the community's resources in order to make appropriate referrals.

Older children whose cardiac status is close to normal usually grow appropriately. Excessive weight gain, particularly in less active children, is a significant problem. Prevention or intervention at the earliest sign that the child is becoming overweight may be easier and more effective than treatment efforts once obesity is established.

Delayed Development and Psychological Problems

As a group, children with congenital heart disease have lower IQ scores than their siblings or physically normal children. Usually the differences are mild, typically averaging 5 to 10 IQ points. Differences are larger in children with cyanotic heart disease. Often, delayed motor development is seen initially, but many overcome delays and appear normal as they become older. As in any chronic illness, threats to the psychological well-being of the child resulting from being different, being subjected to surgery and other invasive interventions, and anxiety about being ill and possibly dying are present and place the child and family at risk. It is important to be alert for evidence of the development of a "vulnerable child syndrome." The generalist should take the lead in monitoring motor, intellectual, and psychological development as part of the ongoing care of the child and provide further evaluation and early intervention whenever deviations from normal are suspected.

MANAGEMENT OF CHILDREN WITH SPECIFIC CARDIAC LESIONS

Box 133-3 lists the categories of specific cardiac lesions to be discussed in this section.

Lesions with Excessive Pulmonary Blood Flow (Left-to-Right Shunts)

As a group these lesion (ventricular septal defects, atrial septal defects, atrioventricular defects, and patent ductus arteriosus) cause increased pulmonary blood flow that can result in CHF or pulmonary hypertension.

Children with small membranous or muscular *ventricular septal defects* are often followed for up to a year or longer

---

Box 133-3. Lesions to Be Considered in Management of Heart Disease

1. Lesions with *excessive* pulmonary blood flow (left-to-right shunts): ventricular septal defect, atrial septal defect, atrioventricular septal defect, patent ductus arteriosus
2. Lesions with *inadequate* pulmonary blood flow: tetralogy of Fallot, pulmonary stenosis, pulmonary atresia
3. Left-sided obstructive lesions: aortic stenosis, coarctation of the aorta, interrupted aortic arch
4. Regurgitant lesions: mitral insufficiency, aortic insufficiency
5. Complex lesions: transposition of the great vessels
6. Single ventricle lesions
7. Coronary artery abnormalities (including aneurysms from Kawasaki disease)
8. Cardiomyopathies: dilated and hypertrophic

---

while awaiting spontaneous closure. Complete closure occurs in approximately 40% to 50% of these children; in some children the defect will become smaller without completely closing. Infants in this age group are seen every 2 to 3 months for well-child care, so following the child's growth and murmur can be done conveniently during these visits. If the murmur disappears and closure is confirmed by echocardiography, the child does not require further follow up or subacute bacterial endocarditis (SBE) prophylaxis. Children with remaining small defects will be asymptomatic but do require SBE prophylaxis. Occasionally, patients with hemodynamically small ventricular septal defects will develop other important complications, including prolapse of the aortic valve into the defect with resultant aortic regurgitation or the development of obstructive muscle in the right ventricular chamber resulting in subpulmonary stenosis.

Children with large defects, for whom closure is planned, will often have surgery delayed until the child reaches a certain size. During this interval, which may last for several months or more, the generalist should monitor for feeding problems resulting in failure to grow appropriately and for evidence of CHF. On occasion it will be necessary to use concentrated formulas or nasogastric feeding for the child to gain weight. Restriction of volume of oral feedings is unnecessary; it is extremely unlikely that an infant will "eat himself into failure." Typically, these children will be receiving diuretics, and some will be on digoxin.

Three types of *atrial septal defects* are recognized. *Secundum defects* (those in the midportion of the atrial septum) are usually diagnosed in patients with an asymptomatic murmur. Approximately 50% of secundum atrial septal defects diagnosed in the first year of life will close spontaneously or will become clinically insignificant. Follow-up in the first few years of life for these children is directed toward determining whether closure has occurred, because these defects seldom close beyond 2 or 3 years of age. Some cardiologists believe that patients with large atrial shunts are at increased risk for recurrent pulmonary infections, but other complications are rare. Moderate or large defects that are present after 3 years of age require surgical or transcatheter closure to prevent long-term complications. *Primum defects*, which involve the portion of the atrial septum nearest to the atrioventricular valves, do not close spontaneously and are almost always associated with mitral valve abnormalities. These defects require surgical intervention. Following surgery, these children must be monitored for development of significant and progressive mitral regurgitation. The least common form of atrial septal defect, the *sinus venosus defect*, is typically associated with anomalies of pulmonary venous drainage that must be redirected at the time of surgical closure. The primary care clinician should be aware that these patients are at risk for sinus node dysfunction, superior vena caval obstruction, and stenosis of one or more pulmonary veins, usually from the right lung.

Endocardial cushion or *atrioventricular defects* are commonly, but not exclusively, found in children with Down syndrome. These lesions result in varying degrees of atrial and ventricular shunting. Associated symptoms depend on the size and location of the shunt. CHF in infancy is common in patients with large ventricular communications. Significant atrioventricular valve regurgitation may be a superimposed and complicating feature. Following surgical repair, these patients should be followed carefully for the development of conduction abnormalities such as heart block They may also develop late progressive mitral regurgitation.

Patients with *patent ductus arteriosus* (PDA) diagnosed beyond the neonatal period are usually recognized because of the characteristic murmur. A large PDA may result in symptoms of CHF. In some cases, there may be very significant left ventricular enlargement and, occasionally, mitral regurgitation. Patients with an audible ductal murmur should be referred to a pediatric cardiologist. PDAs are closed either surgically or by transcatheter techniques. Children with an isolated patent ductus who have undergone successful ductal ligation or closure do not require long-term follow-up.

Lesions Characterized by Inadequate Pulmonary Blood Flow

Tetralogy of Fallot with Pulmonary Stenosis or Pulmonary Atresia

The pathophysiology of tetralogy of Fallot (TOF) includes both decreased pulmonary blood flow and cyanosis. Anatomically TOF consists of right ventricular hypertrophy, overriding aorta, anterior malalignment ventricular septal defect, and obstruction of the right ventricular outflow tract. Correction of TOF can be either by an *initial complete repair* or a *staged repair* followed in 3 to 18 months by a complete repair (Chapter 134). Children whose repair will be staged first have an operation to create a systemic to pulmonary artery shunt to allow for growth. Timing of the complete repair depends on adequate growth and development of increasing cyanosis as the shunt is outgrown. The primary care physician needs to follow these children carefully to detect increasing cyanosis, decreasing growth rate, or the development of other problems that could compromise the success of the definitive surgery.

Pulmonary Stenosis and Subpulmonary Stenosis

Decisions regarding the need for and timing of treatment for *pulmonary stenosis* depend on severity. Valvar pulmonary stenosis that is more than mild in degree will usually be detected in the newborn because of a prominent and typical murmur. If the obstruction is sufficiently severe, the infant will demonstrate systemic cyanosis from right-to-left atrial shunting, usually an indication for balloon dilation of the pulmonary valve within the first few days of life. Less severe obstruction presents as an asymptomatic murmur. Unlike aortic stenosis, valvar pulmonary stenosis seldom progresses after the first few months of life. Mild obstruction in early childhood will probably continue indefinitely. Patients whose pressure gradient across the pulmonary valve exceeds 40 to 50 mm Hg are candidates for balloon dilation. This procedure is very safe and effective, usually resulting in lasting relief of obstruction. Patients whose gradient is not sufficiently severe to require balloon dilation will almost never have cardiac symptoms, and their activity should not be restricted. Endocarditis prophylaxis is required for all.

Subpulmonary stenosis, unlike valvar obstruction, is often progressive and is frequently associated with other intracardiac abnormalities such as a ventricular septal defect, TOF, or with more complex cyanotic heart disease. Because of its muscular and progressive nature this lesion generally requires surgical resection.

Left-Sided Obstructive Lesions: Aortic Stenosis and Coarctation of the Aorta

Valvar aortic stenosis is progressive. The rate of progression is quite variable. In some children, the gradient across the aortic valve may increase significantly over a period of 6 to 12 months. In others, the stenosis remains virtually unchanged throughout childhood and into young adult life. Factors influencing the rate of progression are unclear. Most patients with valvar aortic stenosis eventually develop aortic regurgitation. The generalist should be aware that most children with aortic stenosis, even severe stenosis, are asymptomatic. Decisions regarding intervention are based on an echocardiographic estimate of the gradient across the valve. Intervention by balloon dilation of the valve ideally is undertaken prior to the development of clinically evident problems. The generalist must ensure that these patients are being followed at regular intervals by a pediatric cardiologist. Symptoms include dyspnea on exertion, exertional, chest pain, and rarely, syncope. Of these, only exertional dyspnea is commonly encountered in childhood. Physical findings suggesting increasing stenosis include the characteristic ejection murmur becoming louder, longer, higher pitched, and peaking later in systole and, in severe stenosis, a thrill at the right upper sternal border. A thrill in the suprasternal notch is common even in patients with mild aortic stenosis and does not have the same prognostic implications as one at the sternal border. Surgical treatment of aortic stenosis is described in Chapter 134. All patients with aortic stenosis require SBE prophylaxis. Long-term anticoagulation is required for those who have had an artificial valve placed. Because of a small but significant risk of sudden death with exercise, patients with a gradient that exceeds 30 mm Hg stenosis are restricted from competitive athletics. Because of the risk of gradually worsening regurgitation or restenosis, these children require long-term follow-up with their cardiologist.

Follow-up of children who have had either balloon or surgical correction of *coarctation of the aorta* should be directed toward the problems of restenosis and the development or persistence of hypertension. Both of these problems are detectable by regular measurements of blood pressure in the arms and legs, and the generalist must share the long-term surveillance with the cardiologist. A blood pressure discrepancy of more than 20 mm Hg between the arm and leg or a significant delay in pulse transmission between the radial and femoral pulses ("femoral lag") suggests significant restenosis. Some patients who are normotensive at rest develop hypertension with exercise. Exercise limitations and clearance for participation in competitive sports in these patients should be made in conjunction with a cardiologist. A treadmill exercise tolerance test to evaluate the blood pressure response to exercise may be required. Because aneurysmal dilation of coarctation repair sites in some young women during pregnancy has been reported, intensive prenatal cardiovascular monitoring is indicated. SBE prophylaxis is indicated for all patients who have had a coarctation repair.

Interrupted aortic arch is repaired in the early infant or newborn period, and the associated ventricular septal defect is often closed at the same time. The generalist should ensure that the infant has been evaluated for manifestations of the 22q deletion syndrome, including fluorescence in situ hybridization (FISH) testing, and obtain the results of the evaluation. Long-term follow-up is similar to that of patients with coarctation, that is, monitoring for evidence of significant narrowing at the sight of repair.

Regurgitant Lesions: Aortic and Mitral Regurgitation

Left-sided valvular incompetence results in a volume load on the left ventricle. *Aortic regurgitation* is often seen in association with aortic stenosis, either as a result of valvotomy or as part of the natural history of a dysplastic aortic valve. Less commonly, bacterial endocarditis or rheumatic heart disease may result in significant regurgitation. *Mitral regurgitation* is a common postoperative complication following repairs of primum atrial septal defect or atrioventricular canal defects. Patients with mitral valve prolapse or congenital mitral valve abnormalities may occasionally exhibit significant mitral regurgitation. Endocarditis and rheumatic fever can also result in mitral regurgitation. Most patients with mitral or aortic regurgitation have minimal symptoms. Even though they may become somewhat short of breath with vigorous exercise, they should be encouraged to remain active. Those patients with moderate to severe regurgitation should be restricted from competitive sports participation. Most children are treated with afterload reduction, usually with an angiotensin-converting enzyme (ACE) inhibitor. Regular, long-term cardiology follow-up is required for periodic echocardiographic evaluation of left ventricular size and function. Surgical intervention is required for progressive enlargement of the left ventricle or a decrease in systolic function. Those who have a mechanical prosthesis are treated with chronic coumadin therapy and are at risk for both bleeding and embolic complications. Patients with a dilated left ventricle secondary to valvular regurgitation are at some risk for arrhythmias, both pre- and postoperatively. SBE prophylaxis is indicated for all patients with aortic or mitral regurgitation.

Transposition of the Great Vessels

Patients with simple transposition of the great vessels are profoundly cyanotic within a few hours of birth and are operated on immediately. The favored current surgical approach is the arterial switch operation in which the aorta and pulmonary arteries are repositioned to connect them to the appropriate ventricle. Complications associated with this procedure include development of supravalvar aortic or pulmonary stenosis, particularly if the vessel sizes were dissimilar. Supravalvar obstruction is characterized by a typical ejection murmur in the pulmonary or aortic location. Some patients also develop clinically significant aortic regurgitation through what had been their pulmonary valve. The most challenging aspect of the operation is

the transplantation of the coronary arteries from the aortic root to what had been the pulmonary root. Problems with the coronary arteries are usually apparent at the time of the surgery, but late coronary complications can arise. Exertional dyspnea or chest pain should raise the possibility of coronary artery compromise in patients who have had arterial switch operations. Decisions regarding exercise limits should be made following a complete evaluation by a cardiologist with treadmill stress testing. Those planning competitive athletics may require myocardial perfusion imaging and cardiac catheterization. Some adolescents or young adults may have had *atrial switching* surgery instead of an arterial switch. This was a common surgical procedure prior to the mid-1980s and may still be done in certain circumstances. The typical operations of this type, the Senning and Mustard operations, leave the right ventricle as the systemic ventricle. Generalists following such patients should monitor for the late complications of sinus node abnormalities, progressive tricuspid (systemic) valve regurgitation, and right ventricular failure. These patients require lifelong cardiology follow-up. All patients who have had surgery for transposition require SBE prophylaxis.

Lesions with Single Functional Ventricles

Many complex cardiac malformations result in some type of single ventricle physiology with only one functionally adequate pumping chamber that must supply both the systemic and pulmonary circulations. The single ventricle may be the right as in the hypoplastic left-sided heart syndrome or the left as in conditions such as tricuspid atresia when the right ventricle is incapable of normal function. Newborns with these conditions depend on a patent ductus that is kept open pharmacologically. These infants require a series of surgical procedures in the first year or two of life (e.g., Norwood, bidirectional Glenn, and Fontan) for hypoplastic left-sided heart syndrome. During the period between surgeries, the generalist should monitor these infants to ensure adequate weight gain. Following a shunt procedure (Blalock-Taussig), patients must be carefully followed for sudden decrease in systemic oxygen saturation, indicating possible clot formation within the surgical shunt or a pulmonary infection. Following the *bidirectional Glenn* procedure, most infants and children maintain oxygen saturation between 80% and 85%. They may become significantly more cyanotic when active, particularly when vigorously using the lower extremities, which increases inferior vena caval return. A pulmonary infection can also significantly decrease oxygen saturation. Upper extremity or facial edema caused by restricted superior venal caval blood flow may indicate stenosis at the surgical site. The generalist needs to consider all patients who have had the *Fontan* operation, the final surgical palliation for patients with single ventricle, as medically fragile. The systemic saturation following a Fontan operation usually ranges between 85% and 95%. The long-term outcome for children who have had a Fontan procedure is unknown, although many children treated in this fashion have done well for many years. Prescribed exercise limitations are usually unnecessary for young children who will limit their own activities. Older children may benefit from exercise testing to determine their capacity and to provide guidelines for the patient and parents. SBE prophylaxis and long-term follow-up with a cardiologist are mandatory.

Cardiomyopathy: Dilated and Hypertrophic

The underlying cause of most cases of *dilated cardiomyopathy* is unknown, although many are probably the result of an unrecognized myocarditis. Cancer survivors who have been treated with doxorubicin (Adriamycin) account for some cases of dilated cardiomyopathy in childhood and adolescence. Regardless of the cause, these children are sometimes surprisingly asymptomatic despite their profoundly reduced ventricular function. Treatment is symptomatic and includes afterload reduction in the form of an ACE inhibitor, an inotropic agent such as digoxin, and a diuretic such as furosemide. The primary care physician who is following a patient with dilated cardiomyopathy should be aware that cardiac function will progressively deteriorate in most children. As a result of the dilated chambers, systemic or pulmonary emboli may occur, causing sudden worsening, arrhythmias, or sudden death. Symptoms or signs suggesting an arrhythmia require a prompt referral for investigation. Because patients with dilated cardiomyopathy tolerate febrile illnesses poorly, prompt, aggressive evaluation must be undertaken. Illnesses that may cause dehydration increase the risk of thrombus and embolus formation. The generalist may need to undertake early but careful rehydration (because volume overload will be poorly tolerated) in this situation. Although usually sporadic, dilated cardiomyopathy may occasionally be familial; siblings and other family members should be evaluated for evidence of the disease. Although some patients recover from dilated cardiomyopathy, the usual course is progressive, with heart transplantation as the only option. Exercise is usually not well tolerated as the children become symptomatic; prior to this phase, reasonable limitations on exercise should be advised. SBE prophylaxis is indicated for all patients.

Patients with *hypertrophic cardiomyopathy* may also be relatively asymptomatic at presentation. Murmurs are common and may be the reason for initial referral. About half of the cases are familial. Siblings and other family members of an index patient should be thoroughly evaluated. Treatment of patients with hypertrophic cardiomyopathy with medications such as calcium-channel blockers or beta-adrenergic agents is controversial, and recommendations vary among pediatric cardiologists. Because arrhythmias are a common feature of this condition, periodic Holter monitoring may be indicated. The primary care provider should monitor patients for easy fatigability, breathlessness, and anginal type pain, symptoms caused by increasing obstruction of the outflow tract. Surgical intervention may be performed in an effort to reduce these obstructive symptoms. Patients with hypertrophic myopathy are at risk for sudden death from arrhythmias and should be restricted from significant exercise, including competitive athletics. Surgery to remove obstructing tissue does not reduce the risk of sudden death. As in the dilated form, these patients poorly tolerate intercurrent illnesses with fever or dehydration. Early recognition and judicious intervention can be lifesaving. SBE prophylaxis is indicated.

Problems Involving the Coronary Arteries

Anomalous origin of the left coronary artery from the pulmonary artery typically results in symptoms leading to diagnosis and surgical treatment in the first months of life. Surgical correction is challenging and has a relatively high immediate postoperative mortality rate. Decreased perfusion of the myocardium from narrowing at the surgical site can develop. Manifestations include anginal pain, cardiomegaly, and CHF. The diagnosis and treatment of *Kawasaki disease* (KD) is discussed in Chapter 60. Some KD patients develop giant aneurysms or other abnormalities of the coronary arteries. In some cases these problems will regress, but if they do not, the children are at risk to develop clots and stenosis of these vessels. A generalist following a patient who is known to have aneurysms from KD should recognize that chest pain in such a patient may represent myocardial ischemia. Prompt evaluation and referral are indicated.

Additional Resources, CD-ROM

Bibliography

Mini-index of Related Topics

SUGGESTED READINGS

Garson A Jr, Bricker JT, Fisher Neish SR (eds): The Science and Practice of Pediatric Cardiology, 2nd ed. Baltimore, Williams & Wilkins, 1998.
Park MK: Pediatric Cardiology for Practitioners, 4th ed. St. Louis, Mosby, 2002.

134 Long-term Management after Cardiac Surgery

Gregory B. Di Russo

ROLE OF THE GENERALIST

1 Understand the timing and procedures for surgical treatment of congenital cardiac disease.

2 Provide primary care and preventive care for patients with surgically repaired congenital cardiac disease.

3 Ensure appropriate follow-up, particularly as children with congenital conditions make transition from pediatric to adult care.

FUNDAMENTALS

Successful management of patients who have undergone or who are in the process of undergoing repair of congenital heart defects depends on an understanding of the underlying lesion, the goals of the repair, and the physiology of the operated patient. Addressing a few simple questions can determine the most important issues for each patient.

1. Is the circulation separated? Are there any intracardiac or extracardiac connections that allow mixing of oxygenated and deoxygenated blood? (Intracardiac communications include atrial and ventricular septal defects.)

2. Is there excessive, inadequate, or balanced pulmonary blood flow? Blood will follow the path of least resistance, so in the absence of restriction to pulmonary blood flow (e.g., pulmonary stenosis, pulmonary artery banding), mixing lesions will result in excessive pulmonary blood flow.

3. Is there an obstructive lesion present? The prototypical right-sided obstructive lesion is tetralogy of Fallot, in which pulmonary blood flow is limited by stenosis at one or more of the following levels—infundibulum (muscular, outlet portion of the right ventricle), pulmonary valve, or pulmonary arteries. The analogous left-sided lesion is Shone complex, in which stenosis may exist at the level of the mitral valve, subaortic region of the left ventricle, aortic valve, or descending aorta (typical aortic coarctation). Obstructive lesions may recur once treated by surgical or catheter-based techniques.

4. Does the patient have an implant or conduit? Unfortunately, the ideal valve or conduit does not exist. That device would be inexpensive, available in a wide range of sizes, have "biocompatible" features, and grow with the patient. Patient growth and conduit failure mandate replacement when the physiologic needs of the patient cannot be met. Examples include right ventricle/pulmonary artery conduits, systemic/pulmonary artery shunts, and prosthetic valves. Knowing whether or not the patient's repair has incorporated a nonviable implant helps the clinician to understand the need for and timing of future interventions.

Answers to these questions help clarify how the child's heart disease is contributing to the present condition.

MEDICAL MANAGEMENT

The details of medical management for children with cardiac disease are covered in Chapter 133. This section addresses medical management of anticoagulation and illnesses commonly seen in the postoperative period.

Anticoagulation

Following cardiac surgical procedures, patients may require anticoagulation. The most stringent use of anticoagulation follows implantation of a mechanical prosthesis. Risk for valve thrombosis is significant and can result in hemodynamic compromise or peripheral embolization (e.g., stroke). Anticoagulation is also used for atrial arrhythmias, known intracardiac thrombus, systemic venous or arterial thrombosis, and hypercoagulable states, including following Fontan connection. Few specific guidelines exist for anticoagulation in children, so extrapolations from adult data are necessary.

Aspirin

Aspirin (acetylsalicylic acid) inhibits platelet aggregation through its inhibition of cyclooxygenase. Common uses following surgery for congenital heart disease include patients with Fontan connection (with or without fenestration), systemic/pulmonary artery shunt placement, or prosthetic valve replacement. Common complications of aspirin are bleeding, especially from the gastrointestinal tract, gastrointestinal symptoms (nausea, dyspepsia, vomiting), and sensitivity in patients with asthma, chronic urticaria, and chronic rhinitis. Aspirin use during viral illnesses has been associated with the development of Reye's syndrome.

Ideal aspirin dosing for children has not been established. The current recommendation is a single daily dose of 5 to 10 mg/kg/day. Duration of therapy depends on the indication. Discontinuation should be decided collaboratively with the cardiologist and cardiac surgeon. Because the antiplatelet effects of aspirin last 7 to 10 days, the drug should be stopped 7 to 10 days prior to any surgical procedure, providing the patient's status permits.

Coumadin

Coumadin (warfarin sodium) prolongs the prothrombin time (PT). In response to variability in the measurement of PT in different laboratories, the international normalization ratio (INR) was developed to correct for laboratory variability. The recommended INR for patients with mechanical cardiac prosthesis is 2.5 to 3.5, a value that balances risk of hemorrhagic complications and adequate anticoagulation to avoid thrombosis. Pediatric dosing recommendations are not well established. A loading dose of 0.1 mg/kg/day (not to exceed 10 mg/day) for 3 to 5 days is recommended, followed by a maintenance dose of approximately 0.05 mg/kg/day. Individual dosing may vary significantly. The INR should be monitored prior to loading and then on a daily basis after the second dose. Dosing can be very difficult because of dietary variation, vitamin K levels in formulas, and noncompliance. Drug interactions affect therapeutic levels by altering absorption, excretion, protein binding, or metabolism. The INR must be monitored frequently, particularly when concurrent medications are adjusted, added, or discontinued. Hemorrhagic complications occur in as many as 48% of patients. Coumadin is a known teratogen.

Intercurrent Illnesses

Respiratory Illness

Patients with congenital heart disease may tolerate acute or chronic respiratory illness poorly. Chronic respiratory disease can result in increased pulmonary vascular resistance and cor pulmonale. Right ventricular hypertrophy and eventually failure can develop from chronically increased pulmonary vascular resistance. Increased pulmonary vascular resistance is poorly tolerated in the early postoperative period when right ventricular compliance is decreased. Neonates and patients whose right ventricle was hypertrophied prior to surgery are particularly vulnerable. Increased pulmonary vascular resistance with a noncompliant right ventricle increases right atrial and systemic venous pressure and increases right-to-left shunting in patients with residual atrial communication. This shunting will cause or exacerbate cyanosis. In the absence of atrial shunting, patients can develop right-sided heart failure and decreased cardiac output. Patients with single ventricle physiology, with Glenn or Fontan connection, may do particularly poorly with increased pulmonary vascular resistance, because pulmonary blood flow is passive.

Increased pulmonary vascular resistance requires aggressive treatment of the underlying cause, if any can be found, and supplemental oxygen, which will lower pulmonary vascular resistance. In severe cases, patients may require mechanical ventilation, sedation, and even paralysis.

Gastrointestinal Illness

Gastroesophageal reflux disease (GER) is common and may occur more frequently in children with congenital heart disease because of associated anomalies such as tracheoesophageal fistula or neurologic impairment (for management of GER, see Chapter 87). Patients who have congenital heart disease have limited ability to tolerate aspiration of gastric contents. Pneumonia and chronic lung disease are serious issues for this group of patients. Patients who have had surgical procedures involving the aortic arch or ductus arteriosus are at risk for injury to the left or, more rarely, the right recurrent laryngeal nerve, increasing the potential for silent aspiration.

Fluid losses from gastroenteritis may be poorly tolerated in the patient who has undergone repair of congenital heart disease. Diuretics can exacerbate dehydration associated with gastroenteritis and may limit the tolerance for fluid loss. In some cases, diuretics should be discontinued in patients at risk of dehydration while there is ongoing fluid loss or inadequate oral intake. Fluid replacement therapy should be instituted early in the course of such illnesses.

Infectious Illness

All patients have an increased propensity for infectious illness in the weeks following surgery.

Asplenia, which may accompany cardiac disease, predisposes patients to bacteremia. Many clinicians recommend antibiotic prophylaxis with amoxicillin and pneumococcal vaccine for these patients. Any asplenic patient who develops a fever higher than 38.0°C (100.4°F) should be seen promptly because of significant risk of developing overwhelming bacterial sepsis (see Chapter 167). Polysplenic patients should be evaluated for splenic dysfunction, and if present, these patients should be treated as if asplenic.

SURGICAL TREATMENT

Timetables for Specific Lesions

The timing of primary or reoperative surgery for an individual patient depends on a number of factors including concurrent illness, associated anomalies, and institutional experience. Individual patient variation may dictate a different course of action and improvements in understanding of the natural and "unnatural" or operated history of these diseases may change the timing of interventions. Timing and repair of tetralogy of Fallot, pulmonary atresia, and complex cardiac lesions is found on the CD-ROM.

Inadequate Pulmonary Blood Flow

Pulmonary Stenosis

Anatomically, pulmonary stenosis with intact ventricular septum comprises a broad spectrum of diseases, ranging from the asymptomatic child who presents with a murmur at a well-child visit to a critically ill infant who is dependent on patency of the ductus arteriosus to maintain adequate pulmonary blood flow. Symptomatic newborns and infants require immediate intervention. Critical pulmonary stenosis is preferentially treated with catheter-based balloon valvuloplasty. Early surgical intervention may be required if the balloon procedure is unsuccessful. Right ventricular outflow tract reconstruction or a systemic/pulmonary artery shunt will increase pulmonary blood flow. A significant recurrence rate following balloon valvuloplasty of the pulmonary valve may be treated with repeated balloon valvuloplasty or surgery depending on anatomic factors, response to previous balloon procedures and institutional experience. Infants and children with severe pulmonary stenosis (valve gradient greater than 80 mm Hg or right ventricle [RV] pressure greater than systemic) and all symptomatic patients should undergo balloon valvuloplasty. Asymptomatic patients with moderate stenosis (valve gradient 25 to 80 mm Hg or RV pressure equal to systemic pressure) may be followed by a cardiologist for progression of disease, manifested by increased echocardiographic gradient or development of symptoms. Mild pulmonary stenosis (valve gradient less than 25 mm Hg or RV pressure greater than systemic) does not usually need treatment but should also be followed.

Excessive Pulmonary Blood Flow

Lesions resulting in excessive pulmonary blood flow (left-to-right shunt) include atrial and ventricular septal defects, atrioventricular septal defects, and patent ductus arteriosus. These lesions can result in congestive heart failure from excessive pulmonary blood flow. They can also cause irreversible pulmonary hypertension that occurs as early as 9 to 12 months of age in patients with large defects.

Ventricular Septal Defects

Infants presenting in the first months of life with congestive heart failure from a moderate to large ventricular septal defect (VSD) should undergo surgical closure. Elective closure of moderate to larger VSDs should be performed at 6 to 12 months of age in order to prevent development of irreversible pulmonary hypertension. Smaller defects, also called "restrictive" or "pressure restrictive," are less likely to cause symptoms; their repair may be delayed to 2 to 3 years of age to allow for spontaneous closure. This decision must be made only after complete echocardiographic assessment of the lesion, as auscultation is an inaccurate means to assess the degree of shunt from an intracardiac defect. The presence of new aortic insufficiency or its progression with an associated VSD is an indication for surgical closure regardless of the size of the defect or the presence of symptoms.

Occasionally, a patient with complex or multiple VSDs will be considered for pulmonary artery banding. This procedure limits the pulmonary blood flow by placing a restrictive bend around the main pulmonary artery. The band is removed when the defects close spontaneously or at 6 to 24 months of age, at the time of surgical closure of the defect(s). The management of complex or multiple VSDs may also include catheter-based placement of an occlusive device.

Surgical survival rate is currently 97% to 98%, with an increased mortality rate among patients with multiple defects, associated left-to-right shunts, and extracardiac abnormalities. Complications include complete heart block, right bundle branch block, and residual defect.

Atrioventricular Septal Defects

Atrioventricular septal defects (AVSDs), also called atrioventricular canal defects, include the complete form in which ventricular and atrial level shunts are present and the partial form in which only the atrial component is present. The intermediate or transitional form has a small, pressure-restrictive VSD component. In the absence of a ventricular level shunt, the lesion (which may be called an ostium primum atrial septal defect) may be treated like an atrial septal defect, with elective closure at 3 to 5 years of age. Complete defects should be closed at any age in patients with congestive heart failure not controlled with medication. Asymptomatic patients can safely undergo repair at 2 to 6 months of age. Palliative pulmonary artery banding will reduce the typically large left–to-right shunt and may improve symptoms in a patient with congestive heart failure from AVSD. However, early complete repair at 6 to 8 weeks of age is the practice in some institutions.

Survival rate for primary repair is 94% to 99%. Complications of surgery include arrhythmias (including heart block requiring pacemaker implantation), left atrioventricular valve regurgitation, and pulmonary hypertension.

The left atrioventricular valve (functionally the "mitral" valve) is abnormal in all patients with AVSD, as is the left ventricular outflow tract. Patients must be followed regularly for the development of atrioventricular valve regurgitation as well as subaortic stenosis. Some patients will eventually need operative intervention for one or both of these problems.

Atrial Septal Defect

Defects in the atrial septum include patent foramen ovale, ostium secundum, ostium primum, and sinus venosus defects. All may occur as isolated lesions or in combination with other cardiac defects. Sinus venosus defects are particularly associated with ipsilateral anomalous pulmonary venous drainage and primum defects with cleft left atrioventricular valve.

A small atrial septal defect or patent foramen ovale typically results in a small degree of left-to-right shunting. The need for closure is controversial in the absence of symptoms but is warranted when the patient experiences paradoxical embolus causing a stroke. As experience develops with catheter-based closure devices, the risk-to-benefit ratio may weigh more in favor of closing smaller asymptomatic defects.

Moderate to large defects resulting in cardiomegaly or symptoms of congestive heart failure should be closed. Asymptomatic moderate to large defects should be closed electively at 3 to 5 years of age. At that age, the procedure can be performed safely with a minimally invasive approach and is generally well tolerated.

Surgical closure of an isolated atrial septal defect is performed with very low morbidity and mortality rates and is considered curative; the recurrence rate is very low. Complications are uncommon but include patch dehiscence, residual defect, pulmonary venous stenosis, and regurgitation of the left atrioventricular valve (mitral valve).

Patent Ductus Arteriosus

Persistent patent ductus arteriosus (PDA) may result in congestive heart failure; may worsen necrotizing enterocolitis, abnormal cerebral blood flow, or respiratory distress in premature infants; and may lead to irreversible pulmonary hypertension. Other complications are infective endocarditis and ductal aneurysm. Symptomatic lesions should be closed at the time of diagnosis and after the first few months of life in the asymptomatic patient. Spontaneous closure after the first year of life occurs in only 0.6% cases per year. Closure of an inaudible or "silent" PDA is controversial.

Current techniques for ductal closure include (1) open surgical ligation, with or without division, via thoracotomy, (2) thoracoscopic ligation, and (3) catheter-based ductal closure with an intraluminal device. The recurrence rate is lowest following ligation and division, but persistence or recurrence of ductal flow may occur following closure with any technique. In addition to persistent ductal flow or recanalization, surgical complications include injury of the recurrent laryngeal nerve, chylothorax, and accidental ligation of the aorta or left pulmonary artery. Surgical mortality rate approaches zero, and life expectancy is normal following closure of isolated PDA.

Left-Sided Obstructive Lesions

Left-sided obstructive lesions include aortic stenosis at the valvar, subvalvar, and supravalvar levels and aortic coarctation. Isolated mitral stenosis is a rare congenital lesion (Fig. 134-1).

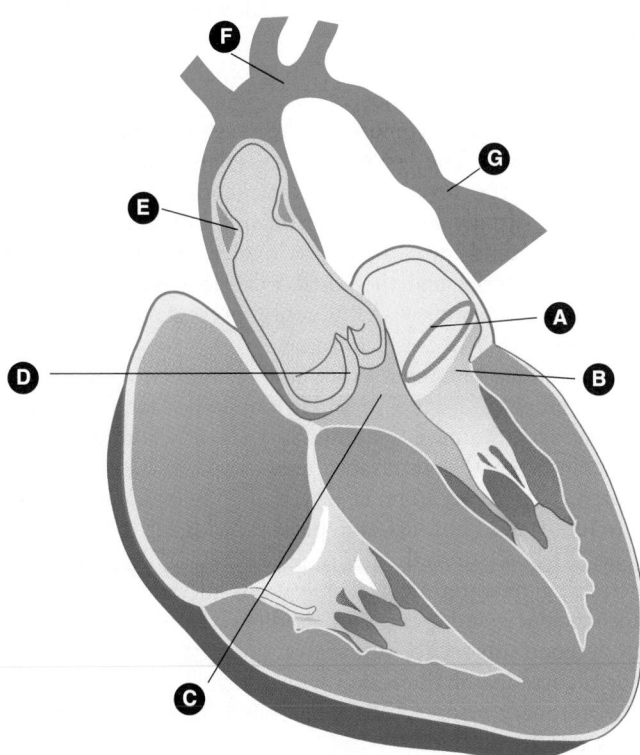

Figure 134-1. Levels of left-sided obstruction. *A,* Supra-annular mitral ring. *B,* Valvar mitral stenosis. *C,* Subaortic stenosis. *D,* Valvar aortic stenosis. *E,* Supravalvar aortic stenosis. *F,* Aortic arch hypoplasia. *G,* Aortic coarctation.

Aortic Coarctation

The infant with aortic coarctation may present as a critically ill neonate whose lower body perfusion is severely compromised owing to ductal closure or as a previously asymptomatic patient who is developing increasing feeding intolerance and tachypnea. Aortic coarctation in infants is frequently associated with other cardiac defects, including bicuspid aortic valve, ventricular septal defect, atrial septal defect, and transposition of the great vessels. Older patients with aortic coarctation are typically asymptomatic with upper extremity hypertension and may occasionally complain of leg cramps and cold feet. Aortic coarctation must be ruled out in any child with hypertension. This is most simply done by confirming equal blood pressure in all four extremities.

In the symptomatic neonate, medical therapy with prostaglandin E1 (PGE1) is started in an effort to open the ductus arteriosus and re-establish perfusion to the lower body. The presence of any associated cardiac defects is determined, and the patient is taken to the operating room for coarctation repair. Asymptomatic infants should undergo elective repair at 3 to 6 months of life. Older children and adults should undergo repair following diagnosis.

Surgical repair, with or without concomitant repair of associated defects, depending on their nature and the preference of the surgeon, is the treatment of choice for neonates. Older children and adults may be candidates for catheter-based procedures, though the current experience is limited, and this mode of therapy is controversial.

Mortality rate following neonatal repair of isolated aortic coarctation ranges from 2% to 9%. Recurrence or persistence of coarctation is defined as a 20 mm Hg gradient across the area of the repair. This occurs in 5% to 20% of patients and is more frequent in patients treated at an earlier age. Recurrence is treated with catheter-based balloon dilatation, patch aortoplasty, or ascending to descending conduit placement. Other complications include injury to the recurrent laryngeal nerve, chylothorax, and aneurysmal dilatation.

Long-term follow-up is necessary for surveillance of recurrence of coarctation, hypertension, and the development of aortic aneurysms, as well as for the monitoring of associated lesions such as bicuspid aortic valve, which can develop progressive stenosis or insufficiency. Performance of exercise testing may help assess the role of residual coarctation in a hypertensive patient following coarctation repair.

Aortic Stenosis

Aortic stenosis can be separated into valvar aortic stenosis, subaortic stenosis, and supravalvar aortic stenosis. More than one level of obstruction may be present in this anatomic region, also referred to as the left ventricular outflow tract (LVOT).

Subvalvar Aortic Stenosis

Subvalvar aortic stenosis represents a broad group of anatomic obstructions to the portion of the left ventricle immediately below the aortic valve. This region includes a portion of the mitral valve and muscle of the left ventricular free wall and the interventricular septum. Muscle, mitral valve tissue, and fibrous tissue contribute to subaortic stenosis. As the narrowing progresses, compensatory left ventricular hypertrophy exacerbates the problem.

Indications for surgery vary among centers, with some centers advocating surgery in the presence of a low pressure gradient (<40 mm Hg) from the left ventricle to the aorta. A gradient of 40 to 50 mm Hg is considered an indication for surgery, as is the development or progression of aortic insufficiency, even in the face of a minimal gradient.

Relief of subaortic stenosis may consist of resection of muscle, fibrous tissue, and accessory mitral valve tissue from the subaortic area, through the aortic valve. Associated aortic valve stenosis is addressed and may require valve replacement. Patching of the ventricular septum or mitral valve replacement occasionally may be necessary.

Complications of surgery include persistent LVOT gradient, aortic valve insufficiency, complete heart block, and iatrogenic ventricular septal defect. The recurrence rate depends on associated lesions and is significantly higher in patients who have associated aortic valve disease. Outcome is also dependent on the specific morphology of the narrowing; longer, "tunnel" stenosis is usually associated with a higher mortality rate. Operative survival rate ranges from 89% to 100% and recurrence occurs in 4% to 56% of cases.

Valvar Aortic Stenosis

Valvar aortic stenosis is the most common form of aortic stenosis. It is typically related to fusion of one or more commissures of the normally trileaflet aortic valve, resulting in a bicuspid or even unicuspid valve. The majority of patients are initially asymptomatic, but approximately 10% of patients will be symptomatic in the first year of life.

Criteria for surgical intervention depend on the age of the patient. An infant with congestive heart failure from critical aortic stenosis is a candidate for surgery. The most common procedures are open surgical valvotomy (typically with cardiopulmonary bypass), closed surgical valvotomy, and percutaneous balloon aortic valvotomy. Which of these procedures is best is controversial, with each having its advocates. Older patients may be candidates for valve repair but may require valve replacement.

The choice of valve for replacement in children has to take into account growth potential and the need for anticoagulation. Prosthetic valves (e.g., St. Jude Medical, CarboMedics) require lifelong anticoagulation to avoid thrombus formation, and the valves do not grow. The advantage of these valves is excellent durability, even in children. In the growing patient, however, the valve will need to be replaced as the child "outgrows" the valve. Typically, anticoagulation is with warfarin (Coumadin), but some some groups have used antiplatelet agents for anticoagulation in children. Bioprosthetic valves are tissue valves made from bovine or porcine material and do not require long-term anticoagulation. They tend to degenerate quickly in children and also do not grow. Human allograft (or homograft) valves are banked valves explanted from cadavers. Pulmonary autograft replacement of the aortic valve (also called the Ross procedure) involves removing the native pulmonary trunk from the patient and using it to replace the aortic valve. The pulmonary valve is then replaced with an allograft pulmonary valve. The operation is more complex than prosthetic aortic valve replacement. Anticoagulation is not required and there is evidence that the "neoaortic" valve grows.

Following successful relief of valvar aortic stenosis in the infant, the patients must be followed closely for recurrent stenosis and aortic insufficiency. These complications can be insidious because left ventricular function may be well preserved. Any neurologic symptom, such as syncope, must be addressed promptly and should be presumed to have a cardiac origin until proved otherwise.

Patients with recurrent stenosis may be followed if they have mild or moderate stenosis before the decision is made to intervene or reoperate. Restrictions of activities in patients with recurrent stenosis should be similar to those for patients with primary mild or moderate stenosis.

Operative mortality rate for infant aortic valvotomy has been as high as 50% but has steadily improved, with the current mortality rate being less than 15%, even in the first months of life. Risk of death is ongoing, with a 10-year survival rate of 74% and a reintervention rate of over 40% at 10 years. Children operated at an older age have better overall survival with fewer reinterventions and a better 10-year survival rate (approximately 95%), falling to 80% at 20 years. Aortic valve replacement in children is associated with overall mortality rates of 5% to 8% and 15% to 20% reoperation rate as late as 20 years. Early and midterm results of the Ross procedure are comparable to or better than those for mechanical or allograft valve replacement.

Percutaneous balloon aortic valvotomy can be performed with very low procedural mortality rate and good midterm results. The need for surgery following this procedure ranges from 50% to 75%.

Supravalvar Aortic Stenosis

Supravalvar aortic stenosis is the least common form of aortic stenosis. The lesion may be isolated to a small area just above the level of the aortic commissures, it may extended distally to involve aortic arch branch vessels, and it may extend proximally to involve the ostia of the coronary arteries and the aortic valve leaflets. Supravalvar pulmonary stenosis is commonly present, especially in patients with Williams syndrome.

Indications for surgery vary among centers; resting pressure gradient of 50 to 75 mm Hg is an indication for surgery in the asymptomatic patient. Surgical procedures involve patching open the supravalvar area to relieve the narrowing. Surgical mortality rate is less than 5% in patients with discrete lesions but higher in patients with the diffuse type. The 20-year survival rate is as high as 77%, with 34% requiring reoperation. Complications include aortic valve insufficiency and persistent gradient. Patients who have undergone surgery for supravalvar aortic stenosis are at risk for recurrence of the lesion with possible progression into the coronary arteries. Main or branch pulmonary arteries may also be involved.

Rheumatic Fever (see also Chapter 60)

Rheumatic fever remains a significant cause of valvular heart disease in some parts of the world. The mitral valve is involved in 85% of cases, the aortic valve in 54%, and the tricuspid and pulmonary valves are involved in fewer than 5%. The mitral valve may develop stenosis or regurgitation. Aortic valve involvement in children typically manifests as insufficiency with little or no stenosis. Stenosis may develop chronically. The goal of surgery for rheumatic valve disease is to leave the patient with a hemodynamically satisfactory result. Ideally, this goal is accomplished by a valve repair rather than replacement because the latter will often require re-replacement as the patient grows. Repair of rheumatic mitral valve disease is possible in many patients with isolated stenosis or regurgitation, but is much less likely when both stenosis and regurgitation are present. Mitral valve repair or replacement can be performed with approximately 5% operative mortality rate. Mechanical replacement is associated with a risk of reoperation of 5% at 10 years. Repair has a 28% risk of reoperation at 10 years. Aortic valve repair and repalcement for rheumatic aortic valve disease has a 3% to 8% mortality rate.

Complications of valve repair include persistent or recurrent stenosis, regurgitation, or endocarditis. Valve replacement is limited by the size of the patient. A small child will not accept a valve that will tolerate the flow needed for adult size. Thus, any valve replacement in a growing child must take into consideration the child's growth and the likelihood of reoperation to replace the prosthesis. Additionally mechanical prostheses require anticoagulation. Bioprosthetic valves, made from bovine or porcine materials, do not routinely require chronic anticoagulation.

Aneurysm

An aneurysm is the enlargement of a blood vessel or cardiac structure. Aneurysms can occur primarily, as in Marfan syndrome and other connective tissue disorders; as the result of another process, such as infection; or in relation to surgery or catheter-based therapy. The focus of this section is the management of aneurysms that occur following cardiac surgery.

Aneurysms following cardiac surgical procedures can occur at sites of surgical incisions, at anastomotic sites, and in prosthetic or biologic material. Whenever an aneurysm in present, one must consider the possibility of distal obstruction causing increased pressure that contributes to the aneurysm's growth. Pseudoaneurysm or false aneurysm occurs when the full thickness of arterial wall is not involved in the aneurysmal process. This typically occurs from a small leak at the site of a surgical anastomosis. As blood leaks out, it is trapped by surrounding structures; eventually an aneurysm develops and the communication with the blood vessel or cardiac chamber can enlarge. Although aneurysm formation following pediatric cardiac surgery is unusual, aneurysm formation has been reported at sites of coarctation repair, cannulation for cardiopulmonary bypass, and right ventricular outflow tract patching.

Few guidelines exist regarding indications for resecting aneurysms that develop following cardiac surgery, so each case must be considered individually. Any aneurysm that is increasing in size or is causing symptoms should be resected. Unresected aneurysms tend to increase in size, may rupture, may serve as a source for distal thromboembolization, or impinge on surrounding structures. Aneuryms in the neck or groin may be obvious to the physician and aneurysms of the heart and great vessels may be noted only on chest radiograph or echocardiogram. Any significant change in a chest radiograph that cannot be attributed to a specific process (such as lobar pneumonia) should undergo further evaluation with echocardiography, after which magnetic resonance imaging and computed tomography can be considered.

Pacemakers

This section addresses the surgical issues of pacemaker implantation. Though the devices continue to decrease in size, the implantation of a pacemaker system in smaller patients requires placing a relatively large generator in a protected pocket. Pocket infections pose a serious problem, especially when the patient is "pacemaker-dependent." Approximately 1% of patients will have a serious infection requiring removal of the pacemaker system and replacement with a new system. Some superficial infections respond to intravenous antibiotic therapy and will not require surgery. Wound complications tend to occur within 2 months of implantation, but late infections are known to occur. Noninfectious complications related to the generator include erosion of the generator through the skin and migration of the generator. Each of these is treated with pacemaker pocket revision, which may include placing the generator in a new location or developing a deeper, submuscular pocket that places muscle between the generator and the skin. Complications relating to the pacemaker leads include lead dislodgment, which usually occurs early after implantation, and lead fracture, which is a later complication, most likely related to repeated mechanical trauma. These problems require lead repositioning or, in the case of lead fracture, replacement.

Routine Follow-up

Individual practices will manage patient follow-up according to what works in the individual setting. As far as the early postoperative care is concerned, a cardiologist and a cardiac surgeon should be involved in the decision to discharge a patient from the hospital and should together provide discharge instructions to the patients and families. Mechanisms should be in place so that contact can be made directly to the cardiology or cardiothoracic surgery services; it is not up to the family to distinguish between "medical" and "surgical" issues, only to recognize that a problem exists.

Cardiac surgeons will often see patients for a single postoperative visit 1 to 2 weeks after hospital discharge. The primary issues for the surgical visit are wound healing and management of activity in the postoperative period. Surgeons also participate in the management of postoperative medications to a varying degree.

In the first 6 weeks after a thoracic or cardiac procedure, patients should be limited in the activities involving their upper extremities. Lifting should initially be limited to 5 to 10 lb, depending on the patient's age, and gradually increased at the discretion of the surgeon. Children should refrain from hanging on bars and swinging, as this will place excessive stress on the chest. Trampolines, bicycle riding, and any activity that could result in a fall may jeopardize healing of the sternum and should be avoided for 6 weeks.

Walking, including hills and outdoor walking, should be encouraged, because it will improve lung function. The sternotomy or thoracotomy incision will have gained nearly full strength within 6 weeks unless there has been significant impairment to healing from poor nutrition, infection, or prolonged hospitalization. At that time, it is no longer necessary to impose limits on activity though some patients may limit themselves.

Transition of Care

Because of the improved outcome for patients with congenital heart disease the transition to adult care is a growing issue. An increasing number of patients with operated congenital heart disease are growing to adulthood and require ongoing care. Although the current recommendations are for regional adult congenital heart surgery centers to care for this group of patients, such a network of centers is not yet in place. Ideally, the network would consist of centers with cardiologists specially trained in treating adults with congenital heart disease and cardiovascular surgeons with an interest in the surgical problems affecting this group. These regional referral centers would have working relationships with adult and pediatric cardiologists in their respective regions, and patients would be followed by a primary cardiologist as well as by a physician caring for adults with congenital cardiac disease at the center.

Such regional centers are well established in Canada and the United Kingdom, but few dedicated adult congenital heart programs exist in the United States. Nevertheless, excellent care for these patients is available and can be administered by a combination of adult and pediatric physicians and surgeons. The role of the generalist is to identify the regionally available professional individuals with an interest in adults with congenital heart disease. These professionals may include pediatric cardiologists, adult cardiologists, and adult or congenital heart surgeons.

A bit of extra time communicating with patients and their cardiologists will help take full advantage of regionally available resources. In most cases, it is unimportant *who* administers the care so long as it is delivered. This organized plan of care includes schedules for medication management, diagnostic studies (catheterization, echocardiogram, blood work), and future interventions. The patient, primary care provider, and cardiologist should all understand the potential need for future intervention, signs and symptoms that are of concern, and the relevance of the specific heart disease in relation to other medical problems.

Additional Resources, CD-ROM

Tetralogy of Fallot	Text, figure
Pulmonary atresia	Text
Single ventricle	Text, figure
Complex cardiac lesions	Text
Bibliography	

Mini-index of Related Topics

	CH.
ACUTE CARDIAC RHYTHM DISORDERS	59
INFECTIOUS DISORDERS OF THE HEART	60
NUTRITION IN CHILDREN WITH CHRONIC DISEASES	130
LONG-TERM MEDICAL MANAGEMENT OF CHILDREN WITH HEART DISEASE	133
CHRONIC RHYTHM DISORDERS	135
PEDIATRIC CARDIAC TRANSPLANTATION	136
DISORDERS OF THE CARDIOVASCULAR SYSTEM IN THE NEWBORN	203

SUGGESTED READINGS

Moran AM, Daebritz S, Keane JF, Mayer JE: Surgical management of mitral regurgitation after repair of endocardial cushion defects: Early and midterm results. Circulation 2000;102(19 suppl 3):160–165.

Najm HK, Williams WG, Chuaratanaphong S, et al: Primum atrial septal defect in children: Early results, risk factors, and freedom from reoperation. Ann Thorac Surg 1998;66(3):829–835.

Serraf A, Lacour-Guyet F, Bruniaux J, et al: Surgical management of isolated multiple ventricular septal defects: Logical approach in 130 cases. J Thorac Cardiovasc Surg 1992;103:437–442.

Yau TM, El-Ghoneimi YA, Armstrong S, et al: Mitral valve repair and replacement for rheumatic disease. J Thorac Cardiovasc Surg 2000;119(1):53–60.

135 Chronic Rhythm Disorders

Nicole K. Boramanand and James C. Perry

ROLE OF THE GENERALIST

1. Differentiate benign arrhythmias from potentially lethal arrhythmias in children with structurally normal hearts and congenital heart disease.

2. Understand medical management of atrial and ventricular arrhythmias in children with structurally normal hearts and with congenital heart disease.

3. Understand the role of radiofrequency catheter ablation as curative management for certain arrhythmias and the need for appropriate referral.

4. Understand medical management of long Q-T syndrome (LQTS), be aware of physical restrictions placed on these children, and assist with adherence.

5. Recognize the potential effect many medications (prescription and over the counter) will have on atrial and ventricular arrhythmias.

6. Recognize that many common over-the-counter medications and prescription drugs are contraindicated in children with LQTS.

7. Recognize what activity restrictions placed on children with anti-bradycardia/tachycardia devices and assist with adherence.

8. Recognize factors that influence prognosis for children with arrhythmias.

Table 135-1. Rhythm Disturbances in Children

Heart Condition	Supraventricular Arrhythmias	Ventricular Arrhythmias
Structurally normal heart	Atrial flutter Atrial ectopic tachycardia Reentrant SVT (AVNRT, PJRT, AVRT) Wolff-Parkinson-White syndrome	PVCs* AIVR* LQTS (torsades de pointes) Idiopathic VT/VF
Congenital heart disease	Reentrant tachycardia Intra-atrial reentry tachycardia Micro-reentry tachycardia Atrial flutter Atrial ectopic tachycardia Occasional reentrant SVT	Incisional reentrant VT Poly/monomorphic VT
Cardiomyopathy	Atrial ectopic tachycardia	Poly/monomorphic VT

*Benign arrhythmias not requiring treatment.
AIVR, automatic ideoventricular rhythm, AVNRT, atrioventricular nodal reentry tachycardia; LQTS, long QT syndrome; PJRT, permanent junctional reciprocating tachycardia; PVCs, premature ventricular contractions; SVT, supraventricular tachycardia; VF, ventricular fibrillation; VT, ventricular tachycardia.

Although the initial approach to understanding childhood cardiac arrhythmias may appear a daunting task, the majority of children with rhythm disturbances fall into one of several categories. First, they can be separated based on the presence or absence of structural heart disease, including both congenital heart disease (CHD) and cardiomyopathies. These children then can be differentiated into those with nonlethal arrhythmias and those with actual or potentially lethal ones (Table 135-1).

Children with structurally normal hearts can also have both nonlethal and potentially lethal cardiac arrhythmias. Those with nonlethal types generally have a fair response to medical management, the arrhythmias are amenable to definitive cure by radiofrequency catheter ablation, and the children have a favorable prognosis with little to no long-term effect on their quality of life. Potentially lethal arrhythmias in children with structurally normal hearts may be controlled medically, but in an unpredictable fashion. Many are not candidates for curative catheter ablation procedures and go on to require implantable cardioverter-defibrillators (ICDs) or pacemakers in attempts to reduce

their risk of syncope and sudden death. These children obviously have more psychosocial issues and the impact of their diagnosis on their quality of life can be quite significant.

Children with CHD are at increased risk of developing arrhythmias from the superimposition of surgical myocardial scars on abnormal hemodynamics. Some can be controlled with antiarrhythmic medications and pacemakers. Although some patients are candidates for radiofrequency ablation, the initial and long-term success of the procedure is variable. As these children reach adulthood, many have increased risk for sudden death and may require ICDs as part of their long-term management. The psychosocial implications of device therapy are significant in these children as well.

The spectrum of long-term management of children with arrhythmias is varied and is dependent on the presence of underlying structural heart disease and the severity and lethality of the underlying arrhythmia mechanism.

ARRHYTHMIAS IN CHILDREN WITH STRUCTURALLY NORMAL HEARTS

Nonlethal Atrial Arrhythmias
Most arrhythmias in children with structurally normal hearts are supraventricular tachycardias (SVTs). The underlying mechanism and time of presentation are age-dependent.

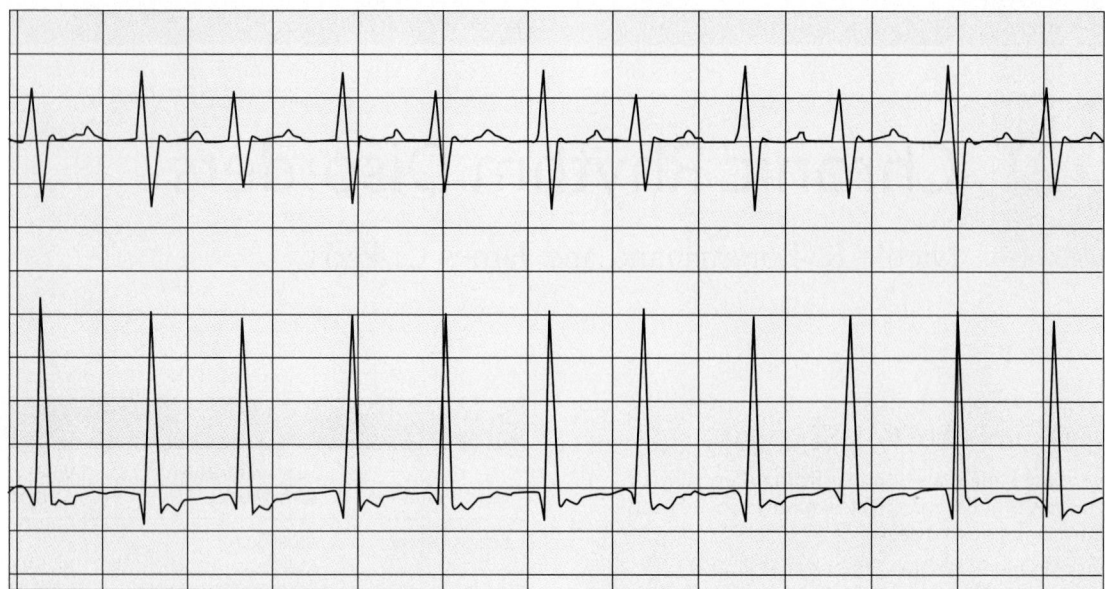

Figure 135-1. Rhythm strip demonstrating supraventricular tachycardia at a rate of 240 bpm. Note the retrograde P waves immediately following the QRS complex seen best on the lower strip *(arrows)*.

Many children will present with reentrant forms of SVT in the first 3 months of life. This SVT is accompanied by the presence of a narrow QRS complex tachycardia at a rate of approximately 220 to 270 bpm. Often a retrograde P wave can be seen in the ST segment or T wave of the electrocardiogram (ECG) during SVT (Fig. 135-1). Of the infants presenting with SVT, 93% will stop having episodes by at least 8 months of age. One third of all patients will have a recurrence of their SVT at a mean age of 8 years.

Atrial flutter is a less common neonatal arrhythmia. The diagnosis is made by the presence of a rapid atrial rate (260 to 400 bpm) often with fixed 2:1 or variable atrioventricular (AV) conduction (Fig. 135-2). Initial management involves acute termination of the tachycardia, followed by appropriate antiarrhythmic therapy for chronic, long-term management. Studies have shown that infants with atrial flutter have an excellent prognosis with rare recurrence and may not require medical management at all after the rhythm is terminated as a newborn.

The most common mechanisms of tachycardia in children are SVT from reentry with an accessory pathway (either manifest as Wolff-Parkinson-White syndrome or concealed) or to reentry without an accessory pathway, most commonly AV node reentry tachycardia (AVNRT). Episodes tend to be paroxysmal. One form of SVT known as permanent junctional reciprocating tachycardia (PJRT) is incessant and caused by a slowly conducting bypass tract. Control of the arrhythmia is crucial in preventing the development of a tachycardia-induced cardiomyopathy. Most SVTs can be controlled to some extent medically. Elimination of the arrhythmia substrate by curative techniques is the only way to truly control arrhythmia.

Figure 135-2. Atrial flutter with variable atrioventricular (AV) conduction. Note the classic "sawtooth" flutter pattern best appreciated in leads II, III, and aVF.

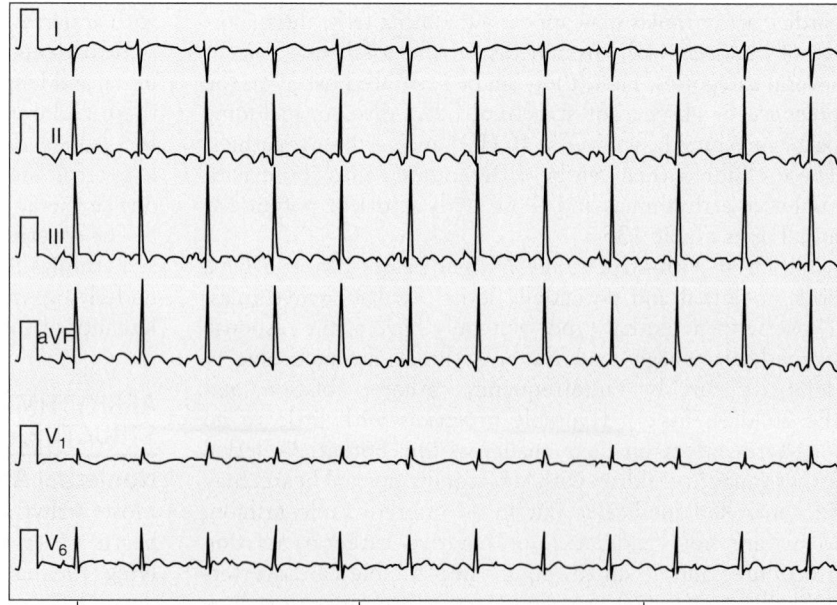

Atrial ectopic tachycardias (AET) also occur. The diagnosis is often made by notation of a persistently elevated heart rate for age. Occasionally, children have congestive heart failure secondary to a tachycardia-induced cardiomyopathy. Atrial rates can vary from 120 to 240 bpm with 1:1 AV conduction or more advanced degrees of AV block. AET is difficult to control medically, and a curative radiofrequency catheter ablation procedure is indicated.

Nonlethal Ventricular Arrhythmias

Children are often referred to a pediatric cardiologist for an irregular rhythm noted during a routine physical examination and the presence of premature ventricular contractions (PVCs) on the surface electrocardiogram (ECG). Even frequent PVCs that suppress at higher heart rates (as determined by 24-hour Holter or exercise stress test) are considered benign.

Life-Threatening Arrhythmias

Life-threatening arrhythmias in children with structurally normal hearts are primarily ventricular in origin. The most common is torsades de pointes (TDP), a polymorphic ventricular tachycardia most often associated with the long Q-T syndrome (LQTS, Fig. 135-3). A complete discussion of the genetics and pathophysiology of LQTS is beyond the scope of this chapter. Briefly, defects in cardiac ion channels regulating potassium and sodium influx and efflux can cause a prolongation of cardiac repolarization. This results in the prolonged Q-T interval seen on the surface ECG and increases the vulnerability of cardiac cells to afterdepolarizations that can lead to TDP, ventricular fibrillation, and sudden death. Children are often diagnosed after a syncopal or seizure episode has prompted a cardiology referral. Occasionally, LQTS is discovered after a family member is diagnosed with the disease or if there is a history of sudden death. Medical management remains the initial mainstay of therapy, but some children require pacemaker or ICD implantation if symptoms persist despite therapy. Children with LQTS have significant exercise and lifestyle restrictions. Additionally, many over-the-counter and prescription medications (that affect potassium channels and prolong the Q-T interval) should be avoided in these individuals.

Rarely, a child may have idiopathic ventricular fibrillation without evidence of structural heart disease or LQTS. Combined medical management and device therapy are the treatment of choice in these individuals. Similar to patients with LQTS, they will have significant restrictions, and caution should be exercised when using certain medications and anesthetic agents.

ARRHYTHMIAS IN CHILDREN WITH STRUCTURALLY ABNORMAL HEARTS AND CARDIOMYOPATHIES

Atrial Arrhythmias

Postoperative patients with Mustard, Senning, and Fontan repairs develop late atrial arrhythmias. These patients often have sinus node dysfunction increasing the likelihood of premature atrial contractions (PACs) and early junctional beats that initiate tachycardia. Many patients require pacemakers for slow rates, especially when antiarrhythmic agents cause exacerbation of sinus bradycardia. Atrial arrhythmias in the postoperative patient can induce dangerous ventricular arrhythmias or lead to myocardial dysfunction.

Ventricular Arrhythmias

Children who have undergone repair of right-sided heart obstructive lesions and some with single ventricle physiology are at increased risk of developing ventricular arrhythmias. These arrhythmias are poorly tolerated and patients can experience rapid hemodynamic compromise and sudden death.

Children with hypertrophic cardiomyopathy, dilated cardiomyopathy, or arrhythmogenic right ventricular dysplasia (ARVD) are at risk for development of ventricular arrhythmias. In ARVD, normal ventricular myocardium is often replaced by fatty tissue.

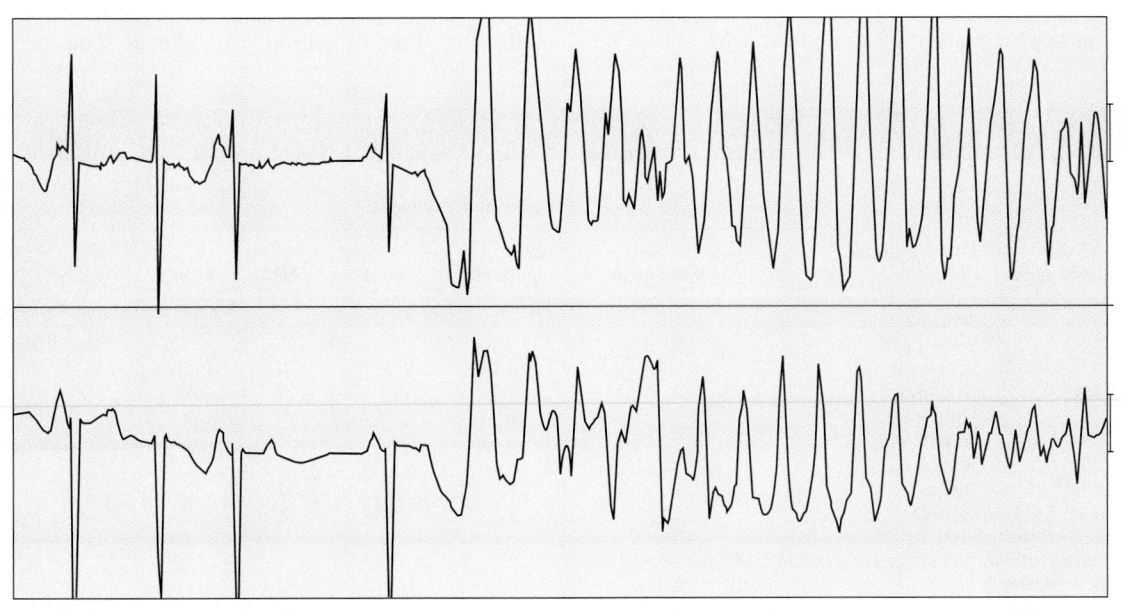

Figure 135-3. Torsades de pointes in a patient with long Q-T syndrome (LQTS).

TREATMENT

Structurally Normal Hearts (Table 135-2)
Supraventricular Tachyarrhythmias

Therapy of SVT is based on the mechanism of tachycardia. Infants with neonatal atrial flutter are often treated with digoxin. Digoxin (6 to 10 µg/kg/day) is used to slow conduction through the AV node and may decrease initiating PACs. Propranolol (2 to 5 mg/kg/day) may be effective and is divided into four daily doses owing to neonatal metabolism. If digoxin and propranolol are not effective in suppressing atrial flutter, sotalol is an alternative. DL-Sotalol has both class III repolarization and beta-blocking properties. In neonates, 2 to 5 mg/kg/day is divided into three doses. Drug-induced torsades de pointes is a theoretical concern.

For infants and children with Wolff-Parkinson-White (WPW) syndrome, digoxin may be contraindicated because it may shorten the antegrade refractory period, resulting in an increased risk of ventricular fibrillation during atrial tachyarrhythmias. This risk may range from 1% to 5%. Initial medical management of these children should consist of β-blocker therapy. If a Holter monitor or stress test (older patients) demonstrates normalization of the QRS complex (implying a long antegrade refractory period of the pathway), digoxin may be used. For resistant SVTs, flecainide is often used as a second-line antiarrhythmic. Flecainide, a class 1C sodium-channel blocker, decreases conduction velocity over the accessory pathway. Initiation of this drug should take place in an inpatient setting with continuous telemetry. Dosing is 80 to 150 mg/m^2 and trough levels should be drawn preceding the fifth dose. Other useful drugs include the class III drugs sotalol and amiodarone. Infants and children with SVT without preexcitation can be started on digoxin as initial medical therapy. The subsequent algorithm for choice of antiarrhythmic medication thereafter is similar to that for children with WPW syndrome.

Given the safety and success of radiofrequency catheter ablation performed in experienced pediatric centers, children with SVT can be referred to a *pediatric* electrophysiologist for curative ablation, especially once they are over age 5 years or approximately 15 kg body weight.

Children with atrial ectopic tachycardia are managed initially with digoxin, followed by β-blocker therapy or sotalol. Flecainide can also be used, but may be contraindicated in patients with dilated cardiomyopathy. Control of the arrhythmia results in regression of the cardiomyopathy.

Ventricular Arrhythmias

Management of children with LQTS is challenging. If the child has an identified LQTS gene for one of the known channel mutations, some mutation-specific management can be considered. However, the mainstay of treatment for children with LQTS is β-blocker therapy. Atenolol and propranolol are commonly used, although nadolol and metoprolol can be used as well. In children with a known sodium-channel defect, mexiletine may be been effective in shortening the Q-T$_c$.

Children with LQTS and pause-dependent ventricular arrhythmia are referred for pacemaker implantation. Children with LQTS and 2:1 AV block or congenital complete AV block are also candidates for pacemaker implantation. There is no clear consensus about the use of ICDs in LQTS. Children who have syncope or aborted cardiac death despite therapy are candidates for ICD implantation, as well as those with a family history of sudden death and noncompliant patients.

Congenital Heart Disease and Cardiomyopathies (Table 135-3)
Atrial Arrhythmias

Treatment of atrial arrhythmias in patients with congenital heart disease is complex. Many patients have more than one arrhythmia, and medical management alone is rarely successful. Most patients are managed on digoxin plus another drug, such as amiodarone or sotalol. Amiodarone has several potential systemic side effects, including hypo- and hyperthyroidism, decreased hepatic function, and pulmonary fibrosis. Because amiodarone is highly protein-bound, it increases the serum level of other protein-bound drugs such as digoxin and Coumadin. Doses of these drugs must be adjusted to avoid potential toxicity. Amiodarone is also highly lipid-soluble, and full clearance of the drug following discontinuation can take as long as 5 months.

Table 135-2. Antiarrhythmic Drug Choice in Arrhythmia Management—Structurally Normal Hearts

Vaughn Williams Class	Antiarrhythmic Drug	Atrial Arrhythmias						Ventricular Arrhythmias	
		AET	Atrial Flutter	AVRT (non WPW)	WPW	PJRT	AVNRT	LQTS	VT/VF
Class IA	Procainamide	X	X						
Class IB	Mexiletine							X	X
Class IC	Flecainide			X	X	X			
Class II (β-blockers)	Propranolol	X		X	X	X	X	X	X
	Atenolol	X		X	X	X	X	X	X
Class III	Amiodarone		X						X
	Sotalol	X	X						
Class IV	Verapamil					X	X		†
Other	Digoxin	X	X	X	X*	X	X		

*Used only if accessory pathway demonstrates long antegrade effective refractory period.
†Occasional need for left-sided VT.

AET, atrial ectopic tachycardia; AVNRT, atrioventricular node reentry tachycardia; AVRT, atrioventricular reentry tachycardia; LQTS, long QT syndrome; PJRT, permanent junctional reciprocating tachycardia; VF, ventricular fibrillation; VT, ventricular tachycardia; WPW, Wolff-Parkinson-White syndrome.

Table 135-3. Antiarrhythmic Drug Therapy in Congenital Heart Disease and Cardiomyopathy

Vaughn Williams Class	Antiarrhythmic Drug	Atrial Arrhythmias		Ventricular Arrhythmias
		Atrial Reentry Tachycardia	*AET*	*VT/VF*
Class IA	Procainamide	X*		
Class IB	Mexiletine			X
Class IC	Flecainide	‡	‡	
Class II (β-blockers)	Propranolol		X	X
	Atenolol		X	X
Class III	Amiodarone	X*	X	X
	Sotalol	X*	X	
Class IV	Verapamil	†		
Other	Digoxin	X	X	X

*Often in combination with digoxin.
†Occasionally used for ventricular rate control. May adversely affect ventricular function.
‡Flecainide is contraindicated in patients with structural heart disease and atrial arrhythmias.
AET, atrial ectopic tachycardia; VT, ventricular tachycardia.

Both sotalol and amiodarone require inpatient initiation of drug therapy. Owing to reports of sudden death in patients with CHD and atrial arrhythmias, the use of flecainide in this population is controversial.

Patients with underlying sinus node dysfunction may be referred for pacemaker implantation prior to antiarrhythmic therapy. A dual-chamber pacemaker with a competent atrial lead also allows for overdrive pacing of the arrhythmia, saving the patient's family and the hospital valuable time and resources.

Persistent tachycardia despite medical or pacemaker therapy can prompt referral for catheter ablation. With the recent development of three-dimensional electroanatomic catheter mapping, electrical activation can be superimposed on a three-dimensional structure, allowing accurate localization of arrhythmia circuit(s) and improving outcomes. Information about circuit location can be used to guide intraoperative ablation if the child requires further surgical intervention for hemodynamic considerations.

Ventricular Arrhythmias

Medical management is required in all patients, and some may need pacemaker or ICD implantation. β-Blockers are often used in combination with mexiletine, a class IA antiarrhythmic. Amiodarone is also used. Pacemaker implantation is indicated in cases of drug-induced sinus bradycardia or in children with pause-dependent VT.

CHD patients whose clinical tachycardia suggests a single focus are candidates for catheter ablation. Sustained polymorphic VT or VT that is unstable often prompts referral for ICD implantation. In these children, dual-chamber ICDs offer benefit in terms of synchronous dual-chamber pacing and in diagnostic evaluation. Many patients have both atrial and ventricular arrhythmias, and analysis of device-stored intracardiac electrocardiograms allows the cardiologist to make necessary changes in medical therapy or device programming. Management of children with poor ventricular function may include an ICD as a bridge to heart transplantation.

Children with cardiomyopathy and VT are also candidates for ICD implantation. Children with obstructive cardiomyopathy may benefit from dual-chamber pacing, thereby decreasing the gradient across the left ventricular outflow tract. Although this result has not been uniformly proved, this procedure may benefit the child who requires an ICD.

CONSIDERATIONS FOR THE PEDIATRIC PRIMARY CARE PROVIDER

Many common over-the-counter cold medications contain β-agonist or sympathomimetic agents that may trigger arrhythmias. Some local anesthetic agents used by dentists contain epinephrine, another trigger for arrhythmia. Parents should be urged to consult with pharmacists before selecting a decongestant or antitussive medication.

The importance of vigilant medication monitoring in patients with LQTS cannot be overstated. Before prescribing any medication, the effect of the drug on the Q-T$_c$ should be investigated; this information can be found in the PDR (Physicians' Desk Reference) as well as the drug insert. A list of drugs that prolong the Q-T$_c$ is listed in Table 135-4. Use of herbal supplements should be discouraged in the child with LQTS. Because they are not subject to Food and Drug Association (FDA) approval, the safety, efficacy, and pharmacokinetics of these supplements are not known. These precautions should also be observed when treating siblings of the child with LQTS. Even a sibling who has a normal ECG, may be a carrier of the defective gene. Challenge with a Q-T$_c$ prolonging drug may produce the LQTS phenotype in a previously asymptomatic individual.

History of arrhythmia is not a contraindication to immunization. These children, especially those with underlying CHD, should receive immunizations according to schedule.

POSTOPERATIVE CARE

Post-Electrophysiology Study and Radiofrequency Ablation

In most pediatric centers, electrophysiology studies (EPS) are performed as outpatient procedures. Postprocedure care is generally limited to mild pain management and activity limitations for the initial 1 to 2 days. Owing to the femoral catheter entry sites, patients are kept supine for 4 to 6 hours immediately following the procedure. Children

Table 135-4. Drug That Prolong the Q-T Interval or Induce Torsades de Pointes

Drug (Trade Names)	Drug Class (Clinical Usage)	Prolonged Q-T Interval	Induced TDP
Amiodarone (Cordarone)	Antiarrhythmic (heart rhythm)	Yes	Yes
Arsenic trioxide (Trisenox)	Anticancer (leukemia)	Yes	Yes
Bepridil (Vascor)	Antianginal (heart pain)	Yes	Yes
Chlorpromazine (Thorazine)	Antipsychotic/antiemetic (schizophrenia/nausea)	No	No
Cisapride (Propulsid)	GI stimulant (stimulates GI motility)	Yes	Yes
Clarithromycin (Biaxin)	Antibiotic (bacterial infection)	No	No
Desipramine (Norpramin)	Antidepressant (depression, others)	Yes	No
Disopyramide (Norpace)	Antiarrhythmic (heart rhythm)	Yes	Yes
Dofetilide (Tikosyn)	Antiarrhythmic (heart rhythm)	Yes	Yes
Doxepin (Sinequan, Zonalon)	Antidepressant (depression, pain, other)	No	No
Droperidol (Inapsine)	Sedative/Hypnotic (anesthesia adjunct)	Yes	Yes
Erythromycin (E.E.S., Erythrocin)	Antibiotic/GI stimulant (infection/GI motility)	Yes	Yes
Felbamate (Felbatrol)	Anticonvulsant (seizures)	No	Yes
Flecainide (Tambocor)	Antiarrhythmic (heart rhythm)	Yes	Yes
Fluoxetine (Prozac, Sarafem)	Antidepressant (depression)	Yes	Yes
Foscarnet (Foscavir)	Antiviral (HIV infection)	Yes	No
Fosphenytoin (Cerebyx)	Anticonvulsant (seizures)	Yes	No
Gatifloxacin (Tequin)	Antibiotic (bacterial infection)	Yes	No
Halofantrine (Halfan)	Antimalarial (malaria infection)	Yes	Yes
Haloperidol (Haldol)	Antipsychotic (schizophrenia, agitation)	Yes	Yes
Ibutilide (Corvert)	Antiarrhythmic (heart rhythm)	Yes	Yes
Imipramine (Tofranil)	Antidepressant (depression, pain, other)	No	No
Indapamide (Lozol)	Diuretic (stimulates urine and salt loss)	Yes	No
Isradipine (Dynacirc)	Antihypertensive (high blood pressure)	Yes	No
Levofloxacin (Levaquin)	Antibiotic (bacterial infection)	No	Yes
Levomethadyl (Orlaam)	Opiate agonist (narcotic dependence)	Yes	No
Mesoridazine (Serentil)	Antipsychotic (schizophrenia)	Yes	No
Moexipril/HCTZ (Uniretic)	Antihypertensive (high blood pressure)	Yes	No
Moxifloxacin (Avelox)	Antibiotic (bacterial infection)	Yes	No
Naratriptan (Amerge)	Migraine treatment	Yes	No
Nicardipine (Cardene)	Antihypertensive (high blood pressure)	Yes	No
Octreotide (Sandostatin)	Endocrine (acromegaly/carcinoid diarrhea)	Yes	No
Paroxetine (Paxil)	Antidepressant (depression)	No	Yes
Pentamidine (Pentam, NebuPent)	Anti-infective (Pneumocystis pneumonia)	Yes	Yes
Pimozide (Orap)	Antipsychotic (Tourette's tics)	Yes	No
Probucol (Lorelco)	Antilipemic (lowers cholesterol)	Yes	Yes
Procainamide (Procan, Pronestyl)	Antiarrhythmic (heart rhythm)	Yes	Yes
Quetiapine (Seroquel)	Antipsychotic (schizophrenia)	Yes	No
Quinidine (Cardioquin, Quinaglute)	Antiarrhythmic (heart rhythm)	Yes	Yes
Risperidone (Risperdal)	Antipsychotic (schizophrenia)	Yes	No
Salmeterol (Serevent)	Sympathomimetic (asthma, COPD)	Yes	No
Sertraline (Zoloft)	Antidepressant (depression)	Yes	Yes
Sotalol (Betapace)	Antiarrhythmic (heart rhythm)	Yes	Yes
Sparfloxacin (Zagam)	Antibiotic (bacterial infection)	Yes	Yes
Sumatriptan (Imitrex)	Migraine treatment	Yes	No
Tacrolimus (Prograf)	Immune suppressant	No	No
Tamoxifen (Nolvadex)	Anticancer (breast cancer)	Yes	No
Thioridazine (Mellaril)	Antipsychotic (schizophrenia)	Yes	Yes
Tizanidine (Zanaflex)	Muscle relaxant	No	No
Venlafaxine (Effexor)	Antidepressant (depression)	Yes	No
Ziprasidone (Geodon)	Antipsychotic (schizophrenia)	Yes	No
Zolmitriptan (Zomig)	Migraine treatment	Yes	No

Adapted from www.torsades.org; last updated April, 2001.

can generally return to their preprocedure level of activity on the third or fourth post-EPS day. Children with left-sided arrhythmia substrates who have undergone ablation are usually required to take aspirin for 2 weeks to decrease the small risk of clot formation and subsequent thromboembolus. Children *without* underlying CHD do not require subacute bacterial endocarditis (SBE) prophylaxis and should not be restricted from physical activity in any fashion. In the otherwise healthy child, freedom from arrhythmia at 1-year follow-up is considered curative and the patient can be discharged from cardiology care.

Post-Pacemaker Implant

Pacemaker implantation involves implantation of the pulse generator and introduction of atrial or ventricular leads. Depending on the age, size, and absence or presence of certain congenital heart lesions, leads can be transvenous or epicardial. Placement of the pulse generator for a transvenous system is subpectoral or axillary. Immediate postoperative care generally consists of pain management and antibiotics. For new leads, patients generally are seen for their first pacemaker clinic visit 4 to 6 weeks post-implant. Capture thresholds for pacing are lowest at the time of implant, peak at 2 to 3 weeks post-implant, and reach chronic values by 4 to 6 weeks. Following the initial visit, if there are no complications, the child will be re-evaluated in the clinic every 6 months. The pacemaker is "interrogated" at each visit to evaluate lead capture and sensing thresholds as well as remaining battery longevity. Pacing parameters and settings are continuously adjusted to meet the hemodynamic demands of the patient.

Children with pacemakers are permitted to participate in most sports and physical activities. Because of the potential for damage to the pacemaker leads, participation in contact sports is not permitted. Parents of younger children and toddlers are advised to prohibit activities that increase the likelihood of trauma to the abdomen, such as bending over swings and monkey bars. Lead fracture in a pacemaker-dependent child can be a life-threatening emergency. For this reason, parents and adults having frequent contact with such a child should be instructed in basic cardiopulmonary resuscitation and life support.

Modern appliances such as toasters, microwaves, and hairdryers do not interfere with pacemaker function. Patients are advised to keep cellular telephones at least 6 to 12 inches from the pacemaker. Magnetic resonance imaging (MRI) scans are contraindicated in all pacemaker patients.

Post-ICD Implant

Follow-up care after ICD implantation is identical to that for pacemaker implantation. Most patients will have exercise restrictions based on the underlying arrhythmia diagnosis. Additionally, many states have driving restrictions for patients who have recently undergone ICD implantation. Adolescents of driving age and young adults should consult their cardiologist about the laws governing driving in their state.

The cardiologist should be contacted for any child receiving an ICD shock. Interrogation of the device will provide diagnostic information about the rhythm treated and is crucial to guiding medical therapy and subsequent device programming. Pacemaker-dependent patients and those with ICDs should wear an identification (Medic-Alert) bracelet or necklace.

LIFESTYLE ISSUES

Structurally Normal Hearts
Supraventricular Tachycardia

The effect of SVT on a child's lifestyle is related in large part to the unpredictable nature of episodes. For children with rare, self-limited episodes, there is minimal interference with activity or quality of life. Children who have episodes triggered by activity or exercise may voluntarily decrease activity levels in an attempt to prevent SVT. Long, sustained SVT that does not respond to simple vagal maneuvers often prompts an emergency room visit; if the episode occurs at school, EMS may be called to transport the child. This event can draw unwanted attention from peers and fear on the part of medically untrained school personnel. Some children undergo multiple medication trials to control their SVT, occasionally requiring a 3- to 5-day hospital admission. For these reasons, the child with

recurrent SVT is an excellent candidate for curative radiofrequency ablation.

Ventricular Arrhythmias

The diagnosis of LQTS has significant lifestyle and psychosocial implications for both the child and family. These children are otherwise healthy and have been participating in a full complement of activities, some of them competitive. Once diagnosed, these children are immediately restricted from participation in competitive sports. Participation in recreational activities is dependent on the child's clinical presentation and genotype (if available): guidelines are determined by the cardiologist on a patient-to-patient basis. For the previously healthy patient, these restrictions seem unnecessary and even cruel. As LQTS is a life-threatening illness, anxiety is associated with its unpredictable nature.

Medication compliance can become an issue with older school-age children and adolescents. Because they don't "feel sick," patients are often noncompliant with their antiarrhythmic regimen. Compliance is especially a concern because a significant number of fatal events have been reported following abrupt discontinuation of β-blocker therapy. Owing to their developmental stage, adolescents often will not adhere to physical activity restrictions for fear of being "different" from their peers. Patients with LQTS who require ICDs as part of the management of their condition have additional anxiety related to potential therapy from the device, including shocks or antitachycardia pacing. These individuals have a heightened awareness of their own mortality and may benefit from psychological counseling.

Atrial and Ventricular Arrhythmias: Congenital Heart Disease and Cardiomyopathy

The natural history of patients with certain congenital heart lesions predicts development of arrhythmias in the years following repair. By this time, these children have undergone numerous procedures, including interventional and diagnostic cardiac catheterizations and staged surgical repairs, each requiring hospitalization. The additional diagnosis of an arrhythmia can be frustrating to the child and family trying to cope with an already complicated medical condition. Not only will the child require additional follow-up and routine testing, but additional hospitalizations for initiation of certain antiarrhythmic drugs and catheterization procedures may be necessary as well. New onset of arrhythmias may suggest worsening hemodynamic insufficiency and can be an indication for surgical revision.

For patients with pacemakers, pulse generator longevity ranges from 3 to 8 years, requiring device replacement on a regular basis. Toddlers and young school-age children may also require lead replacement as they grow.

Despite maximal antiarrhythmic therapy, patients may still experience breakthrough episodes of arrhythmia. Because of poor hemodynamics, these episodes may not be well tolerated and will prompt emergency room visits. The child with a pacemaker and competent atrial lead can be overdrive paced with minimal discomfort. Otherwise, DC cardioversion is indicated. Frequent emergency room and cardiology clinic visits are disruptive to the child's and family's schedules and can interfere with normal functioning.

Congenital heart patients who require ICDs have the attendant lifestyle concerns previously mentioned. Progressive deterioration of hemodynamic function may increase the frequency of arrhythmias, leading to frequent device-delivered therapy. These patients are often heart transplant candidates and will require close follow-up and supervision.

PROGNOSIS

Structurally Normal Hearts

Supraventricular Tachycardia

The prognosis for children with SVT and structurally normal hearts is excellent. Control may be achieved with antiarrhythmic therapy until the child is referred for radiofrequency catheter ablation. The success of the procedure is related to institution experience and location of the underlying substrate. Long-term success in over 90% of patients should be expected. If the substrate is close to the child's His bundle, ablation may not be attempted.

Children who have undergone successful radiofrequency ablation are considered cured. They should have no activity restrictions and should be considered normal from a medical and insurance standpoint.

Ventricular Arrhythmias

The prognosis of patients with LQTS is variable and is largely related to genotype, positive family history, and symptomatology or aborted sudden death. Patients with LQT3, a sodium-channel defect, have an increased incidence of sudden death despite β-blocker therapy. Patients with LQT1, the slowly rectifying potassium-channel defect, respond well to β-blocker therapy, although it is not entirely protective. Patients with family members who have died suddenly are also at increased risk for sudden death. Abrupt discontinuation of β-blocker therapy puts the child at significant risk for ventricular arrhythmia from resultant rebound tachycardia. The noncompliant family or adolescent may require ICD implantation to prevent episodes of TDP and sudden death.

Atrial Arrhythmias: Congenital Heart Disease

The development of atrial arrhythmias often occurs in the adolescent or young adult with CHD. Given the relatively recent growth of this population, their long-term prognosis has not been established. These patients are at risk for sudden death from rapid conduction of atrial arrhythmias to the ventricle. When possible, radiofrequency ablation should be attempted, or the patient should be referred for surgical intervention and revision.

Ventricular Arrhythmias: Congenital Heart Disease and Cardiomyopathy

The prognosis of CHD patients with VT depends on the underlying arrhythmia substrate. Monomorphic VT suggests a single ectopic focus that may be amenable to radiofrequency ablation, either in the catheterization laboratory or at the time of surgical revision in the operating room. These patients will have clinical improvement but remain at risk for future arrhythmias. Polymorphic VT is poorly tolerated and these patients will require ICDs. These arrhythmias are generally a sign of worsening hemodynamics and ventricular function and the ICD is ultimately a "bridge" to heart transplantation.

Ventricular arrhythmias in patients with cardiomyopathy are generally multifocal and are not candidates for radiofrequency ablation. These patients require ICDs and may have frequent shocks.

SUMMARY

Rhythm disturbances in children range from benign to life-threatening and occur with or without concomitant structural heart disease. The long-term management of these patients can be challenging from medical and behavioral perspectives. Close communication between the managing pediatric cardiologist and the primary care provider is paramount to appropriate management and anticipatory guidance of the patient and family.

Mini-index of Related Topics

SUGGESTED READINGS

Kanter RJ, Garson A Jr: Atrial arrhythmias during chronic follow-up of surgery for complex congenital heart disease. PACE 1997; 20:502–511.

Kugler JD, Danford DA, Deal BJ, et al: Radiofrequency catheter ablation for tachyarrhythmias in children and adolescents. N Engl J Med 1994;330:1481–1487.

Perry JC: Pharmacologic therapy of arrhythmias. In Deal BJ, Wolff GS, Gelband H (eds): Current Concepts in the Diagnosis and Management of Arrhythmias in Infants and Children. Armonk, NY, Futura Publishing, 1998, pp 267–308.

Pfammatter JP, Paul T, Lehmann C, et al: Efficacy and proarrhythmia of oral sotalol in pediatric patients. J Am Coll Cardiol 1995; 26:1002–1007.

Towbin JA, Vatta M: The genetics of cardiac arrhythmias. PACE 2000;23:106–119.

136 Pediatric Cardiac Transplantation

Chuck Norlin

ROLE OF THE GENERALIST

1 Know the conditions for which cardiac transplantation is indicated.
2 Understand the process, implications, and complications of cardiac transplantation.
3 Support and advise families in decisions related to transplantation.
4 Collaborate with the transplant team in the ongoing care of the child.
5 Provide health maintenance care with attention to transplant-related issues.
6 Provide acute care and triage with attention to transplant-related problems.
7 Identify and collaborate in managing immunosuppression-related complications.
8 Provide ongoing support for the patient and family.

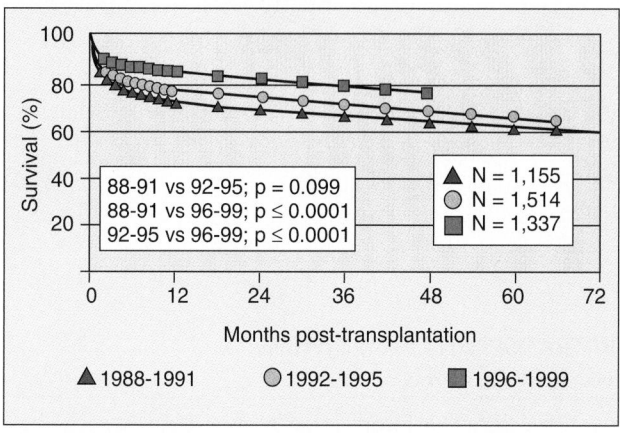

Figure 136-1. Pediatric heart transplantation actuarial survival by era. (Modified from Boucek MM, Faro A, Novick RJ, et al: The Registry of International Society for Heart and Lung Transplantation: Fourth official pediatric report—2000. J Heart Lung Transplant 2001;20:41, with permission from Elsevier Science.)

Since its introduction in the late 1970s, pediatric cardiac transplantation (PCT) has proved to be a successful life-saving and quality of life–enhancing procedure. Though PCT must still be considered palliative owing to continued problems with complications of immunosuppression and rejection, survival rates are improving. Overall, about 60% of PCT patients are alive 9 years after transplant, and the predicted 5-year survival rate for those transplanted after 1996 is above 70% (Fig. 136-1). With improving survival and expanding indications, primary care providers increasingly will be called upon to provide routine and acute care for PCT patients and to collaborate with the transplant team.

BACKGROUND AND STATISTICS

Since 1993, the number of PCTs performed in the 51 transplant centers in the United States has remained constant at 263 to 277 per year (see the list on the CD-ROM). As of January 2001, 1647 patients under 20 years of age have been transplanted. Waiting times for PCT vary by candidate age group and have been generally increasing. In 1999, the median wait time was 75 days for infants; 49 days for 1- to 5-year-olds; 92 days for 6- to 10-year-olds; and 104 days for 11- to 17-year-olds. Twelve percent of pediatric patients listed in 1999 died while they were waiting for a donor; however, the death rate for the most seriously ill was 25% to 30%.

ALLOCATION OF HEARTS FOR TRANSPLANT

Since 1986, the United Network for Organ Sharing (UNOS) has maintained the computer-based allocation program for matching donor organs with recipients. The allocation scheme for PCT reflects the priority for patients with more severe disease and for local organ transfer to minimize donor heart ischemic time. Allocation priority is based on the following criteria:
1. Medical urgency status (Box 136-1)
2. ABO blood typing (those with blood type O face the most competition)
3. Waiting time within status since registered
4. Distance between donor and recipient

INDICATIONS FOR TRANSPLANTATION

Congenital heart disease leads to about 45% of PCTs. Of those patients, infants with lethal congenital heart disease are the most common, the majority having aortic atresia or variants of hypoplastic left heart syndrome (HLHS), for which the Norwood procedure offers an alternative to PCT. Another 45% of PCTs are performed for cardiomyopathies. Retransplantation accounts for about 3%, with the most common indications being primary graft dysfunction, refractory acute rejection, and cardiac allograft vasculopathy. The remaining indications include valvular abnormalities and coronary artery disease.

Box 136-1. Pediatric Medical Urgency Status Codes

Status 1A

The patient must meet at least one of the following requirements:

- Requires assistance with a ventilator, mechanical assist device, or balloon pump
- More than 6 months old with pulmonary hypertension over 50% of systemic
- Requires infusion of high-dose or multiple inotropes
- Life expectancy is less than 14 days

Status 1B

- Requires infusion of low-dose single inotropes
- Less than 6 months old and does not meet status 1A criteria
- Exhibits growth failure

Status 2

Is a patient of any age who does not meet criteria for status 1A or 1B

Status 7

Is temporarily inactive with regard to organ allocation

PRETRANSPLANT EVALUATION AND MANAGEMENT

Box 136-2 lists the information required about each PCT candidate. All routine immunizations should be given prior to PCT if feasible. A history of malignancy or evidence of prior infection with the pathogens listed warrants attention for the patient's lifetime of immunosuppression.

The transplant program often manages pretransplant clinical care but, particularly for status 2 patients, the generalist may continue to provide acute care and ongoing counseling. While waiting, patients must remain within an hour of the transplant center and must be accessible 24 hours a day. Families are usually very stressed during this time: they put their lives on hold, are interrupted by false alarms, wait for the call, and hope it doesn't come too late.

Box 136-2. Pretransplant Evaluation

All relevant medical history, including immunization status

Anthropometric data to determine size compatibility for donor hearts

ABO blood type and, sometimes, panel reactive antibodies (significant elevations of which are associated with higher rates of allograft loss and posttransplant death)

Laboratory data reflecting kidney, liver, and bone marrow function

Serologic tests reflecting status of infection with human immunodeficiency virus, hepatitis viruses, cytomegalovirus, Epstein-Barr virus, *Toxoplasma gondii*, and syphilis (*Treponema*)

Purified protein derivative (PPD) skin test

Consultation with indicated specialists, including pediatric dentistry

Full cardiopulmonary data to assist with accurate diagnosis, prognosis, identification of contraindications or risk factors, and information to guide the transplant surgeon

Psychosocial evaluation to assess family resources and support, ensure understanding of the implications of PCT, and anticipate emotional or compliance problems

TRANSPLANTATION PROCEDURE

When the call comes, events move fast. The patient is admitted to the intensive care unit, immunosuppressive drugs are begun, and he or she is taken to the operating room before the donor heart arrives. Surgery may last from 4 to 8 hours, much of it on cardiopulmonary bypass. The recipient's atria are mostly left intact, resulting occasionally in two unsynchronized P waves on the electrocardiogram (ECG). The donor heart is denervated and unable to signal pain to the recipient or respond to neurologic stimuli, though later there is occasional reinervation in PCT. Donor factors, including injury related to the cause of the donor's death, may affect graft survival and patient morbidity. Latent infection, particularly with cytomegalovirus (CMV) or *Toxoplasma*, may be transmitted with donor tissue or blood, putting the new immunosuppressed host at risk.

Following PCT, the patient must remain in close proximity to the transplant center for 3 to 6 months. He or she will be seen twice weekly and then weekly until stable. Monthly visits with the transplant team, or a more proximate pediatric cardiologist, will often continue for a year or more, moving toward quarterly or semiannual visits for life.

IMMUNOSUPPRESSIVE THERAPY

The goal of immunosuppression in PCT is to maintain sufficient suppression of humoral and cellular immunity to prevent rejection while minimizing adverse effects and the risks of an overly suppressed immune system. Immunosuppressive drugs require close monitoring and attention to interactions, particularly with commonly used drugs such as macrolide antibiotics and ibuprofen. Immunosuppression in PCT generally consists of cyclosporine A (CsA) or tacrolimus, azathioprine or mycophenolate mofetil, and perhaps a corticosteroid (Table 136-1). Dosage and serum drug levels are maintained high in the first few months following PCT. After a prolonged rejection-free period, dosage is adjusted to attain gradually lower drug levels. Tables 136-2 and 136-3 list adverse effects and drug interactions.

Both CsA and tacrolimus inhibit lymphocyte proliferative and cytotoxic responses by suppressing calcineurin. They require ongoing monitoring of drug levels, with dosage adjustment in response to diarrhea and drug-drug interactions. CsA is available in two forms, the original (Sandimmune) and a microemulsion preparation (Neoral), that differ considerably in bioavailability and cannot be used interchangeably.

Azathioprine is a purine antagonist that interferes with RNA synthesis, but its action in allograft protection remains obscure. Azathioprine's primary side effect is dose-related leukopenia, which may occur late in therapy. The leukocyte count must be monitored, aiming for counts of 4000 to 8000 and reducing dosage promptly if the count falls below 2000.

Mycophenolate mofetil inhibits proliferation of both T and B lymphocytes. Diarrhea and vomiting are common side effects that may respond to lower dosage. Corticosteroids have multiple sites of action and are a mainstay of initial therapy and in acute rejection. Sirolimus, a new agent that inhibits T lymphocyte activation and proliferation, is being used increasingly in patients with recurring rejection.

Table 136-1. Immunosuppressive Medications—Pharmacokinetics (Maintenance)

Drug	Usual Dosage	Frequency	Target Blood Level	Metabolic Pathway
Cyclosporin A	3–10 mg/kg/d (higher in infants)	q8–12h	100–350 ng/mL	Cytochrome P-450 3A4 and other pathways
Tacrolimus	0.05–0.3 mg/kg/d	q12h	5–15 ng/mL	Cytochrome P-450 3A4 and other pathways
Azathioprine	1–2 mg/kg/d	qd	NA (WBC > 4000)	To oxymercaptopurine, then oxidized in RBCs and liver
Mycophenolate mofetil (MMF)	600 mg/m^2/dose	q12h	1.5–4 mcg/mL (of MPA)	Glucuronyl transferase, urinary excretion
Corticosteroids	Wide range	q12–24h	NA	Multiple pathways

MPA, mycophenolic acid; NA, not applicable; RBCs, red blood cells; WBC, white blood count.

GRAFT REJECTION

Monitoring for graft function and rejection varies among centers, but the basic evaluation at each visit will include history, height and weight, vital signs, physical and cardiac examination, and an echocardiogram. Rejection is often asymptomatic. Most presenting signs and symptoms are nonspecific (Box 136-3). An endomyocardial biopsy may be used to confirm and quantify rejection.

Most rejection episodes occur in the first few months following transplantation, with a peak in the second month. Most PCT patients experience rejection in the first year, with an average of 1.5 episodes. Absence of acute rejection in the first year may predict lower risk of late rejection. Treatment for rejection involves increased immunosuppression (increased levels of or switching drugs, pulse steroids, and other measures for refractory cases) and supportive care. Late rejection can be difficult to treat and may portend graft loss. Late rejection should prompt consideration of noncompliance, reported in up to 20% of PCT patients. Some degree of chronic rejection may be present in all transplanted hearts and is the primary factor in late graft loss.

COMPLICATIONS

Opportunistic infection is the most common complication in the first 6 months after PCT, when immunosuppression is greatest. Many centers prescribe prophylaxis with nystatin for fungi, trimethoprim/sulfamethoxazole for *Pneumocystis*, and ganciclovir or acyclovir for those receiving CMV-positive hearts. Optimal dosage and duration for prophylaxis is unknown. Sixty percent of serious infections are bacterial with peak incidence, along with fungal infections (7%), in the first month. Serious infections with CMV (18%) and other viruses (13%) peak in the second month. Though uncommon after 6 months, the risk of unusual or unusually severe infection persists for life. Patients should avoid exposure to cat feces (toxoplasmosis), kittens (cat-scratch fever), and reptiles *(Salmonella)*. Standard endocarditis prophylaxis for dental, upper respiratory, gastrointestinal, and genitourinary tract procedures is recommended.

Over a third of PCT patients have hypertension that requires therapy at 3 years posttransplant, most likely as an adverse effect of CsA, tacrolimus, or corticosteroid therapy. Therapy may include angiotensin-converting enzyme inhibitors or calcium-channel blockers. Cyclosporin-related gingival hyperplasia resulting in problems with tooth eruption or dental hygiene should prompt referral to a pediatric dentist and when severe may require gingivectomy or a switch to tacrolimus.

Tremors, dysesthesias of the palms and soles, seizures, or altered mental status from CsA or tacrolimus occur in up to 25% of patients in the postoperative period. Persistent neurotoxicity is uncommon, but may be seen more often with tacrolimus. Hypercholesterolemia occurs in more than 10% of PCT patients at 3 years, but little is known about its implications. Treatment with HMG-CoA reductase inhibitors may be indicated for high levels.

Table 136-2. Immunosuppressive Drugs: Selected Side Effects

Drug	Common Side Effects	Uncommon Side Effects (or Seen) with Prolonged Use
Cyclosporin A	Hypertension Nephrotoxicity Hirsutism Gingival hyperplasia Fine hand tremor Hypomagnesemia	Cramping Headache Diarrhea/nausea/vomiting Paresthesias Flushing Gynecomastia
Tacrolimus	Nephrotoxicity Hypertension Glucose intolerance Tremor Hypomagnesemia Headache Diarrhea	Neurotoxicity Red blood cell aplasia Hypertrophic cardiomyopathy Hirsuitism Gingival hyperplasia
Azothioprine	Leukopenia Thrombocytopenia Nausea/vomiting	Diarrhea Hepatotoxicity Pancreatitis Alopecia
Mycophenolate	Diarrhea Vomiting Leukopenia Headache	Anemia Bone marrow suppression Fever
Corticosteroids	Emotional lability Increased appetite/weight gain Hypertension (with CsA/tacrolimus) Glucose intolerance (diabetes mellitus) Gastritis/ulcer disease Hypercholesterolemia	Cushingoid habitus Adrenal suppression Impaired wound healing Growth retardation Myopathy Osteoporosis Cataracts Atherosclerosis Psychosis Pseudotumor cerebri

Table 136-3. Immunosuppressive Medications: Drug Interactions

Drug	Increased Levels	Decreased Levels	Enhanced Toxicity
Cyclosporin A and tacrolimus	Grapefruit juice Erythromycin and other macrolides Fluconazole/ketoconazole Theophylline Calcium-channel blockers Metaclopramide Prednisolone Cimetadine Loratidine	Phenobarbital Phenytoin Rifampin Carbamazepine Trimethoprim Isoniazid	NSAIDs Aminoglycosides Trimethoprim Acyclovir/gancilovir Digoxin Furosemide Amphotericin B
Azathioprine			Allopurinol Captopril/enalapril
Mycophenolate	Phenytoin Theophylline Salicylates Acyclovir/ganciclovir Probenecid	Cholestyramine Antacids	
Corticosteroids	Estrogens	Barbiturates Carbamazepine Phenytoin Rifampin Isoniazid	

NSAIDs, nonsteroidal anti-inflammatory drugs.

Box 136-3. Acute Rejection: Associated Findings

Symptoms

Irritability
Lethargy
Poor feeding
Sleep disturbance

Physical Findings

Pallor
Cyanosis
Tachycardia
Tachypnea
Fever
Jugular venous distention
Rales
Hepatosplenomegaly
New murmur
Gallop rhythm
New arrhythmia

Echocardiogram Findings

Reduced fractional shortening
Reduced wall thickening
Increased diastolic wall thickness
New pericardial effusion
New mitral regurgitation

Electrocardiogram

Reduction in QRS voltages
Change in QRS axis
Arrhythmia

Chest X-ray Findings

Cardiomegaly
Pulmonary edema
Pericardial effusion

Close to 5% of PCT patients will demonstrate renal dysfunction after 3 years, secondary to CsA or tacrolimus. Lifelong monitoring of renal function is necessary and minimizing medication dosage may lessen chronic renal failure. About 3% of PCT patients will develop insulin-dependent diabetes. Steroid therapy increases the risk, but both CsA and tacrolimus can cause glucose intolerance in the absence of steroids. Anemia is common in PCT patients, though the etiology is unclear; the red blood cell (RBC) profile is similar to that found in the anemia of chronic disease. Magnesium wasting is common with CsA (less so with tacrolimus) and most patients will require magnesium supplementation to maintain normal levels.

Malignancy is reported in up to 8% to 10% of PCT patients at 5 years. Posttransplant lymphoproliferative disorder (PTLD), a unique complication of immunosuppression usually related to infection with Epstein-Barr virus (EBV), may present with gastrointestinal, pulmonary, tonsillar, or other symptoms or findings. It often responds completely to reduction of immunosuppression, but can be fatal despite aggressive therapy. Acyclovir prophylaxis may be warranted after primary EBV infection. Both CsA and tacrolimus may increase sun sensitivity. Extra caution should be taken to minimize sun exposure and the risk of skin cancer.

Cardiac allograft vasculopathy (CAV), reported in up to 10% of PCT patients at 5 years posttransplant, is the leading cause of death after the first year post-transplantation. CAV is an accelerated coronary artery disease with multiple contributing etiologies. With denervation of the heart preventing sensation of ischemic pain, the symptoms of CAV include congestive heart failure, "silent" myocardial infarction, and sudden death. Effective methods of prevention are unknown and the only proven therapy is retransplantation.

HEALTH MAINTENANCE AND PRIMARY CARE

Routine health maintenance care is important for all PCT patients. Ongoing attention to growth and development, behavioral and emotional issues, and family functioning may identify problems when they can be optimally managed. No live vaccines should be given, but all other immunizations, including influenza vaccine, should be given according to current recommendations. Immunization of PCT patients with 7-valent pneumoccocal conjugate vaccine, in addition to the 21-valent pneumoccocal vaccine after age 2, may be warranted.

Normal growth and development is common in PCT, but may vary depending on pretransplant risk factors and degree of illness and disability, posttransplant complications, and steroid therapy. Feeding and nutrition issues are common among infants who never had normal feeding patterns and in some older children who were severely debilitated prior to PCT.

The frequency of common infections in PCT patients is not different from that in the general population and most are tolerated well. Otitis media and viral respiratory and gastrointestinal infections may be approached much as they would in other children (avoiding drug-drug interactions). However, unusual severity, duration, or presentation should prompt a more extensive evaluation, careful management, and early consultation with rejection as a possibility with nonspecific findings. RSV and rotaviral infections may be prolonged, though usually not more severe. Prolonged marrow suppression from parvovirus may result in significant anemia. An episode of chickenpox when immunosuppression is greatest warrants varicella immune globulin (VZIG) and acyclovir, though close monitoring alone may serve for infection when immunosuppression is less.

Issues of adolescence (rebellion, independence, body image, self-esteem) are challenging for the PCT patient on chronic medications, with chronic illness and perhaps physical changes caused by drugs. Noncompliance is a significant and life-threatening problem during adolescence.

Numerous resources and organizations are available to assist patients and families with knowledge and support as they pursue PCT and manage life afterward (see the CD-ROM). Participation in local camps and the national Transplant Games are particularly popular.

OUTCOMES

Overall, PCT patients have very good quality of life and are capable of full-time school attendance and work without disability. Allowing for the prior risk associated with congenital heart disease and missed school because of illness, PCT patients are likely to have normal cognitive function and school performance. Though exercise testing would suggest persistent suboptimal performance, many patients are able to compete successfully in all sports. PCT patients who have survived 5 years have an 80% chance of surviving another 5 years, 67% for surviving 10 years.

COLLABORATION

Caring for PCT patients is challenging and rewarding. Collaborating with the transplant team is an essential aspect of this care. Frequently, the transplant coordinator is the pediatrician's best, and most available, ally. The generalist should not hesitate to detail her or his desire and ability to participate actively in the management of PCT patients.

 Additional Resources, CD-ROM

Bibliography	

Mini-index of Related Topics

	CH.
■ LIVER TRANSPLANT	142
■ RENAL TRANSPLANT	175
■ ANTI-INFLAMMATORY AND IMMUNOMODULATORY THERAPY	286

SUGGESTED READINGS

Addonizio LJ: Current status of cardiac transplantation in children. Curr Opin Pediatr 1996;8:520–526.

Boucek MM, Shaddy RE: Pediatric heart transplantation. In Allen HD, Gutgesell HP, Clark EB, Driscoll DJ (eds): Moss and Adams' Heart Disease in Infants, Children, and Adolescents Including the Fetus and Young Adult, 6th ed. Philadelphia, Lippincott Williams & Wilkins, 2000, pp 395–407.

Chinnock R, Sherwin T, Robie S, et al: Emergency department presentation and management of pediatric heart transplant recipients. Pediatr Emerg Care 1995;11(6):355–360.

Gajarski RJ, Kearney DL, Price JK, Denfield SW: Update on pediatric heart transplantation: Long-term complications. Texas Heart Inst J 1997;24(4):260–268.

Nevins TE: Overview of new immunosuppressive therapies. Curr Opin Pediatr 2000;12:146–150.

137 Congenital Anatomic Disorders of the Gastrointestinal Tract

Peter Lee and Samuel A. Kocoshis

ROLE OF THE GENERALIST

1 Refer patients with congenital disorders of the gastrointestintal tract for surgical intervention in a timely and appropriate manner.
2 Distinguish between Hirschsprung disease and functional constipation.
3 Recognize complications from Hirschsprung disease.
4 Recognize symptoms of Meckel diverticulum and indications for laparotomy.
5 Recognize symptoms of disorders of intestinal rotation and indications for emergent intervention.

Although most congenital disorders of the gastrointestinal tract are readily apparent at birth, a subset of congenital abnormalities can be delayed in their presentation. These disorders may manifest sometime during childhood or, in some cases, in adulthood. Complications from these conditions can be quite dramatic and result in significant gastrointestinal bleeding, obstruction, perforation, or ischemia. Such intestinal catastrophes may result in short-bowel syndrome, which carries its own set of long-term management issues. This chapter focuses on the potential complications and long-term management of Hirschsprung disease, Meckel diverticulum, and disorders of intestinal rotation.

HIRSCHSPRUNG DISEASE

Hirschsprung disease, or congenital aganglionic megacolon, is a disorder of intestinal motility resulting from a loss of enteric neurons in the submucosal and myenteric plexus. Failure of migration of ganglion cell precursors in utero causes a disruption of inhibitory parasympathetic neurons and inhibition of relaxation in the affected segment of intestine. This contracted segment is usually limited to the rectosigmoid but may involve the entire colon or even the colon and small bowel (total aganglionosis).

Clinical Presentation

Only 15% of infants with Hirschsprung disease are diagnosed within the first month of life with classic symptoms of acute intestinal obstruction. The remainder present variably with a history of delay in passage of meconium, or symptoms of constipation, abdominal distention, or vomiting. Although 60% of cases of Hirschsprung disease are diagnosed by 1 year of age, those with short or ultra-short segment disease may not be diagnosed until childhood or adolescence. The older child or adolescent may have a history of chronic, severe constipation or intermittent intestinal obstruction. The presence of abdominal distention, diarrhea, fever, or shock is indicative of Hirschsprung enterocolitis (toxic megacolon) and is associated with a high mortality rate.

Diagnosis

Several important symptoms and signs distinguish Hirschsprung disease from functional constipation (Table 137-1). A history of normal growth and of fecal soiling is consistent with functional constipation. Children with functional constipation frequently exhibit retentive behavior, attempting to keep from passing large-caliber stools that they retain within a dilated rectal canal. They may contort their bodies to maximally tighten their buttocks or they may "dance" around the house when they feel a defecatory sensation. Other retentive behaviors include back-arching, squatting in a corner, or running back and forth throughout their homes.

Most patients with functional constipation lack abdominal distention. A digital rectal examination revealing a large amount of stool within the rectal vault is very suggestive of functional constipation. Patients with Hirschsprung disease grow poorly, have abdominal distention, and have a relatively empty vault on rectal examination.

Although the presence of a transition zone on contrast barium enema is highly suggestive of Hirschsprung disease, definitive diagnosis is confirmed with rectal biopsy that shows absence of ganglion cells or enhanced acetylcholinesterase staining of nerve fibers. Because of ease of

Table 137-1. Comparison of Features of Hirschsprung Disease and Functional Constipation

Hirschsprung Disease	Functional Constipation
Poor growth	Normal growth
No fecal soiling	Fecal soiling
No stool in rectal vault	Large amount of stool in rectal vault
Abdominal distention	Stool withholding behavior

performance and a favorable safety profile, suction rectal biopsy is the preferred biopsy technique. If tissue samples are inadequate by this technique, a full-thickness surgical biopsy may be mandatory. Absent relaxation of the internal anal sphincter after insufflation of a rectal balloon on manometric assessment is also confirmatory, if available. Because of the minute length of the internal anal sphincter, the procedure is technically difficult (especially in young infants).

Acute and Long-Term Management

A variety of procedures are now available for treatment of Hirschsprung disease, including the modified Swenson, Duhamel, or Soave pull-through. In the Swenson pull-through procedure, the aganglionic rectosigmoid is removed and the remaining ganglionic bowel is reanastomosed to the rectal cuff. The Duhamel procedure involves a side-side anastomosis of proximal bowel to a longer aganglionic rectal stump. In the Soave procedure, the rectal mucosa is stripped and the ganglionic proximal bowel is then pulled through the remaining rectal sleeve and reanastomosed.

The long-term management of patients with Hirschsprung disease requires monitoring for possible complications after surgical correction. Recurrent obstruction, fecal incontinence, and enterocolitis are some of the most common potential complications. Causes of recurrent obstruction include residual aganglionosis from an inadequate repair, acquired aganglionosis from presumably further ischemic injury to enteric neurons, or the development of anal stenosis. The presence of a transition zone on contrast barium enema helps differentiate anal stenosis from aganglionosis. Anal stenosis is easily managed with repeated dilations and rarely requires reoperation, but acquired aganglionosis will require resection of the affected segment.

A more troublesome long-term issue with Hirschsprung disease is postoperative fecal incontinence. Some patients simply have overflow incontinence from constipation that should respond to laxative therapy. However, some patients appear to have abnormalities in anorectal function. Loss of internal anal sphincter relaxation or decreased rectal sensation on anorectal manometry are two prominent features in these patients. Biofeedback, periodic enemas, or intrasphincteric botulinum toxin injection may be useful in this situation to maintain an empty rectosigmoid.

Hirschsprung enterocolitis during the initial presentation of disease, or even postoperatively, has been associated with an increased mortality rate. Abdominal distention and pain associated with fever, diarrhea, or shock are typical features of enterocolitis. Initial medical management should focus on the stabilization of any hemodynamic or electrolyte disturbances. Broad-spectrum antibiotics and colonic irrigation with warm saline are also warranted.

MECKEL DIVERTICULUM

Meckel diverticulum is a relatively common congenital abnormality of the gastrointestinal tract occurring in approximately 2% of the general population. Most cases of Meckel diverticulum, however, are asymptomatic and found incidentally during laparotomy for other indications. Some controversy exists over whether asymptomatic cases

of Meckel diverticulum should be resected because only a minority of patients will develop complications. Although complications arising from Meckel diverticulum may occur at any age, the majority develop within the first 2 years of life and include intestinal bleeding, obstruction, and inflammation.

Meckel diverticulum occurs as a result of an incomplete separation of the vitellointestinal duct at 6 weeks' gestation with the formation of a diverticulum on the antimesenteric border of the ileum. A spectrum of vitellointestinal duct remnant malformations is possible and ranges from a fibrous band connecting the terminal ileum with the umbilicus to a completely patent connection with the umbilicus. The diverticulum is located 50 to 75 cm from the ileocecal valve and may contain either ectopic pancreatic or gastric tissue.

Clinical Presentation

Intestinal bleeding is the most common presentation in children. Ulceration from acid or pepsin production in ectopic gastric mucosa may occur within the diverticulum or, more commonly, at its base in the adjacent terminal ileal mucosa, which is especially vulnerable to acid-induced injury.

Patients typically present with intermittent episodes of painless rectal bleeding. This presentation can be mistaken for milk protein enterocolitis in infants or juvenile polyps in older children. In some cases, the diverticulum can become inflamed and mimic appendicitis or, if in association with rectal bleeding, inflammatory bowel disease. The diagnosis can be established with technetium-99m pertechnetate scanning. Technetium pertechnetate is taken up by both normal as well as ectopic gastric mucosa. A positive scan should reveal an abnormal collection of signal in the right lower quadrant. However, the sensitivity of this technique is only 80%, and a negative scan should not preclude laparotomy when indicated (Box 137-1).

Intestinal obstruction is another complication. The diverticulum may serve as a lead point for intussusception among patients presenting with colicky abdominal pain and the passage of current jelly stools. An air contrast enema or ultrasound examination should be diagnostic. Obstruction resulting from the volvulus of bowel around a duct remnant or a diverticulum within an indirect hernia sac are less frequent complications.

In cases of symptomatic Meckel diverticulum, definitive treatment involves surgical excision of the diverticulum. Whenever the base of the diverticulum is large or necrotic

---

Box 137-1. Indications for Laparotomy in Meckel Diverticulum

1. Positive technetium-99m pertechnetate scan
2. Intermittent episodes of painless rectal bleeding when milk protein enterocolitis in infants and juvenile polyp in older children has been excluded
3. Intestinal obstruction from intussusception with Meckel diverticulum as leading point
4. Suspected volvulus around vitellointestinal duct remnant and Meckel diverticulum
5. Suspected inflammation or perforation of Meckel diverticulum

bowel is present from ischemic injury after intussusception or volvulus, resection of the involved area will also be necessary.

DISORDERS OF INTESTINAL ROTATION

During the fifth week of embryogenesis, the developing intestine leaves the abdominal cavity and undergoes a 270-degree counterclockwise rotation around the axis of the superior mesenteric artery. It returns to the abdominal cavity by the 11th week; and fixation of the cecum, ascending colon, and descending colon to the posterior abdominal wall occurs. Abnormalities of intestinal rotation include nonrotation, malrotation, and reversed rotation and have the potential for serious complications such as intestinal obstruction and ischemia.

Of the three types of abnormal rotation, malrotation is the most common and has the highest risk of associated morbidity and death. Malrotation results from an arrested or incomplete rotation of the developing intestine. This results in an abnormal placement of the small and large intestine that are suspended by a narrow mesentery that is not fixed and free to rotate. The age at diagnosis can be quite variable and depends on whether it is found incidentally or because of a specific complication (Box 137-2). Duodenal obstruction from extrinsic compression by peritoneal bands (Ladd bands) typically presents as bilious vomiting in infancy. Midgut volvulus is another serious complication occurring when the intestine rotates around its mesentery causing intestinal obstruction, vascular compromise, bowel ischemia, and eventual infarction. The association of bilious vomiting with rectal bleeding is an ominous sign and should prompt immediate evaluation.

Reversed rotation is relatively rare and results in the duodenum being anterior to the superior mesenteric vessels rather than posterior. Colonic obstruction from internal herniation is the most common complication.

Nonrotation, as its name implies, is the failure of the midgut to rotate with the small intestine remaining on the right side of the abdomen and the large intestine on the left. Fortunately, the vast majority of these patients will remain asymptomatic and will not require surgical correction.

Box 137-2. Indications for Referral for Suspected Disorder of Intestinal Rotation

1. Bilious vomiting in infancy
2. Bilious vomiting with rectal bleeding
3. Abnormal position of ligament of Treitz on upper gastrointestinal contrast study in any patient with persistent vomiting
4. Abnormal location of the cecum on barium enema in any patient with suspected intestinal obstruction

Evaluation

Diagnostic evaluation for malrotation is primarily radiographic in nature unless circumstances dictate urgent laparotomy for suspected midgut volvulus with bowel compromise. Contrast studies of the intestinal tract will reveal an abnormal position of the ligament of Treitz, and if followed to the large intestine, the cecum can be visualized in the right upper quadrant rather than the normal right lower quadrant location. A barium enema may also demonstrate the abnormal location of the cecum. Infants with duodenal obstruction from Ladd bands may also have a "double bubble" sign visible across the epigastrium on an abdominal radiograph. The two bubbles represent the dilated duodenum and stomach.

Treatment

Surgical intervention usually involves the division of any Ladd bands, reduction of the malrotated bowel, broadening of the mesentery, and conversion of the malrotation to a nonrotation. Any portion of bowel that has had a significant ischemic insult will also require resection of the involved segment. Fixation of the bowel is generally not necessary to prevent reoccurrence.

Additional Resources, CD-ROM

Positive Meckel scan	Figure
Bibliography	

Mini-index of Related Topics

	CH.
SHOCK	28
APPROACH TO THE CHILD WITH CONSTIPATION	83
MALABSORPTION DISORDERS	138
DISORDERS OF THE GASTROINTESTINAL TRACT AND LIVER	204

SUGGESTED READINGS

Kleinhaus S, Boley SJ, Sheran M, et al: Hirschsprung's disease—a survey of the members of the Surgical Section of the American Academy of Pediatrics. J Pediatr Surg 1979;14(5):588–597.

Landman GB: A five-year chart review of children biopsied to rule out Hirschsprung's disease. Clin Pediatr 1987;26(6):288–291.

Nurko S: Complications after gastrointestinal surgery: A medical perspective. In Walker WA, Durie PR, Hamilton JR, et al (eds): Pediatric Gastrointestinal Disease. St. Louis, Mosby, 1996, pp 2067–2094.

Seagram CG, Louch RE, Stephens CA, et al: Meckel's diverticulum: A 10-year review of 218 cases. Can J Surg 1968;11(3):369–373.

Yazbeck S: Gastrointestinal emergencies of the neonate. In Roy CC, Silverman A, Alagille D (eds): Pediatric Clinical Gastroenterology. St. Louis, Mosby, 1995, pp 63–67.

138 Malabsorption Disorders

Conrad R. Cole and Samuel A. Kocoshis

ROLE OF THE GENERALIST

1 Recognize malabsorption.
2 Distinguish malabsorption from maldigestion.
3 Determine the etiology of malabsorption.
4 Initiate appropriate laboratory evaluation in suspected malabsorption disorder.
5 Manage malabsorption appropriately.
6 Recognize conditions that require emergent, urgent, and elective referral to a gastroenterologist.

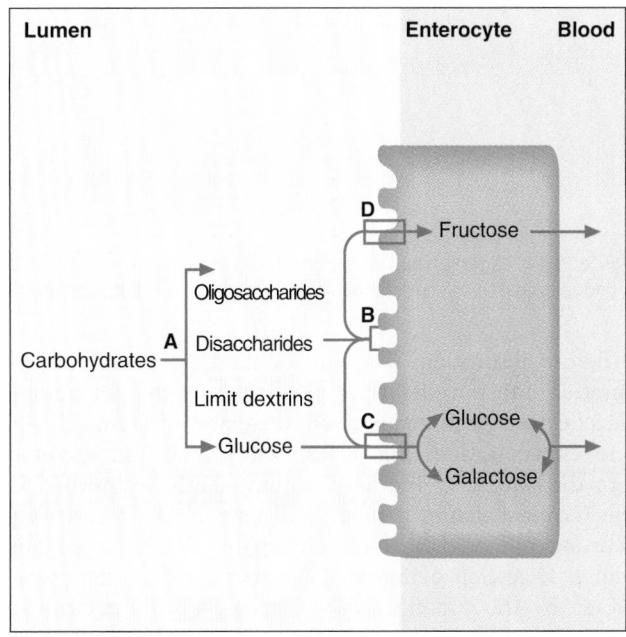

Figure 138-1. Digestion and absorption of dietary carbohydrates. *A,* Salivary and pancreatic amylase. *B,* Disaccharidases located on intestinal brush border. *C,* Glucose-sodium-ATPase transporter. *D,* Fructose transporter.

DEFINITION

Malabsorption is "abnormal intestinal absorption of dietary constituents leading to excessive loss of nutrients in the stool" and may be caused by a digestive defect, mucosal abnormality, or lymphatic obstruction. Malabsorption can produce excessive losses of dietary fat, carbohydrate, protein, vitamins, and minerals individually or in combination. Malabsorption disorders are characterized by specific hydrolysis or transport defects, intestinal villous atrophy, exocrine pancreatic insufficiency, and the short-bowel syndrome. The clinical presentation of these disorders varies with the dietary constituent most affected. Maldigestion occurs when specific enzymes are unavailable and nutrients cannot be processed for absorption.

FUNDAMENTALS

Carbohydrates constitute the major component of most diets. They consist mainly of starch (60% of ingested carbohydrate in older children), sucrose, and lactose (100% of ingested carbohydrate in infants exclusively fed milk). Digestion and absorption of carbohydrate start in the mouth where mastication breaks down food particles to create a greater surface area for the action of salivary amylase. Only starch molecules (glucose polymers of high molecular weight) require intraluminal digestion by salivary and pancreatic amylase (Fig. 138-1). Salivary and pancreatic amylases act on starch to release disaccharides, oligosaccharides, and branched limit α-dextrins. The final hydrolysis occurs on the brush border of the enterocytes where disaccharidases (lactase, sucrase-isomaltase, and glucoamylase) act on them to yield glucose, galactose, and fructose. These sugars are absorbed into the enterocyte by carrier-mediated transport. The glucose-sodium-ATPase (adenosine triphosphatase) transporter SGTA1 transports glucose, and fructose is transported by glucose transporter proteins (GLUTS). Once within the enterocytes, the transported molecule dissociates from the carrier. Glucose, fructose, and galactose then move by simple diffusion into the bloodstream.

Digestion and absorption of protein begin in the lumen of the stomach. Gastric acid denatures protein and activates pepsinogen. Pancreatic proteases are secreted as proenzyme forms (trypsinogen, chymotrypsinogen, proelastase) and activated by enterokinase, a glycoprotein situated on enterocyte brush border of the proximal small bowel. Active endopeptidases (trypsin, chymotrypsin, and elastase) and exopeptidases digest ingested protein to amino acids or oligopeptides (Fig. 138-2). Oligopeptides are further digested by brush border aminopeptidases into single amino acids, dipeptides, and tripeptides. Single amino acids and peptides enter the enterocyte by specific transport systems. Di- and tripeptides are digested by cytoplasmic peptidases into amino acids, which pass through the enterocyte rapidly to the bloodstream.

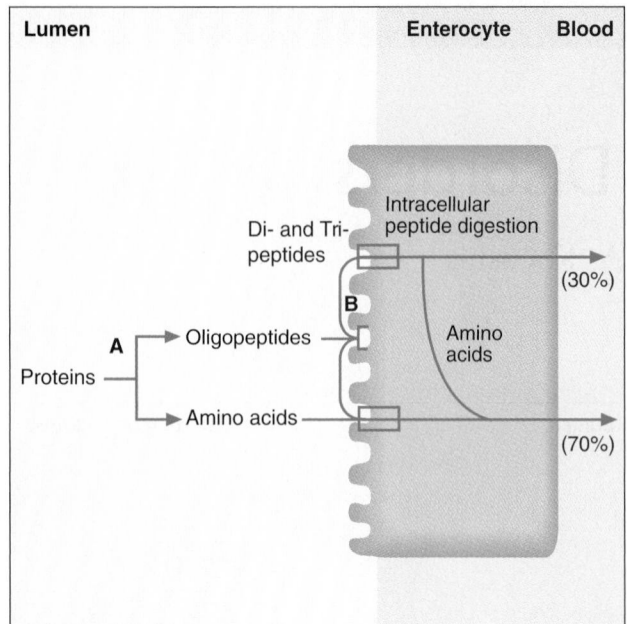

Figure 138-2. Digestion and absorption of dietary proteins. *A,* Endopeptidases: trypsin, chymotrypsin, and elastase. *B,* Enterokinase.

Before absorption, fats must be made soluble by incorporation into micelles (Fig. 138-3) within the gut lumen. Micelle formation requires an adequate intraluminal bile acid concentration. Bile acids, synthesized and secreted into the lumen by the liver, are efficiently reabsorbed in the terminal ileum, a process that maintains a relatively constant bile acid pool (enterohepatic circulation of bile acids). Digestion of ingested fat starts within the gastric lumen by the action of gastric lipase, which requires an acidic milieu for optimal activity and hydrolyzes long-chain (LCT) and medium-chain (MCT) triglycerides. Gastric

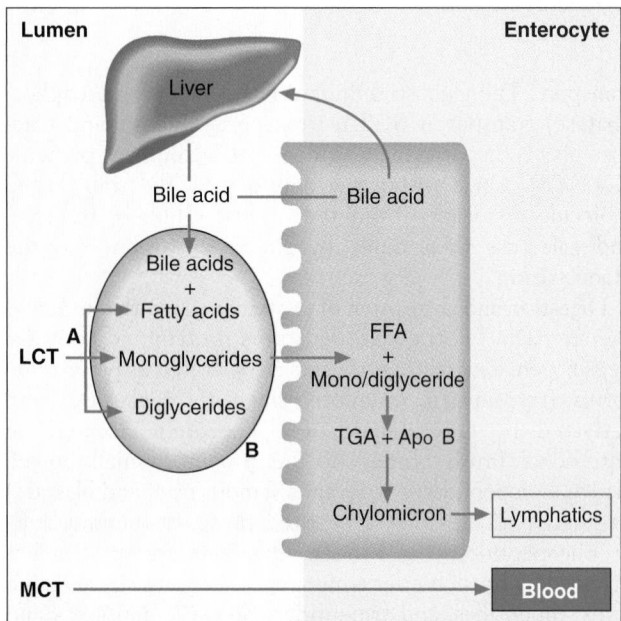

Figure 138-3. Digestion and absorption of dietary triglycerides. *A,* Lingual, gastric, and pancreatic lipase. *B,* Mixed micelle. Apo B, apoprotein B; FFA, free fatty acids; LCT, long-chain triglycerides; MCT, medium-chain triglycerides; TGA, triglycerides.

lipase is very important in neonates whose pancreatic lipase activity is low.

In the small intestine pancreatic lipase acts on the fat-water interface. Bile salts increase the interface by emulsifying the ingested lipids. In the presence of bile salts, pancreatic lipase acts on the outer ester bonds and releases free fatty acids and 2-monoglycerides. Free fatty acids and 2-monoglycerides are solubilized in bile salt micelles, forming mixed micelles that diffuse through the luminal surface of the brush borders, liberating the products of lipolysis. Within the enterocytes, free fatty acids combine with mono- and diglycerides, resynthesizing triglycerides. At low concentrations, free fatty acids enter enterocytes by attaching to a fatty acid binding membrane protein with high affinity for long-chain fatty acids. Chylomicron is formed within the Golgi body of the enterocyte and then released by exocytosis into the intercellular spaces to enter the lymphatics and the thoracic duct and then the systemic circulation. MCT is not re-esterified within the enterocyte, bypassing the lymphatics, to directly enter the bloodstream.

PATHOPHYSIOLOGY

Categories of malabsorption include (1) defects of hydrolysis or transport, (2) disorders of villus atrophy, (3) protein-losing enteropathy, and (4) short-bowel syndrome. Exocrine pancreatic disorders are discussed in other chapters. Malabsorption defects and their associated disease entities are listed in Table 138-1.

Congenital deficiency of enzymes or acquired loss of enzyme or the ability to transport from mucosal injury are defects of hydrolysis and transport that result in malabsorption of carbohydrates. Maldigested and unabsorbed carbohydrates are osmotically active substances, drawing water into the lumen of the gut, increasing stool volume, and stimulating peristaltic activity. Unabsorbed sugars are

Table 138-1. Absorption Defects and Specific Diseases

Defect	Disease
Stomach	
Hypochlorhydria	Protein-energy malnutrition
Decreased production of intrinsic factor	Pernicious/megaloblastic anemia
Pancreas	
Impaired secretion of pancreatic enzymes	Cystic fibrosis, Shwachman-Diamond syndrome, chronic pancreatitis, chronic protein-energy malnutrition
Liver	
Cholestasis	Fat-soluble vitamin deficiencies, fat malabsorption
Enterocyte	
Sucrose-isomaltase deficiency	Impaired digestion/malnutrition
Lactase deficiency	Impaired digestion, diarrhea
Glucoamylase deficiency	Starch malabsorption, diarrhea
Selective defect in glucose-galactose sodium cotransport	Glucose-galactose malabsorption Protein-energy malnutrition
Enterokinase deficiency	Congenital chloride diarrhea
Selective defect in chloride transport	
Impaired production of apolipoprotein B	Abetalipoproteinemia

fermented in the colon by bacteria producing hydrogen gas and short-chain fatty acids. Patients present with large volume, acidic diarrhea. Sucrase-isomaltase deficiency, the most common primary carbohydrate malabsorption disorder, is inherited as an autosomal recessive disorder (prevalence of 3% to 10% among Alaskan and Canadian indigenous peoples) and presents during infancy shortly after sucrose-containing formulas or fruits are introduced to the diet. Although congenital lactase deficiency is rare, acquired hypolactasia is very common. Prevalence varies from 15% to 75% among people of European ancestry and exceeds 80% among Asians, African Americans, and people of Semitic background.

Secondary loss of brush border disaccharidase activity occurs in any disease with mucosal injury. Lactase is the most readily depleted and the slowest to recover after mucosal damage. Glucoamylase, which digests starch and glucose polymers, is the most resistant to depletion. Glucose-galactose malabsorption is very rare, but occurs in cases of congenital transporter mutations or from severe villus injury.

Celiac disease is the most common disorder of villus atrophy among Western Europeans and North Americans of European descent with a prevalence of approximately <1 in 133 to 1 in 300. Epidemiologic evidence links celiac disease closely with type I diabetes mellitus and with trisomy 21. Celiac disease is an autoimmune enteropathy triggered by the ingestion of gluten-containing grains (e.g., wheat, barley, and rye) in genetically susceptible individuals. Age at presentation depends on the age of exposure to gluten in the diet. Although sensitivity to offending foods is lifelong, symptoms may be minimal, especially during adolescence and adulthood. Clinical presentation varies by age at onset (Table 138-2). Toddlers present with diarrhea, growth failure, and anorexia; older children present with symptoms related to chronic malnutrition (delayed puberty, anemia, and rickets). Neuropsychiatric problems, constipation, anasarca, and cutaneous disorders have also been described.

Intractable diarrhea of infancy is a syndrome rather than a disease (symptoms listed in Box 138-1). Protracted diarrhea of infancy is usually due to specific immune deficiency, food protein sensitization, or infection of the gastrointestinal tract, and usually responds to bowel rest. Diseases that cause intractable diarrhea of infancy include (1) microvillus inclusion disease, (2) tufting enteropathy (intestinal epithelial dysplasia), (3) syndromic diarrhea, and (4) autoimmune

Box 138-1. Intractable Diarrhea of Infancy

1. Diarrhea of more than 2 weeks' duration with stool volume greater than 100 mL/kg/day
2. Age younger than 2 years
3. Three or more negative stool cultures for bacterial pathogens
4. Life-threatening persistent symptoms

or immune enteropathy. Microvillus inclusion disease and tufting enteropathy usually present in the neonatal period. Syndromic diarrhea usually presents after 1 month of age. Patients (generally born small for gestational age) have abnormal facies (prominent forehead, broad nose, and hypertelorism), brittle unmanageable hair, and a subtle defect in antibody production. Autoimmune and immune enteropathy present after 3 months of age.

Protein-losing enteropathy (PLE) occurs with many gastrointestinal disorders. Although malabsorption of protein from enterokinase deficiency and pancreatic insufficiency mimic PLE, they are due to maldigestion. Gastrointestinal disorders with PLE induce direct transudation of protein into the intestinal lumen, leading to massive fecal loss of protein nitrogen and results in growth failure, hypoproteinemia, and peripheral edema. Congenital enterokinase deficiency, reported in only a few children, presents early in infancy with intractable diarrhea and malnutrition. Because enterokinase is an essential activator of pancreatic trypsinogen, there is a complete absence of pancreatic proteolytic activity.

Short-bowel syndrome is defined as malabsorption produced by small bowel of length less than two thirds of normal. Malabsorption is almost always present in infants if the small intestine is less than 100 cm long. Although the small intestine may be congenitally short (intestinal atresia, gastroschisis), the majority of cases result from surgical resection (necrotizing enterocolitis, malrotation, midgut volvulus, Crohn's disease, venous and arterial occlusion). Inadequate absorptive surface and abnormal bowel function causes malabsorption that correlates with the extent and anatomic level of the resection. Infants usually have a better prognosis than do older children or adults after extensive small bowel resection because of their greater potential for adaptation, a gradual process associated with substantial increase in villus height with modest bowel lengthening.

Because bile acids and vitamin B_{12} are absorbed in the ileum, ileal resections result in significant nutritional consequences. The ileocecal valve is a physiologic sphincter that controls the rate of delivery of chyme from the small bowel to the colon and prevents bacterial backwash and subsequent bacterial overgrowth into the small intestines. Bacterial overgrowth causes deconjugation of bile salts and subsequent fat malabsorption. The colon slows intestinal transit time and improves absorption of fluid and electrolytes. Colonic bacteria ferment unabsorbed complex carbohydrates to short-chain fatty acids that provide a source of calories by colonic salvage. Fermentation in the colon of malabsorbed carbohydrates can lead to the production of excess D-lactic acid if the patient is colonized with D-lactate-synthesizing organisms. D-Lactic acidosis will then result.

Table 138-2. Clinical Presentation of Celiac Disease by Age of Presentation

Infant (8–12 months)	Toddler	Older Child
Acute growth failure	Gradual growth failure	Anorexia
Severe anemia refractory to oral treatment	Anorexia	Weight loss
Diarrhea	Diarrhea	Diarrhea
	Occasional constipation	Constipation
Moderate abdominal distention	Abdominal pain	Infrequent abdominal pain
	Anemia	Delayed puberty
	Rickets	

EVALUATION

Malabsorption disorders tend to present with similar signs and symptoms: chronic diarrhea; pale, foul-smelling, bulky stools; abdominal distention; and growth failure. Congenital disorders of mucosal structure and function (e.g., congenital chloride-losing diarrhea, microvillus inclusion disease, tufting enteropathy) are frequently associated with in utero diarrhea, resulting in polyhydramnios. Symptoms may not develop until the introduction of new foods in children with other disorders (e.g., celiac disease, allergic enteropathy, congenital sucrase-isomaltase deficiency).

An outline of the progression of diagnostic studies is presented in Figure 138-4. A careful history of the time of the onset of symptoms and the relationship to diet is very important. If a dietary component is the cause of malabsorption, repetition of symptoms should occur with reintroduction of the substance, and improvement should occur with removal of the offending agent. The timing, looseness, frequency, size, color, and smell of the stools can be helpful in formulating a differential diagnosis. The presence of in utero polyhydramnios and large volume stools in the neonatal period favors a congenital disorder. Onset after gluten is introduced in the diet suggests celiac disease, and persistence after an acute infection suggests postinfectious diarrhea. A 5-day prospective diary of dietary intake should always be obtained.

The physical examination should include anthropometric measurements (weight, height, head circumference, body mass index). Prior growth data are important to determine alterations in growth velocity. The usual growth pattern associated with malabsorption and malnutrition demonstrates an initial decrease in weight followed by a deceleration in height velocity. Figure 138-5 illustrates a typical patient who was eventually diagnosed with celiac disease. The examination should also focus on the skin, mouth, neurologic findings, evidence of hepatosplenomegaly, and perianal and rectal examinations. Signs of malnutrition include lethargy, decreased subcutaneous tissue, edema, depigmentation of the skin and hair, abdominal distention, and muscle wasting. Occasionally features present in the physical examination such as digital clubbing (cystic fibrosis, celiac disease), rectal prolapse (cystic fibrosis), and facial features (Johnson-Blizzard syndrome) may be helpful in making a specific diagnosis.

The most useful laboratory investigation is analysis of a fresh stool sample for consistency, pH, presence of reducing sugars, presence of fecal leukocytes, and analysis for occult blood. The stool sample should also be submitted for culture of enteric pathogens and analysis for parasites. Fecal

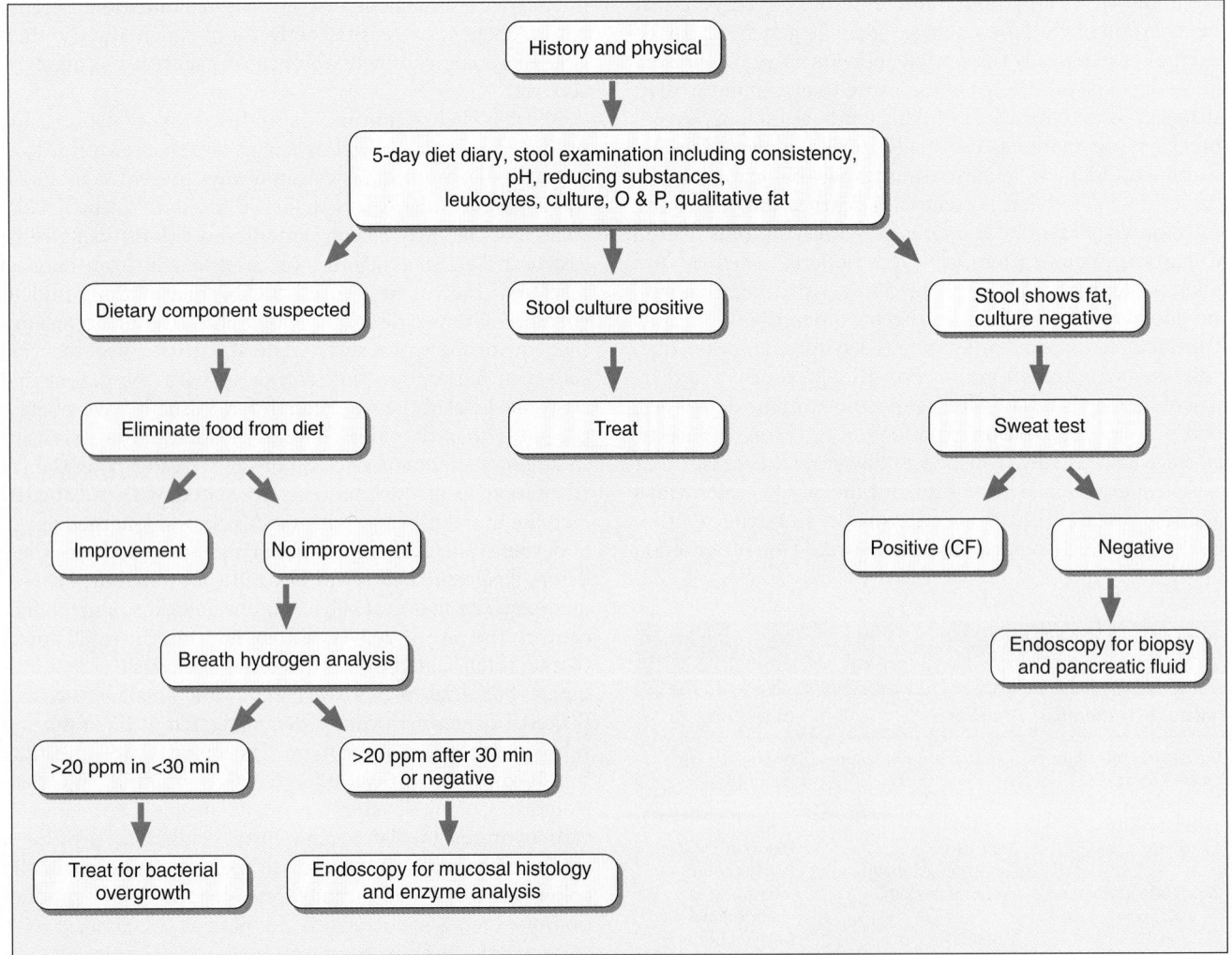

Figure 138-4. Stepwise approach to evaluate a patient with diarrhea. CF, cystic fibrosis; O, ova; P, parasites.

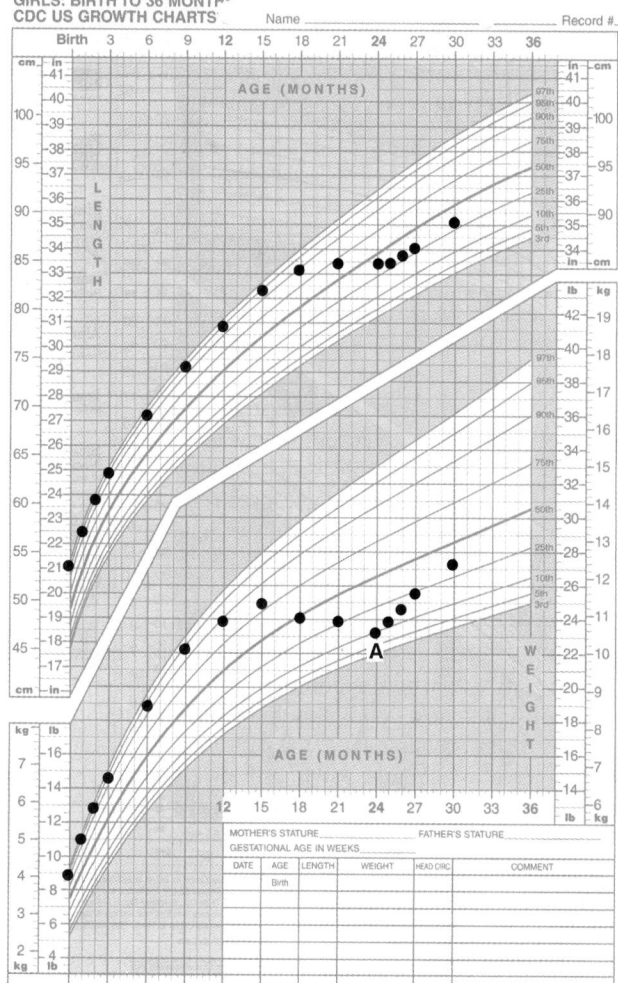

GIRLS: BIRTH TO 36 MONTHS
CDC US GROWTH CHARTS   Name _____   Record # _____

Figure 138-5. Growth pattern of celiac disease. The patient depicted on this chart shows that body weight gain and height progression slowed after 15 months of age. Diagnosis was made at age 24 months *(point A)* and appropriate therapy initiated.

be valid. Steatorrhea is more severe in pancreatic insufficiency than in intestinal mucosal disorders. Table 138-3 lists the differential diagnoses of steatorrhea and suggested evaluation.

If protein loss is suspected, then stool should be examined for presence of α_1-antitrypsin, which is resistant to digestion and, if present in the stool, suggests PLE. Alanine aminotransferase (ALT) and gamma glutamyltranspeptidase (GGTP) are used to document hepatic injury or biliary obstruction. Radiologic bone age can reveal delay in skeletal development, present in vitamin D deficiency and various malabsorption disorders.

Carbohydrate malabsorption is suspected if there is evidence of reducing sugars in the stool and the stool is excessively acidic (pH < 5.6). Breath hydrogen test can also be used to assess carbohydrate malabsorption. A documented rise in breath hydrogen over 20 ppm 90 minutes or more after the ingestion of 2 g/kg body weight of the suspected offending sugar implies malabsorption. An early rise in hydrogen after ingestion of any sugar suggests small intestine bacterial overgrowth.

Endoscopy and biopsy by a gastroenterologist are the gold standard for documenting mucosal enzyme content and villus injury. As injury can be patchy, multiple biopsies must be obtained from the duodenum and jejunum. Pancreatic fluid can also be obtained for pancreatic enzyme analysis after stimulating the pancreas with cholecystokinin (CCK). Patients with symptoms suggestive of intractable diarrhea of infancy should be referred to a pediatric gastroenterologist for further evaluation that should include an endoscopy and histologic examination. Patients with suspected celiac disease should also be referred for diagnostic biopsy. Attempts to initiate gluten-free diets without histologic confirmation frequently lead to erroneous diagnoses, thereby committing some children to unnecessary, lifelong dietary restriction.

MANAGEMENT

Appropriate management of a malabsorption disorder is directed to the cause of malabsorption. Malnutrition and vitamin or trace element deficiency should be treated vigorously to stimulate catch-up growth and maintenance of normal growth. Supplemental pancreatic enzymes are

fat analysis is very important for documenting malabsorption. This test can be done qualitatively with Sudan stain or quantitatively by 72-hour fecal fat analysis. Red blood cell folate and serum carotene levels can also be used as screening tests for fat malabsorption, but the child must be receiving folate and carotene in the diet for blood levels to

Table 138-3. Differential Diagnosis and Evaluation of Steatorrhea

Disease	Clinical Characteristics	Findings
Gluten enteropathy	Endoscopic biopsy	Small bowel villus injury
	Serologic tests	
	Antigliadin IgG	Elevated, can be used to follow adherence to diet
	Antigliadin IgA	
	Tissue transglutaminase	
Cystic fibrosis	Sweat chloride	Elevated chloride
Shwachman-Diamond syndrome	Complete blood count	Anemia
		Neutropenia
Intestinal lymphagiectasia	Complete blood count	Lymphopenia
	Serum protein	Hypoalbuminemia
		Hypogammaglobinemia
	Fecal α_1-antitrypsin	Present in stool
	Endoscopic biopsy	Dilated lacteals, villus distortion
Inflammatory bowel disease	Erythrocyte sedimentation rate	Elevated
	Small bowel biopsy	Patchy inflammation

required in cystic fibrosis and Shwachman-Diamond syndrome. Fat-soluble vitamins (vitamins A, D, E, and K) are utilized in an attempt to overcome malabsorption in cystic fibrosis and cholestatic liver diseases. Dietary medium-chain triglycerides can improve fat absorption in patients with impaired fat digestion and absorption.

In patients with mild to moderate malabsorption, a slow continuous infusion of formula through a nasogastric or gastrostomy tube may increase absorption. Parenteral nutrition is customarily required in intractable diarrhea of infancy, short-bowel syndrome, and significant protein energy malnutrition (Chapter 294). If evidence strongly suggests PLE, the patient should be referred to the gastroenterologist for further and more invasive testing.

Patients with gluten enteropathy require lifelong avoidance of all gluten, including wheat, rye, oats, barley, spelt, teff, triticalice, amaranth, quinoa, and millet. Patients and families must learn to read all food labels carefully (Chapter 130). Consultation with a nutritionist is advisable. The combined use of serum antigliadin IgG (highly sensitive), IgA (highly specific), and antiendomysial IgA levels can be used to monitor patient compliance because they should decline after the introduction of gluten-free diet.

Ideally, patients with short-bowel syndrome should be managed in a multidisciplinary setting where they have access to gastroenterologists, nutritionists, home care specialists, social workers, pediatric surgeons, and transplant surgeons. By definition, these children initially cannot maintain adequate nutrition entirely by the enteral route. They receive most of their nutrition parenterally. Attention to fluid, electrolyte, and nutritional management is very important in these patients.

Many variables contribute to the chronic diarrhea of short-bowel syndrome. Large volumes of fluid and electrolyte normally secreted by the upper gastrointestinal tract are not reabsorbed in this condition and may result in dehydration, hyponatremia, hypokalemia, hypomagnesemia, and acidosis. Depending on the size of the infant, a continuous gastric or jejunal infusion of an elemental formula at full strength (0.67 kcal/mL) should be give at a rate of 1 to 3 mL/hour. This practice, termed trophic feeding, is important because exposure to enteral feedings contributes to adaptive growth of the small bowel and stimulates biliary flow and gallbladder emptying. This reduces the incidence of cholestasis induced by total parenteral nutrition (TPN). The rate of formula infusion

Table 138-4. Management of Children with Rare Malabsorptive Disorders

Malabsorptive Disorder	Management
Intestinal lymphangiectasia	TPN, surgical resection, antiplasmin therapy, octreotide, small bowel transplantation
Microvillus inclusion disease	TPN, small bowel transplantation
Autoimmune enteropathy	Immunosuppression, TPN, small bowel transplantation
Tufting enteropathy	TPN, small bowel transplantation

TPN, total parenteral nutrition.

can be slowly advanced as tolerated. During this period, oral diet should be advanced slowly using small, frequent feedings in order to establish appropriate feeding behavior. Provision of large quantities of oral feedings may induce a dumping syndrome. Stool output greater than 40 to 50 mL/kg/day suggests that enteral feedings should not be advanced.

As the bowel begins to adapt, the amount of oral feedings and enteral feedings tolerated will increase. Solids can be initiated at the usual recommended age. The nutrient composition of these foods should be high in fats or protein because when broken down, they create less osmotic load. Beyond creating an excessive osmotic load in the small intestine, carbohydrates promote small bowel bacterial overgrowth.

Box 138-2 describes Shwachman-Diamond syndrome. Table 138-4 outlines therapies for patients with microvillus inclusion disease, autoimmune eneropathy, and tufting enteropathy. Treatment of disaccharidase deficiency is avoidance.

LONG-TERM SEQUELAE OF MALABSORPTION DISORDERS

The long-term effects of malnutrition are related to its duration and the age at which it develops. Learning disabilities may result if malnutrition occurs within the first 2 years of life. Delayed sexual maturation occurs in chronic malnutrition and celiac disease. T-cell lymphoma and other neoplasms are possible in longstanding gluten enteropathy, especially with poor adherence to diet. Digestive tract tumors and fibrosing colonopathy are reported in cystic fibrosis. Long-term prognostic factors for infants with short-bowel syndrome are listed in Box 138-3.

Box 138-2. Clinical Features of Shwachman-Diamond Syndrome

- Autosomal recessive
- Failure to thrive from malabsorption, onset by 4 months of age
- Growth failure
- Metaphyseal chondrodysplasia, can be associated with dwarfism
- Delayed puberty
- Respiratory problems associated with pneumonia and recurrent otitis media
- Bone marrow hypoplasia with thrombocytopenia and anemia
- Can have myelodysplasia and acute myelogenous leukemia

Box 138-3. Long-Term Prognostic Factors for Infants with Short-Bowel Syndrome

- Underlying etiology of short bowel syndrome
- Presence of complications associated with total parenteral nutrition (TPN)
- Tolerance of enteral feeds
- Length of remaining small bowel
- Presence of terminal ileum
- Presence of ileocecal valve
- Presence of colon

SUGGESTED READINGS

Fasano A: Celiac disease: The past, the present, the future. Pediatrics 2001;107:768–772.

Ghishan FK: Chronic diarrhea. In Behrman RE, Kliegman RM, Jenson HB (eds): Nelson's Textbook of Pediatrics, 16th ed. Philadelphia, WB Saunders, 2000, pp 1171–1176.

Schmitz J: Maldigestion and malabsorption. In Walker WA, Durie PR, Hamilton JR, et al (eds): Pediatric Gastrointestinal Disease, 3rd ed. Hamilton, Canada, BC Decker, 2000, pp 40–58.

Talsusan-Soriano K, Lake AM: Malabsorption in childhood. Pediatr Rev 1996;17:135–142.

Ulshen M: Malabsorptive disorders. In Behrman RE, Kliegman RM, Jenson HB (eds): Nelson's Textbook of Pediatrics, 16th ed. Philadelphia, WB Saunders, 2000, pp 1159–1171.

SECTION 4   CHRONIC MEDICAL CARE: *Disorders of the Gastrointestinal Tract*

139 Inflammatory Bowel Disease

Kathleen M. Campbell and William F. Balistreri

ROLE OF THE GENERALIST

1. Recognize various presentations of inflammatory bowel disease.
2. Initiate the workup for inflammatory bowel disease.
3. Refer all patients with inflammatory bowel disease to the pediatric gastroenterologist for assistance in long-term management.
4. Participate in ongoing, coordinated partnership with specialists.
5. Screen for complications of primary disease and complications of treatment.
6. Promote normal growth and development.
7. Assist in managing the psychosocial impact on patients and their families.
8. Provide patient education and support.

Table 139-1. Comparison of Ulcerative Colitis and Crohn Disease

Feature	Ulcerative Colitis	Crohn Disease
Site of disease	Colon, continuous from rectum, +/– backwash ileitis	Patchy involvement from mouth to anus
Extent of inflammation	Mucosal only	Transmural
Radiologic features	Loss of normal haustral pattern, pseudopolyps	"Skip" lesions, thickened bowel loops, fistulas, deep ulcers, serosal fat
Pathologic features	Mucosal and submucosal inflammation only, cryptitis, crypt abscesses, goblet cell depletion	Transmural inflammation, noncaseating granulomas, prominent lymphoid tissue, fibrosis
Intestinal complications	Toxic megacolon, colonic adenocarcinoma, strictures	Strictures, fistulas, abscesses, bowel obstruction

Clinical Features	Frequency	
Diarrhea	95%	85%
Rectal bleeding	90%	20%
Abdominal pain	90%	85%
Weight loss	40%	75%
Growth failure	15%	45%
Fever	15%	50%
Perianal disease	10%	30%

Ulcerative colitis and Crohn disease are chronic intestinal inflammatory disorders characterized by alternating periods of relapsing and remitting disease activity. Although the two share some common characteristics, they are distinct diseases, differentiated by the location and characteristics of the gastrointestinal inflammation. Table 139-1 compares the two diseases. In a minority of children (10% to 15%), the distinction between Crohn disease and ulcerative colitis cannot be made at presentation, although it may become clear as the disease progresses. These patients are considered to have indeterminate colitis.

The initial presentation of inflammatory bowel disease can be quite subtle with nonspecific symptoms. The primary care practitioner must recognize the presentation of the disease and understand the potential complications, treatment modalities, and possible outcomes.

FUNDAMENTALS

Epidemiology

The onset of inflammatory bowel disease (IBD) occurs during childhood in 15% to 25% of patients with IBD. The age of onset has a bimodal distribution, with peaks between 15 and 25 years, and again between 50 and 60 years. The typical age at diagnosis of Crohn disease is 11.5 to 13 years, and for ulcerative colitis it is 10 to 19 years. Ulcerative colitis is more common than Crohn disease in children younger than 10 years of age. The increasing incidence of Crohn disease, currently about 15 per 100,000, supports the role of environmental factors in development of the disease. The incidence of ulcerative colitis is stable at approximately 4 per 100,000.

The strongest risk factor for the development of IBD is having a first degree relative with IBD. Crohn disease and ulcerative colitis tend to occur in the same families and may share some common genetic predisposition. Siblings of patients with childhood onset IBD have a 4% to 5% chance of developing IBD in their lifetime. Offspring of patients with Crohn disease have a 9% chance of developing IBD, but if both parents are affected, children carry a greater than 35% risk. With Crohn disease specifically, onset of disease occurs earlier in affected children than in the affected parent; the average difference in age at diagnosis is 15 years.

Clinical Features

Ulcerative colitis is characterized by bloody diarrhea; in general, systemic manifestations are less likely than in Crohn disease. The clinical features of ulcerative colitis can be divided into three typical forms, distal colonic involvement, pancolitis, and fulminant colitis. Table 139-2 describes signs and symptoms of each of these entities. Clinical features of Crohn disease vary widely, depending on the area of intestine involved, the severity of the inflammation, and the presence of complications. Inflammation is limited to the terminal ileum in about 30% of patients, involves the ileum and colon in 60%, and is limited to the colon in 10% to 20%. Gastroduodenal inflammation is present

in 30% to 40%. Crohn disease with primarily colonic involvement may have features identical to ulcerative colitis, but upper gastrointestinal tract disease may manifest as vomiting and epigastric pain. Small bowel involvement frequently is manifest by crampy abdominal pain, which may be localized to the right lower quadrant in ileal disease. Systemic manifestations of fever, fatigue, weight loss, growth failure, and pubertal delay are more common in Crohn disease.

Both Crohn disease and ulcerative colitis may have a myriad of extraintestinal manifestations that may precede the onset of intestinal symptoms. Extraintestinal features are slightly more common with Crohn disease than with ulcerative colitis and tend to be associated particularly with colonic involvement. Arthritis and arthralgias occur in 10% to 20%. Joint involvement varies from a nondestructive, migratory arthritis involving large joints, to sacroileitis or asymptomatic ankylosing spondylitis, which occurs more frequently in patients with histocompatibility gene HLA-B27. Erythema nodosum and peripheral arthritis correlate with active intestinal disease. Pyoderma gangrenosum, another skin manifestation, has no correlation with intestinal disease and tends to occur more frequently in ulcerative colitis (see Figs. 79-7 and 79-8). Hepatobiliary manifestations, such as primary sclerosing cholangitis and autoimmune hepatitis, are found more commonly in ulcerative colitis than in Crohn disease. Other extraintestinal manifestations of IBD are uveitis, calcium oxalate renal calculi, glomerulonephritis, and hypercoagulability. Cholelithiasis may follow ileal dysfunction in Crohn disease or resection that interrupts the enterohepatic circulation of bile salts.

Complications

Complications of IBD in pediatric patients are a significant component of the morbidity and mortality rates associated with the disease. One third of patients with Crohn disease develop fistulas between loops of bowel, bowel and bladder, bowel and vagina, or bowel and abdominal wall or perineum. Perianal complications (fistulas, skin tags, anal fissures, abscesses) are specific to Crohn disease, may precede other signs of intestinal Crohn disease or develop during exacerbations of colitis, and are often recalcitrant to standard medical therapy (Fig. 139-1). Adhesions, strictures, intra-abdominal abscesses, and complete or partial small bowel obstruction can also complicate Crohn disease. More than 50% of patients with Crohn disease will eventually require surgery for these or other complications.

Table 139-2. Patterns of Involvement in Ulcerative Colitis

Distal Colonic Involvement	Pancolitis	Fulminant Colitis
■ 30% of patients	■ 40–50% of patients	■ 10% of patients
■ Onset may be insidious		
■ Diarrhea (+/– tenesmus)	■ Tenesmus/urgency, bloody diarrhea	■ Grossly bloody diarrhea (>6/day)
■ Rectal bleeding		
■ +/– pain	■ Abdominal tenderness	■ Abdominal tenderness, +/– distension
■ Usually no fever	■ Fever	
■ Usually no weight loss	■ Weight loss	
	■ Mild anemia	■ Hematocrit <30%
		■ Serum albumin <3 g/dL
		■ Leukocytosis

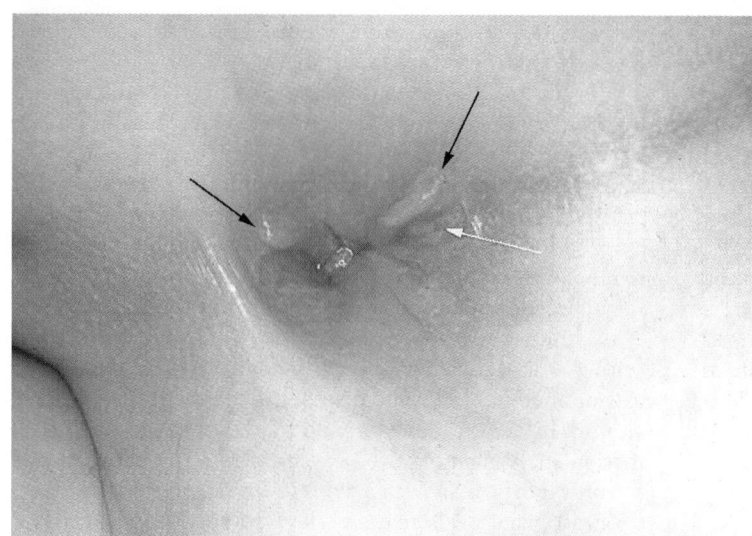

Figure 139-1. Fleshy perianal skin tags *(black arrows)* and fissures *(white arrow)* may be the only physical signs of Crohn disease and should alert the health care provider to the possibility of inflammatory bowel disease in a patient with chronic abdominal pain, growth failure, rectal bleeding, or related symptoms. (Photograph courtesy of Dr. James Heubi, Children's Hospital Medical Center, Cincinnati, Ohio.)

Fulminant colitis and toxic megacolon (Fig. 139-2) are the most serious complications of ulcerative colitis. These represent medical emergencies and require immediate hospitalization and evaluation by a pediatric gastroenterologist and surgeon (see the Acute Care Issues section of this chapter). Malnutrition, usually from inadequate intake, is present at diagnosis in 85% of pediatric patients with Crohn disease and 65% of pediatric patients with ulcerative colitis. Malabsorption, protein-losing enteropathy, and increased energy expenditure associated with active inflammation also play a role in weight loss and poor nutritional status. Anorexia, beyond that expected from intestinal disease, is especially profound in patients with Crohn disease.

Growth impairment is more common in patients with Crohn disease than in those with ulcerative colitis. Boys are more vulnerable because their growth spurt occurs later and lasts longer than that of girls. Impairment of linear growth may be the first sign of Crohn disease, with almost 50% of children having decreased height velocity that antedates their gastrointestinal symptoms. Osteoporosis does not commonly develop in children and adolescents with ulcerative colitis without corticosteroid treatment, but is a frequent problem in Crohn disease. Chronic inflammation, decreased calcium intake, vitamin D deficiency, malabsorption of fat-soluble vitamins, and corticosteroid use all play a role. The accumulation of bone mass peaks in girls at age 13 and in boys by age 14.5. Achieving adequate mineralization in childhood is an important defense against bone disease in later life.

Pathogenesis

The pathogenesis of IBD is not completely understood, but immunologic, environmental, and infectious factors are thought to play a role. The predominant theory is that, in susceptible individuals, inflammation is initiated by the host response to intraluminal antigens (microbial or dietary), and is perpetuated by an abnormal or dysregulated immune system. The cytokine response in Crohn disease and ulcerative colitis is markedly different. Crohn disease is associated with T_H1 (type 1 helper T cell) cytokines such as interferon-γ (IFN-γ), tumor necrosis factor-α (TNF-α), and interleukin 12 (IL-12). Ulcerative colitis is not associated with a T_H1 response, but more closely resembles a T_H2 response with increased IL-5 and IL-10. These

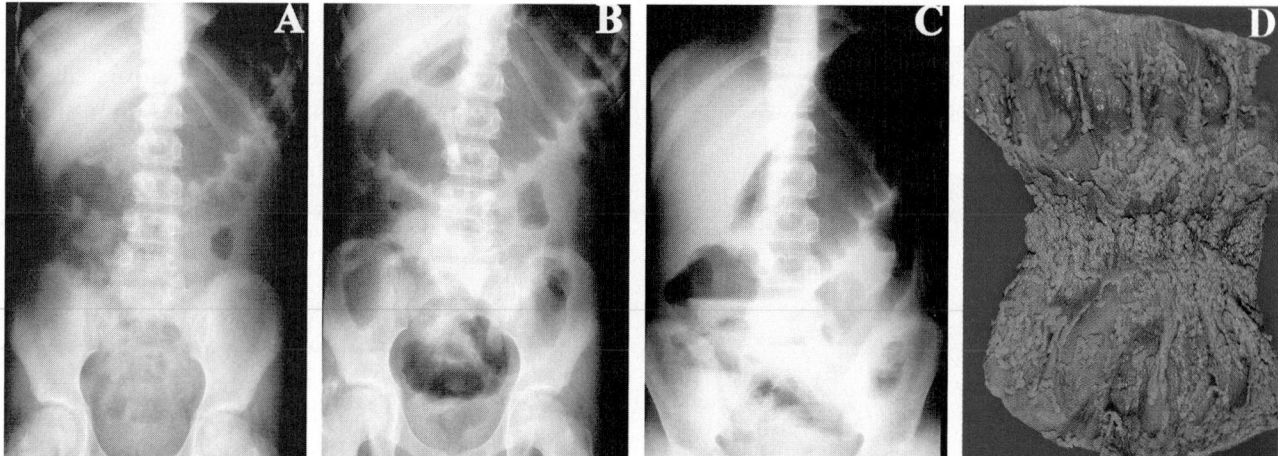

Figure 139-2. This patient with ulcerative colitis presented with severe abdominal pain, fever, and dehydration. Plain films of the abdomen show progressive colonic dilatation on admission **(A)**, at 24 hours **(B)**, and at 48 hours **(C)**. After failing to respond to 5 days of maximum medical therapy, he underwent total colectomy **(D)**. (Photographs courtesy of Dr. James Heubi, Children's Hospital Medical Center, Cincinnati, Ohio.)

proinflammatory cytokines promote inflammation and stimulate electrolyte secretion, contributing to diarrhea. In Crohn disease, diarrhea is also caused by malabsorption, loss of bile salts from the terminal ileum, and bacterial overgrowth in the small bowel with subsequent bile salt deconjugation.

The local production of TNF-α is also believed to play a role in the initiation and propagation of Crohn disease. TNF-α stimulates the production of other proinflammatory cytokines, up-regulates adhesion molecules, and stimulates fibroblast proliferation, thereby perpetuating the inflammatory response. Levels of TNF-α are increased in the intestinal mucosa of patients with Crohn disease, and TNF-α blockade has proved to be an effective treatment. Mucosal T-cell resistance to apoptosis may also contribute to perpetuation of the inflammatory process.

PRESENTATION AND EVALUATION

The diagnosis of IBD requires careful evaluation of a combination of typical symptoms, physical examination findings, and laboratory, radiologic, endoscopic, and histologic features, as well as the exclusion of other disorders, particularly enteric pathogens. A detailed history and physical examination are essential to the diagnosis. Findings that should alert the primary care practitioner to the possibility of IBD are listed in Box 139-1. Presenting symptoms vary from readily apparent gastrointestinal symptoms (abdominal pain, bloody diarrhea) to growth failure and subtle extraintestinal manifestations. The diagnostic time lag, that is, the length of time from symptom onset to diagnosis, is considerable in both Crohn disease and ulcerative colitis (6 to 7 months). The most frequent presenting symptoms of IBD are abdominal pain, diarrhea, hematochezia, and weight loss. Less frequent symptoms include fever, arthritis, malaise, and growth failure. Patients with Crohn disease who present with growth failure have the longest diagnostic time lag.

The clinical presentation of ulcerative colitis is frequently straightforward: bloody diarrhea with mucus, often accompanied by tenesmus and urgency. Abdominal pain is usually related to, and relieved by, defecation. The most frequent presenting symptoms of Crohn disease are abdominal pain, diarrhea, and weight loss. The abdominal pain is frequently more severe than that associated with ulcerative colitis, may occur at any time of day, and may awaken the patient from sleep. It may be localized to the right lower quadrant in those with ileal or ileocolonic disease, or may be periumbilical in those with colonic or isolated small bowel disease. Diarrhea is seen in about 50% of patients with Crohn disease. Perianal disease (fissures, fistulas, tags) occurs in approximately 25%. Occasionally, Crohn disease may present with small bowel obstruction secondary to acute inflammation or postinflammatory strictures.

IBD should be considered in the differential diagnosis of any child with growth failure. A careful search must also be made for extraintestinal manifestations of IBD, as these may precede the onset of intestinal symptoms.

Laboratory features associated with IBD include anemia (either iron deficiency anemia secondary to chronic blood loss or anemia of chronic disease); decreased serum folate, vitamin B_{12}, and iron levels; and markers of chronic inflammation such as an elevated erythrocyte sedimentation rate or thrombocytosis. With a protein-losing enteropathy, stool α_1-antitrypsin levels may be elevated and the serum albumin level may be low. Hypoalbuminemia may also result from malnutrition. Stool should be examined for blood and ova and parasites and cultured, looking for *Salmonella*, *Shigella*, *Campylobacter*, *Escherichia coli*, *Aeromonas hydrophila*, and *Yersinia*. Assays for *Clostridium difficile* toxin should rule out pseudomembranous colitis. If hepatobiliary complications are present, serum aminotransferases and gamma-glutamyltransferase levels may be elevated. These findings are all nonspecific markers of disease, and normal laboratory values do not rule out IBD.

Although there are no specific laboratory tests for IBD, several commercially available serologic markers may aid in the diagnosis. Antineutrophil cytoplasmic antibodies (ANCA) are found in 60% to 70% of patients with ulcerative colitis. The most common pattern is perinuclear ANCA (pANCA), which has also been associated with an ulcerative colitis–like subtype of Crohn disease. Anti-*Saccharomyces cerevisiae* antibodies (ASCA) are found in 60% to 70% of patients with Crohn disease. These antibodies are not pathogenic, but appear to be markers of underlying immune dysregulation. Although these measures are not sufficiently accurate for broad-based population screening, they may be helpful in identifying IBD in symptomatic patients, and in distinguishing ulcerative colitis from Crohn disease.

Radiologic studies can also be helpful in the diagnosis of IBD. Plain films of the abdomen may suggest complications such as toxic megacolon and small bowel obstruction. Radiographic findings are described and illustrated on the CD-ROM. Although contrast studies are frequently helpful, they are dangerous in patients with fulminant colitis, and are contraindicated when there is colonic dilatation. Other radiology studies that can be useful in identifying complications and assessing extent of inflammation include computed tomography (CT) scan and ^{99m}Tc-labeled white blood cell scan.

Every patient in whom the diagnosis of IBD is being seriously considered needs to be referred to a pediatric gastroenterologist for upper endoscopy and colonoscopy. Colonoscopy is more sensitive than barium enema at identifying mild mucosal disease, and upper endoscopy is necessary to exclude upper tract Crohn disease. Endoscopic and biopsy findings in Crohn disease and ulcerative colitis are described on the CD-ROM.

> **Box 139-1.** Red Flags of Inflammatory Bowel Disease in the History and Physical Examination
>
> - Decreased growth velocity
> - Delayed sexual maturation
> - Perianal disease (skin tags, abscesses, fissures, "hemorrhoids")
> - Unexplained weight loss, fever, or anemia
> - Small bowel obstruction in absence of previous surgery
> - Right lower quadrant mass or tenderness
> - Digital clubbing
> - Recurrent painless oral ulcers
> - Family history of inflammatory bowel disease

Table 139-3. Differential Diagnosis of Crohn Disease and Ulcerative Colitis

Crohn Disease
Infectious ileocolitis
   Yersinia
   Giardia
   Histoplasmosis
   Tuberculosis
   Campylobacter
Appendicitis
Anorexia nervosa
Intestinal lymphoma
Behçet disease
AIDS-associated enteropathy
Irritable bowel syndrome
Peptic ulcer disease
Vasculitis
Fissures, hemorrhoids, condyloma

Ulcerative Colitis
Infectious colitis
   Salmonella
   Shigella
   Escherichia coli O157
   Campylobacter
   Entamoeba histolytica
   Clostridium difficile
   Aeromonas
   Cytomegalovirus
Schönlein-Henoch purpura
Hirschsprung enterocolitis
Radiation proctitis/colitis
Hemolytic-uremic syndrome
Allergic/eosinophilic colitis
Meckel diverticulum
Polyposis
Hemorrhoids

In the process of arriving at a diagnosis of IBD, it is necessary to rule out other disorders. The differential diagnoses of Crohn disease and ulcerative colitis are given in Table 139-3.

MANAGEMENT

Goals in the management of IBD are as follows:
1. Inducing and maintaining remission of disease while promoting appropriate growth and development
2. Minimizing the psychosocial impact of the disease
3. Identifying patients who are not responding to their current therapy
4. Avoiding complications of the disease and its therapy

The generalist should participate in an ongoing, coordinated partnership with the specialist to coordinate care and support the goals of disease management, screen for complications of primary disease and treatment, and provide patient education and support. Mainstays of treatment include nutritional management, pharmacotherapy, and surgery.

Nutrition

Nutritional management of IBD includes providing adequate caloric intake to ensure normal growth and development and to allow catch-up growth. Nutrition therapy may be either primary or adjunctive in Crohn disease and is adjunctive only in ulcerative colitis. As primary therapy for acute Crohn disease, exclusive enteral nutrition offers

additional benefit to corticosteroids in decreasing intestinal inflammation. Using nightly enteral feeds (given via a nasogastric tube) to supplement an ad lib diet has been associated with prolonged disease remission and improved growth.

Supplementation with omega-3 polyunsaturated fatty acids (found in fish oils) is a popular adjunct to standard nutritional therapy and exerts an anti-inflammatory effect by modulating cytokine synthesis. Unfortunately, rapid relapse is common when nutritional therapy is discontinued. Specific dietary management is found in Chapter 130.

Pharmacotherapy

Medications frequently used in IBD and common side effects are listed in Table 139-4. 5-ASA agents are the mainstays of therapy for mild to moderate ulcerative colitis and can often be used to induce and maintain remission in mild disease. They are also useful in patients with mild to moderate Crohn disease, especially with colonic involvement. Although the oral preparations of 5-ASA are appropriate for pancolitis or proximal disease, distal colitis or proctitis may respond to topical therapy with ASA-containing enemas or suppositories.

Corticosteroids are the first line of therapy in patients with moderate to severe Crohn disease, regardless of the site of disease, and are useful for moderate to severe ulcerative colitis or in those who have failed to respond to aminosalicylates. For treatment of severe inflammatory bowel disease (including fulminant colitis and toxic megacolon) intravenous steroids may be necessary, in addition to antibiotics, bowel rest, and blood and albumin infusions. Although they are extremely effective at inducing remission, steroids have little to no role as maintenance therapy. Among patients with Crohn disease who initially respond, more than one third will develop steroid dependency within 1 year. Twenty percent of patients with Crohn disease will be resistant to steroids. In ulcerative or Crohn colitis, hydrocortisone enemas or foam may be used to reduce the dose of systemic steroids necessary to control distal disease.

Immunomodulatory agents are used in patients who have a poor response to steroids, or who are steroid-dependent. The purine analogs azathioprine and 6-mercaptopurine (6-MP) may be useful to induce remission; however, their use is limited by their delayed onset of action, which is 3 to 6 months. Recent evidence indicates that beginning 6-MP at the time of diagnosis of Crohn disease may decrease the time to remission, and may increase the likelihood of becoming steroid-free. Adverse effects associated with the purine analogs are listed in Table 139-4.

Methotrexate is primarily used in patients who do not respond to or cannot tolerate 6-MP or azathioprine. It has been effective at both inducing and maintaining remission in steroid-dependent Crohn disease. Cyclosporine, a calcineurin phosphatase inhibitor more commonly used in organ transplantation, has little use in Crohn disease but has been efficacious in treating acute severe colitis unresponsive to steroids. It is not considered as maintenance therapy in either Crohn disease or ulcerative colitis.

Antibiotics have no role in treatment of uncomplicated ulcerative colitis, although they may be useful when there is an overlying infection. In Crohn disease, antibiotics can be extremely useful in a maintenance regimen, and are

Table 139-4. Medications Frequently Used in Inflammatory Bowel Disease

Medication	Dose	Side Effects
Corticosteroids	1.0 mg/kg/day qd or divided bid; usually decreased by 5 mg/week when disease under control	Hypertension, hyperglycemia, mood changes, decreased bone mineralization, decreased linear growth, acne, adrenal suppression, cataracts, cushingoid features, hirsutism
Aminosalicylates		
Sulfasalazine (colonic release)	50–75 mg/kg/day divided qid	Hypersensitivity reactions, headache, rash, abdominal pain, nausea, vomiting, diarrhea, hemolysis, folate deficiency
Mesalamine Asacol (ileal release) Pentasa (release throughout small bowel and colon)	25–50 mg/kg/day divided tid	Headache, rash, exacerbation of colitis
Olsalazine (colonic release)	25 mg/kg/day	Same as for mesalamine
6-Mercaptopurine (6-MP)	1–2 mg/kg/day	Nausea, rash, arthralgias, myelosuppression, infections, macrocytosis, pancreatitis
Azathioprine	2–3 mg/kg/day	Same as for 6-MP
Methotrexate	15–25 mg/week IM, SC	Nausea, vomiting, mouth ulcers, myelosuppression, megaloblastic anemia, neuropathy, hepatotoxicity, teratogenic
Infliximab	Fistulas: 5 mg/kg IV at 0, 2, 6 weeks No fistulas: 5 mg/kg × 1, then ~q8–12 weeks as needed	Infection, acute or delayed hypersensitivity reaction, lupus-like reaction
Metronidazole	10–20 mg/kg/day divided tid	Anorexia, nausea, vomiting, neuropathy, disulfiram-like effect, neutropenia, metallic taste

of particular benefit in the treatment of perianal disease. The most commonly used agents are metronidazole and ciprofloxacin, which may prevent the perpetuation of inflammation. Metronidazole can be used following bowel resection to delay anastomotic recurrence. Unfortunately, disease almost always relapses with discontinuation of therapy, and the side effects are significant.

A better understanding of the pathophysiology of Crohn disease has led to the development of biologic agents and novel therapies that target specific disease pathways. Infliximab, a murine-human chimeric monoclonal antibody to TNF-α, has proven to be efficacious in the treatment of moderate to severe Crohn disease refractory to conventional therapy and in fistulizing Crohn disease. Other forms of anti-TNF-α therapy include humanized monoclonal antibody CDP-571 and etanercept. Thalidomide has been used in patients with moderate to severely active Crohn disease, particularly fistulizing disease. Because of its side effects and teratogenic potential, thalidomide is generally reserved for use in patients in whom all other medical therapy has failed.

Other novel therapies currently under investigation for use in IBD include anti-inflammatory cytokines such as IL-10 and IL-11, anti-sense oligonucleotides, anti-α-4 integrin antibody (Antegren), growth hormone, tacrolimus, and mycophenolate mofetil.

Surgery

Total colectomy, which is curative for patients with ulcerative colitis (see Fig. 139-2), is generally indicated in the face of life-threatening blood loss, toxic megacolon, fulminant colitis not responsive to maximum medical therapy, steroid dependence, unacceptable treatment side effects, or mucosal dysplasia. The procedure of choice is the ileal pouch–anal anastomosis, which can be performed either as a primary operation or in a staged approach. Colectomy has a signifi-

cant impact on quality of life and body image, especially in children and adolescents. Up to 40% of children will develop inflammation of the surgically created pouch (pouchitis).

Surgery is not curative in Crohn disease, and because disease recurrence at the surgical site is very common, surgery should be avoided in the absence of specific indications, which include localized disease unresponsive to medical therapy, perforation, stricturing with bowel obstruction, fistulas, and intractable bleeding. Perianal disease often requires drainage of perianal abscesses, fistulotomy if perianal fistulas are severely symptomatic and unresponsive to medical therapy, and even diverting colostomy in severe, recalcitrant perianal disease. The risk of recurrence of Crohn disease after surgery is greater than 50% by 5 years, and this risk increases with each subsequent surgery.

CHRONIC CONDITION COMANAGEMENT

As with all children who are being managed by a health care team, the family should understand whom they should call for medical problems. The generalist, as the primary care provider, must recognize medical and surgical emergencies, referring patients to the appropriate specialists as needed. The generalist should also coordinate ongoing care, monitor patients for complications of the disease and adverse side effects to medications, provide health maintenance, and treat common acute illnesses.

Acute Care Issues

Fulminant colitis and *toxic megacolon* are medical emergencies in children with IBD. They present with severe abdominal tenderness and altered peristalsis. The diagnosis of toxic megacolon is confirmed with radiologic evidence of significant colonic dilatation (colonic diameter >6 cm in adults), accompanied by fever, tachycardia, electrolyte disturbances, hypoalbuminemia, and dehydration. Both of these disorders are associated with a high risk of perforation. Aggressive medical management is warranted, including bowel decompression, intravenous steroids and broad-spectrum antibiotics. Failure to respond to these measures within days constitutes one of the indications for colectomy.

Acutely ill children, and those with severe colitis, may require hospitalization for intravenous steroids, intravenous antibiotics, hydration, bowel rest, parenteral nutrition, or introduction of supplemental feeds.

Side effects of medications commonly used in the treatment of IBD are listed in Table 139-4. The generalist must be aware of the medications that a patient is currently using, their side effects and drug interactions, and must monitor the patient carefully.

Health Maintenance

Careful attention needs to be paid to ensure that patients with IBD receive regular preventive health care. Immunizations should be kept up to date. Monitoring of growth and adherence to medical and psychosocial recommendations are particularly important.

Psychosocial

Children and adolescents with IBD experience many of the psychosocial complications of chronic disease, including behavior problems, psychiatric disorders, depression, and social isolation. Up to 50% of children with IBD suffer from psychiatric disease, predominantly emotional disorders. Because depression is commonly encountered, generalists must recognize the symptoms and provide appropriate treatment and referral.

Treatment of IBD in children should include both medical and psychosocial approaches. The health care team should provide education and support to patients and families. This support helps to minimize stresses that may hinder recovery or contribute to disease exacerbations. Creating a knowledgeable and caring environment for the child or adolescent also helps to minimize adverse social impact of the disease, promote compliance with therapy, and improve overall outcome. Patient support groups are an excellent resource for educational and social opportunities. A list of excellent resources for patients and families is found on the CD-ROM.

OUTCOME

Although IBD is typically marked by periods of relapsing and remitting disease activity, most children have the potential for a full, active life with good general health. Seventy percent of children who have ulcerative colitis will enter remission within 3 months of initiating therapy. About 50% remain in remission over the next year; however, up to 25% who present with severe disease and 10% who present with mild disease require colectomy within 5 years. Children who present with proctitis have a high likelihood of developing more extensive disease.

Crohn disease is associated with a high morbidity rate but low mortality rate. Most patients have continuous activity or intermittent symptoms throughout their life, and relapses commonly occur when therapy is discontinued.

Complications of the inflammatory process increase with time, with approximately 70% of patients eventually requiring surgery. Frequent relapses and disease progression are difficult to manage, from both a medical and a psychosocial standpoint.

The risk of colorectal cancer in both Crohn disease and ulcerative colitis is significant. In Crohn disease, the cumulative risk after 20 years of disease is 8%. The risk of colon cancer in ulcerative colitis is approximately 12% by 10 to 25 years after onset of disease, and increases by 10% to 20% per decade. The most important risk factors for the development of adenocarcinoma are duration and extent of colitis. The presence of sclerosing cholangitis is also a risk factor.

FOLLOW-UP

Frequency of subspecialty follow-up of patients with IBD depends on the course and activity of the disease. Intervals should be no longer than every 6 to 12 months when in remission. From the time of initial diagnosis until the patient is stabilized, and during disease exacerbations, weekly visits may be necessary. In addition to the interval history and physical examination, subspecialty follow-up will frequently include screening laboratory tests. These tests vary, depending on disease location, activity, and known complications, but may include a complete blood count with differential, liver panel, and drug metabolite levels. Patients who have colonic disease of more than 8 to 10 years' duration should also undergo annual to biannual screening colonoscopy to look for evidence of dysplasia, which is an indication for colectomy.

◉	**Additional Resources, CD-ROM**
Radiographic findings of inflammatory bowel disease	Table, figures
Endoscopic findings of inflammatory bowel disease	Table, figures
Biopsy findings of inflammatory bowel disease	Table, figures
Resources for patients and families	Text
Bibliography	

SUGGESTED READINGS

Balistreri WF: Hepatobiliary complications of inflammatory bowel disease: Overview of the issues. Inflamm Bowel Dis 1998;4(3):220–224.

Dubinsky MC, Lamothe S, Yang HY, et al: Pharmacogenomics and metabolite measurement for 6-mercaptopurine therapy in inflammatory bowel disease. Gastroenterology 2000;118(4):705–713.

Hampe J, Cuthbert A, Croucher PJ, et al: Association between insertion mutation in NOD2 gene and Crohn's disease in German and British populations. Lancet 2001;357(9272):1925–1928.

Hoffenberg EJ, Fidanza S, Sauaia A: Serologic testing for inflammatory bowel disease. J Pediatr 1999;134(4):447–452.

Hyams JS: Inflammatory bowel disease. Pediatr Rev 2000; 21(9): 291–295.

Present DH, Rutgeerts P, Targan S, et al: Infliximab for the treatment of fistulas in patients with Crohn's disease. N Engl J Med 1999; 340(18):1398–1405.

SECTION 4 CHRONIC MEDICAL CARE: *Disorders of the Gastrointestinal Tract*

140 Pancreatic Disorders

Stavra A. Xanthakos and Samuel A. Kocoshis

ROLE OF THE GENERALIST

1. Diagnose and manage acute and chronic pancreatitis.
2. Recognize manifestations of pancreatic insufficiency and when to refer to specialist.
3. Understand management of pancreatic disease caused by cystic fibrosis.
4. Recognize spectrum of congenital and hereditary pancreatic disorders.
5. Recognize spectrum of pediatric pancreatic tumors.
6. Refer to specialist if needed for procedures and medical management.

The pancreas is composed of approximately 80% exocrine and 2% endocrine tissue. The remainder of the organ is composed of supporting structures, including the excretory ducts, blood vessels, nerves, and lymphatic vessels. Exocrine function is carried out by acinar cells that synthesize, store, and secrete the digestive enzymes. Endocrine function, mainly regulation of glucose homeostasis, is carried out by special cells located in the islets of Langerhans. An overview of major exocrine and endocrine functions of the pancreas is given in Table 140-1. Diseases of the pancreas are rarer in children than in adults. Many patients with pancreatic dysfunction require referral to gastrointestinal specialists for further evaluation and management, unless they have acute, nonrecurrent pancreatitis (see also Chapter 91).

Table 140-1. Overview of Pancreatic Functions

Tissue	Function
Exocrine	**Synthesize, Store, and Secrete Digestive Enzymes**

Proteolytic enzymes
  Trypsinogen
  Chymotrypsinogen
  Proelastase
  Procarboxypeptidases A and B
	Activated in duodenum to yield trypsin, chymotrypsin, elastase, carboxypeptidases A and B
	Cleave peptide bonds of proteins to yield oligopeptides and free amino acids

Lipolytic enzymes
  Lipase
  Phospholipase A$_2$
  Carboxylesterase lipase
	Hydrolyze triglycerides
	Presence of bile salts important for full activity

Amylolytic enzyme Amylase Trypsin inhibitor	Hydrolyzes starch and glycogen Inactivates trypsins that are activated autocatalytically in the acinus
Endocrine	**Synthesize and Release Hormones Active in Glucose Regulation and Growth**
A cells	Glucagon
B cells	Insulin
D cells	Somatostatin
PP cells	Pancreatic polypeptide

PANCREATITIS

The differential diagnosis of acute pancreatitis in children is extensive and varied (Table 140-2). Although investigation does not always reveal the cause, the most frequently identified etiologies in pediatric patients are trauma, medications, and viral infections. Less common entities include

954

Table 140-2. Differential Diagnosis of Acute Pancreatitis

Category	Disorders

Systemic	Infections
	  Viral: mumps, coxsackie B,
	    echovirus, influenza A and B,
	    varicella, Epstein Barr, rubeola,
	    hepatitis A and B, rubella
	  Bacterial: typhoid fever, *Escherichia*
	    coli, Mycoplasma, leptospirosis
	  Parasitic: malaria, ascariasis, and
	    Clonorchis sinensis (duct
	    obstruction)
	Inflammatory and vasculitic disorders
	  Collagen vascular diseases
	  Henoch-Schönlein purpura
	  Hemolytic-uremic syndrome
	  Kawasaki disease
	  Inflammatory bowel disease
	Sepsis/peritonitis/shock
	Transplantation

Mechanical/structural	Trauma (blunt injury, child abuse,
	  endoscopic retrograde
	  cholangiopancreatography)
	Perforation (duodenal ulcer)
	Anomalies (pancreas divisum,
	  choledochal cyst, stenosis)
	Obstruction (stones, parasites, tumors)

Metabolic disorders and toxins	Hyperlipidemia Hypercalcemia (primary or secondary) Cystic fibrosis Malnutrition (refeeding) Renal disease Hypothermia Diabetes mellitus Organic acidemia Drugs/toxins

hyperparathyroidism, hypertriglyceridemia, α_1-antitrypsin deficiency, cystic fibrosis and the cystic fibrosis carrier state (strongly associated with recurrent pancreatitis), and pancreatic or ductal anatomic abnormalities. Pancreatitis in adults is usually related to alcoholism or biliary tract disease.

Several pathogenic mechanisms seem to act in concert to produce pancreatitis. In familial pancreatitis, mutation in the trypsinogen binding domain results in high pancreatic concentration of active trypsin, leading to autodigestion. Mechanical, toxic, or metabolic injury to the pancreas can also block intrapancreatic inactivation of proteases. Anatomic anomalies or masses can obstruct the flow, leading to local edema, hemorrhage, thrombosis, ischemia, inflammation, and necrosis. Free radical formation appears to play a role in edema formation, but its role in pathogenesis of necrosis is unclear. Increased levels of superoxide radicals and lipid peroxides and depletion of ascorbic acid have been noted in adults with acute pancreatitis.

Diagnosis

The most common complaint associated with acute pancreatitis is epigastric abdominal pain. The pain is generally acute in onset, with variable intensity and duration. Pain can also occur in other abdominal locations, worsening gradually or being intermittent and colicky. In children, radiation to the back is less common than in adults. Associated symptoms often include nausea, vomiting, and anorexia. Meals may exacerbate the pain and nausea.

On inspection, the child may appear quiet, irritable, or ill. He may prefer a curled position with flexed knees and hips. Examination most often reveals epigastric tenderness, with diminished bowel sounds. Rebound tenderness and guarding may be present if the inflammation has spread to the peritoneum. In severe hemorrhagic pancreatitis, the periumbilical area (Cullen sign) or flank (Grey Turner sign) may take on a bluish cast. In very severe cases, the child may present in shock. A palpable abdominal mass consistent with a pseudocyst may be present. Other signs are jaundice, ascites, and respiratory distress from pleural effusions.

No single laboratory test is pathognomonic for acute pancreatitis. Serum amylase is the most widely used screening test, but may be normal in children with pancreatitis. Amylase rises within hours of onset of acute pancreatitis and can remain elevated for 2 to 5 days. Elevation of amylase or lipase more than three times normal is considered suspicious for pancreatitis; however, the degree of elevation is not proportional to the severity or duration of pancreatitis.

Although extrapancreatic amylase (salivary, ovarian, intestinal, tumor-derived) may be elevated under other pathologic conditions, fractionating amylase isoenzymes to determine the proportion of pancreatic amylase is no more helpful than checking the serum lipase level.

Serum lipase levels are also elevated in most cases of acute pancreatitis. Lipase is more specific than amylase and is usually normal in conditions that cause elevated serum amylase, such as parotitis and some carcinomas. Lipase may remain elevated for up to 14 days. However, lipase is found in other tissues as well (salivary and gastric). Measuring both amylase and lipase increases both sensitivity and specificity.

Both amylase and lipase may be incorporated within immunoglobulin complexes in patients with a variety of inflammatory or autoimmune conditions, such as systemic lupus erythematosus or chronic infection. These immune complexes, termed "macroenzymes," are poorly cleared by the kidney and can cause spurious enzyme elevation in the absence of pancreatitis. The course of elevated amylase or lipase levels does not correlate with the clinical course or prognosis of the patient. If the patient is not improving clinically, prolonged elevation of amylase or lipase heightens suspicion for a pseudocyst.

Other laboratory abnormalities sometimes found in children with pancreatitis include elevated glucose, leukocytosis, mild hypertriglyceridemia, hyperbilirubinemia (10% of patients), elevated alkaline phosphatase and gamma-glutamyltranspeptidase, hypocalcemia (25% of patients), and hypoalbuminemia (25% of patients). Hemoconcentration and azotemia may occur from dehydration.

Evaluation

A new scoring system for pediatric patients has been developed to guide prognosis. Eight parameters are included: age under 7 years, weight under 23 kg, admission white blood count over 18,500, admission lactate dehydrogenase over 2000 U/L, 48-hour trough Ca^{2+} under 8.3 mg/dL,

48-hour trough albumin under 2.6 g/dL, 48-hour fluid sequestration over 75 mL/kg, and 48-hour rise in blood urea nitrogen over 5 mg/dL. When the cutoff for predicting a severe outcome was set at three criteria, the sensitivity of this system was 70% versus 30% and 35%, respectively, for the Ranson and Glasgow criteria, and the negative predictive value was 91% versus 85% for the adult scoring systems. Although many cases of pancreatitis can be managed by the generalist, patients who carry a high severity score are best served by referral to a pediatric gastroenterologist or surgeon.

During the first episode of acute pancreatitis in childhood, the more common causes should be sought. The possibility of abdominal trauma, both recent and remote, accidental and nonaccidental, should be explored. Medication history should be reviewed. If clinical symptoms suggest an antecedent or ongoing viral infection, viral causes should be sought. The history taker should question the parents and patient regarding a family history of metabolic disorders or hereditary conditions associated with pancreatitis. Hypercalcemia, hypertriglyceridemia, and hypercholesterolemia, which may be signs of endocrinologic or hereditary disorders, should be excluded. Because cystic fibrosis (CF) may sometimes present with pancreatitis, a sweat chloride test should be obtained, even if the child does not have respiratory symptoms. Many patients with pancreatitis from CF have a CF transmembrane conductance regulator (CFTR) mutation and are less likely to have pancreatic insufficiency or lung disease at the time of presentation. Recent epidemiologic evidence linking the CF carrier state with idiopathic chronic or recurrent acute pancreatitis has prompted some to advocate checking for CFTR mutations in all patients with pancreatitis.

Radiographic imaging should be performed to evaluate for trauma, or biliary or pancreatic duct abnormalities. Plain radiographs of the abdomen provide little diagnostic information. Dilated loops of small bowel near the pancreas may be visible. A plain film is used to evaluate for bowel perforation or obstruction. The most useful imaging tests are abdominal ultrasonography (US) and computed tomography (CT). US may reveal increased pancreatic dimensions and hypoechoic parenchyma. In diagnosing acute pancreatitis among children, the positive predictive value (PPV) of US is 0.93 and the negative predictive value (NPV) is 0.78. CT with contrast offers better definition of the pancreas. The ideal imaging technique is rapid intravenous infusion of contrast material with thin sections through the pancreas. Helical pancreatic images enable excellent visualization of the entire gland. A normal pancreas may be seen in a subset of patients with mild pancreatitis. In more severe cases the scan can reveal increased size and texture changes consistent with inflammation, pseudocysts, abscesses, calcifications, edema, peritoneal exudate, and bowel distention. CT is the study of choice in children who have suffered blunt abdominal trauma.

Endoscopic retrograde cholangiopancreatography (ERCP) can be performed safely in children with chronic or recurrent pancreatitis. ERCP is seldom required in acute pancreatitis and is relatively contraindicated because it may worsen symptoms. If traumatic duct disruption is suspected, it may be necessary. Other indications include detecting sphincter of Oddi dysfunction or primary or secondary duct abnormalities.

As computer software improves, magnetic resonance cholangiopancreatography (MRCP) will complement current imaging techniques, enabling identification of pancreatic and bile duct lesions.

Treatment

Treatment of acute pancreatitis is supportive. Pain control, fluid resuscitation, and nutritional support are the mainstays of therapy. Oral intake is stopped for a few days because of nausea, vomiting, and in more severe cases, gastrointestinal ileus. A nasogastric tube to suction is placed if ileus or severe vomiting is present, primarily for patient comfort. In most cases, intravenous rehydration is initiated. Pain should be controlled, if necessary with intravenous narcotics.

Patients who are not fed for more than 7 to 10 days can be treated with total parenteral nutrition (TPN). Intravenous amino acid and lipid infusions do not appear to stimulate pancreatic secretion, and intravenous glucose infusions suppress pancreatic exocrine secretions. Pancreatic exocrine secretions are stimulated by intragastric and intraduodenal feedings, particularly those high in fat content.

Jejunal feedings have been advocated in the management of pancreatitis after the initial ileus has resolved. These feedings, by bypassing the duodenum and the ligament of Treitz, trigger significantly less exocrine pancreatic secretion both in animals and in healthy human subjects. Total enteral nutrition is as safe and effective as TPN and far less costly. If enteral nasojejunal feedings are started, elemental formulas such as Peptamen (that contains medium-chain triglycerides and partially hydrolyzed protein) or Vivonex (with a very low fat and protein content) are more easily digested and minimize pancreatic exocrine stimulation.

Insufficient data are available to conclude whether early resumption of enteral nutrition has a direct effect on survival or incidence and severity of complications in acute pancreatitis. Patients should resume oral eating when pain has subsided, bowel sounds are present, amylase and lipase levels have returned to near normal, and hunger returns. A clear liquid, low-fat diet is initiated for the first 24 hours. If well tolerated, the diet may be advanced to low-fat solids over the next 24 hours. Fat should form less than 20% of the calories consumed. Antioxidant supplements (vitamins A, C, and E, selenium, and methionine) seem to have decreased pancreatic inflammation and edema, but data are controversial.

Attempts to rest the pancreas pharmacologically have not proved helpful in adults. Agents used have included histamine-2 (H$_2$) blockers, atropine, calcitonin, glucagon, somatostatin, and fluorouracil, but there is no evidence that they improve symptoms.

Additional treatment goals are to stop any causative agents if possible (medications and toxins) and treat any complications. Antibiotic coverage does not appear to change the course of uncomplicated pancreatitis unless necrotizing pancreatitis or infection occurs. Electrolytes, glucose, calcium, and lipids are monitored, as are blood pressure and urinary output. Surgery should be reserved for exploration if peritonitis ensues, removal of obstruction of the main pancreatic ducts or common bile duct, drainage of cysts and abscesses, and débriding of necrotic tissue.

Most cases of acute pancreatitis resolve within 3 days. Moderate to severe cases should be watched closely for evidence of organ failure which can result from shock owing to third space losses, toxins from the pancreas that reach systemic circulation, or cytokine production. If clinical symptoms and signs persist, possible complications should be investigated. The incidence of complications in children is significant, approximately 15%. Early complications include multisystem organ failure of the pulmonary, cardiovascular, or renal systems. Pancreatic or peripancreatic necrosis or infection may occur. Late complications occur after the second week and include pseudocysts and abscesses. Rare complications include jejunal infarction, splenic vein rupture or thrombosis, subcutaneous fat necrosis, pancreatic insufficiency, and diabetes mellitus. Mortality was reported as 21% in one small series of 61 children.

Blunt trauma, particularly injury from a bicycle handlebar, is the most common cause of pancreatic pseudocyst formation (65% of cases). Twenty-five percent of cysts resolve without surgical intervention. If the cyst fails to resolve or symptoms persist, percutaneous external catheter drainage or surgical excision is required.

CHRONIC PANCREATITIS

Several classification systems have been developed to define and characterize chronic pancreatitis. The Marseille classification system was devised in 1963 with revisions in 1984 and 1988. Summarized, the system defines acute pancreatitis as an inflammatory condition of the pancreas with clinical, histologic, and functional resolution once the inciting factor has been removed. Chronic pancreatitis is defined by permanent irreversible morphologic changes with or without clinical or functional impairment. Chronic or acute relapsing pancreatitis should prompt an assiduous search for the etiology (Table 140-3). The most common cause of recurrent pancreatitis worldwide, juvenile tropical pancreatitis, is seldom seen in North America.

Table 140-3. Differential Diagnosis of Chronic Pancreatitis

Category	Disorder
Nutritional	Juvenile tropical pancreatitis
Congenital	Hereditary pancreatitis
Metabolic	Cystic fibrosis (with pancreatic sufficiency)
	Hyperlipidemia
	Familial hyperchylomicronemia
	Homocystinuria
	Hyperparathyroidism
	Hypercalcemia
Anatomic	Pancreas divisum
	Choledochal cyst
	Cholelithiasis
	Sphincter of Oddi dysfunction
	Sclerosing cholangitis
	Trauma
	Idiopathic fibrosis

Hereditary pancreatitis (HP) is the second most common cause of chronic or recurrent pancreatitis and the second most common hereditary disease of the pancreas (following cystic fibrosis). HP is a chronic idiopathic inflammatory disorder of the pancreas. Over 100 family groups with more than 500 affected individuals have been described. The disorder is marked by recurrent episodes of pancreatitis and occurs equally among boys and girls. Pancreatic duct stones are often found, as is a positive family history and absence of other known causes of pancreatitis. Over half of patients present before age 5 (58%), but the disorder may go unrecognized for many years, with age of diagnosis between 6 and 15 years in 25% and between 16 and 20 years in 17%. Inheritance is autosomal dominant with variable penetrance. Gene mutations affect the structure or enzymatic activation of trypsinogen, preventing binding of trypsin with elastase inhibitors. Selective groups of patients with HP appear to have antioxidant deficiencies, and supplementation with antioxidants such as selenium or vitamin E may be beneficial in therapy.

Chronic or recurrent pancreatitis can result from other inherited causes, such as cystic fibrosis, hyperlipidemia, homocystinuria, hyperparathyrodism, familial hypocalciuric hypercalcemia, and familial hyperchylomicronemia.

Anatomic abnormalities, such as pancreas divisum or choledochal cysts, may cause recurrent pancreatitis. Pancreas divisum, which is the most common anatomic abnormality associated with pancreatitis, occurs in 6% of routine autopsies in adults. Children with recurrent pancreatitis should be referred to a pediatric gastroenterologist for further evaluation. The episodes of pancreatitis are managed in a supportive fashion as described for acute pancreatitis.

In patients with chronic pancreatitis, a previously normal ERCP does not obviate the need for a follow-up study if symptoms are worsening, as fibrotic duct strictures may obstruct the pancreatic duct at any time during the course of the pancreatic process. Therapeutic ERCP enables extraction of common duct stones, sphincterotomy, and bile or pancreatic duct stent placement.

PANCREATIC INSUFFICIENCY

Pancreatic insufficiency results from deficiencies in one or more digestive enzymes produced by the pancreas. Numerous hereditary disorders that impair the exocrine functions of the pancreas have been described (Table 140-4). The most common of these is CF, followed by the Shwachman-Diamond syndrome. The primary care practitioner must recognize the symptoms of pancreatic insufficiency. Symptoms invariably include growth failure and in most cases, steatorrhea, which is due to malabsorption of carbohydrates, proteins, and fat. Infants or children with these symptoms should be screened for CF, the most common cause. If the sweat chloride assay is negative, these patients should be referred to a pediatric gastroenterologist to screen for more rare hereditary disorders, some of which are listed in Table 140-4. In several of these rare disorders, a characteristic constellation of signs and symptoms may be present.

Table 140-4. Diseases Causing Pancreatic Insufficiency

Disorder	Mode of Inheritance	Incidence
Cystic fibrosis	Autosomal recessive	1 in 1900–3700 in whites, 1 in 17,000 in African Americans
Shwachman-Diamond syndrome	Autosomal recessive	1 in 10,000–20,000
Johanson-Blizzard syndrome	Autosomal recessive	Less than 40 cases described
Pearson marrow-pancreas syndrome	Mitochondrial deletion	Unknown
Pancreatic aplasia/hypoplasia	Unknown	Unknown
Isolated pancreatic enzyme deficiencies: lipase, lipase-colipase, colipase, amylase, trypsinogen	Unknown	Unknown

Management

Treatment is supportive and consists of nutritional management and pancreatic enzyme replacements. These patients often need 120% to 150% of the recommended daily allowance of nutrients, vitamins, and minerals to grow. Once supplemented with pancreatic enzymes, they should have unrestricted dietary fat and should also be supplemented with fat-soluble vitamins. There is no reference standard for the optimal dosage of pancreatic enzyme replacements, but now that acid-resistant microspheres and microtablets inside acid-resistant capsules are available, the dose necessary to treat steatorrhea is lower than it has been in the past.

Fibrosing colonopathy was reported in pediatric patients with CF taking high-dose pancreatic enzyme supplements (24,000 to 30,000 units lipase/capsule) for over 1 year. Some centers recommend limiting lipase to 2500 units/kg/dose. Now that enzyme dosage has been restricted, this complication is rarely, if ever, observed.

SPECIFIC DISORDERS OF THE PANCREAS

Cystic Fibrosis

Cystic fibrosis (CF) is the most common cause of exocrine pancreatic dysfunction in children and should be considered in all patients who present with signs of pancreatic insufficiency whether or not they have signs of chronic lung disease.

About 85% of patients with CF have pancreatic insufficiency (PI) with clinically evident steatorrhea. Steatorrhea becomes apparent when the production of lipase falls by about 98%. The remaining 15% of patients have sufficient pancreatic exocrine function initially, although 10% to 20% eventually develop insufficiency. These patients tend to be diagnosed at an older age, have lower sweat chloride levels, are less likely to have had meconium ileus in infancy, and have better nutritional status.

The pancreatic insufficiency seen in CF is secondary to decreased chloride secretion in the lumina of pancreatic ducts. The decreased concentration of chloride ion indi-rectly leads to insufficient secretion of pancreatic fluid because of impaired exchange for bicarbonate ion. Beginning in utero, this leads to plugging and obstruction of pancreatic ducts and eventually to destruction of the organ.

CF may lead to pancreatitis in patients with pancreatic insufficiency or sufficiency. Pancreatitis can be the presenting feature of CF. Destruction of pancreatic tissue can lead to endocrine dysfunction and diabetes late in the course. Diabetic ketoacidosis is uncommon.

The diagnosis of cystic fibrosis is typically made by sweat chloride testing. Greater than 99% of patients have abnormally high sweat chloride concentrations. The test may be falsely positive in malnutrition and falsely negative in hypoalbuminemia and edema. Genotype analysis for the 20 to 30 most common CF mutations is available when insufficient sweat can be obtained.

Shwachman-Diamond Syndrome

Shwachman-Diamond syndrome is the second most common cause of pancreatic insufficiency in children. The reported incidence is 1 in 10,000 to 20,000 live births. Inheritance is autosomal recessive. Clinical manifestations include stunted but steady linear growth (less than the third percentile), steatorrhea usually evident in infancy, cyclic neutropenia, and metaphyseal dysostosis in the femur, tibia, and ribs. Other associations include dental abnormalities, thoracic dystrophy, dermal ichthyosis, hepatomegaly or hepatosplenomegaly, kidney dysfunction, abnormal lung function, diabetes mellitus, delayed puberty, developmental retardation, thrombocytopenia, and anemia.

Confirmatory tests include an increased stool fat and low to undetectable pancreatic enzymes following a pancreozymin-secretin test. In some patients, steatorrhea will improve in adulthood. Twice weekly blood tests should be performed during a 3-week period to screen for cyclic neutropenia. The neutropenia can occur as often as every 1 to 2 days. Bone marrow aspiration may show hypoplasia, fatty infiltration, and arrest of myeloid maturation. The pancreas is universally lipotic on radiographic or histologic evaluation.

Patients with Shwachman-Diamond syndrome are at increased risk for bacterial infections and orthopedic complications. Neutrophil abnormalities such as defective motility and abnormal chemotaxis may explain the increased susceptibility to infection. Hematologic associations reported include aplastic anemia and leukemia. Pancreatic insufficiency may lead to malnutrition and growth failure.

Treatment is largely supportive. To minimize malabsorption and growth failure, oral pancreatic enzymes and fat-soluble vitamins are prescribed. These patients should be carefully monitored for infection and appropriate antibiotic coverage prescribed as indicated. Bone marrow transplantation has been attempted as a curative option.

Johanson-Blizzard Syndrome

Johanson-Blizzard syndrome is an autosomal recessive inherited disorder. Clinical features include pancreatic insufficiency, nasal alar hypoplasia, no permanent teeth, short stature, congenital deafness, psychomotor retardation, ectodermal scalp defects, rectourogenital malformations

Table 140-5. Fat-Soluble Vitamin Replacement

Vitamin	Recommended Daily Dose
A	5000–10,000 IU
D	400–800 IU
E	50–200 IU
K	5 mg twice weekly

such as imperforate anus, and hypothyroidism. The most common presentation is growth failure from malabsorption from pancreatic insufficiency. The pancreatic insufficiency is caused by an acinar cell defect that results in decreased production of trypsin, colipase, and total lipase.

Pearson Marrow-Pancreas Syndrome

Pearson marrow-pancreas syndrome was initially described in four children with severe macrocytic anemia, with low reticulocyte counts, and variable neutropenia and thrombocytopenia either simultaneously or subsequently in the neonatal period. Three of the patients had evidence of exocrine pancreatic insufficiency. No endocrine pancreatic abnormalities were detected. Other findings observed in later reports included marked hepatomegaly, cirrhosis, steatosis, photosensitivity and patchy erythematous skin lesions, ataxia, proximal muscle weakness, external ophthalmoplegia, pigmentary retinopathy, diabetes mellitus, and renal tubular disease. The disorder is diagnosed by analyzing for large mitochondrial DNA rearrangements.

Isolated Enzyme Deficiencies

Isolated pancreatic enzyme deficiencies are extremely rare. All share the hallmarks of pancreatic insufficiency: malabsorption, maldigestion, and steatorrhea. Some of these disorders may have unique symptoms such as sideroblastic anemia, edema, and hypoproteinemia. If the diagnosis of CF is excluded in a patient with the clinical signs and symptoms of pancreatic insufficiency, he or she should be referred to a pediatric specialist for evaluation for one of the hereditary pancreatic exocrine disorders. Table 140-5 lists vitamin replacement of fat-soluble vitamins.

CONGENITAL ANOMALIES

Pancreas Divisum

Many congenital pancreatic anomalies arise from failure of complete rotation and fusion during embryogenesis. The most common congenital anomaly of the pancreas is pancreas divisum, in which the embryonic ventral duct never fuses with the dorsal duct to form the main pancreatic duct. Therefore, the dorsal duct becomes the main pancreatic duct draining into the duodenum via the accessory papilla. In children with pancreatitis, pancreas divisum was identified in 7.5% of children with pancreatitis and in 19% of children with recurrent or chronic pancreatitis. Pancreas divisum has been reported in association with recurrent acute pancreatitis or chronic pancreatitis, but in many patients this anomaly remains silent. In symptomatic patients, ERCP balloon dilation of the accessory papilla, papillotomy, or stenting has been effective.

Annular Pancreas

During rotation of the ventral pancreas in embryogenesis, a portion may encircle the duodenum. It is the most common anatomic anomaly causing duodenal obstruction in infants. Annular pancreas may lead to duodenal obstruction at any age, most often in infancy. It may be associated with several other congenital anomalies: Down syndrome, intestinal malrotation, duodenal bands, cardiac anomalies, Meckel diverticulum, imperforate anus, spinal defects, and cryptorchidism. Signs of an upper gastrointestinal obstruction in infants include a history of polyhydramnios, abdominal distention, feeding difficulties, and bile-stained emesis. Signs in older children include nausea, vomiting, upper abdominal pain, postprandial fullness, weight loss, and gastrointestinal bleeding.

Plain abdominal radiographs in infants may show a double bubble sign consistent with duodenal obstruction. An upper gastrointestinal barium study reveals a dilatation of the duodenum proximal to a smooth, symmetric filling defect. The anomaly is confirmed by laparotomy. Treatment is surgical.

Ectopic Pancreas

Ectopic pancreas is a condition in which normal pancreatic tissue is found in an anatomically aberrant area. The reported incidence is 0.5% to 14% at autopsy and 0.2% at surgery. It is usually asymptomatic, but can produce symptoms based on its location. Ectopic pancreas is located in the upper gastrointestinal tract in 70% of cases: 25% within 5 cm of pylorus, 30% in duodenum, 15% in jejunum. More rarely, it has been reported in Meckel diverticulum, appendix, ileum, ileal or gastric duplication, rectum, liver, gallbladder, umbilicus, mediastinum, bronchogenic cysts, pulmonary sequestrations, hiatal hernia, and fallopian tube. It can present at any age with epigastric abdominal pain or distention, gastrointestinal bleeding, biliary obstruction, cholecystitis, or intussusception. There is a long-term risk of malignant transformation. Asymptomatic ectopic pancreatic tissue should be observed. If symptoms persist after ruling out other coexisting diseases such as peptic ulcer or gastroesophageal reflux disease, excision should be considered. If coincidentally discovered during an operation, it should be prophylactically excised.

Pancreatic Agenesis, Aplasia, Hypoplasia, and Dysplasia

Complete agenesis is rare and incompatible with life. Partial agenesis results from abnormal dorsal bud development. In pancreatic hypoplasia, the pancreas is normal in size, but the tissue is marked by reduced duct number and decreased terminal differentiation with increased fatty infiltration. In dysplasia, the parenchyma is disorganized with dilated ducts and increased fibromuscular proliferation. Clinical presentation is varied. These disorders can be silent if sufficient pancreatic function is present. However, pancreatic exocrine or endocrine insufficiency may result in in utero growth retardation or postnatal growth failure, insulin-responsive hyperglycemia, neonatal death, or malabsorption and steatorrhea.

Diagnosis can be confirmed by abdominal US, CT, angiography, or ERCP and confirmed at surgery or autopsy or by a cholecystokinin secretin stimulation test. These anomalies can be associated with other disorders or syndromes such as chromosomal anomalies, hepatic or renal dysplasias, and sideroblastic anemias.

Choledochal Cysts

Congenital choledochal cysts or cystic dilatations of the extrahepatic or intrahepatic biliary tree have been reported in association with pancreatitis. Most choledochal cysts are diagnosed before age 10. Classic symptoms include right upper quadrant abdominal pain, jaundice, and a palpable right upper quadrant mass, although this triad may not always be present. Diagnosis is confirmed by a hepatic US, CT scan, or a nuclear study of the biliary tree. Complete resection with creation of a Roux-en-Y hepatojejunostomy is the recommended treatment because there is an increased risk of carcinoma in the unresected cyst mucosa.

Congenital Cysts

True pancreatic cysts are very rare. They may produce no symptoms or may cause abdominal pain or bowel or biliary obstruction. Typically, pancreatic cysts are solitary, although multiple cysts may be seen in polycystic kidney disease, cystic fibrosis, and von Hippel–Lindau syndrome. If symptomatic, surgical resection or drainage may be indicated. Generally, though, no intervention is recommended for patients with multiple cysts.

TUMORS OF THE PANCREAS

Pancreatic tumors are very rare in children. Lymphoma can involve the pancreas. Most pancreatic tumors present with abdominal pain and elevated serum levels of pancreatic enzymes, mimicking simple acute pancreatitis. Children with insulinomas present with hypoglycemia and irritability. Such cases emphasize that pancreatic imaging is essential in patients who present with hyperamylasemia or hyperli-

pasemia. Some patients may also present with a palpable abdominal mass. Tumors can be identified by abdominal CT scan or by US. The decision to embark on radiation therapy, chemotherapy, or surgical excision should be individualized according to the type and stage of the tumor, in consultation with experienced pediatric oncologists and surgeons.

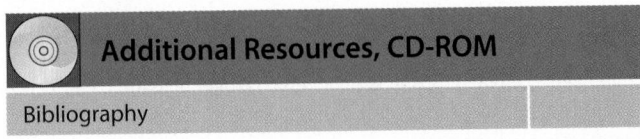

Additional Resources, CD-ROM

Bibliography

Mini-index of Related Topics

SUGGESTED READINGS

Etemad B, Whitcomb DC: Chronic pancreatitis: diagnosis, classification and new genetic developments. Gastroenterology 2001;120:682–707.

Hsu RK, Draganov P, Leung JW, et al: Therapeutic ERCP in the management of pancreatitis in children. Gastrointest Endosc 2000;51:396–400.

Lerner A, Branski D, Lebenthal E: Pancreatic diseases in children. Pediatr Clin North Am 1996;43:125–156.

Sharer N, Schwartz M, Malone G, et al: Mutations of the cystic fibrosis gene in patients with chronic pancreatitis. N Engl J Med 1998;339:645–652.

Thompson DR: Narcotic analgesic effects on the sphincter of Oddi: A review of the data and therapeutic implications in treating pancreatitis. Am J Gastroenterol 2001;96:1266–1272.

141   Liver and Biliary Tract Disorders

Stephen L. Guthery and William F. Balistreri

ROLE OF THE GENERALIST

1. Recognize the manifestations of chronic liver disease.
2. Recognize the complications of chronic liver disease.
3. Distinguish emergent and elective referrals of children with chronic liver disease.
4. Stabilize patients with life-threatening complications and transport to tertiary center for definitive care.
5. Understand the natural history of biliary atresia.
6. Determine the conjugated/direct bilirubin in any jaundiced infant older than 14 days.
7. If otherwise clinically stable, refer infants with newly diagnosed cholestasis within 1 week of its discovery.

Chronic liver disease includes a spectrum of clinical conditions caused by a variety of hepatic disorders, including cholestasis, portal hypertension, and end-stage liver disease. The extent to which a generalist manages children with chronic liver disease depends on the clinician's experience and proximity of subspecialty care. Familiarity with the clinical consequences of chronic liver disease is important to all primary care providers, because they play an integral role in the recognition of life-threatening complications of chronic liver disease and recognition of the less urgent but important complications.

Clinical care of children with chronic liver disease can be divided into the diagnosis of the underlying condition and the management of the complications. One essential concept is that whatever the underlying disease, the management of the complications is similar. For example, while the pathophysiology of cholestasis in children with the Alagille syndrome and primary sclerosing cholangitis are fundamentally different, the management of chronic cholestasis in both diseases is identical: Both require optimization of nutritional status, supplementation of fat-soluble vitamins, and treatment of pruritus. The generalist need not necessarily be well versed in the causes of each clinical condition, but should be familiar with the management and complications of each, and must recognize associated emergencies.

These clinical conditions—portal hypertension, chronic cholestasis, and end-stage liver disease—all represent common manifestations of a variety of underlying diseases. Portal hypertension may exist in isolation or in combination with chronic cholestasis, and the converse may occur. Each may develop over time in a given patient. For example,

infants with biliary atresia have chronic cholestasis at diagnosis and will uniformly develop portal hypertension and end-stage liver disease in the first year of life without intervention. Thus, time, the underlying etiology, and the effectiveness of the intervention determine whether a patient will develop portal hypertension, cholestasis, or end-stage liver disease.

FUNDAMENTALS

A frequent problem encountered in children with chronic liver disease is the interpretation of "abnormal" liver function tests. This term should be uniformly discarded because it neither clearly communicates nor defines the precise abnormality. Most often, the term is used to describe elevated serum aminotransferase levels, or more specifically, elevations in alanine aminotransferase (ALT) and aspartate aminotransferase (AST). Both enzymes are important in amino acid metabolism, are released from damaged tissue, and are frequently elevated with hepatocellular damage. Although present in the liver, AST is found in many tissues and is less specific for hepatic injury. ALT is more specific for hepatocellular damage than AST but is also present in muscle. Although isolated elevations of serum aminotransferase levels are rarely helpful in determining the underlying etiology of the liver disease, they may alert the clinician to the presence of chronic liver disease and are important for monitoring disease activity in those with established liver disease. Autoimmune hepatitis, chronic viral hepatitis, drug-induced hepatitis, cystic fibrosis, Wilson's disease, and nonalcoholic steatohepatitis may all present with isolated AST and ALT elevations, and all are monitored by measuring serum levels of these enzymes. These biochemical abnormalities may be the only manifestation of chronic liver disease in these patients.

Cholestasis (Table 141-1) is frequently characterized by jaundice, and is defined by an elevated serum conjugated bilirubin level or elevated serum bile acids. Cholestasis is abnormal bile flow, and when chronic, it has several physiologic and clinical consequences. Abnormal bile flow disrupts nutrient fat absorption. This malabsorption may result in malnutrition and fat-soluble vitamin deficiency. Ocular symptoms, rickets, neuropathy, or bleeding dyscrasias should alert the clinician to the presence of vitamin A, D, E, and K deficiencies. Cholestasis often causes intense pruritus (Fig. 141-1), probably as a result of deposition of bile acids in the skin. For many children, pruritus is the most debilitating symptom of their chronic liver disease. Chronic

Table 141-1. Manifestations, Complications, and Etiology of Chronic Cholestasis

Clinical Manifestations

Jaundice
Pruritus
Diarrhea

Complications

Malnutrition
Fat-soluble vitamin deficiency
Fractures
Cirrhosis

Causes

Biliary atresia
Total parenteral nutrition cholestasis
Cystic fibrosis
α_1-Antitrypsin deficiency
Alagille syndrome
Familial intrahepatic cholestasis syndromes
Primary sclerosing cholangitis
Inborn errors of bile acid metabolism

cholestasis frequently leads to hepatocyte damage, leading to hepatic fibrosis and sometimes cirrhosis, and ultimately end-stage liver disease.

The most common cause of chronic cholestasis in children is biliary atresia. Biliary atresia is caused by the inflammatory destruction of the intra- or extrahepatic bile ducts. It presents in early infancy with cholestatic jaundice, and definitive diagnosis is made by liver biopsy and cholangiography. Most important, early recognition and appropriate

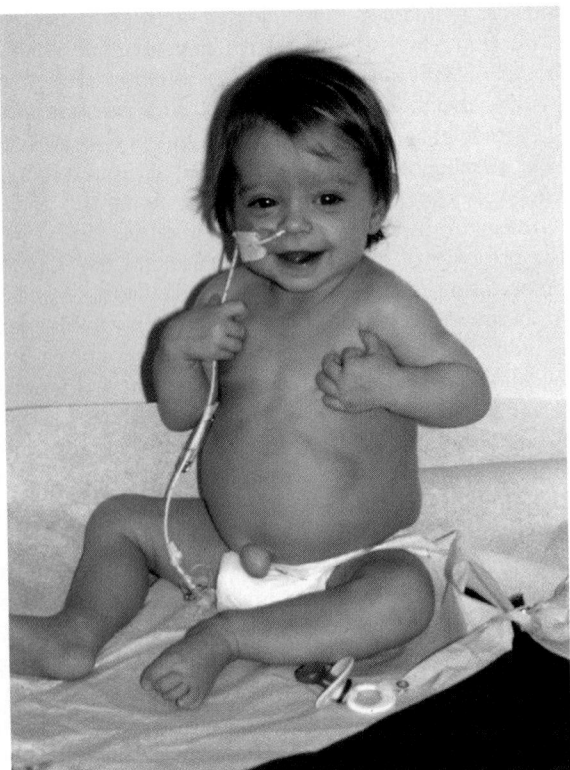

Figure 141-1. Chronic liver disease in 10-month-old infant with chronic cholestasis from biliary atresia. Note jaundice and pruritus (note excoriation of forehead and active scratching). An enteral feeding tube is in place to treat malnutrition. Abdominal distention is due to ascites secondary to portal hypertension. (Photo by Stephen L. Guthery, MD.)

referral significantly affect outcome. The most common reason for delay in diagnosis is mistaking cholestatic jaundice for physiologic jaundice. Because early diagnosis of biliary atresia has a direct influence on outcome, all babies older than 14 days with jaundice should have a fractionated bilirubin to determine the contribution of unconjugated and conjugated bilirubin to the total bilirubin. Those with conjugated hyperbilirubinemia should undergo an aggressive search for the etiology.

Alagille syndrome is a primarily cholestatic disorder. This heterogenous syndrome is variably characterized by a distinctive facies and cardiac, ocular, renal, and vertebral abnormalities. α_1-Antitrypsin deficiency, cystic fibrosis, various inborn errors of bile acid metabolism, total parenteral nutrition-associated cholestasis, panhypopituitarism, and familial intrahepatic cholestatic syndromes all may present with chronic cholestasis.

Portal hypertension is a clinical entity characterized by the presence of splenomegaly, varices, and/or ascites (Table 141-2). The fundamental cause is an alteration of the portal circulation because of elevated right-sided heart pressure, hepatic vein obstruction, abnormalities in the hepatic parenchyma such as cirrhosis, or portal vein obstruction. Varices are dilated veins formed at the areas where the systemic and the portal venous systems form collateral vessels: the esophagus, stomach, anterior abdominal wall, and rectum are common locations (Fig. 141-2). Variceal hemorrhage is a life-threatening consequence of portal hypertension requiring emergent intervention. *Ascites* is a collection of transudative fluid in the peritoneal cavity. Infected ascites, called spontaneous bacterial peritonitis, can be life-threatening, and requires immediate intervention.

Any underlying condition that can cause cirrhosis may result in portal hypertension. Chronic liver congestion either from right ventricular heart failure or hepatic vein obstruction (also called the Budd-Chiari syndrome) may eventually lead to portal hypertension. Portal vein thrombosis is a common cause of portal hypertension in children, and may occur without an identifiable cause, as a complication of umbilical vein catheterization, or an underlying hypercoagulable state.

End-stage liver disease is the final common pathway in progressive liver disease. It is characterized by a combination of portal hypertension, severe cholestasis, intractable ascites, and hepatic synthetic dysfunction as evidenced by hypoalbuminemia and prolonged prothrombin time, and

Table 141-2. Manifestations, Complications, and Etiology of Portal Hypertension

Clinical Manifestations

Splenomegaly
Ascites
Varices

Complications

Spontaneous bacterial peritonitis
Variceal hemorrhage

Causes

Extrahepatic (portal vein thrombosis; splenic vein thrombosis)
Intrahepatic (cirrhosis)
Suprahepatic (Budd-Chiari syndrome; right ventricular heart failure)

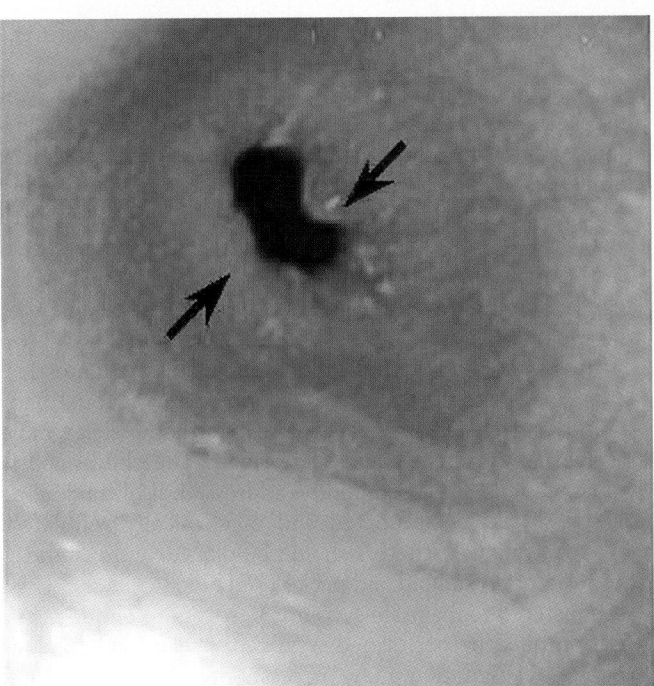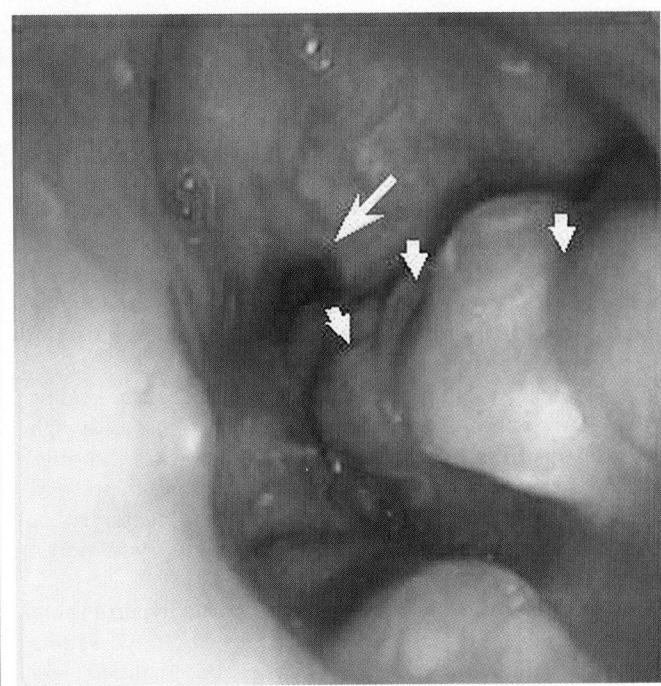

Figure 141-2. Endoscopic view of esophageal varices in a 7-year-old child with portal hypertension caused by cirrhosis. *Left,* A normal esophagus with gastroesophageal junction in center *(arrows). Right,* Esophagus with multiple varices. The largest is evident at 9 o'clock *(arrowheads).* The gastroesophageal junction is evident in the center of the photograph *(arrow).*

failure to thrive in young children. Children with end-stage liver disease may develop hepatorenal syndrome, a type of renal insufficiency caused by physiologic and systemic changes in end-stage liver disease. Similarly, they may develop hepatopulmonary syndrome, which is pulmonary insufficiency caused by changes in the pulmonary vascular bed as a result of end-stage liver disease. Finally, children with end-stage liver disease may have variable neuropsychiatric abnormalities, which may range from subtle findings to frank obtundation.

DIAGNOSIS

This discussion concentrates on the diagnosis of the complications of chronic liver disease. These complications may be considered separately as manifestations of chronic cholestasis and portal hypertension.

Chronic cholestasis is manifested by jaundice, pruritus, malnutrition, and fat-soluble vitamin deficiency, and the diagnosis of each is readily established. Elevated serum conjugated bilirubin levels or elevated serum bile acid levels define cholestasis. Irritability may be a sign of pruritus in the young child, but older children will be able to communicate a history of itching. It is not unusual for children to scratch themselves to the point of excoriation, providing physical evidence of the severity. Because of fat malabsorption, diarrhea is common. Loss of subcutaneous fat or decreased muscle mass suggests malnutrition. Among the fat-soluble vitamins, a deficiency in vitamin K is most commonly clinically apparent. A history of easy bruising or bleeding should be sought and, if present, should alert the clinician to the possibility of vitamin K deficiency. On physical examination, the patient may have ecchymoses and petechiae. A prolonged prothrombin time is often present.

Increased bruising, bleeding, and prolonged prothrombin time with severe hepatic dysfunction does not improve with the administration of vitamin K. If the child is clinically stable, all these complications of chronic cholestasis and their management may be discussed with the specialist on a nonemergent basis, preferably within a few days of their development.

Because of abnormalities in their biliary tract, some children—such as those with biliary atresia—are at risk for developing bacterial cholangitis. Worsening jaundice and the presence of fever are both manifestations of cholangitis. Laboratory evidence of cholangitis includes elevated conjugated bilirubin levels. Leukocytosis provides evidence for cholangitis, although many patients with chronic liver disease will have neutropenia at baseline values because of splenomegaly. Blood cultures are warranted, although they are rarely positive. Because of the inability to make a definitive diagnosis, cholangitis is often suspected on clinical grounds alone and treated empirically.

The clinical consequences of portal hypertension include ascites, esophageal varices, and splenomegaly. A history of feeding difficulties or vomiting may indicate new-onset or worsening ascites. Abdominal distention, increased respiratory rate, umbilical hernias in young children, and scrotal edema in boys are all signs of ascites. The presence of fever in a patient with ascites must be assumed to be due to spontaneous bacterial peritonitis (SBP) unless proved otherwise. As in cholangitis, the child may have a history consistent with acute systemic illness, and may or may not appear systemically ill on physical examination. Children with SBP may have leukocytosis. Blood cultures may or may not be positive. Abdominal paracentesis and analysis of the ascitic fluid is the diagnostic procedure of choice. Paracentesis with a white blood count of more than 500 cells/dL is consistent with SBP. Although not always present, positive Gram stain or a positive culture is diagnostic.

A history of hematemesis, hematochezia, or melena must alert the clinician to the presence of variceal hemorrhage. This is a medical emergency and immediate steps should be undertaken to ensure adequate initial management and appropriate emergent referral. The child may have a variety of signs suggestive of hypovolemic shock, from isolated tachycardia to cardiovascular collapse. Laboratory measures vary depending on the cause and extent of the underlying liver disease. A normal hemoglobin does not exclude the occurrence of significant blood loss.

Splenomegaly can result in hypersplenism, often leading to a relative thrombocytopenia and neutropenia. Although neutropenia from hypersplenism is less important clinically, thrombocytopenia may contribute to bleeding, if present. However, platelet transfusions are rarely necessary as part of the routine management of patients with portal hypertension.

In addition to severe cholestasis and portal hypertension, end-stage liver disease is characterized by worsening hepatic dysfunction, neuropsychiatric abnormalities, and electrolyte disturbances. The development of end-stage liver disease is frequently gradual rather than abrupt. However, the clinical condition of these patients is often quite tenuous, and they may become sick quite quickly. It is vital for the child's generalist physician and pediatric gastroenterologist to form a partnership, relying on good communication, to optimize care for these patients. The only therapeutic intervention available for end-stage liver disease is liver transplantation.

Worsening hepatic dysfunction is manifested by severe jaundice and coagulopathy not improved with vitamin K administration. Any historical symptoms suggestive of changes in mental status—(i.e., poor nutritional intake, irritability, lethargy) should be noted, and hepatic encephalopathy must be considered. Hepatic encephalopathy may occur with acute liver failure, and neuropsychiatric changes may occur with chronic liver disease. They may range from subtle behavioral changes to frank obtundation. Physical examination findings are usually significant for the stigmata of end-stage liver disease, including asterixis, ascites, and caput medusae. Unlike in adults, hepatic encephalopathy may be difficult to diagnose in young children.

Hyponatremia may be present, but because it is chronic, it should not be treated aggressively. An elevated serum creatinine may indicate renal insufficiency caused by the hepatorenal syndrome or as a complication of diuretic therapy. Cyanosis, clubbing of the extremities, and hypoxia are all of concern in the hepatopulmonary syndrome. The development of hepatorenal or hepatopulmonary syndrome is an ominous sign.

Any suspicion of cholangitis, spontaneous bacterial peritonitis, variceal hemorrhage, or hepatic encephalopathy should warrant emergent communication with the specialist.

MANAGEMENT

The generalist plays an integral role in managing patients with chronic liver disease. Frequently it is a child's pediatrician or family physician who must distinguish emergent, urgent, and nonurgent conditions and communicate the details to the tertiary center (Table 141-3).

The goals in managing any patient with chronic liver disease are fourfold: (1) identify life-threatening complications, (2) treat other complications, (3) help both the family and child cope with chronic illness, and (4) and manage the underlying hepatic disorder. Clearly the fourth goal is the responsibility of the pediatric gastroenterologist. The generalist and the gastroenterologist must work together on the first three goals to optimize management of these patients.

Life-threatening complications include gastrointestinal hemorrhage caused by varices, spontaneous bacterial peritonitis, and cholangitis. Gastrointestinal hemorrhage must be managed prudently and aggressively. The child's ability to maintain an airway should be addressed: if obtunded, he or she should be intubated and mechanically ventilated. Two intravenous catheters should be placed, and volume in the form of crystalloid and packed red blood cells should be administered to maintain systemic perfusion. Volume resuscitation must be performed with care because overzealous volume resuscitation may increase portal vein pressure, thereby increasing variceal bleeding. A nasogastric tube should be placed to assess rate of bleeding and minimize the risk of aspiration. Some centers rely on octreotide to attempt to pharmacologically control hemorrhage. This agent does not replace airway management, volume expansion, or nasogastric tube decompression. Finally, emergent (e.g., following initial stabilization) communication with and transport to a pediatric tertiary care center should be arranged for definitive care. Once hemodynamically stable, the child should undergo endoscopic therapy to control hemorrhage.

Spontaneous bacterial peritonitis (SBP) is infected ascites not caused by bowel perforation. A child with ascites and fever should be considered to have SBP until proved otherwise. Both blood and ascitic fluid should be obtained for cultures, and empiric antimicrobial therapy should be initiated. Although the most common bacterial agent isolated from children with SBP is *Streptococcus pneumoniae*, gram-negative enteric organisms may also cause SBP. Cholangitis also requires empiric antibiotic therapy and should be suspected in any child with biliary tract abnormalities (such as biliary atresia), fever, and worsening cholestasis. Suspected SBP and cholangitis should be treated

Table 141-3. Timing of Communication with Pediatric Gastroenterologist

Emergent (Immediately)
Gastrointestinal hemorrhage
Fever and worsening jaundice
Encephalopathy
Fever and ascites
Renal or pulmonary insufficiency

Nonemergent (within 24–48 Hours)
New-onset ascites without fever
Worsening jaundice
Malnutrition/failure to thrive
Easy bruising
Pruritus

964

as an emergency and comanaged with a pediatric gastroenterologist, for both have implications for long-term prognosis and liver transplantation.

Fat-soluble vitamin deficiency should be prevented by the administration of supplemental vitamins A, D, E, and K in the setting of cholestasis. Aggressive nutritional management, often with nasoenteral feedings, should be instituted. Pruritus may be managed primarily with antihistamines, although rifampin and ursodeoxycholic acid are helpful in some patients. Finally, chronic ascites is managed with a combination of diuretics and dietary salt restriction. Suspicion of malnutrition, fat-soluble vitamin deficiency, and pruritus may be communicated to a pediatric gastroenterologist on a nonurgent basis. All these therapies should be initiated in concert with a pediatric gastroenterologist.

OUTCOME AND FOLLOW-UP

The outcome of children with chronic liver disease is variable, and depends on the underlying liver disease, effectiveness of the therapeutic intervention, and the severity of complications. In adults, poor outcome depends on underlying liver disease, and the risk of death from end-stage liver disease increases with increasing serum bilirubin, serum creatinine, and prolongation of the prothrombin time. Although not well studied in children, these factors are likely to be similarly prognostic.

The outcome of children with biliary atresia has improved significantly since the development of the Kasai hepatoportoenterostomy and the success of liver transplantation. Without the Kasai procedure, biliary atresia is uniformly fatal. Of those undergoing the Kasai procedure, 35% to 45% will not require early transplantation. Notably, a successful Kasai procedure is related to early diagnosis of biliary atresia and the experience of the center performing the operation. The remaining children require liver transplantation. With both the Kasai and liver transplantation, the overall survival of children with biliary atresia is on the order of 80% to 90%.

Whatever the underlying etiology, good clinical care unquestionably improves the outcome and the quality of life of the child with chronic liver disease. An integral part of good clinical care is recognition of the complications of chronic liver disease, and prudent communication with specialists.

Mini-index of Related Topics

SUGGESTED READINGS

Balistreri WF: Liver disease in infancy and childhood. In Schiff ER, Sorrell MF, Maddrey WC, Schiff L (eds): Schiff's Diseases of the Liver, 8th ed. Philadelphia, Lippincott-Raven, 1999, pp 1357–1512.

Balistreri WF: Manifestations of liver disease. In Behrman RE, Kliegman R, Jenson HB (eds): Nelson Textbook of Pediatrics, 16th ed. Philadelphia, WB Saunders, 2000.

Balistreri WF: Pediatric hepatology: A half-century of progress. Clin Liver Dis 2000;4(1):191–210.

D'Agata ID, Balistreri WF: Evaluation of liver disease in the pediatric patient. Pediatr Rev 1999;20(11):376–390.

Rudolph JA, Balistreri WF: Optimal treatment of biliary atresia: "Halfway" there! Hepatology 1999;30(3):808–810.

142 Liver Transplant

Valeria Cohran and William F. Balistreri

ROLE OF THE GENERALIST

1 Recognize the complications of end-stage liver disease.
2 Know the indications for liver transplantation.
3 Know the different types of immunosuppression and possible drug interactions.
4 Recognize signs and symptoms of lymphoproliferative disease.
5 Recognize the long-term complications of liver transplant.
6 Provide primary, preventive, and acute care for patients with liver transplants.

Because patients with liver transplants are living longer and often reside a distance from the transplant center, the primary care provider plays an integral role in their health care. The primary care clinician managing these patients must recognize acute liver failure, initiate the evaluation, and know when to refer to a specialist.

FUNDAMENTALS

Orthotopic liver transplantation is a proven medical therapy for patients with end-stage liver disease caused by a wide variety of disorders (Box 142-1). In 1999, approximately 4500 liver transplants were performed in the United States; 6% were performed in children. However, 21,267 patients were registered for transplantation and 1756 patients died without receiving an organ. Advances in medicine have allowed these patients to live longer and be placed on the organ waiting list. Unfortunately, the supply of donor organs has remained constant while the number of patients awaiting transplant has increased.

The advent of living related donation has reduced the waiting time for some patients. In this procedure, a left

Box 142-1. Common Indications for Liver Transplant

- Biliary atresia
- Progressive familial intrahepatic cholestasis (PFIC)
- Alagille syndrome
- Metabolic disease (i.e., α_1-antitrypsin deficiency)
- Malignancy
- Drug-induced liver failure
- Acute liver failure

lateral segment of an adult liver of a first-degree relative, usually a parent, is transplanted to the patient. Because of the morbidity and mortality associated with this procedure, donors undergo stringent medical testing for unrecognized medical problems.

INDICATIONS

The most common indications for liver transplantation in children are biliary atresia, progressive familial intrahepatic cholestasis (PFIC), Alagille syndrome, metabolic disease such as α_1-antitrypsin deficiency, malignancy, drug-induced liver failure, and acute liver failure (see Box 142-1).

Biliary atresia, a progressive fibro-obliterative obstruction of the biliary tree, is the leading indication for pediatric liver transplantation. Despite the Kasai procedure that attempts to establish biliary drainage, approximately two thirds of patients progress to biliary cirrhosis with portal hypertension and require transplantation. Progressive familial intrahepatic cholestasis types I through III result from defects of bile acid synthesis or transport. This more recently recognized family of disorders can lead to progressive liver disease and eventual liver failure.

Alagille syndrome is a multisystem disorder characterized by complex cardiac disease, vertebral abnormalities (such as butterfly vertebrae), posterior embryotoxon, and liver disease. The progressive cholestasis can lead to intractable itching and portal hypertension. Although patients with this disorder have successfully undergone liver transplantation, the complex cardiac disease can prevent a successful transplant.

α_1-Antitrypsin deficiency is a metabolic liver disorder that can be treated with liver transplantation. This disorder is found in whites of Northern European ancestry. α_1-Antitrypsin deficiency is the most common metabolic disorder leading to liver transplantation in children.

Acetaminophen (APAP) is one of the most commonly encountered hepatotoxins. An overdose of APAP can induce liver failure that can require transplantation. Other drugs such as minocycline or methotrexate can also lead to significant liver dysfunction.

Two less common indications for transplantation are hepatoblastoma and hepatocellular carcinoma. Liver transplantation is performed when these tumors are nonresectable because of their location in the liver. The tumor mass is initially treated with chemotherapy. If there is no evidence of metastases and the tumor mass is stable or decreasing, the patient is eligible for transplantation.

Chemotherapy may be given after transplant if metastases are a concern.

CLINICAL PRESENTATION OF LIVER FAILURE

Acute liver failure can occur in previously healthy patients. The precipitant could be viral infections, drugs, metabolic liver disease, previously unrecognized liver disease, or idiopathic liver failure. A thorough history should be taken in the hopes of identifying a possible etiology. A family history of liver disease, psychiatric or autoimmune disorders, unexplained deaths or liver disease are important details to elicit. Any drug usage, including over-the-counter medicines and herbal supplements, must also be noted. For patients with multisystem disorders, such as seizures and muscle weakness, mitochondrial disorders should be included in the differential diagnosis. Wilson's disease should be considered in an adolescent with hemolysis and jaundice.

A physical examination is helpful in differentiating the patient who needs immediate referral to a tertiary center or who can be referred on a nonurgent basis (Table 142-1). Vital signs could reveal elevated temperature, tachycardia, or hypotension. Jaundice and scleral icterus are common physical examination findings. Lymphadenopathy can be seen, especially in an infectious process such as infectious mononucleosis or cytomegalovirus. Hepatomegaly, splenomegaly, or ascites can be found on abdominal examination. A firm liver edge is more indicative of chronic liver disease than acute liver disease. A thorough neurologic examination is also imperative. Encephalopathy is manifested as increasing lethargy, asterixis, unresponsiveness, or personality changes. Neurologic findings are very important indications of cerebral edema that can lead to coma and death. A skin exanthem could be indicative of a drug reaction or a viral illness.

Patients with chronic liver disease can have physical findings such as clubbing of the extremities, vascular spiders, caput medusa, and palmar erythema. Cutaneous xanthomas can be seen, especially in patients with Alagille syndrome. The liver edge may be firm or even hard. Splenomegaly is typically present in patients who have developed portal hypertension.

Laboratory data can determine the severity of liver dysfunction. Serum aminotransferase levels, alanine aminotransferase (ALT), and aspartate aminotransferase (AST) are useful to assess the degree of hepatocyte injury. Serum alkaline phosphatase and gamma glutamyltransferases (GGT) levels are often elevated in obstructive processes such as biliary atresia. A crucial test, which must be performed in patients with jaundice and suspected liver failure, is the prothrombin time (PT). The PT is an index of the synthetic function of the liver. If a patient has elevated serum aminotransferase levels and an elevated PT, consultation with a specialist is urgent. Elevated ammonia levels may be seen in patients with mental status changes. However, a patient's mental status may not directly correlate with the degree of hyperammonemia or encephalopathy. Factor VII is a clotting factor made in the liver that has a half-life of 6 to 8 hours, the shortest of all coagulation factors in the liver. A serum level under 10% indicates significant liver dysfunction.

Table 142-1. Indications for Urgent Referral to a Tertiary Care Center

Urgent Referrals to Pediatric Gastroenterologist

Symptoms	Diagnostic Evaluation
Bleeding in patient with end-stage liver disease	CBC, PT, PTT, and upper endoscopy
Conjugated hyperbilirubinemia in a neonate	Ultrasound, LFTs, PT, PTT
New-onset jaundice	Ultrasound, LFTs, PT, PTT, viral serologic tests
New-onset ascites	Ultrasound, LFTs, PT, PTT, peritoneal tap
Fever in patient with end-stage liver disease manifested by ascites	Peritoneal tap, ultrasound, LFTs, PT, PTT

Keys to an Essential History

Febrile illness
Drug usage including over-the-counter medicines
Family history of liver disease, autoimmune disease, unexplained deaths
Detailed past medical history including seizures and muscle weakness
Prenatal history in neonate

Immediate Consultation with Transplantation Center

Fever: elevated temperature >38.5°C for more than 24 hours without obvious explanation, abdominal pain, headaches, or seizures associated with fever
Medication: new prescriptions or over-the counter medicines being prescribed
Hypertension: newly elevated systolic or diastolic blood pressure >95th percentile for age
Neurologic: unusual headaches, seizures, visual disturbances
Respiratory: persistent cough, respiratory distress, abnormal chest x-ray
Gastrointestinal: diarrhea for more than 24 hours, vomiting for more than 12 hours; gastrointestinal bleeding, severe persistent pain
Liver: acute change in serum aminotransferases
Renal function: acute change in serum creatinine or electrolytes
Hematologic: persistent neutropenia, leukopenia, anemia, or leukocytosis
Surgery: before any elective surgery; as soon as possible or before emergency surgery
Other: when questions arise

CBC, complete blood count; LFTs, liver function tests; PT, prothrombin time; PTT, partial thromboplastin time.

An autoantibody panel evaluates possible autoimmune disease. A negative result does not eliminate autoimmune disease from the differential diagnosis. Autoimmune hepatitis can be seen with other disorders such as autoimmune hemolytic anemia or inflammatory bowel disease.

Electrolyte and glucose disturbances can be present with liver dysfunction. A glucose infusion rate of 6 mg/kg/min is usually adequate to maintain normal glucose levels in a patient with liver failure. Hypoglycemia is caused by lack of insulin degradation, inadequate glycogen stores, and inadequate gluconeogenesis. Hyponatremia is common, especially with ascites. The kidneys sense a relative vascular fluid depletion and conserve fluid leading to the hyponatremia. Renal insufficiency with oliguria or azotemia can also be present.

Liver biopsy, the next step in evaluation of a patient with liver disease, can be done by a percutaneous method using the Menghini needle or via a surgical procedure. If coagulopathy is present, a surgical liver biopsy is done to prevent uncontrolled bleeding, which may present later with the percutaneous method. An experienced pathologist should review the biopsy to aid with the diagnosis. If Wilson disease or mitochondrial disorders are suspected, specialized tests need to be done and coordinated with the pathologist prior to the biopsy. The goal of the evaluation is to find a cause of the liver failure.

Supportive therapies for liver failure include vitamin K, intravenous glucose and fluids, and oral lactulose. Bleeding can be treated with platelets or fresh frozen plasma. If the liver failure is drug-related, the offending agent must be withdrawn.

In those who do not recover hepatic function despite medical therapy, the decision must be made regarding whether the patient should be listed for liver transplantation.

EVALUATION FOR TRANSPLANTATION

If the patient's condition is reversible by transplantation, a series of laboratory and radiologic evaluations should be initiated to determine if the patient is a good surgical candidate for transplantation. The radiologic tests evaluate the patient's vascular anatomy. The vasculature of the native liver is defined using ultrasound or magnetic resonance imaging to help determine the technical approach to transplantation.

Multiple studies for viral infections including human immunodeficiency virus (HIV) should be obtained. A full assessment of the patient's nutritional, hematologic, and renal status must also be completed.

The surgical technique of liver transplantation is very intricate. The most delicate portion of the surgery is removal of the native liver. Portal hypertensive collaterals and adhesions require the surgeon to exercise extreme care. The rupture of the collaterals can lead to massive irreversible bleeding.

Once the native liver is removed, the vascular supply to the liver is occluded. After attaching the new liver to needed blood vessels, bile ducts are reconstructed, starting with a Roux-en-Y jejunal limb or end-to-side choledocho-jejunostomy. Each separate bile duct must be reimplanted into this Roux-en-Y loop for proper drainage. Transplantation is completed with closure of the abdomen, which can be delayed if increased abdominal pressure is a concern. Access to the intraperitoneal space is easier if a complication such as hepatic artery thrombosis occurs.

During the immediate postoperative period, fluid and electrolyte balance is monitored closely. Appropriate antibiotics and antiviral agents are administered. Immunosuppression is also initiated.

MANAGEMENT

Immunosuppressive therapy is the cornerstone of liver transplantation. Cyclosporine and tacrolimus are the main immunosuppressive agents used in liver transplantation. Both agents work by blocking the T-cell response that leads to T-cell proliferation.

Tacrolimus has become the primary immunosuppressant utilized in pediatric liver transplantation centers. It is also used in rescue therapy in unresponsive rejection in patients treated with cyclosporine. The liver metabolizes tacrolimus and cyclosporine almost entirely through the cytochrome p-450 system. As a result, both share a common drug interaction profile (Table 142-2). Nephrotoxicity is an important side effect of these drugs, so other nephrotoxic drugs, such as aminoglycosides and nonsteroidal anti-inflammatory drugs should be used sparingly. Renal tubular dysfunction can lead to hypomagnesemia, hyperkalemia, or mild acidosis. Treatment of electrolyte disturbances includes supplemental bicarbonate, magnesium, or reduction in potassium-sparing diuretics. Hypertension, alopecia, and headache are other known side effects. High serum levels of either agent have been associated with neurotoxicity such as seizures. Cardiomyopathy associated with tacrolimus is a rare side effect that can be resolved by using cyclosporine as the primary immunosuppressant.

Steroids such as Solu-Medrol or prednisone are another integral part of the immunosuppression regimen. Glucocorticoids inhibit the functions of leukocytes and macrophages, inhibiting their response to various antigens such as those of foreign tissue. In the immediate postoperative period, transplant patients receive large doses of steroids that are tapered over a 6- to 9-month period. Glucocorticoid usage has both long- and short-term sequelae. Hypertension is a common side effect and can be treated with diuretics and calcium-channel blockers. Insulin may be required to treat severe cases of hyperglycemia. Acne, cushingoid facies, and weight gain are other common side effects. These effects can be especially devastating to the adolescent patient and can lead to noncompliance. As the steroid doses are tapered, these side effects can resolve.

Table 142-2. Common Immunosuppressants

Drug	Mechanism	Side Effect
Cyclosporine (Neoral)	Inhibits T-cell synthesis of interleukins	Nephrotoxic, hyperglycemia, hyperlipidemia, excessive hair growth, posttransplant lymphoproliferative disease
Tacrolimus (Prograf)	Inhibits T cell synthesis of interleukins (10–100 times more potent than cyclosporine)	Nephrotoxic, hypertension, alopecia, headache, seizures, posttransplant lymphoproliferative disease
Glucocorticoids (steroids)	Inhibit cytokine production and chemotaxis	Hyperglycemia, hypertension, cushingoid facies, striae
Mycophenolate mofetil (CellCept)	Inhibits purine synthesis	Diarrhea
Rapamycin	Blocks the response of T cells to cytokines	Nephrotoxic, hyperlipidemia, hypertension

The complications from a liver transplant can be divided into immediate and long-term. Immediate complications include primary nonfunction of the graft, hepatic artery thrombosis, portal vein thrombosis, rejection, and infection. Primary nonfunction of the graft in which the new liver does not resume synthetic activity requires emergent retransplantation.

Vascular compromise of the hepatic artery, the main supply of blood to the transplanted liver, can lead to necrosis and failure of the graft. Thrombosis of this vessel can lead to hepatic necrosis and biliary strictures. Surgical thrombectomy or anticoagulant therapy reinstitutes adequate blood supply. Because of these potentially devastating consequences, daily Doppler ultrasound examinations are performed to assess vascular flow to the transplanted liver in the immediate postoperative period.

Rejection, an immune reaction to the presence of a foreign organ or tissue, can be acute or chronic. Acute rejection can present with symptoms of fever, abdominal pain, acholic stools, prolonged PT, jaundice, and elevated serum aminotransferase levels. A liver biopsy must be performed if there is any suspicion of rejection.

Acute rejection is defined as (1) portal tract inflammation with polymononuclear neutrophils, eosinophils, or lymphocytes, (2) bile duct inflammation, and (3) inflammation in the vasculature. Once rejection is diagnosed, patients are treated with a bolus of corticosteroids, and immunosuppressants are maintained at higher levels. In the rare patient who has steroid-resistant rejection OKT-3, a monoclonal antibody, is used. This antibody has been shown to be 90% successful in inducing remission. A liver biopsy may be repeated at any time during therapy to assess histologic response, especially if the serum aminotransferase levels are not declining.

Because of the degree of immunosuppression, infection can be a life-threatening complication of transplantation. Bacteria, yeast, and viral infections can cause significant morbidity and even death. Patients are at high risk for bacterial infections from central vascular access lines and peritoneal drains placed during or after transplantation. Dormant viral infections can become overwhelming from significant immunosuppression. Prophylactic antibiotics and antiviral agents are instrumental in postoperative care.

The viruses of the most concern are Epstein-Barr virus (EBV) and cytomegalovirus (CMV). A primary infection or reactivation of these viruses can present with fever, rash, or elevated serum aminotransaminases. Ganciclovir and acyclovir both inhibit EBV DNA replication. Unfortunately, neither of these drugs can affect B cells with latent infection. Protocol at one center requires that patients receive intravenous ganciclovir initially in the immediate post-operative phase. They are changed to oral acyclovir prior to discharge. Patients who are seronegative for CMV and EBV and who receive a seropositive organ are treated with a full 14-day course of intravenous ganciclovir and CytoGam, a gamma globulin product that contains high titer anti-CMV antibodies. These patients are at especially high risk for developing overwhelming viral infection.

Intravenous antibiotics, such as third-generation cephalosporins, are continued while the abdominal drains and central lines are in place. If the initial cultures are negative and all the drains and central lines have been removed, antibiotics are usually stopped within 3 to 4 days after transplantation.

Fluconazole and nystatin are used for antifungal prophylaxis. Because the normal gut flora contains yeast, patients who undergo multiple surgical interventions are at risk for invasive fungemia. After the immediate postoperative period, nystatin is initiated. Unlike fluconazole, nystatin does not interfere with tacrolimus levels.

Pneumocytis carinii is an opportunistic infection that can be seen in any immunocompromised patient. Bactrim is the prophylaxis of choice for this parasitic infection. Sulfa reactions including headaches, rashes, or bone marrow suppression are common side effects that require the use of aerosolized or intravenous pentamidine. Children younger than 3 years of age rarely tolerate aerosolized pentamidine and therefore receive intravenous drug. Dapsone is another less used prophylactic medicine. Both pentamidine and dapsone have been associated with pancreatitis.

Late complications from liver transplantation include acute and chronic rejection, biliary strictures, lymphoproliferative disease, and developmental delay.

Chronic rejection, which can occur at any time after transplantation, is characterized by decreasing bile ducts, worsening cholestasis, and inflammation in the arterioles. Unresolved acute rejection, elevation in serum GGT, jaundice, and increased alkaline phosphatase levels are warning signs. Chronic rejection is not responsive to steroid boluses and can lead to failure of the graft and retransplantation.

A different immunosuppressive medicine such as mycophenolate mofetil (CellCept) or rapamycin (Rapamune) is initiated when chronic rejection is suspected. CellCept is an antiproliferative agent, which works by inhibiting purine synthesis. A major side effect of this drug is diarrhea. Rapamycin, which is similar to tacrolimus, blocks the response of T cells to cytokines. Resistant chronic rejection has been a leading indication for this drug in the pediatric liver transplant population. Because rapamycin has been associated with hepatic artery thrombosis in adults, its use is becoming rarer.

Biliary duct strictures are common postoperative complications related to the technical difficulties associated with reduced size grafts and insufficient vascular flow. Because bile ducts receive their vascular supply from the hepatic artery, any reduction in hepatic artery flow can lead to a subsequent stricture. Bile leaks can also occur requiring drainage either by radiologic or surgical techniques. These collections are prone to infections from bacteria in the biliary tree.

Posttransplant lymphoproliferative disease (PTLD) results from a latent or new EBV infection resulting in an abnormal proliferation of B lymphocytes. This disease can be fatal. Table 142-3 lists presentations of PTLD. Common symptoms include elevated serum aminotransaminase levels, gastrointestinal blood loss, bone marrow suppression, and an abdominal mass. Bone marrow suppression can be significant, leading to anemia, neutropenia, and thrombocytopenia. Adenotonsillar enlargement is a more subtle

Table 142-3. Multiple Presentations of Posttransplant Lymphoproliferative Disease

Symptoms	Diagnostic Evaluation
Unexplained fevers	Cultures and viral serologic tests
Gastrointestinal bleeding	Immediate consult with transplant center, stabilize patient and transfer if needed to transplant center.
Easy bruising	CBC, PT, PTT, notify transplant center
Diarrhea	Stool studies for infection, notify center
Jaundice	LFTs, PT, PTT, ultrasound, notify transplant center
Lymphadenopathy, tonsillar enlargement	Viral serologic tests, notify transplant center

CBC, complete blood count; LFTs, liver function tests; PT, prothrombin time; PTT, partial thromboplastin time.

presentation of PTLD. Lymphoproliferative disease *must* be considered when a transplant recipient has new onset snoring or sudden enlargement of tonsils. Neurologic changes, such as severe headache or seizures, also suggest lymphoproliferative disease. If a head computed tomography scan reveals an intracranial mass, the patient should be thoroughly evaluated for evidence of malignancy and infection such as EBV.

Liver transplant recipients are at high risk for EBV infection because of the lack of prior exposure to EBV and the high degree of immunosuppression. Patients who are seronegative for EBV at the time of transplant undergo frequent monitoring for an EBV infection. Seropositivity does not indicate true disease.

When the patient begins to have concerning symptoms, a thorough evaluation should be initiated. Endoscopy is performed looking for gastrointestinal involvement, such as ulcers, and a full-body computed tomography scan is done to search for lymphadenopathy or masses. Initial therapy is reduction of immunosuppression. Tacrolimus levels are maintained between 4 and 8 ng/mL. Intravenous ganciclovir and CytoGam are the next therapy if there is no significant response. Frank masses often require surgical resection and chemotherapy. Central nervous system involvement may even require radiation therapy.

CHRONIC CONDITION COMANAGEMENT

As fewer centers perform liver transplantation, patients may travel further distances for this procedure. After the immediate postoperative period, the patients may be discharged within 3 to 4 weeks after transplantation. The generalist may be the first clinician to see these patients once they become ill. The transplant center and the primary care provider must maintain a strong working relationship in caring for these patients.

Like any other patient, immunizations are important and should be kept on schedule. Live virus immunizations are avoided in the transplant population. Fear of activating the virus in the patient is a major concern.

The primary care clinician should manage well-child care and ill visits. In treating bacterial infections, the treating clinician must remember that any medicine prescribed

for a transplant patient has the potential to interact with the immunosuppressive agents (see Table 142-2). Careful monitoring of immunosuppressant levels must be done in order not to precipitate an episode of rejection.

Education

Significant liver disease, especially during the first year of life, can lead to developmental delay. Patients may fail to attain various motor skills from a number of complications such as significant ascites, prolonged hospitalizations, and liver enlargement. After transplantation, the hope is that these patients will display catch-up and attain appropriate developmental milestones. However, some patients will not be successful. The primary care provider must monitor intellectual development. These patients may benefit from supportive programs with speech therapist, physical therapist, and occupational therapist. Referral to the appropriate educational specialist will maximize the patient's learning potential.

Psychosocial Factors

Patients, especially adolescents, who have often spent long periods of time in the hospital are at risk for depression. Noncompliance with immunosuppressive agents can lead to rejection and eventual failure of the graft, a major cause of rejection in the adolescent transplant patient. Recognizing the warning signs of depression (see Chapter 247) should alert caretakers that the patient should be referred to an appropriate mental health specialist. In the younger patient, it may be the caregiver who displays signs of depression or anger. The primary care physician should contact the transplant center if there is any suspicion of noncompliance by the caregiver or the patient.

Follow-up

Liver transplantation has prolonged the lives of thousands of pediatric patients. The transplant center and the primary care physician work as a team to manage the care of these special patients. The advent of living related donation and split liver donation has increased the number of pediatric liver transplants done each year. Early referral of patients with liver disease to a pediatric gastroenterologist should lengthen these patients' lives and hopefully delay the need for transplantation. By working with the primary care physicians, transplant centers around the country hope to enhance the quality of life for these patients.

Mini-index of Related Topics

SUGGESTED READINGS

Alonso MH, Ryckman FC: Current concepts in pediatric liver transplant. Semin Liver Dis 1998;18(3):295–307.
Arya G, Balisteri WF: Pediatric liver disease in the United States: Epidemiology and impact. J Gastroenterol Hepatol 2002; 17(5):521–525.

Bucuvalas JC, Ryckman FC: Long-term outcome after liver transplantation in children. Pediatr Transplant 2002;6(1):30–36.
McDiamid SV: Management of the pediatric liver transplant patient. Liver Transplant 2001;7(11 suppl 1):S77–S86.
Ryckman FC, Alonso MH: Causes and management of portal hypertension in the pediatric population. Clin Liver Dis 2001; 5(3):789–818.

SECTION 4 CHRONIC MEDICAL CARE: *Disorders of the Head and Neck*

143 Craniofacial Disorders

Carol D. Berkowitz

ROLE OF THE GENERALIST

1 Identify the different forms of cleft lip and palate.
2 Evaluate a child for the problems (ear infections, speech disorders, malocclusion) associated with cleft lip and palate.
3 Recognize the association between cleft lip/palate and different genetic syndromes.
4 Recognize microtia and know the appropriate management plan.
5 Diagnose craniosynostosis and implement an appropriate management plan.
6 Participate on a craniofacial team as a pediatric consultant.
7 Recognize the psychosocial issues related to craniofacial anomalies.
8 Refer to psychosocial services and parent support groups.

Craniofacial anomalies are frequent malformations that are often present at birth and easily identifiable on physical examination during the neonatal period. Other conditions such as craniosynostosis develop during the first few months of life either as a result of an intrinsic impairment of bony growth along the cranial sutures or as a result of environmental factors such as infant position in utero or after birth.

CLEFT LIP AND PALATE

Fundamentals

Clefts occur because of a defect in closure of the facial and palatal structures during embryogenesis. Facial development begins at 7 to 9 weeks postconception as mesodermal tissue moves from a lateral position to a more medial one.

Normally lateral and medial portions of the facial structures meet and fuse. Failure of this fusion results in cleft deformities. The lip and the palate form independently and are under different controls. The lip develops earlier than the palate, forming at about 7 weeks, while the palate develops at 9 weeks. The vast majority of clefts result from a failure of normal fusion, but occasionally a vascular "accident" may interrupt normal blood flow to the facial structures causing tissue necrosis. Sometimes other structures of the body are similarly affected. When portions of the extremities are affected, resulting in digital amputations, the syndrome is referred to as amniotic band syndrome.

The overall incidence of cleft lip with or without cleft palate is 1:600 to 1:1200. The incidence of clefts among whites is 1:600 to 1:700 and about 1:2000 in African Americans. Clefts of the lip with or without palatal clefts occur twice as frequently in boys as in girls. Isolated cleft palates are less common (1:2000 to 1:2500) and occur twice as frequently in girls as in boys. The overall recurrence risk for a second affected child is 4% to 7%. If one parent is affected with a cleft lip with or without a cleft palate, the risk of having an affected offspring is 3% to 4%. If the parent has an isolated cleft palate, the risk of having an affected offspring is 6% to 7%. Once a couple has an offspring with a cleft, the recurrence risk for another affected sibling is 9%.

Clefts may occur with about 250 genetic syndromes, but only 20% of children with clefts have a syndrome. The presence of a syndrome may affect the risk of recurrence. For instance, Van der Woude syndrome is inherited in an autosomal dominant manner. Affected individuals may have cleft lip with or without cleft palate, isolated cleft palate, or lip pits (Fig. 143-1). Cleft palate, micrognathia, and glossoptosis are components of Pierre Robin sequence. A proposed mechanism for this sequence is that cervical vertebral anomalies reduce the ability of the infant to extend his neck in utero. The head stays flexed, and the tongue protrudes through the unfused palate, preventing its closure. Growth of the mandible is inhibited and the base

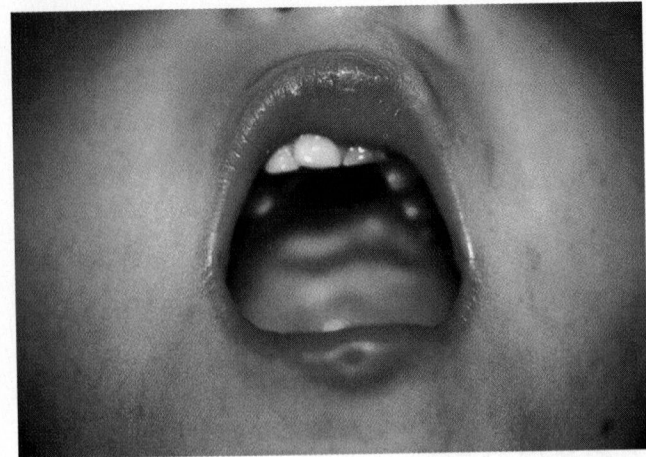

Figure 143-1. Lip pits in a child with van der Woude syndrome.

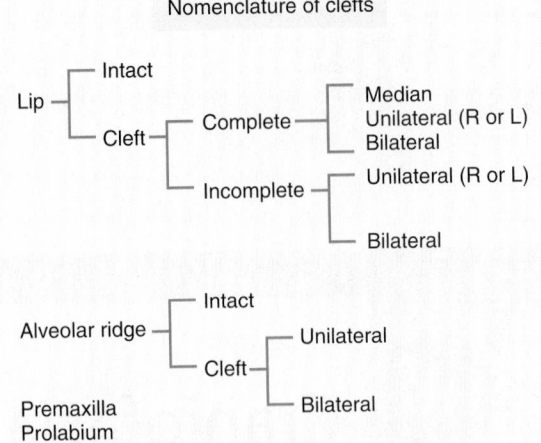

Nomenclature of clefts

Figure 143-2. Nomenclature of clefts.

of the tongue does not descend down the throat. Although various genetic factors may influence the occurrence of facial clefts, there appears to be a link between the presence of clefts and transforming growth factor alpha.

Because children with clefts may have other anomalies, detection of a cleft mandates a careful physical examination. Common anomalies associated with clefts may involve the face, skeleton, or heart (Box 143-1). Teratogens associated with clefts include hydantoin, alcohol, warfarin, trimethadone, thalidomide, and aminopterin.

Diagnosis

Most clefts are readily discernible on physical examination. The pediatric clinician should be facile at defining and describing the clefts (Fig. 143-2). Clefts may be restricted to the lip or the palate or may involve both structures. Clefts that are confined to the alveolar ridge are said to affect the primary palate, whereas those that affect the soft palate posterior to the incisor foramen affect the secondary palate. Clefts may be unilateral or bilateral. Midline clefts are rare and are usually associated with central nervous system anomalies such as holoprosencephaly and endocrine disturbances such as diabetes insipidus.

Clefts are classified as complete if they extend all the way through and into the nares, or incomplete if a band of tissue separates the nostril from the cleft (Fig. 143-3). Children with bilateral clefts have a midportion of the face that remains separated from the lateral portions. The prolabium is the midportion of the lip that contains the

Cupid's bow, the normal curved central portion of the lip. The premaxilla is the midportion of the alveolar ridge. The size of the premaxilla is determined by the number of tooth buds that it contains. There can be central as well as lateral incisors in the premaxilla. Sometimes there will be other facial anomalies such as lip pits, preauricular ear tags, or coloboma affecting the eyelids. The presence of other anomalies suggests the possibility of a genetic syndrome.

A submucous cleft involves the muscle layers below the mucous membrane of the soft palate. The physical examination may reveal the presence of a bifid uvula (Fig. 143-4).

Box 143-1. Anomalies Associated with Clefts	
Nasal glioma or meningoencephalocele	Aniridia
Persistent buccopharyneal membrane	Cleft larynx
Congenital neuroblastoma	Polydactyly
Congenital heart disease	Anencephaly
Thoracopagus twins	Foot deformities
Congenital oral teratoma	Oral duplication
Forearm bone aplasia	Spina bifida
Lateral proboscis	Aplasia of trochlea
Sacral agenesis	Laryngeal web

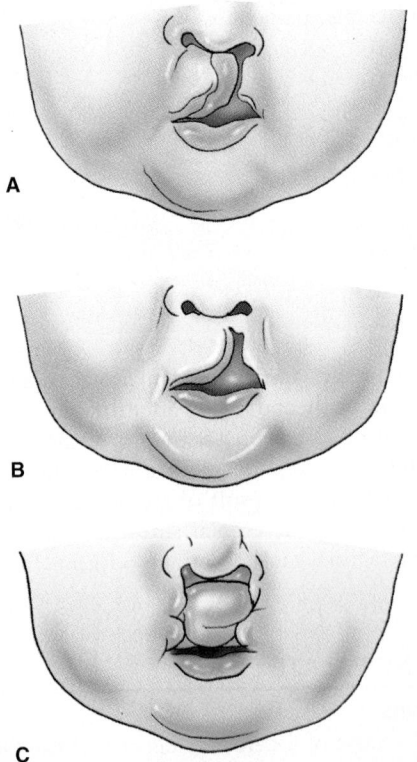

Figure 143-3. A–C, Clefts of the primary palate. (From Berkowitz CD (ed): Pediatrics: A Primary Care Approach, 2nd ed. Philadelphia, WB Saunders, 2000, p 208.)

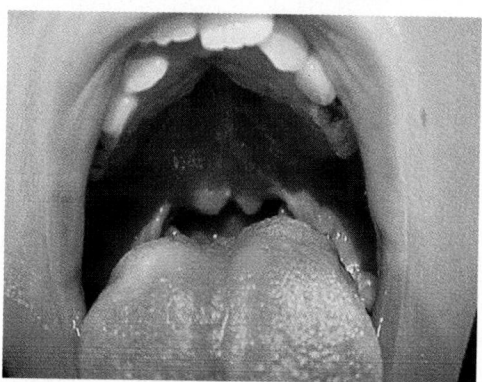

Figure 143-4. Bifid uvula.

Primary care providers must conduct a careful pharyngeal examination in the newborn nursery to make certain the uvula is singular and mobile. Infants with submucous clefts may experience nasal regurgitation. As they get older, they are at risk for recurrent ear infections and hypernasal speech, which may be exacerbated with adenoidectomy. Children with submucous clefts may have a bluish line through the length of the soft palate (zona pellucida) and a palpable notch at the junction on the hard and soft palates.

Primary care providers must be knowledgeable about other problems that children with clefts experience. Some children have difficulty feeding or gaining weight. Appropriate weight gain is important so that surgery can proceed in a timely manner. Children with clefts also may have recurrent bouts of otitis media, predisposing them to hearing impairment. Speech may be affected by hearing problems or articulation difficulties secondary to velopharyngeal incompetency or insufficiency or dental malocclusion. The child may have medical problems related to their other anomalies or medical conditions and may experience psychosocial problems particularly related to issues of self-esteem.

Management

Although surgery provides anatomic correction of the anomaly, medical management is crucial to ensure normal growth and development. Most children with cleft lip or palate are managed by craniofacial teams, which include reconstructive surgeons, pediatricians, otolaryngologists, speech pathologists, dentists, orthodontists, prosthodontists, social workers, and psychologists. The generalist needs to make an early referral to the craniofacial team, but must remain involved in the care of the affected infant and should provide primary care, health maintenance, and care for acute illness.

Management during the newborn period involves counseling the parents about the anomaly and referring them to appropriate parent support groups. Close follow-up of infant weight gain is very important. The generalist should be familiar with various bottles and nipples that help facilitate feeding. Infants should be fed orally if possible. Because sucking is important for normal development of the lip and jaw, nasogastric tubes should not be used unless the infant is neurodevelopmentally unable to suck. Infants with clefts are capable of breast-feeding. The breast may serve as an occlusive device to seal off the cleft. More often, however, women who wish to offer their infants breast milk

pump their breasts and give their milk to their infants in a bottle. Long black nipples, referred to as lamb's nipples, are no longer recommended. Soft nipples, such as those used to feed premature infants, are usually well tolerated. These nipples may be used in conjunction with flat compressible plastic bottles that can be squeezed during feeding to facilitate milk flow. Formula can be concentrated to 22 to 25 kcal per ounce.

The scheduling of surgery depends on the type of anomaly. For clefts involving the lip, the "rule of 10s" is followed. The first surgical procedure is scheduled when the infant is 10 weeks old, weighs 10 lb and has a hemoglobin concentration of at least 10 g/dL. Infants may require lip revisions over time, depending on the severity of the initial anomaly. For infants with bilateral complete clefts, application of a device to approximate the edges of the lateral aspects of the lips to the prolabium may be necessary. Infants are now referred for presurgical maxillary orthodontia. They are custom-fitted with nasal and alveolar molding plates, which are then worn prior to their surgical repair (Fig. 143-5).

The palate is usually repaired at around 12 to 18 months. Sometimes pressure equalization tubes (PETs) are inserted to reduce the frequency of otitis media and to address conductive hearing losses. Many children with cleft palates require speech therapy. Orthodontics may be begun even when the child has mixed dentition of primary and secondary teeth.

Support groups for parents are particularly helpful following the birth of an affected infant. Information about the availability of such groups locally can be obtained from the Foundation for Faces of Children (www.facesofchildren.org), the National Association for the Craniofacially Handicapped, or from the Cleft Palate–Craniofacial Association. Psychosocial support and coordination of community services is also needed. Parents may require help in accessing additional insurance for medical or surgical procedures, speech therapy, and orthodontia.

Outcome

In general, reconstructive surgery produces cosmetically aesthetic results involving the lip. Palatal repair diminishes or eliminates nasal regurgitation of liquids and may improve

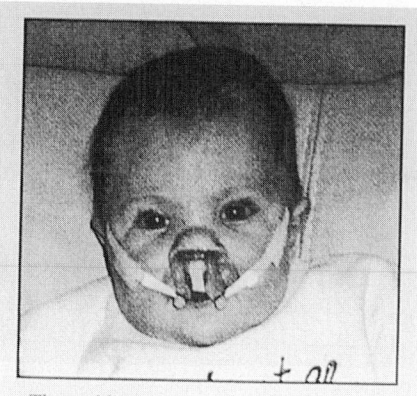

The molding plate reduces the severity of the cleft.

Figure 143-5. Infant with molding plate.

speech. Sometimes the palate functions inadequately following surgery (a condition referred to as velopharyngeal incompetence, or VPI) and additional procedures such as palatal lengthening may be necessary. Some children with VPI can be adequately managed with prosthetic devices such as speech bulbs (Figs. 143-6 and 143-7).

Because of the propensity to otitis media, children with clefts may develop conductive hearing losses. Episodes of otitis media should be treated appropriately. Some craniofacial teams routinely place PETs at the time of the initial lip repair.

Speech problems may persist despite anatomic correction. Some children require speech therapy through much of their school years. Many children can achieve a normal speech pattern when they are speaking slowly and carefully. Children with clefts may also experience persistent feelings of low self-esteem in spite of parental reassurance and counseling.

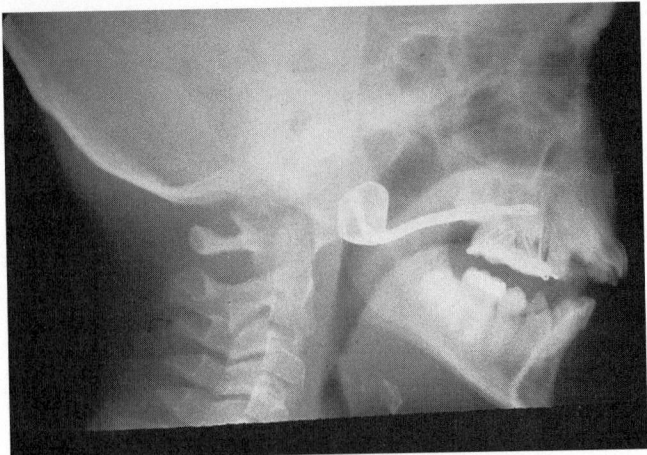

Figure 143-7. X-ray showing speech bulb in place.

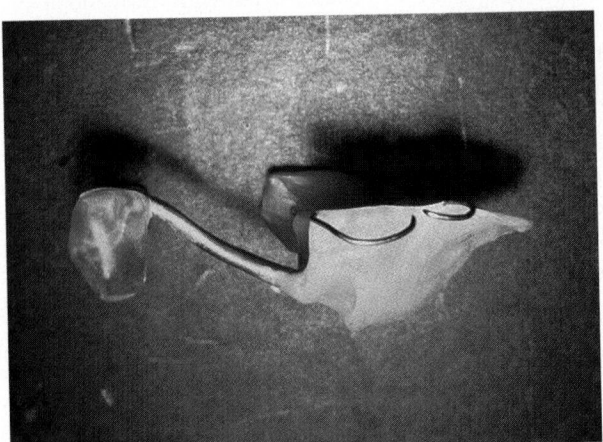

A

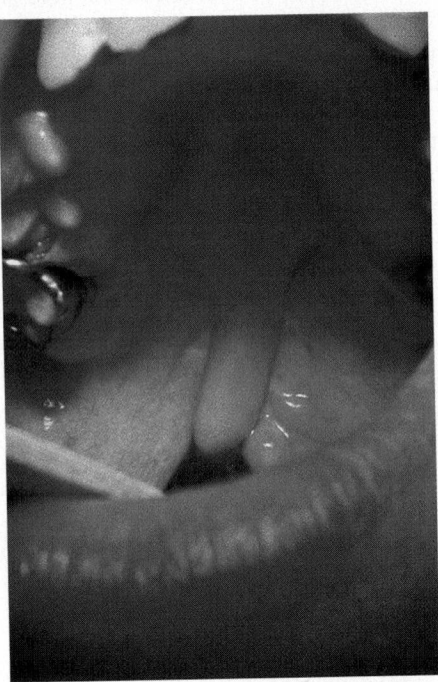

B

Figure 143-6. A, Speech bulbs used in the management of velopharyngeal incompetence. **B,** Speech bulb in place in patient.

Follow-up

Children with clefts require frequent follow-up visits during the initial months of life to ensure that they are gaining weight in an appropriate manner. As they get older, they need to be assessed for adequacy of speech and language development. During the school years, the child's self-esteem and academic progress must be monitored.

Surgical refinement of initial repairs is often necessary. Nasal reconstruction is carried out during adolescence to correct laterally slanted or downwardly displaced nasal tips. Once the adolescent has reached the reproductive years, genetic counseling about the chance of similar deformities in offspring should be addressed.

MICROTIA

Fundamentals

Microtia is maldevelopment of the auricle resulting in a small external ear with an atretic appearance, most often with an absent external auditory canal (Fig. 143-8). Cryptotia is a condition in which the auricle has an abnormal appearance with the helix folded over. Dystotia refers to abnormal placement of the ear on the cheek.

The external ear develops during the 12th week of gestation. Microtia results when a vascular accident occurs disrupting this development. The incidence of microtia is 1:6000 to 1:8000. Microtia may be seen in association with other syndromes, including Treacher Collins syndrome, an autosomal dominant condition with midfacial hypoplasia and an antimongoloid slant to the eyes, and Goldenhar syndrome. Other features of Goldenhar syndrome are hemifacial microsomia, epibulbar dermoids, hemivertebrae, micro-ophthalmia, renal anomalies, and cardiac anomalies.

Diagnosis

The diagnosis of microtitia is readily apparent on physical examination in the neonatal period. Most cases are unilateral and involve only one ear. The infant should be examined for the presence of other anomalies that suggest a genetic syndrome. Findings such as hemifacial microsomia may not be readily apparent in the newborn period. Although some recommend that infants with microtia

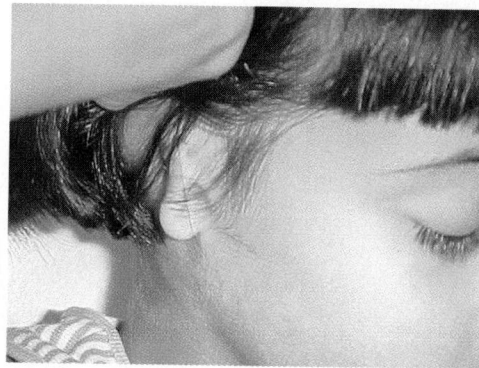

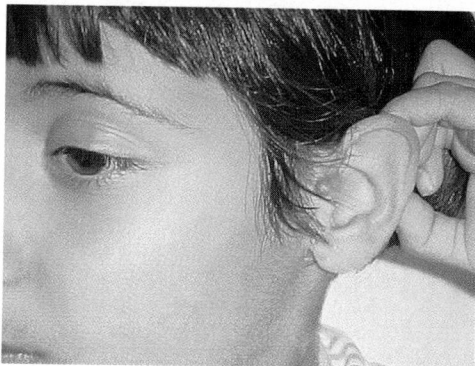

Figure 143-8. A, Abnormal ear: microtia. **B,** Normal ear of same child.

undergo a renal ultrasound to determine the status of the kidneys, the yield of routine evaluation is limited. Because the middle ear ossicles are usually malformed in children with microtia, computed tomography (CT) scan is recommended to evaluate middle ear structures.

Management

Children with microtia require baseline audiometric evaluation. Most children with isolated microtia should be referred to a craniofacial team for coordination of care. Surgical reconstruction is usually delayed till 5 years of age when the ear has reached 90% of its adult size. Repair before entry into kindergarten is recommended.

Children with microtia usually have normal hearing on the unaffected side, have normal speech development, and do not need hearing aids or speech therapy. In girls, the microtia may not be readily apparent because of the child's hairdo. In boys, coverage by the hair is not as easy during all fashion periods. Because children with microtia may suffer from problems of embarrassment and low self-esteem, the primary care clinician should question the child about friends and school.

Outcome

Cosmetically acceptable results are usually achieved with reconstructive surgery using either cartilage or a prosthesis. The helix of the ear is usually reconstructed sufficiently to allow for eyeglasses, if necessary, to be adequately balanced. Hearing on the affected side is not restored by the reconstruction of the external ear.

Follow-up

Pediatric follow-up is required for routine health maintenance, with emphasis on issues related to self-esteem. Follow-up by the craniofacial team will ensure that further reconstruction to achieve acceptable results is scheduled in a timely manner.

CRANIOSYNOSTOSIS

Fundamentals

Craniosynostosis refers to premature closure of the sutures of the skull, resulting in deformation of the head and the potential for impairment of growth of the brain. The incidence of craniosynostosis is 1:2000 to 1:3000. Its etiology is uncertain. Craniosynostosis can be seen in conjunction with genetic syndromes with other anomalies, such as polydactyly and syndactyly. True craniosynostosis involves bony fusion of the suture.

Sometimes a deformation appears that is related to positioning either in utero or after birth. In recent years, since the American Academy of Pediatrics "Back to Sleep" campaign, the incidence of positional plagiocephaly has increased. Positional plagiocephaly is not associated with premature closure of the sutures. Some infants with plagiocephaly have an associated torticollis secondary to a hematoma involving the sternocleidomastoid muscle. Treatment of children with positional plagiocephaly is different from those with closure of the sutures.

Craniosynostosis is categorized on the basis and extent of the suture involvement. When a single suture is involved, the condition is referred to as simple craniosynostosis. Compound craniosynostosis involves multiple sutures. Primary craniosynostosis occurs when the problem is related to the suture itself, and secondary craniosynostosis occurs when it is related to the growth of the brain.

Diagnosis

The diagnosis of craniosynostosis is suspected on physical examination (Fig. 143-9). The appearance of the skull suggests which sutures are involved. In cases of simple craniosynostosis, growth of the skull continues in a plane parallel to the affected suture. Isolated fusion of the sagittal suture results in scaphocephaly in which the head has an elongated, boat-like appearance. Brachycephaly, a shortened wide head, results from coronal suture synostosis. A triangular shape to the head occurs with premature closure of the metopic suture, the suture that extends from the nasal bridge to the anterior hairline. Plagiocephaly, flattening of the occipital area, can occur as a result of positioning as related to the "Back to Sleep" campaign, or torticollis, or may occur with early fusion of one or both lambdoidal sutures. Infants with positional plagiocephaly secondary to torticollis usually exhibit unilateral occipital flattening with contralateral malar flattening reflecting the fact that the infant holds the head preferentially toward one direction. Children should also be evaluated for strabismus, because ocular muscle paresis may be associated with head-tilt.

Sutures should be carefully palpated to determine if they appear to be overriding. The neck should also be palpated

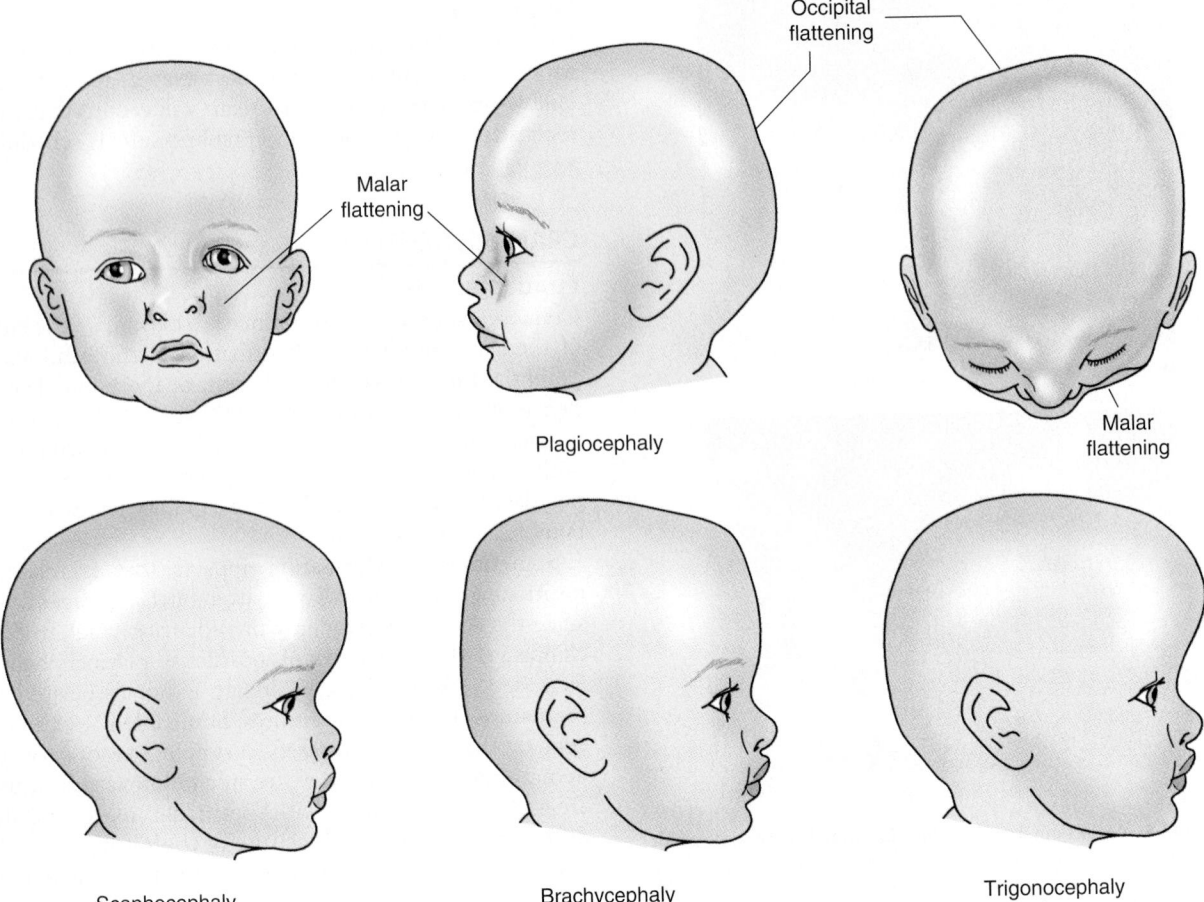

Malar flattening

Occipital flattening

Plagiocephaly

Malar flattening

Scaphocephaly

Brachycephaly

Trigonocephaly

Figure 143-9. Different types of craniosynostosis. (From Berkowitz CD (ed): Pediatrics: A Primary Care Approach, 2nd ed. Philadelphia, WB Saunders, 2000, p 210.)

for torticollis or an appreciable hematoma in the sternoclei-domastoid muscle. The child should also be carefully examined for other anomalies suggestive of a genetic syndrome.

Diagnostic studies include routine skull radiographs to assess the sutures, CT or magnetic resonance imaging (MRI) scan of the brain to determine if there are anomalies of the central nervous system, and three-dimensional CT scan of the skull. The latter imaging study accurately assesses whether the sutures are fused and helps differentiate positional deformities from those with premature fusion.

Children with suspected craniosynostosis should have their head circumference measured routinely and their development assessed to determine if both are progressing normally. Abnormal neurodevelopment suggests that the craniosynostosis might be secondary to an intrinsic brain problem and surgical correction would not be appropriate. A child whose development has been normal and who then seems to be deteriorating raises concern that the craniosynostosis may be having a negative effect on brain growth. Current studies suggest that brain growth may predispose to craniosynostosis but that the reverse, craniosynostosis, unless it involves all sutures, does not affect the ability of the brain to grow.

Management

Management depends on the diagnosis. In children with positional plagiocephaly related to torticollis, neck stretching exercises improve the tendency to place the head in the

same position. In addition, the infant can be placed in an infant seat rather than in a recumbent position. Bright, colored objects should be placed in the infant's crib on the side opposite to the infant's preferred direction of gaze to encourage the infant to hold his or her head in the opposite direction. Children with positional plagiocephaly may also be treated with a molding helmet referred to as a dynamic orthotic craniotomy device or DOC (Fig. 143-10). These helmets exert pressure on the skull thereby encouraging growth in all directions.

When craniosynostosis is due to premature fusion of the sutures, surgery may be indicated. The decision to proceed with surgery is complicated, and should be made by a craniofacial team. Factors that are considered include which suture(s) are involved, whether the facial features including the orbits and the eyes are affected, and the degree of the resulting deformity. Surgery is complicated, and usually involves the combined efforts of a reconstructive surgeon and a neurosurgeon.

Outcome

Positional plagiocephaly responds well to stretching exercises and DOC devices. Minor asymmetries may become less apparent as children grow older and their hair becomes more abundant. Surgery can produce dramatic improvement in the cranial abnormality. The unfused sutures must be kept apart to prevent refusion and the reappearance of the deformity.

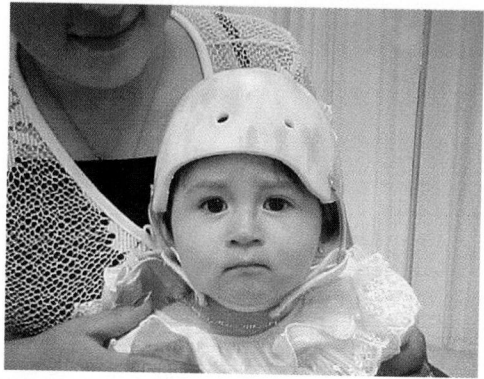

Figure 143-10. Child with a dynamic orthotic craniotomy device (DOC).

Follow-up

Infants with craniosynostosis should continue to have their head circumference assessed to be certain that growth is proceeding in a normal manner. Their development should also be monitored to ensure normal progress.

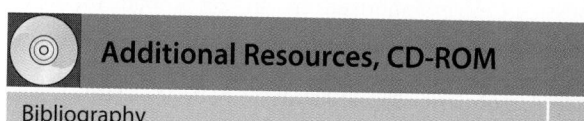

Additional Resources, CD-ROM

Bibliography	

SUGGESTED READINGS

Balasubrahmanyam G, Schere NJ, Martin JA, Michal ML: Cleft lip and palate: Keys to successful management. Contemp Pediatr 1998;15:133–153.

Bardach J, Morris HL: Multidisciplinary Management of Cleft Lip and Palate. Philadelphia, WB Saunders, 1990.

Keating RF: Craniosynostosis: Diagnosis and management in the new millennium. Pediatr Ann 1997;26:600-612.

Nagata S: A new method of total reconstruction of the auricle for microtia. Plast Reconstr Surg 1993;92:187–201.

Rohan AJ, Golombek SG, Rosenthal AD: Infants with misshapen skulls: When to worry. Contemp Pediatr 1999;16:47–70.

SECTION 4   CHRONIC MEDICAL CARE: *Disorders of the Head and Neck*

144 Care of the Blind Child

William Walker Motley III and Michael C. Struck

ROLE OF THE GENERALIST

1. Understand total blindness, legal blindness, partially sighted, and visual impairment.
2. Recognize common etiologies of infantile and acquired blindness.
3. Recognize the impact of blindness on child development.
4. Participate in a team approach for care of the blind child.

DEFINITION

Visual impairment is a condition in which an individual has less than normal vision with optimal optical correction. The level of impairment can vary with the diagnosis and severity of illness. Blindness is defined simply as the absence of sight. Total blindness exists when one is unable to perceive light with either eye. Legal blindness requires vision worse than 20/200 in the better eye, or a visual field of less than 20 degrees. Partially sighted refers to those individuals with vision better than 20/200, but worse than 20/70. Although 20/70 vision is the legal criterion in most states for assistance and disability, many children have functional visual impairments (i.e., nystagmus) that do not meet this criteria. Providers of health care for children must be familiar with educational options, community resources, and social networks available to their patients with visual impairment.

Epidemiologic studies of blindness and vision loss in childhood in the United States are limited. Studies in Europe and westernized countries estimate the prevalence of severe visual impairment at 1 to 4 per 10,000 children. The prevalence of partially sighted children is estimated to be 5 to 10 times this figure. The incidence of congenital blindness in Canada is reported as 3 per 10,000 live births.

FUNDAMENTALS

The treatment of vision loss in childhood involves preventing disease (e.g., rubella), management of established disease (e.g., retinopathy of prematurity) to prevent progression, and restoration of vision in those children already affected (e.g., congenital cataracts). Box 144-1 lists the avoidable and treatable causes of vision impairment.

Blindness may result from congenital or acquired disorders. Conditions causing visual impairment can be divided into those presenting in infancy and those affecting older children. Infants may have poor vision in both eyes secondary to abnormalities of the optical media (cornea, aqueous humor, lens, and vitreous humor), retina, optic nerve, or central nervous system. Systemic disorders such as metabolic diseases, congenital infections, and albinism may cause severe visual impairment by affecting various ocular structures. Table 144-1 lists many causes of infantile blindness.

DIAGNOSIS OF SPECIFIC CONDITIONS

Cataracts may cause blindness by obscuring the optical image, which over time results in deprivation amblyopia. A cataract is an opacity of the crystalline lens, which may occur in as many as 1 in 10,000 infants. Although early surgical intervention for bilateral cataracts often results in very good visual acuity, 14% to 25% of patients may be legally blind after bilateral cataract treatment. Patients may present with leukocoria, strabismus, or nystagmus. The primary care provider may detect even small lens opacities by ophthalmoscopic examination of the red reflex. Prompt referral to an ophthalmologist is essential. Surgical treatment may be indicated within days of diagnosis.

Leber congenital amaurosis (LCA) is a bilateral retinal dystrophy responsible for approximately 10% of congenital blindness. LCA is inherited in an autosomal recessive pattern. Severe visual impairment is present at birth but may not be detected until 2 to 3 months of age, when nystagmus is noticed. Visual acuity in patients with LCA is usually 20/200 or worse but tends to remain stable over time. The patient with LCA may demonstrate a positive oculodigital sign of Franceschetti whereby visual pathways are stimulated by pushing or rubbing the eyes with a finger or fist. The pupils are poorly reactive to light and paradoxical pupillary constriction may occur in the dark. The fundus examination may appear normal or may reveal diffuse retinal pigmentary changes. Optic atrophy may be present. LCA is associated with polycystic kidney disease, osteoporosis, kyphoscoliosis, cleft palate, seizures, mental retardation, and hydrocephalus.

Achromatopsia (rod monochromism) is a bilateral congenital disorder whereby retinal tissue contains essentially no cone photoreceptors. Inheritance of the condition occurs in an autosomal recessive pattern. The lack of cone photoreceptors usually results in visual acuity of approximately 20/200. The patient has true color blindness in that all colors are seen as shades of gray. Patients prefer dim lighting, which affords more functional vision by rod photoreceptors.

Congenital stationary night blindness (CSNB) is a bilateral retinal disorder with multiple inheritance patterns. The patient with autosomal recessive or X-linked CSNB may present early in infancy with nystagmus and a normal funduscopic examination. Visual acuity is in the range of 20/200 with poor dark adaptation in autosomal recessive and X-linked forms of CSNB. Visual function is usually stable over time.

Retinopathy of prematurity (ROP) occurs when a child is born before development of the retinal vasculature is complete. In premature infants the posterior retina may be vascularized while the peripheral retina is avascular. Growth of fine, weak blood vessels at the junction of the vascular and avascular retina is called neovascularization. The abnormal vessels from neovascularization may extend from the retina into the vitreous and produce traction on

Table 144-1. Causes of Infantile Bilateral Blindness

Cause of Blindness	Diseases
Corneal opacity	Sclerocornea
	Congenital hereditary stromal dystrophy
	Congenital hereditary endothelial dystrophy
	Infectious corneal ulcer
	Trauma
Anterior segment dysgenesis	Axenfeld-Reiger syndrome
	Peter anomaly
Cataract	
Norrie disease	
Retinopathy	Leber congenital amaurosis
	Achromatopsia (rod monochromism)
	Congenital stationary night blindness
	Retinopathy of prematurity
	Retinoschisis
	Coloboma
Optic neuropathy	Opic nerve hypoplasia
	Optic atrophy
	Coloboma
Central nervous system	Cortical visual impairment
	Delayed visual development
Congenital infection/TORCH* syndrome	
Albinism	

*TORCH describes a group of infections: toxoplasmosis, other agents, rubella, cytomegalovirus, herpes simplex.

the retina, retinal detachment, and severe loss of vision during infancy or childhood.

Some degree of ROP occurs in about 50% of infants with birth weight 1000 to 1250 g, about 75% of those 750 to 999 g, and 90% of those weighing less than 750 g. Treatment of patients at the time of significant neovascularization includes laser photocoagulation or cryotherapy of the avascular retina. A scleral buckling procedure or vitrectomy may be required for retinal detachment.

Visual function may be severely impaired by congenital infections including toxoplasmosis, rubella, cytomegalovirus, herpes simplex, and syphilis. Toxoplasmosis causes a focal necrotizing retinochoroiditis. Approximately 68% of infected newborns develop bilateral atrophic scars of the macula. Infants with congenital rubella commonly have bilateral cataracts and may have microphthalmia (small disorganized eye). Cytomegalovirus causes retinochoroiditis in 15% of infants with systemic symptoms. Neonatal herpes may cause conjunctivitis, keratitis (corneal lesions), retinochoroiditis, and cataracts. Typical ocular manifestations of syphilis are keratitis, choroiditis, and cataract.

In optic nerve hypoplasia development of the nerve tissue is interrupted prior to the 13th week of gestation. The optic nerve appears small and vision may be severely impaired. Bilateral optic nerve hypoplasia may be accompanied by nystagmus. A magnetic resonance imaging (MRI) scan of the brain is recommended for patients with bilateral optic nerve hypoplasia to investigate for midline defects. Bilateral optic nerve hypoplasia associated with absent septum pellucidum and pituitary dwarfism is known as the de Morsier syndrome. An endocrine evaluation is indicated for patients with an absent septum pellucidum.

Other congenital optic nerve anomalies include optic nerve coloboma and morning glory disk anomaly. Both conditions may result in severe bilateral visual impairment. Optic nerve coloboma results from incomplete closure of the embryonic fissure and may be part of a CHARGE syndrome (coloboma, heart disease, choanal atresia, growth retardation, genital hypoplasia, and ear or hearing disorders). The etiology of morning glory disk anomaly is unknown. Basal encephalocele has been associated with morning glory disk anomaly.

Optic atrophy is a disorder in which the optic disk appears pale with a normal diameter. Optic atrophy results from an insult to the anterior visual pathway and subsequent loss of the axons that normally pass through the optic disk. Atrophy of the optic nerve may result in mild to severe vision loss in one or both eyes. Bilateral optic atrophy present before 2 years of age may cause nystagmus. Atrophy may be congenital or acquired and causes include intracranial tumors, previous episode of meningitis or optic neuritis, hereditary disorder, hydrocephalus, perinatal hypoxia, and porencephaly.

Cortical visual impairment results from an insult to the optic radiations or the occipital cortex. Vision loss may be severe, but total blindness is uncommon. Cortical visual impairment in infants may be due to perinatal or postnatal hypoxia, intracranial hemorrhage, cerebral dysgenesis, trauma, hydrocephalus, intrauterine infection, encephalitis, meningitis, and metabolic disorders. Cortical visual impairment is rarely present without other systemic or neurologic

abnormality. Examination usually reveals normal ocular structures but optic atrophy may be present. Improvement in vision over time is variable.

Delayed visual maturation (DVM) is diagnosed when an infant with a lack of age-appropriate visual function and normal ophthalmic and neurologic examinations subsequently develops improved vision over time. Infants with DVM are sometimes initially thought to have cortical visual impairment but neuroimaging studies reveal no cerebral abnormality. Children with delayed visual maturation tend to have global developmental or speech/language delay.

Congenital nystagmus is typically noted by 3 months of age. Congenital motor nystagmus is one type of congenital nystagmus in which visual acuity may be relatively good. Sensory nystagmus may have poor visual prognosis when associated with Leber congenital amaurosis, achromatopsia, blue cone monochromatism, congenital stationary night blindness, optic atrophy, optic nerve hypoplasia, albinism, and deprivation amblyopia.

Albinism is a group of disorders in which melanin is reduced solely in the eye (ocular albinism) or in association with pigmentary defects of the skin and hair (oculocutaneous albinism). Albinism is inherited in an autosomal recessive or X-linked recessive pattern. Infants may present with nystagmus at 2 to 3 months of age. Visual acuity ranges from 20/40 to 20/400 and tends to be worse in patients with less pigmentation. On examination the iris appears light blue. Owing to decreased pigmentation, a pink light reflex may be transmitted through the iris when examined with an ophthalmoscope. Decreased pigmentation of the fundus and prominent choroidal vessels are present on funduscopic examination. Hermansky-Pudlak and Chediak-Higashi syndromes result in albinism as well as life-threatening platelet bleeding disorder and recurrent infections.

ACQUIRED VISUAL IMPAIRMENT IN CHILDHOOD

Children may become visually impaired later in childhood as a result of progression of congenital disorders or new onset of acquired diseases. Box 144-2 lists diseases that typically cause vision loss acquired after infancy.

Box 144-2. Causes of Childhood Bilateral Blindness

Stevens-Johnson syndrome
Meesman corneal dystrophy
Cataract
Glaucoma
Retinitis pigmentosa
Juvenile macular degeneration (Stargardt disease, fundus flavimaculatus)
Dominant optic atrophy
Leber optic neuropathy
Tumors
   Intracranial
   Orbital
   Intraocular
Trauma (globe, optic nerve, central nervous system)
Metabolic diseases

Table 144-2. Metabolic Diseases as Causes of Childhood Bilateral Blindness

Disorder	Cause of Blindness
Cystinosis	Corneal opacities
Hyperornithemia	Atrophy of choroid and retina
Galactosemia	Cataract
Abetalipoproteinemia	Retinal degeneration, neurologic
Lecithin-cholesterol acyltransferase deficiency	Corneal opacities
Subacute GM₂ Gangliosidosis	Retinal degeneration, optic atrophy
Neiman-Pick disease	Optic atrophy
Hurler syndrome	Corneal opacities, glaucoma, retinal degeneration
Hunter syndrome	Corneal opacities, retinal pigment degeneration
Adrenoleukodystrophy	Optic atrophy
Refsum disease	Retinitis pigmentosa, cataract

Glaucoma is a progressive optic neuropathy associated with increased intraocular pressure. Patients with glaucoma may present within the first year of life with cloudy cornea, enlarged corneal diameter, tearing, or photophobia. Older children and adolescents tend to present with vision loss. Uncontrolled glaucoma may result in severe constriction of the visual field or total blindness. Progressive enlargement of the optic cup is typical of uncontrolled glaucoma. Glaucoma diagnosed in infancy is usually treated surgically. In older children, surgery is often reserved for cases that are refractory to medical management.

Dominant optic atrophy is an autosomal dominant bilateral deterioration of the optic nerves. Onset typically occurs at approximately 10 years of age and may cause severe bilateral loss of visual acuity and peripheral visual fields. Leber optic neuropathy is a bilateral disease of the optic nerves, usually with onset during the second to fourth decades of life. Male-to-female ratio is 9:1. Visual acuity may decrease to 20/200 or worse bilaterally.

A variety of systemic metabolic diseases may affect the eyes bilaterally, resulting in vision impairment. Table 144-2 lists metabolic diseases and associated ocular manifestations that tend to cause vision loss after infancy.

DEVELOPMENT IN VISUALLY IMPAIRED CHILDREN

Sighted and visually impaired children have basic developmental differences. A sighted child receives a continuous stream of visual information that allows organization of space, facilitates mobility, provides feedback while performing motor tasks, and fosters interaction with people and objects in his or her environment. Visual impairment deprives the child of visual information, which in turn stifles incidental learning such as observational learning, reinforcement, and instantaneous reproduction. The developmental delay of the visually impaired child depends on severity of blindness, cause of vision loss, age at onset of impairment, and confounding conditions such as mental retardation, deafness, seizures, and cerebral palsy. Generalizations about development of otherwise healthy children with congenital visual impairment may not apply to development of children with acquired blindness and neurologic disorders.

This discussion is limited to otherwise healthy children with infantile blindness.

Elements of childhood development include motor/locomotor, sensory (tactile, auditory), language/cognitive, social, and personality development. Blind children tend to have delays in motor development including reaching, crawling, and walking. Reaching to a sound stimulus may occur at 8 to 12 months, crawling at almost 1 year of life, and unassisted walking at 18 to 24 months. Visual perception of objects and people stimulates a child to move. Conversely, a lack of visual stimulation reduces a child's motivation to move. Motor development is also restricted by an inability to see and imitate the movements of others. Fluent movement development may be delayed by the lack of visual feedback.

A visually impaired child's perception of his or her environment is dependent on sensory development involving tactile, auditory, and residual visual function. Development of tactile function is not strikingly different between blind children and sighted children. Auditory milestones reported for blind infants are smiling at a parent's voice at 3 to 5 months of life and an adverse response to a stranger's voice at 8 months. At 14 months the blind infant may be able to track and find an object dragged across a rug. Visually impaired children can be trained to use their residual vision more effectively than they would spontaneously.

Cognitive development in blind children is slower than in sighted children in part because of exposure to less information (e.g., visual information) about the world. Blind children often must experience the environment through verbal descriptions. The cognitive milestone of searching for hidden objects is delayed in blind children, often until after 3 years of age, compared to 9 months for sighted children. Limited locomotor activity of blind children limits exposure to environment. Language development, including babbling, production of words, and development of grammar and vocabulary, is similar between blind and sighted children. Social development of blind children is delayed in the areas of attachment, identification, eating, toilet training, and dressing.

Four types of parental attitudes toward blindness have been described: fear, guilt, disgrace, and punishment. Modes of parental adjustment include acceptance, denial, overprotection, and rejection of the child. Parents experiencing guilt and frustration may withdraw from the infant and reduce nonvisual stimulation. Tactile communication such as holding and cuddling is often decreased between the blind child and caregiver. A blind child's requests for attention from parents are ignored more often than those of a sighted child. If parents frequently ignore the child's requests for attention, the blind child may develop a sense of inability to control his or her environment, which in turn leads to a withdrawal. Parents who engage in overprotective behavior may limit the child's development of independence and access to his or her environment. Parents may experience depression and may require counseling.

MANAGEMENT

The generalist should engage a team approach for care of the blind child. Care providers include parent, primary care provider, ophthalmologist, orientation and mobility (O/M)

specialist, teacher of the visually impaired (TVI), physical/occupational therapist (PT/OT), and speech therapist. Evaluation by an ophthalmologist is indicated for infants and children with suspected vision loss. A visually impaired infant or child should be evaluated by a local agency for the visually impaired if available. Early intervention programs are important in training parents and children to facilitate development. Parents are important teachers and may impact a blind child's development by providing nonvisual sensory stimulation, physical exercises, and positioning. Parents can provide tactile, auditory, and kinesthetic activities while feeding, cuddling, and playing games. O/M specialists train visually impaired children to move safely in their environments using auditory, olfactory, and tactile clues. O/M specialists may recommend modification of the home and school to facilitate mobility. A TVI may be the

child's primary teacher or a consultant working with a regular or special education teacher. A PT or OT specialist may be consulted for evaluation and treatment of gross motor, fine motor, and sensory integration skills. A speech therapist can evaluate the child's speech and language skills and recommend appropriate learning activities.

The following are some practical suggestions to keep in mind when working with a visually impaired infants and children. Speak softly to the infant before touching or examining to allow him or her to associate voice with change. The infant has no visual warning of physical contact and therefore should be touched gently. Look for verbal or physical signs of responsiveness rather than eye contact. Address older children by name when entering the room and every time a response or an answer to a question is desired. Give verbal explanations before and during examination procedures and allow the child to touch instruments when possible. See Box 144-3 for resources that may be helpful to blind children, parents, and physicians.

Box 144-3. Some Helpful Resources for Blind Children, Parents, and Physicians

American Foundation for the Blind

11 Penn Plaza, Suite 300
New York, NY 10001
(800) 232-5463
www.afb.org

American Printing House for the Blind, Inc.

P.O. Box 6085
Louisville, KY 40206-0085
(800) 223-1839
http://aph.org/

Blind Children's Center

4120 Marathon Street
Los Angeles, CA 90029-3584
(800) 222-3566
www.blindchildrenscenter.org

National Association for Parents of Children with Visual Impairments

P.O. Box 317
Watertown, MA 02471
(800) 562-6265
www.spedex.com/NAPVI/

National Federation of the Blind/National Organization of Parents of Blind Children

1800 Johnson Street
Baltimore, MD 21230
(410) 659-9314
www.nfb.org

Additional Resources, CD-ROM

Bibliography

Mini-index of Related Topics

	CH.
DISORDERS OF THE EYE	62
APPROACH TO THE CHILD WITH VISUAL IMPAIRMENT	68
THE PRIMARY CARE MEDICAL HOME FOR CHILDREN WITH SPECIAL HEALTH CARE NEEDS	124
CONGENITAL DISORDERS OF THE CENTRAL NERVOUS SYSTEM	176
INFECTIOUS DISEASES IN THE NEONATE	209
SPECIAL EDUCATION	306

SUGGESTED READINGS

Robers M: First Steps: A Handbook for Teaching Young Children Who Are Visually Impaired. Los Angeles, Blind Children's Center, 1993.

Teplin SW: Visual impairment in infants and young children. Inf Young Children 1995;8(1):18–51.

Warren DH: Blindness and Early Childhood Development. New York, American Foundation for the Blind, 1977.

145 Care of the Deaf Child

Steven Barnett, Lilah M. Katcher, and Murray L. Katcher

ROLE OF THE GENERALIST

1   Recognize the impact of hearing loss on a child's and family's life.

2   Recognize that hearing loss has a context and meaning that varies with each child and family, and their meaning may differ from that of the clinician.

3   Recognize the social implications of medical interventions.

4   Appreciate similarities and differences in family issues with deaf children and hard-of-hearing children.

5   Recognize the impact of delayed language exposure on language development.

6   Assist families to maximize their children's access to language and information.

7   Provide appropriate information and support for families with deaf children so they can make the best decisions.

8   Recognize the barriers to communication between clinicians and deaf children and adolescents.

9   Overcome barriers to communication through collaboration with the deaf child and the family.

DEFINITIONS

The word "deaf" has various meanings, some involving different aspects of hearing level, speech discrimination, speech skills, language preference, and cultural affiliation. For the purpose of clarity and consistency in this chapter, "deaf" refers to hearing loss that profoundly limits the ability to hear and understand speech, even with amplification. This is a functional rather than an audiometric definition. Two children with very similar audiograms may have very different functional outcomes. The reasons for these differences are often unclear.

People who are "hard of hearing" are defined here as those with hearing loss who are able to get some linguistically useful information from sound, with or without amplification. Although some of the information in this chapter will be helpful for clinicians working with families with a hard-of-hearing child, the chapter's focus is on working with children with more severe hearing loss.

FUNDAMENTALS

Congenital deafness occurs in approximately 1 per 1000 births. Of adults deafened in childhood, 40% became deaf prelingually (before age 3 years). Some estimate that 50% of cases of childhood deafness have a hereditary component. Despite this, 90% of deaf children have two normally hearing parents.

Childhood deafness is not associated with increased mortality or biomedical morbidity rates, but there are social morbidities: adults deafened as children have less education and lower income on average than adults in the general population. Adults deafened in childhood are also less likely to go to the doctor than adults in the general population and may have limited health-related knowledge. They also report more communication difficulties with their doctors than non-English–speaking immigrants to the United States. The median reading level of deaf high school graduates in the United States is between grades four and five. Clinicians working with families with deaf children should focus on diminishing these negative social consequences.

Physiology of Hearing

Hearing is the translation of sound waves into electrical messages that the brain can interpret. Sound waves are funneled by the external ear into the external auditory canal (Fig. 145-1). The sound waves vibrate the tympanic membrane, causing the ossicles of the middle ear to move. The stapes presses on the oval window of the cochlea, causing vibration in the fluid of the inner ear. The cochlea is lined with rows of hair cells, and vibrations in the fluid in the cochlea cause the hair cells to bend, stimulating firing of the fibers of the eighth cranial nerve. Neurons transmit sound information from the cochlea to the auditory cortex along the auditory pathway. Information about sound pitch and loudness comes directly from the cochlea, while sound location is processed in the central nervous system by comparing information from each cochlea. Sensorineural hearing loss is caused by factors in the inner ear or central nervous system. Conductive hearing loss is caused by factors affecting the outer or middle ear.

Sound and Speech

Hearing ability is mapped on an audiogram (Fig. 145-2). The vertical axis represents hearing level (loudness) in decibels and the horizontal axis is sound frequency (pitch)

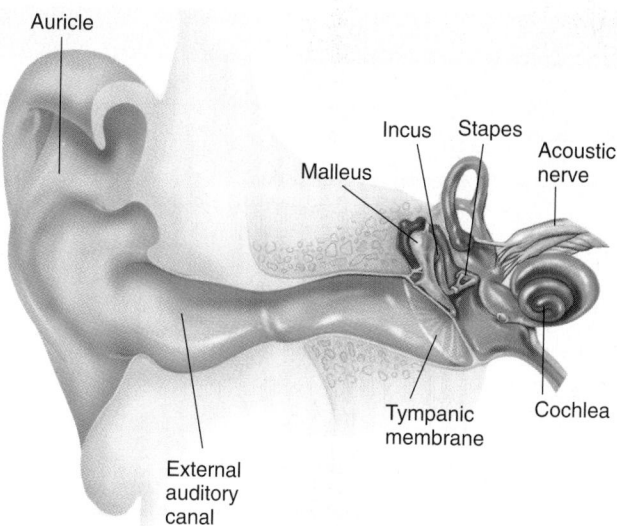

Figure 145-1. Anatomy of the auditory system.

measured in hertz. Speech sounds fall into an area of the audiogram called the "speech spectrum" or "speech banana." Children's access to spoken language can be partially estimated based on where the map of their hearing ability falls in relation to the speech spectrum. It is unlikely that a child will be able to hear speech sounds that are "above" the graph of his hearing level (i.e., have a lower absolute decibel level). Showing parents the speech spectrum and their child's audiogram may help them to better understand why their child reacts to some sounds but not others.

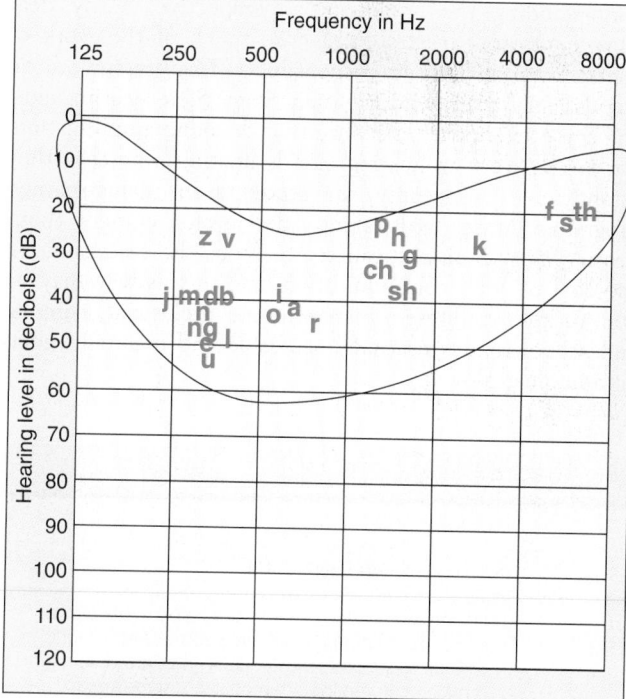

Figure 145-2. Audiogram with speech spectrum. The banana-shaped area (speech spectrum) delineates the frequency and loudness of normal conversational speech.

Language Acquisition

Language acquisition is easiest when a child is exposed to language at a young age (see Chapter 5, which discusses normal development). Both age at onset and age at diagnosis of deafness are important factors in the language development of a deaf child. Earlier diagnosis can alert families that they need to visually augment communication to help their deaf child develop language. Only 30% of English sounds are visible on the lips, so speech reading alone is probably insufficient language exposure for a deaf child. Children reared in homes with American Sign Language (ASL) can achieve normal language developmental milestones.

DIAGNOSIS

The mean age at diagnosis of congenital hearing loss of moderate to profound intensity in the United States has been 30 months. Risk factors (Box 145-1) are present in approximately half of children with congenital hearing loss. Table 145-1 describes hearing tests for children. All children with a risk factor should have their hearing tested. Identifying children with hearing loss who have no risk factors is more challenging. Universal newborn hearing screening has not been adequately studied to demonstrate effects on long-term outcomes, although it is supported by some professional organizations and legally mandated in many states. Clinicians need to be vigilant for signs of hearing loss, including loss of babbling, speech and language delay, and parental concern about hearing. Because it is difficult to predict which children will benefit from amplification, even children with a profound hearing loss warrant a trial with hearing aids.

MANAGEMENT

Supporting the Family

After the diagnosis of deafness in their child, parents may need to mourn and clinicians should be supportive. Early on, parents often feel they have insufficient information with which to process the diagnosis and make family

---

Box 145-1. Risk Indicators for Hearing Loss, Birth Through Age 2 Years

- Parental or caregiver concern regarding hearing, speech, language, or developmental delay
- Family history of hearing loss
- Congenital infections associated with hearing loss (herpes, syphilis, rubella, cytomegalovirus, toxoplasmosis)
- Postnatal infections associated with hearing loss (bacterial meningitis)
- Head/neck malformations or other physical examination findings or conditions associated with hearing loss
- Neonatal intensive care for 48 hours or more
- Head trauma
- Recurrent or persistent otitis media with effusion (at least 3 months)

Adapted from Joint Commission on Infant Hearing: Year 2000 position statement: Principles and guidelines for early hearing detection and intervention programs. Pediatrics 2000;106(4):798–817.

Table 145-1. Hearing Tests in Children

Test	Description	Type	Youngest Age
Otoacoustic emission (OAE)	Tests sound detection at the level of the cochlea at different frequencies	Screening	1 day (including preterm infants)
Auditory brainstem response (ABR), also called brainstem auditory evoked response (BAER)	Tests sound detection to the level of the midbrain at different frequencies	Screening or diagnostic	1 day (including preterm infants)
Visual reinforcement audiometry	Observe a child's response to sounds (response to sound is rewarded by a visual reinforcer)	Diagnostic	6 months
Conditioned play audiometry	A child is taught to "play" (e.g., drop a block into a box) in response to tones of different frequency and loudness	Diagnostic	2 yr
Speech audiometry	Test provides information about communicative abilities, can be presented in an open-set or closed-set (e.g., picture pointing) format	Diagnostic	3–3.5 yr
Pure-tone audiometry	A child is taught to raise a hand in response to tones of different frequency and loudness	Screening or diagnostic	4–5 yr

decisions. Later, parents may be overwhelmed by information from various sources, each presenting a different approach to rearing a child with deafness, and each reporting that its method is the best choice. Primary care clinicians can help by pointing out that no one educational or communication method has been demonstrated to be clearly superior to others (Table 145-2; see also CD-ROM Tables 145-2 and 145-3).

Primary care clinicians can support the parents as experts of their own family's strengths and needs. Clinicians can remind parents that the important goals are to facilitate good communication within families for all members and to maximize the deaf child's access to language and information. Parents should be encouraged to examine established family communication patterns so that they can be modified in ways to be more inclusive. For example, dinner table seating arrangements may need to be adjusted so that the deaf child can see everyone and be included in family discussions. Family members should be encouraged to learn the sign language or sign system that the deaf child is learning. Parents will need to be more aware of lighting to ensure visual access to information. Children usually must look up at speaking adults. Bright light behind the head of the speaker may interfere with reading facial expressions because the child's pupils will constrict and the speaker's face will be in shadows. If aware of the location of overhead lighting or the sun, parents can adjust their position to improve visual communication access. Other factors that impede reading facial expressions and speech are cigarettes, gum, and other items in the mouth, facial hair, and poor eye contact (Table 145-3). Assistive devices in the home can be used to help the child detect sounds that others hear, such as doorbells, smoke alarms, and alarm clocks (Table 145-4).

Changes in the environment as the family adjusts to the needs of the deaf child will affect siblings. Clinicians need to be sensitive to siblings and ask them about their experiences, feelings, and adjustment process.

Clinicians are more likely to see families and children during family life-cycle transitions, such as adolescence. For example, deaf teens may choose not to wear their hearing aids. Family and school systems may find this behavior stressful, and the clinician may be asked to intervene. If the clinician, like many other hearing adults, has difficulty communicating with the deaf adolescent, he or she may inadvertently "take sides" against the deaf adolescent before understanding the adolescent's perspective. Many deaf adolescents feel frustrated that so much of the work of communication is their responsibility. Many receive little linguistically useful information from their hearing aids, and some experience discomfort with sound amplification. For some, wearing hearing aids is another way that they "stand out," especially for students in mainstreamed programs. Rather than taking sides in an argument about hearing aids, clinicians can try to focus the discussion on the goal of good communication, and in this way may be able to help facilitate a plan with the adolescent, parents, and school that is mutually agreeable and maintains good communication.

Table 145-2. Educational Approaches when Working with Deaf Children

Approach	Description	Concerns
Bilingual	Children are taught in American Sign Language (ASL), and English is taught as a second language	Requires teachers fluent in ASL
Total communication	Uses aural, oral, and visual methods to communicate; communication methods vary based on the skills and needs of the individuals trying to communicate	Total communication programs often try to use signed and spoken languages simultaneously; because it is difficult to simultaneously speak and sign while remaining fluent in both modalities, some are concerned that the child may not develop fluency in either a spoken or signed language
Oral	Emphasizes the development of lipreading and speaking skills	Limited language exposure may delay or hinder development of normal language skills

Table 145-3. Factors That Interfere with Visual Communication

Category	Example
Environmental factors	Obstructed view of speaker Lighting and shadows that limit ability to see speaker (speaker is "backlit") Being in a group with multiple potential speakers Visual distractions and background noise
Speaker characteristics	Obscured mouth or face (facial hair, cigarette, poor eye contact) Distorted mouth or face (speaking slowly with exaggerated mouth movements, chewing) Facing away from the listener
Communication characteristics	Topic or words unfamiliar to the listener
"Listener" characteristics	Distractions such as stress and pain

Special Case: The Deaf Child with Deaf Parents

Many family issues are different when a deaf child is born to deaf parents. Although over 90% of deaf couples have hearing children, many welcome the birth of a deaf child. Deaf children with deaf parents are exposed to visual communication at an early age, and often have normal language development, including babbling in sign language. Deaf children with deaf parents are less likely to feel deficient or abnormal because of their deafness, and have, through their parents and their parents' friends, deaf adult role models. Understanding the nature of each parent's hearing loss and his or her perspective on deafness may help the clinician in caring for their deaf child.

MEDICAL MANAGEMENT

Because some cases of deafness are associated with specific syndromes, clinicians should observe the deaf child carefully for associated abnormalities (Table 145-5). Aspects of the history and physical examination may suggest a hereditary etiology for the child's hearing loss (Table 145-6). If a referral is warranted, genetic counselors can advise families about the likelihood that other family members would be affected. Identifying a particular syndrome may help clinicians and families in the ongoing management of the child's and the siblings' health.

Even if no syndrome is identified, clinicians need to monitor aspects of the deaf child's health more closely than for a child with normal hearing. Regular ophthalmologic examinations are warranted because of both the association of hearing loss with eye abnormalities and the potentially devastating effect of vision loss in a person who is deaf. Because hearing loss can be associated with other neurologic problems, primary care clinicians should monitor deaf children for appropriate developmental milestones. Working with qualified professional sign language interpreters can help clinicians evaluate the child's language development in ASL.

Some experts believe that deaf children are at increased risk for sexual abuse. Clinicians should be vigilant for signs and symptoms that suggest abuse (see Chapter 269). Part of a deaf child's vulnerability to sexual predators is the lack of fluent communication with most adults. Regularly working with interpreters can help establish the clear communication and safe environment necessary for a deaf child to disclose abuse to the clinician.

Working with interpreters can also help clinicians teach the deaf child about health and health care. Hearing children often learn about medical care by observing the interactions

Table 145-4. Nonauditory Ways to Indicate or Substitute Sound

Modality	Description	Examples
Vision	Signal lights or other devices can be programmed to indicate occurrence of a sound or to signal one's attention without using sound	A flashing computer screen can indicate that the computer program made a sound. Lights can signal: Telephone ring Doorbell chimes A crying baby Smoke detector or fire alarm Alarm clock
Vibration	Vibration devices can be programmed to indicate the occurrence of a sound or to signal one's attention without using sound	Pagers Alarm clocks that shake the bed Vibrating watch alarm Vibrotactile aids are worn by the user and vary vibration frequency with the sound pitch; they sometimes help some people with speechreading
Touch	Use the sense of touch rather than vibration or sight to indicate sound or to signal one's attention without using sound	Hearing dogs trained to notify their owner of the occurrence of particular sounds Alarm clock that turns of fans Tapping to get a person's attention
Language	Convert auditory language to visual language or communicate language without using sound	Captioned movies, television shows, computer programs Computer-aided real-time transcription (CART) captions live presentations Voice recognition software E-mail Teletypes (TTY) for typed communication via normal telephone lines Telephone relay services typing what one person says for another person to read on a TTY English-ASL (American Sign Language) interpreters

Table 145-5. Syndromes Associated with Childhood Deafness

Syndrome	Etiology	Prevalence in Deaf Children	Findings (Often Variably Expressed)
Usher (multiple types)	Autosomal recessive	3–10%	**Hearing loss:** moderate to profound, stable or progressive Vision: retinitis pigmentosa (variable onset and severity)
Pendred	Autosomal recessive, autosomal dominant (variable expression)	5%	**Hearing loss:** profound sensorineural (congenital onset) Endocrine: euthyroid goiter (mean age at onset 8–10 yr)
Waardenburg (multiple types)	Autosomal dominant (variable expression)	1–5%	**Hearing loss:** variable severity, stable or progressive Hair: white forelock Face: appearance of widely spaced eyes, heterochroma irides, high broad nasal root, hyperplasia of the medial eyebrow Skin: spotty hyperpigmentation
Alport (multiple types)	X-linked dominant, autosomal dominant, autosomal recessive	1%	**Hearing loss:** progressive sensorineural (onset usually after age 10 yr) Renal: hematuria (progressive glomerulonephritis) Eye: cataracts, "oil droplet" appearance of red reflex
Treacher Collins	Autosomal dominant (variable expression)	0.7%	**Hearing loss:** stable conductive Face: craniofacial malformations
Jervell and Lange-Nielsen	Autosomal recessive	0.3%	**Hearing loss:** profound sensorineural (congenital onset) Cardiovascular: prolonged Q-T interval, syncopal episodes, sudden death due to fatal arrhythmia
Osteogenesis imperfecta (multiple disorders)	Autosomal dominant		**Hearing loss:** conductive, sensorineural or mixed, onset often after age 10 yr, stable or progressive Musculoskeletal: bone fragility Eye: blue sclerae
Down	Trisomy 21		**Hearing loss:** conductive, sensorineural or mixed; usually not progressive See Chapter 158
Neurofibromatosis (type 2)	Autosomal dominant		**Hearing loss:** onset often after age 10 yr, progressive sensorineural Skin: café au lait spots Nerves: acoustic neuromas and other schwannomas
Sickle cell disease	Autosomal recessive		**Hearing loss:** sensorineural of varying severity, sometimes worse during sickle cell crises; may affect up to 45% of homozygous people See Chapter 159
Congenital rubella	Viral infection (prenatal)		**Hearing loss:** stable sensorineural, severe to profound, may be asymmetric General: low birth weight Eye: cataracts Cardiac: congenital heart disease Gastrointestinal: hepatomegaly Hematologic: splenomegaly, purpura
Congenital syphilis	Spirocete infection (prenatal)		**Hearing loss:** sensorineural, progressive, often symmetric and fluctuating Skin: rash Hematologic: anemia Head: saddle nose; dental abnormalities Neurologic: central nervous system abnormalities
Cytomegalovirus (CMV)	Viral infection (prenatal)		**Hearing loss:** mild to profound, onset may occur after birth, may be asymmetric and progressive General: low birth weight Head: microcephaly Eye: chorioretinitis, optic atrophy Gastrointestinal: hepatomegaly, jaundice Neurologic: central nervous system abnormalities, cerebral palsy, mental retardation Hematologic: splenomegaly, petechiae
Toxoplasmosis	Parasitic infection (prenatal)		**Hearing loss:** sensorineural, often progressive General: fever, poor feeding Eye: chorioretinitis, retinopathy Gastrointestinal: hepatomegaly, jaundice Hematologic: thrombocytopenia, purpura, splenomegaly
Kernicterus	Elevated level of circulating unconjugated bilirubin (neonatal)		**Hearing loss:** often high frequency, mild to severe See Chapter 198

Table 145-6. Pertinent History and Physical Examination when Working with a Deaf Child

Examination	Findings
History (pre-, peri-, and postnatal)	Exposure to ototoxic medications, history of illnesses, trauma or exposure to infectious agents that are associated with hearing loss
Family history	Hearing loss, pigment abnormalities (including the hair and iris), eye abnormalities, poor vision or blindness, goiter, kidney disorder, cardiac dysrhythmias, syncope, sudden death
General appearance	Morphology, body habitus
Skin	Skin pigment, texture, skin tags, petechiae
Head	Dysmorphic features (symmetry, shape, skin tags)
Hair	Color, texture, white forelock
Eye	Spacing, shape, color, retina, eyebrows, eyelids, cataracts, vision
Ear	Malformation, position, symmetry, preauricular pits, sinuses or tags, canal patency
Nose	Morphology
Mouth	Morphology, tooth development
Neck	Morphology, thyroid, cysts, fistulas
Abdomen	Organomegaly
Genitals	Hypogonadism
Extremities	Morphology of limbs and digits
Neurologic system	Developmental abnormalities, mental functioning, balance, gait

between their parents and doctor. A deaf child is unable to overhear these discussions. As a result, adults deafened as children may not know much of their own family health history and may not be familiar with the usual course of a medical interview. Efforts should be made to make all health care communication accessible from an early age.

During a clinical encounter, there are three primary communication goals: (1) clear communication between the clinician and parent (or other adult caretaker); (2) clear communication between the clinician and deaf child; and (3) involvement of the deaf child in "overhearing" the communication between the clinician and parent (and anyone else present). These goals are difficult to achieve when a parent is expected to assume the additional role of interpreter. Working with medically experienced, qualified interpreters allows family members (including the deaf child) to focus on the content of the communication with the clinician, rather than on the process of making communication accessible (see CD-ROM Table 145-3 for organizations that may help clinicians identify resources for local interpreters).

In addition to interpreters, primary care clinicians will need to work collaboratively with other professionals when caring for a family with a deaf child. Teachers, audiologists, speech-language pathologists, ophthalmologists, otolaryngologists, other specialist physicians, family therapists, and genetic counselors can help with diagnosis and ongoing care. Because most hearing people do not socialize with adults deafened in childhood, many deaf children have never met a deaf adult. Working with adults deafened in childhood, regardless of their profession, can introduce the deaf child to role models and offer the family ideas regarding a deaf child's potential (some organizations listed in CD-ROM

Table 145-1 may be able to help match families with deaf adults in their area).

ON THE HORIZON

Currently there is no medical treatment for deafness. Research on hair cell injury and rejuvenation may lead to treatments, and genetic research may lead to ways to identify and treat those susceptible to hearing loss.

Cochlear implants are a surgical intervention gaining notoriety for their potential use in children with hearing loss. A surgeon inserts an electrode array into a cochlea of a deaf person. The electrode array is attached to the implant body, which sits under the skin in a well that is carved into the skull behind the ear. A receiver is worn behind the ear much like a hearing aid, and sound is transmitted from the receiver along a wire to a speech processor, which either fits behind the ear or can be worn clipped onto clothing like a pager. The speech processor analyzes the sound and sends information along a wire to a coil behind the ear that is held in place by a magnet on the skull. The information is transmitted transcutaneously to the implant body, and the information is then sent into the cochlea via the electrode array. Professionals experienced with cochlear implants help determine over time the optimal speech processor programming for the individual. With training, some deaf people can learn to understand some speech.

Cochlear implant studies in young children are limited. Outcomes frequently studied are speech perception and production. Research to date has not adequately examined how these outcomes affect or reflect educational or economic achievement, or happiness. Accompanied with the appropriate follow-up with professionals experienced with children with cochlear implants, a cochlear implant may be an appropriate intervention in some families. Parents should be told about the limitations of the research, and need to be aware that a 22-channel electrode array cannot replace the function of the more than 10,000 hair cells to make their child hear normally.

OUTCOME

With appropriate stimulation and support, a deaf child without other neurologic conditions should develop normally. Primary care clinicians should monitor the well-being of the child and family and should inquire about the quality of the family's communication. In addition, clinicians will want to pay attention to the child's language skills. Normal development includes reading ability, but does not necessarily include speaking and lipreading skills.

FOLLOW-UP

More frequent primary care visits will help clinicians to keep track of input from the different professionals involved in the deaf child's care. During these visits, the clinician can assess the development and well-being of the child and family, and assist in sorting through information so that the child and family can make the best decisions for themselves. For children with cochlear implants, clinicians will want to check for the latest vaccination recommendations.

The enzyme is normally present in liver, kidney, and intestinal mucosa, and glycogen accumulates in these organs. Both glycogen and fat are stored in excess in the liver. Symptoms are massive hepatomegaly, often already present at birth, growth retardation, profound hypoglycemia, lacticacidemia, hyperlipidemia, and hyperuricemia. Type IB also has a defect of white blood cells. Long-term complications include gout, hepatic adenomas, osteoporosis, renal disease, and short stature. Early death was the rule prior to effective treatment.

Current management includes nocturnal nasogastric infusion of glucose and oral administration of uncooked cornstarch to maintain euglycemia.

Glycogen storage disease type II (*Pompe disease*, or alpha glucosidase deficiency) is a classical lysosomal storage disease, discussed in Chapter 149.

Glycogen storage disease type III, or debrancher enzyme deficiency, occurs in both a hepatic and a more common mixed form. The hepatic form looks like a somewhat milder case of type I GSD disease but with elevated liver enzymes and resolution of the hepatomegaly in adolescence. Cirrhosis of the liver and renal tubular acidosis occur rarely. In the mixed form, a myopathy is also present with elevated creatine kinase. Hypotonia and weakness are variable in infancy and childhood but become more problematic with age. Cardiomyopathy is usually a late complication.

Like the other glycogen storage diseases, this disorder is an autosomal recessive condition. Diagnosis is confirmed by enzyme analysis on liver or muscle biopsy. Management is similar to that for GSD type I. A high-protein diet may help the muscle disease.

Glycogen storage diseases types IV, VI, and IX are disorders of the phosphorylase system (types VI and IX) and branching enzyme deficiency (type IV) and are rarer hepatic glycogenoses. All have marked hepatomegaly and mild fasting hypoglycemia.

Muscle Glycogen Storage Diseases

The most common muscle enzyme defects of glycogenolysis are myophosphorylase deficiency (GSD V or McCardle disease) and phosphofructokinase deficiency (GSD VII). Symptoms are caused by inadequate fuel for muscle function. ATP is rapidly depleted and ADP is degraded to form uric acid. Elevated creatine kinase and uric acid levels occur, especially with exercise. Exercise intolerance, the usual initial symptom, may not occur until adulthood. Other symptoms are weakness, stiffness, cramps, and muscle pain. Diagnosis is suggested with an exercise test and confirmed by muscle biopsy with enzyme assays.

Mitochondrial Fatty Oxidation Defects

An increasing number of disorders of fatty acid oxidation are now being recognized. Nearly all present in infancy or early childhood, most commonly as an acute life-threatening event with hypoketotic hypoglycemia. Some forms also have chronic muscle weakness, acute or exercise-induced muscle weakness, rhabdomyolysis, or cardiomyopathy. Oxidation of fatty acids has four components: the carnitine cycle, the beta oxidation cycle, the electron transfer pathway, and the ketone synthesis pathway.

Disorders of the Carnitine Cycle

Carnitine is necessary to shuttle long-chain fatty acids into the mitochondria. Several defects are known.

Carnitine transporter defect: A severe carnitine deficiency results from a defect in sodium-dependent transport of carnitine across the plasma membrane. Cardiomyopathy and generalized weakness result. Carnitine treatment is effective.

Carnitine palmitoyl transferase-1 (CPT-1) deficiency presents with the typical hypoketotic hypoglycemia of many fatty acid oxidation disorders. The muscle form of the enzyme is apparently not involved. Elevated levels of plasma carnitine and severe abnormalities of liver function are common during attacks.

Diagnosis is confirmed by enzyme assay. Treatment is avoidance of fasting and prompt treatment of hypoglycemic episodes with glucose infusion.

Carnitine/acyl carnitine translocase deficiency is a very rare disorder with fatal neonatal cardiomyopathy in most cases.

Two forms of *carnitine palmitoyl transferase-2 deficiency* have been described. Patients with the milder form of the disorder have attacks of rhabdomyolysis beginning in adolescence or young adulthood. The severe form presents in the neonatal period with life-threatening coma, cardiomyopathy, and weakness. Hypoketotic hypoglycemia without dicarboxylic aciduria is present. There may be brain and kidney malformations. Diagnosis requires enzyme studies.

Beta Oxidation Defects

Defects of the acyl-CoA dehydrogenases involve a series of enzymes with overlapping, chain-length specific function. Understanding of the range of clinical phenotypes, pathogenesis, treatment, and long-term prognosis is rudimentary for all but the medium-chain acyl-CoA dehydrogenase deficiency (MCADD). All are autosomal recessive conditions, but some patients may have compound heterozygosity for multiple defects. Presumptive diagnosis is made by analysis of the acyl carnitine profile and determination of the chain length of metabolites present in abnormal amounts. Confirmatory enzyme analyses or DNA testing are available for some disorders.

Patients with short-chain acyl-CoA dehydrogenase deficiency are rare and have had a variety of symptoms. Very long chain acyl-CoA dehydrogenase deficiency usually produces severe disease with chronic cardiomyopathy, weakness, and episodes of hypoglycemic coma associated with fasting, but some patients have milder disease or primarily skeletal muscle involvement. In some families, overwhelming neonatal decompensation and death have occurred. Treatment is avoidance of fasting, low-fat diet, and use of medium-chain triglycerides to replace some of the dietary fat. Use of carnitine supplementation is controversial.

Medium-chain acyl-CoA dehydrogenase deficiency (MCADD) is the single most common disorder of fatty acid oxidation, occurring in 1 in 15,000 live births. Although many affected individuals may never develop symptoms, those with the most common mutation frequently develop hypoketotic hypoglycemia with fasting. Depending on the age of the child, some cases have been classified as SIDS and others as Reye syndrome. Usually an episode of illness leads to decreased feeding in the infant or young child, most commonly between 3 months and 2 years of age. Lethargy, nausea and vomiting, and elevation of free fatty acids occur before hypoglycemia is prominent. The child rapidly becomes comatose with hypoglycemia, inappropriately low ketones, hyperammonemia, and elevated liver enzymes. Death during the first episode occurs in about 25% of cases but is unusual after a diagnosis has been made. Children who have experienced an attack frequently have neurologic sequelae including developmental disability, behavioral problems, cerebral palsy, and seizures. Attacks become less common after early childhood.

Diagnosis can be suspected based on the excretion of characteristic organic acids. The acyl carnitine profile is characteristic and both enzymatic and DNA testing is available. Unfortunately, metabolite testing may be uninformative when the child is well. Expanded newborn metabolic screening using tandem mass spectroscopy detects this disorder, and it is hoped that it will prevent most deaths and disabilities. Treatment is by avoidance of fasting. Moderate fat restriction and carnitine supplementation are sometimes used.

3-Hydroxyl acyl-CoA dehydrogenase deficiencies: Three enzymes, long-chain enoyl-CoA hydratase, 3-hydroxyacyl-CoA dehydrogenase, and beta keto acyl thiolase are combined in a single trifunctional protein. Some patients have isolated deficiency of the dehydrogenase, often called long-chain hydroxyacyl-CoA dehydrogenase deficiency (LCHADD). This disorder is not rare. Considerable heterogeneity has been reported.

Features may include fulminant liver failure, cardiomyopathy, rhabdomyolysis, and fasting hypoketotic hypoglycemic encephalopathy. A pigmentary retinopathy occurs by late childhood. Mothers carrying affected infants frequently have severe toxemia of pregnancy, often with acute fatty liver or the HELP syndrome (hemolysis, elevated liver enzymes, and low platelets syndrome). Diagnosis is by acylcarnitine profile with confirmation by enzyme analysis and DNA studies. Treatment is to avoid fasting, reduce fat in the diet, and consider medium-chain triglycerides and carnitine supplementation. Experimental treatments to prevent blindness are in progress.

Disorders of Ketone Body Metabolism

Ketone bodies are important sources of energy during fasting and other lipolytic stress. Acetoacetate is produced by ketogenesis and 3-hydroxybutyrate and acetone are derived from acetoacetate.

Ketogenic defects involve disorders of mitochondrial hydroxymethylglutaryl-CoA (HMG-CoA) synthase and HMG-CoA lyase. Deficiencies cause episodic hypoketotic hypoglycemia and coma, sometimes resulting in death or neurologic sequelae. These autosomal recessive disorders are diagnosed by the specific pattern of urine organic acid excretion. Avoidance of fasting is usually effective treatment.

Ketolytic defects involving deficiencies of succinyl-CoA, 3-ketoacid-CoA transferase, and mitochondrial acetoacetate CoA thiolase (beta ketothiolase) cause episodes of ketoacidosis. Neurologic damage may occur and a death in an undiagnosed sibling suggests that episodes may sometimes be lethal. Mild protein restriction, avoidance of fasting, and prompt treatment of episodes are indicated.

Hyperlactic Acidemias and Disorders of the Tricarboxylic Acid Cycle (Congenital Lactic Acidosis)

Disorders of pyruvate metabolism and the tricarboxylic acid cycle (TAC) affect gluconeogenesis, lipogenesis, and amino acid synthesis. Symptoms usually involve the central nervous system and are often difficult to diagnose. Manifestations are frequently present at birth and do not require intake of specific nutrients to become apparent.

Disorders of Pyruvate Metabolism

Pyruvate carboxylase deficiency occurs in three forms. The most severe presents as profound neonatal lactic acidosis with seizures, coma, and abnormal muscle tone. Survival beyond a few months is rare. The most common presentation is at several months of age with developmental delay and other neurologic problems including seizures, spasticity, microcephaly, and feeding problems. Failure to thrive is common and renal tubular acidosis may be present. There may be mild hepatic enlargement and intermittent or chronic lactic acidosis. Some individuals have the anatomic and brainstem changes seen in Leigh syndrome. A milder form with attacks of lactic acidosis and mild neurologic impairment has also been described.

All three forms are autosomal recessive disorders. The diagnosis should be considered whenever there is lactic acidosis and neurologic symptoms, especially if hypoglycemia, hyperammonemia, or ketosis is present. Enzyme studies on leukocytes or liver are necessary to confirm the diagnosis. Treatment includes a high-carbohydrate diet and avoidance of fasting, but the prognosis is poor for severely affected children.

Phosphenolpyruvate carboxykinase deficiency is rare; few cases are known. The presentation is similar to other disorders of pyruvate metabolism.

Pyruvate dehydrogenase complex diseases are the most common disorders of pyruvate metabolism. The pyruvate dehydrogenase complex (PDHC) has three components. Most cases are due to a defect in the first component. Symptoms of all three overlap. Central nervous system symptoms are most often progressive. The most common features are developmental delay and hypotonia, often with seizures and ataxia. Defects of respiratory control with periodic apnea, agenesis of the corpus callosum, and microcephaly are characteristic. In a minority of cases brain imaging shows the neuropathologic findings of Leigh disease.

Although most of the genes for the components of PDHC are autosomal, the E1-alpha subunit gene is on the X chromosome and accounts for most cases of PDHC deficiency. A disproportionate number of affected males have more severe disease than heterozygous females. Diagnosis is suggested by lacticacidosis with a normal lactate-to-pyruvate ratio. Measurement of cerebrospinal fluid levels or performance of loading tests is sometimes necessary to detect the elevated lactate levels. Enzyme studies are required for confirmation. Treatment with a ketogenic diet has shown some promise, but the prognosis is generally poor.

Table 148-1. Common Disorders of Protein Metabolism

Type of Defect	Specific Disorder
Aminoacidopathies	Hyperphenylalaninemias (e.g., PKU) Tyrosinemias (types I, II, III) Homocystinuria Nonketotic hyperglycinemia
Organic acid disorders	Branched-chain ketoacidurias (maple syrup urine disease, isovaleric acidosis, 3-hydroxy-3-methylglutaryl CoA dehydrogenase deficiency) Disorders of propionate and methylmalonate Glutaric acidemia type I
Urea cycle defects	Ornithine transcarbamoylase deficiency Carbamoyl phosphate synthetase deficiency Argininosuccinic acid synthetase deficiency Argininosuccinic acid lyase deficiency Arginase deficiency
Transport defects	Cystinuria Lysinuric protein intolerance

produce amino acids, especially alanine and glutamine. The alanine is used for gluconeogenesis. In the fed state, excess amino acids can be used to synthesize either triacylglycerols that are converted to fats or glucose for storage as glycogen.

Excess nitrogen is converted to urea by the urea cycle, again mainly in the liver. Waste nitrogen occurs in the body as ammonia or the ammonium ion, which are interconvertible. Muscle cells can generate ammonium ion by way of the purine nucleotide cycle. Ammonium can be formed from glutamate or several other amino acids. Glutamate plays a pivotal role in amino acid synthesis and degradation. It provides nitrogen for amino acid synthesis by obtaining it from other amino acids or directly from ammonium ion by the glutamate dehydrogenase reaction. When amino acids are degraded and urea is formed, glutamate receives nitrogen from other amino acids and allows it to enter into the urea cycle.

The major disorders of protein metabolism are the aminoacidopathies, organic acid disorders, and urea cycle defects. Disorders of amino acid transport also occur. Aminoacidopathy is the name given to a disorder resulting from inability to metabolize a specific amino acid such as phenylalanine (phenylketonuria) or homocysteine (homocystinuria). Organic acid disorders occur when the metabolic defect is in a step after deamination of the amino acid, and the resulting accumulation of metabolites is as the organic acid derivatives. Branched-chain ketoacidemia (maple syrup urine disease) is actually an organic acid disorder, as are methylmalonic and propionic acidemias. Disorders of the formation of urea from waste nitrogen are called urea cycle disorders. Table 148-1 lists common disorders of protein metabolism.

SIGNS AND SYMPTOMS

Most disorders of protein metabolism present with a picture of acute intoxication from accumulation of metabolites that are substrates for the dysfunctional enzyme. Several relatively common disorders, however, result from chronic damage to various tissues or organs from metabo-

lites that do not cause acute symptoms, such as the brain damage of phenylketonuria, liver and kidney damage of type I tyrosinemia, and disorders of clotting found in homocystinuria. These disorders have in common a symptom-free period of days to months or even years followed by clinical signs of acute intoxication (e.g., vomiting, lethargy, coma, liver failure, thromboembolic events, ataxia, seizures) or chronic end-organ failure (e.g., developmental delay, ectopia lentis, liver dysfunction)

Measurement of the metabolites as amino acids, organic acids, or ammonia is relatively easy.

COMMON INBORN ERRORS OF PROTEIN METABOLISM

Diagnosis

When a patient presents with acute symptoms, screening studies (see Chapter 146) should be obtained and further investigations are then based on the initial results, as shown in Table 148-2.

Patients with chronic neurologic problems, failure to thrive, speech and language abnormalities, or hair and skin changes should have serum or plasma amino acids and urine organic acids measured after review of their presentation with a consultant. Ectopia lentis is a reason for measurement of plasma homocysteine and methionine. Disorders of amino acid transport are usually suspected on the basis of measurement of quantitative urine amino acids. Suspicion of a disorder of protein metabolism may come from a positive newborn metabolic screening test. If an inborn error is suspected on the basis of these studies, referral to a metabolic specialist is recommended. Definitive diagnosis often requires enzyme studies or DNA analysis and treatment is usually, at least in part, dietary.

Management

Prompt emergency management of metabolic crises in disorders of protein metabolism is imperative if long-term disability and death are to be prevented. A protocol should be provided by the consultant with guidelines for hospital admission or transfer to a tertiary center. Guidelines for emergency management are summarized in Box 148-1.

Patients with inborn errors of protein metabolism should be managed jointly with a metabolic service providing a multidisciplinary team approach. Specialized nutritional services are virtually always required. Frequent monitoring is necessary both to assess the disease and to ensure

Table 148-2. Evaluation for Disorders of Protein Metabolism with Acute Presentation

Screening Abnormality	Further Studies
Metabolic acidosis	Lactate Ammonia Urine organic acids Serum or plasma amino acids Consider acyl carnitine profile, urine orotic acid
Liver failure	Ammonia Urine for succinylacetone Serum or plasma amino acids

Box 148-1. Guidelines for Emergency Management of Metabolic Crises in Disorders of Protein Metabolism

- Correct hypoglycemia and electrolyte imbalances with appropriate intravenous solutions.
- Hydrate, hydrate, hydrate.
- Remove sources of protein from the diet and administer nutrition through enteral feedings of the special medical food or a protein-free formula if possible.
- Provide adequate calories to prevent catabolism and maintain glucose levels above 100 mg/dL (use insulin if needed).
- Support respirations.
- Provide appropriate hemodynamic support.
- Correct bleeding problems.

adequate nutrition. Acute deterioration and metabolic crises occur frequently in the organic acid disorders and urea cycle defects. Complications are common, especially progressive neurologic deterioration, strokes, pancreatitis, and chronic renal insufficiency.

The metabolic specialist will often request regular laboratory monitoring. The use of a laboratory experienced in these studies is essential, and consistency is important to assess disease progression. The requested tests may be unusual and available at only a few sites. Use of a laboratory without the necessary expertise results in poor patient care and unnecessary expense. Conditions for obtaining specimens may be quite specific and necessary for reliable results.

Dietary management has been the mainstay of treatment for most disorders of protein metabolism. Various medications also serve to enhance enzyme activity, replace absent cofactors, scavenge toxic compounds, block certain reactions, or treat secondary complications. The principles of dietary therapy have been developed by long experience with treating phenylketonuria. Patients whose disorder results from an enzyme deficiency in the metabolic pathway of an essential amino acid can be treated by controlling the amount of that amino acid, or amino acids, consumed. Sometimes simple protein restriction is enough, but more commonly special medical foods must be used in which the offending amino acid(s) are removed from the product and the remaining amino acids are included along with varying

amounts of fat, carbohydrates, vitamins, and minerals. The amount of the excluded amino acids required for growth and repair are supplied by carefully regulated amounts of natural protein. Adequate calories to prevent catabolism must be provided. These diets are frequently unpalatable, and most patients with organic acid disorders require gastrostomy feedings. The highly artificial nature of the diet requires regular monitoring for nutritional adequacy and vitamin and mineral status. Diets are adjusted based on metabolic monitoring studies, which should be performed at least monthly. Nutritional deficiencies have been seen in many patients with inadequate dietary monitoring and include osteopenia, rashes, abnormal hair, anemia, and visual deficits.

In addition to dietary therapy, supportive care and specific medications are frequently necessary for metabolic patients. Therapy for the more common disorders is summarized in Table 148-3.

Treatment with currently available strategies is unsatisfactory for many of these disorders. Individuals suffer metabolic crises and multisystem complications. Liver transplantation has been effective in several urea cycle defects, although central nervous system damage has usually occurred prior to transplantation. Transplantation of liver and kidney has been attempted in some organic acid disorders with generally disappointing results, but further studies are needed to assess the role of transplantation. New drugs are under development, and gene therapy has been attempted unsuccessfully in ornithine transcarbamylase deficiency.

Patients receiving restricted diets should have regular monitoring of serum or plasma amino acids, albumin or prealbumin, hematocrit, vitamin and iron levels, as well as assessment for bone density and trace minerals. Measurement of essential fatty acids is a research procedure and is sometimes recommended. The growth pattern should be assessed regularly. Additional monitoring may be recommended to measure metabolites such as ammonia and plasma organic acids. Assessment of the function of sensitive organs (such as kidney and liver) may also be necessary.

Many inborn errors of metabolism are managed using investigational drugs or research protocols. In some cases there is long experience with the regimens, such as in the

Table 148-3. Therapy for Selected Disorders of Protein Metabolism

Disorder	Diet	Adjunctive Therapies
Phenylketonuria	Phenylalanine restricted	Usually unnecessary; tetrahydrobiopterin should be tried and is needed in cases due to cofactor deficiency; neurotransmitters and folinic acid may be required, depending on the enzyme defect
Tyrosinemias	Restricted in tyrosine and phenylalanine	NTBC in type I (hepatorenal)
Homocystinuria	Restricted in methionine	Pyridoxine, betaine, antiplatelet agents
Nonketotic hyperglycinemia	None	Anticonvulsants, sodium benzoate, dextromethorphan
Branched-chain ketoaciduria	Restricted in leucine, isoleucine, and valine	Trial of thiamine
Propionic acidosis	Restricted in methionine, tryptophan, isoleucine, and valine	Carnitine, trial of biotin, metronidazole, nitrogen scavengers
Methylmalonic acidosis	Restricted in methionine, tryptophan, isoleucine, and valine	Trial of vitamin B_{12}, carnitine, nitrogen scavengers
Glutaric academia I	Consider protein restriction	Prompt treatment and support during infections
Urea cycle disorders	Protein restriction, essential amino supplementation	Arginine, nitrogen scavengers (sodium benzoate, sodium phenylacetate, sodium phenylbutyrate)

case of nitrogen scavengers for hyperammonemia, and in others many questions still remain. The primary care provider can help families decide whether they wish to participate in experimental treatments by evaluating research protocols, discussing theoretical and practical considerations with other specialists not involved in the research, and acting as an advocate for the child and family. In some cases the experimental treatments are the only hope for survival, but the long-term outcome of such survival is frequently unknown. The pediatrician often knows the family and its resources, values, and competing interests better than the specialist and has no vested interest in the proposed therapies.

Most inborn errors of protein metabolism are autosomal recessive disorders, with the notable exception of ornithine transcarbamylase deficiency. The latter is X-linked and about 20% of heterozygous girls are symptomatic. The clinician should provide appropriate genetic counseling or make a referral for counseling. Most metabolic clinics have a regular genetic counselor who is knowledgeable about treatment and reproductive options, prognosis, and carrier testing.

Outcomes

The outcomes in various inborn errors of protein metabolism are variable. Well-managed phenylketonuria results in healthy, normally functioning adults, who differ little from their unaffected siblings if treatment is continued throughout adult life. Improvements in therapy and earlier diagnosis promise better outcomes in other conditions. Nonetheless, many of these disorders have serious long-term complications and continue to threaten acute deterioration with complications and possible death despite optimal management. In many cases the small number of surviving adults precludes statements about what can be expected over a lifetime.

Pregnancies have been reported in several disorders. The fetal damage caused by elevated maternal levels of phenylalanine in phenylketonuria (PKU) is well documented. Excellent metabolic control seems to be compatible with good fetal outcome, however, and adolescents and young women with PKU need to know about the importance of optimal control prior to pregnancy. In other disorders, the mother has sometimes experienced easier management during pregnancy, but in some cases there have been maternal deaths associated with the stress of labor and delivery.

For some disorders, liver transplantation has been curative. Because of the uncertainties of outcome and effectiveness of treatment, careful counseling should be provided to families at risk for these conditions or who have an affected child who has suffered serious damage prior to diagnosis. Counseling should also be provided by both the specialist and the primary physician if a child dies with an inborn error of metabolism diagnosed either before or after death.

SPECIFIC DISORDERS

Hyperphenylalanemias

The best-known disorder of amino acid metabolism is phenylketonuria.(PKU), which occurs in about 1 in 15,000 births. PKU is an autosomal recessive condition that usually results from defective activity of the enzyme, phenylalanine hydroxylase. This enzyme converts excess phenylalanine to tyrosine and requires a biopterin cofactor, tetrahydrobiopterin. Affected individuals are normal at birth, but the blood phenylalanine level rises quickly thereafter. Classical disease is defined by a blood phenylalanine level greater than 1200 µmol/L (20 mg/dL) on a regular diet. Lesser elevations are common and are also frequently seen in disorders of cofactor synthesis or metabolism. Phenylalanine hydroxylase is coded for by a gene on chromosome 12. Hundreds of different mutations have been described.

Patients begin to show developmental delay in the first year of life. Most untreated individuals will be severely or profoundly retarded, nonverbal, hyperactive, and often autistic. Seizures are common. Eczema and decreased pigmentation are the major non-neurologic findings. Individuals with lesser degrees of hyperphenylalaninemia are at risk for mental retardation and learning problems. Those with cofactor defects will have progressive neurologic deterioration despite dietary treatment. All infants with a positive newborn screening test for phenylalanine should have studies of biopterin, and other causes of phenylalanine elevation, which include liver disease and transient tyrosinemia of the newborn, should be excluded.

Treatment is highly successful when begun immediately after birth when diagnosis is made as a result of newborn screening. Diet may also be useful in older, retarded patients. Dietary management requires careful control of phenylalanine intake to allow for growth while preventing accumulation of toxic levels of phenylalanine and its metabolites. Blood phenylalanine levels must be monitored regularly. Because a nutritionally adequate diet using only natural foods is impossible, a special medical food (formula) is prescribed to meet amino acid, vitamin, and mineral requirements, and provides a portion of the carbohydrates and fats required as well. Treatment should be lifelong. Discontinuation is associated with a slow decrease in intellect, often with other neurologic problems. When phenylalanine levels are elevated, patients have poor attention, hyperactivity, anxiety, and mood disorders.

Phenylalanine crosses the placenta and is concentrated in the fetus. It is teratogenic at maternal levels of 300 µmol/L (6 mg/dL) and above. Maternal PKU is a syndrome associated with microcephaly, intrauterine growth restriction, mental retardation, congenital heart disease, a typical dysmorphic appearance, and esophageal abnormalities. Young women with PKU and lesser degrees of hyperphenylalaninemia must be carefully counseled about the need for tight metabolic control when undertaking a pregnancy.

Disorders of Tyrosine Metabolism

Five disorders of tyrosine catabolism are known: tyrosinemia I (hepatorenal tyrosinemia), tyrosinemia II (oculocutaneous or Richner-Hanhart syndrome), tyrosinemia type III (which is often asymptomatic, but may be associated with mental retardation), hawkinsinuria (described in only four families), and alkaptonuria. Oculocutaneous albinism is caused by a deficiency of tyrosinase in the melanocytes but will not be discussed here. Transient tyrosinemia of the newborn is common in premature infants with high-protein intake. Elevated levels of tyrosine are also seen in severe liver disease.

Hepatorenal tyrosinemia is a severe disorder affecting the liver, kidney, and nervous system. Rickets results from the renal disease, and renal failure may occur. Sepsis is common. Liver dysfunction is associated with a coagulopathy and hypoalbuminemia, but jaundice and elevation of transaminases may be relatively mild. Attacks of abdominal pain, acute peripheral neuropathy, and hypertension may be life-threatening. Untreated patients die of liver failure, cirrhosis, or hepatic carcinoma. The disorder is autosomal recessive and caused by a deficiency of the enzyme fumarylacetoacetase.

The compounds which accumulate in fumarylacetoacetase deficiency are the precursors of succinylacetone, which is elevated in urine and plasma. Measurement of urine succinylacetone is the usual means of making the diagnosis.

Treatment of this condition was disappointing prior to 1992, when NTBC (2-[2-nitro-4-trifluoromethylbenzoyl]-1,3-cyclohexanedione) was introduced. A combination of therapy with NTBC, which prevents accumulation of the toxic metabolites, and dietary restriction of tyrosine and phenylalanine has been very successful. Early diagnosis and treatment may prevent hepatic carcinoma, but late-diagnosed patients are still at risk for this life-threatening complication, and careful monitoring is necessary.

Hereditary tyrosinemia type II, an autosomal recessive disorder that results in plasma tyrosine levels above 1200 μmol/L, is caused by deficiency of tyrosine aminotransferase. Symptoms are corneal ulcerations and painful blisters of the palms and soles, which become hyperkeratotic over time. Some patients have had mental retardation. Individuals may become symptomatic in infancy or at any age.

Treatment by dietary restriction of phenylalanine and tyrosine is almost always successful.

Tyrosinemia type III, a poorly understood disorder, is caused by deficiency of 4-hydroxyphenylpyruvate dioxygenase and has been associated with mental retardation.

Alkaptonuria, one of the original four inborn errors of metabolism described by Archibald Garrod, is caused by a defect of the enzyme homogentisic acid dioxygenase. The presence of homogentisic acid in the urine causes it to turn dark on standing or when alkalinized. The manifestations are darkening of cartilage in ears, nose, and joints. Severe arthritis, which occurs in adulthood, may be incapacitating. Valvular heart disease may also occur. No definitive treatment is known, and dietary management is difficult because of the lack of symptoms until the fourth or fifth decade.

Homocystinuria

Homocystinuria owing to deficiency of cystathionine β-synthase is the most common disorder of sulfur-containing amino acids. Symptoms include dislocation of the lens of the eye, skeletal problems (joint enlargement with mild contractures, osteoporosis), arachnodactyly, thromboembolic episodes (stroke), and mental retardation. The clinical spectrum is wide. The diagnosis may not be made until unexplained thromoembolic episodes lead to severe secondary damage. About half of all patients have a pyridoxine-responsive form of the disorder, which has a generally better prognosis.

Urine screening by the cyanide-nitroprusside test is unreliable for diagnosis of homocystinuria. Newborn screening, performed in some states, misses the milder cases. Measurement of methionine, homocystine, and cysteine-homocysteine disulfide in plasma is necessary for diagnosis and may be difficult. Enzymatic confirmation of the diagnosis is recommended.

All patients should be tested empirically for pyridoxine responsiveness. In nonresponsive or only partially responsive patients, a diet low in methionine and high in cystine is recommended. Betaine is also given and antiplatelet agents are recommended. The outcome in nonpyridoxine-responsive patients is generally poor, although early diagnosis and treatment are clearly beneficial in preventing mental retardation and delaying complications.

Nonketotic Hyperglycinemia

Nonketotic hyperglycinemia, a devastating central nervous system disorder caused by a defect in the glycine cleavage system, is autosomal recessive and occurs in a classical neonatal lethal form and as a nonlethal infantile or later onset form. Atypical cases also occur and are poorly understood. The typical newborn with this condition begins to deteriorate within the first 48 hours of life with lethargy, poor feeding, seizures, and apnea. Hiccoughs are common. The more common findings of metabolic disease—acidosis or hyperammonemia—are absent. Coma and death usually ensue, although some infants will survive if supported by ventilator therapy for days or weeks. Thereafter, seizures are relentless and psychomotor progress is minimal. Late onset patients may have severe seizures disorders and retardation or lesser degrees of neurologic impairment. A transient, nongenetic form of this condition with a good prognosis has been described.

Diagnosis is made by finding elevated glycine levels in the plasma, excluding ketotic hyperglycinemia by measuring urine organic acids, and demonstrating accumulation of glycine in the cerebrospinal fluid (CSF). In nonketotic hyperglycinemia, the CSF-to-plasma glycine concentration ratio is greater than 0.09. Valproate therapy is the most common cause of elevated glycine levels in older patients.

Treatment of this condition is unsatisfactory. Some patients clearly suffer prenatal brain damage of a severe degree. Efforts to reduce glycine levels with dietary therapy and administration of sodium benzoate has minimal if any clinical benefit. Strychnine, ketamine, and dextromethorphan have all had some effect in reducing seizures in some patients, but the long-term outcome remains poor.

Sulfite oxidase deficiency is another cause of intractable seizures beginning in the newborn period and has no known treatment as well as a dismal prognosis.

Glutaric Acidemia Type I

Glutaric acidemia type I is a disorder of lysine metabolism caused by the autosomal recessive deficiency of glutaryl-CoA dehydrogenase. Infants appear normal at birth, although megalencephaly with dilated ventricles is common. The neurologic manifestations, dystonia and dyskinesia, appear during infancy and early childhood in most affected individuals, usually in association with an intercurrent infection. Damage is usually progressive, with the symptoms worsening with each infectious episode. Patients are frequently diagnosed with cerebral palsy.

There is good evidence that early supplementation with carnitine and prompt, aggressive treatment of infections with fluids, glucose, and insulin can prevent developmental of symptoms. Lysine-restricted diets may be helpful.

Organic Acidemias

The organic acidemias as a group clinically have much in common. The most common disorders are branched-chain ketoacidemia (maple syrup urine disease), isovaleric aciduria, propionic aciduria, and the methylmalonic acidurias. They usually present early with acute ketoacidosis and resulting symptoms, but late-onset, intermittent and mild, progressive examples also are seen. Infants present with poor feeding, lethargy progressing to coma, posturing, and apnea. Seizures may occur.

In branched-chain ketoaciduria, acidosis is less pronounced than in the other disorders. Hyperammonemia occurs with isovaleric, propionic, and methylmalonic acidemias. Bone marrow depression is common. Later onset cases usually have recurrent episodes of metabolic decompensation or failure to thrive with developmental delay.

Each of these disorders is autosomal recessive. Diagnosis is made by the characteristic pattern of urine organic acid excretion or by acyl carnitine profile followed by enzyme studies for confirmation. Some types are responsive to specific vitamin cofactors.

Treatment for these conditions is complicated because of the frequency of metabolic crises associated with increased stress and infection. The mainstay of treatment is a highly specialized diet limiting one or more essential amino acids, depending on the diagnosis. Many patients require gastrostomy feedings owing to anorexia and the unpleasant taste of the special metabolic foods. Catabolism must be prevented. Pharmacologic doses of specific cofactors may be helpful depending on the specific genetic defect. Carnitine supplementation may be needed, as well as scavengers for hyperammonemia. Prompt emergency management of crises is crucial.

Unfortunately, patients with organic acid disorders often suffer from secondary complications despite optimal treatment. Pancreatitis, basal ganglia strokes, bone marrow suppression, renal disease, and cardiomyopathy are frequently seen. Neurologic impairment is most often secondary to damage during the initial presentation, and many patients do well developmentally with comprehensive management. The complications of these conditions are not well understood, and although liver transplantation has been used in some cases, complications have not always been prevented.

Urea Cycle Disorders

Disorders of the urea cycle have been observed involving all five of the enzymatic steps. All are autosomal recessive except ornithine transcarbamoylase, which is X-linked. Hyperammonemic encephalopathy is the common symptom of all except arginase deficiency, which usually manifests as a progressive spastic quadriparesis. Neonatal and later onset forms occur for most of the disorders, and girls with ornithine transcarbamoylase deficiency often present as late-onset or recurrent disease.

Typically the affected infants are normal at birth but become ill rapidly thereafter with poor feeding, vomiting, lethargy and irritability, tachypnea, progressing rapidly to coma and respiratory failure. Older individuals may present with episodic nausea, vomiting, and altered levels of conciousness that tend to resolve when feeding is interrupted and intravenous therapy given. Stress, high-protein intake, and infections often precipitate episodes of metabolic decompensation.

Hyperammonemia can be detected only by measuring blood ammonia levels. When hyperammonemia is present, it may be massive. In the presence of concomitant acidosis, an organic acid disorder is likely. When the infant is alkalotic or not acidotic, a urea cycle disorder is likely. Severe liver dysfunction is the major nongenetic cause of hyperammonemia and has been seen with herpetic infections and severe shock. Transient hyperammonemia of the newborn is a rare, poorly understood condition most common in premature or stressed infants. Disorders of fatty oxidation may also present with hyperammonemia, and valproate therapy is a common reason for milder elevations. Many cases of alleged Reye syndrome are actually inborn errors of metabolism.

The diagnosis of a disorder of the urea cycle depends on measurement of ammonia, organic acids, and plasma amino acids and orotic acid. Enzymatic confirmation is recommended. Babies with ornithine transcarbamoylase deficiency are usually boys with elevated glutamine, alanine, and orotic acid. Carbamoyl phosphate synthetase deficiency causes elevated glutamine and alanine with normal orotic acid. Citrullinemia, caused by a deficiency of argininosuccinate synthetase, has markedly elevated citrulline levels, and argininosuccinic aciduria, caused by argininosuccinate lyase deficiency, has elevated citrulline and markedly elevated argininosuccinic acid. Arginine is low in all urea cycle defects except arginase deficiency.

Treatment of these disorders requires a low-protein diet and other adjunctive therapy. In all but the mildest cases, nitrogen scavengers, sodium benzoate, sodium phenylacetate, and sodium phenylbutyrate are needed to provide an alternative pathway for waste nitrogen excretion. Prompt diagnosis and recognition are necessary to prevent severe and ongoing brain damage. Dialysis is frequently required to treat coma. Nitrogen scavengers are used as rescue drugs, as well as for long-term maintenance. Despite aggressive treatment, most patients suffer repeated crises with progressive central nervous system (CNS) damage or death. For this reason, liver transplantation from a parent or unrelated donor has been used in a number of individuals with encouraging results.

Transport Disorders

Cystinuria, a disorder of dibasic amino acid transport, is an autosomal recessive disorder. The only symptom is renal stones. Cystinosis is a lysosomal storage disease (see Chapter 99).

Lysinuric protein intolerance is a rare, autosomal recessive disorder with a defect in transport of dibasic amino acids in the intestine and the kidneys. As a result, the patients become deficient in arginine, ornithine, and lysine, which are required for the urea cycle. Symptoms mimic urea cycle defects and include failure to thrive, hepatosplenomegaly, hypotonia, osteoporosis, and anemia plus immunologic defects. Problems often become obvious with weaning from breast milk and beginning a higher protein diet. Diagnosis requires measurement of urine and plasma amino acids. Treatment is dietary, and the prognosis is generally good if diagnosis is made early.

Mini-index of Related Topics

SUGGESTED READINGS

Blau N, Duran M, Blaskovics ME, Gibson KM: Physician's Guide to the Laboratory Diagnosis of Metabolic Diseases, 2nd ed. New York, Springer, 2002.

Fernandes J, Saudubray JM, van den Berghe G (eds): Inborn Metabolic Diseases, Diagnosis, and Treatment, 3rd ed. New York, Springer, 2000.

Scriver CR, Beaudet AL, Sly WS, et al: The Metabolic and Molecular Bases of Inherited Diseases, 8th ed. New York, McGraw-Hill, 2001.

SECTION 4 CHRONIC MEDICAL CARE: *Metabolic Disorders*

149 Lysosomal Storage Disorders

Gregory M. Enns and Robert D. Steiner

ROLE OF THE GENERALIST

1 Recognize the symptoms and signs suggestive of lysosomal storage disorders.

2 Obtain appropriate screening laboratory studies.

3 Arrange consultation with metabolic disease specialist for definitive diagnosis and management.

4 Refer family for genetic counseling.

5 Coordinate care with appropriate specialists.

6 Monitor head circumference, growth, development, and nutritional parameters.

7 Assist in arranging appropriate educational services and developing the individualized health plan for the child's school.

8 Monitor for the complications associated with a particular disorder, in conjunction with appropriate specialists.

9 Be aware of anesthesia risks for children undergoing surgical procedures.

10 Coordinate supportive measures and palliative care.

11 Assist in arranging hospice care if needed.

12 Provide ongoing psychological support and guidance.

Lysosomes are cytoplasmic intracellular organelles that contain a variety of hydrolytic enzymes responsible for the stepwise degradation of complex macromolecules, including glycosaminoglycans (GAGs), sphingolipids, glycoproteins, and glycogen. Lysosomal storage disorders (LSDs) are caused by dysfunction of one or more of these enzymes with resultant progressive accumulation of substrates that are normally degraded within lysosomes. When a lysosomal enzyme is deficient, the particular substrate (or substrates) degraded by a given enzyme accumulates in organs where it is synthesized, including brain, liver, spleen, and bone. Therefore, depending on the tissue specificity of the involved enzyme, various organ systems may be affected, leading to the diverse symptoms encountered in these disorders. As the stored materials increase within target cell lysosomes, impairment of the affected organs occurs.

LSDs are individually rare with incidences ranging from approximately 1 in 50,000 to disorders with only a few published case reports. Collectively, the overall incidence is estimated to be 1 in 7000 to 1 in 10,000 births. There are over 50 recognized LSDs corresponding to nearly every step in the catabolism of complex macromolecules. LSDs include mucopolysaccharide, oligosaccharide, sphingolipid, glycogen, and glycoprotein degradation disorders, disorders of transport of enzymes into lysosomes, neuronal ceroid lipofuscinoses, and defects of egress of products from the lysosomes. Classification of LSDs is based on the type of stored metabolite in a given condition. However, nomenclature may be confusing in some instances, because there are several classes of stored substance in some disorders (leading to the same disease being classified under different headings) and different names have been used for the same disorder based on historical precedent. For example, sialidosis has been referred to both as a mucolipidosis and a glycoproteinosis. The important point is that all such disorders have lysosomal dysfunction in common and are, therefore, classified as LSDs. A classification scheme and clinical features of the lysosomal storage diseases are presented in Table 149-1.

CLINICAL PRESENTATION

Although the LSDs are associated with a variety of clinical findings that may be present as early as in utero or as late as adulthood, in most cases these diseases have three characteristic clinical phases. Clinical findings are absent or

Table 149-1. Classification and Clinical Features of the Lysosomal Storage Diseases

Disorder (Type)	Enzyme Defect	Clinical Features
Mucopolysaccharidoses (MPS)		
Hurler syndrome (MPS IH)	α-L-Iduronidase	Mental retardation, coarse features, hydrocephalus, corneal clouding, organomegaly, airway disease, heart disease, hearing impairment, dysostosis multiplex*
Scheie syndrome (MPS IS)	α-L-Iduronidase	Normal intelligence, stature, and lifespan, corneal clouding, aortic valve disease, mild coarse features
Hurler-Scheie syndrome (MPS IH/S)	α-L-Iduronidase	Features intermediate between MPS IH and MPS IS
Hunter syndrome (MPS II)	Iduronate sulfatase	Mental retardation, absent corneal clouding, hearing impairment, dysostosis multiplex,* coarse features
Sanfilippo syndrome type A (MPS IIIA)	Heparan N-sulfatase	Mental retardation, relatively later onset of coarse features, relatively mild organomegaly, behavior and sleep abnormalities
Sanfilippo syndrome type B (MPS IIIB)	α-N-acetylglucosaminidase	Similar to MPS IIIA
Sanfilippo syndrome type C (MPS IIIC)	Acetyl-CoA:α-glucosaminide acetyltransferase	Similar to MPS IIIA
Sanfilippo syndrome type D (MPS IIID)	N-acetylglucosamine-6-sulfatase	Similar to MPS IIIA
Morquio syndrome type A (MPS IVA)	N-acetylgalactosamine-6-sulfatase	Normal intelligence, severe skeletal manifestations, corneal clouding, hearing impairment, atlantoaxial instability
Morquio syndrome type B (MPS IVB)	β-Galactosidase	Similar to MPS IVA
Maroteaux-Lamy syndrome (MPS VI)	N-acetylgalactosamine-4-sulfatase	Normal intelligence, corneal clouding, variable coarse features, organomegaly, heart disease, dysostosis multiplex,* spinal cord compression
Sly syndrome (MPS VII)	β-Glucuronidase	Wide range of severity, nonimmune fetal hydrops, variable severity of mental retardation, coarse features, organomegaly, dysostosis multiplex*
Hyaluronidase deficiency (MPS IX)	Hyaluronidase	Normal intelligence, short stature, nodular periarticular masses
Disorders of Lysosomal Enzyme Localization		
I-cell disease (mucolipidosis II)	N-acetylglucosamine-1-phosphotransferase	Similar to MPS I, but earlier presentation and no mucopolysacchariduria
Pseudo-Hurler polydystrophy (mucolipidosis III)	N-acetylglucosamine-1-phosphotransferase	Milder than I-cell disease
Sphingolipidoses		
GM₂ Gangliosidoses		
Type A (Tay-Sachs disease)	β-Hexosaminidase A	Rapidly progressive neurodegeneration, cherry red spot, absent organomegaly, milder forms exist, relatively common in Ashkenazi Jewish population
Type O (Sandhoff disease)	β-Hexosaminidase A and B	Similar to Tay-Sachs disease
Type AB (GM₂ activator deficiency)	GM₂ activator	Similar to Tay-Sachs disease
Niemann-Pick disease		
Type A	Sphingomyelinase	Rapidly progressive neurodegeneration, organomegaly, failure to thrive, cherry red spot, relatively common in Ashkenazi Jewish population
Type B	Sphingomyelinase	Normal intelligence, organomegaly, pulmonary disease (alveolar infiltration, dyspnea, bronchopneumonia)
Type C	Defect in cholesterol esterification	Broad clinical spectrum, progressive neurodegeneration, upward gaze palsy, variable organomegaly, fatal neonatal liver disease
Gaucher disease		
Type 1	β-Glucosidase	Normal intelligence, organomegaly, bone disease, avascular necrosis of the hip, relatively common in Ashkenazi Jewish population
Type 2	β-Glucosidase	Severe neurodegeneration, opisthotonus, organomegaly, nonimmune fetal hydrops, panethnic
Type 3	β-Glucosidase	Intermediate between types 1 and 2, prominent organomegaly, relatively common in Northern Sweden

Table 149-1. Classification and Clinical Features of the Lysosomal Storage Diseases—cont'd

Disorder (Type)	Enzyme Defect	Clinical Features
Sphingolipidoses—cont'd		
Fabry disease	α-Galactosidase A	Pain and paresthesias in extremities in childhood or adolescence, angiokeratomas,[†] renal failure, corneal and lens opacities, heart disease
Metachromatic leukodystrophy	Arylsulfatase A	Progressive neurodegeneration, late-infantile, juvenile, and adult forms, quadriparesis, blindness
Saposin B deficiency	Sulfatide activator protein	Similar to metachromatic leukodystrophy
Multiple sulfatase deficiency	Multiple sulfatases	Similar to metachromatic leukodystrophy, mucopolysaccharidosis features
Globoid cell leukodystrophy (Krabbe disease)	β-Galactocerebroside	Progressive neurodegeneration, prominent long tract signs, blindness, deafness, absent organomegaly
Farber lipogranulomatosis	Acid ceramidase	Painful joints, subcutaneous nodules, hoarseness, variable neurologic and visceral involvement
Sialic Acid Disorders		
Sialidosis (mucolipidosis I)	Neuraminidase	Variable features ranging from similar to MPS I to cherry red spot, myoclonus in adolescence
Galactosialidosis	Neuraminidase and β-Galactosidase (secondary to protective protein/cathepsin A deficiency)	Variable features including nonimmune fetal hydrops, coarse features, mental retardation, organomegaly, cherry-red spot, myoclonus
Infantile sialic acid storage disease	SLC17A5 deficiency	Coarse features, profound mental retardation, hepatosplenomegaly in infancy, panethnic
Salla disease	SLC17A5 deficiency	Mental retardation, ataxia with presentation in early childhood, relatively high incidence in Finland
Sialuria	Uridine diphosphate–N-acetylglucosamine 2-epimerase lack of feedback inhibition	Massive overexcretion of sialic acid, coarse features, hepatosplenomegaly, relatively mild intellectual impairment and skeletal involvement
Mucolipidosis IV	Mucolipin-1	Mental retardation, corneal clouding, retinal degeneration, absent organomegaly, secondary neuraminidase deficiency, relatively common in Ashkenazi Jewish population
Oligosaccharidoses (Glycoproteinoses)		
GM₁ Gangliosidosis	β-Galactosidase	Coarse features, severe psychomotor retardation, hepatosplenomegaly, blindness, failure to thrive, dysostosis multiplex,* seizures, cherry-red spot in 50% of infantile onset type
α-Mannosidosis	α-Mannosidase	Mental retardation, coarse features, organomegaly, lens and corneal opacities, dysostosis multiplex*
β-Mannosidosis	β-Mannosidase	Mental retardation, respiratory infections, hearing impairment
Fucosidosis	α-L-Fucosidase	Mental retardation, coarse features, angiokeratomas,[†] dysostosis multiplex*
Sialidosis	See Sialic Acid Disorders	See Sialic Acid Disorders
Galactosialidosis	See Sialic Acid Disorders	
Schindler disease	α-N-acetylgalactosaminidase	Variable features ranging from infantile neuroaxonal dystrophy to mild impairment, angiokeratomas[†]
Aspartylglucosaminuria	Aspartylglucosaminidase	Mental retardation, coarse features, osteoporosis, relatively common in the Finnish population
Neuronal Ceroid Lipofuscinoses (NCL)		
Infantile NCL (Santavuori-Haltia disease)	CLN1, palmitoyl-protein thioesterase deficiency	Onset after 6 months: seizures, neurologic deterioration, macular degeneration, brain atrophy, choreoathetosis
Late infantile NCL		Onset 2 to 5 years: myoclonus, ataxia, neurologic deterioration, macular degeneration +/– pigmentary retinopathy
Jansky-Bielschowsky disease	CLN2, pepinase deficiency	
Finnish variant	CLN5	
Variant/atypical variant	CLN6	
Juvenile NCL (Batten disease)	CLN3, battenin	Onset 4 to 8 years: myoclonus, macular degeneration, pigmentary retinopathy, slurred speech
Adult NCL (Kufs disease)	Unknown	Onset in adolescence or adulthood: myoclonus, psychosis
Other Lysosomal Storage Disorders		
Wolman disease	Acid lipase	Hepatomegaly, steatorrhea, adrenal calcification, usually fatal before 1 year
Cholesterol ester storage disease	Acid lipase	More mild disorder than Wolman disease
Cystinosis	Cystinosin	Most common cause of renal Fanconi syndrome in childhood, growth failure, rickets, retinopathy, corneal crystals
Pycnodysostosis	Cathepsin K	Dysmorphic appearance, short stature, osteosclerosis, pathologic fractures
Pompe disease (glycogen storage disease type II)	α-Glucosidase (acid maltase)	Cardiomegaly, hypotonia, early demise, more mild forms with proximal weakness also exist

*Multiple skeletal abnormalities apparent on radiographs (see text).
†Punctate, dark red to blue telangiectasias.

Estimates of the prevalence of growth hormone deficiency are highly varied, with frequencies reported from 1:350,000 to 1:3500 children. Growth hormone deficiency is usually idiopathic, but may be accompanied by multiple anterior and some posterior pituitary hormone deficiencies. It is occasionally associated with inheritable deletions/ mutations of the Prop-1 or Pit-1 genes, with midbrain malformations including septo-optic dysplasia, with spina bifida, or with clinical findings including palatal clefts, double hair whorls, and single central incisor. Congenital growth hormone deficiency may present with antenatal or postnatal linear growth failure. While linear growth velocity is an important diagnostic clue, some patients with demonstrable deletions in the growth hormone gene may present with normal velocity but with stature more than 2 standard deviations below the mean for family.

Recently, hypothalamic growth hormone deficiency has been described in up to 80% of patients with Prader-Willi syndrome. A combination of growth hormone deficiency/ resistance has been recognized in a significant number of patients born small for gestational age who fail to achieve normal growth percentiles by age 2 years.

Some patients with congenital growth hormone deficiency may not present until later childhood. All patients with acquired growth hormone deficiency present in later childhood. Acquired growth hormone deficiency may be isolated or may occur in conjunction with other pituitary hormone deficiencies, and can be the result of central nervous system (CNS) tumor, trauma, hypoxia, CNS irradiation, or chemotherapy. The effects of trauma or hypoxia may not be apparent for several years. The loss of pituitary function after irradiation may not appear for decades. Because acquired growth hormone deficiency may occur at the time of expected onset of puberty and, especially in conjunction with hypogonadotropic hypogonadisim, may mimic constitutional delay of growth and adolescence, clinicians must be vigilant to avoid misdiagnosing patients with significant CNS or other occult disease.

Initial screening for growth hormone deficiency requires the exclusion of chronic disease, hypothyroidism, and chromosomal abnormality (Turner syndrome). Because growth hormone is released intermittently, random growth hormone levels are of no diagnostic value. Instead, insulin-like growth factor 1 (IGF-1) and insulin-like growth factor binding protein 3 (IGF BP-3) should be measured. Unfortunately, IGF-1 may be suppressed in poorly nourished patients, and overlap between the normal and abnormal ranges is considerable, especially in younger children. A study of 201 children (average age 9.9 +/– 4.2 years), using –2 standard deviations as the lower limit of normal, found IGF-1 had a sensitivity of 34% and specificity of 72% with a positive predictive value of 22%. In this study IGF BP-3 had a sensitivity of 22% and specificity of 92% and a positive predictive value of 52%. Thus, although low levels strongly suggest growth hormone deficiency, normal IGF-1 and IGF BP-3 levels should not be used to exclude growth hormone deficiency when other clinical and laboratory findings are present. Emotionally deprived or severely undernourished children can also have the biochemical appearance of growth hormone deficiency.

Ultimately, the diagnosis is reached using a combination of growth and laboratory data, and interpretation of growth hormone stimulation testing. Patients with suspected growth hormone deficiency or insensitivity should be referred to an endocrinologist. An endocrinologist should direct the evaluation and the possible use of growth hormone therapy for patients with Turner syndrome, Prader-Willi syndrome, those who were small for gestational age, and patients with chronic renal failure and other diagnoses that require high-dose steroid therapy.

The one consistent symptom of glucocorticoid excess in growing children is linear growth failure. Because many patients with exogenous Cushing syndrome are neurasthenic, they may fail to demonstrate the classic Cushing phenotype. Primary care providers should remain alert to the possibility of Cushing syndrome, especially of iatrogenic origin.

Disorders of puberty can result in linear growth failure. Hypogonadism may accompany pituitary failure or may occur in isolation and may mimic constitutional delay. True isosexual central precocious puberty or conditions that mimic it (congenital adrenal hyperplasia, McCune-Albright syndrome) may result in premature epiphyseal fusion and, despite tall stature for age when young, may ultimately lead to short adult stature. The most severely affected children are those with CNS injury that results in combined growth hormone deficiency and sexual precocity. Because these patients frequently maintain normal growth velocity at the expense of a rapidly advancing bone age, the clinician can be mistakenly reassured. Most commonly these patients have a history of trauma, including surgery, irradiation, or spina bifida. A similar clinical picture may occur in the obese child whose secondary hyperinsulinism results in premature epiphyseal fusion.

Tall Stature

The most frequent cause of tall stature is benign familial polygenic inheritance, but children with genetic abnormalities resulting in tall stature must be recognized. Although children with Marfan syndrome who have the classic findings of arachnodactyly and superior lens dislocation may be easily spotted, some patients may present with familial autosomal dominant tall stature and double-jointedness. Making the diagnosis requires a very focused examination with specific criteria. Homocystinosis with developmental delay and metabolic abnormalities and Sotos' syndrome with macrocephaly are more easily recognized.

Children with sexual precocity or pseudoprecocity may initially present with tall stature. Androgen insensitivity may also mimic genetic tall stature. These patients may present with partial masculinization, with labial masses, or as tall adolescent girls who fail to develop pubic hair or to menstruate. Finally, patients with growth hormone excess/ gigantism may present with linear growth acceleration with or without the stigmata of acromegaly.

DIAGNOSTIC EVALUATION

The initial evaluation of the patient with abnormal linear growth is clearly the task of the primary care provider. These providers should initiate the diagnostic evaluation by recognizing clinical signs and symptoms associated with the varying etiologies of tall and short stature, reviewing the details of history and physical examination as suggested, and by performing the appropriate laboratory evaluation and then referring to the appropriate specialist for completion or confirmation of that evaluation. Although the long-term management of such conditions as chronic renal failure, inflammatory bowel disease, celiac disease, Turner syndrome, and growth hormone deficiency are usually the province of the specialist, their recognition falls to the primary care provider, who should ultimately coordinate the care provided by different specialists.

History

Although the differential diagnosis of short stature is lengthy, and laboratory investigations may ultimately prove to be complex, the primary care provider has an excellent opportunity to screen patients by means of a short list of questions (Box 150-4). Careful measurement and the accumulation of appropriate growth data may readily answer the first four questions. The gathering of family health and growth history data may require a bit more detective work and may be facilitated by sending parents home with an appropriate family questionnaire (Questions 5 through 9). Questions 10 through 13 can be addressed in the course of a routine physical examination. In the case of question 13 the family or pediatric care provider has an opportunity to assess family dynamics that is rarely afforded the specialist.

Physical Examination

When measurement or history suggests a growth problem, the primary care provider should perform a thorough examination that searches for the key physical findings enumerated in Table 150-1. These clinical findings are helpful in pinpointing for the cause of short stature, but their presence or absence is by no means conclusive.

Laboratory Evaluation

A child who is unusually short or tall for family, or who is accelerating or decelerating across growth percentiles, warrants laboratory investigation. For the short child, initial assessment for chronic disease should be performed promptly with the tests indicated in Box 150-5. In addition, history and physical examination may prompt other more specific tests outlined in Box 150-6. Once a specific diagnosis is entertained, referral to the appropriate specialist for

confirmation and assistance with management should be considered. Sometimes a diagnosis may not be as simple as its initial presentation suggests. Renal tubular acidosis may be the presenting symptom of Fanconi syndrome. Secondary hypothyroidism may be the presenting symptom of panhypopituitarism with or without a brain tumor.

Evaluation of the patient with tall stature is somewhat more difficult. A patient who is unusually tall for family or who, after the age of 2 years, is accelerating across growth percentiles should be evaluated for sexual precocity and conditions that mimic it (congenital adrenal hyperplasia).

Table 150-1. Noteworthy Physical Findings in Growth Disorders*

System	Finding
Head, eyes, ears, nose, throat	Microcephaly/macrocephaly
	Double or anterior hair whorl
	Small optic disk (septo-optic dysplasia)
	Visual impairment/abnormal visual fields (septo-optic dysplasia, tumor)
	Roving nystagmus
	High arched palate/central incisor (midline defect)
	Delayed/advanced puberty
	High arched/cleft palate (midline defect, a syndrome)
	Hypertelorism (midline defect, a syndrome)
	Hypernasal voice (growth hormone deficiency)
	Midface hypoplasia (syndrome or growth hormone deficiency)
	Cherubic faces (growth hormone deficiency)
Neck	Webbing (Turner syndrome)
	Goiter (hypothyroidism)
Thoracic	Pectus deformity
Cardiovascular	Hypertension
	Murmur
	Cyanosis
Abdominal	Distention
	Hepatomegaly
	Splenomegaly
	Pain
	Marasmus
Genitourinary	Tanner stage
Musculoskeletal	Abnormal upper to lower segment ratio
	Increased carrying angle
	Clinodactyly

*It is vital to recognize that these findings should raise suspicion but that their presence or absence is by no means conclusive.

Box 150-4. Useful Screening Questions for Growth Disorders

1. How tall is the child?
2. How long was the child at birth?
3. Is the child short for family or population?
4. How much does the child weigh?
5. How much did the child weigh at birth?
6. What is the child's growth velocity?
7. How tall are the parents?
8. Are the parents healthy?
9. What was the timing of the parents' puberty?
10. What is the patient's dental age?
11. Is the patient's growth proportionate?
12. Is there evidence of a syndrome?
13. Is there evidence of deprivation?

Box 150-5. Initial Laboratory Assessment for Short Stature

Chronic Disease Screening

Complete blood count with differential
Erythrocyte sedimentation rate (ESR)
Electrolytes, blood urea nitrogen (BUN), creatinine
Calcium, magnesium, phosphate
Liver function tests
Glucose
T_4, thyroid-stimulating hormone (TSH)
IgA/IgA tissue transglutaminase antibodies

Tests Indicated from History and Physical Examination

Sweat chloride
IgG subclasses
Renal ultrasound

154 Disorders of the Adrenal Glands

Nicholas Jospe

CONGENITAL ADRENAL HYPERPLASIA

Fundamentals

Congenital adrenal hyperplasia (CAH) is a group of autosomal recessive disorders with a deficiency of one of the enzymes necessary for cortisol synthesis by the adrenal cortex. The enzymatic defect results in increased adrenocorticotropic hormone (ACTH) secretion. The increased ACTH causes adrenal hyperplasia and overproduction of the adrenal precursors proximal to the enzyme block, and deficiency of the adrenal steroids distal to the disrupted enzymatic step (Fig. 154-1). Although several enzymes are necessary for steroid synthesis, 90% of cases are caused by deficiency of 21-hydroxylase enzymatic activity.

Virilization is the hallmark of 21-hydroxylase deficiency and is caused by excessive adrenal androgen production, most markedly of androstenedione, and its peripheral conversion to testosterone. Virilization can present in newborns with ambiguity of the external genitalia, in later childhood with early pubarche, or in mild cases, in early adulthood with hirsutism. Complete deficiency of 21-hydroxylase activity causes the "classic," or severe form of the disorder that presents infancy with simple virilizing (25%) or salt-wasting (75%) forms. Partial deficiency of 21-hydroxylase activity, the "nonclassic" form, is milder, without ambiguous genitalia, and presents later in childhood or young adulthood. Other forms of CAH result from deficiency of different enzyme activities within the adrenal gland, and can cause virilization in affected female fetuses (enzyme activities 4 and 5 in Fig. 154-1) or undervirilization of affected male fetuses (enzyme activities 1, 2, 3, or 8 in Fig. 154-1).

Immediate recognition of severe CAH is crucial. The most crucial clinical issues are the potential for death within the first few weeks of life from the addisonian crisis (shock, hypotension, and hypoglycemia following days or weeks of failure to thrive and weakness) and salt-losing crisis, with hyponatremia and hyperkalemia that are not present at birth but evolve over days and weeks. An increasing number of states are screening for 21-hydroxylase deficiency. Screening can identify infants at risk for adrenal salt-losing crisis and identify incorrect male gender assignment in very virilized female fetuses.

Presentation and Initial Evaluation
Classic or Severe 21-Hydroxylase Deficiency

Table 154-1 highlights clinical signs that may indicate CAH in the newborn. The practitioner must always suspect the severe classic form of CAH in any newborn with ambiguity of the external genitalia (Fig. 154-2). Because the appearance of the genitalia is not diagnostic, any newborn with these findings should be urgently evaluated for CAH. The diagnosis must also be suspected in a male infant who presents at a few weeks of age with dehydration, shock, failure to thrive, vomiting, spitting up, or formula changes without relief of symptoms, and hyponatremia (Na < 130 mg/dL) with hyperkalemia (K > 6 mg/dL). No other disorder presents with this combination of electrolyte abnormalities. Because of the ambiguity of the external genitalia (clitoromegaly, partial posterior fusion labioscrotal folds, single urogenital sinus), the diagnosis of 21-hydroxylase deficiency is usually made prior to a salt-losing crisis in female infants. Although newborn screening for CAH will detect the deficiency, screening is not universal. Practitioners must remain attentive to this possible diagnosis in male infants.

The hallmarks of the salt-losing crisis are vomiting, lethargy, shock, severe hyponatremia, hyperkalemia, and acidosis. Infants with pyloric stenosis, another cause of vomiting in the neonatal period, usually present with hyponatremia and hypokalemia. Other features include increased pigmentation of skin creases and genitalia, particularly the labia majora or scrotum.

If CAH is suspected, referral to a pediatric endocrinologist for assistance in diagnosis is recommended. Serum 17-hydroxyprogesterone and androstenedione are useful for initial evaluation by the generalist, but careful attention must be paid to age- and gender-specific norms in

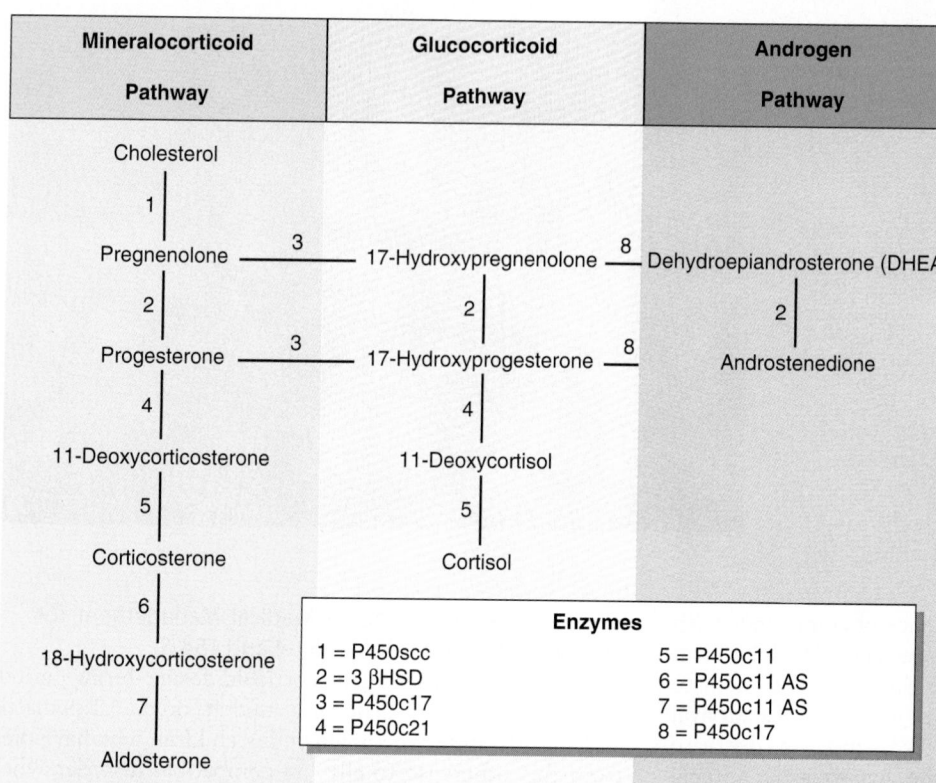

Mineralocorticoid Pathway	Glucocorticoid Pathway	Androgen Pathway

Cholesterol

1

Pregnenolone —— 3 —— 17-Hydroxypregnenolone —— 8 —— Dehydroepiandrosterone (DHEA)

2   2   2

Progesterone —— 3 —— 17-Hydroxyprogesterone —— 8 —— Androstenedione

4   4

11-Deoxycorticosterone   11-Deoxycortisol

5   5

Corticosterone   Cortisol

6

18-Hydroxycorticosterone

7

Aldosterone

Enzymes

1 = P450scc	5 = P450c11
2 = 3 βHSD	6 = P450c11 AS
3 = P450c17	7 = P450c11 AS
4 = P450c21	8 = P450c17

Figure 154-1. Adrenal steroidogenesis.

interpreting values. Electrolytes must be carefully followed. They are normal in the first days of life but trend toward hyponatremia and hyperkalemia within 5 to 10 days when salt loss is present. The specialist will conduct an ACTH stimulation test. The diagnosis is confirmed by demonstrating markedly elevated baseline and ACTH-stimulated levels of serum 17-hydroxyprogesterone. Baseline androstenedione, and dehydroxyepiandrosterone (DHEAS) and testosterone will also be measured. Plasma renin activity is also elevated.

Table 154-1. Indications of "Classic" or Severe 21-Hydroxylase Deficiency

Females
Ambiguous genitalia
Clitoromegaly
Partial posterior fusion labioscrotal folds
Single urogenital sinus
Signs of salt-losing (see below) if present

Males
Dehydration and/or shock
Failure to thrive
Vomiting, spitting up or formula changes without relief of symptoms
Hyponatremia (Na < 130 mg/dL) with hyperkalemia (K > 6 mg/dL)

Salt-Losing Type
Vomiting
Lethargy
Shock
Severe hyponatremia (Na < 130 mg/dL)
Hyperkalemia (K > 6 mg/dL)
Acidosis

Milder Nonclassic 21-Hydroxylase Deficiency

Table 154-2 highlights signs of the milder nonclassic form of 21-hydroxylase deficiency. CAH should be suspected with a postnatal presentation of androgen excess. Clinical signs are male penile or female clitoral enlargement, and in both genders, accelerated height gain with tall stature in childhood relative to genetic growth potential, acne, early onset of pubic hair and axillary hair, advanced skeletal maturation, and hirsutism. Later features in girls include masculinized body habitus, temporal hairline recession, amenorrhea, infertility, and polycystic ovary syndrome (PCOS). Adolescent girls or young adult women may present with disordered puberty and infertility. Skeletal maturation measured by bone age exceeds the height age advancement. Ultimate stature in undiagnosed or inadequately treated children is shorter than expected for the genetic target.

Referral to a pediatric endocrinologist is recommended whenever a patient has signs of androgen excess. Laboratory studies demonstrate normal or mildly elevated baseline levels of serum 17-hydroxyprogesterone and supranormal ACTH-stimulated 17-hydroxyprogesterone. A single determination of androstenedione, and DHEAS and testosterone will also be moderately elevated.

Management

Severe Classic Congenital Adrenal Hyperplasia

The generalist must pay meticulous attention to coordinating the care of children with this disorder (Table 154-3). Following diagnosis, patients should be referred to a tertiary care center and a pediatric endocrinologist. Families must be thoroughly educated regarding whom to call and what to

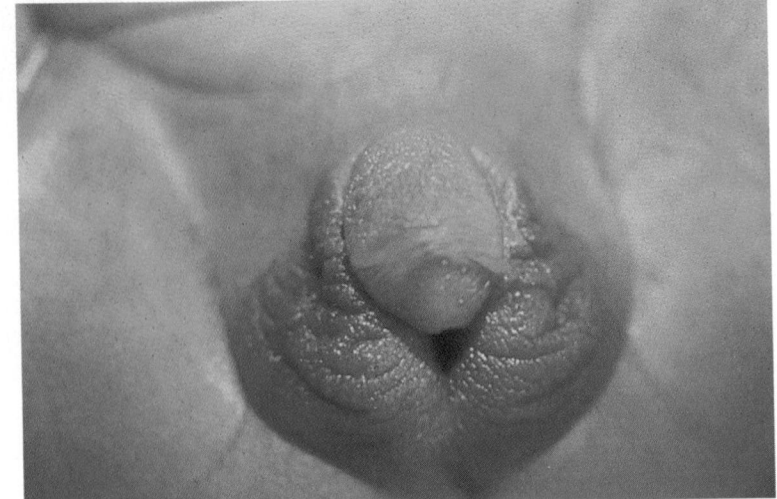

Figure 154-2. Ambiguity of the genitalia secondary to congenital adrenal hyperplasia.

do for acute illness and the importance of compliance with follow-up and treatment with the specialist. The long-term goals of therapy are highlighted in Box 154-1. Immediate goals in infancy and early childhood are to ensure survival and provide precise glucocorticoid therapy to decrease ACTH, appropriately suppress the hyperplastic adrenal gland, and stop the overproduction of adrenal androgens. Usually, hydrocortisone (10 to 20 mg/m² per 24 hours) is administered orally in three divided doses. The doses must be individualized with frequent adjustments in dosage because of growth and immediate attention to periods of stress. Overtreatment results in relative obesity and growth retardation; undertreatment results in progressive virilization and bone age advancement. Although virtually all affected subjects require therapy with glucocorticoid, only those with the salt-losing form of CAH require mineralocorticoid therapy. This therapy is provided as 9α-fluorohydrocortisone (0.05 to 0.3 mg daily) and oral sodium chloride (1 to 3 g). Ongoing care, commonly managed by the specialist, requires measuring 17-hydroxyprogesterone, androstenedione, and plasma renin activity. The 17-hydroxyprogesterone level should not be suppressed to normal levels, but to levels at which androstenedione (and testosterone) are also in the normal range for age.

Table 154-2. Signs and Symptoms of Mild or Nonclassical Congenital Adrenal Hyperplasia by Age of Onset

Age	Sign
Infancy through late childhood males	Penile enlargement
Infancy through late childhood females	Clitoral enlargement
Early through late childhood	Accelerated height gain
Late childhood	Acne
Early through late childhood	Early onset of pubic hair and axillary hair
Early adolescence to adulthood	Amenorrhea or oligomenorrhea
Adulthood in females	Masculinized body habitus females, infertility, polycystic ovary syndrome, temporal hairline recession

Severe Classic Form: Acute Medical Management for Intercurrent Illness (Tables 154-4 and 154-5)

The need for increased glucocorticoid dosing during periods of stress cannot be sufficiently underscored. All pediatric endocrinologists have known young children who have died from this otherwise totally life-compatible disorder when insufficient attention has been paid to stress and the need for increasing the replacement dosage of glucocorticoids. The primary care provider usually will be called first regarding acute illness and stress management. Mild stress,

Table 154-3. Management of Classic Congenital Adrenal Hyperplasia

Category	Specific Management
Coordination of care	Newborn: initial referral for assistance in diagnosis
	Referral to pediatric endocrinologist and tertiary care center for long-term management of condition
	Assist pediatric endocrinologist with referral and follow-up for patients who require surgical intervention
	Communicate regularly with specialists
Parent education	Instruct parents as follows:
	Whom to call when child is sick
	What to do in an emergency
	Importance of regular health maintenance visits
	Importance of regular follow-up with specialist
	Adherence
Acute illness	Adequately treat stress (see Box 154-3)
	Treat underlying illness appropriately
	Consult pediatric endocrinologist regularly for any questions regarding treatment of acute illness
	Refer patients who are not responding adequately to treatment
Health maintenance	Ensure immunization, including pneumococcal and annual influenza
	Regularly monitor growth and provide growth data to pediatric endocrinologist
	Monitor adherence with long-term treatment
	Carefully follow development

Box 154-1. Goals of Therapy for Classic Congenital Adrenal Hyperplasia

- To achieve normal growth
- To achieve normal pubertal development
- To achieve normal sexual function
- To discuss establishment of a satisfactory gender identity
- To discuss fertility issues

such as a simple upper respiratory infection (URI), requires no intervention. Moderate stress, such as an upper respiratory infection with fever, or mild gastroenteritis, requires doubling the glucocorticoid doses. Severe stress from illness managed on an outpatient basis (mild dehydration from gastroenteritis, pneumonia) requires tripling to quintupling of the usual doses. Any concerns regarding inadequacy of oral absorption from vomiting, diarrhea, or ileus should prompt the practitioner to institute parenteral hydrocortisone, using doses of 30 to 50 mg/m^2/day in four divided doses. The families need to have parenteral hydrocortisone at home, and must be familiar with intramuscular injection or else live virtually within minutes of the practitioner's office. Table 154-5 lists recommendations for glucocorticoid and mineralocorticoid therapy for adrenal insufficiency and hypocortisolemia under a variety of conditions.

Severe Classic Form: Surgical Management

Female infants with ambiguity of the external genitalia require surgical consultation with a pediatric surgeon, gynecologist, or urologist for discussion and management. The overall surgical goal is reduction clitoroplasty that reduces the clitoris (not a clitorectomy), and vaginoplasty with correction of the urogenital sinus. Figure 154-3 shows pre- and postsurgical reduction clitoroplasty. Controversies about genitoplasty in affected female infants make it difficult for families to feel comfortable with decisions regarding constructive surgery. The primary care provider will need to assist families in these matters. Helpful information can be obtained from the Intersex Society of North America website http://www.isna.org.

Table 154-4. Management of Acute Illness in Children with Congenital Adrenal Hyperplasia

Degree of Illness	Treatment
Mild stress (URI, immunization)	No intervention
Moderate stress (URI with fever, otitis media, mild gastroenteritis)	Double glucocorticoid dose
Severe stress, but manageable as outpatient (pneumonia, gastroenteritis with mild dehydration)	Triple to quintuple glucocorticoid dose
Severe stress with concerns about absorption of glucocorticoid (vomiting, diarrhea with moderate dehydration, ileus)	Parenteral hydrocortisone*

*Note that all parents should have parenteral hydrocortisone at home and know how to give an intramuscular injection or should live within minutes of care source.
URI, upper respiratory infection.

Table 154-5. Therapy for Adrenal Insufficiency/Hypocortisolemia

Circumstance	Medication Dose
Usual glucocorticoid maintenance therapy	PO hydrocortisone (10 to 20 mg/m^2 per 24 hours) in 3 divided doses
Usual glucocorticoid maintenance therapy in older adolescents and adults	PO dexamethasone 0.5 (0.25–0.75) mg
Usual glucocorticoid maintenance therapy	PO prednisone 4 mg/m^2/24 hours in 2 divided doses
Usual mineralocorticoid maintenance therapy	9α-fluorohydrocortisone (0.05 to 0.3 mg daily)
Salt supplementation in infancy	Sodium chloride (1 to 3 g)
Moderate stress glucocorticoid replacement when PO route unreliable	IM hydrocortisone 30–50 mg/m^2/day in 4 divided doses
Severe stress glucocorticoid replacement when PO route unreliable	IM hydrocortisone 50–75 mg/m^2/day in 4 divided doses
At all times, once independent	Medic-Alert tag or bracelet or necklace or wallet card

IM, intramuscular; PO, by mouth.

Nonclassic Form: Medical and Surgical Management

Diagnosis and therapy are needed to preclude any further bone age advancement in childhood. Therapy is also indicated to prevent development of severe acne, hirsutism, menstrual irregularities, and infertility. In childhood, oral hydrocortisone is required. After puberty, single daily therapy with oral dexamethasone, 0.5 mg daily in the evening, may be possible. The risk from the stress of undercurrent illness is much less in this form of CAH. Female subjects with milder nonclassic 21-hydroxylase deficiency do not require surgical treatment unless clitoromegaly is severe or the posterior labia majora are fused.

Outcome

CAH is a completely life-compatible disorder and longevity should be normal. With the appropriate attention to monitoring and dosage adjustment by the specialist, the outcome in CAH is excellent. Monitoring for signs of cortisol excess includes attention to reduced growth and increased weight gain (subtle features of Cushing syndrome) and for signs of androgen excess (pubertal development with signs of adrenarche). Osseous maturation by bone assessment should be determined annually. Glucocorticoid therapy must be continued indefinitely in all patients who have the classic forms of CAH. Surgical correction is most often performed within the first year of life.

Follow-up

Short stature can occur in affected subjects who are undiagnosed or are diagnosed as having CAH but are inadequately treated or who have not adequately adhered to treatment. Disordered puberty, menstrual irregularity, infertility, and difficulty with sexual function may occur as a consequence of inadequate adherence. In young adulthood, surgical revision of vaginoplasty may be necessary if

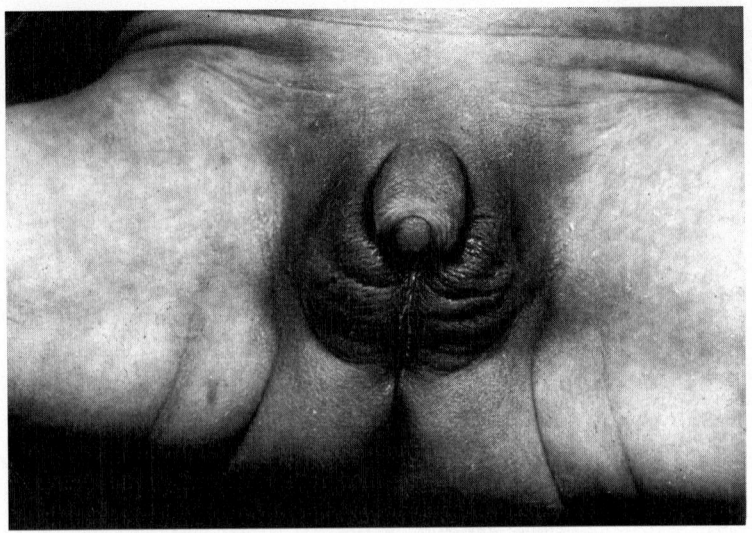

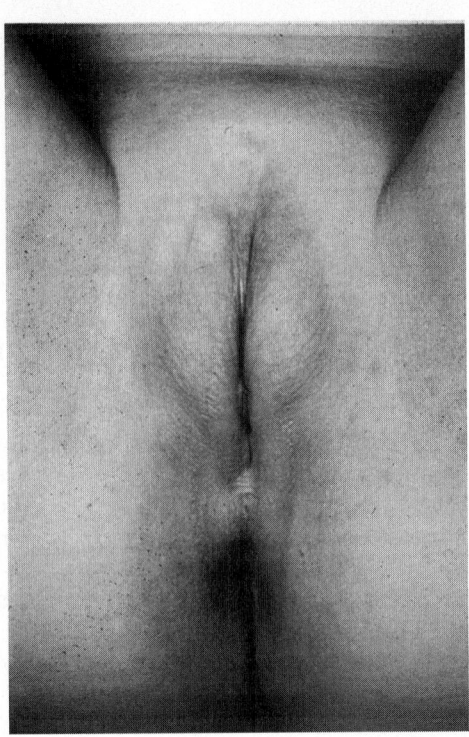

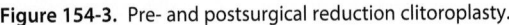
Figure 154-3. Pre- and postsurgical reduction clitoroplasty.

the initial vaginal reconstruction is considered inadequate. Cross-gender development and gender change from female to male have been reported.

Once a child is diagnosed with CAH, future pregnancies in the family can be monitored. Prenatal therapy, while experimental, is available. Prenatal administration of glucocorticoids to the mother will reduce the virilization of the external genitalia of any affected female fetus. Prior to becoming pregnant again, a mother can be referred to a research center or tertiary care center for discussion regarding the 1:4 risk of having another affected fetus (and thus 1:8 for an affected female fetus) and discussion regarding prenatal therapy. CAH can be rapidly and reliably diagnosed prenatally by gene analysis.

ADRENAL HYPOFUNCTION

Adrenal hypofunction is adrenal insufficiency or hypocortisolemia. Hypocortisolemia may be relative or absolute, depending on the level of endogenous glucocorticoid secretion by the adrenal gland. Hypocortisolemia may result from loss of adrenal function (primary hypocortisolemia) or from lack of pituitary ACTH stimulation to the adrenal gland (secondary hypocortisolemia). Adrenal insufficiency also includes deficiency of mineralocorticoid secretion.

Fundamentals

The most common cause of adrenal insufficiency is suppression of hypothalamic-pituitary-adrenal function by chronic administration of pharmacologic doses of glucocorticoids (Table 154-6). Patients are at jeopardy if adequate stress doses of glucocorticoids are not provided or if a patient who has been suppressed has not received an appropriate weaning schedule. Inhaled corticosteroids cause little adrenal suppression, and although they may have long-term

effects on bone and growth, their use does not raise the concern of acute adrenal insufficiency.

Adrenal insufficiency can be secondary to hypopituitarism, which may be congenital in the newborn or follow a catastrophic CNS event such as intraventricular hemorrhage. Adrenal hypoplasia is a rare familial condition in which the adult adrenal cortex does not develop normally. In children and adolescents, primary adrenal insufficiency usually results from autoimmune destruction of the adrenal cortex. Autoimmune adrenal insufficiency is commonly associated with other autoimmune entities in the polyglandular syndrome and can be coupled with any of the following: hypoparathyroidism, autoimmune thyroid disease (hyper- or hypothyroidism), diabetes mellitus, atrophic gastritis, pernicious anemia, and chronic mucocutaneous candidiasis. Adrenal insufficiency can be secondary to infectious agents, acquired immunodeficiency syndrome (AIDS), or hemorrhage. Adrenoleukodystrophy and adrenomyeloneuropathy are rare causes of adrenal insufficiency. Adrenoleukodystrophy presents with progressive neurologic dysfunction and primary adrenal insufficiency and progresses rapidly to dementia, mental retardation, blindness, and quadriplegia. Adrenomyeloneuropathy begins in adolescence and early adulthood with weakness, spasticity,

Table 154-6. Glucocorticoid Therapy That Can Lead to Adrenal Suppression*

Therapy with more than 25 mg/m²/day oral hydrocortisone for more than 3 weeks or 0.7–1 mg/kg/day
Therapy with more than 12 mg/m²/day parenteral hydrocortisone for more than 3 weeks or 0.3–0.5 mg/kg/day
Therapy with more than 4–6 mg/m²/day oral prednisone for more than 3 weeks, or 0.1–0.15 mg/kg/day on average
Therapy with any dose of dexamethasone for more than 3 weeks

*Note that patients who are suppressed require weaning over 4 to 6 weeks.

and distal polyneuropathy. Secondary adrenal hypofunction may also follow from hypopituitarism in childhood or adolescence. Drugs such as ketoconazole may induce a degree of relative hypocortisolemia.

Presentation and Initial Evaluation of Glucocorticoid Deficiency

Adrenal insufficiency must be considered in the differential diagnosis when a patient presents with symptoms of weakness, fatigue, weight loss, or gastrointestinal complaints. Signs and symptoms include failure to thrive, postural hypotension, a decreased sense of well-being, gastrointestinal disturbances, anorexia, nausea, vomiting, abdominal pain, weakness, fatigue, lethargy, confusion or coma, and abnormal glucose metabolism (low). Patients with adrenal insufficiency consistently have chronic malaise, lassitude, fatigability, weakness, weight loss, and anorexia. They may have increased pigmentation on the backs of hands, elbows, and knees, hand creases, buccal mucosa, genitalia, umbilicus, axillae, and nipples. Scars and freckles may be especially pigmented. Exposed areas of the skin are the most intensely affected. Failure of a suntan to disappear may be the first clue to the condition. Buccal mucosa pigmentation is usually bluish brown.

Because men derive most of their androgens from the testes, adrenal androgen deficiency is evident only in women, manifesting with decreased pubic and axillary hair and decreased libido. Decreased adrenal epinephrine secretion may contribute to postprandial hypoglycemia. The lack of cortisol negative feedback increases hypothalamic corticotropin-releasing hormone (CRH) and arginine vasopressin (AVP) synthesis and secretion, leading to increased synthesis and secretion of pituitary ACTH and other proopiomelanocortin (POMC)-related peptides: this induces increased pigmentation visible as noted previously.

If the generalist suspects adrenal hypofunction, then blood cortisol, ACTH, and renin can be measured in blood. Cortisol is low (and will not increase normally with acute or chronic ACTH stimulation) and ACTH and renin levels are high. All patients with abnormal tests should be referred to a tertiary care center for short ACTH stimulation test

Presentation and Initial Evaluation of Mineralocorticoid Deficiency

Decreased renal potassium and hydrogen ion excretion and reduced sodium retention are characteristic findings of mineralocorticoid deficiency. Contraction of intravascular volume, hypotension, and dehydration are observed. Electrolyte abnormalities, hyponatremia, and hyperkalemia present as intense salt craving. Volume depletion is compounded by reduced peripheral vascular adrenergic tone from glucocorticoid deficiency and can lead to vascular collapse and shock. Hyperkalemia from potassium retention can cause cardiac arrhythmias and death. A mild acidosis contributes to the hyperkalemia from the potassium shift from the intracellular to the extracellular space. Azotemia and hypercalcemia may also be present.

Laboratory tests should include electrolytes, plasma renin and aldosterone, and urinary electrolytes. Hyponatremia and hyperkalemia are evident, along with increased plasma renin and decreased aldosterone. Urinary excretion of sodium and chloride is increased; urinary potassium is decreased.

Management

The management of adrenal hypofunction includes replacement of glucocorticoids and mineralocorticoid (see Table 154-5) with particular attention to risk for adrenal crisis.

Acute Care Management

Adrenal crisis is a life-threatening emergency that requires immediate and appropriate treatment. Fluid resuscitation includes 0.9% saline solution or 5% dextrose in saline to reverse hypotension and electrolyte abnormalities. Dexamethasone sodium phosphate or a soluble form of injectable cortisol (e.g., hydrocortisone sodium succinate) should be injected intravenously immediately (see Table 154-5). Dexamethasone is preferred, because its effect lasts 12 to 24 hours and it does not interfere with measurement of plasma or urinary steroids during subsequent ACTH stimulation tests. Because dexamethasone has no mineralocorticoid activity, it does not provide adequate protection against hyponatremia and hyperkalemia in cases of total adrenal hypofunction.

Long-term Management

Patients need to know (1) the nature of their hormonal deficit and the rationale for replacement therapy, (2) their maintenance medications, (3) how to change their medications during minor illnesses, (4) when to consult their primary care practitioner or their specialist, and (5) when and how to inject parenteral glucocorticoid for emergencies.

Outcome

The potential outcome for patients who are appropriately diagnosed and managed is excellent, with normal longevity.

Follow-up

The specialist will monitor skeletal maturation by bone age determination, and will adjust replacement and emergency medications based on body surface area and by monitoring for any of the signs and symptoms of overtreatment and undertreatment, such as height and weight gain.

ADRENAL HYPERFUNCTION

Fundamentals

The hallmark of hyperfunction of the adrenal cortex (Cushing syndrome) is abnormally high blood levels of endogenous cortisol. This exceedingly rare syndrome most often results from an adrenocortical tumor. More than 50% of cortical tumors occur in children 3 years of age or younger, and 85% occur in children 7 years or younger. These tumors often overproduce other steroids (androgens, or estrogens, or aldosterone). Other causes of hypercortisolism include ACTH-independent Cushing syndrome with nodular hyperplasia and adenoma formation. In older children, ACTH-dependent Cushing syndrome may present with bilateral adrenal hyperplasia from pituitary adenomas (microadenomas). The most frequent cause of Cushing syndrome is prolonged therapy with exogenous ACTH or glucocorticoids.

Presentation and Evaluation

The common findings of Cushing syndrome in children are generalized rather than centripetal obesity and slowed or arrested linear growth. A decline in height velocity is often the first indication of glucocorticoid excess. Obesity with maintenance of height gain or tall stature is almost incompatible with a diagnosis of Cushing syndrome. Other features of the cushingoid phenotype are facial fat accumulation leading to a moon face, a buffalo hump, loss of subcutaneous fat, and purple striae. In older children, weakness is common. Psychiatric symptoms occur in more than half of the patients. Some patients appear euphoric or manic, particularly during the early course of the disease. School performance can deteriorate, while other subjects tend to be tireless overachievers, often ranking near the top of their class in school. An adrenocortical tumor must be considered if any of the following signs and symptoms are present: hirsutism, hypertrichosis on the face and trunk, pubic hair, acne, deepening of the voice, and enlargement of the clitoris in girls. These signs and symptoms in any child under age 6 warrant immediate referral. In addition to excessive cortisol secretion, adrenocortical tumors may produce excess androgens, thereby offsetting the growth arresting features of glucocorticoids and allowing near preservation of height gain. Hypertension is common.

Initial Evaluation

The initial laboratory test by the generalist is serum cortisol or urinary excretion of cortisol. In Cushing syndrome, the diurnal rhythm of cortisol secretion is lost, and cortisol levels in the evening are usually elevated. Urinary excretion of free cortisol may be measured, and is almost always increased in Cushing syndrome above normal values of 20 to 90 µg/24 hours. Urinary excretion of cortisol metabolites, the 17-hydroxycorticosteroids, is usually increased (>5 mg/m^2/24 hours). In questionable cases, a single-dose dexamethasone suppression test may be helpful. A dose of 0.3 mg/m^2 given at 11 P.M. should result in a fall in plasma cortisol level to less than 5 µg/dL the next morning in normal children.

Magnetic resonance imaging (MRI) with gadolinium is the method of choice for investigating for pituitary adenomas. Further studies to determine whether Cushing syndrome is ACTH-dependent or -independent, usually within the purview of the specialist, include corticotropin-releasing hormone (CRH) testing and the two-step dexamethasone suppression test. Likewise limited to specialty centers is bilateral inferior petrosal blood sampling to measure concentrations of ACTH before and after CRH administration to localize the pituitary tumor. If an adrenocortical tumor is suspected on the basis of androgenic features, DHEAS, androstenedione, testosterone, and aldosterone should be measured and a computed tomography (CT) scan of the adrenal glands is obtained.

Management

Transphenoidal surgery is the method of choice for pituitary adenomas. Adrenocortical carcinomas require immediate adrenalectomy, and chemotherapy is needed if all tumor tissue is not removed.

Outcome

Because adrenocortical carcinomas frequently metastasize, the prognosis is often unfavorable despite treatment. There is no effective chemotherapy or long-term effective inhibitor of adrenal steroidogenesis. The outcome is better for pituitary adenoma.

Follow-up

The specialist will monitor skeletal maturation by bone age determination, will adjust replacement and emergency doses based on body surface area, and will monitor any signs and symptoms of overtreatment and undertreatment, such as height velocity decrease and weight gain.

PHEOCHROMOCYTOMA

Fundamentals

Pheochromocytoma is a catecholamine-secreting tumor that most commonly arises in the adrenal medulla. It may be inherited as an autosomal dominant trait or as part of the multiple endocrine neoplasia (MEN) type 2A or with other syndromes.

Presentation and Initial Evaluation

Signs and symptoms of pheochromocytoma are sustained rather than paroxysmal hypertension headache, palpitations, abdominal pain, weakness, exhaustion, dizziness, pallor, vomiting, and sweating. Features on physical examination include papilledema, hemorrhages, or exudates. The diagnosis is established by documenting elevated blood or urinary levels of catecholamines and their metabolites, predominantly norepinephrine. A 24-hour urine collection, not a spot urine test, is taken for homovanillic acid (HVA), vanillylmandelic acid (VMA), metanephrines, and unconjugated (free) catecholamines. Imaging studies may be obtained by the practitioner or following referral to the specialist and include ultrasonography, CT, or MRI.

Management

These tumors require surgical removal with careful attention to preoperative α- and β-adrenergic blockade.

Outcome and Follow-up

Removal is usually curative and the prognosis is good. Because the multiple endocrine neoplasia can be familial, practitioners should refer family members for genetic counseling.

Mini-index of Related Topics

SUGGESTED READINGS

Collett-Solberg PF: Congenital adrenal hyperplasia: From genetics and biochemistry to clinical practice, Part 1. Clin Pediatr 2001; 40(1):1–16.

Collett-Solberg PF: Congenital adrenal hyperplasia: From genetics and biochemistry to clinical practice, Part 2. Clin Pediatr 2001; 40(3):125–132.

Intersex Society of North America. Available at: http://www.isna.org/.

Leinung MC, Zimmerman D: Cushing's disease in children. Endocrinol Metab Clin North Am 1994;23(3):629–639.

Levine L: Congenital adrenal hyperplasia. Pediatr Rev 2000;21:159–171.

Ten S, New M, Maclaren N: Clinical review 130: Addison's disease 2001. J Clin Endocrinol Metab 2001;86(7):2909–2922.

SECTION 4   CHRONIC MEDICAL CARE: *Disorders of the Endocrine System*

155

Diabetes Mellitus

Joan MacCracken

ROLE OF THE GENERALIST

1 Recognize the early signs and symptoms of type 1 and type 2 diabetes mellitus.

2 Understand insulin treatment, blood glucose monitoring, nutritional needs, and behavioral aspects of diabetic care.

3 Diagnose acute diabetic ketoacidosis.

4 Stabilize, manage, or refer the patient with diabetic ketoacidosis for intensive treatment.

5 Provide health maintenance and health supervision for children with diabetes mellitus.

6 Communicate with the pediatric diabetes team.

7 Manage acute complications of severe hypoglycemia and intercurrent illnesses.

8 Ensure that suggested annual laboratory evaluation and screening occur.

9 Advocate for the child and family at the day care or school by encouraging American Diabetes Association (ADA) guidelines for a specific diabetes care plan.

10 Screen children at high risk for type 2 diabetes.

DEFINITIONS

Diabetes mellitus is a state of relative or absolute insulin deficiency that results in the body being unable to utilize carbohydrates for energy. Lipolysis ensues. An osmotic diuresis with glucosuria occurs, and free fatty acids and ketones accumulate. The most common form of diabetes among children and adolescents is type 1 diabetes mellitus, also known as insulin-dependent diabetes mellitus (IDDM). IDDM is an insulin deficiency from an autoim-

mune process that destroys the insulin-producing pancreatic beta cells. Type 2 diabetes mellitus, also known as non–insulin-dependent diabetes (NIDDM), results from insulin resistance and a relative insulin deficiency. The incidence of type 2 diabetes has been increasing dramatically. Table 155-1 lists characteristics of diabetes mellitus.

Type 1 diabetes is caused by a combination of genetic and environmental factors. HLA DR3 and HLA DR4 genotypes are present in over 90% of whites with IDDM. The causal relationship of environmental factors is not well understood, but certain viral, nutritional, and toxic agents may be precipitating agents. The incidence of type 1 diabetes varies worldwide, with the incidence in Scandinavian countries being approximately 35 times higher than that of Japan and Korea. Male-to-female distribution is equal. Seasonal

Table 155-1. Characteristics of Type 1 and Type 2 Diabetes Mellitus in Children and Adolescents

Features	Type 1	Type 2
Autoantibodies	Present	Absent
Age at diagnosis	All ages	Usually at puberty
Diabetic ketoacidosis at onset	Common	Less common
Obesity	Less common	Very common
Family history	Infrequent	Frequent
Gender distribution	Male = female	Female > male
Highest prevalence	Whites	African Americans, Latinos, Native Americans
Polyuria, polydipsia, weight loss	Common	Less common
Diagnosis on routine physical	Uncommon	Common
Acanthosis nigracans	Rare	Common
Hypertension	Less common	Common
Vaginal infection	Rare	Common
Dyslipidemia	Less common	Common

Table 155-2. Types of Human Insulin

Type of Insulin	Onset	Peak	Duration
Rapid-acting			
Lispro	<2.5 min	0.5–1.0 hr	2–3 hr
Fast-acting			
Regular	0.5 hr	2–3 hr	3–6 hr
Intermediate-acting			
NPH	2–4 hr	4–8 hr	10–14 hr
Lente	2–4 hr	4–12 hr	12–18 hr
Long-acting			
Glargine*	0.5 hr	None	24 hr†

*Glargine is clear and may not be mixed with other insulins.
†Significant intrapatient variability exists.

variations also occur, with more cases diagnosed in the winter months.

FUNDAMENTALS

Insulin

Insulin has been the cornerstone of treatment of type 1 diabetes mellitus since its discovery in 1921. Beef and pork insulins were used until the more recent synthesis of human insulin analogs. Currently available insulins vary in their duration and peak of action (Table 155-2). A larger dosage of regular and NPH insulins will alter both the duration and the timing of the peak. Regular insulin binds to itself in the subcutaneous tissue and must break down before complete absorption. However, Lispro, a bioengineered human insulin, is more rapidly absorbed and gives a more consistent time of peak and duration regardless of the dosage. The fast acting insulins can be given immediately before the meal or just after, whereas regular insulin should be given 15 to 20 minutes before the meal. Currently, the most common method of insulin administration is subcutaneous by injection. However, the use of insulin pumps in children is rapidly increasing.

INITIAL DIABETIC MANAGEMENT

Forty percent of children and adolescents with IDDM are diagnosed in diabetic ketoacidosis. Astute parents and physicians can diagnose the onset of diabetes before the child's condition progresses to severe, life-threatening diabetic ketoacidosis. Many parents seek prompt medical attention because they recognize the symptoms of increased thirst and urination, new-onset enuresis, fatigue, and weight loss. A urine dipstick will reveal glucose, with or without ketones. Confirmation with a plasma glucose evaluation is necessary. Box 155-1 provides guidelines for early suspicion and diagnosis of diabetes. *It is imperative to think about diabetes mellitus in a child who is not improving during an acute illness. Home glucose monitoring machines should not be used to confirm the diagnosis.* Finger sticks can be contaminated and the machines are not accurate enough for diagnostic purposes.

Box 155-2 lists diagnostic criteria for type 1 diabetes mellitus. The diagnosis should be confirmed by a repeat test with any of the three methods listed. Usually the diagnosis is obvious.

Box 155-1. Guidelines for Early Suspicion and Diagnosis of Diabetes

1. Consider the possibility of new-onset diabetes in a child who is sick and not improving.
2. Remember to think about osmotic diuresis and do not assume that if child is urinating, the child is hydrated; worry about dehydration.
3. Ask about the recent onset of weight loss, polyuria, and polydipsia.
4. Remember that a family history of type 1 diabetes is not usually present.
5. Consider doing a urinalysis; it just might save a child's life.
6. Home blood glucose machine values are not accurate enough to use for diagnostic purposes and may give false positive readings.

Triage and Diabetic Ketoacidosis

Once the diagnosis has been confirmed, the generalist must determine how ill the child is and coordinate the care. The first determinations concern whether immediate intensive care management is necessary and who shall provide the initial stabilization and subsequent management and education. Management of acute diabetic ketoacidosis is described in detail in Chapter 42. If the patient is diagnosed before the onset of acute ketoacidosis, the initial diagnosis and initiation of insulin should be done in the hospital unless a very experienced and immediately available pediatric diabetes team is organized to handle this care in an outpatient setting.

Transition Care

Once the patient has been stabilized, diabetes education should be ongoing. The minimal knowledge for discharge must be an understanding of survival skills: monitoring blood glucose, giving insulin injections, and recognizing signs and symptoms of hypoglycemia. Initial contact with a pediatric diabetes team is essential. If such a team is not available at the local hospital, a referral of the child and family for consultation after discharge is advisable. The team will have extensive experience with diabetic education, psychosocial support of families, and interacting with schools and other agencies to advocate for the diabetic child. The team can be a resource for the primary care provider if, for reasons of distance, finances, or patient

Box 155-2. Diagnostic Criteria for Type 1 Diabetes Mellitus

Symptoms of the following:
1. Polyuria
2. Polydipsia
3. Unexplained weight loss
and/or the following:
4. Random glucose concentration equal to or greater than 200 mg/dL
5. Fasting plasma glucose level equal to or greater than 126 mg/dL*
6. 2-hour plasma glucose level equal to or greater than 200 mg/dL during an oral glucose tolerance test

* Fast is defined as at least 8 hours with no caloric intake.

preference, the primary care clinician must provide the majority of the diabetic care for the child.

The initially hospitalized patient may require an average of 1 U/kg/day, although this dosage may vary, depending on the severity of the insulin deficiency. A few weeks after initial diagnosis, most, but not all, patients experience a dramatic drop in insulin requirements. This "honeymoon phase" is defined as a period when the insulin requirement is less than 0.5 U/kg/day. Dosages must be adjusted downward to prevent significant hypoglycemia. Failure to educate the family regarding this possibility can lead to low blood sugars with subsequent seizures. In young children very low doses of insulin may be required. A small dosage of intermediate-acting insulin in the morning may be sufficient until the honeymoon phase ends. Because the family may want to believe the diabetes is going away permanently, discontinuing injections is rarely a good idea.

Acute Psychosocial Concerns

Diabetes has an impact on every aspect of a child and family's lifestyle. Guilt, uncertainty, fear, and anxiety—ingredients for significant psychological problems in the families with children with diabetes—are virtually always present. These issues must be addressed to help families understand and cope with the disease.

Families come to the startling realization that theirs and their child's life will never be the same. Questions of why and how can be daunting, the times of juggling the multiple components that affect blood sugar frustrating, and the uncertainty of the future worrisome. The initial reactions within the family unit should be anticipated. Guilt appears and parents question whose side of the family caused this or wonder if they fed their child too much sugar. The family may become angry, taking it out on the bearer of bad news. They will be frustrated by receiving no good answer for why this has happened. Disturbing images of past associations may emerge. Fatigued and exhausted, parents may be over-whelmed with information overload, a sense of futility, and sadness. These issues should be anticipated and recognized by the primary care provider and handled with compassion, sensitivity, experience, and support. The parents will need some time to mourn in private. If counseled alone, parents can let down their defenses and grieve for the loss of their previously healthy child.

GENERAL PRINCIPLES OF CHRONIC CARE MANAGEMENT

Appropriate and continued education is the keystone to successful management. This educational effort can be very time-consuming, but it is imperative. The generalist must have a solid understanding of the basic aspects of diabetes management in order to provide excellent care to the patient and family and to communicate with the specialist.

Glucose Regulation
Insulin Dosage

With a variety of insulins available (see Table 155-2), insulin schedules can be tailored to patients' individual lifestyles. Good glucose regulation requires frequent administration of insulin. Few patients can be adequately controlled with

---

Box 155-3. Storage and Care of Insulin

1. Refrigerate insulin to prolong potency.
2. Do not freeze or expose to heat.
3. If kept at room temperature, discard after 1 month.
4. Fast-acting insulin is *clear*. If particles are present in solution, discard the insulin.
5. Long-acting insulin is *cloudy*. If lumps are present in solution, discard the insulin.

---

a single daily injection. Combinations of multiple types of insulins in one syringe are used in an attempt to have their peaks correspond more closely to the body's endogenous insulin response to meals. Fixed-ratio insulins are seldom used in pediatrics.

Insulin requirements change over time. The honeymoon stage can end abruptly. More commonly, the insulin required to maintain acceptable blood glucose levels gradually increases. In the prepubertal child the insulin requirements range from 0.5 to 0.8 U/kg/day and in the adolescent the range is 0.75 to 1.2 U/kg/day. Regimens must be tailored to the individual patient. Factors that influence insulin needs include caloric intake, amount of exercise, pubertal stages with increased insulin resistance, chronic stress factors, and individual sensitivities. Initial insulin administration can begin with giving two thirds of the total dosage in the morning, with a 3:1 or 4:1 ratio of intermediate-acting to short-acting insulin, and giving one third in the evening, with a 1:1 ratio of NPH/regular or lispro. Recently, a schedule of rapid acting and long acting insulin analogs is being used.

Storage and Administration of Insulin

Box 155-3 details the storage of insulin. Box 155-4 describes injection of insulin. Very sharp thin disposable needles reduce the pain of injection. Two lengths of needles allow for variation in subcutaneous tissue thickness. The volumes available are 0.3 mL (30 U), 0.5 mL (50 U), and 1.0 mL (100 U). The smaller volume syringe allows for adjustment

---

Box 155-4. Insulin Injection

1. When drawing mixed dosage, draw up fastest acting insulin first.
2. Use needle length appropriate to thickness of subcutaneous tissue.
3. Use smaller volume syringes for small adjustments of insulin dosage.
4. If insulin has been refrigerated, warm insulin briefly by holding syringe for a few moments.
5. Inject into subcutaneous tissue by pinching skin and holding needle at a 90-degree angle (perpendicular to surface), except in some very thin small children.
6. Avoid intramuscular injection.
7. Rotate injection sites, using arms, anterior and lateral thighs, buttocks, and abdomen.
8. If anticipating exercise, use the abdomen for injection.
9. Maintain sterility; if reusing syringes, recap without wiping with alcohol.
10. Use a hard plastic sharps container to dispose of needles and syringes.

of small dosages by a unit or two. Prescriptions should include brand, volume, and needle size (e.g., BD 30 U, 0.3 mL, Ultrafine 2 insulin syringe). Syringes can be reused, but this dulls the needle and increases risk of infection. Rules and regulations regarding needle disposal in towns and counties vary. Primary providers should check with the local health department to be able to advise patients. Whether there are other regulations, used syringes must be disposed of in a hard plastic container.

Poor injection technique can lead to loss of some insulin. Common injection sites are the back of the upper arm (avoiding the deltoid muscles), the anterior and lateral thighs, the buttocks, and the abdomen. Rotation of the sites is important to avoid lipohypertrophy. A consistent site location for the same time of day avoids variability in absorption. Insulin injected into the abdomen is more quickly absorbed than from the buttocks, and the arms and legs are in between. Exercise of the injected extremity increases absorption.

Home Monitoring

Self-monitoring blood glucose (SMBG) is the standard method of following day-to-day control. Results should be used to modify treatment plans to obtain near-normal blood glucose levels. Machines are small, quick, and require a small amount of blood. Their internal memories allow retrieval of blood glucose values, give averages, and may be downloaded for evaluation. Although at least 4 data points a day are optimal (readings from before each meal and at bedtime), many find this too big a burden. Work closely with families or teens to figure out what regimen of testing is possible for them. Arrangements should vary depending on the current level of control, the school schedule, support systems, the history of hypoglycemic episodes, and the patient's and family's concept of burden. Occasionally, families and teenagers may do more tests than seems reasonable. A child must not become a pin cushion because an overly anxious parent or baby-sitter constantly needs to know the blood glucose level. Addressing their fears is very important.

SMBG is a tool for diabetes control. However, often the data presents the frustrating reality that insulin replacements are not as physiologic as the normal pancreatic response. Data must be used in a nonjudgmental fashion. Box 155-5 lists guidelines for assisting patients and families with home glucose monitoring. Children and teenagers, wishing to please their parents or the health care provider,

Box 155-5. Guidelines for Helping Patients Manage Results of Home Glucose Testing

1. Do not become judgmental in the review; avoid referring to numbers as "good" or "bad."
2. Refer to numbers as "high," "low," or "in range."
3. Work through the data cooperatively with family or patient; for example, ask the patient to evaluate the data and ask him- or herself, "Is my nighttime dosage appropriate?"
4. Highlighting numbers in the logbook can help distinguish useful patterns.
5. Encourage families and patients to modify insulin doses when patterns become apparent.
6. Encourage weekly evaluations and adjustments.

Box 155-6. Indications for Measuring Urinary Ketones*

1. Acute illness
2. Physiologic stress
3. Blood glucose > 300 mg/dL for two or more consecutive readings
4. Abdominal pain, nausea, or vomiting

*Note that urinary ketone testing may have false readings with some medications.

often improve their records by writing in false numbers or omitting the high ones. Blood glucose machines with memories make attempts to alter records futile. The family or teen needs to understand the numbers are to help them. If the collected numbers are not used to improve control and adjust insulin dosages, then why do them? Unfortunately, some patients make no adjustments until they return to the clinic. Those who are fearful of self-adjusting insulin are strongly encouraged to contact their health care provider for assistance.

Urinary ketone monitoring is important. Box 155-6 lists indications for testing ketones. Early detection of ketones may prevent ketoacidosis (see later discussion of sick day management). The urinary ketone strips can give false negative readings if exposed to air or moisture for too long. Ketone tests using the nitroprusside-containing reagents have been shown to give false positive readings in the presence of some medications such as captopril. Some home monitor machines can test blood ketones by measuring β-hydroxybutyic acid.

ACUTE COMPLICATIONS

Hypoglycemia

Hypoglycemia is a very common. Blood glucose under 60 mg/dL is considered hypoglycemia, but symptoms may appear above that level. Hunger, shakiness, sweatiness, rapid heart rate, and pallor are caused by a counterregulatory hormone response. Headache, drowsiness, confusion, behavioral changes, loss of consciousness, and seizures are caused by low blood sugar in the brain. Hypoglycemia may be asymptomatic. A rapid drop in blood sugar may cause symptoms even though the level is not below 60 mg/dL. With repeated episodes of hypoglycemia, a blunting of the epinephrine response may occur, causing loss of autonomic symptoms such as tachycardia and sweating (hypoglycemic unawareness). Testing is the only way to document the blood sugar level. *If immediate testing cannot be performed, empiric treatment will do no harm and may prevent severe symptoms.* The most common causes of hypoglycemia are too much insulin, inadequate food, or unanticipated exercise.

In children, especially those younger than 5 years, repetitive hypoglycemia may cause significant neurocognitive impairment. Although hypoglycemia appears to have no long-term consequences in adults and older children, the immediate consequences can be detrimental, including potential for loss of consciousness in precarious situations like driving, the patient's embarrassment at requiring assistance, the subsequent fear of tight control of blood sugar, and the possible acquisition of hypoglycemic unawareness.

Mild cognitive dysfunction and electroencephalographic (EEG) abnormalities have been described in early-onset diabetes (below age 5) with hypoglycemic seizures. Three to 7 years after diagnosis, children diagnosed before age 5 performed less well on fine motor skills and attention tasks. Visual spatial function also appeared to be impaired compared to siblings and those diagnosed after age 5. Several studies have shown impairment of IQ, memory, eye-hand coordination, and school performance, particularly in those with a history of severe hypoglycemia and seizures.

Fear of hypoglycemia is very real and affects many decisions of parent or patient. Once a child or teenager has experienced a severe hypoglycemic reaction, the usual clinical result is an increase of hemoglobin (HbA_{1c}) with the patient allowing higher blood glucose numbers to prevent a recurrence. The clinician should determine what range of blood glucose the patient or parents feel comfortable with, particularly at night. Fifty percent of severe reactions occur during the night or before breakfast. Levels below 115 to 120 mg/dL at the presupper and 11 P.M. reading predict potential nocturnal hypoglycemia.

About 50% of diabetic patients experience nocturnal hypoglycemia, with half of the episodes being asymptomatic. Common times for onset of nocturnal hypoglycemia are between 2 A.M. and 3 A.M. and between 11 P.M. and midnight. Clues to nocturnal hypoglycemia include waking with a headache or drowsiness, nightmares, or bedwetting. Palatable cornstarch snacks prolong carbohydrate availability through the night. Use of the more rapid-acting insulin, lispro, has been helpful in children prone to hypoglycemia. Delayed hypoglycemia may occur 4 to 10 hours after strenuous exercise. Teenagers must be taught that alcohol ingestion also may cause hypoglycemia.

Children with total daily insulin doses greater than 0.8 U/kg/24 hours and adolescents with total daily doses greater than 1.3 U/kg/24 hours run a higher risk of significant hypoglycemic events. In some closely monitored pump patients, despite lower HbA_{1c} levels, the rate of severe hypoglycemic events is 50% lower than in those on multiple dose injections. In general, however, the lower the HbA_{1c}, the greater the risk of hypoglycemia. In the Diabetic Control and Complications Trial (DCCT) intensive treatment increased the risk of severe hypoglycemia by threefold compared to the conventional treatment group.

Box 155-7 describes the steps for treating mild to moderate hypoglycemia. Treatment of hypoglycemia requires intake of easily available carbohydrate. For mild symptoms with blood sugar above 60 mg/dL, fruit or crackers may be

---

Box 155-7. Treatment of Mild to Moderate Hypoglycemia

Glucose level >60 mg/dL with mild symptoms:
   Fruit or crackers
Glucose level <60 mg/dL with mild to moderate symptoms:
   10 to 20 g carbohydrate, such as 4 to 6 oz orange juice, 6 to 8 oz milk, 2 tbsp raisins
or
3 or 4 glucose tablets, Insta-Glucose, or cake frosting
Wait 10 minutes, recheck blood glucose, repeat if necessary.

Box 155-8. At-Home Sick Day Management Rules

1. Monitor blood glucose levels more frequently, perhaps every 2 hours.
2. Check ketones every 4 hours.
3. Give usual dosage of insulin even if child is not eating (give carbohydrate in liquids).
4. Encourage fluids to prevent dehydration and wash out ketones.
5. Try antiemetic suppositories if vomiting is part of the illness; repeat only once.
6. If blood sugar and ketones are elevated, more insulin more often is required.
7. Communicate with your health provider to discuss insulin doses and possible infection.
8. Intravenous fluids will be necessary if vomiting persists or ketones do not clear.

---

eaten. With the blood sugar below 60 mg/dL, liquids are recommended (milk, juice, or regular soda). Depending on the size of the child, 10 to 20 g of carbohydrate should be ingested (4 to 6 oz of orange juice, 6 to 8 oz of milk, 2 tablespoons of raisins). Glucose tablets (3 or 4), Insta-Glucose, or cake frosting may also be used. Wait 10 minutes for the blood sugar to increase and symptoms to improve. If necessary, repeat the process. With severe hypoglycemia and loss of consciousness or convulsions, glucagon, a pancreatic hormone that raises blood sugar, should be used. Glucagon emergency kits should be available and instructions reviewed well before they are needed. The kits contain 1 mg/mL of glucagon. Doses should range from 0.3 mL, 0.5 mL, to 1 mL, depending on the size of the child, and are given either by subcutaneous or intramuscular injection. If there is no improvement, the dose should be repeated. Glucagon may cause vomiting. It may be stored at room temperature, but expiration dates should be checked. A child who requires frequent use of glucagon is receiving too much insulin. Glucagon should be required rarely or not at all.

Acute Illness and Sick Day Management

Children and adolescents with diabetes do not have a higher incidence of acute illnesses, but when ill, they require more care. Diabetic ketoacidosis remains the number one killer of children with diabetes. Prompt preventive steps will help to reduce the incidence of diabetic ketoacidosis. Box 155-8 describes sick day rules that, when promptly employed, may prevent development of significant ketoacidosis. Patients should contact their physician when these rules are initiated.

Ketoacidosis develops when insufficient insulin is available, either from a relative insulin resistance from counterregulatory hormonal responses to stress or illness, or from an absolute deficiency caused by missed injections, defective or outdated insulin, or inappropriately low doses. *Hyperglycemia that does not abate over a few hours or the presence of urinary or serum ketones should raise the level of concern.* Symptoms of acute illness must be recognized and attended to. Blood sugar levels should be checked more frequently, perhaps as often as every 2 hours. Ketones should be checked at least every 4 hours. Fluids must be encouraged. Solid food is not required; calories should be provided in liquid form. Instruct families not to worry about the fat and protein in the meal plan, but to concentrate on replacing the carbohydrate equivalent with sugared fluids. *Except in very rare circumstances, the insulin dosage should be maintained or increased. The insulin dosage should be withheld only with documented hypoglycemia and then only with close monitoring of blood glucose levels.*

With hyperglycemia and small amounts of ketones, insulin should be increased and given at the usual times. Encourage intake of both caloric and noncaloric fluids. With hyperglycemia and moderate to large ketones, the dose of insulin should be both increased and given more frequently. The usual dosage of morning intermediate-acting insulin should be given. The rapid-acting insulin should be increased by 20% to 25% of the total morning dosage. For example, if the morning dosage is 7 U NPH and 3 U regular, increase the rapid-acting insulin by 2 U; so the morning dosage would be 7 U NPH and 5 U regular insulin. The usual timing of insulin injection may be maintained with glucose monitoring, or lispro or regular insulin can be repeated every 2 to 4 hours. Readjustments in the dosage may be necessary, depending on the blood glucose. It may take several hours for urinary ketones to decrease. Insulin injections may be necessary throughout the night to avoid progression to diabetic ketoacidosis and prevent hospitalization. When parents understand the continued need for and benefits of low dose, frequent insulin injections, they accommodate the request.

With a second vomiting episode, 12.5 to 25 mg promethazine HCl (Phenergan) suppositories are recommended. Within half an hour, small sips of fluids should be reintroduced. The dosage can be repeated *once* in 4 to 6 hours. Ketones can cause vomiting that is not well controlled by antiemetics. Antiemetics should be used only in the initial stages of acute gastrointestinal illness. Under no circumstances should antivomiting medication be given more than twice. Uncontrolled vomiting requires intravenous hydration. The family should be instructed to go to the emergency department. In some circumstances, rehydration in the emergency department may be all that is required. Treatment of significant ketoacidosis is described in Chapter 42.

SURGERY AND DIABETES MANAGEMENT

Management of diabetes during surgery depends on the extent and the duration of the surgery. For brief outpatient procedures, such as dental extractions, reduce the intermediate-acting insulin by one half, withhold the short-acting insulin, and check the blood sugar level frequently (every 2 hours). Give extra short-acting insulin as necessary. When patients tolerate oral feedings, they may be given short-acting insulin with the next feeding and the standard evening dose may be restarted. Alternatively, both intermediate-acting insulin and the short-acting insulin may be withheld, frequent blood sugars checked, and injections of short-acting insulin given as needed. Ketones must be checked also.

For longer procedures or those requiring general anesthesia, both insulin and glucose should be given intravenously.

Standard protocols for adjustments of glucose infusion rate and insulin dosage changes have been developed and work well as long as the patient is taking nothing by mouth.

EXERCISE AND DIABETES

Vigorous exercise in type 1 diabetes patients should *not* be discouraged. The metabolic state of the athlete must be monitored to prevent hypoglycemia or hyperglycemia and ketosis. The amount of insulin in the body at the time of exercise plays a significant role in determining which may occur. Tailoring the diabetes treatment to fit the activity requires concerted effort. Coaches and athletic trainers must be knowledgeable to support the athlete's participation and safety. The athlete must learn to adjust insulin dosage and carbohydrate ingestion to mimic function of the pancreas and liver of healthy athletes.

Participation in sports and exercise has many positive social aspects. Exercise can significantly delay the onset or lessen the severity of type 2 diabetes. Although benefit of exercise for control in type 1 diabetes remains controversial, most patients feel it improves their quality of life.

Sports or other physical activities must be carefully considered when loss of motor control or minimal inattention might endanger the diabetic patient or others. Some experts believe that activities such as the scuba diving, sky diving, rock climbing, and car racing are too dangerous for those with diabetes, even with frequent monitoring.

Significant hypoglycemia is a risk, both during the event and for several hours after. In general a 25% to 50% reduction in insulin may be necessary for anticipated, strenuous, prolonged exertion. Fifteen to 30 g of carbohydrate may be required for each 30 to 45 minutes of strenuous activity. Glucagon must be available for administration by others should the affected athlete become disoriented, combative, or unconscious. Glucose gels should also be available but should not be administered if the patient cannot swallow.

Athletes with type 1 diabetes have run Ironman triathlon races, captured Olympic gold medals, and played in the World Series. Physicians must educate their patients, encourage participation, and support their dreams.

LONG-TERM COMPLICATIONS AND ASSOCIATED CONDITIONS

Important findings from the DCCT has resulted in even greater emphasis on attaining near normoglycemia. The study demonstrated that with improved metabolic control, the risk for complications can be significantly decreased. Nephropathy, retinopathy, neuropathy, celiac disease, and thyroiditis are discussed on the CD-ROM.

Diabetic Monitoring and Health Maintenance (Table 155-3)
Physical Examination
Growth parameters are important clues to health. If all is well, children with diabetes will follow along normal percentiles. Table 155-4 details the common causes of poor or excessive growth in diabetic children. Blood pressures should be obtained at every visit and compared to norms for

Table 155-3. Diabetic Monitoring and Health Maintenance

Parameter	Frequency of Measurement
Height, weight, blood pressure	Every 3 months
Injection sites	Every 3 months
Palpation neck	Every 3 months
Examination of hands and feet	Every 3 months
Skin	Every 3 months
Dilated ophthalmic examination	Annually after 5 years of disease or at onset of puberty
HbA$_{1c}$	Every 3 months
Microalbuminuria	Annually in children with disease for 5 years or at the onset of puberty
Lipid profiles	Annually
Thyroid-stimulating hormone	Annually

children and adolescents. Any consistent elevation above normal for age should be noted and evaluated and treated (see CD-ROM Chapter 174, especially CD-ROM Tables 174-1 and 174-2).

Injection sites should be checked at each visit. The patient is usually aware of the overuse of certain preferred spots. Lipohypertrophy can be both visualized and palpated by running one's finger along the skin to see whether it meets with resistance, and if resistance is noted, strong recommendations for avoiding these areas and rotating sites should be made. Injection sites occasionally become infected. Strongly discourage injecting through clothing. Hives noted at the injection site may signal latex allergy. Very few children are actually allergic to the purified insulins.

The neck should be palpated at each visit. The thyroid is enlarged in approximately 20% to 30% of patients. Examination of the hands may reveal limited joint mobility, manifested with a positive prayer sign (failure of the palmar surfaces of interphalangeal joints to approximate when the hands are placed palms together) suggesting restricted digital extension. The hands may appear waxy and tight. Wrist extension can be limited also. With improved control, fewer children have these findings, which may be associated with microvascular complications and poorer outcomes.

Dermatologic findings include necrobiosis lipoidica diabeticorum and acanthosis nigricans. Necrobiosis lipoidica diabeticorum usually occurs in the third and fourth decades of life in the diabetic population, but may be seen in adoles-

Table 155-4. Common Causes of Poor or Excessive Growth

Growth Parameter	Possible Cause
Poor height gain	Extremely poor diabetic control Hypothyroidism
Rapid height gain	Onset of puberty, usually requires increasing insulin and nutritional adjustments
Excessive weight gain	Overinsulinization Overeating, exogenous obesity
Poor weight gain	Celiac disease Unsuspected ketosis from insufficient insulin Hyperthyroidism

cents. It is characterized by reddish brown or violet plaques, most commonly located on the shin but occasionally found on the arms, trunk, scalp, or face. No successful treatment is known. Acanthosis nigricans consists of velvety dark brown plaques, usually on the sides or back of the neck, axillae, or groin, and is generally associated with obesity and insulin resistance and suggests type 2 diabetes (see Fig. 79-1).

After 5 years of diabetes children should have a thorough, dilated ophthalmologic examination. Adolescents should have this examination as soon as possible.

Follow-up Laboratory Studies

Glycosylated hemoglobin, or HbA$_{1c}$, is the gold standard for monitoring glycemic control. The rate of production of glycosylated hemoglobin is directly proportional to mean blood glucose levels over 2 to 3 months. The nonenzymatic step of glycosylation of hemoglobin is irreversible and remains throughout the 120-day life of the red blood cell. Using the DCCT reference method, data suggest that a HbA$_{1c}$ of 8.0 is equivalent to a mean blood glucose level of 180 mg/dL and that with each change of 1.0 in HbA$_{1c}$, the average mean blood glucose changes by 30 mg/dL. For example, 7.0 would be 150 mg/dL and 9.0 would be 210 mg/dL. Regular measuring of glycosylated hemoglobin allows observation of significant deviations from desired control. Measurement is recommended every 3 months. Values between 7.0 and 8.0 are considered excellent. Goals for HbA$_{1c}$ should be adjusted individually. The relationship between HbA$_{1c}$ and risk of long-term complications is directly proportional. Encourage adolescents to do their very best to reduce this value. A value of 9.0 is much better than 12.0. Every improvement decreases the risk of long-term complications.

Microalbumin should be screened annually in children with diabetes after 5 years of disease or at the onset of puberty. A timed sample of 12 or 24 hours is recommended. Spot testing for initial screening may be done. Glomerular damage can be reversed with improved glycemic control. If microalbuminuria persists despite improved control, treatment with angiotensin-converting enzyme (ACE) inhibitors is appropriate.

Annual lipid profiles should also be obtained. Patients with diabetes, particularly with a strong family history of heart disease and dyslipidemia, need important nutritional counseling to reduce cholesterol, low-density lipoprotein (LDL), and possibly triglycerides. Poor diabetes control can cause elevated lipids. Improving diabetic control improves the lipid profile. Medication may be appropriate for extremely high cholesterol levels.

Screening with thyroid-stimulating hormone (TSH) for thyroid disease is recommended yearly. The TSH can be elevated with relatively few symptoms. A thyroid antibody test at the time of diagnosis may flag those at higher risk of developing hypothyroidism.

Adherence

Adherence to the difficult regimens that are required for diabetic control is challenging. Box 155-9 describes some helpful hints to encourage the patient's adherence to

---

Box 155-9. Some Helpful Hints to Encourage Adherence to the Diabetes Plan

1. Make sure everyone has the same understanding about exactly what is expected.
2. Look for opportunities to praise and reward good self-care.
3. Negotiate with the teenager to establish reasonable and achievable intermediate goals.
4. Have frequent family meetings and include self-care on the agenda.
5. Plan and expect some difficult times when extra help may be needed to accomplish the goals.
6. Use nonverbal cues like signs, Post-its, and calendars to encourage adherence instead of nagging or coaxing.
7. Rotate responsibilities between the parents for supervising and encouraging adherence, but be very clear about which parent is on call.
8. At school find a mutually chosen adult who can help guide the teenager.
9. Make every attempt to leave diabetes out of other family problems.
10. A referral to a mental health professional may be necessary if adherence to the negotiated plan is consistently poor for 3 to 6 months and the HbA$_{1c}$ is significantly elevated or hospitalizations or emergency room visits have been necessary.

Adapted from Wysocki T: Ten keys to helping your child grow up with diabetes. Alexandria, Va, American Diabetes Association, 1997.

---

the diabetes plan. Additional information is found in Chapter 279.

LONG-TERM ASPECTS OF PSYCHOSOCIAL MANAGEMENT

Long-term aspects of psychosocial management are essential in the care of children and adolescents with diabetes. Family issues, school issues, and management of the teenage years are discussed on the CD-ROM. Risk factors for adolescents are discussed, particularly smoking, because it significantly increases the risk of long-term vascular complications and must be discouraged.

DIABETES MELLITUS TYPE 2 IN CHILDREN AND ADOLESCENTS

Over the last few decades the incidence of type 2 diabetes mellitus has increased in the United States, particularly among Native Americans, African Americans, and Hispanics. As the incidence of obesity in children and adolescents increases at almost epidemic proportions, so has the incidence of this non–immune-mediated diabetes. Obesity is the major risk factor for type 2 diabetes. Depending on the population studied, recent reports suggest a range from 8% to 45% of newly diagnosed diabetes is type 2. Behavioral, social, environmental, and genetic risk factors play a role in the etiology of this disorder.

Table 155-1 compares type 1 and type 2 diabetes mellitus. At the time of diagnosis, clinical presentations may be indistinguishable from those seen in patients with type 1 diabetes. Although typically, type 1 patients are not obese, with the increasing incidence of obesity, up to 20% of type 1 patients are now overweight at diagnosis. In type 2 diabetes, 85% of the children are either overweight or obese. Type 2 patients do not usually develop ketoacidosis, but recent studies indicate that ketonuria is seen in about 30% and ketoacidosis may be present in as many as 25% of patients subsequently diagnosed as type 2. The clinical picture over time gives the appropriate diagnosis. Family history of type 1 diabetes is present in only 5% of type 1 patients. In type 2 patients, 75% to 100% of the patients have a first- or second-degree relative with type 2 diabetes. Occasionally, the relative's disease is not discovered until the child is diagnosed.

Acanthosis nigricans and polycystic ovarian syndrome are seen in type 2 patients and are associated with insulin resistance and obesity. Hypertension and lipid abnormalities are also seen frequently in type 2. Children with type 2 diabetes are usually over the age of 10 and in middle to late puberty. There have been cases of prepubertal children with type 2 diabetes. Girls have a slightly higher incidence than boys. Autoantibodies, frequently seen in type 1 patients, are not present in type 2 patients. C-peptide and insulin levels are elevated or normal.

Type 2 diabetes seems to result from a combination of insulin resistance and insulin hyposecretion. Impaired insulin action is thought to be the initial defect, followed later by relative inadequate insulin secretion. The concept of glucose toxicity—hyperglycemia begets more hyperglycemia—suggests that the hyperglycemia occurring from the ineffective action of insulin poisons the beta cell and decreases insulin secretion. When the hyperglycemia is treated, insulin secretion improves for a time.

Treatment of type 2 diabetes varies, depending on clinical presentation. If ketonuria or ketoacidosis occur, insulin treatment is necessary. Asymptomatic patients with mildly elevated (just above 126 mg/dL for fasting, or just over 200 mg/dL for random glucose) may be initially managed with medical nutrition therapy (dietary adjustments) and increased exercise. Exercise has been shown to decrease insulin resistance. Oral hypoglycemic agents have been tried. Metformin is the first FDA-approved alternative to insulin for children 10 years and over with type 2 diabetes. A rare side effect of metformin is lactic acidosis, which occurs mainly in patients with compromised renal function. The most common side effect is gastrointestinal upset. Insulin has been used in children with type 2 diabetes, but may lead to continued weight gain and is not more effective than oral medications. Newer drugs continue to enter the marketplace.

Because type 2 diabetes may have a long preclinical course, a high index of suspicion is necessary to make an early diagnosis. The generalist must know the indications for screening (Box 155-10). In adults significant lifestyle changes (improved eating habits and increased exercise) have been shown to decrease eventual cardiovascular morbidity. Initiating these changes in the formative second decade of life may not be easy, but may significantly improve long-term quality of life for these children as adults. Helpful websites for diabetes education and support are found in Box 155-11.

Box 155-10. Criteria for Screening for Type 2 Diabetes in Children

When:
Initiate screening at age 10 years or younger if puberty has begun; repeat every 2 years.

Who:
Those who are overweight, BMI >85th percentile for sex and age, weight >120% of ideal weight for height plus any two of the following risk factors:

1. Race/ethnicity is Hispanic, Native American, African American, or Asia/Pacific Islander
2. Family history of type 2 diabetes in first- or second-degree relative
3. Signs of insulin resistance or conditions associated with insulin resistance (polycystic ovary syndrome, hypertension, dyslipidemia, acanthosis nigricans)

What:
Test for fasting plasma glucose (no caloric intake for at least 8 hours); a level equal to or greater than 126 mg/dL is diagnostic if reconfirmed on a different day.

Box 155-11. Helpful Websites for Diabetes

- American Diabetes Association, 1660 Duke Street, Alexandria, VA 22314, www.diabetes.org.
- Juvenile Diabetes Foundation, 23 East 26th St. NY, NY 10012, www.jdfcure.org.
- The On-Line Community for Kids, Families and Adults with Diabetes. Available at: www.childrenwithdiabetes.com. (This is a very helpful site that offers up-to-date information and support.)

 Additional Resources, CD-ROM

Nutritional management of diabetes mellitus	Text, tables
Long-term complications and associated conditions	Text
Long-term aspects of psychosocial management	Text
Insulin pumps	Text, table
Future trends and research	Text
Bibliography	

Mini-index of Related Topics

SUGGESTED READINGS

American Diabetes Association: Type 2 in children and adolescents (consensus statement). Pediatrics 2000;105:671–680.

American Diabetes Association: Care of children with diabetes in the school and day care setting. Diabetes Care 2001;24(suppl 1):108–112.

Plotnick LP, Henderson R: Clinical Management of the Child and Adolescent with Diabetes. Baltimore, Johns Hopkins University Press, 1998.

Wysocki T: Ten Keys to Helping Your Child Grow Up with Diabetes. Alexandria, Va, American Diabetes Association, 1997.

156 Presentation and Evaluation of Genetic Disorders

Michael J. Bamshad

ROLE OF THE GENERALIST

1   Recognize children who may have a genetic condition.

2   Perform an efficient and appropriate screening evaluation of a child who may have a genetic condition.

3   Suggest a preliminary diagnosis (or group of diagnoses) of a child with a genetic condition.

4   Coordinate the care of children with genetic conditions, including appropriate referrals to specialists.

5   Deliver primary, preventive, and acute care to children with genetic conditions.

6   Provide care during intercurrent illnesses.

7   Provide ongoing psychosocial support for the family.

8   Explain genetic information to families and patients.

FUNDAMENTALS

The contribution of genetic variation to health and disease has become increasingly clear since the 1990s. In the past, various conditions were divided into those that are "genetic" versus those that are "nongenetic" (disorders "caused" by the environment, e.g., infections, teratogens). This distinction has become increasingly blurred. Disorders caused by mutations in a single gene (e.g., cystic fibrosis, sickle cell disease) can be heavily influenced by the environment, and diseases produced by environmental exposures (e.g., AIDS secondary to infection with HIV-1) can be substantially modified by an individual's genetic constitution. Most conditions can be considered genetic *and* environmental.

Although the perception that genetic conditions are immutable is still common, some can be effectively treated. Some (e.g., isolated cleft lip) need only limited intervention while others (e.g., trisomy 21) require chronic, ongoing management, often of a multidisciplinary nature. Prevention of conditions that manifest later in life requires appreciation of genetic predisposition during childhood. An understanding of the preliminary evaluation of children with genetic disorders is essential for generalists to provide individualized health supervision and care.

Genetic disorders and birth defects contribute substantially to pediatric morbidity and mortality. Birth defects are the leading cause of death in infancy (>20%) in the United States. Cardiovascular malformations are the leading cause of premature mortality caused by congenital anomalies. Genetic diseases also account for a large proportion of pediatric hospital admissions. Population-based studies suggest that birth defects and genetic disorders account for approximately 10% of hospitalizations and approximately 30% of all hospitalization charges. Approximately 7% of pediatric admissions are for single-gene and chromosomal disorders, another 15% to 20% for congenital malformations. Approximately 35% of deaths in a children's hospital are caused by a genetic condition and/or birth defect. Recent therapeutic advances are substantially prolonging survival of children with birth defects and/or genetic diseases. Generalists will care for a burgeoning patient population of older children and young adults with genetic disorders.

DIAGNOSIS AND EVALUATION

The generalist is the ideal health care provider to identify children at high risk for a genetic disorder, to arrange for diagnostic evaluation and counseling, and to provide long-term care. Circumstances that suggest a child may have a genetic disorder are listed in Box 156-1. Because there are thousands of different genetic conditions, and the ability to diagnose and treat these disorders is always changing, a single health care provider cannot be an expert on all genetic conditions. A logical and systematic approach to the evaluation of children with genetic conditions can substantially improve the care provided by the generalist.

Box 156-1. Conditions Suggesting a Child May Have a Genetic Disorder

1.   Family history of genetic disorder
2.   Abnormal prenatal or newborn screening result
3.   Multiple congenital anomalies; distinctive or rare physical characteristic
4.   Neurodevelopmental delay
5.   Chronic multiorgan dysfunction
6.   Acute life-threatening event
7.   Defect of growth or stature
8.   Perinatal or neonatal death

Establishing a specific diagnosis for a child with a genetic condition is important for the child, the family, and health care professionals. The diagnosis of a well-characterized disorder, even if the etiology is unknown, facilitates the provider's ability to give anticipatory guidance to patients and their families, including predictions of future manifestations and outcomes, use of appropriate screening tools for anticipated problems, and guidelines for routine care and educational interventions. Establishing a diagnosis often provides information on the pattern of inheritance of a condition and estimated risk of recurrence, and defines options for the management of future pregnancies. A specific diagnosis may also eliminate the need for additional diagnostic testing.

The initial evaluation of a child who may have a genetic condition should include detailed obstetrical, medical, and family histories, a comprehensive physical examination, and laboratory, physiologic, or imaging studies. The family history can be particularly useful and is usually more extensive than is commonly obtained for most patients (Box 156-2). Obtaining a family history is easier when a summary of the pedigree is available as parents are being interviewed (Box 156-3 provides instructions on drawing a pedigree). The pedigree helps prioritize questions to be asked and organizes the information obtained into meaningful patterns that may suggest a specific diagnosis. Examination of photographs of the parents, siblings, and extended family members taken when they were children is useful, especially when attempting to determine whether a physical characteristic is a diagnostic clue or part of the phenotypic background of the family or both (i.e., when a parent or relative is unknowingly affected as well).

Family history should be obtained by first asking general, open-ended questions. Sometimes asking questions that are less direct can facilitate the interview. For example, to explore whether anyone in the extended family had developmental delay or mental retardation, ask whether a child has relatives who did not graduate from high school, cannot drive a car, cannot live by themselves, have never been employed. Also ask about consanguineous mating. Various explanations can account for a positive response to any of these questions. The next step is to follow general questions with more specific queries.

Obstetrical history should include information about the duration of the pregnancy, the level of prenatal care, performance of prenatal tests (e.g., serum α-fetoprotein level, fetal ultrasonography), complications of the pregnancy, quantity and quality of amniotic fluid, exposures to over-the-counter and prescription medications and illicit drugs,

frequency and vigor of fetal movements, and chronic or acute medical problems experienced during the pregnancy. The pregnancy history should also include information about labor and delivery.

Because many genetic conditions are associated with abnormal cognitive development and/or birth defects that produce sensory or motor deficits, a comprehensive developmental history is also important. Comparison of the dates at which milestones were achieved among siblings is often helpful as an added control for family background and environment.

The physical examination is the cornerstone of the evaluation of children for most genetic conditions. Primary care providers must be observant and skilled at differentiating between "normal" and "abnormal" physical findings, rather than identifying every specific morphological variant. Abnormal findings may be clues to the diagnosis of a genetic condition. Many of the key physical findings are found on the most noticeable parts of the body—the head and the limbs.

The approach toward examination of the face and limbs is slightly different from that used to examine other areas of the body or organ systems. General relationships among the features of the face or the limbs should be examined and then each feature studied separately. For the face this means looking first at the relationships among the ears, forehead, eyes, nose, midface, philtral folds, lips, mouth, jaw, and neck to form a "gestalt" (i.e., a subjective impression of the overall pattern of relationships), and subsequently examining each of the aforementioned parts individually. Queries to think about during the examination are listed in Box 156-4. For example, if the ear of an infant appears set too low on the side of the head, is it because the ear is too small or rotated posteriorly, or is the superior helix overfolded? Each of these findings can be perceived as an ear that is set too low on the head of an infant, even when the position of the ear is appropriate. On the other hand, an ear with a normal size and structure but positioned at the angle of the mandible is an ear genuinely set too low. This distinction can serve as a clue for diagnosis.

Box 156-3. Recommendations for Drawing a Pedigree

1. Record at least three generations.
2. Include relatives of both parents.
3. Include all pregnancies and their outcomes.
4. Identify affected and unaffected individuals.
5. Include date of birth and causes of death of each individual.

Box 156-2. Important Elements of a Family History

1. Ancestry/ethnic origin
2. Presence of birth defects (e.g., cleft lip, neural tube defect)
3. Learning problems, developmental delay, mental retardation
4. Early (<55 yr old), sudden, or unexplained deaths, miscarriages
5. Unusual dietary habits
6. Cancer
7. Consanguinity
8. Known genetic disorders

Box 156-4. Queries to Consider While Doing a Physical Examination

- Does a particular characteristic (e.g., a very small chin, upslanting palpebral fissures) make the face look different from what might be anticipated based on the facial appearance of the parents and siblings?
- Are there specific characteristics that when juxtaposed with one another make a face look particularly distinguishable?
- If a physical feature appears different compared to normal, what is the specific relationship of that feature to other features that is abnormal?

Examination of the limbs should be similar to assessment of the face. The general relationships among the parts of the hand (e.g., length of digits, spacing between digits) should be studied first and then each part examined individually. The thumb is a particularly complex element of the hand. Anomalies of the thumb include low-set thumbs (usually hypoplastic with an underdeveloped thenar eminence), tapered thumbs, bifid thumbs, and triphalangeal thumbs (three phalanges instead of two). Observing the character of the flexion creases on the digits can also be valuable. Flexion creases develop between the 8th and 10th week of gestation, and perturbations of the flexion creases (e.g., hypoplasia, absence) may reflect an abnormality of fetal movement in the first trimester of gestation. The character of the flexion creases can help differentiate between congenital contractures caused by an intrinsic abnormality (e.g., amyoplasia) versus those that are caused by an extrinsic force (e.g., oligohydramnios). For example, an infant with amyoplasia will lack flexion creases while a child with multiple congenital contractures from oligohydramnios that developed in the third trimester of pregnancy will have normal flexion creases.

Each abnormal physical characteristic should be classified as a minor or major abnormality. Minor anomalies include both qualitative characteristics (e.g., size of the nasal tip) that can be challenging to judge as normal versus abnormal, and quantitative characteristics such as the distance between the right and left inner canthal folds. Measurement of quantitative features can subsequently be compared to normative data controlled for age, gender, ethnic background, and continent of origin (i.e., Africa, Asia, or Europe). The latter is important because the mean measurements of many morphological characteristics can vary substantially among individuals of recent European, Asian, and African ancestry. For example, short palpebral fissures are a consistent finding in children with fetal alcohol syndrome (FAS). However, variation in length of the palpebral fissures is wide among individuals of European, Asian, or Native American ancestry. Comparison of the length of the palpebral fissures of a child in whom the diagnosis of fetal alcohol syndrome is being considered must be to the appropriate normative data. Many minor anomalies (e.g., posterior polydactyly) are minor malformations that result in structural changes that have no intrinsic medical significance (unlike major malformations).

The recognition of minor and major anomalies helps the primary care provider determine the next step in the evaluation process. Studies indicate that about 10% of newborns have two or more minor anomalies. Most do not have a specific syndrome diagnosis, and are unlikely to experience further physical and/or developmental problems. However, minor anomalies can also help the clinician decide whether a more severe defect of a body part or organ may be present. For example, the presence of a deep sacral dimple, particularly with an overlying patch of hair or a hemangioma, should prompt further investigation for spinal dysraphism. Pits in the skin or tags of skin near the external ear should bring to mind specific syndrome diagnoses (e.g., branchial-oto-renal syndrome) and are also associated with an increased risk of hearing loss. Because many purported associations have been overstated and probably have little significance (e.g., accessory nipples and renal defects), caution should be exercised.

REFERRAL AND MANAGEMENT

Once a genetic diagnosis is entertained, the most productive and cost-effective next step is referral to a clinical geneticist. Clinical geneticists can often confirm or exclude a diagnosis by using only clinical criteria, suggest a focused set of diagnostic tests, provide an overview of a condition, explain the natural history and management options of a condition, and provide specialized genetic counseling. A typical comprehensive evaluation by a medical geneticist can require 1½ to 2 hours to complete, an evaluation that is impractical in the setting of a busy general pediatrics clinic.

Whether children or their parents are first informed of a diagnosis by the primary care provider or by a consultant should be decided on a case-by-case basis. Information about a possible or confirmed diagnosis should be fully disclosed to the family promptly and in a context where preliminary counseling is available. This so-called "informing interview" has been the focus of considerable investigation, and guidelines to make the interview more effective have been proposed (Box 156-5). The most important information imparted during this interview is an explanation of the diagnosis and the natural history of the condition. Explaining the logic used to deduce a specific diagnosis or conclude that the diagnosis is unknown is helpful. Explanation of the characteristics of the natural history should be conducted in an optimistic tone while maintaining realistic predictions about outcomes. Parents need to be informed that predictions are generalizations, that specific outcomes are uncertain, and that there are often exceptions to generalizations (e.g., children with trisomy 18 or 13 who live beyond 1 year of age).

Although a clinical geneticist may perform the informing interview, in most cases the generalist should remain the primary care provider. The generalist's role is especially important because children with genetic conditions are often referred to many different specialists. The generalist must oversee and coordinate care among the specialists.

Box 156-5. Guidelines for an Effective Informing Interview

1. Inform both parents together.
2. Inform them in a private setting and minimize distractions such as siblings, beepers, and hospital technology (monitors, ventilators).
3. Avoid unnecessary delays in imparting news of the diagnosis.
4. Have adequate information to answer common questions and plan sufficient time to answer questions and address concerns.
5. Focus on the child and not on the disease (use child's name, hold child, make positive statements about the child).
6. Avoid medical jargon.
7. Try to avoid providing too much information and give parents enough time to process the information.
8. Provide written information, information about resources, and a follow-up plan.
9. Anticipate a follow-up meeting if the diagnosis is unexpected.

Subsequently, the generalist and clinical geneticist can work together to create an individualized management plan for a child's health maintenance and supervision. Specific health maintenance guidelines for many common disorders have been developed. These guidelines, frequently available from clinical geneticists, focus on preventive care, well-known concerns, and common complications.

For some common conditions, multidisciplinary teams of care providers can be found at children's hospitals, academic medical centers, and health departments. These teams generally consist of professionals who can address the medical, psychological, genetic counseling, social, nutritional, functional, and educational needs of a child at a single clinic visit. The generalist should interpret the recommendations of the team for the family and assist in implementing appropriate recommendations. Explicit definition of the responsibilities of each component of the health care team (family, generalist, specialty clinics) is important to prevent omissions in care and to ensure that families know whom to contact in specific circumstances, particularly who is responsible for caring for a child during an acute illness related to the underlying genetic condition. These decisions are best coordinated and executed by the primary care provider. The generalists must make a concerted effort to remain engaged in the care provided to a child with special needs and communicate effectively with the family and specialists.

Parents will often develop an expertise about their child's condition beyond that of most health care providers with whom they are likely to interact, especially in emergency situations. Parents should be encouraged to keep an accurate, up-to-date, and comprehensive record of evaluations, test results, and management protocols for their child. Children with special health care needs should also be provided with a summary document specifying their diagnosis, treatment information, potential acute complications, plans for emergency management, and source for consultation. These facilitate the efforts of parents to be strong, informed advocates for their children.

In the case of genetic conditions for which death is frequent during childhood, the primary care provider is often the most appropriate professional to support the family and to arrange for postmortem exam and/or diagnostic studies. These studies are especially important when a genetic condition is suspected but not yet confirmed. In some cases DNA or other tissues may be banked for future investigation. Because of the significance for future pregnancies or siblings (e.g., estimation of the recurrence risk), an accurate diagnosis of a genetic condition may be the most significant service that clinicians can provide.

Regardless of whether a specific diagnosis or a specific etiology for the condition is proposed, one of the most important elements of managing a child with a genetic condition is to provide families with information about the implications of the condition. Communicating this information and providing psychotherapeutic input is known as genetic counseling (Box 156-6). Genetic counseling attempts to facilitate informed and autonomous decision making, integrate genetic information into a framework useful for individuals/families, provide individuals/families with insight about the potential consequences of their

---

Box 156-6. Usefulness of Genetic Counseling to Families

1. Comprehend medical facts, including the diagnosis, probable course of the disorder, and the available management.
2. Appreciate the way heredity contributes to the disorder, and the risk of recurrence in specified relatives.
3. Understand the alternatives for dealing with the risk of recurrence.
4. Choose the course of action that seems to the family members to be appropriate in view of their risk, family goals, and ethical and religious standard, and act in accordance with that decision.
5. Make the best possible adjustment to the disorder in an affected family member and/or to the risk of recurrence of that disorder.

---

decisions, and improve the emotional well-being of those affected and their families. One widely held professional standard is to provide this counseling in a nondirected fashion. This standard reflects the personal nature of the family's decision-making process (especially reproductive decisions) and the reluctance to judge the worthiness of the life of an individual with a genetic condition. Many parents are influenced by the nature of the information provided to them and the manner in which it is provided.

The task of educating and counseling parents to empower them and permit them to function as integral members of the management team is primarily the responsibility of clinical geneticists and genetic counselors, although nurse specialists and in some countries social workers also provide genetic counseling. Genetic counselors are medical professionals who are specifically trained to counsel individuals and families about genetic disorders. They provide genetic counseling in a wide variety of clinical settings (e.g., prenatal, pediatric, cancer) and are becoming more common in research and commercial environments.

Genetic counselors can explain the nature of genetic tests and interpret test results. Despite the widespread availability of geneteic testing, the clinical indications for many tests remain quite limited. Whether and how a test result affects risk estimation or case management must be considered. The interpretation of many genetic tests is complex, often with important implications for family members of an affected individual (e.g., inference of carrier status). Families should consider unforeseen risks of genetic testing (e.g., how will a test result affect insurance eligibility or employment opportunities). Too few genetics providers are available to counsel individuals and families about the ever-increasing number and availability of genetic tests. In the future many genetic tests for conditions commonly encountered by generalists will be ordered and interpreted by primary care providers who must be knowledgeable about fundamental genetics concepts and their application to clinical practice (see Chapter 9).

 Additional Resources, CD-ROM

Bibliography

SUGGESTED READINGS

Cassidy SB, Allison JE: Management of Genetic Syndromes. New York, Wiley-Liss, 2001.

Frias JC, Carey JC: Mild Errors of Morphogenesis. Adv in Pediatr 1996;43:27–75.

Jones KL: Smith's Recognizable Patterns of Human Malformation, 5th ed. Philadelphia, WB Saunders, 1997.

Jorde LB, Carey JC, Bamshad MJ, White RL: Medical Genetics, 3rd ed (Revised Reprint). St. Louis, Mosby, 2003.

Wilson GN, Cooley WC: Preventive Management of Children with Congenital Anomalies and Syndromes. Cambridge, Cambridge University Press, 2000.

SECTION 4   CHRONIC MEDICAL CARE: *Genetic Disorders*

157 Chromosome and Single Gene Disorders

Mary Beth Dinulos

ROLE OF THE GENERALIST

1. Recognize the high prevalence of chromosome disorders.
2. Understand chromosome organization, classification, and nomenclature.
3. Recognize the uses and limitations of cytogenetic studies in the diagnosis of chromosome abnormalities.
4. Recognize the phenotype of common chromosome abnormalities.
5. Refer children with suspected or confirmed chromosome abnormalities to clinical geneticist for assistance with diagnosis and management.
6. Manage acute and preventive care issues in children with chromosome abnormalities, using Internet resources and published guidelines.
7. Coordinate care for medical conditions associated with chromosome abnormalities.

Cytogenetics is the study of chromosomes, their structure, and their inheritance. Approximately 1 in 150 newborns has a chromosome abnormality, and at least 50% of first trimester miscarriages have a detectable chromosome abnormality. Chromosome abnormalities are a significant cause of pregnancy loss, mental retardation, and birth defects.

FUNDAMENTALS

The human genome consists of 6 to 7 billion base pairs of DNA organized into 23 pairs of chromosomes with those numbered 1 through 22 referred to as autosomes and the 23rd pair designated the "sex chromosomes" (XX = female, XY = male). A karyotype is an ordered set of chromosomes, arranged from largest to smallest, with the exception of the sex chromosomes, which occupy the lower right-hand corner (Fig. 157-1). Each chromosome has a characteristic banding pattern, which aids in its identification. The band level noted on the chromosome analysis report is an important factor in determining the quality of the study. A higher band level yields a more informative study. Subtle rearrangements may not be detected at a 450 band level, a typical level for amniocentesis, but may be visible at a 750 band level, normal-high resolution blood study. A standardized system of karyotype nomenclature has been defined. Table 157-1 gives examples of nomenclature for common chromosome abnormalities.

Each chromosome is composed of hundreds to thousands of genes. There is an estimated 30,000 to 40,000 genes in the entire human genome. Each gene is composed of DNA. A change or mutation in a gene may result in a recognizable genetic disorder. These disorders are referred to as single gene or Mendelian disorders.

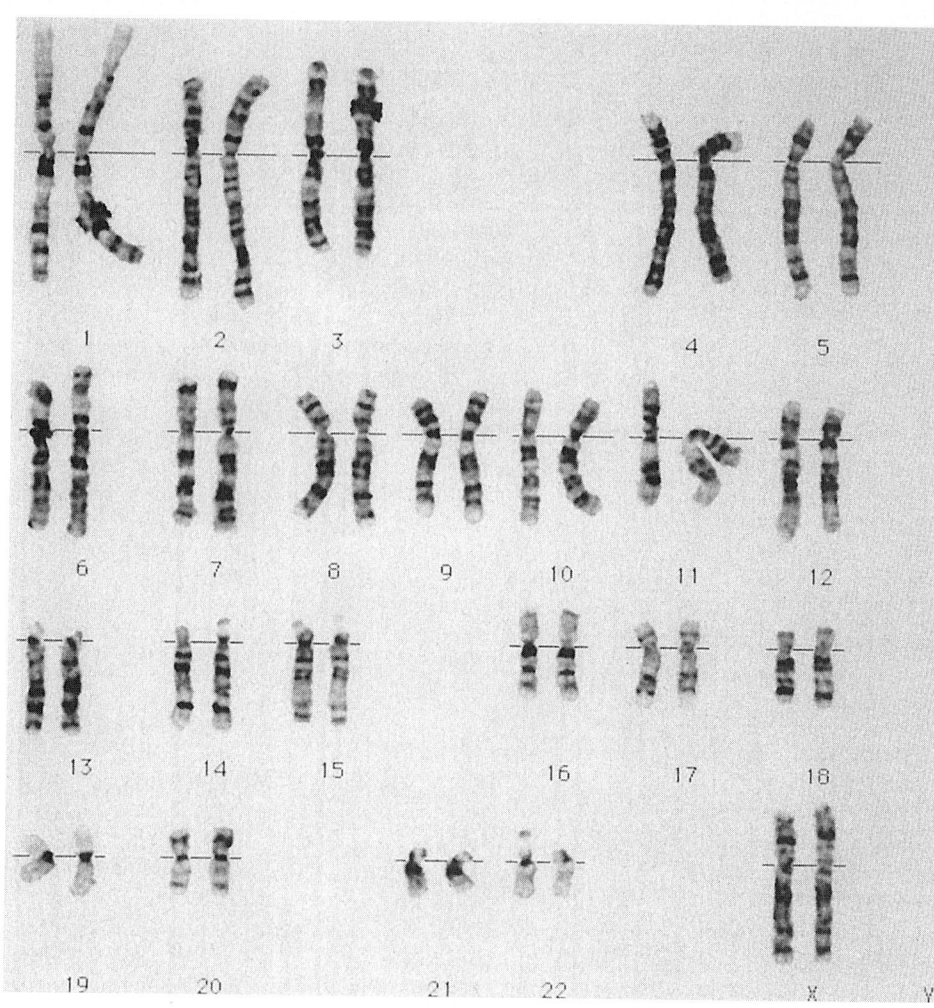

Figure 157-1. A G-banded karyotype of a normal female. Note that the chromosomes are arranged from largest to smallest, with the sex chromosomes in the lower right-hand corner. (From Jorde LB, Carey JC, Bamshad MJ: Medical Genetics, 3rd ed. St Louis, Mosby, 2003.)

NUMERICAL CHROMOSOME ABNORMALITIES

Chromosome abnormalities are classified into two major groups: numerical and structural. Numerical abnormalities are due to extra or missing chromosomes (aneuploidy) or multiples of the haploid set (polyploidy). Aneuploidy may involve either autosomes or sex chromosomes. Most cases of aneuploidy are due to maternal nondisjunction. Autosomal chromosome imbalances are characterized by multiple birth defects, growth retardation, mental retardation, and sometimes early fetal or neonatal demise. Sex chromosome abnormalities are quite common, tend to exhibit a less severe phenotype, and have a better prognosis.

Table 157-1. Standard Nomenclature for Chromosome Karyotypes

Karyotype	Description
46,XY	Normal male chromosome constitution
47,XX,+21	Female with trisomy 21, Down syndrome
47,XY,+21[10]/46,XY[10]	Male who is a mosaic of trisomy 21 cells and normal cells (10 cells scored for each karyotype)
46,XY,del(4)(p14)	Male with distal deletion of the short arm of chromosome 4 band designated 14
46,XX,dup(5)(p14p15.3)	Female with duplication of the short arm of chromosome 5 from bands p14 to p15.3
45,XY,(der)(13;14)(q10;q10)	A male with a balanced Robertsonian translocation of chromosomes 13 and 14. Karyotype shows that one normal 13 and one normal 14 are missing and replaced with a derivative chromosome
46,XY,t(11;22)(q23;q22)	A male with a balanced reciprocal translocation between chromosomes 11 and 22; the breakpoints are at 11q23 and 22q22
46,XX, inv(3)(p21;q13)	An inversion on chromosome 3 that extends from p21 to q13; because it includes the centromere, this is a pericentric inversion
46,X,r(X)	A female with one normal X chromosome and one ring X chromosome
46,X,i(Xq)	A female with one normal X chromosome and an isochromosome of the long arm of the X chromosome

From Jorde LB, Carey JC, Bamshad MJ, White RL: Medical Genetics, 3rd ed. St. Louis, Mosby, 2003.

Table 157-2. Presenting Signs and Symptoms of Turner Syndrome by Age at Presentation

Newborn	■ History of fetal hydrops ■ Nuchal thickening ■ Lymphedema of hands and feet ■ Congenital heart disease (bicuspid Aortic valve, coarctation of aorta) ■ Feeding problems
Childhood/adolescence	■ Short stature ■ Delayed puberty ■ Amenorrhea or oligomenorrhea ■ Lack of secondary sexual characteristics ■ History of congenital heart disease ■ Webbed neck with low posterior hairline ■ Broad chest with widely spaced nipples ■ Widened carrying angle of arms (cubitus valgus) ■ Structural renal abnormalities
Adulthood	■ Above phenotypic features ■ Infertility

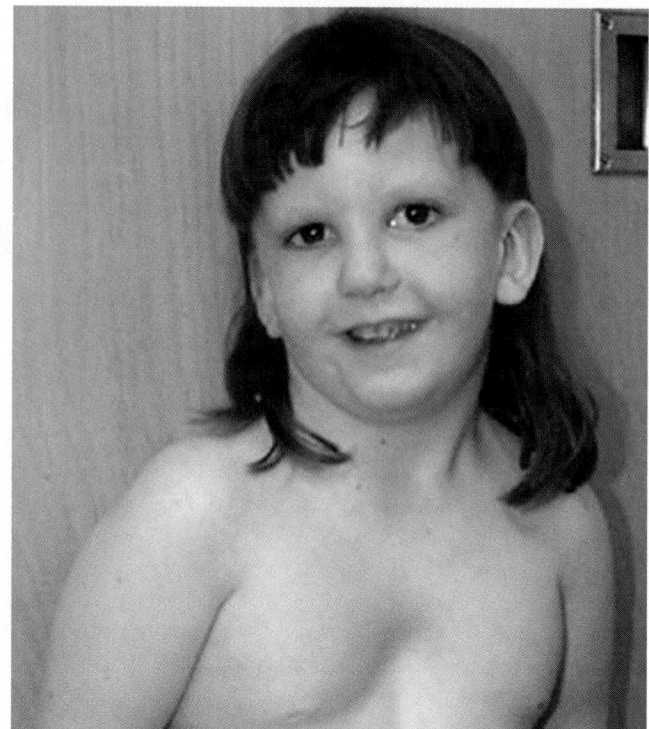

Figure 157-2. Turner syndrome (45,X).

Down Syndrome, Trisomies 18 and 13. Down syndrome (trisomy 21) is the most common trisomy (see Chapter 158). Trisomy 18 (Edwards syndrome) and trisomy 13 (Patau syndrome) are the second and third most common trisomies. Both have a high rate of morbidity and mortality. Their salient features and management issues are discussed on the CD-ROM.

Turner Syndrome. Table 157-2 lists the presenting signs and symptoms by age of presentation of girls with Turner syndrome. Its incidence is approximately 1 in 2500 to 5000 live female births. Various X chromosome abnormalities responsible for the Turner syndrome phenotype are listed in Table 157-3. Cardinal features are short stature and gonadal dysgenesis with resultant amenorrhea and/or oligomenorrhea, lack of secondary sexual characteristics, and infertility (Fig. 157-2). Associated abnormalities include congenital heart disease, structural renal abnormalities, hypothyroidism, and recurrent ear infections. Intelligence is usually normal, but some girls may have difficulty in spatial perception. Typically, growth hormone production is normal. Table 157-4 outlines management issues. Referral to a medical geneticist is highly recommended when Turner syndrome is suspected or has been newly diagnosed.

Klinefelter Syndrome. The presenting signs and symptoms by age at presentation of Klinefelter syndrome are listed in Table 157-5. Klinefelter syndrome is the most common sex chromosome abnormality with an incidence of

approximately 1 in 600 live male births. The karyotype is typically 47,XXY. Rarer forms with multiple X chromosomes do exist (i.e., 48,XXXY and 49,XXXXY). Cardinal features of Klinefelter syndrome include tall stature, learning disabilities (specifically, language problems), testicular dysgenesis (hypogonadism, infertility), and gynecomastia. Risk of breast cancer and extragonadal germ cell tumors is increased in 47,XXY boys. Management is outlined in Table 157-6.

47,XYY Boys. The incidence of 47,XYY boys is approximately 1 in 1000 newborn males. Presenting signs and

Table 157-3. X Chromosome Abnormalities Associated with the Turner's Syndrome Phenotype

45,X	50%
45,X/46,XX	30–40%
45,X/46,XY*	*increased risk for gonadoblastoma
46,XXp- 46,X,i(Xq) 46,X,i(Xp)	10–20%

Table 157-4. Management of Girls with Turner Syndrome

Short stature	■ Turner syndrome growth grids ■ Referral to endocrinologist to discuss growth hormone therapy at age 4 years or after ■ Encourage physical activity and healthy diet to avoid obesity
Gonadal dysgenesis	■ Ovarian hormone replacement therapy at approximately age 14 years
Congenital heart disease	■ Echocardiogram at diagnosis and thereafter as recommended by the cardiologist ■ Routine blood pressure screening ■ Antibiotic prophylaxis for valvular disease
Renal abnormalities	■ Renal ultrasound at diagnosis
Hypothyroidism	■ Thyroid function tests every 1–2 years beginning at age 10 years, or earlier if growth abnormal
Learning problems	■ Routine developmental screening ■ Monitoring school performance
Neoplasia (gonadoblastoma)	■ Prophylactic gonadectomy in girls with a Y chromosome

Table 157-5. Presenting Signs and Symptoms of Klinefelter Syndrome by Age at Presentation

Newborn	■ Subtle hypotonia
Childhood	■ Slightly delayed milestones
	■ Learning disabilities (language and sensorimotor integration problems)
	■ Shyness, immaturity
	■ Normal testicular volume
Adolescence	■ Decreased athletic ability
	■ Learning difficulties
	■ Initial normal prepubertal development, then cessation with resultant hypogonadism and infertility
	■ Gynecomastia
	■ Tall stature
Adulthood	■ Hypogonadism and infertility
	■ Autoimmune disorders

Box 157-1. Presenting Signs and Symptoms of 47, XYY Males

- Large teeth
- Severe cystic acne in adolescence
- Tall stature
- Learning disabilities
- Poor fine motor coordination
- Behavior abnormalities (ADHD, temper tantrums)

symptoms are listed in Box 157-1. These boys may be taller than average but otherwise have a normal phenotype. Puberty and fertility are normal. IQ may be slightly below that of their siblings. Behavior problems (such as attention deficit hyperactivity disorder [ADHD]) are common; however, they are not at increased risk to commit violent crimes, as once thought. Management is similar to that of any child with a learning disability or with behavior problems.

47,XXX Girls. The incidence of 47,XXX is 1 in 1000 live female births. Box 157-2 lists presenting signs and symptoms. These girls may have learning difficulties and slight reduction in IQ compared to their siblings. They may have tall stature but an otherwise normal phenotype. Fertility is usually normal. Management is similar to other children with learning disabilities.

STRUCTURAL CHROMOSOME ABNORMALITIES

Chromosome abnormalities involving chromosomal rearrangements, deletions, or duplications are called structural chromosome abnormalities. Deletions are typically associated with birth defects, growth retardation, and mental retardation. Two common deletion syndromes are cri-du-chat syndrome (5p-) and Wolf-Hirschhorn syndrome (4p-), which are discussed on the CD-ROM.

Microdeletion Syndromes. 5p- and 4p- are abnormalities easily detectable under the light microscope. However, some deletions are very small and not visible by routine chromosome analysis. Introduction of fluorescence in situ hybridization (FISH) in the early 1990s has revolutionized the field of cytogenetics. Submicroscopic deletions or duplications and subtle chromosome rearrangements can be detected using this technique.

Velocardiofacial Syndrome. Velocardiofacial syndrome (VCFS) is the most common microdeletion syndrome with an estimated incidence of approximately 1 in 2000 to 4000 live births. Individuals with VCFS have a small deletion of the long arm of one chromosome 22 (22q11.2). Presenting signs and symptoms of VCFS are listed in Table 157-7. The phenotype is quite variable and the facial features may be subtle, especially in the newborn period. The diagnosis should be suspected when two or more of the characteristic features are present. Referral to a medical geneticist would be warranted at this point. Management of VCFS is dependent on the system involvement and outlined in Table 157-8.

Williams Syndrome. Williams syndrome is due to a submicroscopic deletion of the long arm of one chromosome 7 (7q11.23), which encompasses the elastin (ELN) and lim kinase 1 (LIMK1) genes. The incidence of Williams syndrome is approximately 1 in 10,000 to 20,000 live births. Box 157-3 lists the presenting signs and symptoms of Williams syndrome. Although the facial features are distinctive (Fig. 157-3), the diagnosis may not be evident until early childhood when the characteristic personality and behavior are present. Referral to a medical geneticist is warranted when the diagnosis is suspected. Management of children with Williams syndrome is listed in Table 157-9.

Prader-Willi Syndrome. Prader-Willi syndrome (PWS) is a multisystem mental retardation syndrome with an

Table 157-6. Management of Klinefelter Syndrome

Testicular dysgenesis	■ Obtain FSH, LH, and testoterone levels at 12–13 years of age
	■ Consider testosterone therapy in mid to late adolescence
Gynecomastia	■ Consider mastectomy if psychologically warranted
	■ Regular breast examination in adult men
Learning disabilities	■ Routine assessment of developmental milestones
	■ Monitor for learning disabilities in childhood
	■ Early intervention

Box 157-2. Presenting Signs and Symptoms of 47, XXX Females

- Tall stature
- Poor coordination
- Learning disabilities (difficulties in verbal learning and expressive language)
- Behavior problems (depression, conduct disorder, problems with interpersonal relationships)

newborn hearing screening, and the usual newborn metabolic screening tests. The risk of congenital hypothyroidism is increased.

For most babies with Down syndrome, newborn care is routine and uncomplicated. Even those with congenital heart defects do not usually appear ill and usually do not have heart murmurs initially. Some may have brief oxygen requirements, and delayed stimulation of hepatic enzymes may prolong physiologic jaundice. Care needs are dictated by the same indicators of health status as in any newborn. Some babies may have difficulty establishing feeding or initiating breast-feeding because of decreased oral motor tone and a weaker suck. Breast-feeding should not be discouraged, since it is successful in most cases.

Parents will need access to accurate and thorough information. Some parents are more comfortable with textbook-style reading material while others may prefer the accounts of experiences written by other parents. Many parents benefit from early contact with veteran parents who are often trained for this role by a local parent-to-parent organization. The Internet contains a rich source of useful, but generally unedited information, and opportunities for contact with other parents. All families should be provided information about and support for referral to early intervention services. Down syndrome babies are universally eligible. Some families with lower income may be eligible for Supplemental Security Income (SSI) benefits and for associated public health insurance programs.

MANAGEMENT

Longitudinal studies have not revealed any long-term differences in social and psychological outcomes for the parents and families of children with Down syndrome compared to those with typical children. One of the sources of resilience among families involves absorbing the issues of Down syndrome into the fabric of family life and sustaining a hopeful, positive attitude about the future. Primary health care providers should strive to sustain these coping strategies. Evidence-based research and consensus among experts has resulted in standards of preventive health care for children with Down syndrome that involve specific additions to the usual periodic screening, immunizations, and anticipatory guidance that applies to all children. Table 158-1 provides a summary of preventive care issues in a chart format that can be copied and used as a reminder in a patient's medical record.

Table 158-1. Down Syndrome Preventive Care Overview

Concern	Clinical Expression	When Seen	Prevalence	Management
Congenital heart disease	Complete AV canal Septal defects Mitral prolapse	Newborn or first 6 weeks; later for mitral prolapse	40–50%	Pediatric cardiology consultation; echocardiogram; surgery; dental prophylaxis
Hypotonia	Reduced muscle tone; increased range of joint movement; motor function problems	Throughout life; tends to improve with age	100%	Guidance by physical therapy early intervention program
Delayed growth	Usually near or below third percentile of general population for height	Throughout life	100%	Nutritional support; DS growth charts check heart/thyroid
Developmental delays	Some global delay, degree varies; specific processing problems; specific language delay	First year; monitor throughout life	100%	Early intervention Individual educational plan Language interventions
Hearing problems	Middle ear problems (fluid and infections) Sensorineural hearing loss	Audiology consult every 6 months until age 2, then annually	50–70%	Audiology, tympanometry ENT consultation Myringotomy tubes if needed
Vision problems	Refractive errors Strabismus Cataracts	Eye exam in 1st month; then annually	50% 35% 15%	Pediatric ophthalmologic consultation and appropriate treatment
Cervical spine problems	Atlantoaxial instability Skeletal anomalies May cause spinal cord injury	Initial x-ray screen at age 3 for AAI	15%	Orthopedic; neurology; neurosurgery; avoid high-risk activity; surgery if spinal cord compression
Thyroid disease	Hypothyroidism (rarely hyperthyroidism)	Some congenital; check annually	15%	Endocrinology consultation; replacement therapy
Overweight	Excessive weight gain	Late preschool; adolescence/adult life	Common	Lifestyle changes around food/exercise; thyroid function; depression
Seizure disorder	Generalized or myoclonic; hypsarrhythmia	Any time	5–10%	Neurology consultation, EEG, medication
Emotional problems	Behavioral changes; depression	Adolescence; young adult	Common	Inclusive education; counseling; support transition from school to work
Dementia	Loss of adaptive skills; seizures; mood lability; rapid decline common	After age 40	20%	Neuropsychological testing; neurology consultation; psychopharmacologic management (NSAID, anticholinergic)

Variable occurrence of: celiac disease; gastrointestinal anomalies; Hirschsprung; leukemia; alopecia areata; diabetes; sleep apnea; hip dysplasia.

After careful evaluation for congenital problems in the newborn nursery, children with Down syndrome need continuous careful reassessment for problems with hearing and with vision. Hearing should be tested by the most accurate means possible by a qualified audiologist at 6-month intervals until age 2 and annually thereafter. Though the hearing loss is usually acquired from middle ear effusion or infection, 10% of individual with Down syndrome have congenital sensorineural hearing loss. Because acquired hearing loss can occur at any age, ongoing surveillance is necessary. A pediatric ophthalmologist should assess eye anatomy and vision on an annual basis. Because the risk for treatable thyroid disease is increased, at least a T_4 and TSH should be obtained annually. At about 3 years of age x-rays of the neck should be obtained looking for atlantoaxial instability. Fifteen percent will demonstrate possible instability that requires careful follow-up for neurologic signs of myelopathy, restriction from activities that place chronic stress on the neck (trampolines, some gymnastic activities, collision sports, competitive diving, and the butterfly stroke in swimming), and caution during general anesthesia requiring intubation.

The incidence of obstructive sleep apnea may be as high as 50% in children and adults with Down syndrome. Children with periodic nocturnal awakening, unusual sleep postures (e.g., sleeping in a sitting position or with the forehead resting on the knees), prominent snoring, somnolence or fatigue in the afternoon, or observed, brief apneic spells during sleep should be referred for a sleep study or home nap study. Treatments for this condition include weight loss, positioning on the side during sleep, tonsillectomy, or use of a positive airway pressure device.

Children with Down syndrome are at higher risk for all autoimmune conditions including autoimmune thyroiditis, alopecia areata, celiac disease, rheumatoid arthritis, and type 1 diabetes mellitus. Ten percent develop seizures; myoclonic seizures are the most common in childhood. Seven percent to 10% of children with Down syndrome also develop autism.

Nearly all are shorter than their peers. Both regular and Down syndrome growth curves should be used to monitor physical growth during well-child care. Growth curves developed from a population of individuals with Down syndrome may underidentify obesity in adolescents with Down syndrome.

No specific medical treatments will alter or ameliorate the effects of the Down syndrome genotype. However, many nonconventional and complementary interventions have been promoted as therapies for Down syndrome. Parents need to be supported in their exploration of these options and in their decisions to use any safe interventions. Nutritional supplementation with a variety of vitamins, minerals, and amino acids has been promoted to "correct" alleged nutritional and metabolic deficiencies. Such approaches have been the subjects of speculation since the early 1950s. During the 1980s several well-designed, controlled studies failed to demonstrate any health or functional benefits of these therapies. Cognition- or memory-enhancing medications such as piracetam have been studied. So far these drugs have proven to be safe but have shown no measurable benefit in the treatment of Down

syndrome. Facial plastic surgery was popularized during the 1980s in Germany and Israel based on the hypothetical benefits of "normalizing" the appearance of a child with Down syndrome. Outcome studies failed to demonstrate any functional or social advantages for children following cosmetic surgery. Surgery such as tongue reduction is rarely justified and may be misguided in view of the normal tongue size in most individuals. No improvement in speech production or intelligibility has been seen following tongue reduction procedures.

Nearly all children with Down syndrome in the United States are eligible for special education services from their local school district between the ages of 3 and 22 years. Most young children with Down syndrome do very well in appropriately supported regular classroom settings. Supports include frequent special education consultation with the classroom teacher and a full-time paraprofessional classroom aide or assistant to implement curricular modifications. Most children will require regular speech and occupational therapy. By age 16, formal transition planning for adulthood should begin, including vocational planning and visioning about adult living situations. Pediatric primary care providers will also need to help youth with Down syndrome and their parents plan for adult health services and the transition to adult health care providers. The website of the National Down Syndrome Society (www.ndss.org) contains additional information regarding transition from child to adult life.

During and after the period of transition to adulthood, young adults with Down syndrome are particularly at risk for demoralization and depression. In some communities, there is a bureaucratic and philosophical disconnect between the inclusive and comprehensive life of a public school student and the limited sometimes regressive supports offered to adults with disabilities. An adult with Down syndrome may find waiting lists for adult services and supports, less challenging and more menial work opportunities, and living situations that fail to continue the promise of optimal growth and independence. Friends from high school have gone on with their lives in postsecondary school, careers, marriages, or military service, leaving the person with Down syndrome more isolated. Model opportunities for appropriate vocation education, supported employment, and community living are increasing, but these opportunities do not exist everywhere. Such circumstances may underlie affective and functional changes consistent with depression. Sometimes they are mistaken for the beginning of an organic brain syndrome or dementia. Treatment of depression requires an accurate diagnosis, advocacy for improved services and supports, and the appropriate use of antidepressant medication.

The increased life expectancy of the individual with Down syndrome should be appreciated, but increased life span has revealed issues of aging that were not apparent a generation ago. Though some body systems age more slowly (e.g., atherosclerosis does not occur), the central nervous system is uniquely vulnerable to the pathogenetic processes associated with Alzheimer-type dementia. By age 40, all individuals with Down syndrome have neuropathologic findings considered hallmarks of Alzheimer-type dementia (amyloid plaques and neurofibrillary tangles). Interestingly, only about 20% of adults with Down syndrome develop clinical dementia. Nevertheless, the risk for dementia is far higher than in the general population with the average age of onset in the early 50s. A number of longitudinal studies of individuals with Down syndrome of various ages have begun testing the potential of antioxidants, nonsteroidal anti-inflammatory agents, and acetylcholinesterase inhibitors to prevent the progression of this neuropathologic process.

OUTCOMES

Important developments in recent decades have brightened and expanded the prospects for individuals with Down syndrome and their families. Nearly every child with Down syndrome is raised in a normative lifestyle among loving family members. Even when parents decide the challenges of raising a child with Down syndrome are too great, adoption is an alternative. There is a waiting list of interested families. Advances in health care for the treatment of life-threatening complications, condition-specific preventive health care, and anticipatory guidance have improved the health and longevity of nearly all individuals with Down syndrome. Early intervention and inclusive approaches to special education services have ensured optimal development of knowledge, skills, and understanding of societal roles. Finally, communities have welcomed children and

adults with Down syndrome as participating and contributing citizens capable of productive work and considerable independence.

Primary health care providers are ideally positioned to provide a Medical Home for children with Down syndrome and their families. Table 158-2 lists useful sources of information available on the Internet. Primary health care providers should be important sources of information, care coordination, advocacy, and longitudinal support for the child and family.

Additional Resources, CD-ROM

Bibliography	

Mini-index of Related Topics

SUGGESTED READINGS

American Academy of Pediatrics Committee on Genetics: Health supervision for children with Down syndrome. Pediatrics 2001;107(2):442–449.

Cohen W: Health care guidelines for individuals with Down syndrome: 1999 revision. Down Syndrome Quarterly 1999;4:1–15.

Cohen W, Nadel L, Madnick M (eds): Down Syndrome: Visions for the 21st Century. New York, John Wiley and Sons, 2002.

Cooley WC: Non-conventional therapies for Down syndrome: A review and framework for decision-making. In Cohen W, Nadel L, Madnick M (eds): Down Syndrome: Visions for the 21st Century. New York, John Wiley and Sons, 2002.

Cooley WC, Graham JM: Down syndrome: An update and review for the primary pediatrician. Clin Pediatr 1991;320:233–253.

Table 158-2. Useful Resources about Down Syndrome on the Internet

Web address	Content
www.denison.edu/dsq	Online version of *Down Syndrome Quarterly,* a journal published by the Down Syndrome Medical Interest Group; contains the latest version of the Preventive Medicine Checklist for Down Syndrome
www.growthcharts.com	Down syndrome growth charts available for downloading
www.ds-health.com	Excellent, well-edited compendium of current articles, information, and advice related to health care issues in Down syndrome
www.ndss.org	Website of the National Down Syndrome Society with links to many other resources; an important connection for parents
www.woodbinehouse.com	Website of the publisher of a series of books about Down syndrome written for the lay reader; *Babies with Down Syndrome: A New Parent's Guide* is one of the best books for new parents
www.familyvillage.wisc.edu	General website for families of children with disabilities with information about diagnosis, health care, schools, adult services, and more

159 Chronic Anemia

Howard A. Pearson and Karen Ann Kalinyak

ROLE OF THE GENERALIST

1   Provide appropriate screening for anemia.

2   Diagnose chronic anemia and refer to hematologist if assistance is needed in determining the cause of anemia.

3   Provide primary care for patients with chronic anemias, including preventive care and appropriate treatment and triage for acute illness.

4   Comanage patients with chronic anemias with a pediatric hematologist, assuring that patients have appropriate referral and follow-up.

Anemia is a reduction in the hemoglobin (Hb) or hematocrit (Hct) of the peripheral blood below the range of normal. The correlation between Hb and Hct is Hct/3 = Hb and Hb × 3 = Hct. The lower limit of normal is arbitrarily set as two standard deviations below the mean of Hb and Hct at any given age. Table 159-1 lists hemoglobin, hematocrit, and mean corpuscular volume (MCV) levels at birth, during the first decade of life, and after puberty and by gender differences. Laboratory reports that reference only adult values will erroneously report levels of Hb and Hct that are normal in children as low. Black children have Hb levels about 0.5 g/dL lower than white children.

The definition of anemia as a Hb or Hct value two standard deviations below the normal mean level implies that about 2.5% of normal children may be classified as being anemic and track at their low level over extended periods of time. Some individuals have Hb and Hct values in the lower part of the normal range that may increase after treatment with hematinics or after the resolution of an infection or inflammatory process.

Anemia can be further classified as mild, moderate, severe, and critically severe (Table 159-2). Children with severe and critically severe anemia may require hospitalization and should usually be managed at least initially in consultation with a pediatric hematologist.

For this discussion, chronic anemia is defined as anemia that persists for more than 3 months.

FUNDAMENTALS

Two mechanisms may result in anemia: underproduction (aregenerative anemia) and increased destruction (hemolytic anemia) (Table 159-3). If not enough red blood cells (RBCs) are produced to balance the number of RBCs reaching the end of their survival, Hb and Hct will decrease. Anemia also results when RBCs are destroyed faster than they are produced. Differentiating between hemolytic anemias and aregenerative anemias is crucial for diagnosis.

Hemolysis refers to an increased rate of RBC destruction leading to a survival time that is less than the normal 100 to 120 days. In chronic hemolytic states, anemia is usually present because the rate of RBC destruction and production are not completely balanced. If the degree of hemolysis is fully compensated by increased RBC production, then hemoglobin level will be normal and the reticulocyte count will be persistently elevated.

Table 159-1. Hemoglobin, Hematocrit, and Mean Corpuscular Volume by Age

Age	Hemoglobin Mean (g/dL)	Hemoglobin Low Limit (g/dL)	Hematocrit Mean (%)	Hematocrit Low Limit (%)	Mean Corpuscular Volume Mean (fL)	Mean Corpuscular Volume Low Limit (fL)
Birth	16.5	13.5	51	42	108	98
8 weeks						
Preterm	8.8	7.1	26	21		
Term	11.0	9.0	35	27		
6 months	11.0	9.5	33	28		
1 year	12.0	10.5	36	33	78	80
6 years	12.5	11.0	37	34	81	75
Adult						
Female	14.0	12.0	42	36	90	80
Male	15.5	13.5	47	41	90	80

Values derived from Nathan DG, Orkin SH, Look AT, Ginsburg D (eds): Nathan & Oski's Hematology of Infancy and Childhood, 5th ed. Philadelphia, WB Saunders, 1997, Appendix 1, p ix.

Table 159-2. Classification of Anemia by Severity

Level of Anemia	Hemoglobin (g/dL)	Hematocrit (%)
Mild	9–10.9	27–32
Moderate	7.0–8.9	21–26
Severe	5–6.9	15–20
Critically severe	<5	<15

In most chronic hemolytic states, RBCs are destroyed extravascularly in the reticuloendothelial (RE) tissues of the spleen, liver, and bone marrow. Many patients with chronic hemolysis are jaundiced with elevated serum levels of unconjugated (indirect) bilirubin. Efficient hepatic conjugation and clearance of bilirubin can result in normal serum bilirubin levels, and hyperbilirubinemia and clinical jaundice are not necessary to consider a diagnosis of hemolysis. Chronically increased rates of bilirubin metabolism and biliary excretion, characteristic of chronic hemolysis, may result in gallstones composed of calcium bilirubinate that are usually multiple, faceted, and radiopaque.

Primarily intravascular hemolysis is characteristic of some immune-related, drug-induced, or microangiopathic hemolytic anemias. Patients with hemolysis are often anhaptoglobinemic. Free hemoglobin is liberated into the plasma, where it combines with haptoglobin. The haptoglobin-hemoglobin complex is then cleared by RE tissues. When the rate of clearance exceeds the rate of hepatic haptoglobin synthesis, the level of serum haptoglobin decreases below the normal range (20 to 200 mg/dL). Low or absent levels of serum haptoglobin are also seen in hemolytic states in which RBC destruction is primarily extravascular. In acute intravascular hemolysis the binding capacity of haptoglobin for hemoglobin may be exceeded. Unbound, free hemoglobin excreted by the kidney results in hemoglobinuria, indicated by a positive test for occult blood without RBCs in the urine. In chronic intravascular hemolytic states, hemosiderin may also be present in the urine.

RBC production is most easily assessed by the reticulocyte count. Reticulocytopenia almost always indicates that inadequate numbers of RBCs are being released from the bone marrow to sustain Hb and Hct levels. Normal RBCs live for about 100 days, so about 1% of senescent RBCs are removed from the circulation each day and in the steady state about 1% of new RBCs are released from the bone marrow each day. Newly released RBCs contain reticulum

Table 159-3. Mechanisms that Cause Anemia

Mechanism	Effects
Underproduction of RBCs	Decreased Hb
	Decreased reticulocytes
	Decreased marrow RBC precursors
Increased destruction of RBCs	Decreased Hb
	Increased reticulocytes
	Increased marrow RBC precursors
	Increased bilirubin
	Decreased haptogobin
	Abnormalities of RBC on blood smear

Hb, hemoglobin; RBC, red blood cell.

for 1 to 2 days, so the normal reticulocyte count is 1.0 to 2.0% of the RBC, or erythrocyte, count. The normal absolute reticulocyte count is 40 to 75×10^9/L. Low values ($< 30 \times 10^9$/L) indicate erythrocyte underproduction, and high values (100×10^9/L) suggest marrow erythroid hyperplasia often associated with chronic hemolysis. Transiently high reticulocyte counts are seen after acute blood loss or hemolysis and after institution of specific therapy for iron, folic acid, or vitamin B_{12} deficiency.

Examination of the bone marrow is often indicated in aregenerative anemias to assess the numbers and morphology of the erythroid precursors. The normal proportion of myeloid to erythroid precursors (M/E ratio) is 2:1 to 4:1. Marked reduction of erythroid precursors is characteristic of pure RBC anemias such as the Diamond-Blackfan syndrome and transient erythroblastopenia of childhood. In chronic hemolytic anemias, the marrow M/E ratio is reversed. Replacement of the bone marrow in leukemia and marrow aplasia in aplastic anemia are associated with anemia and reduction in neutrophils and platelets. Low levels of erythropoietin (EPO) occur in end-stage renal disease, an aregenerative anemia that responds to erythropoietin therapy.

PRESENTATION AND EVALUATION

The evaluation of a chronically anemic child must include a careful history, exploring the diet, the presence of infection or chronic disease, medications, and other environmental exposures and the patient's past and family history and ethnicity.

The diet during infancy is particularly relevant to iron deficiency. Infants who have been fed only whole cow milk or non–iron-fortified cow milk formulas are at risk for developing iron deficiency. Although the iron present in human milk appears to be better absorbed than that in cow milk, the amount is insufficient to meet the requirements for growth, and infants consuming only breast milk may develop iron deficiency after 9 to 12 months of age.

The age of the child when anemia is discovered may be diagnostically important. Iron deficiency anemia is most common at 12 to 24 months of age and during adolescence, especially in girls. Abnormalities of the RBC membrane and RBC enzymopathies often present in the newborn with hyperbilirubinemia. Infants with major β-globin chain hemoglobin disorders such as sickle cell disease and thalassemia have normal hematologic values in the neonatal period and do not become anemic until 3 to 6 months of age or older. Many hemolytic anemias are genetically determined. An inherited anemia such as hereditary spherocytosis may be suggested by a family history of neonatal hyperbilirubinemia, anemia, jaundice, splenomegaly, splenectomy, or gallstones. A family history indicating dominant inheritance suggests a defect of the erythrocyte membrane, whereas recessive inheritance is characteristic of many enzymopathies.

In the differential diagnosis of anemia in children, the relative frequency of various etiologies should be considered. Iron deficiency and the anemia of acute and chronic infections are by far the most common causes of anemia in children. Next in frequency are genetic conditions such as hereditary spherocytosis. Sickle cell diseases are prevalent in African Americans, and thalassemia is common in people of Mediterranean or Southeast Asian ethnicity.

The most important physical finding of anemia is pallor, but this finding is often subtle and may be evident only when the degree of anemia is relatively severe (Hb < 7.0 g/dL). Anemia is best appreciated by pallor of the mucous membranes and conjunctivae, particularly in dark-skinned children. The red color of the lines in the palms of the hands disappears when the hemoglobin falls below 7.0 g/dL.

Children may tolerate even fairly severe degrees of anemia well when it develops slowly, because of compensatory processes that maintain oxygen delivery. These mechanisms include an increase in cardiac output and a shift in the oxygen dissociation curve secondary to increased levels of 2,3-diphosphogluconate that are evoked by anemia. Children with severe iron deficiency anemia may have few symptoms. Children with sickle cell anemia who chronically have hemoglobin levels of 6.5 to 7.5 g/dL usually have normal activity and few symptoms of anemia. Tachycardia is present only when anemia is severe or of sudden onset.

Some chronic anemias of childhood have associated abnormalities on physical examination. These include the thumb abnormalities seen in children with Fanconi and Diamond-Blackfan anemias and neurologic abnormalities associated with chronic vitamin B_{12} deficiency.

Jaundice and yellow sclerae suggest a hemolytic process, although some children with chronic hemolytic anemias are not clinically jaundiced. The spleen is frequently enlarged in children with chronic hemolytic anemias. Signs and symptoms of systemic diseases such as fever, weight loss, and lymphadenopathy are of diagnostic importance. In anemias associated with marrow aplasia or replacement, the other formed elements of the blood are also reduced. Thrombocytopenia may be manifested by easy bruising and petechiae. Neutropenia may be accompanied by bacterial infections of the skin and respiratory tract.

The initial evaluation of an anemic child should include a complete blood count (CBC) using age-appropriate standards to determine whether the child is really anemic. Electronic blood cell counters accurately measure white blood cell, red blood cell, and platelet numbers. They also measure Hb, Hct, the mean corpuscular volume (MCV), and the mean corpuscular hemoglobin (MCH). Most cell counters also measure the RBC distribution width (RDW), which assesses the variability of the size of the RBCs evident as *anisocytosis* on the peripheral blood smear.

The MCV indicates whether the RBC population is macrocytic, microcytic, or normocytic. Age values must be used in childhood. In addition to cell size, the blood smear should be evaluated for specific morphologic abnormalities such as spherocytosis, RBC fragmentation (schizocytes), target cells, sickled cells, and others that indicate a specific diagnosis. The CBC also indicates whether the white blood count and differential and platelet counts are normal. The reticulocyte count helps differentiate between aregenerative and hemolytic anemias.

Several questions can be answered by the history, physical examination, and preliminary laboratory studies and often suggest a specific diagnosis and the need for additional diagnostic studies or referral (Box 159-1).

Box 159-1. Questions to Ask When Evaluating Laboratory Studies

Is the child *really* anemic based on age-appropriate normal values for hemoglobin?

Is the red blood cell macrocytic, normocytic, or microcytic based on age-appropriate values for mean corpuscular volume?

Is the anemia aregenerative or hemolytic based on reticulocyte count?

Are there abnormalities of the neutrophils or platelets?

Are there specific abnormalities of the red blood cell on peripheral blood smear?

DIAGNOSIS OF CHRONIC ANEMIAS IN CHILDHOOD

Diagnosis based on history, physical examination, and basic laboratory studies are the key to management. Children with non-nutritional chronic anemias should be referred to a pediatric hematologist for diagnosis and initial management. Some of these conditions respond to specific and limited therapies, and others require chronic interventions with multiple RBC transfusions or specific hematinic stimulants. Other types of anemia do not respond to therapy but are not so severe that they require intervention; however, children with these conditions must be monitored and treated if the degree of anemia worsens. The most common diagnostic categories are based on RBC size and morphology and whether the anemia is aregenerative or hemolytic.

MANAGEMENT AND COMANAGEMENT ISSUES

Long-term management of patients with chronic anemia depends on the underlying diagnosis. Once a chronic or non-nutritional anemia is suspected, referral to a pediatric hematologist for assistance with diagnosis and management is indicated. Management and treatment of the anemia should be accomplished by the hematologist. The generalist should provide primary care, including preventive and acute care, for these patients. One consideration for all anemic patients is modifying acute care in the presence of a pulmonary infection or disorder. The reduced oxygen-carrying capacity of these patients must be factored into both the diagnostic and treatment process.

Although some chronic anemias require no treatment, the more severe anemias often require repeated transfusions with continued chelation therapy to avoid hemosiderosis and subsequent damage to the cardiovascular and endocrine systems. Patients with Blackfan-Diamond syndrome may be treated with chronic steroid administration. The generalist must be aware of the complications of chronic steroid administration and consider this during both health maintenance visits and when the patient is being seen for an acute illness. These patients may also eventually undergo stem cell transplantation.

Patients with sickle cell disease require meticulous coordination of care between the generalist and specialists. Prevention of serious complications is essential. Care must be taken to ensure maintenance of immunizations, particularly with pneumococcal, *H. influenzae*, and hepatitis B vaccines. Prophylaxis with oral penicillin V to prevent pneumococcal infections is indicated for children under the age of 5 years with sickle cell disease. Patients and parents should be instructed to seek medical attention promptly for acute illness, particularly for fever. Complications of sickle cell disease include acute splenic sequestration, painful episodes, vaso-occlusive events, and aplastic episodes that can be acutely life-threatening. Treatment of these complications is described later in this chapter and should be guided by the assistance of a pediatric hematologist.

SPECIFIC ANEMIAS

Microcytic Anemias

Microcytic anemias include iron deficiency anemia, the thalassemias, anemia from chronic inflammation, and anemia from lead poisoning. Table 159-4 describes laboratory findings in microcytic anemias.

Iron Deficiency Anemia (see also Chapter 92)

Iron deficiency anemia is most frequently caused by inadequate intake of dietary iron and is most prevalent in infants between 9 and 24 months of age and in adolescent girls. The child usually has few symptoms unless the anemia is severe. Chronic blood loss can also result in iron deficiency anemia. Chronic, occult bleeding lesions of the gastrointestinal tract such as peptic ulcers, Meckel diverticulum, and hemangiomas as in Rendu-Weber-Osler syndrome occasionally present as iron deficiency anemia. In tropical countries, bleeding from hookworm infestation is a frequent cause of iron deficiency anemia.

The diagnosis of iron deficiency anemia requires that the patient have a microcytic, hypochromic anemia as indicated by RBC indices on the CBC. The RDW is characteristically elevated (>15%). Studies of iron status reveal low serum iron and increased total iron-binding capacity (TIBC). The serum ferritin level is below 12 µg/L. Erythrocyte zinc protoporphyrin levels are increased. Serum transferrin receptors are increased. Management includes elimination of bleeding lesions or parasites when present. Anemia is treated with oral iron medication, given in a divided dose of elemental iron, 4 to 6 mg/kg/day, usually produces a prompt hematologic response. An increase in Hb of at least 1 to 2 g/dL is considered to confirm a diagnosis of iron deficiency anemia. Iron medication is given until the anemia has been corrected and then is continued at a reduced dose for several months to replenish iron stores.

Failure to respond is almost always a consequence of not taking the medication. A parenteral iron medication, iron dextran, is available, but its use is rarely indicated. Rare instances of genetic syndromes of iron malabsorption of have been reported as a cause of microcytic anemia.

Thalassemias

Thalassemias are a heterogeneous group of inherited anemias of varying severity. Thalassemias are classified genetically, based on the defective synthesis of specific chains comprising the various normal hemoglobin components. Thalassemia generally comes to the attention of a clinician from the presence of microcytosis detected by automated blood cell counts. Iron deficiency should first be excluded, because it is the most common cause of microcytosis and is treatable. If the serum iron concentration is not abnormal, the proportion of Hb A_2 should be measured by hemoglobin electrophoresis or high performance liquid chromatography (HPLC). If the proportion of Hb A_2 is greater than 3.5%, the diagnosis is β-thalassemia.

Thalassemia trait is a chronic, mild, familial microcytic anemia. The thalassemia mutations predominantly occur in specific ethnic groups. About 3% to 5% of Italian and Greek Americans and 0.5% of black Americans carry a β-thalassemia gene. The gene also has a relatively high prevalence in people from Middle Eastern countries, Southeast Asia, and the Indian subcontinent and Pakistan.

The hematology of β-thalassemia trait includes a hemoglobin level that is about 2 g/dL below the normal age-related hemoglobin so most children with β-thalassemia trait have hemoglobin levels of 9 to 10 g/dL. The MCV is greatly decreased and averages about 65 fL. Most individuals with β-thalassemia trait have elevated (>3.5%) of hemoglobin A_2. Fetal hemoglobin levels are slightly elevated (3.0% to 5.0%) in about half of all cases. RDW is normal. Although thalassemia trait is often mistaken for iron deficiency anemia, studies of iron status, including serum ferritin and transferrin saturation, RBC zinc protoporphyrin and serum transferrin receptors are normal. No hematologic response occurs after iron therapy.

Homozygous β-thalassemia is usually associated with clinical thalassemia major. In most of these patients, the anemia is so severe that regular RBC transfusions are necessary. Regular RBC transfusions inevitably result in iron overload that must be treated with chronic iron chelation

Table 159-4. Selected Laboratory Features of Microcytic Anemias (MCV <70 fL)

Diagnosis	Hb (g/dL)	Serum Iron (Fe) (mg/dL)	TIBC (µg/dL)	Ferritin (ng/mL)	ZPP (µg/100 mL)	RDW (%)	Other Features
Normal	12–14	30–135	300–400	20–53	<35	11–15	
Iron deficiency	↓ to ↓↓	↓	↑	↓	↑	↑	Response to iron
β-Thalassemia trait	↓	N	N	N	N	N	↑ Hb A_2 (3.5%), no response to iron, similar blood findings in family
α-Thalassemia trait	↓	N	N	N	N	N	≤ Hb A_2 and F, no response to iron, similar blood findings in family
Chronic infection	↓	↓	↓	N to ↑	N	N	Systemic illness, ↑ ESR, no response to iron

ESR, erythrocyte sedimentation rate; Hb, hemoglobin; RDW, red blood cell distribution width; TIBC, total iron-binding capacity; ZPP, zinc protoparphyrin.

(deferoxamine) to prevent hemosiderotic damage to the heart and endocrine systems and early death. About 10% of patients with homozygous β-thalassemia are able to maintain hemoglobin levels above 7.0 g/dL (thalassemia intermedia). Regular RBC transfusions may not be necessary in these patients.

α-Thalassemia trait is caused by genetic deletions that reduce synthesis of the α-chains of hemoglobin. Because there are four α-globin genes in humans, two α-globin genes must be deleted to manifest α-thalassemia trait. α-Thalassemia trait occurs in about 3% of African and Caribbean Americans and is also prevalent in Southern China and the Philippine Islands. Slight reductions in hemoglobin level and MCV characterize α-thalassemia trait. Levels of Hb A_2 and Hb F are normal. Iron studies are normal and there is no response to iron therapy. A diagnosis of α-thalassemia trait is usually made by excluding iron deficiency and β-thalassemia trait, and is likely when the same hematologic findings are present in a first-degree relative.

In persons from Southeast Asia, deletions of three and four α-globin genes may occur, resulting in much more severe anemic syndromes called hemoglobin H disease and fetal hydrops syndrome associated with hemoglobin Bart's. These more severe α-thalassemias do not occur in African and Caribbean Americans.

Anemia of Chronic Inflammation and Infection

The basic mechanism of the anemia of chronic inflammation and infection is an inability to mobilize iron from tissue storage sites into the plasma, where it can be delivered to hematopoietic cells in the bone marrow for hemoglobin synthesis. This block is probably caused by inflammatory cytokines. The anemia is usually mild or moderate, although in some chronic inflammatory states such as systemic rheumatoid arthritis, hemoglobin levels may be as low as 7.0 g/dL.

Serum iron levels and transferrin saturation are low, however, in contrast to iron deficiency anemia in which serum iron-binding capacity is decreased or normal. Normal levels of serum transferrin receptors is a good discriminator between iron deficiency anemia and the anemia of chronic inflammation. Serum ferritin levels are normal or increased, indicating normal or increased iron stores. Serum ferritin levels may be further increased because serum ferritin levels increase as an acute phase reaction in inflammatory states. Serum transferrin receptor levels are normal in the anemia of inflammation and infection but are increased in iron deficiency anemia.

There is no specific therapy for the anemia of chronic inflammation. Iron therapy is ineffective. If the underlying inflammatory process can be controlled, anemia usually improves.

The chronic anemia that accompanies end-stage renal disease results from lack of production of erythropoietin by the damaged kidneys and can be treated with regular injections of recombinant erythropoietin.

Anemia of Lead Poisoning

Chronic lead poisoning inhibits heme synthesis and at very high levels of blood lead (>40 to 60 μg/dL) microcytic anemia may occur. In addition to elevated blood lead levels, greatly elevated blood zinc protoporphyrin (ZPP) levels are found. It should be noted that lead poisoning and iron deficiency often occur together, and lead poisoning should always be considered in a young child with iron deficiency and vice versa (see also Chapter 109).

Macrocytic Anemias

Macrocytic anemias are unusual in pediatric practice. The most common cause of RBC macrocytosis is treatment with cancer chemotherapeutic agents. However, it may also be a consequence of deficiencies of folic acid or vitamin B_{12} (see Chapter 92). These vitamins are necessary for normal RBC maturation and their deficiency causes aregenerative macrocytic anemia with distinctive *megaloblastic* changes in the bone marrow. Dietary folic acid deficiency may result from inadequate dietary intake, but the vitamin is nearly ubiquitous, being present in dairy, animal, and plant foods. Intestinal malabsorption may also contribute to a deficiency. In the past folic acid deficiency occurred because of cow milk formulas that had been processed and heated, destroying the vitamin. Adequate amounts of folic acid to prevent deficiency are present in today's commercial formulas as well as in whole cow milk and breast milk. Goat milk, however, contains very little folic acid. Infants fed exclusively goat milk, usually because of allergy to bovine proteins, are at risk of deficiency and resultant macrocytic anemia. A diagnosis is based on determination of folic acid levels in the serum and RBCs. Therapy with folic acid therapy and adjustment of the diet are usually sufficient to correct the anemia.

Vitamin B_{12} deficiency is usually a consequence of malabsorption or underutilization of the vitamin because of genetically determined abnormalities such as juvenile pernicious anemia, abnormalities of specific receptors in the terminal ilium (Immerslund syndrome), or to abnormalities of vitamin B_{12} transport proteins in the blood. It has also been described in infants exclusively breast-fed by vitamin B_{12}–deficient mothers, usually strict vegetarians (vegans). Diagnosis can be made by direct measurement of serum vitamin B_{12} levels. Diagnosis and management of these rare diseases require the input of pediatric hematologists. Most patients require long-term, parenteral vitamin B_{12} therapy.

Chronic severe macrocytic anemia may be seen in congenital hypoplastic anemia (Diamond-Blackfan syndrome). Affected children develop severe anemia during the first few months of life. The anemia is aregenerative, very few RBC precursors are present in the bone marrow, and reticulocytes are very low or absent. About two thirds of these children respond to continuous corticosteroid therapy. Children who do not respond require regular RBC transfusions. In refractory cases stem cell transplantation may be considered.

Hemolytic Anemias

The RBC is a relatively simple cell. It consists of a complex membrane and cytoskeleton, a cytoplasm largely made up of hemoglobin, and a variety of enzymes necessary for maintaining the ionic balance of the cell and maintaining hemoglobin in the divalent Fe^{2+} form necessary for oxygen transport and resisting oxidant stresses to the RBC. Almost all hemolytic anemias are caused by inherited abnormalities of the RBC membrane, hemoglobin, or enzymes.

Red Blood Cell Membrane Abnormalities

Genetically determined abnormalities of the RBC membrane include hereditary spherocytosis (HS), hemolytic ellipto-cytosis (HE), and its variant pyropoikilocytosis. These conditions are usually dominantly inherited and are caused by structural abnormalities of spectrin or ankyrin, essential proteins of the RBC cytoskeleton and membrane. Instances of what appear to be new mutations, as well as recessive transmission, have been described.

HS and HE are often manifested in the newborn period by hemolytic anemia and hyperbilirubinemia. Exchange transfusion may be necessary to prevent kernicterus. Management of infants with HS and HE requires long-term monitoring of the level of hemoglobin and the effects of anemia on growth and activity. In some patients the anemia is so severe that RBC transfusions are necessary. However, most affected patients are able to compensate for the hemolytic process by increasing RBC production (sometimes as much as six- to eightfold) and so maintain hemoglobin levels of 7.0 to 10 g/dL. If the anemia is interfering with growth or normal activity, splenectomy will correct the anemia. When possible, surgery should be delayed until after 5 or 6 years of age, when the risk of severe post-splenectomy infections decreases substantially. Patients who are not splenectomized should have periodic ultra-sonography for gallstones.

Red Blood Cell Enzyme Abnormalities

The nonspherocytic hemolytic anemias are caused by recessively inherited RBC enzyme deficiencies. The most common of these disorders is RBC pyruvate kinase (PK) deficiency. The severity of anemia in PK-deficient patients varies considerably. Some severely affected children may benefit from splenectomy. Other RBC enzymopathies are unusual. Diagnosis usually requires consultation with a reference laboratory where assays of all the RBC enzymes are performed.

Hemoglobinopathies

More than 500 mutations of human hemoglobin have been described. Most of them are infrequent, but some hemo-globinopathies have relatively high frequency in certain ethnic groups and populations. The most common hemo-globinopathies are Hb S, Hb C (which predominantly occurs in African Americans), and Hb E (which is frequently seen in Southeast Asians). These hemoglobins occur frequently in the heterozygous or trait form and are of little clinical consequence. However, homozygosity or double heterozygosity may be associated with chronic hemolytic anemia.

The most common symptomatic hemoglobinopathy is sickle cell anemia (Hb SS disease). Box 159-2 describes issues of co-management in children with sickle cell disease. In the United States this occurs primarily (but not exclusively) in African and Carribbean Americans. The diagnosis is usually made in the newborn period by genetic screening programs, which are conducted in 43 states. Affected infants have only hemoglobins F and S in their

---

Box 159-2. Co-management Issues in Sickle Cell Disease

- Perform appropriate evaluation of infants with positive sickle cell screening tests.
- Suspect diagnosis and perform appropriate evaluation in states without sickle cell screening.
- Refer patients with sickle cell disease for specialty care and co-management.
- Provide preventive care and regular immunization and immunization with protein conjugate pneumococcal vaccine.
- Follow growth and development.
- Follow for adherence to prophylactic therapy with penicillin.
- Provide emergency care and stabilization for vaso-occlusive crises and aplastic crises followed by appropriate specialty referral.

---

blood; no Hb A is present. By 3 to 6 months of age, most affected infants have developed a moderately severe hemolytic anemia (Hb 6.5 to 8.5 g/dL; reticulocytes 5% to 15%). Vaso-occlusive episodes do not usually occur during the first 6 to 12 months.

Most children tolerate their anemia fairly well, although their growth is slower than normal. The most serious clinical problems that these children may develop in early childhood are pneumococcal sepsis and meningitis. This risk can be greatly decreased by continuous prophylactic therapy with penicillin, and more recently by early immunization with the protein conjugate pneumococcal vaccine.

Some children with sickle cell disease have pain on an almost daily basis. Occasionally, they will have a painful crisis that requires hospitalization for treatment. Specific guidelines for treatment of pain in children with sickle cell disease is found in Chapter 128.

Vaso-occlusive events present with acute pain. They can be severe, causing ischemic damage, including bone marrow or bone infarction, splenic infarcts, pulmonary infarction, and cerebrovascular occlusion. Ischemic damage may also affect the heart, kidneys, and liver. Priapism can occur from obstruction of the venous outflow. Dehydration and acidosis should be treated promptly with intravenous fluids, but overhydration should be avoided.

These children may also have acute episodes when the degree of anemia becomes much more severe and require intervention with blood transfusions. Acute sequestration of large amounts of blood in the spleen is evident by very low hemoglobin levels (Hb 1 to 2 g/dL) and massive splenomegaly. Blood transfusions to correct the severe anemia and hypovolemia are usually effective, but because these severe episodes may recur, splenectomy is often indicated.

Parvovirus B19 infections in patients with severe hemolytic anemias, including Hb SS disease, may be followed by *aplastic crises*, characterized by more severe anemia and reticulocytopenia because the virus destroys RBC precursors in the bone marrow. Aplastic crises last for 10 to 14 days and then terminate because the patient produces antibodies to the virus. However, RBC transfu-sions may be necessary until recovery occurs.

SUGGESTED READINGS

Abshire TC: Sense and sensibility: Approaching anemia in children. Contemp Pediatr 2001;18:104–113.

Andrews NC: Disorders of iron metabolism. N Engl J Med 1999; 341:1986–1995.

Ezekowitz RA: Hematologic manifestations of systemic diseases. In Nathan DG, Orkin SH, Look AT, Ginsburg D (eds): Nathan and Oski's Hematology of Infancy and Childhood, 6th ed. Philadelphia, WB Saunders, 2003, Chapter 49.

Walters MC, Abelson HT: Interpretation of the complete blood count. Pediatr Clin North Am 1996;43:599–622.

SECTION 4   CHRONIC MEDICAL CARE: *Disorders of the Blood*

160 Bone Marrow Dysfunction

Richard S. Lemons

ROLE OF THE GENERALIST

1 Recognize presenting symptoms of childhood acquired and constitutional aplastic anemias.

2 Develop a rational diagnostic approach for evaluating signs and symptoms of bone marrow dysfunction in children.

3 Refer appropriately to a pediatric hematologist for assistance in diagnosis, treatment, and long-term management of bone marrow dysfuntion in children.

4 Understand the prognostic factors and general types of treatments for children with bone marrow dysfunction.

5 Assist in the outpatient management of children with bone marrow dysfunction.

6 Evaluate common acute symptoms of bone marrow dysfunction in children, such as fever, bleeding, and anemia.

7 Recognize and treat potential life-threatening complications of aplastic anemia in children.

FUNDAMENTALS

Hematopoiesis is a complex process by which pluripotent stem cells respond to an array of stimuli and controls to give rise to committed hematopoietic progenitors that ultimately differentiate and replicate to produce functional mature blood cells. The microenvironment and external stimuli are part of a complex system regulating normal hematopoiesis. Bone marrow dysfunction may result from perturbations of the microenvironment or changes in external stimuli or as a constitutional alteration or deficiency of a normal stem cell function.

Bone marrow dysfunction can be classified as affecting a single or multiple cell lineages. Primary bone marrow dysfunction must also be differentiated from infiltrative processes that affect bone marrow function such as storage diseases (e.g., Gaucher disease), malignancies originating in the bone marrow (i.e., leukemias) or metastasizing to the bone marrow (e.g., solid tumors), or other causes such as megaloblastic anemia or myelofibrosis.

Aplastic anemia is aplasia of the bone marrow resulting in peripheral blood cytopenias. Hypoplastic anemia affects only erythropoiesis, such as in Diamond-Blackfan syndrome. Aplastic anemia may be acquired or inherited, as in Fanconi syndrome. Exposure of children to high doses of ionizing radiation and certain insecticides (e.g., chlordane and DDT), drugs (e.g., chloramphenicol and sulfonamides), and chemicals (e.g., benzene) is known to result in development of acquired aplastic anemia. Aplastic anemia may also occur following viral hepatitis. Most cases of childhood aplastic anemia are idiopathic with no known cause or risk factor. Approximately 100 new cases of acquired aplastic anemia are diagnosed in children in the United States annually.

DIAGNOSTIC APPROACHES TO BONE MARROW DYSFUNCTION

The presentations of patients with bone marrow dysfunction are usually related to the underlying changes in the bone marrow. For example, patients with hypoplastic anemia or isolated red blood cell aplasia present with signs and symptoms of anemia. Patients who present with cytopenias secondary to a systemic disease process often present with manifestations related to the underlying disease. Patients with leukemia or metastatic solid tumors often have organomegaly, palpable tumor mass, pain, fever, or bleeding. Once bone marrow dysfunction is suspected, referral to a pediatric hematologist is indicated for assistance with diagnosis.

Aplastic Anemia

Box 160-1 outlines the diagnosis and management of aplastic anemia.

Signs and Symptoms

Patients present with findings related to aplasia of the bone marrow including anemia, bleeding, and fever and infections secondary to neutropenia. Early on, patients may present with fatigue, pallor, bleeding, and bruising from anemia and thrombocytopenia. With progression of the disease, patients may develop tachycardia and lightheadedness from severe anemia or bleeding. Neutropenia can cause fevers and life-threatening infections.

Diagnosis

Severe aplastic anemia is defined as a hypoplastic bone marrow biopsy with less than 25% normal cellularity and the presence of two of the following three findings: an absolute neutrophil count (ANC) less than 500/µL, platelet count less than 20,000/µL, and corrected reticulocyte count of less than 1%.

Fanconi Anemia

Box 160-2 summarizes the diagnosis and management of Fanconi anemia.

Signs and Symptoms

First described in three brothers by Fanconi in 1927, patients usually present at age 5 to 10 years with cytopenias leading to pancytopenia and physical abnormalities. Initial presenting symptoms may be similar to those with acquired aplastic anemia, but with age, these patients show physical findings of short stature and skin pigment changes. Other physical findings are renal anomalies in about one

Box 160-1. Diagnosis and Management of Bone Marrow Dysfunction from Aplastic Anemia

Presenting Signs and Symptoms
- Anemia
  Pallor
  Fatigue
  Tachycardia and lightheadedness
- Thrombocytopenia
  Bruising
  Bleeding
- Neutropenia
  Fevers
  Infections (can be life-threatening)

Diagnosis
- Refer to pediatric hematologist for bone marrow studies.

Treatment by Specialist
- Initial supportive care
- Bone marrow transplantation when possible
- If transplant not possible, antithymocyte globulin (ATG) and immunosuppression including steroids and cyclosporin
- Growth factors (G-CSF)

Generalist Role in Management
- Provide regular health maintenance.
- Monitor blood cell counts regularly.
- Transfuse symptomatic patients with leukocyte-depleted, irradiated platelets or packed red blood cells.
- Assess and treat patients with fever and neutropenia.

third of patients, café au lait spots, abnormality of the thumb, hypogonadism, and cardiopulmonary abnormalities. Approximately half of the patients have no structural abnormalities.

Diagnosis

Laboratory findings may initially reveal mild thrombocytopenia, anemia, and leukopenia, but severe pancytopenia occurs with time. Red blood cell volume is high. The bone marrow aspirate and biopsy are hypocellular with fatty infiltration. Diagnosis is confirmed by chromosome breakage analysis showing chromatid breaks, gaps, and other abnormalities in metaphase preparations from phytohemagglutinin-stimulated peripheral blood leukocytes. Breakage may be apparent in routine cultures but is markedly enhanced upon exposure to diepoxybutane (DEB) or mitomycin C. Prenatal diagnosis is possible using fetal fibroblasts. Inheritance is autosomal recessive.

Diamond-Blackfan Anemia

Box 160-3 summarizes the diagnosis and management of Diamond-Blackfan anemia.

Signs and Symptoms

Patients with Diamond-Blackfan anemia (DBA) usually present at birth or early infancy with pallor and anemia. The platelet count and white blood cell count and differential are normal, so the patient will have findings related to isolated anemia.

Presenting Signs and Symptoms
- Anemia
  Pallor
  Fatigue
  Tachycardia and lightheadedness
- Thrombocytopenia
  Bruising
  Bleeding
- Neutropenia
  Fevers
  Infections (can be life-threatening)
- Physical findings
  Short stature
  Renal anomalies (33%)
  Café au lait spots
  Abnormalities of thumb
  Cardiac abnormalities
  Hypogonadism

Diagnosis
- Refer to pediatric hematologist for bone marrow studies.
- Refer for chromosome analysis.

Treatment by Specialist
- Initial supportive care
- Androgens
- Bone marrow transplantation when possible

Generalist Role in Management
- Provide regular health maintenance.
- Monitor blood cell counts regularly.
- Transfuse symptomatic patients with leukocyte-depleted, irradiated platelets or packed red blood cells.
- Assess and treat patients with fever and neutropenia.

Diagnosis

Over 90% of patients present in the first 6 months of life with pallor and a macrocytic anemia with reticulocytopenia. Bone marrow examination reveals a decrease or absence of erythroid progenitors with normal cellularity. The remaining erythroid precursors show maturation arrest.

Box 160-3. Diagnosis and Management of Diamond-Blackfan Anemia

Presenting Signs and Symptoms
- Patients usually present at birth or early infancy with pallor and anemia.
- Over 90% of patients present in the first 6 months with pallor and a macrocytic anemia with reticulocytopenia.

Diagnosis
- Refer to pediatric hematologist for bone marrow studies.

Treatment by Specialist
- Ensure annual follow-up assessments.

Generalist Role in Management
- Provide regular health maintenance.
- Monitor blood cell counts regularly.
- Ensure follow-up with hematologist.

Fetal hemoglobin is commonly increased in DBA. Serum levels of iron, ferritin, folate, and erythropoietin are increased. About one quarter of patients have a physical abnormality such as short stature or cardiac or renal abnormalities.

The presence of circulating or cellular inhibitors has been proposed, although experimental data suggest a defect in the erythroid stem cell in DBA. In vitro culture of bone marrow from patients with DBA shows decreased erythroid colonies. Families with multiple affected siblings have been reported, but the parents are usually normal.

TREATMENT, SIDE EFFECTS, AND OUTCOMES

Acquired Aplastic Anemia

Supportive care is the initial goal of treatment at diagnosis. If bleeding is present at diagnosis, transfusion of platelets, preferably single donor pheresis, is given. Packed red blood cells are transfused if the patient is clinically symptomatic from anemia. All blood products should be leukocyte-depleted by filtration and irradiated. Blood products from family members should be avoided to minimize the risk of graft rejection in the event of an allogeneic bone marrow transplantation. Prophylactic antibiotics are not indicated if the patient is afebrile, has no history of recent fever or infection, and does not have an identifiable source of infection on physical examination. If the patient is neutropenic and is febrile or has a source of infection, blood cultures and other appropriate cultures as clinically indicated should be obtained. Prompt initiation of broad-spectrum antibiotics should be given, similar to those that are given for a febrile, neutropenic cancer patient. Antifungal therapy should be considered in patients who are febrile for more than 5 days after receiving broad-spectrum antibiotics.

If the patient has siblings, complete human leukocyte antigen (HLA) typing should be performed at diagnosis. Matched sibling bone marrow transplant is curative in severe aplastic anemia, with a 80% to 95% long-term disease-free survival rate if performed in a minimally transfused patient free from infection.

Patients without a matched sibling can be treated successfully with antithymocyte globulin (ATG) and immunosuppression including steroids and cyclosporin. Responses can be seen in up to 90% of patients, although relapses are common as the immunosuppression is tapered or stopped. Growth factors such as granulocyte colony-stimulating factor (G-CSF) can be beneficial in improving the absolute neutrophil count in neutropenic patients, reducing the risk of life-threatening infections. G-CSF can be administered initially at 5 µg/kg/day subcutaneously. If no response is seen in 1 to 2 weeks, the dose can be increased to 10 µg/kg/day. If a satisfactory response is seen, the time interval between doses can be increased to every other day or less often as tolerated. Steroids alone are seldom beneficial over the long term. Androgens are no longer used, except rarely in patients who are refractory to immunosuppression and who are unable to undergo a bone marrow transplant (BMT). Chemotherapy such as high-dose cyclophosphamide has been successful in treating a subset of patients.

Fanconi Anemia

Bone marrow transplantation is the only curative treatment in Fanconi anemia, although the toxicities potentially can be significantly greater than in patients with a malignancy. The preparative regimen used for transplant in Fanconi anemia patients is significantly altered from that used in malignancies because of the marked toxicities and life-threatening complications experienced by these patients. Supportive care is the treatment of choice at diagnosis while workup for possible BMT is undertaken. Transfusion of platelets and packed red blood cells is given based on clinical findings. All blood products should be leukocyte-reduced by filtration and irradiated. Blood products from family members should be avoided so as to minimize the risk of graft rejection in the event of an allogeneic BMT. Patients who are neutropenic and febrile are treated similarly to cancer patients with fever and neutropenia using broad-spectrum antibiotics. Androgens such as oxymethalone are the main initial therapy and induce a clinical response in 50% of patients, lasting up to several years. Relapses are common once the androgens are stopped. Side effects of androgen therapy can be significant and must be closely monitored.

Nearly 10% of Fanconi anemia patients develop acute myeloid leukemia or rarely acute lymphocytic leukemia. An additional 5% to 10% of patients develop liver or solid tumor cancers. The risk of development of cancer increases dramatically with increasing age.

Diamond-Blackfan Anemia

Corticosteroids are the initial therapy with prednisone given at 2 mg/kg/day. Some patients do not respond to this dose but will respond to higher doses of 4 to 5 mg/kg/day. Approximately 20% to 30% of patients are refractory to steroids. With administration of steroids, increase in erythroid progenitors is found in the bone marrow followed in several weeks by an increase in the absolute reticulocyte count and subsequent inprovement in the anemia. With improvement in the hematocrit, the dose of steroids can be slowly tapered to a low maintenance dose of 0.5 to 5 mg per day or every other day. A few cases of severe Diamond-Blackfan anemia successfully treated with BMT have been reported. Androgen therapy is only occasionally beneficial. Spontaneous remissions have been reported. In patients refractory to steroids, chronic transfusion therapy is used, although long-term side effects can be significant.

COORDINATION OF CARE BETWEEN PEDIATRICIAN AND PEDIATRIC HEMATOLOGIST

The pediatrician plays a crucial role in the diagnosis, initial treatment, and long-term management and follow-up of patients with bone marrow dysfunction. Prompt recognition of the signs and symptoms of patients with acquired or constitutional aplastic anemia can lead to a referral to a pediatric hematologist, resulting in a timely diagnosis before life-threatening complications develop. Early diagnosis and implementation of supportive care and definitive treatment can significantly improve long-term outcome in both acquired and constitutional aplastic anemia. Most patients with bone marrow dysfunction will require a bone marrow aspiration or biopsy as part of their diagnostic workup. This procedure is best performed by a pediatric hematologist so that the appropriate definitive ancillary tests can be performed on the marrow sample such as immunophenotyping, cytogenetic analysis, or in vitro culture assays. The risk of life-threatening complications including bleeding, fever, neutropenia, and infection increase with increasing symptoms and prolonged delays in diagnosis and implementation of appropriate supportive care.

The pediatrician can assist in the management of patients with bone marrow dysfunction by monitoring regularly obtained blood cell counts; transfusing symptomatic patients with leukocyte-depleted, irradiated platelets or packed red blood cells; and assessing and treating patients with fever and neutropenia.

Patients with DBA can be managed almost entirely by the pediatrician in consultation with the pediatric hematologist. Annual follow-up assessments with a pediatric hematologist are recommended. Management and follow-up of patients with aplastic anemia, either acquired or constitutional, is enhanced by the involvement of the pediatrician. Monitoring of blood cell counts, regular assessments of the clinical status of the patients, and intervention and treatment of fever and neutropenia or bleeding are important roles for the pediatrician.

Effective and timely communication between the pediatrician and pediatric hematologist are crucial for achievement of the best possible outcome in patients with bone marrow dysfunction.

Mini-index of Related Topics

SUGGESTED READINGS

Nathan DG, Orkin SH: Nathan and Oski's Hematology of Infancy and Childhood, 6th ed. Philadelphia, WB Saunders, 2003.

Pizzo PA, Poplack DF: Principles and Practice of Pediatric Oncology, 4th ed. Philadelphia, Lippincott-Raven, 2002.

161

Long-term Care of Children with Hemophilia

Gregory Thomas

ROLE OF THE GENERALIST

1   Provide a medical home for patients with hemophilia.

2   Understand the genetics of hemophilia and be able to provide basic genetic counseling.

3   Treat routine bleeding episodes.

4   Recognize potentially serious bleeding episodes and provide appropriate triage and management.

5   Refer hemophilia patients to a comprehensive hemophilia treatment center.

6   Provide immunizations, health maintenance, acute care, and coordination of care.

7   Work in collaboration with the hemophilia treatment center to provide patient and family education about hemophilia and to facilitate the patient's transition to independent management of the disease.

DEFINITION

Hemophilia A and hemophilia B are hereditary clotting factor deficiencies that result in excessive bleeding. Hemophilia A is due to a deficiency of factor VIII and occurs in approximately 1 in 6000 live male births. Hemophilia B (also called Christmas disease) is due to a deficiency of factor IX and occurs in approximately 1 in 25,000 live male births. The genes for both factor VIII and factor IX are located near the end of the long arm of the X chromosome. Hemophilia A and hemophilia B are inherited as X-linked recessive disorders and usually affect only boys and men. Hemophilia in girls and women is due to extreme lyonization (inactivation of one of the two X chromosomes), hemizygosity for the X chromosome (Turner syndrome), or inheritance of two hemophilia genes. Most patients with hemophilia have other affected family members, but approximately 30% of newly diagnosed patients have no family history of hemophilia and the hemophilia is presumably due to a spontaneous mutation. A negative family history does not rule out hemophilia.

FUNDAMENTALS

Factor VIII and factor IX activity levels are reported in units in which 1 unit is defined as the amount of clotting factor present in 1 mL of normal plasma and 1 unit/mL is

Table 161-1. Classification of Severity of Hemophilia by Percentage of Normal Clotting Factors

Classification	Level of Normal Clotting Factor Activity
Severe hemophilia	<1%
Moderate hemophilia	1–5%
Mild hemophilia	5–30%

equivalent to 100% activity. The normal range for factor VIII or IX activity is from 50% to 150%. The severity of hemophilia depends on the amount of circulating clotting factor present (Table 161-1). Of patients with hemophilia A, 70% have severe disease, 15% have moderate disease, and 15% have mild disease. In hemophilia B, 50% of patients have severe disease, 30% have moderate disease, and 20% have mild disease.

The risk of bleeding is related to the severity of disease. Patients with severe hemophilia often bleed following circumcision and may have intracranial hemorrhage in the newborn period. The diagnosis of severe hemophilia is usually made within the first year of life. As patients with severe hemophilia grow older, they experience spontaneous bleeding into muscles or joints, bleed when undergoing dental work, have hematuria, and are at high risk of intracranial bleeding. Patients with moderate hemophilia also may have bleeding after circumcision, but neonatal intracranial hemorrhage is uncommon. Patients with moderate hemophilia may have bleeding following surgery or major dental work and can have bleeding into muscles and joints with minor trauma. Intracranial hemorrhage is uncommon. Patients with mild hemophilia often have few bleeding problems and the diagnosis may not be made until later in childhood or even until adulthood. Bruising and oral bleeding are common, and bleeding into muscles or joints may occur with major trauma, but other significant bleeding is rare.

CLOTTING FACTOR CONCENTRATES

The cornerstone of therapy for hemophilia is clotting factor replacement, which can be accomplished using several different products, including fresh frozen plasma, cryoprecipitate, plasma-derived clotting factor concentrates, and recombinant clotting factor concentrates. The use of fresh frozen plasma or cryoprecipitate generally is not recommended for most hemophilia patients because of the large volume required to achieve an adequate clotting factor level and because these products usually have not undergone a viral purification process.

Plasma-derived clotting factor concentrates are prepared from pooled plasma obtained from thousands of donors. The risk of viral transmission with these products is greatly reduced by donor screening and viral inactivation methods including pasteurization, dry heat, solvent detergent, and affinity purification using monoclonal antibodies. The purity of plasma-derived clotting factor concentrates is determined by the amount of residual contaminating plasma proteins in the final product. Ultrapure and high purity plasma products contain little or no contaminating proteins. Intermediate purity products contain other plasma proteins, including fibrinogen and von Willebrand factor, and can be used to treat some types of von Willebrand disease as well as hemophilia.

Recombinant clotting factor concentrates are manufactured using genetic engineering and recombinant DNA technology. The gene for factor VIII or factor IX is cloned into mammalian cells in tissue culture and expression of the transfected gene leads to secretion of clotting factor into the tissue culture medium. The clotting factor is purified from the tissue culture medium using ion exchange and affinity chromatography. Recombinant factor VIII was licensed for general use in 1992 and recombinant factor IX was licensed in 1997. Recombinant factor products have been shown to be as safe and effective as plasma-derived factors. In contrast to some plasma-derived factor IX concentrates, there is no increased risk of thrombosis with recombinant factor IX.

The first-generation recombinant factor VIII products (e.g., KoGENate, Recombinate) used human albumin to stabilize the final product. Second-generation recombinant factor VIII products are now available (e.g., KoGENate FS, Helixate FS, ReFacto) that are stabilized with sucrose instead of albumin in the final product. However, these products do utilize albumin in the tissue culture medium. Current recombinant factor IX products (e.g., Benefix) are not manufactured with human albumin.

No cases of HIV (human immunodeficiency virus), hepatitis B, or hepatitis C transmission with plasma-derived clotting factor concentrates have been documented since 1990. However, other viruses that do not have a lipid envelope, including parvovirus B19 and hepatitis A, may not be inactivated by current purification techniques. There are also theoretical concerns that new infectious agents such as prions, the cause of Creutzfeldt-Jakob disease (CJD) and other transmissible spongiform encephalopathies, might escape eradication with current manufacturing processes. For these reasons the Medical and Scientific Advisory Council of the National Hemophilia Foundation recommends that recombinant factor products "be considered the treatment of choice for individuals with hemophilia." Which type of factor product to use should be an individualized decision made in conjunction with the family and will depend on cost, previous exposure to factor concentrates, and HIV and hepatitis C status, but in general children should receive recombinant clotting factor products whenever possible.

DIAGNOSIS

Hemophilia should be suspected in boys with increased bleeding symptoms, regardless of family history of hemophilia. Approach to bleeding is discussed in more detail in Chapter 95.

A factor VIII or factor IX activity level should be drawn from the umbilical cord at the time of delivery of a male infant if there is a family history of hemophilia and the mother is a possible carrier. The diagnosis of hemophilia A can be made reliably in the newborn period because the normal level of factor VIII activity present at birth is similar to normal adult levels. Type 3 or type 2N von Willebrand disease can be confused with hemophilia A, so additional testing should be done to rule out von Willebrand disease. The diagnosis of hemophilia B may be less certain because the level of factor IX activity (and all other vitamin K–dependent clotting factors) is low at birth and may not reach normal adult levels until 6 to 9 months of age. An extremely low factor IX activity (e.g., <5%) is highly suggestive of hemophilia B, but a mildly low factor IX activity level (e.g., 20% to 30%) may be developmentally normal and will increase during the first year of life. It may be necessary to repeat the factor IX activity level to determine whether an infant has a persistently low factor IX activity level consistent with the diagnosis of hemophilia B. Because the specific gene mutation can be identified for most cases of hemophilia, other family members at risk to carry the affected gene can be screened.

Prenatal testing can be done to determine the carrier status of women who may be at risk because of a family history of hemophilia or to determine whether a fetus of a woman known to be a carrier of hemophilia A or hemophilia B is affected. A woman is considered to be an obligate carrier of hemophilia if her father has hemophilia, if she has given birth to two previous boys with hemophilia, or if she has given birth to one previous boy with hemophilia and there is a family history of hemophilia on her side of the family. Prenatal testing can be done by direct mutation analysis of the factor VIII or factor IX gene or by linkage analysis using restriction fragment length polymorphisms (RFLP). Fetal samples can be obtained by chorionic villous sampling at 10 to 12 weeks of gestation or by amniocentesis at 15 to 16 weeks of gestation. These techniques are not without risk to the fetus. Families should be referred to a genetic counselor prior to any prenatal testing to provide counseling about risks and benefits and to recommend appropriate diagnostic testing.

MANAGEMENT

Because the risk of intracranial hemorrhage in an infant with hemophilia born by vaginal delivery is small, routine cesarean section for a woman known to be a carrier of hemophilia is unnecessary. However, the delivery should be done with the least amount of trauma possible. Vacuum extraction and fetal scalp monitors should not be used and prolonged delivery should be avoided.

When deciding on appropriate management of bleeding in a hemophilia patient it is useful to divide bleeding episodes into routine types of bleeding and serious life- or limb-threatening types of bleeding (Table 161-2).

Table 161-2. Classification of Bleeding Episodes

Bleeding Episode	Types of Bleeding
Routine bleeding episode	Uncomplicated joint or muscle bleeding Oral bleeding Nosebleed Hematuria
Serious bleeding episode	Central nervous system bleeding (brain or spinal cord) Bleeding in the throat, possibly compromising the airway Bleeding causing a limb compartment syndrome Iliopsoas muscle bleeding Intra-abdominal bleeding

Bleeding into Joints

The most common type of bleeding in patients with moderate or severe hemophilia is bleeding into joints or muscles. These bleeds may occur spontaneously with little or no known trauma. The most common joints to be involved are the knees, ankles, and elbows. Patients with hemophilia often develop a "target" joint from repeated episodes of bleeding into the same joint. A destructive cycle may develop in which bleeding into a joint causes iron deposition in the synovium and articular cartilage and release of inflammatory cytokines, leading to villous hypertrophy of the synovium. The inflamed synovium is very friable and is more likely to rebleed, causing further damage to the joint. Ultimately, this causes degeneration of cartilage and bone, resulting in chronic arthritis.

Early symptoms of a joint bleed may include a feeling of tingling and warmth in the joint, mild pain, and limitation of motion. There may be no external physical signs of an early joint bleed, and in young children the only clue may be nonspecific irritability or decreased use of the affected limb. If the bleeding progresses, the joint becomes hot and swollen with little or no motion without significant pain. The goal of therapy is early recognition and treatment of bleeding episodes before significant signs and symptoms develop. Early joint bleeds should be treated with an infusion of clotting factor calculated to increase the factor level to 50% to 60%.

In addition to infusion of factor concentrate, the joint should be rested or immobilized until the swelling decreases, and application of ice packs, compression with an elastic wrap, and elevation (RICE) may help decrease swelling as well. Physical therapy should be instituted as soon as the swelling decreases to maintain range of motion and to prevent atrophy of the muscles supporting the joint.

Aspiration of blood from the joint is rarely indicated and may only make the joint worse by creating another site of bleeding. If joint aspiration is considered necessary (e.g., to rule out infection), then the procedure should be done by an orthopedic surgeon experienced in the treatment of hemophilia and only after adequate clotting factor replacement.

Bleeding into Muscles

Symptoms of bleeding into a muscle include warmth, swelling, localized tenderness, and pain with contraction of the muscle. Any muscle may be subject to bleeding, but common sites include the upper arms, thighs, and calves. Young children may experience buttock and perineal bleeds from falls or rough activity. A significant amount of blood loss can occur in large muscles, resulting in anemia. Bleeding into muscles in the closed fascial spaces of the forearm or calf may cause a compartment syndrome. Pressure on nerves and blood vessels from these hematomas can result in neuropathy or ischemia and permanent impairment if inadequately treated. If a compartment syndrome is suspected, the patient should receive an infusion of clotting factor calculated to raise the factor level to 100% and then be referred to a medical center experienced in the treatment of hemophilia.

Bleeding into the iliopsoas muscle also may lead to significant loss of function. The femoral nerve exits the lumbar spine and passes between the iliacus and the psoas muscles. Bleeding into these muscles can compress the femoral nerve, resulting in paresthesias of the anterior thigh, weakness of the quadriceps muscles, and possible permanent loss of function. Iliopsoas bleeding may cause pain symptoms that can be confused with bleeding into the hip joint. Patients with an iliopsoas bleed will complain of pain in the hip and may prefer to have the hip joint in a position of slight flexion. Active flexion or passive extension may cause significant pain. In addition, patients may complain of numbness on the anterior aspect of the thigh. Rotation of the hip is not as painful as flexion or extension, and this finding may help distinguish an iliopsoas bleed from bleeding into the hip joint. Diagnosis of an iliopsoas bleed can be confirmed by pelvic ultrasound or abdominal computed tomography (CT) scan. Patients with an iliopsoas bleed should be referred to the hemophilia treatment center. Treatment of an iliopsoas bleed requires bedrest and clotting factor replacement to maintain a factor level of 50% to 100% for several days.

Mucous Membrane Bleeding

Oral bleeding and nosebleeds are common in patients with hemophilia. Falls in toddlers learning to walk may result in injuries to the lip, tongue, or frenulum. Oral bleeding may also occur when teeth are erupting or with loss of baby teeth. An infusion of clotting factor calculated to increase the factor level to 30% to 50% and the use of an antifibrinolytic agent (e.g., Amicar [Table 161-3]) is often necessary to control bleeding. Once bleeding is controlled, a soft diet should be used until the site of bleeding is well healed. Milk products promote clot breakdown and should be avoided until the bleeding site is healed. Nosebleeds will often stop with direct external pressure, but clotting factor infusion may be required. For recurrent nosebleeds, petroleum jelly (Vasoline) applied to the membranes of the anterior nares or nasal decongestants (e.g., Afrin, Neo-Synephrine) also may be helpful.

Hematuria

Gross hematuria is common in patients with moderate or severe hemophilia. This bleeding can be a frightening symptom but usually is not serious. The etiology often remains unknown but hematuria can be precipitated by infection, kidney stones, trauma, or the use of nonsteroidal anti-inflammatory drugs. Initial management should include

Table 161-3. Dosing of Factor Concentrates

Type of Bleeding	Desired Factor Level*
Joint/muscle	50–60%, may need more than one dose
Oral mucosa	30–50%, antifibrinolytic agents useful
Surgery	100%, then 50–100% for 10–14 days
Central nervous system	100%, then 50–100% for 10–14 days
Prophylaxis	50–60%, 3x/wk for factor VIII, 2x/wk for factor IX

*Factor VIII: number of units to infuse = weight (kg) × desired level (%) × 0.5.
Factor IX: Number of units to infuse = weight (kg) × desired level (%).

bedrest and increased fluid intake for 24 to 48 hours. If the hematuria persists, infusion of clotting factor calculated to increase the level to approximately 50% may be necessary. Use of antifibrinolytic agents (e.g., Amicar) is contraindicated because of the risk of causing clots in the collecting system and obstructive hydronephrosis.

Intracranial Hemorrhage

Intracranial hemorrhage (ICH) remains the most common cause of death from bleeding in patients with hemophilia. ICH may occur following little or no known trauma. Young children are particularly prone to falls and trauma that result in blows to the head. It is often difficult to determine how significant was the head trauma and whether intervention is needed. The signs and symptoms of increased intracranial pressure from bleeding may not appear for 24 to 48 hours following known trauma because the bleeding is due to oozing and a slow accumulation of blood. Therefore, the absence of symptoms does not rule out ICH. If the trauma is observed and known to be minor (e.g., tripping and falling onto a carpet or padded surface), and the child is stable without symptoms, no therapy may be necessary. If the child seems stable without symptoms but the amount of trauma is uncertain, it may be reasonable to give the child an infusion of factor concentrate calculated to increase the factor level to 100% and observe closely without further evaluation.

Urgent evaluation in an emergency department is required for any head trauma with loss of consciousness, falls onto a hard surface such as concrete or playground equipment, and falls with added momentum such as falling off a moving bicycle or skateboard. Patients with significant headache, vomiting, mental status changes, or neurologic symptoms following head trauma should also receive immediate attention. Any patient with hemophilia suspected of having an ICH should receive factor replacement calculated to increase the activity level to 100% *before* any imaging or further evaluation is done. Following infusion of factor concentrate, an emergency CT scan can be done to rule out intracranial bleeding. Depending on the degree of trauma or the child's symptoms, admission to the hospital for observation may be indicated. If an ICH is documented the patient should receive clotting factor replacement to maintain a factor level of 50% to 100% for 10 to 14 days. Hemophilia patients with a past history of intracranial bleeding are at increased risk for subsequent ICH, and prophylactic infusions for up to 6 months to prevent rebleeding are often recommended.

Intra-abdominal Bleeding

Signs and symptoms of intra-abdominal bleeding include abdominal muscle pain or tenderness, flank pain, bloody emesis, or blood in the stool. Forceful coughing or protracted vomiting can precipitate abdominal bleeding. Trauma to the abdomen may result in injury to the liver, spleen, or kidneys, or bleeding into muscles of the abdominal wall. Blood loss into the abdominal cavity may result in significant anemia. Patients suspected of intra-abdominal bleeding should be evaluated in the emergency department and receive factor replacement calculated to increase the activity level to 100% *before* further evaluation is done.

The amount of clotting factor to infuse depends on the type of hemophilia the child has and the kind of bleeding for which the clotting factor is being administered (see Table 161-3). When using factor VIII, 1 unit of clotting factor per kilogram of body weight will raise the plasma level approximately 2%. Factor IX has a larger volume of distribution, and therefore, 1 unit of factor IX per kilogram will raise the plasma level approximately 1%. The final dose of factor should be rounded to the nearest whole vial size. Clotting factor concentrates are very expensive and infusing more than the calculated dose has no adverse consequences, so the whole vial should be infused and factor should not be wasted.

For routine joint or soft tissue bleeding, increasing the plasma factor activity level to 50% to 60% is usually adequate to control bleeding. Thirty to 50% factor activity is adequate for oral bleeding. In cases of life-threatening bleeding such as ICH or prior to surgery it is desirable to raise the plasma factor level to 100% and then maintain it at 50% to 100% for several days. As a general rule of thumb, infusion to 50% factor activity is adequate for treatment of most routine bleeding episodes, and correction to 100% activity is necessary for life- or limb-threatening bleeding episodes and occasionally in some cases of muscle or joint bleeding if there has been delay in initiating therapy.

Ancillary therapies include DDAVP (1-deamino-8-D-arginine vasopressin) and antifibrinolytic agents. In patients with mild hemophilia A, intravenous or intranasal DDAVP causes release of endogenous factor VIII and von Willebrand factor from endothelial cells. This may increase the level of clotting factor in the blood enough to control mild bleeding (Table 161-4). In cases of oral bleeding, epistaxis, or menorrhagia, use of antifibrinolytic agents such as epsilon-aminocaproic acid (Amicar) is often helpful. By inhibiting fibrinolysis, these agents stabilize clots

Table 161-4. Ancillary Therapy

Indication	Drug and Dosage
In hemophilia or von Willebrand disease	DDAVP (1-deamino-8-D-Arginine vasopressin): Intravenously: 0.3 μg/kg (maximum dose 25 μg) Nasal (Stimate): 150 μg (1 squirt) if <50 kg, 300 μg (2 squirts) if >50 kg
For oral bleeding, epistaxis, or menorrhagia	Epsilon-aminocaproic acid (Amicar) Orally: 50–100 mg/kg q6h (maximum dose 5 g)

that have already formed. The use of antifibrinolytic agents is contraindicated in cases of renal or urinary tract bleeding.

OUTCOME

The most common long-term problems in patients with hemophilia have been chronic viral infections (e.g., HIV, hepatitis B, hepatitis C), chronic hemophilic arthropathy, or the development of inhibitors to infused clotting factor concentrates. However, the incidence of these chronic problems is decreasing with current treatment protocols. The risk of infusion-related viral infections has been virtually eliminated by the use of recombinant clotting factor concentrates, donor screening, and viral inactivation methods for plasma-derived products.

The incidence of significant chronic arthropathy is decreasing with the use of home infusion programs and primary and secondary prophylaxis. Secondary prophylaxis involves regular infusions of clotting factor concentrate given to prevent bleeding once the patient has begun to experience joint bleeding, or has developed a target joint. Secondary prophylaxis often is used for a limited period of time to allow a specific target area to heal. The goal of secondary prophylaxis is to arrest joint damage. However, prospective studies have shown that while secondary prophylaxis can stabilize or improve clinical symptoms, chronic joint changes may continue to progress radiographically.

In primary prophylaxis scheduled infusions of factor concentrate are begun before any joint bleeding has occurred and may be continued indefinitely. The rationale for primary prophylaxis is based on the observation that patients with mild or moderate hemophilia rarely have spontaneous joint bleeding and that over their lifetime are much less susceptible to chronic joint disease. It was assumed that if the factor level could be maintained at greater than 1% of normal (equivalent to moderate or mild disease), chronic joint problems could be prevented. Primary prophylaxis has been common in Europe for many years and recent data show that it does prevent or significantly decrease the incidence of chronic joint damage in hemophilia patients. A review of primary prophylaxis in Sweden over a 25-year period showed that patients who began primary prophylaxis prior to the onset of any joint bleeding continued to have normal joints, both clinically and radiographically.

Typically, patients with hemophilia A receive prophylactic infusions three times per week, and patients with hemophilia B receive infusions twice per week. Potential drawbacks to primary prophylaxis include the significant increase in cost of treatment and the frequent need for central venous catheters in young children. Currently, the World Federation of Hemophilia and the Medical and Scientific Advisory Committee of the National Hemophilia Foundation recommend that, "prophylaxis should be considered optimal therapy for children with severe hemophilia A and B."

A synovectomy may be indicated in patients who develop a target joint and continue to experience recurrent joint bleeding episodes despite secondary prophylaxis. Elimination of the inflamed synovium may break the cycle of chronic inflammation and rebleeding. Typically this is done as an arthroscopic synovectomy or as a radionucleotide synovectomy. The radionucleotide technique is the least invasive and involves injecting a radioisotope into the joint space that causes shrinkage and ablation of the inflamed synovium.

A major complication of the treatment of hemophilia with clotting factor concentrates is the development of an inhibitor. Inhibitors are alloantibodies that neutralize infused factor VIII or factor IX. Inhibitors develop in approximately 25% to 30% of patients with hemophilia A and in 1% to 5% of patients with hemophilia B, typically within the first 20 exposure days to exogenous factor. The presence of an inhibitor should be suspected if standard doses of factor replacement fail to control bleeding episodes. Management of hemophilia patients with an inhibitor is frequently complicated, and these patients should be referred to a hemophilia treatment center. Bleeding in patients with a low titer inhibitor can often be managed with larger than normal doses of factor replacement. Patients with a high titer inhibitor are treated with so-called bypassing agents, including factor IX complex concentrates, both activated and unactivated, or recombinant factor VIIa. Long-term eradication of an inhibitor can often be accomplished by immune tolerance induction protocols followed by indefinite prophylaxis.

FOLLOW-UP AND COMANAGEMENT ISSUES FOR PRIMARY CARE PROVIDERS

Primary care providers (PCPs) should provide a medical home for patients with hemophilia, providing coordination of care, timely referrals, acute and emergency care in consultation with specialists, and health maintenance. All newly diagnosed patients with hemophilia should be referred to a comprehensive hemophilia treatment center (HTC). These centers provide clinical expertise in pediatric and adult hematology, orthopedic surgery, dentistry, nursing, genetic counseling, social work, and physical therapy and offer integrated, multidisciplinary care for patients with bleeding disorders including diagnosis, clinical management, patient education, counseling, and assistance with financial or insurance issues. A recent study from the Centers for Disease Control (CDC) demonstrated a significant decrease in mortality rate in patients with hemophilia who receive their hemophilia care in a comprehensive HTC compared to hemophilia patients who do not receive medical care in an HTC.

Close collaboration between the PCP and the HTC is necessary for optimal treatment of patients with hemophilia. The diagnosis of hemophilia in a child often results in feelings of shock, grief, fear, and guilt in the parents. The family may already have a relationship with a PCP, who can play a key role to help calm the parent's fears and help them cope with the diagnosis.

The PCP is often the first to evaluate a possible bleeding episode, particularly if the patient does not live close to the HTC. The PCP should be familiar with the general management of bleeding episodes and know which types of bleeds require referral to an emergency department or the HTC (Box 161-1). The PCP can review instructions provided by

(leukemia cutis) and cranial nerve infiltration resulting in palsy are uncommon. Central nervous system (CNS) disease is present at diagnosis in about 5% of children with ALL but does not affect prognosis. Two percent to 5% of pediatric ALL cases are in infants younger than 1 year old. Infant ALL is a distinct biologic disease that differs from ALL in children older than 1 year in age. These patients often present with very high white blood counts (WBCs) and organomegaly and have a different leukemic blast immunophenotype. Infant ALL outcomes have been significantly lower than those of older children, which has resulted in risk-based intensive treatment to improve the survival in the infant age group. Congenital ALL is very uncommon and is diagnosed before the infant is 4 weeks old. Congenital leukemia can be either lymphoid or myeloid and is treated similarly to infantile leukemia.

Treatment is risk based and is initially assigned based on age and WBC at initial presentation. Outcomes for standard risk ALL (age 1–9 years and initial WBC < 50,000/μL) approaches 85% long-term survival. High-risk patients (age 10 years and older or WBC > 50,000/μL) with ALL have a long-term disease-free survival of greater than 70%.

Characterization of lymphoblasts by morphology, immunophenotype, genetic, and biologic studies has shown that ALL is a heterogeneous disease. The morphologic classification of the French-American-British (FAB) group describes three categories of lymphoblasts based on specific criteria including size, nuclear shape, nuclear cytoplasmic ratio, inclusions and character of chromatin, and presence of cytoplasmic granules. L1 lymphoblasts are small with scant cytoplasm and inconspicuous nucleoli and are present in about 85% of children with ALL. L2 lymphoblasts are larger with more cytoplasm and prominent nucleoli, are present in about 14% of childhood ALL, and are the most common lymphoblasts in adult ALL. L3 lymphoblasts have very prominent and characteristic cytoplasmic vacuolization, have deep blue cytoplasm, and morphologically are identical to Burkitt lymphoma cells. Immunophenotyping of leukemic blasts from the bone marrow is commonly conducted to confirm the diagnosis and establish the stage of maturation of the leukemic cells, and may affect determination of the treatment plan. Early pre-B-cell ALL is the most common type of ALL in children. T-cell ALL occurs more commonly in children older than 10 years of age and is often associated with a mediastinal mass and large tumor burden. Patients with mature B-cell ALL (L3) usually have extensive disease, large tumor burdens, and abnormal chemistries, including elevated uric acid and phosphorus, at presentation as a result of tumor lysis.

ACUTE MYELOID LEUKEMIA

Acute myeloid leukemia (AML), the second most common type of childhood leukemia, accounts for about 20% of acute leukemias or about 400 to 500 cases annually in the United States. AML is thought to arise from clonal proliferation of a bone marrow myeloid precursor cell that determines the FAB type (M0–M7) of AML. AML is most common during the first 2 years of life and again in the teenage years. Children may have signs and symptoms of fatigue, lethargy, fever, bleeding, or bone pain. Symptoms

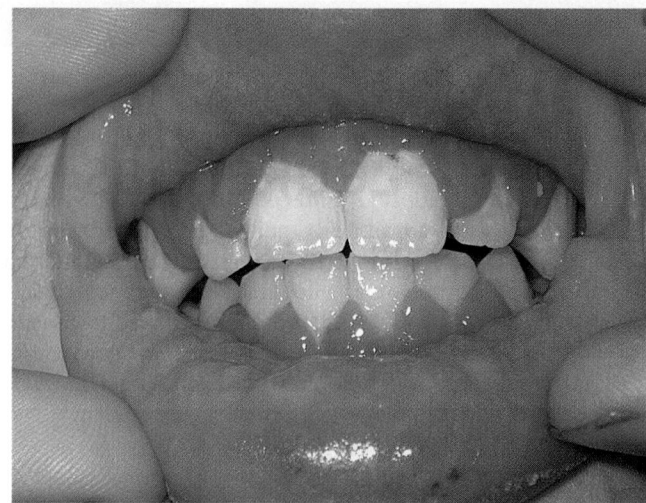

Figure 162-2. Gingival hyperplasia associated with AML subtypes M4 (myelomonocytic) and M5 (monoblastic).

may have been present for a month and usually increase in severity until the diagnosis is made. Some patients present acutely ill with fever, sepsis, and bleeding. Hepatosplenomegaly and lymphadenopathy can be present but are usually not as pronounced as in children with ALL. Chloromas or granulocytic sarcomas, localized masses or growths of leukemia blasts in the skin, orbit, or other sites, can be the only site of disease or can be present in addition to bone marrow disease. As shown in Figure 162-2, gingival hyperplasia may be present and is associated with AML subtypes M4 (myelomonocytic) and M5 (monoblastic).

The initial white blood cell count in patients with AML can be normal, elevated, or low. Coagulation abnormalities resulting in a consumptive process and disseminated intravascular coagulopathy (DIC) may be present at diagnosis. Patients with acute promyelocytic leukemia, subtype M3, often present with severe bleeding and DIC as a result of release of procoagulants or thromboplastins from the leukemic blasts. CNS disease at diagnosis can be present in up to 20% of children with AML but does not affect prognosis. Risk factors for development of AML include neurofibromatosis 1 (NF1) and previous maternal fetal loss.

JUVENILE MYELOMONOCYTIC LEUKEMIA AND MONOSOMY 7

Juvenile myelomonocytic leukemia (JMML) is an uncommon group of disorders accounting for less than 2% of leukemia in children. These disorders were formerly placed in the category of juvenile chronic myelogenous leukemia (JCML) to distinguish this type of disorder from adult type CML (chronic myelogenous leukemia). Patients with JMML are almost always younger than 5 years old, present with impressive hepatosplenomegaly that can result in respiratory compromise, and frequently have involvement of other tissues including skin, lung, and intestines. Peripheral blood counts usually reveal anemia, thrombocytopenia, and an elevated white blood cell and absolute monocyte count. The median survival with chemotherapy has historically been 6.5 months with a 5-year survival of 5%.

Monosomy 7 syndrome (Mo7) presents with many of the same signs and symptoms as JMML. Patients with Mo7 usually have an increased number of infections compared to JMML patients and, unlike JMML, can convert to an acute leukemia phase. Children with neurofibromatosis 1 have a 200- to 500-fold increased risk of developing Mo7, JMML, or AML than that of their peers. The mean survival for Mo7 is 32 months with a 5-year survival of 40%.

CHRONIC MYELOGENOUS LEUKEMIA

Adult type CML is uncommon in children and accounts for less than 3% of all leukemia in children. CML presents with splenomegaly, often massive, elevated WBC with an increased monocyte count, weight loss, lethargy, and fatigue. CML is a clonal disorder of a stem cell containing a specific chromosome translocation, t(9;22), designated the Philadelphia chromosome. Patients usually present in the chronic phase. This can last from a few months to several years before transforming into the accelerated phase followed by the blast crisis phase, which can be refractory to treatment.

DOWN SYNDROME, LEUKEMIA, AND TRANSIENT MYELOPROLIFERATIVE DISORDER

Children with Down syndrome (DS) have a 10- to 20-fold increased risk of developing leukemia over that of the general population. ALL and AML occur about equally in DS children although AML M7, acute megakaryocytic leukemia, is the most common type of AML in this group. Hypotheses regarding why DS predisposes to development of leukemia include developmental errors, immune deficiency, or altered DNA repair. Children with DS and AML or JMML have a much better outcome with less intensive therapy than children without DS. The survival for DS children with AML is about 80%, similar to the survival for ALL. DS children with leukemia have similar presenting signs and symptoms as children without DS.

Transient myeloproliferative disorder (TMD) occurs in newborns, particularly those with DS, and is characterized by an increased proliferation of myeloblasts. In one study, the mean age at presentation was 4 days with a range of 0 to 34 days with a WBC of 73,000 with 57% blasts. The blasts in TMD are clonal in origin and can have cytogenetic abnormalities. TMD can be difficult to distinguish from AML although TMD resolves spontaneously without treatment aside from supportive care. However, up to 30% of children with DS and TMD will develop AML (M7) at 1 to 3 years of life.

DIAGNOSIS OF LEUKEMIA

Most cases of childhood leukemia are diagnosed or at least suspected by the generalist during examination of an ill child. A child with leukemia is typically seen several times by the primary care provider before a definitive diagnosis is made, presenting with common signs and symptoms of childhood illnesses. The chief complaint may be fatigue, petechial rash (see Fig. 162-1), recurrent fevers, or recurrent epistaxsis. Most generalists will diagnose only one or two cases of leukemia in their lifetime. Tentative diagnosis is made by a thorough history, physical examination, and perhaps a complete blood count (CBC) with differential. If leukemia is suspected, the primary care provider should refer the patient to a pediatric hematologist for evaluation.

Acute Lymphoblastic Leukemia

Signs and Symptoms. The most common symptoms in children with ALL (see Table 162-1) are fever, lethargy, fatigue, malaise, petechial rash, bleeding, bone pain, weight loss, and abdominal pain. About two thirds of children have palpable lymphadenopathy, hepatomegaly, or splenomegaly. Symptoms may be present for up to a month prior to the diagnosis.

Evaluation. For the generalist, the single most important laboratory test is a CBC with differential, which may show abnormalities in one or more cell lines. Anemia and thrombocytopenia are common, or a very low, normal, or elevated total WBC with immature lymphocytes or lymphoblasts can be seen. Rarely, patients may present with a normal CBC but with symptoms of a systemic disease such as generalized bone pain and fevers. The WBC differential often reveals neutropenia and immature or "atypical" lymphocytes. With significant tumor burden, manifested by a markedly elevated WBC, hepatosplenomegaly, mediastinal mass, or significant palpable lymphadenopathy, chemistries including uric acid, blood urea nitrogen (BUN), creatinine, calcium, phosphorus, and potassium may be abnormal from rapid cell turnover and cell death. Patients with T-cell leukemia often present with a large tumor burden from a mediastinal mass and organ involvement.

Lymphadenopathy, splenic or liver enlargement, skin infiltrates, petechiae, bleeding, gum hypertrophy, or testicular involvement in boys may be present on physical examination.

Definitive diagnosis is made by a bone marrow aspiration to document the presence of leukemic lymphoblasts. A diagnosis of acute leukemia requires more than 25% blasts in the bone marrow. If the bone marrow is too tightly packed to obtain an aspirate sample, a bone marrow biopsy is required. Immunophenotyping of the leukemic cell population by flow cytometry can assist in classification of the leukemia. Leukemic cell blasts are stained with monoclonal antibodies against specific cell surface antigens. Analysis of the pattern of expression aids in classifying the leukemic subtype, cell of origin, and stage of maturation or differentiation of the leukemia. Chromosome or cytogenetic analysis is performed to identify chromosome abnormalities in the leukemic cell population. Cytogenetic changes are present in more than 80% of cases of ALL. Specific chromosome alterations are important to identify early in treatment because they can affect treatment decisions.

A chest x-ray is obtained to evaluate for a possible mediastinal mass, which commonly occurs in patients with T-cell leukemia, and to identify the unusual patient with a pleural effusion, pulmonary edema, pneumonia, or a leukemic pulmonary infiltrate. Plain radiographs (which are no longer routine) in about half of patients with ALL reveal bone abnormalities, the most commonly showing generalized rarefaction of bones or transverse radiolucent bands in the metaphyses of long bones.

All patients with ALL must have a diagnostic lumbar puncture to determine if CNS leukemia is present. CNS involvement is defined as a WBC greater than 5/μL with blasts present. The diagnostic tap is often delayed until final diagnosis of acute leukemia is made so that intrathecal chemotherapy can be given at the same time.

Other important laboratory tests performed by the specialist include a complete chemistry panel to evaluate the creatinine, blood urea nitrogen, electrolytes, glucose, calcium, phosphorus, magnesium, uric acid, and liver function. If the patient has had any bleeding episodes or evidence of a coagulopathy, a coagulation panel (prothrombin time [PT], partial thromboplastin time [PTT], fibrinogen) is recommended.

Acute Myeloid Leukemia

Signs and Symptoms. Patients with AML can present with findings similar to those of children with ALL. Most common signs and symptoms include fever, pallor, bleeding, malaise, bone pain, and abdominal distention. Lymphadenopathy is uncommon in children with AML and less than half of the patients have an enlarged liver or spleen. AML occurs almost equally in girls and boys. About half of the cases occur in children older than 10 years of age. Symptoms may be present for a month prior to diagnosis although the symptoms usually progress in severity with time.

Diagnosis. A CBC with differential often reveals thrombocytopenia, anemia, neutropenia, and an abnormal (high or low) WBC. Coagulopathy, present in about one in five patients with AML, is documented by a low fibrinogen, presence of fibrin split products, elevated D dimer, and prolonged promthrombin time or partial thromboplastin time. Liver function tests and blood urea nitrogen, creatinine, calcium, phosphorus, uric acid, and electrolyte values should be obtained.

Definitive diagnosis is made by analysis of a bone marrow aspiration. Examination of the morphology of the marrow leukemic blasts and immunophenotyping using flow cytometry determines the FAB subtype of AML (M0–M7). Cytogenetic analysis of the marrow blasts aids in identifying common chromosome abnormalities, particularly those that might affect treatment plans and outcome. Patients with M3 AML, acute promyelocytic leukemia (APL), have a classic t(15;17) translocation present in the leukemic blasts. It is important to diagnose APL early in the course of the disease because it is the only form of childhood AML treated with a different regimen.

Physical examination should document gum hypertrophy, found in M4 or M5 AML, enlargement of the liver or spleen, skin involvement, lymphadenopathy, abdominal distention from organomegaly, ileus or infection, sites of bleeding, neurologic status, and respiratory compromise.

A chest x-ray is recommended for all patients with AML to evaluate for a mediastinal mass, pneumonia, pulmonary edema, pleural effusion, or leukemic infiltrate.

All patients with AML must have a diagnostic lumbar puncture to determine if CNS leukemia is present. CNS involvement is currently defined as a WBC greater than 5/μL with blasts present. The diagnostic tap is often delayed until the final diagnosis of acute leukemia so that intrathecal chemotherapy can be given at the same time.

Juvenile Myelomonocytic Leukemia and Mo7

Signs and Symptoms. JMML and Mo7 occur in children younger than 5 years of age and are more common in boys than girls. Both diseases can present with hepatosplenomegaly and skin rash. JMML can also be associated with failure to thrive and lung infiltrates. Mo7 patients commonly have a history of multiple bacterial infections. Laboratory data reveal abnormal CBCs with leukocytosis, anemia, thrombocytopenia, and monocytosis. Elevated fetal hemoglobin is found in 60% to 90% of children with JMML and 25% with Mo7. Blast transformation can occur in about 40% of children with Mo7 but is rare in JMML.

Diagnosis. Physical examination is important for determining the extent of lymphadenopathy and hepatosplenomegaly. The spleen is often massive and can result in respiratory compromise. CBCs reveal anemia, thrombocytopenia, and leukocytosis with an elevated absolute monocyte count. A bone marrow examination differentiates JMML and Mo7 from AML. Cultures of bone marrow samples can be helpful in diagnosing JMML and Mo7. Elevations of fetal hemoglobin are commonly seen in these disorders. Cytogenetic analysis of the bone marrow sample should also be performed.

Chronic Myelogenous Leukemia

Signs and Symptoms. Children with CML often present with pallor, fever, bleeding and bruising, bone pain, and abdominal distention from hepatosplenomegaly. Patients can also have findings related to hyperleukocytosis including respiratory distress, neurologic abnormalities, papilledema, retinal hemorrhage, and decreased urine output.

Diagnosis. The CBC can show a mild anemia with marked leukocytosis, elevated monocyte count, and thrombocytosis. Peripheral blood white blood cell differential shows cells at all stages of differentiation with an increase in the number of basophils and eosinophils. The mean platelet count is 500,000/mm^3. Lactic acid dehydrogenase (LDH), uric acid, and phosphorus may be elevated. Bone marrow examination usually shows hypercellularity with myeloid hyperplasia. The leukocyte alkaline phosphatase activity of the granulocytic population is reduced in CML compared to an inflammatory response.

CML usually presents in the chronic phase in which cells show continued ability to differentiate. Conversion to the blast phase can occur within months to years. Blast phase is associated with the loss of ability of the leukemic cells to differentiate. Blast conversion can occur in either the myeloid or lymphoid lineage and clinically resembles acute leukemia.

Down Syndrome, Leukemia, and Transient Myeloproliferative Disorder

Signs and Symptoms. Patients with DS with acute leukemia present with the same signs and symptoms as discussed for ALL and AML. TMD occurs in the first 90 days of the newborn period and can have features similar to those in an infant with AML. Patients may have hepatomegaly, splenomegaly, lymphadenopathy, peripheral blasts (nonerythroid), and cardiac or pleural effusions.

Diagnosis. The diagnostic workup is the same as described for ALL or AML.

THERAPY

Cooperative group clinical trials have resulted in very impressive improvements in the outcome of children with leukemia so that acute leukemia is now a curable disease in most children.

Acute Lymphoblastic Leukemia

The main treatment for childhood ALL is chemotherapy in a sequence of phases. Most of the treatment can be delivered in the outpatient setting after diagnosis, education, and initial treatment are completed. The first phase, lasting 4 to 5 weeks, is designed to induce complete clinical remission. Agents used are intravenous vincristine, oral prednisone, or dexamethasone and the enzyme asparaginase given as an IM injection. High-risk patients also receive anthracycline as a fourth drug. Chemotherapy is instilled via lumbar puncture using one or all of the following drugs: cytosine arabinoside, methotrexate, and hydrocortisone. The leukemic cells are very sensitive to these chemotherapy drugs at diagnosis and rapidly undergo cell death with 95% to 98% of children achieving a remission. Bone marrow examinations may be performed 7 and 14 days after initiation of treatment to determine the rapidity of treatment response. The rate of clearing leukemic blasts from the bone marrow may be prognostic of long-term survival. Risk-based treatments are assigned based in part on the rate of response to initial chemotherapy. By the end of induction at 4 or 5 weeks, the bone marrow examination is expected to be a remission marrow, called M1, with less than 5% leukemic blasts present.

The second treatment phase is consolidation, lasting about 4 weeks, with intensification of CNS treatment using intrathecal chemotherapy. Oral and intravenous chemotherapeutic agents may also be administered. The third phase is interim maintenance with oral and intravenous chemotherapy followed by delayed intensification, which consists of reinduction and reconsolidation chemotherapy. This intensive phase resulted in marked improvement in long-term outcomes in clinical trials in the 1980s. In some risk groups, the interim maintenance and delayed intensification phases are repeated a second time. Patients then move to the maintenance phase, which consists of lumbar punctures with intrathecal chemotherapy several times each year, monthly intravenous vincristine with a short course of oral steroids, oral antimetabolites mercaptopurine given daily, and methotrexate weekly. Modifications or additions to the therapy are recommended for some patients with high-risk features, slow response to initial therapy, or unfavorable chromosome findings. In the Children's Oncology Group trials, chemotherapy lasts approximately 3.3 years for boys and 2.3 years for girls. CNS treatment involves lumbar punctures with intrathecal chemotherapy. Cranial irradiation for treatment or prophylaxis of CNS ALL resulted in late-term neuropsychological side effects and is used only in certain very high-risk patients.

After completion of chemotherapy, the pediatric oncologist and primary care provider should follow children closely for signs of relapse and monitor growth, performance, and development in school, vocation, and social activities.

Relapse of the leukemia can occur during or following completion of therapy, most commonly occurring in the bone marrow, CNS, or testicles in boys. It may present as bone pain, headaches, vision changes, vomiting, anemia, bleeding, fevers, or pancytopenia. The time of relapse from the first complete remission can be prognostic in terms of long-term outcome and influences choice of therapy for reinduction. Patients with late relapses after completion of chemotherapy have better outcomes and tolerate therapy better than those who relapse early during therapy. Patients with CNS relapse receive weekly intrathecal chemotherapy until the blasts clear. CNS relapse patients require systemic reinduction because they have a high rate of bone marrow relapse if not treated systemically. Testicular relapse should be confirmed by biopsy and treated with focal radiation therapy to the testes and systemic reinduction chemotherapy. Testicular relapse portends bone marrow relapse. Patients with bone marrow relapse usually require reinduction chemotherapy with a more intensive regimen. HLA typing should be performed on the patient, siblings, and parents to determine availability of a matched donor for possible bone marrow transplantation (BMT).

BMT is not used for treatment of newly diagnosed ALL, as the cure rate with conventional chemotherapy can be as high as 85%. The exception is newly diagnosed patients who are found to have unfavorable cytogenetic abnormalities, such as the t(9;22), present in their leukemic blasts. BMT may be a therapeutic option for recurrent disease based on the site of recurrence (i.e., CNS or bone marrow), time of recurrence, and availability of a suitable bone marrow donor.

Acute Myeloid Leukemia

Treatment regimens for AML have been developed from pediatric clinical trials over the past 30 years. Through the use of intensively timed chemotherapy, the outcome of children with AML has improved significantly. Chemotherapy is used to induce a remission in patients with AML. The treatment plan is markedly different from that used for ALL. Commonly, cytosine arabinoside, an anthracycline, and etoposide are administered intravenously on days 0 to 3 with oral thioguanine and dexamethasone. The therapy is repeated on day 10 for an additional 4 days. The patient is then observed in the hospital for potential toxicities and side effects until the peripheral counts begin to recover, usually 4 to 7 weeks after initiation of treatment. This intensively timed chemotherapy results in a remission induction rate of 75% to 80% and improved long-term survival. Upon recovery from induction cycle 1, a second identical cycle of chemotherapy is given. Patients then receive a consolidation course of intensive chemotherapy. Allogeneic BMT in first remission is recommended for patients with a matched sibling or parent donor. Those without a matched related donor receive intensification chemotherapy. Maintenance chemotherapy has not been shown to be of benefit in treatment of AML. Intrathecal chemotherapy is an integral component of the treatment plan. The entire treatment is approximately 6 to 8 months' duration, much shorter but much more intense than ALL therapy. Intensive timing induction chemotherapy followed by an allogeneic BMT has approximately a 70% 3-year disease-free survival (DFS) whereas induction, intensification, and consolidation chemotherapy has a 55% 3-year disease-free survival.

Acute promyelocytic leukemia (FAB M3) contains the t(15;17) translocation in the leukemic blasts. The nuclear receptor for all-trans-retinoic acid (ATRA) is interrupted by the breakpoint and translocated or juxtaposed to a portion of the PML gene on chromosome 15 resulting in a new fusion protein that responds to ATRA. Patients with APL are now treated with oral ATRA that causes the malignant promyelocytes to differentiate and mature into granulocytes. The coagulopathy associated with many patients with APL improves within the first few days. Patients also receive chemotherapy but tolerate the treatment with fewer side effects because of the actions of ATRA, resulting in decreased morbidity and mortality and improved outcomes.

After completion of therapy, patients are monitored for recurrent leukemia and late side effects. A patient's CBC, growth and development, learning and school performance, social interactions, and vocational performance should be followed as well.

Relapse in AML portends a bad prognosis. If the patient has not received a BMT, reinduction with intensive chemotherapy and BMT is an option. An unrelated matched donor can be used, although risk of side effects and toxicities is increased from an unrelated versus a related donor. For the relapsed patient who has undergone a BMT, reinduction chemotherapy with a donor lymphocyte infusion can aid in controlling disease and symptoms.

Juvenile Myelomonocytic Leukemia and Monosomy 7

The response of these diseases to chemotherapy has been poor. Encouraging results from the use of intensive chemotherapy, biologic modifiers such as cis-retinoic acid, and BMT have recently emerged, even in very young children. Research is under way to determine the role and effectiveness of other biologic agents, including a farnesyl transferase inhibitor, in treatment of these diseases.

Chronic Myelogenous Leukemia

The initial treatment for patients with CML with hyperleukocytosis is oral hydroxyurea to reduce the WBC. The hydroxyurea is titrated to lower the WBC and maintain it in a normal range. Studies have demonstrated the efficacy of interferon used either alone or with hydroxyurea during the chronic phase to reduce leukocytosis and organomegaly and perhaps delay progression from the chronic to blast phase. BMT is the preferred and potentially curative treatment for this disease. Outcomes with BMT depend on the phase at the time of transplant, duration of the chronic phase, and degree of organomegaly. Superior outcomes are achieved when BMT is performed in the first chronic phase, with poorer outcomes in the accelerated and second chronic phase, and worst outcomes when performed in blast crisis. Biologic agents including STI-571, an inhibitor of the Bcr-Abl fusion protein produced from the t(9;22)

Philadelphia chromosome, are being used to treat CML. This agent is being used in patients in blast crisis, accelerated phase, or in chronic phase after failure of interferon-alpha therapy.

Down Syndrome, Acute Leukemia, and Transient Myeloproliferative Disorder

Patients with DS and ALL are stratified and treated identically to children with ALL without DS. DS patients with AML have a very good outcome, comparable to children with ALL. The current treatment for DS children with AML is less intensive than that used for non-DS children with AML. The timing, number of chemotherapy drugs, and doses are all less intensive. BMT is not recommended for DS patients with AML in first remission because of the high cure rate with chemotherapy alone.

DS patients with TMD are observed and given supportive care. Chemotherapy is not recommended unless there is significant organ compromise such as respiratory compromise from organomegaly or side effects from the hyperleukocytosis. Transfusion of platelets and packed red blood cells is recommended as necessary. Treatment of fevers and infections with appropriate antibiotics and antifungals is recommended. Patients must be monitored long term after resolution of symptoms because they can subsequently develop AML.

Complications, Toxicities, and Side Effects of Therapy
(Box 162-1)

Metabolic Disorders. The major toxicities at the initial presentation of acute leukemia are related to metabolic changes caused by the disease. Tumor lysis syndrome occurs with high tumor burdens. Intracellular products are released during high cell turnover or as a result of chemotherapy. Hyperuricemia can cause uric acid nephropathy, hyperkalemia, and hyperphosphatemia with secondary hypocalcemia that results in renal impairment or failure and nephrocalcinosis. Box 162-2 lists interventions to prevent or treat these complications. Vigorous hydration with good urine output often results in a decrease in the peripheral WBC in patients with hyperleukocytosis. In cases of severe hyperleukocytosis, a double volume blood exchange or leukopheresis is recommended. Transfusion of platelets or

---

Box 162-1. Complications, Toxicities, and Side Effects of Therapy

- Tumor lysis syndrome
  Hyperuricemia
  Uric acid nephropathy
  Hyperkalemia
  Hyperphosphatemia with secondary hypocalcemia
- Infection
  Septicemia
  Pneumocystic carinii pneumonia
  Varicella
  Herpes simplex
- Bleeding and anemia
- Cardiac toxicity
- Secondary malignancy

packed red blood cells may be needed for severe thrombocytopenia, bleeding, and anemia. Caution must be used in transfusing packed red blood cells in patients with hyperleukocytosis so as not to significantly increase the blood viscosity.

Infection. Fever and neutropenia with risk of infection can be a serious and life-threatening complication at diagnosis secondary to the leukemia or during treatment as a result of myelosuppression from the chemotherapy. Patients with newly diagnosed leukemia often present with fever, which may result from the leukemia or infection. These patients should have blood cultures and be considered for treatment with intravenous antibiotics pending results of cultures. In patients with neutropenia and fever following chemotherapy, obtain blood cultures and a CBC. Patients with the indicators listed in Box 162-3 should have blood cultures and receive a broad-spectrum intravenous antibiotic (e.g., ceftazidime) for at least 48 hours, pending culture results and resolution of the fever for a period lasting at least 24 hours. The patient then continues receiving the antibiotics until the absolute neutrophil count (ANC) reaches 500. If the patient has a skin cellulitis, perirectal tenderness or inflammation, or pneumonia, antibiotics such as nafcillin, vancomycin, an aminoglycoside, and metronidazole may be added for further antibacterial coverage. If oral thrush is present, fluconazole may be added. If the fevers persist, it is usual to make empiric changes in antibiotic therapy. Persistent fevers for 4 to 5 days require further examination of the patient, possible computed tomography (CT) scans of the sinuses, chest, abdomen, and pelvis, and consideration of adding amphotericin B for fungal coverage. Granulocyte transfusions are rarely used today for treatment of infections in immunocompromised patients.

Acetaminophen can be safely administered to children with fever with normal liver function while the underlying cause is being investigated. Ibuprofen and aspirin are not recommended for children with cancer because of the potential effects on platelet function, especially in patients at risk of developing thrombocytopenia from their therapy.

Pneumocystis Carinii *Pneumonia.* Patients undergoing chemotherapy have a compromised immune function and are at risk of developing *Pneumocystis carinii* pneumonia (PCP). Patients routinely take prophylaxis during treatment and for an additional 6 months after completion of chemotherapy (Box 162-4).

Varicella and Herpes Infections. Patients undergoing chemotherapy who have not had varicella but who have a significant exposure to someone with varicella may be treated within 96 hours of the exposure with varicella-zoster immune globulin (VZIG). Immunocompromised patients who develop varicella or herpes virus infections may be treated with acyclovir. Patients with leukemia have been safely given live attenuated varicella vaccine. Other live virus vaccines are not recommended because patients with cancer are more susceptible to viral infections and because those receiving chemotherapy are unlikely to mount a sufficient immune response.

Bleeding and Anemia. Patients may have anemia, thrombocytopenia, or bleeding at initial presentation or they may develop these following chemotherapy. Platelets may be transfused for bleeding or significant thrombocytopenia and are administered at 10 to 15 cc/kg up to 1 pheresis unit. Packed red blood cells are usually administered at 10 to 15 cc/kg for anemia secondary to cancer or chemotherapy. For significant anemia (e.g., hematocrit < 15% or with evidence of cardiovascular compromise), consider administering the transfusion slowly as 5 cc/kg over 4 hours followed by additional transfusions as needed.

Cardiac Toxicity. Patients receiving anthracycline chemotherapy are at risk of developing cardiac toxicity with functional impairment. The risk of damage is related to total dose received but may not appear for years after receiving the drug. Patients receiving these drugs are monitored with periodic echocardiograms during and after completion of therapy. The cumulative dose of anthracyclines must be closely monitored to minimize toxicity and possible long-term cardiac abnormalities.

Secondary Malignancy. Any patient treated with chemotherapy for a malignancy is at risk for a secondary cancer 8 to 10 years later. The second cancer is usually therapy-related AML that is often refractory to standard treatment. The risk in adults is approximately 1 in 800. The risk in children is not yet known.

Outcomes

Survival for children with leukemias has significantly improved over the previous 20 years with long-term survival of up to 85%. Therapies are now used based on the risk

Table 162-2. Risk Categories as Defined by the National Cancer Institute (NCI) and Survival Rates for ALL

Risk Category	Survival Rate
Standard-risk leukemia (60% of patients)	85%
■ 1 through 9 years of age	
■ Initial WBC < 50,000/µL	
High-risk leukemia	>70%
■ Age 10 or older (regardless of initial WBC)	
or	
■ Initial WBC > 50,000/µL (regardless of age) at presentation	

features at time of presentation and initial response to therapy. Risk features for ALL include the initial WBC and patient age at the time of presentation (Table 162-2). Approximately half of all children who relapse with ALL are from the standard-risk group, although they tend to relapse later and survive longer than children in the high-risk group. On current treatment regimens, CNS relapse occurs in about 5% of standard-risk ALL patients, usually between 1 and 3 years from diagnosis. Bone marrow relapse or testicular recurrence in boys can occur during or following therapy.

Specific chromosome alterations in the leukemic blasts at diagnosis unfavorably affect treatment. These changes include presence of the Philadelphia chromosome t(9;22), t(4;11), hypodiploidy (<44 chromosomes), and in standard-risk patients a balanced t(1;19). Therapy in these patients is intensified with consideration of BMT in first remission. Infants with acute leukemia have poorer outcomes depending on the biologic and genetic features of the leukemic blasts.

Patients with AML have a 3-year disease-free survival of approximately 65% to 70% with chemotherapy followed by allogeneic BMT, and 50% to 55% with chemotherapy alone.

Patients with JMML have had a poor prognosis, with 5-year survival of 5% and 40% for monosomy 7. Outcomes of current therapies using chemotherapy, biologic modifiers, and BMT are encouraging and, it is to be hoped, will result in improved survival rates.

Children with CML are currently treated with hydroxyurea, 5TI-571, and BMT if a suitable donor is available, with survival surpassing 50% depending on the stage of the disease.

COORDINATION OF CARE WITH THE PEDIATRIC ONCOLOGIST

The pediatric oncologist should perform initial evaluation, diagnosis, and implementation of a therapeutic treatment plan for a child with leukemia in consultation with the primary care provider (Box 162-5). Knowledge of the most current pediatric clinical trials and treatment plans is crucial for choosing the best therapy. Important diagnostic, biologic, and genetic tests of the bone marrow or blood in patients with leukemia often affect the choice of the risk-based therapy. Over 70% of children with cancer are enrolled in a national cooperative group, National Cancer Institute sponsored, clinical trial. Therapeutic, biologic, and epidemiologic clinical trials have resulted in research studies to identify the best treatments and elucidate the causes of cancer in children. Fewer than 3% of adults are enrolled in a clinical trial.

Most of the therapy for patients with ALL can be given in the outpatient setting either in a pediatric cancer center or by a community pediatrician in collaboration with a pediatric oncologist. Patients with AML, on the other hand, receive nearly all of their therapy in the inpatient setting because of the intensity of the treatments and the life-threatening side effects of the disease and therapy. As the treatment and care move more to the outpatient setting, collaboration between the pediatric oncologist and primary care provider is crucial to successful treatment and management of the underlying disease, toxicities, and side effects of the therapy. Families and patients often prefer to receive some of their therapy and management near their home, from the primary care physician who frequently has had a long and close association with the family. The primary care provider can play an important role in monitoring laboratory values such as CBCs, administering chemotherapy, and evaluating patients for signs of toxicities and fevers.

After leukemia patients with fever and neutropenia have received initial treatment and are doing well, they can be discharged to complete antibiotics at home. Home care and the primary care provider can assist the family in completing the prescribed course of antibiotics. The primary care clinician can obtain regular blood counts, usually twice weekly, and monitor treatment side effects. Many cancer patients require supplemental enteral or parenteral nutrition at some time during their therapy.

Regular physical examinations and evaluations are important. Since patients with leukemia can develop significant and life-threatening complications, including infection, pancreatitis, pneumonia, coagulopathy, thrombosis, stroke, and liver toxicity, the pediatric oncologist should maintain regular and frequent communication to optimize the care of the child with leukemia.

The specialist and the multidisciplinary pediatric oncology team can also provide assistance with psychosocial issues and intervention. They can support spiritual beliefs, identify financial concerns, assist in finding additional resources, enlist social support systems and home care, and provide advanced care planning and palliative care when necessary. The multidisciplinary team at a pediatric children's hospital with a pediatric cancer program can assist in providing comprehensive care across the continuum in the hospital, clinic, generalist's office, and home.

Box 162-5. Roles of the Primary Care Clinician in Comanaging Children with Cancer

- Schedule regular physical examinations and evaluations to monitor for complications of the disease or of therapy.
- Communicate frequently and regularly with oncologist.
- Provide emergency care, stabilize patient, and refer to oncologist.
- Monitor blood counts.
- Administer chemotherapy under supervision of oncologist if patient lives far from medical center.
- Supervise home health care administration of antibiotics after febrile, neutropenic patient is discharged from hospital.
- Administer supplemental enteral or parenteral nutrition under supervision of subspecialist when needed.
- Provide psychosocial support to patient and family.

CONCLUSION

Patients presenting with leukemia can have predictable signs and symptoms that can be recognized by the pediatrician who should make a diagnosis and refer the patient to a pediatric oncologist. Early recognition of leukemia and consultation and referral to a pediatric oncologist enable initiation of therapy prior to development of severe and potentially life-threatening complications of the underlying disease. The primary care physician should continue to play an important and collaborative role in the management and follow-up of children with leukemia.

Mini-index of Related Topics

SUGGESTED READINGS

Keene N: Childhood Leukemia: A Guide for Families, Friends, and Caregivers. Sebastopol, Calif, O'Reilly, 1997.

Nathan DG, Orkin SH: Nathan and Oski's Hematology of Infancy and Childhood, 6th ed. Philadelphia, WB Saunders, 2003.

National Childhood Cancer Foundation website. Available at: http://www.nccf.org.

Pizzo PA, Poplack DF: Principles and Practice of Pediatric Oncology, 4th ed. Philadelphia, Lippincott-Raven, 2002.

SECTION 4 — CHRONIC MEDICAL CARE: *Cancer*

163 Lymphomas

Robert E. Goldsby and Richard S. Lemons

ROLE OF THE GENERALIST

1 Diagnose and manage lymphadenopathy appropriately.

2 Distinguish malignant lymphadenopathy from reactive or infectious lymphadenopathy.

3 Refer a child with lymphadenopathy to a specialist when assistance is needed for diagnosis and medical management.

4 Diagnose a mediastinal mass.

5 Know the differential diagnosis of an enlarged spleen.

6 Understand the distinctions between Hodgkin disease and non-Hodgkin lymphoma.

7 Understand the differences between leukemia and lymphoma.

8 Assist in the management of patients with lymphoma.

DEFINITIONS

Lymphomas are the third most common malignancy in children in the United States after leukemias and brain tumors, representing more than 10% of pediatric cancers. Lymphomas are cancers of lymphoid tissue. Lymphoid tissue is distributed throughout the human body in the lymph nodes, spleen, thymus, and bone marrow. If more than 25% of the malignant cells are in the bone marrow, the cancer is classified as leukemia (Chapter 162). Lymphomas usually present with lymphadenopathy, splenomegaly, and/or mediastinal masses. Leukemias may have similar findings but also have symptoms of marrow dysfunction such as fatigue (anemia), infections and fevers (neutropenia), and/or bruising and bleeding (thrombocytopenia).

Childhood lymphomas are categorized in two clinico-pathologically distinct entities, non-Hodgkin lymphoma (NHL) and Hodgkin disease (HD) (Table 163-1). In the United States NHLs account for 60% and Hodgkin disease for 40% of childhood lymphomas. Each category is further classified by integrating clinical, morphologic, immunophenotypic, and cytogenetic information (see Table 163-1).

Lymphadenopathy is enlargement of the lymph nodes. The distribution of lymph node involvement can be localized, regional, or generalized. The location, timing, and character provide clues to the pathogenesis of disease. Lymphadenopathy can be related to infection, inflammation, or, less commonly, malignancy. Lymphomas can present with localized or generalized lymphadenopathy. Hodgkin disease generally spreads in a contiguous fashion. NHL can spread in a noncontiguous fashion. Lymphomas can arise in the anterior or middle mediastinum as a consequence of mediastinal lymphadenopathy or thymic infiltration. Lymphoma can cause splenomegaly by infiltrating the spleen. Other causes of splenic enlargement are portal hypertension and infections.

FUNDAMENTALS

Lymphoid tissues are the site of preparation, processing, and proliferation of lymphocytes, the main workhorse of acquired immunity. B cells and T cells, the two major types of lymphocytes, are derived from progenitor cells in the bone marrow. B cells differentiate in the bone marrow, whereas T-cell progenitors migrate to the thymus in the superior anterior mediastinum to complete the maturation process. The normal thymus is enlarged during the neonatal period and slowly decreases in size during the first year of life.

B-cell and T-cell lymphocytes are morphologically indistiguishable but functionally differently. Each has a specific pattern of cell surface markers that correlates with the stage of maturation. B-cell lymphocytes respond to specific antigenic stimuli by maturing into antibody or immunoglobin (Ig) producing plasma cells that provide humoral immunity. T-cell lymphocytes express antigen specific T-cell receptors (TCRs) and interact with antigen presenting cells to signal a cytotoxic effect or cell-mediated immunity. The Igs and TCRs are heterodimeric polypeptides with an almost unlimited repertoire of antigen recognition.

Lymphocytes circulate in the blood and are recycled in the lymph through a meshwork of lymphatic vessels. These vessels drain lymph into lymph nodes, then into the thoracic duct, and ultimately into the superior vena cava. The lymph node functions as an antigen trap, enlarging with infection or inflammation from a responsive lymphocytic proliferation and from recruitment of other immune cells or, less commonly, with malignant infiltration.

The spleen, the largest lymphoid tissue, plays important immune functions. The spleen traps foreign materials in the blood and allows immune cells to respond and react to the intruder. The spleen can be enlarged from infections, chronic hemolysis, inflammatory diseases, hepatic disease, or infiltrative diseases (storage diseases and malignancy).

Lymphoma Biology

Lymphomas are a heterogeneous group of neoplasms that arise from the clonal proliferation of lymphoid precursor cells in the lymphoid tissues. Lymphoid neoplasms arise from a series of genetic changes that transform the immune cell from normal to neoplastic. Investigation of chromosomal translocations has lead to tremendous strides in understanding the biology of lymphomagenesis. The biologic features of the lymphoma cells are important in defining the type of lymphoma and the appropriate therapy.

Non-Hodgkin Lymphoma

There are three main categories of pediatric NHLs: Burkitt, lymphoblastic, and large cell lymphoma. Each category has its own biological characteristics. Burkitt lymphoma is commonly associated with nonrandom chromosomal translocations that juxtapose c-myc next to the highly active immunoglobulin genes in these precursor B cells and cause deregulation and overexpression of c-myc protein, a transcription factor that stimulates lymphomagenesis.

The majority of lymphoblastic lymphomas are of T-cell origin. These lymphomas share similar morphology, immunophenotype, and genetic alterations with T-cell leukemia that likely represents a different form in a spectrum of a single disease. T-cell leukemia/lymphomas have fewer cytogenetically detectable chromosome abnormalities than Burkitt lymphomas (less than 25% versus more than 90%). Most of these translocations place a proto-oncogene, usually a transcription factor, under the control of a T-cell receptor regulatory domain. This results in aberrant expression of the proto-oncogene, similar to c-myc

Table 163-1. Classification of Common Childhood Lymphomas

Morphology	Clinical Presentation	Phenotype	Genetic Alteration
Non-Hodgkin Lymphoma (60%)			
Burkitt (small noncleaved cell lymphoma) (50%)	Intra-abdominal (sporadic) Jaw (endemic)	B cell	Ig:Myc translocation
Lymphoblastic lymphoma (35%)	Mediastinal	T cell	TCR: transcription factor translocation
Large cell lymphomas (15%)	Variable	T, B, or null	ALK:NPM fusion protein
Hodgkin Lymphoma (40%)			
Classic Hodgkin (Reed-Sternberg cells)	Cervical adenopathy, mediastinal, contiguous spread	Usually B cell	p53 mutations Bcl-2 family EBV

overexpression in mature Burkitt lymphomas. The aberrant expression of transcription factors presumably activates target genes involved with cell cycle regulation and differentiation.

The morphology of a subset of large cell lymphomas (LCLs) called anaplastic large cell lymphoma (ALCL) has a characteristic translocation, t(2:5)(p23:q35), that results in a fusion between the promoter sequences of the ubiquitously expressed nucleolar phosphoprotein (NPM) gene on 5q35 and a protein tyrosine kinase gene, anaplastic lymphoma kinase (ALK), on 2p23. Overexpression of the truncated anaplastic lymphoma kinase, which is normally not expressed in lymphoid cells, may contribute to the lymphomagenesis.

Two major conditions may predispose individuals to developing the genetic events that lead to NHLs. Epstein-Barr viral infection is associated with subsequent development of NHL. People with primary and secondary immunodeficiency syndromes have an increased incidence of NHL. The mechanism by which these conditions predispose individuals to the molecular events involved in lymphomagenesis is unclear.

Hodgkin Disease

Despite tremendous advances in the treatment of Hodgkin lymphoma, the biologic basis of this disease has remained elusive. The Reed-Sternberg (RS) cell, the malignant cell of Hodgkin disease, usually represents less than 1% of the tumor mass. These large, bizarre, binucleate cells probably originate from B-cell lymphocytes in germinal centers of lymphoid tissues, but they occasionally appear to be of T-cell lineage. RS cells secrete numerous cytokines that activate T cells. They produce additional cytokines promoting tumorigenesis and inducing the systemic "B" symptoms (fever, night sweats, and/or weight loss) so commonly seen in this disease. Overproduction or imbalance of cytokines may play a significant role in the genesis of Hodgkin disease. Unlike NHLs, no consistent chromosomal rearrangements are identified in patients with Hodgkin disease. Familial predisposition has been reported. Accumulated evidence suggests that Epstein-Barr virus (EBV) may play a role in the pathogenesis of Hodgkin disease.

EVALUATION OF PATIENTS WITH LYMPHADENOPATHY, SPLENOMEGALY, OR MEDIASTIAL MASS

Approach to Lymphadenopathy

Lymphadenopathy, common in children, can be the first manifestation of a serious condition such as lymphoma. The site, extent, duration, and character can be used to determine an appropriate investigation and when to refer to other specialists.

Lymphadenopathy can be generalized or localized. The cervical lymph node region is the most common site of localized lymphadenopathy. Cervical lymph node enlargement is usually secondary to infectious adenitis (Fig. 163-1A). Inguinal adenopathy is also common often due to infectious adenitis. Less common sites should be carefully evaluated. Axillary or epitrochlear adenopathy without

evidence of regional inflammation or infection may require further investigation or, at a minimum, very close follow-up. Supraclavicular or mediastinal adenopathy always requires further investigation and referral to a pediatric oncologist.

Generalized adenopathy, a manifestation of a number of diseases, must be evaluated (see Fig. 163-1B). Infections with Epstein-Barr virus (mononucleosis), cytomegalovirus (CMV), HIV, or other viruses can cause generalized adenopathy. Bacterial infections usually cause localized adenopathy. However, *Salmonella*, *Brucella* (brucellosis), and *Borrelia* (Lyme disease) infections may be accompanied by generalized adenopathy. Toxoplasmosis can resemble mononucleosis. Disseminated tuberculosis can exhibit generalized adenopathy. Noninfectious causes of generalized adenopathy include connective tissue disease (juvenile rheumatoid arthritis), serum sickness, storage diseases (Gaucher disease and Neimann-Pick disease), sarcoidosis, and malignancies. Patients with malignancies disseminated through the lymph nodes generally have other symptoms or physical findings.

Rapidly progressing lymphadenopathy is a feature of malignancy, but can also be seen with infectious adenopathy. If the lymph node enlargement progresses during a

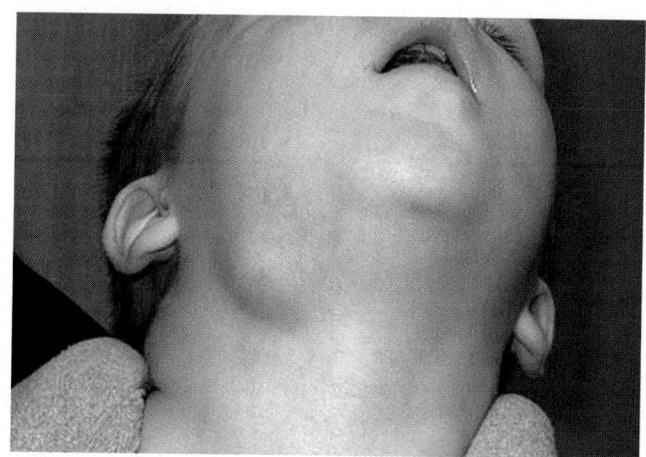

A

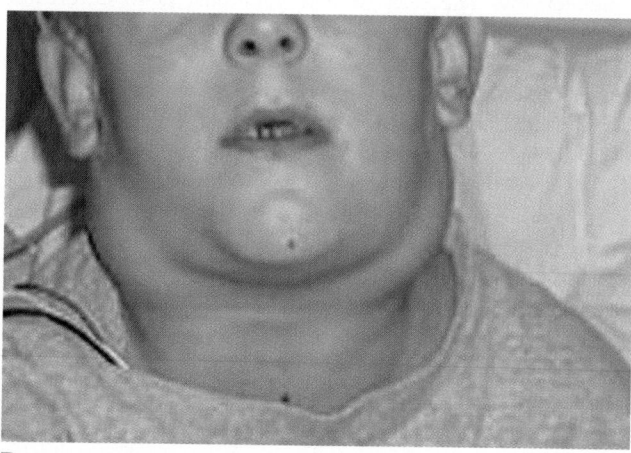

B

Figure 163-1. A, Large lymph node with overlaying erythema in a child with infectious cervical lymphadenitis. **B,** Massive cervical lymphadenopathy in a child with lymphoblastic lymphoma.

course of observation or antibiotics, then a biopsy is often warranted. Lymphadenopathy that persists for more than a month without diminution should be evaluated.

Malignancy is more of a concern with lymph nodes that are immobile, matted, and nontender. Infected lymph nodes are usually tender and may have erythema of the overlying skin. Cervical and inguinal nodes that are smaller than 1 cm are common, usually reactive, and of little consequence. Axillary and epitrochlear lymph nodes that are larger than 0.5 cm should be followed closely. Supraclavicular lymph nodes, regardless of size, mandate further evaluation.

Regional lymphadenopathy without other concerning features may be observed or treated empirically with a course of antibiotics (e.g., amoxicillin clavulanate [Augmentin], cephalexin [Keflex]). A skin test for tuberculosis (PPD) may be of value. If a malignant process is suspected, additional tests should include a complete blood count, chemistries including lactic acid dehydrogenase (LDH) and uric acid, and liver function tests. A chest x-ray may also be warranted. If the lymphadenopathy is highly suspicious, a biopsy is required. Fine-needle aspiration may be easier and provide a quicker answer, but it does not allow examination of the lymph node architecture, limits material for diagnostic evaluations, and may miss localized disease within the lymph node.

Generalized lymphadenopathy must be evaluated. Radiographic imaging of the chest and abdomen may be necessary to assess the presence of mediastinal, liver, or spleen involvement. Screening laboratories might include a complete blood count (CBC), chemistries including LDH and uric acid, and liver function tests. Bone marrow evaluation is warranted for any patient with evidence of marrow abnormalities on complete blood count and lymphadenopathy. Other tests depend on patient history and physical examination.

Approach to Splenomegaly

Enlargement of the spleen can occur in a number of benign processes or as a consequence of malignancy, particularly leukemia and lymphoma. Sophisticated imaging techniques can aid in defining the pathology and reduce the need for splenectomy. The task for the generalist is to determine when and what additional investigations are needed.

Many infections that cause lymphadenopathy can also cause splenomegaly, including malaria (massive splenomegaly), syphilis, and abscess of the spleen. Other diagnostic considerations include hemolytic anemia, congestive splenomegaly (i.e., splenic vein thrombosis, hepatic fibrosis, or cirrhosis), cysts, connective tissue diseases (i.e., juvenile rheumatoid arthritis, systemic lupus erythematosus), and metabolic diseases (i.e., Gaucher disease, Neimann-Pick disease, and others). Malignant splenomegaly is usually caused by lymphoma or leukemia (chronic myelogenous leukemia [CML] often presents with massive splenomegaly). Hamartomas can also cause splenomegaly.

A thorough history, physical examination, and appropriate imaging usually provide the diagnosis. Consultation with radiology to determine the best imaging approach may be of value. Screening laboratories for patients with suspected malignancy are similar to those for patients with lymphadenopathy. Radiologic evaluation may be necessary to differentiate splenomegaly from other abdominal masses. Ultrasound with Doppler flow analysis may help define congestive splenomegaly. Computed tomography (CT) or magnetic resonance imaging (MRI) scan may be necessary for diagnosis and staging, but should be done in coordination with a pediatric oncologist.

Approach to Mediastinal Mass

Mediastinal disease may be clinically indicated by respiratory compromise or discovered by screening chest x-ray. Symptoms may include cough, dyspnea, orthopnea, stridor, and/or hoarseness. An associated superior vena cava syndrome may be present with swelling and plethora of the face, neck, and upper extremity. The differential diagnosis of mediastinal disease depends on the location (Table 163-2). Lymphoma and leukemia must be ruled out in a child with anterior or middle mediastinal mass. Nearly half of the patients with Hodgkin disease or lymphoblastic lymphoma have mediastinal disease at diagnosis.

Approach to the evaluation of a mediastinal mass must be modified to avoid respiratory collapse when signs of respiratory compromise are present. Chest x-ray is the quickest method to assess mediastinal involvement (Fig. 163-2A). CT of the chest (see Fig. 163-2B) defines the location, characterizes the mass, and provides additional clues for diagnosis (see Chapter 164). Chest CT can indicate airway compression and the risk of an adverse respiratory event. Pulmonary function tests (PFTs) may also predict risk for respiratory failure with sedation. General anesthesia is contraindicated if pulmonary function tests are less than 50% predicted. Occasionally, emergent radiation can be used to treat patients with mediastinal masses and airway compromise even before a tissue diagnosis is made.

Table 163-2. Mediastinal Masses	
Position	**Mass**
Anterior mediastinum	Normal thymus (newborn period)
	Reactive thymus
	Teratoma (most common mass in the newborn)
	Cysts
	Cystic hygroma
	Hamartoma
	Lymphoblastic lymphoma
	Thymoma (indistinguishable from lymphoblastic lymphoma)
	Hodgkin lymphoma
	Leukemic involvement
	Hemangioma
Middle mediastinum	Vascular rings
	Pericardial cysts
	Bronchogenic cysts
	Hemangioma
Posterior mediastinum	Neuroblastoma
	Ganglioneuroblastoma
	Bronchogenic cysts
	Esophageal duplication
	Lipomatosis
	Hemangioma
	Hernia

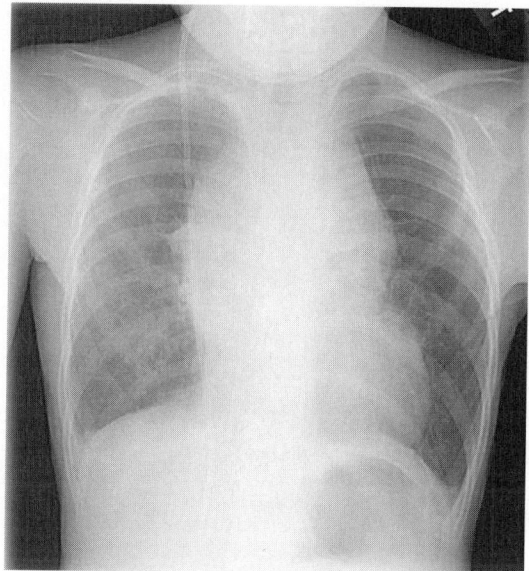

A

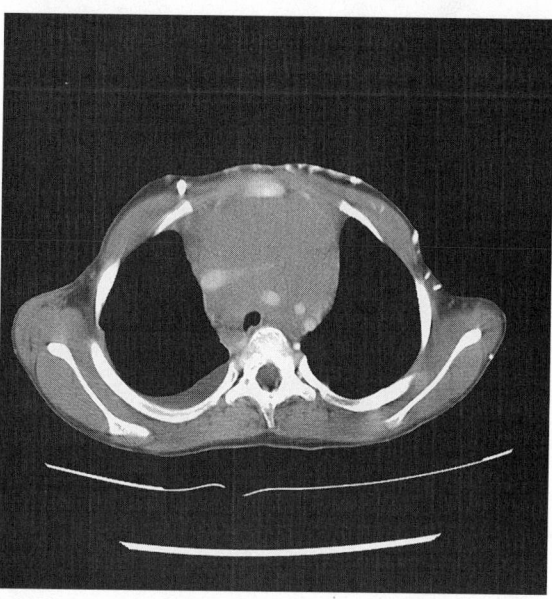

B

Figure 163-2. Chest x-ray **(A)** and chest CT **(B)** showing mediastinal disease and a small right-sided pleural effusion in a child with lymphoblastic lymphoma.

DIAGNOSIS OF LYMPHOMA

Each type of lymphoma has a characteristic clinical presentation. Tissue biopsy to diagnose the lymphoma precisely and staging evaluation to define the extent of disease are necessary to determine therapy and outcome.

Clinical Presentation

Burkitt (Small Noncleaved Cell) Lymphomas

The two forms of Burkitt lymphoma have distinct clinical presentations. Sporadic Burkitt lymphoma, the predominant form in the United States, tends to arise in gastrointestinal lymph nodes. Patients with sporadic Burkitt lymphoma often present with abdominal symptoms including pain, nausea, and vomiting. Symptoms often mimic a surgical abdomen, such as appendicitis or bowel ob-

struction. They can also present with symptoms of sepsis or gastrointestinal bleeding from obstruction, perforation, or intussusception of the bowel. Primary tumors of the head and neck, especially the jaw, characterize the endemic form of Burkitt lymphoma that is common in Africa. Pleural effusions or bone marrow involvement is more common with the sporadic form of Burkitt. Orbital or paraspinal disease is more common with the endemic form. Headaches, signs of meningismus, or cranial nerve palsies suggest central nervous system (CNS) involvement, which occurs in approximately 15% of cases.

Lymphoblastic Lymphoma

Children with lymphoblastic lymphoma often present with thymic disease and/or marked lymphadenopathy. Patients can present with cough, dyspnea, or shortness of breath related to airway compromise associated with mediastinal disease and/or pleural effusions. The lymphoma can compress the superior vena cava causing swelling of the face, neck, and right upper extremity, a condition known as superior vena cava (SVC) syndrome. Other less common sites of involvement are abdomen, kidney, bone, and skin. CNS involvement is rare.

Large Cell Lymphoma

LCLs have the most varied spectrum of clinical presentations. Children can present with isolated or disseminated disease. Isolated skin disease or lymphomas arising in unusual sites are often LCLs. Clinical presentation tends to parallel the immunophenotype with B-cell LCLs presenting similarly to small noncleaved cell lymphomas and T-cell LCLs presenting similarly to lymphoblastic lymphomas.

Hodgkin Lymphoma

Hodgkin disease often presents as painless lymphadenopathy. Cervical lymph nodes are the most common site. The disease tends to spread in a contiguous fashion. Mediastinal lymphadenopathy is common. Splenic infiltration can also occur. Extranodal disease, such as bone marrow and hepatic infiltration, is relatively rare. Approximately 25% of patients present with "B" symptoms: night sweats, fevers, or weight loss. Pruritis and fatigue are also relatively common systemic symptoms. The stage of disease largely determines treatment and outcome. The presence of bulky disease also affects treatment.

Pathology

Biopsy of the involved site confirms the diagnosis. The morphology, immunophenotype, and cytogenetics of the material are evaluated to define the specific lymphoma. The typical morphology for each different type of lymphoma is shown in Figure 163-3. Details regarding the pathologic diagnosis are available on the CD-ROM.

Evaluation and Staging of Lymphomas

After a thorough history and physical examination, patients with a suspected lymphoma should have screening laboratory evaluation and appropriate imaging. Laboratory tests that may be helpful in initial evaluation include a complete blood count with a differential and selected chemistries (Table 163-3). The complete blood count may show

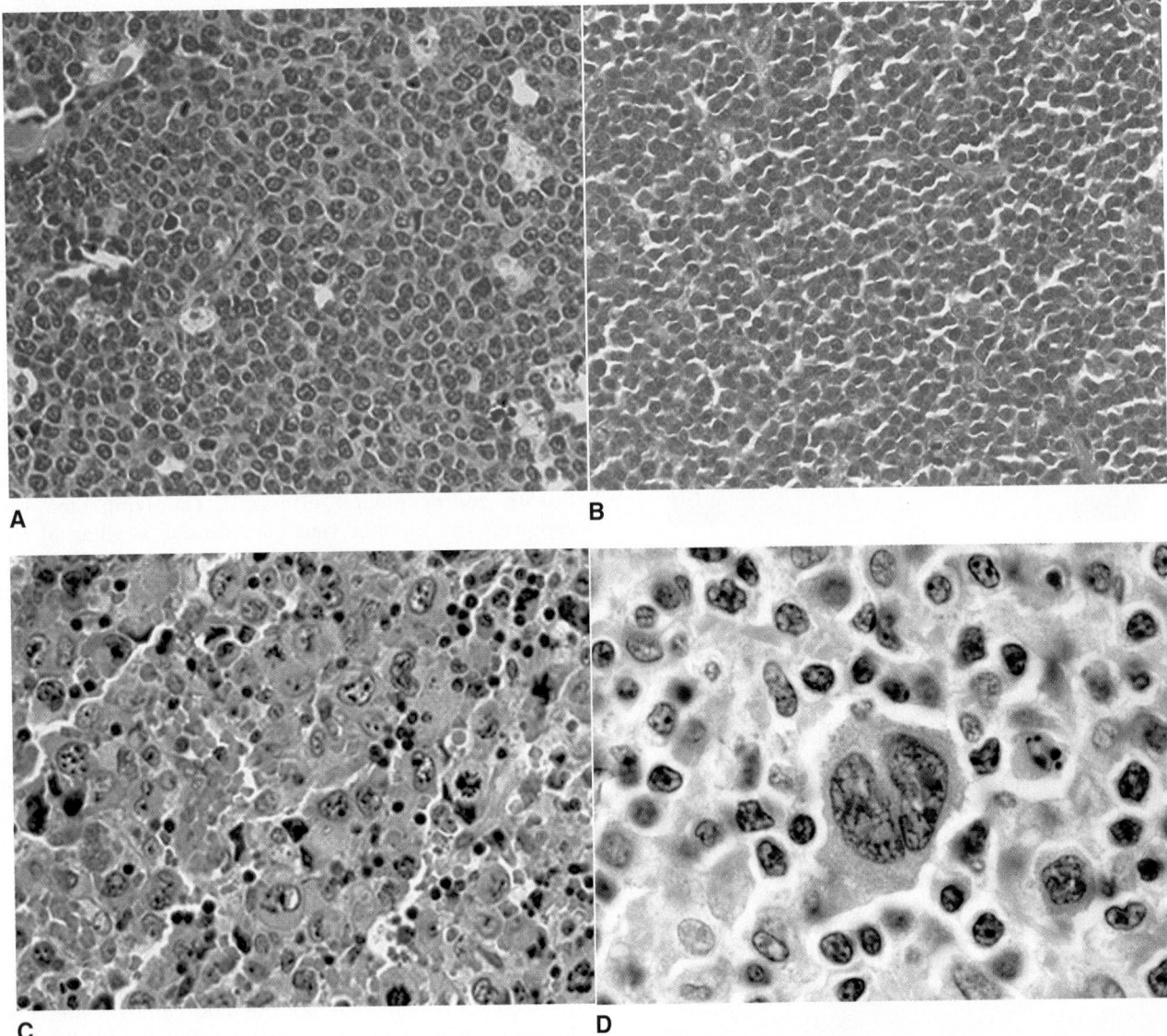

Figure 163-3. A, Burkitt lymphoma showing the classic starry sky pattern. **B,** Lymphoblastic lymphoma demonstrating homogeneous population of lymphoblasts. **C,** LCL exhibiting characteristic pleomorphic morphology. **D,** Classic Reed-Sternberg cell in Hodgkin disease.

cytopenias and lymphoblasts suggesting the diagnosis of leukemia. The presence of atypical lymphocytes may be more indicative of a viral process. The chemistries should include electrolytes, renal and liver function tests, lactic acid dehydrogenase, and uric acid. An elevated potassium, uric acid, and/or phosphate level may suggest looming tumor lysis syndrome, a serious complicating factor in newly diag-

nosed lymphoma. Tumor lysis is more commonly associated with Burkitt lymphoma.

Any child with concerning lymphadenopathy should have a chest x-ray to rule out mediastinal involvement. Any child with a suspicious abdominal mass should have a radiographic evaluation (see Chapter 164).

Staging of the lymphoma after diagnosis requires additional tests. The primary purpose of staging is to ensure appropriate risk-based therapy. General lymphoma staging is defined in Table 163-4. Hodgkin disease can be subclassified into "A" or "B": "B" signifies the presence of B symptoms (10% weight loss, unexplained fevers, or drenching night sweats). Radiographic imaging is a major determinant of staging for both types of lymphoma, generally requiring CT scans of the neck, chest, abdomen, and pelvis. Other scanning modalities may be useful. Gallium scans, often positive in patients with Hodgkin disease, provide a useful marker for follow-up. Positron emission tomography (PET) scan can detect lymphomas or assess residual posttherapy masses. Splenectomy is *not*

Table 163-3. Initial Screening Tests in a Child with a Suspected Lymphoma

Evaluation	Test
Laboratory tests	Complete blood count with differential
	Electrolytes including potassium, calcium, and phosphate
	Renal function (BUN, creatinine)
	Liver function tests (total bilirubin, AST, ALT)
	LDH
	Uric acid
Radiograph	Chest x-ray

Table 163-4. Staging of Pediatric Lymphomas

Stage	Description
Stage 1	Lymphoma involving one lymph node or one extranodal site
Stage 2	Lymphoma involving two or more lymph node areas on the same side of the diaphragm, or a single extranodal site with regional lymph node involvement on the same side of the diaphragm
Stage 3	Lymphoma involving lymph nodes on both sides of the diaphragm. Lymphoma may also involve an area or organ near the lymph node areas and/or spleen
Stage 4	Lymphoma involving extralymphatic sites (e.g., bone marrow, CNS, liver)

necessary in the staging evaluation of children with lymphoma. Bone marrow evaluation is an essential part of the evaluation for all patients with non-Hodgkin lymphomas and high-stage Hodgkin disease. Patients with non-Hodgkin lymphoma must have a lumbar puncture to assess CNS involvement.

MANAGEMENT

The primary care provider should refer all children and adolescents with a suspected lymphoma to a pediatric oncologist. Expedited referral allows rapid diagnosis, biologic assays to determine risk-based therapy, and initiation of therapy. Urgent medical triage is required for patients with respiratory compromise, metabolic abnormalities, or neurologic manifestations.

Acute Management Issues

Respiratory Compromise. Any patient with a suspected lymphoma and respiratory distress should be transferred to a tertiary medical center with pediatric oncology as soon as medically feasible. Tests and procedures that can adversely affect respiratory status must be limited prior to transfer. A chest x-ray is a quick and relatively simple test that may define the etiology of the respiratory symptoms. Do not force into a prone position a child who is more comfortable sitting up. CT scan may be deferred until the child is transferred to the tertiary hospital. Phone consultation with the pediatric oncologist will help define the best approach regarding management, stabilization, and transfer. Emergent radiation therapy is occasionally required prior to definitive diagnosis.

Metabolic Abnormalities. Because lymphomas, especially Burkitt lymphoma, grow rapidly, tumor lysis may be present at diagnosis or, more commonly, develop within the first few days of therapy. The electrolyte abnormalities of tumor lysis syndrome include hyperkalemia, hyperuricemia, and/or hyperphosphatemia. Tumor lysis can lead to renal dysfunction or failure as a consequence of uric acid or calcium phosphate precipitates in the kidney. Initial therapy includes hydration at 2 times maintenance (3000 cc/m^2/24 hours) with alkalization fluids and no potassium added (i.e., D$_5$¼NS with 40 meq Na HCO$_3$/L). Maintaining a urine pH of 7.0 to 7.5 helps promote uric acid and phosphate excretion. Allopurinol can be initiated to help process the uric acid. Urate oxidase is now being used to quickly lower uric acid levels in patients exhibiting tumor lysis. Aluminum hydroxide (Amphojel) can bind phosphate and reduce phosphate levels. An electrocardiogram (ECG) and medical management of hyperkalemia may be warranted (see Chapter 42). Hyperkalemia with a potassium level of less than 6.5 meq/L can usually be treated with oral sodium polystyrene sulfonate (Kayexalate) that binds to and eliminates potassium via the bowels. When the potassium level is above 6.5 meq/L, the treatment is intravenous therapy with calcium gluconate, loop diuretics, insulin, and/or sodium bicarbonate. Occasionally, patients with renal failure will need dialysis during the initial phases of therapy.

Neurologic Manifestations. The most common neurologic manifestations in children with lymphoma, headaches, signs of meningimus, and/or cranial nerve palsies are from CNS involvement. Spinal cord compression is a rare complication of lymphoma, but it requires emergency attention. Patients with signs and symptoms of spinal cord compression need magnetic resonance imaging of the spine to define the site and degree of compression. Therapy for spinal cord compression may include steroids, decompressive laminectomy, and/or emergent radiation. Discussion with the pediatric oncologist facilitates the most appropriate initial treatment.

GENERAL ASPECTS OF LYMPHOMA THERAPY

After the diagnosis, patients are treated with chemotherapy or chemotherapy and radiation. Chemotherapy is type-specific and stage-specific. Various combinations of agents are used in sequential fashion. Radiation is used to treat compression of vital organs or to achieve local control of the lymphoma in certain patients with Hodgkin disease.

Comanagement Issues
Common Acute Care Issues in Therapy

Fever and Neutropenia. Fever in immunocompromised patients may be the first sign of a life-threatening infection. A fever is defined as a single oral temperature of 38.5°C or a temperature higher than 38.0°C on two occasions more than 1 hour apart within a 24-hour period. The absolute neutrophil count (ANC) is an indicator for risk of severe bacterial infection. A patient with a fever and an ANC less than 500 must be immediately evaluated, blood cultures obtained, and IV antibiotics administered. Initial hospitalization for observation is generally warranted even if a source of infection, such as otitis media, is identified. If the ANC is more than 500, inpatient hospitalization depends on the results of the evaluation. Pediatric patients with central lines and fevers require blood cultures from each lumen to ensure that the line is not infected. Filgrastim (Neupogen [granulocyte-colony stimulating factor, G-CSF]) is commonly used to accelerate the recovery of neutrophil counts, but should be initiated only with the recommendation of the pediatric oncologist. Coordination with the pediatric oncologist is important to ensure the most appropriate management.

Mucositis. Mouth sores are a common complication of cancer therapy. They may be a direct consequence of therapy or arise from an infection. Chemotherapy agents that commonly cause mucositis include anthracyclines (daunomycin and doxorubicin), methotrexate, and dactino-mycin (Actinomycin D). Herpes and yeast are common infectious causes of mouth sores. Patients with fever, uncontrolled pain, dysphagia, lethargy, signs of dehydration, or bleeding should be evaluated immediately. Treatment includes hydration, pain management, and evaluation and treatment of possible infections.

Abdominal Pain. The differential diagnosis of abdominal pain is vast. In the immunocompromised host it can represent serious, life-threatening pathology. Serious side effects of chemotherapy include esophagitis, gastritis, ulcers, pancreatitis, typhlitis, cholecystitis, hepatitis, intus-susception, ileus, small bowel obstruction, and kidney stones. Patients with severe diffuse or localized pain, fever, neutropenia, injury to the abdomen, bloody stools, or bilious emesis require immediate evaluation. Coordination with the pediatric oncologist is necessary to facilitate appropriate care.

Nausea and Vomiting. One of the common side effects of therapy is chemotherapy-induced nausea and vomiting. Patients who develop lethargy, bloody or bilious vomiting, or signs of dehydration require immediate evaluation. Treatment includes rehydration and the use of antiemetics. An evaluation to identify other sources of nausea and vomiting should be undertaken if emetogenic agents have not been recently used.

Health Care Maintenance. Maintaining adequate nutrition during chemotherapy is a significant challenge in children with cancer. Children receiving intensive chemotherapy regimens are frequently unable to maintain adequate caloric intake and often require either intravenous or enteral nutritional support. Malnutrition complicates healing, reduces the amount of chemotherapy that can be tolerated, and increases the risk of infections. If children undergoing chemotherapy show limited weight gain or weight loss, supplemental nutrition should be considered (see also Chapter 30).

Immunizations for children undergoing immunosup-pressive chemotherapy are generally not recommended. Live virus vaccines can be harmful and the effectiveness of other vaccines is limited in the immunocompromised cancer patient. Siblings of children with cancer can continue to receive their full complement of immunizations as recommended by the American Academy of Pediatrics with the exception of the live polio vaccine. Siblings should receive the inactivated polio vaccine. Siblings can be given the MMR and varicella vaccines because these vaccines are not transmitted after vaccination. Influenza vaccination is recommended for children undergoing cancer therapy and for other members of their households. Nonlive vaccines can be resumed 6 months after the completion of immuno-suppressive therapy, and live vaccines can be safely given 1 year after the completion of immunosuppressive therapy. Patients do not need to be revaccinated; they need to receive only the vaccines that were omitted during their cancer therapy.

Exposure to chickenpox requires special mention because primary infection in an immunocompromised host can lead to severe dissemination of the virus. An exposure is defined as close contact with someone who has unscabbed chickenpox lesions or who develops the illness within 48 hours after the contact. Children who are receiving chemotherapy or are less than 6 months from completing therapy need to have varicella zoster immune gobulin (VZIG) (125 units for every 10 kg with maximum of 625 units) if they have not previously had chickenpox or have not been previously immunized with the varicella vaccine. Additionally, steroids should be avoided during the 28-day potential incubation period. The family of children who have had a significant chickenpox exposure should be instructed to call immediately if the child develops signs or symptoms of chickenpox. The treatment of chickenpox infections in children with a compromised immune system requires parenteral antiviral therapy.

Regular dental care during chemotherapy may help prevent infection, but certain precautions must be taken. Routine dental care should be done only when the ANC is above 1000 and the platelet count is adequate (>100K). Any child with a central line or other hardware should receive bacterial endocarditis prophylaxis prior to oral manipulations including teeth cleaning. Oral amoxicillin (50 mg/kg with maximum of 2 g) 1 hour prior to the procedure is the standard regimen. Follow-up guidelines are available to help facilitate proper long-term care (www.survivorshipguidelines.org).

TREATMENT

Burkitt (Small Noncleaved Cell) Lymphomas

Tremendous progress has been made in the treatment of mature B-cell lymphomas over the past 50 years. Dr. Burkitt was the first to discover that children afflicted with the lymphoma that bears his name respond dramatically to chemotherapy. Over the past 5 decades, the treatment intensity has increased with a corresponding increase in cure.

Nearly all patients with stage 1 or resected abdominal stage 2 disease are cured with two cycles of multiagent chemotherapy that includes cyclophosphamide, vincristine, prednisone, and doxorubicin. Overall, patients with advanced Burkitt lymphoma have a greater than 80% chance of cure with aggressive therapy. Patients with the most aggressive disease, which includes patients with extensive bone marrow *and* CNS involvement, have a worse prognosis (30%). Aside from these patients, the morbidity and mortality associated with therapy equal the risk of relapse. Therefore, efforts are being made to reduce the intensity of therapy based on stage and response to therapy. Newer targeted therapies, such as Rituximab, are also being evaluated.

Lymphoblastic Lymphomas

Localized lymphoblastic lymphoma is relatively rare. Patients with localized lymphoblastic lymphoma are currently treated using a standard acute lymphoblastic leukemia protocol or with shorter and more intensive regimens, such as CHOP therapy, and have an excellent chance of cure (80% to 90%). Disseminated lymphoblastic lymphoma is treated similarly to high-risk acute lympho-blastic leukemia (ALL) (see Chapter 162). Treatment course generally lasts 2 years and uses intrathecal chemotherapy for CNS prophylaxis. Radiation is used emergently to relieve airway compromise, but it is not essential to treat the primary site. With aggressive therapy, patients with disseminated lymphoblastic lymphoma have an event-free survival rate of 70% to 80%.

Large Cell Lymphomas

Like the other NHLs, LCLs usually present with advanced stage (III or IV) disease. LCLs have a relatively good prognosis when treated with intensive multiagent chemotherapy. The treatment is less intensive than the treatment for Burkitt lymphoma and the duration (≈1 year) is shorter than that of lymphoblastic lymphoma treatment.

Hodgkin Disease

Treatment of Hodgkin disease is also stage dependent. Localized Hodgkin disease is treated with fewer cycles of chemotherapy with or without reduced dose irradiation. Patients with bulky mediastinal disease, defined by greater than one third the maximal diameter of the chest, generally require combined multiagent chemotherapy and radiation. Patients with advanced disease are treated with combination chemotherapy with or without radiation depending on growth status and gender. Commonly used treatment regimens include the combination of cyclophosphamide, vincristine, prednisone, and procarbazine or doxorubicin, vinblastine, bleomycin, and dacarbazine. More than 90% of all children and adolescents with newly diagnosed Hodgkin disease are cured with current therapy. Clinical trials are attempting to reduce late effects such as organ damage, secondary malignancies, and infertility.

Recurrent Lymphoma

The prognosis for patients with recurrent lymphoma is generally poor. Reinduction therapy depends on the timing of recurrence and prior therapy. Patients should be treated with alternative intensified chemotherapy and possible bone marrow transplantation.

OUTCOME

The treatment of Hodgkin disease and non-Hodgkin lymphoma is truly one of the success stories of modern medicine. With treatment based on type and staging, the vast majority of these patients are cured. When patients relapse, therapy is less effective despite intensification. With new insight into the biology of these cancers, other effective and directed therapies will become available.

Additional Resources, CD-ROM

Pathology of Lymphomas	Text

Mini-index of Related Topics

SUGGESTED READINGS

American Academy of Pediatrics: Guidelines for the pediatric cancer center and role of such centers in diagnosis and treatment. Pediatrics 1997;99:139–141.

Hudson MM, Donaldson SS: Treatment of pediatric Hodgkin's lymphoma. Semin Hematol 1999;36:313–323.

Hudson MM, Donaldson SS: Hodgkin's disease. In Pizzo PA, Poplack DG (eds): Principles and Practice of Pediatric Oncology, 4th ed. Philadelphia, Lippincott, 2001, pp 637–656.

Magrath IT: Malignant non-Hodgkin's lymphoma in children. In Pizzo PA, Poplack DG (eds): Principles and Practice of Pediatric Oncology, 4th ed. Philadelphia, Lippincott, 2001, pp 661–696.

National Cancer Institute. Available at: http://cancer.gov.

164 Solid Tumors of Infancy and Childhood

Lars M. Wagner

FUNDAMENTALS

Extracranial solid tumors account for approximately 40% of all childhood cancers. Because of the wide variety of tumors and presentations, the diagnosis of malignancy may be difficult to establish quickly. Difficulty in making a diagnosis is increased because cancer is rare in children. Symptoms of cancer are common ones that usually have benign, not malignant, causes. Generalists will see many more patients whose abdominal pain is caused by constipation rather than neuroblastoma. As with other disorders, a thorough history and meticulous physical examination are essential to identify patients who require further evaluation. The classic symptoms, physical findings, and ages of presentation of several common solid tumors are summarized in Table 164-1. Quick recognition of these presenting features by the primary care provider, followed by appropriate diagnostic testing, allows for timely referral to the oncologist and rapid initiation of treatment. Even though the oncologist determines the treatment plan, the generalist must provide easily accessible care and support for oncology patients throughout the course of their illnesses. The primary care provider is involved in both the initial diagnosis and long-term management of patients with childhood solid tumor.

NEUROBLASTOMA

Neuroblastoma is the most common type of cancer in infancy and is second only to brain tumors as the most common type of childhood solid tumor. Roughly 550 new cases of neuroblastoma are diagnosed annually in the United States. The median age at diagnosis is 22 months, and 75% of patients are diagnosed by 5 years of age. Primary tumors are most commonly found in the abdomen along the sympathetic chain ganglia, particularly in the adrenal gland. These tumors usually present as a firm, irregular, nontender abdominal mass. Another common location is the posterior mediastinum; a chest x-ray ordered for other reasons is often the route of discovery of the tumor in these patients. Findings at diagnosis may range from an asymptomatic abdominal mass in patients with localized disease to fever, pallor, and bone pain in children with widespread metastases.

The clinical course may vary widely between patients, ranging from spontaneous regression in patients younger than 1 year to progressive dissemination and resistance to therapy in older infants and children. By analyzing histologic and genetic factors, oncologists are now able to divide

Table 164-1. Classic Presenting Features of Common Childhood Solid Tumors

Tumor	Median Age at Diagnosis	Usual Presenting Symptoms
Neuroblastoma	22 months	Abdominal or mediastinal mass
Wilms tumor	3.5 (unilateral) 2.5 years (bilateral)	Abdominal mass or distension
Rhabdomyosarcoma	Usually <6 years Small peak in adolescents	Painless mass in head or neck Vagina, prostate, or bladder Extremity or paratesticular mass
Ewing sarcoma	Adolescents	Bone pain, soft tissue swelling, fever
Osteosarcoma	Adolescents	Extremity pain, soft tissue swelling
Retinoblastoma	2 years (unilateral) 8 months (bilateral)	Leukocoria, strabismus

patients into low-, intermediate-, and high-risk groups. Such distinctions allow for more appropriate tailoring of therapy and have reduced unnecessary toxicity for patients who require minimal treatment. Patients with low-risk disease are usually younger than 1 year of age and have localized disease that may be cured with surgery alone. Patients with intermediate-risk disease are typically older than 1 year and have more extensive abdominal disease that requires surgery and chemotherapy for successful treatment. Patients with high-risk disease are older than 1 year, have widespread metastases, and have DNA amplification of the N-*myc* oncogene, which portends a particularly poor prognosis despite aggressive therapy with autologous bone marrow transplantation.

WILMS TUMOR

Wilms tumor accounts for nearly all renal malignancies in childhood, and represents 5% to 6% of pediatric cancers. The typical age of presentation for unilateral tumors is approximately 3.5 years, which is slightly older than the median age at diagnosis for neuroblastoma. Approximately 5% of patients have bilateral tumors, and these are usually diagnosed earlier in life. Wilms tumors most commonly present with either abdominal swelling or the presence of an abdominal mass, which is frequently noted by parents while bathing or dressing the child. Abdominal pain, fever, hematuria, and hypertension may also be seen at presentation. Some patients develop anemia from hemorrhage into the tumor. Other associated physical findings include aniridia, partial or complete hemihypertrophy, and genitourinary abnormalities.

Wilms tumors typically arise as a solitary mass within the kidney, resulting in compression and distortion of remaining normal tissue. This intrarenal origin usually can be appreciated on imaging studies, and helps distinguish Wilms tumor from neuroblastoma. The primary care provider should promptly refer patients with such masses to a pediatric oncologist and/or surgeon, where further workup can determine the presence of pulmonary or hepatic metastases. For children with typical imaging findings of unilateral Wilms tumor, a nephrectomy with abdominal lymph node sampling is usually performed. This procedure confirms the diagnosis and stage, and provides local control of the tumor. After surgery, patients receive multiagent chemotherapy, and radiation for those with advanced stage disease. The most important prognostic factors are stage and histology; however, even patients with distant metastases may have long-term survival with appropriate therapy.

RHABDOMYOSARCOMA

Rhabdomyosarcoma arises from embryonic skeletal muscle and represents slightly more than half of all the soft tissue sarcomas seen in children. In children younger than 5 years, these tumors are usually found in the head and neck, prostate, bladder, and vagina. By contrast, teenagers frequently have tumors in the extremities or in paratesticular tissue. The most common presenting feature is a mass, which may cause pain or other local symptoms depending on the site.

When located in the extremities, the swelling may first be noticed after trauma and assumed to be a hematoma; however, as the mass continues to grow, a malignant process is eventually suspected. A properly performed surgical biopsy confirms the diagnosis and defines the histologic subtype. Care must be taken to distinguish rhabdomyosarcoma from other types of soft tissue sarcomas because the treatment and expected outcome may be quite different.

Prognosis is related to the site and histologic type of the primary tumor, presence of metastases, and ability to obtain good local control with surgery and/or radiation. Of patients with completely resectable tumors, 80% to 90% have long-term survival with treatment that includes surgery, chemotherapy, and often radiation. Young patients with periorbital tumors have a particularly high rate of cure. However, older children who have alveolar histology and disseminated disease in the lungs or bone marrow at diagnosis continue to have poor outcomes, with fewer than one third of these children having long-term survival.

BONE TUMORS

Osteosarcoma and Ewing sarcoma represent the two most common bone tumors in children. Both tumors occur most frequently in adolescence, although some patients with Ewing sarcoma may be quite young. There is a striking disparity among race in patients with Ewing sarcoma, with less than 2% of patients being black. While there is some overlap in primary site between these tumor types, osteosarcoma usually occurs in the extremities, particularly around the knee or shoulder. In contrast, Ewing sarcoma may involve the flat bones, often of the pelvis or ribs. Both tumors may have extensive soft tissue components, and some Ewing sarcomas arise exclusively from extraosseous tissue and not bone.

The main symptom for both tumors is pain at the primary site. Intermittent fevers are more commonly seen with Ewing sarcoma. Although there are radiographic features considered classic for each disease, not all tumors display these characteristics. The diagnosis is frequently confused with osteomyelitis, eosinophilic granuloma, or a benign bone cyst; therefore, a surgical biopsy properly performed by an experienced surgeon is necessary to confirm the diagnosis. Ewing sarcoma must be distinguished from other so-called "small round blue cell tumors of childhood," including neuroblastoma and non-Hodgkin lymphoma. Recent advances in cancer genetics have shown that both Ewing sarcomas and peripheral primitive neuroectodermal tumors (PNETs) are characterized by similar chromosomal translocations. While these tumors differ in the degree of histologic differentiation, their clinical behavior is similar; thus primitive neuroectodermal tumors are now classified together with Ewing sarcomas.

Treatment for these tumors always includes chemotherapy, which is necessary to treat the micrometastatic disease that is likely present in most patients at diagnosis. Ewing sarcoma is relatively sensitive to radiation therapy, and this modality can be used either with surgery or as an alternative to surgery to obtain local control of the tumor. Unfortunately, osteosarcoma rarely responds to radiation, and requires some type of surgical resection to be treated effectively. New techniques such as limb-sparing surgery can be offered to selected patients as an alternative to amputation.

The outcome for patients with these tumors depends primarily on the extent of disease at diagnosis and the ability to eradicate tumor at the primary site. Many patients with localized disease enjoy long-term survival, whereas the outcome remains poor for those with lung or bone marrow metastases at diagnosis.

RETINOBLASTOMA

Retinoblastoma is a congenital tumor of the eye that occurs almost exclusively during infancy. Unilateral tumors are usually discovered around age 2, whereas the 25% of patients with bilateral tumors are diagnosed at an average of 8 months of age. Leukocoria is the most common initial finding, although strabismus and other eye abnormalities may also occur. When primary care providers suspect this diagnosis, they should promptly refer patients to a pediatric ophthalmologist or oncologist. Because these tumors rarely metastasize, the main concern is the preservation of useful vision, particularly in patients with bilateral tumors. Treatment options depend on the size and location of the tumor(s), and range from radiation, cryotherapy, and photocoagulation to enucleation. In some clinical trials, patients with extraocular metastases have received chemotherapy, but it is not routine treatment for patients with localized disease. Long-term survival after retinoblastoma is excellent for patients with localized tumors, but remains poor for the less than 10% of patients with extraglobal extension at the time of diagnosis.

The genetic changes seen with retinoblastoma have been well characterized, and serve as an excellent model of a tumor suppressor gene (i.e., a gene whose loss or mutation allows for the development of a malignancy). For all patients with bilateral tumors and for 15% of patients with unilateral tumors, the retinoblastoma gene is mutated or deleted. This change predisposes these patients not only to retinoblastoma, but also to the development of osteosarcoma later in life. Every patient with retinoblastoma should receive thorough genetic analysis and counseling.

DIAGNOSIS OF SOLID TUMORS

A significant number of malignancies may be first identified by primary care providers performing routine examinations. Even when the chief complaint involves a different organ system, careful palpation of the abdomen should be a routine part of the office visit, especially with young children. Most experienced clinicians can recall cases of Wilms tumor or other malignancies discovered in such an incidental fashion.

When a mass is suspected or found on physical examination, further evaluation with imaging studies are indicated. Physicians need to appreciate the strengths and weaknesses of various imaging modalities, and to approach the workup of patients with masses in a systematic fashion. Suggested diagnostic approaches to children who present with signs or symptoms of solid tumors are discussed in the following sections.

Abdominal Masses

Signs and Symptoms. A palpable abdominal mass is the most common presentation of malignant solid tumors in childhood. Although there are some benign causes of abdominal masses such as renal cysts or constipation, all masses should be investigated to ensure that a malignancy is not missed. The evaluation begins with a thorough history, particularly focusing on urinary and gastrointestinal symptoms (Box 164-1). The physical examination may be quite challenging in children who are young or in pain; accordingly, every effort should be made to relax or distract the patient in order to achieve an adequate examination. For masses suspected to be stool or bladder, a repeat examination after defecation or voiding is essential. A rectal examination often gives important information in identifying pelvic masses.

Evaluation. Imaging studies are indicated for any child with a suspicious abdominal mass, regardless of its size, consistency, or mobility. The first study is often a radiograph of the abdomen in two views, which can easily identify masses caused by fecal impaction and constipation. Plain films can also identify calcified masses in the adrenal gland, a common finding with neuroblastoma. If the plain film is not informative, an ultrasound or computed tomography (CT) scan of the abdomen should be obtained. Ultrasonography is attractive because it is noninvasive, does not expose the patient to ionizing radiation or contrast, and can often be done the same day with no patient preparation. In most instances, ultrasound can quickly identify the presence or absence of a mass, suggest its likely origin, and provide descriptive information such as whether the mass is cystic, solid, or mixed. If a suspicious mass is identified on ultrasound, particularly if it is a solid mass, then further anatomic information should be obtained with either CT or magnetic resonance imaging (MRI). However, coordination of these studies is best done in consultation with a pediatric oncologist and/or surgeon, as many CT or MRI studies done at community hospitals are repeated once a patient arrives at a tertiary care center. A sequence of suggested steps in the evaluation of an abdominal mass is listed in Box 164-2.

Other important aspects of the diagnostic workup of abdominal masses include a urinalysis and urine culture, serum blood urea nitrogen (BUN) and creatinine measurements, and a complete blood count. An elevated serum lactate dehydrogenase (LDH) level may be helpful in identifying states of rapid cell turnover, as is often seen at diagnosis in patients with advanced solid tumors. Measurement of specific tumor markers may be helpful in

---

Box 164-1. Important Symptoms in Children with Abdominal Masses

Abdominal pain (location, characterization, chronicity, relieving factors)
Vomiting
Change in stool consistency or color
Recent changes in weight
Changes in urination (frequency, dysuria, hematuria)
History of urinary tract infections

certain circumstances. If neuroblastoma is suspected because of the young age of the patient or the presence of calcification on imaging, urine should be sent for the catecholamine metabolites homovanillic acid (HVA) and vanillymandelic acid (VMA), which are elevated in up to 90% of cases. For testicular or pelvic masses, or when teratomatous features are seen on imaging, elevated serum levels of α-fetoprotein (AFP) and β-hCG may help diagnose germ cell tumors. Finally, children with masses arising from the liver should have measurement of the α-fetoprotein, which is elevated in 90% of hepatoblastomas and 50% of hepatocellular carcinomas.

Mediastinal Masses

Signs and Symptoms. While many mediastinal masses cause respiratory symptoms such as chest pain, cough, or shortness of breath, even sizable masses are sometimes completely asymptomatic. Occasionally, there may be swelling of the face or upper extremities caused by compression of the superior vena cava.

Evaluation. Prompt consultation with a pediatric oncologist is indicated for any patient with a mediastinal mass. Chest x-ray findings of a mediastinal mass require careful clinical assessment of the respiratory status in an attempt to identify patients with impending airway compromise. Special attention should be given to patients who have tachypnea or hypoxia at rest, or who are uncomfortable laying supine. Most malignant mediastinal masses in children involve the anterior or middle mediastinum, and are caused by non-Hodgkin lymphoma, Hodgkin disease, or leukemia, particularly T-cell acute lymphoblastic leukemia (ALL) in teenagers. Posterior mediastinal masses are less common. Occasionally, they are incidentally discovered in young children, which is a presentation and location that is classic for neuroblastoma. Such tumors may be associated with Horner syndrome (characterized by unilateral ptosis, miosis, and absence of facial sweating).

Box 164-3 details several steps to be taken after a mediastinal mass is identified. Laboratory tests important in the assessment of anterior or middle mediastinal masses include a complete blood count with differential and lactate dehydrogenase, serum electrolyte, and uric acid levels. Patients with rapidly growing tumors such as non-Hodgkin lymphoma may have tumor lysis syndrome prior to starting

therapy, and early identification of this problem allows for appropriate intervention. Imaging with CT can help define the nature of mediastinal masses, assess airway impingement, and identify pleural effusions that could be tapped for diagnostic or therapeutic purposes. For posterior mediastinal masses, MRI may help define the relationship of the mass to the vertebral column and spinal cord.

Extremity Pain or Masses

Signs and Symptoms. Most extremity pain in children is caused by known trauma and resolves in a relatively short time. Also common are the so-called "growing pains" in which well children ranging from preschoolers to early adolescents have bilateral lower extremity pain that characteristically occurs at night before falling asleep. Symptoms that indicate a diagnosis other than "growing pains" are unilateral pain, pain that awakens a child late at night, or pain that limits activity the next morning.

Evaluation. Any child with persistent bone pain should be evaluated with radiography, particularly if the pain is out of proportion to the injury or is associated with a mass or limitation of range of motion. If plain films are suggestive of a malignancy, a pediatric oncologist and/or surgeon must be quickly involved to coordinate further diagnostic imaging studies (usually MRI) and arrange for biopsy. Because of the variety and overlap in imaging appearances of musculoskeletal lesions, a biopsy is always necessary for evaluating these patients. Proper biopsy location and technique are crucial and should be performed by a physician experienced with pediatric malignancies; improperly performed biopsies may not be informative and may compromise further efforts at surgical resection.

Bone metastases from neuroblastoma or large cell lymphoma can also present with a radiographic and clinical appearance similar to primary bone tumors, underlying the importance of a careful workup and biopsy. Because metastatic involvement of the bone marrow by neuroblastoma or leukemia can certainly cause significant hip or leg pain, a complete blood count is essential in evaluating such problems.

Eye Abnormalities

Signs and Symptoms. Leukocoria, defined as a whitish appearance to the pupil, is usually the first finding noticed with retinoblastoma. Leukocoria is seen when a large intraocular tumor causes total retinal detachment, and the retrolental mass becomes visible through the pupil. Other eye abnormalities found with retinoblastoma include strabismus, orbital inflammation, hyphema, fixed pupil, and heterochromia iridis. These may appear in isolation or in combination with leukocoria. Visual loss is an infrequent complaint because these patients are very young and unable to describe unilateral decreased vision. However, parents may report asymmetry or absence of the red reflex noted in family photographs. The primary care physician is crucial in the early recognition of retinoblastoma, as many of the above initial abnormalities can be picked up during well-child examinations in the first 2 years of life.

Evaluation. Any patient with a suspected retinoblastoma should be promptly evaluated by a pediatric ophthalmologist who has experience in the management of this problem. Ultrasonography of the eye and either CT or MRI of the brain and orbits are often performed to confirm the diagnosis and define the extent of involvement.

THERAPY

The usual treatment for most pediatric solid tumors combines the modalities of surgery, radiation, and chemotherapy. Almost all solid tumors require a biopsy to confirm diagnosis and obtain tissue for prognostic information such as histologic typing or N-*myc* gene amplification. For some tumors, such as Wilms tumors, complete resection is attempted prior to starting other therapies. For other tumors, such as Ewing sarcoma and osteosarcoma, chemotherapy is offered first in hopes of shrinking the tumor and making surgical resection more feasible and less morbid. New surgical techniques such as limb-sparing procedures have given many patients with extremity bone tumors an alternative to amputation.

Radiation therapy is used for many solid malignancies as another way to achieve local control of the primary tumor. A notable exception to this is osteosarcoma, which is relatively radioresistant. Radiation is often incorporated after surgical resection of bulky disease, and may be given in conjunction with chemotherapy. Long-term effects of radiation include growth and functional abnormalities, as well as the risk of second malignancies within the radiation field.

Solid tumor patients treated with chemotherapy invariably receive multiple agents, in order to overcome existing resistance and to prevent the development of acquired resistance. Table 164-2 lists the five most common types of chemotherapy given to children with solid tumors, and describes side effects that deserve special attention. All agents listed cause hair loss, and all except vincristine have been associated with varying degrees of nausea and blood count suppression, with the attendant risks of infection and bleeding. While many of these agents are best given in the oncology clinic or as an inpatient, vincristine can easily be given by intravenous push in the primary care provider's office. Any time vincristine is given through a peripheral vein and not a central venous line, care must be taken that the medicine does not extravasate into the skin, as it can be a dangerous vesicant. If this complication is suspected, the oncologist should be contacted at once to help with management.

OUTCOME

Survival following treatment of pediatric solid tumors has improved tremendously over the decades. For many patients with localized solid tumors and favorable histologic features, the chance of long-term survival is 70% or higher. The prognosis is particularly good for most children with retinoblastoma, Wilms tumor, and periorbital rhabdomyosarcoma. However, patients with solid tumors who have distant metastatic disease at diagnosis continue to fair poorly, with long-term survival rates of 30% or less. Notable exceptions to this are patients with Wilms tumor, a disease in which even stage IV patients with favorable histology have estimated survival rates of up to 80%. Similarly, children under 1 year of age with stage 4S neuroblastoma have an excellent prognosis even with little or no therapy. It should be noted that the factors cited here are dramatically simplified and may be influenced by other clinical and pathologic factors.

COORDINATION OF CARE WITH THE ONCOLOGIST

As the majority of patient care continues to shift from the inpatient to the outpatient setting, primary care providers assume an increasingly important role in caring for oncology patients, particularly in less populated areas. The benefits of familiarity and convenience that the generalist provides are often greatly appreciated by patients and their families,

Table 164-2. Commonly Used Chemotherapy Agents for Children with Solid Tumors

Class of Agents	Examples	Other Names	Special Toxicities or Concerns*
Vinca alkaloids	Vincristine	Oncovin	Neuropathic pain and neuropathies Constipation Vesicant if extravasated
Epidophyllotoxins	Etoposide	VP-16, VePesid	Secondary leukemia
Anthracyclines	Doxorubicin	Adriamycin	Acute or chronic heart failure Vesicant if extravasated Mucositis
Alkylating agents	Cyclophosphamide, ifosfamide	Cytoxan, Ifex	Hemorrhagic cystitis, infertility Secondary leukemia
Platinum agents	Carboplatin, cisplatin	Paraplavin, CDDP	Nephrotoxicity Hearing loss

*In addition to the common toxicities of nausea and blood count suppression seen with all of the above agents except vincristine.

who frequently spend long periods of time away from home at tertiary care centers. The primary care provider, in coordination with the oncologist, can play a pivotal role in obtaining laboratory tests, administering medicines, and evaluating patients for common complaints such as fever.

Chemotherapy for solid tumors is often administered over 1 to 5 days, followed by a rest period of up to 3 weeks to allow for blood count recovery. During this rest period, patients receiving intensive chemotherapy are often placed on granulocyte-colony stimulating factor (G-CSF, Neupogen), which is a recombinant human cytokine that stimulates proliferation and maturation of myeloid progenitor cells. This drug is usually given subcutaneously by the parents each day until the absolute neutrophil count has sufficiently recovered to at least $1000/\mu L$ following its chemotherapy-induced nadir. When patients are receiving granulocyte-colony stimulating factor, blood counts are routinely checked twice a week, and the primary care provider can advise when this medication can be stopped. Also during this time patients may have anemia and/or thrombocytopenia that necessitates transfusion; primary care providers are strongly encouraged to consult with an oncologist prior to arranging for this, as oncology patients require blood products that have been irradiated and leukofiltered.

For some patients with solid tumors, chemotherapy results in loss of potassium, magnesium, phosphate, and bicarbonate in the urine. This condition, termed Fanconi syndrome, is usually treated with oral supplementation of the appropriate electrolytes. For those patients unable to take oral supplements, or who have renal insufficiency and require daily home intravenous fluids, these supplements can be given intravenously. The primary care provider can help arrange for routine measurements of serum electrolytes and help modify supplementation in conjunction with the oncologist.

Fever is a common occurrence in patients with solid tumors, and may result from various causes. Patients who develop fever while on therapy should be seen promptly by a physician; often, it is the primary care provider who sees the patient first and does the initial assessment. Any oncology patient being evaluated for a new fever should have the absolute neutrophil count (ANC) determined, as patients with fever higher than 100.3°F and absolute neutrophil count less than $500/\mu L$ are routinely hospitalized for broad-spectrum antibiotics and observation. Because of the significant risk of bacteremia, especially in patients with central venous lines, blood cultures should also be part of the routine evaluation of febrile oncology patients.

CONCLUSION

The common solid tumors of childhood often have predictable presenting symptoms and physical findings that the alert primary care provider can readily identify. Prompt recognition of tumors and early consultation with a pediatric oncologist may help children be able to start treatment before metastases develop. Most children with localized solid tumors can be effectively treated with current therapeutic regimens. Even after diagnosis, the primary care provider can play an integral role in delivering care to children both during and after therapy.

SUGGESTED READINGS

Coffin CM, Dehner LP, O'Shea PA: Pediatric Soft Tissue Tumors. Baltimore, Williams & Wilkins, 1997.

Crist WM, Kun LE: Common solid tumors of childhhod. N Engl J Med 1991;324:461–471.

Lanzkowsky P: Manual of Pediatric Hematology and Oncology, 3rd ed. San Diego, Calif, Academic Press, 1999.

National Children's Cancer Fund, an organization providing information to parents and physicians website. Available at: http://www.nccf.org.

Pizzo PA, Poplack DG: Principles and Practice of Pediatric Oncology, 3rd ed. Philadelphia, Lippincott-Raven, 1997.

165 Brain Tumors

Diane Puccetti

ROLE OF THE GENERALIST

1   Recognize genetic conditions that predispose a child to developing a central nervous system (CNS) tumor.

2   Recognize the common signs and symptoms present in a child with a brain tumor.

3   Promptly and accurately evaluate a child with a suspected CNS lesion.

4   Refer the child to the appropriate specialist for diagnostic procedures and initiation of treatment.

5   Understand the multiple modalities of treatment for children with CNS tumors, which vary with the age of the child, location of tumor, and histology of the lesion.

6   Provide ongoing primary care, acute care, and health maintenance.

7   Assist the family in coping with the diagnosis and the long-term sequelae associated with the treatment.

Tumors of the nervous system are the most common solid tumors in childhood, and now surpass acute lymphoblastic leukemia as the most common type of childhood malignancy. These primary CNS lesions occur in 2.5 to 4 per 100,000 children at risk per year. Childhood brain tumors are the leading cause of cancer-related morbidity and mortality. The proportion of cancer deaths from CNS tumors has nearly doubled during the past 25 years. Approximately 30,000 to 40,000 children develop CNS tumors each year throughout the world with about 2200 children diagnosed per year in the United States. The majority of these childhood brain tumors are primary CNS lesions. They differ significantly from those arising in adults in their incidence, location, histology, and response to treatment.

FUNDAMENTALS

The majority of children diagnosed with brain tumors have no specific risk factors. There are several genetic disorders, including neurofibromatosis type I, tuberous sclerosis, and Li-Fraumeni syndrome, that place those affected at a higher risk of developing a central nervous tumor, but these account for a minority of newly diagnosed children. Therapeutic irradiation to the head is another known but uncommon risk factor. The genetics of childhood brain tumors and nonrandom chromosomal deletions have

implicated tumor suppression genes in tumorgenesis in some histologies, such as frequent loss or deletions of chromosomes 10q, 11, and 17p in medulloblastoma and loss of 22q 11.2 in atypical teratoid/rhabdoid tumors.

The peak incidence of childhood CNS tumors occurs in children younger than 5 years of age. The overall incidence is inversely proportional to age and the condition occurs in boys more than girls by a ratio of 55% to 45%. A little more than half of the CNS malignancies are astrocytomas, about 20% are primitive neuroectodermal tumors (PNETs), approximately 20% are other gliomas, and about 10% are ependymomas. The incidence of astrocytomas remains relatively independent of age, while PNETs, ependymoma, and other glioma each have an inverse relationship to age.

For children younger than 10 years of age, the cerebellum is the most common site of malignancy within the CNS. The cerebrum and the brainstem account for the second and third most common sites with near equal frequency. In children 10 years and older, the incidence of cerebral malignancies increases (the cerebrum is the most common location in adults) and the incidence of malignancies in the cerebellum and brainstem decreases.

PRESENTATION AND INITIAL EVALUATION

The presenting signs and symptoms of a child with a brain tumor are variable and dependent on the age, the developmental level, and the site of origin of the mass (Table 165-1). Presenting signs and symptoms include evidence of increased intracranial pressure (ICP) and/or focal neurologic signs. The classic triad of increased ICP is morning headaches, vomiting, and lethargy. Acute onset and rapid progression is not a frequent occurrence, but must be evaluated immediately. Subacute signs of increased ICP are more commonly seen and include fatigue, personality changes, academic problems in school, and vague intermittent headaches in school-age children. Children in the first few years of life will experience irritability, anorexia, developmental delay, and regression of intellectual and motor abilities. Because chronically increased pressure may result in macrocephaly in younger children, surveillance of head circumference is important.

A history of progressive headache especially when associated with vomiting or ataxia requires a full evaluation. A complete history is essential, with particular attention to details regarding the headache such as type of pain, location, presence upon waking, pattern of increasing

Table 165-1. Signs and Symptoms of Brain Tumors by Age and Location

Signs and Symptoms by Age	
Older Children	**Infants/Toddlers**
Declining school performance	Irritability
Personality change	Anorexia
Intermittent headache	Developmental delay/regression
	Increasing head circumference

Signs and Symptoms by Location	
Infratentorial	**Supratentorial**
Ataxia	Headache
Facial weakness	Seizure
Hearing loss	Hemiparesis
Cranial nerve deficit(s)	Hyperflexia
Headache	Behavior problems
	Nystagmus
	Visual symptoms

frequency, and/or severity of pain. Other key information includes presence of vomiting (especially without nausea), blurred or double vision, balance problems, weakness, academic problems, or behavioral changes. Infants' and toddlers' symptoms are less specific and include irritability, vomiting, anorexia, and loss of developmental milestones.

The physical examination should include assessment of vital signs and measurement of head circumference in young children. The skin should be examined for neurocutaneous lesions, such as café au lait spots (neurofibromatosis, see Fig. 74-5) or hypopigmented nevi (tuberous sclerosis, see Fig. 74-14). The fundi should be evaluated for presence of papilledema (Fig. 165-1), passive swelling of the optic disk caused by increased ICP. The cranial nerves should be tested. A cranial nerve VI palsy either unilateral or bilateral is a sign of ICP. Evidence of visual field cuts, presence of nystagmus, or a gaze palsy require further evaluation. Assessments of strength, tone, reflexes, and

balance, including finger-to-nose testing as well as gait, complete the examination.

The most common presenting signs and symptoms of brainstem and cerebellar tumors are balance problems, cranial nerve dysfunction, truncal unsteadiness, and symptoms of increased ICP. The most common symptom of cerebral tumors is headache, with seizures the second most common symptom of a mass lesion in this area. Hemiparesis, clonus, and hyperreflexia may also be present. Change in visual acuity or evidence of pituitary dysfunction implies a lesion in the visual pathway or other midline structures.

A child with a worrisome history plus any physical findings compatible with evidence of ICP should undergo an immediate assessment and simultaneous referral to a pediatric oncologist, pediatric neurosurgeon, or pediatric neurologist. Radiographic evaluation should include a computed tomography (CT) scan of the head for rapid investigation of possible mass lesion with hydrocephalus (especially for a child who is medically unstable) and magnetic resonance imaging (MRI) may be indicated for better delineation and for purposes of surgical planning. For the child with a presumed CNS lesion who is medically stable, MRI of the head with and without contrast is the radiologic study that best evaluates the posterior fossa and the brainstem. Referral to a specialist can occur after a positive scan.

Table 165-2 compares CT and MRI scanning for evaluation of brain tumors. The CT scan when performed with and without contrast medium can detect about 95% of CNS tumors. MRI is an important diagnostic tool with a greater sensitivity in detecting infiltrating lesions, there is no bone artifact as with CT scan, and it is superior at detecting leptomeningeal spread of some tumors. Positron emission tomography (PET) provides metabolic images of the brain. This is useful in distinguishing radionecrosis from recurrent or residual tumor. MRI spectroscopy, which is currently under study, is another noninvasive method for monitoring tumor metabolism.

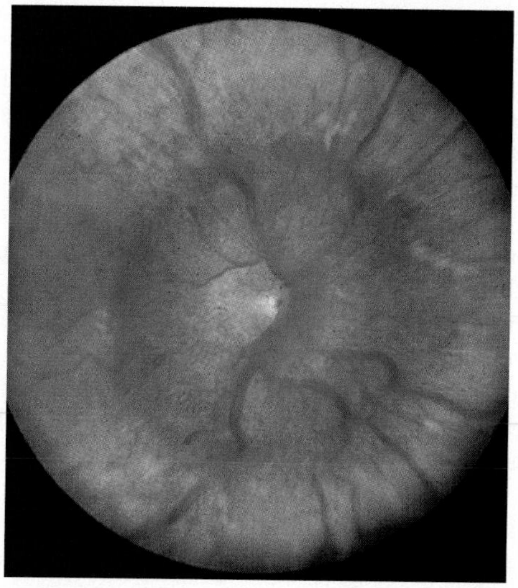

Figure 165-1. Acute papilledema, characterized by blurred disk edges, an absent physiologic cup, and intraretinal exudates. (From Zitelli BJ, Davis HW: Atlas of Pediatric Physical Diagnosis. St. Louis, Mosby, 1997.)

Table 165-2. Neuroimaging Modalities

Computerized Tomography Performed with and without Contrast	
Advantages	**Disadvantages**
Can detect 95% of CNS tumors	Radiation exposure
Duration 10 to 20 minutes	May miss early tumors, primarily low-grade glial lesions
Does not usually require sedation	Bone artifacts
Less costly	

Magnetic Resonance Imaging Performed with and without Contrast	
Advantages	**Disadvantages**
Greater sensitivity in detecting tumors	May be difficult to distinguish tumor from infiltrating lesions, edema, or scar
No bone artifact	Sensitive to movement artifact
Better visualization of the brainstem	Longer scanning time
Can detect leptomeningeal disease	Sedation may be required
	More costly

MANAGEMENT

The role of the generalist in the acute management of brain tumors is to provide emergency care for patients who present with life-threatening increased ICP and to refer them to appropriate specialists. Acute management of life-threatening ICP includes initiation of dexamethasone (0.5 to 1 mg/kg for the first dose and then 0.25 to 0.5 mg/kg/day divided into 4 daily doses) to decrease preoperative peritumoral edema. If seizures have occurred, if the lesion is in an epileptogenic area, or if the surgical approach is likely to cause seizures, an anticonvulsant such as sodium phenytoin should be administered.

Initial treatment for those who present without life-threatening ICP is urgent. If the child is medically stable and has evidence of a brain lesion on scans, a prompt consultation with a specialist should occur. The initial discussion with the pediatric specialist should include a description of the child's symptoms and physical findings, and the radiographic findings including any evidence of midline shift, edema, or hydrocephalus. This information will be useful in determining the medical urgency of the situation. For the specialist's evaluation of the child, the primary care provider should provide radiographic studies and copies of pertinent medical records (including growth charts).

Role of the Pediatric Neurosurgeon

Surgical intervention is the primary treatment for all newly diagnosed brain tumors and should ideally be performed by a pediatric neurosurgeon who devotes the majority of his or her practice to children. If hydrocephalus is present, the clinical severity and likelihood that tumor resection will remove the obstruction determine whether treatment is necessary. A cerebrospinal fluid (CSF) diversion procedure should be performed if the child's level of consciousness is depressed. Placement of an external ventricular drain will allow temporary diversion of CSF flow until tumor removal re-establishes CSF flow. Less than one third of children with tumors located in the midline posterior fossa require a permanent shunt postoperatively. Because intra-axial surgery for tumors outside the posterior fossa does not usually re-establish CSF flow when the tumor location is midline, hydrocephalus is treated with either a CSF shunt or an endoscopic third ventriculostomy.

Nearly every child with a brain tumor undergoes a biopsy, either open or stereotactic (for deep lesions in eloquent areas of the brain or tumors for which resection is not feasible), with the following exceptions: diffuse brain stem tumors and chiasmal gliomas. The latter tumors have characteristic MRI features, and biopsy results rarely influence treatment.

Extent of tumor resection correlates with survival rate for the following tumors: malignant astrocytomas, cerebral PNETs, and medulloblastoma, with total or near-total resection affording a longer survival. This correlation is not as clear-cut for low-grade gliomas, and an increased morbidity is possible with overly aggressive resection.

Role of Chemotherapy in Treatment of Central Nervous System Tumors

Chemotherapy has been the newest weapon utilized in the battle against childhood CNS tumors. Previously, the erroneous belief that the blood-brain barrier (BBB) prevented any penetration of chemotherapy into the CNS and the historical dismal prognosis for childhood brain tumors dampened any enthusiasm for adding chemotherapy to treat these disorders. Because research over the past 2 to 3 decades has supported the efficacy of chemotherapy, it has become an important therapeutic tool. While the BBB limits penetration to compounds that have a small molecular weight, are un-ionized, and are highly lipophilic, the BBB is not uniformly intact in CNS tumors, as evidenced by the variable amount of enhancement produced by the water-soluble contrast agents used in neuroimaging in CNS tumors. These areas of BBB disruption are commonly seen in the central portions of most tumors, while the BBB is more intact in the tumor periphery.

Chemotherapy has had the biggest impact in the treatment of medulloblastoma, which was previously treated with surgery and radiation therapy alone. Chemotherapy is now the standard of care for all children diagnosed with this type of CNS tumor. Chemotherapy has also been used to replace or decrease the dose of radiation therapy needed to cure certain CNS tumors. Decisions regarding chemotherapy are made using the same considerations for radiation therapy: tumor type and location, amount of residual tumor after surgery, metastatic potential, and age of the child. A list of common agents, their main side effects, and adverse drug interactions are listed in Table 165-3.

Stem cell rescue, utilizing high-dose chemotherapy, is another potential treatment for a select group of patients. This procedure is specifically used in younger patients with high-risk malignant tumor types or patients with recurrence after conventional therapies.

Role of Radiation Therapy

Radiotherapy has been a mainstay of treatment for children with brain tumors for decades. For tumors that have a propensity to spread throughout the CSF pathways, the target volume is the whole brain and the craniospinal axis, while localized tumors that do not share that propensity are more focally targeted. The decision to include radiotherapy as a treatment modality takes into consideration the following factors: tumor type and location, amount of resection, metastatic potential of the tumor, and the age of the child. To lessen or avoid altogether the deleterious cognitive sequelae that occur after irradiation of the supratentorial region, especially in young children, chemotherapy is used instead of or to decrease the amount of radiation therapy. Whether maintaining previous survival rates is possible without radiation is an ongoing area of study.

Radiotherapy advances have improved the ability to deliver this modality with greater precision, thereby diminishing the effects on the surrounding normal brain tissue. These techniques coupled with improvements in neuroimaging have lead to more targeted treatment. The acute and late complications of radiation therapy are listed in Table 165-4.

The Role of the Generalist

As with all children who are being managed by a health care team, the family should understand whom they should call for medical problems. The generalist, as the primary care provider, must recognize medical and surgical emergencies and refer patients to the appropriate specialists as needed.

Table 165-3. Chemotherapy Agents Used in Treating CNS Tumors

Common Agents	Side Effects	Adverse Drug Interaction
Vincristine	Peripheral neuropathy, constipation	Intraconazole, Zidovudine
Cisplatin	Hearing loss, nephrotoxicity, electrolyte imbalance	Phenytoin, carbamazepine, nephrotoxic drugs
Carboplatin	Myelosuppression, allergic reaction	Phenytoin
Cysclophosphamide	Myelosuppression, hemorrhagic cystitis	Allopurinol, digoxin, succinylcholine
CCNU	Myelosuppression, pulmonary fibrosis	Cimetidine
Etoposide	Myelosuppression, hypotension, secondary malignancy	Warfarin, cyclosporine
Procarbazine	Myelosuppression, nausea/vomiting, tremors, seizures	MAOI drugs, carbamazepine, phenobarbital
BCNU	Myelosuppression, nausea/vomiting, pulmonary fibrosis	Phenytoin, cimetidine
Ifosamide	Myelosuppression, nausea/vomiting, nephrotoxicity	Warfarin
Agents Currently under Investigation		
Irinotecan	Myelosuppression, diarrhea, nausea/vomiting	Dexamethasone
Topotecan	Myelosuppression, diarrhea, nausea/vomiting	
Methotrexate	Myelosuppression, renal/hepatic toxicity, nausea/vomiting	NSAIDs or salicylates, amoxicillin/penicillin, TMP-sulfa, doxyclycline, cyclosporine, phenytoin, thiazide diuretics, omeprazole, theophylline
Temozolomide	Nausea, vomiting, fatigue, myelosuppression	Valproic acid
Mafosfamide	Myelosuppression, hemorrhagic cystitis	

The generalist should also coordinate ongoing care, monitor patients for complications of the disease and adverse side effects to medication, provide health maintenance, and treat common acute illnesses.

A child with a CNS tumor who develops signs and symptoms of increased ICP, or new/worsening neurologic deficits should have an immediate evaluation by a specialist who, guided by the history and examination, can order the appropriate radiologic studies. If the symptoms are compatible with increased ICP, a CT scan of the brain (without contrast) can assess ventricular size to rule out obstructive hydrocephalus. If the child has a ventricular peritoneal shunt and CT evidence of enlarging ventricle, consultation with a pediatric neurosurgeon is indicated. The neurosurgeon is likely to order further radiologic studies to assess the integrity of the shunt (shunt series obtained by plain film). The surgeon may perform a percutaneous tap of the shunt reservoir to ascertain the CSF pressure. Dependent on the findings, a MRI of the brain may be necessary to assess the status of the tumor. Reinstitution of dexamethasone may be necessary if there is increased ICP, increased edema from the tumor, or treatment-associated radiation necrosis.

The primary care provider should manage acute illnesses in concert with the specialist, particularly for the child receiving chemotherapy, given the serious nature of infections in the potentially neutropenic child and the need for rapid initiation of broad-spectrum antibiotics in this scenario. Table 165-3 lists the common side effects and potentially harmful drug interactions of commonly used chemotherapeutic agents. Children undergoing chemotherapy may be taking other medications for supportive care, such as TMP-sulfa (trimethoprim/sulfamethoxazole) for pneumocystic prophylaxis, fungal therapy, and anticonvulsants in some instances.

Children with CNS tumors may suffer long-term effects as a result of the very treatment that cured their tumor. The CNS lesion and/or the therapy given including radiation therapy, surgery, and chemotherapy all lend themselves to the development of long-term sequelae, accounting for a high likelihood of morbidity (see Chapter 166). These may include cognitive problems, endocrine dysfunction, vision and hearing loss, psychosocial difficulties, and the risk of a second treatment-related malignancy.

OUTCOME

Treatment is dependent on the child's age, tumor location, and histology of the tumor. Prognostic variables include age at diagnosis, tumor location, absence or presence of metastatic disease, amount of postoperative residual tumor, and histology.

While the overall cure rate for childhood cancer has been steadily increasing with cure rates approaching 80%, the population of patients enduring childhood brain tumors lags behind with an overall survival of 67%. Within this group of children, there is a diverse prognostic range from less than 10% to more than 90%. Even comparing a group of children with the same histological tumor type yields a diverse prognosis.

Several prognostic variables can more accurately predict an individual's chance of cure. Younger children, especially those under 3 years of age, have poorer outcomes. The presence of metastatic disease, residual postoperative tumor, and certain histologic subtypes are also indicators of a poorer prognosis.

The details of treatment specifically recommended for common childhood brain tumors and the associated prognosis are included on the CD-ROM.

Table 165-4. Radiation Therapy

Acute Side Effects

Erythema, nausea and vomiting, mucositis, diarrhea, alopecia, somnolence syndrome

Long-term Side Effects

Growth hormone deficiency, thyroid or gonadal dysfunction, secondary malignancy, cognitive sequelae, alopecia, spinal growth deficiency, radiation necrosis, vasculopathy

FOLLOW-UP

Comprehensive follow-up is essential for monitoring the child for possible relapse and accurately identifying any long-term effects of therapy. The primary care provider must address both of these issues and provide appropriate care.

Surveillance radiologic studies are necessary for early detection of recurrent tumor. Asymptomatic recurrences may have a better prognosis because good surgical resection is an important prognostic factor. A thorough clinical history and neurologic examination in addition to the radiographic studies provide an accurate assessment of the child's condition.

The primary care provider must carefully monitor the child's growth, endocrine system, vision and hearing, and in a subgroup of children the cardiac and pulmonary systems. Thorough assessment of the child's emotional well-being and school performance is also necessary. Neuropsychological testing should be considered the standard of care for children who have a history of hydrocephalus, previous exposure to methotrexate, or irradiation to the whole brain, supratentorium, or posterior fossa that may scatter to the temporal lobes. Children who are not in one of these categories but who are struggling with school performance also benefit from a neuropsychological assessment.

Just as the optimum treatment strategy for a child with a brain tumor requires the coordination of many specialists, the ongoing management and follow-up should be an integrated, multidisciplinary approach. Many centers have established pediatric brain tumor clinics for this very reason. Childhood brain tumor survivors deserve individuals advocating on their behalf as they make the transition back into society.

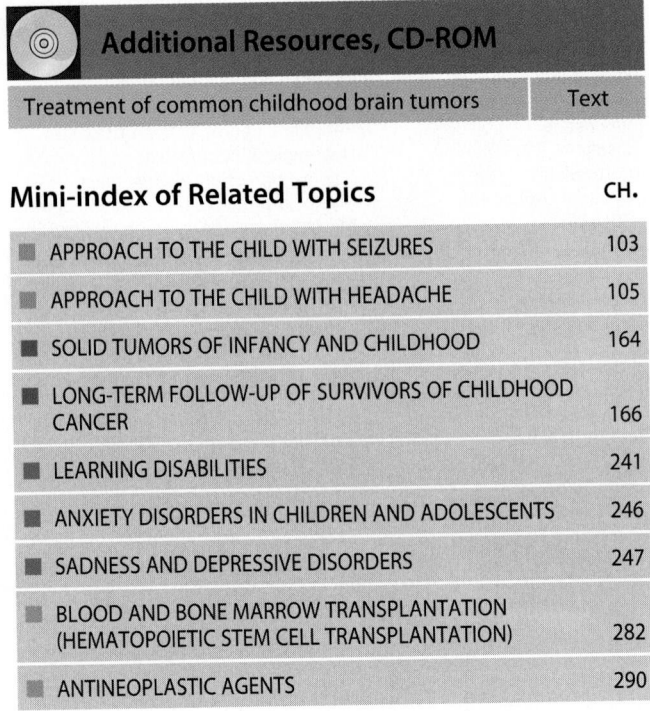

Additional Resources, CD-ROM

Treatment of common childhood brain tumors	Text

Mini-index of Related Topics

SUGGESTED READINGS

Bleyer WA: Epidemiologic impact of children with brain tumors. Childs Nerv Syst 1999;15(11–12):758–763.

Habrand J-L, De Crevoisier R: Radiation therapy in the management of childhood brain tumors. Childs Nerv Syst 2001;17(3):121–133.

Packer RJ: Childhood medulloblastoma: Progress and future challenges. Brain Dev 1999;21(2):75–81.

Pollack IF: Pediatric brain tumors. Semin Surg Oncol 1999;16(2):73–90.

Strother DR, Pollack IF, Fisher PG, et al: Tumors of the central nervous system. In Pizzo PA, Poplack DG (eds): Principles and Practice of Pediatric Oncology, 4th ed. Philadelphia, Lippincott Williams & Wilkins, 2002, pp 751–824.

166 Long-term Follow-up of Survivors of Childhood Cancer

Sara Chaffee

ROLE OF THE GENERALIST

1   Maintain a Medical Home for the survivor of childhood cancer.

2   Recognize general long-term and late effects of treatment on specific organ systems.

3   Anticipate potential long-term and late effects of specific chemotherapeutic agents.

4   Anticipate potential long-term and late effects of treatment of specific childhood cancers.

5   Anticipate possible long-term educational and psychosocial effects of treatment.

6   Assure appropriate follow-up.

DEFINITION

By the year 2010 as many as 1 in every 250 young adults will be a survivor of childhood cancer. Survival of childhood cancer can no longer be considered to be a "rare" occurrence. This growing population of survivors is at increased risk for a number of treatment-related health complications. Seventy-three precent of young adult survivors are described as having at least one late effect; half of these survivors have two or more late effects of treatment, with 30% to 40% of the effects described as moderate to severe. Individuals who have survived 5 years or more from the time of diagnosis have an approximately 11-fold excess in mortality compared to their peers in the general population. Among 5-year survivors of childhood cancer, risk of death from the original cancer is 6% to 7% and risk of treatment-related death is 2%. The increased mortality risk is lifelong. The average generalist might be expected to care for as many as 5 to 10 survivors. The generalist must be able to anticipate, identify, and ameliorate late effects experienced by those survivors for whom they provide primary care. The generalist must have sufficient background to use information gained from the history and physical examination to piece together a broad treatment summary in order to address immediate health care issues.

FUNDAMENTALS: ANTICIPATING LATE EFFECTS

The majority of childhood cancers are treated with a combination of local control (surgery and/or radiation therapy) and systemic control (chemotherapy). Historical information about the combination and sequence of ther-

apy, in addition to the physical examination, may provide important clues about the diagnosis and stage of the underlying malignancy. With access to this knowledge, the health care provider can obtain more individualized information about the therapy and predict possible late effects. Table 166-1 lists common childhood malignancies with common historical and current treatments.

When taking a history and the names of chemotherapeutic agents are not available, the physician may be able to identify them by their route of administration, by color, by acute side effects, and by tests used to screen for side effects. Commonly used antineoplastic agents are described in Chapter 290. The occurrence of late effects of chemotherapeutic agents depends on the dose intensity, cumulative dose, developmental stage of the specific organ at the time of exposure, and cumulative stresses associated with treatment, growth, and aging. Many chemotherapeutic agents have unique toxicities affecting specific organs or tissues acutely over the long term.

Survivor memories of radiation therapy may include having to lie very still, sometimes in a restraining device, alone in a very large room under a very large machine. The unavoidable exposure of normal tissues to radiation affects their growth, development, and function, especially in younger children. The late effects of radiation therapy are primarily a consequence of progressive, irreparable injury to small blood vessels that compromises parenchymal function. Late effects of radiation visible on physical examination could include hypoplasia of bone or muscle in the radiation field, a change in skin pigmentation or permanent loss of hair in the radiation field, or chronic otitis and dry cerumen in the ear canal.

The physical examination may also provide information about the surgical treatment of a cancer. The location of the scar may be indicative of a particular type of cancer, or the possibility of a missing organ. The number of scars may suggest an intensity of therapy. A small scar on the chest accompanied by a prominent chest wall vascular pattern suggests the prior presence of a central line and a deep venous thrombosis.

COMMON CHILDHOOD CANCERS

(See the CD-ROM for additional information.)

Knowledge of the specific underlying malignancy allows the generalist, with the help of appropriate references, to outline an individualized treatment plan in enough detail

Table 166-1. Common Childhood Malignancies with Common (but Not All-inclusive) Historical and Current Treatments

Malignancy	Surgery	Chemotherapy	Radiation Therapy
Non-Hodgkin lymphoma	Biopsy	Anthracyclines Vincristine Methotrexate Glucocorticoids Antimetabolites Intrathecal chemotherapy Possibly alkylators	Occassionally

Hodgkin disease	Biopsy	Combinations that may include
		  several of the following:
		    Alkylators
		    Vincristine
		    Vinblastine
		    Bleomycin
		    Cytarabine
		    Glucocorticoids
		    Epipodophyllotoxin
		    Cisplatin
			Commonly

Rhabdomyosarcoma	Biopsy and/or definitive procedure	Stage-dependent and may include
		  combinations of the following:
		    Anthracyclines
		    Dactinomycin
		    Vincristine
		    Cyclophosphamide
		    Ifosfamide
		    Epipodophyllotoxin
			Commonly; stage-dependent

Soft tissue sarcoma	Biopsy and/or definitive procedure	Anthracyclines Ifosfamide	Commonly; stage-dependent
Osteosarcoma	Biopsy and then definitive procedure	Cisplatin Anthracyclines Methotrexate Ifosfamide Epipodophyllotoxin	Rarely

Ewing family tumors
  (peripheral primitive
  neuroectodermal tumors
  [PNETs])
	Biopsy and/or definitive procedure	Ifosfamide
		Cyclophosphamide
		Anthracyclines
		Epipodophyllotoxin
		Dactinomycin
			Commonly

Wilms tumor	Biopsy and/or definitive procedure	Vincristine Dactinomycin Anthracyclines Cyclophosphamide Ifosfamide Epipodophyllotoxin	Commonly; stage-dependent
Neuroblastoma	Biopsy and/or definitive procedure	Cisplatin Carboplatin Cyclophosphamide Ifosfamide Anthracyclines Epipodophyllotoxin	Commonly; stage-dependent
Germ cell tumors	Biopsy and/or definitive procedure	Cisplatin Epipodophyllotoxin Bleomycin	Rarely
Hepatoblastoma	Biopsy and/or definitive procedure	Vincristine Cisplatin Carboplatin	Rarely
Acute myelogenous leukemia	Rarely	Cytarabine Anthracyclines Thioguanine	Rarely

and accuracy to predict possible late effects. Historical information about the treatment of a malignancy is important since therapies have changed over the course of time. It has been possible to minimize therapy in certain diagnoses (e.g., low-stage Wilms tumor) and still maintain good outcome. This approach to treatment may decrease the severity of late effects. In other diagnoses (e.g., high-risk leukemia) the therapy has been intensified and individuals diagnosed and treated more recently are likely to experience more severe late effects.

The most common general categories of childhood cancers are acute lymphocytic leukemia (ALL), which accounts for about one fourth of all cancers diagnosed in individuals younger than 19 years of age, and central nervous system (CNS) malignancies, which account for about one fifth of all cancers in the same age group. Generally, ALL is treated with multiple types of chemotherapeutic agents, including intrathecal chemotherapy, and sometimes with craniospinal radiation, over the course of approximately 30 to 36 months. Many CNS tumors are treated with radiation doses as high as that tolerated by normal tissues, with treatment volumes as large as the whole brain. Knowledge of the treatment of leukemia and CNS malignancies provide the generalist with basic understanding of potential health problems that are commonly seen in survivors of childhood cancer.

Specific Effects of Therapy on Organs and Organ Systems

Details of specific effects on organs and organ systems by the type of therapy and specfic agents can be found on the CD-ROM. The affected organ or organ system may have been directly impacted by the cancer or may have been an "innocent bystander" that became involved as a result of the effects of local or systemic therapy on normal tissues. Exposure effects may initially be subclinical, and unmasked later by growth and/or aging processes. Periodic screening tests for organ function may be appropriate.

Chemotherapeutic agents and classes of agents have organ-specific effects. Both the acute and long-term severity of any particular effect may depend on the factors listed in Box 166-1. The systemic effect of chemotherapy may have a significant impact on any tissue with accelerated growth during the time of exposure.

Several well-described late effects of specific agents have acute and profound effects on the individual. Anthracycline exposure may cause a cardiomyopathy that can be abruptly unmasked by a growth spurt, isometric exercise such as weight lifting, exposure to anesthesia, or pregnancy. Those who need to undergo general anesthesia or who are pregnant require increased monitoring for cardiac effects. Bleomycin may cause pulmonary scarring and progressive pulmonary failure, which may become evident with pulmonary infections and/or exposure to oxygen. Anesthesiologists must be informed of prior treatment with bleomycin so they can appropriately limit intra-anesthetic oxygen exposure.

Radiation therapy may affect the growth and function of any malignant or normal tissue in the field of exposure. Box 166-2 lists factors that affect severity of radiation injury.

Exposure of normal tissues to two or more modalities of therapy may compromise organ function more profoundly than exposure to a single modality. The combination of radiation and surgery may cause increased scarring, affecting the appearance and function of the involved organ or the normal tissue. The combination of radiation and chemotherapy increases the functional damage to any exposed tissue.

Box 166-1. Factors Affecting Severity of Acute and Long-Term Effects

- Dosing of the agent including the following:
  Intensity of each dose
  Dosing schedule
  Cumulative dose of the agent
- Severity of complications associated with acute side effects
- Individual's genotype and phenotype
- Age at the time of exposure
- Preexposure and postexposure life/health experiences

Box 166-2. Factors Affecting Severity of Injury from Radiation

Radiation factors
  Dose
  Treatment volume
  Schedule
  Energy of the radiation
Patient factors
  Age
  Developmental status
  Underlying disease or abnormalities
Tumor factors
  Size
  Systemic effects

Second Malignancies

Any individual who has received chemotherapy and/or radiation therapy as treatment for a childhood cancer is at risk of developing a second malignant neoplasm (SMN). The risk is 10 to 12 times that of age-matched controls. The incidence ranges between 8% and 12% at 20 years. The lifelong incidence of SMNs is, as yet, unknown. The malignancy may have developed as a consequence of the therapy (secondary malignancy) or may be a second primary malignancy. Genetic conditions listed in Box 166-3 are associated with an increased risk of multiple primary cancers.

Certain types of therapy and specific primary malignancies are associated with a higher rate of SMNs. Much of the information about SMNs in children comes from long-term studies of survivors of Hodgkin disease. Follow-up of these individuals suggests that the actuarial estimate for SMNs is about 4% at 10 years, rising to 26% at 30 years. Several classes of chemotherapeutic agents, alkylators and epipodophyllotoxins, are known to be leukemogenic. Myeloid leukemias may occur between 2 to 3 and 5 to 10 years after exposure. Rapidly growing tissues such as bones and soft tissues are extremely susceptible to the carcinogenic effects of radiation. The most common radiation sarcomas are osteogenic sarcoma, fibrosarcoma, malignant fibrous histiocytoma, and chondrosarcoma. Girls who have received radiation to developing breast tissue are at an extremely high risk for developing breast cancer as young women. Thyroid cancer and central nervous system cancers may also develop in the radiation field. Radiation therapy may induce second malignancies in slower growing epithelial tissues such as the lung and gastrointestinal tract, but these types of cancer take a very long time to develop and

---

Box 166-3. Genetic Conditions Associated with Increased Risk of Multiple Malignancies

Hereditary retinoblastoma
Neurofibromatosis
Familial adenomatous polyposis
Hereditary nonpolyposis colorectal cancer
Multiple endocrine neoplasia
Li-Fraumeni syndrome

SUGGESTED READINGS

Keene N, Hobbie W, Ruccione K: Childhood Cancer Survivors. Sebastopol, Calif, O'Reilly, 2000.

Oeffinger KC, Eshelman DA, Tomlinson GF, et al: Grading of late effects in young adult survivors of childhood cancer followed in an ambulatory adult setting. Cancer 2000;88:1687–1695.

Oeffinger KC, Eshelman DA, Tomlinson GF, et al: Providing primary care for long-term survivors of childhood acute lymphoblastic leukemia. J Fam Pract 2000;49:1133–1146.

Schwartz CL: Long-term survivors of childhood cancer: The late effects of therapy. Oncologist 1999;4:45–54.

Schwartz CL, Hobbie WL, Constine LS, Ruccione KS: Survivors of Childhood Cancer. St Louis, Mosby, 1994.

SECTION 4   CHRONIC MEDICAL CARE: *Disorders of the Immune System*

167 Management of the Child with Asplenia

Carol S. Bruggers

ROLE OF THE GENERALIST

1. Recognize the conditions associated with hyposplenism and asplenism.

2. Recognize morphologic red blood cell abnormalities associated with hypofunctional spleen.

3. Immunize hyposplenic/asplenic patients against *Pneumococcus*, *Haemophilus influenzae*, and *Neisseria meningitidis*.

4. Provide appropriate antibiotic prophylaxis.

5. Recognize the clinical prodrome associated with overwhelming sepsis.

6. Provide immediate, aggressive medical intervention when fever occurs.

7. Assume that no infection is trivial.

8. Assist in consideration of splenic conservation surgery when applicable.

Normal splenic function has become increasingly appreciated. Overwhelming bacterial infection, particularly by encapsulated organisms, has been reported following surgical splenectomy for diverse conditions, congenital asplenia, and functional asplenia. Hypersplenism can result in abnormal, premature removal of physiologically normal hematopoietic cells from the circulation, creating significant pathophysiology that may need to be treated by splenectomy. Although the risk for overwhelming infection is greatest in infants and young children and during the first few years following splenectomy, overwhelming sepsis resulting in death has been reported decades after splenectomy. Generalists must understand the physiologic consequences of splenectomy and must follow medical care guidelines to prevent overwhelming bacterial sepsis in those without a functioning spleen.

THE NORMAL ANATOMY AND PHYSIOLOGY OF THE SPLEEN

The spleen's unique anatomy and composition are central to its physiologic functions that involve the circulatory, reticuloendothelial, and immune systems. The splenic artery branches into segmental arteries as it enters the hilum. These arteries branch into trabecular vessels that give rise to central arteries, which enter the encasing splenic white pulp at nearly right angles. This flow pattern skims off the plasma and soluble substances. With arterial narrowing, the rate of blood flow is reduced and the cellular elements are progressively concentrated as they enter the red pulp. Most of the substance of the spleen is red pulp, which consists of the splenic cords and large, thin-walled sinuses.

The spleen's immunologic functions are crucial (Table 167-1 and Box 167-1). Nearly 50% of the body's T cells and 10% of B cells reside in the spleen. The spleen plays a central role in the generation and modulation of specific

Table 167-1. Functions of the Spleen

Immunologic	Antibody production and immune system modulation
	Clearance of IgG and complement-opsonized cells and particles
Filtering	Removal of senescent red blood cells
	Culling red blood cell inclusions
	Howell-Jolly bodies
	Siderotic granules
	Heinz bodies
	Malarial parasites
	Removal of deformed red blood cells
	Sickle cell disease
	Red blood cell membranopathies (hereditary spherocytosis)
	Red blood cell enzymopathies (pyruvate kinase deficiency)
	Acanthocytes (abetalipoproteinemia)

antibody formation in response to circulating antigens in the blood. The spleen's reticuloendothelial cells, monocytes and macrophages, perform filtering and clearance functions, including antigen processing and removal of antibody-coated and complement-sensitized cells. Reticuloendothelial cells also (1) remove senescent or otherwise abnormal red blood cells in the hemoconcentrated red pulp (culling); (2) remove opsonized particulate material in the sinusoids by phagocytosis (filtering); and (3) selectively remove intraerythrocytic inclusions, such as Howell-Jolly bodies (pitting).

PATHOPHYSIOLOGY

Significant pathophysiologic changes may occur with "normal" splenic function, hypersplenism, and asplenia. A normally functioning spleen can cause significant, occasionally life-threatening cytopenias if hematopoietic cells are abnormal (abnormalities of red blood cell membranes, hemoglobin structure, and enzymopathies) or through immune-mediated processes (immune-mediated thrombocytopenia and autoimmune hemolytic anemia). If these conditions are life-threatening, excessively prolonged, or resistant to medical management, surgical splenectomy may be warranted.

Hypersplenism can be caused by diverse pathophysiologic conditions involving either the spleen or the liver. Liver diseases that result in vascular obstruction from cirrhosis or portal hypertension can dramatically increase the amount of blood flowing through the splenic cords and

Box 167-1. Evidence of Functional and Anatomic Asplenia

Hematologic
  Howell-Jolly bodies—persistent nuclear remnants
  Abnormal red blood cell morphology—spherocytes, fragments, sickled cells
  Pits or vacuoles in red blood cell submembrane cytoplasm
Radiologic studies
  Labeled red blood cell scan
  Technetium-99m sulfur colloid scans
  Ultrasonography
  Computed tomography

cause slowed flow and sludging through the spleen. Physiologically normal red blood cells, platelets, and white blood cells are then prematurely removed from the circulation. Infiltrative splenic processes such as hematopoietic malignancies, metabolic storage diseases, and histiocytic disorders are also associated with congested, slowed blood flow, premature removal of hematopoietic cells, and resulting peripheral cytopenias and functional hyposplenism.

Table 167-2 lists conditions associated with asplenia or functional hyposplenism. Asplenia can be either anatomic, following surgical resection or if congenitally absent, or functional in nature, as is seen in sickling hemoglobinopathies.

OVERWHELMING SEPSIS IN ASPLENIA

The major medical concern for patients who are functionally or anatomically asplenic is overwhelming bacterial infections by encapsulated organisms, a condition asso-

Table 167-2. Conditions Associated with Anatomic and Functional Asplenia

Conditions Associated with Anatomic Asplenia
Surgical Removal
Following trauma associated with splenic rupture
Anatomic defects
  Cysts
  Hemangiomas
Congestive splenomegaly from hepatic pathology
  Hepatic fibrosis
  Metabolic storage diseases (Gaucher disease)
  Biliary atresia
  α_1-Antitrypsin deficiency
Malignancies
  Chronic myelogenous leukemia
  Hodgkin disease
Infiltrative histiocytic disorders associated with hypersplenism
  Langerhans cell histiocytosis
  Virus-associated hemophagocytosis
  Familial hemophagocytosis syndrome
Hematologic disorders
  Red cell membrane disorders
  Hemoglobinopathies (sequestration in sickle cell disease)
  Red cell enzymopathies
Refractory immune-mediated disorders
  Chronic immune-mediated thrombocytopenia
  Autoimmune hemolytic anemia
Congenital Asplenia
Familial nonsyndrome
Ivenmark syndrome
Cardiac and digestive tract disorders

Conditions Associated with Hyposplenism
Hemoglobinopatheis
  Hb SS, Hb SC, Hb S, β-thalassemia
Connective tissue disorders
  Systemic lupus erythemotosus
  Polyarteritis nodosa
  Rheumatoid arthritis
Gastrointestinal disease
  Celiac sprue
  Ulcerative colitis
  Liver disease
Other
  Dermatitis herpetiformis
  Irradiation for cancer
  Sarcoidosis
  Immunodeficiency
  High-dose corticosteroid therapy

Table 167-3. Organisms Associated with Overwhelming Sepsis in Asplenia or Hyposplenia

Prevalence	Organisms
Most common	*Streptococcus pneumoniae*
	Haemophilus influenzae type b
	Neisseria meningitidis
Less common	*Escherichia coli*
	Staphylococcus
	Pseudomonas
	Salmonella
	Other streptococci
Rare but reported	*Plasmodium* (malaria)
	Babesia
	Capnocytophaga canimorsus (infection from dog bite)

ciated with very high morbidity and mortality rates (Table 167-3). The exact frequency of overwhelming sepsis associated with anatomic or functional asplenia is uncertain, but appears to vary with the duration of time following splenectomy and the age of the individual at the time of splenectomy (Table 167-4). The reason for the splenectomy, immunization status of the patient at the time of splenectomy, and the use of prophylactic antibiotics following splenectomy also appear to influence the risk for overwhelming sepsis.

The prodrome usually begins with nonspecific symptoms, including fever, myalgia, vomiting, and malaise. However, rapid progression usually occurs wihin hours to rigors, disseminated intravascular coagulation, diffuse purpura and fulminant septic shock, cardiovascular collapse, respiratory distress, coma, and death within hours.

The reason for the splenectomy appears to influence the risk of sepsis, and the associated morbidity and mortality. In a large retrospective study overwhelming sepsis occurred in 4% of patients who had undergone splenectomy and was lethal 2% to 3% of cases. Patients with thalassemia were at the greatest risk of postsplenectomy sepsis. In another retrospective study the overall average mortality rate was 50%. In patients with hematologic malignancies, the mortality rate was 69%, compared to 46% for patients following trauma or nonmalignant hematologic etiologies. *Streptococcus*

Table 167-4. Overwhelming Sepsis in Asplenic-Hyposplenic Conditions

Condition	Total Number of cases	With Sepsis N (%)	Fatal Sepsis N (%)
Incidental splenectomy	1768	17 (1.0)	11 (0.6)
Idiopathic thrombocytopenic purpura	1271	20 (1.5)	17 (1.3)
Sickle cell disease	105	2 (1.9)	0 (0)
Trauma	1444	36 (2.4)	29 (2.0)
Transplantation	120	4 (3.3)	1 (0.8)
Hereditary spherocytosis	1376	49 (3.6)	31 (2.3)
Hodgkin disease	1256	84 (6.7)	51 (4.1)
Portal hypertension	267	23 (8.6)	14 (5.2)
Thalassemia	265	35 (13.2)	15 (5.6)
Total	7872	270 (3.5)	169 (2.1)

Adapted from Hansen K, Singer DB: Asplenic-hyposplenic overwhelming sepsis: Postsplenectomy sepsis revisited. Pediatr Dev Pathol 2001;4:105–121.

pneumoniae was the infectious agent in 90%. Most patients had not been immunized against *Pneumococcus* but were taking prophylactic antibiotics.

Retrospective studies support the efficacy of pneumococcal immunization in decreasing the incidence of overwhelming postsplenectomy sepsis, but immunization failures do occur. Prophylaxis with antibiotics with or without immunization has unequivocally been shown to significantly decrease the incidence of postsplenectomy infection and death. In a prospective, multicenter, randomized trial of children younger than 5 years of age with sickle cell anemia, the risk of pneumococcal infection was reduced by 84% in the group taking penicillin compared to the group taking placebo.

Immunization Recommendations

Three licensed formulations of pneumococcal vaccines are available. Two vaccines, Pnu-Immune and Pneumovax, contain purified pneumococcal capsular polysaccharides from 23 *S. pneumoniae* serotypes and are designed to provide potential protection against 85% to 90% of infections caused by pneumococci in children in the United States. Limited immunogenicity in young children up to 10 years of age and persistent nasopharyngeal carriage *S. pneumoniae* remain significant problems with these preparations. A heptavalent pneumococcal protein conjugate vaccine, Prevnar, was recently licensed and shows very good immunogenicity, even in infants. Currently, the Committee on Infectious Diseases of the American Academy of Pediatrics recommends that Prevnar be administered to all children at high risk of pneumococcal infection at the youngest age possible, including those with functional, anatomic, and congenital asplenia. The Committee also recommends that these same children be immunized with the 23-valent polysaccharide vaccine to expand serotype coverage.

Children with anatomic or functional asplenia should also be immunized with the protein conjugated vaccine against *H. influenzae* prior to splenectomy, if they have not already been immunized in infancy. This vaccine is very immunogenic, even in infants, and has resulted in a marked decrease in the frequency of invasive *H. influenzae* infections. Finally, children two years of age or older who are asplenic or for whom a splenectomy is planned should also be immunized with quadravalent meningococcal vaccine.

Prophylactic Antibiotic Recommendations

The duration of prophylactic antibiotic administration in children with functional or anatomic asplenia remains controversial and largely unstudied. The risk of overwhelming sepsis is a lifelong problem, with most episodes occurring 10 to 30 years following splenectomy. Recommendations range from 2 years following splenectomy to lifelong administration, depending on associated factors, including the reason for splenectomy, age at the time of splenectomy, and the duration of time elapsed since splenectomy. Major issues are potential for emergence of penicillin-resistant strains of pneumococcus, difficulty maintaining long-term compliance, and the possible lack of true benefit. Literature supports continued antibiotic prophylaxis for a minimum of 2 to 5 years following splenectomy. If discontinued, patients and clinicians must remember that the risk of overwhelming postsplenectomy sepsis is lifelong in some individuals. Erythromycin is the drug of choice for those who cannot take penicillin or amoxicillin.

The Committee on Infectious Disease of the American Academy of Pediatrics recommends that prophylactic antibiotics be administered to children with functional or anatomic asplenia who are younger than 5 years of age. Prophylactic antibiotics may be discontinued in children with sickle cell disease at age 5 years, provided they have not undergone splenectomy, are receiving comprehensive medical care, and have not had prior episodes of pneumococcal bacteremia. These children and their families must be instructed to seek medical care for all febrile events. Because the safety of discontinuation of prophylaxis in children with asplenia from other causes is unknown, some experts continue to recommend prophylaxis throughout childhood.

The incidence of invasive *H. influenzae* infection is less common, although children with anatomic or functional asplenia are at increased risk. Antibiotic prophylaxis may not be necessary if children have been properly immunized with a protein conjugated Hib (*H. influenzae* type b) vaccine, because the excellent immunogenicity of these vaccines has been demonstrated in infants and young children with and without splenic function.

MEASURES TO REDUCE THE INCIDENCE OF POSTSPLENECTOMY SEPSIS

Education of patients and clinicians is essential to reduce the incidence of overwhelming sepsis in patients with hyposplenism-asplenism. Education must include recognition of (1) medical conditions associated with splenic dysfunction; (2) the prodrome associated with the onset of overwhelming sepsis, and (3) the need for prompt medical intervention at the earliest sign of possible infection (Box 167-2). Spleen-conserving approach should be considered when possible, such as partial splenectomy in hereditary spherocytosis, storage diseases, and anatomic cysts; partial splenic embolization in cases of hypersplenism related to hepatic disease; and heterotopic autologous splenic transplantation following trauma.

Box 167-2 summarizes management of patients with asplenia or hyposplenia. Important issues include the following:

1. Immunization at least 2 weeks prior to anticipated splenectomy with pneumococcal protein conjugate vaccines (Prevnar) and polyvalent polysaccharide vaccine to expand serotype coverage, quadravalent polysaccharide meningococcal vaccine, and protein conjugated Hib vaccine if not yet given in infancy
2. Prophylactic penicillin, amoxicillin, or erythromycin for at least the first 2 years following surgical splenectomy
3. Prophylactic penicillin, amoxicillin, or erythromycin in all children with sickle cell disease until the age of 5 years
4. Antibiotic prophylaxis prior to dental procedures (see Tables 60-2 and 60-3)
5. Strict malarial prophylaxis when traveling in areas highly endemic for malaria, as well as areas where malaria infection is possible though not very likely

---

Box 167-2. Treatment of the Asplenic/Hyposplenic Patient

Immunization prior to splenectomy
1. Protein conjugated pneumococcal vaccine (Prevnar)
2. Polysaccharide pneumococcal vaccine (Pneumovax, Pnu-Immune)
3. Protein-conjugated *Haemophilus influenzae* type b (Hib) vaccine
4. Quadravalent polysaccharide meningococcal vaccine

Antibiotic prophylaxis
1. Penicillin 125–250 mg orally twice daily
2. Amoxicillin 125–250 mg orally twice daily
3. Erythromycin* 250 mg orally daily
4. Malarial prophylaxis when traveling to endemic areas

Dental procedure prophylaxis (see Tables 60-2 and 60-3)
Standby antipneumococcal antibiotic supply
Treatment of febrile illness
1. Prompt medical evaluation (blood culture, broad-spectrum antibiotic)
   Ceftriaxone, 75 mg/kg/day, maximum 4 g
   Cefotaxime, 100 mg/kg/day IV in three divided doses, maximum 12 g/day
   Vancomycin,† dose dependent on age and renal function
2. Close inpatient or extended outpatient observation

Referral to specialists for associated hematologic, cardiac, or gastrointestinal abnormalities

---

*In penicillin-allergic individuals.
†In areas with high prevalence of resistant pneumococcus.

---

6. Patient education in the following areas:
   - Recognition of the prodrome, which may be nonspecific and mild: myalgias, headache, low-grade fever, emesis diarrhea, abdominal pain
   - Wearing a warning bracelet
   - Carrying a laminated warning card including information that the patient is asplenic, with the physician's name and phone number
   - Keeping antibiotic available to be taken at earliest sign of infection

Table 167-5 indicates the role of the primary care provider and the other specialists who may be involved in the care of children with these conditions. As with all chronic illness, the primary care provider must provide continuity of care, coordinate care with specialists, and provide acute care and health maintenance.

Table 167-5. Chronic Condition Comanagement of the Child with Asplenia

Primary care provider
1. Prior to splenectomy, minimize risk of sepsis:
   Immunization
   Patient education
2. Following splenectomy, prevent postsplenectomy sepsis:
   Prophylactic antibiotics
   Recognizing the prodrome of overwhelming sepsis
   Immediate and aggressive treatment of febrile episode
Specialists for conditions associated with the primary underlying problem:
   Hematologist
   Cardiologist
   Gastroenterologist

SUGGESTED READINGS

American Academy of Pediatrics Committee on Infectious Diseases: Policy statement: Recommendations for the prevention of pneumococcal infections, including the use of pneumococcal conjugate vaccine (Prevnar), pneumococcal polysaccharide vaccine, and antibiotic prophylaxis. Pediatrics 2000;106:362–366.

Lortan JE: Management of asplenic patients. Br J Haematol 1993;84:566–569.

Pearson HA:. The spleen and disturbances of splenic function. In Nathan D, Orkin SH (eds): Nathan and Oski's Hematology of Infancy and Childhood, 2nd ed. Philadelphia, WB Saunders, 1998, p 1914.

Working Party of the British Committee for Standards in Haematology Clinical Haematology Task Force: Guidelines for the prevention and treatment of infection in patients with an absent or dysfunctional spleen. BMJ 1996;312:430–434.

SECTION 4   CHRONIC MEDICAL CARE: *Disorders of the Immune System*

168 Complement Disorders

Timothy R. La Pine and Harry R. Hill

ROLE OF THE GENERALIST

1. Recognize the signs and symptoms suggesting complement immune deficiency.
2. Order appropriate laboratory tests to differentiate complement immune deficiency from infection or other immune deficiency.
3. Arrange consultation with an immunologist.
4. Arrange genetic consultation as indicated.
5. Assist specialists with laboratory studies to monitor treatment during infections.
6. Assist the specialists with family education.
7. Be available to assist the family with school and other psychosocial issues.

The complement system is part of the innate immune system that defends against initial pathogen invasion, providing protection when previous exposure has not occurred. The complement system bridges the innate and the adaptive immune systems (T cells and B cells), helps to defend against pyogenic bacterial infections, and disposes of immune complexes and the products of inflammatory injury (Box 168-1). Major complement functions are (1) amplification of leukocyte-associated inflammatory responses; (2) anaphylactoid responses through histamine release; (3) chemotaxis and activation of neutrophils and macrophages; (4) opsonization of foreign microbes and antigens; and (5) cytolysis of target cell membranes (Box 168-2).

Box 168-1. Physiologic Effects of Complement

1. Bridge the innate and adaptive immune responses.
2. Defend against pyogenic bacterial infections.
3. Dispose of immune complexes and the products of inflammatory injury.

The complement system is made up of a series of more than 30 plasma and regulatory membrane proteins. The system functions as a cascade, similar to the coagulation system, with activation of each component, depending on activation of the prior component(s) in an orderly sequence. Any defect in complement component production can result in immune deficiency. Complement defects should be considered in patients with recurrent infections with encapsulated bacteria (e.g., *Streptococcus pneumoniae* and *Haemophilus influenzae*) and with *Neisseria* species, with collagen vascular–like disease and lupus-like disease (e.g., nephritis, arthritis, and facial rashes), and with hereditary or isolated angioedema usually of the face extremities and gastrointestinal tract.

Box 168-2. Major Complement Functions

1. Amplification of leukocyte-associated inflammatory responses
2. Anaphylactoid responses through histamine release
3. Chemoattraction and activation of neutrophils and macrophages
4. Opsonization of foreign microbes and antigens
5. Cytolysis of target cell membranes

FUNDAMENTALS

The complement system functions as a highly ordered system of activation and inactivation of specific serum and membrane-bound complement proteins that follow logical rules. Because the complement proteins were numbered in the order of their discovery, rather than by their functional sequence within the cascade, the nomenclature can be confusing. An understanding of the interactions of the complement components during inflammation, however, allows prediction of many of the clinical effects observed in complement deficiency states.

The complement cascade comprises the classical pathway, activated by binding of antibody, and the alternative pathway, initiated by the direct attachment of activated C3 to the surface of bacteria, viruses, fungi, and virus-infected cells (Table 168-1). These pathways eventually join into a common pathway that contains an amplification loop and the membrane attack complex. The classical pathway begins when antibody binds to a cell's surface and ends with the lysis of the cell. The serum proteins described in the classical pathway include C1 through C9, with C4 being out of order. C1 activation begins the classical pathway and is composed of q, r, and s subcomponents. It is followed by C4 and C2 and then C3, which in turn activates in sequence C5 through C9, the membrane attack complex of the complement cascade. The alternative pathway functions in the absence of antibody. The serum proteins in the alternative pathway are called factors. Their numbers are followed by a letter, such as factor B.

The complement proteins on cell membranes can be receptors for activated complement proteins or can serve as proteins that regulate the complement system itself. They often have multiple names. During the activation of the complement cascade several serum complement proteins are cleaved. These activated complement protein fragments are designated with lower case suffixes "a" and "b" (for example, C3 is cleaved into two fragments, C3a and C3b). The "a" fragment usually designates the smaller fragment of the cleaved protein. The classical and alternative pathways join in the common pathway that includes the C3 amplification loop and the membrane attack complex. Once the alternative pathway is triggered, an amplification loop is activated, inducing more C3b formation. Surface-bound C3b, in conjunction with activated C4b2a of the classical pathway or C3bBb of the alternative pathway, serves as activator of C5, which initiates formation of the membrane attack complex (C5b, C6, C7, C8, C9) and lyses the cell membrane.

All activated components of the complement system are tightly controlled by regulatory proteins. C1 esterase inhibitor inhibits the classical pathway by inactivating C1 esterase. Factors I and H regulate the alternative pathway. Factor I inactivates C3b, and factor H dissociates Bb from C3b. Both inhibit the alternative pathway. Regulation of the formation of the membrane attack complex on cell membranes is controlled by two membrane-bound complement proteins: (1) decay accelerating factor regulates the formation of C3 convertase and (2) CD59 is the membrane inhibitor of reactive lysis.

The major effects of active complement components are anaphylatoxic (C3a and C5a), opsonic (C3b, iC3b), chemotactic (C5a), and cytolytic activity (membrane attack complex, C5 to C9).

The complement system contributes significantly to neonatal defense against infection. The production and function of complement proteins is quantatively and qualitatively different in the newborn compared to adults. Complement protein synthesis in the developing human fetus occurs between 8 and 19 weeks of gestational age. Complement proteins are produced in decreased quantity with decreased functional activity depending on the gestational age of the fetus. Few, if any, maternal complement components cross the placenta. Preterm and term infants are markedly deficient in complement activities compared to adults. The neonate and especially the preterm infant usually have profound deficiencies in opsonic and chemotactic activity, which are crucial to host defense. The cellular and humoral factors important for generation of complement activities are also deficient in newborns. For example, most newborns have low levels of IgM, which does not cross the placenta. Opsonization of bacteria and certain viruses whose antibodies are of the IgM class may be reduced in newborns because of insufficient IgM to activate the classical pathway of complement.

The genetics and heritability for nearly all the complement deficiencies have been described. Genes for several complement components are found within the major histocompatibility complex class III region on chromosome 6. Complement deficiencies are inherited as autosomal recessive disorders with two exceptions. C1 inhibitor deficiency is inherited in an autosomal dominant fashion, and properdin deficiency is inherited as an X-linked recessive disorder.

SIGNS AND SYMPTOMS

Interactions of the complement components during inflammation predicts the clinical effects observed in complement deficiency states. The major effects of active complement components are anaphylatoxic (C3a and C5a), opsonic (C3b, iC3b), chemotactic (C5a), and cytolytic activity (membrane attack complex, C5 to C9). Any defect in the production or function of these complement components can lead to specific clinical disorders that are characterized by the specific component deficiency (Table 168-2). Complement defects should be considered in patients with recurrent infections with encapsulated bacteria (e.g., *Streptococcus*

Table 168-1. Activation of the Complement System

Classical Pathway

Activated by immune complexes, antigen-antibody complexes.

IgG1, IgG2, and IgG3 can activate the complement, which occurs as C1 binds to the Fc portion of immunoglobulins.

IgM is a much more powerful activator of complement. One IgM molecule can activate the classical complement pathway, whereas hundreds of IgG molecules may be necessary.

IgA, IgE, and IgD do not cause classical pathway activation.

Alternative Pathway (Properdin System)

Activated in the absence of antibody.

Initiated by direct attachment of activated C3 to the surface of gram-negative and gram-positive bacterial cell walls, complex polysaccharides, lipopolysaccharides, cobra venom, fungi, viruses, parasites, and IgA and IgE aggregates.

Table 168-2. Clinical and Functional Features of Complement Component Deficiencies

Complement Deficiency	Functional Defect	Clinical Association
Classical pathway: C1q, C1r, and C1s, C4, C2	Defective immune complex clearance Defective immunoregulation Failure to activate the classical pathway	Systemic lupus-like symptoms Infections with encapsulated bacteria
Alternative pathway: Factor B	Defective immune complex clearance	Infections with encapsulated bacteria
Late-acting components: C3	Important in both classical and alternative pathways	Autoimmune disease Severe infections with encapsulated bacterial and *Neisseria* species
Properdin, membrane attack complexes (C5–C9)	Impaired opsonization Impaired chemotaxis Critical for cell lysis	
Membrane-bound regulators: Delay accelerating factor CD59	Failure to prevent formation of membrane attack complex	Paroxysmal nocturnal hemoglobinuria
Serum regulating proteins: C1 inhibitor	Failure to activate the classical pathway Overactivation of the alternative pathway	Hereditary angioedema Pyogenic infections
Factors H and I	Impaired degradation of C3	Autoimmune diseases

pneumoniae and *Haemophilus influenzae*) and with *Neisseria* species, with collagen vascular–like disease and lupus-like disease (e.g., nephritis, arthritis, and facial rashes), and with hereditary or isolated angioedema usually of the face, extremities, and gastrointestinal tract (Box 168-3).

Deficiencies of the early components of the classical pathway result in a high incidence of collagen vascular–like and lupus-like disease (C1q, C1r, C1s, C4, or C2 deficiency). Patients who lack these components often present with some combination of recurrent infection (usually pneumococcal), arthritis, skin rash, and glomerulonephritis. The clinical disorder most likely results from suboptimal removal of circulating immune complexes from the circulation from failure to attach C3b and iC3b to the particle. Patients with late complement deficiencies have recurrent infections with *Neisseria* species. Patients with a defect in the alternative pathway (deficiency of factor B) present with recurrent infections with encapsulated bacteria.

Patients with a defect in the alternative pathway (deficiency of factor B) present with recurrent infections with encapsulated bacteria. Those with deficiencies in late-acting components (C3 and membrane attack complexes C5 to C9) may present with symptoms of autoimmune disease and with recurrent severe pyogenic infections from pneumococci and meningococci.

DIAGNOSIS

If a complement deficiency is suspected, evaluation in collaboration with a pediatric immunologist is most efficient. The first screening test to order is total hemolytic complement (CH$_{50}$ and CH$_{100}$). The functional status of

---

Box 168-3. Signs and Symptoms of Complement Disorders

- Recurrent infections with encapsulated bacteria (e.g., *Streptococcus pneumoniae* and *Haemophilus influenzae*) and with *Neisseria* species
- Collagen vascular–like disease and lupus-like disease (e.g., nephritis, arthritis, and facial rashes)
- Hereditary or isolated angioedema, usually of the face, extremities, and gastrointestinal tract

---

the classical and common pathways is measured by the total hemolytic complement assay. The CH$_{50}$ measures the ability of the patient's serum to lyse 50% of a standard sheep erythrocyte suspension. The amount of complement in the patient's blood is reflected by the number of sheep cells lysed. The CH$_{100}$ is a radial hemolytic assay that records 100% hemolysis. A normal CH$_{50}$ or CH$_{100}$ indicates that components C1 through C9 are present; they do not quantitate any particular complement component.

Other general tests of complement activity are liposome immunoassays, which use a color change to indicate complement-mediated lysis of liposomes, and enzyme immunoassays, which use monoclonal antibodies to detect the formation of C5b through C9 in wells coated with immune complexes or aggregated immunoglobulin.

The alternative pathway hemolytic assay uses rabbit red blood cells to activate and assess the function of the alternative pathway. Rabbit erythrocytes are potent activators of the human alternative pathway. Patients with deficiencies of the components of the alternative pathway, as well as patients with deficiencies of C5 to C9 will fail to lyse rabbit erythrocytes.

Accurate immunochemical assays for specific complement components are not widely available. The individual complement component assays are often performed by rate nephelometry. This assay use antibody that is raised specifically against the human complement factor in question and then is added to the patient's serum. The resulting Ab-complement complexes will cause measurable light scattering (nephelometry) that is proportional to the amount of complement in the serum (e.g., C2, C3, C4, C5, C1 esterase inhibitor, factors B, I, and H). Note that in complement defects that are characterized by dysfunctional proteins (e.g., C1 esterase inhibitor deficiency type 2 and C1q deficiency) the specific immunochemical component assays may demonstrate normal component concentrations, but they are reduced in functional activity.

MANAGEMENT

The generalist is the primary care provider and must coordinate the recommendations of the specialists involved. This role includes communicating a health care plan to the families, providing ongoing health care surveillance, recognizing and treating medical emergencies, and assisting with family support.

Treatment of most complement-deficient patients should be directed at their specific clinical manifestations. No specific therapy replaces or restores complement function. Patients with early complement defects usually present with recurrent infections with encapsulated bacteria (e.g., *Streptococcus pneumoniae*, *Haemophilus influenzae*) and may benefit from antibiotic prophylaxis and immunization with polyvalent pneumococcal or *Haemophilus influenzae* vaccine. Patients with late complement defects are at risk for infections with *Neisseria* species and should be immunized with the polyvalent meningococcal vaccine. Patients with C1 esterase inhibitor deficiency may respond to antifibrinolytic agents and androgen administration. Concentrates of C1 esterase inhibitor have also been employed to treat acute attacks. The benefit of plasma infusions or specific complement infusions to treat complement-deficient patients has not been demonstrated in clinical trials.

It is important to consider the type of immune deficiency and the most likely etiologic agents of infection. For example, patients with congenital absence of their terminal complement components often have infections with *Neisseria meningitides* or *Neisseria gonorrhoeae*. Patients with known terminal complement defects should receive the appropriate intravenous antimicrobial therapy for these organisms. In addition, the administration of fresh frozen plasma may be beneficial by supplying the missing complement components. Guidelines for emergency management are summarized in Box 168-4.

SPECIFIC COMPLEMENT DEFICIENCIES

C1 Esterase Inhibitor Deficiency

C1 esterase inhibitor deficiency of hereditary angioedema was the first complement deficiency described. This familial syndrome is characterized by recurrent episodes of swelling (angioedema) and is inherited in an autosomal dominant fashion. The gene for C1 esterase inhibitor deficiency is encoded on chromosome 11. Two forms of the deficiency have been described. C1 esterase inhibitor deficiency type I represents 85% of the cases and is characterized by decreased or absent C1 protein production. Type II represents 15% of the cases and is characterized by dysfunctional C1 esterase inhibitor protein. In C1 esterase inhibitor deficiency activated C1 is not regulated, and C4

and C2 levels are low from continuous activation and consumption. The mediators responsible for producing the edema are incompletely understood.

The attacks of swelling usually first appear during adolescence and persist through life. They are episodic in nature, developing over 4 to 6 hours and persisting for 2 to 4 days with spontaneous resolution. The swelling is nonpainful, nonpruritic, nonerythematous, and nonpitting. It commonly involves the extremities, face, and gastrointestinal tract. Laryngeal swelling with airway occlusion can be life-threatening in these patients. Afflicted individuals have less than 25% of normal functional activity of C1 esterase inhibitor.

The incidence of angioedema has shown to be reduced with plasma infusions (which contain C1), specific purified C1 esterase inhibitor concentrate infusions, and treatment with antifibrinolytic agents. Androgen administration promotes increased levels of C1 esterase inhibitor, with some patients achieving normal levels and absence of clinical symptoms, which return when the medication is stopped. The exact mechanisms of androgen responsiveness are unknown at this time.

C1q Deficiency

The C1 complement complex contains three subunits (C1q, C1r, and C1s). The C1q subunit is composed of three polypeptides (C1qA, C1qB, C1qC), which are encoded by genes on chromosome 1. Individuals with C1q deficiency have reduced levels of total hemolytic complement as well as reduced C1 functional activity. There are two forms of C1q deficiency. The first form appears to result in a production defect and C1q is not detected by either immunochemical analysis of functional assays. The second form appears to result from defective production so that C1q is present by immunochemical analysis but functional activity is not detected. The most common clinical features of C1q deficiency are lupus-like symptoms, however, patients with C1q deficiency also have an increased frequency of infections with pyogenic organisms owing to their inability to activate the classical complement pathway.

C1r and C1s Deficiency

The genes for C1r and C1s are closely linked on the short arm of chromosome 12. Patients with C1r and C1s deficiency, like the C1q-deficient patients, have reduced to absent levels of total hemolytic complement activity with reduced activity of C1. The most common clinical features of C1r and C1s deficiency is lupus-like symptoms, although pyogenic infections and glomerulonephritis have also been reported

C2 Deficiency

C2 deficiency is an autosomal recessive trait and is the most commonly reported complement deficiency. The incidence of homozygous C2 deficiency is 1 in 28,000 to 40,000. The heterozygous carrier rate is estimated at 1.2% of the general population based on screening of normal blood donors.

Patients can have recurrent pneumonia, bacteremia, or meningitis caused by *S. pneumoniae* (present in about two thirds of reported infections), *H. influenzae*, and *N. meningitidis*. Autoimmune or rheumatic complications are present in about half of the patients. The lupus-like disease in C2-deficient patients is characterized by early onset, marked photosensitivity, low-titered or absent antinuclear antibody, and a low incidence of renal involvement.

C3 Deficiency

C3 deficiency is transmitted by autosomal recessive inheritance. C3 is positioned at the junction of the classical and alternative complement pathways and has an important role in the opsonization of most encapsulated bacteria, generation of C3a and C5a, and initiation of the membrane attack complex.

Patients with total C3 deficiency usually have severe episodes of infection including recurrent pneumonia, sepsis, meningitis, and peritonitis. The most common pathogens isolated are *S. pneumoniae*, *H. influenzae*, *N. meningitidis*, and *S. aureus*. Lupus-like illness and glomerulonephritis occur in 15% to 21% of the patients.

C4 Deficiency

The fourth component of complement exists as two isotypes (C4A and C4B) encoded for by genes within the major histocompatibility complex class III region on chromosome 6. The deficiency is transmitted by autosomal recessive inheritance. Deficiencies of one or the other isotype are relatively common among immune deficiencies with heterozygous individuals being identified in 10% to 15% of the general population. Complete deficiency of C4 is the result of being homozygous and deficient for both isotypes, which is uncommon.

The most common manifestations of complete C4 deficiency are lupus-like symptoms. Because activation of the alternative pathway may be sufficient for host defense against many pathogens, deficient patients generally have few infectious complications.

C5 to C9 Deficiency

Some individuals with deficiencies of C5 to C9 are completely asymptomatic, whereas others have unusual susceptibility to recurrent *Neisseria* infections (*N. meningitidis* or *N. gonorrhoeae*). Deficiency of the terminal complement components are also transmitted by autosomal recessive inheritance. Recurrent episodes of meningococcemia, meningococcal meningitis, and disseminated gonococcal infections have occurred in about 50% of reported patients. The rate of C5 to C9 deficiency in patients with disseminated *Neisseria* infections may be as high as 10% to 15%. In contrast to early complement component deficiencies, autoimmune diseases are only occasionally diagnosed in these patients.

Factor I and Factor H Deficiencies

For the most part, factor I and factor H deficiencies are similar. These deficiencies are inherited as autosomal recessive traits. Factor I is encoded by a gene on chromosome 4q, and the gene encoding factor H lies within the regulators of complement activation (RCA) gene cluster on chromosome 1.

Affected individuals have recurrent infections and some have hemolytic anemia and urticaria. In both of these deficiencies C3 is synthesized normally, but turnover is rapid because the alternative pathway cannot be adequately controlled. As a result there is continuous activation and cleavage of native C3 through the alternative pathway, resulting in the production of C3b. Patients with factor I and factor H deficiency, therefore, have a secondary deficiency of C3 and markedly reduced serum levels of C3, most of which is in the form of C3b. The total hemolytic complement activity and alternative pathway complement activity are also significantly reduced. Patients with both factor I and factor H deficiency are predisposed to infections with encapsulated bacteria, and *Neisseria* infections are common. Although glomerulonephritis is common in patients with C3 deficiency and factor H deficiency, renal disease has not been described in factor I deficiency.

Properdin Deficiency

Properdin deficiency is the only deficiency of complement that is transmitted by X-linked recessive inheritance. In some families properdin levels are undetectable, but in others activity can be as high as 10% of normal. The serum of patients with properdin deficiency is unable to activate C3 via the alternative pathway, resulting in an increased susceptibility to meningococcus infections. Patients with properdin deficiency have an intact classical pathway and normal levels of C3. Factors A, B, and D of the alternative pathway are present in normal concentrations as well. Properdin acts to stabilize the alternative pathway C3 convertase (C3bBb). Affected patients have recurrent pyogenic infections and fulminant meningococcemia. Isolated cases of lupus have been described.

Decay Accelerating Factor and CD59 Deficiency

Paroxysmal nocturnal hemoglobinuria is characterized by spontaneous episodes of red blood cell lysis. Erythrocytes, leukocytes, and platelets from these patients can be shown to have an increased sensitivity to lysis by complement because of cell membrane defects. Two molecules restrict the formation of the membrane attack complex on cell surface membranes. They are decay accelerating factor, which regulates the formation of C3 convertase, and CD59, the membrane inhibitor of reactive lysis. Deficiencies in these regulators of complement can contribute to red blood cell fragility and paroxysmal nocturnal hemoglobinuria.

Mini-index of Related Topics   CH.

SELECTED READINGS

Frank MM: Complement deficiencies. Pediatr Clin North Am 2000;47(6):1339–1354.

Sullivan KE, Winkelstein JA: Genetically Determined Deficiencies of the Complement System. In Ochs HD, Smith CIE, Puck JM (eds): Primary Immunodeficiency Diseases. New York, Oxford University Press, 1999, pp 397–416.

Walport MJ: Complement: First of two parts. N Engl J Med 2001; 344:1058–1066.

Walport MJ: Complement: Second of two parts. N Engl J Med 2001; 344:1140–1144.

169 Phagocytic and Leukocyte Abnormalities

Timothy R. La Pine and Harry R. Hill

ROLE OF THE GENERALIST

1. Recognize the signs and symptoms suggesting phagocytic immune deficiency.
2. Order appropriate laboratory tests to differentiate phagocytic immune deficiency from infection or other immune deficiency.
3. Arrange consultation with an immunologist for genetic counseling.
4. Arrange genetic consultation as indicated for assistance with diagnosis and management.
5. Assist specialists with laboratory studies and monitor treatment during infection in patients with phagocytic immune deficiency.
6. Assist the specialists with family education.
7. Be available to assist the family and patient with school and other psychosocial issues.

The phagocytic system includes polymorphonuclear leukocytes (neutrophils and eosinophils) and mononuclear phagocytes (circulating monocytes, tissue macrophages, and fixed macrophages). Major phagocytic functions include adherence to endothelial cells, aggregation, diapedesis, chemotaxis, attachment, phagocytosis, and degranulation, leading to pathogen destruction. The phagocytic system is responsible for defense against extracellular bacterial or fungal invasion in association with opsonins, antibodies, complement, and some acute phase proteins.

FUNDAMENTALS

Phagocytic cell development occurs when stem cells mature into neutrophils and monocytes within the fetal bone marrow by 5 months of gestation. This process is regulated by granulocyte (G) and monocyte (M) colony-stimulating factors (GM-CSF, G-CSF), interleukin 3 (IL-3), and interleukin 6 (IL-6). Neonatal neutrophils are not completely functional and show decreased activation, chemotaxis, degranulation, and killing abilities. During development the bone marrow stores of undifferentiated stem cells become committed to the myeloid lineage through interactions with stem cell factors, IL-3, and GM-

CSF. G-CSF and IL-6 act later to stimulate the differentiation of these myeloid precursors into mature neutrophils. The circulating half-life of neutrophils is approximately 8 hours and the tissue half-life is approximately 2 days. Any disruption in bone marrow function leads to a rapid decrease in neutrophil pools, resulting in a predisposition to infection. Following release from bone marrow stores, mature neutrophils must adhere to capillary endothelium and migrate through the endothelial cell surface to extravascular sites of infection. At the site of inflammation, neutrophils are further activated by bacteria and bacterial products as well as other inflammatory mediators to engulf invasive pathogens. Once ingested, superoxide radicals and other cytotoxic degranulating agents direct pathogen killing. Any alteration or disruption in this process, from neutrophil production and migration to pathogen annihilation, renders a host susceptible to infection, particularly with bacteria and fungal pathogens.

Neutrophils are one of the first lines of defense against bacterial invasion. Neutrophil disorders include defects in neutrophil production, leukocyte adhesion deficiency, Chédiak-Higashi syndrome, chronic granulomatous disease, and Job syndrome (hyperimmunoglobulinemia E syndrome).

PRESENTATION AND EVALUATION

Phagocytic and leukocyte immune defects should be considered in patients with signs and symptoms listed in Box 169-1. Assessment of phagocytic function requires complex, specialized testing that is most accurately and efficiently accomplished by referral to a pediatric immunologist. Box 169-2 lists tests used in the laboratory assessment of phagocytic function.

Box 169-1. Signs and Symptoms That Suggest a Phagocytic Disorder

1. Cutaneous bacterial abscesses, perirectal and oral ulcers, gingivitis, cellulitis, and mucocutaneous candidiasis
2. Frequent pneumonias, otitis media, and sinusitis
3. Osteomyelitis
4. Periodontitis and lymphadenitis
5. Granulomatous lesions

Box 169-2. Laboratory Assessment of Phagocytic Function

1. Complete blood cell count with absolute neutrophil count
2. Measurement of surface expression of selectins and integrins by flow cytometry
3. Chemotactic assays: Boyden chamber assay, under-agarose assay, migration assay, Rebuck skin window
4. Respiratory burst assays: nitroblue tetrazolium (NBT) dye reduction, dihydrorhodamine fluorescence, cytochrome C reduction
5. Phagocytosis and killing assays: colony count reduction

MANAGEMENT

Management of the primary disorder is best accomplished in conjunction with a specialist, and depends on the etiology of the disorder. The generalist is the primary care provider and must coordinate the recommendations of the specialists involved. This work involves communicating a health care plan with the families, providing ongoing health care surveillance, recognition and treatment of medical and surgical emergencies, and assistance with family support and education. Generalists can help families to adhere to proscribed regimens, such as assisting in the management of the eczematoid eruptions of Job syndrome and maintenance of prophylactic antibiotics when prescribed (see Chapter 279). It is particularly important that these children receive regular health maintenance with special attention paid to growth, development, safety issues, nutrition, and appropriate immunization.

Careful emergency management of acute issues is crucial. It is important to consider the type of immune deficiency and the most likely etiologic agents of infection. For example, patients with chronic granulomatous disease often develop severe pneumonias and other infections caused by *Staphylococcus* and a variety of other pathogens such as *Nocardia* and *Aspergillus*. Initial treatment consists of antibiotics directed against staphylococci and especially drugs that are known to penetrate into cells. The use of nafcillin or oxacillin along with agents such as rifampin or an aminoglycoside may provide the best coverage. Box 169-3 describes initial management and stabilization of acute disorders in these patients. Consultation with the specialist should be accomplished as soon as possible.

Box 169-3. Initial Stabilization of Serious Acute Illness in Patients with Granulocytic and Leukocyte Disorders

1. Admit for intravenous hydration and antibiotics.
2. Isolate the patient.
3. Pan-culture–this must include any indwelling catheters.
4. Remove any indwelling catheters as indicated.
5. Treat with broad-spectrum antibiotics.
6. Treat respiratory distress and shock as indicated.
7. Correct electrolyte imbalance, particularly hypocalcemia.
8. Screen for and correct coagulopathy.

SPECIFIC PHAGOCYTIC AND LEUKOCYTE DISORDERS

Neutrophil Production Defects

Neutropenia is defined as an absolute neutrophil count less than 1500 cells/μL, and clinically significant neutropenia occurs with absolute neutrophil counts of less than 500 cells/μL. Neutropenia can be either acquired or congenital in origin. Acquired neutropenias can be due to (1) bone marrow stem cell suppression, as in the case of pharmacologic toxicity; (2) increased neutrophil adherence to the microvasculature, as observed with complement activation and in severe burn patients; and (3) increased neutrophil destruction, as in hypersplenism or in cases of autoimmune or alloimmune neutropenia. Acquired neutropenia has also been associated with vitamin B_{12} or folate deficiency. Primary or metastatic bone marrow malignancy can present with neutropenia, and transient neutropenia can follow viral infections (Epstein-Barr virus, cytomegalovirus, parvovirus, and human immunodeficiency virus) or immunizations.

Congenital neutropenia consists of inherited neutrophil production defects. In the newborn, neutropenia may be a sign of sepsis. Kostmann syndrome or congenital agranulocytosis is one of a few of the inherited neutropenias. Neutrophil counts are reduced from birth. Bone marrow stores in these patients show maturational arrest of the promyelocytes and myelocytes. Kostmann syndrome is associated with an increased risk for acute myeloid leukemia. Defects in the G-CSF receptors are accountable for some, but not all, cases of Kostmann syndrome. Despite the defect in G-CSF receptor signaling, more than 90% of these patients respond to exogenous recombinant G-CSF. In patients refractory to G-CSF, stem cell transplantation from an HLA-matched siblings has shown to be beneficial. Cyclic neutropenia is another form of congenital neutropenia and is characterized by regular fluctuations in circulating neutrophil pools, which occur on 21-day cycles.

Treatment of cyclic neutropenia with recombinant G-CSF enhances absolute neutrophil counts but does not eliminate the cycling of cell counts, indicating that the underlying disorder is not solely associated with a G-CSF response. It is suspected that cyclic neutropenia arises from dysregulation of GM-CSF–responsive multipotent stem cell progenitors and neutrophil-specific G-CSF–responsive myeloid progenitors. Recently, cyclic neutropenia has been linked to a mutation in a gene located on chromosome 19p, which encodes neutrophil elastase. Other congenital disorders associated with neutropenia include Shwachman-Diamond syndrome, a rare autosomal recessive disorder that usually manifests in infancy characterized by exocrine pancreatic insufficiency, short stature, bone marrow dysfunction, and associated neutropenia. Numerous other features have been described in Shwachman-Diamond syndrome, including metaphyseal dysostosis, epiphyseal dysplasia, rib abnormalities, hematopoietic dysfunction, liver disease, growth failure, renal tubular defects, insulin-dependent diabetes mellitus, and psychomotor retardation. These patients respond to treatment with recombinant G-CSF or bone marrow transplantation and are also predisposed to leukemic transformation. Metabolic diseases (glycogen storage disease Ib and Gaucher disease) are also associated with neutropenia in the newborn period.

Leukocyte Adhesion Deficiency

Neutrophil adherence and migration through capillary endothelium is a critical early event in the acute inflammatory response. The adhesive interaction between neutrophils and endothelial cell surfaces is regulated by two novel families of glycoproteins: the integrins and the selectins. The beta-2 integrins are membrane-bound glycoprotein receptors found on the surface of neutrophils. The beta-2 integrins CD11/CD18 are required for neutrophil adherence to endothelial cell surfaces.

The selectins are also membrane-bound glycoproteins that mediate neutrophil adhesion to endothelial cells. These include L-selectin, which is found on the surface of neutrophils, P-selectin, and E-selectin, which are expressed on the surface of activated endothelial cells. The interaction between beta-2 integrins and the selectins serves to regulate neutrophil responses during inflammation. In general, P-selectin and E-selectin on the activated endothelial cells surface and L-selectin on the neutrophil cell surface function to facilitate neutrophil rolling and tethering to activated capillary endothelium. Once this tethering has occurred and the neutrophil itself is activated, the beta-2 integrin CD11/CD18 receptors on the neutrophil form a tight adhesion with the endothelial cell surface that facilitates neutrophil polarization leading to migration.

Two types of leukocyte adhesion deficiency (LAD) have been described. The first type is congenital beta-2 integrin CD11/CD18 deficiency (LAD-1). A second type, LAD-2, has been described resulting from a deficiency in the sialyl Lewis X, the neutrophil ligand for E-selectin, on endothelial cells. The deficiency of the CD11/CD18 complex (LAD-1) is transmitted as an autosomal recessive trait. The gene encoding CD18 has been mapped to chromosome 21. The underlying defect results from heterogeneous mutations affecting the CD18 gene, which impair its synthesis.

This disorder is characterized by frequent infections, poor wound healing, leukocytosis, and a history of delayed umbilical cord separation. Patients suffer from recurrent bacterial skin abscesses, otitis media, periodontitis, omphalitis, and perirectal abscesses, pneumonia, and sepsis. The striking feature of these infections is the almost total absence of leukocytes in the lesion. The prevalent invading microorganisms are *Staphylococcus aureus*, group A streptococci, *Proteus mirabilis*, *Pseudomonas aeruginosa*, and *Escherichia coli*. Based on severity, two phenotypes, severe and moderate, have been defined. The severe form is associated with a complete absence of the CD11/CD18 expression, but the moderate form demonstrates about 10% to 20% of normal expression. The degree of deficiency is closely related to the severity of the patient's clinical manifestations. Patients with these severe forms of leukocyte adhesion deficiency usually die within the first years of life. In contrast, patients with some expression of the adhesive glycoproteins usually have a mild disease course and can survive into adulthood.

The diagnosis is made by assessing the expression of CD11b or CD18 on the patient's neutrophils by flow cytometry. Further confirmation can be made by assessing the expression of these cell surface glycoprotein after exposure to a degranulating stimuli. The expression of these glycoproteins is increased fivefold to 20-fold after stimulation with the degranulating agent. This method is also helpful in identifying symptom-free heterozygous carriers in whom the expression of the glycoprotein is about half of that seen in normal carriers.

Treatment consists mainly of early, aggressive antibiotic therapy to reduce bacterial infections. During severe infections, granulocyte infusions in addition to antibiotics have shown therapeutic benefit. Bone marrow transplantation has been successful in treating some patients. Gene therapy, aimed at replacing the defective CD11 or CD18 genes in the patient's myeloid precursor cells may be available in the future. In vitro correction of CD18-deficient lymphocytes by retrovirus-mediated gene transfer has been accomplished. A transfection efficiency of about 5% to 10% may be sufficient to change the disease course from severe to moderate.

Job Syndrome

Job syndrome of hyperimmunoglobulinemia E and recurrent infections is transmitted by autosomal dominant inheritance with incomplete penetrance. It is characterized by extremely high IgE levels (often greater than 1000 to 2000 IU/mL), recurrent serious infections, and chronic eczematoid dermatitis usually beginning early in infancy. The infections primarily involve the skin and sinopulmonary tract and usually present as recurrent furunculosis, cutaneous abscesses, bronchitis, pneumonia, chronic otitis media, and sinusitis. Some skin abscesses are cold without classic signs and symptoms of inflammation (redness, heat, pain).

The most common infecting organisms include *Staphylococcus aureus* and *Candida albicans*. Infections caused by *Haemophilus influenzae*, group A streptococci, gram-negative pathogens, and fungi are also observed. Pneumatoceles, bronchiectasis, and bronchopleural fistula formation are not uncommon after episodes of acute or chronic pneumonia. Chronic mucocutaneous candidiasis, primarily involving the mouth, nails, skin, and vagina, is found in about one half of the patients. Associated features include coarse facial features with broad nasal bridge and broad nasal ali, growth retardation, osteoporosis and bone fractures, keratoconjunctivitis, asymmetric sterile polyarthritis, and eosinophilia. In addition to the markedly elevated IgE concentrations, other immunologic abnormalities include elevated specific anti-*Staphylococcus aureus* and anti-*Candida* IgE antibodies and intermittent defects in neutrophil chemotaxis, low antibody response to booster immunizations, and poor antibody and cell-mediated responses to newly encountered antigens. The underlying defect is most likely associated with T-cell abnormality characterized by inadequate production of interferon-gamma, which normally suppresses IgE production. The intermittent neutrophil chemotactic abnormality, which may have a major role in the pathogenesis of the recurrent abscesses seen in these patients, most likely results from this interferon-gamma deficiency.

Differentiation of patients with severe Job syndrome from those with atopic dermatitis is sometimes difficult and depends on the recurrence of abscesses along with classic facial features. Management consists of controlling the pruritic eczematoid dermatitis with emollient creams, topical steroids, and antihistamines. Prophylactic oral dicloxacillin or trimethoprim sulfamethoxazole for *Staphylococcus aureus* infections or oral fluconazole to prevent *Candida albicans* infection usually benefit the patients. Intravenous immunoglobulin therapy should be reserved for patients with confirmed IgG subclass deficiency and poor antibody formation, a finding rarely observed in our experience. Plasmapheresis has been attempted in a few patients who do respond to more conservative therapies with variable results.

Reported experimental immunotherapies include the use of Levamisol, ascorbic acid, cimetidine, and transfer factor. Interferon-gamma therapy has been shown to increase these patients' neutrophil chemotaxis response in vitro and to decrease eczema and respiratory secretions in vivo.

Chronic Granulomatous Disease

Chronic granulomatous disease (CGD) is a group of genetic disorders characterized by recurrent infections with catalase-positive microorganisms of the respiratory tract, skin, and soft tissues. Symptoms usually appear by 2 years of age. CGD has X-linked (65%) or autosomal recessive (35%) inheritance.

This defect is due to lesions in the membrane-associated NADPH-oxidase necessary for the production of oxygen radicals, which are required for intracellular killing. This results in the inability of phagocytes to generate superoxide anion, hydrogen peroxide, and other radicals needed to kill catalase-positive bacteria. The catalase-negative bacteria including pneumococcal, streptococcal, and *H. influenzae* species rarely cause serious infections in these patients. CGD should be suspected in any patient with subcutaneous abscesses or furunculosis associated with abscess formation in a lymph node, the liver, or the lung, or in patients with infections with organisms normally of low virulence (*Staphylococcus epidermidis*, *Serratia Marcescens*, *Aspergillus* species) that are catalase-positive. The underlying defect in X-linked CGD is due to the defect in a gene encoded on the X-chromosome that has been identified as the cytochrome B heavy chain (91 kD) gene. Autosomal recessive forms of CGD can be caused by the absence of the cytosolic phox 47, the cytosolic phox 67, or the cytochrome light chain (p22) encoded on chromosomes 7, 1, and 16, respectively.

The diagnosis of CGD is demonstrated by an absent or greatly diminished respiratory burst by stimulated phagocytes. Available assays include nitroblue tetrazolium dye reduction, dihydrorhodamine fluorescence, chemiluminescence, measurements of oxygen consumption, and production of superoxide anion and hydrogen peroxide. A documented inability of blood granulocytes to kill ingested catalase-positive bacteria confirms CGD. Symptom-free carriers of the X-linked form of CGD can be identified by determining the respiratory burst activity of their neutrophils, which is approximate half that of normal, and by genetic analysis.

Prenatal diagnosis can be made during the second trimester by sampling fetal blood cells with nitroblue tetrazolium or dihydrorhodamine fluorescence, which serves as a screen for superoxide production. Molecular reagents prepared from cloned DNA may also prove to be clinically useful for prenatal diagnosis in the future.

Prophylaxis with trimethoprim-sulfamethoxazole may prolong infection-free intervals by preventing infections, especially with *Staphylococcus* species. Therapy also includes treatment with interferon-gamma, which has decreased infections by as much as 70%, and bone marrow transplantation including the use of minitransplants to established chimerism, which to date has been of limited success and should be reserved for those patients who cannot optimally be treated in other ways. Patients with CGD may be excellent candidates for gene therapy.

Chédiak-Higashi Syndrome

The Chédiak-Higashi syndrome is an autosomal recessive disorder, which is characterized by recurrent pyogenic infections, a bleeding tendency caused by platelet storage pool deficiency, partial oculocutaneous albinism, and giant granules in the cytoplasm of many cells, particularly leukocytes. The underlying defect results from abnormal cell membrane fluidity, which leads to abnormal granular fusion as well as other defects, including the inability of neutrophils to move normally, concentrate serotonin in the platelets, and express normal lytic functions. Symptoms generally begin in early childhood with recurrent pyoderma, subcutaneous abscesses, otitis, sinusitis, severe periodontal disease, bronchitis, and pneumonia. The most common microorganisms are *Staphylococcus aureus*, and beta-hemolytic streptococci. Approximately 85% of the patients have an associated organ infiltration by histocytes and atypical lymphocytes. Hepatomegaly, lymphadenopathy, and neurologic abnormalities, along with pancytopenia and a bleeding tendency, are also seen in patients with Chédiak-Higashi syndrome.

The diagnosis is made by identification of the characteristic giant cytoplasmic granules in the patient's leukocytes or microscopic examination of hair shafts for giant melanosomes. Prenatal diagnosis is made possible by measuring large acid phosphatase positive lysosomes in cultured amniotic fluid cells, chronic villus cells, or fetal blood leukocytes.

In addition to prophylaxis with antibiotics, the management of patients with Chédiak-Higashi syndrome includes prompt treatment of acute infections with antimicrobial agents; high doses of ascorbate may also be beneficial. Bone marrow transplantation may be curative. Splenectomy has been used for the treatment of patients unresponsive to other forms of therapy and has resulted in clinical, hemologic, and immunologic improvement.

Mini-index of Related Topics

SUGGESTED READINGS

La Pine TR, Hill HR: Patients with recurrent infections and leukocyte abnormalities. In Wilson WR, Sande MA (eds): Current Diagnosis and Treatment in Infectious Diseases. Stamford, Conn, Lange, 2001, pp 356–370.

Puck JM: Primary immunodeficiency diseases. JAMA 1997;278:1835–1841.

Rosenzweig SD, Uzell G, Holland SM: Phagocytic disorders. In Stiehm ER, Ochs HD, Winkelstein JA (eds): Immunologic Disorders in Infants and Children, 5th ed. Philadelphia, Elsevier/Saunders, 2004, pp 618–651.

Stiehm ER, Ochs HD, Winklestein JA (eds): Immunologic Disorders in Infants and Children, 5th ed. Philadelphia, WB Saunders, 2004.

Yang KD, Quie PG, Hill HR: Phagocytic system in primary immune deficiency disease, a molecular genetic approach. In Ochs HD, et al (eds): Primary Immunodeficiency Disorders: A Molecular and Genetic Approach. New York, Oxford University Press, 2002, pp 82–96.

SECTION 4   CHRONIC MEDICAL CARE: *Disorders of the Immune System*

170 T- and B-Lymphocyte Disorders

Timothy R. La Pine and Harry R. Hill

ROLE OF THE GENERALIST

1 Recognize the signs and symptoms suggesting T-lymphocyte and B-lymphocyte immune deficiency.

2 Order appropriate laboratory tests to differentiate T- and B-lymphocyte immune deficiency from infection or other immune deficiency.

3 Arrange consultation with an immunologist for assistance with diagnosis and management.

4 Arrange genetic consultation as indicated for genetic counseling.

5 Assist specialists with laboratory studies and to monitor treatment during infections.

6 Assist the specialists with family education.

7 Be available to assist the family and patient with school and other psychosocial issues.

FUNDAMENTALS

With the exception of IgA deficiency, which is estimated to occur in 1 in 500 live births, immune deficiencies are rare. Although frequent infections in children are much more commonly related to exposure, generalists must have a high degree of suspicion so that children with these disorders can be diagnosed and appropriate therapy instituted.

T and B lymphocytes orchestrate both the cellular and humoral immune responses (see Chapter 10). A critical and delicate balance of cellular and humoral immune function is essential for complete immunologic responsiveness to invasive microbial pathogens. Any alteration in immune function or regulation may render a host susceptible to recurrent or life-threatening infections. The specific components of immune responsiveness are complex, requiring the close cooperation between a variety of cellular elements of both the T-lymphocytic and B-lymphocytic systems. Understanding specific functional mechanisms involved in lymphocyte production, activation, and migration; antibody and cytokine production; and pathogen annihilation is essential to appropriately evaluate a patient with suspected T- or B-lymphocyte immune deficiency.

The T-lymphocyte system effects and regulates delayed hypersensitivity reactions. The major function of the T-lymphocytic system is host defense against intracellular pathogens (fungi, viruses, protozoa, and intracellular bacteria such as mycobacteria and *Listeria* species). The T-lymphocytic system is involved with tumor surveillance, delayed hypersensitivity reactions, and graft-versus-host disease. The T-lymphocytic system orchestrates pathogen annihilation through antigen-dependent cellular interaction. Box 170-1 lists specific causes of T-cell immune deficiency disorders. Any defect in T-cell immunity is also associated with variable degrees of B-cell deficiency because most of the maturation, differentiation, and activation processes of B cells require T-cell help.

B-lymphocyte defects are the most frequently encountered primary immune deficiency syndromes, with IgA deficiency being the most common immune deficiency. B lymphocytes produce antibodies to the protein and carbohydrate antigens present on microorganisms, toxins, or other antigenic agents that are potentially harmful to

---

Box 170-1. Causes of T-cell Immune Deficiency Disorders

- Defects in maturation, differentiation, and activation of lymphopoietic stem cells
- Thymic defects including the thymic micro environment and associated humoral factors
- Specific T-lymphocyte defects
- Defective production of cytokines
- Defective expression of cytokine receptors
- Defective production of the regulatory proteins needed for T-cell activation
- Destruction of T cells

the host. Any defect in the maturation and differentiation of B cells (from the lymphopoietic stem cells to plasma cells and their secondary immunoglobulins) or T cells and their receptors or secretory cytokines may result in B-cell immune deficiency syndromes.

DIAGNOSIS AND EVALUATION

T- and B-lymphocyte abnormalities should be suspected in patients with the symptoms listed in Box 170-2. Deficiencies of the T-cell lymphocyte system should be considered in patients with symptoms listed in Box 170-3. Signs and symptoms associated with B-cell abnormalities are listed in Box 170-4. Initial evaluation of children with suspected immunologic defects begins with a thorough history. Pertinent information regarding infections includes the frequency and location of infections, exposure history (day care), recurrence of severe infections, unusual infections with opportunistic organisms, severe infections that are usually mild, and difficulty clearing infections. Other pertinent facts include family history, history of immunizations and reactions, and history of atopic disease. On physical examination, particular attention should be paid to growth parameters, dysmorphic features, skin rashes, telangiectasias, presence of thrush, absence of lymphoid tissues or enlarged lymph nodes, hepatosplenomegaly, signs of arthritis, and subcutaneous nodules.

Initial screening laboratory tests that may be helpful include complete blood cell count with differential, platelet count, and erythrocyte sedimentation rate. Screening tests for delayed hypersensitivity are helpful if a T-cell abnormality is suspected. In normal individuals, intradermal injections of *Candida*, mumps, diphtheria, tetanus, and other protein antigens cause induration (not just redness) within 24 to 48 hours, as committed T-cells produce cytokines, which recruit lymphocytes and macrophages to the injection site. Screening tests for suspected B-cell abnormalities include serum immunoglobulins, isohemagglutinins, and antibody titers to tetanus, diphtheria, *Haemophilus influenzae*, and pneumococci. Other tests that might be indicated, depending on the history, include chest x-ray, sinus x-ray, stool for ova and parasites, and human immunodeficiency virus (HIV) testing.

Patients with abnormal screening test and signs and symptoms of immune deficiency (see Box 170-2) should be referred to a specialist for assistance in diagnosis and long-

---

Box 170-2. Clinical Indicators of Possible T- or B-Lymphocyte Disorders

- Increased frequency of viral, fungal, and bacterial infections compared to patients of similar age and exposure risk
- Infections from common, usually nonpathogenic organisms
- Infections of prolonged duration that require prolonged antimicrobial therapy
- Incomplete clearing between infectious episodes
- Infections requiring surgical intervention
- Multiple complicated infections that involve different organ systems
- Infections with unusual or opportunistic organisms

Box 170-3. Clinical Indicators of Possible Defects of the T-Lymphocyte System

- Systemic illness after vaccination with live virus or with *Mycobacterium* species (bacille Calmette-Guérin vaccine)
- Chronic oral candidiasis and mucocutaneous candidiasis persisting after 6 months of age with resistance to therapy
- Graft-versus-host disease after blood transfusions
- Persistently low absolute lymphocyte counts
- Hypocalcemia or tetany with DiGeorge syndrome facies
- Intracellular infections (caused by bacteria, protozoa, viruses, or fungi)

---

term management. Laboratory tests commonly used by immunologist to diagnose T- and B-cell immune difficiency syndromes are listed in CD-ROM Boxes 170-1 and 170-2.

MANAGEMENT

Management of T- and B-cell disorders depends on the specific deficiency. The generalist is the primary care provider and must coordinate the recommendations of the specialists involved. This work involves communicating a health care plan with the families and recognition and treatment of medical and surgical emergencies. The generalist should be available to respond to acute care treatment issues, provide health care maintenance, and assist with family support and education.

It is important to consider the type of immune deficiency and the most likely etiologic agents of the infection. For example, patients with T-cell abnormalities should be considered for infections with fungal species and undergo screening of the kidneys and eyes for signs of occult infection. Patients with the Wiskott-Aldrich syndrome are particularly susceptible to infections with *Streptococcus pneumoniae*, *H. influenzae*, and other encapsulated bacteria. In the antibody-deficient patient, intravenous gamma globulin has been shown to reduce the severity of the illness and improve survival. Box 170-5 describes the initial emergency treatment of acute serious illness in patients with T- and B-cell disorders.

SPECIFIC T-CELL DISORDERS

Severe Combined Immune Deficiency
The most severe form of leukocyte immune deficiency consists of the syndromes of severe combined immune deficiency (SCID). This immune deficiency category includes a spectrum of X-linked, autosomal recessive, and

---

Box 170-4. Clinical Indicators of Possible Defects of the B-Lymphocyte System

- Decreased humoral immunity with variable to absent antibody isotype production
- Recurrent gastrointestinal or sinopulmonary infections
- Recurrent bacterial pneumonia or meningitis and severe sepsis
- Enteroviral or other viral infections
- Nodular lymphoid hyperplasia, autoimmunity, and malignancy

1. Admit for intravenous hydration and antibiotics.
2. Isolate the patient.
3. Pan-culture–this must include any indwelling catheters.
4. Remove any indwelling catheters as indicated.
5. Treat with broad-spectrum antibiotics.
6. Treat respiratory distress and shock as indicated.
7. Correct electrolyte imbalance, particularly hypocalcemia.
8. Screen for and correct coagulopathy.

sporadic genetic defects characterized by the inability to mount a normal T-lymphocyte (cell-mediated) and B-lymphocyte (humoral) immunity. These syndromes include X-linked SCID, adenosine deaminase deficiency, ZAP-70 deficiency, and other signaling defects that are characterized by onset of viral, bacterial, fungal, or protozoal infections before 6 months of age. Patients with SCID usually suffer from failure to thrive, persistent oral candidiasis, recurrent diarrhea, pneumonias (usually interstitial and often caused by *Pneumocystis carinii*) in the first months of life. Several immunologic defects are associated with similar clinical patterns. Seventy-five percent of the patients with SCID are male.

When SCID is suspected, infants should be referred to an immunologist. Infants lacking both T- and B-cell immunity, whose T lymphocytes are phenotypically normal but are unable to respond appropriately, should be evaluated by an immunologist for specific defects listed in CD-ROM Box 170-3. X-linked SCID, adenosine deaminase deficiency, and ZAP-70 deficiency are discussed in detail on the CD-ROM.

Purine Nucleoside Phosphorylase Deficiency

Purine nucleoside phosphorylase (PNP) deficiency is an extremely rare autosomal recessive disorder characterized by a deficiency in the enzyme purine nucleoside phosphorylase, which is associated with marked T-cell immune deficiency, with a relatively intact humoral immunity. These patients usually have recurrent viral, bacterial, and fungal infections. Two thirds have neurologic disorders ranging from developmental delay or muscle spasticity to severe mental retardation. Bone marrow or stem cell transplantation is the only successful therapy. Enzyme replacement therapy as well as viral gene transfer is currently being investigated as a promising future therapy in purine nucleoside phosphorylase deficiency.

DiGeorge Syndrome

DiGeorge syndrome is a polytropic developmental defect consisting of congenital aplasia or dysplasia of the thymus and parathyroid glands, leading to lymphopenia with decreased T-cell populations as a result of monosomy of chromosome 22q-11 (Chapter 157). T-cell immunity in DiGeorge syndrome is variable and ranges from diminished T-cell numbers to complete absence of T-cell immunity. Some DiGeorge syndrome patients have normal B-cell immunity as measured by normal concentrations of immunoglobulin and normal antibody responses after immunization. Other patients, however, have low immunoglobulin levels and fail to make specific antibody in response to immunization. Natural killer cell activity is normal in DiGeorge syndrome patients.

Treatment of patients with DiGeorge syndrome has included the implantation of fetal thymic tissue, fetal thymic epithelium, or fetal thymus in a diffusion chamber, all of which have demonstrated very limited success. Bone marrow transplantation, which provides the donor postthymic T cells to reconstitute the patient's immunity, has been used successfully to treat some patients with DiGeorge syndrome.

Wiskott-Aldrich Syndrome

Wiskott-Aldrich syndrome is an X-linked recessive disease characterized by recurrent pyogenic infections within the first years of life. Thrombocytopenia is characterized by small poorly functioning platelets. Eczema is also present at some time in most patients. Wiskott-Aldrich syndrome patients have low serum concentrations of IgM. IgA and IgE concentrations are high, and the IgG level is normal, elevated, or only slightly depressed. These patients are unable to produce antibody in response to polysaccharide antigens. T-cell numbers and function progressively decrease in this disorder, leading to profound leukopenia. Patients have increased susceptibility to autoimmune disorders and malignancy. Prenatal diagnosis can be made by fetal blood sampling with analysis of thrombocyte numbers and size. An analysis of the pattern of X-chromosome activation can detect carriers. Bone marrow or stem cell transplantation may correct the immunologic defect and platelet disorders.

Ataxia-Telangiectasia

Ataxia-telangiectasia, an autosomal recessive disorder, is thought to be a specific gene defect affecting mitogenic signal transduction, meiotic recombination, and cell cycle control. The defect can result in recombination errors that interfere with the rearrangement of T-cell and B-cell genes and the inability to repair damaged DNA. The defects observed in DNA repair in these patients after x-irradiation result in a high incidence of chromosomal translocation, specifically in chromosomes 7 and 14. Ataxia-telangiectasia is characterized by progressive cerebellar ataxia, oculocutaneous telangiectasia, chronic sinopulmonary disease, and a high incidence of malignancy. Clinically progressive ataxia becomes apparent when the child begins to walk. Telangiectasia develop between 2 and 8 years of age, predominantly on the bulbar conjunctivae as well as the exposed flexor surfaces of the arm and neck. Nearly 70% of the patients have a selective IgA deficiency and more than one half have an associated IgG2 subclass deficiency. Eighty percent of the patients have depressed or absent IgE levels.

The most notable T-cell abnormalities include leukopenia, a decrease in helper-inducer T-cell/cytotoxic-suppressor T-cell ratios, and a decrease in the total number of cytotoxic-suppressor T-cells. Serum α-fetoprotein level, which is persistently elevated in these patients, is a nonspecific aid in the diagnosis. Therapy consists of intravenous immunoglobulin using IgA-depleted preparations. Gene therapy for ataxia-telangiectasia is currently under investigation. Mothers of infants with ataxia-telangiectasia are at increased risk for the development of breast cancer.

SPECIFIC B-CELL LYMPHOCYTE DEFECTS

Selective IgA Deficiency

The incidence of selective IgA deficiency is about 1 in 400 to 1 in 1000 births. A gene located in the major histocompatibility complex class III region on chromosome 6 recently has been implicated in both selective IgA deficiency and common variable immune deficiency, suggesting a relationship between these two disorders. The cause of selective IgA deficiency appears to be a terminal block in B-cell differentiation into plasma cells capable of secreting the IgA isotype.

Symptoms of selective IgA deficiency are recurrent infections of the respiratory and gastrointestinal tracts, autoimmune disease, allergy, and malignancy. Approximately two thirds of the patients do not have an increased susceptibility to infection, presumably because of the protective effects of the IgG and IgM immunoglobulins.

Selective IgA deficiency has been defined as a serum IgA concentration of less than 5 mg/dL in severe deficiency and less than 2 SD below the mean of age-matched control subjects in partial deficiency. In some IgA-deficient patients, secretory IgA is low but present. Serum concentrations of IgA may return to normal within 4 years of diagnosis. These patients have normal T-cell immunity. Therapy is not possible in patients with selective IgA deficiency because the half-life of IgA is short, about 7 days. The intravenously administered IgA is not transported to the mucosal surfaces, and presence of anti-IgA autoantibodies in IgA-deficient patients may cause anaphylactic reactions when blood components containing IgA are transfused. About 20% of IgA-deficient patients with frequent infections have an associated IgG2 subclass deficiency. Some of these patients benefit from treatment with intravenous administration of immunoglobulin containing very low levels of IgA.

Bruton Agammaglobulinemia

Bruton agammaglobulinemia is an X-linked recessive disease that affects only boys and men. The underlying defect is an arrest in the differentiation of pre-B cells caused by the absence of Bruton tyrosine kinase, which functions in B-cell differentiation. Immunoglobulins of all classes and circulating immunoglobulin bearing mature B cells are absent. The absence of plasma cells in lymphoid tissue and the absence of functional serum antibody are hallmarks of the disorder. Clinically the defect is characterized by recurrent pyogenic infections, usually beginning around 5 to 6 months. Affected individuals may not be symptomatic before 6 months of age because of the presence of transplacentally acquired maternal IgG antibodies. Infections are usually caused by encapsulated bacterial pathogens, including *S. pneumoniae, Neisseria meningitidis,* and *H. influenzae* type b. Sinopulmonary infections are predominant. There is an unusual susceptibility to persistent echovirus or coxsackievirus infection, including lethal meningoencephalitis as well vaccine-associated poliomyelitis.

Approximately half of the patients have family histories of affected male siblings or maternal male relatives who are affected. Female carriers do not exhibit antibody deficiency and can be detected by analyzing the unbalanced pattern of X-chromosome inactivation in peripheral blood mononuclear cells. Prenatal diagnosis of suspected patients is facilitated by sex determination of the fetus and direct sampling of fetal blood or by DNA markers. Therapy consists of the administration of intravenous immunoglobulin and surveillance for infection, for lymphoreticular and other malignancies, and for autoimmune disorders.

X-Linked Hypogammaglobulinemia with Normal to Increased IgM Concentrations

Patients with this immune deficiency have an increased IgM concentration, recurrent pyogenic infections, autoimmune disease, and lymphoproliferative disease, especially of IgM surface-bearing B-cell lymphomas of the gastrointestinal tract. The hyper-IgM syndrome can be inherited in an X-linked or an autosomal recessive fashion. The underlying cause of X-linked hyper-IgM syndrome is a deficiency in expression of T-cell CD40 ligand, which specifically binds B cells and drives immunoglobulin isotype switching. The gene for CD40 ligand has been cloned and mapped to Xq-26. Concentrations of serum IgM and in some cases IgD are increased, and IgG, IgA, and IgE are decreased or absent. T-cell numbers and function, other than the absence of the CD40 ligand, appear to be normal.

Neutropenia is commonly associated with this disease and nearly half of these patients have hepatosplenomegaly. Chronic liver disease and lymphomas are long-term clinical abnormalities seen in this disorder. Some patients have increased susceptibility to opportunistic infections such as *P. carinii* pneumonia. Prenatal diagnosis can be performed by DNA analysis or flow cytometry for the CD40 ligand on the T cells. Bone marrow and stem cell transplantation have recently been attempted in the treatment of hyper-IgM syndrome. Replacement therapy with recombinant soluble form of the CD40 ligand or gene therapy may be developed for these patients in the near future.

Common Variable Immune Deficiency

B cells do not differentiate into plasma cells in common variable immune deficiency (CVID) or acquired hypogammaglobulinemia. This lack may be due to a primary B-cell defect (failure to glycosylate and secrete immunoglobulins) or a failure of helper T-cell factor production, or an increase in specific suppressor T-cell effects. The immunologic defect is seen in B cells, macrophages, and immunoregulatory T cells. CVID is characterized by markedly decreased serum immunoglobulin levels, normal or nearly normal numbers of circulating immunoglobulin-bearing mature B cells, and impaired antibody responses. The defect in T-cell immunity includes abnormalities of activation and lymphokine production that usually progress with age. Many patients (11%) with CVID have first-degree relatives with selective IgA deficiency or CVID. Susceptibility group of genes for both CVID and selective IgA deficiency are located within the major histocompatibility complex class III region of chromosome 6. In both disorders exogenous factors that act intrinsically or extrinsically on genetically susceptible individuals appear to determine the degree of expression of the immunoglobulin genes.

Patients with CVID commonly have chronic diarrhea and associated malabsorption. They may have recurrent bacterial sinopulmonary infections associated with chronic, progressive bronchiectasis. Autoimmune disease, hepatitis, gastrocarcinoma, and lymphoreticular malignancy have been observed in older patients. Nodular intestinal lymphoid hyperplasia and a sarcoid-like syndrome associated with hepatosplenomegaly are additional features of this disease. Sporadic cases of X-linked agammaglobulinemia can be differentiated from CVID in male infants with recurrent infections and significant hypogammaglobulinemia by the absence of mature immunoglobulin B cells in the peripheral blood or X-chromosome inactivation analysis of the patient's mother. Management of CVID involves immunoglobulin replacement therapy, antimicrobial therapy, pulmonary drainage, and possibly immunomodulatory therapies, including the use of recombinant IL-2 conjugated with polyethylene glycol.

Additional Resources, CD-ROM

Laboratory assessment of T-cell immunity	Box
Laboratory assessment of B-cell immunity	Box
Evaluation of suspected severe combined immunodeficiency (SCID)	Box
X-linked SCID	Text
Adenosine deaminase deficiency	Text
Zap-70 deficiency	Text
Bibliography	

Mini-index of Related Topics

SUGGESTED READINGS

Bordignon C, Notarangelo LD, Nobili N, et al: Gene therapy in peripheral blood lymphocytes and bone marrow for ADA immunodeficient patients. Science 1995;270:470–475.

La Pine TR, Hill HR: Patients with recurrent infections and leukocyte abnormalities. In Wilson WR, Sande MA (eds): Current Diagnosis and Treatment in Infectious Diseases. Stamford, Conn, Lange, 2001, pp 356– 370.

Ochs HD, Stiehm ER, Winkelstein JA (eds): Antibody deficiencies. In Immunologic Disorders in Infants and Children, 5th ed. Philadelphia, Elsevier/Saunders, 2004, pp 365–462.

Puck JM: Primary immunodeficiency diseases. JAMA 1997;278:1835–1841.

171 Human Immunodeficiency Virus Infection

Joseph A. Church

ROLE OF THE GENERALIST

1 Identify children and adolescents at risk for human immunodeficiency virus (HIV) infection.

2 Diagnose HIV infection in children 18 months of age or older with appropriate antibody assay (ELISA) interpretation.

3 Initiate postnatal antiretroviral therapy in newborns identified prenatally as at risk for HIV.

4 Refer HIV-infected children and at-risk newborns for multidisciplinary center management.

5 Comanage, in selected cases, HIV-infected patients, recognizing that the potential risks of complications are related to T-cell numbers and HIV virus load.

6 Advise mothers on the risks of HIV transmission from breast milk and the potential risks of administration of live virus vaccines.

7 Provide long-term follow-up for uninfected children exposed to HIV or antiretroviral drugs, observing for hematologic, metabolic, and neurologic complications.

8 Recognize the social and legal implications of school and community disclosures of HIV diagnosis.

9 Consistently practice standard precautions for all patients in the office setting.

10 Counsel families with regard to HIV risk from needle stick injuries that may occur outside the medical setting.

Table 171-1. Laboratory Criteria for Surveillance Case Definition of HIV Infection

1. Adults, adolescents, children 18 months of age or older
   A. Confirmed positive test for HIV antibody
   or
   B. Positive virologic test:
      HIV nucleic acid (DNA or ANA detection)
      HIV p24 antigen test
      HIV isolation (culture)
2. Children younger than 18 months of age
   A. Positive results on two separate specimens (excluding cord blood) using any of the following HIV virologic tests:
      HIV nucleic acid (DNA or RNA detection)
      HIV p24 antigen test
      HIV isolation (culture)

From Centers for Disease Control and Prevention: Guidelines for national human immunodeficiency virus case surveillance, including monitoring for human immunodeficiency virus infection and acquired immunodeficiency syndrome. MMWR Morb Mortal Wkly Rep 1999;48(RR):29–31.

The clinical disorder acquired immunodeficiency syndrome (AIDS) represents the most serious clinical consequences of retrovirus-induced immune dysregulation. The disease is caused by a retrovirus, human immunodeficiency virus-1 (HIV-1). The pathophysiology of the disorder is characterized by both immune deficiency and pathologic immune activation.

The Centers for Disease Control and Prevention (CDC) has defined HIV infection in children according to the age at which maternal antibody is likely to represent a significant influence on standard assays (Table 171-1). The CDC also has developed a specific classification system to describe the clinical (Table 171-2) and immunologic (Table 171-3) features of the disease in children. The clinical and immunologic categories are combined to provide a pediatric HIV classification (Table 171-4). The classification system defines patients at their worst clinical and immunologic states. The assigned class does not change even if a patient improves with treatment. Many patients with "AIDS/category 3" are now clinically well and immunologically competent.

First described in 1981 as "gay-related immune deficiency" (GRID), the current term *acquired immunodeficiency syndrome (AIDS)* was adopted in 1982. The first cases of pediatric AIDS were reported in 1983. Other major events in HIV/AIDS history are outlined in CD-ROM Table 171-1.

FUNDAMENTALS

Pathogenesis

HIV is a member of the *Lentivirus* genus of the Retroviridae family. An appreciation of virus structure and replicative cycle is essential for understanding the pathogenesis of HIV-associated disease and the potential for therapeutic intervention. The virus envelope consists of a lipid bilayer studded with virus-specific glycoproteins and variable host cell proteins (Fig. 171-1). A glycoprotein of 120 kd molecular weight (gp120), a crucial feature of the HIV surface membrane, plays an essential role in determining HIV target cell tropism and interacts with CD4 and chemokine receptors on the surfaces of its target cells: "helper" T cells, monocytes, macrophages, and microglia (macrophage-related cells) in the brain.

Table 171-2. Clinical Categories and Criteria for Children with HIV Infection

Category	Description of Criteria
Category N	Not symptomatic
	No surgery or treatment considered a result of HIV infection
	Only one condition tested in category A
Category A	Mildly symptomatic
	Two or more of the following:
	Lymphadenopathy
	Hepatomegaly
	Splenomegaly
	Diarrhea
	Nausea
	Recurrent or persistent upper respiratory tract infections, sinusitis, otitis media
	No condition in categories B and C
Category B	Moderately symptomatic
	Symptomatic conditions other than those listed in categories A and C
	May include, but not limited to
	Anemia (<8.5), neutropenia (<1000), thrombocytopenia (<100,000 ≥30 days)
	>2 months thrush in child >6–12 months of age
	Single episode of bacterial meningitis, pneumonia, sepsis
	Specified herpes virus infection
	Cardiomyopathy
	Nephropathy
	Diarrhea (recurrent/chronic)
	Lymphoid interstitial pneumonitis (LIP)/pulmonary lymphoid hypertrophy (PLH)
Category C	Severely symptomatic (except for LIP, meets criteria of case definition of acquired immunodeficiency syndrome, AIDS)
	Specified opportunistic infections (abbreviated list):
	Pneumocystis carinii pneumonia (PCP)
	Mycobacterium avium complex (MAC/MAI)
	Disseminated *Mycobacterium tuberculosis*
	Histoplasmosis
	Candidiasis (esophageal or pulmonary)
	Severe bacterial infections (multiple or recurrent, two or more infections over 2 years)
	Specified lymphomas
	Wasting syndrome
	Encephalopathy

From Centers for Disease Control and Prevention: 1994 revised classification system for human immunodeficiency for human immunodeficiency virus infection in children less than 13 years of age. MMWR Morb Mortal Wkly Rep 1994;43(RR12): 1–10.

Table 171-4. Combined Clinical and Immunologic Classification of Pediatric HIV Infection*

Immunologic Category	Clinical Categories (Signs/Symptoms)			
	N: None	A: Mild	B:† Moderate	C:† Severe
1. No evidence of suppression	N1	A1	B1	C1
2. Evidence of moderate suppression	N2	A2	B2	C2
3. Severe suppression	N3	A3	B3	C3

*Children whose HIV infection status is not confirmed are classified by using the above grid with a letter E (for perinatally exposed) placed before the appropriate classification code (e.g., EN2).
†Both category C and lymphoid interstitial pneumonitis in category B are reportable to state and local health departments as acquired immunodeficiency syndrome (AIDS).

From Centers for Disease Control and Prevention: 1994 revised classification system for human immunodeficiency virus infection in children less than 13 years of age. MMWR Morb Mortal Wkly Rep 1994;43(RR12):1–10.

target cell nucleus where it integrates into the host-cell genome. In this form it constitutes a "provirus," which may remain hidden inside the infected cell for prolonged periods of time. Activation of the infected host cell initiates proviral DNA transcription, production of HIV-specific genomic RNA and messenger RNA, and translation of viral messenger RNA to virus-specific proteins. Virus-specific proteins are processed and assembled, and free virions bud and are released from the infected cell surface. Over 10 billion virus particles are produced daily.

The host cell targets of HIV are crucial components of the immune system. When confronted with pathogens, these cells normally produce a coordinated, protective effector response. The molecular signals that activate normal cell responses to pathogens are read by the HIV proviral DNA as signals to initiate replication.

Three pathologic consequences of HIV infection induce recognizable patterns of clinical disease: progressive immunologic attrition and immune deficiency, central nervous system infection, and uncontrolled immune activation (Fig. 171-3). Because functional CD4+ T cells are required for the generation of protective, antigen-specific T-cell and antibody responses, T-cell loss and impaired T-cell production eventually induce an acquired, combined immune deficiency. Progressive susceptibility to opportunistic infections results. Although the neurons in the central nervous system are not specific targets for HIV, it infects and activates local microglial cells in the brain. These activated macrophage-like cells generate a variety of cytokines that cause

Following tight adhesion of the virus to target cells, the respective membranes fuse through the action of another viral membrane protein, gp41. Viral RNA along with virus-specific reverse transcriptase enters the cytoplasm of the target cell (Fig. 171-2). Viral genomic RNA is "reversely transcribed" to DNA, which is then transported to the

Table 171-3. Immunologic Categories of HIV Disease Based on Age-Specific CD4+ T-Lymphocyte Counts

Immunologic Category	Age of Child		
	<12 Mo mL (%)	1–5 Yr mL (%)	6–12 Yr mL (%)
1. No evidence of suppression	≥1500 (≥25)	≥1000 (≥25)	≥500 (≥25)
2. Evidence of moderate suppression	750–1499 (15–24)	500–999 (15–24)	200–499 (15–24)
3. Severe suppression	<750 (15)	<500 (<15)	<200 (<15)

From Centers for Disease Control and Prevention: 1994 revised classification system for human immunodeficiency virus infection in children less than 13 years of age. MMWR Morb Mortal Wkly Rep 1994;43(RR12):4.

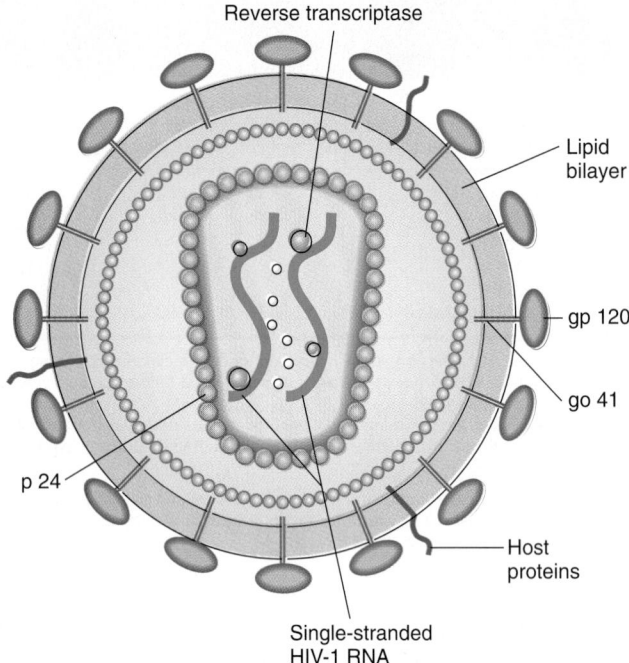

Figure 171-1. Schematic diagram of an HIV virion.

activation-induced programmed cell death of neurons in close proximity to the infected cells, resulting in signs and symptoms of neuroencephalopathy. HIV may also induce an inappropriate and uncontrolled activation of infected target cells, producing a variety of proliferative disorders, such as lymphoid interstitial pneumonitis, lymphadenopathy, and hepatosplenomegaly, and systemic features of chronic infection, including fatigue, fever, and wasting.

Epidemiology
Vertical transmission of HIV from mother to newborn has always been the primary route of transmission to infants, although before 1985 HIV was transmitted to a significant number of children through contaminated blood products.

Maternal risk factors for HIV differ significantly by geographic area in the United States. Injecting drug use among women of childbearing age is a major risk factor. In the developing world, heterosexual transmission from infected men to women is responsible for the vast majority of HIV infections in women. Untreated, approximately 20% of infected women will transmit HIV infection to their newborn. Three general models have been proposed for this transmission (Fig. 171-4). In intrauterine transmission the placenta is invaded and HIV infects the unborn fetus. Intrapartum transmission late in the third trimester or during labor and delivery is believed to be the route of transmission in over 80% of infected infants. Breast-feeding transmits HIV to approximately 15% of otherwise uninfected newborns at risk. Most factors that increase the risk for maternal-fetal transmission of HIV are related to the state of the maternal HIV disease, including increased maternal symptoms, reduced maternal CD4+ T cells, and increased maternal plasma virus levels. Additional factors are premature delivery, premature rupture of membranes, amnionitis, instrumentation at delivery, and vaginal delivery in a mother who has not been treated.

Although new adult infections in the United States remain stable at about 40,000 cases per year, the number of babies born with HIV infection has dropped from an estimated 1600 in 1994 to less than 200 in the year 2001. This dramatic decline has been due to intense public health efforts to identify HIV-infected pregnant women, to counsel against breast-feeding by these women, to initiate or maintain effective antiretroviral therapy of infected women, and to provide postnatal prophylaxis to their newborn infants.

Antepartum and intrapartum zidovudine (AZT) treatment of the mother and a 6-week postnatal zidovudine treatment course of the newborn infant has been shown to reduce the risk of maternal-HIV transmission by two thirds. This regimen is now recommended as minimal intervention in all HIV-positive pregnant women and their newborns. Addition of lamivudine or nevirapine to the newborn's regimen has theoretic advantages.

Figure 171-2. Replicative cycle of HIV.

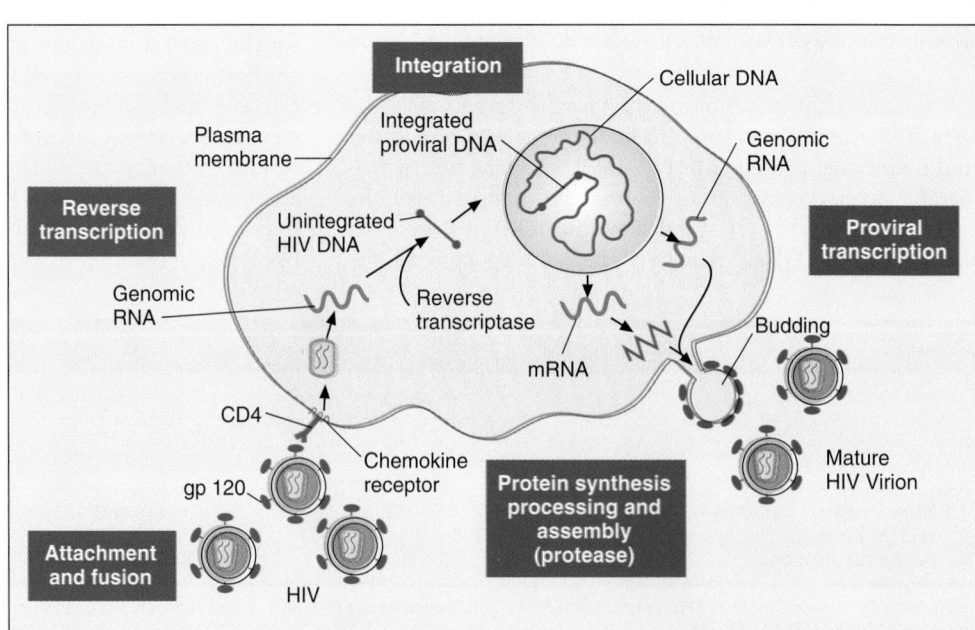

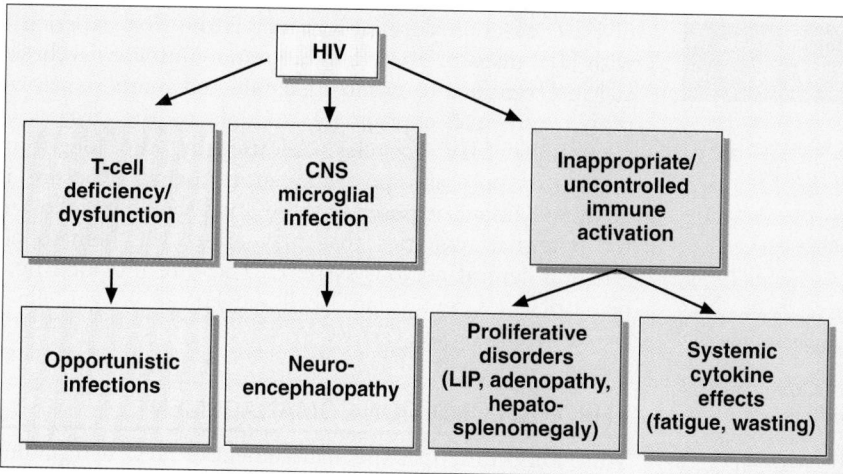

Figure 171-3. Pathophysiologic processes in HIV infection. LIP, lymphocytic interstitial pneumonia.

The CDC estimates that half of all new cases in the United States are younger than 25 years of age. Adolescents at risk for HIV infection are those that engage in "adult" high-risk behaviors including multiple sexual partners, male homosexual encounters, and injection drug use.

DIAGNOSIS

HIV infection causes a remarkable spectrum of clinical manifestations. Infected children may display few or no symptoms for more than 10 years before developing a complication suggestive of a compromised immune status. HIV testing should be considered in children presenting with signs or symptoms of immune dysfunction and in selected asymptomatic children and adolescents (Table 171-5).

The standard HIV antibody assays, including enzyme-linked immunosorbent assay (ELISA) and western blot assay, detect primarily IgG antibodies with a very high degree of sensitivity and specificity. After 18 months of age, these assays are highly specific for the diagnosis of HIV infections. Virtually all infants born to HIV-positive women will have positive antibody test results because of the active transport of maternal IgG across the placenta. Because

maternal antibody may remain detectable in some uninfected children for up to 18 months of age, a child younger than 18 months of age is considered to be HIV-infected only if he or she has positive test results on two separate occasions (excluding cord blood testing) with tests that directly measure virus or viral components, including HIV culture, polymerase chain reaction (PCR) for HIV DNA, and p24 antigen assay. HIV DNA PCR is the preferred virologic method for diagnosing HIV infection during infancy. HIV can be reasonably excluded in infants with two or more negative HIV DNA PCR tests, two of which are performed at 1 month of age or older, and one performed at 4 months of age or older.

Table 171-5. Indications for HIV Testing of Infants

Symptomatic Patients

Failure to thrive
Development delay or regression
Symptoms of congenital toxoplasmosis, rubella, cytomegalovirus, herpes (TORCH) infections
"Opportunistic" infections (including thrush in a child over 1 year old, or recurrent, severe vaginal yeast infection)
Recurrent, severe bacterial infections
Chronic or recurrent diarrhea
Hepatomegaly
Splenomegaly
Lymphadenopathy
B-cell or CNS lymphoma
Extrapulmonary mycobacterial infection
Unexplained:
   Wasting
   Neuro-encephalopathy
   Myopathy
   Hepatitis
   Cardiomyopathy
   Nephropathy

Asymptomatic Patients

HIV+ parent
Parent at high risk (sex, drugs)
Blood transfusion before June 1985 or in a country where blood not screened
International adoptees
History of sexual abuse
Adolescent with history of multiple sex partner, sexually transmitted diseases, or illicit injection drug use

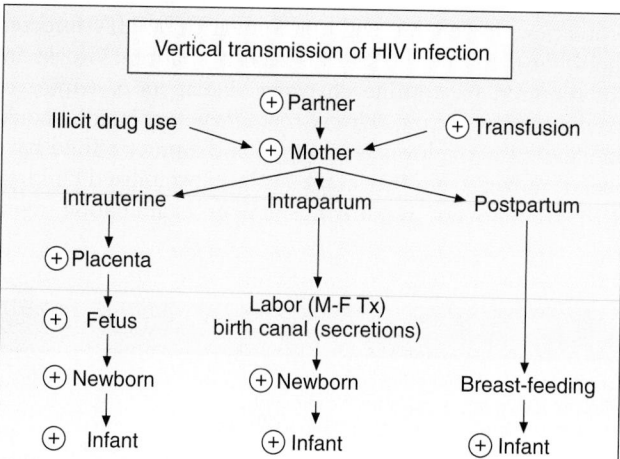

Figure 171-4. Mechanisms of HIV transmission from mother to infant. M-F Tx, maternal-fetal transmission.

Table 171-6. Management of the Newborn at Risk for HIV Infection

Antiretroviral therapy
    Zidovudine (AZT): beginning 8–12 hours after birth, oral administration of zidovudine (AZT) syrup at 2 mg/kg of body weight per dose every 6 hours for 6 weeks
    Consider an additional agent in high-risk newborns:
    ■ Lamivudine (3TC) 2 mg/kg of body weight per dose every 12 hours for 6 weeks
    or
    ■ Nevirapine 2 mg/kg of body weight at birth (if mother has not received this drug); one additional dose at 48–72 hours of age
Avoid breast-feeding
Obtain blood for HIV DNA polymerase chain reaction (PCR) within 48 hours of age; repeat at 2 weeks and at 1 month of age
Begin *Pneumocystis carinii* pneumonia prophylaxis at 6 weeks of age with trimethoprim (TMP)-sulfamethoxazole 5 mg TMP/kg body weight once daily or twice a day 3 days per week

From Public Health Service Task Force Perinatal HIV Guidelines Working Group: Summary of the updated recommendations from the Public Health Service Task Force to reduce perinatal human immunodeficiency virus-1 transmission in the United States. Obstet Gynecol 2002;99(6):1117–1126.

MANAGEMENT OF THE HIV-EXPOSED NEWBORN

Crucial components of the management of the newborn born to an HIV-infected mother include antiretroviral therapy, avoidance of breast-feeding, testing to determine the infant's HIV infection status, and prophylaxis for *Pneumocystis carinii* pneumonia (Table 171-6). Zidovudine should be started at 8 to 12 hours after birth and should be given at 2 mg/kg per dose every 6 hours for 6 weeks. In infants born to mothers who have had little or no prenatal care, or whose own clinical or virologic status suggests an increased likelihood of transmission, a second agent may be added. Lamivudine (3TC) may be given at 2 mg/kg every 12 hours for 6 weeks along with the zidovudine. Alternatively, nevirapine 2 mg/kg may be given at birth if the mother has not received nevirapine in the immediate perinatal period; a single additional dose may be given at 48 to 72 hours of age. The infant's mother should be counseled against breast-feeding. An initial laboratory evaluation includes HIV DNA PCR on cord or peripheral blood within 48 hours of birth. DNA PCR should be repeated at 2 weeks and at 1 month of age. At 6 weeks of age, prophylaxis with trimethoprim-sulfamethoxazole should be initiated to prevent *P. carinii* pneumonia.

REFERRALS

All HIV-infected pregnant women should be managed in perinatal centers where the care of high-risk pregnancies seamlessly proceeds to the care of at-risk newborns. Because of the complexity of current (and very rapidly developing) anti-HIV therapy, all children demonstrated to be infected with HIV should be referred to a pediatric HIV/AIDS center. Pediatric HIV center management for these infants provides significant advantages for the medical, psychosocial, and other supportive aspects of patient care. Uninfected infants born "at risk" also benefit from HIV center care. In many families, the identification

of HIV infection during pregnancy is the first experience with HIV disease. These families require intense psychosocial interventions to ensure that infected mothers receive proper care and appropriate referrals to the myriad of community HIV agencies. Additionally, the long-term impact of pre- and postnatal antiretroviral exposure is unknown. Infants exposed to these drugs should be followed for potential toxicities that may affect the hematopoietic and central nervous systems. The care provided by a pediatric HIV center and T-cell and HIV RNA guidelines are described on the CD-ROM.

CHRONIC CONDITION COMANAGEMENT

Table 171-7 describes the management of HIV. Two guiding principles must be considered in the long-term comanagement of children with HIV: The lower a patient's T-cell count, the more likely that the acute process is a serious one, and close communication between the comanaging generalist and the HIV specialist is crucial.

Office Infection Control

Occupational HIV infection can be effectively prevented. "Standard precautions" focus on the specific types of potentially infected body fluids rather than on individual patients and include protection from sharps injuries, or mucous membrane contamination with selected body fluids including blood, genital secretions, cerebrospinal fluid, or body fluids likely to be contaminated with blood. Unless visible blood contamination is apparent, specific barrier protection (gloves and gowns) is not indicated for feces, urine, vomitus, nasal secretions, saliva, and sweat. HIV transmission occurs approximately once in 250 to 500 injuries with HIV-contaminated sharps. Transmission risk is increased with exposure to larger amounts of virus, either by fluids with high levels of HIV or by exposure to large volumes of contaminated body fluid. Table 171-8 lists CDC guidelines for provision of postexposure prophylaxis following percutaneous injuries or mucous membrane or nonintact skin exposures. Emphasis must be placed on safe handling of needles, avoidance of recapping used needles, and use of puncture-resistant containers for disposal of used sharps. For minor surgical procedures such as wound suturing, double gloving provides some additional degree of protection. In general, children known to be HIV-infected should be managed the same as healthy children. Gloves are not required for routine changing of diapers or wiping of nasal secretions. In the delivery room, newborn infants should be handled with gloves until blood and amniotic fluid have been removed from the infant's skin. Hospitalized children with HIV do not require hospital or examination room

Table 171-7. HIV Disease Management

Antiretroviral drug therapy
Prophylaxis against opportunitic infections
Selective use of intravenous immunoglobulin
Nutritional support
Social support
Psychological support

Table 171-8. Recommended Postexposure Prophylaxis (PEP) in the Health Care Setting

Type of Exposure	HIV Status of Source	Prophylaxis
Perentaneous injuries		
Less severe	HIV+, Class 1*	Two drugs
	HIV+, Class 2†	Three drugs
	Unknown	NA (consider two drugs)
More severe	HIV+, Class 1 and Class 2	Three drugs
	Unknown	NA (consider two drugs)
Mucous membrane or nonintact skin		
Small volume	HIV+, Class 1*	Consider two drugs
	HIV+, Class 2†	Two drugs
	Unknown	NA (consider two drugs)
Large volume	HIV+, Class 1*	Two drugs
	HIV+, Class 2†	Three drugs
	Unknown	NA (consider two drugs)

*Class 1: asymptomatic HIV infection or low viral load.
†Class 2: symptomatic HIV infection, AIDS, acute seroconversion, or known high viral load.
NA, not advisable.

From Centers for Disease Control and Prevention: Updated US Public Health Service guidelines for the management of occupational exposure to HBV, HCV, and HIV. MMWR Morb Mortal Wkly Rep 2001;50(RRII):1–42.

isolation unless they have other conditions that require such isolation.

Day Care and School Issues

HIV-infected children should be admitted without restriction to schools and childcare facilities and allowed to participate in all activities that their health allows, including competitive sports. Informing childcare and school personnel of a child's HIV infection is not required. Schools and day care facilities must have guidelines to manage potential exposures to blood or blood-containing materials.

Potential HIV Exposures Outside the Medical Setting

There are no national guidelines for the management of potential HIV exposures outside the medical setting. Accidental needle stick injury from discarded needles and syringes found in the urban environment generate significant anxiety. The efficacy of providing postexposure prophylaxis in such cases has not been proved. A decision to initiate antiretroviral therapy must be based on the assessment of risk of infection and potential adverse effects of the prescribed medications. Postexposure prophylaxis is an accepted practice for health care workers with occupational injuries and after sexual assault from sources known or likely to be HIV infected. Consultation with physicians trained in the assessment of risk and initiation of prophylaxis is strongly recommended.

Psychosocial Issues

Family centered social support is crucial for children with any catastrophic disease. HIV disproportionately affects poor children, particularly in African-American and Latino communities. Affected families have extensive material needs. Transportation to medical visits, arrangement for medical care of other HIV-infected family members, emotional support of uninfected family members, advice on legal issues surrounding immigration and guardianship issues, and assistance in securing food, shelter, and clothing are all needs that must be addressed.

Acute Care Issues
Adverse Effects of HIV Medications

Adverse medication reactions are very common in HIV patients and may develop acutely or after prolonged exposure to various drugs. The primary side effects associated with these agents are listed in Table 171-9. The long-term impact of antiretroviral agents on metabolism and bone is concerning. HIV-associated lipodystrophy affects adults and has been noted in children. This is associated with increased abdominal girth, increased dorsocervical fat pad, and peripheral fat loss characterized by thinning of the extremities and buttocks. Further metabolic complications may include insulin resistance and diabetes, and hyperlipidemia with elevated cholesterol and triglyceride levels. Osteopenia is an emerging complication. Adverse effects are more common in patients on long-term therapy or with other complications of HIV disease.

Fever

Although potentially a sign of an underlying malignancy or of HIV infection itself, fever is usually an indication of secondary infection. A "routine" infection must be differentiated from an "opportunistic" infection. Risk for developing an opportunistic infection is directly related to the degree of the immune suppression in an individual child. An opportunistic infection is less likely, the closer the CD4 count is to "normal." One to 2 days of fever with symptoms of a routine childhood infection is not alarming in children whose T-cell counts are "good" or better. High-risk indicators that should prompt consultation with the child's HIV physician are high-grade fever associated with marked T-cell depletion, marked elevation of HIV RNA, or indwelling central venous catheter.

Oral Lesions

HIV-infected children with dental and gingival disease, such as aphthous ulcers, herpes stomatitis, and oral candidiasis, should be referred to a pediatric dentist in a timely fashion. Aphthous ulcers may be difficult to differentiate from lesions of herpes simplex virus. Empiric therapy with

Table 171-9. Primary Side Effects Associated with Antiretroviral Agents

Antiretroviral Classes and Agents	Primary Side Effects and Toxicities
Nucleoside Reverse Transcriptase Inhibitors (NRTIs)	
Zidovudine (Retrovir; ZDV; AZT)	Anemia, neutropenia, nausea, headache, insomnia, muscle pain, and weakness
Lamivudine (Epivir; 3TC); Emtricitabine (Emtriva)	Abdominal pain, nausea, diarrhea, rash, and pancreatitis
Stavudine (Zerit; d4T)	Peripheral neuropathy, headache, diarrhea, nausea, insomnia, anorexia, pancreatitis, increased liver function tests (LFTs), anemia, and neutropenia
Didanosine (Videx; ddl)	Pancreatitis, lactic acidosis, neuropathy, diarrhea, abdominal pain, and nausea
Zalcitabine (Hivid; ddC)	
Abacavir (Ziagen; ABC)	Nausea, diarrhea, anorexia, abdominal pain, fatigue, headache, insomnia, and hypersensitivity reactions
Tenofovir (Viread, TNV)	Nausea, diarrhea, vomiting
Non-nucleoside Reverse Transcriptase Inhibitors (NNRTIs)	
Nevirapine (Viramune; NVP)	Rash (including case of Stevens-Johnson syndrome), fever, nausea, headache, hepatitis, and increased LFTs
Delavirdine (Rescriptor; DLV)	Rash (including case of Stevens-Johnson syndrome), nausea, diarrhea, headache, fatigue, and increased LFTs
Efavirenz (Sustiva; EFV)	Rash (including cases of Stevens-Johnson syndrome), insomnia, somnolence, dizziness, trouble concentrating, and abnormal dreaming
Protease Inhibitors (PIs)	
Indinavir (Crixivan; IDV)	Nausea, abdominal pain, nephrolithiasis, and indirect hyperbilirubinemia
Nelfinavir (Viracept; NFV)	Diarrhea, nausea, abdominal pain, weakness, and rash
Ritonavir (Norvir; RTV)	Weakness, diarrhea, nausea, circumoral paresthesia, taste alteration, and increased cholesterol and triglycerides
Atazanavir (Rayataz, ATV)	
Saquinavir (Fortovase; SQV)	Diarrhea, abdominal pain, nausea, hyperglycemia, and increased LFTs
Amprenavir (Agenerase; AMP); fosAmprenavir (Lexiva)	Nausea, diarrhea, rash, circumoral paresthesia, taste alteration, and depression
Lopinavir/Ritonavir (Kaletra, LPV/r)	Diarrhea, fatigue, headache, nausea, and increased cholesterol and triglycerides
Entry Inhibitor	
Enfuvirtide (Fuzeon, T-20)	Injection site reactions; household exposure to contaminated needles

From Centers for Disease Control and Prevention: Updated US Public Health Service guidelines for the management of occupational exposure to HBV, HCV, and HIV. MMWR Morb Mortal Wkly Rep 2001;50(RR-11):13.

acyclovir and cautious observation suffice in patients with "good" T-cell counts and mild symptoms. Oral candidiasis in children over 1 year of age indicates significantly impaired T-cell function. Therapy consists of oral fluconazole or itraconazole to clear the acute candidiasis. Prophylaxis against recurrence with twice daily nystatin may be considered. Long-term use of systemic antifungal agents may be required as T-cell numbers deteriorate.

Rashes

Skin lesions affecting children with HIV include hypersensitivity reactions, infectious lesions, and nonspecific eruptions. Drug-induced rashes affect a high proportion of HIV-infected children. Development of a typical maculopapular, pruritic rash 10 days to 4 weeks following introduction of a new antiretroviral regimen points to one of the drugs as the cause. All the antiretroviral agents should be discontinued until the eruption has cleared. HIV-positive children often develop large local reactions to mosquito and flea bites. Antipruritics and topical antibiotics can reduce excoriation and secondary infection. Warts (verruca vulgaris), molluscum contagiosum, and perinatal condylomata are seen more commonly in HIV-infected children and may require aggressive interventions if T-cell counts are low. Herpes zoster (shingles) may be misidentified early in its course as an impetiginous eruption. Failure to initiate proper antiviral therapy may result in disseminated varicella or scarring of the affected areas. Hospitalization for parenteral administration of acyclovir is usually indicated. In patients with a lesser degree of immunocompromise,

outpatient treatment with oral valicyclovir or famciclovir may be considered. The skin of children with prolonged HIV disease may have subcutaneous tissue atrophy, ichthyosis, erythema, exfoliative dermatitis, thinning hair, and nonspecific macules and papules. Many of these changes will reverse with new, effective antiretroviral regimens.

Abdominal Pain

Abdominal pain in a patient with HIV may be caused by common etiologies such as dyspepsia, routine gastroenteritis, and even appendicitis. Abdominal discomfort may be associated with unpalatable antiretroviral agents. Pancreatitis is a frequent complication of antiretroviral drugs, especially in children who have had long-term disease or who have had pancreatitis previously. Acute pancreatitis is a life-threatening complication. The patient must be hospitalized, placed on intravenous fluids and nutrition, and adequately treated for pain. Hepatosplenomegaly may be associated with diffuse abdominal pain. Organomegaly and abdominal lymphadenopathy are frequently seen in disseminated *Mycobacterium avium* complex infections in children whose T-cell counts are very low for a prolonged period of time.

Lymphadenopathy

HIV infection is often characterized by generalized lymphadenopathy, often with parotitis, which when directly related to HIV, responds to antiretroviral therapy. Focal bacterial parotitis may complicate focal long-term parotid gland swelling and is treated with standard antibiotics. High-grade B-cell lymphomas may present as a rapidly progressive local adenopathy in subjects regardless of T-cell level.

Diarrhea

Antiretroviral therapy, the most common cause of diarrhea in HIV-infected children, is usually treated symptomatically with loperamide or diphenoxylate with atropine. Because risk for serious infectious enteritis is increased, screening may be indicated for *Salmonella*, *Shigella*, and *Campylobacter*, and parasitic infections with *Giardia lamblia* and *Cryptosporidium*. *Clostridium difficile* and intestinal candidiasis are complications of long-term prophylactic antibiotics. Nonspecific enteritis commonly seen in children with long-term HIV disease may be associated with malabsorption and wasting. Alternative routes of nutritional support are indicated in such patients.

Respiratory Distress

Children with HIV infection, even those with T-cell counts sufficient to avoid opportunistic infections, are at increased risk for pneumonias and upper respiratory tract infections with "routine" organisms including *Streptococcus pneumoniae*, *Moraxella catarrhalis*, and *Haemophilus influenzae*. They are also at increased risk for reactive airway disease. More than 30% require bronchodilators or more intense therapy for asthma. Differentiation between an acute asthma attack and an acute infectious process is essential. HIV-infected children under 1 year of age or who have T-cell counts in the "not good" range are at increased risk for *P. carinii* pneumonia and should receive prophylactic antibiotics. Adherence to long-term prophylaxis may wane over time. Children with *P. carinii* pneumonia usually present with a progressive cough, often with dyspnea and shortness of breath on exertion. If no adventitious sounds are heard on auscultation and a chest x-ray fails to show interstitial infiltrates, oxygen saturation should be measured. Demonstration of oxygen desaturation is an indication for immediate hospitalization and diagnostic bronchoalveolar lavage.

Health Maintenance
Breast-feeding

In the United States, HIV-positive mothers, regardless of their own viral load, should not breast-feed their infants. The 15% chance of infecting the newborn via breast milk far outweighs the benefits.

Immunizations

Children with HIV infection should receive all standard immunizations except for live poliomyelitis virus vaccine and varicella vaccine. Clinically stable patients with good T-cell counts may receive the measles-mumps-rubella (MMR) vaccine. A more conservative approach is to administer inactivated polio vaccine, tetanus toxoid, and *H. influenza* type b (Hib) conjugate vaccine at 2, 4, and 6 months of age and then measure tetanus and Hib-specific antibodies. If the infant generates protective antibodies, then an MMR vaccine may be given safely at 12 to 15 months of age. Failure of an HIV-infected infant to generate protective

antibodies to routine immunizations is an indication for intravenous immunoglobulin (IVIG) replacement therapy. Varicella vaccine is probably safe for children with normal T-cell numbers, but should not be given to other HIV-positive children. Parents should be advised to obtain medical attention immediately if their child is exposed to wild-type varicella for consideration of administration of varicella-zoster immune globulin (VZIG). If a child develops varicella, antiviral therapy should be immediately initiated.

Growth and Development

Children with HIV often have suboptimal growth related to the long-term infection with HIV, episodic complications of immune deficiency, and nutritional compromise secondary to reduced caloric intake or excessive intestinal loss. Every effort must be made to maintain normal growth patterns using dietary supplements and appetite stimulants as indicated. These are best managed by the patient's HIV specialist. Developmental issues are very common in children with HIV. Over 80% of the patients followed at one center have demonstrable deficits in behavioral, emotional, or cognitive realms. Close monitoring of school performance and early intervention for behavior and cognitive impairment is essential. The emotional impact of HIV as a stigmatizing chronic disease only becomes more stressful for children as they get older and enter the teen years. Every effort should be made to get these children into therapeutic situations with individual counseling or group therapy as indicated. Antidepressants are commonly required and should be directed by a psychiatrist familiar with the management of HIV-associated emotional disorders.

SUGGESTED READINGS

American Academy of Pediatrics, Committee on Pediatric AIDS: Evaluation and medical treatment of the HIV-exposed infant. Pediatrics 1997;99:909–917.

American Academy of Pediatrics, Committee on Pediatric AIDS and Committee on Infectious Diseases: Issues related to human immunodeficiency virus transmission in schools, child care, medical settings, the home, and community. Pediatrics 1999;104:318–324.

Centers for Disease Control and Prevention–National Prevention Information Network. Available at: www.cdcnpin.org.

HIV/AIDS Treatment Information Service. Available at: www.hivatis.org.

Merchant RC, Keshavarz R: Human immunodeficiency virus

postexposure prophylaxis for adolescents and children. Pediatrics 2001;108:e38.

National Pediatric and Family HIV Resource Center. Available at: www.pedhivaids.org.

Shearer WT, Hanson IC (eds): Medical Management of AIDS in Children. Philadelphia, WB Saunders, 2003.

172 Chronic Genitourinary Tract Disorders

Brent Snow

ROLE OF THE GENERALIST

1   Diagnose congenital and chronic disorders of the urinary tract.

2   Follow bladder and kidney function.

3   Treat urinary tract infections.

4   Help families of patients with chronic urinary tract infections comply with treatment recommendations.

5   Refer patients with chronic genitourinary tract disorders to specialists when appropriate and coordinate care.

Production, collection, and excretion of liquid waste are the urinary functions of the genitourinary (GU) system. The pathophysiologic effects of congenital abnormalities on these functions can be the result of the anomaly itself or secondary from mechanical obstruction or neuropathic dysfunction. The major complication of chronic disorders of the urinary system is renal damage. Long-term management consists of correction of anatomic defects, management of voiding dysfunctions, and prevention and treatment of urinary tract infections.

Children with congenital abnormalities require ongoing follow-up with specialists, particularly urologists and nephrologists. The generalist plays an important role in diagnosing disorders of the genitourinary system and coordinating care, assuring that these children receive appropriate acute and preventive care.

VESICOURETERAL REFLUX

Fundamentals

Vesicoureteral reflux is backflow of urine from the bladder through the ureter toward the kidney during either bladder filling or emptying. Primary vesicoureteral reflux develops during the second trimester of pregnancy, resulting from inadequate intramural ureteral tunnel length within the bladder. Reflux can also be caused by anatomic abnormalities of the ureter that affect the competency of the ureterovesical junction, such as ureteral duplication or ureterocele. Secondary reflux or acquired reflux is caused by increased bladder pressure from obstruction, inflammation, or in some cases, by surgical procedures that involve the ureterovesical junction.

Clinical Evaluation and Management

Children with the risk factors listed in Box 172-1 should be evaluated for vesicoureteral reflux with a voiding cystourethrogram. Because vesicoureteral reflux spontaneously resolves over time in mild to moderate cases, reflux is discovered more frequently in younger patients than in older patients with indications for evaluation.

The International Reflux Classification grades the reflux on a scale of I to V (Fig. 172-1) and is used to predict resolution of vesicoureteral reflux. It distinguishes patients at high risk for continued vesicoureteral reflux so they can be guided toward early surgical repair. Spontaneous resolution of vesicoureteral reflux correlates fairly well with the International Reflux Grading System (Table 172-1). The goal of vesicoureteral reflux management is to maintain good kidney function by prevention of pyelonephritis and kidney scarring. Vesicoureteral reflux and infections are the most common cause of kidney damage during childhood.

Box 172-1. Risk Factors for Vesicoureteral Reflux

1. Antenatal hydronephrosis
2. Urinary tract infections
3. Voiding disorders, including neurologic bladder impairment
4. Siblings of patients with vesicoureteral reflux
5. Offspring of parents who had vesicoureteral reflux as children

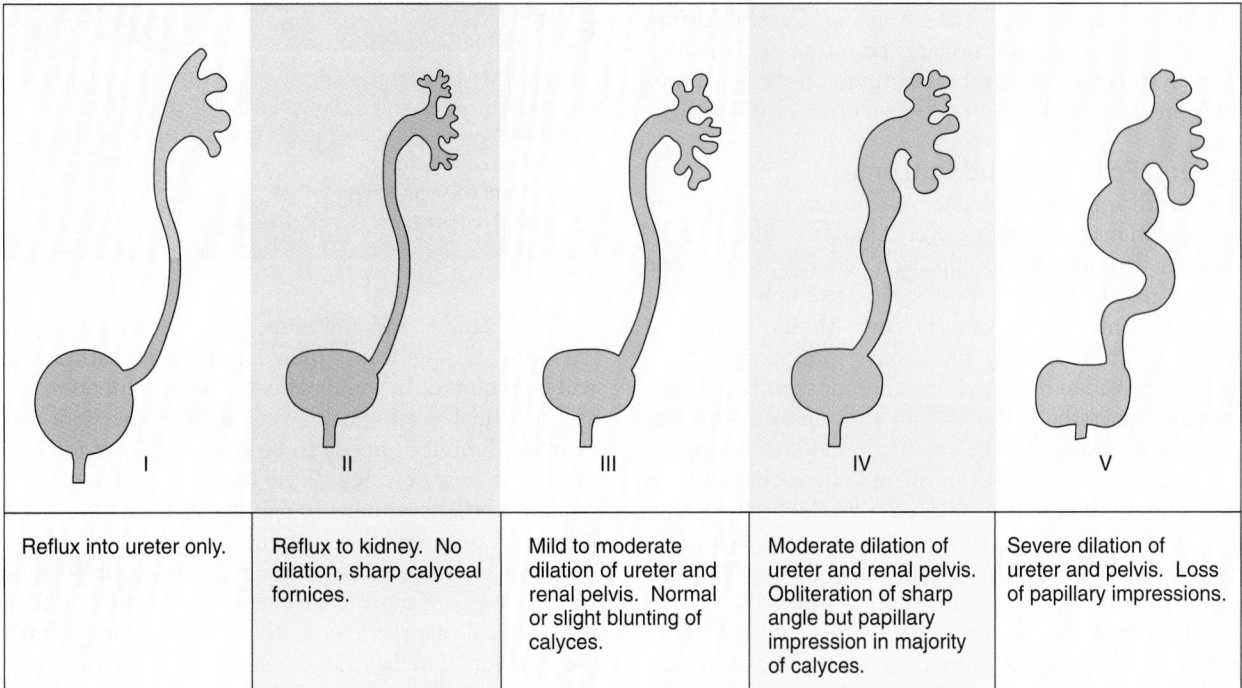

I	II	III	IV	V
Reflux into ureter only.	Reflux to kidney. No dilation, sharp calyceal fornices.	Mild to moderate dilation of ureter and renal pelvis. Normal or slight blunting of calyces.	Moderate dilation of ureter and renal pelvis. Obliteration of sharp angle but papillary impression in majority of calyces.	Severe dilation of ureter and pelvis. Loss of papillary impressions.

Figure 172-1. International reflux classification.

Long-term management consists of intervention to prevent urinary tract infection until vesicoureteral reflux resolves spontaneously or is surgically corrected. Because severe reflux is unlikely to resolve spontaneously, patients with grade V and many with grade IV are surgically corrected upon discovery. Box 172-2 lists indications for surgical intervention.

Long-term prophylactic antibiotics are the mainstays of medical management. The ideal antibiotic for prophylaxis is one that is effective in the urinary tract against urinary pathogens, is absorbed high in the gastrointestinal tract so that it does not alter lower gastrointestinal flora, has low potential for selection of resistant bacteria, and has minimal side effects. Sulfa medications such as sulfamethoxazole or sulfa-trimethoprim combinations have been used with good success, as has nitrofurantoin. Because kidneys concentrate the medication prior to excretion, the required dosage for effective prophylaxis in the urinary tract is usually one quarter the amount needed to treat an infection.

After diagnosis of vesicoureteral reflux and the initiation of prophylactic antibiotics, periodic surveillance of the urine is needed to ensure that the dose of prophylactic antibiotics is sufficient to prevent infection. Urine culture is recommended monthly for the first 3 months, quarterly for the first year, and whenever a child with reflux has a fever. Because discontinuation of prophylactic antibiotics is based on resolution of vesicoureteral reflux, bladder imaging is recommended annually. Because complete resolution of reflux, not the interval grade of reflux, guides treatment decisions, nuclear cystogram is the imaging study of choice. Because time to resolution of vesicoureteral reflux averages nearly 3 years after diagnosis, effective medical management to avoid surgery requires vigilance and patience.

Experience suggests older children have kidney damage less often following infections. Some experts are interested in stopping prophylactic antibiotics in these patients. Because data are sparse, this approach should be used cautiously at this time.

Children with reflux must be carefully observed for voiding dysfunction as they grow and develop. Bladder

Table 172-1. Average Percentage of Reflux Resolution 5 Years after Diagnosis

IRC Grade,* Age at Diagnosis	Reflux Resolution
Grade I	91.8%
Grade II	80.6%
Grade III unilateral, age 0–24 mo	70%
Grade III unilateral, age 25–60 mo	51.3%
Grade III unilateral, age 61–120 mo	43.6%
Grade III bilateral, age 0–24 mo	49.3%
Grade III bilateral, age 25–60 mo	30.5%
Grade III bilateral, age 61–120 mo	12.5%
Grade IV, unilateral	58.5%
Greade IV, bilateral	9.9%

*International Reflux Classification. See Figure 172-1 for more detailed description of grades I through V.

Box 172-2. Indications for Surgical Intervention in Patients with Vesicoureteral Reflux

High-grade reflux unlikely to resolve
Persistent urinary tract infections despite prophylactic antibiotics
Poor compliance with prophylactic antibiotics
Reflux that persists in girls at puberty
Failure of kidney growth, presence of new kidney scars, or deterioration of renal function
Parents highly unreliable to keep follow-up appointments
Failure to thrive in young children with high-grade vesicoureteral reflux

instability is common with toilet training. Careful history taking for dribbling and urinary retention is essential. Voiding dysfunction should be promptly treated to lower bladder pressures and allow rapid resolution of the reflux.

Long-term Follow-up and Outcome

Patients with mild to moderate vesicoureteral reflux may meet indications for surgery over time (see Box 172-2). When boys with mild reflux approach puberty, prophylactic antibiotics may be stopped. Surgery is contemplated only if urinary tract infections ensue. Because of the high likelihood of recurrent urinary infections, surgical correction should be considered in girls as they approach puberty. During pregnancy the risk is not only for urinary tract infections, but also pyelonephritis and further kidney damage.

One third of the siblings of an index patient who has vesicoureteral reflux will also have reflux. Siblings younger than 3 to 5 years of age should undergo radiologic evaluation. If they have vesicoureteral reflux, they should be managed in a similar fashion to patients who were discovered with symptoms. Three quarters of children born to women who had reflux during childhood have reflux, regardless of whether the mother's reflux was surgically corrected or spontaneously resolved.

NEUROGENIC BLADDER

Fundamentals

Neurogenic bladder is caused by interruption of the innervation of the bladder. Because the nerves to the bladder arrive through the sacral roots, bladder impairment most commonly results from neurologic birth defect or injury. Impairment of bowel control is commonly associated with bladder impairment and must also be considered in the medical management.

Neurologic bladder deficits are lifelong. Medical issues include urinary incontinence or retention, urinary tract infection, and damage to the upper urinary tract. In the past patients with spinal cord impairment often died from acquired kidney scarring and renal failure from urinary tract infections and their complications. This problem does not occur with adequate medical management. Social issues related to bladder and bowel dysfunction must also be addressed. Urinary and fecal continence must be managed aggressively for social acceptance.

Clinical Evaluation and Management

Children with the disorders listed in Box 172-3 should be evaluated for the possibility of neurogenic bladder dysfunction. Appropriate studies include voiding cystourethrogram to evaluate bladder emptying and to detect vesicoureteral reflux, and a renal ultrasound to evaluate the upper urinary tract. Urodynamic studies that determine the bladder pressure during filling and emptying are invaluable in determining the course of treatment and follow-up. Bladders that empty well and have low pressures can be followed less frequently. Those that empty poorly and have high pressures are at significant risk for kidney damage and require close surveillance including urine checks for infections, frequent ultrasounds of the kidneys, and periodic bladder x-rays.

> **Box 172-3.** Causes of Neurogenic Bladder
>
> 1. Myelodysplasia (spina bifida)
> 2. Occult spinal dysraphism, including tethered cord, lipomeningocele, diastematomyelia, abnormal nerve roots
> 3. Spinal cord tumors
> 4. Central nervous system tumors
> 5. Spinal cord trauma

If the bladder does not empty completely and the residual urine is significant, then intermittent catheterization will be required. In some patients, bladder function returns as the spinal cord shock from birth, surgery, or trauma resolves. Emphasis needs to be placed on individualization of care because few neurologic lesions are alike.

Many patients with neurologic injuries have vesicoureteral reflux. Vesicoureteral reflux may resolve if bladder pressures can be lowered. Indications for vesicoureteral reflux surgery are similar to those for primary reflux after maximal medical management of the neurologic impairment. If bladder function has not been maximized, then surgical efforts to correct reflux may fail.

As patients reach toilet training and school age, every effort must be made to establish continence. Urinary continence can be established through frequent timed voidings, anticholinergic medications, and intermittent catheterization. If, despite an optimal regimen of medications and intermittent catheterization, patients are not acceptably continent, then surgical options should be considered. Surgery for urinary continence is directed at the sphincter and bladder neck area. Bladder augmentation procedures to enlarge bladder capacity and lower the bladder pressures are sometimes necessary. After bladder augmentation, intermittent catheterization is generally still required for emptying, but is usually well tolerated and well received because of the patient's desire to be continent. Patient compliance is an essential part of attaining continence. Some children may not reach a level of maturity or have enough motivation to be compliant with these regimens until the end of the teenage years.

Outcome and Follow-up

One of the most important caveats of neurologic bladder impairment in children is that growth and development may change the bladder dysfunction. Early efforts may control the bladder physiology until a successful balance has been reached. However, growth may stretch nerves, spinal cord tethering may occur, or bladder fibrosis may develop. Under these conditions asymptomatic bladder pressure increases may cause significant kidney and bladder damage. Frequent periodic review of the neurologically impaired bladder is necessary to avoid these problems, maintain good bladder function at low pressures, and maintain good kidney function.

PRUNE BELLY SYNDROME

Fundamentals

Prune belly syndrome is a triad of deficient abdominal wall musculature, abnormal urinary tract dilation, and bilateral undescended testicles (Fig. 172-2). Pulmonary function

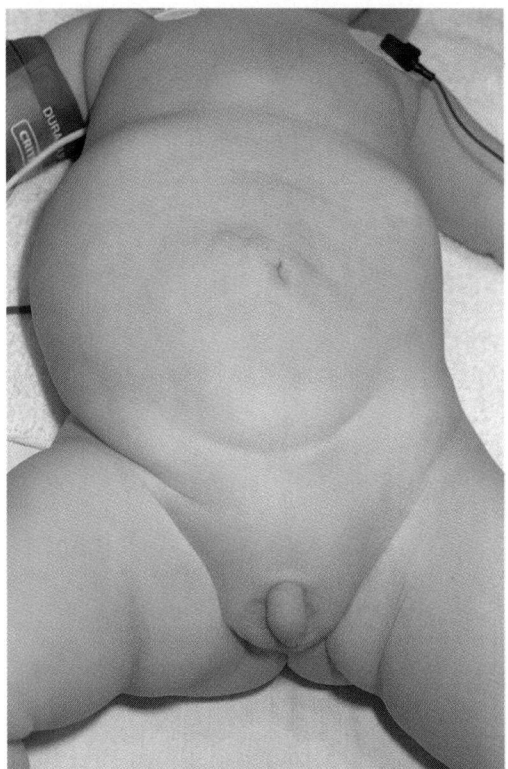

Figure 172-2. A newborn boy with prune belly syndrome. Note the lax abdominal musculature and undescended testicles.

may also be a concern in the perinatal period. Kidney function may be diminished, causing oligohydramnios and secondary pulmonary hypoplasia. Even in patients who have well-developed lungs, pulmonary toilet is impaired because of inadequate musculature of the abdominal wall. Urinary tract dilation is a developmental anomaly and is not secondary to obstruction.

Evaluation and Management

Management goals are preservation of kidney function and bladder emptying, and prevention of urinary tract infection. Vesicoureteral reflux occurs in most patients. Principles of reflux management should be applied, with particular attention to adequacy of urinary tract drainage. Patients with prune belly syndrome can void on their own if post-voiding residuals are not too great. Residuals must be checked promptly after voiding because the upper urinary tract is dilated and will drain immediately into the bladder after the bladder is emptied. If the bladder empties completely, then intermittent catheterization is unnecessary. If bladder emptying is inadequate or kidney function is abnormal or deteriorates, patients should be referred to pediatric urologists and nephrologists for assistance with concurrent care. Intermittent catheterization may be necessary. Constipation and stool retention, common among patients with prune belly syndrome, also interferes with bladder emptying and should be aggressively treated.

Surgical correction of massively dilated ureters is not as successful as with normal ureters. The kidneys are not as likely to be damaged in urinary tracts with balanced pressures. For these reasons, surgery is considered only if kidney

function deteriorates. Undescended testicles are usually placed into the scrotum during the first year of life. Plication of the abdominal wall is done for cosmetic purposes as these children approach school age.

Outcome and Follow-up

Adults with prune belly syndrome have normal sexual function but are infertile. Tumors of the testes develop sporadically. Kidney function may deteriorate in some patients, requiring renal dialysis and renal transplantation. Lifelong careful surveillance of urinary and kidney function and meticulous follow-up and management are essential to maintain health in these patients.

POSTERIOR URETHRAL VALVES

Fundamentals

Initial diagnosis, evaluation, and management of newborns with posterior urethral valves is described in Chapter 205. Patients with posterior urethral valve have a wide spectrum of involvement. In some, ablation of the posterior urethral valves is sufficient treatment. Kidney and bladder function return to normal, and only periodic evaluation is necessary. However, half of these patients have vesicoureteral reflux that can be massive. Approximately 20% of the patients will have a *v*alve *u*nilateral *r*eflux and *d*ysplasia or VURD syndrome with a functionless dilated kidney. If the bladder function returns to normal, then a nephroureterectomy is generally performed. Reflux resolves in about half of the 30% of patients who continue to have reflux after the newborn period, and half undergo reimplant surgery with the same considerations of other refluxing patients.

Patients who have had congenital bladder outlet obstruction may have bladder dysfunction as a result of detrusor hypertrophy and hyperplasia and increased amounts of type 3 collagen and elastin. Up to one third will have persistent bladder dysfunction throughout childhood.

Evaluation and Management

Long-term complications of posterior urethral valves are vesicoureteral reflux, continued bladder dysfunction, and chronic renal failure. Reflux management is the same as for other patients. In some patients with posterior urethral valves, however, bladder function remains abnormal, pressures remain high, and the upper urinary tracts remain dilated. These children must be diagnosed and treated so that renal function is not silently lost. Recurrent urinary tract infections, difficulty in toilet training, and continued urinary leakage are indicators of bladder dysfunction and should be evaluated. Urodynamic evaluation of the bladder pressures show high pressures during filling and even higher pressures during emptying. Referral to a pediatric urologist for obstruction evaluation is indicated. Continued bladder dysfunction is managed by frequent timed voidings, anticholinergic medications, careful attention to bowel habits, and aggressive treatment of constipation when it occurs. Urinary diversion with a vesicostomy may be considered in some patients.

Kidney function should be carefully followed and periodically evaluated. Diuretic renal scans should be obtained to evaluate differential kidney function and drainage because upper urinary tracts often remain dilated. Toilet-trained children who experience continued bladder dysfunction and urinary leakage should be evaluated to determine how well the kidneys concentrate urine. Many have a concentrating defect that results in high urinary volumes and exacerbates bladder dysfunction. If the bladder dysfunction persists after anticholinergic medications and timed voidings, clean intermittent catheterization may be required. Bladder augmentation may be necessary to reduce the bladder pressure and enlarge the bladder volume.

BLADDER EXSTROPHY

Fundamentals

Bladder extrophy occurs when the cloacal membrane rupture is delayed. The symphysis pubis is widely separated. At birth the open bladder is on the ventral lower abdominal wall (Figs. 172-3 and 172-4). The ureters enter the bladder perpendicularly and the umbilicus is tethered to the top part of the exstrophic bladder. Immediate surgery is required to close the bladder and reconstruct the external genitalia. Almost all patients have vesicoureteral reflux after the bladder is closed. Reflux should be managed as with other patients, except that surgical correction for the reflux can be scheduled at one of the stages of bladder exstrophy repair. After initial closure usually no further surgery is necessary until the time of toilet training when most patients require surgery at the bladder neck to achieve continence.

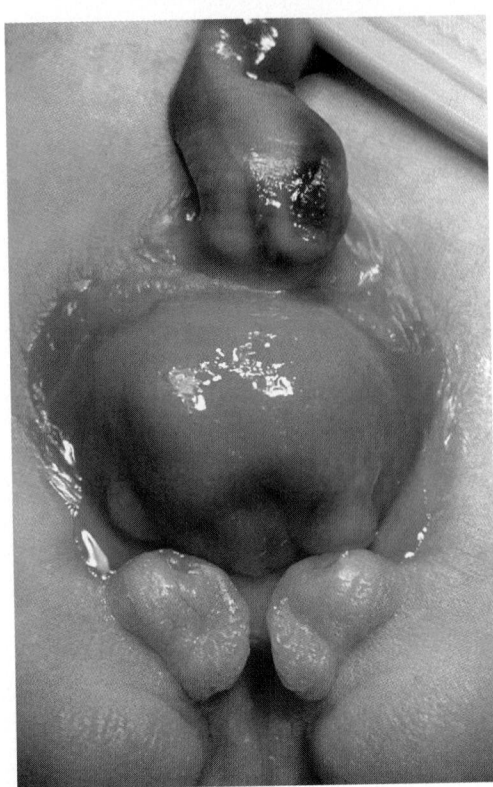

Figure 172-4. A baby girl with bladder exstrophy and epispadias. The labia are separated and the umbilicus is adjacent to the superior edge of the bladder epithelium.

Because the bladder did not fill and empty during fetal development, normal voiding patterns are difficult for these patients to learn. At times the bladder may have high pressure and poor compliance, causing elevated bladder pressures during filling and leakage. Timed voidings and anticholinergics can be used to attempt to establish normal bladder function. Often exstrophic bladders are small in capacity and high in pressure. Bladder augmentation may be required to allow better storage of urine.

Reconstruction of genitalia for boys may not be completed at the time of newborn closure. Epispadias closure is a difficult surgical procedure. Urethrocutaneous fistula is a common complication after surgery. Multiple operations may be required to have a well-healed watertight reconstructed penis and urethra.

Because the internal and external rings are not in their normal anatomic position as a result of the diastasis pubis, inguinal hernias are more common in patients with bladder extrophy, and careful surveillance is important. Hernias should be repaired when found.

When the patients reach puberty, monsplasty is often necessary because the hair-bearing region had been displaced as a newborn by the bladder. Cosmetic repair is accomplished through rotational skin flaps to bring the hair to a more normal position over the genitalia.

Outcome and Follow-up

Repair of bladder extrophy is one of the most challenging surgical reconstructions in pediatric urology, often taking multiple operations over many years. Close

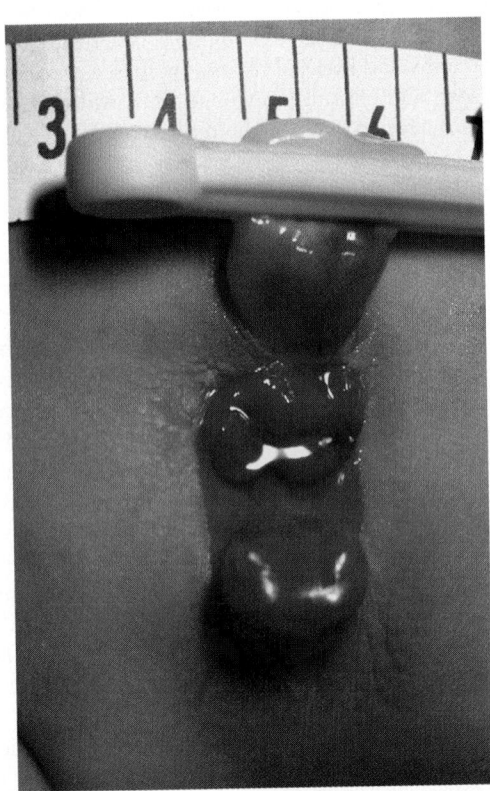

Figure 172-3. A baby boy with bladder exstrophy and epispadias. The urethra is open from the bladder to the tip of the penis and the umbilicus is displaced inferiorly at the top edge of the bladder.

coordination between pediatric urologists and generalists is necessary to provide the best medical care and brightest outlook.

Mini-index of Related Topics

SUGGESTED READINGS

Bauer, SB: Neurogenic dysfunction of the lower urinary tract in children. In Walsh PC, Retik AB, Vaughan ED, Wein AJ (eds): Campbell's Urology, 7th ed. Philadelphia, WB Saunders, 1998, pp 285–289.

Coplen DE, Snow BW, Duckett JW: Prune belly syndrome. In Gillenwater JY, Grayhack JT, Howards SS, et al: Adult and Pediatric Urology, 3rd ed. St. Louis, Mosby-YearBook, 1996, pp 2297–2316.

Elder JS, Peters CA, Arant BS Jr, et al: Pediatric vesicoureteral reflux guidelines panel summary report on the management of primary vesicoureteral reflux in children. J Urol 1997;157(5):1846–1851.

Gonzales ET: Posterior urethral valves and other urethral anomalies. In Walsh PC, Retik AB, Vaughan ED, Wein AJ (eds): Campbell's Urology, 7th ed. Philadelphia, WB Saunders, 1998, pp 2069–2084.

Grady RW, Mitchell ME: Complete primary repair of exstrophy: Surgical technique. Urol Clin North Am 2000;27(3):569–578.

SECTION 4 CHRONIC MEDICAL CARE: *Disorders of the Genitourinary System*

173 Long-term Management of Renal Disorders

Paul T. McEnery and C. Frederic Strife

ROLE OF THE GENERALIST

1. Diagnose renal and urologic conditions that can cause chronic renal insufficiency (CRI).
2. Coordinate care of children with chronic renal insufficiency.
3. Refer patients with CRI to specialty centers for long-term management.
4. Provide preventive health care with particular attention to growth, nutrition, and development.
5. Monitor renal function and ensure follow-up with specialists as necessary.
6. Provide acute care, considering effects of all medications on renal function and hypertension.
7. Assist in psychosocial support of children and families.

Chronic renal insufficiency (CRI) is the irreversible loss of more than 50% of the glomerular filtration rate (GFR) with resultant metabolic and hormonal derangements and accumulation of uremic toxins. During the past 30 years medical and surgical therapies and diagnostic testing have evolved with tremendous advances to maximize the potential for achieving normal health status in children with CRI. With the potential for normal life expectancy for these patients, coordination of care between the primary care provider and nephrologists and urologists is essential to the long-term well-being of patients with these disorders.

The complexity of medical practice, the explosion of new information, and the inevitable differences of opinion between experts, as well as both physicians and parents, require an absolute need for frequent and open communication between the medical team of specialist, generalist, and family. The standard guidelines from the American Academy of Pediatrics for preventive and routine pediatric health care must be accomplished. Alterations to that schedule need to be resolved through consultation and guidance with the specialist.

Children having renal dysplasia or urologic deformities and a GFR between 100% and 50% of normal, except for a concern for adequate hydration, would be expected to require no specific alteration or limit to their diet, activities, or dosing of medication compared to normal children. Values for normal serum creatinine for age and GFR, estimated by a creatinine clearance (C_{Cr}), are given in Table 173-1. The GFR, based on body surface area, can also be estimated from the child's serum creatinine and height by

Table 173-1. Normal Values for Renal Function by Age

Age (Term Infants)	Creatinine (mg/dL)	Creatinine Clearance (mL/min/1.73 m²)
1 week	0.5	20–30
2 weeks	0.4	35–45
8 weeks	0.4	70–80
1 year	0.5	90–110
1–20 years	0.5–0.9	90–130

Table 173-2. Schwartz Formula*: Estimation of Glomerular Filtration Rate

Patient	Age	k
Normal infant	Up to 1 year	0.45
Girls	1–12 years	0.55
	13–20 years	0.57
Boys	1–12 years	0.55
	13–20 years	0.7

*Length-height × constant (k)/serum creatinine = C_{Cr} (mL/min/1.73 m²).
Schwartz GJ, Gauthier B: A simple estimate of glomerular filtration in adolescent boys.

use of the "Schwartz formula" (Table 173-2). Depending on the degree and type of renal impairment (congenital/structural or metabolic versus glomerular disorders) the need for specialist involvement varies. Failure of growth (length/height or head circumference), unexplained fevers, change in general well-being (daytime naps, continued lack of appetite, worsening school performance and concentration), and hypertension are the usual signs and symptoms suggesting progression of CRI and the need for increased involvement and direct care by the specialist.

Early recognition of neonatal renal, ureteral, and bladder structural abnormalities by means of prenatal ultrasonography has greatly improved the care of children with major renal disorders. Pediatric urology or nephrology consultation and direct care can be accomplished at birth or shortly thereafter. Guidelines for medical/surgical care are still being established, but the goal remains to avoid infections, resolve ongoing injury from obstruction, ameliorate the consequences of hyperfiltration, and reduce the effects of retained uremic by-products.

Most children with a diagnosis of renal dysplasia (CPT code 753.15) and moderate renal impairment can maintain an adequate electrolyte and metabolic status, normal hemoglobin, and healthy bones and achieve reasonable growth through the early years of life. During the initial 2 years of life, brain volume more than doubles and achieves approximately 80% of its final adult size. Children with CRI early in life are at a significant risk for development of microcephaly, seizures, brain atrophy, and mental retardation. Adequate nutrition and hydration must be maintained. Nutritional deficiencies, which can be difficult to diagnose, must be addressed to avoid long-lasting effects when evaluating well-being in children with CRI. When necessary, peritoneal dialysis and nasogastric/gastrostomy feedings can be provided in a home environment if a committed group of family providers to support the child and one another are available.

Renal transplantation, the ultimate goal for all children with severe renal impairment, and dialysis, a means of maintaining or preparing children for that event, are further treatment options for progressive CRI.

PROGRESSION AND PATHOGENESIS OF CHRONIC RENAL DISORDERS

Chronic renal failure is invariably progressive. Metabolic derangements result from the accumulation of uremic toxins and metabolic and hormonal adaptations to glomerular and tubular loss. These adaptations produce a process known as compensatory adaptation in which signs and symptoms of renal failure progress, yet the resulting GFR is greater than expected from the injured kidneys. With continuing glomerular loss, glomerular perfusion increases from dilatation of afferent and efferent arterioles to the remaining nephron units. The dilatation of the efferent vessel is less than that of the afferent, leading to an increase in pressure within the glomerular capillary, resulting in an increase in GFR of the kidney as a whole, termed hyperfiltration. This adaptation is thought to be responsible for release of inflammatory and growth factors, causing progression of glomerular sclerosis and atrophy in nephron units (Fig. 173-1).

Adaptation of tubular function also occurs as GFR decreases. Glomerular tubular balance is preserved as each tubule adjusts handling of water and solutes. In normal health status, approximately 99% of the water and sodium filtered by the kidney is reabsorbed. In early stages of renal compensation, tubular handling of water, minerals, and solutes is minimally altered. As renal function declines, tubular function may be compromised, resulting in an inability to conserve salt or water. Regulation of water and sodium may be impaired in children with renal dysplasia characterized by high urine volume and result in difficulty in handling excesses or deficiencies of both or either. As the GFR decreases from normal to 50% of normal, hypertrophy and hyperplasia of remaining nephron units compensate for atrophic areas, achieve functional adaptation, and maintain normal glomerular tubular balance. Although with GFR of

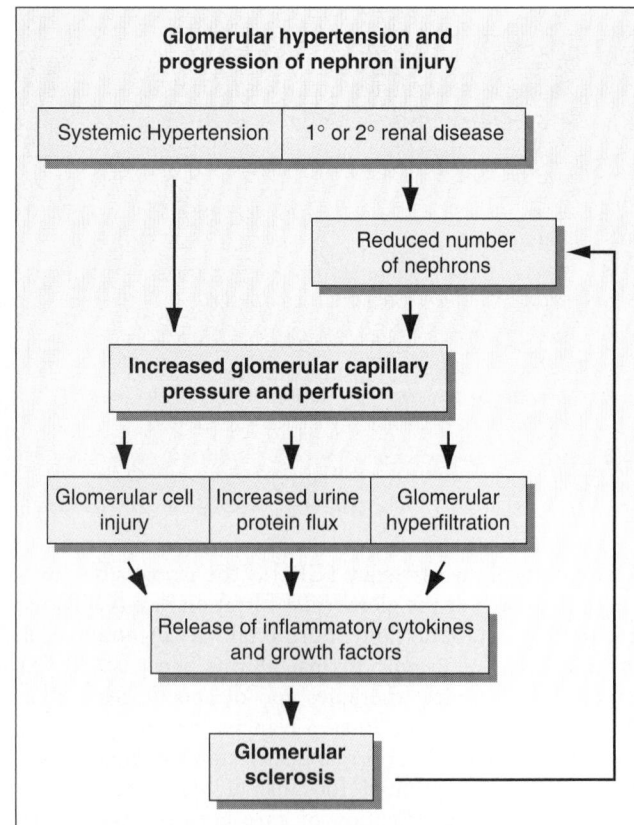

Figure 173-1. Glomerular hypertension and progression of nephron injury.

50% to 25% of normal biochemical alterations are mild, in this range irreversible changes seem be initiated, leading to further loss of nephron units and CRI. As the GFR becomes less than 50% of normal, retention of urea, creatinine, and other waste products causes development of acidosis and loss in production in the renal hormones calcitriol and erythropoietin. At this stage of CRI metabolic acidosis is present because of the tubular inability to reabsorb bicarbonate, synthesize ammonia, and secrete fixed acids. Tubular secretion of potassium is impaired and the colon increases its capacity for excretion of uremic waste products. Impaired patient well-being is not seen until the remaining nephron population is reduced to below 25%. As glomerular/tubular sclerosis and atrophy continue, end-stage renal disease (ESRD) evolves.

In the absence of medical therapy for CRI, acidosis, hyperkalemia, hyponatremia, hypocalcemia, and hyperphosphatemia are common and can result in growth retardation, anemia, osteodystrophy, and hypertension. Specialized treatment centers are essential for these chronically ill children to address the children's and families' social, psychological, financial, and medical/surgical needs in a coordinated process. Multiple treatment options are available for each developing problem of CRI. No choice is final and the autonomy of the family in the decision-making process must be respected. Yet, the consensus in pediatric care of children with progressive CRI is that renal transplantation is the preferred mode of treatment of children with ESRD.

DIAGNOSIS OF CHRONIC RENAL DISORDERS

Patients and families deal best with their illness when they know the diagnosis and can become educated about the disease process and possible therapeutic options. The patient history and urinalysis remain most important in formulating appropriate diagnoses and determining if the disease process is acute or chronic. Renal/bladder ultrasound continues to be the simplest imaging study to define renal anatomy. Serum creatinine is the best screening test for renal function and may be supplemented with a timed urine collection for calculation of creatinine clearance. Measurement of serum complement proteins C3 and C4 are very helpful in diagnosing hypocomplementemic glomerulonephritides. Serum albumin and IgG measurements identify patients with proteinuria that affects total body concentrations of these proteins. Although evaluation is relatively straightforward, assimilation and interpretation of the results to reach a clear diagnosis or to determine the need for a renal biopsy or surgical intervention often requires the assistance of a specialist in pediatric nephrology or urology.

According to the North American Pediatric Renal Transplant Cooperative Society (NAPRTCS) Chronic Renal Insufficiency registry more than 50% of chronic renal disorders in childhood are congenital or inherited, with most patients having obstructive uropathy or renal dysplasia (Table 173-3). Congenital structural defects of renal position, size, or architecture are most commonly discovered during prenatal ultrasound examinations (Table 173-4). The finding of congenital renal abnormalities often leads to early identification of known syndromes (Box 173-1). In a vari-

Table 173-3. Causes of Chronic Renal Insufficiency in Children

Category	Percentage of All Causes	
Congenital	46%	
Obstructive uropathy		23%
Dysplastic/hypoplastic kidneys		21%
Inherited	6.1%	
Polycystic kidney diseases		4.1%
Medullary cystic disease/nephronophthisis		1.2%
Tubular (cystinosis)	1.5%	
Acquired renal disorders	28%	
Reflux nephropathy/chronic pyelonephritis		10%
Glomerular diseases		
Focal segmental glomerulosclerosis		8%
Glomerulonephritides		
Primary		6%
Systemic		4%
Infarct/hemolytic-uremic syndrome	5.4%	
Other/unknown	13%	

Adapted from North American Pediatric Renal Transplant Cooperative Society (NAPRTCS) 2001 Annual Report, The EMMES Corp., 401 N. Washington St. Suite 700, Rockville, Md 20805, pp 13–15.

ety of inherited disorders renal involvement is known to be commonly present, but may not become evident for many years (e.g., tuberous sclerosis, glycogen storage disease, dominant polycystic kidney disease).

Chronic renal diseases can also be related to tubular abnormalities. Most of these disorders are the result of specific enzyme defects that cause cell dysfunction. In Fanconi syndrome, patients typically have proximal tubular dysfunction with abnormal reabsorption of bicarbonate, potassium, phosphorus, sodium, amino acids, and glucose. These patients have excess wasting of electrolytes in the urine, leading to poor growth, electrolyte imbalance, acidosis, and rickets. Diseases that present with Fanconi syndrome include cystinosis, galactosemia, tyrosinemia, glycogen storage diseases, and Lowe syndrome. Cell dysfunction, especially in cystinosis and Lowe syndrome, can lead to cell death and slow development of renal insufficiency. Patients with distal renal tubular acidosis rarely develop renal insufficiency unless their tubular dysfunction is associated with severe and progressive nephrocalcinosis or renal stone disease.

Acquired chronic renal disorders fall into two major categories: renal scarring associated with urinary tract infection (UTI) with or without vesicoureteral reflux (VUR) and glomerular disorders related to glomerulonephritis, nephrotic syndrome, or thrombotic/ischemic injury. The American

Table 173-4. Prenatal Ultrasound Screening for Renal Abnormalities

Abnormality	Defect
Abnormal renal position	Horseshoe kidney
	Pelvic kidney
	Absent kidney
Abnormal renal size	Dysplasia/hypoplasia (small)
	Duplicate kidney (large)
	Tumor
Abnormal renal archetecture	Cystic kidney
	Hydronephrosis/hydroureter

Box 173-1. Syndromes with Frequent Associated Renal or Urinary Tract Abnormalities

Syndromes Commonly Associated with Obstructive Uropathy

- Myelomeningocele with neurogenic bladder
- OEIS complex (omphalocele, cloacal extrophy, *imperforate anus, spinal dysraphism*)
- Posterior uretheral valves (and associated syndromes)
- Potter sequence (oligohydramnios from any genitorenal anomaly)
- Prune belly syndrome
- VATER association (vertebral defects, imperforate *anus,* tracheoesophageal fistula, *radial* and *renal* anomalies)

Syndromes with Frequent Associated Renal Abnormalities

- Branchial-otorenal (earpit deafness) syndrome—renal dysplasia
- Denys-Drash (Frasier) syndrome—pseudohermaphroditism, Wilms tumor, mesangial sclerosis
- Down syndrome—renal microcystic disease
- Neurofibromatosis—renal artery stenosis, usually segmental
- Tuberous sclerosis—angiomyolipomas, polycystic kidneys

Box 173-2. Common Presentation of Children with Glomerular Diseases

Acute Nephritic Syndrome

Gross hematuria, proteinuria, ± hypertension, ± nephritic syndrome

- Acute poststreptococcal glomerulonephritis (rarely progresses to renal insufficiency)
- IgA nephropathy
- Rapidly progressive glomerulonephritides
- Membranoproliferative glomerulonephritis types I and II (dense deposit disease)

Nephrotic Syndrome

Heavy proteinuria, swelling, ± microscopic hematuria

- Minimal change disease (rarely progresses to renal insufficiency)
- Mesangial proliferative glomerulonephritis
- Focal segmental glomerulonephritis
- Congenital nephrotic syndrome
- Membranous nephropathy

Asymptomatic Microscopic Hematuria and Proteinuria

- Hereditary glomerulonephritis (Alport syndrome)
- Membranoproliferative glomerulonephritis type III
- IgA nephropathy (especially older adolescents)

Academy of Pediatrics Committee on Quality Improvement recommends evaluation of children under 2 years of age after the first febrile UTI with renal ultrasound and voiding cystourethrogram (VCUG).

VCUG is used to identify VUR and ureteroceles and to evaluate uretheral patency in male patients. Acquired renal scarring related to UTI occurs most commonly in children younger than 2 years old and is often, but not always, associated with VUR. Renal scarring most often results from a congenital ureteral defect leading to VUR (reflux nephropathy) or from obstructive uropathies and should not be considered as an acquired cause of renal insufficiency. Recent research indicates that at least half of young children who develop pyelonephritis with resulting renal scarring do not have VUR. Following their first UTI, 30% to 40% of young girls have VUR, which is mild to moderate (grades I to III) in 85%.

The purpose of the ultrasound is to identify structural abnormalities, gross parenchymal scarring, hydronephrosis, and hydroureter. Ten to 20% will have gross renal scarring, suggesting previous undetected pyelonephritis or congenital renal malformation. Therapeutic intervention such as use of prophylactic low-dose antibiotics to prevent recurrent UTI and ureteral reimplantation to prevent reflux must be considered; however, evidence that these measures will prevent progressive renal scarring is lacking. The degree of loss of renal parenchyma (scarring) has not been demonstrated to be related to the extent of loss of renal function.

Acquired glomerular diseases are most often discovered by the generalist performing a urinalysis either because of patient symptoms (swelling, gross hematuria, hypertension) or as part of a health maintenance examination (Box 173-2). In most instances childhood nephrotic syndrome presents in the toddler age group with generalized swelling. The diagnosis is suspected by finding heavy proteinuria (3 to 4+) with minimal or no microscopic hematuria. Low serum albumin and elevated serum cholesterol confirm the presence of nephrotic syndrome. Patients with steroid-responsive nephrotic syndrome rarely progress to renal insufficiency. Patients with less common forms of nephrotic syndrome that are often resistant to steroid treatment (mesangial proliferative glomerulonephritis, focal segmental glomerulosclerosis, and membranous nephropathy) may progress over time to renal insufficiency.

Glomerulonephritis most often presents to the primary care provider with the onset of gross hematuria (brown or dark, smoky urine). Some patients may have only microhematuria and proteinuria on routine urinalysis. Microscopic examination of the urine can identify granular, white blood cell, and red blood cell casts that confirm glomerular origin of the hematuria. The finding of microscopic hematuria without proteinuria does not usually indicate glomerulonephritis. However, if in addition to microscopic hematuria, persistent proteinuria develops, the clinician should suspect a more chronic form of glomerulonephritis and measure serum creatinine, serum proteins, and C3. Measurement of C3 concentration (Table 173-5) is crucial

Table 173-5. Relation of C3 Concentration to Type of Glomerular Disease

Low C3 Concentration

Acute poststreptococcal GN
Membranoproliferative GN
Systemic lupus erythematosus GN
GN associated with chronic bacteremia

Normal C3 Concentration

IgA nephropathy (SHP)
Rapidly progressive GN
    Idiopathic
    ANCA+
    Anti–basement membrane GN (Goodpature syndrome)
Membranous nephropathy
Hereditary nephritis (Alport syndrome)

GN, glomerulonephritis; SHP, Schänlein-Henoch purpura.

to diagnosis and for planning management. For example, acute poststreptococcal glomerulonephritis is the most likely diagnosis in a child between the ages of 3 and 10 years who presents with an acute onset of gross hematuria associated with a low serum C3 concentration. However, if the C3 concentration does not return to normal within 6 to 8 weeks, an alternative diagnosis must considered (see Table 173-5) and confirmed with a renal biopsy. If the initial C3 level is normal and family history or physical findings do not contribute to a diagnosis, a renal biopsy will usually be necessary. IgA nephropathy is the most common diagnosis in older children. This disorder occurs predominantly in boys and men, especially in those with recurrent gross hematuria in association with upper respiratory infections.

Renal thrombosis or ischemia is a less common cause for CRI in children. Diarrhea-related hemolytic-uremic syndrome (HUS) is the most common cause for acute renal failure in young children. Approximately 10% of children who have had diarrhea-associated HUS develop CRI.

MANAGEMENT OF CHRONIC RENAL INSUFFICIENCY

Progression and presentation of symptoms of renal impairment vary considerably in children with glomerular versus congenital/structural/metabolic causes of CRI. Infants and toddlers with dysplastic or structural abnormalities and a serum creatinine level greater than 1.0 mg/dL during the first year of life will usually progress to CRI or ESRD by the end of the first decade of life. Children with severe glomerular disorders can have rapid progression to CRI or ESRD at any age, but with unremitting or progressive glomerular disorders, many progress to ESRD during the stage of rapid growth during their adolescent years.

Hypertension is rare in the children with tubular/dysplastic renal diseases until ESRD, but is common in children with glomerular or cystic renal diseases and is a major cause for frequent medical observation and adjustment in medication. In children with immunologic glomerular disorders, in addition to hypertension, the scope of care often includes multiple immunosuppressive medications. Management of these complex patients is optimized through specialized pediatric nephrology care and study protocols at centers interested and capable of accumulating the necessary excellence to achieve improved outcomes. Hypertension should be managed to maintain the systolic and diastolic pressures at or below the 95th percentile for age, height, and gender. Dietary counseling, prescription of long-acting antihypertensive medication, and the use of a pill box for medication dispensing all aid compliance with the therapeutic regimen. All clinicians must be aware of the secondary effects of over-the-counter medications and antibiotics commonly used for childhood illnesses. These agents should be checked for interaction and adverse physiologic effects in children with moderate to severe renal impairment. With progression of CRI, dietary indiscretion or medications may cause dangerous hyperkalemia or hypertension.

Evidence for autonomous glomerular injury through hyperfiltraion is often signaled by the development of mild proteinuria, suggesting that, in addition to other medications, an angiotensin-converting enzyme inhibitor (ACEi) is indicated to reduce hyperfiltration and slow progressive loss of nephron units. Although some advocate reducing hyperfiltration by the addition of essential amino acids to a low-protein diet of high biologic value, growing children need adequate intake of proteins, calories, and minerals and prescription of a low-protein diet is uncommon. The current recommended protein and calorie intake for children with CRI is 100% of the daily recommended dietary allowances (RDAs) (Table 173-6). The goal is to maintain the blood urea nitrogen (BUN) level below 60 to 70 mg/dL, serum bicarbonate at 20 mEq/L or greater, serum calcium between 10 and 11 mg/dL, and phosphorus at 4.5 to 5.5 mg/dL. A rise in serum phosphorus above 5.5 mg/dL indicates the need to reduce dietary phosphorus and add medication that will bind phosphorus in the gut (calcium carbonate, calcium acetate, sevelamer HCl).

The failing kidney, as an endocrine organ, slowly reduces production of the renal hormones erythropoietin, resulting in anemia, and calcitriol (dihydroxyvitamin D, resulting in osteodystrophy). Virtually all children with advancing renal impairment will require replacement with calcitriol and erythropoietin. Correction of anemia improves many symptoms of renal insufficiency, including fatigue, exercise tolerance, sleep, appetite, concentration, and overall well-being. During the early stages of CRI when the GFR is between 50% and 25% of normal, the generalist has the greatest opportunity to minimize the deleterious effects of chronic renal disease on the skeleton, brain, heart, and hemopoietic systems.

SCHEDULING OF CARE BY GENERALISTS AND SPECIALIST PEDIATRICIANS

The reciprocal of the serum creatinine followed over an extended period and plotted against lapsed time over years can yield a straight line. This line can be used with a fair degree of accuracy in assisting the clinician, medical team members, and family in frank discussions and an optimistic attitude regarding the progressive course of renal impairment and the scheduling of treatment in ESRD care of children. Disruptions in daily family life with dietary restrictions, medication compliance, and the switch from a conservative treatment course to aggressive management with renal replacement therapy in the form of dialysis or transplantation or both need to be addressed early in the

Table 173-6. Recommended Dietary Allowances (RDA) of Protein and Calories for Patients with Chronic Renal Insufficiency

Age	Protein (g/kg)	Calorie (kcal/kg)
0–6 months	2.2	108
6–12 months	1.5	98
1–3 years	1.2	102
4–6 years	1.2	90
7–10 years	1.0	70
11–14 years	1.0	45–55
15–18 years	0.9	40–45
Adult	0.8	40

Table 174-1. Factors Influencing Blood Pressure in Childhood

Physical
Age
Weight
Height
Gender
Small gestational age

Familial
Race (relationship uncertain)
Genetics (relationship uncertain)

Environmental
Family influence
Diet (salt)

CD-ROM Tables 174-1 and 174-2). Contrary to adult studies in which hypertension is more prevalent in African Americans compared to whites, no significant difference in the prevalence of hypertension according to race has been found in children. High intake of dietary sodium has been linked to increased blood pressure. However, the effect of sodium intake differs in individuals with increased susceptibility to salt among blacks. The presence of genetic influence is well documented, with at least 20% to 40% of the blood pressure variability explained by familial factors. Low birth weight has recently been found to be associated with elevated blood pressure.

Measurement of Blood Pressure in Children

Accurate measurement of blood pressure in children requires careful attention to the environment and use of standard procedures and equipment. Children 3 years of age and older should have their blood pressure checked during routine and emergency visits. Blood pressure should be measured at least twice on each occasion in the child's right arm, after at least 3 to 5 minutes of rest in the seated position. Use of clinical sphygmomanometer is the gold standard for measurement of blood pressure in a child. Systolic blood pressure is determined by the onset of the first Korotkoff sound. The fifth Korotkoff sound (disappearance of Korotkoff sounds) is used to define diastolic blood pressure. The choice of appropriate cuff size is very important. Too small a cuff for the arm leads to falsely high blood pressure. Figure 174-1 illustrates determination of proper cuff size. If two cuffs could be chosen, the larger cuff should be selected. The cuff should be inflated to at least 20 mm Hg above expected systolic blood pressure (disappearance of the radial pulse) and deflated at the rate of 2 to 3 mm Hg per second.

Automated blood pressure devices are used increasingly. Most machines use an oscillometric method to measure systolic and mean arterial blood pressures and calculate the diastolic blood pressure. They are easy to use, allow measuring blood pressure in newborns and infants, and are free from observer bias, but have problems with calibration. Because published normative blood pressure data are based on the auscultation method, using those standards when blood pressure is obtained with an automated device may be inappropriate.

Ambulatory blood pressure monitoring (ABPM) overcomes some limitations of causal blood pressure measure-

ment. Multiple measurements of blood pressure during a 24-hour period more accurately reflects the continuous nature of blood pressure. ABPM assesses blood pressure in the patient's normal environment, both awake and asleep. ABPM might better identify patients with "white coat hypertension," when the blood pressure is falsely high in the office setting from stress or anxiety. After completing ABPM, mean 24-hour and mean daytime and nighttime systolic and diastolic blood pressure data can be compared against gender- and height-specific 95th percentile norms derived from normative pediatric ABPM data. Blood pressure load is a calculated ABPM parameter, the percentage of blood pressure readings that exceed the 95th percentile of normal for the individual patient. Percentage of sleep decline in blood pressure can be determined. Normally blood pressure decreases at least 10% (dipping) during night hours; if blood pressure declines less than 10%, this pattern is called nondipping. In adults, nondipping has been associated with hypertensive end-organ injury.

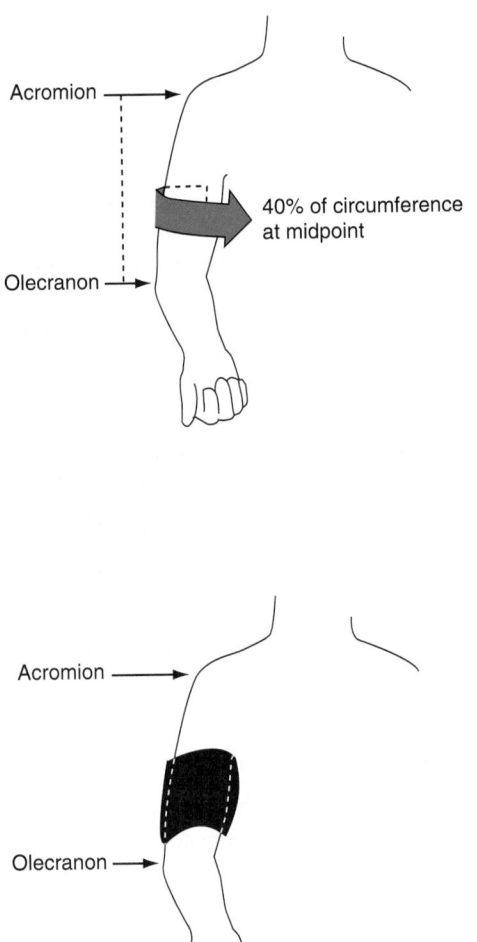

Figure 174-1. Determination of proper cuff size: The cuff bladder should cover 80% to 100% of the circumference of the arm. The width of the bladder cuff should be approximately 40% of the circumference of the arm measured at a point midway between the olecranon and acromion. (From Update on the 1987 Task Force Report on High Blood Pressure in Children and Adolescents: A Working Group Report from the National High Blood Pressure Education Program. Pediatrics 1996;98:651.)

DIAGNOSIS

Causes of Blood Pressure Elevation In Children

Table 174-2 lists the many causes of elevated blood pressure in children. Hypertension can be classified as primary, or essential, with no identified cause, and secondary, when cause of hypertension can be identified. The etiology of hypertension in children is age-dependent. The prevalence of secondary hypertension is inversely related to the child's age. Younger patients are most likely to have secondary forms of hypertension. The most likely causes of hypertension according to age group are listed in Table 174-3. The prevalence of secondary hypertension increases directly with the severity of hypertension, because essential hypertension is usually mild or moderate. Renal causes such as renal artery thrombosis, renal artery stenosis, congenital renal malformations, polycystic kidney disease, and coarctation of the aorta are most common causes of hypertension in children up to 6 years. In children 6 to 10 years old renal parenchymal and renovascular diseases remain the most frequent causes of increased blood pressure. The prevalence of essential hypertension increases with age; after 10 years of age it becomes the leading cause of elevated blood pressure. The pathophysiology of essential hypertension is not well understood, but likely involves genetic, environmental, and lifestyle influences. Obesity is emerging now as a significant cause of essential hypertension in pediatric patients.

Table 174-2. Causes of Hypertension in Children*

Cardiovascular
Coarctation of the aorta
Systemic arteritis (Takayasu arteritis, Schönlein-Henoch purpura)
Arteriovenous fistula
Radiation aortitis
Subacute bacterial endocarditis

Renal
Structural abnormalities (obstructive uropathy, reflux nephropathy)
Acute or chronic glomerulonephritis
Cystic kidney disease
Dialysis-related
Acute and chronic renal failure

Oncologic
Pheochromocytoma
Adrenal adenocarcinoma
Wilms tumor
Neuroblastoma

Endocrine
Hyperthyroidism
Congenital adrenal hyperplasia
Cushing syndrome
Liddle syndrome
Primary aldosteronism

Neurologic
Guillian-Barré syndrome
Increased intracranial pressure
Familail dysautnomia

Drug-Induced
Steroids
Sympathomimetics (decongestants)
Oral contraceptives
Cocaine
Calcineurin inhibitors (cyclosprine)

*The most common type of hypertension is essential hypertension, which is of unknown cause.

Table 174-3. Most Common Causes of Hypertension According to Age Group

Age Group	Cause
Neonates and young infants	Renal artery or venous thrombosis Coarctation of aorta Renal artery stenosis Congenital renal abnormalities Bronchopulmonary dysplasia
1–6 years	Renal parenchymal disease Renal artery stenosis Coarctation of aorta
6–10 years	Renal parenchymal disease Renal artery stenosis Essential hypertension
11–18 years	Essential hypertension Renal parenchymal disease

Medical History and Physical Examination

A careful history and physical examination can provide clues to detect secondary causes of hypertension or alternatively to make a diagnosis of essential hypertension (Table 174-4). Family history should address a history of essential hypertension; cardiovascular, endocrine, and renal diseases; and stroke. The history of inherited conditions such as polycystic kidney disease and neurofibromatosis should also be asked. Medical history should focus on birth history and neonatal course (prematurity, bronchopulmonary dysplasia, and the use of umbilical catheters), history of urinary tract infections (reflux nephropathy), hospitalizations, and other medical problems. All medications, including home remedies and nonprescription pills, should be listed. The use of decongestants (e.g., pseudoephedrine, phenylpropanolamine) is a frequent problem. In adolescents, history of using oral contraceptives, smoking, alcohol, and street drugs should be explored. Review of systems and physical examination (see Table 174-4) should be directed by associated signs and symptoms. The recognition of hypertension in infants is not always simple. They usually present with symptoms and signs of congestive heart failure such as increased irritability, respiratory distress, feeding problems, or failure to thrive. Boxes 174-1 and 174-2 list red flags, symptoms that should alert the clinician to the possibility of hypertension.

Diagnostic Approach to Hypertension in Children

When a child is found to have an elevated blood pressure, prior to further evaluation the clinician should consider the patient's age, sudden onset and severity of hypertension, presence of any symptoms of increased blood pressure, evidence of end-organ damage, and family history. The primary goal of the investigation should be identification of secondary and potentially correctable causes of hypertension.

For older overweight children with a family history of hypertension, with mild to moderate elevation of blood pressure, and no indications from the history and physical examination of a secondary cause, few diagnostic tests are required. Hypertension should be confirmed by two or three repeated blood pressure measurements above 95th percentile over a 1-month period. Screening studies in these children include urine analysis, urine culture, and serum creatinine. If one of these studies is abnormal, a renal

Table 174-4. Physical Examination Findings Suggestive of Hypertension

System	Findings/Disorders
Body habitus	Obesity: Cushing syndrome, steroids, essential hypertension
	Failure to thrive: chronic renal disease
	Thinness: hyperthyroidism
Head and face	Round face: Cushing syndrome
	Elfin face: Williams syndrome
Eyes	Fundal changes
	Proptosis: hyperthyroidism
Neck	Goiter: hyperthyroid goiter
	Bruit
Heart	Enlargement: cardiac failure
Lungs	Rales: congestive heart failure
Abdomen	Masses: Wilms tumor, neuroblastoma, obstructive uropathy
	Hepatomegaly: cardiac failure
	Hepatosplenomegaly: autosomal recessive polycystic disease
	Bruit: renal artery stenosis, arteriovenous malformation
Pelvis	Masses: obstructive uropathy
Genitalia	Ambiguous, virilized: congenital adrenal hyperplasia
Extremities	Disparity in blood pressure: coarctation of aorta
	Edema: renal disease
	Rickets: chronic renal disease
Skin	Neurofibromas
	Café au lait spots: pheochromocytoma
	Tubers: tuberous sclerosis
	Rashes: Schönlein-Henoch nephritis
	Pale: chronic renal disease

ultrasound should be performed. In obese children, fasting lipid profile should be performed to evaluate for elevated plasma triglycerides and low-density lipoprotein (LDL) cholesterol. Assessment of chronic elevation of blood pressure and end-organ damage includes echocardiography to evaluate the presence of left ventricular hypertrophy and ophthalmologic examination for retinal abnormalities. Chest x-ray and electrocardiogram are not as effective as echocardiography in evaluating end-organ effects.

A younger child with more severe hypertension and the presence of symptoms is predictive of secondary hypertension. The evaluation of these children should be guided by suspected problem and performed by the specialist. For example, the child with suspected coarctation of the aorta should have echocardiographic evaluation; the child with suspected pheochromocytoma would have 24-hour urine collection for catecholamines performed as well as localization (imaging) studies using MRI (magnetic resonance

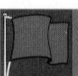 **Box 174-1.** Red Flags: Symptoms of Hypertension in Infants: Alerts to Cardiac Failure

Failure to thrive
Feeding problems
Irritability
Respiratory distress
Cyanosis
Seizures

 Box 174-2. Red Flags: Symptoms of Hypertensive Emergencies: Alerts to Hypertensive Encephalopathy

Severe headache
Vomiting
Seizures
Ataxia
Changes in mental status
Visual disturbances

imaging) or ^{123}I-MIBG (metaiodobenzylguanidine) scan. In case of suspected renovascular disease, renal angiography is a gold standard procedure for children.

The pediatric provider must recognize hypertensive emergencies (see Boxes 174-1 and 174-2) presented as hypertensive encephalopathy with severe headache, vomiting, seizures, ataxia, stupor, and visual disturbances. Immediate treatment should be initiated, including rapid control of blood pressure. Treatment approach of hypertensive encephalopathy is found in Chapter 40.

MANAGEMENT

Specific recommendations for treatment of elevated blood pressure are based on the patient's clinical situation. In case of hypertensive emergencies, the goal of the therapy is to lower blood pressure by 25% to 50% within 1 hour after initiation of the treatment. Too rapid reduction of blood pressure may be dangerous, especially in patients with increased intracranial pressure. In case of chronic hypertension the goal is to reduce blood pressure to a level below the 95th percentile, and ideally below the 90th percentile.

The initial therapy of mild elevation of blood pressure when hypertension is most likely essential and without end-organ damage consists of nonpharmacologic intervention, or so-called lifestyle modification. This approach includes diet modification with low caloric intake and salt restriction and an exercise program. The combination of weight loss and improved physical fitness has been shown to significantly reduce blood pressure in children with essential hypertension.

Children with severe or symptomatic hypertension, as well as those who have evidence of end-organ damage or failed nonpharmacologic intervention, require initiation of pharmacologic therapy. Antihypertensive drug therapy can be divided into two groups: hypertensive emergencies (see Chapter 40) and chronic hypertension. In cases of chronic elevation of blood pressure, individualization of therapy must be strongly considered (Box 174-3). The initial drug choice is based on the mechanism and severity of hypertension, patient's demographics and compliance issues, previous history of side effects, the presence of other medical problems, and concomitant drug therapy. One of the most important considerations is pediatric safety and efficacy data. Unfortunately, for many antihypertensive medications these data are not available in children. There is also lack of age-related data for dose selection and dosing interval as well as drug formulations for young children who are unable to swallow pills although liquid preparations are available for some medications. Drug therapy usually starts with a low dose of a single agent. The dose is titrated

LONG-TERM SEQUELAE

Persistent and poorly controlled hypertension is a significant risk factor for myocardial infarction, stroke, peripheral vascular disease, and end-stage renal disease in adults. In children, long-term consequences of hypertension are not known. However, there is increasing evidence of a link between childhood onset of hypertension and adult morbidity and death from end-organ damage. For example, hypertensive children frequently have left ventricular hypertrophy and retinal vascular abnormalities, markers of prolonged elevation of blood pressure. Of particular importance is the management of overweight children, because hypertension of childhood is directly related to the problem of obesity in children.

FOLLOW-UP

Children who have been diagnosed with hypertension need careful follow-up. In general, the primary care provider is able to manage children with mild essential hypertension:

1. The emphasis should be directed toward nonpharmacologic intervention.
2. If in 6 months good control of blood pressure has not been achieved, drug therapy should be offered. After

until blood pressure goals are achieved. If adequate blood pressure control is not achieved on a single agent, a second agent should be added. Angiotensin-converting enzyme (ACE) inhibitors and calcium-channel blockers (CCB) are the most common antihypertensive medications prescribed currently for all pediatric ages. The wide use of these medications is based on their effectiveness and relatively low rate of side effects. The classification, preparations, and dosages of most commonly used antihypertensive drugs are summarized in Table 174-5.

Table 174-5. Commonly Used Drug Therapy for Chronic Hypertension in Pediatric Patients

Drug	Child Dose*	Dosing Interval	Adolescent/Adult Dose	Adverse Effects
Angiotensin-Converting Enzyme Inhibitors				
Enalapril	0.1–0.5 mg/kg/day	12–24 hours	2.5–40 mg/day	Hypotension, hyperkalemia, decreased renal function, cough
Lisinopril	Not established	12–24 hours	2.5–40 mg/day	Same as above
Quinapril	Not established	12–24 hours	10–80 mg/day	Same as above
Captopril	0.5–2 mg/kg/day	8 hours	12.5–50 mg/dose, max 450 mg/day	Same as above
Calcium-Channel Blockers				
Nifedipine (extended release)	0.25–2 mg/kg/dose	12–24 hours	30–90 mg/dose, max 180 mg/day	Flushing tachycardia, hypotension
Amlodipine	0.1–0.3 mg/kg/dose	12–24 hours	2.5–20 mg/day	Same as above, peripheral edema
Isradipine	0.05–0.15 mg/kg/dose	8–12 hours	2.5–5 mg/dose, max 20 mg/day	Same as above
Felodipine (extended release)	0.1 mg/kg/day	12–24 hours	2.5–5 mg/dose, max 20 mg/day	Same as above
Diltiazem	1.5–2 mg/kg/day	8–12 hours	60–180 mg/day, max 360 mg/day	Arrhythmia, AV block, bradycardia
Diuretics				
Chlorothiazide	5–10 mg/kg/dose	12–24 hours	250–1000 mg/day	Hypokalemia, increased serum uric acid and glucose
Hydrochlorothiazide	0.5–2.0 mg/kg/dose	12–24 hours	25–100 mg/day	Same as above
Furosemide	0.5–2.0 mg/kg dose	12–24 hours	20–80 mg/dose	Hypercalciuria, hypokalemia
Spironolactone	1–3 mg/kg dose	6–12 hours	25–100 mg/dose	Hyperkalemia, arrhythmia
β-Blockers				
Atenolol	0.8–1 mg/kg/dose	24 hours	25–50 mg/dose, max 100 mg	Bradycardia, AV block, fatigue
Propranolol	0.5–2 mg/kg/day	6–12 hours	40 mg/dose, max 480 mg/day	Same as above, bronchospasm, hypoglycemia
Labetalol	1–3 mg/kg/day	6–12 hours	100–400 mg/day	Same as above
α-Blockers				
Clonidine				Drowsiness, rebound hypertension
Oral	0.05–0.6 mg/day	8–12 hours	0.2–1.2 mg/day	
Transdermal	Not established	1 week	0.1–0.3 mg/day	

*Use child dose until age 12 or when dose/kg reaches adult minimum.
Av, atrioventricular.

initiation of pharmacologic treatment, the patient needs to be seen by the primary care provider within 2 weeks. The dose of medication should be adjusted every 2 weeks until blood pressure control is adequate. Once blood pressure control has been achieved, twice a year follow-up is sufficient.

3. After 6 months of normal blood pressure, the dose of medication may be tapered down during a 1- to 6-month period of follow-up until the patient is off pharmacologic therapy. The patient must then be followed carefully for another 6 months and annually to ensure that the blood pressure remains normal.

4. If there is no response to a 1-month trial of antihypertensive therapy, referral to the specialist is necessary.

5. Recommendations for athletic participation depend on the severity of hypertension. American Academy of Pediatrics published guidelines for sport participation using the 26th Bethesda Conference on heart disease and athletic participation and of the second Task Force on Blood Pressure Control in Children as a basis. Children with hypertension below the 99th percentile and without end-organ damage have no limitations for competitive sport activity. Children with severe hypertension (>99th percentile) with no target-organ damage are restricted from competitive sports and high static activity until blood pressure is under control. High static activities include field events (throwing), gymnastics, karate/judo, water skiing, weight lifting, body building, downhill skiing, wrestling, cycling, decathlon, rowing, and speed skating. Participation of children with target-organ damage should be determined on an individual basis according to the severity of both end-organ damage and hypertension.

Additional Resources, CD-ROM

Blood pressure levels for 90th and 95th percentiles	Tables
Bibliography	

Mini-index of Related Topics

	CH.
■ PROMOTING PHYSICAL ACTIVITY	19
■ HYPERTENSIVE CRISIS	40
■ APPROACH TO THE CHILD WITH HEADACHE	105
■ NUTRITION IN CHILDREN WITH CHRONIC DISEASES	130

SUGGESTED READINGS

Flynn JT: Neonatal hypertension: Diagnosis and management. Pediatr Nephrol 2000;14:332–341.

Jung FF, Ingelfinger JR: Hypertension in childhood and adolescence. Pediatr Rev 1993;14:169–179.

National High Blood Pressure Education Working Group on Hypertension Control in Children and Adolescents: Update on the Task Force Report (1987) on High Blood Pressure in Children and Adolescents: A Working Group Report from the National High Blood Pressure Education Program. Pediatrics 1996;98:649–658.

Sinaico AR: Hypertension in children. N Engl J Med 1996;335:1968–1973.

Sorof JM, Portman RJ: Ambulatory blood pressure monitoring in the pediatric patients. J Pediatr 2000;136:578–586.

175 Renal Transplant

Michael Chobanian

ROLE OF THE GENERALIST

1   Maintain role as primary care provider to ensure continuity of care both physically and emotionally for children who are transplant recipients.

2   Recognize rejection, tolerance, and compatibility.

3   Identify unique clinical situations of the transplant recipient such as infections, cancer, cardiovascular disease, bone disease, growth and development, and sexual maturation.

4   Recognize drug-drug interactions, utilization of live versus killed vaccines, and long-term effects of immunosuppression.

5   Know when to refer patients to transplant specialist and how to help in evaluating prospective recipient candidates.

6   Understand outcomes and long-term consequences of solid organ transplantation, including donor awareness.

7   Help implement a plan for renal transplantation in children with end-stage renal disease.

8   Monitor growth, development, cardiovascular stability, and psychosocial behavior in children awaiting transplant.

9   Coordinate care of children awaiting renal transplant.

Renal transplantation has evolved from an experimental therapy in which only those unfit for dialysis were considered as potential recipients into the major renal replacement therapy for all children with end-stage renal disease (ESRD). Because a well-functioning kidney leads to a quality of life that cannot be surpassed by any mode of dialysis, every effort should be made to attain a functioning graft in all children. Recipient selection is now limited by very few exclusionary criteria in children.

Because of dismal outcomes of children younger than 1 year of age, age has been an exclusion criterion. More recent data regarding outcomes of children receiving living versus cadaveric donor kidneys demonstrate excellent 5-year actual patient and graft survival rates in children who received living donor kidneys versus cadaveric kidneys. Improvement came from living related adult-size kidneys, placed and maintained in the child of at least 10 kg bodyweight. Current recommendations state that transplantation should be deferred until the recipient is at least 2 years of age with a weight of 10 kg, unless a living related donor is available.

The unique objective of any renal replacement therapy is to afford the child every opportunity to achieve growth and development conducive to receiving a graft. How to achieve that objective is well summarized in Chapter 173 and can only underscore the importance of pediatric nephrologic backup for the primary pediatrician.

In the child older than 2 years of age and of appropriate weight, referral for transplantation requires screening records and tests, which in part can be performed by the primary care provider. These records include growth charts, immunization records, neurodevelopmental assessments, nutritional assessments, psychological assessments, cognitive and school assessments (when available), family history, and social history. This historical record provides the basis for the selection of the potential recipient. For example, although not an absolute exclusionary criterion, the teenager with repeated noncompliance behavior or involvement in high-risk behaviors (early sexual activity, tobacco or drug abuse) may require a "written contract" between the patient and the transplant center for a designated period of time prior to proceeding with the pretransplant workup. The primary care provider's role is vital in this agreement process.

Referrals to a particular transplant center are based on the preference and confidence between the primary care provider and family. Referrals should be made when both the primary care provider and family feel the need to explore transplantation as an option. This is especially important when considering a preemptive transplant. Once the child has less than 30% functional renal capacity remaining (based on a creatinine clearance or the Schwartz equation; Table 173-2) patients should be referred to either a pediatric nephrologist or a transplant center. Decisions made prior to this point are difficult unless the child has acute renal failure with concomitant chronic renal insufficiency or a known renal disease that inevitably results in ESRD (e.g., congenital nephrotic syndrome). Children with chronic renal insufficiency should be followed in part by a pediatric nephrologist.

Because urologic anomalies are commonly associated with renal parenchymal dysplasia/hypoplasia, and account for the largest number of pediatric cases resulting in ESRD, a functioning urinary reservoir (whether a natural bladder or intestinal conduit) must exist prior to transplantation. Early intervention by a pediatric urologist working in conjunction with a pediatric nephrologist and the child's primary care provider are essential. Nephrectomy of either or both native kidneys is avoided unless there is an inherent risk of malignancy (e.g., Deny-Drash syndrome and associated Wilms tumor). Even if the bladder has been dysfunctional prior to transplantation, the likelihood of successful micturition with or without intermittent bladder catheterization remains high. Formal urodynamic testing and x-ray analysis (voiding cystourethrogram) can be performed under the direction of a pediatric urologist at the child's primary care provider's facility. Documentation of true urinary tract infections and identification of infective organisms with their respective antibiotic sensitivities are of vital importance to the transplant team in selecting posttransplant urinary tract infection prophylaxis, if necessary (see Chapter 172).

Special consideration regarding transplant is required for the child with chronic renal insufficiency progressing toward ESRD who has renal osteodystrophy, nephrotic syndrome, or prior malignancies or is currently dialysis-dependent (see Chapter 173). Control of hyperparathyroidism and the bone disease of ESRD before transplant is essential because of the difficulties in achieving growth potential after transplant. The child on hemodialysis or peritoneal dialysis remains at risk for bone disease and ultimately reduced growth potential owing to calcium, phosphorus, parathormone (PTH), vitamin D, and acid-base metabolism. Utilization of pretransplant recombinant human growth hormone (rhGH) is effective only if the child's mineral metabolism remains in balance. In the child with nephrotic syndrome, control of proteinuria is paramount. Large nondiscriminate losses of large-molecular-weight proteins can lead to malnutrition. Risk of thrombosis, vitamin deficiencies, and infections can continue unless the diseased kidneys are removed or they become sclerosed, particularly in children whose ESRD was the result of congenital nephrotic syndrome or focal segmental glomerulonephritis. Children with ESRD secondary to Wilms tumor should have a 2-year tumor-free period. Individuals who have undergone transplantation without this waiting period are at increased risk for recurrent malignancy and overwhelming sepsis from prolonged chemotherapy. Those children who have had other malignancies must also have an observed tumor-free period. Most waiting periods are at least 2 years. Invasive urogenital cancer and melanoma require 5-year tumor-free follow-up periods. This time obviously can be problematic for the child on a cadaveric waiting list.

The role of the primary care provider is implementing a plan toward providing renal transplantation as an option for the patient. Monitoring of neurodevelopment, psychosocial behavior, and cardiovascular stability remains the most important. Loss of cognitive and developmental milestones are common in the young child with uremia. Aggressive programmatic interventions, such as early childhood physical therapy, occupational therapy, and speech therapy, can make important contributions to the child's neurodevelopmental outcome after transplant. Seizures requiring anticonvulsants occur in approximately 10% of children with ESRD. When the transplant is either scheduled or imminent, anticonvulsant drugs that do not interfere with immunosuppressive agents must be initiated prior to the transplant and appropriately adjusted after transplant.

Psychiatric disorders that are controlled are not absolute contraindications to transplant, but involvement of the child's primary care provider, psychiatrist, and psychologist is essential.

The stress of the transplant process is greatest at the cardiovascular level. Hypertension and fluid imbalances are common in the child with ESRD and must be regulated prior to the transplant itself. Risk factors such as salt-sensitivity, familial hyperlipidemia, familial diabetes and early cardiovascular deaths, uncontrolled hypertension, obesity, syndrome X, and poor cardiovascular conditioning increase the risk in the transplanted child for premature cardiovascular disease and shortened graft survival. The primary care provider is vital in assuming the role of long-term manager of all these issues prior to, during, and long after the transplant. The guidelines for management can be originated only at the transplant center; the implementation, documentation, and maintenance of the posttransplant health care plan resides at the level of the primary care provider through coordination with the transplant team.

DONOR REQUIREMENTS

Donation today involves relatively little beyond consideration for a healthy adult individual with a compatible blood group and an unrestricted motivation. An absolute restriction of donation is that of age. Donors must be 18 years or older. In rare instances, an older related teen who is younger than 18 years old, who has successfully petitioned the courts, and who is free from a psychosocial disorder has been used as a donor with parental consent. Blood group matching is also an absolute requirement between eligible donor and recipient but does not include Rh and the minor blood groups. Only ABO blood group compatibility is necessary (Table 175-1). Histocompatibility matching remains an important consideration only when multiple donors are available to the recipient. Again, the six antigen-matched kidney remains the most likely organ to last decades for the recipient. Parents are haplotypic matches (half matches) for their children and, in general, are the most likely to proceed as eligible donors for all the obvious reasons.

Donor workup includes a complete medical evaluation, which can immediately rule out the at-risk donor. Risks for poor outcome are listed in Box 175-1. Laboratory screening tests for the donor that provide invaluable information for minimizing risk to the potential recipient are listed in Box 175-2. Chest radiograph, electrocardiogram, and psychosocial evaluation can also provide insightful information for the transplant team. A helical computed tomog-

Table 175-1. ABO Blood Type Matching for Renal Transplantation

Donor Blood Type	Recipient Blood Type
A	Can accept A or O
B	Can accept B or O
O (universal donor)	Can accept O
AB (universal recipient)	Can accept A, B, O, or AB

Box 175-1. Risk Factors for Poor Donor Outcome

- Hypertension
- Diabetes
- Proteinuria (>150 mg/m² body surface area)
- Recurrent kidney stones, glomerular filtration rate <80 mL/min, hematuria
- Urologic anomalies
- Chronic obstructive pulmonary disease (COPD)
- Recent/remote malignancy
- Obesity (BMI >32%)
- History of thrombosis
- Psychiatric illness
- Strong family history of sudden death, renal disease, hypertension, or diabetes

raphy (CT) urogram is then performed to identify which kidney is structurally the most advantageous to remove from the donor. Selection of the donor ultimately rests with the family and transplant team. The primary care provider can best serve as mediator and guide for the interested donor when historical information or concerns about either the donor's motivation or psychosocial stability are addressed directly to the transplant team.

There are specific issues related to cadaveric donors when the recipient is a child. Age of the donor is an essential consideration. Data from a wide number of sources have prompted exclusion of kidneys from cadaveric donors younger than 3 years old and caution in use of organs retrieved from donors between the ages of 3 and 6 years. Because donor age is critical, the favorable donor remains between 16 and 40 years old. This may be in part due to the fact the human kidney loses 1% of its functional capacity each year after age 32. Ideal donor age is between 21 and 22 years old. Size of the living donor is also essential. Reports of living donations into recipient children less than 10 kg body weight continue to accumulate, based on the technical expertise of specific centers. Structurally large grafts provide additional risks of ischemia and maintenance of renal perfusion pressure from an otherwise small individual.

The decision to proceed with the best possible form of transplant (living versus cadaveric donor) is based on outcomes. Current data suggest a distinct advantage of the living donated organ versus the cadaveric one. However, not every recipient is fortunate enough to know a compatible donor, and thus must be placed on a cadaveric waiting list during which accumulation of time is the greatest burden to the child on ESRD. While the patient is "active" on the

Box 175-2. Donor Laboratory Screening Tests to Reduce Risk for Recipient

- Complete blood cell count
- Chemistry panel
- Human immunodeficiency virus (HIV)
- Hepatitis B and C, cytomegalovirus, Epstein-Barr virus
- Glucose tolerance or Hb A$_{1c}$
- Fasting lipid profile

waiting list, maintenance of health is essential and regular reports of infections, nonrenal/ESRD hospitalizations, and new untoward effects of drugs as well as psychosocial issues must be reported to the transplant center.

CHOICE OF IMMUNOSUPPRESSION

Immunosuppressive regimens are transplant center specific owing to protocols and programmatic success, but in general, most regimens utilize a "triple" therapy combination involving steroids, a calcineurin inhibitor (cyclosporin or tacrolimus), and an antiproliferative agent (azathioprine or mycophenolate mofetil). The addition of a calcineurin inhibitor has improved graft survival by as much as 20% to 25%. Additional immunosuppressive agents (e.g., sirolimus, brequinar, mizoribine) have not been adequately studied in the pediatric transplant population and are used only during "rescues" from acute steroid-resistant rejections.

Ultimately the final choice of the immunosuppressive regimen is made by the transplant team, the patient, and the family. Concerns over body image, changes which occur with both prednisone and cyclosporine, may force a more rapid taper of prednisone and the use of tacrolimus, which avoids the hypertrichosis and gingival hyperplasia seen in patients taking cyclosporin. If the patient is receiving a second or even a third transplant and a past history of acute rejection resulting in sensitization is factored in, triple therapy with antibody induction may be necessary. The child who received a cadaveric kidney may require a lower dose of calcineurin inhibition in an attempt to salvage renal perfusion pressure, whereas the "obese" child may benefit from a more rapid steroid tapering to avoid the almost 20% gain in body weight seen in the first year after transplant. More than half of all transplant centers use antibody induction in pediatric recipients considered at greatest risk of rejection, especially those of younger age and who have been previously sensitized by either organ transplantation or blood transfusions.

CADAVERIC VERSUS LIVING DONOR ORGANS

Within an 11-year period between 1987 and 1998, roughly 6000 children received 6500 kidney transplants. The vast majority of patients were older than 12 years, and more than half were white and male. More than half of the transplants performed since 1995 were from living donors. This number indicates both the importance of finding a suitable organ and the willingness of donors. It also reflects concerns regarding the prolonged waiting times for those on the list for a cadaveric organ.

Unfortunately the national trend since the early 1990s has been for prolonged waiting times with fewer available organs and more potential recipients. Generally, children are favored under the guidelines set forth by the United Network for Organ Sharing (UNOS), the national registry clearinghouse for all organ procurement organizations. Addition of the child's name on his or her transplant center's list enables the child to acquire priority points. These points are assigned based on age (younger age carries higher priority points for children under 16 years old), waiting time, HLA match, and center location versus procurement center. In general, in the nonsensitized child, waiting times have averaged less than a year for the child less than 5 years old to up to 2 years or more for those between 11 and 18 years old. Obviously the sensitized child may wait longer because of the higher likelihood of a positive crossmatch with a potential cadaveric donor. Regional differences also become important if assigned organ preferences are made for the youngest of children.

Advantages of living organs versus cadaveric organs seem to be mounting, especially in the pediatric population. There is up to a 20% increase in graft survival during all years for living versus cadaveric kidneys. This advantage likely reflects the lack of cold ischemic time, lower acute rejection rates, and the selection of better donors, including age and HLA matching.

REJECTION

Three major forms of rejection have been identified: hyperacute, acute, and chronic. Each has distinct pathologic findings, yet only one, acute, can be treated.

Rejection can be manifested with various signs or symptoms. The typical fever, constitutional symptoms of malaise, arthralgias or myalgias, graft tenderness, diminished urine output, edema, excessive weight gain, or hypertension may appear later in the course of rejection rather than as presenting features. Changes in creatinine of greater than 0.2 mg/dL warrant investigation under most circumstances. Unfortunately, because the measurement of creatinine in and of itself can be in error of 0.2 mg/dL, the smallest child is left with only the clinician's high index of suspicion every time a change in creatinine occurs. Any concern parents may have regarding their transplanted child may indicate the earliest changes of rejection, such as headache, vague abdominal pain, leg pain, or visual changes. Of course, drug toxicity, urinary tract infection including extraureteral obstruction secondary to a urinoma or lymphocele, or simple dehydration can account for the subtle change in creatinine as well as the accompanying signs or symptoms.

The gold standard to diagnose rejection of any form is the percutaneous renal transplant biopsy, performed using real-time ultrasound guidance. For children older than 12 years of age, light sedation can be used to alleviate the anxiety associated with the procedure. For the younger child, heavy conscious sedation under the direction of the pediatric anesthesiologist or intensivist is mandatory. Accurate processing of the specimen requires that the procedure be accomplished at a transplant center or that arrangements be made to ship the sample to the transplant center's pathology department.

Hyperacute rejection occurs when preformed cytotoxic antibodies cause rapid (immediate up to 2 or 3 days later) vascular thrombosis resulting in a nonurine producing graft. Because of the severity of the reaction, nephrectomy is indicated to avoid the extensive cytokine release and resultant systemic vascular collapse. This type of rejection has been rendered a rarity because of the sophistication of the final crossmatch between recipient and donor which can now detect both T- and B-cell positivity through flow cytometry.

Acute rejection can occur via a cell-mediated or antibody-mediated mechanism. Acute rejection occurs when insufficient immunosuppression is present, permitting cellular rejection by increasing numbers of lymphocytes found in the tubular interstitium, not the glomerulus of the nephron (classic "tubulitis"). This most common form of rejection is the most responsive to treatment with either Solu-Medrol pulses (for 3 or 5 days) or antibody therapy (OKT3, Atgam, or thymoglobulin). In a rarer form, the antibody-mediated acute rejection, an arteritis with necrosis, thrombosis, and endotheliitis, dominates the pathologic picture. This form of rejection almost always necessitates antibody therapy with variable outcomes. If success is defined as a return to prerejection serum creatinine level, then less than 50% are successful if steroid pulses are used. However, 90% success rates are achieved using OKT3. Success involves changing immunosuppressive therapy (e.g., by converting from cyclosporin to tacrolimus) or adding mycophenolate mofetil, or doing both, as part of the maintenance regimen.

Chronic allograft nephropathy is a term preferred over chronic rejection because it represents the multifactorial causes of long-term graft dysfunction. The causes may be secondary to recurrent acute immune-mediated rejection episodes or may be nonimmunologic, such as chronic drug toxicity, reflux (which all transplanted kidneys have), infections, nephrosclerosis, or endogenous renal disease (e.g., ischemic nephropathy or urate nephropathy). No known treatment is available, but minimizing calcineurin inhibition drug levels, adding alternative adjunct therapies (nondihydropyridine calcium-channel blockers or angiotensin-converting enzyme inhibitors), or switching immunosuppressives while regulating blood pressure or uric acid metabolism should be undertaken. Despite success in defining newer immunosuppressive regimens, rejection rates in children are higher than their adult counterparts. In the North American Pediatric Renal Transplant Cooperative Study, over 5000 transplants in children have resulted in 43% of living donor and 68% of cadaver donor patients having had at least one rejection episode within the first year compared to less than 40% in adults. The current national average of an acute rejection episode during the first year after transplant is approximately 20% for adults 18 years or older.

SPECIFIC DRUG SIDE EFFECTS

Clearly, like any other condition which requires long-term steroid use, the prominent cushingoid features and side effects render the benefits at times questionable. Growth retardation, hypertension, chemical diabetes, hyperlipidemia, cushingoid facies/habitus, acne, hypertrichosis, osteoporosis, aseptic necrosis of hips and tibia, delayed wound healing, myopathy, pancreatitis, peptic ulcer disease, psychiatric disturbances (euphoria/depression, overt psychosis), and increased intracranial pressure are the most frequently encountered side effects. In attempts to minimize those risks, reducing dosages of prednisone to 0.10 to 0.15 mg/kg/day by 6 months has been a common goal. More recently, deflazacort (a less potent steroid than prednisone), has been used and schemes to move toward alternate-day dosing have been attempted. As noted earlier, up to a 20% increase in body weight can be expected in the first year if steroid dosing is not closely observed.

Azathioprine can induce marrow immunosuppression, liver toxicity, pancreatitis, increased gastrointestinal symptoms, and increased risk of infection and cancer. Mycophenolate mofetil has marrow toxicity and gastrointestinal disturbances as its two most prominent side effects. Recent data suggest it is a superior drug over azathioprine in the at-risk rejection patient.

Cyclosporin and tacrolimus are classic nephrotoxins and have distinct pathologic changes that mimic rejection but can be discerned only through biopsy. Drug level monitoring is a helpful guide, but levels do not accurately reflect the risk of developing toxicity. Both drugs have been implicated in posttransplant hemolytic-uremic syndrome. Other side effects of calcineurin inhibitors include magnesium wasting, renal tubular acidosis (type 4), hypertension, liver toxicity (cholestasis and "transaminitis"), neurotoxicity including tremors, seizures, and a peculiar abnormality known as leukoencephalopathy, which mimics multiple microinfarcts on CT scan or magnetic resonance imaging (MRI). With cyclosporin hyperlipidemia is more difficult to control than with tacrolimus, but chemical diabetes is more frequently encountered in the patient taking tacrolimus. Important considerations need to be made when drugs that utilize the liver and intestinal cytochrome P-450 system and calcineurin inhibitors are concomitantly used. Cytochrome P-450 metabolized drugs can lower or raise immunosuppressive levels of either cyclosporin or tacrolimus. Any drug prescribed ought to be discussed with the patient's transplant center prior to starting it. Something as simple as grapefruit juice has been implicated in increasing levels.

Antibody therapy can result in a systemic cytokine release syndrome referred to as the "shake and bake" syndrome. Hyperpyrexia, chills, fever, rigors, erythroderma, hyper- or hypotension, palpitations, tachycardia, hyperpnea, fluid retention, and pulmonary or cerebral edema can all occur to varying degrees. Obviously, as part of their pharmaceutical effectiveness, severe neutropenia can result creating the risk for more dramatic types of infections, such as *Pneumocystis* or disseminated cytomegalovirus infection, in the at-risk patient. Antibody therapy, which is used either as an induction regimen or as a treatment for steroid-resistant rejection, is given only in the hospital for several doses rather than on an outpatient basis, in order to monitor the patient's response.

OUTCOMES

Current data from North American Pediatric Renal Transplant Cooperative Study and the U.S. Renal Data System (USRDS) reveal patient survival rates for 1, 2, and 5 years at 97%, 96%, and 94%, respectively, if this is the patient's first graft. Only 1% to 2% differences exist between children receiving living donor kidneys and those receiving cadaveric organs. Of course, as stated previously, the survival rate is lower in the younger than 2 year old group, with overwhelming infection and then cardiovascular disease being the two major causes of death (over 50%). Slightly fewer than 50% die with a functioning graft. Again, the role of the primary caregiver in maintaining a high awareness of an infectious risk and cardiovascular conditioning cannot be emphasized enough.

Recent data suggest that despite increasing living donations, no further changes have demonstrated improved outcomes through data collected up to 2000. A disturbing recent finding is a clear-cut racial difference demonstrating that graft survival is 50% lower in African Americans in the younger age groups than their white counterparts.

Mini-index of Related Topics	CH.
■ CHRONIC GENITOURINARY TRACT DISORDERS	172
■ LONG-TERM MANAGEMENT OF RENAL DISORDERS	173
■ HYPERTENSION	174
■ ANTI-INFLAMMATORY AND IMMUNOMODULATORY THERAPY	286

SUGGESTED READINGS

Benfield MR, Current status of kidney transplant: Update 2003. Pediatr Clin North Am 2003;50(6):1301–1334.
Davis ID, Bunchman TE, Grim PC, et al: Pediatric renal transplantation: Indications and special considerations: A position paper from the Pediatric Committee of the American Society of Transplant Physicians. Pediatr Transplant 1998;2(2):117–129.

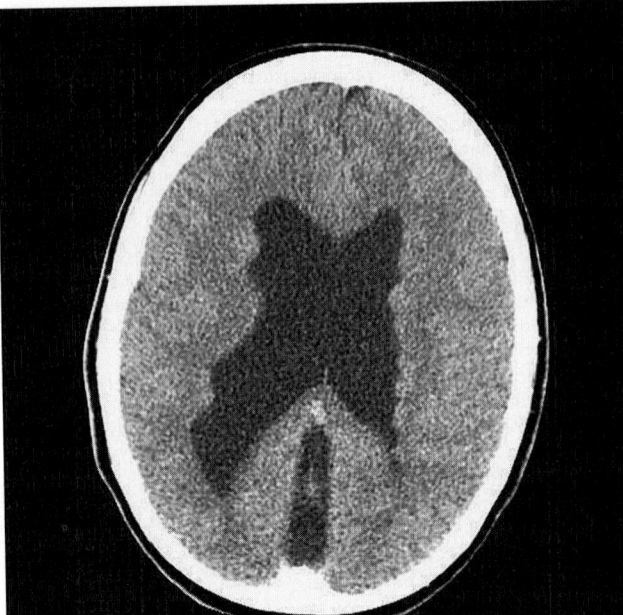

Figure 176-2. CT of a child with macrocephaly shows enlarged lateral ventricles and features of periventricular nodular heterotopia, a developmental CNS disorder.

subarachnoid (pacchionian) granulations, or noncommunicating, which indicates cerebrospinal fluid obstruction, usually at the level of the aqueduct of Sylvius. When hydrocephalus warrants surgery, a ventriculoperitoneal shunt is placed. The radiopaque shunt components consist of a proximal catheter placed into the body of the lateral ventricle, a valve and a pumping chamber placed beneath the scalp, tubing burrowed subcutaneously through the scalp, neck, chest, and abdomen, and a distal catheter that enters the peritoneal cavity for drainage of cerebrospinal fluid.

Ventriculoperitoneal shunts frequently require revision for malfunction or infection. Signs of shunt malfunction or shunt infection include lethargy, irritability, anorexia, vomiting, opisthotonic (extensor) posturing, or seizure activity (Box 176-3). Fever can be an inconsistent feature. Shunt infections, typically caused by *Staphylococcus epidermidis*, usually occur within the first 3 to 6 months after shunt placement, so infection should be considered in shunted infants during this vulnerable period. Infants with suspected shunt infection or malfunction require emergent

Box 176-3. Symptoms and Signs of Shunt Malfunction or Infection

Lethargy
Irritability
Poor oral intake
Vomiting
Fever
"Setting sun" sign
Seizures
Opisthotonic posturing

referral to an experienced neurosurgeon for replacement of the shunt.

The prognosis for infants with neonatal hydrocephalus depends on several factors, including the thickness of the cranial mantle, the presence of additional CNS anomalies, the avoidance of shunt infection, and the rapid recognition and therapy for shunt malfunction. Recent studies suggest that infants with hydrocephalus have favorable prognoses when hydrocephalus is managed aggressively in the neonatal period. Overall, the majority of shunted infants have normal or near normal intellectual outcomes when examined at school age.

Microcephaly. Infants with occipital-frontal circumferences below the 10th percentile have microcephaly, a feature reflecting deficient brain growth. Because the most common cause of microcephaly is familial small heads, parental head circumferences should be measured. If the parental head circumferences are normal (average of 54.5 cm for women and 57 cm for men) or large, infants should undergo stepwise evaluations for potential underlying disorders (see Box 176-1). The diagnostic evaluation should consist of an imaging study, ophthalmologic examination, karyotype, plasma amino acid analysis, and appropriate studies for infectious agents associated with deficient brain growth. Because CT detects calcifications, it is the preferred imaging modality for infants with microcephaly (Fig. 176-3). Infants with CT features suspicious for migrational disorders (e.g., lissencephaly) may also require imaging by MRI. Plain skull radiographs have no role in the evaluation of the infant with microcephaly.

Neonates with microcephaly should be evaluated for intrauterine infections (see Chapter 209). Numerous chromosomal and syndromic conditions can be associated with microcephaly. Such infants display systemic features distinct from those of intrauterine infection, such as

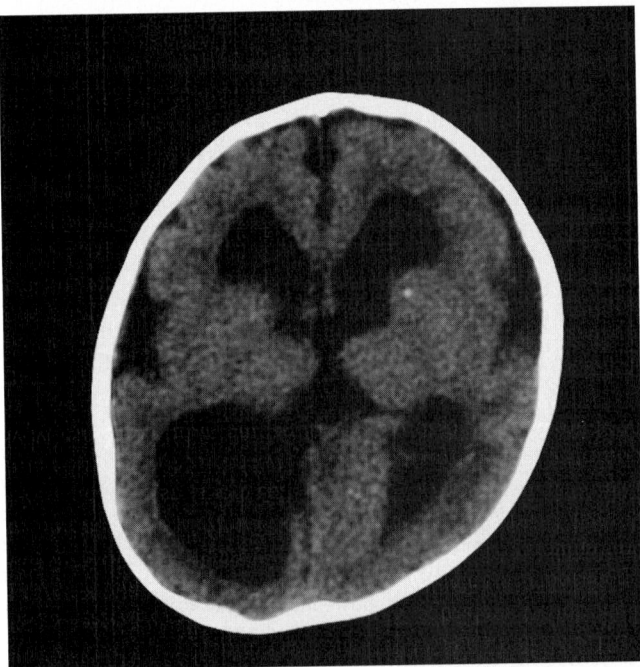

Figure 176-3. CT shows microcephaly with calcifications.

dysmorphic appearance or anomalies of the heart, skeleton, eyes, or other systems. Infants with suspected genetic conditions require a karyotype and consultation with a pediatric geneticist. Additional investigations, such as a neuroimaging study (preferably an MRI), abdominal ultrasound, and ophthalmologic, orthopedic, and cardiologic consultations, may be necessary, depending on the constellation of physical findings. Microcephaly may also be a sign of cerebral malformations such as lissencephaly or holoprosencephaly.

Misshapen Heads. Infants with craniosynostosis, premature fusion of cranial sutures, usually present in the perinatal period with misshapen heads. The precise shape depends on the location of suture fusion. Because bone growth proceeds perpendicular to the suture, fusion of the sagittal suture, the most common location of craniosynostosis, causes occipital-frontal elongation (scaphocephaly), whereas fusion of the coronal sutures causes occipital-frontal shortening (brachycephaly). Premature fusion of a lamboid suture causes asymmetric flattening occipitally and prominence of the opposite side of the forehead (plagiocephaly). Premature fusion of the metopic suture in the midline of the forehead causes ridging of the forehead and a triangular appearance to the cranium (trigonocephaly). Certain syndromic or medical conditions are associated with specific patterns of craniosynostosis (see Table 176-1).

Craniosynostosis can be suspected clinically, based on an abnormal head shape in early infancy. Because skull radiographs have low sensitivity, spiral CT is preferred for detection of craniosynostosis. Management depends on the severity of head deformity and the magnitude of suture closure. Infants with nonsyndromic fusion of a single cranial suture, such as the sagittal, usually have no long-term neurodevelopmental sequelae as a direct consequence of craniosynostosis. The decision to pursue surgical correction should be made in consultation with the family and an experienced neurosurgeon. By contrast, infants with fusion of multiple sutures, including those with Crouzon disease, frequently experience complications of chronically increased intracranial pressure, such as vision or hearing loss, developmental delay, and cerebral palsy, when untreated. Consequently, such infants require timely referral to a neurosurgeon for early and aggressive surgical management.

Surgery consists of a craniectomy performed parallel to the affected suture. Inert material is inserted within the surgically induced skull defect to inhibit bone growth. Infants with craniosynostosis should undergo surgery within the first 6 months of life; this highlights the need for early referral to a neurosurgeon. The American Academy of Pediatrics "back-to-sleep" campaign has led to an epidemic of positional plagiocephaly, a benign, acquired condition that begins in late infancy and improves as the infant develops and assumes a more erect posture. Occasionally, severe positional plagiocephaly requires application of a "helmet" to restore a more normal head shape or causes secondary craniosynostosis that may necessitate surgical intervention.

Neural Tube Defects. The neural tube defects anencephaly and myelodysplasia represent the most serious of the birth defects affecting the CNS. Anencephaly, congenital absence of the brain, skull, and scalp, indicates failure of closure of the anterior neuropore. Infants with anencephaly have low set ears, flattened nasal bridge, cleft palate, microophthalmia, or corneal clouding and may have systemic defects, such as congenital heart disease, pulmonary hypoplasia, or renal anomalies. The incidence of anencephaly in the United States averages approximately 1 per 1000 births.

The diagnosis is suspected when mothers have elevated serum and amniotic fluid α-fetoprotein levels, and it can be confirmed in utero by prenatal ultrasound. Clinical criteria for the diagnosis include (1) absence of a large portion of the skull, (2) absence of scalp over the skull defect, (3) exposed fibrotic tissue within the scalp defect, and (4) absence of cerebral hemispheres. Most infants with anencephaly are stillborn or die within the first 28 days. Because the brain stem may function, albeit temporarily, infants with anencephaly may breathe, move, and have primitive reflexes, such as sucking, rooting, and swallowing. Given the severity of the brain defect and associated grim prognosis, the management should consist of comfort care only. Anencephalic infants rarely serve as satisfactory organ donors.

Defects of the Spinal Cord. Myelodysplasia, reflecting defective closure of the posterior neuropore, ranges in

Table 176-1. Disorders Associated with Craniosynostosis

Disorder	Craniosynostosis	Other Features
Crouzon syndrome	Multiple, causing oxycephaly (tall skull) and microcephaly	Shallow orbits producing a characteristic facial appearance; mild mental retardation
Apert syndrome	Lambdoid and coronal, causing tall forehead or oxycephaly	Shallow orbits; small nose; syndactyly; mental retardation
Carpenter syndrome	Coronal, lambdoid, and sagittal causing brachycephaly and oxycephaly	Brachydactyly, syndactyly, clinodactyly of the hands; mental deficiency
Hypophosphatasia	Multiple, causing microcephaly	Low serum alkaline phosphatase; vision and hearing loss; certain types lethal in infancy
Hyperthyroidism	Premature fontanel closure, causing microcephaly	Elevated free T_4 and low TSH
"Back-to-sleep" syndrome	Positional plagiocephaly, causing asymmetric occipital flattening and protrusion of the forehead on the opposite side	None

severity from occult spina bifida, the radiographic detection of an incomplete vertebral arch (usually of L5-S1) without neurologic symptoms, to myeloschisis, a rare condition in which the entire spinal cord is exposed as a result of complete failure of neural tube closure. Meningocele, posterior protrusion of connective tissue without neural elements, and myelomeningocele, exposure of connective tissue and neural elements of the spinal cord, represent intermediate but potentially severe defects of spine and spinal cord development.

Meningoceles or myelomeningoceles are often suspected or diagnosed antenatally by detecting elevated maternal serum levels of α-fetoprotein or by performing prenatal ultrasonography. At birth the anatomical defects are readily apparent. Because these lesions require urgent management, the generalist has an important role in providing initial therapy and parental education. Management begins with the application of moist, sterile dressings to open defects and immediate referral to a pediatric neurosurgeon for primary closure of the lesion. Closure within 24 to 48 hours of birth reduces the risk of infection and improves long-term neurologic outcome.

Hydrocephalus, a common feature in children with myelomeningocele, results from a Chiari malformation (type II), a posterior fossa anomaly consisting of downward displacement of the cerebellar tonsils and vermis and elongation of the medulla caudally through the foramen magnum (Fig. 176-4). All infants with myelomeningocele should undergo neuroimaging studies in the perinatal period; head ultrasound provides useful preliminary information regarding ventricular size. Infants with myelomeningocele and hydrocephalus require ventriculoperitoneal shunting. This procedure, coupled with early closure of the spinal defect, improves substantially the neurodevelopmental outcome for infants with myelodysplasia. Long-term

medical complications and management of myelomeningocele are described in Chapter 177.

Diastematomyelia, tethered cord, intraspinal lipoma, and sacral agenesis represent rare defects of spinal cord development. Intraspinal anomalies such as tethered cord, lipoma, or diastematomyelia are often suggested by the presence of congenital foot deformities or hairy patches, dimples, or soft tissue masses in the lumbosacral region. However, dimples or pits below the top of the intergluteal fold rarely indicate occult spinal dysraphism. Children with tethered cord often present in early childhood with gait disturbance, perineal pain, foot deformity, and bladder dysfunction.

Sacral agenesis, a potential complication of maternal diabetes, reflects regression of neural and bony elements in the lumbosacral region. Infants with this condition have foot deformities, constipation, and neurologic abnormalities consisting of motor and sensory dysfunction of variable severity involving the lower extremities and sacral region. Neurogenic bladder occurs commonly in children with sacral agenesis and requires management comparable to that of myelomeningocele. Sacral agenesis can be detected by obtaining plain radiographs of the lumbosacral spine and precisely characterized by MRI.

Other Congenital Disorders of the Central Nervous System. Disorders originating during the subsequent stages of embryonic neural development include holoprosencephaly, schizencephaly, lissencephaly, agenesis of the corpus callosum, and cortical dysplasia. Certain infants with these disorders may be recognized in the perinatal period because of dysmorphic features, poor feeding, seizures, congenital microcephaly, or other neurologic abnormalities, but more often they come to the attention of the generalist later because of delayed development, abnormal postnatal head growth, or abnormalities of vision and muscle tone. Infants with these disorders should be referred to a pediatric neurologist and geneticist for confirmation of the diagnosis.

Agenesis of the corpus callosum can be inherited as an autosomal recessive or dominant trait or be the result of syndromic or chromosomal conditions. The disorder is usually not evident in the neonatal period unless the infant has seizures, macrocephaly, or abnormalities of tone or eye movement. MRI, particularly in the sagittal and coronal planes, detects the absence of this structure. Although the neurodevelopmental prognosis for infants with agenesis of the corpus callosum varies, most will have cognitive delays and many have seizures.

Holoprosencephaly results from impaired cleavage of the forebrain (prosencephalon) during the second month of intrauterine development. Schizencephaly consists of focal clefts in the cerebral hemispheres connecting the lateral ventricle(s) with the subarachnoid space. Lissencephaly represents a heterogeneous disorder of neuronal migration that ranges in severity from an agyric or smooth cerebral cortex to a brain with incomplete gyration and pachygyria. The infants with heterotopia or cortical dysplasia occasionally present in the neonatal period with seizures. Each of these rare brain defects is best diagnosed by MRI. Table 176-2 describes characteristics of these disorders.

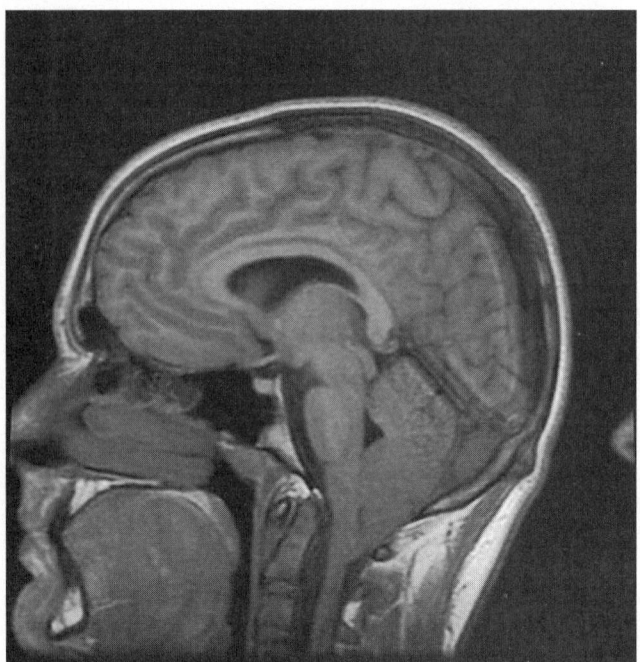

Figure 176-4. Chiari malformation.

Table 176-2. Clinical Features of Rare Congenital Brain Defects

Disorder	Etiology	Clinical Features	MRI or CT Features
Holoprosencephaly	Trisomy 13 or 18; 13q-, 18q- Maternal diabetes	Microcephaly Midface hypoplasia Single central incisor Seizures Failure to thrive Spasticity	Fusion of cerebral hemispheres; classified as alobar, semilobar, or lobar, depending on degree of fusion
Schizencephaly	Genetic Environmental	Microcephaly Spasticity Developmental delay Seizures Hydrocephalus Cognitive delay	CT or MRI demonstrates size and extent of cleft
Lissencephaly	17p13.3 deletion	Miller-Dieker syndrome Microcephaly Bitemporal narrowing Long philtrum Ear anomalies	Agyric or smooth cerebral cortex to incomplete gyration and pachygyria
	9q31 mutation	Fukuyama congenital muscular dystrophy	
	XLIS gene mutation (Xq22.3-q23) Intrauterine CMV		
Heterotopia and cortical dysplasia	Unknown except periventricular nodular heterotopia, from filamin A mutation	Seizures Developmental delay	Variable degree of cortical or subcortical abnormality

Mini-index of Related Topics

SUGGESTED READINGS

Clark GD: Brain development and the genetics of brain development. Neurol Clin 2002;20:917–939.
Liptak GS, Serletti JM: Pediatric approach to craniosynostosis. Pediatr Rev 1998;19:352–358.
Northrup H, Volcik KA: Spina bifida and other neural tube defects. Curr Probl Pediatr 2000;30:313–332.

177 Spina Bifida

Gregory S. Liptak

ROLE OF THE GENERALIST

1. Recommend folic acid to all women of childbearing age who are considering conceiving.
2. Recommend that all children known prenatally to have meningomyelocele (MM) be delivered at a center with a neonatal intensive care unit.
3. Recognize the signs of occult spinal dysraphism (OSD) and refer the infant for definitive evaluation of the spinal cord.
4. Recognize that MM is *not* a progressive condition and deterioration of a child is usually due to a problem that is treatable.
5. Recognize secondary conditions that complicate MM.
6. Actively participate in an interdisciplinary team to prevent complications and optimize the child's functioning.

DEFINITION OF THE CONDITION

The term *neural tube defects* (NTDs) refers to a group of malformations of the brain, spinal cord, and vertebrae. Figure 177-1 shows the three major NTDs. Anencephaly and encephalocele are discussed in Chapter 176. Spina bifida refers to a split in the vertebral arches. Approximately 10% of the population has an asymptomatic split in the vertebral arches, spina bifida occulta, an anomaly that typically has no clinical significance and is believed to be genetically different from the other NTDs.

Figure 177-1. The most common conditions characterized as NTDs.

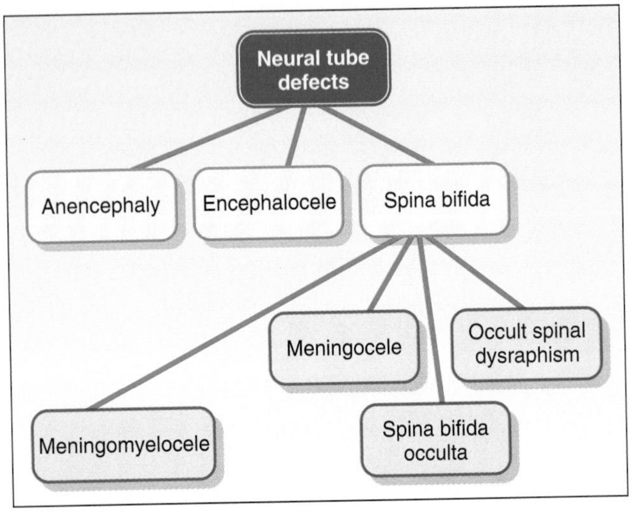

FUNDAMENTALS

Occult Spinal Dysraphism

Many infants have visible anomalies on the lower back. The most common anomaly is a small sacral or coccygeal dimple. If this is in the midline, the bottom of the dimple is visible (e.g., through an otoscope), and the child is neurologically normal, the lesion does not need to be investigated further. However, if the dimple is cephalad to the sacral region or is not in the midline, it may represent a dermal sinus tract and may be associated with OSD. Other birthmarks commonly associated with OSD include hemangiomata, flame nevi, tufts of hair, dermal sinuses, or small lumps (masses) (Fig. 177-2). A dermal sinus may serve as a tract for bacteria into the spinal canal, which can lead to meningitis. In OSD the spinal cord may be tethered to surrounding tissue or may be split (diastematomyelia or diplomyelia), both of which can lead to subsequent neurological damage as the child grows. The spinal cord may have a lipoma bound to it, which also can lead to neurological damage.

Infants who have these stigmata on their backs should have a thorough neurological evaluation and imaging of the underlying soft tissue and spinal cord using magnetic resonance imaging (MRI), or ultrasonography if the radiologist is experienced. The primary care provider should refer any child who is found to have an underlying abnormality of

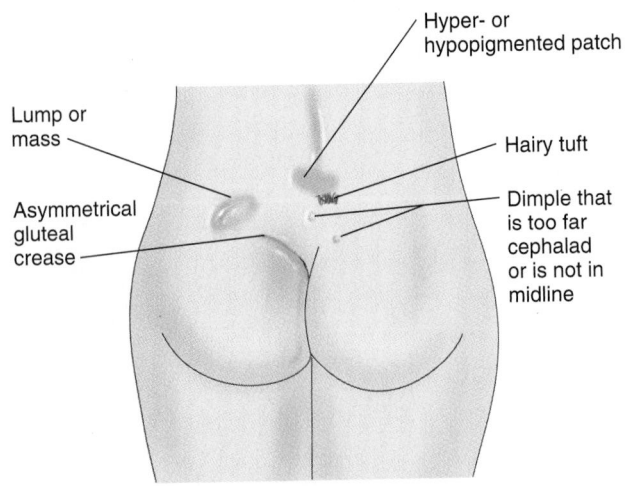

Figure 177-2. Signs of OSD.

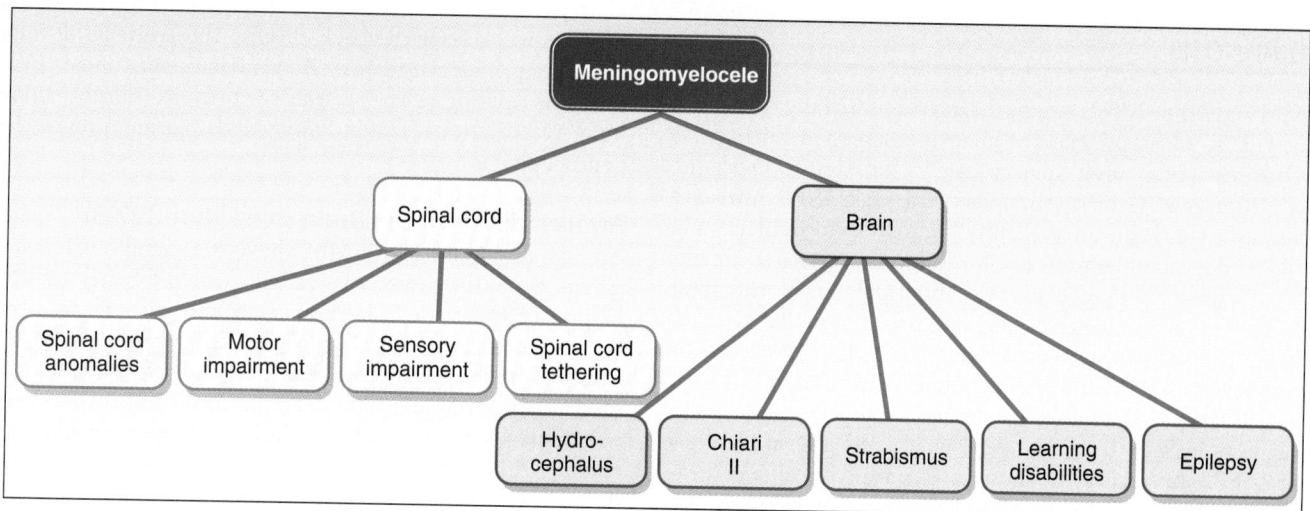

Figure 177-3. Conditions associated with motor and sensory impairments in MM.

soft tissue or cord to a pediatric neurosurgeon, since most clinicians believe that surgical treatment should be performed early, even in asymptomatic infants, to prevent progressive neurological damage.

Meningocele and Meningomyelocele

A menigocele presents as open vertebral arches, open skin, and underlying soft tissues with the meninges of the spinal cord exposed, but with a normal underlying spinal cord. This defect does not typically produce paralysis or loss of sensation. Because the defect is associated with other anomalies of the brain including hydrocephalus, however, a cranial ultrasound, computed tomography (CT) scan, or MRI scan is indicated.

If the vertebral arches and overlying soft tissue are open and the spinal cord is malformed, the child has MM (meningomyelocele, or myelomeningocele). This disorder is associated with a complex array of symptoms shown in Figures 177-3 and 177-4, and has been called the most complex birth defect compatible with life. Spina bifida and MM are not just disorders of the spine. Children with MM

have other abnormalities of the brain, including abnormal migration of cells.

In the United States, the prevalence of MM is approximately 60 in 100,000 births and has been falling; in Wales and Ireland, the prevalence is three to four times higher. This variability is a reflection of both genetic and environmental factors. Girls are three to seven times more likely to have MM. Maternal exposure to valproic acid, carbamazepine, isotretinoin, alcohol, and hyperthermia have been linked to the occurrence of MM. Maternal obesity and diabetes also increase risk.

Although the etiology of MM is uncertain, daily supplemental doses of folic acid can reduce the incidence of new cases of NTDs in the general population by more than 50%. Folic acid also reduces the recurrence risk in affected families by 70%. *All women who are contemplating a pregnancy should take 0.4 mg (400 mcg) of supplemental folic acid per day while they are trying to conceive and during the first trimester.* Women who have NTD or have a first-degree relative with an NTD should take 4 mg per day around the time of conception and through the first trimester.

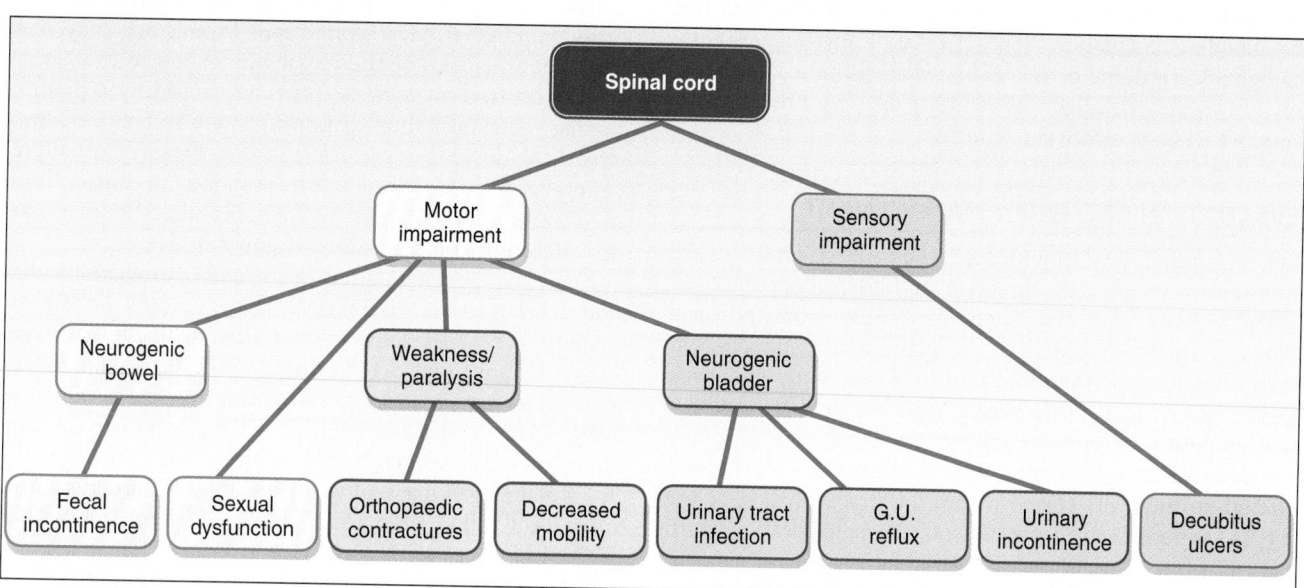

Figure 177-4. Conditions associated with spinal cord and brain impairments in MM.

DIAGNOSIS

MM and other NTDs can be diagnosed prenatally by several methods. Most pregnant women are screened during the 16th to 18th week of pregnancy for serum levels of α-fetoprotein (AFP). An open MM leaks AFP into the amniotic fluid and subsequently the maternal circulation. If the AFP level is elevated, a high-resolution ultrasound should be obtained to detect specific abnormalities of the fetal head (lemon and banana signs) and back consistent with an NTD. If NTD is suspected, amniocentesis is indicated to test levels of AFP and acetylcholinesterase (ACH) as well as karyotype. Acetylcholinesterase in the amniotic fluid suggests leakage from an open spinal cord. Elevated levels of AFP and acetylcholinesterase with abnormal ultrasonographic findings makes the diagnosis of NTD in the fetus quite certain. Chromosome analysis of the amniotic fluid will indicate syndromes such as trisomy 13 that may be associated with NTDs. About 50% of parents in the United States terminate the pregnancy if MM is detected. Some evidence suggests that delivery of the child by cesarean section at a center with a neonatal intensive care unit may decrease the severity of subsequent paralysis. Prenatal surgery to repair the lesion is available experimentally through the National Institutes of Health (NIH) (www.spinabifidamoms.com).

The diagnosis of MM is apparent at birth. The manner in which the family is informed of the diagnosis is critical. For the clinician meeting the family for the first time, (1) congratulate family members on the birth of their baby! Then (2) determine their understanding of the child's condition. Ask them what they believe contributed to the child's condition. (3) Deliver the news. Address the family's need for information by giving simple, focused bits of information. Use clear language that families can understand. Address the child's immediate medical risks and discomforts. Give families written information to which they can refer later. (4) Respond to their feelings; listen, acknowledge, legitimize, explore, and empathize with them. (5) Provide support. Minimize the family's aloneness and isolation; let family members know that they will not be abandoned. Maintain hope. (6) Ask if anything that the caregivers are doing or not doing worries them. (7) Agree on a specific, detailed follow-up plan. (8) Offer group support when they are ready for it.

EVALUATION AND EARLY MANAGEMENT

When an infant is born with MM, the top two priorities are to prevent spinal cord infection and to protect exposed spinal nerves and associated structures from physical damage. The lesion should be protected with a nonadherent sterile dressing or the child's entire lower body and back can be placed in a sterile plastic bag. The child born with a leaking lesion should be started on antibiotics to cover *Staphylococcus* and gram-negative bacteria. The lesion should be surgically closed within the first few days of life by an experienced neurosurgeon, in collaboration with plastic surgery if necessary. If the child is medically unstable, surgery can be delayed for at least a week. The infant should be evaluated for hydrocephalus, hydronephrosis, and orthopedic abnormalities as soon as practical. Typically within a week after the back closure, these infants develop worsening hydrocephalus. A ventriculoperitoneal (VP) shunt is customarily placed to prevent cerebrospinal fluid (CSF) from accumulating and causing progressive hydrocephalus.

Abnormalities of the Brain (see Figure 177-3)

Almost all children with MM above the sacral level have a Chiari type II (previously called Arnold-Chiari) malformation of the brain. The brainstem and part of the cerebellum are crowded and displaced downward toward the neck, as if the spinal cord had been pulled downward in utero. Symptoms and signs of spinal cord compression from the Chiari malformation include difficulty swallowing, choking, hoarseness, stridor, breath holding, apnea, disordered breathing during sleep, spasticity in the arms, and opisthotonos. Rare instances of sudden death from cardiorespiratory arrest have been reported. The Chiari II malformation is invariably associated with hydrocephalus. Of children who have MM, 70% to 80% have Chiari malformation and hydrocephalus. Symptomatic Chiari malformations can be treated by surgical decompression, in which part of the occiput and the arches of some of the cervical vertebrae are removed to provide additional space for the brainstem. A malfunctioning ventriculoperitoneal shunt may exert pressure on the brainstem leading to symptoms of Chiari malformation. All children who have symptomatic Chiari malformations should have evaluation of their ventricular shunts, including neuroimaging such as a CT scan.

Disordered breathing during sleep, including obstructive sleep apnea, central apnea, and central hypoventilation, occur frequently in individuals with MM. A formal sleep study can diagnose specific problems. Treatment for disordered sleep depends on the breathing disorder. Tonsillectomy with adenoidectomy can relieve upper airway obstruction and may unmask an underlying central apnea. Posterior fossa decompression, continuous positive airway pressure (CPAP), bilevel positive pressure ventilation (BiPAP), or tracheotomy with mechanical ventilation, especially during sleep, may be used to help the child.

Strabismus, present in about 20% of children with MM, often requires surgical correction. Strabismus may result from abnormalities of the visual gaze center in the brain or from increased intracranial pressure caused by a malfunctioning ventricular shunt. Approximately 15% of individuals with MM develop a seizure disorder. Seizures usually are generalized tonic-clonic and respond to antiepileptic medication (see Chapter 180). A blocked shunt or shunt infection must be considered if new seizures occur.

Many children with spina bifida and hydrocephalus have nonverbal learning disabilities. They typically have better reading than math skills and may have difficulty with executive functions, such as the ability to organize, plan, initiate, sequence, sustain, inhibit competing responses, and pace work. Many of these individuals will know how to do something such as catheterize themselves, but will have difficulty planning and actually carrying it out. These disabilities often lead to impaired social skills and interactions. About 30% of children with MM have attention deficit disorder, which may be related to their learning disabilities, and about 30% of these children respond to methylphenidate (Ritalin).

Abnormalities of the Spine and Spinal Cord
(see Figure 177-4)

Almost 90% of children with MM above the sacral level have scoliosis and kyphosis that worsen with age. This is related to the abnormal formation of the vertebral bodies and differential muscle function. Scoliosis greater than 25 degrees requires orthopedic intervention, including use of an orthosis (body jacket, or TLSO) and surgery (see Chapter 53).

The degree of motor paralysis and sensory loss in MM depends on the location of the defect in the spinal cord (Table 177-1). Children with defects at the thoracic or high-lumbar level have paralysis and loss of sensation in the legs and lower abdomen. Children with low-lumbar lesions usually can flex their hips and extend their knees and ankles but typically have weak or absent ankle-toe flexion and hip extension. Children with sacral lesions usually have only mild weakness of their ankles or toes. The loss of motor and sensory function is not always symmetrical. The higher the level of the MM and the greater the muscle weakness, the more ambulation will be impaired. Although children with lumbar-level lesions walk with support, as they approach adolescence and their center of gravity and relative strength change, most rely increasingly on wheelchairs for mobility. Contractures around a joint may occur either because of uneven muscle function (e.g., hip flexion without hip extension) or complete paralysis around a joint with prolonged immobility (e.g., the child with thoracic-level lesion who sits in a wheelchair all day). Obesity is common in older children and adolescents with MM and can impair mobility.

Spinal cord tethering can lead to loss of function in a child with MM. A tethered spinal cord usually results from scarring at the site of the initial surgery to close the back. Pressure or stretch on the tethered cord leads to local hypoxia and diminished motor functioning. Signs and symptoms of tethered cord include back pain, change in bowel or bladder function, new orthopedic contractures (e.g., clawing of the foot), increasing weakness (with deterioration of gait), and spasticity of the legs with increase in deep tendon reflexes. A malfunctioning ventriculoperitoneal shunt may mimic signs and symptoms of tethered cord. All children who present with neurological deterioration should first be evaluated for structure and function of the ventricular shunt with imaging of the head (CT or MRI scan) with or without plain radiographic imaging of the shunt (shunt series) from head to abdomen. The posterior fossa (for Chiari malformation) and spinal cord should be also evaluated by performing MRI with flow of the head and MRI of the spine.

Neurogenic Bladder and Bowel

Because the bladder, the urethra, and rectum are all innervated by sacral-level nerves (S2-4), bladder and bowel dysfunction are present in virtually all children with MM. Even children with sacral lesions usually have bladder and bowel problems. The neurogenic bladder has two major dysfunctions: failure to store urine and failure to empty the urine once the bladder is full. Retention of urine predisposes the child to infection of the bladder and/or kidneys. The combination of a tight bladder outlet and increased tone in the bladder may also produce kidney damage over time, especially if urine infections occur.

To detect early structural damage, ultrasonography at regular intervals should begin in infancy. Bladder function may also be evaluated using a cystometrogram. To avoid permanent kidney damage, elevated pressure should be reduced by clean intermittent catheterization (CIC) at least four times a day to drain urine. Vesicostomy is indicated in some infants for whom CIC is not successful. Because neurogenic bladders are susceptible to infection, long-term prophylactic oral antibiotics such as cephalexin, nitrofurantoin, or cotrimoxazole may be necessary to prevent infections. Alternatively, antibiotics such as Neosporin can be instilled directly into the bladder through the catheter. Attempts to achieve urinary continence using CIC are generally begun at 3 to 4 years of age. About 70% of children who receive a combination of CIC and medications (like oxybutinin or pseudoephedrine) achieve continence during elementary school. Obesity can make CIC difficult to accomplish, especially for girls.

If CIC and medication are unsuccessful in producing continence, surgical interventions may be helpful. Bladder augmentation procedures increase the bladder capacity with a flap of bowel or stomach. Appendico-vesicostomy uses the appendix to connect the bladder to the abdominal wall, permitting catheterization. These approaches are often used simultaneously (see Chapter 172).

Table 177-1. Level of Lesion in Spina Bifida in Relation to Bracing in Childhood and Prognosis for Mobility in Adulthood

Level of Lesion	Motor Function	Bracing in Childhood	Prognosis for Adult Ambulation
Thoracic or high lumbar (T7 to L2)	Hip flexion absent or weak. No function below that level.	Parapodium can provide upright posture. Parapodium, HKAFO*, or RGO† for mobility.	Usually require wheelchair. May be household ambulators with bracing.
Mid lumbar (L3-4)	Hip flexors present. Some quadriceps function. No function below the knee.	Bracing to the knees usually needed. Mobility requires crutches.	Most will require wheelchair. Household ambulation common, but not community ambulation.
Low lumbar (L5) or sacral (S1-2)	Hip flexors and quadriceps function. Some gastrocnemius function. Weak intrinsic muscles of the feet. Weak hip extension.	Will ambulate with minimal bracing, such as AFOs‡, and usually without crutches.	Community ambulation is typical.

*Hip-knee-ankle-foot orthosis
†Reciprocal gait orthosis
‡Ankle-foot orthosis

postnatal or childhood cerebrovascular accidents and stroke. Each of these results not only in hypoxic injury from interruption of blood flow, but also to shearing injury of cortical tissue and the necrolytic effect of free blood on otherwise healthy brain tissue.

The *third* category of central nervous system insult is central nervous system infections, especially with organisms that can cause significant encephalitis, including the so-called TORCH infections (toxoplasma, rubella, cytomegalovirus, herpes). These remain important considerations because of their protean presentation and because the morbidity from some, especially herpes, can be reduced with antiviral agents. *Streptococcus* (group B), *Escherichia coli*, and *meningococcus* are examples of bacterial organisms that can be especially damaging to the central nervous system. Mechanisms of injury include ischemia as direct cytotoxicity and postinfectious scarring and disruption of normal cell function.

Degenerative injuries comprise the *fourth* category of central nervous system insult associated with cerebral palsy. These include a number of metabolic etiologies that involve both intrinsic intracellular dysfunction and the accumulation within the central nervous system of metabolites that are toxic to otherwise normal upper motor neurons. The emergence of clinical features of cerebral palsy in a child for whom no history of ischemia is identified should alert one to the possibility of an inborn error of metabolism, neurometabolic disorder, including mitochondrial disorders, or progressive demyelinating disease (affecting the axonal component of the upper motor neuron unit).

The *fifth* category includes malformations of the central nervous system, notably schizencephaly, holoprosencephaly, and congenital porencephalic cysts. Depending on the pattern of motor impairment, other malformations may be suspected, including Chiari II malformation, vascular malformation syndromes, and heterotopic migration abnormalities. In children whose recognized syndromes do not ordinarily include features of cerebral palsy, health care providers should suspect additional central nervous system pathology when these features are present.

Finally, two or more of the sources described in the previous five categories of central nervous system insult may combine to cause cerebral palsy. This is especially true when infection or metabolic derangement result in concomitant ischemia. In many cases ischemia can represent an important "final common pathway" in the evolution of cerebral palsy.

CLINICAL PRESENTATION

The diagnosis of cerebral palsy is never an accurate one when it is based on isolated aspects of a child's development. Particularly in newborns and infants, the motor examination, although important, has relatively poor predictive value when performed without equal attention to the quality of their movements, their level of alertness, temperament, speech and language, and feeding skills. When history indicates a high risk, the clinician should always have a heightened concern, and developmental delay will usually prompt careful consideration of this

diagnosis. In the setting of significant delays on screening examination, without a supporting history but when there are significant delays in any screening domain, it is best to begin with a working diagnosis of developmental delay and pay close attention to the variables outlined in Table 178-1.

MANAGEMENT AND NATURAL HISTORY

In each life epoch of a child with cerebral palsy, primary care management should include careful attention to three general areas. The generalist caring for children with cerebral palsy needs to pay attention to all three, both during general health maintenance and in times of illness or changes in health status. The three areas are as follows:

- General health considerations and a primary care "healthwatch"
- Developmental/educational/vocational assessment and support
- Orthopedic and orthotic care

Expected outcomes and indicators are summarized in Table 178-2.

Families of children and young adults with cerebral palsy face the challenges of a lifetime balancing great personal sacrifice and attention to detail with the desire to create as normal and natural family life for their children as possible. Each stage in the child's life involves seeking normal opportunities, while at the same time making provisions and contingencies to accommodate the child's special needs. A sensitive and astute generalist will see parents as true partners in the care of their patients, and almost always seek their opinions and wisdom concerning their children's primary care needs. Family centered care means respecting the dignity and knowledge of families, not relying on them to do work that health and social support networks should be doing. The overarching goal in serving children with cerebral palsy and their families is to assist families in making the right choices for their children, and to help them decide on the kinds of interventions they will implement and what assistance they need at different times in their lives.

Four basic but major supports and services available to children with cerebral palsy based on the diagnosis alone, with which the generalist should be especially familiar, are: Early Intervention, special education, Children with Special Health Care Needs (CSHCN) state programs, and Supplemental Security Income (SSI). These services are described on the CD-ROM materials for this chapter and in Chapters 125 and 127.

OUTCOME

The primary mutual goal of practitioner and family for children with cerebral palsy is to help them achieve the highest quality of life and maintain the best possible level of function. While these are straightforward goals, in the course of each child's life, issues of access to services, intercurrent illness, nutrition, surgery, educational planning, and transitional planning for adulthood can often be distracting

Table 178-1. The Clinical Presentation of Cerebral Palsy

Clinical Pattern	Predominant Features	Distinctive Features	Typical Physical Correlation
Common Clinical Subtypes			
Increased tone	Spastic quadriplegia	Four extremity involvement	Hyperreflexia, spasticity Hypertonia Ankle clonus Upgoing plantar reflexes
	Spastic hemiplegia	Upper and lower extremity involvement	Hyperreflexia Spasticity Hypertonia Ankle clonus Upgoing plantar reflexes
	Spastic diplegia	Bilateral lower extremity involvement	Hyperreflexia Spasticity Hypertonia Ankle clonus Upgoing plantar reflexes
	"Asymmetric"	E.g., diplegia/upper extremity hemiplegia	As above in affected limbs
Decreased/very low tone	Hypotonic/atonic	Usually generalized, involving trunk and all extremities	Motor exam may be mixed with hyperreflexia and low tone, upgoing plantar reflexes
"Fluctuating tone"	Dystonic	Usually generalized, involving trunk and all extremities. Tone may seem "improved" when child is at rest, then child may suddenly extend, arch, grimace when stimulated or startled.	Physical exam varies considerably. May see features typical of children with lower or even near-normal tone, then have dramatic shifts to hypertonia, extensor posturing, and generalized tremor.
Disregulated movement	Ataxia, dyskinetic mixed	Unsteady gait, poor balance and coordination, usually in setting of trunk and four extremity involvement	Provoking movement (e.g., reaching for toy, walking) will amplify disregulation.
	Athetosis	Distinctive movement disorder, usually generalized	May note disregulated movement at rest, but usually brought out by intentional movement
Other Clinical Features to Note on Examination			
Congenital microcephaly	>2 standard deviations below mean	Implies possible decelerated brain growth in utero	Disproportionate head size in relation to linear height further suggestive of CNS growth disorder
Abnormal posture and general movement	Asymmetric tonic neck reflex Asymmetric "position of comfort"	Tone-related postural disturbances, persistence may lead to torticollis but is distinct from it	Persistence of the tonic neck reflex or patterns of asymmetry are clues of either hemiplegia or more generalized spastic form of CP.
Abnormal DTRs	Hyperreflexia especially when associated with hypertonia	Disinhibition	Decreased DTRs may be present initially, then change over time to increased DTRs in CP.
Level of activity Degree of arousability response to visual stimuli and sounds	"Blunted" or attenuated affect	Diffuse cortical involvement possible	Parents report of responsiveness important. Response to voices assesses visual and auditory responsiveness.

180

Long-term Management of Seizure Disorders

Alan B. Silken

ROLE OF THE GENERALIST

1 Educate family about seizures, medications, and lifestyle changes.
2 Manage recurrent seizures.
3 Manage medication side effects.
4 Manage drug interactions.
5 Order appropriate follow-up laboratory tests.
6 Consult pediatric neurologist when appropriate.

Chronic management of seizure disorders falls into three basic areas: (1) educating the family and child, (2) managing recurrent seizures, and (3) managing medication side effects and drug interactions when multiple antiseizure medications are used.

While the generalist will be pivotally involved in the ongoing management of a child with seizures, the pediatric neurologist can provide unique support. A referral to the specialist is appropriate when families are overwhelmed and distraught by the diagnosis and for assistance with diagnosis, treatment, and comanagement of children with seizure disorders. The pediatric neurologist can offer a broad perspective and may have more in-depth answers to families' concerns. Whenever a pediatric neurologist is available, care should be coordinated between generalist and specialist. This is especially true since the advent of many new antiseizure medications. While recurrence of a seizure or appearance of an adverse medication effect does not necessarily dictate a change in medication, the pediatric neurologist can be invaluable in helping to devise a rational

Box 180-1. When to Call the Pediatric Neurologist

Status epilepticus
Uncertain etiology for seizures or intractable seizures
First-line antiseizure medication not effective
Complex side effects or drug interactions
Complex seizure syndromes such as infantile spasms, Lennox-Gastaut syndrome, juvenile myoclonic epilepsy, neurocutaneous disorders, and other conditions
Cognitive, learning, and developmental concerns in a child with seizures
Assistance needed for support of the family

treatment plan. Box 180-1 lists indications for consulting with a pediatric neurologist.

EDUCATING THE FAMILY AND CHILD

The term *epilepsy*, derived from the Greek "to take hold of," is the source of much confusion, fear, and myth among both clinicians and families. Once the diagnosis has been established (see Chapter 103), educating parents and the child is an essential early and ongoing task. A common, often unspoken, fear is that epilepsy indicates mental retardation resulting in seizures or that seizures lead to mental retardation. Anticipating and correcting these misconceptions early in the management plan, even in apparently "enlightened" families, facilitates a trusting doctor-patient relationship, improves compliance with treatment, and allows families to focus on the real issues confronting them. Because *epilepsy* is a broad, nonspecific term that encompasses all seizure types, this chapter employs the more specific term *seizure disorder*, which is also a preferable term to employ with families once they understand that the term *epilepsy* is often misused.

Parents will have many questions: What do I tell my child? What activities can he or she do? How does this affect learning and sports? Is it contagious or inherited? What are the side effects of medication? Why does my child need medication? Are the seizures harming my child's brain? Why did this happen at this age? Will it affect my child's ability to have children? When will it end?

Many parents search the Internet for answers. Box 180-2 lists helpful resources. Clinicians must guide parents to reliable sources of information about seizure disorders. If parents raise concerns about what they have read online, ask them to print out the information and bring it to an office visit for review in order to separate fact from fiction. If the clinician's practice has a professional website, providing links to reliable, accurate health care websites for patients is appropriate. While the family's questions must be clearly answered in reasonable segments over time, parents can be overwhelmed with information when they are coming to grips with the reality that their child has a chronic illness. Assuming the child has not been diagnosed with a catastrophic seizure syndrome, begin with a brief description of what a seizure is, emphasizing that the brain is acting on the body, and that with rare exceptions, seizures do not cause brain damage. Inform family members that seizures can be well controlled with a wide choice of safe medications, and that their child can live a normal life span with little change in activities. Febrile seizures, absence seizures, and benign Rolandic seizures have a familial predisposition. If other relatives with a seizure disorder have had a good outcome, the clinician can reassure families that the long-term prognosis is good. Family members should also be made aware that catastrophic seizures in a relative do not necessarily mean their child is destined to a poor prognosis.

ENHANCING THE LIFESTYLE OF SEIZURE PATIENTS

The diagnosis of seizure disorder in a child is a major life-altering event for any family. Parents will immediately express concern about how their child's lifestyle will change, and what the consequences for the family will be. While antiseizure medications allow for an essentially normal childhood, many aspects of the child's life will be altered by the inherent anxiety of anticipating an unpredictable event. Although risks of injury from seizures exist, the vast majority of childhood seizure disorders are well controlled with medication. Commonsense precautions, which apply to any child, should be used, including the use of bicycle helmets, supervision while swimming or climbing, and a raised consciousness about a child's whereabouts. More risky activities, such as scuba diving, should probably be curtailed in seizure patients. While most seizures are brief and resolve without problem, that would not be the case if the child were under water.

For teenagers, driving is a frequent concern. This must be discussed responsibly, since a benign seizure takes on far greater risks if it occurs while the patient is driving. All states have specific laws regarding the length of seizure-free time required before driving is allowable (see Box 180-2). Beyond the legal issue, all teenagers are inexperienced drivers and when that is combined with the often variable compliance of that age group in taking medication, the risk of seizure as a cause of automobile accident increases significantly.

Irresponsible and illegal use of alcohol, common among teenagers, represents a special risk to teens with seizure disorders. Alcohol does not normally induce seizures, but it may lower the seizure threshold in patients with known seizure disorders. Alcohol withdrawal is a potent cause of seizures in chronic alcoholism. There is no medical evidence that marijuana causes seizures or withdrawal seizures, but alcohol is often abused together with marijuana. Other illicit drugs, especially central nervous system stimulants such as cocaine and amphetamines, can cause seizures.

Special issues for girls with seizure disorders deserve discussion. The incidence of polycystic ovaries, dysmenorrhea, and anovulatory cycles is increased with seizure disorders. Hypothalamic regulation of pituitary hormones may be affected in some patients by temporal lobe seizures that involve the limbic system. An increased frequency of seizures during the menstrual period, clinically termed "catamenial seizures," is presumed to be due to a hormonal effect on neuronal activity and can be difficult to control with antiseizure medications. Acetazolamide (Diamox) may be somewhat effective in these patients. The interaction between antiseizure medications and oral contraceptives should be discussed with adolescent girls and their families. Many antiseizure medications, especially those that induce hepatic enzymes, can significantly reduce oral contraceptive blood levels and result in contraceptive failure (Box 180-3). When antiseizure medication is initiated in a patient on oral contraceptives for birth control purposes, a change in oral contraceptive dose or an additional form of birth control should be considered.

The risk of a seizure in school needs to be acknowledged. The school nurse must be aware of the child's diagnosis and medication. Complex partial and absence seizures may be subtle, and can be mistaken for inattentiveness or even defiant behavior. Adverse effects on cognitive function including attention, memory, and processing speed are seen with many anticonvulsant medications. The teacher is the primary observer in monitoring for these medication effects. A plan for periodic communication with the teacher could include a regular teacher conference, a written communication book, or use of e-mail. A child with a seizure disorder should not be restricted from any regular school activities, including competitive sports, unless the seizures are not controlled or present an obvious danger. Contact sports, such as football and boxing, deserve special mention. The risk of a posttraumatic seizure is always present in contact sports, but despite the prevalence of concussion in these sports, seizures remain uncommon. The risk is greater in the child who already has a seizure disorder, and families must be willing to take that risk if their children participate

Box 180-3. Anticonvulsants That Reduce Blood Levels of Oral Contraceptives

Reduce Blood Levels

Phenytoin
Phenobarbital
Carbamazepine
Ethosuximide

Reduce Blood Levels to a Lesser Extent

Oxcarbazepine
Topiramate

in a contact sport. Ultimately, the parents and the child must make the final decision about activities, but the clinician is responsible for informing them about the risks.

A small number of children may have photosensitive seizures, which increases risk of seizure when exposed to certain photic stimuli. Stimuli include strobe lights of certain frequency or color and intense, colored cathode ray tubes of computer monitors and video games. Because of media reports regarding this phenomenon, video game and computer screen manufacturers have modified equipment to greatly reduce the risk of seizure in photosensitive patients. The majority of seizure patients are not photosensitive. Standard electroencephalogram (EEG) procedure includes photostimulation with a variable frequency strobe light, which enables diagnosis of photosensitivity.

Once a child is stabilized on antiseizure medication, a common reason for a recurrent seizure is failure to take medication. Poor adherence can be documented by history or by obtaining serum drug concentration determinations. If compliance is good, the next most likely cause for a breakthrough seizure is sleep deprivation. Illness, fever, fatigue, and stress are other risk factors for increased or breakthrough seizures. Beware the formerly well-controlled college freshman who becomes variable in remembering to take medication, begins experimenting with alcohol, and pulls an all-nighter—the "breakthrough triad" of noncompliance, alcohol, and sleep deprivation.

The clinician should also discuss dietary issues with families of children with seizure disorders. Regular, balanced meals are important in avoiding hypoglycemia, dehydration, and inadequate vitamin intake, all of which can provoke seizures. Some antiseizure medications, especially phenytoin and phenobarbital, and oral contraceptives, may block folate absorption. B vitamins, particularly vitamin B6 (pyridoxine), are especially important to healthy neuronal function. Pyridoxine deficiency is a serious though uncommon cause of seizures in newborns. The use of dietary carnitine supplementation is indicated in specific groups at risk for carnitine deficiency. Groups at risk are infants and young children on valproate, children with metabolic defects affecting carnitine metabolism, children on valproate with elevated ammonia levels or risk factors for hepatotoxicity, and children on the ketogenic diet. Otherwise healthy children on valproate do not require carnitine supplementation. Intravenous carnitine therapy is indicated in cases of acute valproate-induced hepatotoxicity.

MANAGING THE TREATMENT OF SEIZURES

Managing Seizure Medications

Since this chapter eschews the term *epilepsy* in favor of the more specific *seizure disorder*, and since many seizures in childhood are not convulsive, the often-used terms *antiepileptic drug (AED)* and *anticonvulsant* are discarded in favor of the more generic term *antiseizure medication*.

Pharmacodynamics: Getting the Medication into the Child

As noted, one of the most common reasons for recurrent seizures is noncompliance. Finding a medication formulation that children tolerate is an important ingredient in improving compliance. Intravenous administration of medications is covered in Chapters 33 and 103. Oral medications are available in regular tablets, chewable tablets, capsules, liquid suspension, and sprinkle formulations. Many regular tablets are unpleasant when chewed, but chewable tablets, while flavored, may contain sugar equivalent to the amount in a piece of candy. Some capsules can be opened and mixed with food (Carbatrol brand of carbamazepine), whereas others must be swallowed whole (ethosuximide). Liquid formulations expire sooner than tablets, may be unevenly distributed in the bottle, and can be light sensitive (carbamazepine, valproic acid, ethosuximide, phenobarbital, phenytoin). Pharmacodynamics are significantly affected by the formulation, since liquids will generally be absorbed more quickly, but have a shorter half-life. Sprinkles often have the most consistent pharmacodynamics, are usually well tolerated by young children, and have little unpleasant taste. They may result in a gritty or sandy quality to the stool (Depakote and Topamax sprinkles). Extended release capsules provide consistent blood levels, but the capsules must be swallowed intact (Tegretol XR). Rectal formulations may have a special role in the chronic management of seizures, since the efficacy of diazepam rectal gel (Diastat) has been well demonstrated. It can be safely administered by a parent in the event of seizure. It has also been shown to be effective in the prevention of recurrent febrile seizures.

Pharmacokinetics: Efficacy, Side Effects, and Drug Interactions

The guiding principle of antiseizure medication management is to use the least amount of the fewest number of medications possible without sacrificing seizure control. Doses are gradually increased until seizures are controlled or adverse effects appear. This is no small task, given the wide range of seizure types and individual variations in metabolism in children who are constantly changing in weight, activity, and diet. The end result is a need for continual monitoring of a child's seizure disorder within the context of general well-child care. For this reason, all children with ongoing seizure disorders should be referred for neurology consultation (preferably with a pediatric neurologist) at least once a year. Many pediatric neurologists willingly assume the management of seizure disorders. However, the management of many common seizure syndromes, including febrile seizures, benign Rolandic seizures, and absence seizures, is well within the capabilities of the generalist. A neurology consultation can always be obtained if breakthrough seizures occur or if there are complex medication issues. Consultation is suggested if a child is being managed with one of the new generation antiseizure medications, since the generalist may not yet have had adequate experience with the most recent medications. Box 180-1 lists conditions and occurrences that indicate the need for referral to a pediatric neurologist.

Choosing the Right Medication

Many new antiseizure medications are now available. While there are few absolute rules in selecting the right medication, certain guidelines can provide some rational relief to the bewildered. A basic understanding of seizure classifi-

Table 180-1. Paroxysmal Events Resembling Seizures

Event	Age range
Vaso-vagal spells, syncope	Adolescent
Night terrors	3 mo–6 yr
Paroxysmal dyskinesia (paroxysmal choreo-athetosis)	Infancy through adolescence
Shuddering spells	Infancy through 6 yr
Choking spells	Infancy
Tics	3 yr through adult
Breath holding spells	6 mo–6 yr
Atypical behaviors	Any age

cation is described in Table 180-1 and in Tables 103-1, 103-2, and 103-3.

Generalized seizures include primary generalized tonic-clonic (grand mal), juvenile myoclonic, and absence (petit mal) seizures. Valproate remains the drug of choice for primary generalized convulsions and is highly efficacious for absence seizures. Ethosuximide is specifically indicated for absence seizures, but should not be used in mixed seizure disorders since it can worsen other seizure types.

Partial seizures include complex partial (formerly called *temporal lobe* and *psychomotor* seizures), which have focal onset and altered consciousness, and simple partial, which do not alter consciousness. Carbamazepine has been the drug of choice and remains very effective. Oxcarbazepine is as effective with fewer side effects, but is not available in as many child-friendly formulations. Phenytoin is often the first drug started in the emergency department setting because it can be administered intravenously. Changing from phenytoin to another medication may be desirable for long-term management because of the incidence of adverse cosmetic effects. Among the newer antiseizure medications, gabapentin and tiagabine have shown efficacy in partial seizures.

Many of the newer antiseizure medications are described as "broad spectrum," a term meant to describe antiseizure medications that show efficacy for both generalized and partial seizures. These include lamotrigine, levetiracetam, topiramate, and zonisamide. The other advantage of the recently developed antiseizure medications is a relatively low side-effect profile with few drug interactions.

Side Effects

The therapeutic range for most antiseizure medications is quite narrow, with little margin between subtherapeutic and toxic doses. For this reason, many seizure patients are managed with medication levels on the brink of adverse effects (Table 180-2). While the guiding principle of antiseizure medication is to employ monotherapy whenever possible, many children require polypharmacy for adequate seizure control. This significantly complicates the medication management due to the high degree of interaction among antiseizure medications. Side effects and drug interactions are largely related to the specific hepatic metabolism and protein binding properties of each medication. Medications with minimal hepatic metabolism and low protein binding have fewer problems.

While the mechanism of action is not known for all antiseizure medications, they all reduce neuronal electrical irritability and thereby prevent the excessive electrical discharging that leads to a seizure. If the blood level is too low, this effect is inadequate and seizures may occur. If the blood level is too high, even normal neuronal electrical activity may be suppressed, and dose-related side effects such as drowsiness may occur.

Other side effects may not be dose dependent. Most of these involve hepatic toxicity, with symptoms including nausea, vomiting, and abdominal pain. Severe hepatic toxicity has been well recognized in children younger than age 2 years treated with valproate. As a result, valproate is not

Table 180-2. Antiseizure Medications and Common Adverse Effects

Medication	Primary Use	Abbr.	Primary Serious AE	Common AE	Blood Tests to Monitor
Carbamazepine (Tegretol, Carbatrol)	Partial sz (1st line)	CBZ	Neutropenia	Dizziness, lethargy	CBC, LFT
Ethosuzimide (Zarontin)	Absence sz	ESM	Blood dyscrasia, Stevens-Johnson syndrome (rare)	Lethargy	None
Gabapentin (Neurontin)	Partial sz	GBP	None	None	None
Lamotrigine (Lamictal)	Partial sz	LTG	Toxic rash	None	None
Levetiracetam (Keppra)	Adjunctive	LEV	None	Drowsiness, dizziness	None
Oxcarbazepine (Trileptal)	Partial sz	OXC	None	Drowsiness, nausea	None
Phenobarbital	Infants	PB		Sedation, behavior problems	None
Phenytoin (Dilantin)	Generalized sz Partial sz	PHT	Erythema multiforme	Gingival hyperplasia	None
Tiagabine (Gabitril)	Partial sz	TGB	None	Dizziness, lethargy	None
Topiramate (Topamax)	Adjunctive	TPM	Kidney stone (rare), secondary acute angle glaucoma (rare)	Dizziness, fatigue, headache, nystagmus, inattention, kidney stones (rare)	Consider UA
Valproate (divalproex sodium) (Depakote, Depakene)	Generalized sz (1st line)	VPA	Hepatic toxicity pancreatitis	Nausea, vomiting, lethargy	LFT
Zonisamide (Zonegram)	Partial sz	ZNS	Stevens-Johnson syndrome (rare)	Drowsiness, dizziness headache, kidney stones (rare)	None

Sz, seizure

recommended in very young children, especially if they are on concomitant medications. Polypharmacy is associated with a higher risk of adverse effects at any age compared to monotherapy. Bone marrow suppression (carbamazepine), severe hepatic toxicity (valproate, felbamate), and Stevens-Johnson syndrome (lamotrigine, especially when combined with valproate) are rare idiosyncratic adverse effects. Kidney stones have been found with chronic use of some antiseizure medications (topiramate, zonisamide) and a few cases of secondary closed angle glaucoma have been reported (with the use of topiramate). Polycystic ovary syndrome was thought to be increased with long-term use of valproate, but recent studies do not support that finding.

A few antiseizure medications are notable for the absence of both serious and mild toxicity (gabapentin, levetiracetam) because they are excreted primary through the kidneys rather than being metabolized by the liver. Because oxcarbazepine is not metabolized to toxic epoxide metabolites, the incidence of dizziness is lower than with carbamazepine.

A primary concern in school-age children is the possibility of adverse cognitive effects of medications. Major offenders include phenobarbital, phenytoin, and, to some degree, valproate. Preferred medications for avoiding problems in attention, memory, and alertness include gabapentin and levetiracetam, providing they are effective. Uncontrolled seizures interfere with learning more than any antiseizure medication.

Teenagers are especially sensitive to cosmetic side effects, chiefly phenytoin (dry skin, gingival hyperplasia, acne) and valproate (weight gain). Topiramate is a good choice when weight loss is a desirable side effect.

Medication Interactions

The two primary issues in medication interactions in children with seizure disorders are interaction between antiseizure medications and interaction with other medications. Interactions between antiseizure medications can be complex and are listed in Table 180-3. With few exceptions, antiseizure medications have complex hepatic metabolism involving the P450 enzyme system. When choosing to add a second medication, a primary consideration must always

be the anticipated pharmacokinetic effects of one drug on another. Carbamazepine in particular is a potent inducer of hepatic enzymes, resulting in accelerated metabolism of other drugs subject to hepatic metabolism. This effect includes the autoinduction of carbamazepine itself, which may result in subtherapeutic blood levels despite high-dose therapy. This problem, common among teenagers, can also make the transition from carbamazepine to oxcarbazepine a complex process.

A lowering of the seizure threshold may occur with centrally acting stimulant medications, including caffeine and decongestants containing pseudoephedrine. Studies have not found an increased seizure frequency in children with seizure disorders who are treated with methylphenidate or dexamphetamine for attention disorders. Of special concern is the teenage girl on oral contraceptives. Hepatic enzyme–inducing antiseizure medications can reduce oral contraceptive effectiveness if higher strength pills are not used.

Discontinuing Antiseizure Medications (Box 180-4)

While seizure disorders certainly can be lifelong, generalists and pediatric neurologists can be optimistic with parents that their child's seizures may resolve. This possibility of "growing out of seizures" is quite high in some particular circumstances, but very low in some specific seizure syndromes. Few controlled studies of discontinuing seizure medications are available. In an otherwise healthy child with normal growth and neurologic development who is seizure-free for 2 to 4 years with a normal EEG, withdrawal of seizure medication has about a 75% chance of being successful. The key issue is that the child does not have any identifiable neurologic deficit, developmental disorder, or structural brain abnormality. Family history of epilepsy or seizures reduces the likelihood that seizure medication can be successfully discontinued. The age of the child may be a factor as well. Although studies have not shown a statistical confirmation, some pediatric neurologists believe on the basis of their clinical observation that the risk of recurrent seizures is higher during adolescence. The reasons are unclear, but the phenomenon could be related to growth, hormones, or adherence.

Table 180-3. Drug Interactions of Antiseizure Medications

Medication	Metabolism	Increases Levels of	Decreases Levels of
Carbamazepine (CBZ)	Hepatic	None	CBZ, TGB, LTG*, TPM, OXC, PB, PHY, ZNS
Gabapentin (GBP)	Renal excretion	None	None
Lamotrigine (LTG)	Hepatic; 10% renal	None	VPA
Levetiracetam (LEV)	Renal excretion	None	None
Oxcarbazepine (OXC)	Hepatic; active metabolite 27%	PHT	CBZ, LTG*, PB, PHT, TGB, ZNS
Phenobarbital (PB)	Hepatic; 25% renal	None	PB, TGB, LTG*, OXC, PHT, VPA, ZNS
Phenytoin (PHT)	Hepatic	None	CBZ, TGB, LTG*, TPM, OXC, PB, VPA, ZNS
Tiagabine (TGB)	Hepatic	None	None
Topiramate (TPM)	Unknown; 65% renal	PHT*, PB*	CBZ, OXC, TGB, ZNS
Valproate (VPA)	Hepatic	CBZ*, TGB, LTG, PHY, PB	TPM, OXC, ZNS
Zonisamide (ZNS)	Hepatic; 35% renal	None	None

*Indicates highest degree of interaction possible
Note: (1) Carbamazepine levels may decrease as doses are increased due to autoinduction. This is a common problem in adolescents. (2) Phenytoin level is both reported to increase or decrease when oxcarbazepine is added.

Metabolism data from Leppik IE: Issues in the treatment of epilepsy. Epilepsia 2001;42(Suppl 4)1–6. Some drug interaction data from Oesterheld JR, Osser DN: P450 Drug interactions version 132. Available at http://www.mhc.com/Cytochromes.

A. Criteria

1. Previously healthy
2. No neurodevelopmental delay
3. No structural brain abnormality
4. No seizures in 2–4 years (on or off medication)
5. Recent normal EEG

B. Technique

1. Wean antiseizure medication gradually (this can be done by reducing the daily dose by 50% each week).
2. Monitor closely once off medication.
3. Repeat EEG in 3 months.
4. For teenagers, no driving is allowed during this time.

C. Assessment

1. If EEG remains normal and no seizure recurrence in 6 months, medication withdrawal is most likely successful.
2. If seizures recur, resume antiseizure medications.

Some specific seizure types resolve in childhood. Benign Rolandic seizures usually resolve by age 12 to 14 and are not seen in adults. Uncomplicated absence (petit mal) seizures often resolve in adolescence. Posttraumatic seizures may resolve, especially if they occur within 2 weeks of the head injury. Posttraumatic seizures with onset later than 2 weeks have a greater likelihood of continuing. Febrile seizures rarely occur after age 6 years. It is highly unlikely that medication can ever be withdrawn in juvenile myoclonic epilepsy (JME), which is usually lifelong. For guidelines to withdrawing antiseizure medications, see Box 180-4.

Nonpharmacologic Approaches to Treatment
Ketogenic Diet

Although the idea of treating seizures with a specialized diet may be appealing, the only clearly beneficial diet for treatment of seizures is the ketogenic diet. This diet may be indicated in children with seizures arising from specific metabolic disorders, such as glucose transporter disorders, pyruvate dehydrogenase deficiency, and cerebral glycolysis disorders. The diet has also been effective in myoclonic seizures and other refractory seizure disorders. The long-chain triglyceride diet induces ketosis and should be initiated in hospital. This diet is not easy to follow and improved seizure control can be variable. However, in some specific children with intractable seizures, the ketogenic diet can be an effective, worthwhile approach. If the ketogenic diet is considered, the clinician should refer the patient and family to an experienced pediatric neurologist.

Vagus Nerve Stimulator

A relatively new approach to seizure management involves the surgical placement of an electrical stimulator device on the left vagus nerve. While the exact mechanism of action is not fully understood, vagus nerve stimulation, often in conjunction with antiseizure medication, has been shown to significantly reduce seizure frequency. A pediatric neurologist may consider referral for this approach in patients with intractable seizures who are able to participate in the active management of the device. While the device provides automatic nerve stimulation at regular intervals, it can also be manually controlled by means of a magnetic "wand" when a patient experiences an aura prior to a seizure event.

Surgery for Seizures

In the past several years remarkable progress has been achieved in the evaluation and treatment of select intractable seizure patients. Successful surgical removal of "seizure-triggering" neuronal tissue has been achieved in both focal and generalized seizure disorders. Patients who have failed to respond to multiple antiseizure medications should be evaluated by a pediatric neurologist for potential referral to a seizure surgery program.

MANAGING SPECIFIC COMMON SEIZURE DISORDERS

Some seizure disorders or seizure syndromes are very difficult to treat, such as Lennox-Gastaut syndrome and infantile spasms. These complex seizure syndromes are best managed through consultation with a pediatric neurologist and are not discussed in this chapter. The generalist is likely to be confronted with several common seizure types: febrile seizures, complex partial seizures, and primary generalized seizures, including absence (petit mal) and tonic-clonic (grand mal). Management of these seizure disorders are discussed in CD-ROM Chapter 180 and in Chapter 103.

CHRONIC MANAGEMENT OF LONG-TERM ISSUES
Blood Tests

Obtaining blood levels of antiseizure medications should not be relied on as the best measure of an effective dose. Control of clinical seizures should be the primary goal. In some patients, seizure control can be achieved at low therapeutic levels or even at levels that are not in the "therapeutic range." With some exceptions, antiseizure medications have a relatively narrow therapeutic range. Small changes in dose can result in toxic blood levels. This is especially true of medications that have nonlinear pharmacokinetics, such as phenytoin. Obtaining medication blood levels can be useful in determining appropriate changes in dosage. However, blood levels can be confusing for medications that have autoinduction. If, for example, increasing the dose of carbamazepine results in a decreased blood concentration, consider the possibility of autoinduction, rather than assuming that the patient is noncompliant.

Once antiseizure medication has been prescribed, a blood level should be obtained in 10 to 14 days. This initial level provides a baseline for the individual patient that can serve as a guide for future changes in dosage. If a child is doing well and without seizures on a given dose, regular blood level testing is not mandatory. A repeat blood level might be appropriate if there is a significant change, such as a recurrent seizure or a marked increase in the child's weight.

Blood levels do help to confirm that the patient is compliant with the medication. One of the most common causes of recurrent seizures is failure to take the prescribed antiseizure medication. Once on medication, if the patient has a breakthrough seizure, a blood level determination can be helpful in assessing the cause of the seizure.

Many of the newer antiseizure medications do not have well-defined therapeutic levels, and blood level determinations may not be routinely available. Medications in this category include gabapentin, levetiracetam, oxcarbazepine, tiagabine, topiramate, and zonisamide.

Routine monitoring of liver function and complete blood count in patients on antiseizure medications should be individualized. Most hematologic and hepatic toxic effects are seen soon after initiation of medication, most often within the first 6 months of treatment. However, idiosyncratic reactions can occur at any time, even a week after normal blood testing. Therefore, routine blood testing can result in false reassurance. It is more important to consider obtaining baseline studies before starting therapy, especially for medications with known toxic risks. For example, if valproate is to be used in children younger than age 2, baseline liver function tests are appropriate.

Repeat Electroencephalograms

Once medication is begun, a follow-up EEG in several months is appropriate. This establishes whether the electrical seizure activity is altered by treatment. While EEGs may improve as a result of treatment, the recording does not usually normalize completely. Once a child is on a stable medication regime, EEG should be repeated annually. A yearly EEG will be helpful once a child has been seizure-free for several years and a plan to taper off medication is being considered. If an EEG has not been obtained for many years and then a normal EEG is obtained, how long the child has had a normal tracing is unknown. Repeat EEG is also indicated with a recurrent seizure or a change in seizure characteristics.

Imaging Studies

Imaging of the brain is indicated in all children who have had a seizure for which they are being treated with antiseizure medication. Imaging is also indicated for focal seizures and recurring seizures. Imaging is not necessary for simple febrile seizures and for typical uncomplicated absence seizures confirmed by EEG. Clinical judgment should be used for benign Rolandic seizures. Magnetic resonance imaging (MRI) is the preferred imaging study for seizures. If a computed tomography (CT) scan of the brain is chosen, contrast medium should be used to exclude a vascular etiology of the seizures.

Lumbar puncture is not routine in the workup of seizures. Clinical judgment should be used, especially in febrile seizures.

OUTCOME AND PROGNOSIS

Most lifelong seizure disorders begin in childhood. Families need to understand that children may not "grow out" of seizures. Long-term studies indicate that in an otherwise healthy child, with normal growth and development, the likelihood of successfully coming off antiseizure medication is as high as 75%. This assumes a seizure-free period of 2 to 4 years with a normal EEG. Some specific seizure types have an excellent prognosis, and the generalist and pediatric neurologist can be optimistic with parents. Simple febrile seizures rarely occur beyond age 6. Benign Rolandic seizures usually end by age 12 to 14. Absence seizures often do not continue beyond adolescence. Other idiopathic seizures in healthy children may resolve during adolescence.

Some seizure types have a more ominous prognosis. Infantile spasms often lead to lifelong mixed seizure types. Juvenile myoclonic seizures usually require lifelong treatment. Children with a history of developmental abnormalities and seizures are less likely to be able to discontinue antiseizure medications. Seizures associated with specific conditions such as tuberous sclerosis, neurofibromatosis, and severe head injury are likely to be lifelong.

While the chronic management of seizure disorders in children requires ongoing diligence on the part of the generalist, with appropriate pediatric neurology consultation, most children enjoy a normal childhood with few modifications in their lifestyle. Conscientious care, common sense, and anticipatory guidance serve as the foundation of high-quality management of children with seizures.

Additional Resources, CD-ROM

Management of specific seizure disorders and syndromes	Text

Mini-index of Related Topics

SUGGESTED READINGS

Browne TR, Holmes GL: Primary care review article: Epilepsy. N Engl J Med 2001;344(15):1145–1151.
Drug interaction data. Available at: http://www.mhc.com/Cytochromes/index.html.
Glauser TA: Integrating advances in pediatric epilepsy treatment options into clinical practice. Neurology 2002;58(suppl 7):12.
Holmes, GL: Diagnosis and management of seizures in children. In Major Problems in Clinical Pediatrics, Vol 30. Philadelphia, WB Saunders, 1998.
Leppik IE: Pharmacological treatment of epilepsy: Current trade-offs and the role of levetiracetam. Epilepsia 2001;42(suppl 4):44–45.
Matching the medicine to the patient. Epilepsia 2001;42(suppl 8):37–38.

181 Myopathies and Neuropathies

Richard E. Nordgren

Neuromuscular disorders include diseases that involve the anterior horn cell, peripheral nerves, neuromuscular junction, and the muscle itself. The term *myopathy* means any disorder of muscle, whether primary or secondary to some other disease process, whereas the term *muscular dystrophy* means a disease of muscle that is congenital and has a genetic basis. Motor neuron disorders include diseases, whether congenital or acquired, that involve the anterior horn cells. Neuromuscular junction diseases may be inherited or acquired, the latter usually from autoimmune dysfunction or from toxins. Peripheral nerve disorders can be inherited, can be secondary to trauma, or can be acquired (infectious, postinfectious, nutritional, secondary to metabolic or toxic etiologies).

FUNDAMENTALS OF DIAGNOSIS

The primary care provider should be familiar with the signs and symptoms of neuromuscular disorders in order to recognize the possibility of neuromuscular disease in patients. The majority of pediatric-age patients with neuromuscular disorders present in one of the following three ways:

1. *An infant with severe weakness or hypotonia.* Spinal muscular atrophy type 1, congenital myotonic dystrophy, some of the metabolic myopathies, myasthenic syndrome, and botulism are the disorders that most frequently present in this way.
2. *An acute or subacute development of weakness.* The clinician should consider Guillain-Barré syndrome,

dermatomyositis, toxins with either peripheral nerve, neuromuscular junction, or muscle involvement, and medication side effects that can present with either a neuropathy or a myopathy. Asymmetrical weakness or monoparesis suggests poliomyelitis, brachioplexopathy, or lumbar plexopathy.
3. *Gradually progressing weakness.* The clinician should consider muscular dystrophies, dermatomyositis, spinal muscular atrophy, and nonacute peripheral nerve disorders. If the patient also has fatigability, neuromuscular junction disorders may be a possibility, whereas if there is muscle cramping, various metabolic myopathies may be operational.

After examination, it should be possible to localize which part of the neuromuscular system is involved (i.e., anterior horn cell, peripheral nerve, neuromuscular junction, or the muscle itself). The predominant symptom in all neuropathies and myopathies is weakness. History should determine the duration of the problem, the distribution of the weakness, associated symptoms such as pain, cramping, sensory loss, fatigability, and urine changes, and family history of neuromuscular disorders. General physical examination should focus on signs of underlying disorders that can present with weakness, in particular, looking for skin lesions such as those seen in dermatomyositis. Neurologic examination should determine the degree of weakness, the distribution of the weakness, changes in or the presence or absence of the deep tendon reflexes, and the presence or absence of sensory findings. Table 181-1 lists signs and symptoms that are helpful in determining types of neuromuscular disorders.

Preliminary blood tests include complete blood count (CBC), erythrocyte sedimentation rate (ESR), creatine phosphokinase (CPK), and liver function tests. X-ray of the chest, electrocardiogram (ECG), and pulmonary function studies may also be appropriate. All of these tests will be helpful when the child is referred to a specialist for more extensive evaluation.

ROLE OF THE GENERALIST IN CARING FOR CHILDREN WITH NEUROMUSCULAR DISORDERS

After the specialist has evaluated the child and made a diagnosis, the primary care provider should ensure that the patient is referred for other evaluations including cardiology, physiatry, and orthopedics consultation. Genetic counseling may also be very important for the family. Often this all can be done through the Muscular Dystrophy Association clinics.

Table 181-1. Signs and Symptoms in Neuromuscular Disorders

Disorder	Distribution of Weakness	Deep Tendon Reflexes	Sensory Exam	Comments
Primary muscle disorders including dermatomyositis	Proximal (major exception myotonic dystrophy)	Preserved early in disorder	Normal	Rash may suggest dermatomyositis
Neuromuscular junction	Variable, often ocular and/or bulbar involvement	Usually preserved	Normal	Fatigability in myasthenia gravis
Peripheral nerves	Distal or in distribution of specific nerve, root	Usually absent in distribution of weakness	Usually involved in distribution of area of weakness	
Anterior horn cell	Variable, often diffuse	Absent in area of weakness		Reflexes often increased in ALS, an unusual disorder in children

In diagnosed patients, primary care providers need to monitor medical regimens such as anticholinesterase agents in myasthenia gravis, steroids in Duchenne dystrophy and dermatomyositis, and acetazolamide in periodic paralysis. They also need to ensure that appropriate electrocardiograms and pulmonary function tests (PFTs) are performed and immunizations including annual flu shots are kept up to date. Generalists also need to monitor modalities such as physical therapy, occupational therapy, and speech therapy. In addition, they play an important role in making sure that an appropriate school program is implemented. This is essential because many neuromuscular conditions have accompanying learning disabilities and behavioral problems. It is also very important that the patient receive appropriate adaptive devices that are then well maintained (AFOs, wheelchairs, vans). As the child's disorder progresses, many decisions need to be made by the child and family such as feeding tubes, tracheostomy, home respiratory support, and end-of-life decisions (see Chapter 129). The primary clinician's role in this decision-making process cannot be underestimated! Table 181-2 lists issues of comanagement between the generalist and the specialist and Table 181-3 lists specific issues related to health maintenance in children with neuromuscular disorders.

SPECIFIC MYOPATHIES AND NEUROPATHIES

Anterior Horn Cell Disorders
Anterior horn cell disorders include spinal muscular atrophies and poliomyelitis.

Spinal Muscular Atrophy
Spinal muscular atrophies present with weakness, hypotonia, and fasciculations. The deep tender reflexes are usually severally depressed or lost and there are typically no sensory findings. Spinal muscular atrophy (SMA) has been classified into three types, depending on the age of onset and severity. Patients with type 1 (Werdnig-Hoffman syndrome) usually present within the first 6 months of life. The infant is severely hypotonic and often lies with legs in the characteristic froglike position. Paradoxical respirations can also be noted in which the diaphragm contracts but because of extremely weak intercostal musculature the abdomen rises and the chest wall collapses. Patients with this variant of spinal muscular atrophy frequently need a feeding tube and vigorous pulmonary toilet. Most patients with this disorder succumb within the first 2 years of life. Spinal muscular atrophy type 2 presents at 6 to 18 months of age. Many of these children eventually sit up and some

Table 181-2. Comanagement Issues in Patients with Neuromuscular Disorders

Disease	Issues
Spinal muscular atrophy	Referral to MDA clinic Coordinate care with neurologist, physiatrist, pulmonologist, orthopedist. Refer family for genetic counseling. Ensure supportive care. End-of-life care
Hereditary neuropathies	Refer family for genetic counseling. Referral to physiatrist, physical therapy Referral to podiatrist when needed
Myasthenia gravis	Coordination of care with neurologist
Muscular dystrophies	Referral to MDA Clinic Ensure genetic counseling. Coordinate care with neurologist, physiatrist, orthopedist, cardiologist, pulmonologist. End-of-life care

Table 181-3. Health Maintenance Issues for Children with Specific Neuromuscular Disorders

Health Maintenance	Intervention
Duchenne's muscular dystrophy	Annual influenza vaccine Monitor cognitive development and school situation. Management of pulmonary and cardiac complications End-of-life care
Myotonic dystrophy and congenital myotonic dystrophy	Annual influenza vaccine Monitor cognitive development and school situation. Ensure cardiology involvement.
Spinal muscular atrophy	Annual influenza vaccine Management of pulmonary complications End-of-life care
Chronic inflammatory demyelinating polyneuropathy	Monitor ongoing treatment (IVIG, immunosupressants, plasmapheresis) with neurologist.

eventually walk. The prognosis is variable, with some patients surviving to the second or third decade. The pattern of weakness may be variable, with some muscle groups preserved and others severely involved. Often, reflexes are preserved when a muscle group is preserved. Many children with this disorder have minipolymyoclonus, a regular small amplitude movement that is most prominent in the distal extremities. Spinal muscular atrophy type 3 (Kugelberg-Welander disease) usually presents after 18 months of age, and is much slower in progression than the other forms of spinal muscular atrophy. Patients eventually ambulate and usually have a normal life span.

Patients with spinal muscular atrophy show a pattern called "grouped atrophy" on muscle biopsy. In recent years, genetic testing has been developed for diagnosis of the disorder. Major deletions at the 5q11.2–13.3 focus have been found. The survival motor neuron (SMN) gene at 5q13 has been found to show deletions in approximately 95% of spinal muscular atrophy patients, and the neuronoapoptosis inhibitory protein gene, which also maps to the 5q13 region, has been found abnormal in 67% of patients with spinal muscular atrophy.

Spinal muscular atrophy is usually a recessive disorder. If the disease is suspected, blood testing of DNA for the survival motor neuron deletion is the first diagnostic test that should be done. Muscle biopsy is no longer necessary to confirm the diagnosis in most patients. Genetic testing has been performed in utero in affected families. A severe form of spinal muscular atrophy called infantile neuronal degeneration presents at birth with contractures, severe muscle weakness, and cranial nerve involvement. Infants with this disorder usually survive for only a short time. Some of these children have also been found to have the survival motor neuron deletion, which is important for genetic counseling.

In some families, spinal muscular atrophy can be inherited as a dominant disorder or as an X-linked recessive disorder. Kennedy disease is a rare disorder that affects spinal bulbar musculature and can cause gynecomastia.

Paralytic Poliomyelitis

Paralytic poliomyelitis has been largely eliminated in the United States. Rare cases are seen when only the oral form of the polio vaccine (OPV) is used or when a nonimmunized adult comes in contact with a patient who recently received the oral polio vaccine. Recent recommendations that the Salk vaccine be given intramuscularly before the institution of the oral polio vaccine prevent infants and exposed adults from developing the disorder from the oral attenuated live vaccine. The disorder usually presents with asymmetrical weakness, muscle atrophy, hyporeflexia, and often fasciculations. There is often pain in the affected extremities, but there is no sensory loss. Usually during the onset of the disorder, there is a fever, irritability, and possible signs of meningial irritation. The cerebrospinal fluid (CSF) shows cells and diagnosis of the disease is achieved via positive stool cultures. Other Enteroviruses including coxsackie virus rarely cause a similar clinical picture. Treatment is supportive care.

Late onset GM2 gangliosidosis can include weakness from involvement of the anterior horn cells. The diagnostic test for this disorder is hexosaminidase-A levels.

Peripheral Nerve Disorders

In addition to weakness, patients with peripheral nerve disorders present with absent or diminished reflexes in the distribution of the peripheral nerve involvement. If the process is diffuse, the sensory involvement and weakness are prominent distally rather than proximally. If the nerve involvement is secondary to a radicular lesion or a peripheral nerve injury, the weakness and sensory loss are in the anatomic distribution for the particular lesion. Sensory examination can be difficult to perform on very young children or in uncooperative patients.

Peripheral nerve disorders can be categorized in several groups. Hereditary sensory and motor neuropathies (Charcot-Marie-Tooth and related disorders) are usually progressive disorders involving the peripheral nerves with no obvious underlying metabolic problem. The acquired disorders include injuries to the peripheral nerves, inflammations and infections of the peripheral nerves, toxins that involve the peripheral nerves, and metabolic disorders involving the peripheral nerves. The primary care clinician must be aware of the various presentations of toxic and inflammatory conditions since there are treatments that can alter the course of the disorder.

Hereditary Neuropathies

The hereditary neuropathies include a large number of disorders that have sensory, motor, and autonomic dysfunction. They frequently have a distal atrophy of the legs and a pes cavus deformity of the feet. These disorders are constantly being reclassified as new genetic information is obtained, but Box 181-1 summarizes some of this information based on inheritance and the primary abnormality in the peripheral nerves. The most common conditions are Charcot-Marie-Tooth types 1 and 2, which present with weakness of the extremities and a foot deformity. Dejerine-Sotas or type 3 is similar to Charcot-Marie-Tooth and is a hypomyelinating disorder. Usually it is more severe and more progressive than types 1 and 2. These disorders can be dominant, recessive, or X-linked and specific testing including neurophysiologic studies, nerve biopsy, and genetic testing may confirm a specific diagnosis.

Acquired Neuropathies

The acquired neuropathies include injury to various nerves. In the newborn, Erb paralysis (an upper plexus injury) and Klumpke paralysis (lower plexus injury) still occur. Repetitive stress injuries such as carpal tunnel syndrome are somewhat unusual in children.

Inflammatory Neuropathies

The inflammatory neuropathies include acute inflammatory demyelinating polyneuropathy (Guillain-Barré syndrome or acute inflammatory demyelinating polyneuropathy [AIDP]) and chronic inflammatory demyelinating polyneuropathy. Primary care clinicians must recognize Guillain-Barré syndrome since it has specific treatment. The classic presentation is weakness in the lower extremities progressing to the upper extremities accompanied by sensory symptomatology, depressed or absent reflexes, and possibly cranial nerve palsies. Variations in this classic presentation include asymmetry of weakness and the Miller Fisher

Box 181-1. Classification of Hereditary Motor and Sensory Neuropathies

Type I (HSMN Type I) Myelin Defect

Autosomal dominant:
> Type Ia: duplication 17p11.2–12 or point mutation PMP-22 gene
> Type Ib: point mutation 1q22–23
> Type Ic: unknown

Autosomal recessive:
> Linkage to several gene loci in different families

Type II (HSMN Type II) Axonal Deficit

Autosomal dominant:
> Type IIa: linkage to 1p35–p36
> Type IIb: linkage to 3q13–q22
> Type IIc: associated with diaphragmatic and vocal cord paralysis, gene locus unknown
> Type IId: linkage to 7p14

Autosomal recessive:
> Infantile type with respiratory failure
> Axonal type with early childhood onset

Type III (HSMN Type II or Dejerine-Sotas) Hypomyelinating Disorder

Usually a dominant disorder
Frequently same gene locus as HSMN types Ia, Ib, Id

Hereditary Sensory and Autonomic Neuropathies

Type I: linked to 9q22.1–22.3, dominant
Type II: unknown gene, recessive
Type III: (Riley-Day syndrome), linked to 9q31–33, recessive
Type IV: possibly related to TRKA (a receptor for tyrosine kinase growth factor), recessive
Type V: gene locus unknown, probably recessive, patients have abnormal pain and temperature sensation, other modalities preserved. Biopsy shows absent small myelinated fibers but normal large fibers

syndrome, which presents with cranial nerve involvement and ataxia. Autonomic dysfunction is a frequent manifestation of these disorders and can be life-threatening if not recognized. Patients who have any evidence of fluctuating blood pressure or other autonomic problems should be managed in an intensive care unit where they can be closely monitored. The hallmark of Guillain-Barré syndrome is an elevated cerebrospinal fluid protein without a cellular response in the spinal fluid. The protein elevation may occur well into the disease course and may be absent early in the illness; this so-called cytoalbuminemic dissociation is not necessary for the diagnosis. Neurophysiologic studies are helpful in the diagnoses and prognosis of an acute inflammatory demyelinating polyneuropathy. Patients who have axonal involvement have a much worse prognosis than patients with only a demyelinating process. *Campylobacter jejuni* is an etiology that usually has the axonal form of the disorder. Management of acute inflammatory demyelinating neuropathy includes respiratory support when necessary and close monitoring for an autonomic dysfunction. Both human immune globulin and plasmapheresis have been found to be efficacious in the treatment of the disorder.

Chronic inflammatory demyelinating polyneuropathy (radiculoneuropathy) (CIDP) is a relapsing form of inflam-

matory neuropathy. It is quite difficult to distinguish acute inflammatory demyelinating neuropathy from chronic inflammatory demyelinating polyneuropathy with the first episode of a polyneuropathy. However, cranial neuropathies are unusual in chronic inflammatory demyelinating polyneuropathy. Patients with chronic inflammatory demyelinating polyneuropathy can be treated with intravenous immune globulin (IVIG) or plasma exchange. Long-term corticosteroids and other immunosuppressants may also be used.

Facial Weakness

Facial weakness in children invokes a wide differential (Box 181-2). The most common cause is Bell palsy, but there are many other conditions presenting with facial weakness. Lyme disease and severe hypertension should be considered as an etiology, especially if involvement is bilateral.

Peripheral Neuropathies

Infectious agents that can involve the peripheral nerves include HIV, herpes zoster, and leprosy. Nutritional deficiencies causing a neuropathy include thiamine deficiency and pernicious anemia. Many toxins can affect the peripheral nerve system including lead, mercury, organophosphates, and medications. Primary care providers should be aware of the so-called intensive care weakness, a diffuse weakness that follows prolonged intensive care hospitalization, usually with respiratory support. This can be secondary to a peripheral neuropathy or a myopathy and has been associated with neuromuscular blocking agents and corticosteroids. An elevated creatine phosphokinase suggests a muscle disorder; electrical studies may also be helpful. A muscle biopsy is necessary in some situations to distinguish between a neuropathic and a myopathic process. While the weakness in this condition is usually severe, the prognosis for eventual recovery is quite good in young patients.

Many neurometabolic conditions can involve the peripheral nerves.

Neuromuscular Junction Disorders

Neuromuscular junction disorders present in children of any age. Infantile botulism can present from 2 weeks to 6 months of age; there is usually a history of constipation and poor feeding. The patient often develops trouble swallowing and then muscle weakness with loss of deep tendon reflexes (DTRs) occurs. Patients usually have diffuse hypotonia, a very weak cry, large pupils that react sluggishly, and ptosis. The diagnosis is confirmed by isolation of organisms from the stool. Respiratory support is often required. Untreated, the disease can last several weeks and the use of immune globulins usually shortens the course of the disease. This disorder has been associated with the infant ingesting honey or being near construction or agricultural sites where a lot of dust is created.

Transitory neonatal myasthenia gravis develops in infants of affected mothers from transfer of fetal antiacetylcholine receptor antibody from the mother to the fetus. The major symptoms are difficulty with feeding and hypotonia, though respiratory depression can also occur. Any woman with known myasthenia should be considered at risk of delivering a baby with transitory neonatal myasthenia and anticipatory treatment should be available. The diagnosis

Box 181-2. Facial Weakness in Childhood

Congenital, Structural Weakness

Chiari malformation
Depressor anguli oris muscle absence (cardiofacial syndrome)
Inner ear and/or facial nerve malformations
Möbius syndrome
Syringobulbia

Genetic Weakness

Facioscapulohumeral dystrophy
Familial cranial neuropathy (recurrent)
Fazio-Londe disease
Myasthenia gravis (nonimmune-mediated)
Myotonic dystrophy
Nemaline myopathy

Infectious, Inflammatory Weakness

Basilar meningitis
Bell palsy
Epstein-Barr infection (infectious mononucleosis)
Guillain-Barré syndrome
Miller Fisher syndrome
Mycoplasma pneumoniae infection
Lyme disease (*Borrelia* species infection)
Otitis media and mastoiditis
Parotitis
Poliomyelitis
Ramsay Hunt syndrome (herpes zoster)
Sarcoidosis
Trichinosis
Tuberculosis

Trauma, Nerve Compression

Forceps pressure during delivery
Cleidocranial dysostosis
Histiocytosis X
Hyperostosis craniolis interna
Increased intracranial pressure
Petrous bone fracture
Pressure from maternal sacrum

Metabolic Conditions

Hyperparathyroidism
Hypothyroidism
Idiopathic infantile hypercalcemia
Osteopetrosis

Neoplasms

Brainstem glioma
Parotid gland tumors

Vascular Weakness

Arterial hypertension
Vascular syndromes of the cranial nerves

Other

Idiopathic cranial neuropathy
Melkersson-Rosenthal syndrome
Multiple sclerosis
Myasthenia gravis (immune-mediated)
Myasthenia gravis (transient neonatal)

From Swaiman KF, Ashwal S: Pediatric Neurology: Principles and Practice, 3rd ed. St. Louis, Mosby, 1999.

is more difficult when the mother is not known to have the disease. If suspected, the disorder can be diagnosed by injection of neostigmine hydrochloride. Edrophonium might also be considered, but its effects are transitory and detection of improvement may be difficult in an infant. The condition is self-limited, rarely lasting longer than 2 months.

Immune myasthenia gravis can occur in childhood and presents with abnormal fatigability of the muscles, often with ptosis, double vision, and limb weakness. The diagnosis can be confirmed by EMG studies with repetitive stimulation, the use of edrophonium hydrochloride to demonstrate improvement of the fatigability or detection of anticholine receptor antibodies. The treatment includes the use of anticholinesterase agents, consideration of prednisone, azathioprine, and/or thymectomy.

Congenital myasthenic syndromes are hereditary nonimmune disorders of neuromuscular transmission. Often these conditions do not respond to anticholinesterase inhibitors. There are both presynaptic and postsynaptic defects in this heterogeneous group of disorders and very specialized testing at a few medical centers is necessary to delineate which type the patient my have. These conditions can present in infancy or later in childhood. Thymectomy and immunosuppression are usually not beneficial treatments.

Other agents that can affect the neuromuscular junction include anticholinesterase drugs and particular organophosphate insecticides, some nerve gases, and some snake and spider venom. Tick paralysis is very important to recognize because removal of the tick results in rapid improvement of the disorder. The paralysis in this case is due to a neurotoxin from the saliva of a female tick that prevents release of acetylcholine at the neuromuscular junction.

Muscle Diseases/Disorders

Muscular dystrophies are inherited muscle diseases that involve striated muscle but can also involve smooth muscle of the heart and gastrointestinal tract (Table 181-4).

Duchenne Muscular Dystrophy

Duchenne muscular dystrophy is an X-linked recessive disorder that presents with proximal muscle weakness, usually accompanied by pseudohypertrophy of the calves. Age of onset is between 3 and 5 years. Reflexes remain until the muscles become quite weak and contractures develop. Facial musculature is usually spared. Most patients lose ambulation before the age of 10 and do not survive much past the mid-20s. The daily use of steroids may prolong the period of ambulation. In addition to the striated muscle problems, patients frequently have a cardiomyopathy and later in the course can develop cor pulmonale. The incidence of cognitive problems, usually mild, is high.

Table 181-4. Clinical Features of Muscular Dystrophies

Disorder	Inheritance	Clinical Manifesations	Diagnostic Testing
Duchenne	X-linked	Progressive symmetrical muscle weakness Onset 3–5 years Pseudohypertrophy of calf muscles Often developmental delay Ambulatory age 8–10 Usually die in 20s	Markedly elevated CPK Mutation of short arm of X chromosome in region Xp21 Muscle biopsy has absent dystrophin
Becker	X-linked	As above except onset usually after age 7 Ambulation often until 30s	Same as above except biopsy has decreased but present dystrophin
Myotonic	Autosomal dominant	Distal weakness Myotonia Typical facial features Mental retardation common Cardiac conduction problems Diabetes GI motility problems Maternal inheritance frequently results in congenital myotonia	Myotonia on EMG Abnormal CTG repeats chromosome 19 Severity of disease correlates with the number of repeats, 5–37 normal range
Facioscapulohumeral	Autosomal dominant	Weakness facial muscles and scapular stabilizers Diagnosis most common age 10–20 Gradual weakness upper and lower extremities High-frequency hearing loss Asymptomatic retinal vasculopathy Normal life span	Deletion chromosome 4q35

The creatine phosphokinase is markedly elevated and persists until atrophy is severe. Muscle biopsy shows changes typical of a muscular dystrophy, and with special staining, dystrophin is absent. The Duchenne muscular dystrophy gene, located at the Xp21 band of the X chromosome, is responsible for the production of dystrophin. Deletion can be detected in approximately 65% of boys with Duchenne dystrophy. If this deletion is present, the carrier state can be detected in girls at risk. If not present, linkage analysis can detect a very high percentage of girls who are carriers. Some carriers have manifestations of the disorder, although usually much milder than in boys with the disorder.

Becker Muscular Dystrophy

Becker muscular dystrophy, a milder form of X-linked recessive muscle disease, is also associated with abnormalities of the Xp-21 locus responsible for the production of dystrophin. The age of onset is much later than Duchenne dystrophy and ambulation is maintained much longer. Becker dystrophy can be compatible with a normal life span. A muscle biopsy is necessary to distinguish Becker from Duchenne dystrophy. In Becker dystrophy, dystrophin (which is absent in Duchenne dystrophy) is present in muscles though in reduced amounts.

Myotonic Dystrophy

Myotonic dystrophy is an autosomal dominant disorder caused by increased CTG trinucleotide repeat expansions and chromosome 19 q13.3. There appears to be a relationship between the number of the repeats and the severity of the disease. Normally, up to 37 repeats are present at this region. In myotonic dystrophy the number can range from 50 to several thousand. The severity of the disorder is also

related to the gender of the affected parent. The patient typically develops a distal weakness associated with myotonia. Facial appearance is typical with temporalis wasting, a facial diplegia, and often tenting of the upper lip. Myotonic dystrophy also affects many other organ systems. The heart is frequently involved, with progressive heart block developing. These patients need to be followed closely by a cardiologist and have electrocardiograms done at regular intervals. In addition, patients frequently develop cataracts. Male patients typically have premature balding and gonadal atrophy. Patients frequently develop diabetes associated with high insulin levels. There is often smooth muscle involvement with intestinal and esophageal motility problems. Varying degrees of intellectual compromise are present. Retardation is especially frequent in children with congenital myotonia. Myotonia can be altered by some medications, including phenytoin, carbamazepine, quinidine, and quinine; however, most patients are not bothered significantly by the myotonia itself but rather by the progressive distal weakness.

Congenital myotonic dystrophy is the severe form of the disease presenting in patients whose mothers have the disorder. The disorder should be considered in any hypotonic infant, especially if there is arthrogryposis (congenital contractures). These infants often have a characteristic tenting of the upper lip as well as facial weakness and swallowing problems. They may need respiratory assistance but typically outgrow this problem. Myotonia is not usually detectable in the infant. If the disorder is suspected, the mother should be examined, especially evaluated for myotonia, which may not be obvious clinically but may show up on electrical studies. Gene testing can be done but the results take time. These infants need orthopedic follow-up for treatment of their contractures. They frequently have intellectual and developmental problems, often functioning in the retarded range. In addition to these neonatal issues, they develop the same problems as patients with a later onset form of the disorder.

Facioscapulohumeral Dystrophy

Facioscapulohumeral dystrophy (FSHD) is an autosomal dominant disorder that presents with weakness of the facial muscles and the scapular stabilizers. Ankle dorsiflexors may also be involved early in the disease. Presentation can occur at any age, but the diagnosis is usually made in the second decade. The course is slow, most patients gradually develop weakness in the upper arms and lower extremities, and there frequently is asymmetry in the distribution of the weakness. Patients with this disorder usually have a normal life span, and ambulation is maintained in the majority of patients with this disorder. There typically is no cardiac involvement but high-frequency hearing loss and a usually asymptomatic retinal vasculopathy are often present. Genetic testing is available and most families have a deletion on chromosome 4q35.

Limb Girdle Muscular Dystrophy

Limb girdle muscular dystrophy is no longer a diagnosis, but a descriptive term that includes a number of heterogeneous disorders that present with proximal muscular weakness that is usually progressive. Many of these disorders are associated with abnormalities in the dystrophin-glycoprotein complex in the muscle cellular membrane. These disorders should be suspected in a girl with a Duchenne or Becker clinical phenotype, or in a boy with a Becker or Duchenne phenotype with a muscle biopsy demonstrating normal dystrophin. Special testing is necessary for diagnosing these disorders and accurate diagnosis is important in regard to genetic counseling and prognosis. The management of these disorders is quite similar to that of other muscular dystrophies and there is no specific treatment for any of these disorders at this point in time.

Congenital Myopathies

The congenital myopathies are a heterogeneous group of disorders that usually present with weakness that either progresses very slowly or is not progressive at all. Many of these disorders are diagnosed by muscle biopsy with histochemistry. They are almost always inherited diseases. It is extremely important to be aware of the close association with congenital myopathies with central core disease (which is an autosomal dominant disorder) and malignant hyperthermia. If a patient is diagnosed with central core disease, everyone in the family should be considered at high risk for malignant hyperthermia. No specific treatment is available for this group of disorders but diagnosis is very important, especially from a genetic and prognostic point of view.

Metabolic Myopathies

Metabolic myopathies include a large number of disorders that are individually somewhat unusual in occurrence, but in total affect a significant number of pediatric patients. These include disorders of mitochondria, disorders of glycogen metabolism, and disorders of lipid metabolism. They should be suspected in any severally hypotonic infant, especially if there are respiratory and feeding problems or if there is evidence of a cardiomyopathy. In older patients, these disorders often present with muscle cramping and trouble with exercise. Usually the creatine phosphokinase is elevated in these disorders and an EMG may be helpful for diagnosis. A muscle biopsy may be necessary to diagnose these disorders and the biopsy should include special staining including staining for glycogen and histochemistry, electron microscopy, and a frozen sample, which can then be available for DNA or other specialized testing.

"Channel" Disorders

The "channel" disorders include the various periodic paralyses (hyperkalemic and hypokalemic as well as normokalemic periodic paralyses). All of these disorders present with episodic weakness. Strenuous exercise, carbohydrate overload, and changes in potassium levels can trigger weakness in patients with these disorders. Hypokalemic periodic paralysis is strongly associated with thyroid disease, especially among Asian patients. Myotonia is also considered a channel disorder but the most common form of myotonia, myotonic dystrophy, is discussed under the muscular dystrophies. Myotonia congenita and paramyotonia congenita are diseases with myotonia, but they do not have the multisystem problems seen in myotonic dystrophy and progressive muscular weakness is not usually a prominent feature in these conditions.

Inflammatory Myopathies

The inflammatory myopathies include dermatomyositis, polymyositis, and infectious myopathies including viral myositis, tuberculosis, trichinosis, and toxoplasmosis. Dermatomyositis usually has proximal muscle weakness, stiffness, and pain. It can present in a fulminate fashion but typically is more insidious in onset. Characteristically, there is a rash over the upper eyelids, which spreads to the periorbital and malar regions. The rash frequently involves the extensor surfaces of the knuckles, elbows, and knees. There often is an accompanying dysphagia. Muscle biopsy shows a diagnostic perifascicular atrophy. In addition to the rash, a high percentage of patients develop calcium deposits in the subcutaneous tissues and joint contractures. The disorder usually responds to treatment with corticosteroids and if this regimen is not successful, other immunosuppressive agents such as methotrexate should be considered. Plasmapheresis and human immune globulin have also been reported to be effective in the disorder. Physical therapy to prevent contracture is a very important part of the treatment of the disorder. Polymyositis is quite unusual in children.

Other Acquired Myopathies

Other acquired myopathies include muscle weakness associated with systemic disease including malnutrition, thyroid disorders, corticosteroids, electrolyte disturbances, and toxic myopathies from alcohol, amphetamines, chloroquine, cimetidine, heroin, licorice, lovastatin, salicylates, sulfasalazine, vincristine, and zydovudine.

SUGGESTED READINGS

Andersson PB, Rando TA: Neuromuscular disorders of childhood. Curr Opin Pediatr 1999;11:497–503.

Hilton T, Orr RD, Perkin RM, Ashwal S: End of life care in Duchenne muscular dystrophy. Pediatr Neurol 1993;9:165–177.

Katirji B, Kaminski HJ, Preston DC, et al: Neuromuscular Disorders in Clinical Practice. Boston, Butterworth Heinemann, 2002.

Neuromuscular disorders. In Swaiman KF, Ashwal S: Pediatric Neurology: Principles and Practice, 3rd ed. St Louis, Mosby, 1999.

SECTION 4   CHRONIC MEDICAL CARE: *Disorders of the Respiratory System*

182   Cystic Fibrosis

Ronald L. Gibson

ROLE OF THE GENERALIST

1. Recognize the diverse presenting signs and symptoms of cystic fibrosis (CF).

2. Refer newly diagnosed patients with CF to an accredited CF center for evaluation.

3. Provide appropriate primary care and health maintenance for children with CF.

4. Encourage patients with CF to make quarterly clinic visits at a CF center and coordinate their care with specialists.

5. Monitor nutritional and pulmonary status of CF patients at regular visits.

6. Recognize and treat or refer patients with common conditions and complications associated with CF.

7. Know common pathogens of minor acute respiratory illnesses to guide treatment.

8. Refer the medical management of CF patients with significant illnesses to a specialist at a CF center.

   • The roles of the generalist and the multidisciplinary specialist CF care team may vary with geographic regions and philosophy of care considerations.

DEFINITION

Cystic fibrosis (CF) is the most common life-shortening, recessive genetic disease in whites. It is an autosomal recessive disorder caused by mutations in the gene encoding the CF transmembrane conductance regulator (CFTR) protein, a regulated cell membrane chloride channel (Fig. 182-1). Mutations in the CFTR protein result in defective electrolyte transport across CF epithelia, and the altered luminal fluid properties contribute to pathogenesis in multiple organs (Box 182-1). Thus, CF is a multisystem disease affecting the lungs and upper respiratory tract, gastrointestinal tract, pancreas, liver, sweat glands, and genitourinary tract. Pulmonary disease is the primary cause of morbidity and death.

FUNDAMENTALS

Prevalence and Genetics

The incidence of CF is approximately 1 in 2000 to 1 in 4000 live births in most European and European-derived populations. CF affects approximately 30,000 persons in the United States. The carrier frequency is about 1 in 22 to 1 in 28 whites. CF occurs less frequently in native Asians, Africans, African Americans (~1 in 15,000), and Asian Americans (~1 in 31,000), although reliable incidence figures are not available.

CF mutations are classified into four categories based on the type of CFTR dysfunction (Fig. 182-2). Class I mutations have premature termination of translation with little or no full length functional CFTR (i.e., W1282X, prevalent in Ashkenazi Jews), or alternative splicing leading to reduced protein production. Class II mutations have defective protein processing and intracellular degradation with reduced apical cell surface expression; they are the most common, including the ΔF508 allele. Class III mutant proteins traffic to the apical membrane but with reduced channel activity from abnormal gating. Class IV mutations, the least common, have defective regulation of chloride conductance despite being present on the apical membrane (i.e., R347P). Such mutations that result in a significant

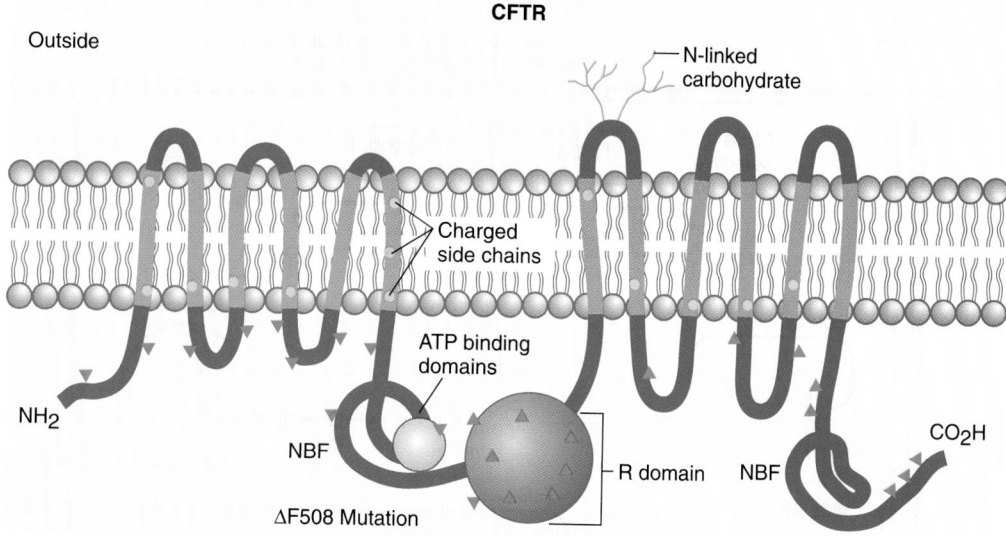

Figure 182-1. Cystic fibrosis is an autosomal recessive disorder caused by mutations in the gene encoding the cystic fibrosis transmembrane conductance regulator (CFTR) protein, a regulated cell membrane chloride channel. CFTR contains two nucleotide binding domains (NBF) that bind and hydrolyze adenosine triphosphate (ATP), two dual sets of membrane-spinning segments that form the channel, and a central regulatory (R) domain. The most common mutation in CFTR, ΔF508, is located in NBF1.

amount of CFTR function may in certain contexts result in only mild pulmonary disease. The variability in pulmonary disease among patients with identical genotypes suggests a role for environmental factors and modifier genes.

Lung Disease

The primary cause of morbidity and death in patients with CF is chronic endobronchial infection and neutrophilic inflammation, with progressive obstructive lung disease and bronchiectasis (Fig. 182-3A and B). This accounts for approximately 80% of deaths in CF. The onset of respiratory symptoms in CF is variable, but most patients with CF have pulmonary signs and symptoms in infancy or as toddlers. Infants and young children with CF already have

---

Box 182-1. Cystic Fibrosis Transmembrane Conductance Regulator Protein

- More than 900 disease-associated mutations have been reported in the CFTR gene.
- The most common mutation, deletion of phenylalanine at position 508 (ΔF508), accounts for nearly 70% of mutations in whites.
- Fifty-three percent of patients in the 2001 U.S. CF Foundation Patient Registry are homozygous for ΔF508, 36% are heterozygous for ΔF508, and 12% have no ΔF508 or both alleles are unidentified.
- Only four other mutations account for more than 1% of CF alleles in patients worldwide.
- CF mutations are classified into four categories based on the type of CFTR dysfunction. ΔF508 is a class II mutation with the great majority of misfolded protein being degraded prior to reaching the apical cell surface.
- Future therapies are likely to be directed toward class-specific CFTR mutations.
- Class of CFTR mutation correlates with pancreatic function, but the relationship to severity of lung disease is less certain and more complex

---

neutrophil-dominated lower airway inflammation and endobronchial infection.

The mechanisms by which CFTR dysfunction leads to viscous secretions, chronic endobronchial infection, and neutrophilic-dominated lower airway inflammation are not completely understood. In the CF airway epithelia, mutations in CFTR result in two aberrant transport processes (Fig. 182-4). First, there is marked reduction in apical membrane chloride permeability that is not responsive to cyclic adenosine monophosphate (cAMP) agonists. Second, the activity of apical sodium channels is approximately doubled compared to non-CF epithelia. The prevailing hypothesis is that the CF airway surface fluid is isotonic and low in volume, resulting in viscous lower airway secretions and reduced mucociliary clearance. Defective CFTR in the CF airway is also associated with a heightened, proinflammatory response to noxious stimuli compared to non-CF lungs. In addition, the respiratory tract in CF patients is ultimately persistently infected with bacterial pathogens that augment the chronic and intense inflammatory response, resulting in copious purulent secretions and lung damage. Other potential theories for early and persistent airway infection with *Pseudomonas* include increased affinity of CF epithelium for *Pseudomonas*, reduced local innate host defenses to clear the bacteria, and abnormal submucosal gland function contributing to suboptimal mucociliary clearance. The vicious circle of chronic infection and inflammation with poor clearance of the viscous mucus results in progressive destruction of the lower airways and bronchiectasis (see Fig. 182-3B).

Common CF pathogens are *Staphylococcus aureus*, nontypable *Haemophilus influenzae*, and gram-negative bacilli including *Pseudomonas aeruginosa* (Fig. 182-5). Data from respiratory tract cultures guide antimicrobial therapy during outpatient and inpatient treatment. *S. aureus* and *H. influenzae* are the predominant pathogens in early childhood. By 1 year of age, 15% to 20% of children with

Box 182-2. Criteria to Consider in Assessing Pulmonary Exacerbation*

- Decreased FEV_1 of >10% from baseline
- Increased cough
- Increase or change in sputum
- Fever
- Weight loss of >5%
- Reduced exercise tolerance
- Decrease SaO_2 from baseline
- New finding on chest radiograph
- Increased respiratory rate or work of breathing
- School or work absenteeism in last week
- New finding on chest physical examination

*Patients who meet 3 of these 11 criteria can be diagnosed with pulmonary exacerbation, but there are no accepted standardized criteria.

Box 182-4. Key Features of Cystic Fibrosis–Related Diabetes Mellitus

- CFRDM is becoming a more frequent complication as lifespan for CF patients increases.
- Insulin-dependent CFRDM occurs in ~3% of patients 18 years old or younger, but in over 15% patients older than 18 years.
- Fatigue and weight loss, secondary to glucosuria, can be presenting symptoms.
- CFRDM patients have more beta cells than patients with type I diabetes mellitus, and a much lower risk of diabetic ketoacidosis.
- Acute pulmonary exacerbation is associated with greater insulin resistance and increased risk of significant glucose intolerance.
- Systemic glucocorticoid treatment can exacerbate glucose intolerance in CF.
- Preliminary data suggest a reduced survival time for CF patients with CFRDM; this highlights the need for screening and management for this CF complication.

cells from fibrosis and fatty infiltration of the pancreas (Box 182-4).

DIAGNOSIS

Newborn Screening

Newborn screening for CF is controversial and is available in only a limited number of states. Evidence indicates linear growth is impaired, at least through 10 years of age, for those patients diagnosed by standard clinical and laboratory testing compared to those diagnosed by newborn screening. A Centers for Disease Control Workshop recently concluded that improved growth alone was not sufficient to mandate newborn screening for CF as U.S. public health policy. Screening methods that incorporate CF mutational analysis will detect carriers approximately three times more

Box 182-3. Key Features of Gastrointestinal Disease in Cystic Fibrosis

- Pancreatic insufficiency (PI) results in fat and protein maldigestion, leading to distended abdomen, and frequent bulky, greasy stools.
- Maldigestion and failure to thrive are the second most common presenting symptoms for the diagnosis of CF (43% of patients in the United States).
- Malabsorption of fat-soluble vitamins is common manifestation of PI.
- Meconium ileus (MI) occurs in approximately 15% to 20% of CF patients at birth and is often diagnostic of the illness.
- Recurrent and chronic abdominal pain is common in patients with CF; the clinician must consider broad differential diagnoses based on history and physical examination.
- Distal intestinal obstruction syndrome (DIOS) occurs in 10% to 20% of patients with CF throughout their lives. DIOS is associated with subacute or acute crampy abdominal pain caused by inspissated, bulky intestinal content.
- Hepatic disease, focal biliary cirrhosis, is often clinically silent until emergence of complications from portal hypertension; this highlights the importance of screening for liver disease in CF patients.
- Recurrent pancreatitis can occur primarily in pancreatic sufficient patients.

frequently than standard testing of newborns with CF. This result would require a marked increase in genetic counseling resources. Evidence that early intervention improves pulmonary outcome would increase the impetus for a national program.

Clinical Diagnosis

CF remains primarily a clinical diagnosis that is confirmed by laboratory testing. Early diagnosis of CF requires the clinician to have a high index of suspicion for patients with clinical characteristics consistent with the multiple presentations of this protean disease. The recent availability of CFTR mutational analysis and measurement of nasal potential difference have broadened the spectrum of CF to include less severe clinical disease. The diagnosis of CF is based on two criteria: the presence of at least *one* clinical characteristic and laboratory evidence of CFTR dysfunction (Box 182-5).

The sweat test used to establish the diagnosis of CF must be done by the pilocarpine iontophoresis method. The sweat gland is composed of two regions, the secretory coil and the reabsorptive duct. The secretory coil is not affected by CF, and secretes isotonic NaCl in normal volumes with cholinergic stimulation. The reabsorptive sweat duct is chloride impermeable in CF owing to mutant CFTR, and thus both sodium and chloride reabsorption are prevented, resulting in elevated concentrations of sodium and chloride in sweat from CF patients.

Many general hospitals use screening tests for CF that measure chloride conductance with a different range of normal values. If a patient with clinical findings consistent with CF has a "normal" screening test for CF at a general hospital, the patient should be referred to an accredited CF center for a pilocarpine iontophoresis sweat chloride test.

Clinical Presentations

The median age of diagnosis for CF is 6 months, and 90% of patients are diagnosed by age 8 years (Fig. 182-6). Chronic respiratory symptoms, failure to thrive, steatorrhea, and meconium ileus are the most common clinical presentations of CF. However, because of the protean

Box 182-5. Diagnosis of Cystic Fibrosis

Clinical Features

- Chronic sinopulmonary disease may be accompanied by persistent infection of the airways with CF pathogens with cough, wheeze/rales, sputum production, obstructive lung disease, digital clubbing, and nasal polyps.
- Gastrointestinal abnormalities including meconium ileus, pancreatic insufficiency, distal intestinal obstruction syndrome, rectal prolapse, failure to thrive, focal biliary cirrhosis, hypoproteinemia-edema, fat-soluble vitamin deficiencies.
- Salt loss syndromes may be due to excessive NaCl losses from sweat glands (hypochloremic metabolic alkalosis).
- Obstructive azoospermia may be due to congenital obstruction or anomalies of the vas deferens.

or

- CF in a first-degree relative or a positive newborn screening test result.

plus

Laboratory Criteria

- Two abnormal (>60 mEq/L) pilocarpine iontophoresis sweat chloride values

or

- Two CF mutations

or

- An abnormal nasal potential difference pattern

---

nature of CF there are numerous presenting signs and symptoms (Table 182-1).

MEDICAL MANAGEMENT

Specialty Care

The majority of patients diagnosed with CF in the United States are managed by a multidisciplinary team at one of more than 100 CF centers accredited by the CF Foundation. The care team consists of physicians, nurses, dietitians, respiratory therapists, social workers, and genetic counselors. The specialty CF care team should evaluate all new or suspected diagnoses of CF. Patients with an established

diagnosis of CF are encouraged to attend scheduled CF clinic visits on a quarterly basis to detect changes in clinical status early, foster compliance, provide ongoing CF education, and provide support to families and patients. Patients with more severe disease may have more frequently scheduled visits, and all patients with a significant change in clinical status may be seen for acute visits at the CF center. The roles of the generalist and the specialty, multidisciplinary CF care team may vary with geographic area. Bidirectional communication between the primary care provider and the specialty team is vital to optimizing patient care.

All new or suspected cases of CF undergo a comprehensive evaluation to review history, examination, and laboratory findings to confirm the diagnosis of CF. The initial role of the CF team is to support and educate the family as well as start necessary therapies, such as pancreatic enzyme supplements, fat-soluble vitamins, and bronchodilators, chest physiotherapy, and antibiotics. Newly diagnosed patients are often seen on a monthly basis until the child's condition has stabilized and basic CF education has been completed. Genetic counseling must be offered to all families with newly diagnosed cases of CF.

Key Medical Management Issues
Maintenance Care

Maintenance care at the CF center involves a comprehensive assessment of the patient's clinical status per established guidelines published by the CFF (Box 182-6).

The routine visit includes an interval history with focus on gastrointestinal and sinopulmonary symptoms, physical examination, and laboratory tests for comparison to best baseline status. A query for intercurrent illnesses, additional medication use, and potential CF complications also occurs. Trend analyses of growth and pulmonary status are crucial for decisions in clinical management.

Complications

Pulmonary exacerbation is generally treated under the supervision of a CF center with 10 to 21 days of intravenous antibiotics (aminoglycoside and β-lactam for

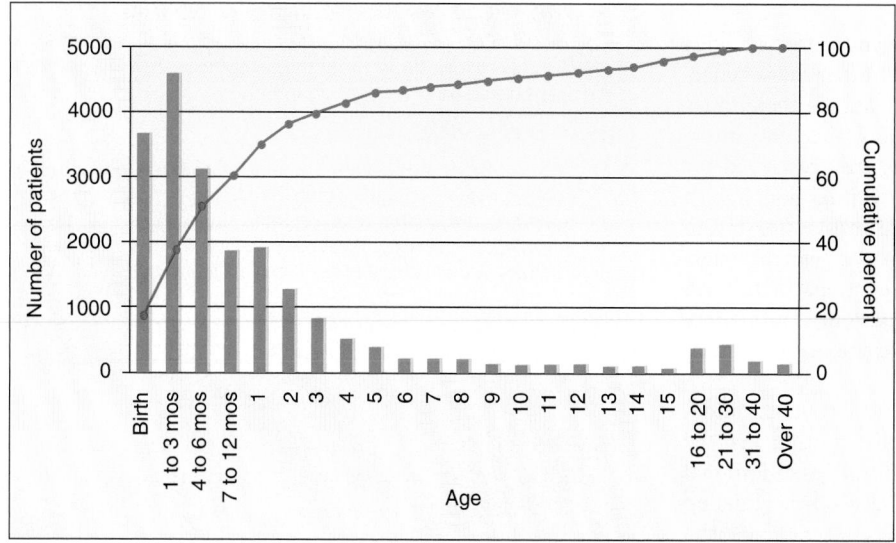

Figure 182-6. Age at diagnosis for CF patients in the United States. (From Cystic Fibrosis Foundation Registry, 2001 Annual Report to the Center Directors, Cystic Fibrosis Foundation, Bethesda, Md.)

Table 182-1. Presentations of Cystic Fibrosis

Common Presentations (>10% of cases)

Chronic respiratory symptoms (recurrent bronchitis/pneumonia/
    wheezing/bronchiectasis)
Failure to thrive/steatorrhea
Meconium ileus
Family history

Less Common Presentations

Nasal polyps/chronic sinusitis
Rectal prolapse
Intussusception
Electrolyte imbalance with metabolic alkalosis
Edema and hypoproteinemia
Liver disease (obstructive cholestasis, biliary cirrhosis)
Male infertility/azoospermia
Prenatal/newborn screening

Pseudomonas aeruginosa), aggressive chest physiotherapy, enteral nutritional supplements, serial monitoring of weight, chest examination, activity tolerance, serum aminoglycoside levels, blood urea nitrogen (BUN) and creatinine levels, and serial lung function tests. Treatment duration is based on observing a plateau in clinical and lung function improvement; patients with more severe pulmonary disease require more prolonged treatment for pulmonary exacerbation. Home intravenous antibiotics are used to complete therapy for pulmonary exacerbation in school-age children under special circumstances, and more routinely in adults. Patients should be seen at the CF center during and 2 to 4 weeks after completion of intravenous antibiotic treatment to ensure improvement and continued stability.

The management of the first isolation of *Pseudomonas* from the respiratory tract in young children with CF is controversial. The Danish CF Center, the United Kingdom, other European CF Centers, and some U.S. CF centers treat the first isolation of *Pseudomonas* with aggressive antibiotic therapy regardless of signs or symptoms of pulmonary disease. Although there is increasing evidence that *Pseudomonas* can be eradicated from respiratory tract cultures of young children with CF, many clinicians feel improved clinical outcomes and more data on the risks of bacterial resistance and emergence of other pathogens are needed before routinely adopting such an aggressive treatment strategy.

Chronic endobronchial inflammation and infection with *Staphylococcus aureus* and *Haemophilus influenzae* is generally treated with maintenance airway clearance techniques three times a day, bronchodilators, mucolytics, and intermittent oral antibiotics. Oral antibiotics are prescribed for minor acute illnesses (upper respiratory infections) with persistent increases in cough and sputum production but in the absence of significant changes in appetite, weight, exercise tolerance, or lung function. However, patients with nonpseudomonal lung infection can experience pulmonary exacerbations that require inpatient treatment with intravenous antibiotics.

Patients with chronic pseudomonal endobronchial infection are treated as just described, and in addition may be prescribed intermittent, maintenance antipseudomonal antibiotics. Alternate month, preservative-free inhaled tobramycin is used by most U.S. CF centers once the patient has chronic symptoms and mild decreases in lung function. The threshold to initiate alternate month inhaled tobramycin is evolving and some physicians start intermittent treatment earlier in the course of disease. The Danish CF center and some European centers are strong proponents for aggressive treatment of chronic pseudomonal infection with prolonged courses of inhaled colistin and oral ciprofloxacin, and scheduled hospitalizations for intravenous antibiotics. The clinical outcomes and adverse events (bacterial resistance, emergence of new pathogens) from aggressive early intervention of pseudomonal infection are active areas of investigation.

Chronic sinusitis and nasal polyposis can result in significant morbidity. Patients may experience headache, sinus pressure, epistaxis, nocturnal cough, and with nasal obstruction from polyps can have reduced taste or appetite and sleep disruption. Maintenance topical steroids and intermittent oral antibiotics directed at CF pathogens are used, but if symptoms persist, a referral to an otolaryngologist is recommended to consider further imaging (sinus computed

Box 182-6. Monitoring at Routine Visits at a Cystic Fibrosis Center

Nutritional/Gastrointestinal

- Height, weight, nutritionist evaluation at each visit; and anthropomorphic measurements on an annual basis
- Review of appetite, stool frequency and character, abdominal symptoms at each visit; liver function tests, vitamin levels, and assessment of risks for osteopenia on an annual basis
- Examination for abdominal masses or tenderness, hepatosplenomegaly

Sinopulmonary

- Review of cough (frequency/severity), sputum production and character, exercise tolerance, nocturnal symptoms, and headache/nasal congestion at each visit
- Evaluation for nasal polyps, nasal obstruction, sinus tenderness, anteroposterior chest wall diameter, adventitious breath sounds (rales/wheeze) or retractions, cyanosis or desaturation, digital clubbing
- Respiratory tract cultures (oropharyngeal/sputum) one to four times per year or with any change in clinical status
- Pulmonary function tests, for patients over 5 years of age, on a quarterly basis or with a change in clinical status
- Chest radiograph every 2 years or with a significant change in clinical status, sinus radiographs/computed tomography scans based on severity of symptoms

Review of Potential Complications

- CF-related diabetes mellitus (annual random blood glucose if patient >14 years, and fasting blood sugar or oral glucose tolerance test if abnormal), chronic sinusitis, chronic DIOS, episodic arthropathy, screening laboratory tests for renal function (annual blood urea nitrogen, creatinine)

Review of Therapies and Compliance

- Pancreatic enzyme dosages, enteral supplements, vitamins, bile salts, bronchodilators, mucolytics, oral and inhaled antibiotics, and airway clearance techniques

Psychosocial Issues

- School or work, insurance, stress of chronic illness, patient/family education tomography scan) and endoscopic sinus surgery. Despite surgical treatment for chronic sinusitis and polyps, the symptoms and signs are often recurrent.

DIOS (distal intestinal obstruction syndrome) can be a subacute or acute complication. Patients with chronic, recurrent crampy abdominal pain need complete evaluation because it is often a symptom of suboptimal treatment of pancreatic insufficiency, intercurrent viral illness, or dehydration. Abdominal radiographs can reveal constipation. Treatment includes optimizing pancreatic enzyme supplementation, review of diet and hydration, laxatives such as lactulose or Miralax, and sometimes the addition of H_2 blockers to optimize the function of pancreatic enzyme supplements. Acute DIOS with signs and symptoms of intestinal obstruction requires evaluation at a CF center and hospitalization with possible surgical consultation. Treatment requires intravenous hydration and attempts to relieve obstruction with isotonic contrast enemas (Gastrografin) or nasogastric/oral administration of GoLytely. Modification in pancreatic enzyme replacement therapy and maintenance laxative therapy may be necessary after stabilization.

Focal biliary cirrhosis with elevated serum liver enzymes can present in school-age children and adolescents without specific symptoms. The diagnosis is generally made with screening laboratory tests. Patients with elevated serum liver enzymes, at least two times the upper limit of normal for age, are treated with ursodeoxycholic acid to promote biliary flow. The impact of this treatment on preventing progressive liver disease is not well established. Rarely, patients progress to multilobar cirrhosis with portal hypertension and varices. Such patients should be referred to a gastroenterologist at a CF center.

CFRDM can present insidiously in adolescents with weight loss, fatigue, polydipsia, and polyuria; CFRDM can be exacerbated by pulmonary exacerbations. A random blood sugar over 200 mg/dL requires further evaluation with a fasting blood sugar or an oral glucose tolerance test to establish the diagnosis of CFRDM. Referral to an endocrinologist is recommended upon diagnosis of CFRDM. Oral agents have not been proved to be effective in the management of CFRDM. Management includes ongoing input from a dietitian at a CF center, as typical American Diabetes Association (ADA) diets are *not* recommended. Insulin is used chronically or during pulmonary exacerbations to manage hyperglycemia and to optimize nutritional status and host defenses against pulmonary infection.

Health Maintenance

Health care maintenance is a shared responsibility between the primary care provider and the CF center. Primary care visits should include a review of the major history and examination issues monitored at routine CF center visits (see Box 182-6). Routine immunizations are recommended as per the American Academy of Pediatrics; respiratory syncytial virus passive immunization is suggested for children with CF who are younger than 2 years of age with evidence of pulmonary disease (on maintenance pulmonary medications). Children with CF may have delayed pubertal development secondary to their suboptimal nutritional status. There should be no exercise/activity limitations imposed on children with CF, except possibly limiting contact sports in children with portal hypertension and splenomegaly. School staff need to be aware of chronic medication needs and the severity of lung disease that may require modifying participation in physical education classes. Maintenance of an exercise program can improve general health status and respiratory function, but benefits are lost when compliance falls off. Issues with adherence/compliance should be addressed (see Chapter 279).

Psychosocial Management

Psychosocial support is vital to help patients with CF and their families cope with the burden of chronic disease. A social worker is an integral member of the CF multidisciplinary care team. Support from care providers is especially important during times of acute stress such as the time of diagnosis, first lower respiratory tract infection, first hospitalization for pulmonary exacerbation, acquisition of *Pseudomonas*, increased frequency of pulmonary exacerbations, and the terminal phase of the disease. At each outpatient visit, psychosocial issues that may be addressed include coping with the daily routine of multiple medications, compliance, family dynamics, mental status, school performance, educational/vocational plans, financial stresses, insurance issues, and transition to an adult CF care center.

Patient response to the diagnosis of CF varies with age, severity of disease, and the family's response. Open, honest communication with both patients and family is crucial for ongoing CF education and in response to questions regarding prognosis. Information should be delivered with guarded optimism to provide hope when appropriate. Adolescence can be a difficult period, with delayed physical maturation affecting appearance, with medical needs extending dependency on parents, and with prognosis compromising life goals. Most patients make appropriate adjustments at home and in school with family and care provider support.

OUTCOMES

CF is a life-shortening disease with median estimated survival at 33.4 years per the 2001 U.S. CCF Patient Registry. Median survival time has steadily increased over the past 60 years (Fig. 182-7). There is an unexplained gender gap, with female patients having a shorter median survival compared to male patients. The primary cause of death (approximately 80%) is progressive obstructive lung disease and bronchiectasis (see Fig. 182-3B). Pulmonary function declines with age (Fig. 182-8); forced expiratory volume (FEV_1) is currently the best predictor of clinical status. Predictors of survival are under active investigation to aid in the counseling of patients regarding possible lung transplantation. Some data suggest that a FEV_1 less than 30% predicts a 50% 2-year survival, but this threshold has recently been challenged. Bilateral lung transplantation remains an uncommon treatment option with complicated medical and psychosocial issues. From 1996 to 2001, the number of lung transplantations performed in CF patients has been stable at 125 to 150 per year (2001 CFF Registry). Transplant complications are now the second leading cause of death in CF (~10% per 2001 CFF Registry).

183 Long-term Care of the Child with Bronchopulmonary Dysplasia

Adam A. Rosenberg and Jan E. Paisley

ROLE OF THE GENERALIST

1. Actively participate in the discharge planning process from the nursery of the infant with chronic lung disease (CLD).

2. Discharge infants from the nursery according to criteria that need to be attained by the infant with CLD.

3. Distinguish the infant with mild CLD from those with more severe disease based on symptoms, chest x-ray findings, and oxygen requirement.

4. Recognize and manage complications of prematurity that may affect the infant with CLD.

5. Coordinate the multidisciplinary follow-up necessary in the infant with CLD.

6. Provide primary care for children with CLD, including routine immunizations according to American Academy of Pediatrics guidelines.

7. Initiate and maintain good disease prevention practices to minimize the frequency of intercurrent illnesses in children with CLD.

8. Maintain close vigilance during intercurrent illnesses and recognize those infants requiring readmission or referral for a higher level of care.

9. Provide psychosocial support for the child with CLD and primary caretakers.

Box 183-1. Clinical Criteria for Chronic Lung Disease at a Postconceptual Age of 36 Weeks

- Persistent supplemental oxygen requirement
- Abnormal chest radiograph
- Required positive pressure ventilation during the first 1 to 2 weeks of life

Although advances in perinatal and neonatal medicine have decreased mortality rate and severity of early lung disease in the premature infant, the incidence of chronic lung disease (CLD) has not significantly changed. With more extremely low-birth-weight survivors, a greater number of infants are being discharged from intensive care nurseries with a diagnosis of CLD. Bronchopulmonary dysplasia (BPD) was initially described as four clinical/radiologic stages occurring in sequential order in preterm infants with hyaline membrane disease. Now a "new" CLD is described in which infants do not necessarily pass through the four classic stages of BPD. Infants of the lowest gestational ages at birth are particularly susceptible. CLD is currently defined as a persistent supplemental oxygen requirement with an abnormal chest radiographic examination at 36 weeks' postconceptual age in an infant who required positive pressure ventilation during the first 1 to 2 weeks of life (Box 183-1). The disease can occur in premature infants who have not had significant respiratory distress syndrome (RDS) but who required oxygen, endotracheal intubation, and assisted ventilation for apnea and bradycardia or who had non-surfactant deficiency related pulmonary insufficiency. CLD can also develop in full-term infants with neonatal pneumonia, meconium aspiration, congenital diaphragmatic hernia, and other congenital anatomic abnormalities requiring mechanical ventilation.

The incidence of CLD is inversely related to gestational age and birth weight and is dependent on the definition used. Infants younger than 28 weeks of gestation or weighing less than 1200 g at birth are at the highest risk for developing CLD. Using the definition of an oxygen requirement at 36 weeks, the Vermont Oxford Network incidence of CLD in 2002 was 80% for infants 501 to 600 g; 64% for those weighing 601 to 800 g; 41% for those who were 801 to 1000 g; and 24% for those 1001 to 1200 g. The National Institutes of Health Neonatal Network reports a somewhat lower, but still impressive, incidence (35% at 501 to 750 g, 26% at 751 to 1000 g, and 12% at 1001 to 1250 g).

DIAGNOSIS

The majority of infants with CLD have mild CLD (Table 183-1), requiring persistent oxygen supplementation without the need for other medications. Tachypnea, when present in these infants, is usually only mild, and they do not manifest increased work of breathing, bronchospasm, or transient desaturation episodes. These infants can usually maintain their oxygen saturation concentrations above 80% on room air (RA) trials. They are usually not at increased risk of poor growth, pulmonary hypertension, or cor pulmonale from their lung disease. Long-term care for these infants is not substantially different than that for a well premature infant, and they can be managed effectively by a generalist.

Table 183-1. Clinical Features in Infants with Mild versus Severe Chronic Lung Disease

Clinical Finding	Mild CLD	Severe CLD
Tachypnea (RR > 2 SD above the mean for age)	Occasionally present	Present
Increased work of breathing (retractions, nasal flaring, use of accessory muscles)	Absent	Often present
Wheezing, rhonchi, or rales	Absent	Occasionally present
Increased anteroposterior diameter of the chest	Absent	Occasionally present
Oxygen saturation on room air after 40 minutes	≥80%	<80%
Chest x-ray	Mild hyperexpansion, streaky fibrosis	Hyperexpansion, atelectasis localized cystic areas
Pulmonary hypertension; right ventricular hypertrophy	Absent	Occasionally present
Recurrent hypoxemic episodes	Absent	Present
Rick for growth failure	Low	High

CLD, chronic lung disease; RR, respiratory rate; SD, standard deviation.

Infants with more severe CLD (see Table 183-1) are at increased risk of complications and require referral to a specialist. Physical examination findings often present in infants with severe CLD include tachypnea, intercostal retractions, nasal flaring, cough, audible wheeze, rhonchi or rales, expiratory grunting, pectus excavatum, and increased anteroposterior diameter of the chest. Tachypnea is difficult to assess secondary to the change in respiratory pattern with the infant's activity and state of consciousness. The most reliable respiratory rates are taken during sleep or a quiet awake state. Tachypnea in infants is defined as respiratory rate greater than 45 per minute (>2 standard deviations above the mean). Tachypnea can result from decreased vital capacity of the lung, ventilation/perfusion mismatching, pulmonary edema, or CO_2 retention. Intercostal retractions and nasal flaring are a result of decreased pulmonary compliance and increased work of breathing. Coughing, wheezing, and rhonchi are symptoms of increased airway resistance, often from bronchospasm or partial airway obstruction from mucous plugging. Rales can be a symptom of pulmonary edema or pneumonia. Expiratory grunting can indicate impending respiratory failure as the infant attempts to maintain lung volume by increasing end-expiratory pressure with an expiratory grunt. Many children with severe CLD have expiratory grunting during times of stress or when they need increased ventilation such as during feeding, playing, or crying. Pectus excavatum can develop as a molding effect from longstanding sternal retractions. The anteroposterior diameter of the chest can be increased from airway obstruction and air trapping from bronchospasm or mucous plugging.

The diagnostic evaluation of the infant with CLD requires careful assessment of signs and symptoms when the infant is well to establish a baseline. A change can indicate worsening CLD related to fluid overload or pulmonary hypertension or, more commonly, an intercurrent respiratory infection. Infants and children with CLD are prone to increasing respiratory distress and reactive airways disease symptoms from lower respiratory infections. Hospitalization rate is increased in the first 2 years of life from these illnesses. Chest x-ray findings in children with CLD are variable. Hyperexpansion, lucency of the peripheral lung fields, segmental atelectasis, peribronchial thickening, and cystic areas are common findings. An x-ray examination may not be helpful in times of illness owing to the preexisting radiographic findings. A baseline film should be taken prior to nursery discharge to be used for future comparison. In school-age children with continued respiratory symptoms, pulmonary function testing is indicated.

Clinicians should be aware of a variety of conditions in infants and children with CLD related to the degree of lung disease as well as prematurity (Box 183-2). Stridor is not a common symptom in an infant with CLD. Inspiratory and expiratory stridor may represent laryngotracheomalacia, usually caused by prolonged endotracheal intubation in the nursery. This condition should slowly improve with time and not progress except acutely with an upper respiratory illness or as a complication of gastroesophageal reflux. Progressive stridor during inspiration may indicate subgottic or tracheal stenosis. Significant stridor should be evaluated by a pediatric pulmonary specialist, who may recommend diagnostic bronchoscopy.

Episodes of severe cyanosis occur only in those infants with the most severe CLD. These episodes are often precipitated by irritability and agitation. They may be caused by airway collapse from tracheomalacia, bronchomalacia,

Box 183-2. Conditions Associated with Chronic Lung Disease and Prematurity

1. Upper airway obstruction
   - Laryngotracheal malacia
   - Subglottic stenosis
2. Failure to thrive
   - Increased caloric demand
   - Gastroesophageal reflux
   - Short-bowel syndrome
3. Recurrent sinus, ear, and lower respiratory tract infections
4. Reactive airways disease
5. Pulmonary hypertension, right ventricular hypertrophy, cor pulmonale
6. Systemic hypertension
7. Developmental delays and issues
   - Motor delays
   - Cognitive delays
   - Behavioral disorders
   - Sensory integration problems
   - Feeding disorders
8. Retinopathy of prematurity
   - Refractive errors
   - Strabismus
9. Hearing loss

laryngomalacia, or bronchospasm. Other factors that can precipitate episodes of cyanosis are gastroesophageal reflux with aspiration and pulmonary hypertensive crisis with right-to-left shunting or ventilation-perfusion mismatching. Intermittent more subtle episodes of hypoxemia occur commonly in infants and children with severe CLD during sleep, during exercise, during feedings, or at rest. If frequent, they can significantly impair growth and development. Agitation, anxiety, lethargy, tachypnea, or tachycardia are other symptoms of intermittent or chronic hypoxemia. Episodes of hypoxemia increase the risk of developing chronic pulmonary hypertension, right ventricular hypertrophy, and cor pulmonale. Physical findings are listed in Box 183-3. Diagnostic evaluation in the child with recurrent hypoxemic episodes despite supplemental oxygen or who desaturate rapidly to less than 80% in room air should include either an electrocardiogram or an echocardiogram to look for right ventricular hypertrophy and evidence of pulmonary hypertension. If a child with CLD is not improving, an evaluation by a pediatric cardiologist may reveal an occult lesion such as an atrial septal defect. The child with CLD must also be followed carefully for the development of systemic hypertension with routine blood pressure measurements.

Failure to thrive and poor growth are common in infants with CLD. These infants need significantly higher calorie intake because of their added work of breathing and need for healing and repair of lung tissue. The situation is complicated by reduced intake secondary to respiratory compromise or a medical requirement for fluid restriction to 150 mL/kg/day or less. Infants and children with CLD are particularly susceptible to gastroesophageal reflux and aspiration. Hyperinflation of the lungs causes low mean pleural pressure and traction on the walls of the esophagus, encouraging reflux of gastric contents into the esophagus, especially during episodes of coughing or crying. An infant with CLD who has an intermittently worsening course may be suffering from chronic aspiration. Infants in whom either failure to thrive or worsening pulmonary status may be related to gastroesophageal reflux should undergo evaluation with pH probe testing and laryngoscopy.

Children with CLD are also prone to chronic or recurrent ear or sinus infections related to distortion of anatomy during prolonged endotracheal and nasogastric intubation. Both the ears and the sinuses should be carefully evaluated in a febrile illness and, if indicated, sinus films or computed tomography (CT) scan of the sinuses obtained.

Box 183-3. Cardiac Complications of Chronic Lung Disease: Pulmonary Hypertension, Right Ventricular Hypertrophy, Cor Pulmonale

Signs and symptoms
- Prominent second heart sound
- Precordial heave
- Tachycardia
- Recurrent hypoxic episodes despite supplemental oxygen
- Rapid desaturation in room air

Diagnostic evaluation
- Electrocardiogram or echocardiogram

Infants with significant CLD are at added risk of neurodevelopmental complications. Early in infancy, gross motor skills tend to lag because physical activity is limited from decreased exercise tolerance and the physical limitations of their oxygen tubing. Poor nutrition and growth can be a factor in their development. In the first 6 months after nursery discharge, these infants may exhibit lower sensory thresholds to sound, light, and position shift. Careful attention to these issues will minimize parental frustration. The increased rate of neurodevelopmental sequelae may be more closely related to gestational age at birth. These children require careful regular assessment of developmental progress corrected for prematurity (until 2 years of age) at regular office visits. Multidisciplinary evaluations are indicated for those with inadequate progress. This can include physical, occupational and speech therapy evaluations, infant developmental testing, and comprehensive preschool motor, speech, and cognitive assessments. Specialty consultation may be required for toddlers and children with sensory integration issues, attention deficit disorder, and other behavioral issues.

Ophthalmology follow-up should continue for sequelae from retinopathy of prematurity, and audiology follow-up should be arranged for infants who did not pass their nursery hearing screen.

Psychosocial issues must be addressed. The status of the home to which the child will go must be considered. Is there adequate space for equipment, access to a telephone, electricity, and access to transportation for health maintenance or emergency visits? Support for the primary in-home caretaker needs to be provided by relatives, friends, and health professionals (e.g., visiting nurses). Whenever possible, services such as physical and occupational therapy should take place in the home. Many families need assistance in accessing services to which the child is entitled. Social work input is very helpful. The psychological state of the child and parents needs to be monitored, with mental health referrals made as needed.

MANAGEMENT

The central role of the primary care provider is to coordinate care among multiple specialists, provide basic health care maintenance, be familiar with the infant's baseline condition and examination so that appropriate care can be provided when the child is ill, and provide focused goals that can be communicated to the family.

Outpatient management of the infant with CLD begins with planning the nursery discharge. Planning should begin well in advance of the intended discharge to allow adequate time for teaching, and for arrangement of necessary equipment and services. Criteria for a safe hospital discharge are elaborated in Box 183-4. The decision and criteria utilized to provide supplemental oxygen in the home, use of tube feedings, and types of monitoring equipment vary nationwide. In general, infants with CLD who cannot maintain consistent oxygen saturation levels at or over 92% awake, while feeding, and while sleeping require continuous supplemental oxygen via nasal cannula.

Decisions about home cardiorespiratory or oxygen monitoring depend on severity of associated apnea and

Criteria for Nursery Discharge of the Infant with Chronic Lung Disease

1. Adequate weight gain is achieved on full enteral feeds taken by mouth. In some special cases, a discharge on partial tube feedings may be entertained.
2. Stable body temperature is maintained outside an isolette.
3. Infant is free of apneic and bradycardic spells that require intervention for at least 1 week. If spontaneously resolving spells are still occurring, home cardiorespiratory monitoring should be used.
4. Supplemental nasal oxygen is needed for all infants unable to maintain pulse oximetry saturations over 92% awake, feeding, and sleeping.
5. Infants on oxygen must maintain saturations over 80% for 40 minutes in room air. Those unable to meet this criterion should have home oximetry while unattended.
6. Social work evaluation is done to ensure a safe home environment with adequate space, utilities, phone access, and transportation.
7. Complete teaching about medical needs, oxygen use, and medication administration.
8. Complete predischarge conference in which all medical issues are addressed and outpatient appointments coordinated. Follow-up with the primary care provider should occur in 7 to 10 days.
9. Age-appropriate immunization is completed. In RSV season, first dose of palivizumab is given.

bradycardia spells and degree of desaturation in room air. Resolution of apnea of prematurity is dependent on gestational age at birth and current postconceptual age (PCA) (Fig. 183-1). Babies of 28 weeks of gestation generally cease having spells by 37 weeks' PCA, while those born at younger gestational ages experience spells for a longer period of time. Spells requiring intervention subside about 1 week prior to spontaneously resolving spells (Fig. 183-2).

Decisions about the need for home cardiorespiratory monitoring can be made using these data. Infants free of spells requiring intervention for a week can be discharged, but should have cardiorespiratory monitoring while the infant is unattended at home until the provider is sure all spells have completely resolved. Pulse oximetry monitoring is indicated for those infants who desaturate in room air with oxygen saturation levels below 80%. This form of monitoring should be continued until the infant has a mature respiratory drive (44 weeks PCA) or demonstrates arousal when oxygen saturation level falls.

The initial outpatient visit with the primary care provider should occur within 1 week of hospital discharge to ensure a smooth transition from hospital to home. Frequency of visits thereafter depends on the severity of the infant's lung disease and other complications of prematurity. Initially the child should be seen at 1- to 4-week intervals, with visits becoming less frequent as the overall condition improves. General goals of comprehensive management are presented in Box 183-5.

Health care maintenance for the infant with CLD involves similar elements as that for the well child. Growth, complete with plots on a standard curve, and neurodevelopment should be assessed regularly. Both growth and development should be "corrected" for prematurity until 2 years of age. Correction is done by subtracting the number of weeks born before term from the infant's chronologic age. Nutrition is of the utmost importance. These infants have increased caloric demands proportional to the severity of the underlying lung disease. In some infants intake is diminished from fatigue, poor oromotor coordination, or nipple aversion. Caloric intake should be adequate to allow continuous growth along a consistent curve. Fluid restriction should be avoided unless no other means are available to prevent a worsening of pulmonary status from fluid

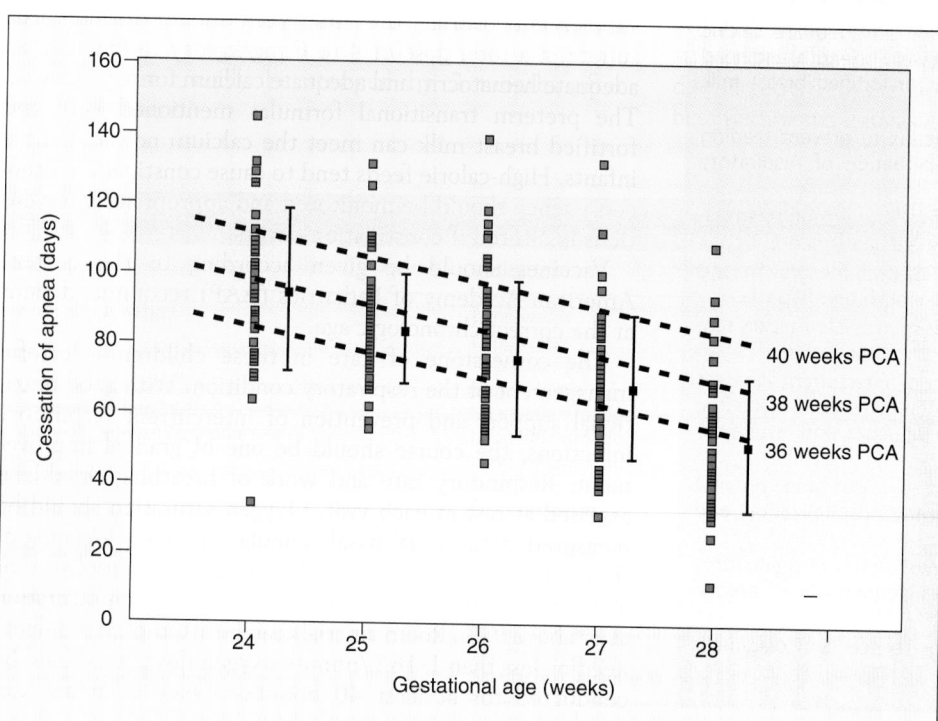

Figure 183-1. Individual and mean (± standard deviation) values for the last postnatal day with a documented apnea and/or bradycardia event by gestational age at birth. PCA, postconceptual age. (From Eichenwald EC, Aina A, Stark AR: Apnea frequently persists beyond term gestation in infants delivered at 24 to 28 weeks. Pediatrics 1997;100:354–359.)

Box 183-7. Indications for Specialty Referral for the Child with Chronic Lung Disease

- Infants with severe chronic lung disease can benefit from multidisciplinary neonatal follow-up
- Upper airway obstruction—pulmonology
- Complicated reactive airway disease—pulmonology
- Cardiovascular complications—cardiology
- Failure to thrive—neonatology; nutrition
- Short-bowel syndrome—gastroenterology
- Recurrent ear and sinus infections—otolaryngology
- Retinopathy of prematurity—ophthalmology
- Hearing loss—audiology
- Motor delay—physical therapy
- Fine motor delay; feeding problems—occupational therapy
- Speech delay—speech therapy
- Behavioral disorders—psychology

sion with some of these preparations is a concern, and efforts should be made to wean infants from these drugs within a few months of hospital discharge. These agents do have an important role in the long-term management of reactive airway disease in those infants who develop this complication. In summary, the goal of the primary care provider should be to discontinue respiratory medications in these infants as soon as is safely feasible after discharge.

The primary care clinician for the infant with CLD must be cognizant of associated conditions (see Box 183-2) that require careful surveillance and management. Specific indications for which the generalist might seek consultation are outlined in Box 183-7. The nutritional status of these infants can be further compromised by significant gastroesophageal reflux that can lead to emesis as well as symptoms of feeding refusal. Management consists of simple interventions such as prone head elevated position after feeds and thickening of feedings. The addition of ranitidine at 2 mg/kg per dose two or three times per day or omeprazole at 1 to 2 mg/kg/day to decrease stomach acidity can reduce symptoms. Prokinetic therapy may be attempted in refractory cases, but treatment with metaclopromide hydrochloride only is suboptimal. Infants who fail medical management with continued failure to thrive or pulmonary exacerbations due to aspiration are candidates for a Nissen fundoplication with placement of a gastrostomy tube.

Short-bowel syndrome, usually secondary to necrotizing enterocolitis, is another concern for optimal nutrition. These infants will often require prolonged use of easy-to-digest feeds such as Pregestimil. In some cases prolonged administration of at least partial intravenous nutrition may be necessary. These patients should be managed in conjunction with a pediatric gastroenterologist.

Cardiac complications associated with CLD include systemic hypertension and cor pulmonale. Blood pressure should be measured at each clinic visit. The systemic hypertension usually originates from high renin and can be managed effectively with Captopril with the dose titrated between 0.1 and 0.5 mg/kg per dose to achieve adequate blood pressure control. After several months on therapy with good blood pressure control, efforts can be made to

wean the medication because many of these infants become normotensive over time. The development of cor pulmonale should be preventable. Cor pulmonale occurs only in severe cases of CLD and can be minimized by provision of adequate supplemental oxygen to maintain normal oxygen saturation and thus normal pulmonary vascular pressure. When right-sided heart failure does develop, management is supplemental oxygen and diuretics.

Anemia of prematurity can be treated with supplemental iron. Compromised respiratory status in these infants should not be exacerbated by anemia. If symptomatic anemia with tachycardia and poor feeding develop (usually at a hematocrit <25%), a trial of erythropoietin injections at 400 IU/kg/day for 7 to 10 days can be attempted. Serial hematocrit and reticulocyte counts should be used to assess the effectiveness of therapy.

Neurodevelopment must be carefully monitored. Appropriate referrals should be made for physical, occupational, and speech therapy. Early intervention with therapies to enhance neurodevelopment and a careful preschool evaluation to establish an appropriate educational program are particularly important. Behavioral disorders should be managed in conjunction with a psychologist. Retina examinations for follow-up of retinopathy of prematurity should be coordinated with an ophthalmologist and be carried out until the retina is fully vascularized. Subsequent visits should occur at least yearly to assess visual acuity. Audiology referral for retesting and fitting of hearing aids is indicated for infants in whom hearing loss is detected prior to their hospital discharge.

Infants with CLD are at markedly increased risk from intercurrent viral infections, particularly during the first winter after hospital discharge. Parents should be instructed on hygiene practices to minimize disease transmission and to avoid high-risk circumstances. Exposure to crowds, day care settings, and young children should be avoided to the extent possible. Household visitors should be screened for illness. Second-hand cigarette smoke should be avoided. Specific measures include administration of flu vaccine to all infants older than 6 months (two doses a month apart in year 1 and then yearly thereafter) and palivizumab (Synagis) injections to prevent RSV infections according the recommendations of the American Academy of Pediatrics (Box 183-8).

Box 183-8. Indications for Palivizumab (Synagis) Prophylaxis against Respiratory Syncytial Viral (RSV) Infections

- Palivizumab is administered monthly during RSV season at a dose of 15 mg/kg intramuscularly.
- Consideration should be given to providing the initial dose to infants discharged during RSV season prior to hospital discharge.
- Prophylaxis should be considered for infants and children younger than 2 years of age with chronic lung disease who have received therapy for their disease within 6 months of the start of RSV season.
- Patients with more severe lung disease may benefit from prophylaxis for two RSV seasons.

OUTCOME AND FOLLOW-UP

Outcomes in premature infants with and without CLD have been extensively reported. Pulmonary outcome with CLD is generally favorable over time. There is an increased incidence of rehospitalization, particularly in the first year after hospital discharge. The most common reasons for readmission are intercurrent viral illnesses with or without a reactive airway component, and failure to thrive. These infants and children do have a higher incidence of reactive airway disease than premature infants without CLD. In many cases, symptoms diminish with increasing age. Pulmonary function testing in children older than 7 years of age does reveal testing abnormalities including decreased 1 second forced expiratory volume (FEV_1), decreased forced expiratory flow between 25% and 75% vital capacity, and evidence of reactive airways. In addition, there may be persistent chest x-ray abnormalities including hyperinflation, localized areas of overdistention, and interstitial or pleural thickening. However, most of these children are not symptomatic and do not report exercise intolerance.

Information about the neurodevelopmental outcome of infants with CLD is mixed. As a rule, neurodevelopmental outcome is dependent on gestational age and neurologic complications in the newborn period. Infants born at lower gestational ages and those with grade 3 and 4 intraventricular hemorrhages or periventricular leukomalacia are at increased risk of handicap. In some reports, CLD has been noted as another risk factor for neurodevelopmental handicap. As previously noted, the incidence of CLD is higher at lower gestational ages, as is intraventricular hemorrhage. Thus, neurodevelopmental outcome is likely predicted by severity of the neonatal course rather than CLD itself.

Mini-index of Related Topics

SUGGESTED READINGS

Barrington KJ, Finer NN: Treatment of bronchopulmonary dysplasia. A review. Clin Perinatol 1998;25:177–202.

Groothuis JR, Rosenberg AA: Home oxygen promotes weight gain in infants with bronchopulmonary dysplasia. Am J Dis Child 1987;141:992–995.

Panitch HB: Bronchopulmonary dysplasia. In Dozer AJ (ed): Primary Pediatric Pulmonology. Armonk, Futura Publishing, 2001, pp 163–186.

Stein MT, Gorski P, Vaucher Y, et al: "What can I do to enhance the development of a premature with chronic lung disease?" Pediatrics 2001;107:966–970.

Vaucher Y: Bronchopulmonary dysplasia: An enduring challenge. Pediatrics Rev 2002;23:349–358.

184

General Approach to the Child with Suspected Rheumatologic Disease

Murray H. Passo and Paul Rosen

ROLE OF THE GENERALIST

1   Identify conditions that mimic rheumatologic diseases that require urgent intervention.

2   Initiate evaluation for a suspected rheumatic condition.

3   Monitor growth parameters in patients with rheumatic disease.

4   Ensure appropriate immunizations to the immunocompromised patient.

5   Evaluate new symptoms that may be part of the emerging rheumatologic disease.

6   Assist in monitoring and managing adverse reactions of treatment.

7   Evaluate and treat interim infection.

8   Collaborate with specialists in supporting family coping and well-being.

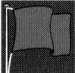

Box 184-1. Red Flags in Musculoskeletal Pain

- Fever, acute joint pain, and swelling → suspect infection
- Pseudoparalysis in a single limb → strongly suspect infection
- Bone pain, especially at night → possible malignancy
- Stiffness after immobility → hallmark—inflammatory arthropathy

Bone pain, especially at night, must be evaluated for possible malignancy or infection.

The hallmark of inflammatory arthropathies is pain and stiffness after immobility, chiefly in the morning. Pain aggravated by activity may be from a mechanical, anatomic problem. Multisystem symptoms suggest a rheumatologic condition. Because autoimmune diseases are dynamic, changing with new symptoms emerging over time, the diagnosis often can be established only after several months.

FUNDAMENTALS

The diagnosis, evaluation, and long-term care of children with rheumatologic diseases require astute observation and collaboration between generalists and specialists. Musculoskeletal pain is frequently the initial complaint for which patients with these conditions seek medical care. The first essential step is to determine whether the complaint represents a focal, benign condition or an urgent systemic process that can cause permanent tissue injury or death. Biopsychosocial conditions commonly manifest as musculoskeletal pain. A patient's primary care provider may have the insights, experience, rapport, and familiarity with the child and family that are essential elements to distinguish organic disease from biopsychosocial disorders.

This chapter provides a basis for *pattern recognition* of the urgent signs and symptoms of serious rheumatologic disease, as well as the features of the less damaging but important pain syndromes of children with musculoskeletal pain (Box 184-1). Infection must be excluded when a patient presents with fever and arthritis in a single joint. "Pseudoparalysis," or refusal to actively move the affected joint, indicates an acute process requiring urgent attention.

DIAGNOSIS AND INITIAL EVALUATION

The diagnosis of rheumatic disorders is usually made by recognizing a pattern of signs and symptoms. Table 184-1 outlines crucial elements of the history and physical examination. Simultaneously conducting a careful and complete history with the physical examination can be efficient and allow the practitioner to corroborate objective findings related to symptoms. Because rheumatic conditions have such varied presentations and manifestations, a thorough history of the chronology and sequence of events in the illness is essential. The cardinal signs and symptoms of arthritis are swelling, stiffness, pain, warmth, and erythema (Fig. 184-1). Characterization of the pain and a complete review of systems are essential. Meticulous physical examination is necessary to determine signs of systemic disease and to establish objective findings that support symptoms elicited in the history. A thorough examination of the entire body and *all* joints yields the highest number of clues to establish the diagnosis.

Joint complaints are not specific to "rheumatic" disease and should be considered in the context of the review of systems. Other diagnoses, particularly malignancy or infec-

Table 184-1. Findings of the History and Physical Examination that Suggest Rheumatic Disease

System	Description
History	
Pain	Frequency
	Duration
	Location—as precisely as possible
	Intensity (quantity)
	Quality—description of "how it feels"
	Aggravating/alleviating factors
	Associated symptoms
	Previous treatments, beneficial or not
	Effect on function
Review of Systems and Matched Concomitant Physical Examination	
Constitutional symptoms	Fever, weight loss, altered growth parameters, delayed sexual maturation, fatigue
Headache	Vascular, muscle contraction
Ocular	Redness, drainage, visual changes, pain, dryness
Oral	Mouth sores, dry mouth, sore throat, chronic sinus congestion
Chest, cardiorespiratory	Pain, dyspnea, orthopnea, cough, hemoptysis, palpitations
Gastrointestinal	Dysphagia, gastroesophageal reflux, anorexia, pain, diarrhea, hematochezia/melena
Genitourinary	Genital lesions, dysuria, pigmenturia
Neurologic	Cognitive changes, seizures, weakness, paresthesias, abnormal movements
Vascular	Raynaud's phenomenon, cyanosis, ischemia, claudication, thrombosis, nail fold capillary telangiectasia
Psychological	Sleep problems, depression, mood changes, behavior problems
Musculoskeletal (Carefully Discern Origin of each Feature)	
Swelling	Effusion, synovial/capsular thickening, soft tissue induration
Tenderness	Focal bony, tendon, ligament, synovium, allodynia (diffuse hyperesthesia)
Pain on motion	Recreating symptom
Erythema	
Warmth	
Range of motion	Passive versus active
Key Findings	
Limb-length inequality (asymmetric joint involvement, accelerated on side of inflammation)	
Muscle atrophy adjacent to joint(s) affected by arthritis, currently or previously	
Bone overgrowth secondary to hyperemia adjacent to physis	

hemoglobinopathy, or hemolysis. Thrombocytosis is found in chronic inflammation, whereas thrombocytopenia is seen in SLE and leukemia.

Serum albumin reflects the degree and duration of inflammatory disease because of its inverse relationship to the other acute phase proteins. Low levels usually reflect chronic inflammation or protein loss from the gastrointestinal tract or kidneys. The erythrocyte sedimentation rate reflects a rise in fibrinogen and other acute phase proteins but is *not* disease specific. It may be normal in some cases of active arthritis. The C-reactive protein is a liver synthesized protein that is reflective of an active inflammatory state and is often used to monitor infection and juvenile rheumatoid arthritis. Baseline liver enzymes and renal function tests are useful, especially when starting medications that may cause toxicity to these organ systems. The urinalysis is central to identifying hematuria and proteinuria, the clues to renal injury from lupus and vasculitis.

The antinuclear antibody and rheumatoid factor tests help to classify disease categories and are helpful to anticipate course and complications. The antinuclear antibody (ANA) test is positive in virtually all patients with lupus and related autoimmune diseases, such as mixed connective tissue disease. The ANA is useful in the context of juvenile rheumatoid arthritis, in which a positive result correlates with an increased risk of developing uveitis. The majority of young children with arthritis will have a negative rheumatoid factor. In the older child with polyarthritis, a positive rheumatoid factor indicates high risk of a progressive, destructive course of disease. The tests must be interpreted in the context of the individual patient. Patients with arthralgia but no objective evidence of disease and a positive antinuclear antibody test rarely develop a rheumatic disease (Box 184-2). High titers of antinuclear antibodies in patients who exhibit objective signs and symptoms suggests SLE or mixed connective tissue disease.

Immunoglobulin levels should be measured if rheumatologic diseases are suspected. Low levels of immunoglobulins are seen in immune deficiency disorders, especially selective IgA deficiency, which is highly associated with auto-

tion, must be considered and excluded before starting corticosteroid or other immunosuppressant therapy that could mask or aggravate an underlying disease.

A diagnosis of rheumatic disease is rarely made by laboratory tests alone, but common laboratory tests can be helpful (Table 184-2). Three components of the complete blood cell count are informative: red blood cells, white blood cell count and differential, and platelet quantitation. Leukocytosis is common in systemic juvenile rheumatoid arthritis and infection. Leukopenia is common in leukemia and systemic lupus erythematosus (SLE). Anemia is common with chronic inflammatory states, blood loss,

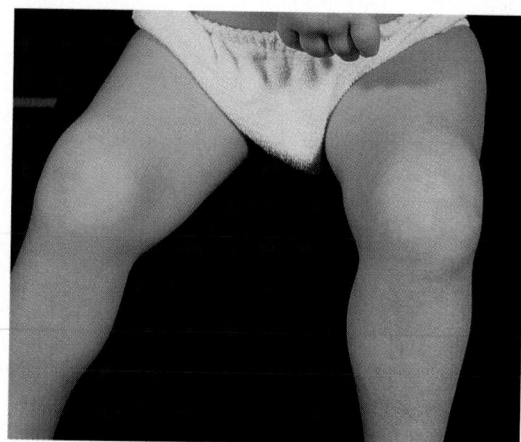

Figure 184-1. Juvenile rheumatoid arthritis. Bilateral swollen knees. Note the extension of fluid above the patella into the suprapatellar bursa and the marked distention of the knee capsule blunting the definition of the medial patellar space.

Table 184-2. Laboratory Tests in Diagnosis and Management of Rheumatic Disorders

Test	Value	Causes
Complete blood cell count	Leukocytosis	JRA Infection
	Leukopenia	SLE Leukemia
	Anemia	Chronic inflammation Blood loss Hemoglobinopathy Hemolysis
	Thrombocytosis	Chronic inflammation
	Thrombocytopenia	SLE Leukemia
Serum albumin	Hypoalbuminemia	Chronic inflammation Renal or gastrointestinal protein loss
Erythrocyte sedimentation rate	Elevated	Rise in fibrinogen and other acute phase reactants; may be normal even with active arthritis
C-reactive protein	Elevated	Active inflammation, used to monitor JRA
Liver enzymes, renal function tests	Elevated	Used to monitor toxicity of medications
Antinuclear antibody	Present	SLE Mixed connective tissue disease With JRA indicative of risk for uveitis
Rheumatoid factor	Present	Indicative of high risk for progressive, destructive, course in JRA; usually negative in young children with JRA
Immunoglobulins	Decrease	Immunodeficiency
Complement (C3, C4)	Low levels	Active disease, SLE
	Increased levels	Chronic inflammatory disorders

JRA, juvenile rheumatoid arthritis; SLE, systemic lupus erythematosus

immune diseases. Complement components C3 and C4 measure disease activity in patients with systemic lupus erythematosus. Low levels, especially of C3, are associated with active disease. Complement levels are elevated in other chronic inflammatory diseases, such as juvenile rheumatoid arthritis.

Radiographic imaging is an important tool in the evaluation of rheumatic disease. Plain film radiographs can show joint effusion. Joint space narrowing (inferring cartilage loss) and subchondral bone erosion are late findings. Radionucleotide bone imaging can localize a focus of inflammatory or destructive disease when the history and physical examination are inconclusive. If a bone scan is positive, radiologists may recommend further imaging, such as magnetic resonance imaging (MRI) or computed tomography (CT).

MANAGEMENT

When a rheumatic disease is suspected or recently diagnosed in a child, the family may experience a flood of emotions. Anticipation of the initial questions provides the basis for first discussions with the family and child (Box

184-3). General statements, briefly described in the next paragraphs, can be made after the diagnosis is suspected. Further explanations are necessary for specific diagnoses. Anticipate unasked questions and provide explanation and guidance, irrespective of lack of inquiry.

Family members are usually concerned about whether the disease is hereditary. Current hypotheses suggest that autoimmune processes are the result of complex genetic traits triggered by unknown environmental events. In rare cases, autoimmunity is associated with a defined syndrome, a known genetic defect, or an immune deficiency. Some families have multiple affected members with a variety of different autoimmune diseases, such as inflammatory bowel disease, hypothyroidism, and type 1 diabetes mellitus. Psoriasis and SLE are examples of diseases that cluster in

Box 184-3. Commonly Asked Questions by Parents Regarding Rheumatic Diseases

1. What caused the arthritis to develop?
2. Did the disease come from a toxic exposure?
3. Are siblings at risk for developing the same illness? (Is there a genetic etiology, is it "my fault"?)
4. Will my child outgrow the arthritis?
5. Will there be a permanent disability or crippling?
6. Should my child be treated differently than other children?
7. What are the safest, most effective treatments?

Common Unasked Questions by Parents

1. Does my child have a malignancy?
2. Where can I get more information (associations, websites)?
3. Are there effective alternative and complementary therapies?
4. Who should I listen to for advice?

Box 184-2. Diagnostic Dilemma: The Child with a Positive Antinuclear Antibody Test

1. If *no* objective abnormalities, then likelihood of autoimmune disease is very low.
2. Take a comprehensive approach with history and physical examination.
3. Scrutinize for evidence of systemic signs or symptoms.
4. Reevaluate if new signs or symptoms emerge or objective arthritis develops.

some families. However, it is rare to have siblings with juvenile rheumatoid arthritis or other autoimmune disease. In most cases of rheumatic disease, future siblings are at only slightly greater risk.

OUTCOME

The clinical course of a rheumatic disease is variable, usually falling into one of three general categories. The group with the most optimal outcomes go into remission after months or years of disease activity. Some patients have a chronic course marked by periods of "flare" of disease activity alternating with periods of disease improvement or quiescence. A minority of patients suffer an unrelenting, severe course in which the disease is persistently active.

The vast majority of children with a rheumatic disease live active lives, attend school, participate in sports, and are employed as adults. They are productive members of society. The overall goal is to control the disease, maintain good function, minimize psychosocial consequences, and prevent deformity and organ injury. When the disease is under control, continued responsibilities, especially school activities, are essential, and the child should resume normal activities within the limitations of the physical status.

Careful attention and constant surveillance are essential to avoid adverse effects of treatment.

Mini-index of Related Topics CH.

SUGGESTED READINGS

American College of Rheumatology Ad Hoc Committee on Clinical Guidelines: Guidelines for the initial evaluation of the adult patient with acute musculoskeletal symptoms. Arthritis Rheumatism 1996;39(1):1–8.

Cawkwell GD, Passo MH: Pursuing the source of musculoskeletal pain. Contemp Pediatr 1994;11(2):72–90.

Henrickson M, Passo MH: Recognizing patterns in chronic limb pain. Contemp Pediatr 1994;11(3):33–62.

Malleson PN, Sailer M, Mackinnon MJ: Usefulness of antinuclear antibody testing to screen for rheumatic diseases. Arch Dis Childhood 1997;77:299–304.

Passo MH: Aches and limb pain. Pediatr Clin North Am 1982;29(1):209–219.

SECTION 4 CHRONIC MEDICAL CARE: *Rheumatologic Disorders*

185 Juvenile Rheumatoid Arthritis

Murray H. Passo and Paul Rosen

ROLE OF THE GENERALIST

1 Evaluate patients with joint pain.
2 Diagnose patients with juvenile rheumatoid arthritis (JRA) or refer to specialist for assistance in diagnosis.
3 Recognize the proper sequence of management of patients with JRA.
4 Diagnose comorbid conditions in patients with JRA.
5 Diagnose complications of JRA or its treatment.
6 Provide appropriate primary and preventive care for patients with JRA.
7 Refer patients with JRA to specialists as needed for evaluation and management.
8 Assist patients with JRA in addressing psychosocial and lifestyle issues.

DEFINITIONS

The nomenclature for the forms of juvenile arthritis is controversial. Internationally, juvenile arthritis is termed juvenile idiopathic arthritis (JIA). In the United States it is still referred to as juvenile rheumatoid arthritis (JRA). Table 185-1 demonstrates the classification systems, along with characteristics of each subtype. The generalist should be aware of these differences in nomenclature when researching information from different sources. The diagnosis of JRA poses challenges, which are listed in Box 185-1.

Juvenile rheumatoid arthritis is a heterogeneous group of chronic arthritides, with onset of disease before 16 years of age and objective evidence of arthritis, lasting a minimum of 6 weeks' duration, in at least one joint. The disease is divided into three major *onset* subtypes, characterized by signs and symptoms in the first 6 months: systemic, polyarticular, and pauciarticular.

Table 185-1. Juvenile Rheumatoid Arthritis Subtypes

ACR	ILAR	Sex Ratio (F:M)	Age (Years)	No. of Joints	Systemic Features	Laboratory Markers	Outcomes
Systemic	Systemic arthritis	1:1 or <1:1	All ages, 50% <5	Many	Fever, rash, pericarditis Hemophagocytic syndrome (MAS)	Marked anemia, leukocytosis	Guarded, 25% severe growth retardation, amyloidosis
Pauciarticular, early onset	Oligoarthritis	4:1	<6	<5	Iridocyclitis	+ANA	Limb length irregularity, blindness, cataracts, glaucoma
	Extended oligoarthritis	>2:1		>5	Iridocyclitis	+ANA	Slow cartilage and subchondral bone injury
Polyarticular Seronegative	Polyarthritis, RF–	>2:1	1–3 8–12	>5	Low-grade fever	RF–, ANA+	Variable prognosis
Seropositive	Polyarthritis, RF+		>8	>5	Nodules, Felty syndrome vasculitis, Sjögren syndrome	ANA+, RF+	Poor, precocious cartilage destruction
Pauciarticular, late onset	Enthesis related	Male predominant	>8	Variable	Spondylitis, acute iritis, inflammatory bowel disease	HLA B-27+ in 60–70%	
Psoriatic arthritis*	Psoriatic arthritis	Female predominant		Variable	Psoriasis, iridocyclitis	ANA+	Variable

*Separate diagnostic disease.
ACR, American College of Rheumatology classification; ANA, antinuclear antibody; HLA, human leukocyte antigen; ILAR, International League of Associations for Rheumatology classification; MAS, macrophage activation syndrome; RF, rheumatoid factor.

FUNDAMENTALS

The clinical presentation of JRA is variable. All patients have objective arthritis, defined as joint swelling or pain with loss of motion (Fig. 185-1; see also Fig. 184-1). Additional signs of arthritis are warmth and tenderness, but rarely erythema. Erythema suggests more intense, acute inflammation, such as infection, acute rheumatic fever, or, rarely, gout. Stiffness after immobility is the hallmark of inflammatory arthropathy. Morning and after napping or, sitting are the times of greatest stiffness. Pain is not universally expressed. Because many young children never complain or exhibit discomfort, diagnosis may be delayed.

Systemic onset JRA is accompanied by intermittent, hectic fevers (103° to 105°F); evanescent, nonpruritic, salmon-colored rash (Fig. 185-2); generalized lymphadenopathy (60%); and hepatosplenomegaly (60%). Patients with systemic onset JRA may not develop arthritis until weeks or months later, making the diagnosis difficult. Patients with a pauciarticular or polyarticular course will not develop the high fever, rash, and other systemic features later. In the systemic onset subgroup, young children often appear toxic when febrile and markedly uncomfortable with myalgia, arthralgia, and malaise. Pleuropericardial inflammation is common, but myocarditis is rare.

Polyarticular JRA involves five or more joints and may affect both large and small joints. Patients with polyarticular JRA may have low-grade fever and less pronounced systemic features. This subtype is divided into two subgroups determined by presence of a positive or negative rheumatoid factor test. The patients in the seronegative subgroup have a somewhat less aggressive arthropathy; however, cartilage injury frequently ensues years later. The seropositive subgroup is the childhood equivalent of adult rheumatoid arthritis, affecting mostly older girls and causing severe destructive arthropathy. These patients occasionally exhibit the features of adult rheumatoid

---

Box 185-1. Diagnostic Challenges for Juvenile Rheumatoid Arthritis

1. Exclude infectious, neoplastic, and postinfectious causes of arthritis.
2. Classify arthritis in subtype of JRA.
3. Identify children at high risk for anterior uveitis.
4. Identify children at risk for macrophage activation syndrome: ↑ AST/ALT, ↓ platelets, ↓ white blood cells, disseminated intravascular coagulation, altered mental status.
5. Monitor local and generalized growth disturbances.

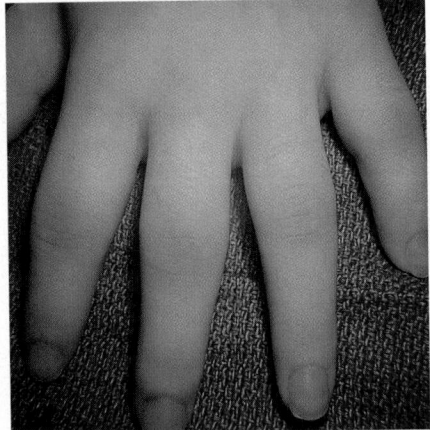

Figure 185-1. Polyarticular juvenile rheumatoid arthritis. Swollen proximal interphalangeal joints (PIP) are noted in all four fingers

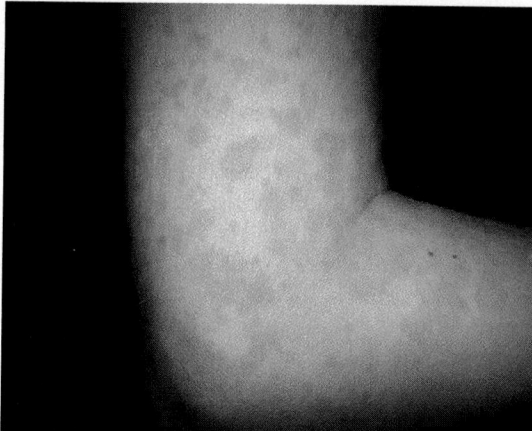

Figure 185-2. Systemic juvenile rheumatoid arthritis. Classic salmon-colored, evanescent rash, giving the maculopapular appearance of "urticaria-like" lesions, is seen in this particular case.

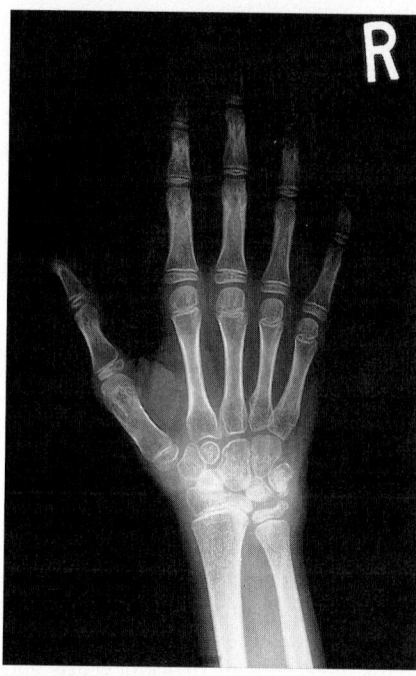

Figure 185-4. Pauciarticular juvenile rheumatoid arthritis seen in a radiograph of the right hand in an 8-year-old girl. Note the periarticular osteoporosis, crowding of the carpal bones, decreased joint space in the radiocarpal joint, and the accelerated maturation of the ulnar epiphysis and ulnar styloid.

arthritis, such as subcutaneous rheumatoid nodules over extensor surfaces (Fig. 185-3); Sjögren syndrome, with dry mouth, dry eyes, and parotid swelling; and Felty syndrome, with neutropenia and splenomegaly.

Pauciarticular JRA, defined as arthritis affecting four or fewer joints, is subdivided into two clinically defined subgroups, early onset and late onset. The early onset subgroup is predominantly female, usually under 6 years of age. The disease is characterized by arthritis in the knees, wrists, ankles, elbows, and small joints (Fig. 185-4). Patients in this group are at highest risk to develop chronic iridocyclitis (Fig. 185-5). This form of uveitis is a chronic, nongranulomatous anterior chamber inflammation, which is often asymptomatic and potentially vision threatening. The late-onset subgroup is mostly composed of older male patients, with arthritis in large weight-bearing joints such as the hips, knees, and ankles. Patients in this group are also subject to *enthesitis*, inflammation of the ligament, tendon, and fascia insertion sites on bone. Typical points of involvement of entheses are the Achilles tendon and plantar fascia insertions on the calcaneus. These patients may develop sacroiliitis that evolves into more classic ankylosing

spondylitis during later adolescence or early adulthood and are better classified as having a spondyloarthropathy. Older patients may develop acute iritis, which commonly presents as a painful red eye. A third, less defined, group of patients with pauciarticular involvement is ANA (antinuclear antibody) and HLA B-27 negative and does not fit into the classic early or late onset subgroups.

The cause of JRA is unknown; however, the basic pathophysiology of JRA is partially understood. In the inflamed JRA joint, there is an infiltration of inflammatory cells in the synovium, including lymphocytes, plasma cells, and monocytes, and excessive synovial fluid is produced. As inflammation persists, the chronically inflamed synovium becomes hypertrophic, thickened to palpation, and encroaches on the edges of the cartilage. A complex interaction of cytokines and proteinases potentially degrades

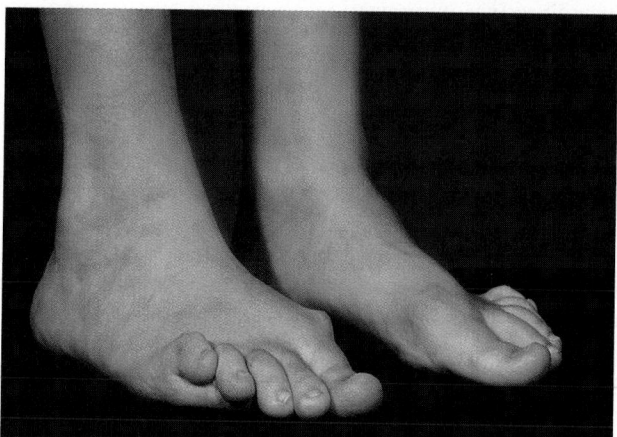

Figure 185-3. Seropositive polyarticular juvenile rheumatoid arthritis. Note the rheumatoid nodule over the right foot great toe metatarsophalangeal joint (MTP). Also note the cock up toe deformities and hallux valgus deformities in this patient with chronic, longstanding rheumatoid factor positive disease. Additionally, her right ankle and midfoot are swollen.

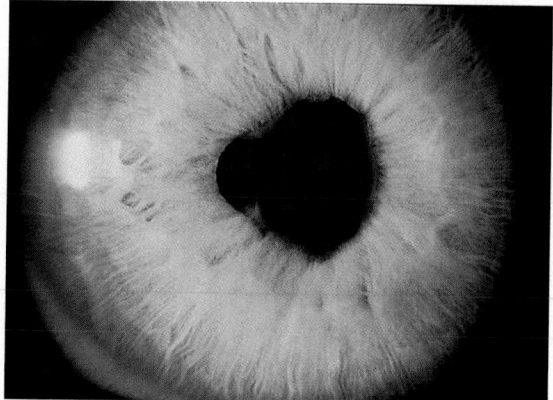

Figure 185-5. Pauciarticular juvenile rheumatoid arthritis. Iridocyclitis is seen in a patient with pauciarticular JRA. Note irregular pupil with synechiae projecting posteriorly toward the lens. (From Zitelli BJ, Davis HW: Atlas of Pediatric Physical Diagnosis. St. Louis, Mosby, 1997.)

cartilage and threatens the integrity of the underlying bone and infrastructure of the joint.

Both environmental and multiple complex genetic risk factors play a role. Associations with certain class II major histocompatibility complex (MHC) alleles have been established. These alleles are different in the subtypes of JRA, suggesting different triggers or pathogenesis. Despite the genetic role for JRA, the family history is rarely positive for other members with JRA, and it is uncommon for families to have more than one child affected by arthritis.

DIAGNOSIS

JRA is a clinical diagnosis based on the presence of arthritis in the subgroups previously described and the exclusion of the other causes of arthritis in childhood. Laboratory tests will not establish the diagnosis. The erythrocyte sedimentation rate is often elevated; however, up to 40% of patients have normal results, which does *not* exclude the presence of inflammation. Most patients with JRA have a negative ANA and rheumatoid factor. A positive ANA indicates a greater risk for development of iridocyclitis and the need for ophthalmologic slit-lamp examinations every 3 to 4 months. A positive rheumatoid factor test, typically in the adolescent girl with arthritis affecting small and large joints, is predictive of a progressive, often pernicious and destructive, course.

MANAGEMENT

The management of JRA is multidisciplinary, with goals as listed in Box 185-2. The pharmacologic strategy is more aggressive and additive than prescribed in the 1980s. The generalist needs to be aware of the sequence of management, possible comorbid conditions, and complications of the disease and treatment.

First-line pharmacologic treatment for JRA begins with administration of a nonsteroidal anti-inflammatory drug (NSAID, see Chapter 286). Initiation of NSAIDs is an important early step for the generalist. Approximately half of the patients will have improvement of their arthritis within 2 months of treatment with an NSAID. The commonly used NSAIDs include naproxen, ibuprofen, tolmetin sodium, and diclofenac. Salicylates are rarely prescribed because of risks of toxicity and Reye syndrome; however, these products are the oldest agents and can be measured in the serum. The most commonly employed NSAID by pediatric rheumatologists is naproxen because it can be given twice a

---

Box 185-2. Management Goals for Juvenile Rheumatoid Arthritis

1. Reduce pain and inflammation.
2. Preserve joint function.
3. Maintain growth and nutrition.
4. Minimize medication side effects.
5. Maintain global functioning.
6. Foster positive self-esteem.
7. Minimize osteoporosis.
8. Obtain regular surveillance for iridocyclitis.

---

day and is available in both liquid and tablet form. Most children tolerate naproxen without gastrointestinal upset if the medication is given with food. A photosensitive eruption called pseudoporphyria is a common adverse reaction to naproxen, especially in fair-complexioned children. This skin condition appears like a papulovesicular eruption that evolves into scabs. Additionally, the skin is fragile and easily traumatized, resulting in shallow scars. Development of pseudoporphyria requires changing to a different NSAID. The new cyclooxygenase (Cox) 2 inhibitors are being evaluated for efficacy and safety. Children taking NSAIDs should have a complete blood count, urinalysis, and liver and kidney function screening every 4 months to monitor for toxicity.

When arthritis persists, or when disease advances to more joints, methotrexate is commonly added as a second-line agent. The NSAID is continued in conjunction with methotrexate. Methotrexate is administered orally or parenterally (subcutaneous injection) once a week. Onset of effect is 4 to 8 weeks. Methotrexate should not be given to the child with significant intercurrent infection. Establishing varicella status (after infection or immunization) is important before initiation of methotrexate. Development of chickenpox must be treated aggressively with acyclovir. Withholding methotrexate after significant chickenpox exposure is prudent. Administration of varicella zoster immune globulin (VZIG) should be considered if the patient is on corticosteroids. Epstein-Barr virus infection is also hazardous and may be associated with a lymphoproliferative disorder when the patient is concomitantly treated with methotrexate. Live virus vaccines should be deferred while the patient is on corticosteroids or methotrexate.

Arthritis improves with methotrexate therapy in about 70% of patients. The most common side effects are nausea, abdominal pain, headache, and malaise, which usually occur within 48 hours of the dose and last less than 24 hours. Aphthous mouth sores are a side effect that can be largely prevented with folic acid supplement, 1 mg daily. Liver fibrosis is a potential adverse effect that can be monitored by measurement of liver transaminases every 4 to 6 weeks. Liver fibrosis is minimized by abstinence from ethanol and avoidance of other liver injury, such as infection. Declining alcohol-containing beverages is a major area of discussion with the older patients. Prior to starting methotrexate in an older child, the clinician must counsel female patients against pregnancy while on the drug. Temporary infertility is possible in both genders, but permanent sterility is not reported. Risk of malignancy is considered extremely rare.

For severe joint involvement that does not respond to NSAIDs and methotrexate, tumor necrosis factor (TNF-α) inhibition offers effective treatment in modifying disease activity. Like methotrexate, these TNF-α mediators should not be given while the patient has an intercurrent infection, and live virus vaccines should not be given.

Systemic corticosteroids are given to patients with systemic onset JRA for serious systemic manifestations. Use of corticosteroids is minimized in most patients because of concern for the complications of growth retardation, osteoporosis, and cataracts. Intra-articular corticosteroids often provide good results without causing the severe systemic side effects, and the therapeutic effect may last 6 months or more.

An integral component of therapy for JRA is physical and occupational therapy (see Chapters 304 and 305). An exercise program is instituted that maintains range of motion of the joints while adjacent muscles are stretched and strengthened; thus, joint contracture deformities are prevented.

OUTCOME

The effects of chronic inflammation of the joints are variable, especially between the subtypes of JRA. Patients with pauciarticular JRA have a less destructive course and slower radiographic progression. In more severe disease, particularly seropositive polyarticular onset JRA, joint radiographs reveal advanced disease indicated by bone erosions in an average of 2.5 years.

Patients with systemic onset JRA are subject to the development of a cytokine-mediated complication called macrophage activation syndrome (MAS) triggered by infection or medications. The patient will present with high fevers, altered mental status, toxic appearance, and possible hypotension. Features that distinguish MAS from a systemic JRA flare include leukopenia, thrombocytopenia, elevated liver transaminases, evidence of coagulopathy, hypofibrinogenemia, and *low* or normal erythrocyte sedimentation rate. The diagnosis is confirmed by bone marrow aspirate or biopsy demonstrating hemophagocytosis. Prompt recognition of this condition is essential, as there is a high mortality rate. Expeditious, high-dose intravenous corticosteroids are necessary to treat MAS. In refractory cases, addition of cyclosporin may be life saving.

In the majority of patients whose JRA is treated early and aggressively, the functional outcome is good. Nonetheless, the disease often remains active or recurs in adulthood in approximately half of the patients. The prognosis is somewhat subtype-dependent, with systemic and seropositive polyarticular onset patients being the most severely affected. Referral to a pediatric rheumatologist is important to establish the diagnosis, craft a treatment plan, and ensure long-term management of the arthritis.

FOLLOW-UP

When the disease process is well controlled, the frequency of follow-up examinations can be reduced to about every 3 to 4 months. Ophthalmologic slit-lamp examination for iridocyclitis should be performed every 3 to 4 months in JRA patients with positive ANA. Screening for iridocyclitis in ANA-negative patients is done every 6 months for patients with polyarticular JRA and yearly with systemic disease. The generalist is responsible for well-child care and acute and primary care. Particular attention should be paid to treatment of infections, administration of immunizations, and avoidance of live virus vaccine if the patient is immunosuppressed.

The extent of comanagement of the long-term care of these patients depends on the distance between the home and rheumatologist, the comfort of the generalist, and the severity of the patient's illness. The most important issue is that each patient has readily available access to a vigilant, knowledgeable primary care provider who can assess new symptoms, identify adverse drug events, and serve as a communication link to the rheumatologist for interim events. Because the primary care provider has special insights into the family dynamics and has had continuity of care over time, psychosocial care and counseling regarding lifestyle issues and adherence is often the domain of the primary care clinician.

Mini-index of Related Topics

SUGGESTED READINGS

Gedalia A, Person DA, Brewer EJ Jr, et al: Hypermobility of the joints in juvenile episodic arthritis/arthralgia. J Pediatr 1985;107(6):873–876.

Giannini EH, Cawkwell GD: Drug treatment in children with juvenile rheumatoid arthritis. Pediatr Clin North Am 1995;42(5):1099–1125.

Olson JC: Juvenile ideopathic arthritis: An update. WMJ 2003;102:45–50.

Petty RE, Southwood TR, Manners P, et al: International League of Associations for Rheumatology classification of juvenile idiopathic arthritis, second revision, Edmonton, NJ 2001. J Rheumatol 2004;31(2):390–392.

Schaller JG: Juvenile rheumatoid arthritis. Pediatr Rev 1997;18(10):337–349.

186 Systemic Lupus Erythematosus and Juvenile Dermatomyositis

Murray H. Passo and Paul Rosen

ROLE OF THE GENERALIST

1. Consider diagnosis in patients with fever of unknown origin or with multisystem organ dysfunction.

2. Diagnose patients with systemic lupus erythematosus (SLE) or refer to a specialist for assistance in diagnosis.

3. Diagnose complications of SLE or juvenile dermatomyositis or treatment.

4. Provide appropriate primary and preventive care for patients with SLE or juvenile dermatomyositis.

5. Refer to specialists as needed for evaluation and management.

6. Assist in addressing psychosocial and lifestyle issues.

SYSTEMIC LUPUS ERYTHEMATOSUS

Definition

Systemic lupus erythematosus (SLE) is the prototype of autoimmune disease. The disease has a broad clinical spectrum, with potential to cause multisystem organ damage, including severe nervous system injury, cytopenias, end-stage renal disease, and polyserositis.

Fundamentals

SLE is a female-predominant disease that affects African Americans, African Caribbeans, and Asians at a higher frequency than whites. Onset of symptoms is uncommon before 5 years of age. Disease prevalence progressively increases during adolescence and young adulthood. Although the etiology of SLE still eludes researchers, known triggers for disease expression include Epstein-Barr virus and parvovirus B19 infection. SLE is a polygenic disease, and it is common for other family members to have an autoimmune disease or positive antinuclear antibody (ANA) test.

Diagnosis

Criteria for diagnosis are listed in Table 186-1. SLE should be suspected with fever of undetermined origin or in patients with evidence of multisystem organ dysfunction. The most common presenting signs and symptoms are fever, fatigue, weight loss, rash (sometimes malar, Fig. 186-1), and arthralgia/arthritis. The arthritis is polyarticular, symmetric,

nondeforming, and nonerosive. Virtually any skin rash is possible, but the "butterfly" malar rash is most common (55%).

The diagnostic classification criteria and goals for SLE are listed in Boxes 186-1 and 186-2. SLE can be diagnosed with a sensitivity of 96% and a specificity of 96% in the presence of at least four of the criteria listed. SLE can be difficult to diagnose because the expression of the disease often evolves over months or years. New symptoms should be thoroughly evaluated. Several manifestations of SLE are especially deleterious (see Box 186-2). Progressive cognitive dysfunction with memory loss is difficult to identify but should be considered, especially in the context of school or social failure. Renal involvement with hematuria, proteinuria, and sometimes hypertension may emerge at any time. Autoimmune hemolysis and thrombocytopenia are common and often of sudden onset. Patients with antiphospholipid antibodies are at risk for thrombosis, either venous or arterial. These patients are at high risk for spontaneous abortion during pregnancy.

The laboratory hallmark of the disease is the ANA test, especially the antibodies to double-stranded or native

Table 186-1. 1997 Revised Criteria for Classification of Systemic Lupus Erythematosus

Criterion	Definition
Malar rash	Fixed erythema, flat or raised, over the malar eminence
Discoid rash	Erythematous raised patches with keratotic scaling and follicular plugging
Photosensitivity	Skin rash as a result of unusual reaction to sunlight
Oral ulcers	Oral or nasopharyngeal ulceration, usually painless
Arthritis	Nonerosive arthritis involving two or more peripheral joints, characterized by tenderness or swelling
Serositis	Pleuritis or Pericarditis
Renal disorder	Persistent proteinuria or cellular casts
Neurologic disorder	Seizures or psychosis
Hematologic disorder	Hemolytic anemia or leukopenia or lymphopenia or thrombocytopenia
Immunologic disorder	Anti-DNA antibody or Anti-Sm or positive finding of antiphospholipid antibodies based on abnormal serum level of IgG or IgM anticardiolipin antibodies, or positive test for lupus anticoagulant
Antinuclear antibody	Abnormal titer

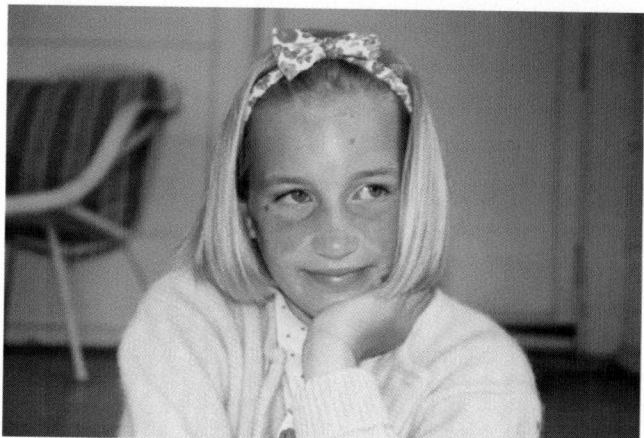

Figure 186-1. Systemic lupus erythematosus. Malar butterfly rash in a 12-year-old, newly diagnosed patient with lupus. Coincidentally, this rash was found after the first sunny spring weekend, illustrating the marked photosensitivity of this patient.

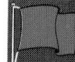

Box 186-2. Red Flags in Systemic Lupus Erythematosus

1. Fever—evaluate for infection and disease activity concomitantly
2. Chest pain—pleurisy, pericarditis, pulmonary infarction
3. Dyspnea—pneumonitis, alveolar hemorrhage, pleural effusions, congestive heart failure
4. Headache—vascular headaches common, beware of cerebrovascular accident
5. Altered mental status—cerebritis
6. Serious cutaneous signs—vasculitic lesions, palpable purpura, infarction
7. Thrombosis—antiphospholipid antibody syndrome, venous or arterial
8. Icterus—autoimmune hemolysis, autoimmune hepatitis
9. Petechiae—thrombotic thrombocytopenia, autoimmune thrombocytopenia

DNA. The ANA test is reported as a titer, usually a multiple of 1:40, maximum 1:5120. The ANA profile will report antibodies to SSA(Ro), SSB (La), RNP, Sm, and ds DNA. There may be autoantibodies against cytoplasmic proteins, lymphocytes, neutrophils, erythrocytes, and platelets.

Management

Management starts with education about the manifestations of the disease and precautions to be observed (Box 186-3). Patients may be photosensitive and need to be advised to avoid prolonged sun exposure and to use sunscreen and photo-occlusive clothing. First-line medical management includes nonsteroidal anti-inflammatory drugs (NSAIDs), hydroxychloroquine, and corticosteroids. Hydroxychloroquine is an antimalarial drug that is anti-inflammatory and also lowers cholesterol, reduces hypercoagulability, and is somewhat photoprotective. Corticosteroids are important; however, a goal is to minimize the use of long-term administration. When a patient incurs the more serious effects of the disease, such as neuropsychiatric symptoms, cardiopulmonary involvement, or nephritis, high-dose corticosteroid, usually prednisone at a dose of 2 mg/kg/day, and immunosuppressive drugs are added to the regimen. Cyclophosphamide is given intravenously in monthly doses to suppress the progression of serious organ damage. The generalist must be aware of potential adverse effects of these medications, especially infection, and carefully monitor patients for complications. Patients should be immunized against hepatitis B, *Streptococcus pneumoniae*, and influenza. Meningococcal vaccination should also be considered. No live virus vaccines are given during immunosuppression.

Female patients should be advised about contraception and family planning. Pregnancy is contraindicated while receiving immunosuppressive therapy. Contraceptives containing estrogen are contraindicated in patients with antiphospholipid antibodies, as well those who smoke tobacco, which may aggravate risk of thrombosis. Estrogen-containing contraceptives are controversial, as these drugs may aggravate or cause a flare of disease activity in female-predominant diseases in which hormonal influences on disease are likely. Additional management issues focus on control of hypertension, hyperlipidemia, glucocorticoid-induced osteoporosis, and depression.

Outcome

The prognosis is 80% survival over 10 years of disease. Patients with significant renal involvement are at more risk for poor outcomes. Other risk factors for poor outcome are noncompliance, poor socioeconomic status, and cognitive deterioration. Patients with SLE are subject to precocious atherosclerosis and premature death associated with coronary artery disease and stroke.

Follow-up

Patients should be followed regularly, questioned about any new complaints, and a complete review of systems and physical examination conducted. Laboratory monitoring includes serial complete blood count (CBC) with differential, urinalysis, renal function tests, and anti-dsDNA antibody titers. Hypocomplementemia usually correlates with disease activity. Complement components C3 and C4

Box 186-3. Management Goals for Systemic Lupus Erythematosus

1. Provide photoprotection.
2. Decrease inflammation; prevent end-organ injury/failure.
3. Preserve renal function; provide blood pressure management.
4. Identify patients at high risk for thrombo-occlusive events.
5. Advise female patients about family planning; preserve gonadal function.
6. Minimize osteoporosis.
7. Evaluate and treat hyperlipidemia.

Box 186-1. Diagnostic Goals and Challenges for Systemic Lupus Erythematosus

1. Evaluate each organ system carefully for immune injury.
2. Remain vigilant for emerging new symptoms.
3. Control disease while minimizing medication adverse effects.

may be decreased with active disease, especially in the patient with nephritis. A urinalysis that shows protein or blood should be further evaluated with a 24-hour urine collection for total protein. When nephritis is present, collaboration with a nephrologist is important. Histologic classification of renal injury by kidney biopsy can guide management decisions for cytotoxic therapy. Comanagement focuses on evaluation of fever for infection versus lupus flare, adherence to medication and photoprotection, close attention to nutrition and blood pressure monitoring, psychosocial adjustment, and lifestyle management.

JUVENILE DERMATOMYOSITIS

Definition

Juvenile dermatomyositis (JDM) is an immune-mediated inflammatory disease that affects skin and striated muscle. The classic presentation is skin rash and weakness, predominantly proximal, but distal muscles are also involved, though to a lesser extent. The typical skin rash is present on the face, with heliotrope, a violaceous discoloration over the eyelids, and a facial erythema similar to SLE. Extensor surfaces of the elbows, knees, and hands are often involved.

Fundamentals

This autoimmune disease results in diffuse angiopathy involving small arteries, venules, and capillaries. Perivascular infiltration with lymphocytes, plasma cells, and macrophages, and an occlusive vasculopathy are often seen in the muscle biopsy. Occlusion of small vessels of the skin results in infarction and ulceration. Muscle histologic examination shows intersitial inflammatory infiltrates, perifascicular atrophy, and myonecrosis.

The disease incidence is about 4 in 1 million in the 1- to 14-year-old age group, with a mean age at onset of approximately 6 years. A viral trigger has been suggested; however, the etiology remains unknown. Current evidence supports a genetic contribution to susceptibility to JDM. Recent genetic research suggests that the severity of disease expression is related with the TNF-α gene.

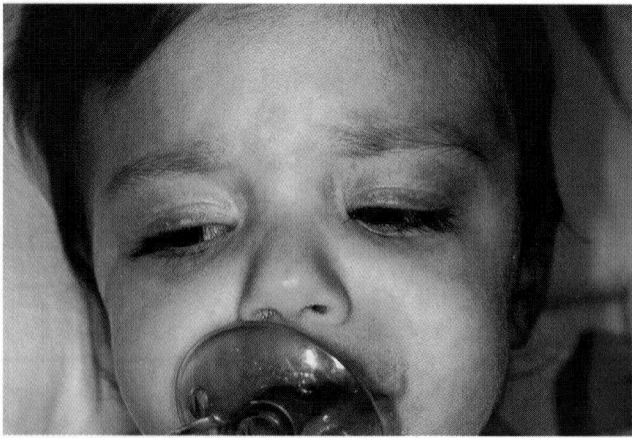

Figure 186-2. Dermatomyositis, heliotrope, violaceous discoloration of the eyelids, with mild edema. Note also the rash present on the forehead, malar distribution, and perioral region.

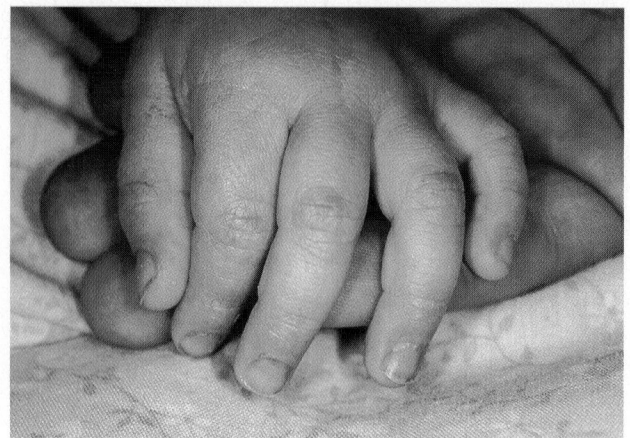

Figure 186-3. Dermatomyositis. In the same patient seen in Figure 186-2, Gottron's papules are noted over the extensor surfaces of the proximal and distal interphalangeal joints. Also note the periungual erythema.

Diagnosis

Onset of the disease may be acute or insidious, with cutaneous manifestations alone for months. The rash is often confused with a photosensitive eruption or psoriasis (Fig. 186-2). Classically, JDM presents with facial rash and swelling, fatigue, edema over affected muscle groups, and proximal muscle weakness. Gottron's papules are erythematous maculopapular plaques on the extensor surface of the metacarpophalangeal (MCP), proximal interphalangeal (PIP), and distal interphalangeal (DIP) joints, knees, elbows, and medial malleoli (Fig. 186-3). Cutaneous ulceration and dilated capillaries around the cuticles (nail bed telangiectasias) are visible evidence of internal vasculopathy. Patients develop fatigue, reduced endurance, and weakness. Manual muscle strength testing should be done to assess for weakness. Constitutional symptoms include fever, arthralgia, myalgia, abdominal pain, and dysphagia. It is important to assess the respiratory function, swallowing mechanism, and quality of voice to identify the patient at risk for aspiration or pulmonary insufficiency (Boxes 186-4 and 186-5).

Laboratory evaluation of JDM investigates for evidence of muscle injury. Box 186-6 lists the enzymes and other parameters that may be abnormal in JDM. Abnormal results are useful parameters to follow for improvement with treatment. Electromyography, previously a mainstay of physiologic evaluation of muscle inflammation, is now less frequently used. Magnetic resonance imaging (MRI) is useful in locating muscle involvement. Heterogeneous muscle involvement is displayed by patchy enhancement of muscle groups, with inflamed areas interspersed with normal muscle. The site for muscle biopsy is guided by MRI

Box 186-4. Diagnostic Goals and Challenges in Juvenile Dermatomyositis

1. Differentiate JDM from other forms of myositis.
2. Identify risk for aspiration, gastrointestinal perforation, or respiratory compromise.
3. Maximize range of motion and strength.

Box 186-5. Red Flags in Dermatomyositis

Cutaneous ulceration
Abdominal pain
Vomiting
Dysphagia
Dysphonia
Deteriorating muscle strength

Box 186-7. Management Goals in Juvenile Dermatomyositis

1. Provide skin care and photoprotection.
2. Preserve muscle strength, range of motion.
3. Monitor for dysphagia.
4. Monitor for calcinosis.
5. Minimize osteoporosis.

to sample an area of abnormal muscle. Additional investigations include upper gastrointestinal imaging for esophageal dysmotility and reflux, pulmonary function testing, and cardiac evaluation with electrocardiography and echocardiography. Sensitive video-endoscopic upper pharyngeal function tests are done to evaluate for aspiration in patients with severe dysphagia with dysphonia.

Management

A multidisciplinary approach should be employed (Box 186-7), with goals to suppress inflammation, maximize function, and prevent complications. Dermatomyositis is treated with high-dose corticosteroids, often given parenterally (methylprednisolone, 30 mg/kg, maximum 1000 mg) for the first few doses, and followed by high-dose oral steroids, usually prednisone 2 mg/kg/day. The steroids are slowly tapered over several months or years. Methotrexate or cyclosporin may be added as a steroid-sparing agent. In refractory cases in which the disease remains active, additional intervention may be necessary, including monthly intravenous gamma globulin infusions or monthly intravenous pulses of cyclophosphamide.

Essential components of management include physical therapy and occupational therapy for range of motion exercises, and muscle strengthening can be initiated when the inflammation is controlled. Photoprotection with sunscreen and occlusive clothing should be used for all sun exposure to prevent cutaneous flare.

Careful attention to glucocorticoid-induced osteoporosis, excessive weight gain, hypertension, and gastrointestinal complications are the key issues at follow-up. As with all immunosuppressed patients, immunization with Pneumovax and influenza vaccines is important. Avoidance of live virus vaccines and monitoring for and management of varicella exposure are important. Comanagement focuses on attention to immunizations, intercurrent infections, vigilance for abdominal and pulmonary complications, and adherence to medications and photoprotection.

Box 186-6. Surveillance Laboratory Tests in Juvenile Dermatomyositis

Aspartate aminotransferase (AST) (previously SGOT)
Alanine aminotransferase (ALT) (previously SGPT)
Lactic dehydrogenase (LDH)
Creatine kinase
Aldolase
von Willebrand factor antigen (factor VIII–related antigen)
Neoptrin

Outcome

In general, there are three main disease courses in JDM. Approximately one third of patients have a mild, unicyclic course. These patients are typically treated with corticosteroids (with or without methotrexate) for 18 to 24 months. In these patients, the disease goes into sustained remission with treatment. The second course is one of chronic, relapsing polycyclic flares. The disease activity waxes and wanes, so that chronic therapy, with adjustments of corticosteroids and addition of second-line anti-inflammatory drugs, is necessary. A minority of patients undergo a more severe, unremitting progressive form of the disease, despite treatment with continuous high-dose steroids, immunosuppression, and intravenous immunoglobulin (IVIG). Morbidity is usually secondary to skin ulceration, weakness, joint contractures, and gastrointestinal complications. Gastrointestinal complications include gastroesophageal reflux, pneumatosis intestinalis, bleeding, and perforation. Perforation is treacherous because symptoms may be masked and the patients may not localize the pain on examination secondary to immunosuppression. Careful attention to abdominal symptoms is mandatory. Calcinosis occurs in approximately 30% to 40% of patients, with calcium deposition in soft tissues occasionally to the extent that patients are entrapped in an exoskeleton. Mortality rate is markedly reduced in the postcorticosteroid era but remains about 5% in recent years.

Mini-index of Related Topics

SUGGESTED READINGS

Hochberg MC: Updating the American College of Rheumatology revised criteria for the classification of systemic lupus erythematosus. Arthritis Rheumatol 1997;40:1725.

Klein-Gitelman M, Reiff A, Silverman ED: Systemic lupus erythematosus in childhood. Rheum Dis Clin North Am 2002;28:561–577.

Lang BA, Silverman ED: A clinical overview of systemic lupus erythematosus in childhood. Pediatr Rev 1993;14(5):194–201.

Pachman LM: Juvenile dermatomyositis: Pathophysiology and disease expression. Pediatr Clin North Am 1995;42(3):1071–1098.

Rennebaum R: Juvenile dermatomyositis. Pediatr Ann 2002;31:426–433.

187 Fibromyalgia and Other Idiopathic Pain Syndromes

Murray H. Passo and Paul Rosen

ROLE OF THE GENERALIST

1 Evaluate children and adolescents who present with pain carefully.

2 Distinguish causes of pain that require urgent evaluation and intervention from idiopathic pain syndromes.

3 Provide an accurate diagnosis of idiopathic pain syndromes.

4 Provide a reasonable treatment and management plan for idiopathic pain.

5 Consult with a specialist when assistance is needed for diagnosis or management of idiopathic pain.

FIBROMYALGIA

Fibromyalgia is characterized by diffuse musculoskeletal pain, fatigue, disordered nonrestorative sleep pattern, and morning stiffness. Patients are often sedentary and complain of other systemic symptoms, such as recurrent headaches, abdominal discomfort, dizziness, Raynaud phenomenon, and subjective joint swelling. Coexistent migraine, irritable bowel syndrome, and dysmenorrhea are common. The physical examination is essentially normal, without objective signs of arthritis or systemic disease. The hallmark of the diagnostic musculoskeletal examination demonstrates typical tender points in well-defined anatomic areas, especially trapezius, parascapular, paralumbar, anterior chest wall, greater trochanter, gluteal areas, and medial fat pad of the knees (Fig. 187-1). Girls are more often affected than boys. The condition is rarely manifested until later school age, and becomes increasingly common during the teenage years. Other family members may have the condition as well. There may be associated stressors, depression, or a precipitating primary illness, such as infection, that cause lifestyle changes and sleep disturbance. Often, there is no identifiable trigger. The patient may begin to have difficulty falling asleep and may awaken several times during the night. In the morning, the patient feels exhausted from the nonrestorative sleep. With increasing fatigue, the patient may become more sedentary. With lack of exercise and chronic fatigue, muscle aches further inhibit activity, and pain exacerbates poor sleep. Thus, a cycle of disordered

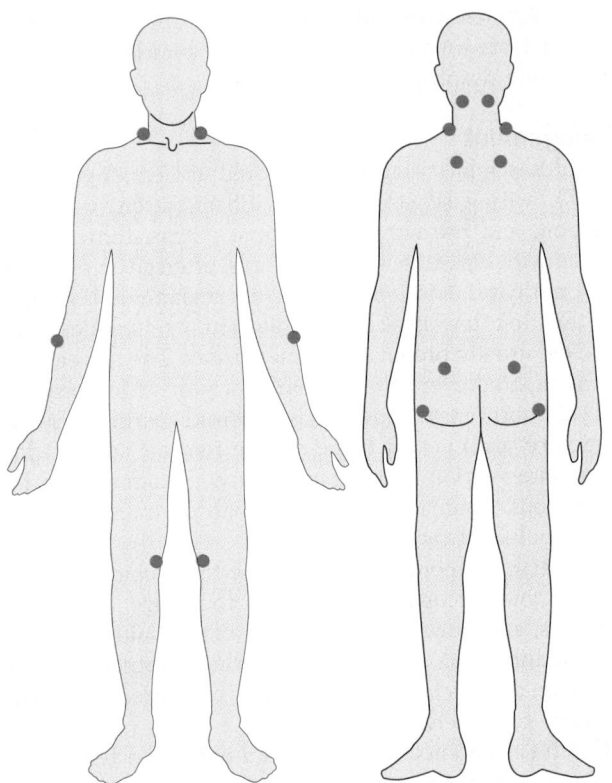

Figure 187-1. Location of tender points in fibromyalgia.

sleep, chronic fatigue, lack of exercise, and musculoskeletal pain is established. Diagnostic goals and challenges of fibromyalgia are listed in Box 187-1.

Patient frustration builds when significance of symptoms is minimized. Acknowledgment of the condition and explanation of all the symptoms is an initial step in the treatment. The next step in altering fibromyalgia is breaking the cycle described previously by improving sleep hygiene. Patients are advised not to eat or watch television in bed. A regular bedtime and waking time should be set. A small dose of an agent such as amitriptyline (10 to 40 mg) or cyclobenzaprine (10 mg) may be given at bedtime to help induce sedation and reestablish a regular sleep pattern.

An aerobic cardiovascular conditioning exercise program must also be initiated. The key point is to have the patient choose an activity that will be enjoyable, albeit these patients are usually sedentary and may need significant motivation. Enlisting family members into the exercise program may hasten participation. A starting regimen may be 10 minutes a day for 4 days a week. The patient may initially experience an increase in musculoskeletal pains. Gradually, the patient increases exercise time to 30 minutes a day of intense cardiovascular exercise 4 to 5 days a week. Musculoskeletal pain may be treated with non-narcotic analgesics. Full attention to essential responsibilities is important. Some patients are overcommitted and may need to cease some of their activities to allow exercise and sleep time.

Psychological factors often play a role in fibromyalgia. Consultation with a psychologist, especially in refractory cases, is helpful. Cognitive behavioral therapy is a useful adjunct to sleep and exercise therapy. Because improvement can take several months, and the patient and family need to be aware of this difficult period which requires continued adherence to the treatment regimen without the reward of immediate improvement. A relapsing course is typical. Limited studies indicate that children and adolescents have a better prognosis than adults.

OTHER IDIOPATHIC PAIN SYNDROMES

The childhood idiopathic pain syndromes are classified by different authorities by many names. Identification by pattern recognition is possible in most cases by history and physical examination.

Growing Pains

Growing pains are transient, self-limited, episodic musculoskeletal pains that occur in children, usually during preschool through teenage years. The pain is bilateral and typically occurs in the calves, thighs, and occasionally the upper extremities. These pains may occur during the day, but typically are felt in the late afternoon or evening and commonly awaken the child from sleep. The pains may be severe. The child awakens the next day without pain, limp, or stiffness. Physical examination must be normal, showing no evidence of objective disease. Treatment with analgesics and massage may be helpful. Reassurance for the parents that this a benign condition is mandatory. Limited laboratory evaluation, including complete blood count and sedimentation rate, is indicated by clinician preference or in atypical cases. Limb radiographs are normal, but usually unnecessary.

Reflex Sympathetic Dystrophy

Reflex sympathetic dystrophy (RSD) is a localized idiopathic pain amplification syndrome that usually affects a single distal limb. It often begins with localized, minor trauma. The patient may have been immobilized because of suspected fracture or sprain. The pain does not resolve as would be expected over a few days, but rather persists for weeks and intensifies. The patient refuses any active or passive movement of the affected limb, usually a hand or foot, which subsequently becomes edematous. Typically, the affected extremity has vasoreactive color changes, such as pallor, blanching, or hyperemia. The sensory response over a localized area becomes so distorted that normal stimuli are perceived as being extremely painful. Light stroking of the skin causes pain with a dramatic wince (allodynia) and withdrawal reaction. The area of tenderness may be in a glove or stocking distribution. There is no definable dermatome distribution.

This condition is treated with intensive physical or occupational therapy, depending on the body part involved. The therapist uses desensitization techniques to introduce gentle stimuli, thus allowing the limb to be touched and moved. Immobilization is contraindicated. An aggressive approach to maintaining range of motion and gradually regaining use of the limb is mandatory. A psychological evaluation is important to help uncover any psychological stressors. The role of the generalist is prompt identification of these patients and referral for evaluation and expeditious management.

Hypermobility Syndrome

Children with joint laxity may experience recurrent musculoskeletal pain. The hypermobility pain syndrome is often postexertional. Hypermobility of the joints is manifested by (1) passive hyperextension of fingers so that they are parallel to the forearm; (2) hyperextension of the elbow or knee 10 degrees or more; (3) forward flexion of the lumbar spine with the knees fully extended so that the patient's palms touch the floor; and (4) passive apposition of the thumb to the forearm. The examination must exclude Ehlers-Danlos syndrome, Marfan syndrome, and other conditions with hypermobility or laxity of joints and connective tissues. The patients may have transient, short-lived joint effusion. Persistent joint effusion should be aspirated and analyzed for inflammatory cells, because children with juvenile rhematoid arthritis may have concomitant hypermobility. Treatment includes a physical therapy program for strengthening the muscles around the lax joints. Analgesics may be necessary. Prognosis is generally good, but is guarded in patients with marked laxity, which may predispose to frequent trauma and progress to precocious osteoarthritis.

FOLLOW-UP

The generalists should identify objective evidence of pain syndromes by diagnostic tender points, evidence of hypermobility, or the classical pain pattern in order to establish an accurate diagnosis, provide a reasonable explanation to the patient, and provide an appropriate treatment plan. Consultation with a rheumatologist may offer support and confirmation to strengthen the diagnosis and plan of management. The primary care provider may also have insight into preexisting or indolent psychosocial issues that commonly aggravate these idiopathic pain syndromes.

Mini-index of Related Topics

SUGGESTED READINGS

Cules-Reed SN, Brawley LR: Fibromyalgia, physical activity, and daily functioning: The importance of efficacy and health-related quality of life. Arthritis Care Res 2000;13:343–351.

Gedalia A, Person DA, Brewer EJ Jr, et al: Hypermobility of the joints in juvenile episodic arthritis/arthralgia. J Pediatr 1985;107(6):873–876.

Kashikar-Zuck S, Graham TB, Huenefeld MD, et al: A review of biobehavioral research in juvenile primary fibromyalgia syndrome. Arthritis Care Res 2000;13:388–397.

Sherry DD, Weisman R: Psychologic aspects of childhood reflex neurovascular dystrophy. Pediatrics 1988;81(4):572–578.

Simms RW: Fibromyalgia syndrome: Current concepts in pathophysiology, clinical features, and management (review). Arthritis Care Res 1996;9(4):315–328.

Wilder RT, Berde CB, Wolohan M, et al: Reflex sympathetic dystrophy in children. J Bone Joint Surg 1992;740A(6):910–919.

SECTION

NEWBORN CARE

5

188 Standards for Routine Prenatal Care

Jeffrey J. Ridgeway

The origins of prenatal care can be traced to the early 1900s with social reformers and nurses in Boston. In 1901, the Boston Infant Social Services Department began a series of outreach visits by nurses to area patients planning a home birth. Based on these programs, an outpatient clinic was established in Boston in 1911 to deliver prenatal services. By 1929, the Ministry of Health of Great Britain issued guidelines for the prenatal care of pregnant women. Prenatal care now is one of the most widely used components of the health care system.

Prenatal care focuses on the reduction in pregnancy-associated mortality. The Centers for Disease Control and Prevention and the American College of Obstetricians and Gynecologists have defined *pregnancy-associated mortality* as the death of a woman, from any cause, while she is pregnant or within 1 year of pregnancy. This definition includes not only deaths attributable to the pregnancy itself, but also any other medical condition encountered during the pregnancy, and usually is measured as the number of deaths per 100,000 women of reproductive age. Another measure used is the *maternal mortality ratio*, defined as the number of maternal deaths per 100,000 live births, a more realistic measure in many parts of the world.

Direct maternal deaths result from the pregnancy itself, including death from hemorrhage, infectious disease, hypertension/preeclampsia, thromboembolic events, ectopic pregnancy, amniotic fluid embolism, anesthesia complications, and complications from procedures such as abortion or cesarean section. Indirect maternal deaths result from other medical conditions that are aggravated by the pregnancy and cause the death of the mother. These conditions include but are not limited to some forms of cardiovascular disease, diabetes mellitus, systemic lupus erythematosus, and asthma. In the United States, direct and indirect maternal deaths declined for most of the 20th century.

Nonmaternal deaths result from trauma or the use of illegal drugs. These causes have been increasing in the United States. A survey of maternal deaths showed that direct and indirect causes of maternal mortality were responsible for 37% of the deaths reported. Injuries accounted for 38% of these deaths. These were divided into homicide (36%), motor vehicle accidents (32%), drug use (13%), suicide (8%), and other causes (11%). Early identification of risk factors for these problems has become a primary focus of prenatal care in the United States.

The true cost-effectiveness of prenatal care has been debated in more recent years, because of an increase in the preterm birth rate despite concurrent increases in the use of prenatal care. Prenatal care is a part of a broader obstetric health care system for pregnant women, however, that has proved successful in reducing maternal mortality and morbidity. Studies document the effect of psychosocial interventions on increasing birth weights and preventing preterm birth and show that increased numbers of prenatal visits are associated with a significantly decreased risk of poor maternal or fetal outcome. Prenatal care must be considered as a component of an overall strategy to decrease maternal mortality and morbidity.

Prenatal care has three main goals: (1) treatment of medical issues, (2) assessment for psychosocial risk factors and planned intervention, and (3) education of the patient about pregnancy and childbirth. Prenatal care is administered by a variety of personnel, including physicians, nurse-midwives, and nurse practitioners, in a variety of settings. Use of alternative health care professionals can allow for prenatal care to be tailored to the patient's specific needs, while maximizing the efficient use of limited health care resources.

PRECONCEPTION CARE

An early component of a successful prenatal care strategy is the identification of the patient at high risk who might benefit from early referral or treatment of a problem before or during pregnancy. Many women attend a preconception visit to review risk factors, including age-related risks, family and genetic conditions, drug and medication effects, and existing medical conditions that may endanger the mother or fetus.

Risk Factors

Teen Pregnancy

Teen pregnancies, although declining in number, account for 13% of all births in the United States. Most are unplanned pregnancies. Young mothers face significant challenges and barriers to access to prenatal care early in the pregnancy, includijng transportation, adequate medical insurance, social support, and child care issues while in school. Increased incidence of neonatal complications, most notably fetal growth restriction and preterm birth, contributes to reported higher infant mortality rates in this population. Adequate prenatal care of teenage patients is vital.

Advanced Maternal Age

A patient with advanced maternal age (>35 years old at the time of delivery) poses a different set of challenges for the caregiver. Complications common in this group include hypertensive disorders and growth restriction. These women have five times the risk of maternal death as women younger than 35 years of age. An increased incidence of chromosomal abnormalities in women older than age 35 warrants genetic testing by amniocentesis or other methods. Women older than age 35 should be counseled about the risks of aneuploidy and the available methods of detection of abnormalities throughout the pregnancy. They should be encouraged to begin consideration of their options should an aneuploid fetus be detected. An increase in nonchromosomal abnormalities is observed as maternal age increases beyond 30 years old (Fig. 188-1). The risk of genetic abnormalities also increases in fathers older than age 55 at the time of conception.

Family History

A thorough history of the patient's family should be obtained at the preconception visit, with particular attention paid to any genetic or inherited conditions. An increasing array of genetic testing is available for problems such as cystic fibrosis, thalassemias, and sickle cell disease. Psychosocial screening for problems including drug and alcohol abuse or domestic violence should be performed. Financial counseling may be undertaken during this process, ensuring that the patient has access to prenatal care despite any social or financial obstacles.

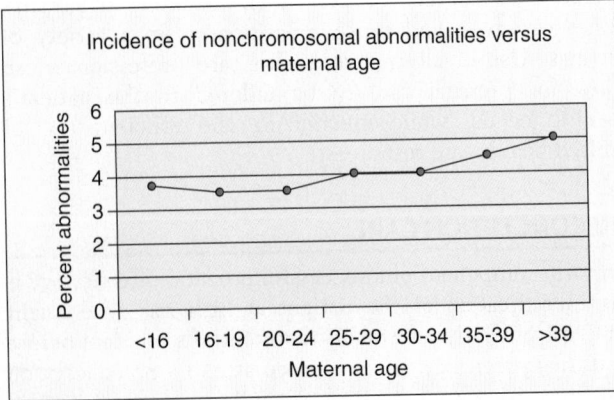

Figure 188-1. Maternal age versus incidence of nonchromosomal abnormalities. (Adapted from Hollier LM, Leveno KJ, Kelly MA, et al: Maternal age and malformation in singleton births. Obstet Gynecol 2000;96:701. Copyright 2000. Reprinted wit permission from the American College of Obstetricians and Gynecologists.)

Medical History

A complete personal medical history is essential in identifying pregnancy-related risk factors. An obstetric history includes full-term deliveries, preterm births, spontaneous abortions, or other adverse pregnancy outcomes. A history of preterm labor is a strong risk factor for future preterm delivery, and a complete history of the exact nature of the delivery is essential. A patient with a prior cesarean section may be a candidate for a vaginal delivery. These options should be discussed as early as possible. Particular attention should be paid to a history of a second-trimester delivery because an incompetent cervix manifests as painless dilation of the cervix or sudden delivery of an infant during this time period with few or no contractions. If identified early, the outcome can be altered significantly by early placement of a cervical cerclage to suture the cervix closed during the current and subsequent pregnancies. A history of glucose intolerance or gestational diabetes during a previous pregnancy may recur even later in the woman's life. Patients with preexisting diabetes often have improved outcomes by optimizing their glucose control before conception. Elevated hemoglobin A_{1C} concentrations in the first trimester place a patient at a significantly higher risk of congenital malformations. Other important medical problems can be evaluated and treated before conception, including hypertension and many autoimmune disorders. A complete list of the patient's medications should be obtained to avoid any possible teratogenic exposure.

Neural Tube Defects

Patients considering pregnancy should be counseled regarding the need for prenatal vitamins with folic acid before conception. Many neural tube defects are associated with a mutated tetrahydrofolate reductase gene and altered folic acid metabolism. Mothers who have had a previously affected infant with a neural tube defect who take at least 4 mg of folic acid daily before conception reduce their risk of a neural tube defect by 72%. The current Centers for Disease Control and Prevention recommendations call for all women of childbearing age who are considering pregnancy to take 0.4 mg of folic acid daily, and women who have had a previously affected infant should increase their consumption to 4 mg daily. Prenatal screening studies that should be completed before pregnancy are the assays for rubella immune status, hepatitis B infection, and varicella exposure. A woman who has not been vaccinated previously or immunized after natural exposure may benefit from vaccination before pregnancy. These vaccines are attenuated live viruses, so theoretical concerns for fetal infection should be weighed against the risk of fetal acquisition of the disease and possible injury.

FIRST TRIMESTER

Dating of Pregnancy

For patients without a preconception visit, the initial visit should occur as soon as pregnancy is confirmed. This initial visit should encompass all of the previously noted screening and history elements, a complete medical and family history, and events and symptoms related to the current pregnancy. Accurate dating of gestational age is essential.

The average full-term gestation is about 40 weeks dated from the first day of the last normal menstrual period. An accurate menstrual history often is all that is needed for early accurate dating of the pregnancy. An irregular menstrual cycle or inaccurate history of menses makes dating difficult. Naegele's rule, a useful method of calculating the date of delivery from the menstrual calendar, calculates the estimated date of confinement (EDC) by adding 7 to the date of the first day of the last menstrual period and counting backward 3 months to obtain the precise date. Although this estimate is useful, only about 5% of all pregnancies actually deliver on the calculated due date. A pregnancy usually is considered full term after 37 weeks and postdates after 42 weeks.

Ultrasound dating of gestational age can be more accurate than the menstrual history, especially if cycles are irregular. Transvaginal ultrasonography can detect the gestational sac and fetal tissues at 5 weeks' estimated gestation age (EGA) with identified fetal cardiac activity present at 6 weeks. A generally reliable early measurement of fetal gestational age is the crown-rump length, the length from the top of the head to the caudal end of the fetus. If this date differs from that predicted by menstrual history by more than 1 week, the EDC often is changed to reflect the ultrasound dating. As a rule, the earliest ultrasound is the most accurate and is used as the benchmark by which in utero growth of the fetus later is measured. An accurate EDC still can be obtained in the second trimester by measurement of the fetal head circumference, biparietal diameter, abdominal circumference, and femur length. As the pregnancy progresses, the margin of error for fetal weight and gestational age increases significantly.

Pregnancy can be accurately dated by bimanual examination of the uterus until about 15 weeks' EGA. After 20 weeks' EGA, measurement of the distance from the pubic symphysis to the uterine fundus in centimeters usually reflects the gestational age in weeks. Because fundal height measurements can be affected by multiple factors, any abnormal measurements should be confirmed with ultrasonography.

Physical Examination

The initial physical examination of a pregnant patient should be as comprehensive as possible, including a pelvic examination and breast examination. Most women also should receive a Papanicolaou smear and screening for sexually transmitted diseases, especially gonorrhea and chlamydia. Additional laboratory testing includes blood type, antibody screen, rubella immune status, rapid plasma reagin, hepatitis B surface antibody, human immunodeficiency virus testing, urinalysis with culture and sensitivity, and complete blood count. Fetal heart tones can be auscultated by Doppler beginning at approximately 10 weeks but no later than 15 weeks. Any delay in detection of fetal heart tones also should prompt an ultrasound evaluation.

Education

A major component of prenatal care in the first trimester is education of the patient about her pregnancy and encouragement of her to modify any behavior that may put her or her fetus at risk. Nutritional management is of specific concern during pregnancy. Pregnant women should consume an extra 300 calories per day as a part of a balanced diet to meet the metabolic needs of the fetus and placenta. Vitamin and mineral requirements increase during pregnancy. These needs are met usually through the intake of supplemental vitamins (Table 188-1). Because most women's diets do not contain adequate iron to accommodate the pregnancy, additional supplementation is required. Total weight gain recommended during pregnancy is approximately 25 to 35 lb, but this figure can be modified to 40 lb for underweight women or to 15 to 25 lb for overweight women. Body weight should be obtained at every visit during the prenatal period. Should an inadequate weight gain be noted, referral for nutritional counseling is appropriate. Delivery of a low-birth-weight infant has been associated with inadequate weight gain in pregnancy. Alternatively, excessive weight gain may be an early indication of a hypertensive disorder of pregnancy. Nausea and vomiting, especially "morning sickness," is experienced in many pregnancies during the first trimester and should be considered when evaluating a patient's nutritional status. Symptomatic therapy may be necessary to allow adequate caloric intake during the early gestational period.

Most patients should be able to maintain normal activity levels throughout their gestation, including maintaining employment as long as there are no job-related hazards or excessive levels of physical exertion. Women should be advised to discontinue any activity that causes them discomfort or strain. Sexual activity may be maintained throughout the pregnancy, although some patients may experience changes in comfort or desire. These activity guidelines may be modified for patients who are at risk of complications, especially patients at a high risk of preterm labor.

Aneuploidy Screening

The first trimester is ideal for screening for aneuploidy in the high-risk population. First-trimester nuchal skin-fold thickening has been associated in multiple studies with an increased risk for fetal trisomy. Measurements greater than

Table 188-1. Recommended Daily Dietary Allowances for Women

Nutrient	Nonpregnant	Pregnant
Kilocalories/day	2200	2500
Protein (g)	55	60
Vitamin A (μg)	800	800
Vitamin D (μg)	10	10
Vitamin E (μg)	8	10
Vitamin K (μg)	55	65
Vitamin C (μg)	60	70
Folate (μg)	180	400
Niacin (mg)	15	17
Riboflavin (mg)	1.3	1.6
Thiamine (mg)	1.1	1.5
Pyridoxine B_6 (mg)	1.6	2.2
Cobalamin B_{12} (mg)	2.0	2.2
Calcium (mg)	1200	1200
Phosphorus (mg)	1200	1200
Iodine (μg)	150	175
Iron (mg)	15	30
Magnesium (mg)	280	320
Zinc (mg)	12	15

From National Academy of Sciences: Recommended Dietary Allowances, 10th ed. National Academy Press, Washington, DC, 1989.

Table 188-2. Recommendations for Care During Pregnancy

Gestational Age	Parameters to Be Checked
First visit	Blood type, antibody screen, RPR, hepatitis B surface antibody, rubella antibody titer, HIV, Pap smear, STD screening, hemoglobin and hematocrit, urinalysis
15–20 wk	Maternal serum marker screening, amniocentesis if desired, ultrasound
26–30 wk	1-hr glucose tolerance test, hemoglobin and hemotocrit, administration of Rh immune globulin if necessary
36 wk	Group B streptococcus screen

HIV, human immunodeficiency virus, Pap, Papanicolaou; RPR, rapid plasma reagin; STD, sexually transmitted disease.

the 95th percentile for gestational age are considered predictive, with a 69% sensitivity for Down syndrome. When this finding is combined with maternal age and biochemical markers, such as pregnancy-associated plasma protein A and serum free β-human chorionic gonadotropin, the sensitivity of detection for trisomy 21 can be increased to 80%. These screening methods may obviate the need for early amniocentesis or chorionic villus sampling.

Chorionic Villus Sampling

Chorionic villus sampling is an early method of detection of fetal chromosomal abnormalities. A small sample of the developing placenta is biopsied and cultured and then karyotyped for major chromosomal defects. The technique can be done either transvaginally or transabdominally under ultrasound guidance. The success rates and fetal loss rates for this procedure are generally accepted to be slightly greater than for amniocentesis. An association with fetal limb defects has resulted in a decrease in popularity of this diagnostic method.

Prenatal Visit Schedule

When the patient's risk factors have been established, an overall plan for prenatal visits can be outlined. Low-risk women without pregnancy complications usually are seen every 4 weeks until 28 weeks. Between 28 and 36 weeks, visits are planned every 2 weeks, increasing to every week from 36 weeks until delivery. Each visit should include a weight, blood pressure, dipstick urine for protein and glucose, assessment of fetal activity or movement, and auscultation for fetal heart tones. Specific care requirements are summarized in Table 188-2.

SECOND TRIMESTER

By the second trimester, many early symptoms have abated by the midpoint. The "quickening" or first movement of the fetus usually is felt around the 16th to 20th week of gestation. By the 20th week of gestation, much of the organ development of the fetus has occurred, allowing more specific anatomic screening of the fetus for anomalies.

Serum Markers

Maternal serum screening is done at 15 to 20 weeks of gestation. The typically used "triple screen" measures maternal hormone levels of α-fetoprotein, β-human chori-

onic gonadotropin, and unconjugated estriol. In some cases, an inhibin A is added to the assay. The values are reported most often as multiples of the median for the given population. Combined with maternal age, a risk ratio can be calculated for Down syndrome, neural tube defects, or trisomy 18. Triple screens generally have a sensitivity of 65% to 70% for detection of Down syndrome, 80% to 90% for neural tube defects, and 60% for trisomy 18. The levels of these analytes in the maternal serum also are affected by maternal weight; race; presence of insulin-dependent diabetes; smoking; and the use of assisted reproductive technology, such as in vitro fertilization. All of these factors must be considered when calculating the patient's true risk. Serum screening for twin pregnancies also is possible, but the sensitivity is low.

Amniocentesis

Although the triple screen is an effective tool when applied to a large population, the low specificity of the test makes it difficult to provide precise answers to families. When borderline or abnormal test results are obtained, more specific testing may be required. During amniocentesis, a 20-gauge or 22-gauge spinal needle is inserted under direct ultrasound visualization, and amniotic fluid is removed for testing. For genetic diagnoses, cells found in the amniotic fluid (known as *amniocytes*) can be grown in culture and a karyotype analysis performed. This analysis allows for diagnosis of most major aneuploidies, including Down syndrome, trisomy 13, and trisomy 18. Other, more specific testing may be available for certain genetic conditions, including polymerase chain reaction analysis of DNA isolated from the amniocytes. Aspirated fluid can be tested for α-fetoprotein (for neural tube defects) and bilirubin levels in mothers with isoimmunization to red blood cell Rh, Kell, and Duffy antigens. Depending on the severity of the hemolysis and the condition of the fetus, delivery or intrauterine transfusion may be indicated. The risk of amniocentesis at most high-risk centers is a fetal loss rate of 1/200 to 1/400 within 2 weeks of the procedure. It is imperative that women undergoing amniocentesis be aware of these risks before consenting to it.

Ultrasound

An ultrasound screening examination usually is performed around 18 to 20 weeks of gestation to evaluate the developing fetus for major anomalies. Routine diagnostic ultrasound in the second trimester is not yet considered indicated in all pregnancies but continues to be used widely throughout the United States and Europe in low-risk women. In the second trimester, the fetus is well developed, allowing many anatomic details to be studied more easily. Fetal bones are not yet fully ossified, and many internal details can be seen clearly. Accurate dating of the pregnancy can be established with a margin of error of about 10 days.

Although a routine ultrasound during the second trimester detects most major fetal structural anomalies, not all can be diagnosed with this modality. Major anomalies that can be detected at this gestational age include anencephaly, hydranencephaly, spina bifida, omphalocele, gastroschisis, holoprosencephaly, hydronephrosis, ventriculomegaly, cystic hygroma, congenital diaphragmatic hernia, hydrothorax, cleft lip and palate, and major structural limb abnormalities. Abnormalities of fetal biometry (measurement of fetal structures to determine weight or gestational age or both) may point to some diagnoses and are clinically useful. Many congenital heart defects also can be detected after 18 weeks, although doing so may require a targeted fetal echocardiogram with special equipment. Some ultrasound markers, such as heart defects, duodenal atresia, hydrops, and increased nuchal skin thickness, may point to specific syndromes, such as Down syndrome. Care must be taken when counseling a patient about any of these ultrasound findings not to increase falsely the fears of an aneuploid fetus; although relatively sensitive, these findings are not always specific. Amniocentesis can be considered for definitive diagnosis.

A slight decrease in blood pressure in the early second trimester is not unusual. During this time, the fetus often can be palpated through the abdominal wall and the presenting part detected. The patient is asked about symptoms of preterm labor at each visit, including contractions, cramps, bleeding, loss of amniotic fluid, or other indicators of pregnancy difficulty. The presence of preterm labor can be evaluated with a speculum examination or sterile digital examination of the cervix. Transvaginal ultrasound of cervical length tends to decrease to less than 2.5 cm if a patient is at risk of delivering a preterm infant. Similarly a cervical swab for fetal fibronectin can help identify women at high risk of preterm delivery.

THIRD TRIMESTER

The third trimester largely is spent preparing for the birth of the infant. The lower limit of infant viability in the United States is approximately 24 weeks' gestational age. By the third trimester, the infant is considered viable and capable of independent survival. Visits become more frequent as the need to screen for preterm labor and preeclampsia increases.

Glucose Tolerance Testing

Glucose tolerance screening usually is performed at 24 to 28 weeks' gestational age. Patients with strong risk factors for gestational diabetes, such as obesity, a history of unexplained stillbirth, glucosuria, or a family history of diabetes, can be screened earlier at the caregiver's discretion. Gestational diabetes is believed to be caused by placental growth and the resultant infusion of higher concentrations of glycogenic hormones in the maternal system. The typical screen is a 1-hour glucose tolerance test following consumption of a 50-g load of glucose. Values of 140 mg/dL or higher are considered abnormal. The sensitivity is improved if the patient fasts before the study. Approximately 14% of low-risk patients tested are found to be positive by this screen. A positive screening should be followed up with a 3-hour glucose tolerance test. A 100-g glucose load is consumed, and the plasma glucose is measured at fasting, 1 hour, 2 hours, and 3 hours after administration. If two of the four measurements are abnormal, the diagnosis of gestational diabetes is made. Gestational diabetes occurs in approximately 2% to 3% of all pregnancies.

Patients diagnosed with gestational diabetes should receive extensive dietary counseling by a nutritionist. Home glucose monitoring is initiated, and dietary control is attempted for 1 or 2 weeks. If dietary control fails, glyburide or insulin is indicated for optimal control. Patients with gestational diabetes have a higher risk of a poor perinatal outcome, including macrosomia or large-for-gestational-age infants with a resultant increased risk for shoulder dystocia at delivery. Strict glucose control may decrease these risks. Patients should be counseled regarding their higher risk of developing type 2 diabetes later in life, which may be 50% within 20 years.

Rh Disease

Rh-negative women are at risk for sensitization to fetal Rh-positive red blood cells if sufficient fetal blood gains access to the maternal circulatory system during delivery or other invasive procedures, such as dilation and curettage or amniocentesis. The risk is approximately 16% with routine vaginal delivery. Women who are Rh negative are given Rh immune globulin (RhoGAM) within 72 hours of delivery. Fetal blood also may cross the placenta before term, and approximately 1% to 2% of patients become sensitized to the Rh antigen prenatally. Rh immune globulin given at 24 to 28 weeks diminishes this risk to 0.1%.

Fetal Monitoring

In some pregnancies, more intensive monitoring of fetal health is indicated during the third trimester. In the nonstress test, the fetal heart rate is monitored electronically for 20 to 30 minutes and examined for periodic accelerations, especially after fetal movement, maternal ingestion of glucose-containing fluid, or acoustic stimulation of the fetus. Some patterns, especially decelerations in the fetal heart rate, may indicate a fetus in danger of intrauterine asphyxia from various causes. In a contraction stress test, the fetal heart rate is monitored continuously after the patient is given a dilute solution of oxytocin or nipple stimulation to induce contractions. Changes in the fetal heart rate are noted when coordinated uterine contractions begin. A biophysical profile uses multiple ultrasound parameters to determine the overall state of the fetus, including the amniotic fluid volume, fetal body movement, fetal limb extension and flexion, and fetal breathing movements. A nonstress test also is performed as a part of this assessment.

Ultrasound is used to follow fetal growth during the third trimester. Estimation of fetal growth can be difficult as the fetus approaches term, when individual genetic characteristics begin to affect the final fetal weight. The relative decrease of amniotic fluid as term approaches and continued ossification of the fetal bones make ultrasound measurements less accurate. At term, manual assessments of size are most accurate.

Group B Streptococcus Screening

At about 36 weeks' gestational age, screening for group B streptococcus (GBS) is performed. GBS, normal genital flora, is the leading source of serious neonatal infection. Appropriate screening and timely treatment can decrease neonatal morbidity and mortality in susceptible mothers and fetuses. Cultures are obtained from the vaginal walls, introitus, and perirectal area. If GBS is detected, the patient is given chemoprophylaxis during labor with intravenous penicillin or ampicillin. Alternative screening techniques use risk factor identification. A patient is treated as a GBS carrier if there is preterm labor (<37 weeks) or membrane rupture greater than 18 hours or if she has had a prior infant with GBS sepsis or a urine culture that grew GBS during the pregnancy. Most clinics use a combination of screening cultures and risk factors to evaluate patients for GBS.

The frequency of clinic visits is increased for patients after 36 weeks. Each clinic visit is similar to the visits in the second trimester. Blood pressure, weight, dipstick urinalysis, fetal heart tones, and uterine fundal height all continue to be measured. A digital cervical examination may be performed for patients suspected to be in labor. Patients should be advised to come to the hospital for evaluation if they have contractions less than 5 minutes apart, the contractions are strong, they are leaking amniotic fluid or bleeding, or they do not feel fetal movement for a prolonged period.

Mini-index of Related Topics

SUGGESTED READINGS

Cunningham FG, Grant NF, Leveno KJ, et al: Williams Obstetrics, 21st ed. New York, McGraw-Hill, 2001.
Gabbe SG: Obstetrics: Normal and Problem Pregnancies, 4th ed. Philadelphia, Churchill Livingstone, 2002.

SECTION 5   NEWBORN CARE: *Perinatal Care*

189 Prenatal Factors Affecting the Newborn

Jeffrey J. Ridgeway and Sterling K. Clarren

ROLE OF THE GENERALIST

1   Recognize the three periods of critical development and the effects of teratogens during each period.
2   Know the potential teratogenic effects of medications, alcohol, tobacco, drug abuse, radiation, and occupational exposures.
3   Recognize and manage newborns with fetal alcohol syndrome and exposure to drugs of abuse.
4   Recognize and manage newborns with congenital defects secondary to exposure to teratogens.

DEFINITIONS

A *birth defect* is defined as any major deviation from normal morphology or function that occurs before delivery. The current rate of birth defects in the United States has remained steady for almost a decade at about 3%. Most congenital abnormalities are secondary to noninheritable factors, including environmental factors, medications, infections, or physical factors that affect the mother while pregnant. The science of studying and understanding the etiology of birth defects is called *teratology*, and substances that cause birth defects are called *teratogens*.

FUNDAMENTALS

The mechanisms by which teratogens affect the developing fetus are varied. At the cellular and molecular level, the teratogenic agent can cause gene mutations, chromosomal abnormalities, enzyme inhibition or alteration of function, changes in membrane characteristics, interference with cell division, or cellular death. These cellular changes can result in alterations in structural characteristics of organs, functions of tissues, and growth and development of the fetus as a whole. Three important times during development are known as the critical development periods. The *preimplantation period* from fertilization until implantation is the first critical development period. During this time, the fertilized egg divides to become a zygote and prepare for implantation. Exposure to a teratogen during this period results in an "all-or-none" effect; either too many cells are damaged, and implantation cannot occur, or the dividing cells continue to develop and compensate for the damaged cells. The second through the eighth week of development is the *embryonic period*, which is an important time for organogenesis.

Teratogens that have an effect during this period are likely to affect development of individual organ systems, possibly even inhibiting their growth completely. Many major fetal birth defects are caused by exposure to teratogens during this period. The third critical period for development is the *fetal period*, which occurs from about 9 weeks of gestation until delivery. During this period, further growth and maturation of organ systems occur, and teratogens still can have major effects. Overall growth and development of the fetus can be affected, resulting in intrauterine growth restriction or decreased amniotic fluid levels. Understanding these three critical periods of development can help tremendously in counseling a patient who has been exposed to a potentially teratogenic agent during pregnancy.

SPECIFIC TERATOGENS

Medications

The U.S. Food and Drug Administration has strict criteria for testing new medications before release to the public, including testing for effects on pregnancy in animals and sometimes humans. Teratogenic effects are often species specific. A drug that has little or no effect on pregnancy in mice or rats still may have effects in humans. The Food and Drug Administration has developed a classification system for medication use during pregnancy based on the evidence available for each drug. This classification system does not reflect a ranking order of safety. Class C medications in pregnancy are not safer than class D medications; they just may have fewer studies available to evaluate the effects. Many medications may have few side effects at one dose, but little research has been done on the effects of higher doses of medication. Ultimately the physician and patient must weigh the benefits of using a drug against the risk of side effects or possible birth defects.

Steroids

Estrogens and progesterones are components of most oral contraceptives. Fetuses commonly are exposed to these medications early in pregnancy as women continue to take them before the pregnancy is diagnosed. Studies have not confirmed any definite risks for these medications with the notable exception of diethylstilbesterol. Diethylstilbesterol is associated with multiple abnormalities in female fetuses and increased risk of specific types of cancers later in life, particularly vaginal clear cell adenocarcinoma. Developmental defects include abnormal vaginal development, structural abnormalities of the cervix and vagina, and uterine abnormalities including a T-shaped uterus. Although diethylstilbesterol use has been rare in recent decades, women should be screened for exposure early in pregnancy. Androgenic steroid exposure early in pregnancy can lead to masculinization of female fetal genitalia. Most progesterones used in oral contraceptives are derived from androgenic sources.

Many steroids are used for problems in pregnancy, such as asthma. These drugs cross the placenta. Prednisone and prednisolone are deactivated by the placenta, making them the drugs of choice for treating asthma or rheumatologic conditions. Low doses of the drug cross the placenta when administered by inhalation. Steroids also can be used to accelerate fetal lung maturity if premature delivery is a concern. Betamethasone and dexamethasone are used because they cross the placenta in appreciable quantities.

Anticonvulsants

Women with seizure disorders have an increased rate of birth defects, including cleft lip and palate, congenital heart defects, and neural tube defects, regardless of exposure to medications. The risk of these malformations seems to increase with the use of anticonvulsants, especially if more than one medication is given or high doses must be used. Phenytoin is associated with a specific syndrome of craniofacial and digital anomalies in 7% of exposed infants. Carbamazepine has been associated with a similar syndrome, but the effect does not seem to be as clear as with phenytoin. Valproic acid carries a 1% to 2% risk of spina bifida but does not seem to be associated as strongly with cleft lip or palate. Other anticonvulsants, such as trimethadione and paramethadione, are associated with major malformations and are not recommended for use in pregnancy.

Anticoagulants

Warfarin and its derivatives have been associated with a specific syndrome consisting of nasal hypoplasia, eye abnormalities, mental retardation, and stippling of long bones in approximately 5% of infants exposed in early pregnancy. In addition, fetal and maternal hemorrhage has been noted in patients taking warfarin later in pregnancy. Unfractionated heparin is a large molecule and does not cross the placenta, making it the drug of choice for anticoagulation in pregnancy. Because the efficacy of low-molecular-weight heparins in pregnancy is questioned, they currently are not recommended.

Psychiatric Medications

Although most psychiatric medications are not associated with specific birth defects, data regarding the effects of these medications on the developing fetal brain are lacking. Patients who use these medications are at increased risk to abuse alcohol and other nonprescription agents, making studies difficult. Lithium has been associated with major cardiac malformations, particularly Ebstein anomaly; however, other, more recent studies show no appreciable risk. Lithium is continued during pregnancy if the risks warrant its use. Women taking lithium should be offered prenatal cardiac echocardiography to rule out major cardiac anomalies.

Antidepressants are used commonly during pregnancy. Tricyclic antidepressants have a questionable association with fetal limb defects. Multiple large studies have shown no increased risk of birth defects with selective serotonin reuptake inhibitors such as fluoxetine (Prozac). Information regarding monoamine oxidase inhibitors, uncommonly used today, is inconclusive.

The risks of fetal malformations associated with the use of antipsychotic medications seem to be low. There seems to be an association of schizophrenia with increased risk of birth defects regardless of medication ingestion. The most commonly used agents, phenothiazines, also are used often in early pregnancy to treat nausea. Extensive evidence indicates no increased risk of fetal malformations. Often the benefits of these medications far outweigh any concerns during pregnancy.

One of the most recognized human teratogens is thalidomide, an antianxiety drug widely used in the 1950s. Thalidomide produces specific limb malformations, including complete absence of limbs, in about 20% of infants exposed prenatally. Other associated anomalies include bone defects, ear malformations, and cardiac abnormalities. Other tranquilizers, such as benzodiazepines, are not associated with any risks of fetal malformation, but infants exposed to these agents near delivery should be examined closely for hypotonia.

Antibiotics

The most frequently used antibiotics in pregnancy are the penicillins and related agents. These drugs do not seem to be associated with any fetal birth defects. Cephalosporins have a long track record of safety in pregnancy. The aminoglycosides, such as gentamicin, have been associated with congenital deafness in fetuses exposed during the first trimester. Nitrofurantoin is concentrated in urine and does not seem to cause birth defects. The tetracyclines are known to cause inhibition of bone growth and a brownish discoloration of teeth and generally are avoided during pregnancy. Quinolones have affinity for bone and are avoided for theoretical concerns. Metronidazole and clindamycin have been used extensively to treat bacterial vaginosis in pregnancy. No increased risk of fetal anomalies has been shown. The macrolides are generally considered safe. Sulfonamides do not cause any increase in birth defects if given in the first trimester. If given in the third trimester, they can displace the bilirubin molecule from its carrier protein, increasing bilirubin levels in fetal blood and potentially causing the buildup of bilirubin in the basal ganglia of the developing fetal brain.

Antituberculosis drugs, such as isoniazid, rifampin, and ethambutal, also have a long history of use in pregnancy with no evidence of teratogenicity. The most widely used antiviral drug, acyclovir, seems to be safe throughout gestation and has been used to treat herpes outbreaks. Antifungal agents seem to be safe, with no associated fetal effects among the most common topical drugs, such as clotrimazole. Fluconazole, an oral or intravenous agent used to treat fungal infections, has been associated with limb deformities when used at high doses in early pregnancy, but normal doses later in gestation seem to be safe.

Antihypertensives and Cardiac Medications

The most widely used drug for treatment of hypertension in pregnancy is α-methyldopa. Extensive physician experience with this drug over many years has revealed no teratogenic side effects. Likewise the vasodilating agents clonidine and hydralazine have shown no increase in birth defects over many years of use. Although β-adrenergic blocking agents have not been linked to major birth defects, there has been an association with lower birth weights and an increase in intrauterine growth restriction in infants exposed during gestation. Close ultrasound monitoring of fetal weight is mandatory for patients taking these drugs. Angiotensin-converting enzyme inhibitors have been linked to severe deformities, such as craniofacial abnormalities,

hypoplastic lungs, and oligohydramnios, in exposed infants and generally are not used in pregnancy. Calcium channel blockers are used by some to treat hypertension in pregnancy and largely are regarded as safe for use. Diuretic agents, such as furosemide or hydrochlorothiazide, are not used commonly during pregnancy, although they have shown no teratogenic potential. The potassium-sparing diuretic spironolactone generally is avoided because of its potential for feminization of male fetuses. Digoxin is regarded as safe for pregnancy. The drug crosses the placenta, or it can be administered directly to the fetus to treat some arrhythmias.

Antihistamines and Asthma Medications

Antihistamine medications often are ingested during pregnancy as treatments for the symptoms of colds and flu. Most are considered safe, although retrospective studies have raised concern about an increased risk of gastroschisis in patients who took pseudoephedrine in the first trimester and an increased risk of birth defects in patients who took phenylpropanolamine in the first trimester. The most common antihistamine is diphenhydramine, which can be used to control nausea and is not associated with any adverse fetal effects. First-trimester use of these drugs should be limited to situations in which the symptoms are extreme.

Asthma is one of the more common medical complications of pregnancy. Many of the medications used to treat this disorder, such as theophylline, cromolyn sodium, β-agonists, and steroids, are inhaled and do not reach the fetus in high doses. Oral or intravenous versions of these drugs, especially steroids, also are useful and can be administered safely.

Antiemetics

Over-the-counter treatments for nausea and vomiting during gestation include vitamin B_6, doxylamine, and diphenhydramine. Other medications include metoclopramide, which has shown no increase in birth defects in animals or humans, and phenothiazines, which are used commonly despite a questionable relationship to increased birth defects in retrospective studies. Another medication, ondansetron, which formerly was limited to nausea from chemotherapy, has been used more recently to treat hyperemesis gravidarum in pregnancy with some success. This drug has shown no increased risk of fetal malformations in studies.

Analgesics

Some reports have shown that more than half of all pregnant women ingest some form of analgesic during pregnancy. The most common of these is acetaminophen, which has no demonstrated increase in birth defects with widespread use. Aspirin, ibuprofen, naproxen, and indomethacin do not seem to be associated with any malformations. These medications have been shown, however, to cause premature closure of the ductus arteriosus and decreased amniotic fluid volume when used in pregnancy. Although some indications still exist for these drugs to be used as tocolytics or to treat polyhydramnios, their use as pain relievers generally is limited. Narcotic analgesics often are used for pain relief during labor, especially meperidine and morphine. Other narcotics include codeine, propoxyphene, hydrocodone, oxycodone, and butorphanol. Although effective for pain control, the possibility for neonatal withdrawal symptoms or respiratory depression exists. These medications are potentially addicting and may be used illicitly during pregnancy.

Chemotherapy Agents

Chemotherapy drugs by design affect quickly reproducing tissues. Most anticancer drugs do not seem to have adverse fetal effects, although the data are limited. Drugs that do increase the risk of fetal malformations fall into two distinct categories. The alkylating agents include cyclophosphamide and are associated with multiple fetal malformations, especially from exposure during early pregnancy. These malformations are thought to be the result of cell death and DNA damage in surviving tissues and include limb hypoplasia, cleft lip and palate, imperforate anus, and intrauterine growth restriction with microcephaly. The other major category of chemotherapy drugs associated with fetal malformations is the antimetabolites. This category includes methotrexate and aminopterin, both of which affect folate acid metabolism. Methotrexate is used occasionally to treat ectopic pregnancy in addition to its uses as an antineoplastic agent. A dose of 10 mg/wk can result in serious fetal developmental abnormalities, including limb abnormalities, micrognathia, small low-set ears, abnormal calvaria ossification, and craniosynostosis.

Alcohol

Alcohol is a potent teratogen that can affect numerous organ systems but most commonly affects the central nervous system. The specific mechanisms that lead to ethanol-related teratogenesis are unknown. Ethanol teratogenesis is related to the dose of alcohol that is ingested, the timing in gestation of exposure, apparent maternal metabolic factors, and variable fetal ability to resist damage. Alcohol is teratogenic alone. Exposure to other substances, such as cigarettes and street drugs, or nutritional deficiencies are not necessary to produce embryonic or fetal damage. At this time, no exposure pattern can be guaranteed to damage every fetus, and no exposure pattern be guaranteed to be absolutely safe. Women who drink at least weekly through the first trimester to levels of inebriation (peak blood alcohol levels >100 mg/dL) place their infants at the highest risk.

The fetal alcohol syndrome (FAS) is neither the aggregate of individuals exposed to alcohol in pregnancy nor all of those damaged by alcohol in pregnancy. Rather it is a group of children whose full spectrum of anomalies defines a specific, recognizable pattern of malformation that is likely due to alcohol exposure in utero. Recognition of FAS is important for the affected child and the birth mother.

The hallmark features of FAS are minimally a characteristic set of facial features and evidence of brain damage. The characteristic facial appearance is primarily due to short palpebral fissures (generally well below −2 standard deviations from the mean) and a flattened philtrum and thin upper lip vermilion (Fig. 189-1). Other facial anom-

alies may be present, such as ptosis, a small jaw, or malformed ears. These anomalies do not differentiate the face of FAS adequately, however, from many other birth defect syndromes without the small eyes and unusual upper lip.

The damage from alcohol teratogenesis is ubiquitous in the brain. There may be alterations in neuronal numbers, malpositions of neurons (heterotopias), decreases in white matter, problems with dendritic proliferation, or abnormally low or high neurochemical levels. These abnormalities may be severe enough in 10% to 15% of patients that they result in microcephaly or abnormalities that can be seen on brain imaging. In most cases, the lesions are microscopic and not detectable by current static imaging techniques. Sometimes the lesions are manifest neurologically with seizure, spasticity, or other hard neurologic signs. More frequently, the problems can be detected only by psychometric assessments of intelligence, memory, language, judgment, and attention. Only about half of the children with significant brain problems have intelligence quotients in the mentally retarded range. In most patients with FAS, the diagnosis cannot be confirmed in infancy because it is impossible to affirm with confidence that the brain is damaged.

Growth deficiency in length and weight originally was touted as a frequent abnormality in alcohol teratogenesis. It would seem that the prenatal growth deficiency associated with alcohol exposure occurs in the third trimester, and women who stop drinking by the middle of pregnancy generally do not have smaller infants. Normal size at birth does not mean that facial anomalies or brain damage has not occurred.

In a small percentage of children exposed to alcohol, major organ malformations are found, such as cleft lip and palate, cardiac defects, and renal malformations, or minor bony anomalies. The presence or absence of these findings does not alter the essential need to detect the face and brain changes as the basis for making the diagnosis.

FAS is estimated to occur in 1 to 3 infants per 1000 live births, making it a significant cause of brain damage and lifetime disability. Many children exposed to ethanol in gestation do not meet the criteria for FAS but have some degree of brain dysfunction. The range of disability can be just as severe as in FAS. Many terms have been used to describe this condition, including *fetal alcohol effects, alcohol-related birth defects, alcohol-related neurobehavioral disorder, fetal alcohol–related conditions,* and *fetal alcohol spectrum disorders.* No prevalence rates have been established for this condition, but it may be 10 times as frequent as FAS.

Whatever term is used to describe adverse outcomes associated with gestational alcohol exposures, the important point is that individuals exposed to alcohol who may or may not meet the criteria for FAS are at risk for numerous problems in brain function that may have a serious effect on learning, adaptation, and social development. These difficulties may be anticipated but usually cannot be diagnosed in infancy. Factors that place the infant "at risk" for this type of damage are listed in Box 189-1.

The families of children at risk for FAS or alcohol-related conditions should be told of this risk. The infant should be placed in an appropriate, nurturing environment with a good infant stimulation program and followed in the

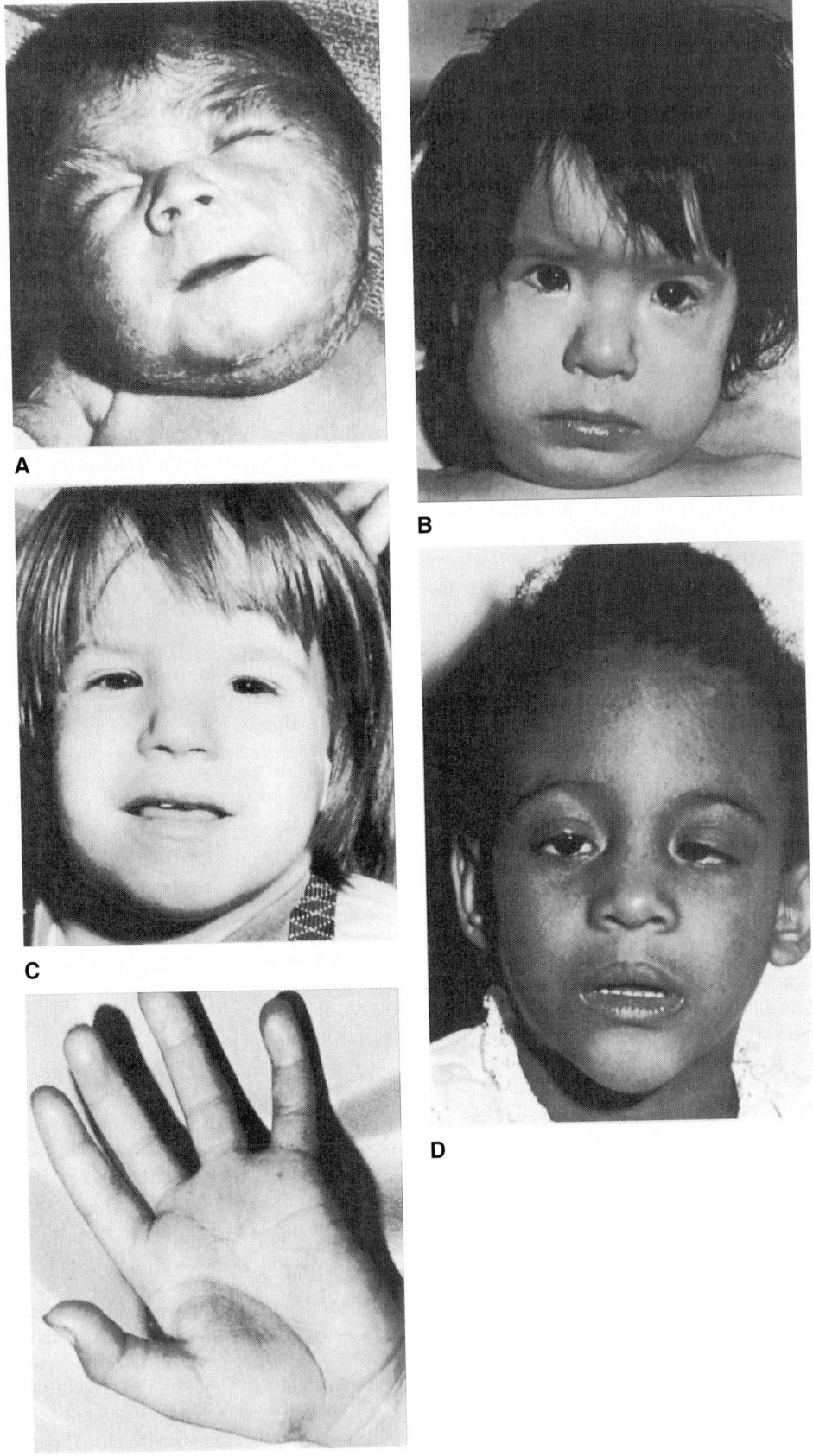

Figure 189-1. Fetal alcohol syndrome. At birth (**A**); 1 year (**B**); 2 years, 6 months (**C**); and 3 years, 9 months (**D**). Note the short palpebral fissures for all children, strabismus (**B** and **D**), ptosis of the eyelid (**D**), and facial hirsutism in the newborn (**A**). The hand shows mildly altered upper palmar crease patterning (**E**). (**A** from Jones KL, Smith DW: Recognition of the fetal alcohol syndrome in early infancy. Lancet 1973;2[7836]:999–1000; **B-E** from Jones KL, Smith DW, Ulleland CN, Streissguth P: Pattern of malformation in offspring of chronic alcoholic mothers. Lancet 1973;1[7815]:1267–1271.)

- Maternal history of high-risk drinking behavior in pregnancy
- Physical evidence of brain damage (e.g., microcephaly, structural anomalies on a brain image)
- Physical stigmata of the face of fetal alcohol syndrome or other major malformations

same manner as infants at risk for other developmental conditions. In contrast to many other conditions, the child remains at risk for 6 to 10 years before it can be concluded fully that he or she does or does not have significant processing difficulties. Many of these children suffer further injuries to their development after birth as a result of neglect, abuse, or a lack of understanding that they may have an underlying disability. Early recognition of the condition or the risk of the condition and close follow-up may prevent these additional adverse circumstances and the further brain damage that they engender.

Thirty years after the seminal publications on FAS, evidence indicates the condition is not becoming less common. Most people are aware that alcohol use in pregnancy might be dangerous. What makes some women persist in this apparent irrational behavior? Studies suggest that the mothers of individuals with FAS have serious problems of their own. As a group, they have a high rate of a lifetime of physical, emotional, and sexual abuse and a high rate of mental health disorders, including depression, manic-depression, phobias, and schizophrenia; perhaps half of them have alcohol-related brain damage themselves. They generally have small social support networks. They are likely to lose their children for abuse or neglect, placing a burden on the foster care system. They also are likely to have more affected children. Early recognition of an infant as having FAS or as being at risk for FAS or alcohol-related neurodevelopmental problems should lead to the recognition of the birth mother as a patient, too. These women deserve emergent attention and referral for substance abuse interventions, mental health interventions, and social service support.

Tobacco

Tobacco abuse during pregnancy is more common than alcohol abuse. Studies on the subject are hampered by confounding factors, such as education and socioeconomic status. Evidence seems to indicate significant risks are associated with cigarette use during pregnancy. Women who smoke are twice as likely to have a spontaneous abortion as nonsmokers. Smoking has been linked to an increase in the rate of small-for-gestational-age infants and prematurity. There also seems to be a dose-response relationship between the amount of tobacco smoked and the perinatal mortality rate, probably from increased risk of placental abruption, placenta previa, preterm labor, and prolonged rupture of membranes. Most complications are thought to result from the vasoconstricting effects of nicotine, but other compounds present in tobacco smoke also may play a role. Secondary smoke intake seems to affect the developing fetus also, with a noted increased risk of small-for-gestational-age infants in those exposed.

All pregnant women should be screened for tobacco use and counseled about the effects of smoking during pregnancy. Women who significantly decrease or stop smoking in early pregnancy have been found to have infants of average birth weight. Because of the addictive properties of nicotine, smoking cessation is not easy for most women. Nicotine patches or gum may help, but the fetus still is exposed to some of the effects of nicotine if these are used. Bupropion, an antianxiety medication, has been approved for use in smoking cessation. Data on its success in pregnancy are limited.

Drug Abuse

Substance abuse among pregnant women is much more prevalent than previously thought. Drug screening programs have shown that 10% to 15% of pregnant women use illicit drugs during pregnancy. Studies are difficult because of the confounding factors, especially race, socioeconomic status, and education level. Many patients abuse multiple drugs, making precise risk estimates more difficult. Illicit drugs may have impurities that also can affect the fetus.

Marijuana

Marijuana is a hallucinogen that usually is smoked in cigarette form. Although high doses of marijuana have been shown to have teratogenic effects in animals, no association with any specific fetal malformations has been shown. Similar to tobacco, ingestion of marijuana is associated with increased risk of a small-for-gestational-age infant.

Cocaine

Cocaine is associated with multiple risks if taken during pregnancy. It can be inhaled, melted and injected, or smoked in solid form. The drug is a stimulant and affects maternal heart rate and central nervous system function. It has been linked to increased risk of cardiac and central nervous system defects if taken in the first trimester. Use later in pregnancy is associated strongly with placental abruption and intrauterine growth retardation.

Narcotics

Narcotics often are used during pregnancy for pain relief during labor or for medical conditions. They are highly addictive, and many women use them outside of the prescribed indications. Although the drugs are not associated with an increased risk of birth defects, the potential for neonatal respiratory depression and withdrawal symptoms is high.

Heroin

The risk of major fetal malformations does not seem to be increased by heroin use in pregnancy. Similar to other narcotics, the potential exists for neonatal withdrawal symptoms and respiratory depression. Several reports have shown that developmental delays and behavioral disturbances are more common in infants exposed to heroin. An analogous narcotic, methadone, often is used to treat narcotic dependence and has not shown any teratogenic effects in pregnancy.

Lysergic Acid Diethylamide and Phencyclidine

Lysergic acid diethylamide (LSD) and phencyclidine (PCP) are not used commonly today. The limited data available indicate that neither LSD nor PCP is associated with major malformations in the fetus.

Radiation

Ionizing radiation was the first identified human teratogen. The main risk seems to be microcephaly and growth restriction in infants exposed in the first trimester. Additional evidence was obtained from survivors of the atomic bombs detonated in Japan during World War II. From these data, a direct relationship between the amount of ionizing radiation and the risk of anomalies was established. Other effects also have been established in the offspring of women exposed to radiation in pregnancy, including approximately a 50% increased risk of childhood leukemia. No data exist regarding radiotherapy for cancer during pregnancy and the associated risks.

Diagnostic radiation is given at significantly lower doses than therapeutic radiation. Radiologic studies that deliver less than 5 rad to the fetus during the first trimester are not believed to be teratogenic. Most radiographic studies deliver only a few millirads at a time, making them safe to use if necessary. These doses can be modified by shielding the maternal abdomen during the procedure. Although there is concern about doses of 5 to 10 rad during the first trimester, no definite risk to the fetus occurs unless the dose is 10 rad or more. As a general rule, radiologic studies may be performed at any point in pregnancy if necessary, but the doses administered to the fetus must be monitored carefully, and abdominal shielding should be used when possible.

Occupational Exposures

Pregnant women can be exposed to a variety of chemicals and substances through their jobs. In the United States, the Occupational Health and Safety Administration sets standards for many commonly found chemicals in the workplace. Regulation outside of the United States is not comparable. Occupational exposure screening should be performed on immigrants recently moved to a new area.

Lead

Lead has been used in the past as an embryotoxic agent for the purpose of early first-trimester abortions. In addition to early fetal demise, other effects include intrauterine growth retardation, mental retardation, and developmental delay. These effects usually are seen at higher levels than those currently allowable in the United States today, and lead fetotoxicity is rare.

Mercury

Most mercury exposures during pregnancy occur from the ingestion of contaminated seafood or from occupational exposures in the health care fields. Mercury easily crosses the placenta, and fetal levels are nearly as high as those of the mother. To date no conclusive evidence has been found that links mercury exposure to fetal malformations or adverse pregnancy outcomes.

Organic Solvents

Patients may be exposed to organic solvents at work or through recreational drug use. Contamination of drinking water in some areas has been reported. Organic solvent exposure does not seem to be associated with major fetal malformations. Risk apparently is increased if a woman develops symptoms from the exposure.

Nitrates

Nitrates are found in many fertilizers and are used often in agriculture. Nitrate exposure increases the risk of cleft lip and palate and neural tube defects. This risk seems to be related directly to the dose of the exposure.

Mini-index of Related Topics   CH.

SUGGESTED READINGS

Cunningham FG, Grant NF, Leveno KJ, et al: Williams Obstetrics, 21st ed. New York, McGraw-Hill, 2001.

Gabbe SG: Obstetrics: Normal and Problem Pregnancies, 4th ed. Philadelphia, Churchill Livingstone, 2002.

Jones KL: Smith's Recognizable Patterns of Human Malformation, 5th ed. Philadelphia, WB Saunders, 1997.

190 Labor Management

Jeffrey J. Ridgeway

ROLE OF THE GENERALIST

1 Recognize normal and abnormal patterns of labor and their effects on the fetus.

2 Recognize consequences of labor problems on the newborn.

3 Understand the various types of obstetric anesthesias and their effects on the newborn.

4 Understand types of fetal monitoring and the causes and consequences of abnormalities.

5 Understand the process of normal spontaneous vaginal deliveries.

6 Understand operative delivery.

DEFINITION

Labor is defined as the onset of regular uterine contractions with progressive dilation of the cervix. When the cervix reaches full dilation (usually 10 cm for a normal full-term delivery), the contractions of the uterus propel the fetus through the cervix and vagina to effect delivery. Understanding the normal progression of labor and delivery can help clinicians diagnose problems early so that risk of harm to the fetus or mother during this process can be minimized. This process can be different for primiparous women (women in the process of their first delivery) and multiparous women (women who have had one or more deliveries previously).

FUNDAMENTALS

Three recognized stages of normal labor are recognized. The first stage begins with the onset of regular uterine contractions and continues until the cervix reaches full dilation. The second stage begins when full dilation is reached and continues until delivery of the infant. The third stage begins after delivery of the infant and ends with delivery of the placenta and membranes. The first stage is subdivided into three phases based on the rate of cervical dilation. The latent phase begins with regular uterine contractions and ends when the rate of cervical dilation is maximal. The duration of this phase varies and may take 20 hours in a primiparous patient. This phase is followed by the phase of maximal cervical dilation. During this period, the cervix dilates rapidly, usually beginning at 2 to 3 cm dilation but

sometimes beginning as late as 5 cm dilation. After this phase, a short phase of deceleration of cervical change is noted. The deceleration phase is marked by a slowing of cervical change and concludes with full cervical dilation.

An understanding of the process of cardinal movements or mechanisms of labor is essential. This process facilitates the delivery of the head. Failure to achieve some of the cardinal movements results in arrest of normal labor and may require intervention. The first movement is *engagement*. During engagement, the biparietal diameter of the fetal head (the largest transverse diameter) descends below the inlet of the pelvis. If the lowest point of the fetal head can be palpated at or below the level of the ishial spines, engagement has taken place. This important milestone during labor usually means that the fetal head is small enough to fit through the maternal bony pelvis. The second cardinal movement is *descent* of the fetal vertex through the pelvis caused by regular uterine contractions. During descent, the third cardinal movement, *flexion*, occurs, characterized by flexion of the head so that the fetal chin touches the thorax. The fourth cardinal movement, *internal rotation* of the fetal head, usually implies that the head changes from a transverse position (the occiput pointing either right or left) to an anterior or posterior position. Flexion and rotation serve to present the smallest possible diameters of the fetal head to the birth canal. When the fetus has descended to the introitus and the fetal occiput is crowning, the fifth cardinal movement, *extension*, occurs. The fetal head extends as it descends under the pubic symphysis and usually results in delivery of the entire fetal head. After delivery of the head, external rotation results in the fetus assuming the correct "face-forward" position with regard to the position of the rest of the body. The final cardinal movement, *expulsion*, refers to the delivery of the shoulders and body of the infant as a result of continued maternal uterine contractions.

LABOR

Abnormal patterns of labor can take several forms. The latent phase of labor usually takes a maximum of 14 hours for multiparous patients or 20 hours for nulliparous patients. A longer latent phase than normal can signal labor problems. Disorders of the active phase of labor fall into two categories. In primary dysfunctional labor, the rate of dilation of the cervix is less than 1.2 cm/hr in nulliparous patients or 1.5 cm/hr in multiparous patients. This problem often is due to inadequate uterine contractile forces, and labor can be augmented with oxytocin or artificial rupture of the membranes (amniotomy). In a secondary arrest, cervical dilation halts for 2 hours or more. Inadequate or uncoordinated uterine contractions can be responsible, and the condition often responds to augmentation of labor. Cephalopelvic disproportion, in which the fetal head is unable to descend into the maternal pelvis from its size or position, also can cause secondary arrest.

When the second stage of labor is reached, the fetal presenting part should descend through the pelvis by 1 cm/hr in nulliparous patients or 2 cm/hr in multiparous patients. The second stage of labor should be approximately 1 hour for multiparous patients or 2 hours for nulliparous patients. These time limits may be extended by 1 hour for patients laboring with an epidural anesthesia. Abnormal patterns in the second stage can signal inadequate uterine contractions, cephalopelvic disproportion, or inadequate maternal pushing efforts. These problems can be corrected by augmentation of labor, or the patient may be evaluated for an operative vaginal delivery.

Abnormalities of the third stage of labor require a different approach. During this time, the placenta separates from the uterine wall and is delivered. The three signs that herald this delivery are lengthening of the umbilical cord from the perineum, a gush of blood from the uterus, and firming of the uterine fundus. The third stage of labor should take a maximum of 30 minutes from the time of delivery of the infant. Longer times can signal problems, such as placenta accreta, and should be evaluated promptly. In some cases, the delivering personnel may have to perform a manual extraction of the placenta and membranes by reaching into the uterus.

AUGMENTATION AND INDUCTION OF LABOR

Augmentation of labor can be accomplished in a variety of ways. One of the most common is by artificial rupture of the fetal membranes, or amniotomy, performed by perforating the chorioamniotic membranes using a hook or small clamp. The fetal head should be engaged in the maternal pelvis before this to prevent umbilical cord prolapse, a life-threatening emergency for the fetus that requires immediate cesarean section. In patients with a favorable cervix, amniotomy alone has been shown to result in vaginal delivery in 88% of cases. Risks of amniotomy include prolapsed cord, prolonged rupture of membranes with increase in neonatal infection, change in fetal position with removal of fluid, and potential rupture of a fetal vessel that is presenting in front of the fetus.

Labor can be augmented with intravenous infusion of a dilute solution of oxytocin. Oxytocin is a hormone produced in the maternal hypothalamus that acts on receptors in the myometrium of the uterus to produce uterine contractions. A continuous infusion of this hormone has been shown to increase the frequency and strength of contractions. Risks of oxytocin infusion include uterine hyperstimulation with resulting fetal bradycardia and possible water intoxication at higher doses because of the hormone's antidiuretic effects. Patients undergoing augmentation of labor with oxytocin are monitored closely with fetal heart tracings and uterine contraction monitors.

Other methods of labor augmentation are not as well established. Often prostaglandins help induce cervical ripening and can increase the sensitivity of the uterus to oxytocin in late pregnancy. Mechanical methods of cervical dilation also can help to augment or induce labor. These methods can cause discomfort for patients during insertion and should be accompanied by appropriate anesthesia.

FETAL MONITORING

Evaluating fetal well-being during the stresses of labor and subsequent delivery always has been a considerable challenge. Doppler ultrasound is the primary modality used for monitoring the fetus in labor with intact membranes. When the membranes are ruptured, external fetal monitoring may be performed or an internal fetal scalp electrode may be applied to allow direct recording of the fetal electrocardiogram. Simultaneous external monitoring of uterine contractions evaluates the fetal heart rate during stressful events. In the event of membrane rupture, an intrauterine pressure catheter may be placed to accomplish the same goal. Monitoring attempts to evaluate the fetal acid-base status during labor. The fetal heart rate reflects fetal brain activity, which is highly sensitive to fetal acidosis. Acidosis can be affected by many factors, including placental function and uterine blood flow. Although nonspecific, monitoring fetal heart rate currently is the most effective method of monitoring when membranes are intact.

Rate, decelerations, and variability are monitored. The rate is usually 120 to 160 beats/min. A sustained elevation in fetal heart rate can signal infection in the fluid and membranes (chorioamnionitis) or fetal arrhythmia. Sustained decelerations indicate a variety of fetal problems and are often the reason for rapid action to save the fetus. The fetal heart rate should vary. Fetal accelerations are periods of at least 15 seconds' duration during which the fetal heart rate increases by at least 15 beats and then returns to the baseline. If fetal heart rate accelerations occur at least twice in 20 minutes, the fetal heart rate is considered "reactive." A reactive fetal heart rate is a sign of a well-oxygenated fetus. Loss of the fetal heart rate variability is an ominous sign—often one of the final signs of impending fetal asphyxia.

Transient changes in fetal heart rate usually take the form of decelerations for variable lengths of time. Early decelerations are shallow, U-shaped dips in the fetal heart rate; occur symmetrically with a contraction; and usually are caused by compression of the fetal head with resultant vagal stimulation as it passes through the cervix. Early decelerations are normal. Variable decelerations, the most common type of transient fetal heart rate change during labor, usually result from fetal umbilical cord compression and are more common after amniotomy. These are sharp drops in the heart rate that occur at any time in relation to the contraction. The depth of the drop varies. Longer and deeper variables are associated with fetal acidosis and should be acted on. Many methods of intrauterine resuscitation can be employed for fetuses with variable decelerations, including amnioinfusion (infusion of normal saline into the uterine cavity), which can relieve some of the compression of the umbilical cord. Late decelerations are the most ominous sign of fetal asphyxia. These are shallow, U-shaped dips in the fetal heart tracing below the baseline that begin about 30 seconds after the onset of a contraction and may even follow the peak. Late decelerations indicate compromise of the fetal-placental unit and, if persistent, the need for immediate delivery.

Fetal pulse oximetry is a newer, yet unproven, adjunct for monitoring. A monitor is inserted along the fetal cheek that allows continuous tracking of fetal oxygenation by measuring the light absorption pattern of hemoglobin in the capillaries of the skin.

OBSTETRIC ANESTHESIA

Intravenous narcotic anesthesia is one of the first medications offered to women in labor who desire pain relief during labor and delivery. It is easy to administer and can be given repeatedly or continuously. The medication also affects the fetus and can cause abnormalities of fetal heart rate patterns or difficulty with the first spontaneous breaths that an infant will take. Concern about allergies to narcotics may make this choice less desirable if others are available.

Epidural anesthesia is accomplished by inserting a needle into the patient's spine below the level of the spinal cord and threading a small catheter into the epidural space. An infusion of either local anesthetic or narcotic is delivered through the catheter directly to the nerve roots, resulting in pain relief or total numbness from the level of the catheter down. Because the fetus does not receive large quantities of medication, the risk of fetal depression is avoided. A continuous infusion of medicine allows for patient comfort for procedures such as operative vaginal delivery or cesarean section. Maternal hypotension (from blockade of sympathetic nerve roots) is a common short-term complication. The technique requires skilled anesthesia personnel. The slight risk of an epidural hematoma or abscess can result in permanent paralysis for the patient. Available data indicate that an epidural given when the patient achieves active labor does not increase the rate of operative deliveries.

Spinal anesthesia requires the insertion of a needle directly into the subarachnoid space of the spinal cord. A single dose of local anesthetic is given. This approach gives the patient a dense block for a short time and often is used for cesarean sections or in combination with an epidural catheter placement. One risk is that a higher block than expected will occur. If too much medication is given, blockade of motor nerves higher than those in the pelvis results. In rare situations, spinal anesthesia can extend all the way up to the motor nerves for the diaphragm, and the patient may have to be intubated and ventilated until the anesthetic wears off. The major disadvantage to spinal anesthesia is the temporary nature of the block; in contrast to epidural anesthesia, a catheter is not placed for continuous infusion of medication.

If the patient does not desire epidural or spinal anesthesia, other methods of pain relief can be discussed. A paracervical block occasionally can be given to patients to relieve some of the pain associated with cervical dilation. Local anesthetic, 5 to 6 mL, is injected at the 3-o'clock and 9-o'clock positions around the cervix. The duration of pain relief varies with the anesthetic used. Readministration during labor often is needed. The pudendal block delivers local anesthetic directly to the pudendal nerve, which travels posterior to the ischial spine and supplies sensory innervation for the perineum and perianal area. This technique provides a lighter block but usually gives enough anesthesia for operative vaginal deliveries if necessary.

NORMAL SPONTANEOUS VAGINAL DELIVERY

When the fetal vertex has reached the perineum, the attendants should prepare for vaginal delivery of the infant. If no significant complications are expected, the perineum should be prepared in a relatively sterile manner, with appropriate drapes used with iodine to clean the introitus. If time allows, a quick catheterization of the maternal bladder can help facilitate delivery and avoid posterior displacement of the fetal head with subsequent laceration of the perineum. As the head delivers, gentle pressure on the mother's perineum can help to prevent further lacerations. Allowing the fetal vertex to sit on the perineum for a few minutes can stretch tissues and prevent laceration.

After the head is delivered, the fetal neck is palpated for a nuchal umbilical cord and reduced. If the cord cannot be reduced, it must be double-clamped and cut on the perineum. The infant's mouth and nose should be suctioned with a bulb syringe or deep suctioning device if necessary to remove meconium. Gentle downward pressure on the fetal head usually facilitates delivery of the shoulder and body. The delivering personnel should assess the infant's condition. A vigorous infant can be cleaned and the umbilical cord cut on the maternal abdomen. Depressed infants must be moved quickly to the warming bed and appropriate personnel summoned for resuscitation.

Meconium in the amniotic fluid may complicate a vaginal delivery. The consistency of the meconium is important in determining management of the delivery. Light meconium usually is not associated with acute fetal stress and does not require any special care at delivery. If moderate or thick meconium is detected antepartum, an intrauterine pressure catheter may be placed and an amnioinfusion of normal saline given to dilute the meconium. Deep suctioning of the infant on the perineum can help to clear the meconium from the airway before the first breath is taken.

Delivery of the placenta and membranes typically takes place within 30 minutes and often occurs without any intervention on the part of delivering personnel. If delivery of the placenta and membranes is not timely, the operator may have to remove the remaining products of conception manually. A dilation and curettage can be performed if manual removal is unsuccessful. Placenta accreta, a placenta that is attached abnormally to the myometrium of the uterus, usually has to be removed operatively, often with a hysterectomy.

Significant blood loss at delivery occurs after delivery of the placenta and membranes. Gentle massage of the uterine fundus through the patient's abdomen usually quickly decreases the bleeding. If bleeding continues, uterotonic medications, such as oxytocin, prostaglandins, or methylergonovine derivatives, may be helpful. In extreme circumstances, surgical management of postpartum hemorrhage may be necessary, such as uterine or hypogastric artery ligation or postpartum hysterectomy.

Lacerations of the perineum are common in vaginal deliveries, particularly in nulliparous patients. A first-degree laceration is superficial and penetrates only the vaginal mucosa. These lacerations can be repaired with a few superficial sutures to bring together the tissue. A second-degree laceration penetrates the vaginal mucosa and the muscular layer underneath, and each layer must be repaired. A third-degree laceration goes further and damages the capsule of the anal sphincter muscle, which must be repaired separately. A fourth-degree laceration penetrates the anal sphincter capsule and musculature and extends through the rectal mucosa. These must be repaired carefully with special attention paid to closing all the rectal mucosa defect to avoid serious wound infection. Patients should be watched closely and placed on stool softeners. Any evidence of infection or incontinence should be evaluated immediately.

Episiotomy is a deliberate incision in the perineum as the infant is delivering. Usually the incision made is directly posterior and is approximately as extensive as a second-degree laceration. Evidence has shown significantly increased blood loss at delivery in women with episiotomy compared with lacerations. The risk of a fourth-degree extension seems to be higher when episiotomy is performed. Episiotomy is no longer a common practice.

MALPRESENTATION

Malpresentation of a fetus refers to any position of the infant in which the vertex is not the first part presenting to the maternal pelvis. Malpresentations cause many problems and in some cases are contraindications to labor. A fetus presenting with the face or a brow instead of the vertex may not progress in labor. Delivery is often difficult, and operative delivery may be required. Occasionally a fetal extremity, usually a hand or arm, presents alongside the fetal head during delivery. This situation, known as a *compound presentation*, usually does not preclude vaginal delivery, although extensive lacerations can occur.

Cord prolapse is an obstetric emergency and can result in significant morbidity or mortality of the infant if not handled appropriately. Cord prolapse, more common with transverse or breech lie, is caused by a loop of the umbilical cord presenting in front of the presenting part of the fetus. It may be recognized by fetal heart rate deceleration and is an indication for emergent cesarean section. As preparations for operative delivery are made, an attendant should support the presenting part of the fetus and prevent compression of the loop of cord. The effectiveness of this maneuver may be gauged by the presence or absence of a continued pulse in the cord.

The management of a fetus in breech presentation is controversial. Breech infants have significantly increased morbidity for the infant over a cephalic delivery, even in the hands of experienced providers. The possibilities for injury arise in two areas. The first is passage of the aftercoming fetal head through the bony pelvis. If the infant's body delivers but the head is delayed, the results can be disastrous. The second problem comes when the fetal head passes through the cervix. This problem can be especially difficult in preterm deliveries, in which the fetal head is larger relative to the body, and the cervix can close down around the head more tightly. An incision in the cervix may be needed to dislodge the head, with resulting blood loss from the cervical laceration. Vaginal delivery is still an accepted method of delivery of a smaller second twin because a larger cephalic first twin dilates the cervix and prevents most of the previously noted problems.

A peculiar obstetric emergency occurs when the fetal head delivers but the shoulders fail to deliver immediately, a complication called *shoulder dystocia*. When diagnosed, all maternal pushing or attempts at downward traction of the fetal head by the operator must be aborted. The maternal hips are flexed back on the patient's abdomen, and suprapubic pressure is applied to the fetal shoulder to facilitate delivery under the pubic symphysis. If this approach is not successful, a corkscrew maneuver may be attempted. Other options include the delivery of the posterior arm of the infant, effectively delivering the posterior shoulder along with it and negating the shoulder dystocia. As a last resort, the fetal head can be pushed back into the maternal birth canal and the patient prepared for emergency cesarean section. This maneuver is associated with considerable morbidity for the fetus and should be used only when all other options have been exhausted. A shoulder dystocia carries with it a 5% to 10% risk of damage to the fetal brachial plexus and subsequent Erb palsy. Although shoulder dystocia occurs more often in women with diabetes or large infants, attempts to predict this complication largely have failed.

OPERATIVE VAGINAL DELIVERY

For any operative delivery, certain criteria must be met, including full dilation of the cervix and rupture of the amniotic membranes. The American College of Obstetricians and Gynecologists classifies deliveries using forceps or vacuum into different categories based on stratification of risk. An outlet delivery is one in which the fetal head is visible at the introitus without separating the labia, the skull has reached the pelvic floor, and the fetal head does not need to be rotated more than 45 degrees. A low pelvic delivery applies to situations in which the vertex is at +2 station or more without being visible at the introitus or when rotation of greater than 45 degrees is performed at a lower station. A midpelvic delivery is classified as a delivery when the fetal vertex is at higher than +2 regardless of the degree of rotation.

Forceps use for delivery is declining in the United States. Forceps are metallic instruments that may be placed around the infant's head during labor for traction to facilitate delivery. Adequate anesthesia and an accurate knowledge of the position of the infant's head are required for a successful forceps delivery. The neonatal risks are considerably less than those for vacuum delivery; the most common complication is temporary erythema or indentations on the sides of the face. The risks to the mother are significant laceration and increased risk of urinary incontinence later in life.

Vacuum extraction of the fetal head can be used in emergent situations to accomplish delivery. Today's vacuum extraction devices are soft plastic cups with flexible handles with suction that can be controlled carefully to the operator's needs. Good anesthesia is optimal for a vacuum delivery, but in emergent situations these deliveries can be performed with minimal or no anesthesia without much discomfort to patients. The vacuum is folded and inserted into the vagina, and then the cup is applied to the fetal vertex. Although rotation of the infant's head is not possible with a vacuum extractor, the flexible handle allows the head to rotate as it would normally during delivery even as traction is applied. The amount of vacuum time must be recorded carefully because longer times have been associated with increased risk to the fetus. This mode of delivery poses minimal risks to the mother other than laceration if a portion of maternal vaginal tissue becomes entrapped in the vacuum. The risk to the fetus is increased over forceps, however, including risks of cephalhematoma, chignon, and subgaleal bleed. Vacuum extraction is more often unsuccessful than a forceps delivery. If suction is lost, forceps use after the vacuum is controversial because multiple studies have shown that fetal outcomes are worsened when both are used during delivery.

CESAREAN SECTION

Cesarean section is defined as the delivery of the infant through an abdominal incision. Until the middle of the 20th century, cesarean section was considered a highly morbid procedure with a low rate of survival for the mother. With antibiotics and improved surgical techniques, the mortality of the procedure has decreased considerably to roughly the same as a vaginal delivery. Cesarean sections are indicated in many different situations, such as a breech presentation or acute fetal distress. The rate has increased substantially in the United States in the last 30 years, a phenomenon that many have blamed on the use of increased electronic fetal monitoring.

The procedure can vary greatly depending on the situation at the time of delivery. The abdominal incision usually is made in a vertical or horizontal manner, and then the layers of subcutaneous tissue and fascia are divided to reach the uterus. The type of uterine incision (hysterotomy) varies with circumstances. A low transverse incision (made in a transverse fashion across the lower segment of the uterus) is preferable to give the patient a chance of future vaginal delivery. If the infant is preterm and the lower uterine segment is not developed fully, a vertical incision may be made that extends from the lower uterine segment into the upper portion of the uterus. When the incision is made, the infant's head is elevated to the opening and delivered with slight fundal pressure. After delivery, the uterus is pulled out of the patient's abdomen if possible and the uterine incision closed. The blood loss at cesarean section is on average more than a vaginal delivery, and risks of damage to the bowel and bladder are increased.

Vaginal delivery after cesarean section is controversial. The main risk is separation of the scar on the uterus during the strong contractions that accompany labor. This catastrophic event carries a high mortality rate for the mother and the fetus. Separation is most common with a prior vertical incision or an incision that extends into the upper, more muscular section of the uterus. Incisions confined to the lower portion of the uterus, which has fewer muscle fibers and does not contract strongly during labor, are much less likely to rupture. These patients may be counseled that a vaginal birth is an option, but must be fully aware of the risks and benefits before delivery. Otherwise, a repeat cesarean section is indicated.

Mini-index of Related Topics CH.

SUGGESTED READINGS

Cunningham FG, Grant NF, Leveno KJ, et al: Williams Obstetrics, 21st ed. New York, McGraw-Hill, 2001.
Gabbe SG: Obstetrics: Normal and Problem Pregnancies, 4th ed. Philadelphia, Churchill Livingstone, 2002.

191 Delivery Room Management and Transitional Care

William A. Engle and David W. Boyle

ROLE OF THE GENERALIST

1   Recognize normal and abnormal cardiopulmonary transition of the newly born infant.

2   Provide resuscitation and transitional needs required by healthy and sick newborns.

3   Anticipate, diagnose, and treat common disorders that occur in the newborn after initial stabilization.

4   Ensure availability of a team of caregivers capable of providing extensive neonatal resuscitation at every delivery.

5   Provide prenatal and postnatal counseling for parents and families of healthy and sick newborns.

Management of newly born infants in the delivery room and during the first hours of life requires an understanding of dramatic physiologic events during transition from fetal to postnatal life. If the major physiologic changes in cardiopulmonary dynamics are interrupted by maternal disease, perinatal complications, neonatal illness, or congenital anomaly, the result may be delayed transition or asphyxia or both that require immediate life-support interventions. Approximately 5% to 10% of newborns require active resuscitation after birth; 1% to 10% require assisted ventilation. Outcome of more than 1 million newborns throughout the world can be improved with implementation of the relatively simple resuscitative measures outlined in the Neonatal Resuscitation Program (Fig. 191-1).

FUNDAMENTALS

Physiologic transition after birth is highly dependent on a series of complex events. The fetus depends on maternal-placental circulation for oxygen, nutrients, and waste removal. At birth, the series circulatory pattern of the fetus must transition to the parallel circulatory pattern of the normal neonate, child, and adult (Fig. 191-2). This transition rapidly progresses with the onset of breathing, which triggers two major events—clearance of intrapulmonary fluid and increase in pulmonary blood flow. Separation of the placenta results in loss of the low-resistance placental circulation and an increase in systemic vascular resistance.

After onset of ventilation, pulmonary vascular resistance decreases, resulting in increased pulmonary blood flow, increased blood flow into the left atrium, and increased left atrial pressure. The ductus venosus, foramen ovale, and ductus arteriosus close, separating the pulmonary and systemic circulations into parallel circulations. These transitions occur during the first minutes to hours of life and are complete by 2 to 4 weeks of age.

When pathophysiologic events prevent the normal decrease in pulmonary vascular resistance, the foramen ovale and ductus arteriosus fail to close. Hypoxemia results from mixture of pulmonary and systemic circulations through these open channels. Inability to effect a decrease in pulmonary vascular resistance is termed *persistent pulmonary hypertension*, which is a common pathophysiologic pathway in many diseases that compromise the pulmonary and cardiac systems of newly born infants.

Pathophysiologic aberrations, especially asphyxia, often result in dysfunction of multiple organ systems. The asphyxiated fetus redistributes cardiac output to the brain, heart, and adrenal glands by intense vasoconstriction. The initial fetal response to asphyxia is a vigorous effort to breathe with preservation of heart rate and blood pressure. If asphyxia continues, primary apnea accompanied by bradycardia with preservation of blood pressure follows. If delivered at this stage, the newly born infant often responds quickly to tactile stimulation. If asphyxia continues, the fetus resumes breathing efforts with irregular gasping followed by secondary apnea, bradycardia, hypotension, and end organ injury. The newborn delivered during the stage of secondary apnea usually requires vigorous resuscitative efforts to recover. Fetal complications associated with asphyxia and other perinatal problems (e.g., premature labor, maternal illness, maternal medications, and congenital anomalies) must be anticipated, identified, and treated during the first minutes and hours of life (see Chapter 192).

Metabolic and endocrine changes precipitated at birth include a surge in cortisol, catecholamine, and thyroid hormone levels; nonshivering thermogenesis; and loss of nutrient supply from the placenta, especially glucose. Preventing heat loss by drying the newborn infant can minimize cold stress and associated increased metabolic activity. Wet linen should be removed, and the infant should be placed in warmed blankets or skin-to-skin on the

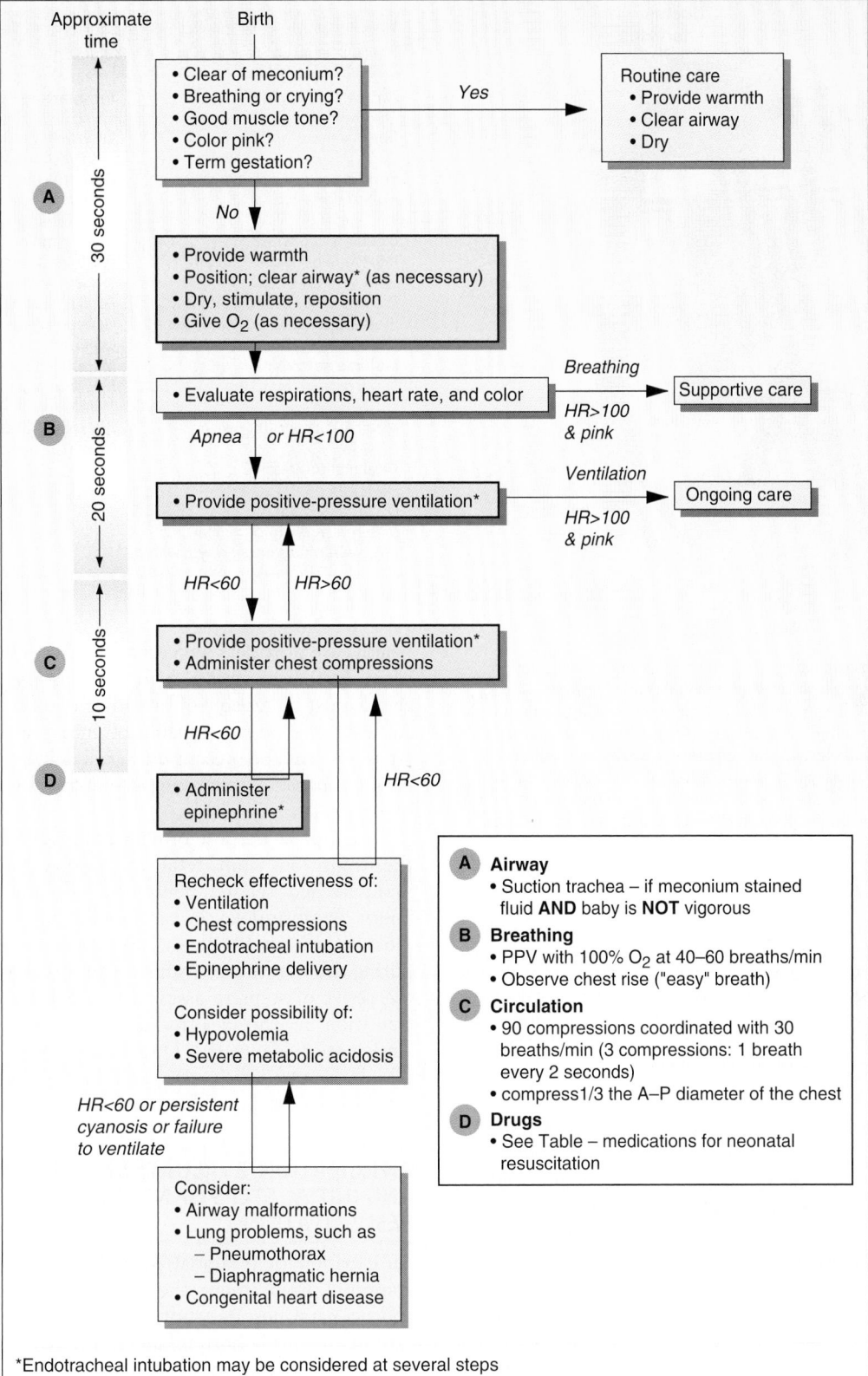

Figure 191-1. Neonatal Resuscitation Program developed collaboratively by the American Academy of Pediatrics and American Heart Association. A-P, anteroposterior; HR, heart rate; PPV, positive-pressure ventilation. (Braner D, Kattwinkel J, Denson SE, et al: Textbook of Neonatal Resuscitation, 4th ed. Elk Grove Village, Ill, American Academy of Pediatrics, 2000, Neonatal Resuscitation Program Reference Chart. Reproduced by permission of the American Academy of Pediatrics.)

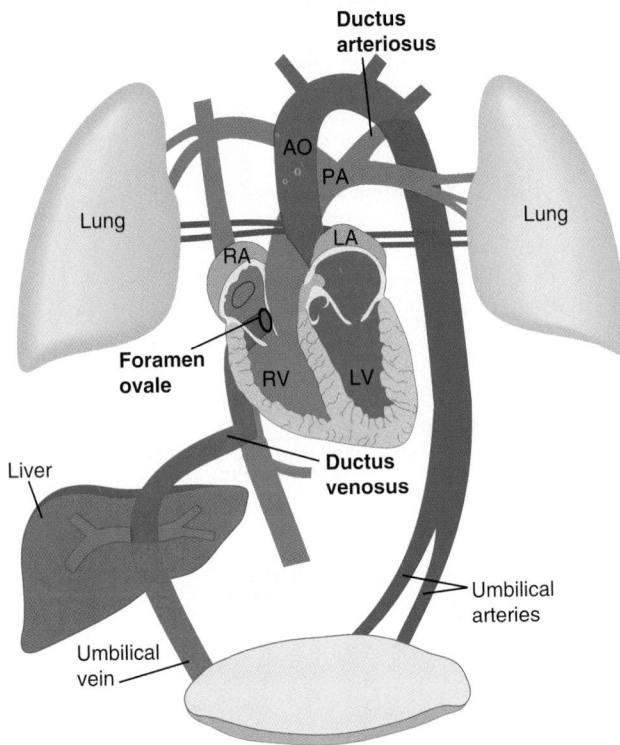

Figure 191-2. Fetal circulation. (1) Fetal cardiopulmonary circulation. Blood flows through a *series* of vascular shunts and cardiac structures, through the umbilical vein and *ductus venosus* into the right atrium. Blood is diverted through the *foramen ovale* and passes from the left atrium (LA), left ventricle (LV), and aorta (Ao) to supply the heart, brain, and right upper extremity with the most well-oxygenated and nutrient-dense blood from the placenta and returns by way of the superior and inferior vena cavae to the right atrium (RA) and into the right ventricle (RV)/pulmonary artery (PA). It is diverted across the *ductus arteriosus* into the descending aorta through the umbilical arteries back to the placenta. (2) Transition from fetal to adult circulation. A decrease in pulmonary vascular resistance after the onset of ventilation results in increased pulmonary blood flow, increased blood flow into the LA and increased left atrial pressure. Right atrial pressure decreases with loss of blood flow from the umbilical vein/ductus venosus; this is associated with placental separation and *ductus venosus closure*. With increased left atrial pressure and decreased right atrial pressure, the *foramen ovale* closes. An increase in oxygen tension flowing through the ductus arteriosus in the newly born infant triggers functional *closure of the ductus*.

mother's chest or abdomen. A wet newborn can lose 2°C in core temperature in 20 minutes. Newborns requiring resuscitation should be placed under a preheated radiant warmer to improve thermoregulatory balance.

Loss of nutrient supply may result in hypoglycemia and symptoms of jitteriness, lethargy, hypotonia, and seizures, particularly in a stressed, cold, newborn infant. Early feeding helps mitigate the risk for hypoglycemia in healthy newborns. Sick newborns who cannot feed enterally may need intravenous glucose within the first minutes to hours.

GOALS OF RESUSCITATION OF THE NEWLY BORN INFANT

The need for significant resuscitation can be predicted about 60% of the time. Because the remaining 40% of resuscitations are unanticipated, knowledge and skills to perform neonatal resuscitation must be learned by all

Table 191-1. Anticipation of High Risk for Neonatal Resuscitation in Newly Born Infants

Antipartum Factors	Intrapartum Factors
Chronic maternal illness	Emergency cesarean, forceps, or vacuum-assisted delivery
Pregnancy-induced hypertension	Abnormal presentation
Isoimmunization	Abnormal labor: premature, prolonged, or precipitous
Bleeding or anemia	Chorioamnionitis
Prior fetal or neonatal death	Prolonged rupture of membranes
Preterm or postterm gestation	Fetal heart rate abnormalities
Premature rupture of membranes	General anesthesia
Maternal infection	Uterine tetany
Multiple gestation	Maternal narcotics <4 hr
Small or large for dates	Meconium-stained amniotic fluid
Medications or drug use	Abruptio placentae or placenta previa
Fetal malformation	
Diminished fetal activity	
No prenatal care	
Maternal age <16 or >35 yr	
Polyhydramnios or oligohydramnios	

health care providers who care for newborns in the delivery room. In the anticipated high-risk delivery, a team of caregivers must be capable of providing extensive resuscitation. At least one person capable of initiating neonatal resuscitation should be present during all deliveries, and a second person capable of performing a complete resuscitation should be immediately available.

The primary purpose of neonatal resuscitation is to assist the transition from fetal to postnatal life, preventing asphyxia and related neurologic and multisystem organ injury. Because delay in cardiopulmonary transition is the most significant life-threatening transitional phenomenon during the first minutes after birth, providers must master the series of steps to assess and support cardiopulmonary transition in the healthy and sick newly born infant. Anticipation (Table 191-1), preparation for delivery (Table 191-2), accurate evaluation, and prompt resuscitative interventions are the keys for successful resuscitation.

ANTICIPATION, EVALUATION, ASSESSMENT, AND INITIAL STEPS OF NEONATAL RESUSCITATION

Anticipation of potential need for resuscitation requires communication among the delivering physician, obstetric and neonatal hospital staff, and physicians responsible for care of the newly born infant. If a pregnancy is considered high risk for either mother or fetus, delivery at a high-risk obstetric and neonatology center is recommended. Interhospital transfer of the mother may be required, or, if a high-risk newborn is born in a nonspecialty hospital, transfer of the sick neonate may be required. Verbal communication and chart review by the staff and physicians responsible for care of the newly born infant should include gestational age, significant maternal illness, maternal medications and drugs, peripartum complications, maternal screening results, family history, and fetal evaluation.

Table 191-2. Preparations for Delivery

Communication and Consultation

Consultation with physicians and staff responsible for care of the newly born infant

Maternal chart review

Prenatal counseling

Equipment and Supplies for Neonatal Resuscitation

Suction equipment: bulb syringe, mechanical suction and tubing, suction catheters (5 Fr, 6 Fr, 8 Fr, 10 Fr, 12 Fr), feeding tube (8 Fr), 20-mL syringe, meconium aspiration device

Manual resuscitator (bag) and mask equipment: neonatal bag (<750 mL) with pressure-release valve or pressure manometer (must be able to deliver FiO_2 0.9–1.0), newborn and preterm facemasks, oxygen with flowmeter

Intubation equipment: laryngoscope with no. 0 and no. 1 straight blades, spare batteries and bulbs, endotracheal tubes (2.5–4.0 mm ID, 2.0 mm ID tubes may be needed for extremely preterm infants, usually weighing <500 g), stylet, scissors, tape, alcohol sponges, CO_2 detector, laryngeal mask airway (optional)

Medications

Antibiotics, surfactant, prostaglandins, emergency red blood cells if indicated, epinephrine (1:10,000 or 0.1 mg/mL)

Normal saline, Ringer lactate

Naloxone hydrochloride (0.4 mg/mL or 1 mg/mL, use single concentration within an institution to avoid dosing error)

Dextrose (10%, 5%)

Sodium bicarbonate 4.2% (0.5 mEq/mL)

Vascular access supplies: umbilical vessel catheterization trays with 3.5 Fr and 5.0 Fr catheters (2.5 single-lumen and 4.0 Fr double-lumen catheters are optional), syringes (1, 3, 5, 10, 20, and 50 mL), intravenous catheters (22-, 24-, 26-, 27-gauge), and tubing connectors

Miscellaneous supplies: 23- and 25-gauge butterfly needles for thoracentesis; 18- and 20-gauge, 1.5-, 2.0-, and 3.0-inch angiocatheters for thoracentesis, paracentesis, or pericardiocentesis; chest tube suction devices; radiant warmer; personal protective equipment and gowns; firm resuscitation surface; warmed linens; stethoscope; cardiac and oxygen saturation monitors; oropharyngeal airways; continuous positive airway pressure device (optional); mechanical ventilator (optional); sterile bowel bags

CO_2; carbon dioxide; FiO_2, fraction of inspired oxygen; ID, inside diameter.

Parental knowledge, psychosocial issues, and content of counseling by the delivering physician and specialists also should be shared.

Anticipation of high-risk deliveries allows time for prenatal counseling and preparation by physicians and neonatology staff. Because time for prenatal counseling and preparation does not exist with unexpected illness, all caregivers of newborn infants must be skilled in initiation of resuscitation. Preparation includes ensuring all equipment is immediately available and in good working order. The team of caregivers must be capable of providing a complete resuscitation and working together in complicated resuscitations.

INITIAL EVALUATION

Initial evaluation begins with visual inspection of signs to determine if the transition to the extrauterine environment is proceeding normally (see Fig. 191-1). Resuscitative decisions are based on presence of meconium-stained amniotic fluid or skin, respiratory and physical vigor (respiratory efforts and muscle tone), cry strength, color, and gestational age. For a term infant who is pink and with no meconium staining, strong respiratory efforts and cry, and appropriate muscle tone, routine care consists of wiping the mouth and nares to clear the airway, drying, providing warmth, and ensuring reunion with mother and family. Early breast-feeding and skin contact with the mother may reduce the risk of temperature and glucose instability and enhance family cohesiveness.

INDICATIONS FOR CONTINUING EVALUATION AND RESUSCITATION

Further evaluation and potential resuscitation are indicated when there is meconium staining, weak respiratory efforts, low neuromuscular tone, persistent cyanosis, and prematurity. First the infant is placed under a radiant warmer, and simultaneous evaluation of respiration, heart rate, and color is completed rapidly. Concurrently the caregiver warms the infant (i.e., radiant warmer, drying, removal of wet linen, prewarmed blankets) and establishes the airway by positioning supine or on the side with the head in a neutral or slightly extended position and clearing the airway (see Fig. 191-1). In the absence of meconium staining, gentle suctioning of mouth and nasopharynx with either a bulb syringe or a suction catheter (8 Fr to 10 F with <100 mm Hg negative pressure) may be indicated. With copious secretions, the head may need to be positioned to the side. Gentle tactile stimulation is provided simultaneously with drying and removal of wet linen. All of these initial steps in resuscitation should be completed within 30 seconds after birth.

MECONIUM STAINING AND INDICATIONS FOR TRACHEAL SUCTIONING

If the amniotic fluid or skin is stained with meconium (12% of deliveries), the caregiver must decide whether to suction the trachea to prevent postnatal meconium aspiration syndrome. Intrapartum suctioning of the mouth, nose, and pharynx after delivery of the infant's head by the delivering physician may reduce the risk of postnatal meconium aspiration syndrome. Despite suctioning at the perineum, approximately 25% of newly born infants who are meconium stained and depressed (i.e., absent or depressed respiratory efforts, hypotonia, or bradycardia [heart rate <100 beats/min]) have meconium in the trachea. In this situation, the caregiver intubates the trachea and uses a "meconium aspiration" device until the trachea is clear. Tracheal suctioning may need to be repeated to clear the airway. Sometimes the infant's heart rate and oxygen saturation decrease to such a level that tracheal suctioning must be aborted and positive-pressure ventilation initiated despite persistence of some meconium. Even with thick particulate meconium, if the infant is vigorous and active, tracheal suctioning is not recommended because of the risk of inducing bradycardia, apnea, vomiting, and upper airway trauma. The exception is an initially vigorous, meconium-stained infant who becomes apneic or develops respiratory distress soon after birth. In this circumstance, intubation and suctioning before initiation of positive-pressure ventilation is recommended. Gastric suctioning to prevent aspiration of swallowed meconium should be delayed until tracheal suctioning is completed and respiration stabilized.

INDICATIONS FOR OXYGEN AND POSITIVE-PRESSURE VENTILATION

When the airway is clear, regular and unlabored respiratory efforts, a heart rate greater than 100 beats/min, and pink oral mucous membranes are expected. With respiratory distress or apnea, repositioning the head and placement of a towel under the shoulders may open and clear the airway. Drying the infant usually stimulates spontaneous ventilation in infants with primary apnea or poor respiratory drive. Further tactile stimulation may be provided by gently rubbing the feet or back. If the infant is cyanotic, free-flow oxygen delivered by face mask (5 to 10 liters per minute) may help when respiratory efforts are re-established.

Ventilation is the key to successful resuscitation. Box 191-1 lists indications for initiating positive-pressure ventilation using a bag and mask (40 to 60 breaths/min, fraction of inspired oxygen [FIO$_2$] 1.0 for 30 seconds). The decision to provide bag-mask ventilation should be made within 30 seconds of birth. The goal is to correct ineffective respiration, bradycardia, or cyanosis. During positive-pressure ventilation, chest excursion is adequate when there is just enough movement of the chest to hear breath sounds by auscultation or move the chest wall slightly. Large chest wall excursion is evidence of overventilation and increases risk for pneumothorax, other air leaks, initiation of chronic lung disease, and compromise of venous return and cardiac output. If bag-mask ventilation is ineffective, the caregiver should check for an adequate seal, reposition the head, and suction the oropharynx. If ventilation is still ineffective, the caregiver should open the mouth or use higher ventilatory pressures and recheck equipment function. Bradycardia and cyanosis usually respond to establishment of ventilation. Currently, 100% oxygen still is recommended when given with a bag and mask.

If respiratory efforts are labored, the clinician must decide whether to begin bag-mask ventilation, continuous positive airway pressure, or mechanical ventilation. In infants with labored respiratory efforts, a trial of continuous positive airway pressure may avert the need for mechanical ventilation. Intubation and bag–endotracheal tube ventilation or mechanical ventilation is indicated if bag-mask ventilation is ineffective or respiratory distress fails to stabilize with continuous positive airway pressure. If respiratory efforts improve significantly, bag-mask ventilation should be withdrawn as tolerated.

Table 191-3 lists indications for endotracheal intubation during the first minutes of resuscitation. Primary reasons for endotracheal tube placement are for tracheal suctioning of meconium, ineffective or prolonged bag-mask ventilation, airway stabilization for chest compressions, or the specific problems listed that require mechanical ventilation.

Laryngeal mask airways can be effective in ventilating term infants in whom bag-mask ventilation is ineffective or if endotracheal intubation is not successful. Laryngeal masks may not be effective in preterm infants and infants with respiratory distress in whom high peak inspiratory pressures are required for adequate ventilation. Laryngeal mask airways are not intended to replace tracheal suctioning in the meconium-stained and depressed neonate.

INDICATIONS FOR CHEST COMPRESSIONS

If effective positive-pressure ventilation is established and bradycardia (heart rate <60 beats/min as determined by palpation of the base of the umbilical cord or auscultation) persists during resuscitation of the neonate, chest compressions usually are indicated (Box 191-2). Rarely an infant does not respond to positive-pressure ventilation because of congenital heart block. Most of these infants have adequate initial cardiac output, perfusion, and oxygen saturation without chest compressions. Unless pre-natal testing indicates congenital heart block, bradycardia should be attributed to hypoxia. Chest compressions should be initiated while positive-pressure ventilation is continued to establish perfusion, especially to the brain, and reverse myocardial insufficiency, acidosis, peripheral vasoconstriction, and tissue hypoxia.

Chest compression to a depth of one third the anteroposterior diameter of the chest is required to establish adequate perfusion. The force should be sufficient to gener-

---

Table 191-3. Indications for Endotracheal Intubation and Laryngeal Mask Airway

Endotracheal Intubation

1. Suctioning meconium from trachea if meconium-stained skin or amniotic fluid *and*
2. Absent/depressed respiratory efforts, hypotonia, or heart rate <100 beats/min
3. Ineffective or prolonged (several minutes) bag-mask ventilation
4. Improved coordination of positive-pressure ventilation and chest compressions
5. Epinephrine administration
6. Special situations: extreme prematurity, surfactant administration, congenital diaphragmatic hernia, apnea unresponsive to bag-mask ventilation, severe hydrops fetalis, hyaline membrane disease, pulmonary hypoplasia

Laryngeal Mask Airway*

1. Ineffective bag-mask ventilation
2. Failed endotracheal intubation

*Optional due to limited information about use during neonatal resuscitation.

Box 191-1. Indications for Positive-Pressure Ventilation

- Apnea or gasping respirations unresponsive to gentle tactile stimulation
- Bradycardia (heart rate <100 beats/min) even when breathing
- Persistent central cyanosis despite 100% free-flow oxygen

Box 191-2. Indications for Chest Compressions

- Heart rate <60 beats/min despite 30 seconds of positive-pressure ventilation
- Absence of known congenital heart block

ate a palpable pulse and may be underestimated from concern about rib and sternum injury. The two-thumb encircling hands technique is recommended, although the two-finger technique is acceptable. Coordination of ventilation and chest compressions is recommended with a 3:1 ratio of chest compressions to ventilations so that 90 compressions and 30 ventilations are performed each minute. This 0.5-sec/event is a more rapid pace than used in older children and adults. When the heart rate responds and exceeds 60 beats/min, chest compressions should be discontinued. Positive-pressure ventilation is continued until the heart rate is greater than 100 beats/min, and spontaneous respirations are established.

OROGASTRIC TUBE PLACEMENT

Because gastric distention can compromise ventilation significantly, placement of an orogastric tube is recommended if positive-pressure ventilation using a bag and mask is required for more than 2 minutes or if marked gastric distention occurs. Gastric decompression may be beneficial in preterm infants within the first 2 minutes of positive-pressure ventilation with a mask.

INDICATIONS FOR MEDICATIONS DURING NEONATAL RESUSCITATION

If the heart rate remains less than 60 beats/min despite 30 seconds of positive-pressure ventilation with 100% oxygen and chest compressions, medications should be given (Table 191-4). The primary drug used during neonatal resuscitation is epinephrine given as a 1:10,000 solution (versus 1:1000 solution used for adults). Epinephrine is particularly beneficial in elevating peripheral vascular resistance, cardiac contractility, and heart rate, all of which improve perfusion pressure to the brain and heart during chest compressions. The dose administered by intravenous (peripheral or low umbilical venous line) or intratracheal routes is 0.1 to 0.3 mL/kg (0.01 to 0.03 mg/kg) every 3 to 5 minutes. When given through an endotracheal tube, distribution may be improved by following with 0.5 to 1 mL of normal saline or diluting the dose to a total 1 mL before placement into the endotracheal tube. Epinephrine should not be given by intramuscular route and usually should not be given more frequently than every 3 to 5 minutes to avoid postresuscitation hypertension. High-dose (>0.03 mg/kg) epinephrine is not recommended in the newborn.

Pallor, diminished peripheral and central pulses, tachycardia, and slow capillary refill indicate hypovolemia in the sick newborn. Perinatal risk factors for hypovolemia include asphyxia, vaginal bleeding, abruptio placentae, abnormal placentation, twin-twin transfusion syndrome, severe isoimmunization, fetal maternal blood, and chorioamnionitis. Volume expansion with normal saline, Ringer lactate, or O-negative red blood cells (if blood loss is suspected) is recommended. Albumin-containing solutions are less acceptable alternatives during the acute phase of resuscitation. Vascular access is best attained through the umbilical vein. Peripheral veins, umbilical artery, and intraosseous sites can be used. Volume expansion is 10 mL/kg intravenously over 5 to 10 minutes initially, with the dose repeated as needed. Caution is warranted to avoid volume overload, pulmonary edema, heart failure, and intracranial hemorrhage, especially in preterm neonates.

Naloxone is recommended for newborns with respiratory depression whose mothers received narcotics within 4 hours of delivery. Naloxone may be given intravenously, intratracheally, intramuscularly, or subcutaneously at a dose

Table 191-4. Medications for Neonatal Resuscitation and Stabilization

Medication	Concentration	Dose/Route	Rate/Precautions/Caveats
Acute Phase of Resuscitation			
Epinephrine	1:10,000	0.1–0.3 mL/kg ET or IV	Rapid injection
Volume expansion Normal saline Ringer lactate O-negative RBCs		10 mL/kg IV	Flush ET tube with 0.5–1.0 mL of saline Infuse over 5–10 min
Postresuscitation Phase and Stabilization			
Sodium bicarbonate	0.5 mEq/mL	2 mEq/kg IV only	Slow infusion (1 mEq/kg/min) Give when effective ventilation is established
Naloxone	0.4 or 1.0 mg/dL	0.1 mg/kg IV, ET, IM, SC	Maternal narcotics within 4 hr of delivery Do not give if maternal narcotic abuse is suspected
Glucose Phenobarbital	D10W (10% glucose)	2 mL/kg/IV 20 mg/kg/IV	Follow with IV glucose infusion Slow infusion (1 mg/kg/min) Watch for respiratory depression
Dopamine		2–20 µg/kg/min IV	For hypotension unresponsive to volume expansion
Surfactant		Preparation dependent	For surfactant deficiency with hyaline membrane disease, perhaps meconium aspiration, persistent pulmonary hypertension, and congenital diaphragmatic hernia
Prostaglandin E$_1$	500 µg in 100 mL of D5W, D10W, or saline solution	0.03–0.1 µg/kg/min	Risks: apnea, hypertonia, seizures, hyperthermia

D5W, 5% dextrose in water; D10W, 10% dextrose in water; ET, endotracheal; IM, intramuscular; IV, intravenous; SC, subcutaneous.

of 0.1 mg/kg. Because naloxone solution is supplied in two concentrations, 0.4 mg/mL and 1 mg/mL, the dose administered may be 0.25 mL/kg or 0.1 mL/kg. Naloxone is contraindicated in infants whose mothers are chronic users of narcotics because of risk for acute withdrawal symptoms. Because the duration of naloxone action may be shorter than that of the narcotic effect, infants who receive naloxone should be monitored for recurrent respiratory depression. Cardiorespiratory monitoring in the transitional or special care nursery for a minimum of 4 hours is advisable.

Sodium bicarbonate generally is not recommended during the acute phase of resuscitation. Paradoxical intracellular acidosis may depress cardiac and neuronal activity. When ventilation is established, sodium bicarbonate given judiciously by intravenous route (1 to 2 mEq/kg over at least 2 minutes) may be considered during a prolonged resuscitation unresponsive to other therapy. Efficacy of epinephrine is not enhanced with alkalinization.

POSTRESUSCITATION EVALUATION AND MANAGEMENT

Neonates who require initial resuscitation may have an underlying illness, congenital anomaly, prematurity, or asphyxia. Discontinuation of resuscitative efforts is reasonable if there is no heart rate after 15 minutes of complete and adequate resuscitation (Apgar score of 0). Likelihood of death or severe disability in these infants is extremely high. Continued resuscitative efforts are warranted for depressed infants who show signs of recovery.

After the initial resuscitative measures, effectiveness of ventilation, chest compressions, medications, and, if not previously performed, endotracheal intubation should be rechecked. If the response to resuscitation is poor, hypovolemia and acidosis should be considered and treated. If hypotension does not respond adequately to volume expansion, dopamine infusion should be considered. Occasionally, hypotension is a complication of pneumothorax or other intrathoracic air leak. In this situation, thoracentesis (Fig. 191-3) may be lifesaving. Doses of indicated medications and routes of administration are listed in Table 191-4. Seizures may complicate hypoxic-ischemic encephalopathy and require phenobarbital administration. Hypoglycemia, hypocalcemia, anemia, polycythemia, disseminated intravascular coagulation, and abnormal blood gas values should be identified and treated. Hypoglycemia usually is responsive to initiation of intravenous glucose followed by an infusion of 3.5 to 7 mg/kg/min or 5% to 10% dextrose in water at 100 mL/kg/day and serial glucose measurements. Calcium gluconate (1 to 2 mL/kg) or calcium chloride (0.35 to 0.7 mL/kg) provides approximately 10 to 20 mg/kg/dose of elemental calcium when given by intravenous infusion over 10 to 30 minutes. Normal ionized calcium levels during the first days of life range from 1.1 to 1.4 mmol/L (4.5 to 5.6 mg/dL) with a nadir in total calcium levels during the first 2 days of life of 1.5 mmol/L (6.1 mg/dL). If total calcium levels are low, ionized calcium levels, if available, should be assessed before calcium supplementation. The benefits versus risks (e.g., bradycardia, subcutaneous infiltrate) of intravenous calcium supplementation should be weighed before administration, especially if given through a peripheral vein. Calcium is not indicated during the acute phase of neonatal resuscitation.

Anemia, polycythemia, and disseminated intravascular coagulation may need to be treated with red blood cell transfusion, partial exchange transfusion, or platelet and fresh frozen plasma transfusion. Acidosis must be determined to be respiratory, metabolic, or mixed. Mild-to-moderate respiratory acidosis may improve cerebral blood flow, whereas metabolic acidosis unresponsive to ventilation and volume expansion is detrimental. Blood gas values help guide adjustments in ventilation and the decision to treat metabolic acidosis with sodium bicarbonate; perfusion and adequate ventilation must be acceptable before giving sodium bicarbonate. Vitamin K prophylaxis, eye care, and hepatitis B vaccination also should be provided as per hospital protocols.

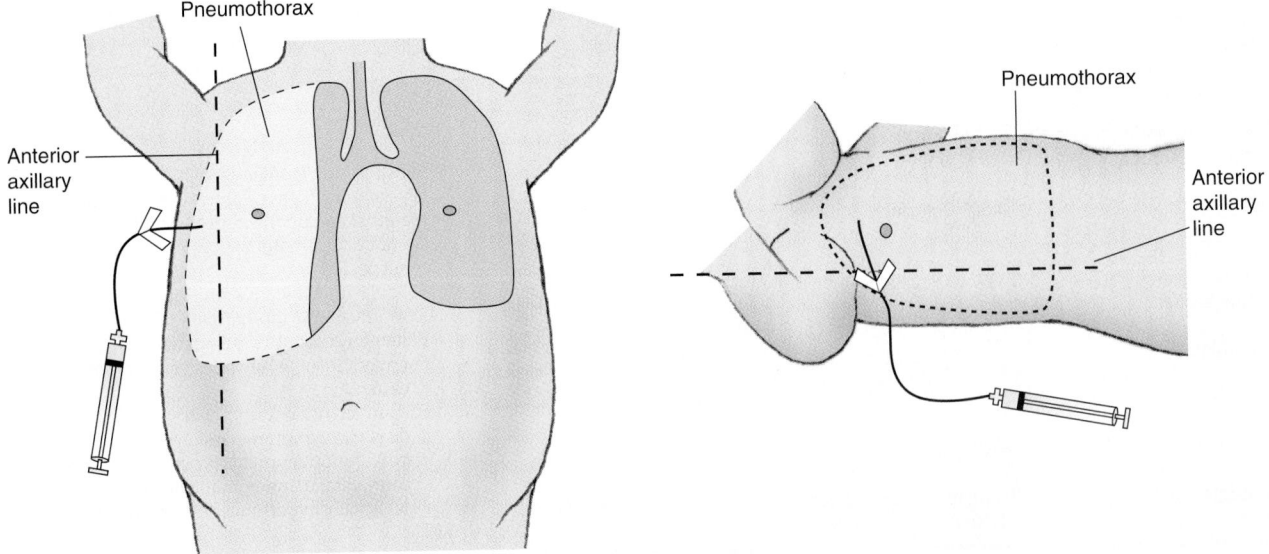

Figure 191-3. Thoracentesis.

SPECIAL CIRCUMSTANCES IN THE DELIVERY ROOM

Candidacy for Resuscitation

Although prenatal diagnosis of fetal abnormalities allows parents and caregivers to plan for care at delivery and prenatal transfer of some patients to specialty facilities, caregivers of newborn infants must be prepared to stabilize, identify, and treat disorders that present at the time of delivery (Tables 191-5 and 191-6). When prenatal diagnostic evaluation and counseling have not been done, and uncertainty exists about candidacy for resuscitation, the clinician should intervene first, stabilize the patient, and then gather more information and plan and consult with parents, subspecialty pediatricians, and other parental support persons regarding further intervention.

Prenatal diagnosis of infants with trisomy 18 and trisomy 13—both usually lethal within the first months of life—allows parents and caregivers to plan care at delivery. Infants who weigh less than 400 g, are less than 23 weeks'

gestation, or have anencephaly have extremely high mortality risks. An acceptable alternative to initiation of resuscitation measures in these cases is to provide simple comfort measures and parental and family support.

Life-Threatening Circumstances in the Delivery Room

See also Table 191-5.

Apnea

Central apnea may be secondary to asphyxia, infection, prematurity, respiratory exhaustion from underlying lung disease, intracranial anomalies or bleeding, metabolic imbalances, hypothermia, or hyperthermia. Central apnea also may be associated with maternal narcotics, hypermagnesemia, or general anesthesia. Interventions for central apnea are gentle tactile stimulation and positive-pressure ventilation. Naloxone, correction of temperature and metabolic disturbances, continuous positive airway pressure, and mechanical ventilation also may stabilize the infant. Use of methyl-

Table 191-5. Life-Threatening Problems and Care Considerations for the Newly Born Infant after Initial Resuscitation*

Select Differential Diagnoses	Diagnostic and Therapeutic Considerations
Central Apnea	
Asphyxia	High risk for seizures and multisystem organ failure
Maternal narcotics	Naloxone, intubation
Hypermagnesemia	No specific antagonist
Maternal general anesthesia	Bag-mask ventilation for 5–10 min may avoid intubation
Obstructive Apnea	
Choanal atresia	Oral airway
Vocal cord paralysis/edema	Observation, racemic epinephrine, helium-oxygen gas mixture, laryngeal mask airway
Upper airway anomaly	Laryngeal mask airway, tracheostomy
Micrognathia	Prone position, oral airway, laryngeal mask airway
Respiratory Disease	
Pneumothorax	Thoracentesis, nitrogen washout, high-frequency ventilation
Congenital diaphragmatic hernia	Immediate intubation, orogastric tube, high risk for persistent pulmonary hypertension, and pneumothorax, consider surfactant
Pulmonary hypoplasia	Low threshold for intubation, high risk for pneumothorax, high-frequency ventilation
Hyaline membrane disease	Continuous positive airway pressure, surfactant
Transient tachypnea	Supportive therapy, increased risk after cesarean birth
Pneumonia/sepsis	Antibiotics, volume resuscitation
Persistent pulmonary hypertension	Oxygen lability, pre/postductal difference in oxygen saturation, hyperventilation, consider surfactant and inhaled nitric oxide
Meconium aspiration	Tracheal suctioning, consider surfactant
Congenital heart disease	Cyanosis unresponsive to oxygen, pulmonary compliance often normal, prostaglandin infusion
Hydrops/anasarca	Thoracentesis, paracentesis, pericardiocentesis, pulmonary hypoplasia, pleural effusions, high-frequency ventilation
Diminished Pulses, Pallor, Poor Perfusion, Bradycardia	
Asphyxia	Volume resuscitation, dopamine
Acute blood loss	Volume resuscitation, emergency red blood cell transfusion
Sepsis	Volume resuscitation and antibiotics
Hypoplastic left heart syndrome, aortic atresia/stenosis, severe coarctation of the aorta	Widely patent ductus arteriosus may allow cardiovascular compensation for days to weeks, prostaglandin E1, dopamine, judicious volume expansion
Congenital diaphragmatic hernia	Cardiovascular compromise with mediastinal shift and/or complicating pneumothorax; see Respiratory Distress above
Tension pneumothorax	See Respiratory Distress above
Hypertrophic cardiomyopathy	Vasopressors may worsen left ventricular outflow tract obstruction, infant of diabetic mother
Congenital heart block	Often asymptomatic, maternal collagen disease
Hypothermia	Overhead warmer, warmed blankets, kangaroo care
Seizures	
Hypoxic-ischemic encephalopathy; metabolic disturbances	Phenobarbital, intravenous glucose or calcium

*Subspecialty consultation is often recommended.

Table 191-6. Non–Life-Threatening Problems and Care Considerations for the Newly Born Infant after Initial Resuscitation

Select Differential Diagnoses	Diagnostic and Therapeutic Considerations
Bilious and/or Copious Gastric Secretions, Abdominal Distention, Excessive Oral Secretions	
Esophageal atresia	Inability to pass orogastric tube, urgent surgical gastric decompression
Bowel obstruction or ileus	Orogastric decompression
Renal mass	Risk for pulmonary hypoplasia, pneumothorax, flattened facies, low-set ears, clubfeet (Potter syndrome)
Meconium ileus	Risk for cystic fibrosis, surgical consultation
Bowel perforation	Paracentesis, surgical consultation
Hepatosplenomegaly	Hemolytic anemia, congenital infection
Gaseous distention	Positive-pressure ventilation
Congenital Anomalies	
Gastroschisis, omphalocele	Sterile "bowel bag," volume expansion, positioning, latex precautions, midline anomaly evaluation, temperature control
Meningomyelocele	Latex precautions, sterile occlusive dressing and/or sterile bowel bag
Multiple congenital anomalies	Multisystem evaluation
Ambiguous genitalia	Multisystem evaluation, family support, postpone choice of first name or choose gender-neutral name
Bladder or cloacal extrophy	Sterile bowel bag, saline dressing, latex precautions
Congenital Anomalies	
Patent ductus arteriosus	Murmur present after fall in pulmonary vascular resistance, often after leaving delivery room
Congenital heart disease	Heart murmurs unusual immediately after birth, high index of suspicion for congenital heart disease, prostaglandin, chest radiograph, echocardiogram
Jitteriness	
Hypothermia	Radiant warmer, warm blankets, kangaroo care
Hypoglycemia	Early feeding and/or intravenous glucose
Hypocalcemia	Intravenous calcium
Jaundice, Yellow Skin Discoloration	
Isoimmune hyperbilirubinemia	Evaluation recommended if jaundice present before 24 hr of age, anemia, phototherapy, see Hydrops/Anasarca (Table 191-5)
Meconium staining	Risk for asphyxia and meconium aspiration

or cyanosis and respiratory distress during initial oral feedings or when the mouth is closed. If the newborn cannot compensate by mouth breathing, an oral airway or endotracheal intubation may be lifesaving. Stridor or increased work of breathing with inadequate or absent breath sounds may indicate vocal cord paralysis (may follow difficult vaginal delivery and brachial plexus injury), vocal cord edema (may follow endotracheal intubation for meconium), laryngotracheal anomaly/malacia, or significant micrognathia with pharyngeal obstruction by the tongue. If respirations are labored and accompanied by cyanosis or bradycardia, treatment with prone positioning, endotracheal intubation, tracheostomy, racemic epinephrine, oxygen, or a helium/oxygen mixture may support the infant until definitive diagnostic evaluations or referrals can be made.

Respiratory Distress

Respiratory distress in the delivery room is associated with many intrinsic pulmonary and cardiac disorders and upper airway anomalies. Severe respiratory distress caused by tension pneumothorax, congenital diaphragmatic hernia, and pulmonary hypoplasia requires immediate stabilization and intervention. Signs of spontaneous pneumothorax are respiratory distress; coarse crackles on auscultation; absent or diminished breath sounds, often unilateral in location; and shift of the heart sounds to the contralateral chest cavity. Transillumination using a fiberoptic light and chest radiograph are helpful. Transillumination, a bedside assessment, eliminates the time required to obtain and read chest radiographs. Initial resuscitation measures, thoracentesis (see Fig. 191-3), and chest tube placement may be required. Nitrogen washout treatment of pneumothorax in infants without significant respiratory distress or bradycardia can be attempted by placing the infant in an oxygen hood with FIO_2 1.0 for up to 24 hours.

Signs of congenital diaphragmatic hernia are severe respiratory distress, unilateral absence of breath sounds, and shift of heart sounds to the contralateral chest cavity (usually to the right because 80% of diaphragmatic hernias are left-sided). Other clues include scaphoid abdomen and absent transillumination on the ipsilateral side of the hernia. Chest radiographs often are diagnostic. If diaphragmatic hernia is suspected in the delivery room, immediate intubation and placement of an orogastric tube is recommended.

Pulmonary hypoplasia presents with severe respiratory distress and symmetric but diminished breath sounds. High positive pressures are required in the most severe cases. Transillumination is negative, unless the course is complicated by pneumothorax. Initial resuscitation, positive-pressure ventilation, thoracentesis for complicating pneumothorax, and mechanical ventilation often are required. In performing diagnostic and therapeutic interventions, pathology associated with pulmonary hypoplasia must be considered, including oligohydramnios, renal anomalies, abdominal mass, congenital diaphragmatic hernia, ascites, hydrops, pleural effusions, lung mass, or idiopathic pulmonary hypoplasia.

Hyaline membrane disease, transient tachypnea, meconium aspiration, pneumonia, and persistent pulmonary hypertension require early recognition and treatment to prevent hypoxemia and acidosis. Acuity of illness and

xanthines generally is reserved for preterm infants in whom other causes for apnea after delivery have been excluded.

Obstructive apnea may present as cyanosis or bradycardia associated with increased work of breathing, poor air movement, or absent breath sounds. Choanal atresia is suggested by absence of air movement through the nares by auscultation, inability to pass a catheter through the nares, urgency of resuscitation in these conditions are high but usually are not as urgent as with apnea, tension pneumothorax, congenital diaphragmatic hernia, or pulmonary hypoplasia. Supportive care and specific treatments, such as oxygen, positive-pressure ventilation, continuous positive airway pressure, mechanical ventilation, antibiotics, and surfactant, may be indicated.

Congenital heart disease also may present with respiratory distress in the delivery room. Signs of cyanotic cardiac lesions are cyanosis, heart murmur, and unlabored tachypnea. Many ductal-dependent cardiac lesions present hours to days after birth when the ductus arteriosus closes. Indications of persistent pulmonary hypertension include cyanosis, systolic heart murmur (tricuspid insufficiency), and tachypnea (often labored and associated with respiratory disorders, such as meconium aspiration, transient tachypnea, pneumonia, sepsis, and hyaline membrane disease). Clinical differentiation between the more common persistent pulmonary hypertension and cyanotic congenital heart disease is often possible within the first minutes to hours of life. Clinical differentiation in the delivery room is based on an increase in PaO_2 (>100 mm Hg) or oxygen saturation (>95%) with a trial of supplemental oxygen or hyperventilation or both. A difference in preductal and postductal oxygen saturations and lability in oxygenation favor the diagnosis of persistent pulmonary hypertension. If cyanosis persists, echocardiographic examination usually is diagnostic. If cyanosis in the delivery room persists despite oxygen and mechanical ventilation, a diagnosis of ductal-dependent congenital heart disease and treatment with prostaglandin E-1 should be considered.

Diminished Pulses, Pallor, Poor Perfusion, and Bradycardia

Pulses that are difficult to palpate, pallor, delayed capillary refill (poor perfusion), and bradycardia often indicate shock. Hypovolemic shock associated with acute blood loss during delivery, asphyxia, and overwhelming sepsis may require volume expansion with normal saline, Ringer lactate, or red blood cell transfusion and dopamine infusion. The volume of fluid administered to expand intravascular volume and when to add dopamine in the delivery room must be based on clinical response and physician judgment. Guidelines cannot be more specific because of large variability in clinical situations and treatment response of the newborn infant.

Shock also can be secondary to pneumothorax, congenital diaphragmatic hernia, and respiratory disorders that compromise cardiac output and venous return. Effective treatment in these conditions requires specific interventions that address the underlying cause (e.g., thoracentesis, intubation, gastric decompression with an orogastric tube, adjustment in positive-pressure ventilation, pericardiocentesis, and paracentesis). Cardiogenic shock associated with asphyxia, septic cardiomyopathy, and congenital heart disease may require volume expansion, dopamine infusion, or prostaglandin infusion in the delivery room after initial resuscitation. Subsequent therapies must be based on the underlying cause of shock.

Diminished or absent pulses also may be the presenting findings for infants with coarctation of the aorta, hypoplas-

tic left heart syndrome, aortic valve stenosis, hypoplastic aortic arch, and hypertrophic cardiomyopathy. Other signs include respiratory distress, pallor, cyanosis, and heart murmurs. Four-extremity blood pressures may be helpful, but can be normal if the ductus is widely patent. If there is concern about these lesions, the clinician can perform serial four-extremity blood pressures, a repeat physical evaluation, a chest radiograph, and an echocardiogram. Neonates with hypoplastic left heart and single ventricle often present with cyanosis, heart murmur, and respiratory distress and are at risk for excessive pulmonary blood flow and diminished systemic blood flow as pulmonary vascular resistance decreases. Oxygen and mechanical ventilation may be needed to treat hypoxia and persistent pulmonary hypertension. If interventions that lower pulmonary vascular resistance (oxygen, mechanical ventilation) result in worsening perfusion, poor capillary refill, diminished pulses, and hypotension, hypoplastic left heart or single ventricle should be considered. If the addition of dopamine or other vasopressor agents results in worsening perfusion, a diagnosis of hypertrophic cardiomyopathy is possible, especially in an infant of a diabetic mother.

Bradycardia most often indicates asphyxia, shock, and impending death when present in the delivery room. Acute resuscitation is necessary to increase heart rate and cardiac output. Other potential causes for bradycardia include hypothermia, hypocalcemia, and congenital heart block. Treatments include use of a radiant warmer, calcium infusion, electrocardiogram, and chronotropic agents (e.g., isoproterenol, epinephrine).

Non–Life-Threatening Conditions Requiring Specific Delivery Room Interventions

See also Table 191-6.

Bilious or Copious Gastric Secretions, Abdominal Distention, or Excessive Oral Secretions

Bilious or copious gastric secretions or abdominal distention should prompt concern about bowel obstruction. When bowel obstruction is suspected, orogastric tube placement to low intermittent (feeding tube) or continuous (Replogle tube) suction is warranted until a diagnosis is established. If oral secretions are copious, swallowing dysfunction or esophageal atresia should be considered. Esophageal atresia can be confirmed by an inability to pass a catheter into the stomach and a chest radiograph (which includes the neck) that shows the catheter curled in the proximal esophageal pouch. Because the most common type of esophageal atresia includes a fistula from the trachea to the distal esophagus, gastric distention may occur, especially in neonates who require positive-pressure ventilation. Prompt referral for gastric decompression with a gastrostomy tube is recommended.

Abdominal distention may follow resuscitation requiring bag-mask ventilation or be associated with other conditions (e.g., renal mass or obstruction, bowel obstruction, volvulus, meconium ileus, imperforate anus, hepatosplenomegaly). Gastric decompression with an orogastric tube to straight drainage or suction should be provided in the delivery room. Diagnostic and therapeutic evaluation should be performed promptly.

Abdominal Wall Defects

Gastroschisis and omphalocele are obvious anomalies that require immediate intervention with orogastric tube placement, fluid resuscitation (150 to 200 mL/kg/day), antibiotics, and placement of the lower body into a sterile "bowel bag" at the time of delivery. Omphalocele is associated with other anomalies in about 50% of cases. A complete physical examination with evaluation of midline structures and monitoring of blood glucose (Beckwith-Wiedemann syndrome) is warranted. Careful positioning of the infant with gastroschisis is important to maximize bowel perfusion because the unsupported bowel has a tendency to twist and kink the vascular supply. Latex precautions and immediate referral for surgical intervention are indicated. Temperature monitoring is essential.

Meningomyelocele

Meningomyelocele, encephalocele, sacral dimples, and sacrococcygeal teratomas are detected easily on examination of the back and spine. If a meningomyelocele is open, the infant is placed in the prone position, and the lower body and meningomyelocele are put into a sterile bowel bag to minimize infection and fluid loss. An alternative is to place a protective sterile dressing moistened with normal saline over the meningomyelocele. Evidence for hydrocephalus and other anomalies should be sought. Latex precautions are particularly important in these infants.

Multiple Congenital Anomalies, Ambiguous Genitalia, and Bladder/Cloacal Exstrophy

Newborn infants with multiple dysmorphic features or ambiguous genitalia require extensive evaluation, multidisciplinary consultation, and sensitive, honest parental counseling. Resuscitation should be provided, unless a lethal diagnosis has been established prenatally and a plan of comfort care established by parents and caregivers. After stabilization, a complete physical examination, urgent radiographic studies, and parental counseling regarding suspected diagnoses and potential outcomes should be provided. If a specific diagnosis and outcomes prediction requires further investigation and consultation, a diagnostic, therapeutic, and consultation plan for the parents and family may be comforting. The clinician needs to estimate the duration of the diagnostic phase and acknowledge empathetically the family's grief. Families should be advised to consider gender-neutral names if they decide to choose a first name in an infant with ambiguous genitalia before sex has been determined. Bladder/cloacal exstrophy requires a saline-moistened protective dressing, bowel bag, and latex precautions.

APGAR SCORE—A TOOL FOR COMMUNICATION

The Apgar score was developed to communicate the clinical status of newborn infants during the first minutes of life. The five categories scored are respiratory effort, heart rate, color, reflex irritability, and muscle tone (Table 191-7). Although several of these categories also are used to make decisions about neonatal resuscitation, resuscitation begins at the time of birth, if needed. By 90 to 120 seconds of age in depressed newly born infants, resuscitation should be well into its course. Apgar scores should not be used to guide the

Table 191-7. Apgar Scores

Sign	Score		
	0	1	2
Heart rate	Absent	<100	≥100
Respiratory effort	Absent	Slow, irregular	Good, crying
Muscle tone	Limp	Some flexion	Active movement
Reflex irritability (catheter in nares or tactile stimulation)	No response	Grimace	Cough, sneeze cry
Color	Blue or pale	Pink body and blue extremities (acrocyanosis)	Pink body and extremities

need for resuscitation. Apgar scores are assigned at 1 and 5 minutes and then every 5 minutes until the Apgar score is greater than 7.

OUTCOME OF NEONATAL RESUSCITATION

Although outcomes of resuscitation are specific to the causes, most neonatal conditions presenting in the delivery room are amenable to supportive, medical, or surgical interventions. Asphyxia may complicate the birth of infants with a variety of problems. Families can be reassured that most depressed neonates recover and have an excellent chance for normal growth and neurodevelopment. Although Apgar scores are primarily a communication tool to describe a newborn's physiologic status at specified times after birth, many clinicians broadly assess the risk of neurodevelopmental disability based on Apgar scores. An Apgar score of 0 at 15 minutes almost uniformly predicts death or severe disability. More than 60% of neonates with an Apgar score of 1 at 1 minute survive, however, and greater than 60% of survivors have a normal outcome. Neonates with Apgar scores greater than 5 usually have normal growth and neurodevelopment.

SUMMARY

Newborn infants frequently need resuscitative intervention to help transition from the fetal to postnatal environment. Outcomes for survival and neurodevelopment are disease specific but are generally good. The Neonatal Resuscitation Program sponsored by the American Academy of Pediatrics and American Heart Association provides excellent educational and technical material for all caregivers responsible for care of newly born infants. Physicians, nurses, and respiratory care clinicians who work with newly born infants should participate in this knowledge and skills course.

Mini-index of Related Topics

SUGGESTED READINGS

Braner D, Kattwinkel J, Denson SE, et al (eds), for American Academy of Pediatrics and American Heart Association: Textbook of Neonatal Resuscitation, 4th ed. Elk Grove Village, Ill, American Academy of Pediatrics, 2000.

Evidence Evaluation Worksheets, Neonatal Resuscitation Program, 2001. Available at: http://www.aap.org/profed/nrp/nrpmain.html.

Hauth JC, Merenstein GB (eds), for American Academy of Pediatrics

and American College of Obstetricians and Gynecologists: Guidelines for Perinatal Care, 4th ed. Elk Grove Village, Ill, American Academy of Pediatrics, 1997.

Hertz D: Principles of neonatal resuscitation. In Polin RA, Yoder MC, Burg FD (eds): Workbook in Pediatrics, 3rd ed. Philadelphia, WB Saunders, 2001, pp 1–27.

Wiswell TE, Gannon CM, Jacob J, et al: Delivery room management of the apparently vigorous meconium-stained neonate: Results of the multicenter, international collaborative trial. Pediatrics 2000;105:1–7.

SECTION 5   NEWBORN CARE: *Perinatal Care*

192 Birth Injury and Asphyxia

Adam A. Rosenberg

ROLE OF THE GENERALIST

1   Recognize perinatal conditions that increase risk for traumatic or hypoxic-ischemic injury.

2   Recognize promptly serious traumatic injury and the clinical manifestations of neonatal seizures, and institute early and effective treatment.

3   Recognize the multiorgan consequences that result from perinatal asphyxia to allow appropriate diagnosis and multisystem management.

4   Be able to use the severity classification of neonatal hypoxic-ischemic encephalopathy and identify infants with a degree of multiorgan dysfunction or hypoxic-ischemic encephalopathy who require consultation or referral to a tertiary care center.

5   Recognize traumatic conditions, including subgaleal bleeding and extensive intracranial bleeding, that require emergent treatments, consultation, or referral to a tertiary care center.

6   Know the outcome and long-term sequelae of traumatic and hypoxic-ischemic birth injury, and coordinate comprehensive follow-up for these sequelae.

Birth injuries are injuries sustained during the labor and delivery process. These injuries can be divided into injuries from physical trauma during the birth process *(traumatic birth injury)* and injuries from lack of oxygen *(hypoxic-ischemic injury* and *perinatal asphyxia)*. These types of injuries can occur separately or in combination.

TRAUMATIC BIRTH INJURY

Traumatic injuries often result from discrepancy between the size or position of the fetus in relation to the birth canal or from an unusually rigid pelvis that has not been adapted

gradually to the size of the fetal head. Although birth injury accounts for fewer than 2% of neonatal deaths and still-borns, six to eight injuries per 1000 live births are reported. Improvements in obstetric care have consistently decreased the frequency of birth injury as a cause for perinatal mortality. Predisposing factors for traumatic birth injury are listed in Table 192-1. Clinicians should be especially aware of poorly controlled diabetic pregnancies with macrosomic or large-for-gestational-age fetuses. Cesarean section does not eliminate the possibility of birth trauma, especially when prior attempts at delivery with vacuum extraction or forceps or both have occurred. Table 192-2 summarizes common types of injuries. Many injuries, such as soft tissue trauma, are minor, but others, such as liver laceration, subgaleal bleeding, or large subdural blood collections, are life-threatening and require prompt recognition and intervention. Traumatic birth injury can result in physical and neurodevelopmental handicaps.

Table 192-1. Risk Factors for Traumatic Birth Injury

Rigid birth canal
    Primiparous
    Older multipara
    Small malformed pelvis
Failure of adequate birth canal adaptation
    Breech position
    Precipitous delivery
Large infant relative to size of birth canal
    Macrosomia
    Cephalopelvic disproportion
    Shoulder dystocia
Other
    Abnormal presentations (face, brow, transverse)
    Use of vacuum or forceps, difficult rotations
    Prematurity

Table 192-2. Traumatic Birth Injuries

Type of Injury	Examples
Soft tissue injuries	Abrasions, bruising, fat necrosis, lacerations
Extracranial bleeding	Cephalhematoma, subgaleal
Intracranial bleeding	Subarachnoid, epidural, subdural, cerebral, cerebellar
Nerve injuries	Facial, cervical nerve roots (brachial plexus palsies, phrenic), Horner syndrome, recurrent laryngeal
Spinal cord injuries	
Fractures	Clavicle, humerus, femur, skull
Dislocations	
Torticollis*	
Eye injuries	Subconjunctival and retinal hemorrhage
Solid organ injury	Liver, spleen

*Secondary to bleeding in the sternocleidomastoid muscle.

Head Trauma
Fundamentals and Diagnosis
The spectrum of traumatic injury to the head is wide. Minor trauma includes injuries from intrauterine fetal scalp electrodes, lacerations, bruising over the presenting part, and caput succedaneum (Fig. 192-1). Caput succedaneum is localized scalp edema from the pressure of the head applied to the dilating cervix. The edema is soft, is superficial, crosses suture lines, and resolves over the first few postnatal days. Cephalhematomas are localized subperiosteal collections of blood that occur in 0.2% to 2.5% of live births. The incidence is increased substantially in forceps deliveries. Cephalhematomas are caused by rupture of blood vessels that traverse from the skull to the periosteum. The bleeding is subperiosteal and is limited by suture lines in the skull (see Fig. 192-1). The most common site for these collections is over the parietal bones. Cephalhematomas are most often unilateral. Cephalhematomas manifest as a firm, tense mass that enlarges after birth. Rarely is the degree of blood loss sufficient to cause either hemodynamic instability or anemia. Linear skull fractures beneath the hematoma have been reported in about 5% of cases but are of no major consequence except in the unlikely event of formation of a leptomeningeal cyst. This cyst is indicated by a widening fracture accompanied by an extracranial, enlarging, fluid-filled mass. Most cephalhematomas resorb in 2 weeks to 3 months, leaving some residual circular calcification at the base. Depressed skull fractures can be seen in neonates but rarely require surgical elevation because of the resilient nature of neonatal bone, resulting in a "ping-pong" deformity without discontinuity. The fracture can be confirmed with plain skull films. Because depressed fractures can be associated with intracranial bleeding, computed tomography (CT) of the head is indicated, especially if neurologic symptoms are present.

Subgaleal hemorrhage occurs beneath the scalp in the subaponeurotic space (see Fig. 192-1). The galea aponeurotica extends from the occiput to the eyebrows in the anteroposterior direction and laterally to the insertion of the temporalis fascia. The injury results from traction on the scalp shearing the emissary veins between the scalp and intracranial venous sinuses. The most common risk factor is a difficult vacuum or forceps extraction. These bleeds are characterized by boggy fluid collections with a ballotable fluid wave beneath the scalp with bleeding extending to above the eyes back to the insertion of the trapezius muscles. The ears are pushed forward with a large subgaleal fluid collection. In contrast to caput succedaneum, this fluid collection increases in size after birth. The infant's occipitofrontal circumference increases 1 cm with each 40 mL of blood. The space is large, allowing extensive blood loss with shock and anemia. These infants can present early in life with pallor, tachycardia, tachypnea, mottling, delayed capillary refill, hypotension, and hypotonia. Over the first few hours of life, the hematocrit decreases, and shock and its treatment lead to dilution and consumption of clotting factors. A clinical coagulopathy may exacerbate blood loss further.

Traumatic intracranial hemorrhages include epidural; subdural; subarachnoid; and, less commonly, intraventricular, intracerebral, and intracerebellar bleeds. Bleeding within the brain is more common in preterm infants. Epidural bleeds (see Fig. 192-1) are rare. Linear skull fractures in the parietotemporal region are present in most cases. Irritability, lethargy, and seizures progress to signs of increased intracranial pressure (full fontanelle, hypertension, and bradycardia) ultimately with unilateral pupil dilation indicating uncal herniation. Diagnosis is confirmed by CT scan showing a characteristic convex, lenslike appearance of the epidural blood collection.

Three major varieties of subdural bleeds have been described: (1) posterior fossa hematomas from tentorial laceration with rupture of the straight sinus, vein of Galen, or transverse sinuses (Fig. 192-2) or from occipital osteodiastasis (a separation between the squamous and lateral portions of the occipital bone); (2) falx laceration, with rupture of the inferior sagittal sinus (see Fig. 192-2); and (3) rupture of the superficial bridging cerebral veins. Clinical symptoms are related to the location of the bleeding; occur within 24 hours of birth; and include focal or generalized seizure activity, altered level of consciousness, irritability, and focal neurologic signs.

Posterior fossa collections lead to signs of brainstem compression or signs of increased intracranial pressure from obstruction of spinal fluid flow. Initial signs are altered level of consciousness, lateral deviation of the eyes not altered by a doll's eyes maneuver, and unequal pupils. Lower brain-

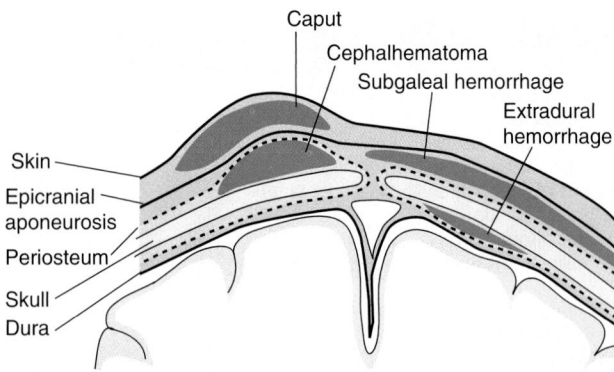

Figure 192-1. Sites of extracranial and extradural hemorrhages in the newborn. (Adapted from Pape KE, Wigglesworth JS: Haemorrhage, Ischemia and the Perinatal Brain. Philadelphia, JB Lippincott, 1979.)

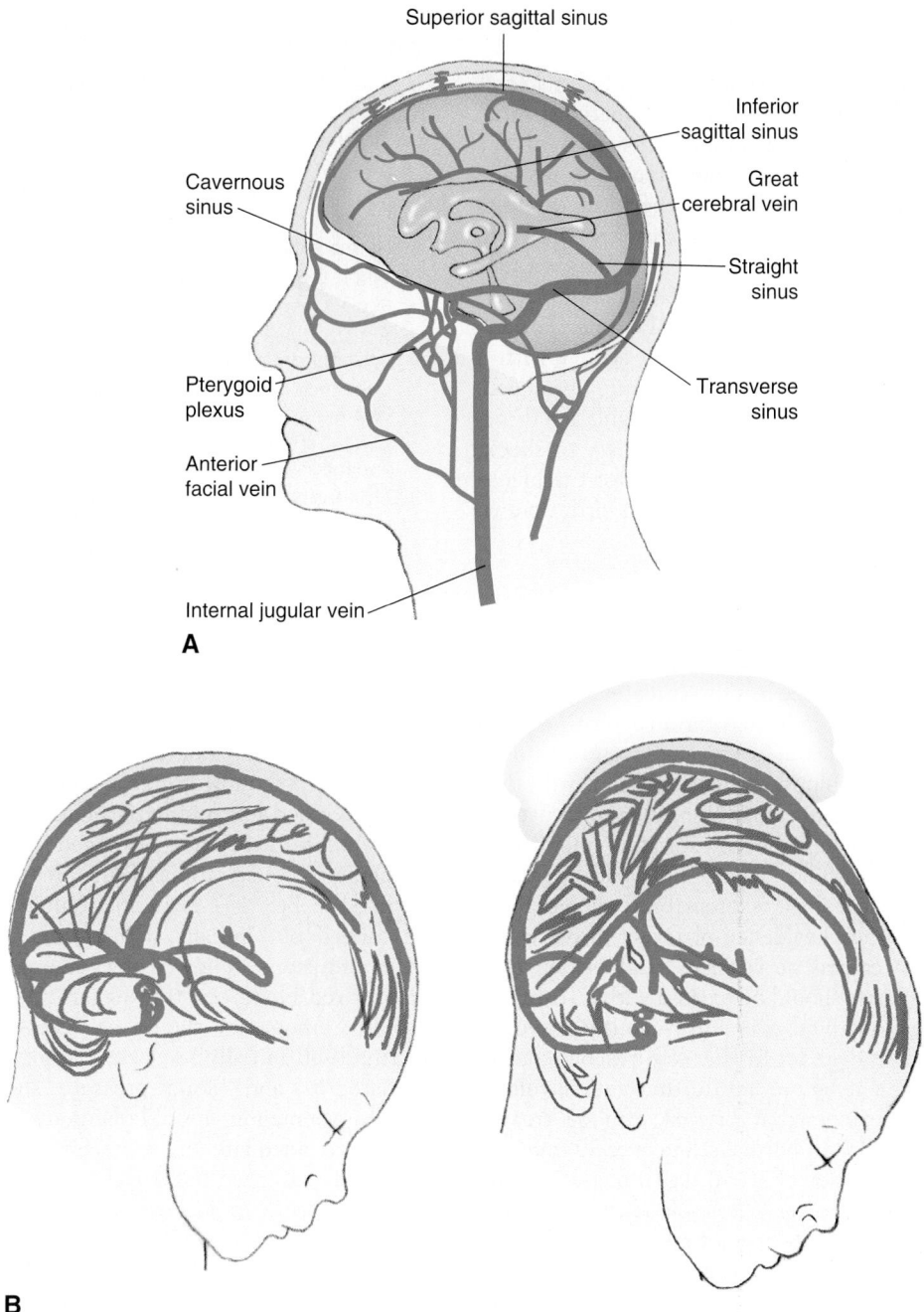

Figure 192-2. A, Major cranial veins and dural sinuses. **B,** The mechanism of tentorial hemorrhage after vacuum extraction. Traction in the occipital-frontal direction produces stress on the vertical axis of the falx and tentorium with kinking of the deep venous drainage of the brain. (**A,** Adapted from Intracranial hemorrhage: Subdural, intracerebellar, intraventricular (term infant), and miscellaneous. In Volpe JJ [ed]: Neurology of the Newborn, 4th ed. Philadelphia, WB Saunders, 2001, p 397. **B,** Adapted from Hanigan WC, Morgan AM, Stahlberg LK, et al: Tentorial hemorrhage associated with vacuum extraction. Pediatrics 1990;85:534–539.)

stem signs can follow, including apnea and bradycardia. Falx tears can cause bilateral cerebral signs (e.g., seizures and focal weakness) or can be asymptomatic. If the bleeding extends infratentorially, signs of brainstem compression evolve. Hemorrhage over the cerebral convexities is the most common site of subdural bleeding and presents with focal or multifocal seizures and focal cerebral signs. In rare circumstances, the accumulation of blood can be large enough to increase intracranial pressure and lead to uncal herniation. Limited subarachnoid bleeding may be asymptomatic; when bleeding is more extensive, irritability and seizures alternate with normal interictal periods. Other, less

common sites of traumatic bleeding are intracerebellar (associated with occipital osteodiastasis), which presents with signs of brainstem compression, and intraventicular, which usually presents with seizures.

Focal intracranial pathology does not always present with focal seizure activity. Neonatal seizures are most commonly subtle, characterized by mouth (sucking) movements; abnormal eye blinking or tonic horizontal deviation; boxing, hooking, or bicycling movements of the limbs; and respiratory (apnea) and heart rate (sudden episodes of tachycardia or bradycardia) abnormalities. Other types of seizures seen in newborns include focal and multifocal (involves more than one site and is asynchronous and migratory) clonic episodes.

Helpful diagnostic tests to evaluate suspected intracranial bleeding include repeated clinical examinations; serial hematocrits to assess blood loss; and brain imaging with CT for epidural, subdural, or subarachnoid blood. A bedside ultrasound examination, although easy to perform, can miss significant blood collections located in close proximity to the skull. A lumbar puncture can be done in infants without signs of increased intracranial pressure. Xanthochromia, red blood cells, and an increased protein level support a diagnosis of intracranial bleeding. Coagulation screen with a prothrombin time, partial thromboplastin time, fibrinogen, and platelet count helps assess congenital coagulation disorders, diffuse intravascular coagulation secondary to shock, and isoimmune thrombocytopenia as causes for the bleeding, especially in cases without overt history of birth trauma.

Management

The management of traumatic head injuries consists of recognition, monitoring, and treatment of serious consequences. The generalist with careful diagnosis and observation can manage many of the less life-threatening injuries. Referral or consultation is indicated for difficult-to-control seizures; depressed skull fractures; any posterior fossa, subdural, or epidural blood collection; and subgaleal bleeding (Box 192-1). Infants at risk for intracranial pathology should have continuous cardiorespiratory monitoring for apnea, periodic breathing, hypotension, and heart rate irregularities. Serial neurologic examinations should focus on level of consciousness, evidence of focal muscle weakness, brainstem or cranial nerve signs, and evidence of seizure activity. Seizures should be treated with a 10-mg/kg loading dose of phenobarbital given intravenously. A second 10-mg/kg dose can be given for further seizures, but consultation should be sought before any further anticonvulsant administration. Hypovolemia, if present, can be treated with a 10-mL/kg infusion of normal saline over 30 minutes, repeated twice more (a total of 30 mL/kg) if blood pressure and perfusion do not improve. Whole-blood or packed red blood cell transfusions usually are not necessary with most traumatic intracranial bleeds. Continued hypotension after 30 mL/kg should trigger consultation and an evaluation for coagulopathy and myocardial performance. Hematocrit should be followed serially, and the infant should be monitored for the development of jaundice. Infants who develop signs of increased intracranial pressure from convexity subdural bleeds or epidural collections require acute surgical drainage of the blood. Posterior fossa bleeds with

---

Box 192-1. Traumatic Birth Injuries: Indications for Referral

- Traumatic head injury with difficult-to-control seizures
- Posterior fossa subdural bleed; epidural bleed
- Subgaleal bleeding
- Depressed skull fracture
- Suspected spinal cord injury
- Brachial plexus injuries that do not resolve; persistent diaphragmatic paralysis requiring mechanical ventilation
- Displaced long bone fracture; any femur fracture

Box 192-2. Management of Subgaleal Bleeds

- Immediate placement of central venous access with an umbilical venous line
- Placement of an umbilical arterial line for blood draws and blood pressure monitoring
- Aggressive replacement of volume losses in 10- to 20-mL/kg infusions
- Normal saline
- Whole blood or packed red blood cells
- Replacement of coagulation factors and platelets
- Anticipation of 40-mL blood loss for each 1 cm increase in occipitofrontal circumference
- Correction of metabolic acidemia with 1 to 2 mEq/kg of sodium bicarbonate
- Careful attention to oxygenation with supplemental oxygen and mechanical ventilation
- Monitoring of serial hematocrits and coagulation studies (disseminated intravascular coagulation screens)
- Accurate monitoring of volume infused and urine output

---

evidence of progressive brainstem compression must be drained emergently. Consultation with a neurosurgeon should occur in the case of a depressed skull fracture. These fractures can be observed or can be elevated externally (e.g., with an obstetric vacuum). Surgical elevation rarely is indicated.

Acute blood loss and hypovolemia from subgaleal bleeding is a life-threatening emergency that should prompt immediate consultation. Principles of stabilization are outlined in Box 192-2. Acute volume resuscitation should be carried out initially with normal saline as 10-mL/kg bolus infusions followed by emergent whole-blood or packed red blood cell transfusion. O-negative blood available for emergency should be accessed and fresh frozen plasma used initially for a developing coagulopathy. Serial hematocrits and blood pressure should be monitored closely. Maintaining a stable hemodynamic status is crucial to ensure adequate organ perfusion. Pressors should be added (dopamine, 5 to 20 µg/kg/min) if volume alone is not sufficient or if cardiac decompensation coexists.

Traumatic Nerve and Spinal Cord Injuries
Fundamentals and Diagnosis

Brachial plexus injuries occur in 0.5 to 2/1000 live births and are caused by stretching of the cervical nerve roots from traction on the neck during delivery. Upper arm palsy (Erb-Duchenne) is the most common injury and is caused by damage to the fifth and sixth cervical nerve roots. Isolated lower arm palsies (Klumpke) that result from damage to the eighth cervical and first thoracic nerves are rare. Damage to all the nerve roots results in total arm paralysis. Because these are stretch rather than avulsion injuries, recovery of function usually occurs over the first several weeks or months of life. Diagnosis is based on the presence of unilateral arm weakness. In Erb paralysis, the arm is limp at the side and internally rotated with flexion of the fingers ("waiter's tip" position). Loss of finger extension can be confirmed by stroking the back of the hand. The presence of a grasp reflex differentiates Erb palsy from total arm paralysis. The presence of tachypnea and an oxygen requirement suggests brachial plexus injuries associated with damage to the nerve roots that form the phrenic nerve and control diaphragmatic function. Other clinical indications are asymmetric chest motion during respiration and diminished breath sounds on the side of the paralysis. The diagnosis is suggested by an elevated hemidiaphragm on a chest x-ray and can be confirmed by an ultrasound examination showing either lack of movement or paradoxical movement of the diaphragm. In addition, damage to the sympathetic outflow via nerve root T1 can result in an associated Horner syndrome with miosis and ptosis. Finally, fractures of the clavicle and humerus and shoulder dislocations may be associated.

Facial nerve injury is the most common neonatal traumatic nerve injury (1% of live births) caused either by pressure on the facial nerve from the sacral promontory as the infant passes through the birth canal or by forceps application. The injury is commonly related to intrauterine position. Clinically, motion is lost on the affected side of the face with an open eye, drooping of the mouth, lack of expression, and an inability to wrinkle the brow. Facial nerve palsy needs to be distinguished from a congenital hypoplasia of the depressor anguli oris muscle causing a localized movement abnormality of the corner of the mouth.

Spinal cord injuries are rare but catastrophic. They are associated with midforcep rotations and difficult breech extractions causing excessive longitudinal or lateral traction or rotation. The type of lesion varies from localized hemorrhage in the anterior cornua to complete destruction of the cord at one or more levels. Epidural bleeding of the cervical cord has been described as well. Clinical presentations include (1) stillbirth or rapid neonatal death, (2) respiratory failure, and (3) generalized weakness. Clues to this diagnosis include paralysis and areflexia of the lower extremities with variable upper extremity involvement, a distended bladder, and patulous anus. These injuries should be considered in the differential diagnosis of infants with generalized hypotonia. Radiographs of the neck should be performed to rule out vertebral fracture or dislocation amenable to neurosurgical decompression. A bedside ultrasound examination can identify swelling and hemorrhage in the cord. Magnetic resonance imaging (MRI) can establish the diagnosis and rule out a potentially treatable lesion, such as an occult dysraphic state.

Management

Most nerve palsies resolve spontaneously as swelling around the nerve roots ceases. For infants with persistent weakness related to brachial plexus injuries, physical therapy to preserve joint mobility and avoid muscle tightness is indicated, beginning at about 7 to 10 days of age. Infants with diaphragmatic paralysis can be managed symptomatically with oxygen supplementation or mechanical ventilation if needed for respiratory failure. Surgical diaphragm plication should be considered for infants who remain ventilator dependent for 6 to 8 weeks. The only indicated management for a facial nerve palsy is to preserve moisture in the eye on the affected side with liquid tears or lid closure. Infants with suspected spinal cord injury should be stabilized and referred to a tertiary care center for further evaluation and management. Initial stabilization should include maintenance of adequate oxygenation and perfusion using mechanical ventilation and volume infusions as needed. The bladder should be decompressed with an indwelling catheter, the spine stabilized, and the infant sedated.

Bone and Soft Tissue Injuries

The clavicle is the most commonly fractured bone during delivery. The incidence varies from 0.5% to 1.5% of live births. Most occur during a normal, spontaneous, vaginal delivery. The incidence is increased with shoulder dystocia and breech extractions that require vigorous manipulations. The most common long bone fracture is of the humerus. Clinical signs include crepitus, pain, swelling, and decreased limb movement. Nondisplaced fractures can be asymptomatic. X-rays to document clavicular fractures are unnecessary. Fractures of the humerus and clavicle can be associated with brachial plexus palsies. Treatment other than limiting mobility of the affected arm often is not needed. Humeral fractures may require immobilization for 2 to 4 weeks, and orthopedic input should be sought. The femur is the most common bone fractured in the leg. Treatment of these fractures requires traction, suspension, and casting by an orthopedic specialist.

Injury to the soft tissues is the most common traumatic birth injury, including petechiae, bruising, and subcutaneous fat necrosis. Petechiae from delivery usually are present over the head, neck, and upper thorax. These are present after birth, do not progress, and are not associated with other bleeding. If any of these clinical points is questionable, a platelet count should be checked. Severe vaginal or scrotal edema and bruising can be seen in breech deliveries. Edema and bruising usually resolve spontaneously, but severe scrotal swelling merits a urology referral because drainage of a hematoma around the testes may be needed in a few cases. Subcutaneous fat necrosis is characterized by a localized area of induration from local ischemia secondary to trauma. The induration with red or purple discoloration usually presents late during the first week of life and resolves by 6 to 8 weeks. Most superficial injuries are related to difficult extractions from the breech position, shoulder dystocia, and use of the vacuum and forceps. Although common, most of these injuries are minor and of importance primarily because of an increased risk for significant hyperbilirubinemia.

Outcome and Follow-up of Traumatic Birth Injuries

The outcome of traumatic birth injury is related to the severity of the initial injury. Superficial soft tissue injuries resolve with the only sequelae being localized infection (scalp electrode) and neonatal hyperbilirubinemia from bruising and cephalhematoma. Subcutaneous fat necrosis can cause symptomatic hypercalcemia at 3 to 4 weeks of age that presents with vomiting, weight loss, decreased feeding, and irritability. Serial calcium determinations should be carried out in these infants over the first month of life. Fractures of the clavicle and humerus rarely are displaced and most commonly resolve without fixed immobilization. In 85% of cases, brachial plexus nerve injuries completely resolve over several days to 4 weeks. In the remainder, some sequelae can be anticipated, and close follow-up is essential. Physical therapy is useful, and patients should be evaluated for possible surgical intervention for nerve root repair if function does not return by 3 months of age. Facial nerve injuries generally resolve over the first week of life. Spinal cord injuries all result in death or paralysis with dependence on long-term care. Long-term ventilation of these infants must be considered in that context.

Infants with subarachnoid bleeding and convexity subdural bleeds generally develop normally without future seizure problems. Occasionally, hydrocephalus or persistent focal neurologic findings result. Posterior fossa subdural blood collections can result in death related to brainstem compression, hydrocephalus, and long-term neurodevelopmental sequelae among survivors. Many survivors of intracerebellar and intraventricular bleeding have neurodevelopmental sequelae. The prognosis for subgaleal bleeding correlates with the degree of brain ischemia after delayed or incomplete correction of blood loss and hypotension.

Birth trauma and asphyxia may occur together. In these cases, prognosis also depends on the degree of the associated hypoxic-ischemic insult suffered perinatally. All infants at risk for neurodevelopmental sequelae should have close monitoring of developmental milestones. Physical and occupational therapy evaluations and preliminary developmental screening at 1 and 2 years of age with the Bayley Scales of Infant Development are indicated if milestones are not being reached. For older survivors, a preschool evaluation of development and school readiness should be done. Infants discharged from the hospital on anticonvulsants should be followed for further seizures. If they remain seizure-free for 3 to 6 months, medication can be discontinued. Some recommend discontinuation only after a normal electroencephalogram is obtained.

PERINATAL ASPHYXIA

The incidence of perinatal asphyxia varies between 1% and 5% and increases with lower gestational age. Risk for perinatal asphyxia depends on conditions specific to the mother (e.g., diabetes, hypertension), fetus (e.g., multiple gestation, intrauterine growth retardation, congenital anomalies), placenta (e.g., placenta previa, abruptio placentae), and labor and delivery (e.g., prolapsed cord, oligohydramnios caused by membrane rupture, abnormal fetal presentations). The physician must be prepared to intervene on behalf of the infant to reestablish ventilation and cardiovascular stability rapidly to minimize the risk or effect of hypoxic-ischemic encephalopathy and multiorgan failure. Hypoxic-ischemic encephalopathy is the neurologic syndrome that follows an asphyxial insult and occurs in 1 to 2/1000 live births. Multiorgan failure is the result of hypoxia and ischemia on organ function. Outcome is related to the severity of the neonatal postasphyxia syndrome. Close neurodevelopmental follow-up is paramount in these infants.

Fundamentals

Perinatal asphyxia occurring during the intrapartum period includes evidence of fetal distress during labor with depression at birth requiring vigorous resuscitation. The fetal circulatory response to acute hypoxemia has been well described in experimental animals and humans (Fig. 192-3). During the sequence of events depicted in Figure 192-3,

blood flow to the kidneys, gastrointestinal tract, liver, muscle, and lungs decreases. Blood is redirected preferentially to the brain and myocardial circulations. This situation is maintained until hypoxemia is severe enough to cause myocardial depression and circulatory collapse. The pattern of organ injury after acute asphyxia can be predicted by these responses. Table 192-3 lists the elements of the possible multiorgan dysfunction present in these infants. Infants who have brain injury related to perinatal asphyxia almost uniformly manifest multiorgan injury that must be anticipated, appreciated, and managed vigorously and proactively. The features of this neurologic syndrome are presented in Table 192-4. The syndrome evolves gradually over the first 72 hours of life. Infants with mild neurologic symptoms recover rapidly, whereas infants with more severe injuries have more protracted symptoms. As cerebral edema worsens over the first 72 hours, the neurologic syndrome can become more severe and challenging. Seizures, if they occur, usually have their onset in the first 12 hours of life. Characteristically the seizures are subtle, focal, or multifocal clonic in type. The time to recovery of normal neurologic function is predictive of outcome.

Diagnosis

As with traumatic birth injury, the postasphyxia syndrome needs to be anticipated in any infant with fetal distress who requires significant resuscitation. These at-risk neonates must be monitored carefully for central nervous system and

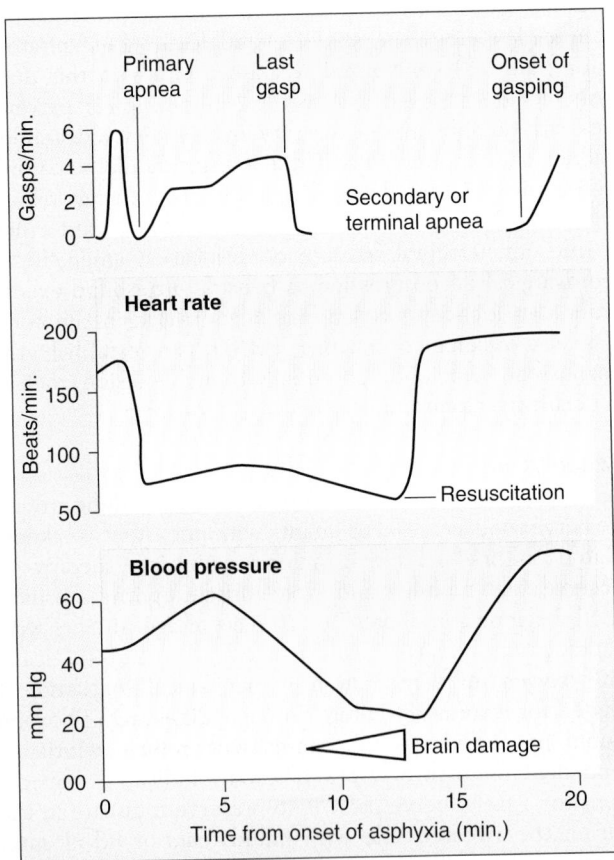

Figure 192-3. Schematic depiction of changes in rhesus monkeys during asphyxia and resuscitation. (Adapted from Birth asphyxia, resuscitation, and brain damage. In Dawes GS: Foetal and Neonatal Physiology. Chicago, Year Book Medical Publishers, 1968, p 141.)

Table 192-3. Multiorgan Dysfunction after Perinatal Asphyxia

Organ System	Clinical Features
Pulmonary	Respiratory distress due to
	Secondary surfactant deficiency
	Meconium or amniotic fluid aspiration
	Persistent pulmonary hypertension
	Shock lung
	Pulmonary hemorrhage
Cardiac	Tricuspid valve insufficiency
	Cardiogenic shock
Renal	Acute tubular necrosis with oliguria
	Acute cortical necrosis
	Asphyxiated bladder syndrome
Gastrointestinal	Gut ischemia
	Necrotizing enterocolitis
	Gastrointestinal bleeding
	Hepatic
	Elevated liver enzymes
	Abnormal clotting studies
	Cholestasis
	Hyperammonemia
Hematologic	DIC, polycythemia, thrombocytopenia
Metabolic	Hypoglycemia
	Hypocalcemia
	Hyponatremia
	Hyperkalemia
	Acidemia
Adrenal	Hemorrhage with insufficiency
Central nervous system	Cerebral edema, seizures, bleeding
	Syndrome of inappropriate ADH secretion

ADH, antidiuretic hormone; DIC, disseminated intravascular coagulation.

multiorgan hypoxic injury. Infants with severe perinatal hypoxia leading to this syndrome almost uniformly exhibit multiorgan dysfunction with central nervous system injury. An exception is an infant who suffers a hypoxic injury well before birth who survives the insult with recovery of most organ function with the exception of the brain.

The perinatal courses of infants at risk for the postasphyxia syndrome are characterized by the presence of any or all of the features listed in Table 192-3. Some degree of pulmonary dysfunction from amniotic fluid or meconium aspiration, transient surfactant production defect, pulmonary hemorrhage, or persistent pulmonary hypertension occurs in 25% of these infants. These respiratory complications present as respiratory distress with the need for supplemental oxygen and ventilatory support. Clinical evaluation to confirm the diagnosis of pulmonary hypertension in infants with high oxygen requirements includes a chest

x-ray for infiltrates and an echocardiogram to evaluate myocardial performance and pulmonary pressure. Preductal and postductal ascertainment of oxygen saturation also can aid in the diagnosis of pulmonary hypertension when a right-to-left ductal shunt indicates persistence of this fetal pattern of blood flow. In this circumstance, the preductal oxygen saturation is higher (usually by >10%) than the postductal value because high pulmonary pressures force unoxygenated blood across the ductus, diluting lower body oxygenated blood.

Myocardial injury can be indicated by a tricuspid regurgitation, systolic murmur, or systemic hypotension caused by myocardial failure and is seen in 25% of infants with the postasphyxia multiorgan syndrome. Oliguria persisting for 24 to 48 hours has been reported in 10% to 40% of infants with perinatal asphyxia. Hematuria is common, as are elevatons in serum creatinine. A transient ileus may be seen, but severe gastrointestinal injury with bleeding or necrotizing enterocolitis is rare. Screening assessment of liver function tests, a coagulation profile, whole-blood glucose, and serum calcium are other useful diagnostic tests.

The neurologic syndrome of hypoxic-ischemic encephalopathy can be divided into mild, moderate, and severe categories. The essential features of these classes are shown in Table 192-4. An electroencephalogram also is useful in assessing the severity of the neurologic syndrome. Moderately affected infants show decreased amplitude and frequency, often with associated seizure activity. The more ominous burst-suppression pattern or an isoelectric recording usually is present in severely affected infants. More recently, a single-lead cerebral function monitor has been used to assess the severity of the neurologic injury at the bedside. Imaging of the brain with CT or MRI is a useful adjunct. Early in the course of severe neurologic injury, there is evidence of cerebral edema with loss of gray-white tissue differentiation and the development of small slitlike ventricles. After 7 to 10 days, early evidence of brain atrophy can be seen. Focal infarcts or intraventricular or parenchymal hemorrhages can be associated findings.

Management

Management of the postasphyxia syndrome should be focused on a careful assessment of potentially affected organs and the degree of central nervous system dysfunction. Appropriate supportive measures are indicated with

Table 192-4. Classification of Hypoxic-Ischemic Encephalopathy

	Mild	Moderate	Severe
Level of consciousness	Hyperalert	Lethargic or obtunded	Stuporous
Muscle tone	Normal	Mild hypotonia	Flaccid
Posture	Mild distal flexion	Strong distal flexion	Decerebrate
Suck	Weak	Weak or absent	Absent
Moro reflex	Strong, low threshold	Weak, incomplete, high threshold	Absent
Oculovestibular response	Normal	Overactive	Weak or absent
Tonic neck reflex	Slight	Strong	Absent
Pupillary response	Mydriasis	Miosis	Variable, often unequal
Respiratory	Normal	Periodic breathing	Apnea
Cardiac	Tachycardia	Bradycardia	Variable
Seizures	None	Common; focal or multifocal	Variable; often difficult to control
Duration	<24 hr	2–14 days	Hours to weeks

Adapted from Sarnat HB, Sarnat MS: Neonatal encephalopathy following fetal distress: A clinical and encephalographic study. Arch Neurol 1976;33:696.

serial monitoring of existing and developing complications. Basic management principles are presented in Box 192-3. A generalist can manage mildly affected infants effectively, but severe symptoms merit the input of a specialist. General therapeutic tenets include modest fluid (free water) restriction at 60 mL/kg/day for renal and central nervous system reasons, ensuring maintenance of effective organ perfusion with isotonic fluids or pressor therapy. Glucose should be controlled carefully, keeping the blood glucose values between 50 and 100 mg/dL. Metabolic acidemia should be slowly and carefully corrected, and adequate oxygenation, ventilation, and blood pressure should be maintained to avoid secondary cerebral ischemia; medical control of seizure activity and careful surveillance for end organ abnormalities are warranted. Many new and, in some cases, investigational drugs and other therapies (e.g., hypothermia) are available to these infants in many tertiary care facilities.

Outcome

In all but the most severely affected infants, multiorgan dysfunction of the postasphyxia syndrome resolves completely. Neurodevelopmental handicap and seizure disorders occur in many fetuses exposed to perinatal hypoxic-ischemic brain injury. A variety of markers have been examined to predict outcome. Meconium in the amniotic fluid and nonreassuring fetal heart rate tracings have not proved to be good predictors of outcome. Low Apgar scores are predictive of death or cerebral palsy only with scores less than 3 after 15 minutes of resuscitation (Table 192-5). Umbilical arterial cord pH predicts an adverse neurodevelopmental outcome at levels less than 6.9. The most accurate predictor of outcome is the severity of the neonatal neurologic syndrome (Table 192-6).

Infants with mild encephalopathy all survive, and most are developmentally normal on follow-up. Moderate encephalopathy carries a 5% mortality risk and a 15% chance of late disability. More severe encephalopathy carries a 100% risk of death or disability. Other predictors of a poor outcome include inability to control seizures, a burst-suppression pattern on an electroencephalogram not related to anticonvulsants, and selected brain imaging abnormalities. Generally, infants who recover completely have a normal examination and are feeding well by 1 week of age. The long-term sequelae of intrapartum asphyxia include cerebral palsy (spastic, quadriplegia, and chorioathetoid varieties) with or without associated cognitive deficits and epilepsy. As a rule, asphyxiated term infants show tone and motor handicaps because of injury to the motor cortex, thalamus, basal ganglia, brainstem, and periventricular regions. The areas of the brain particularly vulnerable to injury are regions of watershed blood supply that are particularly prone to ischemia.

Follow-up

Close neurodevelopmental follow-up for evidence of cerebral palsy and cognitive deficits is important during the early recovery period from perinatal asphyxia. As with traumatic birth injuries, appropriate referrals for physical and occupational therapy should be made. Careful assessment of feeding abilities, ongoing seizure activity, hearing, visual acuity, and head growth needs to be done regularly. These infants are at risk for failure to thrive from inadequate oral intake on a neurologic basis and from severe

Table 192-5. Apgar Score as a Predictor of Outcome from Perinatal Asphyxia

Apgar Score of 0–3	Death in First Year (%)	Cerebral Palsy in Survivors (%)
1 min	3	1
5 min	8	1
10 min	18	5
15 min	48	9
20 min	59	57

Adapted from Nelson KB, Ellenberg JH: Apgar scores as predictors of chronic neurologic disability. Pediatrics 1981;68:36–44.

Box 192-3. Goals of Management for Perinatal Asphyxia

1. Restrict fluids to 60 mL/kg/day for renal failure and cerebral edema.
2. Maintain blood glucose in the normal range of 50 to 100 mg/dL (may need higher glucose concentrations than 10% dextrose in water).
3. Support oxygen delivery with oxygen, red blood cells, blood pressure support, and mechanical ventilation as needed. Monitor therapy with pulse oximetry and arterial blood gases. Keep arterial carbon dioxide tension in the normal range of 35 to 45 mm Hg. Dilutional partial exchanges with normal saline for hematocrits >65% are advised.
4. Support blood pressure with volume replacement and pressors as needed. The initial pressor of choice is dopamine, 5 to 20 μg/kg/min.
5. Give nothing by mouth until normal intestinal function and hunger are documented.
6. Control seizures with phenobarbital; initial loading dose is 20 mg/kg. Continue to administer phenobarbital to a total dose of 40 mg/kg. If seizures are refractory to single-drug therapy, fosphenytoin (10 to 20 mg/kg) can be added and lorazepam (0.1 mg/kg/dose).
7. Consider neuroprotection in moderate-to-severe cases of hypoxic-ischemic encephalopathy with 40 mg/kg of phenobarbital.
8. Central venous and, in some cases, arterial access should be established for monitoring and infusion of drugs and fluids.
9. Careful surveillance for clinical and laboratory evidence of organ dysfunction and neurologic status should be ongoing; accurate input and output should be recorded.

Table 192-6. Outcome from Perinatal Asphyxia; Relation to Severity of Hypoxic-Ischemic Encephalopathy

HIE Severity	No. of Patients	Deaths (%)	Cerebral Palsy or Cognitive Deficits (%)	Normal (%)
Mild	115	0	0	100
Moderate	136	5	24	71
Severe	40	80	20	0
All	291	13	14	73

HIE, hypoxic-ischemic encephalopathy.

Adapted from Robertson C, Finer N: Term infants with hypoxic-ischemic encephalopathy: Outcome at 3–5 years. Dev Med Child Neurol 1985;27(4):473–484; Thornberg E, Thiringer K, Odeback A, Milsom I: Birth asphyxia: Incidence, clinical course and outcome in a Swedish population. Acta Paediatr 1995;84(8):927–932.

gastroesophageal reflux. Infants may require home tube feedings and at some point require placement of a gastrostomy tube with or without fundoplication. Adequate medical and social support services should be sought.

Mini-index of Related Topics

SUGGESTED READINGS

American College of Obstetricians and Gynecologists, American Academy of Pediatrics: Neonatal Encephalopathy and Cerebral Palsy: Defining the Pathogenesis and Pathophysiology. American College of Obstetricians and Gynecologists. Washington, DC, 2003.

Mangurten HH: Birth injuries. In Fanaroff AA, Martin RJ (eds): Neonatal-Perinatal Medicine: Diseases of the Fetus and Infant, 6th ed. St. Louis, Mosby, 1997, p 425.

Piazza AJ: Postasphyxial management of the newborn. Clin Perinatol 1999;26:749–766.

Volpe JJ: Hypoxic-ischemic encephalopathy: Clinical aspects. In Volpe JJ (ed): Neurology of the Newborn, 4th ed. Philadelphia, WB Saunders, 2001, p 331.

Volpe JJ: Intracranial hemorrhage: Subdural, primary subarachnoid, intracerebellar, intraventricular (term infant), and miscellaneous. In Volpe JJ (ed): Neurology of the Newborn, 4th ed. Philadelphia, WB Saunders, 2001, p 397.

Volpe JJ: Perinatal trauma. In Volpe JJ (ed): Neurology of the Newborn, 4th ed. Philadelphia, WB Saunders, 2001, p 813.

SECTION 5   NEWBORN CARE: *Perinatal Care*

193 Stabilization and Transport of Ill Newborns

Carl Bose

ROLE OF THE GENERALIST

1   Develop criteria, in collaboration with obstetric care providers, which define the limits of obstetric and neonatal care in the community hospital.

2   Understand the responsibilities of the community hospital and its personnel during the transport of a neonate and prepare the hospital to fulfill these responsibilities.

3   Recognize the features of the transport environment that increase the complexity and risk of care during transport, and stabilize infants in preparation for transport using strategies that minimize the impact of these features.

4   Provide high-quality, short-term care of a neonate before transport.

5   Support the emotional needs of the family of a transported neonate.

6   Manage convalescing infants after back transport.

7   Support the education and training of nursery staff to stabilize infants optimally in preparation for transport.

A regionally coordinated system of perinatal health care requires that each hospital providing obstetric and neonatal services assess its resources and capabilities and define the limits of its scope of practice. During the antepartum or intrapartum period, each mother should be evaluated to determine whether her care or the predicted care of her newborn exceeds the capabilities of the hospital. When this occurs, the mother should be referred to a center capable of delivering more complex care. Ideally, mothers always would deliver in hospitals capable of providing the care required for their neonates. Even in the best systems of regionalized perinatal care, neonatal illness cannot always be predicted, however, and mothers may present too late in the intrapartum period to permit safe maternal transfer. Under these circumstances, personnel in the community hospital must assume the burden for resuscitation, for recognition of critical illness in the neonate, and for stabilization in preparation for transport. Optimal preparation requires that personnel understand the regulatory and other responsibilities of the referring hospital, understand the hazards of the transport environment, identify and treat the usual emergent problems, and know when and how to contact consultants for advice.

RESPONSIBILITIES OF THE COMMUNITY HOSPITAL AND ITS PERSONNEL

The responsibilities of a community hospital and its personnel related to the transfer of a neonate to another hospital are dictated by standards of medical care and ethics. These responsibilities also are mandated by Federal law for hospitals that have Medicare provider agreements under regulations delineated in the Emergency Medical Treatment and Active Labor Act (EMTALA). This act requires that hospitals provide medical screening for all patients. Stabilization must be provided for emergency medical conditions. Patients may be transferred to another hospital only after the emergency condition is stable except when transfer of an unstable patient is necessary for survival. This section provides recommendations for fulfilling the requirements of EMTALA, and other responsibilities, with the understanding that some legal requirements may vary based on local or state regulations (Box 193-1).

Criteria for Transfer

Hospitals providing obstetric services should develop criteria for transfer of mothers and neonates based on their resources, personnel, and level of competence in perinatal care. These criteria should be developed collaboratively by medical and nursing obstetric and pediatric care providers and should become part of hospital policy. Except when an emergent problem (e.g., impending delivery) makes the risks of maternal transport greater than delivery in the community hospital and subsequent neonatal transport, mothers should be referred on the basis of these criteria.

Anticipatory Planning

The transport of a critically ill neonate is rarely a scheduled event. The inability to anticipate the event does not mean, however, that it should not proceed in an orderly fashion. Established protocols for referral of neonates should provide information about each center to which a patient might be referred, including the following:

1. Available services
2. Criteria for referral
3. Telephone numbers for consultation and referral
4. Distance and usual response time

Box 193-1. Responsibilities of a Referring Physician Related to the Transfer of a Neonate to Another Hospital

1. Provide short-term care for all emergent problems.
2. Locate a center capable of providing for all of the anticipated needs of the patient.
3. Obtain an agreement for receipt of the patient from a qualified physician.
4. Arrange for transfer of the patient using a service with sufficient expertise.
5. Determine the mode of transportation.
6. Obtain consent for transfer from a parent or guardian whenever possible.
7. Support the emotional needs of the family.

Note: Many of these responsibilities are fulfilled best in collaboration with the receiving physician.

---

5. Type of transport personnel and their capabilities
6. Type of transport vehicles
7. Protocols for preparation of patients

Community hospitals should consider developing formal agreements with regional centers that include this information and denote the circumstances under which patients can be transferred without prior administrative approval.

Stabilization and the Decision to Transfer

All hospitals with obstetric services assume responsibility for providing resuscitation and stabilization of neonates delivered in their hospital, regardless of the size or condition of the newborn. To satisfy this requirement, a provider specifically trained in newborn resuscitation should attend every delivery. Nursery personnel, in conjunction with consultants from a regional center, should be prepared to provide short-term care for usual medical emergencies. A physician with pediatric experience and training should be responsible for determining whether a neonate could receive adequate long-term care in the community hospital or should be transferred to another hospital.

After a decision to transport an infant has been made, community hospital personnel have a mandated responsibility to stabilize the patient in preparation for transport. The Omnibus Budget Reconciliation Act (OBRA) of 1989 formally defines stabilization of an emergency medical condition as providing "such medical treatment of the condition as may be necessary to assure, with reasonable medical probability, that no material deterioration of the condition is likely to result from or occur during the transfer of the individual from a facility." Also the Joint Commission on Accreditation of Healthcare Organizations (JCAHO) mandates that "a hospital is capable of instituting essential lifesaving measures and implementing emergency procedures that will minimize further compromise of the condition of any infant, child, or adult being transported."

Consent

The referring physician is responsible for informing the parents or legal guardians of the need and reason for transfer and for obtaining consent. To avoid abandonment of the patient, the referring physician must contact a receiving hospital and identify a receiving physician *before* transfer. *Abandonment* is defined as "the unilateral termination of a physician-patient relationship by the physician, without the patient's consent and without giving the patient sufficient opportunity to secure the services of another competent physician." Under Federal law, the referring hospital assumes liability for the medical integrity and adequacy of the receiving hospital and the medical appropriateness of the patient's transfer. Abandonment also includes a referral that results in any degradation in the quality of care. These acts also state that patients may not be transferred solely for financial reasons.

Responsibility for Transport

A collaborative decision between the referring and the receiving physicians must be made regarding who will assume the responsibility for transport. Three options usually exist: (1) local ambulance service, (2) local ambulance with personnel from the referring hospital, or (3) transportation and personnel provided by the receiving hospital. The selection should be based on the appropriate balance between the needs of the patient and the resources of each type of provider. Because many families bear all or a portion of the costs of transport, cost should be a consideration when more than one provider or mode of transportation can satisfy the patient's needs. The referring physician is responsible for ensuring that the skills and equipment available during transport meet the anticipated needs of the patient. This responsibility usually can be dispatched most efficiently by using a transport service with documented expertise in the transport of neonates. For most critically ill neonates, ideal care occurs when personnel at the referring hospital devote their energy to providing emergent short-term care, and the responsibility for transport is left to the receiving hospital. When the referring hospital chooses to transport the patient, they must understand that they assume full responsibility for the patient until arrival in the receiving hospital.

Mode of Transportation

In many areas, physicians also have a choice between air and ground transportation. The advantage of air transportation is the reduction in travel time. Air transport should be reserved for situations in which reduction of a critical period of time during transport is likely to reduce morbidity or mortality. During neonatal transport, the critical period often ends with the arrival of the transport team because they usually are capable of administering all necessary short-term therapies. Under these circumstances, the advantage of air transport is appreciated only when air transportation markedly reduces the one-way travel time from the receiving to the referring hospital. The risks and costs of this option should be weighed carefully when distance and medical condition do not suggest a significant benefit.

Communications and Decision Making

The referring physician is responsible for providing complete historical information about the patient to the receiving physician, including the medical history of the mother, antenatal and intrapartum history, birth and early neonatal history, current vital signs, interventions performed and patient response, and results of laboratory and radiographic evaluations. Receiving physicians often make recommendations regarding stabilization of the patient. Whenever feasible, referring physicians should comply with these recommendations. They are not obliged, however, to follow recommendations deemed medically unsuitable in view of developments in the patient's condition or because of limitation of resources at the community hospital. The referring physician should notify the receiving physician of any recommendation that is not followed, and alternate management should be discussed.

When the transport team arrives, providers in the community hospital are responsible for delivering a concise report and for supplying requested medical, nursing, or technical support to the transport team. The referring physician should be physically present until the team arrives and should transfer care personally to the transport team or designate another physician to transfer care.

TRANSPORT ENVIRONMENT

Under most circumstances, the same basic therapies used in tertiary care centers can be delivered during transport. Some features of the transport environment may compromise the ability to deliver many of these therapies, however. Using strategies that minimize the impact of the environment may improve outcome. For this reason, individuals who participate in the preparation of infants for transport, in addition to individuals providing care during transport, must understand the transport environment.

Table 193-1 lists the distinguishing features of the transport environment, the effects of these features on patients and providers, and strategies to minimize the impact of these features. Strategies in which community providers have a significant role are listed in Table 193-1. In contrast to most adult trauma transport services, a "swoop and scoop" approach is contraindicated for neonatal transport. Unless the immediate needs of the patient can be met only

Table 193-1. Features of the Transport Environment: Effects and Preventive Strategies

Feature	Effect	Strategies to Minimize Impact
High sound levels	Desaturation in preterm infants Impairs ability of care providers (e.g., auscultation ineffective, communication difficult)	Use extensive electronic monitoring
Vibration	Motion artifact on monitors Indwelling devices less stable	Use monitors that are resistant to artifact Increase attention to securing devices* (e.g., additional adhesive tape) Use devices that are more stable* (e.g., plastic intravascular catheters versus metal intravenous needles)
Inadequate lighting	Impaired use of visual diagnostic aids Procedures difficult to perform	Use extensive electronic monitoring Prepare patient in anticipation of in-transit problems*
Changes in barometric pressure with ascent	Expansion of gas in closed space Decreased partial pressure of oxygen	Vent closed spaces* Oxygenate with extra margin of safety Limit ascent in some situations
Limited space and services	Limited number of care providers Limited availability of ancillary services and tests (e.g., radiography)	Perform all anticipated tests before transport* Ensure high skill level of transport personnel Provide communication link between vehicle and consultants

*Indicates strategies in which providers in referring hospitals should participate.

by sophisticated interventions in the receiving hospital (e.g., surgical intervention, inhaled nitric oxide), all necessary time should be devoted to stabilizing the patient in the referring hospital. Preparation should include not only care for the identified problems, but also anticipation of problems that may arise during transport.

PREPARATION OF A PATIENT FOR TRANSPORT

Basic Preparation
Referring hospitals should direct immediate attention to three critical areas: (1) respiration, including airway management and ventilation; (2) circulation, including the treatment of hypotension and shock; and (3) vascular access.

Respiration
The decision to intubate and mechanically ventilate a patient usually is based on objective evidence of respiratory failure. The threshold for intervention should be lower, however, for neonates requiring transport. This more aggressive approach to airway management is justified because the transport environment impairs the identification of respiratory failure and the ability to intubate and confirm appropriate tube placement. For example, an infant with a $PaCO_2$ of 55 mm Hg might be observed without ventilatory support in the inpatient setting but probably should be intubated and ventilated in preparation for transport. In addition, patients without overt signs of respiratory failure but in whom deterioration can be reasonably anticipated should be intubated in preparation for transport.

All delivery services and newborn nurseries should be supplied with equipment to intubate neonates. Table 193-2 lists the appropriate laryngoscope blade, endotracheal tube size, and insertion distance for infants based on body weight. Neonatal patients should be premedicated using an opiate analgesic (morphine or fentanyl), unless they are obtunded or in extremis. Apparatus to provide positive-pressure ventilation and suction should be available before sedation and intubation is attempted.

Neonatal intubation can be challenging, especially for personnel not experienced in neonatal airway management. Intubation of the esophagus is common and may result from insertion of the laryngoscope blade into the esophagus (Fig. 193-1). Careful withdrawal of the blade should bring the glottis into view. The glottis is more difficult to visualize

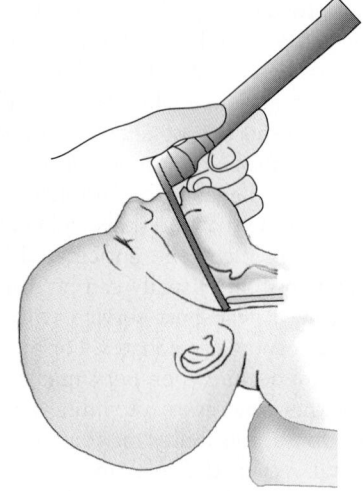

A   Laryngoscope inserted too far

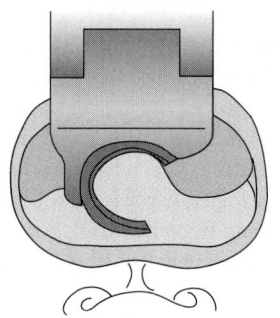

B   You see the walls of the esophagus surrounding the blade

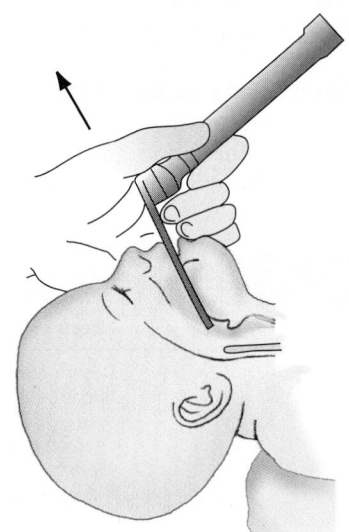

C   Withdraw the blade slowly until the epiglottis and glottis are seen.

Figure 193-1. Inability to visualize the glottis because of insertion of the laryngoscope blade into the esophagus. **A,** Laryngoscope inserted too far. **B,** The esophageal wall appears in the field of vision. **C,** The problem is corrected by slow withdrawal of the laryngoscope. (Adapted from American Academy of Pediatrics and American Heart Association: Textbook of Neonatal Resuscitation. Elk Grove Village, Ill, American Academy of Pediatrics, 2000, pp 5–21. Reproduced by permission of the American Academy of Pediatrics.)

Table 193-2. Intubation of Neonates: Equipment and Insertion Distance of Tube

Body Weight	Laryngoscope Blade Size*	Tube Size†	Insertion Distance‡
<500 g	0	2.0	6.0
500 g–1 kg	0	2.5	6.0–7.0
1–2 kg	0	3.0	7.0–8.0
2–3 kg	0 or 1	3.0–3.5	8.0–9.0
3–4 kg	1	3.5–4.0	9.0–10.0
>4 kg	1	4.0	10.0

*Miller (straight) blade.
†Size in mm; cuffed tubes should not be used.
‡Distance in cm from lip to tip of tube.

in neonates compared with older children because it is in a more ventral position. This problem can be minimized by avoiding overextension of the neck, by lifting the laryngoscope in the direction of the axis of the handle instead of rotating the blade, and by applying gentle pressure to the cricoid (Fig. 193-2).

The position of the tip of the endotracheal tube should be estimated by auscultation and confirmed with a chest radiograph as soon after insertion as possible (Fig. 193-3). A radiograph should be obtained even when reassuring signs of a successful intubation are present (condensation on the wall of the tube, symmetric chest rise/breath sounds, and positive carbon dioxide detection). Right main stem intubation is common in neonates and when prolonged increases the likelihood of pneumothorax (Fig. 193-4). The stomach should be emptied through a nasogastric tube if the infant has been fed within 4 hours of intubation.

Most neonates are ventilated during transport with time-cycled, pressure-limited ventilators using intermittent mandatory ventilation. The quality of each breath is deter-

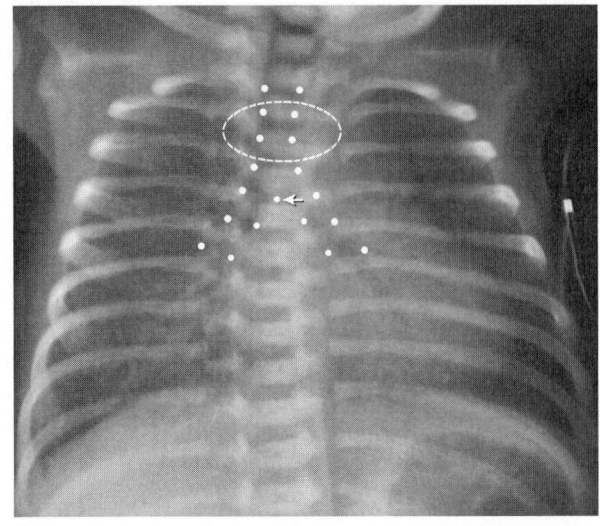

A

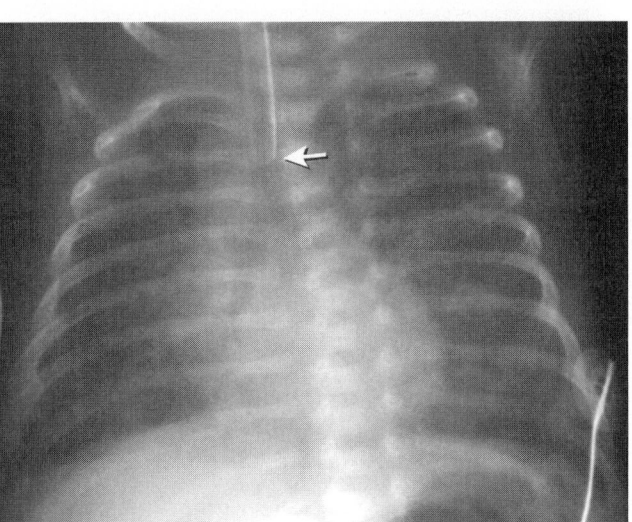

B

Figure 193-3. Chest radiographs show correct positioning of the endotracheal tube. **A,** The tracheal shadow is outlined. The *circle* indicates the correct position of the tip of the endotracheal tube. The *arrow* indicates the carina. **B,** Intubated infant. The *arrow* indicates the tip of the endotracheal tube in midtrachea. (Adapted from Karlsen K: Transporting Newborns the S.T.A.B.L.E. Way. [www.stableprogram.com.] Park City, Utah, 2001, p 49.)

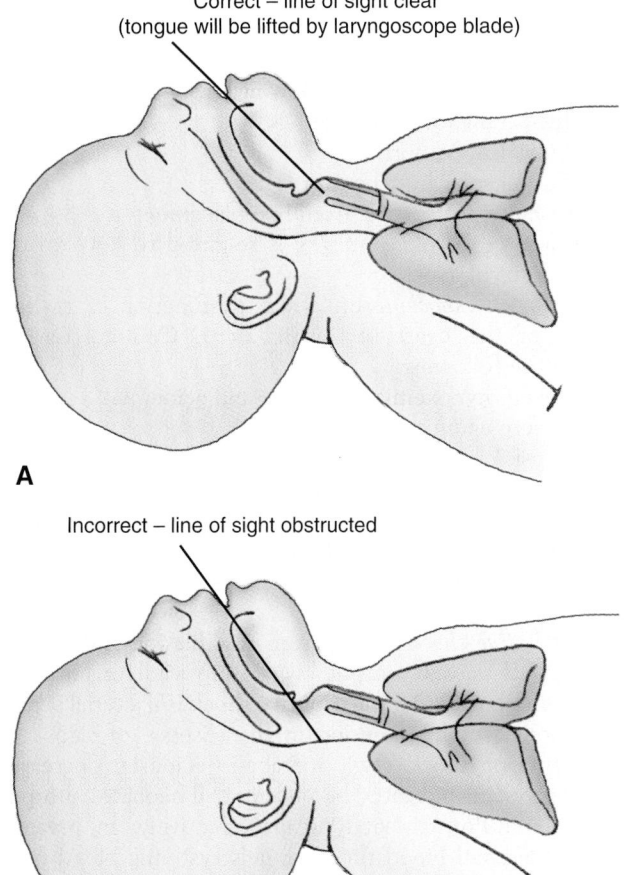

Correct – line of sight clear
(tongue will be lifted by laryngoscope blade)

A

Incorrect – line of sight obstructed

B

Figure 193-2. Difficulty visualizing the glottis because of hyperextension of the head. **A,** The correct position of the head places the glottis in the line of sight after gentle displacement of the tongue in the ventral direction. **B,** Overextension of the head causes the glottis to be out of the line of sight. (Adapted from American Academy of Pediatrics and American Heart Association: Textbook of Neonatal Resuscitation. Elk Grove Village, Ill, American Academy of Pediatrics, 2000, pp 5–21. Reproduced by permission of the American Academy of Pediatrics.)

mined by setting a peak inspiratory pressure (PIP), an end-expiratory pressure (PEEP), and an inspiratory time (T_I). The clinician also must set the fraction of inspired oxygen (FIO_2) and ventilator rate. Suggested initial ventilator settings for infants with varying severity of lung disease are listed in Table 193-3.

The adequacy of oxygenation and ventilation should be assessed immediately after the initiation of ventilation by observing the degree of chest expansion and the change in the color of mucous membranes. This assessment should be followed by blood gas analysis. Although arterial blood is the most accurate source for blood gas analysis, capillary and venous blood are acceptable alternative sources of blood for measurement of PCO_2 and pH. Adequacy of oxygenation can be assessed using pulse oximetry. The target ranges for oxygenation and ventilation of neonates are listed in Table 193-4. Overventilation is a common error that may have serious consequences. The blending of humidified oxygen and air to deliver the minimum FIO_2 required to achieve adequate oxygenation is desirable, particularly in a premature infant in whom hyperoxia may result in retinal damage.

Circulation

Maintenance of adequate circulation is essential for normal organ and cellular function. Low blood pressure (hypotension) and inadequate tissue perfusion (shock) may cause decreased systemic oxygen transport, resulting in organ dysfunction, tissue damage, and ultimately death. There are three general categories of shock: (1) hypovolemic, (2) cardiogenic, and (3) distributive.

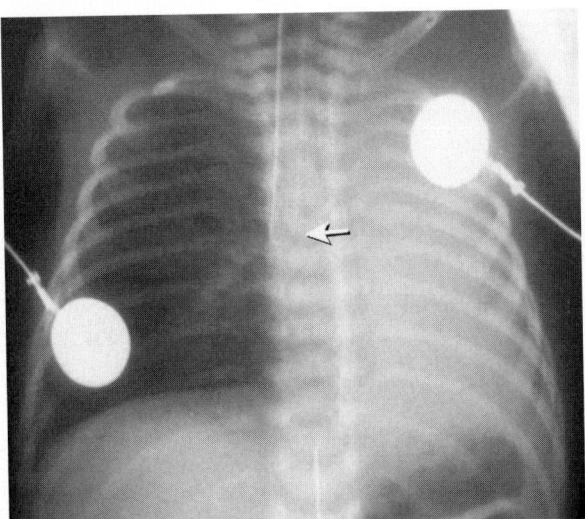

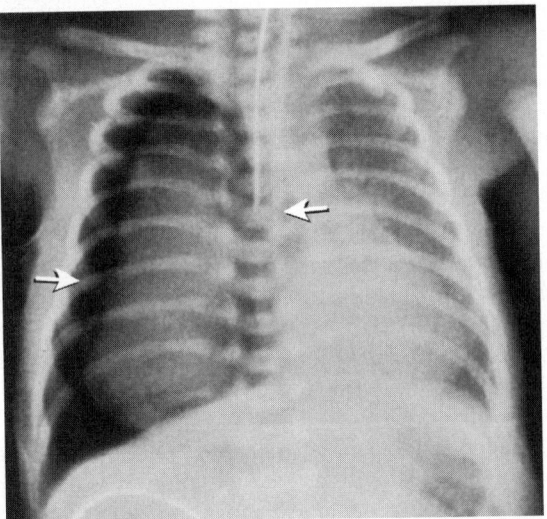

Figure 193-4. Chest radiographs show incorrect endotracheal tube position. **A,** The *arrow* on the right indicates the tip of the endotracheal tube in the right main stem bronchus. **B,** The *arrow* on the left indicates a right pneumothorax, presumably resulting from right main stem bronchus intubation. (Adapted from Karlsen K: Transporting Newborns the S.T.A.B.L.E. Way. [www.stableprogram.com.] Park City, Utah, 2001, p 51.)

Table 193-3. Suggested Initial Ventilator Settings for Neonates Ventilated with Time-cylced Pressure Limited Ventilation

	Disease Severity		
	Mild	Moderate	Severe
PIP (cm H_2O)	18	24	28
PEEP (cm H_2O)	4	4	5
T_1 (sec)	0.4	0.4	0.3
Rate (/min)	20	30	40

PEEP, positive end-expiratory pressure; PIP, peak inspiratory pressure; T_1, inspiration time.

Hypovolemic shock most often results from acute blood loss. In the immediate neonatal period, causes include the following:

1. Abruptio placentae
2. Placenta previa
3. Vasa praevia
4. Umbilical cord accidents
5. Fetomaternal hemorrhage
6. Acute twin-to-twin transfusion

Thereafter, shock may result from closed space hemorrhages. Causes include the following:

1. Intracranial hemorrhage
2. Subgaleal hemorrhage
3. Subcapsular liver hemorrhage
4. Vascular perforation from line placement

Acute loss of 20 to 30 mL/kg is required to develop the clinical signs of shock.

Cardiogenic shock results from dysfunction or malformation of the heart (or aortic arch). Common causes include the following:

1. Severe hypoxemia, ischemia, and acidemia
2. Severe anemia
3. Sepsis
4. Hypoplastic left heart syndrome
5. Coarctation of the aorta or interrupted aortic arch
6. Prolonged tachyarrhythmias
7. Congenital heart block
8. Cardiomyopathies

Distributive shock results from vasodilation and maldistribution of cardiac output away from vital organs. The most common cause of distributive shock is bacterial sepsis.

Treatment of hypotension in the absence of signs and symptoms of shock (e.g., metabolic acidosis, decreased urine output) is indicated because not all neonates autoregulate blood flow to vital organs effectively. In preterm infants, cerebral blood flow parallels systemic blood pressure, and mild hypotension may risk cerebral hypoperfusion and ischemia.

The range of normal blood pressure varies directly with gestational age. A simple guideline for the treatment of hypotension is to maintain the mean arterial blood pressure above the numerical gestational age. The most effective treatment of hypotension is to eliminate the underlying cause. When this approach is not immediately possible, it is advisable to attempt to restore blood pressure initially with the administration of a blood volume expander. Either whole blood or packed red blood cells should be given to infants if

Table 193-4. Target Ranges for Oxygenation and Ventilation

	Oxygenation*		Ventilation	
	Arterial Po$_2$	Sao$_2$	Arterial Pco$_2$	Capillary Pco$_2$
Premature infants	50–70 mm Hg	93–98%	35–50 mm Hg	40–55 mm Hg
Term infants	60–100 mm Hg	96–100%	35–50 mm Hg	40–55 mm Hg

*Capillary Po$_2$ not reliable.

blood loss or closed space hemorrhage is suspected. An isotonic crystalloid solution (e.g., lactated Ringer solution) should be used in other situations. A 10-mL/kg bolus should be administered over 15 to 30 minutes. This volume should be administered a second time if hypotension persists and hypovolemic shock is suspected.

An inotropic agent should be administered to infants who have cardiogenic shock or who are unresponsive to volume expansion. Dobutamine appears to be the agent of choice. A constant infusion should be administered initially at 5 µg/kg/min and should be titrated to 10 µg/kg/min until an adequate blood pressure has been achieved. Immediate consultation is advised if an infant is unresponsive to these therapies, and higher doses are considered.

Vascular Access

Establishing peripheral vascular access in a neonate can be technically challenging. In infants less than 1 week old, intravascular lines placed through the umbilicus are the preferred alternatives for arterial and venous access. The temporary placement of an umbilical venous catheter 1 to 2 cm below the level of the skin is the most rapid way to obtain vascular access. An umbilical venous catheter located in this position can be used to draw emergent laboratory values (e.g., complete blood count, blood culture, blood gas analysis) and to administer isotonic fluids and most medications in emergency situations. It is not a sufficiently stable form of access, however, during transport. By contrast, an umbilical venous catheter with the tip located near the junction of the inferior vena cava and the right atrium is ideal for all infusions during stabilization and transport. When a deep venous line is placed, the position of the tip of the catheter should be determined radiographically before use to ensure that medications are not being infused into distal hepatic vessels or the portal vein. An umbilical artery catheter is desirable when frequent blood gas analysis is anticipated or central blood pressure monitoring is indicated. An umbilical artery catheter should not be used for the administration of inotropic agents or hypertonic fluids.

In neonates, intravascular lines should be infused only with the use of pumps. Open "drips," even with volumetric drip chambers, should not be used because of the risk of fluid intoxication from inadvertent administration of large boluses. The amount of fluid administered should be monitored carefully and recorded.

OTHER PROBLEMS

The stabilization and transport of critically ill neonates is complicated by their dependence on extrinsic factors to maintain homeostasis. This situation is particularly true of preterm infants. The following aspects of care deserve special consideration.

Thermal Regulation

Humans conserve body temperature by several mechanisms, including (1) shunting blood from the skin and periphery to the core, (2) increasing basal metabolic rate, (3) voluntary muscle activity, (4) shivering, and (5) nonshivering thermogenesis. With the exception of nonshivering thermogenesis, all of these mechanisms are less effective in neonates. Although older patients can maintain normal core body temperature effectively when subjected to a wide range of environmental conditions, neonates, particularly premature infants, are limited in this regard. Even in conditions in which a neonate can maintain normal body temperature, this often is accomplished at the expense of increased oxygen consumption.

Neonates should receive care in a neutral thermal environment, a set of conditions in which core temperature remains normal and oxygen consumption is minimal. This environment is provided best on or within a thermocontrolled bed specially designed for neonates. These come in two varieties—an open platform heated with an overhead radiant heat source and a closed plastic incubator heated with a convection heater. Although not satisfactory for transport, open incubators with radiant heaters are ideal for the care of critically ill neonates in the nursery because they permit simultaneous access by several caretakers. All warming devices that are not servo-controlled should be used with extreme caution with frequent monitoring of the infant's body temperature to avoid hyperthermia. Skin probe temperatures should be confirmed with axillary temperatures.

Neonates lose body heat in four ways: (1) evaporation, (2) conduction, (3) convection, and (4) radiation. Preterm infants are particularly susceptible to heat loss compared with term infants because of a relatively large surface-to-body mass ratio, skin that is more permeable to water vapor, and their paucity of subcutaneous tissue. Provisions to minimize heat loss include the following:

1. Infants should be dried thoroughly to avoid evaporative heat loss. This is crucial immediately after delivery. Drying should not be delayed under any circumstances. If emergent procedures are necessary, another caretaker should dry the infant simultaneously.

2. Infants should be placed on a prewarmed surface to avoid conductive heat loss. The temperature of these surfaces or auxiliary heat sources (e.g., hot water bottles) should not exceed 104°F because of the risk of thermal injury. Chemical heat packs specifically designed for newborns are ideal because their heat output is limited within this range.

3. When treating an infant in an open crib or platform warmer, the room temperature should be increased to avoid convective heat loss. The infant should be located away from drafts (e.g., heat/air conditioning vents).

4. Infants not warmed by radiant heat should be clothed to the extent that it does not interfere with care and should not be placed near cold surfaces (e.g., exterior windows) to avoid radiant heat loss. At a minimum, a hat should be placed on the head.

Glucose Homeostasis

During fetal life, the placenta and maternal circulation closely regulate metabolic homeostasis. In healthy full-term neonates, homeostasis is maintained by the infant's autoregulatory mechanisms. These mechanisms often fail during acute illness or after preterm birth. The most common metabolic abnormality in the newborn is hypoglycemia. At birth, blood glucose in the neonate is approximately 60% to 70% of the maternal level. Within 1 to 2 hours, the level decreases to approximately 40 mg/dL. This decline may be accentuated in premature infants, acutely ill infants of any gestational age, and certain other high-risk infants (e.g., infants of diabetic mothers).

Because of the risk of hypoglycemia, all neonates should receive glucose-containing fluids in preparation for transport. In infants with birth weight greater than 1000 g, 10% dextrose infused at a rate of 80 mL/kg/day should be used. In smaller infants, 5% dextrose should be used because they are likely to develop hyperglycemia with high glucose intake. In these infants, the infusion rate should be increased to approximately 100 mL/kg/day to compensate for excessive insensible water loss. In all infants at risk for hypoglycemia, measurement of blood glucose should be repeated at frequent intervals, at least every 2 hours.

Risk of Infection

Signs and symptoms of infection in a neonate are often nonspecific and may be indistinguishable from signs and symptoms associated with other diseases. Infection should be presumed as a cause of illness in any sick neonate. Broad-spectrum antibiotics should be administered, unless the presenting signs and symptoms can be attributed with reasonable certainty to a cause other than infection. Antibiotics also should be administered after most premature births because uterine and placental infection is a common cause of preterm labor. The only exception is when an infant is delivered prematurely for an indication unrelated to infection (e.g., severe preeclampsia). Antibiotics should be administered as soon as possible because early treatment decreases the risk of mortality and morbidity. It is preferable to collect a blood culture before the initiation of antibiotics, but therapy should not be withheld because of difficulties in collecting blood.

PSYCHOLOGICAL MILIEU OF TRANSPORT

There is virtually no way to eliminate the parental anxiety associated with neonatal transport. A few techniques may help families cope with this anxiety, however. It is essential to provide the family with as much information as possible about the nature of their infant's illness, the therapies and equipment that will be used, the center to which the infant will be transported, and the professionals who will provide care. If this information is provided by a transport team from the receiving hospital, a member of the referring hospital staff should be in attendance during this discussion to prepare them for dealing with questions that arise after the departure of the transport team. When possible, this information should be provided verbally and in written form.

It almost always is advisable to arrange contact between parents and an infant before departure from the referring hospital. Visitation should be encouraged even when an infant is critically ill or when parents are reluctant to view their infant. A photograph of the infant should be left with the family.

NEONATAL BACK TRANSPORT

Overcrowding of tertiary neonatal centers remains a problem in some regions of the United States. One strategy for managing this problem has been to transport convalescing infants to community hospitals before discharge home (back transport). The potential benefits of back transport include the following:

1. It preserves the resources of centers with specialty care for critically ill patients.
2. It improves the use of community hospital resources, and helps prepare local personnel for the care of acutely ill patients.
3. It familiarizes primary care providers with infants before discharge home.
4. It improves relationships between specialty centers and community hospitals.
5. It improves family visitation and promotes family-infant bonding.
6. It reduces the total cost of medical care.

The potential disadvantages associated with back transport include the following:

1. Parental anxiety and loss of continuity of care
2. Hazards and cost of transport
3. Variable reimbursement by third-party payers for the transport
4. Occasional need for readmission to a specialty center
5. Loss of the opportunity in specialty centers to participate in convalescent care

Back transport should be considered an option for all infants who no longer require the unique resources of a specialty center and for whom the center is not the site of primary care. If community hospitals anticipate receiving infants after back transport, care providers should be prepared to manage the typical problems of convalescing neonates and their families, including the following:

1. Thermal regulation
2. Gavage feeding
3. Monitoring growth and nutrition
4. Apnea monitoring
5. Methylxanthine therapy
6. Oxygen administration
7. Assistance with lactation

A community hospital may not be prepared to manage all of the problems of convalescing infants. Candidates for back transport should be limited to infants whose needs can be met by the community hospital. The decision to accept a patient should be a collaborative one between the referring and receiving physicians and a member of the nursing staff of the receiving hospital.

Mini-index of Related Topics

SUGGESTED READINGS

Blake WW, Murray JA: Heat balance. In Merenstein GB, Gardner SL (eds): Handbook of Neonatal Intensive Care, 4th ed. St. Louis, Mosby, 1998.

Bose CL, Gordon PV: Neonatal and pediatric transport. In Tintinalli JE, Kelen GD, Stapczynski JS (eds):. Emergency Medicine: A Comprehensive Study Guide, 5th ed. New York, McGraw-Hill, 2000.

Hauth JC, Merenstein GB (eds), Committee on the Fetus and Newborn, American Academy of Pediatrics and Committee on Obstetrical Practice, American College of Obstetricians and Gynecologists: Guidelines for Perinatal Care, 4th ed. Elk Grove Village, Ill, American Academy of Pediatrics, 1997.

Hodson WA, Truog WE: Principles of management of respiratory problems. In Avery GB, Fletcher MA, MacDonald MG (eds): Neonatology, Pathophysiology and Management of the Newborn, 5th ed. Philadelphia, Lippincott Williams & Wilkins, 1999.

Petleft G, Sewell S, Merenstein GB: Regionalization and transport in perinatal care. In Merenstein GB, Gardner SL (eds): Handbook of Neonatal Intensive Care, 4th ed. St. Louis, Mosby, 1998.

MacDonald MG, Ginzburg HM (eds), Task Force on Interhospital Transport, American Academy of Pediatrics: Guidelines for Air and Ground Transport of Neonatal and Pediatric Patients, 2nd ed. Elk Grove Village, Ill, American Academy of Pediatrics, 1999.

194 Routine Care of the Full-Term Newborn

Jacinto Hernandez and Elizabeth Thilo

ROLE OF THE GENERALIST

1 Promote and facilitate normal adaptation to extrauterine life.

2 Detect significant medical problems.

3 Evaluate and treat medical problems in the newborn period.

4 Promote bonding between newborn and mother.

5 Refer when appropriate to specialists for assistance in evaluation and management.

The initial evaluation, assessment, and management of a newborn must be directed toward promoting and facilitating normal adaptation to extrauterine life and early detection of significant medical problems so that they can be evaluated and treated appropriately.

EVALUATION AND CARE DURING THE TRANSITIONAL PERIOD

Birth is an obligatory change of environments. In adjusting to extrauterine life, a newborn infant experiences a complex series of biologic, physiologic, and metabolic changes. These complex changes are essential for survival. Every infant must complete this process of transition successfully to survive in the extrauterine environment. For a small percentage of infants, transition is never achieved; for a slightly larger number, transition is delayed or complicated; but for most, transition is so smooth it appears uneventful.

During the first few hours after birth, the normal infant progresses through a fairly predictable sequence of events, recovering from the stress of delivery and adapting to extrauterine life. The intrapartum and the immediate neonatal events result in sympathetic discharges that are reflected in changes in heart rate, color, respiration, motor activity, gastrointestinal function, and body temperature of the infant. Figure 194-1 shows Desmond's classic description of the

Table 194-3. Assessing the Adequacy of Breast-Feeding: Early Follow-up Visit

Timing of visit	2–3 days after discharge
Feeding history	Frequency of nursing: every 1.5–3 hr, 8–12 feeds per day
	Duration of nursing: approximately 15 min per breast
	Finish at first breast before going on to the second?
	Alternate which breast is first?
	Observe nursing interaction
	Position comfortable?
	Baby latches on correctly?
	Audible swallowing without smacking or other extraneous noises?
Elimination history	Stool color, number: yellow, at least 4 per day by day 4–5
	Urine output, color: dilute, colorless, at least 6–8 wet diapers/day after milk is in
	Dark urine, "brick dust" urine, and scant or meconium stools after day 4–5 indicate inadequate breast milk intake
Physical examination	Assess general health: color, jaundice, hydration, level of consciousness
	Unclothed weight (g): should not be more than 8% below birth weight
	General examination: heart murmur, pulses, perfusion

because a mother cannot judge her infant's color or weight adequately. Risk factors for failed breast-feeding are listed in Box 194-6. Occasionally, failed breast-feeding is associated with severe sequelae in otherwise healthy, term infants, including hyperbilirubinemia severe enough to cause encephalopathy (kernicterus) and hypernatremic dehydration severe enough to cause cerebral sinus thrombosis, cerebral infarction, or death. These are truly tragic outcomes that should be prevented easily by appropriate vigilance.

Box 194-6. Risk Factors for Failed Breast-Feeding

Maternal Factors

- Anatomic breast problems
  - Marked asymmetry, tubular breasts
  - Lack of breast enlargement during pregnancy
- Previous breast surgery, especially periareolar incisions
  - Breast reduction
  - Some augmentations
- Flat or inverted nipples
- Previous poor milk production
- Excessive nipple pain, excessive unrelieved engorgement
- Failure of milk to "come in" by 4th day postpartum

Infant Factors

- Prematurity (<38 weeks' gestation)
- Low birth weight (<6 lb)
- Oral defects (i.e., cleft palate, partial or complete; micrognathia)
- Neuromotor problems with poor tone
- Excessive jaundice, especially requiring phototherapy
- Difficulty latching on; poor arousal to feed in hospital
- Infant separated from mother for >24 hours
- Weight loss >7–8% from birth weight
- Failure to have yellow stools by 4th day of life

Several hospital practices can foster, or interfere with, successful breast-feeding. Mothers and infants should room-in together to facilitate frequent nursing. Supplemental formula should be avoided unless medically indicated (e.g., to treat hypoglycemia), and, if given, the amount should be limited to 15 to 30 mL per feed, given after nursing if possible. The use of pacifiers should be avoided. If inadequate breast milk production is suspected because of excessive weight loss or jaundice or because of inadequate latch-on and emptying of the breast, the mother should begin using a breast pump, preferably electric, to achieve complete emptying and to encourage better milk production. If the infant becomes significantly jaundiced and inadequate breast milk production is suspected, the mother should be instructed to begin pumping her breasts, and the infant can be supplemented with either the expressed breast milk or formula. There is no need to interrupt nursing, although pumping the breasts and supplementation of the infant's intake are crucial.

Other common problems are encountered during breast-feeding. A blocked milk duct leads to formation of a tender, firm lump in the affected area of the breast. Local massage while breast-feeding and warm compresses can help relieve the obstruction. If the lump persists for days or weeks, an alternate diagnosis must be sought. Mastitis occurs in about 3% of nursing mothers during the first several weeks postpartum. In addition to local symptoms of inflammation, there often are systemic flulike symptoms, including fever, chills, body aches, and malaise. Empirical antibiotic therapy with dicloxacillin or a cephalosporin is indicated. Breast-feeding should continue. If direct nursing is too painful to the affected breast, use of an electric breast pump is recommended. Breast abscess should be suspected if symptoms persist after several days of antibiotic therapy or if fluctuance is detected. Surgical drainage or aspiration under ultrasound guidance is required. Sore nipples from incorrect latch-on (early) or, with superinfection, especially from yeast (later), are seen frequently. Lanolin cream is useful in the former case, along with appropriate intervention to ensure better latch-on. Candidal infection is suspected if the infant is seen to have thrush or diaper dermatitis or if the mother has been treated with antibiotics. The mother and infant should be treated. Breast pumping is useful if the pain precludes direct nursing temporarily.

Many mothers must return to work but desire to continue nursing. They should use a breast pump, preferably electric, once or twice per day at the workplace and refrigerate the milk for use in bottle-feeding the infant within 24 hours in the day care setting. Direct nursing while the mother and infant are together mornings, evenings, and weekends continues. This practice can be quite successful, although there is a greater likelihood that early weaning will occur.

EARLY DISCHARGE OF THE NEWBORN INFANT

The trend for several years has been toward shorter hospital stays for well mothers and infants, with typical stays today of 24 to 36 hours after a normal vaginal delivery and 48 to 72 hours after a cesarean section. Discharge at 24 to 36 hours of age seems safe and appropriate for most infants if there are no contraindications (Box 194-7) and a follow-

Box 194-7. Criteria for Early Newborn Discharge

- Contraindications to early newborn discharge
  - Jaundice at ≤24 hours
  - Mother treated with antibiotics in labor for group B β-hemolytic streptococcus prophylaxis
  - Known or suspected narcotic addiction or withdrawal
  - Physical defects requiring evaluation
  - Oral defects (clefts, micrognathia)
- Relative contraindications to early newborn discharge (infants at high risk for feeding failure, excessive jaundice)
  - Prematurity or borderline prematurity (<38 weeks' gestation)
  - Birth weight <2700 g (6 lb)
  - Infant difficult to arouse for feeding; not demanding regularly in nursery
  - Medical or neurologic problems (e.g., Down syndrome, hypotonia, cardiac problems)
  - Twins or higher multiples
  - ABO blood group incompatibility or severe jaundice in previous child
  - Mother whose previous breast-fed infant gained weight poorly
  - Mother with breast surgery involving periareolar areas (if attempting to nurse)

up visit at 48 to 72 hours after discharge is ensured. Most infants with severe cardiorespiratory disorders and infections are identified in the first 12 to 24 hours of life.

The American Academy of Pediatrics recommends a follow-up visit within 48 to 72 hours for any newborn discharged before 48 hours of age. Infants who are small or slightly premature—especially if breast-feeding—are at particular risk for inadequate intake, which often is associated with a rapid rise in serum bilirubin. Suggested guidelines for the follow-up interview and physical examination are presented in Box 194-8.

Box 194-8. Guidelines for Early Outpatient Follow-up Evaluation

History

- Rhythmic sucking and audible swallowing for at least 10 minutes total per feeding?
- Infant wakes and demands to feed every 2–3 hours (at least 8–10 feedings per 24 hours)?
- Do breasts feel full before feedings and softer after?
- Are there at least six noticeably wet diapers per 24 hours?
- Are there yellow bowel movements (no longer meconium)—at least four per 24 hours?
- Is infant still acting hungry after nursing (frequently sucks hands, rooting)?

Physical Assessment

- Weight, unclothed: should not be >8–10% below birth weight
- Extent and severity of jaundice
- Assessment of hydration, alertness, general well-being
- Cardiovascular examination: murmurs, brachial and femoral pulses, respirations

CIRCUMCISION

Circumcision is an elective procedure to be performed only in healthy, stable infants. The procedure is described in Chapter 301. Care of infants with a bleeding circumcision is described in Chapter 199.

HEARING SCREENING

Normal hearing is crucial to normal language development. Significant bilateral hearing loss is present in 1 to 3 infants per 1000 in the well nursery. All infants should be screened for hearing loss by auditory brainstem evoked responses or evoked otoacoustic emissions as early as possible. Parents need to be advised of the possibility of hearing loss and offered ready referral in suspect cases.

Additional Resources, CD-ROM

Assessment of gestational age	Figure
Intrauterine growth curves	Figure
Bibliography	

Mini-index of Related Topics

SUGGESTED READINGS

Avery GB (ed): Neonatology: Pathophysiology and Management of the Newborn, 4th ed. Philadelphia, JB Lippincott, 1999.

Desmond MM, Rudolph AJ, Phitaksphraiwan P: The transitional care nursery: A mechanism for preventive medicine in the newborn. Pediatr Clin North Am 1966;13:651–668.

Fletcher MA: Physical Diagnosis in Neonatology. Philadelphia, Lippincott-Raven, 1998.

Padbury JF (ed): Neonatal adaptation: The transition to postnatal life. Semin Perinatol 1988;12:95–172.

Powers NG, Slusser W: Breastfeeding update 2: Clinical lactation management. Pediatr Rev 1997;18:147–161.

Thureen PJ, Deacon J, O'Neill P, Hernandez J (eds): Assessment and Care of the Well Newborn. Philadelphia, WB Saunders, 1999.

195 The Ill Newborn: Early Identification and Stabilization

Richard A. Molteni

Identification of an ill newborn is an essential skill of the pediatric provider. Because of the rapidity of deterioration and the subtlety of the changes often shown by the neonatal patient, this is a crucial assessment skill that must be exercised by the pediatrician or family practitioner. The neonatal period is the most hazardous period in the human lifetime. Missing subtle changes in the immediate postnatal period leads to serious morbidity or mortality.

The key to effective management in the neonatal period is based on a keen knowledge of normal fetal growth and development, prenatal indicators of fetal compromise or disease, signs of fetal compromise in labor, and normal progressions of neonatal transition after birth. This chapter concentrates on the high-level identification of a sick neonate and a single system of evaluation and stabilization that is acceptable in most infants. Unique, although common, situations in which special conditions and therapies apply are pointed out and identified. Complete discussions of each of these conditions are found in other chapters.

ANTICIPATING DISEASE FROM THE PRENATAL HISTORY

Fetal health and fetal growth are closely connected. The essential component of nutritional support, oxygen exchange, and waste removal for the fetus is a healthy placenta. Slow or impaired growth implies placental dysfunction—a placenta that has failed to grow, has become infarcted, has separated from the uterine wall, has become infected, or has become hydropic. Poor growth (nutritional transfer) also is associated with diminished oxygen delivery and can be associated with acute hypoxemic injury (especially during labor) or chronic hypoxemic and ischemic injuries that are apparent only after birth. A fetus with unexplained fetal heart rate changes during labor and an unplanned cesarean section must be evaluated carefully for this complication. At times, this recognition may be difficult because the infant's weight plots as appropriate for gestational age (AGA), confusing the association. When the newborn's weight is compared with length (weight-to-length ratio or ponderal index), however, impaired growth is recognized; this long thin infant represents growth restriction in utero.

Under normal prenatal circumstances, nutritional deprivation initially impairs fetal weight; secondarily, fetal length; and only when severe and prolonged, head circumference (brain growth). Recognizing this uterine effect allows the clinician to appraise the newborn more carefully for the additional effects that follow on this restriction after birth, including hypoglycemia, temperature instability and hypothermia, polycythemia and hyperviscosity, delayed feeding, and other mild neurologic abnormalities. More chronic and profound effects include low neutrophil counts, diminished platelet levels, abnormal liver and clotting studies, elevated creatinine levels, and thickened brawny skin edema (sclerema). Other physical findings seen with fetuses that are undergrown include poor subcutaneous tissue, long fingernails (often with chronic meconium staining), absent or diminished breast tissue, and hyperalert appearance. With obstetric monitoring tools (ultrasound combined with nonstress tests and biophysical profiles), these latter types of changes are seen only in completely unmonitored pregnancies and mothers without prenatal care. Common prenatal warning signs that should be looked for are listed in Table 195-1.

ANTICIPATING NEONATAL DISEASE BY EVALUATION OF THE TRANSITIONAL PERIOD

In addition to the prenatal warning signs, a newborn's behavior during the immediate postnatal period, termed the *transitional period*, is extremely important in the timely identification of the sick neonate. During normal transition to extrauterine life, there are three well-defined stages through which a normal neonate progresses. Failure to follow the expected course is a strong indication of an abnormal neonate or a neonate showing the first signs of an

Table 195-1. Common Prenatal Warning Signs for Illness in Newborns

Sign	Conditions in Newborn
Oligohydramnios	Severe placental insufficiency, congenital renal aplasia or dysplasia, pulmonary dysplasia
Polyhydramnios	Spina bifida, high intestinal obstruction, severe neurologic lesion impairing fetal swallowing
Membrane rupture before labor	Infection, large amniotic fluid volume, placental abruption
Fetal tachycardia	Fetal infection, fetal anemia, maternal drug ingestions, maternal fever
Absent, diminished fetal movements	Fetal neurologic injury, neuromuscular defect, hypoxemia
Maternal diabetes	Fetal anomalies, hypoglycemia, polycythemia, macrosomia with birth injury
Maternal bleeding	Abruptio placentae, placenta previa, and vasa praevia or cord traction injury may have associated fetal anemia or hypovolemic shock
Maternal smoking	Small-for-gestational-age infant with hypoglycemia, polycythemia
Materal drug (cocaine) use	Fetal and neonatal strokes
Forceps delivery	Mechanical injuries, skull fractures, brain lacerations, subarachnoid and subdural bleeding
Vacuum extractor	Bruising and bleeding of the scalp ("chignon"), subgaleal hemorrhage
Pitocin	Hyperstimulation of the uterus with fetal hypoxia, uterine rupture

impending postnatal emergency. Nursing and pediatric providers must be aware of this normal pattern and establish nursery protocols and flow sheets that allow for early recognition of abnormalities in the expected progression and pattern.

In the immediate postnatal period, a neonate should be hyperalert, crying, plethoric, tachycardic, tachypneic, abdominally distended, and retracting; on examination, there are rales, positive bowel sounds, and jittery tremulous activity. The neonate is difficult to console, although he or she does act hungry and usually feeds if offered the breast or bottle. This constellation of findings at any other time during the postnatal period would be concerning for cardiac or respiratory disease, neurologic injury, polycythemia, infection, or other metabolic conditions. For the first 30 to 45 minutes of life, this is normal activity as the neonate reacts to the enormous stimulation of the extrauterine environment. At the same time, the newborn infant is clearing the normal lung fluid and as a result shows signs of increased work of breathing; the infant cries and swallows air and begins the process of expanding alveoli, exchanging fluid-filled alveoli for air-filled sacs. Prenatal blood flow patterns begin to change, and blood is rerouted from the foramen ovale to the pulmonary bed as pulmonary artery pressure begins to decrease. The peripheral vasculature bed begins to clamp down, replacing the low resistance circuit of the placenta. Central pinkness slowly replaces the initial dark ruddy color, respiratory and heart rates begin to decrease, the work of breathing declines, and blood pressure and oxygen saturation steadily increase.

Neonatal abnormalities can be identified early either by failure of this pattern to be seen immediately after birth or by failure of this pattern to disappear by 45 to 60 minutes of life (Table 195-2). In the former situation, a quiet, pale, poorly reactive neonate with low respiratory rate and heart rate implies an infant who is sleepy (maternal medications), who is neurologically impaired (prenatally), or who has sustained a traumatic brain injury during delivery. A quiet, pale, poorly perfused, and mottled infant with limited spontaneous movement but with tachycardia and tachypnea implies fetal infection and septic shock or fetal anemia with hypovolemic shock. Rarely does a newborn present with cardiogenic shock in the immediate postpartum hours. The exception is congenital cardiac disease in which diminished or absent pulmonary blood flow is combined with an absence of available shunts (e.g., pulmonary atresia with intact septum). Other cyanotic cardiac lesions may present with blue discoloration, but in every other way the infant may appear to be progressing through a normal first stage of transition. The neonate who continues with tachypnea, tachycardia, and increased work of breathing beyond this initial interval should be evaluated for cardiac or pulmonary disease.

Respiratory distress that begins and persists from birth is rarely hyaline membrane disease (primary surfactant deficiency). Except at the smallest birth weights, these infants appear normal or only minimally affected at birth and show progressive respiratory distress over the next 2 to 4 hours. Distress from birth implies a lung lesion present at birth (e.g., pulmonary hypoplasia, congenital diaphragmatic hernia, cystic adenomatoid malformation) or a condition initiated at or immediately before birth (e.g., clear amniotic fluid, blood, or meconium aspiration).

When either of these abnormalities of the first stage of transition is appreciated, the practitioner must come to the nursery to evaluate the history and examine the newborn. A complete blood count, glucose value, chest radiograph, and venous blood gas analysis represent the minimal laboratory evaluation necessary to begin an investigation. A neonate who is not progressing through this first phase after birth is at risk for serious neurologic disease and should not

Table 195-2. Signs of Illness in the Newborn during First 30 to 45 Minutes of Life

Sign	Illness
Decreased activity, quiet, poorly reactive	With low respiratory and heart rate: Maternal medications Prenatal neurologic impairment Traumatic brain injury during delivery With tachypnea and tachycardia: Fetal infection with septic shock Fetal anemia and hypovolemic shock
Cardiogenic shock (rare)	Diminished or absent pulmonary blood flow combined with an absence of available shunts (e.g., pulmonary atresia with intact septum)
Respiratory distress	Lung lesion present at birth, including: Pulmonary hypoplasia Congenital diaphragmatic hernia Cystic adenomatoid malformation Condition initiated at or immediately before birth: Clear amniotic fluid, blood, or meconium aspiration

be fed at this point. The infant should be monitored closely for apnea and seizures and should be assumed to be at risk for vomiting and aspiration (consider a nasogastric tube). There is little indication for an emergent brain imaging study at this time. If symptoms persist, a head ultrasound is indicated, however, with later computed tomography or magnetic resonance imaging if this screening study is abnormal or symptoms do not improve.

The second stage of transition begins variably at 30 to 60 minutes after birth. This stage is characterized by a sleepy quiet newborn with a paucity of spontaneous movement. Infants typically are in deep sleep and difficult to arouse for more than a few moments. Their respiratory rates are low, and they have long pauses (although usually <10 seconds) and periodic breathing patterns. They have no retractions, grunting, flaring, or other signs of respiratory work. Their breath sounds are clear, and there are no rales or wheezes. Their cardiac rates are low, and if the monitor is set too low (e.g., 100 beats/min), occasionally the monitor alarm may go off. Earlier murmurs, if present, typically have disappeared or are becoming less audible. Bowel sounds are less prominent; infants are not hungry and are not passing stools. Forcing feedings in this stage may lead to emesis. Their skin, although pink, is quite pale. Acrocyanosis is disappearing. Capillary refill times and blood pressures are normal. If an infant's caretakers were not aware that the infant was in this stage of transition, serious concern for infection might lead to a septic workup and unnecessary antibiotic therapy, a metabolic evaluation might be obtained, a cardiac workup might be considered, and a neurologic evaluation or consultation might be requested. Only careful continued monitoring is required, however.

In another 2 to 3 hours, healthy newborns wake up and vigorously demand to be fed. All of these concerns are allayed when infants take to breast-feeding or bottle-feeding well. If the period of deep sleep were to continue beyond this 2- to 3-hour period, however, serious concern for all of the aforementioned possibilities would be warranted. Evaluations for infection (complete blood count and blood, urine, and spinal fluid cultures), anemia (hematocrit and, if low, reticulocyte count, blood type, and Coombs test), metabolic disease (glucose, calcium, and bicarbonate), and neurologic disease (head ultrasound) should be seriously considered.

The third stage of transition begins as the neonate wakes from the second stage and demands to be fed. Failure to wake normally and exhibit hunger represents a serious risk for underlying disease. The third stage is characterized by behavior and patterns considered normal neonatal behavior at home. The neonate establishes a pattern of sleep, wake, and feeding cycles that become ever more predictable and routine. In this third stage, the neonate progresses from deep sleep, to quiet awakening (wiggles, groans, stretches, yawns), loud fussing, and crying from hunger; quiet feeding with intense focusing on the mother or caretaker; a postfeeding quiet alert period in which interest in the maternal face, sound, and smell leads to optimal bonding; and finally light and deep sleep. The length of the cycle varies by infant, but the pattern should remain the same. Failure of any of these components to be seen is worrisome for underlying disease. An infant who fails to develop this pattern of quiet alert bonding is at risk for neurologic disorders, including vision and hearing disorders. An infant who fails to attain deep sleep is at risk for cardiac or pulmonary disease, metabolic disturbances (e.g., hyperthyroidism), drug withdrawal, trauma (e.g., brain bleed, fracture), or pain. A neonate who awakens but shows no hunger is at risk for infection or abdominal disease (e.g., obstruction, volvulus, esophageal or gastric irritation). Although great variability may be seen in this pattern in the first 1 or 2 days of life, there should be a consistent change in behavior of the neonate with increasing age that mimics more closely the pattern described. Failure to establish a normal feeding pattern and failure to attain the normal third stage of transition is adequate reason to maintain the mother-child dyad in the hospital beyond 24 or 48 hours for further observation and testing.

ANTICIPATING NEONATAL DISEASE BY POSTNATAL AGE

Another useful and reliable tool to aid the practitioner in categorizing the likely reasons for a neonate's signs and symptoms is the infant's postnatal age at the time the abnormal findings are first recognized. Prenatal onset can be suspected by any of the following characteristics: poor intrauterine growth with fetal growth restriction and placental insufficiency; slowing, cessation, or change in type of fetal activity in utero; diminished quantity of amniotic fluid; nonreactive nonstress test or falling total score for the biophysical profile; immature lecithin/sphingomyelin ratio or absence of phosphatidylglycerol in a fetus not treated with betamethasone; and fetal heart rate pattern that shows little or absent long-term variability, persistent fetal tachycardia, or recurrent late decelerations. Abnormalities on the prenatal ultrasound view of the fetal head or four-chamber view of the fetal heart, polyhydramnios, maternal gestational or insulin-dependent diabetes, premature or prolonged rupture of the membranes, maternal group B streptococcus or herpes colonization, and maternal fever in labor all are high-risk associations. These conditions represent only a portion of the problems that can affect the fetus in the 9 months before birth. The signs and symptoms the neonate exhibits, if not attributable to late effects from labor and delivery, will thave been present for some time before birth. Careful questioning of the mother and a thorough review of the prenatal record are required to make this important association. When the association is made, however, a significant amount of unnecessary evaluation and therapy can be avoided.

Neonates who acquire a condition during the intrapartum period (labor and delivery) have symptoms present at birth and initially are difficult to distinguish (without the appropriate prenatal history) from infants who acquired their condition during gestational development. Intrapartum acquired conditions can be divided into infective, traumatic, metabolic, and hypoxemic. Some of these conditions can be catastrophic, such as complete abruption of the placenta, a prolapsed cord, or a torn vasa praevia. Some conditions may represent the cumulative effects of a dysfunctional placenta, a prolonged labor, oxytocin overstimulation, severe variable decelerations after membrane rupture, or an early chorioamnionitis after a prolonged rupture of the membranes and labor.

These neonates commonly are born with a low Apgar score and require vigorous resuscitation. If significant fetal blood loss is present, infants have hypovolemic shock, which requires immediate fluid resuscitation. Assuming that the resuscitation is successful, the major symptoms may be delayed many hours as the organs that have been less essential in utero while connected to the placenta (kidney, lung, gastrointestinal tract, liver) now must take over nutritive, oxygenation, metabolic, and clearance functions postnatally. Brain swelling usually is delayed 8 to 12 hours, as are seizures. Secondary inappropriate antidiuretic hormone secretion complicates the electrolyte abnormalities and brain swelling. Early hyperglycemia can be followed by hypoglycemia. Delayed or low urine output results in unexpected weight gain and secondary hyponatremia and hyperkalemia. Renal cortical injury can be seen with low urine blood flows, hematuria, and elevations in blood urea nitrogen and creatinine. Tubular injury is seen with inability to dilute or concentrate the urine, impaired excretion of hydrogen ion and the volatile acids, and with appearance in the urine of large molecules (e.g., albumin and macroglobulin) and a series of ions that would be reabsorbed if the tubule were functioning normally. Early and excessive hypotonic fluid therapy accentuates the overhydration and hyponatremia. Abnormal liver function tests, accentuation of normal bilirubin elevations, impaired albumin production, hyperammonemia, and clotting factor deficiencies all can be seen. Mucosal sloughing of the gastrointestinal tract can produce bloody mucus, atony, distention, necrotizing enterocolitis, and perforation. The lung can develop shock lung, secondary surfactant production, or persistence of the normal high prenatal pulmonary pressure—leading to ongoing cyanosis and hypoxemia. The cardiac muscle can have temporary pump dysfunction or ischemia of the chordae tendinae of the valves or ischemia of the posterior ventricular wall. Persistence of fetal blood flow channels (ductus arteriosus and foramen ovale) follows the elevated pulmonary artery pressures. The marrow may show elevation of nucleated blood cells if the hypoxemic or anemic stress was present for some days or more before delivery. Postnatal disseminated intravascular coagulation can be identified by declining platelet counts, an abnormal smear with fragmented red blood cells, and clotting and bleeding abnormalities. The number and severity of organs affected and the time to recovery of function help to define the severity and the length of the intrapartum exposure.

Traumatic injuries can be sustained by the fetal skull and brain, long bones, internal organs (e.g., the liver), skin and soft tissues, and umbilical cord. Although forceps use has diminished, the use of the vacuum extractor to effect delivery and avoid cesarean section has increased. This instrument has been associated with subgaleal bleeding, a form of hemorrhage that rapidly can exsanguinate the neonate. Rapid recognition (scalp swelling that is diffuse and not limited by suture lines) is crucial to prevent morbidity and death. Forceps are associated with skull fracture, brain contusion and laceration, and subdural and subarachnoid bleeding. The latter two conditions can lead to significant blood loss and hypovolemic shock, in addition to major

neurologic deterioration and seizures. In contrast to hypoxemia experienced during labor, seizures are seen soon after birth when serious brain trauma has occurred.

Metabolic emergencies primarily are seen in infants of diabetic mothers (low blood glucose), infants with intrauterine growth restriction, premature infants, and infants with a few, less common disease states (e.g., nesidioblastosis and Beckman-Wiedemann syndrome). Infection poses the primary risk to a neonate in the immediate (first 12 hours) period after birth. Although group B streptoccocus has been the predominant organism for a few decades, gram-negative organisms still account for a significant percentage of these infections. Infection must be on every pediatric provider's mind when evaluating infants in the nursery. Mortality rates still are high, and morbidity is even greater. Morbidity and mortality increase dramatically as gestational age decreases. Morbidity and mortality also mount sharply based on the timing of antibiotic introduction to the neonate. Most serious bacterial infections leading to sepsis occur within the first 24 hours of life, and the majority of those in the first 12 hours. Acquired bacterial infections after scalp electrode site contamination, skin abrasion, or cord infection can occur much later, and the source should be apparent. Early infection can be found and confirmed if a careful examination of the placenta is done or the mother had prolonged rupture of the membranes with intrapartum fever and an elevated white blood cell count or a positive vaginal culture for group B streptoccocus. In these situations, the placenta is shown to have evidence of villitis, placentitis, and invasion of the blood vessels on the placental surface, the chorion, the amnion, and the umbilical cord itself (funisitis).

In some high-risk situations, the initial white blood cell count may be misleading. If the fetus has been allowed to labor, it would be expected that the neonatal white blood cell count (stress demargination) would be quite high (≥20,000), especially if labor augmentation was used because of lengthening membrane rupture. In addition, a significant stress-related shift to the left in the neutrophil series would be expected. Often with early infection, however, the white blood cell count is determined to be "normal" when the total count (e.g., 12,000) and the percentage of polymorphonuclear neutrophils were low (e.g., 40%) when the stresses of labor were considered. In retrospect, this finding provided evidence that the bone marrow's expected response had been suppressed by the infection. If the white blood cell count is followed over the next 12 hours, further reductions in the white blood cell count and polymorphonuclear neutrophil count occur to severe neutropenic levels. A concomitant decrease in the platelet count also is seen. Identifying this subtle abnormality of the white blood cell count early is essential to initiate therapy in a timely fashion.

Newborns who do not show this type of deterioration in the first 12 hours after birth but who become ill at 24 to 48 hours rarely are infected with bacteria. Rather, these newborns typically have serious cardiac disease that has been masked by continued patency of the ductus arteriosus and foramen ovale. These neonates have ductal-dependent lesions of the left side of the heart—hypoplastic left heart syndrome, coarctation of the aorta, interrupted aortic arch, aortic atresia or severe aortic stenosis, and other complex cardiac defects in which the ductus provides a source for right-to-left flow into the descending aorta. These infants have no sign of heart disease (most have no or unimpressive murmurs) and progress normally through transition, feed well, are pink, and for all purposes appear to be healthy. Their deterioration begins with a subtle increase first in respiratory rate and then in heart rate. Their feeding begins to decline, and they show fatigue at the end of shorter feedings. They may have diaphoresis with feeds and they are less interested in their surroundings and begin to sleep poorly. They show limited feeding interest when they do awaken. Eventually these infants begin to show skin mottling, a pale gray undertone, and then cyanosis. On chest radiograph, most have significant enlargement of the cardiac shadow and marked increase in vasculature. Time is now of the essence, and the rapid introduction of prostaglandin is necessary to reopen the ductus and preserve blood and oxygen flow (and with it organ function) to all organs supplied by the descending aorta.

Less common than infection and cardiac disease, genetically determined metabolic disease in neonates presents typically later than the aforementioned conditions but often with the same catastrophic appearance. The later appearance of metabolic disease has much to do with the change in body weight the normal neonate experiences over the first few postnatal days. Normal newborns are slow to establish an effective feeding volume. To compensate, they are born with excessive water and salt. The normal formula-fed infant loses 5% to 6% of the body weight before beginning a steady pattern of gain, usually at 20 to 30 g/day. The breast-fed infant commonly loses 6% to 8% of birth weight before steady gains begin. Because the total intake is low for the first few days, the appearance of serious congenital metabolic disease is delayed until sufficient protein intake has been achieved. Typically, this occurs around the 3rd or 4th postnatal day. Diminished levels of consciousness, tachypnea and hyperpnea, loss of feeding interest, hypoglycemia, developing metabolic acidemia, and hyperammonemia constitute the most frequent signs. When the diagnosis is suspected, fluid rehydration, correction of academia, and rapid transfer to a tertiary site is essential to characterize the defect appropriately and initiate specific corrective therapy or dialysis. Serum electrolytes and urine and blood for plasma amino acids and organic acids eventually lead to the correct diagnosis. Until that time, empirical therapy (fluid, electrolyte, bicarbonate) combined with sodium benzoate suffices, unless dialysis is thought to be useful.

Beyond the 5th day of life, with the exception of hyperbilirubinemia and concomitant dehydration in many infants, few perinatal conditions appear regularly in the later newborn period. One that should be kept in mind, however, is herpesvirus infection. Acquired during the time between rupture of the membranes and delivery, herpes infection commonly does not present until the 7th to 10th postnatal day, or earlier if there has been prolonged rupture or a high viral exposure (primary herpes). The disease can be limited to the skin or the eye, be confined to the central nervous system, or be present in an overwhelming septic form. Infants with the last-mentioned form present and appear similar to newborns in the first 24 hours of life who have acquired a serious bacterial infection during delivery. They cease feeding, develop lethargy, may be hypothermic or hyperthermic, show poor capillary refill and skin mottling, develop tachypnea and tachycardia, have evidence of pneumonia, and often show petichiae or frank ecchymosis. Laboratory values show evidence of thrombocytopenia and disseminated intravascular coagulation, liver function abnormalities, a progressive acidosis, and abnormalities of the central nervous system including seizures. Polymerase chain reaction (PCR) diagnosis and rapid introduction of acyclovir are essential for survival and diminished morbidity.

INITIAL EVALUATION AND CARE OF THE SICK NEWBORN

The delivery room resuscitation of the neonate is discussed in Chapter 191. Stabilization and transport are discussed in Chapter 193. The remainder of this chapter discusses appropriate initial evaluation and treatment of conditions that require expert stabilization and preparation for transport.

Infant Sick from Birth

If a neonate was depressed at birth or required prolonged and significant resuscitation to develop an effective cardiac output and ventilatory pattern, it is unlikely that the neonate will have a completely benign postnatal course. If the ventilation, oxygenation, or cardiac output does not normalize in the first 30 minutes, arrangements should be made for transport to a tertiary care center. Whether or not the neonate is transported, the initial treatment of this diverse group of sick neonates is similar. First, complete baseline vital signs are obtained on admission to the nursery, including blood pressures and oxygen saturation. The infant is maintained in an open warmer with a servo-controlled skin temperature set to 36.5°C. Next, venous access is obtained if the infant is well saturated. If poor saturation, irregular respirations, or apnea is seen, the infant first is intubated and ventilated, and then venous access is obtained. In the interim, the nurse can attempt a peripheral venous line. When the infant is intubated (and during preoxygenation), the clinician uses a hand bag with a manometer and notes the pressure that it takes to see acceptable chest rise and to hear good breath sounds. If lung disease is a component of the infant's illness, it is likely that this pressure requirement will increase as lung compliance decreases or pulmonary edema or pneumonia progresses. The healthy lung requires only 15 to 20 mm Hg to ventilate after normal lung fluid has been reabsorbed. Whatever pressure is necessary is used to attain lung rise. In term and near-term infants, a 3.0 or 3.5 endotracheal tube is used. Proper position in the midtrachea is ensured by auscultation and by chest radiograph. The tube is suctioned, and any fluid is sent to the laboratory for culture. If there is significant gastric distention from previous bag-and-mask inflations, an oral or nasal gastric tube is placed first to decompress the stomach. If distention is not present, the gastric tube is placed when intubation has been completed. Placement of both is confirmed on the same radiograph. If a ventilator is being used, the clinician begins at pressures of 20 to 25 mm

Hg at 30 to 40 breaths with an inspiratory time of 0.3 to 0.35 seconds. The clinician begins at 100% inspired oxygen and weans steadily based on the oxygen saturation readings.

If perfusion was poor in the delivery room or on return to the nursery, the clinician first places an umbilical venous line. If the line passes easily in the term infant, it requires 10 to 15 cm to reach the superior vena cava and right atrium. If this line passes easily to this length, samples for the initial blood studies (listed subsequently) are drawn, and this line is used for initial isotonic fluid infusions or other resuscitative drugs. If there is any difficulty in passing the catheter or the operator is inexperienced, it is passed 2 to 3 cm into the umbilical vein until blood flow is obtained. The catheter is tied in the vessel at this point and used for subsequent draws and any further fluid therapy and volume pushes. The position of a deep line is confirmed with a chest radiograph.

When venous access has been obtained, samples for the following baseline studies are drawn: venous blood gas, type and hold, complete blood count with platelets, glucose, and blood culture. The newborn's electrolytes are in equilibrium with the mother's at birth. Unless there are no maternal values available, or there is reason to suspect that the mother's values may be abnormal, there is no reason to obtain them at this point. If infection is a serious risk, a bladder tap or catheterized urine for culture also is obtained. A spinal tap is not necessary at this point in the stabilization. After intubation, a tracheal aspirate is obtained for culture. Initial antibiotic doses should be ordered with ampicillin and gentamicin or ampicillin and cefotaxime.

Initial fluid therapy should use 10% dextrose in water. If the first glucose value comes back high, 5% dextrose in water can be used and 10% dextrose in water substituted as the glucose value decreases. Especially in an infant who has been depressed at birth, the possibility of poor urine output must be considered and free water minimized until adequate urine output has been shown. The initial fluid load should not exceed 50 to 60 mL/kg (even under a radiant warmer) to prevent accentuation of cerebral and pulmonary edema. If perfusion or blood pressure decrease or acidemia increases, isotonic fluid expansion (normal saline, Ringer lactate, or 5% albumin) should be used instead of increasing the glucose solution. If the total fluid load is diminished below this level, glucose levels need to be monitored. With a central umbilical catheter, glucose concentration of 20% or more can be used at free water infusion rates as low as 30 mL/kg/day (insensible water loss). After the water is given, in the absence of urine output, only dialysis or time will remove it. Push infusions of isotonic solutions can be given at any time low volume is in question.

Capillary refill time, blood pressure, and acid-base status determine the need for further volume therapy. When 30 to 40 mL/kg has been exceeded, cardiac and pulmonary status should be evaluated carefully before further fluid is given. The chest radiograph is repeated to look for increased heart size or wet lungs. If either abnormality is present, the clinician should change to low-dose pressor therapy (dopamine or dobutamine) beginning at 5 μg/kg and increasing to 20 μg. If the effect is still suboptimal, a second agent is added, and the volume infusion is repeated. Blood pressures and venous blood gases are followed for

pH, P_{CO_2}, P_{O_2}, and bicarbonate. The ventilator rate or pressure is increased if the P_{CO_2} increases; the peak pressure or the inspiratory time is increased if the inspired oxygen need continues to increase. If the bicarbonate level continues to decrease, small, slow infusions of sodium bicarbonate (1 to 2 mEq/kg) should be considered for correction. The hematocrit should be followed closely. If the need for volume was not due to septic or cardiogenic shock, blood loss may be the most likely cause. The hematocrit takes 2 to 4 hours or more to equilibrate if the bleeding occurred close to the time of delivery.

With the presence of pulse oximetry, there is no urgency for an umbilical arterial line for accurate oxygen monitoring. Oxygen saturations are maintained in the 95% to 98% range. If constant blood pressure monitoring is essential or the provider is familiar and skilled in the placement of an umbilical arterial line, this could be performed at this point. An easy placement rule (for a high line that is safe and effective) is one third of the neonate's crown-to-heel length plus 2 cm. The position is confirmed with a radiograph to ensure it is above the diaphragm.

The clinician should request that the placenta be sent to pathology for gross and microscopic evaluation. The maternal record should be copied and sent with the neonatal record to the receiving nursery.

Special Situations and Conditions

When polyhydramnios and upper intestinal obstruction is suspected, the diagnosis can be made easily by determining the volume of fluid in the stomach in the delivery room. Quantities greater than 25 mL are consistent with obstruction. After removing this fluid, the provider should instill approximately 50 cc of air in the stomach. If there is duodenal obstruction, the air passes to the first portion of the duodenum only and produces the typical double bubble. No matter where the obstruction or the timing of its recognition, these infants should be placed on NPO (nothing per mouth) status, with maintenance fluids (glucose solution is sufficient because they have excess salt supplies for the first 2 to 3 postnatal days). A large-bore nasal or oral gastric tube should be placed and connected to intermittent Gomco suction. Antibiotics, in the absence of a perforation, are not required.

Higher intestinal obstruction, such as esophageal atresia with or without a tracheoesophageal fistula, becomes apparent soon after birth and in the transitional period. The infant has constant volumes of clear secretions at the mouth that do not resolve with intermittent suctioning. The secretions may spill into the upper airway, and occasional desaturation and bradycardic spells are frequent. Some clinicians prefer to intubate all of these infants to prevent spillover aspiration. The major risk is from below, however, if there is a fistula present (identified by air in and beyond the stomach). As pH falls, this fluid drains into the lung producing a chemical pneumonitis. Maintenance of the infant on the abdomen in a slight head-up position should be combined with a Replogle tube in the upper airway connected to constant drainage. The infant should be NPO and continued on maintenance fluids. The use of antibiotics varies by locale and should be determined after consultation with the receiving surgeon.

Neonates with omphalocele and gastroschisis present special problems in heat and water loss and contamination and secondary infection. Neonates with gastroschisis and ruptured omphalocele should be placed on higher free water concentrations (approximately 120 mL/kg/day), and their sodium (a sign of overhydration or underhydration in the first few postnatal days) should be monitored closely. At higher free water concentrations, hyperglycemia and an osmotic diuresis can occur. When higher glucose concentrations ($\geq$10% dextrose in water) are used, blood or urine glucose (or both) should be followed. Sterile, warm, saline-soaked Kling bandages work well, particularly when covered with clear plastic wrap. This same therapy is appropriate for neonates with open spinal lesions (meningomyelocele).

Patients with congenital diaphragmatic hernia are extremely challenging and commonly require massive ventilatory support to oxygenate and ventilate effectively. Hand bagging at higher pressures sufficient to lower the PCO_2 and produce a respiratory alkalosis may aid in lowering pulmonary vascular resistance and dilating the pulmonary artery, improving oxygenation. All patients require sedation (e.g., midazolam) and analgesia (e.g., morphine or fentanyl), and many are successfully ventilated and oxygenated only after paralysis (e.g., pancuronium). Patients are at high risk for pneumothorax; sudden or progressive deterioration should be assumed to be a result of this complication until proved otherwise. Although brief improvement can be obtained with a needle in the midclavicular line at the second or third interspace, these leaks are persistent and require chest tube placement. Placing an intercatheter connected to a three-way stopcock allows intermittent removal of air until the chest tube can be placed. Bicarbonate infusions to produce a metabolic alkalosis to match the respiratory one also may be helpful. These neonates should be prepared for emergent transfer as soon as possible.

Neonates who are believed to have cardiac disease (cyanosis, mottling, large heart, tachypnea, tachycardia, poor perfusion, enlarged heart, engorged vasculature) should be considered to have ductal-dependent lesions until proved otherwise. Discrepant blood pressure in the lower limbs and signs of lower body organ dysfunction (intestine, liver, kidney) provide supportive data and together should lead the provider to begin prostaglandin therapy before transport to the cardiac center. Care should be taken in these infants *not* to use supplemental oxygen. Oxygen dilates the pulmonary vasculature bed and leads to further left-to-right flow through the lung, flooding it and further diverting flow away from the aorta and the organs most in need of oxygen when the duct has been reopened with prostaglandin.

OUTCOME

The outcome of an ill newborn depends on the underlying condition, the promptness with which it is recognized, and timely institution of treatment. The generalist must be able to distinguish symptoms of illness and meticulously follow a careful, logical approach to the initial evaluation and stabilization of ill newborns, with appropriate triage to other providers and facilities that are appropriate to the level of care needed.

Mini-index of Related Topics	CH.
PRENATAL FACTORS AFFECTING THE NEWBORN	189
DELIVERY ROOM MANAGEMENT AND TRANSITIONAL CARE	191
BIRTH INJURY AND ASPHYXIA	192
STABILIZATION AND TRANSPORT OF ILL NEWBORNS	193

SUGGESTED READINGS

Committee on Infectious Diseases, American Academy of Pediatrics: 2000 Red Book: Report on the Committee on Infectious Diseases. Elk Grove Village, Ill, American Academy of Pediatrics, 2000.

Hauth JC, Merenstein GB (eds), American Academy of Pediatrics and American College of Obstetricians and Gynecologists: Guidelines for Perinatal Care, 4th ed. Elk Grove Village, Ill, American Academy of Pediatrics, 1997.

Hodson WA, Truog WE: Principles of management of respiratory problems. In Avery GB, Fletcher MA, MacDonald MG (eds): Neonatology, Pathophysiology and Management of the Newborn, 5th ed. Philadelphia, Lippincott Williams & Wilkins, 1999.

Kattwinkel J, Short J, Denson S (eds), American Academy of Pediatrics and American Heart Association: Textbook of Neonatal Resuscitation, 4th ed. Elk Grove Village, Ill, American Academy of Pediatrics, 2000.

Rudolph AM: Congenital Diseases of the Heart: Clinical-Physiological Considerations, 2nd ed. Armonk, NY, Futura, 2001.

196

Special Issues in the Care of the Ill Premature Infant

Robert D. White

ROLE OF THE GENERALIST

1   Identify, treat, and refer, when indicated, medical problems as they arise.

2   Provide ongoing management of stable or improving medical conditions.

3   Anticipate and provide for medical needs at discharge.

This chapter provides guidance regarding issues the generalist must master to care for premature infants. In some cases, the generalist needs to recognize and initiate treatment and then refer to a specialist. In others, the generalist assumes care of an infant after the acute phase of a particular problem is over and continues care through discharge from the hospital and beyond.

ENVIRONMENT OF CARE

The neonatal intensive care unit (NICU) evolved as a place where lifesaving support was provided for large numbers of critically ill and recovering infants. It is a noisy, busy place where infant sleep, family concerns, and pain control often received inadequate emphasis. These issues were of secondary concern during an era when infants were thought to be oblivious to much that was done to them or around them. Understanding has grown regarding how significant the surroundings are to successful treatment of premature infants, making this a priority in any discussion of the special needs of premature infants.

The in utero setting is strikingly different from a typical NICU. The infant is in a fluid-filled environment where sound, movement, taste, smell, and touch all are intimately determined by the mother and mediated by the uterus and amniotic fluid. Diurnal cycles of activity, heart rate, and many hormones are well established before term; neurologic development of the areas of the cortex responsible for interpreting sensory input proceeds in a carefully sequenced and regulated manner. Preterm delivery interrupts this process, in some ways irretrievably, but evidence is accumulating that the NICU can be made more appropriate for preterm infant development through a threefold approach (Box 196-1).

The nursery is each infant's bedroom. In adult and pediatric intensive care units, the syndrome of intensive care unit psychosis is well recognized, caused by near-constant unpleasant auditory, visual, and tactile stimulation and loss of day/night cues. All of these aspects contribute to significant sleep deprivation. Infants are programmed to sleep more than 20 hours a day, a prerequisite for optimal tissue repair and growth. Nursery environment and practices that interfere with extended periods of infant sleep should be minimized or eliminated whenever possible.

Nursery policies should encourage extensive parental-infant interaction. The mother's touch, smell, and sounds become familiar to the infant throughout pregnancy, and although it is impossible to replicate this outside of the uterus, extended time spent skin-to-skin between the parent and the infant is beneficial to both. Parents who assist in the care of their NICU infant become comfortable and competent in their infant's care more quickly, and the infant may be ready for discharge sooner as a result.

Unpleasant procedures should be minimized and conscientious and safe pain control provided in the NICU. Clustering interventions so that the infant can sleep in at least 2- to 3-hour segments is usually possible when the infant is medically stable. Necessary treatments that cause significant discomfort or instability should be preceded by analgesia whenever possible. Many newer agents are now available that are safe for use in ill premature infants. Efforts to make the nursery a place where extensive family involvement is welcomed, where infant sleep is protected, and where the frequency and discomfort of procedures is limited would ensure that the environment of care is supportive rather than constituting an additional risk and stress to the ill premature infant.

Box 196-1. Factors Important to Neonatal Intensive Care Unit Environment

1. Recognize the nursery is the infant's bedroom.
2. Encourage extensive parental-infant interaction.
3. Minimize unpleasant procedures, and provide conscientious and safe pain control.

SPECIFIC CONDITIONS OF THE RECOVERING PREMATURE INFANT

Anemia of Prematurity

A physiologic anemia, or perhaps better termed *pseudoanemia*, occurs in many healthy premature infants for whom the combination of fetal hemoglobin (with excellent oxygen uptake) and good lung function provides adequate oxygen supply to the tissues until the hemoglobin level decreases to less than 8 or 7 g/dL. True anemia, defined as a hemoglobin level inadequate to ensure adequate tissue oxygenation, can occur from causes that are not unique to the premature infant, including congenital infection, hemorrhage at or near the time of birth, hemolysis, and repeated blood sampling. Other factors more common or unique to premature infants that contribute to anemia are shortened erythrocyte life span, rapid body growth, and transient end organ unresponsiveness in the kidney (erythropoietin production) or bone marrow (red blood cell production) or both. The diagnosis of anemia of prematurity requires a decision whether clinical or laboratory evidence, or some combination of the two, should be used to define anemia.

Other, potentially pathologic causes of anemia must be excluded carefully by a complete blood count, with differential and a smear, combined with a routine screen for hemoglobinopathies. Clinically significant anemia in premature infants is suggested by flattening of the growth curve, increased episodes of apnea, elevated respiratory or heart rate, and elevated reticulocyte count. None of these signs and symptoms have been shown reliably to define an infant who would respond to transfusion. Some clinicians prefer to transfuse before these signs and symptoms appear, especially if the infant has significant ongoing respiratory difficulties or oxygen requirement, choosing a hemoglobin level to transfuse routinely the recovering premature infant.

Guidelines for caring for a stable, growing premature infant in detecting and managing anemia of prematurity err on the more conservative side. The infant's hemoglobin or hematocrit should be monitored weekly. When the hemoglobin decreases to less than 8 g/dL, more extensive monitoring is justified, including a reticulocyte count and vigilance for impaired growth or increased respiratory difficulties or apneic spells. If the hemoglobin decreases to less than 7 g/dL or if clinical symptoms develop, transfusion should be considered. Stable premature infants usually can be transfused safely with 20 to 40 mL of packed red blood cells over 6 to 8 hours without respiratory compromise or fluid overload. Cytomegalovirus-negative blood should be used or comparable precautions taken to minimize the risk of transfusion-acquired infection.

Erythropoietin use can reduce the number of transfusions needed for some premature infants. Efforts to decrease blood sampling loss through microtechniques and transcutaneous monitoring can reduce successfully the incidence of anemia and need for erythropoietin therapy in the premature infant. Preventive measures include limitation of the amount and frequency of blood draws, combined with adequate nutrition and special attention to appropriate provision of vitamins and, after the first month of life, iron in the diet.

Apnea of Prematurity

Apnea is common in infants born before 32 weeks' gestation. It is remarkable that apnea is not a universal problem in premature infants because repetitive breathing pauses are the rule in utero. Apnea from impaired central nervous system regulation of respiration is called *central apnea.* Central apnea can be exacerbated by other factors that cause central nervous system depression or malfunction, including seizures, hydrocephalus, sepsis, hypoxia, sedative or narcotic medications, or severe electrolyte abnormalities. *Obstructive apnea*, also common in premature infants, is related to the immature development and muscular control of the nasopharyngeal and hypopharyngeal structures. *Combined apnea* includes features of both.

Diagnosis of apnea of prematurity requires exclusion of central, obstructive, and combined apnea and other causes of apnea, including gastroesophageal reflux, patent ductus arteriosus (PDA), and nasal congestion. In practice, onset of apnea in the first week of life in an infant less than 35 weeks' gestation for whom sepsis and metabolic abnormalities can be excluded is assumed to be apnea of prematurity. Careful clinical observation for other causes of apnea should continue because gastroesophageal reflux and seizures can be exacerbated by some pharmacologic treatments for apnea.

Mild, self-limited apnea does not require treatment. More serious apnea requiring frequent interventions is treated most often with methylxanthines (aminophylline, theophylline, or caffeine), at times in combination with nasal cannula delivery of air or oxygen or with continuous positive airway pressure. Occasionally, very small premature infants require mechanical ventilation for apnea in the first weeks of life. Apnea generally improves with increasing postconceptual age, becoming mild beyond 32 weeks and typically resolving by 35 weeks.

This time course usually allows for weaning of mechanical and medical support by the time an infant is otherwise ready for discharge; an apnea-free period of at least 1 week after all supportive treatment has been discontinued is considered sufficient to document resolution of this problem, although occasionally infants can have an exacerbation of apnea with infections acquired or immunizations received after discharge.

While treatment with methylxanthines continues, monitoring of drug levels and symptoms suggesting toxicity should be considered. If an infant's apnea is well controlled and there are no indications of toxicity, such as tachycardia, irritability, or emesis, determination of levels probably is not necessary. If symptoms consistent with toxicity are noted or if a previously stable infant acutely deteriorates, drug levels should be checked to ensure that the dose being administered still is appropriate.

A few infants with persistent apnea, especially infants with congenital or acquired abnormalities of the brain, require medical treatment and monitoring up to and sometimes even beyond term. These infants are candidates for home therapy, which is discussed in Chapter 197.

Patent Ductus Arteriosus and Heart Murmurs

The PDA is a normal finding in the fetus and persists in most infants for a few hours or days after birth. In some premature infants, a PDA may be the source of significant problems in the first week of life and occasionally beyond. Clinical and laboratory diagnoses of a PDA are based on the presence of continued blood flow through the PDA connecting the aorta to the pulmonary artery. When flow is turbulent, the characteristic heart murmur is present. The murmur progresses from ejection-type to holosystolic and eventually spills over into diastole when the gradient between aortic and pulmonary pressures becomes great enough. The murmur can be absent, especially in very small and ill premature infants in the first week of life when pulmonary artery resistance is high, limiting the flow through the PDA, or the ductus is so widely open that flow is not restricted (similar to the situation in utero). In the former situation, arterial pulses and the pulse pressure may be normal; in the latter situation, the runoff or arterial steal is sufficient to cause an active precordium and bounding pulses. Findings on the chest x-ray vary with this physiology. The initial x-ray may show a normal heart and lung fields and then progress to cardiomegaly with increased vascularity and pulmonary edema as the amount of left-to-right flow through the PDA increases.

Echocardiography is the gold standard for diagnosis of a PDA. In a healthy, growing infant with no murmur and normal pulses and blood pressure, detection of a PDA is of little consequence because treatment would not be indicated. Even an ill premature infant in the first week of life with mild respiratory symptoms does not routinely require echocardiography in the absence of a murmur or other symptoms suggesting a PDA. When bounding pulses, active precordium, widened pulse pressure, cardiomegaly, or increased pulmonary vascularity is present or a murmur or severe respiratory symptoms exist (even if other causes of these symptoms are present), an echocardiogram is indicated.

A premature infant who develops a heart murmur after the first week of life may have a newly opened or reopened PDA, some other form of heart disease, functional or anatomic peripheral pulmonic stenosis, significant anemia, or a normal heart. A murmur may coincide with the development of anemia. Peripheral pulmonic stenosis, a condition rarely of clinical significance, is characterized by a blowing systolic ejection murmur loudest in the back and axillae. When any physical findings apart from the murmur are present, echocardiography and consultation with a pediatric cardiologist are indicated.

Treatment of a symptomatic PDA in a premature infant has undergone significant change over time, from early surgical intervention to repeated courses of indomethacin before surgery is considered. Indomethacin usually is successful in constriction or closure of the PDA. If factors that enhance patency of the PDA persist after treatment (e.g., severe respiratory distress, sepsis, fluid overload, and perhaps anemia), recurrence of symptoms is likely. Box 196-2 lists contraindications for use of indomethacin with a PDA. Infants whose PDA does not require treatment or who have a persisting murmur without symptoms after treatment do not need further monitoring in the hospital because the PDA usually closes by term; even in infants in whom the PDA does not close, endocarditis prophylaxis is not necessary.

Box 196-2. Use of Indomethacin in Closure of Patent Ductus Arteriosus

Contraindications

- Renal insufficiency
- Thrombocytopenia

Administration

- *Should not* be given through an umbilical artery catheter
- *Should not* be given by rapid intravenous push

Retinopathy of Prematurity

Retinopathy of prematurity (ROP) is characterized by the disruption of normal vascularization of the retinae in infants born before or early in the third trimester of gestation. Previously thought to be exclusively due to excessive oxygen administration, ROP now is recognized as a complication of extreme prematurity with multiple contributing factors. Most retinal vascularization occurs during the third trimester. The premature infant is exposed to pharmacologic agents and factors atypical of the intrauterine environment, such as oxygen free radicals, acute inflammatory responses, perturbations of cerebral blood flow, and a distorted physical environment. The incidence and severity of ROP are correlated most strongly with the extent of prematurity, with the disorder being rare and generally mild in infants born after 28 weeks' gestation and common and often severe in infants born before 24 weeks' gestation. The more premature the infant, the more delayed is onset.

Although ROP cannot be prevented, clues have allowed development of screening methods that identify nearly all cases of severe ROP in time for treatment. Infants less than 32 weeks' gestation should be screened for ROP by 4 to 6 weeks of age by a trained ophthalmologist; most require repeated examinations until the retinae are fully vascularized near term. Table 196-1 and Figures 196-1 and 196-2 describe the stages of ROP. When ROP is extensive or accompanied by plus disease, which is an indication of an active neovascularization process, surgical intervention with laser or cryotherapy is considered, and referral to specialty care is indicated.

In infants who do not require surgery and in most infants who do, the process that causes progression of ROP tends to diminish in the weeks just before term, but careful follow-up through the preschool years of all infants with ROP is necessary because the incidence of myopia and other visual problems is higher in this population.

Table 196-1. Stages of Retinopathy of Prematurity

Stage	Clinical Description
0	ROP absent
1	A line of demarcation at the edge of the developing vasculature, signifying the start of an abnormal pattern of vascularization
2	Line of demarcation begins to develop a three-dimensional character, creating a ridge on the retina
3	Fibrovascular elements, or neovascularization, have begun to invade the vitreous

ROP, retinopathy of prematurity.

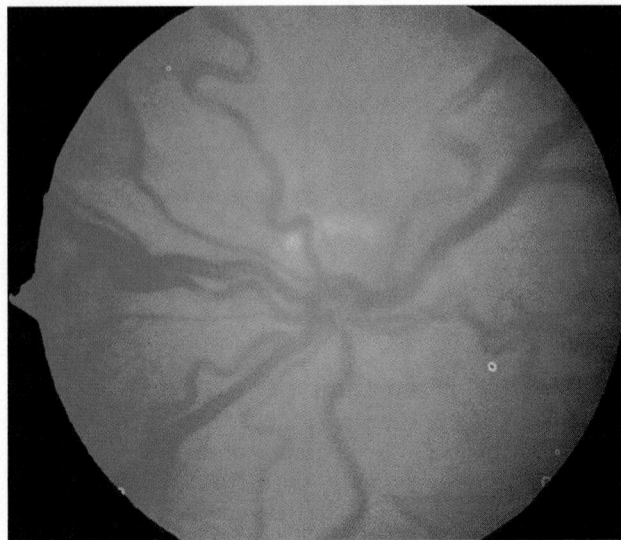

Figure 196-1. Vessel tortuosity. (From Clark DA, Thomson JE, Barkemeyer BM: Atlas of Neonatology: A Companion to Avery's Diseases of the Newborn. Philadelphia, WB Saunders, 2000, p 283.)

Necrotizing Enterocolitis

In necrotizing enterocolitis (NEC), the degree of prematurity is the most important risk factor. Age of onset is inversely related to the degree of prematurity—that is, the younger the infant is at the time of birth, the later in life NEC is likely to present. NEC can present from day 1 until well into the 2nd month of life in very premature infants. Although many complications of prematurity tend to correlate with a high risk for NEC, including sepsis, PDA, and maternal abruption, none is highly predictive. NEC often has occurred in stable, growing infants who would be considered low risk.

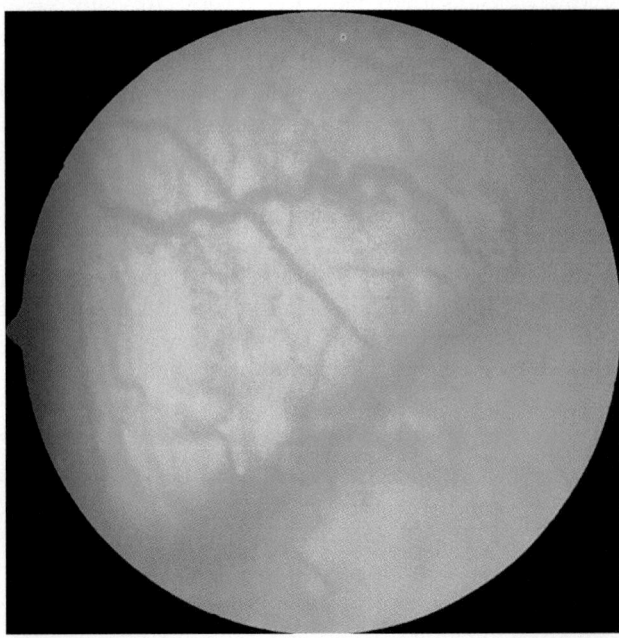

Figure 196-2. Vascular ridge with peripheral avascular zone. (From Clark DA, Thomson JE, Barkemeyer BM: Atlas of Neonatology: A Companion to Avery's Diseases of the Newborn. Philadelphia, WB Saunders, 2000, p 283.)

Sometimes a nursery experiences a cluster of cases of NEC, suggesting a possible infectious cause. Whatever the primary cause, damage to the fragile intestine of the premature infant rapidly leads to infectious complications and often intestinal necrosis and perforation.

The diagnosis of NEC should be considered in any premature infant with unexplained signs and symptoms of ileus. Most often, it presents with symptoms of acute abdominal distention, gastric residuals (often bile-stained), diminished bowel sounds, and heme-positive or grossly bloody stools. Presence of discoloration or rigidity of the abdomen on examination and thickened bowel walls, pneumatosis intestinalis, or portal venous air on the abdominal x-ray distinguish this from more benign conditions. The complete blood count often shows neutropenia or thrombocytopenia. Hyponatremia also is common, and if large areas of bowel necrosis exist, acidemia and hyperkalemia are usually present.

Immediate management of an infant with NEC is supportive and should be instituted in conjunction with referral for specialty care. Feedings should be stopped, and an oral or nasal gastric tube should be placed to suction. After appropriate cultures, broad-spectrum antibiotic therapy (including coverage for anaerobes) should be initiated. Third-space fluid losses after inflammation and ileus may compromise blood pressure and organ perfusion, requiring volume expansion or pressors or both. Some infants experience sufficient compromise of respiratory status from abdominal distention or apnea that ventilatory support is required. Intestinal perforation with the presence of free air confirmed on a cross-table or decubitus film of the abdomen is a clear indication for surgical intervention, although some infants who are considered too small or unstable for immediate laparotomy may be stabilized temporarily by placement of a peritoneal drain. At surgery, involvement of the bowel may be limited, allowing primary resection and reanastomosis. More extensive disease necessitates removal of a sizable portion of bowel and placement of an ostomy and mucous fistula. Other infants have extensive disease and progressive septic shock, incompatible with life.

The search for a cause of this apparently capricious disease has led to many theories and suggestions for prevention; many center on how feeding should be managed in premature infants. Delay of feedings until a high-risk infant is stable and use of dilute milk and slow advance of feeding volumes have not been been shown to eliminate the risk of NEC. Small feedings in the first few days of life (trophic feedings) followed by steady advance of isotonic milk, preferably breast milk, creates no added risk of NEC, with the benefit of earlier establishment of good caloric intake.

Seizures

The cause of seizures in preterm infants is similar to that in term infants, although the relative incidence of each cause is different. Seizures can occur as the result of intracerebral and intraventricular hemorrhage (IVH), hypoxic-ischemic encephalopathy (HIE), birth injury or congenital malformation of the brain, infection, or metabolic disorders (especially hypoglycemia or hypocalcemia) or, as in other age groups, may be idiopathic. Rare causes include drug toxicity or withdrawal and congenital epilepsy syndromes. Because of the immaturity of the premature brain, seizures often are subtle. Many infants have no physical manifestation at all, and many manifest only apnea. Unmistakable tonic-clonic spasms are rare, but a careful observer often first suspects seizures in an infant exhibiting a staring, fixed gaze; chewing motions of the mouth; or repetitive tonic posturing of a single or multiple extremities.

In the presence of obvious seizure activity in a premature infant, the diagnostic assessment is straightforward. A sepsis workup, including spinal tap, and metabolic evaluation, including glucose, sodium, and calcium, should be done immediately. A brain imaging study (computed tomography scan or head ultrasound for infants who are too unstable to leave the nursery) should be completed as soon as feasible. An electroencephalogram provides confirmatory evidence but is most useful as a means of following the success of treatment and determining when anticonvulsant therapy might be terminated safely.

A more difficult challenge involves deciding which infants with apnea require evaluation for seizures. Most apnea in the preterm infant is not due to seizures, yet waiting for more specific signs of a seizure may allow the disorder to go undetected and untreated for an extended period. Clinical judgment, with consultation when uncertain, must be used. Sepsis or a metabolic abnormality usually is detected through other clinical signs or monitoring tests, but seizure-induced apnea secondary to HIE or IVH could be attributed mistakenly to prematurity. A useful rule of thumb in this setting might be to consider apneic episodes that do not respond to usual supportive measures for apnea of prematurity, especially in infants with a history of HIE or IVH, as deserving of a screening electroencephalogram. If the electroencephalogram is equivocal, a therapeutic trial of phenobarbital can be a useful diagnostic tool.

Phenobarbital continues to be the initial drug of choice for seizures in premature infants. The loading dose is 20 to 30 mg/kg, and subsequent management should be coordinated with a neurologic specialist. Some children require anticonvulsant therapy only for the acute stage of their illness, whereas others require treatment for several months or years.

Intraventricular Hemorrhage and Periventricular Leukomalacia

IVH and periventricular leukomalacia (PVL) are conditions that show a striking predilection for very-low-birth-weight infants. These complications are unusual beyond 28 weeks' gestation and are common and more likely to be severe in infants less than 24 weeks' gestation. IVH and PVL arise from disruption of blood flow in the tissues and capillary beds adjacent to the lateral ventricles of the premature brain (the so-called subependymal germinal matrix), where growth and metabolic activity are robust, yet blood vessels are thin and fragile at the end of the second trimester.

The basic presentations for IVH may exist separately or together. *Grade I* bleeding is limited to the germinal matrix, *grade II* bleeding extends into the ventricle, and *grade III* bleeding causes dilation of the ventricle. *Grade IV* IVH occurs within the parenchyma of the brain and is considered to represent a hemorrhagic infarction. As the necrotic tissue is resorbed, the infarcted area eventually may communicate with the lateral ventricle, forming a porencephalic cyst.

Early signs and symptoms of IVH range from silent in most cases of germinal matrix (grade I) hemorrhage to serious or life-threatening in some cases of intraparenchymal (grade IV) hemorrhage. Extensive bleeding can lead to a rapid decline in the hemoglobin level with volume loss and hypotension, seizures, apnea, and prolonged elevation of serum bilirubin. Late complications are related primarily to the development of obstructive hydrocephalus from protein occlusion of the subarachnoid villi and require referral for specialty care.

The diagnosis of IVH is made by screening ultrasonography performed in the 2nd week of life or sooner if symptoms warrant. Bleeding after 10 days of age is rare so that a normal ultrasound at that time usually negates the need for further studies, unless unusual findings (e.g., seizures, rapid head growth, sudden unexplained decrease in hemoglobin) appear. An abnormal screening ultrasound requires a follow-up plan, which should be established in consultation with a specialist. Careful clinical monitoring of head circumference for the development of hydrocephalus is essential. Grades I and II IVH are not associated with a significant increase in risk for developmental problems after discharge, whereas grades III and IV IVH carry a higher risk for mental retardation, cerebral palsy, and other developmental and behavioral difficulties. This latter group of children requires close monitoring and developmental support throughout the preschool years.

PVL is an ischemic injury to the white matter surrounding the ventricle that is difficult to detect on early ultrasonography and may be missed in some affected children. Similar to IVH, PVL is more common with increasing prematurity and carries a high risk for the later development of cerebral palsy. PVL is detected most often during brain imaging for other conditions and has no known treatment.

Mini-index of Related Topics

SUGGESTED READINGS

Albanese C, Rowe M: Necrotizing enterocolitis. Semin Pediatr Surg 1995;4:200–206.

Anand KJS, and the International Evidence-Based Group for Neonatal Pain: Consensus statement for the prevention and management of pain in the newborn. Arch Pediatr Adolesc Med 2001;155:173–180.

Bhatia J: Current options in the management of apnea of prematurity. Clin Pediatr 2000;39:327–336.

Committee on Infectious Diseases, American Academy of Pediatrics: 2003 Red Book: Report on the Committee on Infectious Diseases, 26th ed. Elk Grove Village, Ill, American Academy of Pediatrics, 2003.

Fielder A, Levene M: Screening for retinopathy of prematurity. Arch Dis Child 1992;67:860–867.

Gilstrap LC, Oh W (eds), American Academy of Pediatrics and American College of Obstetricans and Gynecologists: Guidelines for Perinatal Care, 5th ed. Elk Grove Village, Ill, American Academy of Pediatrics, 2002.

Scher M: Seizures in the newborn infant: Diagnosis, treatment and outcome. Clin Perinatol 1997;24:735–772.

Vohr B, Ment L: Intraventricular hemorrhage in the preterm infant. Early Hum Dev 1996;44:1–16.

White R: Enhanced neonatal intensive care design: A physiological approach. J Perinatol 1999;16:381–384.

SECTION 5   NEWBORN CARE: *Perinatal Care*

197 Continuing Care of the Growing Premature Infant

Robert D. White

ROLE OF THE GENERALIST

1 Provide ongoing management of stable or improving premature infants.

2 Ensure optimal nutrition and growth.

3 Initiate immunizations when an infant's hospital stay exceeds the first 2 months of life.

4 Perform indicated screening examinations, with referral to an appropriate specialist if abnormal screening results are obtained.

5 Anticipate and arrange for medical needs at discharge.

Management of the stable growing premature infant in the days or weeks preceding discharge from the hospital is focused on two priorities—achieving and maintaining optimal nutrition and anticipating discharge needs.

NUTRITION

Many premature infants receive inadequate nutrition during the crucial first weeks after birth. Their immature intestine does not permit full caloric feedings to be given enterally, often for several weeks. The provision of adequate caloric intake via intravenous alimentation during this time frequently is constrained by the need for fluid restriction, hyperglycemia, or hyperlipidemia. As a result, nearly all infants born before 32 weeks' gestation enter their 2nd month of life below the 50th percentile for weight. Many infants are well below the 10th percentile. When more serious, acute medical problems have been stabilized, providing optimal nutrition becomes a high priority. The infant still is in a critical phase of brain growth. Maturation of other organs proceeds best when the infant is in a consistently anabolic state.

The optimal nutritional substrate for the growing premature infant is fortified breast milk. Breast milk is digested more easily than premature formulas and provides the infant with the greatest protection against infection and the optimal delivery of trace elements (Box 197-1). Because a premature infant's needs exceed those of the full-term infant on a weight-for-weight basis, breast milk alone provides inadequate protein, sodium, calcium, phosphorus, and vitamin D. Human milk fortifiers can be added to meet these requirements when breast milk is given to the infant in amounts of at least 150 mL/kg/day, and preferably 180 mL/kg/day. Because cytomegalovirus can be excreted in breast milk and premature infants receive inadequate protective antibodies because of their abbreviated time in utero, breast milk provided to these

Box 197-1. Advantages of Breast Milk for Nutrition of the Preterm Infant

- It is highly digestible.
- It contains multiple anti-infective properties not present in formulas.
- It contains trace elements and nutrients not present in formulas.
- Breast-feeding enhances maternal-infant bonding.

Table 197-1. Composition of Various Milk Sources (per 100 cal)

Milk Source		Cal/oz	Osmolality (mOsm)	Protein (g)	Ca (mg)	P (mg)	Na (mg)	Iron (mg)	Vit D (IU)
Breast, preterm		20	255	2.1	37	19	37	0.2	3
+ fortifier	Similac	24	329	3	175	98	49	0.6	150
(1 packet/25 cc)	Enfamil	24	290	3.2	146	81	49	1.9	200
Enfamil Premature 20 cal		20	230	3	165	83	58	0.5	240
Enfamil Premature 24 cal		24	270	3	165	83	58	0.5	240
Similac Special Care 20 cal		20	211	2.7	180	100	43	0.4	150
Similac Special Care 24 cal		24	246	2.7	180	100	43	0.4	150
NeoSure		22	224	2.6	105	62	33	1.8	70
Standard term formula		20	270	2.1	78	53	27	1.8	60
Standard soy formula		20	180–200	2.5	105	80	40	1.8	60
Pregestimil		20	280	2.8	115	75	47	1.88	50

Note: All figures are approximations to be used for comparison only. Treatment decisions should be based on current data from the manufacturer.

infants should be frozen, pasteurized, or obtained from cytomegalovirus-seronegative donors. Most medications taken by nursing mothers do not constitute contraindications to use of breast milk, although the physician should check the status of any unfamiliar medication.

Several formulas have been developed for premature infants that meet their needs for a highly digestible formula with higher concentrations of protein, minerals, and vitamins than are given to term infants. Table 197-1 lists the contents of formulas and of breast milk. These can be substituted safely and effectively when breast milk is unavailable; when given in a 24-cal/oz preparation, 150 to 160 mL/kg/day provides infants with the 120 cal/kg/day needed for optimal growth. Preparations of 20 cal/oz need to be given at 180 mL/kg/day to meet the same goal.

Whether breast milk or formula is used, all infants should be monitored on a weekly basis for common metabolic abnormalities (Box 197-2). Metabolic acidosis, hyponatremia, hypercalcemia or hypocalcemia, hyperphosphatemia or hypophosphatemia, and elevated alkaline phosphatase all are typical in these patients and may require frequent adjustments of specific components of the formula.

Even after an infant's acute medical problems have been surmounted, providing adequate calories enterally can be difficult. Gastroesophageal reflux is a typical complication noted when bolus feedings approach the optimal volumes for growth; strategies that have been employed to minimize this problem include higher calorie, lower volume feedings; frequent, small feedings (e.g., every 1 to 2 hours); continuous feedings; transpyloric feedings; and use of metoclo-

pramide. In addition, generic interventions, such as thickening or concentrating the milk and elevating the head of the bed, have proved successful in some patients (Box 197-3). Although occasional small emeses rarely interfere with adequate nutrition or lead to aspiration pneumonia in a healthy, growing premature infant, emeses can occur in association with infection or increasing apnea or respiratory distress and in those settings should be viewed with concern.

Although nearly all infants born before 32 weeks' gestation and most born before 35 weeks' gestation are unable to receive nipple feedings at birth, when the infant has shown readiness (e.g., good non-nutritive suck, minimal respiratory instability with handling), oral feedings can be considered. A typical approach to instituting oral feedings is to offer a bottle once a day. When the infant has shown ability to take a satisfactory amount within 30 minutes, the frequency of oral feedings is advanced gradually over the next several days or weeks until all feedings are taken by mouth.

Infants whose mothers intend to breast-feed can be started in a similar fashion, but establishing the adequacy of their intake is more problematic. Some nurseries employ prenursing and postnursing weights to estimate the amount of the infant's intake; others maintain at least one bottle feeding a day to get a sense of how much an infant is taking; still others, recognizing that these approaches have definite limitations, make no direct effort to establish how much a infant is taking during breast-feeding, but simply evaluate weight gain and increase the frequency of breast-feeding gradually as long as the infant is maintaining satisfactory growth.

There is not yet a consensus on the appropriate target for growth in a stable premature infant. Achieving intrauterine growth rates seems like a reasonable standard, and prema-

Box 197-2. Weekly Metabolic Monitoring in the Growing Preterm Infant

- Length
- Head circumference
- Hemoglobin or hematocrit
- Calcium
- Phosphorus
- Alkaline phosphatase
- Sodium
- Albumin or total protein
- Total carbon dioxide or bicarbonate

Box 197-3. Management Strategies for Gastroesophageal Reflux in the Preterm Infant

- Frequent small feedings (every 1–2 hours)
- Continuous feedings
- Transpyloric feedings
- Elevate head of bed
- Thickened or concentrated feedings
- Metoclopramide (Reglan)

ture infants have shown the ability for "catch-up" growth when their medical condition stabilizes. Another rule of thumb is that premature infants should gain approximately 1% to 2% of their body weight each day. A 1-kg infant should gain 10 to 20 g/day, and by the time the infant reaches 1500 g, he or she should be gaining 15 to 30 g/day. Daily increases above or below the targets are normal, but sustained growth significantly below or above the targets should be the cause for concern and investigation.

Head growth should be followed on at least a weekly basis and should parallel the intrauterine curve; growth of the head circumference of less than 1 cm/wk on a sustained basis, if not secondary to a recognized congenital malformation or a perinatal insult, is highly suggestive of nutritional inadequacy. Infants with chronic lung disease often can achieve acceptable growth in weight and head circumference, yet they fall well off the normal curve for length. This situation suggests inadequate nutrition, particularly in the provision of adequate minerals and vitamin D.

When a premature infant has shown optimal weight gain on oral feedings, he or she usually is ready for discharge. Feeding issues for the breast-fed infant center around when it is appropriate to discontinue the human milk fortifier; in most cases, the infant can be weaned from this as a natural consequence of receiving all of his or her nutrition directly from the breast. In some cases, supplementing breast feedings with breast milk and added human milk fortifiers may be desirable even after discharge. An infant with a markedly elevated alkaline phosphatase receiving high levels of minerals or a mother who is unable or unwilling to nurse full-time may benefit from this approach. Infants of mothers whose breast milk supply has dwindled also can receive formula supplementation, but the possibility of improving the mother's milk supply should be explored by referring her to a lactation consultant. Infants who continue to receive breast milk as their primary source of nutrition after the human milk fortifier is discontinued should receive an alternative source of vitamin D through the first year of life.

Formula-fed premature infants should be transitioned from their initial formula to one intended for home use that still contains enhanced levels of protein and minerals. Current evidence suggests that these special premature formulas should be used throughout the first year of life to allow the infant to restore the acquired nutritional deficit.

Most infants for whom reflux was a problem early in their course can be weaned from antireflux measures before discharge. The use of frequent small feedings, antireflux medications, and positioning techniques can be discontinued well in advance of discharge so that the infant's tolerance of larger volume feedings can be shown.

IMMUNIZATIONS

Premature infants should be immunized on the same schedule as full-term infants because they usually are able to mount an adequate immune response to vaccines by 2 months' postnatal age. Hepatitis B immunization in premature infants whose mothers are hepatitis B surface antigen negative also should be initiated at 2 months of age, rather than at birth.

SCREENING FOR PROBLEMS OF PREMATURITY NEAR THE TIME OF DISCHARGE

Routine screening tests for some of the more serious complications of prematurity (e.g., intraventricular hemorrhage, retinopathy of prematurity) are discussed in Chapter 196. Most premature infants also should be screened shortly before discharge for hearing and developmental problems.

Hearing screening now is standard practice for all newborns in many states but in states where it is not standard, premature infants still constitute a high-risk group who should be screened routinely. Although an abnormal screen may be due to persistent middle ear fluid, occult otitis media can be seen in this population, whose eustachian tube function often is compromised. If otitis media can be excluded, an abnormal hearing screen should be followed up with a diagnostic-level brainstem auditory evoked response or otoacoustic emission and then a referral to a pediatric otolaryngologist if the test is abnormal. A normal hearing screen at discharge for a premature (or full-term) infant does not preclude hearing problems later, so vigilance during well-child visits throughout the first 2 years of life is essential until language skills are well established.

Screening the premature infant for developmental problems at the time of discharge can be problematic. Success in oral feeding by 35 to 36 weeks' postconception is the easiest and a useful criteria to define the basic integrity of the central nervous system; additional reassuring findings in the history and physical examination at that stage include the absence of apnea or seizures, normal muscular tone and reflexes, and the infant's ability to fix his or her gaze on a face for brief periods. More extensive neurologic testing has been formalized and studied by many investigators, but use of these instruments requires special training and provides only an indication of risk, not assurance of normalcy or diagnosis of delay. Nevertheless, the availability of a skilled developmental therapist to complete this testing near the time of discharge can be helpful to show to parents their infant's capabilities and may be useful when making referrals to agencies providing developmental support to the infant and family after discharge.

DISCHARGE PLANNING

Many concerns should be addressed in the days leading up to discharge to ensure a safe transition to home. Perhaps the greatest concern to parents assuming the care of a previously critically ill, extensively monitored infant is the risk of sudden infant death syndrome (SIDS). The incidence of SIDS is higher in premature infants than in the general population. The distinction between this problem and apnea of prematurity is not always clear to families and has been the source of confusion within the medical profession as well, complicating the decision of discharge with home apnea monitoring.

Infants in whom medical treatment for apnea (e.g., caffeine or theophylline) has been discontinued and who have been free of apneic episodes for more than 1 week before discharge do not need home monitoring. Infants who continue to have occasional episodes of apnea within the week before discharge or who still are on oxygen at the time of discharge should be considered for monitoring. The family and all other caregivers for the infant should learn cardiopulmonary resuscitation and exhibit knowledge of the monitor and how to respond to an apneic episode. The home must be assessed carefully for adequate electrical wiring and the availability of a telephone to ensure that help can be summoned quickly should the infant have a serious apneic episode at home.

Parents should understand that a home monitor does not prevent SIDS and that appropriate precautions (e.g., "back to sleep"; avoidance of heavy bedding and pillows; avoidance of exposure to cigarette smoke; use of an approved crib, avoiding a sofa, waterbed, or recliner for sleep) are the best way to avoid SIDS. When the infant has been apnea-free for a sufficient period, discontinuing the monitor 1 or 2 days before discharge also is helpful as a signal to families that their infant really will be safe without extensive home monitoring.

Prevention of respiratory syncytial virus (RSV) infection is a significant concern during the winter months. The injection of monoclonal antibody against RSV has lessened, but not eliminated, this risk for premature infants; additional measures that can be protective include limiting exposure to other preschool children who may be infected, frequent hand washing by caregivers who care for multiple infants or who may themselves be ill, and avoidance of cigarette smoke.

Thermoregulation of a premature infant is often more of a concern to families than caregivers realize, with a tendency to overbundle infants even in warm environments. Families should understand that before discharge, the infant's ability to maintain his or her temperature already has been shown at temperatures comfortable to adults. Overbundling is not necessary and may constitute a hazard for hyperthermia, apnea, and SIDS.

Safety measures, such as the use of a car seat and "child-proofing" the home, that are routine for full-term infants merit extra emphasis in the preterm infant approaching discharge. Because most car seats are not designed for preterm infants, these infants first should be placed in their car seat while oxygen saturation is monitored in the nursery before discharge and adjustments made, if necessary, to their seating arrangement.

Mini-index of Related Topics

SUGGESTED READINGS

Committee on Infectious Diseases, American Academy of Pediatrics: 2003 Red Book: Report of the Committee on Infectious Diseases, 26th ed. Elk Grove Village, Ill, American Academy of Pediatrics, 2003.

Gilstrap LC, Oh W (eds), American Academy of Pediatrics and American College of Obstetricians and Gynecologists: Guidelines for Perinatal Care, 5th ed. Elk Grove Village, Ill, American Academy of Pediatrics, 2002.

Hay WW Jr, Lucas A, Heird WC, et al: Workshop summary: Nutrition of the extremely low birth weight infant. Pediatrics 1999;104:1360–1368.

Schanler R, Shulman R, Lau C: Feeding strategies for premature infants: Beneficial outcomes of feeding fortified human milk versus preterm formula. Pediatrics 1999;103:1150–1157.

198 Jaundice

Ashima Madan and David K. Stevenson

ROLE OF THE GENERALIST

1   Distinguish between physiologic and pathologic jaundice in a newborn.
2   Know the differential diagnosis of jaundice in the newborn period.
3   Recognize the need for early follow-up in certain cases (e.g., premature and near-term infants, breast-feeding infants, infants discharged before 48 to 72 hours, infants with blood group incompatibility or a high bilirubin level at discharge).
4   Initiate appropriate diagnostic workup to determine the cause of jaundice.
5   Initiate treatment for hyperbilirubinemia and its underlying cause in a timely fashion.
6   Recognize the need for referral to a specialist when appropriate.
7   Recognize early signs of neurotoxicity and kernicterus.
8   Provide appropriate discharge advice and follow-up care after discharge.

DEFINITION

Jaundice is a yellowish discoloration of the skin caused by deposition of the pigment, bilirubin. In a newborn, jaundice usually is apparent when the serum total bilirubin (STB) level reaches 5 mg/dL. Newborn jaundice occurs in 60% to 80% of term infants and is a normal phenomenon reflecting adaptation to extrauterine life. Hyperbilirubinemia, an excess accumulation of bilirubin in the circulation, is a relative state and is defined best by reference to an hour-specific STB level that is at or above the 95th percentile for a given population of neonates.

Physiologic jaundice is caused by an increased production of bilirubin and a delay in the maturation of hepatic proteins or enzymes that are necessary for the uptake, conjugation, and excretion of bilirubin. Before birth, unconjugated bilirubin is removed and eliminated from the fetal circulation by the placenta. After birth, production of bilirubin increases secondary to the relatively large red blood cell mass and associated shorter red blood cell life span. Because bilirubin must be metabolized by the infant's liver and eliminated in stool, any delay in stooling results in decreased elimination and increased enterohepatic circula-

tion of bilirubin. Each of these factors leads to a normal increase in STB levels soon after birth.

Under certain conditions, lipid-soluble, unconjugated bilirubin crosses the immature blood-brain barrier and is deposited in the basal ganglia of the brain, resulting in kernicterus or acute bilirubin encephalopathy. Although many factors are related to the development of acute bilirubin encephalopathy, the major variable is height of the unconjugated serum bilirubin level. The occurrence of injury is not related, however, to a linear increase in total bilirubin levels. Prematurity, acidosis, decreased albumin levels, hypoxia, and sepsis increase the risk for injury. Kernicterus presents with a wide spectrum of clinical signs. Lethargy, poor feeding, hypotonia, and an absent Moro reflex are seen early in the process. In severe cases, these findings are followed by hypertonia, opisthotonos, high-pitched cry, fever, and convulsions. Survivors often have cerebral palsy of the choreoathetoid type, deafness, mental retardation, and other neurologic defects. Bilirubin encephalopathy is most likely to develop 3 to 7 days after birth. Risk factors for recent cases are male gender, breast-feeding, gestation less than 38 weeks, and discharge before 72 hours of age. Hemolysis also is associated with increased risk for kernicterus.

FUNDAMENTALS

Bilirubin Physiology in the Fetus and Newborn

The physiology of bilirubin metabolism in the fetus and newborn is illustrated in Figure 198-1. Bilirubin is produced predominantly from the breakdown of heme derived from senescent red blood cells and from turnover of heme-containing enzymes. Heme oxygenase catalyzes heme into equimolar amounts of biliverdin and carbon monoxide (CO). Unconjugated bilirubin, produced by the action of biliverdin reductase on biliverdin, is bound to albumin and transported to the liver. Unbound or free bilirubin moves variably into tissues, such as the brain and the skin. Deposition of unbound bilirubin in the tissues depends on the binding capacity of albumin, affinity of the tissue, and pH of the blood. At the liver cell membrane, unconjugated bilirubin dissociates from albumin, enters the hepatocyte, and binds to an intracellular protein. It is conjugated into water-soluble monoglucuronides or diglucuronides by the catalytic action of uridine diphosphoglucuronate glucuronosyltransferase (UGT), secreted into the bile ductules, and finally eliminated with bile into the intestine. Conjugated bilirubin

and s
serum
patho
Lab
levels
signs
direct
carboi
the de
in equ
heme
of her
and a
tion is
or cho
if the
Scre
bilirub
of nev
discha
nomog
infants
photot
high bi
who ar
STB le
or prec
multice
ETCO
effectiv
alone.
a norm
efficier
and an
follow-
the pre
such a
periphe
degree
neous r
employ
reduce
infants

MANAC

Prevent
instituti
caloric
educatic

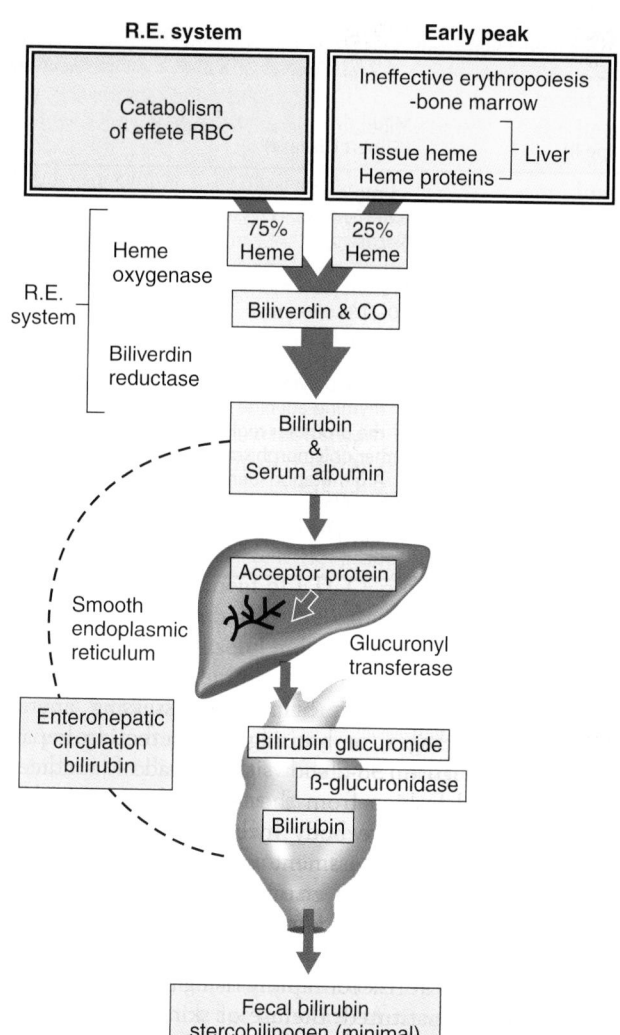

Figure 198-1. Bilirubin metabolism in the newborn. CO, carbon monoxide; RBC, red blood cells; RE, reticuloendothelial. (From Maisels MJ: Jaundice in the newborn. Pediatr Rev 1982;3:305–319. Copyright 1982. Reproduced with permission from *Pediatrics in Review*.)

or its bacterial degradation product, stercobilin, is excreted in meconium and stool. The intestinal enzyme β-glucuronidase can unconjugate bilirubin, which may be reabsorbed into the circulation (the enterohepatic circulation).

Incidence and Epidemiology

Hyperbilirubinemia occurs in approximately 8% of newborns, with 6% to 7% reaching STB levels greater than 12 mg/dL and less than 2% having levels of 20 mg/dL or greater. Hyperbilirubinemia is much more common in premature infants and infants between 35 and 37 weeks' gestation. It also is more prevalent in full-term breast-fed infants, infants with hemolysis secondary to blood group incompatibilities, infants of East Asian or Mediterranean descent, infants of diabetic mothers, infected infants, polycythemic infants, and infants with a sibling who had jaundice (Box 198-1).

Recognition of variations in peak STB levels of different racial groups is important for the management of infants with jaundice. In term breast-fed newborns of European or African ancestry, STB levels peak at 72 to 96 hours and then

Box 198-1. Risk Factors for Hyperbilirubinemia

- Race or ethnic group: Asian, Native American, Mediterranean
- Diabetes mellitus (including gestational)
- Rh incompatibility, ABO incompatibility, other Coombs-positive hemolytic conditions
- Use of oxytocin in hypotonic solutions during labor
- Instrumentation during labor
- Breast-feeding
- Premature infants and near-term infants 35 to 37 weeks' gestation
- Infants with a sibling who had jaundice
- Polycythemia
- Cephalhematoma, hidden bleeding, or bruising

gradually decrease to adult values over a few weeks. Native American and East Asian infants have a different pattern of physiologic jaundice characterized by a more rapid increase in STB levels during the first few days and a higher peak level, which reaches its maximum approximately 1 week later.

Etiology

Unconjugated or indirect hyperbilirubinemia can be caused by a myriad of conditions and is found frequently among otherwise healthy breast-fed newborns. Breast-feeding jaundice is most common in preterm or term infants who nurse fewer than eight times in 24 hours and have difficulty in establishing an effective feeding pattern. They typically weigh less than nonjaundiced infants, stool and void less frequently, and do not receive supplementation with formula. Poor feeding results in a catabolic state, which is known to cause increases in STB. Breast milk jaundice syndrome is an elevation in unconjugated bilirubin that typically presents after the 2nd week of life and can persist for several months in a small percentage of infants. STB levels decrease with cessation of nursing for 24 hours.

The second most frequent cause of hyperbilirubinemia is increased bilirubin production from breakdown of red blood cells secondary to ABO, Rh, or minor blood group incompatibilities; polycythemia; or extravasated blood. Hemolysis from ABO incompatibility is seen in approximately 10% of A-positive or B-positive infants born to O-positive women. Hemolysis from Rh sensitization is seen less commonly, but typically is more severe than that of ABO incompatibility. Hemolysis also is caused by red blood cell enzyme defects (glucose-6-phosphate dehydrogenase [G6PD] or pyruvate kinase deficiency) and by structural red blood cell membrane defects (hereditary spherocytosis). Congenital infections from cytomegalovirus, rubella, or toxoplasmosis also are associated with increased hemolysis, causing jaundice that usually presents around the time of birth.

Infants of diabetic mothers are more likely to become hyperbilirubinemic from polycythemia, ineffective erythropoiesis, or decreased elimination of bilirubin. Increased enterohepatic circulation caused by decreased caloric intake, pyloric stenosis, intestinal obstruction, and endocrine disturbances are other causes of neonatal jaundice. Urinary

Table 200-1. Characteristics of Fetal, Neonatal, and Adult Red Blood Cells

Characteristic	Fetal Red Blood Cell	Neonatal Red Blood Cell	Adult Red Blood Cell
Size (MCV in fL)	120–130	108–118	82–92
Shape	Many abnormal shapes	Many abnormal shapes	Few abnormal shapes
Life span (days)	30–50	60–90	110–120
2,3-DPG content (mol/L)	2–4	4–6	9
Fetal hemoglobin content (%)	95–98	70–80	2–10

2,3-DPG, 2,3-diphosphoglucerate; MCV, mean cell volume.

higher than the mean mean cell volume of 108 fL in term infants (Table 200-1).

Reticulocyte counts are slightly higher, averaging 6% to 10%. Nucleated RBCs number 1000 to 1500/mm³. There is an inverse relationship between nucleated RBCs and gestational age. Nucleated RBCs are cleared rapidly from the circulation during the first postnatal days, although a few still may be observed in small preterm infants at 7 days. Variations in RBC size and shape are greater than variations observed in term infants. RBC survival is considerably shorter than in term infants.

Erythropoietin concentrations gradually increase until birth. Erythropoietin measurements made on cord blood from infants of laboring and nonlaboring mothers and from infants undergoing labor stress may reflect hypoxic stress during labor and delivery. An increase in nucleated RBCs often is associated with chronic in utero hypoxic stress; however, acute stress (<24 hours) may be associated with elevated erythropoietin concentrations alone. Serum erythropoietin concentrations at birth normally range from 10 to 100 mU/mL.

Immediately after birth, increased oxygenation results in systemic oxygen delivery that far exceeds the tissues' demand for oxygen. Lacking the hypoxic stimulus, serum erythropoietin concentrations decrease, and erythropoiesis rapidly declines. The hemoglobin concentration decreases over the first 2 to 3 months of life as the infant gains weight, remains stable over the next several weeks as erythropoiesis is reinitiated, and then rises at 4 to 6 months of age in response to a greater erythropoietin stimulus. Term infants tolerate these changes in hemoglobin and hematocrit without consequence. Preterm infants experience a greater decline in hemoglobin than term infants, and the decrease appears proportional to the degree of prematurity. Hemoglobin concentrations between 7 and 8 g/dL occur commonly in preterm infants who have not undergone significant phlebotomy losses.

Transfusions affect erythropoiesis in newborns. Erythropoietin concentrations and reticulocyte counts are lower at any given hemoglobin concentration for infants who undergo exchange transfusion or multiple transfusions.

DIAGNOSIS OF ANEMIA

The approach to anemia in the newborn period often requires rapid investigation, laboratory evaluation, and treatment. The infant must be assessed immediately to determine whether acute or chronic anemia is present because treatment varies significantly. Clinical signs and symptoms of acute and chronic anemia are presented in Table 200-2. Infants who are critically ill and present in shock from anemia most likely have suffered massive hemorrhage, and volume replacement and patient stabilization is crucial to avoid organ damage and death. The ABCs of newborn resuscitation should be followed. Initial steps include stabilizing the infant's airway, administering oxygen if needed, and determining the infant's cardiovascular and intravascular volume status. Immediate volume expansion should begin with normal saline when a significant, acute hemorrhage is suspected. A transfusion of type O, Rh-negative blood ("trauma" blood) is needed in the first hour if massive hemorrhage has occurred, and repeat transfusions of crossmatched packed RBCs may be necessary to treat lactic acidosis, if oxygen delivery to the tissues is significantly compromised.

When the infant is stable, information can be gathered to determine the cause of anemia. The first source of information is the maternal chart. Any family history of anemia, bleeding, "low" blood counts, transfusions, jaundice, or unusual hematologic indices should be noted. Ethnicity of both parents should be obtained because some inherited disorders (glucose-6-phosphate dehydrogenase [G6PD] deficiency, thalassemias, and sickle cell disease) are more prevalent in specific ethnic groups.

Table 200-2. Acute versus Chronic Anemia in the Neonate

Clinical Characteristics	Acute Anemia	Chronic Anemia
General appearance	Pale, hyperalert, "stunned" gaze	Pale, normal neurologic examination
Cardiovascular	Tachycardic, weak pulses, low blood pressure	Normal, rarely may have congestive heart failure with hepatomegaly, normal or increase blood pressure
Respiratory	Tachypneic, no oxygen requirement	Normal, rarely may be tachypneic with an oxygen requirement if congestive heart failure is present
Hematologic		
Hemoglobin	May be normal, drops over 24 hr	Low at birth
Morphology	Macrocytic normochromic (normal)	Microcytic hypochromic anemia

A thorough pregnancy history should include information on vaginal bleeding, trauma, infection or exposure to infected individuals, and any prescribed or nonprescribed drug use during the pregnancy. Exposure to substances that increase oxidative stress and hemolysis in G6PD-deficient mothers must be determined (naphthalene—found in moth balls—and fava beans). Maternal cocaine or crack use before delivery increases the potential for placental abruption, fetal infarction, and postinfarction hemorrhage. Notable maternal laboratory values include blood type and antibody screen, maternal hepatitis, syphilis status, and rubella status. Prenatal infectious exposures, including parvovirus, cytomegalovirus, and varicella, should be noted.

Detailed information regarding labor and delivery sometimes can be difficult to obtain, especially if the route of delivery was not anticipated (e.g., an emergent cesarean section for fetal distress). Episodes of decelerations, fetal tachycardia, or other fetal heart rate abnormalities, such as loss of beat-to-beat variability, should be noted. Notable historical information includes length of labor; vaginal bleeding; evidence of placenta previa, vasa praevia, or placental abruption; route of delivery (including use of forceps, vacuum, or other manipulations); and information regarding the placenta (cord hematoma, cord rupture, chorioangioma, velamentous insertion of the cord). The placenta should be examined if possible. The presence of multiple gestations, especially if associated with discordant growth, should be documented.

Box 200-1. Estimating Fetal Blood Loss by Kleihauer-Betke Stain

Information to Gather

1. Maternal weight
2. Maternal hematocrit
3. Infant weight
4. Kleihauer-Betke stain results

Assume

Average maternal blood volume is 75 mL/kg at term (normal adult blood volume = 60 mL/kg); average fetal-placental blood volume is 120 mL/kg at term.

Example

You are given a Kleihauer-Betke stain result of 4%. This means that 4% of the RBCs on the mother's peripheral smear contain fetal blood. If the mother weighs 80 kg and her hematocrit is 35%, her RBC volume can be calculated as:

80 kg (weight) × 0.35 (hematocrit) × 75 mL/kg (blood volume) = 2100 mL (RBC volume)

If 4% of this RBC volume is fetal, the estimated fetal RBC mass transferred into the maternal circulation is:

2100 mL × 0.04 = 84 mL

If the infant weighs 3 kg and had a prehemorrhage hematocrit of 45%, the fetoplacental RBC volume can be calculated as:

3 kg × 0.45 × 120 mL/kg = 162 mL

The infant would have hemorrhaged 84 mL of 162 mL, or 52% of his or her RBC volume, into the maternal circulation. This would be considered a massive fetomaternal hemorrhage.

RBC, red blood cell.

The timing of presentation of anemia is important. Infants with significant acute blood loss immediately before or during delivery may be anemic and hypovolemic at birth, whereas infants with chronic hemorrhage or hemolysis from isoimmunization may not be immediately symptomatic. Infants with intrapartum internal trauma and hemorrhage (adrenal, renal, splenic, or hepatic) may be asymptomatic initially and then deteriorate rapidly. Attention to details of the infant's transition period may be lifesaving; for example, an infant with an increase in heart rate and respiratory rate during stage two of transition may be experiencing volume loss and metabolic acidosis from ongoing hemorrhage.

The initial laboratory evaluation of an anemic infant includes a complete blood count with RBC indices and peripheral smear, a reticulocyte count, a direct Coombs test, and a bilirubin determination if jaundice is evident. A Kleihauer-Betke (KB) stain of maternal blood is helpful in identifying fetal cells in the maternal circulation (Box 200-1). With minimal laboratory tests, a thorough history, and a physical examination of the infant and the placenta, most causes of anemia in the newborn period can be determined. Figure 200-1 presents an approach to the differential diagnosis of anemia in the newborn period.

HEMORRHAGE IN THE NEWBORN PERIOD

Hemorrhage can occur at various times during the fetal and neonatal period and commonly is broken down into prenatal, perinatal, and postnatal hemorrhage (Box 200-2).

Prenatal Hemorrhage

Maternal and fetal circulating cells may cross the placental barrier at varying times during pregnancy. The passage of fetal RBCs into the maternal circulation is termed *fetomaternal hemorrhage* (FMH). Some degree of FMH occurs in approximately 50% to 75% of pregnancies, usually occurring after the first trimester. The volume of fetal blood transferred into the maternal circulation is usually relatively small, on the order of 0.01 to 0.1 mL. About 1 pregnancy in 400 is associated with a FMH of 30 mL or greater, and about 1 pregnancy in 2000 is associated with a FMH of 100 mL or more.

Sensitization is the initial exposure of an individual to a specific antigen that results in an immune response. The overall risk to a mother of blood group sensitization occurring with FMH in an Rh-incompatible pregnancy is 16% if the fetus is Rh positive, ABO compatible with the mother. This risk decreases to 1.5% if the fetus is Rh positive but ABO incompatible, owing to the destruction of ABO-incompatible cells early during transfer. Fetal transfer of cells to the mother also can occur during abortions (about a 2% incidence of transfer with spontaneous abortion and a 4% to 5% incidence if abortion is induced).

The KB stain of maternal blood evaluates the acid elution of hemoglobin from RBCs. Fetal hemoglobin resists acid elution to a greater degree than adult hemoglobin. Maternal cells appear clear (termed *ghost cells*), whereas the contaminating fetal cells appear pink. Box 200-1 presents an

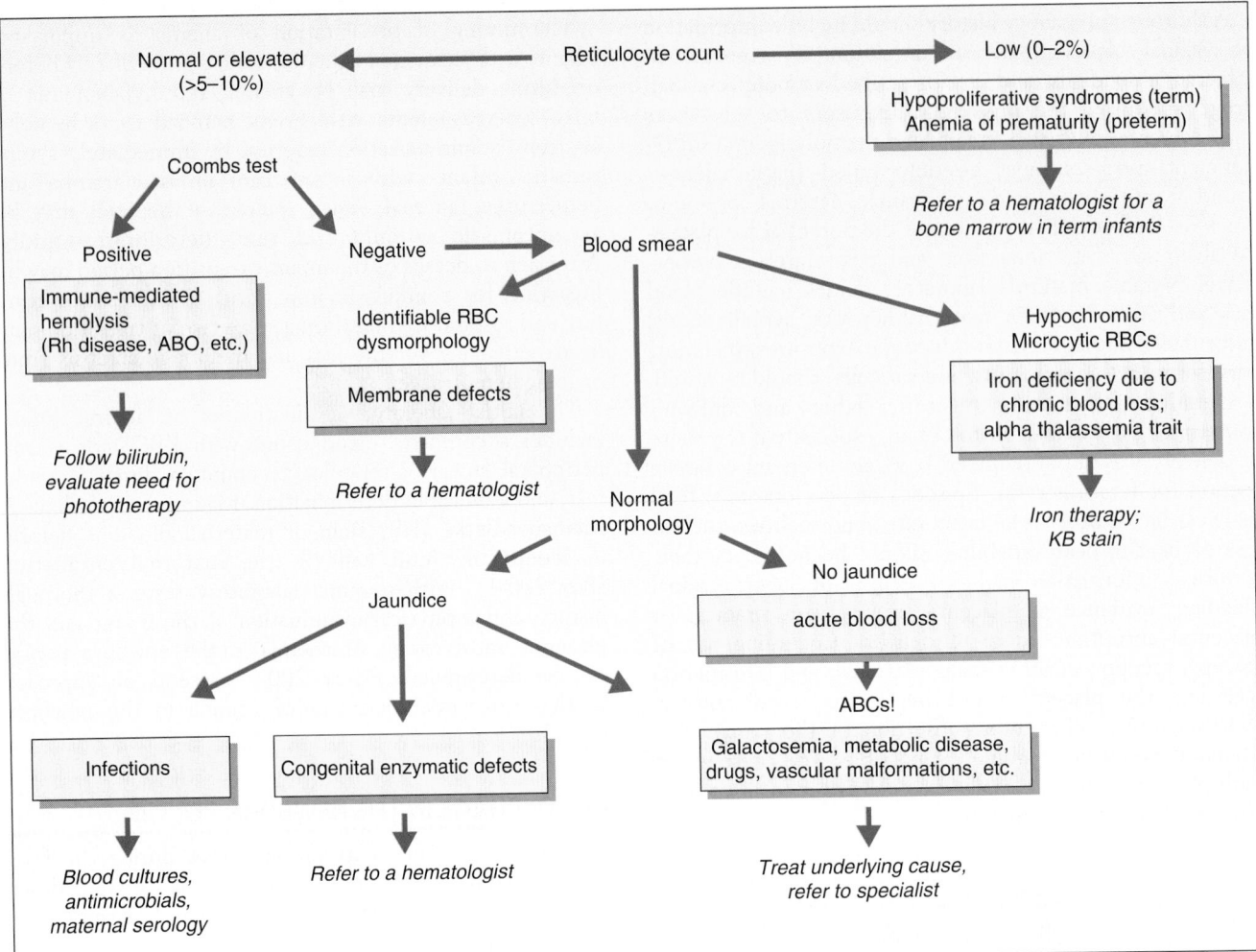

Figure 200-1. Algorithm for the differential diagnosis of anemia in the newborn period. After obtaining a thorough maternal history (including pregnancy, labor, and delivery history) and performing a physical examination and minimal laboratory evaluation (hemoglobin, reticulocyte count, blood type, direct Coombs test, peripheral smear, red blood cell [RBC] indices, and bilirubin), this algorithm assists the general pediatrician in differentiating anemia as hemorrhagic, hypoproliferative, or hemolytic and further differentiating immune-mediated from non–immune-mediated hemolysis. ABCs, airway, breathing, and circulation; KB, Kleihauer-Betke.

example of estimating the volume of fetal blood loss based on a KB stain.

Another method for detection of FMH involves flow cytometry using anti–hemoglobin F antibodies. Diagnosis of a small-volume FMH may be difficult when the mother and infant are ABO incompatible because fetal cells are cleared rapidly from the maternal circulation by maternal anti-A or anti-B antibodies. Results of KB stains obtained from mothers with increased fetal hemoglobin synthesis, such as mothers with sickle cell disease, thalassemia, and hereditary persistence of fetal hemoglobin, are not reliable. In these cases, other measures should be taken to detect FMH.

Severe FMH occurs in 1 in 1000 deliveries and has been associated with decreased fetal movements and diminished long-term variability and a fetal sinusoidal heart rate pattern. In one review, for a period ranging from 1 to 7 days, fetal movements were noted to be absent in 10% to 15% of cases. Two thirds of the infants died either in utero or during the neonatal period. A sinusoidal heart rate pattern was reported in 15% of cases and was associated with decreased fetal movement in 40% of the cases. No significant difference was found between cases with a FMH of

greater than 200 mL and cases with a FMH of less than 200 mL.

Decreased neonatal blood volumes are associated with a maternal history of vaginal bleeding, vasa previa, placenta previa or placental abruption, nonelective cesarean section, and deliveries associated with cord compression. Significant FMH has been described after trauma, and fetal hemorrhage into the placenta has been associated with placental chorioangioma.

Infants need rapid evaluation and treatment if a significant hemorrhage is suspected. An infant with massive hemorrhage presents with pallor, tachycardia, and tachypnea but may not have a significant oxygen requirement. Hemoglobin concentrations can be extremely low at birth (4 to 6 g/dL). A significant metabolic acidosis often is present as a result of poor perfusion.

Other causes of pallor in the newborn period can be evaluated when the infant is stable. Infants with shock, hypoxemic ischemic injury, and chronic anemia from hemolysis also can present with pallor. These diagnoses can be distinguished from acute hemorrhage based on differences in clinical signs and symptoms (Table 200-3).

Box 200-2. Causes of Hemorrhage in the Perinatal Period

Before Delivery

- Chronic or acute twin–twin transfusion syndrome
- Chronic or acute fetomaternal hemorrhage
- Hemorrhage into amniotic fluid after periumbilical blood sampling
- Traumatic amniocentesis
- Maternal trauma
- Trauma after external cephalic version

During Delivery

- Placental abruption
- Placenta previa
- Vasa praevia
- Trauma or incision of placenta during cesarean section
- Ruptured normal or abnormal (varices, aneurysms) umbilical cord
- Cord or placental hematoma
- Velamentous insertion of the cord
- Nuchal cord

During or after Delivery

- Subgaleal hemorrhage
- Cephalhematoma
- Intraventricular/intracranial hemorrhage (prematurity, trauma, isoimmune thrombocytopenia)
- Hemorrhage associated with disseminated intravascular coagulation/sepsis
- Organ trauma (liver, spleen, adrenal, renal)
- Pulmonary hemorrhage
- Iatrogenic blood loss (phlebotomy, central line accidents, arterial line accidents)

The clinical picture with chronic blood loss is usually mild, and infants respond to conservative therapy with iron alone. Asphyxiated infants are pale and floppy and may have poor peripheral circulation. Hemoglobin is stable, but it may decrease if disseminated intravascular coagulation and internal bleeding occur or if excessive volume replacement is provided.

Twin–twin transfusion syndrome (TTS) is a complication of monochorionic twin gestations and occurs in 5% to 30% of these pregnancies. The perinatal mortality rate can be 70% to 100%, depending on severity and timing of presentation. In TTS, placental anastomoses allow transfer of blood from one twin to the other. Approximately 70% of monozygous twin pregnancies have monochorionic placentas. Although vascular anastomoses are present in almost all instances of monochorionic placentas, not all of those develop TTS.

Acute TTS results in twins of similar size but with hemoglobin concentrations that vary by more than 5 g/dL. In chronic TTS, the donor twin becomes progressively anemic and growth retarded, whereas the recipient twin becomes polycythemic, macrosomic, and sometimes hypertensive. Both infants can develop hydrops fetalis. The donor twin becomes hydropic from profound anemia, whereas the recipient twin becomes hydropic from congestive heart failure and hypervolemia. The donor twin often has low amniotic fluid volumes, whereas the recipient twin has increased amniotic fluid from significant differences in blood volume, renal blood flow, and urine output.

Chronic TTS can be diagnosed by serial prenatal ultrasounds measuring cardiomegaly, discordant amniotic fluid production, and fetal growth discrepancy of greater than 20%. After birth, the donor twin may be hemodynamically stable or may require transfusions and can experience neutropenia, hydrops from severe anemia, growth retardation, congestive heart failure, and hypoglycemia. The recipient twin is often the sicker of the two, experiencing hypertrophic cardiomyopathy, congestive heart failure, polycythemia, hyperviscosity, respiratory difficulties, hypocalcemia, and hypoglycemia. Neurologic evaluation and imaging are important because the risk of antenatally acquired neurologic cerebral lesions is 20% to 30% in both twins. Morbidities include multiple cerebral infarctions, hypoperfusion syndromes from hypotension, and periventricular leukomalacia. Long-term neurologic follow-up is indicated for all TTS survivors.

Prenatal treatment consists of close monitoring and in some cases reduction amniocenteses to decrease uterine stretch and prolong the pregnancy. The average survival rates with serial reduction amniocenteses range from 40% to 70%. Selective fetocide of the hydropic twin also has resulted in the survival of the healthier twin in some studies. Treatment in utero has occurred during some pregnancies using laser surgery to ablate bridging vessels, resulting in improved survival rates of around 50%, with approximately 70% of the pregnancies having at least one survivor. The survival rate without morbidity in the surviv-

Table 200-3. Pale Newborn: Anemia versus Asphyxia

Organ System	Hemorrhagic Anemia	Hemolytic Anemia	Asphyxia
Neurologic	Normal or hyperalert/hyperirritable ("catecholamine response")	Normal	Abnormal transition period, hypotonic, decreased arousal state, seizures in first 12–48 hr of life
Respiratory	Tachypnea, no oxygen requirement	Normal	Respiratory distress, oxygen requirement
Cardiovascular	Tachycardia, hypotension	May vary from normal to congestive heart failure and hydrops, depending on degree of anemia	Bradycardia or normal heart rate; variable blood pressure
Hematologic	Drop in hematocrit/hemoglobin	Anemic from birth, hepatosplenomegaly, jaundice, positive Coombs test	Hematocrit/hemoglobin remains stable over time; may develop thrombocytopenia and DIC from hypoxic injury to marrow

DIC, disseminated intravascular coagulation.

ing twin is approximately 50%, however. Meta-analyses have found no differences in outcome between amnioreduction, fetoscopy, septostomy, or close observation for fetuses with TTS.

Perinatal Hemorrhage

Obstetric complications, such as vasa previa, placenta previa, placental abruption, hemorrhage during percutaneous umbilical blood sampling, incision or tearing of the placenta during cesarean section, and cord evulsion of normal or abnormal umbilical cords, can result in significant neonatal blood loss. Newborns also may undergo significant blood loss back into the placenta, termed a *fetoplacental hemorrhage*. Finally, placental anomalies, such as a multilobed placenta and placental chorioangiomas, may be a source of hemorrhage during the perinatal period.

Placental abruption occurs when there is premature separation of the placenta from the uterus. Prolonged rupture of the membranes, severe fetal growth restriction, chorioamnionitis, hypertension (before pregnancy and pregnancy-induced), cigarette smoking, maternal abdominal trauma, advanced maternal age, and male fetal gender are potential risk factors for placental abruption. The incidence of abruption increases with decreasing gestation. Mortality is 0.8 to 2 per 1000 births, or 15% to 20% of the deliveries in which significant abruption occurs.

Women with a history of a previous cesarean birth and increased parity are at increased risk of having a pregnancy complicated by *placenta previa*, a condition in which part or all of the placenta overlies the cervical os. Cigarette smoking is associated with a 2.6-fold to 4.4-fold increased risk of placenta previa. *Vasa praevia* (anomalous vessels overlying the internal os of the cervix) can be diagnosed prenatally with transvaginal color Doppler. Vasa praevia should be suspected in any case of antepartum or intrapartum hemorrhage. Although uncommon (1 in 3000 deliveries), the perinatal death rate is high, ranging from 33% to 100% when the condition is undetected before delivery. Infants are often stillborn.

Infants born after placental abruption or placenta previa may be anemic, but also may present with signs of hypoxia. In these infants, it is important to monitor changes in hematocrit and neurologic signs. The need for postnatal transfusions in these infants generally is associated with the volume of maternal hemorrhage. The infant's hemoglobin should be measured at birth and at 12 to 24 hours whenever there is evidence of placental abruption, placenta previa, or unusual vaginal bleeding. A KB stain can be performed on maternal blood to determine if fetal hemorrhage occurred. Monitoring mothers with a history of second-trimester or third-trimester bleeding with Doppler flow ultrasound may decrease the incidence of severe anemia and fetal loss in newborns by detecting placental abnormalities.

Cord rupture from excess traction on a shortened or abnormal umbilical cord usually occurs on the fetal side. Cord aneurysms, varices, and cysts all can lead to formation of a weakened cord. Cord infections also can weaken the cord and increase the risk of rupture. Infants born precipitously may be at increased risk for hemorrhage from a ruptured cord.

Hematomas of the cord occur infrequently (1 in 5000 to 6000 deliveries) but can be a cause of fetal blood loss and may be associated with significant perinatal mortality. Intrauterine death may occur as a result of compression of the umbilical vein and arteries by the hematoma. Cord hematomas can result from trauma caused by percutaneous umbilical blood sampling and can be associated with a high maternal α-fetoprotein. Hematomas of the cord can be diagnosed accurately in utero by ultrasound and differentiated from other lesions of the placenta and cord. The lesion can be associated with poor fetal growth and FMH.

Velamentous insertion of the umbilical cord occurs when the umbilical cord enters the membranes distant from the placenta and is present in approximately 0.5% to 2% of pregnancies. Blood vessels left unprotected by Wharton jelly are more likely to tear. Rupture of anomalous vessels in the absence of traction or trauma can occur even if the cord itself attaches centrally or paracentrally. The fetal mortality remains high in this condition, often because detection by routine ultrasound is rare.

Postnatal Hemorrhage

Blood loss into the placenta, termed *fetoplacental hemorrhage*, is one of the most common causes of a low birth hematocrit in a neonate. Of the 120 mL/kg of blood in the fetoplacental unit, a large residual volume remains in the placenta, and blood continues to flow in the direction of gravity after birth. Fetoplacental hemorrhage occurs when the infant is held above the placenta after birth; for this reason, infants born by cesarean section have smaller blood volumes than infants born vaginally. In addition, infants can lose 10% to 20% of their total blood volume when born with a tight nuchal cord, which allows blood to be pumped through umbilical arteries, while constricting flow through the umbilical vein.

Blood loss into the subgaleal space can occur during difficult deliveries requiring vacuum or forceps assistance, such as face presentation, occiput posterior presentations, and shoulder dystocias. Subgaleal hemorrhage is potentially life-threatening and must be recognized as early as possible to prevent significant morbidity or mortality. The hematomas occur when emissary or "bridging" veins are torn, allowing blood to accumulate in the large potential space between the galea aponeurotica (the epicranial aponeurosis) and the periosteum of the skull. The subgaleal space extends from the orbital ridge to the base of the skull and can accommodate an infant's entire blood volume (80 to 90 mL/kg of blood).

Subgaleal hematomas may form because of preexisting risk factors (e.g., coagulopathy or low platelets), but vacuum extraction itself is a risk factor for the development of subgaleal bleeding. The diagnosis should be considered when a ballotable fluid collection in dependent regions of the infant's head is coupled with signs of hypovolemia. Treatment requires rapid restoration of blood volume and control of bleeding. Exsanguination from subgaleal hemorrhage has been reported; the mortality is high if the hemorrhage goes unrecognized. A rule of thumb for estimating the volume of blood in the subgaleal space is 38 mL of blood has been lost for every 1-cm increase in head circumference.

Infants undergoing vacuum extraction have an increased risk for subgaleal hemorrhage. The duration of vacuum application is thought to be the best predictor of scalp injury, followed by duration of second stage of labor and paramedian cup placement. Of infants with reported subgaleal hemorrhages, 80% to 90% had some history of vacuum-assisted or instrument-assisted delivery. A cesarean section does not preclude the use of vacuum or forceps, and significant hemorrhage still can occur via this route of delivery. Limiting the frequency and duration of vacuum assistance in high-risk infants may decrease the incidence of subgaleal hemorrhage, however.

Anemia appearing after the first 24 hours of life in a nonjaundiced infant may result from occult hemorrhage or from birth trauma that causes visible hemorrhages, such as a cephalhematoma. Breech deliveries may be associated with renal, adrenal, liver, or splenic hemorrhage into the retroperitoneal space. Delivery of macrosomic infants, such as infants born to diabetic mothers, also may result in organ damage from hemorrhage.

Adrenal hemorrhage, in addition to causing anemia, may result in circulatory collapse from the loss of organ function. The incidence of adrenal hemorrhage is 1.7 per 1000 births. Adrenal hemorrhage also can affect surrounding organs. Intestinal obstruction and kidney dysfunction have been reported. Diagnosis can be made using ultrasound: Calcifications or cystic masses are noted. Adrenal hemorrhage can be distinguished from renal vein thrombosis by ultrasound. Renal vein thrombosis generally results in a solid mass. Occasionally, these entities may coexist. Infants with renal vein thrombosis may have gross or microscopic hematuria and may go on to develop renal failure and hypertension.

The newborn liver is prone to iatrogenic rupture, resulting in a high morbidity and mortality. Infants may appear asymptomatic until the liver ruptures and hemoperitoneum occurs. Iatrogenic liver rupture can occur in term and preterm infants and has been associated with breech extractions and with chest compressions during cardiopulmonary resuscitation. Surgical intervention involving vascular tamponade has been reported to save some infants; however, the mortality remains high.

Splenic rupture can result from birth trauma or distention caused by extramedullary hematopoiesis, such as that seen in erythroblastosis fetalis. Abdominal distention and discoloration, scrotal swelling, and pallor are clinical signs of splenic rupture. These signs also may be seen with adrenal hemorrhage or hepatic rupture.

Other rare causes of hemorrhage in the newborn include hemangiomas of the gastrointestinal tract, vascular malformations of the skin, and hemorrhage into soft tumors, such as giant sacrococcygeal teratomas. Occult intra-abdominal hemorrhage can occur with fetal ovarian cysts, which usually are benign and resolve spontaneously.

The management of hemorrhage in the neonatal period depends on the cause, timing, and extent of hemorrhage. Infants with chronic hemorrhage, such as infants with TTS or FMH, may have had time to compensate for a gradual decrease in hemoglobin and may be minimally symptomatic (see Table 200-2). These infants require iron supplementation to replace iron stores depleted by blood loss;

however, they are less likely to require an immediate transfusion or volume expansion. Infants who have had an acute hemorrhage require volume expansion to improve circulation and organ perfusion. The decision to administer an immediate transfusion of O-negative "trauma" blood should be made carefully. Immediate transfusions benefit infants with a significant metabolic acidosis and oxygen requirement, generally reflecting a greater than 40% acute blood loss.

Regardless of whether the blood loss was acute or chronic, iron therapy is indicated. Infants with acute blood loss may receive iron in the form of transfused blood; however, the replacement does not equal the amount of iron lost. Infants who have had chronic blood loss are iron deficient at birth, and replacement therapy should begin immediately using oral doses of 6 to 10 mg of elemental iron/kg/day.

Treatment of anemic infants with modalities beyond volume expansion, transfusion, and vitamin and iron supplementation depends on the comfort level of the practitioner. The use of recombinant erythropoietin to stimulate erythropoiesis has become more common in neonatal intensive care units, but its role in the newborn nursery and in outpatient treatment still is being evaluated.

Follow-up of infants who have experienced a moderate or significant hemorrhage includes ongoing evaluation of satisfactory iron replacement; this is accomplished by evaluating the RBC indices after 6 to 8 weeks of iron therapy. Mean cell volume within the normal range reflects adequate replacement. Continued replacement is determined by the extent of the original hemorrhage and the erythropoietic response of the infant.

HEMOLYTIC ANEMIA

Anemic infants with elevated reticulocyte counts (>5% to 10%) have evidence of stimulated erythropoiesis, and their anemia is due to either chronic hemorrhage or hemolysis. Hemolytic anemia is a common cause of decreased hematocrit values in the newborn period and can be divided into two major subtypes (Table 200-4). *Immune-mediated hemolysis* occurs when destruction of RBCs is caused by maternal immunoglobulin G (IgG) that crosses the placenta and recognizes an antigen on the fetal RBC. *Non–immune-mediated hemolysis* occurs when the life span of the RBC is shortened because of characteristics or factors that can be either intrinsic or extrinsic to the RBC. The average life span for a term neonatal RBC is 60 to 90 days, approximately one half to two thirds that of an adult RBC. Remarkably shorter RBC life spans (35 to 50 days) are found with increasing prematurity (see Table 200-1). The shortened RBC life span of the preterm and term neonate may be explained by some of the characteristics specific to newborn cells, which include a rapid decline in intracellular enzyme activity and adenosine triphosphate, loss of membrane surface area, increased mechanical fragility and susceptibility to peroxidation, and decreased levels of intracellular carnitine.

A positive Coombs test is evidence for immune-mediated hemolytic anemia. The direct Coombs test evaluates the presence of antibody on the surface of neonatal

Table 200-4. Causes of Hemolysis in the Fetal and Neonatal Period

Immune-Mediated Hemolysis
Rh incompatibility (anti-D antibody)
ABO, c, C, e, G incompatibility
Minor blood group incompatibility:
    Fya (Duffy), Kell group, Jka, MNS, Vw
Drug-induced (penicillin, methyldopa,
    cephalothin)
Maternal autoimmune hemolytic anemia
 	
Non–immune-Mediated Hemolysis
Congenital Erythrocyte Enzyme Defects
Glucose-6-phosphate dehydrogenase
    deficiency
Pyruvate kinase deficiency
Hexokinase deficiency
Glucose phosphate isomerase deficiency
Pyrimidine 5′ nucleotidase deficiency
Erythrocyte Membrane Disorders
Spherocytosis
Elliptocytosis
	Stomatocytosis
	Pyropoikilocytosis
	Other membrane disorders
	Hemoglobin Defects
	α-Thalassemia syndromes
	γ-Thalassemia syndromes
	α and γ chain structural anomalies
	Drug-induced
	Valproic acid
	Infection
	Bacterial sepsis (*Echerichia coli*, group B
	    streptococcus)
	Parvovirus B19
	Congenital syphilis
	Congenital malaria
	Congenital TORCH infections (toxoplasmosis,
	    cytomegalovirus, rubella, disseminated
	    herpes)
	Other congenital viral infections
		Disseminated Intravascular Coagulation
		Macroangiopathic and Microangiopathic
		Hemolysis
		Cavernous hemangiomas
		Arteriovenous malformations
		Renal artery stenosis or thrombosis
		Other large vessel thrombi
		Severe coarctation of the aorta
		Severe valvular stenoses
		Associated with Systemic Disease
		Galactosemia
		Lysosomal storage diseases
		Prolonged metabolic acidosis from metabolic
		    disease (amino acid and organic acid
		    disorders)
		Transfusion reactions
		TAR syndrome

TAR, thrombocytopenia–absent radius.

RBCs. A blood type should be obtained on the infant, and maternal serum should be evaluated for antibodies. Immune-mediated RBC destruction is the most common cause of hemolytic disease in the newborn period. *Rh isoimmunization* refers to the transplacental passage of maternal antibodies directed against the D antigen on fetal RBCs, resulting in fetal RBC hemolysis (Fig. 200-2). Fetuses can have significant hemolysis and anemia. The anemia sometimes is severe enough that it results in *erythroblastosis fetalis* and *hydrops* in the fetus.

Hydrops refers to the presence of excess extracellular fluid in two or more areas of the fetoplacental unit, including generalized edema of the skin (≥5 mm), polyhydramnios, placental edema, pleural effusions, pericardial effusions, and ascites. In the case of Rh isoimmunization, the cause of hydrops is fetal anemia from severe hemolysis, or *immune-mediated hydrops*. Anemia leads to high-output cardiac failure, myocardial dysfunction, venous congestion

from extramedullary hematopoiesis in the liver, hepatic dysfunction resulting in decreased protein production, and ultimately decreased intravascular oncotic pressure.

Non–immune-mediated hydrops is differentiated from immune-mediated hydrops and can be caused by multiple disorders (Table 200-5), including disorders of the cardiovascular system, such as arrhythmias and structural cardiac defects; chromosomal defects or syndromes; infections, such as congenital syphilis, parvovirus, or cytomegalovirus; non–immune-mediated anemia; and thoracic lesions. In approximately one third of the cases, no etiology for non–immune-mediated hydrops is discovered. In contrast

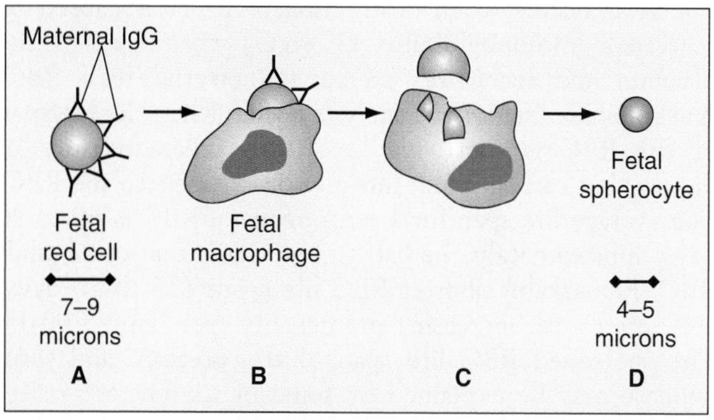

Figure 200-2. Immune-mediated red blood cell (RBC) membrane loss resulting in spherocytosis. The process of membrane loss leading to smaller, more compact RBCs (spherocytes) is shown. **A,** Antigens on the fetal RBC are recognized by maternally derived IgG antibodies. **B,** Fetal macrophages are activated to attack the antibody-coated RBC. **C** and **D,** When parts of the RBC membrane are phagocytized by the macrophage (**C**), the RBC is left with a decreased surface area and increased density (**D**), resulting in the production of spherocytes, which have smaller mean cell volumes and higher mean corpuscular hemoglobin concentrations.

Table 200-5. Causes of Nonimmune Hydrops in the Fetus

Disorder	Incidence (% of Cases)	Survival (%)

Cardiovascular
    Tachyarrhythmias, bradyarrhythmias,
      hypoplastic left heart, endocardial
      cushion defect
	15–26	20–35

Chromosomal anomalies
    Trisomy 18, trisomy 21, monosomy X
      abnormal karyotype
	8–16	0–8

Syndromes
    Mucopolysaccharidoses, skeletal
      dysplasia, arthrogryposes
	10	0–11

Infections
    Parvovirus B19, syphilis,
      cytomegalovirus, adenovirus
	2–4	0–50

Anemias
    α-Thalassemia, enzyme defects,
      membrane defects, fetomaternal
      hemorrhage, twin–twin transfusion
      syndrome
	2–6	0–50

Congenital intrathoracic masses
    Cystic adenomatoid malformation,
      pulmonary sequestration,
      diaphragmatic hernia, lobar
      emphysema, bronchogenic cyst
	2–13	0–60

Other Genitourinary, tumors	1–3	0–10
Idiopathic	22–35	10–50

to immune-mediated hydrops, non–immune-mediated hydrops is associated with a poor prognosis. Despite advances in prenatal diagnosis and treatment, mortality is 80% to 93%.

With improved prenatal monitoring and neonatal technology, three fourths of infants born with immune-mediated hydrops survive. Since the development of Rh immunoglobulin (Rhogam) in 1968, the incidence of isoimmunized pregnancies has decreased from 1% to less than 0.1%. Of fetuses that are isoimmunized, approximately 10% require an intrauterine transfusion. Infants born after in utero transfusion generally are known to the perinatologists and neonatologists, who should provide close follow-up. These infants sometimes are born prematurely, which places them at risk for morbidities associated with prematurity but effectively ends the transfer of anti-D antibody across the placenta.

A few infants with Rh hemolytic disease remain undiagnosed until after birth. When the diagnosis is suspected or confirmed, steps should be taken to monitor the infant's serum bilirubin closely and provide appropriate care (Box 200-3). Infants can develop hyperbilirubinemia at a much faster rate than infants with ABO incompatibility, and evaluation and ongoing medical management are essential during the acute phase of the illness. Infants receiving optimal phototherapy who continue to have an increase in indirect serum bilirubin greater than 0.5 mg/dL/hr require additional therapy. This therapy may involve administration of intravenous immunoglobulin or placement of central lines for double-volume exchange transfusion. Intensifying medical management beyond phototherapy should be done in consultation with a neonatologist, and the generalist should consider transfer of care to a neonatal intensive care unit at this point.

Because of the increased incidence of kernicterus since the 1990s, the criteria for exchange transfusion have undergone review. Guidelines for exchange are listed in Box 200-3. The purpose of a double-volume exchange transfusion is threefold. First, it removes 70% to 90% of the infant's Rh-positive RBCs, replacing them with Rh-negative cells that will not undergo immune-mediated hemolysis. Second, it removes approximately 25% of the total bilirubin and decreases serum bilirubin concentrations. Because most of the total bilirubin resides in the extravascular space, the serum bilirubin can be expected to rebound after the initial decrease with exchange transfusion. Finally, an exchange transfusion decreases the total maternally derived anti-D antibody so that ongoing hemolysis is diminished. Similar to total bilirubin, a fraction of antibody resides in the tissues, so continued hemolysis occurs.

Exchange transfusions should be performed only by pediatricians experienced with the procedure and knowledgeable about the risks and side effects that can occur. Potential metabolic problems include hypoglycemia, hypocalemia, acidosis, and hyperkalemia. Cardiac effects include volume overload, arrhythmias, and cardiac arrest. Hematologic abnormalities that can occur include bleeding from heparinization, graft-versus-host disease, neutropenia, and thrombocytopenia. Finally, hazards associated with line placement include perforation, embolization, thrombosis, necrotizing enterocolitis, and infection.

Box 200-3. Role of the Generalist When Immune-Mediated Hemolysis Is Suspected or Confirmed

The approach to the jaundiced infant must be altered when immune-mediated hemolysis in the neonatal period is confirmed prenatally or suspected after delivery. Rh isoimmunization causes brisk hemolysis, resulting in rapid elevation of serum bilirubin that often exceeds the level of clinical (visible) jaundice, especially in infants born prematurely. Consultation with a neonatologist should be sought in these instances, particularly if the infant requires exchange transfusion.

Information to Gather

1. Maternal prenatal history (previously affected children, Rh sensitization, ultrasounds, amniocenteses, in utero transfusions, most recent fetal hematocrit, medications received [e.g., intravenous immunoglobulin or steroids])
2. Maternal blood type and Coombs test
3. Infant blood type and Coombs test
4. Red blood cell indices (hematocrit, mean cell volume, mean corpuscular hemoglobin concentration, red blood cell distribution width index, reticulocyte count)
5. Bilirubin values, including the hour of life at which they were drawn

Treatment and Monitoring

1. Monitor direct and indirect serum bilirubin concentrations every 4 hours for a minimum of three to four measurements to calculate rate of increase of indirect bilirubin.
2. Start phototherapy when indirect bilirubin reaches
   4 mg/dL at birth (cord blood)
   10 mg/dL at 12 hours of age
   12 mg/dL at 18 hours of age
   14 mg/dL at 24 hours of age
   15 mg/dL at 48 hours of age
3. Consult with neonatologist: Consider intravenous immunoglobulin (500 mg/kg) if rate of increase of indirect bilirubin is >0.5 mg/dL/hr.
4. Consult/transfer care to neonatologist: Perform double-volume exchange transfusion if rate of increase of indirect bilirubin is >0.5 mg/dL/hr with optimal phototherapy, the infant's hematocrit is <30%, and the indirect bilirubin reaches
   20 mg/dL in a healthy infant >2500 g birth weight
   18 mg/dL in an ill infant >2500 g birth weight
   17 mg/dL in an infant 2000 to 2500 g birth weight
   15 mg/dL in an infant >1500 to 2000 g birth weight (these infants may be in an intensive care unit)
   12 mg/dL in an infant >1000 to 1500 g birth weight (these infants should be in an intensive care unit)

Follow-up after Discharge

1. Monitor infant for clinical signs of anemia (e.g., tachycardia, poor feeding, new murmur); obtain hematocrit as necessary every 1 to 2 weeks until the infant reaches 3 months of age or until the hematocrit begins to increase.
2. Ensure adequate iron supplementation for erythropoiesis (2 to 6 mg/kg/day elemental iron).
3. Consult with neonatologist: Consider subcutaneous erythropoietin (250 U/kg three times a week) to maintain hematocrit during the late anemia of Rh hemolytic disease.

Follow-up

Infants with Rh hemolytic disease often have anemia at birth and the first weeks of life secondary to ongoing, antibody-mediated hemolysis. These infants also can develop a late anemia at 1 to 3 months of age, which is due to diminished erythrocyte production. Infants with the late anemia of Rh hemolytic disease may require transfusions until anemia spontaneously resolves, generally by 3 or 4 months of age. The incidence of late anemia seems to be much higher in infants who receive intrauterine transfusions. When an infant has been discharged, follow-up is required until the anemia resolves. Follow-up may require hematocrit checks for 2 to 3 months if an infant has symptoms suggesting anemia.

During the period of decreased circulating antibody and delayed endogenous erythropoietin production, administration of exogenous erythropoietin has been effective as an alternative to erythrocyte transfusion because this anemia is characterized by low serum concentrations of erythropoietin but erythroid progenitors that are responsive to recombinant erythropoietin. Some infants have avoided rehospitalization for transfusions with erythropoietin administration. Consultation with a neonatologist or hematologist familiar with the use of erythropoietin in neonates is suggested.

With the introduction of RhoGam (anti-D immunoglobulin), the incidence of Rh hemolytic disease has been reduced drastically, such that ABO incompatibility now represents a more common etiology for severe neonatal hemolysis. ABO incompatibility represents a spectrum of hemolytic disease in newborns, ranging from infants with little or no evidence of erythrocyte sensitization but evidence of hemolysis to infants with severe hemolytic disease in which erythrocyte sensitization is markedly present. Infants with significant hemolysis and jaundice may have only weakly positive Coombs tests because of the configuration of antigens present on the neonatal RBC.

A negative Coombs test (or matching blood types) does not rule out completely immune-mediated hemolysis, and minor blood group incompatibilities should be considered. Anti-Kell anemic fetuses have lower reticulocyte counts and total serum bilirubin levels than do comparable anti-D anemic fetuses. The level of hemolysis caused by anti-Kell antibodies is less than that caused by anti-D antibodies; however, fetal erythropoiesis is suppressed by direct effects of anti-Kell antibodies on erythroid progenitors.

A negative Coombs test in a jaundiced infant occurs with nonimmune hemolytic anemias, and further workup is required to determine a specific etiology. Infants may have normal or elevated reticulocyte counts and may not present with symptomatic anemia at birth. RBC enzyme deficiencies, such as G6PD, pyruvate kinase, and hexokinase deficiencies, may lead to increased hemolysis. Male infants of Mediterranean or Asian descent are at increased risk for G6PD deficiency; however, female infants also can manifest this disease. Abnormalities in RBC morphology, such as spherocytosis and elliptocytosis, result in accelerated membrane loss and a shortened life span. These structural defects can be determined by evaluating the peripheral smear. The presence of spherocytes on the peripheral smear occurs in immune-mediated hemolytic disease as well (see Fig. 200-2); the diagnosis of hereditary spherocytosis should be made only after further tests have been performed. Testing for osmotic fragility can be done after the newborn period, when the infant is not acutely hemolyzing RBCs.

If the cause of hemolytic anemia has not been determined, other causes of hemolytic disease in the newborn

should be evaluated. Hemoglobinopathies (other than β-hemoglobinopathies, which never present in the newborn period) can present with hemolysis in the first months of life. Maternal medications, such as valproic acid, can lead to fetal hemolysis. Other, less common causes of hemolytic anemia include galactosemia, lysosomal storage diseases, and amino acid disorders. Prolonged metabolic acidosis, transfusion reactions, thrombocytopenia–absent radius syndrome, and osteopetrosis all can present with hemolytic anemia in the newborn. Macroangiopathic and microangiopathic hemolytic anemias can occur with vascular malformations, such as coarctation, hemangiomas, and large vessel thromboses.

Treatment of hemolytic anemia is based on the etiology of the hemolysis. Immune-mediated disorders resolve with time, as the maternally derived antibody is consumed. Although a late anemia associated with Rh hemolytic disease can prolong follow-up, treatment is symptomatic. Infants with severe anemia and evidence of immediate need of improved oxygen delivery to tissues should receive a packed RBC transfusion. Infants often develop an indirect hyperbilirubinemia requiring phototherapy. Jaundice can be severe enough to require immunoglobulin therapy and double-volume exchange transfusion. These treatments would be performed while the newborn was still hospitalized. Follow-up of an infant with Rh hemolytic disease, ABO incompatibility, or minor blood group incompatibility involves documenting resolution of the infant's anemia (see Box 200-3). Generally, infants are not iron deficient, but sufficient iron should be available in the diet to support active erythropoiesis. Outpatient therapy with subcutaneous erythropoietin has been evaluated in infants with late anemia and seems to be effective in stimulating erythropoiesis. Consultation with a neonatologist or pediatric hematologist familiar with dose and scheduling is helpful in arranging this treatment.

Treatment of non–immune-mediated hemolysis also is dictated by the cause of the anemia. Infants in whom an intrinsic RBC defect is suspected should be referred to a pediatric hematologist for evaluation and long-term management because these conditions require lifelong follow-up. The underlying systemic causes of hemolysis, such as galactosemia, require lifelong follow-up by the generalist and specialists as needed.

HYPOPROLIFERATIVE ANEMIAS

Anemic term infants with low reticulocyte counts (<2%) have evidence of decreased erythropoiesis (Table 200-6). Although the peripheral smear may present clues to the diagnosis, in most cases a bone marrow aspiration is required to diagnose hypoproliferative anemias presenting in the newborn period.

Anemia of Prematurity

In preterm infants, adaptive mechanisms to the extrauterine environment are incomplete. Erythropoietin concentrations in anemic preterm infants still are significantly lower than concentrations found in adults, given the degree of their anemia. This normocytic, normochromic anemia, termed the *anemia of prematurity*, commonly affects

Table 200-6. Syndromes Involving Hypoproliferative Anemia in the Newborn Period

Syndrome	Features, Inheritance, and Mapping
Congenital dyserythropoietic anemias	Type I (rare), megaloblastoid erythroid hyperplasia and nuclear chromatin bridges between nuclei; type II (common), hereditary erythroblastic multinuclearity, positive acidified serum (HEMPAS) test, increased lysis to anti-i; type III, erythroblastic multinuclearity (gigantoblasts), macrocytosis Mapped to: type I, 15q15.1–q15.3; type II, 20q11.2; type III, 15q21
Diamond-Blackfan syndrome	Steroid-responsive hypoplastic anemia, often microcytic after 5 mo of age; inheritance: AR; sporadic mutations and AD inheritance described; mapped to 19q13.2, 8p23
Dyskeratosis congenita	Hypoproliferative anemia usually presenting between 5 and 15 yr of age Inheritance: X-linked recessive, locus on Xq28; some cases with AD inheritance
Fanconi pancytopenia	Steroid-responsive hypoplastic anemia, reticulocytopenia, some macrocytic RBCs, shortened RBC life span; cells are hypersensitive to DNA cross-linking agents Inheritance: AR, mapped to multiple genes: complementation group A, 16q24.3; C: 9q22.3; D2, 3p25.3; E, 6p22–p21; F, 11p15; G; 9p13
Osteopetrosis	Hypoplastic anemia from marrow compression, extramedullary erythropoiesis; lethal form due to reduced osteoclasts AR form: mapped to 16p13, 11q13.4–q13.5; AD form: mapped to 1p21
Pearson's syndrome	Hypoplastic sideroblastic anemia, marrow cell vacuolization caused by pleioplasmatic rearrangement of mitochondrial DNA Inheritance: X-linked or AR
X-linked α-thalassemia/mental retardation (ATR-X and ATR-16) syndromes	ATR-X, hypochromic, microcytic anemia; mild form of hemoglobin H disease ATR-16, more significant hemoglobin H disease/anemia present Inheritance: ATR-X, X-linked recessive, mapped to Xq13.3; ATR-16, mapped to 16p13.3, deletions of α-globin locus

AD, autosomal dominant; AR, autosomal recessive; RBC, red blood cell.

infants of 32 weeks' gestation or less and is the most common anemia seen in the neonatal period. Anemia of prematurity is not responsive to the addition of iron, folate, or vitamin E. Some infants may be asymptomatic, whereas others show signs of anemia that are alleviated by transfusion. These signs traditionally include tachycardia, increased episodes of apnea and bradycardia, poor weight gain, increased oxygen requirement, and elevated serum lactate concentrations that decrease after transfusion.

Multiple studies evaluating the use of recombinant erythropoietin to prevent and treat anemia of prematurity have been done. Erythropoietin is successful in preterm infants in stimulating erythropoiesis, and transfusion requirements are decreased. Success rates in preventing transfusions in preterm infants depend in part on transfusion criteria and the frequency of phlebotomy. Regardless of treatment, anemia of prematurity resolves by 6 months of age and requires no long-term follow-up.

With the exception of anemia of prematurity, anemia in the newborn period is rarely the result of impaired RBC production. Although classified as a congenital anemia, *Diamond-Blackfan syndrome* characteristically is not recognized until after 2 to 3 months of age. It is estimated, however, that 10% to 25% of affected infants have mild anemia at birth. Rarely, hydrops fetalis has been reported in conjunction with this syndrome.

Congenital dyserythropoietic anemia is a rare disorder marked by ineffective erythropoiesis, megaloblastic anemia, and characteristic abnormalities of the nuclear membrane and cytoplasm seen on electron microscopy. Three types have been described; type II congenital dyserythropoietic anemia is the most common form, characterized by erythroblastic multinuclearity and positive acidified serum test results (HEMPAS anemia). Congenital dyserythropoietic anemia can manifest in the newborn period with megaloblastic anemia, early jaundice, hepatosplenomegaly,

and intrauterine growth retardation. Treatment for this disorder consists of supportive therapy and close observation for side effects of long-term transfusions. Splenectomy in some patients with severe anemia has been helpful.

Fanconi anemia is an autosomal recessive disorder characterized by marrow failure and congenital anomalies, including abnormalities in skin pigmentation, gastrointestinal anomalies, renal anomalies, and upper limb anomalies. Approximately one third of patients have no obvious congenital anomalies. Most patients present in early childhood, but newborns with Fanconi anemia have been reported, usually when obvious congenital anomalies are present. Patients generally have steroid-responsive hypoplastic anemia, reticulocytopenia, macrocytic RBCs on peripheral smear, and shortened RBC life span. Treatment of Fanconi anemia is similar to that for Diamond-Blackfan syndrome; marrow transplantation has been successful.

Osteopetrosis is a rare autosomal recessive disorder characterized by defects in osteoclastic function, resulting in a decreased bone marrow space. Developmental delay, ocular involvement, and neurodegenerative findings occur in association with hypoplastic anemia, although patients also may present with hemolytic anemia. Longitudinal studies in the United States and Europe have shown variability in outcome, although survival beyond 5 to 6 years is less than 30%. Patients presenting with early hematologic and visual impairment have an even shorter life expectancy. Limited treatment options for this disorder include marrow transplantation and administration of calcitriol and interferon gamma.

Pearson marrow-pancreas syndrome is a disorder involving the hematopoietic system, exocrine pancreas, liver, and kidneys. Patients present in infancy with macrocytic anemia, sometimes associated with neutropenia and thrombocytopenia. Bone marrow transplantation has not been reported in these patients, and the disorder is considered fatal.

Except for anemia of prematurity, the previously described hypoproliferative anemias generally require referral to a pediatric hematologist for evaluation and treatment. Recognition of impaired erythropoiesis in a term infant should prompt the generalist to obtain further assistance with diagnosis and long-term management.

FETAL/NEONATAL ANEMIA FROM CONGENITAL INFECTION

Infections before and after birth can lead to anemia through any of the common mechanisms—hemorrhage, hemolysis, or hypoproliferative disease. Neonatal sepsis from group B streptococcus, *Escherichia coli*, and other perinatal organisms may result in hemolysis, disseminated intravascular coagulation, and hemorrhage. Infants often are jaundiced and have hepatosplenomegaly, although the degree of hyperbilirubinemia does not always reflect the degree of anemia. Infants may have an elevated direct bilirubin as well, possibly from infectious involvement with the liver. Bacteria such as *E. coli* produce hemolytic endotoxins, causing increased RBC destruction, often associated with a microangiopathic process. Appropriate antibiotic therapy should be instituted when these symptoms are present and continued until a cause is determined or until it becomes clear that the infant dos not have a bacterial infection.

Fetal and neonatal infection with parvovirus B19 can cause severe anemia, hydrops, and fetal demise. The fetus or neonate generally presents with a hypoplastic anemia, but hemolysis also can occur. The virus replicates in erythroid progenitor cells and shuts down erythropoiesis, resulting in aplastic anemia. In utero transfusions for hydropic fetuses have been investigated but are not successful in all patients. Experimental treatment with intravenous immunoglobulin during aplastic crises has led to resolution of the anemia.

Congenital viral infections from cytomegalovirus, toxoplasmosis, rubella, and herpes simplex are associated with hemolytic anemia and should be considered in the workup of an infant with non–immune-mediated hemolysis. Congenital syphilis also may present with hemolytic anemia, despite negative testing in the mother. Initial maternal screening for syphilis may be negative despite overwhelming infection—a condition termed the *prozone effect*. This effect occurs when a higher than optimal amount of antibody in the tested sera prevents the flocculation reaction seen in positive reagin test results. Serum dilution is necessary to make the correct diagnosis. In cases of non–immune-mediated hydrops, nontreponemal testing should be repeated using serum dilutions to prevent a missed diagnosis of syphilis in women with negative syphilis serologic results.

Other infections associated with neonatal anemia include malaria and human immunodeficiency virus (HIV). Congenital malaria may occur in areas such as New York City, where imported cases of malaria are increasing. Congenital HIV infection can be asymptomatic in newborns, but infants born to mothers taking zidovudine may have a hypoplastic anemia caused by side effects of the drug.

Treatment of anemia secondary to congenital infections begins with appropriate antimicrobial therapy and management of associated organ disorders, such as hepatic, pulmonary, or renal disease. Depending on the mechanism causing anemia, treatment can involve transfusions, nutritional therapy, or administration of specific or nonspecific immunoglobulin. Anemia resulting from congenital infection generally resolves within 4 to 6 weeks, and follow-up entails documenting normal RBC indices.

Mini-index of Related Topics CH.

SUGGESTED READINGS

Alcock GS, Liley H: Immunoglobulin infusion for isoimmune haemolytic jaundice in neonates. Cochrane Database Syst Rev 2002; 3:CD003313.

Christensen RD: Expected hematologic values for term and preterm neonates In Christensen RD (ed): Hematologic Problems in the Neonate. Philadelphia, WB Saunders, 2000, pp 117–136.

Goldberg MA, Dunning SP, Bunn HF: Regulation of the erythropoietin gene: Evidence that the oxygen sensor is a heme protein. Science 1988;242:524–528.

Merck: Committed to Bringing Out the Best in Medicine. Available at: http://www.merck.com/pubs/mmanual/section19/chapter260/260h.htm.

Ohls RK: Evaluation and treatment of anemia in the neonate. In Christensen RD (ed): Hematologic Problems in the Neonate. Philadelphia, WB Saunders, 2000, pp 137–170.

Supski DW, Gurushanthaiah K, Chasen S: The effect of treatment of twin-twin transfusion syndrome on the diagnosis-to-delivery interval. Twin Res 2002;5:1–4.

201

Neonatal Erythrocytosis (Polycythemia)

Robert D. Christensen and Darlene A. Calhoun

ROLE OF THE GENERALIST

1 Recognize neonatal erythrocytosis.
2 Determine the etiology of erythrocytosis.
3 Manage complications of erythrocytosis, including hyperviscosity and hypoglycemia
4 Refer patients with erythrocytosis to appropriate specialist when assistance is needed for management or procedures.
5 Ensure follow-up for all patients with erythrocytosis, including long-term care with a high-risk neonatal follow-up program

DEFINITIONS

The terms *polycythemia*, *erythrocytosis*, and *hyperviscosity* sometimes are used incorrectly as synonyms. *Polycythemia*, which literally means "many cells," indicates an abnormal increase in the circulating concentration of erythrocytes. The terms *polycythemia rubra vera* and *polycythemia vera* refer to a disorder in which the concentrations of leukocytes, platelets, and erythrocytes all are increased. The neonatal variety of polycythemia does not involve elevations in all of these elements.

The term *hyperviscosity* indicates that the blood is abnormally viscous. This condition is distinct from polycythemia because hyperviscosity can occur in the absence of polycythemia, and not all polycythemic patients are significantly hyperviscous. Increases in white blood cells, platelets, and plasma proteins have been associated with hyperviscosity. Viscosity, expressed in centipoise, is:

$$\frac{\text{Shear stress (dynes/cm}^2)}{\text{Shear rate}}$$

Shear stress refers to the frictional forces within a fluid, whereas *shear rate* is defined by the velocity of flow at a given radius. The shear rate in the aorta is approximately 230 seconds^{-1}, whereas it is only 11.5 seconds^{-1} in small arterioles and venules. As the shear rate decreases, the viscosity increases. At low shear rates, such as occur in the microcirculation, blood with a high hematocrit virtually may stop flowing.

Increase in the circulating concentration of erythrocytes is the most common cause of hyperviscosity, but it is not the only cause. The term *erythrocytosis* is preferred to either polycythemia or hyperviscosity for the relatively common condition in neonates. *Erythrocytosis* simply denotes an increased concentration of erythrocytes in the circulating blood and, in contrast to polycythemia, is not confused with *polycythemia vera*.

FUNDAMENTALS

Sampling Site

Measurements of erythrocyte concentrations in the blood of neonates vary predictably according to the vascular source from which the blood sample is obtained. Erythrocytes are more concentrated when the blood is obtained from the capillaries than when drawn from a vessel or an indwelling catheter; this is a result of rouleaux formation and the movement of the red blood cells through the vessel wall. Capillary blood obtained from a poorly perfused site erroneously might suggest erythrocytosis because erythrocyte counts obtained from such sites are 5% to 25% higher than counts simultaneously obtained from a vessel. Warming the extremity before lancing can produce a better correlation between capillary and vascular values. Although capillary hematocrits can correlate poorly with venous hematocrits, the latter correlate significantly with arterial hematocrits ($r = 0.95$, $P < 0.001$)

Time of Blood Sampling Relative to Delivery

The hematocrit generally increases over the first 4 to 12 hours after delivery, partially from hemoconcentration of the erythrocytes received at delivery from a placental transfusion. The magnitude of increase in erythrocyte values over the first hours of life varies, in part, in proportion to the volume of the placental transfusion received. The hematocrit, similar to the hemoglobin concentration and erythrocyte count, begins to decline after 12 hours of life, and by the end of the 1st week of life, the hematocrit is close to the original cord blood value.

Hemoglobin, Hematocrit, and Erythrocyte Count

The hemoglobin concentration and the hematocrit are different measurements of the same biologic variable. The hemoglobin concentration is a direct measurement, whereas the hematocrit generally is a calculated value, making hemoglobin concentration the preferred variable.

Many studies have reported a "normal range" of hemoglobin values from the umbilical cord blood of healthy term infants (see CD-ROM Table 201-1). The summation of these reports indicates an overall average hemoglobin, at term, of 16.8 g/dL (range 13.7 to 20.1 g/dL). Values less than 13.7 g/dL could be considered *anemic*, and values greater than 20.1 g/dL (corresponding with a hematocrit of 0.60 to 0.61) could be considered *erythrocythemic*.

The normal hemoglobin in female fetuses can be determined by the formula: 7 + the gestational age in months. A female infant delivered at 7 months' gestation would be expected to have a hemoglobin concentration of 7 + 7, or 14 g/dL. This relationship does not hold true for male fetuses, who reach a value of about 16 g/dL by 32 weeks' gestation and then remain constant through term. Postmature infants have higher hemoglobin concentrations than do infants delivered at term if placental insufficiency and chronic hypoxemia occur. The hematocrit, similar to the hemoglobin concentration and the erythrocyte count, normally increases during the first hours of life and then slowly declines so that by the end of the first week of life it is near the original cord blood value.

Modern hospital laboratories use aperture-impedance instruments that calculate the hematocrit by electronically measuring the mean red blood cell volume and multiplying this number by the electronically measured erythrocyte concentration. Other types of cell counters calculate the hematocrit using laser optics, correlating the magnitude of a light pulse generated by passing a red blood cell through a laser with the cell's volume. When hematocrit values obtained by centrifuging and values obtained through electronic methods are used on an individual patient, a consistent difference between the two occurs. Neonates tend to have a slightly higher "spun" hematocrit than "automated" hematocrit. The reason involves the phenomenon of "trapped plasma" in the spun hematocrit determinations. When it is clinically important to follow the hematocrit closely, this difference between spun and automated values should be recognized, and a consistent method should be employed.

Erythrocyte Count

The erythrocyte count, or number of erythrocytes in a volume of blood, is determined electronically by a particle counter. Many children's hospital clinical laboratories express the erythrocyte count as *cells/μL of blood*, whereas most adult clinical hematology services express the count as *cells/L of blood*. Cells/μL (usually × 10^6) and cells/L (usually × 10^{12}) are equivalent.

Reticulocyte Count

Reticulocytes are erythrocytes that have been released recently from the bone marrow into the blood and still contain organelles. Normally, these are erythrocytes that have been in the circulation for 24 hours of less.

A reticulocyte count helps to assess the level of erythrocyte production because high reticulocyte counts signify increased erythropoiesis, and counts of 0 signify a low level of effective erythropoiesis. A reticulocyte "percentage" is the percent of erythrocytes that stain as reticulocytes. A limitation of this method is that it fails to account for

differences in the absolute number of erythrocytes. Reporting the reticulocyte count as an *absolute number* gives a clearer comparison of effective erythropoiesis despite differences in hematocrit.

On the 1st day of life, normal term infants have reticulocyte percentages of 4% to 7% and absolute reticulocyte counts of 200,000/μL to 400,000/μL. Infants delivered prematurely have higher reticulocyte counts than infants born at term. Values of 6% to 10% and 400,000/μL to 550,000/μL are common in low-birth-weight infants. In healthy neonates, reticulocytes decrease markedly over the first few days of life. By the 4th day of life, the percentage may be 0% to 1%, with an absolute count of 0/μL to 50,000/μL.

Hyperviscosity

Three major factors determine the viscosity of blood: (1) the hematocrit, (2) the deformability of the erythrocytes, and (3) the plasma viscosity. Extremely high concentrations of leukocytes or platelets can result in increased viscosity, although we have not observed hyperviscosity in neonates with extremely elevated blood neutrophil counts (leukemoid reactions, 85,000/μL). Reduced plasma volume, increased plasma proteins, and endothelial factors can augment the plasma viscosity. In neonates, the hematocrit seems to be the parameter that determines the viscosity, however. The relationship between hematocrit and viscosity is nearly linear to a hematocrit of 65% and is exponential thereafter.

DIAGNOSIS

Presenting signs and symptoms of neonatal erythrocytosis are listed in Table 201-1; these include a distinctive ruddy appearance, termed *rubeosis*, and a slow refilling of the capillaries after pressing on the skin (Fig. 201-1). Reports indicate that about half of neonates who have hematocrits greater than 0.65 are symptomatic. It is difficult to distinguish, however, whether these symptoms are related primarily to increased viscosity or are secondary signs of diminished organ blood flows of the fetal condition that led to the elevation in hematocrit and viscosity. The most consistent signs, other than rubeosis and poor perfusion, are lethargy, hypotonia, poor sucking, and easy startle. Hypoglycemia occurs in 15% to 40% of cases. Hypocalcemia also can be a problem (occurring in about 10%). Thrombocytopenia is common (30% to 40%), but tends not to be

Table 201-1. Common Laboratory Findings and Clinical Signs Associated with Neonatal Erythrocytosis

Laboratory	Clinical
Hypoglycemia (15–40% of cases)	Rubeosis
Hypocalcemia (10% of cases)	Poor capillary perfusion
Thrombocytopenia (generally mild; 75–150 μL)	Weak suck
	Lethargy
	Tachypnea
	Hypotonia
	Tachycardia
	Easily startled
	Jitteriness
	Hepatomegaly

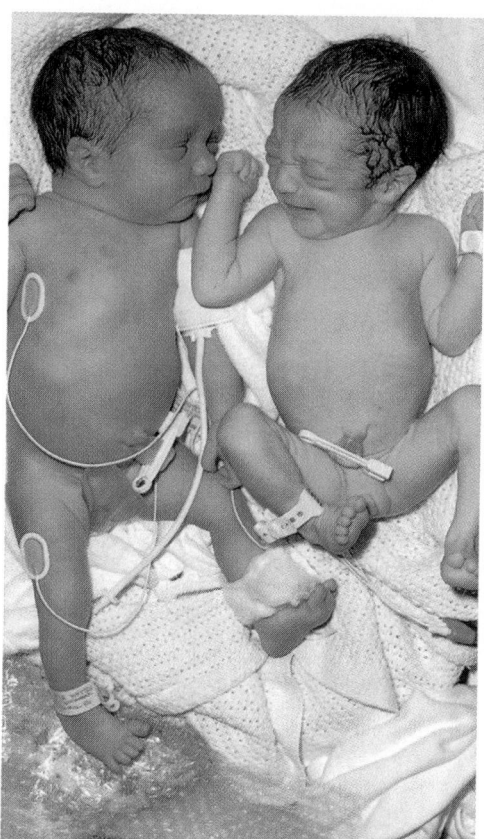

Figure 201-1. An acute transfer of blood occurred between these twins with one born anemic and the other polycythemic. Urgent transfusion of the anemic infant is needed; a partial exchange of the recipient twin is needed if the infant is symptomatic with a packed cell volume of greater than 60% or if asymptomatic with a packed cell volume greater than 65% to 70%. The exact packed cell volume at which an exchange transfusion is indicated is hotly debated, with some long-term studies showing no adverse effects of untreated asymptomatic polycythemia. Most authorities agree, however, that a packed cell volume greater than 70% is an absolute indication for an exchange transfusion. (From Markiewicz M, Abrahamson E [eds]: Diagnosis in Color: Neonatology. St. Louis, Mosby, 2000, p 20.)

severe, with counts generally between 75,000/μL and 150,000/μL. Thrombocytopenia may serve as a marker for severity of hyperviscosity.

Evaluation of the maternal history should include questioning about diabetes; smoking; prenatally diagnosed intrauterine growth restriction; pregnancy-induced hypertension or HELLP (hemolysis, elevated liver enzymes, and low platelet count) syndrome; pulmonary, renal, or cardiac disease; placental transfusion from delayed cord clamping; and the possibility of twin–twin transfusion syndrome. Physical examination should include careful monitoring of vital signs during the transitional period (tachycardia and tachypnea are relatively common); routine morphometric measurements (macrosomia and intrauterine growth restriction are common); examination looking for rubeosis, capillary refill, and hepatosplenomegaly; and repetitive evaluations of tone, suck, and startle reflex.

Neonates who have rubeosis and poor perfusion should have a complete blood count done using a central (not capillary) site, a platelet count, blood glucose, and ionized calcium. Diagnosis of neonatal erythrocytosis/hyperviscosity syndrome generally depends on the hematocrit/hemoglobin

concentrations. Measurements of viscosity generally are not available in most hospitals. In neonates with any of the symptoms listed in Table 201-1, who have a central hematocrit greater than 0.70, the diagnosis of erythrocytosis can be made with confidence. Some authors have advocated using a hematocrit of 0.68 and some have recommended 0.65 as the "trigger" value for treatment of symptomatic neonates. Because the effect of treatment on long-term outcome is unclear, most recommend treatment for neonates with a central hematocrit greater than 0.70.

MANAGEMENT

When it has been decided that the degree of erythrocytosis constitutes a significant risk to the neonate, the goal is to reduce the blood viscosity rapidly and safely. Although reduction can be attempted by diluting the blood via infusion of low-viscosity fluid, removal of erythrocytes by partial exchange transfusion with equivalent crystalloid replacement is the recommended treatment. Increased fluid intake through feeding seldom is sufficient for a symptomatic neonate because erythrocythemic neonates generally are poor feeders. Gavage feeding large amounts to these neonates carries the additional risk of necrotizing enterocolitis because the mesenteric circulation likely is compromised by the hyperviscosity. The time required for enteral fluids to diminish the blood viscosity is long. These considerations make partial exchange transfusion a more appropriate approach.

Partial exchange transfusion is a relatively safe and rapid means of decreasing the blood viscosity and resolving the clinical symptoms. The goal of the partial exchange is to lower the hematocrit to 0.60. The volume to be exchanged is calculated from the following formula:

$$\text{mL to be removed} = \text{blood volume} \times \frac{\text{observed hematocrit} - 60}{\text{observed hematocrit}}$$

Accuracy of the blood volume estimate is not needed; the blood volume simply is estimated to be 100 mL/kg, and the volume to be removed is calculated by:

$$\text{Patient wt (kg)} \times 100 \text{ (mL/kg)} \times \frac{\text{observed hematocrit} - 60}{\text{observed hematocrit}}$$

For a neonate weighing 3 kg with a hematocrit of 80% (0.80) the volume to be removed is $300 \times 0.25 = 75$ mL.

The following method for the partial exchange is simple. The clinician places an umbilical venous catheter if it passes the ductus venosus (tip at the level of the diaphragm on chest x-ray) or an umbilical arterial catheter if the umbilical venous catheter cannot be placed properly. After the catheter is in place, four syringes are prepared: one empty and three containing 25 mL (each) of sterile normal saline (total 75 mL). The empty syringe is attached first to the umbilical venous catheter via a three-way stopcock, in such a way as to avoid any infusion of air. The empty syringe is used to withdraw 25 mL of blood, after which the syringe is removed, capped, and replaced by one of the three syringes containing sterile normal saline. The 25 mL of saline is infused slowly. When the syringe has been emptied into the patient, that same syringe is used to withdraw 25 mL of blood; then it is removed from the stopcock and capped. The second saline-containing syringe is attached and its contents are infused slowly; then 25 mL blood is withdrawn into the syringe, and it is removed from the stopcock and capped. The third and final saline-containing syringe is attached and infused. However, to keep the total amount of saline "in" plus blood "out" to equal one another (isovolemic), blood is not withdrawn into the final syringe; 75 mL of normal saline is infused, and 75 mL of blood is withdrawn. The catheter is removed after the procedure.

The partial exchange transfusion procedure reduces the hematocrit immediately, generally to within 5% of the target value. Reports indicate that immediate improvement occurs in capillary perfusion, cerebral blood flow, and cardiac function. The effect of the procedure on long-term outcome is unclear. Possible reasons for this uncertainty are that damage done from hyperviscosity already might have occurred before the exchange or that the damage might be the result of something other than the hyperviscosity. Despite these unresolved issues, we advocate a partial exchange transfusion, using the aforementioned methods, for any neonate with rubeosis, poor capillary refill, and venous hematocrit greater than 0.70.

⊚ Additional Resources, CD-ROM

Umbilical cord blood hemoglobin concentrations	Table
Procedure for partial exchange transfusion	Text
Bibliography	

Mini-index of Related Topics

SUGGESTED READINGS

Acunas B, Celtik C, Vatansever U, Karasalihoglu S: Thrombocytopenia: An important indicator for the application of partial exchange transfusion in polycythemic newborn infants? Pediatr Int 2000; 52:343–347.

Drew JH, Guaran RL, Chello M, Hobbs JB: Neonatal whole blood hyperviscosity: The important factor influencing later neurologic function is the viscosity and not the polycythemia. Clin Hemorheol Microcirc 1997;17:67–72.

Linderman R, Haga P: Evaluation and treatment of polycythemia in the neonate. In Christensen RD (ed): Hematologic Problems of the Neonate. Philadelphia, WB Saunders, 2000, pp 171–184.

Roithmaier A, Arlettax R, Bauer K, et al: Randomized controlled trial of Ringer solution versus serum for partial exchange transfusion in neonatal polycythemia. Eur J Pediatr 1995;154:53–56.

Wong W, Folk TE, Lee CH, et al: Randomized controlled trial: Comparison of colloid or crystalloid for partial exchange transfusion for treatment of neonatal polycythemia. Arch Dis Child Fetal Neonatal Ed 1997;77:F115–F118.

202 Thrombocytopenia, Bleeding Disorders, and Disorders of Coagulation in Newborn Infants

Cynthia Edstrom

ROLE OF THE GENERALIST

1 Recognize clinically significant bleeding and the specific patterns that occur in the newborn period.

2 Recognize the presentations and clinical findings of thrombocytopenia in the newborn.

3 Recognize the presentations and clinical findings of thrombosis in the newborn.

4 Initiate evaluation of newborns with evidence of bleeding, thrombocytopenia, and thrombosis.

5 Resuscitate and stabilize an acutely bleeding infant.

6 Stabilize an acutely ill infant with suspected thrombosis.

7 Transfer an infant with bleeding or thrombosis to a tertiary neonatal intensive care unit for further evaluation and treatment.

8 Ensure appropriate follow-up, including monitoring for complications of bleeding or thrombosis, performing and coordinating follow-up testing to ensure adequate diagnosis, and coordinating ongoing care with pediatric hematologists and other specialists.

Problems of hemostasis are more common during the newborn period than at any other time during childhood. The frequency of hemostatic disorders in newborn infants is due in part to physiologic immaturity of the hemostatic system. An overview of hemostasis and the clotting cascade is presented in Chapter 95. The specific components of the clotting cascade and mechanisms of hemostasis in newborn infants are the same as those of older children and adults. The levels of clotting factors are different in the newborn, however, and vary with gestational age. In particular, many of the procoagulant vitamin K–dependent factors (factors II, IIV, IX, and X) are present at comparatively low levels in term newborns, and preterm infants have even lower levels. Factor VIII levels are the same in newborns and in older children, but factor IX levels are low. These differences in factor levels affect the ability to diagnose hemophilias and other hemostatic abnormalities during the newborn period. Besides differences in procoagulant factor levels, levels of many factors involved in coagulation inhibition (e.g., protein C and protein S) and fibrinolysis (the

process of breaking down clots) are lower in newborns than in older children and adults. Because of the varying levels of procoagulant and anticoagulant factors in newborn infants, hemostasis can become unbalanced during illness, resulting in either excessive bleeding or excessive clotting. Normal ranges for hemostatic factors are established for newborn infants and can be found in the references listed in Suggested Readings.

Thrombocytopenia is a frequent problem in sick neonates and has many causes. The platelet counts of newborns tend to be slightly lower than those of adults but usually remain within the range of 150,000 to 400,000/mm^3—considered normal for older children and adults. Thrombocytopenia is defined as a platelet count less than 150,000/mm^3. Whether platelet counts of 100,000 to 150,000/mm^3 are abnormal for neonates is unclear but does demand close attention by the clinician. Counts less than 100,000/mm^3 are abnormal, however, and require monitoring and further investigation. The role of platelets in hemostasis and definitions of platelet function and disorders are covered in Chapter 95.

Minor bleeding is common in newborn infants. Streaks of gross blood in "spit up" gastric contents, bruising at a venipuncture site, oozing from a heel-stick site, and oozing or bleeding after circumcision are familiar problems for the generalist. These types of bleeding most often are caused by benign conditions, such as emesis of swallowed maternal blood, difficulty in performing a venipuncture, or application of inadequate pressure after a procedure. Clinically significant bleeding suggesting a problem with hemostasis may present in the same manner, however. More commonly, clinically significant bleeding or oozing occurs from several sites; is more severe than expected given the clinical condition; is difficult to stop or control; and frequently is accompanied by poor perfusion and unstable vital signs, such as tachycardia and decreasing blood pressure. A normal newborn generally has about 80 mL of blood per kilogram of body weight. Loss of seemingly small amounts of blood may be clinically significant in a newborn. The acute loss of 4 mL of blood represents 5% of the total blood volume for a 1-kg infant.

Although bleeding and coagulation problems are fairly frequent in newborns, thromboembolic problems are encountered infrequently but often are serious. Thromboembolic

Box 202-1. Thrombophilias Associated with Neonatal Thromboembolic Problems

- Factor C deficiency
- Factor S deficiency
- Antithrombin III deficiency
- Factor V Leiden
- Prothrombin G20210A
- Activated protein C resistance
- Methylenetetrahydrofolate reductase T677T genotype
- Lipoprotein (a)
- Antiphospholipid/anticardiolipin antibodies (transplacental acquisition)
- Plasminogen activator inhibitor–1 promoter polymorphism (4G/5G or 4G/4G)

Box 202-2. Sites of Bleeding in the Newborn

- Circumcision (see Chapter 199)
- Intravenous line, venipuncture, or heel-stick sites
- Skin—bruising, petechiae, oozing from surgical sites or line insertion sites
- Umbilicus
- Intracranial (intraventricular, subarachnoid, subdural, intracerebral)
- Gastrointestinal tract (heme positive or gross blood in stool, emesis, gastric aspirate)
- Pulmonary, tracheal
- Scalp (subgaleal, subperiosteal)
- Liver—subcapsular, parenchymal
- Renal or bladder

disease occurs when the factors that inhibit or counteract the effects of clotting are inadequate. Most thromboembolic problems in newborns occur in sick infants and in association with centrally placed intravascular catheters. In addition, infants at risk for thromboembolic problems include infants with congenital heart disease, infants of diabetic mothers, small-for-gestational-age infants, infants with neonatal sepsis, infants with asphyxia, infants with Extra-Corporeal Membrane Oxygenation, infants with polycythemia, and infants with inherited thrombophilias. Inherited thrombophilias, similar to hemophilias, are genetic predispositions to excessive clotting. Box 202-1 lists thrombophilias reported in infants with thromboembolic problems.

FUNDAMENTALS

When a newborn presents with bleeding, the generalist first must decide whether the bleeding is clinically significant or benign. Clinically significant bleeding occurs in the newborn and can vary from mild oozing in the umbilicus to frank, life-threatening hemorrhage from sites such as the lungs, gastrointestinal tract, circumcision, or brain. Sites of bleeding are listed in Box 202-2. Bleeding after circumcision is discussed in Chapter 199.

Infants presenting with bleeding may be well appearing or ill appearing. Well-appearing infants typically have bleeding or oozing as the primary problem. Bleeding typically occurs from blood sampling sites, from the umbilicus, or after circumcision. In contrast, ill-appearing infants usually have concurrent serious conditions, such as shock, sepsis, asphyxia, trauma, or extreme prematurity. Bleeding may be profuse with resultant hypotension and tachycardia. Bleeding often is intracranial, from endotracheal or gastric tubes, from intravascular line sites, and from the gastrointestinal tract, and often bleeding occurs at multiple sites. Causes of bleeding in well-appearing and ill-appearing infants are summarized in Table 202-1. Bleeding in a well-appearing newborn is most often from congenital factor deficiency, immune-mediated thrombocytopenia, or congenital thrombocytopenia. Bleeding in an ill-appearing newborn is most commonly a consumptive process, such as disseminated intravascular coagulation (DIC), thrombocytopenia from peripheral platelet destruction, or liver failure.

Vitamin K deficiency bleeding (also called h*emorrhagic disease of the newborn*) occurs primarily in the newborn period, and almost all cases occur within the first year of life. Newborn infants are vulnerable to vitamin K deficiency bleeding because little vitamin K crosses the placenta, the intestinal flora is poorly developed and produces little vitamin K in the first weeks of life, and breast milk contains sufficient vitamin K only if taken in adequate amounts. Vitamin K is an essential cofactor for the vitamin K–dependent procoagulant factors II, VII, IX, and X. Hemostasis depends on the presence of adequate amounts of vitamin K. For these reasons, vitamin K prophylaxis is recommended for all infants at birth. Infants who are to be formula fed or who are to receive total parenteral nutrition also should receive vitamin K prophylaxis, even though formula and total parenteral nutrition contain vitamin K.

Three forms of vitamin K deficiency bleeding are recognized: early, classic, and late. The early form manifests within 24 hours of birth with generalized hemorrhagic symptoms. This form is a rare cause of neonatal bleeding and is associated with maternal medications. Implicated medications include carbamazepine, phenytoin, barbiturates, some cephalosporins, rifampin, isoniazid, and warfarin.

Table 202-1. Causes of Bleeding in the Newborn

Well-Appearing Newborn	Ill-Appearing Newborn
Inherited factor deficiency (hemophilia, von Willebrand)	Consumptive coagulopathy/disseminated intravascular coagulation (septic, hypovolemic, or cardiogenic shock)
Immune thrombocytopenia	Thrombocytopenia related to increased destruction (sepsis, necrotizing enterocolitis, congenital infection, asphyxia)
Vitamin K deficiency bleeding	Liver disease/liver failure
Congenital thrombocytopenias related to decreased production	Medications—indomethacin, heparin
Congenital disorders of platelet function	Vitamin K deficiency bleeding
	Thrombocytopenia related to decreased production (preeclampsia, small for gestational age)
	Inherited factor deficiency (hemophilia)

Table 202-2. Types of Vitamin K Deficiency Bleeding

Type	Timing	Cause	Evaluation	Treatment
Early	≤24 hr of birth	Maternal medications	Maternal medication history Rule out other causes of bleeding	Vitamin K Supportive Referral to NICU
Classic	2–7 days	Failure to receive vitamin K prophylaxis Inadequate intake of vitamin K Physiologic low production of vitamin K	PT, PTT, fibrinogen, and platelet count Give vitamin K IV or SC and assess response	Vitamin K Supportive Referral to NICU
Late	2 wk–6 mo	Inadequate intake of vitamin K (exclusively breast-fed) Inadequate absorption (hepatobiliary disease)	PT, PTT, fibrinogen, and platelet count LFTs Ultrasound of liver and gallbladder Consider PIVKA-II testing if available Give vitamin K IV or SC and assess response	Vitamin K Supportive Consult hematology PICU referral if bleeding serious

LFTs, liver function tests; NICU, neonatal intensive care unit; PICU, pediatric intensive care unit; PIVKA-II, protein induced by vitamin K absence; PT, prothrombin time; PTT; partial thromboplastin time.

The classic form, the most common form of vitamin K deficiency bleeding, usually occurs in infants who are exclusively breast-fed, have inadequate intake, and either did not receive vitamin K prophylaxis or received inadequate doses of vitamin K at birth. Prematurity, asphyxia, any illness that results in feeding delay, liver disease, and other serious illnesses increase the risk. Infants present at 2 to 7 days of life with bleeding or oozing, often from many sites. The classic form can be prevented by administration of intramuscular or oral vitamin K prophylaxis at birth.

Late-onset vitamin K deficiency often presents as intracranial or other catastrophic hemorrhage. This form of vitamin K deficiency is caused by inadequate intake from low vitamin K content in exclusively breast-fed infants or by inadequate absorption secondary to hepatobiliary disease. Most cases of vitamin K deficiency caused by inadequate intake probably can be prevented by a single intramuscular injection of vitamin K at birth. Repeated doses of oral vitamin K are required for prevention of the late form of vitamin K deficiency bleeding. Countries that have adopted oral vitamin K prophylaxis have reported increasing numbers of cases of late-onset vitamin K deficiency bleeding. Table 202-2 summarizes presentation, evaluation, and treatment of the three forms of vitamin K deficiency bleeding. Prophylaxis and treatment regimens for vitamin K deficiency bleeding are presented in Table 202-3.

Although not unique to the newborn period, DIC is a common cause of abnormal bleeding in sick newborn infants. DIC occurs when processes such as hypoxia, sepsis, shock, and other serious illnesses excessively activate coagulation processes. These illnesses presumably stimulate excessive expression of tissue factor and cytokines, with resultant activation of all aspects of the hemostatic system. The end result is consumption and depletion of procoagulant, anticoagulant, and fibrinolytic factors. Clinically an infant with DIC is usually critically ill. Typically, DIC is recognized when oozing is observed from venipuncture, intravenous, and heel-stick sites. Blood may be observed when suctioning an endotracheal tube or aspirating gastric contents. Urine and stool are often heme occult positive. Bleeding can occur from any site and can be profuse. No single test establishes the diagnosis of DIC. Most infants with DIC have prolonged prothrombin time (PT) and partial thromboplastin time (PTT) values, depletion of fibrinogen, and increased D dimers. Thrombocytopenia frequently is present, and a blood smear demonstrates fragmented red blood cells. D dimers measure the breakdown of cross-linked fibrin (the final step in clotting) and increased D dimers are highly suggestive of DIC. D dimers can be increased in the absence of bleeding, however, and in healthy newborns. The diagnosis of DIC is made based on combined clinical and laboratory assessments. Successful treatment of DIC depends on accurate diagnosis and effective treat-

Table 202-3. Recommendation for Vitamin K Administration

Indication	Dose*	Route	Contraindications	Precautions
Prophylaxis: Term newborn	1 mg	IM		
Prophylaxis: Term newborn—alternative (healthy, exclusive breast-feeding)	2 mg with first feed. Repeat at 1, 4, and 8 wk	Oral	Preterm Ill Cholestasis Receiving antibiotics Diarrhea	No approved oral formulation in United States Increased cases of hemorrhagic disease in countries using oral formulations, especially if receive only a single dose
Prophylaxis: Preterm newborn <1000 g	0.3 mg	IM		Give slowly
Treatment: Hemorrhagic disease	1–10 mg slow IV push	IV		Reference Neofax for precautions Anaphylaxis-type reactions, shock, cardiac arrest reported in adults

*Neofax2002.

From Magnum B, Young TE (eds): Neofax 2002. Battle Creek, Mich, Acorn Publishing, 2002.

ment of the underlying disorders. Management of bleeding during DIC is discussed later in the management section.

Bleeding is a common presentation of neonatal liver disease and can occur at any time during the course of the illness. The liver is the primary source for production of most coagulation factors, including factor V, the vitamin K–dependent factors, and fibrinogen. Diseases causing cellular damage, impaired function, or failure of the liver result in inadequate production of hemostatic factors with resultant bleeding. Thrombocytopenia frequently is present and may be profound, requiring multiple platelet transfusions. Secondary vitamin K deficiency occurs, particularly in patients with biliary disease, as a result of impaired intestinal absorption of vitamin K. Infants with coagulopathy and liver disease often have prolonged PT values, thrombocytopenia, and decreased factor V levels. Because factor VIII is produced in the vascular endothelium, factor VIII levels usually are normal in infants with liver disease, helping to distinguish liver disease from DIC. Causes of liver disease in newborns include asphyxia, bacterial or viral sepsis, congenital infections, metabolic diseases, shock, hydrops, and complications of total parenteral nutrition. The presentations, diagnosis, and treatment of liver diseases are discussed further in Chapter 90.

Inherited factor deficiencies, such as hemophilia A and B, von Willebrand disease, and other factor deficiencies, can present with neonatal bleeding. The common presentation of an inherited factor deficiency is bleeding in an otherwise healthy infant, particularly after circumcision. Bleeding in an ill-appearing infant also can be caused by an inherited factor deficiency, however, especially when bleeding is more severe than expected by the clinical illness. Catastrophic intraventricular hemorrhage in a stable 31-week premature male infant with mild respiratory distress syndrome might suggest an inherited factor deficiency. Hemophilia A and B, von Willebrand disease, and other factor deficiencies are discussed in Chapters 95 and 161.

Thrombocytopenia is frequent in the newborn period. Causes of neonatal thrombocytopenia are presented in Table 94-3. Neonatal thrombocytopenia can present in many ways: as an incidental finding on a complete blood count in a well-appearing infant, as mild-to-severe bleeding in a well-appearing or ill-appearing infant, or as part of a constellation of findings in a critically ill infant. Thrombocytopenia occurs frequently in neonatal infections, particularly accompanying fungal infections and congenital viral infections. Thrombocytopenia is a frequent, and often early, finding in association with necrotizing enterocolitis, presumably from sequestration and destruction of platelets.

Thrombocytopenia also occurs frequently in premature infants born after pregnancies complicated by pregnancy-induced hypertension, particularly small-for-gestational-age premature infants. Thrombocytopenia related to pregnancy-induced hypertension usually presents at birth, develops shortly after birth, or develops within the first few days of life, often is accompanied by neutropenia, usually reaches a nadir within 2 to 4 days of life, and commonly resolves by 7 to 10 days of life. The thrombocytopenia usually is mild and requires no treatment. Occasionally, thrombocytopenia

related to severe pregnancy-induced hypertension is more profound and prolonged, however, and requires platelet transfusions.

Thrombocytopenia occurs in many chromosomal disorders, including Turner syndrome and trisomies 13, 18, and 21 (Down syndrome). Thrombocytopenia accompanies many other congenital and genetic disorders, including Noonan syndrome, Wiskott-Aldrich syndrome, Alport syndrome, thrombocytopenia–absent radius syndrome, and some inborn errors of metabolism. An infant with thrombocytopenia who is dysmorphic or has unexplained metabolic aberrations may have a congenital or genetic disorder needing further evaluation. Neonatal alloimmune and autoimmune thrombocytopenias usually present with bleeding in an otherwise well-appearing infant and are discussed further in Chapter 94.

Thromboembolic complications in newborns can occur in many different organ systems and in infants with many medical problems. Prenatal onset in mothers with thrombophilias and in those with primary or secondary placental disease also must be considered. Because thrombotic complications in newborns commonly occur in sick and premature infants, most are patients in a neonatal intensive care unit (NICU) at the time the complications develop. Table 202-4 summarizes presentations of newborns with thrombotic complications and common locations of thrombi. Long-term follow-up and care of most of these patients with neonatal thrombotic complications are provided and coordinated by the generalist. Occasionally the generalist encounters an infant born with an unexpected thrombotic condition. These conditions are rare but serious. Conditions that may be encountered by the generalist include acute

Table 202-4. Locations and Presentations of Thromboses in Newborn Infants

Site	Presentation
Line associated: arterial (aorta)	Blanching
	Poor perfusion—toes, legs, buttocks
Line associated: venous (IVC, SVC)	Swelling
	Oozing of fluids from line entry site
	Skin discoloration
	Chylothorax
Intracardiac	Cardiac failure
	Arrythmia
	Recurrent septicemia
	Hypoxia
	Embolic phenomena
Renal artery	Hypertension
	Anuria
Renal vein	Hematuria
	Flank mass
	Thrombocytopenia
Central nervous system	Seizures
	Poor feeding
	Lethargy
	Tone changes
	Focal neurologic deficit
Purpura fulminans	Dermal vascular thromboses
Femoral or brachial artery	Blanching
	Cool, pulseless extremity

IVC, inferior vena cava; SVC, superior vena cava.

thromboses of the arteries to extremities following direct trauma or stretch injuries, stroke following central nervous system thrombi, venal vein thrombosis, vascular thrombi following polycythemia and hyperviscosity, and purpura fulminans. Infants with acute arterial thrombosis in the extremities present with a pale, pulseless, cool extremity. These infants need to be transported emergently to a tertiary level NICU for surgical treatment because these thromboses can result quickly in loss of the limb or death. Stroke or central nervous system thromboses can present in asphyxiated term infants who present with seizures, lethargy, or focal deficits. Purpura fulminans is a rare condition in which infants are born with diffuse dermal vascular thromboses that often develop significant necrosis. Most infants with purpura fulminans have homozygous protein C or protein S deficiency, but occasionally purpura fulminans occurs in infants with severe sepsis and DIC. Immediate consultation with a neonatologist and expedited transfer to a tertiary NICU with neonatologists and pediatric hematologists experienced in the care of infants with thrombic disorders is essential to avoid serious morbidity or death.

INITIAL EVALUATION, SAMPLE COLLECTION, AND DIAGNOSIS

Table 202-5 lists possible initial laboratory evaluations for an infant presenting with bleeding. Infants with significant bleeding should be referred urgently to tertiary NICU care. While initiating transport and stabilizing the infant, obtaining a complete blood count with platelet count, PT, PTT, and fibrinogen is helpful. If the generalist performs coagulation screening tests, correct sample collection is vital. PT, PTT, fibrinogen, D dimer, and most other coagulation tests are performed on citrated plasma (light blue–top tubes). The ratio of citrate to blood must be 1:9 for the results to be meaningful. The tubes must be filled to the indicator line with blood. Many laboratories have 2.7- or 4.5-mL tubes as standard sizes; however, 1.8-mL tubes also should be available if requested, or the laboratory should be able to make a special tube by measuring a specific amount of citrate in a capillary tube and drawing an indicator line on the tube (e.g., 0.1 mL of citrate is added to a tube, and then 0.9 mL of blood is added). Some laboratories have 0.9-mL tubes available. Coagulation testing equipment should be able to perform PT, PTT, D dimer, and fibrinogen on 1.8 mL or less of blood.

To obtain the sample, the generalist should use the smallest available tube size. The generalist performs a venipuncture or draws from an intravascular line before using any heparin-containing solutions. Coagulation tests should not be drawn by heel puncture because this process activates coagulation factors and gives unreliable results. If heparin from flush or heparin-containing intravenous fluids are present and unavoidable, the contamination can be counteracted by the laboratory. The generalist orders "hepabsorbed" testing or notifies the laboratory directly that heparin contamination of the sample is a concern. Omitting heparin from fluids and flush solution used in an actively bleeding patient should be considered. When the sample is drawn and placed in the appropriate tube, the sample is mixed gently by inverting several times to prevent clotting (clotting renders the sample useless); then the tube is sent immediately to the laboratory for processing. The sample tube should not be shaken vigorously because hemolysis renders the sample useless. In the laboratory, the sample immediately should be centrifuged and the plasma separated.

Full diagnostic evaluation of infants with bleeding disorders, thrombocytopenia, or thrombotic disorders is likely to take place at a tertiary NICU. The diagnostic evaluation for hemophilias, von Willebrand disease, and other, rarer coagulopathies is discussed in Chapter 95, and platelet disorders are discussed in Chapter 94. Pertinent history and physical findings to aid in the differential diagnosis of neonatal thrombocytopenia are presented in Box 202-3. The diag-

---

Table 202-5. Initial Evaluation of the Newborn with Bleeding

Well-Appearing Newborn	Ill-Appearing Newborn
CBC with differential and platelet count	CBC with differential and platelet count
PT, PTT, fibrinogen	PT, PTT, fibrinogen, D dimer
Consider factor VIII and IX	Consider liver function panel or total/direct bili, ALT, AST
Careful family history	Workup and treat underlying condition, such as sepsis, PPHN
	Careful prenatal and intrapartum history
	Placental pathology

ALT, alanine aminotransferase; AST, aspartate aminotransferase; CBC, complete blood count; PPHN, persistent pulmonary hypertension of the newborn; PT, prothrombin time; PTT, partial thromboplastin time.

Box 202-3. Pertinent History and Physical Findings for Differential Diagnosis of Neonatal Thrombocytopenia

Prenatal/Family History

- Preeclampsia, pregnancy-induced hypertension, intrauterine growth restriction
- Maternal medications—quinine, hydralazine, thiazide diuretics, tolbutamide
- Maternal thrombocytopenia
- Family history of excessive bleeding

Perinatal/Neonatal History

- Risk of bacterial or fungal sepsis, congenital viral infection
- Asphyxia
- Bleeding
- Small for gestational age

Physical Examination

- Septic shock presentation—hypoperfusion, hypotension, cardiopulmonary failure
- Dysmorphic—features suggesting trisomy 13, 18, or 21; Turner syndrome; thrombocytopenia–absent radii syndrome; other dysmorphic features
- Bleeding—type and source
- Presence of a central line

nostic approach for evaluation of a thrombosis at the referral center depends on the suspected location of the clot. Angiogram is considered the gold standard for evaluating neonatal thromboses. Ultrasound and echocardiography are used more commonly in practice, however. Central nervous system thromboses usually are diagnosed by magnetic resonance angiogram. Infants with diagnosed thromboses are likely to be evaluated for some or all of the thrombophilias listed in Box 202-1.

MANAGEMENT

Emergency management of the bleeding circumcision is discussed in Chapter 199. The initial steps in the emergency management of a bleeding infant are listed in Box 202-4, and guidelines for specific therapies based on laboratory results and clinical condition are presented in Table 202-6. As in any emergency situation, the generalist's initial attention is to airway, breathing, and circulation. Hypotension and hypoperfusion should be stabilized initially with lactated Ringer solution or normal saline, 10 mL/kg intravenously, usually given over 20 minutes while awaiting the availability of specific blood product treatment (see Table 202-6). Uncommonly, O-negative blood may be needed if blood loss was severe and oxygen delivery is compromised. Intravascular access needs to be secured (see Chapter 295). When providing bolus fluids to premature infants at risk for intraventricular hemorrhage, particular care must be taken to avoid infusing fluids more rapidly than necessary. Most infants with significant bleeding need urgent transfer to a tertiary NICU for further treatment and evaluation.

Management of an infant with thrombocytopenia depends on the underlying condition. Infants with active

---

Box 202-4. Emergency Management of the Bleeding Infant

1. Apply direct pressure if bleeding from circumcision or skin puncture site.
2. Assess airway, breathing, and oxygenation status, and intervene as needed.
3. Assess perfusion—capillary refill, pulses, heart rate, and blood pressure.
4. Treat hypoperfusion with 10 mL/kg of lactated Ringer solution or normal saline intravenously over 5 to 20 minutes depending on clinical status; the infusion may be repeated while awaiting blood products (intravenous access necessary—consider umbilical venous catheter).
5. If infant is critically bleeding (pale, tachycardic, hypotensive), order O-negative blood emergently (cytomegalovirus-negative, irradiated blood preferred).
6. Activate transport system.
7. Obtain complete blood count with platelet count before giving blood if possible. Consider obtaining prothrombin time, partial thromboplastin time, and fibrinogen.
8. Question available family members about any bleeding tendencies in family.
9. In a previously well-appearing infant with a family history of bleeding, consider obtaining factor VIII and factor IX levels.
10. See Table 202-6 for further therapy.

---

bleeding and platelet counts less than 100,000/mm^3 warrant platelet transfusion. One approach to platelet transfusion trigger levels in thrombocytopenic patients without active bleeding is presented in Chapter 193.

Emergency management of an infant with a suspected acute thrombotic event consists of standard resuscitation, including support of airway, ventilation, and circulation, followed by emergent transfer to a tertiary NICU. Depending on the location and severity of the thrombus,

---

Table 202-6. Guidelines for Specific Treatment of Active Bleeding in the Newborn Infant

Test Results/Condition	Treatment	Amount	Comments
Platelet count <100,000	Platelet transfusion	15 mL/kg nonpooled, nonpacked	Obtain maternal platelet count and maternal bleeding history
Platelet count >100,000, continued bleeding	FFP	10–15 mL/kg	
Fibrinogen <150 mg/dL	Cryoprecipitate	Probably 2–5 mL/kg for small neonates; one unit (5–20 mL) for larger neonates raises the fibrinogen by about 100 mg/dL	Dosage not clearly established for neonates
PT, PTT prolonged, fibrinogen >150 mg/dL	FFP	10–15 mL/kg	
PT prolonged; platelets, fibrinogen, PTT normal	Vitamin K	1–10 mg slow IV push	Give slowly; see Table 202-3
Continued significant bleeding; platelets, fibrinogen, PT, PTT normal	Consider FFP; consider vitamin K	See above	
Hematocrit <25, ongoing significant loss	PRBCs	10–20 mg/kg	CMV negative, irradiated preferred; O negative or type and crossmatch
Hematocrit 25–35	Consider PRBCs	10–20 mg/kg	CMV negative, irradiated preferred; O negative or type and crossmatch
Continued life-threatening hemorrhage despite multiple blood product replacements	Consider factor VIIa (NovoSeven)	Consult hematology/neonatology	Experimental, consider calling manufacturer (NovoNordisk)* before giving

*NovoNordisk A/S, Denmark, can be contacted at NovoNordisk: A Focused Healthcare Company. Available at: www.novonordisk.com.
CMV, cytomegalovirus; FFP, fresh frozen plasma; PRBCs, packed red blood cells; PT, prothrombin time; PTT, partial thromboplastin time.

treatment at the referral center may consist of supportive care and observation, thrombolysis of the clot with an agent such as tissue plasminogen activator, or anticoagulation with heparin or low-molecular-weight heparin.

OUTCOME

The outcome for infants with neonatal bleeding disorders, thrombocytopenia, or thrombotic disorders depends on the underlying condition and the organ systems affected. Few long-term data are available regarding outcome of newborns after thrombotic disorders.

FOLLOW-UP

The generalist has a crucial role in the follow-up of patients with neonatal bleeding disorders, thrombocytopenia, and thrombotic disorders. The generalist provides well-child and preventive care and must monitor for complications, coordinate ongoing care with appropriate specialists, and ensure that adequate workup and diagnosis have been completed. Because of the changing nature of coagulation factor concentrations over the first year of life, abnormal coagulation tests often must be repeated in close cooperation with the pediatric hematologist to ensure accurate diagnosis. If no specific diagnosis or cause of bleeding has been identified, the generalist must monitor the patient closely for recurrent bleeding that might merit further workup. Examples of bleeding that would merit workup include epistaxis, hemarthroses, bleeding after tooth loss or dental work, and menorrhagia in an adolescent girl.

Specialist involvement depends on the nature of the problem. All patients with congenital bleeding disorders, most patients with congenital thrombocytopenias, and all patients with neonatal thrombosis should be followed in consultation with a pediatric hematologist. Patients with self-limited conditions, such as DIC or thrombocytopenia related to infection or pregnancy-induced hypertension, generally do not need ongoing follow-up by a hematologist. Depending on the underlying conditions, these infants might need ongoing follow up with a multispecialty developmental follow-up team comprising neurology, cardiology, or other specialists.

Neonates who have thrombotic complications may have postthrombotic complications, such as postphlebitic syndrome. This condition consists of swelling, pain, and collateral vessel development in a body area, such as an extremity, affected by a previous thrombus. The generalist is in an ideal position to recognize these and other complications and to make appropriate referrals.

Mini-index of Related Topics

SUGGESTED READINGS

Andrew M, Paes B, Milner R, et al: Development of the human coagulation system in the healthy premature infant. Blood 1988;72:1651–1657.

Calhoun DA, Christensen RD, Edstrom CS, et al: Consistent approaches to procedures and practices in neonatal hematology. Clin Perinatol 2000;27:733–753.

Edstrom CS, Christensen RD: Evaluation and treatment of thrombosis in the neonatal intensive care unit. Clin Perinatol 2000;27:623–641.

Edstrom CS, Christensen RD, Andrew M: Developmental aspects of blood hemostasis and disorders of coagulation and fibrinolysis in the neonatal period. In Christensen RD (ed): Hematologic Problems of the Neonate. Philadelphia, WB Saunders, 2000, pp 239–271.

Sola MC, Del Vecchio A, Rimsza LM: Evaluation and treatment of thrombocytopenia in the neonatal intensive care unit. Clin Perinatol 2000;27:655–679.

203 Disorders of the Cardiovascular System in the Newborn

Troy Johnston

ROLE OF THE GENERALIST

1 Recognize newborns with cardiovascular disorders.
2 Stabilize newborns with cardiovascular disorders, particularly newborns with ductal dependent lesions.
3 Refer newborns with cardiovascular disorders to a pediatric cardiologist.
4 Recognize acute arrhythmias in newborns.
5 Stabilize newborns with arrhythmias.
6 Refer newborns with arrhythmias for assistance in diagnosis, treatment, follow-up, and long-term management.

The broad topic of cardiovascular disorders that present in the newborn period includes many specific congenital heart lesions and arrhythmias. Despite this often-confusing collection of disorders and terminology, cardiovascular disorders can be classified into categories that aid in diagnosis and management. A combination of clinical presentation and anatomy provides the most useful categorization. Most disorders are in the categories of *acyanotic heart disease*, *cyanotic heart disease*, and *arrhythmias*. Congestive heart failure and low cardiac output are two other clinical manifestations of congenital heart disease. Often the only clue to the presence of congenital heart disease is the finding of a murmur.

An understanding of ductal dependency is key to effective treatment of newborns with congenital heart disease. Patency of the ductus arteriosus may be required to maintain adequate pulmonary or systemic blood flow. Recognizing which patients may require ductal blood flow is essential to effective stabilization. The initiation of prostaglandin E_1 is an effective palliation that can stabilize hemodynamic status before definitive treatment.

FUNDAMENTALS

Cyanosis is the blue coloration of the skin that becomes discernable when the absolute concentration of reduced hemoglobin is 5 g/dL (corresponding to a saturation of 70%). Experienced observers can detect cyanosis at levels of 3 g/dL of reduced hemoglobin (saturation of 80% to

85%). Figure 203-1 shows the face of a cyanotic infant. Cyanosis is noted best in the mucous membranes and nail beds. *Hypoxemia* is below-normal oxygenation of the arterial blood. Cyanosis may indicate hypoxemia, but it may be present when the arterial saturation is normal. To understand why cyanosis is present or absent, the hemoglobin must be measured. Cyanosis appears at higher oxyhemoglobin saturations in polycythemic infants. The higher the total concentration of hemoglobin, the easier it is to have 3 to 5 g/dL of desaturated hemoglobin. In anemic infants, severe hypoxemia is present before cyanosis becomes apparent. Alterations in pH, temperature, and the ratio of adult to fetal hemoglobin also can influence the presence of cyanosis. Acidosis, fever, or higher concentrations of adult hemoglobin shift the oxygen dissociation curve to the right, making cyanosis evident at higher saturations.

Congestive heart failure is a clinical syndrome that results when the heart is unable to circulate sufficient blood to meet the metabolic needs of the body. This may be the result of structural problems, abnormalities in myocardial performance, severe anemia, or arteriovenous malformations that can lead to congestive heart failure from volume overload. The signs and symptoms of congestive heart

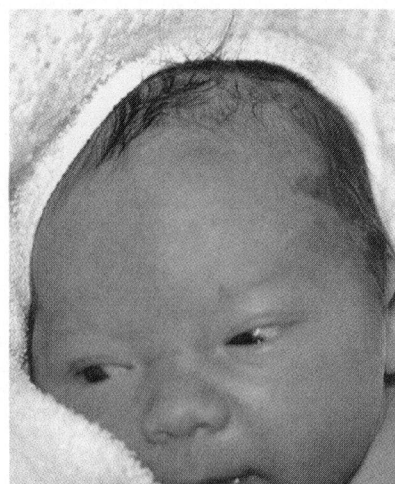

Figure 203-1. This infant was 4 hours old and had transposition of the great arteries. The infant's oxygen saturation was 20%, which did not change when 100% inspired oxygen was given. (From Markiewicz M, Abrahamson E [eds]: Diagnosis in Color: Neonatology. St. Louis, Mosby, 2000, p 91.)

failure are produced largely by the effects of compensatory mechanisms. Congestive heart failure activates the sympathetic nervous system, resulting in catecholamine-mediated increase in heart rate, myocardial contractility, cardiac output, and vascular tone. Decreased renal perfusion activates the renin-angiotensin axis resulting in the kidneys retaining salt and water. Increased intravascular volume initially results in increased cardiac output by increasing preload. Pulmonary and systemic venous congestion and increased myocardial energy consumption are secondary deleterious effects of these compensatory mechanisms. Clinical presentation can be the result of low cardiac output or of the compensatory mechanisms.

Clinical presentation varies with age. Although the underlying pathophysiology may be similar, cardiac disorders present differently in infancy and childhood. The primary symptoms in infants are feeding difficulties. The effort to feed in the presence of mild hypoxemia and tachypnea is often insurmountable. Diaphoresis, especially while feeding, is caused by the increased autonomic nervous system activity attempting to improve cardiac output. Infants with significant congestive heart failure can be irritable.

Tachypnea, tachycardia, and hepatomegaly are hallmark physical findings of congestive heart failure. Tachypnea is usually the result of increased interstitial fluid in the lungs, either from pulmonary edema (elevated pulmonary venous pressure) or from increased volume of pulmonary blood flow (large left-to-right shunts). Increased autonomic nervous system activity causes tachycardia. Increased systemic venous pressure results in hepatic congestion and subsequent hepatomegaly. Findings on cardiac examination depend on the underlying cause of congestive heart failure.

A murmur may be the only sign of congenital heart disease in infancy. A murmur in the presence of cyanosis or congestive heart failure increases the likelihood of underlying cardiovascular disease. A murmur in the absence of other findings more often is innocent. The risk for congenital heart disease in the presence of a systolic murmur is greatest if the murmur is heard in the first 24 hours of life. This risk decreases by 6 months. Innocent murmurs always are associated with normal heart sounds. With the exception of the venous hum, which usually is not heard in neonates, innocent murmurs are always systolic. They generally are less harsh and less intense than pathologic murmurs. They usually have a limited area of transmission and usually are of short duration.

Diagnostic tests useful for determining the presence of cardiovascular disease include the 12-lead electrocardiogram (ECG) and chest radiograph. The ECG is used to diagnose arrhythmias and may provide clues to the presence of cardiac defects. It may show chamber enlargement or hypertrophy. The cardiac silhouette should be assessed on a chest x-ray. Cardiomegaly always is present with congestive heart failure. The pulmonary vascular markings also give an indication of the amount of pulmonary blood flow. These markings may be normal, increased, or decreased. The shape of the cardiac silhouette and mediastinum may provide clues. The sidedness of the aortic arch also should be noted.

Echocardiography provides an accurate anatomic diagnosis. Accurate interpretation of pediatric echocardiograms requires review by a pediatric cardiologist. Telemedicine has improved access to accurate and timely interpretation of echocardiograms, particularly for infants initially evaluated in centers distant from a pediatric cardiologist. Cardiac catheterization now is less important as a diagnostic tool and today is more commonly used to achieve nonsurgical correction of congenital lesions.

DIAGNOSIS

The ability to recognize cardiovascular disease correctly relies on careful assessment. The findings associated with cardiovascular disorders often are obvious if the condition is severe, but they may be subtle. Objective assessment is necessary. The ability to recognize cyanosis, congestive heart failure, and poor cardiac output is crucial. The accuracy of the diagnostic evaluation leads to more appropriate and timely referral.

Cyanotic Heart Lesions

Severe cyanosis is easily recognizable. Saturations less than 80% usually produce easily identifiable central cyanosis. Significant, but not severe, cyanosis can be missed easily on visual inspection alone. Transcutaneous oximetry is a mandatory component of evaluation of infants with suspected cardiovascular disease. Measuring a preductal (right arm) and postductal (either foot) saturation can give information about the presence of a right-to-left shunt at the ductus arteriosus. A lower postductal saturation is consistent with this phenomenon. An arterial or venous blood gas also provides information about ventilation and acid-base status.

After cyanosis is recognized, the fundamental question that must be answered is etiology. The most common clinical issue is differentiating pulmonary disease from cardiac disease. History can be useful in this determination. Cyanosis in premature infants often is associated with respiratory distress syndrome. Risk factors for sepsis increase the likelihood of bacterial pneumonia. Fetal distress is associated with respiratory syndromes or shock lung. Other congenital defects and chromosomal abnormalities are associated more often with congenital heart disease. A family history of congenital heart disease increases the likelihood of cardiovascular disorders.

Physical examination findings can assist in diagnosing the cause of cyanosis. Tachypnea, although present with cardiac and pulmonary disorders, is usually less severe and less likely to be associated with increased work of breathing in infants with congenital heart disease. Abnormal findings on auscultation that suggest a cardiac etiology are a single second heart sound, a pathologic heart murmur, clicks, or a gallop.

The arterial blood gas in patients with congenital heart disease is more likely to be associated with normal or low PCO_2. A hyperoxia test further helps differentiate pulmonary from cardiac causes of cyanosis. After an arterial blood gas is obtained in room air, the infant should be placed in 100% oxygen for 10 minutes. A repeat arterial blood gas is done. If the PO_2 increases to greater than

150 mm Hg, pulmonary disease is more likely. Most infants with cyanotic heart disease cannot increase PO_2 significantly. If the PO_2 remains virtually unchanged, transposition of the great arteries or obstructed pulmonary venous return is more likely.

Anatomically, congenital heart disease that results in cyanosis can be placed into three categories: (1) Pulmonary and systemic circulation may be independent. (2) Pulmonary blood flow may be inadequate. (3) The pulmonary and systemic circulations may be mixed. Classification based on the degree of cyanosis and the radiographic findings is more useful clinically.

Transposition of the great arteries with intact ventricular septum produces pulmonary and systemic circulations that are in parallel. The aorta arises from the right ventricle, and the pulmonary artery arises from the left ventricle. There must be at least one site of bidirectional shunting to allow survival after birth. Shunting may occur at the level of the ductus arteriosus or the atrial septum through a patent foramen ovale or atrial septal defect.

The clinical presentation is usually notable for otherwise normal-appearing infants with severe cyanosis. The incidence of associated congenital abnormalities is low. There is an association with large-for-gestational-age infants and infants of diabetic mothers. The cyanosis is present from birth. Poor mixing, particularly as the ductus arteriosus closes, can lead to worsening hypoxemia and metabolic acidosis. Tachypnea is invariably present, but usually without increased work of breathing. Auscultation is notable for a single second heart sound.

The chest radiograph reveals normal or slightly enlarged cardiac silhouette. The pulmonary vascular markings are normal to decreased. The abnormal location of the great arteries leads to a narrow mediastinum and the classic description of the "egg on a string" appearance. The ECG is usually normal.

Tricuspid valve atresia usually produces cyanosis as a result of decreased pulmonary blood flow. The absence of the tricuspid valve is associated with a small right ventricle. The pulmonary valve and arteries are usually normal in size, but may be small. The systemic venous return must cross the atrial septum, and there is usually a stretched patent foramen ovale or large atrial septal defect. Pulmonary blood flow is most often through a ventricular septal defect. The ventricular septal defect is usually small and restrictive, limiting pulmonary blood flow. Rarely the ventricular septum is intact, and pulmonary blood flow is solely from the patent ductus arteriosus.

The clinical presentation is usually notable for severe cyanosis. Auscultation often reveals a holosystolic murmur characteristic of the ventricular septal defect. The second heart sound is single because of low-velocity pulmonary blood flow. The chest radiograph shows a normal-to-enlarged cardiac silhouette. The amount of pulmonary blood flow determines the size of the cardiac shadow. The pulmonary vascular markings usually are decreased. The ECG has a leftward and superior QRS axis (0 to −90 degrees). There is right atrial enlargement. There are often decreased right-sided forces in the precordial leads.

Pulmonary valve atresia with an intact ventricular septum presents with severe cyanosis immediately after

birth. Because the pulmonary blood flow is ductal dependent, there may be an acute decompensation as the ductus arteriosus closes. The right ventricle is often hypoplastic. There is obligatory right-to-left shunt at the atrial level. Auscultation may reveal no significant murmur. There may be a loud holosystolic murmur in patients with severe tricuspid valve regurgitation. The second heart sound is single. The cardiac silhouette usually is normal to enlarged. The pulmonary vascular markings are decreased to normal. The ECG usually shows a normal QRS axis between 0 and 120 degrees. There is dominance of left-sided forces in the precordial leads. There is usually right atrial enlargement.

Tetralogy of Fallot is a result of anterior and superior deviation of the conal septum. This is the portion of the ventricular septum that separates the ventricular outflow tracts. The degree of displacement of the conus varies from mild to severe and includes pulmonary valve atresia. The variable anatomic obstruction leads to a variable amount of right ventricular outflow tract obstruction and a variable presentation for infants with tetralogy of Fallot. The more severe the obstruction, the more severe the cyanosis present. These infants may be small for gestational age, and there often are associated congenital anomalies. Auscultation reveals a high-frequency systolic ejection murmur loudest at the left upper sternal border. If there is pulmonary valve atresia, the right ventricular outflow tract murmur is absent, but a continuous murmur, from the patent ductus arteriosus or aortopulmonary collaterals, is often present. The second heart sound usually is single because of low pulmonary blood flow. The chest radiograph shows a normal-sized cardiac silhouette with decreased pulmonary vascular markings. The cardiac shadow may be "boot shaped." The main pulmonary artery segment usually is diminished or absent, giving rise to concavity of the pulmonary trunk area compared with the usual convexity. Additionally, the apex of the heart usually is upturned from right ventricular hypertrophy. Approximately 25% of patients with tetralogy of Fallot have a right aortic arch. The ECG usually shows right-axis deviation and right ventricular hypertrophy.

Ebstein anomaly of the tricuspid valve is an abnormality of the septal and posterior leaflets. The valve is deformed and has a variable amount of displacement into the right ventricle and attachment to the ventricular septum. The "atrialized" portion of the right ventricle is the portion above the adherent tricuspid valve leaflets. The tricuspid valve usually is incompetent. Less commonly, the tricuspid valve is stenotic. There may be associated cardiac malformations, and there usually is an atrial level communication. Infants usually present with cyanosis. The degree of cyanosis is variable. Tachypnea is present in proportion to the degree of cyanosis. Auscultation usually does not reveal a significant murmur. Third and fourth heart sounds may be present. The liver often is enlarged, especially if there is significant tricuspid valve regurgitation. The chest radiograph usually shows cardiomegaly, which may be impressive. The pulmonary vascular markings usually are decreased. The ECG usually shows marked right atrial enlargement. There is right-axis deviation and often right bundle-branch block. A shortened P-R interval and preexcitation may be present because of the association with Wolff-Parkinson-

White syndrome. Conversely the P-R interval may be long in the absence of Wolff-Parkinson-White syndrome.

Total anomalous pulmonary venous return is defined as the pulmonary veins draining to the right heart. The abnormal drainage may be supracardiac, with the most common connection consisting of a vertical vein that drains into the innominate vein. The drainage may be cardiac to the coronary sinus. Alternatively the drainage may be infracardiac to the inferior vena cava. In this case, the drainage is via a vein that passes through the diaphragm to the portal venous drainage. The presence of an atrial level shunt is required to fill the left heart. If there is obstruction to pulmonary venous return, cyanosis results. Infracardiac drainage always is associated with obstruction. Obstruction is less common with supracardiac and cardiac drainage. Infants with obstruction are tachypneic and often in severe respiratory distress. The clinical presentation may be confused with respiratory distress syndrome. The physical examination usually reveals a critically ill infant. Auscultation usually does not reveal murmur. Hepatomegaly is present. The chest radiograph shows a normal to slightly enlarged cardiac silhouette. Pulmonary edema may produce "white-out" of the lung fields. The characteristic "snowman" appearance is present if there is supracardiac drainage without obstruction. The heart in this case usually is enlarged, and the mediastinum is widened, producing the snowman shape. The ECG shows right atrial enlargement. There is right ventricular hypertrophy. An umbilical venous blood sample will show systemic oxygen levels in neonates with intracardiac connections,

Truncus arteriosus may present with cyanosis. The usual presentation is that of congestive heart failure, so this lesion is discussed with other left-to-right shunt lesions.

Acyanotic Heart Disease

Acyanotic cardiac abnormalities present with congestive heart failure. Left heart obstructive lesions usually present with seriously impaired systemic blood flow. The lesions with left-to-right shunts usually present with less critical congestive heart failure. Presentation with cardiovascular collapse in the first days of life usually indicates ductal dependent systemic blood flow until proven otherwise.

Lesions with Low Systemic Output

The primary lesions that depend on ductal flow are *hypoplastic left heart syndrome, critical aortic valve stenosis, coarctation of the aorta,* and *interrupted aortic arch.* The clinical presentation is similar for the obstructive lesions. Infants initially appear normal. When the ductus arteriosus closes, rapid clinical deterioration occurs. Initially, signs may be subtle, such as lethargy, poor feeding, tachypnea, and tachycardia. Poor perfusion may become more evident with weak pulses, mottled skin, and increased capillary refill time. As pulmonary edema increases, respiratory distress increases, followed by development of grunting, nasal flaring, and wheezing. Right heart failure results in hepatomegaly. Diminished venal flow leads to oliguria and poor mesenteric flow to abdominal distention and ileus.

Cardiac examination reveals a prominent right ventricular impulse. Pulses and blood pressure may be decreased throughout. Presence of differential pulses is a clue to diagnosis. Aortic valve stenosis and hypoplastic left heart syndrome usually result in decreased pulses in all extremities. Differential in the pulses of the arms and legs is a sign of coarctation or interrupted aortic arch. Auscultation may reveal an early systolic click in aortic valve stenosis. There is a single second heart sound in hypoplastic left heart syndrome. Gallops often are present.

Cardiac silhouette and pulmonary vascularity are increased on the chest radiograph. Pulmonary blood flow may be increased in addition to pulmonary edema. The ECG shows right-axis deviation. Right atrial enlargement and right ventricular hypertrophy are present. There may be a paucity of left-sided precordial forces.

Lesions with Left-to-Right Shunts

Lesions that produce left-to-right shunt are *atrial septal defects, atrioventricular septal defects* (endocardial cushion defects), *ventricular septal defects,* and *patent ductus arteriosus.* Left-to-right shunting is present with arteriovenous malformations. Atrial septal defects rarely produce congestive heart failure in the first year of life. The clinical presentation of congestive heart failure from volume overload usually does not occur in the first week of life. The one exception is a large arteriovenous malformation, which may produce symptoms earlier than cardiac sources of shunting. Auscultation over the cranium and the abdomen can lead the clinician to that diagnosis.

The onset of symptoms usually is slow over the first weeks of life as pulmonary vascular resistance decreases. The primary symptoms of congestive heart failure in infants are related to feeding (Box 203-1). Tachypnea usually interferes with feeding so that the infant stops frequently, appears to tire easily, and may become diaphoretic. Classic physical findings include tachypnea, tachycardia, and hepatomegaly. Precordial activity is increased. Auscultatory findings may be subtle. A large ventricular septal defect or atrioventricular defect may not generate a loud murmur if the velocity left-to-right flow is low. Auscultation over the anterior fontanelle and the liver is useful to identify the bruit associated with an arteriovenous malformation. Bounding pulses and a large pulse pressure are signs of a large patent ductus arteriosus. Diastolic pressure is lower from runoff into the pulmonary circulation.

The chest radiograph in infants with left-to-right shunts shows cardiomegaly and increased pulmonary vascularity. Areas of atelectasis may be present. The ECG is rarely normal in infants with congestive heart failure and may show chamber enlargement or hypertrophy. Atrioventricular septal defects often have a superior QRS axis.

Box 203-1. Signs and Symptoms of Heart Failure in Newborns

- Infant stops frequently when feeding
- Infant appears to tire easily with feeding
- Infant becomes diaphoretic when feeding
- Tachypnea
- Tachycardia
- Hepatomegaly
- Increased precordial activity

Mixing Lesions

Lesions with admixture of the pulmonary and systemic venous return and increased pulmonary blood flow present with congestive heart failure with mild cyanosis. *Total anomalous pulmonary venous return* without obstruction, *truncus arteriosus, transposition of the great arteries* with a large ventricular septal defect, and *single ventricle conditions* are examples of mixing lesions. The cyanosis may be mild enough to be noticeable only with crying. The symptoms and signs of congestive heart failure are similar to the signs for left-to-right shunts. Auscultation usually is abnormal. Flow murmurs usually are present in all of these patients, especially pulmonary outflow murmurs. The second heart sound is single in patients with truncus arteriosus and transposition of the great arteries.

The chest radiograph usually shows cardiomegaly and increased pulmonary vascular markings. The ECG is usually abnormal, but not specific. There may be chamber enlargement or hypertrophy.

Myocardial Dysfunction

Myocarditis, cardiomyopathies, hypoxemic-ischemic injuries, and anomalous left coronary artery from the pulmonary artery all can present with congestive heart failure. The myocardial performance is inadequate because of myocardial dysfunction resulting from infection, metabolic disease, or ischemia. The presentation may be precipitous. The symptoms and signs are similar to those for congestive heart failure of any etiology. Auscultation may reveal a gallop rhythm and in the presence of tricuspid valve chorda tendinae injuries an audible mumur. The chest radiograph usually shows cardiomegaly and possibly pulmonary edema. The ECG is usually abnormal, but not specific. Chamber enlargement and voltage criteria for hypertrophy often are present. The classic ECG with anomalous origin of the left coronary artery from the pulmonary artery is abnormal Q waves in leads I and aVl and the left precordial leads. They may have changes in the ST segments and T waves consistent with myocardial ischemia.

Arrhythmias

Arrhythmias are common in neonates. The most common arrhythmias are benign (Table 203-1) and include sinus tachycardia, premature atrial contractions, premature ventricular contractions, and sinus arrhythmia. Arrhythmias may compromise cardiac output, however, and sustained tachyarrhythmias may induce myocardial dysfunction. Arrhythmias are classified as slow rhythms, or bradyarrhythmias (Table 203-2), and fast rhythms, or tachyarrhythmias (Table 203-3). To diagnosis an arrhythmia accurately, a 12-lead ECG is necessary.

Sinus arrhythmia is phasic variation in the heart rate. The variation often is related to the respiratory cycle and is more common at slower heart rates, so it may be present only during sleep in the neonate. It is a normal variant. If the ECG shows a normal P-wave axis, no other evaluation is necessary.

Premature atrial contraction is a common, usually benign finding in the neonate. The morphology of the P wave of the premature beat is usually different than the sinus beats, and the QRS complex is identical to the sinus beats. Occasionally, if the premature beat comes early enough, there may be no associated QRS. The premature atrial contractions may be frequent. Rarely, electrolyte abnormalities, myocarditis, or structural heart disease is present. A central line in the atrium may cause premature atrial contractions. If the infant is healthy, and there are no risk factors, no further evaluation is necessary.

Premature ventricular contractions are rare in neonates. The reason to obtain an ECG in a neonate with an irregular rhythm is to differentiate between atrial and ventricular ectopic beats. The ECG shows a different QRS morphology of the ectopic beats without an associated P wave. The neonate with premature ventricular contractions should be evaluated for metabolic abnormalities, long Q-T syndrome, myocarditis, drug toxicities, and structural heart disease. Isolated premature ventricular contractions with uniform morphology (i.e., they all look alike) do not require any additional evaluation or therapy. They usually resolve over the first several months of life. If they persist or if they are multiform, further evaluation is recommended.

Bradyarrhythmias

Second-degree atrioventricular block is an intermittent loss of atrioventricular conduction. The two variations are Mobitz type I (Wenckebach) and Mobitz type II. Mobitz type I is defined as gradual lengthening of the P-R interval followed by loss of conduction and a dropped beat. Mobitz type I block does not require further evaluation or treatment. Mobitz type II is intermittent loss of conduction without lengthening of the P-R interval. Mobitz type II may

Table 203-1. Benign Arrhythmias in the Neonate

Arrhythmia	Description	Management
Sinus arrhythmia	Benign arrhythmia Phasic variation in heart rate	If P wave axis normal, no further evaluation necessary
Premature atrial contractions	Benign arrhythmia P wave morphology different from normal beat QRS complex same as normal beat	Rarely associated with electrolyte abnormalities, myocarditis, or structural heart disease If no risk factors present, no further evaluation necessary If central line in place, consider movement. Evaluate for atrial thrombus
Premature ventricular contractions	No P wave Abnormal QRS complex	Evaluate for metabolic abnormalities, prolonged Q-T syndrome, myocarditis, structural heart disease Review medications and classes If isolated premature ventricular contractions have uniform morphology of QRS complex, no further evaluation necessary

Table 203-2. Bradyarrhythmias in Neonates

Arrhythmia	Description	Management
Second-degree heart block	Intermittent loss of atrioventricular conduction	No further evaluation or treatment
Mobitz type I (Wenckebach)	Gradual lengthening of P-R interval followed by loss of conduction	Cardiac referral for observation; may progress to complete heart block
Mobitz II	Intermittent loss of conduction without lengthening of P-R interval	
Complete or third-degree heart block	Failure of atrial impulses to be conducted to ventricle	If heart structurally normal, suspect maternal lupus erythematosus or other collagen vascular disease Refer to cardiologist for evaluation and management Treat congestive heart failure if present

progress to complete heart block and is more concerning than type I second-degree heart block.

Complete or third-degree heart block is failure of atrial impulses to be conducted to the ventricle. There is dissociation of the atrial and ventricular impulses. The atrial rate is usually in the range of normal with a separate slow ventricular escape rate. The onset of complete heart block is usually prenatal. Neonates with structurally normal hearts often are infants of mothers with lupus erythematosus or other collagen vascular diseases. The mother may have no symptoms; the presence of neonatal complete heart block and a structurally normal heart should result in a thorough evaluation for rheumatologic disorders in the mother.

Infants with complete heart block and a structurally normal heart are usually asymptomatic. Signs and symptoms of congestive heart failure may be present. Infants with structural heart disease and complete heart block have a poorer prognosis. Occasionally these are detected prenatally and can be associated with fetal hydrops. Prenatal maternal

treatment with digitalis can be useful. Progression of fetal congestive failure necessitates an early elective delivery.

Tachyarrhythmias

The most common arrhythmia in neonates is supraventricular tachycardia. Most use an accessory pathway between the atria and the ventricle. The onset and termination usually are sudden. The heart rate usually is greater than 250 beats/min. These high rates often are transiently tolerated in neonates, but if they persist the infant eventually develops signs and symptoms of congestive heart failure. Most of these patients have structurally normal hearts, but a few may have associated congenital heart disease, in particular Ebstein anomaly.

The ECG confirms the diagnosis. The most typical finding is a narrow-complex tachycardia with a rate greater than 200 beats/min. The P wave is usually not present. Heart rates of less than 220 beats/min are more likely to be sinus tachycardia. The presence of a normal P wave is

Table 203-3. Tachyarrhythmias in Neonates

Arrhythmia	Description	Management
Supraventricular tachycardia	Sudden onset Heart rate >250 beats/min Eventually develop signs and symptoms of congestive heart failure Narrow-complex tachycardia P wave usually absent Heart rate constant	Usually heart structurally normal, but may have Ebstein anomaly If infant not critically ill, attempt vagal maneuvers Adenosine may be used; verapamil contraindicated Unstable patients require synchronized cardioversion Consultation with pediatric cardiologist Prophylactic therapy with β-blocking agents
Atrial ectopic tachycardia	Incessant tachycardia Originates in atrium, but ectopic from sinus node Gradual onset and termination Congestive heart failure if persists Narrow QRS complex P wave morphology different from normal sinus Rate often varies	Referral to pediatric cardiologist β-blocking agents Radiofrequency ablation
Atrial flutter	Reentrant tachycardia Heart usually structurally normal Heart rate usually >300 beats/min Variable ventricular response, commonly 2:1 or 3:1 conduction Often characteristic flutter waves, best seen in lead II Narrow QRS complex	Referral to pediatric cardiologist Synchronized cardioversion or overdrive pacing
Ventricular tachycardia	Wide QRS complex, but complex may not appear that wide QRS morphology always different compared with sinus QRS	Often associated with electrolyte abnormalities, metabolic disorders, myocarditis, structural heart disease Requires emergent therapy with cardioversion

consistent with sinus tachycardia. Supraventricular tachycardia produces a constant heart rate. Variability in the heart rate is more consistent with sinus tachycardia.

A less common tachyarrhythmia in neonates is atrial ectopic tachycardia. It is an incessant tachycardia that originates in the atrium but from a site ectopic from the sinus node. The onset and termination usually are gradual. This rhythm may produce signs of congestive heart failure if it persists. The ECG shows a narrow QRS complex tachycardia with a P-wave morphology that is different from normal sinus. Additionally the rate often varies.

Atrial flutter is a reentrant tachycardia originating within the atrium. It is rare in neonates. When it does occur, it is usually in the presence of a structurally normal heart. The atrial rate is often fast, usually greater than 300 beats/min. The ventricular response is variable. Commonly, there is 2:1 or 3:1 conduction producing ventricular rates one half to one third the atrial rate. Depending on the combination of the atrial rate and the ventricular response rate, congestive heart failure may be present. The faster the ventricular rate, the more likely cardiac output will be compromised. The ECG often shows characteristic flutter waves. They may be seen best in lead II. There is a narrow QRS complex. If there is 2:1 conduction, the P waves may be hard to visualize. Giving a dose of adenosine to block the atrioventricualr node transiently allows for diagnosis. During the time when there is no ventricular response, the flutter waves are seen clearly.

Ventricular tachycardia is a wide-complex tachycardia that is rare in neonates. The QRS complex may not appear that wide in the neonate. The QRS morphology is always different compared with the morphology present during sinus rhythm. The rate should be faster than the sinus rate. It may be confused with supraventricular tachycardia with aberrant conduction. If the QRS is wide, ventricular tachycardia should be the diagnosis until proved otherwise. Ventricular tachycardia often is associated with electrolyte abnormalities, metabolic disorders, myocarditis, or structural heart disease. It may be secondary to long Q-T syndrome, and the Q-T$_c$ interval should be checked during sinus rhythm.

MANAGEMENT

Identification of ductal dependency is the key to appropriate management of most congenital heart disease. The mainstay of appropriate stabilization, whether the systemic or the pulmonary blood flow is dependent on the ductus arteriosus, is the administration of intravenous prostaglandin E$_1$ (Box 203-2). If cardiology consultation is not readily available, empirical treatment of an infant with suspected heart disease is appropriate. Prostaglandin E$_1$ can be infused in a peripheral intravenous line, but a central line is preferred. If an umbilical venous catheter cannot be obtained, two peripheral lines are recommended. The usual starting dose is 0.05 to 0.1 µg/kg/min. It is common practice to start at the higher dose and decrease the dose. The infusion rate should not be decreased if there has not been a documented improvement in the infant. If the child is cyanotic, there should be an increase in the saturation. Infants with systemic obstruction should have improvement in cardiac

---

Box 203-2. Management of Ductal Dependent Congenital Heart Disease

1. Provide immediate cardiac consultation if available.
2. Administer intravenous prostaglandin E$_1$.
   Central line administration is preferred.
   Starting dose is 0.05 to 0.1 µg/kg/min.
   Usually start at higher dose and then decrease.
3. Prostaglandin is contraindicated in the presence of total anomalous pulmonary venous return with obstruction.
4. Observe for central apnea, fever, hypotension.
5. Intubate infants who require transportation to a cardiac center.

---

output. Prostaglandin E$_1$ is contraindicated if total anomalous pulmonary venous return with obstruction is present.

Prostaglandin E$_1$ is associated with side effects, the most serious of which is central apnea. It is prudent to intubate infants who require transportation to a cardiac center. The risks of having to treat apnea during transport are higher than elective intubation. Prostaglandin E$_1$ also may cause fever; however, evaluation for sepsis should be performed. Attributing a fever to prostaglandin E$_1$ without a negative sepsis workup is not recommended. The infusion rate does not have to be reduced for increased temperature. Prostaglandin E$_1$ also may cause hypotension, which can be treated with volume or a reduction in the prostaglandin infusion rate. Adjustment of the dose is performed best after accurate definition of the heart lesion has been accomplished.

Cyanotic Heart Disease

Oxygen for cyanotic infants is not contraindicated. Oxygen is a potent pulmonary vasodilator and may increase pulmonary blood flow; this may be beneficial for patients with decreased pulmonary blood flow. The goal of oxygen therapy is to correct hypoxemia, not cyanosis. The oxygen saturation need not increase to normal range. High saturation may indicate excessive pulmonary blood flow that is unnecessary and possibly deleterious.

Intubation and mechanical ventilation often is required when prostaglandin is infused. High positive end-expiratory pressure (PEEP) increases pulmonary vascular resistance and in general should be avoided. PEEP should not be avoided in the presence of total anomalous pulmonary venous return and obstruction. These patients do not tolerate increased pulmonary blood flow because of the obstruction to pulmonary venous return. Increasing pulmonary vascular resistance may be beneficial.

Cyanotic infants require adequate oxygen carrying capacity to avoid hypoxemia. A hemoglobin level of 15 g/dL is beneficial. Transfusion of packed red blood cells should be considered to correct relative anemia. Diuretics and inotropic support may be needed, but only if signs of poor cardiac output are present.

Acyanotic Heart Disease
Lesions with Low Systemic Output

Initiation of prostaglandin E$_1$ is the primary management for stabilization of infants with obstruction to systemic output. In contrast to cyanotic patients, more emphasis needs to be placed on balancing systemic and pulmonary blood flow. The goal for patients with ductal dependent systemic output is to maintain adequate systemic output and avoid excessive pulmonary blood flow. Intubation and control of ventilation is necessary. High PEEP can be helpful. In addition to increasing pulmonary vascular resistance, it also may help reduce pulmonary edema, allowing improved pulmonary gas exchange.

Oxygen should be avoided. If systemic blood flow is ductal dependent, increasing pulmonary blood flow decreases systemic blood flow. Infants with this anatomy and resultant physiology may benefit from fractional inspired oxygen levels lower than room air. This can be accomplished by low concentration of blended nitrogen. Low oxygen saturation does not imply hypoxemia. The ideal oxygen saturation for these patients is 80%. Pulmonary and systemic flows usually are well balanced at this saturation.

Congestive heart failure from obstruction usually responds to diuretic therapy, particularly if renal function has not been impaired. Therapy with diuretics is performed best after the specific diagnosis has been obtained and the patient is stabilized. Inotropic support often is required to increase cardiac output. Dobutamine and dopamine are the most appropriate initial therapy if poor cardiac output is present. If there is evidence of poor myocardial function, dobutamine as a continuous infusion of 5 to 10 μg/kg/min is an appropriate therapy. Dobutamine is a more potent inotrope than chronotrope, which is beneficial when myocardial performance is decreased. In acute cardiac failure, the benefit from digoxin is limited. Additionally, in clinical settings in which renal function and metabolic homeostasis are often compromised, digitalis toxicity is more likely. Digoxin is not a component of acute therapy for stabilization of these infants.

Anemia should be treated with a blood transfusion. Increasing oxygen carrying capacity is useful in patients with cardiac failure. Hemoglobin of 15 g/dL is an appropriate goal if transfusion is performed.

Lesions with Left-to-Right Shunts

Acute cardiac failure from excessive pulmonary blood flow (excluding ductal dependent lesions) regardless of the specific lesion usually responds to supportive therapy. Critically ill infants should be intubated. Mechanical ventilation reduces the work of breathing. The use of PEEP may reduce pulmonary blood flow and alleviate pulmonary edema. If there is sufficient interstitial pulmonary fluid to cause ventilation-perfusion mismatch, oxygen may be beneficial. Oxygen use should be cautious because the pulmonary vasodilatory effects may contribute to congestive heart failure by increasing pulmonary blood flow.

Diuretic therapy is appropriate. Intravenous furosemide as an initial therapy at a dose of 1 mg/kg should be instituted. In the presence of poor cardiac output, intravenous inotropic support should be instituted. Dopamine or dobutamine is often first-line therapy and should be started at the usual dose of 5 to 10 μg/kg/min. Digoxin therapy is not helpful for the management of acute cardiac failure. Its benefit is limited to patients with chronic cardiac failure. Anemia should be corrected. Transfusion of packed red blood cells has been shown to decrease congestive heart failure.

Mixing Lesions

Mixing lesions should be treated similar to left-to-right shunt lesions. The etiology of the cyanosis is mixing of systemic and pulmonary venous return and not decreased pulmonary blood flow. The cyanosis is usually mild. Oxygen is often not necessary. Increasing the fractional inspired oxygen level may worsen cardiac failure because of increased pulmonary blood flow.

Myocardial Dysfunction

The treatment of congestive heart failure from myocardial dysfunction is similar to treatment of congestive heart failure from large left-to-right shunts. Oxygen should not worsen congestive heart failure in the absence of large left-to-right shunts. Inotropic support with dobutamine is preferential in infants because of the lack of chronotropic effects. Phosphodiesterase inhibitors also are often useful. Milrinone has inotropic effects and systemic vasodilatory effects. The combination of direct myocardial effect and reduction of systemic afterload often is helpful in the management of these patients.

Arrhythmias
Bradyarrhythmias

Bradyarrhythmias rarely require emergent therapy. Patients with Mobitz type II second-degree heart block require referral to a pediatric cardiologist. Complete heart block that is associated with symptomatic bradycardia and congestive heart failure requires treatment. Therapy includes isoproterenol for inotropic and chronotropic effects. Pacing also may be required; this can be accomplished with placement of transcutaneous electrodes. Pacing also can be accomplished with a temporary transvenous or transesophageal pacing system.

Tachyarrhythmias

Supraventricular tachycardia is terminated by breaking the reentry circuit at the atrioventricular node. If the neonate is not critically ill, vagal maneuvers may be attempted first. The placement of a bag or glove containing a mixture of ice and water is often effective. The mouth and nose should not be covered, and pressure should not be placed on the eyes. Contact with the upper face should be maintained for approximately 20 seconds. A rhythm strip should be performed during this maneuver. Adenosine is an effective agent at termination, and it may be used in a stable infant with intravenous access. Adenosine should be given rapidly through an intravenous line preferably placed in an upper extremity. Intravenous verapamil is contraindicated in neonates. If the infant is unstable, synchronized cardioversion is required. The initial dose is 0.5 J/kg; if ineffective, it may be increased to 1 to 2 J/kg.

Because of a high recurrence risk, prophylactic therapy usually is recommended. The β-blocking agents are usually the preferred treatment. The use of digoxin has decreased, and it is contraindicated in patients with preexcitation. Digoxin may increase the conduction through the accessory

Table 204-1. Differential Diagnosis of Neonatal Intestinal Obstruction

Diagnosis	Symptoms	Workup
Upper Tract Obstruction		
Esophageal atresia (usually with TEF)	Feeding intolerance, excess secretions, drooling, aspiration, NGT will not pass	Chest x-ray with NGT in place, with or without UGI, ECHO NGT will not pass
Gastric duplication	Feeding intolerance, palpable mass	Ultrasound, UGI
Lactobezoar	Prematurity, hypertonic feeds, delayed emptying, mass	UGI
Gastric volvulus	Acute pain and retching, bilious emesis	X-ray, UGI
Pyloric stenosis	Nonbilious projectile emesis, 3–8 weeks old, palpate olive fluid waves	Ultrasound, UGI
Focal antral foveolar hyperplasia	Gastric obstruction with PGE therapy, immune deficiency	UGI, endoscopy
Antral or pyloric web/atresia	Congenital gastric obstruction, bullous skin lesions	Prenatal ultrasound, x-ray, UGI
Duodenal atresia	Usually bilious emesis, antenatal diagnosis, trisomy 21	Prenatal ultrasound, x-ray (double-bubble), microcolon on BE
Lower Tract Obstruction		
Jejunoileal atresia	Bile emesis, distention	AXR, BE (microcolon)
Meconium ileus	Bile emesis, distention Family history of cystic fibrosis	AXR, BE (colon pellets with inspissated stool in ileum)
Distal meconium obstruction or plug	Bile emesis, distention	AXR, BE (small left colon with proximal plug), with or without rectal biopsy
Midgut volvulus/malrotation	Bile emesis, examination may be normal	AXR, UGI, or BE
Hirschsprung's disease	Bile emesis, distention, failure to pass meconium in 24 hr	AXR, BE (transition zone), rectal biopsy
Imperforate anus	Abnormal perineal examination	AXR, renal and sacral ultrasound, ECHO

AXR, abdominal x-ray; BE, barium enema; ECHO, echocardiography; NGT, nasogastric tube; PGE, prostaglandin E; TEF, tracheoesophageal fistula; UGI, upper gastrointestinal.

segment is usually at the level of the third thoracic vertebra, just above the tracheal carina, and more than 90% have an associated tracheoesophageal fistula (TEF). The frequency is 1 in 3000 to 4000 births with a slight male predominance. Approximately 40% of neonates with esophageal atresia weigh less than 2500 g at birth. The lower the birth weight, the greater the frequency of associated anomalies.

Intrauterine ultrasound confirms polyhydramnios and may reveal the absence of a fluid-filled stomach in the left upper quadrant after 16 weeks' gestation (40%). In 60%, the stomach is filled via the trachea. Intrauterine magnetic resonance imaging has increased the diagnostic sensitivity by revealing the proximal pouch of the esophagus.

There are five basic forms of esophageal atresia and TEF. The most common (85%) is atresia with a distal TEF. Isolated atresia without a TEF and isolated "H-type" TEF without atresia occur in 3% to 5%. The final two forms, also seen in 3% to 5%, are atresia with a proximal fistula and atresia with a proximal and a distal fistula. More than 50% of neonates with esophageal atresia and TEF have other significant midline defects. The most common complex is called *VACTERL* (*v*ertebral, *a*nal, *c*ardiovascular, *t*racheal, *e*sophageal, *r*enal, and *l*imb malformations).

The diagnosis of esophageal atresia is established by the inability to pass an orogastric tube into the stomach. Chest and abdominal radiographs confirm that the tube is in the dilated proximal esophageal pouch. In unclear cases, a small amount of barium may be injected into the esophagus by an experienced radiologist, but this must be removed promptly. Attention should be paid to the abdominal gas pattern on x-ray. A gasless abdomen suggests an isolated or distal atresia, whereas a markedly dilated stomach with no distal air indicates an associated duodenal atresia, which can lead rapidly to gastric perforation. These infants require emergent surgical intervention. Because associated anomalies are frequent, the neonate also should have x-rays of

the spine, echocardiogram of the heart, ultrasound of the kidney, and a careful anal examination.

The most crucial components of initial management include prevention of primary aspiration from the pouch, prevention of gastroesophageal reflux through the fistula, and minimizing gaseous distention of the gastrointestinal tract through the fistula. A 10 Fr flexible suction tube (e.g., a Replogle tube) is placed into the pouch for intermittent suction of secretions. The infant should be positioned in modified Fowler position (head up) to keep gastric contents from entering the fistula. Most neonates are able to breathe spontaneously and should be allowed to do so. Intubation and positive-pressure ventilation can exacerbate a ventilatory crisis. The tidal volume selectively enters the gastrointestinal tract through the fistula, which has a much lower resistance than the newborn lung.

Primary surgical repair generally is undertaken during the first 24 to 48 hours of life. The success of primary surgical repair in otherwise healthy neonates is excellent. Results can be affected by birth weight less than 1500 g and by significant associated anomalies, especially cardiac. Very sick neonates should undergo ligation of the fistula and placement of a gastrostomy for decompression, with delayed repair of the atresia.

There are significant postoperative concerns in the neonate with esophageal atresia. Dysphagia is common because the esophagus below the level of the fistula does not have normal motility, and gastroesophageal reflux is universal. Tracheomalacia usually is present, at least in the first several months; reactive airway disease may persist for several years. Stricture of the esophagus can occur from gastroesophageal reflux or, less commonly, vascular compromise. These children present with dysphagia after solid foods and may have large pieces of food trapped at the stricture that require endoscopic removal and stricture dilation. If an infant has persistent feeding intolerance, an

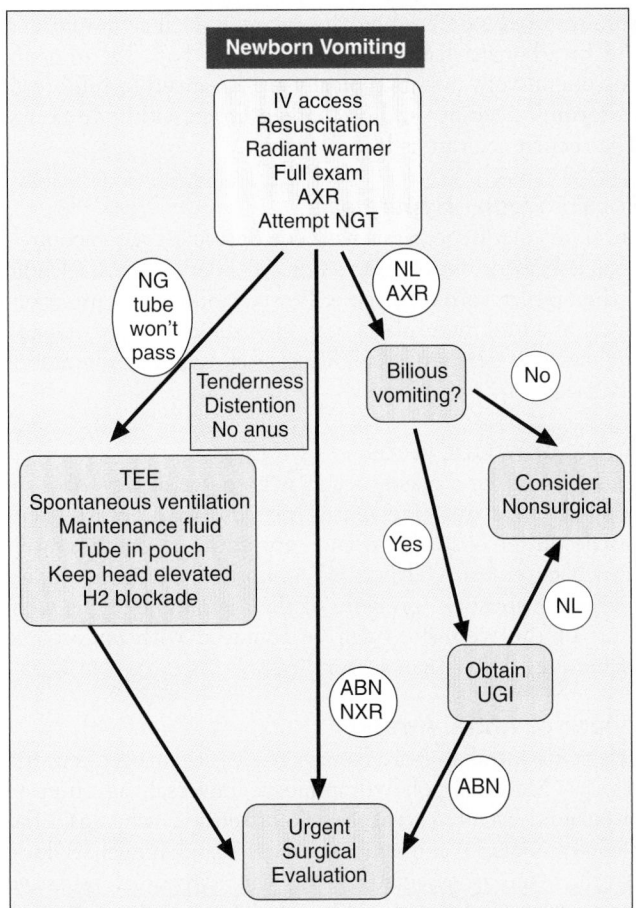

Figure 204-1. Approach to a neonate with emesis. AB, abnormal; ABN NXR, abnormal abdominal x-ray; AXR, abdominal x-ray; N, normal; NGT, nasogastric tube; NL AV, normal abdominal x-ray; TEE, tracheoesophageal fistula; UGI, upper gastrointestinal series.

upper gastrointestinal series should be obtained to exclude malrotation, as this study would not have been possible preoperatively.

Acute Gastric Perforation

Acute gastric perforation in the neonate may be traumatic, ischemic, or spontaneous. All forms present with acute vascular collapse and radiographic evidence of free air in the abdomen. Most have hematemesis and progress quickly to sepsis and respiratory failure. Traumatic perforation of the stomach (or esophagus) usually arises after passage of a nasogastric tube, although cases after positive-pressure ventilation have been reported. Ischemic perforation develops after 2 to 4 days in neonates with birth asphyxia, sepsis, or necrotizing enterocolitis. Rare cases of spontaneous perforation occur in otherwise healthy neonates in the first week of life. All neonates with gastric perforation require immediate vascular access to meet fluid and vasopressor needs until urgent surgical intervention is achieved. The surgical outcome depends on the underlying issues, with term infants generally doing well if treated in a timely fashion.

Gastric Duplication

Gastric duplication accounts for less than 4% of enteric duplications. Approximately 30% present in the neonatal period, with 50% diagnosed by 1 year. The clinical presen-

tation is feeding intolerance mimicking pyloric stenosis, with a palpable mass frequently noted in the epigastrium. Contrast studies are required to define the preoperative anatomy and exclude other duplications in the more distal bowel.

Lactobezoars

Lactobezoars usually present 5 to 10 days after initiation of feedings, developing most commonly in premature infants on hypercaloric feedings of greater than 24 cal/oz with increased medium-chain triglycerides or in neonates receiving antacids. The clinical presentation is abdominal distention, delayed gastric emptying, emesis, or a palpable epigastric mass. Radiographic contrast studies confirm the extent and location of the lactobezoar. Conservative therapy with lower osmolar feedings usually is successful. Rarely, endoscopic disruption is needed, and very rarely surgery is required for removal.

Gastric Volvulus

Gastric volvulus may present with acute obstruction, pain, and retching with or without emesis in the neonatal period, but it is more common in infancy and early childhood. Similar symptoms are seen in infants with paraesophageal hernias, in which the stomach herniates through the hiatus next to a normal gastroesophageal junction. Gastric volvulus may be associated with malrotation and asplenia. Vascular compromise leads to rapid gastric necrosis and perforation with potential loss of the entire stomach. These infants need emergent surgical intervention with aggressive fluid resuscitation. A chronic form with early satiety and gastroesophageal reflux may be encountered in older children.

Congenital Microgastria

Congenital microgastria, a hypoplastic tubular stomach, is rare, presenting in the first 48 hours with profound feeding intolerance, intractable gastroesophageal reflux, dumping syndrome, and diarrhea. It usually occurs in association with distal atresias, duplications, malrotation, situs inversus, or Hirschsprung disease. Congenital microgastria is diagnosed by radiographic contrast studies and managed in the neonatal period by continuous infusion nasogastric feedings.

Pyloric Stenosis

Pyloric stenosis, first described in 1717, occurs in 1 to 3 per 1000 births, with a 4:1 male predominance. More than 90% are full-term neonates. The frequency of pyloric stenosis in white neonates is far in excess of that seen in black or Asian neonates. If a mother has pyloric stenosis, 19% of her sons and 7% of her daughters also are expected to have it.

Presentation is usually at 2 to 8 weeks of age. Rarely an intrauterine ultrasound study reveals gastric distention in retrospect. Only 4% of patients present after 3 months of age. Classic symptoms include nonbilious, projectile emesis with a mobile palpable "olive" in the right upper quadrant. If the pyloric olive is felt, no further diagnostic evaluation is needed. Although contrast studies can be done to exclude other potential origins, the diagnosis now usually is confirmed, when necessary, by abdominal sonography. Sonographic features are a pyloric muscle thickness of greater than

4 mm extending over a channel of 17 mm. The contrast study reveals either a single "string sign" or a double "railroad track sign" of the stenotic pylorus and can exclude other diagnoses, including gastric duplication, antral web, antral inflammation from eosinophilic gastritis or chronic granulomatous disease, and extrinsic compression of the pylorus (Fig. 204-2). Associated secondary features include hiatal hernia and a transient unconjugated hyperbilirubinemia. About 5% have intestinal malrotation, obstructive uropathy, or both, so the sonographer is encouraged to image the kidneys along with the pylorus.

Pyloric stenosis is a metabolic rather than a surgical emergency. These children typically are profoundly dehydrated, with marked hypochloremic alkalosis and potassium depletion. Correction of these abnormalities *must* occur before surgery.

Infants are given nothing by mouth, although a nasogastric tube is not needed unless vomiting is persistent. Rehydration is accomplished typically with intravenous normal saline boluses until urine output is restored. Infants then can be placed on 1.5 times maintenance with ½ normal saline and dextrose. Potassium should be added because the alkalosis does not resolve until adequate potassium reserves are restored. General anesthesia may be

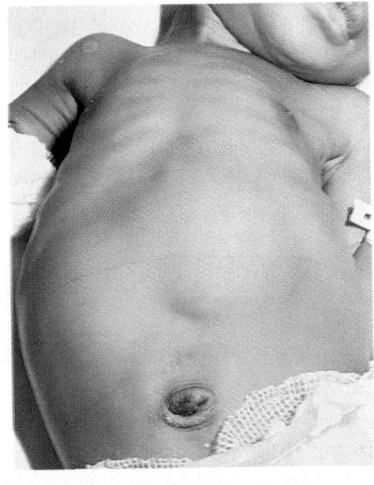

A

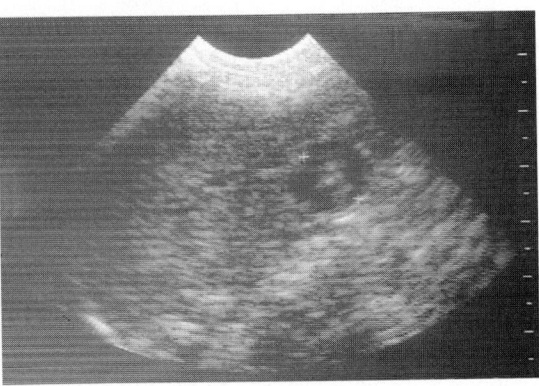

B

Figure 204-2. A, Pyloric stenosis may cause epigastric distention by the obstructed stomach. This patient also has a visible wave of peristalsis, which moves from left to right. **B,** Ultrasound of the upper abdomen shows the thickened pyloric muscle, indicated by cursors. (From Zitelli BJ, Davis HW: Atlas of Pediatric Physical Diagnosis. St. Louis, Mosby, 1997.)

administered safely when the infant is well hydrated and the bicarbonate has decreased to less than 30 mEq/dL. Postoperatively, infants typically are advanced to full breast or formula feedings and discharged home within 48 hours. The recurrence rate is low.

Focal Foveolar Hyperplasia

Focal foveolar hyperplasia has been described as an acquired neonatal gastric outlet obstruction secondary to prostaglandin E therapy for cardiac disease. Prostaglandins also are implicated in antral hyperplasia seen in eosinophilic gastritis and the immune deficiency condition of chronic granulomatous disease.

Antral or Pyloric Webs

Antral or pyloric webs occur with a frequency of 1 in 100,000 neonates. Newborns present with intermittent gastric outlet obstruction and symptoms of feeding intolerance or emesis. Ultrasound is normal; contrast studies reveal a "windsock" prolapse of the membrane of the web. Lysis of the web often can be achieved with endoscopic techniques rather than surgery.

Pyloric or Antral Atresia

Pyloric or antral atresia accounts for less than 1% of enteric atresias. Maternal polyhydramnios is universal. Intrauterine ultrasound usually reveals gastric distention, whereas a flat plate radiograph confirms a gasless distal bowel. Pyloric atresia often is associated with the autosomal recessive form of junctional epidermolysis bullosa with its cutaneous feature of vesiculobullous lesions.

Duodenal Atresia

Duodenal atresia is encountered with a frequency of 1:7500 live births. More than 30% occur in the context of trisomy 21. The diagnosis often is suspected on the prenatal sonogram, especially in the third trimester, with polyhydramnios and the characteristic double bubble of a dilated stomach and first portion of the duodenum. In nearly all cases, the atretic segment is distal to the ampulla of Vater, producing the double bubble and bilious emesis that may be documented by bilious amniotic fluid. Feeding intolerance and bilious emesis develop in the first 24 hours. When duodenal atresia is suspected, 20 mL of air is injected via nasogastric tube into the stomach; then an abdominal x-ray with the double bubble documents a gasless distal bowel. The nasogastric tube is left in place to suction secretions, and intravenous fluids and nutrition are initiated. If the diagnosis is not made antenatally, it is necessary to exclude midgut volvulus as the cause of duodenal obstruction; this usually is accomplished with a contrast enema to document a normal hepatic flexure and cecum. Otherwise, surgical exploration should be performed urgently. With intrauterine diagnosis, surgical intervention can be delayed until other anomalies have been excluded and stabilized. Additional investigations should address the 25% frequency of associated significant cardiac disease by echocardiogram and 10% frequency of renal disease by ultrasound. At the time of surgery, the bowel is evaluated carefully for additional problems because 25% of infants have other intestinal abnormalities.

Jejunoileal Atresias

Jejunoileal atresias can occur with equal frequency throughout the small intestine. They can affect varying lengths of bowel and have multiple locations. The atretic segment occasionally may represent most of the intestine. These atresias are believed to be a consequence of an ischemic event in late pregnancy. Associated intestinal anomalies, other than malrotation or gastroschisis, are unusual.

Intrauterine ultrasound may show polyhydramnios, the severity of which is correlated with the the level of atresia (i.e., the higher the level of atresia, the greater the severity). Dilated proximal bowel loops with a diameter greater than 7 mm may be seen. Although polyhydramnios is a feature of high intestinal atresia, less than 10% of intrauterine polyhydramnios is caused by bowel atresia.

A newborn with a jejunal or ileal atresia is distended shortly after birth. Aspiration of the stomach yields a volume of 25 mL or more, relative to the 5-mL fluid content of a normal neonate's stomach. Because the ischemic event may have been late in gestation, these newborns can pass normal meconium in the first 24 hours. Recent in utero perforation may present as meconium peritonitis with massive ileus and peritoneal calcifications at birth. These disorders are seen commonly with meconium ileus.

Meconium Ileus

Meconium ileus is a distal small bowel obstruction diagnosed with a contrast enema, typically using dilute contrast medium (Gastrografin) and showing a microcolon with pellets of dried meconium proximally. The distal ileum is distended with tenacious meconium, which often is loosened by the hypertonic contrast medium. If the obstruction is relieved by one or more enemas (roughly 40%), the meconium ileus is considered uncomplicated.

Most patients require laparotomy because of persistent obstruction or the presence of meconium peritonitis from intrauterine ileal perforation. The sterile meconium initiates an intense inflammatory peritonitis with dense adhesions, calcifications, and ascites. Most neonates present with early obstruction with distention noted in the delivery room. Meconium peritonitis is the presenting manifestation of 15% of children with cystic fibrosis, and sweat tests are required in all newborns with complicated meconium ileus. Many infants with complicated meconium ileus are found to have a segment of distal small bowel atresia, presumably secondary to an intrauterine volvulus. This loss of small bowel complicates long-term nutritional management.

Preoperative preparation of neonates with meconium ileus requires close attention to volume maintenance, especially after the hypertonic contrast enema, which can induce a profound hypovolemia. Infants also are prone to hypothermia with extended exposure in the radiology suite. Postoperative management is complicated not only by the enteric compromise, but also by the other pulmonary and biliary complications of cystic fibrosis.

Distal Meconium Obstruction

Distal meconium obstruction, frequently called *meconium plug* or *small left colon syndrome*, typically is a self-limited obstruction of the distal colon from viscous but otherwise normal meconium. It often is encountered complicating the neonatal course of premature infants, infants with chronic magnesium exposure, infants with hypothyroidism, and infants of diabetic mothers.

The diagnosis is made by contrast enema, which shows a small but otherwise normal rectum and distal colon with more proximal dilation. The enema characteristically induces the passage of a large "plug" of meconium, after which the infant should start a normal stooling pattern. If the neonate has any residual evidence of obstruction or delayed stooling, further evaluation to exclude aganglionosis must be done. In contrast to meconium ileus, meconium plug syndrome is not associated with cystic fibrosis.

Midgut Volvulus

Midgut volvulus must be the initial consideration in all infants with bilious emesis without an antenatal diagnosis of intestinal obstruction. It is a surgical emergency with a high morbidity and mortality if not recognized and treated promptly.

Midgut volvulus, in the context of intestinal malrotation, occurs in 1:6000 live births. Of neonates born with malrotation who ever become symptomatic, 50% to 75% do so in the first month, and 90% become symptomatic in the first year. Approximately half of children present with an extrinsic duodenal obstruction secondary to Ladd bands, and half present acutely with bilious emesis progressing with ischemic injury to transmural necrosis and sepsis. The diagnosis is established by upper contrast studies showing the position of the ligament of Treitz to the right of the midline. Malrotation of the cecum is a less consistent finding, so the contrast enema may be normal. Malrotation is encountered in 50% of neonates with duodenal atresia; 30% of neonates with jejunal atresia; and most infants with omphalocele, gastroschisis, and diaphragmatic hernia.

If malrotation or midgut volvulus is suspected, surgical consultation must be obtained immediately. Adequate intravenous access must be obtained because these patients may deteriorate rapidly. Nasogastric suction also is necessary to minimize the distention. A long period of preoperative preparation is not warranted because the ongoing bowel ischemia frequently frustrates all resuscitation efforts and mandates emergent exploration. Even if the bowel is found to be viable, the intraoperative and postoperative course of these patients is often complicated.

Hirschsprung Disease

Hirschsprung disease is due to the absence of intramural ganglion cells in the myenteric and submucosal plexus of the distal colon with variable degrees of continuous extension into the more proximal bowel and occurs in 1 in 5000 births. Of infants, 80% have disease limited to the rectosigmoid with a transition zone shown on lateral views of the barium enema. In contrast, 3% have involvement of the entire bowel with no transition zone. The risk for a second involved child increases from 3% with rectosigmoid disease to 25% in a girl with long segment disease. Mutations of the long segment of the *RET* gene produces an autosomal dominant inheritance. Increased associations with trisomy 21, deletion of chromosome 13q, Smith-Lemli-Opitz syndrome, Waardenburg syndrome, and Laurence-Moon-Bardet-Biedl syndrome have been reported.

The diagnosis is suspected in neonates with distal bowel obstruction, abdominal distention, and failure to pass meconium. Virtually all term normal newborns pass their first meconium within 48 hours. Failure to do so can be documented in greater than 90% of patients with Hirschsprung disease and should prompt further workup. Contrast enema ideally should be performed *before* a digital rectal examination because this can obscure the characteristic transition zone. The diagnostic gold standard is suction or full-thickness rectal biopsy, which reveals absence of ganglion cells and presence of hypertrophied nerve trunks and increased tissue acetylcholinesterase. Although unusual in the newborn period, enterocolitis of the prestenotic colon can be the presenting sign.

Surgical evaluation focuses on confirmation of the transition zone, the level at which ganglion cells begin to appear, and defining comorbid complications or enterocolitis. In otherwise healthy infants with a transition zone at or below the distal descending colon, decompression with dilation and enemas is generally effective. These infants are candidates for primary corrective surgery without colostomy. Otherwise, a colostomy is performed at the level of the histologically confirmed transition zone followed by delayed pull-through. Many infants with Hirschsprung disease have some degree of colonic dysfunction, even after the pull-through. Constipation is common and occasionally can be associated with recurring bouts of enterocolitis.

Imperforate Anus

Imperforate anus is diagnosed in 1 in 4000 live births. The hindgut fails to descend completely and join properly with the proctodeum. Although the anal sphincter muscles are present, they frequently are attenuated, and the rectum does not pass through them. Instead the rectum ends in a fistula anteriorly. In male infants, 90% of the rectal fistulae end somewhere on the urinary tract ("high defects"), whereas 90% of female infants have a "low defect," with a fistula to the perineum or vestibule.

More than 50% of neonates with imperforate anus have associated midline anomalies—28% genitourinary, 8% significant cardiac disease, and the rest with some component of the VACTERL syndrome discussed in association with TEF earlier. Cardiac echocardiogram and abdominal and pelvic sonograms are performed routinely before surgical decisions.

Surgical evaluation involves identifying the location of the fistula and the presence of any other anomalies. Otherwise healthy infants with perineal or vestibular fistulae can undergo primary anoplasty, often without a protective colostomy. An interval of dilation often is employed in girls before primary repair is performed. Infants with higher fistulae typically undergo colostomy formation so that radiographic and possibly endoscopic evaluation can be performed to determine the exact level of the fistula. Girls with a high defect, or persistent cloaca, can have particularly complex anatomic concerns.

The long-term outcome depends mostly on the type of defect. Patients with a low defect and a normal sacrum typically have some long-term constipation but are continent. Higher defects are associated with increasing degrees of fecal incontinence. Both conditions can be managed with diet, medication, and careful follow-up.

ABDOMINAL WALL DEFECTS

The two most common forms of abdominal wall defects in newborns are gastroschisis and omphalocele. Both forms commonly are diagnosed antenatally by ultrasound. Elevation of amniotic fluid α-fetoprotein may be noted in gastroschisis and omphalocele (higher in gastroschisis). The immediate management of abdominal wall defects is shown in Figure 204-3.

Gastroschisis

Gastroschisis is a relatively small (<4 cm) defect in the anterior abdominal wall, usually superior and to the right of the umbilical cord, which usually is intact. It occurs after formation of the abdominal wall and typically is not associated with chromosomal or midline defects. The bowel, but not the liver, herniates into the amniotic fluid because there is never a protective sac. The intestines generally are malrotated, and there typically is a severe serosal inflammation that causes thickening and shortening of the bowel and mesentery. Because of the tight ring, portions of the bowel may become atretic.

Gastroschisis is a true surgical emergency. In the delivery room, the infant should be placed in a clear plastic bag up to the chest to minimize heat and water loss and to allow visualization of the bowel. The bowel must be kept moist. Intravenous access should be established to replace the profound fluid losses, which can approach 300% of maintenance. Nasogastric suction must be initiated promptly to prevent distention of the bowel. Antibiotics are begun. There is no need to spend further time stabilizing or eval-

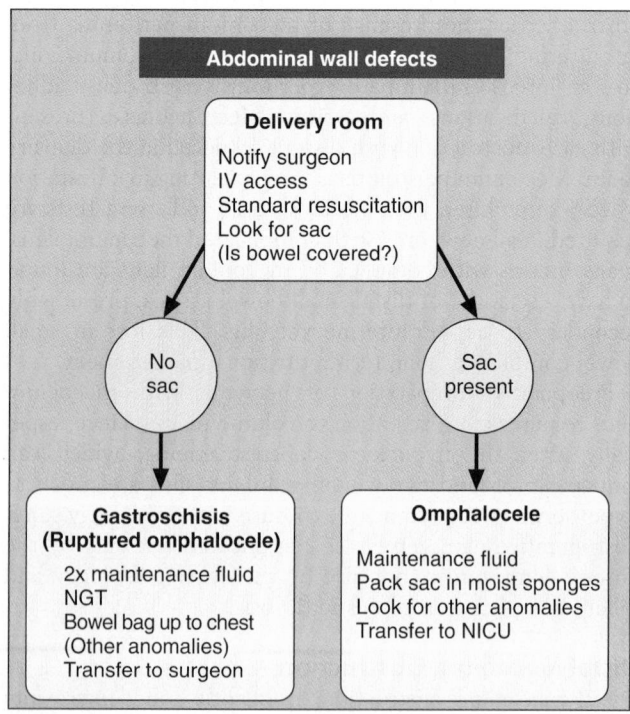

Figure 204-3. Immediate management of abdominal wall defects. NGT, nasogastric tube; NICU, neonatal intensive care unit.

uating for associated concerns. They need to be taken to the operating room for reduction. Although data suggest that bowel inflammation progresses rapidly at the end of gestation, preterm delivery currently is not advised. The mode of delivery does not affect the outcome of these infants.

Omphalocele

Omphalocele is a congenital malformation of the abdominal wall in which the umbilical ring fails to form. This creates a large (typically >4 cm) defect that generally is covered with a sac, to which the umbilical cord attaches. Omphalocele frequently is associated with other midline defects and with chromosomal anomalies (trisomy 13, trisomy 18, and Beckwith-Wiedemann syndrome). The defect also may include the chest wall (ectopia cordis) or the lower abdominal wall (exstrophy of the bladder).

Unless the sac is ruptured, omphalocele typically is not associated with the serositis or the fluid and heat loss seen with gastroschisis. In the delivery room, the sac is kept moist with saline-soaked gauze, and an orogastric tube is placed for decompression. The surgical correction is deferred until associated concerns are addressed, recognizing that the long-term prognosis is determined primarily by the associated anomalies.

NECROTIZING ENTEROCOLITIS

The most common acquired enteric disease in the nursery is necrotizing enterocolitis, documented in 2 to 5 per 1000 live births and 2% to 4% of admissions to the neonatal intensive care unit. Of symptomatic infants, 90% are premature. Risk factors in premature infants include repeated doses of maternal steroids, perinatal asphyxia, significant pulmonary or cardiac disease, exchange transfusion, use of umbilical catheters, and hyperosmolar oral feedings. In term infants, risk factors also include hypoglycemia, prolonged rupture of membranes, and chorioamnionitis. The absolute cause of necrotizing enterocolitis is unknown; a triad of selective bowel ischemia, intraluminal nutrition, and microbial contamination is implicated.

Infants present with feeding intolerance, increased gastric residuals, bilious vomiting, abdominal distention, and heme-positive or bloody stools. Abdominal tenderness, abdominal wall erythema, and ascites may follow. Infants may exhibit decreased activity, temperature instability, and respiratory distress or apnea. The peripheral blood count may be elevated or depressed with increased immature forms and thrombocytopenia. Acidosis is common. The typical radiographic features progress from ileus to focal bowel wall thickening to pneumatosis intestinalis, which may include portal vein air, to perforation and free air in the abdomen.

When suspected, feedings are discontinued, nasogastric decompression is begun, and intravenous antibiotics are initiated. This protocol is followed for 7 to 10 days with careful monitoring for progression of disease and serial examinations by the primary care physician and consulting surgeon. Although surgical consultation should be obtained early, the preferred management approach is nonoperative.

Infants with bowel perforation indicated by pneumoperitoneum, diffuse abdominal wall cellulitis, or paracentesis showing feces or bile should have emergent surgery. Relative indications for surgery include signs of bowel necrosis, such as localized abdominal wall erythema, a persistent dilated bowel loop on x-ray, or mass on examination, and signs of ongoing sepsis, such as persistent neutropenia or thrombocytopenia, acidosis, hyperkalemia, respiratory failure, or hemodynamic instability. Surgical intervention is limited to management of the perforation and resection of all clearly necrotic bowel. Areas of questionable viability are left to be reassessed later as necessary. Preservation of bowel length and control of sepsis are the primary goals of surgery in necrotizing enterocolitis.

Regardless of the intervention, recurrent episodes of necrotizing enterocolitis may complicate refeeding. Compromised bowel may exhibit signs of malabsorption and dysmotility. Postoperative stricture formation is seen commonly, 3 to 6 weeks postoperatively, with 70% in the colon and 15% in the ileum.

ABDOMINAL MASSES

Most abdominal masses in neonates are benign. Many are diagnosed on antenatal sonogram, which remains the diagnostic procedure of choice for cystic and solid masses that are palpable at birth. Table 204-2 lists the differential diagnosis of neonatal abdominal masses by location. Multicystic kidneys, hydronephrosis, hydroureter, and

Table 204-2. Differential Diagnosis of Neonatal Abdominal Mass

Retroperitoneal	Pelvic	Intra-Abdominal
Renal	**Ovarian**	**Hepatic**
Hydronephrosis	Physiologic cyst	Choledochal cyst
Multicystic dysplastic kidney	Hemorrhagic cyst	Hepatoblastoma
Mesoblastic nephroma	Teratoma	Hemangioendothelioma
Renal vein thrombosis	Germ cell tumor	Hematoma
Wilms tumor		
Subcapsular hematoma		
Adrenal		**Enteric**
Adrenal hemorrhage		Mesenteric cyst
Adrenal abscess		Omental cyst
Neuroblastoma		Meconium cyst
Teratoma		Enteric duplication
		Sacrococcygeal teratoma

mandatory. To the general pediatrician, these conditions lead to a level of involvement that includes early suspicion, referral, diagnosis, and long-term comanagement.

Mini-index of Related Topics

SUGGESTED READINGS

Ashcraft KW (ed): Pediatric Surgery, 3rd ed. Philadelphia, WB Saunders, 2000, pp 267–294.

D'Agata ID, Balistreri WF: Evaluation of liver disease in the pediatric patient. Pediatr Rev 1999;20:376–389.

Damato N, Filly RA, Goldstein RB, et al: Frequency of fetal anomalies in sonographically detected polyhydramnios. J Ultrasound Med 1993;12:11–15.

Kays DW: Surgical conditions of the neonatal intestinal tract. Clin Perinatol 1996;23:353–375.

Shneider BL: Genetic cholestasis syndromes. J Pediatr Gastroenterol Nutr 1999;28:124–131.

SECTION 5   NEWBORN CARE: *Disorders of the Genitourinary System*

205 Disorders of the Genitourinary System in the Newborn

Jordan Symons and Richard Grady

ROLE OF THE GENERALIST

1 Recognize disorders of the genitourinary system by prenatal diagnosis and physical examination.

2 Recognize risks for complication from disorders of the genitourinary system, and monitor for and treat complications.

3 Perform appropriate studies to evaluate disorders of the genitourinary system.

4 Refer to a specialist for further management of disorders of the genitourinary system.

5 Participate in ongoing follow-up for disorders of the genitourinary system before and after referral to the specialist, including education of the family.

Prenatal imaging techniques have changed greatly the approach to newborn genitourinary abnormalities. Because many anomalies now are diagnosed before birth, some parents are aware of a structural defect prenatally that previously might have gone unnoticed even after delivery. Consequently the general pediatrician needs to be prepared to advise parents regarding abnormalities of the genitourinary system even before the infant is born.

Despite the influence of prenatal diagnosis, the importance of physical examination of the newborn cannot be overemphasized. Not every newborn undergoes prenatal imaging, and many abnormalities cannot be detected by current imaging techniques. Careful examination of the external genitalia for the presence of abnormalities is an essential part of newborn care.

Table 205-1. Indications and Timing of Referral for Genitourinary Abnormalities in the Newborn

Condition	Indications for Referral	Timing
Hypospadias	Simple, all cases	Before 6 mo of age
	Severe	Immediately on detection
	With cryptorchidism or possible intersex	Urgent, immediately on detection
Hydronephrosis	Minimal, low-risk infants detected on prenatal ultrasound	2–5 days after birth
	Males with bilateral hydronephrosis, massive hydronephrosis, findings suggestive of severe obstruction, reflux, or other genitourinary abnormality	Urgent, immediate referral
Posterior urethral valves	All cases when suspected	Immediate, urgent referral
Ambiguous genitalia	All cases	Immediate, urgent referral
Cryptorchidism	Unilateral	Before 6 mo of age
	Bilateral	Urgent, immediate referral

The generalist provides the important link between the specialist and the family. Good communication is essential for adequate care to ensure that all of the needs of the patients and families are met. Many disorders of the genitourinary system require referral and ongoing follow-up with a specialist (Table 205-1). The generalist plays an essential role in coordinating the overall care of the child.

HYPOSPADIAS

Definition

Hypospadias is a condition in which the urethra opens along the ventral surface of the penis, rather than at the tip of the glans, and is an event of arrested development because the male urethra normally passes through this state during embryogenesis. Hypospadias results from failed closure of the urethral folds, which should fuse under the influence of testosterone to create the urethra of the penis and the median raphe of the scrotum.

Fundamentals

Hypospadias has a variable presentation, with the urethral opening appearing anywhere from the glans penis, to more proximal locations along the shaft, all the way to the perineum (Fig. 205-1). An incomplete prepuce with a dorsal hood configuration typically accompanies a hypospadic urethra. The foreskin may be intact in 10% of cases (megameatus intact prepuce [MIP] variant). Ventral chordee, a downward deflection of the penis, often accompanies hypospadias and is more pronounced in severe cases. Hypospadias is associated with undescended testes and with inguinal hernia. Intersex states must be considered in any apparent male with more severe forms of hypospadias

and in any male with hypospadias and cryptorchidism. Boys with proximal hypospadias may have an enlarged prostatic utricle, a müllerian duct remnant that arises at the level of the verumontanum. It can cause difficulty with urethral catheterization and sometimes serves as the source of chronic urinary tract infections. Other abnormalities of the upper urinary tract are associated rarely with hypospadias. Hypospadias occurs in about 1 in 300 live male births. Reports suggest that the incidence of hypospadias is increasing. Maternal risk factors include advanced age, vegetarianism, and diabetes mellitus.

Diagnosis

The physical findings of distal or glanular hypospadias can be subtle. Most other cases of hypospadias can be noted readily on physical examination of the newborn genitalia (Fig. 205-2). The foreskin generally is not retracted during the newborn examination. As a result, MIP variant hypospadias may not be detected unless a newborn circumcision is done. Careful evaluation for the presence and location of gonads is essential in infants with hypospadias. Although advances in ultrasound technology now allow the antenatal detection of some cases of proximal hypospadias, most remain undiagnosed until the physical examination after birth.

Management

Except in the mildest forms of hypospadias, the surgeon uses a portion of or the entire foreskin to repair this congenital defect. For this reason, circumcision of a newborn male with hypospadias must be avoided. In the case of a MIP variant, the urethral anomaly typically is not detected until after circumcision. MIP variant can be repaired without the use of foreskin so the infant may be

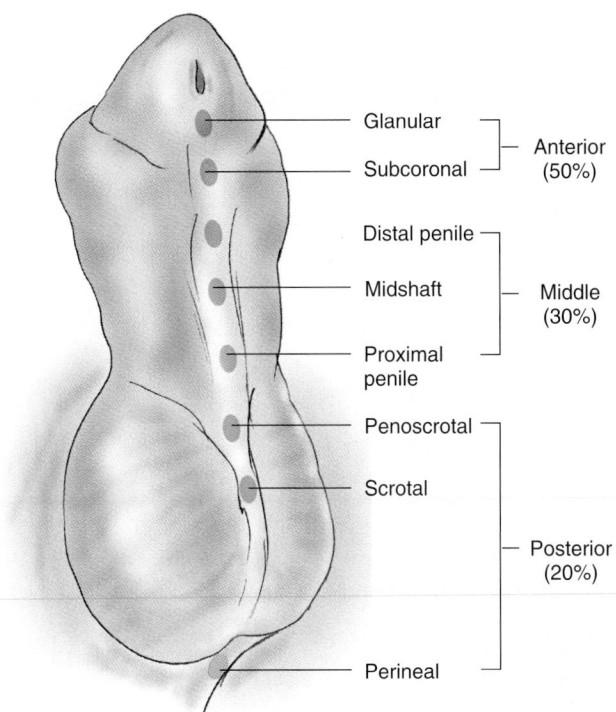

Figure 205-1. Summary sketch of hypospadias locations. (Redrawn from Duckett JW: Successful hypospadias repair. Contemp Urol 1992;4:42–55. Copyright © 1992 Foerster.)

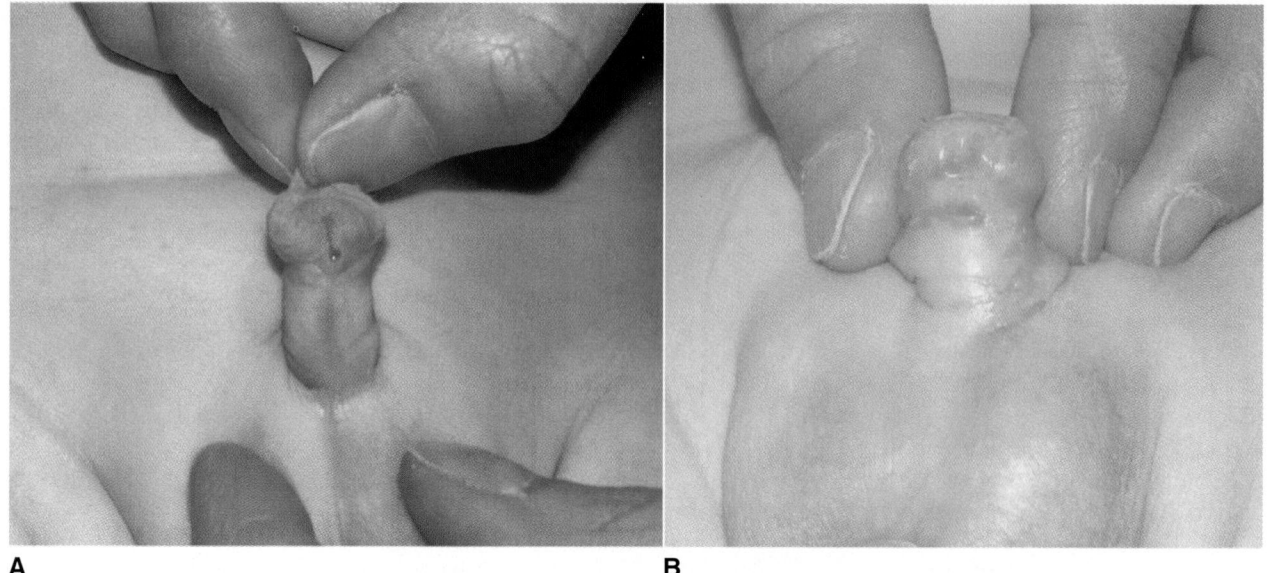

A

B

Figure 205-2. **A** and **B,** Hypospadias on physical examination.

referred for hypospadias repair after the circumcision. In cases of proximal hypospadias or hypospadias associated with cryptorchidism, one should consider an intersex state (Box 205-1). Because the differential diagnosis of intersex states includes congenital adrenal hyperplasia, appropriate evaluation must be done in a timely manner. Simple cases of hypospadias can be referred to a pediatric urologist for outpatient evaluation. More severe cases or cases with possible intersex warrant prompt evaluation at the time of diagnosis.

The optimal time to hypospadias repair is before 2 years of age. Many pediatric urologists prefer to operate between 6 and 12 months of age. Patients tolerate the perioperative course better at this age. Also, this timing allows any complications of hypospadias repair to be corrected before the boys begin toilet training. An otherwise healthy male infant can undergo extensive hypospadias repair as an outpatient with a clinic appointment typically 1 week after the operation. The goals of surgical repair involve correction of the chordee, reconstruction of the urethra and glans penis, and skin coverage of the penile shaft.

Outcome and Follow-up

Modern hypospadias repair yields excellent functional and cosmetic results. More proximal lesions and larger defects are more difficult to repair and have a higher complication rate, including urethrocutaneous fistula and urethral stricture formation. Most children who undergo distal hypospadias repair have no long-term sequelae. Boys with more severe forms of hypospadias may require several operations to correct the hypospadias and chordee completely. Late complications of hypospadias operations include recurrent chordee, urethrocutaneous fistula formation, and urethral stricture. These occur in a few boys who undergo surgical correction. Boys who do not have hypospadias corrected typically cannot direct their urinary stream and need to sit to urinate.

Although data are limited, the available data suggest that boys who have undergone successful hypospadias repair have normal sexual function and do not have impaired fertility as adults even after multiple operations. If chordee is present, this anomaly may interfere with sexual intercourse later in life. Severe forms of hypospadias also can decrease fertility because the ejaculate exits from the base of the penis.

Box 205-1. Anomalies or Syndromes Associated with Cryptorchidism

- Androgen insensitivity syndrome
- Mixed gonadal dysgenesis
- True hermaphroditism
- Aarskog syndrome
- Beckwith-Wiedemann syndrome
- Cockayne syndrome
- Cornelia de Lange syndrome
- Fraser syndrome
- Lowe syndrome
- Smith-Lemli-Opitz syndrome
- Klinefelter syndrome
- Noonan syndrome
- Prader-Willi syndrome
- Cystic fibrosis
- Maternal diethylstilbestrol exposure
- Omphalocele
- Gastroschisis
- Prune-belly (Eagle-Barrett or triad) syndrome
- Cloacal exstrophy
- Cerebral palsy
- Upper lumbar myelomeningocele

HYDROURETERONEPHROSIS

Definition

Hydronephrosis refers to dilation of the renal pelvis and calyces, whereas *hydroureteronephrosis* includes dilation of the ureters; neither term defines a specific etiology for the dilation, which can result from several possible causes. Hydronephrosis is a common finding on prenatal ultrasound, reported in 1 in 500 routine prenatal studies. Although hydronephrosis can be a clue to urologic abnormalities, the isolated finding of hydronephrosis can occur in the absence of urinary obstruction or other significant renal or urologic pathology.

Fundamentals

Obstruction to urinary flow can cause dilation of the collecting system. Depending on the location of the obstruction, there is either hydronephrosis or hydroureteronephrosis (Fig. 205-3). Obstruction at the ureteropelvic junction (UPJ) causes hydronephrosis. The UPJ is a common location for urinary obstruction. Distal obstruction, at the ureterovesicular junction (UVJ), leads to hydro*ureter*onephrosis.

Even more distally, obstruction can occur at the level of the bladder outlet. Posterior urethral valves (PUV) are the most common cause of obstruction at this level. Bladder outlet obstruction typically causes bilateral hydroureteronephrosis. The bladder itself may be abnormal, with thickening of the bladder wall and dilation of the posterior urethra (the "keyhole sign" seen on ultrasonography). These findings in a male infant suggest PUV. Vesicoureteral reflux is another important cause of hydro*ureter*onephrosis in newborns.

Because bilateral hydronephrosis has profound implications for global renal function, evaluation of this condition should be performed expediently. Bilateral UPJ or ureterovesicular junction obstruction can occur. Bilateral hydroureteronephrosis can occur secondary to distal obstruction (e.g., PUV, ureterocele).

Antenatally diagnosed hydronephrosis is the second most common abnormality noted in utero after cardiac abnormalities. In utero, hydronephrosis may be a consequence of normal fetal development. The fetal urinary system is thought to be more distensible than the postnatal system.

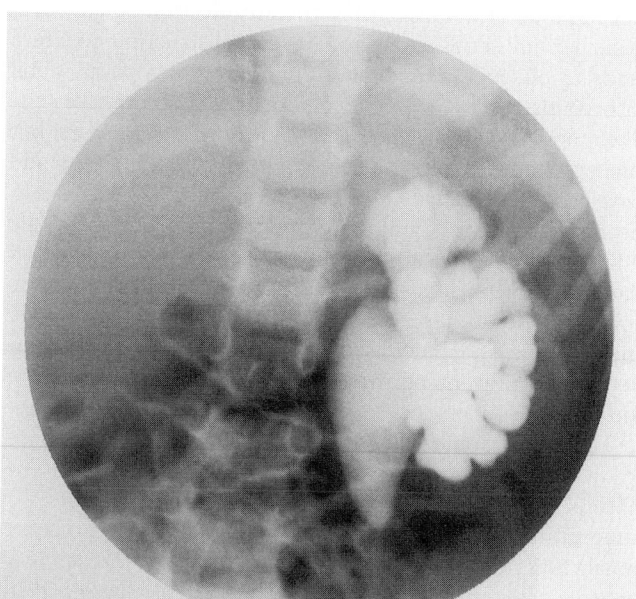

Figure 205-3. Obstruction at ureteropelvic junction causing hydronephrosis.

In addition, fetal urinary flow rates are much higher than the rates seen immediately after birth. Transient kinks ("fetal ureteral folds") in the ureters also generally resolve as genitourinary development progresses. Many prenatally diagnosed cases of hydroureteronephrosis resolve after birth.

Diagnosis

Prenatal ultrasound commonly diagnoses hydronephrosis (Fig. 205-4). Hydronephrosis noted on prenatal ultrasound should be re-evaluated after birth (see Fig. 205-4). Most low-risk newborns with prenatal hydronephrosis should have a repeat ultrasound of the kidneys and bladder done at 2 to 5 days of age. Ultrasound performed earlier may miss some cases of hydronephrosis because of the relative oliguria present in the first 24 to 48 hours of life. Exceptions include male infants with bilateral hydronephrosis, in whom there would be concern for bladder outlet obstruction owing to PUV, or any infant with massive hydronephrosis or additional genitourinary findings suggesting severe obstruction, reflux, or other abnormality. These high-risk patients should be referred for urgent evaluation.

Voiding cystourethrogram (VCUG) is recommended for any patient in whom there is a possibility of vesicoureteral reflux or bladder/urethra abnormality. Repeat VCUG is recommended in patients with persistent hydronephrosis. For low-risk patients, VCUG can be done at about 1 month of age; oral antibiotic prophylaxis should be used pending the result of the study. VCUG should be part of the urgent evaluation of most high-risk patients. Infants should undergo a cycling VCUG to improve the sensitivity of the study. Excretory studies can be used to evaluate for the presence of ureteral obstruction. These studies are particularly useful for identifying UPJ obstruction.

The preferred imaging technique for newborns in this setting is the radionuclide renogram, with MAG3 as the radiopharmaceutical. Evaluation of tracer excretion before and after a dose of intravenous furosemide can show the presence and the degree of urinary obstruction. The renogram also shows the relative function of each kidney. Because the renogram is safe, provides superior imaging in the newborn, and provides additional information regarding function, intravenous pyelography is not recommended in this setting. High-risk patients should have an evaluation of renal function by checking blood urea nitrogen and serum creatinine.

Management

Because of the increased risk of urinary tract infection, newborns with hydronephrosis should receive antibacterial prophylaxis. Amoxicillin (12.5 mg/kg/day orally) is the most common agent used. Sulfa-containing antibiotics are contraindicated in newborns because of concerns of displacement of bilirubin from its albumin carrier by sulfas. Recommendations vary regarding duration of antibiotic therapy. Although there is controversy regarding the appropriate length of antibacterial prophylaxis and the indications for discontinuation, we recommend placing all infants who have antenatal hydronephrosis on suppressive antibiotic therapy until the VCUG is done because of the 20% incidence of associated vesicoureteral reflux (sometimes in the contralateral system) in these patients.

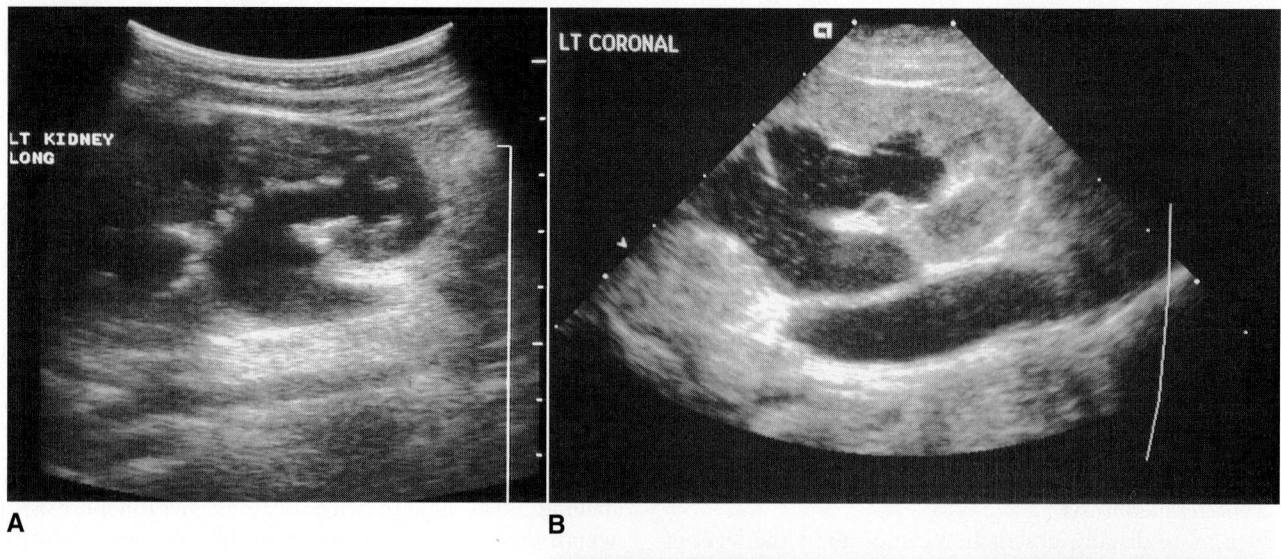

Figure 205-4. A-C, Prenatal and postnatal ultrasound studies showing hydronephrosis.

High-risk patients, including male infants with bilateral hydroureteronephrosis at risk for PUV or any infant with high-grade hydroureteronephrosis, warrant specialty evaluation immediately after birth. Low-risk patients, with only mild isolated collecting system dilation, can receive antibacterial prophylaxis and the imaging study sequence outlined previously; positive or persistent findings in these patients warrant referral. If a neonate has persistent hydronephrosis on postnatal ultrasound without evidence of vesicoureteral reflux by VCUG or clear obstruction by furosemide-enhanced renography, the infant should undergo serial ultrasound studies every 3 to 4 months for the first year of life and semiannually to annually thereafter. These studies allow the physician to monitor renal growth and changes in the degree of hydronephrosis, permitting early intervention for patients who show progressive hydronephrosis and poor renal growth.

Outcome and Follow-up

The outcome for hydroureteronephrosis in a newborn depends on the diagnosis and the severity of disease. Patients with bladder outlet obstruction can have significant renal impairment and urologic dysfunction owing to developmental abnormalities that result from high intravesicular pressures in utero. Severe obstruction in utero leads to oligohydramnios and pulmonary hypoplasia. Fetal intervention may improve pulmonary outcome or the likelihood of carrying the fetus to term in severe cases, but such procedures carry considerable risk to the fetus and have not been shown to reduce renal morbidity. There is, however, great variation in presentation and outcome. Male infants with PUV are the most common examples of patients with bladder outlet obstruction. Mild-to-moderate forms of hydronephrosis from narrowing at the UPJ may resolve spontaneously; others require surgical intervention to prevent permanent, progressive damage to the kidney.

The radiographic finding of hydroureteronephrosis also is known as *megaureter* when it occurs in isolation. The natural history of megaureter is gradual improvement over time in most cases. The degree of obstruction and relative renal function should be assessed first by furosemide-enhanced renography, however, before embarking on serial evaluations with ultrasonography. These children also should undergo VCUG to determine if they reflux urine into this system (refluxing megaureter).

Follow-up for newborns with hydronephrosis may be exclusively with the generalist or may involve coordinated care in consultation with a specialist. Given the risks for infection with these patients, the generalist must be particularly vigilant for urinary tract infection when patients develop fever. The generalist always should consider obtaining a sterile urine specimen for culture, especially before starting antibiotics for some other presumed indication. Patients on prophylactic antibiotics as conservative management who have breakthrough urinary tract infection may do better with surgical correction. Antibiotic prophylaxis should continue for all patients who are at increased risk for ascending infection into the kidney. This includes any patient with documented or suspected vesicoureteral reflux. The generalist must coordinate the care of these infants with the multiple specialists involved. Repeat imaging studies (e.g., ultrasound, VCUG) may be indicated depending on the clinical situation.

POSTERIOR URETHRAL VALVES

Definition

PUV are recognized as an important cause of obstructive uropathy in newborn boys. This disorder is the most common obstructive abnormality affecting both kidneys in boys. Valves result from abnormal integration of the wolffian (mesonephric) ducts into the prostatic urethra. This abnormal integration produces mucosal folds within the urethra causing variable amounts of obstruction at the bladder outlet. PUV occur in a clinical spectrum of severity.

Fundamentals

Early detection of PUV improves outcome. Patients with mild-to-moderate obstruction should have the valves ablated in the newborn period. Early ablation seems to improve bladder function and may preserve renal function. Patients with more severe obstruction may require treatment for renal failure in addition to valve ablation. Any child with PUV is at increased risk for urinary tract infection and requires appropriate monitoring. In addition, one third of patients with PUV have vesicoureteral reflux. Some boys show unilateral vesicoureteral reflux into a dysplastic kidney; this is known as *vesicoureteral reflux dysplastic kidney* and seems to protect the nonrefluxing system from damage through a "pop-off effect" of pressure relief.

Bladder function may not be normal in patients with PUV. Some patients require a specific voiding program, possibly including catheterization; this is especially true for boys who are not detected to have PUV until later in life. The best long-term outcomes are seen in patients who are detected and treated at the earliest possible time. PUV are an important cause of chronic renal failure in children. In the past, half of children with PUV died before reaching young adulthood; 25% died within the first year. Modern neonatal and nephrologic care now can support these chil-

dren with dialysis and kidney transplantation. Early recognition also has improved outcomes of this "silent killer." Infants with more severe forms of obstruction are at risk for pulmonary hypoplasia at birth because of in utero obstruction to fetal urinary flow and subsequent oligohydramnios and impaired fetal breathing activity.

PUV can have a broad range of presentation, from severe fetal bladder outlet obstruction with renal failure and severe lung dysfunction at birth to extremely mild forms that may present only with urinary tract infection or voiding dysfunction in later years. Bladder dysfunction from an obstructive cystopathy, causing poor or incomplete bladder emptying and associated vesicoureteral reflux, may lead to an increased risk of urinary tract infection in these patients.

PUV can cause primary bladder dysfunction. In the most severe cases, these children require a specialized voiding or clean intermittent catheterization program to ensure adequate emptying of the bladder, reducing the risk of urinary tract infection and additional kidney injury. These children also ultimately may require bladder augmentation to improve the urinary compliance in the bladder. Early valve ablation increases the potential, however, to achieve normal bladder function. There is a strong correlation between PUV and vesicoureteral reflux. One third to one half of patients with PUV also have vesicoureteral reflux. The incidence of PUV is thought to be 1 in 5000 to 1 in 8000 male births. Exact numbers are difficult to ascertain because of the highly variable presentation.

Diagnosis

Prenatal ultrasound may suggest the diagnosis of PUV. The diagnosis should be considered in any male infant with bilateral hydronephrosis. Dilation of the bladder and posterior urethra produces a characteristic ultrasound finding on longitudinal view of the lower urinary tract known as the keyhole sign. The index of suspicion is raised further in the presence of bladder distention and oligohydramnios. In this setting, there is a high correlation with pulmonary hypoplasia. Palpable abdominal masses resulting from the distended bladder and hydronephrotic kidneys are consistent with bladder outlet obstruction owing to PUV. Infants with pulmonary hypoplasia may have respiratory distress; the most severely affected infants may present with Potter syndrome.

A newborn who is suspected of having PUV should have a renal and bladder ultrasound and a VCUG. Ultrasound may reveal variable hydroureteronephrosis bilaterally. Contrast VCUG reveals the urethral abnormality and shows dilation and elongation of the posterior urethra, bladder wall thickening or trabeculation, and possible vesicoureteral reflux (Fig. 205-5). Because of the necessity of defining the bladder and urethral anatomy, radionuclide cystography should not be used.

Cystoscopic examination confirms the presence of PUV and its sequelae—dilation and enlargement of the posterior urethra and bladder hypertrophy. PUV are categorized as type I, II, or III based on their appearance. All PUV may be treated endoscopically by direct visualized valve ablation (transurethral resection of valves).

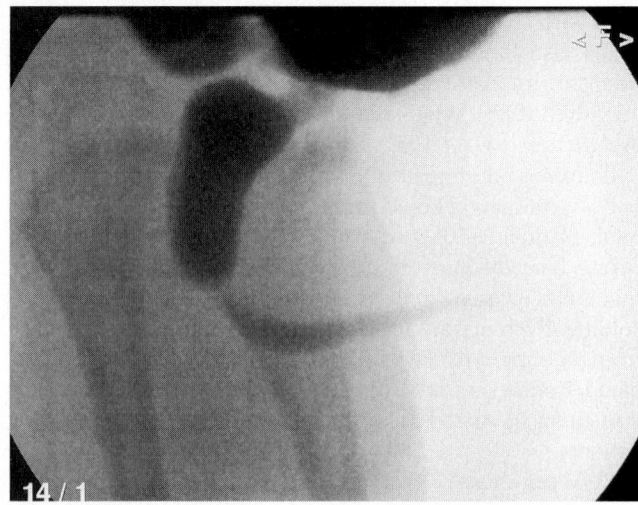

Figure 205-5. Voiding cystourethrogram showing posterior urethral valves correlated with ultrasound findings in Figure 205-4.

Management

Patients with PUV require referral to a pediatric urologist and nephrologist for definitive therapy of the valves and ongoing management of residual renal and bladder problems. Bladder outlet obstruction should be relieved initially by placing an indwelling catheter through the urethra. Bladder neck hypertrophy and posterior urethral dilation can cause the catheter to coil in the urethra. If there is any question of proper catheter placement, fluoroscopic examination should be used to confirm catheter location. The patient should receive antibacterial prophylaxis or, if there is evidence of urinary tract infection, appropriate therapy.

Early surgical intervention for *most* male infants with PUV entails transurethral valve ablation alone. Occasionally a child continues to have severe hydroureteronephrosis and a persistently elevated creatinine value despite valve ablation. If catheter drainage improves this situation, the infant should be reexamined under anesthesia to confirm valve ablation; creation of a vesicostomy may be considered. If catheter drainage does not improve the situation, percutaneous nephrostomy tube placement may assist in diagnosis and short-term management, with later consideration for percutaneous ureterostomy or pyelostomy. Long-term studies have not shown any clinical value to upper urinary tract diversion because damage to the kidneys is largely irreversible; however, it may assist in short-term fluid management.

Renal insufficiency should be addressed with conservative management before and after correction. Initial serum creatinine in a newborn reflects maternal renal function and placental function. Placement of the urinary catheter allows for observation of the infant's renal function in the absence of obstruction. Serum creatinine should be monitored closely, especially for patients who present with severe obstruction and renal insufficiency. Conservative management or dialysis support should be coordinated with the pediatric nephrologist.

After placement of the urinary catheter, the infant may have a postobstructive diuresis, with large fluid and electrolyte losses. Appropriate attention must be paid to fluid balance and serum electrolyte levels. Strict monitoring of input and output and daily weights assists in tracking the patient's status. Obstructive uropathies such as PUV adversely affect the concentrating ability of the kidneys. This can be a chronic condition that results in high-volume urine output and chronic constipation secondary to dehydration. Antibiotic prophylaxis is essential for an infant with PUV. Amoxicillin, 12.5 mg/kg/day, can be used for the first 6 to 8 weeks of life. Nitrofurantoin or sulfamethoxazole/trimethoprim typically is used after this time.

Outcome and Follow-up

Outcome for children with PUV is highly variable, depending on the severity of the obstruction and how early it is relieved. Many patients born with PUV have had significant renal parenchymal damage before correction, which could lead to the development of long-term renal dysfunction and kidney failure. If treated early in infancy, PUV is likely to have a minimal impact on later bladder function. Male infants born with pulmonary hypoplasia and renal insufficiency can accommodate to some degree. A nadir serum creatinine of greater than 0.8 mg/dL at 1 year of life is predictive, however, for the need for renal replacement therapy later in life. Even patients with successful neonatal management may have ongoing issues related to bladder dysfunction and vesicoureteral reflux that have an impact on ultimate outcome.

Patients treated for PUV should have a repeat VCUG at 1 month posttreatment to confirm adequate valve ablation. Serial ultrasound studies allow the physician to assess renal growth. Infants with PUV may require specialized nutritional support because of their renal injury. Some boys have decreased urinary concentrating ability that requires a high fluid intake to keep up with the obligate fluid losses. This increased fluid intake often occurs at the expense of other caloric needs. Some of these children require gastric tubes to allow overnight feeding and rehydration to ensure normal growth. Fluid and electrolyte balance requires observation immediately after relief of the obstruction in the phase of diuresis and later when defects such as decreased urinary concentration, renal tubular acidosis, or other renal tubular anomalies may become evident.

These children should undergo urodynamic evaluation if ultrasound or VCUG suggests adverse upper or lower urinary tract changes or if they fail to go through toilet training successfully at an age-appropriate time. Because these patients may be at risk to develop progressive renal failure, it is wise to perform interval monitoring for hypertension, proteinuria, and changing renal function. The frequency of this monitoring depends on the severity of the obstruction and the level of residual renal function. Ongoing coordination with the urologist and nephrologist is needed, especially for children with more severe forms of obstruction.

AMBIGUOUS GENITALIA

Evaluation and management of ambiguous genitalia is challenging medically and socially. The generalist needs to be sensitive to the medical and social challenges in these situations, when the infant's gender may not be obvious (Fig. 205-6).

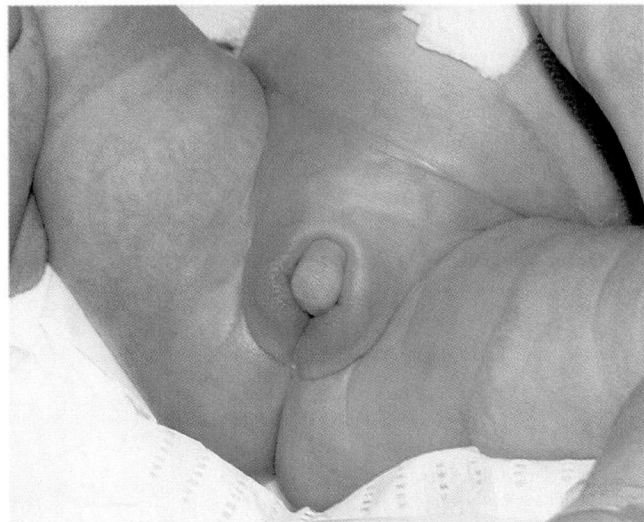

A

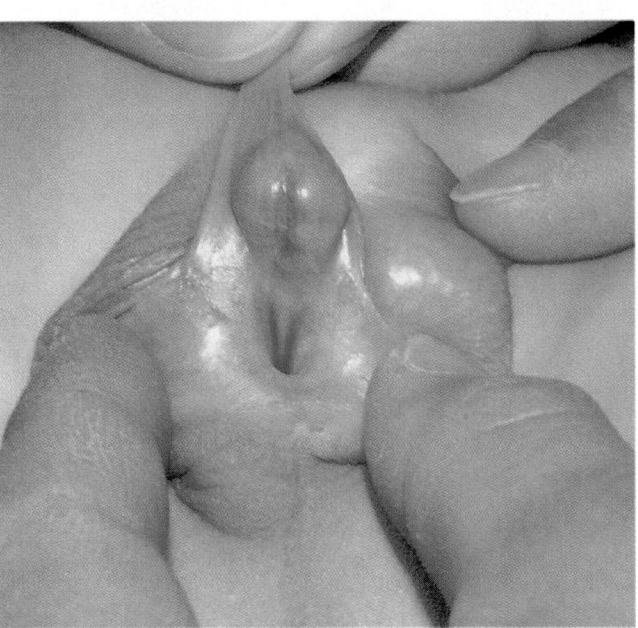

B

Figure 205-6. A and **B,** Newborns with ambiguous genitalia.

Definition

The term *ambiguous genitalia* includes many different developmental abnormalities of the external sexual structures. Genotypic females may be highly androgenized and may appear to have male genitalia, whereas an XY infant may have female genitalia. Any infant in whom there is discordance between the appearance of the external genitalia and the karyotype may be considered to have ambiguous genitalia.

Fundamentals

Table 205-2 lists categories and characteristics of disorders with ambiguous genitalia.

Diagnosis

Careful physical examination of the newborn genitalia is essential. The most important part of the examination is palpation for the presence or absence of gonads in the labioscrotal compartment. A gonad that has descended into this compartment is likely a testis and the patient a karyotypic male, although there are exceptions (e.g., SRY+ XX male and uterine hernia inguinalae). In the absence of a palpable gonad in a phenotypic male, no definitive sex assignment should be made. Additional findings to be noted on physical examination include phallus size, location of urethral opening, appearance and pigmentation of labiosacral folds, and other associated anomalies.

Ultrasound may be a useful tool for the identification of internal gonads, although pelvic ultrasonography generally is not considered sensitive enough to confirm their absence if gonads are not visualized. Ultrasound also can be used to document the presence of uterine structures in an externally virilized female but is typically useful only immediately after birth, when the maternal estrogen effect increases the thickness of the endometrial lining. Magnetic resonance imaging with gadolinium and laparoscopic exploration of the pelvis are the most accurate methods to evaluate pelvic anatomy in these patients and should be used when indicated. Improved magnetic resonance imaging technology makes this an increasingly attractive imaging modality to evaluate these infants. Genetic evaluation by karyotype should be performed as soon as possible. Infants born with ambiguous genitalia should undergo a metabolic evaluation including serum electrolytes (after birth and several days later if congenital adrenal hyperplasia is a possibility), serum testosterone, dihydrotestosterone, follicle-stimulating hormone, luteinizing hormone, and estrogen. Particular care must be taken to identify patients with endocrinologic abnormalities that can be rapidly life-threatening, such as salt-wasting syndromes with congenital adrenal hyperplasia. Evaluation of serum chemistries for evidence of hyponatremia or hyperkalemia should be done if there is a suspicion of such abnormalities.

Management

Careful communication with the family is essential in cases of ambiguous genitalia. It is vital to avoid definitive sex assignment until data are collected. Gender-specific pronouns should be avoided when speaking to the family about the infant until a decision is made by the family regarding the sex of rearing. Rapid diagnosis is important not only to assist the family through the stress of ambiguity, but also to ensure that potentially life-threatening conditions, such as congenital adrenal hyperplasia, are recognized. Consultation with specialists is required to plan for appropriate medical and surgical management.

Outcome and Follow-up

Timing and extent of surgical correction for ambiguous genitalia are controversial. It is important to inform families fully about the complex psychosocial issues related to surgical correction in addition to the medical risks and benefits.

Long-term hormonal management may be indicated for some patients. This therapy is particularly important for infants with congenital adrenal hyperplasia, who require replacement for glucocorticoid and mineralocorticoid deficiency.

Table 205-2. Categories and Characteristics of Disorders with Ambiguous Genitalia

Diagnosis	Defect	External Appearance	Karyotype, Internal Status
Female Pseudohermaphroditism Congenital adrenal hyperplasia Progestin induced Maternal androgen induced Indeterminate	Fetal exposure to virilizing substances Congenital fetal metabolic defect Coming from the mother	Virilization depends on extent of androgen exposure in utero; mild clitoromegaly to fully male-appearing phallus No palpable gonads	46,XX Ovarian tissue only Müllerian structures present
Male Pseudohermaphroditism Androgen insensitivity Androgen receptor defect (5α-reductase)	Several possible defects Defective androgen synthesis Target tissue insensitivity to androgen Failure of müllerian regression Other uncertain causes	Variable presentations Near-normal male Inguinal hernias Cryptorchidism	46,XY Testicular tissue only Wolffian structures present Müllerian structures may be present
Vanishing testis syndrome Persistent müllerian duct syndrome Indeterminate		Small phallus Hypospadias Intermediate genitalia Near-normal or normal female	
Mixed gonadal dysgenesis	Development defect	Usually incompletely virilized male Small phallus Cryptorchidism Hypospadias	Most 46, XY/45,XO Testis, streak gonad present Müllerian structures may be present on the side of the streak gonad
Pure gonadal dysgenesis	Developmental defect	Often initially normal; infertility, lack of sexual development noted later	46,XX; 46,XY; 45,XO Bilateral streak gonads Underdeveloped müllerian structures
True hermaphroditism	Developmental defect	Variable presentations Female with clitoromegaly Male with hypospadias, undescended testes	46,XX (approximately 70%); remainder 46,XY or mosaic Testicular and ovarian tissues are present (separate or as ovotestis) Wolffian and müllerian structures may be present
Others Cloacal exstrophy Aphallia Microphallus	Developmental defect	External male genitalia severely compromised Cloacal exstrophy—bifid phallus and scrotum	46,XY Testes present Wolffian structures present

The ultimate success for an infant with ambiguous genitalia may depend as much on the quality and extent of psychosocial support as on sophisticated medical and surgical management. Complex family dynamics have a profound impact on children born with ambiguous genitalia. Honest and informed communication between the family and the health care provider is important to create trust and understanding around this emotionally charged issue. The generalist must play a central role during follow-up care for the infant with ambiguous genitalia because many consulting services typically are involved, including medical genetics, endocrinology, urology, and psychiatry. Long-term psychosocial support for the family and the child should be provided. Patient-based support groups are an excellent resource for the children and families. For patients requiring ongoing medical management for hormonal replacement, the generalist also needs to be an active participant.

CRYPTORCHIDISM

Definition

Testicular descent is a complex multistage process. The testis initially begins to develop in utero on the gonadal ridge in the retroperitoneum. During the last trimester of pregnancy, it migrates to the scrotum. Testicular descent is controlled by a variety of mechanical and hormonal factors. Interruption of this process leads to cryptorchidism, or "hidden testis" (Fig. 205-7).

Fundamentals

A combination of mechanical, developmental, and hormonal factors contributes to the normal descent of the testis. Defects in any of these processes may lead to cryptorchidism. Testes may fail to descend in any clinical syndrome in which there is a defect in androgen synthesis or activity or mechanical problems with the abdominal wall. The incidence of cryptorchidism is approximately 3% in term infant boys. Most of these undescended testes later migrate into the scrotum, such that the incidence at age 18 years is only 0.8%. Cryptorchidism is more common in premature infants, appearing in 30% of premature boys.

In humans, normal spermatogenesis cannot occur at the warmer body temperatures found in the abdomen. For this reason, the longer a testis remains in the abdominal cavity, the greater the likelihood of reduced fertility. Significant histopathologic changes in the cryptorchid testis begin to occur at 12 to 15 months of age. Fertility evaluation in men who underwent orchidopexy shows decreased fertility with abnormal semen parameters. Fertility is significantly more compromised when both testes are cryptorchid.

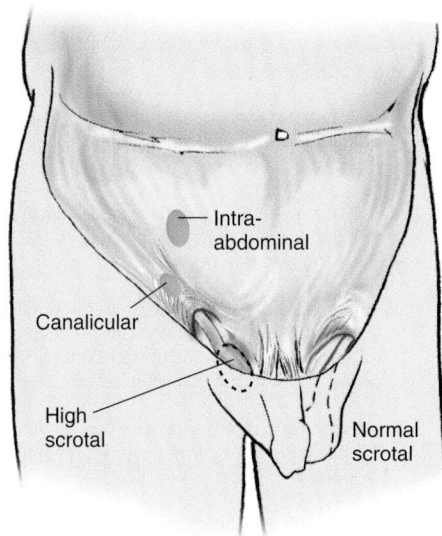

Figure 205-7. Schematic showing range of testes locations.

Undescended testes are 35 to 48 times more likely to develop malignancy than normal testes. Higher cryptorchid testes (i.e., intra-abdominal) are at greater risk for malignant degeneration. Approximately 10% of testicular cancers arise in cryptorchid testes. Orchidopexy decreases the risk for later malignant degeneration. The overall risk remains relatively low with less than one tumor per 2500 cases of cryptorchidism. Testosterone production in cryptorchid testes typically is within normal limits for age even through puberty. More subtle alterations in hormonal function can occur and are likely responsible in part for the decreased fertility seen in these patients.

Diagnosis
Undescended testes are noted at the time of newborn examination. Most patients have cryptorchidism as an isolated finding. Uncommon anomalies associated with cryptorchidism are listed in Box 205-1.

Management
Because a testis that has not descended by 1 year of age is likely to remain cryptorchid, and the cryptorchid seminiferous tubules begin to degenerate by age 2 years, treatment for cryptorchidism should occur within the first year of life. Nonpalpable testes should be evaluated by 6 months. There is only a minimal chance of spontaneous descent of an intra-abdominal testis, and a testis in a high intra-abdominal position may require two operations to bring it down to the scrotum. Most pediatric urologists perform a laparoscopic evaluation for nonpalpable testis to distinguish between an absent or vanishing testis and an intra-abdominal testis. Laparoscopic orchidopexy can be performed at the same time if an intra-abdominal testis is identified.

Intervention to correct cryptorchidism can be hormonal or surgical. Hormonal therapy, using injected human chorionic gonadotropin or intranasal gonadotropin-releasing hormone, can stimulate migration of undescended testes. Clinical studies show success rates of approximately 40%

with low undescended testes and retractile testes. Surgical correction involves mobilizing the undescended testis and placing it in the scrotum. New laparoscopic techniques allow this procedure to be performed in a minimally invasive fashion for an intra-abdominal testis. Inguinally located cryptorchid testes are approached surgically through a groin incision.

Outcome and Follow-up
Long-term outcome varies depending on the location of the testis and how many testes are affected. Most series report success rates with orchidopexy of greater than 90% for undescended testes located in the inguinal region. Intra-abdominal testes are brought down with less success; results vary from 70% to 90% success. Orchidopexy decreases the risk for malignant degeneration in cryptorchid testes. If the orchidopexy is performed after 2 years of age, it is unlikely to affect fertility positively. Bringing the testis to the scrotum does allow for easy examination and a more normal cosmetic appearance regardless of when it is done.

Given the increased risk for malignancy in an undescended testis, regardless of whether it is brought down to the scrotum, the importance of testicular self-examination should be stressed as the boy goes through puberty. For a patient with isolated cryptorchidism, a fertility evaluation generally is not performed until it becomes clinically apparent that the couple is having difficulty achieving a pregnancy. In contrast, patients with some syndromes associated with cryptorchidism (i.e., prune-belly syndrome) routinely have poor fertility and may wish to be evaluated before attempting to achieve a pregnancy.

LOW-PREVALENCE GENITOURINARY ANOMALIES

Definition
The generalist occasionally sees uncommon genitourinary anomalies when providing care to newborns. A complete listing of all such anomalies is beyond the scope of this chapter. Table 205-3 lists a few of these low-prevalence anomalies to provide the generalist with a brief overview.

Fundamentals
Low-prevalence anomalies such as those listed in Table 205-3 can have a broad range of presentations from asymptomatic to severe. Several of these anomalies can be noted on prenatal ultrasound. Renal agenesis and cystic kidney disease are readily apparent. Prune-belly syndrome and cloacal abnormalities also typically are noted on antenatal studies because of the dilation of the genitourinary system. The exstrophy-epispadias complex is detected prenatally in less than 50% of cases. The characteristic findings are more subtle and can be missed by an ultrasonographer unfamiliar with this anomaly. Some anomalies can be associated with multiorgan involvement and are recognized as established syndromes or associations. Cloacal exstrophy and cloacal anomalies in particular are associated with an increased incidence of abnormalities affecting the nongenitourinary systems.

Table 205-3. Low Prevalence Genitourinary Anomalies Seen in the Newborn

Name	Abnormality	Special Considerations
Renal dysplasia Cystic kidney disease	Abnormal differentiation or organization of renal tissue; unilateral or bilateral, diffuse or segmental; may result in variably sized cysts within kidney	In unilateral disease, increased risk of vesicoureteral reflux into the normal kidney
Polycystic kidney disease	Diffuse cystic involvement of both kidneys, without dysplasia; there are autosomal recessive (ARPKD) and autosomal dominant (ADPKD) forms	ARPKD may present in neonatal period with greatly enlarged kidneys, decreased function; ADPKD less likely to present in neonates
Exstrophy-epispadias complex	Spectrum of anterior abdominal wall abnormalities resulting in herniation of the urethra, bladder, or colon secondary to premature disruption of the cloacal membrane	Instantly recognizable at birth, this congential defect ranges from cloacal exstrophy (most severe) to distal epispadias (least severe); urinary continence, sexual function, and fertility are affected.
Eagle-Barrett (prune-belly) syndrome	Severe congenital anomaly characterized by a dilated urinary tract, abdominal wall laxity, abdominal muscle deficiency, renal dysplasia, cryptorchidism	Broad spectrum of presentations; most severe forms also can have gut malrotation, oligohydramnios, lung hypoplasia
Cloacal and urogenital sinus anomalies	Spectrum of anomalies resulting from arrested development of the primitive genitourinary system	Highly variable presentation
VATER/VACTERL association	Renal anomalies, such as agenesis, ectopy, or obstruction associated with vertebral, intestinal, cardiac and limb anomalies	Can be associated with chromosomal abnormalities; broad spectrum of disease

Diagnosis

Prenatal ultrasound often provides the first indication of an uncommon genitourinary anomaly. A complete family history should be obtained. A thorough physical examination may confirm prenatal findings or may uncover an unexpected congenital anomaly (Fig. 205-8). Postnatal imaging studies, such as renal ultrasound, may clarify further the extent of abnormalities suggested by prenatal studies or postnatal physical examination. A postnatal ultrasound examination should be performed for any infant with the previously noted anomalies. Genetic studies may be indicated for anomalies with a specific genetic basis but are recommended as a matter of routine. Children with cloacal exstrophy often undergo karyotype evaluation to confirm gender. Biopsy rarely is indicated for diagnosis of neonatal genitourinary anomalies.

Antenatally diagnosed ovarian cysts are the second most common source of abdominal masses in newborns, accounting for 20% of all newborn abdominal masses. The incidence has been estimated at 1 in 2625 pregnancies. Cysts are thought to develop in response to placental human chorionic gonadotropin, fetal gonadotropins, or maternal estrogen. Antenatally diagnosed ovarian cysts are rarely malignant. Most are follicular, serous, or theca lutein in origin.

Management

Management of low-prevalence anomalies depends on the specific abnormality and the severity of the presentation. All patients require appropriate fluid management and correction of any metabolic derangements that may result from the anomaly in question. Some patients may have significant involvement of other organ systems as part of a syndrome or association. Most of these patients require consultation and possible referral to a pediatric nephrologist or urologist, either to diagnose and manage the more severe abnormalities or to allay parental concerns and establish a plan for long-term follow-up for anomalies with less severe manifestations. Cloacal anomalies and the exstrophy-epispadias complex anomalies require urgent consultation with a pediatric urologist.

In the neonatal period, many antenatally diagnosed cysts can be managed expectantly with serial ultrasound if the cyst is simple and the infant is asymptomatic. In one series, nearly two thirds of cysts managed by observation resolved spontaneously over 1 year. The most serious complication of expectant management was torsion, which occurred in 30% of infants and required emergency laparotomy. Symptoms included vomiting, fussiness, anemia, and an acute abdomen. Half of the infants had no symptoms other than increasing mass size. A complex or enlarging cyst is worrisome for torsion or hemorrhage and requires surgical management.

Outcome and Follow-up

Outcome for these anomalies is highly variable and depends on the specific abnormality and its severity. Some patients have mild manifestations that have little effect on the patient's long-term health. A patient with mild unilateral renal hypoplasia may be at increased risk for hypertension in adulthood but otherwise asymptomatic. By contrast, bilateral renal involvement with resultant pulmonary disease, as might be seen in Eagle-Barrett syndrome or severe renal hypoplasia, may not be compatible with long-term survival. Patients with unusual anomalies require coordination between the generalist and the specialist for ongoing care.

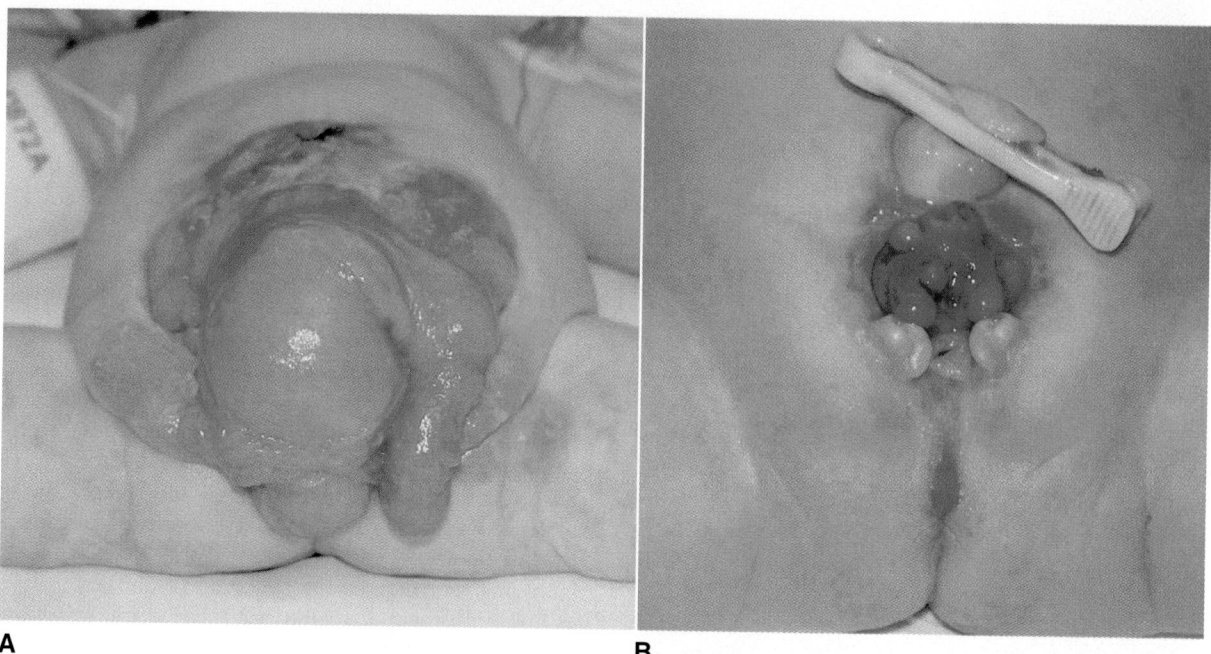

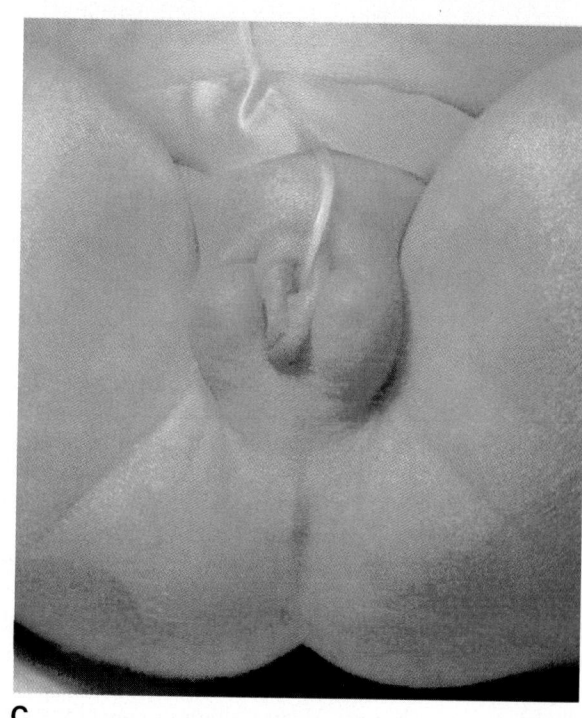

Figure 205-8. Bladder exstrophy **(A)**, prune-belly syndrome **(B)**, and cloacal anomaly **(C)**.

SUGGESTED READINGS

American Academy of Pediatrics: Timing of elective surgery on the genitalia of male children with particular reference to the risks, benefits, and psychological effects of surgery and anesthesia. Pediatrics 1996;97:590–594.

American Academy of Pediatrics: Committee on Genetics, Section on Endocrinology, and Section on Urology: Evaluation of the newborn with developmental anomalies of the external genitalia. Pediatrics 2000;106:138–142.

Baskin LS: Hypospadias and urethral development. J Urol 2000; 163:951–956.

Mayr JM, Lawrenz K, Berghold A: Undescended testicles: An epidemiological review. Acta Paediatr 1999;88:1089–1093.

Roth JA, Daimond DA: Prenatal hydronephrosis. Curr Opin Pediatr 2001;13:138–141.

206 Disorders of Calcium Metabolism

J. Ross Milley

ROLE OF THE GENERALIST

1   Recognize the normal transition of calcium metabolism during the immediate newborn period.

2   Recognize newborns at high risk to develop hypocalcemia.

3   Diagnose newborns with hypocalcemia.

4   Make appropriate treatment decisions in newborns with asymptomatic hypocalcemia, weighing benefits of treatment versus risks.

5   Treat newborns with acute symptomatic hypocalcemia

6   Treat newborns with late-onset hypocalcemia

7   Refer patients to appropriate specialists for assistance in diagnosis, treatment, and long-term management for underlying endocrine and cardiac conditions

DEFINITION

A single range of normal calcium concentrations does not define abnormal calcium values at all ages. Total serum calcium ranges from 8.5 to 10.5 mg/dL in adults to 7 to 12 mg/dL in normal full-term infants at less than 1 week of age. Even lower values of serum calcium concentration are usual in premature infants. Defining normal calcium values is complicated by the fact that the ionized fraction of calcium in blood is the physiologically active form. The proportion of the ionized component of total serum calcium varies with serum albumin. Higher albumin concentration increases calcium binding and lowers ionized calcium concentration at any given total serum calcium. Measurement of ionized calcium has become more readily available and reliable. Because the physiologically important fraction of the compound in the blood is measured, use of this measurement is preferable to that of total serum calcium.

Definitions of neonatal hypocalcemia range from 2.5 to 4.8 mg/dL (0.62 to 1.20 mmol/L). In two studies, the lower range of normal calcium concentrations was 4.2 to 4.4 mg/dL (1.05 to 1.10 mmol/L). Using statistical grounds to define normal ionized calcium concentration, a serum concentration of less than 4.4 mg/dL (1.10 mmol/L) can be considered as the lower limit in term infants.

The relationship of total serum calcium to the ionized fraction is modified by several physiologic variables. Increases in serum pH or serum bicarbonate increase the binding of calcium to albumin and decrease ionized calcium concentrations at any given level of total serum calcium. Serum phosphate concentration and increasing serum magnesium decrease the proportion of total serum calcium that is ionized. Citrate (e.g., from blood transfusions, including exchange transfusions) and free fatty acids (given as lipid infusions) also alter the relationship of total serum calcium concentration to its ionized fraction.

FUNDAMENTALS

Clinical ability to diagnose and manage neonatal disorders of calcium metabolism depends directly on understanding the normal transition from fetal life. Prenatally calcium concentrations are related to the rapid accretion of calcium into the fetal skeleton (Fig. 206-1). Before birth, fetal calcium concentrations are higher than maternal levels through a constant uptake of calcium across the umbilical circulation from the placenta. The direct consequence of these high fetal calcium concentrations is that fetal parathyroid hormone and 1,25-dihydroxycholecalciferol concentrations are low, and serum calcitonin concentrations are high. As a consequence of this hormonal milieu, the rate of fetal accretion of calcium into bone is remarkably accelerated.

At birth, the continuous supply of calcium from the mother across the placenta is interrupted. Because exogenous intake of minerals is not immediately available, the normal newborn is without adequate supplies of calcium (and other minerals) for several days. The endocrine system does not adapt to this decreased exogenous supply as rapidly as severing the umbilical cord cuts off calcium intake. Over the first 24 hours of life, parathyroid hormone concentrations increase, from normally low fetal levels to values more in keeping with mobilization of calcium from endogenous stores, such as bone. Concomitantly, serum 1,25-dihydroxycholecalciferol levels increase to normal adult levels. Finally, serum calcitonin levels, already increased in fetal life, rise after birth to levels higher than in adults. The cause for this remarkable rise probably is related to the stress of birth, perhaps mediated through increased hormone concentrations, such as cortisol or catecholamines.

The endocrine milieu of the immediately newborn infant is such that bone formation continues and mobilization of calcium from bone osteoclastic activity is inhibited despite decreased exogenous calcium availability. This same hormonal balance inhibits the intestinal absorption of calcium

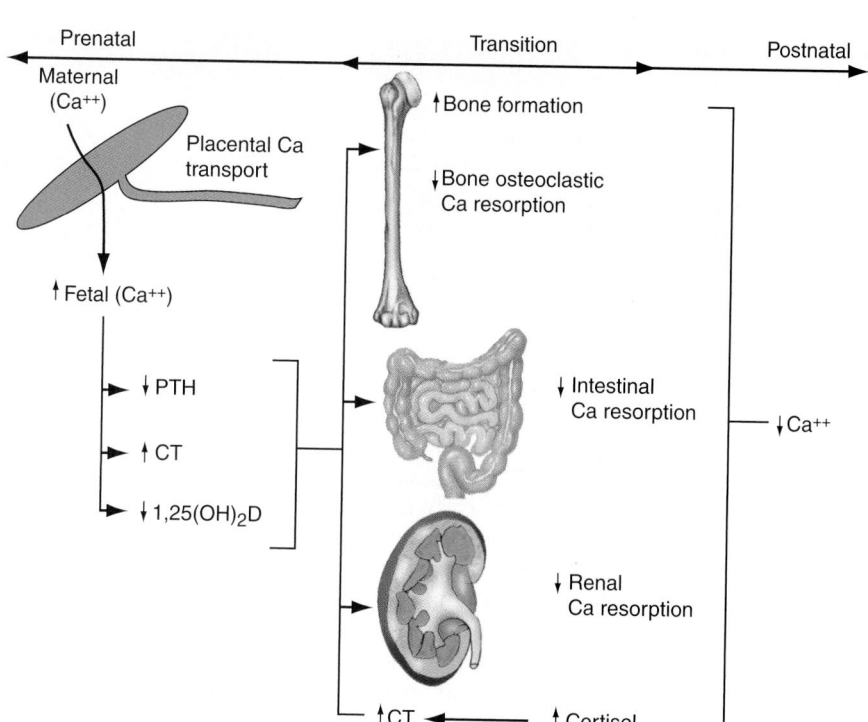

Figure 206-1. The transition from fetal to neonatal calcium metabolism. Ca, calcium; CT, calcitonin; 1,25(OH)$_2$D, 1,25-dihydroxycholecalciferol; PTH, parathyroid hormone.

and increases renal calcium excretion. As a result of these changes in endocrine regulation, the normal neonate undergoes a 24- to 48-hour period of decreased serum calcium concentration. At the end of this period, the serum calcium concentration stabilizes (generally >8 mg/dL in the term infant), and thereafter, as enteral intake increases, serum calcium concentration rises so that by 1 week of age the values are similar to those found later in childhood.

DIAGNOSIS

Disorders of calcium metabolism that lower neonatal calcium concentrations generally fall into two major categories (Table 206-1). "Early" neonatal hypocalcemia usually results from factors that exaggerate the normal decrease in calcium concentrations during transition from fetal to neonatal life. These factors define a population of infants at risk for neonatal hypocalcemia in whom appropriate monitoring may reveal hypocalcemia before it becomes symptomatic. "Late" hypocalcemia occurs in infants greater than 2 days of age. Infants with late hypocalcemia may or may not be defined as at risk before the onset of the signs and symptoms.

Three major groups of term infants are at risk for early neonatal hypocalcemia. Term infants with significant perinatal depression may have increased calcitonin production secondary to an exaggerated birth stress response. These

infants also may receive additional alkali therapy, contributing to an exaggerated postnatal hypocalcemic response. Infants of diabetic mothers may have a functional hypoparathyroidism induced by magnesium deficiency that considerably prolongs the normal course of neonatal hypocalcemia and may be refractory to calcium therapy until their magnesium deficiency is corrected. In mothers who receive certain anticonvulsants during pregnancy, specifically phenobarbital and phenytoin, the hepatic breakdown of vitamin D and its metabolites may be enhanced, increasing their risk for neonatal hypocalcemia. Neonatal hypocalcemia may be mitigated by vitamin D supplementation of these mothers.

The incidence of neonatal hypocalcemia increases with decreasing gestational age. Preterm infants often have a combination of delayed parathyroid hormone production, persistent production of calcitonin, and a relative end organ resistance to 1,25-dihydroxycholecalciferol. Delayed introduction of feeding (exogenous calcium intake) also can exacerbate hypocalcemia.

Late hypocalcemia is encountered in infants greater than 2 days of age. With magnesium deficiency, neonatal hypocalcemia resolves only when magnesium is replaced. Replacement of calcium alone may exacerbate the hypomagnesemia through competition of calcium with magnesium for reabsorption in the kidney and absorption in the intestine.

Late, sometimes prolonged hypocalcemia has been reported as a complication of unusual dietary intake. Excessive phosphate intake, most notoriously associated with intake of whole cow milk, has induced late infantile hypocalcemic tetany. Although this disorder is unusual in developed countries because of the availability of infant formulas with lower phosphate content, it continues to be problematic in areas where cow milk feedings are used. Infusion of substances that chelate serum calcium also can

Table 206-1. Causes of Neonatal Hypocalcemia

Early (≤2 days)	Late (>2 days)	Iatrogenic
Prematurity	High phosphate intake	Chelating agents
Maternal diabetes	Hypomagnesemia	
Perinatal depression	Hypoparathyroidism	
Maternal anticonvulsants		

induce neonatal hypocalcemia. Citrate present in blood products causes sufficient chelation during exchange transfusions to decrease serum calcium concentration notably.

Late neonatal hypocalcemia also is encountered in hypoparathyroidism, which can be grouped into three major categories. Congenital primary hypoparathyroidism is usually encountered as an X-linked or autosomal dominant condition, either in association with ring chromosomal abnormalities or as part of DiGeorge syndrome. In this syndrome (and the closely related velocardiofacial syndromes), agenesis of the parathyroid glands occurs secondary to incomplete development of the pharyngeal arches, causing varying degrees of parathyroid and thymic hypoplasia and conotruncal cardiac defects, facial malformations, and learning disabilities. Because partial variants of DiGeorge syndrome have been described, infants with congenital hypoparathyroidism need evaluation for possible cardiac anomalies and immune deficiencies. Conversely, infants with conotruncal cardiac defects merit a careful examination for potential congenital hypoparathyroidism and consequent hypocalcemia, especially before undergoing transfusion or operative intervention. Hypoparathyroidism also occurs secondary to maternal hyperparathyroidism or hypercalcemia of any cause. Because the newborn condition is due to an abnormal maternal endocrine milieu, the condition generally resolves spontaneously in days to several weeks.

A condition termed *transient congenital hypoparathyroidism* has been described. It lasts several weeks to months with classic features of hypocalcemia, hyperphosphatemia, and low serum parathyroid hormone. The condition resolves spontaneously.

In many infants, hypocalcemia is discovered in the absence of clinical manifestations (or nonspecific clinical findings) when a serum calcium level is obtained because infants are known to be at risk. Because calcium plays a vital role in transmission of nerve impulses and muscle contractility, these organ systems manifest the consequences of significant hypocalcemia. Central nervous system symptoms of hypocalcemic neonates include "jitteriness" and "hyperactivity." More classic tetany and seizure activity (either generalized or focal), although uncommon, does occur. Central nervous system symptoms are recognized more frequently in term infants than in preterm infants. Because calcium has important effects on myocardial contractility, severe cardiac contractile dysfunction may occur with severe or prolonged hypocalcemia. Intravenous calcium infusion rapidly improves myocardial performance.

Hypercalcemia occurs much less frequently than neonatal hypocalcemia and often is iatrogenic in nature. Excessive calcium administration, either as part of parenteral nutritional support or during treatment of hypocalcemia, should be excluded before extensive investigation of other rare causes of neonatal hypercalcemia are undertaken. The neonatal severe form of primary hyperparathyroidism is an autosomal recessive disorder in which inactivation of the calcium-sensing receptors results in extreme parathyroid enlargement and remarkable hypercalcemia. Although partial parathyroidectomy has been attempted, generally total parathyroidectomy is required to achieve manageable

---

Box 206-1. Conditions Associated with Hypercalcemia

- Iatrogenic
- Idiopathic infantile hypercalcemia
- Subcutaneous fat necrosis
- Hyper–prostaglandin E syndrome
- Severe infantile hypophosphatasia

---

calcium homeostasis. Other unusual causes of neonatal hypercalcemia are listed in Box 206-1.

TREATMENT

Treatment of early neonatal hypocalcemia is controversial. The need for treatment may be complicated by coexisting factors, such as asphyxia or hypoglycemia, conditions that have similar clinical manifestations. More important, hypocalcemia may be asymptomatic and in most infants is self-limited. Recommendations vary regarding intervention in cases of asymptomatic hypocalcemia identified in infants who are at risk. In most cases, hypocalcemia resolves spontaneously without long-term consequences. Symptoms may be silent, however. Because significant depression of myocardial performance may occur before heart rate and blood pressure are notably affected, it has become common practice to treat asymptomatic term infants whose ionized calcium concentrations are less than 4.40 mg/dL (1.10 mmol/L).

Serious complications of treatment demand that decisions to treat asymptomatic infants be weighed against the risks. Rapid infusion of intravenous calcium can lead to bradycardia, other cardiac arrhythmias, and myocardial failure. Because extravasation of calcium solutions during intravenous infusion can cause severe cutaneous necrosis, special attention must be paid to peripheral intravenous sites during calcium infusion. Many centers prohibit intra-aortic (umbilical arterial) calcium infusion because it may contribute to the development of necrotizing enterocolitis by inducing mesenteric artery spasm. Calcium cannot be administered simultaneously with sodium bicarbonate because calcium carbonate precipitates from these solutions.

Maintenance calcium is initiated at dosages ranging from 45 to 90 mg/kg/day of elemental calcium by continuous intravenous infusion, starting at the lower end of this range and increasing as needed. Calcium is available as chloride and gluconate salts. The latter is preferred and is available as a 10% solution that may be given orally or intravenously; 1 mL of 10% solution contains 100 mg of calcium gluconate, which approximately equals 9 mg of elemental calcium. An oral preparation also is available in syrup form (Neo-Calglucon). Enteral calcium treatment is not appropriate for initial treatment in many at-risk infants. Because this preparation has a high sugar content and high osmolality, its use preferably is reserved for older infants.

Acute Symptomatic Hypocalcemia

Infants with arrhythmia, pump failure, or central nervous system symptoms in association with low serum calcium concentration warrant immediate therapy, consisting of 9 to 18 mg of elemental calcium per kg given by intravenous infusion over 5 minutes (1 to 2 mg of 10% calcium gluconate/kg). This dose should not be given more quickly than approximately 1 mg/min with careful observation of the heart rate and the intravenous site. Symptoms should resolve within 10 minutes. If not, the dose may be repeated one time. After the initial dose, a maintenance infusion of calcium should be begun approximating 75 mg/kg/24 hours. Thereafter, the infusion of calcium should be weaned gradually over 3 days to prevent rebound hypocalcemia. Treatment rarely is necessary for more than 4 to 5 days unless other complications are present.

Late-Onset Hypocalcemia

Treatment of late-onset hypocalcemia varies by the etiology. Because hypocalcemia does not respond to therapy unless any associated magnesium deficiency is corrected, infants with hypocalcemia and coincident hypomagnesemia should receive magnesium sulfate solution, intravenously or intramuscularly, followed by maintenance therapy with supplemental intravenous or oral magnesium. Generally, infants require treatment for 1 to 2 days to resolve the hypomagnesemia.

When symptomatic late-onset hypocalcemia is associated with hyperphosphatemia, the acute hypocalcemia should be treated as stated earlier with bolus and then constant infusion of intravenous calcium supplementation. Meanwhile the renal phosphate load must be reduced. The infant should receive a low-phosphate formula or human milk to decrease phosphorus intake. It may be necessary to increase the calcium-to-phosphorus ratio of the milk with oral calcium supplementation to minimize renal phosphate load appropriately. Calcium supplementation should not be needed for more than 2 to 4 weeks, but serum calcium and phosphorus need to be monitored at least weekly while making changes in calcium supplementation. Finally, if the clinician suspects primary, secondary, or transient hypoparathyroidism, he or she should consult with and endocrine specialist for assistance with diagnosis, treatment, and long-term management.

OUTCOME

Hypocalcemia with seizures may be a significant life-threatening event in infants who often are experiencing other simultaneous life-threatening difficulties. In contrast to neonates whose seizures are caused by hypoglycemia, hypocalcemia does not seem to induce long-term structural damage in the brain. As a consequence, the outcome for hypocalcemia is excellent. Conditions predisposing to hypocalcemia, most notably asphyxia, may have independent consequences unrelated to the hypocalcemia itself.

FOLLOW-UP

Infants with transient early-onset neonatal hypocalcemia (whether symptomatic or asymptomatic) generally do not require specific follow-up when the condition has resolved. Mild hypocalcemia (compared with adult norms) is the expected consequence of the normal transition from fetal to postnatal life. Many risk factors for early hypocalcemia simply increase the duration or the severity of the hypocalcemia but do not change the transient nature of the difficulty. In rare cases, early-onset neonatal hypocalcemia does not prove to be transient. In these cases, appropriate follow-up by a pediatric endocrinologist is needed to diagnose and manage infants appropriately. Similarly, some of the causes of late-onset hypocalcemia may be identified as dietary or procedural. In this case, there is little need for follow-up when the acute problem has resolved.

Mini-index of Related Topics   CH.

SUGGESTED READINGS

Demari S, Mimouni FB, Tsang RC: Disorders of calcium, phosphorus and magnesium metabolism. In Fanaroff AA, Martin RJ (eds): Neonatal-Perinatal Medicine: Diseases of the Fetus and Neonate, 6th ed. St. Louis, Mosby, 1997, pp 1463–1476.

Leatherby L, Kirby ML: Cardiac development and perinatal care of infants with neural crest-associated conotruncal defects. Semin Perinatol 1996;20:473–481.

Mimouni F, Tsang RC: Pathophysiology of neonatal hypocalcemia. In Polin RA, Fox WW (eds): Fetal and Neonatal Physiology. Philadelphia, WB Saunders, 1992, pp 1761–1767.

Mimouni F, Tsang RC: Neonatal hypocalcemia: To treat or not to treat? J Am Coll Nutr 1994;13:408–415.

207 Disorders of the Thyroid

J. Ross Milley

ROLE OF THE GENERALIST

1   Ensure appropriate neonatal screening for thyroid disorders.

2   Recognize abnormal screening tests.

3   Perform laboratory evaluation on all infants with possible congenital hypothyroidism in conjunction with a pediatric endocrinologist.

4   Recognize signs and symptoms of congenital hypothyroidism and of congenital hyperthyroidism.

5   Ensure timely and appropriate treatment of infants with congenital hypothyroidism, with the assistance of or a referral to a pediatric endocrinologist.

6   Ensure adequate follow-up of infants with congenital hypothyroidism.

7   Stabilize newborns with congenital hyperthyroidism, and provide adequate treatment with the assistance of or referral to a pediatric endocrinologist.

DEFINITION

Disorders of neonatal thyroid function are divided into two categories—hypothyroidism and hyperthyroidism. Congenital hypothyroidism is especially important. A common pediatric endocrine disorder, congenital hypothyroidism, is one of the most common causes of preventable cognitive compromise. Congenital hypothyroidism epitomizes a pathophysiologic process for which screening is justified during the neonatal period. Screening was introduced in the early 1970s, when measurement of the thyroid hormones thyroxine (T_4) and thyroid-stimulating hormone (TSH) could be analyzed on the spots of whole blood then collected for screening for phenylketonuria. Congenital hypothyroidism has been confirmed in 1:3000 to 1:4000 live births. Screening has been remarkably successful in the early detection of infants with the classic types of congenital hypothyroidism, allowing treatment in a timely fashion and preventing mental retardation. Screening also has revealed a series of transient disorders of thyroid function, the significance of which remains unclear. As a consequence, there have been a variety of therapeutic approaches to these infants. This chapter summarizes understanding of the etiology of congenital hypothyroidism and hyperthyroidism and presents a rigorous and well-founded approach to the treatment of these disorders.

FUNDAMENTALS

Hypothyroidism

Table 207-1 lists the abnormalities of thyroid development, function, and regulation. The most common etiology of congenital hypothyroidism (accounting for approximately 75% to 85% of cases) is thyroid dysgenesis—aplasia, hypoplasia, or ectopia. Failure of the anatomic development of the thyroid gland may be either complete or partial. Infants with ectopic thyroid usually have a remnant of undescended thyroid tissue situated in the midline between the base of the tongue and the gland's normal location. This tissue may undergo compensatory hypertrophy as hormone production becomes inadequate and manifests as a mass in the midline. Partial thyroidal agenesis, whether in normal or ectopic position, accounts for 60% to 80% of infants and children with hypothyroidism. The specific pathogenesis of thyroid dysgenesis is unclear. Many factors suggest the possibility of an underlying genetic defect. The disorder is more common in girls (approximately 2:1 female-to-male ratio). Familial forms of congenital hypothyroidism and other thyroid disorders are recognized. Congenital hypothyroidism occasionally occurs in twins and siblings. Frequency of certain HLA types is increased with congenital hypothyroidism, and the incidence of congenital hypothyroidism is lower in black infants compared with white or Hispanic infants.

Inborn errors of the T_4 synthesis or metabolism involving one or more enzyme deficiencies constitute the second most common cause of congenital hypothyroidism (approximately 10% of cases) (Box 207-1). One such defect is

Table 207-1. Causes of Neonatal Hypothyroidism

Permanent	Transient
Primary	Primary neonatal hypothyroidism
Defective embryogenesis	Hypothyroxinemia
Agenesis	Hyperthyroxinemia
Dysgenesis (including ectopia)	Euthyroid sick syndrome
Inborn errors (see Box 207-2)	
Peripheral resistance to thyroid hormones	
Thyroid resistance to TSH	
Goiter	
Maternal goitrogen ingestion	
Endemic (iodine deficiency)	
Secondary	
Hypothalamic/pituitary disorders	

TSH, thyroid-stimulating hormone.

Box 207-1. Inborn Errors of Thyroxine Synthesis or Metabolism

- Iodide-trapping defects
- Iodide organification defects
- Iodotyrosine coupling defects
- Deiodination defects
- Defects in thyroglobin synthesis

impaired hormonal secretion that increases hypothalamic secretion of TSH. The increase in TSH concentrations usually leads to thyroid hyperplasia, which often manifests as goiter. Although the mode of transmission for some inborn errors of thyroid hormone synthesis has not been delineated fully, errors that have been described all are autosomal recessive.

In some patients, the peripheral tissues are resistant to the action of thyroid hormones. These patients are clinically hypothyroid but have elevated levels of thyroid hormones. These patients require significantly greater amounts of thyroid hormone replacement to ameliorate clinical symptoms.

In other neonates, the thyroid gland itself may be unresponsive to the actions of TSH. These infants do not develop a goiter. Although serum TSH is elevated, exogenous TSH stimulation causes no increase in thyroid response.

Goitrous congenital hypothyroidism occurs for two major reasons. Maternal ingestion of antithyroid drugs—specifically iodides, thiocarbamides, and potassium perchlorate—may lead to neonatal hypothyroidism. Neonatal goiter has been associated with the maternal perinatal administration of large amounts of inorganic iodide antiseptics. A second cause of congenital goitrous hypothyroidism is the prevalence of large geographic areas with deficient dietary iodine. Even in such areas, the incidence of neonatal goiter is relatively low, suggesting other environmental factors must be superimposed on iodine deficiency to cause occasional severe hypothyroidism.

Although hypothyroidism secondary to hypothalamic or pituitary defects is unusual in neonates, these defects are detected in thyroid screening programs that measure low T_4 and TSH. Low serum T_4 and low or normal serum TSH level characterize the disorder. These patients normally respond to thyrotropin-releasing hormone infusion. Thyrotropin-releasing hormone deficiency secondary to pituitary aplasia is associated strongly with anencephaly or other severe brain malformations. These infants are likely to experience neonatal hypoglycemia from associated growth hormone and adrenocorticotropic hormone deficiencies, polyuria from antidiuretic hormone deficiency, and small phallus with gonadotropin deficiencies.

Congenital hypothyroidism may be transient in some neonates. The results of neonatal screening tests from patients with transient congenital hypothyroidism may be indistinguishable from the results of infants with permanent hypothyroidism. Transient primary neonatal hypothyroidism occurs in many situations. Although seen in healthy term infants, premature infants are most susceptible, with the incidence of the disorder increasing with decreasing gestational age. This condition may be confused with transient hypothyroxinemia of prematurity.

A second cause of transient primary neonatal hypothyroidism is transplacental passage of antithyroid drugs (which also can cause permanent hypothyroidism as noted earlier). Cases have been reported following the excessive use of iodine-containing antiseptics on the mother or her infant (e.g., on mucous membranes when iodine-containing antiseptics are used on an infant with omphalocele) and when iodine-containing dyes have been injected into the amniotic cavity. Maternal antibody-mediated congenital hypothyroidism from transplacental passage of a thyrotropin receptor blocking antibody is the most frequent cause of transient neonatal congenital hypothyroidism, accounting for 5% to 10% of cases. This condition represents maternal autoimmune thyroid disease, with recurrence in future pregnancies. The course of their hypothyroidism is transient, resolving as maternal antibody is degraded over 3 to 6 months.

Transient hypothyroxinemia is noted in many premature infants. The likely cause is a physiologically appropriate immaturity of the hypothalamic pituitary axis. This condition is characterized by normal or low TSH levels but lower than usual total or free T_4 levels. In some instances, maternal dietary supplementation of iodine may be slightly deficient, resulting in low free T_4 levels accompanied by high TSH levels. Premature infants born in areas in which iodine deficiency is endemic are exposed to the combined risk of transient tertiary and primary hypothyroidism. Repeat evaluation of T_4 levels in these infants shows that they normalize by approximately 3 to 4 months of age.

Transient hyperthyrotropinemia is characterized by elevated neonatal serum TSH levels but normal T_4 and free T_4 levels. Infants usually are asymptomatic, and the cause usually is unknown. The disorder has been reported in infants of mothers receiving antithyroid medications or iodine. The incidence of this disorder is higher in infants with Down syndrome. Laboratory abnormalities usually resolve spontaneously but occasionally may be associated with permanent congenital hypothyroidism. Continued close monitoring is warranted. If increased TSH persists for more than 3 months, a more vigorous workup for congenital hypothyroidism (see later) is indicated.

Critically ill infants (most often premature infants with respiratory distress syndrome) are reported with low serum triiodothyronine (T_3) levels and low or normal T_4 levels. This constellation of findings (characterized as the *euthyroid sick syndrome*) gradually ameliorates as the primary illness improves. These infants should be followed carefully with serial determinations of thyroid function to ensure that other disorders of thyroid metabolism that can occur in premature infants do not complicate the illness.

Hyperthyroidism

The predominant cause of neonatal hyperthyroidism (Box 207-2) is transplacental passage of TSH receptor stimulating antibodies from the mother (Graves disease). This process may occur whether Graves disease is active in the mother or previously treated with thyroidectomy or radioiodine ablation. The effects on the fetus are not uniform, however, and mothers with detectable antibodies

- Maternal Graves disease
- Generalized (peripheral and pituitary) resistance to thyroid hormone
- Isolated (pituitary only) resistance to thyroid hormone

| Box 207-3. | Early (within 6 weeks) Clinical Manifestations of Hypothyroidism in Athyrotic Infants |

- Neurologic symptoms
  - Lethargy
  - Hypotonia
  - Poor feeding
- Respiratory symptoms (airway myxedema)
  - Respiratory distress
  - Perioral cyanosis
  - Hoarse cry
- Prolonged jaundice
- Periorbital edema
- Large fontanelles
- Pallor
- Mottled skin
- Constipation
- Hypothermia

may give birth to normal infants. Neonatal hyperthyroidism in infants without detectable TSH receptor stimulating antibodies occurs uncommonly (see Box 207-2).

DIAGNOSIS

Hypothyroidism

Most infants with primary hypothyroidism have low serum T_4 values and high serum TSH concentrations; however, 10% to 20% of infants with congenital hypothyroidism have T_4 values in the low-normal range. Consequently, whether TSH or T_4 should be the initial thyroid hormone screened to detect congenital hypothyroidism has been debated. Presently, primary TSH screening is used in most of Europe, Japan, and Australia. Most states in the United States and some provinces in Canada initially screen T_4. Essentially all of these programs use the filter paper spot technique obtained from capillary blood specimens from a heel stick at 2 to 5 days of age.

The various screening programs in North America have shown an incidence of congenital hypothyroidism of 1:3500 to 1:4000 live births. Racial differences are noted, with increased incidence among whites and Hispanics and a markedly decreased (approximately 1:32,000) incidence in blacks. The female-to-male ratio is approximately 2:1. Prevalence of transient hypothyroidism varies geographically with iodine intake.

The clinical signs and symptoms of congenital hypothyroidism are manifested unreliably early in life. Even in completely athyrotoxic infants, the classic features of congenital hypothyroidism for the most part are absent at birth and occur only gradually over the first 1 to 2 months of life. In patients with a functional remnant of ectopic thyroid tissue, the clinical manifestation may take additional months or years to develop.

The early manifestations outlined in Box 207-3 are, with the exception of large anterior and posterior fontanelles, relatively nonspecific. After the first week of life, prolonged physiologic jaundice is associated specifically with hypothyroidism. More classic features associated with congenital hypothyroidism occur only after approximately 6 weeks of age (Box 207-4). The most notable clinical manifestation of certain forms of congenital hypothyroidism is neonatal goiter. These goiters may be extremely large and asymmetric or small enough to escape notice on anything other than a detailed examination. The thyroid gland should be palpated in all newborns to detect neonatal goiter. The infant should be prone with the neck extended. The thyroid cartilage should be used as a landmark for palpation inferior and lateral to the thyroid isthmus and lobes.

Given the extreme importance of early identification on ultimate cognitive outcome, the laboratory evaluation of newborns with possible congenital hypothyroidism should

be conducted in consultation with a pediatric endocrinologist. Infants with abnormal screening tests should undergo without delay confirmatory measurements of a free T_4 (range 0.8 to 2.2 ng/dL at 0 to 1 month) and TSH (range 0.4 to 15 mU/L at 1 to 6 days; 0.4 to 10 mU/L at 1 to 3 weeks) on a sample obtained by venipuncture. When the diagnosis of congenital hypothyroidism has been confirmed, the timing and further workup as to specific etiology must be directed by a pediatric endocrinologist. If and when to test to find the ultimate etiology is controversial. Delay in treatment while further workup is undertaken should occur only under the direction of specialists. The most likely reasons for further testing include borderline thyroid function test results, discerning permanent from transient hypothyroidism, and cases of congenital hypothyroidism that are likely to be genetic in origin that deserve genetic counseling before further pregnancies.

Box 207-5 outlines the tests commonly used to determine the underlying cause of congenital hypothyroidism. Because thyroidal dysgenesis is the most common cause of congenital hypothyroidism, tests to determine the location

| Box 207-4. | Late (after 6 weeks) Clinical Manifestations of Hypothyroidism in Athyrotic Infants |

- Typical facies
  - Depressed nasal bridge
  - Narrow forehead
  - Puffy eyelids
  - Large tongue
  - Large and patent fontanelle
- Thick, dry, coarse skin
- Coarse hair
- Abdominal distention
- Umbilical hernia
- Hyporeflexia
- Bradycardia
- Hypotension with narrow pulse pressure
- Anemia
- Goiter

Box 207-5. Laboratory Evaluation of Suspected Congenital Hypothyroidism

To Confirm Diagnosis

- Free thyroxine
- Thyroid-stimulating hormone

To Determine Underlying Cause (if Indicated)

- Imaging (location and size of thyroid)
  - Radionuclide scan
  - Ultrasound
- Function
  - Radioiodine uptake
  - Thyroglobulin (serum) concentration
- Thyroxine synthesis deficiency suspected
  - Radioiodine uptake and perchlorate discharge
  - Salivary and serum radioiodine concentrations
- Autoimmune thyroid disease suspected
  - Maternal and neonatal serum thyrotropin receptor blocking antibody concentrations
- Iodine excess or deficiency suspected
  - Urinary iodine concentration
- Fetal hypothyroidism suspected
  - Knee radiograph for skeletal maturation

of the thyroid are done initially, including localization of the thyroid with uptake of radioactive tracers and thyroid sonography. Other, more specialized tests may be needed to detect specific inborn errors of thyroid synthesis. If results are positive, these tests may be followed by testing for specific gene mutations. If maternal autoimmune thyroid disease is suspected, determination of TSH receptor blocking antibody in the mother and infant is warranted.

Hyperthyroidism

In contrast to neonatal hypothyroidism, neonatal hyperthyroidism often is clinically apparent at birth or within the first 24 hours of life. Infants may be irritable, jittery, and excessively active. Other symptoms include sweating, tachycardia, hypertension, increased appetite, intrauterine growth retardation, lack of weight gain, goiter, and exophthalmos. Although goiters almost always are present in infants with thyrotoxicosis, the size may vary from quite large and clinically obvious to sufficiently small to escape notice. In severe neonatal hyperthyroidism, hyperthermia, arrhythmias, and high-output cardiac failure may occur and, if untreated, may lead to death.

Classically the hyperthyroidism subsides spontaneously after weeks to months as the titer of the TSH receptor stimulating antibody decreases. Although the goiter may persist after other signs of hyperthyroidism have ameliorated, it too gradually returns to normal size. The classic course of this syndrome may be modified by maternal treatment. Infants may be euthyroid or even hypothyroid at birth, becoming more typically hyperthyroid only after several days as the antithyroid agents are cleared.

The evaluation of infants with signs and symptoms of hyperthyroidism or infants with a maternal history of Graves disease before or during pregnancy should include physical examination and determination of free T_4 and

TSH. Assay for TSH receptor stimulating antibodies supports the diagnosis of neonatal thyrotoxicosis and serial determinations assist decision making regarding decreasing or stopping therapy.

MANAGEMENT

Hypothyroidism

All newborn infants with congenital hypothyroidism (whether or not they have goiter) should be treated as quickly as possible. Some infants, although they have a normal free T_4, also may warrant initial treatment. Specifically, infants with ectopic thyroid dysgenesis routinely should be treated, given the nearly universal later development of overt hypothyroidism. Infants with mild idiopathic hyperthyrotropinemia with consistently normal free T_4 values may be followed closely without treatment.

Treatment is with levothyroxine (Table 207-2). This form of thyroxine is absorbed reliably and has relatively uniform potency. The recommended initial dose for levothyroxine therapy is 10 to 15 µg/kg/day. Lower initial dosage of levothyroxine has been associated with decreased full-scale and verbal IQ scores. At this initial dosage, the serum free T_4 levels should approach the upper half of the normal range (1.4 to 2.3 ng/dL). Decreases in dosage may be needed if free T_4 exceeds the noted desired range, TSH decreases to less than 0.05 mU/L, or clinical symptoms of thyrotoxicosis develop.

Hyperthyroidism

Treatment of neonatal hyperthyroidism is with antithyroid medications. Propylthiouracil (5 to 10 mL/kg/day in three divided doses) is used to inhibit thyroid hormone synthesis and T_4 deiodinization. Iodine supplementation (Lugol solution, 1 drop three times daily) is used to suppress thyroid hormone synthesis and thyroid hormone secretion. Because circulating T_4 has a half-life in neonates of approximately 3 to 4 days, little or no clinical response to these medications should be expected for the first days of therapy. Many of the signs and symptoms of hyperthyroidism—most notably the cardiovascular manifestations—are related closely to increased adrenergic response. Consequently, β-adrenergic blockers (propranolol, 2 mg/kg/day) can alleviate many of the life-threatening effects of neonatal thyrotoxicosis on the cardiovascular system. Effects of this agent are evident within hours. In infants with severe cardiac failure, digitalization may also be necessary. In severe cases, prednisone (2 mL/kg/day) may be added to suppress deiodinization of T_4 to T_3. Finally, although typical congenital hypothyroidism secondary to neonatal Graves disease remits as

Table 207-2. Recommended Thyroxine Dosages for Age

Age	Thyroxine (µg/kg/day)
Initial dose	10–15
0–3 mo	8–12
3–6 mo	7–10
6–12 mo	6–8
1–3 yr	4–6
3–10 yr	3–5

maternal antibody decreases, hypothyroidism secondary to some other etiologies is more persistent and may require thyroid ablation.

OUTCOME

Hypothyroidism

Before the era of systematic screening at birth, the diagnosis of congenital hypothyroidism was based on clinical findings alone. During this era, the incidence of congenital hypothyroidism was estimated to be significantly lower than at present (1:5000 to 1:10,000). More importantly, because of the lack of specificity of the clinical signs and symptoms of early congenital hypothyroidism, the diagnosis often was delayed. During this era, it became obvious that early diagnosis was paramount if any hope of normal intellectual function was to be preserved (Fig. 207-1). Even when therapy prevented severe mental retardation, infants with congenital hypothyroidism frequently had neurodevelopmental outcomes that included deficient fine motor abilities and learning disabilities, especially with mathematic function. School success was particularly affected.

With routine neonatal screening, now in place since the 1980s, it is apparent that infants with congenital hypothyroidism who are treated adequately attain IQ values similar to those of matched controls. Nevertheless, some treated patients may exhibit an increased incidence of significant impairment of coordination and fine motor skills. The severity of these latter abnormalities correlates with initial serum T_4 levels and imply a prenatal effect. These neurologic deficits can impair school and social performance and suggest the need for psychometric evaluation of these children throughout early and later childhood.

Hyperthyroidism

In instances, where neonatal hyperthyroidism has been recognized appropriately and treatment has been initiated, the condition is self-limited and no long-term sequelae have

Table 207-3. American Academy of Pediatrics Recommendations for Follow-up of Infants with Congenital Hypothyroidism

Age	Frequency
Initiation of treatment	2 and 4 wk later
1 yr	Every 1–2 mo
2–3 yr	Every 2–3 mo
>3 yr	Every 3–12 mo through puberty

Goals: Serum T_4 (or free T_4) in the upper normal range and TSH suppressed (<10 mU/L)
Prevent overtreatment
Clinical evaluation may be at less frequent intervals

T_4, thyroxine; TSH, thyroid-stimulating hormone.

From American Academy of Pediatrics, AAP Section on Endocrinology and Committee on Genetics, and American Thyroid Association Committee on Public Health: Newborn Screening for congenital hypothyroidism: Recommended guidelines. Pediatrics 1993;91:1203–1209.

been noted. However, the cranial sutures in these infants may close prematurely and radiographic examination of the skull is recommended at 6 to 12 months of age.

FOLLOW-UP

Given the important effects of neonatal thyroid status on ultimate developmental outcome, the American Academy of Pediatrics has recommended especially close follow-up for the first 3 years of life (Table 207-3). These recommendations include initiation of replacement therapy as soon as possible. Thereafter, thyroid function should be checked every 1 to 2 months for the first year and every 2 to 3 months for the second and third years of life. Thyroid function also should be evaluated after every change in dose and whenever therapeutic adherence is a concern. At 3 years of age, the diagnosis should be re-evaluated to decide whether the hypothyroidism is permanent or transient, if transient hypothyroidism remains a possibility. After 3 years of age, treatment of congenital hypothyroidism becomes similar to that for other forms of acquired hypothyroidism, and dosage would be expected to decrease based on more occasional monitoring of T_4 and TSH status.

Mini-index of Related Topics   CH.

SUGGESTED READINGS

DeLange F: Neonatal hypothyroidism: Recent developments. Bailliere Clin Endocrinol Metab 1988;2:637–652.
DeLange F: Neonatal screening for congenital hypothyroidism: Results and perspectives. Horm Res 1997;48:51–61.
LaFranchi S: Congenital hypothyroidism: Etiologies, diagnosis, and management. Thyroid 1999;9:735–740.
Rose SR: Thyroid disorders. In Fanaroff AA, Martin RJ (eds): Neonatal-Perinatal Medicine: Diseases of the Fetus and Infant, 7th ed. St. Louis, Mosby, 2002, pp 1392–1416.
Van Wassenaer AG, Kok JH, de Vijlder JJ, et al: Effects of thyroxine supplementation on neurologic development in infants born at less than 30 weeks' gestation. N Engl J Med 1997;336:21–26.
Zimmerman D: Fetal and neonatal hyperthyroidism. Thyroid 1999; 9:727–733.

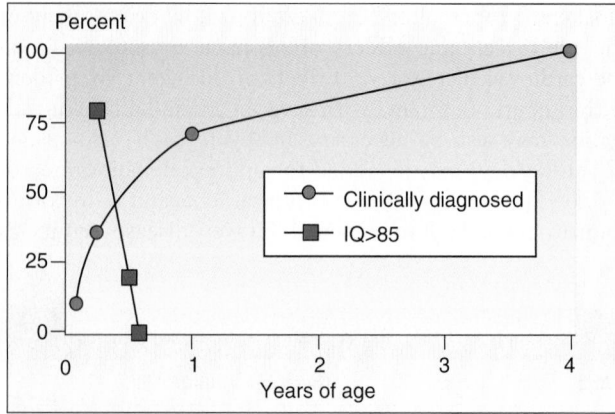

Figure 207-1. The incidence over time of untreated infants with hypothyroidism who eventually present with IQ greater than 85% is shown with the incidence of these infants diagnosed by clinical symptoms. The minimal number of infants who are diagnosed before irreversible intellectual compromise indicates the need for early screening.

208 Infants of Diabetic Mothers

David Lawrence and Henry T. Akinbi

Five percent of infants are delivered to mothers with diabetes mellitus. When maternal blood glucose levels are not controlled adequately during pregnancy, infants of diabetic mothers (IDM) are at significant risk for neonatal morbidities, including birth trauma from macrosomia, hypoglycemia, respiratory distress, and congenital anomalies. The incidence of diabetes in adolescents has increased by 50% since 1994. In the United States, 21% of 11- to 18-year-old obese adolescents have impaired glucose tolerance, a prediabetic condition. With the epidemic of obesity in American youths, the incidence of diabetes during pregnancy could double in 10 years. Most of the complications in IDM are preventable; others could be anticipated and managed appropriately to ensure uneventful transition to extrauterine life.

FUNDAMENTALS

Glucose is the major fuel used by the fetus for growth and development. Before birth, the fetus depends on a continuous transplacental flux of glucose from the mother. In the last trimester, increasing amounts of glucose are stored by the fetus as hepatic glycogen or converted to lipids for deposition of brown adipose tissue, an important source of energy in the immediate postnatal period. Pregnancy is associated with relative insulin resistance and increased levels of counterregulatory hormones (human placental lactogen, cortisol, progesterone, and prolactin). These factors predispose to diabetes. During pregnancy, the requirement for insulin increases threefold in diabetic women, and hepatic ketone production increases significantly. Diabetes mellitus during pregnancy may result in significant morbidity and mortality to the fetus and the neonate.

Epidemiology

Diabetes complicates 3% to 5% of all pregnancies. Gestational diabetes mellitus (GDM), defined as impaired glucose tolerance with onset or first recognition during pregnancy, accounts for 80% to 90% of these cases. GDM is diagnosed in the presence of two or more abnormal maternal plasma glucose values in a 1-hour oral glucose tolerance test after ingestion of 50 g of glucose (Table 208-1). Neonatal hypoglycemia is a common complication of GDM and is most commonly defined as a blood glucose level less than 40 mg/dL in term or preterm infants. This value is derived from analyses of measured blood glucose levels and their correlation with adverse neurodevelopmental outcomes at levels less than 40 mg/dL.

The severity of maternal diabetes is described using the modified White classification (Table 208-2). The risks of complications to the mother and fetus increase with increasing severity of disease. These risks of perinatal mortality and neonatal complications are reduced dramatically when plasma glucose levels are maintained at less than 100 mg/dL during pregnancy. Diabetes in pregnancy is associated with a twofold (3% to 5%) increase in perinatal mortality, and congenital anomalies are significantly greater relative to nondiabetic pregnancies (6% to 12% versus 2% to 3%). This excess mortality is primarily attributed to congenital malformations, respiratory distress syndrome, and extreme prematurity.

Overall, the incidence of diabetes parallels the rates in the general population and varies with different ethnic groups (Table 208-3). The incidence of GDM is 0.5% in gravidae who are younger than 20 years old and increases with advancing maternal age to 8% in gravidae 35 to 39 years old. Other risk factors for GDM include high prepregnancy weight, high body mass index, increased parity, previous infant who weighed greater than 9 lb, family history of diabetes, and history of repetitive miscarriages, neonatal death, or congenital malformations.

Pathophysiology

Glucose tolerance deteriorates during pregnancy with a twofold increase in fasting plasma insulin levels in the third trimester compared with levels in nonpregnant women.

Table 208-1. American Diabetes Association Recommended Criteria for Gestational Diabetes

Time	Glucose Level (mg/dL)
Fasting plasma glucose	≥105
1 hr	≥190
2 hr	≥165
3 hr	≥145

From American Diabetes Association: Position Statement: Gestational diabetes. Diabetes Care 1993;16(suppl 2):5.

coexist in IDM. Associated hyperviscosity may lead to intravascular thrombosis of the renal or adrenal veins in the IDM. Renal vein thrombosis presents as a flank mass, hematuria, and hypertension.

Congenital anomalies are more common in IDM, especially in poorly controlled diabetic mothers. These anomalies include ventricular septal hypertrophy and other cardiac anomalies (e.g., atrial septal defect, ventricular septal defect), gastrointestinal (e.g., left microcolon), and skeletal (e.g., sacral agenesis).

APPROACH TO DIAGNOSIS

The key point in diagnosis is a history of GDM. Possible complications of IDM should be anticipated. Infants who are depressed at birth should be monitored closely for signs of perinatal injury and respiratory distress. IDM should be examined carefully for congenital anomalies with special attention to the respiratory, cardiac, renal, gastrointestinal, and musculoskeletal systems. Signs of birth injury, such as clavicular fractures and Erb palsy, should be sought. Patients with suspected cardiac anomalies should be evaluated accordingly.

Of particular importance in the immediate newborn period are acute metabolic and hematologic derangements, including hypoglycemia, hypocalcemia, hypomagnesemia, polycythemia, and hyperbilirubinemia. The nadir of blood glucose usually occurs 2 to 4 hours after delivery. Often, hypoglycemic infants are asymptomatic. IDM should be screened for hypoglycemia and polycythemia within 2 hours of delivery or at the onset of symptoms. Follow-up testing is dictated by the initial results and intervention applied. Caring for IDM involves careful observation for symptoms of metabolic derangement, screening tests, and prompt management in the immediate postnatal period. IDM should be observed closely for hyperbilirubinemia and may not be ideal candidates for discharge from the nursery before 48 hours of age.

MANAGEMENT

Hypoglycemia

Asymptomatic infants with mild hypoglycemia (blood glucose 20 to 40 mg/dL) must be given oral feedings of formula or nursed on the breast promptly. Subsequently, blood glucose level should be monitored in 30 minutes and 2 hours after feeding to ensure normoglycemia is maintained. Regular feedings can be maintained in a scheduled fashion. If the blood glucose cannot be maintained at greater than 45 mg/dL after a feeding of formula or breastfeeding or if an infant is symptomatic, consideration should be given to continuous intravenous glucose infusion. For intravenous glucose therapy, an initial bolus of 2 mL/kg 10% dextrose in water is recommended. This bolus should be followed by continuous glucose infusion at a rate of 6 to 7 mg/kg/min. Large boluses of glucose should be avoided because they may result in rebound hypoglycemia. While vascular access is being obtained, it is appropriate to offer the infant oral feedings of formula if the child is alert and otherwise neurologically normal. In an emergency, intravenous access may be obtained via umbilical vein catheteri-

zation. As the blood glucose levels stabilize, the glucose infusion is weaned gradually, while oral feedings are increased. Infants who fail to respond to conventional therapy for hypoglycemia should be evaluated for other causes of neonatal hypoglycemia, such as islet-cell hyperplasia, Beckwith-Wiedemann syndrome, hypopituitarism, and hereditary congenital metabolic disorders.

Polycythemia and Hyperbilirubinemia

Infants with pathologic signs of polycythemia or asymptomatic infants with hematocrits greater than or equal to 70% should be considered for partial exchange transfusion, a procedure in which a portion of the infant's blood is removed and replaced with an equal volume of normal saline to decrease the hematocrit to about 50%. Treatment of hyperbilirubinemia depends on the level of total serum bilirubin and may require phototherapy or rarely double-volume exchange transfusion.

Hypocalcemia and Hypomagnesemia

Symptomatic hypocalcemia (seizures, tetany) should be treated with a slow intravenous bolus of 10% calcium gluconate, 4 mL/kg given over 10 minutes with continuous cardiac monitoring. Symptomatic hypomagnesemia should be treated with intravenous or intramuscular magnesium sulfate, 25 mg/kg per dose every 6 hours until normalization. Hypocalcemia and hypomagnesemia are transient and do not warrant aggressive correction in asymptomatic infants.

Management of Other Complications

Respiratory distress should be managed based on its severity. It is mild in most cases and can be managed with supplemental oxygen delivered through a head hood or nasal prongs. Rarely, respiratory distress may be severe enough to warrant continuous positive airway pressure, endotracheal intubation, surfactant replacement, and mechanical ventilation. Hypertrophic cardiomyopathy rarely requires specific therapy because it usually resolves spontaneously. In rare cases, a β-blocker may be indicated. Care should be taken before administering inotropes to IDM because of the risk of outflow obstruction. IDM with congenital abnormalities of the renal, gastrointestinal, or musculoskeletal systems should be referred to the appropriate specialist for further management.

CONCLUSIONS

IDM are at risk for significant morbidities from birth trauma, respiratory distress, metabolic derangement, and congenital malformations. The closer to physiologic range the mother's blood glucose is maintained, the better the neonatal outcome. Most neonatal complications are preventable through preconception counseling of diabetic women of childbearing age, scrupulous control of blood glucose during pregnancy, routine use of fetal ultrasound to measure fetal size and anatomy, and anticipation and management of neonatal complications. IDM require close surveillance and interdisciplinary collaboration among obstetricians, nutritionists, perinatologists, pediatricians, and sometimes endocrinologists.

SUGGESTED READINGS

Cowett RM: The infant of the diabetic mother. In Cowett RM (ed): Principles of Perinatal-Neonatal Metabolism. New York, Springer-Verlag, 1991.

Expert Committee on the Diagnosis and Classification of Diabetes Mellitus: Report of the Expert Committee on the Diagnosis and Classification of Diabetes Mellitus. Diabetes Care 1997;20:1183–1197.

Persson B, Hanson U: Neonatal morbidities in gestational diabetes. Diabetes Care 1998;21:S79–S84.

SECTION 5 NEWBORN CARE: *Infectious Diseases*

209

Infectious Diseases in the Neonate

David M. Coulter

ROLE OF THE GENERALIST

1 Diagnose newborns with congenital infections.
2 Provide acute treatment for newborns with congenital infections.
3 Coordinate long-term care of newborns with congenital infections.
4 Diagnose newborns with acute bacterial infections.
5 Stabilize and treat newborns with acute bacterial infections.
6 Refer ill newborns to appropriate care centers and specialists when needed for assistance with diagnosis, treatment, and management.

Infection is an important cause of morbidity and mortality in the neonatal period. Infections can be transmitted to the fetus from the maternal circulation via the placenta, can ascend through the birth canal infecting the fetus before the onset of labor or during the labor process, or, less commonly, can be acquired by the neonate after delivery. Maternal infections may have additional indirect adverse effects on the fetus. Cytokines produced during chorioamnionitis can reach the preterm fetus directly or may lead to vasoconstriction of placental vessels and produce hypoxemia or hypotension or both and subsequent brain injury. This chapter is divided into two broad areas: (1) infections acquired before the intrapartum period, so-called congenital infections, and (2) infections that arise around labor and during neonatal life. Human immunodeficiency virus and hepatitis B, infections that do not have immediate effects on the neonate but carry substantial risk of morbidity and mortality later in life, are discussed in other chapters.

ACUTE EARLY-ONSET BACTERIAL INFECTION

A newborn infant, especially a premature infant, is uniquely vulnerable to bacterial infection. Because all aspects of host defenses are impaired in neonates, bacterial infections in a newborn are more likely to become disseminated rather than remain localized. Early clinical signs of sepsis often are subtle and nonspecific. The mortality rate in infants with bacterial sepsis is high. Clinicians must remain extremely vigilant to make a prompt diagnosis and institute effective therapy. Case Study 209-1 describes the course of a newborn with early-onset bacterial infection.

Some infants who develop sepsis have definable risk factors for infection, but many do not. The fact that a woman is negative for group B streptococcus (GBS) earlier in pregnancy provides no assurance that she will remain so. The infant in Case Study 209-1 had no apparent risk factors for sepsis (e.g., preterm labor, prolonged rupture of membranes, maternal fever during labor, or instrumental delivery). She was ill immediately after birth, however. Although transient tachypnea was a likely diagnosis, it is a diagnosis of exclusion. In any situation in which a newborn has an abnormal transition or an unexplained deterioration in his or her clinical condition, sepsis must be considered a possibility. In the case study, failure to improve by 1 hour of age should have prompted a complete blood count (CBC) as part of an initial evaluation of possible infection. A normal CBC may occur during the transition from leukocytosis to granulocytopenia and is not reassuring. A follow-up CBC may be necessary to rule out sepsis. The infant's

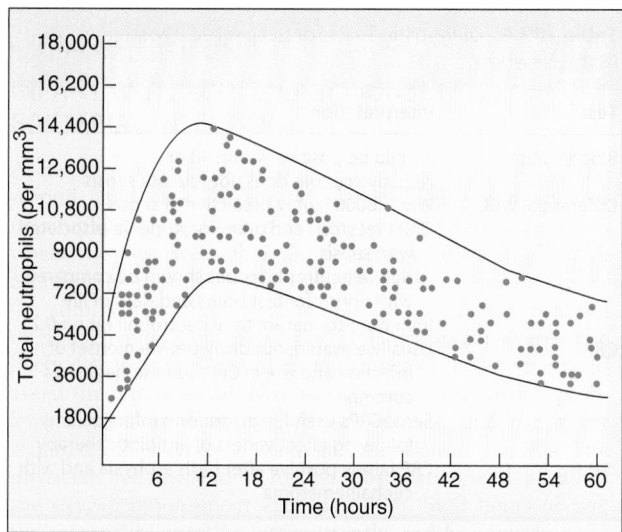

Figure 209-1. Absolute neutrophil count during the first hours and days of life (From Manroe BL, Weinberg AG, Rosenfeld CR, Browne R: The neonatal blood count in health and disease: I. Reference values for neutrophilic cells. J Pediatr 1979;95:89–91.)

not uncommon in infants who are infected based on clinical findings and other laboratory tests. Bacterial infection has been diagnosed at autopsy in infants who had negative blood cultures. A negative blood culture does not rule out sepsis.

Leukocytopenia (white blood cell count <6000) is highly predictive of bacteremia. Granulocytosis and granulocytopenia are associated with sepsis. Granulocytopenia is an ominous prognostic sign. The range of normal for the absolute neutrophil count varies during the first hours and days of life. Values should be compared with the norms for term infants described in Figure 209-1. An elevated immature-to-total neutrophil ratio (>0.2) also is associated with sepsis. Toxic granulation of neutrophils is another sign of bacterial infection. Normal values for these indices do not exclude a diagnosis of sepsis. Serial tests are more informative than single measurements.

C-reactive protein (CRP), an acute phase reactant, usually becomes elevated during bacterial sepsis. There is a delay between the onset of infection and an increase in CRP, so initial false-negative tests are common. Serial CRP determinations can be useful in diagnosing sepsis and may aid in defining duration of therapy. Preliminary data suggest that antibiotic therapy can be stopped when the CRP becomes normal. False-positive CRP levels occur after birth asphyxia and with cephalhematomas.

Treatment

Early aggressive empirical use of broad-spectrum antibiotics in infants with clinical illness is the key to preventing mortality from neonatal sepsis. Therapy should be tailored to treat the organisms that usually cause these infections. Current recommendations are ampicillin and gentamicin. Use of cephalosporins for routine sepsis coverage is discouraged because of the probable development of resistance to these drugs when they are used commonly in nurseries and because they do not cover *Listeria monocytogenes*. They may be appropriate in certain clinical situations, such as

renal failure (reduced nephrotoxicity) or CNS infection with susceptible organisms (enhanced cerebrospinal fluid [CSF] penetration).

Along with new recommendations for intrapartum antibiotic prophylaxis, the CDC published a management algorithm for infants whose mothers had been treated with antibiotics before delivery (Fig. 209-2). Adherence to this approach spares some patients antibiotic treatment, while ensuring that patients with a definable risk of bacterial infection receive appropriate therapy.

Culture results may modify the choice of antibiotics. The recommended duration of therapy is 7 to 10 days, unless there is focal infection, such as meningitis. There is no scientific basis to define duration of treatment. Shorter courses may be reasonable if the CRP normalizes. Research currently in progress may clarify this issue.

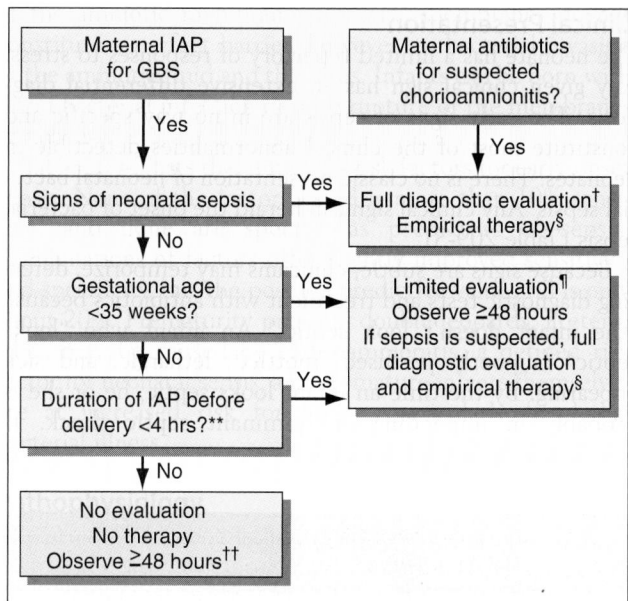

Figure 209-2. Sample algorithm for management of a newborn whose mother received intrapartum antimicrobial agents for prevention of early-onset group B streptococcal disease* or suspected chorioamnionitis. This algorithm is not an exclusive course of management. Variations that incorporate individual circumstances or institutional preferences may be appropriate.
*If no maternal intrapartum prophylaxis (IAP) for group B streptococcus (GBS) was administered despite an indication being present, data are insufficient on which to recommend a single management strategy.
†Includes complete blood count and differential, blood culture, and chest radiograph if respiratory abnormalities are present. When signs of sepsis are present, a lumbar puncture, if feasible, should be performed.
§Duration of therapy varies depending on results of blood cultures; cerebrospinal fluid findings, if obtained; and the clinical course of the infant. If laboratory results and clinical course do not indicate bacterial infection, duration may be only 48 hours.
¶Complete blood count with differential and blood culture.
**Applies only to penicillin, ampicillin, or cefazolin and assumes recommended closing regimens.
††A healthy-appearing infant who was 38 or more weeks' gestation at delivery and whose mother received 4 or more hours of intrapartum prophylaxis before delivery may be discharged home after 24 hours if other discharge criteria have been met and a person able to comply fully with instructions for home observation will be present. If any one of these conditions is not met, the infant should be observed in the hospital for at least 48 hours and until criteria for discharge are achieved.
(From Centers for Disease Control. Prevention of perinatal group B streptococcal disease. MMWR Morb Mortal Wkly Rep 2002;51[RR-11]:1.)

Adjunctive therapy can improve outcomes. According to a meta-analysis, intravenous immunoglobulin reduces mortality in infants who are granulocytopenic, a group at increased risk of fatal sepsis. It also speeds resolution of granulocytopenia. Preliminary data suggest that use of colony-stimulating factors also may improve outcome in granulocytopenic infants. These data are not yet sufficient, however, to recommend use of these cytokines outside of prospective studies. Other supportive therapy is directed at specific organ system dysfunction.

LATE-ONSET SEPSIS

Infections presenting beyond the first days of life are considered late-onset infections. Previously healthy term infants may present with signs of focal infection (e.g., pneumonia, gastroenteritis, omphalitis, skin lesions, osteomyelitis) or nonspecific findings (e.g., respiratory distress, poor feeding, lethargy, irritability, seizure, apnea, jaundice). In this age group, meningitis and urinary tract infections are more common than in the immediate neonatal period, so the initial diagnostic assessment should include a lumbar puncture and urine culture obtained by bladder tap or aseptically obtained catheter specimens. Bag urine specimens usually are contaminated and have virtually no value. Urinalysis is useful if positive, but pyuria often is absent in neonatal urinary tract infection, so negative results are uninformative. Ampicillin resistance is more common in infants with late-onset, gram-negative infections whose mothers received intrapartum ampicillin prophylaxis for GBS.

Although bacterial pathogens frequently are responsible, viral etiologies must also be considered. During the first 2 weeks of life, specimens from the eye, nasopharynx, and rectum should be sent for herpes simplex virus (HSV) polymerase chain reaction (PCR) or culture or both. Neonatally acquired HSV infections typically present at 3 to 5 days of life and often mimic bacterial sepsis. In this age group, empirical antibiotic coverage should include antiherpetic therapy (see Case Study 209-2).

GBS, most commonly a problem of term infants, with onset from 1 to 12 weeks of life, also can affect premature infants. Typically, affected infants have an unremarkable neonatal course before presenting with fever, tachypnea, poor feeding, or nonspecific CNS signs of irritability or lethargy. Most of these infants are thought to have been colonized with GBS during delivery. Late-onset infections have occurred, however, after prolonged treatment with appropriate antibiotics in the immediate neonatal period, suggesting that recolonization with the organism may play a role in pathogenesis. In contrast with early-onset sepsis, meningitis is much more common in late-onset disease. A lumbar puncture is essential in assessment of any infant who presents with possible sepsis beyond the first days of life.

Although *Staphylococcus aureus* currently is an uncommon nursery pathogen, this organism was the cause of multiple outbreaks of infection in nurseries during the first half of the 20th century, peaking in the 1950s. The cyclic nature of *S. aureus* nursery infections remains unexplained. The organism usually is acquired from the hands of nursery personnel, so meticulous attention to hand washing is a mainstay of preventive techniques. As few as 10 organisms can produce cord colonization. Most infants in nurseries are colonized within the first 5 days of life. Vertical transmission is rare. Despite ubiquitous carriage of the organism, infection in the nursery is uncommon. Typically, infants develop skin infection (including the umbilical cord or circumcision site) or pneumonia 2 weeks to 2 months after discharge. *S. aureus* can cause the typical neonatal sepsis syndrome. Skin manifestations of infection include bullous impetigo and, less commonly, scalded skin syndrome. Toxic shock syndrome in newborns occurs but is rare. Nosocomial infection with this organism is more common in neonatal intensive care unit (NICU) patients with indwelling catheters, surgical incisions, or endotracheal tubes.

L. monocytogenes is a gram-positive rod, but its morphology depends on the culture medium. In Gram stains of amniotic fluid, it can appear as chains of gram-positive cocci and be misidentified as streptococci. *Listeria* is common in the natural environment and is a frequent pathogen of farm animals, causing abortion and CNS infections. Most human infections are associated with contaminated food, particularly chicken, and dairy products such as homemade soft cheese. Maternal infections have protean manifestations, ranging from a mild flulike illness to frank sepsis. The organism has a predilection for the fetoplacental unit in humans and animals. It can reach the fetus via the placenta or by an ascending route. Similar to GBS, neonatal infection can present early, during the first days of life, or late, after 1 week of age. *Listeria* causes a typical neonatal sepsis syndrome, clinically indistinguishable from infection with other bacteria. Nosocomial transmission can occur in nurseries. Ampicillin is the drug of choice for neonatal listeriosis. Resistance to gentamicin has been reported, and resistance to cephalosporins is typical. The possibility of *Listeria* infection provides a strong rationale for continued use of ampicillin in the initial treatment of suspected neonatal sepsis.

Mycoplasma species are ubiquitous organisms in fetal and neonatal infection and in premature birth. *Mycoplasma hominis* and *Ureaplasma urealyticum* can cause chorioamnionitis. *Ureaplasma* is a cause of neonatal pneumonia, particularly in premature infants less than 34 weeks' gestation. Data conflict concerning the role of these organisms in the cause of bronchopulmonary dysplasia. A predominance of evidence seems to implicate *Ureaplasma*, however, as a causative agent or cofactor in the lung injury that leads to bronchopulmonary dysplasia. *Mycoplasma* and *Ureaplasma* can cause CNS infection in neonates.

Diagnosis of mycoplasmal infection is by culture, though PCR methods are under development. The presence of the organisms in normally sterile loci together with symptomatic disease is considered sufficient to diagnose infection.

Treatment is controversial. No prospective studies are available to make evidence-based decisions regarding treatment. Positive cultures in the absence of clinical illness do not warrant treatment. Many practitioners treat premature infants with worsening lung disease if these organisms are present in a tracheal aspirate. Treatment of infants who have positive CSF cultures without pleocytosis is controversial. Erythromycin is the drug of choice, but it does not penetrate the CNS. Chloramphenicol would be a

Bacteriuria in a specimen obtained by bladder tap or aseptic bladder catheterization is diagnostic of urinary tract infection. Bag urine specimens always are contaminated by perineal organisms and are unreliable. Urinalysis frequently fails to show pyuria. Blood cultures are often positive. After resolution of the acute infection, radiologic imaging is indicated to identify vesicoureteral reflux or anatomic abnormalities. Current recommendations are to obtain an ultrasound assessment followed by a voiding cystourethrogram. Renal scans have been recommended for situations in which ultrasound suggests renal parenchymal damage or in which there is grade 3 or greater vesicoureteral reflux (see Chapter 172).

Therapy

Initial intravenous therapy to treat the expected organisms consists of ampicillin and gentamicin except in hospitalized infants at risk for coagulase-negative staphylococcal infections. Focused therapy depends on culture and sensitivity results.

Omphalitis

Bacterial colonization of the cord stump normally occurs in the first hours of life. Multiple organisms have been cultured from this site, but staphylococci predominate. Colonization and the consequent inflammatory response seem necessary for cord separation. Colonization can progress to cellulitis or more invasive infection, such as arteritis, ascending venous infection and portal venous thrombosis, and necrotizing fasciitis. The last-mentioned entity usually has a polymicrobial etiology with staphylococci present and comes with a high mortality rate.

Diagnosis

Expanding erythema and induration characterize early omphalitis (Fig. 209-3). Blood cultures are indicated. Aspirated material from the advancing edge of the process may yield the infecting organism. Necrotizing fasciitis, infection spreading along subcutaneous planes and fascial sheaths, presents as rapidly spreading erythema and induration, sometimes in association with blue/black skin discoloration, vesicles, bullae, and signs of acute illness.

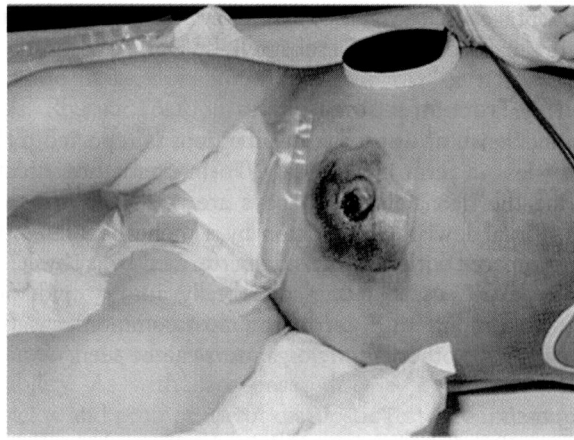

Figure 209-3. A neonate with fatal omphalitis from *Clostridium perfringens*. (From Hart CA, Broadhead RL: Color Atlas of Pediatric Infectious Disease. St. Louis, Mosby-Year Book, 1992, p 24.)

Treatment

Broad-spectrum coverage, including an antistaphylococcal agent, is the initial approach. Topical agents have been used when only mild erythema is present, but evidence of efficacy is lacking. Signs of necrotizing fasciitis mandate referral to a tertiary center. Surgical therapy consists of wide resection of all involved tissue. This complication often is fatal.

Ophthalmia Neonatorum

Neonatal conjunctivitis is common, often caused by *Chlamydia trachomatis* or *Neisseria gonorrhoeae*. Infection is acquired through transmission of these bacteria from the genital tract of the infected mother. Acquisition of *C. trachomatis* occurs in approximately 50% of vaginally born infants if the mother is infected, with 25% to 50% contracting conjunctivitis and another 5% to 20% developing pneumonia 1 to 3 months after birth. The incubation period of *N. gonorrhoeae* is much shorter, with infection usually appearing within 2 to 5 days of birth. Gonococcal conjunctivitis also can be acquired later in infancy through inoculation by contaminated fingers of adults.

Diagnosis

Presentation of *C. trachomatis* can be variable, ranging from mild conjunctival injection with a slight mucoid discharge to purulent exudates, chemosis, and pseudomembrane formation (Fig. 209-4). The conjunctiva may be friable and bleed when swabbed. Gonococcal conjunctivitis begins with mild inflammation with serosanguineous discharge, which then progresses to a thick, purulent discharge within 24 hours with chemosis. If treatment is delayed, infection can spread to the deeper layers of the conjunctiva and the cornea. *N. gonorrhoeae* also can cause scalp abscess and disseminated infection.

Pneumonia from *C. trachomatis* presents between 1 and 3 months of age, usually with an insidious onset of persistent, staccato cough and tachypnea without fever. Rales without wheezing may be present on physical examination—a sign that can be helpful in distinguishing chlamydial pneumonia from respiratory syncytial viral pneumonia.

Purulent discharge from the eye should be examined by Gram stain for the characteristic intracellular gram-negative diplococci of *N. gonorrhoeae* and sent for culture. Because *Chlamydia* species are obligate intracellular organisms, epithelial cells obtained from a conjunctival scraping must be included in the culture specimen. Nucleic acid amplification methods, such as PCR and ligase chain reaction, are more sensitive than cell culture. Presence of intracytoplasmic inclusion bodies on Giemsa stain of conjunctival scrapings is diagnostic but is less accurate, with its sensitivity dependent on the quality of specimen collection and the examiner's expertise.

Infants with chlamydial pneumonia may have a peripheral eosinophilia (>400 cells/mm^3). Chest x-ray shows hyperinflation with minimal interstitial or alveolar infiltrates.

Treatment

Recommended treatment for *C. trachomatis* conjunctivitis is oral erythromycin (50 mg/kg/day in four divided doses) for 2 weeks to clear the conjunctivitis and reduce the risk

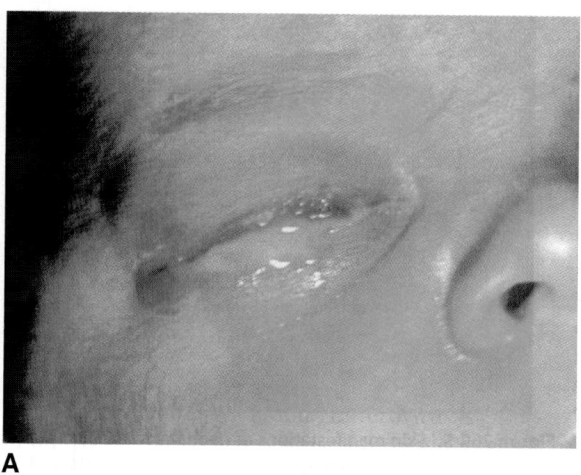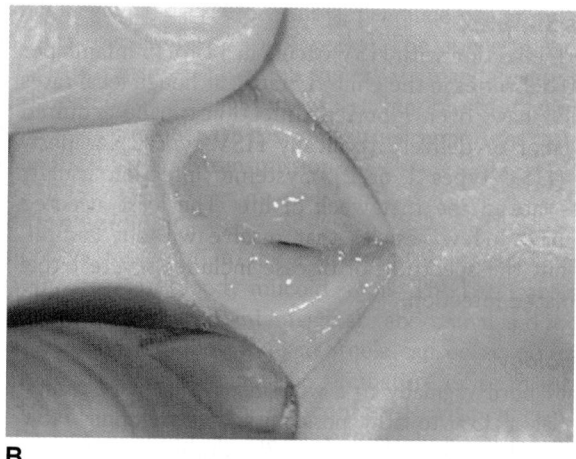

Figure 209-4. A, A neonate with a purulent ocular discharge from *Chlamydia trachomatis*. **B,** A neonate with the eyelid everted to show palpebral inflammation from *C. trachomatis*. (From Hart CA, Broadhead RL: Color Atlas of Pediatric Infectious Disease. St. Louis, Mosby-Year Book, 1992, p 22.)

of later pneumonia. An association between oral erythromycin and idiopathic hypertrophic pyloric stenosis has been reported in infants younger than 6 weeks of age. Because the risk has not been confirmed and alternative therapies not yet studied, the American Academy of Pediatrics continues to recommend use of erythromycin.

Infants with clinical evidence of infection with *N. gonorrhoeae* should be hospitalized. For ophthalmia neonatorum, recommended antimicrobial therapy is ceftriaxone (25 to 50 mg/kg intravenously or intramuscularly, not to exceed 125 mg) given once. A single does of cefotaxime (100 mg/kg given intravenously or intramuscularly) is an alternative. If infection is disseminated, recommended therapy is ceftriaxone (25 to 50 mg/kg intravenously or intramuscularly, given once per day) for 7 days. If the infant is hyperbilirubinemic, cefotaxime (50 mg/kg/day given intravenously or intramuscularly in two divided doses) for 7 days is recommended. Documented meningitis should be treated for 10 to 14 days.

Prevention
The best prevention for *C. trachomatis* and *N. gonorrhoeae* is prenatal screening and treatment of pregnant women. Eye prophylaxis with 1% silver nitrate solution, 0.5% erythromycin ointment, or 1% tetracycline ointment are equally effective in preventing gonococcal ocular infection. Topical antibiotics and silver nitrate have not been shown to be effective in preventing either conjunctivitis or nasopharyngeal colonization with subsequent risk of pneumonia from *C. trachomatis*.

Outcome
Outcome of *Chlamydia* infection is excellent, although some infants may require a second course of treatment. If ophthalmia from *N. gonorrhoeae* is not treated promptly and adequately, corneal ulceration, rupture, and blindness may follow.

Other Focal Bacterial Infections
Osteomyelitis, septic arthritis, and other focal infections are relatively rare. Other focal infections are covered in chapters on the specific organ system involved (e.g., Chapter 54).

ACUTE VIRAL INFECTIONS

Case Study 209-2 describes an acute viral infection in a newborn. The most likely diagnosis in this infant was bacterial pneumonia. Beyond the first day of life, however, the possibility of neonatal viral infections also must be entertained. Routine empirical antibiotic therapy should be planned to cover likely bacterial pathogens and possible HSV infections. Prompt institution of treatment with acyclovir could have altered the outcome in Case Study 209-2.

CASE STUDY 209-2

ACUTE VIRAL INFECTION IN A NEWBORN

A healthy primiparous 24-year-old married woman had a normal pregnancy and an uncomplicated vaginal delivery at term. The infant was discharged home at 48 hours of age, feeding well and in good condition. The mother brought him to the pediatrician's office on the 5th day of life because he was breathing rapidly and seemed warm. The infant had a temperature of 38°C and was tachypneic with mild retractions. On arrival at the children's hospital, the infant's oxygen saturation in room air was 83%. He was still febrile with mild respiratory distress. Chest x-ray showed asymmetric, nonhomogeneous infiltrates. The white blood cell count was 26,000 (57% polymorphonuclear neutrophils, 22% bands). Lumbar puncture results were normal. After bacterial cultures were obtained, the infant received ampicillin and gentamicin. Over the next 12 hours, his condition progressively deteriorated. He required mechanical ventilation. The pulmonary infiltrates became more dense and homogeneous. Jaundice developed, his platelet count fell, and liver function tests were consistent with hepatitis. After viral cultures were obtained, he was started on acyclovir. Neither the mother nor the father had any history of herpes infection. His subsequent clinical course consisted of progressively worsening pulmonary function, coagulopathy, and circulatory failure, and he died 2 days later. Viral cultures grew herpes simplex type II.

Infected individuals are believed to be able to transmit the virus during the period beginning 2 days before the appearance of the characteristic rash and ending 5 days after its onset or when all lesions are crusted. The virus is spread by respiratory droplets and direct contact with vesicles. The presence of an infected individual in a nursery represents potential infection for infants in direct contact with the individual or exposed to respiratory droplets. Premature infants born before 28 weeks' gestation are at particular risk because they have not received maternal antibody transplacentally. Similarly, any infant whose mother has not had chickenpox or been immunized to the disease is at risk.

Pathophysiology

Varicella zoster virus can cause severe, life-threatening disease in neonates, although typical chickenpox is more common. Severe disease is characterized by large numbers of vesicles, pneumonia, and hemorrhagic complications.

Treatment

Prevention is the best therapy. Infected individuals should be kept out of nurseries. If a mother develops varicella, separation from the infant during the period of transmissibility is recommended, even if passive immunization is used. Nursery exposure is defined by the presence of an infected person in the same two- to four-bed room, the presence of an infected person in adjacent beds in a large unit, face-to-face contact with an infected person, or direct contact with an infected person.

Varicella-zoster immune globulin administered to susceptible infants after exposure can reduce the risk of infection and may decrease severity. It is not indicated for healthy, full-term infants. Varicella-zoster immune globulin is available through the American Red Cross. Acyclovir may reduce the severity of disease. Based on its minimal toxicity, acyclovir treatment of exposed infants may be reasonable. It must be given intravenously. One publication reported effective prophylaxis when newborns whose mothers had chickenpox within 2 weeks of delivery were given intravenous immune globulin and acyclovir.

CONGENITAL INFECTIONS

Congenital infections are infections acquired before the perinatal period. Infections acquired by the fetus early in gestation may result in fetal loss. Some organisms can produce chronic infections in the fetus that have profound lasting effects. Although most of these organisms are viruses, some bacteria and parasites cause illnesses that fall into this category. These are the so-called *TORCH* infections (*t*oxoplasmosis, *o*ther, *r*ubella, *c*ytomegalovirus [CMV], *h*erpes). This acronym has become increasingly obsolete with the recognition that so many "other" organisms can cause chronic fetal infection. Klein and Remington suggested the update *TORCHES CLAP* (Table 209-5). Box 209-1 lists some of the organisms that can cause congenital infections, listed in order of prevalence in the United States. This chapter discusses only organisms encountered commonly in developed countries.

Table 209-5. Congenital Infectious Agents of TORCHES CLAP

Toxoplasma gondii	TO
Rubella	R
Cytomegalovirus	C
Herpes simplex	H
Enteroviruses	E
Syphilis	S
Chickenpox	C
Lyme disease	L
AIDS	A
Parvovirus B19	P

AIDS, acquired immunodeficiency syndrome.

Despite the broad range of organisms from viruses to parasites, similarities among the illnesses that result from this fetal infection are remarkable. The earlier in gestation the infection begins, the worse the long-term effects. Very early infection can result in fetal loss or stillbirth. Later infections may cause fetal growth retardation or hydrops fetalis, microcephaly, ocular abnormalities, hepatosplenomegaly, and petechiae. Infections acquired later in gestation can be asymptomatic at birth and the infection or its effects (e.g., hearing loss) may not become manifest weeks to years later. Suspicion of congenital infection with one member of this group mandates assessment for others to ensure that the appropriate diagnosis is made.

Cytomegalovirus

CMVs are the largest members of the herpesvirus family. They are species specific and are distributed widely in mammals. Characteristic of infected tissues are enlarged cells with inclusions in the nucleus and cytoplasm.

Epidemiology

CMV is the most frequently diagnosed congenital infection in the United States, where about 1% of infants have viruria at birth. Less than 15% of these infants have clinical signs of CMV infection. The virus is endemic in all human populations. Transplacental infection can occur during the viremia of primary maternal infection, during the viremia of secondary maternal infection with a new strain of CMV, or during reactivation of latent infection. Typically, primary or secondary maternal infection is asymptomatic. The most severe fetal involvement seems to result from primary

Box 209-1. Organisms Causing Congenital Infections, Listed by Prevalence

- Cytomegalovirus
- *Toxoplasma gondii*
- Rubella
- *Treponema pallidum*
- Varicella zoster
- Human immunodeficiency virus type I
- Herpes simplex
- Parvovirus
- *Borrelia burgdorferi*
- *Plasmodium*
- *Trypanosoma cruzi*

maternal infection. Of women who contract primary CMV infection, however, only 30% to 40% transmit the virus to their fetus.

Pregnancy is the only definable risk factor for reactivation of latent disease. Mere isolation of the virus during a pregnancy does not define risk of fetal involvement. New data suggest that the risk of fetal infection is determined in part by the affinity of maternal antibodies for specific viral antigens. Viruria in healthy, asymptomatic neonates presents a significant risk of transmission to susceptible health care workers. The 10% to 20% prevalence of viruria in older infants highlights the risk of transmission to childcare workers and hospital personnel. Nosocomial transmission of the virus among infants in a nursery is rare. Neonates can become infected during delivery, rarely from virus in breast milk, or from transfusions. The risk of transfusion transmission of CMV is reduced by leukocyte depletion and irradiation of donated blood. Because of the high prevalence of CMV carriage in many areas, selection of CMV-negative donors may be impractical.

Pathogenesis

About one third of infants with symptomatic CMV infection are born prematurely. The virus infects multiple organ systems. The worst sequelae are caused by CNS infection. CMV causes a focal encephalitis followed by gliosis and calcification, typically in a periventricular distribution. Inner ear involvement results in hearing loss, the most common sequela of congenital CMV infection. Chorioretinitis occurs in less than 20% of symptomatic infants. CMV hepatitis produces typical laboratory evidence of moderate hepatic cellular injury and cholestasis. Marrow involvement manifests as thrombocytopenia that may persist for a prolonged period. Renal infection results in persisting viruria without evidence of renal dysfunction. About 25% to 30% of infants with clinically apparent congenital CMV have a distinctive defect of the dental enamel. The teeth have a yellow discoloration, are fragile, and chip easily. Primary dentition is much more severely involved than secondary teeth. Severe pneumonitis is frequent in neonatally acquired CMV but relatively rare in congenital infection. About one quarter of boys with congenital CMV infection have inguinal hernias.

Diagnosis

Typical presenting signs of CMV infection at birth are petechiae, hepatosplenomegaly, and jaundice (Fig. 209-6). The most severely affected infants are growth restricted and have microcephaly. Laboratory evaluation reveals thrombocytopenia, moderate elevations of transaminases, and conjugated hyperbilirubinemia.

Growth of CMV from urine specimens obtained during the first 2 weeks of life establishes the diagnosis of congenital CMV. PCR is useful to detect viral DNA in CSF. Besides urine culture, the initial assessment of an infant with suspected congenital CMV infection should include skull x-rays to detect calcifications, lumbar puncture, ophthalmologic examination, baseline neurologic assessment, and hearing screening. The differential diagnosis includes congenital rubella syndrome, congenital toxo-

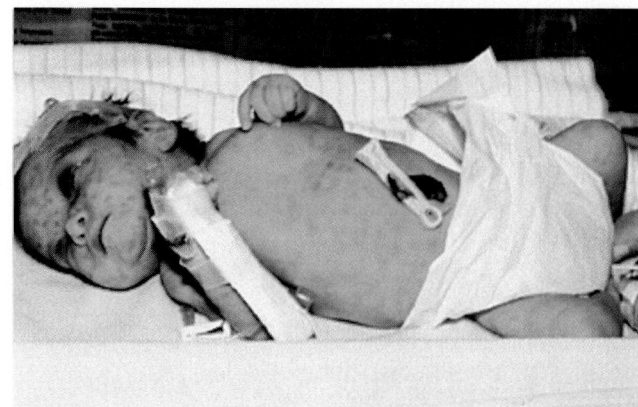

Figure 209-6. Newborn with symptomatic congenital cytomegalovirus infection. This 3-day-old infant was born with hepatosplenomegaly, jaundice, ecchymosis, petechiae, and purpuric skin lesions. (From Mandell GL: Atlas of Infectious Diseases, Vol XI. Pediatric Infectious Diseases. Philadelphia, Churchill Livingstone, 1999, p 12.10.)

plasmosis, congenital syphilis, neonatal HSV infection, and bacterial sepsis. Isolated conjugated hyperbilirubinemia or thrombocytopenia has a much broader range of diagnostic possibilities. Imaging reveals periventricular intracranial calcifications.

Treatment

At present, there is no treatment for congenital CMV infection. Drugs effective against other herpesviruses have not shown efficacy against CMV. Gancyclovir is under investigation for this use. Treatment reduces viral load substantially, but so far there are no data concerning changes in prognosis.

Prognosis

Mortality in seriously affected infants approaches 30%, and risk of long-term sequelae in infants who have symptomatic CMV infection is high. Sensorineural hearing loss is present in almost 60% of survivors. Infants who have microcephaly, intracranial calcifications, and chorioretinitis have the worst neurologic prognosis. There is no clear relationship between an adverse neurologic outcome and neonatal CMV disease characterized by transient organ dysfunction (petechiae, hepatosplenomegaly, premature birth). Hepatitis and thrombocytopenia may take months to resolve. Despite marked thrombocytopenia, severe hemorrhage is uncommon. Infants who have asymptomatic CMV infections have a much lower risk of sequelae. Of these children, 10% to 15% develop abnormalities in the first 2 years of life, most commonly hearing loss. More severe sequelae also occur.

Toxoplasmosis

In the United States, 1 to 8 infants per 1000 births are infected with toxoplasmosis. The organism, *Toxoplasma gondii*, is ubiquitous in the world but is slightly more prevalent in warmer climates.

Epidemiology

Prevalence of *T. gondii* infection is related to dietary habits. In Paris, the high rate of conversion to seropositivity during pregnancy has been attributed to the French preference for raw or undercooked meat. The cat is the domestic reservoir that accounts for most infections during pregnancy in the United States. Oocytes from cat feces contaminate food or water. Parasitemia in the mother, often asymptomatic, results in transplacental passage to the fetus. When a woman becomes infected, she can become a chronic carrier of the parasite, but transmission to the fetus does not occur in this state.

Pathogenesis

Toxoplasma is an obligate intracellular protozoan. The tachyzoite, the actively reproducing stage, multiplies rapidly in host cells and then induces cell lysis. Its offspring invade adjacent cells, and the process is repeated. The end result is areas of necrosis surrounded by an inflammatory response. The organism is capable of persisting in the form of tissue cysts. These cysts can reactivate if immunodeficiency develops later in life. Severe fetal involvement is rare in infections that begin after the first half of pregnancy.

Diagnosis

The clinical spectrum of congenital toxoplasmosis is broad. Severely affected infants may have multisystem involvement. Typical signs include hydrocephalus, chorioretinitis, hepatosplenomegaly, petechiae, and seizures. Fever, jaundice, and pneumonitis are seen less frequently. Infants with this degree of involvement represent only 10% of all congenital infection, however. About two thirds of infected infants have no clinical signs at birth, but more thorough investigation of these infants often reveals CSF abnormalities (elevated protein, pleocytosis), chorioretinitis, or intracranial calcifications (Fig. 209-7).

The diagnosis can be established during pregnancy, but a high index of suspicion is required. The illness is symptomatic in only 10% to 20% of adults. In countries with a relatively low incidence of toxoplasmosis, serologic testing of pregnant women is not routine. If the disease is diagnosed in a pregnant patient, fetal assessment is indicated. The diagnosis of fetal infection rests on the growth of the

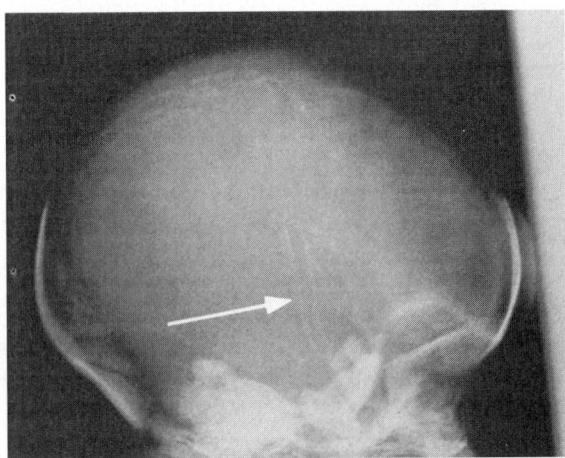

Figure 209-7. Lateral skull x-ray of a child with congenital toxoplasmosis. Intracerebral calcification is clearly visible. (From Hart CA, Broadhead RL: Color Atlas of Pediatric Infectious Disease. St. Louis, Mosby-Year Book, 1992, p 18.)

organism in mice from samples of fetal blood or amniotic fluid. Serologic tests also can be helpful. Fetal ultrasound may identify hydrocephalus or ascites.

Pathologic examination of the placenta can diagnose congenital toxoplasmosis. About 70% of infected infants have the organism in their blood during the first week of life. Serologic testing can establish the diagnosis. The double sandwich IgM enzyme-linked immunosorbent assay detects about 75% of congenitally infected infants. IgA enzyme-linked immunosorbent assay has diagnosed infection when the IgM serology was negative. Testing for toxoplasmosis using IgG antibodies requires serial testing over several months. PCR for the B1 gene is more sensitive than other methods. Lumbar puncture and cranial imaging seeking the characteristic punctate calcifications also are indicated.

Treatment

Toxoplasmosis can be prevented. Pregnant women should be cautioned about avoiding ungloved contact with cat feces or litter boxes, forgoing raw or undercooked meat and careful hand washing after handling raw meat.

The disease is treatable when a prenatal diagnosis is established. Neonatal disease is treated for at least 1 year with combinations of drugs, including folate antagonists and antibiotics. Pyrimethamine and sulfadiazine are used in older patients. Clindamycin can replace sulfa. For neonates, folinic acid supplementation is used in conjunction with sulfadiazine. Caregivers are reminded that sulfa drugs should not be used in jaundiced neonates because they increase the risk of bilirubin encephalopathy. Corticosteroids may be indicated to reduce the local inflammatory response to the organism, but their use is considered controversial.

Prognosis

Earlier infection leads to worse outcomes. The prognosis for severely affected infants is believed to be so poor that termination of pregnancy has been considered a reasonable option. Drug therapy prenatally and during the first year of life has made substantial improvements, however, in the outlook for infected infants with clinical signs of toxoplasmosis at birth. Nonetheless, published experiences describe significant CNS sequelae (seizures, developmental delays) despite treatment. In the absence of treatment, many infants without initial clinical signs develop symptomatic disease, in particular, neurologic signs (seizures, spasticity, mental retardation) and eye disease later in life. Even late-trimester infection can cause long-term CNS sequelae. Ocular involvement develops in most and has been reported to occur 10 years after birth.

Syphilis

Treponema pallidum is a motile, gram-negative spirochete. It cannot be grown in culture media. Fetal infection was rare in the United States for the 3 decades ending in the 1980s and became progressively more frequent in association with the epidemic of crack cocaine use. A 1998 initiative by the CDC to eliminate syphilis in the United States reduced the rate of congenital syphilis from 27.8 per 100,000 live-born infants in 1997 to 13.4 in 2000. Cases of congenital syphilis were associated with lack of prenatal care, maternal age younger than 19, and illicit drug use. Racial/ethnic minorities in the South were disproportionately affected.

Epidemiology

In adults, *T. pallidum* gains entrance to the body via breaks in epithelial barriers, most commonly from sexual activity. Shared needles account for much of the transmission among intravenous drug abusers. The fetus becomes infected via the placenta from organisms in the maternal circulation; this can occur during the initial episode of secondary syphilis or during subsequent relapses during the latent stage. Although transmission is most common during the second half of pregnancy, it can occur during the first trimester. Fetuses infected early in gestation may die before birth or can have severe neonatal illness. Fetuses who are infected during the third trimester—most neonates with congenital syphilis—may be asymptomatic at birth. These infants usually develop clinical signs of syphilis during the first weeks of life, although the disease can remain occult until puberty.

Pathophysiology

The organisms are carried initially to the fetal liver, where they reproduce and are disseminated to the rest of the body. Their most common loci of invasion are the brain, skin, bones, and mucous membranes of the mouth and anus, although treponemes may be found in virtually any tissue. Placental infection produces focal villitis and placental arteritis. Although this causes abnormal placental blood flow and increased vascular resistance, most infants do not have intrauterine growth restriction. In the fetus, the organism produces a relatively low-grade inflammatory response in infected tissues.

Diagnosis

Severe, early-onset disease may present as stillbirth or hydrops fetalis. Common neonatal presenting signs include hepatosplenomegaly, anemia, jaundice (conjugated and unconjugated), and generalized lymphadenopathy. Syphilis produces a variety of skin lesions. The fluid of bullous lesions, often present on the palms and soles, abounds in living spirochetes and is highly contagious (Fig. 209-8). Petechiae also are common, and the "blueberry muffin" lesions of extramedullary hematopoiesis may be seen. Less common manifestations include severe pneumonitis, myocarditis, and gastrointestinal dysfunction. Despite the frequency of CNS involvement, neurologic signs usually are not present. Elevated CSF protein and a mononuclear pleocytosis indicate CNS infection, however. Osteochondritis and periostitis are present on long bone films in 80% to 90% of infected infants who have other clinical signs at birth. These lesions give rise to the later appearance of pseudoparalysis of an extremity.

Asymptomatic congenital syphilis may present as rhinorrhea at 2 to 3 weeks of life. Initially clear, the discharge becomes mucopurulent and then bloody. Signs of infection also may develop later in infants who are untreated or treated inadequately after birth.

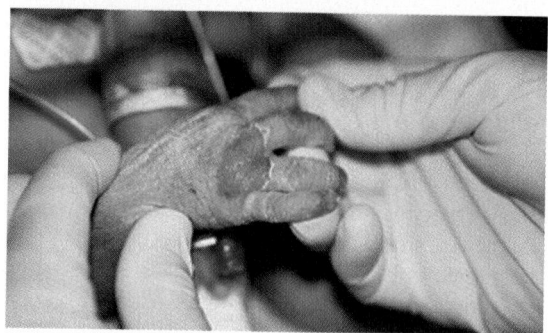

Figure 209-8. Skin manifestations of congenital syphilis. (From Mandell GL: Atlas of Infectious Diseases, Vol XI. Pediatric Infectious Diseases. Philadelphia, Churchill Livingstone, 1999, p 12.13.)

Diagnosis

Visualization of the organism under a darkfield microscope in scrapings from lesions or in body fluids is diagnostic. PCR techniques for treponemal DNA in these specimens eventually may prove more sensitive. Other confirmatory tests include IgM titers for antibody directed specifically against *T. pallidum*. A positive CSF Venereal Disease Research Laboratory (VDRL) is not specific for neurosyphilis because the antibody can enter CSF passively.

Further diagnostic assessment is indicated to identify characteristic lesions and to establish the presence of CNS disease and involvement of other systems. A lumbar puncture should be performed, and the CSF should be sent for cell count, protein, and VDRL testing. To identify all infants with CNS syphilis, additional testing of CSF must include IgM immunoblotting and PCR assay. CNS infection is indicated by pleocytosis (>24 white blood cells/mm^3) and protein concentration greater than 150 mg/dL in term infants or greater than 170 mg/dL in premature infants. Some experts recommend lower cell counts (>4 white blood cells/mm^3) and protein levels (>40 mg/dL) to minimize the likelihood of false-negative results. A positive CSF VDRL result without accompanying abnormalities of cell count and protein concentration merely may reflect movement of IgG into the CSF. Other testing should include assessment of liver function, CBC, and x-rays of the long bones.

Treatment

Treatment of the infected mother with penicillin cures most infected infants. Treatment of penicillin-allergic patients still is debated. Erythromycin is recommended, but treatment failure remains a problem. Fewer data are available on other antibiotics. Most treatment failures occur during late pregnancy. Failures are associated with high VDRL titers at treatment and delivery, earlier maternal stage of syphilis, shorter intervals between treatment and delivery, and delivery of an infant at less than 36 weeks' gestational age. Penicillin is the drug of choice to treat the infected fetus or neonate. If the CSF VDRL remains positive at 6 months of age, a second course must be given.

Prognosis

The extent of injury to the fetus or neonate at the time treatment begins defines the prognosis. Treatment in the first trimester of pregnancy can eliminate sequelae.

Interstitial keratitis may require glucocorticoid therapy. The bone lesions eventually heal.

Borrelia burgdorferi

Borrelia burgdorferi, a tick-borne spirochete and the agent of Lyme disease, causes multisystem illness in older patients. Maternal-fetal transmission has been described, causing a clinical picture similar to congenital syphilis. The incidence, nature, and extent of fetal and neonatal disease attributable to Lyme borreliosis currently are under active investigation.

Epidemiology

The organism is widespread in the North American hemisphere, and its range worldwide probably is substantially more extensive than currently recognized. *Borrelia* infects a variety of animal species in different habitat areas. It is transmitted to humans via arthropod bites. The most common transmitters are ticks, but other species, including flies and mosquitoes, have been implicated.

Pathophysiology

Most pregnant women are seronegative, even in Lyme disease endemic areas. Lyme *Borrelia* causes a multisystem illness with a plethora of clinical manifestations in adult patients. The disease begins as a focal skin infection at the site of the initial insect bite. It progresses through a spirochetemic phase during which the organism reaches the fetus transplacentally. First-trimester fetal infection can cause fetal demise with relatively late fetal loss between 15 and 25 weeks. Spirochetes have been described at autopsy throughout the body. There is only a minimal inflammatory response. Congenitally infected infants can have involvement of virtually any organ system.

Diagnosis

Disease manifestations are protean, without clinical findings specific for or strongly suggestive of congenital Lyme *Borrelia* infection. In addition to the usual findings caused by chronic congenital infections, infection early in gestation has been associated with congenital heart lesions, although some studies indicate that the risk of heart lesions is not increased.

Diagnostic testing for Lyme borreliosis is under vigorous investigation. Current tests have a variety of problems. The CDC has published standards for diagnosis of Lyme disease during pregnancy. These standards continue to evolve, and the interested reader is referred to current updated recommendations. There are similar difficulties with the diagnosis in neonates.

Treatment

Doxycycline is the drug of choice in patients older than 8 years of age, but it is contraindicated in pregnancy. Amoxicillin is the alternative. Antibiotic therapy reduces the severity of congenital Lyme borreliosis, but it does not eliminate it in all cases. Recommendations for treatment continue to evolve.

Malaria

Malaria rarely is acquired in North America. Cases have occurred with limited transmission from travelers or recent immigrants with active infections. Fewer than 10 cases of congenital malaria occur each year in this country.

Epidemiology

Malaria remains endemic in many areas of the world. The ease and rapidity of travel increase the likelihood that individuals with active infection will return to the United States. Domestic mosquitoes are capable of transmitting the parasites. *Plasmodium malariae* may persist as an asymptomatic erythrocytic disease for decades after untreated or partially treated initial infections. The parasite can cross the placenta and infect the fetus. Pregnancy makes women more susceptible to malaria and increases the density of parasitemia, promoting transplacental passage. High levels of maternal anti-*Plasmodium* antibodies reduce the risk of transmission.

Pathophysiology

Infection frequently is confined to the placenta. The spectrum of fetal illness runs the gamut from early fetal demise to delivery of an asymptomatic term infant. Typically, clinical illness in the infant appears between 2 and 4 weeks of age, but it has been described on the first day of life. Unexplained fever is the most common presentation. Anemia and splenomegaly are other common signs.

Diagnosis

The triad of fever, anemia, and splenomegaly occurs in 80% of cases. A more subtle presentation, unexplained fever, also can occur, however. Thick blood smears may be negative in mother and infant. Negative *Plasmodium*-specific antibody testing rules out current or previous maternal infection. PCR can be used in antibody-positive patients to diagnose active infection and to determine the infecting species. A travel and residence history of the parents and close relatives is an essential part of the evaluation of any infant with unexplained fever. The mother also should be asked about any history of transfusions with blood products.

Treatment

Chloroquine is the drug of choice for sensitive organisms. There are other choices for resistant strains of *Plasmodium falciparum*, and the interested reader is referred to specialty texts or the CDC website.

Herpes Simplex

HSV are widely prevalent in North America. Approximately 10 million people are chronically infected, and each year another 0.5 million new cases occur. The combination of chronic fetal infections and acute disease in the neonatal period produces 700 to 1000 neonatal cases a year in the United States. The virus has two types with distinct but overlapping predilections for sites of infection. HSV-1 predominantly infects the upper airway, but it can infect the genital tract. HSV-2 causes most herpetic genital infections and is responsible for 70% to 85% of neonatal and fetal infections.

HSV gains entry through breaks in skin or mucosal structures. The initial infection often is asymptomatic. The virus can produce local illness and can infect nerve endings. From there, it migrates centrally to ganglia, where it can reproduce and spread further or remain latent. Intermittent reactivations of latent virus result in recurrent surface illness. Primary HSV infection, defined as symptomatic illness in the absence of serologic evidence of prior infection, poses the greatest risk of transmission to the fetus or neonate. Viral shedding from the genital tract can persist for 2 to 3 months after resolution of clinical symptoms. Chronic fetal infection acquired transplacentally or by ascending infection early in gestation accounts for about 3% of infected infants.

Diagnosis

The clinical spectrum of chronic fetal HSV infections ranges from fetal demise to minor skin lesions. Infection early in pregnancy usually causes fetal death. The virus causes encephalitis with resultant hydrancephaly, hydrocephalus, or microcephaly. Additional clinical findings are typical of other chronic fetal viral infections and include retinitis, pneumonia, hepatosplenomegaly, hepatitis, and thrombocytopenia. Infected infants are categorized by the extent of organ involvement. The mildest cases are restricted to SEM infections. The second level of severity includes CNS infection, with or without SEM infection. The most severely infected infants have multiorgan infection—liver, lung, skin, or adrenals. The CNS also can be infected in these infants.

Stringent diagnostic criteria include isolation of HSV and exclusion of other organisms that cause a similar clinical presentation (CMV, toxoplasmosis, syphilis, or rubella). Specimens for viral culture and PCR should be obtained from skin lesions, the eye, the nasopharynx, and the rectum. CSF also should be sent for these tests. Specimens for herpes viral culture should not be frozen. Direct immunofluorescence can identify the virus in scrapings from the bases of skin lesions. Other cytologic techniques (Tzanck preparation) are only 60% to 70% sensitive, so negative results are not informative. Serologic tests have little value. PCR of CSF for HSV DNA is useful to diagnose CNS infection.

Treatment

Acyclovir is the drug of choice for neonatal HSV infections. Although there is no proof of efficacy in chronic infections, the possibility remains that therapy would prevent further progression of acute infection. This result is particularly desirable in infants who present only with skin findings. Because the drug has virtually no toxicity, logic would favor therapy. Newer antiherpetic agents so far have not shown advantages over acyclovir. Treatment improves the overall prognosis substantially.

Prognosis

The most important sequela of HSV infection is brain injury. Infants who have had intrauterine encephalopathy can be expected to have a bleak prognosis. The more severe the degree of neonatal disease, the worse the prognosis. Merely having SEM infection increases the risk of poor developmental outcome.

Rubella

Effective immunization largely has eliminated congenital rubella from North America. The incidence of congenital rubella is currently about 1% of prevaccine levels. It remains prevalent in other parts of the world, however, and unimmunized immigrant groups increase the pool of susceptible women. The few cases that occur in the United States each year are attributable to failure to vaccinate or represent imported cases. Because it is routine to measure maternal rubella titers early in pregnancy, obstetricians have the opportunity to ensure that susceptible women are immunized immediately after delivery before they are at risk of another pregnancy. As a fail-safe, pediatricians should verify that immunization is given.

Rubella occurs in winter and spring. About 10% to 20% of women of childbearing age are susceptible, and the infection most commonly occurs in situations in which they live and work in close proximity to their peers. Colleges, cruise ships, hospitals, and religious enclaves have been the sites of vaccine era outbreaks.

Pathogenesis

The fetus becomes infected during maternal viremia. Passage to the fetus is efficient early in gestation (80% in the first trimester), and the risk of fetal infection decreases progressively as the pregnancy progresses. The earlier in gestation infection occurs, the worse the injury to the fetus. The full-blown congenital rubella syndrome occurs after infection during the first 8 weeks of pregnancy. Infection during the first 8 weeks causes cataracts; infection at the end of the third trimester can cause heart defects. Retinal injury or deafness can arise from infection before the end of the second trimester, but sequelae are uncommon beyond the first trimester.

Several viral effects may mediate fetal injury. Vascular injury may cause hypoxic tissue damage. The virus affects receptors for growth factors. Also, cells infected with the rubella virus reproduce more slowly. The result is decreased cell numbers and a growth-retarded fetus. Ongoing viral infection may cause cell death directly or injure the fetus indirectly by immune-mediated mechanisms.

Rubella immunization during pregnancy carries a theoretical risk to the fetus, estimated by the CDC at 1.6%. Of 226 susceptible women vaccinated during the first trimester, 2% of the infants had asymptomatic infection. None had clinical findings. Vaccination during pregnancy currently is not considered an indication for pregnancy termination.

Diagnosis

The typical infant with congenital rubella infection is born growth restricted at term. Birth defects occur in at least 50% of infants infected during the 1st month, 20% to 30% of infants infected during the second month, and 5% of infants infected during the third and fourth month. Common findings include a large fontanelle, cataracts, hearing defects, chorioretinitis, glaucoma, a purpuric rash, thrombocytopenia, hepatosplenomegaly, and cardiac defects. Peripheral pulmonary arterial stenoses are virtually universal. Other associated lesions are patent ductus arteriosus and septal defects. Extramedullary hematopoiesis in the skin creates the raised, purple lesions of the so-called blueberry muffin infant. There is a plethora of other less common manifestations of the disease. X-rays of the long bones may show linear zones of increased lucency ("celery stalking") and increased opacity in the metaphyses.

217 History and Physical Examination

Melissa Weddle

Adolescence is a time of rapid biological and psychosocial change. Despite being a period of rapid change, adolescence is a time of relative physical health with generally few scheduled doctor visits. Many adolescents seek health care only for acute illness or when required for camp or sports participation. An annual preventive care visit can provide a vital opportunity for the generalist to identify factors that place the adolescent at health risk, to provide counseling regarding prevention of health risk behaviors, and to intervene when health risk factors are identified. In addition, the preventive health care visit can provide an opportunity for the health care provider to reinforce positive behaviors, to offer information to assist with responsible decision making, and to assist the adolescent in assuming responsibility for health care.

PERIODICITY

Because adolescence is a period of rapid and complex change, an annual health maintenance visit is optimal. This permits the adolescent to develop and maintain a relationship with the primary care provider and for the provider to promote healthy behaviors and to identify early risk taking.

For many adolescents, the acute care visit can serve as an opportunity for targeted preventive health care. For example, the adolescent who has an upper respiratory infection should be asked about smoke exposure and, if the response is positive, counseled about health risks. All adolescents who present for sports or camp physicals should receive a full preventive health visit. This is a unique opportunity to screen for the range of health care issues discussed later.

THE ENVIRONMENT

The health care provider who sees adolescents should offer a space that is adolescent-friendly. This may include having a waiting area with teen reading material and an examination room with appropriate décor. If adolescents are interviewed in a room filled with toys and cartoon characters, they might feel that the provider is not attuned to adolescent issues. In addition, there should be adequate time in the schedule to conduct the visit in an unhurried way. If an adolescent feels that the provider is rushed, questions and concerns are less likely to be revealed. For providers in a busy practice, it might be most appropriate to schedule extra time for the adolescent visit or to schedule the preventive health care visit as the last appointment of the session.

CONFIDENTIALITY

At the start of the visit, it is important to explain policies regarding confidentiality to both the adolescent and the parent. The provider needs to identify any limitations to confidentiality, for example, whether all visits generate a billing statement to the adolescent's parents. It is important to mention that confidentiality does not extend to behaviors that place the adolescent or others at serious risk.

PROCESS

The purposes of taking a careful history are to obtain information about any concerns the adolescent and parent may have, to identify factors that may either protect or predispose the adolescent to illness or injury, and to identify ongoing health problems (Box 217-1). Information may be obtained by questionnaire or entirely by interview. The parent and/or adolescent may be given a questionnaire, and the provider may focus the interview on the positive responses. When the adolescent is given a questionnaire, adequate privacy must be offered.

The parent's role in the visit will vary according to the adolescent's development and preference. The early adolescent might be more comfortable with the parent in the room for the entire visit. For the middle or late adolescent, it generally works well to conduct the first part of the interview with the parent present, send the parent out for the more sensitive questions and examination, and invite the parent back at the end to discuss the assessment. It is best to discuss with the adolescent before the parent's return what information will be shared with the parent. Many adolescents assume responsibility for their own health care and may come without a parent. Whatever the age, the office visit can be an opportunity to gradually increase an adolescent's responsibility in managing his or her own health care.

The interview is the time to develop rapport with the adolescent. The interview should be conducted while the adolescent is fully clothed. Communication style and word choice can affect the amount of information the adolescent provides. It is important to limit the use of medical terminology and to explain terms the adolescent might misinterpret. For example, one way to inquire about contraception might be to ask, "Do you use any kind of birth control, like condoms, birth control pills, birth control shots?"

Some adolescents might feel that questions are invasive. It can be helpful to provide an explanation of why questions are being asked, to explain that the adolescent is not being singled out: "I ask these questions of all these patients I see." Sensitive questions can first be asked in the third person, particularly of young adolescents or new patients. For example, the health care provider might say, "There are some teens your age who are using marijuana and other drugs. Do you know any kids who smoke weed?" before moving on to "Have you ever smoked weed?" In addition, questions should be asked in a nonjudgmental way that does not suggest a norm. For example, rather than asking a girl whether she has a boyfriend as a prelude to sexual history, it is better to ask whether she has been in a sexual relationship. If the answer is positive, the next question could be "With male partners, female partners, or both?"

COMPONENTS OF THE HISTORY

At the start of the interview, one should obtain the parent's and adolescent's concerns, remembering that these might be different. If the adolescent's chief concern is acne and the parent's is school truancy, the provider needs to address the acne to develop trust and credibility for treating the other issues. A past medical history should be obtained, asking about chronic disease and recurrent illness (Box 217-2). The provider should ask about medications, asking specifically about over-the-counter medications, herbal medications, oral contraceptives, and injectables (e.g., DepoProvera). As with the younger child, allergies and history of hospitalizations and surgeries should be documented. History of injuries and trauma should be documented, particularly asking about role of intoxication or personal violence. Immunization history should include specific information about hepatitis B, MMRs, tetanus booster, and varicella status.

Important components of the family history (Box 217-3) include cardiovascular disease (heart attack or stroke before age 55, sudden death, arrhythmias, hypertension, and elevated cholesterol or triglycerides). It is important to ask about family members with asthma, clotting disorders, diabetes, alcohol and drug abuse, and psychiatric disorders including history of suicide. In addition, the adolescent should be asked about exposure to tuberculosis.

Review of systems should include information about diet, asking specifically about eating habits that place the adolescent at risk for osteoporosis, iron deficiency, and atherosclerosis. Questions should address calcium intake, iron intake, fat consumption, and vegetarian diet (Box 217-4). The provider should inquire about weight loss methods and history of weight gain or loss. For young women, it is important to ask about body image, how she feels about her current weight/size. For girls, it is important to obtain a gynecologic history, including age of menarche, frequency and regularity of menses, duration of menses, dysmenorrhea (including medications taken), last menstrual period, and tampon or pad use (Box 217-5). For all adolescents, the last dental visit should be documented.

The psychosocial portion of the history is best obtained by asking the least sensitive questions first and then moving to the more sensitive questions. The HEADSS format can provide a useful structure for this (Box 217-6). Questions about home include who lives at the home, relationship to the patient, family members not living at home, and feelings of safety at home. Education questions include school attended and grade level, performance, attendance, best and worst subjects, attitude toward school, special education needs, and career goals. Additional questions can include asking about best and worst subjects and about favorite and least favorite subjects. It is also useful to compare performance this year to performance in the previous year, looking for changes that could signal learning or behavioral issues.

Box 217-4. Review of Systems: Nutrition

- Calcium, iron, fat intake
- Vegetarian diet
- Weight loss methods
- History of weight loss or gain
- Body image

Activities includes questions about level of physical activity, sports participation, job, special interests or hobbies, peer relationships, activities with friends, and sleep patterns. Drug questions include asking about tobacco use (including smokeless tobacco), alcohol, and other drugs. If a positive response is obtained, it is important to characterize use. The CAGE questionnaire is one useful tool to screen for problem use, and others are described in Chapter 234. With respect to sexuality, it is important to first ask about any history of sexual activity. For adolescents who have not been sexually active, it is important to explore feelings and plans. For those who have been or are sexually active, important information includes age at first intercourse, gender of partner(s), and history of sexually transmitted diseases. Sexually active girls should be asked about the most recent screen for sexually transmitted diseases and Papanicolaou smear, prior pregnancies, and outcomes. In addition, both boys and girls should be questioned about use of methods to prevent sexually transmitted diseases and pregnancy. Finally, the adolescent should be asked about feelings of safety in current relationships and about any history of sexual abuse or rape.

Family history of depression, suicide, and other mental health problems will have been already been asked. At this point, the provider can ask about personal history of depression or other mental health problems. When the adolescent reports disordered sleep, substance abuse, multiple somatic complaints, or chronic fatigue or has experienced a recent loss, depression should be suspected. A reasonable order of questions to ask about current depression is listed in Box 217-7. If the adolescent reports feelings of self-harm, immediate psychiatric evaluation is required.

The primary health provider should screen for safety risks, including seat belt use, bicycle helmet use, and presence of guns in the home. If there are guns in the home, questions should address where they are kept, whether they are locked, and whether ammunition is kept separate from the gun. For some adolescents, it might be important to ask whether they carry weapons and whether they have been involved in physical fights. For adolescents who have identified health risk behaviors, it is important to ask about time spent in detention, foster homes, or homeless shelters.

Box 217-5. Review of Systems: Gynecologic

- Age of menarche
- Frequency and regularity of menses
- Duration of menses
- Dysmenorrhea (including medications taken)
- Last menstrual period
- Tampon or pad use

Box 217-6. HEADSS

Home: Household composition, relations with parents and siblings (including those who live elsewhere), feelings of safety, presence of guns

Education: Level, grades this year compared with last, best and worst subjects, attitude toward school, attendance, special education needs, career goals

Activities: Exercise, sleep, sports participation, job, hobbies and special interests, peer relationships, gang membership, weapon carrying, history of physical fights

Drugs: Alcohol and other drug use, tobacco use

Sex: Feelings toward same or opposite sex, types of sexual practices, age at first intercourse, gender of partner(s), number of lifetime partners, age of partner, history of sexually transmitted diseases, last screens

Suicide/depression: Feelings about self, history of depression or other mental health problems, suicidal thoughts, suicide attempts

PHYSICAL EXAMINATION

Adolescents are often more uncomfortable with the physical examination than either children or adults would be. It is generally best to start with the least embarrassing areas, saving the most sensitive part of the examination until last. If the provider talks through the examination, explaining each step, the examination may be less stressful for the adolescent.

For adolescents, as with younger patients, it is important to obtain a height and weight and to compare these to previous measurements. For the adolescent younger than age 18, these measurements should be graphed onto a growth chart. Calculating a body mass index (BMI) is a useful tool to assess for overweight and underweight, correlating well with body fat content. An adolescent who has a BMI greater than or equal to the 95% for gender and age is overweight. Those with a BMI between the 85th and 95th percentiles are at risk for becoming overweight. Those who have gained two or more BMI points from the previous should be evaluated further. Adolescents who have lost 10% of their previous weight or who have a BMI at the fifth percentile or lower should be questioned further about possible eating disorders and underlying organic disease.

Blood pressure should be checked annually. Percentile curves for age are shown in Chapter 174. Elevated blood pressure is defined as either systolic or diastolic pressure above the 95th percentile for age and sex. A single blood pressure elevation warrants return for a repeat reading. If pressure is elevated on three separate occasions, further

Box 217-7. Progressive Screening Questions for Adolescents Suspected of Having Significant Depression and Suicidal Thoughts

- Do you ever feel down?
- How do you make yourself feel better?
- Have you ever thought about hurting yourself?
- Have you ever made a plan?
- Have you ever attempted to hurt or kill yourself?
- Do you feel like hurting yourself now?

evaluation is indicated. Adolescents with at least three blood pressure readings between the 90th and 95th percentiles should be counseled about weight reduction (if obese) and exercise.

In general, the physical examination of the adolescent is like that of the school-age child. Only points specific to the adolescent will be included here. General appearance including affect and eye contact should be noted. Skin should be examined for acne, scars, tattoos, and piercing. Mouth examination should include observation of dentition with notation of caries and gingivitis. Visual acuity should be measured. The neck should be examined for thyroid size, masses, and lymphadenopathy.

A complete musculoskeletal examination is recommended for adolescents who are involved in competitive athletics. Recommendations for scoliosis screening vary. Though sensitivity is examiner-dependent, the forward bend test is the most common scoliosis screen. In this test, the child bends forward at the waist, dangling arms toward the floor. The observer views the spine from the back, looking for asymmetry of the ribs or lumbar soft tissue.

Girls should have breasts assessed for Tanner stage and masses. Finding nodularity on examination is common and is a cause for reassurance. The majority of discrete masses are benign, most of them fibroadenomas. They may be observed for 2–3 months before referral, because most resolve without intervention. Masses that require immediate referral are hard, nonmobile, and associated with skin changes or nipple discharge. Any nipple discharge requires evaluation. There is controversy regarding teaching breast self-examination to adolescents. Some providers believe that this can cause unnecessary worry. Others believe that it is worthwhile, a possible benefit being increased comfort with one's body.

Boys should be assessed for presence of gynecomastia. About two thirds of boys are affected, and the gynecomastia may be unilateral or bilateral. The two sides may be enlarged simultaneously or sequentially. Boys might worry that they have cancer or that they are developing breasts. They can be counseled that most cases resolve within two years. Surgical referral should be considered for those who have persistent gynecomastia into late adolescence and those who report that the gynecomastia interferes with their lives. External genital examination should include assessment of Tanner stage. Testicular examination should include checking for masses, varicoceles, and hernias. One checks for hernias by inserting an index finger into the external inguinal ring while the patient coughs. As with the breast self-examination, there is controversy about teaching testicular self-examination.

Sexually active girls should receive a pelvic examination with Papanicolaou smear within 3 years of onset of sexual activity or at age 21 if not yet sexually active. The examination includes inspection of the external genitalia, vagina, and cervix, and palpation of the cervix, uterus, and adnexa. Pelvic examination should be considered for those who have primary or secondary amenorrhea, severe dysmenorrhea, or irregular menses.

Mini-index of Related Topics   CH.

SUGGESTED READINGS

Beach RK: Routine breast exams: A chance to reassure, guide, and protect. Contemp Pediatr 1987;70:100.

Elster AB, Kuznets NJ(eds): AMA Guidelines for Adolescent Preventive Services (GAPS) Recommendations and Rationale. Baltimore, Md, Williams & Wilkins, 1994.

Gotlieb E (ed): Practicing Adolescent Medicine: A Collection of Resources. Elk Grove Village, Ill, American Academy of Pediatrics, Section on Adolescent Health,1994.

Green M (ed): Bright Futures: Guidelines for Health Supervision of Infants, Children, and Adolescents. Arlington, Va, National Center for Education in Maternal and Child Health, 1994.

Joffe A: Why adolescent medicine? Med Clin North Am 2000; 84:769–785.

U.S. Preventive Services Task Force: Guide to Clinical Preventive Services, 2nd ed. Baltimore, Md, Williams & Wilkins, 1996.

218 Health Maintenance in Adolescents

Melissa Weddle

ROLE OF THE GENERALIST

1   Provide preventive health counseling for adolescents who do not engage in risk-taking behavior.

2   Provided targeted health counseling for adolescents who engage in risk-taking behavior.

3   Recommend appropriate laboratory testing for an individual adolescent.

4   Provide appropriate immunizations.

5   Include appropriate parental involvement in the adolescent's health care.

Health maintenance refers to interventions made by the primary health care provider to develop and sustain a state of emotional and physical well-being. For adolescents, this can include immunizations, laboratory testing to screen for health risk factors, and counseling about prevention or modification of risk behaviors. The annual preventive health care visit provides an opportunity to provide these services. Acute care visits are also opportunities for targeted preventive health care.

The leading causes of morbidity and mortality in adolescents are modifiable behaviors and hence are preventable. Many lifestyle patterns that are established in adolescence persist into adulthood, placing the adolescent at long-term risk. Counseling about health behaviors, including discussion of diet, exercise, sexuality, and drug and alcohol use, constitute a significant portion of the preventive health visit. In addition to risk-taking behaviors, the adolescent may have physical findings (e.g., obesity, hypertension) or a family history that places him or her at risk (e.g., family members with early onset cardiovascular disease). During a health maintenance visit, the primary health care provider can impact both immediate and long-term health.

Prevention, a major goal of the health maintenance visit, can be primary, secondary, or tertiary. Primary prevention refers to preventing health risk behaviors. Positive reinforcement for protective behaviors is a method of primary prevention. Secondary prevention refers to altering existing health risk factors before disease or injury has developed. Tertiary prevention is modifying or preventing sequelae of established disease. The adolescent preventive health visit focuses on primary and secondary prevention, helping the adolescent to assume increasing responsibility for his or her own health care, and often reassuring the adolescent of his or her own normality.

PRINCIPLES OF HEALTH COUNSELING

Counseling must be tailored to the individual. Information provided is very different for an adolescent who is contemplating engaging in a high-risk behavior than for one who already displays health risk behaviors. During the preventive health visit, positive behaviors and responsible decision making should be reinforced. The health care provider should use the health maintenance visit to identify and reinforce protective and healthy behaviors.

In counseling, the adolescent's developmental level must be considered. For the immature adolescent who is still quite dependent on parents, the counseling will be very different than that for the adolescent who has a job and is making most of his or her own decisions. In the former case, the adolescent might prefer having a parent present for most of the visit. Counseling may be provided to the parent and to the parent and child together. In the latter case, most, if not all, counseling is directed to the adolescent. Health counseling should consider the adolescent's culture. The approach used should be respectful and culturally sensitive.

At a time when adolescents develop increasing autonomy but are still dependent on parents, communicating a management plan to both can be challenging. Adolescents may resent parental involvement, yet some outcomes are likely to be more successful if parents understand their own role in the behaviors. For example, encouraging an adolescent to adopt a healthier eating pattern is more likely to be successful if the parent is encouraged to make healthier foods available in the home. The level of parental involvement depends on whether the parents are appropriately supportive of their adolescent, whether counseling regards confidential topics, and whether the patient is mature enough to assume responsibility for some or all aspects of health care.

Increasing health care knowledge does not necessarily lead to behavior change. In counseling about behavior change, it is important to identify barriers to change, plan strategies to overcome those barriers, and develop a plan to provide ongoing reinforcement. When the adolescent is reluctant to change, the provider should discuss how to access services if assistance is desired.

COMPONENTS OF HEALTH MAINTENANCE

Normal Growth and Development

For the early adolescent, anticipatory guidance should be provided about physical changes, including rapid growth, body hair, acne, menstruation, and wet dreams. Boys with gynecomastia and girls with asymmetric breast development should be reassured about the normality of these findings. Adolescents may have unvoiced concerns about their height and weight. Reassurance that they are within a wide range of normal can be helpful.

Peer Pressure

An increased role of peers as an influence on decision making is a normal aspect of adolescent development. For some adolescents, peers may exert a positive influence; for others, peers may contribute to risk-taking behavior. Discussion of peer pressure should start in early adolescence, with discussion of ways to resist it when risk might be involved.

Nutrition

Nutrition counseling should be tailored to the individual adolescent. Adolescents who have diets with high fat content might need a discussion about ways to substitute healthy foods for high-fat items. Taking the "fat is bad" approach is generally not helpful. A more flexible approach advising moderation is more likely to be accepted. For the many adolescents who have inadequate calcium intake, it is important to increase calcium intake, either by adding calcium-containing foods to the diet or by supplementation. The vegetarian or vegan adolescent should be counseled about adequate protein, vitamin B_{12}, and iron intake. For obese adolescents or those who require substantial changes to develop a healthy diet, referral to a nutritionist who has experience working with adolescents is appropriate.

Exercise

Talking about benefits of regular exercise is important for adolescents who have low levels of exercise. The adolescent might have ideas about ways to increase physical activity that are compatible with his or her current lifestyle. Suggestions could include walking rather than getting a ride, walking up stairs, or following an exercise tape.

Injury Prevention

All adolescents should be asked about seat belt use. For those who bicycle or ride motorcycles, helmet use should be discussed. Alcohol use while operating motor or recreational vehicles or swimming should be discouraged. Adolescents should be strongly counseled to avoid riding with someone who has been drinking or using drugs. Both parents and adolescents should be asked about guns in the home and should be counseled about gun safety both within and outside the home. Parents should be advised

that having a gun in the home always poses a risk and that the safest storage is to lock up guns in a separate place from locked ammunition. Children and adolescents should not have access to the key to the gun case or to the ammunition.

Violence

Adolescents who participate in a culture in which physical violence is used to resolve conflict often carry weapons for protection. As with counseling about other behaviors, saying "Don't do it" is not enough. Exploring with those adolescents their insights into ways of avoiding injury from violence can be helpful. Whenever possible, adolescents should be counseled to avoid places where violent behavior is likely to occur. For adolescents who are amenable, referral to a counselor or program might be appropriate to help develop tools for conflict resolution without violence.

Sexuality

Responsible sexual behavior should be promoted before an adolescent initiates sexual activity. Exploration of the views and plans of the adolescent who is not sexually active is important. Those who plan to wait should be supported and encouraged. For these adolescents, one should review sexually transmitted disease and pregnancy prevention and how to access services should they be needed.

For the both the heterosexual and homosexual sexually active adolescent, prevention of sexually transmitted disease must be discussed. "Safer sex" by consistent condom use should be promoted, and ideally, condoms should be provided. Proper use of a condom should be illustrated with a model, and potential risks of oral and anal sex should be discussed. Communication with partners should be discussed, and limiting the number of partners should be encouraged. Abstinence should be presented as an option, including examples of ways to show affection other than intercourse.

For both male and female adolescents in a heterosexual relationship, discussion of pregnancy prevention is essential. For adolescents who are using no or ineffective contraception but are amenable to starting effective contraception, those services should be provided that same day. Emergency contraception should be discussed, including how to obtain it. A prescription may be provided for emergency contraception. The male partner in a heterosexual relationship should be counseled about his responsibility in pregnancy prevention and advised to discuss this with his partner(s).

For all adolescents, the role of alcohol in placing one at risk for unwanted and unsafe sex should be reviewed. In addition, the importance of sex being wanted and consensual should be discussed.

Tobacco Use

Most adolescents try cigarettes at least once. Although some experiment and then stop, many become addicted. Adolescents who smoke are much more likely to continue to smoke throughout adulthood. Nicotine dependence can occur through use of smokeless tobacco, such as snuff and chewing tobacco. Smoking has been described as the single most preventable cause of death.

Prevention efforts should focus on preventing adolescents from smoking and, for those who already smoke, involvement in a cessation program. Most adolescents are aware of health risks of smoking but might not be concerned about long-term risks. It may be more effective to counsel about immediate negative effects of smoking, such as bad breath and decreased athletic performance. Effective cessation efforts include initiating the discussion, offering nicotine patches or gum and/or setting a quit date, and arranging follow-up. It can be helpful to identify barriers to cessation and develop strategies to overcome these barriers.

Alcohol and Other Drugs

As with other risk-taking behaviors, all adolescents should receive guidance about potential dangers and ways to refrain from use of alcohol and other drugs. Most adolescents will experiment with psychoactive substances. When use of alcohol or other drugs is reported, the health care provider must determine whether the use is low-intensity, experimental use, or abuse/dependency. For adolescents who indicate problem use, a referral for in-depth evaluation is indicated.

Emotional and Psychological Health

Changing family dynamics during adolescence can result in family conflict. Change in peer relations and academic challenges that often accompany the transition to junior high or high school can be stressful. Adolescents who develop physically later or earlier than peers may be teased by peers. Unexpected change, such as divorce or family relocation, are stressful events. The primary care provider can explore with the adolescent ways to relieve stress, review signs that indicate stress is interfering with normal functioning, and advise the adolescent how to seek help.

Parents

Including the parent in preventive health counseling is important. It has been shown that adolescents who feel more connected to their families are less likely to engage in health risk behaviors. Information to parents should include anticipatory guidance about normal physical and emotional development, peer pressure, change in communication patterns, conflicts about independence, and risk-taking behavior. The health care provider might want to tell parents about their adolescent's strengths. Some parents might need information about setting limits, monitoring their adolescent's activities, and communicating with their adolescent.

Laboratory Screening

Laboratory testing is targeted to the individual (Table 218-1). Vegetarians, female athletes, and adolescents who have had a recent weight loss or have a history of menorrhagia should be screened for anemia.

Girls who have been sexually active with male partners should be screened for gonorrhea and chlamydia. Current recommendations support performing a Pap smear within 3 years of sexual activity onset or at age 21 for those who have not yet become sexually active. Sexually active boys

Table 218-1. Indications for Laboratory Testing in Adolescents

Hemoglobin or hematocrit	Menorrhagia, nutritional risk, female athletes, chronic weight loss
Urinalysis	Not routinely indicated
Varicella titer	No history of varicella infection or immunization
Papanicolaou smear	Females who have been sexually active with males
Chlamydia and gonorrhea screens	Females who have been sexually active with males, sexually active males
Syphilis screen	Sexually active males and females who have who have had multiple or recurrent STDs, sex with more than one partner in the past 6 months, those who have exchanged sex for drugs
HIV Ab	Same groups as for syphilis screen, history of intravenous drug use
Hepatitis B and C	History of intravenous drug use

may be screened for gonorrhea and chlamydia by urine DNA amplification tests. Syphilis and HIV screening should be offered to adolescents who have had multiple or recurrent sexually transmitted diseases, sex with more than one partner in the past 6 months, those who have exchanged sex for money or drugs, or boys who have had sex with male partners. HIV testing should be offered confidentially with provision of pretest and posttest counseling.

Varicella titer should be obtained in adolescents who have no or uncertain history of varicella infection or immunization. Because about 80% of adolescents without a history of varicella infection are actually immune, screening is cost-effective. If the adolescent is unlikely to return, initiation of the two-dose vaccine series at the visit is preferable.

Universal cholesterol screening for adolescents is currently not recommended but should be done if the adolescent (1) has a parent or grandparent who has been diagnosed at age 55 or younger with atherosclerosis, myocardial infarction, angina, peripheral vascular disease, cerebrovascular disease, or sudden cardiac death or (2) has a parent with a cholesterol level of 240 or higher. Providers should consider screening adolescents who are at higher risk of coronary heart disease: those who smoke cigarettes, have high blood pressure, or are overweight. Health care providers may choose to measure cholesterol levels in adolescents with an unknown parental or grandparental history.

For adolescents who have a history of intravenous drug use, screening for HIV and hepatitis B and C should be offered. A PPD should be administered for adolescents who are at increased risk of acquiring tuberculosis infection (Box 218-1).

Immunizations

A tetanus booster can be given at age 11 or 12 or if at least 10 years have past since the last one. Immunization records should be reviewed to determine that the adolescent has received two MMRs and the hepatitis B series. For adolescents who have a negative varicella titer, the varicella vaccine is recommended. For adolescents who will be

Box 218-1. Tuberculin Skin Test (TST) Recommendations for Infants, Children, and Adolescents

Immediate TST is indicated in the following cases:
1. Contacts with confirmed or suspected infections tuberculosis
2. Radiographic or clinical findings suggestive of tuberculosis disease
3. Immigration from endemic countries (Asia, Middle East, Africa, Latin America)
4. Travel history to endemic country or significant contact with persons from such countries

TST should be considered in the following cases:
1. Parents immigrated (with unknown TST status) from endemic countries
2. Travel to endemic area and/or household contact with persons from endemic country
3. Reside in high-prevalence area (Note that rates in any area of the city may vary by neighborhood or even block to block.)

From American Academy of Pediatrics: Tuberculosis. In Pickering L (ed): Red Book: 2003 Report of the Committee on Infectious Diseases, 26th ed. Elk Grove Village, Ill, American Academy of Pediatrics, 2003, p 646.

starting college and living in a dormitory, the meningococcal vaccine may be offered. The hepatitis A vaccine is recommended for boys who are sexually active with male partners or for adolescents who reside in areas with a high prevalence of hepatitis A. See Table 218-2 for immunization recommendations.

Table 218-2. Recommended Immunizations for Adolescents

MMR	At least two doses after first birthday
Tetanus and diphtheria	Booster at 11 to 12 years or if at least 10 years since last one
Hepatitis B	All adolescents
Varicella	If no history of disease or if negative titer
Meningococcal	Consider for college freshman living in dormitories
Hepatitis A	For adolescents living in areas with elevated rates of hepatitis A and sexually active males having sex with males

SUGGESTED READINGS

Cohen DA, Nsuami M, Martin DH, Farley TA: Repeated school-based screening for sexually transmitted diseases: A feasible strategy for reaching adolescents. Pediatrics 1999;104:1281–1285.

Davis BJ, Voegtle KH: Culturally Competent Health Care for Adolescents. Chicago, Ill, American Medical Association, 1994.

Elster A (ed): AMA Guidelines for Adolescent Preventive Services (GAPS) Recommendations and Rationale. Baltimore, Md, Williams & Wilkins, 1994.

Green M (ed): Bright Futures: Guidelines for Health Supervision of Infants, Children, and Adolescents. Arlington, Va, National Center for Education in Maternal and Child Health, 1994.

Hoffman AD: Communicating with adolescents and their parents. In Hofmann AD, Greydanus DE (eds): Adolescent Medicine, 3rd ed. Stamford, Conn, Appleton & Lange, 1997, pp 40–50.

Joffe A, Radius SM: Health counseling of adolescents. Pediatr Rev 1991;12:344–351.

National Cholesterol Education Program Expert Panel on Blood Cholesterol Levels in Children and Adolescents: Highlights of the Report of the Program Expert Panel on Blood Cholesterol Levels in Children and Adolescents. Washington, DC, U.S. Department of Health and Human Services, 1993.

219 Sports and the Adolescent

Wendi A. Johnson and Gregory L. Landry

ROLE OF THE GENERALIST

1 Know that the highest yield area in the PPE is the history and how to take that history.

2 Perform an appropriate PPE physical examination.

3 Know what skill performance is appropriate before return to play after an injury.

4 Counsel adolescents in sports about overuse sports injuries.

5 Be aware that many of the overuse injuries in teens are related to midfoot hyperpronation and know how to treat those injuries.

There are more opportunities than ever before for both male and female adolescents to participate in sports with almost 7 million high school participants in organized sports. With some of these opportunities comes pressure to train and compete year-round. Although acute injuries bring athletes in to see their physicians, increased intensity and duration of training for sports have led to an increasing number of overuse injuries. The win-at-all-costs attitude in some sports puts athletes at risk for high-risk behaviors such as anabolic steroid use and eating disorders. This chapter addresses the preparticipation evaluation, playability of athletes, and management of overuse injuries to the apophyses.

PREPARTICIPATION EVALUATION

Most of the time, adolescent athletes are healthy, and their only interaction with health care workers might occur at their preparticipation evaluation (PPE). Fortunately, most states require medical clearance of student athletes before they may take part in junior high or high school sports competition. The main goal of the PPE is to help the athlete participate safely. This means identifying injuries or conditions that might affect participation in sports or affect the overall well-being of the adolescent. There are some issues that are unique to the PPE compared to the health supervision visit of the nonathlete. Thorough discussions of the health supervision visit appear elsewhere, so this discussion will address only the most cogent points for athletes. Whether performed in the private office or utilizing a team of examiners at the school, the history is the highest-yield area of the evaluation.

HISTORY

It is helpful to have a standard history form to distribute prior to the examination for the parent to review or update. The most important screening questions should be included on the written form, but some of the important personal issues such as sexual behavior and substance abuse may be more appropriately addressed verbally in the private office.

One of the goals of the PPE is to prevent sudden death. Although it is difficult to identify the athlete who is at risk, questions in the history will identify up to 30% of those at risk. Box 219-1 lists the key questions related to sudden cardiac death. "Yes" answers to any of these questions may warrant a further cardiac evaluation even if the cardiovascular examination is normal.

Has the athlete ever had a concussion? It is important to define this term as ever being dazed, "dinged," or knocked out. The biggest risk factor for a concussion is having had a previous concussion. Have there been more than one? How severe was the injury? These questions are especially important if the athlete is competing in a collision sport such as football, soccer, or ice hockey.

Is there shortness of breath and/or cough after exercise? Exercise-related cough is a relatively sensitive marker for exercise-induced asthma, and further evaluation of allergies and possible asthma should be pursued. Exercise-induced chest pain and wheezing are less frequent symptoms of exercise-induced asthma.

It is helpful to ask the athlete his or her current weight and desired weight. Most boys want to be bigger, and most girls want to weigh less. We usually ask the athlete verbally how she or he is going to achieve the desired weight, especially if there is a significant discrepancy. This discussion can give the examiner a feel for the athlete's comfort with his or her body.

For the girls, how many menstrual periods have they had in the past 12 months? Amenorrhea or oligomenorrhea puts the athlete at risk for stress fractures and loss of bone mineral density. This group should also be asked about

Box 219-1.	Key Questions Related to Sudden Cardiac Death

1. Does the athlete have the same exercise tolerance as peers?
2. Has the athlete ever fainted with exercise?
3. Has you the athlete ever felt light-headed or dizzy with exercise?
4. Is there a family history of sudden nontraumatic death in anyone younger than age 50?

calcium intake because if it is low, it further increases the risk of loss of bone mineral and subsequent injury.

Has the athlete ever sustained a musculoskeletal injury? What was the treatment and was the injury rehabilitated? The orthopedic history is the most likely area to produce significant findings that can affect playability. The most important risk factor for a musculoskeletal injury during the season is having had a previous injury to that area.

EXAMINATION

Blood pressure and pulse should be obtained to detect the rare, severely hypertensive patient or the one who needs to be monitored. Exercise is beneficial to individuals with mild hypertension, and only an extreme measurement would warrant disqualification. Most dysrhythmias are benign. If premature ventricular contractions are noticed, it is helpful to document the effect of exercise on their frequency. This can be done by having the athlete run in place or up and down stairs for a minute or so. Premature ventricular contractions that go away with exercise are benign. The cardiac examination is low yield compared to the cardiac history but should be performed carefully to pick up any pathologic murmurs. The most common cause of sudden cardiac death is hypertrophic cardiomyopathy. Hypertrophic cardiomyopathy may produce a systolic murmur, which is worse with squatting or with a Valsalva maneuver.

The highest-yield area of the physical examination is the musculoskeletal examination. Any injury in the history warrants a more detailed examination of that body part. Whenever possible, the findings should be compared to the uninjured side to determine what is normal for the individual athlete. Physical fitness assessment with some kind of exercise test is not feasible in all settings, but it can help to determine evidence of off-season training and increased risk of injury if poor flexibility or poor strength is demonstrated.

PLAYABILITY

Following the history and examination, the disposition should be clear to the athlete and his or her parents. This is best communicated verbally and in writing. Frequently, the athlete is cleared to play but the health care provider has recommended a consultation with a specialist or recommends treatment with a medication. The health care provider should be mindful of the benefits of exercise and make efforts to help the youngster participate rather than focusing on a small risk as a reason for disqualification. There are few conditions that are absolute contraindications to participation in sports. Certain cardiac conditions, for example, significantly limit the number of activities in which the athlete can safely participate. A disqualification might be temporary pending further testing, as in the athlete who has characteristics of Marfan syndrome or the one with exercise-associated syncope, both of which need further cardiac evaluation. Some conditions that traditionally disqualified an athlete from football, such as a single kidney, no longer warrant disqualification. Because of the Americans with Disabilities Act, many physically challenged athletes legally must be allowed to play. For the athlete with

a single kidney, most attorneys recommend a written informed consent before allowing the athlete to play.

The American Academy of Pediatrics has produced charts that classify sports by strenuousness and degree of contact and identify particular exercise and sport considerations for specific medical conditions. These charts can be found on the CD-ROM and can be quite helpful in addressing playability issues (see CD-ROM Tables 219-1 to 219-5).

GENERAL PRINCIPLES OF PLAYABILITY

Caring for the athlete is often not different from caring for any other patient until the question arises "When can I play?" Sometimes the athlete has unrealistic expectations of returning to play or is concerned about pressure from the coach or teammates to return to action. We emphasize a functional examination to determine playability and to help the adolescent to pay attention to signals from the body in regard to playability. In general, before the athlete is allowed to play after an injury to the extremity, the joint(s) must have full pain-free range of motion, and there should be nearly full strength of the involved muscles. The athlete must be able to perform activities resembling the sports activity. In running sports, the athlete must first be able to run full speed without pain or limp and then run full speed and change directions both ways without pain or limp. We provide a written program so that the criteria for return to competition are clear and the athlete can work toward a goal (Box 219-2).

OVERUSE INJURIES

As was mentioned previously, adolescents are sustaining an increasing number of overuse injuries. With acute injuries, there are often obvious findings because of macro-level tissue

---

Box 219-2. The Running Program

This can be handed out to the athlete so that the criteria for return to competition are clear and the athlete can work toward a goal.

Running Program

1. Jog ¼ to ½ mile. Stop immediately if limping or if there is pain. Wait until tomorrow to start the program again. If there is no pain or limp during your jog, you may proceed to the following:
2. Three or four 40-yard sprints at half speed. If no pain or limp, then do the following:
3. Three or four 40-yard sprints at three quarter speed. If no pain or limp, then do the following:
4. Three or four 40-yard sprints at full speed followed by four to six full-speed starts. If no pain or limp, then do the following:
5. Six to eight 40-yard cutting (changing directions) at half speed every 5 to 10 yards. Then do the following:
6. Six to eight 40-yard cutting at full speed.

   After every workout, ice should be applied immediately to the injured area. (Do not stand around.)

   Once you can perform all of the above tasks with no pain and minimal swelling, you may return to competition. If you short-cut this program, you are only fooling yourself, risking reinjury or possibly a more serious injury and a much longer time out of competition.

trauma. With overuse injuries, there is repetitive microscopic tissue damage that is exceeding the body's ability to heal. This can lead to tenderness of the area without swelling or other findings on examination.

The treatment of these injuries usually requires *relative* rest. Since the athlete is overusing the extremity, he or she must do less, but this does not always require total rest for any period of time. For example, the swimmer with a sore shoulder might need to cut her yardage in half and learn appropriate exercises for her rotator cuff for a minimum of 4 to 6 weeks. She will not be as well served by being required to rest completely for more than a few days.

APOPHYSITES

Overuse injuries appear to be on the rise in young athletes. Among the most common overuse injuries are injuries to various apophyses, the traction growth plates that usually correspond to bony prominences at tendinous attachments (Fig. 219-1). Although described as apophysites, implying considerable inflammation, these injuries are usually due to repetitive microtrauma of fibrocartilage. The most common apophyses to be affected with corresponding eponyms are the calcaneal (Sever), tibial (Osgood-Schlatter), and iliac.

Calcaneal Apophysitis

The calcaneal apophysis closes around the seventeenth year of life. Calcaneal apophysitis is epidemic in youth soccer players, usually between the ages of 8 to 14. It is unusual to see Achilles tendonitis in childhood, because the apophysis undergoes microscopic breakdown under stress instead of the tendon being injured. This is due to overuse of the plantar flexor mechanism, not from bruising of the calcaneus. Many of the children are running in shoes with little or no arch support. Unlike many running shoes, soccer shoes for children rarely have such support. Quarter-inch heel lifts provide some relief, but for children who have significant ankle valgus, that is, midfoot hyperpronation (Fig. 219-2), arch supports or new shoes with better arch supports are often helpful. Some of the children have poor calf flexibil-

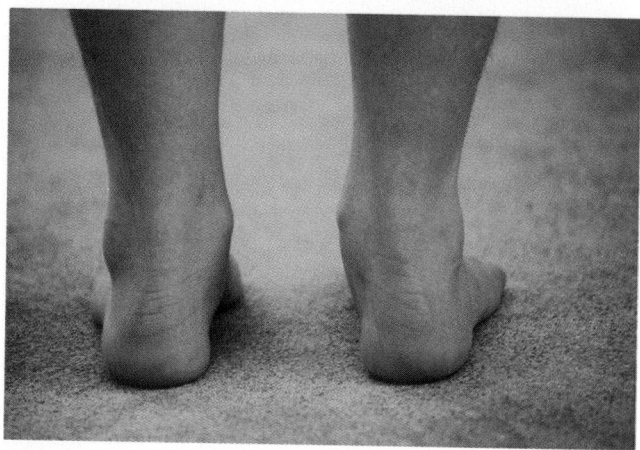

Figure 219-2. Hyperpronation. This young athlete has marked bilateral ankle valgus and midfoot pronation. She is at risk for a variety of overuse syndromes with this degree of hyperpronation.

ity and need to work on stretching the heel cords. Ice and analgesia are used as needed for comfort. In general, as long as the youngster is not limping, play may continue. If there is limping or favoring of one heel, it is time to stop and ice down.

Osgood-Schlatter Disease

Osgood-Schlatter disease (OSD) occurs between the ages of 11 and 15 years, with earlier onset in girls. Factors in the history can often suggest OSD (Box 219-3). The athlete usually reports pain with running and jumping activities and exquisite pain if they bump the tender, prominent tibial tubercle. There is an association of OSD and growth spurts, probably because of the concomitant loss of muscular flexibility, especially of the hamstring muscles. On examination, there is point tenderness of the tibial tubercle with localized swelling, poor quadriceps bulk, and poor hamstring flexibility. Athletes with OSD also are likely to be hyperpronators on gait analysis. Radiographs are usually not indicated but should be considered if the injury is acute or if there is an effusion of the knee joint, which would be indicative of some other injury. Management includes attention to better arch support in sport shoes for the athlete with hyperpronation. Most athletes with OSD will benefit from a diligent hamstring-stretching program, ideally taught by an athletic trainer or physical therapist. Any work on quadriceps strengthening risks worsening the condition and should be addressed when the athlete is asymptomatic.

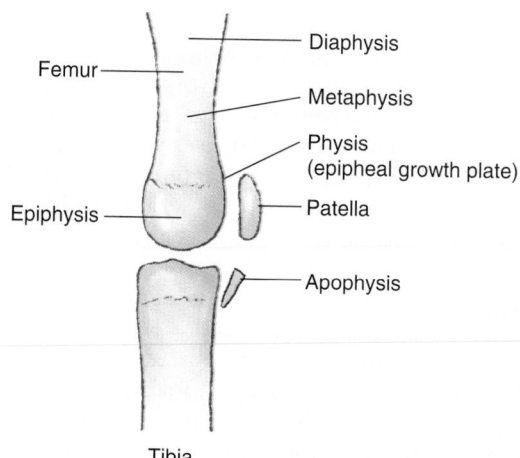

Figure 219-1. The apophysis is a traction growth plate and is located at the tibial tubercle for the patellar tendon. The pressure physis is located between the epiphysis and metaphysis on long bones.

Labels in figure: Femur — Diaphysis; Metaphysis; Physis (epipheal growth plate); Epiphysis — Patella; Apophysis; Tibia

Box 219-3. Factors Contributing to Osgood-Schlatter Disease

Excessive running
Excessive jumping
Running or jumping on hard surfaces
Direct trauma to the tibial tubercle
Tight hamstring muscles
Midfoot hyperpronation

Iliac Apophysitis

Iliac apophysitis occurs in running athletes who present with dull, achy hip pain associated with activity. It may be bilateral. On examination, the athlete localizes the tenderness to the iliac crest and most commonly the anterior superior iliac spine. There may be reduced hip flexor flexibility. Any pain with hip rotation should make the examiner think of another diagnosis, and radiographs should be obtained to rule out hip joint pathology. Treatment of the iliac apophysitis includes relative rest and diligent stretching of the hip flexors. Ice and an analgesic may be used for comfort.

SUMMARY

An increasing number of adolescents participate in sports, sustaining an increasing number of overuse injuries. Adolescents will likely visit with a health care provider for the preparticipation evaluation or for an overuse injury. Knowledge of the principles of sports medicine will continue to be important in the care of active adolescents.

Additional Resources, CD-ROM

AAP charts on sports medicine	Tables 219-1 to 219-5
Bibliography	

SUGGESTED READINGS

American Academy of Family Physicians, American Academy of Pediatrics, American Medical Society for Sports Medicine, American Orthopedic Society for Sports Medicine, American Osteopathic Society for Sports Medicine: Preparticipation Physical Evaluation, 2nd ed. New York, McGraw-Hill, 1997.

Micheli LJ, Fehlandt AF: Overuse injuries to tendons and apophyses in children and adolescents. Clin Sports Med 1992;11(4):713–726.

SECTION 6   ADOLESCENT CARE: *General Approach to the Adolescent*

220

Legal and Ethical Issues in Adolescent Health Care

Alain Joffe

ROLE OF THE GENERALIST

1 Understand the core concepts of consent and confidentiality.

2 Know and apply the three key elements of consent.

3 Know the particular state laws about consent and confidentiality.

4 Discuss confidentiality issues with patients.

5 Know the limits of confidentiality, especially with regard to state laws.

Adolescents occupy an ambiguous place in society. As they pass through adolescence, they achieve adult physical and cognitive capabilities well before the law or their parents are prepared to accept them fully as adults. Relatively mature in mind and body, many young people engage in behaviors that society often view as being reserved for adults. When seeking health care pertaining to these behaviors, adolescents wish to be treated as adults. In contrast, many parents believe that they are entitled, in fulfilling their role as parents, to participate in their teenager's health care and make decisions for or with the teenager. The situation is even more complex when an adolescent is living on his or her own or in circumstances in which parents are not acting in the adolescent's best interests. These differing perspectives give rise to a number of legal and ethical issues, centering primarily on consent and confidentiality.

CONSENT

Western culture and its health care system place great value on the related principles of respect for persons and patient autonomy. It is generally accepted that adult patients should be free to either consent to or refuse the recommendations of their health care providers. Consent has three essential components (Box 220-1): that it be freely given, that the individual have all the relevant (from the patient's perspective) information necessary to make an informed decision, and that the individual have the capacity (competence) to make a decision based on the information provided. Most controversies concerning consent by adolescents revolve around whether adolescents are competent to make health care decisions and whether the adolescent or his or her parents should make the decision.

Less than 20 years ago, Chief Justice Warren Burger wrote, "Most children, even in adolescence, simply are not able to make sound judgments concerning many decisions, including their need for medical care or treatment." Developmental psychologists have demonstrated just the opposite. Early in adolescence, teenagers tend to be quite concrete in their thinking and lack the future orientation and abstract reasoning ability that would permit them to understand the significance of information presented to them and assess the risks and benefits of various treatment options. As adolescents mature, they acquire increasingly sophisticated cognitive capabilities. Research demonstrates that by age 14, adolescents demonstrate reasoning abilities regarding health-related matters similar to those of adults. Affording young people increasing autonomy in making their own health care decisions fosters this development and helps them achieve the important developmental goals of separating from parents and consolidating an individual identity.

Recognition of this developing capacity and of the many adolescents who are either living on their own or will not seek care for potentially serious health care conditions if parental consent is a prerequisite has moved the courts beyond Justice Burger's assessment. Most state legislatures have enacted minor consent statutes, specifically granting adolescents (regardless of age) the authority to consent on their own for advice about or treatment of emergencies, sexually transmitted infections, pregnancy, contraception (excluding sterilization), and drug abuse. Since infection with the hepatitis B or human immunodeficiency virus (HIV) is usually related to sexual or drug use behaviors, minors in some states also have the legal capacity to consent to vaccination against hepatitis B or be tested for HIV without parental consent. Many states also permit adolescents to seek care for mental health–related problems at age 16. Because the exact wording of these laws varies from state to state, clinicians should review their state's statutes carefully before treating an adolescent. To date, no provider has been successfully sued by a parent for treating a minor age 15 or above without parental consent if the care was consistent with accepted medical standards. State regulations regarding abortions are more complex, often requiring consent of a parent or permission of a judge ("judicial bypass"). Some states do permit minors to consent to abortion if, in the opinion of the physician, parental notifi-

---

Box 220-1. Key Elements of Consent

1. It is freely given.
2. The individual has all the relevant information necessary to make an informed decision.
3. The individual has the capacity (competence) to make a decision based on the information provided.

Box 220-2. Mature and Emancipated Minors

Mature Minor

1. Age 15 or older
2. Demonstrates some indication of maturity

Emancipated Minor

1. Living on his or her own and/or financially independent
2. Married
3. In the military
4. Pregnant or parenting

---

cation would not be in the best interests of the minor (e.g., would lead to physical or emotional abuse).

Courts have increasingly acknowledged the right of "mature minors" to give consent on their own behalf. Mature minors must be 15 years of age or older and demonstrate some indication of maturity, such as making one's own appointments, getting to or paying for appointments independently, following up on recommendations, and/or displaying an understanding of the risks or benefits of varying treatment options (Box 220-2). The mature minor doctrine is most easily applied when an adolescent consents to treatment that is clearly in his or her best interests, when there is no clear choice among competing options, or when the minor's wishes are in accord with those of his or her parents. More challenging are situations in which a minor refuses potentially life-saving treatment, either in agreement with his or her parents (as in the case of a teenager of the Jehovah's Witness faith who refuses a blood transfusion) or in conflict with their opinion. If a minor over the age of 14 demonstrates a clear understanding of the consequences of refusal, appears to be acting free of parental pressure, and shows no indication that his or her competence to consent is diminished in any way owing to illness or medication, it is difficult to argue against granting the minor's wishes.

States also generally recognize the right of emancipated minors to give their consent. Emancipated minors are those living on their own and/or financially independent, married minors, those in the military, and pregnant or parenting teenagers.

A direct corollary of respecting the adolescent's capacity and right to consent (or refuse) would preclude drug-testing them without the adolescent's knowledge and permission. The emerging field of presymptomatic genetic testing will require careful reexamination of an adolescent's right to be informed of and accept or refuse such testing.

CONFIDENTIALITY

Respect for persons and their privacy dictates that information shared by patients with clinicians remain confidential unless there is a legal requirement to disclose it or unless the information reveals a serious threat to the adolescent's or another person's health. An argument for confidentiality can also be constructed on utilitarian grounds: Granting confidentiality increases the likelihood that patients will reveal very personal or potentially embarrassing information. Survey research has demonstrated that adolescents would not seek care for a variety of situations, particularly those related to sexual behaviors, if information were shared with parents. In one study, fewer than 20% of adolescents would seek care for contraception, sexually transmitted infections, or drug use if parental knowledge of the visit were mandatory. If reassured about confidentiality, 50% more would seek care for these conditions. More recent research indicates that adolescents are more likely to disclose sensitive information if clinicians make explicit statements about confidentiality. Conversely, there is no evidence to suggest that mandating parental involvement improves communication among teenagers and parents or improves health outcomes. The American Academy of Pediatrics, the American College of Obstetricians and Gynecologists, the American Medical Association, and the National Medical Association have all endorsed the concept of confidentiality for adolescents, noting that "ultimately, the health risks to adolescents are so compelling that legal barriers and deference to parental involvement should not stand in the way of needed care." Whether this important principle can be maintained in an era when third-party payers are increasingly scrutinizing medical records and requiring extensive documentation remains to be seen.

Both teenagers and physicians often misunderstand the concept of confidentiality. In one study, only one third of adolescents knew of their right to seek confidential care, and 11% could not choose the correct definition of "confidential" from four possible word choices. Among a random sample of 786 primary care physicians, only 21% reported discussing confidentiality at every visit, and 11% never discussed it at all. Among those who discussed the topic, 64% offered *unconditional* confidentiality. Since there are certain circumstances in which the law (sexual abuse) or the principle of beneficence (the adolescent discloses participation in a behavior that poses a significant risk to his or her health) requires that confidentiality be broken, clinicians should be careful how they discuss this concept. Clinicians should make an explicit statement about confidentiality at the beginning of the visit and describe, in general terms, its limits. They should also

reassure the adolescent that if the clinician believes that confidentiality must be broken, he or she will tell the adolescent first and involve the adolescent in the process of doing so.

The foregoing discussion should not be interpreted to mean that the practice of adolescent health care generally excludes parents from participating in their son's or daughter's health care. Parents can provide important information about the psychosocial functioning of their son or daughter, and most adolescents actively involve their parents in their health care. Conversely, clinicians often assist the reluctant adolescent to involve a parent (or another adult) when it appears that it is in the best interests of the teenager to do so. However, it is the reassurance about confidentiality that creates the environment in which this process can move forward.

Additional Resources, CD-ROM

Bibliography

Mini-index of Related Topics   CH.

- ETHICAL AND LEGAL ISSUES IN PEDIATRICS   260

SUGGESTED READINGS

Alderman EM, Fleischman AR: Should adolescents make their own health-care choices? Contemp Pediatr 1993;10:65–82.

Council on Scientific Affairs: Confidential health services for adolescents. JAMA 1993;269:1420–1424.

Ford CA, Milstein SG, Halpern-Felsher BL, Irwin CE Jr: Influence of physician confidentiality assurances on adolescents' willingness to disclose information and seek future health care: A randomized controlled trial. JAMA 1997;278:1029–1034.

Hofman AD: A rational policy toward consent and confidentiality in adolescent health care. J Adolesc Health Care 1980;1:9–17.

Sigman GS, Silber TJ, English A, Epner JEG: Confidential health care for adolescents: Position paper of the Society for Adolescent Medicine. J Adolesc Health 1997;21:408–415.

221 Risk and Resilience

Amy J. N. Plumb and Patricia K. Kokotailo

ROLE OF THE GENERALIST

1   Identify risk factors in adolescents.
2   Identify resilience and protective factors
3   Recognize that risk, resilience, and protective factors are affected by age, developmental status, and family and social contexts.
4   Counsel adolescents and families regarding risk reduction.

FUNDAMENTALS

The American Heritage Dictionary defines risk as "the possibility of suffering harm or loss; danger." Risk taking can be defined as participating in potentially health-compromising activities with little or no understanding of the potential negative consequences. Risk-taking behaviors include those activities that can directly or indirectly cause suffering or harm. They are dangerous to the health and well-being of the individual. The most common examples of risk-taking behavior are smoking, illegal drug use, alcohol consumption, sexual activity, and operating motor vehicles—activities that can cause adverse outcomes such as cancer, brain damage, and death. They can also cause harm by association, that is, the person killed in the car crash might not be the driver of the car. Many of these behaviors are linked, and the effects are compounded. Alcohol has been linked to 50% of motor vehicle accidents that cause injury to adolescents. An individual using drugs and/or alcohol might not make the same choices about engaging in sexual behavior and certainly does not have the same ability to operate an automobile as when he or she is not under the influence.

Vulnerability, a term that is now more frequently used in discussions of risk behaviors, is an interactive process between the social contexts of young people's lives and a set of underlying behaviors that, when present, place the young person at risk for negative outcomes such as injury and unwanted pregnancy. Vulnerabilities may result from biologic factors (e.g., chronic illness), cognitive factors (e.g., how the adolescent perceives risk), and familial factors (e.g., being reared in an abusive family). An adolescent's level of vulnerability can be described by the observed risk behaviors and outcomes.

For some activities, the level of risk associated with an activity may vary with the age, developmental status, and the participants' social and environmental situation. There are, however, risks involved in all daily activities that everyone assumes while going about one's routines. Driving a car to work 5 miles on a sunny day, with no one else on the road, is inherently less risky than making that same drive at midnight during an ice storm when the driver has forgotten his or her glasses. The underlying physical and emotional health of the individual can play a role in determining the level of risk. Smoking cigarettes is dangerous for everyone but more immediately dangerous for someone with cystic fibrosis or a pregnant adolescent. Table 221-1 lists adverse outcomes of common adolescent risk-taking behaviors.

Some risk-taking activities can be made less dangerous with proper equipment and precautions. For example, the use of helmets when riding bikes or motorcycles can reduce the risk of injury and death. Seat belt use can diminish the morbidity and mortality associated with car crashes. Using these safety measures can prevent about 30% of deaths and 60% of injuries.

Participating in sports can cause injury. Football, wrestling, and gymnastics have the highest potential for injury. Swimming is the leader for risk among recreational activities.

Resilience, the ability to recover quickly from illness or change, is what enables some individuals to withstand the social forces and behaviors that could cause them harm. Resilience, along with resources, assets, and protective factors, arise from individual, familial, and social environments in which a young person lives. Resilient people have good

Table 221-1. Connection between Risk-Taking Behaviors and Adverse Outcomes

Risk-Taking Behavior	Adverse Outcome
Smoking	Lung irritation, coughing, addiction
	Chronic lung disease, heart disease
	Cancer, death
Illegal drug use	Mood alteration, mental slowness, addiction
	Cardiac arrhythmia, death
Alcohol use	Mood alteration, chronic liver failure
	Addiction, malnutrition, death
Sexual activity	Sexually transmitted diseases
	Fertility problems
	Pregnancy
	Emotional trauma (if not consensual)
Driving motor vehicles	Unintentional injuries, death

communication skills, easygoing temperaments, good problem-solving skills and sense of humor, empathy, and a balanced perspective and are spiritual. Protective factors also include intelligence. While some characteristics of resilience seem to be genetic, some may be learned and affected by environment. Nurturing the qualities that can enhance resilience is important to decrease the effects and prevalence of risk-taking behaviors and their associated outcomes (Boxes 221-1 and 221-2).

In addition to the personal qualities of resiliency listed above, resilient adolescents have been found to have at least one close relationship with a caring, competent adult who recognizes values and rewards prosocial behavior. Parents, teachers, relatives, and neighbors can all serve as protective adult figures. This concept has strengthened interest in improving various social programs aimed at improving adolescents' well-being. Many programs that involve adolescent work, juvenile justice, education, and social legislation place a focus on adult mentorship, social skills training, volunteerism, and community service.

ADOLESCENT RISK

Risk taking in adolescence is common. Adolescents are trying to define who they are as they move from childhood to adulthood. They endure the pressures of school, friends, family, and society during a time when their sense of self is not well developed. Their life experience does not give them the breadth of knowledge to fully understand the consequences of their behavior. Depending on their psychological stage of development, they might still feel invincible and not have the ability to think abstractly or far into the future. Compounding these difficulties, the parents and adults to whom the teenager looks for role modeling might themselves be participating in risk-taking behaviors. The

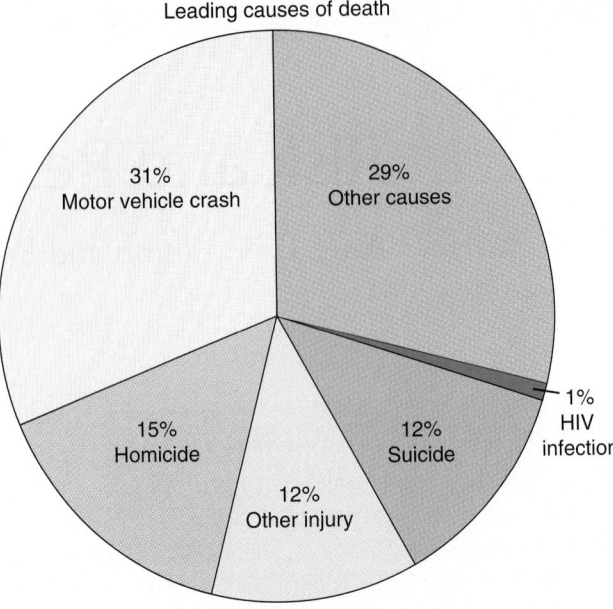

Leading causes of death

Figure 221-1. Leading causes of death in youths ages 10 to 24. (From Centers for Disease Control and Prevention: Youth Risk Behavior Surveillance System 2001 Information and Results; Summary Results: United States and by State. Available at: www.cdc.gov/nccephp/dash/yrbs/2001/summary_results/index.htm.)

adolescent might not know how to access adults who could be good role models to help guide them.

In the United States, the leading causes of death among adults are heart disease, cancer, cerebral vascular accidents, and unintentional injuries. Nearly three quarters (70.6%) of all deaths among youths and young adults aged 10–24 years result from only four causes: motor vehicle crashes (31.4%), other unintentional injuries (12%), homicide (15.3%), and suicide (11.9%) (Fig. 221-1). Adolescents are relatively inexperienced and might not have the driving skills needed. They might be distracted by friends and loud music. Not wearing a seat belt and being under the influence of drugs or alcohol add to the level of risk and potential injury. Peer pressure to experiment with drugs and alcohol is common. In 2003, 29% of twelfth-graders in the United States admitted to binge drinking (the consumption of five or more drinks in a row) in the previous 2 weeks, according to the national *Monitoring the Future Study*. Teens are also at risk for infections and unplanned pregnancy through sexual intercourse: 47% of boys and girls in high school in the United States state that they have ever had intercourse, and 63% of those state that they used a condom at the last intercourse (Box 221-3).

APPLICATION TO PRACTICE

The primary care provider can play an important role in helping adolescents to negotiate some of the perils that they face. The physician can be a source of accurate information about health, illness, and disease. He or she can help to identify youths who are at risk as well as the factors that are associated with resiliency. This can be done through direct questioning of the adolescent and reviewing the family and social history and past medical history (Boxes 221-4 and 221-5).

Many unintentional injuries, attempted overdoses, and self-harm events present to the emergency department, not to primary care offices. It is important to obtain these records to look for clues or patterns to the patient's behavior. The primary care physician might have known the patient since birth. This can be a distinct advantage. In this circumstance, the physician will know the family and social support systems so important to fostering resilience in children. It is important to identify adolescents who are at risk and provide support and praise to those who are not choosing to participate in risk-taking behaviors.

History

Questions about the patient's as well as his or her friends' activities should be asked to screen for risk-taking behaviors. It might be more comfortable for the patient if the

---

Box 221-4. Evaluating Risk: Questions to Ask

Do you and/or your friends participate in any behaviors you think are risky? If yes, what are they?

Do you smoke (cigarettes/marijuana)?

How do you drink alcohol?

Have you ever tried drugs or used prescription medicine that was not yours?

Are you sexually active? If so, how many partners have you had?

When you drive cars, boats, or ATVs, are you ever under the influence of drugs or alcohol?

Have you ever gotten into a car with a driver who was under the influence of drugs or alcohol?

Do you use a seat belt in the car? How often?

Do you wear a bike helmet? How often?

Are there guns in your home? Are they locked?

Do you feel safe with your boyfriend/girlfriend or the person you are seeing?

Box 221-5. Evaluating Resiliency: Questions to Ask

How is your relationship with your parents?

What do you like to do with your friends?

What activities in your school or community are you involved in?

Is there an adult besides your parents with whom you can talk? If so, who is he or she?

---

primary care provider asks questions about friends' behavior first. Specifically, the provider should question the patient about his or her own experience with tobacco, alcohol, drugs and sexual intercourse. The provider should also ask about use of seat belts in the car and, if they are driving, who is in the car with them. Some states have graduated driving laws for new teenage drivers. These might allow new drivers an excuse not to have friends with them in the car, which can be an added distraction. Usually, these questions should be asked when the physician is alone with the adolescent. It is important to establish the confidential nature of this time with the patient. Unless the adolescent reveals issues regarding immediate self-harm or abuse, the information can be kept confidential. Factors associated with increase risk should also be explored (Box 221-6).

Physical Examination, Laboratory Tests, and Screens

No specific physical examination is linked to diagnosing an adolescent at risk. However, there might be clues to some of the behaviors that could cause harm. When performing the physical examination, the provider should look closely at the skin for unusual bruises or scars. Has the adolescent tried to harm himself or herself, or are there needle marks? Is the patient clean and well groomed or disheveled and dirty? What is the patient's sense of self-confidence? Does the patient make eye contact? Does the patient smell of cigarettes or marijuana?

Laboratory tests are available to screen for drug use, but they are not necessarily useful in the routine office setting. The presence or absence of these substances on a given day might not reflect the person's risk status. These tests are most beneficial in the acute emergency department setting when the patient is medically ill or unconscious.

Management

Prevention, both primary and secondary, is a key to managing risk issues with adolescents. If an adolescent is not engaging in risky behaviors, the provider should discuss the

---

Box 221-6. Factors Associated with Increased Risk

Lack of close relationship with parents

Minimal parental supervision

Family chaos

School transitions

Peers who participate in risky behaviors

Illicit substance use availability

Male gender

Lack of concern about consequences of behavior

normative nature of many risk activities with the parents and young person, the risk of increasing participation in such activities, and the consequences of activities. Parental role modeling, such as wearing seat belts or not drinking and driving, can send powerful messages to a teen. The provider should discuss the comorbidity of alcohol use and illicit drug use, the danger of alcohol or drug use and driving, and the dangers of substance use and sexual activity. It is also advisable to explore the difficulty in making good choices about safety while under the influence of alcohol and illegal or prescription drugs.

The long-term implications of risk-taking activities may be difficult to understand, so finding immediate outcomes to risk-taking behavior is important. The provider should, for example, talk about the accident that occurred recently in his or her neighborhood when the teenagers driving were killed in a car crash. Although engaging in early sexual intercourse with multiple partners increases the chance for a woman to have cervical cancer, the more immediate threat might be pregnancy or HIV infection.

If an adolescent who is at risk or already engaging in risky behaviors is identified, the provider should talk with the adolescent about his or her behavior (Box 221-7). The provider should try to help adolescents find alternative activities and give them resources for counseling or therapy. Emphasizing delaying riskier activities, such as sexual activity, can be a good strategy, buying time for an adolescent to gain more cognitive maturity and resistance skills. The provider should involve the patient in the plan and involve the parent whenever possible. It is also important to identify resilience factors, and encourage families to strengthen those aspects that can help the adolescent to avoid risky behaviors.

A clinician should know his or her community resources and medical facilities to facilitate referral. Ongoing consultation and follow-up, especially in aftercare, are important roles of the clinician. Serving in an advocacy role, through local, state, or national organizations, and supporting risk reduction legislation are possible roles for providers. Local advocacy in promoting positive activities for youth through such groups as scouts, church groups, and community organizations can also serve to modify risk factors for youth.

Box 221-7. Risk Reduction Messages

Don't drink alcohol or use drugs.
Don't smoke cigarettes.
Practice sexual abstinence.
Practice safe sex if you are sexually active.
Use a seat belt in the car.
Use a bike helmet or motorcycle helmet.
Be aware that having a gun in the home always poses risks.
Avoid people who have guns illegally.
Learn how to solve conflicts without violence.
Use protective equipment (helmets, mouth guards, face protectors) for sports.
Learn to swim.
Wear life jackets for boating and water sports.
Learn first aid and CPR.

Mini-index of Related Topics

SUGGESTED READINGS

Blum RW, McNeely C, Nonnemaker J: Vulnerability, risk and protection. J Adolesc Health 2002;31S:28–39.

Grunbaum JA, Kann L, Kinchen SA, et al: Youth Risk Behavior Surveillance: United States, 2003. MMWR Morb Mortal Wkly Rep 2004;53(SS-2):1–96.

Johnston LD, O'Malley PM, Bachman JG, Schulenberg JE: Monitoring the Future—National Results on Adolescent Drug Use: Overview of Key Findings, 2003. (NIH Publication No. 04-5506.) Bethesda, Md, National Institute on Drug Abuse, 2004. Available at: www.monitoringthefuture.org.

Resnick M, Bearman P, Blum R, et al: Protecting adolescents from harm: Findings from the National Longitudinal Study on Adolescent Health. JAMA 1997;278(10):823.

222 Chronic Illness in the Adolescent

Maria Britto

ROLE OF THE GENERALIST

1 Provide primary and preventive health care, including anticipatory guidance.

2 Know areas of increased need in preventive care for this population.

3 Know resources available in the community for adolescents and young adults with chronic conditions and disabilities.

4 Coordinate care with specialists and community-based resources.

5 Prepare the adolescent and family for transition from child-oriented to adult-oriented health care.

6 Assist the adolescent with self-management and with adherence to medical regimens.

In the past 30 years, the proportion of adolescents with chronic conditions has risen markedly, with recent estimates of 12%–18% of adolescents living with some chronic condition and 6%–8% having a limitation in daily activity because of that condition. Although much of the increase is attributable to increased survival of those with formerly lethal conditions, the incidence of some conditions has also increased. Examples are survivors of improved neonatal care (e.g., children with cerebral palsy) and the increase of type 2 diabetes mellitus in adolescents.

PREVENTION

Youth with chronic conditions face the dual challenges of adolescent development and coping with their condition and its treatment. They engage in risky behaviors at rates similar to or slightly lower than those of the general adolescent population. They may have additional health concerns such as delayed maturation, difficulty in becoming independent from parents, or impaired fertility. Preventive care for these adolescents is extremely important, yet those with chronic conditions are less likely than healthy peers to receive routine preventive health care and anticipatory guidance. Too often, attention to preventive care is diverted to disease-related issues, or preventive care is lost through lack of coordination of care between the primary care clinician and the specialists.

For adolescents who are receiving both specialty and generalist care, the generalist should collaborate with the specialist regarding both chronic condition management and preventive care. The characteristics of the condition, coupled with the preferences of the family and the providers will determine whether responsibility for the chronic condition is shared between the primary care and specialty provider or whether the specialist will assume essentially all responsibility for management of the chronic condition. Responsibility for preventive care may vary in a similar manner. Clear delineation of these responsibilities must be communicated to all providers and the family to avoid duplications and omissions in services. Clear lines of communication and responsibility are especially important when there is a transition of the adolescent's care from pediatric providers to family physicians, internists, or other adult health care providers.

Most preventive care needs of adolescents with chronic conditions are similar to those of healthy peers and can follow well-established guidelines such as GAPS (Guidelines for Adolescent Preventive Services) and Bright Futures, but additional issues are usually present. Chronic conditions may speed up, delay, or have no effect on pubertal growth and maturation. Adolescents with spina bifida and with some genetic syndromes such as McCue-Albright syndrome often enter puberty early. More commonly, chronic conditions are associated with pubertal delay. For some conditions, such as diabetes mellitus, delay is associated with poor metabolic control. In others, such as cystic fibrosis, pubertal delay is intrinsic, even among those with good nutrition and mild lung disease. Anticipatory guidance regarding likely delays or advances and strategies for dealing with atypical pubertal timing should occur during late childhood and early adolescence.

Children and adolescents with chronic conditions, especially those with cognitive disabilities, are less likely than others to be asked about future plans and career goals. Regular inquiries throughout childhood and adolescence can help families develop visions of their adolescents as independent adults. Adolescents with chronic conditions might have additional challenges in development of appropriate romantic relationships. Adolescents with cognitive disabilities need developmentally appropriate counseling regarding good touch/bad touch, appropriate hugging, and so on. Those with physical disabilities might require assistance with comfortable means of physical intimacy. Adolescents are often quite inventive, and peer-to-peer support, through groups or informal contacts, can be helpful. The primary care clinician might not have the time or resources to provide detailed education for these concerns but can refer families to community resources such as the ARC (formerly the Association of Retarded Citizens).

In addition to the usual health promotion and risk behavior counseling, special attention should be paid to lifelong physical activity and recreation, since adolescents with chronic conditions may be less likely to engage in these behaviors and might require adaptive equipment. Another topic of special importance for some groups, such as adolescents with diabetes, is eating disorder screening. These adolescents both are at increased risk of disordered eating and may suffer serious short-term consequences from manipulating their insulin or diet to control weight. Substance use, even infrequent or experimental use, can be particularly risky for some adolescents with chronic conditions. For example, patients who are prescribed methotrexate for rheumatoid arthritis are at increased risk for liver damage if they consume alcohol. In prescribing any medication for any adolescent, potential interactions with substances that are frequently used by adolescents must be considered, especially alcohol. Psychiatric or behavioral comorbidity associated with chronic conditions varies greatly. It is essential to screen for depression and consider disease- and medication-related depression.

Reproductive health counseling can also be more complicated in this population. Condoms and other barrier methods are appropriate for all sexually active adolescents, regardless of their medical conditions. Those with latex allergy, common among individuals who have had multiple procedures, should be cautioned to use nonlatex condoms. Hormonal contraception, particularly estrogen-containing methods, may be relatively contraindicated in those with hypercoaguable states such as sickle cell disease or systemic lupus erythematosus. Adolescents who are at risk for low bone density, such as those with cystic fibrosis or impaired mobility, should be counseled about the risk of bone loss associated with injectable progestins. Some adolescents, such as boys with cystic fibrosis and those who have undergone pelvic irradiation for cancer, will be at high risk for infertility. Depending on the level of complexity and the provider's comfort with these issues, a referral to an adolescent medicine specialist or a gynecologist with expertise in medically complicated adolescents might be indicated.

Screening tests are generally the same as those for the healthy population. In some instances, however, the chronic condition may be associated with increased risk of premature or severe comorbid disease, and screening should be instituted early. For example, because systemic lupus erythematosus is associated with an increased risk of accelerated cardiovascular disease, screening for lipid abnormalities should start soon after diagnosis.

Immunizations are particularly important for adolescents whose condition puts them at increased risk from vaccine-preventable diseases. Essentially all adolescents can receive killed or recombinant vaccines such as hepatitis B and tetanus vaccine. Those who are immunocompetent but likely to become immunosuppressed (for example, an adolescent with juvenile arthritis who might require steroids or methotrexate in the future) should receive catch-up MMR and varicella vaccine as soon as possible. Pneumococcal vaccine should be given to all adolescents who have chronic pulmonary or cardiovascular disease or diabetes, if it was not given earlier. Those who are at very high risk (e.g., those with functional asplenia or renal failure) should receive a second pneumococcal vaccine by early adolescence. Influenza vaccine is administered in the fall of each year to those at increased risk. Hepatitis A vaccine should be given to those with chronic liver disease.

ADHERENCE

Problems with adherence in adolescents are often attributed to developmental factors such as a sense of invulnerability, the need to establish independence, the propensity for risk taking, or the lack of a future orientation. While these factors undoubtedly influence treatment adherence and self-management, empirical studies clearly relating developmental factors to adherence are sparse. In fact, reported levels of adherence with treatment regimens for chronic health conditions among adolescents are similar to those reported for adult populations. Between 30% and 60% of adolescents and adults fail to receive the full benefit of prescribed medications owing to nonadherence. Family, individual, and regimen factors have been determined that may identify those at high risk for adherence problems (Table 222-1). Adolescents with multiple risk factors and a history of chronic nonadherence likely will require a team effort to address the underlying issues and to create effective adherence plans. However, many adolescents can be helped in the primary care setting using simple intervention strategies.

Although accurately assessing adherence is the first step toward improving it, doing so has proved difficult. Physicians' global estimates are quite inaccurate in comparison with more invasive, labor-intensive, and costly methods such as pill counts, electronic monitoring devices, and blood or urine drug assays. A patient's prior level of adherence and the patient's own predications of his or her likelihood of adhering to a given regimen (especially if it is low) are better correlated with adherence than is physician assessment. Asking youths and families about their past experience with similar regimens and their willingness to undertake a new one is a reasonable first step. In assessing adherence to an ongoing regimen, more specific questions provide better information than global ones. Questions should be nonjudgmental, should ask about very specific aspects of the treatment regimen, and should have a short time frame, such as the last day or the last week. Additional questions such as "What keeps you from doing your exercise?" or

Table 222-1. Risk Factors for Adherence Problems	
Factor	**Problem**
Family factors	Dysfunctional families
	Familes with high levels of other activities reducing treatment regimen supervision
	Low family education
Patient factors	Adjustment or coping problems
Disease and regimen factors	Fluctuating course of disease
	High complexity of regimen
	Multiple side effects of regimen

"What gets in the way of taking your pills?" might help to identify modifiable barriers to adherence.

The most common reason given by patients for nonadherence is simple "forgetting." A second common cause is conflict between the regimen and the patient's usual daily routine. In prescribing a new regimen or changing an existing one, it is best to make only one change at a time. Adherence declines markedly with each additional dose of medication or action required per day. Choose medications that can be given the fewest times per day. Help the adolescent and family to identify stable, predictable times of the day to which medication can be linked. For example, if the adolescent always brushes his or her teeth in the morning, couple taking medication to that activity. Whenever possible, avoid the need to take medication at school. The more the adolescent participates in determining his or her medication schedule, the more likely it is that the adolescent will be able to adhere to it. In-office modeling and rehearsal, particularly of complicated maneuvers such as metered-dose inhaler use, can also help. Although adolescents are in the process of becoming independent adults, continued parental involvement and monitoring of treatment regimens have clearly been shown to improve adherence.

While there are no "magic bullets" for improving adherence, a number of strategies have been shown to be effective. One important strategy is to ensure that adolescents and their families have easy access to their health care provider. This includes readily available information and support by phone, through the Internet, or other means and easy access to appointments. A consistent contact in the physician's office, such as a primary nurse who knows the adolescent and his or her treatments, also helps.

For patient- and family based interventions, combined strategies have been generally more effective than strategies with a single focus. Educational or cognitive interventions are those based on improving knowledge. These may include one-on-one or group teaching, written and audiovisual materials, and phone interventions. These often focus on learning about the disease or condition, learning what needs to be done to control it, setting goals for desired outcomes (such as a hemoglobin A1C below 8 for an adolescent with diabetes), understanding expected benefits of treatment, knowing expected side effects and how to reduce them, and instruction and modeling of the regimen itself.

Behavioral interventions must balance adolescents' need for developing autonomy with their need for continued parental and professional monitoring. Token economies and other strategies that are effective for younger children gradually become less appropriate for adolescents. Prompts, such as beeping watches, can serve to cue the adolescent to take a medication or do a treatment but do not require active intervention from others. They serve to reinforce the adolescent's sense of autonomy and self-efficacy. Repackaging of medication (such as daily pillboxes) and dose schedule modification also allow the adolescent to take control of his or her treatment. Contracting, usually undertaken as a joint venture between the provider, the adolescent, and the parents, can set bounds on the adolescent's allowable behavior and create guidelines for parental intervention. Discipline-related interventions that are appropriate for most adolescents include parental monitoring of their adherence behavior, positive reinforcement of desired behaviors, ignoring of trivial or minor problems, structuring the environment to promote adherence (for example, placing medications on the dining table if the adolescent is to take them with breakfast), and consistent consequences for serious negative adherence behavior. Not surprisingly, these interventions are similar to effective discipline approaches for adolescents in all areas of life.

Affective interventions are those that are applied to feelings, emotions, social relationships, or social support. Some, such as peer-to-peer support networks, may be helpful to all adolescents with chronic conditions, whether they have current adherence problems or not. Others, such as family counseling and home visits, are usually reserved for those with greater difficulties.

TRANSITION

Adolescence is a time of transition from dependence on the family of origin to independence and orientation toward a family of one's own. Health care providers tend to think of transition primarily in terms of transfer of medical care from pediatric to adult health care providers. While health care transitions are extremely important, families report that education and vocational planning are their most important transition needs and the ones least likely to be addressed by health care providers (Box 222-1).

Promotion of optimal transition to adulthood starts in early childhood with helping families to develop a vision for their child as an independent adult. Parents of small children with chronic conditions should be asked about their goals and vision for their child. Young children themselves should be asked what they want to be when they grow up. In early adolescence, providers should inquire about family responsibilities, such as chores. All but the most disabled adolescents can accept responsibility for some aspect of family well-being. Appropriate work experiences during adolescence and financial responsibilities, such as handling an allowance, can help to prepare the adolescent for more independent living.

By middle adolescence, inquiries should include specific plans for post–high school vocational training, work, or college. This planning might need to be more detailed than that for adolescents in the general population. While most primary care physicians will not have the resources or expertise to be extensively involved in this planning, they can assist families in many ways. First, they should raise the issue early. Second, the physician can act as the adolescent's health advocate in the school-based transition planning that is mandated by age 14 for all those with an Individualized

Box 222-1. Domains of Transition

- Medical care
- Education
- Vocation/career
- Social/recreation
- Housing/transportation
- Financial management

Education Plan. Third, providers should be aware of transition and vocational resources in their community. Every state has a department of vocational rehabilitation, and many states have programs specifically designed for the transition needs of adolescents and young adults with chronic health conditions. Formal transition programs may be available through community youth-service agencies or through large medical centers.

Transition of medical care is a process that occurs over time. For all adolescents, health care transition should involve a gradual shift in responsibilities and interactions with health care providers from parents to the adolescent. Young adolescents should assume increasing responsibility for self-management of their condition and should increasingly interact directly with their physicians and other health care providers. By middle to late adolescence, most adolescents should spend time alone with their health care providers. They should also, with their parents' help, assume gradual responsibility for negotiating the health care system, such as making their own appointments and calling for their own prescription refills. For many adolescents, transition to an adult-oriented system of care will involve actual transfer of care from a pediatric to an adult health care provider. For others, it will involve an ongoing relationship with a primary care provider (such as a family physician) but with a reorientation of the clinical interactions to reflect the adolescent's increasing maturity. Adolescents and families should be involved in discussions about the timing and processes for undertaking transfer. For situations in which an actual transfer of care will occur, steps that primary care providers can take to ensure successful transfer are summarized in Box 222-2. For

adolescents with multiple physicians, sequential transfers may be helpful. For many adolescents, it might be easier to transfer primary care first. The adult primary care provider can then serve as a bridge to adult specialty services. Family physicians with a particular interest in children and young people with chronic conditions or internal medicine/pediatric physicians may be ideally suited to care for this population. Many adolescents transfer outpatient services first and, when ill, revert initially to a pediatric setting. Adolescents and young adults might move back and forth between pediatric and adult settings for some time during the transition. A brief written summary of the adolescent's major diagnoses, key surgeries, medications, and other health and community care providers is essential to smooth the transition from one provider to another.

Mini-index of Related Topics

SUGGESTED READINGS

American Academy of Pediatrics, American Academy of Family Physicians, American College of Physicians—American Society of Internal Medicine: A consensus statement on health care transitions for young adults with special health care needs. Pediatrics 2002; 110:1304–1306.

Health Care Transitions. (A consortium site for health care and other life transitions for those with disabilities and chronic conditions. Contains an annotated bibliography as well as resource, program, and policy information.) Available at: http://hctransitions.ichp.edu.

Rapoff MA (ed): Adherence to Pediatric Medical Regimens. New York, Kluwer Academic/Plenum Publishers, 1999.

Rosen DS: Pubertal growth and sexual maturation for adolescents with chronic illness or disability. Pediatrician 1991;18:105–120.

Roter DL, Hall JA, Merisca R, et al: Effectiveness of interventions to improve patient compliance: A meta-analysis. Med Care 1998; 36:1138–1161.

Sackett DL, Haynes RB (eds): Compliance with Therapeutic Regimens. Baltimore, Md, Johns Hopkins University Press, 1976.

Box 222-2. Health Care Issues That Are Important for Transition

- Health insurance (especially changes after age 18–21)
- Adult-oriented generalist provider
- Adult-oriented subspecialty care
- Assessment for other disability-based services
- Personal assistance and waivers
- Self-management
- Health care advocacy skills
- Health promotion and prevention

223 Acne

Mark Herron and Sheryll L. Vanderhooft

ROLE OF THE GENERALIST

1 Recognize the four basic pathophysiologic factors of acne vulgaris.

2 Select appropriate treatments for acne based on the morphology of the lesions and severity of involvement.

3 Identify the side effects of medications used to treat acne.

4 Provide appropriate education for the patient with acne to promote compliance with treatment.

5 Identify acne patients who need evaluation for an underlying endocrinologic abnormality.

6 Refer to a dermatologist for treatment of severe, nodulocystic, scarring acne, or acne that is refractory to conventional treatment.

FUNDAMENTALS

Pilosebaceous units, sebaceous glands associated with a hair follicle (see Fig. 71-1), are found everywhere on the body except the palms and the soles. Sebaceous glands develop from a bulge in the hair follicle and are well differentiated alongside the hair follicles at 4 months' gestation. The central cells become lipid producing. Because pilosebaceous units are activated at birth by maternal hormones, newborns have large sebaceous glands. They diminish in size early, are quiescent during most of childhood, and then activate around adolescence. Sebaceous glands begin to enlarge at 10 or 12 years of age and continue to grow until adulthood.

Acne is an inflammatory disease of the pilosebaceous unit characterized by comedones (blackheads and whiteheads), inflammatory papules, pustules, nodules, and cysts. It affects 80% of those between 10 and 30 years (17 million people in the United States) and is the most common skin condition treated by physicians. Although two thirds of teenagers with acne want to discuss acne with their physician, only one third will actually ask to be treated. Acne is not just a disorder of adolescence; it spans all ages and is seen in neonates, infants, prepubertal children, adults, and even the elderly. It may physically and emotionally scar those who suffer from it.

Acne is not caused by poor hygiene or eating sweets or greasy foods. Four basic pathophysiologic factors are involved with the development of acne: excessive sebum production, abnormal follicular keratinization, follicular microflora, and inflammation.

Excessive Sebum Production. Sebum is a mixture of triglycerides, wax esters, squalene, and sterol esters. Sebum production, a result of androgen stimulation of the sebaceous glands, peaks during adolescence and declines after age 20. Adrenarche begins around ages 8 to 9 as dehydroepiandrosterone sulfate is produced, even before the onset of secondary sexual characteristics. Dehydroepiandrosterone sulfate causes enlargement of the sebaceous glands and increases the sebum secretion rate. The severity of acne correlates with the amount of sebum secreted.

Abnormal Follicular Keratinization ("Sticky Pores"). In acne patients, the follicular epithelium is abnormally cohesive from abnormal cell differentiation. Follicular keratin is retained in the follicule when it does not desquamate in a normal fashion, producing a plug known as a microcomedone (see Fig. 71-2), the precursor lesion in acne. Obstruction of the pilosebaceous duct prevents the normal transfer of triglycerides, waxy esters, and lipid product of the sebaceous glands to the skin surface.

Follicular Microflora. *Propionibacterium acnes* is an anaerobic gram-positive diphtheroid that colonizes the follicles after adrenarche when sebum production has increased. Although a normal skin flora, the number of these bacteria inhabiting the follicles is higher in patients with acne. The combination of sebaceous oils and desquamated epithelial cells provides a nutritive culture. *P. acnes* will hydrolyze triglycerides to free fatty acids within the pilosebaceous follicles. These fatty acids are irritating, contribute to the obstruction of the follicle, and promote an inflammatory response. The organism also recruits polymorphonuclear leukocytes through its chemoattractant factors. In the process of phagocytosis, leukocytes release hydrolases that rupture the follicular wall, releasing the contents of the follicle into the dermis, which intensifies the inflammatory reaction.

Inflammation. If the clogged pilosebaceous unit is traumatized in any way or if the sebaceous material increases in volume, the thin-walled structure ruptures, releasing sebum into the surrounding dermis. If the rupture and inflammation is near the surface, pustules develop. When rupture and inflammation is deeper, nodules develop. Inflammation that extends beyond the pilosebaceous unit causes nodulocystic acne that can lead to scarring.

Noninflammatory acne is characterized by open and closed comedones. If the opening of the follicle is tight, a closed comedone (whitehead) is produced (see Fig. 71-3). These are small white papules beneath the skin surface. Closed comedones have no surrounding erythema. Open comedones (blackheads) are keratin-filled follicles with a dilated opening (see Fig. 71-4). The blackness of the tip of the open comedone results from the presence of melanin, not dirt.

Inflammatory acne is characterized by erythematous papules, pustules, nodules, and cysts. The most severe form is nodular disease that has undergone suppuration. Scarring occurs in adolescents who have nodular acne; however, any inflammatory lesion may produce scarring.

DIAGNOSIS

Acne during the teen years arises on the face, upper neck, chest, and back, where the pilosebaceous units are densely concentrated. It presents with a combination of comedones (Fig. 223-1) and inflammatory papules and pustules (Fig. 223-2). The inflammatory lesions heal with postinflammatory pigmentary changes, ranging from red to purple macules that eventually turn brown and resolve after several months. This process may be associated with pitted scarring. Acne is often familial; however, it is not possible to predict the severity based on the family history. The peak incidence of acne vulgaris is between 14 to 17 years of age for girls and 16 to 19 years of age for boys. Acne varies seasonally, being more active during the winter than in the summer, leading to the misconception that sun exposure helps clear up acne.

When evaluating the teen with acne, particular attention should be paid to all the over-the-counter and prescription preparations and oral antibiotics the patient has tried. It is also important to identify the cosmetics and hair preparations the patient is using, since these may be contributing to the acne. Girls should be asked about the regularity of their menstrual cycles and whether acne flares premenstrually, a common phenomenon caused by progestins. Any androgenic stimulation worsens acne in boys and girls. A complete medication history is also vital. Medications that can exacerbate acne include androgen-dominant oral contraceptives, systemic corticosteroids, anabolic steroids, phenytoin, and lithium. Examination of the face, chest, and

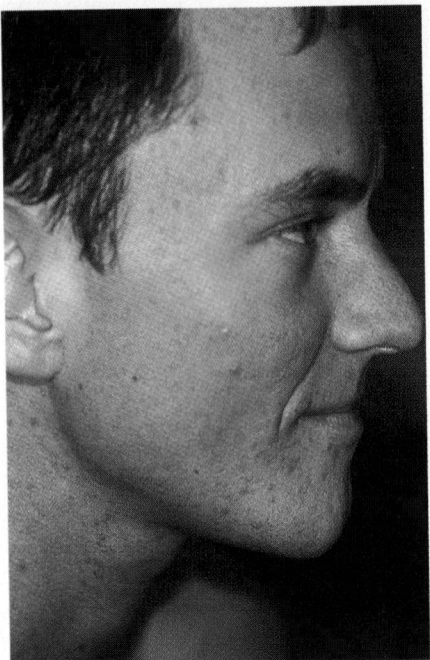

Figure 223-2. Inflammatory acne.

back is crucial to determining the extent of acne. Acne is graded as mild, moderate, or severe depending on the number and extent of inflammatory lesions. Therapy is directed by severity of disease.

Girls with severe or recalcitrant acne should also be evaluated for virulizing signs and symptoms that could indicate an underlying medical problem, such as polycystic ovarian disease, an ovarian tumor, an adrenal tumor, congenital adrenal hyperplasia, or Cushing syndrome. Other signs of virilization include hirsutism, clitoral hypertrophy, decreased breast size, deepening of the voice, increased muscle mass, heightened libido, and irregular or absent menses. Hormonal screening tests include dehydroepiandrosterone sulfate and total free testosterone. Additional tests that may be helpful include follicle-stimulating hormone, luteinizing hormone, prolactin, 17-hydroxyprogesterone, and androstenedione.

CYSTIC ACNE, ACNE CONGLOBATA, AND SAPHO SYNDROME

Cystic acne is the most severe form of acne vulgaris. The predominant lesions are deep-seated nodules that suppurate and resolve with prominent scarring (Fig. 223-3).

Acne conglobata is an unremitting suppurative form of acne seen primarily in men between 18 and 30 years of age. Cysts and abscesses develop interconnecting sinus tracts that burrow beneath the skin surface. These cysts are localized to the forehead, cheeks, and anterior neck. The result is prominent scarring, often with keloid formation.

Synovitis, acne, pustulosis, hyperostosis, and osteitis (SAPHO) syndrome is associated with a variety of inflammatory skin conditions. This rare disorder is characterized by chronic recurrent multifocal osteomyelitis, osteoarticular inflammation, and severe acne. Other cutaneous features include palmoplantar pustulosis, nonpalmoplantar

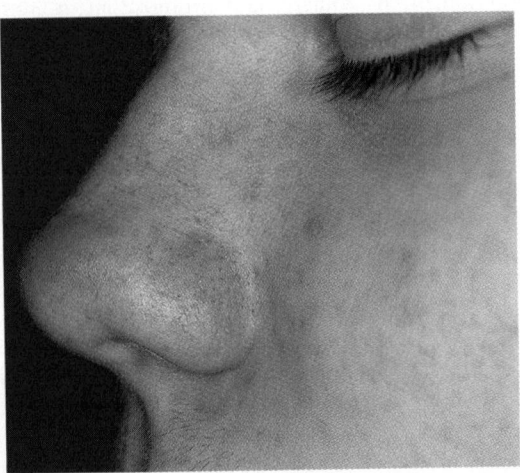

Figure 223-1. Comedonal acne.

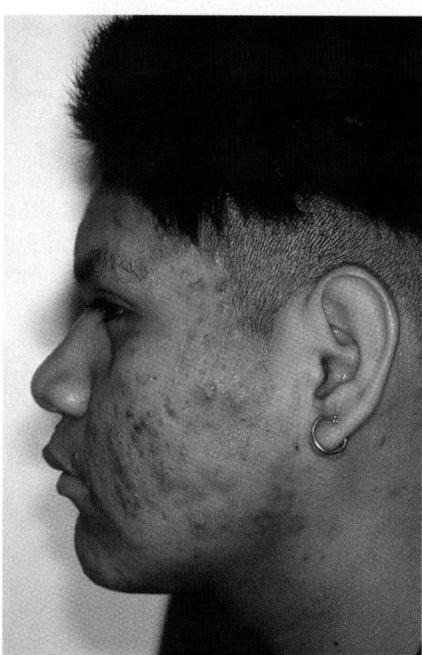

Figure 223-3. Cystic acne.

pustulosis, and psoriasis. This disorder affects children and young adults, particularly boys and young men.

MANAGEMENT

Successful management of acne requires addressing the pathophysiologic factors that cause it, usually a combination therapy with various topical preparations or with topical and systemic medications used together. When selecting topical preparations, the vehicle of the preparation may be as vital to successful treatment as the active ingredient. Creams are best for patients with dry or sensitive skin. For patients with oily skin, gels and solutions are better choices. Note that gels may cause burning and irritation and can prevent some cosmetics from adhering to the skin. Lotions can be used for both dry and oily skin and work well in hair-bearing regions; the propylene glycol in lotions may burn and irritate the skin.

Topical Preparations

Benzoyl Peroxide. Having both bactericidal and comedolytic activity, benzoyl peroxide reduces the population of *P. acnes* on the skin with twice daily usage by inhibiting triglyceride hydrolysis and reducing the proportion of free fatty acids in surface lipids. It acts as a comedolytic by increasing epithelial cell turnover with desquamation.

The effectiveness of benzoyl peroxide is directly dependent on the vehicle. Most of the over-the-counter creams and lotions are less effective than the prescription gels (Table 223-1). Higher concentrations of creams, lotions, and soaps have no advantage over a 5% gel. Increasing to a 10% concentration does not necessarily benefit the patient, but is more likely to cause drying, erythema, and burning and therefore decrease compliance. A single daily application is adequate for most patients, especially if used in combination with a topical retinoid. Water-based formulations are less drying than alcohol-based preparations and tend to cause less stinging, redness, and burning. For patients with dry skin, prescribe water-based preparations. Patients with oily skin tolerate the alcohol- and acetone-based products.

Patients should expect some dryness when using benzoyl peroxide, but any irritation should be addressed by decreasing the frequency of use. Problems with benzoyl peroxide are usually related to overzealous use. Skin irritation is the most common side effect. This occurs more commonly with higher concentration preparations. Regular use leads to tolerance and a decrease of the irritant side effect. Alternatively, incremental therapy can be employed. For this, the patient applies a low-concentration benzoyl peroxide to all acne prone areas every other day and increases the frequency of application to twice daily usage of a 2.5% to 5% preparation for the face; the chest and back can typically tolerate a 5% to 10% gel. Contact allergic dermatitis occurs in 1% of patients using benzoyl peroxide and is a contraindication for future use. Benzoyl peroxide is an oxidizing agent and may bleach shirts, blouses, towels, and sheets. Bleaching of clothing and linens can be avoided by applying the benzoyl peroxide to dry skin in the morning and then reapplying it in the early evening.

Table 223-1. Prescription Benzoyl Peroxide Products

Trade Name	Base	Formulation	Concentration	Size
Benzac	Alcohol	Gel	5%, 10%	60 g
Benzac AC	Water	Gel, wash	2.5%, 5%, 10%	60 g, 90 g
Benzac W	Water	Gel	2.5%, 5%, 10%	60 g, 90 g
		Wash	5%, 10%	8 oz
BenzaClin	Alcohol	Gel	5% (and 1% clindamycin)	25 g
Benzagel	Alcohol	Gel	5% 10%	1.5 oz, 3 oz
Benzamycin	Alcohol	Gel	5% (and 3% erythromycin)	23.3 g, 46.6 g
Benzashave		Shaving cream	5%, 10%	120 g
Brevoxyl	Water	Gel, lotion	4%, 8%	42.5 g, 90 g, 10.5 oz (lotion)
Desquam-E	Water	Gel	2.5%, 5%, 10%	1.5 oz
Desquam-X	Water	Gel, wash	5%, 10%	1.5 oz, 3 oz (gel), 5 oz (wash)
Panoxyl	Alcohol	Gel	5%, 10%	56.7 g, 113.4 g
Panoxyl AQ	Water	Gel	2.5%, 5%, 10%	56.7 g, 113.4 g
Sulfoxyl		Lotion	5% (and 2% sulfur)	60 mL
Triaz	Water	Gel, wash	3%, 6%, 10%	1.5 oz (gel)
				6 oz (wash)
Xerac BP	Water	Gel	5%	45 g, 90 g

Topical Retinoids. These are the most effective comedolytic agents available and are the drugs of choice for treatment of comedonal acne (Table 223-2). Retinoids normalize desquamation of the follicular epithelium, promote drainage of preexisting comedones, minimize rupture of comedones and hence slow the progression of inflammation, and inhibit formation of new comedones. Retinoids also produce follicles that are less anaerobic and increase follicle accessibility to penetration of antimicrobial agents.

The successful use of topical retinoids requires proper patient selection, adequate education, and good compliance. Patients should be instructed to apply an extremely small amount of the topical retinoid to clean and dry skin; topical retinoids should never be applied to wet skin, as this increases the risk of irritation. Patients need to wait 30 minutes after washing the face to apply the retinoid. To increase compliance and decrease irritation, treatment should begin with the lowest strength preparation, which can be titrated to a higher concentration as needed. Initially, application should be two to three times weekly, increasing to use every other night and then to nightly use as tolerated. Topical retinoids make the treated skin more sensitive to sunlight and therefore nighttime application is recommended; a noncomedogenic facial moisturizer with sunscreen can be used during the day.

Improvement may not be apparent for 2 to 3 months. Unfortunately, over half of patients treated with a topical retinoid experience worsening of their acne as comedones are expelled during the first 2 weeks. Patients should be warned they may experience a pustular flare during the first weeks of therapy and should be reassured that this pustular flare is a sign of accelerated resolution of existing acne rather than a treatment failure.

Erythema, peeling, and dryness, the most common side effects of topical retinoids, generally occur when the patient is applying an excessive amount of the preparation. Although after months of treatment the sensitivity and irritation subsides, patients with dry skin may continue to have difficulty. Because of the known teratogenicity of oral vitamin A products in pregnancy, tretinoin and other topical retinoids are listed as pregnancy category C drugs. Studies of 215 women exposed to tretinoin during the first trimester showed no increase in birth anomalies compared to control subjects.

Keratolytic Agents. Salicylic acid is the active ingredient in many popular over-the-counter acne preparations and is available as 0.5%, 1%, or 2% lotions, gels, creams, or washes. Salicylic acid inhibits comedogenesis, reducing plug formation by the follicular epithelium. When used once or twice daily, it is well tolerated. Salicylic acid is as effective as benzoyl peroxide in the treatment of comedonal acne and is an alternative for patients with comedones who cannot tolerate tretinoin.

Sulfur and resorcinol are other keratolytic agents found in over-the-counter acne preparations. These active ingredients also have broad-spectrum antimicrobial activity.

Azelaic acid is a by-product of wheat that has both antibacterial and comedolytic activity. Azelaic acid 20% cream (Azelex) has been approved for the treatment of mild to moderate inflammatory acne and appears to be as effective as benzoyl peroxide, topical erythromycin, and topical tretinoin. Azelaic acid 20% cream should be applied to clean, dry skin twice a day. Skin irritation and erythema is less common with azelaic acid than with benzoyl peroxide and topical tretinoin. Over the course of several months of treatment with azelaic acid, scars and postinflammatory hyperpigmentation caused by acne tend to fade. Because azelaic acid decreases pigmentation, it should be used with caution in patients with darker skin. Azelaic acid is an alternative for patients who cannot tolerate tretinoin.

Topical Antibiotics. Topical antibiotics inhibit the growth of *P. acnes* and exert anti-inflammatory properties by suppressing chemotaxis and decreasing the proportion of free fatty acids in surface lipids. Although their primary action is their bactericidal activity, topical antibiotics may have an indirect effect on comedogenesis. Topical clindamycin and erythromycin are the most frequently prescribed preparations (Table 223-3). Topical tetracycline is less effective against *P. acnes* and can stain the skin. Drug-resistant strains of *P. acnes* are emerging. Resistance to erythromycin is more common than to clindamycin. To counter resistance to topical erythromycin, a combination product containing erythromycin and benzoyl peroxide

Table 223-2. Topical Retinoids for Treatment of Acne

Trade Name	Retinoid	Formulation	Size	Comments
Avita	Tretinoin	0.025% cream, gel	20 g, 45 g	Less irritating formulation of tretinoin
Differin	Adapalene	0.1% gel, cream	15 g, 45 g	Adapalene gel is significantly less irritating than tretinoin gel
		0.1% solution	30 mL	
Renova	Tretinoin	0.05% emollient cream	40 g, 60 g	Less irritating formulation of tretinoin for treatment of facial photoaging
Retin-A	Tretinoin	0.025% cream	20 g, 45 g	Least irritating
		0.05% cream	20 g, 45 g	
		0.1% cream	20 g, 45 g	
		0.01% gel	15 g, 45 g	
		0.025% gel	15 g, 45 g	
		0.05% solution	28 mL	Most irritating
Retin-A micro	Tretinoin	0.1% gel	20 g, 45 g	"Microsphere" delivery system, less irritating than tretinoin 0.1% cream
Tazorac	Tazarotene	0.05%, 0.1% gel	30 g, 100 g	Most irritating retinoid
		0.05%, 0.1% cream	15 g, 30 g, 60 g	

Table 223-3. Topical Antibiotics for Treatment of Acne

Trade Name	Antibiotic	Formulation	Size	Other Ingredients
Akne-mycin	Erythromycin	2% ointment 2% solution	25 g 60 mL	
A/T/S	Erythromycin	2% gel 2% solution	30 g 60 mL	
Benzamycin	Erythromycin	3% gel	23.3 g, 46.6 g	5% benzoyl peroxide—needs refrigeration
BenzaClin	Clindamycin	1% gel	25 g	5% benzoyl peroxide
Cleocin-T	Clindamycin	1% gel 1% solution 1% lotion 1% pledgets	30 g, 60 g 30 mL, 60 mL 60 mL 60/box	
Clindets	Clindamycin	1% pledgets	60/box	
Emgel	Erythromycin	2% gel	27 g, 50 g	
Erycette	Erythromycin	2% pledgets	60/box	
Klaron	Sulfacetamide	10% lotion	60 mL	
Metrogel	Metronidazole	0.75% gel	30 g, 45 g	
Metrocream	Metronidazole	0.75% cream	45 g	
Noritate	Metronidazole	1% cream	30 g	
Novacet	Sulfacetamide	10% lotion	30 mL, 60 mL	5% sulfur
Sulfacet-R	Sulfacetamide	10% lotion	25 mL	5% sulfur
Theramycin	Erythromycin	2% solution	60 mL	Zinc acetate

(Benzamycin) has been formulated. A combination product containing clindamycin and benzoyl peroxide (BenzaClin) is also available. Because resistant strains of *P. acnes* lead to treatment failures, topical preparation may need to be changed periodically. The degree of skin irritation arising from treatment with a topical antibiotic is related to the vehicle. Topical antibiotics are best employed with mild to moderate inflammatory acne. If the acne is more widespread, with facial, chest, and back involvement, systemic antibiotic therapy is indicated.

Sulfur preparations are effective in the treatment of inflammatory acne. Many over-the-counter acne washes and cleansing bars contain sulfur. Some sulfur preparations rarely cause skin discoloration, but have a displeasing odor. The combination of sulfacetamide and sulfur, available by prescription as Novacet and Sulfacet-R, has been shown to decrease inflammatory acne by 83% over 12 weeks of topical application. The sulfacetamide-sulfur preparations do not have the unpleasant side effects of other topical sulfur preparations.

Systemic Antibiotics

Oral antibiotics are indicated for diffuse inflammatory acne or moderate inflammatory acne that does not respond to topical antibiotic therapy (Table 223-4). The addition of systemic antibiotics can hasten the control of inflammatory

Table 223-4. Oral Antibiotics for Treatment of Acne

Name	Dosing	Frequency	Precautions	Adverse Reactions	Drug Interactions
Tetracycline	250–500 mg	Bid	Must be over 8 years old to take. Dairy foods and antacids decrease absorption. Must take on an empty stomach.	Photosensitivity, GI upset, vaginal candidiasis Rare: esophageal ulceration, pseudotumor cerebri Teratogenic	Penicillins, anticoagulants, oral contraceptives
Erythromycin	250–500 mg	Bid		GI upset	Theophylline, digoxin, anticoagulants, terfenadine, astemizole
Minocycline	50–100 mg	Bid	Must be over 8 years old to take. Dairy foods and antacids decrease absorption.	Photosensitivity, vertigo, blue-gray skin pigmentation Rare: systemic lupus–like reaction, hepatitis Teratogenic	Penicillins, anticoagulants, oral contraceptives
Doxycycline	50–100 mg	Bid	Must be over 8 years old to take. Dairy foods and antacids decrease absorption.	Photosensitivity, GI upset Rare: pseudotumor cerebri Teratogenic	Penicillins, anticoagulants, oral contraceptives
Trimethroprim-sulfamethoxazole	80/400 mg 160/800 mg	Bid		Severe drug eruption, bone marrow suppression, hepatitis	Thiazide, warfarin, phenytoin
Amoxicillin	250–500 mg	Bid		Diarrhea	Probenicid

acne and decrease the risk of scarring. Systemic antibiotics are employed for their bactericidal activity, leading to reduction in the population of *P. acnes*. Systemic antibiotics also have anti-inflammatory activity, inhibit neutrophil chemotaxis, and decrease the proportion of free fatty acids in surface lipids. Eight weeks of oral antibiotic therapy are usually required before seeing clinical improvement. Once the inflammation is controlled, the antibiotic should be tapered. Patients whose acne flares with tapering may require long-term antibiotic therapy, lasting months to years.

Tetracycline has the longest and safest history of systemic antibiotic treatment of acne. It is safe and effective and is the least expensive oral antibiotic for acne patients. Tetracycline is taken at a dosage range of 250 to 500 mg twice a day, on average for 6 months before tapering to the lowest possible dosage to maintain the response. Once-daily dosing may be all that is required at that point. Dairy products and antacids bind to tetracycline, which must be taken on an empty stomach. Since tetracycline will stain developing teeth and bones, it should not be prescribed for children younger than 8 years old.

Erythromycin is another safe, effective, and inexpensive oral antibiotic choice. It is taken at a dosage range of 250 to 500 mg twice a day. Because its main side effect is gastrointestinal upset, it should be taken with food. Erythromycin-resistant *P. acnes* can cause a poor response to this treatment.

Minocycline and doxycycline are effective in patients who do not respond to tetracycline or erythromycin. Minocycline is dosed at 50 to 100 mg twice a day. It is the most expensive antibiotic choice for the treatment of acne. Skin pigmentation (see Fig. 74-13) and permanent discoloration of the teeth are well-known adverse effects of minocycline. Minocycline has been rarely associated with autoimmune hepatitis, serum sickness, hypersensitivity reactions, and systemic lupus erythematosus–like syndrome. Although minocycline has been shown to be very effective in the treatment of acne vulgaris, research from the Cochrane Library demonstrates that no reliable random controlled trials support its use as a first-line oral antibiotic in acne treatment. Doxycycline is dosed at 50 to 100 mg twice a day. Minocycline and doxycycline can be taken with food, but administration with dairy products and antacids should be avoided. Doxycycline is most likely to induce a photosensitivity reaction.

Sulfa-containing oral antibiotics are another option for acne patients who do not respond to first-line oral antibiotic agents. Because of the possibility of a severe skin reaction and bone marrow suppression, treatment with a sulfa-containing oral antibiotic must be carefully considered.

Gram-negative folliculitis is a persistent papulopustular eruption that occurs as a complication in patients on prolonged systemic antibiotic treatment for perioral dermatitis and acne vulgaris. Cultures of the pustules will grow gram-negative bacilli and gram-negative rods, including *Escherichia coli*, *Klebsiella*, *Enterobacter*, and *Proteus* species. Patients with this condition often benefit from treatment with oral amoxicillin, although the sensitivities of the cultured organism should guide the choice of antibiotic.

Combination Therapy

Patients with purely comedonal acne benefit from using topical benzoyl peroxide, retinoids, or keratolytics; often a combination of these classes of topical agents is required for successful management. There is no rationale for treating comedonal acne with topical or oral antibiotics. Inflammatory papules and pustules are treated with topical or systemic antibiotics. Most acne patients have a mixture of comedones, inflammatory papules, and pustules. It is common for a patient's treatment regimen to consist of benzoyl peroxide applied in the morning, a topical retinoid in the evening, and a topical or systemic antibiotic used twice daily. Using such combinations, three of the four pathogenic mechanisms of acne are addressed: abnormal follicular keratinization, proliferation of *P. acnes*, and inflammation. Only excessive sebum production goes unchecked with conventional combination therapy.

Hormonal Therapy

Oral Contraceptives. Estrogen-dominant oral contraceptives benefit girls with acne. Estrogens increase the levels of sex hormone binding proteins, leading to a decrease in the circulating active free testosterone and less androgen-induced sebum production. Oral contraceptives with the highest estrogen content have increased side effects and should not be used routinely for acne patients. Since most oral contraceptives contain a combination of estrogens and progestins, attention must also be paid to the progestin component of oral contraceptives in their selection for girls with acne. Progestins with less androgenic activity are favored. The most popular oral contraceptives with a reasonable balance of estrogens and progestins in descending order of benefit to the acne patient are Ortho Tri-Cyclen, Ortho Cyclen, Ovcon 35, Tri-Norinyl, Ortho-Novum, Desogen, Ortho-Cept, and Estro Step. Oral contraceptives containing highly androgenic progestins that should be avoided in acne patients include Alesse, Levlen, Levora, Lo-Ovral, Nordette, Ovral, Ovrette, Tri-Levlen, and Triphasil. The only oral contraceptive that has an FDA-approved indication for treatment of acne is Ortho Tri-Cyclen.

Corticosteroids and Anti-androgens. Low-dose glucocorticoids have an anti-inflammatory effect and also inhibit androgens. However, because of associated side effects, routine use for the acne patient is discouraged. Anti-androgens, such as spironolactone and flutamide, compete with androgens at receptor sites and result in suppressed sebum production. These agents are not routinely used in adolescent girls with acne vulgaris, but may play a role in the treatment of acne in older women, especially those with associated hirsutism.

Isotretinoin (Accutane)

In 1982, the FDA approved the use of 13 cis-retinoic acid (isotretinoin) for the treatment of acne. The use of isotretinoin (Accutane) is best limited to patients with severe nodulocystic scarring acne and inflammatory acne that is not responsive to conventional topical and systemic therapy. For the best chance of inducing remission from acne, isotretinoin must be taken for 20 weeks at a dosage of 1 mg/kg/day. The starting dose is often 0.5 mg/kg/day to allow the patient time to adjust to the drying side effects.

The initiation of isotretinoin can also be associated with severe flaring of the acne. Keeping the dose lower during the beginning of treatment may decrease this. Side effects include significant dryness of the skin, lips, nasal mucosa, and eyes, diminished night vision, photosensitivity, arthralgias, headaches, hair loss, elevation of serum lipids, and transient elevation of hepatic enzymes. It may also cause depression, especially in those already predisposed. The most serious issue is that isotretinoin is a teratogen. A strict pregnancy prevention program must be used for female patients treated with isotretinoin. During therapy it is essential to monitor serum cholesterol; triglycerides; liver function tests; and, in female patients, serum or urine pregnancy tests. Because the medication has such a high side effect profile, the American Academy of Pediatrics advises that isotretinoin be prescribed only by specialists, such as dermatologists.

Surgical Management

The mechanical removal of comedones, when performed properly, promotes the rapid resolution of acne lesions. Mechanical removal of closed comedones prevents rupture of the plugged pilosebaceous unit and subsequent inflammation. Removal of open comedones is desirable for cosmetic purposes. The best results occur when the clinician nicks the surface of the lesions with a sharp, sterile needle and then expresses the contents of plug with a comedone extractor. Poor technique causes damage and inflammation of the surrounding skin and can lead to scarring. When cystic lesions are drained, a larger incision may be necessary. Choosing a sterile needle over a scalpel blade will always minimize the potential for scarring.

Intralesional injection of corticosteroids into inflammatory lesions, particularly nodules and deep-seated cysts, leads to more hasty resolution. With the use of intralesional injections, the incision and drainage of inflammatory lesions can be avoided and the potential for scarring decreases. The injection of triamcinolone acetonide at a concentration of 2.5 to 5 mg/mL may resolve the inflammation within 24 hours. The patient should be aware of the risk of dermal atrophy with steroid injections. Fortunately, most cases of steroid atrophy improve in 6 months to 1 year.

For the treatment of acne scarring, the primary health care provider should refer the patient to a dermatologist with a background in cosmetic procedures or to a plastic surgeon. Skin resurfacing by dermabrasion or laser treatment may remove superficial scars and minimize the appearance of deeper scars. Dermabrasion smooths sharp-edged scars, breaks up fibrotic bases, and unroofs epithelialized sinuses. Deep scars, commonly described as "ice-pick" scars, benefit from punch excision of the pitted scar followed by immediate replacement with a full thickness graft of normal skin. Common donor sites include the posterior scalp and posterior earlobe. Collagen augmentation is suitable for diffusely depressed scars.

PATIENT EDUCATION

Time should be spent dispelling common myths about acne. Acne is not caused by poor hygiene. Blackheads are not caused by dirt stuck in the pores. Scrubbing blackheads will not get rid of them; frequent washing and use of harsh soaps will only irritate the skin. Similarly, alcohol-based astringents will not help remove "dirt." There is no evidence that chocolate, fatty or greasy foods, nuts, junk food, pizza, or soda make acne worse. Sun exposure does not improve acne. Acne is not caused by stress, but certainly existing acne can be exacerbated by it.

Instruct acne patients to wash their faces with water and a mild soap. Since mechanical trauma can make acne worse, warn patients that picking the lesions leads to inflammation and scarring. Oils from hair products, cosmetics, and suntan lotions can worsen acne; direct patients to use oil-free, noncomedogenic cosmetics, moisturizers, and sunscreens. Inform female patients that their acne may worsen the week before menses.

To increase compliance, the primary health care provider should reassure teenagers that acne is treatable with regular use of their medications. It is important to inform them, however, that it can take a minimum of 6 weeks to see improvement whenever the treatment regimen changes. The clinician should avoid prescribing complicated treatment regimens and be sure to outline the proper use of the medications. Discussing the potential side effects of the medications and strategies to reduce irritation from topical preparations as well as encouraging the patient to ask questions are also important components of a successful treatment plan. If noncompliance is an issue, the clinician should not get discouraged but rather should discuss openly with the patient a plan to overcome this obstacle.

OUTCOME

The main goal of treating acne is to minimize new lesion formation and scarring. Early intervention can improve patient outcome by preventing both physical and emotional scarring that commonly complicates acne. Most teenagers are self-conscious about their appearance. They feel socially inhibited by acne lesions. Acne patients may suffer from lower self-esteem, social withdrawal, or depression compared with their clear-complexioned peers. Unfortunately, many clinicians and parents dismiss the clinical significance of acne and acne treatment. Subsequently, teenagers tend to self-medicate with over-the-counter products that are not nearly as effective in treating acne as prescription medications.

FOLLOW-UP

Acne patients should be instructed that treating the acne is a long-term process. Most treatments take 6 to 8 weeks of regular use before beneficial results are appreciated. It is advisable to schedule a return visit at 2 months after therapy has been implemented, and every few months thereafter until the acne is well controlled. The clinician may need to alter specific medications from time to time to maintain a beneficial response. Because flaring of the acne is likely if therapy is discontinued, the clinician should encourage patients to continue treatment until they no longer have a tendency to develop acne lesions. Ongoing education with every visit promotes compliance with medical treatment and improves outcome.

SUGGESTED READINGS

Krowchuk DP: Managing acne in adolescents. Pediatr Clin North Am 2000;47:841–857.

Krowchuk DP: Treating acne: A practical guide. Med Clin North Am 2000;84:811–828.

Krowchuk DP, Lucky AW: Managing adolescent acne. Adolesc Med 2001;12:355–374.

Plewig G, Kligman AM, Jansen T: Acne and Rosacea, 3rd ed. Berlin, Springer-Verlag, 2000.

SECTION 6 ADOLESCENT CARE: *Medical Conditions Manifesting in Adolescents*

224 Adolescents and Sexually Transmitted Diseases

Wendi Ehrman and Steven C. Matson

ROLE OF THE GENERALIST

1. Recognize the role that biologic, behavioral, and societal risk factors play in the susceptibility of adolescents to sexually transmitted diseases.

2. Recognize the signs and symptoms of the more common sexually transmitted diseases.

3. Diagnose sexually transmitted diseases using standard laboratory tests and microscopy.

4. Treat sexually transmitted diseases with the appropriate antimicrobial therapy, taking into consideration extenuating circumstances such as pregnancy and allergies.

5. Refer the patient to an appropriate specialist when there are severe or systemic signs and symptoms or the diagnosis is in question.

6. Understand the potential morbidity of treated and untreated sexually transmitted diseases.

7. Ensure appropriate follow-up of adolescents who have been treated for sexually transmitted diseases.

Sexually transmitted diseases (STDs) are due to an increasing group of more than 30 infectious pathogens that are or can be transmitted through sexual activity. Infection by these pathogens can lead to dozens of more serious clinical syndromes including pelvic inflammatory disease (PID), acquired immunodeficiency syndrome (AIDS), and Fitz-Hugh-Curtis syndrome (perihepatitis). STDs are almost always transmitted from person to person through direct sexual contact including vaginal, anal, or oral intercourse. The parasitic STDs scabies and pubic lice, as well as the herpes simplex and molluscum contagiosum viruses, can be transmitted from direct skin-to-skin or genital-to-genital contact. Other STDs (human immunodeficiency virus [HIV], hepatitis B and C) can be transmitted parenterally through contaminated needles. In addition STDs can be passed to a newborn in utero through the placenta, during passage through the birth canal, or by breast-feeding and can lead to spontaneous abortion, stillbirths, premature rupture of membranes, and preterm delivery.

Adolescents have the highest rate of STDs of any age group. Each year at least 3 million teenagers acquire an

STD. About 25% of all sexually experienced adolescents become infected each year. Young women between the ages of 15 and 24 have the highest number of reported cases of gonorrhea and Chlamydia infections. The reported rate of STDs in adolescents actually underestimates the true prevalence rate because the calculations include all adolescents even though only sexually active teens are at risk.

FUNDAMENTALS

Because of a number of biologic, behavioral, and societal factors, adolescents and young adults are highly susceptible to acquiring sexually transmitted diseases.

Biologic Factors. These include cervical ectopy or the presence of columnar epithelium on the exocervix, commonly seen during adolescence. Columnar cells have been shown to be more susceptible to many sexually transmitted infections when compared to the squamous epithelial cells that gradually replace them in adulthood. Many organisms such as *Chlamydia trachomatis* and *Neisseria gonorrhoeae*, as well as human papillomavirus (HPV) and HIV, more easily infect the columnar epithelium.

Lack of immunity also plays a role in the high rates of STDs in adolescents. Although the role of cellular and humoral immunity in preventing sexually transmitted diseases is unclear, one would assume that prior exposure to organisms would improve the body's ability to prevent clinical infection. For most adolescents, the STDs that they acquire will be their first exposure to that organism. Without any prior immunity the likelihood of infection increases and the severity of infection is often greater.

Behavioral Factors. Adolescent sexual behaviors contribute significantly to the increased risk of STD exposure among this age group and are listed in Box 224-1. Although there has been some leveling off of adolescent sexual activity over the years, the 2003 Youth Risk Behavior Survey (YRBS) documented that 61.6% of high school seniors had been sexually active compared with 46.7% of students overall in grades 9 through 12. Nationwide, 7.4% of students had sexual intercourse before the age of 13 and 20.3% of high school seniors reported having had four or more sexual partners. Condoms continue to be the only reliable method for protection against STDs, yet adolescents remain relatively poor users. According to the 2003 Youth Risk Behavior Survey, 37% of students or their partners had not used a condom during their last sexual intercourse. Reasons for poor use of condoms by adolescents include embarrassment about purchasing condoms, low self-efficacy, a lack of perceived risk of STDs, and low partner support.

Societal Factors. Although the adolescent's right to confidential identification and treatment of STDs is guaranteed by all states, several barriers to appropriate treatment exist. Many practitioners are unfamiliar with the legalities as well as the pathophysiology of sexually transmitted diseases and thus do not provide appropriate services. Discomfort discussing sexuality and sexual issues, lack of time, and lack of training are other major hurdles that prevent primary care providers from adequately assessing and treating adolescents for STDs.

An adolescent's inability to pay for confidential services may also delay care. Many adolescents still lack the necessary information regarding STDs and consequently do not even know that they should be examined for these infections. Finally, adolescents often perceive STD clinics as adult clinics and thus underutilize them.

COMMON SEXUALLY TRANSMITTED DISEASES

Identification of common sexually transmitted infections (Box 224-2) requires knowledge of the typical presentations of each infective agent.

Bacterial Infections

Chlamydia trachomatis. *Chlamydia trachomatis* is the bacterial organism most commonly associated with adolescents. It is an obligate intracellular parasite that cannot be cultured on artificial media. Young people, ages 15 to 19, account for approximately 40% of reported Chlamydia infections. Prevalence has been shown to exceed 10% among adolescent girls and exceed 5% among adolescent boys. These percentages are higher among high-risk (detained, homeless, runaway, low socioeconomic status) youth who are not as likely to access traditional health care settings. Symptomatic girls may present with dysuria, urinary frequency, pyuria, mucopurulent vaginal discharge, cervical friability, or irregular menstrual bleeding. Boys may note a scant urethral discharge and dysuria. Chlamydia can also cause an acute epididymitis presenting as epididymal pain or swelling, testicular pain, and fever. Patients who engage in anal intercourse can have infections characterized by anorectal pain, bloody mucopurulent discharge, and tenesmus. Boys typically become symptomatic within 1 to 3 weeks after exposure. Despite the extent of symptoms, many adolescents will have asymptomatic Chlamydia infections that can be identified only through routine screening of all sexually active youth.

Box 224-1. Sexual Behaviors Increasing Risk of STD Exposure
Early initiation of sexual intercourse
Greater numbers of sexual partners
Higher risk partners
Increased frequency of sexual intercourse
Lack of barrier use
Concurrent substance use

Box 224-2. Common Sexually Transmitted Diseases
Chlamydia
Gonorrhea
Syphilis
Trichomonas
Pubic Lice
Scabies
Genital Herpes
Herpes
HIV

Neisseria gonorrhoeae. This gram-negative diplococcus is the source of another infection found in sexually active adolescents. In the United States young women aged 15 to 19 consistently have the highest rates of gonorrhea. Among young men, the highest rates occur among those aged 20 to 24. African-American adolescents have a disproportionate number of the gonorrhea infections in the United States. Although rates vary across the country, in the year 2001, African American girls (ages 15–19) had a gonorrhea rate 18 times higher than that of non-Hispanic white girls; African American boys of the same age range had a rate 46 times higher than that of non-Hispanic white boys. Symptomatic boys will typically present with a copious purulent urethral discharge and dysuria occurring within 2 to 5 days of exposure (Fig. 224-1). They can also have epididymitis presenting as unilateral epididymal pain and swelling. Girls typically present with vaginal discharge, dysuria, or irregular, heavy vaginal bleeding usually within 10 days of exposure. Pelvic examination often reveals purulent or mucopurulent vaginal discharge as well as cervical inflammation and friability. Women can also develop acute and chronic PID characterized by lower abdominal pain, dyspareunia, and abnormal vaginal bleeding.

Syphilis. Syphilis is caused by a subspecies of the spirochete *Treponema pallidum*. It is an STD that often goes unnoticed by both teens and adults. Syphilis rates have continued to drop in the United States since the epidemic between 1986 and 1990 but remain disproportionately high among certain groups. Among adolescents aged 15 to 19, rates among African Americans remain significantly higher when compared to non-Hispanic whites. Syphilis clinically begins as a painless chancre or ulcer at the inoculation site (Fig. 224-2) that occurs 10 to 90 days after exposure. This primary lesion heals without treatment after 3 to 5 weeks. The second stage of syphilis can occur as the chancre is healing or can be delayed for weeks. Secondary syphilis is characterized by a generalized macular papular rash that frequently involves the palms and soles of the feet (Fig. 224-3). It may also be accompanied by an influenza-like illness. The secondary period can also resolve without treatment and is followed by a latent period that may last for years. Approximately one third of these untreated patients will go on to tertiary syphilis and develop cardiovascular or central nervous system damage

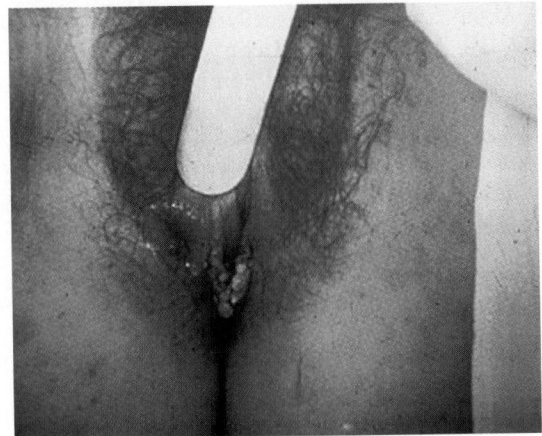

Figure 224-2. Syphlitic chancre.

Bacterial Vaginosis. Bacterial vaginosis (BV) is a nonspecific vaginitis that is the most prevalent cause of discharge in women of reproductive age. It is characterized by an overgrowth and replacement of the normal vaginal flora (*Lactobacillus* species) with a mixture of coccobacilli including *Gardnerella vaginalis, Mycoplasma hominis*, and anaerobic bacteria such as the *Mobiluncus* species. Symptoms of BV typically include a homogeneous, thin, grayish white vaginal discharge that often has an unpleasant "fishy" odor and adheres to the walls of the vagina. However, up to 50% of women who meet clinical criteria for BV are asymptomatic, as are their male partners. The exact transmission of BV is not known but it is more commonly seen in sexually active girls.

BV in pregnant women has been associated with premature rupture of membranes, preterm labor, preterm birth, and postpartum endometritis. BV has also been found in association with PID and postsurgical vaginal cellulitis. Diagnosis is based on clinical criteria requiring at least three of the four signs listed in Box 224-3, one of which is the presence of "clue cells" (epithelial cells coated with bacteria) in a vaginal smear (Fig. 224-4). A gram stain of vaginal fluid looking for the relevant concentrations of bacterial types characteristic of BV can be used for diagnosis (Nugent criteria). Other commercially available tests for diagnosis

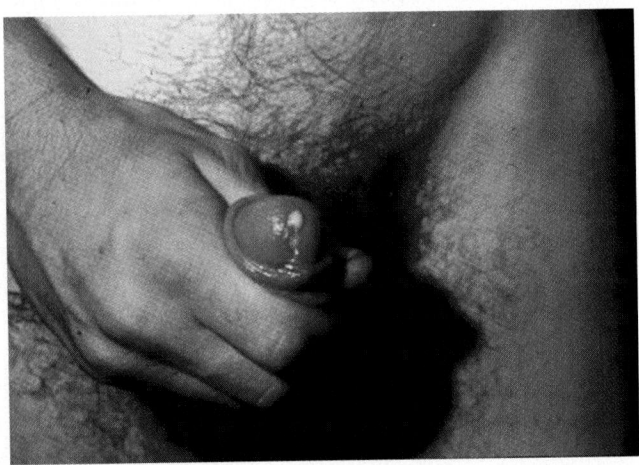

Figure 224-1. Male urethral purulent gonorrheal discharge.

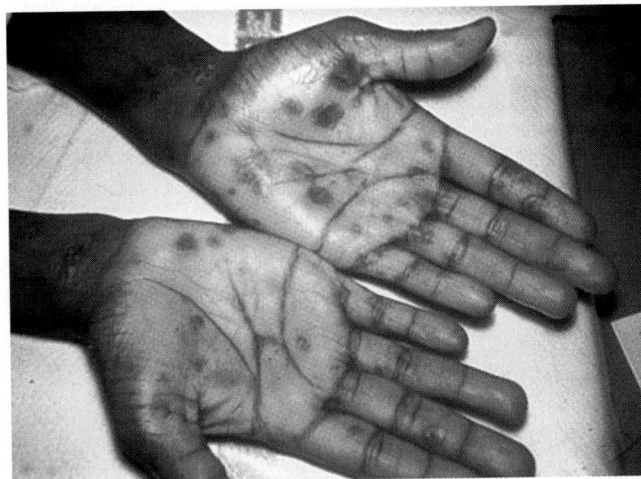

Figure 224-3. Generalized macular popular rash of the palms in secondary syphilis.

include a card test for detection of elevated pH and trimethylamine (FemExam, Pip Activity TestCard) and a DNA probe test looking for high concentrations of *G. vaginalis* (Affirm VP III). Antibiotic treatment includes oral or intravaginal antibiotics. Treatment may be augmented by topical application of vaginal medications that help restore the vaginal pH. No benefit has been found in treating partners and follow-up is usually not necessary if symptoms resolve.

Protozoon/Parasitic Infections

Trichomonas vaginalis. *Trichomonas vaginalis* is a flagellated protozoon that infects the human urogenital tract 4 to 28 days after exposure. There is little known about the current rate of *Trichomonas* infection in adolescents although past studies have shown a prevalence of 6% to 15%. Symptomatic girls present with a frothy vaginal discharge, dysuria, and often irregular menstrual bleeding. On examination the vulva, vagina, or cervix may appear erythematous and edematous. The finding of a "strawberry cervix" or small punctate hemorrhages with ulcerations on the cervix is highly specific for *Trichomonas* infection but seen in only a small percentage of infected women. Boys may present with dysuria but are often asymptomatic. Diagnosis of *Trichomonas* infection indicates the need for evaluation and testing for other STDs.

Phthirus pubis. The pubic louse (*Phthirus pubis*) is one of the sucking lice that are ectoparasites of mammals. Pubic lice are about 1 mm in length and have greatly enlarged claws and middle and hind legs. The highest incidence of pubic lice is in single persons aged 15 to 25. Patients are often unaware of their infestation but may complain of pruritus in the pubic area or even have noted "bugs" in their pubic region. Excessive scratching may lead to superinfection. Small blue maculae may appear on the thighs and abdomen as a result of the louse bites. The demonstration of nits or live organisms (Fig. 224-5) confirms the diagnosis. It is important to remember that patients noted to have pubic lice require a complete evaluation for other STDs.

Sarcoptes scabiei. *Sarcoptes scabiei* is a mite that infects humans by burrowing under the skin, laying eggs, and spreading to new sites. The scabies mite walks rapidly on human skin, covering 2.5 cm per minute. Sexual transmission of scabies is relatively common and should alert the provider to the need for a complete evaluation for other STDs. Symptomatic patients complain of significant pruritus and typically have lesions on the hands, wrists, elbows, and axillae, though lesions may also appear on the genitalia and buttocks.

Viral Infections

Genital Warts. Genital warts are caused by HPV, a small naked virus with a double-stranded DNA genome. After sexual contact, the virus infects the epidermis and begins to replicate. The most common subtypes noted in genital warts are HPV 6, 11, and sometimes 16. Currently, HPV is the most common STD in the United States. Several studies have documented the high prevalence of HPV among adolescents and young adults, with rates of infection ranging from 25% to 50% of sexually active adolescents. Patients may present with a complaint of bumps or sores in their genital area (Fig. 224-6). Routine Papanicolaou testing (Pap smear) of the cervix may reveal changes consistent with HPV such as atypia, koilcytosis, and dysplasia. Evaluation and treatment of abnormal Pap smears is carried out independent of the presence of HPV effect. Any reports of dysplasia or squamous intraepithelial lesions should be investigated further with repeat Pap smears or colposcopic-guided biopsy. HPV DNA testing is now available as an alternative to repeat Pap smears to assist in the management of atypical squamous cells of undetermined significance (ASCUS) or low-grade squamous intraepithelial lesions (LSILs). HPV DNA testing allows for identification of high-risk HPV types that have been associated with high-grade squamous intraepithelial lesions (HSILs) and cervical carcinoma. This testing can be performed independently or as part of a liquid-based

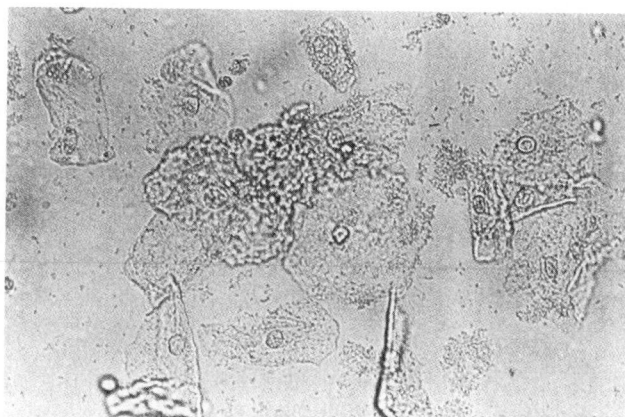

Figure 224-4. Presence of "clue cells" (epithelial cells coated with bacteria) in a vaginal smear.

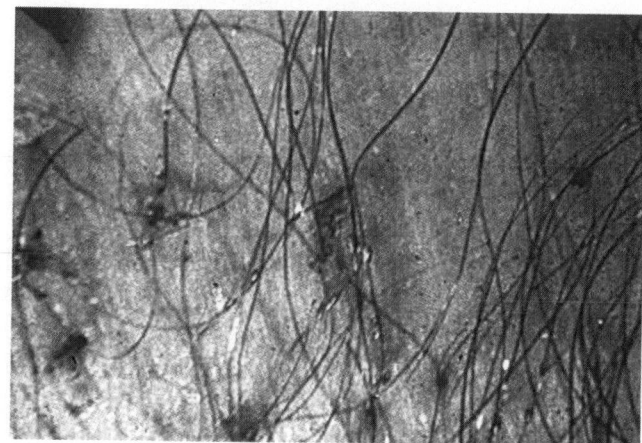

Figure 224-5. Nits on hair follicle found in *Phthirus pubis*.

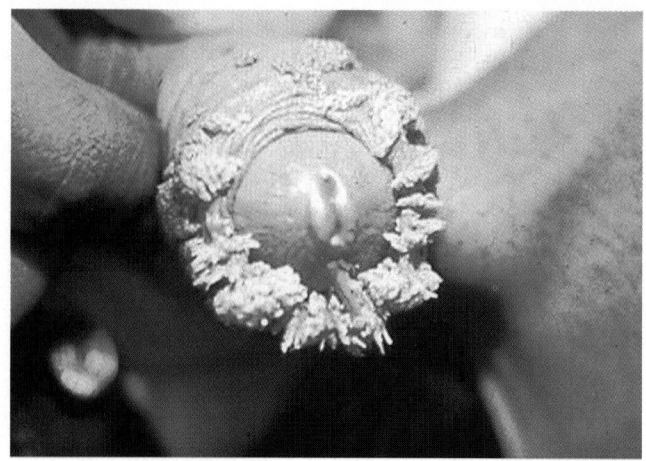

Figure 224-6. Penile lesions of genital warts.

cytology. Patients who have been identified as having high-risk HPV types should be referred for colposcopy.

Herpes Simplex Virus. Herpes simplex virus (HSV) is a double stranded linear DNA virus. Both HSV types 1 and 2 can cause genital HSV infection although type 1 does have a greater predilection for sites above the waist. Most infected individuals never recognize that they are carrying the infection and only a small number experience HSV episodes after an initial genital infection. A recent study revealed that the seroprevalence of HSV-2 in persons 12 and older in the United States was 21.9%. This represented a 30% increase from 1976 to 1980. Initial infection occurs at the site of inoculation usually through mucosa or broken skin. First episodes of genital herpes are usually associated with systemic symptoms such as fever and malaise. There are usually painful eroded ulcers often on the labia of girls (Fig. 224-7) or the penile shaft in boys. Lesions may occur wherever contact has occurred with the infecting virus. Whenever ulcers are noted on examination, HSV infection should be considered. Treatment is most beneficial for primary infections.

Human Immunodeficiency Virus. HIV is a member of a subfamily of the retroviruses called lentiviruses. HIV is an RNA virus that replicates in the host cell via an RNA-directed DNA polymerase, or reverse transcriptase. After an individual is infected with HIV there exists a wide variation in the time until development of AIDS. The median time between infection and disease is 10 years with a range from a few months to 12 years. This period of quiescence may be even longer for those who acquire the infection in their teenage years. The number of adolescents with AIDS from sexual contact is small. However, considering the long period of quiescence after infection, many AIDS patients 20 to 30 years of age must have become infected during their adolescence. One report estimated that 25% of HIV infections were acquired before the age of 22. Homeless and runaway youth and those in correctional facilities have been shown to have appreciable HIV-infection rates in excess of 1%. Adolescent boys who have sex with male partners are at high risk for HIV infection; however, a large number of the HIV infections in adolescents are due to heterosexual transmission.

DIAGNOSIS

Many STDs are asymptomatic and go undetected. In addition, adolescents may not recognize signs and symptoms of STDs. The 1996 Guidelines for Adolescent Preventative Services (GAPS) recommends that all adolescents receive yearly guidance on abstinence and responsible sexual behaviors and that all sexually active adolescents be screened annually for STDs (especially gonorrhea and Chlamydia). Pap testing is now recommended at or within 3 years after the initiation of sexual activity. Testing for syphilis and HIV should be considered if the adolescent has had more than one sexual partner or STD or engages in other high-risk sexual behaviors (i.e., prostitution, sex, and substance abuse). Retesting for STDs should be considered whenever the patient has a new risk factor such as a new partner or if there is a question of whether or not the partner was adequately treated. Recent data suggest that, because of a high rate of reinfection, girls who have tested positive for Chlamydia should be retested at 3 to 4 months after treatment. STD testing should also be done in any sexually active adolescent who presents with complaints of abdominal or pelvic pain, vaginal or urethral discharge, dysuria, genital swelling or pain, genital itching, or genital lesions. Additionally, STD testing should be considered in unexplained arthritis, or pharyngitis where the adolescent admits to engaging in oral sex.

Evaluation for STDs should begin with a thorough history that includes inquiring about any genital complaints, followed by visual inspection and examination of the genital area. The physical examination should include close inspection of the pubic hair for pubic lice and all skin surfaces for other signs of STDs such as ulcerative lesions, burrows, warts, chancres, or other rashes. Careful palpation of the inguinal nodes, testicles, and epididymis for pain, swelling, redness, or lesions may also help identify a sexually transmitted infection.

In symptomatic or high-risk girls, a complete pelvic examination should be performed including laboratory evaluation for gonorrhea and Chlamydia and a saline wet preparation to look for yeast, bacterial vaginosis, and *Trichomonas vaginalis*. Cultures or nonculture swabs for gonorrhea and Chlamydia should be taken from the endocervix by inserting the swab 1 to 2 cm into the os and

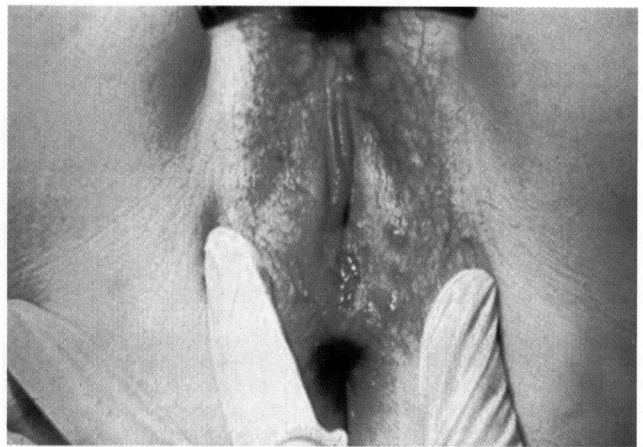

Figure 224-7. Eroded labial ulcers of herpes simplex virus.

rotating several times for 20 to 30 seconds. A Dacron swab or cytobrush should be used for Chlamydia sampling, as wooden stick swabs are inhibitory to Chlamydia. A swab of any vaginal discharge should be taken and immersed in 1 cc of saline solution to examine later microscopically. In addition, a Gram stain from the cervical os can be obtained to identify cervical inflammation (>30 polymorphonuclears [PMNs] per high-power field) or gonorrhea (gram-negative intracellular diplococci) (Fig. 224-8).

In cases where it is not possible to perform a pelvic examination for tests or culture or for asymptomatic screening of young women (especially in institutional settings), urine testing can be used to detect gonorrhea and Chlamydia. If urine testing is used, then consideration should be given to patient- or provider-obtained wet preparations for microscopic examination.

A Pap smear should be performed at or within 3 years of initiation of sexual activity. If the patient is menstruating, the Pap can be delayed until the patient has completed her period, or liquid-based cytology methods (Thin Prep or Surepath) can be used. If the cervix is inflamed and friable, the Pap can be delayed until after the patient is treated for infection. If the patient has engaged in oral or anal sexual activity, STD testing should be considered at all sites of sexual contact.

For boys, screening tests should be collected to search for urethritis. If urethral swabs are to be used for testing, they should be collected before urination. Urination within 1 hour of sample collection can reduce sample sensitivity by washing out infected columnar cells. A small dry calcium alginate swab should be gently inserted 3 to 4 cm into the male urethra and rotated in one direction for at least one revolution for 5 seconds and then placed in the proper media for gonorrhea and Chlamydia testing. A similar swab can also be used to make a gram stain to look for gram-negative diplococci (gonorrhea) or inflammation (>5 PMNs per high-power [× 1000] field). If urethral discharge is present at the meatus, this can be swabbed and plated (Thayer-Martin agar) for gonorrhea. Urine testing can also be used as an alternative to urethral swabs, especially if large groups of young men are being screened. Preferably a first voided urine specimen is collected. Regardless of the type of specimen obtained, examination of the urine for the presence of leukocyte esterase, *Trichomonas*, and white blood cells may assist with the diagnosis. Presumptive treatment for gonorrhea, Chlamydia, and *Trichomonas* should be considered in the presence of leukocyte esterase, *Trichomonas*, or if there are more than 10 white blood cells per high-powered microscopic field.

Although culture is still considered the gold standard for diagnosis with a specificity of 100%, a number of nonculture tests are available for gonorrhea and Chlamydia testing. Nonculture tests include direct fluorescent-antibody (DFA) staining of Chlamydia organisms, immunohistochemical detection of antigen (EIA or enzyme immunoassay), and DNA probes. These tests have the advantages of standardization and easier transport. Although these tests are highly specific, they are less sensitive than the more recently developed nucleic acid amplification tests known as NAATs, which detect and amplify DNA or RNA sequences that are specific for gonorrhea and Chlamydia. Although NAATs are highly sensitive and specific, they typically cost more. They can be used on endocervical and urethral swabs and are the only type of gonorrhea and Chlamydia testing currently approved for urine specimens. The three currently available NAATs are polymerase chain reaction (PCR [Amplicor]), strand displacement amplification (BD [ProbeTec]), and transcription-mediated amplification (TMA [Gen-Probe APTIMA]).

Boys or girls with painful vesicles or ulcerated skin lesions in the genital area should be tested for the herpes simplex virus. Lesions should be unroofed and the bases swabbed. The herpesvirus grows rapidly in culture and the diagnosis can usually be confirmed within several days. Rapid tests such as direct fluorescent antibody staining and enzyme immunoassays are also available. These tests are specific but slightly less sensitive than viral culture. HSV DNA detection by PCR is a sensitive test that is of particular value in evaluating the cerebrospinal fluid for herpes encephalitis.

All sexually active adolescents, especially those with documented STDs, should be counseled regarding HIV and syphilis and offered screening tests. The usual HIV screening test is an HIV enzyme immunoassay. If this test is positive, it is confirmed with an HIV antibody test such as the Western blot. Three rapid HIV screening tests are currently available for use with blood specimens. The most recently approved test, Oraquick, can be performed in an office laboratory setting with blood obtained from a finger stick, oral fluids, or plasma specimens. Test results are available in 20 to 40 minutes. Positives need to be followed up with a confirmatory Western blot or immunofluorescent assay. Syphilis screening is done by serology using either the rapid plasma reagin (RPR) test or the Venereal Disease Research Laboratory (VDRL) test. Because these tests are nontreponemal tests that identify substances present in a variety of other disease processes, false-positive results may occur. A confirmatory treponemal test such as the fluorescent treponemal antibody absorption (FTA-ABS) test is required.

Patients who present with abdominal pain and adnexal tenderness or cervical motion tenderness should be evaluated and treated for PID in the absence of an established etiology. PID involves a spectrum of inflammatory disorders

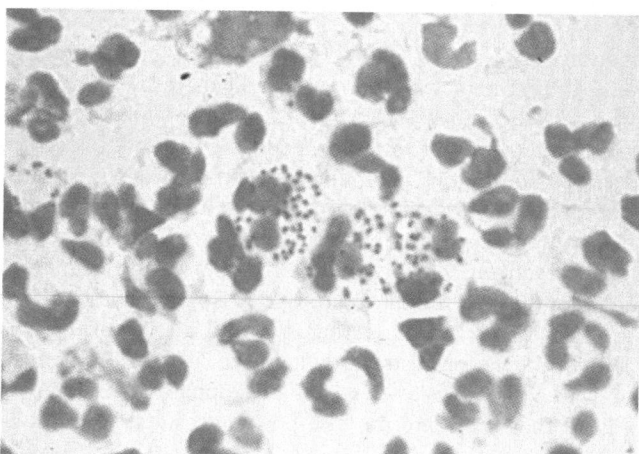

Figure 224-8. Gram-negative intracellular diplococci typical of gonorrhea.

of the upper female genital tract including the fallopian tubes. No one sign, symptom, or laboratory test is sensitive or specific for PID. A lack of or minimal symptoms may cause episodes of PID to be missed. To increase specificity and limit unnecessary morbidity, patients who are suspected of having PID should also be evaluated for fever (>38.3°C or 101°F), vaginal or cervical discharge, presence of white blood cells on saline microscopy of vaginal secretions, sedimentation rate greater than 15 mm/h, elevated C-reactive protein, and laboratory documentation of cervical infection with gonorrhea or Chlamydia. Most patients with PID have evidence of mucopurulent vaginal discharge or have white blood cells present in a saline preparation of vaginal fluid. In cases where the diagnosis remains questionable a more extensive diagnostic evaluation that includes laparoscopy, endometrial biopsy, ultrasound, or magnetic resonance imaging (MRI) may be needed.

MANAGEMENT

Presumptive antibiotic treatment should be considered in any adolescent who is symptomatic (urethral/vaginal discharge, pain, dysuria, genital itching), has *Trichomonas* present in a urine or wet preparation sample, or who has numerous white blood cells in the wet preparation, gram stain, or urinalysis (which does not appear consistent with a urinary tract infection) and cannot be relied on for follow-up. Initial doses of antibiotics to cover gonorrhea, Chlamydia, and *Trichomonas* can be given at the time of presentation in the health care setting.

Patients with obvious genital ulcers can be started on antiviral therapy while awaiting culture results. Any positive finding of lice or nits justifies treatment for pubic lice.

Specific treatments for individual STD treatments are listed in Table 224-1 with alternatives given for special cases such as pregnancy. Compliance is typically a significant issue in adolescents; therefore, single-dose therapy is generally preferred to a longer course of pharmacotherapy.

Patients who are suspected of having PID should be empirically started on antibiotics (see Table 224-1) and considered for hospitalization if (1) a surgical emergency such as an ectopic pregnancy cannot be ruled out, (2) compliance and outpatient follow-up within 72 hours cannot be guaranteed, (3) the presentation is severe (suspected tubo-ovarian abscess or peritoneal signs), (4) the patient is pregnant, (5) the patient is immunodeficient, or (6) the patient has failed to respond to outpatient therapy within 48 hours.

All patients with known or suspected STDs should be counseled on the need for partner notification and partner testing or treatment. Abstinence should be strongly encouraged until both partners are adequately treated and follow-up completed.

OUTCOME

The majority of bacterial and protozoal sexually transmitted diseases can be successfully treated with appropriate pharmacotherapy. However, pelvic inflammatory disease can lead to long-term sequelae such as recurrent infection (up to one third of women), chronic pelvic pain, ectopic pregnancies, and infertility, thus necessitating the need for regular reproductive health care and diligent barrier contraceptive use.

Herpes simplex virus establishes itself as a latent infection in the sensory ganglia of nerves innervating the site of initial infection. Both clinical and subclinical reactivation of the virus occurs in the majority of infected individuals. Viral shedding and subsequent transmission of the virus to a sexual partner can occur even during subclinical recurrence. As a result, adolescents need to be told that herpes is treatable but not curable and that transmission can occur even when they are asymptomatic. Suppressive pharmacotherapy can be used to prevent future outbreaks and ongoing transmission. Adolescents should be counseled about consistent condom use and abstaining from intercourse during outbreaks. A national Herpes Hotline is also available at 919-361-8488 for further information.

Untreated genital HPV may spontaneously regress or remain unchanged, or the warts may increase in size or number. Treatment modalities are usually successful for initial removal of warts but none will eradicate HPV from surrounding normal tissue. As a result, infectivity is probably reduced but not eradicated and recurrences are common. Subclinical cervical HPV infection, detected by colposcopy, biopsy, or DNA testing, is common but does not require treatment unless associated with high-grade squamous intraepithelial lesions or a high-risk type of HPV. In these cases colposcopy with possible biopsy is recommended. Despite these recommendations, cervical cancer is exceedingly rare in young women. In addition most cervical HPV infections among women aged 13 to 22 are transient, with a 70% rate of regression in high-risk types and 90% rate of regression in low-risk types.

Longer healthier life spans are now available with early HIV diagnosis and treatment. Combination antiretroviral therapy can now suppress viral replication to undetectable levels. As a result the occurrence of opportunistic infections has been dramatically lowered and HIV-positive patients can lead healthier lives.

FOLLOW-UP

STD follow-up is suggested after treatment to ensure medication and contraception compliance and to check on notification and treatment of sexual partners. This may also be a good time to obtain a Pap smear (if cervical inflammation has cleared) and to discuss STD prevention. To ensure treatment success some clinicians rescreen patients who tested positive for gonorrhea or Chlamydia. Although there is currently little resistance to the majority of recommended antibiotics (some resistance has been seen to fluoroquinolones), patients may come in with reinfections from new or untreated partners. Because of the high prevalence of repeat Chlamydia infections in young women in the months after initial treatment, it is recommended that they have repeat STD testing in 3 to 4 months. If nucleic acid amplification tests are being used, it is recommended to wait at least 3 to 4 weeks after pharmacotherapy to ensure that there are no false-positive results from detection of residual DNA/RNA after clearance of infection.

Education is imperative to the prevention and successful treatment of STDs in adolescents. Proper knowledge of

Table 224-1. Treatment of Sexually Transmitted Diseases

Organism	Treatment	Alternative Regimens
Chlamydia	Azithromycin (Zithromax) 1 g po × 1 Doxycycline 100 mg po bid × 7 days Ofloxacin 300 mg po bid × 7 days Levofloxacin 500 mg po qd × 7 days	*Pregnancy:* Erythromycin base 500 mg po qid × 7 days or 250 mg po qid × 14 days *Erythromycin ethylsuccinate 800 mg po qid × 7 days or 400 mg po qid × 14 days *Amoxicillin 500 mg po tid × 7 days (only 50% effective) Azithromycin 1 g po × 1
Gonorrhea	Cefixime (Suprax) 400 mg po × 1 Ceftriaxone (Rocephin) 125 mg IM × 1 Ciprofloxacin 500 mg po × 1 Ofloxacin 400 po mg po × 1 Levofloxacin 250 mg po × 1 *Note:* Quinolones should not be used for infections acquired in Asia/Pacific/Hawaii or Pacific coastal states due to increased prevalence of resistance strains in these areas. Consider alternative therapy for men who have had sex with men or for women whose male partners have had sex with men in the past 90 days.	*Penicillin/cephalosporin allergy:* Spectinomycin *Pregnancy:* Spectinomycin, cefixime,* ceftriaxone, or alternative cephalosporin listed below: Certizoxime 500 mg IM × 1 Cefotaxime 500 mg IM × 1 Cefoxitin 2 g IM with probenecid 1 g po × 1 *Other alternatives:* Gatifloxacin 400 mg po × 1 Lomefloxacin 400 mg po × 1 Norfloxacin 800 mg po × 1 Azithromycin 2 g po × 1[†]
Pharyngeal infections	Ceftriaxone 125 mg IM Ciprofloxacin 500 mg po × 1	
Bacterial vaginosis	Metronidazole 500 mg po bid × 7 days Metronidazole gel 0.75%, one intravaginal applicator bid × 5 days Clindamycin cream 2% one intravaginal applicator qhs × 7	*Pregnancy:* Metronidazole 250 mg po tid × 7 days (preferred) Clindamycin 300 mg po bid × 7 days *Other:* Metronidazole 2 g po × 1 Clindamycin 300 mg po bid × 7 days Clindamycin ovules (100 mg) one intravaginally qhs × 3 nights
Syphilis	Duration <1 year (primary, secondary, early latent): Benzathine penicilline G 2.4 million units IM × 1 Latent >1 year, tertiary: Benzathine penicilline G 2.4 million units IM q week × 3	*Nonpregnant, penicillin allergic:*[‡] Doxycycline 100 mg po bid × 14 days Or tetracycline 500 mg po qid for 2 weeks if duration <1 year 4 weeks if duration >1 year *Pregnancy:* Penicillin desensitization
Trichomonas	Metronidazole 2 g po × 1	*Pregnancy:* Metronidazole 2 g po × 1 *Other:* Metronidazole 500 mg po bid × 7 days
Pubic lice[§]	Permethrin (Nix) 1% creme rinse, wash off after 10 minutes Lindane 1% shampoo, wash off after 4 minutes Pyrethrins with piperonyl butoxide, wash off after 10 minutes (RID; Triple X shampoo)	*Pregnancy:* Do not use Lindane
Scabies[§]	Elimite Cream 5%, wash off after 8–14 hours	*Pregnancy:* Use Elimite *Other:* Lindane 1% lotion or 30 g of creme, wash off after 8 hours Ivermectin 200 µg/kg po, repeated in 1 week
Venereal warts (human papillomavirus)	(Patient-applied) Imiquimod 5% cream qhs 3 times a week, for 4–16 weeks, wash off with soap and water 6–10 hours after application or Podofilox 0.5% solution or gel bid for 3 days, off 4 days, may repeat cycle 4 times using no more than 0.5 mL/day	(Provider-administered) Intralesional interferon Laser surgery *Pregnancy:* TCA/BCA
	(Provider-administered) Cryotherapy with Liquid nitrogen; repeat every 1 to 2 weeks as necessary Podophylline resin 10%–25%, to warts; wash off in 1–4 hours, repeat weekly as necessary	Cryotherapy, laser, surgery

*Repeat testing recommended 3 weeks after completion due to decreased efficacy and side effects limiting compliance.
†Effective but expensive and causes a significant amount of gastrointestinal distress.
‡Limited studies suggest Ceftriaxone is effective but optimal dose not defined, however some specialists use: 1 g daily IM or IV for 8–10 days, azithromycin 2 g may also be effective (primary, secondary, and early latent only).
§Bedding and clothing need to be hot-cycle machine-washed and dried, dry-cleaned, or bagged and sealed 72 hours. Symptomatic patients may be retreated in 1 week.

Table 224-1. Treatment of Sexually Transmitted Diseases—cont'd

Organism	Treatment	Alternative Regimens
Venereal warts (human papillomavirus)—cont'd	Bi or Trichloroacetic acid 80%–90% (TCA/BCA) to warts weekly prn; use talc or baking soda to remove unreacted acid if excess amount applied	
Vaginal	Cryotherapy, TCA/BCA	
Anal	Cryotherapy, TCA/BCA, or surgery	
Urethral meatus	Cryotherapy or podophyllin 10–25%	
Cervical	Refer for treatment	
Herpes *Primary infection*	Acyclovir 200 mg po 5 times daily × 7–10 days or 400 mg po 3 times daily for 7–10 days Famciclovir 250 mg po tid for 7–10 days Valacyclovir 1 g po bid for 7–10 days	*Pregnancy:* The safety of these agents has not been established. However, there are no known increases in birth defects. Oral acyclovir has been used in the first clinical episode of herpes during pregnancy and with severe recurrent herpes, and can be given IV in severe cases.
Episodic recurrent infection	Acyclovir 400 mg po tid Or 200 mg po 5 times daily Or 800 mg po bid for 5 days Famciclovir 125 mg po bid for 5 days Valacyclovir 500 mg po bid for 3–5 days or 1 g po qd for 5 days	
Daily suppressive therapy	Acyclovir 400 mg po bid Famciclovir 250 mg po bid Valacyclovir 500 mg or 1000 mg po q	
Severe disease	Acyclovir 5–10 mg/kg IV q 8 hours for 2–7 days or until clinical improvement is observed, followed by oral therapy to complete at least 10-day course	
Pelvic inflammatory disease parenteral treatment	*Regimen A* Cefotetan 2 g IV every 12 hours *or* Cefoxitin 2 g IV every 6 hours *plus* Doxycycline 100 mg po or IV every 12 hours Discontinue parental therapy 24 hours after clinical improvement and continue with Doxcyline 100 mg po bid to complete 14 days of therapy *Regimen B* Clindamycin 900 mg IV every 8 hours *plus* Gentamicin loading dose (2 mg/kg) IV or IM followed by 1.5 mg/kg every 8 hours (may substitute single daily dosing) Discontinue parenteral therapy as above and continue with Doxycycline 100 mg po bid or clindamycin 450 mg po qid to complete 14 days of therapy. *Oral Regimen A* Ofloxacin 400 mg po bid × 14 days *or* Levofloxacin 500 mg po daily × 14 days Oral+Intramuscular Regimen B Ceftriaxone 250 mg IM *or* Cefoxitine 2 g IM with Probenecid 1 g po *or* Other parenteral 3rd generation Cephalosporin *plus* Doxycycline 100 mg po bid × 14 days Metronidazole 500 mg po bid × 14 days can be added to both of the above oral regimens for added anaerobic coverage.	*Alternative Parenteral Regimens* Ofloxacin 400 mg IV every 12 hours *or* Levofloxacin 500 mg IV qd with or without Metronidazole 500 mg IV every 8 hours *or* Ampicillin/Sublactam 3 g IV every 6 hours *plus* Doxycycline 100 mg po or IV every 12 hours

disease presentation and treatment will aid health care providers in providing up-to-date care for these young patients and increase the likelihood that they will make better, healthier sexual choices.

Additional Resources, CD-ROM

Bibliography

Mini-index of Related Topics   CH.

SUGGESTED READINGS

Centers for Disease Control and Prevention: Screening tests to detect *Chlamydia trachomatis* and *Neisseria gonorrhoeae* infections, 2002. MMWR Morb Mortal Wkly Rep 2002;51(RR–15).

Centers for Disease Control and Prevention: Sexually transmitted diseases treatment guidelines, 2002. MMWR Morb Mortal Wkly Rep 2002;51(RR–6).

Grunbaum JA, Kann L, Kinchen SA, et al: Youth risk behavior surveillance: United States, 2003. In Surveillance Summaries, May 21, 2004. MMWR Morb Mortal Wkly Rep 2004;53(SS-2):1–100.

Holmes KK, Sparling PF, Mårdh PA, et al (eds): Sexually Transmitted Diseases, 3rd ed. New York, McGraw-Hill, 1999.

Institute of Medicine/Committee on Prevention and Control of Sexually Transmitted Diseases, Eng TR, Butler WT (eds): The Hidden Epidemic. Washington, DC, National Academy Press, 1997.

Wright TC, Cox JT, Massad LS, et al: 2001 consensus guidelines for the management of women with cervical cytological abnormalities. JAMA 2002;287(16):2120–2129.

SECTION 6   ADOLESCENT CARE: *Medical Conditions Manifesting in Adolescents*

225 Menstrual Disorders

Chris L. Ohlemeyer

ROLE OF THE GENERALIST

1 Distinguish normal menstrual pattern from pathophysiological processes.

2 Determine when excessive uterine bleeding has affected the hemodynamics of a patient and to refer her to an appropriate facility for immediate care.

3 Provide (or offer referral for) a gynecological evaluation of nonurgent patients with abnormal menstrual patterns.

4 Treat primary dysmenorrhea with medications.

5 Diagnose primary and secondary amenorrhea and determine the causes.

6 Refer patients with menstrual disorders to an appropriate specialist for procedures or management when indicated.

7 Establish follow-up criteria for patients with dysmenorrhea and abnormal menstrual bleeding.

8 Offer age-appropriate patient education for dysmenorrhea and abnormal menstrual bleeding.

DEFINITIONS

Menstruation begins at an average age of 12.8 years with a range of 9 to 16 years of age, generally approximately 2 to 3 years after onset of puberty. The menstrual cycle is defined as the time interval between the first day of one menstrual flow to the first day of the next menstrual flow, normally 21 to 40 days. Patterns of irregular menstrual cycles in adolescent girls include too much bleeding, too little bleeding, or painful bleeding. Each should be explored separately for pathological conditions.

Dysmenorrhea is painful menstruation. Primary dysmenorrhea is menstrual pain attributed to normal physiological processes. Secondary dysmenorrhea is menstrual pain caused by a pathologic process, usually pelvic.

Amenorrhea is absence of menstrual periods. Primary amenorrhea refers to when a girl who has no pubertal development has not reached menarche by age 14 years or when a girl who has normal puberty has not reached menarche by age 16. It is cause for concern when a girl does not have onset of menses within 2 years of completing puberty. Secondary amenorrhea is when a female patient who previously had menstrual cycles has not had one for 6 months or a length of time equal to three previous cycles.

Excessive uterine bleeding can be described by several terms. Menorrhagia is menses with heavier flow than normal but lasting the normal 3 to 7 days. Polymenorrhea is menses with normal flow (usually 30–40 mL of blood) but at decreased intervals, that is, bleeding too often. Dysfunctional uterine bleeding in teens refers to abnormal bleeding patterns from an immature hypothalamic-pituitary-gonadal axis.

FUNDAMENTALS

Menarche occurs in most girls by Tanner IV breast and pubic hair development when linear growth is slowing. For menarche to occur, hormone cycling must be established and adequate estrogen present for endometrial proliferation and sloughing. A complex hormonal feedback system regulates menstruation. At the level of the hypothalamus, gonadotropin-releasing hormone (GnRH) is made and released. GnRH causes the pituitary gland to synthesize and release the gonadotropins follicle-stimulating hormone (FSH) and luteinizing hormone (LH). FSH acts at the level of the ovary, causing growth of follicles. These increase estradiol levels, which in turn stimulate growth of the endometrium in its proliferatory phase. This rise in estradiol also causes the LH surge that triggers ovulation. During the second half of the cycle, progesterone produced by the corpus luteum changes the endometrium to its secretory phase. If the ovum is not fertilized, the corpus luteum regresses and estrogen and progesterone levels fall, causing shedding of the endometrial lining. Figure 225-1 reflects the normal changes at the level of the pituitary gland, ovary, and endometrium during the menstrual cycle.

During the adolescent years, ovulation does not always occur with every cycle, because the hormonal feedback system is not fully mature. By 2 years after menarche, 55% to 82% of cycles are ovuatory, increasing to 80% to 90% by 5 years. Anovulatory cycles often differ from normal ovulatory cycles. Changes from the normal parameters for the menstrual cycle (i.e., 21- to 40-day cycle length, 3–7 days flow, and 30–40 cc blood loss) warrant a complete history and physical examination.

With ovulation often comes menstrual pain or dysmenorrhea. Prostaglandin levels are higher in menstrual fluid during ovulatory cycles than anovulatory ones. During luteal and menstrual phases the endometrium secretes prostaglandins, which increase myometrial tone and cause uterine contractions leading to pain. These prostaglandins can also cause headache, nausea, vomiting, diarrhea, and dizziness. Leukotriene, an inflammatory mediator, may also play a role in the development of symptoms of dysmenorrhea. As many as 60% to 92% of adolescent girls have dysmenorrhea with 14% to 42% missing school or other activities because of the pain.

Primary dysmenorrhea can be classified as mild, moderate, or severe. Mild dysmenorrhea usually occurs on the first day of menses and does not interfere with daily activities. Moderate dysmenorrhea occurs on the first 2 to 3 days of menses and may have associated symptoms of diarrhea or headache. Severe dysmenorrhea refers to signif-icant cramping, often associated with nausea and vomiting and interferes with daily activities. Teens presenting with moderate or severe menstrual pain should have a complete history and examination to rule out the causes of secondary dysmenorrhea, shown in Box 225-1.

Premenstrual syndrome (PMS) may occur in adolescent girls. This includes a variety of symptoms (Box 225-2) occurring in the 7 to 10 days prior to onset of menses. The etiology of premenstrual syndrome is unclear at this time.

Causes of primary and secondary amenorrhea in adolescents can be divided into several categories by level of hormonal disturbance such as hypothalamic, pituitary, ovarian, and adrenal problems. Other causes of amenorrhea, usually primary, involve the genital outflow tract. Figure 225-2 outlines the range of etiologies for amenorrhea. Gonadal dysgenesis (Turner syndrome 46,XO) and agenesis of the uterus and vagina are the most common causes of primary amenorrhea. The most common cause of secondary amenorrhea is pregnancy.

Table 225-1 outlines the common causes of excessive bleeding in adolescent girls. When excess uterine bleeding presents at menarche, a bleeding diathesis is most common.

DIAGNOSIS

The most important step in the evaluation of menstrual disorders is taking a complete menstrual history. Included in this should be age at onset of breast and pubic hair development, age at menarche, date of last menstrual period, cycle length and regularity, duration of flow, amount of flow, use of hygiene products, and presence of cramping and other symptoms. A menstrual calendar, such as that shown in Table 225-2, can help teens record their cycles.

Gynecologic information obtained should include sexual, contraceptive, and pregnancy histories. General medical history should focus on chronic medical conditions, use of medications, and eating and exercise behaviors. Family history of menstrual disorders including bleeding problems may be helpful.

The physical examination for menstrual disorders should be complete. Table 225-3 outlines examination components and positive findings that warrant further evaluation. Decisions regarding performing a pelvic examination should be based on the history and physical examination. Often a thorough vulvar examination along with a bimanual examination are adequate for certain diagnoses; a speculum examination may be needed, however.

For a diagnosis of primary dysmenorrhea in teens, laboratory studies are not necessary. If causes of secondary dysmenorrhea are being considered, helpful studies include testing for sexually transmitted diseases or a pelvic ultrasound.

Adolescents presenting with primary amenorrhea with delayed puberty should be evaluated with chromosomal analysis to determine whether Turner syndrome is extant. Other studies include a complete blood count, thyroid function tests, prolactin, FSH, and LH. Low to normal levels of FSH and LH suggest hypothalamic or pituitary causes of amenorrhea whereas a high FSH level suggests an end organ problem such as ovarian dysfunction. Radiologic

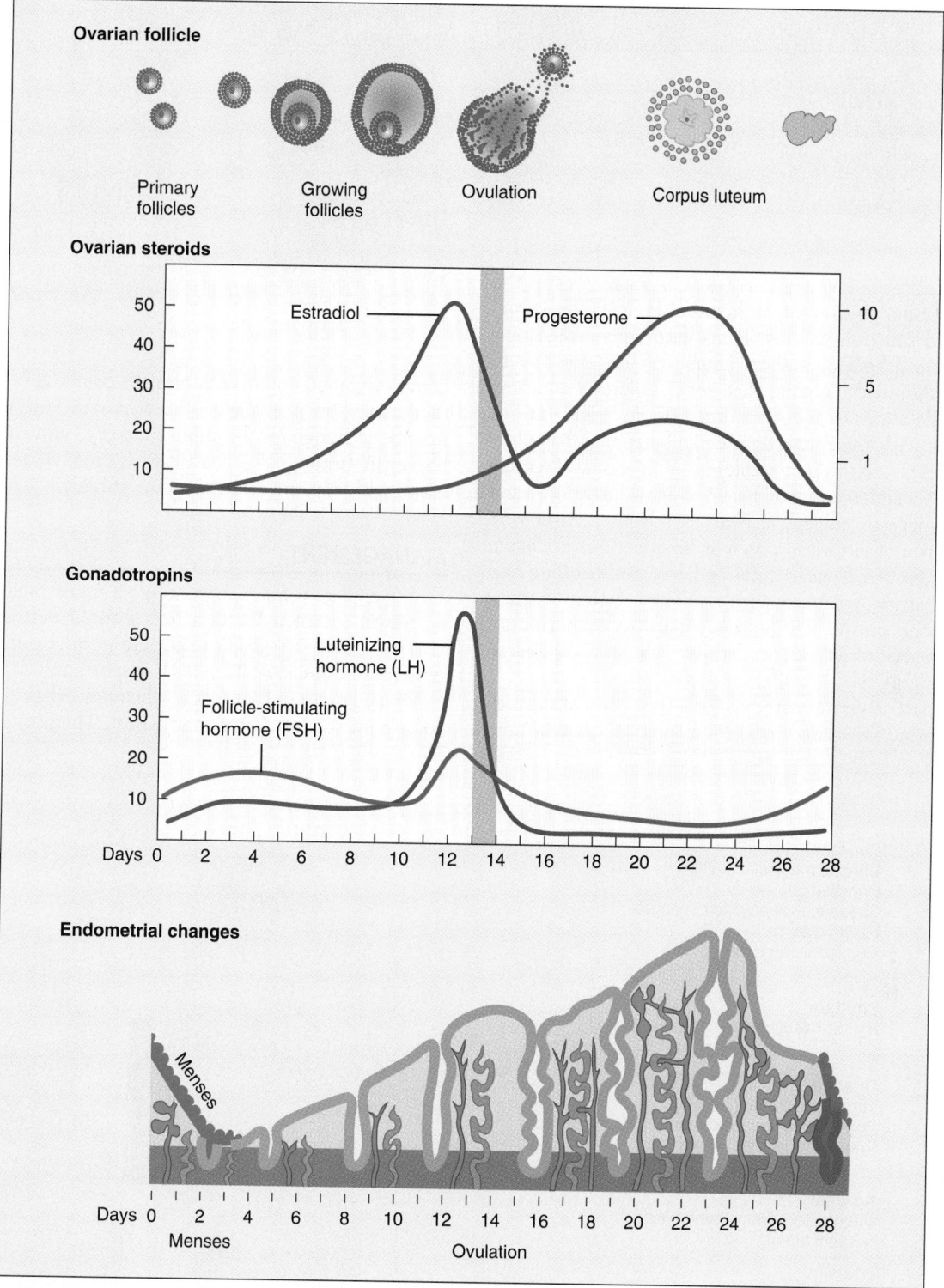

Figure 225-1. Normal changes at the level of the pituitary gland, ovary, and endometrium during the menstrual cycle.

studies may be warranted in some cases. These might include a bone age to look for constitutional delay, a pelvic ultrasound to verify normal anatomy, or neurological imaging (such as magnetic resonance imaging [MRI] of the head) to rule out pituitary or hypothalamic abnormalities.

In girls with some pubertal development, the above studies are helpful at discerning causes. Confirmation of normal genital tract structure is important in order to rule out certain disorders. Patients with findings of lack of axillary and pubic hair, normal breast development, and a blind vaginal pouch with no uterus suggest androgen insensitivity (46,XY). Patients with normal breast and pubic hair development with an absent or blind vaginal pouch and no uterus should be evaluated for congenital absence of the uterus also known as Mayer-Rokitansky-Kuster-Hauser syndrome.

Box 225-1.	Causes of Secondary Dysmenorrhea

Endometriosis
Genital tract obstruction
Pelvic inflammatory disease
Uterine fibroids or polyps
Tumor

Box 225-2.	Premenstrual Syndrome Symptoms

Bloating
Weight gain
Appetite changes
Breast tenderness
Fatigue
Stool changes
Hot flashes/chills
Headache
Mood changes, emotional lability, irritability, depression

In cases of secondary amenorrhea, a pregnancy test is the first step. Other studies might include LH, FSH, prolactin, and thyroid function studies. Teens with amenorrhea may benefit from a trial of a short course of progesterone to initiate withdrawal bleeding that verifies normal anatomy and an adequate estrogen source. Teens who fail to menstruate with the progesterone challenge may have low estrogen levels, as seen in athletes or in cases of eating disorders. Secondary amenorrhea in a teen who is obese and has acne suggests polycystic ovary syndrome. Girls who have evidence of virilization such as hirsutism, severe acne, or clitoromegaly will need total and free testosterone and DHEAS (dehydroepiandrosterone sulfate) testing. If these are abnormal, an ACTH (adrenocorticotropic hormone) stimulation test may be needed to rule out congenital adrenal hyperplasia.

Appropriate laboratory studies for a teen presenting with excess uterine bleeding include a pregnancy test and complete blood count with platelet count. A bleeding time study may be prolonged in teens with von Willebrand's disease, although prothrombin time (PT) and partial thromboplastin time (PTT) are often normal. Confirmation is made with specific clotting factor studies.

MANAGEMENT

The overall goal for management of menstrual disorders is to return menstrual cycles to a normal pattern and flow without pain. Education regarding normal pubertal development and menstrual cycles is important.

Management of primary dysmenorrhea starts with counseling for the patient and family. The primary goal is to

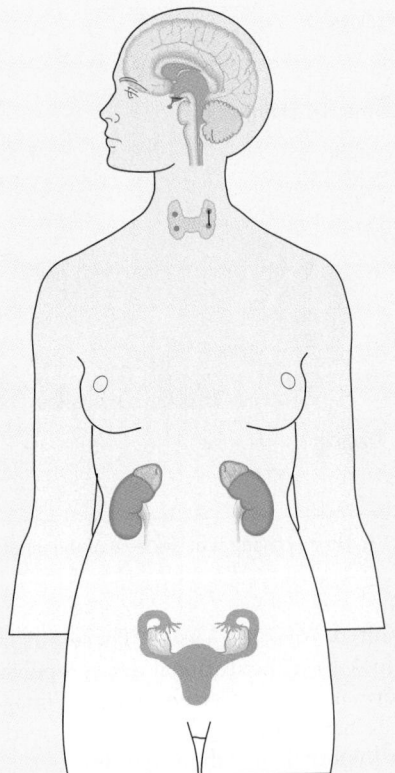

Hypothalmic
Chronic medical condition
Constitutional delay
Stress/exercise/weight changes
Eating disorder
Craniopharyngioma

Pituitary
Hyperprolactinemia

Ovarian
Turner syndrome (46, XO)
Polycystic ovary syndrome
Premature ovarian failure

Adrenal
Congenital adrenal hyperplasia
Adrenal tumor

Structural
Absence of uterus, cervix, and/or vagina
Imperforate hymen
Vaginal septum
Testicular feminization (androgen insensitivity)

Other
Pregnancy
Thyroid disease

Figure 225-2. Causes of primary and secondary amenorrhea.

Table 225-1. Causes of Excess Uterine Bleeding

Bleeding abnormalities	von Willebrand disease
	Idiopathic thrombocytopenic purpura
	Autoimmune hemolytic anemia
	Leukemia
	Other clotting factor or platelet disorders
Pregnancy-related	Threatened, spontaneous, or elective abortion
	Pregnancy
	Postpartum endometritis
Hormonal	Anovulatory cycles
	Polycystic ovary syndrome
	Contraceptive hormones such as oral contraceptives, depot medroxyprogesterone acetate, or levonorgestrel implants
Other	Sexually transmitted diseases
	Thyroid disease
	Systemic illness (renal, diabetes, liver)
	Trauma or sexual assult
	Medications: aspirin, warfarin
	Neoplasms
	Polyps
	Foreign bodies

keep teens pain-free during their menses and maintaining normal attendance in school and outside activities. Teens who keep a menstrual calendar can anticipate the onset of their cycles and initiate use of the appropriate NSAID (nonsteroidal anti-inflammatory drug) (Box 225-3). The important step is to start the medication 24 to 48 hours prior to the onset of menstrual flow and continue it through the few days of menses. If teens become nauseated, have chronic conditions that prohibit NSAID use, or are sexually active, they may benefit from using oral contraceptives. Referral for the evaluation of causes of secondary dysmenorrhea should be done when NSAIDs or oral contraceptive pills do not resolve the pain.

After the initial history, physical examination, and preliminary laboratory or x-ray studies of a teen with primary amenorrhea, the primary health care provider should consider referral to a gynecologist for management and counseling regarding the diagnosis. For a teen with secondary amenorrhea and a negative pregnancy test, administration of progesterone (oral progesterone 10 mg

daily for 5–10 days) is the next step. If menses restarts and laboratory studies are normal, it may be reasonable to follow the menstrual cycle pattern of the patient for several months. However, if there is failure of withdrawal bleeding, menstrual cycles continue to be infrequent, or laboratory studies are abnormal, further investigation or referral to a specialist is advised.

The primary goals in the management of teens who present with excess uterine bleeding are to stop any active bleeding, maintain a normal hemodynamic state, and correct any anemia. Adolescents who present with excess uterine bleeding first need to be assessed for hemodynamic stability. If there is an increased pulse, low blood pressure, dizziness, or orthostatic changes, immediate transfer to a facility that can offer stabilization is warranted. Another step in the office setting is a hemoglobin or hematocrit along with a pregnancy test. Patients with bleeding and a positive pregnancy test should be transferred to a hospital with obstetrical care. Management for hemodynamically stable teens is based on the hemoglobin level (Table 225-4).

OUTCOME

Menstrual irregularities are common during the teen years. The prognosis depends on the etiology of the disorder and its management. Primary dysmenorrhea can generally be controlled with medication to help teens continue with their normal daily activities. Certain causes of secondary dysmenorrhea and primary or secondary amenorrhea may affect the fertility of teen patients. The consulting physician should review this information and discuss it with the adolescent and her family. Teens with bleeding disorders such as von Willebrand disease can become pregnant and deliver safely under close supervision. Prognosis for teens with other types of excess uterine bleeding varies with the cause.

FOLLOW-UP

Continued monitoring of future menstrual cycles is crucial to the management of menstrual disorders in teens. Reviewing the menstrual calendar at each office visit is key to the care of teens with abnormal menses. For patients

Table 225-2. Menstrual Calendar

Month	1	2	3	4	5	6	7	8	9	10	11	12	13	14	15	16	17	18	19	20	21	22	23	24	25	26	27	28	29	30	31
January																															
February																															
March																															
April																															
May																															
June																															
July																															
August																															
September																															
October																															
November																															
December																															

X, normal bleeding; H, heavy bleeding; S, light bleeding/spotting.

Table 225-3. Physical Examination Findings in Teens with Menstrual Disorders

System	Finding
General	Height percentile
	Weight percentile
	Body Mass Index
	Pulse
	Blood pressure
	Dysmorphic features
Skin	Pallor
	Petechiae
	Hair pattern (lanugo/hirsutism)
	Acanthosis nigricans
	Acne
HEENT/neck	Webbed neck
	Thyroid goiter
	Lymphadenopathy
Chest	Breast development (Tanner rating)
	Galactorrhea
Abdomen	Tenderness
	Masses
	Hepatosplenomegaly
Pelvic	Pubic hair development (Tanner rating)
	Patency of hymen
	Discharge
	Lesions
	Cliteromegaly
	Presence of estrogenized vaginal mucosa
	Septum of vagina
	Foreign body
	Polyp
	Uterine tenderness or masses
	Ovarian tenderness or masses
Neurological	Anosmia
	Visual fields

Table 225-4. Management of Excessive Uterine Bleeding

Extent of Bleeding	Management
Mild bleeding (Hgb > 11 g/dL)	1. Reassure and educate patient/family.
	2. Keep a menstrual calendar.
	3. Follow-up for future prolonged bleeding episodes.
Moderate bleeding (Hgb 9–11 g/dL)	1. Consider stopping flow with one of the following therapies:
	a. Provera 10 mg daily for 5–10 days (flow will restart within 1 week of cessation).
	b. Oral contraceptives 1–4 pills daily depending on flow; taper as indicated.
	2. Initiate iron therapy.
	3. Follow closely for bleeding cessation and hemoglobin status.
Severe bleeding (Hgb <9 g/dL)	1. Assess hemodynamic state and refer to ER if unstable.
	2. Oral contraceptives 1–4 pills daily until flow diminishes; taper as tolerated to maintain no flow. Withhold placebos until hemoglobin status is adequate.
	3. Initiate iron therapy.
	4. Follow closely for bleeding cessation and hemoglobin status.

with primary dysmenorrhea, return visits every few months initially, then annually, ensure that management strategies are adhered to help minimize the interference of menstrual pain in the teen's daily life. Teens with secondary amenorrhea who respond to the progesterone challenge can be seen every 3 to 6 months at first to ensure regular cycles. Others need follow-up based on their specific diagnoses. Teens with excess uterine bleeding need closer follow-up, depending on their initial hemoglobin. Once their anemia is resolved and the etiology of their excess bleeding is addressed, they can be seen annually.

Box 225-3. Medications for Primary Dysmenorrhea

Ibuprofen 400–800 mg 3–4 times a day (maximum dosage 3200 mg)

Naproxen (Aleve 220 mg) or Naproxen sodium (Anaprox 275 mg) 2 tablets at onset and then 1 every 6 hours

Anaprox DS 550 mg twice a day

Mefenamic acid (Ponstel 250 mg) 2 tablets at onset and then 1 tablet every 6 hours

 Additional Resources, CD-ROM

Bibliography

Mini-index of Related Topics

SUGGESTED READINGS

Braverman PK, Sondheimer SJ: Menstrual disorders. Pediatr Rev 1997;18(1):17–25.

Emans JS, Laufer MR, Goldstein DP: Pediatric and Adolescent Gynecology, 4th ed. Philadelphia, Lippincott-Raven, 1998.

Harel Z, Lilly C, Riggs S, et al: Urinary leukotriene (LT) E4 in adolescents with dysmenorrhea: A pilot study. J Adolesc Health 2000;27(3):151–154.

Iglesias EA, Coupey SM: Menstrual cycle abnormalities: Diagnosis and management. Adolesc Med 1999;10(2):255–273.

TeensHealth. Coping with common period problems. Available at: http://kidshealth.org/teen/sexual_health/girls/menstrual_problems.html.

226 Gynecologic Disorders

Paula J. Adams Hillard and Helen F. Deitch

ROLE OF THE GENERALIST

1 Develop knowledge, skills, competencies, and comfort with adolescent gynecology.

2 Be sensitive and nonjudgmental regarding adolescent sexuality and risk-taking behaviors.

3 Maintain confidentiality in provision of care for adolescent gynecologic problems.

4 Refer when necessary to colleagues who are sensitive and skilled in addressing the gynecologic problems of adolescents.

5 Provide care for vaginitis, menstrual abnormalities, dysmenorrhea, abstinence/contraceptive counseling, and STDs.

6 Recognize symptoms and initiate evaluation of pelvic pain, polycystic ovary syndrome (PCOS), and adnexal masses and refer patients appropriately.

7 Co-manage pelvic pain, PCOS, and adnexal masses with specialists.

8 Recognize acute gynecologic pain as a possible life-threatening emergency and evaluate it expeditiously to minimize morbidity and mortality.

The role of generalists in caring for gynecologic problems in adolescents should be based on their knowledge, skills, competencies, and comfort in dealing with specific gynecologic conditions within a framework of adolescent physical, psychosocial, psychosexual, and cognitive development. Care must be delivered with a nonjudgmental attitude. It is important to provide facts clearly and concisely in an open, respectful manner with genuine interest in the adolescent's health and well-being, particularly regarding issues of sexuality, risk-taking behaviors, and gynecologic conditions. Clinicians should refer patients to an appropriate colleague if they are unable or unwilling to deal with the complex psychosocial situations and confidentiality issues often associated with gynecologic problems in adolescents. A good consultant should answer questions and see referred patients without judging the abilities of the primary clinician, as many gynecologic problems can be particularly challenging or difficult to evaluate and manage.

This chapter addresses specific gynecologic conditions of adolescents, including pelvic pain (both acute and chronic), polycystic ovary syndrome (PCOS), and adnexal/ovarian masses. Care for some conditions, such as PCOS, requires input from multiple sources, necessitating collaborative management by the primary clinician, a gynecologist, an endocrinologist, and a dietician. Selection of a gynecologic consultant should be based on the gynecologist's experience and expertise with adolescents. While many teens prefer a female clinician for gynecologic care, the physician's sex does not ensure provision of compassionate, clinically competent care. Feedback from patients previously referred to a specific colleague should be used to guide subsequent referrals.

PELVIC AND LOWER ABDOMINAL PAIN

Definition

Anatomically, the organ systems that can cause pelvic pain in adolescent girls are the gastrointestinal tract, the urinary tract, the female genital tract, and the abdominal wall. Acute pelvic pain is intense pain of relatively sudden and recent onset with a sharp increase in intensity and short course. Table 226-1 lists causes of acute pelvic pain. Conditions usually associated with chronic or cyclic pelvic pain may initially present as acute or episodically recurrent pelvic pain. Chronic pelvic pain is defined as pain of more than 6 months' duration, although adolescents may not strictly adhere to the time definition. Chronic pelvic pain may be cyclic and associated with the menstrual cycle, although the pattern may not be easily or readily apparent to the clinician, the adolescent patient, or her family. Table 226-2 lists causes of chronic pelvic pain.

Fundamentals

Acute pelvic pain is often associated with signs of infection or inflammation, including fever and leukocytosis. Pelvic pain can be referred, with the location related to the nerve distribution or dermatome of the innervation of the uterus or ovary. Dysmenorrhea can present with back pain or pain perceived as arising from the anterior thighs. Delay in diagnosing the cause of acute pelvic pain can increase morbidity and mortality. Delay in diagnosis of an ovarian torsion increases the risk of ovarian necrosis. Ruptured ectopic pregnancy remains an important cause of maternal morbidity and mortality. Diagnosing the cause of acute pelvic pain is particularly difficult if the clinician does not consider that the adolescent may be sexually active and at risk for pregnancy-associated conditions or STDs. Figure 226-1 illustrates changes between 1970 and 1995 in the percentage of adolescents who are sexually experienced.

An accurate history, including menstrual and sexual history, is absolutely key to diagnosing gynecologic causes of acute pelvic pain. Table 226-3 lists the elements of an adequate gynecologic history. The clinician should ask questions about menstrual and sexual history in a variety of ways to ascertain accurate information. Questions about sexual activities need to be asked privately with ensurances of confidentiality. Information about the number of sexual partners, date of last intercourse, and types of sexual activities engaged in enables an assessment of STD and pregnancy risk. Questions about the consistency of condom or contraceptive use must be asked sensitively and specifically, using terms the adolescent understands. The type of contraceptives is related to specific gynecologic conditions that cause pain. Oral contraceptives decrease the risk of functional ovarian cysts, and consistent condom use decreases the risks of pelvic inflammatory disease (PID).

Questions regarding menstrual bleeding need to be specific. Many adolescents interpret any bleeding as a "menstrual period." Bleeding in early pregnancy (implantation bleeding) can mimic a menstrual period in timing, but usually is shorter in duration and lighter in flow. A patient may state the date of onset of her last menstrual history, but may neglect to indicate that it was not normal unless queried about the character of the flow. Adolescents often do not keep track of their periods, and may need to be prompted to recall specific events (e.g., the prom or a holiday) in relationship to their bleeding.

Table 226-1. Causes of Acute Pelvic Pain

Organ System	Disorder
Gynecologic	■ Dysmenorrhea
	■ Mittelschmerz
	■ Corpus luteum cyst
	Rupture
	Bleeding into
	Torsion
	■ Ectopic pregnancy
	Rupture
	Tubal distension
	■ Spontaneous abortion
	■ Adnexal torsion
	■ Ovarian tumor
	Rupture
	Bleeding into
	■ PID
	■ Endometriosis
	■ Obstructed genital outflow tract
Gastrointestinal	■ Appendicitis
	■ Acute gastroenteritis
	■ Inflammatory bowel disease
	■ Mesenteric lymphadenitis
	■ Constipation
	■ Irritable bowel syndrome
	■ Meckel diverticulitis
Urinary tract	■ UTI
	Cystitis
	Pyelonephritis
	■ Urinary calculus
	■ Interstitial cystitis
Other	■ Sickle cell crisis
	■ Acute intermittent phorphyria
	■ Psychosocial
	Sexual or physical abuse
	School avoidance
	■ Abdominal wall
	Trigger point/musculoskeletal pain
	Hernia

Table 226-2. Causes of Chronic or Recurrent Pelvic Pain

Organ System	Disorder
Gynecologic	Cyclic/Recurrent
	■ Mittelschmerz (midcycle pain)
	■ Primary dysmenorrhea
	■ Secondary dysmenorrhea
	Endometriosis
	Uterina leiomyomata
	Obstructed genital outflow tract
	■ Recurrent functional ovarian cysts
	■ Endometriosis
	Noncyclic
	■ PID
	■ Ovarian tumor
	■ Obstructed genital outflow tract
Gastrointestinal	■ Inflammatory bowel disease
	■ Constipation
	■ Irritable bowel syndrome
Urinary tract	■ Urinary calculus
	■ Interstitial cystitis
Other	■ Sickle cell crisis
	■ Acute intermittent phorphyria
	■ Psychosocial
	Sexual or physical abuse
	School avoidance
	■ Abdominal wall
	Trigger point/musculoskeletal pain
	Hernia

The timing of pelvic pain in relationship to the menstrual cycle may be an important clue to the diagnosis. Adolescents may experience pain around the time of ovulation (mittelschmerz). Because adolescent menstrual cycles are often not ovulatory and somewhat irregular, this diagnosis is sometimes made in retrospect when the next menstrual period occurs approximately 14 days after the onset of pain. Interpretation of an ultrasound showing a simple cyst should be made in the context of the menstrual cycle. A corpus luteum cyst typically occurs in the second half of the cycle, the luteal phase (see Fig. 225-1).

A history for the purpose of diagnosing the gynecologic causes of pelvic pain in adolescents includes the typical questions listed in Table 226-4.

Presentation and Initial Evaluation of Acute Pelvic Pain

Ovulatory Pain. Pain occurring with ovulation may be difficult to diagnose, although the occurrence of pain midcycle is classic. Typically pain is sudden in onset, unilateral lower quadrant in location, dull and steady in character, exacerbated by movement, and may be alleviated by nonsteroidal anti-inflammatory drugs (NSAIDs). Pain is moderate to severe, but rarely awakens an individual from sleep. It is not associated with fever or other gastrointestinal or genitourinary symptoms. Examination reveals moderate abdominal tenderness and mild guarding, usually without signs of peritoneal irritation (rebound tenderness). Unilateral adnexal tenderness is found if pelvic examination is performed. Because an acute visit with these symptoms is more likely to occur with girls whose cycles have not previously been ovulatory, a complete pelvic examination may sometimes be deferred in the young teen who denies sexual activity. Bimanual examination with palpation of the adnexae is the most important component of the exami-

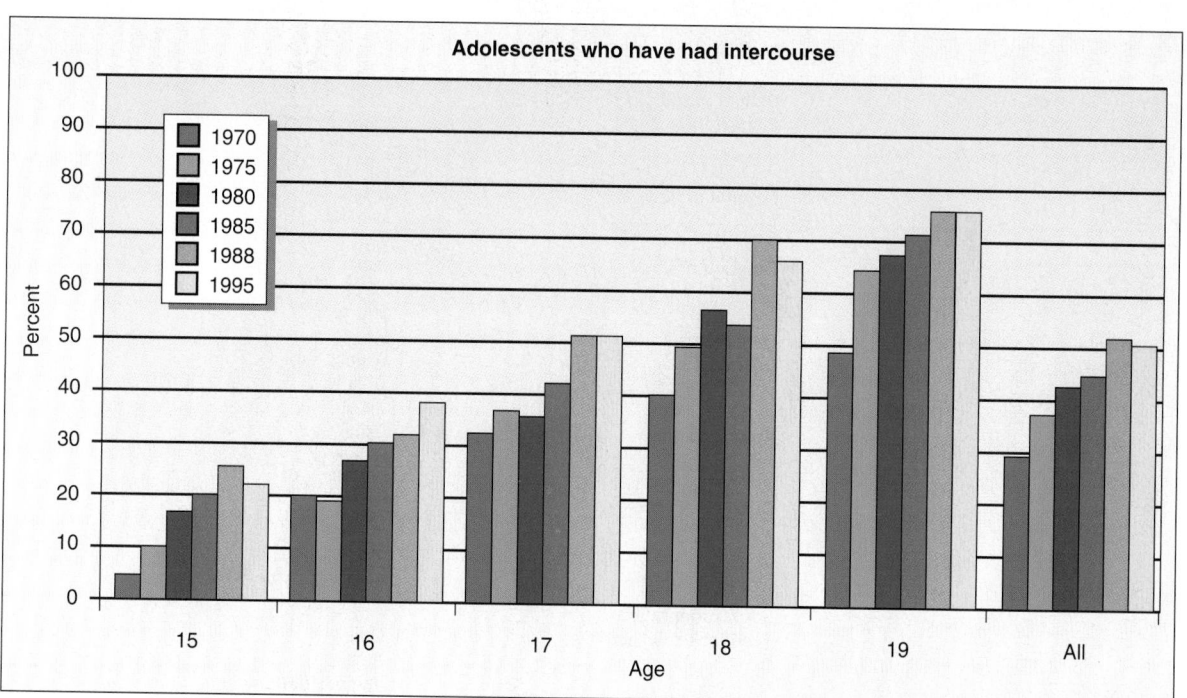

Figure 226-1. Changes in the percentage of adolescents who are sexually experienced. (Data from the National Surveys of Family Growth, CDC.)

nation, and can usually be performed with sensitivity and gentleness, using a single index finger. The speculum examination is rarely helpful for making this diagnosis, and often can be deferred. Pelvic ultrasound is typically normal. Laboratory studies show no leukocytosis, and hematocrit is stable.

Rupture/Hemorrhage into Ovarian Cyst. Rupture of a corpus luteum cyst, or acute hemorrhage into a corpus luteum cyst, occurs in the second half of the menstrual cycle, usually with a history of relatively regular menses with menstrual molimina (dysmenorrhea, breast tenderness, bloating) that suggest ovulatory cycles. The onset of pain is sudden and may awaken the adolescent from sleep. The pain may be severe. It is usually unilateral, dull and steady in character, exacerbated by movement, and not relieved by NSAIDs. It is not associated with fever, although it may be associated with signs of peritoneal irritation, including loose stools. Nausea and vomiting may occur with severe pain. Examination reveals moderate to severe abdominal tenderness, often with voluntary guarding, and sometimes with signs of peritoneal irritation (rebound tenderness). Pelvic examination should be performed in individuals who have been sexually active, but may be deferred or modified in those who have not. The definitive diagnostic test is a pelvic ultrasound, which typically reveals a unilateral multilocular cyst, usually filled with debris (hemorrhage). This mass is often 4 to 5 cm in diameter, but may be as large as 8 to 10 cm. A hemoperitoneum is indicated by the presence of more than a minimal amount of pelvic fluid in the cul-de-sac behind the uterus. There is usually no leukocytosis. Hematocrit is typically stable when there has been hemorrhage into the corpus luteum cyst, but observation over time and repeated hematocrits may be necessary to diagnose clinically significant intraperitoneal bleeding. The usual mechanism of pain with hemorrhage into the cyst is distension of a closed space (the cyst cavity).

Pelvic Inflammatory Disease. Adolescents who have been sexually active who present with the gradual and insidious onset of bilateral lower abdominal and suprapubic pain, typically accompanied by gastrointestinal symptoms of nausea or vomiting, fever, and an abnormal vaginal discharge should be presumed to have PID. Gonococcal or chlamydial PID presents with symptoms around the time of menses, although many factors, including access to clinical care, denial of symptoms, lack of a Medical Home, or unwillingness to disclose sexual activity can result in a delay in presentation or diagnosis. The pain is usually exacerbated by movement. The term *PID shuffle* refers to the gait in which patients walk gingerly and slowly to avoid sudden movements that increase peritoneal irritation. Pain is typically mild to moderate in intensity, and often relieved by NSAIDs, although pain relief may be incomplete, and ongoing therapy is required. Examination reveals moderate abdominal tenderness, often with mild to moderate voluntary guarding, and may include rebound tenderness. Pelvic examination is essential in making the diagnosis, and reveals uterine and bilateral adnexal tenderness, often severe. Pain is increased with movement of the cervix (cervical motion tenderness). The pain of the pelvic examination can result in the "chandelier sign," in which the patient elevates the pelvis and body away from the examiner. Care and gentleness should be used in gauging the pressure required to assess the pelvis during the examination. This degree of pain is not specific to PID. It can also be associated with other adnexal pathology, such as an ovarian torsion. Speculum examination typically reveals a mucopurulent cervical discharge, cervical friability, pain on cervical manipulation, and sometimes vaginal discharge consistent with concomitant trichomoniasis.

Testing for gonorrhea and Chlamydia should be performed. Microscopic examination of the cervical and vaginal discharge reveals leukocytes. A pelvic ultrasound is

Table 226-3. Gynecologic History

Last menstrual period (LMP)	Date of onset	
	Character	Usually expected time
		Early
		Late
	Amount of flow	Usual
		Heavier
		Lighter
	Duration of flow	Usual
		Longer
		Shorter
Previous menstrual period (PMP)	Date of onset	
	Character	Usually expected time
		Early
		Late
	Amount of flow	Usual
		Heavier
		Lighter
	Duration of flow	Usual
		Longer
		Shorter
Regularity of menses	Regular, monthly	Irregular, need dates
Sexual history	Sexual orientation	
	Types of sexual activities	Oral
		Anal
		Vaginal intercourse
		Date of last intercourse
	Parents aware?	
	Number of partners	
	Contraceptive use	Hormonal
		Oral contraceptives
		Missed pills?
		Injectable
		Date last injection
	Barrier	Condom use
		Consistency?
		At last intercourse
		Always
		Ever *not* used?
		Sometimes
		Never
		With all partners?
		Regular partner(s)
		Casual partners(s)
	Barrier plus hormonal	

important to diagnose a tubo-ovarian abscess. Transvaginal ultrasound examination provides more information than does a transabdominal scan. Laboratory studies classically reveal leukocytosis and an elevated sedimentation rate.

Ectopic Pregnancy. A ruptured ectopic pregnancy presents with sudden onset of severe unilateral and supra-pubic pelvic pain, which may be accompanied by signs of intraperitoneal hemorrhage including syncope and shoulder pain from irritation of the diaphragm. Classically, this event occurs after an interval of 6 to 8 weeks of amenorrhea, with symptoms of pregnancy: nausea/vomiting, breast tenderness, excessive fatigue, and urinary frequency. Severe tenderness, guarding, and rebound tenderness are present on abdominal examination. Pelvic examination may reveal signs of pregnancy including cyanosis of the cervix, uterine softening or enlargement, and marked adnexal tenderness. Fullness of the cul-de-sac is present if there is a significant hemoperitoneum.

Classic presentation of a ruptured ectopic pregnancy is fortunately less common than in years past. Easily available and sensitive home and office pregnancy tests can reveal a pregnancy before catastrophic tubal rupture. The more common presentation is less dramatic with symptoms of vague, dull, unilateral lower abdominal pain from tubal distension rather than rupture. Because an adnexal mass may occur in a normal intrauterine pregnancy (a corpus luteum cyst), pelvic ultrasound is necessary to confirm or refute the diagnosis. An intrauterine pregnancy on trans-vaginal ultrasound virtually excludes an ectopic pregnancy;

Table 226-4. Gynecologic Pain History

Onset	Relationship to menstrual period
	Sudden versus gradual
Duration	
Character	Sharp
	Dull
	Crampy
	Constant
	Intermittent
Location	Radiation
Alleviating/exacerbating factors	
Previous similar pain?	
Medications taken	Dose
	Frequency
	Efficacy
Beliefs about etiology	Causative factors
	Related factors

however, absence of an intrauterine gestational sac is associated with both an early intrauterine pregnancy (before about 6 weeks from the last menstrual period) and an ectopic pregnancy. In this situation, the diagnosis rests on the correlation of serum levels of human chorionic gonadotrophin (hCG [quantitative]) with the ultrasound findings. Such a diagnostic distinction is difficult, and should be made in consultation with or by an obstetrician/gynecologist.

Adnexal Torsion. The diagnosis of adnexal torsion is difficult and requires a high index of suspicion. A normal adnexa does not usually twist on its vascular pedicle. More commonly, torsion occurs with an abnormal ovary (a functional or neoplastic cyst). Intermittent torsion results in intermittent severe pain. Typically, pain is acute, sudden, and severe. It may begin during physical activity (e.g., running, gymnastics, a sudden sharp turn). Severe pain may cause nausea and vomiting. Examination reveals moderate to severe tenderness and guarding, often with signs of rebound tenderness. Pelvic ultrasound shows an adnexal mass. Doppler imaging shows decreased or absent blood flow to the ovarian stroma. Doppler studies are neither perfectly sensitive nor specific, but can confirm this difficult-to-make diagnosis, which it is urgent to determine. Timely surgical intervention with laparoscopy can confirm the diagnosis. Ovarian viability is frequent with detorsion when the condition is diagnosed expeditiously.

Laboratory Evaluation and Imaging of Acute Pelvic Pain

Laboratory evaluation of acute pelvic pain requires a small number of tests, with additional testing used to assess conditions included in the differential diagnoses. The only laboratory studies typically required are a qualitative hCG and complete blood count (CBC). Additional studies may be helpful if other abdominal conditions (such as urinary tract disease) are suspected.

Testing for pregnancy, regardless of the stated sexual history, is essential. The consequences of missing a pregnancy-related complication, such as an ectopic pregnancy, can be life-threatening. Urine hCG testing detects pregnancy when the urinary concentration is 25 mIU, a value that is typically present within about 7 to 10 days of conception (not the missed period). Because serum testing detects levels at about 5 to 10 mIU, only a day or so before the urine test, and typically long before a growing ectopic pregnancy becomes symptomatic, a urine test is virtually as sensitive. Easily performed urine tests are commercially available at relatively low cost, and should be used in outpatient settings to facilitate urgent clinical decision making. Quantitative serum hCG level may be appropriate in the diagnosis and management of early pregnancy complications, particularly in distinguishing between an ectopic pregnancy and an early intrauterine pregnancy and its complications (e.g., a spontaneous abortion). Serum quantitative hCG levels can be correlated with the likelihood of visualizing an intrauterine pregnancy using transvaginal or transabdominal pelvic ultrasound, typically at about 6 weeks from the last menstrual period (LMP), and often with an hCG in the range of 1500 mIU/mL.

In inflammation (PID) or bleeding (ruptured hemorrhagic corpus luteum cyst), a CBC with differential can be helpful. An elevated white blood count (WBC) or a left shift may be noted with PID. Adnexal torsion can be associated with a mildly elevated white blood count, and acute bleeding may result in a low hemoglobin/hematocrit.

Imaging Studies. Pelvic ultrasound can give valuable information about ovarian masses or their absence. They can be especially helpful in young teens who have not had a pelvic examination, because a bimanual pelvic examination may be unrevealing or uninterpretable because of either pain or fear. A transabdominal ultrasound examination is usually sufficient to rule out large masses. A transvaginal examination is more sensitive and specific and is usually tolerated by young women who have been sexually active and some cooperative teens who have used tampons. Ultrasound is a more helpful test than computed tomography (CT) in providing information about the character of adnexal masses (cystic, solid, or mixed in echogenicity). Color-flow Doppler examination with the ultrasound examination is essential to evaluate blood flow to the ovaries and can suggest the diagnosis of torsion. While most adnexal masses are benign, some characteristics of ovarian masses are more suggestive of neoplasm (Table 226-5).

Chronic Pelvic Pain

Cyclic Primary Dysmenorrhea. One of the most common causes of chronic or chronic recurrent pelvic pain is primary dysmenorrhea. Primary dysmenorrhea is associated with ovulatory cycles, which may not occur consistently until 1 to 2 or more years after menarche. The mechanism of pain involves the presence of elevated levels of prostaglandins in the endometrium and menstrual fluid, which induces uterine contractility with hypertonus and resulting ischemia. Antiprostaglandin agents (NSAIDs) and combination birth control pills can markedly improve primary dysmenorrhea. These agents, either singly or in combination, are effective in relieving primary dysmenorrhea in most women. Because dysmenorrhea may begin before the onset of bleeding, the association between pain and menses may not be recognized by adolescents who do not keep careful records of their cycles, or who may have somewhat more irregular cycles than older women. Cycle-related pain may occur in association with ovulation, causing the association with the menstrual cycle to be missed unless the pain is carefully charted on a menstrual calendar (Fig. 226-2).

Severe cyclic abdominal/pelvic pain should prompt the consideration of a possible obstructing genital anomaly, such

Table 226-5. Ultrasound Characteristics of Benign Ovarian Masses

- Cystic
- Unilateral
- Unilocular
- No mural nodules or solid components
- Smooth border
- Calcifications consistent with teeth or bone
- Fat density
- No ascites

Menstrual flow chart

Patient _____

Address _____ Phone _____

Year _____

Month	1	2	3	4	5	6	7	8	9	10	11	12	13	14	15	16	17	18	19	20	21	22	23	24	25	26	27	28	29	30	31	No. of days from part of period to beginning of next	Breast exam alone (✓)
Jan.																																	
Feb.																														▓			
Mar.																																	
Apr.																														▓			
May																																	
June																														▓			
July																																	
Aug.																																	
Sept.																														▓			
Oct.																																	
Nov.																														▓			
Dec.																																	

Don't forget to have this chart with you when you call or visit your health care provider

Type of flow
Normal N
Light   L
Heavy   H

Figure 226-2. Menstrual calendar.

as an imperforate hymen or an obstructing vaginal septum. The findings on examination of an imperforate hymen in a menarchal girl who has developed a hematometra and hematocolpos are obvious on genital examination. Such a dramatic presentation of this condition can be prevented by routine examination of the genitalia by primary clinicians and the diagnosis made prior to adolescence. Imperforate hymen is pictured in Figure 226-3. A partially obstructing lesion should be suspected if the menstrual history includes abnormal bleeding between menses, particularly if the bleeding is dark and brownish in color. Pelvic ultrasound is the appropriate test to screen for these disorders. Magnetic resonance imaging (MRI) may be needed to clearly assess the anatomy. While imperforate hymen can be treated by most gynecologists, patients with more complex anatomic abnormalities should be referred to a medical center with experience in managing these unusual conditions.

Secondary Dysmenorrhea. In adult women, a variety of acquired conditions can result in pain with menses, including uterine leiomyomata, other uterine or ovarian tumors, or endometriosis. Leiomyomata, uterine tumors, and ovarian masses are all uncommon in adolescents. Pelvic endometriosis can and does occur in adolescents and should be considered as an etiology for severe dysmenorrhea, cyclic, or even the noncyclic occurrence of pain.

Endometriosis. Endometriosis is ectopic growth of endometrial glands and stroma caused by retrograde flow of endometrial tissue through the fallopian tubes into the peritoneal cavity with implantation. The incidence of endometriosis in one community study was 0.2%. The incidence has been reported to be as high as 60% in adolescents who undergo laparoscopy for evaluation of chronic pelvic pain.

Both genetic and immunologic factors influence susceptibility to endometriosis. Having a first-degree relative

with surgically documented endometriosis increases risk for the condition several-fold. A gentle bimanual pelvic examination to help the patient differentiate between "discomfort" and "pain" or "tenderness" should be performed if the diagnosis is suspected. A speculum examination typically adds little in the absence of sexual

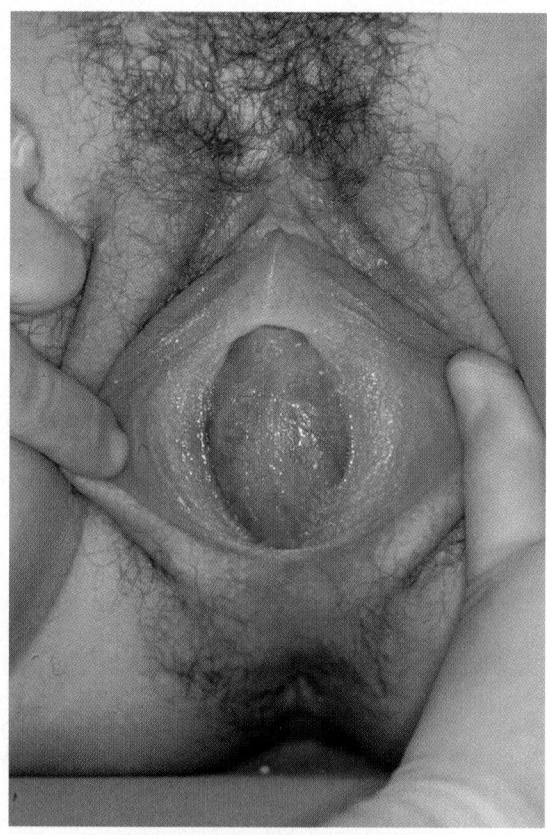

Figure 226-3. Imperforate hymen.

activity (to rule out STDs/cervicitis) or features that would suggest a congenital anomaly. Tenderness posterior to the uterus, particularly along the uterosacral ligaments as demonstrated on rectovaginal examination suggests endometriosis that typically implants in the most posterior portion of the pelvis: the retrouterine Douglas pouch/cul-de-sac. Because peritoneal implants are typically small, imaging studies are usually normal. Most adolescents have not yet developed adhesive disease or scarring from their disease, so that the classic finding in adults—nodules along the uterosacral ligaments or in the cul-de-sac—is unusual in teens.

When primary physicians suspect endometriosis, they should refer the patient to a clinician who frequently evaluates and manages adolescents with this condition. Laparoscopy is necessary to confirm the diagnosis. Therapy with KTP laser ablation of endometriotic lesions may be combined with postoperative medical therapy with GnRH (gonadotropin-releasing hormone) agents.

Ovarian Masses. Uterine or pelvic masses can cause chronic pelvic pain. A mass can result in pressure symptoms—pelvic heaviness, urinary frequency, and constipation. While all pelvic tumors are rare in adolescents, the presence of undiagnosed chronic pelvic pain should prompt consideration of a pelvic ultrasound examination.

Management of Pelvic and Lower Abdominal Pain
Acute Pelvic Pain

All patient presenting with acute pelvic pain must be assessed for presence of a condition that requires emergency surgery: appendicitis, ovarian or adnexal torsion, ruptured corpus luteum cyst with intraperitoneal hemorrhage, or a ruptured tubo-ovarian abscess. If these conditions can be eliminated by the clinical picture (no peritoneal signs on examination, no fever), appropriate imaging studies (pelvic ultrasound with focus on right lower quadrant, pelvic ultrasound with Doppler flow studies, transvaginal pelvic ultrasound examination), or laboratory testing (normal leukocyte count and hemoglobin), then other conditions can and should be managed medically.

After an acute abdomen or other surgical emergency has been eliminated, medical therapy should be instituted. The key to demonstrating menstrual or cycle-related pain is a pain diary. This is a written record in which menses are charted and some notation is made of days on which pain occurs. This can be helpful in pinpointing midcycle ovulatory pain whose cause and patterns of occurrence are not always obvious. Breast tenderness, headache, and bloating are commonly associated with ovulatory cycles, and can also be charted on the same calendar. Menstrual calendars are often available from pharmaceutical companies that make oral contraceptives (useful for charting breakthrough bleeding).

The management of most causes of acute gynecologic pain rests strongly on the use of NSAIDs as primary therapy for pain. Although certain NSAIDs have been marketed as being particularly beneficial for dysmenorrhea, all of the drugs in this class inhibit prostaglandins and result in analgesia if taken in appropriate doses with an appropriate frequency. Some of these medications are available over the

counter (OTC). Many teenagers are unaware that not all OTC medications touted as beneficial for dysmenorrhea contain NSAIDs or even anything with any proven efficacy for this condition. Table 226-6 lists available over-the-counter analgesics used for dysmenorrhea. OTC medications other than NSAIDs do not have demonstrated clinical efficacy. Table 226-7 lists prescription medications commonly used for dysmenorrhea.

Prescription NSAIDs usually provide excellent relief for cycle-related pain (dysmenorrhea, ovulatory pain) or other gynecologic pain when taken in adequate doses at an adequate frequency. Parents or physicians may be reluctant to prescribe them on an ongoing basis, although pain relief is typically needed for a relatively brief period, a few days each month. Taking a few days of NSAIDs beginning a day or so before expected onset of cycle-related pain and continuing every month in the same way (depending on the NSAID chosen and its duration of action) can be helpful. NSAIDs should be taken with food to minimize gastrointestinal symptoms or gastroesophagitis.

Oral contraceptives (OCs) provide excellent relief of dysmenorrhea or cycle-related pain. Although they have been used in this manner for a number of years, this use is "off-label." Oral contraceptives can be used as "second-line" when pain is recurrent, if there are no medical contraindications to their use. Supplementation with NSAIDs may be required. Dysmenorrhea may respond variably to a particular pill formulation. Switching from one pill formulation to another, after an adequate 2- to 3-month trial, may be necessary.

Chronic Pelvic Pain

The medical management of chronic or cyclic pelvic pain begins with a menstrual calendar/pain diary documenting frequency and severity of pain. Adolescents can be asked to quantify their pain on a 1–10 scale, with 1 representing no

Table 226-6. Over-the-Counter Analgesics and Medications Marketed for Dysmenorrhea

NSAIDs	Ibuprofen Motrin 200 mg q 4–6 h; 2 if no relief; not >6/24 h Advil 200 mg Nuprin 200 mg Naprosyn Aleve 220 mg q 8–12 h; 2 as initial dose; not >3/24 h Ketoprofen Orudis KT 12.5 mg
Midol	Acetaminophen 500 mg Parabrom 25 mg
Midol Menstrual Pain and Multi-Symptom	Acetaminophen 500 mg
Menstrual Relief	Caffeine 60 mg Pyrilamine maleate 15 mg
Maximum Strength Midol PMS	Acetaminophen 500 mg Parabrom 25 mg Pyrilamine maleate 15 mg
Pamprin	Magnesium salicylate 250 mg Parabrom 25 mg
Fish oil	

Table 226-7. Prescription NSAIDs Commonly Used for Dysmenorrhea

Drug	Dose
Motrin	Ibuprofen 400 mg q 4–6 h
Anaprox	Naproxen sodium 550 mg, then 275 mg q 6–8 h or 550 mg q 12; maximum 1375 mg/d day 1, then 1100 mg 1 d
Cataflam	Diclofenac 100 mg, then 50 mg tid
Ponstel	Mefenamic acid 500 mg, then 250 mg q 6 h
Toradol	Ketorolac 10 mg q 4–6 h
Vioxx	Refecoxib 50 mg qd
Celebrex	Celecoxib 200 mg qd/100 mg bid

pain, and 10 the worst imaginable pain. Pain ratings may appear to be inflated (e.g., a rating of "10/10" for a teen who appears to be resting comfortably) if an adolescent's worst previous pain experience involved only cuts and scrapes. Clinicians need to be constantly aware that pain may be a manifestation of school avoidance, depression, sexual abuse, or other issues related to sexuality. Asking parents about pain tolerance in other situations can be helpful in assessing the extent of disability. Parents who react to pain in a histrionic or excessively demonstrative manner or who themselves harbor unresolved issues about abuse or sexuality may model inappropriate or exaggerated responses to pain.

If pain continues in spite of adequate dosing and frequency of NSAIDs and oral contraceptives, the primary physician should consider reevaluating the patient. An imaging study may be indicated if one has not previously been performed, and referral to a gynecologist who is experienced in managing pelvic pain in adolescents may be advisable.

Box 226-1. Situations in Which Laparoscopy May Be Indicated

Suspicious pain history
    Primarily cyclic pain with menses or ovulation
    Pain that was initially cyclic, but has become more chronic and noncyclic
    Pain unrelieved by NSAIDs and OCs
History of the following
    Significant disability
    Costly evaluations
    Hospitalizations
Suspicious examination
    Cul-de-sac tenderness
    Uterosacral nodularity
Positive family history of endometriosis
Patient/family concerns
    Extremely anxious
    Need reassurances before additional evaluation can take place
    Psychiatric evaluation or psychological counseling
    Other medical therapies
Other surgical interventions planned
    GI endoscopy
    Appendectomy

Conditions Requiring Surgical Consultation/Management

Patients with chronic pelvic pain, unrelieved by NSAIDs and oral contraceptives, should be evaluated for causes of pain that can be confirmed only by laparoscopic surgery, the most common being endometriosis. Situations in which laparoscopy can be helpful with chronic pelvic pain are listed in Box 226-1.

Follow-up/Referral

Patients with chronic pelvic pain require careful evaluation, management, and follow-up. Patients with a diagnosis of endometriosis require ongoing medical management with chronic hormonal suppressive therapy. Psychological counseling is frequently important to address pain-management strategies and to help avoid detrimental behaviors, such as substance abuse, and depression.

POLYCYSTIC OVARY SYNDROME (PCOS)

Definition

Polycystic ovary syndrome (PCO or PCOS), the most common female endocrinopathy, occurs in about 4% to 10% of adult women. Although the incidence among adolescents is not well established, a careful history from adult women with the condition indicates that symptoms and signs began in adolescence. In adults the condition is underdiagnosed, even when all of the classic features are demonstrated. In adolescents the typical features of anovulatory cycles, irregular menstrual bleeding, and severe acne are frequently attributed to normal adolescence.

The syndrome was originally described by Stein and Leventhal in 1935 and consisted of the clinical findings of hirsutism, obesity, infertility, and enlarged polycystic ovaries. The condition is heterogeneous, with some patients exhibiting the biochemical and hormonal features of the condition but not the classic phenotype. For example, not all individuals with PCOS are obese.

Definitions of the condition vary, without uniformly agreed-upon diagnostic criteria. Features of PCOS are listed in Box 226-2. Other features of the disease, such as polycystic ovaries demonstrated on ultrasound (multiple follicular cysts in a peripheral pattern), are neither perfectly sensitive nor specific, nor diagnostic of the condition or required to make the diagnosis. Some commonly associated metabolic features (insulin resistance and an abnormal lipid profile) tend to occur in older women, but may be present in adolescents. The condition appears to be familial, with some studies suggesting an autosomal dominant mode of genetic transmission with marked variability of phenotypic expression. The male phenotype has premature balding.

Box 226-2. Features of Polycystic Ovary Syndrome

Hyperandrogenism
Chronic anovulation
Absence of specific disease of the ovaries (an androgen-producing tumor such as Sertoli-Leydig cell tumor), the adrenals (a late-onset partial adrenal hyperplasia), or pituitary (Cushing syndrome)

Causes of irregular bleeding and anovulation
  Thyroid dysfunction
  Hyperprolactinemia
  Exercise-induced oligomenorrhea
  Eating disorders
Causes of hirsutism/hyperandrogenism
  Congenital adrenal hyperplasia
  Cushing syndrome
  Tumor
    Ovarian
    Adrenal

Presentation and Initial Evaluation

PCOS must be differentiated from causes of menstrual abnormalities, anovulation, and hyperandrogenism (see Chapter 225). These are listed in Box 226-3. Adolescents can present with a variety of symptoms and signs of PCOS, although menstrual irregularities are a hallmark, and hirsutism and acne prominent features.

Menstrual patterns within the first two gynecologic years can be variable and are typically anovulatory. Evaluation with a careful physical examination and laboratory studies should be considered for those who have long intervals of amenorrhea beyond the first menstrual cycle and other features of the condition. Menstrual dysfunction in adolescents with hyperandrogenism commonly presents as regular monthly menses for a period of time with the subsequent development of oligomenorrhea.

Hirsutism, a common feature of PCOS, can be very distressing to an adolescent. Careful and sensitive questioning is required, as teens and older women with excess facial hair often go to great lengths to hide it. Use of depilatories, shaving, waxing, bleaching, laser hair removal, and electrolysis should be directly inquired about. The required frequency of use of these methods gives some idea of the severity of hirsutism and can be used to monitor the effects of therapy. Patients should be examined completely unclothed to look for subtle midline lower abdominal coarse hairs or periareolar hair that can easily be hidden by clothing.

Moderate to severe or recalcitrant acne, particularly when accompanied by irregular menses or hirsutism, should prompt evaluation for PCOS.

Laboratory Evaluation and Imaging

Laboratory studies that confirm the condition include an elevation of androgens (sometimes only free testosterone or percent free testosterone), an elevated LH (luteinizing hormone)/FSH (follicle-stimulating hormone) ratio, and decreased sex hormone binding globulin (SHBG). Ultrasound imaging of the pelvis and adrenals should be considered when clinical evaluation is difficult, such as in a young patient unable to tolerate bimanual examination, those who are markedly obese, or those with severe hirsutism or markedly elevated androgens in whom a tumor must be ruled out. Polycystic appearance of the ovaries on ultrasound is not diagnostic of the condition. As many as 8% to 25% of normal women have such features. In addition, with early diagnosis, the characteristic ultrasound image may not be present in adolescents who have not had a significant period of anovulation.

Management of PCOS

Management of PCOS is based on the patient's developing a good understanding of the features of the condition and acquiring the motivation to relieve the signs and symptoms. Teens may be motivated by the possibility of improving acne and regularity of periods. Motivating an adolescent to make helpful lifestyle changes can be more difficult. Lifestyle changes can have a positive impact on the risk of developing the medical conditions associated with PCOS, including hyperlipidemia, insulin resistance and type 2 diabetes, endometrial cancer, and early cardiovascular disease. The beneficial impact on fertility is harder to demonstrate, but may be motivating for some teens.

The best therapy for women with PCOS is weight loss for those who are overweight or obese, and weight maintenance for those who are not. Both hyperinsulinemia and hyperandrogenemia are improved with weight loss. Dietary changes can improve hyperlipidemia or an unfavorable lipid profile and are required for weight loss. Emphasis needs to be on healthy lifestyle changes and changes in diet that can be maintained. Regular exercise provides benefit for cardiovascular status and for weight loss and weight maintenance. A baseline lipid profile can be helpful in providing counseling about necessary lifestyle changes.

The mainstay of therapy for patients with PCOS who do not wish to become pregnant involves suppression of ovarian androgen production with combination oral contraceptive pills. OCs improve hirsutism and acne, provide regular menstrual periods, protect the endometrium from hyperplasia, help protect against osteoporosis, and may improve androgenic lipid profiles. Excess hair growth typically slows with the introduction of OCs, allowing permanent hair removal with electrolysis or less frequent application of hair removal products or shaving. A growing body of data suggests that most OCs improve acne in the majority of women and the particular OC formulation may not be significant.

Both lean and obese women with PCOS can have hyperinsulinemia. Women with acanthosis nigricans, a clinical marker for insulin resistance, should be tested. Abnormalities of the ratio of glucose and insulin in the fasting state are evidence of insulin resistance. Insulin-sensitizing agents such as metformin are likely to become important in the therapy of women with PCOS.

Other therapies can improve outcomes, particularly among those with severe hirsutism. Spironolactone, in doses up to 200 mg/day, inhibits the ovarian and adrenal synthesis of androgens, competes for androgens at the hair follicle, and directly blocks 5-alpha reductase activity in the skin. For patients with acne, topical therapies combined with OCs are helpful. Some patients require isotretinoin (Accutane) for severe cystic, scarring acne.

Outcome

Adolescents are often concerned about their future fertility. It should be emphasized to teens at the time of diagnosis that not all girls or women with PCOS have difficulty becoming pregnancy and they should not assume that they are infertile. Metformin is proving useful in the treatment of infertility associated with PCOS. Girls should be told that problems with anovulation are one of the more easily treated causes of infertility.

Care should be taken in describing and explaining the condition to emphasize the opportunities to manage the condition and normalize the metabolic features, thus theoretically lowering the risks. It can be stated that untreated PCOS poses an increased risk of type 2 diabetes, cardiovascular disease including stroke, myocardial infarction, and hyperlipidemia. Risk is also increased for endometrial cancer and possibly breast cancer.

Follow-up

Since lifestyle changes are so important in the management of PCOS, the primary clinician can help reinforce healthy behaviors in the teen, working in conjunction with the gynecologist and the endocrinologist. Regular health care visits are essential to monitor weight and blood pressure, compliance with OC therapy, and compliance with and side effects of metformin if prescribed.

ADNEXAL MASSES

Definition

An adnexal mass in neonates and prepubertal children is any mass, either cystic or solid, of the ovary or paraovarian structures. In pubertal and postpubertal children, development of any mass of the ovary or paraovarian structures (with the exception of simple physiologic cysts less than 3 cm in diameter, i.e., corpus luteum or follicle) is considered abnormal. Approximately two thirds of adnexal masses in childhood and adolescence are non-neoplastic (corpus luteum or simple/follicular cysts), and one quarter of the remaining neoplastic lesions are benign.

Cystic Ovarian Follicles. Cystic ovarian follicles are physiologic and are typically less than 3 cm in diameter. They occur from FSH stimulation of the ovary, resulting in oocyte maturation. A surge in LH in the middle of the menstrual cycle causes release of the egg and follicular collapse. In a postmenarchal adolescent, the finding on an ultrasound of a unilocular cyst measuring less than 3 cm in diameter should be considered a normal finding, and should not be managed as a "cyst." No further management is required. An exaggeration of this normal physiologic process can result in the development of a unilocular follicular cyst, defined as a follicle larger than 3 cm in diameter. Follicular cysts are most often an asymptomatic, incidental finding of examination or ultrasound. They are typically smaller than about 5 cm in diameter.

The corpus luteum forms in place of the ruptured follicle and provides progesterone support for the endometrium in anticipation of implantation of an embryo. If implantation does not occur, the corpus luteum resolves. Rupture of a hemorrhagic corpus luteum cyst can result in hemoperi-

toneum and hemodynamic instability. Bleeding into a cyst or a ruptured corpus luteum cyst can result in pain. Hemorrhagic corpus luteum cysts can reach a size of up to 8 to 10 cm.

Follicular Cysts and Corpus Luteum Cysts. Follicular cysts and corpus luteum cysts are termed functional ovarian cysts and are the most common adnexal masses in postmenarchal adolescents. They will resolve over time without surgical intervention.

Ovarian Neoplasms. Ovarian neoplasms do not spontaneously resolve but will persist or enlarge over time. Ovarian neoplasms can be solid or multilocular or of mixed echogenicity on ultrasound examination. Ovarian tumors account for approximately 1% of all tumors in children and adolescents. Germ cell tumors (both benign and malignant) make up one half to two thirds of ovarian neoplasms in those younger than 20 years of age. In prepubertal girls, most ovarian neoplasms (up to 80%) are malignant. In adolescents, a much smaller percentage of ovarian neoplasms are malignant, probably less than one third. The most common neoplasm in adolescents is the benign cystic teratoma, or dermoid.

Fundamentals

Ovarian Cysts in Childhood. During childhood, the development of small ovarian follicles is not uncommon, and in one series were diagnosed in 68% of asymptomatic, ultrasound-screened, prepubertal children. About 10% of these cysts were larger than 9 mm in diameter. Most simple cysts in prepubertal children are the result of sporadic follicular development and occur when a follicle fails to involute. However, ovarian cysts may be secondary to central precocious puberty or, if the cyst is hormonally active, present with precocious pseudopuberty. A patient with recurrent ovarian cysts and precocious puberty should be evaluated for McCune-Albright syndrome. Hypothyroidism can also be a cause of enlarged, multicystic ovaries.

Adnexal Masses in Adolescents. While ovarian masses are the most common mass found in the area adjacent to the uterus (adnexal area), other conditions may mimic an ovarian mass, including Mullerian abnormalities, ectopic pregnancy, paratubal or paraovarian cysts (embryologic remnants of either the wolffian duct system or Muller ducts). Even a full urinary bladder can mimic a pelvic mass on examination. A palpable pelvic mass may be a pelvic or horseshoe kidney. Box 226-4 lists causes of adnexal masses in adolescents.

Box 226-4. Differential Diagnosis of Adnexal Masses

Ovary: Cyst, neoplasm, torsion, endometrioma, ectopic pregnancy
Tube: Pregnancy, tubo-ovarian abscess, hydrosalpinx, paratubal cyst
Uterus: Mullerian anomaly
GI: Appendiceal abscess
Bladder: Full bladder on examination
Peritoneal inclusion cyst

Box 226-5. Common Presenting Symptoms of Adnexal Masses

Abdominal pain: 56%–78%
Abdominal tenderness: 25%
Vomiting: 10%–18%
Palpable mass: 35%–62%*
Swelling/distention: 5%–34%
Irregular vaginal bleeding: 5%–71%

*31% with abdominal pain, 31% without pain.

From Piippo S, Mustaniemi L, Lenko H, et al: Surgery for ovarian masses during childhood and adolescence: A report of 79 cases. J Pediatr Adolesc Gynecol 1999;12:223–227. Templeman C, Fallat ME, Blinchevsky A, et al: Noninflammatory ovarian masses in girls and young women. Obstet Gynecol 2000;96:229–233. Van Winter JT: Surgically treated adnexal masses in infancy, childhood, and adolescence. Am J Obstet Gynecol 1994;170:1780–1789.

Presentation and Initial Evaluation

Box 226-5 lists common presenting symptoms in a patient with an adnexal mass. Symptoms include abdominal pain, tenderness, and palpable mass. In a prepubertal child, the small size of the pelvic cavity means that as an ovarian mass enlarges, it will become abdominal in location, rather than hidden in the pelvis. Thus an ovarian mass will be palpable on examination. In adolescents, the pelvic cavity is larger, and it is uncommon to palpate an ovarian mass smaller than 8 to 10 cm. Initial evaluation should be aimed at distinguishing adnexal pathology from other intra-abdominal sources, and discerning which adnexal conditions require immediate medical or surgical therapy.

The gynecologic history, examination, and initial laboratory evaluation is very important in evaluating an adnexal mass and is essentially the same outlined for pain earlier in this chapter.

Even if a mass is not palpated on pelvic examination, imaging is advisable in a patient with abdominal or pelvic pain. Ultrasound is the preferred method for imaging suspected adnexal masses. It is relatively inexpensive and has no radiation exposure. Ultrasound can elucidate the size, relationship to surrounding structures, presence or absence of pelvic fluid, and characteristics of the mass. Color-flow Doppler is used to evaluate ovarian blood flow if adnexal torsion is suspected. CT and MRI are not the first modality for imaging for a suspected adnexal mass. CT scan should be used if the ultrasound diagnosis is unsure or for further evaluation of a suspected malignancy. MRI is the best means of imaging a suspected Mullerian anomaly.

Management of Adnexal Masses

Based on the combination of ultrasound findings and physical examination, patients who require emergency surgical intervention can be identified. Adnexal torsion, ruptured ectopic pregnancy, ruptured tubo-ovarian abscess, and ruptured hemorrhagic cyst with falling hematocrit or hemodynamic instability are all surgical emergencies.

The management of childhood adnexal masses depends on the patient's symptoms and ultrasound findings. Ovarian torsion and cyst rupture with hemodynamic instability require emergency surgical intervention. A child with an asymptomatic, simple adnexal cyst should be managed expectantly with serial ultrasounds. Intervention is warranted if the mass is enlarging, if there are ultrasonographic characteristics of malignancy (solid mass, mixed echogenicity, papillations/septations), or with signs of hormonal production (precocious puberty).

Most adnexal masses in adolescents can be managed conservatively. The majority are either a benign neoplasm or functional cysts that will spontaneously resolve. The decision to manage an adnexal mass conservatively should be made either by the primary clinician in consultation with a gynecologist or by a gynecologist upon referral. The actual rate of malignancy is very low in the adolescent population and risk can be determined based on ultrasound findings. Sonographic features that raise concern for malignancy include: nonhyperechoic solid component, central flow in the mass with color-flow Doppler, free intraperitoneal fluid, and the presence of septations. Patients with masses having any of the features listed in Box 226-6 should be immediately referred to a gynecologist.

Both simple and complex cystic masses less than 10 cm can be managed expectantly over the course of 6 to 8 weeks. During this time, the patient should be seen at regular intervals to assess continuing or worsening symptoms and provide reassurance that the mass is most likely benign. Patients with adnexal masses are at an increased risk for torsion and cyst rupture, and should be educated to seek immediate medical care if they develop acute severe pain or vomiting. Oral contraceptives can be started in patients without contraindications to prevent the formation of new functional cysts that may cause confusion at the time of repeat imaging. Oral contraceptives do not increase the rate of resolution of existing cysts. At the end of the observation period, ultrasound should be repeated. Cysts that decrease in size can continue to be managed expectantly, with repeat ultrasounds to document resolution.

If the cyst persists or increases in size, or has characteristics suggesting malignancy, surgical removal may be indicated. Cystic and complex masses with ascites, masses larger than 10 cm, and any solid masses require surgical removal because of the risk of malignancy.

Outcome

Potential sequelae from pelvic surgery are pelvic adhesions that can result in chronic pelvic pain, increased risk for tubal/ectopic pregnancy, tubal infertility, and bowel obstruction. Surgery for functional cysts should be avoided whenever possible to minimize these risks. Every effort should be made to preserve ovarian tissue, even if it appears that there is very little viable ovarian stroma. Normal ovarian tissue can be compressed, particularly with benign

Box 226-6. Ultrasound Characteristics of Malignant Masses

Nonhyperechoic solid component
Central flow in the mass with color-flow Doppler
Free intraperitoneal fluid (ascites)
Septations

cystic teratomas. These cysts are usually relatively easy to separate from normal tissue, so the best efforts of a gynecologic surgeon are warranted in an effort to be conservative. It should not be assumed that "she'll always have the other ovary," because other benign or malignant conditions may subsequently arise.

Follow-up

There are no data to provide guidance about the likelihood of an adolescent who has one functional ovarian cyst (such as a symptomatic corpus luteum) experiencing a recurrent cyst. Anecdotally, it does appear that some individuals, perhaps those with underlying ovarian dysfunction and anovulation, may be more likely to experience a recurrent cyst. Care must be taken, however, to avoid concluding that every twinge of pelvic pain is due to an ovarian cyst. Combination oral contraceptives decrease the risk of ovulation, and thus the risk of functional cysts associated with ovulatory cycles. The data suggest a dose relationship. Cyst suppression may be somewhat better with combination OCs containing higher doses of estrogen, and perhaps with monophasic pills. Progestin-only pills do not decrease the risk of cyst formation. The option of suppressing future cyst development with oral contraceptives should be discussed with parents and adolescents, provided there are no medical contraindications. OCs provide additional benefits, including effective contraception, cycle regulation, decreased dysmenorrhea and menorrhagia, and improvement in acne. In those who have had an ovarian neoplasm, whether benign or malignant, oral contraceptive therapy is more strongly recommended to avoid the significant anxiety of finding a subsequent ovarian cyst, even if it is later proven to be functional and benign.

Mini-index of Related Topics

SUGGESTED READINGS

Davis AR, Westhoff C: Primary dysmenorrhea in adolescent girls and treatment with oral contraceptives. J Pediatr Adolesc Gynecol 2001;14(1):3–8.

Hewit GD, Brown RT: Acute and chronic pelvic pain in female adolescents. Med Clin North Am 2000;84(4):1009–1025.

Propst AM, Laufer MR: Endometriosis in adolescents: Incidence, diagnosis, and treatment. J Reprod Med 1999;44(9):751–758.

Rickert VI, Kozlowski KJ: Pelvic pain: A SAFE approach. Obstet Gynecol Clin North Am 2000;27(1):181–193.

Schroeder B, Sanfilippo JS: Dysmenorrhea and pelvic pain in adolescents. Pediatr Clin North Am 1999;46(3):555–571.

Stafford DEJ, Gordon CM: Adolescent androgen abnormalities. Curr Opin Obstet Gynecol 2002;14(5):445–452.

Strickland JL: Ovarian cysts in neonates, children, and adolescents. Curr Opin Obstet Gynecol 2002;14(5):459–466.

SECTION 6   ADOLESCENT CARE: *Medical Conditions Manifesting in Adolescents*

227 Male Genitourinary Disorders

Corinne E. Lehmann and Frank M. Biro

ROLE OF THE GENERALIST

1 Recognize the common causes of scrotal and testicular swelling in adolescent boys.

2 Make a prompt referral of the painful testis of uncertain diagnosis because the viability of a torsed testis is decreased after 6 hours.

3 Be knowledgeable about the association between epydidimitis and urinary tract abnormalities.

Although many genitourinay disorders present in the neonatal period, especially those associated with congenital abnormalities, the majority of cases present in early to mid-puberty. The most common male genitourinary disorder in adolescent boys is urethritis secondary to sexually transmitted infections, described in Chapter 224.

In the assessment of genitourinary disorders a useful diagnostic approach is to distinguish between acute and nonacute and between painful and nonpainful presentations. Prompt surgical referral of any patient with an uncertain cause for an acute painful testis is important, especially since viability of a torsed testis is decreased after 6 hours. Among the more common disorders, a missed diagnosis of testicular torsion is associated with the highest morbidity, whereas a missed diagnosis of testicular cancer is associated with the highest mortality.

This chapter focuses primarily on the causes and treatment of scrotal and testicular disorders in adolescents. Box 227-1 lists the most common causes of scrotal and testicular swelling, both acute and chronic. With regard to the acute scrotum, recent studies have estimated the etiologies as follows: 14% to 16% from testicular torsion, 14% to 46% from torsion of the testicular appendage, and 35% to 71% from epididymitis.

HERNIA/HYDROCELE/SPERMATOCELE

Hernias and hydroceles can be thought of as a result of a patent processus vaginalis (Fig. 227-1). A spermatocele is a retention cyst of the rete testis, ductuli efferentes, or epididymitis that is filled with fluid containing spermatozoa. In children the patency of the processus vaginalis allows peritoneal fluid to collect between the layers of tunica. In adults an imbalance between the secretory and absorptive properties of the tunica vaginalis is postulated. An indirect hernia arises when peritoneal contents pass through an "open" processus vaginalis or when increased intra-abdominal pressure allows contents through weakened transversalis fascia at the internal inguinal ring. (A direct hernia, less common in children, protrudes through the external inguinal ring.) Little data are available on the incidence of these disorders in adolescence. The incidence of hernias in large pediatric series is 1% to 5%.

A hernia presents as a painless groin bulge, unless it is incarcerated. A direct (medial) hernia must be distinguished from an indirect (lateral) hernia as direct hernias are less likely to strangulate. The hernia orifice can be localized with a vigorous cough or strain. An ultrasound may help differentiate between a hernia and lymph nodes. A hydrocele appears as a cystic mass around the testis that transilluminates. As hydroceles can occur as a result of trauma, infection, or tumor, one must carefully palpate for the testicle. An ultrasound may be helpful. Spermatoceles also transilluminate as a cystic mass above the testis. A spermatocele is often described as a "third testicle."

Hernias require surgical repair secondary to the risk of bowel strangulation and immediate referral if not reducible. There is a 10% to 15% recurrence after surgery. Hydroceles in adolescents usually require a urological evaluation as infection and tumor are concerns. Asymptomatic noncommunicating hydroceles are not treated. Large or painful hydroceles may warrant surgery or aspiration. Spermatoceles are treated in a similar fashion except that surgery is discouraged in the younger patient as it may affect future fertility (the presence of a spermatocele does not). Recurrence of the latter two conditions after surgery is rare.

VARICOCELE

Varicoceles are dilated and tortuous veins of the pampiniform plexus surrounding the spermatic cord. Many theories attempt to explain the pathophysiology of varicoceles; none are proven. Because the majority (85% to 90%) of varicoceles are left-sided, the left spermatic vein is thought to be under more hydrostatic pressure as its course is 10 cm longer than the right spermatic vein and joins the left renal vein at a sharper angle (Fig. 227-2). The right spermatic vein empties into the ascending superior vena cava. A right-sided varicocele should prompt consideration of venous crossover, situs inversus, and venous obstruction. The absence of valves in the testicular vein could lead to increased pressure in the vein, but several autopsy studies have shown that valves can be lacking in normal subjects.

Varicoceles may be associated with ipsilateral testicular atrophy and declining testicular function. Varicoceles raise the temperature of the scrotum and the testis, which is

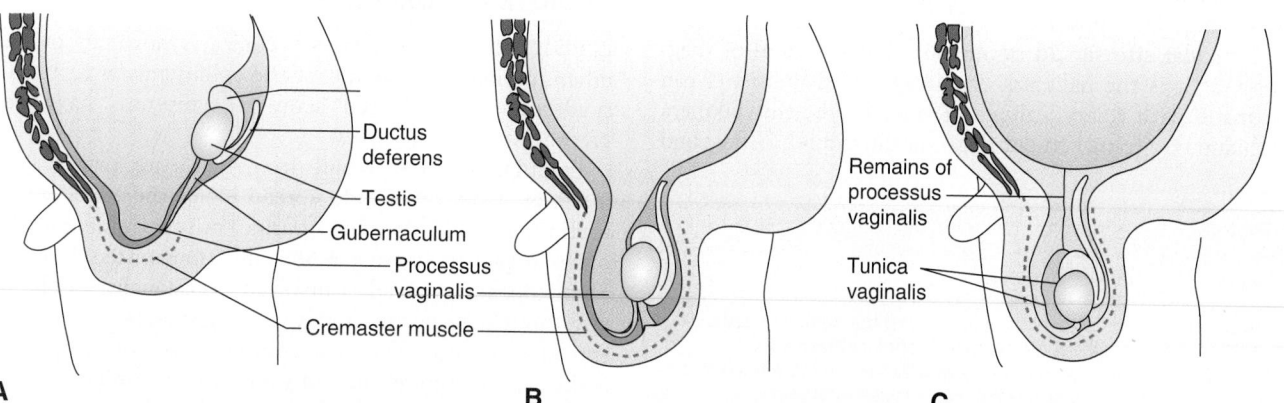

Figure 227-1. Anatomy of hernias: diagram illustrating descent of the testes. **A,** Before descent: The processus vaginalis is present before descent begins; the testis is lying behind the peritoneum. **B,** Descent is nearly complete, but the processus vaginalis is not obliterated. **C,** The processus vaginalis is obliterated except for the terminal portion, which persists as the tunica vaginalis of the adult. (From Gross CM: Gray's Anatomy of the Human Body. Philadelphia, Lea & Febiger, 1966, p 1270, Fig. 17-6.)

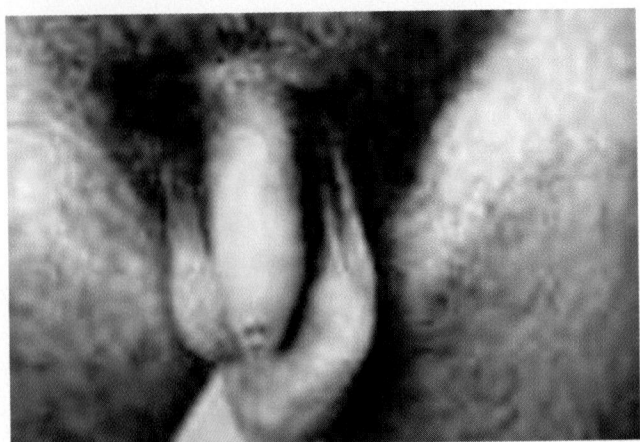

Figure 227-2. Left-sided varicocele.

harmful to spermatogenesis. Other factors such as adrenal vein content reflux, endocrine imbalance (decreased serum testosterone), testicular paracrine imbalance, altered blood flow, and reactive hypoxia may lead to degeneration and sloughing of germ cells or arrest of germ cell maturation, though none of these models has been proven. Some degree of varicocele is present in 15% to 20% of all adult and adolescent boys. Of the adults, only 15% to 20% with a varicocele seek treatment for infertility.

Varicoceles present infrequently in the prepubertal patient and then have a dramatically increased incidence in puberty. Patients may have scrotal swelling, a dull discomfort after prolonged standing, or no symptoms. As adolescents with a varicocele are often asymptomatic, a varicocele can be missed. The pediatric genital examination should include observation and palpation of the testes in the standing and supine position. A grading classification for varicoceles developed by Hudson is shown in Table 227-1.

A right-sided or persistent varicocele (in the supine position) may indicate tumor or obstruction. A horizontal lie to the testicle may also be found in varicocele. Besides physical examination, other methods are used to diagnose varicocele. Venography, the gold standard, is expensive and invasive and should be used with adolescents only in confusing cases or in conjunction with embolization. Other techniques include thermography, Doppler ultrasound, and scrotal scintigraphy. They are not specific for varicocele and have a high false-positive rate.

Testicular size should be measured at the time of diagnosis, as it is the hallmark of damage. Measurements can be made with rulers, calipers, Prader beads, the Takihara orchidometer (punched-out rings), or ultrasound. Ultrasound

is the most accurate. A discrepancy of greater than 2 mL is considered a sign of damage. Semen analysis can be done in the adult, but no standards exist for adolescents. Stimulation of gonadotropin-releasing hormone (GnRH) has been evaluated, with 30% of adolescents responding with elevated levels of luteinizing hormone (LH) and follicle-stimulating hormone (FSH). However, the response was not associated with testicular volume loss and should not be done routinely in adolescents.

Which adolescent should have a surgical repair is controversial. If the patient has bilateral normal size testes, an ultrasound can be done every 6 to 12 months to evaluate a change in size or semen analysis can be completed when the patient is of the appropriate age. Right-sided, large, bilateral, or painful varicoceles should be further evaluated and are surgical candidates. When the testicular volume differential is greater than 2 mL, repairing moderate to large varicoceles can partially reverse growth retardation, suggesting a more aggressive, preventative approach. However, 80% of male patients with varicocele are fertile, and no criteria have been developed to show which adolescent might benefit from repair.

A variety of surgical procedures can be used to repair a varicocele, such as embolization of the spermatic vein, microsurgical varicocelectomy, and testicular vein ligation. For adolescents, the Palomo approach (ligation of the testicular vein and artery above the inguinal ring) has often been performed, as the rate of postoperative testicular atrophy is low. However, the recurrence rate of the varicocele is as high as 16% with this procedure. Many providers use the microsurgical approach, as the long-term effects of testicular artery ligation are not known. With the microsurgical approach, the rate of postoperative hydrocele is low (0% to 7%). A laparoscopic procedure has been successful as well. Recurrence rates of varicocele range from 9% to 16%, usually because of unrecognized collaterals. This rate drops to 6% with intraoperative venography.

One must be cautious in alerting a teenager to the presence of a varicocele as he is probably unaware of the condition. Terminology, options, and the controversy surrounding this situation must be explained carefully and communication with a consulting urologist is crucial.

EPIDIDYMITIS/ORCHITIS

Epididymitis and orchitis are clinical syndromes of pain, inflammation, and swelling of the epididymis or testis. The syndrome is considered acute if symptoms have been present less than 6 weeks.

Epididymitis may result from an acute urinary tract infection with retrograde spread along the vas deferens, urethra, or bladder (reflux of urine) or retrograde migration of an organism causing a sexually transmitted infection. Hematogenous spread is involved occasionally. Orchitis is also thought to occur from ascending infection, metastatic spread, or trauma. The most common cause of epididymitis is the most common cause of genitourinary infections in the respective age group. Coliforms are found mostly in children, while gonorrhea and Chlamydia are the cause in sexually active, heterosexual male patients younger than 35 years old. Chlamydia accounts for two thirds of the latter

Table 227-1. Grading Classification for Varicoceles	
Grade	**Clinical Description**
Subclinical	Not palpable or visible at rest but demonstrated by special tests (such as Doppler ultrasound).
Grade 1	Small: palpable only with Valsalva maneuver (creates impulse distending the intrascrotal veins).
Grade 2	Moderate: not visible but palpable. Described as a bag of worms or squishy tube when palpating the spermatic cord.
Grade 3	Large: visible from the door.

cases. Rare causes of epididymitis include sarcoid, Henoch-Schönlein purpura, and Kawasaki disease. Viruses can be a cause of orchitis, with the finding of parotitis and isolated orchitis diagnostic for mumps.

The clinician needs to ask about voiding symptoms and sexual activity. Pain and scrotal swelling have a gradual onset over hours to days. On examination the epididymis is enlarged, firm, and tender. The adjacent testis should feel normal and have an intact cremasteric reflex. There may be a reactive hydrocele and a swollen spermatic cord. Elevation and support of the scrotum may relieve the discomfort (Prehn sign). Fever, leukocytosis, pyuria, and bacteruria may be present. Pyuria can be an unreliable clinical indicator: 27% to 40% of patients with testicular torsion had pyuria; 15% had swelling of the tail of the epididymis. Urethral secretions should be sampled prior to urination as the organism may be washed away. A Gram stain can be prepared from a calginate swab. Midstream urine should also be gram-stained for gram-negative bacteria. If there is any question of the diagnosis, consultation with a urologist is advisable to help rule out testicular torsion. If Chlamydia or gonorrhea is likely, a urine specimen can be sent for DNA amplification (e.g., polymerase chain reaction or transcription-mediated amplification).

Treatment for epididymitis is antibiotics directed at the suspected organism. For bacteruria the protocol is Bactrim (sulfamethoxazole) or a quinolone, with the length of treatment ranging from 10 to 14 days to 6 weeks. Ceftriaxone followed by doxycycline for 10 days is indicated for sexually transmitted organisms. Bed rest and scrotal support are recommended; sexual partners should be treated, if appropriate. If symptoms do not resolve in 10 to 14 days, a workup for neoplasia should be considered. If the first episode is not related to a sexually transmitted disease, a genitourinary workup should be done to rule out a structural abnormality. Orchitis is usually self-limited, with symptoms residing in 7 to 10 days. Epididymoorchitis is treated similarly to epididymitis.

TORSION OF THE TESTIS/TESTICULAR APPENDAGE

Testicular torsion is the twisting of the spermatic cord and testis on its vertical axis, leading to obstruction of venous return and then arterial flow. Torsion of a testicular appendage is the twisting of a remnant of the Muller duct (appendix testis) or wolffian duct (appendix epididymis). Anatomic abnormality is frequent. The peritoneal investiture of the testis inserts high on the cord rather than on the lower pole. This allows for poor testicular fixation and extreme mobility (the bell-clapper deformity). Most torsions happen intravaginally, within the sac. Appendage torsions are thought to result from gonadotropin-releasing hormone (GnRH) stimulation increasing the size of the remnant. Of all torsions, 65% to 80% occur in boys between the ages of 12 and 18 years, with the peak for a torsed appendage at the onset of puberty. Estimated incidence is 1 in 4000 boys and men younger than age 25.

Up to one third of patients with a torsed testis have had a previous pain episode. Torsion presents with sudden onset of scrotal or lower abdominal pain, although 10% can be painless. The triad of colicky pain, a high-riding testis, and nausea/vomiting are highly suggestive of testicular torsion. On examination, the most sensitive physical finding is an absent cremasteric reflex. Swelling and erythema may be present. Pain at the upper outer pole of the hemiscrotum suggests a torsion of the appendix testis (92% of cases). These conditions can be differentiated by using a pencil eraser tip or tongue depressor to define pinpoint tender areas. Pain with an appendix testis torsion should be localized and without nausea or vomiting; a blue dot sign (Fig. 227-3) on the scrotal skin may be seen. Swelling, erythema, and a reactive hydrocele may be found as well. Dysuria or pyuria is less commonly seen in torsion and suggests an infectious process.

Efficient diagnosis is crucial, as up to 98% of tests can be salvaged if repaired in the first 6 hours. The rate of salvage declines to 20% to 50% in the 6- to 48-hour time window. Imaging is required if the examination is equivocal. Doppler ultrasound has equal sensitivity to nuclear scintigraphy in the adolescent. As swelling is present in both torsion and epididymitis, the radiologist examines testicular blood flow. Flow is decreased in torsion and normal to increased in epididymitis in pubertal boys. Up to 38% of healthy, normal, prepubertal boys do not have identifiable blood flow on ultrasound. Cases have been reported in older boys with normal Doppler flow with a torsion. Thus, clinical and imaging data must be carefully integrated to make the appropriate diagnosis in cases of scrotal pain. If the presentation is typical, one can proceed directly to surgery without imaging. Table 227-2 compares the clinical presentation of testicular torsion with epididymitis.

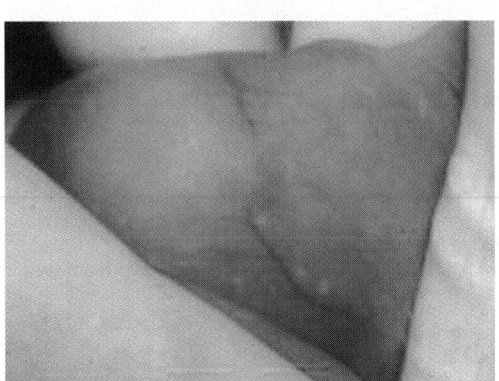
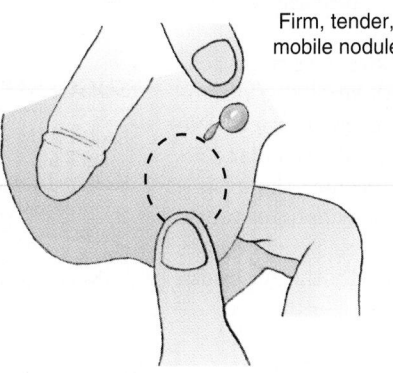

Firm, tender, mobile nodule

Peak incidence: 9–11 years
Diagnosis
 Firm, tender, mobile nodule.
 Blue dot sign.
 Imaging – unnecessary if
 the testis itself is normal:
  size
  shape   } Otherwise:
  consistency   color-Doppler
  nontender   ultrasound
Treatment:
 Bed rest, analgesics, antibiotics.
 Surgical excision – protracted pain.

Figure 227-3. Blue dot sign of appendix testis torsion and area of point tenderness.

Table 227-2. Testicular Torsion Compared to Epididymitis

	Torsion	Epididymitis
Peak age, years	0–1, 12–16	8–15
Duration of symptoms	<12 Hours	12–72 Hours
Similar pain in past	10%	20%
Local tenderness	20%	97%
Normal testicular lie	50%	100%
Color Doppler ultrasound	Decreased flow	Increased/normal flow
C-reactive protein	Normal	4 times elevated

Surgical repair with nonabsorbable sutures is performed for testicular torsion. Most surgeons explore the contralateral testis and perform scrotal fixation if a bell-clapper deformity is present. An experienced clinician may attempt manual detorsion after patient sedation in order to "buy time" until surgery can be done. If the testis does not appear viable, it is removed, as 20% of nonviable testes become infected. One to two thirds of patients may have atrophy of either testicle after successful surgery. Some propose that the injured testis allows the body to form an immunological reaction to sperm, while others believe an abnormality may have existed prior to torsion. Torsion of an appendix testis is treated conservatively with analgesia. Surgery is reserved for persistent pain or intermittent torsion.

TESTICULAR TUMOR

Most testicular tumors in adolescents are seminomas, neoplasms "curable" by surgery and radiation therapy if the tumor is detected in time. The frequency of testicular tumor rises during the ages of 15 to 19, with a peak at ages 25 to 29. Testicular tumor accounts for 1% of all male cancers and is the most common solid male tumor between puberty and age 40. Ten percent of cases are associated with a history of cryptorchidism.

Symptoms may include testicular enlargement and a dragging sensation in the scrotum. Most are found as a painless, firm nodule in the lower pole of the testis. The mass does not transilluminate. Pain, when present, may indicate an advanced tumor with bleeding into the mass.

If cancer is suspected, refer immediately to a urologist. The primary care physician should prepare the patient for the potential workup and the possibility of sperm banking. Usually an ultrasound, tumor markers, baseline laboratory work, and CAT scan of the abdomen and chest are obtained prior to treatment.

The value of teaching adolescent boys testicular self-examination (TSE) has been questioned, similar to discussion regarding breast self-examination in women. No studies confirm the efficacy or specificity of testicular self-examination. Others question whether teaching the examination heightens anxiety in already self-conscious teens, though a recent study did not show elevated anxiety scores in two samples of adolescent boys. Currently the American Academy of Pediatrics recommends regular testicular self-examination for the early detection of cancer.

OTHER CAUSES OF SCROTAL SWELLING

Two to five percent of all scrotal swelling is idiopathic. Onset of edema and erythema that may extend onto the abdominal wall is sudden. It is usually painless and the testis and epididymis should be easily palpated. This entity spontaneously resolves in 48 to 72 hours. Other causes of swelling include spontaneous gangrene, idiopathic fat necrosis, and acute vasculitis (Henoch-Schönlein purpura).

MACROORCHIDISM

Macroorchidism designates testes that are twice the normal testicular volume. Unilateral enlargement can result from compensatory enlargement in those who have an undescended or rudimentary testis on the other side. If there is a firm mass, testicular tumor must be considered. Bilateral macroorchidism may be idiopathic but is found in fragile X syndrome, leukemia, lymphoma, testicular germ cell tumors, precocious puberty, and congenital adrenal hyperplasia.

MICROORCHIDISM

Small testes should be evaluated in relationship to pubertal maturation. Testicular volume should be greater than 3 mL by age 14. If no signs of sexual maturation are found, the hypothalamic-pituitary-adrenal axis must be investigated. In the case of small testes and other normal secondary sexual characteristics, Klinefelter syndrome is the most common disorder (1 in 600 male births). Other considerations include bilateral atrophy after torsion or trauma, mumps orchitis, or other testicular failure.

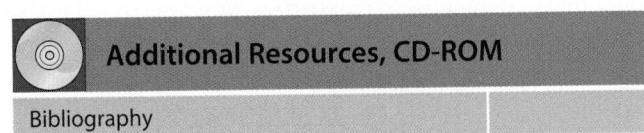

Additional Resources, CD-ROM

Bibliography

Mini-index of Related Topics   CH.

SUGGESTED READINGS

Kadish HA: The tender scrotum. Clin Pediatr Emerg Med 2002; 3:55–61.

Kadish HA, Bolte RG: A retrospective review of pediatric patients with epididymitis, testicular torsion, and torsion of the testicular appendages. Pediatrics 1998;102(1):73–76.

Lewis AG, Bukowski TP, Jarvis PD, et al: Evaluation of acute scrotum in the emergency department. J Pediatr Surg 1995;30(2):277–282.

228 Chronic Fatigue Syndrome

Mark S. Smith

ROLE OF THE GENERALIST

1 Know the clinical definition of chronic fatigue syndrome especially with regard to the level of disability *not* related to ongoing exertion nor substantially reduced by bedrest.

2 Know the organic differential diagnosis of fatigue in adolescents.

3 Know the psychiatric differential diagnosis of fatigue in adolescents.

4 Order selected and appropriate laboratory testing in evaluation of chronic fatigue.

5 Refer fatigued patients for appropriate mental health consultation.

6 Target individual fatigue symptoms with specific therapy with an emphasis on acquiring normal coping skills and social competence.

DEFINITION

The term *chronic fatigue syndrome* (CFS; ICD-9 code: 780.71) has been proposed to describe a group of symptoms occurring together in which profound persistent or recurrent fatigue of longer than 6 months' duration is the predominant symptom. To qualify for the diagnosis of CFS, the chronic fatigue must cause significant functional disability and be unexplained after a comprehensive medical and psychological evaluation. A symposium of clinical researchers in Great Britain has proposed a definition (Oxford criteria) that requires only the presence of chronic disabling fatigue without medical explanation regardless of the presence of additional symptoms. The 1988 Centers for Disease Control (CDC) criteria required the presence of eight additional symptoms to meet CFS criteria and patients who met criteria for psychiatric disorders were excluded from this CFS case definition. The 1994 revised CDC case definition of CFS (Table 228-1) reduced the number of required additional physical symptoms to four and allowed the coexistence of nonmelancholic depression, anxiety, and psychosomatic disorders.

EPIDEMIOLOGY

CFS is predominantly an adult disorder that appears to be relatively uncommon in adolescence and rare in childhood. Adult population-based studies estimate the prevalence of "CFS-like" illness (i.e., not necessarily meeting full criteria) at 200 to 2800 per 100,000 with an approximate 3:1 female-to-male ratio. Scant pediatric data exist, but an increasing prevalence with advancing age has been noted, with estimates of adolescent prevalence ranging from 23 to 116 per 100,000 with an approximate 2.5:1 female-to-male ratio. Studies in referred populations suggest that CFS is relatively increased in the white population with no consistent trend in socioeconomic status. Since most data are from referred populations, it is difficult to ascertain whether ethnic, racial, or socioeconomic factors are of importance, but dismissive terms such as *yuppie flu* are not based on strong epidemiological evidence.

ETIOLOGY

A review of the current evidence suggests that CFS may not be a homogenous disorder and that a single causative factor is unlikely to be found. It is probable that the etiology of

Table 228-1. 1994 CDC Revised CFS Case Definition

I. Clinically evaluated, unexplained, persistent, or relapsing fatigue that meets the following criteria:
   A. Of new or definite onset
   B. Associated with substantial reduction in previous levels of occupational, educational, social, or personal activities
   C. Not the result of ongoing exertion
   D. Not substantially reduced by bedrest
II. Concurrent occurrence of ≥4 of the following symptoms, all of which must have persisted or recurred for at least 6 months and must not have predated the fatigue:
   A. Substantially impaired short-term memory or concentration
   B. Sore throat
   C. Tender cervical or axillary adenopathy
   D. Myalgias
   E. Polyarthralgias
   F. Headache of a new type, pattern, or severity
   G. Unrefreshing sleep
   H. Postexertional malaise lasting ≥24 hours
III. The following conditions exclude an individual from the diagnosis:
   A. Any active medical condition that may explain symptoms
   B. Any past or current diagnosis of a major depressive disorder with psychotic or melancholic features, bipolar affective disorders, schizophrenia, delusional disorders, dementias, anorexia nervosa, or bulimia nervosa
   C. Alcohol or substance abuse
   D. Severe obesity
IV. The following conditions do *not* exclude the diagnosis:
   A. Any condition defined primarily by symptoms that cannot be confirmed by laboratory tests, including fibromyalgia, anxiety disorders, somatoform disorders, nonpsychotic or nonmelancholic depression, neurasthenia, and multiple chemical sensitivity disorder

CFS involves multiple factors with variable expression in any individual case. Although unproven, factors of importance may include: a genetic predisposition to fatiguing illness; psychophysiological vulnerability; precipitating factors such as infectious agents, antigens, or stress; and sustaining factors such as illness attribution that rejects the contribution of psychological factors, maladaptive coping style, and reinforcement of illness behavior.

It has *not* been established that all patients meeting CFS diagnostic criteria have the same condition or that pediatric and adult cases represent the same disorder. It is important to note that although small numbers of adolescents are often included most populations evaluated for etiologic factors are composed of adult CFS patients. While numerous theories have been proposed (Box 228-1), the etiology of CFS is unknown.

Viral Infection. Because of the frequent presence of clinical features that are compatible with the precipitation of illness by acute infection and subtle immunologic findings compatible with immune activation (e.g., activated CD8 cells, reduced natural killer cell activity), there has been major interest in the possible role of latent or persistent viral infection in CFS. Although some cultural belief in the relationship between certain viruses and CFS persists (e.g., "chronic mono"), subsequent well-designed studies have not supported the purported relationship between these viruses and CFS. Multiple RNA and DNA viruses have been considered as causative or sustaining agents in CFS, but to date none has been confirmed in this role. Recently, interest has centered on the potential role of reactivated latent herpesviruses in CFS. The potential role of infectious agents in CFS, while representing an important area of ongoing investigation, remains undefined.

Immune Dysfunction. Hyperactive immunologic responses are known to occur in many medical and psychological disorders in response to allergic, infectious, and stressful stimuli. Immune system activation (e.g., cytokine release) may result in symptoms commonly noted in CFS. Many immunologic studies of CFS patients, using diverse populations and methodologies, have produced inconsistent results in T-cell function, mitogen responses, natural killer cell activity, and cytokine response. While minor immunologic abnormalities do appear to occur frequently in CFS, it is difficult to ascertain whether they are primary, secondary, or epiphenomena.

Hypothalamic-pituitary-adrenal Axis. Some CFS patients have been found to have an exaggerated response to adrenocorticotropic hormone (ACTH) and an attenuated response to exogenous corticotropin-releasing hormone (CRH) suggesting mild centrally mediated hypocortisolism. A recent study utilizing a rigorous design and an intravenous synacthen protocol did not support previous results indicating low adrenal reserve in CFS. Additionally, a double-blind controlled trial of adrenocorticosteroid therapy in CFS did not show a therapeutic effect. Hypothalamic-pituitary-adrenal (HPA) axis perturbations may occur with stress, sleep disturbance, chronic illness, use of certain medications, psychological disorders, and other conditions. Currently, there is no definitive evidence that a disturbance in the hypothalamic-pituitary-adrenal axis plays a major role in the etiology of CFS.

Atypical Anxiety, Depression, and Somatization. Since there is a well-established relationship between anxiety, depression, and fatigue, it is reasonable to consider psychological factors as contributing to either the etiology or maintenance of CFS. It is important to note that in both adults and adolescents who meet current CDC criteria for chronic fatigue syndrome, about half will have concurrent psychiatric diagnoses (predominantly depression, and less often, anxiety disorders). Several adolescent studies have found CFS patients have more internalizing symptoms, somatic complaints, or functional disability than comparison groups of adolescents with chronic disorders such as arthritis, cancer, or cystic fibrosis. Although adolescents with CFS who do *not* have concurrent psychiatric diagnoses often endorse symptoms such as decreased energy, difficulty with concentration and memory, and sleep problems, they do not often endorse depressed or anxious mood, self-deprecating thoughts, anhedonia, or suicidal ideation. Psychological factors appear to be of major importance in at least half of adolescents with CFS, but their etiologic role is unclear.

Sleep Disorder. Although sleep abnormalities have been demonstrated in several small studies of CFS patients, no definitive pattern has emerged. CFS patients have been found to spend more time in bed, sleep less efficiently, and have more frequent nocturnal awakenings than healthy controls. One study found that adolescents with CFS showed significantly higher levels of sleep disruption than healthy controls.

Neuromuscular Dysfunction. A number of earlier studies suggested metabolic and physiologic abnormalities of neuromuscular function in CFS. Recent studies have shown normal intracellular lactate content with exercise, normal muscle biopsies, unrevealing single fiber electromyographic responses, normal maximal voluntary and electrically stimulated contraction, and submaximal isometric contraction in CFS patients. Current research therefore suggests that abnormal peripheral neuromuscular function is not an important central component of muscle fatigue in CFS.

Orthostatic Intolerance. Recently, there has been considerable research interest in the concept that subclinical, persistent, or intermittent orthostatic intolerance might be the cause of symptoms in many CFS patients. Adult studies using tilt-table and other autonomic nervous system tests have produced conflicting results. However, tilt-table studies have been more consistent in adolescents indicating an increased incidence of postural orthostatic

---

Box 228-1. Etiology of CFS

- Unknown
- Prominent theories include the following:
    - Persistent latent viral infection
    - Subtle immune system activation
    - Impaired hypothalamic-pituitary-adrenal axis
    - Atypical depression, anxiety, or somatoform disorder
    - Sleep disorder
    - Abnormal neuromuscular function
    - Orthostatic intolerance

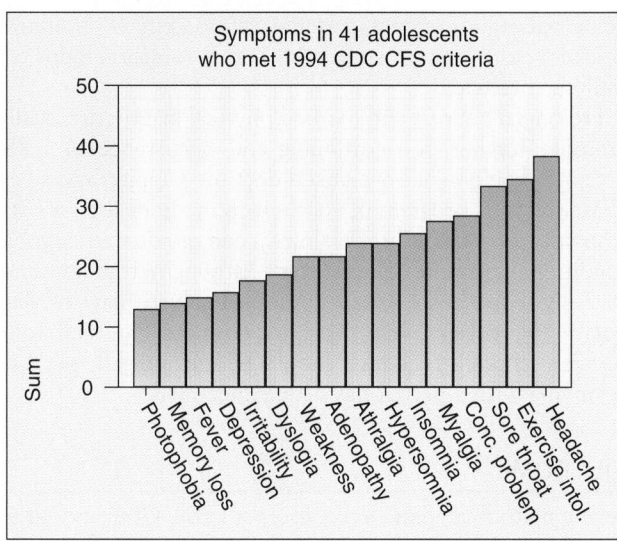

Figure 228-1. Symptoms in adolescents with CFS.

tachycardia (POTS), orthostatic hypotension, and disturbances of consciousness or syncope in those with CFS when compared with normal adolescents. It has been hypothesized that subacute or chronic dysregulation of autonomic control of orthostatic blood pressure and heart rate precipitated by an event such as a viral infection may be important in CFS. Additionally, vascular abnormalities that may be related to either autonomic dysfunction or abnormalities in local circulatory regulation have been demonstrated in adolescent POTS. Inactivity with consistent bedrest (or microgravity) in otherwise healthy adults has been shown to produce orthostatic blood pressure responses. To date the possible role of deconditioning has not been adequately assessed in adolescents with CFS.

PRESENTATION

The onset of CFS in children and adolescents reportedly follows an acute febrile illness in approximately two thirds of cases whereas one third may develop symptoms insidiously. The clinical course is persistent in approximately half of the cases and intermittent with remissions and relapses of several months' duration in the other half. Figure 228-1

displays the symptoms reported by adolescents with CFS evaluated in the University of Washington Adolescent Clinic. In addition to profound disabling fatigue, common symptoms in descending order include: headache, exercise intolerance, sore throat, difficulty concentrating, insomnia, hypersomnia, myalgia, generalized weakness, and arthralgia. Functional disability usually impairs all spheres of activity and decreased school performance and marked absenteeism are often dramatic.

EVALUATION

Figure 228-2 is a diagram of the evaluation of CFS. The physical examination in children and adolescents with CFS is generally unremarkable. Routine supine to standing blood pressure measurements usually do not reveal orthostatic changes, although tilt-table testing may demonstrate orthostatic intolerance. Growth and development and pubertal progression are unaffected by CFS. Although common in adults with CFS, more than a few positive fibromyalgia tender points are uncommon in adolescent patients. Complaints of concentration and memory difficulties are common, but neurological and mental status examination is usually normal. The results of adult CFS neurocognitive studies are ambiguous, but some studies have found evidence of cognitive processing difficulty. No well-designed neurocognitive studies of children and adolescents with CFS have been published.

Since careful psychosocial evaluation demonstrates anxiety, depressive disorders, or both in approximately half of adolescents with CFS, mental health consultation is appropriate in most cases. While fatigue is a common complaint in anxiety and depression, many adolescents with CFS do *not* meet criteria for psychiatric disorders. When present with CFS, it may be difficult to ascertain if anxiety and depression are primary or secondary conditions. A few pediatric studies have suggested that certain personality traits such as perfectionism and maintaining unrealistic performance standards are common in adolescents with CFS. Although malingering appears to be rare in children and adolescents with CFS, the level of school absenteeism is very high in comparison with other common pediatric disorders. The role of school avoidance has not been

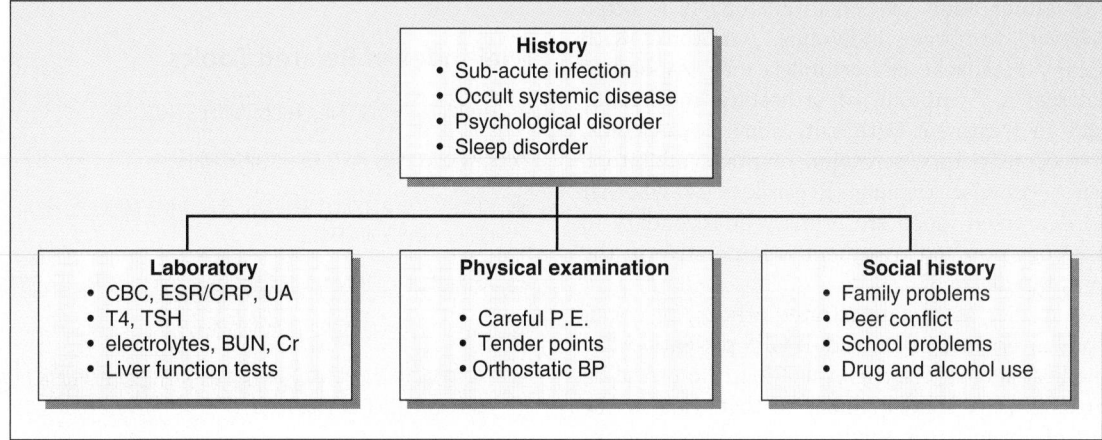

Figure 228-2. Diagram of the evaluation of CFS.

systematically evaluated, but seems an unlikely primary explanation in the majority of cases.

A selected laboratory evaluation including complete blood count, acute phase reactant, TSH, electrolytes, BUN, creatinine, LDH, ALT (amino alanine transferase), AST (aspartate amino transferase), and urinalysis is indicated in the evaluation of unexplained chronic fatigue in children and adolescents. Unless specifically suggested by history and physical examination, other laboratory studies such as ANA (antinuclear antibody), viral titers, immunoglobulins, and cortisol are rarely useful in establishing the diagnosis of pediatric CFS. Neuroimaging studies of adult CFS patients have produced ambiguous results and are not routinely recommended. Cardiovascular tilt-table testing may be useful in patients with symptoms suggestive of orthostatic intolerance.

After careful review of history, physical examination, and selected laboratory data, the differential diagnosis of CFS in children and adolescents should include the medical and psychosocial conditions known to be associated with persistent fatigue disorders (Box 228-2).

MANAGEMENT

Although the prognosis for the vast majority of children and adolescents with CFS is good, a prolonged course is common and functional disability is often marked. Controlled studies to date have not identified any specific treatment that has been shown to result in the complete resolution of either adult or pediatric CFS. It is often useful, however, to target individual symptoms with specific therapy. Headache and arthralgia may respond to nonsteroidal agents. Symptoms of orthostatic intolerance may respond to treatment with salt, mineralocorticoids, peripheral vasoconstrictors, serotonin reuptake inhibitors, and resistance exercise training. Regardless of whether anxiety and depressed mood are primary or secondary to CFS, their recognition and treatment is imperative in the management of pediatric CFS.

Controlled studies have demonstrated efficacy of cognitive behavioral interventions with adult CFS patients. After a careful medical and psychiatric evaluation, the use of an adaptive, rehabilitative model similar to that used in the management of chronic pain syndromes is appropriate for pediatric CFS. The primary care physician should tactfully point out unintentional parental reinforcement of illness behavior and make suggestions for reinforcement of wellness behavior.

Prolonged bedrest and marked physical inactivity actually promote further deconditioning and persistence of CFS. Patients should avoid prolonged daytime napping and sleep phase shifts. A program of gentle incremental exercise with emphasis on strength, flexibility, and graduated aerobic conditioning should be instituted. Although often administratively expedient, total home schooling may further isolate the patient and serve to promote the sick role. Regular school attendance should be encouraged, perhaps beginning with a partial-day attendance plan.

OUTCOME

Few longitudinal data exist for pediatric CFS and most reports result from the evaluation of referred patients in academic centers. These reports indicate that although symptoms may persist for months to several years patients and their parents describe a satisfactory outcome in the majority of cases. Roughly half report complete recovery, a third report marked improvement with some residual symptoms, and the remainder report persistent CFS symptoms that are unchanged or worse.

FOLLOW-UP

The proper management of pediatric CFS requires close follow-up to re-evaluate symptoms and monitor and re-enforce the treatment plan. At each visit the clinician should address specific symptom control and conduct a careful medical assessment (including weight) to detect any change or new findings. Monitoring of mood, coping efforts, and psychosocial status and the provision of supportive counseling are also important components of follow-up. Adherence to recommendations for increased physical activity and school attendance may be particularly problematic and require periodic re-evaluation and program modification. Given the data indicating an ultimate favorable prognosis for most cases of pediatric CFS, an optimistic stance by the health care provider seems appropriate and should include advising patients and their parents that the majority of pediatric CFS patients improve with time.

Mini-index of Related Topics

SUGGESTED READINGS

Breau LM, McGrath PJ, Ju LH: Review of juvenile primary fibromyalgia and chronic fatigue syndrome. J Dev Behav Pediatr 1999;20(4):278–288.

Cavanaugh RM: Evaluating adolescents with fatigue: Ever get tired of it? Pediatr Rev 2002;23(10):337–347.

Jordan KM, Landis DA, Downey MC, et al: Chronic fatigue syndrome in children and adolescents: A review. J Adolesc Health 1998;22:4–18.

Richards J: Chronic fatigue syndrome in children and adolescents: A review article. J Clin Child Psychol 2000;5(1):31–51.

Wright JB, Beverley DW: Chronic fatigue syndrome (Current Topics). Arch Dis Child 1998;79(4):368–374.

SECTION 6   ADOLESCENT CARE: *Sexuality and the Adolescent*

229 Contraceptive Methods and Counseling

Nava Stoffman and S. Jean Emans

ROLE OF THE GENERALIST

1 Obtain a reproductive health history (including sexual activity) and provide services (physical examination, Pap smear, screening for sexually transmitted diseases) to adolescents.

2 Be knowledgeable about the advantages, disadvantages, and contraindications of each contraceptive method.

3 Provide counseling about all contraceptive methods to adolescent patients.

4 Monitor adherence, satisfaction, and possible side effects of contraceptive methods.

STATISTICS OF SEXUAL ACTIVITY AND TEEN PREGNANCY

Teen pregnancy remains a major problem in the United States. The high rates of sexual activity coupled with inconsistent contraceptive use have resulted in a pregnancy rate approximately twice as high as in Great Britain and Canada; three times as high as in Sweden; and four times as high as in France. Four in 10 young women become pregnant at least once before they reach the age of 20 years old—nearly 1 million adolescents a year. Sexually transmitted diseases (STDs) remain epidemic among teens. Although clinicians, family members, and school personnel should promote postponement of sexual activity, it is essential for clinicians to be knowledgeable about rates of sexual activity and available contraceptive methods.

In the 2003 Youth Risk Behavior Survey, 46.7% of high school students (grades 9 to 12) reported having had sexual intercourse at least once; 48% of boys and 45.3% of girls were sexually experienced. The use of condoms during last intercourse ranged from 67.5% in 9th grade to 57.4% in 12th grade among those currently sexually active. The use of birth control pills among currently sexually active students rose from 8.7% for those in 9th grade to 22.6% in 12th grade. Young teenagers rarely make a specific request for contraceptives from their primary health care provider unless they know that the topic can be discussed confidentially. An older adolescent is much more likely to seek gynecologic and contraceptive care. Young men are frequently neglected in contraceptive counseling, and a history of sexual activity and condom use should be a routine part of their preventive health care.

CONSIDERATIONS IN PRESCRIBING CONTRACEPTION

The most effective contraception is abstinence. However, in sexually active adolescents, the contraceptive method would ideally be safe, effective, reversible, inexpensive, convenient, private, and have few side effects. Clearly this method does not exist, and every decision about selection of a birth control method is a compromise. However, every method of contraception for adolescents is safer than pregnancy. Factors that clinicians should consider when prescribing a female contraceptive method include personal characteristics of the user such as her age, educational level, socioeconomic status, parity, social context, and how much she wants to avoid a pregnancy. Characteristics of the method such as ease of use, cost, and side effects are factors that should also be taken into account. Parameters of the health care system providing the methods will influence choice: Is access easy? Is counseling age-appropriate? Are methods explained? Are all the choices offered, including backup emergency contraception? In order to assess the adolescent's knowledge and concerns regarding contraceptive methods, the clinician should ask general questions such as those in Box 229-1.

SCREENING MEDICAL QUESTIONS AND PHYSICAL EXAMINATION

The clinician providing contraceptive care to adolescent girls should obtain a complete gynecologic history (Box 229-2). It is also important to ask whether they will continue using condoms if a hormonal method is initiated because of concern about sexually transmitted disease. Because of possible side effects and contraindications of the different methods, a review of systems history is important to obtain, including a history of weight change (gain, loss, dieting), hirsutism, acne, hypertension, headaches, breast tenderness, nausea/vomiting, and thrombotic episodes. It is important for the clinician to know if the patient has a history of chronic illness or use of medications, tobacco, alcohol, or other substances. A family history of thrombosis, diabetes mellitus, or hyperlipidemia should also be obtained.

Typically the physical examination includes measurement of blood pressure, weight and height, a general assessment, and gynecologic examination. However, the pelvic examination should be thought of as part of preventive health care, not a barrier to the use of hormonal contraception. Screening laboratory tests for preventive health care include a Pap Smear (within 3 years of initiating sexual activity or age 21 years, whichever occurs first), urine or endocervical tests for Chlamydia and gonorrhea, and HIV (human immunodeficiency virus) counseling and testing, if indicated. Hemoglobin and cholesterol/HDL-C are usually performed once during adolescence (hemoglobin is obtained more frequently in adolescents with iron deficiency anemia) and reviewed when considering contraceptive methods.

Table 229-1. Efficacy of Contraceptive Methods: Pregnancy Rate per 100 Woman-Years of Use in First Year

Type	Lowest Expected	Typical Use
Oral contraceptives: combined	0.1	5–8
progestin only	0.5	
IUDs: Copper T 380A	0.6	0.8
Levonorgestrel-releasing intrauterine system	0.1	0.1
150 mg medroxyprogesterone acetate (Depo-Provera)	0.3	3
25 mg medroxyprogesterone acetate/25 mg estradiol cypionate (Lunelle)	0.05	3
Vaginal ring	0.65–1*	
Transdermal contraceptive patch (Ortho-Evra)	1.0*	
Levonorgestrel implant (Norplant)	0.05	0.2
Cervical Cap	9–26	20–40
Spermicides	6–15	26–29
Diaphragm	6	10–18
Condom	3	14
Withdrawal	6	19–27
Periodic abstinence	9	25
No method	85	85
Abstinence	0	0

*Pearl Index in actual clinical trials (similar to oral contraceptives).

Adapted from Trussell J, Hatcher RA, Cates E, et al: A guide to interpreting contraceptive efficacy studies. Obstet Gynecol 1990;76:558–567; Hatcher RA, Trussell J, Stewart J, et al: Achievements in public health, 1900–1999: Family planning. MMWR Morb Mortal Wkly Rep 1999;48(47):1073–1080; Hatcher RA, Nelson AL, Zieman M, et al: A Pocket Guide to Managing Contraception. Tiger, Ga, Bridging the Gap Foundation, 2002.

The various available contraceptive methods and their efficacy are listed in Table 229-1.

HORMONAL CONTRACEPTIVE METHODS

Oral Contraceptive Pills

Many teenagers choose an oral contraceptive because of the low failure rate, the relief from dysmenorrhea, and the ease of use. There are three classes of oral contraceptive pills, cited in Box 229-3. Common pills and their hormone content are listed in Table 229-2.

The majority of oral contraceptives are combination pills containing an estrogen and a progestin. The estrogen contained in the pills is either mestranol or ethinyl estradiol and varies in dose from 20 µg to 50 µg. Mestranol is converted in the liver to ethinyl estradiol (with 50 µg of mestranol roughly equivalent to 35 µg of ethinyl estradiol).

Table 229-2. Common Oral Contraceptives Available in the United States*

Drug	Estrogen	(mcg)	Progestin	(mg)
{ Demulen 1/50 { Zovia 1/50E	Ethinyl estradiol	50	Ethynodiol diacetate	1
{ Ovral { Ogestrel	Ethinyl estradiol	50	Norgestrel	0.5
{ Ovcon-50	Ethinyl estradiol	50	Norethindrone	1
{ Norinyl 1+50	Mestranol	50	Norethindrone	1
{ OrthoNovum 1/50				
{ Norinyl 1+35, Necon 1/35 { OrthoNovum 1/35	Ethinyl estradiol	35	Norethindrone	1
{ Demulen 1/35 { Zovia 1/35E	Ethinyl estradiol	35	Ethynodiol diacetate	1
{ Ortho-Novum 7/7/7	Ethinyl estradiol	35	Norethindrone	0.5 × 7d 0.75 × 7d 1.0 × 7d
{ Ortho-Cyclen	Ethinyl estradiol	35	Norgestimate	0.25
{ Ortho-TriCyclen	Ethinyl estradiol	35	Norgestimate	0.180 × 7d 0.215 × 7d 0.250 × 7d
{ Brevicon { Modicon { Necon 0.5/35	Ethinyl estradiol	35	Norethindrone	0.5
{ Ovcon 35	Ethinyl estradiol	35	Norethindrone	0.4
{ Yasmin	Ethinyl estradiol	30	Drospirenone	3.0
{ Lo/Ovral { Low-Ogestrel	Ethinyl estradiol	30	Norgestrel	0.3
{ Loestrin 1.5/30	Ethinyl estradiol	30	Norethindrone acetate	1.5
{ Nordette { Levlen	Ethinyl estradiol	30	Levonorgestrel	0.15
{ Desogen { Ortho-Cept	Ethinyl estradiol	30	Desogestrel	0.15
{ Loestrin 1/20	Ethinyl estradiol	20	Norethindrone acetate	1
{ Estrostep	Ethinyl estradiol	20 × 5d 30 × 7d 35 × 9d	Norethindrone acetate	1
{ Tri-Norinyl	Ethinyl estradiol	35	Norethindrone	0.5 × 7d 1.0 × 9d 0.5 × 5d
{ Triphasil { Tri-Levlen	Ethinyl estradiol	30 × 6d 40 × 5d 30 × 10d	Levonorgestrel	0.05 × 6d 0.075 × 5d 0.125 × 10d
{ Cyclessa	Ethinyl estradiol	25	Desogestrel	0.1 × 7d 0.125 × 7d 0.150 × 7d
{ Ortho Tri-Cyclen Lo	Ethinyl estradiol	25	Norgestimate	0.180 × 7d 0.215 × 7d 0.250 × 7d
{ Alesse { Levlite	Ethinyl estradiol	20	Levonorgestrel	0.1
{ Mircette	Ethinyl estradiol	10 × 5d 20 × 21d	Desogestrel	0.15
{ Ovrette			Norgestrel	0.075
{ Nor-Q.D. { Micronor			Norethindrone	0.35

*Many other generics are available.

All of the low-dose oral contraceptives have 20 to 35 μg ethinyl estradiol. Most of the progestins used in oral contraceptives, termed 19 nortestosterone derivatives, are related to 19 carbon androgens and are given in varying doses. Progestins can be divided into estrane and gonane progestins, which differ in their bioavailability, serum half-life, and binding affinity. For example, levonorgestrel, one of the gonane progestins, has the highest bioavailability and a long serum half-life, and thus may provide better cycle control than some pills with norethindrone. Unlike the rest of the progestins, the new progestin drospirenone differs in that it is an analogue of spironolactone and exhibits mild antimineralocorticoid properties.

The mechanism of action of the pill includes inhibition of ovulation, endometrial changes, and thickening of cervical mucus. The pill suppresses hypothalamic release of gonadotropin-releasing hormone (GnRH) and thereby reduces follicle-stimulating hormone (FSH) and luteinizing hormone (LH) secretion. The combination pill suppresses ovulation in 95% to 98% of cycles. The progestin-only pill does not inhibit ovulation as efficiently. Additionally, the presence of a progestin early in the cycle results in a thin endometrium with atrophic glands and minimal glycogen stores, which is not suitable for implantation. The progestin component also produces thick, viscid, scanty cervical mucus that is hostile to sperm penetration, slows tubal motility, and may have a direct effect on corpus luteum steroidogenesis.

Selection of a particular combined pill depends on the patient's needs and response, the availability of samples and supplies to family planning clinics and physician offices, and cost. Typical starter pills contain 20 to 35 μg of ethinyl estradiol. Some pills are more estrogen dominant and others more progestin dominant. An oral contraceptive pill with more progestin is helpful in patients with dysmenorrhea, hypermenorrhea, previous breakthrough bleeding, or dysfunctional uterine bleeding. A patient with previous nausea or vomiting on oral contraceptives may benefit from using a 20 μg ethinyl estradiol pill. Progestin-only pills should be offered to patients who cannot tolerate estrogen, have a medical contraindication to estrogen, or women who are breast-feeding. The benefits of the combined pill include effectiveness and relative ease of use, as it is taken independent of coitus. The effect is short acting and so it is rapidly reversible. Benefits resulting from the mechanism of action of the pill include decreased menstrual bleeding and less iron deficiency anemia, decreased dysmenorrhea, and usually regular menstrual periods. Use of combined oral pills has been shown to lower the risk of ovarian and endometrial cancer and hospitalization for salpingitis. A lower risk of ovarian cysts and improvement in acne and hirsutism are additional benefits seen with the use of combined pills.

Progestin-only pills do not have all the benefits of the combined pills and so are usually prescribed when estrogen treatment is contraindicated. Progestin-only pills require taking the pill with a more precise timing compared to combined pills and usually result in more breakthrough bleeding. Progestin pills do not protect from ovarian cysts and are not as helpful as combined oral contraceptives in the treatment of polycystic ovary syndrome (PCOS).

The contraindications to use of combined oral contraceptives include pregnancy, heart attack, stroke, deep venous thrombosis, pulmonary embolism, and retinal thrombosis. Known or suspected cancer of the breast, endometrium, cervix, or vagina or hepatic tumors (benign or malignant) are contraindications as well. Use of the new progestin drospirenone is also contraindicated in renal or adrenal insufficiency and in hepatic dysfunction. In any given patient, assessment should be made to evaluate the benefits versus the risks of taking the pill. The WHO has published guidelines to help simplify the assessment by classifying patients into four groups according to their degree of risk (Table 229-3 and Boxes 229-4 and 229-5).

The occurrence of side effects can lead to noncompliance, and thus should be discussed with teens prior to starting the use of pills. Weight gain is a major concern for many teenage girls, although many studies have shown minimal if any weight gain when oral contraceptives are taken. However, minimal weight gain may occur as a result of fluid retention, or as a result of increased appetite. Teens may lose weight because of self-imposed dieting, nausea, or depression. Healthy nutritional patterns and exercise should be encouraged by the clinician. Weighing the patient at each visit provides important monitoring since even perceived weight gain can lead to noncompliance.

Table 229-3. WHO Guidelines for Use of Oral Contraceptives

Classification	Use with Clinical Judgment	Use with Limited Clinical Judgment
1	Use method in any circumstances	Yes
2	Generally use the method	Yes
3	Use of method not usually recommended unless other more appropriate methods are not available or not acceptable	No
4	Method not to be used	No

From World Health Organization: Improving Access to Quality Care in Family Planning: Medical Eligibility Criteria for Contraceptive Use, 2nd ed. Geneva, WHO, 2000. Available at: http://www.who.int/reproductive-health/publications/RHR_00_2_medical_eligibility_criteria_second_edition/index.htm.

Nausea is generally considered an estrogenic side effect. Many patients will experience mild nausea for the first few days or occasionally for the first cycle or two. If nausea persists, it is wise to reduce the amount of estrogen to a lower dose pill (20 μg ethinyl estradiol).

Breakthrough bleeding is the occurrence of endometrial bleeding while the patient is taking hormonal pills. It occurs most frequently in the first one or two cycles, generally during the second week of the cycle. It usually diminishes with subsequent cycles on the same pill. The patient should be told in advance about the possibility of breakthrough bleeding to avoid anxiety and discontinuation of the pills. Other causes of bleeding could be missed pills, Chlamydia or other sexually transmitted infections, or pregnancy.

Box 229-4. Category 3 WHO Guidelines for Combined Oral Contraceptives

Use of method is usually not recommended in the presence of any of the following, unless other more appropriate methods are not available or not acceptable:

- Smoking (1–15 cigarettes/day) *and* age > 35 years
- Hypertension
  History of hypertension in which blood pressure cannot be monitored
  Adequately controlled hypertension, where blood pressure can be evaluated
  Systolic blood pressure 140–159 or diastolic 90–99* mm Hg
- Postpartum <21 days
- Primary breast-feeding, 6 weeks to 6 months
- Long-term use of enzyme-inducing antibiotics or anticonvulsants (rifampin, phenytoin) because of drug interactions
- History of oral contraceptive–related cholecystitis
- Symptomatic biliary tract disease (not treated by cholecystectomy)
- Known genetic hyperlipidemia (category 2–3)

* These blood pressure ranges are for adults; lower levels corresponding to 95% of age should be used in young teens.

Adapted from World Health Organization: Improving Access to Quality Care in Family Planning: Medical Eligibility Criteria for Contraceptive Use, 2nd ed. Geneva, WHO, 2000. Available at: http://www.who.int/reproductive-health/publications/RHR_00_2_medical_eligibility_criteria_second_edition/index.htm.

Box 229-5. Category 4 WHO Guidelines for Combined Oral Contraceptives

Method is contraindicated in the presence of any of the following:

- Smoking > 15 cigarettes per day *and* age > 35 years
- Hypertension (Systolic blood pressure > 160 or diastolic > 100 mm Hg)
- History of or current deep vein thrombosis or pulmonary embolism
- Complicated valvular heart disease (pulmonary hypertension, atrial fibrillation, history of subacute bacterial endocarditis)
- Migraine headaches with focal neurologic symptoms
- Major surgery with prolonged immobilization
- Active viral hepatitis
- Breast-feeding < 6 weeks postpartum

Adapted from World Health Organization: Improving Access to Quality Care in Family Planning: Medical Eligibility Criteria for Contraceptive Use, 2nd ed. Geneva, WHO, 2000. Available at: http://www.who.int/reproductive-health/publications/RHR_00_2_medical_eligibility_criteria_second_edition/index.htm.

Questions regarding these etiologies should be asked before assuming the cause is breakthrough bleeding. For breakthrough bleeding in the early months of pill-taking, patients can usually be reassured and observed over several months. If the breakthrough bleeding is a persistent problem after the first three cycles or lasts an entire cycle, a change to a more progestin-dominant pill or higher estrogen pill (if the patient was on a very low dose of estrogen) may reduce the bleeding.

A small percentage (1% to 2%) of normotensive individuals have been observed to develop hypertension after starting combined pills, with the risk increasing with age, parity, and obesity. The elevated blood pressure usually returns to normal within 2 to 12 weeks of discontinuing the pills. Progestin-only contraceptives or a lower dose estrogen pill can be utilized.

Scanty or absent withdrawal flow, most commonly associated with progestin-dominant and low-estrogen pills, may develop months or even years after continuous use. If a patient becomes amenorrheic, she should continue taking her pills, and the possibility of pregnancy should be evaluated promptly. The clinician should explain to the patient that the amenorrhea is not harmful and that she can continue taking her pill accompanied by periodic pregnancy tests. If the patient desires a change of pill, selecting one with less progestin or more estrogen is often helpful.

Headaches, which are a common complaint in adolescents, may improve or worsen with the use of oral contraceptives. Patients with headaches, including those with migraines without aura, usually tolerate oral contraceptives well, and some patients whose headaches are related to their menstrual cycle may even benefit from the pills. Use of combined oral contraceptives for patients who have migraine headaches with focal neurological symptoms is a WHO level 4 (see Table 229-3).

Subjective symptoms such as depression, nervousness, or emotional lability have been associated with oral contraceptive use in some studies but not in others. Some patients, perhaps because of a predisposition or intervening life stresses, do feel symptoms of irritability or depression that appear to coincide with the initiation of oral contraceptive use. After other causes for the depression or emotional lability are explored, the clinician can suggest a change to a different pill with less progestin or discontinuing the pill to see if the patient feels better.

The oral contraceptive pill can cause changes in laboratory values. For example, an increase in thyroid-binding globulin (TBG) leads to an increase in measured total T_4 and a decrease in resin T_3 levels and in the TBG index. However, there is no change in free T_4 or in the clinical status of patients. Sex hormone binding globulin also increases, which results in the beneficial effect of reducing free testosterone (helpful for patients with acne, hirsutism, or polycystic ovary syndrome).

Serious side effects are rare among oral contraceptive users. They include thromboembolic disease, cardiovascular accidents, pulmonary embolism, mesenteric artery thrombosis, and retinal artery thrombosis. Fortunately, these side effects appear to be mainly age related. The highest risk of cardiovascular events is in smokers over age 35 years. Diabetes and obesity also appear to increase the possibility of serious side effects. The estimated annual risk for nonfatal venous thrombosis is 4 per 100,000 for healthy women, 10 to 30 per 100,000 for women taking oral contraception, and 60 per 100,000 for pregnant women. Several genetic mutations, factor V Leiden and prothrombin 20210, have been recently identified to increase the risk of thrombosis in combination with oral contraceptives. However, screening in the absence of a family history is not cost effective and many familial factors associated with thrombosis have not yet been identified. Before starting an adolescent on hormonal contraceptives, it is helpful to obtain a personal and family history by asking questions such as those in Box 229-6.

Numerous studies over the past 3 decades have examined the potential relationship between oral contraceptives and a variety of cancers. Most studies have found no increase in overall risk of breast cancer. A recent study of women aged 35 to 64 years with current or former use of oral contraceptives, found no significant increase in the risk of breast cancer. Progression of cervical dysplasia may be associated with long-term oral contraceptive use, but there are many cofounders related to pill users in the studies, including lack of condom use, earlier age of sexual intercourse, and increased surveillance with Pap smears leading

Box 229-6. Personal and Family History Questions for Venous Thromboembolic Risk

Have you or a close family member ever had blood clots in the legs or lungs?

Have you or a close family member ever been hospitalized for blood clots in the legs or lungs?

Have you or a family member taken blood thinner?

Under what circumstances did the clot form? (e.g., cancer, airline travel, obesity, immobility, pregnancy)

From Wallach M, Grimes D (eds): Modern Oral Contraception: Updates from the Contraception Report. Totowa, NJ, Emron, 2000, p 118.

potentially to a detection bias. Previous or current use of combination oral contraceptives reduces the incidence of endometrial cancer and has a strong protective effect against ovarian cancer.

In order to increase the compliance with the chosen contraceptive method, the clinician should emphasize the benefits of the pills other than for contraception, and discuss the side effects to lessen anxiety. The clinician should also provide a concrete demonstration of how to use the pill, including help in planning what time of day to take the pill, how to remember, and what to do if a pill is forgotten. Patients should be able and encouraged to call the health care provider for any questions, and a follow-up visit should be scheduled for 1 to 3 months from the initial visit for evaluation of satisfaction, compliance, and side effects.

Injectable Hormonal Methods

Injectable hormonal methods are the choice of many adolescents who prefer the ease of administration and the privacy. The injected hormones are similar to the pills in their mechanism of action, side effects, and some of the contraindications.

Depot medroxyprogesterone acetate (DMPA) is a synthetic progestin derived from progesterone. A 150-mg dose is injected intramuscularly every 12 weeks. The first injection is given within the first 5 days of menses (with a pregnancy test recommended before initiation). This method can be used when estrogen is contraindicated or not desired, such as with postpartum/lactating women or patients with hypertension, hemoglobinopathy, seizure disorder (it has no interaction with anticonvulsant medication), or mental retardation (to help with menstrual hygiene problems). Most patients experience irregular bleeding for the first 3 to 6 months and then become amenorrheic, which may seem to be an advantage for some women. Weight gain can be a problem, and it has been estimated that women gain about 5 pounds each year for the first 3 years of use. A number of studies have suggested that this contraceptive may have a deleterious effect on bone density, of particular relevance to adolescents. Ongoing studies may better define optimal candidates and age for this method and the degree of rebound if loss occurs. Return to regular periods and fertility can take 1 to 2 years. The occurrence of irregular bleeding may require reassurance, assessment for other gynecologic problems, and short-term treatment with combined oral contraceptives or ibuprofen.

Lunelle is an injectable contraceptive with 25 mg medroxyprogesterone acetate/5 mg estradiol cypionate in 0.5 mL solution given every 28 to 30 days (probably effective when given between days 23 and 33). The first shot is administered during the first 5 days of a normal menstrual period. Withdrawal bleeding usually starts between days 20 and 25. The action, advantages, disadvantages, contraindications, and side effects are similar to those of the combined pills, although menstrual disturbances may occur more frequently, especially in the first few months of use. Return to ovulation and fertility is rapid, in contrast to DMPA. Lunelle is not currently available in the United States.

Vaginal Rings

A new form of contraceptive is the combined vaginal ring (marketed as NuvaRing; Fig. 229-1). The ring placed in the vagina releases 120 µg of etonogestrel and 15 µg of ethinyl estradiol daily. The ring is typically left in the vagina for 3 weeks and then removed for a week to allow withdrawal bleeding. The efficacy is high with a reported failure rate of 0.65 to 1.0 per 100 woman-years of care in a 12-month trial. Cycle control is good, although about 25% experience withdrawal bleeding that extends beyond the ring-free week. The common side effects include headaches, leukorrhea, and vaginitis.

Transdermal Contraceptive Patch

The transdermal contraception patch, marketed as Ortho-Evra, is a 4.5-cm square that releases 150 µg of norelgestromin and 20 µg of ethinyl estradiol daily. It is worn on the abdomen, buttocks, upper torso, or upper arm, and left in place for 7 days. Three consecutive patches are followed by a patch-free week to allow withdrawal bleeding. Side effects include application site reaction, headaches, nausea, breast tenderness, and breakthrough bleeding in the first 2 months. Contraceptive failure rate is approximately 1 pregnancy per 100 woman-years and may be higher in women greater than 90 kilograms.

Subdermal Implants

Levonorgestrel implants (Norplant) slowly release levonorgestrel over 5 years. The pregnancy rate is very low. The implant is inserted through a small incision in the upper or lower arm, immediately postabortion, in the postpartum period, or within the first 7 days of the cycle. This implant is effective in less than 24 hours from administration, and

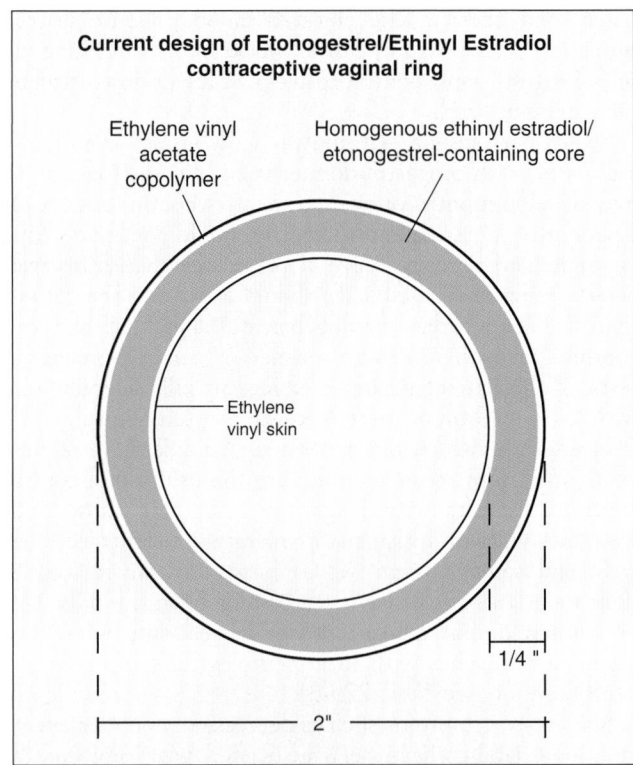

Figure 229-1. Current design of etonogestrel/ethinyl estradiol contraceptive vaginal ring.

there is rapid return of fertility with removal. Irregular periods occur in most women initially and weight gain can be a problem. Subdermal implants are not currently available in the United States, although Norplant 2 (a two rod implant) has recently been approved. A single rod implant that has 68 mg of etonogestrel (Implanon) and maintains contraceptive dose for 3 years is expected to be available in 2005. The pregnancy rate is very low (Pearl Index 0), and bleeding patterns are acceptable.

Emergency Contraception

Emergency contraception, previously known as postcoital contraception or the "morning after pill," is an important method about which all adolescents should be educated. Emergency contraception can be used in situations of unexpected coitus, broken condoms, rape, missed oral contraceptive pills, dislodged diaphragm or cervical cap, exposure to a possible teratogen, and so forth.

There are two hormonal options in emergency contraception. The most commonly used method in the past was the Yuzpe regimen, which utilizes a dose of 100 µg ethinyl estradiol and 1.0 mg of norgestrel (or 0.5 mg levonorgestrel), repeated 12 hours later. The Preven emergency contraceptive kit contains the required medication, a patient education booklet, and a pregnancy test. The main side effect of the Yuzpe regimen is nausea and vomiting from the high dose of estrogen. Taking an antiemetic such as meclizine prior to the first dose of pills decreases nausea. Oral contraceptives with the same dose may be administered as well. The second common option uses only progestin. Plan B is a kit including two pills of 0.75 mg levonorgestrel each, to be taken 12 hours apart starting within 72 hours after the unprotected intercourse. One study found equal efficacy in taking 1.5 mg of levonorgestrel as a single dose. Plan B is more effective and has fewer side effects than the Yuzpe regimen. The mechanism of action of emergency contraception changes throughout the menstrual cycle and includes inhibition of ovulation, disruption of tubal transport, and changes in the endometrial lining. The most important fact is that emergency contraception does not work as an abortifacient: It will not terminate a pregnancy that has already been established. The sooner the medications are taken, the more effective they are, although there is evidence of efficacy up to 5 days after intercourse.

BARRIER METHODS

Barrier contraceptives act by killing or blocking sperm in the vagina and are available in different forms, both for male and female use. The efficacy of these methods depends on correct use by the patient, with incorrect use resulting in lower efficacy than any other contraceptive method.

Male condoms are the most frequently used of all contraceptive methods, either in combination with a hormonal method or as a single method. Concerns about exposure to STDs and specifically AIDS has increased the use of condoms among teens. The importance of using condoms should be discussed in any medical visit in which anticipatory guidance or sexuality related issues are discussed. More than 100 brands of condoms are sold in the United States; they are made of latex (rubber), plastic (vinyl), or natural materials (animal products). Latex is the safest of the three. The most important advantage of the condom is that, excepting abstinence, it is the most effective method to decrease the risks of STDs. Their effectiveness against HIV, Chlamydia, and gonorrhea is high, but the protection against the herpes and human papilloma viruses is lower because there is still exposure (base of penis, vulva, upper thigh) that could lead to transmission of the disease. Additional benefits of the condom are its availability, low price, and immediate effectiveness. It can be used as a backup for other methods or, if used correctly, as a single method. There are no systemic side effects or method-related health risks. The only side effect is an allergic reaction possible in both partners to the latex condom or to spermicide if used. The main limitation is that its efficacy is user dependent. Condoms may reduce the sensitivity of the penis, interfere with the erection, and reduce the overall satisfaction from the intercourse, which can result in lower compliance. Patients should be counseled to use emergency contraception if the condom slips, tears, or breaks.

The female condom is a loose fitting polyurethane sheath with two diaphragm-like rings; the condom is inserted into the vagina. This condom can be used as a backup for other methods and for prevention of STDs. The high price, moderate effectiveness, and need to learn how to insert the female condom make this contraceptive method a less popular method among adolescents than male condoms.

The diaphragm with spermicide has a relatively high failure rate and offers much less protection from STDs than condoms. There are three types of diaphragms: flat spring, coiled wire, and arching spring. A health care provider fits the adolescent with the diaphragm and needs to teach her how to insert it and use it properly. Contraindications include inability to fit the patient or a previous allergic reaction to latex or spermicide. The advantages are the immediate contraceptive effect.

Cervical caps are made of rigid plastic and designed to cover the cervix. Small amounts of spermicide placed in the cap increase efficacy. The mechanism of action is similar to the diaphragm. Problems seen with cervical cap use include odor, vaginal discharge, and difficulty with insertion or removal. An abnormal Pap smear is considered a contraindication to use. Similar to the cervical cap is Lea's Shield, which is shaped like an elliptical bowl with a valve that allows passage of cervical secretions and air.

Spermicides come in different forms: creams, jellies, foams, suppositories, and films. The active ingredient varies, with the most common being nonoxynol-9. Spermicides are not recommended for STD or HIV protection and may, with repeated use, enhance transmission of HIV.

OTHER METHODS

There are currently two available intrauterine devices (IUDs): copper T 380A (ParaGard) and the recently approved levonorgestrel-releasing intrauterine system (Mirena). The mechanism of action in the hormonal intrauterine device includes thickening of cervical mucus, inhibition of the sperm, and changes of the endometrium. The advantages are high efficacy with all types. Decreased menstrual flow and a very low risk of infection are

Box 230-2. Factors Associated with Consistent Contraceptive Use

Academic success
Anticipation of a satisfying future
Being involved in a stable relationship with a sexual partner

PREGNANCY AND CHILDBEARING AMONG ADOLESCENTS

All sexually active teens are at risk for pregnancy. Overall, 40% of sexually active adolescent girls in the United States experience a pregnancy prior to turning 20. Population characteristics of young people at higher risk for pregnancy are listed in Box 230-3. These associations point to a complex interplay of culture, environment, and internal characteristics contributing to pregnancy and childbearing among young people. Comprehensive sexuality education and access to safe and effective means to prevent pregnancy are absolutely crucial for young people who engage in sexual intercourse, but these measures are not sufficient to prevent all pregnancies. A fuller understanding of the complex factors contributing to pregnancy and parenting reveals a need to focus on positive youth development and motivation not to become pregnant rather than assuming that all teen pregnancy is unintended.

Pregnant teens younger than 17 years of age have a higher incidence of medical complications than do adult women, with risk being greatest for the youngest teens (Box 230-4). The incidence of low birth weight and neonatal deaths are two to three times greater among infants of teens compared with those born to adults. While the rates are very low, teens have twice the risk of maternal mortality than do adult women. Similarly, children of teen parents do not fare as well as children of adult mothers (Box 230-5).

Fathers of infants born to adolescent mothers are at risk. One third of these fathers are also adolescents. Adolescent fathers are similar to adolescent mothers in that they are more likely than their peers to be failing school and to be poor. Adolescent fathers who engage in parenting produce better outcomes for themselves, the child, and the child's mother than do teen fathers who do not participate. However, information on teenage marriage does not support

Box 230-3. Populations of Girls at Higher Risk of Pregnancy

Girls who are in the following categories:
- Live in isolated poor communities
- Are not succeeding in school
- Have had many peers and close female relatives who have experienced early pregnancy or parenting
- Have had a previous pregnancy (ending in birth, miscarriage, or elective termination)
- Have had a negative pregnancy test
- Are urban rather than suburban or rural dwellers
- Are ethnic minorities
- Have been victims of child sexual abuse
- Have mothers or sisters who were teen mothers

Box 230-4. Maternal Risks Higher for Pregnant Teens as Compared with Those for Adults

Medical complications
Low birth weight
Neonatal deaths
Maternal mortality
Poor maternal weight gain
Premature birth
Pregnancy-induced hypertension
Anemia
Sexually transmitted diseases
Risk for domestic abuse
Stress
Depression

the belief that simply by encouraging a young couple to marry the attendant risks are alleviated.

Problems associated with early childbearing include school interruption, poverty, limited vocational options, divorce, and repeat pregnancy. Several long-term follow-up studies show that the long-term outcomes are not as negative as once thought. Two decades after childbearing most teen mothers are economically self-sufficient and have completed high school. They do not necessarily have large families. When pregnancy does interrupt education, a history of poor academic performance usually predates the pregnancy. Having a second pregnancy prior to age 18 has a negative effect on high school completion. Factors associated with increased high school completion include being African American, being raised in a small family, the presence of reading material at home, employment of the teenager's mother, and high parental education.

Adolescent pregnancy is a multifaceted problem that requires multidimensional solutions (Box 230-6). Both primary and secondary prevention strategies are important. Prevention strategies need to target teens, including boys, at highest risk for early pregnancy, and must engage parents, grandparents, and entire communities. Some of the most commonly overlooked strategies for primary prevention are quality early child and educational care (such as Head Start and Early Head Start programs) and comprehensive home visiting for vulnerable families.

DIAGNOSIS AND PRESENTATION

The key to early diagnosis of pregnancy is a willingness to consider the possibility. Box 230-7 lists early signs and symptoms of pregnancy. While some adolescents may

Box 230-5. Risks to Children of Teen Parents That Are Higher than for Children of Adult Parents

Developmental delay
Academic difficulties
Behavioral disorders
Substance abuse
Becoming teen parents themselves
Becoming incarcerated

Box 230-6. Components of Successful Pregnancy Prevention Programs

Abstinence motivation
Contraception availability
Comprehensive sexuality education
Positive youth development
Interpersonal skills development
Vocational training
School completion strategies

request an examination because they think they may be pregnant, not all are so clear. Presenting complaints can be specific, such as a missed period following unprotected intercourse, or they may be vague, such as fatigue, nausea, dizziness, or depression. Suicide attempters need to be tested for pregnancy. As with many adolescent issues, the presenting complaint may simply be the ticket to the visit when the real concern is pregnancy. While some young women come with almost certain knowledge that they are pregnant, others may deny any possibility of pregnancy. A study of young women receiving emergency room care indicated that 12% of those found to be pregnant had denied being sexually active.

Menstrual history should be a part of every medical visit for adolescent girls. The most common symptom leading to adolescents suspecting that they are pregnant is a missed period. Menstrual histories are not entirely reliable as indicators of pregnancy, however. One study showed that only 68% of pregnant adolescents report having missed a period. Other signs and symptoms of early pregnancy can include breast tenderness, fatigue, nausea, morning sickness, and frequent urination. All of these may occur prior to even missing a period and often prior to the sixth week of gestation. Common gynecological signs of early pregnancy are softening of the cervix, softening of the uterus, and a bluish purple hue to the cervix and vaginal walls caused by hyperemia. Physical examination alone is an unreliable predictor of early pregnancy. Physical diagnosis of pregnancy becomes more reliable as the gestational age advances. Enlargement of the uterus is usually recognizable by about 8 weeks' gestation with the uterus palpable at the pelvic brim by about 12 weeks' gestation. Using a Doppler, fetal heart tones are generally audible at 12 weeks' gestation and fetal movement is detectable by 20 weeks' gestation.

Pregnancy tests based on the detection of human chorionic gonadotropin (HCG) in maternal urine or serum

Box 230-7. Early Signs and Symptoms of Pregnancy

Missed menstrual period
Breast tenderness
Fatigue
Nausea and "morning sickness"
Frequent urination
Softening of the cervix
Softening of the uterus
Bluish purple hue to the cervix and vaginal walls caused by hyperemia

are the standard for early diagnosis. HCG, a glycoprotein hormone secreted by the trophoblastic cells of the placenta, is composed of an alpha and a beta subunit. The alpha subunit is similar to other human hormones including follicle-stimulating hormone (FSH), luteinizing hormone (LH), and thyroid-stimulating hormone (TSH). The beta subunit is specific to HCG. Testing for the beta subunit allows specific identification of HCG.

The most accurate measure of serum HCG is done by radioimmunoassay, using a highly specific antiserum to the beta subunit. These assays can measure levels as low 2 to 7 mIU/mL (milli international units per mL). The implanted trophoblast begins to secret HCG as early as 7 days after ovulation. In normal pregnancies, HCG levels increase, rapidly reaching 100 mIU/mL in maternal serum by the date of the first missed menses. HCG levels double approximately every 2 days in the first 6 to 7 weeks of pregnancy. The gestational sack is clearly identifiable on vaginal sonography at HCG levels of 1000 to 2000 mIU/mL. In ectopic gestations and spontaneous abortions HCG levels are usually lower than normal and increase at lower than normal rates. Molar pregnancies and multiple gestations are both associated with higher than normal HCG levels. After pregnancy termination, HCG levels decrease gradually. In general most first trimester abortions resulted in negative pregnancy tests by 40 days postprocedure. The benefits of serum pregnancy testing are the ability to acquire both qualitative and quantitative measures. Following quantitative levels of HCG is very important when concerned about the possibility of an ectopic pregnancy or spontaneous abortion.

Home and office-use pregnancy tests are based on the identification of HCG metabolites in maternal urine. Most of this is a beta core fragment of the beta subunit and therefore specific to HCG. The test is qualitative and can either rule pregnancy in or rule it out but does not give a quantitative level of HCG. The most commonly available urine pregnancy tests are ELISA type kits based on highly specific monoclonal antibodies to the beta subunit of HCG. Sensitivity of most urine pregnancy tests ranges from 5 to 25 mIU/mL of HCG. They may be positive as early as 3 or 4 days after implantation and they are positive by the expected date of the missed menses in nearly all normal pregnancies.

While currently available tests are accurate and easy to use, the use of too much or too little urine can lead to false-negative results. Urine pregnancy tests are not impaired by small amounts of hemoglobin, glucose, albumin, or other serum proteins or by most commonly used medications. Grossly bloody specimens and those with proteinuria greater than 2+ may lead to false negatives in some kits. Most urine pregnancy tests have fairly strict timing windows during which the tests should be read as all tests may develop color after the recommended time interval. Refrigerated urine specimens can be used up to 48 hours after collection. Most kits have built-in negative controls.

Bleeding or spotting occurs in 20% to 25% of pregnancies. Ectopic gestation should always be considered when pregnant patients present with bleeding with abdominal pain. Abdominal pain and cramping can also be symptoms of normal gestation perhaps associated with corpus luteal cysts. Spontaneous abortion is defined as a pregnancy

> **Box 230-8.** Risk Factors for Ectopic Pregnancies
>
> History of pelvic inflammatory disease (PID)
> Chlamydial infection
> Prior tubal surgery
> Use of intrauterine devices (IUDs)
> Use of progestin-only methods of contraception (Norplant, Depoprovera, or the minipill)

loss occurring before 20 weeks' gestation. The rate of spontaneous abortion in pregnancies recognized clinically is 20%. An additional 30% of pregnancies are lost prior to implantation and thus prior to a positive pregnancy test.

More than 100,000 ectopic pregnancies occur annually in the United States (2% of all pregnancies). Women over 35 years of age are the most likely to have ectopic pregnancies, but teens have the highest mortality rates. Minority teens have a fivefold higher mortality rate from ruptured ectopic pregnancies compared with nonminority adolescents, probably because youth, and minority youth in particular, present later in pregnancy. Risk factors for ectopic pregnancies are listed in Box 230-8. Users of contraception have lower rates of ectopic pregnancies compared to nonusers of contraception. When pregnancy does occur, however, the odds of an ectopic pregnancy are increased. Classic symptoms of ectopic pregnancy are abdominal pain with late menses. Pain may be unilateral and can range from mild cramps to severe pain. As pregnancy progresses, the pain may be bilateral or diffuse. If the ectopic pregnancy results in tubal rupture, peritoneal signs and shoulder pain may be present. Advanced cases may present with hypovolumic shock caused by blood loss. Fortunately, because of increasing use of sensitive pregnancy testing most ectopic pregnancies are diagnosed prior to becoming emergencies. Quantitative HCG levels and vaginal ultrasounds are important components of diagnosis. In normal pregnancy, a sack is visible on sonography with HCG levels of 1000 to 2000 mIU/mL or approximately 1 week after expected menses. HCG levels double approximately every 48 hours. If the HCG level is more than 1500 mIU/mL and no pregnancy is identified in the uterus, further evaluation is indicated.

The most commonly used of the various options for treating ectopic pregnancy is an IM injection of methotrexate. Approximately 95% of ectopic pregnancies resolve using this method. The remainder require either a second dose of methotrexate or surgical intervention. At any time in the management of ectopic pregnancy, symptoms of syncope or shocks or signs of rupture require immediate surgical intervention. Determination of Rh antibody status is important in all cases of spontaneous abortion and ectopic pregnancy. Prophylactic administration of anti-D gamma-globin is given to women at risk for Rh sensitization.

MANAGEMENT

Options Counseling
Acknowledgment of the life-altering impact of the diagnosis of a pregnancy is important, as is an appreciation of the potential personal and family crises that may ensue. The

news of a positive pregnancy test is often met with mixed emotions that can be very confusing to adolescents. The news of a negative test can likewise be confusing to young people. Because of high rates of subsequent pregnancy among those who test negative for pregnancy, the event of a negative test is an opportunity to explore attitudes and beliefs about sexual activity, pregnancy, and pregnancy prevention, and to discuss both contraception and emergency contraception. It is also an opportunity to discuss alcohol and other drug use in the context of sexual decision making and their role in partner violence and involuntary intercourse. For young women desiring pregnancy or refusing contraception, prescribing a daily folate supplement (400 mcg) reduces the risk of neural tube defects in future pregnancies.

After diagnosing a pregnant adolescent, the clinician should be able to help her garner the support of appropriate adults in her decision making, help her understand her options, and help her act on her decisions either to continue the pregnancy with good prenatal care or to terminate it safely. The adolescent patient and other concerned persons must be given complete information on all available options to help make an informed decision. All pregnancy options benefit from early diagnosis. Issues of confidentiality and consent vary from state to state. It is important for clinicians to become familiar with the laws pertaining to young people in the state in which they practice.

In general, clinicians should encourage adolescents to include their parents or other trusting adults in all decision making. However, since the adolescent patient has the right to a confidential relationship with her physician unless there is evidence of imminent harm to self or others such as suicide, homicide, or abuse, the diagnosis should first be conveyed to the adolescent alone and only with her consent to other people. Clinicians must always be sensitive to the possibility of pregnancy resulting from involuntary intercourse, abuse, or incest, especially among young or developmentally delayed teens. In such cases, child protection services, community sexual assault response services, and local law enforcement agencies may need to be involved.

Discussions with adolescents need to be undertaken at developmentally appropriate levels. This essential requirement assumes that the clinician is able to assess a young person's ability to understand the complex and potentially life-altering consequences of her decisions. Depending on the adolescent's cognitive and psychosocial maturity, this may require varied approaches. Encouraging adolescents to reflect on their choices, their beliefs about parenthood, and their life dreams and plans may help them sort through the situation. These discussions may also help the physician gain a clearer appreciation for the individual's developmental status.

The specific options available vary depending on the gestation of the pregnancy. Usually there are three options: to carry the pregnancy to term and raise the baby, to carry the pregnancy to term and place the baby up for adoption, or to terminate the pregnancy. All three options need to be discussed fully. Decision making is a process that requires time and work and may require several office visits. Whatever the decision, the clinician must follow up with the patient to ensure successful referral to prenatal care or termination services and to address subsequent pregnancy prevention, sexual decision making, and family planning.

Elective Termination of Pregnancy

Elective termination of pregnancy has been legally available to all women in the United States since 1972. Some states have instituted mandatory waiting periods, partner notification, and consent requirements for minors. Most states with mandatory parental consent for minors also have mechanisms for judicial bypass of this requirement. Clinicians must be familiar with the specific laws in the state and community in which they practice. The greatest threat to the availability of safe legal abortion services is usually limited access to providers. Fewer and fewer providers offer termination services. In a growing number of locations, women must travel to obtain them. The rate of elective termination has dropped more than 30% over the past 10 years.

Legally induced abortion is safer than continuing a pregnancy to term. Elective termination does not impair future fertility. The earlier the pregnancy is diagnosed, the greater the range of options for termination method. Women seeking abortion early in pregnancy usually have multiple safe options from which to choose. Second-trimester terminations generally have fewer. Vacuum aspiration is the most commonly used method (more than 90% of all procedures). It is performed primarily in the first trimester. Dilation and evacuation (D&E) is the most commonly used second-trimester method.

Mifepristone or methotrexate used in combination with misoprostol provides an alternative to surgical methods. Mifepristone and misoprostol have recently been approved for use in pregnancies of less than 7 weeks' gestation. Access to mifepristone is limited to providers who have the ability to perform or refer patients for surgical abortion, should this be needed. Mifepristone, a steroid with high affinity for progesterone receptors, acts as a progestin antagonist and stimulates production of prostaglandins by decidua cells. It has been used for the past decade in France, Sweden, the United Kingdom, and China. It is used in conjunction with misoprostol, a prostaglandin analogue, marketed in the United States for gastric ulcer disease. The combination of mifepristone and misoprostol results in complete abortion in 95% of women who are less than 7 weeks' pregnant. By 9 weeks' gestation, it is about 80% effective. The drugs cause uterine contraction, cramping, and bleeding in 80% of women. Median blood loss is 100 mL. Approximately 1% of women using this method experience uterine bleeding that requires curettage. Less than 0.1% require transfusion. Administration of the regimen usually requires three visits. Mifepristone is given orally on day 1. Two days later, the woman returns for misoprostol. Most abortions occur within 4 hours of receiving misoprostol. Women then return to their provider 2 weeks later for follow-up to ensure that a complete abortion has occurred.

Continuing the Pregnancy

If the adolescent chooses to continue her pregnancy, she should be referred for prenatal care. Special comprehensive programs of prenatal care for adolescents have been evaluated and have been shown to be effective among teens in increasing adherence to prenatal care and improving birth outcomes. When available, they are a preferred alternative. Programs for comprehensive home visiting by medical professionals have also been evaluated and shown to be effective and of long-term benefit to teen mothers and their children. These are most effective when begun prenatally. Community resources for pregnant and parenting teens and schools vary widely. Learning about the range of services available in the community enables clinicians to be more effective in counseling youth regarding pregnancy resolution. Local health departments and human service departments can be helpful in gathering this information. Federal law prohibits exclusion of pregnant teens from school. TANF (temporary aid for needy families) has specific resources and requirements for teenage parents.

Adoption is an important option to discuss, although it is the one least often chosen by teens. Fewer than 3% of young women who choose to carry to term opt for adoption. Being familiar with local adoption resources, especially ongoing counseling and social service support throughout the pregnancy, is crucial. Advocates of open adoption (the active involvement of the adoptive parents with the birth mother) believe that adolescents may find this option developmentally more acceptable.

For all young women choosing to carry to term, discussions about lifestyle including attention to nutritional diet, getting plenty of rest, and avoiding alcohol and illicit drugs are very important. Stress reduction strategies and personal safety discussions are crucial as well. Starting prenatal vitamins is also important. The clinician can play a key role in helping teen patients prepare for parenthood and their transition to parenthood.

SUMMARY

Sexual exploration and, for many, sexual intercourse are normative behaviors in adolescence. Unfortunately, in the United States this results annually in nearly 1 million pregnancies in girls younger than 20 years old. Comprehensive sexuality education (including discussions of abstinence), access to reliable contraception, positive youth development, and addressing economic and social disparities contribute to diminution of these rates.

The earlier adolescent pregnancies are diagnosed, the greater the options available and the safer the resolution of the pregnancy, regardless of the option chosen. It is crucial for clinicians to become familiar with the laws regarding adolescent pregnancy and the resources available in the communities in which they practice. The key to early diagnosis is a willingness to consider the possibility of pregnancy. When pregnancy does occur, the clinician plays an important role in delivering the diagnosis, explaining the options available, and lending continuing support of the adolescent and her family to facilitate their follow through on decisions. Remembering that adolescents are sexual beings and including sexual health as part of all encounters with adolescent patients facilitates both primary and secondary prevention.

Mini-index of Related Topics

SUGGESTED READINGS

American Academy of Pediatrics: The adolescent's right to confidential care when considering abortion (RE9614). Pediatrics 1996;97(5):746–751.

American Academy of Pediatrics: Adolescent pregnancy: Current trends and issues. Pediatrics 1999;103(2):516–520.

American Academy of Pediatrics: The care of adolescent parents and their children (RE0020). Pediatrics 2001;107(2):429–434.

Kaufman RB, Spitz AM, Strauss LT, et al: The decline in U.S. teen pregnancy rates, 1990–1995. Pediatrics 1998;102(5):1141–1153.

Polaneczky M, O'Connor K: Pregnancy in the adolescent patient: Screening, diagnosis, and initial management. Pediatr Clin North Am 1999;46(4):649–670.

Tobias B, Ricer R: Counseling adolescents about sexuality. Prim Care 1998;25(1):49–71.

Youth Risk Behavior Surveillance, U.S. 2003. Available at: www.cdc.gov/mmwr.

SECTION 6   ADOLESCENT CARE: *Adolescent Mental Health*

231 Psychosocial Issues of Maturation

Jennifer Johnson

ROLE OF THE GENERALIST

1 Assess psychosocial development at each visit.

2 Adapt interview to stage of psychosocial development.

3 Modify content and presentation of patient education and counseling according to psychosocial and cognitive development.

4 Provide anticipatory guidance to parents regarding adolescent psychosocial development.

5 Identify and provide counseling for parental concerns regarding issues related to psychosocial development.

6 Discuss anticipated changes and stressors.

7 Screen for factors that may adversely influence the developmental trajectory.

8 Identify and encourage positive coping strategies.

CORE PRINCIPLES

Adolescence encompasses not only the physical changes of puberty, but also profound changes in psychosocial functioning and cognition. During this decade of life, roughly from 10 to 21 years of age, childhood is cast aside. The youth develops the capabilities and skills needed to function as an adult. Societal milestones, such as getting a driver's license and graduating from high school, formalize some transitions. Other landmarks are personal: the first kiss, the senior prom, moving away from home.

Many parents view the approach of their child's adolescence with trepidation. In fact, 9 out of 10 adolescents and their families navigate this passage without the "Sturm und Drang" (storm and stress) often ascribed to this period.

Adolescence does require the family to renegotiate roles, responsibilities, and limits. Parents who are experiencing developmental crises of their own or who have difficulty relinquishing control will probably experience greater friction with their adolescent offspring.

The pediatric health care provider can provide valuable anticipatory guidance about the usual course of events, possible variations, and parenting skills that can reduce conflict and enhance the quality of life for adolescents and their families. Parents who are familiar with the "navigational chart" of adolescence can watch for channel markers and provide or seek guidance if the youth appears to be off course. A disagreement over curfew, for example, may "rock the boat." This type of disagreement represents the adolescent's need for autonomy. Repeated truancy, on the other hand, signals that a major course adjustment is necessary to keep the ship off the rocks.

Adolescent development is influenced by a number of factors: biological, cognitive, social, cultural, and environmental. Individual characteristics such as personality and temperament affect the interpersonal interactions of adolescents, which in turn shape their development. Current psychological research conceptualizes processes in adolescent development as progressing through continuous change. Intermittent regression is as normal an aspect of development as is progress. This chapter delineates the changes in functioning that mark the steps toward adulthood, and discusses the roles of these factors in adolescent development.

GROWTH TASKS OF ADOLESCENCE

The transitions prerequisite to assuming an adult role in society are referred to as the "growth tasks" of adolescence (Box 231-1). Each growth task represents an important developmental process.

Adolescence is often described as consisting of three stages: early (10 to 13 years of age), middle (14 to 16 years of age), and late (17 to 21 years of age). Each stage is characterized by typical manifestations of progress in accomplishing the developmental tasks (Table 231-1). Several points should be kept in mind while considering these developmental stages: (1) Differences between stages do not necessarily represent qualitative transformations. (2) Many developmental processes are interdependent so that some transitions tend to occur in temporal proximity. For example, the development of social skills depends on cognitive maturation. (3) There is not necessarily synchrony of stages between developmental tasks. A late adolescent who functions quite independently may still be a "middle" adolescent in terms of sexual identity.

Independence and Autonomy. Separating from parents and parental control (relinquishing dependence) is a prerequisite for independence. The early adolescent begins to separate from the family and strive for independence. A close relationship with a trusted adult outside the immediate family—a favorite teacher or a family friend—may

Box 231-1. Growth Tasks of Adolescence
Achieving autonomy and independence
Forming a distinct self-identity
Developing an identity as a sexual person
Developing new cognitive skills
Acquiring social competence

serve as a bridge to the larger world. The youth tests boundaries and may demand their revision within the context of a well-known environment. Parents can decrease friction by easing or relinquishing control over nonessential matters. Encouraging independence in familiar surroundings helps prepare adolescents to manage the changes in their broader social environment. Ambivalence about independence is common. For example, the young teenager and a friend may go to the movies with the family but insist on sitting apart from the other members.

In middle adolescence the drive for emancipation and independence becomes stronger. Contrary to the "Rebel without a Cause" stereotype, conflict in the family generally does not increase. However, parents who do not loosen the reins in early adolescence are likely to encounter rebelliousness in their middle adolescent.

The late adolescent completes the process of emancipation. He or she "rejoins" the family, participating as an adult rather than a dependent member. Society also acknowledges adult status by permitting 18-year-olds to vote and, in most states, enter into contracts and marry. Complete independence is achieved only when a person becomes financially self-sufficient. This may be delayed until the mid- to late twenties, pending completion of vocational or professional training.

Self Identity. Erikson conceptualized development of an identity as a central task of adolescence. This task is consid-

Table 231-1. Characteristics of Adolescents by Developmental Stage

	Developmental Stage		
	Early	**Middle**	**Late**
Age (years)	10–13	14–16	17–21
Autonomy/Independence	■ Increased independence ■ Control issues produce minor to moderate conflicts with parents	■ Peer group facilitates separation from family ■ Minor to moderate conflicts over control	■ Emancipation completed ■ Accepted as adult member of family and society
Self-identity	■ Adaptation to physical changes of puberty	■ Identification with peer group reinforces self-image ■ Recognition of personal uniqueness; egocentrism	■ Stable identity ■ Individuated from peers ■ Career/vocational exploration
Sexuality	■ Adaptation to physical changes of puberty	■ Exploratory sexual behavior ■ Idealistic romantic fantasies	■ Sexual behavior within context of more durable, meaningful relationship
Social competence	■ Relationships with peers more complex and intimate ■ Same-sex peer group	■ Peer group more important; opposite sex added	■ Individual relationships more important than peer group ■ Idealism
Cognitive skills	■ Beginning of transition from concrete to abstract throught	■ Abstract thinking predominant ■ Time perspective extended (future orientation) ■ Improved decision-making skills	■ Transition from concrete to abstract thought completed ■ Consistent application of abstract thinking to solve problems ■ Long-term plan for future

ered as discovering who you are, what you are all about, and where you are going in life. Rather than a developmental "crisis," the course of individuation is characterized as a series of small transitions.

The rapid physical changes of puberty (linear growth, increase in body mass, and development of secondary sexual characteristics) preoccupy the early adolescent. Adaptation to a changing body includes revision of the adolescent's body image. This explains the hours before the bathroom mirror and the mutual grooming sessions (e.g., trying out hairstyles) that are common in this age group.

The middle adolescent is completing puberty and no longer has to contend with a rapidly changing body. In addition to internalizing a new body image, the middle adolescent begins to explore the *person* inhabiting that body. Various roles are tried out, modified, or discarded. Changes in style of attire and grooming are visible manifestations of these explorations: the tomboy may wear makeup or don a saucy beret. The late-maturing bookworm who ended up with long legs may go out for track. And with a newfound ability to think introspectively (see under Cognitive Skills in this chapter), the middle to late adolescent ponders the personal and social characteristics of the person he or she would like to become.

In late adolescence, a more realistic, stable sense of self emerges. The gifted boy who wanted to become a fighter pilot has accepted the limitations of his poor vision and decided on a career as an aeronautical engineer.

Sexuality. Curiosity about sexual behavior and interest in exploring one's sexuality intensify during puberty. Early adolescents begin by investigating their own bodies. It is also common for early adolescents to explore jointly. Two girls at a sleepover may rub each other's breasts. Boys at a secluded lake may masturbate each other or have a competition to see who can "shoot" the farthest. Such behaviors occur independently of sexual orientation. Parents should be made aware that these behaviors are common and normal.

Middle adolescents begin to explore and express their sexual interest with others to whom they are attracted. Before teenagers begin to date in the traditional sense, they may "get together" in other ways. At parties they may play sex games or pair off. When middle adolescents "go" with someone, the relationships tend to be brief, perhaps lasting only a week. Middle adolescents may utilize such relationships for their own purposes. They may want to test their sexual attractiveness or to try on various aspects of a gender role. In exploring their sexuality, young people may participate in sexual intercourse or other activities that put them at risk for pregnancy and sexually transmitted infections.

At late adolescence, most individuals have developed the capacity for truly intimate, caring, reciprocal sexual relationships. These relationships are more stable, last longer, and involve mutual commitment.

Social Competence. Early in adolescence, the nature of relationships with peers changes. Friendships become more intimate and involved; there is more sharing of thoughts and feelings. Increased cognitive abilities contribute to this growth in social competence. Peer groups are primarily same-sex. In middle adolescence, the peer group and indi-

vidual friendships with peers become more important. Peer groups become larger and more complex and include members of both genders. Peer groups find commonalities in areas of "adolescent culture," such as music and clothing. Generally, adolescents retain the core values and beliefs of their family of origin. In late adolescence, the peer group decreases substantially in importance. Individual relationships take precedence.

Cognitive Skills. The cognitive changes of adolescence include development of the ability to think abstractly and to make decisions based on reasoning (problem-solving skills). The adolescent becomes capable of extending thought beyond the present and into the future.

Most adolescents develop the capacity for abstract reasoning between the ages of 11 and 14 years. This includes thinking hypothetically, applying formal logic, and using abstract concepts. The ability to apply these skills to solve real-life problems is situational. The adolescent's knowledge about the topic, prior experience in solving similar problems, and degree of emotional arousal determine whether he or she is able to employ abstract reasoning in a given situation.

In middle adolescence and late adolescence, practice helps consolidate abstract-thinking skills. Their application is still situational but gradually less so. (Even adults may regress in their thinking when confronted with new, emotionally laden problems.) The adolescent recognizes that a problem may be solved in more than one way. Many youth, in discovering the power of their ability to think, challenge adults to "think outside the box." Many adults find this a refreshing trait. (Someone who takes such questioning personally, of course, will not.)

THE CONTEXT OF ADOLESCENT DEVELOPMENT

Society shares responsibility with the community and family for promoting healthy adolescent development. All young people need a physically and emotionally safe, nurturing environment. Family and school are key in providing adolescents with models for meaningful relationships, along with feelings of belonging and self-worth. Adolescents who feel highly connected to their parents, other family members, and school are less likely to be affected by issues that can delay, disrupt, or even foreclose development. These include emotional distress; suicidal thoughts and behaviors; violence; use of cigarettes, alcohol, or marijuana; and early age at first sexual intercourse.

Adolescents and their families need social systems that support adolescent development of the attitudes and skills necessary to function as a member of society. Renowned psychiatrist David Hamburg identified 10 fundamental requirements for healthy adolescent development (Box 231-2). Many youth in America do not experience an environment that fulfills these requirements. Some thrive nonetheless; others suffer great harm as they strive to accomplish developmental tasks. These issues are discussed in Chapter 221.

Local government, community- and faith-based organizations, health care systems, and the media are also potent mediators of adolescent development. They can collaborate to create an environment that fosters healthy development. For example, a program to reduce the occurrence of unintended pregnancies among unmarried adolescents in part of a South Carolina county was successful through a variety of messages targeted at parents, teachers, public school students, representatives of faith-based organizations, and community leaders. Individual organizations may also provide life skills training that offsets inadequacies in other learning environments. "Life skills" as used here means, for example, conflict resolution, friendship formation, peer resistance, and assertiveness.

DEVELOPMENTAL STRESSORS, PSYCHOLOGICAL FUNCTIONING, AND MENTAL HEALTH

Virtually every adolescent encounters a certain set of stressful developmental challenges that can affect psychological functioning. Some of these are listed in Box 231-3. Some youth manage these transitions better than others do. Those who cope well tend to have higher self-esteem and self-efficacy, and so experience less anxiety. Youth who are

Box 231-3. Universal Developmental Stressors of Adolescence

Puberty
Beginning, end, and change of school (e.g., elementary school to junior high/middle school)
Disagreements with parents over rules
Learning to drive
Sexual exploration
Breaking up with boyfriend/girlfriend
Gainful employment
Graduation from high school
Moving away from home
Matriculation in college

unduly stressed by these transitions often do not recognize that they are. They may present with a variety of symptoms, such as fatigue, headaches, or abdominal pain. The pediatrician can be of great help to these adolescents by discussing the stressful nature of adolescence and helping the patient identify and apply simple coping strategies (see Chapter 250).

In our society, most youth are subject to developmental stressors beyond the universal ones (see Box 231-3). These stressors, which are present in a unique individual constellation, are often present in multiple personal and social settings. Many of these are listed in Table 231-2, as are factors that can lessen their impact. For example, many youth live in poverty or in another adverse environment, surroundings that are not conducive to healthy adolescent development. Concerns over worldwide events such as nuclear war and, more recently, terrorism are common and may be intrusive.

Two Stressors: Pubertal Status and Pubertal Timing

Pubertal status and pubertal timing provide examples of universal and personal stressors that affect psychological functioning in early adolescence. *Pubertal status* refers to the changes experienced concurrently with physical maturation. Advancing pubertal status is thus a universal stressor of adolescence. Boys appear to have improved body image and mood as puberty progresses. Girls, not surprisingly considering our cultural norms, feel less attractive as the pubertal stage advances and they gain weight. They also have more conflicts with their parents. *Pubertal timing* refers to the timing of physical changes relative to others of the same age. The onset of puberty significantly earlier (in girls) or later (in boys) than in same-sex peers is a developmental stressor. This stressor is individual, however, rather than universal.

Boys who experience puberty earlier and girls who experience it later than their peers have better body image and higher self-esteem. Conversely, early maturing girls and late maturing boys are most likely to have poor psychological outcomes. Among other factors, the effects of pubertal timing are greatly influenced by social relationships and roles. The early maturing boy, for example, has increased muscle mass relative to his peers. This not only enhances the masculinity of his appearance; it improves his performance in many sports. The girl who develops breasts before her female classmates feels out of place. She is likely to be teased by her generally prepubescent male classmates, while older boys may make sexual advances for which she is not prepared. Her pubertal weight spurt results in deposition in body fat, which conflicts with her desire for thinness.

Developmental Stressors and Mental Health

The previous discussion of pubertal status and pubertal timing demonstrates how developmental stressors affect psychological functioning. It is not surprising, then, that most adolescents at some time evidence symptoms of psychological dysfunction. The vast majority of adolescents develop normally nonetheless.

Box 232-4. Great Ormond Street Classification for Disordered Eating in Children

Anorexia Nervosa

Determined weight loss
Body image distortion
Morbid preoccupation with weight or shape

Bulimia Nervosa

Recurrent binges and purging
Lack of control over binge/purge behavior
Morbid preoccupation with weight or shape

Food Avoidance Emotional Disorder

Food avoidance (not attributable to another disorder)
Weight loss
Mood disturbance (not meeting criteria for a primary affective disorder)
No body image distortion
No morbid preoccupation with weight or shape
No organic brain disease or psychosis

Selective Eating

Narrow range of foods for at least 2 years
Unwillingness to try new foods
No body image distortion
No fear of choking or vomiting
Low, normal, or high weight

Functional Dysphagia

Food avoidance
Fear of swallowing, choking, or vomiting
No body image distortion
No morbid preoccupation with weight or shape
No organic brain disease or psychosis

Adapted from Nicholls D, Chater R, Lask B: Children into DSM don't go: A comparison of classification systems for eating disorders in childhood and early adolescence. Int J Eat Disord 2000;28:317–324. Copyright © 2000 Wiley Periodicals, Inc., A Wiley Company. Reprinted with permission of John Wiley & Sons, Inc.

tent with eating disorders (see Boxes 232-1 to 232-4). Some patients with eating disorders will be secretive and mistrustful or may lack the capacity to describe their behavior accurately, which makes assessment more difficult. Follow-up visits or additional information from family members or friends may clarify an otherwise ambiguous case. Other characteristics that are common with eating disorders include preference for eating alone, extremely limited food choices, unusual eating habits, excessive fluid intake, excessive chewing of ice or gum, or recent vegetarianism. The typical "layered look" attire of eating disorder patients may also be a helpful diagnostic sign. Patients whose initial presentation is consistent with a diagnosis of an eating disorder do not require exhaustive medical evaluations. On the other hand, when the typical features of eating disorders are absent, alternative medical or psychiatric diagnoses should be fully explored while also considering the possibility of denial or intentional deception. All patients should be screened for suicidal ideation and intentional self-harm, which are especially common among patients with bulimia nervosa.

Nutritional Assessment. Nutritional assessment should include eating and exercise patterns, a history of weight changes or previous dieting practices, and history of any purging behaviors. A careful diet history should be obtained, including overall caloric intake and intake of specific nutrients, especially calcium. Many patients with eating disorders develop obsessional preoccupations with counting calories, fat grams, or with restricting fat or carbohydrate intake. Peculiar eating habits, driven by these or similar obsessions, are common. Weight and height should be measured with the patient undressed and gowned. Body mass index (BMI) (see Chapter 2) must be calculated as it more accurately reflects weight-height relationships than do traditional "growth curves" or standard height-weight tables. Age- and gender-specific percentile tables for BMI are available for both adolescents and adults.

Medical Evaluation. Initial medical evaluation helps to exclude other diagnoses and to identify the extent of systemic and organ-system dysfunction. Patients with eating disorders frequently complain of cold distal extremities, fatigue, mood changes, poor concentration and memory, early satiety, abdominal pain, and constipation. Symptoms or signs of hemodynamic instability should be identified, such as orthostasis, syncope, presyncope, or palpitations. Purging behaviors (vomiting, diuretic use, laxative use) may all cause potentially dangerous electrolyte disturbances. Patients should be examined for stigmata of self-induced vomiting, which include parotid enlargement, soft palate lesions, dental erosions, or calluses of the knuckles (Russell sign). Patients with self-induced vomiting often have symptoms of gastroesophageal reflux disease or concomitant unintentional vomiting.

Essential laboratory studies in all patients include measurement of serum electrolytes, serum calcium, serum magnesium, and serum phosphorus. An electrocardiogram should be done, in particular looking for evidence of a prolonged QTc interval. Fractionation of serum amylase and quantification of the salivary isozyme can be helpful when surreptitious vomiting is suspected. In patients with atypical presentations the laboratory evaluation must be sufficient to rule out other diagnostic considerations. Depending on the specific symptoms and signs, this might include erythrocyte sedimentation rate (ESR), thyroid function studies, serum glucose, serologic testing, or imaging studies of the head or gastrointestinal tract.

MANAGEMENT

Principles of Treatment

The management of eating disorders requires an integrated, comprehensive approach that addresses the psychological, medical, and nutritional aspects of the disease. Psychiatric intervention is aimed at treating the underlying psychopathology, correcting distorted views of eating and body image, and identifying and managing comorbid psychiatric conditions. Nutritional intervention is required to assess the current nutritional status and diet, to provide accurate nutritional information, and to help provide structured dietary recommendations to patients whose dietary judgment is nearly always severely impaired. Medical supervision is required to identify and manage somatic consequences of disordered eating; to guard against life-threatening sequelae of starvation, malnutrition, and purging; and to anticipate and prevent complications of re-feeding. The array of services required to manage patients with eating disorders may be delivered in an eating disorder unit or center, by an interdisciplinary team that includes physicians, mental health professionals, and nutritionists, or by individual health care providers who communicate regularly with each other. However it is provided, the approach should be interdisciplinary and coordinated. It is rare for a patient with an eating disorder to be successfully managed by the pediatrician, therapist, or nutritionist working alone.

The decision to hospitalize a patient for inpatient management of an eating disorder is based on clinical factors, availability of resources, insurance coverage, and patient/family preference. Absolute indications for hospitalization include hemodynamic instability, cardiac arrhythmia, congestive heart failure or cardiomyopathy, and suicidality. Acute food refusal, uncontrollable vomiting, or failure of appropriate outpatient therapy are also indications for inpatient admission (Box 232-5). Most experts agree that once severe malnutrition has occurred, outpatient therapy is unlikely to be effective. In these cases, hospitalization permits behavioral interventions that are difficult to enforce in the outpatient setting, such as explicit written contracts, structured diets, nutritional supplementation, and activity restrictions. These can be useful tools in working with patients whose dysfunctional eating habits are deeply entrenched or where the disorder is compounded by lack of insight, denial, or cognitive deficits attributable to malnutrition. For younger patients, early hospitalization may prevent the development of intractable symptoms and the need for repeated hospitalization.

Adolescents with eating disorders frequently resist the diagnosis and treatment recommendations, which makes intervention efforts difficult and at times ineffective. The clinician must state the diagnosis as unambiguously as possible and support it with as much objective information as possible. Directly linking physical symptoms and signs to the malnutrition or purging that caused them can sometimes help to overcome denial or minimization. Frustration, guilt, and helplessness often characterize the feelings of family members of patients with eating disorders. Family relationships are often strained by well-intentioned but unsuccessful attempts by family members to manage the

problem themselves. Some family members can become confused, frustrated, or angry with the patient for what they see as a lack of commitment to correcting dysfunctional eating habits.

The management of eating disorders typically requires protracted efforts over an extended period of time. Early in therapy, frequent visits are helpful in developing a therapeutic alliance to provide nutritional re-education and close medical supervision. As progress is seen, visits can be less frequent and tailored to meet the patient's psychological, nutritional, and medical needs.

Medical Management

Medical complications of eating disorders are common, potentially dangerous, and can affect any organ system. Because patients with eating disorders are so often reluctant to disclose their symptoms, health care providers must be vigilant for early signs of organ system involvement. Furthermore, many of the most serious medical complications of eating disorders may present suddenly and catastrophically. A high index of suspicion and careful medical surveillance are crucial.

Over time, malnutrition leads to a decline in metabolic rate and an inability to maintain body temperature. Patients are cold-intolerant and especially complain of cold hands and feet. Energy level is low, patients are fatigued, and psychomotor retardation may be impressive. Cognitive impairment can be detected by means of formal neuropsychological testing and affects concentration, memory, and problem solving. Structural brain changes have been seen with computed tomography (CT) or magnetic resonance imaging (MRI) scanning. These changes are of uncertain etiology and significance, but presumably arise as a direct effect of malnutrition. More worrisome, there is emerging evidence to suggest these changes may be irreversible. Depression, irritability, and other mood changes are also common.

Cardiovascular changes are among the most frequent complications of eating disorders. Bradycardia occurs as a consequence of decreased basal metabolic rate. Patients are typically asymptomatic despite low heart rates, which may reach the 40s and 30s. Hypotension and orthostatic blood pressure changes are also commonly seen. Electrocardiographic findings include nonspecific ST-segment changes and prolongation of the QRS, PR, and QTc intervals. Prolongation of the QTc interval, which has been associated with an increased risk of sudden cardiac death, is especially common in eating disordered patients who purge, and in settings of hypokalemia or hypomagnesemia. In anorexia nervosa, cardiac adaptation to a lower cardiac output may lead to a functional and reversible mitral valve prolapse.

Gastroesophogeal reflux, Mallory-Weiss tears of the esophagus, and upper gastrointestinal bleeding may occur in any patient whose eating disorder involves vomiting. In patients who restrict their intake, both gastric emptying time and total gastrointestinal transit time increase, causing postprandial fullness and abdominal pain. Constipation is frequent. Though gastrointestinal symptoms usually resolve with re-feeding, this resolution may lag well behind the restoration of normal body weight or the cessation of binge eating and purging. This is significant, since persistent

---

Box 232-5. Indications for Hospitalization

Hemodynamic instability
Cardiac dysrhythmias
Congestive heart failure or cardiomyopathy
Severe hypovolemia
Severe electrolyte disturbances
Severe hematemesis
Severe malnutrition
Acute food refusal
Intractable vomiting
Suicidality
Failure of outpatient therapy

have criticized this as an arbitrary judgment of what constitutes a "serious" suicide attempt. *Self-mutilation* refers to any deliberate act of self-harm in which the person doesn't consciously intend to die, regardless of motive. The term *parasuicidal act* refers to the spectrum of suicide attempts and self-harm, regardless of the motive or perceived lethality. *Suicidal ideation* consists of thoughts of actively killing one's self. *Passive death thoughts* are thoughts about being dead without the self as agent.

When describing a parasuicidal act, description of the level of risk and the potential for rescue is helpful. Risk is the degree of lethality or risk of death, from very low (holding one's breath or making superficial scratches on the wrist) to very high (jumping from a 70-foot cliff or firing a gun at the head). Potential for rescue also ranges from very low (as when the individual is isolated in the wilderness) to very high (as when the individual slowly performs the act in front of others in the hospital).

FUNDAMENTALS

Suicide, the third leading cause of death in youth aged 10 to 19 years, accounts for over 2000 deaths annually. The suicide rate in adolescents older than age 14 has tripled since the 1950s, and is now roughly equal to that of the general population. In adolescents aged 15 to 19 the annual incidence of suicide is approximately 1 in 10,000. The number-one method used in completed adolescent suicides is firearms, with hanging a distant second. In contrast, medication overdose is the leading method used in suicide attempts.

The vast majority of adolescents, including depressed adolescents, do not commit suicide. In this sense suicide is a rare event, an exceptional behavior. This makes suicide unpredictable in individual patients, and means that even with "perfect" clinical management suicide can still occur. Clinicians cannot predict the future behaviors of patients. What clinicians can do is estimate the degree of risk, and use this assessment to make decisions that will lower the risk. Clinicians can play a role in preventing suicide by reducing the risk in their patient population.

Certain patient traits correlate statistically with suicide, over the short term (weeks to months) and over the long term (years). These risk factors are sensitive but nonspecific (i.e., well over half of adolescents who commit suicide have a mood disorder, but most adolescents with a mood disorder will not commit suicide). Risk factors are difficult to quantify and there is a paucity of research on their interactions. The most significant risk factors are listed in Box 233-1.

PRESENTATION AND INITIAL EVALUATION

The level of suicide risk must be assessed in every patient who appears to have any increased risk (Box 233-2). This assessment can be very difficult. A good suicide risk assessment requires time, and clinicians may not anticipate the risk in patients presenting with a separate primary complaint. The inherent uncertainty of suicide can provoke tremendous anxiety in clinicians. If a patient is uncooperative, some clinicians feel resentful or view the patient as

---

Box 233-1. Risk Factors for Suicide in Adolescents

1. Demographics/Past Behaviors
   Male gender*
   Previous suicide attempt or parasuicidal activity (may be higher risk for high lethality, if low rescue potential, or within last year)*
   Psychiatric hospitalization within the last year
   Family history of suicide
2. Psychiatric Diagnoses/Personality Traits
   Active mood disorder*
   Active alcohol or drug abuse*
   Active psychosis
   Antisocial or borderline personality or history of persistent impulsive behavior
   Perfectionistic personality traits
3. Stressors
   Severe anxiety, agitation, or insomnia (potent short-term risk)*
   Feelings of hopelessness or being overwhelmed
   Suicidal ideation, plan, or intent (more risk with plan and expressed intent) peer isolation or recent peer rejection (including romantic breakup)
   School difficulties
   Family dysfunction or marked conflict
   Conflict over sexual identity
   Recent peer suicide or publicized suicide

* Highest risk factors.

---

manipulative or attention seeking. Managing these feelings can help to avoid unconsciously hastening or avoiding the assessment.

Suicide risk assessment is an opportunity. Clinicians with a long-standing primary care relationship are uniquely positioned to obtain crucial history. When conducted carefully, the assessment can be both diagnostic and therapeutic. Asking about suicide will not increase risk or "put ideas in their head." On the contrary, adolescents at risk may be quite relieved to talk frankly about their despair.

Box 233-3 lists important information to obtain in the interview. When asking about suicidal ideation, it is helpful to inquire in a stepwise fashion as described in Box 233-4. This progression can help place positive responses in context, making the adolescent feel less "crazy." Interviewing the family is crucial to a complete assessment and is essential for a reasonable estimation of the risk.

Many clinicians mistakenly rely entirely on the patient's expressed suicidal ideation, without considering other risk factors. Risk factors are multiplicative. Suicidal ideation is only one of many risk factors that correlates with suicide (see Box 233-1). Between 50% and 80% of adolescents report contemplating the idea of suicide at one time or

---

Box 233-2. Patient Presentations That Should Prompt a Suicide Risk Assessment

Presence of mood, thought, or anxiety disorder
Presence of alcohol or drug abuse
Suicidal ideation
Parasuicidal activity of any kind
Marked distress, hopelessness, or loss

Box 233-3. Information to Obtain in a Suicide Risk Assessment

Presence of mood or anxiety disorder

Alcohol and drug use

Current and recent mood, outlook, passive death thoughts, suicidal ideation, intent, and plan

History of previous suicidal ideation and previous parasuicidal activity, including context and precipitants, lethality, rescue

Current stressors, conflicts, or perceptions of failure

School functioning and peer relationships, recent breakups or losses, recent peer suicides

Family psychiatric and suicide history, current family functioning and relations

---

another, so taken alone it is a statistically normal behavior. In the context of a suicide risk assessment, the clinician must take suicidal ideation seriously, while not relying on ideation alone to assess the risk.

Although several standardized instruments for assessing suicide risk exist, most have no information on sensitivity, specificity, or positive predictive values. Furthermore, most have been developed for adults, not adolescents. Standardized suicide risk questionnaires are not a substitute for a clinical interview, and have great potential for misuse in a busy medical practice.

The degree of suicide risk may be estimated as minimal (no or very few risk factors for suicide), low, moderate, or high (multiple risk factors in many domains leading to a substantial likelihood of suicide). Risk factors should be classified and noted as chronic, new, or a mixture of both. These levels are subjective estimates and somewhat arbitrary; there is no validated formula for calculating an exact risk in each individual. Nonetheless, estimating the degree of risk is necessary to guide the immediate disposition of the patient.

MANAGEMENT

When faced with an adolescent at increased risk for suicide, two aspects of management are important. First, the clinician must address the short-term safety of the patient to protect him or her during the period of heightened risk. Second, the physician must initiate treatment for reversible risk factors to reduce the level of risk. The family fills a crucial role in both these aspects. The safety of the patient outweighs concerns about confidentiality. Before the patient returns to the home, the physician must ensure that the family is informed about the relevant risk factors, level

---

Box 233-4. The "Ladder" of Suicide Questions

How bad do you feel? What is it like?

Do you ever wish you were dead?

Have you had thoughts of taking your life? Of hurting yourself?

Have you thought of how you would do it? How close have you come to this?

Do you want to kill yourself? How much of you wants to die, and how much wants to live?

When will you do it?

---

of risk, and the presence of suicidal ideation, plan, or intent. If firearms are present in the home, the clinician should urge the family to remove or disable them.

For patients at low suicide risk, outpatient treatment is usually sufficient for both safety and treatment goals. The risk of suicide should be discussed with patients and their families. They should have a clear place to call or go should the patient's distress or suicidal ideation intensify. Safety and treatment are aided by regular appointments, with clear follow-up set after every visit and telephone follow-up for missed appointments. Reversible risk factors such as depression should be treated aggressively. Consultation or referral to a mental health specialist may not be necessary if the clinician is comfortable with the assessment and treatment of risk factors present.

For patients at moderate or high suicide risk, the primary care provider should arrange immediate consultation with a specialist. Consultation can be helpful to confirm the assessment, guide short-term safety options, and assist with more comprehensive psychiatric treatment if indicated. Consultation may also be needed to access more intensive management options such as inpatient hospitalization. At a minimum, these patients need very close and regular outpatient follow-up along with aggressive treatment.

Sometimes patients with moderate to high risk refuse treatment or refuse to answer crucial questions, after repeated but unsuccessful efforts to engage them. In these cases consultation with a specialist is invaluable. The patient's safety must take precedence. Occasionally, involuntary treatment is necessary. Laws vary by state; in many areas physicians cannot initiate treatment with adolescents older than a certain age who refuse. If necessary, the police may be contacted to ensure the immediate safety and control of the patient. In most jurisdictions police also initiate involuntary treatment when necessary.

No-self-harm contracts are informal verbal or written agreements by adolescent patients that they will not harm themselves or act on their suicidal thinking. Some patients report that making an agreement is helpful in inhibiting parasuicidal behaviors. These contracts may also aid in building a physician-patient alliance, clarifying a crisis plan, and reducing the anxiety of the clinician. They are not legally binding and have not been shown to be universally protective or predictive. While inviting discussion, no-self-harm contracts are not a substitute for sound risk assessment and management.

As with any clinical work, documentation of the risk factors, assessment, and plan are very important. Medicolegally, clinicians are not responsible for predicting the future or successfully guessing which patients are "suicidal." Rather, they must demonstrate that they assessed the risk for suicide when indicated, decided on reasonable management, and obtained consultation if the risk was high or management uncertain.

OUTCOME

The outcome for any individual at risk of suicide is uncertain. The vast majority of adolescents at risk do not commit suicide. Good risk management will decrease but not eliminate this risk and, with time and experience, the generalist may save lives. Aggressive treatment of underlying disorders and psychosocial stressors can reduce morbidity as well as mortality.

FOLLOW-UP

When patients are referred to any aspect of the mental health system, the primary care physician still has an important role to play. The patient and family may reveal information to their primary care physician that they do not reveal to a mental health professional, especially if the relationship with the primary care physician is long-standing. The primary care physician can provide feedback regarding the effectiveness of psychiatric treatments and their interaction with other somatic conditions and treatments. Communication with mental health professionals is crucial, but can be frustratingly difficult. In many areas, a variety of systemic barriers make communication between the physical and mental health systems much more difficult than communication with other specialists. Forming relationships with the local mental health systems and problem-solving if there are any communication barriers can pay huge dividends.

Mini-index of Related Topics

SUGGESTED READINGS

American Academy of Pediatrics, Committee on Adolescence: Suicide and suicide attempts in adolescents. Pediatrics 2000;105:871–874. Available at: www.aap.org/policy/re9928.html.

American Association of Suicidology. Available at: www.suicidology.org/index.html.

National Center for Health Statistics. Available at: www.cdc.gov/nchs/fastats/suicide.htm.

National Center for Injury Prevention and Control (a CDC site). Available at: www.cdc.gov/ncipc/ncipchm.htm.

National Youth Violence Prevention Resource Center. Available at: www.safeyouth.org/topics [select "violence prevention topics," then "suicide"].

SECTION 6 ADOLESCENT CARE: *Adolescent Mental Health*

234 Alcohol, Tobacco, and Other Drug Use

Patricia K. Kokotailo

ROLE OF THE GENERALIST

1. Know the extent and nature of community use of alcohol, tobacco, and other drugs.
2. Recognize the risk factors and signs of substance abuse.
3. Offer appropriate anticipatory guidance and prevention strategies.
4. Evaluate the nature and extent of substance use.
5. Interview adolescents and maintain confidentiality.
6. Refer patients for appropriate substance abuse treatment.
7. Serve an advocacy role in prevention and treatment.

DEFINITION

The definition of substance abuse is complicated by the many different terms that describe alcohol and other drug (AOD) use by adolescents and other youths. Specialists and clinicians variously employ terms such as *use*, *misuse*, *abuse*, *dependence*, and *addiction*. The criteria from the current *Diagnostic and Statistical Manual of Mental Disorders (DSM-IV)* of the American Psychiatric Association provide for strict definitions for diagnosing substance use and dependence and emphasize the concept of a maladaptive pattern of AOD use that leads to clinically significant impairment or distress. Because use of alcohol and illicit drugs is illegal for those younger than 21 years of age, as is the purchase of tobacco products in most states, use can be considered a form of abuse. Regardless of whether AOD use fits the DSM-IV criteria for substance disorders, many experts agree that any AOD use that leads to major impairment or distress in life is a problem and therefore of concern. Some children have also been inadvertent victims of substance abuse through the passive transfer of alcohol and drugs via the placenta during fetal life or postnatally during breast-feeding. The health implications for children and adolescents of passive inhalation of drugs that are smoked has also been reported.

Besides the toxic effects of drugs themselves, there are indirect effects on the health of the adolescent. AOD use is linked with other adolescent risk behaviors such as early sexual activity and the risk of sexually transmitted disease, violence, academic failure, school problems, and delinquency. Intravenous drug use also poses a major hazard for the contraction of acquired immunodeficiency syndrome (AIDS) and other blood-borne diseases. The 2003 Youth Risk Behavior Surveillance System survey, developed by the Centers for Disease Control and Prevention (CDC), found that during the 30 days before the survey, 30.2% of 9th to 12th graders rode with a driver who had been drinking alcohol and 12.1% of students drove a vehicle themselves after drinking alcohol. In 1998 the CDC reported that 38% of all fatal motor vehicle crashes are associated with the AOD use, and a high proportion of homicides and suicides among youth are also AOD related. Both psychiatric symptoms and disorders are common among adolescents who have substance use disorders, and diagnosis can be difficult because it is frequently unclear if symptoms are a consequence of AOD use or part of a comorbid psychiatric disorder. Depression is the most common psychiatric symptom seen in adolescents with substance abuse disorders, but affective disorders are present in a significant minority of patients and may need specific treatment.

EPIDEMIOLOGY

After a long period of decline in drug use from peaks in the late 1970s and early 1980s, drug use rose in the early 1990s among 8th-, 10th-, and 12th-grade students in the United States, as measured by the Monitoring the Future Survey, one of the largest longitudinal surveys of adolescent AOD use and attitudes toward use. During the 1990s the peak rates for use of any illicit drug were in 1996 or 1997; since then, use of any illicit drug has remained fairly level in grades 10 and 12, with a steady, gradual decline among 8th graders. In 2003 use of any illicit drug in the previous year declined for all three grade levels. In 2003 use of several specific drugs, including marijuana, LSD, and methylenedioxymethamphetamine (MDMA, or "ecstasy") declined, although not for all grade levels. Cocaine use has held fairly steady since 1999, but rates are much lower than during the height of cocaine use in the early to mid-1980s and modestly down from recent peaks in the mid-1990s. Over half (51%) of American young people have tried an illicit drug by the time they finish high school.

Marijuana use showed the sharpest increase among illicit drugs in the early and mid-1990s, and now shows some gradual decline or stability in use. Marijuana is still the most widely used illicit drug. In 2003 the annual prevalence rates in grades 8, 10, and 12 were 12.8%, 28.2%, and 34.9%, respectively. The rise in marijuana use in the early and mid-1990s was mirrored by a sharp decline in perceived risks of using marijuana, but in the late 1990s there was some turnaround in this belief. In 2003 the perceived risk of marijuana use increased in all three grades, generating a more positive picture than in previous years.

In the late 1990s and early years of the 21st century, some of the most important increases in drug use were in MDMA use among 8th, 10th, and 12th graders. In 2002 ecstasy use dropped for the first time in recent years and continued to do so in 2003. Ecstasy and other drugs such as methamphetamine, gamma-hydroxybutyrate (GHB), flunitrazepam (Rohypnol), and ketamine are included in the term *club drugs*, which refers to drugs reportedly used at all-night parties and "rave" dance clubs and bars. The decline in use in 2002 was not entirely unexpected, as more young people reported perceiving the drug as dangerous in the preceding year. Ecstasy use was down in 2003 for all three time periods measured (lifetime, annual, and 30-day use) for 8th, 10th, and 12th graders. Declines from 2001 to 2003 ranged from 40% to 50%. Use of other club drugs appears to be either decreasing or at a constant level, but note that many other types of drugs can also be used in club settings.

Ecstasy or MDMA, a form of methamphetamine, has psychostimulant and psychedelic properties. It is an "empathogen" or "enactogen," producing a feeling of great self-awareness and insight. Regular ecstasy use is associated with persistent depression of mood, elevated anxiety, anger and hostility, impulsiveness, sensation seeking, and novelty seeking. The most important acute adverse event after MDMA use is hyperthermia, which contributes greatly to seizures, cerebral hemorrhage, cardiac arrest, rhabdomyolysis, and disseminated intravascular coagulation, all of which can be fatal, and hepatotoxicity, which has required liver transplants. Recent studies show that very high or even moderate doses of MDMA destroy the axons and axon terminals of seratonin-containing neurons. Studies regarding the neurotoxicity of the drug are significant for possible long-term or perhaps even permanent learning and memory problems with prolonged use.

The use of anabolic steroids has been more variable. Use rose sharply among 8th and 10th graders in 1999. In 2002 steroid use remained flat among 8th, 10th, and 12th graders, but at historically high levels. In 2003 use declined. Rates of use have been considerably lower among girls than among boys.

Inhalant use is the intentional inhalation of a volatile substance to induce a euphoric state. Types of substances inhaled include hydrocarbons, propellants, nitrous oxide, and other anesthetics. Gasoline, solvents (such as toluene), or substituted fluorohydrocarbon propellants from aerosol cans can cause brief euphoria when inhaled in a plastic bag or enclosed space. Such practices, occurring among early adolescents seeking an inexpensive "high," are associated with dangerous side effects on the heart, brain, and liver. Cardiac arrhythmias and sudden death, termed *sudden sniffing death*, may be induced by fluorocarbons or halogenated hydrocarbons. Anoxia is a risk. Central nervous system damage, peripheral neuropathy, seizures, liver and renal damage, and coma have all been observed after inhalant use. The use of inhalants declined through the end of the 1990s, but use is still the highest among 8th graders, as compared to 10th and 12th graders.

Cigarette smoking is the single largest cause of preventable morbidity and mortality in the United States, and is truly a pediatric disease, with the great majority of habitual smoking beginning in childhood and adolescence. Data about adolescent smoking can be found in Chapter 22.

Alcohol use remained fairly stable during the late 1990s as measured by the Monitoring the Future Survey, but some declines in use were seen in 2003. The numbers of adolescents using are still alarming. In 2003, 20% of 8th graders, 35% of 10th graders, and 48% of 12 graders used alcohol in the 30 days previous to the survey. Seventy-seven percent of high school students have consumed alcohol by the end of high school and about half (45.6%) have done so by 8th grade. In addition, 58.1% of 12th graders and 20.3% of 8th graders report being drunk at least once in their lives. Binge drinking, or the intake of five or more drinks in a row at least once in a 2-week period, is prevalent but appears to be leveling to declining in recent years.

RISK FACTORS AND PROBLEM RECOGNITION ISSUES

There are a number of risk factors associated with the frequent use of alcohol or other drugs by adolescents. Such risk factors may help to identify adolescents who are most vulnerable to developing problems, but it is also important to examine adolescent AOD use along a continuum. Some adolescents progress to heavy or dependent use from experimental use, but for others, even experimental use can

---

Box 234-1. Risk Factors for Substance Abuse

1. Behavioral factors
   Antisocial behavior
   Aggressiveness
   Negative affect
   Impulsivity
2. Cognitive factors
   Attention deficit disorder
   Learning disabilities
   School problems
3. Psychological well-being
   Depression
   Low self-esteem
4. Family problems
   Family history of alcohol or other drug abuse
   Conflicted families
   Permissiveness or authoritarianism
5. Community factors
   Ready availability of alcohol and other drugs
   Tolerance for use of alcohol and other drugs
6. Other factors
   Early onset of use
   History of sexual abuse
   Association with drug-using peers

Box 234-2. Resiliency and Protective Factors for Substance Abuse

Clear parent-defined conduct norms
Strong attachment of adolescents to parents
Siblings who are intolerant of drug use
Parents who provide praise and encouragement, develop trust, and are sensitive to their children's needs

---

lead to major morbidity or mortality, especially with drinking and driving. It is therefore important to realize that all adolescents are at risk for AOD problems, but that some are at greatly increased risk. Risk factors and resiliency factors are listed in Boxes 234-1 and 234-2, respectively.

As a routine part of health supervision visits, the pediatric physician should assess the risk of AOD use by reviewing risk factors and behaviors with adolescents and their parent(s). A general psychosocial assessment of the adolescent's functioning is felt to be the most important component of screening for AOD problems and related risk behaviors. In order for the clinician to obtain valid information, the adolescent must trust the interviewer and know that confidentiality is operational. Although there are many interviewing techniques that can be employed, and interviewing may be done in conjunction with a screening questionnaire, general interviewing techniques of establishing rapport, interviewing the adolescent alone, using open-ended questions, and progressing from less threatening to more threatening questions are useful. The HEADS psychosocial screen, in which H = home, E = education/employment, A = activities, D = drugs, S = sexuality/suicide, can serve as a guideline for open-ended questions relating to these areas; problems in one area may be related to problems in others. The CAGE mnemonic (Box 234-3) can be used in screening for AOD use in this context, and positive questions can lead to further inquiry about quantity, frequency, and consequences of use. The CAGE questions can be adapted to inquiry about the AOD use of a parent or other person in the adolescent's life, as well. Two other screening tools used with adolescents include the RAFFT and CRAFFT screens (Boxes 234-4 and 234-5). In the recommendations arising from the initial validation of the CRAFFT screen, one positive answer to the screening questions indicates the advisability of further evaluation of the patient by a health profession; two positive answers suggests the need for referral for formal assessment or treatment. Further validation study has concluded that a score of 2 or higher was optimal for identifying any problem, disorder, or dependence. Other brief paper-and-pencil screening tools, such as the Perceived-Benefits-of-Drinking Scale (PBDS) and the Alcohol Use Disorders Identification Test (AUDIT), as well as lengthier instruments may also be helpful screens.

DIAGNOSIS AND MANAGEMENT

Once an adolescent has screened positive for alcohol or other drug problems, assessment is necessary to establish a diagnosis. Assessment is a lengthier procedure that determines the extent rather than the existence of a problem,

Box 234-3. CAGE Screening Questions

Have you ever felt the need to **C**ut down on drinking (drug use)?

Have you ever felt **A**nnoyed by criticism about your drinking (drug use)?

Have you ever felt **G**uilty about something you did or said while you were drinking (using drugs)?

Have you ever taken a morning **E**ye-opener?

Box 234-5. CRAFFT Screening Questions

Have you ever ridden in a **Ca**r driven by someone (including yourself) who was "high" or who had been using alcohol or drugs?

Do you ever use alcohol or drugs to **R**elax, feel better about yourself, or fit in?

Do you ever use alcohol or drugs while you are **A**lone?

Do you ever **F**orget things you did while using alcohol or drugs?

Do your family or **F**riends ever tell you that you should cut down on your drinking or drug use?

Have you ever gotten in **T**rouble while you were using alcohol or drugs?

Adapted from Knight JR, Schrier LA, Bravender TD, et al: CRAFFT: A new brief screen for adolescent substance abuse. Arch Pediatr Adolesc 1999;153:591–596. Copyright © 1999. All rights reserved. Reproduced by permission.

explores comorbidities, and assists in treatment planning. Assessment may include a detailed history, mental status, physical examination, questionnaires, standardized tests, and laboratory screening. Urine drug screening does not provide a definitive diagnosis, but is a spot test for the presence of drug metabolites. Although such testing can be helpful in determining type of drug use and ongoing use and in monitoring abstinence, it is subject to laboratory technical cutoff point specifications, the timing of substance use and subsequent persistence of metabolites in the body, and adulteration of specimens by the patient. Pediatric health care providers must therefore interpret urine tests within a clinical context and use them in conjunction with interviewing. Assessment may be beyond the time and expertise limitations of many pediatricians, but all health care providers need to be able to screen and refer patients for appropriate treatment.

Treatment can be in inpatient and outpatient settings and include such modalities as group and individual therapy, self-help groups, family counseling, structured day programs, and short- and long-term residential therapy. Treatment modalities that involve families have been shown by most research to be more effective. Sustaining abstinence from AOD use requires that adolescents learn about the dangers of drugs, learn refusal skills, avoid drug-using peers, connect with nonusing peers, and develop positive alternatives to AOD use. Health care providers should be involved in follow-up to encourage and monitor abstinence and provide ongoing support and counseling.

PREVENTION

Primary prevention efforts are the most effective in decreasing the prevalence of smoking. The National Cancer Institute has proposed five physician activities, all beginning with the letter A to aid in smoking prevention and cessation for children and adolescents (Box 234-6). During the child's adolescence, the focus shifts to the young person from the family and parents. Cessation techniques include counseling the adolescent with subsequent setting of a quit date and making a contract to quit. Nicotine replacement systems such as nicotine gum and patches can be utilized, but supervision is important (see Chapter 22).

Inclusion of AOD topic discussion as part of anticipatory guidance and screening at visits for issues such as poorly explained trauma, chronic pain, or chronic fatigue as well as at routine health supervision is important. Patient-physician discussion, peer counseling, and computer-assisted interviewing and instruction are effective ways to educate about health risks associated with AOD use. Although pediatric health care providers should advocate for no tobacco, alcohol, or drug use by youth younger than 21 years of age, the most urgent messages in terms of long-term health are not to use tobacco products, not to drink or use drugs and then drive, and not to ride with those who have used drugs or alcohol. Providers can assist adolescents coping with peer pressure; aid parents in developing strategies for anticipating, avoiding, or coping with behavioral issues; and provide supervision and monitoring of behavior. They can also help to strengthen protective factors among adolescents by encouraging their participation in organized school and community activities and the maintenance of family rituals. Office strategies can include providing appropriate pamphlets, posters, and other media information, as well as providing age-appropriate prevention messages for younger as well as older patients. Becoming involved in school and community-wide substance-abuse prevention activities and

Box 234-4. RAFFT Screening Questions

Do you drink or use drugs to **R**elax, feel better about yourself, or fit in?

Do you ever drink alcohol or use drugs when you are **A**lone?

Do you or any of your closest **F**riends drink or use drugs?

Does a close **F**amily member have a problem with alcohol or drug use?

Have you ever gotten into **T**rouble as a result of drinking or drug use (e.g., truancy, bad grades, trouble with the law or parents)?

Adapted from Riggs SG, Alario AJ: Adolescent substance use: Instructor's guide. In Dube CE, Goldstein MG, Lewis DC, et al (eds): The Project ADEPT Curriculum for Primary Care Physician Training. Providence, RI, Project ADEPT, Brown University, 1989, p 26.

Box 234-6. Physician Activities to Aid in Smoking Prevention and Cessation

Anticipatory guidance

Ask

Advise

Assist

Arrange follow-up examination

legislative action are other ways to promote child and adolescent health.

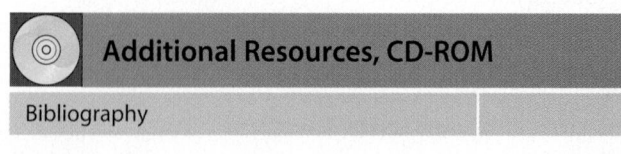

Additional Resources, CD-ROM

| Bibliography | |

SUGGESTED READINGS

American Academy of Pediatrics: Tobacco, alcohol, and other drugs: The role of the pediatrician in prevention and management of substance abuse. Pediatrics 1998;101(1):125–128.

American Academy of Pediatrics: Indications for management and referral of patients involved in substance abuse. Pediatrics 2000; 106(1):143–148.

Fishman M, Bruner A, Adger H: Substance abuse among children and adolescents. Pediatr Rev 1997;18(11):394–403.

Johnston LD, O'Malley PM, Bachman JG, et al: Monitoring the future—National results on adolescent drug use: Overview of key findings, 2003. (NIH Publication No. 04-5506). Bethesda, Md, National Institute on Drug Abuse, 2004. Available at: www.monitoringthefuture.org.

Knight JR, Schrier LA, Bravender TD, et al: CRAFFT: A new brief screen for adolescent substance abuse. Arch Pediatr Adolesc Med 1999; 153(6):591–596.

Knight JR, Sherritt L, Shriser LA, et al: Validity of CRAFFT substance abuse screening test among adolescent clinic patients. Arch Pediatr Adolesc Med 2002;156(6):607–614.

Rogers PD, Heyman RB (eds): Addiction medicine: Adolescent substance abuse. Pediatr Clin North Am 2002;49(2):245–496.

SECTION 6　　ADOLESCENT CARE: *Adolescent Mental Health*

235 Adolescents and Violence

Gwen McIntosh

ROLE OF THE GENERALIST

1　Understand the types, extent, and nature of violence experienced by adolescents.

2　Provide anticipatory guidance on key areas of adolescent violence.

3　Screen for violence among all adolescent patients.

4　Identify and treat, counsel, and refer victims and perpetrators of adolescent violence.

5　Provide medical follow-up and ensure psychosocial follow-up for victims and perpetrators of violence.

6　Advocate for violence prevention programs.

Violence is the threatened or actual use of physical force against a person or group that results in or is likely to result in injury or death. Violent acts are intended to cause physical or psychological harm. Many teens feel the physical and psychological effects of violence in their daily lives. The highest and most rapidly increasing rates of fatal and non-fatal violence are in the adolescent age group. The most common forms of adolescent violence are homicide, suicide, dating violence, and school-associated violence.

U.S. violence rates on the whole are declining, but violence rates among adolescents are increasing. Approximately 25% of all adolescents have been the victims of violence in the previous year. Over the past 20 years, violent victimization crime rates have increased by more than 30% for youths ages 12 to 19. In addition, adolescents are increasingly the perpetrators of violent acts. In the past two decades, the homicide arrest rates among adolescents have increased by over 200% while decreasing by more than 25% in all other age groups.

To effectively address the many forms of violence that are reaching epidemic proportions in the adolescent population, clinicians must be familiar with the major types of violence experienced by teens and be aware of the risk factors associated with violent acts.

FUNDAMENTALS

Homicide is the second leading cause of death for teenagers and young adults in the United States. Adolescent homicide is epidemic in our country; the teen homicide rate has tripled in the past 40 years. The homicide rate for children younger than age 15 in the United States is 6 times the combined homicide rate of 25 other industrialized countries for the same age group. Figure 235-1 compares homicide with the other leading causes of death for teens and young adults.

Firearms are the single greatest risk factor for homicide. Eighty percent of all teen homicides involve firearms. Adolescents have easy access to firearms. A survey of rural

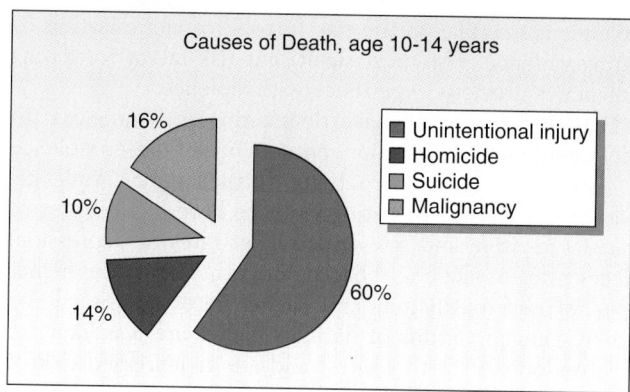

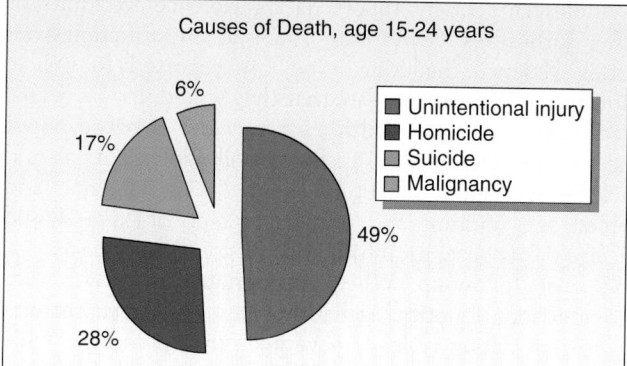

Figure 235-1. Leading causes of death among teens and young adults. (Adapted from the National Vital Statistics System, National Center for Health Statistics, Centers for Disease Control and Prevention. Available at: www.cdc.gov/nchs/about/major/dvs/mortdata.htm.)

and suburban youth showed that 48% of male teens owned a gun and 11% of eighth-grade urban students owned a gun. The average age of gun acquisition is 12.5 years, with most children and teens receiving their guns as gifts. The 2001 Youth Risk Behavior Surveillance indicates that 6% of all high school students regularly carry a gun. For those adolescents who don't already own a gun, access is not limited. Half of all U.S. households contain a firearm and in 25% of these homes, guns are stored loaded and unlocked. As a result, over 9 million adolescents have immediate access to handguns in their own home. One third of teens report they could acquire a gun in less than 1 hour. Presence of a gun in the home is associated with a 3.4-fold increase in the risk of adolescent homicide.

The risk factors associated with homicide victimization summarized in Box 235-1 are the same as the factors for perpetration of homicide with several exceptions. Perpetrators of homicide are more likely to be male and are generally at least 2 years older than their victims. Perpetrators are usually the same race or ethnicity as their victim. In three fourths of adolescent homicide cases, the perpetrator is well known by the victim. The most commonly cited motives for adolescent homicide are drug-related killings, retaliation for a previously perceived threat or injury, and interpersonal altercation.

Several important risk factors associated with adolescent homicide—drugs, gender, and race—merit further discussion. More than 40% of homicide victims ages 15 to 24 have positive blood alcohol levels. Over 40% of juvenile murderers are under the influence of drugs or alcohol at the time

of their offense. Adolescent boys are five times more likely to die of homicide than are adolescent girls. Black adolescent boys are also at increased risk of homicide. Homicide is the leading cause of death for male African Americans ages 15 to 19, accounting for 49% of all deaths in this group. Black male teens have nine times the homicide rate of white male teens.

Prevention begins with office counseling. Health care providers can improve their screening for the presence of firearms in the home; pediatricians currently discuss gun safety with only 11% of their patients. Less than 5% of adolescents have had a physician speak to them about guns. Providers should ask all families about the presence of firearms in the home, provide counseling on the risks associated with firearms, and advocate for the removal of guns from the home. At a minimum, parents should be encouraged to store all guns unloaded and locked. Ammunition should be locked in a separate location. Reducing adolescent access to guns will decrease the teen homicide rate. Health care providers should also seek to identify and refer high-risk adolescents, such as those with a substance abuse problem or a previous history of aggression.

Homicide prevention measures have not been well established or researched. At a state and national level, health care providers can help reduce teen homicide mortality by lobbying for passage of legislation to reduce teen access to handguns and alcohol. Although some people advocate the use of gun safety classes in place of restricted gun access, no published research confirms the effectiveness of gun safety training for teens or for young children.

Suicide. Suicide is a major form of violence in the lives of adolescents. This topic is covered separately in Chapter 233.

Box 235-1. Risk Factors Associated with Adolescent Homicide

Family Factors

Firearm in home
Low income
History of domestic violence
Teenage parent
Divorce

Personal Factors

Male gender
Alcohol/drug use
Poor impulse control
Previous gunshot injury

Social Factors

Ethnic/linguistic heterogeneity
Crowded housing
Racial intolerance
Lack of adult supervision
Social acceptance of violence

Psychological Factors

Aggressive personality
Antisocial behavior
Conduct disorder
Depression

Dating Violence. Dating violence, which is experienced by many teens, is *the threat or perpetration of an act of violence by at least one member of an unmarried couple on the other member in the context of dating.* This broad definition includes sexual assault, physical assault, and emotional abuse. As early as ninth grade, one fourth of male and female students have been the victim of nonsexual dating violence and 8% have been the victim of sexual dating violence. By the late teen years, 30% to 60% of male and female students have been subjected to dating violence and as many as one fourth have experienced extreme violence, such as rape or assault with a weapon. Preliminary data indicates that boys and girls receive and inflict dating violence in roughly equal proportions. However, girls are more likely to inflict minor injuries, to receive major injuries, and to initiate aggression as a form of self-defense.

Sexual assault and rape are extreme forms of dating violence. Twenty percent of high school students have been the victim of rape or forced sex. Female teens are two to three times more likely than male teens to experience rape or forced sex. Many adolescent boys show a high level of acceptance of sexual aggression. Surveys indicate that 60% of high school boys find it acceptable for a boy to force sex on a girl. Thirty percent of male teens and young adults report they continue to make sexual advances after a female partner says no. Changing the attitudes of teenagers with regard to sexual violence is a crucial component to preventing future violence.

Box 235-2 summarizes the risk factors associated with dating and sexual violence. As with many forms of violence, the risk factors associated with the perpetration of dating

violence are similar to the risk factors for victimization by dating violence. The most significant risk factor for dating violence is previous experience with violence.

Dating violence can have devastating consequences for adolescent victims. A major consequence of dating violence is that it serves to perpetuate further dating violence. Adolescent victims of dating violence have higher rates of suicidal ideation and attempts; higher rates of depression; higher rates of alcohol, tobacco, and other drug use; higher rates of self-mutilation; and higher rates of disordered eating. Female victims of dating violence are less likely to use condoms or birth control and are at increased risk of pregnancy and sexually transmitted diseases.

Adolescents rarely report dating violence to adults or other authorities. Fewer than 5% of all cases of adolescent dating violence, including rape, are reported to police. However, 72% of teens state that they would discuss sexual victimization with a health care provider if asked about the subject. The medical history of all adolescents should include screening questions about dating violence and forced sex. Victims and perpetrators of violence should receive risk counseling, information on community resources, and close follow-up. When appropriate, the health care provider should notify legal authorities. Preliminary efforts to prevent dating violence have been disappointing. While intervention strategies have shown sustained improvements in perception of adolescent dating violence norms and conflict management skills, they have failed to show a sustained reduction in the perpetration of dating violence.

School-Associated Violence. School-associated violence is defined as *a threat of violence or an act of violence that occurs on the property of a functioning school, on the way to or from regular school sessions, or while attending an official school-sponsored event.* This definition encompasses a wide range of school violence such as bullying, fighting, assault, and gang violence. It also includes school-associated homicides and suicides.

Each year, adolescents are the victims of more than 2.5 million violent crimes committed at school or while traveling to or from school. One third of all violent crimes against teens occur at school. While bullying is the most common form of violence in middle school, threats, physical fights, and assaults are the most common forms of violence in the high school setting. Figure 235-2 summarizes the types of violent crimes reported by public schools. Other common crimes include theft of property and vandalism. The statistics likely underestimate the true level of violent crime in schools as only a percentage of the crimes or attempted crimes are reported to police.

Physical fights and assaults are a frequent occurrence among high school students. Physical attack or fight without a weapon is the most commonly reported crime in middle schools and high schools. Figure 235-3 depicts the prevalence of school fighting by grade and gender. On average, 15% of high school students engage in fighting behavior while at school. Boys are more likely to engage in fighting than are girls. Younger students, such as those in 9th and 10th grade, are more likely to participate in fights than are 11th- and 12th-grade students. Additional risk

---

Box 235-2. Risk Factors Associated with Adolescent Dating Violence

Personal Factors

Previous history of physical abuse
Previous history of interpersonal violence
Previous history of forced sex
Alcohol/drug use
Minority race
History of pregnancy
Partner of same sex
Poor academic performance
Increased number of sexual partners
Anabolic steroid use
Low self-esteem

Psychological Factors

Aggressive personality
Dominating negotiating style
Suicidal ideation

Family Factors

History of family violence
History of family sexual abuse

Social Factors

Acceptance of dating violence
Lack of adult supervision

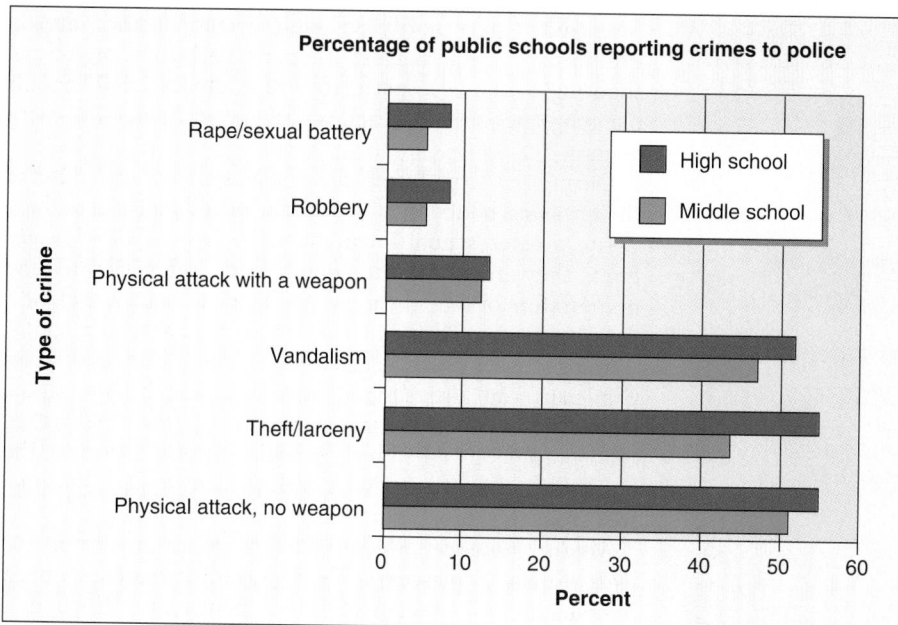

Figure 235-2. Public school violent crime. (Adapted from U.S. Department of Justice, Office of Justice Programs, National Center for Education Statistics/Bureau of Justice Statistics, Indicators of School Crime and Safety 2000. Available at: http://nces.ed.gov/pubsearch/search.asp.)

factors for fighting include gang involvement, minority ethnicity, and alcohol or marijuana use.

Weapons are a major component of school violence. Over 17% of high school students carry weapons such as guns and knives to school. In an average year, 6 U.S. teens die of stab wounds sustained at school and another 16 die as the result of firearm injury. Known risk factors associated with carrying a weapon to school are male gender, gang membership, alcohol and drug use, a history of criminal activity, poor academic performance, and a history of previously being threatened with a gun. Methods currently used to keep weapons out of schools include metal detectors, random locker searches, and the use of clear plastic or mesh book bags. While such measures have increased a sense of security, there is no current evidence that these methods result in fewer weapons assaults and injuries. Recent data indicate that the percentage of students carrying weapons to school

is decreasing and that fewer students are avoiding school out of fear of violence.

Box 235-3 reviews the risk factors associated with school violence. As with many types of violence, the risk factors for perpetrating school violence are similar to the risk factors for school violence victimization. Large urban schools show higher rates of most types of school violence such as vandalism, fighting, larceny, and homicide. While violent school deaths occur in all types of communities, the estimated rate of school homicide in urban school districts is nine times greater than the estimated rate in rural school districts.

School shootings have become a major focus of public attention after several highly publicized multiple victim shootings in the late 1990s. School shootings are not a new phenomenon; the first widely reported episode occurred in 1974. The annual number of school shootings has decreased

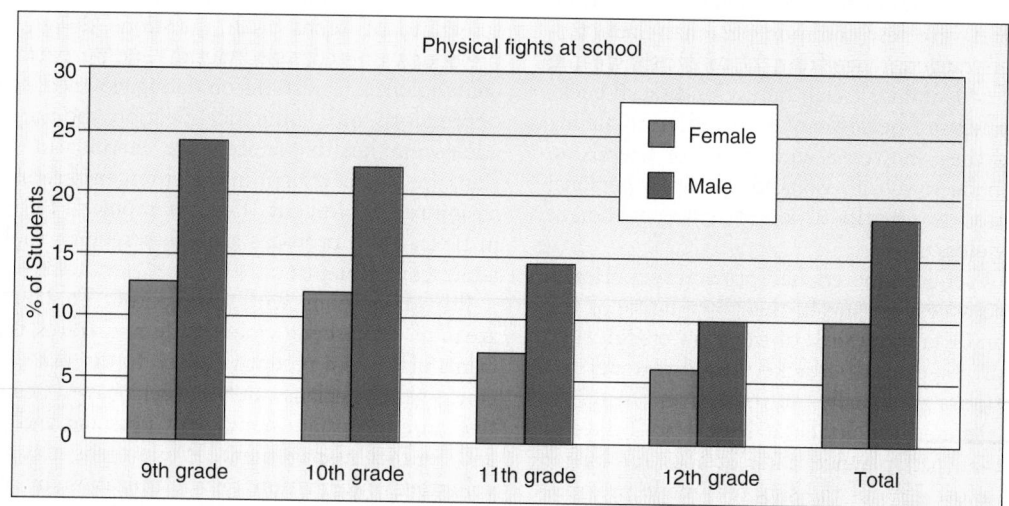

Figure 235-3. Student fights at school. (Adapted from U.S. Department of Public Health and Human Services, Public Health Service, Centers for Disease Control and Prevention, National Center for Health Statistics, National Health Interview Survey—Youth Risk Behavior Surveillance, 2001. Available at: www.cdc.gov/nccdphp/dash/yrbs/2001/index.htm.)

Box 235-3. Risk Factors for School Violence

Personal Factors

Male gender
Alcohol/drug use
Poor impulse control
Gang involvement
Younger age (ages 12–14)
History of weapon carrying
History of fighting
History of aggression

Psychological Factors

Feelings of persecution, victimization
Depression
Previous history of suicidal ideation or attempt
Feelings of social isolation

Family Factors

Poor parental monitoring/supervision
Marital or parental conflict
Exposure to parental violence
Child abuse/neglect

School Factors

Larger schools
Urban schools

---

since 1993; however, the average number of victims per shooting has increased. School shootings can be classified as a form of "targeted violence." Targeted violence is *any incident of violence in which a known attacker selects a particular target prior to attacking.* The target may be an individual, a group of people, or a building. Thirty-seven school shootings have occurred in the past 3 decades resulting in more than 170 student deaths. Student deaths from school shootings are summarized in Figure 235-4.

Students who commit multiple-victim school shootings have been extensively profiled by government agencies to identify common characteristics. All perpetrators of multiple-victim school shootings have been male. Aside from gender there were few common personal characteristics. Perpetrators ranged in age from 11 to 21; they came from a variety of geographic, social, family, and racial backgrounds; their academic performance ranged from failing to excellent; and they showed a wide range of friendship patterns from popular to socially isolated. No single personal feature can be used to identify a potential perpetrator of targeted school violence.

The majority of school shooters had previous experience with guns and had access to guns in their own home or the home of a relative. Over two thirds of the shooters felt they had been bullied, persecuted, attacked, or threatened by others. School attacks are usually not impulsive. Over 75% of the attackers planned the attack at least 1 to 2 days in advance. More than half planned their attacks for longer than 2 weeks. Almost 75% of the shooters made previous suicidal threats or attempts. Importantly, in over three fourths of the cases, the perpetrator told one or more peers of his interest in attacking the school. However, in only two

cases did a peer notify an adult of the planned attack. Preliminary data suggest that perpetrators of school shootings follow a path toward violence that entails planning, acquiring weapons, and communicating with peers.

During the school year, teens spend almost one third of their waking hours on school property. Clinicians can help create a safer school environment in a number of ways. First, they must seek to identify and refer victims and perpetrators of school violence. Clinicians can counsel individual patients and families on conflict management skills, warning signs of violence, and available community resources. Clinicians can also support further research into school violence prevention and intervention programs. Finally, they can continue to advocate for violence prevention in the curricula and for the right of each student to attend school free from the threat of violence.

Media Violence. Media violence has an impact on the lives of many adolescents. The average teen watches almost 3 hours of television a day and spends over 6 hours a day with TV, videotapes, and video games. By the age of 18, the average American child has witnessed over 200,000 overt acts of violence on television. While nearly two thirds of television programming contains violence, less than 15% of television shows contain any type of advisory content code. Violence on television is portrayed in a glamorous fashion. Perpetrators of violence rarely get punished or experience any negative consequences of their violent actions. More than 1000 studies have demonstrated a relationship between media violence and aggressive behavior in children. Health care providers can help to minimize the influence of media violence by encouraging teens to limit television viewing to 1 to 2 hours a day. At the community and state level, physicians can advocate for ratings systems, parental advisories, and an industry-wide reduction in the violent material portrayed in television programming.

DIAGNOSIS

The key to diagnosing adolescent violence remains careful screening of teens with questions designed to identify previously unrecognized victims and perpetrators of adolescent violence. Questions on dating violence, school violence, depression, and homicidal ideation should be part of all adolescent health maintenance examinations. These questions are also pertinent in the emergency room evaluation of an injured adolescent. The mnemonic "FISTS," as detailed in Box 235-4, provides a quick screening tool to assess for adolescent violence.

Providing teens with anticipatory guidance on the key areas of adolescent violence demonstrates that the physician's office is a receptive place to discuss violence-related concerns. Physicians can help teens have a healthier perspective on appropriate nonviolent personal and peer behavior and conflict management. While teens may be hesitant to volunteer information on victimization by violence, data suggest that a high percentage of adolescents would discuss violence with physicians if asked about it. Health care providers have a unique opportunity to identify adolescent

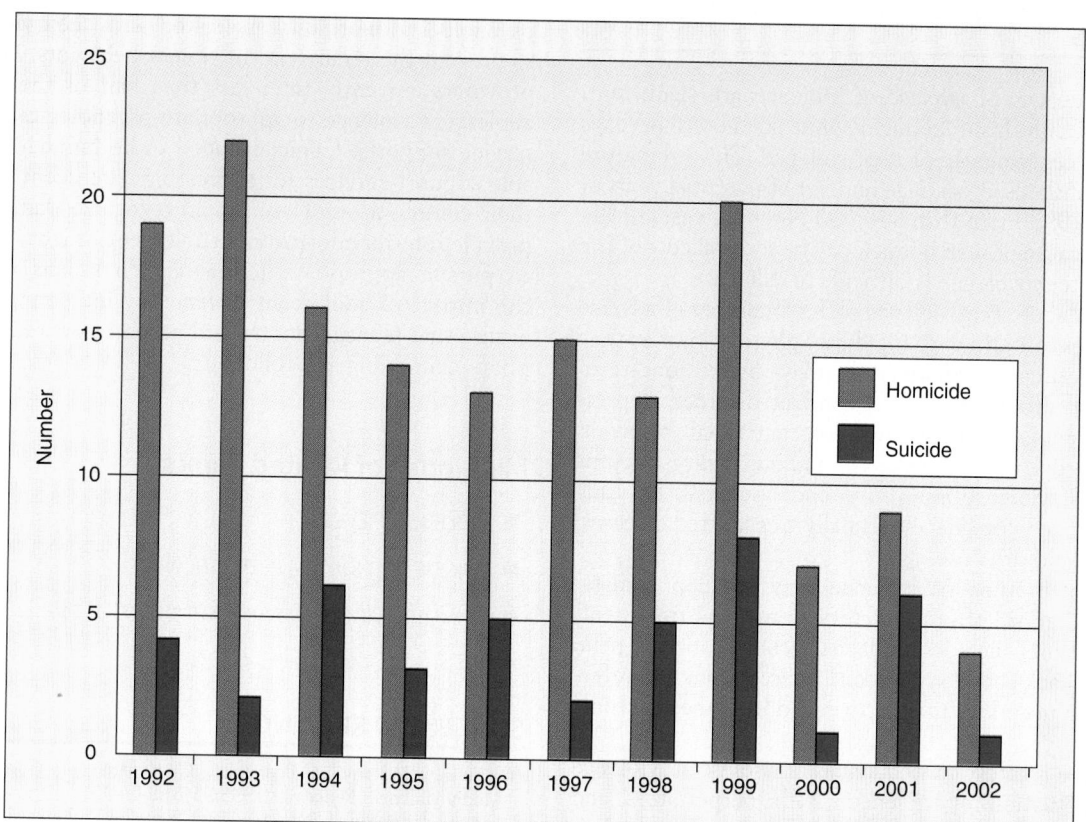

Figure 235-4. Student deaths from school shootings. (Adapted from Stephens R: The National School Safety Center's report on school associated violent deaths: In-house report of the National School Safety Center, 2003. Available at: www.nssc1.org/savd.)

victims of violence and to serve as a resource for these victims.

MANAGEMENT

Management of adolescent violence begins with identifying victims and perpetrators of violent acts. For victims, the health care provider must ensure the diagnosis and treatment of acute physical injuries. The clinician should then conduct a comprehensive psychosocial evaluation of

Box 235-4. FISTS Pneumonic for Assessing Adolescent Violence

Fights: Ask questions such as "How many fights have you had within the past month (year)?
"When was your last pushing or shoving fight?"

Injuries: Ask questions such as "Have you ever been injured in a fight?"
"Has anyone you know been injured in a fight?"

Sexual Violence: Ask questions such as "Have you ever been forced to have sex against your will?"
"Have you ever had a pushing or shoving fight in a dating relationship?"

Threats: Ask questions such as "Have you ever been threatened with a knife or a gun?"
"Have you ever threatened someone with a knife or a gun?"

Self-defense: Ask questions such as "How do you avoid getting into a fight?"
"Do you ever carry a weapon for self-defense?"

both victims and perpetrators of violence. For victims, a complete evaluation should assess premorbid psychological disturbances, the teen's response to the traumatic experience, available family and community supports, and available professional counseling resources. The goal is to reduce the risk of posttraumatic stress disorder, depression, and chronic victimization. As previous victimization is a common risk factor for future perpetration of violent act, efforts should also be directed toward preventing victims from becoming assailants. At the time of discharge from the clinic or emergency department, plans for both medical and psychosocial follow-up should be clearly defined. When appropriate, the health care provider should notify legal authorities.

For perpetrators of violent acts, psychosocial interventions focus on the identification and remediation of coexisting risk factors such as weapons carriage, substance abuse, depression, gang membership, family violence, and previous criminal history. Effective intervention programs require a multidisciplinary approach involving physicians, families, mental health workers, social services, and often the criminal justice system. The goal is identification and modification of characteristics associated with violence, promotion of self-esteem and anger management skills, treatment of substance abuse disorders, and prevention of future violent behavior. Successful programs stress nonviolent problem-solving techniques and conflict resolution skills in conjunction with mentoring programs for positive role modeling and job training.

OUTCOMES

The consequences of adolescent violence are significant. Premature death from homicide and suicide is perhaps the greatest consequence of teen violence. This premature mortality translates into a huge number of potential years of life lost. In 1995 more than 470,000 potential years of life were lost because of teen homicide. The societal cost of the lives lost to teen violence is difficult to calculate.

Victims of adolescent violence suffer a number of adverse consequences in addition to the direct physical injuries they receive. Victims of violence display many long-term psychological problems such as conduct disorder, depression, posttraumatic stress disorder, antisocial behavior, anxiety disorder, low self-esteem, and suicidality. Victims of adolescent violence are also at increased risk for gang involvement, teen pregnancy, sexually transmitted diseases, alcohol use, and drug use.

Adolescent victims of violence may develop somatic complaints that are often refractory to medical treatment. Such complaints include headaches, chronic pelvic pain, and chronic back pain. Psychosocial interventions and referrals are often necessary to effectively address these chronic issues.

One of the greatest consequences of adolescent violence is its perpetuation of violence. Both perpetrators and victims of violence are at risk of committing future violent acts such as interpersonal violence, date rape, gang violence, and homicide. Preliminary data also link adolescent victimization by violence with an increased risk for perpetrating child abuse as an adult.

FOLLOW-UP

Medical and psychosocial follow-up are critical for both the victims and the perpetrators of adolescent violence. The goal of counseling and follow-up is to reduce the long-term psychological morbidity associated with teen violence and to prevent the recurrence of violent behaviors. Health care providers currently refer less than half of the victims of adolescent violence to appropriate psychological and social service supports. Clinicians need to be familiar with available support services for addressing adolescent violence in their communities. They should recognize that when they provide referral information, adolescents might be reluctant to pursue appropriate follow-up. Physicians can reduce the impact of adolescent violence by increasing efforts to ensure that teenage victims and perpetrators receive appropriate counseling and follow-up.

Mini-index of Related Topics

SUGGESTED READINGS

American Academy of Pediatrics, Committee on Communications: Media violence. Pediatrics 1995;95(6):949–951.

American Academy of Pediatrics, Task Force on Violence: The role of the pediatrician in youth violence prevention in clinical practice and at the community level. Pediatrics 1999;103(1):173–178.

Grausz HM, Pelucio MT: Adolescent violence. Emerg Med Clin North Am 1999;17(3):595–602.

Hennes HMA, Calhoun AD (eds): Violence among children and adolescents. Pediatr Clin North Am 1998;45:269–280.

Kaufmann P, Chen X, Choy SP, et al: Indicators of School Crime and Safety 2000. Washington, DC, U.S. Department of Education and Justice, Office of Justice Programs, National Center for Education Statistics (2001-017/NCJ-184176), 2000.

Malik S, Sorenson SB, Aneshensel CS: Community and dating violence among adolescents: Perpetration and victimization. J Adolesc Health 1997;21:291–302.

MENTAL HEALTH CARE

236

Conceptualizing Behavioral and Mental Health Issues in Pediatrics

F. Daniel Armstrong

ROLE OF THE GENERALIST

1. Screen for common behavior problems during well-child visits.

2. Screen for risk factors associated with child behavior problems.

3. Provide anticipatory intervention focused on prevention of behavior problems.

4. Develop and maintain referral network for assessment and treatment of behavioral and mental health problems

5. Evaluate the appropriateness and effectiveness of recommended treatments (pharmacologic, behavioral, and psychotherapeutic) and provide parents with guidance in decision making about mental health treatment

6. Screen for parent or family mental health problems or chronic illness, and make appropriate referrals for parents as indicated.

7. Advocate for children's access to child-competent mental health services.

A significant portion of a general pediatrician's practice is devoted to concerns about behavioral and mental health issues for children. Since the publication of the American Academy of Pediatrics policy statement that defined the "new morbidity," the pediatrician's role in identifying and obtaining appropriate services for children with behavioral problems and significant mental health disorders has expanded with the significant increase in the number of developmental, behavioral, or serious mental health difficulties encountered during general pediatric office visits. Concerns about the ability to deal with these problems appropriately now have reached the national stage.

This chapter was prepared with the support of grants from the Maternal and Child Health Bureau (Leadership Education in Neurodevelopmental Disabilities Program-T73MC00013-10); the Administration for Developmental Disabilities (University Center for Excellence in Developmental Disabilities Education, Research, and Service-90DD0408); and Children's Medical Services of Florida (Contract COQ03).

Pediatricians are the frontline professionals for screening for behavioral problems, providing preventive anticipatory guidance, developing referral sources, evaluating the need for and use of medications, screening for family difficulties, and advocating for access to mental health services for children. These are not easy tasks. Behavioral and mental health problems occur for a variety of reasons and often are multiply determined, and the determination of the seriousness of the problem may depend on the age of the child and normal developmental variations. In addition, risk factors for child behavioral problems may involve other family members, individuals outside the family, and systems that have an impact on the child. Intervention may require direct services to the child, treatment for an adult parent, or family or system intervention.

DEVELOPMENTAL NATURE OF CHILD BEHAVIORAL PROBLEMS

Screening for mental health or behavioral problems in children represents a significant challenge for pediatricians for several reasons. Normal growth and development creates different patterns of behavior that occur at different ages. Developmental perspective is needed to determine whether a behavior (e.g., activity) is a developmentally normal variation or a problem behavior (e.g., hyperactivity). Likewise, behaviors commonly associated with a mental health disorder (e.g., suicidal thoughts) may never occur for a toddler, but other significant behavioral indicators of depression not seen in older children may be observed in the same toddler. It is essential for the general pediatrician to have knowledge of normal behavioral development and developmental variations and age-related problem behaviors. The type of behavior, frequency of occurrence, and intensity are all dimensions that vary with age and overall development.

RISK FACTORS FOR MENTAL HEALTH PROBLEMS IN CHILDREN

Behavior in children varies across situations, and reports of a child's behavior vary depending on who is reporting (e.g., parent or teacher). Determination of whether a behavior is a problem also depends on whether the behavior is of concern to someone else. These factors create a context for understanding behavior and determining whether it constitutes a significant concern for the child. It is inadequate simply to observe a child and make an in-office determination of whether a mental health problem exists (or is likely to exist in the future). A review of risk factors and consideration of their contributions in individual cases is crucial for appropriate screening and referral.

Adults most frequently recognize behaviors that are bothersome or annoying and report these to the pediatrician as concerns. Behaviors that are less overt and more internal, such as anxiety or depression, are reported less frequently as concerns. The pediatrician must evaluate carefully what parents report and what they do not report. Parents who report a high level of concern about the activity level of a preschool child may be accurate reporters. Alternatively the behavior of the child may be developmentally normal, but the parent response to it may represent hypersensitivity, lack of tolerance, or lack of parenting skill. Parents who report concerns about a child's social withdrawal or low activity level may be sensitive to early signs of depression; however, parents who fail to report concerns in the face of indicators obvious to other observers may be limited in their sensitivity to their child's needs. In addition to observing the child's behavior, pediatricians must consider the concerns expressed and concerns not expressed.

Many factors may contribute to the identification of a child behavioral problem or mental health disorder (Box 236-1). Some, such as the co-occurrence of a developmental disability, congenital abnormality, or serious chronic illness, are relatively simple to recognize and consider. Others are not as obvious and constitute a challenge for the general pediatrician.

Social Risk Factors

Poverty and violence are two significant contributors to child mental health problems. Poverty is associated with a variety of challenges to the child and family (Box 236-2)

Box 236-1. Common Risk Factors for Child Behavioral or Mental Health Problems

- Genetic risk factors (e.g., congenital developmental disability)
- Chronic medical illness (e.g., cancer, cystic fibrosis, sickle cell disease, human immunodeficiency virus) and effects of treatment (particularly illnesses affecting the central nervous system)
- Social risk factors
  - Poverty or homelessness
  - Exposure to domestic violence
- Family risk factors
  - Maternal depression and social isolation
  - Separation or divorce
  - Chronic physical or mental illness in family members
  - Substance abuse by a family member
- Skills deficiencies
  - Parenting knowledge or performance deficits
  - Child social skills deficits
  - Masked school failure and learning disability

From Erickson MT: Etiological factors. In Ollendick TH, Hersen M (eds): Handbook of Child Psychopathology, 3rd ed. New York, Plenum Press, 1998, pp 37–61.

Box 236-2. Behavioral and Developmental Risks Associated with Poverty and Violence

Risk Factors

- Family instability
- Lack of access to basic resources
- Lack of access to adequate health care
- Lack of access to pediatric/child mental health care
- Inadequate child supervision
- Transient caregiving
- Child injury
- Child abuse, child neglect, or medical neglect

Associated Developmental and Behavioral Outcomes

- Increased depression
- Increased anxiety
- Increased high-risk health behavior, particularly in adolescents
- Increased cognitive and speech and language developmental delays
- Increased emotional problems

---

that increase the risk of behavior problems for children. Likewise, direct exposure to violence in the home, community, or school can have serious and far-reaching developmental and behavioral consequences. Most pediatricians routinely screen for signs of child sexual and physical abuse, but screening for effects of domestic violence or exposure to community violence is not provided as frequently. Domestic violence occurs at all socioeconomic levels and should be considered in any screening performed by the general pediatrician. It is important for the pediatrician to recognize, however, that these are only risk factors; some parents, even in the face of abject poverty and challenges associated with violence, provide nurturing relationships and oversight that produce resiliency and adjustment in their children.

Family Risk Factors

Perhaps the greatest risk factors for child behavioral or mental health problems are parental depression or social isolation. These two factors are associated with a variety of behavioral and emotional problems for children (Table 236-1). Pediatricians should screen routinely for these factors and offer referrals for treatment. Intervention at this level may offer one of the best primary prevention approaches to child behavioral and mental health disorders.

Other significant family risk factors include separation and divorce of parents, which may affect adversely children's emotional and behavioral well-being for prolonged periods. Separation is acutely disruptive to children, but the process of communication and determination of the nature of the ongoing parenting relationship between divorcing spouses may be a long-term determinant of adjustment or maladjustment in children. Pediatricians should be aware of the impact of divorce on children and provide guidance (and referrals where necessary) to parents to assist them in minimizing the negative impact of the divorce on their children. The marriage may not last, but the parenting relationship extends far into the future. How this relation-

Table 236-1. Behavioral and Developmental Risks Associated with Family Risk Factors

Family Risk Factors	Associated Developmental and Behavioral Outcomes
Parental depression and social isolation	Increased risk of child abuse Decreased environmental stimulation Decreased access to emotional nurturing Increased risk of disruptive and externalized behavior problems
Separation and divorce	Acute behavioral and emotional problems Long-term maladjustment, social difficulties
Parental substance abuse	Decreased positive, increased negative parent-child interaction Inadequate supervision Increased injury risk Increased instability in the home Increased risk of abuse, divorce, domestic violence
Parent chronic illness	Diminished family resources Redirected attention from normal tasks Increased risk of school problems Increased risk of aggression Increased occurrence of sleep problems Increased demands on children

ship is handled may have a profound effect on the child's emotional development.

Parental substance abuse and chronic physical or mental illness are other significant family risk factors (see Table 236-1). The pediatrician always should be aware of potential signs of substance abuse and provide parents with guidance for professional assistance. Similarly, having a family member with a chronic illness, such as cancer, immobility as a result of limb amputation secondary to diabetes, or bipolar disorder, places unusual burdens on children. The pediatrician should be aware of this often-overlooked risk factor and offer guidance or referral for family support.

SKILLS DEFICIENCIES

The behavior observed in most children and families is often the result of the best efforts and application of skills that they know. Most families do not set out to be maladaptive or to have children with behavioral or mental health problems. Lack of skills and knowledge may be a significant determinant of this type of outcome. There are three major types of skills that should be considered in screening and recommending referrals for children.

Parenting Skills

Despite the explosion of popular literature on parenting, many parents are limited in their knowledge or ability to know how to raise their child. Two factors need to be considered. First, parents may not have the necessary knowledge about what approaches are effective and recommended for dealing with common child behavior. Anticipatory guidance and recommendations of professional organizations (e.g., American Academy of Pediatrics Guidance for Effective Discipline, 1998) may be helpful in this regard. Second,

parents may have the knowledge, but lack the skills to implement the knowledge. In this situation, pediatricians may hear a parent describe an understanding of the usefulness of ignoring inappropriate behavior in a toddler, but observe that parent to attend consistently to the inappropriate behavior while in the office. In this case, anticipatory guidance may be helpful, but referral to a parenting skills class may be necessary.

Child Social Skills

Child social difficulties have been associated with behavioral problems, school achievement difficulties, and long-term psychological adjustment in adolescence and adulthood. Social avoidance, withdrawal, bullying, rejection by peers, and more subtle social ignoring by peers all are significant risk factors for child behavioral disturbances. Children who lack the ability to initiate social interaction, who initiate negative interactions with others, or who behave in ways perceived as strange by peers are at the greatest risk. These social behaviors, in many cases, respond well to social skills training interventions. Pediatricians should ask routinely about the number and quality of children's relationships at school and home and refer children with social difficulties for professional assistance.

School Failure

School failure or low academic achievement is a significant problem for children. Learning difficulties often are masked by behavioral disturbances, however, and parents and teachers frequently indicate behavior problems as a primary concern without considering the possibility of a co-occurring learning problem. Pediatricians should be alert to the relationship between learning problems and behavioral problems and refer children for appropriate intellectual and academic evaluation when this kind of relationship is suspected. In many cases, identification of a learning problem, with appropriate academic accommodations, leads to a significant reduction in the frequency and intensity of a child's behavioral problems.

APPROACHES TO SCREENING AND DIAGNOSIS IN PRIMARY CARE

Many checklists can be used to screen briefly for child behavior problems. Most of these checklists have good reliability and validity and can be administered in the office setting (see Chapter 238). Other information from other reporting sources may be needed, however. This may include not only teacher reports using checklists similar to those administered in the office setting, but also information derived from interviews with parents and teachers and, in some cases, observation of the child in office, home, or school settings.

For this information to be useful, a conceptual framework that recognizes the contribution of risk factors, developmental variations, co-occurring conditions, and variability in level of intensity of behaviors is essential. The American Academy of Pediatrics, in collaboration with several other professional organizations, developed the *Diagnostic and Statistical Manual for Primary Care, Child and Adolescent*

Version (DSM-PC) to provide this framework. The DSM-PC provides information to assist the pediatrician in discriminating between developmental variations, problem behaviors, and disorders and provides links to common risk factors that should be included when considering a possible diagnosis. Each classification provides a list of common complaints and the epidemiologic background for each and then provides the pediatrician with contextual guidance for decision making.

TREAT OR REFER CONSIDERATIONS

Screening for child behavioral or mental health problems generally can be accomplished in the office setting using the assistance of nurses or other paraprofessionals. What can be done beyond screening depends on several factors, including the time available, competence of the pediatrician in diagnosing or treating the condition, and complexity of the treatment needed. Pediatricians should become aware of the evidence-based parameters for treatment of various problems. Interventions may include advice, medication, a structured treatment approach, or family therapy; decisions about whether to provide treatment or refer should be based on the pediatrician's ability to provide care that is consistent with current evidence.

Table 236-2. Barriers to Coordination of Care and Strategies for Overcoming Barriers

Barriers	Strategies
Referrals limited by MCO restricted behavioral health panel	Contract with MCOs that offer behavioral health panels that include child mental health providers
	Advocate with MCOs to add providers you know and trust
Child has state/federal insurance with limited/no behavioral/mental health coverage	Join professional groups to advocate for full mental/behavioral health coverage for children
	Support expansion of disciplines (e.g., developmental and behavioral pediatrics, psychology, social work) eligible for reimbursement under state/federal insurance
	Develop network of services using schools and community agencies
Communication with mental health providers is poor or nonexistent	Send request for follow-up with contact information at time of referral
	Inform MCO of need for follow-up and of any failure to receive follow-up
	Schedule periodic meetings with mental health providers to discuss care coordination mechanisms
	Establish collaborative practice that includes shared contracts
Cultural or language barrier exists	Join with other pediatricians and community agencies to develop a network of culturally competent mental health providers (e.g., Spanish speaking, sign language)

MCO, managed care organization.

Often, even if the pediatrician has received appropriate training and can treat certain problems competently, time is not available. Likewise, some problems are beyond the scope of training and experience of the pediatrician and require outside referral. In these cases, it is crucial for the pediatrician to establish a referral network of mental health professionals. At a minimum, this network should be based on knowledge about the competence of the mental health providers to treat the identified problems, an established system of communication between the pediatrician and mental health provider, and a mechanism for coordination of care for complex cases. The establishment of such a network may be difficult in the managed care environment, and pediatricians are likely to have to overcome many barriers to create an effective referral process (Table 236-2).

The collaborative practice model is one approach to dealing with the complexities of referrals for mental health services. In this model, pediatricians and mental health providers (psychologists, psychiatrists, social workers, psychiatric nurses) work together in the same office setting, share screening responsibilities, provide in-office consultation during regular office visits, and operate intervention programs in the pediatric office. As part of the same practice, contracts that pediatricians negotiate with third-party providers include the mental health practitioners as part of the plan, eliminating plan-related barriers to collaboration and communication. One outgrowth of this model is broader acceptance of mental health services by parents and their children, leading to greater likelihood of kept appointments and positive outcomes.

ADVOCACY

One of the great frustrations for pediatricians is the inability to gain access to competent mental health services for children. It is estimated that only 20% of children with mental health needs have access to mental health providers with training and experience in providing child assessment and treatment services. Several factors are related to this problem, including (1) a shortage of providers with competency in child treatment, (2) lack of coverage of mental health services by third-party insurers, (3) lack of mental health coverage by federal insurance (e.g., Medicaid), and (4) no health insurance at all. These problems are not going to disappear, so advocacy on the part of pediatricians is needed to increase access. First, pediatricians can join with mental health professionals in their communities to advocate for private, state, and federal coverage of child mental health services. Second, local efforts to identify funding mechanisms for children who have no coverage can be initiated. Third, pediatricians can develop consultation arrangements with schools, childcare centers, and school health programs to provide early screening and intervention to prevent serious mental health problems. Finally, pediatricians and mental health providers can join together to create funding to train mental health providers to work with children and their families. Progress in these areas increases the chances that the efforts devoted to screening and prevention in the pediatric office will lead to better outcomes in the lives of children.

SUGGESTED READINGS

American Academy of Pediatrics: The pediatrician and the "new morbidity." Pediatrics 1993;92:731–733.

American Academy of Pediatrics: Guidance for effective discipline. Pediatrics 1998;101:723–728.

Erickson MT: Etiological factors. In Ollendick TH, Hersen M (eds): Handbook of Child Psychopathology, 3rd ed. New York, Plenum Press, 1998, pp 37–61.

U.S. Public Health Service: Report of the Surgeon General's Conference on Children's Mental Health: A National Action Agenda. Washington, DC, U.S. Public Health Service, 2000.

Wolraich ML, Felice ME, Drotar D (eds): The Classification of Child and Adolescent Mental Diagnoses in Primary Care. Elk Grove Village, Ill, American Academy of Pediatrics, 1996.

SECTION 7   MENTAL HEALTH CARE: *Theoretical Basis of Mental Health*

237 Family Focused Behavioral Pediatrics: A Primary Care Approach

William Coleman

ROLE OF THE GENERALIST

1. Understand how family structure and function affect child behavior.

2. Apply principles of a family centered approach to behavioral issues.

3. Identify problems suitable for a family focused approach.

4. Develop and apply effective techniques for interviewing families.

5. Provide appropriate follow-up.

6. Refer to an appropriate mental health provider when assistance is needed with diagnosis, treatment, or management.

BACKGROUND

Today, the well-being of American children and adolescents more often is affected adversely by psychosocial problems than by medical illness. Primary care pediatric providers (pediatricians, family practitioners, child psychiatrists, psychologists, pediatric nurse practitioners, physician assistants, and social workers), hereafter termed *clinicians*, increasingly encounter a variety of behavioral/emotional family relationship problems. Clinicians are expected to provide initial assessment and treatment for these problems, which often do not respond to (in fact tend to recur or intensify) traditional child/symptom centered interventions (i.e., the "five R's" [Box 237-1]).

Case Study 237-1 presents a common child-parent problem and the child centered and the family centered

1525

Box 237-1. Five R's: Traditional Child/Symptom Centered Interventions

1. *Reassurance*—emotional support, compliments, encouragement
2. *Readings*—information and education about the issue (e.g., books, pamphlets, handouts, websites), demystification, brief explanations
3. *Rx's*—medications (stimulants, antidepressants, mood stabilizers, antipsychotics)
4. *Recipes*—parenting advice, conventional wisdom, behavioral management techniques (e.g., time-out, rewards)
5. *Resources*—parent support groups, friends, family, church/temple, local/national organizations (e.g., Children and Adults with ADD [CHADD]), referrals (e.g., specialists, medical centers, Department of Social Services)

approaches to the problem. The clinician should consider the family centered approach when (1) these problems seem resistant to the clinician's best efforts or (2) when the family or the clinician, or both, is working too hard and too long and feeling frustrated, tired, and confused. The family focused approach, based on the family systems model, explores the problem and the solution within the family context. The interventions of the family model are not exclusive and usually are used in conjunction with the five R's interventions.

FAMILY FOCUSED APPROACH

A family is characterized by its structure and function, both of which define relationships. The family structure includes the composition and organization of the family in the home, the hierarchy (power structure), the subunits (e.g., parent dyad, siblings), and extended family membership (all who live outside the home). Each member has a position in the family structure. Family function is how the members and the subsystems interact, how they perceive each other, and how they designate and carry out roles and responsibilities. The family system maintains the family balance or stability and helps it adapt to change and stress.

The family systems model envisions the family as a set of connected relationships. Everything that happens to a child occurs, at some level, within the family and always affects the family. Everything that affects the family always affects the child. The family focused approach is an integral part of the biopsychosocial model, which has been shown to be the most effective approach to child and adult health and well-being. Psychosocial factors influence health and behavior as much as biologic factors. Another benefit of the family context approach is that it yields information not readily available from the patient/problem focused biomedical model (Box 237-2).

Visualize a mobile with four or five pieces suspended from the ceiling, gently moving in the air. The whole is in balance, steady yet moving. A breeze (a normal change or a stress) catching only one piece immediately influences the movement of every piece (some more than others), and the pace picks up, with some pieces unbalancing themselves and moving about chaotically for a time. Gradually the

CASE STUDY 237-1

A NONCOMPLIANT, DISRUPTIVE TODDLER, A DEPRESSED MOTHER, AND A SEEMINGLY UNSUPPORTIVE FATHER

During a well-child visit, David, a 2-year-old, is out of control. He runs all around the office, pulling open drawers, spilling supplies on the floor, and opening and slamming the door. His passive, depressed-looking mother angrily and repeatedly, yet ineffectively, tells him to stop. David ignores her and continues his antics. Finally, she gives him a single spank on his behind. He cries and retreats to a corner. Although the mother does not voice a concern, the clinician raises the subject of David's behavior and her need to set limits more effectively.

Child Centered Approach

If the clinician had used traditional child/symptom centered techniques, he might have (1) explained that toddlers tend to be difficult ("the terrible two's"); (2) described briefly several behavioral techniques (time-out, ignoring/extinction, 1-2-3 rule); (3) encouraged her to "be firmer," even suggesting spanking more often; (4) warned her of the ineffectiveness of spanking and that it can "harm David's self-esteem"; or (5) offered her some pamphlets and titles of books on discipline.

Family Focused Approach

Using a family focused approach to understand the interactive nature of the problem (David's behavior and the mother's behavior) and to develop solutions within the family context, the clinician suggested a family meeting with both parents. During the family meeting, the mother again appears unable to set limits, and David is as noncompliant and disruptive as before. The clinician asks the parents if this happens at home and in public (multiple settings). They reply that it does. The father's interactions with David are minimal, and he openly criticizes the mother for not setting limits. The clinician senses that the mother's anger, ineffectiveness, and corresponding criticism she receives from her husband leave her feeling depressed, inadequate, and discouraged. The clinician takes a brief family history, and the mother reveals that she has felt depressed for several years, especially since David was born, but that she has not sought help.

The clinician helps the parents define and agree on a goal, helps them determine how they might cooperate with each other, and offers advice on two appropriate behavior management techniques that they feel they can carry out. Because he also helps them understand that the mother's difficulty in setting limits seems associated with her long-standing depression, the father becomes more sympathetic to his wife's struggles. The clinician also suggests a referral to a therapist for the mother, which she accepts, and suggests that occasionally they see the therapist together, which they accept. Figure 237-1 is brief genogram of the current and desired relationships. Other possible desired relationships might be (1) forging a "close" relationship between the father and David, between the mother and David, or both; (2) forming an "average" relationship between the parents, while they both form a close relationship with David; (3) all family members forming average relationships; (4) all family members forming close relationships; or (5) any combination of these relationships over time.

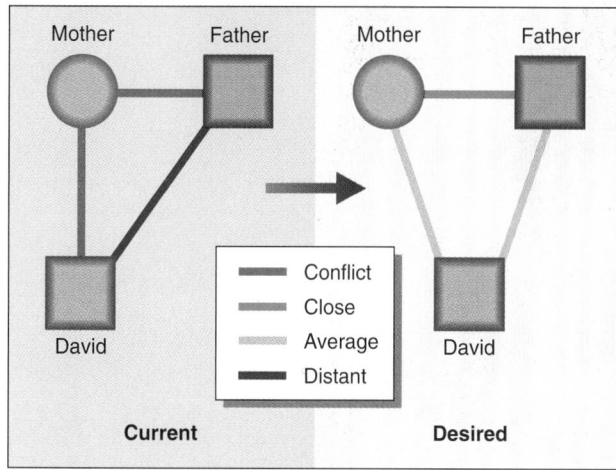

Figure 237-1. David's family: current and desired relationships.

whole exerts its influence on the errant pieces, and balance is restored. Notice also the changeability regarding closeness and distance among the pieces and the importance of vertical hierarchy; they describe the behavior and relationships among individuals in a family.

Family members, in or out of the pediatrician's office, behave much like the individual pieces of a mobile; that is, each is capable of independent behavior, but each is connected to another and to the whole. Any movement by a single member influences and changes the movement of the group as a whole. The concept of homeostatic balance within the family system is most important—balance and movement, movement and balance.

Figure 237-2 depicts a family mobile. In this particular family, the mother is at the top of the hierarchy. The father and the eldest child are approximately on the same level. Next in line is the second eldest child, followed in descending order by the three youngest children. Every member has his or her "place," and their relationships are defined further by their emotional closeness to each other, their roles, and the integrity of the "boundaries," which define

---

Box 237-2. Benefits of a Family Context Approach

Assessing the child's problem within the family context provides the physician with the following:

1. Information not available from the index patient. Every family member has valuable information, perceptions, and beliefs that enhance the physician's understanding of the child and the presenting problem.
2. The opportunity to observe family interactions. Understanding how family members make decisions and communicate is key to understanding the family's patterns of behavior, which may serve to maintain the problem (to serve individuals' roles and maintain the family's "balance").
3. The opportunity to involve the family, the physician's greatest resource, in the treatment. Helping family members cooperate and develop their solutions (a major goal of the meetings) is best accomplished, initially, in family meetings.
4. The opportunity to recognize "warning signs." If the family members cannot or will not cooperate in the meeting, they will not do it at home. This is a signal to the physician to deepen or widen his or her exploration or consider a referral.

---

and protect family subunits (e.g., the parent dyad, the spousal dyad, and various sibling relationships).

IDENTIFYING PROBLEMS SUITABLE FOR A FAMILY FOCUSED APPROACH

Clinicians encounter three levels of psychosocial behavioral problems. Level I problems are predictable and mild and may represent variations of normal development (Box 237-3). To assess and manage level I problems, the clinician, employing a child/symptom perspective, uses good interviewing skills and knowledge of basic child development and behavior and prescribes an array of generic parenting skills and behavioral techniques. Level I problems occur in families that are competent, caring, and capable of problem solving. They require a minimal family assessment and usually resolve with the five R's interventions (see Box 237-1).

Level II problems are suitable for a family focused approach. They include (1) level I problems that have failed to resolve, recur, or intensify (e.g., sleep disorders); (2) child problems that have an apparent psychosocial etiology (e.g., chronic somatic complaints); or (3) parent problems (e.g., parental disagreement over discipline). Level II problems are not exclusive and may exist on a continuum with level I problems (i.e., they often are discovered to be part of, or to evolve from, a level I problem, such as the emotional and family interaction complications of attention deficit hyperactivity disorder). Level II problems often resolve with child centered interventions and family focused approaches (Box 237-4).

Level II problems generally have three characteristics: (1) Children often present as the "symptomatic patient" or the "identified patient" of a disturbed or stressed (not always dysfunctional) family system; (2) relationship problems (e.g., child-parent, parent-parent) invariably are a major issue; and (3) the family, after repeated attempted child centered interventions, feels frustrated, hopeless, and confused. They are "stuck" and need a "map" to create new movement and solutions (Box 237-5).

Level III problems are long-standing, are complex, and tend to occur in families or individuals with multiple problems. Level III problems include substance abuse, severe psychiatric disorders, and failure to thrive. These problems may be revealed by the family during the initial assessment, or they may become apparent after attempted level I or level II interventions have failed (Box 237-6). Level III problems also include common issues that often require a referral for individual advice or guidance (e.g., gay or lesbian adolescent dealing with sexual orientation in a straight world or parents wishing to adopt a child).

The clinician should refer the family or individual to the appropriate agencies and professionals when the clinician has an understanding of them and has gained the family's trust, which ensures an appropriate referral and enhances the likelihood of patient compliance and improved outcome. These referrals might include religious organizations, Department of Social Services, Women's Shelter, Planned Parenthood, clinical psychologists, psychiatrists, and behavioral-developmental pediatricians and a referral

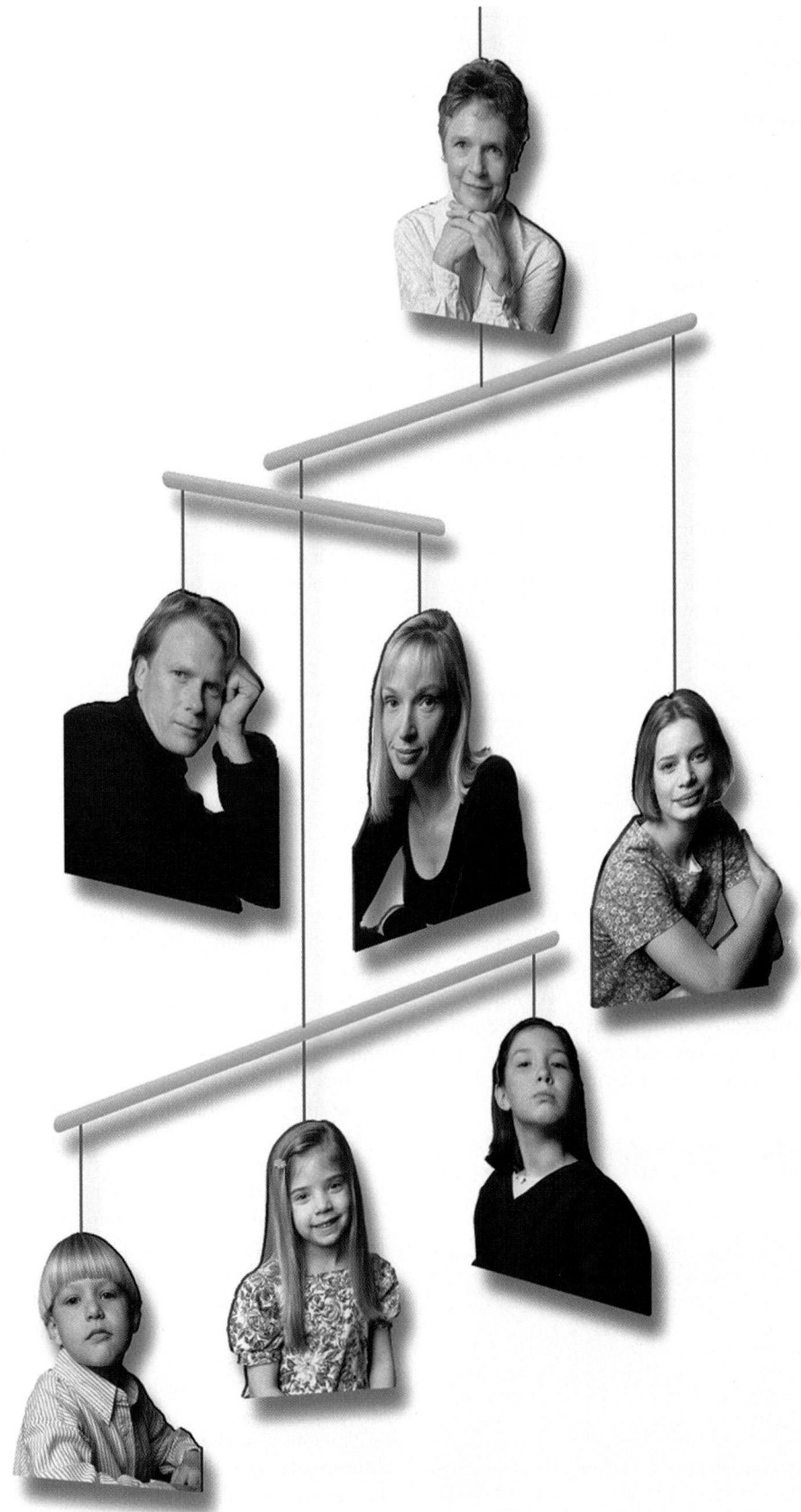

Figure 237-2. The family mobile. (Courtesy of John DeNapoli.)

> **Box 237-3.** Examples of Level I Problems*
>
> - Developmental variations—tantrums, sleep disorders, colic, feeding problems, toilet training, enuresis, encopresis
> - Developmental transitions—toddlerhood, entering school, entering adolescence
> - Mild, predictable behavioral and parenting problems—noncompliance of child, sibling rivalry, parental disagreement, parental difficulty imposing limits
> - Mild emotional and temperament problems—situational/reactive sadness, shy/slow to warm up child, difficult child
> - Attention and learning problems—child with minimal emotional and behavioral complications
> - Peer interaction problems—child has no friends, teases others, acts bossy, bullies or is bullied
> - Family life cycle events—birth of an infant, death of a grandparent, parent "midlife crisis"
>
> *A level I problem may be the initial presentation of a level II problem or the symptom of a level III problem.

to an adult medicine physician for a parent's medical or emotional problems. Often families need a second referral when the first does not "fit" their needs or style. The clinician should continue to follow the child, manage the problems that he or she can, and monitor the family's compliance with the referral and overall well-being.

> **Box 237-4.** Examples of Level II Problems or Indications for a Level II Approach*
>
> - Any level I problem that does not resolve or intensifies despite child/symptom centered interventions
> - Poor compliance with medical regimens, parental requests, household chores
> - Significant parent disagreement/conflict about parenting style and discipline
> - Punitive parenting, including constant threats or use of corporal punishment
> - Family communication-interactive patterns that discourage expressions of affection, acceptance, and approval, resulting in depression or diminished self-esteem
> - Intense parent-child conflict, including a poor "fit" between child and parent temperaments
> - School refusal, separation anxiety, chronic somatic pain complaints (e.g., abdominal pain)
> - Vulnerable child syndrome and overprotected child
> - Mood disorders in a child or in a family member that affect the child
> - Family stresses (losses, changes, transitions), including divorce, formation of stepfamily, death of or illness in a loved one, diagnosis of a developmental delay
> - Initial complaint is centered on family relationships and interactions (e.g., "My daughter and I argue all the time")
> - Single parenting with any attendant stressors on parent or child or both
> - When a referral is needed and the family does not understand or is hesitant
> - Whenever the physician believes a family systems approach is appropriate
>
> *Level II problems often are resolved with child centered and family centered interventions. They also may be the initial presentation of a level III problem (e.g., a severe or complex individual/family problem).

> **Box 237-5.** Level II Problems Do Not Imply Family Dysfunction
>
> All families experience stress and strain at various times and with a range of psychosocial problems. A level II problem does not mean the family is dysfunctional or abnormal. All families need help during these times and usually respond well to a family centered approach.

Clinicians' abilities and interests vary widely. Some clinicians are skilled and comfortable in advising parents how to "behave" during a divorce, what reactions to expect from the child, and how to help the child adjust. The clinician may provide family counseling, facilitating "therapeutic communication" among family members. Other clinicians might choose to refer the family right away.

SUGGESTING A FAMILY MEETING

After the clinician has identified an appropriate problem, he or she should suggest a family meeting in a way that conveys support, understanding, and hope—not blame, incompetence, or psychopathology. The clinician always should "normalize" the situation and allay the family's worries by reminding them that all families need help from time to time. The clinician respectfully states that the family is affected by the problem, that the family is the best resource for understanding the problem, and that family input and participation are needed to resolve it (Box 237-7). The clinician can state the shift from a traditional child focus to a family focus in various ways:

1. "Mr. and Mrs. Wong, a family meeting would be very helpful. It is not intended to focus on any one person or imply blame. Instead we can understand Anita's problem better by getting more information. You are the best resource for that—everyone has something to offer. We need everyone's perspectives and cooperation."
2. "Mr. Greenberg, your family has the best understanding of the issues. When someone has a problem, I find that getting information from other family members help us understand and resolve the problem. The family meeting is the best way to do this."

> **Box 237-6.** Examples of Level III Problems
>
> - Marital/partner conflict, separation, divorce
> - Domestic violence, physical/sexual abuse
> - Alcohol and substance abuse
> - Psychiatric problems in parents or when severe in children
> - High-risk behaviors—juvenile delinquency, school failure/dropout, sexual promiscuity/repeated infections with sexually transmitted diseases, unplanned pregnancies resulting in abortions or many children born close together
> - Any level I/level II problems that do not respond to the physician's interventions or that exceed the physician's abilities, time, interests
> - Common issues requiring support (e.g., gay/lesbian adolescent dealing with sexual orientation in a straight world)

Box 237-7. Suggesting a Family Meeting

The physician suggests a family meeting in a supportive, nonstigmatizing, nonjudgmental manner. The family is looking for leadership and guidance, and as the (temporary) leader, the physician must be confident and directive (at this time). The physician must signal clearly the shift from a child/symptom focus to a family perspective and ensure the family understands and is comfortable with and agrees to that shift.

---

3. After child centered interventions have failed: "Mrs. Garcia, I appreciate all you have done. You have worked very hard, and yet the problem is not getting better. I sense your frustration. We have been focusing on Juanita, but it's not working. She says she's a bad girl. She feels terrible. We need more information to understand the whole situation. A family meeting would be very helpful."

4. "Ms. Raimondi and Julie Ann, I know you would like to see things get better, but from what I hear, everyone is still feeling pretty upset. When I see a family issue like this, the best thing is a family meeting, including Johnny [Julie Ann's brother] and Grandmother [who lives with them]. Everyone shares his or her feelings and thoughts, giving us a much better idea of what's going on. No one is singled out

---

Box 237-8. Clinical Tips for Making the Shift to a Family Centered Focus

1. If possible, do not wait for a family crisis to suggest a family meeting.
2. Call the visit a family meeting, family session, or family visit, not "family therapy."
3. Remind the family that all families need help from time to time.
4. Address the parent's chief complaint; do not imply the meeting is to explore all aspects of the family life or to reconstitute the family.
5. Identify the family leader, and form an alliance with him or her.
6. After requesting a family meeting, permit silence and encourage the family to ask questions. Never force the idea of a meeting or argue with the family. Let them think about it and call you back.
7. Meet with the whole family, but although not ideal, meet with family members who wish to attend when others cannot or will not attend.
8. Do not say you want to refer the family to a mental health professional.
9. Select families carefully. A family that the physician already knows from prior visits and with whom the physician feels comfortable is ideal when beginning to use family meetings.
10. Select problems carefully. Focus on one (apparently) well-defined problem (e.g., parental disagreement over discipline or child noncompliance with parental requests).
11. Remind the family (and yourself) that progress takes time and effort. This attitude allows everyone to set realistic expectations and removes pressure from the physician and the family to do it all now.
12. Remind the family that an initial assessment and intervention plan (working with the family to develop solutions) requires two visits; then two or three follow-up visits are needed.

---

or blamed [Julie Ann had been feeling defensive, angry, and scapegoated]. Then you can begin to work together."

The clinician must make the shift to a family focus in a manner that is clear, worded to fit the family's social-verbal style, sensitive to their normal hesitation, and respectful of their pride and privacy. When stated clearly, sensitively, and respectfully, the family is more likely to accept the suggestion. This family focused form of communication requires special interpersonal and clinical skills (Box 237-8).

INTERVIEWING THE FAMILY

Interviewing the family is not the same as interviewing a parent about a child (a parent "reports" about the child and answers specific clinician-directed questions). Family interviewing is an exploration of the family context, an opportunity for the clinician to join with the family, to observe family interactions, and to get a hint of family life at home. The family invites the clinician to hear, see, feel, share, and understand their inner, private psychosocial life.

The family interview is not just a set of interviewing techniques, but much more. It is an intensely human experience, which can evoke a range of strong feelings in the clinician and the family (ranging from anger, sadness, and hopelessness to love, laughter, joy, and relief). The overall purposes of a family meeting are to help the family adapt to change, cooperate, learn to problem solve, and strengthen the family relationships (good communication; demonstrations of affection, appreciation, and approval; a supportive hierarchy; a sense of family loyalty and connectedness; and a respect for each individual's attributes, differences, and autonomy). The family achieves their goals by agreeing about a problem, defining a goal, mobilizing their strengths, supporting each individual's own needs, and working together. The clinician facilitates this process by "leading by following" or "leading from behind." It is essential to recognize and praise families for their successes and not blame them for their failures.

Successful family interviewing is built on a good relationship between the clinician and the patient, the best single predictor of a good outcome. In this setting, the family (parent and child) is the patient, but the clinician must differentiate between the parent and the child and respect their individual needs. The clinician strengthens this relationship by allowing his or her interviewing to be guided by the dynamics of the therapeutic triad, which evolve from the three simultaneous interactions that occur in any family meeting: clinician-child interaction, family-child interaction, and clinician-family interaction. In this depiction of the therapeutic triad, "family" is the parent(s) or the designated primary provider (Fig. 237-3).

In the therapeutic triad shown in Figure 237-3, the three relationships are depicted with solid bidirectional arrows. In the meeting, the clinician supports the family-child relationship, and the family supports the clinician-child relationship (dotted arrows). The clinician develops and maintains a good relationship with the child and the family, essential ingredients for a successful family meeting.

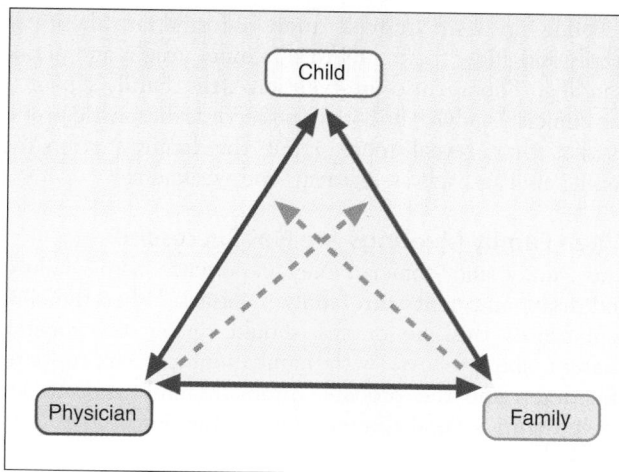

Figure 237-3. The therapeutic triad. (Adapted from Doherty W, Baird M: Family Therapy and Family Medicine. New York, Guilford, 1983, p 13.)

Four Steps of the Family Interview

A family interview loosely follows a four-step sequence: (1) engaging the family, (2) understanding the family and its concerns, (3) working with the family, and (4) concluding the interview (Box 237-9). This sequence is intended to facilitate the formation of a therapeutic alliance with the family, observations of family interaction, gathering of information, and working with the family. The interview does not always need to follow this sequence. The clinician should be flexible and creative, while modifying the interview format to create a "good fit" between his or her style and the family's style and to address adequately the family's concern within the time constraints of the visits.

A complete first family meeting (initial assessment and treatment plan) usually requires 45 to 60 minutes. Most office practitioners and academic center clinicians might need to divide the meeting into two separate visits. The first visit would include step 1 (engaging) and step 2

Box 237-9. Four Steps of a Family Interview

- Step 1. Engaging the family
  - The start of forming a therapeutic alliance between the physician and the family (each and every member)
- Step 2. Understanding the family and its concerns (assessment phase)
  - Understanding the family composition, hierarchy, and patterns of behavior
  - Understanding the family's concern
- Step 3. Working with the family (the problem-solving phase)
  - The physician facilitates (but does not direct or prescribe) changes in the family's behavior and interactions to create their own solutions and to achieve their stated goals
  - The physician explores the family's strengths and past successes
- Step 4. Concluding the meeting
  - Emphasizing positives
  - Summarizing the meeting
  - Getting family feedback about their impressions of the meeting
  - Ending on a hopeful note

(understanding), and the second visit would include step 3 (working) and step 4 (concluding).

Engaging the Family (3 to 5 minutes)

The first step, engaging the family, proceeds as follows:

- The greeting: warm welcome; expression of appreciation for them attending the meeting; each member is addressed by his or her proper name; members choose their seating arrangement, which might reveal family relationships
- Social conversation: brief informal conversation to put family at ease; each member is engaged; something special is learned about each; the visit is personalized; each member is made to feel involved; each member is given the opportunity to talk and share
- Who's in charge: the clinician's identification of the family leader and establishment of a good relationship with him or her
- Explanation of the purpose of the meeting (may need repeating, especially for family members whom the clinician is meeting for the first time): the clinician shifts to a family focus to understand the problem; everyone is given the opportunity to give input and participate; cooperation is encouraged; problem-solving strategies (behaviors) are developed
- Estimation of the number of visits: the clinician tells the family the time frame—two visits for the initial interview and two to four shorter follow-up visits. Establishing a time frame helps the family relax and "pace" themselves and sets realistic expectations for the visit (e.g., "In this first visit, we'll discuss your concern, your views, and your goals. In the second visit, we'll work together on ways to help you go where you want to.").

Understanding the Family and Its Concerns (20 to 25 minutes)

The second step, understanding the family, proceeds as follows:

- Family composition and structure: who lives in the home; other members not in home
- Family patterns of interactions (process—*how they interact*): verbal and nonverbal communication and body language; sibling relationships; how the family adapts and cooperates in the meeting; emotions (e.g., fear, anger, guilt, disappointment, sadness, resentment, level of worry) and how they communicate them
- Family concern (content—*what they talk about*): onset, duration, intensity of problem; impact on child and family function, beliefs, perceptions, interpretations, expectations
- Psychosocial family history: mood disorders; substance abuse; domestic violence; learning, behavioral, or attentional problems
- Social history: marital/partner status and satisfaction; sexual orientation; job/financial status; recent stresses and losses; family activities and rituals (e.g., holidays, birthdays, weekend events, family reunions)
- Identification of interactions that maintain the problem

- Parenting history: When asked to reflect on their own upbringing, how they were raised as children, parents often gain insights into their parenting practices.

Working with the Family (20 to 25 minutes)

The third step, working with the family, proceeds as follows:

- Identification of past successes, recent interventions, and outcomes; explore reasons and perceptions about success and failure
- Identification and use of family strengths: network of support (family, friends, religious and social organizations); satisfying and fulfilling marriage/partnership; sense of humor; family connectedness; healthy children and parents; access to health care; adequate financial support
- Helping the family achieve the following: adapt to change; cooperate and develop own solutions; learn to problem solve without clinician's guidance; define individual and collective responsibilities; set appropriate expectations so that everyone can contribute and feel valued
- Offers of advice and interventions if and when appropriate
- Making referrals if and when appropriate

Concluding the Meeting (3 to 5 minutes)

The final step, concluding the meeting, proceeds as follows:

- The clinician always starts with positives: summarizing the meeting; acknowledging what's right, what's working (e.g., the family's willingness to attend the meeting, to share concern and associated feelings [anger, sadness, disappointment]); acknowledging the family's motivation to do better and be happier, sense of commitment, apparent or expressed love for one another.
- The clinician reviews the family's expectations, solutions, and plans; compliments them.
- The clinician encourages the family to respond (questions, clarifications) and to communicate with each other.
- The clinician asks for family feedback: "Did this meeting address your concerns? Was it helpful? Why? Why not? Are you willing to return?"
- The clinician (as leader) schedules another meeting or suggests that it is time or nearing time to end the meeting (this assumes the family is doing better). At the final meeting, the clinician assures the family of his or her continued interest and availability.
- The clinician schedules the next meeting.
- The clinician suggests a referral if appropriate.
- The clinician always ends with positives, complimenting the family again and closing on an appropriately hopeful note.

Follow-up Visits

Follow-up visits are essential. Follow-up visits are the only reliable way for the clinician to know how the family is doing and if he or she really helped the family to help itself. The visits provide a measure of the clinician's skills and effectiveness.

Follow-up visits provide more information about the family and allow the family to gain more insight and understanding. Therapeutic interventions (the family's plan or the clinician's advice or both) also serve as diagnostic probes in that they reveal more about the family's strengths, coping abilities, self-assessment, and weaknesses.

When Family Meetings Are Not Successful

The family and clinician may experience some failures and disappointment with family meetings. When the clinician senses this, he or she should review the meeting content and process (with family input, if appropriate) and determine the probable problems and work to improve them. Several common family meeting problems are listed:

- Unrealistic expectations and goals exist. The clinician or the family or both expect too much progress or expect it to happen too quickly, or the family fails to realize how much work is entailed.
- The clinician fails to appreciate the complexity and severity of problem and underestimates the immense difficulty for the family to change chronic, entrenched interaction patterns.
- The clinician fails to appreciate that families often perpetuate a child's problem/symptom as a way to preserve family balance, maintain members' individual roles and beliefs, and to avoid confronting another painful problem (e.g., marital dissatisfaction or alcoholism).
- The clinician does not have the skills or experience or is unwilling to confront a variety of difficult families—chaotic and loud; discouraged and hopeless; disrespectful of and ignoring time limits of the visit (arrive late, want more time); angry (argumentative or sullen).
- The clinician has a "rescue fantasy" and feels compelled to "save" the family. The family is disappointed when the clinician cannot fulfill the promise to save it.
- The clinician fails to search for strengths, redeeming features, and positives in the family; he or she does not help the family identify or mobilize its strengths. The meetings are dominated by problem-talk, and the family becomes discouraged and depleted of creativity.
- The clinician takes sides and becomes part of a dysfunctional system. The clinician is drawn into "the battle," joins in family arguments, and loses all objectivity and credibility.
- The clinician (trained in the biomedical model) rushes in with well-intentioned advice and directives before he or she has understood the family and its concern and gained its trust. The advice is premature, often inappropriate, unwanted, resented, and sometimes counterproductive. It undermines a central purpose of the family meeting: to help the family develop its own solutions and to feel more competent.
- The clinician fails to protect his or her own personal, social, and emotional life; schedules too many patients; cannot say no; and loses control of his or her time. Eventually the clinician burns out and becomes ineffective and dissatisfied.

- The family problems are so severe that assistance or services are required beyond those that a primary care clinician can provide in his or her office.

Mini-index of Related Topics

SUGGESTED READINGS

Allmond BW, Tanner JL: The Family Is the Patient. Baltimore, Lippincott Williams & Wilkins, 1998.

Coleman WL: Family-Focused Behavioral Pediatrics. Philadelphia, Lippincott Williams & Wilkins, 2001.

Coleman WL, Taylor EH (eds): Family-focused pediatrics: Issues, challenges and clinical methods. Pediatr Clin North Am 1995; 42:1–239 (entire issue).

Green M (ed): Bright Futures: Guidelines for Health Supervision for Infants, Children, and Adolescents. Arlington, VA, Maternal and Child Health Bureau, 1994.

Schmitt B: Pediatric counseling. In Levine MD, Carey WB, Crocker AC (eds): Developmental-Behavioral Pediatrics, 3rd ed. Philadelphia, WB Saunders, 1999, pp 748–755.

238 Obtaining Information: Parent and Child Interviewing and Rating Scales

Terry Stancin and Susan K. Santos

ROLE OF THE GENERALIST

1 Recognize patients with mental health problems.

2 Refer children and adolescents with clinically significant mental health problems for therapy.

3 Conduct thoughtful, systematic parent and patient interviews.

4 Understand and use appropriate rating scales and questionnaires in assessing a child's mental health status.

5 Integrate identification of patient issues with treatment and management.

Mental health issues are recognized as a leading cause of morbidity among children and adolescents. Epidemiologic studies have shown that 11% to 20% of school-age children attending pediatric clinics have one or more diagnosable mental health disorders. Approximately half of all pediatric office visits involve some behavioral, psychosocial, or educational concern.

Failure to recognize mental health problems in a pediatric patient may lead to inappropriate diagnostic testing and place children at high risk for future psychosocial morbidity. Primary care providers (PCPs) fail to identify and refer most children and adolescents with clinically significant mental health problems. There are many possible reasons for underidentification of mental health problems during the pediatric office visit. Only one third of parents (or caregivers) with a psychosocial concern about their child discuss this issue with their child's PCP; this may be secondary to the parent's reluctance to raise concerns or the lack of opportunity to do so during the office visit. When psychosocial issues are raised, the PCP responds less than half of the time; this may be due to time constraints present in the office setting, the PCP's lack of training in dealing with mental health issues, or limited availability of mental health services.

PCPs serve a crucial role as "gatekeeper" of mental health needs for children. The PCP is expected to identify psychosocial and behavioral concerns, make a diagnosis, and determine appropriate treatment and referral. Clinical interview strategies that target mental health issues and behavioral rating scales are important tools to facilitate the diagnosis and management of psychosocial complaints.

Table 238-1. Sample Interview Questions for the Pediatric Patient

	Preschool	School Age	Adolescent
Home/Family	Who in your home do you get along with the best (the worst)? With whom do you have the most fun? When do you feel sad? What makes you afraid? If you could make a wish come true, what would you wish?	What does your family do for fun? Draw me a picture of your family and tell me about it. How often do you feel sad, worried, or scared? If you woke up one morning and a miracle happened, what would be different?	How do you get along with your family? Do you feel like your family listens to you? How often do you feel sad, worried, or scared? Have you ever been hit, punched, or kicked by a family member?
School	What do you like about going to day care/preschool? How do you feel about starting school? What worries you about starting school?	What do you like/dislike about your teacher? What do you like/dislike the most about school? Tell me about a time when you got into trouble at school. How easily do you learn things compared with other kids at school?	How many times this year have you cut school or been suspended? How easily do you learn things compared with other kids at school? Have you ever had a learning problem or needed any special help in school?
Peer Relationships	Do you have a best friend? What are your favorite things to do with your friends? Tell me about a time when you had trouble with another kid.	Do you have a best friend? What do you and your friends do for fun? How would other kids describe you?	How would other kids describe you and your group of friends? Have you recently changed the group of friends you hang out with? Why? How many friends do you have that really understand you and whom you can count on?

what would be different if they woke up one morning, a miracle happened, and all his or her problems were gone. Similarly the child can be asked, "If you found a genie in a bottle and were granted three wishes, what would you wish?"

As they mature, teenagers can offer more insight into their condition. Ideally the interview should begin with the parent and the teenager, and then the PCP should seek consent to see the patient alone. Even the presence of a sibling or friend may make the patient less open. It is crucial to ensure the teenager understands that confidentiality will be maintained. The PCP always should inform the teenager, however, that the parents will be notified if there is a life-threatening concern (e.g., suicidal or homicidal ideation, psychosis, eating disorder, or sexual abuse). It is important to assessing substance use, sexual activity, and mood in confidence. A good way to initiate these discussions is to inquire about peer activity first and then make the questions more specific to the patient. When discussing drug use, the interviewer may start by saying, "A lot of teenagers your age use drugs: how is it at your school?" After discussing this issue, the clinician can ask, "Have you ever been placed in a position where someone has offered you drugs? What did you do about that?" These questions can lead into a discussion about the patient's drug habits and allow the PCP to give the appropriate anticipatory guidance. When trying to assess if the teenager is depressed, the clinician can start by saying, "A lot of teenagers often feel sad or blue; do you often feel this way? How often do you have these feelings?" Addressing the concern in the context of a common problem may make the teenager more comfortable discussing the issue.

Situations that warrant an urgent mental health evaluation include concerns about psychosis, suicidal ideation, and homicidal ideation. When assessing whether a patient is suicidal, it is best to ask the patient directly, "Do you have thoughts about hurting or killing yourself?" If the patient acknowledges suicidal intent, the PCP can determine the risk by asking the patient about a specific plan, previous attempts, access to firearms, and access to medications in the home. Homicidal thoughts can be addressed by saying, "When people get angry, they sometimes think about hurting others; do you ever think about that?" Schizophrenia and bipolar disorder can present in adolescence. If psychosis is suspected, the patient can be asked questions such as the following: "Do your ears or eyes ever play tricks on you; do you hear or see things that others don't?" "Do your thoughts race by so fast that you cannot think?" "Do you feel like other people are plotting to hurt you?"

RATING SCALES AND QUESTIONNAIRES

Child mental health professionals have long used standardized behavioral rating scales that can be completed by a parent or teacher to collect information about a child's problem behaviors. Although physicians have been encouraged to consider using rating scales and other instruments to identify and monitor developmental and behavioral problems, most have not embraced their use for routine practice.

Some confusion related to terminology exists regarding use of rating scales. Concepts of behavioral screening and assessment are confused easily because some instruments have been suggested for both practices. By definition, *screening* practices are intended to identify patients in need of further evaluation and assessment, whereas *assessment* relates to the more comprehensive process leading to diagnosis and intervention.

Rating scales and questionnaires offer several advantages as methods of obtaining behavioral data. Because most scales can be completed by a parent outside of the examination room (in the waiting room or at home before an appointment) and can be scored by clerical staff, rating scales are efficient methods for collecting information. Most scales have been standardized so that comparisons to normative standards can be made. Material and scoring costs are minimal. Rating scales are an excellent way to collect the opinions of multiple observers, especially teachers. Some scales allow for an objective way to monitor and quantify effectiveness of therapeutic interventions. The American Academy of Pediatrics clinical practice guidelines for evaluating attention deficit hyperactivity disorder (ADHD) discussed the option of using ADHD-specific rating scales to help in the evaluation of the disorder.

There are disadvantages to using rating scales and questionnaires in addition to advantages. First, interpretation of results must take into account the fact that caregiver perceptions are subject to bias. Norms may not exist for the population being screened/assessed (e.g., parents from a different cultural group). There may be considerable new administrative demands placed on office staff to administer questionnaires properly. Proper scoring and interpretation of results requires training and expertise to ensure the valid use of tests.

A variety of rating scales and questionnaires are available to pediatricians. Some are broad-based, multidimensional measures (e.g., Child Behavior Checklist), some are problem focused (e.g., ADHD Rating Scale or the Child Depression Inventory), and others are global screening measures (e.g., Pediatric Symptom Checklist). There are measures that rely on parents and others that were developed for obtaining teacher perceptions (e.g., Teacher Report Form) or child self-ratings (Youth Self-Report Form). Specific common rating scales and questionnaires can be found in CD-ROM Chapter 244. Some instruments may be downloaded from the Internet and used free of charge (e.g., the Pediatric Symptom Checklist), although most must be purchased from test distributors.

Sound clinical practice dictates that behavioral screening and assessments be done within the context of a clinical evaluation that includes a thorough history, direct observation, physical examination, and other diagnostic tests. If rating scales are used as part of this procedure, they should be psychometrically sound, acceptable to parents, accurate, and cost-effective, and they should fit into the practice setting. Users of standardized behavioral instruments should become knowledgeable about psychometric issues (i.e., reliability, validity, sensitivity, specificity) and should recognize differences between tests in terms of readability, response format, scoring, completion times, and norms. This information assists the PCP in the selection of instruments and limits potential misuses and invalid interpretation of results. It may be advisable for the PCP to collaborate with a pediatric psychologist when developing screening and behavioral assessment practices. A knowledgeable pediatric psychologist can assist the PCP greatly in selecting procedures that best suit the population and practice needs.

Although standardized screening methods have been shown to increase the rate of identification of children with behavioral problems in primary care settings, comparative studies have not been conducted that would recommend any one method over the others. There is a lack of evidence to support the assumption that the use of screening measures leads to increased recognition, evaluation, and interventions. Ultimately, increasing the repertoire of behavioral treatment options known to pediatricians and integrating psychological services with primary care services may be necessary for greater recognition and intervention.

INCORPORATING RATING SCALES INTO PRACTICE

There are many ways to incorporate rating scales into office practice. If global behavioral screening is the goal, brief questionnaires can be mailed to parents in advance and brought to appointments or completed in the waiting room. For parents with poor reading or English skills, rating scales could be completed via interview. It may be reasonable in some settings to incorporate measures into routine intake forms or to use computer-assisted methods. A series of guides that are suited to office practice was published in the appendix of *Guidelines for Health Supervision III* (available from the American Academy of Pediatrics, Publications Department, 141 Northwest Point Boulevard, PO Box 972, Elk Grove Village, IL 60009-0927, and from the Academy's website, www.aap.org). These guides communicate information about normal aspects of development to parents and patients and provide a checklist of psychosocial and health concerns. Although the American Academy of Pediatrics checklists have not been validated psychometrically as screening measures, they may be useful to alert the clinician about issues to address during an office visit.

If rating scales are being used to clarify further specific concerns (e.g., possible ADHD), appropriate instruments targeting relevant symptoms can be completed during or after a visit. Assessment practices may be adapted depending on the level of expertise and preferences of the PCPs. Some PCPs with more expertise and interest may wish to conduct their own further evaluation, whereas others may wish to refer directly to behavioral specialists.

All tests can be scored by hand using scoring templates, guides, or instructions. Brief measures, such as the Pediatric Symptom Checklist, can be scored in seconds. Other measures are self-scoring (e.g., Child Depression Inventory). Others are scored best by computer (e.g., Child Behavior Checklist). When working with schools, it may be possible to request that scoring of teacher data be done by the school psychologist rather than office staff.

INTEGRATION OF IDENTIFICATION WITH TREATMENT

When a mental health concern is identified during the interview or with the assistance of a specific rating scale, a partnership between the PCP, parent, and patient (depending on age) is crucial in establishing the success of the therapeutic plan. In particular, it is important for the clinician to respect an adolescent's independence and ability to participate in the decision-making process. When determining specific therapy for a patient, it is important to determine whether the plan is acceptable to the parent. If the parents do not agree with the plan or the therapy is

1. *The easy child:* high rhythmicity, tendency to approach, high adaptability, positive mood, low or moderate intensity
2. *The difficult child:* low rhythmicity, tendency to withdraw, low adaptability, negative mood, high intensity
3. *The slow-to-warm-up child:* tendency to withdraw, low adaptability, frequent negative reactions of low intensity; such children are often considered to be shy

through parent report measures), and to provide further empirical evidence of the biologic basis of certain temperamental traits.

To aid in the assessment of the temperamental traits described by Chess and Thomas, Carey and others developed parent report questionnaires, such as the Infant Temperament Questionnaire (for infants 4 to 8 months old), the Toddler Temperament Scale (for children 1 to 3 years old), the Behavioral Style Questionnaire (for children 3 to 7 years old), and the Middle Childhood Temperament Questionnaire (for children 8 to 12 years old). To date, these scales have found their greatest utility in research or specialty settings.

Associations between physiologic and temperamental differences contribute to a growing body of research on the biologic basis for temperamental characteristics in infants. Kagan's research has shown consistent behavioral differences between what he termed *inhibited* and *uninhibited* infants and children. Behaviorally inhibited (i.e., shy) children also had faster and more stable heart rates, pupils that were more dilated, and morning cortisol levels that were higher than uninhibited children. In addition, twin studies that have shown greater concordance in temperamental traits for monozygotic than for dizygotic same-sex twins provide further support for the biologic etiology of temperament.

The nine temperamental traits (see Box 239-1) initially described by Chess and Thomas are a useful context for viewing the personality of the infant and young child. Whether the child shows a greater or lesser degree of each of these traits (with the exception of mood) is not inherently "good" or "bad." Parents and pediatricians should exercise caution in interpreting the common patterns of temperament outlined in Box 239-2, which are well described in the lay parenting literature. What is easy or difficult for one parent may not be so for another. The key issue is whether there is a *goodness-of-fit* between the child and the caregiver. Problems arise when there is a mismatch between the child's temperamental traits and the traits of the caregiver or when the situational context is suited better to a different temperamental profile. A high activity level in a toddler or preschool child may be viewed positively by a parent who enjoys active play with the child, especially if that parent is not required to provide long periods of supervision for the child. Difficulties first may be seen when a highly active child is placed in a group context, such as day care or kindergarten, where there is less opportunity for and tolerance of highly active play. Children who show high-intensity reactions often are described as exuberant and exciting; these same children are likely to be equally intense in their displays of displeasure and negative emotion, leading to intense temper tantrums and outbursts. High task persistence may frustrate parents who find it difficult to distract their children from pursuing misbehaviors (e.g., a toddler who is intent on exploring the electrical outlets in the house despite attempts at distraction and refocusing); yet this same level of task persistence, when applied to educational tasks such as learning to read, is associated with academic success.

Because the relationship between the child and caregiver is not static, what is felt as a good fit during a particular developmental period or stage may not be as compatible at another age or stage. A parent and infant may have a good fit when the infant is totally dependent on the parent, but as that child becomes a toddler or teenager and strives for more autonomy, the parent's expectations may not yield as good a match. A good parent-child fit does not mean, however, that there is continuous harmony and no stress in the relationship. Occasional stress is normal and promotes healthy personality development.

Temperamental traits represent innate personality characteristics that are persistent features throughout at least the first few years of life. Although efforts to change completely a child's temperamental profile are about as successful as efforts to change the personality of a spouse, the child's temperamental characteristics can and are modified over time. Despite evidence of biologic predispositions, it is well accepted that personality is neither entirely predetermined nor fixed. Psychological development is characterized by continuity and change, and in any individual case, a linear one-to-one prediction from early to later life is unreliable. Instead, personality traits are shaped by experiences at each successive developmental stage, allowing an individual's personality to evolve throughout one's lifetime.

ANTICIPATORY GUIDANCE

Parents often are made to feel that they somehow can create a particular type of child through effective or creative parenting. When parents instead understand that temperamental traits are, at least in part, innate characteristics of the child, they can disavow the sense of personal blame. Parents also should be helped to appreciate that mismatches in temperamental traits between themselves (or other caregivers) and their child do not represent inherent problems in their child's personality.

The goal in providing anticipatory guidance to parents about temperament is to help them understand and appreciate the child's temperamental characteristics and personal preferences. Box 239-3 lists books that can be helpful to parents. Parents can be helped to find strengths in their child's personality and to work, with patience, tolerance, and a degree of humility, to modify the features that are most maladaptive.

In addition, a better understanding of the child's temperamental profile helps parents anticipate situations that will pose a unique challenge for their child and identify means to modify the situation to minimize the challenges or to provide additional support. Parents who recognize that their child is "slow-to-warm-up" may arrange for a new babysitter to visit with the child before the first evening they plan to leave the child alone with the sitter. Parents with a child with a high activity level might wish to select a day care setting that provides more opportunities for active play, whereas parents with a child who has low adaptability may select a more structured setting.

Pediatricians frequently are confronted with parental concerns about their children's behavior. Often, these concerns relate to normal temperamental variations that may be misperceived by the parents as behavioral abnormalities. Children who are highly avoidant may show relative intolerance to the introduction of new foods, which may be labeled as a feeding disorder or a behavioral problem. An understanding of the etiology of the conflict between the child's temperamental traits and the parents' behavioral expectations can serve as the basis for appropriate intervention.

A preexisting appreciation of the child's temperamental characteristics also allows pediatricians to individualize their advice on child care so that recommendations anticipate and address the temperamental profile of the child. General guidelines for child rearing do not work equally well with all children. Children respond differently to toilet training and the use of time-out, and guidance for parents in these areas should be tailored, to the extent possible, to the child's most likely reactions. A pediatrician with a long-standing relationship with the parents is also in the unique position to identify potential conflicts between the caregivers' and child's temperament that may interfere with optimal interactions. Suggesting that parents ignore

bedtime protests from a child who is intense, slow-to-adapt, and highly persistent may be ill advised, particularly if the parent has a low threshold of responsiveness and low task persistence.

Children's temperamental traits also affect the way they respond to and manage illness. The pediatrician should be concerned if a normally active and intense child who withdraws from new situations (e.g., pediatric visits) is suddenly seemingly cooperative and quiet during a visit for an acute illness; atypical behavior should raise the concern of a more serious illness. Similarly, temperamental characteristics manifest themselves in the way children approach the management of chronic illness. For example, a child who is rhythmic, adaptable, and persistent may learn and adjust more easily to a management routine for diabetes mellitus.

Mini-index of Related Topics

SUGGESTED READINGS

Carey WB: Clinical use of temperament data in pediatrics. J Dev Behav Pediatr 1985;6:137–142.

Chess S, Thomas A: Temperament in Clinical Practice. New York, Guilford, 1995.

Chess S, Thomas A: Temperament. In Lewis M (ed): Child and Adolescent Psychiatry: A Comprehensive Textbook, 2nd ed. Baltimore, Williams & Wilkins, 1996.

Chess S, Thomas A: The development of behavioral individuality. In Levine MD, Carey WB, Crocker AC (eds): Developmental-Behavioral Pediatrics, 3rd ed. Philadelphia, WB Saunders, 1999, pp 89–99.

Kagan J: Temperamental contributions to social behavior. Am Psychol 1989;44:668–674.

Kagan J: Temperament and the reactions to unfamiliarity. Child Dev 1997;68:139–143.

Kagan J, Snidman N: Temperamental factors in human development. Am Psychol 1991;46:856–862.

Table 240-3. Pros and Cons of Using the Diagnosis of Mental Retardation

Pros	Cons
Groups children with similar characteristics	Groups children with different characteristics
Focuses on realistic expectations	Label can be an excuse
Helps meet eligibility criteria for federal and state programs, early intervention	May limit services or access to insurance
Defines needs	Can limit expectations
Can help to understand some behaviors	Negative connotations of labels
Is needed to get coverage Medicaid, SSI	May limit access to health insurance
Improves access to parent support groups	Patients with same etiology may have different profile and outcome
The disability should be identified before one can search for an etiology	Diagnosis can be, and frequently is, misused
Diagnosis helps to increase knowledge	The meaning of the diagnosis can have different meanings based on past experience and professional and cultural background
Giving a name can help to relieve anxiety and confusion	
Helps to provide proactive guidance, anticipate secondary problems	People with mild mental retardation find the diagnosis demeaning when applied to them

SCREENING

Early detection, diagnosis, and treatment of cognitive disorders can have lasting effects on children and their families. The pediatrician is in a unique position to detect, diagnose, and initiate treatment. Periodic developmental screening should be performed as recommended by the American Academy of Pediatrics and required under Medicaid regulations for Early Periodic Screening, Diagnosis, and Treatment. A wide variety of acceptable screening tests are applicable for pediatric practice (Table 240-4).

A practical approach to developmental surveillance is to use every encounter to ask about the parents' concerns about development and their estimates of the child's developmental age, supplemented by informal schedules of developmental milestones and red flag symptoms and periodic use of formal screening tests. For surveillance purposes, delay can be quantitated using the *developmental quotient* (DQ = developmental age/chronologic age). A cognitive DQ greater than 0.8 can be considered normal; 0.7 to 0.8, suspicious; and less than 0.7, abnormal. This approach allows the pediatrician to *quantify degrees of delay* for children with DQ less than 0.7, rather than grouping them together as "abnormal," as most screening tests do. These approaches are often in close agreement and should be seen as complementary.

PREVALENCE

The prevalence of mental retardation generally is regarded as falling between 1% and 3% of the population. Statistically, about 3% would be the expected prevalence if one assumed an entirely normal distribution of cognitive functioning in a population. Several factors serve to modify this expectation, however, including definition used in identifying cases (IQ versus IQ and adaptive level); age of population (school-age children are identified more easily than preschoolers or adults); location, socioeconomic status, and cultural makeup; and whether samples are drawn from direct surveys of geographically defined populations, service delivery systems, or case registries. In general, overall prevalence noted in more recent studies in developed countries trends toward the lower end of the traditional range.

Prevalence studies of mental retardation usually do not subdivide cases into the clinical categories of mild, moderate, severe, and profound. Instead most useful studies make a distinction between *mild mental retardation* (IQ 50 to 70) and *severe mental retardation* (IQ <50). Severe mental retardation is present in about 3 to 5 per 1000 children, a prevalence level that has been fairly consistent across studies and over time. Variability in the prevalence of mild mental retardation has varied much more widely. Reported prevalences range from 2 per 1000 children to 23 per 1000 children. Variation in reports of prevalence for mild mental retardation accounts for the wide range of prevalences reported for mental retardation in general. It is generally safe to conclude, however, that in any large population, subgroup prevalence increases with increasing IQ.

In the United States, prevalence consistently varies with socioeconomic, racial, and cultural factors, with higher prevalences noted in populations with lower socioeconomic status and African-American and Latino populations. The direct and indirect effects of poverty and cultural isolation and their causes cannot be disentangled from the effects, if any, of race and culture. This relationship between poverty and mental retardation prevalence seems to operate largely at the level of mild mental retardation. Greater degrees of mental retardation do not seem to be influenced greatly by poverty or related variables.

ETIOLOGY

Etiology varies with severity of mental retardation. The greater the severity, the more likely an identifiable organic etiology would be detected. In severe mental retardation (IQ <50), only about 25% to 40% of children do not have an identifiable etiology. Detected etiologies include prenatal (e.g., chromosomal disorders, single-gene defects, congenital infection, central nervous system malformations), perinatal (e.g., infection, hypoxia-ischemia), postnatal (e.g., injury, central nervous system trauma), or multiple-stage etiologies (e.g., sequelae of prematurity). In contrast, more than half (50% to 62%) of children with mild mental retardation (IQ 50 to 70) do not have an identifiable organic cause; this does *not* mean they do *not* have an organic etiology. Organic factors tenuously or not at all associated with poverty, race, or culture may be involved. In recent decades, there has been increased understanding of the effects of maternal use of alcohol and more recently tobacco on the developing fetus. Fragile X syndrome, the most common heritable form of mental retardation, now is noted to have a broader range of disability than the originally reported severe mental retardation in boys; milder degrees of retardation in boys and girls are recognized. The relationship between low levels of lead burden and subsequent

Table 240-4. Developmental Screening Instruments

Test	Age (mo)	Time of Administration (min)	Sensitivity	Specificity	Comments
Denver II Denver Developmental Materials, Denver	0–72	15–20	Variable	Low for language, good for motor	Personal social, fine motor/adaptive, gross motor and adaptive
Batelle Developmental Inventory Screening Test (BDIST) Riverside Publishing Co, Chicago	7–48	10–30	Moderate to high	Moderate (better with use of cutoff at 2 SD below the mean)	Fine and gross motor, adaptive, language (expressive and receptive), adaptive, and cognitive skills
Parents' Evaluations of Developmental Status (PEDS) Ellsworth & Vandermeer Press, Ltd, Nashville	0–84	5	Good	Good	Language (expressive and receptive), fine motor, gross motor, behavior, social, learning
Bayley Infant Neurodevelopmental Screening (BINS) The Psychological Corporation, San Antonio	3–24	10–15	High	High	Directly elicited items. Assess neurologic processes (reflexes and tone), neurodevelopmental skills (movement, symmetry), and developmental skills (object permanence, imitation, language)
Ages and Stages Questionnaires (ASQ) Paul H. Brookes, Baltimore	4–48	10–15	High	High	One form every 2 mo until 2 yr, every 3 mo until 3 yr, then every 6 mo. Each form contains 30 items in 5 areas: communication, gross and fine motor, problem solving, and personal-social
Developmental Screening Questionnaires Paul H. Brookes, Baltimore	0–48	5	Moderate to high	High	Simple directions and pictures help parents to indicate children's skills. Separate forms for each age range
Child Developmental Inventory (CDI) Behavior Science Systems, Minneapolis, MN	3–72	10	Good	High	Pass-fail. Developmental parental questionnaire with 60 yes/no questions: social, self-help, gross motor, fine motor, and language

reduction in IQ and adaptive performance are becoming clearer. Similarly, controversial data suggest that maternal ingestion of fish containing high levels of methylmercury compounds may have adverse neurodevelopmental outcomes. These are factors that may have relatively small but reproducible deleterious effects on subsequent neurodevelopment. Even small effects on a normally distributed variable in a large population increase the number of individuals whose variable falls beneath any arbitrary cutoff (e.g., IQ<70). From a population perspective, the prevalence of mild mental retardation especially may be driven by such factors.

In much the same manner, the effects of early experience on brain development and behavior may influence mental retardation prevalence through seemingly small effects. A clearer understanding of the broad range of interrelated organic and environmental mechanisms and etiologies for mild mental retardation and related neurodevelopmental disabilities is expected to emerge in the coming years and replace the overly general and potentially pejorative concept of "sociocultural mental retardation." Physicians are cautioned against immediately ascribing the *direct influence* of poverty, race, or culture as the primary cause of mild mental retardation.

When a developmental diagnosis of mental retardation has been made or is suspected, consideration of an etiologic diagnosis is necessary. Often the medical history, including family history, and physical and neurodevelopmental exam-

inations suggest an etiology or at least a category of etiologies (e.g., prenatal, perinatal, postnatal, infectious, genetic, toxic). Laboratory, imaging, and related studies and specialty consultations should be guided by data from the history and examination. "One-size-fits-all" laboratory panels are not warranted. An exception is DNA testing for fragile X syndrome. Fragile X syndrome is the most common heritable cause of mental retardation and can present in a variety of manners in boys and girls. Although typical dysmorphic features are described, they are by no means always present. All children with unexplained mental retardation should have DNA testing for the fragile X repeat abnormality. Brain imaging should be considered when motor disabilities coexist or when there are craniofacial, multiple somatic, or neurocutaneous abnormalities; seizures; or suggestion of neurodegeneration. In almost all settings, magnetic resonance imaging is preferred over computed tomography because of the better resolution. Functional neuroimaging remains investigational at this time. Cytogenetic studies are warranted when there are multiple, even minor, somatic anomalies; family history of neurodevelopmental disability; or history of fetal loss. Several genetic disorders may be detected using fluorescent in situ hybridization probes if the clinical situation warrants. Metabolic studies should be considered when there is poor growth, episodic vomiting, seizures, movement disorder, loss of skills, sensory abnormality, hepatosplenomegaly, or unusual rashes. A specialist best directs further investigations.

Table 240-5. Common Problems Often Affecting Children with Mental Retardation—cont'd

Area	Main Issue	What to Do	Helpful References
Family—cont'd	Siblings	Assess the impact on siblings Incorporate siblings in the discussion. Provide individualized time for the siblings. Show them that you are concerned about them, too Help parents to keep a balanced view of the entire family	
Finance	Family support	Ask about health insurance Consider help from Medicaid, SSI, Title V services (states' Children with Special Health Care Needs Services) Medicaid waiver resources may be available for technology-dependent children or children with severe medical problems Tax-deductible expenses: transportation, lodging, and meals for medical purposes; diapers; respite caregivers	Rosenfeld LR: Your Child and Health Care: A "Dollars & Sense" Guide for Families with Special Needs. Baltimore, Paul H. Brookes, 1994

*These problems are more frequent in children with severe and profound mental retardation. Relevance varies with age of the child.

SUGGESTED READINGS

Batshaw ML (ed): When Your Child Has a Disability. Baltimore, Paul H. Brookes, 2001.

Capute AJ, Accardo PJ (eds): Developmental Disabilities in Infancy and Childhood, 2nd ed. Baltimore, Paul H. Brookes, 1996.

Shonkoff JP, Phillips DA (eds), National Research Council and Institute of Medicine, Committee on Integrating the Science of Early Childhood Development: From Neurons to Neighborhoods: The Science of Early Childhood Development. Washington, DC, National Academy Press, 2000.

Wallace HM, MacQueen JC, Biehl RF, Blackman JA (eds): Mosby Resource Guide to Children with Disabilities and Chronic Illness. St. Louis, Mosby, 1997.

241 Learning Disabilities

Jane N. Hannah

EVOLUTION OF LEARNING DISABILITIES

Kirk is credited with formulating and publishing the earliest definition of *learning disability* in 1962 in his book, *Educating Exceptional Children;* however, Hinshelwood and Morgan described childhood learning disabilities in case reports in the late 1800s. Morgan reported the existence of developmental dyslexia in the *British Medical Journal* in 1896. Early in the evolution of learning disabilities, much of the research stemmed from the work of Orton from the 1920s and 1930s. These investigators attempted to identify a single processing deficit (e.g., visual perceptual deficits, auditory-perceptual deficits and associated language deficiencies, deficits in intersensory integration) that would account for all learning disabilities. We now recognize that the category of learning disabilities is not a single disorder but encompasses seven areas: (1) listening comprehension, (2) oral expression, (3) basic reading skills, (4) reading comprehension, (5) written expression, (6) math calculation, and (7) math reasoning.

The first official published definition of learning disability was developed in 1968 out of the National Advisory Committee on Handicapped Children, which was chaired by Kirk. The committee's recognition of a learning disability as a handicapping condition was based on advocacy rather than scientific evidence. It was adopted into the federal definition of learning disability in the Rules and Regulations for the Education for All Handicapped Children Act of 1975 (PL 94-142) and has been modified only slightly since 1975: "The term 'specific learning disabilities' means a disorder in one or more of the basic psychological processes involved in understanding or using language, spoken or written, that may manifest itself in imperfect ability to listen, think, speak, read, write, spell, or do mathematical calculations. The term includes such conditions as perceptual disabilities, brain injury, minimal brain dysfunction, dyslexia, and developmental aphasia. The term does not apply to children who have learning problems that are primarily the result of visual, hearing, or motor disabilities, of mental retardation, of emotional disturbance, or of environmental, cultural, or economic disadvantage. In making determination of eligibility, a child shall not be determined to be a child with a learning disability if the determination is lack of instruction in reading, math, or limited English proficiency."

Since the inception of PL 94-142, there has been a significant increase in the number of school-age students served under the Individuals with Disabilities Education Act (IDEA), with the number of students classified with learning disabilities increasing by 37.8% in 10 years, greater than for any other high-incidence disability. In the 1996–97 disability census, it was reported that 51.1% (or 2,676,299 children) of children with 1 of the 12 disabilities listed in the IDEA were classified with a learning disability. This increase has prompted many state departments of education to investigate the need for changes in their diagnostic criteria. Meanwhile, researchers are investigating approaches to prevent and treat learning disabilities.

Because approximately 75% to 80% of students who are classified with a learning disability have a significant deficit in language and reading, most of the research has been in the general area of reading and in particular basic reading skills (i.e., dyslexia). Consequently, 100 years after Morgan reported developmental dyslexia in the medical literature, the understanding of dyslexia has evolved from a poorly understood disorder to one that is, as Shaywitz and colleagues put it in their 1996 *Neuroscientist* article, "at the cutting edge of scientific accomplishments." These advances should lead to improved methods to diagnose the condition and improved instructional approaches to prevent and treat learning disabilities. Research in other areas of learning disabilities has been less well developed, and understanding of these conditions is limited. It is speculated that only 5% to 10% of children within the entire learning disability sample have a nonverbal learning disability. Since the 1990s, understanding of the nonverbal learning disability has increased, but much more research is needed before understanding matches that of dyslexia.

ETIOLOGIES OF LEARNING DISABILITIES

Individuals with learning disabilities are a diverse group with a variety of strengths and weaknesses because of the way in which they process information. It is believed that the causes of a learning disability can be genetic and environmental. Because most of the research has been in the area of dyslexia, understanding of the causes of dyslexia is more advanced. Dyslexia and normal reading ability are influenced significantly by heredity. The evidence suggests that 27% to 49% of parents and 40% of siblings of children with dyslexia are affected. In 1991, Pennington suggested that genetic markers on chromosomes 15 and 6 possibly might influence reading ability. While to date, no single gene has been reliably identified, several genes that lie on chromosomes 2, 3, 6, 7, 15, and 18 continue to be suspect.

Since the 1990s, researchers have investigated the deficits linked to dyslexia and have identified that dyslexia is caused by a core deficit in phonologic processing, which underlies deficits in word recognition and decoding. Consequently, there is little evidence to support the hypothesis that dyslexia is caused by deficits in visual processing as previously thought. Frequently, children with dyslexia may show subtle deficits in spoken language (e.g., immediate word recall or syntax), however, which result in problems in reading comprehension. Additionally, these children may have comorbid skill deficits in spelling, written expression, or memorization of math facts, and they are usually slow readers and poor spellers into adulthood. By understanding the impact of heredity on reading development, children can be referred for preventive care partly based on family history.

Less is known of the environmental causes of learning disabilities. It is recognized, however, that risks associated with the sociologic environment (large family size, low socioeconomic status, poor language models) affect reading problems. Although it has been speculated that infectious or toxic environmental insults may result in learning disabilities, this evidence has been weak.

In Pennington's review of the literature on right hemisphere or nonverbal learning disorders (e.g., specific math and handwriting problems), he reported that Turner syndrome and fragile X syndrome in girls may be a possible genetic cause of these disorders. He further speculated that there likely are other genetic influences on these disorders that have yet to be discovered. In the research that has been completed, the core deficit in specific math disabilities has been linked to problems in spatial cognition. Less is known about the environmental causes of these disorders; however, possible causes include moderate-to-severe closed head injury, cranial radiation, unsuccessfully treated hydrocephalus, and congenital absence of the corpus callosum.

SYMPTOMS OF LEARNING DISABILITIES

Preschool Children

Preschool children who later may be diagnosed with learning disabilities in reading or other language areas often have delays in the acquisition of speech, show articulation errors, have difficulty naming the letters and colors, have problems executing one- and two-step directions, and missequence syllables (e.g., "aminals" for "animals"). These children also may use physical measures to solve problems with peers because of their limited language skills. For children who might have learning disabilities classified in the nonverbal area, it is more difficult to identify markers in the preschool years. Generally, it is thought that these children resist activities that require fine motor skills (e.g., puzzles, building toys, drawing, coloring), and they tend to prefer verbal activities (e.g., talking to adults, reading, listening to stories). Until further research is completed, however, this area remains difficult to predict in the preschool years.

Elementary School–Age and Middle School–Age Children

When children attend school, other symptoms appear, with the best predictor for reading skills being phonologic awareness. To read fluently, the child must be able to develop an understanding of the alphabetic system and the translation of these skills to the application of phonics in reading words. They must be able to perceive and segment these sounds in words (e.g., hear the difference in "hat" and "cat"). Poor readers labor to sound out unknown words and are poor spellers within the context of their writing because they attempt to spell words through memorization rather than phonics. While attempting to read, they expend so much mental energy decoding the words that little energy remains to extract meaning from what has been read. In addition, these children often have deficient word retrieval skills, overuse fillers in their conversation (e.g., "like," "you know"), and have problems making use of inflectional endings (e.g., "-ed," "-ing"). Many times, these children are described as being shy because of their difficulty with word finding.

Children with nonverbal learning disabilities often are not identified until much later in their schooling because their deficits do not interfere with the acquisition of skills in the early grades as do deficits in the reading and language areas. Symptoms in school may include difficulty with handwriting (e.g., copying from the board, spatial orientation of letters to each other and to the lines on the page, and slow and labored handwriting), weaknesses in pragmatic language (i.e., functional language with peers), difficulty with time and money concepts, and weak eye-hand coordination.

With any learning disability, children may exhibit physical symptoms, such as headaches, stomachaches, depression, anxiety, or a reluctance to go to school. If these physical symptoms occur only on school days, it is possible that a child might have a learning problem.

Adolescents

Children who are highly intelligent may escape detection of a learning disability until they are older; however, the impact of the learning disability still is present. The individual's slow rate of reading and difficulty with spelling are found to be the most clinically significant predictors of a reading disability in adolescence and adulthood. For an adolescent with a nonverbal learning disability, more emotional or motivational problems may be the expressed concern of parents or teachers. The adolescent may show poor peer relations, an overdependence on one or both parents, oppositional behavior with parents and teachers that is associated with the completion of written work, and difficulty with mathematics despite good reading and spelling skills.

ADVANCES IN THE NEUROBIOLOGY OF LEARNING DISABILITIES

Functional neuroimaging studies in dyslexia began in the late 1980s. Soon afterward, magnetic resonance imaging and positron emission tomography provided technology for studying the brain structure and function in learning disorders. Through this technology, it has been suggested that most physically healthy children with dyslexia are expected to have normal computed tomography and magnetic resonance imaging studies and that dyslexia is not associated with macroscopic lesions on the brain. Although functional studies have shown a variety of differences in activation in the left posterior language regions that affect reading, it also is speculated that anomalies may be variably distributed, and additional subcortical structures (e.g., the thalamus) may be affected. This technology has helped clinicians to understand how early brain development occurs and then how it responds once reading develops. Scientists hope to be able to map and quantify the particular neural network that affects reading and extend the understanding, treatment, and prevention of learning disabilities.

EFFICACY OF INTERVENTIONS FOR LEARNING DISABILITIES

In reviewing studies completed over 33 years on more 30,000 children, Lyon reported that for 90% to 95% of poor readers, prevention and early intervention programs that combine instruction in phoneme awareness, phonics, fluency development, and reading comprehension strategies, provided by well-trained teachers, could increase reading skills to average levels. Lyon reported that if this instruction was delayed until children were in third grade, approximately 75% would continue to have reading difficulties throughout high school.

Researchers have provided strong evidence that phonologic coding is essential to learning to read and that the root cause of dyslexia is a deficit in this skill. For children with dyslexia, remedial instruction in phonologic coding is crucial if they are to learn to read. Often, traditional phonics programs fail because children have not acquired the prerequisite phoneme awareness skills. Consequently the instruction must be individualized to each child's specific deficits and level of skill development. This instruction must be sustained over a sufficient time and be taught systematically by well-trained teachers. Although the development of phoneme awareness and phonics skills is necessary to learning to read, other skills are needed for a child to acquire meaning from what is read. For this to occur, children must read fast enough to understand what is read. To obtain this fluency, children must read large amounts of material at the independent reading level (95% accuracy) so that sufficient practice can occur without frustration. In addition to phonologic coding instruction and activities to foster fluency, children's reading skills are influenced by other factors, including (1) the frequency with which they are read to as young children; (2) their experiences with

word play (e.g., nursery rhymes), language patterns, and word usage (semantic and syntactic structures that help predict meaning); (3) their background knowledge; (4) their ability to reason verbally; and (5) their ability to remember verbal information (Box 241-1).

The current knowledge on the etiology and treatment approaches for individuals with nonverbal learning disabilities is sparse. Some families have found, however, that the diagnosis itself is helpful because the problem takes on new meaning. The evaluation may have been initiated because of a concern about behavior or motivation. After the diagnosis is made, it is possible to focus on the great stressor that may be causing or exacerbating the problem behaviors. For children in elementary school, occupational therapy may be helpful, and in later grades, computers, additional time to complete assignments, and modified/shortened written assignments often are helpful. To date, there is no evidence to suggest that children can overcome math disabilities completely. Instruction in step-by-step procedures to solve math problems, in using verbal mediation to help with math problem solving and handwriting, and in providing guidance in course selection and career paths may be beneficial.

Generally, grade retention is not a recommended remedial tool for children with learning disabilities. It usually has a negative effect on achievement and social-emotional adjustment. There is also a high correlation between children who are retained and children who later drop out of school.

There are many unsubstantiated treatments or "cures" that parents may want to pursue. It is wise to express concern to the parent when these treatments are tried in lieu of proven treatments. Some of these unproven treatments are eye movement exercises, Irlen lenses or colored transparencies, visual therapies, chiropractic, megavitamins, dietary treatments, sensory/motor integration, and electroencephalographic biofeedback.

FEDERAL LEGISLATION THAT IMPACTS SPECIAL EDUCATION SERVICES TO STUDENTS WITH LEARNING DISABILITIES

The IDEA of 1990, amended in 1997, was formerly the Education of all Handicapped Children Act of 1975, or PL 94-142. The IDEA established the particular services, procedural safeguards, and requirements for identifying and serving children with disabilities. *Learning disabilities* is 1 of 12 disabilities listed in the IDEA. According to these regulations, public schools have an affirmative duty to locate, identify, and evaluate "all children who have disabilities or who are suspected of having disabilities and are in need of special education and related services." The public school is required to evaluate only children who are suspected of having disabilities; consequently, not all children who are referred for an assessment receive one.

If there is concern about a child's progress and a learning disability is suspected, the parent needs to be assisted in following these steps:

1. The parent meets with the child's teacher to discuss the concerns. It may be helpful for the generalist to send a letter of concern to the teacher or principal before this meeting. If the concerns are warranted, the teacher proceeds to the next step.
2. Personnel from the school convene a student support team that consists of educators and sometimes the parents to discuss the type of interventions or modifications or both needed in the classroom for the child to make progress.
3. Interventions and modifications begin in the classroom for a specified time period.
4. If these interventions are not sufficient to meet the child's needs, the student support team suggests that the school complete a psychoeducational assessment.
5. After testing, the school convenes an individualized education plan (IEP) team meeting, which consists of educators, assessment specialists, parents, other individuals who work or interact with the child, and sometimes the child. The IEP team determines if the child is eligible for special education services. If the child is eligible, goals in the IEP are written to target all deficit areas.
6. When the child is eligible for special education services, an IEP team meeting is held at least one time per school year to monitor his or her progress and modify or add services and goals to the child's IEP as needed.
7. A child remains eligible for special education services until another evaluation by the IEP team determines that the child no longer meets eligibility criteria.

MANAGEMENT

Recognizing the symptoms of a learning disability early in the child's development can make a life-altering difference in a child. The expected role of primary care clinicians in managing the patient's care is not to diagnose a learning disability but to identify the symptoms and to refer the patient to appropriate professionals for diagnosis and treatment.

The process of identification should include a thorough medical, gestational, developmental, family, and school history. The medical examination is likely to provide little information that suggests a possible learning disability; however, the examination may detect other conditions that are interfering with school performance (e.g., sleep apnea caused by enlarged tonsils, eating or sleep problems, migraines, seizures, vision or hearing problems, substance abuse, tic disorder, or possible genetic conditions). The developmental history should include questions about the symptoms listed earlier in this chapter. A thorough family history is useful in the identification process because of the hereditary factors associated with learning disabilities. The school history should include more than just the child's grades. Often a child with learning disabilities spends hours completing work that may take other students 30 minutes to complete, or the child needs extensive help from a parent or tutor. Consequently the child's grades may show little evidence of academic struggle. Inquiries should be made about struggles in completing homework, peer relations, behavior in school, and school absences to gain greater insight into the child's problems.

A brief screen to assess phonologic awareness if problems in reading are evident also can be included (Box 241-2). A screen of phonologic awareness can be assessed in the first semester of kindergarten in about 15 minutes. Lyon reported that these instruments can predict with 80% to 90% accuracy children who will become good readers and children who will have difficulty.

For children with disabilities related to mathematics and handwriting, there may be some confusion with right-left directionality or in understanding mathematical concepts.

Box 241-3. Suggested Readings for Parents

1. Lelewer N: *Something's Not Right: One Family's Struggle with Learning Disabilities*. Acton, Mass, VanderWyk & Barnham, a Division of Publicom, 1994.
2. National Center for Learning Disabilities: *Our World* (quarterly publication). New York, National Center for Learning Disabilities (381 Park Avenue South, Suite 1420, New York, NY 10016).
3. Stevens S: *The Learning Disabled Child: Ways That Parents Can Help*. Winston-Salem, NC, John F. Blair Publisher, 1990.
4. Vail PL: *About Dyslexia: Unraveling the Myth*. Rosemont, NJ, Learning Press, 1990.

Box 241-4. Suggested Readings for Children

1. Gehret J: *Learning Disabilities and the Don't Give Up Kid*. Fairport, NY, Verbal Images Press, 1990. (For children in grades 1–3.)
2. Janover C: *Josh, a Boy with Dyslexia*. Burlington, Vt, Waterfront Books, 1988. (For children in grades 2–5.)
3. Levine MD: *Keeping a Head in School: A Student's Book about Learning Abilities and Learning Disorders*. Cambridge, Educators Publishing Service, 1990. (For children 9 to 15 years old.)

Box 241-2. Screening Tools

- Comprehensive Test of Phonological Processing (CTOPP): ProEd Publishers, Austin, Texas
- Texas Primary Reading Instrument (TPRI): Barbara Foorman, University of Texas at Houston (a 15-minute screening tool for grades K–2)

Asking a young child to draw a picture and relay information about the picture can help to determine the child's word retrieval and fine motor skills. Some of this information can be obtained from adolescents by talking about favorite movies, music, or sports.

After the information from the history and screen has been obtained, the parental concerns should be discussed, and a referral should be made to appropriate specialists for diagnosis and treatment. If the child cannot receive a free assessment from the school, information about local agencies that can provide the services should be provided to the parents. Ongoing information on the efficacy of interventions and ways to access special education or independent services within their community also is useful to families. Box 241-3 lists suggested reading for parents. Box 241-4 lists suggested readings for children. Box 241-5 lists other useful resources and support groups.

OUTCOME AND FOLLOW-UP

Identification and appropriate treatment are crucial to children with learning disabilities. When children go undiagnosed and untreated, they are at greater risk for dropping out of high school, getting into trouble with juvenile authorities, failing to obtain gainful employment after high school or being able to attend college, and abusing alcohol and other substances. In contrast, children who are at risk for a reading disability can become average readers if (1) the deficits are detected early (before third grade), and (2)

Box 241-6. Outcome

1. Outcome is significantly better the earlier the learning disability is identified and appropriate intervention is begun.
2. Gains are greater if the remedial treatment is targeted to the deficiencies, treatment is delivered by well-trained instructors, treatment is intense, and duration of treatment is sufficient.
3. Outcome is improved when course selection and college and career choices are appropriate for the student.

Box 241-7. Follow-up Care by the Generalist

1. Refer for annual educational testing early in the treatment.
2. Refer for a comprehensive psychoeducational assessment every 3 years.
3. Provide periodic eye and audiologic screenings.
4. Interview parents and child to screen for possible comorbid conditions.

appropriate intervention is begun and sufficiently sustained. Otherwise, approximately 75% of students who are poor readers in third grade are poor readers in high school. Older students and adults can be taught to read, but the time and cost are enormous. More research on the etiology and treatments for children with learning disabilities in math and written expression is needed before treatment recommendations and outcomes can be documented with greater certainty (Boxes 241-6 and 241-7).

Learning disabilities are chronic, with lifelong implications. After the diagnosis has been made, continued management is required. It is recommended that the child have annual individual educational testing during the first 2 years of treatment to monitor academic progress. A comprehensive assessment typically needed only once every 3 or 4 years if educational progress has been monitored carefully. It is important to monitor the child's physical, school, and emotional and social development and refer to appropriate professionals if other concerns present (e.g., depression, anxiety).

Mini-index of Related Topics   CH.

SUGGESTED READINGS

Francks C, Fisher SE, Olson RK, et al: Fine mapping of the chromosome 2p12–16 dyslexia susceptibility locus: Quantitative association analysis and positional candidate genes SEMA4F and OTX1. Psychiatr Genet 2002;12:35–41.

Grigorenko EL: Developmental dyslexia: An update on genes, brains, and environments. J Child Psychol Psychiatry, 2001;42:91–125.

Lyon GR: Toward a definition of dyslexia. Ann Dyslexia 1995;45:3–27.

Lyon GR, Cutting LE: Learning disabilities. In Marsh E, Barkley R (eds): Treatment of Childhood Disorders, 2nd ed. New York, Guilford Press, 1998, pp 468–498.

Pennington BF: Diagnosing Learning Disorders: A Neuropsychological Framework. New York, Guilford Press, 1991.

Shaywitz SE, Shaywitz KP, Pugh KR, et al: The functional organization of the brain for reading and reading disability (dyslexia). Neuroscientist 1996;2(4):245–255.

Shaywitz SE, Shaywitz KP, Skudlarski P, et al: The neurobiology of developmental dyslexia as viewed through the lens of functional magnetic resonance imaging technology. In Lyon GR, Rumsey JM (eds): Neuroimaging: A Window to the Neurological Foundations of Learning and Behavior in Children. Baltimore, Paul H. Brookes, 1996, pp 79–94.

242 Speech and Language Skills and Language Disorders

Heidi M. Feldman

ROLE OF THE GENERALIST

1   Distinguish normal developmental processes from delays and disorders of speech and language.

2   Diagnose language and speech delays and disorders.

3   Initiate a workup of causes of language and speech delays and disorders.

4   Refer children with delays and disorders of speech and language to the appropriate services.

5   Coordinate care for children with delays and disorders of language and speech within the health care sector and among other services, such as early intervention, rehabilitation, and speech and language therapy.

6   Counsel parents regarding the management and support of children with language and speech delays and disorders.

7   Ensure appropriate long-term follow-up of children with language and speech delays and disorders.

DEFINITIONS

Language is an elaborate, rule-governed system of symbolic communication. *Symbols*, such as spoken and written words, are signs that have an arbitrary relation between the sign itself and what it designates. In contrast, *signals*, such as the whistle of the teapot, the mating call of an animal, and the tears of a child who skinned his or her knee, provide communication but are tied intimately to their meaning. *Receptive language* refers to the ability to understand this symbolic communication. *Expressive language* refers to the ability to produce symbolic communication. *Speech* is the oral or verbal output of the language system. Most language is conveyed through speech. *Sign language* also qualifies as a language, however. Although signs in sign languages may have originated from action or pantomime, they have become arbitrary and socially agreed-on symbols. As evidence of their symbolic nature, individuals who are unfamiliar with the language cannot guess their meaning.

Language is distinctively human. No other species seems to have the generative capacity to create a potentially infinite number of messages that relate to abstract concepts and hypothetical situations as well as to concrete needs. Children learn language early in life; the major develop-

ments are completed before a child enters kindergarten. Language skills play a key role in the development of social relationships and in the development of higher mental processes, such as learning, memory, and reading. Language assessment as a routine aspect of health maintenance is legitimately within the realm of general pediatric care.

Language disorders are persistent delays or deficits or both in the development of language skills. Characteristics of language disorders include limited vocabulary, misuse of words and their meanings, difficulty expressing ideas, immature grammatical patterns, and difficulty following directions or conversation. *Speech disorders* are persistent delays or deficits in the development of speech skills and voice quality. Characteristics of speech disorders include disruptions in the flow or rhythm of speech; problems with the way sounds are formed; difficulty with the planning and production of speech sounds; problems with the pitch, volume, or quality of the voice; and poor intelligibility. Language and speech disorders may influence cognitive, academic, social, and emotional development. Assessment of the causes of delay or deficit, management, and referral are skills appropriate to the general pediatrician.

FUNDAMENTALS

Normal Development

Table 242-1 reviews key milestones in receptive and expressive language. Infants are born with a set of perceptual biases that facilitate the learning of language. Awake and alert infants, only minutes after birth, typically turn to look at the source of a sound. They show preferences for high-pitched female voices over low-pitched male voices and for the voice of their mother over the voice of another woman. They focus on the features of the human face. These early capacities are assessed as part of neonatal assessments, such as the Brazelton Neonatal Assessment Scale, and can be shown to parents to encourage them to speak to their infants.

Early expressive communication consists of cries and differentiation of the infant cry in different states, such as hunger or fatigue. By 2 months of age, infants produce sounds for social purposes and not merely to express physical needs or desires. *Cooing*, the earliest form of vocalization, comprises continuous musical vowel sounds without syllabic boundaries. Some cooing may be heard in infants with hearing loss, suggesting that it is a biologically

Table 242-1. Milestones of Language Development and Indications for Evaluation

Age of Acquisition	Child's Receptive Skills	Child's Expressive Skills	Abnormal Findings or Red Flags for Full Assessment
Birth–2 mo	Responds to sound and voice Shows social interest in faces and people	Cries Varies crying	Lack of response to sound at any age Lack of interest in interaction with people at any age Lack of any drive to communicate after 4 mo of age
2–4 mo		Differentiates crying for pain, hunger Coos (musical sounds) Reciprocal cooing and turn-taking	
4–9 mo	Deliberately turns head toward sound Responds appropriately to tone of voice Responds to name	Babbles (uses repetitive consonant/vowel sounds)	Loss of the early ability to coo or babble Poor sound localization or lack of responsiveness to sound
9–12 mo	Comprehends verbal routines, such as "wave bye-bye" Responds appropriately to "no" Understands pointing	Points for needs and for interesting objects or actions Gestures Creates complicated babbling called *jargon*, which sounds like sentences	Poor comprehension of verbal routines, such as wave bye-bye, by 12 mo Pointing for wants or needs, but no pointing at interesting objects or actions
10–16 mo	Points to body parts or objects to show comprehension Understands more words than produces Follows single-step command	Produces single words Has vocabulary that grows gradually to 30–50 words	Failure to use words, add new words, or loss of most words previously learned Failure to point to body parts or follow single-step commands
18–24 mo	Comprehends simple sentences Points to pictures in response to words	Experiences vocabulary spurt Concurrently begins to use two-word phrases	Minimal comprehension and limited symbolic play, such as doll or truck play <30 words in expressive vocabulary at 24 mo
24–30 mo	Understands personal pronouns Understands negatives Understands some prepositions such as *in* and *on*	Uses two-word utterances Shows good intelligibility for familiar people such as family members Greater mastery of nouns and verbs than grammatical words or markers	<50 words at 30 mo No two-word utterances when vocabulary is >50 words More than half utterances are unintelligible to family after age 2 yr
30–36 mo	Follows 2-step commands Identifies objects by use	Converses through asking and answering questions	Frequent immediate or delayed repetition of what others say (echolalia) Rote memorization with failure to generate novel sentences
36–48 mo	Knows colors Knows what to do if hungry, tired, thirsty Answers yes/no, which, and what questions	Shows good intelligibility for unfamiliar adults Full, well-formed sentences Shows some developmental dysfluency	More than a quarter of utterances are unintelligible to strangers after age 4 yr Consistent use of only short, simple sentences Repetition of individual sounds of words or other signs of stuttering
4 yr	Understands same/different Follows 3-step command	Tells stories Knows colors and numbers Enjoys rhyming Pronounces all basic consonants correctly	Persistent stuttering Inability to express thoughts and ideas Poor comprehension
5 yr	Comprehends most of what is said, limited only by conceptual development		Errors in consonants such as *b, p, d, t, p, k, m, n, l, r, w, s* by 5 yr
7 yr		Pronounces all speech sounds correctly	Immature production blends such as *st, sh, sp* at 7 yr

prepared behavior that does not require auditory feedback for initiation or maintenance. Infants 2 to 4 months old often engage in *reciprocal cooing.* They respond to the vocal input of an adult or child with these musical sounds, wait for responses from the other person, and then emit additional cooing. *Babbling* begins at approximately 6 months of age and comprises consonant and vowel sounds, such as "ma-ma" and "da-da." The addition of consonants to the vowel sounds creates syllable boundaries. Babbling progresses from a single repeated syllable to more varied sounds. Gradually the infant produces strings of babbling that possess the sounds, rhythms, and intonation of sentences of the language. This sophisticated babbling has been called *jargon* and characterizes expressive skills of 9- to 12-month-old

infants. Infants of this age also use gestures, such as head nods, pointing, and open palm, to express specific meanings.

Early receptive communication abilities begin at about 6 months of age, when the infant begins to respond reliably to his or her own name. By about 9 months of age, infants learn to associate motor movements to particular verbal stimuli. They open and close their hand when asked to "wave bye-bye," or they spread wide their arms when asked "how big is the baby." These *verbal routines* reflect increasing abilities to understand strings of speech.

True receptive and expressive language skills begin at about 1 year of age. From about 12 to 18 months of age, children remain in a *one-word stage.* Vocabulary growth is slow. Their word forms often are simplified, consonant-vowel combinations, such as "wa-wa" for water or "bow-wow" for dog. Words sometimes are applied too narrowly, such as the use of "dog" for only one particular animal, or too broadly, such as the use of "dog" for all types of animals. During this developmental era, language comprehension is in advance of language production. Children can point to the name of a body part and follow a single-step command. Children provide evidence of symbolic thinking in their pretend play.

At about the time when the child reaches a vocabulary of 30 to 50 words, usually between 18 and 24 months of age, the *two-word stage* typically begins. The most dramatic feature is the rapid pace of learning. From a rate of one to two words per week, the vocabulary begins to grow by four to five words per day. Often a single exposure to a new word is adequate for learning. Mature forms replace the simplified consonant-vowel combinations. The child simultaneously begins to combine two words into phrases or sentences. The reason for the short sentence length seems to be an output limitation. Children often seem to have more than two words that they would like to say, but they need to concatenate a series of two-word phrases to accomplish this goal. For example, they will request help in dressing like this: "Mommy sock. Sock on. Mommy put." Their comprehension and symbolic skills also advance. They point to a picture in response to a word and comprehend simple sentences.

After 24 to 30 months of age, sentence length limitations seem to resolve, and language begins to resemble a telegram. Meaningful words are reliably included, but nonessential grammatical words and markers often are left out. This phase has been dubbed *telegraphic speech* because of the resemblance of child sentences to telegrams. Grammatical words, such as pronouns, negatives, and prepositions, are understood before expressed.

Gradually the child masters grammatical constructions and builds sentences of increasing complexity. The child begins to ask questions, use pronouns, and tell stories. Table 242-1 lists many accomplishments in this developmental sequence. By school age, the main milestones of language development have been accomplished. For some children, there is continued development of the speech sound system until about 7 years of age.

Speech and Language Disorders

A rough estimate of children's language developmental rate can be calculated by dividing the age of their developmental accomplishments by their chronologic age. If a 24-month-old child is functioning at the level of an 18-month-old child, the developmental rate is 75%. In general, if children are functioning at or less than 75% of the expected rate, the delay is clinically significant and should prompt further evaluation. Table 242-1 includes some abnormalities or red flags that warrant full evaluation at various ages from birth to 7 years old.

Language and speech delays affect 10% to 15% of 2-year-olds and about 5% of children at the time of school entry. It is extremely difficult to distinguish toddlers who will catch up in language development, the so-called late bloomers, from children with developmental language disorders. Early

Table 242-2. Common Misconceptions about Language Development

Misconception	Actual Findings
Boys are significantly delayed compared with girls "He's just a boy" "His dad didn't speak until age 3"	Boys as a group are mildly delayed (1–2 mo behind) compared with girls
Second- and third-born children are delayed in language compared with first-born children "They do not need to speak" "His older sibling speaks for him" "Her parents anticipate her needs"	Second- and third-born children are not consistently delayed in language. Most children have a strong motivation to communicate as soon as they can, similar to their motivation to walk, climb, and perform in other ways
Children from bilingual households are delayed in language development "She's so confused by the clatter"	Children from bilingual households may show minor delays in language development. They also may show language mixing in the early stages of language development, particularly if their parents use both languages

identification and treatment for all children with delays is strongly recommended, even though some children are destined to outgrow their delays.

Many myths about language development are responsible for delays in the identification and evaluation of children with significant problems. Table 242-2 lists three common misconceptions about language development. The first is that boys are considerably slower in language development than are girls. In various studies, the average difference in vocabulary size or grammatical skills between girls and boys is slight, equivalent to 1 to 2 months. Additionally, boys are more at risk for language disorders. If a boy's rate of development less than 75% of the average, the delay should not be attributed simply to his sex. The second myth is that second-born or third-born children in a family are delayed substantially compared with first-born children because others speak for them. Children experience intense motivation to learn to speak. If they can learn, they rarely are deterred even in the context of accommodating adults or loquacious siblings. The same standards should be applied to all children regardless of birth order. The third myth is that children in bilingual families experience delays in learning language. On average, children exposed to two languages may show minor delays and language mixing during the one-word and two-word stages. The separation of the two languages occurs earlier for children who have clear environmental cues about which language is being spoken than for children with considerable language mixing in the environment. If one parent reliably speaks the first language and the other speaks the second, or if one language is spoken at home and the other in preschool, children have an easier time segregating the languages. Children from bilingual homes also may have language disorders, however. Children with significant delays merit a full evaluation.

The quality of the environment influences the rate of language development. Children who live in poverty are far more likely to have language delays than are children in middle-class environments. The source of the difference at least in part seems to be a difference in exposure to verbal language. Children from lower socioeconomic status homes are likely to hear fewer words than children from middle-class homes hear. They are more likely to be exposed to direct commands, such as "shut the window," than to indirect requests, such as "would you mind shutting the window." Not only does the polite form have more words than the command, but it also puts the auxiliary verb, "would," at the front of the sentence, where it is perceptually salient. These features may improve the perception and production of complex grammatical forms. Literacy programs for children who live in poverty may be successful at improving language skills and reading because they increase the child's exposure to verbal language from an early age. A literacy program that is suitable to the pediatric office is called Reach Out and Read.

Table 242-3 lists and describes various language and speech disorders. Clinicians evaluating children should make an effort to characterize the type of disorder. Often the assistance of a speech and language clinician assists in this process. The differential diagnosis of the disorder varies by its categorization.

Differential Diagnosis of Language and Speech Delays

The most common cause of speech and language delays is hearing loss. In evaluating hearing, it is important to determine the threshold at which children reliably detect sounds of different frequencies. The amount of energy in a sound is measured in decibels (dB) and relates to the

psychological experience of loudness. The frequency of the sound is measured in hertz (Hz) and relates to the perception of pitch. The speech range generally is considered 1000 to 2000 Hz. Figure 242-1 includes three audiograms showing normal hearing, sensorineural hearing loss, and conductive hearing loss. Figure 242-1A is a normal audiogram. Normal children have a threshold of 10 to 20 dB. Figure 242-1B shows sensorineural loss. Sensorineural hearing loss typically affects the high frequencies, often including the speech range. A mild loss is considered a threshold of 21 to 40 dB; a moderate loss, 41 to 70 dB; a severe loss, 71 to 90 dB; and a profound loss, greater than 90 dB. Conversational language is typically at 55 to 60 dB. If a child has a hearing threshold greater than 60 dB at 1000 to 2000 Hz, the child misses most conversational language. Children with a mild hearing loss of 30 dB in the speech range might experience conversational language like a whisper.

Figure 242-1C is an audiogram of conductive hearing loss. In this case, the loss is mild and in the low-frequency range. The most common cause of conductive hearing loss is otitis media. Whether variable and intermittent hearing loss associated with otitis media is associated with persistent speech and language disorders is a controversial topic. The prevalence of otitis media is higher among children living in poverty. They have multiple reasons for language delays. A study designed to address the issue of causality randomly assigned children with persistent middle ear effusion to obtain tympanostomy tubes after 3 continuous months of bilateral effusion or to wait for 6 additional months before the decision to place tympanostomy tubes. The study found that even though the delayed treatment group had a greater number of days of effusion, there were no differences in speech, language, cognition, or behavior at age 3 years.

The second major cause of delays and disorders of language and speech is disorders of the central nervous system. Most commonly, delays in speech and language development are the presenting complaint of general developmental delays. If these overall delays persist throughout preschool years, the child may be classified as having a cognitive impairment, learning disability, or mental retardation at a later age. The underlying etiology of cognitive impairment is variable and often multifactorial. Language delays and disorders also are components of known disorders associated with central nervous system abnormalities. Children with Down syndrome have language delays beyond what is expected for their level of intelligence. Children with traumatic brain injury, seizure disorders, and anticonvulsant medications may present with speech and language delays or disorders. Communication delays and disorders have been reported in the aftermath of prematurity and other perinatal problems. Table 242-4 lists conditions associated with cognitive impairment and a recognizable pattern of speech and language functioning.

The third condition in the differential diagnosis of language and speech delays is autistic disorder. Autism is characterized by three cardinal features: (1) qualitative impairment in social interactions, manifested by impairments in the use of nonverbal behavior, failure to develop peer relationships, and a lack of social or emotional

Table 242-3. Definitions of Selected Language and Speech Disorders

Disorder	Description
Language Disorders	
Receptive and expressive language disorder	Delays in language comprehension and expression out of proportion to cognitive skills
Expressive language disorder	Delays in language expression out of proportion to cognitive skills
Reading disorders	Difficulties with reading, written expression, or spelling
Speech Disorders	
Phonologic or articulation disorders	Substitution of simple (1) for complex sounds (y) ("lellow" for "yellow") or single consonants (s) for consonant blends (sk) ("see" for "ski")
Persistent or progressive hoarseness	Result of persistent harsh vocal quality or nodules
Stuttering	Dysfluencies that are frequent, persistent, and accompanied by tension, involving repetitions of parts of words, prolonging sounds, or opening the mouth to speak without words being produced
Dysarthria	Weakness and discoordination of the muscles of the lips, tongue, and other body parts used for speech, affecting the clarity and intelligibility of speech
Developmental verbal dyspraxia	Inability to plan, sequence, and execute volitional speech sounds, resulting in variability in words over trials

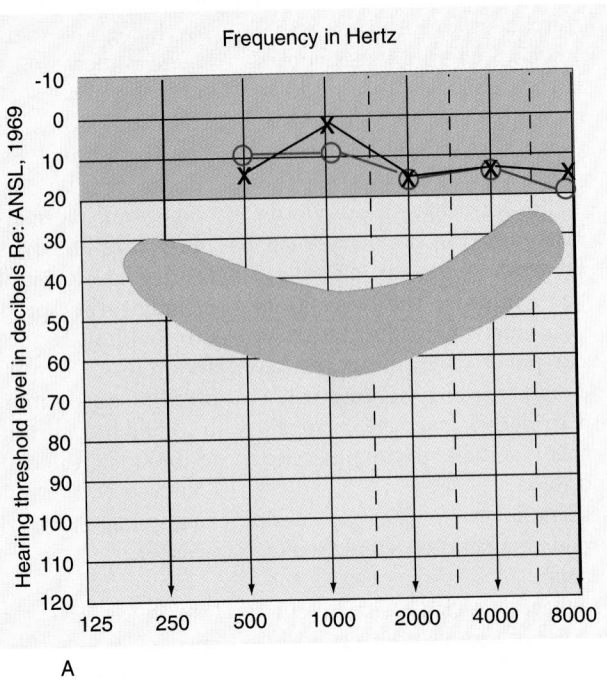

A

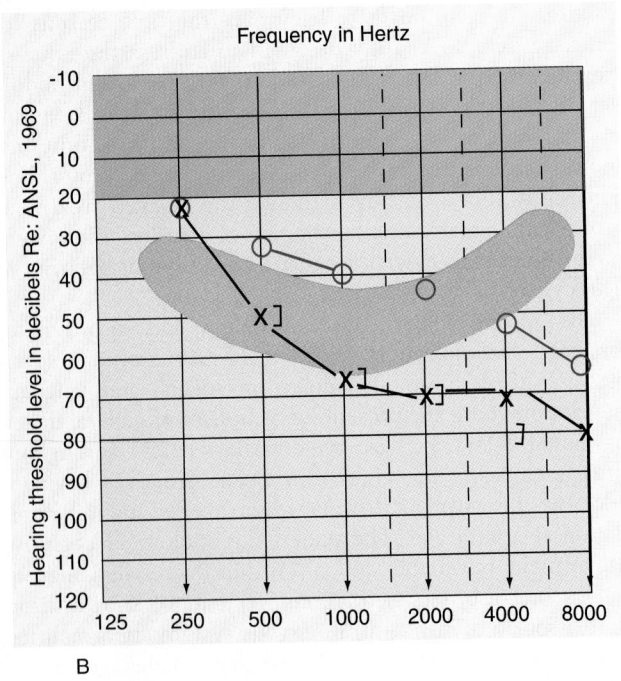

B

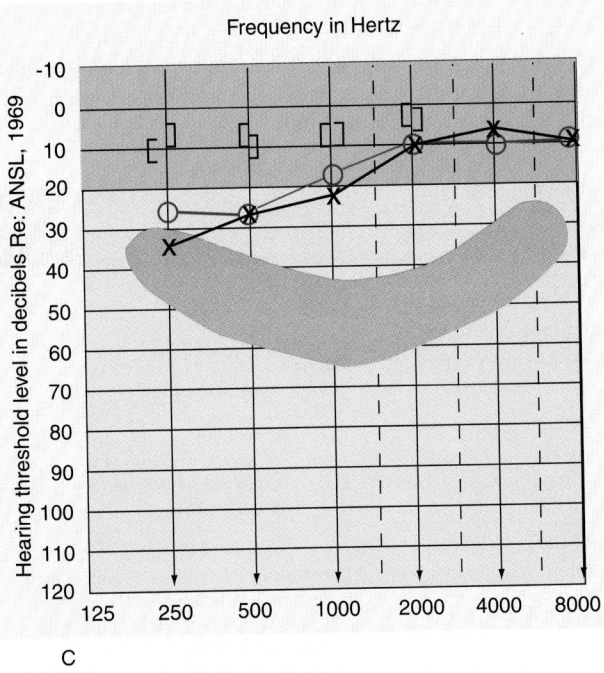

C

Figure 242-1. On all the audiograms, the letter X indicates the threshold for the left ear, and the letter O indicates the threshold for the right ear. Brackets indicate the threshold for bone conduction. The red section shows the frequency and energy levels for most speech sounds. **A,** Normal audiogram with a threshold of 15 dB from low to high frequencies. **B,** Sensorineural hearing loss in the moderate (right ear) to severe (left ear) range. **C,** Mild conductive hearing loss in the low frequencies, characteristic of otitis media with effusion. Bone conduction thresholds are normal in this case.

reciprocity; (2) qualitative impairment in communication, such as total lack of spoken language, inadequate speech, or stereotypic or repetitive use of language; and (3) restricted, repetitive, and stereotypic patterns of behavior, such as preoccupations, inflexible adherence to routines, and repetitive motor movements. The characteristics of autism fall along a spectrum. Table 242-5 describes the manifestation of communication issues at three points on this spectrum.

At the extreme end, children are completely nonverbal and noninteractive and unable to focus on the same objects as their communicative partners. At the mild end of the spectrum, children may show awkward social skills and stilted or robotic communication. Early diagnosis and treatment is associated with improvement in social and communication skills. Referral for early intervention should be considered at the earliest possible time.

Table 242-4. Selected Conditions Associated with Cognitive Impairment and Abnormalities in Speech or Language

Conditions	Specific Diagnosis	Characteristic Findings
Perinatal problems	Prematurity	Cognitive impairment/learning disability
		Delays/disorders in speech and language
Neurologic disorders	Periventricular leukomalacia/cerebral palsy	Motor disability; strabismus
		Cognitive or learning disability
		Delays/disorders in speech and language
	Landau-Kleffner syndrome	Deterioration in language and communication at age 3–7 yr
		Abnormal EEG over temporal lobe
	Spina bifida	Learning disorders
		Cocktail party syndrome—verbosity, loose associations, superficial meaning
Chromosomal disorders	Down syndrome	Cognitive impairment
		Expressive language impairment greater than expected for cognitive level
	Fragile X	Cognitive impairment
		Social deficits/poor eye contact
		Anxiety
		Speech and language deficits
	Kleinfelter syndrome (47, XXY)	Hypotonia
		Cognitive impairment/learning disability
		Speech and language deficits
Genetic disorders	Velocardiofacial syndrome	Learning disability/cognitive impairment
		Blunt or inappropriate affect
		Psychotic illness
		Nasal voice
	Williams syndrome	Cognitive impairment
		Speech and language skills better than expected for a cognitive level
		Cocktail party speech—see above
Severe psychosocial deprivation	Child abuse	Speech and language deficits
	Child neglect	Behavior and emotional problems
		Cognitive impairment/learning disability

In the absence of any of the aforementioned causes, the most common diagnosis is *developmental language disorders* or *specific language impairment*. This condition is characterized by delays in language receptive and expressive skills or expressive skills without or with minimal cognitive impairment. Although the precise cause of specific language impairment is not known, it seems to have a strong genetic component. Children with a parent or sibling with speech, language, or reading disorders are at high risk for a similar delay. The precise genetic etiology and pathophysiology are under investigation. It is highly likely that multiple causes and patterns will be found.

The most common speech problems are unintelligibility or immaturity. The distinction between the more common phonologic disorder and developmental verbal dyspraxia relates to the nature of the errors. In the phonologic disorder, the child makes consistent errors in the formation of speech sounds. In developmental verbal dyspraxia, a problem in the planning, sequencing, and forming of speech sounds exists, and the child makes inconsistent errors. Another important distinction in the analysis of speech is stuttering versus developmental dysfluency. Transient developmental dysfluency is common in children 3 to 4 years old and typically includes the repetition of entire syllables, words, or phrases. Stuttering that is destined to be long lasting typically involves the repetition of individual sounds, prolongation of sounds, excessive pauses, or the development of unusual compensatory behaviors.

PRESENTATION AND INITIAL EVALUATION

Figure 242-2 presents an algorithm for the identification and evaluation of speech and language disorders. Language and speech disorders may present to a clinician in one of

Table 242-5. Communication Characteristics of Children with Autistic Disorder

Domain	Severe (Low Functioning)	Moderate	Mild (High Functioning)
Vocabulary	Nonverbal	Limited vocabulary	Decent vocabulary
			Limited interests
Grammar	Nonverbal	Short phrases	Mix of simple and complex sentences
		Simple, telegraphic sentences	
Pragmatics (social and conversation abilities)	No joint focus of attention	Echolalia	Flat intonation
		Poor conversational abilities	Robotic quality
			Indifference to other person's needs
Comprehension	None to poor	Limited	Adequate for words and sentences
		Concrete interpretation	Poor comprehension of humor, metaphor, emotional content

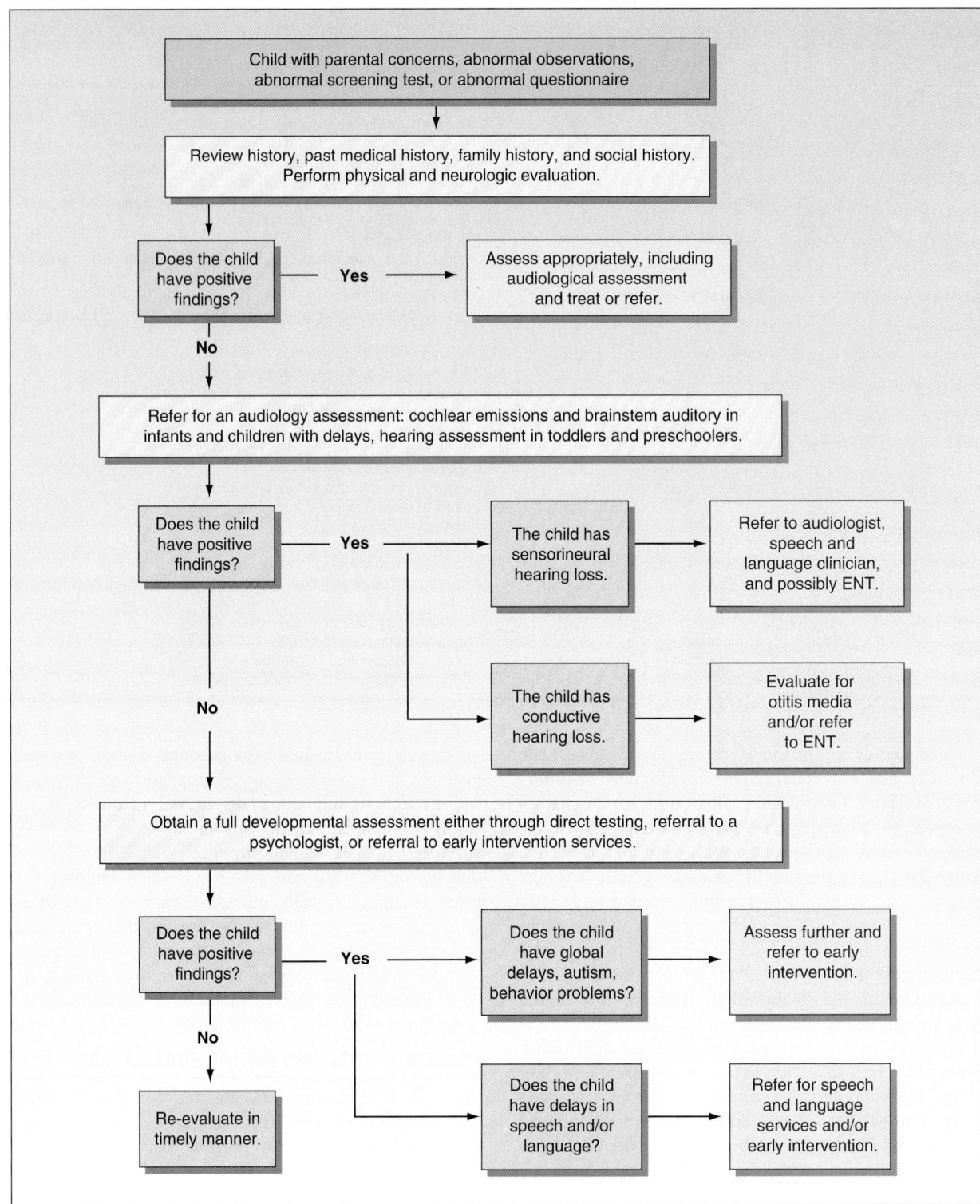

Figure 242-2. Algorithm for evaluating speech and language delays and disorders. ENT, ear, nose, and throat.

three ways. First, parents may raise concerns about their children. The parents have the best opportunity to evaluate the children because they interact with them for long periods in their natural environment. Their concerns should be taken seriously. Second, clinical observation in the clinical setting may serve as an appropriate method for detecting language and speech disorders. Children near the age of 2 often are shy and noncommunicative around strangers, however, particularly in the pediatric office if they remember immunizations and other painful procedures. For these reasons, it is important to check with the parents about whether behavior in the office is a valid indication of behavior in the home, preschool, or school environment. Third, screening tests are appropriate to detect language delays and disorders in asymptomatic children. The Early Language Milestone, second edition, and the Clinical Adaptive Test/Clinical Linguistic and Auditory Milestone Scale are screening measures specifically designed to screen language and speech. These instruments are extremely appropriate for the pediatric office. Because these procedures take time, the staff in the office may need to determine the most efficient methods for obtaining the screening data. The Denver II can be used to assess developmental status across four domains but cannot be used legitimately to screen specifically for speech and language skills. A comprehensive parent-report inventory, the MacArthur Communicative Development Inventories, can be given to parents to complete before or at a health maintenance visit to obtain a full assessment. These assessments are more accurate when children are older than 1 year of age.

If parents or clinicians are concerned about language delays, screening is not necessary because the child is already symptomatic. Similarly, screening is not appropriate for children in high-risk categories, such as children who were born weighing less than 1000 g. These children warrant full assessment. Many clinicians use measures developed for screening for case finding, however, and to increase the information they have about the child.

The medical assessment of a child with abnormal language or speech development or of a child who fails a screening test begins with a full history, in this case a detailed historical description of the speech and language findings. Table 242-6 lists some of the usual findings and the main elements of differential diagnoses for speech and language abnormalities.

The assessment proceeds with a past medical history, family history, developmental history, social history, and physical and neurologic examinations. Positive findings direct the next steps of assessment. A history of regression of skills may warrant obtaining metabolic screening tests. Past medical history of prematurity or trauma might indicate the need for neuroimaging. A history of staring spells or unusual movements might suggest the need for an electroencephalogram. A family history of first-degree or second-degree relatives with similar problems may suggest the need for genetic testing. A social history suggesting child abuse or neglect warrants a comprehensive home and family assessment. Physical findings, such as dysmorphic features or neurologic abnormalities, often require additional laboratory testing.

For all children with speech and language disorders, an audiologic assessment is essential to rule out hearing loss. Infants, young toddlers, and older children with significant delays are assessed with brainstem audio evoked responses or otoacoustic emissions. Toddlers, who do not tolerate headphones, may be tested in a sound field, but the evaluation does not provide information on each ear separately. Children older than age 3 years undergo conventional audiometry. If sensorineural hearing loss is documented, the child should be referred to an audiologist and a language clinician for assessment of the utility of hearing aids and the most appropriate mode of communication. An ear, nose, and throat evaluation may reveal the cause of hearing loss. If conductive hearing loss is identified, it is important to determine if it is due to a transient problem, such as otitis media, or a permanent problem, such as anatomic abnormalities of the ossicles. Referral to an otolaryngologist is advisable for conductive hearing loss with no evidence of otitis media with effusion.

Children with language and speech delays should undergo a developmental assessment that includes evaluation of motor, cognitive, and social abilities and speech and language skills. These assessments allow differentiation of global developmental delays (mental retardation in older children) and autism from developmental language disorders, speech disorders, and normal findings.

MANAGEMENT

Clinicians who routinely screen children in terms of language development may recognize language delays before they are apparent to parents and caregivers. Early detection allows for early treatment and increases the likelihood of good outcomes.

Clinicians should refer a child with language or speech disorders to other professionals for treatment. The nature and intensity of intervention vary as a function of diagnosis. Referral for early intervention or educational services is appropriate for children with global delays, autism, or behavior problems in addition to language or speech disorders. In most states and locations, some services can be obtained free of charge through the early intervention or educational system, depending on the child's age and degree of delay. Referral for language therapeutic services is

Table 242-6. Description of Language and Speech Findings and Possible Underlying Causes

	Possible Underlying Condition
Language Findings	
Comprehension of language below age level	Hearing loss
Production of language below age level	Cognitive impairment/mental retardation
	Autism
	Specific language impairment—receptive and expressive
Normal comprehension	Slow expressive language development
Production of language below age level	Specific language impairment—expressive
Adequate verbal language	Poor phonologic awareness
Poor reading for level of intelligence	Poor verbal memory
Poor spelling skills	Late manifestation of specific language impairment
Speech Abnormalities	
Poor intelligibility	Hearing loss
	Phonologic or articulation disorder
	Developmental verbal dyspraxia
	Other speech motor abnormality
Immature sounds, such as difficulty with consonant blends and *r, l, y, z, s*	Phonologic disorder
Abnormal voice	Vocal chord abnormalities, such as nodules or vocal abuse
Resonance and nasality	Adenoidal hypertrophy (hyponasality)
	Velopharyngeal insufficiency (hypernasality)
	Submucous cleft palate (hypernasality)
Smoothness and rhythm of speech	Developmental dysfluency
	Stuttering

appropriate for children with isolated language or speech delays or disorders. Children who present with stuttering generally show the best improvement if intervention by a speech and language pathologist begins early.

Speech and language services may or may not be available through state programs depending on the rules for eligibility. Many health insurance programs do not reimburse for communication therapy for a child with developmental problems. Advocacy to find and pay for appropriate services falls to the primary care clinician.

For most children, therapy involves improving the language environment and allowing the child to practice weak skills. Sometimes therapy is handled best in an individual session. Because communication is a social function, however, in many cases, therapy may be offered in groups or in classrooms. Classrooms composed of children with and without developmental delays provide children with language or speech problems with normal peers as models. Inclusive early intervention is particularly helpful for improving communication skills.

In some children with poor prognosis for competent verbal language, therapy entails introduction of alternative or assistive communication systems. Children with moderate, severe, or profound hearing loss usually are taught sign language. Sign language in these children facilitates verbal language learning. Sign language also has been used to provide initial access to communication in children with a variety of developmental disorders. Children with Down syndrome are exposed to sign language at young ages because of the predictable impairments of verbal communication. They tend to shift to verbal language naturally and readily when able to do so. Children with difficulty with verbal and motor development may be introduced to other forms of assistive communication. Young children with autism who may not recognize the value of communication may be treated with a picture communication system.

Children who are referred for treatment require close monitoring over time. Children who are normal in the full assessment should be monitored closely to ensure that developmental problems do not arise over time. Children with delays and disorders should be monitored over time to assess developmental progress in language and speech and to assess for the development of other disorders, such as reading disability or neuropsychiatric conditions.

OUTCOMES

Multiple factors predict the outcome of early intervention or speech and language services for children with delays or disorders in speech and language skills. The underlying cause of the problem and the nature of the disorder are key variables. Early therapeutic services should be considered as preventive. These services generally are effective in improving communication abilities and ameliorate the child's quality of life and prognosis for later adaptive functioning. They may not cure the disorder completely, however.

Children with early speech and language disorders, even children who show good progress during the preschool years, are at risk for later difficulties with the development of reading, writing, and spelling. Ongoing surveillance of their developmental progress into school age is important to detect early reading difficulties and should lead to early intervention for children with delays.

Speech and language disorders also frequently are associated with behavior problems. Approximately half of children with communication disorders also exhibit behavior problems or psychiatric disorders. For these reasons, it is important to arrange for comprehensive evaluations and close follow-up of children with speech and language delays and disorders into the school-age years.

 Additional Resources, CD-ROM

Bibliography

Mini-index of Related Topics

SUGGESTED READINGS

Coplan J, Gleason JR: Quantifying language development from birth to 3 years using the Early Language Milestone Scale. Pediatrics 1990;86:963–971.

Hart B, Risley TR: Meaningful Differences in the Everyday Experience of Young American Children. Baltimore, Paul H. Brooks, 1995.

Needlman R, Bauchner H, Zuckerman B: Literacy and the pediatrician. Pediatr Rev 1990;11:259–260.

Rescorla L, Mirak J: Normal language acquisition. Semin Pediatr Neurol 1997;4:70–76.

Wachtel RC, Shapiro BK, Palmer FB, et al: CAT/CLAMS: A tool for the pediatric evaluation of infants and young children with developmental delay: Clinical Adaptive Test/Clinical Linguistic and Auditory Milestone Scale. Clin Pediatr 1994;33:410–415.

243 Autism Spectrum Disorders

Lisa A. Ruble and Wendy L. Stone

ROLE OF THE GENERALIST

1 Recognize early social communicative behavioral symptoms of autism.

2 Conduct screenings for autism at all well-child visits.

3 Refer families and young children to appropriate diagnosticians for a comprehensive assessment when the child exhibits no babbling, pointing, or other gestures by 12 months of age; single words by 16 months of age; or two-word spontaneous phrases by 24 months of age (exclude echolalia).

4 Refer families and young children to appropriate diagnosticians when there is loss of any language or social skills at any age.

5 Conduct formal audiologic assessment and lead screen (if pica present).

6 Evaluate carefully alternative treatment approaches with families.

7 Assist families in obtaining other services.

Autism is recognized as one of the most complex neurodevelopmental disorders. The diagnosis and treatment of autism require specialized skills, and the etiology remains unknown. Autism involves an alteration of normal brain development before birth. The specific impairments result in qualitative differences in development of social and communicative behaviors and restricted, repetitive, and stereotypic patterns of behaviors, interests, and activities. Specific diagnostic criteria are available in the *Diagnostic and Statistical Manual of Mental Disorders, fourth edition, text revised* (DSM-IV-TR). Many researchers believe that the social impairment represents the core feature that distinguishes autism and autism spectrum disorders from other developmental disorders, such as language disorder or attention deficit hyperactivity disorder. The social impairment has an early onset, significantly impairs all individuals regardless of their level of functioning, and is predictive of outcome and employment success in adulthood.

Autism first was described in 1943 by Kanner, an Austrian psychiatrist. For many years after Kanner's description, autism erroneously was thought to be a disorder caused by the child's reaction to parental rejection. Empirical research long since has dispelled such psychoanalytic theories. Today, autism is recognized as a lifelong developmental disorder that becomes evident in infancy or early childhood. Described as the third most common developmental disability, autism affects approximately 1 of 600 children. Taking into account milder forms of autism, such as Asperger syndrome and pervasive developmental disorder not otherwise specified (PDD-NOS), the actual incidence may be 1 of 160 children. Autism occurs about four times more often in boys than in girls. No ethnic or racial boundaries exist in the incidence of autism. Every pediatrician should expect to encounter at least several children with autism in his or her practice.

FUNDAMENTALS

The causes of autism continue to elude scientists. Researchers are reaching a consensus, however, that there are multiple causes resulting in the characteristic triad of behavioral symptoms. Hypotheses have centered on genetic, neuropathologic, and environmental sources. Genetic research has indicated a sibling ocurrence rate of 3% to 7% and a monozygotic twin concordance rate of 60% for autism and 92% for the broader phenotype (including social and communication impairments). Dizygotic twin studies have identified concordance rates of 0% to 30% for autism and the broader phenotype. A polygenic model of inheritance has been proposed, involving a range from 3 to 20 genes. Linkage studies of genetic markers have implicated all but two chromosomes, numbers 14 and 20, again emphasizing the complexity of autism.

Neuropathologic evidence from postmortem analysis of microscopic brain tissue and neuroimaging studies has provided neither consistent nor specific findings for autism. Researchers have revealed many abnormalities, all implicating the prenatal period as the time of insult. Cerebellar hypoplasia, reduced size and number of Purkinje cells, reduced neuronal cell size and dendritic growth, increased cell-packing density in limbic structures, and shortening of the brainstem associated with abnormal facial and superior olivary nuclei have been reported.

For many years, researchers have investigated environmental causes of autism. It is hypothesized that the environment may play a part in the multifactorial etiology for autism, including a genetic predisposition. Maternal rubella and thalidomide exposure are examples of environmental associative agents. The measles-mumps-rubella vaccine was reported to be associated with an increased risk of autism. No evidence has validated this hypothesis, however.

This chapter discusses issues related to individuals with autism in general and young children in particular. We discuss children younger than 3 years old separately in each section to emphasize the need for early identification and early intervention.

DIAGNOSIS

Autism is one of five disorders described in the DSM-IV-TR under the rubric of *pervasive developmental disorders* (PDDs). The other PDDs are Asperger syndrome, PDD-NOS, Rett syndrome, and childhood disintegrative disorder (Table 243-1).

Asperger syndrome and PDD-NOS are associated most closely with autism. Asperger syndrome is diagnosed when the child has average intelligence with an impairment in social development and a restricted range of interests and activities. Children with Asperger syndrome meet early language milestones within the broad range of single words by age 2 years and communicative phrases by age 3. Their social communication skills remain problematic, however. Debate centers on whether Asperger syndrome is a separate disorder or simply a milder form of autism.

PDD-NOS is diagnosed when a child shows impairment in social development and either problems in communication or restricted, repetitive patterns of behaviors and interests. This diagnosis is used for children showing a later onset or some subclinical features of autism.

The remaining two PDDs are unique from the previous descriptions. Both disorders describe a period of normal development followed by a loss of skills. Rett syndrome is neurodegenerative and affects mostly girls. After a period of normal development during the first years of life, the onset is characterized by a loss of purposeful hand skills and often accompanied by hand wringing. Gross motor, language, cognitive, and social interaction skills also are affected. A genetic mutation has been identified for Rett syndrome.

Childhood disintegrative disorder is diagnosed after a period of at least 2 years of normal development followed by a profound loss of language, social, and motor skills. In contrast to Rett syndrome, children with childhood disintegrative disorder have a longer period of normal development. Childhood disintegrative disorder is extremely rare, and little research is available on this disorder.

In addition to differentiating autism from other PDDs, the diagnostician must consider differential diagnosis of autism from mental retardation, language disorder, and obsessive-compulsive disorder. To complicate the clinical picture further, other comorbid conditions often are associated with autism. Mental retardation occurs in about 65% to 85% of individuals with autism. Medical conditions, such as fragile X syndrome, neurofibromatosis, and tuberous sclerosis, and other syndromes, such as Down syndrome, Cornelia de Lange syndrome, and Tourette syndrome, are associated with autism in about 10% of cases. About 50% of children with autism are nonverbal or minimally verbal, and 25% to 30% develop seizures by adulthood. These associated conditions are not unique or invariant causes of autism.

Clinicians base the diagnosis of autism on the presence of the triad of behavioral symptoms as identified through observation or parental report. No medical or genetic tests currently are available to confirm the diagnosis of autism. Table 243-2 lists suggestions for identification of autism.

One obstacle to accurate diagnosis is the persistence of stereotypes, such as the child with autism as one who does not display affection or attachment to parents. The observation of a child clinging to or hugging a parent in the office or waiting room does *not* rule out a possible diagnosis of autism. Other stereotypes or misconceptions are listed in Table 243-3. A second obstacle in making the diagnosis is the heterogeneity in symptoms from individual to individual. Table 243-4 provides examples of behavioral features associated with different levels of severity.

Pediatricians are advised to refer children suspected of having autism to specialists with experience in diagnosing autism. Often these specialists are available in tertiary care clinics. A comprehensive evaluation using a multidisciplinary team approach is necessary. The multidisciplinary team often comprises a physician, clinical psychologist, and speech-language pathologist. Other clinicians, such as occupational therapists and educational specialists, may offer important information for treatment planning. A comprehensive diagnostic approach helps identify the multiple treatments required for children with autism.

Several publications are available to assist pediatricians in making screening and diagnostic decisions. The American

---

Table 243-1. Major Diagnostic Features for Pervasive Development Disorders

Feature	Autistic Disorder	Asperger Syndrome	Childhood Disintegrative Disorder	Rett Syndrome	PDD-NOS
Social impairment	Present	Present	Present*	Present	Present
Language/communication impairment	Present		Present*	Present	Present†
Repetitive interests and activities	Present	Present	Present*		Present†
Onset before 36 mo	Present			Present	
Average intelligence		Present			
Period of normal development			Present	Present	
Loss of skills in several areas			Present	Présent	

*At least two of these three features must be present.
†At least one of these two features must be present.
PDD-NOS, pervasive development disorder–not otherwise specified.

Table 243-2. Identification of Autism: Suggestions for Health Care Providers

Don't	Do
Expect to make a formal diagnosis of autism during an office visit	Recognize the constellation of symptoms and refer to a multidisciplinary team of specialists for diagnosis
Expect the behavioral manifestations of autism to be the same from one child to another	Recognize that variability in symptom expression can occur as a function of age, intellectual functioning, and language development
Rule out the possibility of autism in a child who shows affectionate behavior toward parents	Ask parents about other aspects of social relating, such as social limitation, affective expression, peer interactions, and empathy
Wait to refer a 2-year-old child who is exhibiting a pattern of deficits in social reciprocity, communication, and play	Refer the child for assessment and early intervention as soon as autism is suspected
Disregard parental expression of frustration, confusion, or distress	Become familiar with community resources for supportive counseling, behavior management, and respite care, and make referrals as necessary

Academy of Neurology and the Child Neurology Society published a set of practice parameters for screening and diagnosis of autism. The American Academy of Pediatrics published a technical report geared toward pediatricians. The National Academy of Sciences and the National Research Council has released a report on the state of the scientific evidence of the effects of early educational intervention on young children with autism spectrum disorders (see Suggested Readings).

EARLY IDENTIFICATION

Although most parents of children with autism report concerns regarding their child's development within the first 2 years, many children remain undiagnosed until age 4 or 5 years. This late diagnosis delays or prevents participation in specialized early intervention programs, which have been shown to improve outcomes for children with autism. Pediatricians should learn to recognize early signs of autism in young children to make appropriate referrals as soon as possible. An early diagnosis is essential for developing effective educational intervention programs. Parents who have accurate knowledge about their child also are better positioned to seek out appropriate information; to gain support and advice from specialists and other parents; and to advocate in local, state, and national arenas for services and research.

There now is evidence that the diagnosis of autism can be made accurately and reliably by experienced clinicians in 2-year-olds. The prominent behavioral features of autism in young children are in the social and communication domains; restricted activities and interests are less reliable indicators of autism in young children. Delayed language milestones and parental concerns about children's auditory responsiveness and hearing ability are common early signs that require referral for audiologic and speech and language

evaluation. Examples of other red flags for autism in children younger than age 3 are listed in Box 243-1 and can be found on the CD-ROM.

Most social and communication characteristics reflect *negative* symptoms, or the *absence* of behaviors that are associated with typical development. Negative symptoms are much more difficult to recognize than positive symptoms, such as hand flapping, which are more salient. The identification of any of these key behaviors during an office visit should be followed up with questioning of the parent to determine the pervasiveness of the behavior in other settings and with other people.

The early social and communicative deficits characteristic of autism are not all-or-none phenomena. One should not expect parents to report a total absence of social or communicative behavior. Many parents become adept at eliciting socially responsive behavior from their children, often through physical activities, such as rough-and-tumble play. Careful querying often reveals, however, that parents of children with autism go to great lengths and expend considerable effort in attempting to elicit the same social behaviors that occur so naturally and spontaneously in typically developing infants.

The development of screening instruments for the early identification of autism is a new area of investigation that

Table 243-3. Common Misconceptions about Autism

Misconceptions	Facts
Autism is an emotional disorder	Autism is a neurobiologic disorder
It is difficult to distinguish between autism and childhood schizophrenia	Autism and schizophrenia differ on several important features, including age of onset, cognitive level, course, and family history
Autism occurs more commonly among higher SES and educational levels	Autism appears to be evenly distributed across all SES and educational levels
Autism exists only in childhood	Autism is usually a lifelong disorder
With the proper treatment, most autistic children eventually "outgrow" autism	Many characteristics and behaviors associated with autism can improve substantially with early intervention
Children with autism do not show social attachments, even to parents	Children with autism can and do form social attachments, although their relationships typically lack a sense of reciprocity
Children with autism do not show affectionate behavior	Children with autism can and do show affectionate behaviors, such as hugging and kissing
Most children with autism have special talents or abilities	Many children with autism have unevenly developed cognitive skills, but few have savant capabilities
Most children with autism have normal intellectual abilities	65–85% of children with autism function intellectually within the range of mental retardation
Children with autism are more intelligent than scores from appropriate tests indicate	By age 4, IQ scores are accurate, stable, and predictive when appropriate instruments and assessment strategies are used

SES, socioeconomic status.

Table 243-4. Characteristics of Autism at Different Levels of Severity

	Mild Impairment	Moderate Impairment	Severe Impairment
Social behavior	Shows clear social interest but limited reciprocity. Seeks social interactions, but relationships may be hampered by limited understanding of the perspective and feelings of others	Shows enjoyment in a limited number of social routines, especially those involving physical activities or satisfaction of needs. Shows little interest in interacting with peers, although may engage in parallel play or chasing games	Shows limited social awareness and interest. Social interactions may be restricted to simple routines with familiar adults. Shows little social initiation and inconsistent responsiveness to others
Language and communication	Speaks in complete sentences, but language may be rigid or inflexible. Conversational skills may be limited by persistence on particular topics and poor understanding of nonverbal cues. May show comprehension problems and difficulty with abstract concepts	Verbalizations may contain a combination of functional speech, jargon, and immediate and/or delayed echolalia. Initiation of communication is for the purpose of satisfaction of needs rather than for the purpose of social interaction	Uses no functional speech. Nonverbal communication is limited and may include using others' hands as tools
Repetitive activities	Shows some behavioral rigidity and inflexibility. May have circumscribed areas of interest and specific routines or rituals that interfere only minimally with daily activities	Resists changes in routines or interruption of activities. Shows repetitive play with toys and may have motor stereotypies, such as rocking or spinning	Shows extreme resistance to changes in activities and routines. Stereotyped motor behaviors may be persistent and difficult to interrupt. May focus on sensory aspects of toys or other objects

seems promising. Table 243-5 presents examples of screening measures.

MANAGEMENT

Autism is a lifelong disorder with no known cure. The needs of families, caregivers, and individuals with autism change and persist throughout the patient's lifetime. Also, because there is no cure, families have many questions regarding treatment. The selection of a treatment approach is a highly charged and controversial issue in autism. Some researchers have claimed to cure children with autism who participated in an intensive 40 hours per week program. This assertion has left many parents of children with autism vulnerable to expensive and controversial treatments. Because pediatricians should expect such questions regarding treatment, three treatment approaches are described: educational, pharmacologic, and alternative treatments.

Educational and Behavioral Intervention

The most effective intervention approaches are educational and behavioral; these approaches ameliorate the behavioral symptoms and teach adaptive behaviors but do not correct

Box 243-1. Characteristics of Autism in Children Younger than 36 Months Old

- Limited use and understanding of gestures such as pointing and following a point
- Limited attempts to direct the attention of others, such as holding up a toy to show a parent
- Reduced use of eye contact during interactions
- Difficulty imitating the actions of others, such as waving goodbye
- Reduced interest in interacting with other children
- Failure to smile at others responsively
- Failure to show off or attempt to please parents
- Limited ability to play with a variety of toys in a creative and flexible manner

the underlying neurologic disorder. One notable behavioral intervention is applied behavior analysis. *Applied behavior analysis* is a broad term that incorporates many specific teaching strategies, including discrete trial training, structured teaching, and incidental teaching. Evidence exists that all these strategies are effective in educating children with autism, and to date, no single teaching approach has been proved more efficacious than others. The goal of applied behavior analysis is to apply systematic teaching techniques to increase desirable behaviors and decrease undesirable behaviors. The selection of teaching strategy should be based on several factors, including an assessment of the child's strengths, weaknesses, and preferences and the skill to be taught. It is likely that an integrated methodologic approach that combines the various teaching strategies is best.

Early Intervention

In 1990, the Federal Individual with Disabilities Education Act mandated early intervention for children with disabilities from birth to age 3 years, resulting in the development of early intervention programs in each state. After age 3 years, the local school system assumes responsibility for providing special educational services. Referral to these systems for intervention is crucial after a diagnosis. It is necessary for pediatricians to be aware of their local early intervention system and how services are accessed.

Despite the presence of controversy regarding specific teaching approaches for young children with autism, information regarding "best practices" is available to help guide the development of appropriate early intervention programs and to inform families. Participation in a meaningful, goal-directed program in which the child is engaged in productive activities for at least 25 hours per week is important. Teaching can occur in a specialized or regular education classroom or at home. Target skills for young children include learning to attend, imitate, play, communicate, and engage in reciprocal social interactions. A low ratio of children to instructors is necessary, as is a

Table 243-5. Description of Screening Tools*

Screener	Description	Target Age
Checklist for Autism in Toddlers (CHAT; Baron-Cohen, Allen, & Gillberg, 1992)	Parent report and observation tool. Designed for primary care settings. 14 items total. Nine parent report and 5 observation items	18 mo
Modified Checklist for Autism in Toddlers (M-CHAT; Robins, Fein, Barton, & Green, 2001)	Parent report tool. Designed for primary care settings. An extension of the CHAT. 23 items total	24 mo
Screening Tool for Autism in Two Year Olds (STAT; Stone, Coonrod, & Ousley, 2000)	Interactive observation tool consisting of 12 activities. Designed for child-find personnel	24–36 mo
Pervasive Developmental Disorders Screening Test (PDDST; Siegel, 1998)	Parent report tool. Combined of 3 stages; stage 1 designed for primary care setting	Birth–36 mo (for stage 1)

*See the CD-ROM for contact information.

highly structured and predictable teaching environment. When problem behaviors occur, it is necessary to take a functional problem-solving approach that involves analyzing the purpose of the behavior from the child's viewpoint. It also is necessary that a transition plan from early intervention services or preschool be developed to ensure a smooth transfer into special education programs. Finally, family involvement is crucial in any intervention approach.

Pharmacologic Approaches

Pharmacologic treatments have not been studied to the same extent as educational and behavioral approaches, and little research has examined the combined effect of pharmacologic and behavioral approaches. Medications do not treat the core symptoms of autism but can alleviate associated problem behaviors. An estimated 50% of individuals with autism are treated with medications to improve attention and reduce overactivity, aggression, self-injurious behavior, agitation, anxiety, or depression and to alleviate sleeping problems or compulsive rituals. Psychotropic medications are discussed in Chapter 288. When medication is being considered for treatment of problematic behavior, it also is necessary that a behavioral assessment from a trained specialist be conducted. This information can be used to determine the cause of the problem behaviors and to develop a behavioral plan that considers modification of the child's environment as well.

Alternative Approaches

Many alternative approaches to autism treatment have been promoted (Box 243-2). More often than not, these treatments receive sensational media coverage before their efficacy is evaluated scientifically, and parents may go to great effort and expense to obtain treatment. In some cases,

even with subsequent empirical study revealing the treatment to be inert, parents choose to continue the treatment. Parents of children with autism seem to be particularly vulnerable to the claims of unproven treatments, perhaps because autism is a behaviorally diagnosed disorder with serious impairment of function and no known cause or cure. The pediatrician is often in a position to help parents evaluate alternative treatments (Box 243-3).

Advising Parents

Before treatment options are discussed with families and caregivers, the clinician must be aware that any treatment approach for children with autism must be individualized. Because of the heterogeneity of the disorder, the diagnosis of autism does not dictate a specific treatment. It is also necessary that the quality of life of the child and family be taken into account. Some intervention approaches may be invasive or disruptive to the family structure, routine, and relationships. Helping families to select intervention programs based on a mutual understanding of the goals of therapy and outcomes is important (Table 243-6). The pediatrician must adopt a delicate balance between supporting parental efforts to seek help for their children and making sure that the children continue to receive interventions with demonstrated efficacy and safety. Caution should be applied when considering any treatment (see the CD-ROM).

Box 243-2. Examples of Alternative Treatment Approaches

- Facilitated communication
- Auditory training
- Secretin infusions
- Mercury chelation
- Dietary supplements, such as megavitamins or tree bark extracts
- Dietary restrictions, such as elimination of casein or gluten or both

---

Box 243-3. Questions to Consider When Evaluating Interventions

Be cautious of interventions that do the following:

- Offer a cure for autism
- Promise to be effective for all children
- Claim to improve all of the symptoms of autism
- Require family members to suspend their belief system and adopt another (e.g., asks them to "believe" in things that do not make common sense or tells them that the treatment will not work unless they believe in it)
- Consist of a general "package" or predetermined curriculum that is not tailored to the needs of the individual child
- Fail to provide routine and periodic assessments of the child's progress and the treatment's effectiveness
- Claim to be the "best" treatment for the child or the "only" treatment the child needs

Table 243-6. Specialized Services Often Needed by Families

Type of Service	Purpose
Educational intervention	To teach individuals the broad range of necessary skills to function as independently as possible in their school, home, and community settings
Speech and language therapy	To increase child's communication and language skills
Occupational therapy	To increase child's fine and gross motor development and address other issues, such as sensory processing problems
Behavior management training	To train caregivers or provide direct assistance in the development and implementation of positive behavioral support plans
Case management	To help coordinate services and increase communication across providers
Counseling and support	To support caregivers
In-home personal assistance	To teach the adaptive behavior skills in the home and community setting
Respite care	To provide relief and support to families

FOLLOW-UP

Identifying children at young ages is the essential first step toward providing appropriate early intervention services and improving outcomes. The pediatrician is the first professional who encounters young children with autism. Helping families recognize early symptoms, referring families for evaluation, and monitoring children's coordination of services are vital activities for the pediatrician.

Box 243-4. Activities to Assist Families

1. Refer the child to specialists when appropriate for diagnostic evaluation, behavioral evaluation, or medication evaluation.
2. Support parents by writing letters:
   For services at school, such as special education services, occupational or speech and language therapy, social skills groups, or extended year programming
   For insurance companies indicating necessity of services, such as speech and language therapy, parent training, or individual/family therapy
3. Provide parents with current information on the National Autism Society of America (ASA) at 1-800-3AUTISM and parent organizations and local ASA chapters in the area.
4. Provide case management to the fullest extent possible and refer families to the State Department of Mental Heath and Mental Retardation for more extensive case management and other services.

Pediatricians are challenged to ensure that children and families receive the unique and multiple interventions required. Families often have to interact with multiple service providers and specialists, such as psychologists, speech-language pathologists, occupational therapists, educators, and behavioral consultants. A coordinated treatment approach that involves collaboration in planning, implementing, and evaluating services is necessary.

The health care needs of children with autism and their families include the provision of case management and individual and family support. The pediatrician is ideally positioned to act as a case manager for families and children and to ensure coordination of treatment. A list of national resources is available on the CD-ROM. Practitioners can identify state and local services by contacting their local Autism Society of America chapters. Box 243-4 lists activities that can assist families of children with autism.

Additional Resources, CD-ROM

Red flags for autism	Text

SUGGESTED READINGS

American Psychiatric Association: Diagnostic and Statistical Manual of Mental Disorders, 4th ed, text revision (DSM-IV-TR). Washington, DC, American Psychiatric Association, 2000.

Committee on Children with Disabilities: The pediatrician's role in the diagnosis and management of autistic spectrum disorder in children. Pediatrics 2001;107:1221–1226.

Dawson G, Osterling J: Early intervention in autism. In Guralnic MJ (ed): The Effectiveness of Early Intervention. Baltimore, Paul Brookes, 1997, pp 307–326.

Filipek PA, Accardo PJ, Ashwal S, et al: Practice parameter: Screening and diagnosis of autism. Neurology 2000;55:468–479.

Lord C, McGee J (eds): Educating Children with Autism. Washington, DC: Committee on Educational Interventions for Children with Autism, Division of Social and Behavioral Sciences and Education, National Research Council, 2001.

244 Attention and Hyperactivity Problems and Attention Deficit Hyperactivity Disorder

Kimberly A. Worley and Mark Wolraich

ROLE OF THE GENERALIST

1 Screen for behavioral concerns at well-child visits and other patient contact times.

2 Pursue evaluation for attention deficit hyperactivity disorder (ADHD) if screening or concern of a parent, teacher, or the physician indicate symptoms of hyperactivity, impulsivity, and inattention are impairing the child's academic functioning, psychosocial functioning, or both.

3 Understand the comprehensive DSM-IV criteria necessary to make the diagnosis of ADHD.

4 Gain knowledge on delineating comorbid diagnoses that can complicate treatment and prognosis of ADHD.

5 Understand treatment options for ADHD.

6 Design and implement a comprehensive individualized management plan for a child with ADHD.

7 Ensure appropriate follow-up in titration and maintenance phases.

8 Refer to a specialist if time, reimbursement, comorbid diagnoses, or refractory cases prohibit the child from receiving optimal care.

DEFINITION

The *Diagnostic and Statistical Manual of Mental Disorders, fourth edition* (DSM-IV), defines attention deficit hyperactivity disorder (ADHD) as "a persistent pattern of inattention and/or hyperactivity-impulsivity that is more frequent and severe than is typically observed in individuals at a comparable level of development." ADHD is a developmental disorder of inattention or hyperactivity-impulsivity or both, meaning children with the disorder may have difficulty filtering external stimuli, inhibiting motor impulses, anticipating events, and adjusting behavior based on feedback about misconduct. It is the most common and most controversial behavioral chronic health condition that affects children today.

The core symptoms of ADHD—inattention, hyperactivity, and impulsivity—are common behavioral characteristics of all children at some time or another. When these symptoms impair a child's academic and psychosocial functioning, evaluation and management are indicated. Struggling with the inability to plan ahead, sit still, finish tasks, or interpret social cues may lead to poor academic achievement, troubled personal relationships, and low self-esteem. Thorough evaluation and prompt diagnosis are important to provide a child with the appropriate treatment plan, which may include behavior changing strategies, medication, and educational options. Appropriate management goals to reduce inattention, hyperactivity, and impulsivity and to improve psychosocial and educational impairment are key to providing the affected child an environment so that he or she may learn to adapt and reach his or her fullest potential.

There are three subtypes of ADHD: (1) primarily inattentive type, (2) primarily hyperactive-impulsive type, and (3) combined type. Distinguishing between the subtypes is accomplished by identifying the core symptoms of inattention, hyperactivity, and impulsivity as defined in the DSM-IV (Boxes 244-1 and 244-2). Some of these symptoms are present in every child, and adult for that matter, at one time or another. Certain criteria must be met for the symptom to be considered significant (Box 244-3). It is especially important to note the presence or absence of impairment. A child theoretically could have all 18 core ADHD symptoms, but if the child is able to function in everyday activities without difficulty, he or she would not meet the criteria for ADHD. The symptoms must be

---

Box 244-1. DSM-IV Inattention Symptoms

- Often makes careless mistakes
- Often has difficulty sustaining attention
- Often does not seem to listen
- Often does not follow through on tasks
- Often is not organized
- Often avoids sustained mental effort
- Often loses things
- Often is distracted easily
- Often is forgetful

Data from Diagnostic and Statistical Manual of Mental Disorders, 4th ed (DSM-IV). Washington, DC, American Psychiatric Association, 1994.

- Often fidgets or squirms
- Often inappropriately leaves seat
- Often inappropriately runs or climbs
- Often has difficulty playing quietly
- Often is "on the go"
- Often talks excessively
- Often blurts out answers
- Often has difficulty waiting for turn
- Often interrupts or intrudes on others

Data from Diagnostic and Statistical Manual of Mental Disorders, 4th ed (DSM-IV). Washington, DC, American Psychiatric Association, 1994.

Box 244-4. Common Comorbid Diagnoses

- Oppositional defiant disorder
- Anxiety disorder
- Learning disorder
- Mood disorder
- Conduct disorder
- Substance use disorder
- Tic/Tourette syndrome
- Developmental coordination disorder
- Motor dysfunction
- Language disorder
- Sleep disorder

causing significant problems in the child's social, academic, or home life. To assess impairment properly, obtaining direct information from the people involved with the child in different settings is crucial. This usually means obtaining reports from the parents/caregivers and teachers. If the child is home schooled or if the two reports differ significantly, it may be helpful to request reports from other caregivers, including coaches and scout leaders. Children often behave differently in different settings. It is important to review behavioral and impairment information from different sources to obtain the most accurate picture of the child and to develop the correct diagnosis.

Many conditions coexist with ADHD (Box 244-4). Screening for comorbid conditions during the evaluation process is important because the existence of a comorbid diagnosis may direct treatment options and prognosis.

ADHD is a complicated condition. Each child may present with different impairments. When the correct diagnosis has been determined, a comprehensive individualized treatment plan should be developed based on information gathered during the evaluation process and the child's impairment areas. The goal of treatment is to minimize functional impairments and may involve behavioral therapy, medications, education modifications, and referral to appropriate specialists as deemed appropriate. It is important that the child, parents, teachers, and clinician have a means of communication to enable proper evaluation and monitoring of the prescribed treatment. Treatment goals should be set based on the needs of the child, and a specific monitoring strategy should be determined and implemented. Suggestions to accomplish this huge task are discussed in the diagnosis section.

Box 244-3. Criteria for Diagnosis of Attention Problems

- Symptoms occur often, to a degree inconsistent with the child's developmental age.
- Certain symptoms have been present for at least 6 months.
- Certain symptoms have been present before age 7 years.
- Symptoms cause significant impairment for the child academically or psychosocially in two or more settings (home, school, leisure, or legal areas).
- Symproms are not attributed solely to another condition (e.g., pervasive developmental disorder, sensory impairment, child abuse, mental retardation, schizophrenia, mood disorder, anxiety disorder).

FUNDAMENTALS

Researchers have noted the symptoms of ADHD in every country and culture studied. The prevalence, reported in the DSM-IV, is 3% to 5% of school-age children. The male-to-female ratio varies cross-culturally from 1:1 to 10:1. The difference may be explained in part because boys tend to exhibit more hyperactive and impulsive behaviors and are more aggressive, leading to earlier referral because of behavioral problems. Girls display more internalizing behaviors (inattentive subtype) and are diagnosed later with academic difficulties.

ADHD symptoms have been baffling parents and health care providers for many years. In 1848, Hoffman, a German physician, wrote a children's book. Two of the characters, Fidgety Phil and Henry Who Looks in the Air, gave us our first literary description of a hyperactive and an inattentive child. In 1902, Still described children with ADHD symptoms in lectures to the Royal College of Physicians. He believed these children had a "defect in moral control." He explained the "problem resulted in a child's inability to internalize rules and limits, and additionally manifested itself in patterns of restlessness, inattentive, and over-aroused behaviors." After a worldwide influenza epidemic in 1917, some children recovering from encephalitis were described as having symptoms of restlessness, inattention, impulsivity, easy arousability, and hyperactivity. In 1937, a stimulant, Benzedrine, was noted to improve these behaviors in affected children, and in 1957, methylphenidate was released for commercial use. As research continued and more became known about children with these troubling symptoms, there have been multiple name changes, including minimal brain damage, minimal cerebral dysfunction, hyperactive child syndrome, and attention deficit disorder with or without hyperactivity.

ADHD currently seems to have a multifactorial etiology. Research has not shown consistently that food allergies, too much television, poor home life, poor parenting, or poor schools cause ADHD. These factors may exacerbate ADHD symptoms and impairment, however.

Approximately 20% of children who have ADHD also have a diagnosis that can be associated with an organic etiology (Box 244-5). The other 80% are thought to have a polygenic basis. The heritability evidence of ADHD has been provided by studies involving adoption, twins, siblings, and parents. Neuroimaging, neuropharmacology, and neuro-

Box 244-5. Diagnoses That May Predispose a Child to Develop Attention Deficit Hyperactivity Disorder

- Prenatal alcohol/drug use
- Prematurity
- Low birth weight
- Birth complications
- Central nervous system infections
- Central nervous system trauma
- Genetic disorders
  - Klinefelter syndrome
  - Turner syndrome
  - Fragile X syndrome
  - Williams syndrome
  - Neurofibromatosis type 1
  - Inborn errors of metabolism
- Tourette syndrome

physiology studies have raised the possibility of biologic basis for ADHD. Magnetic resonance imaging and positron emission tomography studies have shown a reduced size in ADHD subjects versus controls in the basal ganglia, cerebellar vermis, and frontal lobes. These areas are thought to regulate attention. The basal ganglia helps inhibit automatic responses. The vermis is thought to regulate motivation. The prefrontal cortex helps one filter out distractions. Investigating the brain's response to stimulants has implicated the dopaminergic system as a possible basis. Dopamine can inhibit or modify the activity of other neurons. If the dopamine transporter gene is affected, the transporter can recycle dopamine before it has a chance to bind to the dopamine receptor. If the dopamine receptor gene is affected, the receptor can become less sensitive to dopamine. These advances in research are not yet clinically useful because of the wide variation of size and function in individuals with and without ADHD such that the degree of overlap makes any of the assessments inaccurate for individual clinical evaluation.

DIAGNOSIS

If a caregiver, teacher, or physician expresses concern that symptoms of inattention, hyperactivity, or impulsivity are causing significant impairment in a child's academic, psychological, or social performance, an evaluation for ADHD is indicated. Many other diagnoses may present with similar symptoms or be present along with ADHD (Table 244-1). It is important to do a thorough evaluation to consider these issues. The correct diagnosis determines the course of treatment, guides treatment monitoring, links treatment to prognosis, and determines if special educational services or treatments for coexisting diagnoses are required.

Reviewing the child's behavioral, academic, psychosocial, developmental, birth, medical, and family history, looking for signs and symptoms of other disorders instead of or in addition to ADHD, is essential to making the correct diagnosis. Laboratory evaluation is unnecessary unless indicated by history. It is essential to gather information from primary caregivers, teachers, and the child when possible. This information comes in various forms—direct interviews, behavioral rating scales, medical records, school grades, and previous testing results including psychoeducational testing. Thorough medical and neurologic examinations are warranted.

To ensure the most accurate diagnosis, the evaluation should include assessing for the specific criteria as listed in the DSM-IV (see Boxes 244-2, 244-3, and 244-4). The DSM-IV criteria define three subtypes of ADHD: (1) primarily inattentive type (six of nine inattentive symptoms present), (2) primarily hyperactive-impulsive type (six of nine hyperactive-impulsive symptoms present), and (3) combined type (six of nine inattentive and six of nine hyperactive-impulsive symptoms present). Not only must the requisite number of core symptoms be present; they must also be developmentally inappropriate for the child's age and the cause of significant impairment in the child's academic and psychosocial performance. Possible presentations of ADHD throughout the life cycle are summarized in Table 244-2. The degree of functional impairment indicates whether an affected individual requires medication management as a teenager and ultimately as an adult. The information concerning core symptoms and impairment must be obtained directly from two sources. Parents and teachers usually are the best resources. Direct interviews and rating scales frequently are used (see the CD-ROM). Including all 18 core ADHD symptoms in the information gathered from home and school and using rating scales is an effective way to make the diagnosis. Children behave differently in different environments; this may lead to discrepancies between parent, teacher, and physician observations and should not be surprising. This is why it is important to have information about the child in multiple settings when making the diagnosis.

Research indicates 50% or more children with ADHD have a comorbid condition accompanying the ADHD symptoms (see Box 244-5). An important aspect of evaluating a child for ADHD includes assessing for possible comorbid conditions. Family history, social history, direct interview, rating scales, physical examination, and neurologic

Table 244-1. Differential Diagnosis

Developmental disorder	Learning disability
	Mental retardation
	Pervasive developmental disorder
Medical	Anemia
	Lead intoxication
	Medications
	Asthma
	Antiepileptic
	Allergy
	Seizure disorder
	Sensory deficits
	Hearing
	Vision
	Sleep apnea
	Substance abuse
	Thyroid disease
Psychosocial	Adjustment disorder
	Mood disorder
	Depression
	Manic-depression
	Psychotic disorder
	Anxiety

Table 244-2. Attention Deficit Hyperactivity Disorder Symptoms and Presentation through a Lifetime

Life Stage	Symptoms	Possible Presentation
Preschooler	Hyperactivity Impulsivity	Motoric hyperactivity Aggressiveness
Elementary school–age child	Inattention Distractibility Frustration Boredom Poor social skills	Underachievement Lack of motivation Class clown Difficulty following class rules
Older school-age child	Poor organizational skills Difficulty learning from mistakes	Difficulty completing homework independently
Teenager/college student		Increased social problems Trouble with long-term projects
Adults		Trouble juggling demand of marriage/family and work Trouble interacting with colleagues Difficulty keeping a job Difficulty managing money

examination may raise concern that a coexisting condition is present. The information gathered combined with the physician's clinical judgment and experience should determine whether further evaluation, testing, or referral is necessary. For the child to receive the most appropriate care, dealing with each concern addressed is imperative. If a child is having trouble at school—daydreaming, not turning in homework, and receiving poor grades—and family history reveals a parent was in special education classes, a referral for intelligence and achievement testing may be indicated. Several scales exist that screen for comorbid diagnoses. Information about these scales can be found on the CD-ROM and in Chapter 238.

TREATMENT

Treating ADHD is challenging. It takes communication and commitment from the clinician, parents, educators, and child. The multidisciplinary team, guided by the clinician, develops an individualized treatment plan. The plan is based on the child's core symptoms, functional impairment, psychosocial environment, and comorbid diagnoses.

Education is the first step in treatment. It is important the child, family, and teacher gain an understanding about the condition. Accepting ADHD as a chronic condition that a child is born with and that is not caused by a "bad child" or "bad parenting" helps the team focus on ways to deal with improving impairments instead of focusing on negative performances. Each child may present with different impairments and require different interventions. The clinician should be able to provide information to the child, family, and teacher about current knowledge of the diagnostic process, etiology, treatment, medications, parenting techniques, teaching tips, social skills, and learning issues and how these affect the child growing up with ADHD, the family members living with the child with ADHD, and the classroom with the child with ADHD. This information can be provided through a variety of resources, including trained staff, handouts, suggested reading lists, Internet websites, local and national support groups, and community programs such as parent training classes. Understanding ADHD and the impact it has on a child's life at home, at school, and in leisure activities is the first step in providing

a way to cope with the condition and one step closer to helping minimize impairment so that a child may reach his or her full potential.

Behavioral therapy can be an important component to managing ADHD. As with any chronic condition, the management requires persistence and expectations of slow-steady progress. The child's specific impairment areas should be determined. With input from the management team, specific goals based on these impairments should be selected. A feasible approach is to choose two to three goals to work on at home and two to three goals to work on at school. When goals are selected, exact expectations for success should be determined. A suggested goal is an improvement from baseline of 20%. If a child is not completing the five assignments he or she is given daily, a goal to complete one assignment a day is appropriate. The goals should be individualized, attainable, and specific enough to be measured. One approach to accomplish this is by using a report card completed at set intervals (daily during titration). This report card allows communication between the home, the school, and ultimately the clinician to ensure a better quality of care for the child. (An example of a report card with directions on usage is included on the CD-ROM.) Other effective techniques include established routines; defined rules; clear, direct commands; and consistent discipline with more positive than negative feedback. Behavior modification is, however, labor intensive. It requires consistency, and progress may be slow.

The primary medical management is stimulant medication. Stimulants are effective in 70% to 80% of children. The benefits while taking stimulants are well documented and include reducing the core symptoms of ADHD and improving behavior, academic productivity and accuracy, parent-child interaction, and aggression. These improvements do not remain when the medication is discontinued. Side effects always are a concern. They usually are mild and can be controlled by modifying the dose and distribution time (Table 244-3). It rarely is necessary to discontinue the medication because of side effects. Table 244-4 lists stimulant medications with dosage information. (Pemoline [Cylert], a stimulant used for ADHD in the past, is known to cause liver toxicity in rare cases and now is prescribed infrequently.) In contrast to most medications, stimulant

Table 244-3. Possible Modifications to Minimize Medication Side Effects

Side Effect	Modifications to Deal with Side Effects
Decreased appetite	Give after meals
	Change diet (calorie-dense food for breakfast)
	Brief drug holidays
Sleep problems	Reduce/eliminate afternoon dose
	Change to short-acting drug if using long-acting one
	Establish bedtime routine
Irritability	Decrease dose, try another stimulant
Headaches	Decrease dose, try another stimulant
Stomachaches	Decrease dose, try another stimulant
Dysphoria	Decrease dose, try another stimulant
Behavioral rebound	Decrease afternoon dose
	Try sustained-release and extended-release preparations
	Combine sustained-release with a short-acting preparation
Growth suppression	Monitor height and weight
	Determine parental height history
	Give drug holidays
Tics	Observe at lower dose and with no medication to determine if tics are truly drug related
	If mild, discuss risk/benefits with parents/child
	Switch stimulants
	If after a sore throat, consider strep association
Psychosis/mania	Stop stimulant

Note: If stimulant is not working or side effects are intolerable, try another stimulant or preparation. If other stimulants do not work or create intolerable side effects, consider second-line drugs or referral to a mental health or developmental/behavioral specialist.

effectiveness is not based on an mg/kg basis. Current recommendations are to start at the lowest dose possible and titrate up based on information gathered from parents and teachers about medication effectiveness.

Initial medication titration can be done in weekly intervals by phone or office visits. Screening for side effects and attainment of target goals give the best measurement of medication effectiveness. This information is obtained best from parents and teachers using behavior rating scales, side-effect scales, and report cards (see the CD-ROM). When the best dose is determined (the dose at which the child is having maximal success in achieving target goals and having

fewest side effects), monitoring can be stretched to monthly and ultimately quarterly office visits. With each monthly refill request, it is helpful to check on adherence, impairment, and side effects (a sample form to do this is included on the CD-ROM). If concerns arise, it is important to re-evaluate the child and request information again from the school and parents concerning the 18 core symptoms and functional impairment.

If after adequate trials of two to three stimulants or stimulant preparations, a best dose for the child has not been achieved, the original diagnosis and management plan should be examined. Is a comorbid diagnosis complicating treatment? Are the target outcomes realistic? Are the family, child, and school adhering to the treatment plan? These questions need to be addressed before moving to the next step in treatment. Second-line medications should be tried only if the physician is familiar with them. These medications include antidepressants and α-adrenergics. Adequate studies to evaluate the use of these medications for ADHD are considerably more limited than the information available on stimulant medications, and the potential side effects can be more serious. The discussion of these drugs is beyond the scope of this chapter. If a child has not responded despite adequate titration and management goals, and the physician is unfamiliar with second-line medications, referral for a more extensive evaluation to mental health or behavioral clinicians is appropriate. Likewise, if a significant comorbid condition, such as major depressive disorder, is present, the clinician may want to consider referral to a mental health clinician.

School interventions may be indicated. Children may be eligible to receive services under Section 504 of the Rehabilitation Act or the Individuals with Disabilities Education Act. Section 504 encourages accommodations be provided for the child when necessary. These modifications could include preferential seating, reduced assignments, clear and direct rules, and a classroom behavioral program. The Individuals with Disabilities Education Act applies for children whose impairment significantly affects their academic performance or who have a learning disability and qualify for special education services. Examples of other services that may be needed include occupational therapy,

Table 244-4. Attention Deficit Hyperactivity Disorder Medications

Medication	Brand Name	Starting Dosage Recommendations (mg)	Dosing Intervals	Onset	Duration (hr)	Maximum Dose (mg)
Mixed salts of amphetamine	Adderall	2.5–5	qd–bid	20–60 min	6	40
Dextroamphetamine	Dexedrine/Dextrostat	2.5–5	bid–tid	20–60 min	4–6	40
	Dexedrine Spansule	5	qd–bid	>60 min	>6 +	40
Methylphenidate	Concerta	18	qd	20–60 min	12	72
	Methylin	5	bid–tid qd–bid	20–60 min	3–5	60
	Methylin ESR	20		1–3 hr	2–6	60
	Ritalin	5	bid-tid qd–bid	20–60 min	3–5	60
	Ritalin-SR	20		1–3 hr	3–8	60
	Metadate ER	10	qd	1–3 hr	3–8	60
	Metadate CD	20	qd	20–60 min	8	60

bid, twice daily; qd, daily; tid, three times daily.

physical therapy, speech therapy, assistive technology, and individual therapy. The school and parents should determine the extent and type of services needed and list them in the child's individualized education plan. More detailed information about section 504 and the Individuals with Disabilities Education Act is included on the CD-ROM.

ADHD is a complex chronic condition. Having an understanding of the diagnostic criteria, treatment options, and monitoring techniques is the first step in offering affected children and their caregivers the treatment and hope required for good outcomes. Although ADHD is a chronic condition, some people with this condition have learned to build on their strengths and become successful adults. Our ultimate goal as caregivers should be to give every child the opportunity to do the same.

Additional Resources, CD-ROM

ADHD Initial Evaluation Summary	Form
ADHD Diagnostic Parent Rating Scale	Form
Teacher Behavior Evaluation Scale	Form
Daily report card	Form
Daily report card instructions	Text
Teacher follow-up information	Form
Parent follow-up information	Form
Bibliography	Text

Mini-index of Related Topics

SUGGESTED READINGS

American Academy of Pediatrics: Clinical practice guideline: Diagnosis and evaluation of the child with attention-deficit/hyperactivity disorder. Pediatrics 2000;105:1158–1170.

American Academy of Pediatrics Subcommittee on Attention-Deficit/Hyperactivity Disorder and Committee on Quality Improvement: Clinical practice guideline: Treatment of the school-aged child with attention-deficit/hyperactivity disorder. Pediatrics 2001;108:1033–1044.

Pliszka S, Greenhill L, Crismon M, et al: The Texas Children's Medication Algorithm Project: Report of the Texas Consensus Conference Panel on medication treatment of childhood attention-deficit/hyperactivity disorder: Part I. Attention-deficit/hyperactivity disorder. J Am Acad Child Adolesc Psychiatry 2000;39:908–919.

Pliszka S, Greenhill L, Crismon M, et al: The Texas Children's Medication Algorithm Project: Report of the Texas Consensus Conference Panel on medication treatment of childhood attention-deficit/hyperactivity disorder. Part II: Tactics: Attention-deficit/hyperactivity disorder. J Am Acad Child Adolesc Psychiatry 2000;39:920–927.

245

Aggressive/Oppositional Behaviors (Oppositional Defiant and Conduct Disorders)

John E. Lochman, Tammy DeShazo Barry, and Karen L. Salekin

ROLE OF THE GENERALIST

1   Understand the developmental trajectory of aggressive and oppositional behaviors and the definitions that form the framework for diagnosis and treatment.

2   Distinguish between developmentally appropriate levels of oppositional behaviors and early symptoms of a behavioral disorder.

3   Identify children with a possible behavioral disorder, and refer to an appropriate mental health specialist for diagnosis and treatment.

4   Recognize the range of assessment tools used by mental health specialists in diagnosing a behavioral disorder, and know what type of information to anticipate in an assessment report.

5   Educate parents in the efficacy of various psychosocial interventions for behavioral disorders.

6   Provide long-term follow-up to ensure that parents have sought appropriate assessment and intervention when indicated.

7   Prescribe medication for mood stabilization when warranted.

According to the *Diagnostic and Statistical Manual of Mental Disorders, fourth edition* (DSM-IV), oppositional defiant disorder (ODD) and conduct disorder (CD) are classified as disruptive behavior disorders that usually are diagnosed first in childhood or adolescence. Both disorders are characterized by the presence of problematic behaviors that are repetitive and persistent and result in significant impairment in social, academic, or occupational functioning (Table 245-1).

Of the two disorders, ODD is considered to be less problematic than CD in relation to overall functioning. The essential feature of ODD is a recurrent pattern of negativistic, hostile, and defiant behavior that is present for at least 6 months. The disorder is usually evident before 8 years of age (not later than early adolescence) with an onset that is gradual, with problems first becoming evident in the home environment. ODD has been found to be more common in families in which at least one parent has a

history of mood disorder, ODD, CD, attention deficit hyperactivity disorder, antisocial personality disorder, or a substance-related disorder. It also has been found in families in which serious marital discord is present. ODD has been found to be more prevalent in boys before puberty but the rates for both genders are similar during the post-pubertal period (2% to 16%). In some cases, the pattern of disruptive behavior ends during or shortly after adolescence. In other cases, ODD does not represent a distinct entity but instead evolves into CD, a disorder that sometimes is associated with long-term problems of adulthood (e.g., antisocial personality disorder). Defiance and hostility are not by themselves indicative of the disorder. These behaviors also are traits associated with normal development and often are present in children who successfully meet the developmental demands of childhood and adolescence. The diagnosis of ODD should be made only if these behaviors occur more often than would be expected for individuals of similar age and developmental level.

Similar to ODD, CD is characterized by a repetitive and persistent pattern of disruptive behavior. The behavior pattern associated with CD is one in which the basic rights of others are violated or the individual violates major age-appropriate societal norms and rules. According to the DSM-IV diagnostic criteria (see Table 245-1), the disruptive behaviors fall into four major types: (1) aggression toward people and animals, (2) destruction of property, (3) deceitfulness or theft, and (4) serious violation of rules. Studies have shown that CD has genetic and environmental components. CD has been found to be more common in families in which at least one parent (biologic or adoptive) has a history of antisocial personality disorder or in which a sibling has a history of CD. The disorder also is more common in families in which a biologic parent has a history of mood disorder, alcohol dependence, schizophrenia, CD, or attention deficit hyperactivity disorder. Although the course of the disorder is variable, onset can occur at 5 or 6 years of age but more typically is seen during late childhood or early adolescence. Estimated rates of CD are 6% to 16% for boys and 2% to 9% for girls, with the prevalence in boys being three times greater than in girls.

One of the most problematic characteristics of either disorder is the stability of the symptoms over the course of

Table 245-1. Oppositional Defiant Disorder and Conduct Disorder (DSM-IV)

	Oppositional Defiant Disorder	Conduct Disorder
Threshold	≥4 criteria must be present for a period of at least 6 mo	≥3 criteria must be present for 12 mo, with at least 1 of the criteria present during the past 6 mo
Criteria	A. Often loses temper B. Often argues with adults C. Often actively defies or refuses to comply with adults' requests or rules D. Often deliberately annoys people E. Often blames others for his or her mistakes or misbehavior F. Is often touchy or easily annoyed by others G. Is often angry or resentful H. Is often spiteful or vindictive	A. Often bullies, threatens, or intimidates others B. Often initiates physical fights C. Has used a weapon that can cause physical harm to others D. Has been physically cruel to people E. Has been physically cruel to animals F. Has stolen while confronting a victim G. Has forced someone into sexual activity H. Has deliberately engaged in fire setting with the intention of causing serious damage I. Has deliberately destroyed the property of others J. Has broken into someone else's home, building, or car K. Often lies to obtain goods or favors or to avoid obligations L. Has stolen items of nontrivial value *without* confronting a victim M. Often stays out at night against parental rules (beginning before the age of 13 yr) N. Has run away from home overnight at least twice while living in the parental/parental surrogate home (once *if* the period of absence was lengthy) O. Often truant from school (beginning before the age of 13 yr)
Typology	Not applicable according to DSM-IV system	Childhood onset: Onset of at least one criterion before the age of 10 yr Adolescent onset: Absence of any criteria before the age of 10 yr Unspecified onset: Unknown time of onset
Severity	Not applicable according to DSM-IV system	Mild: Few conduct problems and the problems associated result in minor harm to others (e.g., lying, truancy) Moderate: More than minimal criteria are met, and the effects of the behavior are substantial, although not severe (e.g., stealing without confronting a victim) Severe: Many conduct problems present, or behaviors result in considerable harm to others (e.g., forced sex, physical cruelty)
Rule-out	The diagnosis is *not* made if any of these are true: 1. The behaviors occur exclusively during the course of a psychotic disorder, mood disorder, or ADHD 2. The person meets criteria for adjustment disorder 3. If ≥18 yr old, the criteria are not met for antisocial personality disorder 4. The conduct problems are considered to be typical for someone of this age, gender, and level of functioning 5. The individual meets the criteria for CD	The diagnosis is *not* made if any of these are true: 1. The behaviors occur exclusively during the course of a psychotic disorder, mood disorder, or ADHD 2. The person meets the criteria for adjustment disorder 3. If ≥18 yr old, the criteria are not met for antisocial personality disorder

Comorbidity	ADHD symptoms
	  75–90% of children with CD may have co-occurring ADHD
	  Longitudinal evidence suggests that children with comorbid conduct problems and ADHD symptoms are at greater risk for serious antisocial behavior in adolescence and adulthood than youth with conduct problems alone
	Internalizing disorders
	  Children with conduct and depressive problems are more likely to use substances in adolescence compared with to youth with conduct problems alone
	  Internalizing symptoms may partially mediate the relation between early conduct problems and later substance use
	Learning problems
	  Children with ODD and CD tend to have problems achieving academically
	  The reason for these difficulties and the potential ramifications in terms of the developmental course of conduct problems remain unclear
	  Adolescents who begin exhibiting conduct problems seem to have learning difficulties that are not accounted for merely by presence of ADHD
	  Children with disruptive behaviors are at greater risk for dropping out of school, which increases their likelihood of gravitating to a deviant peer group in their neighborhood	

ADHD, attention deficit hyperactivity disorder; CD, conduct disorder; ODD, oppositional defiant disorder.

From American Psychiatric Association: Diagnostic and Statistical Manual of Mental Disorders, 4th ed, text revision (DSM-IV-TR). Washington, DC, American Psychiatric Association, 2000.

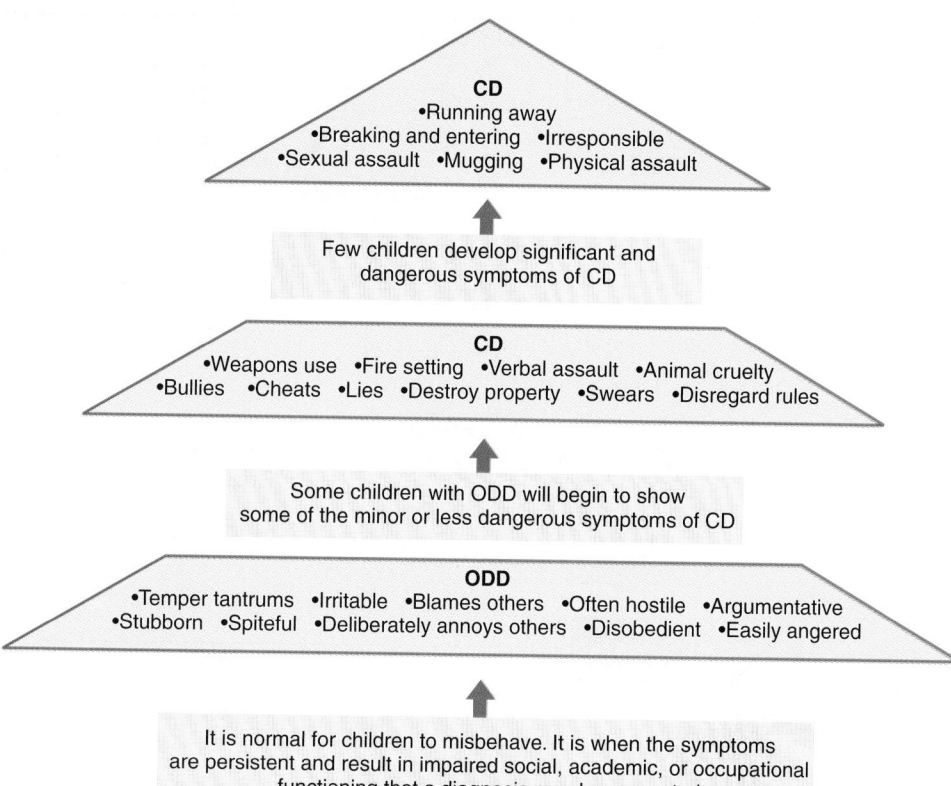

Figure 245-1. Possible developmental progression of disruptive behavior problems. CD, conduct disorder; ODD, oppositional defiant disorder.

childhood, adolescence, and adulthood. CD may be one of the most enduring forms of psychopathology in children and, when evident in early childhood, is expected to be preceded by physical aggression and poor peer relationships. Children are more at risk for continued aggressive and antisocial behavior if they display aggressive behavior in multiple settings and if they develop "versatile" forms of antisocial behavior by early to mid-adolescence. Longitudinal research has indicated that ODD precedes CD (especially the childhood-onset form of CD) and that CD is often a precursor of antisocial personality disorder in adulthood (Fig. 245-1). It is estimated that approximately half of children with CD develop significant antisocial personality disorder symptoms. Two factors that predict the development of antisocial personality disorder are the number of CD symptoms the child exhibits and early age of onset of symptoms. Finally, children with ODD and CD may have other comorbid diagnoses and problem areas. Common areas of comorbidity are summarized in Table 245-1.

RISK AND CAUSAL FACTORS

The developmental trajectory leading to childhood-onset CD may start early among infants whom exhibit irritable, difficult-to-soothe temperaments and whom are less adaptable to change. A model of developmental trajectories, which has received substantial empirical support, indicates that children progressively can accumulate sets of risk factors for later antisocial behavior (Fig. 245-2). At any point in the trajectory, children can move off of the trajectory, as a result of a variety of factors, such as benign school or home environments, constructive peer relationships, or psychosocial treatment. The role of an alert pediatrician in recognizing the child's movement on this path and in referring and initiating early intervention can be a key force in diverting children off this trajectory. If the children instead continue to progress up the trajectory toward serious CD, they accumulate a collection of additional risk factors. As this "developmental stacking" of risk factors occurs, it becomes progressively more difficult to alter the children's trajectory through psychosocial treatments and preventive interventions.

Ecologic Models

Ecologic models of child development have suggested that children's behavior is the result of individual characteristics (e.g., irritable temperament) and of social and contextual influences that radiate out around the child (Fig. 245-3). Social contexts that are most proximal are contexts in which the child spends the most time and which are likely to have the most impact on the child's behavior (e.g., family environment, school environment, and peer groups). Children's broader environments, such as their neighborhoods

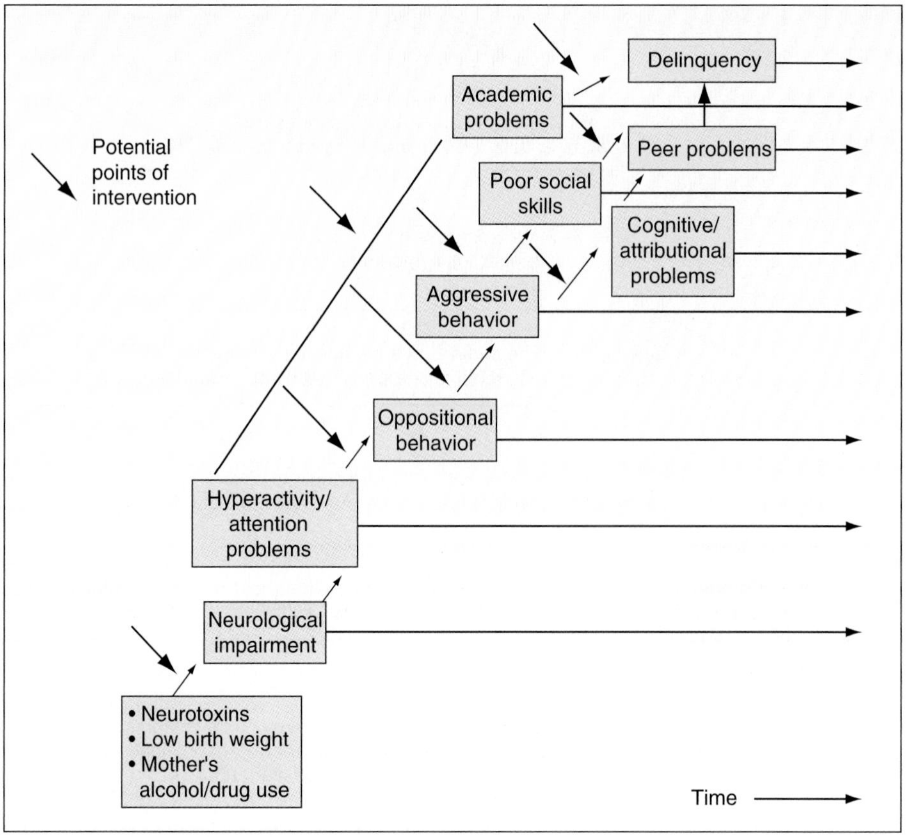

Figure 245-2. Hypothesized maximal developmental sequence of stacking of problem behaviors in children with disruptive behavior disorders. (Adapted from Loeber R: Development and risk factors of juvenile antisocial behavior and delinquency. Clin Psychol Rev 1990;10:1–41.)

and medical clinics, social agencies, and recreation centers within their communities, also can affect them, but often in an indirect way. Typically this indirect effect occurs because the stresses produced by these community and family forces lead to disruptions in the parents' efforts to raise and discipline their children. The ecologic model also stresses the importance of understanding how these systems interact with each other and how these interactions between systems influence the children's behavioral development. Parents' abilities to interact in positive, proactive ways with school personnel (crossing the family and school systems) can assist children's positive behavior, and, similarly, parents and physicians' abilities to interact in positive, open ways can assist the assessment and referral of children who have behavioral problems.

Development of Conduct Disorder
Early Risk Factors

In early stages of the developmental trajectory leading to CD, temperamentally difficult children are at risk for failing to develop positive attachments with caretakers, for displaying high rates of hyperactive behavior and poor attentional control in the preschool years, and for becoming involved in increasingly coercive interchanges with parents and later with teachers. Life course–persistent delinquents, or "early starters," are at risk early in life because of a set of biologic, family, and broader community risk factors that can exacerbate these coercive parent-child relationships in the preschool years. In some children, family dysfunction, consisting of preexisting problems such as severe marital conflict, parental psychopathology or drug abuse, parental

criminal behavior, or poverty, may be sufficient to initiate a sequence of escalating aversive behaviors between parents and children. Poor, crime-ridden neighborhoods that have limited resources and weak social cohesion also add to the environmental risk factors leading to seriously aggressive behavior.

Parenting Practices

As the coercive interaction style develops between a parent and an increasingly aggressive child, a set of maladaptive parenting practices becomes apparent and serves to maintain and increase further the child's aggressive behavior throughout the preschool and elementary school years. Parents who have low levels of warmth and involvement with their children, use rigid control and harsh punishment, and have inconsistent and unclear expectations for their children have children who are likely to become increasingly aggressive. As children become older and move into middle school and high school, parents who do not monitor or supervise their children's activities well contribute to children's increasingly antisocial behavior. This behavior occurs in part because parents fail to prevent their children's involvement in deviant peer groups, which become a major proximal risk factor for serious adolescent conduct problems.

Peer Difficulties

As the aggressive behavior becomes developed in the preschool years at home, children begin to generalize their use of coercive behaviors to other social interactions, leading to increasingly aggressive behavior with peers and

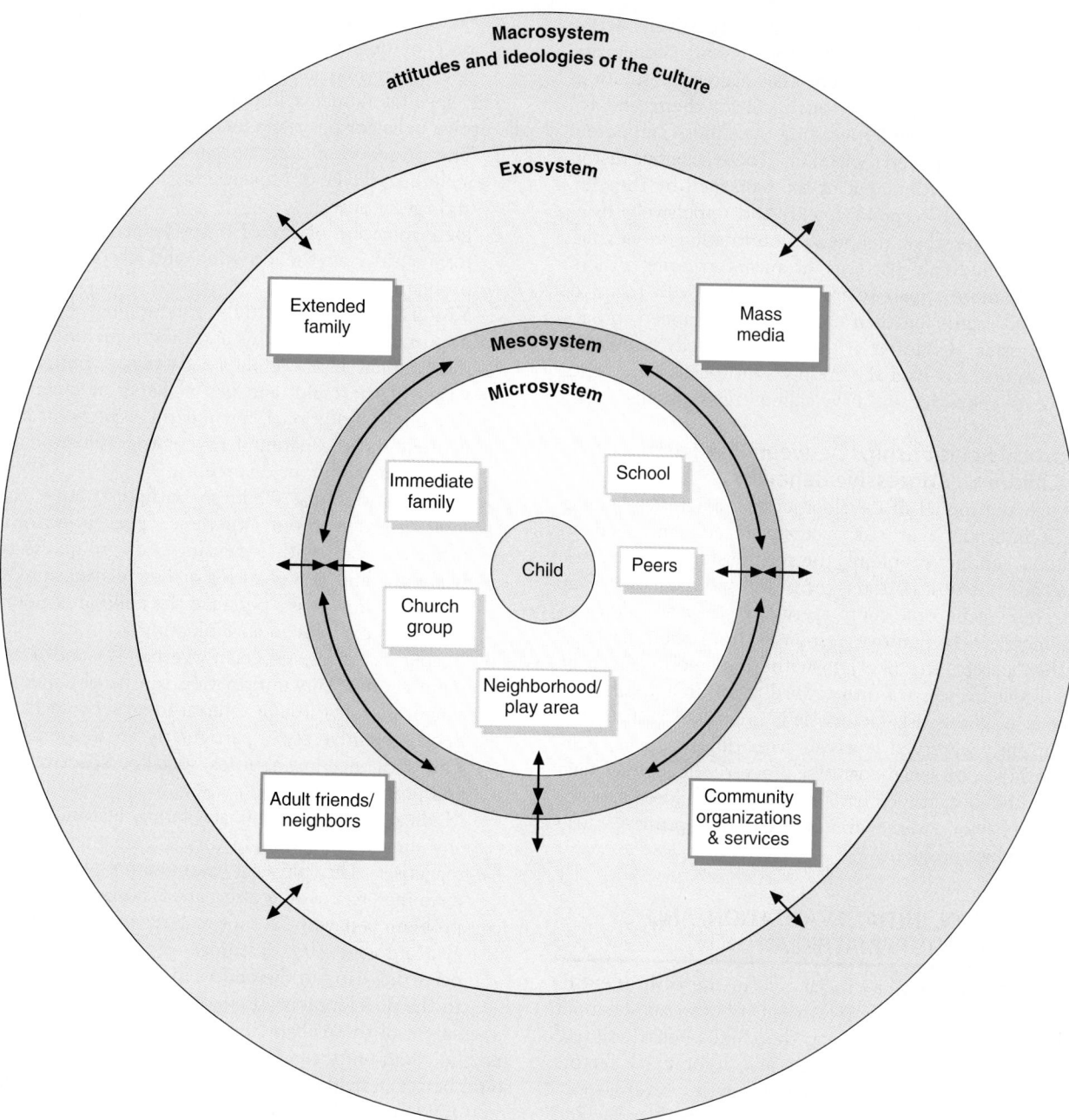

Figure 245-3. Oppositional defiant disorder and conduct disorder considered within Bronfenbrenner's ecologic model of development.

adults by early elementary school and to dysfunctional social-cognitive processes. Because of their aggressive behavior, these children often are rejected socially by their peer group and, as a result, can become more withdrawn and isolated and lacking in social skills. Aggressive children who are rejected by their peer group are likely to have greater difficulty adjusting to middle school, to have poorer academic progress, and to show more severe behavioral problems than are aggressive children who manage to maintain some peer relationships.

Children with conduct problems usually are rejected continuously from prosocial peer groups during the elementary school years, and as they enter adolescence, they tend to turn to deviant peer groups as a means of social support and affiliation. When involved in a deviant peer group, youths' risks for committing antisocial acts increase by two to four times.

Social-Cognitive Distortions and Deficiencies

Aggressive children have been found to have difficulties processing social information, and these social-cognitive problems contribute to their social rejection and maintain their aggressive behavior. Compared with nonaggressive children, aggressive children (1) pay more attention to hostile social cues; (2) have hostile attributional biases, in which they erroneously perceive hostile intentions from others in ambiguous social situations; (3) have dominance-oriented and revenge-oriented social goals; (4) think of solutions to social problems that are excessively action oriented and lacking in verbal assertion and cooperation strategies; (5) have expectations that aggressive solutions will produce the greatest personal gain for them; and (6) have difficulty successfully enacting their more competent ideas because of impaired social skills. These cognitive distortions and cognitive deficiencies are worsened by the children's tendency to respond quickly and impulsively, using automatic rather than deliberate information processing. Aggressive children's patterns of misinterpreting others' behavior is more apparent among children with reactive, anger-based aggression than children with planned, proactive aggression. Children with more planned, calculated aggression are part of a subgroup of antisocial adolescents who are psychopathic and have callous, unemotional traits.

Reciprocal Relationships between Risk Factors and Children's Aggressive Behavior

Although the model of developmental trajectories leading to CD indicates that risk factors precede and lead to children's conduct problems, the relationship between risk factors and outcomes often is reciprocal and recursive. That is, as children become more aggressive, they are likely to elicit increasingly punitive responses from their parents, and their parents are likely to withdraw emotionally over time, displaying less warmth toward them. In assessing the presence of these risk factors, it is crucial to realize that the currently observed levels of parenting practices, peer relationships, and social-cognitive processes likely may have deteriorated because of earlier levels of children's problematic behavior and may not be the only or primary cause of the conduct problems.

PRESENTATION, INITIAL EVALUATION, AND REFERRAL BY THE PEDIATRICIAN

The pediatrician plays a crucial role in the early identification, prevention, and treatment of various conduct problems by carefully assessing the child's behavioral and social functioning and the family and community factors that maintain children's problem behavior. After assessment, proactive parent education about this disorder and about parenting strategies and referral to treatment can occur. Before discussing referrals and types of assessment tools that may be useful, it is important to consider a few main points important to any clinical evaluation:

1. Disruptive behavior disorders are a heterogeneous grouping; the assessment needs to be tailored to the specific presenting problem and child being evaluated.
2. Patterns of behaviors associated with disruptive behavior disorders often vary based on context (e.g., school versus home). Recognition of this fact highlights the importance of using multiple informants and multiple modalities during the evaluation.
3. Behaviors associated with disruptive behavior disorders may not be seen during an evaluation (e.g., because of low frequency or social desirability). For this reason, gathering information at multiple points in time is useful in determining the diagnosis.
4. The development of disruptive behaviors is often the result of a complex interaction of multiple causal

factors. As such, it is important to consider a multitude of domains related to child functioning when developing a conceptual framework of the problem.

The specific domains important to the assessment of disruptive behavior disorders include the following:

1. The presence of core symptoms (see Table 245-1), including degree of impairment, situational variability, and age of onset
2. Determination of age of onset (especially important for considering the duration and chronicity of the problem behaviors)
3. Various aspects of family functioning: Particularly important aspects of this assessment include parental involvement in the child's activities, parental supervision of the child, and use of harsh or inconsistent discipline. Additional meaningful aspects of family context include parental psychiatric adjustment and marital instability or divorce.
4. Peer relationships: Children with disruptive behavioral disorders often experience peer rejection and often associate with a deviant peer group. As such, how the child perceives his or her relationships with peers and how peers perceive the child are important factors to examine in an evaluation.
5. Academic status, especially verbal IQ and achievement scores: This information can be obtained from school files or through referral to a psychologist.
6. Social-cognitive style, particularly attributional style: This cues encoding abilities, social perspective-taking, and problem-solving.
7. Medical, developmental, and family histories: As with any clinical evaluation, history is crucial to an accurate diagnosis. The physical examination can alert the examiner to possible alternative explanations for the problem behaviors. A thorough developmental history also informs the examiner of any circumstances occurring early in the child's life that may be relevant to the development of conduct problems.

Assessment of these characteristics of the child, the family, and the community can lead the health provider to understand better individual differences within children exhibiting ODD and CD symptoms. Understanding of these individual differences and of subtypes of conduct problem children can lead to more effective referrals and psychosocial treatment plans using identified efficacious treatments.

If a behavioral disorder is suspected, the pediatrician should refer the child to a mental health specialist for a comprehensive assessment. An important consideration in the referral process is whether the professional (i.e., psychiatrist, psychologist, social worker) to whom the patient is referred is likely to use empirically supported assessment tools and treatment programs. A shift toward increased interdisciplinary practice has provided pediatricians the opportunity to work directly with mental health professionals in developing a diagnostic and intervention plan for children presenting with aggression and disruptive behavior problems. Likewise, pediatricians in private practice often can follow a multidisciplinary model by contracting with mental health professionals to assess their patients on a consultant basis (e.g., for specialized clinic appointments).

ASSESSMENT OF OPPOSITIONAL DEFIANT DISORDER AND CONDUCT DISORDER BY MENTAL HEALTH SPECIALISTS

When a child is referred for an evaluation for ODD or CD, several types of assessment tools are used by mental health specialists to gather comprehensive information from multiple informants across multiple domains of functioning. Commonly used assessment instruments are behavioral rating scales and structured interviews (see Chapter 238). The mental health professional typically uses direct behavioral observation, which can supply data about the child's behaviors without the filter of the perceptions of others. When a child presents with disruptive behaviors and externalizing symptoms, it is important also to consider other possible comorbid problems, such as depressive symptoms and attentional difficulties, which also can be assessed through these types of diagnostic instruments.

When possible, clinicians collect peer-referenced data to obtain valuable information regarding the nature of the child's peer relationships. Vignettes and hypothetical situations also are used to assess social-cognitive processes, whereas intellectual and academic achievement tests are used to conduct a psychoeducational assessment (Table 245-2 lists examples of assessment instruments often included in a comprehensive diagnostic battery). In addition to making a differential diagnosis, the use of a comprehensive assessment battery is important in determining which symptoms are primary and which are secondary, an important first step in formulating an effective treatment plan. The mental health professional compiles all assessment information gathered into a clinical report, which outlines the case formulation and treatment plan for the child. In doing so, the clinician follows a multistep strategy for integrating information, including (1) documenting any clinically significant findings regarding the child's adjustment; (2) seeking convergent findings across sources and methods; (3) explaining any existing discrepancies among sources and methods; and (4) developing a profile for the child, including his or her strengths and weaknesses.

TREATMENT OF OPPOSITIONAL DEFIANT DISORDER, CONDUCT DISORDER, AND AGGRESSION

After a comprehensive diagnostic assessment, the mental health professional has the essential information required to develop and implement an individualized treatment plan for the child. Empirically supported treatments for children with ODD and CD have been identified through controlled, randomized clinical trials. There are several systematic reviews of the treatment research literature for children with ODD and CD, which have revealed several programs with well-established positive effects (see the Suggested Readings). Cognitive-behavioral interventions have been shown to be effective in reducing disruptive and aggressive behavior, and interventions that focus on children and parents produce broader positive effects and better maintenance of improvements over time than do interventions that focus on either the child or the parent alone.

Cognitive-behavioral therapy for children presenting with aggression, ODD, or CD may include training in self-instruction, social problem solving, perspective taking, imagery, and relaxation. The focus is on the deficient and distorted social-cognitive processes identified in aggressive children. In addition, the therapist is likely to work with the parents to teach positive parenting techniques and to target improvement in the application of parenting skills that have been shown to decrease aggressive and disruptive behaviors in children (e.g., reinforcement of positive behaviors; ignoring minor disruptive behaviors; implementing negative consequences, such as time-out and response costs; and setting up clear rules and expectations). Consultation with personnel at the child's school regarding school-based behavior modification (e.g., home-school note program, behavioral check chart) also may be warranted. Treatment is most effective when modifications are consistent across situations.

Family therapy also has been shown to produce significant improvements in parenting practices and reductions in children's aggressive, conduct problem behavior. Although the behaviorally disordered child may be the "identified patient," a family therapist treats the family as an interactive system. This therapy can be accomplished through several routes, including reorganizing the boundaries of the family's subsystems, restructuring the family's circular interactional patterns, and conducting a functional analysis of the family's behaviors in an effort to teach the family new responses to achieve desired outcomes.

Finally, research on intensive prevention programs directed toward young high-risk children, such as the Fast Track, Anger Coping, and Coping Power Programs, shows that disruptive and aggressive behavior, ODD, and CD can be reduced through early intervention that targets the correlates of these externalizing behaviors (e.g., child's social competence, parenting practices). Likewise, intervention programs targeting aggressive adolescents already displaying many problem behaviors (e.g., Anger Control Training, Adolescent Transitions Program) also decrease disruptive behaviors.

FOLLOW-UP BY THE PEDIATRICIAN

The pediatrician should remain actively involved with the patient while the treatment of ODD or CD is being provided. Because parents tend to have low motivation to seek treatment, the pediatrician should encourage and monitor their follow-through and should be aware of overall goals of intervention and reinforce the family (parents and child) for reaching those goals. During the course of follow-up, the pediatrician should consider the individual differences of children who present with ODD and CD and recognize that the course of treatment will vary. Not all children respond well to treatment. In addition to referral for psychosocial treatments, in some cases, the pediatrician may determine that medication for mood stabilization is warranted. Finally, as noted earlier, pediatricians working in a multidisciplinary setting are actively involved in the follow-up of children diagnosed with disruptive behavior disorders.

Table 245-2. Recommended Battery of Assessment Tools

Type	Respondent	Examples	Advantages	Disadvantages
Omnibus rating scales	Child	Behavior Assessment System for Children–Self Report of Personality (BASC-SRP) Minnesota Multiphasic Personality Inventory–Adolescent (MMPI-A) Youth Self Report (YSR)	Can gather similar information from multiple informants A lot of data in a short period of time; efficient Easy to administer Often includes a straightforward computer-based scoring program Allows for the detection of low-frequency behaviors	Does not always provide enough coverage of core symptoms to differentiate among subtypes Rarely includes information regarding the severity, age of onset, and situational variables related to the problem behaviors Not always tied to diagnostic criteria Sometimes involves excessive item overlap
	Parent	Behavior Assessment System for Children–Parent Rating Scale (BASC-PRS) Child Behavior Checklist (CBCL) Connors Parent Rating Scales	Allows for screening for the presence of comorbid disorders Often have good normative data (can determine if behaviors are developmentally appropriate) Interpretive flexibility due to the numerous scales available	
	Teacher	Behavior Assessment System for Children–Teacher Rating Scale (BASC-TRS) Teacher Report Form (TRF)		
Domain-specific rating scales	Child	Reynolds Child Depression Scale (RCDS) Child Depression Inventory (CDI) Revised Child Manifest Anxiety Scale (RCMAS) Harter's Perceived Competence Scale for Children	Can gather similar information from multiple informants Time efficient Easy to administer Often have good normative data (can determine if behaviors are developmentally appropriate)	Does not always provide enough coverage of core symptoms to differentiate among subtypes Rarely includes information regarding the severity, age of onset, and situational variables related to the problem behaviors Not always tied to diagnostic criteria
	Parent	Attention Deficit Disorders Evaluation Scales (ADDES)–Home Version Social Skills Rating System (SSRS)		
	Teacher	Attention Deficit Disorders Evaluation Scales (ADDES)–School Version Social Skills Rating System (SSRS)		
Structured interviews	Child and parent	Diagnostic Interview Schedule for Children (DISC) Diagnostic Interview for Children and Adolescents (DICA) Child Assessment Schedule for Children (CAS)	Can gather similar information from multiple informants Allows for collection of detailed information Often provides enough coverage of core symptoms to differentiate among subtypes of disorders Allows for a screening for the presence of comorbid disorders Gathers information regarding the severity, age of onset, and situational variables related to problem behaviors Often tied to diagnostic criteria May include normative information	Usually time-consuming to administer May require specialized training of the interviewer Often does not include normative data
Direct observation	Clinician	Behavior Assessment System for Children–Student Observation System (BASC-SOS) Child Behavior Checklist–Direct Observation Form (CBCL-DOF) Dodge's Observation of Peer Interactions	Not filtered through the perceptions of others (e.g., parents, teachers) Provides in-depth information Similar data can be collected across various settings and multiple time periods Sensitive to treatment effects	Can be time-consuming to conduct Usually does not include normative data Can have low reliability (avoided by having well-trained observers) Standard method of assessing

Data from Kamphaus RW, Frick PJ: Clinical Assessment of Child and Adolescent Personality and Behavior. Needham Heights, Mass, Allyn & Bacon, 1996; and Lochman JE, Dane HE, Magee TN, et al: Disruptive behavior disorders: Assessment and intervention. In Vance B, Pumareiga A (eds): The Clinical Assessment of Children and Youth Behavior: Interfacing Intervention with Assessment. New York, Wiley, 2002.

Table 245-2. Recommended Battery of Assessment Tools—cont'd

Type	Respondent	Examples	Advantages	Disadvantages
Direct observation—cont'd	Clinician—cont'd	Structured observation of academic and play settings Clinician-designed systematic observation schedule		antecedents and consequences of behaviors not always established
Peer-referenced assessment	Peers	Sociometric data for which classmates rate other classmates (including target child) on variables including "liked most" and "liked least" Additional variables (e.g., "fights most," "can't pay attention") may be included for supplementary data Peer Nomination Inventory of Depression (PNID)	Provides information important for subtyping socialized versus undersocialized children with conduct problems Provides data about peers' perceptions of a child without the filter of the teacher (teacher ratings) or the target child (self-report ratings)	Can be time-consuming to administer Informed consent typically must be obtained from the peer group before administering the nominations/ratings Important to ensure that classmates do not know the assessment is focused on one individual Often requires teacher participation and sometimes raises teachers' concerns Not a great deal of normative data for these measures
Vignettes	Child	Problem Solving Measure for Conflict (PSM-C) Child Attribution Measure	Provides insight into the child's current repertoire of problem-solving strategies	Can be time-consuming to administer and score (often have to apply elaborate coding techniques)
Intellectual tests	Child tested	Examples of Full Batteries: Wechsler Intelligence Scale for Children–3rd edition (WISC-III); Stanford-Binet–4th edition; Kaufman Assessment Battery for Children (K-ABC) Examples of abbreviated batteries: Wechsler Abbreviated Scales of Intelligence (WASI); Kaufman Brief Intelligence Test (K-BIT)		
Academic achievement tests	Child tested	Examples of full batteries: Wechsler Individual Achievement		

Additional Resources, CD-ROM

Bibliography	

Mini-index of Related Topics

SUGGESTED READINGS

Campbell M, Cueva JE, Adams PB: Pharmacotherapy of impulsive-aggressive behavior. In Cloninger CR (ed): Personality and Psychopathology. Washington, DC, American Psychiatric Press, 1999, pp 431–455.

Dodge KA: Conduct disorder. In Sameroff AJ, Lewis M, Miller SM (eds): Handbook of Developmental Psychopathology, 2nd ed. New York, Kluwer Academic/Plenum Publishers, 2000, pp 447–463.

Forness SR, Kavale KA, Walker HM: Identifying children at risk for antisocial behavior: The case for comorbidity. In Gallimore R, Bernheimer LP, MacMillan DL, et al (eds): Developmental Perspective on Children with High-Incidence Disabilities: The LEA Series on Special Education and Disability. Mahwah, NJ, Lawrence Erlbaum Associates, 1999, pp 135–155.

Lochman JE, and Conduct Problems Prevention Research Group: Screening of child behavior problems for prevention programs at school entry. J Consult Clin Psychol 1995;63:549–559.

Reich W, Herjanic B, Welner Z, Gandhy PR: Development of a structured psychiatric interview for children: Agreement in diagnosis comparing child and parent interviews. J Abnorm Child Psychol 1982;10:325–336.

Rey JM, Walter G: Oppositional defiant disorder. In Hendren RL (ed): Disruptive Behavior Disorders in Children and Adolescents, Vol 18, No 2, Review of Psychiatry Series. Washington, DC, American Psychiatric Press, 1999, pp 99–132.

Robins LN: A 70-year history of conduct disorder: Variations in definition, prevalence, and correlates. In Cohen P, Slomkowski C, Robins LN (eds): Historical and Geographical Influences on Psychopathology. Mahwah, NJ, Lawrence Erlbaum Associates, 1999, pp 37–56.

246 Anxiety Disorders in Children and Adolescents

John S. March

ROLE OF THE GENERALIST

1 Differentiate normal from pathologic anxiety.

2 Identify patients at high risk for anxiety or who have an anxiety disorder.

3 Treat with or provide a mental health referral for cognitive-behavioral therapy.

4 Treat with first-line medications or, if necessary, refer for pharmacotherapy.

5 Provide ongoing follow-up to increase treatment adherence.

Box 246-1. Treatment Planning

1. Conduct a comprehensive baseline evaluation, including rating scales and, if indicated, laboratory measures.
2. Carefully consider the question of differential therapeutics to identify potential targets for medication treatment as distinct from psychosocial treatments where possible.
3. Establish risk-to-benefit ratios for each treatment, and obtain informed consent.
4. In general, begin with cognitive-behavioral therapy either alone (mild to moderate, no or mild comorbidity) or in combination (severe, multiple comorbidities) with medication.
5. Define indicators for each important outcome domain to track potential benefits and side effects better.
6. Where possible, start only one medication at a time to minimize confusion with respect to tracking outcome.
7. When adjusting treatments, consider dose-response (intensity) and time-response (temporal) characteristics of the chosen medication in relationship to the patient's psychiatric disorder.
8. Using an evidence-based stages-of-treatment model, establish a defined end point at which a decision is made about whether the expected benefit has occurred and whether additional treatment can or should be implemented.

Because anxiety disorders in children and adolescents cause major suffering and disrupt normal psychosocial and academic development, they are second only to disruptive behavior disorders as a cause of referral for mental health care in children and adolescents. This chapter discusses the diagnosis and treatment of common anxiety disorders in general pediatrics.

If at any point in the sequence of treatment outlined in the Role of the Generalist box and Box 246-1 (i.e., from a comprehensive assessment through initial and downstream treatment options), the generalist pediatrician cannot provide optimal care, referral for specialty consultation is warranted. Depending on the level of interest and knowledge possessed by the pediatrician and on the complexity of the patient, it is appropriate to refer for assistance in the management of the patient or to transfer care directly to the specialist, who may be a child and adolescent psychiatrist, a psychologist, a developmental-behavioral pediatrician, or a behavioral neurologist. Given heterogeneity of practice and quality of care, it is crucial that referral be made to a clinician with specialty expertise in the care of anxious children.

ANXIETY DISORDERS

Definition

Most fears occurring during childhood are developmentally appropriate to the context in which they occur. *Anxiety*, in contrast to normal worry, usually refers to developmentally inappropriate fears (e.g., panic attacks in a child or adolescent) or to developmentally appropriate fears that produce excessive distress or dysfunction (e.g., separation anxiety and school refusal in a preschool child). Phobias are fears that are attached to specific objects and that usually provoke avoidance, such as the fear of snakes or heights. Anxiety typically is more diffuse than either a normative fear, such as fear of separation, or a specific phobia, such as fear of the dark, in that anxiety is attached to a myriad of different situations and triggers.

DSM-IV Anxiety Disorders

With the aim of increasing reliability and validity, the *Diagnostic and Statistical Manual of Mental Disorders, third edition*, introduced a categorically defined subclass of anxiety disorders of childhood and adolescence. In deleting avoidant disorder and adding overanxious disorder under

This work was supported in part by NIMH Grants 1 R10 MH55121-02 and 1 K24 MHO1557-02 to the author and by generous contributions from the Gorrell family.

the *generalized anxiety disorder* rubric, the *Diagnostic and Statistical Manual of Mental Disorders, fourth edition* (DSM-IV) refined these constructs and established a greater degree of continuity—developmental and nosologic—with the adult anxiety disorders. Table 246-1 summarizes the characteristics, onset, course, and important features of the DSM-IV anxiety disorders affecting children and adolescents.

Comorbidity

Comorbidity among the anxiety disorders and between the anxiety disorders and other internalizing and externalizing disorders complicates diagnosis and treatment. A wide variety of specific phobias commonly accompany the other anxiety disorders. Nighttime fears, resistance to going to bed, difficulty falling asleep alone or sleeping through the night alone, and nightmares involving separation themes are more common than not in children with separation anxiety. Phobic symptoms are common triggers for panic/separation anxiety and are responsible for many of the avoidance and ritualized anxiety-reducing behaviors seen in anxious children. Anxious children also show high rates of comorbid depression. In younger children, generalized anxiety disorder precedes depression in approximately two thirds of cases and may form the nidus for recurrent affective illness if left untreated. Children and adolescents with anxiety and depression have a significantly worse long-term prognosis, with a higher than expected risk for suicide. Finally, about 25% of children with an anxiety disorder have a comorbid externalizing disorder, particularly attention deficit hyperactivity disorder or oppositional defiant disorder.

Course

To understand the course of anxiety disorders, the severity and prevalence of normal fear and worry, which follow a prescribed developmental pattern, must be considered first. Certain specific phobias, such as nighttime fears, are age dependent in that they are much more common in preschool children and elementary school–age children. When present in older children, however, these fears more reliably indicate pathologic anxiety. Other fears, such as fears about self-presentation and consequently social phobia, become more common as children mature into adolescence. Although separation anxiety disorder typically has

Table 246-1. Anxiety Disorders

Disorder	Defining Characteristic	Prominent Symptoms	Age of Onset	Prevalence (%)	Course	Comment
Separation anxiety disorder	Intense fear of being separated from home and/or important attachment figures	Fear of leaving home or being separated from parent. Stomachaches, headaches, or sick feelings	Early childhood	4	Remission common	Predicts panic disorder as a teenager
Panic disorder	Unprovoked panic attacks	Fear of losing control, going crazy, dying; rapid heart rate, hyperventilation, shaking, sweating, nausea	Adolescence	1	Chronic	Fear of having a panic attack leads to agoraphobia (e.g., presenting as school refusal)
Generalized anxiety disorder	Perfectionistic "worriers" who constantly ask for reassurance	Worry about past or future events. Tense, restless, on edge, headaches	Middle childhood	2–5	Chronic	Associated with depression
Social anxiety disorder	Fear of embarrassment and/or rejection in social and/or performance settings	Fear of saying or doing something foolish or embarrassing. Blushing, sweating, shaking. Dysfunction related to avoiding social interchange	Early or middle childhood; commonly adolescence	5	Chronic	Shyness "warms up"; social anxiety does not
Selective mutism	Refusal to talk (despite normal language) to other than "safe" friends and adults	Fear of speaking	Early childhood	<1	Chronic	Age-specific variant of social anxiety disorder
Specific phobias	Common, tightly circumscribed fears that are unreasonable in degree or nature	Situations, such as fear of the dark or heights, natural phenomena such as thunderstorms and water, or "objects," such as snakes and spiders, monsters, bugs or small animals, and blood or hypodermic syringes and needles	Early childhood more common	20	Remission common	Phobias cause problems by provoking avoidance of the feared object or situation or by inducing extreme anxiety if forced to confront the phobic object or situation

From American Psychiatric Association: Diagnostic and Statistical Manual of Mental Disorders, 4th ed, text revision (DSM-IV-TR). Washington, DC, American Psychiatric Association, 2000.

been seen as a relational disturbance, more recent evidence suggests that separation anxiety disorder may represent an age-specific presentation of panic disorder in younger children. As with panic disorder, separation anxiety disorder typically begins with somatic/autonomic complaints, with symptoms escalating to full panic and activation of important attachment mechanisms as a means of coping with panic-level anxiety. The fear of not being able to escape to a safe place in panic disorder is similar to the need to have a parent immediately available in separation anxiety disorder; both involve acute proximity seeking as a means of arousal/fear reduction. In this context, the course of anxiety disorders in children can be summarized as follows: (1) Separation anxiety and specific phobias occur early; (2) social anxiety and panic occur early but peak in adolescence; (3) single disorders tend to be episodic; (4) comorbid anxiety disorders, which describe two thirds of anxious children not counting the specific phobias, tend to be more chronic than single disorders; (5) early onset, comorbidity, and the presence of generalized worry predict comorbid depression; and (6) anxiety disorders in childhood strongly predict anxiety and depressive disorder in adulthood.

ASSESSMENT

The cornerstone of pharmacologic and psychosocial management of pediatric anxiety disorders is a thorough diagnostic assessment, including a clinical interview and a multimethod, multi-informant, multidomain scalar evaluation that includes not only anxiety, but also comorbid conditions, such as depression or attention deficit hyperactivity disorder.

Most anxious children present for mental health care because of problematic behaviors either in their relationships or in the school setting. Starting with the presenting complaint, the clinician's task is to understand these behaviors in the context of the constraints to normal development that underlie them and in doing so construct a differential diagnostic hierarchy that informs a thoughtfully constructed treatment regimen. In this sense, the task of the psychiatric diagnostician is similar to that of the pediatric endocrinologist confronted with a patient with polyuria and polydipsia. Based on the presenting complaint and probabilities attending important demographic factors, the pediatric endocrinologist identifies the most likely diagnosis and all important intercurrent conditions and psychosocial risk and protective factors that might influence the outcome of treatment in the process of reaching a decision regarding differential therapeutics.

Of the assessment technologies available to the child psychiatrist, psychologist, or general pediatrician, gender-normed, age-normed, and race-normed rating scales offer the most efficient way to collect information regarding internalizing and externalizing behavioral disturbances at home and school. Excellent scales with good psychometric properties are available for self-report or parent report of developmental history, conduct problems, fear, anxiety, and depression. The parent and child assessment inventory used in the Program in Child and Adolescent Anxiety Disorders

Table 246-2. Anxiety Disorders Assessment Battery*

Instrument	Type of Information
Conners/March Developmental Questionnaire (CMDQ)	Demographics, developmental, medical and treatment history, other risk and protective factors
Conners Parent Rating Scale (CPRS)	Parent-rated general psychopathology
Multidimensional Anxiety Scale for Children (MASC)	Self-reported anxiety
Children's Depression Inventory (CDI)	Self-reported depression

*From MultiHealth Systems. Available at: www.mhs.com.

at the Duke University Child and Family Study Center is presented in Table 246-2.

Although some anxiety symptoms, such as refusing to attend school in a patient with panic disorder and agoraphobia, are readily observable, others are open only to child introspection and to child self-report. A self-report measure of anxiety, such as the Multidimensional Anxiety Scale for Children, when combined with a parent-report general psychopathology measure, such as the Conners Parent Rating Scale, increase clinician efficiency by facilitating accurate assessment of the probability that a particular child will or will not have symptoms within a specific symptom domain. Typically, self-report measures use a Likert-scale format in which a child is asked to rate each questionnaire item in an ordinal format anchored to frequency or distress/impairment or a combination of the two. A child might be asked to rate "I feel tense" on a four-point frequency dimension that ranges from almost never to often. Besides assessing an overall construct (e.g., anxiety), child self-report measures, such as the Multidimensional Anxiety Scale for Children, provide useful information at the factor (e.g., physical anxiety symptoms) and item (e.g., suffocation anxiety) level. Self-report measures are easy to administer, require a minimum of clinician time, and economically capture a wide range of important anxiety dimensions from the child's point of view. In addition, to differentiate normal from pathologic anxiety, gender, race, and age norms are necessary. Much like hypertension is the extreme of blood pressure and presages multiple adverse medical outcomes, anxiety disorders can be conceptualized dimensionally, rendering rating scales for anxiety similar to the sphygmomanometer—an essential tool for screening for children "at risk" or who already have a clinically significant anxiety disorder.

TREATMENT

With the emergence of a rich psychopathology literature covering all the important domains of child and adolescent symptoms, the care of anxious children has moved away from nonspecific interventions toward problem-focused treatments keyed to specific DSM-IV diagnoses. In particular, since the 1990s, diverse, sophisticated, empirically supported, cognitive-behavior therapy (CBT) and pharmacologic treatment strategies have emerged that cover the range of childhood-onset anxiety disorders.

Prevention

Some children identified either on clinical examination or through school or other community screening procedures are found to have anxiety that is "worrisome" but that is not yet at the point of clinical disorder. In many cases, these children have an internalizing temperament and, not coincidentally, parents with a similar temperament and perhaps anxious or depressive (or both) disorders. Using the cognitive-behavioral tools described subsequently, preliminary evidence suggests that early intervention consisting of (1) normalizing fear thoughts, (2) reducing parental reinforcement of inappropriate worry, and (3) encouraging exposure to fearful stimuli can reduce current distress and prevent development of clinical disorder.

Treatment Planning

Box 246-1 summarizes the general approach to the effective treatment of anxious children beginning with a review of demographic, developmental, treatment, and psychiatric/medical history; review of findings from normed rating scale data; review of school records and previous mental health treatment records; a clinical interview of the child and his or her parents covering Axis I through V of the DSM-IV; a formal mental status examination; and in some cases, a specialized neuropsychologic evaluation. Having completed a thorough initial evaluation, key decision points in the everyday treatment of patients with anxiety disorders include the following four elements:

1. With respect to selecting the initial treatment, the clinician must make a judgment about the relative benefits and risks of single (CBT or drug) versus combined treatment over the short-term and long-term. Besides relative effectiveness, the feasibility, acceptability, and tolerability of the treatment also must be considered.

2. Most patients improve substantially with current initial treatments. Clinical experience and the empirical literature suggest, however, that many patients do not normalize with monotherapy, especially when functional outcomes rather than symptoms are considered. When a primary disorder remits, secondary problems often come to the fore. Combining CBT and drug treatments becomes more common as treatment progresses, and the limits of initial treatment become apparent.

3. When a patient is a treatment responder, it is crucial from a personal and public health perspective to know how long to continue treatment and at what dose and visit schedule before trying, if appropriate, to discontinue treatment. If discontinuation is desirable, and it may not be in the face of persisting symptoms or previous relapses, CBT may show enhanced durability relative to medication management, unless drug treatment is continued.

4. When a patient has had two trials of different medications and, where appropriate, combinations of medications and optimal psychosocial treatment, and when these trials are adequate in dose and duration and the patient still shows little or no improvement, it is justifiable to label the patient as treatment resistant. In this situation, newer treatments, treatments with a lower probability of success, heroic treatments, and riskier combinations of treatment may be warranted.

Cognitive-Behavioral Therapy

Given the absence of solid empirical data to guide the ordering of treatments, most clinicians treating anxious children and adolescents should begin with CBT, which has considerably more empirical support, and advance to a pharmacologic interventions only if the patient is not rapidly responsive to CBT. Historically, behavioral therapy evolved within the theoretical framework of classic and operant conditioning, with cognitive interventions assuming a more prominent role with the increasing recognition that person-environment interactions are mediated powerfully by cognitive processes. Behavioral psychotherapists work with patients to change behaviors and to reduce distressing thoughts and feelings. Cognitive therapists work first to change thoughts and feelings, with improvements in functional behavior following in turn.

Although CBT for a specific disorder, such as panic disorder and social phobia, differs in important details, virtually all cognitive-behavioral interventions for anxiety share five qualities: (1) an emphasis on psychoeducation; (2) a detailed behavioral analysis of the problem and the factors that maintain or extinguish it; (3) problem-specific cognitive interventions, such as restructuring anxious thoughts; (4) hierarchy-based graded exposure to feared stimuli; and (5) relapse prevention and generalization training at the end of treatment. The major techniques used in CBT for pediatric anxiety disorders are summarized in Table 246-3.

Pharmacotherapy

Chapter 288 discusses the drugs most commonly used to treat anxious children and adolescents. Randomized evidence suggests that selective serotonin reuptake inhibitors are the agents of choice when long-term drug treatment is anticipated. Either alone or in combination with a selective serotonin reuptake inhibitor, high-potency benzodiazepines may be an appropriate brief treatment for acute anticipatory and situation-related anxiety symptoms, such as those seen in acute separation anxiety disorder. Buspirone is a potentially useful agent in generalized anxiety disorder, and its relatively benign side-effect profile and low abuse potential make it an attractive choice particularly in an adolescent population at risk for substance abuse. Targeted propranolol may be useful to treat the cardiovascular aspects of performance anxiety in patients with social phobia. Tricyclic antidepressants and neuroleptics should be avoided when possible because of their lack of demonstrated efficacy and high potential for serious side effects. In every patient, careful attention to dose-response relationships (the intensity dimension) and time-action effects (the temporal dimension) is crucial to maximize benefit and minimize side effects.

Combining Treatments

The exact place of medication strategies alone and in combination with psychosocial interventions is unclear. Given that early intervention with CBT is the preferred

Table 246-3. Techniques Used in Cognitive-Behavioral Therapy for Anxiety Disorders

Term	Definition	Examples
Cognitive restructuring	Active altering of maladaptive thought patterns, replacing negative thoughts with more constructive adaptive cognitions and beliefs	Challenging aberrant risk appraisal in the patient with panic disorder or helplessness in the patient with depression
Define a stimulus hierarchy	A list of phobic stimuli ranked from least to most difficult to resist using fear thermometer rating scores	Unique list of exposure targets ranked by fear thermometer score. An individual patient may have one or more hierarchies, depending on the complexity of symptoms (e.g., a particular patient may have separate hierarchies for social fears and for separation anxiety)
Exposure	Exposure principle states that anxiety will decrease after prolonged contact with the phobic stimulus in the absence of real threat. Exposure may be contrived (sought out contact with feared stimuli) or uncontrived (unavoidable contact with feared stimuli)	For example, a patient with fear of heights goes up a ladder: the first time it is scary; the tenth time it is boring
Extinction	By convention, extinction usually is defined as the elimination of problem behaviors through removal of parental positive reinforcement. Technically, extinction often means removing the negative reinforcement effect of the problem behavior so that it no longer persists	Refusal to reassure the anxious patient. Refusal by the mother to cave-in to the anxious oppositional child's tantruming by withdrawing a command
Negative reinforcement	Termination of an aversive stimulus (e.g., anxiety), which when stopped, increases or stamps in the behavior (e.g., reassurance seeking) that removed the aversive stimulus	Scratching an itch produces more scratching. Similarly, although reassurance produces short-term relief of anxiety, continued reassurance increases rather than allays anxiety over the long run. Gradually minimizing inappropriate reassurance by the parent blocks this negative reinforcement and so is an important part of treatment
Prompting, guiding, and shaping	External commands and suggestions that increasingly direct the child toward more adaptive behavior that then is reinforced. Typically, shaping procedures are rapidly faded in preference to generalization training	Gradually encouraging and helping the social phobic youngster to talk in class and with other children
Positive reinforcement	Imposition of a pleasurable stimulus to increase a desirable behavior	Praising the selectively mute youngster who talks to the teacher
Punishment	Imposition of an aversive stimulus to decrease an undesirable behavior	Time-out because of unacceptable behavior or overcorrection (as in extra chores to make restitution for aggressive behavior). Typically, punishment makes anxiety disorders worse
Restructure the environment	Changes in setting or stimuli that decrease problem behaviors and/or facilitate adaptive behavior	Intervening to protect the anxious child from punishment by the teacher or teasing by peers
Generalization training/relapse prevention	Moving the methods and success of problem-focused interventions to targets not addressed specifically in treatment	Exposure in imagination for developmentally appropriate fears, even those not particularly bothersome or not specifically addressed in treatment. Anticipate triggers for re-emergence of symptoms; practicing skillful coping in advance

strategy for many, if not most, children, factors leading to early medication intervention might include unavailability of CBT, patient preference, and severe or multiple comorbidities or suicidality. For many patients with moderately severe–to–severe symptoms, most clinicians believe that the combination of CBT and medication is most likely to lead to durable symptom remission, although empirical evidence for this assertion is largely lacking.

SUMMARY

Despite limitations in the research literature with regard to long-term outcome of treated versus untreated patients; how best to combine CBT and pharmacologic treatment; effectiveness across divergent cultural, age, and ethnic groupings; and optimal assessment procedures, the empirical literature nonetheless is generally positive regarding the benefits of short-term CBT and pharmacotherapy for anxiety disorders in children and adolescents. The short-

term benefits of treatment do not translate, however, into long-term benefit across all domains of outcome. At this stage of understanding, it is likely that targeted CBT, alone or in combination with psychotropic medication, skillfully applied across time affords the most plausible basis for sustained benefit in anxious children and adolescents.

Mini-index of Related Topics

SUGGESTED READINGS

Bernstein GA, Shaw K: Practice parameters for the assessment and treatment of children and adolescents with anxiety disorders: American Academy of Child and Adolescent Psychiatry. J Am Acad Child Adolesc Psychiatry 1997;36(10 suppl):69S–84S.

March J: Anxiety Disorders in Children and Adolescents. New York, Guilford Press, 1995.

March J: Manual for the Multidimensional Anxiety Scale for Children (MASC). Toronto, MultiHealth Systems, 1998.

Rapee R, Spense S, Cobham V, Wignal A: Helping Your Anxious Child: A Step-By-Step Guide for Parents. San Francisco, New Harbinger, 2000.

Rapee R, Wignal A, Hudson J, Schniering C: Treating Anxious Children and Adolescents: An Evidence Based Approach. San Francisco, New Harbinger, 2000.

Research Unit on Pediatric Psychopharmacology Anxiety Study Group: Fluvoxamine for the treatment of anxiety disorders in children and adolescents. N Engl J Med 2001;344:1279–1285.

SECTION 7   MENTAL HEALTH CARE: *Emotions and Moods*

247 Sadness and Depressive Disorders

Mary A. Fristad and Dory P. Sisson

ROLE OF THE GENERALIST

1 Differentiate normative and pathologic responses to negative life events.

2 Identify patients at high risk for depressive disorders.

3 Screen for suicidal risk.

4 Provide mental health referrals.

5 Treat, if appropriate, with first-line pharmacologic agents.

6 Provide ongoing follow-up to increase treatment adherence and reduce relapse risk.

Depression is among the most common of psychiatric disorders, with prevalence rates of 0.4% to 2.5% in children and 0.4% to 8.3% in adolescents. The lifetime prevalence rate of major depressive disorder (MDD) in adolescents is 15% to 20%, which is similar to adult rates. In children, the rates of MDD in boys and girls are approximately equal. Sex differences become evident in adolescence, when the female-to-male ratio is 2:1.

Symptoms of depression can be seen in infancy. The mean length of a major depressive episode is 7 to 9 months, which is especially problematic for children because this time period can represent an entire school year. Most children and adolescents (90%) recover from their depression by 1.5 to 2 years after the onset, but many have protracted illnesses. Recurring episodes are common, with 40% of children relapsing within 2 years and 70% relapsing within 5 years. Childhood depression is associated with an increased risk for adult mood disorders, highlighting the importance of early intervention. Additionally, children,

particularly adolescents, with mood disorders are at a high risk for suicidal ideation and suicide attempts. Suicide is currently the third leading cause of death in 10- to 19-year-olds.

The cause of depression currently is understood best as a combination of genetic and psychosocial factors. Twin and adoption studies show that genetic factors account for at least 50% of the variance in the transmission of mood disorders. The impact of environmental factors is equally important, and individuals at high genetic risk may be more sensitive to adverse environmental effects.

The strongest single risk factor for MDD is a family history of mood disorders. Children of depressed parents are three times more likely than children of nondepressed parents to develop an episode of major depression. They also are at increased risk for general psychopathology, including anxiety and disruptive behavior disorders such as attention deficit hyperactivity disorder (ADHD). Studies have suggested that what may be inherited is a vulnerability to depression and anxiety and that certain environmental stressors may be required for the manifestation of one or more of these disorders.

The family environment of depressed individuals is characterized by more conflict, more abuse, more communication problems, more rejection, less support, and less expression of affect than the families of normal controls. The precise relationship between stressful family interactions and childhood depression currently is not established. Parents may be modeling maladaptive coping styles for the child, which then predisposes the child to respond to stress in a way that leads to depression. Alternatively, poor family functioning may be a nonspecific stress that triggers depression in predisposed individuals. Conversely, a depressed child may be contributing to family problems by creating conflicts and exhibiting behavior that is difficult to control. Finally, some combination of the previously mentioned interactions may contribute synergistically to a depressogenic cycle of family interactions.

Another risk factor for depression is a negative cognitive style of interpreting and coping with stressful situations. Depressed children and adolescents have cognitive distortions, negative attributions, hopelessness, a feeling of lack of control over circumstances, and low self-esteem. Longitudinal studies show that even after remission, formerly depressed children have lower self-esteem, which predicts future episodes.

DIAGNOSIS

The same criteria are used to diagnose mood disorders in children as adults; however, certain features are seen more commonly in children than in adults. Young children are less likely to report dysphoria and hopelessness, but rather may appear depressed. Children display more anxiety, irritability, and somatic complaints. Adolescents are more likely to display seasonal affective disorder, premenstrual dysphoric disorder, and atypical depression (i.e., psychomotor retardation, increased sleep, increased appetite). Social withdrawal, excessive worrying, behavioral problems, and self-esteem problems also are seen frequently in children and adolescents with depression.

Transient depressive reactions are common in children, and sadness is a normal reaction to a real or perceived loss. The death of a family member or pet, a family move, a school transition, or a broken-off relationship all can create a sense of loss in a child, who may display sadness, tearfulness, loss of interest in activities, and sleep or appetite changes. These mood disturbances usually are transitory, however, lasting several days to 1 or 2 weeks at the most, except for bereavement, in which a grief reaction of several months is considered normal (Box 247-1). These normal, transitory depressive responses to life events can be distinguished from a clinical disorder based on the severity and chronicity of symptoms. When many depressive symptoms cluster (i.e., occur at the same time); persist for longer than 2 weeks; and interfere with school functioning, family life, or peer relationships, they are more likely to represent a clinical disorder rather than a transient mood disturbance in response to a stressful life event.

MDD must be distinguished from a mood disorder resulting from a general medical condition. The latter diagnosis is assigned if the depressive symptoms are a consequence of a specific medical condition (e.g., multiple sclerosis, hypothyroidism, diabetes, cancer). A substance-induced mood disorder is distinguished from MDD when a substance (an illicit drug, a medication, or toxin exposure) is the cause of the mood disturbance. Dysthymic disorder and MDD are differentiated based on the number, severity, and chronicity of symptoms. Dysthymic disorder is the "low-grade fever of mental health," with duration of 1 or more years. Symptoms are fewer in number but must be present and impair function for 12 months or longer. Children with dysthymic disorder often appear pessimistic, with low energy and irritability, but have fewer symptoms

such as anhedonia (a loss of interest or pleasure in daily activities). Differentiating ADHD from depression can be difficult at times because of overlapping symptoms of poor concentration and restlessness. Establishing age of symptom onset is crucial to classify these symptoms correctly. ADHD symptoms, by definition, must be present by age 7. If the child is older than 7 and presents with a recent onset of symptoms similar to ADHD, the diagnosis of depression should be considered. A second, common clinical scenario is a child with ADHD who develops a secondary depressive disorder, possibly in response to the stress of social, academic, and family based impairments resulting from the ADHD symptoms. Finally, some children present for an initial assessment with symptoms of ADHD and a mood disorder. In this case, care must be taken to determine whether the impaired concentration and psychomotor agitation noted as part of the depression have exacerbated from the child's usual baseline functioning, which would not be considered "normal" because of the concomitant ADHD.

The presence of comorbid diagnoses in children is the rule rather than the exception; 40% to 70% of young people with depression have one or more comorbid diagnoses, and 20% to 50% have two or more. Box 247-2 lists common comorbid conditions. Anxiety disorders frequently occur in depressed children and adolescents; they usually develop before the major depression. Depression also occurs commonly with disruptive behavior disorders. In depressed adolescents, personality disorders (i.e., a stable, inflexible, maladaptive pattern of relating to the environment) may seem apparent but usually remit when the depression remits. This phenomenon reminds clinicians to be cautious about diagnosing Axis II conditions (i.e., personality disorders) while the teenager is in the midst of an Axis I condition (i.e., depression). Eating disorders, such as anorexia and bulimia, can co-occur. Academic problems and learning disorders also are seen commonly in depressed children. It is important to be aware of potential bidirectional influences of cognitive functioning and mood (i.e., the impaired concentration, apathy, and low energy of depression can interfere with school performance, whereas preexisting learning disabilities can contribute to feelings of worthlessness in school-age children and adolescents). Children and adolescents with several comorbid diagnoses are at risk for increased severity and duration of symptoms, more suicidality, worse social impairment, and increased substance abuse.

Instruments used to screen children and adolescents for mood disorders include self-report questionnaires and behavior checklists. Self-report questionnaires specifically designed to assess depressive symptoms include the Children's Depression Inventory, the Beck Depression Inventory, the Reynolds Child Depression Scale, the Reynolds Adolescent Depression Scale, and the Children's Depression Scale. Omnibus behavior checklists that assess a broad array of internalizing and externalizing symptoms, including depression, include the Revised Behavior Problem Checklist, the Conners Parent Rating Scale, the Child Behavior Checklist, the Conners Teacher Rating Scale, the Teacher Report Form, and the Youth Self-Report. To make a diagnosis of depression, however, a direct interview with

Box 247-1. Diagnostic Criteria for Mood Disorders

Major Depressive Disorder

- Must have either of the following for ≥2 weeks:
  - Depressed or irritable mood most of the day, most days
  - Loss of interest or pleasure in most activities
- Must have four of the following for ≥2 weeks:
  - Weight loss, failure to make expected weight gains, or excessive weight gain
  - Insomnia or hypersomina
  - Psychomotor agitation or retardation
  - Fatigue or loss of energy
  - Feelings of worthlessness or guilt
  - Poor concentration
  - Suicidal or morbid ideation
- Symptoms cause distress; interfere with family, school, friends, or work; or both
- Symptoms are *not* due to other drugs or illness
- Symptoms do *not* directly follow the loss of a loved one
- There has never been a manic episode

Dysthymic Disorder

- Sad or irritable mood lasting 1 year
- Two or more of the following symptoms, while depressed:
  - Poor appetite or overeating
  - Insomnia or hypersomnia
  - Low energy or fatigue
  - Low self-esteem
  - Poor concentration or difficulty making decisions
  - Feelings of hopelessness
- During the year of the disturbance, the person has never been without the symptoms for more than 2 months at a time
- No major depressive episode has occurred during the year
- Symptoms are *not* due to other drugs or illness
- There has never been a manic episode

Double Depression (Major Depressive Disorder/Dysthymic Disorder)

- Major depressive disorder superimposed onto dysthymic disorder

Seasonal Affective Disorder

- A seasonal pattern can be applied to major depressive disorder or bipolar disorder if the onset and remission of the episodes occur at characteristic times of the year
- Most common pattern:
  - Fall/winter: depression with increased sleep and appetite, carbohydrate craving, psychomotor retardation
  - Spring/summer: nondepressed or manic

Adjustment Disorder with Depressed Mood

- A response to an identifiable stressor
- Results in depressed mood, tearfulness, or feelings of hopelessness
- Symptoms develop within 3 months after the onset of the stressor
- Symptoms do *not* represent bereavement

Bereavement

- A grieving reaction to a loss
- Symptoms appear similar to a major depressive episode:
  - Sadness
  - Insomnia
  - Poor appetite
  - Weight loss
- Diagnosis of major depressive disorder is not given unless the symptoms are still present 2 months after the loss
- Certain symptoms are *not* characteristic of a "normal" grief reaction:
  - Guilt about things other than action taken or not taken by the survivor at the time of the death
  - Thoughts of death other than feeling that he or she would be better off dead or should have died with the deceased or would like to "visit" the deceased
  - Morbid preoccupation with worthlessness
  - Marked psychomotor retardation
  - Prolonged and marked functional impairment
  - Hallucinatory experiences other than thinking that he or she hears or transiently sees the deceased

Depression Not Otherwise Specified

- Depressive features do not meet criteria for major depressive disorder, dysthymic disorder, or adjustment disorder with depressed mood
- There is inadequate or contradictory information about the depressive symptoms, such that no more specific diagnosis can be made

Bipolar Disorder–Depressed

- Currently (or most recently) in a major depressive episode
- There has been at least one manic episode previously:
  - At least 1 week of elevated, expansive, or irritable mood
  - During the period of mood disturbance, at least three of the following symptoms are present (four if the mood is only irritable):
    Grandiosity
    Decreased need for sleep
    Increased talking
    Racing thoughts
    Distractible
    Increased activity or agitation
    Foolish or reckless behavior

---

the child or adolescent is crucial. This information should be substantiated or supported by information obtained through an interview with the parent.

Suicidal risk should be assessed in all patients suspected of having a mood disorder. The presence or absence of suicidal ideation (thoughts about suicide), intent (the desire to die), plans, and attempts should be ascertained. When assessing plans and attempts, it is important to consider the level of lethality and the severity of intent. A child with limited knowledge of a medicine's toxicity might make a low-lethality attempt even though the intent to die was high. If suicide risk is determined to be high, the child or adolescent needs to be treated in a restrictive setting, such as an inpatient psychiatric unit.

Box 247-2. Common Comorbidities

- Anxiety disorders (separation anxiety, generalized anxiety disorder, social phobia, specific phobias, panic disorder, obsessive-compulsive disorder, posttraumatic stress disorder, or acute traumatic stress disorder)
- Attention deficit hyperactivity disorder
- Oppositional defiant disorder
- Conduct disorder
- Substance abuse
- Eating disorders
- Learning disorders

MANAGEMENT

Ideally the generalist should refer the child or adolescent to a mental health specialist who is knowledgeable about childhood mood disorders for diagnosis, psychosocial treatment, and any necessary environmental interventions (e.g., school placement adjustments). The therapist should complete a thorough evaluation; then provide treatment, as appropriate, to the individual child or his or her family or both; and intervene with the school as needed.

Generalists frequently contend with the "can'ts" (i.e., families for whom the barriers to treatment make psychosocial intervention difficult or impossible to arrange) and the "won'ts" (i.e., families who do not pursue treatment because of stigma or negative beliefs about the mental health profession in general or the efficacy of interventions in particular). Regarding the former, if intervention with a qualified therapist is truly not available, because of financial hardship, transportation limitations, or inflexible parental work schedules, some assistance might be attainable during the school year via a school guidance counselor. Although such a person probably would not have access to the family unit and may have more limitations on the depth of work that can be accomplished, the child at minimum has a safe haven where he or she can vent feelings and problem solve about conflict areas. Regarding the latter (i.e., "won'ts"), some simple education about the progress that has been made in children's mental health in the 1980s and 1990s may result in a parent's willingness to try professional assistance (much resistance stems from the experiences of previous generations, in which treatment truly was less efficacious).

Despite the generalist's best efforts to refer, which are complicated further by a lack of child and adolescent psychiatrists and other well-trained children's mental health specialists in many communities, the generalist often is called on to provide first-line diagnostic and biologic interventions. Medication safety has improved substantially since the 1990s, and the number of available agents likewise has increased dramatically. See Chapter 288 for a detailed overview of psychotropic medications.

Frequent medication monitoring is recommended until a safe and efficacious dosage regimen is established. Alternatively the generalist can refer the child to a child and adolescent psychiatrist for medication evaluation and management. If the child presents with complications (e.g., bipolar disorder–depressed, failure of first-line interventions), the child also should be referred to a child and adolescent psychiatrist.

OUTCOME

A single major depressive episode is not associated with additional problems, but patients with recurrent episodes have minor impairment even when not officially "in episode." Psychosocial problems after a major depressive episode include risk of increased suicidality, negative attributions, drug and alcohol use, subclinical depressive symptoms, impaired relationships, impaired global functioning, early pregnancies, and other health problems. A major depressive episode seems to leave the child or adolescent with a "psychosocial scar," sensitizing him or her to future stressors and subsequent depressive episodes. Childhood-onset depression is associated with a range of negative sequelae and functional impairments. School and academic problems are common, as are cognitive difficulties, such as poor self-esteem and dysfunctional beliefs. Interpersonal difficulties may take the form of peer rejection, social withdrawal, or incompetence in social problem solving. The deleterious long-term impact of these problems should not be underestimated and support the need for aggressive identification and treatment.

Children and adolescents with MDD are at an increased risk of developing bipolar disorder; 20% to 50% "switch" into mania and develop bipolar I disorder (periods of MDD and mania) within 5 years after the onset of depression. Risk factors for switching include a childhood onset of the depressive episode, symptoms of psychomotor retardation or psychosis, a family history of bipolar disorder, a strong family history of depressive disorder, and pharmacologically induced hypomania (i.e., a period of mania that is not severe enough to meet criteria for a manic episode). In adolescents, the conversion to bipolar II (periods of MDD and hypomania) is associated with early-onset depression, atypical depression, seasonal affective disorder, protracted depressive episodes, comorbid substance abuse, and high rates of psychosocial problems. The clinical presentation of bipolar II disorder in adolescents may be misdiagnosed as a disruptive behavior disorder or a personality disorder, so careful assessment is particularly crucial.

FOLLOW-UP

While the child or adolescent is in a current major depressive episode, frequent medication checks by the generalist (or specialist, if the child has been referred to a child and adolescent psychiatrist) are necessary. Ongoing treatment by a children's mental health professional is important. Between episodes, the generalist must be alert for a recurrence. The generalist serves an important function in referring back to the mental health professional if subsyndromal symptoms result in functional impairment or if a relapse occurs.

 Additional Resources, CD-ROM

Bibliography

Mini-index of Related Topics

SUGGESTED READINGS

American Academy of Child and Adolescent Psychiatry: Summary of the practice parameters for the assessment and treatment of children and adolescents with depressive disorders. J Am Acad Child Adolesc Psychiatry 1998;37:1234–1238.

American Psychiatric Association: Diagnostic and Statistical Manual of Mental Disorders, 4th ed, text revision. Washington, DC, American Psychiatric Association, 2000.

Birmaher B, Ryan ND, Williamson DE, et al: Child and adolescent depression: A review of the past 10 years: Part I. J Am Acad Child Adolesc Psychiatry 1996;35:1427–1439.

Hovey JD, King CA: The spectrum of suicidal behavior. In Marsh DT, Fristad MA (eds): Handbook of Serious Emotional Disturbance. New York, Wiley, 2001, pp 284–303.

Wilens TE: Straight Talk about Psychiatric Medications for Kids. New York, Guilford Press, 1999.

SECTION 7 MENTAL HEALTH CARE: *Emotions and Moods*

248 Obsessive-Compulsive Disorder: Cognitive-Behavioral and Psychopharmacologic Treatments

Daniel T. Gustafson and Bruce J. Masek

ROLE OF THE GENERALIST

1. Distinguish obsessions from normal childhood worries, and distinguish compulsions from normal childhood rituals.

2. Refer to specialists as needed for cognitive-behavioral therapy or psychopharmacologic therapy or both.

3. Collaborate in appropriate cases with a provider of cognitive-behavioral therapy by managing psychopharmacologic therapy.

4. Support the patient and family by demystifying the disorder, encouraging appropriate treatment, and engaging in long-term follow-up.

In recent years, effective cognitive-behavioral therapy (CBT) and psychopharmacologic therapies have been developed for a potentially intractable condition, obsessive-compulsive disorder (OCD). The rate of identification of child and adolescent OCD remains low, however. Pediatricians, in their capacity as frontline diagnosticians, are positioned to reverse this trend.

Obsessions are intrusive thoughts or actions that generate anxiety. Among children and adolescents, obsessions often involve fears of contamination, unacceptable impulses, harm befalling oneself or others, or a perceived need for exactness. *Compulsions* are behaviors or thoughts undertaken to alleviate obsessive anxiety. Compulsions involve behaviors such as excessive hand washing, checking for danger, touching objects in a proscribed manner, and ordering rituals. A need for precision in the execution of compulsions may result in a child becoming "stuck" on activities for extended periods (e.g., rewriting words until each letter is perfect). Compulsions also may take the form of covert mental acts, such as counting rituals, praying, and repeating words silently. Although the clinical presentation of compulsions often fits one of these subtypes, they also can be highly idiosyncratic.

Children affected by OCD are psychologically impaired, often spending hours a day locked in cycles of obsessive worry and ritualized coping. Parents eventually tire of the haze of distraction, odd mannerisms, and repetitive actions that characterize the disorder. Despite high levels of impairment, however, it is common for years to pass before OCD is identified and treated because the disease often is misdiagnosed or endured in secrecy.

Historically, misdiagnosis and secrecy led to the misperception that OCD was a rare condition. Point-prevalence of OCD among adolescents now is estimated at 1%, and lifetime prevalence is 1.9%. OCD may begin as early as preschool age. Peak onset of the disorder among boys is between 13 and 15 years of age, but onset is later among girls (20 to 24 years old). One third to one half of adults with OCD develop the disorder during childhood. Across the life span, a slightly greater proportion of sufferers are female.

FUNDAMENTALS

OCD now is thought to be a classic example of a neurobehavioral disorder because biochemical and psychological factors exert an influence on the development and maintenance of the disorder. Early biochemical explanations for the disorder—described collectively as the *serotonin hypothesis*—arose from the observation that OCD symptoms decrease on administration of serotonin reuptake inhibitors and return to premorbid levels when medications are discontinued. Genetic studies have indicated that OCD and Tourette syndrome in some cases may reflect different expressions of the same gene or gene sequence. Neuroimaging research has identified abnormalities in cortical to basal ganglia linkages among OCD patients; there abnormalities are reduced by either psychopharmacologic therapy or CBT.

In an important discovery for pediatricians—specialists who are all too familiar with streptococcal infections—there is preliminary research evidence that the etiopathogenesis of a subtype of OCD is linked to group A β-hemolytic streptococcal (GABHS) infections. This group of OCD and tic disorders, which collectively have been named *pediatric autoimmune neuropsychiatric disorders associated with streptococcal infections (PANDAS)*, is characterized by dramatic pediatric OCD or tic symptom onset, associated GABHS infection, and neurologic abnormalities. Common neurologic abnormalities include hyperactivity or adventitious movements. After sudden onset of symptoms, the clinical course of PANDAS is characterized by a gradual resolution of symptoms (usually within 1 to 3 months). The pattern may be repeated with subsequent streptococcal exposures. Although the natural history of PANDAS is not well understood, it generally is thought to remit fully before adulthood. Researchers are investigating a hypothesis that occurrence of the condition may increase the risk for adult OCD.

Psychological research on the causes of OCD has focused on behavioral and cognitive explanations. One area of behavioral research shows that obsessive-compulsive symptoms are developed through a two-stage classic conditioning process. First, individuals come to associate certain situations or thoughts with emotional distress. Second, the individuals learn that specific rituals allow them to escape or avoid the conditioned distress. The more effective the compulsion is at reducing distress, the stronger it grows. Research on the cognitive underpinnings of OCD has found that patients (1) overestimate risk of danger; (2) exaggerate their sense of personal responsibility to avoid dreaded outcomes; (3) attempt to cope through perfectionistic control over their thoughts and actions; and (4) may have difficulty processing needed information due to their arousal, repetition of rituals, or possible neuropsychologic deficits (e.g., if a person has checked to see if the door is locked 50 times, it may be difficult to form a salient memory of the last time the door was checked).

OCD usually endures in the absence of treatment. The course of the disorder varies widely, however. Some children experience only small fluctuations in an otherwise chronic symptom presentation, whereas others experience periods of exacerbation and remission. Studies are under way to determine whether this variability in symptom expression may reflect subtypes of the disorder. The prognosis improves significantly for patients who receive appropriate treatment.

DIAGNOSIS

The first diagnostic challenge for the pediatrician is to differentiate normal obsessive-compulsive behaviors from OCD. Most children exhibit some obsessive-compulsive behaviors. Normal obsessive-compulsive behaviors include detailed bedtime rituals, "don't step on a crack" rules, perfectionistic tendencies, and actions associated with "good luck" (e.g., tapping bat on home plate before every pitch).

Five factors help differentiate normal obsessive-compulsive behaviors from OCD: (1) Normal behaviors usually resolve by puberty, whereas the disorder usually does not emerge until later childhood or adolescence. (2) OCD behaviors frequently, by description, seem bizarre. (3) When OCD symptoms superficially resemble normal behaviors, they still can be distinguished by their intensity, frequency, and impact on the child. (4) Children with OCD typically are either angry or defensive when confronted about their OCD behaviors. (5) Normal obsessive-compulsive behaviors often contribute to the child's sense of mastery and independence; by definition, OCD symptoms never improve a child's functioning.

When OCD symptoms have been identified, the next diagnostic challenge is to assess the extent to which they impair the child's functioning. Impairment is defined in the *Diagnostic and Statistical Manual of Mental Disorders, fourth edition* (DSM-IV), in terms of marked distress and time consumption (>1 hour a day) or significant interference with the child's daily routine, academic performance, or social relationships.

The DSM-IV further stipulates that adults diagnosed with OCD understand at some time during the course of the disorder that their obsessions or compulsions are excessive or unreasonable. This diagnostic requirement is not applied to children. More recent research has called into question, however, the extent to which even adults with OCD regard their obsessions or compulsions as unreasonable with studies showing their beliefs often are closely held.

When assessing OCD symptoms, the pediatrician sometimes detects logical links between compulsions and specific obsessive thoughts, such as a contamination fear being relieved through compulsive hand washing. Some obsession-compulsion pairings lack an obvious thematic connection, however. These compulsions stem from the alleviation of obsessive anxiety on a specific occasion. A child may establish an esoteric obsession-compulsion pairing when fears of catastrophic injury to a parent are controlled successfully by repeating a proscribed hand movement.

A small proportion (approximately 2%) of individuals with OCD experience obsessions but not compulsions. This unusual symptom presentation can be challenging to diagnose because these children do not show the overt compulsive behaviors that may call attention to more typical expressions of OCD.

When OCD symptoms are present but initially appear to fall short of an OCD diagnosis, the pediatrician is advised not to rule out the diagnosis prematurely. There are numerous reasons why obsessions and compulsions often are endured in secrecy. Topics that the child considers extremely embarrassing or distressing are hallmarks of obsessive thinking. Most compulsions are abandoned reluctantly because the child may believe his or her compulsions are the only way that disaster can be forestalled and anxiety controlled. Consequently, it usually takes time for trust to develop between the pediatrician and child before the full constellation of symptoms is known.

There is a high degree of comorbidity between OCD and many other psychological disorders. Epidemiologic studies of individuals diagnosed with OCD have found a lifetime incidence of specific phobia in 30%, social phobia in 20%, and panic disorder in 15%. There is also an association between OCD and the following disorders:

1. Bulimia—33% of individuals with bulimia have a history of OCD.
2. Depression—30% of individuals diagnosed with OCD also meet criteria for a major depressive episode.
3. Tourette syndrome—35% to 50% of Tourette syndrome patients also are diagnosed with OCD. Proportionally fewer people with OCD as the primary diagnosis also carry a concurrent Tourette syndrome diagnosis (5% to 7%). Approximately 20% to 30% of patients with OCD report a current or past history of tics.

Given the high rates of comorbidity, there are distinctions between OCD and other psychological disorders that aid differential diagnosis. Depressed people often ruminate obsessively, but in contrast to OCD patients, they rarely attempt to ignore or suppress their thoughts. Among people with eating disorders, obsessions typically focus on eating, thinness, and body dysmorphic beliefs. Although the thoughts and behaviors of OCD patients often are bizarre, they do not show other symptoms of psychotic disorders, such as hallucinations, thought insertion, loosening of associations, and inappropriate affect. In contrast to OCD, generalized anxiety tends to focus on realistic daily worries. Repetitive behaviors seen in tic disorders and Tourette syndrome differ from OCD compulsions in that they are perceived as involuntary and typically are not used to neutralize obsessive fears.

OCD and phobia patients may experience phobic avoidance of situations that evoke anxiety (e.g., shaking hands with a person who has acquired immunodeficiency syndrome). Phobic anxiety tends to be relieved, however, when a person escapes the feared situation. In contrast, the pervasive obsessional fears of OCD patients often are not eliminated by avoidance.

Because of naming similarities, OCD often is confused with obsessive-compulsive personality disorder. The conditions are quite dissimilar and are rarely comorbid among children and adolescents. In contrast to OCD, obsessive-compulsive personality disorder is not characterized by the presence of obsessions and compulsions. As delineated in the DSM-IV, individuals affected by obsessive-compulsive personality disorder may be perfectionistic, preoccupied with rules, excessively devoted to work, morally strident, unable to throw out worthless belongings, reluctant to delegate, miserly, and rigid.

MANAGEMENT

The current consensus among psychiatrists and psychologists is that psychological therapy is usually a necessary component of effective and durable OCD treatment. Psychopharmacologic treatment also is indicated in many, but not all, cases. Figure 248-1 is a treatment algorithm developed by the Expert Consensus Treatment Guidelines for OCD working group.

In most cases, CBT is the psychological therapy of choice. The behavioral component of CBT involves exposure and response prevention. Through exposure and response prevention, patients learn to face feared thoughts and situations gradually. Sustained and frequent exposure to particular fears (e.g., touching a soiled piece of clothing that normally would prompt feelings of contamination), in the absence of compulsion-based anxiety management (e.g., remaining in contact with the clothing and not washing hands), leads to habituation of anxiety. Treatment effectively reverses the classic conditioning process, as the association between the obsession and anxiety is undermined, and patients learn they can manage their residual anxiety without the aid of compulsions. The cognitive component of CBT involves teaching patients to self-monitor and alter their thinking process as they (1) assess risk, (2) ascribe personal responsibility, and (3) determine causal relationships. A patient might be taught to evaluate systematically the likelihood her mother would be killed by a tornado if she did not perform a counting ritual.

Individuals who experience obsessions, but not compulsions, present a unique challenge to the treating cognitive-behavioral therapist. The absence of rituals means patients are less suited to traditional exposure and response prevention treatment. Specialized CBT approaches have shown promise with this group, however.

Given the psychological demands of CBT, it is important for pediatricians to help motivate patients to commit to therapy. Therapy typically involves 12 to 20 weekly or biweekly sessions, with each session lasting 50 to 75 minutes. To increase motivation and overcome mental health stigma, it may be helpful to speak of an "OCD coach," rather than a "therapist." Children often respond to analogies between the exposure and response prevention treatment process and overcoming other anxieties, such as riding a roller coaster or jumping off a diving board. Children are likely to feel a similar sense of pride and freedom when they overcome their OCD fears.

Clinical research has not shown the superiority of one serotonergic agent over another in combating OCD. The pragmatics of medication selection emphasize side-effect profiles and risk of drug interactions. In part due to their lower side-effect profiles, the current preference is to use

SUGGESTED READINGS

Ellingrod VL: Pharmacotherapy of primary obsessive-compulsive disorder: Review of the literature. Pharmacotherapy 1998;18:936–960.

Geller DA, Biederman J, Jones J, et al: Obsessive-compulsive disorder in children and adolescents: A review. Harv Rev Psychiatry 1998;5:260–273.

March JS, Mulle K: OCD in Children and Adolescents: A Cognitive Behavioral Treatment Manual. New York, Guilford Press, 1998.

Todorov C, Freeston MH, Francois B: On the pharmacotherapy of obsessive-compulsive disorder: Is a consensus possible? Can J Psychiatry 2000;45:257–262.

Wilhelm S: Cognitive therapy for obsessive compulsive disorder. J Cogn Psychother 2000;14:245–259.

SECTION 7   MENTAL HEALTH CARE: *Emotions and Moods*

249 Helping Children Deal with Terrorism

David J. Schonfeld

ROLE OF THE GENERALIST

1 Understand children's likely reactions to terrorism.
2 Advise parents, schools, and communities how to help children cope with terrorist events.

Much of what is known about how children respond to acts of terrorism is based on an understanding of the psychological impact of natural and humanmade disasters. Humanmade disasters, especially when there is an underlying human intent to cause harm, often result in more psychological distress than natural disasters. Acts of terrorism, the major aim of which is not to cause physical harm but instead to instill a state of terror in victims, should be expected to have predominantly psychological and emotional impact. Box 249-1 lists potential symptoms of adjustment reactions to acts of terrorism. Parents often underestimate the extent of children's reactions to a crisis situation, especially related to internalizing symptoms, as children may attempt to withhold complaints of these symptoms because of concerns that the symptoms are abnormal or inappropriate or because they wish to protect their parents who also may be upset. Parents are more likely to be aware of and report behavioral symptoms they have observed in their children.

How children perceive and react to a terrorist attack depends in large part on their cognitive, social, and emotional developmental levels. Somatization in the

---

Box 249-1. Potential Symptoms of Adjustment Reactions to Terrorism

■ Sleep problems—difficulty falling asleep or sleeping alone, nightmares, and trauma-related dreams
■ Separation anxiety and school avoidance
■ Anxiety and trauma-related fears
■ Generalized irritability
■ Difficulties with concentration and deterioration in academic performance
■ Regression—developmental (e.g., secondary enuresis) and social
■ Depression; a sense of foreshortened future or pessimism regarding the future
■ Avoidance of previously enjoyed activities
■ Onset of, or increase in, substance abuse
■ Somatization
■ Symptoms consistent with the diagnosis of posttraumatic stress disorder

Box 249-2. Factors That May Affect Adversely the Nature and Degree of Reaction to a Terrorist Event

- Direct victimization of self or others close to child in terrorist attack, especially if injury or death is involved, or direct witnessing
- Child's perception (whether or not accurate) that his or her life was in jeopardy
- Exposure to horrific scenes (including indirectly through media)
- Separation from parents or other important caregivers (especially for preschool-age children) as result of event
- Loss of property or belongings; disruption in routine/environment
- Prior psychopathology or traumatic experiences
- Parental difficulty in coping
- Lack of supportive family communication style
- Lack of community resources and support

context of bioterrorism is likely affected by children's perceptions of the symptoms suffered by victims or potential victims of the known or alleged biologic agents; children's immature understanding of illness causality is likely to shape how they understand and respond to a threat of bioterrorism. Children's responses also are related to their prior experience and preexisting psychological state and the presence of a supportive family network and community resources to facilitate adjustment. Box 249-2 lists some of the factors that may affect adversely the nature and extent of adjustment reactions to a terrorist event.

The goal of short-term interventions with children in the setting of a crisis event is to help them understand and accept the events that have occurred; to identify, understand, and express their emotions; to begin to regain a sense of control and mastery over their life; and to resume developmentally appropriate activities. Children who also need to grieve the death of a family member or friend may benefit from additional bereavement support. To accomplish these tasks, pediatricians can help parents identify and address their children's reactions and facilitate their children's acquisition of coping skills.

ADVICE FOR PARENTS

It is important to create environments within children's homes, at schools, and throughout the community where it is safe for children to ask questions, to come to understand the terrorist events, and, as a family and community, to make meaning together. Children pick up readily on cues from adults when adults are uncomfortable talking about topics. Discussions of terrorist attacks involve complex and emotionally laden issues. In addition, children have a tendency to ask direct and often poignant questions—questions that adults often feel ill equipped to answer and often do not even wish to think about. Children may misinterpret the discomfort of adults as a sign that the questions are inappropriate and assume it best not to pose such questions again. The silence that results is not an indication that children are too young to be aware of or to understand what has occurred or that they are ready to end the discussion.

Similar to adults, children are better able to deal with a crisis event if they feel they understand it. They want and need basic information. Although they are likely to hear about the events on television, at school, or from their friends, much of what they hear will be inaccurate or misunderstood. Adults should start by asking children what they already understand about the situation—not only what has happened, but also what they think it represents for them, their family, and their community. As children explain what they understand, adults should listen carefully for misinformation, misconceptions, and underlying fears or concerns. Terrorist acts remind us all that we are never completely safe, but after a recent act of terrorism, children need, whenever possible, to be reassured honestly of their safety. After explaining to children the steps that are being taken to keep them safe at home, at school, and in their community, it is important to explore what fears may remain. Children's fears may be different than those of adults. To the extent that the children's fears stem from incomplete or inaccurate information or misunderstandings, the fears can be addressed through clarification and honest reassurance.

The amount of information that children find useful depends in part on their age; older children generally want and benefit from additional information. For all children, no matter how old they are, it is best to start with the basic facts and use simple, direct terms. Adults can ask questions of the children regarding what more they would like to know. The goal is to help children feel that they understand what is going on—not to tell them everything that is known; graphic details are not necessary. Television and other media often provide detailed information and unsettling images that are not useful. Especially for younger children, parents should consider limiting the amount of television viewing of coverage of terrorist events. For older children and adolescents, when they do watch television coverage, adults should try to watch along with them and use it as an opportunity to discuss what is being seen and the questions, concerns, and emotions that it raises.

Parents should be prepared that individual children may show a range of reactions to a terrorist attack; the same child may show different reactions at different times and in different settings. Initial responses may range from excitement to anxiety, with many children appearing unaffected or disinterested. There are many reasons that children may appear disinterested. Young children may appear to be disinterested because they do not understand what has occurred or what it represents. Children also have difficulty sustaining strong emotions continuously for long periods. They may allow themselves to deal with their emotions briefly but then turn to play or school work before they allow themselves to become overwhelmed. Older children and adolescents, who are apt to turn to peers to discuss important issues, may be inclined at first to reject adult offers to discuss the terrorist acts. It generally is not a good idea to try to force the discussion; instead, invitations should be extended on several occasions to discuss the events. Children also may appear disinterested because they are afraid to ask questions or to voice their feelings. They may be disinclined to bring up the topic if they think there is nothing they can do to change the situation or to provide practical assistance. Adults should help children think of concrete ways to provide assistance to others within their family and community who might be affected by the terrorist attacks.

Although it is true that children who have coped successfully with a tragic event may emerge from the experience with increased maturity and new coping skills, most children (and adults) react *during* the crisis by acting less maturely, or regressing. Children who had mastered toileting recently may develop secondary enuresis; preschoolers who were confidently independent may become more clingy and manifest separation difficulties. Children also may regress in their social skills when under stress; they may become more demanding or more selfish or have more difficulty sharing or getting along with peers or family members. This regression is often a sign that children are under stress and having difficulty coping. It is not a time to accuse children of being selfish or uncaring, but a time for adults to show more caring and concern. It is helpful to warn parents to expect their children to think more about themselves at times of crisis, at least at first. When children feel their needs are being met, they are more likely to start to think about the needs of others.

Similar to adults, children may look to assign blame for terrorist activities. They also may be angry with the government or at adults they trust to protect them (including their parents) for allowing the terrorist events to occur. As adults model and help children learn how to express other feelings, such as fear, sadness, and helplessness, children may be less likely to express anger. Children should be told that although it is normal to feel angry in the setting of terrorist attacks, it is important to remember that acts of terrorism generally are practiced by a small group of individuals who do not represent a particular country, race, or ethnic group. This topic is especially important to discuss with older children and adolescents who are more aware of and sensitive to racial and ethnic differences.

As adults begin these discussions, children may show that they are upset. It is important to remember that it is not the conversation that is upsetting them, but rather the events. Adults should feel free to pause the conversation to provide support or comfort and offer to continue the discussion at another time. Adults should emphasize that it is healthy to express personal feelings; otherwise, children may try to hide their feelings, and then they are left to deal with them alone. A good way to show children it is okay to express their feelings is for adults around them to share their own feelings and show how to cope with them effectively. Children are more likely to develop effective coping techniques for negative feelings if they have the opportunity to see the coping techniques shown by competent adults in their lives.

BENEFIT OF PRIOR PREPARATION

Planning and preparation for potential terrorist attacks can help minimize the resultant psychological and social consequences. Pediatricians should work with community leaders to promote the development and implementation of community response plans to deal with potential crises, including models for providing trauma-related supportive services in community sites such as schools. In situations of terrorism, pediatricians are ideally suited to reach out to children, families, and their communities to provide guidance, assistance, and support. Pediatricians can work with schools and local agencies to mobilize secondary prevention services, involving the early identification of adjustment reactions and the provision of supportive services in community sites such as schools.

Mini-index of Related Topics

SUGGESTED READINGS

American Academy of Pediatrics. Available at: www.aap.org/terrorism.

American Academy of Pediatrics Committee on Psychosocial Aspects of Child and Family Health: How pediatricians can respond to the psychosocial implications of disasters. Pediatrics 1999;103:521–523.

National Center for Children Exposed to Violence. Available at: www.nccev.org.

Schonfeld DJ: Talking with children about death. J Pediatr Health Care 1993;7:269–274.

Schonfeld DJ, Kline M, and Members of the Crisis Intervention Committee: School-based crisis intervention: An organizational model. Crisis Intervention and Time-Limited Treatment 1994; 1:155–166.

Vernberg EM, Vogel JM: Interventions with children after disasters. J Clin Child Psychol 1993;22:485–498.

Vogel JM, Vernberg EM: Children's psychological responses to disasters. J Clin Child Psychol 1993;22:464–484.

250 Chronic Functional Pain/Somatic Complaints and Associated Disability

Brenda Bursch and Lonnie Zeltzer

ROLE OF THE GENERALIST

1   Identify and treat common functional symptom disorders within a biopsychosocial framework and using a multimodal rehabilitation approach.

2   Refer to a specialist when indicated.

Functional symptoms in children are the result of a dynamic integration of biologic processes, psychodevelopmental factors, and social context. These symptoms may be persistent or recurrent and may fluctuate in severity, quality, regularity, and predictability. Symptoms may occur in single or multiple body regions and can involve single or multiple organ systems. Functional symptoms may include varying amounts of disability, ranging from none to severe. Disability can contribute to the development of secondary or increased symptoms because of abnormal body posturing and prolonged inactivity (Box 250-1).

Nociception is the term used to describe the afferent sensory neural pathways that transmit noxious sensory

---

Box 250-1. Development of a Disability Syndrome

A subset of chronic symptom patients have common and severe difficulties in functioning, regardless of the severity or etiology of their symptoms. These patients experience a downward spiral of increasing disability and symptoms for which acute symptom-focused assessment and treatment strategies have not led to acceptable resolution. When the downward spiral begins, a multifactorial chronic illness model, which also addresses contextual factors, often must be adopted to ensure that comprehensive and appropriate assessment and treatment measures are carried out.

Disability in the above-mentioned definition refers to school absenteeism or severe restriction of functioning in other activities, or both. The initial symptom could be caused by a specific identifiable illness or injury, by a systemic virus, by a developmental challenge, or by a psychosocial stressor. Often it is not possible to identify the trigger. The time frame for development of disability varies dramatically.

---

information to central areas in the brain. Ongoing nociception can result in a sensitization of the peripheral and central nervous systems to produce neuroanatomic, neurochemical, and neurophysiologic changes. Pain perception occurs in certain areas of the cortex (e.g., anterior cingulum, lingula, and somatosensory cortex I and II), and pain perception is the final common pathway of nociception as modified by feelings, thought, arousal, and memory. It is important that assessment and treatment strategies consider this definition and related dimensions.

Traditionally, disability and symptoms in excess of what would be expected given the amount of tissue pathology have been considered psychogenic. Children and families frequently are informed that the symptom has no physiologic basis, with the suggestion that the child is fabricating or exaggerating or that the child is psychologically disturbed.

It is misleading to dichotomize functional symptoms as organic versus nonorganic because all symptoms are associated with, at minimum, neurosensory changes. Likewise, all symptoms are influenced by behavioral, cognitive, and emotional factors. Maintaining the organic versus nonorganic dichotomy can be harmful because it can lead to unnecessary tests, procedures, and medical treatments on the one hand or to a therapeutically detrimental lack of empathy on the other hand. To evaluate and treat functional symptoms efficiently and effectively, the mind/body dualism must be abandoned.

One way functional problems develop is when a recognized or unrecognized significant life event, physical stressor, or developmental challenge surpasses the "at-risk" child's coping abilities. The child's coping inadequacy results in a physiologic stress response (including autonomic nervous system arousal, which affects sensory processing), rendering the child somatically vulnerable. A somatic symptom may result in the child retreating to a dependent role or to avoidance of the stressor, or both. Because retreat from the stressor prohibits mastery over the challenge and serves to strengthen inefficacy beliefs, a progressively declining course ensues with decreasing functioning, increasing distress, and increasing vulnerability to emotional and physical impairment. Well-meaning and concerned family members and health care providers may perpetuate the downward spiral of pain and disability by fostering the dependent role or by contributing to the stress (central nervous system arousal) of the child, or both. As a result of the somatic presentation, however, many reasonable parents question a behavioral or psychiatric diagnosis, especially if they feel blamed for the disorder. Finally, no one is inclined to follow treatment recommendations unless they believe the recommendations will work and that the family is able to follow them.

A rehabilitation approach is recommended as an understandable and useful alternative to the acute illness model of care. Within a rehabilitation model, the focus turns to improving independent functioning and to skills building designed to improve coping and self-efficacy. This means that functioning, rather than symptoms, is tracked to determine whether or not progress is being made. It is contraindicated to inquire about symptoms when the treatment phase has begun. The rationale behind this is that asking about symptoms causes the patient to scan his or her body for somatic cues, reinforcing somatic hypervigilance. As functioning, coping skills, and self-efficacy improve, symptoms or the distress related to the symptoms or both often remit.

Central to a successful approach to treatment is the integration of the various targeted interventions into a consistent and cohesive package. All professionals involved in the case first must agree on (1) what constitutes completion of the evaluation, (2) what language/words to use to describe the problem and plan, and (3) what interventions should be included in a comprehensive biopsychosocial plan.

The family and treatment team often share worries about missing a diagnosis that would be remedied easily with medication or surgery alone. This fear is especially strong when the patient or family exhibits significant distress about the symptoms or disability or both, and a rehabilitation approach seems too slow or difficult. The treatment team must believe that a reasonable evaluation has been completed so that they can refrain from unnecessary assessment that detracts from rehabilitation and continues to focus the family on finding a magic bullet. When the treatment team can agree that enough information is available to construct a treatment plan, it is important that this decision be communicated clearly to the family and that no further evaluation be conducted. The team's comfort with the available information and treatment plan, if communicated clearly, often reduces anxiety in the family, reducing "doctor shopping" and pleas for continued medical testing.

CONCEPTUAL FRAMEWORK AND LANGUAGE

The biopsychosocial model of chronic symptoms is an abstract and complicated model, even to most medical professionals. Confusion can be kept to a minimum if each professional working with the family uses the same language to describe the problem and the plan. One advantage of using a rehabilitation model is that most people already are familiar with the concepts and language associated with either physical therapy or some other kind of rehabilitation.

For some parents to believe that treatment interventions would benefit their child, it is important for them to understand what is known about the mind/body link and how interventions target this link. When explaining the problem to family members, an initial focus on the symptoms and sensory signaling mechanisms is important to reassure them that the symptoms are real. Specifically, it might be helpful for family members to understand that ongoing nociception can result in a sensitization of the peripheral and central nervous systems to produce neuroanatomic, neurochemical, and neurophysiologic changes. Next, it is important to explain how the interacting biologic and psychological systems in the child and the systems in the social environment of the child all affect symptoms and disability. The role of memory and attention in reinforcing chronic symptoms may be included in this portion of the education session. It must be stated explicitly that neither the patient nor the family is to blame for the symptoms and disability, but that there are things the patient and family can do to reverse the downward disabling spiral. Even if parents have difficulty remembering the specifics of how the mind and body interact, the physiologic explanation can be sustaining throughout treatment. The emphasis should be that however the pain or other symptom problem began, it has developed a life of its own as a neural signaling problem. Reachieving balance in this neural sensory signaling system is the overall goal of treatment now that the cause of the problem is known.

The clinician should present the specific treatment goals of the rehabilitation plan, provide treatment options and rationale for each option, and promote active problem solving by requesting that the family decide which treatment options to follow. Ongoing education, review of the diagnoses, repeated description of the rationale for the treatment approach, reminders to track functioning rather than symptoms as an indication of progress, and frequent reassurance that all is proceeding in an expected manner usually are required by families as they progress through the treatment plan.

PRESENTATION AND INITIAL EVALUATION

A thorough evaluation typically is indicated to develop a treatment plan that best targets the biologic, psychological, and social factors that are maintaining the pain, other symptoms, or disability. Whenever possible, conducting a concurrent medical and psychosocial evaluation is suggested to reinforce the importance of the biopsychosocial model, regardless of the cause of the symptoms. It can promote therapeutic alliance and be clinically helpful to spend a considerable amount of time understanding the specific nature of the child's symptoms from the perspective of the child and from the perspective of family members, including siblings, who often are the best observers in the family (Box 250-2 and Table 250-1).

After an extended interview, a determination can be made if additional medical or psychological assessment is indicated. Reports of additional symptoms may prompt further inquiry or specific focus in the physical examination. Additionally, intellectual, academic, or psychological

Box 250-2. Screen for Anxiety

- Fears
- Worries
- Nervousness
- Physical symptoms of panic
- Disruptive repetitive or ritualistic behaviors or thoughts
- Perfectionism
- Significant concerns about germs, safety, competence, or evenness
- Intrusive thoughts
- Flashbacks
- Nightmares
- Lack of memory for a traumatic event
- Restricted affect
- Persistent arousal
- History of witnessing or experiencing a significant trauma, abuse, or other positive or negative major life event

testing may be needed to identify specific problems that might be suspected during the interview but difficult to assess through interview alone.

If the child is academically delayed, has weak social problem-solving skills, or has a previously unsuspected learning disorder, school can be a significant source of stress, even if the child does not report it as such. This situation is especially true among perfectionistic children who strongly identify with being a good student, attempt to maintain high grades, or experience strong internal or external pressure to achieve. Because of the time and expense associated with

Table 250-1. Screen for Depression

Mood
Euthymic ☐ Dysthymic ☐ Depressed ☐ Euphoric ☐ Grandiose ☐ Angry ☐ Irritable ☐ Anxious ☐ Apathetic

Affect
Alert ☐ Appropriate ☐ Happy ☐ Sad ☐ Flat ☐ Blunted ☐ Labile ☐ Incongruent ☐ Lethargic ☐ Angry ☐ Alexithymic

Sleep
WNL ☐ Increased ☐ Decreased ☐ Nighttime wakenings ☐ Not rested

Appetite
WNL ☐ Increased ☐ Decreased ☐ Weight change

Energy
WNL ☐ Increased ☐ Decreased

Interest in Activities
WNL ☐ Decreased

Guilt
Yes ☐ No

Suicidal ideation
Yes ☐ No

Thoughts of death
Yes ☐ No

Concentration
WNL ☐ Impaired

If depressed, for how long?

psychological testing, however, such testing might be reserved for cases in which the child seems to be experiencing an alarming progression of disability; already is significantly disabled; or has been treatment resistant using an intensive, integrated rehabilitation approach to treatment. Testing sometimes can be obtained through the school district if the child is having recognized academic difficulties.

CLINICAL INTERVIEW, SELF-REPORT MEASURES, AND OBSERVATIONS OF SYMPTOM BEHAVIOR

A thorough evaluation should include the domains of questions listed in Box 250-3.

PHYSICAL EXAMINATION

The physical examination should include the following components:

- General appearance (weight, posture, gait, sick versus healthy appearing)
- Emotional state (e.g., flat versus labile, distressed, eye contact)
- Vital signs (height, weight, blood pressure, heart rate, respiratory rate, temperature)
- Laboratory studies (complete blood count, erythrocyte sedimentation rate, urinalysis)
- Muscle spasms and trigger points (especially posterior cervical, suprascapular, paraspinous, and sacroiliac areas)
- Complete neurologic examination, evaluating motor, coordination, and sensory systems, including areas of somatic sensitivity to light touch, funduscopic and visual field examination, and assessment of deep tendon reflexes (Box 250-4)

MANAGEMENT

A multimodal approach is recommended over a single sequential treatment approach. Interventions should address possible underlying sensory signaling mechanisms, specific symptoms, and disability. In general, treatment goals focus on increasing independent functioning (activities of daily living; academic, social, and physical functioning); remediation of specific symptoms, deficits, or problems revealed in the assessment; enhancing communication, especially of non–symptom-related distress, with peers and family members; and facilitating more adaptive problem-solving skills.

Treatment techniques designed to address possible underlying sensory signaling mechanisms and specific symptoms include cognitive-behavioral strategies (e.g., psychotherapy, hypnosis, biofeedback, or meditation), behavioral techniques, family interventions, physical interventions (e.g., massage, yoga, acupuncture, transcutaneous electrical nerve stimulation, physical therapy, heat/cold therapies, occupational therapy), sleep hygiene, and pharmacologic interventions. In general, interventions that promote active coping are preferred over interventions that require passive dependence.

Family interventions can be extensive and sometimes are more important than the patient interventions. Family interventions include helping family members to under-

Box 250-3. Clinical Interview, Self-Report Measures, and Observations of Symptom Behavior

Chief Complaint and History of Present Illness

- Onset and development of the current problem (review results of previous evaluations and treatment attempts, including home remedies and alternative/complementary therapies)
- Locations of symptoms
- Intensity of symptoms at different times and under differing circumstances
- Symptom quality, duration, variability, and predictability
- Exacerbating and alleviating factors
- Impact of symptoms on daily life of patient, including school and concentration, social activities, eating, and sleep (onset and maintenance)
- Other sensations that accompany the symptoms
- Thoughts and behaviors associated with symptoms
- Perceived cause of symptoms and beliefs about what would and would not help
- Coping responses; ability to tolerate the symptoms
- How symptoms have affected the lives of family members
- Congruity between verbal reports of symptoms and related behavior
- How family members react to symptoms displayed during the interview
- Any unusual behavior or use of language during the interview

Review of Symptoms

- Review entire body for symptoms, not just the site of the pain complaint

Past Medical History

- Illnesses, hospitalizations, surgeries, injuries, emergency department visits, allergies

Birth and Early Childhood History

- Developmental milestones of child

Family History

- Who is in the family and who lives at home
- Intensity and types of emotion displayed by the patient and family
- Roles various family members hold and who speaks about which topics
- Child and family history of all somatic and emotional symptoms and diagnoses
- Baseline functioning of the child and of each family member

Social History

- School and school absenteeism, including academic difficulties and challenges, friends, bullies, teachers, tests, grades, classes, and academic aspirations
- Social history of family, especially significant (positive and negative) life events, including changes at school or in living arrangements or the witnessing or direct experience of physical or sexual assault, a robbery, death, or injury

Emotional History

- Depression, panic, anxiety, worries, or fears related to parents, academic achievement or tests, social situations, or school; obsessive-compulsive traits; posttraumatic stress; enuresis or encopresis
- Parents' emotional functioning, marital stress, and coping skills
- Parental behaviors—excessive sympathy and attention for symptoms, external help seeking, strong emotional responses, modeling of symptoms, and support for task avoidance (see Table 250-1 and Box 250-2)

stand the nature of the condition (including relevant medical, cognitive, behavioral, and psychological contributions), facilitating acceptance of a rehabilitation approach, elucidating biopsychosocial factors that likely contribute to the syndrome, altering family patterns that inadvertently maintain or exacerbate the syndrome, helping parents to cope with their own and the child's distress during the rehabilitation process, and developing a plan to ensure adequate support for self-management of symptoms and independent functioning.

Pharmacologic interventions are geared toward quieting the central nervous system arousal and enhancing the regulatory mechanisms of the brain. The specific medication choice depends on the likely neurophysiologic and neurochemical contributors to the symptom. Classes of medications to consider include tricyclic antidepressants (TCAs), selective serotonin reuptake inhibitors (SSRIs), anticonvul-

Box 250-4. Laboratory Test Results That Support a Rehabilitation Approach

- Complete blood count—within normal limits
- Erythrocyte sedimentation rate—within normal limits
- Urinalysis—within normal limits
- Antinuclear antibody—normal or slightly elevated

sants (e.g., gabapentin), muscle relaxants (e.g., baclofen), and low-dose phenothiazines (e.g., thioridazine). Low-dose TCAs, such as amitriptyline, given at bedtime can help with neuropathic and irritable bowel syndrome pain and have the added advantage of facilitating sleep. SSRIs can reduce the anxiety components underlying many functional symptoms in children and facilitate sleep if anxiety is a component in sleep difficulty. Phenothiazines, such as thioridazine (Mellaril), have relatively rapid onset and can play a significant role when anxiety is a major contributor to the symptoms and the SSRI has had insufficient time to be effective. Risperidone can be useful, especially when tics are present as a component of the symptom complex. Benzodiazepines often elicit paradoxical reactions and interfere with restorative sleep more than the other available options. Blocks, trigger point injections, and epidurals often are contraindicated in cases of complex and disabling chronic symptoms because they may stimulate the central nervous system further, exacerbating the problem.

Evidence-based treatments, based on a current literature review, should be used whenever available. In adolescent migraine headache, cognitive behavioral interventions have better evidence for efficacy than triptans, and ibuprofen seems to be more effective than acetaminophen. Most of the currently employed pharmacologic strategies are extrapolated from adult trials without evidence of efficacy in children.

The most significant obstacle can be reluctance to adopt a rehabilitation model. It sometimes is difficult to dispel the strong belief that a medication alone or surgery is the only thing that would help. This belief often is accompanied and exacerbated by the perceived absence of meaningful psychosocial stressors or problems other than the somatic symptoms or the inability to understand how life stressors could be related to a biologic process. Additionally, there may be an intense fear of causing harm or pain to the child by pushing too hard (especially when fears remain that the medical team missed an injury or disease). Finally, family members may have difficulty tolerating the emotional distress of the child and their own distress during rehabilitation.

The treatment team must be able to contain the family's distress and their own distress during assessment and rehabilitation. Evaluating progress by tracking functioning in small increments, rather than by monitoring symptoms, often helps contain anxiety. Weekly appointments with families usually are needed during the treatment phase, and telephone contacts between appointments often are required at first. Just as the goal of the child's treatment plan is to increase independent functioning, the goal of the family's treatment plan is to increase the family's ability to respond appropriately and independently to challenges. If all goes well, the family's dependence on the medical team lessens as they learn how to take responsibility for the rehabilitation program. Close teamwork, high communication among team members, planning for common challenges, and monitoring for team contributions to the problem help rehabilitation progress as smoothly as possible. Referral to a pediatric pain program should be considered for children with complex or refractory problems.

SUGGESTED READINGS

Bennett RM: Emerging concepts in the neurobiology of chronic pain: Evidence of abnormal sensory processing in fibromyalgia. Mayo Clin Proc 1999;74:385–398.

Caplan R: Epilepsy syndromes in childhood. In Coffey CE, Brumback RA (eds): Textbook of Pediatric Neuropsychiatry. Washington, DC, American Psychiatric Association Press, 1998, pp 977–1010.

Krilov LR, Fisher M, Friedman SB, et al: Course and outcome of chronic fatigue in children and adolescents. Pediatrics 1998;102(2 Pt 1):360–366.

Li B, Balint JP: Cyclic vomiting syndrome: The evolution of understanding of a brain-gut disorder. Adv Pediatr 2000;47:117–160.

Zeltzer L, Bursch B, Walco GA: Pain responsiveness and chronic pain: A psychobiological perspective. J Dev Behav Pediatr 1997;18:413–422.

251 Sleep Problems and Disorders

Jodi A. Mindell and Thornton B. A. Mason II

ROLE OF THE GENERALIST

1   Understand developmentally appropriate sleep norms and the impact of sleep disturbances on daytime functioning.

2   Educate parents on proper sleep hygiene for children and adolescents and prevent development of behaviorally based sleep disturbances.

3   Diagnose pediatric sleep disorders, including sleep-disordered breathing, narcolepsy, restless legs syndrome, periodic limb movement disorder, and delayed sleep phase syndrome.

4   Treat infant and toddler sleep disturbances.

5   Refer children and adolescents to an appropriate specialist when expert assistance is needed for assessment and treatment.

6   Ensure long-term follow-up of children with chronic sleep disorders.

A pediatrician's assistance is often sought for sleep problems. Numerous studies have documented that approximately 20% to 30% of all children and adolescents have some type of sleep problem, indicating a widespread prevalence. These sleep issues affect not only the patient, but also the family.

FUNDAMENTALS

Review of Normal Sleep Patterns Across Ages

Infants have polyphasic sleep periods (i.e., many sleep periods throughout the day). A newborn infant typically sleeps 30 minutes to 4 hours, resulting in about seven sleeping and waking periods per day. As infants get older, their sleep begins to consolidate, and they begin to sleep less. Typical newborns sleep 17 to 18 hours a day; by 1 month of age, infants sleep 16 to 17 hours; and by 3 or 4 months of age, infants sleep about 15 hours a day. At 4 months, sleep is consolidated into about three or four sleep periods, with two thirds of sleep occurring at night. By 6 months, sleep duration at night increases, with the longest sustained daily sleep period lasting about 7 hours. Many infants wake for brief periods but can put themselves back to sleep. Many parents who assume their infant is sleeping for 10 to 12 hours continuously may be inaccurate in their assessment. The infant may be waking for brief periods

without disrupting anyone. By 24 months of age, sleep has reduced to about 12 hours per day, with most children continuing to take naps during the day. By 4 years of age, children sleep about 10 to 12 hours per day, consisting of chiefly nighttime sleep with one daytime nap. The amount of sleep gradually decreases throughout childhood and adolescence, although sleep need usually is greater than expected. Adolescents require 8.5 to 9.5 hours of sleep.

Naps are an important aspect of the sleep of infants and young children. As an infant ages, the number of naps decreases. By 4 months of age, most infants are taking either two or three naps per day. By 6 months, most (nearly 90%) infants are taking only two naps per day. By 15 months, almost half of all children are taking just one nap daily, with most children discontinuing naps altogether between the ages of 30 months and 5 years.

Sleep Physiology

Sleep comprises two distinct states: rapid eye movement (REM) sleep and non-REM sleep. Non-REM sleep is divided into four stages, with stages 3 and 4 often referred to as *delta sleep* or *slow-wave sleep;* this is the deepest level of sleep. This deep non-REM sleep occurs in the first 1 to 3 hours of the night, and children have increased deep slow-wave sleep compared with adults. It is difficult to awaken a child from this deep sleep, and when awakened the child often is disoriented and confused. Sleepwalking and sleep terrors occur during deep sleep.

REM sleep incorporates deep sleep and light sleep. REM sleep involves the active suppression of peripheral muscle tone and increased variability in the regulation of blood pressure, heart rate, and respiration. Cortical brain function is extremely active in REM sleep. Most dreaming occurs during REM sleep, and when awakened a person is quickly alert. REM episodes occur in cycles of 60 to 90 minutes in adults (slightly shorter in children) with increasing duration throughout the night. The longest REM episodes occur in the early morning just before awakening, making nightmares most likely to occur in the second half of the night. Another aspect of sleep is that arousals occur throughout the sleep period. These short episodes of wakefulness typically occur five to seven times a night, and children usually return to sleep quickly with no recall of the awakening.

Prevalence of Sleep Problems and Disorders

Across multiple studies, sleep problems have been found to be common, with most studies reporting prevalence rates of 20% to 30%. Many of these problems may not be problematic, such as infrequent sleepwalking or sleep talking, whereas others have a significant impact on sleep and daytime functioning.

Impact of Sleep Disturbances on Daytime Functioning

Sleep deprivation and sleep disturbances affect multiple components of daytime functioning. Studies conducted on school-age children, adolescents, and adults have noted significant impacts of sleep deprivation and sleep disturbances on emotional well-being, cognitive abilities, academic performance, and behavior.

Assessment of Sleep Problems and Sleep Disorders

A thorough assessment of sleep problems for children and adolescents should encompass multiple components. The first step is the completion of a sleep history with all aspects of the sleep-wake cycle evaluated, including evening activities, medications, intake of caffeinated beverages, bedtime, and bedtime routines. During the night, areas to be evaluated include latency to sleep onset, behaviors during the night, and the number and duration of nighttime awakenings. In the morning, the time of awakening, sleepiness, and initial behaviors on arising should be evaluated. During the day, sleepiness, naps, meals, caffeine intake, medications, and feelings of anxiety and depression should be reviewed. Details about abnormal events should be collected, such as night terrors, confusional arousals, respiratory disturbances, seizures, and enuresis. A review of psychological symptoms during the day, including anxiety and depression, is important. Finally, a thorough evaluation should include questioning about school performance, social functioning, and family functioning.

The second step in the evaluation of sleep problems is the keeping of sleep diaries. A typical sleep diary includes information on the time to bed, sleep latency, number and duration of nighttime awakenings, time of arising in the morning, total sleep time, and duration and time of naps. For the most useful information, 2 weeks of baseline sleep diaries should be kept.

When there is a concern about an underlying physiologic problem, polysomnography (PSG) is an essential component in the assessment. Even if the patient does not report any physiologic symptoms, it may be important to evaluate sleep objectively. Many children and parents are unaware of snore arousals or sleep apnea that may be interrupting their sleep and resulting in complaints of insomnia and daytime sleepiness. PSG consists of an overnight sleep study in which oxygen saturation, nasal and oral airflow, thoracic and abdominal respiratory movements, limb muscle activity, and electroencephalogram are recorded.

INFANT AND TODDLER SLEEP DISTURBANCE

Definition

Bedtime struggles and night awakenings are likely among the most common complaints of parents of infants and toddlers. These disturbances occur in approximately 20% to 30% of infants and toddlers.

Box 251-1. Sleep Hygiene Tips for Children and Adolescents

1. Maintain a regular bedtime, waketime, and naptime schedule.
2. Maintain a regular daily schedule of activities.
3. Establish a consistent bedtime routine.
4. Avoid caffeine.
5. Ensure adequate sleep time.
6. Provide a cool, dark, and comfortable bedroom environment.
7. Expose child or adolescent to bright light in the morning hours.

Common Causes of Infant and Toddler Sleep Disturbance

There are many possible causes of infant and toddler sleep disturbance, including perinatal problems (e.g., prematurity), difficult temperament (e.g., less adaptable), and nighttime feedings. The primary cause for night awakenings for most young children is sleep-onset associations, however, in that the manner in which the child falls asleep affects whether he or she is able to return to sleep following normal nighttime awakenings. If an infant is nursed or rocked to sleep at bedtime, he or she requires the same during the night after a normal awakening. Bedtime struggles are often the result of parental difficulties with limit setting, separation anxiety, and sleep scheduling.

Presentation and Initial Evaluation

The usual presentation is a parental complaint of sleep difficulties, at bedtime, naptime, or throughout the night. The pediatrician needs to ensure that no underlying medical condition is responsible for the sleep disturbance, such as gastroesophageal reflux or otitis media. When all other medical conditions are ruled out, an evaluation for the underlying cause is needed. A sleep disorder may result from a negative sleep association, temperament issues, or a more pervasive noncompliance or general behavioral problem.

Management

The first step for any behavioral treatment of infant and toddler sleep disturbances includes the institution of a regularized sleep schedule and a bedtime routine. Next, a behavioral management plan for bedtime struggles and night awakenings needs to be developed, which includes putting the child to bed awake and allowing for the development of positive, independent sleep associations. Bedtime struggles often respond well to the establishment of consistent bedtime routines, which include some allowances for the child to control the situation (e.g., choice between two sets of pajamas) and the inclusion of preferred activities toward the end of the routine. Reward systems can be highly effective with older toddlers and preschoolers. The key to successful intervention is the development of a parenting plan that includes consistency in responding and appropriate guidelines (Box 251-1).

OBSTRUCTIVE SLEEP APNEA

Definition

Obstructive sleep apnea (OSA) is a respiratory sleep disorder that is characterized by repetitive episodes of upper airway obstruction during sleep. These events result in

periodic, distressing paresthesias (described as "crawling" sensations, burning, tingling, aching, stabbing, or itching) that occur mostly between the knees and ankles. These sensations are paired with irresistible urges to move the extremities (usually the legs), and symptoms characteristically are worse in the evening or at night. Consequently, patients with RLS may experience sleep disturbances, especially initiating sleep (Boxes 251-5 and 251-6).

Diagnosis

The diagnosis of PLMS may be suspected in a child with prominent repetitive movements of the legs and sometimes the arms during sleep. PLMS needs to be differentiated from several other sleep-related movements, including normal phenomena such as sleep starts (also known as *hypnic myoclonus*) and phasic REM activity (a type of fragmentary myoclonus). Abnormal movements in the differential diagnosis of PLMS include apnea-related or seizure-related movement. To differentiate PLMS from other movement disorders, overnight PSG generally is needed with recording of leg movements. Periodic leg movement events are reported per hour (PLMS index) and per hour with arousals (PLMS arousal index). Movement episodes may predominate in the first half of the night and tend to occur during stages 1 and 2 of sleep, although they can recur during any period of sleep.

In children, PLMS have been reported in association with fibromyalgia, radiation/chemotherapy management, and Williams syndrome. Previous studies also have shown an association between disturbed sleep with PLMS and attention deficit hyperactivity disorder. Children with sleep disturbances (PLMS) and attention deficit hyperactivity disorder have been reported to show improvement in attention deficit hyperactivity disorder symptoms with medical therapy for PLMD.

The diagnosis of RLS is based on a patient's report of symptoms, including the quality, severity, and time of day when paresthesias appear and the motor responses to these sensations. Primary (idiopathic) RLS has a high familial incidence, and several large pedigrees suggest an autosomal dominant pattern, although no specific gene linkage has been identified. In adults, secondary RLS has been described with many neurologic disorders (including polyneuropathies, myelopathies, and multiple sclerosis), anemia (including iron and folate deficiencies), uremia,

---

Box 251-5. International Classification of Sleep Disorders Diagnostic Criteria for Restless Legs Syndrome

A. A complaint of an unpleasant sensation in the legs at night or difficulty in initiating sleep

B. Disagreeable sensations of "creeping" inside the calves often associated with general aches and pains in the legs

C. The discomfort is relieved by movement of the limbs.

D. Polysomnographic monitoring demonstrates limb movements at sleep onset.

E. No evidence of any medical or psychiatric disorders that account for the movements

F. Other sleep disorders may be present but do not account for the symptom.

Box 251-6. International Classification of Sleep Disorders Diagnostic Criteria for Periodic Limb Movement Disorder

A. A complaint of insomnia or excessive sleepiness. Occasionally the patient will be asymptomatic and the movements are noticed by an observer.

B. Repetitive, highly stereotyped limb muscle movements, which in the leg are characterized by extension of the big toe in combination with partial flexion of the ankle, knee, and sometimes hip

C. Polysomnographic monitoring demonstrates
1. Repetitive episodes of muscle contraction (0.5 to 5 seconds in duration) separated by an interval of typically 20 to 40 seconds
2. Arousal or awakenings may be associated with movements.

D. No evidence of a medical or psychiatric disorder that can account for the primary complaint

E. Other sleep disorders may be present but do not account for the movements (e.g., obstructive sleep apnea syndrome).

---

diabetes, hypothyroidism, and medication use (e.g., tricyclic antidepressants and serotonin reuptake inhibitors).

Referral

Assessment and evaluation of PLMD and RLS should be performed by a sleep specialist. Overnight PSG with leg leads is required for the diagnosis of PLMD and may define better associated features of RLS.

Treatment

For secondary PLMD or RLS, associated medical conditions (e.g., anemia, diabetes, hypothyroidism) or sleep disorders (e.g., OSA) should be addressed first. Successful medical management with dopaminergic agents and with benzodiazepines has been reported; these findings parallel the experience in adults. To date, no randomized, placebo-controlled trials of therapy for PLMS or RLS have been conducted in children. Medications for PLMS and RLS in children probably should be prescribed by a pediatric sleep specialist or pediatric neurologist.

DELAYED SLEEP PHASE SYNDROME

Definition

Adolescents and many younger children enjoy staying up late at night. This becomes problematic, however, when their sleep-wake schedule becomes completely shifted. The end result is delayed sleep phase syndrome, with symptoms of sleep-onset insomnia and extreme difficulty awakening at a desired time in the morning. Approximately 7% of adolescents are sleep phase delayed. Delayed sleep phase syndrome often begins with a tendency to stay up late at night, sleep late, or take late afternoon naps. This process often begins on weekends, holidays, or summer vacations. There is a normal, physiologically based phase delay of approximately 2 hours post-puberty. This tendency is in conflict, however, with early high school start times. Some school districts are considering moving high school start times back. The first school districts that implemented such a program, in the Edina and Minneapolis school districts of Minnesota, have had positive results. For some adolescents, this normal delay becomes extended and entrenched, however, affecting the ability to fall asleep and awaken at usual times. The end result for many children and adolescents with this sleep disorder is difficulty in school, primarily because of chronic absenteeism and tardiness (Box 251-7).

Presentation and Initial Evaluation

The presentation of a child or adolescent with delayed sleep phase syndrome typically includes a significantly shifted sleep schedule and complaints of insomnia (when the patient attempts to fall asleep at a more typical bedtime) and difficulty waking in the morning. The preferred sleep period is usually early morning to early afternoon (e.g., 4 A.M. bedtime, noon wake time), with difficulty adhering to a more regular sleep schedule (e.g., 10 P.M. bedtime, 7 A.M. wake time). Insomnia is likely present only when attempts are made to go to bed earlier than the preferred hour and does not occur if the patient goes to bed at the preferred time. Usually there are few complaints regarding sleep maintenance.

An initial evaluation should exclude other potential sleep disrupters, including OSA and RLS, and other causes of sleeplessness, such as depression or anxiety. Evaluation for school refusal also should be done.

Management

The primary mode of treatment for this disorder is chronotherapy. The first step in this program is stabilizing sleep at the phase-delayed times (e.g., 3:00 A.M. to noon). For the

next week to 10 days, the sleeping period is delayed by 2 to 3 hours every day until the desired sleeping times occur. On night 1, sleep is to occur from 6:00 A.M. to 3:00 P.M. and on night 2 from 9:00 A.M. until 6:00 P.M. The imposed scheduling of sleep must be followed strictly for treatment to be effective. When sleep is occurring at the appropriate times, the new schedule must be adhered to rigidly given that it is easy for these individuals to return to a delayed sleep phase pattern. Additional treatment recommendations include appropriate sleep hygiene (e.g., avoidance of caffeine) and exposure to early morning light. Some adolescents are resistant to treatment, and in those cases psychological issues need to be addressed, with a possible referral to a mental health specialist.

 Additional Resources, CD-ROM

Bibliography

Mini-index of Related Topics

Box 251-7. International Classification of Sleep Disorders Diagnostic Criteria for Delayed Sleep Phase Syndrome

A. A complaint of an inability to fall asleep at the desired clock time, or inability to awaken spontaneously at the desired time of awakening, or excessive sleepiness

B. There is a phase delay of the major sleep episode in relation to the desired time for sleep.

C. Symptoms are present for at least 1 month.

D. When not required to maintain a strict schedule (e.g., vacation time), patients will:
  1. Have a habitual sleep period that is sound and of normal quality and duration
  2. Awaken spontaneously
  3. Maintain stable entrainment to a 24-hour sleep-wake pattern at a delayed phase

E. Evidence of a delay in the timing of the habitual sleep period illustrated on daily logs for at least 2 weeks

F. Laboratory evidence of a delay in the timing of the habitual sleep period by
  1. 24-hour polysomnographic monitoring (or by means of 2 consecutive nights of polysomnography and an intervening multiple sleep latency test) or
  2. Continuous temperature monitoring showing that the time of the absolute temperature nadir is delayed into the second half of the habitual (delayed) sleep episode

G. Does not meet criteria for any other sleep disorder causing inability to initiate sleep or excessive sleepiness

SUGGESTED READINGS

Carskadon MA, Dement WC: Normal human sleep: An overview. In Kryger MH, Roth TR, and Dement WC (eds): Principles and Practice of Sleep Medicine, 3rd ed. Philadelphia, WB Saunders, 2000, pp 15–25.

Chesson AL Jr, Wise M, Davila D, et al: Practice parameters for the treatment of restless legs syndrome and periodic limb movement disorder: An American Academy of Sleep Medicine Report. Standards of Practice Committee of the American Academy of Sleep Medicine. Sleep 1999;22:961–968.

Littner M, Johnson SF, McCall WV, et al: Practice parameters for the treatment of narcolepsy: An update for 2000. Sleep 2001;24:451–466.

Marcus CL: Sleep-disordered breathing in children. Curr Opin Pediatr 2000;12:208–212.

Mindell JA: Empirically supported treatments in pediatric psychology: Bedtime refusal and night wakings in young children. J Pediatr Psychol 1999;24:465–481.

Mindell JA, Owens JA: A Clinical Guide to Pediatric Sleep: Diagnosis and Management of Sleep Problems. Philadelphia, Lippincott Williams & Wilkins, 2003.

Owens JL, France KG, Wiggs L: Behavioural and cognitive-behavioural interventions for sleep disorders in infants and children: A review. Sleep Med Rev 1999;3:281–302.

Thorpy M: Current concepts in the etiology, diagnosis, and treatment of narcolepsy. Sleep Med 2001;2:5–17.

252 Soiling Problems (Encopresis)

Edward Christophersen and Susan L. Mortweet

ROLE OF THE GENERALIST

1   Diagnose encopresis by obtaining an extensive history of the child's stooling habits, including evidence of soiling and constipation.

2   Provide the child and parents with education about encopresis and effective treatment options.

3   Treat constipation through methods that clean out the colon, such as enemas, mineral oil, or oral medications.

4   Assist the child and parent in implementing treatment components that prevent the reoccurrence of constipation and soiling, such as suppositories and oral medications.

5   Assist the child and caregivers in implementing behavioral and dietary changes to encourage successful bowel training and reduce soiling and constipation.

6   Consider the child and parent's strengths and challenges, and provide treatment that encourages adherence to the treatment protocol.

7   Ensure appropriate long-term follow-up until the encopresis is resolved; referral to a pediatric psychologist to assist in behavioral aspects of treatment may be warranted.

Encopresis is the voluntary or involuntary passage of feces on inappropriate places, such as underwear or the floor, in children older than 4 years of age. To be diagnosed with encopresis, a child must have at least one such event per month for at least 3 months. In addition, the behavior cannot be due exclusively to the physiologic effects of a substance, such as a laxative, or to a general medical condition except constipation. The most common type of encopresis is overflow incontinence, in which there is evidence of constipation on physical examination or by history. A less common condition is encopresis without constipation.

Primary or *continuous* encopresis applies to children who have been incontinent their entire life. The *secondary* or *discontinuous* type applies to children who were fully bowel trained once for a minimum of 6 months. The mean age of onset for secondary encopresis has been estimated at 7 years, 4 months. Although the two types of encopresis typically are treated using the same strategies, children with primary or continuous encopresis typically have a better prognosis.

FUNDAMENTALS

The prevalence of encopresis in children has been estimated to range from 1% to 3%, affecting boys three to six times more often than girls. Despite its prevalence, many parents of children with encopresis often think that they are the only family with a child with encopresis. This misconception also may be perpetuated by the popular press, which rarely mentions this condition when discussing common childhood problems.

Although there have been numerous theories offered as to the etiology of encopresis, including coercive toilet training, a history of hostile or violent events, and child abuse, the only etiologic factor that we could find support for in the literature was constipation. Constipation plays a major role in encopresis and in other toileting problems, such as withholding, which can create and exacerbate stooling difficulties. Constipation-related problems, including encopresis and stool withholding (the term used to refer to children who refuse to have a bowel movement in the toilet but who defecate in a pull-up or a diaper), usually are present in children who are referred to gastroenterology clinics.

Constipation-related stooling abnormalities (e.g., frequent small or pebbly stools, infrequent large stools, or both) are not always distressing to the child. The significance of these episodes may be overlooked or underestimated by parents. Constipation also may be misinterpreted by parents and consequently treated improperly. A child's cycle of constipation may be confusing for parents due to the child's "paradoxical diarrhea," which refers to the seepage of feces around hard stool in the rectum that the child has been unable to pass. Although the child is constipated or impacted, symptomatically it appears to the parents as though the child has diarrhea, producing numerous watery, foul-smelling stools. Some parents attempt to treat this type of diarrhea with over-the-counter antidiarrheal agents, an approach that potentially exacerbates the condition.

In addition to having constipation, children with encopresis may have a rectum that is less sensitive to the "call to stool" than is needed for appropriate elimination. They may need excessive pressure in their rectum before they feel the call to stool. Children often complain that they "couldn't feel it [the bowel movement] coming."

DIAGNOSING ENCOPRESIS

As with other childhood disorders, a thorough history of the child and family's physical and mental health should be obtained. The history should include questions about the family medical history; the child's stooling habits; the child's diet history; and information about any previous attempts to deal with the encopresis, including rewards or punishment. Having parents complete a detailed history to be returned before the child's first appointment can increase the efficiency of the initial intake interview. An example of an intake form for encopresis can be found in Christophersen. More specific assessment information that is important to collect is described subsequently.

History of Constipation

When obtaining a history of the child's stooling habits, special attention should be paid to any evidence of prior or current constipation. This historical information should include stooling frequency, stool size, stool consistency, any problems such as bleeding, and any prior interventions attempted by professionals or by parents using home remedies. Many medications, such as pain medications and some anticonvulsants, relax the intestine and may produce or aggravate constipation as a side effect. It also is important to ask parents about any medication-related constipation problems.

Children who have a history of constipation or stool holding also often develop large-caliber stools. The large caliber stools are more difficult to pass, resulting in longer gastric transit times. Longer gastric transit times promote greater dehydration of the stool, producing firmer and harder stools, which inhibit peristalsis. The longer the stool is held in the colon, the greater the likelihood of producing foul-smelling stools. The large, foul-smelling stools stay in the colon, and the child has no bowel movement for days, followed by soiling.

Many parents fail to recognize constipation in their child, apparently assuming that as long as a child has a bowel movement on most days, he or she "couldn't be constipated." Children can have daily bowel movements, however, and still be constipated. A child who is having daily bowel movements, but not expelling all of the waste from the rectum, gradually can accumulate larger and larger amounts of fecal matter. In addition to stooling frequency, bowel movement size and consistency are key indicators of constipation. The clinical interview may be supplemented by a flat plate x-ray of the abdomen. Lack of constipation evidence from the x-ray does not mean, however, that the child does not have a history of constipation, only that the child was not constipated at the time the x-ray was taken.

History of Soiling

Soiling accidents tend to occur at home, typically after school, although children with histories of chronic and frequent soiling may have accidents outside the home and at various times throughout the day. Only rarely do children soil during their sleep. At times, parents can misinterpret soilings as intentional, especially if they occur only at home or when the child is playing. Parents may say, "He just doesn't want to take time to go to the bathroom." We rarely, if ever, find that this is the case. As with constipation, the key indicators of soiling to assess and manage are consistency of the stool and frequency and amount of the soiling incidents. Soiling incidents can be difficult for parents to assess at times, however, because of the smashing of the stool in the underwear from the regular activities of

the child or if the child hides his or her underwear. Parents should be encouraged to provide their best estimate.

History of Diet and Exercise

Children with a long history of constipation may develop a decrease in appetite and lethargy. A history of the child's eating habits and energy level should be obtained. It is important to assess how much daily fiber and dairy products the child is eating and how much exercise he or she gets on a regular basis. Parents and the child should be questioned specifically to provide the best estimate of the child's diet. The health care provider can ask, "If a half-cup of milk is one serving, how many servings of milk do you drink every day?" Parents also need specific questioning for fiber intake because they may not know what types of foods in their child's diet contain fiber.

History of Behavior Problems

Many studies have examined specifically the notion that children with encopresis have emotional or behavioral problems. The use of child-behavior rating scales has revealed no systematic differences between children with encopresis and normal children of the same age and gender. Children with encopresis generally have been found to be similar to their typical peers in terms of their self-perceived psychological functioning, behavioral problems, parent-child relations, and social competence. Given the research that shows the presence of significant physical findings and the absence of research showing consistent behavior problems in most children diagnosed and treated for encopresis, the conclusion seems warranted that encopresis can and should be treated primarily as a dysfunction of the bowel.

Some comorbid behavioral issues or disorders may have a negative impact on the success of treatment of this disorder. Children with attention deficit hyperactivity disorder may not be attentive to their diet or may have difficulty taking time to complete toilet sits. Children with untreated depression may not have the energy or interest to treat their symptoms of encopresis. Children with oppositional behavior may not adhere to the treatment regimen. In the absence of outcome studies of treatments with children who have encopresis and comorbid disorders, we suggest that encopresis and interfering comorbid conditions be treated simultaneously. Children with oppositional behavior or adherence problems may need interventions to address those areas first before treatment for encopresis can be successful. The issue of adherence is addressed further in the treatment section.

Encopresis versus Hirschsprung Disease

A thorough history should help the practitioner differentiate between encopresis and Hirschsprung disease. Hirschsprung disease occurs in 1 out of 25,000 live births, and many of the symptoms are different from those present in encopresis. In contrast to most children with encopresis, children with Hirschsprung disease present with symptoms as a newborn, such as failure to thrive and anemia. Children with Hirschsprung disease also may have loose or tight sphincter tone and obstructive symptoms. Late-onset (>3 years old) also is rare for Hirschsprung disease; most children are diagnosed during infancy.

TREATING ENCOPRESIS: MEDICAL-BEHAVIORAL MANAGEMENT

One of the first approaches to treating encopresis, the "pediatric approach," originally was described by Davidson and included a three-phase treatment protocol. The first phase involved cleansing the child's colon with enemas and giving the child large doses of mineral oil to help the child continue passing stools. The second phase involved decreasing the child's consumption of milk and dairy products to the equivalent of one pint of whole milk daily, due to the aggravating effects of dairy products on constipation. The objective of this phase was to eliminate enemas and encourage regular bowel habits. The third phase involved continuation of the stool habit, while gradually fading out the use of mineral oil. A more recent report of the Society of Pediatric Gastroenterology and Nutrition by Baker and colleagues recommended a similar approach to the treatment of encopresis. Specific treatment components based on the work of these authors are described subsequently. Although historically there has been some concern in the literature for the safety of a mineral oil, increased dietary fiber, and laxative regimen for ameliorating problems with constipation, more recent research by McClung and associates has not detected any negative effects.

Providing Education

The first and perhaps most important step in managing encopresis is providing the parents and child with specific information on encopresis, resulting in the demystification of encopresis and an understanding that it is a common problem for children. Families may benefit from viewing a simple drawing or diagram to explain how abnormal bowel functioning can lead to encopresis. It also is important that the parent and the child be told that the child is not to blame for abnormal bowel functioning and that effective treatment methods are available.

Cleaning Out the Colon

After explaining the mechanics of encopresis to the child and parents, the steps for successful treatment can be introduced. The first step is that of cleaning out the colon. Family members can be told that to help the muscles "heal," the intestines and colon must be empty. Sometimes we liken the situation to a pregnant woman who has to deliver her baby before she can start to heal the stretched muscles of her abdomen.

The most common way to clean out the child's colon effectively, based on the works of Davidson and Levine, is the use of at least one enema. Baker and associates provided a flow chart of the procedures to follow, including whether the patients respond to the procedures. They listed the dosing for the initial cleaning out using mineral oil instead of an enema (1 to 3 mL/kg, up to 240 mL daily). Baker and associates stated correctly that there are no studies comparing the oral route (stool softeners, laxatives, or lubricants) with the rectal route (enemas or suppositories) for relieving constipation and recommended discussing the treatment options with the child and parents. This step in encopresis management is vital. If a child with constipation is not cleaned out adequately, neither the constipation nor the encopresis is likely to resolve. For this reason, we routinely recommend that the clinician be more rather than less aggressive. When deciding between 1 mL/kg or 2 mL/kg of mineral oil or lactulose, initially, it is probably better to use 2 mL/kg.

Keeping the Colon from Reimpacting

When the child's colon is cleaned out successfully, the next step is to keep it from getting too full again. There are several components to this step that can be implemented simultaneously—scheduled toilet sits, oral medications, and suppositories.

Scheduled Toilet Sits

The simplest component is that of a scheduled toilet sit. The child is asked to sit on the toilet for approximately 5 minutes, two or three times a day, to facilitate good bowel habits. Many children have a pattern to their soiling and bowel movements, and the toilet sits should be structured around these times. If the child typically soils after school but before dinner, a toilet sit should be scheduled for right after school to train the child's body to eliminate into the toilet at that time. Adherence to these toilet sits can be enhanced by allowing the child to have a special toy or book that can be played with only during toilet sits. Tangible reinforcers for cooperation, such as stickers or special time with a caregiver, also can be helpful.

Oral Medications

In addition to information about enemas for cleaning out, Baker and associates included a list of recommended dosages for each of the medications that commonly are used in the management of constipation and encopresis on a daily basis. They recommended mineral oil, lactulose, or polyethylene glycol. We usually start with 1 mL/kg and increase the dose to 2 mL/kg of mineral oil if the child's symptoms have not improved after 1 week. Too much mineral oil can result in orange stains in the child's underwear and clothing. Close monitoring is needed to avoid this embarrassing side effect.

Suppositories

Numerous authors, including us, reported favorable outcome data with the use of rectal suppositories as one treatment component. We often recommend that the parents administer one adult glycerine suppository if a certain amount of stool has not been passed for the day. These suppositories are reduced gradually as the child has daily bowel movements. Because no studies could be located that evaluated the relative efficacy of oral treatments (lubricants or laxatives or both) and rectal treatment (enemas or suppositories or both) or a combination of the two for the daily treatment of encopresis, the choice of treatment routes is left to the practitioner and family.

Role of Diet and Exercise

Perhaps one of the most important and most difficult components of the treatment protocol for encopresis is that of the lifestyle changes required in diet and exercise. The American Academy of Pediatrics recommends a daily intake of dietary fiber equivalent to the child's age plus five;

for example, a 5-year-old child should be eating 10 g of dietary fiber (5 + 5) per day. Because most parents do not know how to estimate the amount of dietary fiber that their children eat, parents should be provided with written fiber content information to assist them in preparing meals that have adequate amounts of fiber in them (Table 252-1).

Role of Data Collection: Symptom Rating Sheets

The regimen that is required of parents and children to manage encopresis can be viewed as a complication to the already busy schedule of most families. A parent-report symptom rating sheet as described by Christophersen can facilitate record keeping (Fig. 252-1). When used reliably and mailed to the treatment provider's office, sent by

e-mail with appropriate consent, or brought in for each follow-up appointment, it can be a quick and accurate way of assessing patient progress, making treatment plan modifications, and encouraging treatment adherence.

As shown in Figure 252-1, the symptom rating sheet asks the parent or child to record several things, including the amount and consistency of stooling, bowel movements in the toilet, and daily dietary fiber intake. This form can be used to watch for trends in the child's habits, such as stool frequency and amount. Immediate feedback can be given on improvements and on warning signs that the child may be becoming constipated again. If the stool volume begins to decrease, the child may be becoming constipated again and may require more aggressive management.

Table 252-1. Fiber Content of Selected Foods*

	Serving Size	Dietary fiber (g)		Serving Size	Dietary fiber (g)
Breads and Crackers			**Fruits†—cont'd**		
Fiberich bread	1 slice	3.2	Prunes, dried	4	5.2
Seven-grain bread	1 slice	3	Orange	1 medium	4.5
High-bran "health bread"	1 slice	3	Banana	1 medium	4
Cornbread	1 square (2.5 inch)	3	Apple, with peel	1 medium	3.3
100% whole-wheat bread	1 slice	2.4	Strawberries	1 cup	3.3
Cracked wheat bread	1 slice	2.1	Pear	1 medium	3.1
Whole-wheat crackers	6	2	Cantaloupe	¼ medium	2.5
Rye crackers	3	2	Plums	2	2.5
Whole-wheat croutons	¼ cup	1.5	Apricots	3	2.4
Rye bread	1 slice	1.2	**Nuts and Seeds**		
White bread	1 slice	0.8	Brazil nuts	10	5.5
Cereals			Peanuts	½ cup	5.5
Fiber One	1 cup	24	Almonds	10	3.6
100% bran cereal	1 cup	20	Soy nuts	2 tbsp	3
Corn Bran	1 cup	8	Sunflower seeds	2 tbsp	3
Cracklin' Oat Bran	1 cup	8	Corn nuts	2 tbsp	3
Fruit n' Fiber	1 cup	8	Walnuts	½ cup	3
Granola	1 cup	7	Peanut butter	2 tbsp	2.3
Shredded Wheat and Bran	1 cup	6	Poppy seeds	2 tbsp	2
Raisin Squares	1 cup	6	Sesame seeds	2 tbsp	2
Bran Muffin Crisp	1 cup	6	**Vegetables‡**		
Raisin Nut Bran	1 cup	6	Baked beans	1 cup	18.6
Grape Nuts	1 cup	5.3	Peas	1 cup	11.3
40% Bran Flakes	1 cup	5	Corn	1 cup	9.3
Most	1 cup	5	Broccoli	2 spears	7
Raisin Bran	1 cup	4	Yams, baked with skin	1 medium	6.8
Oatmeal, cooked	¾ cup	3	Brussels sprouts	1 cup	6.5
Shredded Wheat	1 biscuit	3	Green beans	1 cup	3.5
Wheat Chex	1 cup	3	Spinach	1 cup	3.5
Ralston, cooked	¾ cup	2.7	Carrots	1 cup	3.2
Wheaties	1 cup	2	Potatoes, baked with skin	1 medium	3
Cheerios	1 cup	1.8	Tomato	1 medium	3
Flours			Cauliflower	1 cup	2.5
Bran (miller's)	1 cup	48	Cabbage, shredded	1 cup	1.9
Cornmeal, stoneground	1 cup	16.5	Lettuce	1 cup	0.8
100% whole wheat	1 cup	14.4	Celery	1 stalk	0.7
100% rye	1 cup	14.4	**Miscellaneous**		
Rolled oats	1 cup	12	Kidney beans	1 cup	20
All-purpose white flour	1 cup	1.6	Chili	1 cup	17
Fruits†			Macaroni and pasta (whole wheat, cooked)	1 cup	5.7
Figs, dried	2	8	Brown rice	1 cup	4
Apricots, dried	8	7.8	Coconut, shredded	2 tbsp	3
Dates, dried	10	7	Popcorn, popped	1 cup	1
Raisins	½ cup	5.4			

*Many new high-fiber foods come on the market each week, and parents should be instructed to watch for them. Check food labels for actual grams of dietary fiber per serving.
†Fresh, unless otherwise indicated.
‡Fresh, raw, unless otherwise indicated.

BOWEL SYMPTOM RATING SHEET

	Amt. of Medication	# of Supp.	# of Enemas	# of Soilings	# BMs in Toilet	Size/Consistency	Servings w/fiber	Amt. of liquids	Type of Activity	Time Reward	Comments
1											
2											
3											
4											
5											
6											
7											
8											
9											
10											
11											
12											
13											
14											
15											
16											
17											
18											
19											
20											
21											
22											
23											
24											
25											
26											
27											
28											
29											
30											
31											

KEY:

Medication:	# of tablespoons
Size/Consistency:	Approx. no. of cups; H = hard, S = soft formed, D = diarrhea
Amt. of liquids:	No, of glasses of water or juices per day
Activity:	3 = very active, 2 = moderately active, 1 = little activity
Time:	Indicates how parent spent reward time with child

Figure 252-1. Bowel symptom rating sheet.

Strategies for Maximizing Treatment Adherence

As with any treatment explanation, the health care provider must be sure to provide written and verbal information that can be comprehended by the caregiver and preferably the child as well. We have found it useful to show families an encopresis "kit" while explaining the components of the treatment. We show them an enema, have them hold a suppository, and ask them to read a few labels that we have removed from food items. This can help to "demystify" the treatment components and help families feel more confident.

It also is important to tailor the treatment regimen to families' needs and strengths. For a child with oppositional behavior, the starting place may be with general behavioral management strategies and simple data collection using the symptom rating sheet. The parent also may choose to try a few dietary changes while working on helping the child learn to comply better with requests. Similarly a child with depression may need assistance with depressive symptoms before being interested or willing to adhere to the encopresis regimen.

For families who simply may not be able to handle all of the components of the treatment at once, it is best to start with the data collection, scheduled toilet sits, and small dietary changes. When a short history of success with these components is shown, the health care provider can introduce the enemas and medications needed to keep the colon from becoming impacted.

Allowing the parent and child to choose the best times to incorporate the components into their day also facilitates adherence. If they have more time in the evening than the morning to give a suppository and wait for it to take effect, the regimen should be structured to fit that time of day. Similarly, if it is easier to remember to take the mineral oil with breakfast and the bedtime snack instead of with dinner, such accommodations should be considered. This tailoring may be especially important for an older child, who does not want friends to know about his or her problem with soiling. The privacy of taking medication or taking a suppository when all friends, including those of a sibling, have gone home is one respectful way to help a child cope with encopresis management.

As mentioned previously, it can be important for some children that they be reinforced for their cooperation with the encopresis treatment regimen. It can be embarrassing for children to have parents check their stools and to have to sit on the toilet while others are outside playing. Parents should consider reinforcing their child for cooperating with eating more fiber, taking medications and suppositories, allowing parents to look at stools, and participating in scheduled toilet sits. The reinforcement can be special time with a caregiver, stickers, or points to earn preferred activities or toys. Strategies for facilitating treatment adherence at length are discussed in the reference by Christophersen and Mortweet (see the Suggested Readings).

FOLLOW-UP

Parents and children need to know that encopresis treatment is a long-term project. In general, 4 to 6 weeks of consistent treatment may be required before a substantial improvement in symptoms of encopresis is observed. Long-term maintenance is needed to prevent recurring constipation. For these reasons, provisions need to be made for follow-up care that includes, at least during the first month of treatment, daily record keeping of treatments and treatment effects. Patients initially may have to return once every 2 weeks with their symptom rating sheets to discuss the success and problems with the treatment regimen. Intermittent phone calls to answer specific questions often are helpful between appointments. When encopresis is managed, families should be informed that recurrences are common, especially if the family stops following the dietary recommendations or the child has a disruption to the gastric system from illness or surgery. For more complicated patients (e.g., patients with comorbid mental health or adherence problems), a referral to a pediatric psychologist who is trained in the management of encopresis is appropriate. Such psychologists are aware that the encopresis is due to a medical condition, such as constipation, and are more likely to provide proper treatment focused on behavioral aspects of the problem and on adherence and self-esteem issues related to embarrassment about the condition.

Mini-index of Related Topics

SUGGESTED READINGS

Baker SS, Liptak GS, Colletti RB, et al: Constipation in infants and children: Evaluation and treatment. J Pediatr Gastroenterol Nutr 1999;29:612–626.

Christophersen ER: Pediatric Compliance: A Guide for the Primary Care Physician. New York, Plenum, 1994.

Christophersen ER, Mortweet SL: Treatments That Work with Children: Empirically Supported Strategies for Managing Childhood Problems. Washington, DC, APA Books, 2001.

Davidson M: Constipation and fecal incontinence. Pediatr Clin North Am 1958;5:749–757.

Levine MD: Encopresis: Its potentiation, evaluation, and alleviation. Pediatr Clin North Am 1982;29:315–330.

McClung HJ, Boyne LJ, Linsheid R, et al: Is combination therapy for encopresis nutritionally safe? Pediatrics 1993;91:591–594.

253 Day/Nighttime Wetting Problems (Enuresis)

Edward Christophersen and Susan L. Mortweet

ROLE OF THE GENERALIST

1   Diagnose enuresis by obtaining a thorough history of the child's voiding habits and perceived severity of the problem for the child and family.

2   Eliminate physiologic causes of incontinence, and treat physiologic causes of incontinence when present.

3   Provide the child and parents with treatment options, including medication or behavioral interventions.

4   Consider the child's and family's strengths and challenges in adhering to a treatment protocol.

5   Ensure appropriate follow-up until the enuresis is resolved by providing frequent contact and treatment recommendations tailored to the family's needs.

Enuresis is the repeated voiding of urine into the bed or clothes, whether involuntary or intentional. The behavior is clinically significant when manifested either by a frequency of twice a week for at least 3 consecutive months or by the presence of clinically significant distress or impairment in social, academic, or other important areas of functioning. The child must be at least 5 years old, or an equivalent developmental level, and the enuretic behavior must not be due exclusively to the direct physiologic effect of a substance, such as a diuretic, or general medical disorder, such as diabetes, spina bifida, or a seizure disorder. The term *primary enuresis* refers to children who have never been dry at night, and *secondary enuresis* refers to children who were dry at night for a minimum of 6 months and then starting bed-wetting again.

Much less research has been devoted to day wetting, or diurnal enuresis. One definition is the leakage of at least 1 mL of urine at least once a week in a child 5 years old or older. Functional day wetting is incontinence not caused by disease, injury, or congenital malformation and is almost always urge incontinence caused by an unstable bladder. Bacteriuria and day wetting are associated strongly in girls, but not in boys.

FUNDAMENTALS

Day and night wetting can be common in young children. At 5 years of age, 15% to 20% of children have some degree of nighttime wetting. Enuresis generally is a self-limiting condition with a spontaneous cure rate of 12% to 15% per year. At 15 years of age, only about 1% to 2% of teenagers still wet the bed. Prevalence figures for day wetting, at least one incident per week, have been estimated as approximately 3% of 7-year-old girls and 2% of 7-year-old boys.

Numerous, well-known potential physiopathologic causes of incontinence are not considered enuresis, including urinary tract infections, urinary tract anomaly, bladder instability, occult spina bifida, diabetes, and sleep apnea. Most of these causes can be eliminated by complete history, physical examination, and urinalysis. Invasive or complex procedures and imaging rarely are needed.

Although many causes of nocturnal enuresis have been suggested, such as anxiety or problematic conduct, no definitive etiology has been identified. The prevailing opinion is that nocturnal enuresis is a developmental problem. Most children, with time, become continent at night. Enuresis generally is not thought to be a primarily a psychopathologic disorder, although secondary emotional and behavioral problems may develop as a result of trying to cope with enuresis.

DIAGNOSIS

A careful medical history and physical examination, including urinalysis, usually provides sufficient information for the physician to arrive at a diagnosis for nocturnal and diurnal enuresis. The history should include an assessment of the child's voiding patterns, including the severity and perceived severity of the problem and any history of spontaneous resolution. Specific information on prior evaluations and therapies should be obtained. A positive family history of clinical enuresis has been noted frequently, with a much higher incidence when histories of both parents' families are significant for enuresis. Most patients can be screened adequately for behavioral and emotional problems through the use of a thorough interview and common rating scales, such as the Achenbach Child Behavior Checklist or the Behavioral Assessment System for Children, without any initial need for an extensive psychological evaluation. Children with primary nocturnal enuresis usually do not present with significant behavioral comorbidity. Health care providers usually should treat primary enuresis as a common biobehavioral problem without a psychiatric component.

The physical examination should include abdominal, genital, and neurologic assessments to rule out abnormalities of the urinary tract, bladder abnormalities, an ectopic ureter, or an epispadiac urethra (urethral opening on the dorsum of the penis). Urinalysis should include urine specific gravity and dipstick tests, which might suggest the presence of diabetes. Abnormalities in renal concentrating ability should be noted. A urine culture should be obtained only if the patient has symptoms consistent with urinary tract infection or if urinalysis results are positive for the presence of red and white blood cells. Urodynamic and radiologic evaluations are not necessary in children with straightforward primary nocturnal enuresis.

MANAGEMENT

Enuresis secondary to a pathophysiologic process, such as bacteriuria, disease (e.g., diabetes), anatomic abnormalities (e.g., nephropathy), or functional abnormalities (e.g., unstable bladder), may resolve when these problems are treated adequately. After physiologic issues are eliminated as a cause for enuresis, the first line of treatment is use of behavioral management strategies. Pharmacotherapy also is available when behavioral management does not work or as an alternative but generally is not the preferred line of treatment.

Behavioral Management of Nocturnal Enuresis
Bell and Pad or Urine Alarm
For 6 decades, the standard behavioral treatment for nocturnal enuresis has been the bell and pad or urine alarm procedure, originally reported in 1938. Studies indicate the urine alarm treatment initially eliminates enuresis in approximately 75% of individuals, with treatment duration ranging from a mean of 5 to 12 weeks. Relapse rates generally are high. Relapse occurs in 46% of cases, although reinstatement of the procedures usually results in a complete cure. The urine alarm treatment also has been shown to be superior to no treatment, short-term psychotherapy, and imipramine. Box 253-1 summarizes urine alarm procedures that can be described to the family.

Overlearning
A process called *overlearning* also has been used, in combination with the urine alarm, to address nocturnal enuresis. The term *overlearning* refers to training children to a higher criterion than normally is thought to be necessary, in hopes of reducing the relapse rate. In the case of enuresis, a child, after being dry at night from using a urine alarm, is encouraged to drink extra liquids before retiring for the night, until attaining 14 additional consecutive dry nights. Drinking extra fluids should make it more difficult for the child to avoid bed-wetting, training him or her to a higher criterion. Although overlearning usually results in a relapse of wetting, in most cases the relapse lasts only a week or so.

Dry Bed Training
The most promising adaptation of the urine alarm treatment is dry bed training. Dry bed training combines many behavioral procedures, including cleanliness training, positive practice, nighttime awakening, retention-control training, and positive reinforcement. Box 253-2 summarizes dry bed training procedures. Only about 5% of physicians are

---

Box 253-1. Urine Alarm Procedures

1. Contract with the parent and child for a 3-month trial.
2. Have the child keep a diary, starting at least 2 weeks before the first visit, that includes the number of wet nights, the number of episodes per night, and the size of the wet spot.
3. The parent must be part of the alarm system (many children do not arouse on their own to the alarm initially but after a few weeks of parental help begin to respond on their own).
4. Emphasize and reward arousal.
5. See the child at least every 3 weeks initially.
6. Use a decreased frequency of wet nights, a decreased number of episodes per night, and a decreased size of wet spot as signs of improvement.
7. Continue until the child achieves 14 consecutive dry nights (no alarm sound for even a spot of urine).
8. After initial goal is achieved, use overlearning—either 16 oz of fluid before bed or gradual 2-oz increments, increasing as each step is mastered, until 16 oz is reached.
9. Continue overlearning until the child achieves 14 consecutive dry nights.
10. When overlearning is completed, stop the alarm and extra drinking.
11. Relapses can be re-treated successfully in the same manner in many cases.

Adapted from Moffatt ME: Nocturnal enuresis: A review of the efficacy of treatments and practical advice for clinicians. J Dev Behav Pediatr 1997;18:49–56.

---

trained in the use of urine alarm or dry bed training versus almost 100% of physicians who are trained in the pharmacologic management of enuresis. Although clinicians may not have been taught to recommend urine alarm or dry bed training, these techniques are effective and should be instituted before resorting to pharmacologic therapy. Dry bed training also has been shown to be effective with adults, with higher cure rates and lower relapse rates than have been reported with children.

Behavioral Treatment of Diurnal Enuresis
The class of diurnal enuresis that responds best to behavioral interventions is urge incontinence. One of the key variables in the treatment of urge incontinence, awareness of bladder distention and incipient or actual bladder neck descent, is similar to routine toilet training. This distention or descent gives rise to postural changes and limb movements suggesting urinary urgency. The function of these movements seems to be maintenance of bladder neck ascent. When children scissor their legs or compress their thighs, the movements produce upward pressure in the perineal region that lifts the bladder neck and forestalls urination. Children often are unaware of these movements and their function, however. When parents advise their children to go to the bathroom based on their observation of the movements, the children appear unaware of the need to urinate. Routine aspects of parental teaching can be applied to help the child make the necessary connections, initially between bodily movements and need and ultimately between bladder contraction and need, and enable the child to complete or forestall urination based on a plan.

In their classic 1974 book, *Toilet Training in Less than a Day*, Azrin and Foxx recommended a procedure they called

Box 253-2. Dry Bed Training Procedures

1. Use a calendar to record if child is dry or wet from the previous night.
2. At bedtime, do the following:
   Have child feel sheets and notice dryness.
   Have child describe what he or she will do if the urge to urinate occurs.
   Have child describe current need to urinate and do so.
   Have parent express confidence in child's ability to progress.
   Place alarm in bed, connected and tested, and child goes to sleep.
3. Awaken child once during the night and do the following:
   Use minimal prompts, but make sure child is awake.
   Have child feel sheets for dryness; parent praises child for dry sheets.
   Have child go to the bathroom and return to bed.
   Have child feel sheets again and state what he or she will do if the urge to urinate occurs.
   Reset the alarm if sounded, or check for connection.
   Wake at scheduled time regardless whether alarm sounded.
4. Adjust time of nightly awakening, as follows:
   On first night, awaken child 5 hours before the usual wakening time.
   After 6 consecutive dry nights, awaken 1 hour earlier. Continue awakening 1 hour earlier every 6 days until time is 8 hours before usual wakening.
   When dry for 14 nights at 8-hour awakenings, discontinue awakening and discontinue alarm.
5. When alarm sounds, do the following:
   Awaken child.
   Child feels sheets and comments on wetness.
   Child walks to bathroom and finishes wetting.
   Child takes quick bath.
   Child changes into dry clothes.
   Child removes wet sheets and places them in laundry.
   Child remakes bed with dry sheets.
   Child feels bed sheets and comments on dryness.
6. Do not reconnect alarm; child returns to sleep.
7. During the day, do the following:
   Child and parents describe progress to relevant friends or family members.
   Parents repeatedly express confidence in child and praise him or her.
   Parent calls therapist at set times to report progress.

Adapted from Azrin NH, Sneed TJ, Foxx RM: Dry-bed training: Rapid elimination of childhood enuresis. Behav Res Ther 1974;12:147–156.

positive practice for day wetting. This procedure consisted of requiring the child to "practice" going to the bathroom 10 times after each wetting. Box 253-3 describes the steps for positive practice. Positive practice is applicable to children from about 3 years of age to about 8 or 9 years of age.

Pharmacotherapy
Despite the effectiveness of behavioral management strategies, physicians prescribe drug therapy for enuresis more frequently than any other treatment. A broad spectrum of drugs is available for the treatment of nocturnal enuresis. The most common drug used to treat enuresis is imipramine (Tofranil), a tricyclic antidepressant. In one

study of pharmacotherapy, imipramine, in doses of 25 to 75 mg given at bedtime, resolved symptoms in about 43% of pediatric patients, whereas other tricyclic antidepressants had a success rate of 33%. The relapse rate was high, and the final outcome was no better than a placebo or baseline treatment. The U.S. Food and Drug Administration recommends that imipramine be used only as adjunctive therapy for enuretic children 6 years old and older. Imipramine has potentially serious side effects and should be reserved for cases in which more conventional therapies are not practical or effective. A review of the literature on pharmacologic treatment of daytime incontinence concluded that there was no evidence from properly controlled studies that showed tricyclic antidepressants or anticholinergic drugs were of value for a child with daytime wetting.

The efficacy and safety of DDAVP, a hormonal nasal spray used to treat diabetes insipidus, has been examined for treatment of nocturnal enuresis. For studies that had not preselected for DDAVP response, the best estimate for dryness was approximately 25%. The relapse rate, when reported, was high. Only 5.7% of test subjects remained dry after withdrawal of the drug. Based on current

Box 253-3. Positive Practice Procedures

When you find your child with wet or soiled pants, use the following guidelines:
1. Tell child why you are displeased with the wetting or soiling.
   State your displeasure; say something like, "Your panties are wet; you should use the toilet."
2. Have your child do positive practice of self-toileting.
   Tell your child what you are doing and why by saying something like, "You wet your pants. Now you have to practice going to the bathroom." Guide your child quickly to the bathroom.
   Guide your child to lower his or her pants quickly and sit on the toilet/potty.
   After sitting 1 or 2 seconds (do not allow urination), guide your child to raise pants quickly.
   Guide your child back to the area where you discovered the accident for a total of five positive practices from where your child had the accident. Then guide your child to practice from five other parts of the house (from the front door, from the back door) to the bathroom.
   If your child refuses to do the positive practice trials or has a temper tantrum, training should proceed as normal. Continue the positive practice with praise when the child is doing well.
3. Make your child responsible for cleaning up.
   With a minimum of guidance, require your child to remove his or her wet pants.
   Guide your child to put the wet clothing in an appropriate place.
   If needed, have your child take a quick bath.
   Guide your child to put on clean clothes.
4. After correcting child, do not continue to talk about it. Start with a clean slate.
5. Remember to praise and hug your child when he or she urinates in the toilet/potty chair.

Adapted from Azrin NH, Foxx RM: Toilet Training in Less than a Day. New York, Pocket Books, 1974. Copyright © 1974 by Nathan H. Azrin, PhD, and Richard M. Foxx, PhD. Excerpted and adapted by permission of Simon & Schuster Adult Publishing Group, and Georges Borchardt, Inc., for the author.

knowledge, DDAVP is inferior to conditioning alarms as a primary therapy. DDAVP and antidepressants are a second line of management when the alarm has failed or is impractical. For children who are known responders to medication, it can be used for special occasions, such as sleepovers and camps.

Strategies for Maximizing Adherence

As with most interventions, adherence by the patient to the treatment recommendations is vital for its success. Health care providers can maximize the potential for success in adherence by following some simple suggestions. First, they must provide verbal and written information at a level that is understandable to the parent and child, allowing enough time to describe adequately the procedures and their importance. Second, providers must answer any questions the parents and child might have and question further on any potential barriers to success that the parents or child may indicate as concerns. Written summaries of treatment recommendations also are helpful. Each of the boxes in this chapter could be used as examples of written treatment summaries to be provided to patients.

Parents can be asked to keep track of treatment components at home to facilitate adherence and communication about progress. The provider can design a symptom rating sheet similar to Fig. 252-1. This form provides parents with a place to record each of the components of the daily procedures. The parents may be asked to record each time they require their child to complete a positive practice trial. Part of the rationale for these sheets is that each time the parents complete the symptoms for that day, they are reminded of all of the components that they have been asked to address.

FOLLOW-UP

Parents can be asked to follow up on the behavioral interventions by return appointments, by completing and returning symptom recording sheets, or both. Adherence typically is better, particularly with complex regimens, if the parents are provided with the kind of structure discussed in the preceding paragraph.

Mini-index of Related Topics

SUGGESTED READINGS

Cendron M: Primary nocturnal enuresis: Current concepts. Am Fam Physician 1999;57:1205–1218.

Christophersen ER: Pediatric Compliance: A Guide for the Primary Care Physician. New York, Plenum, 1994.

Christophersen ER, Mortweet SL: Treatments That Work: Empirically Supported Strategies for Managing Childhood Problems. Washington, DC, APA Books, 2001.

Glicklich LB: An historical account of enuresis. Pediatrics 1951; 8:859–876.

Luxem MC, Christophersen ER: Elimination disorders. In Netherton S, Holmes D, Walker CE (eds): Child and Adolescent Psychological Disorders: A Comprehensive Textbook. New York, Oxford, 1999, pp 195–223.

Moffatt ME: Nocturnal enuresis: A review of the efficacy of treatments and practical advice for clinicians. J Dev Behav Pediatr 1997; 18:49–56.

SECTION 7   MENTAL HEALTH CARE: *Feeding, Eating, and Elimination Behaviors*

254 Eating Problems and Disorders

Estherann Grace

■ ROLE OF THE GENERALIST

1. Recognize patients with eating disorders.
2. Perform appropriate history and physical examination on patients suspected of having an eating disorder.
3. Diagnose eating disorders.
4. Refer patients with eating disorders to appropriate eating disorders consultants for assistance in diagnosis and long-term management.

FUNDAMENTALS

An estimated 5 million Americans are affected by eating disorders annually. Anorexia nervosa, bulimia nervosa, and binge eating disorder are thought to be the consequence of a cultural obsession with thinness equaling beauty. Previously limited to the affluent upper class, eating disorders cross socioeconomic, racial, and ethnic barriers. In girls age 15 to 19, anorexia nervosa is the third most common chronic disease after obesity and asthma. Bulimia affects approximately 20% of adolescent girls and frequently

Box 254-1. Complications of Eating Disorders

Cardiovascular

- Bradycardia
- Congestive heart failure
- Dysrhythmias
- Electrocardiographic abnormalities
- Ipecac-induced cardiomyopathy
- Mitral valve prolapse
- Pericardial effusion
- Orthostatic hypotention

Dermatologic

- Acrocyanosis
- Brittle hair and nails
- Carotene pigmentation
- Edema
- Hair loss
- Lanugo hair
- Russell's sign

Endocrine

- Amenorrhea
- Diabetes insipidus
- Growth retardation
- Hypercortisolism
- Hypothermia
- Low triiodothyronine syndrome
- Pubertal delay

Gastrointestinal

- Acute pancreatitis
- Barrett esophagus
- Bloody diarrhea
- Constipation
- Delayed gastric emptying
- Esophageal or gastric rupture
- Esophagitis
- Fatty infiltration and focal necrosis of liver
- Gallstones
- Intestinal atony
- Mallory-Weiss tears
- Parotid hypertrophy
- Perforation/rupture of the stomach
- Perimolysis and increased incidence of dental caries
- Superior mesenteric artery syndrome

Hematologic

- Bone marrow suppression
- Impaired cell-mediated immunity
- Low sedimentation rate

Neurologic

- Cortical atrophy
- Myopathy
- Peripheral neuropathy
- Seizures

Skeletal

- Osteopenia
- Osteoporosis
- Osteoporotic fracture

---

continues well into adulthood. Although eating disorders typically present in adolescent girls, 10% of cases are boys. Anorexia and bulimia often coexist: Individuals with anorexia binge and purge, whereas 30% to 80% of bulimics report restrictive eating patterns.

The etiology is unknown. Contributing factors include genetic, neurochemical, psychodevelopmental, and sociocultural. Personal dissatisfaction with their appearance begins for many adolescents as they complete puberty. Surveys reveal 50% of girls by age 18 perceive themselves as fat even though they are normal weight. Age of initiating dieting is decreasing. Studies of 9- to 12-year-olds have found 75% admit to dieting in the past year.

Primary care providers caring for adolescent girls and young women see patients with eating disorders. Knowledge of a community reference base is essential. A base of nutritional and psychological consultants willing to accept patients in treatment when a condition is recognized is essential. Time constraints and insurance restrictions make the services of eating disorders consultants invaluable

(Box 254-1). Box 254-2 lists factors that predict risk for development of an eating disorder.

ANOREXIA NERVOSA

The diagnostic criteria for anorexia nervosa include weight loss in excess of 15% ideal body weight, the relentless pursuit of thinness, distorted body image, and amenorrhea (absence of three consecutive cycles in postmenarcheal adolescent girls and women). Two subtypes of anorexic patients have been identified:

1. Restrictive—individuals who lose weight by decreasing their calorie intake
2. Binge/purge subtypes—individuals who binge and purge (vomiting, laxative use, diuretic use) to control their weight

Diagnosis

Medical assessment of anorexia nervosa focuses on the history of the behavior (i.e., its onset, duration, associated symptoms and signs). Patients frequently report amenorrhea before an actual weight loss sufficient to reduce the percentage of body fat to less than 20%. The patient should be questioned on her weight (maximum/minimum/ideal), satisfaction with how she looks (body image), exercise regimen, diet history, sexual history/orientation, laxatives/diet pills, substance abuse, binge/purge behaviors, and depression symptoms.

The physical examination begins with vital signs and a height and weight with all clothing removed. Box 254-3

Box 254-2. Predictive Factors to Developing an Eating Disorder

- Family history of eating disorders
- Psychological traits of perfectionism, obsessive-compulsive disorder, addictive disorder, depression
- Dissatisfaction with body image and poor self-esteem
- History of sexual abuse

lists physical findings in patients with anorexia nervosa. The appropriateness of the weight is determined by the patient's height, bone structure, and body mass index. Findings on physical examination typical of anorexia nervosa include low body temperature, bradycardia, orthostatic hypotension, dry skin with lanugo hair, acrocyanosis, parotid swelling (secondary to vomiting), abnormal dentition with gum recession, breast atrophy, mitral valve prolapse, scaphoid abdomen with retained stool, ankle and leg edema, and absence of fat pads over the scapulae. The consequences of malnutrition in a patient with anorexia are determined by the severity of the starvation and its duration (see Box 254-1). The associated mortality rate at 0.56% per year is more than 12 times the death rate in the general population of young women.

Young women seeking gynecologic care require screening for anorexia nervosa when they present with a history of amenorrhea for more than three cycles, vague abdominal discomfort associated with constipation, decreased food intake with resultant weight loss, depressed affect, and the characteristic findings on physical/gynecologic examination. Gynecologic examination shows the consequences of reduced estrogen (i.e., atrophic vaginitis). If indicated in the sexually active patient, pregnancy testing and sexually transmitted disease screening are obtained. The differential diagnosis should cover briefly new-onset diabetes; adrenal insufficiency; primary depression; inflammatory bowel disease; abdominal masses, which may cause chronic vomiting; central nervous system lesions, which may cause vomiting; appetite suppression; and a depressed affect. Screening office laboratory studies include complete blood count, electrolytes, glucose, thyroxine, thyroid-stimulating hormone, phosphorus, magnesium, and erythrocyte sedimentation rate.

Treatment

A team approach is recommended to treat a patient with anorexia nervosa. The treatment team consists of a medical provider, a therapist, and a nutritionist. In pediatric patients, a family therapist is recommended to help family members deal with the illness. Some patients prefer working in a group therapy setting. Treatment occurs in an outpatient setting or an inpatient program. Typically, it takes several years to guide the patient to resolution of the eating disorder. Medication has been used over the years.

Box 254-3. Physical Findings in Anorexia Nervosa

- Weight loss to the point of cachexia
- Hypothermia
- Bradycardia
- Orthostatic hypotension
- Acrocyanosis
- Dry, flaky skin with lanugo hair
- Nail destruction
- Scaphoid abdomen with retained stool
- Mitral value prolapse and murmur
- Ankle and leg edema
- Absent fat pad over scapulae

Selective serotonin reuptake inhibitors are the preferred treatment at this time. There are no studies that prove a selective serotonin reuptake inhibitor makes a causal difference in the outcome of the illness. Long-term multicenter trials are currently under way. Clinically, many patients with anorexia have shown an improvement in their depressive symptoms when taking a selective serotonin reuptake inhibitor.

The long-term recovery outcome depends on the individual dealing with the illness. About 50% experience a full recovery, 30% experience a partial recovery, and 20% show no improvement. Patients who show no improvement remain in their anorexia behavioral patterns for life.

BULIMIA NERVOSA

The word *bulimia* originates from the Greek meaning "ox appetite." Patients with bulimia nervosa consume large amounts of food, frequently in secret, and then purge to compensate for the volume consumed. There is an associated perceived lack of control over the amount and type of food eaten. Purging bulimics frequently resort to laxatives and diuretics in a further attempt to reduce the effect of the caloric overload. In contrast to patients with anorexia, who feel elated with control of their intake, bulimics experience depression over their inability to stop the bingeing and purging. Another significant psychological difference between anorexics and bulimics is asking for help. Bulimic patients often are disgusted with their behavior and want help in stopping it, whereas anorexic patients identify with their eating disorder and resist treatment efforts.

Diagnosis

Patients with bulimia nervosa are not recognized easily. They typically are normal to slightly overweight. Consequently, it is important to ask during a patient encounter if there is a history of vomiting or use of laxatives or diuretics to control weight. Bulimia can start at any age and frequently continues well into adult life. The incidence among older women is not known. Because the physical findings can be subtle, in contrast to the obvious weight loss of an anorexic patient, eating behaviors should be included in the review of systems during routine health care. A convenient time to inquire is during the abdominal examination.

The physical examination of a patient with bulimia is frequently normal (Box 254-4). Weight for height is within 10% to 20% of the expected standard. When signs and symptoms are present, they result from the mechanical effects of vomiting and laxative/diuretic abuse. Typical findings include scalp hair loss (diffuse thinning), scleral hemorrhages, gum disease, enamel erosion of the teeth, linear scars on the anterior tonsillar pillars, enlarged salivary glands, scars on fingers (Russell's sign), and increased bowel sounds secondary to laxatives.

Consequences of purging may be life-threatening, particularly hypokalemia and hypophosphatemia. Gastrointestinal malfunctions include pancreatitis, esophagitis and esophageal rupture, Mallory-Weiss lesions, paralytic ileus secondary to laxative abuse, and cathartic colon. Lowered magnesium causes muscle cramps, weakness, and restlessness. Pulmonary

Box 254-4. Physical Findings in Bulimia

- Usually normal weight to slightly overweight
- Thinning of hair (scalp)
- Periodontal disease (gum disease and enamel erosion of teeth)
- Scleral hemorrhages
- Enlarged salivary glands (parotids)
- Scars on fingers (Russell sign)
- Increased bowel sounds (secondary to laxatives)

complications of aspiration pneumonia and pneumomediastinum are due to vomiting.

The laboratory evaluation of a patient with bulimia includes complete blood count, electrolytes, blood urea nitrogen and creatinine, glucose, calcium, phosphorus, and magnesium. An electrocardiogram and rhythm strip is obtained when electrolytes are suspected to be abnormal.

Treatment

Treatment involves a team approach with medical supervision, psychological therapy, and nutritional counseling. The prognosis remains guarded because of the habituation and ease of performing the behavior. A positive family history of bulimia often is found extending back for several generations.

In contrast to anorexic patients, patients with bulimia usually have menstrual cycles, although they may tend to be irregular. Because of the impulsive nature of the bulimic, safe sex may not always be practiced, warranting a careful eating history in patients with sexually transmitted diseases and unplanned pregnancies.

BINGE EATING DISORDER

Binge eating disorder is a variant of bulimia nervosa. The patient with binge eating disorder also consumes large quantities of food, but rather than purging may engage in other inappropriate compensatory behaviors, such as excessive exercise or prolonged fasting. Research has shown that dieting (fasting), chronic restrained eating, and excessive exercise may be important triggers for binge eating disorder. Binge eating disorder is relatively common in the general population. The rates are comparable among black women, white women, and white men, but lower among black men.

Morbid obesity is associated more commonly with binge eating disorder than with bulimia. The incidence of obesity in the United States is rising, with only 40% of the population considered to be at normal weight. The increasing obesity in childhood has altered the definition and

Box 254-5. Physical Findings in Binge Eating Disorder

- Obesity
- Elevated blood pressure
- Acanthosis nigricans secondary to obesity
- Striae usually on abdomen, hips, thighs
- No abnormal findings expected if weight is appropriate for height

management of type 2 diabetes, a complication of obesity. The implications for the gynecologist of an elevated insulin level in an obese young woman with the subsequent risk of polycystic ovary syndrome are obvious.

Diagnosis

Binge eating disorder has a persistent course, often is associated with comorbid psychopathology (depression), and contributes to medical complications. Because a patient with binge eating disorder is not purging, he or she avoids the risks associated with vomiting, laxatives, and diuretics. The consequence of massive caloric intake often results in obesity, however, with its attendant complications. Obese adolescent girls present with menstrual irregularities (a direct effect of their obesity with elevated insulin level contributing to polycystic ovary syndrome). The other deleterious effects of obesity include cardiovascular, pulmonary, and musculoskeletal disease. Essentially no body function is spared the negative outcome of obesity. Box 254-5 lists possible positive findings on physical examination.

Identifying a patient with binge eating disorder requires a history sensitive to the issue of bingeing. The patient with binge eating disorder often has an associated psychological diagnosis; depression is common.

Obese patients with binge eating disorder have the laboratory profile typical of the morbidly obese. The fasting insulin level is elevated. The serum glucose also may be abnormally high if type 2 diabetes has developed. The cholesterol, high-density lipoprotein and low-density lipoprotein cholesterol, and triglycerides may be abnormal. Liver function tests reflect fatty degeneration of the liver when present. For the binge eating disorder patient with normal weight, the body's compensatory mechanisms normalize the laboratory values.

Treatment

Research on the etiology of binge eating disorder suggests that treatment should focus on healthy weight-control techniques, ignoring the media's sociocultural pressures to be thin, eliminating the thin ideal of beauty, and improving self-esteem, particularly of adolescent girls. There has been case-based evidence that selective serotonin reuptake inhibitors decrease the number of binge episodes at least for the first 2 months of treatment. Long-term studies are not available at this time. The mechanism of selective serotonin reuptake inhibitors has not been identified as yet.

FEMALE ATHLETE TRIAD

In 1992, the American College of Sports Medicine coined the term *female athlete triad*, which consists of disordered eating, amenorrhea, and osteoporosis. The disordered eating ranges from severe restricting and purging to obsessive avoidance of fat and chemical preservatives. Amenorrhea in athletes is the absence of three or more consecutive menstrual cycles in a postpubertal adolescent girl or woman. Athletes excessively training before puberty may delay menarche. Oligomenorrhea is a common finding is female athletes. The premature bone loss and inadequate bone formation characterizes osteoporosis in the athlete. These young women experience a reduction in bone mass, the microarchitecture of the bone deteriorates, and the skeleton becomes fragile and results in an increased risk of fractures. Athletes most at risk of developing the triad are those in whom a low body weight and lean physique are desired (gymnast, figure skater, ballet dancer, and runner).

The prevalence of disordered eating in female athletes varies from 15% to 62%. The incidence of premature osteoporosis is unknown. In a young athlete with delayed menarche, immature bone ages have been noted. In ballet dancers with primary amenorrhea, an increased risk of stress fractures and scoliosis has been reported. Female athlete triad disorders can decrease physical performance and cause morbidity and mortality. Further research is needed to identify its causes, prevalence, and consequences.

Diagnosis

Box 254-6 lists physical signs of female athlete triad. Exercise favors bone formation; weight-bearing exercise is most effective. When excessive exercise leads to amenorrhea, however, the benefits are lost. Amenorrhea associated with a low estrogen level results in low bone mineral density. Normal estrogen levels are essential in maintaining normal bone density. Studies show that athletes with regular menstrual cycles have higher bone density than amenorrheic athletes. The impact of anorexia nervosa on skeletal health is significant. Patients with anorexia nervosa have a bone mineral density 25% lower than age-matched controls. Bone density of trabecular bone (spine and femoral neck) may remain low even after recovery to a normal weight. There is a direct correlation between the duration of anorexia and osteoporosis. The demineralization of bones in the too-thin athlete is rapid, often noted within 6 months of onset of weight loss and amenorrhea.

Treatment

The management of the female athlete triad stresses healthy behaviors while supporting the young woman's interest in sports. Athletic participation and exercise are healthy. It is inappropriate to deny participation in sports because of the risk of developing the female athlete triad. When recognized, however, prompt intervention is advised. As with the other eating disorders, proper nutrition is essential, including an adequate intake of calcium (1300 mg daily). Studies have supported a positive relationship between calcium intake and normal bone density. An athlete with amenorrhea poses a particular treatment dilemma. Estrogen deficiency is associated with increased bone resorption and eventual bone loss. Estrogen replacement therapy has not been consistently effective in halting or correcting osteoporosis.

Box 254-6. Physical Findings in Female Athlete Triad

- Typically a fit athletic appearance
- Low percentage of body fat
- Well-developed muscle mass
- Bradycardia without orthostasis
- Low range of blood pressure, but not orthostatic
- Typical effects of low estrogen level on skin, hair, vagina
- Spontaneous fractures or secondary to minimal trauma

Box 254-7. Prognostic Outcomes of Eating Disorder

Good Prognostic Signs

- Young age at onset
- Prompt diagnosis
- Treatment team availability
- Absence of severe family dysfunction

Poor Outcomes

- Older age at onset
- Delay in diagnosis
- Resistance by patient to seek treatment or follow recommendations
- Failure of outpatient and inpatient treatment programs
- Longevity of disordered eating patterns

TREATMENT FOR EATING DISORDERS

A team approach is recommended for the outpatient treatment of all types of eating disorders. The treatment team includes the primary health care provider, individual therapist, nutritionist, and family therapist for the younger adolescent. The team communicates regularly on the patient's progress. For many providers, e-mail has simplified the process. Goals of treatment are identified and negotiated with the patient. The criteria for medical or psychological admission also are identified clearly for the patient and her family. The medical admission usually is based on the failure to comply with the meal plan resulting in further weight loss and a deterioration of vital signs.

A variety of inpatient programs exist throughout the United States. Emphasis is placed on the physical and the psychological needs of the patient. Many inpatient programs also have a step-down program, which allows a gradual reentry of the patient into her usual lifestyle. These day programs provide the additional support needed around meal times.

To date, there are no long-term studies specifically identifying a medication that treats eating disorders. The serotonin reuptake class of drugs has shown to have some benefit in the short term (<4 months) for decreasing bulimic behavior. These drugs also have proved helpful in treating the depression and obsessive-compulsive ideation frequently seen in patients with eating disorders. Large multicenter trials are ongoing.

Estrogen replacement is advocated after 1 year of amenorrhea. The available studies have not confirmed a definitive corrective benefit in osteoporosis. There are other secondary gains, however, to normalizing the estrogen level (improve sense of well-being, muscle strength, decreased libido, sleep disturbance, and night sweats).

For the severely restrictive patient, a multivitamin and calcium supplements are advised. A stool softener also is recommended because anorexic patients often are constipated because of decreased gut motility secondary to starvation. Box 254-7 lists factors associated with the eventual outcome of eating disorders.

PREVENTION

Ideally, eating disorders would never occur, eliminating the need for treatment. Because the definitive etiology is unknown, prevention remains a mystery. The societal factors are present in all women's lives, yet not all women have an eating disorder. A familial tendency and characteristic personality traits have been noted. In general terms, emphasizing a healthy lifestyle, avoiding extremes, and reinforcing the belief that all body types are acceptable provide young women with a positive environment. Extreme thinness as a beauty criterion must end. Primary care providers play a vital role in promoting young women's health. Primary care providers have the opportunity to provide the structured guidance young women need to counteract society's unrealistic expectations. A few simple guidelines for parents of young children are listed in Box 254-8.

Box 254-8. Preventive Measures Guidance for Parents

1. From infancy, avoid using food as a reward.
2. Focus on health, not weight.
3. If weight is an issue in a young child, encourage healthy eating patterns and exercise; discourage fad diets.
4. Foster self-esteem based on the child's self-work, not on his or her weight; reinforce the child's talents; eliminate unnecessary criticism.
5. Share meals in a calm social atmosphere; delay discussion of stressful issues until the meal is over.
6. Communicate concerns openly if there are symptoms of an eating disorder, and seek professional help.

 Additional Resources, CD-ROM

Bibliography

Mini-index of Related Topics CH.

SUGGESTED READINGS

Abraham S, Llewellyn-Jones D: Eating Disorders: The Facts, 4th ed. New York, Oxford University Press, 1997.

Fisher M, Golden N, Katzman D, et al: Eating disorders in adolescents: A background paper. J Adolesc Health 1995;16:420–437.

Powers PS: Initial assessment and early treatment options for anorexia nervosa and bulimia nervosa. Psychiatr Clin North Am 1996;19: 639–655.

Putukian M: The female athlete triad. Clin Sports Med 1998;17: 675–686.

Woodside DB: A review of anorexia nervosa and bulimia nervosa. Curr Probl Pediatr 1995;25:67–89.

255 Sexual Development, Sexual Orientation, and Gender Identity Issues

Sergio R. Russo Buzzini and Melanie A. Gold

ROLE OF THE GENERALIST

1. Promote healthy sexual development in children and adolescents.
2. Recognize normal and abnormal sexual behaviors.
3. Provide appropriate anticipatory guidance for child and adolescent sexual development.
4. Facilitate parent-child understanding and communication about normal childhood sexuality.
5. Offer responsive care to lesbian, gay, bisexual, and transgender youth.
6. Provide assistance and support in negotiating individual, familial, and societal conflicts and problem areas.
7. Refer patients to a health care provider who can provide comprehensive, nonjudgmental care to patients if you are unable to do so because of religious or other personal beliefs.

FUNDAMENTALS

Terms used in the literature to describe sexuality issues often are unclear. For this chapter, the term *sex* is used to refer to the classification as male or female based on external anatomy, such as the penis and testes or vulva. The term *gender* is used to refer to the psychological experience of being male and female (Box 255-1).

In humans and other mammals, genetic sex is determined at fertilization by the sex chromosome of the sperm. The embryonic gonad and the external genitalia are bipotential structures until 6 weeks' gestation with the 46,XX and 46,XY embryos each possessing a set of wolffian ducts and müllerian ducts. The undifferentiated embryonic gonads develop into testes under the influence of testes-determining factor (TDF). The locus for the TDF is the sex-determining region of the Y chromosome (SRY). In the absence of SRY, female differentiation occurs. The fetal testes produce testosterone in the Leydig cells and müllerian inhibiting factor in the Sertoli cells at the time of internal duct differentiation. A fetus with functional testes suppresses the müllerian ductal system and has concomitant development

of the wolffian system. The wolffian ductal system forms the epididymis, vas deferens, and seminal vesicles. A fetus with functional ovaries develops the müllerian duct system to form the fallopian tubes, uterus, cervix, and upper portion of the vagina with concomitant regression of the wolffian duct system (Fig. 255-1).

Timing is crucial for masculinization of external genitalia. Masculinization typically begins at 7 weeks of gestation. If androgens are not present by week 12 or later, full masculinization cannot take place. Although testosterone promotes the growth of the wolffian ducts, dihydrotestosterone, produced by the conversion of testosterone in the skin of the external genitalia, is necessary to develop and masculinize the external genital structures.

The mammalian brain also begins as a bipotential structure with regard to gender and develops under the influence of gonadal steroid hormones. Male sexual differentiation of the brain occurs in the presence of sufficient amounts of

---

Box 255-1. Definitions

1. *Sex*—the classification as either male or female based on external anatomy, such as the penis and testes or vulva
2. *Gender identity*—the personal sense of one's integral maleness or femaleness
3. *Gender role*—behaviors within a culture commonly thought to be associated with maleness or femaleness
4. *Sexual orientation*—the persistent pattern of emotional or physical attraction (or both) to members of the same or opposite sex (included are *homosexuality* [same-sex attractions], *bisexuality* [attraction to members of both sexes], and *heterosexuality* [opposite-sex attractions])
5. *Transsexual*—an individual whose gender identity does not match his or her anatomic sex (often the individual may seek to alter his or her physical appearance to that of the other biologic sex; these individuals may prefer to be called *transgendered*)
6. *Transvestite*—an individual for whom dressing in the clothing of the other sex is experienced as a form of sexual arousal
7. *Homophobia*—the unprovoked fear, distrust, or hatred of lesbian or gay people
8. *Heterosexism*—the institutional and societal reinforcement of heterosexuality as the privileged and powerful norm
9. *Coming out*—the process of recognizing one's homosexuality and sharing that information with others

Table 255-2. Typical Adolescent Sexuality

Age Category	Developmental Issues	Anticipatory Guidance

Early adolescence, 12–13 yr	Concerns regarding menstruation and nocturnal emissions
	Increased curiosity and concern with their own bodies and the bodies of others
	Increased need for privacy
	Sexual fantasies begin and may be a source of emotional discomfort or guilt
	Masturbation becomes more common and may be a source of guilt; normal adolescents may or may not engage in masturbation
	Nonphysical sexual activities (double dates, phone calls) predominate; however, early adolescents may engage in a range of sexual behavior, including open-mouth kissing, sexual fondling, simulated intercourse, sexual penetration behaviors, and intercourse
	Heterosexual and homosexual experimentation are common
	During early adolescence and later adolescence, youth struggle to define when they are ready for sex; what is important in relationships; how to say no to sex; and how do they deal with frustration, rejection, and loneliness
		Discuss advantages of abstinence in youth
		  Offer support and suggestions for managing peer pressure, emphasizing the youth's right to refuse and/or discontinue sexual contact
		Inform adolescents about sexual issues
		  Reproductive anatomy and physiology
		  Sexual functioning (debunking common myths and educating youth regarding alternatives to intercourse)
		  Health consequences of sexual intercourse
		  Relationship between sex, contraception, and pregnancy
		  STD prevention
		  Range of human relationships
		  Components of decision making
		  Importance of self-esteem and respect
		  Emotional aspects of sexual activity
		  Availability of resources to address current and future concerns
		Screen for difficulties in negotiating sexuality that may require multidisciplinary intervention (i.e., unwanted activity, discomfort with recognition of sexual orientation)
		Educate parents regarding adolescent/parent roles and boundaries, role of sexuality in adolescent growth and development, role of values in adolescent decision making, and role of self-esteem in parent-adolescent relationships

Middle adolescence 14–16 yr	High degree of sexual energy and emphasis on contact sexual behavior Sexual behavior may be of an explorative and/or exploitative nature Dating and petting common Coital and noncoital contact may be part of relationships Recognition of same-sex attraction occurs for many gay and lesbian youth. Recognition may precipitate severe depression for youth Consequences of sexual behavior are typically denied General acceptance of body and concern over making body more attractive	Discuss the advantages of abstinence Empower adolescents to report abuse and to refuse unwanted sexual activity Assist adolescents who want to avoid or discontinue sexual activity to plan and practice how they will manage social pressure Assist adolescents who are sexually active or planning to become sexually active to identify strategies for pregnancy and disease prevention Encourage sexually active adolescents to discuss their feelings regarding their experiences with parents and health care providers Discuss connection between sexual activity and intimacy Continue to address educational needs of youth regarding sexuality issues
Late adolescence, 17–21 yr	Shift in sexual behavior from an emphasis on personal needs to intimacy and giving Intimacy in relationships may develop Acceptance of pubertal changes	Discuss advantages of abstinence Remind adolescents that fewer lifetime partners lowers health risks Assist adolescents who want to avoid or discontinue sexual activity to plan and practice how they will manage social pressure Assist adolescents who are sexually active or planning to become sexually active to identify strategies for pregnancy and disease prevention Emphasize appropriateness of saying no to sexual activity Discuss relevant health issues with special populations (gay, lesbian, bisexual, and transgender youth) Continue to address educational needs of youth regarding sexuality issues

Guidelines for abnormal sexual behavior among adolescents are similar to the guidelines used for adults and can be found in the most recent edition of the *Diagnostic and Statistical Manual of Mental Disorders* (DSM-IV-TR) under Sexual Dysfunction, Paraphilias, and Sexual Disorder Not Otherwise Specified. Providers also can help facilitate parent-child understanding and communication about normal childhood sexuality during routine well-child care visits. The pediatrician can play a role in teaching parents to find opportunities to discuss sexual matters by actively inviting questions about sexuality when the child seems ready and by providing information to parents to share with their children when they are asked about sexual matters.

For older children and adolescents, including topics such as love and caring in discussions on sexual matters places sexuality in a broader context. This can shape healthy sexual values and may prevent premature sexual activity.

Pediatricians are increasingly aware of the influence of the media (television, music lyrics, and Internet) on child development. The American Academy of Pediatrics' position on children and the media supports the use of broadcast industry standards to provide guidelines for developmentally appropriate exposure to sexual content. Parents should be encouraged to help their child to understand sexual media content and to discern unrealistic, inaccurate, and misleading portrayals of sexuality. Media depictions of sexuality may serve as the basis for discussion, whereby parents may teach their children to recognize sex as a healthy and natural part of life; to realize that not all affection and touching must lead to intercourse; to identify love, affection, and respect as important components of sexual activity and sexual relationships; to recognize that there are consequences of unprotected sex; to understand that violence is not a part of a loving relationship; and to know that individuals have the right to "say no" and have their wishes recognized and respected.

Parents who repress or project unacceptable thoughts and feelings regarding their own sexual impulses and conflicts may find it difficult to acknowledge or accept their child's normal expression of sexuality. By supporting parents' acceptance of their own sexuality, the pediatrician can facilitate the parents' ability to accept their child's normal expressions of sexuality. Physicians have the opportunity to serve as a role model for parents by showing appropriate openness and initiative in discussing sexual issues with children in the office setting. Asking parents questions about sexual functioning in the review of symptoms of the urogenital or gynecologic portion of the medical interview or the examination can convey that sexual issues are normal and acceptable topics for the pediatrician to discuss with parents and children.

For older children and adolescents, the ideal time for eliciting a sexual history is when the pediatrician is gathering psychosocial information during the medical interview. Introducing the topic of sexuality should be gradual. A helpful place to start can be to ask about sexual attraction or the sexual behavior of peers and the adolescent's attitudes about these behaviors (Box 255-2). Asking abrupt questions about sex without explaining the health reasons for eliciting the information can be anxiety provoking and offensive unless the reason for the visit is of a sexual nature. Never inquiring about sexual attraction or behaviors puts an excessive burden on the adolescent, who may have a sexual concern but feel too embarrassed to bring it up.

In the process of eliciting a sexual history, rapport must be established and caring and respect conveyed for the adolescent and his or her concerns. Before asking questions related to sexuality, the physician should discuss with youth the issue of confidentiality and the limits of confidentiality (e.g., requirements to report sexual abuse and statutory rape and issues about parents' access to medical records). Asking permission to discuss issues related to sexuality and sexual behavior can be a useful way of transitioning to the topic and respecting the patient's right to determine when he or she is ready to discuss it. When exploring issues related to sexual behavior, the physician should ask questions in a manner that does not presume heterosexuality by using words such as *partner* instead of *boyfriend* or *girlfriend*. Sexual attraction and comfort with sexual feelings should be assessed separately from sexual behavior. Individuals who have same-sex attraction may prefer to be called *lesbian* or *gay* rather than homosexual. Permission should be obtained from the patients as to whether they wish information about sexual orientation recorded in the medical record, especially if access to the medical record cannot be limited or privacy cannot be guaranteed. When discussing sexual organs and behaviors, simple and specific

---

Box 255-2. Ways to Ask Questions for an Adolescent Sexual History

Obtaining Patient Permission to Discuss Issues Related to Sexuality

- Is it okay if we discuss some sexual issues and how they relate to your health?
- Are any of your friends having sex? How do you feel about that?

Questions about Sexual Attraction

- When you think of people to whom you are sexually attracted, are they guys, girls, or both, or are you not sure yet?
- Do you feel comfortable with your sexual feelings?

Questions about Sexual Behavior

- Have you ever had the kind of sex where someone did the following:
  - Kissed your mouth with their mouth open?
  - Touched you breasts with their hands or mouth?
  - Put their mouth on your penis/vagina?
  - Put a penis inside your vagina?
  - Put a penis in your rectum or anus?
- Are you satisfied with what you do sexually with your partner?

Questions about Sexual Function

- Do you ever have problems getting sexually aroused, meaning getting an erection (hard) or ejaculating (coming) [for boys] or getting lubricated (wet) or having an orgasm [for girls]?
- Do you ever have pain when you have sex?

Questions about Sexual Abuse

- Has anyone ever touched you in a sexual way that made you feel uncomfortable or was against your will? When did this happen? Was it ever reported to anyone? To whom?
- Does that experience still affect your day-to-day life? Does it ever get in the way of close or intimate relationships with others?

---

language should be used. Pediatricians should avoid using medical or technical language, such as *penetration* and *ovulation*, and avoid slang or words that might offend, such as *promiscuous* or *sodomy*. The pediatrician should ensure that he or she and the patient understand the terminology used in communicating about sexual issues. Box 255-2 gives some examples of appropriate questions that can be used when taking a sexual history from an adolescent. The pediatrician should consider his or her own personal sexual history, beliefs, and attitudes regarding sexuality and the role these may have in how he or she assesses and counsels about sexuality and sexual behavior. Care must be taken to avoid projecting one's own beliefs, attitudes, or discomforts regarding sexuality on parents and youth.

SEXUAL ORIENTATION AND GENDER IDENTITY ISSUES

Development of Sexual Orientation

Much is known about the embryologic development of the genital tract and the influence of hormones on sexual desire, but substantially less is known about the determinants of sexual orientation. Sexual orientation is thought to be formed by a complicated interaction of social, cultural, biologic, economic, and political factors. Despite the fact that sexual

Table 255-3. Stages of Homosexual Identity Development with Suggested Counseling Interventions

Identity Stages	Possible Feelings/Behaviors	Counseling Interventions
Sensitization	Awareness of generalized feeling of being different from or unlike same-sex peers Usually occurs before puberty Gender-neutral or opposite-gender sexual attraction Do not see homosexuality as personally relevant	Provide support and an opportunity to discuss "feeling different" Discourage premature self-labeling Explore and build self-esteem

Confusion	Inner turmoil and confusion associated with same-sex attractions, dreams, and fantasies
	Responses to identity confusion may include denial, avoidance, and redefinition
		All of above, plus
		  Explore fears, anxieties, shame, or guilt
		  Raise awareness of the role of social stigma and issues of internalized homophobia

Acceptance	Self-definition as homosexual
	Increased contact with lesbian, gay, or bisexual peers
	Exploration of homosexual subculture
		All of above, plus
		  Affirm basic self-worth
		  Discourage sexual behavior with adults
		  Encourage safer sex practices (i.e., condom use, limiting number of sexual partners) if sexually active
		Explore coming-out issues
		Supply age-appropriate peer support resources
		Encourage connection with supportive heterosexuals

Pride	Positive self-esteem associated with a lesbian, gay, or bisexual identity	
Commitment	Homosexuality adopted as an identity	Support efforts to bridge gay/lesbian/bisexual self with aspects of identity

is more likely to be associated with symptoms such as depression or suicide attempts. The process of coming out for women is characterized by greater fluidity and ambiguity, perhaps because historically women have been allowed a broader range of emotional experimentation and behavior with other women.

Management

According to the 1993 American Academy of Pediatrics statement on homosexuality and adolescence, therapy directed specifically at changing sexual orientation is contraindicated. However, a recent study of more than 800 adults initially dissatisfied with their sexual orientation has

documented changes in homosexual thoughts and fantasies after psychotherapy or self-help. Large improvements in psychological, interpersonal, and spiritual well-being were reported. This study cannot be generalized beyond the samples used, but it may suggest a need for future research.

Pediatricians can offer responsive care to lesbian, gay, bisexual, and transgender (LGBT) youth by creating a comfortable office environment; serving as a resource for information and referral; and providing assistance and support in negotiating individual, familial, and societal conflicts and problem areas. The health care provider should not seek to identify all gay and lesbian youth, but rather create a comfortable environment in which they may seek

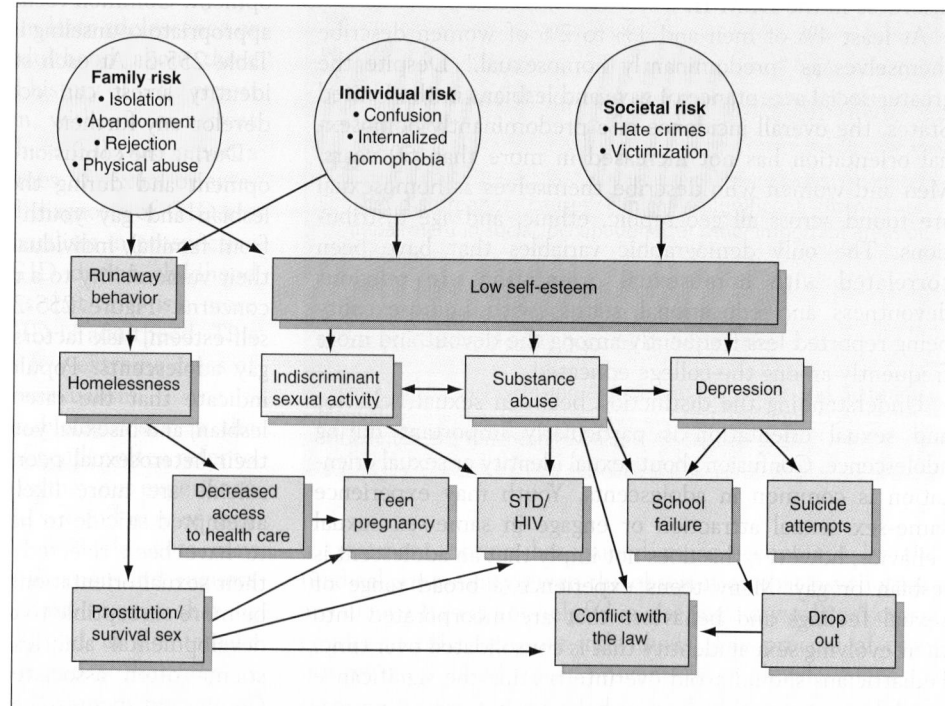

Figure 255-2. Vulnerabilities and risks of lesbian and gay adolescents.

help and support for appropriate medical care. LGBT youth should be accorded the right to disclose their sexual identity at their own pace. Creating an office that is a safe space to come out can be accomplished by providing visual cues, such as gay and lesbian health books, posters, brochures, and fliers in the office waiting room and examining rooms and hiring office staff and colleagues who are comfortable with and accepting of LGBT youth. Removing heterosexist language from forms and including nonheterosexist terms, such as *partner* instead of *boyfriend* or *girlfriend*, can communicate that an office is "gay-friendly." Posting a non-discrimination policy stating that the office appreciates diversity and does not discriminate based on race, age, religion, ability, sexual orientation, gender, or perceived gender signals that all patients will be treated with respect. Posting such a policy also communicates to gay and lesbian parents that their children will be treated in an appropriate nonbiased manner by the pediatrician and the office staff. Health care providers should keep an updated list of LGBT resources available to offer teens, and they should stay current on issues that affect the LGBT community.

Providers can play a key role in dispelling myths and correcting stereotypes with patients and families within the office and the community. Health care professionals should help adolescents transform a stigmatized identity into a positive one through referral to support groups and to mental health services when indicated. Lesbians and gay men who have an integrated positive identity show better psychological adjustment, greater satisfaction, higher self-concept, and lower rates of the risk factors listed in Figure 255-2 compared with individuals who experience conflict with their identity.

Family support is especially important for developing the self-esteem of LGBT youth. Some parents may not be prepared to support their child, however. Poor communication, parental grief or anger, parental fears, religious beliefs, homophobia, misinformation, and stereotyping can create a difficult situation for the teen and his or her family. The role of the pediatrician is to support and advocate for the well-being of the adolescent and to provide information and resources to the adolescent and his or her family when they are requested. The pediatrician should identify when a patient or his or her family is experiencing distress related to sexuality issues and should maintain an up-to-date referral list of mental health care professionals to whom youth and families in crisis can be referred if conflicts over sexuality issues arise.

Health care providers who are unable to offer comprehensive, nonjudgmental care to patients because of religious or other personal beliefs have a moral and legal obligation to refer patients to a health care provider who can offer such care. Physicians should be knowledgeable about the capacity of other health care providers to work with LGBT adolescents before making a referral and should follow-up with the patient to ensure that appropriate care was received.

Sexuality issues are important throughout the life span. Pediatricians are in a key position to provide support and guidance to facilitate healthy sexual development, to reduce morbidity and mortality associated with sexual behavior, and to coordinate with other professionals to meet youth needs.

Additional Resources, CD-ROM

Bibliography	
List of websites and organizational links	

Mini-index of Related Topics	CH.
■ PRINCIPLES OF GROWTH AND MATURATION	4
■ DISORDERS OF SEXUAL DIFFERENTIATION	152
■ DISORDERS OF THE GENITOURINARY SYSTEM IN THE NEWBORN	205

SUGGESTED READINGS

Frankowski BL, American Academy of Pediatrics Committee on Adolescence: Sexual orientation and adolescents. Pediatrics 2004; 113(6):1827–1832.

Friedrich WN, Fisher J, Broughton D, et al: Normative sexual behavior in children: A contemporary sample. Pediatrics 1998;101:E9.

Kinsey AC, Pomeroy WB, Martin CE: Sexual Behavior in the Human Male. Philadelphia, WB Saunders, 1948.

Kinsey AC, Pomeroy WB, Martin CE, et al: Sexual Behavior in the Human Female. Philadelphia, WB Saunders, 1953.

Nicolosi J, Byrd AD, Potts RW: Retrospective self-reports of changes in homosexual orientation: A consumer survey of conversion therapy clients. Psychol Rep 2000;86:1071–1088.

256
Influences of Community on Child Health and Well-being

Tom Tonniges

ROLE OF THE GENERALIST

1. Develop a perspective that enlarges the focus from one child to all children in the community.
2. Recognize that family, educational, social, cultural, spiritual, economic, environmental, and political forces act favorably or unfavorably, but always significantly, on the health of children.
3. Synthesize clinical practice and public health principles directed toward providing health care to a given child and promoting the health of all children within the context of the family, school, and community.
4. Make a commitment to use community resources to achieve optimal accessibility, appropriateness, and quality of services for all children and to advocate especially for children who lack access to care.
5. Integrate the professional role and duty of the pediatrician.

Since the 1970s, child health care professionals have had an increasing awareness of the impact of the community on child health and well-being. In the 1860s, Smith, an early pediatrician who practiced public health, recognized that improved child health would require clean water, improved sanitation, and disease-free food. Medical and pediatric training was through apprenticeships. The pioneers of pediatrics practiced what is now known as *community pediatrics*, the blending of clinical practice with public health practice at the interface of the child and family with the community. In the 21st century, the influences of the community on child health are recognized increasingly as the core for improving the overall health of children.

DEFINITION OF A COMMUNITY

Just as we have begun to develop an understanding of what constitutes the concept of family, we are beginning to recognize that the concept of community can be defined in many different ways. A *community* is a group of people that may be large or small and that share a common interest, set of experiences, or a common place.

A community often is seen as a geographic/political area. It can be a town (Rockport, Maine), part of a town (Cabrini Green in Chicago, Illinois), a county (Dade County, Florida), a region (panhandle of Nebraska), or a frontier (large area of Montana). Often "artificial" geographic/political boundaries can have a significant impact on child health. A child may not be able to access needed medical services provided under public assistance because although the child is geographically close to these services, he or she resides across the border in another state and is not entitled to the services. This child may be forced to travel long distances within the state to get needed services.

A community may represent a specific population. A child with cystic fibrosis and his or her family may have more in common with a similarly affected child and family than with the child and family who live next door. Because of this situation, there has been extensive development of local, state, and national advocacy groups that provide educational, emotional, and other support services for children with special health care needs.

With the advent of the Internet, worldwide virtual communities have developed overnight. From the standpoint of the public, this development is seen as positive. The general public can learn about the newest diagnostic and treatment modalities with the click of a button and connect with the world's experts on any disease or condition. From the child health care professional's perspective, this development has been a challenge. The virtual community allows the public to demand accountability from health care professionals like never before. Child health care professionals have an opportunity to use these new technologies to improve child health.

A community can be defined on a socioeconomic basis. Divorce, death, or change in employment can have an acute effect on a family. These changes can happen quickly and can affect the family's support network and financial status. Similarly, children born into low-income families often are found in communities with poor housing, increased safety risks (e.g., lead, violence), and poor schools. With poverty being a primary determinant of a child's health, a strong community can provide protective factors for the child and family.

A community can be built on a common heritage. Currently the United States is undergoing the largest increase in immigration in its history. Recent immigrants often live in poorer parts of urban communities. Living together frequently provides security, a sense of community, and a challenge in assimilating into the new culture. Often as the children of these families begin to adapt to the when they are viewed as a tool to inform the community and used over time with periodic reporting. This approach allows the community to do the following:

- See where they are making progress and monitor health conditions
- Prioritize the allocation of community resources by informing the resource allocation process of community-based organizations and programs, such as the United Way
- Educate the community
- Galvanize community members to make improvements in specific areas

Most communities develop their own measurements, suggesting that local community members know what are their biggest concerns. Key to the success of a community health report card is connecting the results to a process that leads to improved community health.

The Community Health Status Indicators Project provides local health data in the form of a status report via the World Wide Web. The project is a collaborative effort among the Association of State and Territorial Health Officials, NACCHO, and Public Health Foundation and is supported and funded by the U.S. Department of Health and Human Services Health Resources and Services Administration. The project publishes reports for all 3082 counties in the United States. This project also provides suggestions of peer counties for comparison purposes.

CORE PRINCIPLES OF THE INFLUENCE OF THE COMMUNITY ON CHILD HEALTH

As discussed earlier, all children are affected by their communities. For example, a Native American child born on a reservation, in an urban poor community, or in a small Midwestern town is likely to have different outcomes concerning the potential risk, diagnosis, and treatment of obesity leading to type 2 diabetes.

As communities change, the clinical practice of pediatrics serving any community needs to change with it. If the population living in a given community changes from middle class to working poor, the health care system needs to respond to these changes. In the past, health care professionals have abandoned the community, leaving services available only through hospital-based emergency departments or medical center–based clinics. In recent years, it has been recognized that services need to be community based. Not-for-profit organizations have relocated to the neighborhoods that they have not served historically, and private practices have added services to serve their population of patients more appropriately.

It has become increasingly obvious that for child health to improve, the health of all children in the community needs to be taken into account. To do this, all child health professionals need to participate actively. Communities need for the clinical practice and public health sector to come together to improve child health.

Child health professionals need to use community data for the planning of strategies to improve child health. Community data can give a picture as to the health of the community. Information systems connected to the medical home need to ensure that a child will be up to date on immunizations and that a child will not be missed during newborn heel-stick screening. As the debate continues about the value and need for an individual patient identifier, children still are lost to follow-up. Improved data collection concerning individual information, if done right, provides patient protection, informs public policy, improves accountability, and improves the overall health of the community. Data collected by national groups, such as All Kids Count and Kids Count, have helped to galvanize advocates. With the development of geographic information systems, the ability to use specific data, such as rates, proportions, prevalences, community resource mapping, and other health-related data, will increase.

Most communities have many of the needed resources to improve child health. The Community Access to Child Health (CATCH) Program of the American Academy of Pediatrics is built on the concept that "local people, using local resources, can solve local problems." It has been shown time and time again that organizing and reallocation of available financial and nonfinancial resources often is all that is needed to improve child health significantly.

Finally, federal laws mandate services for children, but services vary because of the inherent differences between communities and priorities (e.g., Title V Children with Special Health Care Needs [CSHCN] programs, Individuals with Disabilities Education Act, Part C). Because of different community values, expectations, and resources, a child with a specific need may be addressed entirely differently.

UNIQUE CONTRIBUTION OF PEDIATRICS TO UNDERSTANDING COMMUNITY HEALTH

Pediatricians should collaborate with families and other child health care professionals to identify and address challenges and barriers to the health and well-being of infants, children, adolescents, and young adults in the communities they serve. Community pediatrics first was recognized by Haggerty in 1968. Haggerty stated, "Community pediatrics is specially, but not exclusively, concerned with children who do not now get adequate medical care." Since that time, there has been an increasing recognition and consensus as to what community pediatrics embodies. The American Academy of Pediatrics statement "The Pediatrician's Role in Community Pediatrics" has provided a framework for pediatrician work in the community.

Attributes of a Community Pediatrician
The following are attributes of a community pediatrician:

- Knowledge of community resources, community leaders, public health issues/community health disparities, effective strategies to reach families in the communities in which they live, and models for community-based and developmentally appropriate practices
- Ability to advocate for family/community-centered care and teach, motivate, inspire, lead, and communicate an idea to other pediatricians, administrators, government officials, and community leaders
- Involvement with or willingness to become involved with community leaders

- Possession of the following personality traits: caring personality and genuine concern, willingness to collaborate, curiosity about the community, charisma/ability to bring people together, willingness to learn, open-mindedness, flexibility, passion to improve child health through change
- Visionary/change-maker quality, ability to see the big picture and areas where change is necessary, ability to think outside the box and the clinic setting and to see children in their environment, ability to think in terms of systems models
- Possession of skills in handling canned presentations to discuss specific health issues for different community groups, ability to integrate services in a way that minimizes duplication, possession of oral and written communication skills, and possession of critical thinking skills/analytical ability
- Willingness to work toward improvement of the social and psychological supports for the families that he or she works with
- Willingness to work to improve the quality of life within the community

The following list addresses the application of the principles discussed so far at the practice level—10 requirements for every pediatrician who seeks to improve child health effectively in his or her community:

1. Apply a strength-based, rather than a deficit-based, view of the community.
2. Recognize the significance of formal and informal associations.
3. Connect to the faith community.
4. Understand the concept of asset mapping.
5. Support families in their role as experts in their children's care.
6. Understand the importance of community social capital.
7. Understand the impact of the various environments that affect child welfare (e.g., child care, preschools, schools).
8. Serve as a catalyst, mentor, and leader for community mobilization.
9. Integrate community-oriented primary care into practice.
10. Explore the use of technology to build the community.

Challenges Faced by Pediatricians

Pediatricians today are faced with many barriers to practicing community pediatrics. With the many financial challenges to providing care and a health care system that in general does not promote or support issues related to community pediatrics, the pediatrician is challenged. Because each community and practice is different, planning and creativity are required on behalf of the health care professional and changes in support provided by government, local, and national organizations and philanthropy are needed. An American Academy of Pediatrics document, "The Future of Pediatric Education: II," recognized that since medical education is geared largely toward treating sick patients, pediatric medical education at all levels must change and must become more focused on the health needs of children in the context of family and community.

Pediatrician Involvement

Examples of pediatrician involvement include the following:

1. Participate in community activities (e.g., United Way allocation committee, local school board).
2. Discuss ways that your office practice can influence child health; ask staff, "Do we have any unmet needs in our community that our office or clinic could address?"
3. Ask families from your practice about what they see as the needs and strengths of the community.
4. Use currently available data to examine the major child health deficits in the community (Kids Count data, CDC data)
5. Hire a parent of a child who makes use of extensive community services to work in your office.
6. Hire staff from diverse backgrounds to help influence child health.
7. Become involved in programs such as the CATCH Program of the American Academy of Pediatrics, which can provide ideas, technical assistance, mentorship, and financial assistance to develop community-based programs.

CONCLUSION

Communities can be defined in many different ways and are in a perpetual state of change. Because of this, the health care system needs to adapt to the needs of children and their parents and other caregivers. The pediatrician, specifically, needs to integrate public health principles with clinical practice to improve child health. Many resources have been developed to help pediatricians and health care professionals identify and act on the assets and the issues facing communities. Pediatric training for the resident and the practicing clinician must provide resources to help them develop the crucial skills needed to practice community pediatrics.

Additional Resources, CD-ROM

Bibliography

Mini-index of Related Topics   CH.

PRINCIPLES OF OFFICE-BASED PRACTICE	8
THE EFFECTS OF CULTURE ON CHILD HEALTH	257
CHILD ADVOCACY	259

SUGGESTED READINGS

American Academy of Pediatrics: Community Pediatrics: An Annotated Bibliography. Elk Grove Village, Ill, American Academy of Pediatrics, 2002.
American Academy of Pediatrics: The future of pediatric education: II. Organizing pediatric education to meet the needs of infants, children,

258 Effects of Poverty

Paul H. Wise and Kenneth L. Fox, Jr.

ROLE OF THE GENERALIST

1   Identify evidence of serious material deprivation in families.
2   Identify special hardships related to childhood chronic illness.
3   Assess adequacy of health insurance coverage.
4   Assess enrollment in public benefit programs, including health insurance plans.
5   Provide high-quality clinical care with dignity.
6   Refer for public program evaluation and enrollment.
7   Refer parents for health care.
8   Support community-based efforts to improve family health and well-being.
9   Inform development of child health policies.

Poverty is the most powerful predictor of child health outcomes. In the United States, poverty is defined most commonly in terms of subsistence—the level at which material resources prove inadequate to maintain physical efficiency. The official "poverty line" for the United States is based on an estimate of subsistence in which the approximate cost of a basic family diet is multiplied by 3 to account for all other material family needs, such as housing and utilities. This estimate is adjusted to account for different family sizes and changes each year only to account for inflation. For 2001, the poverty figure for a family of three was $14,630. Such absolute definitions do not take into consideration how a particular family's income relates to the general distribution of family incomes in a society. Definitions of poverty also have been based on the concept of relative deprivation, in which poverty implies a level of resources so inadequate that the realistic opportunity to pursue essential societal activities or acquire necessary skills is functionally undermined. Absolute and relative definitions are relevant to clinicians, who must confront poverty's threat to subsistence and its broader capacity to weaken, through its subversion of opportunity, the fundamental promise of childhood.

Because poverty has decreased among other segments of the U.S. population over the past several decades, particularly among the elderly, poverty has never been concentrated as deeply in childhood as it is today. Although the figure fluctuates slightly from year to year, approximately one in five children in the United States lives in a family with an income less than the poverty line. Approximately one fourth of these impoverished children live in "extreme poverty," with family incomes less than half of the poverty line. Although poverty rates generally are highest in inner-city neighborhoods, most poor children reside in other urban, suburban, and rural areas. This fact suggests that clinicians should not dismiss the possibility of serious material deprivation among their patient population even if their practice is located in a relatively high-income community.

Trends in child poverty are viewed best as the result of changes in the material well-being of the American family. These changes can be separated into two related developments: (1) changes in demography and (2) changes in parental earning capacity. The demography of the American family has been altered dramatically by the increase in families with only one parent present, primarily women-headed households. This trend primarily reflects high rates of divorce and births to women who are unmarried. Approximately half of all marriages in the United States end in divorce, a rate that has been relatively stable since the 1970s. Currently, almost one in three births in the United States is to a woman who is not married. This proportion represents a dramatic increase over past decades. This increase is important because poverty rates among single-parent households are approximately five times higher than rates among dual-parent households. In addition to these demographic changes, the earning capacity of young families, particularly for unskilled or semi-skilled parents, has deteriorated over the past several decades.

When families cannot meet their children's material needs, the only meaningful alternative for child provision is the state. The primary mechanism of this public provision to children has been the cluster of programs generally labeled "the welfare system." The central welfare program is the Temporary Assistance to Needy Families (TANF). This program was instituted in 1996 and imposed some major changes in traditional welfare approaches in the United States, including maternal work requirements; limits for how long children can receive benefits; and administrative separation of welfare from the Medicaid program, the central health insurance program for poor children. These changes and the expanded authority of state and local officials to modify welfare regulations have made it particularly important for clinicians to understand the impact of local programs on their patients.

FUNDAMENTALS

Poverty can be viewed as elevating the likelihood of poor health by two broadly defined mechanisms: (1) the enhancement of risk for poor health and (2) the reduction of access to effective interventions. Elevated risk can affect health by increasing the probability that an illness or trau-matic event will occur and by increasing the severity with which the illness or injury affects the child. Table 258-1 lists the increased health risks of poverty. This elevated risk can be the product of social conditions that increase harmful exposures, such as inadequate or overcrowded housing, insufficient nutritional intake, unsafe play areas, or severe parental stress. It also may reflect larger community effects, particularly in how parents and children draw strength from neighborhood relationships and the capacity for collective action. Of great importance for the clinician, however, access to efficacious interventions often can reduce the ultimate impact of poverty on child health. When a clinical intervention is highly efficacious, differences in access to it dominate disparities in outcome. When a clinical intervention is of low efficacy, differences in underlying risk dominate disparities in outcome.

Clinicians should never make the mistake of thinking they have nothing to offer poor families. To the contrary, clinicians have an enormous potential to uncouple poverty from its implications for health. For families living in poverty, the primary role of the clinician is to ensure a match of service to need. Clinicians need to be able to identify family needs and have mechanisms in place that can respond with appropriate, effective interventions.

Table 258-1. Relative Risk for Selected Health Problems, Poor versus Nonpoor

Health Problem	Relative Risk
Low birth weight[1]	1.3–2×
Neonatal mortality[2]	1.5–4×
Infant mortality (28 days–1 yr)[3]	1.3–3×
Prone sleep position[4]	2×
Iron deficiency anemia[5]	2–4×
Hunger[6]	7×
Chronic undernutrition[7]	1.5–2×
Plumbism[8]	3–4×
Pneumonia[9]	1.2–2×
Frequent diarrhea or colitis[9]	1.5–2×
Meningitis[10]	2×
Complications of meningitis[10]	2–3×
Complications of appendicitis[10]	2–3×
Diabetic ketoacidosis[10]	2×
Functional visual impairment[11]	2–3×
Impaired hearing[11]	1.5–2×
Untreated cavities/missing teeth[11]	3–6×
Asthma hospitalization[12]	2–4×
Fire mortality[13]	2–4×
Motor vehicle accident mortality[13]	2–3×
Pedestrian mortality[14]	2–6×
Poisoning hospitalization[15]	5×
Accidental injury mortality[16]	2–3×
Child deaths (overall)[17]	3–4×

PRESENTATION AND INITIAL EVALUATION

Because effective interventions exist, it is essential that clinicians recognize the material needs of their patients and families. This evaluation has four components. First, clinicians should seek to identify the impact of poverty on the health and well-being of an individual patient. This includes inquiring as to the adequacy of basic necessities, including housing, food, utilities, safety, child care, and school enrollment. Second, an understanding of how poverty may affect access to health care and the impact of any chronic illness on the child's daily functioning is essential. This component would focus on the adequacy of health insurance, but also might entail questions regarding difficulties with transportation to clinical visits, interference of child medical visits to parental employment, out-of-pocket costs for essential medication or equipment, or barriers to eliminating environmentally based allergic or toxic threats. Third, clinicians who care for children should attempt to identify the presence of any serious unattended health conditions in parents. This is essential because parental health can have a dramatic influence on the health and well-being of children, and parents of young children are likely to have far more contact with their children's clinicians than their own. Fourth, clinicians should ascertain whether their patients are enrolled in public programs designed to assist families in need. Of special concern should be cash assistance, housing subsidies, health insurance, and nutritional support programs.

Rather than inquiring directly about levels of income or wealth, the evaluation of basic material necessities generally should rely on evidence of inadequacy. Simple questions may be asked regarding whether children are forced to skip meals or experience hunger because of an inadequate food supply. Similarly, housing problems can be assessed by inquiring into whether the family has lived in a shelter; has

[1]Starfield, B, Shapiro S, Weiss J, et al: Race, family income, and low birthweight. Am J Epidemiol 1991;134:1167–1174.

[2]Collins J, David R: Differences in neonatal mortality by race, income and prenatal care. Ethnicity Dis 1992;2:18–26.

[3]Centers for Disease Control: Poverty and infant mortality—United States, 1988. MMWR Morbid Mortal Wkly Rep 1995;44:922–927; Starfield, B, Shapiro S, Weiss J, et al: Race, family income, and low birthweight. Am J Epidemiol 1991;134:1167–1174.

[4]Brenner R, Simmons-Morton B, Bhaskar B, et al: Prevalence and predictors of the prone sleep position among inner-city infants. JAMA 1998;280:341–346.

[5]Cook J, Marti K: Differences in nutrient adequacy among poor and non-poor children. Medford, Mass, Tufts University Center on Hunger, Poverty and Nutrition Policy, 1995.

[6]Alaimo K, Olson C, Frangillo E, Briefel R: Food insufficiency, family income and health in US preschool and school-aged children. Am J Public Health 2001;91:781–786.

[7]Miller J, Korenman S: Poverty and children's nutritional status in the United States. Am J Epidemiol 1994;140:233–243.

[8]Brody D, Pirkle J, Kramer R, et al: Blood lead levels in the US population, phase I of the Third National Health and Nutrition Exam Survey (NHANES III, 1988–1991). JAMA 1994;272:277–283; Starfield B: Effectiveness of Medical Care: Validating Clinical Wisdom. Baltimore, Johns Hopkins University Press, 1985.

[9]Hardy A: Incidence and impact of selected infectious diseases in childhood. Vital Health Stat 1991;10:11.

[10]Starfield B: Effectiveness of Medical Care: Validating Clinical Wisdom. Baltimore, Johns Hopkins University Press, 1985.

[11]Newacheck P, Jameson W, Halfon N: Health status and income: The impact of poverty on child health. J School Health 1994;64:229–233; Halfon N, Newacheck P: Childhood asthma and poverty: Differential impacts and utilization of health services. Pediatrics 1993;91:56–61.

[12]Department of Health, New York City, press release, 2001. Available at: www.nyc.gov/html/doh/html/public/press01/pr53–806.html.

[13]Baker S, O'Neill B, Ginsburg M, Li G (eds): The Injury Fact Book. New York, Oxford University Press, 1992.

[14]Baker S, O'Neill B, Ginsburg M, Li G (eds): The Injury Fact Book. New York, Oxford University Press, 1992; Pless I, Verreault R, Arsenault L, (eds): The epidemiology of road accidents in childhood. Am J Public Health 1987;77:358–360.

[15]Children's Defense Fund: Wasting America's Future. Boston, Beacon Press, 1994.

[16]Grossman D: Accidental injuries in children. Future of Children 2000;10:23–52; Starfield B: Effectiveness of Medical Care: Validating Clinical Wisdom. Baltimore, Johns Hopkins University Press, 1985.

[17]Children's Defense Fund: Wasting America's Future. Boston, Beacon Press, 1994; Starfield B: Effectiveness of Medical Care: Validating Clinical Wisdom. Baltimore, Johns Hopkins University Press, 1985.

needs or challenges. Whether for the individual or the group, advocacy occurs on local, regional, state, and national levels.

Type the name of almost any childhood disease in an Internet search engine, and one can discover multitudes of "advocates." Which of these groups of children are in need of advocacy efforts by health care providers? Some may have obvious links to child health issues, whereas other relationships are less clear. Clinicians individually decide how and when to engage in advocacy efforts.

ADVOCACY: TOOLS OF THE TRADE

Thomas Edison said, "Genius is one percent inspiration, ninety-nine percent perspiration." One could say the same thing about child advocacy. Identifying the issue for which to advocate is the easy part. Effective advocacy is hard work and requires skill. Just as medical students must master specific skills necessary for clinical care, clinicians must master skills necessary for child advocacy (Box 259-1).

By definition, child health care providers already possess professional expertise. Humility often prevents clinicians from assuming their deserved role as child health care experts. For pediatricians in particular and child health care providers in general, the title of "pediatrician" is a respected one and identifies the individual as an expert in child health care and as someone with the child's best interest at heart. In all public settings, pediatricians' advocacy efforts are enhanced when they are identified as "pediatrician."

Effective communication skills are paramount to successful advocacy efforts. An effective child advocate has ample opportunity to communicate through personal letters, letters to the editor of the local newspaper, editorials, and articles for the public. Public speaking skills are necessary for committee meetings, medical staff meetings, town meetings, and presentations to various civic groups. Regardless of the venue, it is helpful to begin preparation by understanding the nature of the audience. A show of hands can give insight as to the audience composition and empower them to participate in the process. When the audience comprises nonmedical people, one should refrain from excessive use of medical jargon. Use of cases can be highly effective, but these must be presented in a clear and concise manner. Too much detail can make a "simple" case incomprehensible to

a nonmedical person. All identifying information must be removed and confidentiality preserved. Similarly, statistics that define the scope of an issue help the audience understand the pediatrician's perspective.

Communication style and content need to be tailored to the specific target group. Legislators and their staff are most interested in concise summaries of the issues and the medical remedies to them. Governmental officials, such as county commissioners or representatives from the health department, may be interested in more detailed descriptions of the problem, potential solutions, and, when possible, cost estimates. Parents of children with a common medical condition often want specifics about treatment options or plans for action.

A similar approach is used when meeting with the media. The clinician needs to identify the target audience. It is useful to personalize health care issues by referring to local cases and statistics. Despite the clinician's best efforts, a reporter or editor determines what the public hears or reads. Providing a fact sheet is an effective way to decrease inaccuracies and highlight key objectives. The clinician needs to focus on the children and avoid being sidetracked.

Advocacy is hard work and requires a team approach. In most areas of child advocacy, groups of potential allies exist. Some groups readily welcome the help of a willing and knowledgeable clinician, whereas others are threatened. Even groups that seem opposed to the pediatrician's point of view may become allies. Obvious allies are other health care professionals, parent groups, nongovernmental organizations (NGOs), and community leaders. Politicians and staff from governmental agencies may be allies or the target audience of advocacy efforts. Students from medical schools or local colleges can be willing workers for a cause.

In addition to hard work, persistence, and organization, most advocacy efforts need financing. This may not be just cash, but rather donations of time, space, and materials. When money is needed, potential sources include hospital foundations; community groups, such as the Rotary and Kiwanis clubs; local medical or pediatric societies; and parent groups. Letters to the editor in the local newspaper and displays of supporters' names are two forms of recognition.

Successful advocacy cultivates passion, and passion can foster an inability to compromise. Yet compromise is essential to advocacy. Advocacy groups rarely achieve all of their goals at once. The advocate must recognize when to negotiate and when to pursue an adversarial position.

RESOURCES

There are multiple resources for child advocates to access. Familiar places may be the best place to begin. Hospitals and medical schools have missions consistent with those of pediatric providers. They also have the infrastructure to support advocacy projects, including public relations departments, space, website hosting and other computer resources, graphic arts departments, and money. Before meeting with hospital administrators, the advocate must define the health care issue and its effects on the hospital's patients and community. The presentation should include a plan of action, outlining the hospital's advocacy role. Participating organizations should be recognized.

Box 259-1. Child Advocacy Skills

- Professional expertise
- Communication skills
  - Written
  - Oral
  - Media
  - Internet
- Identification of allies
  - Parents
  - Health care professionals
  - Politicians
  - Community leaders
  - Governmental agencies
  - Nongovernmental organizations (NGOs)
- Identification of winnable issues

Medical and pediatric societies, parent groups, school groups, and religious institutions also are potential resources. Other professional organizations should not be overlooked as allies. Teachers, law enforcement officers, lawyers, judges, social workers, and psychologists are some of the professionals with vested interests in the welfare of children. These professionals can be strong and valuable child advocate allies for pediatricians.

Pediatric providers would be well advised to seek allies beyond the health care professions. In New York State, the Permanent Judicial Commission on Justice for Children has been a model of effective child advocacy. Composed of judges, lawyers, child welfare experts, and pediatricians, the Commission has established walk-in day care centers in county courthouses for participants in court proceedings; improved access for children to early intervention; and trained judges, lawyers, and other child welfare personnel in their role in improving health care for children in foster care.

National and regional professional pediatric organizations provide support for advocacy efforts. The AAP has extensive programs for general strategies for the pediatric child advocate and for specific content areas. Many of these resources are packaged and readily available. The AAP also provides multiple funding opportunities for pediatricians, including pediatricians in private practice. These can be accessed through AAP offices or through the website, http://www.aap.org. Other medical specialty societies and the American Medical Association offer similar services.

Two additional organizations useful to the child advocate have a more educational and academic mission. The Ambulatory Pediatric Association (http://www.ambpeds.org), composed primarily of general academic pediatricians, and the Accreditation Council for Graduate Medical Education (http://www.acgme.org), which is responsible for setting residency training standards, address training issues in pediatric advocacy.

A comprehensive listing of issue-specific advocacy groups is accessible on the Internet, either through search engines or through other advocacy groups, such as the AAP. Local, state, and federal governmental resources are abundant. Local and state health departments and social services departments may be a source for information, personnel, and possibly financing. Websites from federal and state agencies often are a good place to start to find information on funding, existing programs, granting opportunities, and disease statistics.

Case Study 259-1 illustrates the advocacy process, including residency training, communication skills, identifying allies, compromise and negotiation, funding, and use of the media. Child advocacy skills were instrumental in the success of this case. Despite lack of expertise or experience in firearm safety, these young child advocates were acknowledged immediately as the experts in child health care issues. Allies from the medical and nonmedical communities were crucial in developing and implementing the Task Force mission and objectives. Print and broadcast media were employed in communicating the educational messages of gun safety. Finally, when gun rights proponents threatened the existence of the Task Force, compromise led to the identification of the issues important to all members.

CASE STUDY 259-1

CHILD ADVOCACY

As part of their training, pediatric residents at Upstate Medical University were required to participate in a child advocacy project. A group of four residents and one faculty member became interested in addressing gun violence in the community. The group formed the Onondaga County Citizens Task Force on Gun Safety with officials from the County Commission on Aging and Youth; prosecutors; local town, city, county, and state law enforcement personnel; parents of gunshot victims; and clergy.

As the Task Force was defining its mission and goals, members of the National Rifle Association were invited to join. Meetings became adversarial and vitriolic. Task Force members polarized into individuals who viewed gun ownership as a right to be protected and individuals who viewed guns as a source of violence and crime. Little was accomplished. It seemed as if the Task Force was doomed to suffer a premature demise.

Eventually, Task Force members settled on an issue that all could agree on—gun safety. All were able to support the idea that gun owners must be responsible for their firearms, store them in a secure manner, and keep them inaccessible to children. The Task Force looked to the gun owners on the committee for technical advice, such as which gun safety locks were acceptable for securing a firearm. As the Task Force developed educational materials, the gun owners were instrumental in accessing sports clubs for distribution. The sports clubs donated money and display space at their activities.

The Task Force sought out key allies. The hospital administration made significant monetary and personnel contributions, as did the hospital's private foundation. Funds supported the purchase of gun safety locks for distribution to gun owners at venues throughout the county, gun safety magnets, and gun safety bookmarks. Strong links developed with the local media facilitated extensive television and radio coverage. The local cable operator funded and produced three public service announcements and provided free airtime. The newspapers printed editorials, articles, and public service announcements.

Clinicians, whether in general practice or subspecialty areas, possess an impressive array of medical skills. A medical approach is not always sufficient, however, to ensure the health of children. Frequently, pediatric health care providers need to rely on their child advocacy skills to promote and improve the health of children effectively in their practice and their community.

Mini-index of Related Topics

SUGGESTED READINGS

American Academy of Pediatrics. Available at: http://www.aap.org/member/memcore.htm.
Andrews R, Biggs M, Seidel M, et al: The Columbia World of Quotations. New York, Columbia University Press, 1996. Available at: www.bartleby.com/66/.
Dicker S, Schall E: The courts' role beyond the courtroom: A case study of New York's Permanent Judicial Commission on Justice for Children and Early Intervention. Child Leg Rights J 1996;16:14–22.

260 Ethical and Legal Issues in Pediatrics

Lainie Friedman Ross

ROLE OF THE GENERALIST

1 Appreciate the distinction between aspects of decisions based on medical knowledge and aspects based on human values.

2 Appreciate the developing autonomy of children to participate in health care decision making as they mature.

3 Understand state laws that are relevant to the care of adolescents.

4 Understand the basic principles of federal regulations governing the conduct of research with children.

5 Identify local resources, such as an institutional ethics committee, that can assist with case consultation and policy development on ethical issues.

Pediatric medicine and research can raise a broad range of ethical and legal controversies. Yet, the field of medical ethics that has developed since the 1970s often involves a competent adult patient who has the right to accept or refuse any and all medical interventions, including lifesaving therapy. When adults are not competent, decisions are made by a surrogate. Surrogates are supposed to act as the patient would have acted if competent (substituted judgment), or if the patient's wishes are unknown, the surrogate is supposed to act in the patient's best interest.

As in other areas of clinical practice, the principles and tools that are applicable to the adult patient cannot be applied to the pediatric patient without some modification. There are several reasons why this is so. First, although adults are presumed to be competent, children and adolescents generally are presumed incompetent. Although there are some ethical and legal challenges to this presumption, most health care decisions are made for children and adolescents by, or at least with, their parents. The physician-patient relationship must be expanded to include parents. The triad of physician, patient, and parent(s) leads to the following questions:

1. Where lies the primary loyalty of the physician?
2. How can one balance the needs and interests of the child and parents when they conflict?
3. To whom is privacy and confidentiality owed?

Second, although competent patients have the right to accept or refuse all treatment, including lifesaving treatment, surrogate decision makers, even when the surrogates are parents making decisions for their children, are given less latitude. Parents who refuse medically indicated treatment for their children can be taken to court on the grounds of suspected child abuse or neglect, even if their reasons would justify refusal for themselves (e.g., an otherwise healthy Jehovah's Witness adult can refuse a lifesaving blood transfusion after sustaining splenic trauma, but refusal would be overridden if a Jehovah's Witness adult refused the same treatment for his or her otherwise healthy young child).

A third reason that pediatric clinical ethics is different from clinical ethics for adult patients is that the range of issues differs—and not just because children and adults have different medical problems. There are some clinical options that may not be morally appropriate in pediatric patients. Although most accept the right of competent adults to choose to undergo elective plastic surgery because they do not like the size or shape of a particular body part, it is less clear whether parents should be able to consent to esthetic surgery on behalf of children who cannot articulate their own wants or needs. This is at the heart of the opposition to parental requests for tongue reduction in infants and young children with Down syndrome. Or consider another example: Although most reproductive endocrinologists would offer a variety of high-technology solutions to a 40-year-old woman with a 2-year history of infertility, they might not be willing to offer these interventions to a

16-year-old who has been having unprotected sex for 2 years.

Despite the need for a comprehensive examination of the breadth and depth of ethical issues that arise in pediatrics, the focus of pediatric clinical ethics has been on the extreme cases: a premature infant who weighs 500 g, a child with leukemia whose parents refuse chemotherapy, or a child whose sibling needs a kidney transplant. The unique issues that generalists face have not received much scholarly attention, despite the fact that these decisions may have profound effects on a child's physical and mental health and on the emotional, spiritual, and economic elements of family life. This chapter examines a range of controversial cases to understand how ethics is integral to pediatric medicine and research.

MODERN HISTORY OF PEDIATRIC ETHICS

In Western society, the normative nature of medicine and medical practice were recognized at least since the Hippocratic era. The scientific, technologic, and social developments of the 20th century demand a reexamination, however, of physicians' moral obligations to their patients and to the structure of the health care delivery system. This is particularly true for pediatrics because although all societies have had the concept of childhood, there have been major changes in the conception of childhood with respect to its boundaries (when childhood begins and ends), its dimensions (how childhood is viewed jurisdictionally, epistemologically, and politically), and its divisions (the stages that distinguish between infants, children, and adolescents). These different conceptions reflect different cultural and normative values, priorities, and assumptions and confer different rights and responsibilities to parents, children, and the state.

One major shift in the 20th century was the shift in attitude from the child as the property of the parents to the child as a person with at least some rights. This shift influenced how courts adjudicated custody battles and the degree of discretion granted to parents regarding medical decisions. Although parents are the presumptive proxy decision makers for their children, they are required to act in their child's "best interest." What the term *best interest* means is not always clear-cut, and there are many cases in which reasonable persons would disagree as to what is best for a child. The tension exists in part because medical decisions often entail risks and probabilities, and there are wide differences in risk assessment by individuals who are or are not averse to risk, and in part because of different attitudes and values regarding quality of life versus sanctity of life. Yet, even if we could develop consensus regarding what is medically best for a child, parents must determine not only what is medically best for the child, but also what is best for the child all things considered. This means that parents must weigh the child's medical needs and interests with the child's other needs and interests and must balance the child's interests against the interests and needs of other family members. Buchanan and Brock argued that the best interest standard is better understood "as a regulative ideal, not as a strict and literal requirement." Rarely do physicians seek to intervene unless parents are acting contrary to their

child's interests, such that intervention becomes, in the words of Goldstein and colleagues, the "least detrimental alternative." Nevertheless, the "best interest of the child" standard can serve as a reminder that the child and his or her interests ought to be the primary focus of the parents' decision.

Today most pediatric hospitals have ethics committees (or ethics consultants) to help physicians and parents sort through the normative aspects of medical decision making. In part, these committees were spurred on by the Baby Doe regulations of the 1980s. Baby Doe was born with Down syndrome, esophageal atresia, and a tracheoesophageal fistula on April 9, 1982, in Bloomington, Indiana. The parents refused surgical repair and intravenous feedings. The hospital asked the Indiana courts whether to comply, and the courts said to respect the parents' wishes. County prosecutors appealed, seeking to shift custody away from the parents to force medical treatment. Hours before arguments were to be heard by the Supreme Court, the infant died. The Court then dismissed the petition as moot.

Baby Doe was not the first child to receive widespread media attention for parental refusal of treatment. In 1969, an infant with Down syndrome and duodenal atresia was born at Johns Hopkins University Hospital. A documentary about the case aired on television and created some short-lived public indignation. The issue persisted in the medical literature with the 1973 publication of two articles that discussed withholding of treatment of newborns. These publications triggered a divisive debate within the medical community, a debate that was ongoing when Baby Doe was born.

President Reagan was in office when Baby Doe died, and he ordered the Department of Health and Human Services (DHHS) to notify hospitals receiving federal aid that it was unlawful to withhold treatment based on an infant's handicaps under the Federal Rehabilitation Act of 1973. The DHHS then sought to implement their threat by issuing interim final rules in March 1983 and again in January 1984. The latter rules encouraged but did not mandate infant care review committees as a compromise. Although the Baby Doe regulations were challenged successfully, eventually parts of the regulations were incorporated as amendments into the Child Abuse Prevention and Treatment Act of 1984. They allow for the nontreatment of children if (1) the infant is chronically and irreversibly comatose; (2) the provision of such treatment merely would prolong dying, not be effective in ameliorating or correcting all of the infant's life-threatening conditions, or otherwise be futile in terms of the survival of the infant; or (3) if the provision of such treatment would be virtually futile or inhumane. Despite this legislation, there still is controversy regarding when it is permissible to withhold or withdraw medical treatment from children, particularly newborns.

CLINICAL PRACTICE

Children and adolescents receive a wide range of medical care, including preventive health care, the treatment of acute illnesses or injuries, and the treatment of chronic conditions. The care may be sought electively or emergently and may be sought for a wide range of reasons, including the prevention of disease and disability, the enhancement of quality of life, the relief of pain, or the treatment of acute or life-threatening illnesses. Ethical issues arise because of conflict, and there are many potential sources of conflict, including differences in goals or in risk-benefit calculations between the physician and the family, within the family, between the family and the state, or between the physician and the state. Conflict resolution can be informal (in the physician's office through conversation) or may involve third-party intervention (including ethicists and ethics committees, chaplains, social workers, or the courts, as a last resort). Consider the following cases.

An 8-Year-Old Child with Pneumonia

The first step in any conflict is further discussion. Issues to be weighed include efficacy, cost, convenience, attendant risks, and compliance. At first, the scenario in Case Study 260-1 does not seem to be an ethical issue because everyone agrees the child needs antibiotics. The two therapeutic options have different benefits and burdens, however, and the child and her mother's divergent calculations have created a conflict between the parent and child about which the physician may feel indifferent. The mother in Case Study 260-1 may prefer an injection because it is a one-time dose and the child will be ensured appropriate treatment. Cost may or may not factor into her equation. Alternatively, she may prefer the shot to avoid a thrice-daily battle of compliance, based on past experience that her child would be poorly compliant when the symptoms are gone. The child may base her decision on her fear of needles and its attendant discomfort. She may promise her mother and the physician that she will be compliant this time.

In most discussions, parents and children come to consensus. Sometimes their positions are intractable, however. Who, then, should have the final word? In February 1995, the Committee on Bioethics of the American Academy of Pediatrics published recommendations regarding informed consent in pediatric practice. In their document, the Committee stated that children should be included (empowered) to the extent of their capacity. The Committee recommended that persistent conflicts might benefit from third-party conflict resolution, with the physician or professional mediator as the third party. Although this approach may be ideal, there may be some parents who are well meaning but intolerant of third-party scrutiny.

CASE STUDY 260-1

AN 8-YEAR-OLD CHILD WITH PNEUMONIA

An 8-year-old girl presents with fever and cough. On physical examination, she has decreased breath sounds in the left lower lobe, and an infiltrate is seen on chest x-ray. You explain to her and to her mother that antibiotic treatment is medically indicated and propose either a 10-day course of oral antibiotics or one intramuscular injection. The mother requests that you give the child a shot. The child says she does not want a shot and will take the liquid three times daily for 10 days.

These parents may find the physician's attempt to forge consensus as threatening their legitimate parental authority.

In Case Study 260-1, what are the pediatrician's options if consensus is not achieved? If the pediatrician sides with the parent, he or she would have to give the protesting child a painful treatment. What if the child resists? What does this tell the child about her right to participate in medical decision making? To side with the child on the grounds of developing maturity places the parent in an awkward position because she must now buy the medicine and ensure her child's compliance three times a day. What if the parent resists and says, "Okay, doctor, at what time will you come by to give my daughter her medicine?"

Generally, in the case of a therapeutic decision between two medically appropriate therapies, parents have ultimate decision-making authority. Parental autonomy is not absolute, however, and the physician has the right, and perhaps the obligation, to involve children in the decision-making process and to attempt consensus. When that fails, the physician should explain to the child why his or her wishes and requests are being overridden, even if the parents complain that this threatens their autonomy.

A 15-Year-Old Girl with Sexually Transmitted Disease

By the age of 18, more than half of all adolescent girls in the United States have had sexual intercourse, and even more are sexually active. More than 1 million American adolescents become pregnant every year. Many teens do not seek medical or gynecologic care or contraception for months or years after they initiate sexual activity; care often initially is sought because of a pregnancy scare or a sexually transmitted disease (STD) (Case Study 260-2).

Although parents generally have the legal right and responsibility to consent for their children's medical care (diagnosis and treatment), health care related to gynecologic and reproductive health issues are exceptions under the specialized consent statutes that exist in every state. These statutes vary in their scope, but all give adolescents the legal autonomy to seek and consent independently to the diagnosis and treatment of drug and alcohol abuse, the diagnosis and treatment of STDs, and the procurement of contraceptives. Some states even allow minors to consent to abortions without disclosure or consent from the minor's parents. The statutes were designed to encourage adolescents to seek health care for problems that they might deny or ignore or for which they might delay seeking treatment if parental permission were required.

The encouragement of early, responsible sexual health care for adolescents is not value-neutral because there are some (parents and pediatricians) who would argue that any decision except abstinence is morally unacceptable. Physicians should realize that the statutes allow but do not require their participation. Pediatricians have the legal latitude to make a moral decision about whether or not to provide gynecologic care. If they do, their practice must ensure confidentiality as guaranteed by the law.

The specialized consent statutes empower the patient in Case Study 260-2 to seek confidential health care for her STD. It is hoped that the physician who cares for this patient not only would treat her STD, but also would

CASE STUDY 260-2

A 15-YEAR-OLD GIRL WITH SEXUALLY TRANSMITTED DISEASE

A 15-year-old girl presents with a high fever and severe abdominal pain for 1 week. She has some vomiting but no diarrhea. The patient admits that she became sexually active in the last 3 months with her 18-year-old boyfriend. She says she may have a slight vaginal discharge. She denies pregnancy but also admits to using no birth control. Her last period was 3 weeks ago. She consents to a pelvic examination on the condition of strict confidentiality because she knows that her actions are contrary to her parents' moral and religious beliefs and she fears they would prohibit her from seeing her boyfriend. On physical examination, the patient has significant cervical and adnexal tenderness and has a thick foul-smelling discharge. Her uterus does not feel enlarged, and a urine pregnancy screen is negative. You explain that she has pelvic inflammatory disease caused by a sexually transmitted disease and that you will send off cultures to determine the exact infectious cause. You explain that her boyfriend needs to be treated as well. You prepare to treat her with an intramuscular shot of cefoxitin and an oral dose of probenecid. The patient refuses the intramuscular injection and demands an oral course of antibiotics. Given her age, the possibility that she would not be able to tolerate oral medications because of her vomiting, her delay in seeking care, and her request for strict confidentiality, you cannot ensure compliance. You insist on the shot. The patient prepares to leave, saying that she will go to another physician.

discuss with her the options of pregnancy prevention because the statutes also empower her to receive counseling and prescriptions for contraception. It is not clear, however, that the specialized consent statutes allow the patient to refuse the recommended course of treatment because the statutes empower adolescents to seek treatment, but they may not empower them to refuse treatment. This is in contrast with the rights of adult women in similar situations. Although this contrast may seem incoherent, one must realize that the statutes were not passed because adolescents were deemed competent to make these decisions or that they have better decision-making capacity regarding these issues than other health care. Rather, the statutes were a pragmatic solution to a potential public health crisis. The statutes aim to encourage adolescents to seek appropriate care early to avoid the untoward complications of delayed treatment and to decrease adolescent pregnancy. Adolescents still are minors, however, and the law and ethics allow a greater amount of paternalism to protect them from themselves than is permitted with respect to adults. Adolescents are empowered to consent to appropriate medical care but not to refuse it.

What should the physician caring for the patient in Case Study 260-2 do? First, the physician should continue to talk with the patient and explain why he or she feels the need to treat her with an intramuscular injection. The physician should try to convince her to accept the treatment voluntarily. If the patient persists in her refusal, however, the physician can threaten to involve her parents. The physician

is morally correct that he or she needs to ensure that the patient is treated adequately, given the short-term and long-term health risks of untreated pelvic inflammatory disease. Although the threat of parental involvement may persuade the patient to accept treatment, it is clear that her consent is no longer truly voluntary. Yet the justification of treating her without parental permission is less about respect for her autonomy and more about reducing public health problems.

A Newborn with Congenital Heart Defect

Traditionally, trisomy 18 was characterized as a *lethal anomaly*, and infants did not undergo surgical repair (Case Study 260-3). Although no specific definition for *lethal anomaly* exists, most practitioners use it to refer to an infant with severe neurologic compromise and structural anomalies that, if untreated, would cause death within a few months. Examples are trisomy 13, trisomy 18, and anencephaly. The "uncorrected" structural anomalies in these infants include airway anomalies, congenital heart disease, and gastrointestinal defects. As isolated findings, these same structural anomalies often are treated. What makes the former conditions lethal is the combination of severe neurologic compromise and structural anomalies.

Although there are data that show that many infants with trisomy 18 die of untreatable central apnea, part of the lethality of trisomy 18 may be due to the decision not to repair surgically correctable malformations. A review of one hospital experience with prenatally diagnosed hypoplastic left heart syndrome by Allan and colleagues stated that 5 of 24 infants who were brought to term were not offered Norwood stage 1 because of trisomy 18 ($n = 2$), unfavorable cardiac anatomy ($n = 2$), or neurologic impairment ($n = 1$). Beginning in the 1990s, however, some families have begun to demand aggressive treatment for infants with so-called lethal anomalies despite medical recommendations for comfort measures only.

What are the arguments for and against aggressive treatment for infants with trisomy 18? One argument against treatment is based on the physician's assessment that such treatment is futile. The problem lies in the meaning of

CASE STUDY 260-3

A NEWBORN WITH CONGENITAL HEART DEFECT

A 2-kg full-term infant is born to a 22-year-old, gravida 1, para 1 mother who received no prenatal care. The infant develops respiratory problems in the delivery room, for which he is intubated. In the nursery, he is noted to be microcephalic and to have other physical features consistent with trisomy 18. Blood is sent for chromosomal study. A cardiac echocardiogram is performed, which reveals hypoplastic left heart syndrome. The current standard of care is the two-stage Norwood procedure, cardiac transplantation, or comfort care. The neonatal intensive care unit director and cardiac surgeon do not believe that the infant should be listed for a heart transplant or surgically treated if he is found to have trisomy 18. The mother insists that the child undergo a Norwood procedure, regardless of the chromosomal diagnosis.

whenever feasible; d) adequate provisions are made to protect the privacy of children and their parents and to maintain confidentiality of data; e) subjects will be selected in an equitable manner; and f) the conditions of all applicable subsequent conditions are met . . . [including that] adequate provisions are made for the assent of the child and permission of their parents or guardians."

The Commission recommended additional criteria depending on the level of risk and harm that the research entailed, the risk versus benefit of the proposed project, and the comparative risk versus benefit of the alternatives. The Commission required the creation of local institutional review boards to ensure that these safeguards were fulfilled. institutional review boards also were given authority to ensure that provisions were made for the solicitation of consent. For most research, parental permission and the child's assent are necessary.

In the 1990s, the U.S. Food and Drug Administration (FDA) and the National Institutes of Health implemented new policies regarding the participation of children. The FDA and the National Institutes of Health now require that children be included earlier in the research process, contrary to the National Commission's second criteria. One impetus for this move is that many pharmaceuticals and therapies prescribed to children have never been tested in children. A second impetus for this move involves research for life-threatening conditions, such as acquired immunodeficiency syndrome. The lag time between FDA approval of new drugs, often based solely on adult trials, and the initiation of clinical trials in children left many health care planners, health policy analysts, researchers, and advocacy groups frustrated. The FDA incentive has resulted in pediatric labeling information for dozens of new pharmaceuticals.

Placebo-Controlled Asthma Trials

According to the American Academy of Pediatrics Committee on Drugs, placebo-controlled studies are permissible if there is no commonly accepted therapy, if the commonly accepted therapy is of questionable efficacy, or to study incidence and severity of undesirable side effects of add-on treatment to an established regimen (Case Study 260-5). A similar statement regarding the ethics of placebo-based trials can be found in Canadian policy and in the modifications to the Declaration of Helsinki. Using this

---

CASE STUDY 260-5

PLACEBO-CONTROLLED ASTHMA TRIALS

A pharmaceutical company wants to prove that its new inhaled steroid is effective. The company proposes a randomized, double-blind, placebo-controlled, multicenter study of children and adolescents with moderate-to-severe asthma (defined as ≥6 months use of two asthma medicines daily, one of the medicines being an inhaled glucocorticosteroid). To participate in this study, children and adolescents would discontinue glucocorticosteroid at randomization and would be randomized to receive a new inhaled steroid or placebo. Is this research project ethical?

CASE STUDY 260-6

DIABETES PREVENTION TRIAL

The Diabetes Prevention Trial is a multicenter trial to prevent or delay the development of type 1 diabetes mellitus in subjects with a type 1 diabetic first-degree relative. Based on genetic susceptibility, immune markers, and metabolic markers of islet autoimmunity, individuals are classified as being at high risk (>50% risk of developing diabetes mellitus in the next 5 years), moderate risk (25% to 50% risk), modest risk (<25% risk), or low risk (risk comparable to the general population). Individuals characterized as high risk are offered participation in a protocol in which they would be assigned randomly to no treatment or to low-dose insulin twice a day and periodic intravenous infusions. Can this research protocol of exposing healthy children to twice-daily injections and the risks of exogenous insulin (including hypoglycemia) be morally justified?

---

standard, the proposed study is not ethical because it does not provide all subjects with the standard of care.

There is much criticism about the absolute impermissibility of placebos under the Declaration of Helsinki. Without trying to resolve the debate, the question for Case Study 260-5 is whether placebos can be justified in children for a new equivalence drug. Since 1991, U.S. consensus guidelines recommend the use of inhaled corticosteroids in children and adults for the treatment of moderate and severe asthma. As such, such a study would not seem to be justifiable, and instead the pharmaceutical company should compare the new compound against current standard of care. Nevertheless, numerous studies such as the one described in Case Study 260-5 have been published in the 1990s in major journals, involving adult and child subjects.

Diabetes Prevention Trial

To determine whether a research protocol is permissible, Subpart D of the *Federal Regulations* requires that the research be classified according to the degree of risk it entails and whether the research offers the prospect of direct benefit. In Case Study 260-6, although the children in the high-risk group are healthy, they are "at risk" for a serious condition with short-term and long-term sequelae. The working hypothesis for the Diabetes Prevention Trial is that treated subjects would have a 35% reduction in developing type 1 diabetes in the next 5 years. Although the subjects may not benefit, the potential benefit is real, and as such, the research is classified as research that offers the prospect of direct benefit. Such research is permitted if the benefits outweigh the risks, an assessment that is made by the institutional review board and by individual subjects and their surrogates. The benefit-to-risk ratio was satisfied by more than 100 hospitals around the United States, suggesting that at the institutional level, there was belief that the benefits could outweigh the risks. The University of Pittsburgh is not participating. They rejected the proposal on the grounds that the protocol would expose healthy children to the risks of daily medication. They were concerned with the cognitive problems associated with hypoglycemia and considered the risks too great. There also are concerns, discussed in other studies, regarding the potential psychosocial harms associated with so many medical interventions when the children are "healthy."

The research does raise a fundamental question about what it means to be healthy. Is it fair to describe children as healthy if they are at high risk of developing type 1 diabetes in the next 5 years? Surely they are not ill, but are they healthy even if some preliminary metabolic studies are abnormal? It probably is more accurate to classify them somewhere between healthy and ill. In this way, the Diabetes Prevention Trial exemplifies how genetics may require a paradigm shift in the way we think about health and disease. The issue of treating at-risk individuals to prevent disease is not unique to genetics. The ACTG 076 trials sought to reduce the vertical transmission of human immunodeficiency virus (HIV) from pregnant women to their children. It involved the exposure of healthy fetuses and infants at risk for perinatal HIV to antiretroviral therapy (zidovudine) in utero, intrapartum, and postpartum. The Diabetes Prevention Trial and the ACTG 076 trial suggest that the current categories of Subpart D may need to be interpreted to accommodate subjects who have a particular condition and subjects at risk for a particular condition.

Recruitment into the treatment arms of the Diabetes Prevention Trial was slow because most diabetes is not inherited, and only a small percentage of subjects enrolled are found to have the markers associated with an increased susceptibility to diabetes mellitus. Unfortunately, in 2002 the researchers reported that they found no difference in the rate of progression to full-blown type 1 diabetes in the treatment and control groups. The negative results, however, do not change the ethical analysis.

CONCLUSION

Cases in pediatric clinical practice and pediatric research raise procedural and substantive issues—how physicians should approach the case (procedural) and what the final decision should be (substantive). Controversial examples have been presented in this chapter to challenge pediatricians to contemplate the meanings and implications of current policies and practices. Although consensus cannot be expected on all of the cases presented, it is only through dialogue that pediatricians may be able to narrow their differences and promote or modify policies to reflect their shared moral understanding of the obligations and responsibilities of health care providers and researchers with respect to children and their families.

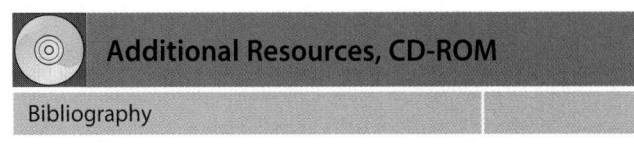

Additional Resources, CD-ROM

Bibliography

Mini-index of Related Topics CH.

SUGGESTED READINGS

American Academy of Pediatrics Committee on Bioethics: Informed consent, parental permission, and assent in pediatric practice. Pediatrics 1995;95:314–317.

Nelson RM: Children as research subjects. In Kahn JP, Mastroianni AC, Sugarman J (eds): Beyond Consent: Seeking Justice in Research. New York, Oxford University Press, 1998, pp 47–66.

Ross LF: Children, Families and Health Care Decision Making. Oxford, Oxford University Press, 1998.

Weir RF: Selective Nontreatment of Handicapped Newborns: Moral Dilemmas in Neonatal Medicine. New York, Oxford University Press, 1984.

Weir RF, Peters C: Affirming the decisions adolescents make about life and death. Hastings Cent Rep 1997;27:29–40.

of Young Children stated, "The single most important activity for building these understandings and skills essential for reading success appears to be reading aloud to children." Despite this statement, a 1996 survey of parents with young children showed that fewer than half of parents with children 3 years old or younger read to their children daily, and 16% of parents did not read to their young children at all.

READING AND SCHOOL SUCCESS

The National Institute of Education estimated that 35% of children nationally enter school not ready to learn to read, with numbers highest among children growing up in poverty. More than one third of the first-graders in the United States read below their grade level, and many of these children continue to struggle with reading all through their school careers, remaining in "slow" reading groups or requiring remedial help. Children who have trouble reading early on are at high risk to proceed through school reading below grade level, despite the extra help they receive. The odds are high that a child who is failing at the end of first grade will be failing at the end of fourth grade. As children advance through school, their reading and written language skills—the ability to use print efficiently and effectively, the ability to get information out of a printed text, the speed and fluency with which children are able to understand and assimilate written material—become decisive in all their subjects and not just in "reading." The educational truism is that a child spends the early grades learning to read and then spends the rest of the school career reading to learn.

Pediatricians increasingly are likely to be consulted about school problems and poor academic performance. By asking regularly about reading skills, in the context of health supervision visits, pediatricians can track a crucial index of academic performance and sometimes anticipate larger school difficulties. It often is helpful to ask a school-age child specifically about out-of-school reading and favorite books to get a sense of whether the child is comfortable and fluent with the printed word, is receiving help and support at home, and is reading on an age-appropriate and grade-appropriate level. It often is enlightening to ask a school-age child to read aloud a sentence or two from a book right in the examination room; although a first-grader may read from word to word, sounding out each one, a third-grader should be able to read a whole sentence fluently, perhaps sounding out only a single unfamiliar word. A fourth-grader who still is reading only picture books and relying heavily on the pictures for prompting information is not ready to cope with information in textbooks. Any indication that reading is a problem deserves prompt attention, either by encouraging parents to press the school for testing and tutoring or by referring the child to a school evaluation clinic. If a child's reading progress is being impeded by an undiagnosed learning disability, more targeted remedial help can make a tremendous difference. Similarly, if reading difficulties are an early signal that a child is having attentional problems, prompt attention to this underlying difficulty may improve the child's reading performance and overall school experience. It is important to emphasize, however, that most children who have trouble with reading do not have learning disabilities, at least under current definitions. Even so, school function assessment and neuropsychiatric testing may help schools teach them more effectively.

Unless corrected, reading failure in the early years of school sets children up for school failure and puts them at higher risk for many of the bad outcomes disproportionately associated with school failure, including chronic absenteeism, truancy, dropping out, substance abuse, and early pregnancy. In all these ways, poor reading skills contribute to bad outcomes in the middle school and adolescent years and to the propagation of cycles of poverty and dependency.

BARRIERS TO EARLY LITERACY DEVELOPMENT

There are many reasons that children may not grow up with the kind of exposure to books and reading aloud that promotes the development of early literacy skills. Time constraints stress many parents, in all socioeconomic groups, and there are alternative sources of electronic entertainment competing for the attention of adults and children. Parents who are not themselves comfortable with books and the written word are unlikely to reach for a children's book as a pleasant way of spending time with a young child. Even parents whose reading skills are adequate may not have been read to when they were young, and they may not understand the importance of reading to young children. To many parents, the idea of reading to an infant or a toddler who is too young to talk seems either uncomfortable or comic—just as some parents do not appreciate the importance of talking to infants who are too young to respond in words. The pediatrician, speaking from the perspective of an expert in healthy child development, can play an essential role in encouraging and modeling developmentally appropriate book-related interactions and in helping parents see the importance of reading to their young children.

For many families, money is in short supply, and books are expensive, especially the board books that are most appropriate for infants and toddlers. Bookstores are not found in the areas where poor families live, and the books available (in pharmacies, chain toy stores, and discount stores) may not be culturally or developmentally appropriate. Surveys of low socioeconomic status families have pointed to what are called "print-poor environments" as risk factors for poor school achievement—that is, children may be growing up in homes where print is not commonly used to transmit information. Without books, newspapers, magazines, pads of paper, writing implements, message boards, notes, e-mail, snail-mail, and alphabetic toys such as magnetic letters and alphabet blocks, young children are deprived of much of the print exposure that is essential for early literacy development. By sending books home with young children, the pediatrician has a chance to modify the home environment and help parents carry out advice about early literacy development.

PEDIATRIC INTERVENTION TO PROMOTE EARLY LITERACY

Literacy promotion in pediatric primary care has met with an enthusiastic reception among pediatricians, particularly among pediatricians who serve lower-income populations.

In taking on the issue of early literacy, child health clinicians are recognizing its important implications for health and development and capitalizing on their special opportunity and access. The nature of pediatric primary care, with multiple visits concentrated in the first several years of life and with strong imperatives toward developmental screening and concomitant discussions promoting child development, offers pediatric providers opportunities to help parents modify the child's early environment.

The Reach Out and Read model was created by pediatricians and early childhood educators who saw the special opportunities that pediatric primary care offered: a chance to see young children many times during the essential early years; the pediatric focus on assessing and assisting age-appropriate motor, language, and cognitive skills; and the role of the pediatrician as a trusted consultant to parents on issues of health and development. Reach Out and Read was created to function in a pediatric primary care environment, taking into account chronic shortages of physician time, support staff, and storage space. Founded in 1989 at Boston City Hospital, the program now has spread to more than 1400 clinics, hospitals, practices, and health centers around the United States. The model has three basic components.

First, pediatricians (and other clinicians providing pediatric primary care) incorporate anticipatory guidance about the importance of books and reading aloud into the health supervision visit. This guidance, which is of necessity brief, is most successful when it is placed in the context of other developmental and behavioral guidance. The parents of a 6-month-old may be advised that just as it is important to talk to infants before they can talk, it also is important to look at books with them and perhaps to point at pictures and name them aloud. The parents of an 18-month-old may need to hear that it is normal for a child to want to hear the same story over and over and over because children this age crave repetition as part of mastering speech and language; the parents of a 2-year-old may need to be reassured that their child's short attention span—too short to listen to a whole book—is normal and no barrier to reading aloud.

Second, this advice and modeling takes place with the gift of a book, given by the pediatrician to the child. Whenever possible, the book should be used to illustrate the guidance, whether by pointing and naming pictures to interest an infant, asking simple questions of a toddler to show parents the technique of dialogic reading (and perhaps to find out something about the toddler's language skills), or engaging a preschooler in the more complex question of what is happening in this picture. Reach Out and Read programs need to choose developmentally and culturally appropriate books, taking carefully into account the needs and preferences of children at each developmental age and stage (Table 261-2). By giving a book at every health supervision visit from 6 months to 5 years of age, a pediatrician can put a total of 9 or 10 books into a child's home before that child starts kindergarten, with each book coming in the context of developmentally appropriate anticipatory guidance.

Third, interventions in the waiting room create a context for literacy and a print-rich environment. Information on library use can be made available, as well as referral information for adult and family literacy programs. Some

Table 261-2. What Children Like in Books

Infants 6–12 months old like the following:
- Board books with photos of other babies
- Brightly colored board books to touch and taste
- Books with photos of familiar objects like balls and bottles

Toddlers 12–24 months old like the following:
- Sturdy board books that they can carry
- Books with photos of children doing familiar things like sleeping or playing
- Goodnight books for bedtime
- Books about saying good-bye and hello
- Books with only a few words on each page
- Books with simple rhymes or predictable text
- Animal books

Preschoolers 2–5 years old like the following:
- Books that tell stories
- Books about kids that look and live like them
- Books about making friends
- Books about going to school or to the doctor
- Books about having brothers or sisters
- Books that have simple texts they can memorize or read

From Literacy Promotion: Research Findings. Reach Out and Read®, www.reachoutandread.org.

clinics make used books available. When possible, volunteer readers in the waiting room read aloud to children who are waiting to be seen, modeling for parents many of the techniques of reading aloud that may be touched on later at the health supervision visit. A volunteer reader may pause and ask a question, such as "Where's the mouse? Who can point to the mouse?" Or a volunteer reader may alter his or her voice with the character, speaking in a squeaky voice when the mouse talks or a deep growl when the bear talks. Parents also can see, by watching the readers, that children do not need to sit in attentive silence when a book is read aloud but can call out answers and suggestions or even jump up and run around and then return to the story. For parents who have not had the experience of being read to themselves, the chance to listen to a story read aloud may illustrate vividly the pleasures that can be linked to children's books. Finally, the waiting room readers may reduce the tension and anger often associated with long waiting room sojourns.

EARLY LITERACY PROMOTION: DEVELOPMENTAL STAGES

Infants (6 to 12 Months)

Although it is important to counsel parents about speaking to infants from birth onward, during the first 6 months of life, young infants are focused on people and faces, rather than on objects. The Reach Out and Read model begins giving books at age 6 months, and the enthusiasm displayed by 6-month-old infants, who can sit up and grasp and manipulate the book and who smile, vocalize, and move their arms and legs to display pleasure, is a powerful reinforcement to a parent who is taking tentative first steps toward looking at books with an infant. Many pediatricians report that parents of infants express surprise and pleasure at their infants' positive reactions to an age-appropriate book. It is important to emphasize to parents that looking at books with an infant is not about teaching the infant to read, but instead is a way of helping the infant grow up enjoying books—and it is that pleasure and attachment that will help

262 Adoption

Mary Allen Staat

ROLE OF THE GENERALIST

1   Inform families of the unique issues faced by internationally adopted children.

2   Review systematically with the family all information provided about a child who is being considered for adoption.

3   Perform a detailed evaluation of the child postadoption with attention to specific issues raised by the background of the child.

4   Provide ongoing evaluation and support for child development and psychosocial issues.

5   Identify resources for consultation and collaboration.

Adoption is becoming increasingly popular. It is estimated that approximately 120,000 children are adopted in the United States each year. Types of adoptions include public, private, kinship, and stepparent adoptions. Public adoptions occur when children in the public child welfare system are adopted through either public government-operated agencies or private agencies contracted by a public agency. There are approximately 520,000 children in foster care in the United States, and of these, 117,000 are eligible for adoption. Data from 1995 found that only 20% of the 100,000 children available for adoption were adopted. Multiple factors are responsible for the low rate of adoption and low proportion of foster care children made eligible for adoption. Improved efforts to facilitate the process of adoption of children from the foster care system are under way; however, many obstacles still remain. Private adoptions occur domestically and internationally. There are no recent statistics on domestic adoptions outside of foster care because states are not required to report these numbers in any systematic manner. Similarly, data on kinship and stepparent adoptions are not available. Statistics for international adoptions come from the U.S. Department of State. International adoptions have increased each year; more than 20,000 children were adopted by U.S. families in 2002. Although children came from more than 20 countries, more than 80% of the children came from seven countries: China (25%), Russia (25%), Guatemala (11%), South Korea (9%), the Ukraine (6%), Kazakhstan (4%), and Vietnam (3%).

There is a growing body of literature on the issues and outcomes of children in foster care. There are only a few studies, however, regarding the outcomes of children who are internationally adopted and even fewer on children adopted domestically outside the foster care system. Institutionalization and impoverished conditions in resource-poor countries place internationally adopted children at an increased risk for many issues. Professionals caring for these children have begun to examine more closely the medical, developmental, and psychological issues of these children. Since the 1990s, many centers have emerged that specialize in the care of internationally adopted children and are available to assist in the care of these children. Foster care is discussed in Chapter 263. Because data are limited on domestic adoption, this chapter focuses on the care of internationally adopted children.

Families are motivated to choose adoption for a variety of reasons. One reason is infertility. For many women, the choice of having a career results in starting a family at an older age, when there are increased rates of infertility and adverse pregnancy outcomes. Single men and women who want to be parents also may choose adoption. Others desire to have a larger family without undergoing additional pregnancies. The desire to provide a family for a child who otherwise would not have one is another motivation for adopting a child. Less commonly, families who experience the death of a child may consider adoption. Increasingly, families are turning to international adoption instead of domestic adoption. With domestic adoption, many families are concerned about involvement by the birth parents. They fear that a birth parent may return to claim the child or become involved in the child's life. In addition, for many prospective adoptive parents, their age, marital status, and number of children already in their family cause concern that they would not be chosen by the birth parent when younger, married, childless couples also often are available. Often, placement of a child can occur much more quickly through international adoption compared with domestic adoption. Although some prospective parents may believe there are fewer health risks associated with international adoption, often the risks are similar and in some cases may be greater, especially in children who have been institutionalized.

With the diversity of reasons for adoption, it is important that the generalist understand and be sensitive to the individual family's reason for adoption to help prepare them for their experience. Physicians can play an important role in the process by assisting families in the planning stages of their adoption and caring for the children after they join their new family.

PREADOPTION CARE

Assisting Families with the Referral Process

Families should be aware of the unique issues that internationally adopted children face so that they can make an informed decision in the adoption process (Box 262-1). Children available for international adoption should be considered an at-risk population because the circumstances that made them available can be associated with a wide range of medical and developmental issues. These children come from resource-poor countries where mothers live in impoverished conditions and often do not have prenatal care. The standard of care for mothers and infants often does not include screening for infectious diseases, such as human immunodeficiency virus (HIV), syphilis, and hepatitis B. There are unknown exposures to drugs, tobacco, and alcohol. Nearly all children have experienced some level of neglect—with their birth family, with a foster family, or in an orphanage. Some children also may have been abused physically or sexually. Often there is little to no information regarding the child's birth parents or medical history, so

---

Box 262-1. Preadoption Review of Referral Information

Birth History
- Maternal history (maternal age, number of pregnancies and outcomes, alcohol or drug use, prenatal care, sexually transmitted diseases, medical or mental health conditions)
- Date of birth
- Gestational age
- Apgar scores
- Birth measurements (weight, length, and head circumference)
- Neonatal medical issues

Growth Parameters
- Head, weight, and length at multiple points in time
- Explanations for poor growth

Developmental Assessment
- Hearing and vision assessment
- Symmetry of reflexes and movements
- Gross motor, fine motor, language, and personal/social skills assessment
- Cognitive assessment in older children

Evaluation of Pictures or Video
- Facial and other body features (for syndromes, especially fetal alcohol syndrome)
- Skin lesions (birthmarks)
- Eyes (strabismus)
- Symmetry and positioning of extremities

Laboratory Evaluation
- Hepatitis B surface antigen, syphilis, and human immunodeficiency virus
- Other studies (anemia, hepatitis C)

Medical Diagnoses
- Recognized medical conditions (i.e., patent foramen ovale, rickets, anemia, limb deficiency, hepatitis B infection, syphilis)
- Unrecognized medical conditions (i.e., perinatal encephalopathy, hypertension syndrome, movement disorder, pyramidal insufficiency)

---

families must develop a level of comfort with never having access to that information. The referral information provided to the family is limited and often insufficient to make an informed decision. Because there is often the opportunity to request additional information, physicians can play an important role in assisting families by systematically reviewing the information provided and then outlining what additional information is needed to evaluate the child. Occasionally, there are requests to communicate with physicians or orphanage directors caring for the children in their birth country to clarify unresolved issues. It is important to understand the expectations of the parents for the child they plan to adopt. Providing an objective assessment of the referral information and outlining a realistic range of possible outcomes for the child helps the prospective parents make the most informed decision possible for their family. Parents commonly may decline a referral; when this happens, parents may grieve or feel guilty for not accepting the referral. It is important that the family's physician provide support to the family if this occurs.

Referrals typically consist of photographs and some general information regarding the child. A videotape sometimes may accompany the referral information. Information often is available about the birth history except in cases in which the child is abandoned, which is nearly always the case in children from China. Unless there is a note with the birth date or the umbilical cord is present, it may be difficult to assess the child's age accurately. Questioning how the age was determined and whether the stated age appears appropriate is important so that one can determine how much emphasis should be placed on the growth parameters and developmental assessment provided. If the child was not abandoned, attempts should be made to obtain as much information as possible about the child's birth history. Data regarding the infant's gestational age, birth weight, length and head circumference, Apgar scores, and maternal history should be evaluated or requested if not provided. Many infants are premature or small for gestational age, and it often is difficult to understand which is the case. The range of outcomes for infants with either condition should be discussed thoroughly with the prospective adoptive parents. The maternal history should include a history of infectious diseases, in particular syphilis and other sexually transmitted diseases, and a history of alcohol, drug, and tobacco use and mental illness. Alcoholism is known to be prevalent in Russia and the former Soviet Union, so the diagnosis of fetal alcohol syndrome (FAS) should be considered particularly for children born in these countries, but should be considered in any internationally adopted child regardless of the birth country. FAS should be considered in any child with poor growth and development and characteristic facial features with or without a maternal history of alcohol use.

Growth parameters, including weight, length, and head circumference measurements, should be obtained from birth and at multiple ages over time. Ideally, measurements within 1 month of the time of the referral should be provided. The measurements should be plotted on U.S. growth charts. Growth charts are available for some countries; however, information regarding how these charts were standardized is lacking, so these charts should not be used routinely. Although many children do not thrive in an orphanage and may not grow well, families should be aware that extremely poor growth may indicate an underlying medical problem and could result in long-term effects on learning and behavior. The significance of microcephaly should be discussed thoroughly with families. Although measurement errors could occur, errors should not be assumed. If the measurements are low, it is important to request repeat measurements done with specific instructions on how to measure the fronto-occipital circumference properly before assuming the measurements provided are incorrect.

A developmental assessment through a report or videotape should address the gross motor, fine motor, language, and personal/social skills of the child and cognitive abilities in an older child. Although mild delays from the orphanage environment or from cultural differences in care are expected, more significant delays may reflect an underlying condition. Attempts should be made to assess the child's ability to see and hear. A child with microcephaly, delayed development, and hearing loss should raise the suspicion of a congenital infection.

Photographs can be helpful in assessing the presence of obvious dysmorphic features; however, often the assessment is limited by the quality of the photographs, the orientation of the child in the photograph, and the child's age and race, especially when attempting to examine for characteristics of FAS. A videotape can provide the opportunity to assess the child's development, facial characteristics, and symmetry of movements. In addition, the child's interaction with caretakers and peers sometimes can be assessed. Often the tapes are only a few minutes in length and are poor quality and may not be representative of the child. The videotapes often are limited in their usefulness because caretakers rarely make an effort to show the child's abilities in age-appropriate activities. If there is a videotape to review, it can be helpful at times because the child may show developmental skills beyond those stated in the written referral and sometimes facial features and movement can be assessed. The child may be sleepy or irritable and may not perform well on the videotape, however, so reviewers should be cautioned not to overinterpret the information provided.

Reports of laboratory studies done in the child's birth country accompany nearly all referrals. Ideally, testing for hepatitis B surface antigen, HIV, and syphilis are done. Although having negative test results is reassuring, families should be aware that the report may not always be accurate. Laboratory errors, reporting errors, or testing during the incubation period could result in a false-negative test. In addition, exposure to HIV or hepatitis B in the birth country after the testing was done could occur. Parents should be educated about the long-term outcomes of these infections should they choose to adopt any child, but in particular if they choose to adopt a child with a history of one of these infections.

Many unfamiliar medications, therapies, and medical and developmental diagnoses often are listed on Russian and Eastern European referrals. Diagnoses such as perinatal encephalopathy, prenatal affect of the central nervous system, and hypertension do not translate into diagnoses known in pediatrics in the United States. Korean records are extremely thorough, whereas records from other countries typically have limited data. For families who choose to adopt a child with special needs, they should be well educated regarding the range of needs the child may have in the future to make an informed decision. Common conditions considered as special needs include prematurity, cleft lip and palate, limb deficiencies, congenital heart disease, and hepatitis B infection. Russian and Eastern European referrals often include diagnoses such as rickets, anemia, hip dysplasia, and open foramen ovale. Except for anemia, however, these diagnoses rarely are confirmed on evaluations in the United States.

Travel Preparation

Most families are required to travel to adopt their child, and in some countries, such as Russia and Bulgaria, families often need to make two trips. For Korean and Indian adoptions and sometimes in other countries, arrangements can be made to have the child escorted to the United States. In developing countries, diseases such as hepatitis B and measles are prevalent. Water and food may not be safe, so diseases such as typhoid, hepatitis A, and traveler's diarrhea also are common. In the case of an unexpected injury and the need for tetanus prophylaxis, tetanus vaccine may not be available or safe. Careful preparation should occur to prepare families for safe travel. Preparation should include education about country-specific risks, receipt of recommended immunizations before travel, provision of medications for traveler's diarrhea, and ensuring means to contact individuals in the United States should problems arise. Table 262-1 outlines general issues to consider when preparing families for travel for international adoption. Because conditions may vary for each country and may change over time, families and physicians should obtain the most recent recommendations to ensure that families are informed appropriately and receive the recommended immunizations and medications for travel.

Preparation for Parenting an International Adoptee

For some families, the adopted child may be the first child, and the new parents need basic advice on how to care for their child. Even for experienced parents, the parenting and childcare skills previously used may not be applicable to an internationally adopted child. Basics regarding safety, sleep, and feeding issues should be addressed before travel, and given an adoptee's early life experiences, these issues may need to be managed differently than in birth children. Anticipatory guidance should include information younger than the child's chronologic age because the child often is younger developmentally, and first-time parents may not have received the guidance for earlier ages.

Families should be aware that their child will need an adjustment period and that there is a wide range in duration of time needed for that adjustment. Some children adapt to their new home and family quickly, whereas others may need months to make the transition. Each child must be given time to grieve losses and adjust to the new environment. Although the adjustments may be more difficult and may take longer in older children, infants may experience difficulties that manifest as feeding and sleeping problems and overt behavioral problems.

Table 262-1. Preparation for International Travel

Country-specific education for parents about the risks involved in travel to their child's birth country
Food and water precautions
Other infectious diseases (scabies, lice, diarrhea, insect-borne infections)
Accidents
Immunize parents and family members who will travel or have close contact with adopted child
  Hepatitis A vaccine—recommended for most travelers >2 years old
  Typhoid vaccine—recommended for most travelers >2 years old
  Hepatitis B vaccine—recommended due to potential exposure from adopted child
  Measles vaccine—recommended if have not received second dose of MMR or born after 1957
  Tetanus booster (Td)—recommended for travelers if have not received booster in past 5–10 yr
  Polio vaccine—recommended for travelers if have not received booster
  Varicella vaccine—recommended if no history of varicella
Preparation for medical issues while abroad
Recognition of issues that may need medical attention
  High fever, rash, difficulty breathing, dehydration
Medical travel kit for family
  Traveler's diarrhea medications for parents
  Antibiotics for child
  Antipyretics for child
  Antiscabies medication for child
Emergency numbers for contact if issues arise
Preparation for caring for child while abroad
Advice on feeding
Advice on sleeping
Discussion about physical conditions commonly seen in adoptees
  Mongolian spots, diaper rashes, posterior scalp molding and balding, scabies, impetigo
Discussion about developmental and psychosocial issues frequently seen in adoptees
Delays in development, attachment issues, irritability, temper tantrums

POSTADOPTION CARE

Internationally adopted children come from resource-poor countries where malnutrition and infectious diseases are prevalent, and prenatal care, including screening for infectious diseases, is uncommon. Postadoption screening, including assessment of overall health and developmental status, is important for early identification of problems so that a management plan can be established. In addition, the generalist should be prepared for long-term management of growth, development, and psychosocial issues.

Initial Evaluation

An initial comprehensive assessment should occur within the first 2 weeks after arrival to the United States or within the first couple of days if there is an acute illness. Records from the child's birth country should be reviewed as outlined earlier in the section on preadoption care. Conditions reported in the record or conveyed to the family should be assessed to determine whether these conditions were diagnosed accurately. Identifying infectious diseases is important for the health of the child and the health of the child's family and community. Developing an immunization schedule to ensure that children are protected against vaccine-preventable diseases is challenging because documentation of immunizations received in the birth country varies, and there have been concerns that even with documentation some children may not have protective antibody to the

vaccines they have received. Box 262-2 outlines the recommended screening and evaluation of an internationally adopted child. Other testing and evaluations may be needed based on medical information from the child's birth country or from findings from the initial or subsequent medical evaluation in the United States. Some specific areas are discussed in more detail subsequently.

Initial Physical Findings

A thorough physical examination should be done with the child fully unclothed to identify scars, bruises, mongolian spots, and other skin lesions. Findings should be documented carefully so that should questions of abuse arise, prior skin findings will have been documented on arrival. If a bone deformity or decreased movement of an extremity is identified, radiographs should be obtained to determine whether the child has fractures. Growth parameters (weight, length, and head circumference) should be taken and plotted on U.S. growth charts. Many children appear thin and malnourished and often have abdominal distention. Many children have flattened, asymmetric skulls from

---

Box 262-2. Postadoption Evaluation of an Internationally Adopted Child

Antibody Testing for Immunization Verification

Children ≥5 Months Old

- Diphtheria IgG antibody (ELISA)
- Tetanus IgG antibody (ELISA)
- Polio neutralizing antibody to serotypes 1–3
- *Haemophilus influenzae* type b antibody
- Hepatitis B surface antibody

Children ≥12 Months Old

- Rubeola (measles) antibody
- Mumps antibody
- Rubella antibody
- Varicella antibody

Testing for Infectious Diseases

- Hepatitis B serology* (surface antigen, surface antibody, and core antibody)
- Hepatitis C antibody*
- HIV ELISA*
- Syphilis serology (MHA-TP and RPR)
- Stool for ova and parasites (three specimens)
- Stool for *Giardia* and *Cryptosporidium* antigen (one specimen)
- Mantoux tuberculin skin test*

Other Testing

- Complete blood count with differential
- Hemoglobin electrophoresis
- Lead level
- Glucose-6-phosphate dehydrogenase assay
- Audiology evaluation
- Ophthalmologic evaluation
- Dental evaluation

*These tests should be repeated 6 months after arrival because of the long incubation periods of these infections.
ELISA, enzyme-linked immunosorbent assay; HIV, human immunodeficiency virus; MHA-TP, microhemagglutination–*Treponema pallidum*; RPR, rapid plasma reagin.

Box 262-3. Common Health Issues among Internationally Adopted Children

- Growth delays
- Microcephaly
- Developmental delays
- Infectious diseases
  - Otitis media
  - Intestinal parasites
  - Tuberculosis
- Anemia
  - Iron deficiency
  - Thalassemia trait
- Rickets
- Lead poisoning
- Dermatologic conditions
  - Infections (scabies, fungal, impetigo)
  - Mongolian spots
  - Scars
  - Eczema
  - Hypopigmented and hyperpigmented lesions (café au lait lesions)
- Dental problems
- Hearing impairment
- Visual problems
  - Strabismus
  - Decreased visual acuity
- Uncertain immunization status
- Attachment issues

positional molding or rickets or both, which resolve over time. Boys are not circumcised, and the parents should be instructed on how to care for an uncircumcised penis. Acute infectious conditions, such as upper respiratory infections, otitis media, impetigo, fungal infections, scabies, and lice, frequently are identified on the initial evaluation. Box 262-3 lists common conditions seen on the initial evaluation, and Box 262-4 lists long-term issues.

INFECTIOUS DISEASE ISSUES

Intestinal Parasites

Intestinal parasites commonly are identified in international adoptees. The prevalence varies by age and birth country, with a higher prevalence in children from Russia and Eastern Europe and older children from any country. Children may be asymptomatic or have symptoms such as diarrhea and bloating. It may be difficult to assess whether children have symptoms, given language barriers and the young age of most children. Screening of all international adoptees regardless of the presence of symptoms is recommended. Screening should include three stool samples for ova and parasite testing collected 2 to 3 days apart because parasites may be shed intermittently, and the yield for recovery increases when three specimens are examined. One specimen should have antigen testing to identify *Cryptosporidium parvum* and to increase the sensitivity for identification of *Giardia lamblia. G. lamblia* is the most common intestinal parasite identified in international adoptees. Other parasites, such as *Blastocystis hominis* and *Dientamoeba fragilis*, also may be identified. Some children harbor helminths,

such as *Ascaris lumbricoides, Trichuris trichiura*, and *Hymenolepis* species; however, these parasites are not as common. Treatment for *G. lamblia, Entamoeba histolytica*, and most helminth infections is recommended. Treatment for *B. hominis* and *D. fragilis* is controversial but should be considered, especially in children who are malnourished or symptomatic. Specific management of these infections is discussed in Chapters 121 and 284. Children with diarrhea also should be examined for bacterial causes and other intestinal parasites not identified through routine ova and parasite testing. Repeat testing several weeks after treatment should be done to ensure that the infection has cleared.

Hepatitis

Hepatitis A and B are endemic in developing countries; although the prevalence of hepatitis C currently is not known for most countries, there is concern that the prevalence is high. Many international adoptees, especially older children, are likely to have been infected with hepatitis A. Routine screening for hepatitis A currently is not recommended for international adoptees. For children who will live in communities where there is a high rate of hepatitis A, however, the hepatitis A vaccine is recommended for children older than 2 years of age. Testing for hepatitis A to document past infection may be considered in adoptees older than 1 year of age to avoid unneccessary immunization.

In resource-poor countries, hepatitis B screening programs to identify mothers who are carriers typically are not in place, and early immunization and administration of hepatitis B immune globulin of exposed infants does not

Box 262-4. Long-Term Issues for International Adoptees

Medical Issues

- Hepatitis B infection
- Hepatitis C infection
- Tuberculosis
- Hearing and vision problems
- Dental problems

Growth Issues

- Global growth delay
- Short stature
- Microcephaly
- Precocious puberty

Developmental Issues

- Persistent developmental delays
- Fetal alcohol syndrome
- Learning disabilities
- Mental retardation
- Sensory integration disorder
- Autism spectrum disorders

Psychosocial Issues

- Attention deficit hyperactivity disorder
- Reactive attachment disorder
- Posttraumatic stress disorder
- Identity issues
- Mental health disorders

occur. Most children have been tested for hepatitis B and have documentation of this testing from their birth country. In addition, many internationally adopted children have documentation of immunization. In a more recent study, the prevalence of chronic hepatitis B infection in a group of internationally adopted children was 3%. In the same study, no children were found to be infected with hepatitis C virus.

All internationally adopted children should be screened routinely for hepatitis B, and screening for hepatitis C should be considered for children adopted from countries where the prevalence is high or if there is a history of receipt of blood products or maternal drug use. This screening should be done regardless of documentation of testing from the child's birth country because testing may be unreliable or may have been done before seroconversion. Hepatitis B surface antigen and hepatitis B surface and core antibody testing should be done to determine whether the child has evidence of past, current, or chronic infection or successful immunization. Hepatitis C antibody testing should be done, but if the test is positive, confirmatory testing is needed because false-positive results occur frequently. If the child has evidence of acute or chronic hepatitis B or C infection, the family should be counseled that the child could transmit the virus to others, and additional testing should be done to evaluate the child's disease state further with the assistance of a pediatric hepatologist. Early screening and identification of infected children helps prevent spread of disease by ensuring that family members are immunized for hepatitis B and use body fluid precautions. Because children could be infected just before their adoption and these infections have a long incubation period, testing 6 months after arrival should be considered. Hepatitis is discussed further in Chapters 90 and 119.

Syphilis

Although syphilis has been reported infrequently in international adoptees, syphilis testing is recommended for all internationally adopted children. Birth country documentation of proven or suspected syphilis is seen frequently in Russian children. Specifics about the extent of disease (i.e., asymptomatic, symptomatic, central nervous system involvement) and treatment (i.e., antibiotic, dose, frequency, and duration) generally are lacking, however. Even in children with a history of syphilis with documentation of treatment, unless the child has complete documentation of the evaluation and treatment, the child should be re-evaluated after arriving in the United States. Screening with nontreponemal tests, such as the rapid plasma reagin (RPR) or the Venereal Disease Research Laboratory (VDRL), identifies children with current infection or children who have been treated and have declining titers. In children who have been infected and have a nonreactive RPR or VDRL, the only evidence of infection (current or past) is a positive treponemal test, such as a fluorescent treponemal antibody absorption or microhemagglutination–*Treponema pallidum*. Screening with a treponemal test is recommended for all international adoptees. Children identified with past or current syphilis should have a thorough evaluation to assess for evidence of neurosyphilis. A child

with syphilis should be managed in consultation with a pediatric infectious disease specialist. Syphilis is discussed further in Chapters 209 and 224.

Human Immunodeficiency Virus

Information regarding the prevalence of HIV in countries where international adoptions occur is limited, and universal screening of mothers and treatment of HIV-positive mothers is uncommon. Nearly all children have documentation of an HIV test done in their birth country. The reliability of the testing is unclear, and there are many scenarios in which initial testing could be falsely negative. HIV testing should be done after the child arrives in the United States and should be considered 6 months later to ensure sufficient time for seroconversion if infection occurred just before arriving in the United States. Although there may be internationally adopted children infected with HIV, a more recent study did not find any children to have HIV infection.

Tuberculosis

Tuberculosis infection is common in international adoptees with 30% of children with latent tuberculosis infection. Shortly after arriving in the United States, internationally adopted children should have a tuberculin skin test (TST) done using the Mantoux method with purified protein derivative. The skin test should be read by a health care professional 48 to 72 hours after placement. Because these children are foreign born coming from countries where tuberculosis is endemic, it is recommended that a TST reading of 10 mm of induration or greater be considered evidence of tuberculosis infection. Many children will have received the bacille Calmette-Guérin (BCG) vaccine. The BCG vaccine is given to children in tuberculosis-endemic countries to prevent tuberculosis. Children may have written documentation of immunization or a characteristic scar in the deltoid area showing BCG vaccine administration. Although the BCG vaccine can cause a reactive TST, reactions are inconsistent and typically not as large as 10 mm induration. A history of receipt of BCG vaccine is not a contraindication to having a TST placed and should not be considered in the interpretation of the TST result. Induration of 10 mm or greater is considered positive and diagnostic of tuberculosis infection. Induration of 5 mm or greater should be used in children who have a known exposure to someone with active tuberculosis. Children with tuberculosis infection should have a thorough physical examination and a chest radiograph to evaluate for tuberculosis disease. Although tuberculosis disease has been reported rarely in international adoptees, a large outbreak in North Dakota was reported because of a lack of appropriate screening in two children from the Marshall Islands. In children who initially have TSTs with less than 10 mm induration, repeating the skin testing 6 or more months after arrival should be considered. This repeat testing is done because at the time of initial testing children may be anergic from malnutrition or may have been infected just before leaving their birth country and may not have had sufficient time to mount an immune response. For children with latent tuberculosis infection, prophylaxis with a 9-month course of isoniazid at 10 to 15 mg/kg/day is

Table 263-1. Age-Specific Guidelines for Foster Care Assessment—cont'd

	Newborn–Toddler	Preschooler	School-age	Adolescent
Follow-up and Care Management	Review of all requested records Rescheduling based on clinical findings and agency policy	Review of all requested records Rescheduling based on clinical findings and agency policy	Review of all requested records Rescheduling based on clinical findings and agency policy	Review of all requested records Rescheduling based on clinical findings and agency policy Birth control, STD education addressed
Foster Parent Anticipatory Guidance	Behavior problems related to visitation, sleep disorders, attachment issues, permanency planning	Behavior problems related to visitation, sleep disorders, attachment issues, permanency planning	Behavior problems related to visitation, sleep disorders, attachment issues, permanency planning	Behavior problems related to visitation, sleep disorders, attachment issues, permanency planning

Developmental, Behavioral, and Mental Health Assessment

An accurate developmental or mental health evaluation may be difficult to perform, especially if out-of-home placement is a recent occurrence. The foster parent, if available, should be questioned about the child's behavior since removal from the home. Despite the sometimes adverse home environments from which these children are removed, each child may view removal from the home as a significant psychological trauma. It should be expected that the child may be tearful, frightened, and withdrawn, depending on the developmental age of the child. Severe emotional distress (uncontrollable crying, suicidal ideation, aggression) requires immediate mental health referral. Most foster parents, although loving and with good intentions, do not have the training to deal with the emotionally fragile child suffering through the trauma of being placed in foster care. Even if the child is reported to be coping well, a reassessment of the child's adjustment to foster placement should occur within 30 days. After the initial shock of separation has subsided, many children display maladaptive behaviors that need to be addressed, and foster families need to be supported through these challenges by the pediatrician and by the foster care agency.

Abused and neglected children are at risk for not having a healthy attachment to anyone, and the consequences of this may be an adult who is unable to trust and love. A child who has had the time and opportunity to form a secure attachment to an adult caretaker may show signs of grief and distress at the separation from the caregiver regardless of abuse or neglect that may have occurred. Visits with the attachment figure (biologic parent or other adult) are important during foster placement to maintain that relationship. These visits should be frequent and long enough to enhance the parent-child relationship. Younger children lack the ability to understand concepts such as "tomorrow" or "next week" and need more frequent visits than older children who have a more developed sense of time. Children with more disordered forms of attachment may appear withdrawn and depressed or inappropriately friendly and willing to be held by strangers. These behaviors should be noted in the assessment and referral made to a mental health specialist. Behavior problems also may be noted before and after visits with the biologic parents. The child may experience anger at the parent who "let them get taken away" and grief when the visit ends and the child is "abandoned" again. The foster family may look to the pediatrician to help put these behaviors into perspective and to explain that these emotions should be respected and discussed with the child in an age-appropriate fashion. Mental health evaluations for all school-age and older foster children should be considered routine because of the high prevalence of behavioral and emotional problems among these age groups.

Using a standardized office developmental screening tool can help document the strengths and weaknesses in the child's development, identify areas of concern, and determine the need for more formal assessments. Two frequently used tests are the Denver Developmental Screening Test–II for ages birth to 6 years, which evaluates performance in gross motor, fine motor, language, and personal/social skills, and the Clinical Adaptive Test/Clinical Linguistic Auditory Milestone Scale (CAT/CLAMS) for ages 1 month to 3 years, which focuses on expressive and receptive language milestones. Language assessment is essential because it is well documented that children in the foster care system are significantly at risk for language delay and other developmental problems. Language evaluation often may need to wait until the foster parent has had more contact with the child to respond to the questions asked on the screening tests. The foster parents can be advised of what is normal language for a particular age group so that at the next visit, more useful historical information may be obtained. Any suggestion of language delay should lead to a hearing evaluation and possibly a speech and language evaluation. If the child is school age or older, the pediatrician can assess whether the child is in the appropriate grade for age and whether school records should be obtained to complete the evaluation.

The Goodenough-Harris Drawing Test (Draw-a-Person Test) for children 3 to 6 years old is a useful tool to screen the child's cognitive skills and visual motor skills. A crayon or pencil and paper can be introduced to the child at the beginning of the evaluation to help alleviate anxiety. The elements of the drawing can be scored to determine if the drawing is age appropriate. A family drawing also can be requested, again as an "ice breaker," but also as a way to get a snapshot of the child's point of view of his or her family and situation. Individual figures in the family drawing can be scored as in the Draw-a-Person Test. If seeing the foster child in a continuity context, a family drawing at follow-up visits can be used to help add to historical data about the child's adaptation to out-of-home care.

Because children in foster care are at high risk for behavioral problems, the routine use of a behavior questionnaire for foster parents to complete may increase the likelihood of identifying problems that need to be addressed. The Child Behavior Checklist is a commonly used tool for this purpose. The foster parent needs to have spent sufficient time with the child for the checklist to be helpful.

When screening for mental health issues in the adolescent, the American Medical Association's mnemonic of HEADSS is helpful in asking and documenting the major aspects of psychosocial behavior (Box 263-2). A depression questionnaire can be given to the adolescent at the time of check-in to screen further for suicide risk. Any child deemed to be at risk for suicide should receive immediate mental health referral.

Laboratory Tests and Imaging

In addition to the age-specific laboratory screening tests performed for routine health supervision, children in foster care may warrant additional screening because of the high risk for health problems in this population. In one inner-city study, newborns discharged to foster care were eight times more likely to be born to HIV-positive mothers than infants discharged home with their mothers. For a newborn or toddler, testing for HIV, hepatitis B, hepatitis C, and syphilis should be considered if maternal records cannot be accessed or are nonexistent. States differ in policies regarding who is authorized to give consent for HIV testing. The pediatrician needs to work with the caseworker to determine the appropriate procedure. Any child suspected of being a victim of sexual abuse, all children with symptoms or physical findings compatible with HIV infection, and all children with a sibling or parent who is HIV infected or at increased risk of HIV infection should be tested for

HIV. All sexually active adolescents and adolescents with a history of illicit substance use should be screened for sexually transmitted diseases, including HIV (with assent of the adolescent). This also is an opportunity for the pediatrician to provide education and counseling about prevention of transmission of HIV and other sexually transmitted diseases. When a foster child is found to be positive for HIV, the foster parents should be educated about the management issues.

A hematocrit or hemoglobin should be obtained in children younger than 6 years of age, starting at age 9 months or earlier if the child was premature or of low birth weight, and in menstruating adolescent girls. Children who are victims of abuse and neglect are at higher risk for lead exposure, and a serum lead test should be performed on foster children from ages 9 months to 6 years at the time of the initial evaluation. A tuberculin skin test at the time of the initial evaluation is recommended for foster children older than age 1 year because of the increased chances of coming from an environment at high risk for tuberculosis and the lack of readily available history to determine exposure. A sickle cell screen should be considered in at-risk infants and for African-American adolescents. Foster children in the newborn-toddler age group may need skeletal radiographs or bone scans or both if there is a history of physical abuse before placement or worrisome signs (e.g., persistent fussiness or crying, refusal to use an extremity) on the physical examination.

Immunizations

The immunization status of the child is important to ascertain. Many children are either unimmunized or underimmunized because they may have had little or no contact with the medical system secondary to the abuse and neglect experienced in their homes. If possible, immunization records should be obtained by caseworkers at time of removal, but this is often not the case. These children should be considered disease susceptible, and appropriate immunizations should be administered at the time of the visit according to the guidelines published each January by the American Academy of Pediatrics (AAP) Committee on Infectious Disease. Before giving the varicella vaccine, the clinician should determine the HIV risk of the child, either through available maternal history or by serum testing.

Management and Follow-up

A working relationship with the caseworker is essential. In many agencies, the caseworker is responsible for arranging the visit to a primary care provider, arranging referrals requested by the physician, and communicating with the biologic parent. The primary care physician should develop a tracking system within the practice for these children that reminds staff to contact the caseworker to check on the progress of the referrals, especially if the child is expected to come back to the practice for further care. The foster parents also can be allies in ensuring that referral appointments are made and kept. Follow-up can be time-consuming, but it is crucial for these high-risk children. Many foster children have never had a primary care continuity experience. A copy of the evaluation of the foster child that includes findings and recommendations for

---

Box 263-2. HEADSS Format for Adolescent Psychosocial Screening

- **H**ome
- **E**ducation
- **E**ating behaviors
- **A**ctivities (including work, peers, gangs, sports, TV, exercise)
- **D**rug (including inhalants)/alcohol/tobacco history
- **S**exual history (including abuse)
- **S**uicidal ideation, attempts, and affect

From AMA Guidelines for Adolescent Preventive Services (GAPS): Recommendations and Rationale. Baltimore, Williams & Wilkins, 1994.

treatment and referrals should be incorporated in the child's social service care plan. Follow-up visits, ideally with the same provider who performed the initial evaluation, should be scheduled based on clinical findings and agency policy. Continuity of primary care allows the pediatrician to support the foster family better. These at-risk children are believed to need a medical evaluation at least twice in the first year of foster care and yearly thereafter. At these follow-up visits, all requested records from previous visits and results of referrals should be reviewed, and appropriate action should be taken. Knowledge of the local foster system, what the responsibilities of the caseworker are, who makes the referrals, and the timing of agency-mandated follow-up visits are essential elements of tracking these children.

ADVOCACY

Pediatricians can act as advocates on a case-by-case basis, pushing for services and placements that serve the best interest of the child. Federal legislation currently requires states to begin terminating parental rights if a child has been in care for 15 of the prior 22 months. The pediatrician should ask the caseworker about the permanency planning for the foster child. The pediatrician should emphasize the importance of limiting the number of placements for children in foster care, especially young children, to provide opportunities for them to form healthy attachment relationships with a trusted adult.

The AAP Committee on Early Childhood, Adoption, and Dependent Care has published recommendations for the general pediatrician in the assessment of children in foster placement, based on work done in the late 1980s between the AAP and the Child Welfare League of America. The standards of the Child Welfare League of America are held up as the bar that state welfare agencies should reach to achieve the level of health services that foster children deserve. These standards emphasize the need for comprehensive medical and mental health assessments of children as they enter the foster care system and continual reassessment as the child remains in the foster system. Pediatricians interested in becoming involved with advocacy for foster

children should be aware of these standards to assess how their state system attempts to meet them. When the bar is not being met, a pediatrician can become an advocate for improving the system by meeting with agency officials and working with local chapters of the AAP, foster parent organizations, and other child advocacy organizations.

Pediatricians need to emphasize to policy makers that foster children have special health care needs. Studies have shown that the cost and use of mental health services by children in foster care were similar to those of children with disabilities. Advocacy for adequate mental health services for foster children is needed in every state.

Additional Resources, CD-ROM

Bibliography	

Mini-index of Related Topics CH.

- CHILD ADVOCACY — 259
- LEGAL ASPECTS OF CHILD ABUSE AND NEGLECT — 267
- CHILD NEGLECT: THE INADEQUATE PROMOTION OF CHILDREN'S HEALTH AND DEVELOPMENT — 268
- PHYSICAL ABUSE AND SEXUAL ABUSE — 269

SUGGESTED READINGS

American Academy of Pediatrics Committee on Early Childhood, Adoption and Dependent Care: Developmental issues for young children in foster care. Pediatrics 2000;106:1145–1150.

Halfon N, Mendonca A, Berkowitz G: Health status of children in foster care: The experience of the Center for the Vulnerable Child. Arch Pediatr Adolesc Med 1995;149:386–392.

Horwitz SM, Owens P, Simms MD: Specialized assessments for children in foster care. Pediatrics 2000;106:59–66.

Simms MD, Dubowitz H, Szilagyi MA: Health care needs of children in the foster care system. Pediatrics 2000;106:909–918.

Szilagyi M: The pediatrician and the child in foster care. Pediatr Rev 1998;19:39–50.

264 Divorce

George J. Cohen and Joseph F. Hagan, Jr.

ROLE OF THE GENERALIST

1 Discuss family interaction as part of well-child care.

2 Recognize indicators of dysfunctional marriage or separation, such as behavioral change in the child or parents or both.

3 Advocate for the child by offering age-appropriate support and explanation of reactions to the problem, particularly sadness, anger, guilt, and feelings of loss.

4 Counsel and support both parents without showing preference, unless there is abuse.

5 If abuse is suspected, refer to a child protection agency.

6 Refer family to resources with expertise in dealing with divorce and its consequences when needed.

Divorce is a remedy to bring an end to unhappy marriages and should serve to protect children from growing up in strife-ridden homes. Yet adjustment to parental divorce is one of the most prevalent psychosocial stressors for children encountered in primary care pediatrics. The divorce rate in the United States has increased more than fivefold in the past century. Approximately 1.1 million children experience parental separation each year, and about 20% experience a second divorce.

EPIDEMIOLOGY

In the United States, 60% of divorces involve children. About one third of divorces occur when involved children are younger than 3 years old. Among children of divorce younger than 6 years old, 40% of divorces occur when children are younger than 1 year old, 20% occur when children are between 1 and 2 years old, and 10% to 15% occur when children are 2 to 6 years old. Approximately 69% of children age 17 or younger live with both parents, 22% live with mother only, and 4% live with father only. Other living arrangements include extended family, stepfamily, and foster care. Only one fourth of nonresident fathers see their children at least once a week, and more than 30% see their children once a year or less frequently.

Divorce is two to four times more frequent if the wife is younger than age 20 compared with wives older than 30. Education beyond high school seems to have a small correlation with decreased frequency of divorce, whereas poverty often is cited as a risk factor. Grounds for divorce

have changed in the United States in the past 100 years. From the 1890s to 1965, adultery as grounds decreased from 25% to slightly more 1% in 1965, desertion from 44% to 14%, and drunkenness from almost 8% to 0.3%, but cruelty increased from 16% to greater than 40%. Other postulated causes for the current high rate of divorce include the theory that men without positive memories of their own fathers have not had appropriate husband role models. Women angry with their mothers may look to their husbands to be their "ideal" mother. Immature needs for instant gratification in either partner, diverse cultural backgrounds, and mental illness in one or both partners are factors in divorce. One half of first marriages and 60% of second marriages end in divorce.

CHILDREN'S REACTIONS TO DIVORCE

Because parents' discord and disagreements and hostility are difficult to conceal from children at any age, children feel the tension, often well before an actual separation occurs. Internalizing and externalizing behavioral problems often appear, even in preschool children. The sense of loss of parental love and of familiar home, school, playmates, standard of living, extended family, and family routines may mean difficult readjustment, insecurity, and distress for the child. More than 50% of children have obvious emotional or behavioral reactions within the first year of parental separation. Continuing parental disagreement about child rearing, child health care, and school choices and parental mental and emotional problems and poverty may lead to children's persisting reactions. Long-term studies show that divorce can limit or delay children's capacity for intimacy and commitment as young adults. Children's reactions vary depending on their age and level of understanding, temperament of the children and parents, temperamental fit, parents' ability to pay attention to children's needs when they are struggling with their own feelings and readjustment needs, and predivorce behavior and functioning of the family. Over time, most children gradually cope and function satisfactorily, although many report at least some residual emotional problems.

Infants and children younger than 3 years old may reflect the preoccupation, grief, and distress of their parents; most often they are fearful, irritable, and tearful and show separation anxiety. They are likely to have sleep problems, somatic symptoms, aggression, or developmental regression. Four- and 5-year-olds often blame themselves for the separation and parental symptoms. They may misperceive

Table 265-1. Development of the Concept of Death in Healthy Children

Approximate Age (yr)	Piagetian Developmental Stage	Approximate Age (yr)	Concept of Death
0–2	Sensorimotor Preverbal Reflex activity > purposeful activity Rudimentary thought	Infancy	Expresses discomfort with separation; fears pain
2–6	Preoperational Prelogical	3	Uses word *dead*, but only to distinguish as *not alive*
	Development of representational or symbolic language	4	Has limited notion; may express no personal emotion but may associate death with sorrow of others
	Initial reasoning	5	Avoids dead things; imagines death as a personified being; believes he or she will always live, only others (especially those older) die
		6	Associates death with "old age"; may be violent and emotional about death, including representations (e.g., magazine pictures), or may display intense curiosity about dead things
6–12	Concrete operational Logical	7	Has great interest in details (e.g., graveyards, coffins, possible causes); seeks answers through observation of decomposition, suspects he or she may die
	Problem solving restricted to physically present, real objects that can be manipulated	8	Is less morbid, more expansive; interested in what happens after death; accepts, with little emotion, that he or she, too, will die
	Development of logical functions (e.g., classification of objects)	9–10	Understands logical and biologic a (e.g., absence of pulse) essentials of death; can understand concrete explanation of death process
>12	Formal operational Abstract Comprehension of purely abstract or symbolic content Development of advanced logical functions (e.g., complex analogy, deduction)	Adolescence	Appreciates meaning of death but does not accept reality of personal death

Adapted from Sahler OJZ, Friedman SB: The dying child. Pediat Rev 1981;3:159–165. Copyright 1981. Reproduced with permission from *Pediatrics in Review*.

conversation. Later, dead becomes distinguished from alive; then, much later, it becomes associated with an irreversible biologic state.

A child's first remembered experience with death often relates to the loss of a pet. Parents should be counseled that immediate replacement of a pet is inadvisable because it reinforces the erroneous notion that everything (and everyone) that dies can be replaced. Immediate replacement also suppresses the heart-wrenching, but necessary, grieving process the child must experience to learn what grief is, how to express it, and that it lessens over time.

Interventions particularly relevant to children this age are focused on correcting misperceptions. The particularly troubling misperception that something they said or did caused the death must be corrected. This belief may be so strong and the child so convinced of personal responsibility that even asking questions about causation may be too threatening. Knowing this, the pediatrician or parents should take the initiative. One way to begin this conversation is to use the third person ("Sometimes when someone dies, children think they made it happen, maybe because they had a 'bad' thought. But everyone knows you can't make someone get sick or die from thoughts or wishes.")

Children this age also need to receive specific information about what "dead" is: "Dead is when a person's heart stops beating. It may look like sleeping but it is very different. When a person dies, the heart and all the other parts of the body, like the lungs and brain, do not work anymore. A dead person doesn't feel cold or hungry."

Children 6 to 12 Years Old

Between age 6 and 12 years, children become increasingly communicative and cognitively sophisticated. Initially, they are painstakingly fair and mete out exact, inflexible justice; by the end of this stage, the need for retribution gives way to understanding the concept of intent. This transition permits them to be less burdened by the concept of illness and death as punishment that is typical of younger children.

Early in this stage, some children seem morbidly attracted to dead things and avidly interested in the physiologic signs of death (e.g., cessation of breathing, changes in skin color). A 7- or 8-year-old may disinter a dead animal repeatedly to follow the progression of physical decomposition. By the age of 9 or 10, the child's use of the word *dead* approximates adult understanding of the term. More importantly, most children this age understand that death is not reserved for "old" people (a popular notion among

5- and 6-year-olds). Dying could happen to them. They also understand that death can be caused by internal events, such as cancer or infection. This understanding is in contrast to typical 6- to 8-year-old children, who associate death with external events, such as ghosts or accidents. Older school-age children understand death as a physical and a spiritual process. Depending on their belief system, they may believe the spirit continues to "live" in heaven or in memories.

Interventions for children this age capitalize on their curiosity and willingness to ask questions. It is most helpful, however, to understand exactly what the child is asking before giving an answer. If a child asks where bodies go after death, it is probably not wise to explain different spiritual belief systems and the concept of "afterlife," unless this is explicitly what the child is asking. As at least one youngster confronted by this barrage has put it, "Just tell me where the body goes. Do they put it in a closet or something before the funeral?"

Adolescents

Psychosocially, adolescents are striving toward identity formation and emotional independence. Cognitively, adolescents generally are capable of abstract thought. Some adolescents are deeply interested in religious or philosophical interpretations of life processes. They may seek to know the meaning of suffering.

Adolescents can conceptualize death as a universal, irreversible process. Because they have the capacity for self-evaluation and insight, adolescents are able to contemplate personal death. Many adolescents find this notion anxiety provoking and attempt to show they are invulnerable by engaging in "death-defying" behaviors. This "it can't happen to me" phenomenon contributes to the high rate of traumatic death among older teenagers and young adults.

Interventions designed for adolescents are most effective when they acknowledge that teens usually prefer to communicate with peers or with nonfamily adults rather than with family members. A peer-group intervention that includes other adolescents undergoing similar experiences is most powerful because the grieving teen learns that the feelings he or she is having are normal, not "weird." Creative writing, music, and art as expressive outlets are more likely to be accepted by teenagers than "counseling" from an adult. Most teenagers argue that depression/sadness/misery associated with grief is normal, and they do not need counseling. The most effective solution is to offer several alternatives and let the teen pursue the approach, formal or informal, that seems most comfortable. The exact method is less important than the outcome.

RITUALS OF DEATH

"Should my child go to the funeral?" is one of the most common questions families ask when someone dies. Some families bring infants to the service; others discourage even young adults from attending. The decision about what is appropriate at a given age may change depending on whether there is an open casket and the manner of death.

The pediatrician should be aware that an invitation to attend a wake or funeral can provide powerful acknowl-edgment to children that their grief is real and their relationship to the deceased was important. Attendance also helps solidify the irreversibility of death and brings closure to relationships. Explaining what will happen and why before the ritual is crucial. A caring, familiar adult who is not emotionally distraught should accompany the child. This adult's specific role is to support the child, answer questions, and model expected behavior. Children should be allowed to leave at any time if they become uncomfortable or bored, not only for their sake, but also for the sake of the other mourners.

Some families incorporate children into the service by having older children read a passage or tell a story. Younger children may carry flowers or put a special object into the casket. One father, whose wife died unexpectedly, walked the hills on his property with his 6-year-old daughter so that they could pick a place together to bury his wife, her mother. The child did not attend the funeral but was present at the burial and helped make the bouquet that was used to mark the burial place.

Although an invitation to attend the wake or funeral is appropriate for almost any child age 4 or older, a child's desire not to attend also must be respected. Alternatives such as a private time to say goodbye or selecting an object to be placed in the casket by someone else should be offered but not demanded. If, at some time in the future, the child expresses regret for not having attended, reassurance that the decision was difficult, that there was no "right" answer, and that the child made the best decision he or she could at that sad and confusing time is essential. The child also can be supported in creative or symbolic expression of what might have been said to the person who died.

OTHER WAYS TO MOURN

Whether a child attends a service or not, other opportunities to mourn must be provided. Art, through drawing pictures, making a memory box, or creating a special picture album, is an excellent outlet for some. As a non-verbal method of communication, art often can express what words cannot. Writing stories or poems about the person who has died can be used to explore sad, ambivalent, and happy memories.

Reading is a major source of comfort to children of all ages. Children's literature is rich with books developed specifically for grieving children and their families to help explain the common beliefs and misconceptions of children of different ages. This literature also provides useful examples of the most appropriate language and concepts to use with a child. Many families ask for information about books they can read or suggest to their children. *Bibliotherapy*, the use of reading materials specifically designed to help a person cope with a difficult situation, can be a highly effective tool for working through grief. Reading stories is a familiar activity for children and serves as a nonthreatening way to enter into discussions that can be viewed from the perspective of the third person before becoming personalized. That is, the reader identifies with characters in the book, experiences the various emotions the characters experience, and discovers that there are many different acceptable reactions to a situation, including his or her own. Examples of books and websites available to professionals and families are included on the CD-ROM under multimedia resources to assist the grieving child.

Attending a peer support group is often more helpful than working individually with a counselor, even for children of early school age. Knowing someone else who has gone through a similar experience is comforting and allows the child to talk about feelings and thoughts that might be perceived as unacceptable to adults.

COMPLICATED GRIEVING

Everyone who has suffered a significant loss must do grief work. Some begin that grief work immediately; others are unable to accept the reality of the death until weeks or months later. Common reactions in grieving people include "seeing" or "hearing" the person who has died; feeling totally exhausted or alone; crying "for no reason"; difficulty sleeping, eating, or making decisions; and worrying about "going crazy." Acute grief that interferes significantly with daily functioning may last several weeks or longer. The symptoms of grief are almost indistinguishable from the symptoms of depression. In adults, the diagnosis of major depressive disorder is reserved for situations in which the symptoms of acute grief are present for more than 2 months. Although distinguishing normal grieving from complicated (pathologic or unresolved) grieving can be difficult, a good rule of thumb is that increasing functional adaptation, even if slow, signifies that the child's grief probably is not pathologic.

Children reflect the processes of the adults around them. It is not unusual for a child to be caught up in the unresolved grief of a parent and to become the identified patient when the parent cannot move forward. Acting out, withdrawal, and anxiety on the part of the child can be markers for a parent's poor adaptation. Because some parents perceive seeking help for their child as more acceptable than seeking help for themselves, it is always appropriate to see parents alone to assess their coping rather than focusing solely on the child. A referral for grief counseling for the parent is likely to free the child from the need to be the call for help.

PEDIATRICIANS AND BEREAVED CHILDREN

A deceptively simple yet highly effective way for the pediatrician to acknowledge the child's grief and extend a natural offer of help is to write a note of condolence to the child. Children often are included in general notes written to the family, but it is uncommon for them to receive personal expressions of sorrow at their loss. Simple language and thoughts are probably best: "I just heard that 'X' died. I know 'X' was very important to you and you will miss [him or her]. I just wanted you to know that I'm thinking of you. If you ever want to talk with me about how things are going or if you have any questions that I might be able to answer, just call me, and I can talk to you on the phone or meet with you. Please give my regards to your family and tell them that I was sorry to hear the news." The note should include a phone number. Some children respond after weeks, months, or even years to this invitation.

CONCLUSION

Almost all children experience loss through the death of a significant person sometime before the end of adolescence. It is essential to acknowledge and attend to their needs as participants in the anticipatory grieving and bereavement processes. Understanding how children conceptualize illness and death at various developmental stages and how to support and comfort them are important roles for the pediatrician. Families should be encouraged to seek advice about how to include children in EOL care and bereavement activities. Children who are included in constructive ways are better able to adapt to their loss immediately and over their lifetime.

◎ **Additional Resources, CD-ROM**

Bibliography

Mini-index of Related Topics   CH.

SUGGESTED READINGS

American Academy of Pediatrics Committee on Psychosocial Aspects of Child and Family Health: The pediatrician and childhood bereavement. Pediatrics 2000;105:445–447.

Corr CA, Corr DM: Key elements in a framework for helping grieving children and adolescents. Illness Crisis Loss 1998;6:142–160.

Geis HK, Whittlesey SW, McDonald NB, et al: Bereavement and loss in childhood. Child Adolesc Psychiatr Clin N Am 1998;7:73–85.

Stanbrook M, Parker K: The development of the concept of death in childhood: A review of the literature. Merrill-Palmer Q 1987; 33:133–157.

Van Riper M: Death of a sibling: Five sisters, five stories. J Pediatr Nurs 1997;23:587–593.

266 Domestic Violence: A Pediatric Perspective

Robert Siegel

Domestic violence has been recognized as a major health problem in the United States. Each year, 1 to 4 million women are abused by their partners. Although a much smaller problem, more than 150,000 men have been abused by their partners. The impact of domestic violence is great. Domestic violence is responsible for one third of women's

---

Box 266-1. Common Clinical and Behavioral Findings in Abused Women

- Bruises, abrasions, lacerations
- Injuries during pregnancy
- Chronic pain
- Symptoms related to stress
  - Anxiety
  - Depression
  - Sleep and appetite disturbances
  - Fatigue
  - Chronic headache
  - Chronic genitourinary complaints
- Substance abuse
- Posttraumatic stress reactions
- Partner attempts to control relationship
  - Limited access to medical care
  - Partner accompanies patient to visits
  - Woman is reluctant to speak or disagree
  - Denial or minimization of violence by partner

---

visits to the emergency department, one quarter of women who attempt suicide, and almost one third of homicides against women. The financial burden also is great, with medical fees, legal fees, and lost wages amounting to more than $5 billion a year in the United States.

In the early 1990s, the American Medical Association (AMA) recognized the importance of the medical community being aware of the medical aspects of domestic violence and suggested that physicians be aware of the signs of domestic violence and screen for this problem in medical settings. Some of the behavioral and clinical findings are listed in Box 266-1.

Although there is no uniformly accepted definition of *domestic violence*, many experts suggest that the term includes all violence by any caretaker or adult partner on any other members of the household, including pets. This chapter focuses on partner violence, particularly men against women because it is the most commonly described form of domestic violence. Risk factors, signs and symptoms, and how to screen for domestic violence in the pediatric setting are discussed.

Since the AMA's campaign of domestic violence awareness, several medical specialty organizations have endorsed screening policies. With screening programs in place, many investigators have reported the benefits of screening in various medical settings, including emergency departments and primary care office settings. In general, women screened in medical settings disclose domestic violence 10% to 40% of the time. Table 266-1 summarizes the results of a sampling of these studies. As can be seen, screening in primary care settings is effective in uncovering abuse.

Women who are pregnant are at high risk for injury. Several factors may play a role and include the woman's increased dependency on her partner, the abuser's perception of increased needs by the pregnant woman, and the possibility of the woman making a move to leave an abusive relationship to protect the infant. Whatever the cause, pregnancy and the immediate period following is a crucial time for health care professionals to screen.

RELATIONSHIP OF DOMESTIC VIOLENCE TO PEDIATRICS

Children are affected profoundly by domestic violence. Family violence often extends beyond the abuse of the partner, and children and even pets in the home are at risk

Table 266-1. Domestic Violence Screening in Specialty Settings

Author	Setting	Old Abuse	New Abuse	Comments
Johnson and Elliott, 1997	Rural family practice	34%	23%	Concluded screening is justified
Canterino et al, 1999	Obstetric	36% old or new		Self-report questionnaire as good as interview
Geary and Wingate, 1999	Obstetric	20%	30.5%	25% had old and new domestic violence
Furbee et al, 1998	Emergency department	51% old or new		3% were in emergency department for abusive injuries

Data from Johnson D, Elliott B: Screening for domestic violence in a rural family practice. Minn Med 1997;80:43–45; Canterino JC, VanHorn LG, Harrigan JT, et al: Domestic abuse in pregnancy: A comparison of a self-completed domestic abuse questionnaire with a directed interview. Am J Obstet Gynecol 1999;181:1049–1051; Geary FH Jr, Wingate CB: Domestic violence and physical abuse of women: The Grady Memorial Hospital experience. Am J Obstet Gynecol 1999;181:517–521; Furbee PM, Sikora R, Williams JM, Derk SJ: Comparison of domestic violence screening methods: A pilot study. Ann Emerg Med 1998;31:495–501.

for physical abuse. The social, physical, and psychological effects of domestic violence on children are enormous (Box 266-2). Virtually any behavioral problem may be precipitated by family violence. In fact, women abused in childhood and adulthood are at risk for maternal depressive symptoms, harsher parenting, and behavioral problems in their children.

SCREENING FOR DOMESTIC VIOLENCE

The American Academy of Pediatrics, similar to several other medical specialty organizations, has endorsed routine screening for domestic violence. The American Academy of Pediatrics recommendations are summarized in Box 266-3. Although there is an extensive screening experience in adult settings (see Table 266-1), studies in pediatric settings are limited. Screening studies in pediatric settings are summarized in Table 266-2. Similar to the adult studies, screening in pediatric settings shows similar rates of domestic violence. Pediatric screening also offers a complement to adult obstetric screening. In a screening study in our primary care office, we found that half of all recent abuse occurred in women with a recent pregnancy. Although all these women delivered in a center in which staff members screen for domestic violence, only half had disclosed their injuries at the time of delivery. This fact reinforces how important it is for pediatric practitioners to do screening.

Box 266-2. Effects of Domestic Violence on Children

- Physical injury
- Posttraumatic stress syndrome
- Anxiety
- Social withdrawal
- Depression
- Suicidal ideation
- Physical aggression
- School problems
- Truancy
- Clinging behavior
- Bullying
- Hyperactivity
- Headaches
- Bed-wetting
- Sleep disturbance
- Failure to thrive

SCREENING RECOMMENDATIONS

Several different screening questions have been used by different investigators. There is little information, however, on which are the best questions to use, in what setting screening should occur, or on who should be asking the questions. Most practitioners use questions selected from the AMA's recommended questions (Box 266-4).

Similar to any other screening test, it is crucial for the practitioner to have a plan or protocol in place in the event of a positive response to screening. The provider should be aware of community services available to battered women. In most communities, these services include women's shelter's and support groups or crisis centers. These organizations are a valuable resource in providing office literature, emergency counseling to victims, and help in risk assessment. The practitioner also should be familiar with the local county child protective services because the children in these settings often are abused or at risk.

When screening, it is recommended always to speak to the woman without the partner present. The questions should be presented in a nonjudgmental manner as a routine set of questions asked of all women who come to office. Most experienced practitioners screen with children older than 3 years of age out of the room. The abuser may be become violent if he is aware that the abused partner has been screened or is taking measures to get out of the relationship. An older child may report to the abuser what was asked and put the mother at risk.

If a woman discloses violence at home, she should be counseled about the services available to her in the community. Questions should be asked about the level of

Box 266-3. Summary of American Academy of Pediatrics Recommendations on Domestic Violence Intervention

1. Residency training programs and continuing education program leaders incorporate education on family and intimate partner violence and its implications for child health into the curricula of pediatricians and pediatric emergency department physicians.
2. Pediatricians should attempt to recognize evidence of family or intimate partner violence in the office setting.
3. Pediatricians should intervene in a sensitive and skillful manner that maximizes the safety of women and children victims.
4. Pediatricians should support local and national multidisciplinary efforts to recognize, treat, and prevent family and intimate partner violence.

Table 266-2. Incidence of Domestic Violence Reported in Pediatric Settings

Study	Incidence (%)	Comments
Wissow et al, 1992	40	Screening in resident continuity clinic
Duffy et al, 1999	32	Pediatric emergency department setting
Siegel et al, 1999	31	Pediatric practice setting
Parkinson et al, 2001	16.5	Pediatric practice setting

Data from Wissow LS, Wilson ME, Roter D, et al: Family violence and the evaluation of behavioral concerns in a pediatric primary care clinic. Med Care 1992;30(5 suppl): MS150–MS165; Duffy SJ, McGrath ME, Becker BM, Linakis JG: Mothers with histories of domestic violence in a pediatric emergency department. Pediatrics 1999; 103:107–113; Siegel RM, Hill TD, Henderson VA, et al: Screening for domestic violence in the community pediatric setting. Pediatrics 1999;104:874–877; Parkinson GW, Adams RC, Emerling FG: Maternal domestic violence screening in an office-based pediatric practice. Pediatrics 2001;108:E43.

risk in the home, whether guns are present, if the mother is afraid to go home, if she is afraid she will be injured that day, or if she is afraid that her children might be injured. Local women's crisis centers and shelters often can supply emergency counseling and be helpful in risk assessment.

Chart documentation is important, but in the pediatric setting, the father of the child often has access to the chart. It is the practice in our office to document the mother was counseled on personal safety rather than using the words *domestic violence* so as not to alert the abuser of screenings and referrals. It should be suggested that the mother may keep brochures on domestic violence hidden from the abuser and have an escape plan if the level of violence escalates.

Although many medical organizations have recommended domestic violence screening, practitioners have been reluctant to screen. Several barriers have been sited in studies and are summarized in Box 266-5. Erickson and colleagues showed that pediatric practitioners underestimate the magnitude of the problem, overestimate the time needed to screen, and often are uneducated on screening methods. These investigators also showed that practitioners

Box 266-4. Possible Screening Questions

1. Are you in a relationship in which you have been hurt physically or threatened by your partner? Have you been in such a relationship?
2. Are you [have you ever been] in a relationship in which you felt you were treated badly? In what ways were you treated badly?
3. Has your partner ever destroyed things that you care about?
4. Has you partner ever threatened or abused your children?
5. Has your partner ever forced you to have sex when you did not want to? Does he ever force you to engage in sex that makes you feel uncomfortable?
6. What happens when you and your partner disagree?
7. Do you ever feel afraid of your partner?
8. Has your partner ever prevented you from leaving the house, seeing friends, getting a job, or continuing your education?
9. If your partner uses drugs or alcohol, how does he act? Is he ever verbally or physically abusive?
10. Do you have any guns in your home? Has your partner ever threatened to use the gun when he was angry?

Box 266-5. Barriers to Domestic Violence Screening

- Lack of physician education
- Fear of "opening Pandora's box"
- Lack of time
- Belief that it is not the physician's role
- Difficulty dealing with women's feelings
- Lack of protocol and resources
- Underestimation of the magnitude of the problem

were 10 times more likely to screen of they had received formal domestic violence training.

Special considerations should be made for high-risk children and adolescents. Universal screening for domestic violence is preferred to targeting high-risk groups because the incidence is about one third in the general population. Children being seen for behavioral and psychiatric problems are thought to be at even higher risk, and these families should be screened. Abused or neglected children are at particularly high risk and merit screening for domestic violence. Most adolescent medicine experts suggest that adolescents be interviewed alone at well visits. This offers an ideal opportunity to screen adolescents themselves.

Several states have developed specific laws for domestic violence screening by health care professionals. Also, some states have mandated reporting laws. Many experts believe mandated reporting laws are problematic in that they potentially violate the physician-patient relationship and further the woman's role as victim. Still, it is crucial that practitioners know their state's laws. State laws are summarized in Box 266-6. State laws and policies are tracked by the Family Violence Fund and can be viewed at their website, http://fvpf.org.

RESOURCES

The practitioner is never alone in dealing with the problem of domestic violence. Local organizations often can assist in developing protocols and making referrals to appropriate community services. A 24-hour domestic violence hotline is

Box 266-6. State Domestic Violence Laws*

- **Training:** Ten states have enacted laws that address domestic violence training. They are Alaska, California, Florida, Kentucky, New Hampshire, New York, Ohio, Oklahoma, Pennsylvania, and Washington.
- **Screening:** Three states have enacted laws that address domestic violence screening. They are California, New York, and Pennsylvania.
- **Protocols:** Eight states have domestic violence protocols in law. They are Alaska, California, Iowa, New Hampshire, New York, Ohio, Pennsylvania, and Texas.
- **Reporting:** Thirteen states have enacted domestic violence reporting laws or reporting laws for gunshot or life-threatening injuries only. They are California, Colorado, Florida, Kansas, Kentucky, Maine, Minnesota, Missouri, New Hampshire, Rhode Island, Texas, Vermont, and Washington.

*Specific state domestic violence laws and polices are tracked by the Family Violence Prevention Fund and can be viewed at their website, http://www.endabuse.org.

Table 266-3. Domestic Violence Internet Sites

Organization	URL	Comments
Family Violence Prevention Fund	http://www.fvpf.org	Has state DV laws and programs
American Medical Women's Association	http://www.dvcme	On-line DV CME program
American Medical Association	http://www.ama-assn.org	Offers access to many DV articles and policies
American Bar Association Commission of Domestic Violence	http:/www.abanet.org/domviol/home.html	Source of statistics and legislation
U.S. Department of Justice	http:/www.usdoj.ogv/vaw	Lists government-funded research and resources
National Coalition Against Domestic Violence	http://www.ncadv.org/	Source of statistics and local program links
Family Peace Project	http://www.family.mcw.edu/ahec/ec/medviol.html	Source of protocols for medical screening and documentation

CME, continuing medical education; DV, domestic violence.

available to battered women. The Internet also provides many informative sites (Table 266-3).

Mini-index of Related Topics   CH.

SUGGESTED READINGS

American Academy of Pediatrics Committee on Child Abuse and Neglect: The role of the pediatrician in recognizing and intervening on behalf of abused women. Pediatrics 1998;101:1091–1092.

Erickson MJ, Hill TD, Siegel RM: Barriers to domestic violence screening in the pediatric setting. Pediatrics 2001;108:98–102.

Knapp JF, Dowd MD: Family violence: Implications for the pediatrician. Pediatr Rev 1998;19:316–321.

Parkinson GW, Adams RC, Emerling FG: Maternal domestic violence screening in an office-based pediatric practice. Pediatrics 2001;108:E43.

Siegel RM, Hill TD, Henderson VA, et al: Screening for domestic violence in the community pediatric setting. Pediatrics 1999;104(4 Pt 1):874–877.

SECTION 8   SOCIAL ASPECTS OF CARE: *Violence and Childhood*

267 Legal Aspects of Child Abuse and Neglect

Donald C. Bross

ROLE OF THE GENERALIST

1. Understand different legal frameworks for managing child abuse and neglect.
2. Know the effects of legal intervention.
3. Report suspected child maltreatment.
4. Document and present information about possible child maltreatment.

The U.S. legal system permits, and in limited ways requires, physicians to participate in various efforts to help maltreated children. Pediatricians as a matter of standard practice consider and respond as appropriate to children's development from all perspectives, including genetic, parenting, and other intrinsic and external influences in children's lives. A "pediatric law" approach considers the development, nurturing, problems, and treatment of children from a legal perspective. Viewed in this way, law is merely another tool that might be brought to bear to help ensure that children's development is maximized and not disrupted. Pediatricians should understand different legal frameworks for managing child abuse and neglect, information about the effects of legal intervention, and the pediatrician's role in documenting and presenting information about possible child maltreatment.

LAW AS A FACTOR IN THE LIVES OF CHILDREN

In the 19th and 20th centuries, universal education, mandatory immunization, requirements for vitamins in food, and restrictions on child labor became standards. Especially during the 20th century, legislation mandated behaviors that previously were private matters solely for parents or businesses to decide. In the past 40 years alone, safety for children in the United States has grown with a mandate for "poison proofing" of some containers with contents dangerous to small children, requirements for car seat belts and infant seats, and a mandate for reporting of suspected child abuse or neglect. Although not the focus here, legislation and judicial decisions also selectively have emancipated persons younger than 18 to allow them to consent to medical care for drug addiction, contraception, abortion, sexually transmitted diseases, and mental illness. The former category of "rights of protection" must be distinguished clearly from the latter category of "rights of choice or emancipation," although both are important and depend to a great extent on the child's physical, mental, and social-psychological competencies. A related and important goal in children's socialization is engendering participation in a government and culture in which respect for law is a central concern.

Imposition of mandatory reporting of suspected child abuse was based on reasoning almost identical to mandatory reporting of suspected infectious diseases to designated state agencies (i.e., the goal was to identify possible vectors of harm to allow prevention of avoidable injury). Given that a confidential relationship exists between physicians and patients, absent another overriding obligation, mandatory child abuse reporting laws remove doubt as to the pediatrician's duty to guard the child's safety over a duty of nondisclosure. Ironically, any duty to smaller children to maintain confidentiality regarding possible abuse or neglect makes little sense. Infants cannot agree to waive the duty of confidentiality, and it is a conflict of interest or a "cover-up" for a caregiver to exercise a right of nondisclosure on behalf of the child, especially if the caregiver is the source of the harm. To reinforce the importance of the duty to report suspected child maltreatment, each of the 50 states immunizes reporters from civil or criminal liability when a report is made, even if the report is wrong, so long as the report was not made either with no basis or with deliberate bad intentions. Such laws are important indicators of a civilization that values children. Similar to mandatory education laws, mandatory reports of suspected child abuse or neglect guarantee that children have a right of access to society.

The legitimization of protection of children from abusive acts by caregivers or others extends to the legal processes that authorize crimes against children to be punished and children in need of protection to be afforded shelter, food,

medical treatment, or other necessary care when it is being denied. The 50 United States do not require that competent adults be given food, medical care, or loving attention, but law must provide children at least minimal support. Children are given a special status enforceable under law as members of a special class and in individual case situations. Although the legal framework for child protection that has developed, especially since the 1960s, has the theoretical potential to benefit children, similar to hospitals of the 19th century, there is still too little information available on the cost-benefit effects of legal intervention on behalf of children. Despite the insufficiency of current data, published data support a conclusion that child protection laws benefit more children than are harmed by intervention.

BALANCING POSSIBLE NEGATIVE AND POSITIVE EFFECTS OF LEGAL INTERVENTION

Available reports of negative effects of legal intervention on behalf of maltreated children almost all are anecdotal, although there are specific examples of egregious errors of evaluation, intervention, and evident psychological harm to children or their parents. Population-based data on this topic are nonexistent, however, and the few studies available are limited in numbers and methodology. A report that children whose cases are criminally filed suffer psychological symptoms for a longer time and symptoms that are more severe could not control for the likelihood that cases filed in criminal court are likely to involve more severe or prolonged abuse. A different study found that sexual abuse cases filed for prosecution were more likely than cases not filed to include the presence of oral-genital contact, use or threat of force, greater duration of abuse, and physical or eyewitness evidence. Still, criminal cases generally are more demanding of victim witnesses than civil cases, including child victim witnesses, although many changes have been made since the 1980s to reduce the courtroom burden on child victim witnesses. In some situations, criminal prosecutors become convinced that an individual is a predator and represents a substantial threat of repeated crimes, meaning the prosecution will continue even if there is psychological risk to the child from testifying. Among positive changes, whether the child is a victim witness or only a witness, protections for child witnesses in criminal cases now have been adopted in federal law and the law of many states.

Although criminal prosecutions are the most visible legal intervention, in reality 4% of cases "substantiated" as child maltreatment by state protective services agencies result in criminal prosecutions. Substantiated cases are more likely to be filed as civil, nonaccusatory child protection proceedings in the juvenile or family courts. Perhaps 10% to 30% of confirmed cases go to the court with the jurisdiction to issue orders of treatment or placement of children and their parents. Few published data exist on the direct effects of child protection agency investigations, including the 20% to 30% that go to family or juvenile court. Asked anonymously, approximately 20% ($n = 176$) of parents involved involuntarily in one state (Iowa) stated that their families were "worse off" after the intervention. Another 20% did not respond to the forced choice question, "My family was better off?" The other 60% reported that their families were "better off" after the intervention.

Several federal acts have conditioned payments to states for child welfare on compliance with regulations to reduce the numbers of children placed in foster care and the time spent by children in foster care, which often has been shown to be too long. These legislative acts assume that at least some children are harmed by mistaken placements and failures to return children to biologic parents or to free children for adoption quickly when safety in the biologic home cannot be ensured. The limited available research provides some basis for believing that children placed and not returned are more benefited than harmed, if measures such as better school performance and reduced trouble with the law are accepted as measures of benefit to the children. At the same time, these children often wish to return to their parents.

Although the possibility that physicians reporting child maltreatment are inordinately inconvenienced has been raised as an issue deserving investigation, the research to establish the extent of the problem has not been undertaken. Physician fears have been identified, but the extent to which these fears are realistic has not been established. Physicians have been sued successfully for failing to report suspected child maltreatment. Because physicians are immunized for reporting suspected child maltreatment cases in all 50 states, the clear ethical and legal priority is reporting of suspected maltreatment when standard differential diagnoses have taken place to the extent feasible.

The research showing positive effects, as contrasted to research indicating that negative results might be limited, also is minimal regarding the broad effects and the case-specific effects. Reporting seems to have been essential, however, for recognition and response to the problem. Before the advent of the battered child syndrome in 1961, there was no national effort to document the existence, let alone the incidence or prevalence of the problem. When reporting laws were passed at the urging of Kempe, a pediatrician, between 1963 and 1968, in all 50 states, the "substantiated" numbers as estimated by the U.S. Department of Health and Human Services rose from none to nearly 1 million cases annually. During the 5 years ending in 1999, reported cases decreased for the first time (by 10%). National random surveys have suggested a decrease in the use of corporal punishment to children over the past few decades. It cannot be proven that these changes in maltreatment or the use of physical punishment are due to the attention to the problem partly fostered by changes in the law, but without the laws it would not be possible to raise the possibility of their positive effect.

The first study suggesting that court-ordered treatment might yield a higher rate of completion of treatment plans and greater likelihood of family preservation was published in 1980, and a subsequent study also suggested positive results. More recent reports have looked at the possibility that racial bias affected court decisions on permanency when parental substance abuse is an issue. A study by Sagatun-Edwards and Saylor found that mothers' behavior was more important for court outcomes than ethnicity, past referrals, or criminal records. A 5-year follow-up of 53 newborns determined by a family court to need a protected status because of positive toxicologies (47 for cocaine) at birth found that only one court adjudicated the infant suffered abuse. When court involvement and social services active involvement ended, 35 infants (66%) had been placed permanently with a biologic mother or father. "Thirteen infants in this study (25%) were never reunited with their parents, and only 6 (11%) were never reunited with relatives." Given a literature that commonly associates substance abuse with child abuse and neglect, MacMahon concluded that the study "suggests that the close monitoring and strict demand for compliance with court orders that ... mothers experienced were appropriate and beneficial to the children." The one mother who abused her child did so after she had failed urine tests over an 18-month period, but the court was convinced by a social worker to return the child. The other 16 of 17 mothers who underwent random testing of their urine were found to have a continuing problem with drugs, and their children were placed permanently with relatives or adoptive parents. As a consequence of court orders, 24 other mothers completed drug rehabilitation for a prolonged period.

LAW AS A NONACCUSATORIAL IMPERATIVE

Experience and limited research to date indicate that neither wholesale rejection nor endorsement of the role of law in managing child abuse and neglect is justified. As it is for most interventions in the lives of children, a case-specific approach is required. One way to consider the role of law is to consider that some types of legal intervention can be considered as especially consonant with health or public health approaches to childhood. Although the purpose of the criminal law is to deter bad conduct through punishment of offenders, relatively few child abuse and neglect cases are handled in this way. Crimes against children merit careful and expert prosecution, but most cases of child abuse or neglect are not managed in this way. A great many inflicted injuries occur that cannot be proven beyond a reasonable doubt or else do not merit severe reactions by authorities.

Within the civil law approach to conflict resolution, there are other types of legal proceedings that are conceptually familiar to health professionals. Public health investigations of disease outbreaks and mental health proceedings related to individuals who might be mentally ill and a direct danger to self or others are specific examples of legal authority to regulate private behavior. These types of laws do not intend the punishment of individuals, however, even though penalties such as loss of business or loss of freedom can be incurred as a result of the state's intervention. The purpose of such legal proceedings is ameliorative, and when courts are not satisfied that the proceedings are ameliorative in nature, any authority to intervene is lost.

For example, assume a situation in which a 2-month-old infant has bilateral subdural hematomas, retinal hemorrhages, and upper arm grab marks while in the care of several adults, including relatives and nonrelatives. Given medical consensus that the child has been abused, it still is possible that despite the medical diagnosis the person harming the child might not be identified. Under such facts, rather than doing nothing, the law can be invoked to recognize that the child needs to be "adjudicated" or determined by a judge or jury as needing a special protected status. Although no one is accused, the parent, guardian, or other caregiver must "respond" to an allegation that this child should not have suffered such harm absent some act of abuse or omission of protective care. When the facts support a finding that the child is in need of *supervision*, is *dependent*, or whatever a particular state defines as the word that means the child is under the court's protection, the judge can be asked to order interventions appropriate and necessary to keep the child safe. Although this order does not necessarily mean placement, either temporary or permanent, it can mean placement, and it can mean monitoring, evaluation, or treatment ordered for the parent before parental care is resumed.

The previously cited studies relate more to civil than to criminal proceedings on child abuse or neglect. Taken together, they convey possibilities for developing case-specific utilization of different types of legal proceedings to prevent and treat child abuse and neglect. As with all interventions for children, the challenge is to improve understanding as to when the various interventions available, including legal measures in this instance, are appropriate.

DOCUMENTATION AND COURTROOM PRESENTATION OF A CHILD'S CONDITION

Given that some children cannot be made safe without legal intervention, physicians working with children might be called to provide evidence in court. For many physicians, it is a process to be dreaded. The time taken from busy practices and the expected intimidation of the courtroom process provide strong disincentives to testify, and even before that possibility occurs, the possibility of being called is a reason for some physicians not to recognize and report child maltreatment. On the positive side, greater than 70% of reported and confirmed cases do not appear in court; in most cases, physicians are not called to testify; and if a pediatrician is called, it is possible to minimize the negative aspects of appearing.

The many pediatricians in the United States who work daily with child abuse and neglect cases are called to court frequently, some nearly every week. They are an important resource to contact before making a first appearance as a pediatric witness. These pediatricians have learned that their most important preparation is to remain true to their training and extensive experience as pediatricians. In other words, the best preparation is to continue to do the best job possible of diagnosis, ruling out alternative diagnostic possibilities and ensuring that any appropriate history, tests, scans, or consultations are undertaken when child abuse or neglect is suspected.

The business-like documentation of the diagnosis of a child's condition is the best possible approach to any eventual courtroom presentation of the same information. In a typical civil or criminal child abuse or neglect case, there is at least one supportive attorney in the courtroom who needs the pediatrician's testimony to help a jury or judge understand why a particular legal outcome is appropriate. The pediatrician is given every opportunity, so long as the person who sought the testimony is competent, to provide a complete recounting of important information. The pediatrician is allowed to provide a complete and accurate story of how he or she came to diagnose a child as being neglected or abused. Only when the pediatrician is finished with providing initial information is any opposing attorney allowed to cross-examine. The opposing attorney attempts to limit the impact of the pediatrician's testimony by attacking the facts or opinion he or she presented; suggesting limits to the pediatrician's training, experience, or credentials; or trying to confuse the issues before the court. The pediatrician is never responsible for any laws, legal rulings, or legal elements of the case. The pediatrician's only responsibility is to ensure, either in the direct presentation of information or in responding to challenges to the information, that the core information of the child's condition as the pediatrician understands it is not being confused or misrepresented. No one can take away the experience of having been there as the child's pediatrician. The best form of advocacy a pediatrician in this role can fulfill is accuracy, with as many facts as possible that speak for a child in ways the child cannot.

Although the pediatrician often is given an opportunity to express opinions, particularly the diagnosis, the underlying facts usually determine legal outcomes. Every human being wants to make up his or her own mind about the circumstances of human behavior, and the more information that a judge or jury understands about a particular child's condition compared with other children, the greater the likelihood that the judge or jury will understand how the pediatrician reached the diagnosis.

SUMMARY

Law is a necessary but not sufficient intervention strategically and tactically for the adequate management of child abuse and neglect. The pediatrician is not responsible for assuming the legal roles of children's counsel or counsel for the people. Without the pediatrician's knowledge about the condition of a child whose life is brought into court, however, there often is no accountability for the child's life.

Courts respond, although inconsistently, to increased scientific knowledge and the facts of particular situations. Research is needed to determine how beneficial effects of the legal system can be maximized for children and iatrogenic trauma minimized. Notwithstanding the imperfection of the legal system, improvements continue to be made, and pediatricians can contribute to improvement in legal protections for maltreated children.

Reporting laws are an example of how pediatricians have encouraged changes in legislation or courtroom responses to children. "Children's trust fund" legislation to pay for prevention of child abuse was the inventive approach of Helfer, a pediatrician. Mandatory child protection teams were another valuable innovation for thoroughness and accountability promoted by pediatricians. Other important improvements remain possible.

Additional Resources, CD-ROM

Bibliography

Mini-index of Related Topics	CH.

SUGGESTED READINGS

Bross DC: Witness preparation for trials related to child abuse or neglect. In King L, Ventrell MR (eds): Improving the Professional Response to Children in the Legal System. Denver, Colo, National Association of Counsel for Children, 2000, pp 143–152.

Dubowitz H, Bross DC: The pediatrician's documentation of child maltreatment. Am J Dis Child 1992;146:596–599.

MacMahon JR: Perinatal substance abuse: The impact of reporting infants to child protective services. Pediatrics 1997;100(5):E1.

Runyan DK, Everson MD, Edelsohn GA, et al: Impact of legal intervention on sexually abused children. J Pediatr 1988;113: 647–653.

Sagatun-Edwards I, Saylor C: Drug-exposed infant cases in juvenile court: Risk factors and outcomes. Child Abuse Negl 2000; 24:925–937.

Warner JE, Hansen DJ: The identification and reporting of physical abuse by physicians: A review and implications for research. Child Abuse Negl 1994;18:11–25.

SECTION 8   SOCIAL ASPECTS OF CARE: *Violence and Childhood*

268 Child Neglect: The Inadequate Promotion of Children's Health and Development

Ari Silver-Isenstadt and Howard Dubowitz

ROLE OF THE GENERALIST

1   Screen children for risk factors for neglect, especially for factors that may not be readily apparent (e.g., maternal depression, parental alcohol or substance abuse, domestic violence, child hunger).

2   Develop a team relationship with social workers or other professionals to assist in evaluation and management.

3   Be aware of local community resources to support families.

4   Assist families in obtaining appropriate resources in the community.

Pediatricians strive to promote the *optimal* health, well-being, and development of children; this includes addressing the enormous problem of child abuse and neglect. The approximately 3 million reports for abuse or neglect to Child Protective Services (CPS) each year belies any idealized assumptions about childhood in the United States. Physical and sexual abuse may be clear in their presentations, often evoking strong responses from physicians and others. In contrast, neglect often is more subtle.

It may present in many ways, and its effects often are insidious. Neglect also has been more difficult to define. Most state laws define neglect as omissions in care when parents or caregivers fail to meet their children's basic needs, resulting in harm or significantly jeopardizing their health and development. Case Study 268-1 illustrates the dilemma pediatricians face when considering child neglect in the primary care setting.

An alternative to the legal definition is to approach neglect from the child's perspective, rather than focusing blame on parents. Neglect occurs when a child's basic need is not met adequately, for whatever reason, resulting in actual or potential harm. Children's basic needs include adequate health care, safety, nutrition, clothing, education, nurturance, supervision, and a home. There may be many reasons contributing to neglect, and these are important to understand for appropriate intervention. Applying this approach to the 6-year-old asthmatic girl in Case Study 268-1, if she is not receiving adequate care and she is experiencing respiratory distress, her medical needs are being neglected. The pediatrician, perhaps with the help of others, needs to understand what is underpinning the noncompliance in order to tailor the response to meet the specific needs of this child and family. This broad and child-

CASE STUDY 268-1

A 6-YEAR-OLD WITH ASTHMA AND POSSIBLE NEGLECT

A 6-year-old girl with moderate persistent asthma presents in respiratory distress. She has had multiple admissions for status asthmaticus and frequent emergency department visits. She finished her last course of steroids last month. The girl's parents smoke at home. The father has asthma. The girl uses her bronchodilator and her inhaled steroid on an as-needed basis. After her last attack, her pediatrician prescribed a different, stronger inhaled steroid than the one that the girl previously had taken. This prescription has not yet been filled.

focused definition encourages consideration of an array of interventions, addressing the child, parental, family, community, and societal factors that may contribute to neglect.

WHY CHILD NEGLECT IS IMPORTANT

Prevalence and Incidence

Neglect is the most prevalent form of child maltreatment in the United States. In 1999, the U.S. Department of Health and Human Services identified nearly 3 million reports of suspected child maltreatment (i.e., abuse and neglect); 826,000 were substantiated. Of the substantiated cases, 482,000, or 58%, were for neglect. These reports represent the "tip of the iceberg." Neglect occurs mostly behind closed doors, unbeknownst to pediatricians and others. It is difficult to estimate the extent of neglected health care. One study based on CPS reports found that 2% of all reports were for medical neglect. Health care providers are unlikely to label many cases of medical neglect as such, however, and relatively few cases are reported to CPS.

Outcomes of Neglect—Morbidity and Mortality

The impact of neglect on children varies greatly, including mental health problems, academic underperformance, poor growth, and sometimes death. Physical manifestations include injuries, ingestions, burns, malnutrition, dental disease, inadequately treated illness, and neurologic deficits associated with severe early deprivation. A study revealed that very-low-birth-weight preterm infants referred to CPS for neglect had smaller head circumferences and inferior cognitive functioning at age 4 than their nonreferred counterparts. Infants who had substantiated reports were in even worse condition. Neglect contributes to behavioral, social, and psychological problems, such as impaired attachment, low self-esteem, and difficulty managing anger. Neglected children also are at risk for delinquent and criminal behavior. Neglect accounts for approximately 50% of the estimated 2000 deaths each year attributed to child maltreatment.

If access to health care and health insurance are considered basic needs in the United States, then 11 million children have their health care neglected by society. Less access to health care is associated with less use of health care, and frequently poor children in poor health are most affected. Malnutrition, lead poisoning, and injuries often are associated with poverty and may be symptoms of neglect.

Legal Mandate to Report Neglect

In all 50 states, pediatricians (and others) are required to report *suspected* child neglect to CPS. Given this mandate to report, how does the pediatrician approach the nuances and the spectrum of child neglect? Pediatricians need to be cognizant of the specifics of state law. There is the inevitable "gray zone" of borderline situations, however, in which discretion may be appropriate in deciding whether to try less intrusive strategies before reporting. It is increasingly clear that reporting to CPS is not a panacea; in some circumstances, alternative approaches may be preferable. Aside from reporting, pediatricians have an opportunity and responsibility to help ensure children's health, safety, and well-being.

DEFINITIONS

At the most basic level, a child requires three components of support: physical, emotional, and educational. *Physical needs* include adequate health care, hygiene, nutrition, shelter, and clothing. *Emotional support* includes nurturance, protection, supervision, and support. *Educational support* requires that children be educated adequately and that special educational needs be addressed appropriately. The prevention of truancy is one form of educational support. Neglect occurs when any of these basic needs of a child are not met adequately. Several considerations have a bearing on definitions of neglect. A child's age or developmental level influences his or her basic needs. A teenager clearly has different needs for supervision than does a preschooler.

ACTUAL VERSUS POTENTIAL HARM

Many situations of neglect do not involve immediate or actual harm, but potential or long-term harm may be a significant concern. The laws of most states consider potential harm in their definitions of child abuse and neglect. Understanding the potentially significant, sometimes life-threatening, harm posed by neglect is an important step in addressing the problem. A child whose asthma medication is not taken regularly may continue to be admitted to the hospital unnecessarily or may have increased periods of respiratory distress.

FREQUENCY AND CHRONICITY

Neglect usually is inferred when the condition is chronic or there is a pattern of unmet needs. A dilemma arises regarding single or rare incidents that may constitute neglect. Some omissions in care are unlikely to be harmful unless they are recurrent, such as the case of a child with a seizure disorder who repeatedly does not receive anticonvulsants; an occasional lapse is unlikely to be significant. An infant left unattended in a bath once for a few minutes could drown, however. This single lapse should be considered as neglect. From a practical standpoint, it often is difficult to establish the duration or frequency of failure to meet a child's need. Medical or pharmacy records that show appointments that have not been kept or prescriptions that have not been filled can help. Sometimes parents or children may disclose how long they have had food shortages or problems accessing health care.

ETIOLOGY

There is no single cause of child neglect. An ecologic theory of multiple *and* interacting contributors has been proposed at the individual (parent and child), familial, community, and societal levels. A toddler with a chronic, toxic blood lead level illustrates this theory. This child's health is being neglected by a lack of protection from lead and a lack of satisfactory treatment. Contributory factors may include the parents' unwillingness to allow treatment, the parents' inability to move to a lead-free home, a landlord's refusal to have the home deleaded, a city's inability to ensure an adequate lead abatement program, and society's limited investment in low-income housing. Regardless of which contributory factors are responsible, a child with a high lead level experiences neglect. An appreciation of the contributory factors is key, however, in planning the optimal interventions.

Community and Societal Factors

Community and societal factors, such as poverty, culture, and religious beliefs, may contribute to child neglect. These factors influence the functioning of families; the attitudes, knowledge, and behavior of parents; and the health care children receive. The community and neighborhood and their resources influence parent-child relationships and are associated strongly with child maltreatment. A community with a rich array of services, such as parenting groups, childcare, and good public transportation, enhances the ability of families to nurture and protect children. Informal support networks and recreational facilities are important in supporting healthy family functioning. In contrast, social isolation contributes to children's neglect.

Poverty has been associated strongly with neglect, including increased exposure to environmental hazards (e.g., lead, violence) and the risk of hunger and malnutrition. Poverty also is associated with diminished access to health care, particularly for the "near-poor," who do not qualify for Medicaid and who lack health insurance. Many American children lack access to mental health services. One major study of youth age 9 through 17 years found that only 38% to 44% of youth meeting stringent criteria for a psychiatric disorder received any mental health service in the prior year. Dental care also is not accessible to many children, particularly children in low-income families. A study of preschoolers found 49% of 4-year-olds had caries, and fewer than 10% were fully treated.

Cultures may differ in their beliefs regarding health care. Children from Southeast Asia may receive the folkloric remedy of Cao Gio for a fever. A hard object is rubbed vigorously, often along the spine, usually resulting in significant bruising. This practice may result in a delay in seeking medical care for a serious illness. Cultural differences also may be less dramatic, such as segments of the population that have no interest in psychotherapy. Similarly, parents

may hold religious views that are antithetical to Western medicine, believing in alternative approaches to health and healing. Sick children may receive prayer from a Christian Scientist faith healer.

These variations in beliefs and practices pose sensitive dilemmas as pediatricians strive to avoid an ethnocentric approach ("My way is right") and cultural relativism (i.e., cultures differ, and all should be accepted). When a practice clearly harms children or when clearly preferable alternatives exist, intervention should ensure that a child's need for effective health care is met adequately.

Family Factors

Poor organization of the home has characterized families of neglected children. Deficient problem-solving skills, poor parenting skills, and inadequate knowledge of children's needs have been associated with neglect. The absence of fathers or their limited involvement in their children's lives may be factors in neglect. Failure to thrive may be the result of "a poor fit" between mother and child, with frustration or anger contributing to feeding problems. A child's passive or lively temperament may displease a parent. In addition, family problems, such as domestic violence or a lack of social support, may contribute to a failure to meet children's basic needs.

Stress also has been associated with child maltreatment. One study found the highest level of stress—concerning unemployment, illness, eviction, and arrest—among families of neglected children compared with abusive and control families. In contrast, a supportive family can buffer the stresses that impair parenting, illustrating the importance of considering risk and protective factors in assessing *and* understanding families.

Parental Factors

Maternal emotional health problems, particularly depression, have been associated with neglect. Intellectual impairment, including severe mental retardation and a lack of education, also has been associated with neglect. High rates of alcoholism and drug addiction have been found in parents of neglected children.

Child Factors

Children may contribute, directly and indirectly, to the neglect of their health. A direct example is an adolescent's denial of diabetes and refusal to adhere to the treatment plan, despite repeated efforts by caring parents. Some children hide the problem by giving few or no clues that they need help. Children with chronic health problems or disabilities have special needs that put them at added risk for failure to meet their needs. Sullivan and Knutson found that disabled children were 3.4 times more likely to be identified as maltreated than were nondisabled peers (31% versus 9%). Although many parents of disabled children are excellent caregivers, others may become overwhelmed.

ASSESSING CHILD NEGLECT

The first step in assessing child neglect is to determine whether a child's basic need or needs are not being met. As with all diagnoses, if pediatricians do not consider neglect, they cannot diagnose it. Related issues are the immediacy of harm or endangerment and the severity of the neglect. Sometimes the risks to a child can be inferred reasonably from data on certain conditions, such as high lead levels. If it is determined that a child's basic needs have not been met, understanding the etiology is key in guiding the intervention. Individual parent and child, familial, community, and societal factors as discussed earlier in the section on etiology must all be considered.

GENERAL PRINCIPLES FOR THE MANAGEMENT OF NEGLECT

The pediatrician should keep in mind the following general principles for the management of neglect:

1. Convey concerns to the family, in a respectful but forthright manner. It is important to focus on the child's needs and to ensure that the child's health care needs are met adequately. Families are more likely to be cooperative when health professionals adopt a supportive stance.

2. Express an interest in helping. This interest fosters the rapport and trust on which successful interventions depend.

3. Address contributory factors, prioritizing those most important and amenable to being remedied. Pediatricians may be able to manage some issues competently and may need to refer others elsewhere.

4. Begin with the least intrusive approach. The approach must fit the underlying problems and risks, but in general it is advisable to respect the importance of a family's privacy and to start with the least intrusive intervention. When faced with a child's failure to thrive, an initial strategy may be to provide guidance on feeding while closely monitoring the child's growth. If the child's growth does not improve, referral to an interdisciplinary program may help. If these efforts do not succeed and parenting problems are suspected as the reason, a referral to CPS may be needed.

5. Be cognizant of state laws regarding the reporting of child neglect. Many instances of neglect, even when recognized as such, are not being reported to CPS. In low-risk situations, it may be appropriate to begin with less intrusive approaches. CPS may have resources, such as parent aides, that would not otherwise be available. A report to CPS does not preclude other efforts to support the family. *CPS needs to be involved* when there is serious harm or risk or when less intrusive interventions have failed. Even when a CPS report is substantiated, most children remain in the care of their parents and are not placed in foster care. Constructive efforts to work *with* families are needed.

6. Recognize that neglect often requires long-term intervention, support, and follow-up. Try to ensure continuity of care as a primary health care provider.

7. Help the family identify specific objectives that they can implement (e.g., the family will always use a car seat), with measurable proximal, intermediate, and distal outcomes (e.g., the family reports routine use of the car seat at the next visit). The objectives should be relevant to the family, reasonable (attainable), and clearly identified, preferably in writing.

8. Engage the family in the development of the plan; solicit their input and agreement. Successful intervention requires working in collaboration with families.

9. Consider the needs of parents, children, and families. Effective programs focus on basic problem-solving skills and families' concrete needs, provide behavioral management, and help address environmental factors. Parents of neglected children often require attention to their own emotional needs in order to nurture their children adequately. Neglected children also may require individual attention. The focus of CPS has been mostly on parents, and few maltreated children receive direct services. Treatment of neglected children may reduce the psychological harm and possibly the intergenerational transmission of neglect. Many interventions appear useful, including therapeutic day care for younger children. It is important that parents be included in their children's treatment and that therapeutic strategies be implemented at home.

10. Build on family strengths. Too often pediatricians focus on problems and ignore strengths. This "deficit approach" impedes more constructive approaches to working with families. A parent's concern for his or her child's well-being can be used to encourage the parent to comply with treatment recommendations.

11. Encourage the use of informal supports (i.e., family, friends). Professionals often think of professionals to provide services, overlooking informal help from family and friends. Health care professionals can encourage a father's involvement in child rearing by inviting him to office visits. Consider support through a family's religious affiliation.

12. Consider the need for concrete services (e.g., Medical Assistance, Temporary Assistance to Needy Families, Food Stamps, and Special Supplemental Nutrition Program for Women, Infants, and Children [WIC]).

13. Be knowledgeable about community resources, and facilitate referrals. Interventions known to be effective should be favored. Because neglectful families often lack basic parenting skills, a behavioral approach usually is preferable to insight-oriented psychotherapy. Primary care providers are in a good position to encourage reluctant or ambivalent families to try such services.

14. Provide support, follow-up, review progress, and adjust plan if needed.

SPECIFIC MANIFESTATIONS OF CHILD NEGLECT

Noncompliance with Health Care Recommendations

One form of neglect is when health care recommendations that would benefit the child are not implemented, resulting in significant risk or actual harm. Some lapses in care, such as missing a follow-up appointment for an ear infection, rarely result in complications in a healthy child. Although parents may be encouraged to adhere to such recommendations, these circumstances should not be construed as neglect.

Assessment

There are many possible contributors to families' failure to adhere to a treatment plan. The pediatrician should consider child factors (e.g., whether the child refused the medicine), parental factors (e.g., whether the parent understood the treatment plan), family factors (e.g., whether there were serious stresses impeding the parent's ability to implement the plan), and community or societal factors (e.g., whether the lack of insurance and cost of the medication were a problem). Other possible contributors include the complexity of the treatment plan (e.g., the need to take a medication four times a day), the nature of the illness (e.g., problems without overt symptoms do not evoke as much concern), and physician-patient communication.

Management

The pediatrician should do the following:
1. Make treatment practical, set priorities, and simplify the approach.
2. Communicate clearly, avoid jargon, ensure caregiver agreement with the plan, give written instructions, and educate to obtain "buy-in" with the plan.
3. Develop a follow-up plan, arrange for home nursing if needed, and consider more frequent appointments to improve compliance.

Delay or Failure in Getting Health Care or Refusal of Medical Care

Another form of neglect occurs when a child is actually or potentially harmed through a delay or failure to obtain health care. Parents are responsible for recognizing their child's health problems. When a child has a medical condition that should be recognizable to a "reasonable layperson" (e.g., overt respiratory distress), and a delay in seeking necessary health care jeopardizes the child's health, medical neglect has occurred. Care must be used in assessing these situations. One naturally would not expect a parent to recognize an asymptomatic child with lead intoxication. One would expect cooperation with the treatment plan, however, when the problem has been identified. Family members' religious background may guide their approach to health care. Parents may refuse regular medical care, preferring to follow practices according to their faith. Jehovah's Witnesses refuse surgery if the need for a blood transfusion is anticipated. The challenge to the primary care provider is to respect a family's religious or cultural approach, while prioritizing a child's essential health care needs. Most states have religious exemptions in their child abuse statutes that state that children who receive treatment by spiritual means are not deemed abused or neglected. The American Academy of Pediatrics has prioritized children's health care needs over parental religious beliefs, however, and there is Supreme Court support for this approach.

Assessment

Learning the caregiver's view of the child's illness and his or her approach to health care helps the primary care provider understand why health care was delayed. Does the family have an alternative approach to health care? Was the child's illness obvious enough that a reasonable layperson would have recognized the need for health care? What is the evidence regarding the alternative method of treatment? Are there studies supporting the parent's approach? Is the child being harmed or at significant risk of being harmed by the alternate approach?

Management

The pediatrician should do the following:
1. Be sure that there is a significant benefit to the medical approach recommended and that significant harm may result from the family's alternative approach before recommending one form of care over another.
2. Educate the family members and patient as to when health care should be sought and the contribution of early care to chances for improved outcome.
3. Approach religious and cross-cultural differences with sensitivity, understand that the family members may not have the authority to override a religious conviction, consider contacting leaders in the family's community who may help with the family, and consider the community's approach to the illness.
4. Avoid *cultural relativism*—viewing all cultural approaches as equally acceptable. Some practices (e.g., female genital mutilation) are not acceptable. Also avoid *ethnocentrism*—assuming that the dominant cultural approach is correct.
5. Involve religious and community leaders to help find a reasonable compromise when religious background impedes treatment. This approach also may be valuable in avoiding future conflicts and reduces the risk that the family members will be ostracized by their community. In some life-threatening situations, court involvement is needed to allow treatment.

Hunger and Failure to Thrive

Neglect of a child's nutritional needs can manifest in a variety of ways, including impaired health and growth and emotional, behavioral, and learning problems. From the child's point of view, inadequate food represents neglect of his or her nutritional needs, even though the parents may not be directly to blame. Children may present with failure to thrive, usually defined as weight/height or height/age less than the 5th percentile or across two major percentiles. The pattern of growth is important, rather than any single measurement. Poor growth may be a late manifestation of inadequate nutrition, however, especially in older children. A hungry child still may grow normally. National data reveal that 10% of U.S. families routinely experience food shortages.

Assessment

Given the prevalence of food shortages for a significant minority of families, there is justification for assessing this as part of primary care, particularly in low-income communities. It is an important issue in evaluating a child with failure to thrive. Is there an underlying medical condition impeding the child's growth? What are the child's eating habits? Is the family eligible for governmental food and other support (e.g., WIC)? What has been done to ensure adequate food or to improve the child's growth?

Recommendations

Exclusion of organic causes is not sufficient to label failure to thrive as *nonorganic* and infer psychosocial contributors. Instead the assessment should include possible psychosocial factors. When psychosocial factors are present and when efforts, such as parent support and education to address them are not successful, a CPS referral may be needed.

Drug-Exposed Newborns and Children

Exposure to illegal drugs, in utero and later, jeopardizes children's health and is a form of neglect. Exposure to legal drugs (e.g., tobacco) with known adverse effects on children's health also can be considered neglect. The high-risk home environment in these situations may pose even more of a risk than the drugs per se.

Assessment

There is a need to clarify the nature and extent of the drug use or exposure. How does the parent perceive his or her use or abuse, and how has he or she tried to address the problem? How does the drug problem affect the child? The parent's interest in obtaining additional help should be assessed.

Management

The pediatrician should do the following:
1. Educate the parent about the actual and potential harm of exposing the fetus and children to drugs.
2. Know the community resources available for drug treatment, and encourage referral.
3. Be positive, hopeful, and persistent. Consider more frequent visits to monitor the situation.
4. Know state laws governing whether a CPS referral is indicated for prenatal drug exposure.

Inadequate Protections from Environmental Hazards

A basic need of children is to be protected from environmental hazards, inside and outside of the home. Avoidable exposure to well-known hazards is a form of neglect. Ingestions; injuries; unsupervised exposure to guns; exposure to domestic violence; and failure to use smoke detectors, car seat belts, or bike helmets all may represent inadequate protection, jeopardizing children's health. Exposing an infant with bronchopulmonary dysplasia to second-hand cigarette smoke threatens the infant's health, constituting a form of neglect.

Assessment

Pediatricians should assess (1) which exposures may be a problem inside and outside the home and (2) parents' understanding of and efforts to address these types of exposure. Have the parents checked the temperature of their hot water heater? Do the parents use walkers? Are dangerous flights of stairs gated?

Management

The pediatrician should educate family members about the risks of environmental hazards. Anticipatory guidance should focus on the specific risks for children at different developmental levels. Specific suggestions to promote children's safety are needed.

Inadequate Nurturance and Affection

An infant's secure sense of attachment to a parent is important for developing trust needed for later relationships. A depressed mother may be unable to respond to her infant when needed and may be unable to respond with warmth and affection. A child who does not receive adequate attention, nurturance, and affection may not develop a secure attachment.

Assessment

It is important to assess the nature of the relationship between parents and child and the extent of emotional support and nurturance. Pediatricians often have a gestalt about the relationship via observation of the parent-child interaction. Is there warmth and affection, irritation, or passivity? Parents may be asked to describe the child's temperament and behavior. Children may be asked in whom they confide if they have a problem or who helps them if they feel sad.

Management

The pediatrician should do the following:
1. Educate the parents on the importance of emotional support and the expression of love.
2. Explain to parent that a crying infant will not be spoiled by being picked up.
3. Remind parents that teenagers too need to know they are loved.
4. Role model supportive behavior in the office (e.g., "I think you're a terrific kid!").
5. Consider referring the child (and the parent) for support services (e.g., Headstart).
6. Consider strategies for addressing problems, such as depression, that may impair the parent's ability to nurture the child.

Inadequate Supervision and Abandonment

Neglect occurs when children are not supervised in accordance with their developmental needs, resulting in clear risks to their health and safety (e.g., when an infant is left unattended in a bath tub, a preschooler is left alone, a teenager is out overnight without parental approval). Abandonment is the extreme form and has been defined as occurring when children are not "claimed" within 2 days. Teenagers may be forced to leave home without safe shelter or sustenance; this, too, can be considered abandonment.

Assessment

The pediatrician should ask about how frequently and for how long children "need to be left alone." Has the child been taught about what to do when left alone should potential dangers occur (e.g., a stranger comes to the door)? Is there always an easily accessible adult to whom the child can turn? What are the family's options for childcare?

Management

The pediatrician should do the following:

1. Teach about the risks of leaving young children without adult supervision (e.g., fires).
2. Teach the parent to teach the child what to do when left alone.
3. Encourage counseling for families in which the teenager has been evicted from the family home.
4. Suggest important considerations in choosing appropriate childcare, such as the ability to "drop in" unannounced.
5. Report to CPS abandoned children and children at significant risk.

Inadequate Hygiene

Standards for personal hygiene are established in a society or community. When these standards are not met, usually in a gross manner (such as when a child exhibits strong body odor), others may notice and disapprove. Peers may tease the child. Alternatively, if many of the child's peers do not meet the standards of hygiene, this may be less of a concern. Occasionally, poor hygiene contributes to health problems, such as when cuts become infected. Sometimes, inadequate hygiene may be a marker of more general neglect of a child's needs.

Assessment

Is the child's poor hygiene a pattern? Does the child identify the hygiene as a problem? Does the parent identify the hygiene as a problem? Is the hygiene related to a medical problem (e.g., encopresis)? Has anyone else asked or commented about the child's hygiene? Does the family have access to appropriate washing facilities? Are the child and family members interested in help? Are there other neglect issues?

Management

The pediatrician should explain to the child and family members the benefits of adequate hygiene and the health and emotional risks of inadequate hygiene. CPS may be able to help if the family does not have adequate washing facilities (e.g., advocate to the family's landlord regarding problematic plumbing). Hygienic food handling should be discussed, and its importance for health should be emphasized.

Inadequate Clothing

A child's basic clothing needs are neglected when the child's clothing is unsuitable for weather conditions or does not fit appropriately (unless fashion dictates the poor fit).

Assessment

Is poverty the issue? Have there been any physical repercussions of the inadequate clothing (e.g., frostbite)? Inadequate clothing may be a marker for other forms of

neglect. Do the child and the parent perceive a problem? Is the family interested in help?

Management

The pediatrician should do the following:

1. Discuss the importance of appropriate protection from the elements.
2. Present the potential problems for the child with regard to mental health issues (the risk of being teased or shunned).
3. Discuss available low-cost options (e.g., consignment shops).
4. Consider CPS referral if the child is significantly at risk (e.g., has no suitable clothing for winter).

Failure to Meet Educational Needs

A child's educational needs are neglected when the child is not being schooled within the community's accepted standards. Home schooling, which has become increasingly popular, should be respected when carried out according to state regulations. Neglect occurs when children miss a significant amount of schooling without a reasonable excuse. Some children may be schooled without adequate attention to their special educational needs. A school system can contribute to the failure to meet children's educational needs.

Assessment

The pediatrician should inquire about how the child is doing in school. How well a child's educational needs are being met can be assessed by asking several questions. Is the child frequently absent? Why? What is being done to ensure participation in school and completion of homework? Is the parent able to advocate for the special educational needs of the child? A call to the child's teacher (with permission) may provide useful insights.

Management

The pediatrician should do the following:

1. Stress the importance of a sound education for success.
2. Help develop strategies to improve school attendance.
3. Support family members in their efforts to advocate for their child's needs in school.
4. Consider formal educational testing and other evaluation services when needed.

Homelessness

The loss of one's home is a major trauma. Many families experience "near-homelessness," needing to stay temporarily with friends and family. These unstable arrangements may have harmful effects on children.

Assessment

Parents may be asked whether they have had problems with their living arrangement. What have they had to do? What are their options, and would they like help?

Management

The pediatrician should refer the family to a social worker or the appropriate local housing assistance resource.

PREVENTION OF NEGLECT: THE ROLE OF PEDIATRIC PRIMARY CARE PROVIDERS

There is a need to screen for risk factors for neglect, especially for factors that may not be apparent (e.g., maternal depression, parental alcohol or substance abuse, domestic violence, child hunger). Many of these problems are sufficiently prevalent and harmful to children to warrant systematic and universal screening during health maintenance visits. Building on a long-standing concern with children's safety and injury prevention, the review of systems can be expanded to consider other potential hazards in children's environments, such as domestic violence. One approach is to use a brief, easy-to-answer screening questionnaire that parents can complete while waiting.

Pediatricians need training and ongoing support to address these problems. Ideally, pediatricians should team up with social workers or other professionals. It is possible for pediatric practices to assess psychosocial risk factors briefly and to provide initial management. Collaboration with other community resources is key, and pediatricians can help facilitate referrals. In addition to acquiring some new skills, pediatricians need to rethink how to optimize the opportunity of a well-child visit, even if it is only 15 minutes.

In addition to systematic screening, pediatric primary care providers must be astute observers of problems, such as parents who appear depressed or high. Pediatric primary care providers need to assess the situation briefly and to offer initial management. The biomedical approach has focused on detecting problems. It is just as important to identify strengths and resources, offering a basis on which to build and intervene. A parent's wish to be a good parent may motivate him or her to seek drug treatment. A teen's wish to play sports may inspire him or her to adhere to an asthma regimen. An understanding of the risks and the strengths in the family is crucial for optimal management and for estimating the risks involved and the likelihood of successful intervention. For children with chronic diseases, health education and support help ensure adequate care. For all children, anticipatory guidance, whether it is about wearing a bike helmet or exposure to domestic violence, is useful in the effort to meet children's basic need to be protected from environmental hazards. Primary care providers' support, monitoring, and counseling are useful in helping families take good care of their children. At times, referrals to other professionals and agencies are necessary for services, such as developmental evaluations, nutritional support (e.g., WIC), Headstart, psychotherapy, or physical protection or home intervention (CPS). Helping a family obtain appropriate services is another valuable role for pediatricians.

ADVOCACY

Child neglect results when basic needs are not met. Contributory factors are at the levels of the child, family, community, and society. Pediatricians can advocate effectively on behalf of children in a variety of ways. Explaining to a parent the safety needs of an increasingly mobile and curious toddler is one form of advocacy. Helping a family obtain services in the community is another form of advocacy, as is remaining involved with a family after a report to CPS is made. Finally, efforts to develop programs in a community and to improve social policies and institutional practices concerning children and families are important forms of advocacy. Improving the care and well-being of children is a great challenge. Much is known about children's needs, and together with colleagues and families pediatricians should strive to meet these needs for all children.

Additional Resources, CD-ROM

Bibliography

Mini-index of Related Topics

SUGGESTED READINGS

Asser S, Swan R: Child fatalities from religion-motivated medical neglect. Pediatrics 1998;101:625–629.

Dubowitz H: Preventing child neglect and physical abuse: A role for pediatricians. Pediatr Rev 2002;23:191–196.

Dubowitz H, Giardino A, Gustavon E: Child neglect: Guidelines for pediatricians. Pediatr Rev 2000;4:111–116

Dubowitz H, King H: Child abuse and neglect: A child-centered, family-focused approach. Pediatr Clin North Am 1995;42:153–166.

Strathearn L, Gary PH, O'Callaghan MJ, Wood DO: Childhood neglect and cognitive development in extremely low birth weight infants: A prospective study. Pediatrics 2001;108:142–151.

Sullivan PM, Knutson JF: Maltreatment and disabilities: A population-based epidemiological study. Child Abuse Negl 2000;24:1257–1273.

269 Physical Abuse and Sexual Abuse

Patti Rosquist and Andrew Sirotnak

■ ROLE OF THE GENERALIST

1   Distinguish physical abuse from accidental injury.
2   Diagnose physical abuse.
3   Diagnose sexual abuse.
4   Report child abuse or neglect.
5   Refer to specialist if needed for procedures or medical management.
6   Recognize conditions mistaken for physical abuse.
7   Prevent physical abuse.
8   Ensure appropriate follow-up.

Child abuse is relatively new to pediatric literature, beginning with the 1962 *Journal of the American Medical Association* article by Kempe and colleagues entitled "The Battered-Child Syndrome." This article remains relevant more than 40 years later, reminding professionals who provide health care to children that child abuse "should be considered in any child exhibiting evidence of fracture of any bone, subdural hematoma, failure to thrive, soft tissue swelling or skin bruising, in any child who dies suddenly, or where the degree and type of injury is at variance with the history given regarding the occurrence of the trauma."

Physical abuse or nonaccidental trauma is a form of child maltreatment that includes inflicted bruising, burns, fractures, and abusive trauma ranging from the abdominal area to the head. These injuries are in contrast to accidental injuries that occur despite the presence of a prudent caregiver. *Sexual abuse* is sexual activity that cannot be understood by the child, is not developmentally appropriate for the child, and is not accepted by law or is against taboos of society. In addition to vaginal, anal, or oral penetration by the genitals, finger, or tongue of another, more subtle fondling, rubbing against a child for sexual gratification, or masturbating in front of a child may be considered sexual abuse.

This chapter provides an overview of the fundamentals encountered when physical abuse, sexual abuse, or neglect are part of the differential diagnosis for a child. In addition to considering the possibility of abuse as part of the differential diagnosis, the fundamentals of reporting abuse and incidence and prevalence of abuse are discussed. Next, key points in the diagnosis of abuse as obtained in a careful history and physical examination are described.

FUNDAMENTALS

Most generalists encounter abuse. Although these are difficult subjects to talk about for most health care providers, it is possible to do so in a direct but nonaccusatory manner. If either physical or sexual abuse is part of the differential diagnosis for a child's condition, abuse is suspected and needs to be reported immediately. In most situations, the medical provider can tell family members about the need to report suspected abuse or neglect before making the report. One may offer that a child's injuries are unexplained, that the medical team is considering all possibilities of causes for the child's injuries, and that one of the possibilities is that someone may have injured the child. The medical provider can inform the family or caregiver that whenever inflicted injuries or neglect is a possibility, health care providers are mandated reporters. In this way, the provider can keep the family informed of developments in the child's medical care without being accusatory. In some cases, however, it is not prudent or possible to discuss reporting ahead of time. There are times when a family is at high risk of leaving against medical advice, and a child may be placed at increased risk of harm if the caregivers are told about reporting. At other times, the possibility of abuse becomes known at a later time. A pediatric radiologist may find healing rib fractures on review of a chest x-ray obtained for possible pneumonia.

When suspected abuse is possibly by a family member, the suspicion generally is reported to the county Department of Human Services in the county where the child lives. At other times, possible abuse by a person not in a position of trust is reported to law enforcement in the jurisdiction where the event probably occurred. It is not unusual to need to call several agencies before reaching the agency responsible for investigating child abuse or neglect for the incident in question. In some instances, it is preferable to tell the caregivers that child abuse is a possibility and that the medical provider is obligated to report the possibility. It is helpful to state clearly that the medical provider does not know the exact source of injury to the child. In other cases, especially when there is concern a family may leave the medical facility before full evaluation, it may be necessary to report without notifying a family.

Almost one third of 3 million reports each year are confirmed as child abuse or neglect. Of these, 20% are physical abuse, and more than 10% are sexual abuse. When prevalence data are reviewed by gender, approximately 30% of men and 20% of women were physically abused as children; almost 13% of women and 4% of men were sexually abused as children. Overall, almost 12 per 1000 children are abused or neglected each year. The youngest children are the most vulnerable, with 43% of maltreated children being younger than 1 year old. Almost 30% of victims of child maltreatment were younger than 4 years old, 25% were 4 to 7 years old, 21% were 8 to 11 years old, and 26% were 12 to 17 years old. Of victims of fatal child abuse, 43% were younger than 1 year old, and 86% were younger than 6 years old. Perpetrators are much more likely to be relatives than nonrelatives. Children from single-parent families and families living in poverty are at greatest risk. Abuse fatalities are significantly underestimated because of incomplete death investigations, inaccurate diagnoses, and limitations of death certificate data. More than 10% of families with a fatality resulting from abuse or neglect had child welfare intervention within the past 5 years. Although it is difficult to report suspected child abuse, it is an important first step in obtaining services with families in need of intervention. Without intervention, abuse tends to continue and in some cases worsen, as evidenced by child fatality statistics.

The history and physical examination are the foundation to making a diagnosis of physical abuse, supplemented by laboratory tests and diagnostic imaging in some cases. In relatively verbal children (≥4 years old), it may be necessary to examine the child without the caregiver present as one might during a routine adolescent examination. In any event, it is helpful to document, in quotation marks with the child's own words, what happened, where it happened, and by whom. Although young children are unable to provide detailed information about timing of an injury, this information can be provided by adolescent patients and adult caregivers if they were present at the onset of symptoms. The clinician should elicit whether or not there is a history of trauma, such as falls, bicycle accidents, or motor vehicle accidents. In past medical history, type of birth; complications; excessive bleeding with circumcision; and any previous trauma, such as previous or fractures, should be documented. In the family history, a history of osteogenesis imperfecta, of "easily broken bones," or coagulopathies should be documented. The social history may be adapted from a detailed adolescent social history (Box 269-1). Physical examination findings may be documented successfully in several ways. In addition to the traditional description, sometimes it is easier to draw or photograph injuries. Commonly ordered laboratory tests and studies are described in the diagnosis section.

In most cases of suspected sexual abuse, the history is especially important because the physical examination is most often normal. Sexual abuse often is a diagnosis based on history. Historical aspects that support a suspicion of sexual abuse include a disclosure of sexual abuse, sexual acting out, or inappropriate sexual knowledge. Nonspecific symptoms that suggest a child may be under stress include enuresis, nightmares, and excessive masturbation. These symptoms are not specific for sexual abuse, however. Children rarely disclose sexual abuse immediately after the event, but rather tend to disclose accidentally or purposefully after a precipitating event or when they feel safe. It is not unusual for children to disclose incrementally, as if testing to find out what sort of consequences would follow

---

> **Box 269-1.** Social History Adapted from Adolescent History: HEADSS Pneumonic
>
> 1. *Home:* Who lives at home? Have you ever seen anyone hurt your mother? Have you ever seen anyone hurt your father? Have you ever seen anyone hurt your siblings? How do you get along with each of them? Does anyone have a gun?
> 2. *Education:* Do you go to school? Where do you go to school? What grade are you in? Have you been held back a grade? Do you get any special help, such as special education or speech therapy?
> 3. *Activity:* What do you like to do for fun?
> 4. *Drugs:* Does anyone get drunk? Does anyone use drugs? What happens then?
> 5. *Sex:* Has anyone ever touched you in a way that made you feel uncomfortable? What would you do if someone did?
> 6. *Suicide:* Do you ever wonder if you might be sad? Have you ever thought about hurting yourself? How? When was the last time? Are you thinking about doing that now?

---

the disclosure. Many of the history-taking techniques listed earlier for physical abuse apply to sexual abuse history taking as well. In the event that a history is obtained from an adult caretaker, it is important not to take the history with the child present. It may be helpful to ask the child about each part of his or her body, including if each part hurts or has been touched. Responses should be noted with quotation marks using the child's exact words. The clinician should not ask leading questions, such as "Who touched you?" Rather, it is appropriate to ask with nonleading questions what happened, with whom, and where. The number of histories and physical examinations needs to be kept to a minimum. The history taking can be deferred to a forensic interviewer or specially trained person, with supplemental medical history taking by the medical provider. Similarly, the genital portion of the examination can be deferred to an experienced sexual abuse medial examiner.

Distinguishing physical abuse from accidental injury begins with considering the diagnosis of nonaccidental injury. Box 269-2 outlines common historical factors that are suspicious for physical abuse. Is the history consistent with the injury? A 3-year-old child running and falling on an outstretched arm is consistent with an injury of acute distal radius and ulna fractures. A 6-week-old infant rolling off a couch is not consistent with massive bilateral retinal hemorrhages and acute subdural hematoma. An absent history might be a nonambulatory infant with no history of trauma presenting with occipital skull soft tissue swelling and findings of a complex occipital skull fracture.

> **Box 269-2.** Historical Aspects Leading to a Suspicion of Physical Abuse
>
> - History not consistent with the injury
> - History absent or evolving
> - Delay in seeking care
> - Triggering event that precipitates loss of control in the caregiver
> - Unrealistic developmental expectations of the child
> - Pattern of increasing severity of injuries

Caregivers often call emergency medical services or present to emergency departments or acute care clinics with concerns about a wide variety of concerns about their child. A delay in seeking care might be the caregiver of a severe burn victim who treats the burn at home for several hours or the caregiver of a child with new-onset apnea and seizures who gives rescue breathing and watches the child's condition deteriorate over 2 days. A common triggering event for abusive head trauma is incessant crying. The "terrible twos" and bowel or bladder accidents are common triggers as well. Occasionally a caregiver displays unrealistic developmental expectations for a child, such as toilet training at 12 months of age. Physical abuse often worsens without intervention, leading to more severe or more frequent injuries.

Physical abuse includes skin manifestations of physical abuse, abusive head trauma, skeletal injuries, and abdominal trauma. Skin manifestations of abuse include inflicted bruises and burns. Most bruises are the result of accidental injuries. These accidental bruises have developmentally appropriate histories and are seen on children who are at least able to cruise around objects. Accidental bruises often are seen over bony prominences, such as the forehead, forearms, elbows, knees, and shins. In other cases, the history may not seem consistent with the injury, or there may be no history at all. Physical abuse is suspected when a child is old enough to give a history of being hit, kicked, or otherwise harmed; there is no history of accidental trauma consistent with the injuries; or there is a history of accidental trauma in children not developmentally able to participate in falls or other common accidents. Although it is not possible to date bruises precisely, the examiner can note if the bruises seem to be of different ages; have a pattern (such as linear or loop); and are on normally protected areas of the body, such as cheeks, neck, back, chest, abdomen, buttocks, genitals, and thighs.

Burns may be accidental, inflicted, or the result of neglect. Children may spill an object containing hot liquid onto them, fall against a hot object, or turn on hot water. At other times, the history provided may not be consistent with the pattern of the burn or the developmental ability of the child. The history of a child playing with a curling iron does not explain multiple burns over arms, chest, and back. The classic dunk scald burn has a relatively straight line at the top of the water line. Sometimes children present with a circumferential extremity burn with a linear edge. In another case, a child may present with a level line at the waist sparing inguinal and popliteal folds. If the burn is suspected to be inflicted or the result of neglect, it should be reported. Investigators visiting the location of the incident and gathering water temperature and other details of the physical surroundings are invaluable. A history may be given that a toddler turned on scalding water, but investigators find the location of the faucet to be out of the child's reach.

Abusive head trauma must be distinguished from accidental injury or illness. As with all forms of abuse, it is imperative that the lesions are taken in the context of history, physical examination, and diagnostic studies. Injuries such as skull fractures, subdural hematoma, and cerebral edema after a witnessed major traumatic event should be consistent with the history. Epidural hematomas can be seen after a relatively minor fall with or without an associated skull fracture. Simple fractures, particularly in the parietal region, can be seen after falls and may be associated with a small, asymptomatic, underlying subdural hematoma. Many disease states may include subdural hematomas, but these follow the natural history of the illness with the associated symptoms and findings. The case of no history of major trauma, no underlying associated illness, and a pattern of injuries such as subdural hematoma and multiple, especially peripheral, retinal hemorrhages suggests the possibility of abusive head trauma.

In the context of a busy pediatric practice, inflicted head trauma such as that seen in shaken baby syndrome is unusual. Nonetheless, the leading cause of severe head trauma in infants is physical abuse. A healthy infant who had been feeding normally without a history of major trauma who presents with a sudden onset of change in mental status should raise a concern over abuse. The history provided may be that the infant suddenly had a decreased level of consciousness, became limp, his or her eyes "rolled back," had apnea, or had seizures. Initially the differential diagnosis is broad. Many of these infants present with no external signs of trauma, so the health care provider must keep the possibility of closed head injury in mind and order appropriate diagnostic imaging, such as computed tomography of the brain. In some instances, the diagnostic image reveals an acute subdural hematoma. In many instances, this is associated with multiple retinal hemorrhages diagnosed by ophthalmology. The plain film pediatric trauma skeletal series or skeletal survey may reveal healing or acute fractures. With this constellation of a previously well child with no history of trauma and a sudden onset of symptoms with the finding of an acute subdural hematoma, the generalist should suspect abusive head trauma. Concurrently with medical and neurosurgical management, the suspicion should be reported to the department of human services and law enforcement immediately.

Skeletal manifestations of physical abuse involve fractures not consistent with the history offered by the caregiver. The generalist's initial suspicion may stem from a history that is not developmentally probable or evidence of multiple fractures of different ages. An acute femur fracture and healing rib fractures in a 6-week-old infant are unlikely to be due to rolling off a countertop. In addition, certain types of fractures are suspicious for nonaccidental trauma because they rarely occur accidentally; these include rib fractures and metaphyseal fractures.

Abdominal trauma may present with nonspecific symptoms, such as vomiting or decreased mental status. Physical findings may be subtle with a small bruise over the liver or spleen or a mildly distended abdomen.

The medical evaluation of a child who may have been sexually abused requires particular care. Keeping in mind that in an ideal evaluation, a child would be interviewed once and examined once, the generalist needs to consider the most experienced person available to obtain the history and perform the detailed genital examination. If a forensic interviewer is available, the medical provider needs to obtain just enough history to determine if sexual abuse is suspected and needs to be reported. Key information includes when an event may have happened. Although sexual abuse often is disclosed some time after an event, it must be determined if acute sexual abuse (within 48 hours) may have occurred, if an exchange of body fluids may have occurred, and if a child has current genital bleeding to plan for necessary laboratory tests to be performed at the time of the examination. An examination under anesthesia may be indicated, particularly in the event of unexplained active genital bleeding. When obtaining this medical history from the child, key information can be obtained by asking nonleading questions, such as "What happened?"; "With what?"; "Where"; and "With whom?" The medical history is not the same thing as the interview and investigation that follow, but rather provides enough information to determine if an examination is urgent. Urgent examinations are indicated in the case of acute sexual abuse with possible penetrating trauma or if the exchange of fluids has occurred; otherwise, the examination is best done later in a clinic setting by the most experienced examiner. Because most children who have been sexually abused have normal genital examinations, the delay in an examination in the case of nonacute sexual abuse usually makes sense. Nonetheless, sexual abuse should be reported to human services or law enforcement immediately when a child discloses sexual activity, engages in sexual acting-out behavior, or expresses developmentally inappropriate sexual knowledge or a provider has other reason to suspect sexual abuse.

After a brief history and reporting, an examination is indicated if there is a history suggesting penetrating trauma. In the context of a complete physical examination, girls can be examined in the supine frog-leg position with genital labial separation and traction. Most children tolerate this technique well. The experienced examiner documents any focal findings, such as bruising or lacerations, and the shape of the hymen in girls, with particular attention to the condition of the edge and approximate width of hymenal tissue. Particularly in the event of an apparent subtle abnormality, such as a hymenal transection or narrowing, it is important to confirm the finding in the knee-chest position. No speculum is used in a prepubertal child to minimize discomfort to the child. During the anal portion of the examination, the tone, perianal rugae, tags, and tears are noted.

Although relatively rare, several conditions may be mistaken for physical abuse. Conditions mistaken for inflicted bruises include bleeding disorders. Family history and screening for an adequate platelet count and normal prothrombin time and partial thromboplastin time help to rule out most of these conditions. It may be necessary to rule out osteogenesis imperfecta or osteopenia in cases of repeated unexplained fractures. Although some cases may be apparent as gracile bones on plain x-rays, it may be necessary to consult a pediatric genetics specialist for assistance with additional workup. In any event, it may be helpful to repeat x-rays looking for additional fractures after a period of out-of-home placement in cases in which children have been placed in foster care. Glutaric acidemia must be considered in young infants with macrocephaly and temporal lobe wasting with subdural hematomas. With respect to sexual abuse, common concerns include genital or anal warts. Transmission and latency are not understood adequately; consequently, infants and toddlers may contract human papillomavirus without a known source. In older children, sexual abuse should be considered, but it is difficult to make the diagnosis of sexual abuse from isolated physical findings without a history. Genital or anal infections, such as group A streptococcus or pinworms, must be considered in children presenting with genital pain, redness, or itching.

Child abuse is managed best with a multispecialty and multidisciplinary team. With so many injuries diagnosed by diagnostic images, the importance of consultation with pediatric radiologists cannot be overstated. Investigations cannot be done without social workers and law enforcement officers. The generalist benefits from knowing regional pediatric specialists in child abuse. Common consultations include ophthalmology, orthopedic surgery, and neurosurgery.

DIAGNOSIS

Child abuse usually is diagnosed by taking into account pertinent positive and negative components of the history together with physical findings, laboratory tests, and other studies. In most cases, history is paramount. Laboratory tests for physical abuse may include platelet count, prothrombin time, and partial thromboplastin time. At times, a supplemental newborn screen, urine organic acids, and serum amino acids are indicated. Children younger than 2 years old with unexplained or poorly explained injuries should have a skeletal survey looking for additional signs of injury. A "babygram" is not adequate. Consultation with other specialists often is desirable. It is helpful to know child abuse specialists to have assistance with patient case reviews and consultation in difficult cases, such as abusive head trauma and sexual abuse or controversial or ambiguous cases.

Future trends should include specific prevention strategies, such as school-based violence prevention programs, home visitation programs, and prenatal parenting classes focusing on parental coping skills. Throughout childhood, health care providers can elicit parental behavior concerns and provide age-appropriate anticipatory guidance. Information about community resources and therapy can be offered to families before abuse occurs.

MANAGEMENT AND REFERRALS

Health care professionals who provide medical care to children play a key role in the management of child abuse. From early referrals for mental health counseling and linking families to community resources to suspecting abuse when a history is not consistent with an injury and reporting suspected abuse, the child's health care provider can facilitate family intervention and child safety. Meanwhile, coordinating specialty care and communicating the complex medical needs of these children to individuals responsible for their care is vital.

OUTCOME

Many abused children can have more unmet medical, developmental, dental, vision, and behavioral and mental health needs than average children and consequently should meet the definition of children with special health care needs set by the American Academy of Pediatrics and the Maternal Child Health Bureau. It is important that all children with special health care needs, including abused and neglected children, have their unmet needs identified and that they are referred for care. For this reason, the medical home with the commitment to care coordination is especially important for these children. Because a significant percentage of these children enter foster care with the possibility of multiple in-home and out-of-home placements, it makes sense that an effort is made to provide some continuity of care despite changes in physical custody. Using the medical home model may increase follow-up for the complex needs of abused children. Most health care providers do not provide all aspects of a medical home, but rather they can seek linkages with other facilities. A rural health care provider may work closely with a physical therapist and orthopedic surgeon after a severe fracture or with a mental health care provider after sexual abuse. It is hoped that current long-term studies will show that early identification of unmet medical and mental health needs and intervention not only would temper the immediate suffering of abused and neglected children, but also would address the increased rates of substance abuse, depression and anxiety, violent behavior, learning problems, and adolescent suicide.

Additional Resources, CD-ROM

Bibliography

Mini-index of Related Topics

	CH.
■ FOSTER CARE	263
■ DOMESTIC VIOLENCE: A PEDIATRIC PERSPECTIVE	266
■ LEGAL ASPECTS OF CHILD ABUSE AND NEGLECT	267
■ CHILD NEGLECT: THE INADEQUATE PROMOTION OF CHILDREN'S HEALTH AND DEVELOPMENT	268
■ MUNCHAUSEN SYNDROME BY PROXY	270

SUGGESTED READINGS

Committee on Child Abuse and Neglect: Guidelines for the evaluation of sexual abuse of children. Pediatrics 1999;103:186–191.

Committee on Child Abuse and Neglect: Shaken baby syndrome: Rotational cranial injuries—technical report. Pediatrics 2001; 108:206–210.

Heger A, Silver J: Evaluation of the Sexually Abused Child. New York, Oxford University Press, 2001.

Kempe CH, Silverman FN, Steele BF, et al: The battered-child syndrome. JAMA 1962;181:17–24.

Reece RM, Ludwig S: Child Abuse Medical Diagnosis and Management. Philadelphia, Lippincott Williams & Wilkins, 2001.

270 Munchausen Syndrome by Proxy

Donna Rosenberg

ROLE OF THE GENERALIST

1   Recognize the warning signs of Munchausen syndrome by proxy.

2   Perform diagnostic tests, refer to specialists, and review medical records as appropriate and possible to distinguish between organic illness and falsified illness.

3   Give correct weight to specialists' opinions, remembering that the generalist is in the best position to put a specialist's opinion in the context of the child's entire medical course.

4   Refer the case to the hospital or community child protection team for consultation, if one is available.

5   Report the case to the Department of Social Services.

6   Review the medical records of siblings or other children in the home for the possibility of Munchausen syndrome by proxy or other abuse or neglect.

7   Be prepared to present medical data at multidisciplinary child protection team meetings or in court.

Munchausen syndrome by proxy (MSBP) is a serious and sometimes fatal form of child abuse. MSBP involves the persistent falsification of illness in a child, by an adult, with the child repeatedly presented for medical care. Typically, multiple investigations of the child are done, and exotic diagnoses are pursued when more usual ones have been excluded. The child's troubles persist, however, with illness that cannot be explained, that does not conform to usual patterns, or that is inexplicably refractory to treatment. Most often the perpetrator is the mother, with whom the pediatrician may have a long-standing relationship in consequence of the "chronic illness" of the child. The length and nature of this relationship, along with the pediatrician's vigorous efforts toward diagnosis and treatment of the child, may inhibit consideration of MSBP in the differential diagnosis. MSBP first was described by Meadow, an English pediatrician, in 1977. Since then, there have been hundreds of additions to the pediatric literature, cataloging the astounding variety of ways by which illness has been falsified.

There are two main strategies for falsifying illness: simulation and production. *Simulation* means faking something, or lying about it, without interfering with the child. Examples of illness simulation include giving a history of a dramatic apneic episode, when apnea never actually occurred, or contaminating a urine specimen with blood and then presenting it as evidence of the child's hematuria. *Production* means interfering with the child in any way. Examples of illness production include the surreptitious suffocation of a child or the introduction of poisons, dangerous and unprescribed medications, or medicines in dangerous quantities. Many mothers simulate and produce illness. Mothers who falsify illness, either through simulation or production, often do so in more than one setting, such as their homes, their cars (often on the way to the physician's office), and the hospital itself. A hospital may be a good place to capture the evidence of illness falsification, but only if the diagnosis is suspected and the child is not placed at untoward risk. If the diagnosis is not suspected and the mother surreptitiously assaults the child in the hospital (e.g., poisons, feces, drugs, or saliva into the intravenous line; suffocation), the child is at risk of serious illness, irreversible damage, or death.

Boys and girls are about equally likely victims. Infants and toddlers are the most common victims of MSBP because they are weak, easily immobilized, and incompletely articulate. As children become older, the risk to the mother of exposure increases with the child's increasing communication abilities. Older children, adolescents, and even adults also may be victims of MSBP, however. Some older victims believe they are genuinely ill because they have been made ill for so long. If one child in a family is a victim of MSBP, successive children also may become victims. In these instances, it is more common for the children to be made ill serially, rather than simultaneously. The elder child's symptoms and signs resolve (or the child dies) close to the time that another, younger child becomes the focus of the mother's malignant attentions.

It is dangerous to be a child victim of MSBP. The risks include pain, suffering, prolonged hospitalization, isolation, developmental delay, psychological disability, mental illness, physical disability or disfigurement, and death. These are the effects of being assaulted by a duplicitous and self-serving mother, of being investigated and treated by well-meaning but misguided physicians, and of being separated from what should have been normal growth and development.

FUNDAMENTALS

The most likely reason that a correct diagnosis of MSBP is delayed is the pediatrician's failure to consider MSBP in the differential diagnosis. The pediatrician must become alert to the warning signs of illness fabrication. Warning signs are those found in a particular condition, but which are not exclusive to it. The main warning signs of MSBP are listed in Box 270-1.

A large array of presenting symptoms, signs, and laboratory findings of MSBP has been documented in the medical literature (Table 270-1). This list is not comprehensive because new presentations of MSBP continue to be described. Overall, certain presentations are more common, including apnea, seizures, diarrhea, vomiting, central nervous system depression, bleeding, rash, and fever. Popular methods of fabrication for these presentations are summarized in Table 270-2, along with their corresponding methods of diagnosis.

The most common presentation of MSBP in infancy seems to be apnea. Features particularly worrisome for MSBP include repeated episodes that begin only in the presence of one individual—usually the mother—and, when the summoned person arrives, the infant is found to be compromised (e.g., gasping, cyanotic, gray). In the evaluation of apnea, as in the evaluation of any symptom, the question for the pediatrician is not merely, "Does the child have an abnormality on physical examination or laboratory investigation that suggests an etiology?" Rather, the pediatrician needs to ask, "Does the abnormality *fully* account for the child's presentation?" In an otherwise healthy child, mild anemia, mild respiratory syncytial virus infection, or mild reflux cannot account for life-threatening episodes of apnea. Often, in reviewing records of children who eventually have been diagnosed correctly with MSBP after a long course of "illness," one sees that the etiology for dramatic symptoms had been ascribed incorrectly to minor abnormalities. There usually are multiple referrals to a variety of pediatric specialists. Often, somewhere along the line, the child victim of MSBP becomes the surgical recipient of a gastrostomy tube or indwelling central venous catheter. Because there now is another access route to the child through which he or she may be poisoned surreptitiously, the child subsequently may develop alarming new symptoms and signs.

Findings associated with MSBP are outlined in Box 270-2. Associated findings are those that frequently coexist with a particular condition, but are not *in themselves* either warning signs or diagnostic features.

Box 270-1. Warning Signs of Munchausen Syndrome by Proxy

1. The child's illness is unexplained and prolonged.
2. The child's illness is of the rare type, but not defined clearly by any reliable diagnostic test.
3. The child presents with symptoms and signs that are incongruent.
4. The child presents with symptoms and signs (especially apnea and seizures) that begin or occur only when one particular caretaker is present.
5. The child's illness has been treated, but the treatment is curiously ineffective or not tolerated.
6. In the child who has died, there is a history of repeated premortem medical visits for unusual, ill-defined, or unpredictable illness.

More commonly than other children, victims of MSBP are found to have living siblings who also are victims of illness falsification. Also, there may be dead siblings, most of whom turn out to have been murdered, but whose deaths originally were misdiagnosed. Commonly, infant sibling homicides have been misattributed to sudden infant death syndrome (SIDS), but the term *SIDS* means only that the review of the clinical history, the death scene investigation, and the forensic autopsy have yielded no cause or manner of death. SIDS is less a diagnosis than it is the absence of a diagnosis. Autopsy findings of infants who have died of suffocation and findings of infants who have died of SIDS may be identical because postmortem signs of suffocation commonly are absent in young children.

Perpetrators of MSBP are usually mothers, although rarely perpetrators may be babysitters, fathers, and others. Most do not have any major psychiatric disorder (e.g., psychosis, dissociation). Many have been found to have some sort of personality disorder, but they are fully aware of what they are doing to the child. Relatively little is known about mothers' motivations for perpetrating MSBP, but they seem to include hatred for the child; using the child to get away from a husband or to get a husband's attention; and using the child to get money, goods, or adoration. Whatever the motivation, perpetrators are highly convincing in their false concern and earnestness, meaning that they are highly manipulative. Perpetrators sometimes themselves manifest features of Munchausen syndrome, although it may not have been diagnosed. They may have some kind of paramedical training and allegedly may have been the victims of unusual events, such as fires or break-ins at their homes. They usually have lied about or staged these events themselves.

DIAGNOSIS

In a child who is presented persistently for medical care, the essence of diagnosis involves differentiating between a natural (and probably rare) disorder and an unnatural/child abuse cause. Failure to diagnose MSBP means that a fundamentally healthy child and his or her siblings could be killed or damaged irreversibly. Conversely the failure to exclude MSBP correctly may mean that necessary treatment is withheld from an ill child or that a family is not offered genetic counseling. When the diagnosis of MSBP is entertained and a diagnostic strategy designed, the diagnosis usually is included or excluded relatively quickly. Child victims of MSBP are not immune from genuine childhood illness; MSBP and real illness may coexist.

The main difficulty in designing a definitive diagnostic strategy revolves around the dilemma of not wishing to expose the child to any more potential risk and yet needing reasonably definitive proof if MSBP exists. The diagnostic strategy (often strategies) must maximize diagnostic capability while minimizing risk to the child.

It is vital to review the entire record and reconsider the differential diagnosis. Has an organic diagnosis been missed? Could the explanation for the child's persistent presentation be attributable to something other than either MSBP or an organic diagnosis? Box 270-3 lists the differential diagnoses for persistent presentation.

Table 270-1. Symptoms, Signs, and Laboratory Presentations of Munchausen Syndrome by Proxy

Head, eyes, ears, nose, throat, mouth
  Bleeding from ears
  Epistaxis
  External otitis
  Hearing impairment
  Nasal excoriation
  Nystagmus
  Otorrhea
  Tooth loss
Respiratory
  Apnea
  Asthma
  Bleeding from upper respiratory tract
  Cyanosis (and other color changes, including pallor)
  Cystic fibrosis
  Hemoptysis
  Respiratory arrest
  Sleep apnea
Cardiovascular
  Bradycardia
  Cardiomyopathy
  Cardiopulmonary arrest
  Hypertension
  Rhythm abnormalities (including bradycardia, tachycardia,
    ventricular tachycardia, and others)
  Shock
Gastrointestinal
  Abdominal pain
  Anorexia
  Bleeding from nasogastric tube/ileostomy
  Crohn disease
  Diarrhea
  Esophageal burns
  Esophageal perforation
  Feculent vomiting
  Feeding problems
  Gastrointestinal ulceration
  Hematemesis
  Hematochezia or melena
  Hemorrhagic colitis
  Intestinal pseudo-obstruction
  Malabsorption syndromes
  Polyphagia
  Pseudomelanosis coli
  Retrograde intussusception
  Vomiting (cyclic or otherwise)
Genitourinary
  Bacteriuria
  Hematuria
  Menorrhagia
  Nocturia
  Polydipsia
  Polyuria and/or impaired urinary concentrating ability
  Pyuria
  Renal failure
  Urination from umbilical micropenis
  Urethral stones
  Urine gravel
Neurologic, musculoskeletal, developmental, psychiatric
  Arthralgia
  Arthritis
  Ataxia

Neurologic, musculoskeletal, developmental, psychiatric—cont'd
  Behavioral/personality change (including anxiety, panic reactions,
    rage, disorientation, and others)
  Developmental delay (failure to attain and/or loss of milestones)
  Headache
  Hyperactivity
  Irritability
  Lethargy
  Morning stiffness
  Psychotic symptoms
  Sleep disturbances (prolonged sleep/other)
  Seizures
  Sexual abuse
  Syncope
  Unconsciousness
  Weakness
Skin
  Abscesses
  Burns
  Eczema
  Excoriation
  Rash
Infectious, immune, allergic
  Allergies (to food and others)
  Bacteremia (unimicrobial and/or polymicrobial)
  Fevers
  Immunodeficiency
  Osteomyelitis
  Septic arthritis
  Urinary tract infection
Abnormalities of growth
  Failure to gain weight or weight loss
Hematologic
  Anemia
  Bleeding diathesis
  Bleeding from specific sites (see system)
  Easy bruising
  Leukopenia
Metabolic, endocrine, fluid, and electrolyte
  Acidosis
  Alkalosis
  Biochemical chaos
  Creatine kinase and aldolase increase
  Dehydration
  Diabetes
  Glycosuria
  Hyperglycemia
  Hyperkalemia
  Hypernatremia
  Hypochloremia
  Hypoglycemia
  Hypokalemia
  Hyponatremia
Other
  Abuse (sexual, physical, other)
  Diaphoresis
  Foreign-body ingestions
  Hypothermia
  Peripheral edema
  Poisonings
  Premature birth

In all cases, the pediatrician needs to check the history, especially whether the past events and diagnoses were real and whether other alleged observers and temporal associations that the mother describes are true. The pediatrician should contact other family members, other physicians, professionals, and agencies that have been involved with the child and mother. The pediatrician should secure and review past medical records and other records that may be relevant (e.g., school records, psychological assessments).

Beyond what should be done in all cases, there are four overall strategies for diagnosis when MSBP is suspected. These diagnostic strategies may be used singly or in combination, depending on the circumstances.

Table 270-2. Selected Methods of Illness Falsification and Their Corresponding Methods of Diagnosis

Presentation	Method of Simulation and/or Production	Method of Diagnosis
Apnea	Manual suffocation	Video monitoring
		Implantable ECG recorder
		Diagnosis by exclusion
		Patient with pinch marks on nose
		Mother caught
	Poisoning	Toxicology (gastric/blood)
	Tricyclic antidepressants	Toxicology of IV fluid
	Hydrocarbon	
Seizures	Lying	Diagnosis by exclusion
	Poisoning	Toxicology of blood, urine, IV fluid, milk
	Phenothiazines	
	Hydrocarbons	
	Salt	
	Tricyclic antidepressants	
	Suffocation/carotid sinus pressure	Witnessed
		Forensic photos of pressure points
Diarrhea	Phenophthalein/other laxative poisoning	Stool/diaper positive
	Salt poisoning	Assay of formula/gastric contents
Vomiting	Emetic poisoning	Assay for drug
	Lying	Hospital observation
CNS depression	Drugs	Assays blood, gastric contents, urine, IV fluid; analysis of insulin type
	Diphenoxylate/atropine (Lomotil)	
	Insulin	
	Chloral hydrate	
	Barbiturates/narcotics	
	Aspirin	
	Diphenhydramine	
	Tricyclic antidepressants	
	Acetaminophen	
	Hydrocarbons	
	Chlordiazepoxide	
	Phenytoin	
	Carbemazepine	
	Suffocation	see Apnea and Seizures
Bleeding	Rodenticide (warfarin) poisoning	Toxicology
	Phenophthalein poisoning	Diapers positive
	Exogenous blood applied	Blood group typing (major and minor)
		^{51}Cr labeling of erythrocytes
	Exsanguination of child	Single-blind study
		Mother caught
	Addition of other substances (paint, cocoa, dyes)	Testing; washing
Rash	Drug poisoning	Assay
	Scratching	Diagnosis of exclusion
	Caustics applied/painting skin	Assay/wash off
Fever	Contamination with infected material	Mother caught
	Materials	Improper taping of IV line discovered
	Saliva	Type of organism growing from infected sites
	Feces	Trial separation
	Dirt	Epidemiology (relative risk assessment)
	Contaminated water	Diagnosis by exclusion
	Coffee grounds	
	Vaginal secretions	
	Others	
	Target tissues	
	Blood	
	Skin	
	Bones	
	Bladder	
	Others	
	Falsifying temperature	Careful charting, rechecking (especially urine for core body temperature)
	Falsifying chart	Careful charting, rechecking
		Duplication (ghost record) of temperature chart in nursing station

CNS, central nervous system; ^{51}Cr, radioactive sodium chromate; ECG, electrocardiographic; IV, intravenous.

Adapted from Rosenberg DA: Web of deceit: A literature review of Munchausen syndrome by proxy. Child Abuse Negl 1987;11:547–563. Copyright 1987. Reprinted with permission from Elsevier.

Box 270-2. Findings Associated with Munchausen Syndrome by Proxy

- A living sibling with current or past, chronic, ill-defined medical problems
- A deceased sibling whose death is not explained clearly
  - *or* whose death followed an ill-defined illness
  - *or* whose death followed an illness that was presumed to exist, but that was unsubstantiated or excluded at autopsy
  - *or* whose cause of death was an illness that rarely is fatal in childhood
  - *or* whose death was related to an accidental intoxication or an unusual accident
  - *or* whose cause of death was signed out as SIDS
- An unrelated child in the same home who previously or subsequently died
- A mother with chronic, ill-defined medical problems
- A mother who is not overly concerned or who seeks publicity or both
- Fires or break-ins at the home
- Pets that have died suddenly or had unusual illnesses

SIDS, sudden infant death syndrome.

Box 270-4. Criteria for a Definitive Diagnosis by Inclusion

1. The test/event is positive for tampering with the child or with the child's medical situation.
and
2. The positivity of the test/event is not credibly the result of miscommunication, misunderstanding, or test error.
and
3. No other explanation for a positive test/event is medically possible.

The first diagnostic strategy is the search for evidence of illness fabrication. One might analyze samples of urine, blood, or vomitus for toxicology and blood group typing. The chain of evidence is important with any samples, and the samples should be preserved if possible so that repeat tests on the same samples can be done if necessary. This diagnostic strategy also may include surveillance of the child in the hospital by the staff, by room searches (the pediatrician should consult a hospital lawyer or law enforcement about the need for a search warrant), or by hidden video monitoring. When video monitoring is used, there must be continuous monitoring with, and recording by, the video units. Plans to intervene immediately and decisively if assault is seen should be in place before starting surveillance. Coordination with hospital security, law enforcement, social services, or all three is generally necessary.

The second diagnostic strategy is the search for evidence of an explanation other than MSBP. Basically, with this strategy, one makes a list of the organic diagnoses that *reasonably* could account for the *totality* of the child's presentation. The point of this diagnostic strategy is to determine if MSBP is the only diagnosis left standing after thorough investigation of the child. MSBP is effectively a diagnosis by exclusion, and this is a powerful diagnostic approach when the contending diagnoses on the differential

definitively and reliably may be included or excluded. Positive test results that suggest a genuine organic etiology must be scrutinized carefully to ensure that they are not false-positive results (e.g., owing to maternal contamination or intervention or as a result of being overcalled). This strategy may be the best one available when neither the opportunity nor the diagnostic test that could capture evidence of commission is possible (e.g., poisoning, suffocation) or if so doing could expose the child to grave risk.

The third diagnostic strategy is trial separation. The only major variable that should be changed during separation is the presence of the suspected caretaker. It is important to have a baseline against which to compare the child's subsequent course during separation. The baseline might be the frequency and type of symptoms reported by the mother (e.g., "He has three to six seizures a day, at least 5 days a week"). Only reversible conditions of the child can be expected to improve, to a degree and at a rate consonant with the condition. Supervised visitation may be reasonable, but no foods, medicines, or candy may be permitted to be given to the child.

The fourth diagnostic strategy is records review. It may be the only diagnostic strategy available in certain circumstances (e.g., if the child is dead). Records review involves the reformulation of a differential diagnosis and its critical re-evaluation, through a minute review of all records. The pivotal facts, although present in the medical records, may have been obscured by the sheer volume of information, and a comprehensive survey of the child's medical presentation may have been overshadowed repeatedly by the immediacy of the crises. A computerized database system for data entry, storage, organization, and retrieval is sometimes indispensable.

When MSBP is considered in the differential diagnosis, the possible outcomes are *definitely MSBP, definitely not MSBP,* or *indeterminate.* The diagnostic criteria for MSBP, by inclusion or by exclusion, are listed in Boxes 270-4 and 270-5. Diagnosis may not be based solely on either warning signs or associated findings. Doing so may result in incorrect diagnosis.

Box 270-3. Differential Diagnosis for Persistent Presentation

- Organic illness
- Anxious parent
- Developmentally delayed parent
- Vulnerable child syndrome
- Psychogenic illness
- Munchausen syndromes

MANAGEMENT

When MSBP is suspected, the tasks for the pediatrician are medical and nonmedical and immediate and longer term. The immediate medical tasks include (1) the treatment of serious and life-threatening conditions (e.g., sepsis, cerebral edema) and (2) the determination of the etiology of the

Box 270-5. Criteria for a Definitive Diagnosis by Exclusion

1. All competing diagnoses have been credibly eliminated, as follows:

   If the child is alive, the competing diagnoses are those that took into account the child's major medical findings* and still do not account for the entirety of the child's presentation.

   or

   If the child is alive, separation of the child from the alleged perpetrator results in resolution of the child's reversible medical problems, in accordance with their degree and speed of reversibility. No variable other than the separation can account logically and fully for the child's improvement.

   or

   If the child is dead, autopsy examination does not reveal a cause of death that is credibly accidental, natural, or suicidal.

   and

2. No findings exclude the diagnosis of Munchausen syndrome by proxy.

*A major medical finding is one that is observed objectively, is sufficiently specific as to help formulate the range of diagnoses, and is verifiable in the record.

child's illness, through physical examination and investigations as appropriate. If poisoning is suspected, the pediatrician should speak with the toxicologist and ask about any special assays that may be necessary, about assays that may be done in-house and assays that would have to be sent out, the best fluid or tissue that should be collected and the quantity, and any special conditions necessary for the transport of the specimen. The pediatrician needs to inquire about the laboratory's chain of evidence procedure and follow it.

There are two immediate nonmedical tasks. First is reporting the case to child protective services. The legal threshold for reporting child abuse is *reasonable suspicion*. The law does not require definitive proof. Failure to report a case of abuse that reasonably should have been suspected may result in civil or criminal liability for the physician. The second task is coordinating with social services and law enforcement as necessary for the immediate protection of the child and for any diagnostic tests that may be decisive (e.g., hidden video monitoring in the hospital).

The longer-term medical tasks are (1) finalizing a diagnosis, whether definitely MSBP, definitely not MSBP, or (as sometimes happens, even when all possible data are gathered) indeterminate, and (2) in some cases, continuing to monitor and treat the child as necessary (e.g., following the child's course during a trial separation; weaning off oral steroids).

The most important longer-term nonmedical task is the clear communication of one's findings to the oversight multidisciplinary child protection team and possibly to the court, either civil or criminal. Cases of MSBP still are quite unlikely to result in criminal action against the perpetrator. The purpose of the civil court is child protection and "treatment" of the perpetrator.

MSBP cases are time-consuming, before and after diagnosis, complex, and often draining. If possible, the pediatrician should seek advice on aspects of diagnosis and treatment specific to the case from a child abuse medical specialist. The American Academy of Pediatrics has a Section on Child Abuse, currently with hundreds of members.

Perpetrators of MSBP tend to be litigious; they bring lawsuits against physicians for malicious reporting of child abuse (when the diagnosis is sound) or for wrongful death (when they themselves have killed the child). As with any other pediatric case, an appropriately thorough medical approach and scrupulous documentation are the best insurance against a successful lawsuit.

SUMMARY

MSBP is a dangerous form of child abuse. If the diagnosis is suspected, its investigation should not be deferred because irreversible damage to the child or homicide may occur in the interim. Perpetrators are dangerous, and no treatment is known to be universally effective, in what is fundamentally a gross disorder of empathy, manifested through the persistent and cruel fabrication of illness.

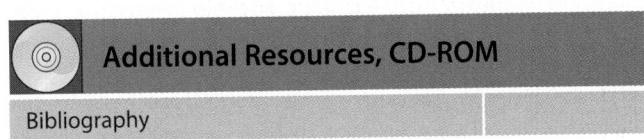

Additional Resources, CD-ROM

Bibliography

Mini-index of Related Topics

SUGGESTED READINGS

Hall DE, Eubanks L, Meyyazhagan LS, et al: Evaluation of covert video surveillance in the diagnosis of Munchausen syndrome by proxy: Lessons from 41 cases. Pediatrics 2000;105:1305–1312.

McClure RJ, Davis PM, Meadow SR, Sibert JR: Epidemiology of Munchausen syndrome by proxy, non-accidental poisoning, and non-accidental suffocation. Arch Dis Child 1996;75:57–61.

Rosen CL, Frost JD, Glaze DG: Child abuse and recurrent infant apnea. J Pediatr 1986;109:1065–1067.

Rosenberg DA: Web of deceit: A literature review of Munchausen syndrome by proxy. Int J Child Abuse Negl 1987;11:547–563.

Waring WW: The persistent parent. Am J Dis Child 1992;146:753–756.

DIAGNOSTICS AND THERAPEUTICS

271

Laboratory Testing of Infants and Children

Gillian Lockitch and Thomas Mock,
with contributions by Eva Thomas, Hilary Vallance,
and Louis Wadsworth

Pediatric laboratories in major medical centers have specialized resources and the capacity to provide routine, complex, and esoteric laboratory tests for infants and children. In these centers specialists in various disciplines of pediatric pathology and laboratory medicine can be consulted on the complexities of investigating disease in infants and children. All physicians treating infants and children must understand the differences between adults and children in regard to laboratory testing and must ensure that testing for their patients is done in laboratories directed by pathologists with expertise in pediatric laboratory medicine. This chapter discusses general principles of laboratory testing in pediatrics, provides information needed to understand ordering and interpretation of frequently ordered tests, and suggests an approach to dealing with unexpected laboratory results.

GENERAL PRINCIPLES OF PEDIATRIC LABORATORY MEDICINE

The actual laboratory analysis is only one component of a much broader diagnostic process. The purpose of the diagnostic process is to answer a question that may relate to screening for or excluding a condition, suggesting or confirming a diagnosis, assessing progression of a disease, or monitoring the effect of treatment. Laboratory testing must take into account preanalytic, analytic, and postanalytic factors to ensure that the answers provided are valid and relevant. Errors in any of these phases can result in an incorrect or misleading result.

Preanalytic components include defining the question, ordering the appropriate test, preparing the patient for testing, collecting the specimen, and transporting it to the laboratory. Analytic factors are directly concerned with the performance of the test, such as specimen handling and processing within the laboratory and the analytic process and quality control. Initial selection of test methods and equipment by the pathologist, establishing the assay linear range, precision and accuracy of the test method, and detection of interferences, are components of the analytic process. Postanalytic factors include result recording and interpretation with correct reference intervals, reporting the result in a timely manner, and interactive follow-up by the laboratory physician with the ordering physician.

Pediatric laboratory medicine encompasses a wide range of developmental and age groups with profound differences in physiologic characteristics that result in important differences in the preanalytic, analytic, and postanalytic phases of testing. The widely differing range of clinical disorders seen at different developmental stages contributes further to the complexity of laboratory testing in this extremely heterogeneous population.

Pediatric laboratories must use phlebotomy staff experienced in the microsampling and skin puncture techniques used for blood collection in infants and young children. Automated diagnostic equipment must use micromethods to minimize the volume of blood or serum/plasma needed. The reporting system should use in-house validated age- and sex-specific reference intervals for all methods and equipment used in the laboratory. Because hospital-based pediatric laboratories deal with a sicker, more abnormal population in comparison to community-based laboratories, they must be staffed by pathologists with special expertise and training in interpretation of pediatric testing.

The ordering physician must be aware of the many factors that can affect test outcome. Pediatric patients should be referred to a laboratory that is prepared for testing infants and children and has appropriate in-house method-specific pediatric reference intervals for all its tests.

The objective of the consultant pathologists who direct pediatric laboratories is to ensure the quality of the diagnostic process. The pathologist must determine that systems are in place to ensure that the correct test is selected for the specific purpose, the correct specimen is collected from the right patient, the test is precisely and accurately performed, and the results are correctly reported to the ordering physician in a timely manner. The pathologist is a valuable resource for the ordering physician.

CRUCIAL CONSIDERATIONS IN PEDIATRIC LABORATORY TESTING

Preanalytic Factors
Defining the Question
Use and interpretation of a test may differ considerably, depending on the test context. To choose the correct tests the physician must be clear about the objective of testing:

screening, diagnosis, prognosis, or monitoring. The pathologists at the laboratory must be provided with sufficient clinical information to ensure that the appropriate test procedure is carried out and results are correctly interpreted.

Screening may involve a formal screening program, such as newborn screening programs for phenylketonuria, congenital hypothyroidism, and other disorders; maternal serum prenatal screening programs for fetal trisomy and congenital anomalies of the neural tube; and screening programs for cystic fibrosis or thalassemia. The objective of tests within a screening program is to identify from a group of individuals of a priori unknown risk, those patients whose a posteriori risk for the given condition is sufficiently high to warrant further investigation.

Panels in screening programs vary with the population being screened. Considerations for introducing new tests into a screening program are that the condition screened for is relatively common in the population being screened, that the test can identify individuals at risk, and that there is an effective treatment. When screening programs are being developed, the clinical sensitivity and specificity of the test are important considerations. The diagnostic efficiency of a test, a combined measure of both clinical sensitivity and specificity, is also considered.

A screening test may also be used in the context of investigating an individual patient for whom clinical presentation or family history may suggest an increased likelihood of disease. Frequently the initial laboratory investigation is guided by an algorithm or guideline developed by expert groups. These initial tests should be of sufficient sensitivity and specificity to rule out or increase the likelihood of a diagnosis. The result of such a screening test may be to halt further need for testing or to lead to further definitive diagnostic testing.

Diagnostic testing is performed to make, confirm, or exclude a diagnosis in an individual. For example, a history may suggest liver disease and enzymes such as alkaline phosphatase (ALKP), gamma glutamyltransferase (GGT), aspartate aminotransferase (AST), or alanine aminotransferase (ALT) may be measured to determine whether liver disease should be further considered. With a persistently high enzyme activity, the physician may proceed to a liver biopsy as a diagnostic test if no other explanation can be advanced.

Both the physician and the patient or family must understand clearly the distinction between a screening test and a diagnostic test, particularly in the context of a screening program. For example, a positive screening test of maternal biochemical marker screening indicates an increased risk for fetal trisomy that justifies amniocentesis. Women may misinterpret this positive screening test as indicating that the fetus is affected, but need to understand that the definitive diagnostic test for the presence or absence of trisomy 21 is cytogenetic analysis of the chromosomes.

Prognostic or evaluative testing is used to judge the severity of an abnormality. Monitoring is used to assess disease progression or improvement or the effect of therapy. Examples may include repeated blood gas analysis to determine respiratory function in neonatal respiratory distress syndrome, or monitoring blood lead levels in a child on chelation therapy.

Selecting the Test

The decision as to whether a new test adds new value to the diagnostics process is made by evaluating its clinical efficiency by considering the clinical sensitivity, specificity, and predictive value of a test. These parameters are calculated from studies evaluating the results of the test in a population of individuals with and without a specific disorder. Test results are considered true if they correctly identify whether the patient has or is free of the disease. False results refer to those that lead to the incorrect interpretation. If a test to detect a disease is carried out in patients with a disease of interest, a patient with the disease will have either a positive result, which would be considered a true positive result (TP), or a negative result, which would be falsely negative (FN) (Table 271-1).

Clinical sensitivity is defined as the ability of a test to detect disease. Clinical specificity is defined as the ability to yield normal results in patients without the particular disease. The predictive value of a positive test refers to the percentage of patients with positive results who have the disease. The predictive value of a negative test refers to the percentage of patients with negative results who do not have the disease.

These parameters of a test can be calculated from results of test evaluation in subjects proved to be affected or free of the disease of interest. The presence or absence of a disease is evaluated in the subjects using a generally accepted gold standard. Controversy often exists in the definition or identification of a sufficient standard. Physicians should be aware that a sensitive test can be used most effectively to rule out a disease. With reference to the equation that follows (Table 271-2), fewer false negatives (i.e., more true negatives = rule out) will lead to increased sensitivity without an alteration in the true positive rate. A specific test can be used most efficiently to rule in a disease (i.e., fewer false positives = more true positives and thus, rule in).

Table 271-1. Test Results: Sensitivity, Specificity, and Predictive Value

Test result accuracy in presence or absence of disease:

	Disease Present (+)	Disease absent (−)
Test Result Positive (+)	True positive (TP)	False positive (FP)
Test Result Negative (−)	False negative (FN)	True negative (TN)

Sensitivity indicates proportion of diseased people correctly identified by a positive test:

$$\text{Sensitivity} = \frac{TP}{TP + FN}$$

Specificity indicates proportion of nondiseased people correctly identified by a negative test:

$$\text{Sensitivity} = \frac{TN}{TN + FP}$$

Predictive value indicates how good a test is at identifying people with the disease (positive predictive value) and without the disease (negative predictive value):

$$\text{Positive predictive value} = \frac{TP}{TP + FP}$$

$$\text{Negative predictive value} = \frac{TN}{TN + FN}$$

Table 271-2. Understanding Diagnostic Test Performance

Sensitivity: The likelihood that the test will be positive in a person with the disease	$\dfrac{\text{True-positive results}}{\text{True-positive + false-negative results}} \times 100$
Specificity: The likelihood that the test will be negative in a person without the disease	$\dfrac{\text{True-negative results}}{\text{True-positive + false-positive results}} \times 100$
Predictive value of positive test: The likelihood that a positive test will be in a person with the disease	$\dfrac{\text{True-positive results}}{\text{True-positive + false-positive results}} \times 100$
Predictive value of negative test: The likelihood that a negative test will be in a person without the disease	$\dfrac{\text{True-negative results}}{\text{True-negative + false-negative results}} \times 100$

These characteristics of tests may help in deciding whether parallel testing (several tests done at the same time) or serial testing is indicated (where the outcome of one test is used to determine whether additional testing is required).

Ordering multiple tests on a single sample increases the likelihood that at least one of the tests will be reported as abnormal. When reference intervals are established for a new test, upper and lower limits for reference intervals are most commonly defined as the values at the 2.5 percentile and the 97.5 percentile. The reference interval includes the central 95% of the population. By definition, therefore, 5% of the values are outside the reference interval. Statistically, therefore, 1 in 20 tests could have a result outside the reference interval in an otherwise healthy individual. Failing to take this into account can send the physician off into a fruitless search for an underlying disease. This is a powerful argument against so-called panel testing, in which a large number of analytes (items to be measured) is ordered without regard to the status of the patient and the perceived clinical usefulness.

Although very useful in describing tests in selected populations in which the diagnosis is made by a "gold" standard, sensitivity and specificity are less useful in characterizing tests in unselected populations, the usual situation the physician confronts because he or she does not know to which category the patient belongs before ordering the test. The positive predictive value and negative predictive value are better suited to guide physicians in determining the presence or absence of disease, because they are calculated using the prevalence (or likelihood of diagnosis) of the disease in the greater population. The positive predictive value provides the physician with the relative likelihood that a positive test result indicates the presence of disease in an individual. The negative predictive value, on the other hand, indicates the relative likelihood that a negative test result suggests the absence of disease. Consider the example in Table 271-3.

Based solely on the result, a physician obtaining a positive result in a patient when the underlying prevalence of the disease in the general population is only 0.1% and the test displays a clinical sensitivity of 90% and a clinical specificity of 90% must recognize that there is only a 0.9% relative likelihood of disease. Follow-up testing would clearly be indicated.

The use of predictive values, although superior to sensitivity and specificity, suffers from the fact that numerical values obtained in most test results are dichotomized simply into positive or negative findings. The magnitude of the abnormal test result and its effect on the likelihood of disease are, therefore, ignored. The use of likelihood ratios predicts the presence of disease at any given test value (likelihood ratio positive = sensitivity/1 – specificity). This would offer the clinician more information than is currently available in the interpretation of numeric results. The drawback to the widespread use of likelihood ratios is the lack of sufficient data (sensitivity and specificity) over the range of results commonly seen.

Given the current limitations placed on the interpretation of laboratory results, a clinician should exercise sound judgment and draw from his or her own experience or that of colleagues. Consultation with clinical and laboratory experts is strongly encouraged. Laboratory results should be used in conjunction with clinical impressions rather than a replacement for clinical judgment.

Evidence-based medicine is defined by Sackett and associates as "the conscientious, explicit and judicious use of current best evidence in making decisions about the care of individual patients." Various multidisciplinary groups have developed clinical practice guidelines from systematic reviews of the literature, assessing the quality and weight of evidence in establishing testing algorithms and guidelines. In theory, review of consistency, clinical effectiveness, and resource implications as a required element of this process should optimize patient care. These testing strategies are intended to influence medical practice and to reduce costs from unnecessary or redundant testing. The success of reflex testing algorithms has been generally accepted to demonstrate the universal application of such strategies. An example is initial testing of thyrotropin (TSH) with free thyroxine (free T_4) provided as a follow-up test only if TSH level is abnormal. However, limitations to these guidelines must also be recognized. One must recognize in specialized pediatric laboratories serving tertiary care institutions that insistence on a primary TSH screen will be inadequate to evaluate children suffering from central hypothyroidism or other pituitary or hypothalamic disorders.

Unusual situations associated with an abnormal test result in the absence of underlying disease must be carefully

Table 271-3. Positive and Negative Predictive Values

For a test with a sensitivity of 90% and a specificity of 90%:

Prevalence (or likelihood)	Positive Predictive Value	Negative Predictive Value
0.1%	0.9%	99.9%
1.0%	8.3%	99.9%
10.0%	50.0%	98.8%

considered. An excellent example of this is a condition called transient hyperphosphatasemia of infancy. This condition, usually seen in children younger than 5 years of age, is characterized by an extremely high serum alkaline phosphatase in the absence of any underlying skeletal or hepatic disorder. The main importance of this condition is the initial alarm caused when the ordering physician receives a result that may be up to 20 times higher than the normal upper reference limit. This often results in a fruitless and expensive search for underlying bone and liver disease.

Test Requisitions

The test requisition or order form is an often overlooked, yet crucial element of the testing process. A well-designed requisition, properly completed, can alert the pathologist to special circumstances or conditions crucial to the interpretation or reporting of the results. Far too often, crucial information that would alert the pathologist to the complexity, urgency, or clinical indication of the test requested is omitted. Other than direct consultation, the requisition should be viewed as the principal mode of communication between clinician and pathologist.

Laboratory requisitions must elicit relevant and necessary information from the clinician. Issues of timed or random specimens, confirmed or suspected diagnoses, and clinical status of the patient have profound implications on how the result is interpreted. Current drugs or other therapy should be indicated on the requisition, such as a cortisol collected during dexamethasone therapy that will almost invariably be suppressed in a normal patient.

Not indicating the need for urgent testing on the requisition could have profound implications on patient outcome. Conversely, the practice of routinely ordering tests "stat" to get rapid results can equally lead to disaster if the laboratory is faced with large numbers of unnecessary "stats" and is unable to prioritize the truly urgent specimens. In emergency situations, the laboratory should be directly alerted.

Preparing the Patient

Spurious or misleading test results are frequently caused by preanalytic factors related to specimen collection or processing. These factors include hemolysis, lipemia, stasis, hemoconcentration, and hemodilution. The test result may be high or low owing to an artifact in the collection method. Physiologic factors responsible for intrapatient variability in test values also alter test results, but in this case the values are a true reflection of the actual concentration in the child's blood. Examples of such physiologic factors include diurnal and circadian variation, exercise, posture, and the effect of food. Age and gender account for many of the most important physiologic changes in test values.

Circadian variation can greatly alter the levels of some analytes. Cortisol, epinephrine, and norepinephrine are highest in the morning; iron is highest in the afternoon; and growth hormone, renin, aldosterone, and parathyroid hormone peak late at night. Measured enzyme activity (alanine or aspartate aminotransferase, alkaline phosphatase, and lactate dehydrogenase) can vary as much as 15% to 50%, depending on the time that the specimen is collected. Urine catecholamine excretion is reduced during bedrest.

Exercise and posture are also important. Enzymes such as creatine kinase may remain elevated for more than 24 hours after vigorous exercise. Posture causes some slight effect. Water shifts from the intravascular compartment on standing up. Slightly higher values occur when blood is collected from a child in the upright position compared to supine. Higher values are seen for protein, albumin, hematocrit, hemoglobin, and erythrocyte and white blood cell counts. Protein-bound analytes such as calcium, bilirubin, and some drugs are also higher. For tests such as renin or aldosterone these effects may be marked, and standardized collection protocols should state whether the subject must be supine, and for how long prior to the collection of the specimen.

If recent eating affects the test results, fasting is required before the specimen is collected. Glucose, potassium, phosphate, and bilirubin generally rise after eating a standard mixed meal. A meal rich in carbohydrates may actually result in a decrease in phosphate. Lesser increases may also be seen in cholesterol, protein, calcium, and uric acid. Alkaline phosphatase may also increase after a lipid rich meal. A 12-hour fast is usually required, but this time is lessened for young children. For infants a 4-hour fasting period is considered sufficient.

Specimen Collection

Specific specimen collection protocols must be developed and used for different test procedures for each type of specimen used in the laboratory. Avoidance of microbial contamination when collecting and processing a blood specimen for blood culture requires a different procedure than that needed to avoid trace element contamination when testing for trace elements present in nanogram amounts. At least the minimal amount of specimen required for an acceptable analysis must be obtained. The laboratory must ensure that the necessary information on requirements for testing is available at specimen collection sites.

Correct identification of the patient is extremely important, especially in a setting in which an adult may not be present. This can be a major source of error in the setting of an intensive care unit or newborn nursery, where correct identification may depend on checking an identification bracelet. The practice of identifying babies as twin A or B can lead to mix-ups.

The specimen container must always be labeled immediately with the patient's name and specimen identification. The microsampling containers used in pediatric laboratories make the pediatric laboratory a difficult problem for large-scale automation. Sample size restrictions and the problem of using bar codes on small containers complicate pediatric blood testing.

The pediatric laboratory must always be conscious of the relatively small blood volume of an infant or young child compared to an adult. Although modern equipment can measure the commonly used analytes on very small (microliter) specimens, the need to preserve blood volume in the small premature or newborn infant mandates the ordering physician to be always conscious of minimizing need for blood replacement. This also places major restrictions on the ability of the pediatric laboratory to develop reference norms for infants. This important problem in the newborn period and especially for premature or low-birth-weight infants is exacerbated by the physiologically high hematocrit of the newborn, which means that less plasma or serum is obtained from a blood specimen. A 10-mL test tube of blood collected from an adult represents less than 0.3% of total blood volume but about 10% of the total blood volume of a 1000-g preterm infant.

Blood specimens may be collected from several types of sites. Skin puncture of the heel is commonly used to obtain blood from infants. Finger puncture may be used in small children. The site should be carefully warmed to increase blood flow and prevent hemolysis. Blood from this source is a mixture of venous, capillary blood and tissue fluids. Excessive squeezing of the puncture site may cause bruising and hemolysis as well as give spurious results.

Extreme care must be used to prevent complications such as infection at the puncture site. Calcaneal osteomyelitis, a complication of heel puncture in the small premature infant, is avoided by careful restriction of puncture site to the outer portions of the heel.

Venipuncture at the antecubital fossa may be used in children older than 2 years. Care must be taken to avoid prolonged stasis from the tourniquet or too rapid removal of blood. Prolonged stasis may cause an artifactual rise in the concentration of some analytes such as potassium and lactate.

The choice of whole blood, plasma, or serum for analysis is dependent on the test and specific method. Although serum and plasma are most commonly used in the clinical laboratory, whole blood is required for some analyses. Whole blood is used for blood gas analysis, for many trace element analyses such as blood lead, and for assays such as free erythrocyte or zinc protoporphyrin and hemoglobin A1c. Whole blood specimens are also used in point of care testing devices for measurement of hematocrit, sodium, potassium, and ionized calcium and may sometimes result in spurious results because of undetected hemolysis. For assays such as erythrocyte enzymes, a red blood cell pellet is prepared from the whole blood sample.

Although serum must be used for certain assays, if plasma can be used, it is usually preferred. To obtain serum, the specimen is collected into a nonanticoagulated container, and must be left for 10 to 15 minutes to allow coagulation to occur prior to centrifugation. For plasma the specimen can be centrifuged immediately. A greater volume of plasma than serum is usually obtained from a given blood specimen. However, plasma specimens may develop fibrin clots on standing or storage and can clog test equipment. For specimens that must be transported to reference laboratories or those that will be stored frozen, serum is often preferable.

If the analysis requires whole blood or plasma, specimens are collected into test tubes, syringes, or microtainers (small plastic tubes) containing anticoagulant. Heparin, in the form of sodium or lithium heparin, is the most commonly used anticoagulant for biochemical analyses. These forms of heparin, however, affect calcium measurements. The preferred anticoagulants for free calcium include lyophilized

low heparin tubes, electrolyte-balanced/calcium-titrated heparin syringes, or lithium-zinc heparin syringes. EDTA (ethylenediaminetetraacetic acid) is used for collection of specimens for hematologic analyses because it preserves the cells. EDTA plasma cannot be used to measure calcium, iron, or enzymes such as creatine kinase or alkaline phosphatase. Specimens for coagulation studies are usually collected in sodium citrate.

Assays of the cellular components of blood include total red blood cell count, white blood cell total and differential count, and platelet count. Examples of assays of red blood cell activity or function include the vitamin-dependent erythrocyte enzyme assays used in evaluating nutritional status for vitamins B_1 (thiamine), B_2 (riboflavin), and B_6 (pyridoxine); and other enzymes such as glutathione peroxidase, superoxide dismutase, or catalase. Red blood cell pellets are prepared from a whole blood sample usually collected in heparin. If these specimens are sent to reference laboratories for testing, they must be kept frozen so that enzyme activity is not lost in transport.

Urine analysis is indispensable in testing for childhood disorders such as neuroblastoma, diseases affecting the glomerulus or tubules of the kidney, and other genitourinary disorders. A pediatric laboratory must be equipped to provide the necessary equipment and guidance to facilitate the proper collection, storage, and transport of urine to the laboratory. The laboratory must provide guidance on the type of specimen to be collected for the test requested. The National Committee for Clinical Laboratory Standards (NCCLS) has produced guidelines on the collection of urine and should be consulted on topics not covered here.

For the collection of urine from pediatric patients, the nursing staff is encouraged to clean and dry the scrotal or perineal area prior to collection to minimize contamination. For random collections a U-bag, which is placed around the infant's genitalia, is often used. Reference to urine creatinine is most often performed to correct for excretion rate. Catheter or suprapubic tap specimens are sometimes collected from critically ill infants and used for microbiologic testing as well as for biochemical testing. Collection from neonates and infants poses obvious problems, particularly for timed specimens. Timed specimens are used to minimize the influence of short-term biologic variation and provide an integrated picture of excretion. Despite this, most laboratories will still assay for urine creatinine to check on completeness of collection. In some populations, particularly adolescents, compliance with collection is often lacking, with implications in testing for drugs, for example. The test report should comment on the completeness of collection with reference to expected urinary creatinine excretion. Special protocols and containers are usually required for urine trace element testing and must be obtained from the laboratory.

Some urine constituents are unstable in unpreserved urine and must be collected with adherence to protocols provided by the laboratory. For many children the parents or caregivers need to help with the collection process and must be educated on the proper procedures to ensure a valid test result. Such tests include the metanephrines and other catecholamines for which an acid preservative is added to the collection container to ensure stability. The parents must be instructed to encourage their children to void into a separate container, which is then emptied into an acid-containing vessel to avoid splashing of the acid. Precautions should be taken to prevent fecal contamination of the urine specimen. The urine should be kept in the refrigerator as an additional measure to ensure stability. Once received by the laboratory the urine volume is measured and tested by dipstick to assess adequacy of pH. Should adjustment be necessary for the test requested, either acid or base is added and the urine is stored in the refrigerator until analysis. For tests run infrequently the urine may be stored frozen and thawed as necessary. The volume requirements for the majority of urine-based tests are such that sufficient volumes can be collected even from infants.

Cerebrospinal fluid (CSF) is collected from children for reasons ranging from diagnosis of meningitis to suspicion of cerebrovascular accident. Diagnosis, treatment, and monitoring of certain malignancies may require examination of CSF. The laboratory plays a crucial role in the management of such patients by measuring glucose, proteins, lactate, and some hematologic parameters in CSF. Protein electrophoresis of CSF is often performed when a demyelinating disorder is suspected. In many cases the interpretation of CSF analytes requires the simultaneous assay of blood analytes to provide the physician a real-time reference against which to interpret the CSF analytes.

Spinal fluid is most often obtained by lumbar puncture, although analysis is sometimes performed on specimens collected from the cervical region during surgery. The site of collection is of relevance and should be indicated on the requisition because some analytes show variation in concentration. As traumatic punctures are not uncommon, it should be recognized that if multiple tests are requested, the order of draw will be important. In general, biochemical testing should be performed on the initial fluid obtained, with microscopic and cytologic testing reserved for specimen collected later. Because the collection of CSF carries risk and is clearly uncomfortable for both the patient and caregiver, the specimens should be processed quickly and treated with extra caution. Some laboratories wish to be consulted prior to collection to ensure that processing of the sample is rapid and timely.

Stool specimens are routinely collected from children for analysis in suspected malabsorption and in the assessment of exocrine pancreatic function, such as occurs in cystic fibrosis. Whereas a random specimen is appropriate for the assessment of stool fat globules, meat fibers, and reducing substances, the collection of a timed specimen is more useful in the assessment of fat malabsorption, a protein-losing enteropathy, or the excretion of hemoglobin precursors in various porphyrias. Most tests require solid specimens for enzyme activity or for α_1-antitrypsin excretion. Some clinicians will request stool electrolytes in the evaluation of unexplained diarrhea. In these cases a liquid stool specimen is necessary and a solid specimen received by the laboratory for electrolyte analysis should be rejected.

In infants, fecal material is often obtained from the diaper itself. For the evaluation of fat excretion, a 72-hour collection is recommended. Participation by the parent and caregiver is often essential to ensure adequate collection. A longer collection period counteracts the periodic variations in fat excretion, providing the physician with a more integrated assessment of fat excretion. This is important in titrating doses of replacement pancreatic enzyme in children with cystic fibrosis. A correctly performed evaluation of fractional fat excretion requires the involvement of nutritionists to ensure that fat intake throughout the collection period is known. Although preservatives are not routinely required for stool collection, patients must keep the collection container refrigerated. Urine contamination of fecal material must be prevented.

The relative ease of collecting saliva in children has led to new tests using this matrix. The concentrations of some drugs or hormones in saliva correlate well with free or unbound levels of the same drugs or hormones in the blood. However, relatively few analytes can be measured reliably for physiologic and method-related reasons. When measuring a substance normally bound to protein, such as cortisol, the free or unbound concentration in saliva may be too low to be measured by many assay systems. Assays that can measure at these low concentrations often involve time-consuming and labor-intensive extraction or purification procedures. Exceptional situations, however, do exist, such as using salivary 17-hydroxyprogesterone to monitor a child with congenital adrenal hyperplasia and severe needle phobia. For the collection of saliva, the mouth is rinsed, an inert material is then chewed to facilitate saliva production. The saliva can be collected or spit out in a tube or glass bottle.

Other fluids (synovial, pleural, or pericardial) or tissues (commonly liver biopsy) may be tested in the clinical laboratory. Procedures for obtaining these fluids will not be covered here. Analysis of liver biopsy tissue for quantitative assessment of iron or copper content is often ordered for assessment of hepatic iron content in thalassemia, neonatal or juvenile hemochromatosis, or copper content in Wilson disease. As with any specimen obtained for analysis of trace element concentration, the physician is advised to consult the laboratory prior to carrying out the biopsy procedure. The laboratory should provide a protocol for collecting the specimen and acid-washed containers for transport and storage.

Transport of Specimens

A specialized pediatric laboratory may serve a large geographic area. Specimens are referred from distant as well as in-house collection sites. The stability of specimens during transport is important in both situations.

Newborn screening blood collection cards mailed into the laboratory to be tested for phenylketonuria, hypothyroidism, galactosemia, and other disorders show remarkable analyte stability provided that temperature extremes are avoided. Most analytes typically measured in a pediatric laboratory show similar stability provided that cells are separated from plasma or serum within 2 hours and the sample is transported either at 4°C or frozen.

In contrast, analytes such as lactate and ammonia can vary markedly with collection, handling, and transport procedures. Spurious results and dangerous misinterpretation can occur when standardized collection and transport procedures are not followed. Blood for ACTH (adrenocorticotropin) and renin assays must be collected in prechilled tubes kept in ice slurry and processed in refrigerated centrifuges. Some hormones such as glucagon and gastrin are best collected in tubes containing a serine protease inhibitor to prevent enzymatic degradation. Studies have shown that handling of specimens without these precautions can lead to artifactual levels within minutes of collection. Samples are best transported in polypropylene or polyethylene containers in a Styrofoam box or similar container. Nonglass containers are less likely to break during transport, and a properly equipped Styrofoam box will maintain the temperature longer.

Analytic Factors

Some analytic factors of laboratory testing are discussed on the CD-ROM, including accuracy, precision, linearity, and common reference standards.

Analytic Interferences

Interference is a process that affects the analysis and causes spurious values. Jaundice, hemolysis, and lipemia are important causes of analytic interference in the newborn or small premature infant. Inadvertent dilution or contamination of a specimen can also give spurious results. An experienced technologist will usually detect specimens that are overtly hemolyzed or lipemic, but often slight degrees may go unnoticed.

Hemolysis increases concentration of many analytes that are at higher concentrations in the erythrocyte than the plasma. The dark red-brown of hemoglobin interferes with many spectrophotometric assays. Hemolysis may also cause spurious results by releasing red blood cell enzymes that degrade proteins, such as insulin, leading to falsely lowered results, an important consideration in the differential diagnosis of neonatal hypoglycemia. Neonatal jaundice, common in the newborn, may affect pediatric laboratory results. Specimens obtained from infants and children receiving parenteral lipid infusions, from children with diabetes or familial hyperlipidemia, may contain a concentration of lipids high enough to interfere with many analyses. It may be necessary to ultracentrifuge such specimens before use in testing. Analytes significantly affected by bilirubin, hemolysis, and lipemia are listed in Table 271-4.

In dehydration or hypovolemia, hemoconcentration may give spuriously high concentrations of analytes such as protein or hemoglobin and mask protein deficiency or anemia. In the intensive care unit, blood is often obtained from intra-arterial or intravenous lines. Inaccurate or spurious results may result if blood is inadvertently diluted or contaminated by intravenous solutions. If unrecognized, this can result in potentially harmful clinical responses. For example, a contaminated specimen read as high blood glucose can be wrongly interpreted as hyperglycemia. Inappropriate insulin therapy may precipitate hypoglycemia. These problems can be avoided by adhering to protocols detailing the amount of blood to be flushed through the line before a laboratory specimen is collected. However, hemodynamic factors may prevent adequate flushing of a

Table 271-4. Analytes Subject to Interferences on Automated Analyzers

Jaundice (Increased Bilirubin)
Albumin
Calcium
Cholesterol
Creatinine
Glucose
Iron
Magnesium
Phosphorus
Proteins
Triglycerides
Uric acid
Alanine aminotransferase
Aspartate aminotransferase
Lactate dehydrogenase

Hemolysis
Albumin
Calcium
Cholesterol
Creatinine
Glucose
Iron
Magnesium
Phosphorus
Proteins
Total bilirubin
Triglycerides
Uric acid
α-Amylase
Alkaline phosphatase
Creatine kinase
γ-Glutamyltransferase

Lipemia
Calcium
Cholesterol
Creatinine
Glucose
Iron
Magnesium
Phosphorus
Proteins
Total bilirubin
Uric acid
Alanine aminotransferase
Aspartate aminotransferase
Creatine kinase

Note: Effects may differ from one analyzer to another. This is not a complete list. Consult laboratory for more details.

line in very small infants. In this case, capillary sampling is preferred.

Communication between clinician and pathologist is vital to identify error from exogenous interfering agents. This reemphasizes the importance of a properly designed requisition that indicates medications or known drug ingestions. Exogenous substances (drugs or medications) can contribute to inaccurate or spurious results, by analytical or physiologic interference. Results can be falsely low or high. For instance, certain drugs and even over-the-counter medications are known to interfere with colorimetric-based reactions such as urine dipstick methodology. Some medications can displace hormone from binding protein, leading to an elevation in free hormone, or alternatively, induce or inhibit enzyme systems used in metabolism. This is a true physiologic event relevant to management of the patient. Different assay systems are affected differently by interfering agents. For commercial, immunologically based assays, these differences are usually attributed to different antibody specificities and concentrations of antibody reactants as well as the assay principle used.

Spurious laboratory results can lead to inappropriate treatment. Unnecessary surgery has been linked to heterophile antibodies in patient serum. Heterophile antibodies, human anti-animal antibodies, and rheumatoid factor can produce erroneous results in immunologically based assays. The prevalence of human anti-mouse antibodies (HAMA) and human anti-rabbit antibody (HARA) is variable. Occupational or recreational exposure to animals or to antibody-containing materials such as used in medical imaging is thought to be the major sources.

Often the only way for laboratory personnel to become aware of inconsistent results is by direct contact from a clinician questioning the validity of a test result. Suspicion may be raised by receiving results incompatible with the clinical picture or when expected relationships (i.e., inverse relationship between TSH and free T_4) are not observed. The laboratory can then initiate testing to rule in or rule out the presence of these interfering antibodies. If interfering heterophile antibodies are detected, reference to the potential for interference in immunologic assays should be made on the patient's record so that the laboratory is alerted for subsequent testing.

Important Interfering Agents in the Neonatal Period

Maternal constituents that cross the placenta can interfere with analysis of some steroid hormones in neonates. An example is that 17-hydroxyprogesterone is falsely elevated in neonatal blood over the first 24 to 48 hours of life. Inappropriate treatment or costly additional investigations can follow if results of early measurement of this analyte are not confirmed. The effects of any maternal administration of steroid on neonatal adrenal function are minimized by delaying the testing until the neonate is 72 hours of age.

Postanalytic Factors

Interpreting the Result

Postanalytic factors deal with interpreting tests and reporting results. Numerous check procedures internal to the laboratory are designed to identify potential errors prior to reporting results. Internal quality control procedures ensure that the analytic procedure was in control. If a problem is found, the test results will not be reported until the concerns are resolved.

Delta checks provide a different form of quality control. When a result is obtained, a delta check determines whether a previous test result for the same analyte has been recorded within a predetermined time period. If so, the two results will be compared to determine whether the difference falls within a predetermined acceptable range. If the difference exceeds this range, both results will be investigated to determine whether there is an acceptable clinical explanation. At this stage the pediatrician may be contacted by the pathologist for additional clinical information that may explain the discrepancy.

The consultative aspect of the diagnostic process cannot be overemphasized at all phases of the diagnostic process. Unnecessary and inappropriate tests and needless specimen collection on children can be avoided if the physician is aware of the role that the laboratory plays in the diagnostic process. Of more immediate concern is the potential for misinterpretation by the physician because of the possibility of errors at various phases of the process. Box 271-1 highlights what the physicians can expect from the laboratory. The laboratory should also be viewed as a resource to recommend testing to clinicians who are not aware of newer tests or recent guidelines.

Reference Values

Reporting a test result in relation to a predetermined reference interval is standard laboratory practice. The reference interval is the interval between a lower and upper reference limit that has been determined by testing healthy individuals that share common characteristics such as age, gender, stage of pregnancy, or ethnic background. Usually the minimum requirements for defining a reference interval are age and gender. Interpreting a test result against an interval expected for individuals of the same age group and gender is essential because concentrations of many analytes measured in infants and children change markedly at different developmental stages.

Box 271-1. Services of a Pediatric Laboratory

Test Information

1. Complete test information readily available printed or on-line
2. For every test the laboratory must provide the following information:
   The test name and commonly used alternate names
   The specimen required for the test
   If plasma, the anticoagulant required (heparin, citrate)
   Requirements such as fasting, timed collections, bedrest
   Reasons that may cause rejection of the specimen for testing purposes
   The minimum volume of specimen required for accurate and precise testing
   Possible interferences with the test method
   Expected time from specimen arrival in the laboratory to result reporting
   Reference intervals: expected range of results for healthy subjects by age range and gender

Reports

1. Result reporting that is accurate, timely, and clear
2. Format of laboratory reports
   Reference intervals
   Interpretation
   Free text commentaries
3. Contact name and numbers for follow-up

Consultation

1. Advice on appropriate testing and test limitations
2. Guidelines and protocols
3. Interpretations of analytic issues

The reference intervals are derived from population-based "normal" data collected from reference ("normal") individuals. The derivation of most population-based reference intervals, whether based on mean ±2 standard deviations or the 2.5 to 97.5 percentile, excludes 2.5% of the healthy population at either end of the range.

Recruiting adults for reference interval studies is not normally a problem for most laboratories. Recruitment of children to obtain samples for testing and establishment of reference intervals is considerably more difficult. Technical, philosophical, and ethical reasons may limit laboratory personnel and clinicians in the correct interpretation of laboratory results in children, especially in infants.

Technical issues include blood volume, problems associated with specimen collection, and the unique physiology of the newborn. Premature infants suffer from respiratory distress syndrome, intraventricular hemorrhage, patent ductus arteriosus, apnea, and altered concentrations of electrolytes, glucose, and bilirubin, making it difficult to define "normal" in this population. Targets for growth-related parameters including nutritional status cannot easily be assigned for premature infants. Interpretation of blood chemistry values is further complicated when a premature infant on parenteral nutrition is compared to a breast-fed infant.

Ethical issues (informed consent, parental consent, and direct benefits) complicate reference value research of healthy children as control subjects. The essential nature of such studies in pediatric laboratory medicine has been acknowledged by federal research agencies. Most reference intervals cannot be transferred from one laboratory to another without a prior evaluation of assay differences. Each laboratory must validate reference intervals for different pediatric age groups for the instruments and methods used and the populations they serve.

Several groups and publications have developed useful information by collaborative studies or by collating the results of studies from pediatric laboratories around the world. Although they provide an indication of how values change with age, they cannot be used directly as reference intervals to evaluate a test performed in another laboratory, which may have used different reagents and equipment.

SPECIAL CONSIDERATIONS

Dynamic or Provocative Testing

An important aspect of pediatric endocrinology laboratory testing is the recognition that basal hormone testing has a limited role in investigation of disease. A random growth hormone measurement, for example, cannot be used to confirm growth hormone deficiency because pulsatile release kinetics and the relationship to meals and exercise can complicate interpretation. The preferred approach to investigating hypothalamic-pituitary-end organ function in pediatric centers is provocative testing. Biochemical response of the end organ or hypothalamus-pituitary to stress or other well-defined stimuli is the only reliable way to quantitate biochemical reserve. This approach assumes that the measured endocrine response shows how the body would respond to a provocative stimulus or stressor

and would therefore demonstrate more conclusively any deficiencies that would be missed by a random measurement.

A definitive diagnosis of certain diseases requires the establishment of an abnormal response to a given stimulus (e.g., response to ACTH in congenital adrenal hyperplasia). A normal response can be used to rule out disease in otherwise difficult cases. Occasionally, provocative testing is used in the follow-up to medical treatment when adequacy of intervention needs to be assessed (e.g., gonadotropin-releasing hormone response in precocious puberty).

This kind of investigation typically involves careful preparation of the patient (fasting, euthyroid status, or sex steroid priming) followed by the administration of one or more chemical or physiologic stimuli under well-defined conditions. Samples are drawn from the patient at predetermined intervals for laboratory testing. This is best done in a specialized testing unit staffed by medical personnel who are involved exclusively in provocative testing to ensure consistency in administration and ensure adherence to protocols. Some protocols require the presence of a physician because complications may occur that require prompt medical attention (e.g., hypoglycemia in the insulin tolerance test). In some cases provocative testing cannot be performed on an outpatient basis. Adherence to protocols is still necessary for accurate interpretation. Any deviations from the protocol necessary to accommodate critical illness made must be evaluated in context. For those children on replacement therapy (e.g., glucocorticoids) consideration must be given to temporarily withholding medication so as not to interfere with the physiologic response. Provocative testing is invasive and potentially hazardous. Physicians must exercise judgment in selecting patients for testing. Screening tests and clinical history should be used judiciously by physicians in requesting provocative testing (e.g., insulin-like growth factor, or IGF-1, in growth hormone deficiency).

Point-of-Care Testing

A variety of point-of-care devices are now capable of performing analyses on whole blood at or near the bedside. Although there currently is a limited repertoire of tests available, instruments can provide blood gases, coagulation testing, and some common chemistry tests. Other devices are designed to be used for only drugs of abuse screening or evaluation of myocardial infarction.

Some clinicians favor point-of-care devices in pediatric medicine because of small blood volume requirement (often less than 100 µL) and rapid result turnaround time. However, little evidence supports enhanced patient outcome with rapidity of results. The cost of point-of-care testing may be higher than laboratory-based medicine because of inappropriate test application or overutilization.

Safe and successful points-of-care programs rely on training, quality assessment, and monitoring provided through the diagnostic laboratory. In each situation the value of point-of-care testing needs to be demonstrated through well-designed randomized controlled trials that show that equally good results will be obtained once usage is broadened to a wider user group.

272 Diagnostic Imaging

Katharine Hopkins

The role of the generalist in diagnostic imaging is increasingly complex, as new imaging techniques and clinical applications revolutionize medical diagnosis (Box 272-1). The generalist, when considering a diagnostic question, must choose between many imaging modalities, balancing diagnostic benefits against risks and rising costs. This chapter provides an overview of pediatric imaging, its common indications and benefits, and discussion of newer applications. Box 272-2 lists the essential components of a pediatric diagnostic imaging facility.

PLAIN RADIOGRAPHY

Plain radiographs are produced by projecting x-rays through the patient onto a recording medium. The conventional recording medium for radiography is x-ray film coated with a silver bromide/silver iodide emulsion that undergoes a chemical change when exposed to radiation. The chemical

change leads to deposition of metallic silver on the film, turning exposed areas black in proportion to the number of x-rays striking the film.

Computed radiography has begun to replace conventional film-based radiography. In computed radiography, a photosensitive electronic plate is used as the recording medium. The amount of radiation striking each point on the plate is converted to a computerized gray-scale digital image. The digital image may be displayed on a high-resolution computer monitor (soft copy), printed onto paper or film (hard copy), and recorded onto magnetic tape or disk for long-term storage.

The term *plain radiography*—whether film-based or digital—indicates that contrast material has not been used in the examination. Plain radiography relies on natural x-ray attenuation differences to demonstrate anatomy and to define abnormalities (Fig. 272-1). Different tissues in the body absorb or scatter x-rays to variable degrees with bone attenuating x-rays more than water, water more than fat, and fat more than air. Table 272-1 lists common indications for plain radiography. Table 272-2 lists contraindications, advantages, and disadvantages of plain radiography.

FLUOROSCOPY AND CONTRAST-ENHANCED RADIOGRAPHY

Fluoroscopy yields real-time radiographic images, allowing assessment of organ motion and function in addition to anatomy. The fluoroscopic detection device is a phosphor-coated screen that fluoresces when irradiated. The fluorescence is amplified electronically and displayed on a television monitor. Some fluoroscopic examinations are performed without contrast material. For others, contrast material is used to increase or decrease x-ray attenuation in areas of specific interest, such as the gastrointestinal or urinary tract.

Indications, contraindications, advantages, and disadvantages of fluoroscopy are described on the CD-ROM (see CD-ROM Table 272-1). The indications, contraindications, advantages, and disadvantages of fluoroscopic contrast agents are also found on the CD-ROM (see CD-ROM Table 272-2).

Gastrointestinal Fluoroscopy
Upper Gastrointestinal Series
The most common pediatric gastrointestinal examination is the upper gastrointestinal series, used to demonstrate morphology of the esophagus, stomach, duodenum, and

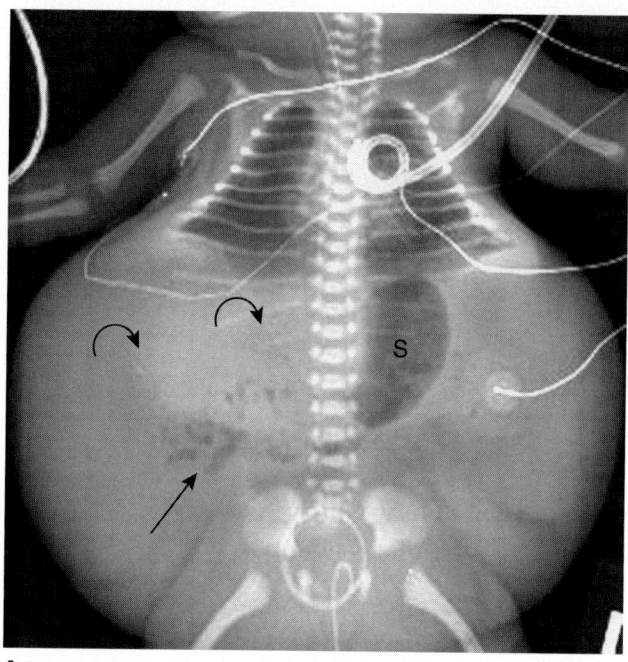

A

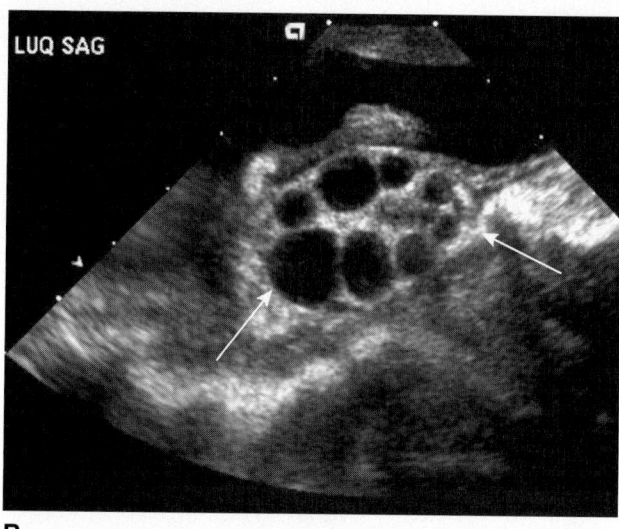

B

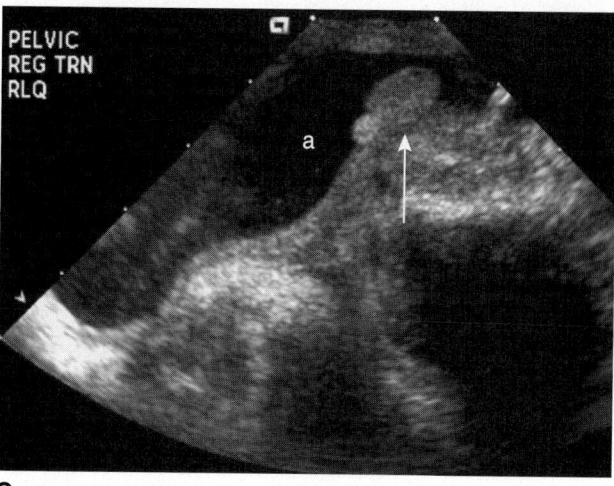

C

Figure 272-1. A plain radiograph **(A)** shows bulging flanks associated with deficient abdominal wall musculature in this newborn male infant with prune belly syndrome. Gas-filled stomach (S) and small bowel *(straight arrow)* are radiolucent. Bones, peritoneal calcifications *(curved arrows)*, and support devices (such as the bladder catheter, chest tube, endotracheal tube, venous catheter, and monitoring leads seen here) are radiopaque. Ultrasonography was used as an adjunct in this case to demonstrate a multicystic dysplastic left kidney **(B,** *arrows)*, undescended right testicle **(C,** *arrow)*, and urine ascites (*a*).

duodenal-jejunal junction as well as esophageal motility, lower esophageal sphincter competence, and gastric emptying.

Although many congenital and acquired abnormalities of the upper gastrointestinal tract are well demonstrated using standard techniques, tracheoesophageal fistulae may be overlooked. Fistulae often fail to opacify after oral contrast administration. To ensure that they are visible, careful injection of contrast material through a naso- or oroesophageal tube may be necessary. Therefore, the radiologist should be informed whenever tracheoesophageal fistula is a credible diagnostic consideration.

Oropharyngeal Motility Study

A detailed assessment of swallowing function is not included in the standard upper gastrointestinal series. For this purpose, a specialized oropharyngeal motility study is necessary, usually performed collaboratively by radiologists and speech pathologists. During the oropharyngeal motility examination, the patient swallows various consistencies of liquid barium, semisolid barium, and, if age-appropriate, barium-coated solids. Fluoroscopy is used to look for evidence of swallowing dysfunction or aspiration.

Small Bowel Follow-Through Examination

Small bowel follow-through examinations are sometimes performed in conjunction with upper gastrointestinal series. Contrast material is followed radiographically through the jejunum and ileum to the ileocecal valve. Because small bowel follow-through examinations take longer to perform than upper gastrointestinal series and result in additional radiation exposure, they should be ordered only when clinical circumstances are compelling.

Contrast and Air Enemas

Contrast enemas are used for assessment of the colon. A rectal catheter is placed, and contrast material is infused into the colon under gravity. Single-contrast enemas—performed with barium sulfate or water-soluble contrast material alone—provide definition of colonic position and caliber. They are used to diagnose stenosis or obstruction involving the colon or distal small bowel. In addition, water-soluble contrast enemas may have therapeutic value in patients with meconium plug, meconium ileus, and meconium ileus equivalent as a result of hyperosmolar effects. For diagnosis of inflammatory bowel disease, polyps, or other mucosal lesions, insufflation of air after barium adminis-

Table 272-1. Common Indications for Plain Radiography

Organ System	Indications
Head and neck	Craniosynostosis
	Sinusitis
	Adenoid hypertrophy
Chest	Acute or chronic lung disease
	Air trapping or atelectasis
	Congenital or acquired heart disease
	Hydro- or pneumothorax
	Pneumomediastinum
	Pulmonary, hilar, mediastinal, or chest wall mass
	Endotracheal tube or vascular catheter placement
Abdomen	Abdominal pain or mass
	Bowel obstruction, ileus, or constipation
	Necrotizing enterocolitis
	Pneumoperitoneum
	Renal or biliary stone disease
	Enteral tube or vascular catheter placement
Musculoskeletal system	Trauma
	Mass
	Infection
	Inflammatory, vascular, or metabolic disease
	Congenital or developmental anomalies (e.g., skeletal dysplasia, scoliosis, hip dysplasia, tarsal coalition, clubfoot)
	Bone age determination
Miscellaneous	Ventriculoperitoneal shunt assessment
	Foreign body localization

tration (air-contrast enema) provides superior mucosal detail.

In recent years, the "air enema," has replaced the contrast enema for diagnosis and reduction of intussusception. It is performed by careful insufflation of air into the rectum. When encountered, an intussusceptum appears as an intraluminal filling defect. Air insufflation reduces intussusception in nearly 80% of cases. If reduction is unsuccessful, surgery is warranted.

Contrast Urography
Intravenous Urography
For intravenous urography, water-soluble contrast material is injected into a vein. Serial radiographs of the abdomen and pelvis demonstrate contrast uptake by the kidneys as well as contrast excretion into the collecting systems and ureters. In children, intravenous urography is used primarily

Table 272-2. Contraindications, Advantages, and Disadvantages of Plain Radiography

Contraindications
None

Advantages
Noninvasive
Widely available
Portable
No sedation required
Excellent bone depiction

Disadvantages
Radiation exposure
Limited soft tissue differentiation

for assessment of urinary calculi. Computed tomography (CT) is now replacing intravenous urography for that application. Cross-sectional imaging has also replaced intravenous urography for diagnosis of renal masses.

Voiding Cystourethrography
The voiding cystourethrogram (VCUG) is performed frequently in children. It involves catheterization of the bladder followed by intravesical infusion of water-soluble contrast material. Intermittent fluoroscopy is performed during bladder filling and voiding. The VCUG allows assessment of bladder size, contour, and function; urethral anatomy; and vesicoureteral reflux (Fig. 272-2).

Miscellaneous Fluoroscopic Examinations
Other contrast-enhanced fluoroscopic studies include the sinogram or fistulogram and the myelogram. The sinogram or fistulogram involves injection of contrast material, usually water-soluble, through an abnormal sinus tract or fistula. Myelography, although less commonly performed since the introduction of magnetic resonance imaging (MRI), is occasionally indicated for diagnosis of nerve root avulsion or spinal cord compression. A needle is inserted into the subarachnoid space, either between two lumbar vertebrae or, less commonly, at the cisterna magna. Cerebrospinal fluid opacification is then achieved by injection of nonionic water-soluble contrast material under fluoroscopy. Myelography is usually performed in conjunction with CT.

ULTRASONOGRAPHY
Ultrasonography derives from technology used for World War II sonar navigation systems. Images are generated with "ultrasound" waves that have frequencies above those audible by the human ear. The waves are transmitted by a transducer into the patient. Tissue interfaces then reflect the waves back to the transducer. Because different tissues have different acoustic properties, they are distinguishable. The reflected waves—or echoes—are recorded and translated by computer into images.

There are several types of sonographic image. Real-time gray-scale imaging is used to depict general anatomy and physiologic motion in two dimensions. Because it enables the ultrasonographer to see images as they are generated, real-time gray-scale imaging permits both dynamic scanning of a moving object and rapid screening of an anatomic region. It is the "work horse" of pediatric ultrasonography and is used for imaging the heart, abdomen, pelvis, scrotum, pleural space, diaphragm, neck, and in some instances, other soft tissues. Because open fontanelles provide an acoustic window, real-time gray-scale ultrasonography may be used in infants to detect and characterize intracranial anomalies. Similarly, absent ossification of the femoral heads allows dynamic sonography of the hips in infants.

Doppler sonography uses the Doppler principle to calculate blood velocity relative to the transducer. The direction and velocity of blood flow may be represented as a waveform (continuous or pulsed Doppler sonography). Alternatively, velocity and direction may be color-coded (color flow Doppler sonography). By convention, the color

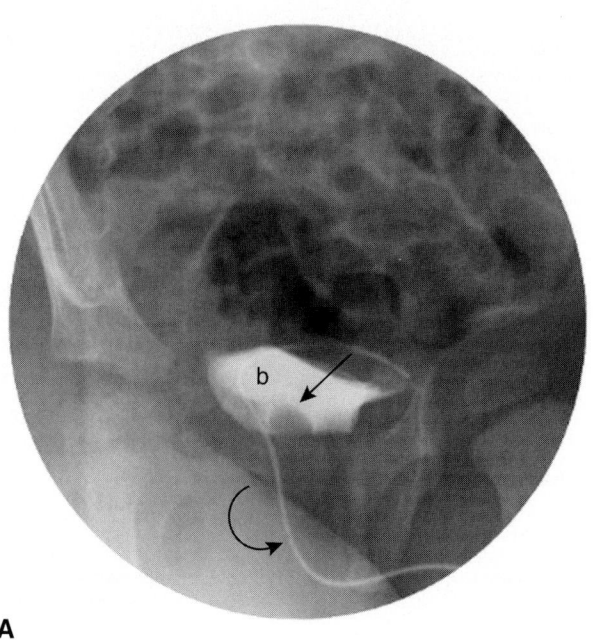

A

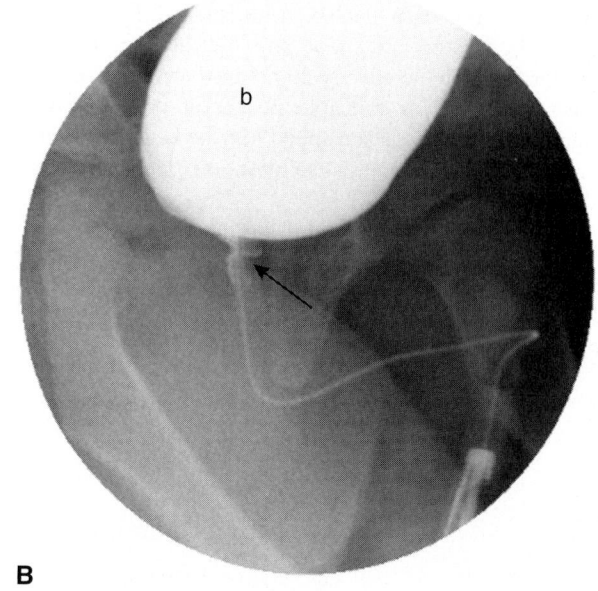

B

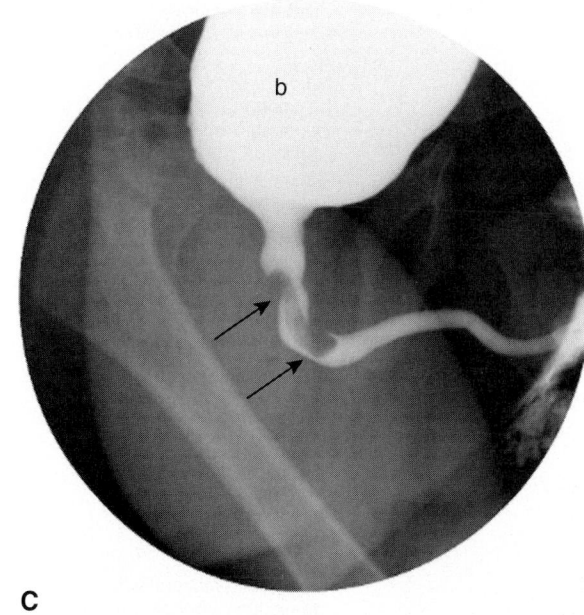

C

Figure 272-2. Voiding cystourethrography reveals the dynamic nature of a benign posterior urethral polyp (22-month-old boy with straining and hematuria). **A,** During early filling of the bladder (*b*), contrast material outlines a mass *(straight arrow)* at the bladder base. A catheter *(curved arrow)* courses through the urethra. **B,** The mass prolapses into the posterior urethra *(straight arrow)* during early attempts at voiding, resulting in intermittent obstruction. **C,** During voiding, the polyp arising from the posterior urethra *(arrows)* is outlined by contrast material.

red indicates flow toward the transducer, and the color blue indicates flow away from the transducer. A newer technique, power Doppler ultrasonography, uses color-coding to show the amplitude of blood flow. It is much more sensitive to blood flow than conventional Doppler sonography. However, it does not reveal the direction of blood flow and is easily degraded by patient motion. Therefore, its role in pediatric imaging is limited.

In the future, vascular sonography will be facilitated by intravenous injection of microbubble-based contrast agents. Such agents are currently under investigation and could potentially improve visualization of blood vessels, vascular organs, tumors, and areas of ischemia. Intravascular echogenicity is increased by microbubbles because of their reflective surfaces. Three-dimensional ultrasonographic techniques have also been developed recently with potential cardiac and musculoskeletal applications.

Tables 272-3 and 272-4 list the indications, contraindications, advantages, and disadvantages of ultrasonography.

COMPUTED TOMOGRAPHY

Computed tomography (CT) uses ionizing radiation and computer data processing to create cross-sectional images (Fig. 272-3). Two types of CT are commonly performed. With "step-and-shoot" CT, cross-sectional images are generated one by one, and the patient is moved incrementally between image acquisitions. With helical (or spiral) CT, image acquisition and patient translation are continuous and simultaneous. Although "step-and-shoot" CT provides sharper image detail, helical CT is considerably faster, able to image entire body parts in a matter of seconds. Helical CT is better tolerated by children and reduces the need for time-consuming and potentially hazardous sedation.

The latest advance in CT technology is multislice CT, introduced in the late 1990s. Multislice CT scanners operate in both step-and-shoot and helical scan modes. They differ from single-slice scanners in that they are able to collect the data for multiple images at once and are considerably faster. Increased speed may be used to reduce scan time, improve image resolution, or lengthen scan

Table 272-3. Indications for Ultrasonography

Organ System	Indications
Head—neonates and infants	Intracranial hemorrhage
	Periventricular leukomalacia
	Hydrocephalus
	Mass
	Congenital anomalies
Spine	Dysraphism
	Tethered cord
Neck	Adenopathy, mass, or abscess
	Fibromatosis colli
Chest	Congenital or acquired heart disease
	Pericardial or pleural effusion
	Diaghragm paralysis
	Chest wall or mediastinal mass
Abdomen	Ascites
	Mass
	Infection
	Pyloric stenosis
	Appendicitis
	Hepatosplenomegaly
	Portal hypertension
	Liver transplant assessment
	Biliary anomalies (choledochal cyst or choledochocele, calculi)
	Duplication or mesenteric cyst
	Pancreatitis and pseudocyst
	Typhlitis
	Mesenteric adenitis
Retroperitoneum	Urinary tract infection
	Hydronephrosis
	Renal mass
	Congenital renal anomalies
	Cystic renal disease
	Urolithiasis
	Renal vein thrombosis
	Hypertension
	Renal transplant assessment
	Adrenal mass or hemorrhage
Scrotum	Cryptorchidism
	Torsion of testicle or appendix testis
	Epipidymo-orchitis
	Hernia
	Hydrocele
	Varicocele
	Mass
	Trauma
Pelvis	Ambiguous genitalia
	Ovarian torsion
	Mass or cyst
	Intrauterine or ectopic pregnancy
	Infection/abscess
	Precocious puberty
	Amenorrhea
	Renal ectopia
Extremities	Developmental dysplasia of hip
	Joint effusion
	Mass
	Abscess
	Foreign body
	Deep vein thrombosis

Table 272-4. Contraindications, Advantages, and Disadvantages of Ultrasonography

Contraindications

None

Advantages

Noninvasive
Portable
Rarely requires sedation
Preferred over computed tomography for body imaging in children because it uses no radiation
Preferred over upper gastrointestinal series for hypertrophic pyloric stenosis
Preferred modality for differentiating solid from cystic masses
Demonstrates pediatric anatomy well because patients are small and thin

Disadvantages

Poor ultrasound wave transmission through air and bone
Limited penetration in obese patients
Operator-dependent image quality
Less sensitive than computed tomography for appendicitis

coverage. Multislice CT reduces the need for pediatric sedation by up to 83%, diminishing risk to the patient, improving department throughput, and reducing costs. Additional advantages include the ability to retrospectively alter slice thickness ("z-filtering") and the ability to create high-quality multiplanar and three-dimensional reconstructions.

To improve lesion conspicuity on CT scans, contrast material may be injected intravenously. In the head, contrast-enhanced CT is used primarily for imaging inflammatory or neoplastic lesions but may be deferred in favor of contrast-enhanced MRI. Neoplastic and inflammatory lesions in the orbits, neck, abdomen, and pelvis are generally imaged with intravenous contrast material as well, although noncontrast images are sometimes useful for revealing calcifications. In the setting of trauma, intravenous contrast is indicated for CT of the neck, chest, abdomen, and pelvis but not for CT of the head, face, spine, or extremities. Intravenous contrast injection for CT of appendicitis is controversial. It is not necessary for CT diagnosis of renal calculi but may provide additional information with respect to ureteral obstruction once calculi have been identified.

The intravenous contrast material used for CT is identical to that used for intravenous urography and has the same contraindications and risks. For CT of the abdomen and pelvis, dilute barium or water-soluble contrast medium may be given by mouth or rectum in conjunction with intravenous contrast material. The intraluminal gastrointestinal opacification that results helps to differentiate normal bowel from abnormal bowel, abscesses, and masses.

Table 272-5 lists the indications for CT. Box 272-3 lists contraindications, advantages, and disadvantages of CT.

MAGNETIC RESONANCE IMAGING

Clinical magnetic resonance imaging (MRI) was introduced in the early 1980s. It relies on the predictable behavior of certain elements within strong magnetic fields. The element most commonly imaged is the hydrogen proton

A

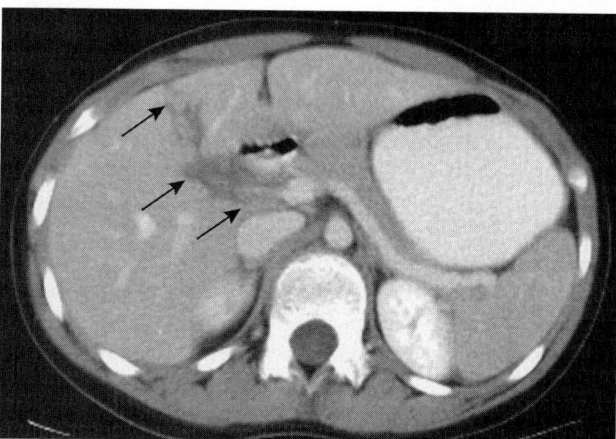

B

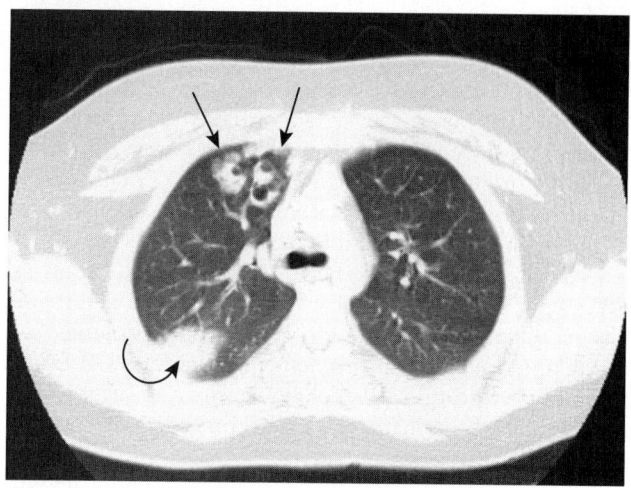

C

(^{1}H), abundant in living tissues. Protons have a positive charge and, when placed in an external magnetic field, become weakly magnetized. In their lowest energy state, they align in the direction of the external field.

To create images, the protons are perturbed out of alignment by bombardment with a radiofrequency pulse. Energy from the radiofrequency pulse is imparted to the protons, which allows them to assume a higher energy state, angled at various degrees to the external magnetic field. Over time, the protons realign with the external field, giving off energy, again in the form of a radiofrequency wave. It is this energy, or "signal," that is captured and amplified to create an image.

Figure 272-3. Because computed tomography (CT) provides exquisite lung, airway, soft tissue, vessel, and bone definition, it has wide-ranging pediatric applications. **A,** In this 13-year-old boy with septic emboli, both cavitary lung lesions *(straight arrows)* and noncavitary lung lesions *(curved arrows)* are identified in the right upper lobe. **B,** Contrast-enhanced CT of the abdomen in a 9-year-old trauma victim shows a low attenuation laceration of the liver *(arrows)*. **C,** Coronal reformatted CT of the ankle reveals intra-articular and physeal extension of a tibial fracture *(arrow)* in a 12-year-old boy.

Table 272-5. Indications for Computed Tomography

Organ System	Indications
Head	Increased intracranial pressure
	Hydrocephalus
	Trauma
	Mass
	Intracranial hemorrhage
	Stroke/hypoxic ischemic injury
	Infection
	Macrocephaly or microcephaly
	Congenital anomalies
	Craniosynostosis
Face and neck	Trauma
	Infection (sinusitis)
	Mass or adenopathy
	Congenital or developmental anomalies (e.g., choanal atresia)
Temporal bone	Trauma
	Infection
	Mass
	Hearing loss
Spine	Trauma
	Scoliosis
	Congenital anomalies
	Mass
Chest	Trauma
	Mass
	Metastatic disease
	Infection
	Acute or chronic lung disease
	Pleural disease
	Congenital anomalies, including vascular ring, pulmonary sling, cystic lesions of lung or mediastinum, and sequestration
	Pulmonary embolus
Abdomen/pelvis	Trauma
	Mass
	Infection/abscess
	Unexplained pain
	Inflammatory bowel disease
	Portal hypertension
	Pancreatitis
	Urinary calculi (preferred over intravenous urography)
	Congenital anomalies
Extremities	Soft tissue or bone mass
	Osteoid osteoma
	Developmental or acquired dysplasia of the hip
	Femoral anteversion
	Leg length discrepancy
	Tarsal coalition
	Fracture

Box 272-3. Contraindications, Advantages, and Disadvantages of Computed Tomography

Contraindications and Precautions

Intravenous contrast material should be avoided in patients with known contrast allergy or renal insufficiency/failure.

Techniques should be modified to reduce radiation exposure in children.

Advantages

Provides cross-sectional images

Is minimally or noninvasive

Allows better soft tissue characterization than conventional radiography

Provides better spatial resolution than ultrasonography and magnetic resonance imaging (MRI)

Is less operator-dependent than ultrasonography

Is more sensitive than ultrasonography for appendicitis, trauma, intracranial abnormalities (especially beyond the neonatal period), lung lesions, and skeletal abnormalities

Is more sensitive than MRI for acute intracranial hemorrhage and calcification, skull fracture, cortical bone lesions, and lung disease

Disadvantages

Results in radiation exposure (more than plain radiography)

Often requires administration of sedatives, gastrointestinal contrast medium, or intravenous contrast

Requires patient transport

Has low sensitivity for leptomeningeal disease/meningitis

Protons in different tissues realign and release "signal" at characteristic rates, known as T_1 and T_2 relaxation times. For example, water has long T_1 and T_2 relaxation times, whereas muscle has intermediate T_1 and T_2 relaxation times. Because of these differences, MRI provides exquisite soft tissue differentiation, even better than that provided by CT. Most neoplasms, inflammatory lesions, and other pathologic tissues have abnormally high water content, resulting in T_1 and T_2 prolongation in comparison to normal tissues.

The term *sequence* in MRI relates to the order in which radiofrequency pulses are administered and received. Sequences are specifically designed to emphasize differences in tissue behavior (Fig. 272-4). For example, sequences may be T_1-weighted or T_2-weighted. Methods are also available for suppressing or accentuating signal from fat, fluid, or blood products. The goal is to increase the conspicuity of abnormalities, thereby improving diagnosis.

A number of contrast agents have been developed for MRI. The most commonly used agent is gadolinium-diethylenetriamine pentaacetic acid (Gd-DTPA). Gd-DTPA shortens T_1 relaxation times and increases signal on T_1-weighted images in areas of inflammation, tumor, or blood-brain barrier breakdown. It is generally injected intravenously at a dose of 0.1 mmol/kg. Dilute Gd-DTPA (0.6%) may also be injected into joints for MR arthrography. Allergic reactions to Gd-DTPA are unusual. Unlike the iodinated contrast agents used for CT, Gd-DTPA is not nephrotoxic.

The future of MRI in pediatric imaging is promising. Diffusion-weighted MRI is an important recent discovery.

It uses an MRI sequence that is sensitive to molecular diffusion. In focal infarcts and diffuse hypoxic-ischemic brain injury, restricted diffusion becomes evident within minutes, long before signal abnormality is apparent on standard MRI sequences. It is expected that diffusion-weighted imaging in infants and children will allow more active stroke management, with earlier diagnosis and intervention than has been possible in the past.

Perfusion MRI is also being studied as a means of assessing pediatric cerebrovascular disease. Perfusion imaging quantifies cerebral blood flow, blood volume, and transit time following intravenous injection of a Gd-DTPA bolus. In the future, MRI techniques such as "arterial spin labeling" may eliminate the need for contrast material injection.

Functional MRI (fMRI) of the brain, also under investigation at this time, localizes focal brain activation in response to directed stimuli. For example, fMRI can identify the discrete areas of visual cortex that are activated by different visual stimuli (e.g., color, patterns, or faces). In the clinical arena, fMRI will have many uses, including mapping of the cerebral cortex prior to tumor or epilepsy surgery. It will also provide crucial information in the study of neurocognitive development and developmental anomalies.

Proton MR spectroscopy is another technique with growing pediatric applications. It provides information about the chemical environment of hydrogen nuclei and is used predominantly to measure the relative concentration of metabolites in the brain. The most important metabolites are *N*-acetylaspartate (NAA), an indicator of neuronal and axonal integrity; choline, a marker of cell membrane turnover; creatine, a marker of high-energy products; and lactate, an indicator of anaerobic metabolism beyond the neonatal period. Specific variations in these metabolites and others characterize metabolic disease, stroke, and hypoxic-ischemic injury.

Box 272-4 and Table 272-6 list the indications, contraindications, advantages, and disadvantages of MRI.

ANGIOGRAPHY

Angiography is the radiographic study of blood vessels. For conventional angiography, iodinated water-soluble contrast agents are injected directly into an artery, and as contrast material flows through the target vasculature, sequential radiographic exposures are made. Angiographic techniques have also been developed for CT and MRI. CT angiography (CTA) involves the rapid acquisition of helical CT data during the arterial phase of a rapid intravenous contrast bolus. MR angiography (MRA) may be performed with or without intravenous Gd-DTPA.

Boxes 272-5 and 272-6 list the indications, contraindications, advantages, and disadvantages of angiography.

NUCLEAR SCINTIGRAPHY

Nuclear scintigraphy is the practice of imaging radiopharmaceuticals. Radiopharmaceuticals are generated by coupling unstable isotopes to compounds that localize in particular organs or diseases. When the unstable isotopes

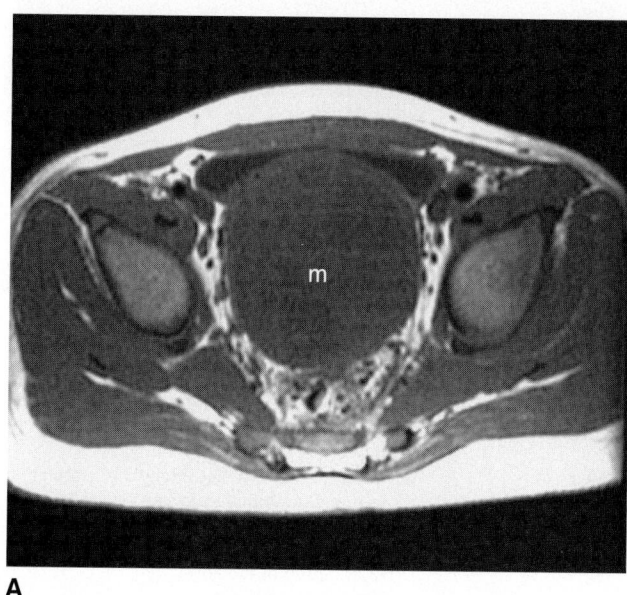

A

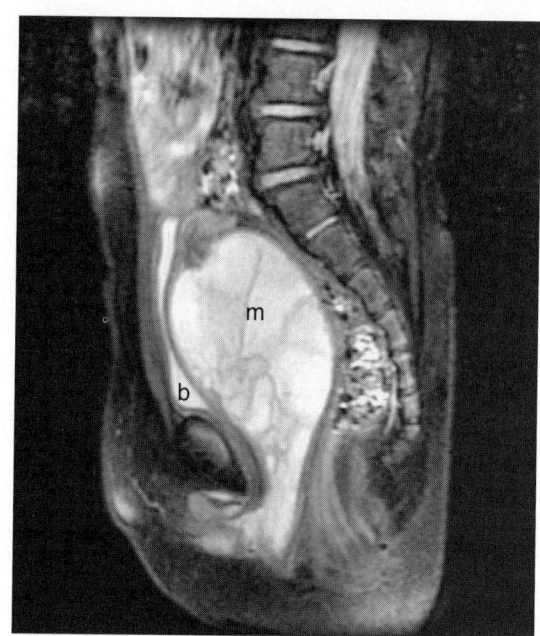

B

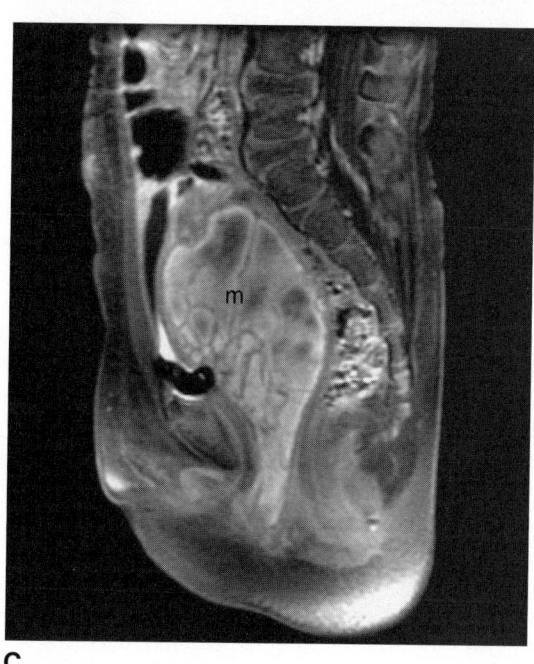

C

Figure 272-4. T$_1$-weighted (**A,** axial) and T$_2$-weighted (**B,** sagittal) magnetic resonance images of the pelvis in an 18–month-old girl reveal a large vaginal rhabdomyosarcoma (*m*, mass; *b*, bladder). The tumor has high water content, resulting in intermediate T$_1$ signal intensity and high T$_2$ signal intensity. Following intravenous Gd-DTPA injection (**C,** sagittal), the tumor enhances heterogeneously (*m*, mass).

decay to a more stable state, they emit radiation. The radiation is then detected externally and translated by computer into an image.

Radiopharmaceuticals are administered to patients by a number of routes—intravenous injection, oral ingestion, and inhalation being most common. The most widely available nuclear imaging techniques include dynamic and static planar scintigraphy and single photon emission computed tomography (SPECT). Dynamic planar scintigraphy generates two-dimensional images over time and provides information about time-dependent phenomena. The functional information that results from dynamic scintigraphy often complements the anatomic information provided by other imaging modalities.

Static planar scintigraphy yields two-dimensional images at a single point in time. Its primary purpose is for local-

ization of disease. Often, static and dynamic planar scintigraphy are combined—such as in the three-phase bone scan (Fig. 272-5)—to provide both functional and anatomic information. When imaging children, optical magnification with a special "pinhole" collimator may be necessary to improve spatial resolution.

SPECT is a technique by which the camera is rotated at least 180 degrees around the patient during imaging. A three-dimensional data set results from which cross-sectional images in axial, sagittal, coronal, and oblique planes may be generated and displayed. Alternatively, the data may be viewed as a three-dimensional volume rendering. Because SPECT removes out-of-plane information, it increases image contrast sixfold, improves lesion detection, and more precisely defines lesion location in comparison to planar scintigraphy.

Box 272-4. Contraindications and Precautions, Advantages and Disadvantages of Magnetic Resonance Imaging (MRI)

Contraindications and Precautions

Strong magnetic, electrical, and thermal effects preclude MRI in patients with cardiac pacemakers, cochlear implants, many other implantable electrical devices, intracranial aneurysm clips, recently placed metallic hardware, and some metallic foreign bodies

Many supportive and monitoring devices must be removed during scanning to prevent serious burns

Advantages

Provides multiplanar cross-sectional images

Provides better soft tissue characterization than all other modalities

Uses no ionizing radiation

Is more sensitive than computed tomography (CT) for intracranial abnormalities except calcification and acute hemorrhage

Is more sensitive than CT for spinal cord injury

Is preferred noninvasive imaging modality for joint disease

Allows noninvasive assessment of cardiac anatomy, function, and blood flow

Disadvantages

Long scan duration (generally ranging from 20 to 60 minutes)

Frequently requires deep sedation

Table 272-6. Indications for Magnetic Resonance Imaging (MRI)

Organ System	Indication
Head	Congenital or developmental anomalies
	Hydrocephalus
	Mass
	Unexplained epilepsy
	Inflammatory/infectious disease
	Stroke/hypoxic ischemic injury
	Intrcranial hemorrhage
	Vascular malformation
	Phacomatoses
	White matter disease
	Neuroendocrine disorders
Face/orbit/neck	Mass
	Infection
Chest	Congenital anomalies (including vascular ring, pulmonary sling, cartilaginous tracheal rings, bronchogenic cyst, etc.)
	Congenital or acquired heart disease
	Coarctation of the aorta
	Venous thrombosis
	Mediastinal or chest wall mass
	Mediastinal or chest wall infection
	Diaphragmatic hernia or eventration
Abdomen/pelvis/ retroperitoneum	Mass or cyst
	Infection
	Vascular anomalies
	Venous thrombosis
	Hemosiderosis
	Hepatosplenomegaly
	Biliary anomalies
	Genitourinary anomalies
Musculoskeletal system	Trauma
	Infection
	Mass
	Osteonecrosis
	Arthritis
	Congenital anomalies (e.g., tarsal coalition)

Positron emission tomography (PET) is a relatively new technique that uses positron-emitting isotopes of biologically active elements to assess regional tissue metabolism. The elements most commonly used are oxygen (^{15}O), nitrogen (^{13}N), carbon (^{11}C), and fluorine (^{18}F). PET cameras are specifically designed to detect coincident gamma rays emitted during annihilation of positrons from these elements. Because of high operating costs associated with PET cameras and poor reimbursement, PET is less widely available than conventional nuclear scintigraphy. Its utilization is growing, however, particularly in the areas of oncology, cardiology, and neurology. In children, its primary applications are diagnosis of lymphoma and other neoplasms and localization of epileptogenic foci.

The indications, contraindications, advantages, and disadvantages of nuclear scintigraphy are listed on the CD-ROM (see CD-ROM Table 272-3 and CD-ROM Box 272-1).

IMAGE MANAGEMENT IN THE COMPUTER AGE

Picture Archival and Communications Systems

The imaging department of the future will not use film or view boxes to the extent used today. Many hospitals are already replacing film with digital picture archival and communications systems (PACS) for more efficient handling of massive amounts of diagnostic imaging data. With PACS, diagnostic images are acquired digitally or converted from analogue to digital form and stored in a computer archive. Computer monitors replace view boxes in the radiology reading room as well as on clinical wards, in the operating room, and in physicians' offices. A major

benefit of PACS is the immediate and simultaneous availability of images in multiple locations. PACS eliminates problems associated with lost films and signed-out film jackets. Moreover, electronic coupling of PACS to the radiology information system (RIS) and hospital information system (HIS) makes patient demographic and historical information more accessible to radiologists. At the same time, it makes radiology images and reports more accessible to practitioners.

Box 272-5. Indications for Angiography

Hemorrhage

Ischemia

Trauma

Aneurysm

Dissection

Mass

Vascular malformations

Thrombotic or embolic disease

Systemic or portal hypertension

Vasculitis/stenosis

Three-Dimensional Display Techniques

Computer workstations with intuitive user interfaces, ultrafast processing, and a number of tools for soft-copy, volumetric image display are now available to radiologists and clinicians—making multiplanar reformations, volume rendering, three-dimensional reconstruction, and virtual or "fly-through" examinations practical in many cross-sectional imaging cases. Delineating spatial relationships better than axial images alone, volumetric images facilitate both interpretation of scans and treatment planning. They expedite communication between radiologists, clinicians, and parents. In addition, they open the door to new and innovative applications, such as CT bronchoscopy and colonoscopy.

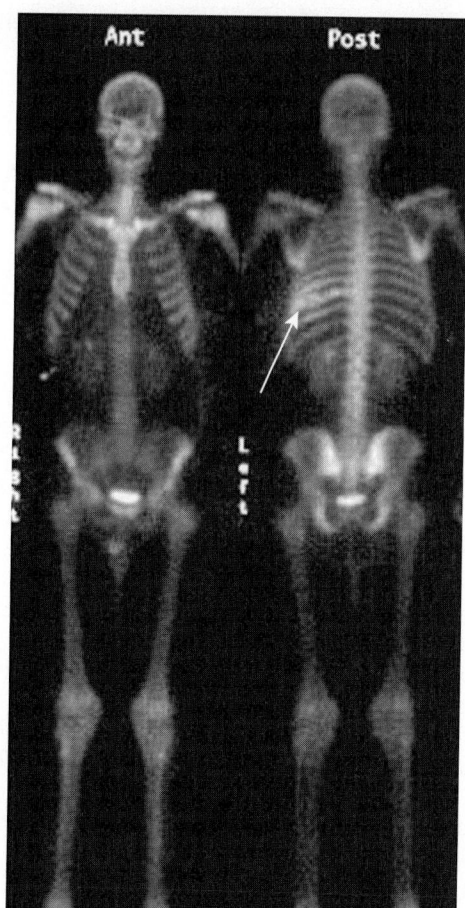

Figure 272-5. Nuclear skeletal scintigraphy in a 16-year-old boy shows increased radionuclide uptake in the left ninth rib *(arrow)* associated with a palpable chest wall mass. Biopsy revealed Ewing sarcoma.

Box 272-6. Contraindications, Advantages, and Disadvantages of Angiography

Contraindications

Contrast allergy

Renal insufficiency/failure

Advantages

Conventional Angiography

Gold standard

Superior to CTA and MRA, especially for diagnosis of small vessel disease and subtle abnormalities

Less susceptible to artifact

Computed Tomography Angiography (CTA)

Less invasive and more accessible than conventional angiography

Less likely than MRA and conventional angiography to require sedation

Rapidly becoming study of choice for diagnosis of pulmonary emboli (probably more sensitive and specific than nuclear ventilation-perfusion scintigraphy)

Magnetic Resonance Angiography (MRA)

Less invasive and more accessible than conventional angiography

Avoids ionizing radiation

May be performed either with or without intravenous contrast injection

Disadvantages

Conventional Angiography

Invasive

Requires radiation exposure

Requires arterial injection of iodinated contrast material

CT Angiograhy (CTA)

Requires radiation exposure

Requires intravenous injection of iodinated contrast material

More susceptible to motion artifact than conventional angiography

Less sensitive than conventional angiography

MRA

More susceptible to motion artifact than conventional angiography

May overestimate severe stenoses

Less sensitive than conventional angiography

Additional Resources, CD-ROM

Indications, contraindications, advantages, and disadvantages of fluoroscopy	Table
Fluoroscopic contrast agents	Table
Indications for nuclear scintigraphy	Table
Indications, contraindications, advantages, and disadvantages of nuclear scintigraphy	Box

SUGGESTED READINGS

Ball WS, Holland SK: Perfusion imaging in the pediatric patient. MRI Clin North Am 2001;9:207–230.

Bydder GM, Rutherford MA: Diffusion-weighted imaging of the brain in neonates and infants. MRI Clin North Am 2001;9:83–98.

Martin E, Marcar VL: Functional MR imaging in pediatrics. MRI Clin North Am 2001;9:231–245.

Pappas JN, Donnelly LF, Frush DP: Reduced frequency of sedation of young children with multisection helical CT. Radiology 2000;215:897–899.

Sivit CJ, Applegate KE, Stallion A, et al: Imaging evaluation of suspected appendicitis in a pediatric population: Effectiveness of sonography vs. CT. AJR 2000;175:977–980.

273 Endoscopy

Kenneth K. Lee

Performed under the right conditions, endoscopy is a powerful diagnostic and therapeutic tool that provides direct nonsurgical access to most of the alimentary tract.

Flexible endoscopy of the upper gastrointestinal (GI) tract (esophagus, stomach, duodenum) and lower GI tract (terminal ileum, colon) is a powerful tool for the assessment of GI disorders. Flexible endoscopy enables a uniquely direct and nonsurgical access to most parts of the alimentary tract. Besides observing most areas of the GI tract mucosa, the trained pediatric endoscopist can perform diagnostic and therapeutic procedures such as biopsy, polypectomy, foreign body removal, esophageal balloon dilatation, esophageal variceal sclerotherapy and variceal banding ligation, ablation of bleeding lesions (electrocautery, thermocoagulation, vessel injection), and gastrostomy placement.

Typical endoscopes are flexible tubes 5 to 12 mm in diameter and 100 to 250 cm in length. These tubes contain multiple optic fibers (fiberoptic endoscopes) or videochip circuitry (video endoscopes) that transmit light images. Videoendoscopic images, digitized through a videoprocessor prior to display on a video monitor, are superior to fiberoptic images. Videoendoscopes have largely replaced fiberoptic endoscopes in modern medical centers, yet the lowest caliber fiberoptic endoscopes are still useful for exam-

ination of small infants, because their caliber is narrower than the smallest-diameter videoendoscopes. Endoscopes are equipped with an instrument channel for biopsy and therapeutic manipulation as well as with air insufflation/water/suction channels to enhance luminal images. Specific endoscopic procedures are listed in Table 273-1.

COMMON ENDOSCOPIC PROCEDURES IN CHILDREN

Esophagogastroduodenoscopy (EGD) and colonoscopy are the two endoscopic procedures most commonly performed in children. Appropriate indications for flexible sigmoidoscopy (FS) are few, as most indications for FS are better served by colonoscopy. For example, both inflammatory (juvenile) and adenomatous polyps in children are often located proximal to the rectosigmoid region and would be missed by FS. Evaluation of suspected inflammatory bowel disease (IBD) requires a complete colonoscopic examination to the terminal ileum (TI). Crohn disease (CD) can affect the colon segmentally and can involve only more proximal areas of the colon inaccessible by FS. This skip pattern, as well as other visual patterns of mucosal inflammation (apthous ulcerations, skip lesions), often distin-

Table 273-1. Endoscopic Procedures and Their Applications

Procedure	Uses	Extent of Visualization
Esophagoduodenoscopy (EGD)	Biopsy Sclerotherapy Variceal banding Esophageal dilation Electrocautery/thermocoagulation/vessel injection Foreign body removal Gastrostomy placement	Esophagus to duodenum
Enteroscopy	Biopsy Ablation of bleeding lesions Polypectomy	Esophagus to proximal jejunum
Flexible sigmoidoscopy	Biopsy Polypectomy Foreign body removal Ablation of bleeding lesions	Rectum to proximal sigmoid
Colonoscopy	Biopsy Polypectomy Foreign body removal Ablation of bleeding lesions	Rectum to cecum and terminal ileum
Endoscopic retrograde cholangiopancreatography (ERCP)	Biopsy of biliary ducts Stent placement Ductal dilation Stone removal Sphincterotomy	Cannulation of ampulla of Vater and visualization of biliary and pancreatic ducts

guishes CD from ulcerative colitis (UC). In addition, many cases of CD involve only the terminal ileum and cecum, both areas inaccessible by FS. Flexible sigmoidoscopy has some useful applications, though: confirmation of the diagnosis of cow milk or breast milk or other protein colitis by biopsy of the rectosigmoid colon, removal of rectosigmoid foreign bodies, and evaluation of mucosal inflammation of a surgically placed ileoanal reservoir (pouchitis) after total colectomy and ileoanal anastomosis in IBD patients.

SPECIALIZED ENDOSCOPIC PROCEDURES IN CHILDREN

Three specialized endoscopic procedures performed in children are endoscopic retrograde cholangiopancreatography (ERCP), enteroscopy, and wireless capsule endoscopy (WCE). Indications for these procedures are few compared to EGD and colonoscopy. ERCP, performed in conjunction with fluoroscopy, involves cannulating the ampulla of Vater with a special side-viewing endoscope. With ERCP, the endoscopist can visualize, biopsy, and dilate the bile and pancreatic ducts and remove stones from the common bile duct and pancreatic ducts. ERCP is indicated for the evaluation of recurrent pancreatitis, sclerosing cholangitis, pancreatic and biliary masses, and biliary obstruction. ERCP is a technically challenging procedure that, in most medical centers, requires the expertise of adult gastroenterologists, who are usually much more experienced with this technique. Few pediatric gastroenterologists are proficient in ERCP because it has so few indications in children. Enteroscopy is an EGD that extends into the proximal jejunum. Indications for enteroscopy include occult GI bleeding in the small bowel (vascular ectasias, arteriovenous malformations), atypical Crohn disease limited to the small intestine, and polyposis disorders involving the small intestine, such as Peutz-Jeghers syndrome. Enteroscopy requires significantly more time and finesse than the standard EGD. Because most endoscopic indications are addressed by EGD and colonoscopy, enteroscopy is rarely performed in children.

WCE utilizes a self-contained capsular device with a video transducer. This capsule is swallowed or placed in the stomach endoscopically and, as it passes through the small intestine, transmits images (two per second) in real time to a portable recording device carried by the patient. This recording occurs up to 8 hours. The image sequence is then downloaded for review. The capsule is excreted with the fecal matter. WCE received FDA approval for general use in August 2001 and for pediatrics in October 2003 and is primarily used to evaluate small bowel lesions, especially those causing occult GI bleeding, undetectable by traditional endoscopy or contrast radiography. WCE has been useful in detecting occult Crohn disease limited to the small bowel and small intestinal bleeding lesions (ulcerations, vascular malformations). The primary drawbacks are risk of capsule retention (estimated to be 1%, especially due to small bowel strictures and diverticula), limited image resolution, inability to perform therapeutic maneuvers, and perhaps most significantly inability to obtain tissue biopsy samples. WCE also does not evaluate the stomach or colon well. For these reasons, WCE does not replace traditional endoscopy for most indications but can be useful for suspected occult small bowel pathology.

ENDOSCOPY INDICATIONS

The indications for endoscopy vary slightly among institutions and gastroenterologists, but generally follow the guidelines outlined in Boxes 273-1 and 273-2. Box 273-3 lists symptoms and disorders for which endoscopy is generally *not* indicated. Using endoscopy, the pediatric gastroenterologist can determine the source for upper and lower gastrointestinal bleeding in 70% to 80% of cases. Studies in adults with GI bleeding suggest that endoscopy performed early upon presentation of GI bleeding may shorten hospital stays and therefore decrease costs. Common causes of upper GI bleeding include peptic ulcers in the stomach and duodenum (Fig. 273-1), esophagitis, gastritis, varices, and Mallory-Weiss gastric prolapse lesions. Etiologies of lower GI bleeding in children include anal fissures, colitis (Fig. 273-2), and inflammatory (juvenile) polyps. An endoscopist can also directly intervene for many causes of GI bleeding: sclerotherapy and band ligation for esophageal varices (Fig. 273-3), sclerosant injection and thermocoagulation for bleeding ulcers and blood vessels, and removal of colonic polyps (Fig. 273-4). EGD is also very effective for the removal of foreign bodies within the upper GI tract. Kim and coworkers surveyed the charts of 80 children in Korea who underwent EGD for foreign body removal and noted that the majority of foreign bodies were coins (Fig. 273-5), batteries, and various sharp and blunt objects, and that these objects were successfully and safely removed in 79 out of 80 patients.

Box 273-1. Indications for Upper Endoscopy

Diagnostic

Dysphagia

Odynophagia

Intractable or chronic gastroesophageal reflux disease (GERD) (including surveillance for Barrett esophagus)

Vomiting

Upper abdominal pain with symptoms of organic disease (weight loss, anemia, fevers, vomiting)

Upper abdominal pain with significant morbidity (limitation of activities of daily living, school absenteeism)

Anorexia/weight loss (unexplained)

Anemia (unexplained)

Chronic diarrhea/malabsorption (includes small bowel biopsy for diagnosis of celiac disease)

Hematemesis

Melena

Hematochezia with hemodynamically significant blood loss

Caustic ingestion (evaluation of degree and severity)

Therapeutic

Foreign body removal from esophagus or stomach

Dilation of esophageal strictures

Esophageal varices—sclerotherapy or banding

Intractable upper gastrointestinal bleeding—sclerosant vessel injection, electrocautery, thermocoagulation leukopenia (particularly for colonoscopy), thrombocytopenia, coagulopathy, neurologic instability, or compromised respiratory function. Both the endoscopist and referring physician must decide whether the benefits of endoscopy outweigh the risks for each patient.

THE ENDOSCOPIST

Endoscopy should be considered as one aspect of a thorough medical evaluation and should be performed only by physicians (pediatric gastroenterologists and surgeons) with proved endoscopic skills and extensive experience in children. The North American Society for Pediatric Gastroenterology, Hepatology, and Nutrition (NASPHAN) has published the recommended minimum numbers of procedures necessary for endoscopic competency. Endoscopic proficiency requires not only high technical skills, but the experience and ability to effectively and efficiently integrate the endoscopic visual and histologic findings into the clinical decision making. A proficient endoscopist must also be able to determine whether potential benefits outweigh the risks of a proposed procedure. Performed properly with appropriate indications, endoscopy is a powerful tool allowing evaluation and treatment of many GI disorders with direct, yet nonsurgical access to most of the alimentary tract.

SUGGESTED READINGS

Boey CC, Goh KL, Hassall E, Magid M: Endoscopy in children with recurrent abdominal pain. Gastrointest Endosc 2001;53(1):142–143.

Eisen GM, Chutkan R, Goldstein JL, et al: Guidelines: Modifications in endoscopic practice for pediatric patients. Gastrointest Endosc 2000;52(6):838–842.

Kim JK, Kim SS, Kim JI, et al: Management of foreign bodies in the gastrointestinal tract: An analysis of 104 cases in children. Endoscopy 1999;31:302–304.

Kavic SM, Basson MD: Complications of endoscopy. Am J Surg 2001;181(4):319–332.

Squires RH, Colletti RB: Medical position paper: Indications for pediatric gastrointestinal endoscopy: A medical position statement of the North American Society of Pediatric Gastroenterology and Nutrition. J Pediatr Gastroenterol Nutr 1996;23:107–110.

Swain P: Wireless capsule endoscopy. Gut 2003;52(suppl IV):48–50.

SECTION 9   DIAGNOSTICS AND THERAPEUTICS: *Diagnostics*

274 Bronchoscopy

Suzanne E. Beck and Daniel V. Schidlow

Bronchoscopy is the examination of the airway by means of an optical instrument. In children, this procedure usually involves the examination of the upper as well as the lower airway; thus, the term *bronchoscopy* is somewhat of a misnomer.

Endoscopic examination of the airway in children helps define anatomic or structural abnormalities, examine dynamic function of the airways, recover secretions for examination and culture, and remove mucous plugs and foreign bodies.

INSTRUMENTS

There are two basic types of bronchoscopic instruments, rigid and flexible. The rigid instrument generally has a larger diameter to allow passage of instruments such as forceps for the removal of foreign bodies and for suctioning. Rigid bronchoscopy requires neck extension and general anesthesia in a controlled setting (operating room) to achieve full relaxation of the child as the instrument is inserted through the mouth and into the airway. The rigid bronchoscope also serves as an endotracheal tube, thereby making assisted ventilation easy to perform during general anesthesia.

Table 274-1. Indications for Bronchoscopy in Children

Indications	Preferred Instrument
Suspicion for foreign body aspiration	Rigid
Suspicion for recurrent oropharyngeal aspiration	Flexible
Chronic or recurrent stridor or croup	Flexible or rigid
Chronic or recurrent wheezing unresponsive to therapy	Flexible
Chronic or recurrent atelectasis or localized pneumonia	Flexible
Pneumonia in an immunocompromised host	Flexible
Hemoptysis or pulmonary hemosiderosis	Flexible

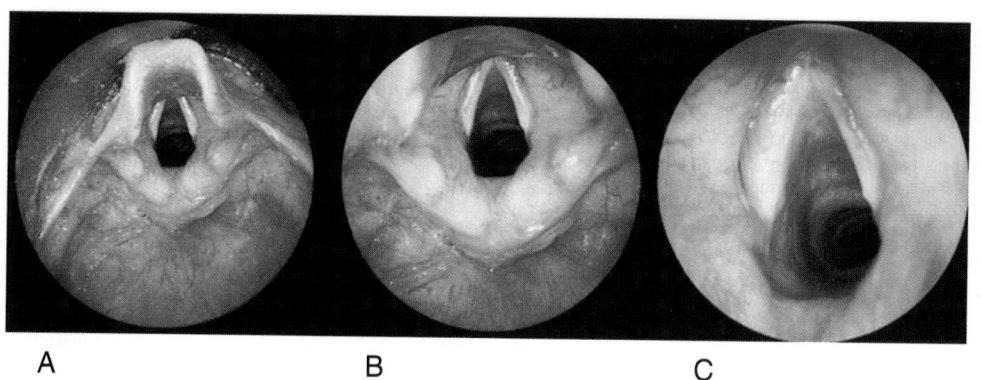

Figure 274-1. Normal larynx. **A,** Overall view of normal laryngopharynx through a flexible fiberoptic pediatric bronchoscope. **B,** Close-up view of normal vocal cords and supraglottic structures. During real-time imaging, normal movement can be appreciated. **C,** Close-up view of normal glottis, subglottis, and upper trachea. During real-time video imaging, normal dynamic function can be observed.

Flexible fiberoptic bronchoscopes allow for examination of airways inaccessible to the rigid bronchoscope. Flexible bronchoscopy often requires only topical anesthesia with minimal sedation. The instrument passes through the nares or mouth or through an artificial airway. Because the flexible bronchoscope is not hollow, the patient must be able to breathe around it. Special adapters make it possible to perform fiberoptic bronchoscopy while a patient is being artificially ventilated.

The smallest available flexible fiberoptic bronchoscope has an external diameter of 2.2 mm, which allows use in neonates and young infants. The smallest flexible bronchoscope with a suction port has an external diameter of 2.8 mm.

Flexible bronchoscopy is particularly useful for examining the dynamics of the airways in conditions such as laryngo-, tracheo-, and bronchomalacia as well as vocal cord dysfunction. Figure 274-1 demonstrates laryngoscopic views of a normal larynx. Figure 274-2 demonstrates laryngoscopic views of laryngomalacia. Flexible bronchoscopy also allows collection of lung specimens through transbronchial biopsy for older children and adolescents with diffuse lung disease or lung transplantation.

Rigid bronchoscopy is a preferable option to surgery to remove foreign bodies and to perform endoscopic laser surgery on subglottic lesions. In the United States, otolaryngologists and thoracic surgeons generally perform rigid bronchoscopy.

INDICATIONS

Indications for bronchoscopy include chronic or recurrent stridor, chronic or recurrent wheezing unresponsive to therapy, chronic or recurrent localized pneumonia or atelectasis, suspicion of foreign body aspiration, evaluation for possible intrinsic obstruction or extrinsic compression of the airway, and recovery of secretions (Table 274-1). Diagnostic bronchoscopy during hemoptysis is controversial because identifying the precise site of the bleeding may not be possible during endoscopic examination of the airway. However, bronchoscopy with bronchoalvelolar lavage is the procedure of choice to diagnose pulmonary hemosiderosis as the suspected cause of hemoptysis.

BRONCHOALVEOLAR LAVAGE

This procedure, performed during bronchoscopy, involves wedging a flexible instrument in a subsegmental bronchus, instilling aliquots of physiologic solution through the instrument followed by suctioning. The purpose of this procedure is to recover fluid for cytologic examination and culture. Table 274-2 lists indications for performing bronchoalveolar lavage (BAL) in pediatric patients and the typical microbiologic and cytologic findings associated with those conditions warranting BAL.

Tracheobronchography has generally been replaced by sophisticated imaging techniques such as high-resolution chest computed tomography and magnetic resonance

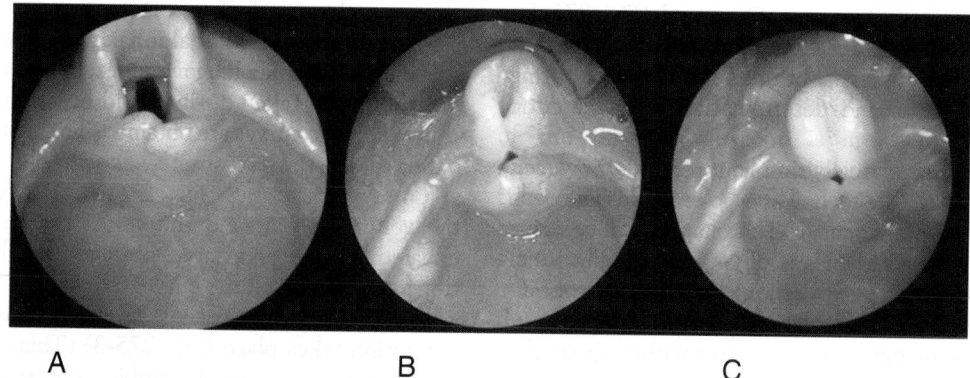

Figure 274-2. Laryngomalacia (floppy airway) is the most common cause of stridor in infants. Inspiratory stridor usually begins shortly after birth and resolves by 2 years of age. Direct endoscopy of the larynx while the patient is breathing spontaneously shows partial inward collapse of the supraglottic structures at the beginning of inspiration (**A**), and the epiglottis curls in on itself and the cuneiform cartilage is sucked into the glottis (**B**). During maximal inspiration, the supraglottis has only a narrow opening, creating the stridulous sound (**C**). During expiration, the supraglottis and glottis are opened.

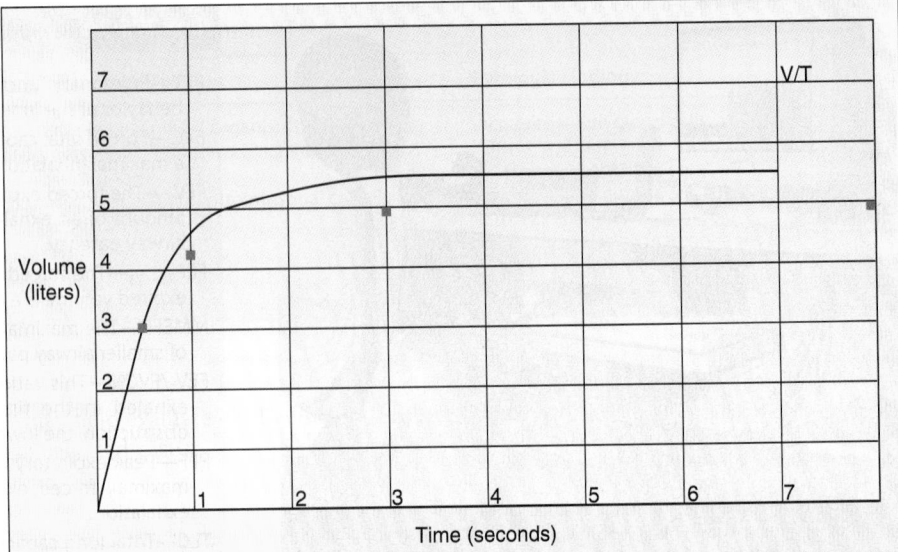

Figure 275-2. Normal spirogram plotting exhaled air volume over time (velocity of air volume exhalation).

of patients with asthma and other pathologic lung conditions.

Handheld spirometers capable of data storage are currently used to monitor early airway obstruction in patients after lung transplantation and in selected patients with obstructive repiratory diseases. Telespirometry, the trans-mission of spirometric values via telephone, is a technology in evolution that shows promise for enhancing outpatient monitoring.

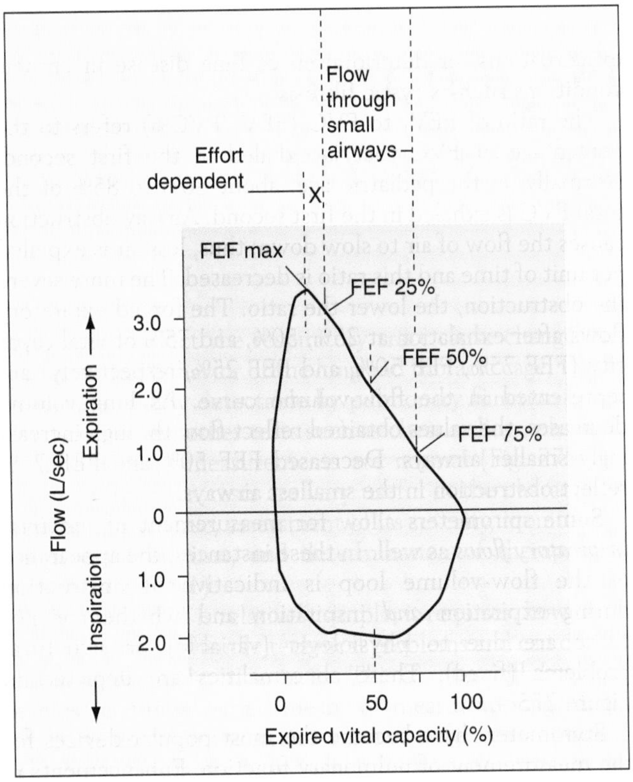

PEAK FLOW MEASUREMENTS

Peak expiratory flow (PEF), or maximal expiratory flow, is the maximum flow achieved during maximal, forced exhalation and occurs at the beginning of exhalation. PEF roughly measures the patency of the larger airways and can be obtained with spirometry or special handheld devices called peak flowmeters.

Peak flowmeters became very popular after publication of the National Institutes of Health guidelines for the management of asthma. These instruments are cheap and simple to use. However, the characteristic flow ranges of children (200 to 400 L/min) are too low to allow accurate measurement by peak flowmeters. Test results are very dependent on effort and technique. Physicians must

Figure 275-3. Normal flow-volume loop, demonstrating relationship of flow to expired vital capacity, obtained by spirometry, with expiratory flow-volume curve above the *x*-axis. The FEF$_{max}$ to FEF$_{25}$ curve is effort-dependent; stronger efforts result in higher values. The FEF$_{25-75}$ curve is "effort-independent," does not change despite force of exhalation, and reflects flow through the small airways.

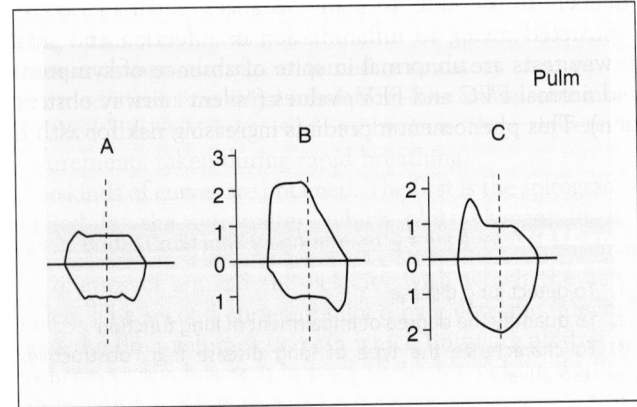

Figure 275-4. Flow-volume loops indicative of obstruction during expiration *and* inspiration caused by physiologic (variable) or structural problems (fixed). *A,* Fixed airway obstruction (tracheal narrowing). *B,* Variable extrathoracic obstruction (laryngeal lesion). *C,* Variable intrathoracic obstruction (asthma).

remember that peak flow values can be normal even when smaller airways are obstructed.

MEASUREMENT OF LUNG VOLUMES

Measuring lung volumes involves having the patient move air via slow inhalation and exhalation (as opposed to forced, quick ones). The values obtained are referred to as "static volumes." The sum of two or more volumes is called a *capacity*. The graph in Figure 275-5 depicts lung volumes and capacities.

Slow vital capacity (SVC) is obtained by exhaling maximally *and slowly* after a maximal inhalation. In situations in which there is significant airway reactivity or obstruction, SVC can be significantly higher than FVC, because the forced exhalation causes airways to collapse.

Total lung capacity (TLC) is the total amount of air that the lungs can hold. Functional residual capacity (FRC) is the air left in the lung after a normal tidal volume exhalation (during regular breathing). Residual volume (RV) is the amount of air left in the lung after a maximum expiration. This portion does not participate in air exchange. The magnitude of the increase in FRC, RV, and the percentage of TLC comprising residual volume (normally 20%, called the RV/TLC) indicate the degree of air trapping in obstructive lung disease.

FRC and RV are best measured by body plethysmography. The patient to be tested sits in an airtight chamber. Changes in pressure within the chamber, caused by the patient breathing against a valve, are translated electronically into volumes. In the past, most laboratories used helium dilution tests to measure FRC, in which the patient breathed helium from a reservoir until equilibration between the lungs and the reservoir occurred. The helium dilution test is slower and less accurate than plethysmography, particularly in patients with widespread airway obstruction.

Of note, the diffusion capacity of carbon monoxide in lungs is useful in the diagnosis and monitoring of uncommon diseases that affect the alveolar-capillary membranes, such as interstitial pulmonary disease. Usually, only specialized laboratories provide this test.

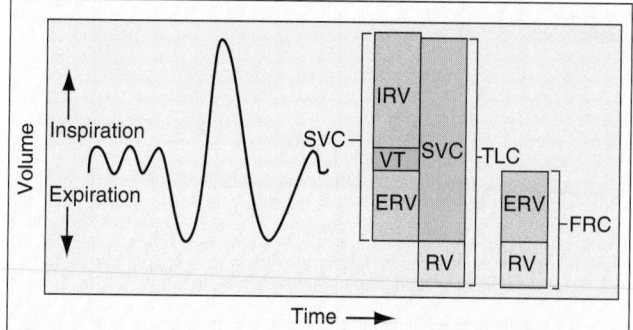

Figure 275-5. Graph depicting lung volumes and capacities. Total lung capacity (TLC) is the sum of the residual volume (RV) and slow vital capacity (SVC). The SVC is the sum of the inspiratory reserve volume (IRV), the tidal volume (TV), and the expiratory reserve volume (ERV). The functional residual capacity (FRC) is the sum of the RV and the ERV.

Table 275-1. Interpretation of Pulmonary Function

Spirometric Measurement	Obstructive Lung Disease	Restrictive Lung Disease
Forced vital capacity (FVC)	N or ↓	↓
Forced expiratory volume at 1 second (FEV₁)	↓	↓
FEV₁/FVC	↓	N or ↑
Forced expiratory flow, 25%–75% (FEF₂₅₋₇₅)	↓	↓
Peak expiratory flow rate (PEFR) or midmaximal expiratory flow rate (MMEFR)	N or ↓	↓
Functional residual capacity (FRC)	↑	↓
Residual volume (RV)	↑	↓
Total lung capacity (TLC)	↑	↓

INTERPRETATION OF PULMONARY FUNCTION TESTS

The two main physiologic categories of pulmonary dysfunction are obstructive and restrictive lung disease (Table 275-1).

The net effect of obstructive disease is reduction in the amount of expired air, especially during forceful exhalation, as noted by decreases in PEFR, FEV₁, MMEFR, and FEV₁/FVC and by increased air trapping. The flow-volume curve, obtained by spirometry, shows a characteristic "scooping." Flows and flow rates are decreased. Asthma is the quintessential obstructive disease in children.

Restrictive disease is characterized by uniform decrease in volumes and flow rates (a physiologically "smaller" lung). Exhalation tends to be short and incomplete. The flow-volume curve, obtained by spirometry, has a normal or close to normal shape but a smaller size. FEV₁/FVC is normal or increased. Conditions that cause restrictive disease in children are relatively uncommon and include thoracic cage deformities, neuromuscular diseases, and diseases that cause lung compliance to diminish ("stiff lungs"), such as chronic interstitial pneumonia and lung fibrosis.

Both obstruction and restriction are present in conditions that have concomitant airway and parenchymal disease such as advanced cystic fibrosis, severe bronchopulmonary dysplasia, and other rare chronic inflammatory diseases of the lung.

Figures 275-6 and 275-7 show flow-volume curves and spirometric values that depict obstructive and restrictive disease, respectively.

Figure 275-8 demonstrates a flow-volume curve depicting both obstructive and restrictive lung disease (e.g., advanced cystic fibrosis)

CHALLENGE TESTING

Symptoms and functional signs of obstruction may be absent in a patient at rest. Challenge testing is indicated for individuals with a history of respiratory dysfunction during exercise, stress, or exposure to environmental agents whose pulmonary function tests, performed under basal circumstances, are normal. Individuals are exposed to situations or

	Predicted	Baseline		Post bronchodilator		
FVC (L)*	3.47	4.07	117%	4.90	141%	20%
FEV1 (L)*	3.07	1.99	65%	3.27	106%	64%
FEV1/FVC	0.87	0.49	56%	0.67	76%	37%
FEF25–75% (L/s)	3.72	0.90	24%	2.08	56%	132%
PEFR (L/s)*	6.53	5.13	79%	7.04	108%	37%

Number of efforts performed: 4   Comments:

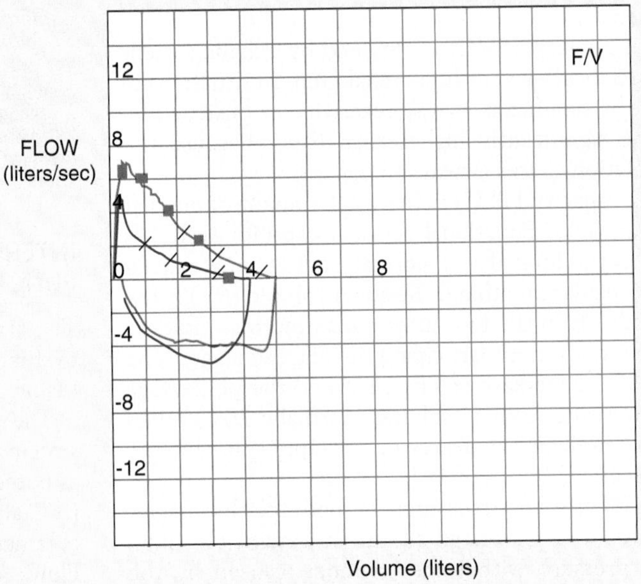

Figure 275-6. Flow-volume curve depicting obstructive lung disease (asthma) and bronchodilator test. At baseline, flow rates at all lung volumes are down. After bronchodilator inhalation, all values significantly increase.

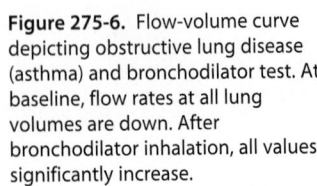

FVC (L)*	1.40	0.88	63%
FEV1 (L)*	1.25	0.80	64%
FEV1/FVC	0.92	0.91	99%
FEF25–75% (L/s)	1.63	1.44	89%
PEFR (L/s)*	2.55	2.45	96%

Number of efforts performed: 3   Comments:

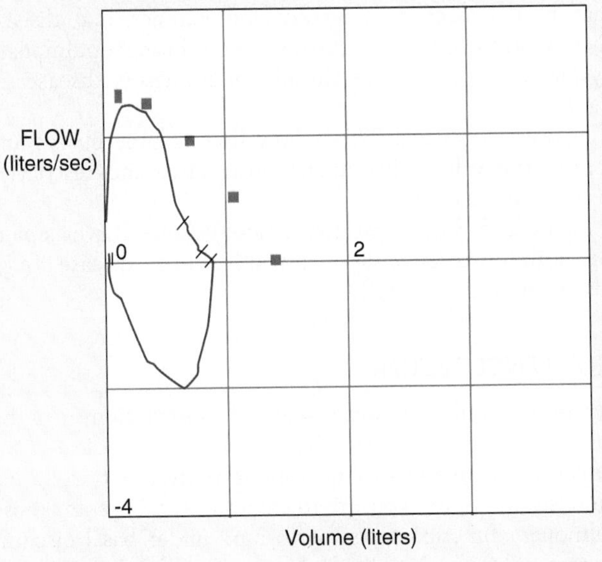

Figure 275-7. Flow-volume curve depicting restrictive lung disease.

FVC (L)*	5.23	3.08	59%
FEV1 (L)*	4.51	1.23	27%
FEV1/FVC	0.85	0.40	47%
FEF25–75% (L/s)	5.02	0.30	6%
PEFR (L/s)*	9.33	6.90	74%

Number of efforts performed: 3   Comments:

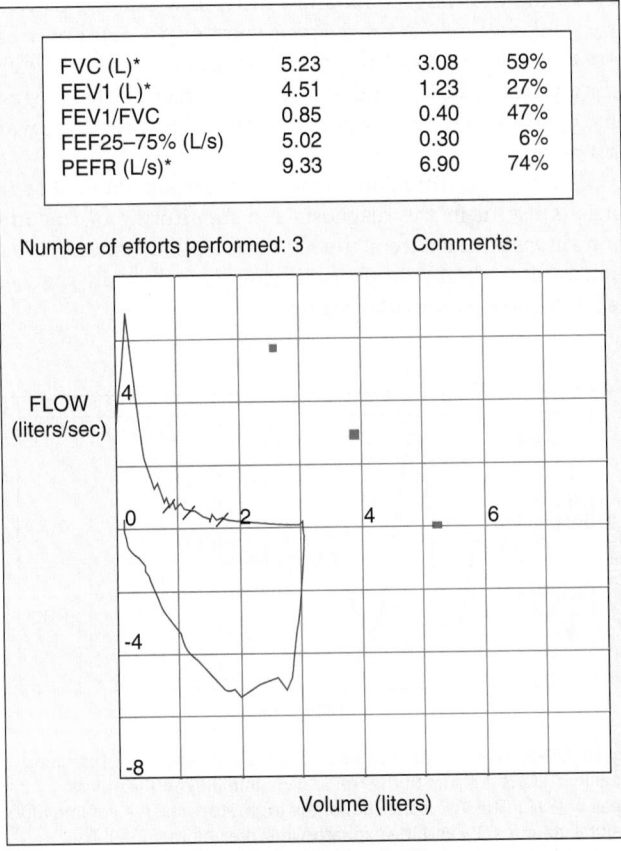

Figure 275-8. Flow-volume curve depicting both obstructive and restrictive lung disease (advanced cystic fibrosis).

substances that induce bronchoconstriction such as cold air, methacholine, or specific allergens. A drop in flow rates and flows of about 10% to 15% or more is considered abnormal.

Challenge testing should not be confused with exercise or stress testing that includes measurement of cardiovascular and respiratory parameters such as blood pressure, cardiac rhythm, and oxygen consumption. A detailed description of stress testing is in Chapter 276.

BRONCHODILATOR TEST

The bronchodilator test measures therapeutic efficacy of bronchodilator medications. The patient first performs spirometry testing to establish degree of airway obstruction and then is given a standard dose of a bronchodilator drug by nebulization or metered-dose inhaler. Approximately 20 minutes later, spirometry is repeated and the two pre- and post-bronchodilator administration values are compared. Improvement of at least 10% (preferably 15%) over baseline value is considered indicative of therapeutic efficacy and is referred to as "bronchodilator responsiveness" (see Fig. 275-6).

It must be remembered that a modest or absent bronchodilator response is not always irrefutable proof of lack of efficacy of bronchodilator treatment. Longstanding endobronchial inflammation can dampen the response to these drugs. Thus, it is advisable to repeat bronchodilator testing over time.

SUMMARY

Pulmonary function testing should be part of the diagnostic and management capabilities of any busy pediatric practice, especially in an era of increasing incidence and severity of asthma in children.

SUGGESTED READINGS

Allen J: Office of Pulmonary Function Testing. In Schidlow DV, Smith DS (eds): A Practical Guide to Pediatric Respiratory Diseases. Philadelphia, Hanley & Belfus, 1994, pp 281–288.

American Thoracic Society: Standardization of spirometry: 1994 Update. Am Rev Respir Crit Care Med 1994;152:1107–1136.

Eid N, Yandell B, Howell L, et al: Can peak expiratory flow predict airflow obstruction in children with asthma? Pediatrics 2000; 105:354–358.

Ferguson AC: Persisting airway obstruction in asymptomatic children with asthma with normal peak expiratory flow rates. J Allergy Clin Immunol 1988;82:19–22.

SECTION 9   DIAGNOSTICS AND THERAPEUTICS: *Diagnostics*

276

Electrocardiography, Echocardiography, and Cardiac Catheterization

Scott Yeager

ELECTROCARDIOGRAPHY

Electrocardiography (ECG), a valuable tool in the evaluation of the child with known or suspected cardiac disease, provides insight into cardiac conduction, rhythm abnormalities, ventricular hypertrophy, and a variety of repolarization abnormalities. ECG is a useful screening test for identifying children with significant structural cardiac abnormalities. Although physiologic principles and basic technique for ECG is identical in all age groups, children present specific technical issues and the interpretation of electrocardiograms in children requires knowledge of age-dependent changes in the electrocardiographic patterns.

Obtaining a technically satisfactory electrocardiogram in children, particularly young children, requires patience and experience. The electrocardiogram is normally obtained with the patient in the supine position, but occasionally the patient will need to sit upright in the parent's lap. Variation from the normal positioning can result in subtle changes in axes and forces and should be noted on the electro-

Table 276-1. Indications for Electrocardiogram

Indication	ECG Effects
Structural abnormality	Axis deviation; hypertrophy
Palpitations	Delta wave; Long Q-T; PR interval; premature beats; P-wave axis
Chest pain	ST segments; ischemic changes; hypertrophy; low voltage
Syncope	Long Q-T; delta wave; heart block; T-wave abnormalities
Drug effects	PR, QRS, Q-T duration; arrhythmias
Metabolic effects	PR, QRS, Q-T duration; arrhythmias; ST-T wave changes
Family history (sudden death, myopathy)	Q-T interval; hypertrophy; T-wave changes

cardiogram. A quiet, calm, and soothing approach to the frightened child usually results in a successful tracing. Technicians uncomfortable with the pediatric patient rarely obtain a good quality electrocardiogram in frightened children. Enlisting the aid of a parent or distracting the child with a mobile, puppets, or bubbles will frequently create an opportunity to obtain a good quality recording.

Pediatric-sized stick-on electrodes are most effective for obtaining adequate skin contact in children. The skin should be cleaned with alcohol if the child has recently been treated with a skin lotion. Electrode stickers must sometimes be trimmed to a smaller size to allow appropriate positioning on the chest. A small area of contact provides greater discrimination between the leads. The electrodes should not be allowed to touch. At least one right-sided chest lead may be useful in pediatric patients to provide a clear assessment of right ventricular forces. Careful confirmation of lead position should be a routine part of electrocardiograms in children. Misplacement of chest or limb leads can simulate a variety of electrocardiographic abnormalities and can be quite misleading. In patients being evaluated for arrhythmias, a 1- or 2-minute continuous rhythm strip following the 12-lead electrocardiogram is often helpful. Table 276-1 lists indications for obtaining an electrocardiogram.

Interpretation

Table 276-2 outlines interpretation of ECG in pediatric patients. Many aspects of pediatric ECG interpretation are the same as in the adult. Standard ECG texts outline how to measure cardiac axes and intervals. However, axes, intervals, and voltages change significantly over the first few days, weeks, months, and years of life. Although the generalist may not be able to "sight read" pediatric electrocardiograms, with the aid of an appropriate pediatric handbook, most tracings can be accurately interpreted. Some general guidelines follow:

- *P waves* will generally be upright and visible in leads 1 and aVF in patients at any age. The P wave is usually most prominent in lead 2 when the patient is in sinus rhythm. A P wave height greater than 3 mm suggests right atrial enlargement. Biphasic P waves are relatively common and do not indicate left atrial enlargement unless the terminal portion of the P wave is deeper than 2 mm and wider than 0.08 second (2 boxes). P waves that are not positive in both leads 1 and aVF may reflect an ectopic atrial pacemaker as the predominant rhythm.

- The *PR interval* changes somewhat with age and heart rate. The PR interval in the normal newborn averages about 0.10 second (2.5 boxes). The PR interval tends to lengthen with advancing age. A typical PR interval in an older child ranges from 0.12 to 0.16 second (3 to 4 boxes). First-degree atrioventricular block is diagnosed when the PR interval is beyond the upper range of normal for age (0.14 to 0.16 second in infants, 0.20 second in older children and adolescents). An abnormally short PR interval may be an indication of a preexcitation syndrome such as Wolff-Parkinson-White syndrome (Fig. 276-1).

- The normal *QRS axis* for a newborn ranges from approximately 90 degrees to 200 degrees. This results in a QRS complex that is primarily positive in lead aVF and negative in lead 1. After birth, there is a leftward shifting of the axis over the next weeks and months such that the QRS complex will be predominantly positive in both leads 1 and aVF by several months of age. A shift of axis to other quadrants in infants and children implies significant underlying structural abnormalities. Precordial voltages in the newborn reflect the normal neonatal right ventricular thickness, and there is a slow progression to left ventricular predominance occurring over the first year or two of life. The normal range of values for the QRS complex is quite wide, and tables of normal voltages at varying ages should be consulted. Normal QRS duration ranges from 0.04 to 0.08 second (1 to 2 boxes) but may be prolonged by conduction abnormalities, metabolic disturbances, and a variety of medications.

- The appearance of *T waves* is quite variable in the first few days of life. Beyond a week or two of age, T waves will usually be upright in both leads 1 and aVF. In the precordial leads, T waves are usually inverted in the right precordial leads and upright in the left precordial leads. After the midteenage years, T waves become

Table 276-2. Electrocardiogram Interpretation

Age	QRS Axis	PR Interval (msec)	T in Lead V$_1$	T in Lead V$_6$	R in Lead V$_1$	R in Lead V$_6$
Birth	90–185	85–130	↑↓	↓↑	6–36	1–11
3 months	30–105	80–110	↓	↑	5–17	6–18
1 year	15–90	90–140	↓	↑	3–15	7–20
5 years	15–90	90–150	↓	↑	2–12	10–24
10 years	15–90	95–160	↓	↑	1–10	10–24
15 years	15–90	100–170	↑	↑	1–9	8–22

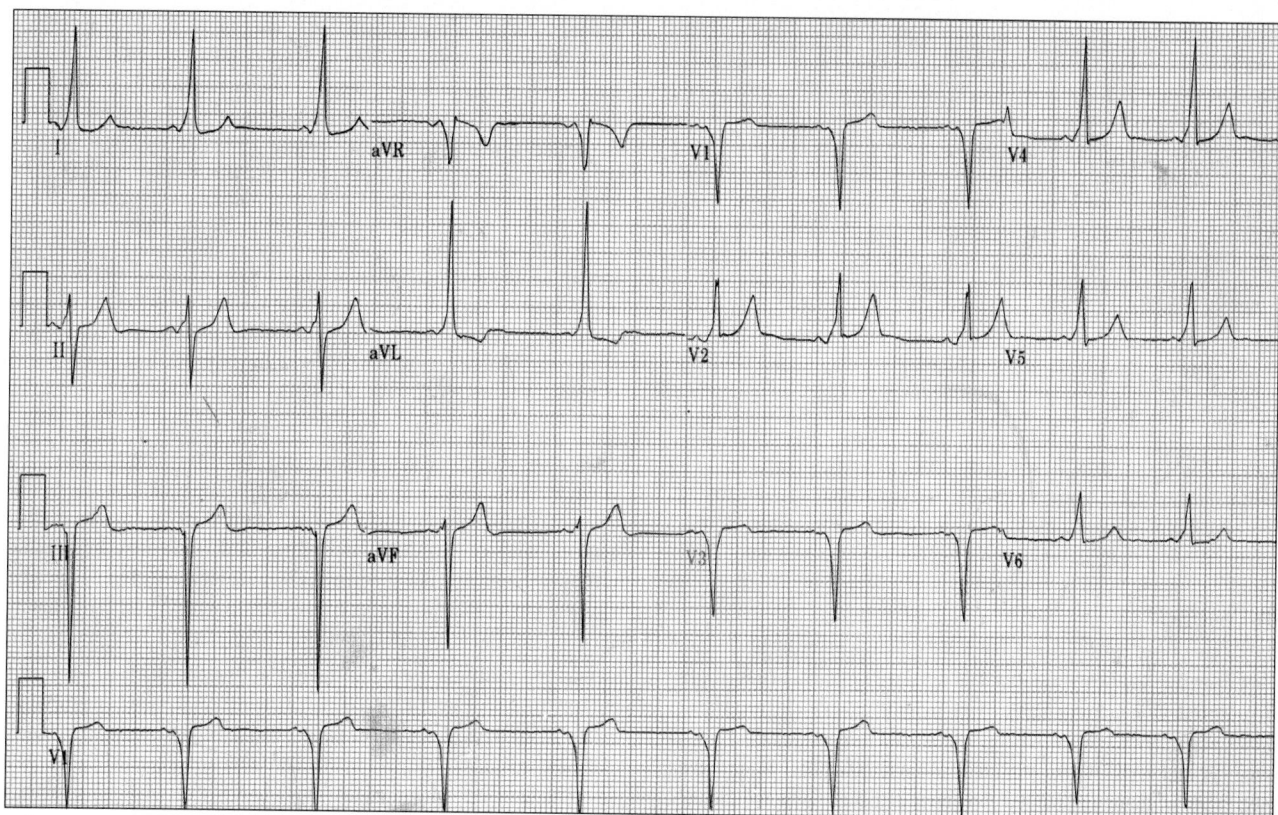

Figure 276-1. A 12-lead electrocardiogram from a 10-year-old with palpitations. The classic features of Wolff-Parkinson-White syndrome are illustrated. The short PR interval and delta wave are most apparent in leads I, II, V₄, V₅, and V₆. There is also a leftward shift in axis, a relatively common finding in Wolff-Parkinson-White syndrome.

upright across all precordial leads. Changes in T waves may reflect a variety of underling metabolic abnormalities. T wave changes commonly accompany inflammatory processes such as myocarditis or pericarditis with ST-segment changes, T-wave flattening, or T-wave inversion. T-wave changes may also indicate abnormal hemodynamic stresses such as aortic or pulmonary stenosis, systemic hypertension, coarctation of the aorta, or coronary artery abnormalities. The T waves are also affected by medications, which can shorten or prolong repolarization. A minor degree of ST-segment elevation, commonly referred to as early repolarization, is a normal feature of the left-sided precordial leads in the adolescent. The Q-T interval (measured from the onset of the QRS complex to the termination of the T wave) normally varies with heart rate and should be corrected before interpretation. The corrected Q-T interval (Q-T$_c$) is determined by dividing the Q-T interval by the square root of the preceding RR interval. The normal range of the corrected Q-T interval is from 0.36 to 0.44 second. A variety of electrolyte abnormalities and medications can affect the corrected Q-T interval. Some patients have familial or spontaneous forms of prolonged Q-T interval, which may predispose to serious ventricular arrhythmias.

Stress Testing

Box 276-1 lists indications for stress testing. Pediatric stress testing is a useful tool for evaluating exercise-related symptoms. The procedure, a continuous 12-lead electrocardio-graphic monitoring during progressive, staged exercise, is performed on a treadmill or a bicycle. The modified Bruce protocol, usually followed in pediatric and adolescent patients, incorporates electrocardiographic monitoring with an automated treadmill that provides progressive exertion from a slow walk on a level surface to moderate running up a significant incline. Sophisticated computers monitor the electrocardiogram, filter motion artifact, and provide trend analysis of ST segments and repolarization changes. The protocol stages progress in 3-minute intervals and are accompanied by periodic blood pressure measurements. Stress tests are performed for symptoms of exertional chest pain or exercise-related arrhythmias and syncope. Stress tests may also be useful for evaluating blood pressure response to exercise, particularly in hypertensive patients or

Box 276-1. Indications for Stress Testing

Exertional chest pain
Exertional syncope
Exertional palpitations
Ventricular ectopy
Diminished exercise tolerance
Exercise-dependent right-to-left shunting
Systemic hypertension
Clearance for competitive sports in patients with
  History of Kawasaki disease
  History of cardiac surgery
  History of structural heart abnormalities

those with residual coarctation of the aorta and in evaluating patients with a perceived decrease in exercise tolerance. Electrocardiographic monitoring can be supplemented with transcutaneous oxygen determination to evaluate the effect of exercise on intracardiac shunting. Stress testing is rarely performed in patients under 8 years of age.

Tilt Testing

Box 276-2 lists indications for tilt testing. Tilt-table testing, a technique for evaluation of syncopal and presyncopal symptoms, is a provocative test involving continuous electrocardiographic monitoring of a patient strapped to a padded platform fitted with a foot rest. The test is initiated when the patient is raised from a supine to a 60-degree upright position while secured to the platform. Continuous electrocardiographic and periodic blood pressure measurements are recorded. The patient is maintained in an upright position for 15 to 45 minutes or until symptoms develop. A positive test elicits hypotension with or without progressive bradycardia and symptoms of syncope or presyncope. Tilt-table tests are often positive in patients with syncope, and may help elucidate the mechanism of symptoms. However, many clinicians do not use tilt testing because results do not alter their initial management in patients with a typical vasovagal history. Tilt testing is sometimes useful in patients with unusual histories, recurrent syncope, or for follow-up testing of patients already receiving medical intervention for symptoms.

Ambulatory Holter Monitoring

Box 276-3 lists indications for electrocardiographic Holter monitoring. Patients with symptoms of palpitations, tachycardia, chest pain, and syncope are frequently evaluated using some form of continuous electrocardiographic moni-

toring. The heart rhythm is continuously monitored for 24 to 48 hours using a magnetic tape cassette recorder worn on a belt or in a backpack. The patient is instructed to press an event marker button when experiencing symptoms, establishing a temporal relationship between electrocardiographic changes and symptoms. Holter monitoring reveals detailed information regarding the onset and termination of arrhythmias, helps quantify ectopy, and can demonstrate intermittent conduction disturbances or interval prolongation. The completed recording is scanned at high speed with sophisticated computer algorithms that identify significant arrhythmias and provide hard copy printouts for more detailed analysis. Holter monitoring is frequently used to evaluate medical interventions in patients with arrhythmias. The principal limitation of Holter monitoring is its relatively short duration and the occasional inability, particularly in younger children, to maintain lead placement for the period of monitoring. However, with appropriate electrode protection and a motivated caretaker, satisfactory Holter monitoring can usually be obtained at any age.

Event Recording

Box 276-4 lists indications for event recording. Event monitors help evaluate infrequent symptoms that could be arrhythmic in origin. These monitors are worn continuously and contain electronic memory. At the time of a symptom, a button is pushed and a segment of rhythm history is stored in memory and several minutes of subsequent rhythm is recorded. The entire recording is then telephone transmitted to a central service for downloading and analysis. Event monitors are typically supplied to the patient for a month or more. Longer term, implantable monitors are also available and can provide more than a year of surveillance. The principal drawback of event monitors is the variable recording and transmission quality and the difficulty of reliably recording the onset and termination of events.

ECHOCARDIOGRAPHY

Echocardiography has been a revolutionary diagnostic tool in pediatric cardiology, allowing detailed anatomic evaluation of cardiac and vascular structures and providing a method for rapid determination of global and regional ventricular function as well as offering significant insight into cardiovascular physiology. Despite its accuracy and versatility, echocardiography still has some limitations. Accuracy of cardiac ultrasound depends on the skill of the operator to obtain a complete and thorough evaluation. Unlike many radiologic procedures, there is no "standard" pediatric echocardiographic study. Variations in cardiac anatomy and limitations in echocardiographic windows heavily influence the quality of the study obtained. Because of the tremendous variation in cardiac anatomy in pediatric patients, a highly experienced ultrasonographer is required to make appropriate adjustments in the study and to obtain all relevant information. A laboratory that may routinely obtain high-quality studies in adults is often quite inadequate for evaluating infants and children with suspected cardiac disease. To be most effective, echocardiography requires close communication between the cardiac sonographer and the cardiologist. In many cases, the cardiologist is present while the study is being performed and will modify the study depending on real-time interpretation. The test is far more sensitive and specific when guided by clinical input. Because cardiac ultrasound is relatively expensive, most pediatric institutions require cardiology consultation before performing an echocardiogram. After evaluation, if further testing is appropriate, echocardiography can be directed based on clinical impressions.

Two-Dimensional Imaging

Cardiac anatomy in children can be displayed, often spectacularly, through two-dimensional real-time images. Sound waves reflecting off cardiac structures are translated into anatomic information that is displayed in shades of gray on a television monitor (Fig. 276-2). Children's small size permits the use of very high frequency sound energy, which, although limited in its penetration into the body, provides much higher resolution of cardiac structures than typical studies in adult patients. In infants and small children, extremely detailed anatomic images can be obtained and, when combined with various Doppler techniques, can provide an almost complete diagnostic evaluation of even the most complex congenital heart abnormalities.

The principal limitations to two-dimensional imaging are created by the extremes of patient size. Very tiny premature infants require specialized, high-frequency probes for adequate imaging. Very large or obese individuals

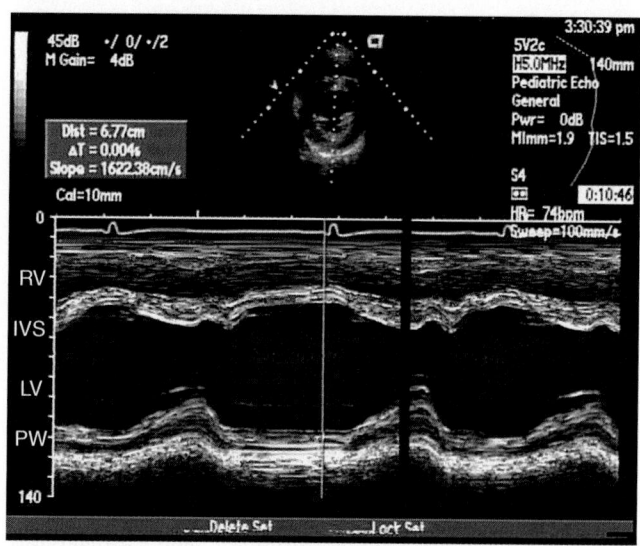

Figure 276-3. M-mode recording of the left ventricle in the same patient illustrated in Figure 276-2. The small image in the upper center portion of the figure is a representation of the left ventricle in cross section with the cursor (dotted line) passing through the middle of the ventricle. The lower panel shows the movement of cardiac structures along the cursor during three cardiac cycles. Left ventricular contraction and relaxation are demonstrated. A quantitative evaluation of ventricular function is determined using this method. IVS, intraventricular septum; LV, left ventricle; PW, posterior wall of the left ventricle; RV, right ventricular outflow tract.

may also have relatively limited imaging windows. In addition, overlying lung will scatter ultrasound energy and prevent adequate anatomic definition. Patients on ventilators or with significant lung hyperinflation may be difficult to study.

Ventricular Function

Echocardiography can provide reasonably sophisticated evaluation of global and regional ventricular function. In patients without regional wall motion abnormalities, a calculation of fractional shortening provides a general indicator of left ventricular function (Fig. 276-3). Normal fractional shortening ranges from about 30% to 36%, which correlates with an ejection fraction of 60% to 70%. Ventricular function can also be expressed as a percentage of area change determined by the planimetered area of the left ventricle in diastole and systole. Alternatively, with the addition of certain geometric assumptions, an ejection fraction can be approximated using echocardiographic images. These calculations assume a standard ventricular shape as well as uniform wall motion.

In the presence of abnormal underlying anatomy and physiology, the determination of ventricular function is often qualitative. Pressure abnormalities that result in flattening of the ventricular septum negate many of the assumptions used for quantitative evaluation of left ventricular performance. Significant volume loading of the right ventricle also changes the ventricular septal behavior, making quantitative analysis unreliable. With abnormal cardiac anatomy or physiology, a qualitative estimation of ventricular performance is usually possible and adequate for clinical management.

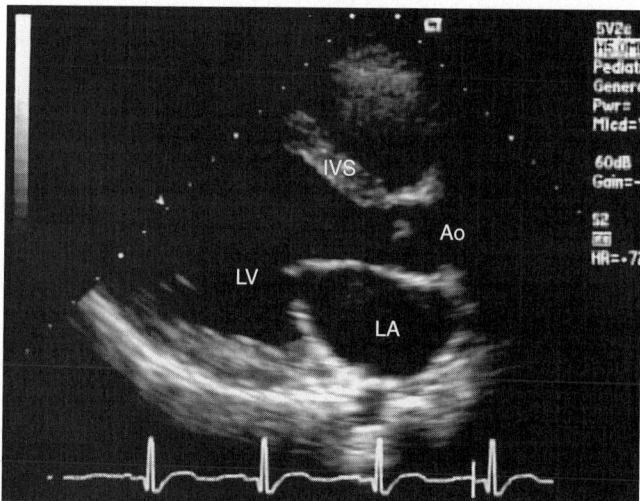

Figure 276-2. Long-axis parasternal view of the left ventricle in a 12-year-old with severe aortic regurgitation. Blood-filled structures appear black on echocardiography, and vessel walls and myocardium appear white or gray. This early diastolic frame demonstrates the aortic valve in a closed position and the mitral valve partially opened. The left ventricle is dilated. Ao, aorta; IVS, intraventricular septum; LA, left atrium; LV, left ventricle.

Doppler Evaluation

The phenomenon of the Doppler shift is utilized to detect the speed and direction of blood movement within the heart, and several different applications of this technology are employed to provide physiologic information.

Doppler interrogation can be performed in a "pulsed" form, which evaluates the direction and speed of blood movement within a small, disk-shaped "sample volume," which can be placed anywhere within the heart or great vessels (Fig. 276-4). This technique allows the operator to determine changes in blood flow direction or velocity associated with different anatomic structures. There are, however, significant technical limitations to the ability of pulsed Doppler to resolve high-velocity flow. When very accelerated blood flow is encountered, continuous-wave Doppler recordings are utilized.

Continuous-wave Doppler provides a measurement of the peak blood velocity encountered anywhere along a single line positioned within cardiovascular structures. In the continuous-wave mode, there is no upper limit to the velocity that can be measured. However, the spatial discrimination available in the pulsed Doppler mode is lost. The operator cannot determine the exact point along the interrogation line at which the highest velocities are encountered. Nonetheless, continuous-wave Doppler is very useful for estimating intracardiac pressures and gradients. The relationship between pressure and flow is a complex one. Under most circumstances, the relationship between pressure and velocity is expressed in a simplified equation as: $\Delta P = 4V^2$, where ΔP is the pressure difference accelerating the flow and V is the peak velocity of flow. For example, if the peak flow velocity measured across a stenotic aortic valve were determined to be 4 m/sec, the estimated pressure difference between the left ventricle and the aorta at peak systole would be predicted as 64 mm Hg. Utilizing this relationship, it is possible to estimate right ventricular pressure in the presence of tricuspid regurgitation, left ventricular to right ventricular pressure gradients in the presence of a ventricular septal defect, left atrial pressure in the presence of mitral regurgitation, and so on.

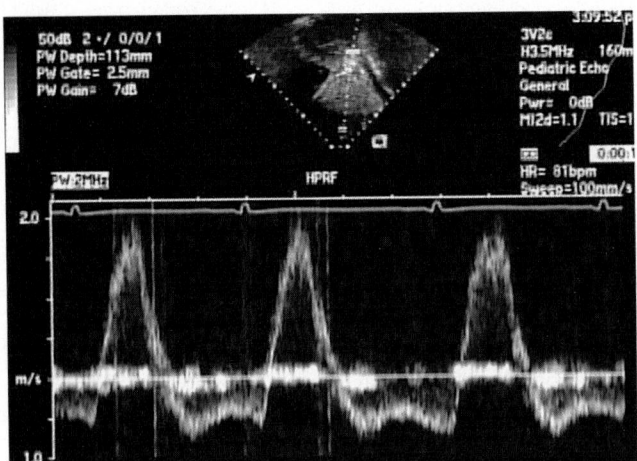

Figure 276-4. A pulsed Doppler recording in the descending aorta in the same patient shown in Figure 276-2. During systole, antegrade flow is demonstrated in the descending aorta with a peak velocity of slightly less than 2 m/sec. During diastole, very prominent reversal of flow occurs as a result of the patient's severe aortic regurgitation.

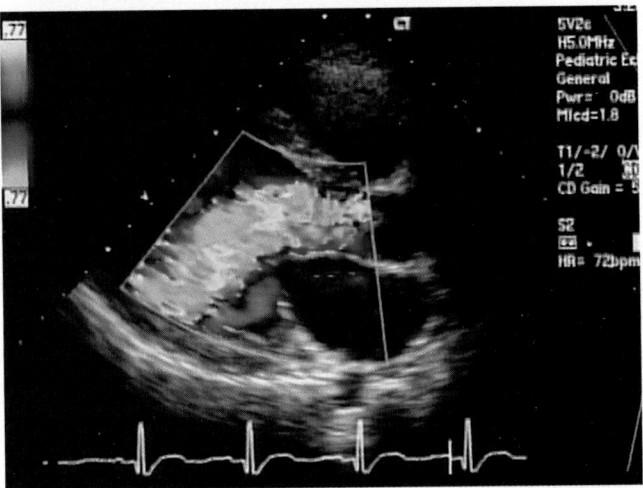

Figure 276-5. Color Doppler from the patient shown in Figure 276-2 demonstrates a broad regurgitant jet of blood flowing back into the left ventricle during diastole, indicating severe aortic regurgitation.

The third application of the Doppler phenomenon is color-flow Doppler. This technology detects blood flow and displays direction and velocity superimposed on a two-dimensional image. Typically, flow away from the transducer is encoded in hues of blue while flow toward the transducer is encoded in red. This method of displaying Doppler information is extremely useful for detecting small intracardiac shunts, regurgitant valves, and small vascular structures (Fig. 276-5). Color-flow Doppler greatly increases the sensitivity of echocardiography for identifying a variety of structural and functional abnormalities.

CARDIAC CATHETERIZATION

Box 276-5 lists indications for cardiac catheterization. Cardiac catheterization involves inserting a long, thin catheter (1 to 3 mm in diameter) into a peripheral blood vessel, either percutaneously or by cutdown, and advancing the catheter into the central circulation. Cardiac access is obtained either antegrade through venous connections or retrograde by way of the aorta. Prior to the development of echocardiography, cardiac catheterization was required in

---

Box 276-5. Indications for Cardiac Catheterization

Diagnostic

Determination of severity of left-to-right shunting
Assessment of pulmonary artery pressure and resistance
Evaluation of regurgitant or stenotic valves
Coronary artery or distal pulmonary artery evaluation
Postoperative assessment

Therapeutic

Balloon atrial septostomy
Balloon dilation of valves and vessels
Coil embolization of vessels
Device closure of intracardiac defects
Stent placement in obstructed outflow tracts and vessels

any infant or child in whom the underlying cardiac diagnosis was in doubt. Critically ill newborns or infants were often rushed to the catheterization laboratory in an attempt to establish an anatomic diagnosis prior to surgical intervention. Because other imaging modalities such as echocardiography and magnetic resonance imaging (MRI) can usually provide detailed noninvasive anatomic imaging, diagnostic catheterization is much less commonly performed. Catheterization is now used primarily to determine specific aspects of cardiovascular physiology. A variety of catheterization-based interventional techniques are now a much more frequent activity than diagnostic catheterization in the pediatric cardiac catheterization laboratory.

Diagnostic Catheterization

Cardiac catheterization can be safely performed in infants and children of any size. Conscious sedation or varying degrees of anesthesia are employed depending on the age of the patient, physiologic circumstances, length of anticipated procedure, and planned interventions. Femoral arterial and venous access is usually obtained using percutaneous techniques. In some circumstances, subclavian or internal jugular access is obtained either because of the loss of patency of femoral vessels or because surgically created vascular connections or anticipated interventions require cardiac access from the upper body. The diagnostic portion of catheterizations usually consists of the measurement of pressure in appropriate cardiac chambers, the determination of oxygen saturation in samples obtained from multiple locations, and cardiac or vascular angiography in which radiopaque contrast material is injected into the circulation to demonstrate anatomic details. Specific angiographic catheters are subsequently introduced to outline anatomic details. Most pediatric cardiac catheterization laboratories employ two independently positioned cameras to record angiography, and they are angled to optimize specific aspects of the underlying anatomic abnormalities. Through pressure recordings and saturation measurements, the physiology can be summarized, including quantitation of intracardiac shunting, determination of pressure gradients, and calculation of systemic and pulmonary resistance (Fig. 276-6). In certain circumstances, the effects of some intervention on the physiology may be of interest. For instance, patients with elevated pulmonary vascular resistance may respond favorably to the administration of 100% oxygen. This information is useful in deciding whether a patient is an operative candidate and for identifying those at risk for postoperative complications.

Most patients with straightforward cardiac anatomy no longer require preoperative or postoperative catheterization. Diagnostic catheterization is sometimes necessary in patients with complex disease, particularly to determine pulmonary artery pressure and resistance and distal pulmonary artery or coronary anatomy.

Interventional Catheterization

Nonelectrophysiologic intervention in the catheterization laboratory is categorized into procedures that create or enlarge a communication or channel between cardiac chambers or within an existing vessel, and those intended to eliminate an existing communication or blood vessel.

Balloon Atrial Septostomy

In this procedure, a balloon-tipped catheter is advanced through the venous system into the right atrium and subsequently across the atrial septum, usually by way of a patent foramen ovale, into the left atrium. The balloon is then inflated and withdrawn forcefully into the right atrium, creating a laceration in the atrial septum itself. The procedure is intended to provide an enhanced communication between the atria in situations in which intracardiac mixing is desirable, such as in the patient with simple transposition of the great vessels without significant intracardiac mixing. The performance of balloon atrial septostomy may be lifesaving in these cases. Less commonly, balloon atrial septostomy may be used under other circumstances such as left atrial outlet obstruction in patients with a small or absent left-sided atrioventricular valve. Balloon atrial septostomy can be performed under fluoroscopic or echocardiographic guidance. Although the procedure is relatively safe and effective in the hands of an experienced operator, significant complications include injury to valves, avulsion of pulmonary veins or the inferior vena cava, and air embolization. In most cases, balloon atrial septostomy is a temporizing procedure that allows optimal preparation for a more definitive resection of the atrial septum.

Beyond the newborn period, the creation of an interatrial communication usually requires other techniques. A transseptal puncture can be performed with the use of a very long needle and catheter system introduced through the femoral vein. Once access to the left atrium is obtained, a guidewire is positioned in the left atrium or a pulmonary vein and a balloon dilation catheter is advanced across the atrial septum and inflated to create a persistent communication of variable size. Creation of an atrial septal defect in an older patient may be desirable because of the development of progressive left atrial outlet obstruction or for patients with right-sided heart obstruction in whom some form of right atrial "pop off" is desirable.

Balloon Valvuloplasty

The development of relatively thin balloon-tipped catheters has revolutionized the management of congenital valvular stenosis. This technique was first applied to stenotic pulmonary valves and subsequently to stenotic aortic valves. Balloon dilation may also be helpful in some types of congenital mitral or tricuspid stenosis and has proved to be a very effective management for rheumatic mitral stenosis in countries where rheumatic fever remains endemic. Predilation physiology is determined, primarily by measurement of cardiac output and resting transvalvular gradient. The stenotic valve is crossed either antegrade with a balloon-tipped catheter (pulmonary, tricuspid, or mitral stenosis) or retrograde utilizing a guidewire (aortic stenosis). With a stiff guidewire in position, an appropriately sized dilation catheter is advanced across the stenotic valve. A balloon diameter equivalent to 80% to 120% of the valve annulus is selected. Larger balloons are utilized in the pulmonary position and smaller balloons in the aortic position. As the balloon straddles the valve, it is inflated and a characteristic waist is usually visible owing to indenting of the balloon at the point of valve leaflet fusion. As the balloon is further inflated, the waist disappears when the

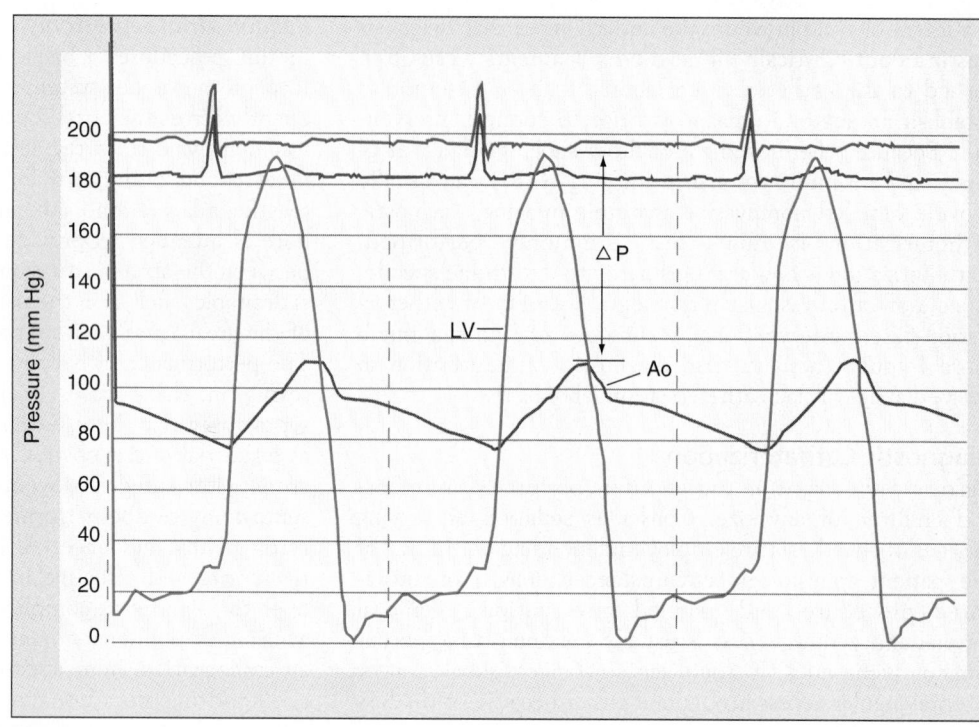

A

Figure 276-6. Pressure recordings determined at cardiac catheterization in a patient with severe aortic stenosis. In the first panel **(A)**, simultaneous left ventricular and aortic pressures are illustrated. The peak left ventricular pressure is approximately 190 mm Hg with a peak aortic pressure of approximately 110 mm Hg leading to a pressure gradient of 80 mm Hg. Following balloon dilation **(B)**, aortic pressure rises to almost 160 mm Hg with a reduction in the peak-to-peak pressure gradient from 80 mm Hg to approximately 30 mm Hg. Ao, aortic pressure; LV, left ventricular pressure; ΔP, peak-to-peak pressure gradient.

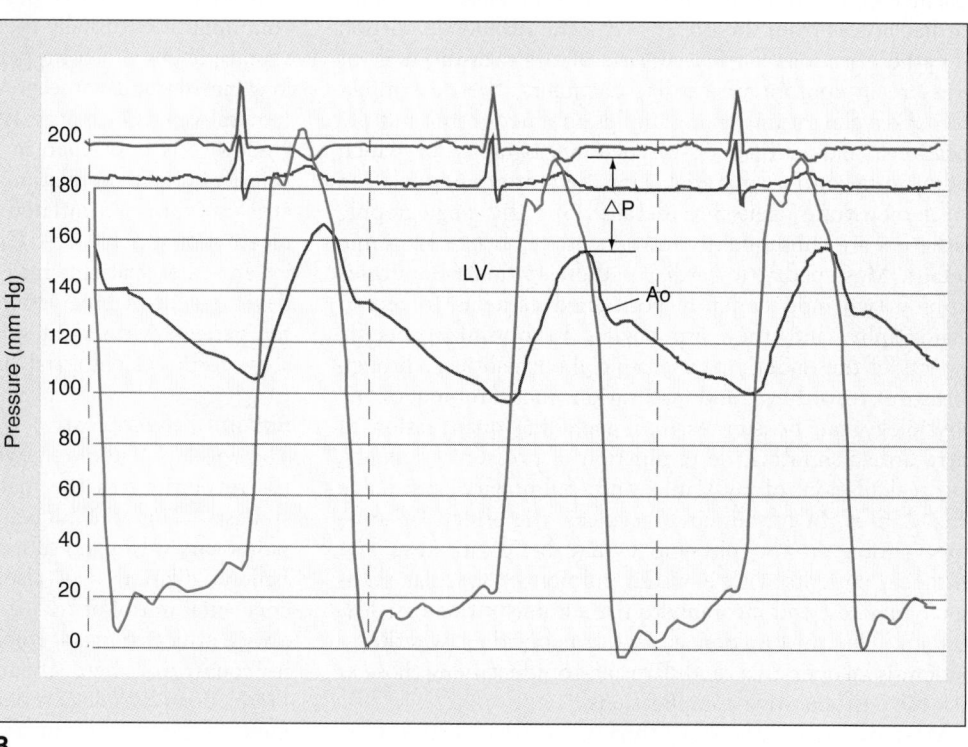

B

valve leaflets separate. Retrograde aortic dilation is technically more difficult because the left ventricle will often eject the inflating balloon before it can fully open within the valve. This is less of a problem using an antegrade approach because the balloon can be stabilized with traction on the catheter. After dilation, postprocedure physiology is determined and the degree of valvular regurgitation induced by the procedure is defined.

Balloon valvuloplasty is a very safe and effective procedure for the management of valvular stenosis. The principal long-term complication of the procedure is the creation of clinically significant valvular regurgitation, a particularly relevant issue for the aortic or mitral valves. Consequently, cautious technique and smaller balloons are indicated when dilating valves on the left side of the heart. Other complications associated with balloon dilation include arrhythmias, balloon rupture, and injury to the peripheral blood vessels because of the relatively large size of the balloon-tipped dilating catheters. Numerous studies demonstrate that the clinical results of balloon dilation are generally equivalent to surgical intervention, both in satisfactory outcome and complications.

Vascular Dilation and Stenting

Hypoplastic or stenotic vessels, either congenital or post-operative, are frequently encountered in association with congenital heart defects. Vessels that are stenotic in a discrete segment or hypoplastic over a short distance are often amenable to dilation with appropriate balloons. Pulmonary arteries are the most commonly dilated. These vessels may be hypoplastic owing to low volume of blood flow during gestation or may have localized scarring and narrowing from prior surgical intervention. Native or post-operative coarctation of the aorta and, less commonly, systemic or pulmonary venous narrowing are also remediable using balloon techniques.

The technique of balloon dilation of peripheral vessels is relatively straightforward, although often the procedure is quite tedious and lengthy because multiple catheter exchanges are required and there may be multiple levels of obstruction. Physiology and detailed angiographic characterization of the narrowing is determined prior to dilation. A balloon two to three times the narrowest diameter of the blood vessel is positioned across the stenosis and fully inflated. Unlike stenotic valves, peripheral vessels often require much higher pressures to fully inflate. High-pressure balloons capable of withstanding inflation pressures of 15 to 20 atm are sometimes used. Following each dilation, pressure measurements and angiograms are performed to assess the results. If hemodynamic and angiographic results are unsatisfactory, a larger balloon is used.

In some circumstances, the elastic nature of the obstruction allows a balloon to inflate easily, but on deflation, the vessel resumes its predilation characteristics. In these cases, a balloon inflatable stent may be useful. These devices consist of a tubular mesh that fits snugly over a balloon and can be positioned across the stenotic region. Upon inflation, the metal mesh expands and locks into a relatively stiff cylinder. Stents can be left in the circulation indefinitely but are often used as a temporizing measure prior to a repeat surgical intervention. Stents have been successfully placed in systemic and pulmonary arterial and venous structures.

Balloon dilation of vessels carries some distinct risks. Inflation of a balloon in a central vessel results in complete obliteration of blood flow and can destabilize hemo-dynamically fragile patients. Use of inappropriate balloon sizes may result in intimal disruption and vascular rupture, sometimes with catastrophic or fatal results. The placement of vascular stents, while theoretically straightforward, may be technically quite difficult. Fracture, migration, or inadvertent deployment in unintended chambers or structures are relatively common complications of stenting procedures.

Closure Devices

A large number of ingenious designs have been developed over the years for the transcatheter closure of blood vessels and septal communications. The most commonly employed device for closure of small or medium-sized blood vessels is the Gianturco embolization coil. These small wire coils have thrombogenic fibers projecting along their length. To embolize a vessel, an appropriate end-hole catheter is positioned in the vessel and a coil is selected of a diameter slightly larger than the vessel at the point of deployment. The coil is pushed from its packaging tube directly into the catheter and advanced through the catheter with the use of a guidewire. As the coil is extruded from the catheter tip, it assumes its predetermined diameter. Multiple coils can be packed together to completely occlude a blood vessel. These coils may also be used to close a small patent ductus arteriosus.

For closure of septal defects or larger blood vessels, a variety of transcatheter devices exist. Most utilize a collapsible wire skeleton and attached occlusive fabric. The device is introduced on one side of a septal defect by advancing through an appropriately positioned catheter. Once a portion of the device has opened on one side of the defect, the catheter is withdrawn and an interlocking or reverse facing portion unfolds on the opposite side of the septum resulting in complete obliteration of the defect. After appropriate position is confirmed by angiography or echocardiography, the device is released. The metal skeleton serves to hold the device in position until endothelialization of the fabric cover or core has been completed. Transcatheter closure devices appear to be an effective alternative to surgical closure of most secundum atrial septal defects. These devices may be helpful in the closure of muscular ventricular septal defects that are difficult or impossible to close using standard surgical approaches. Occasionally, large vessels, valves, and other vascular communications are obliterated using transcatheter methods.

The principal complications associated with the use of closure devices are the result of the rather large delivery systems required, which can result in significant bleeding, vessel injury, or introduction of air into the circulation. Some of these devices embolized early after placement, in most cases the result of using too small a device for the existing opening. Residual shunting around or through the devices is more common than after surgical closure. Some patients have also experienced persistent arrhythmias after placement of these devices in the myocardium.

Nevertheless, these transcatheter closure devices are a valuable adjunct to surgical intervention in some patients with complex cardiovascular abnormalities, and with some refinement of design they are likely to replace certain routine surgical procedures such as closure of secundum atrial septal defects.

Electrophysiologic Testing and Intervention

Box 276-6 lists indications for electrophysiologic testing. Arrhythmia evaluation and treatment is a specific category of diagnostic and interventional catheterization. The introduction of multiple, electrode-tipped catheters to stimulate and map arrhythmias has become commonplace. Through the careful positioning of catheters and recording of the cardiac depolarization sequence, re-entry and ectopic tachycardias can be induced and defined. The presence and location of accessory pathways can be determined and their conduction characteristics clarified. Diagnostic electrophysiologic studies are often performed in patients with Wolff-Parkinson-White syndrome to determine the risk for rapid

Electrophysiologic testing and therapy have become much more sophisticated. The exact nature of arrhythmias can be elucidated, drug efficacy can be tested, and many patients can be cured by the judicious use of catheter techniques. All the diagnostic and therapeutic applications of electrophysiologic diagnosis and intervention in adults are applicable to pediatric patients. In general, most routine testing and intervention is delayed until patients are older than 10 or 12 years of age, although infants and young children can be evaluated and treated if their clinical situation is felt to warrant intervention.

Additional Resources, CD-ROM

Bibliography

ventricular conduction of atrial arrhythmias and, consequently, the likelihood for dangerous ventricular ectopy. Diagnostic studies may also be performed in patients with tachyarrhythmia symptoms that are difficult to control on medications or result in very debilitating symptoms such as syncope or presyncope.

In appropriate patients, a diagnostic electrophysiologic study may proceed to transcatheter ablation of a portion of an arrhythmia circuit or an ectopic focus. This procedure is typically performed in patients with an accessory pathway. With careful electrophysiologic mapping, the approximate location of the pathway is determined and, through radio-frequency heating of the catheter tip, a small burn is delivered to the endocardium with resultant disruption of the underlying aberrant conduction and termination of the arrhythmia risk.

SUGGESTED READINGS

Colan SD: Quantitative applications of Doppler cardiography in congenital heart disease. Cardiovasc Intervent Radiol 1987; 10(6):332–347.
Levine MM: Neurally mediated syncope in children: Results of tilt testing, treatment, and long-term follow-up. Pediatr Cardiol 1999;20(5):331–335.
Rao PS: Interventional pediatric cardiology; state of the art and future directions. Pediatr Cardiol 1998;19(1):107–124.
Rocchini AP: Comparison of risks and short-and long-term results of balloon dilation versus surgical treatment for pulmonary and aortic valve stenosis and restenosis and coarctation and recoarctation of the aorta. Curr Opin Cardiol 1993;5(5):611–618.
Sanders SP: Echocardiography. In Fyler DC (ed): Nadas' Pediatric Cardiology. Philadelphia, Hanley & Belfus, 1992, pp 159–186.

SECTION 9   DIAGNOSTICS AND THERAPEUTICS: *Diagnostics*

277

Electrodiagnostics in Pediatrics

Thomas Koch

ELECTROENCEPHALOGRAPHY

The electroencephalogram (EEG) is an essential part of the diagnostic study of all patients with seizures and those suspected of having seizure. EEG can help in the evaluation of the overall functional integrity of the brain, demonstrating the effects of many systemic disorders on the cerebrum.

Technique

The EEG records spontaneous electrical activity generated by the cerebral cortex, recording the electropotential differences between two points on the scalp under assigned electrodes. An adequate EEG requires a minimum of 10 electrodes placed on the head but most EEGs use 22 electrodes. The electrodes connect to an encephalographic machine that records amplified brain waves as a voltage-versus-time graph. The EEG appears as a number of parallel wavy lines, each line representing a channel or electrical potential between two electrodes. The standard speed of the recording is 3 cm per second. Bipolar recordings measure the electrical activity between two active areas of brain. Referential recordings compare a reference or neutral electrode with an active electrode. Neutral electrode placement is usually on the ear or mastoid. Bipolar recordings permit better localization of electroencephalographic phenomenon. Referential recordings better display patterns of EEG that have widespread distribution. Simultaneous recording of muscle movement, respiratory activity, eye movement, and cardiac activity with the EEG helps define specific portions of the sleep cycle as well as movement artifact.

The completed EEG consists of 150 to 300 or more pages, each representing 10 seconds. The EEG should include notation of movements or other events that may cause artifacts in the recording. The ideal EEG records a patient while awake, asleep, and transitioning between sleep and wakefulness. The routine EEG includes two procedures that may elucidate unusual brain activity. The first is hyperventilation. Having the patient breath deeply for 3 minutes may activate certain seizure types such as absence patterns. Flashing a strobe light approximately 15 inches from the patient's eyes at a frequency of 1 to 20 flashes per second with the patient's eyes open and then closed may also activate seizure patterns. Occipital EEG leads may show waves corresponding to each flash of light (photic driving) or may show abnormal photoconvulsive discharges.

The proper reading of an EEG requires recognition of characteristic age-dependent normal and abnormal patterns, recognition of background rhythm, detection of any changes in rhythm or asymmetries, and differentiating between artifact and true abnormal waves.

Types of Brain Waves

Brain waves, categorized based on their frequency, are classified into four types: alpha, beta, theta, and delta. Alpha waves occur between 8 and 13 Hz, usually in sinusoidal waveform in both occipitoparietal regions, wax and wane spontaneously, and decrease or are suppressed with eye opening or mental activity. The frequency of the alpha rhythm varies individually and increases in frequency as the child matures. Beta waves are faster (18 to 25 Hz) and tend to have a lower amptitude. They are recorded predominantly from more frontal regions and should be relatively symmetric, although some asymmetry may be seen. Theta waves have a frequency of 4 to 7 Hz. They may normally be present over the frontocentral regions and are frequently related to drowsiness. Delta waves are the slowest at 1 to 3 Hz and predominate during sleep.

Normal Electroencephalogram Patterns
Waking Patterns

An important feature of the waking EEG is the dominant background rhythm. The background rhythm should be organized with an anterior-posterior frequency-amplitude gradient. Faster, lower amplitude rhythms predominant over the frontal regions transitioning to slower somewhat higher amplitude rhythms posteriorly (Fig. 277-1). In children this rhythm pattern develops with age. Higher amplitudes tend to be seen in younger children and do not consistently decline until adolescence. A well-developed posteriorly dominant *alpha* rhythm may not be seen until approximately 3 years of age in the majority of children. *Beta* activity is of limited usefulness because asymmetries can occur especially with skull defects and scalp edema. *Beta* activity is also commonly encountered with sedating medications used to premedicate children for an EEG. Approximately 25% of normal children may have posterior *slow waves of youth*, the most common normal *delta* slow activity in the waking EEG of a child. This activity is located primarily over the occipital, parietal, and temporal regions and may have superimposed alpha waves. It will attenuate with eye opening and may be asymmetric. It is rarely seen in children younger than 2 years of age, is maximal between ages 8 and 14 years, and is more common in girls than in boys.

Drowsy and Sleep Patterns

With drowsiness, occipital alpha rhythm disappears and more prominent frontocentral theta and high-voltage paroxysmal rhythmic slow activity develop, a pattern labeled hypnagogic hypersynchrony, a transitional state referred to as stage 1 sleep. With the transition into stage 2 sleep, sharp-wave discharges maximal in amplitude over the vertex (vertex waves) and high-voltage biphasic slow waves

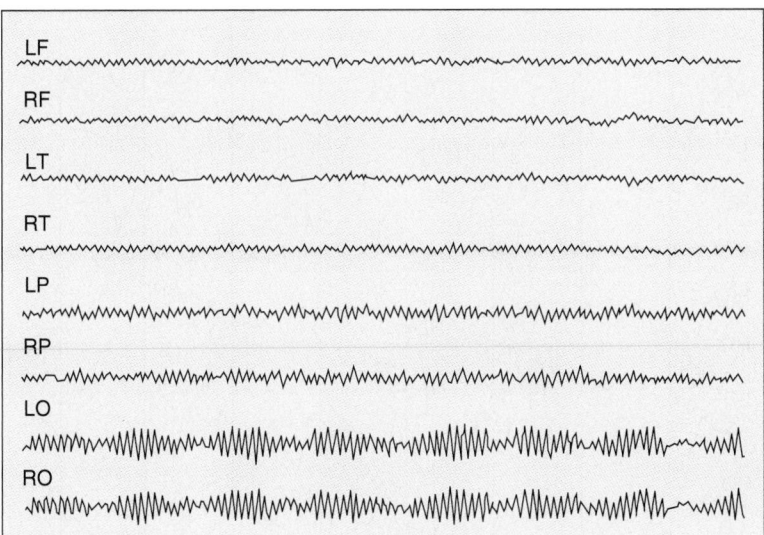

Figure 277-1. Normal electroencephalogram with well-developed posterior alpha rhythm. LF, left frontal; LO, left occipital; LP, left parietal; LT, left temporal; RF, right frontal; RO, right occipital; RP, right parietal; RT, right temporal.

(K complexes) develop. Sleep spindles, bursts of synchronous diphasic waves with a central predominance and a frequency of 12 to 14 Hz, also occur. Sleep spindles may not appear until 3 to 4 months of age and hypnagogic hypersynchrony may not appear until 18 months of age. The duration of sleep spindles is usually less than 4 to 6 seconds. Long duration sleep spindles may be seen in neurologically abnormal children. Positive occipital sharp transients (POSTs) may also occur during this stage of sleep. In deeper stages of sleep (stages 3 and 4), the EEG waveforms become slower until greater than 60% of the record contains delta activity. These stages are frequently called slow-wave sleep. During rapid eye movement (REM) sleep the EEG resembles stage 1 sleep.

Neonatal Electroencephalogram

Interpretation of neonatal EEG is challenging because of its evolving brain wave pattern. Neonatal EEG activity predominates at the vertex, central, and occipital regions. In the normal term infant during wakefulness, the EEG has mixed frequency activity mainly at the 4 to 7 Hz range. Sleep is characterized by a discontinuous pattern of slow activity separated by periods of relative electrocerebral attenuation (trace alternant). This attenuation is more pronounced in the preterm infant. Neonates also frequently have scattered sharp waves in the frontal regions and interhemispheric differences in the amplitude and background frequency.

Specific Findings
Epileptiform Activity

Spikes, sharp waves, and spike-wave discharges, the only forms of EEG activity that correlate with susceptibility to epileptic seizures, have a very high association with clinical seizure disorders. Greater than 80% of children with focal epileptiform discharges have had seizures. This association is even greater if the epileptiform discharges are either multifocal or involve the temporal lobe. The risk of clinical epilepsy is less if they are central (rolandic) or occipital. All epileptiform activity decreases as a function of age. There is no helpful or consistent correlation between the amount of epileptiform activity and the number or intensity of clinical seizures. A single routine EEG may not always demonstrate epileptic activity in an epileptic patient. Subsequent recordings increase the chances of detecting epileptiform activity from 50% to 80% to 90%. A single normal EEG does not exclude the diagnosis of epilepsy in a patient who has had a seizure.

Nonspecific Abnormalities

EEG abnormalities other than epileptiform discharges may be seen in patients with epilepsy and with other nonepileptic neurologic abnormalities. The most common are focal or generalized slowing. Focal slowing may correspond to an underlying focal cerebral lesion and usually warrants further study with neuroimaging studies. Generalized slowing may be associated with a static or reversible encephalopathy and is also seen in many progressive neurologic conditions involving diffuse cortical function. Depending on the clinical situation, further imaging and metabolic studies may be indicated. Less common abnormalities include asymmetry of EEG frequencies and voltage that may be seen with overlying problems with the scalp or skull.

Specific Pediatric Epileptic Syndromes
Infantile Spasms (West Syndrome)

Infantile spasms are typically clustered episodes of generalized massive myoclonus of the infant younger than 2 years of age. They usually have a severe encephalopathy and a severely abnormal EEG. The most characteristic EEG abnormality is called *hypsarrhythmia*, very high-voltage, irregular slow waves with intermixed spikes and polyspikes that occur randomly over the head in an asynchronous fashion (Fig. 277-2). Variations occur and 10% to 15% of infants may have other EEG abnormalities, particularly in older infants. Hypsarrhythmia is more pronounced during slow-wave sleep and may disappear during REM sleep.

Childhood Absence Seizures (Petit Mal Epilepsy)

Typical childhood absence seizures are associated with a characteristic and diagnostic EEG abnormality. With the clinical ictal event there is abrupt onset of a generalized,

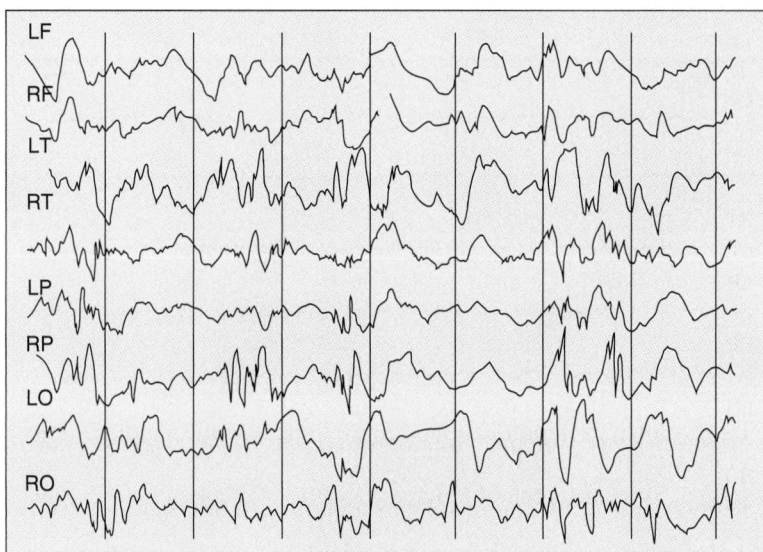

Figure 277-2. Hypsarrhythmia characterized by multifocal sharp waves and spikes in each channel, high-amplitude slow waves, and a poorly organized background rhythm. LF, left frontal; LO, left occipital; LP, left parietal; LT, left temporal; RF, right frontal; RO, right occipital; RP, right parietal; RT, right temporal.

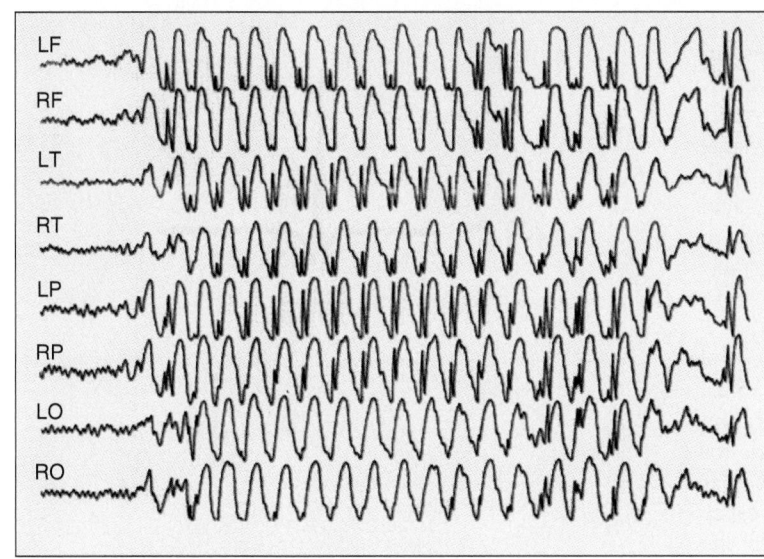

Figure 277-3. Absence electroencephalogram showing a generalized 3 cps spike and wave discharge. LF, left frontal; LO, left occipital; LP, left parietal; LT, left temporal; RF, right frontal; RO, right occipital; RP, right parietal; RT, right temporal.

symmetric stereotyped 3-Hz spike and wave abnormality lasting several seconds and abruptly ending (Fig. 277-3). The background activity before and after the event is usually normal. The clinical and electrical events are often easily precipitated by hyperventilation. Discharge frequencies slightly slower or faster than 3 Hz may be seen with atypical forms of absence seizures.

Lennox-Gastaut Syndrome

The Lennox-Gastaut syndrome is a severe childhood encephalopathy characterized by a difficult seizure disorder with multiple seizure types, mental retardation, and a severely abnormal EEG (Fig. 277-4). The characteristic EEG findings are best seen in children between 2 and 7 years of age and consist of generalized bisynchronous runs of spike, polyspike, and sharp and slow-wave complexes at frequencies of 1.5 to 2.5 Hz. Multifocal spikes and sharp waves frequently occur. Sleep will often activate the epileptic activity. Background activity is almost always abnormal with moderate to severe slowing and poor development of normal age-appropriate patterns. Up to one

third of children may have a preceding history of infantile spasms.

Benign Childhood Epilepsy with Centrotemporal Spikes (Rolandic Epilepsy)

Benign rolandic epilepsy (BRE) is a familial localization-related epilepsy with a characteristic EEG, clinical history, and favorable prognosis. All children with BRE outgrow BRE by 16 years of age. Focal di- and triphasic sharp waves occurring in the central and midtemporal regions are the diagnostic EEG features. These discharges are usually high voltage, tend to occur in clusters, and activate with sleep. On a single EEG they may appear unilateral, but with prolonged recordings or repeated studies they are bilateral, and lateralization may switch from side to side. Generalized spikes and spike-wave activity may occur during sleep. The EEG abnormalities tend to be more impressive than the degree of clinical seizures. Familial studies indicate that the EEG abnormality is genetic with an autosomal dominant pattern, but the epileptic condition appears to have multifactorial inheritance.

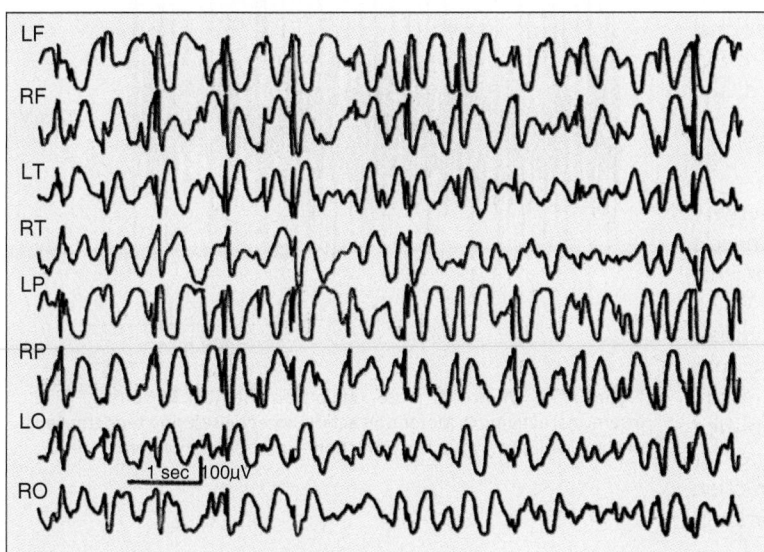

Figure 277-4. Lennox-Gastaut electroencephalogram showing generalized polyspike and sharp and slow-wave complexes on a slow and poorly organized background. LF, left frontal; LO, left occipital; LP, left parietal; LT, left temporal; RF, right frontal; RO, right occipital; RP, right parietal; RT, right temporal.

Juvenile Myoclonic Epilepsy

Juvenile myoclonic epilepsy (JME) is an idiopathic, presumably genetic, generalized epilepsy characterized by generalized 4 to 6 Hz "atypical" spike-wave activity with short bursts of polyspikes and polyspike-waves. Photoparoxysmal responses occur in nearly one third of patients with JME. This condition is very responsive to valproic acid therapy, but unlike rolandic epilepsy, patients tend not to outgrow JME.

ELECTROMYOGRAPHY AND NERVE CONDUCTION VELOCITY

Electrodiagnostics studies utilizing electromyography (EMG) and nerve conduction velocity (NCV) are aids for evaluating the patient with suspected neuromuscular disease. Electrodiagnostic information can help localize pathology along the peripheral nervous system, from the anterior horn cell, to the nerve fiber, the neuromuscular junction, and the muscle. EMG and NCV studies may determine the definitive diagnosis in certain clinical situations or may indicate which studies are necessary for a diagnosis.

Electromyography

Changes in striated muscle membrane polarity can be recorded using a coaxial needle electrode that measures variations in voltage between the tip of an insulated wire and the shaft of the cannula through which it is inserted. The needle electrode allows recording of single motor units rather than the summation of many motor units measured by surface electrodes. The motor unit is the smallest unit that can be activated by a volitional effort. Anatomically, each motor unit consists of a single anterior horn cell, single nerve fiber, and the muscle fibers innervated by that nerve. The number of muscle fibers innervated by a single anterior horn cell varies from 30 for extraocular muscle movement to up to 1700 for limb muscle movement. A needle electrode records between 10 to 20 motor units at one time. The action potential recorded tends to be diphasic or triphasic, measuring 300 μv to 2 mv in amplitude and 4 to 10 msec in duration (Fig. 277-5A). Measurement values of motor unit potentials vary with the size of the motor unit, the muscle tested, and patient age. Well-defined normal motor unit potentials must be established at each EMG laboratory for muscles tested during infancy, childhood, and adulthood.

Normal Electromyogram

A brief burst of electrical activity called insertional activity occurs with insertion of the EMG electrode into the muscle (see Fig. 277-5B). In normal muscle, after the insertional activity there is electrical silence during muscle rest. When the patient contracts slightly, single muscle unit potentials can be seen on the monitor. Measurements and photographs can be obtained for calculations of amplitude and duration. Converting unit potentials to corresponding amplified sound waves may reveal sound patterns distinctive for certain muscle pathologies. Vigorous muscle contraction recruits more motor units, resulting in a blur of markings called an interference pattern (see Fig. 277-5C).

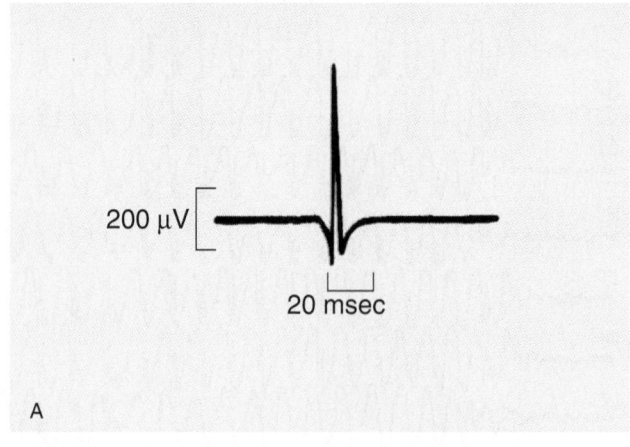

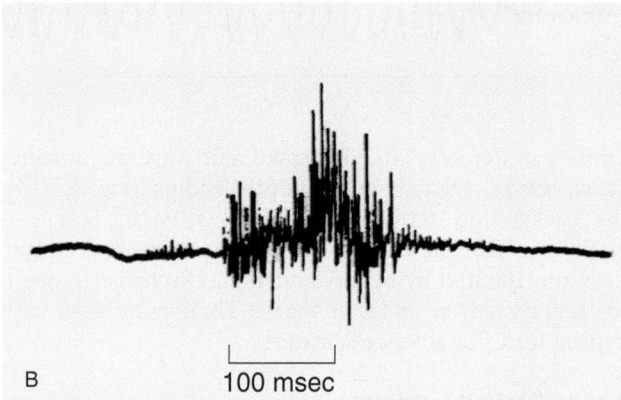

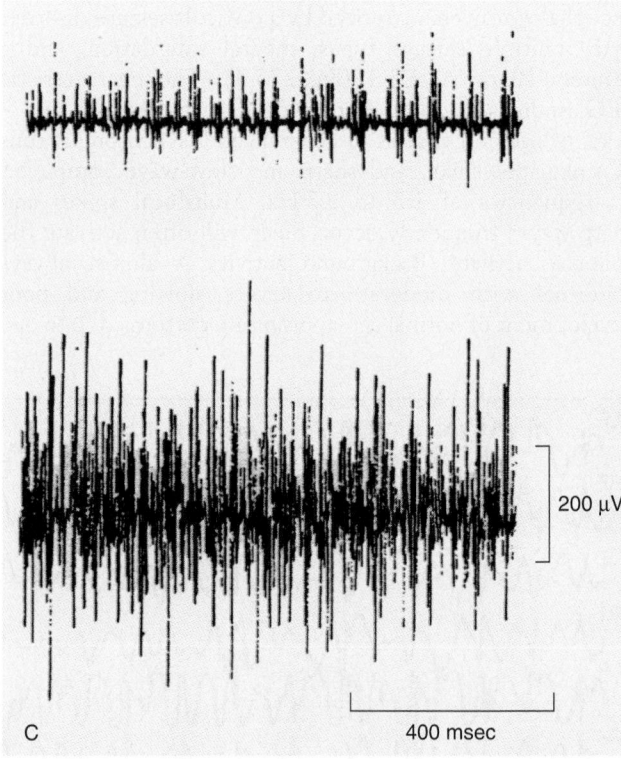

Figure 277-5. A, Normal motor unit action potential. **B,** Normal insertional activity. **C,** Motor unit action potentials during moderate and maximal voluntary muscle contraction—interference pattern.

Abnormal Electromyogram

Increased irritability occurs with *denervation* in the muscle, resulting in abnormally prolonged insertional activity. Collateral sprouting from normal axons innervating denervated cells creates larger and more complex motor units. Because of the loss of axons and motor units the interference pattern with maximal contraction will be decreased. Ten to 20 days after denervation, fibrillations will be seen as small (50 to 100 μv), brief (<2 msec) irritable depolarizations in the resting state. Long duration (100 to 200 msec) positive sharp waves are frequently seen in association with fibrillations.

Primary myopathies such as the muscular dystrophies are characterized by a decreased number of functional muscle cells in a motor unit, manifested by a small amplitude motor unit with short duration. Because most motor units remain active, an interference pattern with maximal contraction will be preserved. In *myotonic disorders* such as myotonic dystrophy or myotonia congenita, movement of the electrode or muscle relaxation frequently results in a high-frequency burst of single cell and single motor unit discharges lasting 15 to 30 seconds. A sound like an old-fashioned "dive bomber" occurs when monitored using sound amplification.

Polymyositis and *dermatomyositis* contain features frequently seen with both denervation and primary muscle disease. Spontaneous fibrillations with positive sharp waves, myopathic action potentials (small amplitude, short duration), and pseudomyotonia with bursts of repetitive action potential, which abruptly cease, form the common triad of action potential wave patterns seen in polymyositis.

Nerve Conduction Velocity Studies

NCV is measured by stimulating a nerve at two separate points and measuring the time to muscle reaction. The difference between the two velocities is the conduction of the nerve. In the pediatric population, the most important factor affecting NCV is age. Infants have slower conduction velocities than older children and adults because of differences in myelin development.

Abnormal Nerve Conduction

Severe neuropathies cause slowed conduction velocities. NCVs are most useful with compression and entrapment neuropathies. The carpal tunnel syndrome is a common example of when the NCV can be diagnostic.

Repetitive Nerve Stimulation

Assessment of the neuromuscular junction conduction can be made by repetitive stimulation of a motor nerve and recording action potentials over the appropriate muscle. If the action potential rapidly decreases in size with repetitive stimulation at rates between 1 and 30 per second, a defect in neuromuscular transmission is suspected. This is typically seen with myasthenia gravis. Infant botulism tends to cause the opposite pattern with an incremental or "staircase" response to repetitive stimulation at 20 to 50 Hz. Initial repetitive nerve stimulation studies for early infant botulism may be falsely negative, so repeating the studies is necessary if there is a high index of suspicion for this disease.

SUGGESTED READINGS

American EEG Society: Guidelines in EEG and evoked potentials: Guideline 7: A proposal for standard montages to be used in clinical EEG. J Clin Neurophysiol 1986;3(suppl 1):26–33.

Binnie CD, Stefan H: Modern electrophysiology: Its role in epilepsy management. Clin Neurophysiol 1999;110:1671–1697.

Browne TR, Holmes GL: Handbook of Epilepsy, 2nd ed. Philadelphia, Lippincott Williams & Wilkins, 2000.

Nordli DR, Pedley TA: The use of electroencephalography in the diagnosis of epilepsy in children. In Pellock JM, Dodson WE, Bourgeois BFD (eds): Pediatric Epilepsy: Diagnosis and Therapy, 2nd ed. New York, Demos, 2001, pp 117–132.

Olney RK: Electrodiagnostic evaluation of neuromuscular diseases. In Berg BO (ed): Principles of Child Neurology. New York, McGraw-Hill, 1996, pp 51–66.

SECTION 9   DIAGNOSTICS AND THERAPEUTICS: *Diagnostics*

278

Allergy and Skin Testing

Edward Kent

Proper use of allergy diagnostic tests requires understanding the relationship of allergen to the immunopathogenesis of the allergic disorder. Gell and Coombs developed a widely accepted classification of immunologic reactions that serves as a useful framework for discussing allergy diagnostics (Table 278-1). Type I responses are IgE-mediated, immediate-type hypersensitivity. Type II describes cytotoxic antibody responses. Type III is antigen-antibody immune complex formation. Type IV is delayed hypersensitivity. Allergic disorders may involve any combination of these responses in the susceptible individual. Although "allergy" may refer to any of these immunologic responses,

Table 278-1. Gell and Coombs Classification of Immunologic Responses

Class	Description	Clinical Examples
Type I	Immediate (IgE mediated)	Anaphylaxis, rhinitis, conjunctivitis, asthma
Type II	Cytotoxic/cytolytic (IgG and IgM antibody mediated)	Autoimmune hemolytic anemia, thrombocytopenia, granulocytopenia from penicillin
Type III	Immune complex mediated	Serum sickness
Type IV	Delayed (cell mediated)	Contact dermatitis

the term *allergy* often refers to immediate hypersensitivity IgE-mediated reactions.

The most useful tests for the diagnosis of allergic disease are determinations for specific IgE antibody. Skin testing is sensitive, safe, rapid, and economical. When skin testing is not available or possible, in vitro testing is useful. The identification of specific allergens assists in diagnosis and management of the allergic diseases.

ROLE OF DIAGNOSTIC TESTS IN ALLERGIC DISEASE

Discovery of IgE antibody to allergens must be correlated with the clinical condition under study. Investigations for specific IgE antibody may help diagnose specific allergens, guide environmental modifications, guide pharmacotherapy, and determine allergen immunotherapy. However, a thorough allergy history is crucial to determining and interpreting allergy diagnostics because the presence of IgE antibody to an allergen does not necessarily demonstrate disease. IgE antibody may exist prior to development of clinical disease, or persist after sensitivity to the allergen has resolved. IgE antibody may also be detected in the absence of any clinically relevant disorder (immunologic allergy without clinical allergy).

IgE antibody should be investigated in disorders in which immediate hypersensitivity responses are relevant to their pathogenesis. Table 278-2 lists disorders that may involve immediate hypersensitivity responses to relevant allergens.

Table 278-2. Disorders in Which IgE Determinations May Be Relevant

Respiratory infection
  Asthma
  Rhinitis
  Conjunctivitis
  Sinusitis
Skin disorder
  Atopic dermatitis
  Urticaria
Systemic disorder
  Food allergy
  Insect sting hypersensitivity
Drug reaction
  Penicillin
  Local anesthetic reactions
  Latex
Anaphylaxis

TESTING FOR IMMEDIATE HYPERSENSITIVITY RESPONSES

Skin testing for detection of specific IgE antibodies is the most widely performed method because of its simplicity, rapid results, low cost, and high sensitivity. Skin testing introduces allergen to mast cells in the skin. If IgE antibody to that allergen is present in the test subject, cross-linking of the IgE onto the mast cell surface occurs, leading to mast cell activation and histamine release. A wheal and flare develop, demonstrating presence of IgE antibody specific for that allergen (Fig. 278-1).

Most allergen extracts have the active allergen suspended in sterile aqueous solutions containing human serum albumin saline diluent (HSA) or plain buffered or phenol saline. Other extract preparations include alum-precipitated extracts (made by precipitating raw resource material or allergenic proteins with a solution of aluminum hydroxide) and alum-precipitated, pyridine-extracted extracts. The concentration of the allergen extract is usually listed in protein nitrogen units per milliliter (PNU/mL) or weight per volume (W/V). In an effort to standardize allergen extracts to better reflect allergenic potency, the Food and Drug Administration (FDA) uses allergy unit (AU) and bioequivalent allergy unit (BAU) designations based on in vivo testing of allergen extracts. The W/V, PNU/mL, AU/mL, and BAU/mL products are not interchangeable. When transferring a patient from one manufacturer's product to another, the dosage should be cut back. The two methods for skin testing are epicutaneous (prick) testing and intracutaneous (intradermal) testing. Box 278-1 compares the two methods.

Epicutaneous (Prick) Testing

Epicutaneous testing introduces a small amount of allergen into cleansed skin by lightly pressing a needle at a 45-degree angle into the superficial epidermis, releasing a drop of allergen, and lifting the skin, thereby producing a "pricking" sensation. The puncture technique, a variation of epicutaneous testing, involves pressing a device into the skin through a drop of allergen, creating a small puncture. Each "prick" or "puncture" must be compared to positive and negative control tests to confirm significant reactions. Histamine or codeine phosphate are appropriate materials for positive control tests; the diluent, usually saline, is appropriate for negative control tests. Comparing the increasing degrees of wheal and flare responses at the test sites to the negative control determines the test score. Tests are interpreted 15 to 20 minutes following allergen application (Table 278-3). Operator technique and patient cooperation

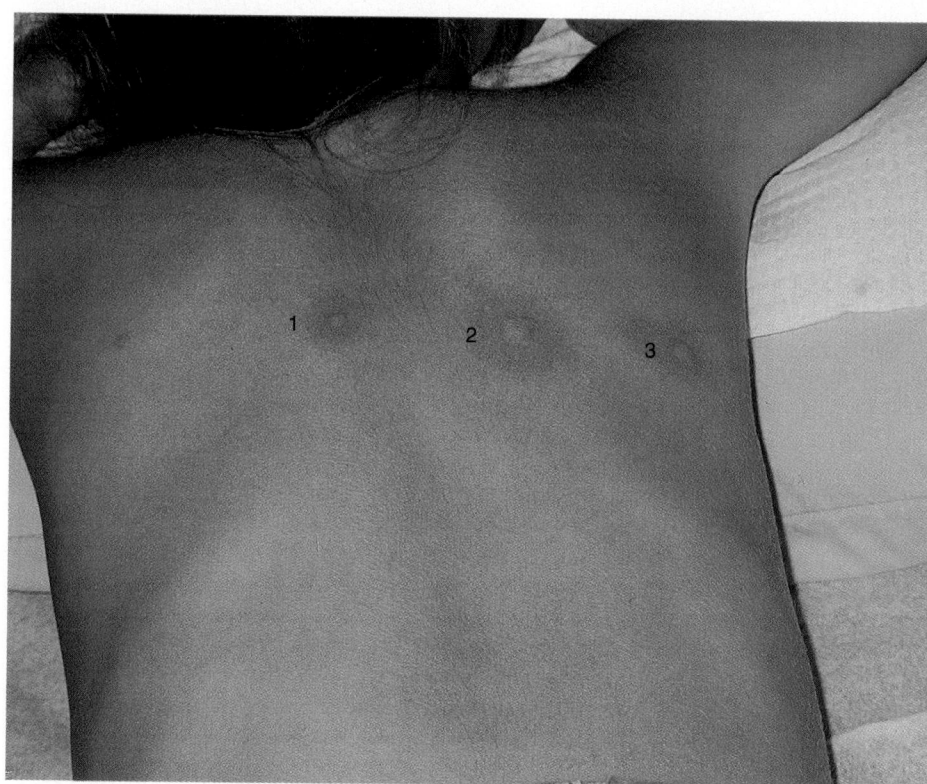

Figure 278-1. Skin test. Wheal and flare reaction more pronounced in *2* than in *1*.

affect results depending on depth of prick or puncture and amount of allergen introduced. The usual sites for epicutaneous testing are the back or forearms. The upper back is more reactive than the forearm.

Epicutaneous testing is quite sensitive for detection of IgE. False-negative rates are about 5% depending on the quality of the allergen extract. The risk of an adverse reaction to prick skin testing is low, with no reported fatalities.

Intracutaneous Testing

Intracutaneous testing has a higher degree of sensitivity, but reduced specificity (increased number of false-positive reactions). Intracutaneous testing is performed when suspicion of sensitivity is present but negative epicutaneous tests have been obtained. Intracutaneous testing is particularly useful when drug or venom sensitivity must be excluded. Intracutaneous testing should be performed only following negative epicutaneous testing to minimize the risk of systemic reaction. Intracutaneous testing is inappropriate

for food allergy testing because it has high false-positive rates for food allergies and it carries an increased risk of systemic reaction in individuals sensitive to food allergens. Systemic reactions occur in approximately 1% to 2% of individuals with intracutaneous testing, primarily in those who did not receive prior prick skin testing.

Intracutaneous testing involves injecting 0.05 mL of allergen into the skin with a 26- to 30-gauge needle. Injecting with the bevel directed downward prevents superficial leakage of the allergen. Allergen injections must be intradermal; deeper subcutaneous injections risk false-negative results. Appropriate positive and negative control sites should be used. Intracutaneous testing is routinely performed on the upper outer arm.

Skin Testing Precautions

Properly performed skin testing is quite safe. However, certain safety precautions are necessary. Skin testing requires the presence of a physician and personnel familiar with treating anaphylaxis and readily available emergency equipment and medications. Testing should be deferred if the patient is experiencing marked asthma signs and

---

Box 278-1. Comparison of Methods for Skin Testing

Epicutaneous (Prick)

Faster
Less painful
Better specificity
Lower risk for causing systemic allergic reaction

Intracutaneous (Intradermal)

More sensitive
More reproducible
More useful for excluding allergen sensitivity

Table 278-3. Skin Test Scores for Epicutaneous Testing

Description	Reaction
No flare, no wheal over negative control	–
Slight flare > negative control, no wheal	+/–
Flare > negative control, no wheal	+
Wheal <3 mm over negative control	++
Wheal ≥3 mm over negative control	+++
Wheal ≥3 mm over negative control and pseudopods present	++++

symptoms. Epicutaneous testing should precede intracutaneous testing. Particular caution must be exercised in utilizing extracts of high potency (peanut, tree nuts) or unknown potency (latex), especially in individuals suspected of high sensitization (history of anaphylaxis). Further dilution of skin test materials or modifications of the prick technique to introduce less allergen may be appropriate for patients suspected of high allergen sensitivity. Pregnancy is a relative contraindication to skin testing because an allergic reaction induced by the testing process may compromise the pregnancy. Skin testing may not be possible in patients with generalized skin disorders (severe atopic dermatitis) if suitable surface area for the testing procedure is unavailable.

Factors Affecting Skin Response

Table 278-4 lists factors that affect skin test response and interpretation of results. Skin test reactivity increases from infancy through adulthood and then declines after approximately age 50 years. Children younger than 2 years of age have a high propensity to develop skin flares with just the application of the skin test. This reaction and the likelihood of poor cooperation make skin testing in this age group difficult. Infants and toddlers rarely sensitize to pollens until later in life, owing to infrequent/inadequate exposure to the seasonal allergens. Perennial inhalant allergens such as animal danders, dust mites, and molds may induce early sensitization. Testing for allergy to perennial allergens may be appropriate for infants and toddlers with severe atopic dermatitis or asthma. Infants and toddlers may also sensitize to foods early in life.

Medications may also affect skin test results. Antihistamines suppress skin test reactivity for variable time periods. The "classic" first-generation antihistamines (e.g., diphenhydramine) suppress skin test reactions for up to 3 days. The newer second-generation antihistamines (loratadine, fexofenadine, cetirizine) must be stopped for at least 3 days or longer before attempting skin testing. The second-generation antihistamine astemizole may suppress skin reactivity for up to 60 days. H_2 blockers, tricyclic antidepressants, prolonged use of topical steroids, and some phenothiazine preparations may also diminish skin test reactivity. Using a positive control substance that should cause a reaction will indicate whether a medication is having an effect on skin test reactivity. Oral steroids do not have a significant effect on skin test reactivity.

Dermatographia may exist in up to 5% of the general population. The process of applying the epicutaneous test will induce a wheal and flare response in these individuals. For patients with dermatographia, mild responses to allergen pricks must be compared to the negative control test results to determine if the test response is significant. On occasion intracutaneous testing may be performed without inducing the dermatographia response.

ALLERGENS SUITABLE FOR SKIN TESTING

Choosing test allergens depends on likelihood of exposure to those allergens in the geographic location specific to the patient's area of residence and travel. Allergen extracts must be of suitable composition and stability.

House dust mites are the major indoor allergens responsible for allergic respiratory disease. The two major dust mite species in the United States causing allergic respiratory disease are *Dermatophagoides farinae* and *D. pteronyssinus*.

Exposure to animal dander is unavoidable in our society. Domestic pets are prevalent in many households. Cat dander allergy is common and cat dander is widespread. Cat dander on students' clothing can spread within a public school to levels similar to those in a home where a cat resides. The major allergen responsible for cat allergy is Fel *d* 1. Cat pelt or cat epithelium serves as a source for testing extracts.

Dog allergy is less common than cat allergy. Dog allergens responsible are less well defined than cat allergens. Can *f* 1 is probably the major dog allergen, which is common to all breeds. Breed-specific allergens may exist as well. Despite claims to the contrary, there is no hypoallergenic breed of dogs. Skin tests are available for other animal danders including horse, rabbit, mice, gerbil, hamster, rat, and guinea pig. However, these tests are not standardized and have variable allergen content. Allergy to any furred animal increases likelihood of allergy to other furred animals.

Airborne pollens are a leading source of morbidity for children and adults with atopic diseases. The anemophilous (wind-pollinated) plants produce widespread dispersion of their pollens into the environment and are responsible for the majority of the pollen-related illnesses (allergic rhinoconjunctivitis, asthma). The entemorphous (insect-pollinated) plants are less common sources for sensitization because exposure to this pollen is limited. The nonvisible pollens from trees, grasses, and weeds are mostly responsible for causing allergic symptoms and not lilacs, roses, and other flowering plants that are commonly mistaken as the sources of pollen-induced symptoms.

Trees pollinate in the late winter and spring and are a major cause of allergy symptoms during that time. Pollinating seasons and responsible allergens vary with geographic location (Table 278-5). In North America, birch, beech, oak, and maple pollen are major sources of sensitization. In Texas and parts of the Southwest, mountain cedar allergies are prevalent. Olive tree pollen is a strong allergen. Allergy is specific for individual tree pollen and does not cross-react with other tree pollens, as is seen with grass allergies.

Table 278-4. Factors Affecting Skin Test Response

Factor	Effect
Age of patient	Infants elderly less reactive
Patient IgE titer	High titer more reactive
Skin test site	Upper back most responsive
Quality of extracts	Unstandardized for many allergens
Storage of materials	Allergen may be temperature sensitive
Nature of the allergen	Fruit/vegetable extracts may not capture labile allergens
Dermatographia	Nonspecific response to testing procedure
Use of medications	Antihistamines, tricyclic antidepressants inhibit skin test response for variable periods
Test method	Epicutaneous more specific Intracutaneous more sensitive
Operator technique	False-positive and false-negative results

Table 278-5. Pollen Seasons in Northern, Central, and Southern United States

Pollen	Northern	Central	Southern
Tree pollen	March–June	February–June	January–June
Grass pollen	May–August	April–September	March–October
Weed pollen	July–October	July–October	July–November
Ragweed pollen	August–October	August–October	August–November

Grass pollens provide widespread and ubiquitous pollen allergens. Pollinating seasons vary markedly with geographic location. The grass pollinating season has a specific start and finish in the North, between mid-May to mid-July, but lasts longer with less defined beginning and end in other areas of the country. Grass pollens are highly cross-reactive, and sensitization to multiple grass species is typical. Common grass pollen allergens include bluegrasses, orchard grass, timothy grass, and red top. In eastern United States, perennial ryegrass and sweet vernal grass allergens are increasingly present. Bermuda grass is primarily a Southern grass.

Weed pollens are common allergens. Ragweed is the major late summer and fall weed pollen allergen. Although the highly visible goldenrod plant appears at the time when ragweed is most abundant and can be a source of pollen allergens, ragweed is the usual culprit of late summer–fall allergies. A heavy frost finishes ragweed pollination season.

Molds or airborne spores and other fungal particles universally occur over nonpolar landmasses, and often form the majority of suspended airborne biogenic debris. Airborne levels may be especially high in areas of field crops. Fungi can survive and sporulate in a wide range of temperatures. Moisture is required for all species, yet some are tolerant to drying. Levels of many ballistospore species will increase with rainfall, fog, and damp conditions. Direct wind can detach spores of other fungi, such as *Cladosporium*, *Alternaria*, *Epicoccum*, and *Helminthosporium*, thereby increasing spore levels when wind speed rises and relative humidity falls. Increased levels of *Alternaria* in the autumn air are associated with asthma exacerbation.

Cockroach allergens can induce allergic respiratory diseases. Frequently, skin test reactivity to cockroach appears in individuals with asthma.

Biting insect reactions are generally not IgE-mediated and represent a direct irritant or toxic effect of the bite. Though rare, biting insects may induce allergic sensitization and IgE-mediated reactions as indicated by reports of allergic antibody reactions for black fly, mosquito, deer fly, and other biting insects. Availability of reliable allergen extracts limits skin testing for biting insects.

Venom of stinging insects, belonging to the Hymenoptera order, including apids, vespids, and formicids, can induce IgE sensitization and cause allergic reactions. Testing materials are readily available for the stinging insects most frequently involved in allergic reactions. Extract materials include honeybee and bumblebee (apids), yellow jackets, yellow- and white-faced hornets, and wasps (vespids). There is also testing material for the fireants (formicids).

Food allergens are frequently associated with atopic dermatitis, anaphylaxis, and urticaria. Because food allergen test materials are not standardized, results of skin testing for food allergy must consider the variability of the potency and quality of the extracts used. In general, the extracts for peanut, tree nuts, cow milk, soy, shellfish, finned fish, chicken eggs, and grains are of high quality. Extracts for many fruits and vegetables are of uncertain quality. Skin testing for allergy to fruits and vegetables may involve using fresh food extracts that allows capture of labile allergens. In prick testing, a testing device first extracts a direct sample of the food and then injects the extract into the patient. The reliability of food prick testing is related to the quality of extract as well as operator training and technique, device used, age of patient, and experience of interpreter. Positive and negative control tests are used to assist in ensuring quality.

Skin testing for drug allergies is limited to those drugs with identifiable antigens. Medications that induce allergic reactions frequently form haptens or metabolic breakdown products that act as antigens. Skin testing with the native drug may not induce reaction because the relevant allergen is absent. The only available antibiotic medication antigens for skin testing are the major and minor metabolic products of penicillin associated with allergic reactions. Skin tests for individual cephalosporins are of unknown sensitivity and specificity.

Skin testing for several general anesthetic agents is possible, and protocols for evaluation of local anesthetic allergy exist. Open challenge with the anesthetic agent should follow negative skin test results if allergy to that anesthetic agent is strongly suspected.

There are currently no standardized skin tests for latex allergy available in the United States. Extracts can be prepared by exposing a latex source (e.g., gloves) to a vehicle (e.g., saline) and using the mixture for skin testing. In addition to unknown sensitivity and specificity, the potency of these extracts is unknown. Testing with these extracts carries the risk of inducing an anaphylactic response in a highly sensitized individual. In vitro testing for latex is available, yet sensitivity and specificity is variable, with the best assays achieving no greater than 85% for both sensitivity and specificity.

IN VITRO TESTING FOR SPECIFIC IgE ANTIBODIES

Tests for detecting allergen-specific IgE antibodies involve placing an allergen in serum to see if IgE antibodies within the serum combine with the allergen. Various methods measure the resulting allergen-IgE antibody complex. The earliest of these tests was called radioallergosorbent test (RAST) and this term is often incorrectly used to refer to any test for serum IgE determination, regardless of method.

Results are expressed in a variety of ways, depending on the particular laboratory. Ratios of test to normal serum may be calculated, with 2.5 or higher considered positive. Class scores of 0 to 5 may be reported, with class 0 nondetectable, and increasing classes demonstrating increasing levels of IgE antibody. Direct specific IgE levels may be reported. One international unit (IU) = 2.4 ng protein. The sensitivity of in vitro tests may vary with the individual allergen tested. There is also variation among laboratories. In some assays sensitivity of 70% to 80% compared to skin tests is reported, whereas in other laboratories correlation of less than 50% exist. In almost all circumstances sensitivity of in vitro tests is less than that of skin tests.

COMPARISON OF IN VITRO AND SKIN TESTING

Skin testing offers rapid and sensitive determination of allergic status and is less expensive than in vitro testing. In certain circumstances, however, in vitro testing may be preferred. The patient may be unable to discontinue medications that may suppress skin test responses. There may be extensive dermatitis with insufficient normal skin surface area to perform testing. Skin testing for food allergy in a patient with exquisite sensitivity to foods may provoke anaphylaxis. Dermatographia may make interpretation of skin testing difficult. Specialist referral for skin testing may be limited. In these circumstances in vitro tests may offer advantages.

OTHER METHODS FOR DETERMINING ALLERGIES

Eosinophil Counts

Eosinophils are primary cells involved in the allergic response. Infiltration of eosinophils into tissues is a characteristic of most allergic disorders. Quantitation of eosinophils from peripheral blood, nasal secretions, and sputum may help the evaluation and management of allergic disease.

Elevation of peripheral eosinophil count is suggestive but not diagnostic of allergic disease. Many patients with allergic rhinitis and asthma will have elevation in their peripheral eosinophil count, although this may occur even in the absence of a direct allergic triggering.

A nasal smear can be useful in evaluating the patient with rhinitis. A preponderance of eosinophils in secretions suggests allergic rhinitis, or nonallergic rhinitis with eosinophilia. Nasal secretions may be collected by having the individual blow the nose into wax paper, then smearing the secretions on a glass slide, and using Giemsa or Wright stain for examination under the microscope.

Sputum eosinophilia often occurs in both allergic and nonallergic asthma, but is of limited diagnostic value.

Mast Cell Mediators

Histamine and tryptase are two of many chemicals released from mast cells upon activation. Measuring serum levels of these mediators may be useful in diagnosis of disorders involving systemic mast cell release such as anaphylaxis and systemic mastocytosis.

Histamine is rapidly released into the circulation following mast cell and basophil activation. It is rapidly cleared from serum and can be detected only shortly after its release. Its presence does not distinguish between mast cell and basophil sources. Tryptase is released specifically from mast cells and therefore serves as a marker of mast cell activation. It can be detected in serum for several hours after the event.

Unproved Techniques

Inappropriate skin tests would include testing for substances that do not induce an IgE response such as tobacco smoke. House dust extracts contain a wide variety of potential allergens, and with the identification of house dust mites as the major dust allergen, testing with preparations made from house dust is no longer appropriate.

In vitro testing for IgG_4 subclasses to foods is purported to demonstrate allergy to these foods. These antibodies naturally occur and exist in all individuals. There is no correlation with any known disease state, and this type of testing is of no proved value. Detection of IgG_4 subclass antibody to specific foods frequently leads to unnecessary dietary restrictions, and therefore may promote nutritional deficiencies.

Other unproved tests of no known value include basophil degranulation assays, cytotoxic food tests, and applied kinesiology.

NONIMMUNOLOGIC RESPONSES MIMICKING ALLERGIC RESPONSES

A number of untoward events may occur upon exposure to inhalants, drugs, insect bites, insect stings, and foods. These events may mimic immunologic hypersensitivity reactions but result from different underlying mechanisms (Table 278-6). Evaluation for IgE antibody is not useful in these situations. Understanding the likely pathogenesis avoids unnecessary diagnostic testing, dietary restrictions, environmental changes, and pharmacotherapy.

Anti-IgE Antibody

Humanized monoclonal anti-IgE antibody has been used in clinical trials for patients with asthma. Administration of the anti-IgE antibody by intravenous and subcutaneous routes has demonstrated an improvement in asthma and reduced medication use to maintain control, primarily in people with severe asthma who require oral steroid therapy. Anti-IgE antibody dosing and administration are still being defined, and its use may expand to other patient indications.

Other atopic diseases may benefit from anti-IgE antibody therapy. For patients with food allergy, anti-IgE antibody therapy might reduce the degree of allergic response upon chance food allergen exposure. Reduction of IgE levels by anti-IgE antibody therapy might also reduce the risk of anaphylactic reaction during administration of conventional immunotherapy.

Peptide Immunotherapy

Immunotherapy is the only available means of altering the host allergic response to inhaled allergens. Subcutaneous injection of allergens to which the patient is sensitive can induce a down-regulation of the immune response directed against those allergens, and thereby reduce patient

Table 278-6. Nonimmune Responses Mimicking Allergy

Circumstance	Symptoms Mimicking Allergy	Mechanism of Response
Milk/dairy ingestion	Cramps and diarrhea	Lactose intolerance
Tobacco smoke exposure	Asthma type response	Irritant
Fish ingestion	Flushing, gastrointestinal symptoms	Scromboid poisoning
Vancomycin infusion	Redman syndrome	Pseudoallergic
Milk ingestion	Nasal congestion	Nonspecific
Chocolate ingestion	Hyperactivity	Caffeine drug toxic response
Insect bite	Swelling and itching	Toxic response
Dust exposure	Rhinorrhea, congestion	Irritant response
Radiocontrast dye exposure	Urticaria, anaphylaxis	Direct mast cell mediator release

symptoms on exposure. These improvements may persist after the completion of the immunotherapy course. The most effective immunotherapy requires administration of high doses of allergens to achieve tolerance. This therapy carries a risk of inducing an anaphylactic response during administration of allergen extracts, which limits its usefulness. Anaphylaxis results when mast cells are activated by allergen binding surface IgE. The beneficial effect of immunotherapy is thought to be the result of a T-cell mediated tolerance to the allergen. Administering small peptide fragments of the native allergen can reduce the risk of inducing an anaphylactic response. These peptides are recognized by the T cell and are able to induce the tolerance effect, but do not bind to IgE, and therefore do not activate the mast cell and cause anaphylaxis. Precise recognition of the relevant peptide segments is necessary for effectiveness.

Another strategy to improve immunogenicity while reducing allergenicity of immunotherapy involves use of immunostimulatory sequence oligodeoxynucleotides. These are repetitive short sequences of bacterial DNA, also known as CpG motifs, and are potent inducers of T_H1 immune responses. They also may prevent T_H2 responses, or divert existing T_H2 responses. Conjugation of immunostimulatory DNA sequences with native allergen may allow for improved immunologic response with a reduced chance of inducing an allergic response.

Peptide immunotherapy and use of immunostimulatory DNA are two strategies that may allow for a safer and more effective means of administering immunotherapy, thereby expanding the role of immunotherapy in the care of allergic disease by intervening at a fundamental level in the allergic response.

T_H1 and T_H2 Hygiene Hypothesis
The incidence of allergic disease has been increasing in Westernized industrial societies. Evidence suggests this may be related to a reduced number of infections and decreased exposure to microbial antigens during childhood, most likely a consequence of indoor plumbing, antibiotic use, change from an agricultural to an industrial society, and cleaner, more energy-efficient homes. Reduced exposure to microbial antigens and products such as endotoxin and immunostimulatory bacterial DNA may lead to a decrease or altered production of regulatory cytokines, thereby altering the balance or degree of T_H1- and T_H2-meditated responses and allowing development of allergic disease. Identifying factors that may promote the development of the allergic immune response may allow for medical intervention at an early and fundamental level.

SUGGESTED READINGS

Kaplan AP: Allergy, 2nd ed. Philadelphia, WB Saunders, 1997.
Middleton E Jr, Reed CE, Ellis EF, et al: Allergy Principles and Practice, 5th ed. St. Louis, Mosby, 1998.

279 Adherence

Doreen Matsui

DEFINITION

Efficacious drug therapy is now available for pediatric patients with many acute and chronic illnesses; however, to benefit from these treatments children must actually take, or be given, their medication. *Compliance*, a term which is often used interchangeably with *adherence*, is most commonly defined as the extent to which a person's behavior, in this instance the taking of prescribed drugs, coincides with medical and health advice. General consensus as to the dividing line between adherence and nonadherence does not exist. It may be more practical to think in terms of what degree of compliance is required for an adequate therapeutic outcome.

Although noncompliance can take many forms, delayed or omitted doses are the most common errors. Discontinuation of medication administration before completion of the course is also common as adherence wanes as symptoms resolve. "Drug holidays," defined as 3 or more drug-free days, are often associated with times of interruption of daily habits such as holidays and weekends and can also be associated with breakthrough clinical events. Improvement in drug compliance, known as the "toothbrush effect" or "white coat compliance," may occur before an anticipated scheduled medical appointment. In addition to whether or not patients take their medications, it may also be important to consider whether patients fill their prescriptions, as the initial step in adherence is to actually obtain the medication.

SCOPE OF PROBLEM OF POOR ADHERENCE

Although the prevalence of medication adherence problems varies depending on the criteria used for defining acceptable adherence and the method of assessment, studies in children suggest that noncompliance is common with an overall rate of approximately 50%, comparable to that reported in adults. Drug compliance is of particular concern with chronic conditions as therapy is often long-term and children without symptoms may be required to take medication to prevent later complications without any immediate benefits noted.

In a nationwide survey of German pediatric patients being treated with oral antibiotics, most commonly for tonsillopharyngitis and otitis media, the overall compliance on the last day of therapy was 69.5%. Medications were forgotten some of the time by 45.2% of children who presented to an emergency department during an acute attack of asthma. Poor compliance with inhaled asthma medication has been confirmed with the availability of an electronic inhaler timer device. Estimates of pediatric patient adherence to anticonvulsant medication regimens for the treatment of seizure disorders range from 25% to 54%. Similar rates of adherence have been shown for regimens in other chronic pediatric medical conditions such as diabetes and cystic fibrosis.

Contrary to what one would think, severity of illness is not a guarantee that prescribed medication will be taken. Even children with life-threatening conditions are at risk of treatment failure because of nonadherence with their drug therapy. Despite the threat and fear of cancer, several studies have reported less than optimal medication compliance in pediatric oncology patients. Likewise, significant noncompliance has been demonstrated in children who have received bone marrow and renal transplants.

CLINICAL CONSEQUENCES OF POOR ADHERENCE

The clinical implications of poor adherence are potentially enormous as this behavior may compromise the efficacy of drugs, resulting in failure to achieve the desired treatment goal. Inappropriate dosage adjustments or changes in medication may adversely affect the well-being of children. Noncompliance is a major cause of drug-related hospital admissions and results in significant financial costs to the health care system. Although the degree of compliance that is required for an adequate therapeutic effect has not been determined for most pediatric regimens, there are several examples of the relationship between poor adherence to drug therapy and unfavorable disease outcome in children. This association has been shown in such varied childhood diseases as asthma, diabetes, sickle cell disease, cancer, and renal transplantation.

FACTORS ASSOCIATED WITH POOR ADHERENCE

Human error is the most likely cause of nonadherence to drug therapy in children and adolescents. Reasons given by parents as to why they were unable to administer medication as prescribed include forgetting, discontinuing medication because symptoms had resolved, misunderstanding instructions, resistance by the child, apparent ineffectiveness or side effects of the medication, and busy schedules. Although it would be useful to be able to anticipate the occurrence of poor compliance, unfortunately, accurate predictors do not exist. Determinants suggested as associated with this behavior include patient and family factors, disease factors, physician factors, and regimen factors.

With respect to patient factors, demographic characteristics such as sex and socioeconomic status have not been consistently related to compliance status. For the most part, adolescents are thought to be less adherent to medication regimens than young children. A dysfunctional family situation may be a risk factor for poor compliance with therapy. The disease being treated may influence adherence; however, as previously discussed, suboptimal compliance has been shown for many pediatric medical conditions, even the more severe and life-threatening ones. In general, compliance with drug therapy for acute diseases is better than for chronic diseases. Lapses in adherence may be more common when treatment is for prophylaxis rather than for symptomatic relief. Knowledge of one's illness and its recommended treatment, although important, does not ensure compliance with medical advice. The health beliefs of children (or their parents), such as their perception of susceptibility to the illness in question, may have an effect on whether prescribed medication is taken. The nature of the relationship between the patient and the physician may be of importance.

Drug regimen factors may have an influential role in adherence to therapy. It is expected that a more complex and demanding regimen will be associated with decreased compliance. Inconvenient medication schedules that disrupt the normal routine are more difficult to follow. For children who attend school or whose parents work during the day, any medication given more than twice daily will probably not be taken as often as prescribed. In a study of 100 children who were prescribed antibiotics to be taken 4 times daily, 36 parents found that the day had elapsed by the time 3 doses had been given. Among preschool children with asthma and prescribed inhaled prophylactic therapy to be administered three or four times daily, it was generally the mid-day doses that were omitted. As compliance tends to decay with time, adherence to long-term regimens is poorer than with short-term ones.

Palatability of the medication may be an important determinant of drug adherence, particularly in the younger age group, as it may influence the ease with which parents are able to give medication to children. Variability in the acceptability of commonly prescribed antibiotic suspensions has been demonstrated.

ASSESSING ADHERENCE IN CLINICAL PRACTICE

To avoid the potentially negative consequences of medication noncompliance, it is essential in clinical practice to identify poor adherence to distinguish those patients who require further counseling or more intensive intervention. Although time and financial constraints may limit the physician's ability to thoroughly examine the area of drug compliance with each patient, it is important to address this issue, in particular in children who have failed to attain their treatment targets. The evaluation of compliance in pediatrics is complicated by the need to look at the behavior of the parent in addition to that of the child.

Unfortunately, although there are a number of techniques available to assess compliance, there is no foolproof method. As a result it is preferable to measure drug compliance using a combination of approaches.

Despite what we would like to believe, physicians are poor predictors of drug-taking behavior, tending to overestimate the adherence of their patients. In clinical practice, patient self-report measures such as interviews, questionnaires, or diaries are commonly used. Relying on patient (or parental) reports may be misleading as patients may be reluctant to admit that they are not following their physician's advice. Self-reports of noncompliance are often more accurate than self-reports of compliance. However, despite its limitations, this method is of value, in particular if it is used as an adjunctive measure. It is most successful if the information is gathered in a nonthreatening and nonjudgmental manner.

Pill counts are occasionally employed, although more often in the research setting. With liquid preparations, commonly used for children, the volume of remaining medication is measured. This method assumes that any medication that is not returned has been ingested, an assumption that is not always justified. Patients may intentionally discard their medication ("pill dumping" or "parking lot effect") to create the false impression that they are taking it. A more direct estimation of adherence is provided by the measurement of drug levels in body fluids, most commonly blood or urine, although detection of the drug reflects only recent drug consumption.

Microelectronic devices are now available for the monitoring of medication compliance. These devices may be useful in differentiating between poor compliance and other reasons for less than expected clinical effect in individual patients and may provide evidence of the correlation between noncompliance and "breakthrough" clinical events. However, their feasibility for widespread use in clinical practice is limited because they are relatively expensive and not readily available to most physicians.

STRATEGIES TO IMPROVE ADHERENCE

When poor compliance is identified, it is important that interventions aimed at improving medication-taking behavior are available for implementation. Strategies to increase adherence to the drug regimen include educational and behavioral modalities (Table 279-1), although a combination of both is usually most successful. If sustained compliance is required, it is necessary to continue the intervention for the duration of therapy as studies have shown deterioration in adherence after an effective strategy is withdrawn.

There are a number of general considerations that the physician should keep in mind in attempting to enhance patient adherence to drug therapy. Meaningful treatment goals should be set in collaboration with children and their parents. It is important that the prescribed regimen is as simple as possible and that clear instructions are provided. The frequency and timing of drug administration, which will be related to the choice of medication, should take into account the patient's usual routine, such as the child's waking hours. Efforts to identify and then, if possible, remove potential barriers to compliance should be

Table 279-1. Strategies to Improve Adherence

	Strategy	Comment
Educational	Verbal or written instructions	Generally more effective for short-term regimens prescribed for acute diseases
Behavioral	Scare techniques	Not recommended as they have not been shown to be helpful
	Self-monitoring, contracting, and reward programs	Employed with chronic disease therapy with good results
	Use of cues and reminder techniques	E.g., clock printed on the prescription label with appropriate times circled or illustrated calendar
	Special container such as pill organizers	Useful tool to aid patients to remember to take their medications

undertaken. In some cases, injection of a long-acting parenteral drug may be the only reasonable option for ensuring that the child receives required medication. If it is determined that compliance with necessary therapy cannot be accomplished by any other means, observed administration of medication may be contemplated. This alternative has been utilized in the drug therapy of tuberculosis and other infectious diseases. Regardless of what approach is taken to improve adherence, it is important that adequate follow-up and reinforcement of compliant behavior are a component of management.

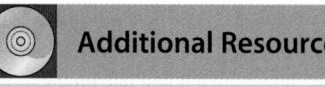
Additional Resources, CD-ROM

Bibliography

SUGGESTED READINGS

Matsui DM: Drug compliance in pediatrics clinical and research issues. Pediatr Clin North Am 1997;44:1–14.
Rapoff MA, Barnard MU: Compliance with pediatric medical regimens. In Cramer JA, Spilker B (eds): Patient Compliance in Medical Practice and Clinical Trials. New York, Raven Press, 1991, pp 73–98.

SECTION 9   DIAGNOSTICS AND THERAPEUTICS: *Therapeutic Interventions*

280   Home Health Care

Thomas Silva and Ann Marie Vovakis

For the pediatric generalist, accessing and coordinating home care services is a challenging and often confusing task. Resources have evolved over the last few years largely as a result of advances in medical technology that allow a growing number of children with chronic conditions to be cared for in the community. Changes in the structure of health care reimbursement have also contributed to the growing number of patients with acute illnesses being managed in the home. For the patient and family this means more care in the home; for the physician this means more direct care of patients.

The trend to community-based services for children began in the mid-1980s. The concepts of "family centered" and "community-based" care evolved. In 1982 passage of the Omnibus Budget Reconciliation Act, which endorsed the "Medicaid Model Home and Community Based Waiver," enabled children to receive home care funding if costs were equal to or less than hospital costs. Children dependent on ventilators and feeding machines were no longer deemed to be permanent hospital residents.

Reimbursement agencies moved to a system of fixed payments to hospitals for diagnosis-related groups, reimbursing hospitals for a fixed sum dependent on the patient's diagnosis rather than length of stay. Patients began reentering the community sooner and sicker. Insurers realized that substantial savings could be gained from supporting home care initiatives.

Continued medical care in the home offers the patient and family an enhanced quality of life during a very stressful period. Services can be limited by poor communication with service providers, poorly trained or unqualified providers, delayed or improper treatment of conditions, and caregiver burnout. Trends in funding and provider availability affect patient access to quality home care services.

AVAILABLE HOME CARE SERVICES

Skilled nursing services are the most commonly used home care service for children. Services are provided in either short-term home visits or for blocks of time, depending on the child's medical needs. Children requiring brief or short-term medical monitoring, or for whom health education is required, can benefit from skilled intermittent nursing visits. Children with more complex medical conditions and ongoing need for skilled intervention may benefit from "block" or private duty nursing. In-home nursing services can help generalists monitor their patients and provide families with support in managing ongoing health and developmental issues.

Skilled intermittent nursing visits (SNVs) typically last 1 to 2 hours each. The nurse monitors the patient's condition, teaches or completes a skilled intervention, and provides support. Services are provided by a licensed nursing agency, usually through a Visiting Nurse Association located in the patient's geographic area or a for-profit nursing agency that specializes in home care. The staff should have training in pediatrics as well as community health. If infusion or phlebotomy skills are required, the provider must specify this upon referral to ensure that the agency can provide a qualified staff person. Local infusion and durable medical equipment (DME) agencies often have staff experienced in starting IVs and drawing laboratory studies. The initial home visit or assessment must be completed by a licensed registered nurse (Box 280-1).

A physician's order is required to initiate services. The order must specify the frequency of visits, skilled intervention to be performed, and expected duration of visits. The nurse remains in communication with the physician through a detailed patient summary, which is required by accreditation agencies and reimbursement sources. If there are changes in treatment, medication, or frequency of visits, the physician must be notified and a written order obtained. A physician's order is necessary to discontinue services once goals have been completed.

Box 280-2 gives examples of appropriate referrals for skilled visits. Skilled visits typically continue until the patient and family reaches the identified goal or until the treatment or condition has stabilized. Some patients may have SNVs reactivated if their condition returns or if new treatments or therapies are prescribed.

Box 280-1. Essential Components of Initial Nursing Home Visit

1. Complete health history of the child including list of health care providers, medications, recent hospitalizations, and treatments
2. Functional assessment of activities of daily living, vision, and hearing
3. Feeding and nutritional assessment
4. Evaluation of the patient and family's understanding of the condition and treatment
5. Formal assessment of medications and compliance issues
6. Physical assessment of the child
7. Performance of any skilled intervention or patient/family education and assessments of burden of care and abilities of caregivers
8. Environmental assessment for safety and accessibility
9. Establishment of goals for subsequent visits
10. Creation of documentation and communication guidelines with the referring provider

---

Box 280-2. Examples of Appropriate Use of Skilled Nursing Visits

- Monitor children with acute or resolving medical conditions (low-birth-weight or premature infants, daily or weekly dressing changes, or wound care management).
- Monitor and educate children with chronic but stable medical conditions (asthma, diabetes, hemophilia, failure to thrive).
- Monitor children with ancillary services (e.g., home health aides).

Private duty nursing (PDN) or "block" nursing is delivered to children with an ongoing need for skilled nursing intervention or those who are dependent on medical technology at least part of each day. Examples are seen in Box 280-3. The need for private duty nursing is determined during hospitalization of a child when physicians and nurses recognize that the level of care involved is too significant for one or two family members to manage on a daily basis. The method of determining private duty nursing hours for pediatric patients is inconsistent. The primary care physician should be involved in the request for nursing hours and is usually responsible for the continued ordering of such hours. Factors considered in the application for approval of PDN hours for pediatric patients are listed in Box 280-4.

Private duty nurses are available through specialized nursing agencies and should have experience in pediatrics and in the requisite technical skills. For children on ventilatory support, the nurse should have experience in pediatrics and in ventilator management and tracheostomy care. Most agencies adhere to the regulation of submitting a complete set of nursing orders to the physician every 3 months for signature. Any treatment or medication changes that occur in the interval period are written as individual orders and are submitted to the physician to sign.

Duration of services depends on the stability of the child's condition, the ability of the family to provide care, and the number of skilled tasks required. Usually the hours are weaned either monthly or weekly so as not to disrupt the care of the child.

Ancillary Providers

Box 280-5 lists typical home care services appropriate for children with different conditions.

Non-nursing providers in pediatric home care include home health aides, rehabilitation specialists (physical therapists, speech therapists, and occupational therapists), respi-

---

Box 280-3. Children with Conditions That Are Appropriate for PDN Services

- Children on mechanical ventilation
- Children with continuous or prolonged use of intravenous nutritional substances or medications
- Children with a daily dependence on other devices for nutritional, elimination, or respiratory support, including tracheostomy care, oxygen support, tube feedings, urinary catheterization, or colostomy care

Box 280-4. Factors Considered in Approval of PDN Hours for Pediatric Patients

1. *Complexity of diagnosis:* Children with multisystem disorders can require almost 24 hours of private duty nursing (PDN) care while those with single system disorders may qualify for less.
2. *Prognosis of the child:* Children with life-threatening conditions may receive 24-hour nursing care for limited periods of time and hospice level care. Patients expected to improve over time may receive only temporary services such as 4 hours daily for 2 to 4 weeks.
3. *Number of medical interventions and medical devices involved* (i.e., suctioning, chest physiotherapy): Frequency of tasks, time required to complete tasks, and number of medical devices required to monitor or treat the child are considered.
4. *Family support:* Important factors are capability of parent(s), marital status, presence and ages of other children in the home, and extended family/friend support. Two caregivers should be trained in the care of a child with complex medical needs in order to maintain a safe environment for the child.
5. *Insurance/funding:* The number of hours recommended by providers may differ significantly from what the insurer will fund. Someone familiar with insurance funding should be part of the process of requesting financial coverage of services. Many children with complex health care needs are placed into "case management" and assigned an individual for the coordination of all covered services. Whoever reports to the insurance case manager must be thorough in presenting the child's medical needs and list of complicating factors. Insurers usually do not take family or social needs into consideration. The number of PDN hours approved may not equal the number of hours received because of staffing issues.
6. *Age of the child:* Younger children may be considered more fragile or unstable.
7. *Length of hospital stay/hospital course:* This can indicate stability of the child's condition.

ratory therapists, nutritionists, and unlicensed caregivers or personal care attendants.

Home health aides (HHAs) are skilled care providers trained in basic health and personal care needs (i.e., bathing, dressing, and feeding). HHA use in pediatrics is generally reserved for those children who have impaired motor function, impaired speech, or cognitive delay, and for those who have severe neurological impairment. HHAs are usually trained in courses that last 4 to 6 weeks sponsored

Box 280-5. Typical Home Care Services Appropriate for Children with Different Conditions

1. Child with quadriplegic cerebral palsy (no gastrostomy, nonambulatory, verbal): SNV once/twice per month to supervise HHA 20 hours per week
2. Child recently discharged from the hospital with gastrostomy tube feedings, neuromotor delay, and recurrent pneumonia: 4–8 hours PDN per day in time-limited fashion
3. Child with tracheostomy (no ventilatory support): 4–8 hours PDN per day depending on stablity and required frequency of suctioning
4. Child with tracheostomy and ventilatory support: 8–24 hours PDN per day depending on type and duration of mechanical ventilation and clinical stability

HHA, home health aide; PDN, private duty nursing; SNV, skilled intermittent nursing visit.

by hospitals, certified agencies, and the Red Cross. They cannot administer medications or provide any "nursing treatments" to the patient. Typically, they are in the home from 2 to 4 hours and can assist the family by completing the tasks for the child that require another individual present. They also work on mobility and transfers and can do light housework. HHAs are provided by local Visiting Nurse agencies. To activate services, a referral must be made to the agency with the patient's diagnosis. A registered nurse or physical therapist must perform the initial evaluation and determine the appropriate level of services. A physician's order is required for HHA services and quarterly renewals are submitted for physician review and signature. The HHA is supervised by a licensed caregiver (registered nurse or physical therapist) every 2 to 4 weeks to ensure proper delivery of care and to monitor the patient's medical condition. Typically, HHA services are long-term. Services can remain in place as long as the child's condition meets criteria and a funding source is available.

Rehabilitation services include physical, occupational, and speech therapies.

Physical therapy (PT) is the most common rehabilitative therapy for children cared for at home. It is beneficial to children with motor impairments or children who require specialized equipment for mobility or transfers. A registered physical therapist must do the initial patient evaluation and treatment plan. Further treatment may be completed by a physical therapy assistant.

Occupational therapy (OT) is useful for the child with fine motor impairment or those unable to perform self-care activities. Occupational therapy services can be provided by a registered therapist or an occupational therapy assistant (OTA).

Speech therapy is indicated for those children with speech or oromotor impairments including children with poor language development, children with structural anomalies such as cleft palate, children with tracheostomies, or children with feeding and swallowing disorders.

All rehabilitative services are available through local Visiting Nurse agencies and may be available through specialized or private agencies. A physician order is required to initiate any rehabilitative service and for ongoing delivery of care. Typically, each visit is 45 minutes to 1 hour and may occur from 1 to 5 times weekly depending on the needs of the child.

Evaluating patients for augmentative communication devices and adaptive equipment is a large part of the job of home therapists. They are resourceful in obtaining insurance coverage for these items and in ensuring that the home environment is physically safe for the child.

Early intervention (EI) provides rehabilitative services to children younger than 3 years of age who either have identifiable developmental impairments or are at risk for these impairments. Depending on the child's level of delay and medical diagnosis, one or all three services (physical, speech, and occupational therapies) may be implemented. At 3 years of age these children qualify for rehabilitative services through their local school districts after a CORE evaluation. Services provided by the local school districts are geared to the child's educational needs and may not relate to the patient's total need for rehabilitative services. Most insurance companies will not pay for additional services at home if a child receives them through school, unless a clear additional benefit is expected.

Personal care attendants (PCAs) are unlicensed caregivers that provide individualized care to children in the home at the direction of a patient or family member. Their work requires no course certification or formal testing. They are hired, trained, and employed by the patient or family. The use of PCAs in pediatrics is growing rapidly, mainly because of the lack of available skilled care providers. The use of PCAs has been shown to be a safe and cost-effective means of providing home care services.

In most states Medicaid covers the cost of PCAs, provided the patient meets functional criteria. PCAs are reimbursed by the families or individuals who employ them. Their services are activated by contacting a registered agency specializing in support services for persons with disability, such as the Association for Retarded Citizens (ARC). This agency sends a nurse clinician to review the medical needs of the patient. The clinical evaluation, which must be verified and signed by the primary care physician, is submitted to the funding source for approval. Patients are allotted hours of PCA services according to their medical and functional needs. In some instances a fiscal intermediary handles reimbursement of the PCA for the family.

PCAs complete a wide variety of tasks ranging from assisting with activities of daily living (meal preparation, bathing, dressing, toileting, transfers, shopping, housekeeping, laundry) to completing skilled nursing care (suctioning, g-tube feedings, medication administration).

The use of PCAs in pediatrics is controversial. In many states, regulations prohibit use of PCAs to complete skilled nursing interventions for children. In all instances state-reimbursed PCA programs must adhere to regulations set forth by that state.

Other Home Care Services

Respiratory care services are available to patients on long-term respiratory management including oxygen or ventilatory support. For ventilator-dependent patients the respiratory therapist monitors clinical progress, institutes treatment changes, and acts as a resource to parents and associated home health care personnel. Respiratory services are reimbursable under limited instances and are generally billed as part of the entire cost of the equipment and supplies provided for the home. When discharging a child with ventilatory support (a child who is ventilator dependent), the identified agency must employ staff with pediatric respiratory experience. Physicians communicate with respiratory care providers in the home through written orders and patient summaries.

Nutritional support services are available through agencies that provide intensive nutritional support devices, formulas, or intravenous medications. Services are generally nonreimbursable but crucial to helping parents and providers ensure that the child receives adequate nutrition and that the most appropriate delivery devices or methods are used. Many chronically ill children have increased or fluctuating caloric needs and may require frequent formula adjustments. Because of changing developmental needs, different methods of delivery or types of equipment may be necessary (i.e., porBox feeding pumps for school attendance). Home care companies that provide nutritional devices communicate with the pediatric clinician through physician orders submitted on a quarterly basis, or more often if new treatments are instituted. A change in equipment may be requested by the child's family or caregiver. Physicians must attend to these orders to ensure that appropriate services and nutritional supplements are being provided.

Laboratory services are provided to patients through a variety of avenues. The primary care physician must specify laboratory data to be obtained and the frequency of services: for example, "SNV $\times$ 2 + 1 prn to check pre- and post-tobramycin levels." The skilled nursing agency can obtain the blood sample, deliver it to the laboratory, and report the results back to the physician. The physician is required to provide a written order to the laboratory or skilled nursing agency. If the patient is receiving parenteral antibiotics or nutrition, the source agency usually has qualified staff obtain the blood sample. A written order is required and can be submitted to the agency pharmacist or nurse coordinator.

Pharmacists play an important role in the care of children at home. They are vital in ensuring the availability of many medications and serve as support to prescribers and caregivers. At-home infusion companies employ pharmacists who are responsible for the ordering and compounding of drugs administered in the home. It is essential that these pharmacists be familiar with pediatric pharmacology and infusion systems.

Additional Modes of Home Care

Respite care is the care of an individual by someone other than the identified primary caregiver. A variety of personnel can deliver respite care. Respite services can be delivered in the patient's home, another home, or a respite care facility. Arranging coverage for respite services can be difficult. Methods vary from state to state. The State Department of Public Health Title V Program or Department of Mental Retardation can provide resources concerning the availability of local respite services. Private funding groups or organizations (e.g., the Cerebral Palsy Foundation) may also have access to respite funds.

The primary care provider should recognize when a patient and family needs respite care and should provide resource information. Children who require a skilled nursing facility to deliver the respite care may need a formal, state-specific evaluation. In this case the facility must obtain physician orders and the child must meet specified medical criteria. Maintaining an individual health plan (IHP) is quite helpful in this process (see under Use of an Individual Health Plan).

Hospice care includes intensive home nursing and social service support for families with a terminally ill child. To activate hospice care a patient must be diagnosed with a terminal illness that is expected to result in death within 6 months. Hospice agencies may be tied to Home Health Care or Visiting Nurse agencies. Hospice care provides up to 24-hour nursing coverage and other flexible support services including home health aides, social workers, family therapists, and volunteer staff for family support. Contact with primary health care providers is close. Specific physician orders are required (e.g., a "Do Not Resuscitate" order). Hospice care agencies have registered nurses on staff who are certified to pronounce death in the home, which is comforting for the family and eliminates the need to transport the body of the deceased to the hospital.

Medical day care facilities are licensed and regulated by states to provide care for technology-dependent children. Children must meet specific medical criteria for enrollment. Staffing ratios are determined according to severity of illness. An individual plan of care is developed in conjunction with the family in collaboration with the primary care physician and specialists. Physician orders are required for the child to attend the day care and for any medications, treatments, or services received there.

Children who attend medical day care benefit from increased socialization with other children and increased stability of services being provided (i.e., staff on site and rare interruption of service because of sick calls). Parents benefit from having consistent caregivers for their child and consistent hours of service. Risk of exposure to infectious agents is increased, however, and in-home services are limited once a commitment is made to this model of care. Typically, parents must use their allotted nursing hours for day care and may not be granted further services in their home if the child is ill and needs to remain at home. Funding for attendance at a medical day care is generally available from public payer sources.

FUNDING SOURCES

Private Funding

Private funding sources include private insurance companies, health maintenance organizations (HMOs), and disease-oriented voluntary organizations. This form of funding previously accounted for the majority of health coverage for children with a serious illness. In 1995 private insurance represented less than 4% of reimbursement for home care costs.

Most children are covered under their parents' private insurance or managed care plan. Home care services are covered benefits in most private insurance plans, but may have a fixed cap or reimbursement amount. Most private insurers cover home care services for brief, self-limited periods and will not cover chronic or custodial care. If a child requires significant home intervention, the family or discharge planner can request that an individual case manager from the private payer be assigned to the client to streamline approval of services, ensure that the child is receiving all available services, and serve as a resource to parents and health care providers. The case manager can rapidly determine what services are not covered under the plan. Children with significant home health care requirements often need a blend of public (Medicaid) and private insurance.

Public Funding

Public funding sources include Medicaid, state-run programs for children with special health care needs (also referred to as Title V programs), the Children's Health Insurance Program, and Medicaid "waiver" programs.

Medicaid is administered at the federal level by the Health Care Financing Administration (HCFA), and at the state level by a public health service agency. Children can receive Medicaid if their parents are eligible for government-sponsored cash assistance programs (formerly known as Aid to Families with Dependent Children), or if they themselves have a disability and qualify for Social Security/disability benefits.

Medicaid covers most home health care services, but each state-controlled agency can modify coverage. Prior approval is usually required for expanded home care services such as private duty nursing. Physician orders and medical reports are reviewed as frequently as every 12 weeks for continued approval and justification of eligibility. To prevent delays and deferrals, health care providers must provide thorough and timely documentation.

Title V programs were initially established in 1936, and were previously referred to as Crippled Children's Services. In 1981 the Omnibus Budget Reconciliation Act was passed. This helped to establish the maternal and child health block grants that consolidated all Title V programs into the state programs for children with special health care needs, Maternal and Child Health Services, and the WIC Programs (the supplemental food program for women, infants, and children). Most Title V programs are administered by state health departments and cover such services as diagnostic testing, rehabilitation services, primary care and immunization programs, and payment for adaptive equipment. Because the state can direct these funds at their discretion, services can vary greatly from state to state.

The Children's Health Insurance Program (CHIP) provides 100% coverage for primary care services and immunizations. Initially parents had to fall below a certain income level; however, income restrictions have been modified in some states to encourage increased enrollment. Short-term home care services are generally covered as if the child were receiving regular Medicaid benefits. If children have a prolonged need for services or develop a chronic health condition, they may qualify for Katie Beckett coverage or Medicaid coverage through Social Security and disability.

Katie Beckett Medicaid waivers grew out of a plea in the early 1980s by the family of Katie Beckett. Katie was a ventilator-dependent child who had been hospitalized for 3 years. Through an exception to policy granted by the federal government in her case, Katie was allowed to retain her Medicaid coverage when she returned home, the rationale being that Medicaid funded care at home was less costly than that which she received while hospitalized. The Health Care Financing Administration then authorized waivers known as Home and Community Based Waivers to states requesting them. To qualify for a waiver program, a state must show that costs of care at home are less than cost of care within an institution. Services covered include: private duty nursing, case management services, experimental medications, respite care, transportation, rehabilitative services, adaptive equipment, preventative services, and long-term care. Children must meet medical criteria to qualify for Katie Beckett waivers. They must have an irreversible chronic condition or one with extensive medical monitoring and daily care. Katie Beckett waivers are not financially restricted.

SSI, the Supplementary Security Income program, provides monthly cash benefits based on family income; qualifies the child for Medicaid health care services (in most states); and ensures referral to the state's Title V Children with Special Health Care Needs program. Qualification criteria are listed in Box 280-6.

The SSI program provides cash benefits that can be used by parents and families as they see fit to meet the needs of the child. Funds may be used for adaptive equipment, specialized services or supplies not covered by insurance, food, clothing, transportation, and respite care. The SSI criteria for determining financial eligibility are complex. Families are asked to submit tax returns and other financial statements for review. In most states if children receive SSI benefits then they automatically qualify for Medicaid coverage.

SSI determinations are based on written information such as hospital records, discharge summaries, laboratory reports, routine health care records, and developmental assessments. The pediatrician's medical report in support of a child's application for SSI should include a detailed medical history; complete findings of physical, intellectual, and developmental examinations; expected duration of the child's impairment; a description of the limiting effects of the child's disability on his or her level of function; and prescribed treatments and therapies. Providers who submit information in a timely manner are reimbursed for their efforts. Inclusion of as much information as possible is important to prevent deferrals.

THE ROLE OF THE GENERALIST

For the pediatric generalist, evaluating patients for home care services can occur at any point in the health care delivery process. When a patient requires home care services, the physician should be aware of the child's physical needs, developmental needs, family structure and supports, available funding sources, and local and statewide services and resources.

The American Medical Association considers the role of the physician in home care not only to manage medical problems, but also to identify the home care needs of the patient, establish and approve the plan of care including short- and long-term goals, provide continuity across all settings, participate when necessary in team and family conferences, and evaluate quality of care.

The generalist should appreciate the components of a complete home care evaluation (see Box 280-1). An evaluation in the home offers a unique window into the daily life

of the patient. It provides an otherwise unavailable opportunity to develop understanding of the child's ability to function in the family.

Initiating a Referral. Any child who has an acute or chronic illness will likely qualify for home care services. The primary or specialty health care provider should conduct a physical evaluation of the child. If services are warranted, the nursing staff caring for the child should make the referral. The agency should have the information listed in Box 280-7 when the referral is first initiated.

Often, an agency requires a signed prescription or faxed physician order before services can commence. The staff person calling the agency should obtain a confirmation that services can indeed be provided and should verify the start-of-care date. Agencies may claim they can staff a case only to find out later that they do not have the resources to do so.

Follow-up. The physician should be contacted once the initial assessment has been made to confirm delivery of services and to approve the treatment plan. A list of orders will be submitted for signature. Periodic communication with the field providers is crucial and a method of communication should be established (i.e., by mail, telephone voice mail, direct paging or e-mail, or through a designated nurse practitioner or nurse). By taking the lead in communicating, the primary health care provider ensures that the patient and family receive the care they require.

Communication and Coordination of Services. Providing comprehensive coordinated care to children with chronic illness can be beneficial to accessing entitlement services, increasing compliance, and decreasing hospitalization. The family needs to be an integral part of this coordination. The pediatric generalist should also assume an integral role. The generalist is in a unique position to ensure that all specialty providers work together to focus on the "whole child" and the family. Children too often receive care that is fragmented.

To provide comprehensive care coordination the primary physician can utilize the guidelines for caring for the child

Box 280-8. Components of the Medical Home as Defined by the AAP

1. The provision of preventative care
2. The ensurance of ambulatory and inpatient care 24 hours/day
3. Strategies and mechanisms to ensure continuity of care
4. Identification of and medically appropriate use of specialty consultation and referrals
5. Interaction with school and community agencies
6. Maintenance of a central record and database containing all pertinent medical information including hospitalizations

in a "Medical Home." As defined by the American Academy of Pediatrics (AAP), the "Medical Home" is characterized by the elements listed in Box 280-8.

Documentation. Several forms of documentation are physician orders, letters of medical justification, prescriptions, and treatment plans. It is helpful to keep a tracking system for these forms as well as create a method for resubmitting forms. Office staff can develop tickler files or home care charts to avoid delaying submission and thus potential delay in services.

Use of an Individual Health Plan. For those children with severe chronic health care needs the use of an individual health plan can be beneficial. This comprehensive document serves to help families and providers by keeping an ongoing record of the child's medical needs including medications, treatments, recent hospitalizations and clinical appointments, baseline review of systems, and actions to take in the event of an urgent and emergent situation. This plan of care can then travel with the patient to appointments as well as serve as a guideline for those caring for the child, including home care staff, schools, specialty care physicians, and on-call staff. Three cases are found on the CD-ROM to illustrate the types of home care services that may be indicated for children with different levels of need (Box 280-9).

SUMMARY

Pediatric home care services can offer enormous benefits to children and families. Families can maintain their integrity in the home as parents can guide the care of their children within their own environment. The children are allowed to grow and develop to their maximum potential. Pediatric physicians can institute treatments and therapeutic changes

Box 280-9. Components of Adequate Short-term Home Care

In the case of short-term home care, the patient can receive adequate care in the home if the following components are in place:

- The family receives proper training and a mechanism for troubleshooting is in place.
- The physician is kept involved in the progress of the patient.
- The home care staff members are competent and knowledgeable about pediatric home care.
- The insurance benefits are verified by the discharging clinician and the home care agency.

in the child's care without having to interrupt the child's routine.

Like other aspects of the health care industry, pediatric home care services are quickly changing. For most patients and their families, these changes have led to greater difficulty accessing and maintaining services. Tighter reimbursement regulations have forced several agencies to cut costs or close their doors. High turnover in home health staff is frustrating for families. Patients and families commonly need to work with new personnel, who may not be familiar with their needs or the products and equipment necessary to maintain the child's health at home. New staff may not be familiar with the reimbursement process, leading to gaps in the approval process. Because of inexperience, lack of reimbursement, lack of time, and a lack of connection with resources, many agencies cannot provide the same level of teaching and case management in the home as they could in the past.

Because of changes in reimbursement structure, many agencies have had to decrease staffing and cap salaries. Fewer well-qualified staff pursue careers in home care. The national shortage of nurses and other home care staff is affecting the quality of care being delivered to patients and families. Patients receiving private duty nursing services may struggle for days without nurses to fill their shifts. The primary care physician must be aware of the present limitations of intensive pediatric home care as this impacts the stability of the child. Where once minor or acute illnesses could be carefully monitored and managed in the home, the child may need more frequent office or emergency room evaluation. Many patients remain hospitalized for longer periods from lack of available home care staff.

One of the largest obstacles to a timely discharge for a technology-dependent child is obtaining approval for home care funding. Public funding groups may take longer to approve services than private insurance agencies.

Because of limited professional support, families are being asked to provide more care and with fewer financial resources. Many suffer from severe fatigue and stress that is related not only to caring for the child, but also to interacting with health care professionals.

Health care professionals need to pay attention to technologic advances that affect patient care; such advances may make the delivery of care in the home more efficient. Physician groups should to continue to lobby for increased financial support for families as well as for health care financing that enhances rather than restricts home care services. Outcome studies are necessary to determine whether it is possible to offer more responsive direct and coordinating services in the home to avert greater costs in the future.

Additional Resources, CD-ROM

Cases	Text
Future trends in home health care	Text
Bibliography	

SUGGESTED READINGS

American Academy of Pediatrics, Ad Hoc Task Force on Definition of the Medical Home: The medical home. Pediatrics 1992;90:774.

American Academy of Pediatrics, Committee on Children with Disabilities: Care coordination: Integrating health and related systems of care for children with special health care needs. Pediatrics 1999; 104:978–981.

Fleming J, Challela M, Eland J, et al: Impact on the family of children who are technology dependent and cared for in the home. Pediatr Nurs 1994;20:379–388.

Jessop DJ, Stein RE: Providing comprehensive health care to children with chronic illness. Pediatrics 1993;93:602–607.

McNeal GJ: Telecommunication technologies in high-tech home care. Crit Care Clin North Am 1998;10:279–286.

SECTION 9 DIAGNOSTICS AND THERAPEUTICS: *Therapeutic Interventions*

281 Technology-Dependent Therapies

Thomas Silva and Ann Marie Vovakis

The number of children who are dependent on medical technology for survival has grown since the 1980s, creating a need for pediatric generalists who are comfortable managing the range of clinical problems that these children present.

WRITTEN HEALTH PLANS

Portable, written health care plans are essential for children with special health care needs. The document should include identifying and family contact data, a current active problem list, active medications and allergies, recent admissions, active consultants and agencies, and a list of predictable complications with which a patient may present. The initial document and subsequent updates should be printed and filed in the patient's office chart, given to the patient to take to appointments, faxed or mailed to specialists for consultations, and should be available to covering physicians after hours. Most children who are assisted by technology on a long-term basis do not have written care plans. An example of an individual health plan (IHP) and a template to create one is given in the CD-ROM.

ROLE OF CARE COORDINATION

Parent groups of technology-assisted children have asked health care providers for enhanced care coordination services both as a quality of life intervention and as a quality indicator for managed care plans. Care coordination functions include the following:

- Active triage of medical problems
- Coordination of prescription refills, durable medical equipment (DME) orders, and the processing of authorization forms
- Creation and maintenance of health care plans and emergency response plans
- Active communication with home health, school health, and rehabilitation staff, teachers, and consultants
- Connection of families with governmental support services or community support services where they exist
- Assurance that the family's goals for medical care and educational and recreational opportunities are paramount

A care coordinator might be a physician, nurse, social worker, or community resource specialist appropriate to the level of the child's technology-dependent therapy. The state's Department of Public Health, Division of Children with Special Healthcare Needs is a good starting point for accessing these services. The National Center for Children and Youth with Disabilities offers access to resources and care coordination in each state. Links to this organization and other helpful websites can be found on the CD-ROM.

COMMONLY USED TECHNOLOGIES

Respiratory Technologies

Nearly all pediatric providers currently manage children who are dependent on respiratory technology, including home nebulizers, oxygen therapy, and tracheostomies and mechanical ventilation.

Indications and Uses

Nebulizers are used to dispense medication into various droplet sizes, which can be deposited in large and small airways. Nebulizers can administer β-adrenergic agonists, mast cell stabilizers, antibiotics, and biologically active enzymes. Oxygen is administered to children with documented hypoxia and to improve growth in some children who attain normal oxygenation only with increased breathing. Tracheostomy is required in children with anatomic abnormalities of the upper airway, severe dysfunctional swallowing, or recurrent pneumonia, and as access for children needing some type of mechanical ventilation. Long-term mechanical ventilation is used for children with a wide variety of causes of respiratory failure. These therapies are

short courses of intravenous nutrition. Their main complication is infection at the entry site, which is best managed by removing the PICC line. These lines can be removed at home or in the office with only 5 minutes of direct pressure after withdrawal.

Central venous catheters are threaded into the great veins of the neck or chest and can protrude through the skin or be completely indwelling. Indwelling catheters are placed by surgeons under general anesthesia. They are completely covered by skin and are accessed in sterile fashion by placing a needle through the skin into a reservoir. Protruding central catheters must be kept scrupulously clean and dry and are monitored twice daily with sterile dressing changes and flushes. Completely indwelling catheters require less daily care and less frequent routine flushes but do not eliminate the pain imposed by phlebotomy.

The potential complications of all of these lines are thrombosis, embolization, and infection. All lines must be checked several times a day for signs of external infection and periodically to ensure that they flush easily. Any central line that does not flush easily should be left alone and the specialist responsible for placing the line should be contacted. Attempts may be made to clear the line with urokinase. PICC lines that do not flush easily should be removed immediately and replaced.

Any child with an indwelling catheter with a significant fever should have blood cultures drawn peripherally and through the line if possible. Clinicians must carefully weigh the decision to "treat through" an infected line versus removing or replacing the line at the first sign of infection.

Feeding and Nutritional Appliances and Procedures

Technologies available to assist children with conditions causing growth failure and malnutrition are intermittent nasogastric feeding, gastrostomy, transpyloric gastrojejunal tubes, and surgically placed jejunostomy. These are indicated when inadequate caloric intake leads to growth failure or dysfunctional swallowing prevents safe oral feeding. Nasogastric feeding is instituted when the condition preventing adequate growth is thought to be temporary and adequate airway protective reflexes exist. Permanent gastrostomy should be considered if supplemental nutrition will be required for longer than 3 weeks. Gastrosotomy with fundoplication or jejunostomy should be considered if refractory gastroesophageal reflux exists. Jejunal feedings can be administered either through a surgical jejunostomy or via a tube threaded through a gastrostomy into the jejunum (transpyloric jejunal feedings).

It is often difficult for parents to decide to shift the focus from oral feeding to gastrostomy. Box 281-5 lists historical triggers that may suggest the need for tube feeding. Before instituting tube feedings all children should undergo a thorough evaluation, which may include the items listed in Box 281-6.

How Therapies Are Administered

Almost all parents of children who are fed via gastrostomy are surprised to learn how simple day-to-day care of the gastrostomy becomes. Ostomy sites should be cleaned with

---

Box 281-5. Historical Triggers That May Suggest the Need for Tube Feeding

1. Mealtimes in excess of 45 minutes
2. Coughing/choking with meals (note symptoms with different textures of ingested foods)
3. Need for extensive adaptive positioning for feedings
4. Sweating/tachypnea after feedings
5. Wheezing/noisy breathing during or 30 minutes after feedings

---

soap and water daily. The site should generally not be covered with gauze or occlusive dressings. Children can be managed with a variety of modes of feeding from 24-hour continuous infusion by pump to bolus feeds given over a 30- to 40-minute period. A wide variety of enteral formulas can be prescribed with the help of a nutritionist. Generally speaking it is preferable that children transition from continuous to bolus feeding for ease of care and the establishment of normal hunger and satiety states. Box 281-7 lists the tasks required of caretakers of children who utilize tube feedings. Boxes 281-8 and 281-9 describe the roles of the generalist before and after the initiation of tube feedings. Children who require enteral feeding should travel with a copy of their IHP as well as an emergency kit that includes all the supplies necessary for an urgent tube change.

Risks and Complications

The complications imposed by feeding technologies can be divided into complications immediate to placement and complications seen during long-term use. The initiation of nasogastric feeding can be complicated by improper placement of the tube into the airway. The position of the nasogastric tube must be carefully assessed by auscultation after every new placement and before each use. Position can always be checked radiographically if any doubt exists. The tubes should be instantly removed if any respiratory distress, choking, or abdominal distension or distress occurs with use.

Percutaneous endoscopic gastrostomy tubes, placed by surgeons in consultation with gastroenterologists, require general anesthesia. The surgical risks of percutaneous endoscopic gastrostomy and surgical gastrostomy are best discussed by the surgeon. Both procedures are reasonably well tolerated. Immediate risk parallels the child's overall risk of anesthesia.

Box 281-6. Evaluation to Consider before Instituting Tube Feedings

1. Direct observation of feeding by a specifically trained speech or occupational therapist with experience in treating children with dysfunctional swallowing
2. Radiologic video assessment of swallowing ability of foods of different textures (thin liquids, thick liquids, purees, soft solids, crunchy solids) to document clinically silent aspiration
3. Attempts at increasing caloric density of ingested food and careful calorie counts
4. Nutritional assessment for total calories, calcium, vitamins, and supplementation if necessary
5. Gastroenterologic evaluation for reflux, maldigestion, and malabsorbtion of nutrients

Risks seen with long-term use include choking or aspiration during feedings, emesis or increased gastroesophageal reflux, gastroesophageal bleeding, skin problems at the ostomy site (granulation tissue, burning from acid leakage, and cellulitis), and dislodgment of the tube.

Many children with gastrostomies have evidence of intermittent low-grade bleeding that may come from irritation at the ostomy site or from ulceration caused by friction of the device against gastric mucosa. This type of bleeding may respond to careful attention to the anchoring of the device, increased antacid use, or Carafate (sucralfate). Clinically significant gastrointestinal bleeding is an emergency and should be treated aggressively.

Granulation tissue is protruding pink or red "mushrooming" tissue that represents a foreign body reaction. It is exacerbated by excessive motion of the tube through the ostomy. Treatment is with intermittent cauterization with silver nitrate or occasional surgical débridement. Burning from leakage of stomach acid is seen as irregular erythema with ulceration at the gastrostomy site; it is best treated by frequent local washing with soap and water, the application

of barrier ointments and stomahesive powder to the skin, and the application of liquid antacid as a wet to dry paint on the skin. The signs of cellulitis (erythema, induration, and pain) around a gastrostomy are identical to the signs on other areas of the body and can be distinguished from acid burns by the presence of induration rather than excoriation. Initial antibiotic coverage should be targeted against gram-positive organisms.

Gastrostomy tubes that fall out must be replaced within hours to prevent healing at the ostomy site. This could require a second surgical procedure. After approximately 6 months, gastrostomy and enterostomy sites should be well healed. Replacing a gastrostomy device at a well-healed site is usually less difficult than most health care providers expect. If a substitute gastrostomy device is not available, a balloon-tipped urinary catheter of the same diameter (usually expressed as "French" units) serves as an adequate replacement. Using clean technique and gloves, the lubricated catheter is gently but firmly inserted into the ostomy. The tube should be advanced 4 or 5 inches, or until stomach contents appear in the tube, before the balloon is inflated with water. The tube should be gently pulled back and taped in place when resistance is met. Usually gastric contents can be aspirated into the tube. Position can be checked by auscultation or x-ray. Patients should be observed for abdominal pain, distention, or feeding intolerance after a gastrostomy change. If the same sized tube cannot be replaced because of stenosis or healing at the site, a smaller tube can usually be placed. Parents should be trained to replace the device at home. In the event that this is not possible, parents should seek medical help immediately if the tube falls out. Health care providers should reinforce that this is not due to great risk for the overall health of the child, but to ensure that the ostomy itself does not "heal" and shut. Box 281-10 lists essential questions to ask if a child requires tube feedings.

Genitourinary Appliances and Procedures, Ileostomy, and Colostomy

Care for children with these technologies is discussed on the CD-ROM.

Positioning and Mobility Devices

There is a vast array of seating and positioning devices, mobility devices, and bracing available for use by Children with Special Health Care Needs (CSHCNs). There is also a wide variety of locations through which these devices can

1. What is the type and size of the tube in use?
2. When was the tube first placed and when was the last tube change?
3. What formula is administered and what are the amounts and rates used?
4. Are there any restrictions on the child's oral feeding?
5. Does the child have a fundoplication or symptoms of gastroesophageal reflux?
6. Where does the child receive specialty care?

be accessed (Early Intervention Programs [EIPs], schools, tertiary care centers). Box 281-11 provides a description of the generalist's role in managing the use of these technologies. The potential complications caused by improper fit or use include worsening hip dysplasia and dislocation, worsening contractures and scoliosis, pressure necrosis, and injuries during transportation.

As with feeding technologies, parents are sometimes reluctant to use these technologies because they do not wish their children to appear different or because they do not want their children to rely on technology but rather on their innate abilities. The decision to employ the technology must carefully balance the child's ability to accomplish a task against the caloric and functional costs of accomplishing that task unassisted. Many children with cerebral palsy are physically capable of walking independently. Because of gait inefficiencies, some of these children expend a tremendous amount of energy to walk even short distances. In addition, some gait abnormalities cause increased risk of acquired arthritis owing to disorders of joint mechanics. The use of a functionally appropriate device such as a walker or wheelchair offers the potential for enhanced mobility at lower cost. This in turn offers the potential for better community mobility and increased opportunities for peer interaction.

Orthotics and Prosthetics

There are many kinds of orthoses, or braces, commonly used in the care of children with neurologic and orthopedic abnormalities. They are generally ordered by a neurologist, orthopedist, or rehabilitation specialist and are fashioned by a physical therapist or orthotist. Orthotics are used to protect or support a joint through a range of motion in a specific activity. They are also used to prevent acquired contractions in joints that are exposed to abnormalities

Box 281-11. The Role of the Generalist in Managing the Use of Positioning/Mobility Technologies

1. Maintain a referral network for these devices.
2. Communicate with the device provider to ensure an adequate schedule for evaluation and reassessment.
3. Review the usefulness of the devices with the family.
4. Monitor for complications and improper use.
5. Recognize that improper fit or use can lead to a number of potentially life-threatening complications.

of tone and posture. They cannot be used to attempt to correct a joint that already has a fixed contracture. Prosthetics are used to replace the function of a missing limb. They are generally fashioned and provided in parallel with orthoses. Caregivers need to pay scrupulous attention to skin care under the orthosis or prosthesis. Any sign of redness, blistering, or ulceration should be reported immediately. Caregivers should receive instructions as to how the devices are applied and removed, how long they should be worn, and for which activities they are needed. These devices are custom built and are carefully crafted for an exact fit on a given patient. Because of this, rapidly growing children may require new orthotics or prosthetics every few months. Actively growing children are at increased risk for complications caused by improper fit. See the CD-ROM for a list of questions parents should ask their orthotics provider.

Parents should be aware that any rash, redness, or signs of chafing on the body (especially near straps or buckles) should be reported immediately. Children who use wheelchairs, orthoses, and prosthetics should be examined in and out of their equipment and should be completely disrobed for part of the examination to evaluate the risk of pressure- and motion-induced skin injury. The use of sling-type seats should be discouraged except for very short-term transportation or transfers because of the increased risk of spine and hip dysplasia associated with these devices.

The hallmark of treatment of pressure-induced injury is decreasing pressure. Adding padding under a brace or belt is often exactly the opposite of what is required. Ulceration is treated with pressure relief and a combination of local dressing changes, local antibiotics, or systemic antibiotics governed by wound cultures. Small ulcers can be treated in a manner similar to the treatment of small second-degree burns, with wet to dry dressing changes and topical antibacterial ointments. Competent surgical specialists should govern the treatment of large or deep ulcers, ulcers over vital structures, and ulcers with exposed bone. The primary health care provider should assist in screening, education, early diagnosis, and prompt treatment in this regard.

Ventriculoperitoneal Shunts

Ventriculoperitoneal and ventriculovascular shunts are siphoning devices that are placed to prevent central nervous system tissue damage from disorders of cerebrospinal fluid circulation. They are commonly placed in infancy or after trauma. Nearly all children with ventriculoperitoneal shunts will require revision in their lifetime. Infection and proximal tubing malfunction are most common within 2 years of initial placement. Distal tubing malfunction is most common when the shunt has been in place for longer than 2 years. The generalist's role is to recognize the early signs of shunt infection and malfunction and respond appropriately.

The cardinal symptoms of ventriculoperitoneal shunt malfunction are well known and include headache, lethargy, depressed mental status, seizure, acute focal neurologic change, vomiting, and fever. However, these symptoms are common and may be present in an otherwise ill child with a functioning shunt. An evaluation in this situation calls for a careful history of the pace and severity of symptom development, a search for an alternative explanation for the symptoms, and a period of active observation. Special attention should be paid to the pattern and symptoms of previous malfunctions. A recently placed shunt (in place for less than 6 months) is far more susceptible to infection or obstruction than an older shunt. Physical examination should include a gentle palpation of the entire length of the tube, noting any swelling in the subcutaneous tissues of the neck. Laboratory evaluation should include peripheral blood cultures and a possible lumbar puncture for opening pressure, cell counts, and cultures. Shunts should be tapped only by neurosurgeons or their trained designates. Shunt series (plain radiographs of the entire length of tubing) are helpful only as a screen for discontinuity of the tubing and should never be used in isolation. A computed tomography (CT) scan of the head is necessary to assess change in the size of the ventricles and should be compared to a clear baseline scan. Some experimental ventriculoperitoneal shunts are equipped with a device that can be programmed to drain at a particular pressure. These can also provide an external pressure reading. In regard to patients with shunts, it is essential for the generalist to know that coagulase-negative *Staphylococcus* is a life-threatening pathogen in this population and should not be assumed to be a contaminating organism.

CONTROVERSIES AND FUTURE TRENDS

Most of the current controversy surrounding the care of children who are dependent on medical technology centers on the rising costs of medical care, the public's continued demand for access to high technology care, and families' increasing involvement in choosing and coordinating their children's health care. The current demand for expert home care services exceeds the supply of trained providers. The need for enhanced respite services, transportation, education, vocational training, and recreation also exceeds supply. Federal law requires local school systems to fund the health care costs required to allow children to safely attend appropriate schools in the least restrictive manner. This places a responsibility on local communities to blend sources of funding, which are not easily blended. Finally, there are obvious ethical issues that arise when scarce resources are proportioned to a small group of individuals. However, Americans continue to demand access to the most advanced high technology care available. Both federal and abundant case law exists to ensure that children with disabilities and chronic illnesses have access to these technologies.

Additional Resources, CD-ROM

Individual health care plan format	Text
Helpful websites for technology dependent care	Text
Example letter of medical necessities	Text
Care of children who require mechanical ventilation, oxygen, or tracheostomy	Text
Care of children with genitourinary appliances	Text
Care of children with ostomies	Text
Bibliography	

SUGGESTED READINGS

Levy SE, O'Rourke M: Technological assistance: Innovations for independence. In Batshaw M (ed): Children with Disabilities, 4th ed. Baltimore, Brookes, 1997, pp 687–709.

Perrin J, Erenberg G, LaCamera R, et al, American Academy of Pediatrics, Committee on Children with Disabilities: Guidelines for home care of infants, children and adolescents with chronic disease. Pediatrics 1995;96(1):161–164.

Porter S, Haynie M, Bierle T, et al: Children and Youth Assisted by Medical Technology in Educational Settings, 2nd ed. Baltimore, Brookes, 1997.

Silva T, Sofis L, Palfrey J: Practicing Comprehensive Care: A Physician's Operations Manual for Implementing a Medical Home for Children with Special Healthcare Needs. Boston, Institute for Community Inclusion/UAP, 2000.

Ziring PR, Brazdziunas D, Cooley WC, et al, American Academy of Pediatrics, Committee on Children with Disabilities: Care coordination: Integrating health and related systems of care for children with special healthcare needs. Pediatrics 1999;104:978–981.

282

Blood and Bone Marrow Transplantation (Hematopoietic Stem Cell Transplantation)

F. Leonard Johnson

TYPES OF TREATMENTS

There are currently three sources of hematopoietic stem cells for transplantation: bone marrow, peripheral blood, and umbilical cord (placental) blood. Transplants are defined as allogeneic (stem cells from another individual), syngeneic (stem cells from an identical twin), or autologous (stem cells from the patient). Allogeneic transplants involve completely or partially matched hematopoietic stem cells from (1) a family member (completely matched sibling transplants are the most common), (2) an unrelated individual registered with an unrelated donor registry, or (3) umbilical cord blood from either either a sibling's or unrelated individual's birth. Potential donors for allogeneic transplantation are identified by tissue typing (HLA typing) which determines compatibility between the donor and recipient at the major histocompatibility complex (MHC).

The degree of compatibility between donor and recipient is commonly defined by identity of at least six antigens located on three major loci of the major histocompatibility complex: HLA-A, HLA-B, and HLA-DR. Each of these loci consists of two antigens (one inherited from each parent). Donors and recipients may be completely matched (six out of six) or partially matched (four or five out of six).

The most common complications of allogeneic transplants are immunological—graft rejection or, most frequently, graft-versus-host disease (GVHD), in which the immunocompetent donor hematopoietic stem cells recognize the patient as foreign.

Autologous transplants do not have this risk of an immunological reaction. Autologous transplants offer the advantage of administering higher, more potentially effective doses of intensive cytotoxic therapy (with chemotherapy, radiation, or both) and then "rescuing" patients with their own marrow or peripheral blood with faster recovery of marrow function. Autologous transplantation cannot be used successfully in patients with genetic disorders or with malignant cells present in the marrow or peripheral blood.

HOW THE THERAPIES ARE ADMINISTERED

Transplant protocols follow four specific steps. The first step is a 4- to 10-day preparative regimen used to prevent graft rejection in all transplants and relapse in transplants for cancer. Step two is the acquisition and infusion of the donor hematopoietic stem cells into the patient. Step three is immunosuppression after the transplant to prevent GVHD. Step four is supportive care related to nutrition, transfusion support, and the prevention of infection (Table 282-1).

The Preparative Regimen

All patients except infants who lack an immune system must be treated with immunosuppression before transplantation to prevent graft rejection. An example of a preparative regimen for a nonmalignant disease (such as severe aplastic anemia) is high-dose cyclophosphamide in combi-

Table 282-1. Examples of Hematopoietic Stem Cell Transplant Protocols

	Nonmalignant Diseases	Malignant Diseases
Preparative regimen (4–10 days)	SCID*: none All other indications: cyclophosphamide ± ATG† ± busulfan ± lymphoid irradiation	Cyclophosphamide + total body irradiation/or busulfan
GVHD prevention (6–9 months) Supportive care	Methotrexate ± cyclosporine ± corticosteroids Total parenteral nutrition Blood product transfusion Trimethoprim-sulfamethoxazole ± intravenous immunoglobulin (IVIG) ± acyclovir	

*Severe combined immune deficiency.
†Antithymocyte globulin.

nation with antithymocyte globulin. In transplants for the treatment of genetic disorders in which the marrow cellularity is normal (e.g., a hemoglobinopathy or metabolic storage disease) cyclophosphamide is combined with busulfan, which more effectively makes space for the transplanted cells. A special preparative regimen may be necessary with some nonmalignant disorders such as Fanconi syndrome (anemia) where patients are particularly sensitive to alkylating agents (e.g., cyclophosphamide and radiation) so very low dose cyclophosphamide, radiation to the lymph nodes only, and the addition of antithymocyte globulin are used.

In transplants for malignant diseases, the preparative regimen must also be effective in destroying all cancer cells before the transplant and is usually more intensive, commonly involving combinations of high-dose chemotherapeutic agents with or without total body radiation. A standard preparative regimen for transplants for the treatment of acute lymphoblastic leukemia is cyclophosphamide plus fractionated total body irradiation. In some patients suffering from myeloid leukemias (acute and chronic), total body irradiation may not be necessary and cyclophosphamide combined with busulfan is a common preparative regimen.

Acquisition and Infusion

Bone marrow is obtained by multiple marrow aspirations from the posterior and anterior iliac crests performed in an operating room under general anesthesia. The volume of marrow collected is based on the size of the patient. Hematopoietic stem cells from the peripheral blood are collected by a series of daily apheresis procedures (usually three to four). Anesthesia is not required. In allogeneic transplants, peripheral blood stem cells are collected after the donor has been treated with granulocyte-colony stimulating factor (G-CSF) to increase the yield of stem cells. Autologous stem cells are also collected after granulocyte-colony stimulating factor treatment when the patient's white cell count has maximally recovered after a course of chemotherapy. Umbilical cord stem cells are obtained by cannulation of the placental blood vessels immediately after birth. The cells are then frozen and stored until required. Umbilical cord stem cells are tested as regular blood products (red cells and platelets) before storage in a blood bank. Once collected and appropriately processed the stem cells are infused into the patient in the same manner as a blood transfusion.

Graft-versus-Host Disease Prevention

The major complication after allogeneic transplantation is GVHD. To prevent GVHD, patients are treated with immunosuppressive agents immediately after the stem cell infusion. A common GVHD prophylactic regimen is a short course of methotrexate for up to 2 weeks combined with cyclosporine given for 6 to 9 months after the transplantation. Prophylactic GVHD regimens also frequently use corticosteroids.

T cells are involved in the pathogenesis of GVHD. T cells are frequently removed from the stem cell source before infusion when administering mismatched bone marrow transplants. T-cell depletion, however, is associated with a higher risk of host rejection in all transplants, and of relapse after transplants for leukemia.

Supportive Care

Advances in supportive care have considerably improved the outcome of hematopoietic stem cell transplantation. Routine use of total parental nutrition ensures adequate nutrition. Red cell and platelet transfusions provide hematologic support during the period of marrow suppression after the preparative regimen. All blood products must be irradiated and leukodepleted before transfusion to prevent donor lymphoid cells from grafting and causing GVHD. Leukodepletion also decreases the risk of infection from cytomegalovirus (CMV). Prophylactic antibiotics and intravenous immunoglobulin (IVIG) administered after transplantation may help prevent infections from *Pneumocystis carinii*, fungi, and herpes viruses, all potential causes of major morbidity and mortality.

INDICATIONS

Table 282-2 lists the spectrum of diseases treated by hematopoietic stem cell transplantation. Table 282-3 compares the benefits of allogeneic versus autologous transplantation for specific diseases.

For nonmalignant diseases, hematopoietic stem cell transplantation can be used to: (1) replace diseased marrow with

Table 282-2. Spectrum of Diseases Treated by Hematopoietic Stem Cell Transplantation

Nonmalignant Diseases
Allogeneic

Immunodeficiency syndromes
  SCID/reticular dysgenesis/Wiskott-Aldrich syndrome
Bone marrow failure syndromes
  Aplastic anemia/Kostmann syndrome/Blackfan-Diamond syndrome/amegakaryocytic thrombocytopenia
Abnormalities of stem cell function
  Glanzmann thrombasthenia
Fanconi syndrome (anemia)
Hemoglobinopathies
  Sickle cell anemia/thalassemia
Metabolic storage disorders
  Hurler syndrome, Hunter syndrome
  Metachromatic/adrenal leukodystrophies, globoid leukodystrophy, Lesch-Nyhan syndrome
Osteopetrosis

Malignant Disorders
Allogeneic

Leukemias
  Poor prognosis/recurrent acute lymphoblastic/acute and chronic myelogenous juvenile chronic myelogenous leukemia
Myelodysplastic syndromes
Disseminated neuroblastoma
Hodgkin/non-Hodgkin lymphomas
X-linked lymphoproliferative disorders
Hemophagocytic syndromes
Refractory anemia with excess blasts

Autologous

Solid Tumors
  Refractory/recurrent Hodgkin and non-Hodgkin lymphoma
  Bone/soft tissue sarcomas
  Brain tumors
  Poor prognosis neuroblastoma

Table 282-3. Indications for Allogeneic and Autologous Stem Cell Support

Disease	Allogeneic Transplant	Autologous Transplant
Leukemia (ALL, AML, CML)	Effective	Controversial; no better than conventional therapy
Lymphomas (Hodgkin disease, non-Hodgkin lymphoma)	Effective	Used rarely and only when marrow not involved
Neuroblastoma (stage IV)	Controversial; studies to define role related to conventional therapy and autologous transplant are ongoing	Controversial; studies to define role related to conventional therapy and allogeneic transplant are ongoing
Bone and soft tissue sarcomas, Wilm tumor, brain tumors	Rarely indicated	Rarely indicated and effectiveness unproven
Aplastic anemia and other cytopenias (not environmentally caused)	Effective	Not indicated
Immune deficiency (e.g., SCID)	Effective	Not indicated
Hemoglobinopathies, thalassemia, sickle cell anemia	Effective	Not indicated
Metabolic storage disorders, Hurler syndrome, metachromatic leukodystrophy	Controversial; may be effective in selected patients	Not indicated

normal stem cells (e.g., in immunodeficiency syndromes, bone marrow failure syndromes, and hemoglobinopathies); (2) replace missing or defective enzymes (e.g., in metabolic storage disorders); or (3) replace individual malfunctioning cells (e.g., osteoclasts in osteopetrosis). Only allogeneic transplantation can be successful in these diseases.

The most common indications for allogeneic transplantation in the treatment of malignant diseases in children are the following:

1. Acute lymphoblastic leukemia, in remission, that had very poor prognostic features at diagnosis (e.g., high white blood cell count or specific chromosomal abnormalities such as 11q23 translocation)
2. Relapsed acute lymphoblastic leukemia, after achieving a second remission
3. Acute myelogenous leukemia in first remission
4. Myelodysplastic syndromes

Allogeneic transplantation may also be indicated in selected solid malignant tumors such as refractory or relapsed (Hodgkin or non-Hodgkin) lymphomas and disseminated neuroblastoma.

The indications for autologous stem cells are very limited. The main impact of high-dose cytotoxic therapy with autologous stem cell support has been in the treatment of lymphomas and specific brain tumors (e.g., recurrent medulloblastoma and glioblastoma multiforme). In malignant diseases with marrow involvement there is no evidence that high-dose cytotoxic therapy with autologous stem cell support is better than conventional therapy. Unfortunately, no method exists at present for completely purging malignant cells from bone marrow or peripheral blood. Gene marker studies have clearly demonstrated that relapse after autologous stem cell transplantation is due to malignant cells present in the autologous stem cell infusion.

The indications for umbilical cord blood transplantation are the same as those for allogeneic transplantations (see under Controversies).

BENEFITS

Allogeneic hematopoietic stem cell transplantation offers children suffering from the nonmalignant diseases noted in Table 282-2 the best, and sometimes the only, chance for cure. Hematopoietic stem cell transplantation can be curative in up to 90% of patients suffering from severe idiopathic aplastic anemia when a matched sibling donor is available. Immunosuppressive therapy is curative in only 30% of such children. Allogeneic hematopoietic stem cell transplantation is the only curative therapy currently available for sickle cell anemia or thalassemia.

The cure rate for a child with acute lymphoblastic leukemia who relapses, particularly during chemotherapy, is less than 10%. Matched sibling allogeneic stem cell transplantation offers a chance for cure for almost half of these patients, and matched unrelated donor transplantation offers a cure rate for one third of patients. Conventional chemotherapy for children suffering from acute myelogenous leukemia (AML) offers a cure rate of approximately 40% to 50%. Marrow transplantation from a matched sibling donor during first remission for acute myelogenous leukemia increases the chance for cure to approximately 70%. Table 282-4 provides an overall summary of current results in allogeneic hematopoietic stem cell transplantation.

RISKS (COMPLICATIONS)

Table 282-5 summarizes the major complications that occur most frequently after blood and marrow transplantation. Immunological complications include host rejection and GVHD. Even with intensive immunosuppression before allogeneic stem cell transplantation, rejection still occurs in approximately 5% to 10% of patients, particularly in transplants for nonmalignant disorders. A second transplant, however, can often be successfully performed in nonmalignant disorders. T-cell depletion of the stem cell source before transplantation increases the risk of rejection.

GVHD occurs in allogeneic stem cell transplantation when the immunocompetent T cells of the donor recognize foreign host antigens. The pathogenesis of *acute GVHD* is not completely defined, but both T-cell and cytokine dysfunction appear to be involved in the process. Clinically acute GVHD causes a generalized maculopapular, erythematous, pruritic skin rash (Fig. 282-1), which is most pronounced on the palms, soles, and behind the ears. Other manifestations of acute GVHD are gastrointestinal

Table 282-4. Summary of Results of Allogeneic Blood and Bone Marrow Transplantation

Stem Cell Source	Indication	Acute GVHD	Chronic GVHD§	Disease-free Survival > 5 years
Matched sibling donor	Nonmalignant disorders	20%	10%	70–90%*
	Malignant disorders	30%	15%	40–70%†
Matched unrelated donor	Nonmalignant disorders	60%	20%	30–50%†
	Malignant disorders	70%	30%	25–40%‡
Umbilical cord blood	Nonmalignant disorders	10–20%	5–10%	50–90%‡
	Malignant disorders	10–20%	10–20%	25–70%‡

*Depends on disease/clinical condition of patients.
†Depends on type of malignancy.
†Depends on closeness of donor-recipient matching.
§Higher incidence of chronic GVHD when allogeneic peripheral blood cells are used compared to bone marrow.

symptoms of cramping abdominal pain and profuse diarrhea and obstructive liver disease from biliary necrosis.

The incidence of acute GVHD depends on the source and compatibility of the hematopoietic stem cells. The risk of acute GVHD is significantly higher (as high as 70% to 80%) in patients whose stem cell source is marrow or peripheral blood from an unrelated donor or whose donor is a four or five out of six HLA-antigen match. GVHD is classified as grade I to IV depending on the degree of involvement of the skin, gastrointestinal tract, and liver. Grades I and II are usually not life threatening and may not need treatment (grade I) or the treatment consists of a short course of corticosteroids. Grades III and IV are life threatening and require intense immunosuppressive therapy and supportive care, often with prolonged hospital-ization for continuing blood product support, total parental nutrition, and treatment of life-threatening infections.

Umbilical cord blood transplantation, particularly in transplants for nonmalignant diseases, has the lowest incidence of both acute and chronic GVHD. Matched sibling cord blood transplants have a lower incidence of significant GVHD than matched sibling marrow transplants. Unrelated umbilical cord blood transplants (particularly a six-out-of-six match) have an incidence of acute GVHD comparable to that seen in the matched sibling setting (see Table 282-4).

Chronic GVHD is a different immunological syndrome from acute GVHD although acute GVHD predisposes to this complication. Chronic GVHD is a multisystem disease with clinical similarities to autoimmune diseases such as juvenile rheumatoid arthritis, systemic lupus erythematosus, or scleroderma. Skin changes include areas of hyperpig-mentation and depigmentation and progression to a scleroderma-like picture with marked fibrosis and joint contractures (Fig. 282-2). Chronic GVHD also causes chronic liver disease, arthritis, bronchiolitis obliterans, and myositis. Immunosuppressive therapy and aggressive physical therapy may prevent or ameliorate some of these problems, particularly joint contractures caused by skin changes.

The incidence of chronic GVHD also depends on the source of donor blood or marrow stem cells. Chronic GVHD is most common in patients undergoing matched unrelated marrow donor transplants and least common in patients undergoing transplants with umbilical cord blood. Allogeneic peripheral blood as the source of stem cells is associated with a higher incidence of chronic GVHD than bone marrow as the source.

One potential advantage of chronic GVHD is an apparent antitumor effect. Patients transplanted for leukemia who develop chronic GVHD have a reduced risk of relapse compared to those patients who do not develop chronic GVHD or whose donor is an identical twin.

Infections after allogeneic marrow transplantation typically fall into a pattern related to time after transplantation. Bacterial and fungal infections are most common in the first month after transplant, secondary to granulocytopenia from the underlying reason for transplantation and the preparative regimen, or secondary to impaired granulocyte function associated with GVHD. *Pseudomonas aeruginosa, Escherichia coli, Klebsiella pneumoniae, Staphylococcus aureus, Staphylococcus epidermidis, Enterobacter* species,

Table 282-5. Major Complications after Blood and Bone Marrow Transplantation

Immunological
  Rejection
  GVHD
    ▪ Acute
    ▪ Chronic
Infection
  Common etiologies
    ▪ Bacterial/fungal/viral especially herpes species and varicella-zoster
  Patterns
    ▪ Early (associated with myelosuppression and acute GVHD)
    ▪ Late (associated with chronic GVHD)
Organ toxicity
  Drug/radiation therapy related
    ▪ Preparative regimen
      ▪ Veno-occlusive disease
      ▪ Specific drug/radiation therapy
    ▪ GVHD prophylaxis/treatment
      ▪ Renal toxicity
      ▪ Gastrointestinal toxicity
      ▪ Long-term effects of corticosteroids
  Immunologically related
    ▪ Acute/chronic GVHD
      ▪ Skin/liver/gastrointestinal tract in acute GVHD
      ▪ Multisystem in chronic GVHD
Relapse in transplants for malignant disease
Late effects of drugs/radiation
  Endocrine
    ▪ Growth retardation
    ▪ Hypogonadism
    ▪ Hypothyroidism
  Increased risk of second malignancies or myelodysplastic syndromes

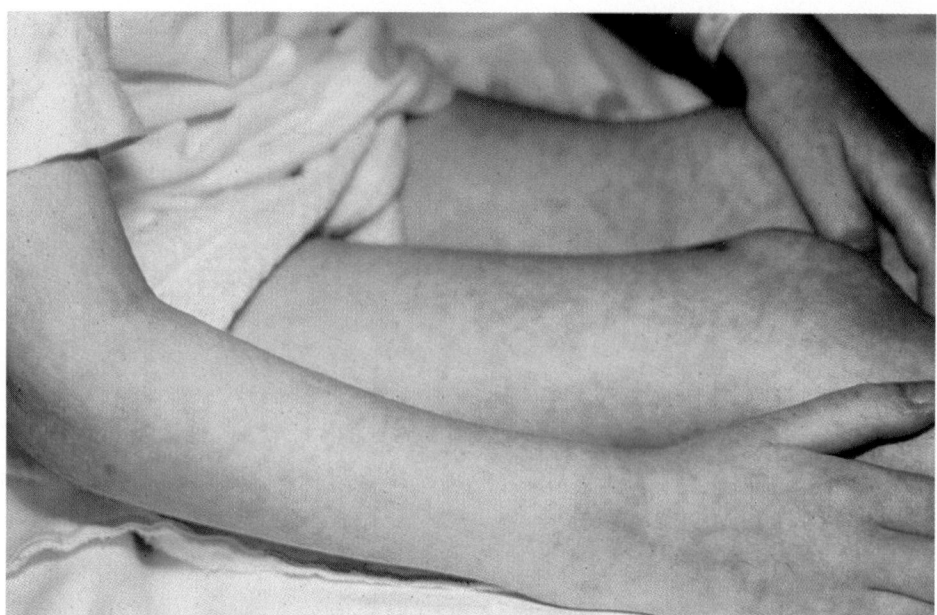

Figure 282-1. The generalized erythematous maculopapular skin rash of acute GVHD.

Candida species, and *Aspergillus* species are the most common pathogens.

Immunosuppression, related to the preparative regimen, acute GVHD, or both, predisposes the patient not only to bacterial and fungal infections, but also to viral infections (particularly herpes viruses, and particularly cytomegalovirus). In the second to third month after transplantation, before trimethoprim-sulfamethoxazole prophylaxis was routine, *Pneumocystitis carinii* pneumonia was a common complication.

In the fourth month and beyond, ongoing acute or chronic GVHD and treatment with immunosuppressive drugs predominantly predispose the patient to herpes virus or other viral infections, particularly varicella-zoster. Patients with chronic GVHD are essentially functionally asplenic and at risk for infections caused by encapsulated bacteria such as *Streptococcus pneumoniae* and *Hemophilus influenzae*. Trimethoprim-sulfamethoxazole or penicillin prophylaxis may help prevent these infections.

Organ toxicity is caused by high doses of immunosuppressive/chemotherapy drugs and radiation that are necessary for successful engraftment and eradication of malignancy in transplants for malignant disease. As many as one in four children develop veno-occlusive disease, secondary to chemotherapy and radiation, after transplantation.

Although patients are susceptible to any of the side effects of the drugs used in the preparative regimen, several complications can be prevented. Aggressive hydration and administration of mesna can protect against drug-induced bladder damage. Drugs given to prevent GVHD, especially

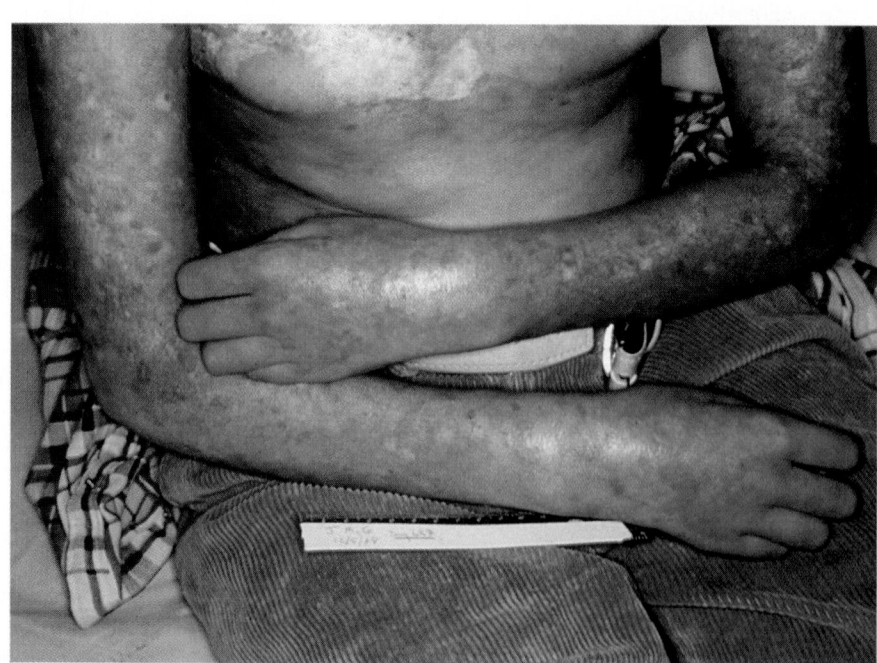

Figure 282-2. The scleroderma-like appearance of chronic GVHD. Note the residual scarring of the skin of the right chest wall from a previous herpes zoster infection associated with the immunoincompetence of chronic GVHD.

corticosteroids and cyclosporine, are also associated with significant organ toxicity. Long-term corticosteroid therapy, used particularly for the treatment of both acute and chronic GVHD, may be associated with aseptic necrosis of multiple joints, secondary diabetes, and hypertension. Cyclosporine may cause significant renal toxicity and hypertension thereby necessitating close monitoring of serum cyclosporine levels. Both acute and chronic GVHD may also cause significant organ damage. Preparative regimen drugs, such as busulfan, and total body irradiation, in particular, may have long-term effects that include endocrine dysfunction, such as growth retardation, hypogonadism, and hypothyroidism, and an increased risk for second cancers. Children undergoing hematopoietic stem cell transplantation require close monitoring for potential late effects many years posttransplantation.

EVIDENCE-BASED EFFECTIVENESS

The overall effectiveness of marrow transplantation depends on three major factors: (1) transplant indication, whether for malignant or nonmalignant disease; (2) clinical condition of the patient at the time of transplant (organ damage before transplant and recurrent cancer before transplant decrease survival rate); and (3) source of hematopoietic stem cells. Table 282-4 summarizes the current results of hematopoietic stem cell transplantation for the treatment of various malignant and nonmalignant diseases.

OUTCOME FOR NONMALIGNANT DISORDERS

Stem cell transplants for nonmalignant disorders such as immunodeficiency and bone marrow failure syndromes are associated with a high cure rate, exceeding 80% in children receiving transplants from a matched sibling marrow or umbilical cord blood donor. The use of matched unrelated donors for these diseases drops the cure rate to 50% to 70% because of increased incidence of GVHD. Children undergoing transplants for a hemoglobinopathy, such as sickle cell disease or thalassemia, and in excellent clinical condition at the time of transplant have better than an 80% chance of cure.

OUTCOME FOR MALIGNANT DISORDERS

Leukemias

Marrow transplantation from a matched sibling allogeneic donor cures up to 40% of children who have relapsed on chemotherapy for acute lymphoblastic leukemia and up to approximately 70% of children with acute myeloblastic leukemia transplanted in first remission. Matched unrelated donor stem cell transplants, associated with the higher incidence of GVHD, are less effective, with overall cure rates of approximately 25% to 30%. The effectiveness of matched umbilical cord blood transplant appears to mirror that of matched sibling donor transplants.

Solid Tumors

The most effective use of blood and bone marrow transplantation for malignant solid tumors appears to be in patients with Hodgkin or non-Hodgkin lymphoma who are either refractory to conventional chemotherapy or have relapsed. In this setting the use of very high dose chemotherapeutic preparative regimens followed by autologous hematopoietic stem cell support has cured up to 60% of patients in some studies. The effectiveness of high-dose cytotoxic therapy and autologous marrow support remains to be determined for other malignant solid tumors including neuroblastoma, brain tumors, and bone and soft tissue sarcomas.

CONTROVERSIES

Graft-versus-Host Disease

GVHD is the major barrier to further progress in the field of stem cell transplantation in children. Currently there is controversy regarding the best preventative approaches and management of this complication. Newer agents and approaches including the use of tacrolimus (FK506), mycophenylate mofetil, and different methods of T-cell depletion appear promising, yet studies to demonstrate their efficacy are often not well controlled.

Role in Metabolic Storage Disorders and Hemoglobinopathies

The role of marrow transplantation in the treatment of metabolic storage disorders and hemoglobinopathies remains controversial. Many of the manifestations of metabolic storage disorders resolve after transplantation, such as the cataracts and hepatosplenomegaly seen in Hurler syndrome, but transplantation does not alter all manifestations, such as the skeletal abnormalities characterizing this disorder. Although most children suffering from sickle cell disease or thalassemia will now live into early adulthood or longer with improvements in supportive care, many still suffer significant morbidity and even early mortality. Hematopoietic stem cell transplantation at a young age remains the only curative therapy for these diseases, but the timing of such therapy raises ethical issues and controversy because of the accompanying transplantation risks and potential mortality.

The Role of Autologous Stem Cells

The role of autologous transplantation in the treatment of malignant diseases also remains controversial. If malignant cells are present in the patient's marrow at the time of stem cell collection, they will cause relapse after transplant. To date there are no effective measures to purge every tumor cell from an autologous stem cell source.

Role of Family-Exclusive Umbilical Cord Blood Storage

Currently "for-profit" companies are encouraging parents to store umbilical cord blood from their child for the child's exclusive use as "insurance" should the child develop any of the diseases discussed in this chapter. Such practice is medically inappropriate for any genetic or other nonmalignant disease. The use of autologous stem cells in leukemia has not produced results superior to conventional therapy. Recent data also indicate that the chromosomal abnormality associated with leukemia occurring later in life is already present at birth, therefore making stored umbilical cord blood ineffective. Given the low incidence of diseases that require treatment by transplantation and the increasing success of conventional treatment in many of these diseases, very few, if any, umbilical cord blood units stored for "family exclusive" use will ever be used. These units would be more effectively used if stored in "not-for-profit" blood banks as a source of hematopoietic stem cells for patients who require treatment by transplantation but do not have a hematopoietic stem cell donor available.

FUTURE TRENDS

Studies are determining whether less marrow-suppressive preparative regimens can achieve a satisfactory rate of engraftment, particularly in nonmalignant diseases. The advantage of less marrow suppression is significantly less patient toxicity and the possibility of performing transplants in the outpatient setting. Better understanding of the pathogenesis of GVHD will lead to better preventive measures and safer transplantation. Because GVHD exerts an antileukemic effect, studies are also under way to see if some degree of GVHD can be utilized to prevent relapse.

Hematopoietic stem cell transplantation is a forerunner to gene therapy. Understanding the specific pathogenesis of diseases currently treated by hematopoietic stem cell transplantation will eventually lead to safer and more effective gene therapy approaches for many life-threatening immunologic, hematologic, and oncologic disorders.

Additional Resources, CD-ROM

Bibliography

SUGGESTED READINGS

Gocer H, Haznedarogo UC, Chal NJ: Acute graft-versus-host disease: Pathobiology and management. Exp Hematol 2001;29:259–277.

Guinan EC, Bierer BE: Principles of bone marrow and stem cell transplantation. In Nathan DG, Orkin SH (eds): Nathan and Oski's Hematology of Infancy and Childhood, 5th ed. Philadelphia, WB Saunders, 1998, pp 336–372.

Gustafsson A, Remberger M, Waniaiski J, et al: Unrelated bone marrow transplantation in children: Outcome in a comparison with sibling donor grafting. Bone Marrow Transplant 2000;25:1059–1065.

Hows JM: Status of umbilical cord blood transplantation in the year 2001. J Clin Pathol 2001;54:428–434.

Johnson FL: Placental blood transplantation and autologous banking—caveat emptor. J Pediatr Hematol Oncol 1997;19:183–186.

Sieff CA: Principles of stem cell therapy. In Nathan DG, Orkin SH (eds): Nathan and Oski's Hematology of Infancy and Childhood, 5th ed. Philadelphia, WB Saunders, 1998, pp 1811–1826.

SECTION 9   DIAGNOSTICS AND THERAPEUTICS: *Pharmacotherapy*

283 Principles of Pharmacotherapy

Susan Ralston

The rational use of drugs in pediatric patients requires a systematic approach and an understanding of the many challenges and characteristics that make pediatric patients unique. Pharmacologic principles must be considered, including a medication's therapeutic index, pharmacokinetics, pharmacodynamics, and adverse reactions that may be unique to specific pediatric age groups. Box 283-1 lists the important principles of pharmacology.

THERAPEUTIC INDEX

A medication's therapeutic index (therapeutic window) refers to the dosage range over which the drug exerts its desired effects compared to the dose that produces toxicity. Drugs with a wide therapeutic index exert a beneficial effect over a wide range of doses requiring very significant overdose to cause toxicity. Examples of drugs with a wide

Box 283-1. Principles of Pharmacotherapy

- *Therapeutic index:* the dosage range over which the drug exerts its desired effect compared to that which produces toxicity
- *Pharmacokinetics:* the absorption, distribution metabolism, and elimination of a medication
- *Absorption:* the passage of a medication from the site of administration to the bloodstream
- *Drug distribution:* the volume within the body into which a drug disperses
- *Drug metabolism:* the conversion of a medication to a form that can eventually be eliminated
- *Drug elimination:* the removal of a medication from the body
- *Pharmacodynamics:* the study of how drugs exert their biologic effects on living tissue
- *Pharmacogenetics:* the study of genetically determined variation in drug response

therapeutic index include penicillins, cephalosporins, and antacids such as the histamine II receptor blockers. Other drugs have a very narrow therapeutic index. For these medications, the correct dose must be given for an individual patient; even then, interindividual variation in metabolism or elimination can lead to undesired effects. Often, drugs with a narrow therapeutic index are monitored through serum concentrations. Examples of medications with a narrow therapeutic index include theophylline, lithium, digoxin, and aminoglycosides. The therapeutic index of a medication is an important consideration in the administration of medications to pediatric patients. Medications for pediatric patients are dosed on the basis of weight or body surface area. It is vital that these calculations are made accurately and precisely in dealing with drugs with a narrow therapeutic index. Furthermore, factors that can affect the elimination of these medications must be considered.

PHARMACOKINETICS

Pharmacokinetics refers to the absorption, distribution, metabolism, and elimination of a drug in an individual. These parameters can vary greatly depending on the drug and the specific individual. The physiologic differences between newborn, infant, child, and adult can influence the absorption, distribution, metabolism, and elimination of a specific drug. Pediatric pharmacokinetics considers the effects of development on the different pharmacokinetic parameters.

ABSORPTION

Absorption is the passage of a medication from the site of administration to the bloodstream. Absorption is measured by the bioavailability (F) of a drug, which can range from 0% for drugs that are not absorbed to 100% for drugs that are completely absorbed. Absorption is dependent on the physical and chemical properties of the medication and the route of administration. All routes beside intravenous are subject to factors that may decrease absorption. Some of these factors are also influenced by physiologic development.

Percutaneous absorption of medications can be affected by developmental factors. Absorption through the skin is inversely proportional to the thickness of the stratum corneum. Premature infants have an immature stratum corneum. In addition, the skin hydration of newborn and preterm infants is higher, and they have a higher body surface area to body weight ratio when compared to adults. All of these factors can contribute to a significant increase in percutaneous absorption of some medications in preterm infants and neonates. Toxicities have been reported in newborns with topical administration of hexachlorophene containing skin cleansers, salicylic acid ointments, and hydrocortisone creams. Furthermore, it has even been shown that therapeutic levels of theophylline can be achieved in premature infants through topical administration.

Intramuscular absorption of medications is affected by developmental factors as well. Small muscle mass, decreased subcutaneous fat, alterations in blood flow, and decreased muscle contraction are factors that make intramuscular absorption of medications unreliable in newborn and premature infants. Some medications may have increased absorption when compared with adults, while others may have decreased absorption. Because of this unpredictability, this route should be avoided in newborns and premature infants whenever possible.

Oral administration, the most common route, varies in absorption owing to age-related factors. Developmental factors that can influence absorption include gastric acid secretion, gastric emptying time, surface area, bacterial colonization, enzyme production, and blood flow. Of these, the two most important factors are gastric pH and gastric emptying time. In premature infants, the gastric pH is elevated owing to immature acid secretion. A term infant has a gastric pH ranging from 6 to 8 at birth, which decreases rapidly over the first day of life. Gastric acid production is then decreased, and a condition of relative achlorhydria exists for several months. This decreased acid secretion could result in decreased absorption of drugs that are weak acids and increased absorption of drugs that are weak bases. Furthermore, drugs that are acid labile might not be degraded and therefore might have increased absorption when compared to adults. Gastric emptying time is also delayed in premature infants. This may result in increased absorption of drugs because of the increased contact with the gastrointestinal mucosa or decreased or delayed absorption of drugs that are absorbed from the proximal bowel. The net effect is the oral absorption of drugs in the neonatal period can differ from that in adults and may be highly variable depending on the chemical properties of the drug.

DRUG DISTRIBUTION

Drug distribution refers to the volume within the body into which a drug distributes. Aside from the characteristics of the drug, several physiologic factors affect how a drug distributes throughout the body. Extracellular and total body water are important. At birth, total body water as a percentage of body weight is around 75% to 80% compared to 60% in adults. The percentage of body weight attributed to extracellular fluid is also markedly increased in the neonate versus an adult. For these reasons, water-soluble medications, such as aminoglycosides, generally have a larger volume of distribution in infants and children. The average volume of distribution for gentamicin is around 0.5 L/kg in a neonate, 0.35 L/kg in a young child, and 0.25 L/kg in an adult. Up to twice the mg/kg dose may be required to achieve the same peak concentration in a neonate compared to an average adult.

Total body fat affects drug distribution, particularly of highly lipid-soluble drugs. The percentage of total body weight accounted for by fat is much lower in a newborn than in an adult.

Protein binding affects drug distribution and is related to the amount of protein, types of protein, binding affinity, and number of binding sites. For drugs that are highly protein bound, only the unbound drug is pharmacologically active. Premature infants and neonates have decreased albumin and other plasma proteins, thereby reducing the number of binding sites available. They may also have drugs displaced from their binding sites through competition with endogenous compounds such as bilirubin. For drugs that are highly protein bound, these factors can lead to significantly higher portions of unbound drug in this population. Because unbound drug is the pharmacologically active component, this can increase the potential for toxicity. Phenytoin, phenobarbital, and salicylates are examples of drugs that are highly protein bound.

DRUG METABOLISM

Metabolism is the major method by which drugs are inactivated in the body and converted to a form that can be eliminated. The most important factor affecting hepatic drug metabolism is enzyme function. The various enzymatic pathways for hepatic metabolism are categorized as Phase I or Phase II reactions. Phase I reactions include oxidation (cytochrome P450), reduction, and hydrolysis; Phase II reactions involve conjugation with a molecule provided by the body, such as glucuronic acid, sulfate, or glycine. Developmental factors affect hepatic drug metabolism. While overall drug metabolism is decreased at birth, the various pathways are present at different levels and mature at different rates. For instance, sulfation is well developed in newborns, but glucoronidation, the process by which chloramphenicol is metabolized, might not reach adult capacity until 3 to 4 years of age. Furthermore, different metabolic pathways may be utilized in neonates or young children and may sometimes compensate for the functional immaturity of others. For example, acetaminophen in the neonate is preferentially metabolized via sulfation rather than glucoronidation as in the adult. The methylation of theophylline to caffeine occurs in newborns but not to any significant extent in adults. In some cases, young children may actually metabolize certain medications faster. For example, theophylline metabolism through oxidation is impaired in the newborn. Over several months to a year, this process matures, and doses will need to be gradually increased. Young children and adolescents have a significantly higher metabolism of theophylline and can require up to twice the mg/kg/day dose of an adult.

DRUG ELIMINATION

Elimination of drugs, which is primarily dependent on kidney function, can be affected by age. The renal elimination of a drug is dependent on glomerular filtration, tubular secretion, and tubular reabsorption. The kidney eliminates drugs through one or some combination of these methods. At birth, all aspects of renal elimination are decreased, and they approach adult values at varying rates. Prior to 34 weeks' gestation, the glomerular filtration rate (GFR) is extremely low. It then begins to increase over the next several weeks. After birth, GFR increases dramatically over the first week of life and then continues to mature over weeks to months. In term infants, GFR is clinically mature at about 1 month of age. In preterm infants, GFR increases more gradually. Maturity of tubular function occurs more slowly and does not approach adult values until

after 6 months. The clinical implication of the immature renal function is a prolonged half-life of drugs eliminated by the kidney in neonates and young infants. Therefore, doses of some drugs, especially those with a narrow therapeutic window, might need to be adjusted for decreased renal function.

PHARMACODYNAMICS

Not all differences in the response to medications seen in pediatric patients are attributable to immaturity of pharmacokinetic parameters. Pharmacodynamics is the study of how drugs produce their biologic effects on living tissue. It refers to an individual's response to a specific drug dose. The pharmacodynamics of a drug includes its interaction with biologic receptors and the mechanism of action of the drug. Differences in binding affinity, number of receptors, and physiologic development account for some altered responses to certain medications in pediatric patients. For example, higher doses of digoxin are required in neonates despite decreased clearance. Increased binding sites on the neonatal erythrocyte and a lower digoxin binding affinity of receptors in the neonatal myocardium explain this phenomenon. There are also physiologic differences in the newborn's heart when compared to an adult. The newborn myocardium has a higher proportion of noncontractile to contractile elements and may be incompletely innervated by the sympathetic nervous system. As a result, dopamine and dobutamine may have a diminished effect, and higher per-kilogram doses may be required.

DISEASE STATES

Several disease states can affect the pharmacokinetics and pharmacodynamics of medications in pediatric patients. Acute or chronic renal failure will decrease the elimination of renally excreted drugs. Renal failure can also change the volume of distribution of some drugs. This can occur through alterations in protein binding because of displacement from uremia or because of an increased fluid status. Similarly, hepatic disease can decrease the metabolism of medications that are inactivated by the liver. Children with hematologic malignancies tend to have altered pharmacokinetic parameters. In general, these children tend to eliminate drugs faster. However, they may also be at increased risk for renal impairment from exposure to nephrotoxic chemotherapeutic agents. Children and adults with burns will also have altered pharmacokinetic parameters. These patients will eliminate drugs faster and have higher volumes of distribution. This may result in higher doses being required to achieve the desired effect. Cystic fibrosis, which typically presents in childhood, is an example of an inherited disease state with altered pharmacokinetic parameters. Individuals with cystic fibrosis tend to have an increased total body clearance of medications. While increased renal clearance accounts for a significant portion of this, the exact mechanism is unknown and also involves increased clearance outside of the kidneys. People with cystic fibrosis tend to have an increased volume of distribution. For these reasons, children with cystic fibrosis have higher dosing requirements than children and adults without this disease

DOSING

All of the principles discussed thus far are important in determining the dose for an individual patient. This is not unique to pediatric patients. However, the range of patients and the varying maturity of the physiologic development across those ages make individualizing doses for pediatric patients a challenge. The doses for most medications in pediatric patients are based on weight. Ideally, these doses have been derived through clinical studies in individuals with ages similar to that of the person who is to receive the therapy. Often, however, they are obtained from less scientific methods. When available, doses based on weight and age variables such as gestational or postnatal age should be utilized. For example, the dose of gentamicin can be individualized for a newborn based on weight and postnatal age to account for the immature renal function and increased volume of distribution. Alternatively, the doses for certain drugs such as acyclovir or chemotherapeutic agents may be based on body surface area. This is probably a more accurate method of dosing medications in children who weigh more than 10 kg. Unfortunately, for many drugs, doses based on body surface area are not published. In addition, this method requires the height of the patient, which is not always readily available. Dosing medications on the basis of body surface area is generally not recommended in infants who weigh less than 10 kg. In this population, doses based on body surface area can overestimate the dose owing to the relatively large body surface area to weight ratio. A final consideration in individualizing the dose for pediatric patients is the indication. As with adults, the dose of a medication may be different depending on its specific indication. For example, in treating meningitis, the dose of antibiotics is higher and given more frequently than for infections outside of the central nervous system.

DRUG DELIVERY

Once the drug, dose, and route are determined, delivery of the medication to the pediatric patient can remain a challenge. Most medications are not manufactured in dosage forms that are convenient for administration to pediatric patients. For example, intravenous administration of some drugs may require drug volumes so small they are not easily measured or delivered accurately. This can require dilutions, which increase the likelihood of an error. Most oral medications are manufactured in capsule or tablet form. This makes delivery to pediatric patients difficult, particularly when they are extended-release or enteric-coated products, which often cannot be crushed or diluted. Furthermore, a child's acceptance of a medication can be challenging. Taste and volume are important considerations in ensuring compliance. Crushing an oral steroid tablet and mixing it with the child's favorite treat may be better accepted than the liquid preparation. When possible, formulations with a higher concentration can be selected so that the volume of drug administered can be reduced.

DRUG EFFICACY

The desired outcome for all medications is efficacy without toxicity. Because of the differences in pediatric patients, some drugs are more toxic in pediatric patients, and some are actually less toxic. The increased toxicity is the most worrisome, and chloramphenicol is the classic example. Decreased metabolism of chloramphenicol by glucoronyl transferase caused increased levels leading to a syndrome of circulatory collapse, or gray syndrome. Tragically, there are many other examples. Decreased elimination of benzyl alcohol has led to metabolic acidosis and neurologic toxicities in preterm infants. Sulfonamides and ceftriaxone displace bilirubin from binding sites, resulting in increased free bilirubin levels, which could lead to kernicterus. For this reason, they are not routinely recommended in infants younger than 2 months of age. The antiepileptic lamotrigine is 10 times more likely to cause severe dermatologic reactions in children than in adults. The use of tetracyclines should be limited or avoided in children younger than 8 years of age to avoid permanent teeth staining, and fluoroquinolones are not recommended in children because of cartilage toxicity and arthropathies seen in animal models. Aside from pediatric specific toxicities, a recent study demonstrated that pediatric patients have three times as many potential adverse effects as adults. This was primarily attributed to the higher potential for errors in pediatric patients, particularly neonates in the neonatal intensive care.

PHARMACOGENETICS

In the future, pharmacogenetics may provide an important tool for improving pediatric pharmacotherapy. Pharmacogenetics describes the study of genetically determined variations in drug response. Certain individuals might be more or less prone to the beneficial or adverse effects of a drug than the general population as a consequence of inherited variations in enzyme activity. The development of phenotyping procedures might allow for determining which patients possess these variations prior to prescribing. If this phenotyping is developed for all age groups, it could provide further information on the variations in enzyme activity that occur during development and at different developmental stages. This knowledge could then be used to truly individualize the dose or therapeutic regimen chosen for an individual. Such advances would improve the ability to safely prescribe medications to pediatric patients.

DRUG LABELING

More data on the pharmacokinetics, pharmacodynamics, and safe use of drugs in pediatric patients may become available. In 1991, only around 20% of drugs in the Physicians' Drug Reference contained pediatric information, and only a small number of the new drugs approved each year contain pediatric labeling. New regulations are attempting to change this. In 1994, the FDA announced plans to mandate pediatric labeling on all new drug applications that might pertain to pediatric patients. Further progress was made in 1997 when a major amendment to the Food, Drug, and

Cosmetic Act was enacted called the Modernization Act. Later, the Pediatric Studies rule was established in 1998. These regulations reinforced the FDA's position for providing pediatric drug labeling in the drug approval process. The Modernization Act also required the FDA to identify drugs that should carry pediatric labeling. Over 300 drugs were identified, including inhaled albuterol, intravenous ampicillin, and methyphenidate in children younger than 6 years of age. In addition, these regulations allow the FDA to issue written requests to manufacturers to voluntarily provide pediatric labeling information. If the information is considered to be highly valuable, the FDA may mandate industry participation. In return for providing the pediatric labeling requirements, the FDA can extend the manufacturer's patent for the drug by 6 months, giving the manufacturer a longer period of exclusivity. Though the effects of these changes are coming slowly, they are positive steps toward improving the safe use of mediations in pediatrics.

Additional Resources, CD-ROM

Bibliography

SUGGESTED READINGS

Berlin CM: Advances in pediatric pharmacology and toxicology. Adv Pediatr 1997;44:545–574.

Gupta A, Waldhauser LK: Adverse drug reactions from birth to early childhood. Pediatr Clin North Am 1997;44(1):79–92.

Rainu K, Bates DW, Landrigan C, et al: Medication errors and adverse drug events in pediatric inpatients. JAMA 2001;285:2114–2120.

Wilson JT: An update on the therapeutic orphan. Pediatrics 1999;104(3):S585–S590.

Yaffe S. ed., Eastrbrook RW, Bouxsein P, et al: Rational Therapeutics for Infants and Children: Workshop Summary. Washington, DC, National Academy Press 2000.

SECTION 9   DIAGNOSTICS AND THERAPEUTICS: *Pharmacotherapy*

284 Antimicrobials

William V. Raszka, Jr.

Today, physicians face an almost bewildering choice of antimicrobial agents, yet important concepts regarding antimicrobial therapy remain the same (Box 284-1). Antimicrobial agents target enzymes or sites present in the microbe that are significantly different or absent from those found in humans (Table 284-1). Selection of an appropriate, effective antimicrobial regimen depends on knowledge of the likely infecting organisms, the spectrum of activity and toxicity for each antibiotic, and both the mechanism of action and resistance to the antibiotic. This chapter will review antimicrobials used to treat bacterial, viral, fungal,

and parasitic diseases that a pediatrician is likely to encounter during practice. Discussion of agents for treatment of viral, fungal, and parasitic diseases is found on the CD-ROM. Additional information about antibacterials is also found on the CD-ROM.

ANTIBACTERIAL AGENTS

Cell Wall Active Agents

Antimicrobial agents in this group take advantage of the fact that almost all bacteria make cell walls while humans do not. The compounds described in this section target microbial enzymes instrumental in making and maintaining the bacterial cell wall. Generally, these agents are bactericidal, well tolerated, and useful in a variety of clinical situations.

Penicillins

The penicillins are a heterogeneous group of β-lactam ring containing drugs that interfere with the terminal steps of bacterial cell wall formation by binding transpeptidases, endopeptidases, and carboxypeptidases located on the cell membrane. These enzymes are collectively known as penicillin binding proteins. The exact mechanism(s) by which the penicillins lead to cell death is not known but

---

Box 284-1. Principles of Antimicrobial Therapy

1. Identify the most likely site of infection.
2. On the basis of the presumed site and clinical epidemiology (e.g., age of patient, immunocompromised), identify the most likely organisms causing disease.
3. Select an antibiotic that will kill or inhibit the growth of the suspected organisms at the suspected site with the least amount of toxicity to the patient.
4. Once the specific organism causing disease has been identified, switch therapy to the narrowest-spectrum antimicrobial with the least toxicity and cost that will kill or inhibit the growth of the organism at the site of infection.

Table 284-1. Antibiotics and Their Targeted Site of Action

Site of Action	Specific Antibiotic or Class of Antibiotics
Cell wall synthesis	Penicillins
	Cephalosporins
	Glycopeptides
	Monobactams
	Carbapenems
	Fosfomycin
	Bacitracin
Protein synthesis	Aminoglycosides
	Tetracyclines
	Macrolides
	Clindamycin
	Chloramphenicol
	Oxazolidinones
	Streptogramins
	Mupirocin
DNA/RNA synthesis or maintenance	Sulfonamides
	Trimethoprim
	Fluoroquinolones
	Rifamycins
Cell membrane integrity	Polymyxins

may involve autolysis and changes in osmotic integrity of the bacteria. Resistance to the penicillins is usually mediated either by enzyme cleavage of the β-lactam ring or by alterations in the penicillin target site of action. As bacteria have developed resistance to various penicillin products, the β-lactam side chains have been modified to either improve access to the target site or resist inactivation by bacteria.

Most penicillins are minimally metabolized and excreted via the kidney. Changes in the dose are required in patients with renal insufficiency. Because penicillinase-resistant penicillins such as oxacillin, nafcillin, and dicloxacillin and the ureidopenicillin, piperacillin, undergo significant hepatic excretion, no dose modification is necessary in patients with renal insufficiency taking these drugs.

Most penicillin products are well tolerated. Hypersensitivity reactions may occur. These are more common following intramuscular dosing and range in severity from fever or a mild nonurticarial rash to anaphylaxis. Antibodies to the penicillin degradation products mediate hypersensitivity reactions. IgM and IgG antibodies usually cause nonurticarial rashes, while IgE antibodies produce urticarial rashes and anaphylaxis. The risk of death from anaphylaxis following penicillin administration is approximately 1/80,000. Testing for penicillin allergy may be difficult, as patients need to be tested against several penicillin breakdown products known as major and minor determinants. Approximately 5% to 15% of patients who are allergic to penicillin are allergic to cephalosporins. Generally, the risk of significant cross-reactivity is greater in patients with severe urticarial rashes or anaphylaxis following penicillin administration. Any of the penicillin products may be associated with hemolytic anemia or neutropenia following prolonged or very high dosing.

Natural Penicillins

The natural penicillins, of which penicillin G is the prototype, were the first of the penicillin products. The penicillins were initially broad-spectrum antibiotics with activity against most gram-positive organisms and anaerobes, but antimicrobial resistance has limited their spectrum of activity. Penicillin remains a highly effective drug for Group A and B streptococci, meningococci in most parts of the world, anaerobic gram-positive organisms, and mouth flora of humans and domestic animals and is the treatment of choice for syphilis (Table 284-2). Penicillin penetrates most tissues except the cerebrospinal fluid. Meningeal inflammation improves cerebrospinal fluid penetration. Four natural penicillins exist, each with a markedly different half-life and achievable peak serum concentration. Table 284-3 lists doses and dosing schedules of penicillin antibiotics used to treat infants and children outside the neonatal period.

Aqueous penicillin G is used when a high serum concentration and rapid effect are desired. With a half-life of approximately 30 minutes, penicillin G is given intravenously every 4 to 6 hours or as a continuous drip. It is used to treat serious infections such as meningitis, sepsis, or endocarditis caused by susceptible organisms and neonatal syphilis. High doses of penicillin G should be used cautiously in the face of significant renal or cardiac dysfunction, as penicillin G is administered as either a sodium or potassium salt. The sodium and potassium forms contain 2.0 mEq and 1.7 mEq/1 million units of penicillin, respectively.

Procaine penicillin G, an equal molar mixture of penicillin and procaine, is indicated when modest drug levels for several hours are needed. Given intramuscularly one to three times a day, procaine penicillin is infrequently used, as other agents are now used to treat *Neisseria gonorrhoeae* infections.

Benzathine penicillin G (Bicillin L-A), a mixture of benzathine and penicillin, is used when low levels of drug are needed for a prolonged time. When it is administered intramuscularly, low penicillin serum levels may persist for 3 to 4 weeks. Benzathine penicillin is indicated primarily for the treatment of streptococcal pharyngitis, early or latent syphilis, and as prophylaxis in those patients with a history of rheumatic fever. A mixture of benzathine penicillin and

Table 284-2. Bacterial Infections for Which Penicillin Is the Drug of Choice or First-Line Therapy

Gram-positives	*Clostridium perfringens*
	C. septicum
	C. tetani
	Erysipelothrix rhusiopathiae
	Streptococcus pyogenes (group A)
	S. agalactiae (group B)
	S. bovis
	S. pneumoniae (penicillin susceptible)
	S. viridans
Gram-negatives	*Capnocytophaga canimorsus*
	Eikenella corrodens
	Kingella kingii
	Neisseria meningitidis
	Pasteurella multocida
	Streptobacillus moniliformis
Others	*Actinomyces* spp
	Leptospira spp
	Treponema pallidum

Table 284-3. Doses and Dosing Schedule of Penicillin Antibiotics Used to Treat Infants and Children outside the Neonatal Period

Type	Generic Name	Route of Administration	Dose (mg/kg/day unless otherwise stated)	Doses/Day	Notes
Natural Penicillins					
	Penicillin G	IV	100,000–400,000 units/kg/day	Continuous or 4–6	Continuous is most cost efficient Maximum dose 24 million units/day
	Penicillin G procaine	IM	25,000–50,000 units/kg/day	1–2	Not to exceed 4.8 million units/day
	Penicillin benzathine	IM	25,000–50,000 units/kg *or* <60 lbs: 300,000–600,000 units (single dose) >60 lbs: 900,000–1,200,000 units (single dose)	1	
	Phenoxymethyl penicillin (penicillin V)	PO	25–50	4	Give on empty stomach Usual adult dose is 250–500 mg every 6–8 hours
Penicillinase-Resistant Penicillins					
	Oxacillin	IV	100–200	4–6	Maximum dose 12 g/day
	Nafcillin	IV	50–200	4	Maximum dose 12 g/day
	Cloxacillin	PO	50–100	4	Adult dosing: 250–500 mg every 6 hours
	Dicloxacillin	PO	25–50	4	Usual maximum dose: 1 g/day
Aminopenicillins					
	Ampicillin	IV, IM, PO	100–400	4	Oral: 50–100 mg/kg/day Endocarditis prophylaxis: 50 mg/kg
	Amoxicillin	PO	25–100	2–3	Larger doses for OM Endocarditis prophylaxis: 50 mg/kg
Ureidopenicillins					
	Piperacillin	IV	100–300	4–6	Maximum dose: 24 g/day
Penicillin plus β-Lactamase Inhibitors					
	Amoxicillin-clavulanic acid	PO	45–90	2–3	Many formulations with various amoxicillin to clavulanate ratios exist. May use 90 mg/kg/day for OM using 14:1 ratio preparation.
	Ampicillin-sulbactam	IV	100–400	4	Not recommended in children <1 year old Dose on ampicillin component Maximum dose: 12 g ampicillin/day
	Piperacillin-tazobactam	IV	240–400	3–4	Not approved for children Dose on the piperacillin component

IM, intramuscular; IV, intravenous; OM, otitis media; PO, orally.

procaine (Bicillin C-R) is sometimes used when an initial high level of penicillin followed by prolonged serum levels is desired.

Penicillin is degraded in the stomach by gastric acid, resulting in low serum levels following oral administration. The potassium salt of phenoxymethyl penicillin (penicillin VK) is more resistant to degradation and achieves higher serum levels. Given four times a day, penicillin VK is indicated for the treatment of streptococcal pharyngitis, some odontogenic processes, and skin infections caused by susceptible organisms. Because absorption and serum concentrations of penicillin VK are less reliable than those of other antibiotics, penicillin is no longer recommended as a prophylactic agent to prevent infective endocarditis.

Penicillinase-Resistant Penicillins

The widespread dissemination of a plasmid-mediated penicillinase has rendered penicillin G ineffective for the treatment of staphylococcal infections. The penicillinase-resistant penicillins possess a side chain that protects the β-lactam ring from destruction by penicillinases. The penicillinase-resistant penicillins include oxacillin, nafcillin, cloxacillin, and dicloxacillin. These are all highly active against methicillin-susceptible staphylococci and active against streptococci. The penicillinase-resistant penicillins are not active against enterococci, methicillin-resistant *Staphylococcus aureus*, penicillin-resistant *Streptococcus pneumoniae*, and gram-negative organisms. Oxacillin and nafcillin are given intravenously every 4 to 6 hours (see Table 284-3). Because both can cause necrosis if infused subcutaneously, intravenous administration should be monitored carefully. Dose modification is indicated in severe hepatic dysfunction but not renal insufficiency, as the liver primarily excretes both drugs. The penicillinase-resistant penicillins are the drugs of choice for the empiric therapy of staphylococcal infections when methicillin-resistant *Staphylococcus aureus* is not suspected. Nafcillin and oxacillin should be used preferentially over vancomycin for the specific therapy of susceptible *Staphylococcus aureus* infections, as they have superior bactericidal activity and cost less. Cloxacillin and dicloxacillin are well-absorbed oral penicillinase-resistant penicillins, although only dicloxacillin has a pediatric indication. Liquid dicloxacillin has an unpleasant taste that may limit compliance. Usually given every 6 hours, these products are used following intravenous therapy and for the primary therapy of soft tissue infections.

Extended-Spectrum Penicillins

Investigators have modified penicillin in an effort to expand gram-negative coverage. The expanded gram-negative activity of extended-spectrum penicillins derives from better penetration through the outer membrane of gram-negative bacteria and higher affinity for penicillin binding proteins. Ampicillin was the first penicillin effective against respiratory and gastrointestinal gram-negative bacilli. Ampicillin is as active as penicillin against streptococcal and meningococcal organisms and more active against enterococci and *Listeria monocytogenes*. Initially very effective against most strains of *Haemophilus*, *Moraxella*, *Escherichia coli*, *Proteus*, *Salmonella*, *Shigella*, and *N. gonorrhoeae*, these organisms have developed β-lactamases that cleave the β-lactam ring of ampicillin and limit its effectiveness. Ampicillin is cleaved by the β-lactamase elaborated by staphylococci.

Ampicillin can be given orally, intramuscularly, or intravenously. Intravenous ampicillin achieves high serum concentrations and penetrates most tissues well. As with penicillin and most β-lactam products, meningeal inflammation improves cerebrospinal fluid penetration. It is usually dosed every 4 to 8 hours (see Table 284-3). Except for the treatment of susceptible *Shigella*, oral ampicillin has largely been supplanted by its close relative, amoxicillin. Amoxicillin is much better absorbed and achieves higher and more reliable serum concentrations. Ampicillin and amoxicillin are most often used for the empiric treatment of upper and lower respiratory tract and suspected *L. monocytogenes* infections, and the specific therapy of streptococci, susceptible gram-negative organisms, and *Borrelia burgdorferi*. Additionally, amoxicillin may be used as a prophylactic agent for the prevention of infective endocarditis.

The carboxypenicillins, carbenicillin and ticarcillin, were developed as antipseudomonal products. These drugs are active against most of the organisms that ampicillin is active against but are also effective against *Pseudomonas aeruginosa* and other multiresistant gram-negative organisms. However, because carboxypenicillin administration at times led to platelet dysfunction and sodium overload, their clinical utility waned as equally effective but less toxic agents were developed.

The ureidopenicillins, mezlocillin and piperacillin, were developed to expand the coverage offered by the carboxypenicillins but without the concomitant toxicity. Piperacillin and mezlocillin have the widest innate spectrum of activity of any of the penicillins. These agents are active against streptococci, enterococci, and respiratory gram-negatives such as *Haemophilus*, *Neisseria*, most Enterobacteriaceae, *Pseudomonas*, and many anaerobes. Neither drug is active against staphylococci or β-lactamase-producing *Haemophilus influenzae*. Penetration into most tissues including the inflamed cerebrospinal fluid is excellent. Piperacillin is given intravenously every 4 to 6 hours (see Table 284-3). No dose modification is necessary in patients with renal insufficiency owing to its significant biliary excretion. Piperacillin and mezlocillin are used to treat *Pseudomonas* and other serious infections caused by gram-negative bacilli. Because a significant percentage of Enterobacteriaceae elaborate a wide spectrum of chromosomally mediated β-lactamases that cleave the ureidopenicillins, neither mezlocillin nor piperacillin is used as a single agent for the empiric treatment of febrile, neutropenic patients or patients with intra-abdominal infections. The ureidopenicillins exhibit in vitro synergistic activity against gram-negative bacilli such as *Pseudomonas* when combined with an aminoglycoside. This combination may be important in neutropenic patients and those in septic shock.

Penicillin and β-Lactamase Inhibitor Combinations

While the extended-spectrum penicillins have expansive activity against gram-negative organisms, they are still quite susceptible to cleavage by β-lactamases. To overcome this problem, they are sometimes combined with a β-lactamase inhibitor. β-lactamase inhibitors are weak β-lactam antibiotics that bind irreversibly to plasmid-mediated β-lactamases, thereby negating the effect of the β-lactamase. Generally, adding a β-lactamase inhibitor to a penicillin expands the spectrum of activity of that drug to include organisms that make simple plasmid-mediated β-lactamases. Hence, addition of a β-lactamase inhibitor to a penicillin expands the activity of the parent drug to include staphylococci (except methicillin-resistant staphylococci), *H. influenzae*, *Moraxella catarrhalis*, *N. gonorrhoeae*, *Bacteroides fragilis*, *E. coli*, and other Enterobacteriaceae. Penicillin-β-lactamase inhibitor combinations, do not, however, have improved activity over the parent penicillin drug against enteric gram-negative bacilli with expanded-spectrum β-lactamases (e.g., *Pseudomonas*, *Enterobacter*, *Citrobacter*) or any organism whose mechanism of resistance does not involve β-lactamase production (i.e., penicillin-resistant *S. pneumoniae*). The three most common β-lactamase inhibitors in clinical use today are clavulanic acid (clavulanate), sulbactam, and tazobactam. Although there are subtle differences between them, they are equivalent clinically.

Three parenteral penicillin-β-lactamase inhibitor combinations are commercially available: ampicillin-sulbactam (Unasyn), ticarcillin-clavulanate (Timentin), and piperacillin-tazobactam (Zosyn). These drugs penetrate into most tissues well, although they are not generally used for the treatment of central nervous system infections. Dosing is similar to that of the parent penicillin product although the dose of piperacillin-tazobactam is often decreased in patients with renal insufficiency (see Table 284-3). Penicillin-β-lactamase inhibitor combinations are effective agents for the treatment of presumed polymicrobial infections. Clinical uses include lower respiratory tract infections, including aspiration syndromes, and gynecologic, intra-abdominal, and complex, soft tissue infections.

Amoxicillin-clavulanic acid (Augmentin) is the only oral penicillin β-lactamase inhibitor combination agent. Amoxicillin-clavulanate comes in many different concentrations of amoxicillin and ratios of amoxicillin to clavulanate. It is useful for treating infections with organisms susceptible to amoxicillin and β-lactamase-producing *H. influenzae*, *M. catarrhalis*, *E. coli*, anaerobes, and *S. aureus*. The most common side effects are gastrointestinal, including nausea, abdominal cramping, and diarrhea. Concurrent administration of food may decrease the likelihood of such events as will use of preparations with a lower concentration of clavulanic. Amoxicillin-clavulanate is commonly used for the empiric treatment of upper respiratory tract infections such as otitis media and sinusitis, lower respiratory tract infections including aspiration syndromes, and is the drug of choice for the treatment of human and animal bites. While amoxicillin-clavulanate does treat *N. gonococcus* infections, it is infrequently used for this purpose. Similarly, although useful in skin and soft tissue infections and urinary tract infections, narrow-spectrum drugs may be more appropriate. Amoxicillin-clavulanate may be given two or three times a day (see Table 284-3).

Cephalosporins

Similar to the penicillin family, the cephalosporins are a heterogeneous group of β-lactam antibiotics with a broad spectrum of activity and an excellent safety profile. First discovered in 1945, the cephalosporins, with the penicillins, are the antimicrobial agents pediatricians are most likely to use in clinical practice. Unlike the penicillins, the cephalosporins contain a six-member ring rather than a five-member ring adjoined to the β-lactam ring. Cephalosporins attach to penicillin binding proteins located on the cell membrane interrupting bacterial cell wall synthesis. Bacteria may develop resistance to cephalosporins by producing hydrolytic enzymes, alterations in specialized channels called porins through which antibiotics must pass to gain access to the target site or alterations in the target site itself.

The safety profile of the cephalosporin family is excellent. Severe, life-threatening reactions are quite rare. Hypersensitivity reactions, usually consisting of nonurticarial rashes, are the most common side effect. The risk of a cross-reaction in a patient who is allergic to penicillin is controversial, as patients who are allergic to penicillin have an increased risk of reactions to even immunologically unrelated products. Approximately 5% to 15% of patients who are allergic to penicillin are allergic to a cephalosporin. In the absence of significant urticaria or anaphylaxis following penicillin administration, cephalosporins may be used cautiously. The development of nonurticarial rashes following use of one cephalosporin does not preclude the use of another cephalosporin.

Most cephalosporins are excreted by the kidney. Patients with renal insufficiency should be given smaller doses of a cephalosporin or a longer dosing interval. The exception is ceftriaxone, which is excreted both by the kidney and liver.

Historically, cephalosporins have been loosely classified by generation from first to fourth based on their spectrum of activity. While sometimes useful, the lines between cephalosporin agents are more blurred than would be suggested by their generation classification. As a rough rule of thumb, first-generation cephalosporin agents are most active against gram-positive cocci. Second-generation cephalosporins are the most varied and possess greater activity than first-generation cephalosporins against certain gram-negative organisms and anaerobes. Third-generation cephalosporins are the most active against gram-negative organisms. Fourth-generation cephalosporins are active against both gram-positive and gram-negative organisms.

First-Generation Cephalosporins

The first-generation cephalosporins all have very similar and excellent activity against both aerobic and anaerobic gram-positive cocci except methicillin-resistant *S. aureus*, penicillin-resistant pneumococcus, and enterococci. They are also active against typical urinary tract pathogens such as *E. coli*, *Proteus*, and *Klebsiella*. First-generation cephalosporins have no significant activity against *Neisseria* species and respiratory pathogens such as *H. influenzae* and *M. catarrhalis*. Several parenteral first-generation cephalosporins exist, although cefazolin is most commonly used (Table 284-4). It is dosed every 8 hours and is an excellent choice for skin, soft tissue, and osteoarticular infections and surgical prophylaxis. Although first-generation cephalosporins penetrate many tissues well, they do not penetrate the cerebrospinal fluid well under any conditions and should not be used to treat central nervous system infections. Many oral first-generation cephalosporins are available (see Table 284-4). Selection is usually dictated by convenience or taste. Cephalexin has a short half-life and is usually dosed four times a day, while cefadroxil, with its long half-life, is given twice daily. These agents are useful for treating streptococcal pharyngitis, skin and soft tissue infections, and urinary tract infections.

Second-Generation Cephalosporins

Unlike the first-generation cephalosporins, the second-generation cephalosporins demonstrate significant variability in activity against bacteria. Compared to first-generation

Table 284-4. Doses and Dosing Schedule of Cephalosporin Antibiotics Used to Treat Infants and Children outside the Neonatal Period

Generation	Generic Name	Trade Name	Route of Administration	Effect of Food on Absorption	Dose Range (mg/kg/day)	Doses/Day	Comments
First Generation							
	Cefadroxil	Duricef	Oral	↓	30	2	Usual maximum dose in children is 2 g/day Adolescent and adult dosing is 1–2 g/day in 1–2 divided doses, maximum dose 4 g/day
	Cefazolin	Ancef, Kefzol	IM, IV		25–100	3	≥1 month Maximum dose: 6 g/day
	Cephalexin	Keflex	Oral	↓	25–100	3–4	
	Cephradine	Velosef	Oral	↓	25–50	2–4	
Second Generation							
	Cefaclor	Ceclor	Oral	↓	20–40	4–3 2–3	≥1 month
	Cefotetan	Cefotan	IM, IV		40–80	2	Not approved for children
	Cefoxitin	Mefoxin	IM, IV		80–160	4–6 3–6	≥3 months
	Cefprozil	Cefzil	Oral		15–30	2	≥6 months 30 mg/kg/day to treat otitis media 15 mg/kg/day to treat pharyngitis 20 mg/kg/day for skin infections
	Cefuroxime	Zinacef	IM, IV		75–150	3	≥3 months
	Cefuroxime axetil	Ceftin	Oral	↑	20–30	3	Not recommended in children <3 months suspension and tablets are not bioequivalent pharyngitis: 20 mg/kg/day otitis media etc.: 30 mg/kg/day
	Loracarbef	Lorabid	PO	↓		2	≥6 months Suspension gives higher serum levels
					15–30		Otitis media and sinusitis: 30 mg/kg Pharyngitis and skin infections: 15 mg/kg
Third Generation							
	Cefdinir	Omnicef	Oral		14	1–2	≥6 months
	Cefditoren	Spectrocef	Oral		200–400 mg/dose	2	>12 years. Approved for pharyngitis, bronchitis, and skin infections. Dose for pharyngitis is 400 mg bid. May lower carnitine level and has milk proteins.
	Cefixime	Suprax	Oral	±	8–10	1–2	≥6 months
	Cefoperazone	Cefobid	IM, IV		100–150	2–3	Not approved for children
	Cefotaxime	Claforan	IM, IV		75–200	3	Maximum dose 12 g/day
	Cefpodoxime	Vantin	Oral	↑	10	2	≥2 months Uncomplicated gonorrhea: 200-mg single dose
	Ceftazidime	Fortaz	IM, IV		75–150	3	Maximum dose 6 g/day
	Ceftibuten	Cedax	Oral	±	9	1	≥6 months

Table 284-4. Doses and Dosing Schedule of Cephalosporin Antibiotics Used to Treat Infants and Children outside the Neonatal Period—cont'd

Generation	Generic Name	Trade Name	Route of Administration	Effect of food on Absorption	Dose Range (mg/kg/day)	Doses/Day	Comments
Third Generation— cont'd							
	Ceftizoxime	Cefizox	IM, IV		150–200	3–4	≥6 months Maximum dose 12 g/day
	Ceftriaxone	Rocephin	IM, IV		50–100	1–2	Maximum dose 4 g/day Uncomplicated gonococcal infection: 125 mg in a single dose
Fourth Generation							
	Cefepime	Maxipime	IM, IV		100–150	3	≥2 months Not approved for meningitis

cephalosporins, second-generation cephalosporins have expanded activity against *H. influenzae*, *M. catarrhalis*, *Neisseria* species, and enteric bacilli. The second-generation cephalosporins remain active against streptococcal species. Although not as active as cefazolin in vitro against methicillin-susceptible *S. aureus*, many second-generation cephalosporins, particularly cefuroxime, are still clinically useful in treating infections with this organism. Cefuroxime is the most commonly used parenteral second-generation cephalosporin in pediatric patients. It is active against aerobic gram-positive cocci except methicillin-resistant *S. aureus* and enterococci, *H. influenzae*, *M. catarrhalis*, *Neisseria meningitidis*, *N. gonorrhoeae*, and most Enterobacteriaceae. It has little intrinsic activity against gram-negative anaerobes or *Pseudomonas*. Cefuroxime is useful in the empiric treatment of upper and lower respiratory tract, urinary tract, and soft tissue infections and bacteremia. Although cefuroxime achieves adequate concentrations in the cerebrospinal fluid, the third-generation cephalosporins have supplanted it in the treatment of meningitis. Two second-generation cephalosporins have expanded anaerobic coverage. Cefoxitin is the most active cephalosporin against *B. fragilis*. It covers many gram-negative bacilli well except for *H. influenzae* and retains fair coverage against aerobic gram-positive cocci. Cefotetan, technically a cephamycin, also possesses excellent activity against anaerobes and, because of a long half-life, may be dosed twice a day. Both these agents are useful in the treatment of aspiration syndromes, polymicrobial gastrointestinal and gynecologic infections including those involving *N. gonorrhoeae*, and diabetic foot infections and as prophylactic agents before pelvic and gastrointestinal surgery.

Several oral second-generation cephalosporins are currently on the market (see Table 284-4). The distinction between second and third generation is particularly blurry in discussing oral agents. Broadly, these agents have activity against methicillin-susceptible *S. aureus*, streptococcal species including modest variable activity against penicillin-resistant pneumococci, respiratory pathogens such as *H. influenzae*, and typical urinary tract pathogens such as *E. coli*, *Proteus*, and *Klebsiella*. Cefaclor, the first orally available second-

generation agent, is now infrequently used. Cefaclor has little activity against penicillin-resistant pneumococcus, has diminished activity against *H. influenzae*, and is associated with a higher rate of hypersensitivity reactions than other cephalosporins. Cefuroxime axetil tablets are well tolerated, although the liquid preparation is somewhat bitter, limiting its acceptance in younger children. Cefprozil is not as active in vitro against β-lactamase producing *H. influenzae* as other oral second- and third-generation cephalosporins but is modestly active against penicillin-resistant pneumococci. Loracarbef, a cephamycin, has good activity against streptococci except penicillin-resistant *S. pneumoniae*, *M. catarrhalis*, and *E. coli*. These agents are used for the treatment of upper and lower respiratory tract, urinary tract, and soft tissue infections (Table 284-5).

Third-Generation Cephalosporins

Third-generation cephalosporin agents are widely used for the treatment of serious bacterial illnesses. As a group, they have enhanced stability against β-lactamases and expanded activity against gram-negative organisms. They are highly active against streptococci but have variable activity against staphylococci and anaerobes. None of the third-generation cephalosporins is active against enterococci, methicillin-resistant *S. aureus*, or *Listeria*. All penetrate the blood-brain barrier in adequate concentrations to treat pyogenic meningitis. Cefotaxime, the first third-generation cephalosporin, has good activity against staphylococci and streptococci, including penicillin-resistant pneumococcus, *Neisseria* species, *H. influenzae*, and most Enterobacteriaceae. It has modest activity against anaerobes and none against *Pseudomonas*. It is approved for use in neonates and is often the third-generation cephalosporin of choice in the treatment of neonatal infections. Cefotaxime dosed intravenously three or four times a day is useful in the treatment of nosocomial infections, presumed sepsis, bacterial meningitis, and serious abdominal, soft tissue, and urinary tract infections. Ceftriaxone has a spectrum of activity similar to that of cefotaxime, but its long half-life allows daily dosing. Ceftriaxone may be given intravenously or intramuscularly. When ceftriaxone for intramuscular injection is prepared,

Table 284-5. Activity of Oral Cephalosporins against Pathogens Associated with Acute Otitis Media, S. aureus, E. coli, and N. Gonorrhea

Cephalosporin	S. Pyogenes	PSSP	PRSP	H. Influenzae	M. Catarrhalis	S. Aureus	E. Coli	N. gonococcus	Notes
Cephalexin	++	++	0	0	0	++	++	0	Not indicated for OM
Cefaclor	++	+	0	+	++*	+	++	0++*	Higher rate of hypersensitivity reactions
Cefprozil	++	++	+	+	++	++	++*	++*	Not approved for UTI in children; Has an indication but β-lactamase-producing H. influenzae has been associated with lower cure rates
Loracarbef†	++	++	0	+	++	+	++	++*	Not indicated for UTI in children <13; Has an indication but β-lactamase-producing H. influenzae has been associated with lower cure rates
Cefuroxime	++	++	+	++	++	++	++	++	Approved for treatment of N. gonorrhoeae; Liquid tastes bitter
Cefixime	++	+	0	++	++	0	++	++	Not indicated for OM due to S. pneumoniae; Approved for treatment of N. gonorrhoeae
Cefpodoxime	++	++	+	++	++	++	++	++	Not approved for UTI in children <13; Approved for treatment of N. gonorrhoeae
Ceftibuten	++	+	0	++	+	0	++	++	Not indicated for OM due to S. pneumoniae; Not approved for UTI
Cefdinir	++	++	0	++	++	++	++*		Not approved for treatment of N. gonorrhoeae; Not approved for UTI; Not approved for treatment of N. gonorrhoeae

*No clinical indication for this organism.
†Loracarbef is a cephamycin.
Note: 0, little or no activity; +, modest activity; ++, excellent activity; absent markings, no in vitro data.
OM, acute otitis media; PRSP, penicillin resistant S. pneumoniae; PSSP, penicillin susceptible S. pneumoniae; UTI, urinary tract infection.

lidocaine solution rather than normal saline is the preferred diluent, as this will decrease the pain associated with intramuscular injection. Ceftriaxone is not usually given to infants under 1 month old because of potential gallbladder sludging and bilirubin displacement. Ceftriaxone is useful in the empiric therapy of pyogenic meningitis, community-acquired pneumonia, bacteremia, urinary tract infection, and nosocomial infections. It is indicated for the treatment of late *Borrelia burgdorferi* infections. Single doses of intramuscular ceftriaxone are effective treatment of *N. gonorrhoeae* infections and uncomplicated acute otitis media and as prophylaxis against meningococcal disease. Ceftazidime has gram-negative coverage similar to that of cefotaxime and ceftriaxone and is active against *P. aeruginosa*. It has less activity against gram-positive organisms than other third-generation cephalosporins. Ceftazidime given intravenously three times a day may be used for infections similar to those treaded by ceftriaxone. Additionally, ceftazidime is used for the empiric therapy of nosocomial pneumonia and presumed bacteremia in febrile, neutropenic patients.

Several oral third-generation cephalosporins, such as ceftibuten, cefdinir, cefditoren, and cefpodoxime, are currently available. Cefixime, an early oral third-generation cephalosporin, was recently reintroduced in the U.S. market (see Table 284-5). Generally, these agents are very effective against group A streptococci, *Neisseria*, *Haemophilus*, *Moraxella*, and most Enterobacteriaceae. Activity against *S. pneumoniae* and *S. aureus* is variable. None of these agents is active against enterococci, methicillin-resistant *S. aureus*, or *Pseudomonas*. These agents are very effective for the treatment of urinary tract infections and bacterial enteritis. While often used for the treatment of upper and lower respiratory tract infections, neither ceftibuten nor cefixime is considered a first-line agent for these infections, as both have modest activity against pneumococcus and no activity against penicillin-resistant pneumococcus. Single doses of cefixime and cefpodoxime are approved for the treatment of uncomplicated *N. gonorrhoeae* infection.

Fourth-Generation Cephalosporins

Cefepime is the only currently licensed fourth-generation cephalosporin. Cefepime not only is extremely active against most gram-negative organisms including *Pseudomonas*, but also retains moderate activity against methicillin-susceptible *S. aureus*. The enhanced activity of cefepime derives from its improved penetration through the bacterial cell wall. Cefepime is not active against enterococci, methicillin-resistant *S. aureus*, or most anaerobes. Cefepime penetrates most tissues well, including the cerebrospinal fluid. Importantly, cefepime might not induce chromosomally mediated β-lactamases to the extent that many third-generation cephalosporins and the carbapenems do. Cefepime is useful for empiric therapy of nosocomial or polymicrobial infections and presumed bacteremia in febrile neutropenic patients.

Other β-Lactam Antibiotics

Carbapenems

Carbapenem antibiotics, first described in the late 1970s, are active against more organisms than any other β-lactam antibiotic. Three are currently available for use: imipenem/ cilastatin (Primaxin), meropenem (Merrem), and ertapenem (Ivanz). Imipenem/cilastin has an indication for use in children older than 12 years and meropenem in children older than 2 months. Ertapenem is not approved for use in children. Imipenem/cilastin is an equimolar mixture of the active antibiotic, imipenem, and cilastin, an inhibitor of a renal brush border dehydropeptidase that cleaves imipenem in the kidney. Meropenem is not hydrolyzed as easily by this enzyme and so is prepared alone. Imipenem/cilastatin and meropenem have excellent activity against most aerobic and anaerobic extracellular pathogens except methicillin-resistant *S. aureus*, *Enterococcus faecium*, *Xanthomonas maltophilia*, *Flavobacterium* species, and *Burkholderia cepacia*. Ertapenem is not active against *Pseudomonas* species or penicillin-resistant pneumococci. The carbapenem antibiotics are not useful for the treatment of some intracellular infections, such as those caused by *L. monocytogenes* or *Legionella pneumophila*. The carbapenems diffuse through porin channels well, bind to somewhat different penicillin binding proteins than penicillin, and are highly resistant to β-lactamase degradation. Resistance to carbapenem antibiotics is uncommon but primarily caused by zinc containing β-lactamases found in some gram-negative bacilli or, more rarely, altered cell wall permeability.

Both imipenem/cilastin and meropenem are given intravenously every 6 to 8 hours. High concentrations are obtained in most tissues. Ertapenem is given once a day. Both imipenem/cilastin, which is almost exclusively excreted in the kidney, and meropenem, which has significant hepatic excretion, need dose modification when given to patients with renal insufficiency. Carbapenems may cross-react with other β-lactam agents and should be used with caution in patients with severe penicillin or cephalosporin allergy. Hypersensitivity reactions occur in approximately 2% to 3% of patients. Neurologic complications, primarily seizures, occur in approximately 1% of patients who are given carbapenem antibiotics. This risk is greater in patients with renal insufficiency or in those receiving high doses. Imipenem/cilastatin, but not meropenem, has been associated with a significantly higher rate of seizures when used to treat patients with pyogenic meningitis.

The broad antibacterial spectrum of the carbapenem antibiotics makes them effective drugs for the treatment of serious nosocomial and polymicrobial infections and infections with potentially highly resistant organisms. These drugs have been very useful in the treatment of complex lower respiratory tract, urinary tract, and pelvic and abdominal infections. The carbapenems may be used as single agents in the management of febrile neutropenic patients. Meropenem, but not imipenem, is approved for the empiric treatment of pyogenic meningitis in children.

Monobactams

Monobactam antibiotics are synthetic compounds that consist of only a β-lactam ring and side chains. The only monobactam drug currently available is aztreonam. Like all products that contain a β-lactam ring, aztreonam binds to the penicillin binding proteins located on the cell membrane interfering with bacterial cell wall synthesis. Aztreonam has a spectrum of activity similar to that of the aminoglycosides in that it is highly effective against most aerobic gram-negative organisms, including *Haemophilus*, most Enterobacteriaceae, and *Pseudomonas*. Exceptions include *B. cepacia*, *X. maltophilia*, and *Acinetobacter* species. Aztreonam is not active against gram-positive organisms. The drug is usually administered intravenously every 6 to 8 hours, and the dose needs to be adjusted in patients with renal insufficiency. Aztreonam is generally quite well tolerated. Allergic reactions are uncommon. Importantly, virtually no cross-reactivity with other β-lactam antibiotics exists, and aztreonam can be used safely in patients with a history of penicillin or cephalosporin allergy. Aztreonam is useful for the treatment of most aerobic gram-negative infections, including those caused by *H. influenzae*, Enterobacteriaceae, *Salmonella*, and *P. aeruginosa*. In pediatric patients, aztreonam is most commonly used in patients with cystic fibrosis or with cephalosporin allergies. It is not approved for the treatment of central nervous system disease.

Other Cell Wall Active Agents
Glycopeptides
The glycopeptides are bactericidal agents that interfere with bacterial cell well synthesis. Unlike β-lactam products, glycopeptides do not bind to penicillin binding proteins on the cell membrane. Instead, both vancomycin, the only glycopeptide currently available for use in the United States, and teicoplanin inhibit peptidoglycan synthesis at an earlier stage by high-affinity binding to a peptidoglycan precursor. They are not affected by alterations in penicillin binding proteins. The glycopeptides are active against most aerobic and anaerobic gram-positive organisms, including enterococci, methicillin-resistant *S. aureus*, penicillin-resistant *S. pneumoniae*, and *Corynebacterium jeikeium*. The glycopeptides are not active against gram-negative organisms, as these large complex molecules cannot penetrate the gram-negative cell wall. Resistance to the glycopeptides is a new phenomenon and is mediated through alterations in the target site.

Following administration, vancomycin penetrates most tissues well except that little vancomycin appears in bile or the cerebrospinal fluid. Therapeutic levels can be achieved in the cerebrospinal fluid only by using large doses (60 mg/kg/day in four divided doses) in the presence of meningeal inflammation. Although vancomycin has a reputation for renal toxicity, new preparations seem to have little intrinsic renal toxicity. However, vancomycin may potentiate the renal toxicity of other drugs if used in combination. Whether vancomycin, independent of other ototoxins, leads to ototoxicity is similarly controversial. Regardless, reports of permanent ototoxicity are rare and are associated with very high serum concentrations. Approximately 2% of patients may develop reversible neutropenia following prolonged dosing regimens. A reaction unique to vancomycin, the "red man syndrome," is a nonallergic reaction, possibly related to histamine release, associated with too rapid intravenous administration. Patients experience erythema of the head and neck. Slowing the infusion from 1 to 2 hours usually corrects the problem. Oral vancomycin is not absorbed and leads to few systemic findings.

Depending on the age of the patient and site of infection, vancomycin is usually given intravenously two to four times a day. Vancomycin dosing needs to be adjusted in patients with renal insufficiency. Except in patients with central nervous system disease or renal insufficiency, monitoring vancomycin levels is infrequently useful, as peak and trough levels do not adequately predict toxicity or clinical efficacy. Measuring levels may be useful in patients with renal insufficiency or when treating central nervous system disease to confirm high serum levels (e.g., 40 μ/dL).

Parenteral vancomycin is indicated for the empiric or specific treatment of infections with resistant gram-positive organisms. Parenteral vancomycin is used for the treatment of infections caused by methicillin-resistant *S. aureus* or coagulase-negative staphylococci, enterococci, and penicillin-resistant *S. pneumoniae*. In children, parenteral vancomycin is most often used with ceftriaxone in the empiric treatment of suspected pyogenic meningitis, in treatment of sepsis in ICU settings, and in febrile patients with neutropenia and a central venous catheter. Indiscriminate vancomycin use should be discouraged. Oral vancomycin is as effective as metronidazole for the treatment of *Clostridium difficile* colitis but is considerably more expensive and has been linked to the emergence of vancomycin-resistant enterococci. Hence, routine use of oral vancomycin is discouraged.

Fosfomycin
Fosfomycin is an unusual bactericidal oral antibiotic that kills bacteria by inhibiting an early step in cell wall synthesis. It is active against Enterobacteriaceae, *Pseudomonas*, and enterococci, including vancomycin-resistant enterococci. Resistance is uncommon and caused by inactivation by a plasmid-mediated enzyme. No cross-resistance with other antibiotics has been reported. Following oral administration, high urine concentrations persist for more than 48 hours. A single 3-gram sachet dissolved in cold water is approved for the treatment of cystitis in adult women. No dosing guidelines are available for its use in patients with significant renal impairment. The drug is not useful for the treatment of bloodstream infections or pyelonephritis.

Antibiotics That Target Bacterial Protein Synthesis
Several different antimicrobial agents take advantage of the difference between bacterial and mammalian ribosomal subunits to inhibit bacterial protein synthesis. The aminoglycosides, macrolides, tetracyclines, lincosamides, streptogramins, oxazolidinones, and chloramphenicol all target binding sites on bacterial ribosomes. Antibiotics that inhibit protein synthesis have been useful in a variety of clinical conditions for many years.

Aminoglycosides
The aminoglycoside antibiotics are bactericidal agents highly active against aerobic, gram-negative organisms. The common parenteral aminoglycosides, gentamicin, tobramycin, and amikacin demonstrate similar bactericidal activity against most Enterobacteriaceae, *Pseudomonas*, *Haemophilus*, *Francisella tularemia*, *Yersinia*, and *Brucella* species. They also possess some activity against methicillin-susceptible *S. aureus*, although the effect may fade after 24 to 48 hours. The aminoglycosides are not active against *Stenotrophomonas*

X. maltophilia, methicillin-resistant *S. aureus*, *B. cepacia*, and anaerobic organisms. Antimicrobial resistance, usually mediated by alterations in the target site or inactivation of the molecule itself, is uncommon. None of the aminoglycosides penetrates the central nervous system well, even in the face of inflammation. Aminoglycosides are not active in vivo in low-oxygen environments such as abscess cavities.

The effectiveness of aminoglycoside microbial killing is dependent on the concentration of antibiotic achieved. Higher serum aminoglycoside concentrations lead to more efficient microbial killing. Even after the serum concentration of the aminoglycoside drops beneath the mean inhibitory concentration of the organism, microbial replication does not occur. The duration of this postantibiotic effect on microbial replication depends on the maximal concentration achieved. Hence, a higher initial aminoglycoside serum concentrations leads to a longer postantibiotic effect.

All parenteral aminoglycosides may cause either renal or otic dysfunction. Nephrotoxicity and cochlear toxicity occurs in 5% to 25% and 3% to 15% of patients, respectively. The likelihood of renal or otic dysfunction developing is dependent on a variety of factors, including genetics, age, glomerular filtration rate, and antimicrobial drug levels. Generally, pediatric patients experience less toxicity than adults do. Maintaining trough antibiotic concentrations in acceptable ranges and avoiding the concomitant use of renal toxic drugs helps to minimize the risk of serious renal injury. Hypersensitivity reactions following aminoglycoside use are infrequently reported.

Aminoglycoside dosing can be complicated (Table 284-6). Dosing needs to be adjusted depending on the patient's renal function and volume of distribution. Traditionally, a loading dose is given followed by maintenance doses. In most situations, the loading dose is similar to the maintenance dose. Patients with extensive burns, congestive heart failure, ascites, or obesity may require higher loading doses of an aminoglycoside. Patients with cystic fibrosis may require twice the usual loading and maintenance doses to achieve appropriate serum levels. Renal insufficiency decreases aminoglycoside excretion. Dosing recommendations are available based on the patient's creatinine clearance, although an alternative approach is simply to follow serum aminoglycoside levels. Traditionally given three times a day either intramuscularly or intravenously, the total cumulative daily dose of an aminoglycoside may also be given as a single dose. Several studies have demonstrated that large, single daily doses of aminoglycosides are as effective as three times daily dosing and may be associated with less renal toxicity. Single daily dosing, however, might not be indicated in patients with impaired renal function or when an aminoglycoside is used as monotherapy. In patients receiving single daily doses of an aminoglycoside, trough concentrations 24 hours after the dose is administered are monitored.

Parenteral aminoglycoside agents are used alone or in combination with other antimicrobial agents in the empiric and specific therapy of serious gram-negative infections. They are not used as single agents in the management of febrile, neutropenic patients. Aminoglycosides have been used in conjunction with β-lactam antimicrobial agents to synergistically kill some bacteria. Synergistic killing has been demonstrated in vitro for the combination of penicillins and aminoglycosides for Group B streptococcus, enterococcal species, and some *Enterobacteriaceae*. Clinical data support the importance of synergistic killing for enterococci and possibly in immunocompromised hosts. In children, aminoglycosides are most often used in the management of suspected neonatal, severe intra-abdominal, nosocomial, and complicated urinary tract infections. Amikacin is less frequently used, given its tremendous expense. Tobramycin is more often used than gentamicin in the management of *P. aeruginosa* infections in patients with cystic fibrosis.

Neomycin and paromomycin are nonabsorbable, oral aminoglycosides sometimes used for bowel decolonization. Paromomycin may be used to treat unusual intestinal parasitic infections. Neomycin is a component of many ophthalmologic, otic, and topical antibiotic preparations. Tobramycin is available in a nebulized form for the management of gram-negative pulmonary infections in patients with cystic fibrosis. Streptomycin, given intramuscularly, is infrequently used to treat sexually transmitted diseases and *Mycobacterium tuberculosis*.

Macrolides

The macrolide group of antibiotics consists of bacteriostatic agents that target the 50S ribosomal subunit. The macrolides that are available in the United States include erythromycin, clarithromycin, and the closely related azalide, azithromycin. Although azithromycin is not technically a macrolide, it will be treated as such in this chapter. Compared to erythromycin, the newer macrolides, clarithromycin and azithromycin, have better pharmacokinetic properties, fewer adverse events, and a somewhat expanded spectrum of activity. As a group, the macrolides have good activity against most aerobic gram-positive cocci, except methicillin-resistant *S. aureus*, penicillin-resistant *S. pneumoniae*, and

Table 284-6. Parenteral Aminoglycosides Doses and Desired Serum Concentration in Infants and Children outside the Neonatal Period

	Amikacin	Gentamicin	Tobramycin
Dose (every 8 hours)	5–8 mg/kg	1–2.5 mg/kg	1–2.5 mg/kg
Dose (single daily dose)	15 mg/kg	5–6 mg/kg	5–6 mg/kg
Targeted trough levels (every 8 hour dosing) (μg/mL)	<10	<2	<2
Target trough levels (single daily dose) (μg/mL)	<1	<1	<1
Targeted peak levels (every 8 hours dosing) (μg/mL)	20–30	5–10	5–10
Targeted peak levels (single daily doses)	N/A	N/A	N/A

the enterococci. This spectrum of activity is not, however, uniform across the world or even the United States. For example, in Japan, many isolates of *S. pyogenes* are resistant to the erythromycin, while fewer than 5% in the United States are. However, in Pittsburgh, Pennsylvania, more than one third of *S. pyogenes* isolates are resistant to erythromycin. All macrolides are active against respiratory pathogens such as *Bordetella pertussis*, *Legionella pneumophila*, and *Chlamydia pneumoniae*. Activity against *H. influenzae* is variable. Erythromycin has no activity, while clarithromycin has moderate activity and azithromycin is reported to have moderate to good activity against *H. influenzae*. The macrolides are active against several organisms associated with sexually transmitted diseases, such as *Chlamydia trachomatis*, *Haemophilus ducreyi*, *Mycoplasma hominis*, and *Ureaplasma urealyticum*. The macrolides are effective against the gastrointestinal pathogens *Helicobacter pylori* and *Campylobacter jejuni*, while only azithromycin has any significant activity against the enteric pathogens *E. coli* and *Shigella*. Clarithromycin and azithromycin, but not erythromycin, are active against *Mycobacteria avium* complex (MAC). As a group, macrolides have little activity against most Enterobacteriaceae and anaerobic organisms.

Resistance to the macrolide antibiotics may be secondary to alterations in the target site, enzymatic inactivation, or efflux mechanisms. Resistance to erythromycin predicts resistance to all the macrolides. Susceptibility testing for the macrolides is somewhat more controversial than with other antibiotics, as the macrolides, particularly clarithromycin and azithromycin, achieve extremely high intracellular concentrations. Most susceptibility testing systems are designed to measure the effectiveness of the antibiotic in an extracellular milieu.

Macrolides may be given orally or intravenously or applied topically. Following oral or intravenous administration, the macrolides penetrate most tissues well, except that none achieve adequate levels in the cerebrospinal fluid under any conditions. Clarithromycin and azithromycin accumulate in most tissues and can achieve high concentrations for prolonged periods of time in pulmonary macrophages and polymorphonuclear leukocytes. Azithromycin is the only macrolide that is widely distributed in brain tissue. The macrolides, except azithromycin, are metabolized in the liver by the cytochrome P450 enzyme system. The dose of erythromycin and clarithromycin should be modified in patients with hepatic, but not renal, disease. Clarithromycin should not be used in patients with severe liver dysfunction, as liver metabolism is required to generate an active metabolite.

Only erythromycin and azithromycin may be given intravenously. Intravenous erythromycin, given four times a day, and azithromycin, given once a day, are used in patients with serious infections who cannot tolerate oral dosing. Intravenous extravasations of erythromycin are painful and can lead to phlebitis and sterile abscesses. Intravenous azithromycin is not yet approved for use in children.

Erythromycin, clarithromycin, and azithromycin are available in both solid and liquid forms for oral administration. Many oral erythromycin preparations exist. These include many formulations of the base with or without acid-resistant coatings and various esters and ester salts that are inherently more acid stable. Besides the base preparations, the common products used are erythromycin ethyl succinate, erythromycin stearate, and erythromycin estolate (Table 284-7). All erythromycin preparations except erythromycin estolate are given four times a day and are absorbed less well if given with food. Erythromycin estolate may be given twice a day and is unaffected by food. Clarithromycin and azithromycin are chemically more stable, are more bioavailable, and allow longer dosing intervals than erythromycin. Neither is affected by food. Clarithromycin is extremely well absorbed and given twice a day. Azithromycin's long half-life and extremely high tissue concentration allows daily dosing for a shorter duration of time than most other antibiotics. Unique among the macrolides, the first dose of azithromycin is often twice that of subsequent doses.

Erythromycin 0.5% ophthalmic ointment may be applied several times a day for the treatment of bacterial conjunctivitis. Topical erythromycin 2% gels or solutions are applied twice a day in the management of acne.

Life-threatening reactions to macrolide antibiotics are quite rare. The most common adverse reaction is gastrointestinal upset. Oral or intravenous administration of erythromycin may cause abdominal cramping, vomiting, or diarrhea by binding to the motilin receptor in the gastroduodenal smooth muscle. The newer macrolides, particularly azithromycin, cause considerably less gastrointestinal disturbance. Allergic reactions, consisting principally of rash, fever, and eosinophilia, occur infrequently with any

Table 284-7. The Doses and Dosing Schedule for Orally Administered Macrolides in Children outside the Neonatal Period

Preparation	Usual dose (mg/kg/day)	Doses/Day	Comments
Azithromycin	5–12	1	Otitis media: 30 mg/kg over 1, 3, or 5 days GABHS pharyngitis: 12 mg/kg/day for 5 days Pneumonia: 10 mg/kg on day 1 then 5 mg/kg/day for days 2–5 Urethral *Chlamydia*: 1000 mg single dose Endocarditis prophylaxis: 15 mg/kg
Clarithromycin	15	2	Endocarditis prophylaxis: 15 mg/kg
Erythromycin base	30–50	4	Food decreases absorption; maximum dose is 2 g/day
Erythromycin estolate	20–50	2–4	
Erythromycin ethyl succinate	30–50	4	Food decreases absorption; maximum dose is 3.2 g/day
Erythromycin stearate	20–40	4	Food decreases absorption

GABHS, *S. pyogenes*.

of the macrolides. Both erythromycin and clarithromycin inhibit the metabolism of many drugs, presumably through their effect on the hepatic cytochrome P450 system. Concomitant macrolide use may lead to elevated serum concentrations of drugs such as theophyline, carbamazepine, valproate, and cyclosporin. Azithromycin rarely causes significant drug interactions because it has a much more limited effect on the cytochrome P450 system.

The macrolide antibiotics are very useful agents for the treatment of upper and lower respiratory tract disease in all age groups, soft tissue infections, and sexually transmitted diseases (Table 284-8). Macrolides have long been used for the empiric treatment of community-acquired pneumonia in children of all ages, as they are effective against penicillin-susceptible pneumococci, C. *pneumoniae*, and *Mycoplasma pneumoniae*, the three most common causes of bacterial pneumonia in the ambulatory pediatric population. Additionally, they are the drugs of choice for the treatment and prophylaxis of B. *pertussis* and C. *trachomatis* infections in children. All macrolides are effective agents for streptococcal pharyngitis in penicillin-allergic patients. Clarithromycin, azithromycin, and the combination agent erythromycin ethyl succinate and sulfisoxazole (Pediazole) are competent agents for the treatment of otitis media and sinusitis. Macrolides are effective for the treatment of skin and skin structure infections such as impetigo. Although active against aerobic gram-positive organisms, the macrolides are infrequently used to treat more serious infections such as osteomyelitis. Macrolides may be used to manage Lyme disease in children younger than 8 years old who are allergic to penicillin.

As a group, the macrolides are useful in treating many sexually transmitted diseases (see Table 284-8). A single oral 1.0-g dose of azithromycin is approved for the treatment of nongonococcal urethritis and cervicitis caused by C. *trachomatis*. Intravenous azithromycin, with or without metronidazole, may be used to pelvic inflammatory disease in adults. If given early in the course, macrolide use may decrease the duration of symptoms associated with C. *jejuni* enteritis. Clarithromycin, combined with a protein pump inhibitor, is effective therapy for H. *pylori* infection. Clarithromycin and azithromycin are effective agents to treat and for prophylaxis against M. *avium* complex disease in HIV-infected and noninfected individuals. Clarithromycin and azithromycin, but not erythromycin, are approved as prophylactic agents to prevent infectious endocarditis. All three drugs, however, may be used to prevent rheumatic fever in penicillin-allergic patients.

Clindamycin

Clindamycin targets sites on the 50S subunit of the bacterial ribosome similar to those targeted by the macrolides. Clindamycin is active against many aerobic gram-positive organisms, anaerobic gram-positive and gram-negative organisms, and several parasites. Clindamycin is effective against methicillin-susceptible S. *aureus*, approximately 50% of methicillin-resistant S. *aureus*, streptococcal species including the majority of penicillin-resistant pneumococci, and gram-positive bacilli such as *Bacillus cereus* and *Lactobacillus*. It is highly active against most anaerobes except possibly C. *difficile*. Although clindamycin is active against the vast majority of B. *fragilis* isolates, some geographic regions may have higher resistance rates. Clindamycin is active against many intracellular pathogens, including C. *trachomatis*, *Toxoplasma gondii*, *Babesia microti*, *Plasmodium* species, and *Pneumocystis jiroveci* (formerly known as *Pneumocystis carinii*). Clindamycin is not active against most aerobic, gram-negative organisms or enterococci. Resistance may be mediated by either modification of the binding site, alteration in the antibiotic, or poor penetration through the cell wall.

Clindamycin may be given orally (75 mg/5 mL) or intravenously three or four times a day (25 to 40 mg/kg/day; maximum intravenous dose is 4.8 g/day; maximum oral dose is 1.8 grams/day). Oral preparations are absorbed rapidly and are highly bioavailable. Food does not significantly interfere with absorption. Following intravenous or oral dosing, clindamycin achieves good tissue levels except in the cerebrospinal fluid. Clindamycin accumulates in abscess fluid, polymorphonuclear leukocytes, and alveolar macrophages. As clindamycin is metabolized in the liver, dosing modification is necessary only in patients with severe hepatic insufficiency or combined hepatic and renal dysfunction. Topical 1% clindamycin available in a gel,

Table 284-8. Clinical Conditions and Organisms for Which Macrolide Therapy May Be Useful

Indication/Organism	Erythromycin	Azithromycin	Clarithromycin
Community-acquired pneumonia	Yes	Yes	Yes
Impetigo	Yes	Yes	Yes
Infective endocarditis prophylaxis	No	Yes	Yes
Malaria prophylaxis	No	Yes	No
Otitis media	No	Yes	Yes
Pelvic inflammatory disease	No	Yes*	No
Sinusitis	No	Yes	Yes
Arcanobacterium haemolyticum	Yes	Yes	Yes
Bordetella pertussis	Yes	Yes	Yes
C. *trachomatis* cervicitis/urethritis	Yes	Yes	No
C. *trachomatis* pneumonia	Yes	Yes	Yes
Campylobacter jejuni infection	Yes	Yes	No
Helicobacter pylori	No	No	Yes*
M. *avium* complex prophylaxis	No	Yes	Yes
M. *avium* complex treatment	No	Yes	Yes

*In conjunction with metronidazole or other agents.

lotion, or solution is applied bid for the treatment of acne vulgaris. Clindamycin 2% vaginal cream is applied vaginally each evening for 3 to 7 days to treat bacterial vaginosis.

The principal adverse events associated with clindamycin are gastrointestinal in nature. Antibiotic-associated diarrhea may occur in up to 20% of patients. Antibiotic-associated colitis caused by toxigenic C. *difficile* occurs in 0.01% to 10% of patients. Clindamycin is the antibiotic most closely associated with this infection, although β-lactam drugs and others may pose a comparable relative risk per dose. Other adverse effects include anorexia, nausea, bitter taste, and, more rarely, reversible elevations of liver function tests. Hypersensitivity reactions are infrequent.

Clindamycin is useful in the treatment of pulmonary aspiration syndromes, pulmonary abscesses, nonmeningeal penicillin-resistant *S. pneumoniae* infections, odontogenic infections, bone infections caused by staphylococcal or streptococcal species, and skin infections in patients with β-lactam allergy and as prophylaxis to prevent infective endocarditis. Combined with an agent that is active against aerobic gram-negative organisms, clindamycin is effective for the treatment of abdominal, gynecologic, and cutaneous polymicrobial processes. On the basis of in vitro data and some clinical experience, clindamycin combined with a β-lactam antibiotic is more effective than a β-lactam antibiotic alone in the treatment of severe, life-threatening *S. pyogenes* or *C. perfringens* infections. Topical clindamycin is useful for the treatment of acne vulgaris and rosacea. Either topical or oral clindamycin is effective for the treatment of bacterial vaginosis. Clindamycin, in conjunction with other agents, is useful in the treatment of *T. gondii*, *Plasmodium falciparum*, and *B. microti* infections.

Tetracyclines

The tetracycline drugs are broad-spectrum bacteriostatic agents that enter bacterial cells through a unique bacteria-specific, energy-dependent transport mechanism and target the 30S ribosomal subunit. The commonly used tetracyclines doxycycline, minocycline, and tetracycline are active against many aerobic, anaerobic, and intracellular bacteria and protozoa. However, the emergence of bacterial resistance has limited their spectrum of activity. Resistance to the tetracycline drugs is usually due to efflux mechanisms but can be secondary to alterations in ribosomal target site, chemical inactivation of the antibiotic, or reduced uptake of the antibiotic. Generally, resistance to one tetracycline predicts resistance to the others.

Many tetracycline products exist. Most pediatricians will use tetracyclines with a shorter half-life of 8 to 9 hours (i.e., tetracycline), or one with a longer half-life of 15 to 18 hours, such as doxycycline or minocycline. Tetracyclines are well absorbed from the gastrointestinal tract in patients who have not recently eaten. The concomitant administration of food, particularly milk, reduces gastrointestinal absorption of tetracycline by 50% and doxycycline by 20%. Following oral or parenteral administration, the tetracyclines are distributed widely throughout the body and are excreted in breast milk. The cerebrospinal fluid concentration, however, is only 10% to 20% of that found in serum. Because most tetracyclines undergo both hepatic and renal excretion, these products generally require little

or no dose modification in patients with renal insufficiency. Doxycycline, however, is generally the tetracycline of choice when treating patients with renal failure.

Most tetracyclines are well tolerated. Approximately 5% of patients taking tetracyclines complain of gastrointestinal upset. Photosensitivity reactions, more commonly seen with doxycycline use, may occur. Occasionally, tetracycline use may be associated with benign, intracranial hypertension. Minocycline frequently causes vestibular symptoms, particularly in women, within days of starting the product. Tetracyclines are not used in children younger than 8 years of age because persistent use may cause permanent discoloration of the teeth and enamel hypoplasia. The degree of enamel staining appears related to the cumulative dose of the tetracycline drug. Similarly, tetracyclines are not given to pregnant or breast-feeding women, as transplacental transfer of the drug or excretion in breast milk may lead to dental or bone abnormalities in the infant. The tetracycline drugs interact with many products, particularly those containing divalent and trivalent cations such as those found in antacids, dairy products, and iron preparations. These products reduce gastrointestinal absorption of the tetracycline. Drugs that induce hepatic enzymes, such as phenytoin or phenobarbital, may decrease serum tetracycline levels. Tetracyclines may decrease the efficacy of oral contraceptives.

The tetracyclines may be given orally or intravenously, usually at the same dose. Oral tetracycline (25 to 50 mg/kg/day) is generally given four times a day except for treatment of acne, when daily or twice daily dosing may be used. Doxycycline (2 to 4 mg/kg/day; usual adult dose 100 to 200 mg daily) is given once or twice a day.

The tetracycline products are now generally considered agents of choice or first-line agents for Chlamydial infections, ehrlichiosis, granuloma inguinale, *H. pylori*, Lyme disease, Q fever, Rocky Mountain spotted fever, and other rickettsial infections. They are useful in the treatment of acne, mycoplasma disease, and *U. urealyticum* infections and the prevention of chloroquine-resistant *P. falciparum* malaria. In children over the age of 8, tetracyclines (most commonly doxycycline) are most often used in the management of Lyme disease, community-acquired pneumonia, ehrlichiosis, and acne. Doxycycline is the only tetracycline drug that is useful for both prevention and treatment of malaria. Tetracyclines are used in children of all ages with suspected rickettsial disease (such as Rocky Mountain spotted fever), since these antimicrobial agents are clearly effective and the duration of treatment is generally too short to cause harm.

Chloramphenicol

Chloramphenicol is a broad-spectrum antibiotic that reversibly binds to the 50S ribosomal subunit. Although used widely around the world, chloramphenicol is mostly of historical interest in the United States, since safer drugs are available. Highly active against most anaerobes, including *B. fragilis*, chloramphenicol is also active against many aerobic gram-positive and gram-negative organisms, rickettsia, Chlamydia, mycoplasma, and spirochetes. Chloramphenicol may be given intravenously or orally. The antibiotic diffuses well into most tissues, particularly the brain and cerebrospinal fluid. The intravenous preparation and the oral suspension are prodrugs requiring hepatic hydrolysis to convert them to the active form. The oral capsule form contains active drug. Both oral forms are very well absorbed and highly bioavailable. Interestingly, higher serum concentrations are achieved following oral than intravenous dosing. Chloramphenicol (50 to 100 mg/kg/day) is given every 6 hours in patients with normal hepatic function.

Chloramphenicol is associated with both idiosyncratic and dose-related toxicity. Approximately 1 in 25,000 to 40,000 patients treated with chloramphenicol, regardless of the preparation and duration of use, may develop fatal idiosyncratic aplastic anemia anywhere from a few days to weeks after administration. Reversible bone marrow suppression of all cell lines is a dose-related phenomenon and involves direct inhibition of mitochondrial protein synthesis. To minimize toxicity, chloramphenicol levels should be monitored in order to maintain serum levels between 10 and 30 mg/mL.

Most recently trained physicians will have little experience with chloramphenicol. It is used in the United States primarily when no other alternatives are available. In the United States, chloramphenicol is most likely to be used to treat central nervous system infections in patients who are intolerant of other medications and patients who cannot take tetracyclines.

Streptogramins

The streptogramins are a new class of antimicrobial agents that inhibit protein synthesis after binding to sites on the 50S ribosomal subunit. The only approved drug in this class is the combination agent quinupristin/dalfopristin (Synercid). The spectrum of activity of quinupristin/dalfopristin is similar to that of vancomycin. It is effective against penicillin-susceptible and penicillin-resistant *S. pneumoniae*, methicillin-susceptible and methicillin-resistant *S. aureus*, and the majority of *E. faecium* strains. Interestingly, the drug has no activity against *Enterococcus faecalis*, making species identification crucial. Resistance may develop through decreased ribosomal binding or efflux mechanisms that pump the antibiotic out of the organism. Cross-resistance to other currently available antimicrobial agents has not been reported. When quinupristin/dalfopristin is given intravenously (7.5 mg/kg/dose every 8 hours), complications include venous irritation, conjugated hyperbilirubinemia, myalgia, and arthralgia. Quinupristin/dalfopristin affects the cytochrome P450 system and can lead to alterations in the serum levels of drugs processed by this system, including cyclosporin and nonsedating antihistamines. The main use for quinupristin/dalfopristin is the treatment of vancomycin-resistant *E. faecium* infection or methicillin-resistant *S. aureus* infections in patients who are intolerant of glycopeptides. Currently, the drug is not approved for children under the age of 16.

Oxazolidinones

The oxazolidinones are a new class of bacteristatic, synthetic antimicrobial agents that block initiation of protein synthesis at the 50S ribosomal subunit. The antimicrobial spectrum of activity of linezolid, the only approved oxazolidinone, is similar to that of vancomycin. It has good

activity against aerobic and anaerobic gram-positive bacteria, including methicillin-resistant *S. aureus*, penicillin-resistant *S. pneumoniae*, and drug-resistant enterococci. Cross-resistance with other currently available antimicrobial agents has not been described. Almost 100% bioavailable, linezolid may be given orally or intravenously twice a day at the same dose. The current recommended dosing schedule is 10 mg/kg/dose every 12 hours for premature (<34 weeks' gestation) infants less than 7 days old, 10 mg/kg every 8 hours for children from birth through 11 years of age, and 600 mg twice a day for children 12 years and older. A 100 mg/5 mL suspension is available. Linezolid does not require dose adjustments for renal or hepatic insufficiency. The principal adverse effects of linezolid include gastrointestinal disturbance and thrombocytopenia. The drug may inhibit monoamine oxidase and should not concurrently be given with over-the-counter cold remedies that contain pseudoephedrine or phenylpropanolamine. Linezolid should be reserved for use treating complicated or severe infections with gram-positive organisms or infections with suspected or confirmed drug-resistant gram-positive cocci.

Antibiotics and Antimicrobials That Affect the Synthesis or Maintenance of Bacterial Nucleic Acid

Antimicrobial agents in this group either directly affect the machinery of bacterial DNA or RNA replication or inhibit metabolic pathways essential to generating DNA precursors. These agents tend to be active against a broad range of bacteria.

Fluoroquinolones

The fluoroquinolones are broad-spectrum bactericidal antimicrobials that target bacterial topoisomerases, including DNA gyrase. Without appropriate topoisomerase activity, DNA replication is unsuccessful. The fluoroquinolones are active against a broad range of bacteria, including aerobic gram-positive cocci, *Enterobacteriaceae*, *Pseudomonas*, and intracellular pathogens such as Chlamydia, mycoplasma, and legionella. Bacterial resistance to the fluoroquinolones is mediated through either altered cell permeability or chromosomal mutations that lead to alterations in the topoisomerases. Fluoroquinolones are not affected by alterations in penicillin binding proteins.

The fluoroquinolones, as a group, are extremely bioavailable. Oral and intravenous doses are the same and have similar clinical efficacy. The newer fluoroquinolones, levofloxacin, gatifloxacin, and moxifloxacin have improved pharmacokinetics compared to ciprofloxacin and allow daily dosing. Following administration, the fluoroquinolones penetrate most tissues well and may achieve therapeutic concentrations in the cerebrospinal fluid. Most fluoroquinolones undergo renal excretion, and all except moxifloxacin require dose modification in patients with renal insufficiency.

The fluoroquinolones are generally well tolerated. A small percentage of patients taking fluoroquinolones complain of dizziness or gastrointestinal upset. Though this is rare, a few patients may have more significant central nervous system disturbance or experience tendon rupture.

Most fluoroquinolones may potentially prolong the QTc interval. Fluoroquinolones that are associated with a significant increase in the QTc interval have been removed from the U.S. market. The fluoroquinolones as a class have been associated with joint arthropathy in immature animals. The arthropathy, generally reversible, is fluoroquinolone and species specific. Although ciprofloxacin has been used in more than 10,000 children worldwide without significant adverse effects, the fluoroquinolones are not approved for use in patients under the age of 18, except for the treatment or prevention of anthrax, because of the potential for arthropathy. Otic and ophthalmic fluoroquinolone preparations, however, are available for use in pediatric patients.

Fluoroquinolones are often classified by generation. Ciprofloxacin, a second-generation product, has excellent activity against aerobic gram-negative organisms, including *Pseudomonas*. Although fluoroquinolones possess good antistaphylococcal activity, activity against streptococcal species and anaerobes is more modest. Levofloxacin and gatifloxacin, third-generation fluoroquinolones, have similar gram-negative activity but also enhanced activity against streptococcal species, including *S. pneumoniae*, and intracellular pathogens such as mycoplasma, Chlamydia, and legionella. Fourth-generation fluoroquinolones, such as moxifloxacin, expand the coverage further to include anaerobic organisms.

In adults, parenteral fluoroquinolones are indicated for the treatment of community-acquired upper and lower respiratory tract, urinary tract, sexually transmitted, and gastrointestinal infections and as prophylaxis against *N. meningitidis*. Although these agents are not approved for such use, pediatricians are likely to use them for similar indications as in adults when alternative agents are not available or intravenous access is difficult to obtain. The most commonly used fluoroquinolone in pediatric patients is ciprofloxacin (20 to 30 mg/kg/day in two divided doses). Otic ofloxacin and ciprofloxacin are approved for the treatment of otitis externa in children older than 1 year of age. Many fluoroquinolone ophthalmic preparations are approved for the treatment of conjunctivitis in children older than 1 year.

Sulfonamides and Trimethoprim

The sulfonamides and trimethoprim act at sequential steps in the folic acid biosynthetic pathway. The sulfonamides are active against a variety of gram-positive and gram-negative organisms, including *Enterobacteriaceae*, *S. pneumoniae*, *Nocardia*, *P. falciparum*, and *T. gondii*. The sulfonamides are not active against *S. pyogenes*, most staphylococcal species, and anaerobes. Trimethoprim is active against many aerobic, gram-positive cocci, including *S. aureus*, most streptococci except *S. pyogenes*, and many *Enterobacteriaceae*. Joint administration as trimethoprim/sulfamethoxazole (TMP/SMX) leads to the synergistic killing of a wide range of aerobic gram-positive and gram-negative bacteria and protozoa, including *Pneumocystis* species, enteric pathogens, *Isospora belli*, and *Cyclospora*. TMP/SMX is variably active against methicillin-resistant *S. aureus* but has little activity against penicillin-resistant *S. pneumoniae* or *S. pyogenes*. Resistance to sulfonamides is mediated through either restricted penetration of the sulfonamides through the cell envelope, hyperproduction of folic acid precursors, or alterations in the sulfonamide target site. Resistance to trimethoprim is generally mediated through alterations in the target enzyme.

Many parenteral sulfonamide preparations exist. The short-acting sulfonamides sulfamethoxazole and sulfisoxazole are most commonly used alone or in fixed combination with other agents. These agents and trimethoprim are all highly bioavailable with similar serum levels following oral and intravenous administration (Table 284-9). TMP/SMX is available in single-strength (80 mg trimethoprim and 400 mg sulfamethoxazole) and double-strength (160 mg trimethoprim and 800 mg sulfamethoxazole) tablets and a suspension that contains 40 mg trimethoprim and 200 mg sulfamethoxazole for each 5 mL. The usual dose of TMP/SMX is 8 to 10 mg/kg/day of the trimethoprim component in two divided doses. Treatment of *P. jiroveci* pneumonia requires 15 to 20 mg/kg/day of the trimethoprim component in three or four divided doses. Following administration, both trimethoprim and sulfamethoxazole penetrate most tissues well, including the central nervous system and cerebrospinal fluid. Dosages need to be adjusted in patients with moderate or severe renal insufficiency.

Table 284-9. Common Parenteral Folate Synthesis Inhibitors

Generic Name	Product Name	Dose (mg/kg/day)	Doses/Day	Youngest Indicated Age	Comments
Sulfisoxazole	Gantrisin	120–150	4–6	2 months	50 mg/kg/day in 1–2 divided doses for prophylaxis
Erythromycin ethyl succinate-sulfisoxazole	Pediazole	50	4	2 months	Dose is based on the erythromycin component
Trimethoprim-sulfamethoxazole	Bactrim Septra	8–10	2	2 months	Dose is based on the trimethoprim component; dose for treatment of *Pneumocystis* is 15–20 mg/kg/day in 3–4 divided doses; dose for pneumocystis prophylaxis is 150 mg trimethoprim/m²/day in 2 divided doses, 3 days/week
Trimethoprim	Primsol	10	2	6 months	Dose for otitis media: 10 mg/kg/day. Dose for treatment of UTI is 4–6 mg/kg/day.
Sulfadiazine		100–200	2–4	0 months	

UTI, urinary tract infection.

The most common adverse reaction to sulfonamide administration is gastrointestinal upset. Approximately 3% to 5% of patients complain of nausea, vomiting, or diarrhea. Hypersensitivity reactions may occur. These are usually mild, consisting of nondescript macular or papular eruptions. However, hypersensitivity reactions may be life threatening. Hypersensitivity reactions occur more frequently in HIV-infected patients. The increased risk of severe hypersensitivity reactions has limited the use of medium- and longer-acting sulfonamides. Prolonged administration of sulfonamides can lead to leukopenia, aplastic anemia, or thrombocytopenia. Because the sulfonamides may displace bilirubin from albumin binding sites, they are not used in children younger than 30 days of age. Fewer adverse reactions follow trimethoprim administration. Hematologic toxicity, though rare, can occur in patients who are predisposed to bone marrow toxicity.

Sulfonamides as single agents are sometimes used for the treatment of urinary tract and *Nocardia* infections and to prevent otitis media. Sulfisoxazole, as a prophylactic agent to prevent otitis media or urinary tract infection, is usually given in a dose of 50 mg/kg/day in two divided doses. Sulfonamides are used to treat toxoplasmosis. Sulfadiazine (100 to 200 mg/kg/day in two to four divided doses) is combined with the folate antagonist pyrimethamine to treat congenital toxoplasmosis. Trimethoprim as a single agent (10 mg/kg/day in two divided doses) may be used to treat urinary tract infections, traveler's diarrhea, and upper respiratory tract infections and is a constituent of several ocular preparations used to treat bacterial conjunctivitis.

Most commonly, pediatricians will use TMP/SMX. Unfortunately, resistance has begun to limit the clinical effectiveness of this drug. An increasing number of *S. pneumoniae*, *H. influenzae*, and *E. coli* isolates are resistant. Resistance among *Shigella* and *Salmonella* species is widespread throughout the world. TMP/SMX is still a reasonable choice for the empiric treatment of uncomplicated upper respiratory tract infections, such as otitis media or sinusitis, in patients allergic to amoxicillin and the empiric treatment of urinary tract infections where the local resistance to *E. coli* is less than 10% to 20%. It remains an excellent drug for the prophylaxis of urinary tract infections and is treatment of choice for *P. jiroveci* pneumonia and for *Cyclospora* and *Nocardia* infections.

Rifampin/Rifabutin

The rifamycins, rifampin and rifabutin, interfere with DNA-dependent RNA polymerase. Although these agents are active against many gram-positive and gram-negative organisms and penetrate most tissues well, rapid emergence of resistance when used alone limits their clinical use. Both drugs affect the cytochrome P450 system and interact with a host of medications (see the later section on antimycobacterial agents). Rifampin and rifabutin are primarily used as antimycobacterial drugs. Rifampin given orally once a day (20 mg/kg/day) for 4 days or twice daily (20 mg/kg/day) for 2 days may be used as prophylaxis following exposure to *H. influenzae* type B and meningococcal disease, respectively.

Miscellaneous Antimicrobial Agents
Nitrofurantoin

Nitrofurantoin is a bactericidal, oral agent that is metabolized by bacteria into toxic intermediates that inhibit multiple bacterial processes, including protein synthesis. Nitrofurantoin has activity against many aerobic, enteric gram-negative bacilli and some gram-positive organisms, including vancomycin-resistant enterococcus. Following oral administration, bloodstream concentrations are very low. The drug is concentrated in the urine, where it reaches therapeutic levels. Anorexia, nausea, and vomiting are the most common side effects and appear to be dose related. Coadministration of nitrofurantoin with food may help to minimize these complaints. Uncommon complications include peripheral neuropathy, alopecia, dermatitis, and hepatic damage. Rare but serious side effects include acute pneumonitis, subacute pneumonitis, and chronic pulmonary reactions. Nitrofurantoin is given four times daily as therapy (5 to 7 mg/kg/day) and once or twice daily as prophylaxis (1 to 2 mg/kg/day). A 5-mg/mL suspension is available. Nitrofurantoin is useful in the treatment of cystitis and urinary tract infection prophylaxis. It should not be used to treat pyelonephritis.

Metronidazole

Metronidazole is a synthetic, bactericidal antimicrobial agent. After entering cells by passive diffusion, the drug is reduced to active metabolites that damage bacterial DNA and other macromolecules and lead to cell death. Metronidazole is extremely active against almost all gram-negative anaerobic bacteria, including *B. fragilis*, and most anaerobic gram-positive bacteria, including *C. difficile*. Additionally, metronidazole is active against the protozoa *Trichomonas vaginalis*, *Entamoeba histolytica*, *Giardia lamblia*, and others. Metronidazole is not effective *against Propionibacterium acnes* or actinomycetes. The development of resistance to metronidazole is quite uncommon and is usually secondary to altered reductive pathways.

Following parenteral administration, metronidazole penetrates most tissues well, including empyema fluid, cerebral abscesses, and the cerebrospinal fluid. Metronidazole may be given intravenously or orally three or four times a day. Highly bioavailable, serum concentrations are similar following oral and intravenous dosing. Primarily metabolized in the liver, the dose of metronidazole should be decreased in patients with hepatic insufficiency. Metronidazole 0.75% gel may be applied vaginally once or twice a day to treat bacterial vaginosis. Metronidazole 0.75% or 1% cream is applied topically twice a day for acne.

The most frequent side effects of metronidazole administration are nausea, anorexia, and metallic taste. Rarely, patients receiving high or prolonged doses may develop reversible central nervous system effects, including seizures, encephalopathy, or cerebellar dysfunction. Patients taking metronidazole should be counseled not to imbibe alcohol so as to avoid disulfiram-like reactions. Because metronidazole metabolites damage DNA, the effect of the drug has been investigated in several different prokaryotic and eukaryotic models. Some would suggest that metronidazole

Table 284-10. Dosage of Parenteral Metronidazole for Various Clinical Indications

Indication	Usual Pediatric Dose (mg/kg/day)	Pediatric Doses/Day	Usual Adult Dose (mg)	Adult Doses/Day
Amebiasis*	30–50	3	750	3
Bacterial infections	30	3–4	500 mg	3–4
Bacterial vaginosis			2000	Single dose
C. difficile colitis	30	4	250 or	4
			500	3
Giardiasis	15	3	250	3
H. pylori[†]	15–20	2	250–500	3
Pelvic inflammatory disease[‡]			500	2
Trichomoniasis	15	3	2000 or	Single dose
			375–500	2

*Taken with iodoquinol.
[†]Taken with other anti-infectives.
[‡]Taken with oflaxacin.

may be mutagenic or carcinogenic. No human data have confirmed these findings, and follow-up studies of women given metronidazole at various stages of pregnancy have failed to show evidence of teratogenicity. However, because of this concern, metronidazole is often avoided during pregnancy, in breast-feeding mothers, and in very young infants.

Metronidazole is used to treat a variety of anaerobic infections and is the drug of choice for anaerobic infections of the central nervous system and gut, including C. difficile colitis. It is best combined with other agents to treat pulmonary aspiration syndromes and polymicrobial enteric or gynecologic infections. Bacterial vaginosis responds to twice a day oral or vaginal dosing for 5 to 7 days. Alternatively, a single 2.0-g oral dose may be used, but this dose is associated with a higher incidence of side effects and relapse. Metronidazole is a component of a triple-drug therapy of H. pylori infection, although resistance of this organism to metronidazole is increasingly common. Patients with overgrowth syndromes respond well to oral metronidazole. The drug is an effective therapy for T. vaginalis, E. histolytica, and G. lamblia infections. Finally, metronidazole has an immunomodulatory effect that is beneficial in some patients with Crohn disease. Metronidazole dosing in children is dependent on the infection being treated but is usually 20 to 30 mg/kg/day in three or four divided doses (Table 284-10).

Antimycobacterial Agents

Antituberculosis agents have radically improved the prognosis of patients with tuberculosis. In contrast to other antimicrobials, antitubercular agents are never used as single agents except for the treatment of M. tuberculosis infection without disease. The agents most commonly used to treat M. tuberculosis are isoniazid, rifampin (or rifabutin), pyrazinamide, and ethambutol (Table 284-11). Clarithromycin and azithromycin are used to treat MAC disease.

Isoniazid

Isoniazid (INH) inhibits the synthesis of mycolic acids in the mycobacterial cell wall. Resistance may develop to isoniazid or any other antitubercular agent if it is used alone. Isoniazid penetrates well into most body fluids. It is metabolized in the liver and excreted in the kidney. Isoniazid is active against most strains of M. tuberculosis and Mycobacterium kansasii but not M. avium complex. The most serious side effect associated with isoniazid therapy is hepatitis. The likelihood of developing hepatitis increases with age. Children less than 20 years old rarely develop significant hepatitis, and routine monitoring of liver function tests is not recommended in this population. Alcohol consumption or large doses of acetaminophen may increase the risk of hepatitis. In patients with poor nutrition or unusual diets, isoniazid may potentiate pyridoxine deficiency and increase the likelihood of peripheral

Table 284-11. Dosages of Commonly Used Antituberculosis Medications

Drug*	Daily Dose[†] (maximum dose in mg)	2×/Week[†] (maximum dose in mg)	How Supplied
Ethambutol	15–25 (2500)	50 (2500)	100, 400-mg tablets
Isoniazid	10–15 (300)	20–30 (900)	100, 300-mg scored tablets
			10-mg/mL syrup
Pyrazinamide	20–40 (2000)	50 (2000)	500-mg scored tablet
Rifampin	10–20 (600)	10–20 (600)	150, 300-mg capsules
			Syrup compounded

*Fixed combination drugs exist including Rifamate (150 mg isoniazid/300 mg rifampin) and Rifater (50 mg isoniazid/120 mg rifampin/and 300 mg pyrazinamide) for use in adults.
[†]Dose in mg/kg/day.

neuropathy. In these patients, 50 mg of pyridoxine per day is recommended. Isoniazid may slow the metabolism of carbamazepine and phenytoin.

Rifamycins (Rifampin and Rifabutin)

The rifamycins inhibit bacterial DNA-dependent RNA polymerase. The rifamycins are active against *M. tuberculosis*, *M. kansasii*, and *M. avium* complex. These drugs are well absorbed orally and achieve good levels in most body fluids, including the cerebrospinal fluid. Rifampin is excreted both in the bile and in the urine. The drug turns most body fluids orange and may permanently discolor contact lenses. The rifamycins may cause hepatitis, neutropenia, and gastrointestinal upset. Higher doses of rifabutin have been associated with uveitis. The rifamycins, particularly rifampin, induce hepatic enzymes of the P450 class and are associated with altered serum concentrations of many drugs. Rifamycin use may increase the metabolism of corticosteroids, oral contraceptives, cyclosporin, azole antifungal agents, clarithromycin, protease inhibitors, verapamil, and phenytoin. Clarithromycin and fluconazole may slow the metabolism of rifampin. Rifampin has been a standard, highly active antitubercular agent for many years. Rifabutin has more recently been approved for the prevention and treatment of *M. avium* complex disease. Rifabutin is not approved for use in patients less than 18 years of age.

Pyrazinamide

Pyrazinamide is an oral agent that inhibits the growth of certain mycobacteria through an unknown mechanism. Hydrolyzed in the liver and partially excreted by the kidney, the dose is often decreased in patients with renal insufficiency. The principal side effects are nausea, vomiting, and, more rarely, hepatotoxicity. Pyrazinamide is most often used in the initial phase of tuberculosis therapy.

Ethambutol

Ethambutol is an oral agent that interferes with mycobacterial cell wall synthesis. It is active against *M. tuberculosis* and approximately one half the strains of *M. avium* complex. The major side effect is optic neuritis, characterized by blurred vision and color blindness. Ocular toxicity is dose related. Ethambutol should be used cautiously in young patients whose vision cannot be easily monitored.

Directly Applied Antibiotics

Antibiotics may be applied to skin and mucosal surfaces. These products achieve high local concentrations without systemic exposure or toxicity. Agents that are too toxic for systemic use are often used to treat wound infections and impetigo and to prevent secondary infections in patients with significant burn injuries (Table 284-12).

Topical Agents
Mupirocin

Mupirocin inhibits protein synthesis by preventing the incorporation of the amino acid isoleucine into protein. Although some staphylococcal isolates have developed resistance, mupirocin generally is highly active against aerobic gram-positive cocci, except enterococci. Mupirocin has poor activity against gram-negative bacteria and has little effect on the normal skin flora, as it is not active against *Corynebacterium*, *Propionibacterium*, or *Micrococcus* species. Mupirocin is well tolerated and infrequently causes dermatitis or pruritus. Mupirocin is used for the treatment of primary skin infections such as impetigo (as an ointment), secondarily infected traumatic skin lesions (as a cream), and the eradication of staphylococcus carriage from the nose (nasal ointment). The cream is usually applied three times a day in children 3 months old or younger, while the ointment is applied three

Table 284-12. Antimicrobial Activity of Topical Antibiotics

Condition and Agent	Staphylococci and Streptococci	Gram Negatives	*Propionibacterium*
Wound infection or prophylaxis			
Bacitracin*	++	0	++
Gentamicin	Staphylococci	++	0
Mupirocin	++	0	0
Neomycin	Staphylococci only	++	0
Polymyxin	0	++	0
Neosporin (bacitracin/neomycin/polymyxin)	++	++	++
Treatment of Burns			
Mafenide acetate	+	++	
Nitrofurazone	++	++	
Silver sulfadiazine	++	++	
Acne therapy			
Clindamycin 10 mg/mL	++	0	++
Erythromycin 2, 3%	++	+	0
Meclocycline 1%	+	+	+
Metronidazole 0.75%	0	0	++
Tetracycline 2.2 mg/mL	+	+	+

*Bacitracin in also used extensively in the management of burns.
Note: +, poor or modest activity; ++, good or excellent activity; 0, no activity.

to five times a day in children 2 months of age or younger.

Neomycin

Neomycin is a topical aminoglycoside antibiotic that inhibits protein synthesis and is active against staphylococci and most gram-negative bacteria, except *P. aeruginosa*. It is not active against other gram-positive organisms or anaerobes. Although neomycin is widely used and inexpensive, allergic contact dermatitis may occur in approximately 1% to 6% of patients. Neomycin should not be applied directly to large areas of compromised skin, as systemic absorption, with potential toxicity, may occur. It is usually applied one to three times a day.

Polymyxin

The polymyxins are positively charged peptides that disrupt bacterial membranes. Polymyxins are active against many gram-negative organisms, including *Pseudomonas*, but lack activity against gram-positive bacteria. Although rarely used systemically or inhaled, they are most frequently used as topical agents. The polymyxins infrequently cause dermatitis, but allergic cross-reactivity with bacitracin may occur. Polymyxin-B sulfate is commonly combined with other topical antimicrobial agents in a petroleum petrolatum base.

Bacitracin

Bacitracin blocks bacterial cell wall formation and is active against most gram-positive organisms, including streptococci, staphylococci, clostridia, and corynebacteria. Bacitracin is inexpensive and nontoxic. Postoperative patients treated with topical bacitracin may be more likely to develop skin sensitization. Topical bacitracin is widely used for the prophylaxis and treatment of minor skin infections, including patients with burn injuries. It is applied to the skin one to five times a day.

Silver Sulfadiazine (Silvadene)

Silver sulfadiazine is a sulfonamide antibacterial agent that is active against many gram-positive, gram-negative, anaerobic, and fungal organisms. Silver sulfadiazine is applied once or twice daily to second- or third-degree burns to prevent and to treat bacterial infections. Its use is contraindicated in premature infants and infants less than 2 months of age. Complications include transient leukopenia and allergic reactions in approximately 5% of patients. Sliver sulfadiazine is usually applied to a thickness of $1/16$ of an inch one or two times a day.

Mafenide Acetate (Sulfamylon)

Mafenide is a sulfonamide antibacterial agent with poor or modest activity against gram-positive and anaerobic organisms but excellent activity against gram-negative organisms, including *Pseudomonas*. Applied to burns, it can reduce the incidence of gram-negative infections. Mafenide application is painful, is associated with allergic reactions in 10% of patients, and can cause metabolic acidosis if large amounts are applied. Mafenide acetate is applied to a thickness of 1.5 mm one or two times day.

Nitrofurazone (Furacin)

Nitrofurazone is a nitrofuran drug that inhibits a number of bacterial enzymes and may damage bacterial DNA. It is active against most gram-positive organisms, including *Clostridia*, and many gram-negatives except *Pseudomonas*. Nitrofurazone is used for topical chemotherapy of wounds, burns, skin infections, and skin grafts. Dermatitis and fungal overgrowth are two potential problems associated with its use.

Otic Preparations

Several topical preparations exist for the management of otitis externa or chronic otorrhea. These agents consist of combinations of anti-infective agents, anesthetics, drying agents, surfactants, cerumenolytics, preservatives, corticosteroids, excipients, and vehicle. Otic preparations are usually placed in the involved external auditory canal several times a day until the process resolves. See the CD-ROM for a table of otic antibiotic preparations.

Ophthalmic Preparations

Several topical preparations exist for the management of ocular conjunctival bacterial and viral infections. See the CD-ROM supplement for ophthalmic antibiotic preparations. Ophthalmic preparations consist of combinations of anti-infective agents and preservatives and are prepared as either solutions or ointments. Most preparations are given several times a day until the process resolves.

Nebulized Antibacterial Agents

Nebulized antibiotics have been used in many parts of the world to treat pulmonary infections. Successful use of a nebulized antibiotic, however, depends on correct particle generation size, compliance, and ability to get the antibiotic to the needed site. Nebulized antibiotics are used to generate high local concentrations of an antibiotic and minimize potential systemic toxicity. Nebulized products are most frequently used in patients with cystic fibrosis. Tobramycin (TOBI) (300 mg/5 mL) is nebulized bid in 28-day cycles and colistin (polymixin E) (1,000,000 units/3 mL of sterile water) nebulized bid are indicated for the treatment of *P. aeruginosa* infections in patients with cystic fibrosis. Pentamidine 300 mg of injectable diluted in 6 mL of water, nebulized monthly is an effective prophylactic agent for *P. jiroveci* pneumonia in HIV-infected individuals who are intolerant of TMP/SMX. Complications include metallic taste, bronchospasm, and cough.

ANTIVIRAL AGENTS

Many parenteral and topical preparations are available to treat viral infections. These agents target viral attachment and entry into host cells or a specific step in viral replication. Effective antiviral agents exist for many of the herpes viruses and influenza. Fewer treatment options are available for other non-HIV viral infections. The following antiviral agents are discussed on the CD-ROM: drugs for herpes virus infections, drugs for influenza virus, ribavirin, and lamivudine. Antiretroviral agents are discussed in Chapter 171.

ANTIFUNGAL AGENTS

While primary care physicians infrequently need to treat invasive fungal disease, most physicians will see children with superficial mucocutaneous fungal infections. This section will deal first with the therapeutic agents used to treat invasive disease followed by a discussion of topical products. Antifungal agents are discussed on the CD-ROM. Specific agents covered are amphotericin B, flucytosine, systemic azole antifungal compounds, and other systemic antifungal agents, such as griseofulvin, terbinafine, caspofungin, and saturated solution of potassium iodide (SSKI). Many topical azole, polyene, and allylamine preparations exist for the treatment of cutaneous fungal infections. These are well tolerated and in many circumstances can be purchased without a prescription.

ANTIPARASITIC DRUGS

Antiparasitic agents are usually classified according to the organism they primarily target. Pediatricians will most commonly use antiparasitic drugs for malaria chemoprophylaxis and the treatment of gastrointestinal infestations. These agents are discussed on the CD-ROM. Agents covered are antimalarial compounds; antiprotozoal therapies including pyrimethamine, sulfadiazine, atovaquone, and pentamidine; and intestinal antiparasitic agents.

◎ **Additional Resources, CD-ROM**	
Agents for treatment of viral, fungal, and parasitic diseases	Text
Otic, ophthalmic antimicrobials	Text
Bibliography	

SUGGESTED READINGS

Brown TJ, McCrary M, Tyring SK: Antiviral agents: Non-antiretroviral drugs. J Am Acad Dermatol 2002;47(4):581–599.
Groll AH, Gea-Banacloche JC, Glasmacher A, et al: Clinical pharmacology of antifungal compounds. Infect Dis Clin North Am 2003;17(1):159–191.
Hessen MT, Kaye D: Principles of selection and use of antibacterial agents: In vitro activity and pharmacology. Infect Dis Clin North Am 2000;14(2):265–279.
Kucers A, Crowe SM, Grayson ML, Hoy JF: The Use of Antibiotics: A Clinical Review of Antibacterial, Antifungal and Antiviral Drugs, 5th ed. Oxford, England, Butterworth Heinemann, 1997.
Root RK: Clinical Infectious Diseases: A Practical Approach. New York, Oxford University Press, 1999.

SECTION 9   DIAGNOSTICS AND THERAPEUTICS: *Pharmacotherapy*

285 Analgesics/Pain Medications/Sedation

Terrence McGraw, Jeffrey L. Koh, and Dan Kovarik

Caring for children and adolescents frequently involves relieving patient pain and/or anxiety as well as controlling uncooperative activity. When choosing a drug or combination of drugs for analgesia and/or sedation, one should consider the effects desired, the logistics of administration, and the risks involved. This chapter discusses pharmacologic analgesia and sedation for the pediatric patient.

ANALGESICS/PAIN MEDICATIONS

Pain and the Nociceptive Pathways

Pain is a conscious, unpleasant sensory and emotional experience associated with actual or potential tissue damage. Nociception refers to the complex anatomic and physiologic correlates of pain. There exists no single "nociceptive pathway." Rather, there are hundreds of sites and pathways within the central nervous system that transmit and modulate nociceptive input.

Damaged tissue initiates sensory signals that travel via small, thinly myelinated or unmyelinated afferent nerves to the spinal cord. Prostaglandins and other substances released by injured tissues may augment the nociceptive signal. Afferent signals arrive at the spinal cord and excite specific spinal nerves. Interneurons, neurotransmitters, and other chemicals, such as endogenous opiates, may augment or diminish the nociceptive signal at this spinal relay site. The evolving signal travels from the spinal cord to the thalamus and higher cortical sensory centers. Again, a number of interneurons, neurotransmitters, and other substances may modify the nociceptive signal at the higher cortical levels.

Analgesic medications work at different anatomic sites along the nociceptive pathway. Mechanisms of action include direct interference with transmission of nerve signals (local anesthetics, anticonvulsants), alteration of the chemical milieu of damaged tissues (nonsteroidal anti-inflammatory drugs), imitation of endogenous opioid modulation of signal transmission (opiates), and alteration of neurotransmitter levels (α-agonists, antidepressants).

Local Anesthesia

Local anesthetics block the conduction of nerve impulses by reversibly blocking the sodium channels of nerve fiber. The degree of blockade is proportional to both the concentration of the local anesthetic and the diameter and amount of myelination of the targeted nerve fiber. Small, thinly myelinated and unmyelinated fibers (e.g., A delta, C, and autonomic fibers) are blocked with lower concentrations of local anesthetics than are large myelinated fibers (e.g., A alpha and motor neurons).

Local anesthetics are weak bases containing both a hydrophilic portion and a lipophilic portion, linked by either an ester (—COO—) or an amide (—CONH—) bond. Examples of ester local anesthetics are procaine, cocaine, and tetracaine. Examples of amide anesthetics include lidocaine and bupivacaine. Plasma cholinesterase metabolizes ester local anesthetics. Several hepatic pathways metabolize amide local anesthetics.

Local Anesthesia Risks

Common routes of local anesthetic delivery include spinal, epidural, and topical and local infiltration. If administered appropriately, local anesthetics do not produce toxic blood levels. However, systemic effects may occur if the total dose of the local anesthetic exceeds a certain amount. Systemic effects depend on amount (e.g., mg/kg) not total volume delivered. The recommended limit for *subcutaneous infiltration* of lidocaine is 5 to 7 mg/kg. Subcutaneous infiltration of bupivacaine should be limited to 2 to 3 mg/kg. There are no universal "maximum" doses for local anesthetics. However, even small fractions of published "maximum" doses of local anesthetics may produce toxic systemic effects if injected intra-arterially or into a highly vascular location. In infiltrating local anesthetic medications into a laceration, it is important to avoid intravascular injection. The peak plasma levels of local anesthetics following injection are therefore dependent on the site of administration (Box 285-1).

The first signs and symptoms of local anesthetic toxicity are generally neurologic and include tinnitus or other perceived sounds, metallic taste, hallucinations, seizures, respiratory arrest, and loss of consciousness. With increasing blood levels, cardiac toxicity ensues. As local anesthetics

depress the rate of depolarization of the cardiac action potential, signs of cardiac toxicity include hypotension, supraventricular tachycardia, atrioventricular heart block, ventricular tachycardia, and cardiovascular collapse. Treatment of local anesthetic toxicity is primarily supportive and includes maintaining a patent airway, ensuring adequate ventilation, and support of circulation ("ABCs"). Bupivacaine-induced ventricular arrhythmias are particularly difficult to treat; these are best treated with phenytoin (5 to 10 mg/kg IV slowly) and/or bretylium (5 to 10 mg/kg IV).

Allergy to amide local anesthetics is extremely rare, but ester anesthetic allergies are more common. Patients with ester anesthetic allergies frequently have a history of allergy to suntan lotions containing PABA. Patients may give a history of "allergy" to local anesthetics because of past reactions to small amounts of local anesthetic and epinephrine intravascularly injected during dental procedures.

Local Anesthetic Infiltration

Sites of action and doses of various local anesthetics are summarized in Table 285-1 (intravenous uses are not included). Lidocaine is a frequently used local anesthetic (e.g., subcutaneous, intradermal, intramuscular) and is widely available and less toxic than other local anesthetics. Duration of action for lidocaine local anesthesia is 1 to 2 hours. Bupivacaine has a much longer duration of action than lidocaine (5 to 10 hours) and is an excellent alternative if there is no risk for significant vascular absorption.

Epinephrine added to local anesthetics in concentrations of 5 to 10 μg/mL (1:200,000 to 1:100,000) may prolong the duration of analgesia. However, combinations of epinephrine and local anesthetics should not be injected into terminal extremities ("fingers, nose, penis, toes"), as blood supply to those areas might be compromised. Pain on injection may be greatly attenuated by using small needles (27 g or 30 g) and by buffering the local anesthetic solution with sodium bicarbonate (sodium bicarbonate:lidocaine = 1:8).

Topical Local Anesthesia

Local anesthetics may be applied topically. Elamax contains lidocaine 4% in a liposomal matrix. EMLA (eutectic mixture of local anesthetics) contains lidocaine 2.5% and prilocaine 2.5%. Applying Elamax or EMLA to the skin with an occlusive dressing prior to performing venipuncture, lumbar puncture, and neonatal circumcision provides effective local anesthesia. Elamax requires a half hour of skin contact; EMLA requires at least 1 hour.

TAC (tetracaine 0.5%, adrenaline [epinephrine] 1:200,000, cocaine 11.8%) is an anesthetic solution that is applied directly to an open laceration. To be effective, TAC should remain in contact with the wound for 15 minutes. One milliliter of TAC typically provides analgesia for a 1-cm laceration. To avoid local anesthetic toxicity (particularly from cocaine), TAC should not be applied to mucosal surfaces. Because it causes vasoconstriction, TAC should not be administered to areas supplied by end arteries. In addition, TAC should not be applied to patients with a history of local anesthetic or suntan lotion allergy. The combination of lidocaine, epinephrine, and tetracaine

---

Box 285-1. Local Anesthetic Absorption and Site of Administration

Relative Order of Absorption

Subcutaneous infiltration < distal peripheral block < brachial plexus block < epidural/caudal block < intercostal block

Table 285-1. Use of Local Anesthetics for Regional Anesthesia

Classification	Topical	Local Infiltration	Peripheral Nerve Block	Epidural	Spinal	Maximum Infiltration Dose (mg/kg)
Esters						
Procaine	No	Yes	Yes	No	No	8
Chlorprocaine	No	Yes	Yes	Yes	No	10
Tetracaine	Yes	No	No	No	Yes	N/A
Amides						
Lidocaine	Yes	Yes	Yes	Yes	Yes	6
Mepivacaine	No	Yes	Yes	Yes	No	5
Bupivacaine	No	Yes	Yes	Yes	Yes	2.5
Etidocaine	No	Yes	Yes	Yes	No	5
Prilocaine	No	Yes	Yes	No	No	7

(LAT) is also effective for topical anesthesia when applied to an open laceration and avoids the use of cocaine.

Iontophoresis may be used with topical local anesthetics. Iontophoresis involves applying a few milliamps of current between the skin surface and subepidermal tissue for 5 to 30 minutes. Studies in children indicate that lidocaine iontophoresis produces effective topical anesthesia for IV placement without dermal toxicity. Electromotive forces pull charged molecules of lidocaine through the skin. Compared to topical placement or infiltration, iontophoretic systems are capable of delivering larger amounts of pharmaceuticals in less time.

Acetaminophen and Nonsteroidal Anti-inflammatory Drugs (NSAIDs)

Acetaminophen

Acetaminophen is the most widely used analgesic drug in the United States. Acetaminophen's analgesic and antipyretic effects are presumably due to acetaminophen's inhibition of cyclooxygenase within the central nervous system, which in turn inhibits prostaglandin synthesis. Dose-response studies with fever indicate that effective blood levels are achieved with oral doses of 10 to 20 mg/kg every 4 hours. Analgesic dose-response studies have not been conducted. Several studies of rectal absorption have demonstrated that effective [antipyretic] blood levels are achieved following a single dose of 35 to 45 mg/kg. Following this initial rectal dose, subsequent doses of 20 mg/kg per rectum ever 6 hours maintain steady blood levels.

While acetaminophen is a relatively weak analgesic, it is an effective adjuvant. For example, in the postoperative patient, acetaminophen administered regularly ("around the clock") lessens both opiate requirements and opiate-induced side effects.

Acetaminophen Risks

Acetaminophen toxicity has been reported with single oral doses of greater than 100 mg/kg in healthy children. Toxicity may be seen following lower doses if acetaminophen is repeatedly administered or if liver disease is present. Blood levels have been reported within the therapeutic range following single rectal administration of up to 60 mg/kg. Hepatic insufficiency is a contraindication for acetaminophen use.

Table 285-2 lists acetaminophen dosages for pain.

NSAIDs

Nonsteroidal anti-inflammatory drugs (NSAIDs), like acetaminophen, inhibit cyclooxygenase and prostaglandin synthesis. However, NSAIDs work both in the central nervous system and peripheral tissues. They are particularly useful in treating pain associated with tissue inflammation. Chapter 286 further discusses NSAIDs and their dosing requirements.

Both acetaminophen and NSAIDs exhibit an "analgesic ceiling"; dosage greater than recommended does not result in a greater degree of analgesia.

Opiates

Opium and opiate derivatives remain the mainstay of treatment for moderate to severe pain. The discovery of naturally occurring opiate-like neuropeptides (endorphins, enkephalins, dynorphins), as well as receptors to these neuropeptides, helped to elucidate the mechanism of action. Opiate medications affect these neuropeptide or "endogenous opiate" receptors, which are located in various areas of the brain (cortex, hypothalamus, amygdala, pons) and spinal cord (substantia gelatinosa). Receptor occupation by either endogenous neuropeptides or pharmaceutical opiates diminishes nociceptive signals. Of note, there is *no* maximum degree of analgesia or "analgesic ceiling" that can be achieved with opiates. Adequate analgesia is usually attained if sufficient amount of opiate is administered. Generally, opiate side effects limit the amount of opiate administration.

Opiates also exhibit a number of systemic effects. These include euphoria, dysphoria (particularly when administered in the absence of pain), sedation, respiratory depression, miosis, decreased gastrointestinal motility (constipation), urinary retention, nausea, vomiting, and pruritus. The physiologic effects generally shared by opiates are listed in Table 285-3.

Table 285-2. Acetaminophen Dosing for Pain

Oral	10–20 mg/kg every 4 hours
Rectal	30–40 mg/kg once, followed by 20 mg/kg every 6 hours

Table 285-3. Physiologic Effects of Opioids

I. Central Nervous System
   A. Analgesia
   B. Sedation
   C. Dysphoria and euphoria
   D. Nausea and vomiting
   E. Miosis
   F. Seizures
   G. Psychomimetic behaviors, excitation
II. Respiratory system
   A. Antitussive
   B. Respiratory depression
      1. Decreased respiratory rate
      2. Decreased tidal volume
      3. Decreased ventilatory response to carbon dioxide
III. Cardiovascular system
   A. Heart rate
      1. Bradycardia (fentanyl, morphine)
      2. Tachycardia (meperidine)
   B. Minimal effects on cardiac output
   C. Vasodilation, venodilation
      1. Morphine >> other opioids histamine release
IV. Gastrointestinal system
   A. Decreased intestinal motility and peristalsis
   B. Increased sphincter tone
      1. Sphincter of Oddi
      2. Ileocolic
V. Urinary system
   A. Increased tone
      1. Ureters
      2. Bladder
      3. Detrusor muscles of the bladder

Opiate Risks

Until recently, fear of causing respiratory depression hampered effective use of opiates in children. In general, opiates are safe to use in children of all ages. Only premature and full-term newborns have reduced clearance leading to prolonged elimination half-life of morphine. By 2 to 4 months of age, a former term infant's metabolism and clearance of morphine are similar to those of adults. By 3 to 6 months of age, infants are no more susceptible to opiate-induced respiratory depression than adults are. Infants younger than 6 months of age should have individual titration of opiate dosing, especially when prolonged use is required. Infants on opiate medication require respiratory monitoring with respiratory support readily available.

The fear that children who are treated with opiates for pain might develop narcotic addiction is unfounded. Addiction is the persistence of obsessive thoughts and compulsive use of a drug despite known adverse effects of the drug. Addiction is often confused with tolerance and withdrawal, which are physiologic phenomena resulting from repeated exposure to opiates. Appropriate modification of dosing schedules can effectively manage tolerance and withdrawal. A number of studies indicate that the subsequent risk of addiction is no higher than that in the general population when children are administered opiates to treat pain.

Opiate Dosing and Delivery

The correct dose of opiates is "enough"—enough to alleviate pain without causing intolerable side effects (e.g., respiratory depression, sedation, pruritus).

Analgesic potency varies greatly among opiates, yet all opiates can achieve an "equipotent" dose. "Unit doses" are a general guide for *starting* opiate analgesia. The unit doses for various opiates are listed in Table 285-4. The effective dose for an individual patient may be less or greater (sometimes much greater!) than a typical unit dose. Intravenous administration is preferred if rapid onset is necessary or if patients do not tolerate oral administration. Once adequate analgesia is achieved, oral administration of opiates can maintain analgesia equal to that achieved by intravenous administration. The only indication for intramuscular administration of opiates is the need for rapid analgesia when easy intravenous access is unavailable.

If intravenous opiate analgesia is required on a regular basis for more than a few hours, opiate administration via continuous infusion or a patient-controlled analgesia device (PCA) is preferred. These delivery methods help to avoid the blood level peaks and valleys associated with toxicity and breakthrough pain. PCAs consist of a push button attached to an opiate-containing infusion pump. Pressing the button delivers a preprogrammed aliquot. Preprogramming of the infusion device also limits dosage frequency. PCAs can deliver continuous infusions either instead of or in addition to bolus doses. PCAs have been used in children as young as 5 to 6 years of age. Under normal circumstances, the patient, rather than a parent or nurse, should push the button as necessary. Typical starting doses for several drugs used in PCAs are listed in Table 285-5.

Opiates, either alone or in combination with local anesthetics, are particularly effective for controlling pain when administered near the spinal cord. Epidural or intrathecal opiates attach to opiate receptors within the spinal cord. Epidural administration of opiates is an effective treatment for the anticipated significant postoperative pain following surgery of the chest, abdomen, perineum, or lower extremities. Typical duration of postoperative epidural therapy is 2 to 5 days. Epidural analgesia helps to facilitate postsurgical recovery, since it achieves maximum analgesia with minimal sedation without interfering with deep breathing exercises, physical therapy, and ambulation. Other indications for epidural analgesia include medical conditions associated with severe pain (e.g., sickle cell disease crises, cancer pain) that are unresponsive to systemic opiates. Only anesthesiologists who are experienced in pain management should administer epidural analgesia (Box 285-2 and Table 285-6).

Morphine

Morphine has been the mainstay of opiate analgesia for over 100 years and is the most commonly prescribed opiate in the postoperative setting. Morphine may be administered via intravenous, oral, epidural, and intrathecal routes. A typical unit dose for intravenous morphine is 0.1 mg/kg every 2 to 4 hours as needed for moderate to severe pain. Alternatively, morphine may be delivered via a PCA. The bioavailability of morphine is approximately 20%. To achieve equivalent analgesia, oral doses are about three to five times the intravenous dose, depending on the patient's prior exposure to morphine. Cancer pain is a frequent indication for oral morphine, which is available in

Table 285-4. Equivalent Opiate Typical Starting Doses

Opiate	Oral Dose	Intravenous Dose	Bioavailability	Comments
Morphine	0.3 mg/kg q3–4h	0.1 mg/kg q2–4h	20–40%	Frequent first choice for parenteral treatment. Injection often results in localized or systemic histamine release.
Hydromorphone	6 mcg/kg q3–4h	15 mcg/kg q2–4h	50–70%	Useful in patients with renal insufficiency/failure. (Metabolites have minimal opiate activity.)
Meperidine	Not recommended	0.75 mg/kg q2–3h	40–60%	Metabolite (normeperidine) can cause seizures, particularly with prolonged use or in patients with diminished renal function.
Methadone	0.2 mg/kg q6–12h	0.1 mg/kg q6–8h	70–90%	Often used in chronic settings (e.g., chronic pain, opiate withdrawal). High bioavailability facilitates changing parenteral to oral administration.
Fentanyl	N/A	1 mcg/kg q0.5–1h	N/A	Short duration of action makes fentanyl most useful for procedure-related pain. Useful in patients with renal insufficiency/failure. (Metabolites have minimal opiate activity.)
Codeine	1 mg/kg q3–4h	N/A	40–70%	Often prescribed in suspension with acetaminophen (codeine 12.5 mg/5 mL, acetaminophen 125 mg/5 mL). Side effects (nausea, constipation, itching) sometimes limit usage. Typical starting dose 0.4–0.5 mL/kg.
Hydrocodone	0.2 mg/kg q3–4h	N/A	40–70%	Available in suspension with acetaminophen (hydrocodone 2.5 mg/5 mL, acetaminophen 167 mg/5 mL). Typical starting dose 0.3–0.4 mL/kg.
Oxycodone	0.1 mg/kg q3–4h	N/A	40–70%	Available in liquid (5 mg/5 mL), tablets (5 mg), and extended-release tablets.

immediate-release and sustained-release preparations. Also, numerous morphine metabolites are active opiates. Patients with hepatic or renal insufficiency requiring morphine might need lower doses and longer intervals between doses.

Morphine, when administered via epidural or intrathecal routes, is an extremely potent analgesic. Epidural and intrathecal morphine is often administered with local anesthetics to children with surgical or cancer pain. Only experienced physicians in facilities with appropriate pediatric support should administer epidural or intrathecal morphine.

Hydromorphone

Hydromorphone is approximately five times as potent as morphine and is a frequent alternative to morphine. A typical unit dose for intravenous hydromorphone is 0.02 mg/kg every 2 to 4 hours as needed for moderate to severe pain. Hydromorphone bioavailability is approximately 50%; an effective oral dose is about two times the intravenous dose. Some practitioners use hydromorphone as the epidural opiate of choice, because it is associated with side effects than morphine. Unlike morphine, the metabolites of hydromorphone are devoid of narcotic

effects. Hydromorphone is a reasonable opiate choice for children with renal insufficiency.

Methadone

Methadone is equivalent in potency to morphine but has a longer half-life (12 to 16 hours) and greater bioavailability (70% to 90%). Consequently, methadone is typically administered every 6 to 12 hours. To achieve equivalent analgesia, oral doses of methadone are 1 to 1.5 times intravenous doses. Methadone's long half-life and ease of conversion from intravenous to oral dosing make it a good choice for painful conditions that are expected to last longer than a week and for weaning a patient off narcotics. Methadone is also available in a liquid preparation, making it very useful for smaller children needing long-term opiate analgesia.

Meperidine

Meperidine is a synthetic opiate whose potency is approximately one tenth that of morphine. The pharmacokinetics and side effects of meperidine are similar to those of morphine. Indications for meperidine include postoperative pain, postanaesthetic shivering, and amphotericin-induced rigors. A typical unit dose for intravenous meperidine is

Table 285-5. Typical Starting Doses for PCAs

Drug	Intravenous PCA Bolus	Lockout Time	Infusion Rate
Morphine	0.01 mg/kg	5–10 min	0.01–0.02 mg/kg/hr
Hydromorphone	2–4 µg/kg	5–10 min	2–4 µg/kg/hr
Fentanyl	0.2–0.4 µg/kg	5–10 min	1–2 µg/kg/hr

0.25 mg/kg for shivering and 1 mg/kg for pain. Meperidine's chief metabolite, normeperidine, is also narcotically active. At toxic levels, normeperidine causes muscle tremors and convulsions. Meperidine is not a good choice for prolonged use or for patients with seizure disorders or renal disease.

Fentanyl

Fentanyl is the synthetic prototype of several recently developed opiates that include sufentanyl, alfentanyl, and remifentanyl. These drugs are notable for their potency (10 to 800 times as potent as morphine), rapid onset, and rapid redistribution and elimination. Their metabolites are not narcotically active. Fentanyl and its analogues block nociceptive stimuli and their associated biochemical and endocrine stress responses while generally maintaining hemodynamic stability. Fentanyl is ideally suited for patients undergoing surgery or critical care. However, fentanyl administered rapidly in doses of greater than 4 μg/kg may cause chest wall rigidity, making even assisted ventilation difficult or impossible. Muscle relaxants or naloxone administration usually counteracts fentanyl induced chest wall rigidity. Patients may rapidly develop tolerance to fentanyl infusion or repeated administration and may require increased dosing to achieve effectiveness (tachyphylaxis). Typical initial doses of fentanyl are 1 to 2 μg/kg intravenous bolus and 1 to 2 μg/kg/hr continuous infusion.

Fentanyl may be administered epidurally as well as via several novel routes, including a topical patch. Fentanyl patches consist of fentanyl embedded in a gel matrix. When applied to the skin, the patch releases fentanyl at a constant rate, resulting in analgesia similar to that induced by intravenous infusions. As with any opiate, fentanyl patches may induce profound hypoventilation and should not be administered to opiate-naive individuals in unmonitored situations. Fentanyl patches are typically administered to patients with long-term opiate requirements who do not have vascular access and are unable to tolerate oral medications. Typical starting doses deliver about 1 μg/kg/hr (e.g., a 25-μg patch for a 25-kg child).

Fentanyl is also available in a flavored solid matrix attached to a handle. This "lollipop" placed in the mouth allows transmucosal absorption of the opiate. (Chewing the preparation is contraindicated.) Transmucosal fentanyl is ideal for providing significant self-limited opiate analgesia in situations when vascular access is unavailable (e.g., reducing fractures, suturing lacerations). The typical starting dose is about 5 μg/kg.

Codeine

Codeine and its analogues (hydrocodone, oxycodone) are primarily oral medications used for the treatment of moderate to severe pain. They are available as tablets or suspension in combination with acetaminophen. Hydrocodone and oxycodone are approximately five and eight times as potent as codeine, respectively. Suspensions of codeine/acetaminophen (12.5 mg/125 mg per 5 cc) and hydrocodone/acetaminophen (2.5 mg/167 mg per 5 cc) are available for children who are unable to swallow tablets. Typical starting dose of codeine/acetaminophen suspension is 5 cc per 10 kg every 4 hours. Typical starting dose of hydrocodone/acetaminophen suspension is 4 cc per 10 kg every 4 hours. Avoidance of acetaminophen toxicity limits the use of codeine/acetaminophen medications. Plain oxycodone is available as 5-mg tablets and 5 mg per 5-mL suspension. A typical starting dose for oxycodone is 0.1 to 0.2 mg/kg every 4 to 6 hours.

Medications for Neuropathic and Chronic Pain (Box 285-3)

Aberrant transmission of nociceptive signals to the central nervous system leads to neuropathic pain. Neuropathic pain is less amenable to treatment with opiates or anti-inflammatory medications. Traumatic or surgical nerve injuries are frequent precursors to neuropathic pain (e.g., phantom limb pain following amputation). Other forms of neuropathic pain have unclear etiologies (e.g., complex regional pain syndrome, reflex sympathetic dystrophy).

Some chronic pain syndromes do not involve neuropathic pain. Examples include fibromyalgia, recurrent abdominal pain syndrome, and some types of recurrent headache.

Several central nervous system medications demonstrate potent analgesia in many patients with neuropathic and/or chronic pain.

Gabapentin

Various anticonvulsant medications (valproate, carbamazepine, phenytoin) effectively relieve neuropathic pain. However, side effects and concerns for long-term toxicity have limited their use. Gabapentin, a newer anticonvulsant medication, appears to be quite promising. Studies suggest that gabapentin is effective for neuropathic pain in children 12 years of age and older. Side effects of gabapentin, which include sedation and dizziness, are generally mild and self-limited, and toxicity rarely occurs with standard doses. The starting dose is typically 300 mg/day (given either 300 mg

Table 285-6. Sample Oral Methadone Weaning Schedule

	QAM	QPM	QHS
Day 1	10 mg	10 mg	10 mg
Day 3	10 mg	5 mg	10 mg
Day 5	5 mg	5 mg	10 mg
Day 7	5 mg	5 mg	5 mg
Day 9	5 mg	None	5 mg
Day 11	None	None	5 mg
Day 13	None	None	None

once a day at bedtime or 100 mg three times a day). Gabapentin may be increased to 2400 mg/day (given 800 mg three times a day) as tolerated. Gabapentin is available as 100-mg, 300-mg, and 400-mg capsules.

Tricyclic Antidepressants

Tricyclic antidepressants provide effective analgesia for neuropathic pain without causing mood alterations. Amitriptyline and nortriptyline are commonly used medications. The starting dose for both medications is 0.25 mg/kg every evening, and doses may be titrated to 2 to 3 mg/kg as tolerated. As in the treatment of depression, a positive response to these medications may take 7 to 10 days. Both medications are available as 10-mg, 25-mg, and 50-mg tablets and capsules; nortriptyline is also available in 10 mg/ 5 cc oral suspension. These medications may cause arrhythmias and conduction disturbances. Side effects of amitriptyline include dry mouth and sedation.

Clonidine

Clonidine is an α-agonist originally marketed to treat hypertension. It stimulates α-adrenoceptors in the brainstem and spinal cord, resulting in reduced sympathetic outflow and reduced pain signal transmission to the brain. The common side effects of sedation, hypotension, and bradycardia limit frequent use of clonidine. It is available in oral, epidural, and transcutaneous preparations.

Future Trends in Analgesia

A number of medications and new drug delivery systems are currently undergoing investigation for the treatment of pain refractory to standard treatment. Drugs include ketamine, dextromethorphan, α-agonists, and anticholinesterase medications. Protein matrix beads containing local anesthetics show promise as an effective delivery system. Such beads placed in wounds or in the epidural space may provide weeks of analgesia.

PROCEDURAL SEDATION

Sedation for procedures requires control of patient anxiety and movement (Box 285-4). Nonpharmacologic techniques for reducing anxiety such as distraction, environment, and age-appropriate information should always be employed to obviate the need for, or reduce the amount of, pharmacologic therapies. Child life specialists may assist with nonpharmacologic techniques when indicated, but such a discussion is beyond the scope of this chapter. The practice of sedation should be viewed as a controlled, progressive slope from *awake*, to *mild sedation (anxiolysis)*, to *moderate sedation*, to *deep sedation/general anesthesia*. Sedation should be a delicate balance between maintaining

---

Box 285-4. Procedural Sedation

Procedural sedation can be an anxiety-provoking experience, but an understanding of the pharmacology of a few sedative agents and some planning can make the event more pleasant for the patient and clinician.

Box 285-5. Fasting Times for Sedation

Infants <6 months: no milk or solids for 4 hours prior to procedure

Infants >6 months and children: no milk or solids for 6 hours prior to procedure

All patients regardless of age may have clear liquids up until 2 hours prior to procedure.

---

the patient in as alert a state as possible while still controlling anxiety and excessive movement.

Sedation should begin with an assessment of the child—the airway, fasting status, physical status (with special attention to hemodynamic, respiratory, neurologic, renal, and hepatic function), and psychological needs—and a discussion with the child's parents or guardians. Sedation should occur only in an area that is suitable for proper monitoring and performance of emergency resuscitation if needed. SOAP is a helpful acronym to ensure that all necessary equipment is available before induction of sedation: *Suction, oxygen* with positive pressure delivery system, *airway* equipment with proper-sized masks, laryngoscopes, and endotracheal tubes, and *pharmacologic* agents for sedation and their reversal, muscle relaxants, and cardiac resuscitation medication and equipment should be at hand. Pulse, respiration, blood pressure, SaO_2, and level of consciousness should be monitored continuously and recorded intermittently throughout the procedure. Children undergoing procedural sedation should be monitored until they are alert and have returned to their baseline level of functioning. The American Academy of Pediatrics provides guidelines for sedation.

Children with significant medical problems that complicate their ability to tolerate sedation require consultation with an anesthesiologist before attempting procedures that involve more than light sedation. Examples include children with diseases that compromise cardiorespiratory systems and children whose anatomy makes intubation difficult if the need arises. Clues to difficult intubation include inability to open the mouth to provide an unobstructed view of the posterior pharynx and presence of a short mandible or neck with limited range of motion. To decrease the risk of aspiration, children undergoing sedation for nonemergent procedures should fast to ensure an empty stomach. See Box 285-5 for recommended fasting times.

Sedation Drugs

The ideal sedation drug has a pleasant route of administration, rapid onset with easy titration and awakening, and no contraindications or side effects and provides both amnesia and analgesia. No such drug exists. Benzodiazepines and barbiturates offer no analgesic properties. Opioids, while excellent centrally acting analgesics, have little amnestic effects and can cause hemodynamic and respiratory depression. The frequent practice of combining different classes of agents may produce a desired response, but adverse side effects may also be enhanced. One should have a good understanding of the effects and pharmacokinetics of the few sedation drugs that provide desired clinical results with few risks to the patient.

The following is a brief review of the major classes of sedatives; Table 285-7 provides routes of administration and dosages. The list is not intended to be comprehensive, and the recommended dosages are subject to change. Always check the manufacturer's package insert or consult an anesthesiologist when using medications that are unfamiliar.

Alpha-2-Adrenergic Agonists

Clonidine was described in this chapter's section on neuropathic and chronic pain. Along with dexmedetomidine, clonidine is gaining popularity as premedications for surgery and light sedation. Cardiovascular effects, mainly hypotension and bradycardia, limit their usefulness in procedural sedation.

Barbiturates

Barbiturates work through barbiturate receptors, a part of the gamma-aminobutyric acid (GABA)-receptor complex that is the major inhibitory neurotransmitter in the brain. With intravenous administration barbiturates have a rapid onset and are easily titratable, making them a good choice for diagnostic studies that require profound sedation and immobility. Barbiturates may induce hyperalgesia, making them a poor choice for painful procedures. Barbiturates also depress respiratory drive and myocardial contractility and cause venodilation with peripheral pooling of blood. Pentobarbital has a 30- to 60-minute duration, making it a popular choice for children undergoing magnetic resonance imaging. Thiopental and methohexital are barbiturates with a short half-life whose roles have largely been replaced by propofol.

Benzodiazepines

Benzodiazepines act by occupying the benzodiazepine receptor that modulates GABA. The benzodiazepine/GABA-receptor complexes in the limbic system modulate arousal, anxiety, and behavioral inhibitions.

Benzodiazepines are the class of sedatives most often called on for procedural sedation in children. They exhibit a mild antiemetic effect and are anticonvulsants, which raise the seizure threshold in patients who are also given local anesthetics. When used by themselves, benzodiazepines have only slight effects on respiration but have a synergistic respiratory effect when combined with opiates, barbiturates, or other central nervous system depressants. The benzodiazepines can also reduce systemic vascular resistance slightly, decreasing arterial blood pressure with little change in cardiac output. Midazolam (Versed), diazepam (Valium), and lorazepam (Ativan) are the three benzodiazepines most commonly used in the United States. Diazepam and lorazepam are less popular for procedural sedation because of their long half-lives and stinging discomfort with intravenous administration. Midazolam has the advantage of rapid onset of action, relatively brief duration, and many routes of administration. However, a child may infrequently become more anxious and excited rather than sedated with midazolam administration. This is probably a disinhibitory effect and can be overcome with higher doses of midazolam or by administration of an opiate.

Flumazenil is a benzodiazepine receptor antagonist that can be titrated to reverse the effects of benzodiazepines. If flumazenil is administered to a patient who is physically dependent on benzodiazepines, it may precipitate a seizure. Because of flumazenil's short elimination half-life the patient should be monitored for possible return of benzodiazepine sedation.

Chloral Hydrate

Chloral hydrate has been used as a hypnotic agent for more than 120 years. Despite its variable onset and recovery times, chloral hydrate is a popular agent for sleep EEG evaluations because this orally administered agent has an extensive history of successful use. Chloral hydrate has an active metabolite, which may account for the occasional return of sedation in a patient starting to arouse.

Etomidate

Etomidate is an ultra-short-acting intravenous sedative hypnotic with minimal cardiorespiratory effects. Etomidate is used for brief deep sedation, frequently causes pain on injection, occasionally produces myoclonus, and suppresses adrenal function if used for more than brief procedural sedation.

Table 285-7. Sedation Drugs

Agent	Dose	Onset	Duration	Notes
Clonidine PO	4 µg/kg	60–90 min	4–6 hr	Bradycardia and hypotension
Methohexital IV	1–2 mg/kg	1 min	5–10 min	Titrate to effect, hiccoughs and myoclonus common
PR	30 mg/kg	5–10 min	45 min	Laryngospasm infrequently
Pentobarbital IV	1–5 mg/kg	1–3 min	1–3 hr	Titrate to effect, best for nonpaintful procedures
Pentobarbital PO	2–6 mg/kg	30–60 min	3–6 hr	Unpredictable onset and recovery
Midazolam IV	0.03–0.1 mg/kg	2–8 min	15–30 min	Titrate to effect, water soluble
IM	0.05–0.1 mg/kg	15–30 min	0.5–1 hr	Cimetidine increases plasma levels
PO/PR	0.5 mg/kg	15–30 min	0.5–1 hr	
IN (intranasal)	0.3 mg/kg	5–10 min	20–40 min	Stings on administration
Chloral hydrate PO/PR	20–100 mg/kg	15–60 min	2–4 hr	Potentiates warfarin, may cause eosinophilia
Etomidate IV	0.1 mg/kg	30 sec	3–12 min	Titrate to effect, stings, may cause myoclonus
Ketamine IV	0.5–mg/kg	30–60 sec	5–15 min	Titrate to effect, tachycardia, salivation, emergence delerium is decreased with benzodiazepine
IM	3–5 mg/kg	3–10 min	20–60 min	Provides analgesia, combine with glycopyrolate 5 µg/kg
Propofol IV	1 mg/kg	15–30 sec	2–10 min	Stings on administration, apnea is common
Remifentanil	0.5–2 µg/kg	15–30 sec	0.5–2 min	Ultra-short-acting opiate analgesic

Ketamine

Ketamine is a dissociative anesthetic agent that is chemically related to phencyclidine (angel dust). Ketamine is a short-acting agent that provides analgesia in addition to amnesia. The patient's eyes often remain open despite deep sedation. Staring eyes with marked nystagmus produces a "lights are on but nobody is home" look that can be disconcerting to parents who have not been not forewarned. Ketamine induces the release of endogenous catecholamines, causing bronchodilation and an increase in heart rate and blood pressure. Ketamine also causes an increase in cerebral blood flow and should not be used in children who may have increased intracranial pressure. An anticholinergic and a benzodiazepine should be used in conjunction with ketamine to decrease salivary gland secretions and prevent emergence delirium.

Opiates

Opiates were described earlier in this chapter. As with benzodiazepines, pharmacokinetics is the major determinant of differences in clinical action. Fentanyl is the opiate most frequently used to provide analgesia for procedural sedation, but remifentanil is an ultra-short-acting opiate that is gaining popularity.

Propofol

Propofol is an ultra-short-acting anesthetic agent that is packaged for injection in a 10% intralipid solution. Propofol's onset of action is within seconds. Since propofol rapidly redistributes throughout the body, the patient usually awakens within a few minutes after propofol infusion is discontinued. Unlike the barbiturates, propofol has analgesic properties, making it a popular choice for brief deep sedation for mildly painful procedures such as bone marrow biopsies. Propofol is a respiratory depressant and frequently induces apnea. It also decreases systemic vascular resistance and cardiac output with a fall in systolic blood pressure. Pretreatment with intravenous lidocaine will reduce the sting propofol causes when administered via a peripheral vein.

Pediatric Office Sedation Problems

Two case examples follow that illustrate sedation procedures in the office setting.

1. A 2-year-old child presents to the office with a 3-cm clean laceration on the forehead. After the family is questioned about medication allergies, a topical mixture of viscous lidocaine, adrenaline, and tetracaine is applied to the wound, and a mixture of aceta-minophen elixir (15 mg/kg) and midazolam (0.5 mg/kg) is orally administered. The child and her parents await the procedure in a quiet examination room for 30 minutes. After 30 minutes, if the child is relaxed and cooperative, the wound is infiltrated with a few milliliters of 1% lidocaine administered through a fine needle via the wound edges. When thoroughly anesthetized, the wound can be irrigated, débrided, sutured, and dressed. If the child remains uncooperative, further sedation options must be discussed with the parents. Assessment of fasting status, airway, and physical status reveals the patient to be at low risk for complications for deep sedation performed in a facility equipped with resuscitation equipment and personnel. Intramuscular ketamine (3 mg/kg) combined with glycopyrolate (0.01 mg/kg) is a good choice, as is intravenously administered opioid or barbiturate. If cardiorespiratory risks of deep sedation are concerning or parents are unwilling to consent, the patient should be referred to a surgical facility.

2. A 6-year-old child presents to the office with a headache and neck stiffness following 3 days of nausea, fever, and malaise. The patient is afraid of doctors and uncooperative on examination. Elamax cream is applied to the patient's back and both antecubital fossa, and the patient waits with the parents for 30 minutes before reexamination. Reexamination confirms the need for spinal fluid and blood examination. The patient's anxiety may be reduced by nonpharmacologic methods or orally administered midazolam. The child's history of nausea or vomiting makes deep sedation a higher risk for cardiorespiratory complications and should be avoided if possible.

SUGGESTED READINGS

American Academy of Pediatrics Committee on Drugs: Guidelines for monitoring and management of pediatric patients during and after sedation for diagnostic and therapeutic procedures: Addendum. Pediatrics 2002;110:836–838.

Anand KJS, Menon G, Narsinghani U, McIntosh N: Systemic analgesic therapy. In Anand KJS, Stevens BJ, McGraw PJ (eds): Pain Research and Clinical Management, 2nd ed, vol 10: Pain in Neonates. Amsterdam, Elsevier, 2000, pp 159–188.

Berde CB, Kain ZN: Pain management in infants and children. In Motoyama EK, Davis PJ (eds): Smith's Anesthesia for Infants and Children, 6th ed. St. Louis, Mosby, 1996, pp 385–402.

Guakroger PB: Paediatric analgesia: Which drug? Which dose? Drugs 1991;41:52–59.

McRorie TI, Lynn AM, Nespeca MK, et al: The maturation of morphine clearance and metabolism. Amer J Dis Child 1992;146:972–976.

286

Anti-inflammatory and Immunomodulatory Therapy

Peter A. Nigrovic and Robert P. Sundel

Rubor, tumor, calor, dolor—redness, swelling, heat, pain—are the four cardinal signs of inflammation noted by the Roman physician Celsus in the first century. Inflammation is an essential component of the body's reaction to infection or injury, without which normal healing is impossible. Occasionally, the inflammatory response may cause more harm than good, either through exuberance or through action against inappropriate targets. When inflammation causes considerable harm, anti-inflammatory therapy becomes necessary.

INFLAMMATION

Inflammation is mediated by the immune system in response to defined triggers. Tissue trauma releases chemical mediators that attract neutrophils, and later macrophages and fibroblasts, to clear up debris and assist with damage repair. These cells and the inflammatory chemicals they release give rise to redness and exudate even in noninfected wounds. Foreign antigens, such as bacterial cell wall components or viral proteins, trigger an even more vigorous response, which varies with the inciting stimulus. Extracellular pathogens tend to elicit neutrophil migration, an appropriate response because phagocytosis is typically central to the elimination of these organisms. Intracellular pathogens or cancers, on the other hand, characteristically incite a lymphocytic response, since lymphocytes are the cells capable of recognizing the surface signs of intracellular infection or neoplastic transformation.

When activated, neutrophils, macrophages, and lymphocytes release cytokines and other mediators. The cytokines that are most important to the inflammatory response are IL-1, IL-6, and TNF-α, which together are responsible for many of the systemic signs and symptoms, including fever, anorexia, and malaise. These cytokines also elicit the *hepatic acute phase response:* down-regulation of housekeeping proteins such as albumin in favor of those important in defense, such as C-reactive protein (an opsonin for certain bacteria), fibrinogen (to assist with clotting), and ferritin (to deprive bacteria of free iron).

Another important class of inflammatory mediators is the arachidonic acid metabolites, including leukotrienes and prostaglandins. Released by inflammatory cells, these mediators contribute to acute erythema and swelling by inducing vasodilation and capillary leak. Prostaglandin E2 is of particular importance because it also sensitizes local nerve endings to pain and, with IL-1, mediates fever via effects on the hypothalamus.

In most situations, the inflammatory response fades away after the inciting stimulus is cleared. Occasionally, the inflammatory stimulus cannot be eliminated, for example, asbestos crystals in the lung or a self-molecule acting as autoantigen. In these situations, ongoing inflammation may result in tissue damage, granuloma formation, scarring, or fibrosis.

ASSESSING SYSTEMIC INFLAMMATION

Cytokines and other mediators released by immune cells account for the clinical picture of systemic inflammation, including fever, malaise, and anorexia. Another clinical manifestation of inflammation specific to children is failure to grow properly despite adequate dietary intake. Careful review of the growth chart often pinpoints the onset of a chronic inflammatory disease.

The blood tests that are most often used to assess the degree of systemic inflammation are the erythrocyte sedimentation rate (ESR) and the C-reactive protein (CRP). The ESR is a rapid and inexpensive proxy for multiple acute phase proteins, especially fibrinogen. Because of their positive charge, these proteins intercalate between negatively charged erythrocytes and facilitate the formation of stacks (rouleaux), which sediment more rapidly than free-floating cells do. CRP is another product of the hepatic acute phase response. The advantage of the CRP is that it rises and falls rapidly with the inflammatory stimulus, while the ESR rises more slowly and remains elevated long after the inflammation resolves. In addition, the ESR is affected by proteins other than acute phase reactants, such as gamma globulins, and by changes with the hematocrit and physical properties of the erythrocytes (e.g., sickling). Despite these disadvantages, ready availability and extensive experience with the ESR make it a useful, if nonspecific, clinical tool.

Inflammatory cytokines are responsible for other manifestations of acute inflammation including leukocytosis, release of immature neutrophils ("bands") from bone marrow, and progressive thrombocytosis. Additional manifestations of prolonged inflammation include normocytic anemia (the anemia of chronic disease) and elevated levels of serum immunoglobulins resulting from nonspecific B-cell stimulation.

PRINCIPLES OF ANTI-INFLAMMATORY THERAPY

Ideal anti-inflammatory therapy would target only aberrant manifestations of the inflammatory response while preserving the surveillance and protective functions of immunity. Unfortunately, the aberration in the immune system that is responsible for specific inflammatory diseases is often unknown, so available agents are generally unable to discriminate harmful from beneficial immune activity, and many drugs have nonimmunologic side effects as well. The result is that risks of immune suppression must be balanced against benefits of controlling inflammation. In many cases, agents other than those commonly used might be effective, but lack of experience has prevented their widespread adoption. A general approach would be the following:

1. *NSAIDs* (nonsteroidal anti-inflammatory drugs) have antipyretic and analgesic effects and therefore are effective for symptomatic relief. They do not meaningfully interrupt the cascade of inflammatory cytokines, however, and generally do not prevent immunologically mediated tissue damage.
2. *Steroids* are employed for rapid suppression of severe inflammation of all types, since they affect almost all inflammatory pathways. Side effects, however, make long-term steroid use highly undesirable.
3. *DMARDs* (disease-modifying antirheumatic drugs, including sulfasalazine, antimalarials, low-dose methotrexate, and leflunomide) are introduced in a limited subset of inflammatory conditions to slow damage from chronic inflammation. The mechanisms of their anti-inflammatory effects are poorly understood.
4. *Steroid-sparing immunosuppressants* are employed when intolerable steroid doses are required for control of inflammation. Steroid-sparing immunosuppressants tend to offer more limited anti-inflammatory effects, allowing gradual replacement of the broadly acting steroids. These agents include cyclosporine, azathioprine, and mycophenolate mofetil.
5. *Biologic response modifiers* (or "biologics") are designer drugs engineered to target specific components of the immune response such as TNF (etanercept, inflix-imab), IL-1 (anakinra), or B-lymphocytes bearing the surface marker CD-20 (rituximab).
6. *Cytotoxic agents and antimetabolites* are required for the most severe or life-threatening illnesses. The principal cytotoxic drug used for inflammatory and autoimmune conditions is cyclophosphamide, though chlorambucil, high-dose methotrexate, and 6-mercaptopurine are also occasionally employed.
7. Other immunomodulatory therapies are useful for selected situations. These include *plasmapheresis, intravenous immunoglobulin (IVIG)*, and *immune ablation* with or without *bone marrow transplantation.*

Each of these categories will be reviewed.

Nonsteroidal Anti-inflammatory Drugs
"NSAID choice depends on dosing schedule, side effect profile, and cost."

The class of NSAIDs includes aspirin and a large number of related agents, including ibuprofen, naproxen sodium, indomethacin, and ketorolac. They are indicated at low to moderate doses for fever, myalgias, and pain and at high doses for anti-inflammatory activity (Table 286-1). Acetaminophen is a related drug that is also effective for fever and pain but does not have anti-inflammatory activity and therefore is not considered an NSAID.

Mechanism of Action
The NSAIDs are inhibitors of the enzyme cyclooxygenase (COX), which converts arachidonic acid to prostaglandin. Prostaglandins are involved in the generation of fever and the sensitization of pain receptors as well as in vasodilation and vascular leak at sites of inflammation. Cyclooxygenase has two isoforms: COX-1 and COX-2. COX-1 is constitutively expressed and is involved in gastric protection and platelet function. COX-2 is induced by IL-1 and appears to mediate most of the prostaglandin-associated symptoms of inflammation. Most traditional NSAIDs inhibit both COX isoforms. However, a new generation of COX-2-specific NSAIDs has been developed. These include celecoxib, rofecoxib, and valdecoxib, which have proven to be effec-

Table 286-1. Selected NSAIDs Useful in Pediatric Inflammatory Disease

NSAID	Total Daily Dose	Interval	Half-Life (hour)	Liquid	Note
Aspirin* NSAIDs	60–100 mg/kg (max 4 g/24 h)	qid	0.25	N	Reye syndrome, more GI effects than most
Choline magnesium trisalicylate (Trilisate)	50 mg/kg (max 2250 mg/24 h)	bid	12	Y	Nonacetylated salicylate similar to aspirin with less GI, hematologic toxicity
*Ibuprofen	30–40 mg/kg (max 2400 mg/24 h)	qid	2	Y	Aseptic meningitis, esp. SLE
Naprosyn*	10 mg/kg (max 1500 mg/24 h)	bid	14	Y	Occasional photosensitization
Indomethacin*	1–3 mg/kg (max 200 mg/24 h)	tid	4	Y	GI, CNS (headache, confusion) (?) better for pericarditis and systemic onset JRA
Tolectin*	15–30 mg/kg (max 1800 mg/24 h)	tid	1	N	May be better for spondylarthropathy
Nabumetone	adult: 1–2 g	qd–bid	26	N	Least GI-toxic standard NSAID
Celecoxib	adult: 100–400 mg	qd–bid	11	N	COX-2-selective. Sulfa moiety
Rofecoxib	adult: 12.5–50 mg	qd	17	N	COX-2-selective. Peripheral edema, hypertension

*FDA approved for use in children.

tive at suppressing inflammation with less gastric toxicity and no effect on platelet function.

Toxicity

NSAIDs are generally well tolerated, but at high doses and with continuous use, they can be associated with toxicity (Box 286-1) Gastric irritation including ulceration and bleeding can occur with all NSAIDs, though the COX-2-selective drugs are significantly less likely to cause this problem. Platelet dysfunction occurs with all COX-nonselective drugs except the nonacetylated salicylates (e.g., salsalate) and may lead to easy bruising or bleeding. The platelet effects are transient with all NSAIDs except aspirin, which acetylates cyclooxygenase irreversibly. Since COX blockade may shunt arachidonic acid down the lipoxygenase pathway, a subset of asthmatic patients (especially those with nasal polyps) may experience worsening bronchospasm on NSAID therapy. In addition, prostaglandins regulate renal blood flow, so cyclooxygenase inhibition, including COX-2-selective blockade, may cause decompensation of renal perfusion in patients with impaired renal function. They may also cause interstitial nephritis even in those with healthy kidneys. Idiosyncratic reactions associated with particular NSAIDs include aseptic meningitis with ibuprofen (especially in lupus patients) and a photosensitive skin rash with naproxen. Reye syndrome is most highly associated with aspirin but has been reported with other NSAIDs.

Clinical Use of Nonsteroidal Anti-inflammatoy Drugs

NSAIDs are indicated on an as-needed basis and at low doses for control of pain, fever, and other systemic symptoms. The response is generally brisk. For inflammation, higher doses are needed and should be prescribed as a standing rather than intermittent dose; the maximum anti-inflammatory effect may require weeks of continuous use. For reasons that are poorly understood, individuals respond differently to various NSAIDs, and one NSAID may work where another has failed, so trials of different agents in this class are reasonable. Although up to 35% of cases of juvenile arthritis may respond completely to treatment with NSAIDs, in general this class of agents does not slow the pace of joint destruction in inflammatory arthritis, even though they provide important symptomatic relief.

Despite differing cyclooxygenase-inhibiting potency in vitro, there are no consistent and reproducible differences in clinical efficacy between NSAIDs. Thus, the choice between particular agents generally comes down to dosing schedule, side effect profile, and cost. Ibuprofen is the customary initial choice in the United States because of its low cost, ready availability, and rapid onset of action. Naproxen has the advantage of twice daily dosing, which not only is convenient, but also allows a child to sleep through the night and awaken with ongoing drug effect. Indomethacin is the most potent COX inhibitor in this class and is a preferred choice for treating pericarditis, ankylosing spondylitis, and systemic juvenile rheumatoid arthritis (JRA). Corresponding to its therapeutic potency, indomethacin also has the highest incidence of gastrointestinal (GI) side effects.

If GI upset or bleeding becomes problematic, use of one of the COX-2-specific agents is reasonable, though the experience in children is small, and these drugs are rather expensive for first-line use. (Note that celecoxib contains a sulfa moiety and is therefore avoided in sulfa-allergic children.) Alternatively, data from adult studies suggest that use of a proton pump blocker such as omeprazole is effective in reducing the gastric and duodenal toxicity of COX-nonselective NSAIDs. In view of the relatively modest therapeutic effects of NSAIDs, however, one must consider carefully whether using additional agents to prevent toxicity is warranted; one might select an agent from a different class of anti-inflammatory medications instead. Monitoring liver function tests and complete blood counts is advised for long-term use of NSAIDs to screen for hepatic toxicity and chronic GI blood loss. Given the small risk of Reye syndrome, aspirin should be generally avoided in children except for defined indications such as Kawasaki disease, desired antithrombotic effects, and acute rheumatic fever. Varicella and influenza vaccinations are recommended for children receiving chronic NSAID therapy.

Corticosteroids

Endogenous glucocorticoids are secreted by the adrenal cortex in a diurnal cycle, peaking in the early morning and trailing off the rest of the day. Physiologically, these hormones play a complicated role in the immune system, suppressing some immune functions while potentiating others. Yet at pharmacologic doses, steroids are the most potent and broad-spectrum anti-inflammatory agents available and have an important role in the therapy of many inflammatory conditions. Their toxicity is equally impressive.

Mechanism of Action

Glucocorticoid hormones bind to a variety of cytoplasmic receptors and migrate to the nucleus, where glucocorticoid-receptor complexes bind to so-called glucocorticoid response elements (GREs) to alter gene transcription. By this mechanism, steroids inhibit nuclear factor kappa B (NFkB), an important link in the production of multiple cytokines including the principal mediators of the systemic immune response (IL-1, IL-6, TNF-α, and IFN-γ) as well as IL-2, the cytokine central to lymphocyte activation. In addition, steroids inhibit phospholipase A2 and therefore block both the prostaglandin and leukotriene arms of the

---

Box 286-1. Toxic Effects of Nonsteroidal Anti-inflammatory Drugs

CNS: Headache, dizziness, aseptic meningitis
Cardiovascular: Hypertension
Pulmonary: Asthma exacerbation
GI: Gastritis and peptic ulcer with GI bleeding, hepatitis
Renal: Renal dysfunction, interstitial nephritis
Heme: Platelet dysfunction with easy bruising, blood dyscrasias
Skin: Rash +/- photosensitivity (piroxicam, naprosyn, others)
Other: Reye syndrome (principally ASA), peripheral edema (especially rofecoxib)

arachidonic acid pathway. They also inhibit neutrophil margination, migration, and production of toxic compounds such as collagenase and elastase. Macrophage function is inhibited directly and by lack of IFN-γ. Thus, steroids dampen the inflammatory response at a variety of different sites.

Toxicity

Unfortunately, steroids can be as toxic as they are effective (Box 286-2). Short-term use, such as for the treatment of an asthma exacerbation, is usually well tolerated, although mood swings may be troublesome. Longer-term systemic use is frequently complicated by secondary Cushing syndrome: moon facies, central obesity, acne, hirsutism, and thinning skin with bruising and striae. Such disfiguring effects may be the source of emotional distress and therefore lead to medication noncompliance, especially in adolescents who are more conscious of their body image. Growth slows, and the loss of height may be permanent if the slow rate of growth persists for more than 6 months.

Steroids increase vulnerability to infections, especially herpesviruses (principally varicella-zoster), but also to mycobacteria, fungi, and bacteria. No data are available in children to quantify this risk, but a meta-analysis of adult trials documented a relative risk of 1.6 for all infections and 2.6 for fatal infections in patients receiving more than 10 mg of prednisone daily. Osteopenia, cataracts, and other problems may also occur, and an Addisonian crisis may supervene if long-term steroids are stopped abruptly. GI bleeding is not generally a consequence of steroids alone, although steroids do potentiate the gastric toxicity of NSAIDs and of physiologic stress.

Clinical Use of Steroids

The choice of agent, dose, and route of administration varies with the condition treated. Inflammation limited to epithelial surfaces often may be treated with topical, intranasal, or inhaled steroids, with the great benefit that absorption and therefore toxicity are limited. Steroid injections into skin, joint, or bursa are also very effective for local inflammation. For diseases requiring systemic immunosuppression, oral or parenteral administration is necessary. The relative potencies and pharmacologic characteristics of commonly used oral and parenteral steroids are listed in Table 286-2. The oral bioavailability of prednisone and prednisolone is nearly 100%, so intravenous administration is indispensable only when patients cannot tolerate enteral medications or when gastrointestinal absorption is impaired (as in vasculitis). In patients with liver disease, hydroxylation of prednisone (an inactive prodrug) to active pred-

> **Box 286-2.** Side Effects of Glucocorticoids
>
> CNS: Mental status changes, pseudotumor cerebri
> Ocular: Cataracts, glaucoma
> Cardiovascular: Hypertension, accelerated atherosclerosis
> GI: GI bleeding, especially on NSAIDs
> Endocrine: Growth failure, central obesity with moon facies, diabetes
> Musculoskeletal: Osteopenia, avascular necrosis of bone, steroid myopathy, joint effusions
> Skin: Skin fragility, bruising, striae, hirsutism
> Infectious disease: Severe herpesvirus infections, Listeria meningitis, disseminated mycobacterial and parasitic infections

nisolone may be impaired, though this is rarely a problem in actual practice.

Experience and custom, rather than data, guide most steroid dosing. Younger patients tend to metabolize steroids faster than older patients, though interindividual differences are large. If inflammation is of recent onset or the triggering stimulus for the inflammation is no longer present, usually only a short course of steroids, for example, 3 to 7 days of prednisone 1 to 2 mg/kg/day divided twice a day for an asthma exacerbation, is required. Life-threatening inflammatory diseases such as systemic lupus erythematosus (SLE), on the other hand, often require continuous, ongoing high doses of steroids to achieve control. In such cases, a slow taper over months is essential to avoid relapse, and a daily maintenance dose is often unavoidable. The use of alternate immunosuppressive medications as steroid-sparing agents is necessary to avoid intolerable side effects. Alternate-day dosing limits side effects but may be insufficiently effective in severe disease. At any given total daily dose, steroids are more potent (and more toxic) when divided two to four times a day. Consolidation into a single daily morning dose, mimicking the typical diurnal cycle of morning cortisol secretion by the adrenal gland, is often an early step in a steroid taper.

In acutely life-threatening conditions such as transplant rejection, central nervous system vasculitis, or pulmonary hemorrhage, "pulse" steroid therapy can help to bring a rapid halt to inflammation. Intravenous methylprednisolone 30 mg/kg to a maximum dose of 1000 to 1500 mg is administered over 1 to 2 hours each day for 1 to 3 days, with cardiovascular monitoring for the rare but potentially fatal complications of bradycardia or hypertension. Since all glucocorticoid receptors are already saturated at much lower doses, the mechanism of action of pulse dose steroids

Table 286-2. Potency and Half-Life of Common Glucocorticoids

Glucocorticoid	Relative Anti-inflammatory Potency	Relative Mineralocorticoid Potency	Half-Life (hours)	
			Plasma	Biologic
Hydrocortisone	1	1	1–2	8–12
Prednisone	4	0.5	1–2	18–36
Prednisolone	4	0.75	2–3	18–36
Methylprednisolone	5	0.5	1–3	18–36
Dexamethasone	25–30	0	2–4	36–54

is uncertain. Direct cell membrane effects have been postulated. In any event, pulse steroids can be remarkably effective, with biologic effects lasting long after the steroids have been metabolized.

Prolonged use of oral steroids, and on occasion even high doses of inhaled or topical steroids, can suppress the hypothalamus-pituitary-adrenal axis. Suppression may last for months, even after steroids have been tapered. In such cases, abrupt discontinuation of steroid or a severe stressor such as infection, trauma, or surgery can precipitate an adrenal (Addisonian) crisis with malaise, fevers, and refractory hypotension. Stress dose steroids, for example, hydrocortisone 25 to 50 mg/m^2 up to 50 to 100 mg three times a day or dexamethosone 1 to 2 mg/m^2 up to 4 mg daily, may be lifesaving. Dexamethosone has the advantage that it does not interfere with cosyntropin testing of the hypothalamus-pituitary axis. Clinically significant adrenal suppression does not occur after short courses of steroids, so it is generally not necessary to taper steroid doses gradually because of fear of adrenal crisis unless a patient has been treated for more than 3 to 6 weeks with more than 2 mg/kg/day. On the other hand, even at lower doses, gradual tapering may be necessary to avoid a flare of the underlying disease even with far smaller doses of steroids.

In general, tapering steroids is generally unnecessary unless a patient has been treated for more than at least 3 weeks with more than 2 mg/kg/day.

The care of the patient on long-term glucocorticoids is outlined in Box 286-3. Every effort should be made to taper the dose. Calcium and vitamin D should be given routinely to slow osteoporosis, and a bisphosphonate such as pamidronate may be considered in patients who develop severe osteoporosis and pathologic fractures. Routine screening for hypertension, glaucoma, and cataracts is important. Steroid acne typically responds well to topical retinoids if benzoyl peroxide is ineffective. A high index of suspicion for infection is important, because steroids can suppress fever and peritoneal signs and can increase vulnerability to atypical infections such as disseminated tuberculosis or pulmonary *Pneumocystis carinii*. Since steroids induce neutrophil release, leukocytosis is an unreliable indicator of infection in children receiving glucocorticoids. However, a significant increase in neutrophils and bands in the white count may indicate developing infection. For patients receiving other immunosuppressants (especially cyclophosphamide) along with steroids, *P. carinii* prophylaxis with TMP/SMX should be considered.

Box 286-3. Care for the Patient on Chronic Steroids

Maintain lowest possible dose.
Consider alternate-day dosing as less toxic alternative.
Consider steroid-sparing agents.
Monitor weight and linear growth.
Monitor blood pressure.
Maintain bone health: calcium, vitamin D, exercise, ± bisphosphonate.
Ophthalmologic evaluation yearly for cataracts and glaucoma.
Proactive therapy for acne.
Pneumocystis carinii prophylaxis if also on cyclophosphamide.

Other Immunomodulatory Agents

Although NSAIDs and steroids are generally sufficient immunomodulators for most situations arising in general practice, further therapy is sometimes needed. Although many of these treatments are not intrinsically very toxic, most primary care providers do not have enough experience with them to feel comfortable in their use. It is worthwhile to review their potential benefits and side effects in order to provide the best care for children. (See Table 286-3.)

Disease-Modifying Antirheumatic Drugs

The first of these alternative immune modulators are the disease-modifying antirheumatic drugs (DMARDs): methotrexate, the antimalarials, sulfasalazine, and leflunamide. The DMARDs are so named because, unlike NSAIDs, they slow the progression of bony erosions in adult rheumatoid arthritis. DMARDs work very well in childhood inflammatory disease and do not cause significant generalized immunosuppression. Similar to steroids, DMARDs demonstrate their clinical benefit slowly, over weeks to months. A patient who stops taking a DMARD before finishing 2 to 3 months of therapy might not fully experience the potential benefits of the drug. Conversely, adverse effects of the medications can persist for many months after the final dose.

Methotrexate (MTX) is the most commonly used DMARD, useful for conditions as diverse as JRA, psoriasis, dermatomyositis, and steroid-dependent asthma. MTX does not appear to be useful for SLE, except perhaps for SLE arthritis. MTX is typically administered orally, though doses above 0.5 mg/kg are best given parenterally (by subcutaneous or intramuscular injection) to optimize absorption.

MTX inhibits dihydrofolate reductase essential for purine synthesis, making MTX useful as an antimetabolite for treating malignancies. However, folate antagonism does not seem to be a significant mechanism of action in the treatment of inflammatory disease, where doses are typically three logs less than those used for cancer. More recently, attention has focused on the effect of MTX on leukocyte release of adenosine, an anti-inflammatory mediator. Methotrexate in very low doses increases adenosine production, and adenosine inhibitors reverse the anti-inflammatory effects of methotrexate in an animal model of arthritis.

Despite its designation as a chemotherapeutic agent, MTX is remarkably safe at anti-inflammatory doses, and its once-weekly administration is convenient. Nausea, irritability, and mucositis can occur, but these are usually preventable with daily oral folate (held on the day of and the day after MTX dosing to prevent antagonism). Other side effects are rare in children, possibly because metabolism of MTX is more rapid in children than in adults, and exposure to other hepatotoxic and pulmotoxic substances (such as alcohol and tobacco) is minimal. Interstitial lung disease occurs only once in 10,000 to 40,000 children, 100-fold less commonly than in adults. Similarly, hepatic cirrhosis can occur but appears to be entirely preventable if liver function tests are monitored every 2 to 4 months, and doses are decreased for any sustained elevation in the AST (aspartate aminotransferase) or ALT (alanine aminotransferase). Myelosuppression may also occur, generally

Table 286-3. Other Immunomodulatory Drugs

Drug	Mechanism of Action	Dose	Principal Toxicities	Monitor
DMARDs (Disease-Modifying Antirheumatic Agents)				
Methotrexate	1. Block folate metabolism and purine synthesis 2. Increase adenosine levels (anti-inflammatory mediator)	10 mg/m² q wk PO/SQ/IV, escalate as tolerated	Hepatitis, nausea, oral ulcers, bone marrow suppression, pneumonitis (rare in children)	LFTs q4–8 wk, periodic CBCs; folate can limit GI and hematologic toxicity
Hydroxychloroquine	? Block lysosome antigen processing	≤7.0 mg/kg/d PO, max 400 mg daily, divided qd–bid	Retinopathy, nausea, rash, agranulocytosis	Ophtho eval q6 mo, CBC, LFTs q3–6 mo
Sulfasalazine	? Increase adenosine levels	Goal: 40–60 mg/kg/d PO divided bid–tid, max 3 g, start slowly	Rash, nausea, leukopenia, hepatitis, headache/CNS, Stevens-Johnson syndrome	CBC + LFTs q mo × 3–4 months then periodically
Leflunomide	Block pyrimidine synthesis	Adult: 10–20 mg qd	Diarrhea, hepatitis, bone marrow suppression, alopecia/rash	LFTs q mo until stable, then q4–8 wk
Biologic Response Modifiers				
Etanercept	Block TNF-α and lymphotoxin	0.4 mg/kg SQ 2/wk, max 25 mg 2/wk	Injection site reactions, infections, cytopenias, ? multiple sclerosis	Sole biologic approved by FDA for children
Infliximab	Block TNF-α	3–5 mg/kg IV q6–8 wk	Infections (esp. reactivation of TB)	None; use with low-dose MTX to inhibit antibodies against drug
Adalibumab	Block TNF-α	Adult: 40 mg sq q 2 wk	Injection site reaction, infection	
Immunosuppressive Agents				
Azathioprine	Active metabolite 6-MP blocks purine synthesis	1–3 mg/kg/d PO qd or divided bid	Bone marrow suppression, infection (esp. zoster), nausea, hepatitis, rash	CBC, LFTs
Cyclosporine A	Block synthesis of IL-2 and other cytokines by inhibiting calcineurin	1–10 mg/kg/d divided bid, max 3.9 daily	Hypertension, nephrotoxicity, hyperlipidemia, diabetes, tremor, seizures, gingival hyperplasia, hirsutism, skin cancer, lymphoma	Blood pressure, UA, CBC, BUN/Cr, glucose, LFTs, K, Mg (not CsA levels) q2 wk × 3 mo then q2–3 mo; *multiple drug interactions*
Mycophenolate mofetil	Block purine synthesis	600 mg/m²/dose bid, max 1 g bid, max 3 g daily	Bone marrow suppression, infections, nausea, diarrhea	CBC
Cyclophosphamide	Alkylate DNA leading to strand breakage	Monthly IV: 500–1000 mg/m² max .1.2 g (with concurrent mesna) PO: 50–100 mg/m²/day	Bone marrow suppression, nausea, alopecia, bladder toxicity, infertility, cardiotoxicity	WBC; periodic UA, BUN/Cr, long-term monitoring for leukemia and bladder cancer. PCP prophylaxis if on steroids

heralded by a gradual increase in red blood cell mean corpuscular volume and preventable by giving higher doses of folic acid. Infection risk is increased minimally.

The antimalarials, of which the most prominent is hydroxychloroquine (Plaquenil), were noted to incidentally benefit arthritis. Their mechanism of action is uncertain but may involve interference with lysosomes (perhaps impairing antigen processing and presentation to T-lymphocytes) and ultraviolet blockade in the skin. In pediatrics, their main use is in mild forms of arthritis, in lupus, and in dermatomyositis, where they are effective for skin and joint disease. Antimalarial medications are generally well tolerated but may cause rash, GI upset, myopathy, and agranulocytosis, among other side effects. The major toxicity is eye disease (maculopathy) that is slowly progressive at any dose (often irreversible), though rare at doses below 7 mg/kg/day. Regular ophthalmologic screening every 6 to 12 months, including testing color vision, is necessary to detect ocular toxicity early enough to prevent visual impairment. Occasional routine monitoring of blood counts and liver function tests may be necessary.

Sulfasalazine (SSZ) was the first "designer drug" for treating arthritis; it was synthesized from a sulfa antibiotic plus aspirin in the 1930s, at a time when arthritis was thought to be due to infection. SSZ's mechanism of action is not understood, since the salicylate moiety is not absorbed from the GI tract and the antibiotic component alone is ineffective for treating arthritis. SSZ may work by up-regulation of adenosine production. SSZ is useful for JRA (except systemic-onset JRA, where SSZ may precipitate hepatitis and DIC in a significant number of patients), psoriatic arthritis, and inflammatory bowel disease. Toxicity includes rash (rarely progressing to full-blown Stevens-Johnson syndrome), leukopenia, abdominal pain, and transaminitis. Gradual dose escalation helps to avoid many of these adverse effects. Recommended monitoring includes periodic checks of blood counts and liver function tests, especially at the start of therapy.

Leflunomide (Arava) is the newest of the DMARDs, and its use in children is limited yet growing. Leflunomide inhibits dihydroorotate dihydrogenase, which blocks uridine (pyrimidine) synthesis and thereby inhibiting leukocyte proliferation in a manner analogous to the effects of methotrexate on purine synthesis. In view of these parallel modes of action, the combination of methotrexate and leflunomide is a logical one. Though no data have demonstrated clinical synergy to date, preliminary experience suggests this is a potent, effective combination. Because leflunamide has a long half-life and can take years to clear the body entirely after being discontinued and because it is highly teratogenic in animals, this agent is relatively contraindicated in women of childbearing age. Side effects include diarrhea and liver toxicity, with several deaths from hepatic necrosis reported. Regular monitoring of liver function tests is mandatory for anyone receiving leflunomide.

Biologic Response Modifiers

An exciting new frontier in anti-inflammatory therapy is the direct antagonism of inflammatory mediators and their cellular targets by using recombinant proteins known as biologic response modifiers (BRM). These agents are called "biologics" because they are engineered to block specific biological functions. Though very effective, BRMs are extraordinarily expensive, typically costing over $10,000 per patient per year.

Etanercept (Enbrel) was the first BRM approved for use in human disease. Etanercept is synthesized in genetically modified hamster ovary cells from two copies of the binding site of the TNF receptor attached to the Fc portion of a human IgG-1 antibody. Injected subcutaneously twice weekly, etanercept removes TNF-α (as well as a second inflammatory cytokine, lymphotoxin) from circulation, interrupting the inflammatory cascade. Infliximab (Remicade) is a humanized mouse monoclonal antibody against TNF-α that is infused IV every 6 to 8 weeks and achieves a similar antagonism of circulating TNF. Etanercept and infliximab can rapidly decrease disease activity in two thirds of patients with active JRA, with infliximab also effective for treating inflammatory bowel disease. The side effect profiles of these drugs are not yet well established, but both agents are immunosuppressive and do lead to an increase in the number and severity of infections. Etanercept has been associated with aplastic anemia and a multiple sclerosis-like condition that appears to be reversible in most cases. Infliximab must be used with methotrexate to block the development of antichimeric antibodies. Recent reports also document a significant increase in the incidence of reactivated tuberculosis with the use of TNF-inhibitors, especially with infliximab. All patients should have appropriate skin testing for tuberculosis before starting one of these agents.

The IL-1 receptor antagonist anakinra (Kineret) was recently approved for the treatment of arthritis. More than 50 other biologic agents are currently under development for the treatment of arthritis, lupus, and other inflammatory diseases.

Immunosuppressive Agents

Occasionally, patients with severe inflammation require high-grade immunosuppression. Clinical examples include vasculitis of the central nervous system or lung, crescentic glomerulonephritis, and any life-threatening inflammatory disease that fails to respond to traditional agents or requires intolerable doses of steroids for control. Transplantation of solid organs or bone marrow sometimes requires powerful immune suppression. High-grade immunosuppressive include cyclophosphamide, cyclosporine A, azathioprine, and mycophenolate mofetil.

Cyclophosphamide (Cytoxan) is an alkylating agent that, by causing DNA breakage, impairs proliferation of leukocytes and neutrophils. Antibody production is variably impaired. In high doses, cyclophosphamide is myeloablative and useful in chemotherapeutic regimens and bone marrow transplantation. Lower doses are used for immunosuppression. In combination with steroids, cyclophosphamide is the cornerstone of treatment for severe nephritis, Wegener granulomatosis, severe fibrosing interstitial lung disease, and life-threatening vasculitis. It is most potent, but also most toxic, when administered as a daily oral dose. Periodic (e.g., monthly) intravenous administration is generally preferred to limit total exposure, though it appears to be less effective in treating some conditions, such as vasculitis, compared to daily administration. The intravenous dosing varies with clinical condition but typically ranges from 500 to 1000 mg/m^2 once a month, adjusted to ensure that the white blood count nadir is no lower than 3000 to 4000 measured 7 to 14 days after administration (although leukopenia per se is not a therapeutic goal).

As with all untargeted immunosuppressive agents, cyclophosphamide administration is associated with significant toxicity. Alkylating agents have their greatest effect on cells with rapid turnover; alopecia (generally partial) and nausea are common side effects. Germ cells are also vulnerable, and infertility may occur in both sexes (men generally more than women). This toxicity occurs in direct proportion to total dose received, the greatest effect being seen in postpubertal patients.

Metabolites excreted in the urine are toxic to the mucosa and may result in severe hemorrhagic cystitis, though ample intravenous hydration, frequent voiding, and antagonism of metabolites with mesna can usually prevent this complication. Cyclophosphamide is also teratogenic. Administered alone, cyclophosphamide does not significantly increase infection risk. Administering cyclophosphamide with high-dose steroids, however, greatly increases patient susceptibility to typical and opportunistic infections, thereby warranting *P. carinii* prophylaxis. Of greatest concern is the increased risk of malignancy, particularly of the skin and bladder. Bladder cytoprotection and avoidance of sun exposure are important protective measures during cyclophosphamide therapy. Leukemia (particularly acute myelogenous leukemia) and lymphoma are the next most common malignancies, occurring years after therapy. These secondary leukemias are unusually resistant to therapy.

Cyclosporine A (CsA) and its newer relative, FK506 (tacrolimus), block lymphocyte proliferation by inhibiting calcineurin, a calcium-dependent cytoplasmic enzyme involved in lymphocyte activation and cytokine production, especially IL-2 production. Since lymphocytes are the principal effector cell of acute and chronic organ rejection, the introduction of CsA was a major advance in transplantation. In the nontransplant setting, CsA is used occasionally as a steroid-sparing agent, especially for the treatment of dermatomyositis and systemic JRA. Administration of CsA is complicated by irregular and unpredictable absorption from the gut, especially in younger children, so monitoring drug levels is important. Side effects include hypertension, nephrotoxicity, GI upset, seizures, glucose intolerance, and increased risk of infection (especially with herpesviruses). CsA and FK506 somewhat increase the risk of squamous cell skin cancer and lymphoproliferative disease, perhaps because lymphocytes are involved in tumor surveillance or because IL-2 enables apoptosis of abnormal cells.

Azathioprine (AZA, Imuran) is another effective anti-lymphocyte drug that is useful in transplantation and as a steroid-sparing agent in inflammatory arthritis, vasculitis, and SLE. Azathioprine is metabolized into 6-mercaptopurine, which inhibits leukocyte proliferation by blocking purine synthesis. Further metabolism of AZA into 6-thioguanine (6-TG) accounts for the majority of drug toxicity, including GI upset and bone marrow suppression. Monitoring of 6-TG levels is sometimes useful, since individual metabolic variation may permit much higher azathioprine doses in some patients. AZA increases the risk of infection, especially with herpesviruses. Use of AZA is also associated with an increased risk of developing certain malignancies, particularly squamous cell skin cancer and non-Hodgkin lymphoma, though this increase is small when azathioprine is not taken in conjunction with other immunosuppressive agents (i.e., the nontransplant patient).

Mycophenolate mofetil (CellCept) is a newer immune suppressant that, like azathioprine, inhibits lymphocyte proliferation by blocking purine synthesis. Mycophenolate mofetil may be more selective in its effect than AZA because it is relatively specific for an enzyme isoform found only in lymphocytes. Mycophenolate is superior to azathioprine in reducing transplant rejection, with a similar toxicity profile (long-term follow-up is not yet available). Given its potency, mycophenolate appears to have a role as a less toxic replacement for cyclophosphamide in the treatment of SLE and lupus nephritis.

Many other immunosuppressant drugs are in development or in clinical trials, though none of these agents has (yet) been studied systematically in autoimmune or inflammatory diseases.

Other Modalities of Immunomodulation

Plasmapheresis is another method for modulating the immune response. Through peripheral or central intravenous access, the patient's blood is filtered to remove plasma. Blood cells are resuspended in replacement fluid (5% albumin or donor plasma) and infused back into the patient. This process allows rapid removal of circulating pathologic antibodies and immune complexes, as well as toxins and inflammatory mediators. Plasmapheresis is essential in conditions such as Goodpasture syndrome, when circulating antibodies quickly damage lung and kidney despite timely initiation of appropriate medications. Plasmapheresis is also useful in thrombotic thrombocytopenic purpura, refractory immune thrombocytopenic purpura, and catastrophic antiphospholipid antibody syndrome. Plasmapheresis has been used as a stopgap measure in numerous conditions. Despite dramatic descriptions of acute reversal of life-threatening cases of SLE, dermatomyositis, and other inflammatory diseases, most studies fail to demonstrate long-term benefit. In the treatment of chronic diseases, a longer-acting immunosuppressant agent must be prescribed to ensure maintaining any short-term benefit first achieved by plasmapheresis.

Intravenous immunoglobulin (IVIG) consists of polyclonal antibodies pooled from thousands of blood donors. Essential for the treatment of hypogammmaglobulinemia and other primary immunodeficiencies, IVIG can also act as a powerful immune modulator. The mechanism of immune modulation is unclear and probably multifaceted. In immune thrombocytopenia purpura, IVIG may block antibody-mediated platelet destruction in part by saturation of Fc receptors. IVIG has also been shown to down-regulate lymphocyte function via binding to inhibitory Fc receptors. IVIG contains anti-idiotypic antibodies that down-regulate autoantibody production as well as clear toxins (as in toxic shock syndrome). In toxic epidermal necrolysis, IVIG blocks keratinocyte receptors involved in apoptosis, possibly explaining the decreased incidence of skin sloughing seen with IVIG therapy. The mechanisms of action of IVIG in numerous other conditions, including Guillain-Barré syndrome and Kawasaki disease, are still unknown.

SUGGESTED READINGS

Denton MD, Magee CC, Sayegh MH: Immunosuppressive strategies in transplantation. Lancet 1000;353:1083–1091.

Gabay C, Kushner I: Acute-phase proteins and other systemic responses to inflammation. NEJM 1999;340(6):448–454.

Stuck AE, Minder CE, Frey FJ: Risk of infectious complications in patients taking glucocorticoids. Rev Infect Dis 1989;11(6):954–963.

287 Antiepileptic Therapy

Thomas K. Koch

The treatment of epilepsy in children requires careful consideration of the risks and benefits of any therapeutic intervention. When to initiate therapy, which treatment option to choose, and for how long to use are decisions that require careful consideration. The goals of treatment remain the control of seizure frequency while limiting side effect risks. Compliance issues unique to each therapy are crucial for success. Current treatment options include pharmacological therapy, the ketogenic diet, the vagal nerve stimulator, and seizure surgery (Box 287-1). This chapter focuses on pharmacological therapy.

Single-drug therapy (monotherapy) accomplishes the optimal pharmacologic therapy. Familiarity with the pharmacologic properties and efficacy of the various antiepileptic drugs (AEDs) is paramount to success in obtaining treatment goals. Since the late 1980s, antiepileptic drug options have greatly expanded. While the established AEDs offer familiarity, the newer AEDs offer diversity, efficacy, and perhaps better safety profiles.

ESTABLISHED ANTIEPILEPTIC DRUGS

Despite the entry of numerous new antiepileptic drugs, most patients still initiate therapy with an established medication because safety and efficacy profiles of these medications in children are well recognized. Furthermore, blood levels of these drugs are easy to obtain, toxicity is easily recognized, and the various drug formulations are well known. Table 287-1 lists the half-life, indications, dosing, and notable side effects of these medications. Table 287-2 lists the currently available formulations for all the major established AEDs.

Phenobarbital

Phenobarbital is the oldest AED prescribed in current practice. Effective for the control of both partial and tonic-clonic seizures, phenobarbital is a good first choice for therapy in infants and newborns. Parenteral phenobarbital is useful for the treatment of status epilepticus. Phenobarbital's long half-life permits single-day dosing, and it is available in both liquid and tablet formulations. Dosing is easy to manage owing to phenobarbital's linear kinetics and readily obtainable blood levels. The major side effects include behavioral changes such as sedation or hyperactivity and impaired cognition. A drug-induced rash is a less common side effect.

Phenytoin

Phenytoin is a well-established and widely prescribed AED, used especially for adults in the United States. Phenytoin is effective for both partial and tonic-clonic seizures and is a first-line therapy for the treatment of status epilepticus. It is available in both oral and parenteral formulations. However, the liquid oral formulation is a suspension plagued by problems with inconsistent concentrations that may lead to underdosing and overdosing. In general, oral phenytoin suspension should not be used. The use of oral phenytoin in children is further complicated by variable intestinal absorption in infants and nonlinear pharmacokinetics with a concentration dependent half-life. The major central nervous system side effects include ataxia, nystagmus, dysarthria, cognitive slowing, and somnolence. Systemic side effects include gingival hypertrophy, hirsutism, acne, hepatic dysfunction, lymphadenopathy, a lupus-like syndrome, and a rash in approximately 5% of patients. Use during pregnancy can cause the fetal hydantoin syndrome. Long-term side effects include osteopenia, folate-deficiency, cerebellar atrophy, and a peripheral neuropathy.

A new parenteral prodrug formulation, fosphenytoin, is gaining popularity for the treatment of status epilepticus. Fosphenytoin has less cardiovascular toxicity and can be administered intravenously more rapidly than phenytoin. Since fosphenytoin is water-soluble and has a balanced pH, it does not cause soft tissue injury if it should extravasate during administration. Fosphenytoin can also be administered intramuscularly, although intramuscular administration is not recommended for the treatment for status epilepticus.

Carbamazepine

Carbamazepine is one of the most important AEDs for the treatment of both partial seizures with or without generalization and tonic-clonic seizures. However, carbamazepine may exacerbate generalized absence and myoclonic seizures. Carbamazepine is a strong hepatic inducing agent and even induces its own metabolism, requiring careful

Table 287-1. Established Antiepileptic Drugs

AED	Half-Life in Children	Indication	Starting Dose	Maintenance	Dosing Schedule	Side Effects
Carbamazepine	8–28 hours Time-dependent kinetics	Partial seizures Tonic-clonic	10 mg/kg/day	20–30 mg/kg/day	bid–tid	Headache, dizziness, hematologic toxicity, rash
Diazepam	15–40 hours	Acute seizures Status epilepticus	0.3 mg/kg	N/A	N/A	Drowsiness, CNS depression, respiratory depression
Lorazepam	6–18 hours	Status epilepticus	0.1 mg/kg	N/A	N/A	Same as diazepam
Ethosuximide	30–40 hours	Absence	10–15 mg/kg/day	20–40 mg/kg/day	bid–tid	Gastric irritation, headache, dizziness, rash
Phenobarbital	30–75 hours 43–217 hours (neonate)	Partial seizures Tonic-clonic Neonatal	3–5 mg/kg/day Load: 15–20 mg/kg	3–5 mg/kd/day	qd	Behavioral/sedation, impaired cognition, rash
Phenytoin	Concentration dependent: 5–14 hours (child) 10–60 hours (neonate)	Partial seizures Tonic-colonic Status epilepticus	5 mg/kg/day Load: 15–20 mg/kg	5–8 mg/kg/day	bid–qd	Cognitive slowing, ataxia, nystagmus, cosmetic, rash
Valproic acid	8–15 hours	All seizures	10–15 mg/kg/day	30–80 mg/kg/day	bid–tid	Tremor, drowsiness, hepatic toxicity, thrombocytopenia, polycystic ovaries, neural tube defects

monitoring of serum levels after initiating treatment. It is available only in oral formulations but can be taken as either a liquid, sprinkles, or a chewable or regular tablet. Major side effects include diplopia, headache, dizziness, nausea, vomiting, and a rash in approximately 5% to 10% of patients. After initiation of therapy, a mild self-limited leukopenia may occur. Hyponatremia may occur, though primarily in elderly adults and rarely in children. There are rare reports of severe blood dyscrasia or toxic hepatitis. Carbamazepine accelerates the hepatic metabolism of a number of medications, including corticosteroids, oral contraceptive pills, valproic acid, and anticoagulants. Phenytoin and erythromycin can inhibit the metabolism of carbamazepine, which may result in toxic carbamazepine levels despite appropriate dosing.

Valproic Acid

Valproic acid is one of the most effective broad-spectrum AEDs in current use for the treatment of a wide range of seizure types. It is a first-line therapy for idiopathic primary

Table 287-2. Antiepileptic Drug Formulations

AEDs	Liquid	Sprinkles	Chewables	Tablets	Parental
Established AEDs					
Carbamazepine	100 mg/5 cc	100 mg, 200 mg 300 mg extended (Carbatrol)	100 mg	200 mg 100/200/400 mg XR extended	N/A
Diazepam (Diastat gel)	2.5/5/10/15/20 mg	N/A	N/A	Not for chronic Rx	5 mg/mL
Ethosuximide	250 mg/5 cc	N/A	N/A	250 mg	N/A
Phenobarbital	20 mg/5 cc	N/A	N/A	15/30/60/100 mg	60 mg/mL 130 mg/mL
Phenytoin	125 mg/5 cc*	N/A	50 mg	30/100 mg extended	50 mg/mL
Valproic acid	250 mg/5 cc	125 mg	N/A	500 mg ER extended	100 mg/mL
Divalproex sodium				125/250/500 mg	
Newer AEDs					
Felbamate	600 mg/5 cc	N/A	N/A	400/600 mg	N/A
Gabapentin	250 mg/5 cc	N/A	N/A	100/300/400/600/800 mg	N/A
Lamotrigine	N/A	N/A	2/5/25 mg	25/100/150/200 mg	N/A
Levetiracetam	N/A	N/A	N/A	250/500/750 mg	N/A
Oxcarbazepine	300 mg/5 cc	N/A	N/A	150/300/600 mg	N/A
Tiagabine	N/A	N/A	N/A	2/4/12/16/20 mg	N/A
Topiramate	N/A	15/25 mg	N/A	25/100/200 mg	N/A
Zonisamide	N/A	N/A	N/A	25/50/100 mg	N/A

*Suspension—see text.

generalized epilepsies and is an important therapy for the Lennox-Gastaut syndrome, infantile spasms, and myoclonic epilepsy. It is available as an oral liquid, tablet, and sprinkle and in extended-release as well as parenteral formulation. Valproic acid can inhibit the hepatic metabolism of a number of medications, most notably other AEDs such as phenytoin, phenobarbital, carbamazepine, and especially lamotrigine. The side effects of valproic acid include sedation, a dose-dependent tremor, weight gain, appetite stimulation, hair loss, menstrual irregularities, amenorrhea, and, in some young women, the polycystic ovary syndrome with obesity and hirsutism. While uncommon, the most significant side effect is hepatic toxicity, which can be seen with greatest frequency in children less than 2 years of age and is unusual in patients over 10 years of age. Sporadically, thrombocytopenia can occur especially in association with intercurrent viral illnesses and pancreatitis. Valproic acid should be avoided during pregnancy because of its association with neural tube defects.

Ethosuximide

Ethosuximide is a good first choice for the treatment of typical absence seizures in children. It is ineffective for myoclonic, partial, and tonic-clonic seizures. Ethosuximide is available as an oral liquid or tablet. The most common side effects of ethosuximide are gastrointestinal, including abdominal pain, nausea, vomiting, and anorexia. Headache and drowsiness may occur, and up to 5% of patients taking this drug may develop a rash.

Diazepam and Lorazepam

Diazepam (Valium) and *lorazepam* (Ativan) are two very important medications for the treatment of acute seizures and status epilepticus. Either can be administered intravenously to effectively abort prolonged seizures, and both are good first choices for treatment of prolonged seizures. While both are equally effective, lorazepam has a longer duration of activity in the central nervous system. Diazepam is now available in a rectal gel preparation (Diastat). This gel allows parents and other family members, at home, to administer diazepam to treat clustered, repetitive, or prolonged seizures in children at risk, including children with a history of prolonged, febrile seizures.

NEW ANTIEPILEPTIC DRUGS

During the 1990s, nine new AEDs became available, offering the clinician therapeutic options, with different safety profiles, for the adjunctive treatment of patients with refractory epilepsy. Table 287-3 lists indications, dosing, and common side effects for the newer AEDs. All of these medications are available only as oral agents. Table 287-2 lists available formulations.

Felbamate

Felbamate (Felbatol) was the first new AED approved for use in the United States since valproic acid became available. Felbamate is effective against a broad spectrum of seizure types, including generalized seizures and partial

Table 287-3. Newer Antiepileptic Drugs

AED	Half-life	Indication	Starting Dose	Maintenance	Dosing Schedule	Side-Effects
Felbamate	14–24 hours	All seizures Lennox-Gastaut	10 mg/kg/day	30–40 mg/kg/day	bid	Headache, weight loss, aplastic anemia, hepatic failure
Gabapentin	5–7 hours Renal elimination	Partial seizures add-on	10 mg/kg/day	30–100 mg/kg/day	tid	Mild: fatigue, dizziness, headache, nausea, behavior
Lamotrigine	15–60 hours*	All seizures Lennox-Gastaut	0.1–1 mg/kg/day	5–15 mg/kg/day	bid	Headache, dizziness, fatigue, tremor, rash—10%, Stevens-Johnson—0.5–1%
Levetiracetam	4–11 hours Renal elimination	Partial seizures Generalized seizures	10–20 mg/kg/day	80 mg/kg/day	bid–tid	Headache, dizziness, nervousness, aggression, sleep disturbance, psychosis
Oxcarbazepine	8–10 hours	Partial Seizures Tonic-clonic	10 mg/kg/day	20–55 mg/kg/day	bid	Headache, somnolence, dizziness, nausea
Tiagabine	4–9 hours	Partial Seizures add-on	0.1–0.2 mg/kg/day	1–2 mg/kg/day	tid–qid	Fatigue, dizziness, tremor, nervousness, confusion, depression
Topiramate	20–24 hours	All seizures Lennox-Gastaut	1–2 mg/kg/day	5–10 mg/kg/day	bid	Cognitive slowing, confusion, fatigue, dizziness, paresthesias, weight loss, renal stones—0.6%, glaucoma—rare
Zonisamide	50–70 hours	All seizures Infantile spasms?	1–2 mg/kg/day	5–10 mg/kg/day	qd-bid	Dizziness, fatigue, headache, nausea, poor concentration, renal stones—0.6%

*Half-life dependent on concurrent medications

seizures with and without secondary generalization. Felbamate is especially helpful in children with Lennox-Gastaut syndrome. Felbamate inhibits the hepatic metabolism of a number of medications, including carbamazepine, phenytoin, and valproic acid. Although its side effects include anorexia, weight loss, insomnia, headache, and nausea, it is reasonably well tolerated. Unfortunately, felbamate has significant bone marrow and hepatic toxicity with reported fatalities secondary to aplastic anemia and hepatic failure. Because of serious safety concerns, felbamate is now limited to treating primarily patients with Lennox-Gastaut syndrome who have exhausted other treatment options.

Gabapentin

Gabapentin (Neurontin) may help to treat partial seizures with or without secondary generalization. However, gabapentin may exacerbate myoclonic and generalized absence seizures. While its efficacy as an antiepileptic appears to be limited, gabapentin appears to be an effective analgesic for neuropathic pain, especially reflex sympathetic dystrophy. Gabapentin may also deliver effective migraine prophylaxis. Gabapentin is not metabolized by the liver and has no inducing or inhibiting effects. Drug interactions are not an issue. Gabapentin is generally well tolerated with only mild and usually transient drowsiness, headache, dizziness, nausea, and occasionally behavioral changes.

Lamotrigine

Lamotrigine (Lamictal) appears to be effective for a wide range of seizures in both children and adults. It is useful for treating both partial and generalized seizures, including generalized absence, and for Lennox-Gastaut syndrome. Lamotrigine is available in multiple sizes and formulations, including chewables for young children. Lamotrigine does not affect the metabolism of other medications including oral contraceptives; however, other medications dramatically alter the half-life of lamotrigine. Enzyme-inducing agents such as phenytoin, phenobarbital, and carbamazepine decrease the half-life of lamotrigine to approximately 15 hours, while valproic acid dramatically prolongs lamotrigine's half-life to approximately 60 hours. The most common side effects of lamotrigine are headache, nausea, dizziness, and, when taken with valproic acid, a mild tremor. Of greatest concern is lamotrigine's association with developing a maculopapular rash. Erythema multiforme, Stevens-Johnson syndrome, and toxic epidermal necrolysis can occur, the risk of the latter being higher in children than in adults. Rapid introduction of the lamotrigine seems to be associated with rash development. A slow gradual titration has dramatically reduced the incidence of serious rash.

Levetiracetam

Levetiracetam (Keppra) appears to be effective for the treatment of partial seizures with or without secondary generalization and for a variety of generalized seizures, including absence and myoclonic. Drug tolerance and possible loss of efficacy may develop over time. Levetiracetam is available in three different sized scored tablets. Since its metabolism is independent of the hepatic cytochrome P450 system, levetiracetam has minimal drug interactions, including with oral contraceptives. The major side effects

are nervousness, headache, dizziness, restlessness, aggressive behavior, and psychosis. Drug-induced psychosis might not immediately disappear with acute discontinuation of the drug. Because of its behavioral effects, levetiracetam should be used carefully in the mentally impaired population.

Oxcarbazepine

Oxcarbazepine (Trileptal) is the 10-keto analogue of carbamazepine. Oxcarbazepine has a spectrum of activity similar to that of carbamazepine but metabolizes in a different manner and tends to have fewer side effects and fewer drug interactions. Oxcarbazepine is available in both liquid and tablet formulations. Oxcarbazepine is not as strong a hepatic enzyme inducer, does not autoinduce its own metabolism, and does not appear to be associated with the blood dyscrasias or rashes that can occur with carbamazepine. Side effects include headache, dizziness, nausea, and somnolence.

Tiagabine

Tiagabine (Gabatril) may be helpful as adjunct therapy for partial seizures. Similar to gabapentin, efficacy appears somewhat limited. Owing to a relatively short half-life, tiagabine should be administered three times per day. It is available as scored tablets of varying sizes. The liver metabolizes tiagabine, yet it does not inhibit or induce hepatic enzymes. Other hepatic inducers such as carbamazepine and phenytoin affect tiagabine levels. The side effects of tiagabine include fatigue, nervousness, dizziness, ataxia, tremor, confusion, impaired concentration, and depression.

Topiramate

Topiramate (Topamax) appears to have a broad spectrum of action with efficacy for both partial and generalized seizures including absence and myoclonic and may provide effective migraine prophylaxis. Topiramate has been approved for use in children with the Lennox-Gastaut syndrome. Topiramate is available in multiple sizes, including sprinkle formulations for children. Side effects include fatigue, dizziness, poor concentration, cognitive slowing, and paresthesias. Anorexia and weight loss may also be seen. Because of a mild carbonic anhydrase inhibitor effect, there is a slight increased incidence of kidney stones with topiramate use (0.6% in children and 1.5% in adults). Topiramate should be used with caution in patients on the ketogenic diet or with a family history of kidney stones or other carbonic anhydrase inhibitor usage. There have also been rare reports of topiramate causing reversible acute-angle glaucoma that presents with sudden decreased vision and eye pain. While topiramate should be introduced using a slow weekly titration schedule to minimize side effects, efficacy can occur even at low doses.

Zonisamide

Zonisamide (Zonegran) also appears to have a broad spectrum of action with efficacy for a variety of partial and generalized seizures. Zonisamide may be particularly helpful for progressive myoclonic epilepsies and possibly infantile spasms. Zonisamide is available as 25-mg, 50-mg, and 100-mg capsules that can be administered once daily. Zonisamide has a long half-life. The liver metabolizes zonisamide, and the kidney clears it. Zonisamide does not induce or inhibit hepatic enzymes, but hepatic inducing drugs do alter its half-life. Zonisamide's primary side effects appear to be somnolence, poor concentration, headache, dizziness, and nausea. A slow gradual titration will minimize these effects. Generally, zonisamide is well tolerated. Zonisamide also has a mild carbonic anhydrase inhibitor effect, thereby giving a slight increased risk of developing renal stones (1%). Similar to topiramate, zonisamide should be administered with caution to patients on the ketogenic diet or other carbonic anhydrase inhibitors or if there is a family history of kidney stones.

Vigabatrin

Vigabatrin appears to have a broad spectrum of efficacy and is widely used outside the United States. It is notably effective in treating infantile spasms, especially in children with tuberous sclerosis. Because of retinal toxicity and the development of tunnel vision in 25% of patients receiving it, vigabatrin is not currently FDA approved and is not available in the United States.

SUGGESTED READINGS

Brodie MJ, Dichter MA: Antiepileptic drugs. N Engl J Med 1996;334:168–175.
Brodie MJ, Dichter MA: Established antiepileptic drugs. Seizure 1997;6:159–174.
Browne TR, Holmes GL: Handbook of Epilepsy, 2nd ed. Philadelphia, Lippincott Williams & Williams, 2000.
Pellock JM: Managing pediatric epilepsy syndromes with new antiepileptic drugs. Pediatrics 1999;104:1106–1116.
Pellock JM, Dodson WE, Bourgeois BFD: Pediatric Epilepsy: Diagnosis and Therapy, 2nd ed. New York, Demos, 2001.

SECTION 9 DIAGNOSTICS AND THERAPEUTICS: *Pharmacotherapy*

288 Psychotropic Agents

G. Scott Waterman and Jeanne Greenblatt

Psychotropic agents are drugs that affect mood, thought, or behavior. This chapter discusses the administration, indications, benefits, risks, controversies, and future trends for psychostimulant, antidepressant, anxiolytic, hypnotic, and antipsychotic drugs. Lithium and anticonvulsant mood-stabilizing drugs are discussed on the CD-ROM.

PSYCHOSTIMULANT DRUGS

Types of Treatment

At the present time, there are a number of psychostimulants available for clinical use (Box 288-1).

How They Are Administered

All psychostimulants are administered orally and are metabolized by the liver. The methylphenidate and amphetamine preparations have rapid and complete absorption from the gastrointestinal tract. Ritalin and Dexedrine are *short-acting agents* that have a maximum time of effectiveness of 4 hours. They require multiple daytime doses in order to provide a consistent daytime clinical response. *Intermediate-acting agents* include Ritalin SR, Dexedrine Spansules, and Adderall. These compounds have onset of action within 60 minutes and peak clinical effect within 1 to 3 hours following administration. These medications usually maintain clinical effectiveness for 5 to 8 hours. One dose of these medications may provide adequate treatment for school time; however, two doses a day are often required for full-

---

Box 288-1. Psychostimulant Drugs

Generic Names

Methylphenidate
D-Amphetamine
Mixed amphetamine salts
Pemoline

Brand names

Ritalin, Ritalin SR, Concerta, Metadate
Dexedrine, Dexedrine Spansule
Adderall
Cylert

---

day coverage. Concerta, Metadate, and pemoline are *long-acting agents*. All of these medications are administered one time a day. Concerta is an extended osmotic controlled-release formulation of methylphenidate, which provides clinical effectiveness for a 12-hour period. Concerta has an osmotic release system within a nondissolving capsule surrounded by a coating of regular (short-acting) methylphenidate. Onset of action occurs within 30 to 60 minutes, and the osmotic pump releases a consistent dose of methylphenidate every hour, leading to consistent blood levels over a 10 to 12 hour period. Metadate is a long-acting form of methylphenidate, which has biphasic peaks at 1.5 and 4.5 hours and has clinical effectiveness lasting 8 to 12 hours. Pemoline is administered as a single oral dose in the morning. Clinical improvement with pemoline is gradual, and clinical response might not be noticed for a number of weeks. Pemoline is not considered a first-line treatment because of its association with hepatic abnormalities and hepatic failure.

Indications

Psychostimulants are indicated for the treatment of attention deficit hyperactivity disorder and narcolepsy in children and adolescents.

Benefits

Approximately 65% to 75% of children treated with psychostimulants demonstrate moderate to marked improvement in the following symptoms:

- Core features of attention deficit hyperactivity disorder (ADHD): inattentiveness, impulsivity, and motor hyperactivity
- Cognition, social function, and aggression
- Performance of repetitive tasks, graphing, and arithmetic
- Social skills through better ability to modulate the intensity of behavior, improved communication, and increased responsiveness. Decreased symptoms can also lead to increased positive interactions and decreased criticism from the child's parents, teachers, and peers.

Risks

The most common side effects of psychostimulant drugs are appetite suppression and sleep disturbance. Sleep can often be improved by lowering or eliminating a late afternoon dose or by using medications to assist with sleep. Appetite suppression can lead to weight loss or temporary delay in height until midadolescence that normalizes by late adolescence. Drug holidays are not necessary, but children using stimulants should have their growth progression monitored regularly. If growth declines significantly, further evaluation is necessary, and discontinuation or a change in medication should be considered. Mild increases in pulse and blood pressure have been observed, and regular monitoring of blood pressure and pulse is indicated. Use of stimulants may exacerbate a preexisting tic disorder. The presence of a tic disorder, however, is not a contraindication to using stimulants in children with ADHD. The use of pemoline has been associated with chemical hepatitis and liver failure. Liver function monitoring is essential if this medication is to be used.

Stimulants are controlled substances that are potentially drugs of abuse. Recent studies, however, have shown that appropriate use of stimulants in children/adolescents with ADHD significantly reduces their risk for substance abuse.

Evidence of Effectiveness

There is more research on the use of stimulants for the treatment of ADHD in children and adolescents than on any other group of medications used in pediatric psychopharmacology. Amphetamines were synthesized in the 1880s and were initially used in the treatment of asthma. In the late 1930s, Bradley treated children on an inpatient psychiatric ward with amphetamine and noted significant improvement in behavior and school performance. In the 1960s, methylphenidate was developed. The efficacy of methylphenidate to treat symptoms of ADHD was verified by using validated parent and teacher rating forms.

Approximately 65% to 75% of children, adolescents, and adults with ADHD respond to treatment with psychostimulants. Double-blind placebo-controlled studies report a placebo response rate ranging between 2% and 39%. Most efficacy research has focused on children in the elementary to middle school years. Evidence strongly suggests, however, that stimulant treatment has similar rates of efficacy in preschoolers, older adolescents, and adults. It is not clear whether those who do not respond to stimulants represent a subtype of ADHD or may have specific patterns of comorbid disorders.

Controversies

The diagnosis and treatment of ADHD in children and adolescents is a highly controversial topic. Much of the controversy in the public media focuses on issues in regard to the safety, efficacy, and use of stimulant medication in children and adolescents. In addition there is concern regarding the use of medication in preschool children with ADHD symptoms. Recent research, however, continues to indicate that ADHD is often underdiagnosed and undertreated pharmacologically.

Trends

The recent availability of longer-acting stimulants, which provide a full day of clinical response with one or two doses, has begun to alter prescribing practices, as these medications reduce the likelihood of children requiring a second dose of medication during their school day. It is likely that a broader array of this type of medication will become available. In addition, the development of effective nonstimulant treatments for ADHD is well underway.

ANTIDEPRESSANT DRUGS

Types of Treatments

Major depressive disorder (MDD) is a common condition in children and adolescents. Recent community-based epidemiologic studies estimate that the lifetime prevalence of MDD is 2% in children and 5% to 8% in adolescents. Please note that the consideration of psychosocial interventions and nonpharmacologic therapies is an essential (and often primary) component in developing a treatment plan for children and adolescents with MDD. This section does not address these highly important issues. Table 288-1 lists the medications that are available to treat major depressive disorder in children and adolescents. This section provides a brief overview of these medications. Please consult a pediatric psychopharmacology text to make specific decisions regarding choosing a specific medication and appropriate dosing of that medication.

How They Are Administered

All antidepressant medications are administered orally. A number of these medications are available in liquid formulations. Appropriate dosing and frequency of administration of these medications vary considerably. In general, however,

Table 288-1. Medications Used in the Treatment of Depression

Tricyclic Antidepressants (TCAs)	Selective Serotonin Reuptake Inhibitors (SSRIs)
Amitriptyline (Elavil)	Fluoxetine (Prozac)
Desipramine (Norpramin)	Sertraline (Zoloft)
Imipramine (Tofranil)	Paroxetine (Paxil)
Nortriptyline (Pamelor, Aventyl)	Fluvoxamine (Luvox)
	Citalopram (Celexa)
Atypical Antidepressants	**Monoamine Oxidase Inhibitors**
Venlafaxine (Effexor)	Phenelzine (Nardil)
Nefazodone (Serzone)	Tranylcypromine (Parnate)
Bupropion (Wellbutrin)	Isocarboxazid (Murplan)
Mirtazepine (Remeron)	

all of these medications should be started at a very low dose and advanced slowly to minimize possible side effects and to allow adequate time to monitor the patient's clinical response to each dose adjustment.

Indications

The use of antidepressant medication is indicated for the treatment of major depressive disorder and dysthymia in children, adolescents, and adults. Many of the antidepressants are also effective in the treatment of other psychiatric illnesses, including generalized anxiety disorder, panic disorder, social phobia, obsessive compulsive disorder, and ADHD.

Benefits

Antidepressants can decrease or eliminate many of the impairing symptoms of major depressive disorder or dysthymia. A positive clinical response to treatment with antidepressant medication may lead to a decrease in irritability, guilt, anxiety, and rumination and improvements in mood, energy level, enjoyment, motivation, concentration, sleep, and appetite. The successful treatment of a mood disorder invariably leads to a significant improvement in the child's or adolescent's level of function.

Risks/Complications

Tricyclic antidepressants (TCAs) are rarely used to treat depression in children and adolescents because of their anticholinergic side effects, possible cardiotoxicity, and the need for invasive monitoring. TCAs are also extremely dangerous in overdose and are likely to be ineffective in the treatment of depression in the pediatric age group. Selective serotonin reuptake inhibitors (SSRIs) all have varying effects on the cytochrome P450 hepatic enzymes. These medications can play a role in drug interactions with both psychotropic and nonpsychiatric medications. Treatment with all antidepressant medications carry the risk of "switching" a person with symptoms of depression to one with symptoms of mania or hypomania. In addition, antidepressants that affect the serotonin neurotransmitter system all have the potential to lead to side effects of "activation." This cluster of side effects consists of agitation, disinhibition, and irritability. Often, activation can be

avoided by starting with low doses of medication and increasing the dose slowly. Mirtazepine often leads to significant weight gain. Monoamine oxidase inhibitors are rarely used in children and adolescents secondary to their potential for precipitating a hypertensive crisis if a tyramine-free diet is not adhered to. In addition, this class of medication is often not a safe choice in adolescents with possible suicidality, impulsivity, or substance use.

Evidence of Effectiveness

Tricyclic antidepressants are the most extensively studied antidepressants. A number of open-label studies have suggested response rates in the range of 75% in the treatment of childhood depression. No randomized controlled trial has demonstrated superiority of TCAs over placebo. It should be noted that the placebo response rate was often over 50% in studies of TCAs. A number of controlled and uncontrolled studies of SSRIs have demonstrated that this class of medications is safe and effective in the short-term treatment of depression, obsessive-compulsive disorder, and many pediatric anxiety disorders. Open-label studies of venlafaxine, nefazodone, and bupropion in children and adolescents have demonstrated improvements in clinical symptoms of depression. Placebo-controlled studies examining the effectiveness of these medications for the treatment of depression in children and adolescents are under way. Open-label and controlled studies have also indicated that bupropion many be helpful as a second-line treatment for ADHD. Monoamine oxidase inhibitors have not been examined closely in children and adolescents, given their significant side effects and the potential to induce hypertensive crisis through not adhering to the prescribed diet. As of 2000, there were no reports on the use of mirtazepine in children and adolescents.

Controversies

Significant controversy exists regarding the association of TCAs, cardiotoxicity, and the risk of sudden death in children and adolescents. TCAs should not be used as antidepressants in the pediatric age group. Other controversies exist in regard to the question of whether antidepressants are overused in our society in general. The efficacy and short- and long-term effects of antidepressant medication in children and adolescents are not fully known, given the dearth of controlled, prospective studies in this age group.

Trends

In recent years, many antidepressants have been developed that are well tolerated and lead to significant clinical improvement in the symptoms of MDD or dysthymia. Newer antidepressants are in development that theoretically may have faster onset of action, more robust efficacy in a greater percentage of patients, and better ability to sustain remission of symptoms.

Many antidepressants are also used to treat conditions other than MDD. This includes treatment of panic disorder, generalized anxiety disorder, social phobia, selective mutism, obsessive-compulsive disorder, attention deficit disorder, enuresis, migraine headaches, chronic pain, and perseverative behaviors.

ANXIOLYTIC DRUGS

Types of Treatments

Among all categories of psychopathology, anxiety disorders are the most prevalent in the adult and pediatric populations. It is not surprising that medications that reduce anxiety are widely prescribed. Not all drugs used to treat anxiety, however, are generally classified as *anxiolytic drugs*. For example, the mainstays of pharmacotherapy for a number of anxiety disorders (e.g., panic disorder, social anxiety disorder, and obsessive-compulsive disorder) are classified as antidepressant compounds, owing to the fact that their original indications were for the treatment of depression.

This section reviews the uses of two types of anxiolytic compounds: benzodiazepines and buspirone. Although there are other classes of medications that remain on the market for the treatment of anxiety (e.g., barbiturates and propanediols), their use in the treatment of pediatric anxiety is not recommended.

How They Are Administered

Some benzodiazepines are available in parenteral form, primarily for use in anesthesia or in the treatment of status epilepticus. When used to treat anxiety, benzodiazepines are given orally. Buspirone is administered orally in two or three daily doses.

Indications

Although anxiety and anxiety disorders are exceedingly common in the pediatric age group, and although anxiolytic compounds are very commonly prescribed, the indications for their use in children and adolescents are not well studied or agreed on.

Potential indications for benzodiazepines include anxiety associated with specific stressful situations that are expected to be transient, such as the anticipatory anxiety that precedes medical or surgical procedures. At least some benzodiazepine compounds (alprazolam and clonazepam specifically) are known to be effective in the treatment of panic disorder in adults and are likely to be helpful in the treatment of that and of similar phenomena in children and adolescents. Youngsters with separation anxiety and anxiety associated with phobic disorders, including anxiety-based school refusal, may benefit from benzodiazepine therapy, though such uses are not well established, and other therapies (pharmacologic and cognitive behavioral) might be more effective. At least on a short-term basis, these medications may be effective in the treatment of insomnia, though nonpharmacologic approaches are generally recommended first and are often beneficial.

Because buspirone is a nonsedating anxiolytic that has no apparent abuse potential, it was hoped that it would fill an important niche. Although it has been shown to be effective in the treatment of generalized anxiety in adults, it has no established indication in the treatment of pediatric anxiety, where it has been inadequately studied. In contrast to the benzodiazepines, whose anxiolytic effects may be seen following a single dose, the onset of therapeutic effects of buspirone is generally at least 2 to 3 weeks after it is initiated. It is therefore of no use on a "prn" basis.

Benefits

Although anxiety is a normal and sometimes even useful emotion under some circumstances and in limited quantities, pathologic anxiety is a very uncomfortable and impairing phenomenon. Its manifestations are many and often include cognitive (e.g., worry, dread, anticipation of adversity) and autonomic (e.g., palpitations, dyspnea, gastrointestinal upset) elements. In addition, self-imposed limitations on the scope of the social and other activities of affected youngsters (i.e., phobic avoidance) frequently complicate the clinical picture of anxiety disorders. Successful treatment ameliorates these symptoms of anxiety. Whether early treatment of anxiety has beneficial effects on the natural history of childhood-onset anxiety disorders needs further study.

Risks

When compared with the compounds that were previously used in the treatment of anxiety and insomnia, such as the alcohol-like drugs (paraldehyde and chloral hydrate), the barbiturates, and the propanediols, the benzodiazepines are remarkable safe, which is why their use has eclipsed that of those other medications. Nonetheless, they have potential drawbacks. Sedation is the most common adverse effect, though patients generally become tolerant to that effect, which is dose-related. A variety of psychomotor tasks may be adversely affected by benzodiazepine compounds, and there is concern that youngsters taking them may thus be less equipped to learn in school, though that has not been demonstrated. A phenomenon known as *behavioral disinhibition* is a potential consequence of benzodiazepines that can include anger and aggressive behavior. Its occurrence appears to be most likely in patients who are predisposed to such outbursts as a result of gross structural brain abnormalities.

With respect to the benzodiazepines, physicians (and the public) tend to be most concerned about the possibilities of abuse of and dependence on these compounds. While these problems are legitimate concerns, they are rare among adults who are prescribed benzodiazepines for the treatment of anxiety. No systematic information is available on this topic regarding the pediatric population, in which avoiding protracted use of these medications, and avoiding their use altogether in adolescents with histories of drug (particularly sedative or alcohol) abuse, is recommended. Particularly after prolonged use, withdrawal symptoms may be seen if benzodiazepines are abruptly discontinued. Such symptoms commonly include anxiety and insomnia but may include seizures. It is therefore advisable that these drugs be withdrawn gradually.

Buspirone is generally well tolerated, with GI upset, headache, dizziness, agitation, insomnia, and fatigue sometimes seen. As was noted above, buspirone has no apparent abuse potential.

Evidence of Effectiveness

As was indicated above, anxiolytic compounds have been inadequately studied in the pediatric population. There are reports in the older literature of beneficial effects, but these are uncontrolled observations in inadequately (by current standards) characterized and likely heterogeneous groups of patients. More recently, there have been a few controlled trials of benzodiazepines (clonazepam and alprazolam) in children and adolescents with anxiety disorders. In aggregate, the results of these studies involving small numbers of subjects are inconclusive.

Case reports and case series have reported favorable effects of buspirone in youngsters with anxiety disorders, but controlled trials are unavailable.

Controversies

Although benzodiazepine compounds are, in most respects, very safe medications, their potential for misuse, the concern that they may cause adverse cognitive effects, and the absence of clear indications for their use in the pediatric population make prescribing them to children and adolescents controversial.

Future Trends

As data accumulate supporting the use of a variety of antidepressant compounds, and of cognitive behavioral psychotherapy, in the treatment of anxiety disorders, the anxiolytic compounds discussed in this section are likely to be prescribed less commonly. For targeted, short-term, or "prn" use in the treatment of anxiety, however, the benzodiazepines will likely remain the safest and most useful drugs for some time to come.

HYPNOTIC DRUGS

Types of Treatments

Hypnotic medications are used for the treatment of insomnia. Difficulty falling asleep or staying asleep is a very common problem with many possible etiologies:

- Primary insomnia
- Secondary insomnia related to the following:
  - Psychiatric disorders or "stress"
  - Pain
  - Sleep apnea
  - Use of medications or drugs of abuse
  - Restless leg syndrome or periodic limb movement disorders
  - Circadian rhythm disturbance

Appropriate medication use is based on understanding the differential diagnosis of insomnia. Treatment of secondary insomnia should initially focus on the treatment of the primary disorder. This often relieves sleep difficulties, and the use of medication can be avoided. Some sleep complaints may resolve with improvement in sleep hygiene. If insomnia cannot be adequately resolved by treating the condition leading to sleep disturbance, hypnotic drugs can be used to induce sleep.

This section briefly reviews sedative-hypnotic medications used in the treatment of sleep difficulties. This includes benzodiazepine and nonbenzodiazepine hypnotics, sedative antihistamines, sedative antidepressants, chloral hydrate, over-the-counter agents, and natural compounds.

This list is most appropriate to consider for use in older adolescents, as these medications have been studied and used primarily in adults. As is often the case, few of these medications have been studied in children and adolescents, and they should be used cautiously and only after behavioral interventions for insomnia have been tried.

Benzodiazepines

Benzodiazepines should not be considered a first-line treatment for insomnia in children and adolescents.

Benzodiazepines with shorter half-lives are often used for treatment of insomnia, as their effects are more likely to wear off by morning.

The type of sleep disturbance should be matched to the characteristics of the sedative. Thus, trouble falling asleep should be treated with a fast-onset, short-acting medication (triazolam). Middle of the night insomnia should be treated with an intermediate-onset, intermediate-acting agent (temazepam, estazolam), and patients with both problems should be treated with a fast-onset, intermediate-acting agent (quazepam).

Sedating Nonbenzodiazepines

Zaleplon, zolpidem, and zopiclone have replaced benzodiazepines as the first-line treatment for insomnia in adults. These agents all have rapid onset and a short duration of action. They have fewer side effects than benzodiazepines. Rebound insomnia, drug dependence, loss of effectiveness with continued use, and possibility of withdrawal are said to be uncommon with these medications.

Chloral hydrate is an effective short-acting sedative.

Sedating Antidepressants

Sedating tricyclic antidepressants can assist with sleep if given at bedtime

Trazodone, mirtazepine, and nefazedone are sedating antidepressants that block serotonin 2A receptors and restore slow-wave sleep. Trazodone has few drug interactions with other psychiatric medications and often is used in combination with medications that can disrupt sleep.

Sedating Antihistamines

Diphenhydramine is often used to treat insomnia due to its sedative effects. It is used in children and adolescents at doses ranging between 12.5 and 100 mg.

Over-the-Counter Agents

Most over-the-counter sleep preparations (or nighttime cold preparations) contain one or more of the following three active ingredients: the anticholinergic agent scopolamine, an anticholinergic antihistamine, or a pain reliever. These medications are generally considered safe and do not lead to dependence or cause rebound insomnia.

Natural Agents

Warm milk contains approximately 2 grams of L-tryptophan, a safe, sometimes effective hypnotic.

Melatonin is a hormone produced by the pineal gland early in the sleep cycle. This substance is available as an over-the-counter preparation. Appropriate doses for children and adolescents are not known and may range between 0.5 and 10 mg.

How They Are Administered

All hypnotic medications used to treat insomnia in children and adolescents are administered orally. Some sedative antihistamines and choral hydrate are available in liquid form. Product labeling and data from sleep laboratories suggest that sedative hypnotic drugs be used for a maximum of several weeks. Short-term insomnia should be treated for a maximum of 3 weeks. It is recommended that chronic treatment for long-term insomnia occur 1 out of every 3 or 4 nights. The need for ongoing hypnotic treatment in patients with long-term insomnia should be re-evaluated every few months.

Indications

At present, approved indications for the use of hypnotic medication include only brief use or occasional use for transitory or short-term insomnia. Long-term insomnia is persistent and disabling. The majority of patients with long-term insomnia have an associated disorder or have insomnia related to drug use or abuse. If treatment of the patient's primary disorder is not effective in resolving insomnia, chronic intermittent treatment may be necessary.

Benefits

Hypnotic medications can induce sleep pharmacologically. If a child or adolescent can fall asleep more easily and obtain adequate restful sleep, an increased level of daytime function often follows.

Risks/Complications

Several problems can occur with using benzodiazepines. These involve using too high a dose, leading to a drugged or sedated feeling during the day; development of tolerance with long-term use; difficulty with memory formation on days following medication use; and the possibility of rebound insomnia or a withdrawal syndrome once the medications are stopped. Tricyclic antidepressants can have anticholinergic side effects. Blood levels and electrocardiograms should be monitored, as tricyclic antidepressants are dangerous in overdose and may lead to cardiac conduction abnormalities. Trazodone has been associated with priapism. Mirtazepine use may lead to significant weight gain. Antihistamines have anticholinergic effects. When taken with other anticholinergic drugs, the use of antihistamines may be problematic. Chloral hydrate can induce hepatic drug-metabolizing enzymes and should be used with caution in patients with renal, cardiac, or hepatic disease. Over-the-counter sleep preparations can cause anticholinergic side effects and difficulties with confusion and memory. Melatonin is not an FDA-approved drug. Its safety and efficacy have not been adequately tested to date.

Evidence of Effectiveness

Benzodiazepines are the most commonly prescribed sedative-hypnotics used in adults. They are very effective as sedative-hypnotics, anxiolytics, muscle relaxants, and anticonvulsants. The appropriate use of benzodiazepines requires the knowledge and ability to balance the possible benefits of these medications against the risks of dependence, rebound insomnia, retrograde amnesia, and possible daytime sedation. Melatonin has been shown to act as an effective hypnotic in studies of insomnia from jet lag or impaired diurnal rhythm. Studies in blind patients have shown that melatonin has been helpful in correcting impaired diurnal rhythms. The antihistamine diphenhydramine has been shown in studies to be effective for sleep difficulties in doses between 12.5 and 100 mg. Patients taking tricyclic antidepressants have been noted in a number of major studies on depression to have improved sleep. The hypnotic effects of TCAs are thought to be independent of their antidepressant effects.

Controversies

There is controversy surrounding the use of these medications, as hypnotic medications can be overused or abused. In addition, the ready availability and usefulness of these medications can lead to situations in which sleep difficulties are treated symptomatically without the physician adequately diagnosing and addressing possible underlying causes of insomnia.

Trends

Newer nonbenzodiazepine sedative-hypnotics, other medications with sedating features, and natural substances have begun to replace benzodiazepines as treatments for insomnia.

ANTIPSYCHOTIC DRUGS

Types of Treatments

The era of modern clinical psychopharmacology was heralded by the introduction in the 1950s of chlorpromazine to treat psychosis. This development is widely credited (not necessarily accurately) with the rapid fall in the population of schizophrenic patients who were chronically hospitalized. It is clear that the advent of effective pharmacotherapy for psychotic illness revolutionized psychiatry, and in the decades since the introduction of chlorpromazine, many more compounds with antipsychotic activity have been marketed.

At this point, it is helpful to classify the available antipsychotic agents into two categories: the traditional neuroleptic drugs (i.e., medications that cause neurological side effects) and the "novel" or "atypical" antipsychotic drugs (i.e., medications that are free, or nearly free, of neurologic side effects). Until relatively recently, the neuroleptic agents were the mainstays of treatment of psychosis. At this point, however, the considerable advantages of the novel antipsychotic compounds have led to their widespread use in a variety of conditions, eclipsing the uses of the traditional neuroleptic drugs.

Prototypic examples of traditional neuroleptic agents include, in addition to the low-potency compound chlorpromazine, the high-potency medication haloperidol. While there are many additional neuroleptic compounds on the U.S. market, they will not be listed here, as their use has fallen significantly—and justifiably—since the introduction of the novel antipsychotic medications.

The novel (or, alternatively, atypical) antipsychotic drugs available in the United States now include clozapine, risperidone, olanzapine, quetiapine, ziprasidone, and aripiprazole (Table 288-2).

Table 288-2. Novel Antipsychotic Drugs

Generic Name	Trade Name	Significant Adverse Effects
Risperidone	Risperdal	Extrapyramidal effects (dose-related),* hyperprolactinemia, weight gain
Olanzapine	Zyprexa	Sedation, weight gain
Quetiapine	Seroquel	Sedation, weight gain
Ziprasidone	Geodon	Nausea, insomnia, QT prolongation
Clozapine	Clozaril	Agranulocytosis, seizures, anticholinergic effects, sedation, weight gain
Aripiprazole	Abilify	Headache, anxiety, insomnia

*Acute dystonia, parkinsonism, akathisia.

How They Are Administered

Several of the traditional neuroleptic compounds are available in parenteral forms. In addition, two of them (fluphenazine and haloperidol) can be given in long-acting depot injections. Nonetheless, when given to children or adolescents, antipsychotic medications are essentially always given orally. In most instances, doses considerably lower than those used to treat adults with psychotic disorders are begun, with gradual upward titration as needed and as tolerated.

Indications

The clearest indication for the use of antipsychotic medication is in the treatment of psychosis. Psychosis (i.e., hallucinations, delusions, or disordered thinking) in children and adolescents may occur in a wide variety of contexts, including schizophrenia, mania, depression, drug intoxication, and delirium, to name the most common. Another indication for the use of these drugs is in the suppression of tics in the setting of a tic disorder such as Tourette syndrome.

Other potential indications include mood disorders, particularly bipolar disorder, not complicated by the presence of psychosis and agitated or aggressive behavior that may occur across a range of diagnostic entities and circumstances. In addition, antipsychotic compounds are used to treat stereotypic, aggressive, and self-injurious behavior associated with autism and other pervasive developmental disorders.

Benefits

Psychosis at any age is extraordinarily frightening and impairing. Onset of psychosis in childhood (relatively uncommon) or adolescence (common) invariably represents an enormous disruption in development and typically portends a chronic and severe illness. Treatment is aimed at reducing or eliminating psychotic symptoms and normalizing development to the extent possible. In addition, there is evidence to support the notion that limiting the duration of psychotic episodes has a favorable effect on the natural history of psychotic illness.

Psychotic symptoms are often divided into "positive" and "negative" varieties. Positive psychotic symptoms include hallucinations and delusions; negative psychotic symptoms include flattened affect, loss of motivation, and social with-drawal, among others. Although antipsychotic medications are generally more effective in the treatment of positive symptoms than in the treatment of negative symptoms, there is some evidence that that disparity in efficacy is less for the novel agents than for the traditional neuroleptic drugs.

Risks

The adverse effects associated with traditional neuroleptic compounds are numerous and, in some instances, severe. Among the high-potency agents (e.g., haloperidol), the predominant adverse effects are neurologic and include acute dystonias, parkinsonism, and akathisia (a subjective sense of restlessness). Among the low-potency drugs (e.g., chlorpromazine), those same neurologic side effects can be seen, but less commonly. However, sedation, weight gain, orthostatic hypotension, and antimuscarinic effects (constipation, urinary hesitancy, blurred vision) are frequently encountered. Galactorrhea or gynecomastia secondary to hyperprolactinemia may occur with any of the neuroleptic medications. The most serious concern with these drugs, however, has been tardive dyskinesia, a movement disorder that is sometimes severe, progressive, and irreversible. The risk of developing tardive dyskinesia is related, among other factors, to total neuroleptic exposure, with larger doses and longer durations of treatment conferring greater risk than smaller doses and shorter durations of treatment.

For the most part, the risks associated with the use of the novel antipsychotic agents are different from those listed above. Although risperidone does have neuroleptic effects (particularly at higher doses) and can cause significant increases in serum prolactin concentrations, the other novel compounds do not. The risk of tardive dyskinesia associated with these drugs cannot yet be fully assessed, though it appears all but certain that that risk is (with the likely exception of risperidone) far lower than that conferred by the traditional neuroleptics. On the other hand, cases of neuroleptic malignant syndrome have been reported to occur in association with at least some of the novel antipsychotic agents as well as with the traditional neuroleptic drugs.

Although more efficacious than the other antipsychotic medications, clozapine carries the risk of agranulocytosis, necessitating very frequent blood drawing for monitoring of white blood cell and absolute neutrophil counts. It also confers a higher risk of seizures than do other antipsychotic medications. All of the novel antipsychotic agents, with the exceptions of ziprasidone and aripiprazole, are associated with weight gain, olanzapine appearing to cause it the most. Weight gain can be profound and accompanied by morbidities such as glucose intolerance and hypercholesterolemia. Ziprasidone, a recently introduced compound, and pimozide, a neuroleptic drug most often used in the treatment of tic disorders, appear most likely to prolong the QT interval on the electrocardiogram, which, in rare instances, may be clinically significant.

Evidence of Effectiveness

Although antipsychotic medications have been used for decades in child and adolescent psychiatry, rigorous studies of their effectiveness in the pediatric population are rare.

High-potency neuroleptics (particularly haloperidol and pimozide) and more recently the novel agent risperidone are generally regarded as effective in suppressing tics. With regard to schizophrenia, antipsychotic agents are without question the treatment of choice. A very small number of studies support the usefulness of traditional neuroleptic medications in the treatment of early-onset schizophrenia. At this point, however, the novel antipsychotic agents are generally preferred, and evidence is accumulating to support the benefits of those drugs, including clozapine. The autism literature supports the use of antipsychotic medications, particularly risperidone most recently, in the management of a range of abnormalities common to children with pervasive developmental disorders. Anecdotal evidence exists to support the usefulness of antipsychotic drugs in the treatment of juvenile bipolar disorder and in the management of agitated or aggressive behavior that is not diagnostically specific.

Controversies

Neuroleptic drugs, particularly chlorpromazine and thioridazine, have ignominious histories in child psychiatry, owing to their excessive use in the past in controlling undesirable behaviors in institutionalized, developmentally disabled youngsters. That legacy led to the practice of resorting to the use of antipsychotic medication to manage nonpsychotic problems only after all other therapeutic options were exhausted. Given the significant morbidity, including but not limited to tardive dyskinesia, associated with neuroleptic medications, such practice was warranted. However, with the advent of the novel antipsychotic agents, whose adverse effect profiles are far more benign and whose range of therapeutic effects may be wider, one wonders whether such reticence might be outdated. Nonetheless, the field clearly needs more data before a significant broadening of the generally accepted indications for antipsychotic medication in children and adolescents can be justified.

As was alluded to above, there is evidence that clozapine is a more efficacious antipsychotic drug than any of the others currently available. Given the severity and catastrophic consequences of early-onset psychosis, and the short- and long-term salutary effects of rapid control of psychotic symptoms, the practice of withholding clozapine pending repeated therapeutic failures with other compounds may not be reasonable.

Future Trends

Data are likely to accumulate over the near future, lending further support to the role of novel antipsychotic medications in the treatment of psychotic, and some nonpsychotic, illnesses in childhood and adolescence. With respect to drug development, success will likely be achieved in the synthesis, testing, and marketing of drugs that have the antipsychotic efficacy of clozapine but without the risk of agranulocytosis. Such medications may be particularly helpful in the treatment of childhood- and adolescent-onset psychotic illness.

Additional Resources, CD-ROM

Lithium and anticonvulsant mood-stabilizing drugs	Text
Bibliography	

SUGGESTED READINGS

Cantwell DP: Attention deficit disorder: A review of the past 10 years. J Am Acad Child Adolesc Psychiatry 1996;35:978–987.

Martin A, Scahill L (eds): Psychopharmacology in Child and Adolescent Psychiatric Clinics of North America, vol 9, no 1. Philadelphia, Saunders, 2000.

Stahl SM: Essential Psychopharmacology. Cambridge, UK, Cambridge University Press, 2000.

Wagner KD: Treatment of childhood and adolescent disorders. In Schatzberg AF, Nemeroff CB (eds): The American Psychiatric Publishing Textbook of Psychopharmacology, 3rd ed. Arlington, Va, American Psychiatric Publishing, 2004, pp 949–1007.

Walsh BT (ed): Child Psychopharmacology. Washington, DC, American Psychiatric Press, 1998.

289 Outpatient Asthma Management

Charles W. Callahan and Daniel V. Schidlow

Asthma is the most common chronic inflammatory disease of the airways, affecting as many as 10% of children in the United States. The recurrent cough and wheezing seen in asthma are due to airway narrowing from smooth muscle constriction, edema, and excessive mucous secretion. The aim of effective asthma therapy is to minimize or suppress symptoms and to eliminate the need for unscheduled visits to the physician's office or emergency room, thus allowing for normal physical and social activity.

Therapy for childhood asthma works. Patients who fail to respond to therapy either do not have asthma or are not receiving appropriate or sufficient ambulatory management. Successful, effective management encompasses more than choosing the "correct" medication. Possible environmental triggers must be identified and addressed. The patient, parent, and caregiver must be adequately educated about essential asthma management (Box 289-1). *Providing all necessary components of asthma therapy is within the scope of a primary care practice.*

Detailed guidelines for the diagnosis and management of asthma in children have been developed and widely accepted. These can be thought of as outlines of "the right things to do" for children with asthma; management focuses on delivering the *right plan* to the *right patient* in the *right place*. Essentially, the three pillars of successful asthma therapy are these:

- Identification of *the right patient*
- Implementation of *the right plan*
- Delivery of the care plan in *the right place*

THE RIGHT PATIENT

As was mentioned before, the right patient proves to have asthma and responds to appropriate therapy. Poor response suggests a wrong diagnosis or inappropriate or insufficient ambulatory management.

THE RIGHT PLAN

Classifying Severity of Asthma

Once the diagnosis of asthma has been established, the next step in all established guidelines is classifying the patient's severity of disease. This classification is based on symptom

---

The views and opinions expressed in this chapter are those of the authors and do not reflect the official policy or position of the Department of the Army, the Department of Defense, or the United States Government.

> **Box 289-1.** Causes of Asthma Therapy Failure
>
> 1. It is not asthma (incorrect diagnosis).
> 2. The patient is not taking the medication.
> 3. The patient is not getting the medication.
> 4. The patient not getting enough medication.
> 5. Persistent trigger in the environment.

frequency and severity as well as physiologic assessment (Table 289-1). The best treatment for an individual patient is based on severity classification.

Monitoring Asthma

Physiologic assessment and monitoring are cornerstones of the management plan. *The goal of therapy is not only relief of symptoms and decreasing frequency of exacerbations, but also normalization of pulmonary function.* Spirometry should be performed on all children with asthma symptoms age 6 years and older and then at periodic intervals thereafter. Children with persistent abnormal spirometry results, despite appropriate management, may be candidates for referral to a specialist to rule out other obstructive pulmonary diseases.

Peak flow monitoring is not indicated or necessary in all children with asthma. Studies show that patients do not consistently use these instruments, despite the fact that patients sometimes record detailed peak flow diaries! In addition, peak flow measurement is insensitive to changes in the smaller airways, the primary site of airways inflammation in asthma. Some patients may benefit from intermittent peak flow monitoring during viral respiratory tract infections or changes in asthma management.

Regular monitoring of pulmonary function should always be tied to a detailed, written asthma action plan. The patient must recognize and track symptoms of asthma by itself or in conjunction with periodic physiologic measurements to determine the effectiveness of the management plan and to make changes accordingly.

Medications

Currently, a broad pharmacologic armamentarium is available for the treatment of asthma, including "reliever" medications for treating acute asthma exacerbations and "controller" drugs for long-term therapy. The medications can be classified into several categories: bronchodilators, mast cell stabilizers, inhaled corticosteroids, methylxanthines, and oral antileukotrienes (Table 289-2).

Table 289-1. Severity Classification of Children with Asthma

Severity of Illness of Asthma	Asthma Treatment	Medication Options
Intermittent Asthma Intermittent symptoms <2 times per week Brief exacerbations (from a few hours to a few days) Nighttime asthma symptoms <2 times per month Asymptomatic and normal lung function between exacerbations PEF or FEV1 >80% predicted with <20% variability	No daily medication needed Short-acting inhaled β₂-agonist prn	Albuterol Oral corticosteroids prn exacerbation
Mild Persistent Asthma Symptoms >2 times per week but <1 time per day Exacerbations may effect activity and sleep Nighttime asthma symptoms >2 times per month PEF or FEV1 ≥ 80% predicted with variability of 20–30%	Daily anti-inflammatory low-dose or mast cell stabilizer *and* Short-acting inhaled β₂-agonist prn	Inhaled corticosteroids, (low dose) *and/or* LTRA Albuterol Oral corticosteroids prn exacerbation

Moderate Persistent Asthma
Daily symptoms
Exacerbations affect activities and sleep
Nighttime asthma symptoms >1 time a week
Daily use of inhaled short-acting β₂-agonist
PEF or FEV1 >60% predicted with >30% variability
	Daily anti-inflammatory medium dose
	   and
	Short-acting inhaled β₂ agonist prn: *or*
	Daily anti-inflammatory low dose *plus*
	Long-acting inhaled β₂-agonist *and*
	Short-acting β₂-agonist prn
		Inhaled corticosteroids (moderate dose)
		   and/or
		Long-acting β-agonist *and/or*
		LTRA; *and* Albuterol
		Oral corticosteroids prn exacerbation

Severe Persistent Asthma Continuous symptoms Frequent exacerbations Frequent nighttime asthma symptoms PEF or FEV1 <60% predicted with >30% variability	Daily anti-inflammatory-high dose *plus* Long-acting inhaled β₂-agonist *and* Short-acting β₂-agonist prn	Inhaled corticosteroids (moderate dose) *and/or* Long-acting β-agonist *and/or* LTRA *and* Albuterol Oral corticosteroids prn exacerbation

*Based on Global Initiative for Asthma: Global Strategy for the asthma management and prevention, NHLBI/WHO workshop report. National Institute of Health, National Heart, Lung and Blood Institute, January 1995.

Bronchodilators

The most commonly used bronchodilator medication is the β-agonist albuterol (Proventil, Ventolin). It is available in solution for nebulizer use (as a 0.5% solution) or in a pressurized metered-dose inhaler (MDI) (90 μg per actuation). The usual dose for children is 1 to 2 puffs of the MDI or 0.5 mL (2.5 mg) of the nebulizer solution, when delivered as rescue therapy for asthma. Tremor and tachycardia are the most common side effects, with rare reports of hypokalemia when higher doses are used. Levalbuterol (Xopenex), a recently introduced nonracemic form of albuterol, appears to be as effective as albuterol in smaller doses with fewer side effects. It is available only in a nebulized form, although the MDI form is currently under review by the FDA. Oral forms of β-agonists are not routinely recommended, as they have poor bioavailability and are frequently associated with side effects. β-Agonist medications delivered by pressurized MDI with mask and spacer are effective even in very small infants.

Ipratroprium bromide (Atrovent) is an atropinergic bronchodilator that is available in both nebulized (002% solution, 500 μg in 2.5 mL is the usual dose) and MDI (18 μg per inhalation) forms. While many use ipratropium in the treatment of acute asthma, its effectiveness in pediatric patients is questionable.

Long-acting β-agonists are also available in metered-dose inhalers (MDIs) and dry powder inhalers (DPIs) (salmeterol xenofolate, Serevent, 21 μg per actuation MDI for children older than 12 years of age or 50-μg inhalation DPI for children 4 years of age and older). The MDI dose is delivered in 1 to 2 puffs once or twice a day, and the DPI dose is 1 inhalation once or twice a day. These agents may be especially helpful for children with nighttime or exercise-induced symptoms and are more effective than long-acting oral β-agonists. Recently, a DPI combining salmeterol with the inhaled corticosteroids fluticasone (Advair) has become available in three different strengths. Formoterol fumarate (Foradil) is also available as a DPI inhaler for children ages 5 and older (12 μg per inhalation twice a day).

Mast Cell Stabilizers

This class of agents has been available for the maintenance treatment of asthma for more than 25 years. Cromolyn sodium (Intal) is the oldest agent of this class. It is an anti-inflammatory agent that is thought to act by stabilizing the membranes and preventing the degranulation of mast cells. Cromolyn is available in nebulized (2.0 mL/20 mg solution three to four times a day) or MDI form (800 μg per actuation, 2 to 4 puffs four times a day). More recently, nedocromil sodium (Tilade) has become available, only in the MDI form (1.75 mg per actuation, 2 puffs four times a day). Both drugs are quite safe, with only very rare incidences of hypersensitivity reactions. Mast cell stabilizers can be used in conjunction or mixed with β-agonists.

Inhaled Corticosteroids

These drugs show great efficacy in asthma control and have replaced the mast cell stabilizers to a great extent as the mainstay of maintenance therapy. Five different inhaled corticosteroids are currently available, and several are to be introduced. They are available as pressurized MDIs and DPIs. The latter formulation has become increasingly

Table 289-2. Pharmacology of Asthma Therapy

Reliever Medications

Bronchodilators

Albuterol	Proventil, Ventolin	Nebulized 0.5% solution, 0.03 cc/kg MDI 90 µg/puff
Levalbuterol	Xopenex	Nebulized 0.63 mg or 1.25 mg in 3.0 mL Older than 12 years 0.63 mg or 1.25 mg three times a day
Ipratroprium bromide	Atrovent	Nebulized 002% solution 500 micrograms in 2.5 mL MDI 18 µg/puff
Salmeterol xenofolate	Serevent	MDI 25 µg/puff MDI for children older than 12 DPI 50 µg/puff DPI for children 4 years and older
Formoterol fumarate	Foradil	12 µg/inhalation DPI for children 5 years and older

Controller Medications

Mast Cell stabilizers

Cromolyn sodium	Intal	Nebulized 2.0 mL/20 mg solution 3–4 times a day MDI 800 µg/puff 2–4 puffs four times a day
Nedocromil sodium	Tilade	MDI 1.75 mg/puff 2 puffs four times a day

Inhaled Corticosteroids

Beclomethasone	Beclovent or Vanceril	MDI 42 or 84 µg/puff 2 puffs, 3–4 times a day 4 puffs twice a day
Fluticasone	Flovent	MDI 44, 110, and 220 µg/puff 1–2 puffs twice a day DPI 50, 100 and 250 µg/puff 1–2 puffs, twice a day
Budesonide	Pulmicort	DPI 200 µg/puff 1–2 inhalations, 1–2 times a day
Flunisolide	Aerobid	MDI 250 µg/puff 2 puffs bid
Triamcinalone	Azmacort	MDI 100 µg/puff 2–3 puffs four times a day

Methylxanthines

Theophylline	Slo-Bid	po 200 mg twice a day Children >6 years and >25 kg Increased to 450, twice a day

Oral Antileukotrienes

Zileuton	Zyflo	Not generally used in children
Zafirlukast	Accolate	po 10 mg twice a day ages 5–11 Po 20 mg twice a day older than 11
Montelukast	Singulair	po 4 mg once a day, 2–5 years po 5 mg once a day 6–14 years po 10 mg once a day >15 years

popular and may replace MDI in the near future as both reliever and controller therapy. (Some data suggest that patients who use both MDIs and DPIs have worse technique with both delivery systems than do those who use exclusively one or the other. It is best to avoid mixing presumably different types of inhaler devices in most patients.)

Beclomethasone (Beclovent or Vanceril) is available as standard (42 µg per actuation) and double-strength (84 µg per actuation) MDIs. The dose is 2 puffs three or four

times a day or 4 puffs twice a day. For many individuals, it is the first-line inhaled corticosteroid. Fluticasone is available in three MDI strengths (Flovent 44, 110, and 220 µg per actuation). All three formulations are given as 2 puffs twice a day. Some data suggest that actuations given once a day may also be effective. DPI is also available (Flovent 50, 100, and 250 µg per actuation).

Other corticosteroids inhalers include Budesonide DPI (Pulmicort 200 µg per actuation, 1 to 2 inhalations, once or twice a day), flunisolide (Aerobid 250 µg per actuation, 2 puffs twice a day), and triamcinalone (Azmacort 100 µg per activation, 2 to 3 puffs four times a day). The relative strength of the inhaled corticosteroids is difficult to gauge. Beclomethasone, triamcinalone, and flunisolide are generally considered first-line therapy, with the more potent agents fluticasone and budesonide considered second line. These latter two agents are dosed once or twice a day, making them more convenient for families to use as well as first-line therapy for specific patients.

The toxicity of inhaled corticosteroids deserves special mention, since this subject appears to be of greatest concern to patients, parents, and providers. Despite the large number of studies published that examine the impact of corticosteroids on growth and adrenal suppression, no study has shown significant side effects with these agents at low (<400 µg/day) dosing. Patients receiving moderate doses (400 to 800 µg/day) may have mild, minimal bone growth suppression, but these effects appear to be reversible and do not affect final adult height.

Patients receiving high-dose corticosteroids (>800 µg/day) may be at risk for significant side effects. Growth should be monitored closely, and consideration should be given for varicella prophylaxis after exposure to varicella in unimmunized children. Some experts also recommend annual eye examination to look for developing cataracts, although there are no data in children to suggest such a clear risk. Additional caution should be taken when children on medium- to high-dose inhaled steroids who also receive frequent bursts of oral steroids, since the risk for steroid side effects may be additive.

Methylxanthines

Once the most widely used therapy for inpatient and ambulatory asthma therapy, theophylline is used only rarely now in either setting. The hidden cost of monitoring drug levels, the potential for systemic toxicity, and the negative aspects of frequent blood sampling in children have led practitioners to use other classes of medications. Theophylline, however, is the only agent that lends itself to easy assessment of adherence. A patient treated with a standard dose of theophylline (200 mg twice a day for children older than 6 years and greater than 25 kg, increased to 450 twice a day) should attain a blood level (8 to 10 µg/dL) within 3 to 5 days. Absence of measurable blood levels suggests that the patient is not adherent with therapy.

Oral Antileukotrienes (Lipoxygenase Inhibitor and Leukotriene Receptor Antagonists)

Oral antileukotrienes are the newest class of medications available for asthma therapy. Zafirlukast (Accolate) was the first leukotriene receptor antagonist available and is dosed

10 mg orally twice a day for ages 5 to 11 and 20 mg twice a day for those older than 11 years. Montelukast (Singulair) is available in three forms: 4, 5, and 10 mg a day for 2 to 5 years, 6 to 14 years, and older than 15 years, respectively. The 4-mg and 5-mg forms are available as chewable pills. Montelukast is the most widely used drug of this class in children with asthma, has the broadest range of indications by age, and has the advantage of once-daily dosing.

All oral antileukotrienes are considered adjunct therapy for children with mild and moderate asthma, although reports suggest that they may increase exercise-induced symptoms. Oral antileukotrienes may also be effective as monotherapy for patients with mild persistent asthma.

Zileutin (Zyflo), a lipoxigenase inhibiter, is not generally used in children.

Chronic Medication Therapy

All published asthma management guidelines demand chronic controller medications in children with persistent asthma. Undergoing chronic therapy may be the most difficult aspect of asthma control for parents and patients to accept. But chronic disease requires chronic therapy, and often parents are more accepting of chronic therapy when the duration of therapy is suggested at the initiation of care, such as a period of 3 to 6 months. The provider should choose the controller medications for an individual patient on the basis of patient-specific considerations including drug cost and frequency of dosing. Initial dosing should be sufficient to ensure symptom control and dosing is either stepped down once a period of symptom resolution is reached or stepped up if symptoms are not controlled.

Immunotherapy

Immunotherapy has long been considered an essential part of asthma therapy. Forty years ago, almost half of all patients with asthma received immunotherapy as a part of their therapy. Today, fewer than 5% of children receive "allergy shots," depending largely on the preference of their provider. Although controversial, this form of therapy appears to help specific children with asthma, usually children with more severe symptoms and specific, identifiable environmental triggers.

A new form of immunotherapy will become available soon. Specific anti-IgE antibody therapy (omalizumab, Xolair) will probably be available as a subcutaneous injection for children with severe allergy and asthma.

Environmental Control

Asthma therapy can fail if the clinician ignores specific aspects of environmental control. Elimination of secondhand tobacco smoke is crucial. The presence of other irritants and allergens must be determined, and the offending agents must be eliminated if possible. Dust mite elimination in the home is important for children with a suggestive history and for children who do not respond initially to appropriate pharmacologic therapy.

Management Plan

A written asthma home management plan should be provided and reviewed at every office visit. Patients and parents often better understand the terms *reliever* for β-agonists and *controllers* for the anti-inflammatory medications. On the reverse side of the management plan, the family should be provided a detailed asthma action plan. This identifies the symptoms (cough, wheezing, dyspnea) or peak-flow values ("yellow zone," 50% to 80% best peak flow, or "red zone," <50% best peak flow) that should provoke more aggressive rescue treatment, including the initiation of corticosteroids, provided to the family at home as a standby medication.

THE RIGHT PLACE

Probably the most important element for successful asthma therapy is delivery of the correct medication to the right place. Pharmacoeconomics, the cost of medical therapy, and lack of convenience may keep families from filling prescriptions. Poor adherence to asthma regimens will keep the child from using the medication. Children should always use a spacer for MDI medications to ensure that the aerosolized medication is suspended in the inhaled air and not deposited in the mouth and oropharynx. Finally, correct MDI technique is key to delivery of the drug to the lung (Box 289-2).

Even after proper instruction, only about one third of children will use the MDI correctly on their first attempt. Only 40% of these children will be using the inhaler correctly at a 2-week follow-up visit. Thus, *MDI technique must be taught, reinforced, and monitored at each visit to ensure effectiveness.* Current data suggest that nebulized therapy, once thought to be the mainstay of asthma therapy for young children and infants, has no particular advantage over using MDIs with spacer and mask. This holds true for therapy delivery to acutely wheezing infants and to those receiving chronic medications at home. Many children's hospitals and practices have replaced nebulizer therapy with MDI therapy, even in the emergency room and on the pediatric ward. MDI therapy is as effective, costs less, and takes less time to administer. Studies also suggest that using MDI bronchodilators on an as-needed basis in hospitalized children, with hourly assessment by nurses or respiratory therapists (instead of using regularly scheduled, around-the-clock administration), decreases length of hospital stay.

FUTURE TRENDS

Future, effective asthma therapy must focus on the child's home and environment. The child and the parents or guardians are the key participants for achieving effective

---

Box 289-2. MDI/Spacer Technique

- Remove cap and shake.
- Take deep breath to full lung volume, then exhale completely.
- Put spacer into mouth, acute MDI.
- Take a slow breath.
- Hold breath for 5–10 seconds.
- Exhale slowly.
  Wait one minute for next puffs.

therapy. Physicians and other health care providers act as team members in the development and implementation of effective care in the patient's home, school, and community.

Ideally, asthma management and training in asthma management should occur where the child lives: in the home, the school, and the neighborhood. This suggests a future role for in-home, electronic monitoring using telemedicine for daily monitoring of children with asthma. Community-based health clinics (e.g., school, church, community center) should work more with the child and parent in the management of the child with asthma. Finally, support groups and the media should further educate for the proper delivery of care.

SUMMARY

Asthma is a disease that can be controlled. The primary care provider can achieve excellent, expert care of children with asthma by using the correct principles of the right patient, the right plan, and the right place.

Additional Resources, CD-ROM

Bibliography

SUGGESTED READINGS

Castro-Rodriguez JA, Holberg CJ, Wright AL, Martinez FD: A clinical index to define risk of asthma in young children with recurrent wheezing. Am J Respir Crit Care Med 2000;162:1403–1406.

Chan D, Callahan C, Moreno C: Decreased asthma hospitalization in children following implementation of a multidisciplinary asthma education and management program. Am J Health Syst Pharm 2001;58:1413–1417.

Childhood Asthma Management Program Research Group: Long term effects of budesonide or nedocromil in children with asthma. N Engl J Med 2000;343:1054–1063.

National Heart, Lung, and Blood Institute: Expert Panel Report II: Guidelines for the Diagnosis and Management of Asthma. NIH Publication No 97-4051. Bethesda, Md, U.S. Department of Health and Human Services, 1997.

Weisberg SC: Pharmacotherapy of asthma in children with special reference to leukotriene receptor antagonists. Pediatr Pulmonol 2000;29:46–61.

SECTION 9 DIAGNOSTICS AND THERAPEUTICS: *Pharmacotherapy*

290 Antineoplastic Agents

Gary R. Jones

The prognosis for children with cancer has markedly improved over the last half of the 20th century. The reasons include refinements in surgical techniques, progress in radiation technologies, and improved supportive care. The most dramatic impact on outcome, such that today over two thirds of children and adolescents treated for malignant diseases are cured, however, is due to the implementation of antineoplastic agents in cancer treatment. Although pediatric hematology/oncology specialists generally develop, evaluate, and prescribe these powerful yet potentially toxic drugs, the general practitioner plays an important role in caring for children receiving chemotherapy. Appropriate care demands a basic understanding of antineoplastic agents, their common uses, and potential side effects.

The oncologist's armamentarium of antineoplastic drugs comes from a variety of sources. The observation of damage to lymphatic tissue in U.S. servicemen exposed to poison gas during World War II led to the use of alkylating agents in the treatment of lymphomas. Clinical deterioration of children with acute lymphoblastic leukemia who were given folic acid led to the clinical development and use of antifolate agents (e.g., methotrexate), and subsequently other antimetabolite drugs (e.g., 6-mercaptopurine) were devel-

oped for cancer treatment. The vinca alkaloids initially used to treat diabetes in mice models were noted to cause marrow suppression. Since the 1950s, animal models of transplantable tumors and malignant cell lines grown in tissue culture have successfully identified a wide range of agents with antitumor effects. Doxorubicin and actinomycin-D are drugs derived from antibiotics produced by a wide array of bacteria, fungi, and plants. Today, the development of potentially powerful and rationally designed antineoplastic agents is based on targeting specific molecular mechanisms and markers of malignant cells.

ROLES FOR ANTINEOPLASTIC DRUGS

Chemotherapy alone can successfully treat some malignancies in children, such as the leukemias and lymphomas, without surgical resection or radiation therapy. Solid tumors usually require combination therapy, including surgery or radiation and chemotherapy. Prior to the 1960s, surgery followed by radiation therapy of the tumor bed was the established method for treatment, and improvements in surgical and radiation techniques led to excellent local tumor control. However, the cancer recurred in the majority of patients owing to development of metastases. The addition of antineoplastic agents provided systemic treatment by effectively destroying microscopic metastatic disease. The term *adjuvant chemotherapy* refers to the administration of chemotherapy following surgery or radiation therapy when residual tumor cells are at a minimum. Adjuvant chemotherapy has been shown to be highly effective in improving the outcome of patients with diseases such as Wilms tumor and soft tissue sarcomas. More recently, antineoplastic drugs are administered prior to definitive local control measures, a technique that is sometimes termed *neoadjuvant chemotherapy*. Neoadjuvant chemotherapy provides early treatment for possibly disseminated disease prior to extensive local control therapy. Neoadjuvant chemotherapy may also decrease the bulk of the primary tumor prior to surgery enabling less extensive surgery. It may also prevent the need for radiation therapy in some patients and may quickly alleviate tumor-related pain. An additional benefit is that neoadjuvant chemotherapy enables assessment of the degree of tumor responsiveness to chemotherapy (by measurement of tumor regression and histological response) prior to surgery, particularly in the treatment of osteosarcomas.

Antineoplastic agents also play a powerful role in palliating cancer-related symptoms and improving the quality of life in patients in whom the cancer disease has progressed and cure is no longer a realistic goal.

Antineoplastic agents may also be administered to specific body sites for which systemic drug therapy might not penetrate sufficiently to eradicate all disease. The central nervous system is one such "sanctuary site." If "prophylactic" therapy is not given, a significant number of patients with acute lymphoblastic leukemia are at risk for central nervous system relapse. Intrathecal injection of chemotherapeutic agents such as methotrexate, cytarabine, and hydrocortisone has become an integral part of successful therapy for children treated for acute leukemias and non-Hodgkin lymphomas.

DEVELOPMENT OF ANTINEOPLASTIC AGENTS

Most antineoplastic agents were discovered or developed on the basis of observed cytotoxic effects on microorganism, animal, or cell culture models. Understanding of the cytotoxic mechanisms for most of these agents came from subsequent research, yet for some classes of drugs, the definitive mechanisms of antitumor activity remain unclear. Some agents, such as the anthracyclines (e.g., doxorubicin), appear to affect multiple cellular mechanisms. Most present-day antineoplastic drugs induce damage to molecular targets such as DNA or disrupt biochemical processes that exist in both malignant and normal cells. The fine line between anticancer efficacy and toxicity to normal tissues may be due in part to differences in the proportion of cells that are in the DNA replication phase of the cell cycle. Subtle differences between cancer cells and normal cells such as specific cell cycle controls, metabolic pathways, repair mechanisms, and rates of drug activation or elimination may affect the degree of molecular damage. Understanding these variations helps to determine which drugs to use, allowing preferential damage to malignant cells while limiting the degree of toxicity to normal tissues.

For most childhood cancers, tumor cells tend to be poorly differentiated or arrested at immature stages of development, features that might make them more susceptible to chemotherapy. Once cancer cell damage occurs, complex molecular and cellular events ultimately lead to cell death. Induction of programmed cell death pathways (apoptosis) is the most likely cause of death of chemotherapy-sensitive cells. However, for some antineoplastic agents, the anticancer mechanism appears to be the induction of cell differentiation or apoptosis without damaging nucleic acid and protein or disrupting biochemical pathways.

Most recently, advances in the development of therapeutic agents exploit molecular processes that are unique or crucial to malignant cell survival. New "designer" drugs target specific types of cancer cells, causing fewer toxic side effects in normal cells. Examples include rituximab, a "humanized" monoclonal antibody to CD-20 used in recurrent B-cell lymphomas, and imantinib (Gleevec, STI-571), a tyrosine kinase inhibitor that is effective in treating chronic myelogenous leukemia and possibly some solid tumors. Some designer drugs also appear to have broader effectiveness. For example, imantinib, which targets the Philadelphia chromosome in chronic myelogenous leukemia, has been shown to be very effective in inducing morphologic and cytogenetic remissions in patients with chronic myelogenous leukemia with minimal toxicity. Imanitinib also appears to be effective in patients with acute lymphoblastic leukemia whose cells contain the Philadelphia chromosome.

ANTINEOPLASTIC DRUG TRIALS

Once identified to have clinical potential, an antineoplastic agent typically undergoes testing in human subjects through a series of phases. Phase I studies are generally designed to determine dose-limiting toxicities, and the agent is given alone at incremental doses to small cohorts of patients. Subsequent Phase II trials involve giving the drug to a larger population of patients at dose levels no higher than the already established maximum tolerated dose to demonstrate clinical efficacy and to further evaluate possible toxic effects. Patients in Phase II studies typically have relapse of their cancer or are no longer responding to standard therapies. Phase III trials complete the evaluation of the drug's clinical efficacy in prospectively randomized clinical trials comparing the outcome in a group of patients treated with the study agent with a control group who did not receive the study agent. These studies require stringent stratification of patients on the basis of age and disease characteristics and often require multicenter or cooperative group participation to attain sample sizes sufficient to show statistical and clinical significance.

Approval for clinical use by the U.S. Food and Drug Administration requires rigorous documentation of side effects and sufficient evidence of medical benefit in one or more types of cancer. Once antineoplastic agents are commercially available, they are incorporated into subsequent clinical trials to determine efficacy at other dose schedules, when combined with other agents, when used for treating other types of cancer, or in differing types of patient populations such as children. Eventually, particular antineoplastic combination regimens become accepted standards of care for pediatric malignancies and become control therapies in subsequent clinical trials of different combinations, dosages, schedules, or new agents. The significant improvement of cure rates for childhood cancers is the direct result of numerous clinical research and cooperative group therapeutic trials conducted over the past four decades. All children who are diagnosed with a malignant disease should participate in ongoing therapeutic trials to ensure access to the best treatment available and to help develop more effective therapies in the future.

ANTINEOPLASTIC AGENTS: DOSING

The dosing and scheduling of specific antineoplastic drugs in children vary considerably depending on the type of malignancy, the chosen combination chemotherapy regimen, and the presence or past history of significant toxicity. Essentially all systemic chemotherapeutic agents are dosed in proportion to the size of the patient, based on the body surface area determined by height and weight. Frequently, drug dosing for infants and younger children is based on weight alone. Some drugs have a recommended maximum dose that should rarely, if ever, be exceeded, regardless of the size of the patient (e.g., Vincristine, maximum dose 2 mg).

Myelosuppression is the most common toxicity of antineoplastic drugs that limits dosing. Most combination chemotherapy regimens are scheduled every 3 to 4 weeks to allow sufficient time for the recovery of neutrophils and platelets before repeating courses. White blood cells and platelets typically decline for several days to a week after intensive combination chemotherapy completion. Recovery of blood counts to levels sufficient for the next course of chemotherapy may take 2 weeks or longer depending on the specific agents used and the patient's condition (e.g., presence of infection). Most protocols require neutrophil recovery of 750 to 1000/mm^3 and platelet counts of 75,000 to 100,000/mm^3 before subsequent course of chemotherapy. Several intensive regimens used in the treatment of acute myeloblastic leukemia (AML) and aggressive sarcomas incorporate subcutaneous injections of granulocyte colony-stimulating factor (G-CSF, Nupogen, filgrastim) in order to decrease the period of neutropenia.

ANTINEOPLASTIC AGENTS: CLASSES

Typical antineoplastic medications include alkylating agents and their related drugs, vinca alkyloids, antimetabolites, asparaginase, topoisomerase inhibitors, and antineoplastic antibiotics. Descriptions of each type of agent and their uses follow. Table 290-1 lists the commonly prescribed antineoplastic agents and their indications, toxicity, and possible place in combination therapy.

Alkylating Agents and Similar Drugs
There are a wide variety of antineoplastic drugs designated as alkylating agents. These drugs vary significantly in their molecular structure, metabolism, and active moieties but have the common propensity to covalently bind to DNA leading to disruption of gene expression and replication

associated with mitosis. Alkylating agents affect cellular repair mechanisms, inducing deletions or point mutations that can further disrupt molecular processes. Unfortunately, these agents have potential carcinogenic effects on normal cells that may lead to treatment-related leukemias and significantly detrimental effects on reproductive function.

Cyclophosphamide is one of the most widely used antineoplastic agents in children with cancer. Although oral preparations are available, this drug is mostly given intravenously. It is frequently employed in the consolidation/intensification phases of acute lymphoblastic leukemia protocols and is commonly utilized in combination with Vincristine and Actinomycin-D or Doxorubicin in regimens for soft tissue sarcomas and Ewing sarcoma. Regimens combining Cyclophosphamide, Vincristine, and prednisone with an anthracycline, methotrexate, or another alkylating agent are the basis of treatment for Hodgkin disease and several types of non-Hodgkin lymphoma (e.g., Burkitt lymphoma). High-dose cyclophosphamide is a commonly used agent in combination with total body irradiation or busulfan administration prior to allogeneic hematopoietic stem cell transplantation. The closely related compound ifosfamide is combined with etoposide or doxorubicin in therapies for aggressive sarcomas. Myelosuppression is the major dose limiting toxicity of these agents. Nausea can be significant with high dosing schedules, and alopecia is common.

Both cyclophosphamide and ifosfamide are metabolized to the active form phosphoramide mustard and acrolein. Acrolein is excreted into the urine and, if it accumulates to high concentrations, can cause irritation to the bladder epithelium leading to hemorrhagic cystitis with risk of fibrosis and chronic bladder dysfunction. This toxicity can be minimized with aggressive hydration, frequent bladder emptying, and the use of mesna (2-mercaptoethane sulfonate), a drug that inactivates the toxic effects of acrolein in the urinary tract.

The platinum compounds cisplatin and carboplatin also induce DNA damage by covalent binding and production of cross-links by platination, a process similar to alkylation. Cisplatinum is commonly used in treatment regimens for osteosarcoma, neuroblastoma, germ cell tumors, and several types of brain tumors. Carboplatin has been combined with ifosfamide and etoposide in the treatment of aggressive or relapsed sarcomas. Cisplatin is less myelosuppressive than carboplatin but is associated with significantly greater nausea, peripheral sensory neuropathy, and hearing loss caused by direct damage to hair cells of the inner ear. Nephrotoxicity associated with cisplatin is accumulative and can be manifested by decreased glomerular function and electrolyte loss, particularly magnesium. Aggressive hydration, electrolyte supplementation, and diuresis with mannitol are commonly employed to minimize these renal effects. Patients receiving cisplatin-based chemotherapy regimens need to be monitored with serial measurements of glomerular filtration rate and audiograms.

Other agents with direct alkylating or similar effects commonly used in pediatric and young adult patients include busulfan, melphalan (both commonly used as preparative agents for allogeneic hematopoietic cell transplantation), procarbazine (an oral agent used in common

Table 290-1. Commonly Prescribed Antineoplastic Agents: Indications, Toxicity, and Possible Combinations

Drug Class	Commonly Used Examples	Acute Toxicity	Long-Term Effects	Examples of Common Combinations/Uses
Alkylating agents		Nausea Myelosuppression Alopecia	Treatment-related leukemia infertility	
	Cyclophosphamide	Hemorrhagic cystitis SIADH		Vincristine/actinomycin-D Cyclophosphamide (VAC) —rhabdomyosarcoma
	Ifosfamide	Hemorrhagic cystitis		Ifosfamide/etoposide—Ewing sarcoma
Platinum-based agents		Nausea Alopecia Hypersensitivity reaction		
	Cisplatin	Renal	Neurosensory hearing loss	Cisplatin/doxorubicin— osteosarcoma
Vinca alkyloids		Alopecia Vesicant-tissue damage associated with extravasation		
	Vincristine	Peripheral neuropathy SIADH		Vincristine, glucocorticoid (e.g., Prednisone) L-asparaginase +/– Daunomycin—ALL induction
	Vinblastine	Myelosuppression		
Topoisomerase inhibitors	Etoposide	Nausea Myelosuppression Hypotension if infused too rapidly	Treatment-related leukemia	Ifosfamide/etoposide Ewing sarcoma
Antineoplastic antibiotics		Nausea Alopecia		
	Doxorubicin/daunomycin	Myelosuppression Vesicant-tissue damage associated with extravasation	Myocardial damage	Daunomycin/cytarabine—AML induction
	Bleomycin	Hypersensitivity reaction skin	Pulmonary fibrosis	Hodgkin disease
Protein synthesis inhibitor	Asparaginase	Hypersensitivity reaction Hyperglycemia due to decreased insulin production Coagulation abnormalities Pancreatitis		Vincristine glucocorticoid (e.g., Prednisone) L-asparaginase +/– Daunomycin—ALL induction

regimens for Hodgkin disease), the nitrosoureas (e.g., lomustine—CCNU), and temozolomide (an oral agent used in recurrent brain tumors).

Vinca Alkyloids
Vinca alkyloids are drugs derived from the periwinkle plant; vincristine and vinblastine are the most commonly used agents in this class. These drugs primarily affect microtubule formation, thereby disrupting normal mitotic spindle development and disturbing cell division.

Vincristine is used in many types of pediatric cancer. It is a key component in the treatment of acute lymphoblastic leukemia, Wilms tumor (combined with actinomycin-D ± doxorubicin), soft tissue sarcomas, neuroblastoma, Ewing sarcoma, lymphomas, and brain tumors. Vinblastine is incorporated in treatment protocols for Hodgkin disease, germ cell tumors, and Langerhan cell histiocytosis.

Unlike many other cytotoxic drugs including vinblastine, vincristine typically does not induce significant myelosuppression, ironic given that myelosuppression in mice led to its use as an anticancer drug in humans. The primary dose-limiting toxicity of vincristine is peripheral neuropathy, manifested by lower extremity weakness, parasthesias, jaw pain, and constipation. Seizures have also been associated with vincristine. These effects are dose dependent, and vincristine's maximum dose is 2 mg. Dose modifications need to be considered in patients with previous toxicity or elevated direct serum bilirubin levels, since vinca alkyloids are eliminated primarily through the biliary system. These drugs generally do not induce significant nausea but do cause alopecia.

Antimetabolites
In contrast to several classes of antineoplastic agents that affect cells by direct interactions with DNA or by disturbing mechanical processes related to replication and mitosis, the antimetabolites are a diverse group of drugs that block specific biochemical pathways or act as chemical analogues that ultimately interfere with the production of DNA.

Methotrexate is a potent inhibitor of the enzyme dihydrofolate reductase leading to diminished levels of reduced folate necessary for the production of thymidine, a basic building block of DNA. Methotrexate is an integral part of acute lymphoblastic leukemia therapy, given by the oral, intravenous or intramuscular route. Methotrexate given intrathecally is an important drug for treating or preventing acute lymphoblastic leukemia (ALL) in the central nervous system. When given at high intravenous doses, such as in treatment regimens for osteosarcoma, lymphoma, or high-risk infant ALL protocols, methotrexate is followed by treatment with folinic acid (leucovorin)

Cytarabine is metabolized by the cell to an active analogue of doxycytidine that incorporates into DNA instead of the normal pyrimidine, thereby interfering with normal DNA replication and repair. Cytarabine in combination with an anthracycline is an important component in the induction therapy of acute myelogenous leukemia. Like methotrexate, cytarabine can be safely and effectively injected into the cerebral spinal fluid space as part of the prophylactic or therapeutic treatment of acute leukemia with central nervous system involvement.

6-Mercaptopurine and 6-thioguanine interfere with purine synthesis and incorporation into DNA, disrupting subsequent replications. These drugs play a major role in maintenance therapy for patients with acute lymphoblastic leukemia. These drugs tend to be tolerated well with minimal myelosuppression and occasional hepatic toxicity associated with elevation of transaminases. Vaso-occlusive disease has been associated with 6-thioguanine.

Fludarabine, another antimetabolite, appears to act as an analogue of adenosine that replaces adenosine in DNA and RNA. It is usually used in the treatment of AML or prior to stem cell transplantation.

Asparaginase

Although asparagine is not an essential amino acid in normal cells, studies in the 1950s showed that malignant cells of lymphoid origin appear to have a decreased capacity for asparagine synthesis. Asparaginase is an enzyme derived from E. coli and Erwinia conotovora that can degrade circulating asparagine, leading to inhibition of protein synthesis by tumor cells. Asparaginase is used primarily in the treatment of acute lymphoblastic leukemia. Since asparaginase is a foreign protein, it can elicit allergic reactions, even anaphylaxis. Although it can be given intravenously, asparaginase given intramuscularly is associated with a lower risk of reaction. Observation of patients up to 30 minutes after an injection of asparaginase is recommended. Asparaginase therapy may also induce hyperglycemia that sometimes requires insulin therapy to correct. Coagulopathies may occur presenting with either increased bleeding or thrombotic events.

Topoisomerase Inhibitors

Topoisomerases are cellular enzymes important for stabilizing strands of DNA in the nucleus. Topoisomerase inhibitors are cytotoxic primarily by preventing the religation of DNA strands. Etoposide is an inhibitor of topoisomerase II and is used in the treatment of a variety of cancers, including Ewing sarcoma, neuroblastoma, germ cell tumors, and relapsing solid tumors. Etoposide is commonly given in combination with Ifosfamide.

Hypotension may occur if the drug is infused too rapidly. A concerning long-term effect of etoposide is the increased incidence of treatment-related acute leukemia. Topotecan is a new topoisomerase I inhibitor that is currently under study for its effect on a variety of pediatric solid tumors. Antineoplastic antibiotics, another class of antineoplastic drugs, work in part by inhibition of topoisomerases.

Antineoplastic Antibiotics

The antineoplastic antibiotics are a fairly broad class of agents that exert their effect by damaging nuclear DNA. Agents such as the anthracyclines (e.g., doxorubicin, daunomycin, idarubicin), actinomycin-D, mitoxantrone, and bleomycin are derived from a variety of bacteria and fungi that produce these compounds as a protection against other organisms in their microenvironment. The antitumor effects of antineoplastic antibiotics may be mediated by several mechanisms. These drugs intercalate into DNA, causing breaks between base pairs in part by interfering with topoisomerases. Some agents, such as the anthracyclines, may increase the production of superoxide radicals that damage intracellular nucleic acid and protein.

Drugs in the anthracycline group are important in the therapy of a broad range of pediatric cancers, including acute leukemias, lymphomas, neuroblastoma, malignant bone tumors, and high-risk patients with Wilms tumor and soft tissue sarcomas. A significant toxic effect of these agents is accumulative damage to the myocardium. Acute heart failure is associated with total accumulated doses above 500 mg/m^2 and with administering anthracycline treatment in combination with radiation therapy to the chest. Myocardial scarring and decreased ventricular wall thickness and function related to anthracycline use might not be clinically evident until years after exposure, particularly in children who are initially treated before 4 years of age. Continuous infusion over 24 or more hours, rather than bolus infusion, may decrease cardiac toxicity, although extending infusion time may increase the extent of mucositis. Dexrazoxane is now used in some regimens to decrease cardiotoxicity.

Bleomycin is used in some Hodgkin disease treatment regimens as well as in the treatment of germ cell tumors. In contrast to other agents in this class, bleomycin is relatively nonmyelosuppressive. Pulmonary fibrosis, leading to dyspnea and hypoxia, is a potential long-term side effect of this drug.

Actinomycin-D is an important agent in the curative treatment of Wilms tumor and rhabdomyosarcoma. This drug may be associated with significant nausea and mucositis. Actinomycin-D can increase radiation sensitivity of normal tissues, increasing hepatic toxicity of the agent.

ANTINEOPLASTIC AGENT REGIMENS FOR COMMON MALIGNANCIES

For a brief review of antineoplastic regimens for the common malignancies, ALL, AML, lymphomas (Hodgkin disease, non-Hodgkin lymphoma), central nervous system tumors, neuroblastoma, Wilms tumor, malignant bone tumors (osteosarcoma, Ewing sarcoma), and rhabdomyosarcoma refer to the CD-ROM supplemental material.

FUTURE TRENDS

Recent advances in the development of therapeutic agents exploit molecular processes unique or crucial to malignant cells. Future drug therapies will target specific cancers while causing fewer or more tolerable, different toxic side effects than the current, "older" cytotoxic agents. Examples of targeted therapies are interference of intercellular communication from the cell surface to the nucleus and development of monoclonal antibodies to cell surface molecules unique to tumor cells.

Other potential cancer treatment strategies include attempts to inhibit formation of blood vessel supply (angiogenesis) to tumors, to induce apoptosis in cancer cells, to decrease chemotherapy agent efflux from tumor cells, and to protect normal tissues from chemotherapy toxicity.

Recent directions of antineoplastic drug development are revolutionary and the resulting new agents will be incorporated into clinical treatment regimens in a more evolutionary fashion. While current cytotoxic agents with their significant toxicities will continue to have an important part in cancer therapy, these new agents will possibly lead to ever more successful cancer therapy with increased cure rates and decreased morbidity.

Additional Resources, CD-ROM

Antineoplastic agent regimens for common malignancies	Text
Bibliography	

SUGGESTED READINGS

Balis FM, Holcenberg JS, Blaney SM: General principles of chemotherapy. In Pizzo PA, Poplack DG (eds): Principles and Practice of Pediatric Oncology, 4th ed. Philadelphia, Lippincott Williams & Wilkins, 2002, pp 237–308.

Bernstein ML, Reaman GH, Hirschfeld S: Developmental therapeutics in childhood cancer: A perspective from the Children's Oncology Group and the US Food and Drug Administration. Hematol Oncol Clin North Am 2001;15(4):631–55.

Brogan PA, Dillon M.: The use of immunosuppressive and cytotoxic drugs in non-malignant disease. Arch Dis Child 2000;83(3): 259–264.

Friedman DL, Meadows AT: Late effects of childhood cancer therapy. Ped Clin North Am 2002;49(5):1083–1106.

Lanzkowski P: Manual of Pediatric Hematology and Oncology, 3rd ed. San Diego, Academic Press, 1999.

SECTION 9   DIAGNOSTICS AND THERAPEUTICS: *Pharmacotherapy*

291

Diagnosis and Treatment of Children with Suspected Metabolic Disease

Gregory M. Enns and Robert D. Steiner

Inborn errors of metabolism may present with a wide array of signs and symptoms at any time during life. Sudden, unexpected death is not an infrequent presentation as well, so inborn errors may be diagnosed postmortem. These disorders should be considered in the differential diagnosis of a previously healthy-appearing child who undergoes an unexplained rapid deterioration. On the other hand, more insidious findings, including developmental delay or regression, various neurologic findings (lethargy, ataxia, seizures, extrapyramidal signs, hypotonia, or hypertonia), feeding intolerance, and failure to thrive, may offer the first clue to the presence of an underlying metabolic disorder. Because inborn errors are individually rare, there is a tendency to consider the possibility of metabolic disease only after more common causes of pediatric distress have been excluded.

However, the aggregate incidence of inborn errors of metabolism is relatively high, as many as one child in every thousand births being affected. When a child suffers an acute catastrophic presentation of an inborn error of metabolism, appropriate therapy must be started immediately, because of the high risk of morbidity or mortality, regardless of the etiology. If treatment is to be helpful in this situation, it must be begun promptly. Therefore, the pediatrician must consider these disorders in all children who have nonspecific features of distress *on initial presentation*. Refer to Chapter 146 for further discussion (Box 291-1).

More than 300 human disorders involving various biochemical pathways have been identified. Examples of inborn errors affecting different steps in intermediary

Box 291-1. The Importance of Basic Laboratory Studies

Although specialized metabolic laboratory testing is required to make a definitive diagnosis, even simple tests, such as the measurement of blood gases, glucose, electrolytes, complete blood counts, lactate, and ammonia and the evaluation of urine for ketones and reducing substances can provide valuable clues to the presence of an inborn error.

metabolism are shown in Table 291-1. Most hospitals and even many tertiary care facilities and academic medical centers do not have the equipment to perform the specialized investigations necessary for comprehensive evaluation of a child suspected of having an inborn error of metabolism, such as quantitative plasma amino acid and acylcarnitine analysis or urine organic acid analysis. Nevertheless, a diagnosis may be suspected and a category of metabolic disease suggested on the basis of the results of simple laboratory studies and the clinical presentation. Initial laboratory investigations for the assessment of the critically

ill child who is suspected of having a metabolic disease are shown in Table 291-2.

LABORATORY EVALUATION

Initial laboratory assessment for inborn errors of metabolism by the primary health care provider should include investigation for normal or increased anion gap (Figure 291-1, Table 291-3), lactic acidosis (Figure 291-2, Table 291-4), hypoglycemia (Figure 291-3), defects in complete blood count, hyperammonemia (Figure 291-4), and appearance of ketones and reducing substances in the urine. Urine odor (Table 291-5) and color may indicate specific inborn error of metabolism. Other simple urine screening tests include the Clinitest (reducing substances), ferric chloride test (oxoacids), dinitrophenylhydrazine (DNPH) test (2-oxoacids), Acetest (ketones), and nitroprusside test (sulfur-containing acids). Causes for urine-reducing substances are listed in Table 291-6. Other compounds that are screened for and the corresponding disorders detected in urine are listed in the CD-ROM supplement.

Table 291-1. Categories of Inborn Errors of Metabolism

Category	Examples	Prominent features
Aminoacidemias	Phenylketonuria	Mental retardation (if untreated)
	Tyrosinemia	Liver disease, renal tubulopathy
	Maple syrup urine disease	Lethargy, coma
Urea cycle disorders	Citrullinemia	Lethargy, coma, hyperammonemia
	Ornithine transcarbamylase deficiency	
Organic acidemias	Methylmalonic acidemia	Lethargy, coma, metabolic acidosis
	Propionic acidemia	
	Isovaleric academia	
Fatty acid oxidation defects	Medium-chain acyl-CoA dehydrogenase deficiency, long-chain 3-hydroxyacyl-CoA dehydrogenase deficiency	Lethargy, coma, Reye-like syndrome, non (hypo)-ketotic hypoglycemia, cardiomyopathy
Carbohydrate disorders	Glycogen storage diseases	Hypoglycemia, hepatomegaly
	Galactosemia	Cataracts, liver disease, E. coli sepsis, ovarian failure, positive urine reducing substances
	Hereditary fructose intolerance	Liver disease, renal tubulopathy, hypoglycemia
	Fructose 1,6-bisphosphatase deficiency	Hepatomegaly, hypoglycemia, lactic acidosis
Lysosomal storage disorders	Hurler syndrome	Hepatosplenomegaly, coarse features
	Hunter syndrome	Dysostosis multiplex, mental retardation
	Gaucher disease	Hepatosplenomegaly (may have gross splenomegaly), bone crises, normal IQ in type II
	Tay-Sachs disease	Macrocephaly, cherry-red spot, development arrest, exaggerated startle reflex
	Fabry disease	Neuritic pain, progressive renal disease, angiokeratomata
Mitochondrial disorders	MELAS	Multisystem (especially neurologic) involvement
	MERRF	
	NARP	
	KSS	
Peroxisomal disorders	Zellweger syndrome	Dysmorphic features, large anterior fontanel, hypotonia, hepatomegaly
	Neonatal adrenoleukodystrophy	Hypotonia, seizures
	X-linked adrenoleukodystrophy	Behavior problems, progressive neurologic impairment, adrenal insufficiency
Purine and pyrimidine disorders	Adenosine deaminase deficiency	Severe combined immunodeficiency
	Lesch-Nyhan syndrome	Choreoathetosis, self-mutilation
	Hereditary orotic aciduria	Megaloblastic anemia, crystalluria
Cholesterol biosynthesis disorders	Smith-Lemli-Opitz syndrome	Dysmorphic features
Metal disorders	Menkes disease	Seizures, hypotonia, kinky hair, lax skin
	Wilson disease	Liver disease, Keyser-Fleischer rings, dystonia
	Acrodermatitis enteropathica	Dermatitis, alopecia

KSS, Kearns-Sayre syndrome; MELAS, mitochondrial encephalomyopathy lactic acidosis and stroke-like episodes; MERRF, myoclonic epilepsy and ragged red fibers; NARP, neurogenic weakness ataxia and retinitis pigmentosa.

Table 291-2. Initial Laboratory Investigation of a Child with a Suspected Inborn Error of Metabolism

Blood tests	Complete blood count
	Blood gases
	Electrolytes, BUN, creatinine, calcium, magnesium
	Glucose
	Lactate, pyruvate
	Ammonia
	Liver enzymes, prothrombin time, and partial thromboplastin time
	Quantitative amino acid analysis
	Carnitine levels (total, free, esterified)
	Acylcarnitine profile
	Plasma for storage at –20°C
Urine	Routine urinalysis
	Metabolic screen (differs in different laboratories)
	Organic acids
	Ferric chloride test, DNPH, Acetest, reducing substances (see text)
	Urine for storage at –20°C

For further discussion of initial laboratory investigation for inborn errors of metabolism, please refer to the CD-ROM supplement.

Specialized Investigation

These investigations are not available in many centers and require specialized equipment and expert interpretation. Nevertheless, children who are suspected of having an inborn error of metabolism should have plasma and urine obtained for these analyses and have the tests sent to a reference laboratory with expertise in biochemical genetic diagnosis. It might be necessary to repeat the metabolic tests outlined in Table 291-2 if the initial studies were inconclusive and obtained during a period of relative good health. Some metabolic disorders may be apparent only if diagnostic samples are obtained when the child is symptomatic or after a period of prolonged fasting (i.e., in a catabolic state).

Specialized investigations include analysis of amino acid, urine organic acid, carnitine, acylcarnitine, very long-chain fatty acid, phytanic acid, bile acid intermediates, plasmalogen, mucopolysaccharide, oligosaccharide, and sialic acid levels.

A brief discussion of each analysis follows. For further discussion, please refer to the CD-ROM supplement.

Amino Acid Analysis

Quantitative plasma amino acid analysis is an important part of the evaluation of a child who is suspected of having an inborn error of metabolism (unless typical features of a lysosomal storage disease are present; see Table 291-1). Different automated technologies are used, including ion-exchange chromatography, high-performance liquid chromatography (HPLC), and, more recently, tandem-mass spectrometry (MS/MS). Characteristic patterns of amino acid elevation or decrease, in conjunction with results from urine organic acid analysis, lead to a diagnosis of a metabolic disease in many cases.

Urine amino acid analysis is performed less frequently but may detect characteristic patterns of dibasic or neutral amino acid elevations seen in specific amino acid transport defects (e.g., Hartnup disease, cystinuria, lysinuric protein intolerance). Sometimes, the urine metabolic screen will include a crude measure of urine amino acids. Generalized aminoaciduria is seen in the renal Fanconi syndrome but may also be present in normal neonates secondary to immaturity of tubular transport.

Secondary abnormalities in the amino acid profile may be present in a variety of disorders, including liver disease, malnutrition, vitamin deficiencies, and renal tubular disease; it can be difficult to determine whether a given detected abnormality is caused by an inborn error of metabolism or a more common acquired condition. However, amino acid analysis is not typically performed in isolation and other clues to the diagnosis of a metabolic condition are often present in the studies described below.

Urine Organic Acid Analysis

The analysis of urine organic acids by gas chromatography–mass spectrometry (GC-MS) is often the key to diagnosing or excluding the presence of an inborn error of metabolism. Diagnostic metabolites may be absent or difficult to detect once therapy has been initiated and metabolic balance has been restored; therefore, the sample is best obtained during the time of decompensation. The sample may be stored frozen without preservatives for later shipment to a specialist laboratory if facilities for testing are not available. Diagnosis is based on pattern recognition of specific organic acid elevations.

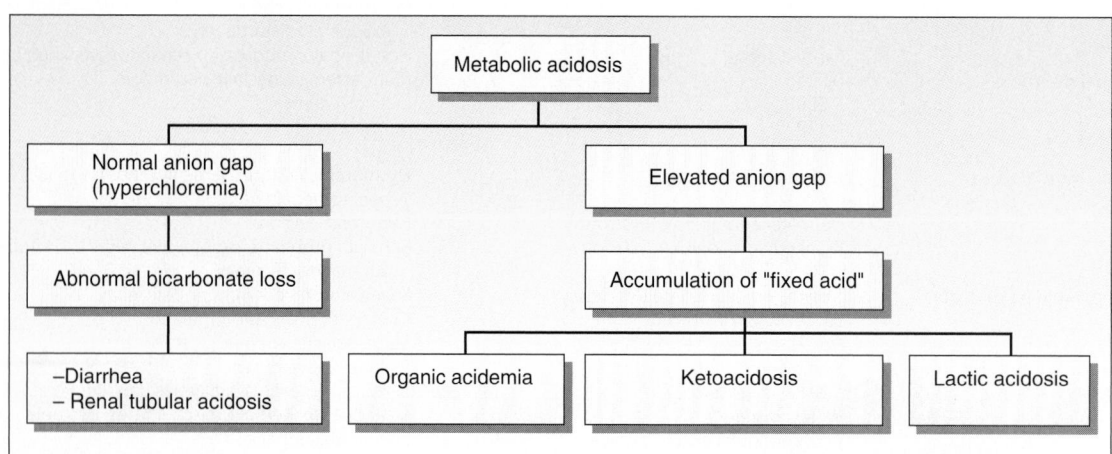

Figure 291-1. Approach to the investigation of metabolic acidosis. (Adapted from Clarke JTR: Acute metabolic illness in the newborn. In A Clinical Guide to Inherited Metabolic Diseases. New York, Cambridge University Press, 1996, p 78, with the permission of Cambridge University Press.)

Table 291-3. Inborn Errors of Metabolism with and without Increased Anion Gap

With Increased Anion Gap

Organic Acidemias

Propionic acidemia
Isovaleric acidemia
Methylmalonic acidemia
Holocarboxylase synthetase deficiency
Multiple acyl-CoA dehydrogenase deficiency
3-Hydroxyisobutyric acidemia
3-Hydroxy-3-methylglutaryl-CoA (HMG-CoA) lyase deficiency

Fatty Acid Oxidation Defects

Short-chain acyl-CoA dehydrogenase (SCAD) deficiency
Medium-chain acyl-CoA dehydrogenase (MCAD) deficiency
Long-chain 3-hydroxyacyl-CoA dehydrogenase (LCHAD) deficiency
Trifunctional protein deficiency
Very long-chain acyl-CoA dehydrogenase (VLCAD) deficiency
Carnitine uptake deficiency
Carnitine-acylcarnitine translocase (CAT) deficiency
Carnitine palmitoyltransferase 2 (CPT-2) deficiency

Congenital Lactic Acidosis

Pyruvate dehydrogenase deficiency
Pyruvate carboxylase deficiency
Mitochondrial respiratory chain disorders

Tricarboxylic Acid Cycle Defects

Fumaric aciduria
α-Ketoglutarate dehydrogenase deficiency

Disorders of Gluconeogenesis

Phosphoenolpyruvate carboxykinase deficiency
Fructose-1,6-bisphophatase deficiency

Without Increased Anion Gap (Renal Tubular Acidosis)

Galactosemia
Hereditary fructose intolerance
Glycogen storage disease, types I and III
Fanconi-Bickel syndrome
Tyrosinemia, type I
Cystinosis
Carnitine palmitoyltransferase 1 deficiency
Mitochondrial respiratory chain disorders
Lowe Syndrome*
Carbonic anhydrase II deficiency†
Wilson disease

*Phosphatidylinositol-4,5-bisphosphate 5-phosphatase deficiency.
†Osteopetrosis with renal tubular acidosis.

Valproate, elemental formulas, and other dietary products (e.g., medium-chain triglycerides (MCT) supplementation) may also lead to the detection of certain organic acids (e.g., octenylsuccinic acid is present in some formulas and adipic acid is an additive in Jello). Intestinal bacterial overgrowth may be severe enough to cause a metabolic acidosis associated with the production of organic acids, especially D-lactic acid. Methylmalonic acid is elevated in vitamin B_{12} deficiency. Drug metabolites may be detected with GC-MS analysis, so providing the testing laboratory with a list of current medications is helpful.

Carnitine Levels

Carnitine (hydroxytrimethylaminobutyric acid) transports long-chain fatty acids across the inner mitochondrial membrane and is therefore essential for the proper function of the fatty acid oxidation cycle. Carnitine is synthesized

by the liver and kidney and is present in the diet, but secondary deficiency is relatively common. Low carnitine levels are common in preterm infants and neonates on total parenteral nutrition without adequate carnitine supplementation for long periods. Patients with some metabolic disorders may also have secondary carnitine deficiency.

In addition to its role in the mitochondrial import of fatty acids, carnitine functions as a "metabolic scavenger" in times of decompensation. In the setting of a metabolic crisis, carnitine forms esters with the unusual, often toxic, metabolites that accumulate in fatty acid oxidation defects or inborn errors of organic acid metabolism. These carnitine esters are then excreted in the urine. Under normal circumstances, the concentration of acylcarnitine esters is low, with most of the plasma carnitine being in a free, unesterified form. An elevation of carnitine esters (an esterified to free carnitine ratio >0.30) may be seen in fatty acid

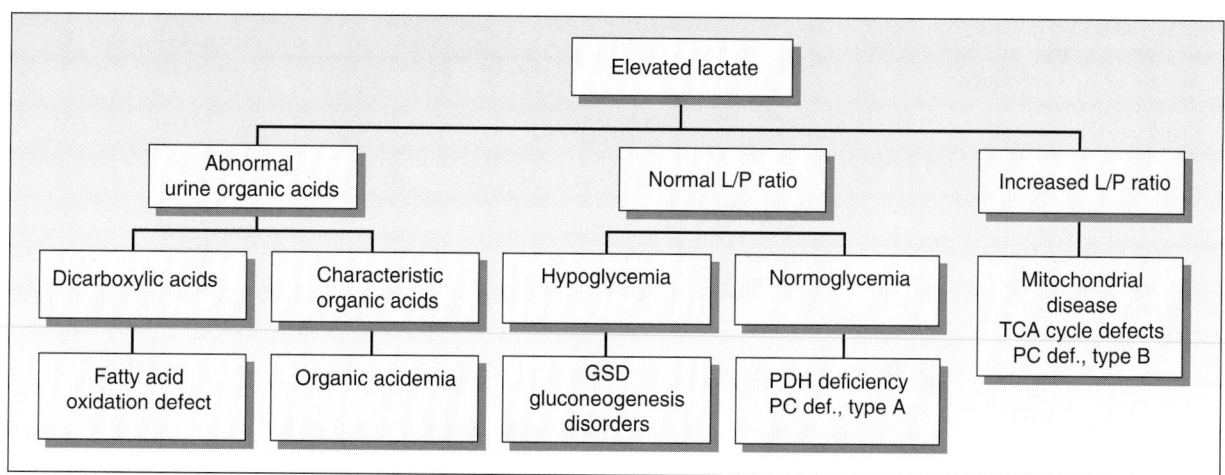

Figure 291-2. Approach to the investigation of lactic acidosis. GSD, glycogen storage disease; L/P, lactate/pyruvate; PC, pyruvate carboxylase; PDH, pyruvate dehydrogenase; TCA, tricarboxylic acid cycle. (Adapted with permission from Scriver CR, Beaudet AL, Sly WS, Valle D (eds): The Metabolic and Molecular Bases of Inherited Disease. New York, McGraw-Hill, 2001.)

Table 291-4. Inborn Errors of Metabolism Associated with Lactic Acidosis

Primary Lactic Acidosis

Defects of pyruvate metabolism
  Pyruvate dehydrogenase deficiency
  Pyruvate carboxylase deficiency
Mitochondrial respiratory chain defects

Secondary Lactic Acidosis

Gluconeogenesis disorders
  Phosphoenolpyruvate carboxykinase (PEPCK) deficiency
  Fructose-1,6-bisphosphatase deficiency
Carbohydrate disorders
  Glycogen storage disease, type I
  Hereditary fructose intolerance
Fatty acid oxidation defects
Organic acidemias
  Holocarboxylase synthetase deficiency
  Biotinidase deficiency*
  Propionic, methylmalonic, isovaleric acidemias
  3-Hydroxy-3-methylglutaryl-CoA (HMG-CoA) lyase deficiency
  Multiple acyl-CoA dehydrogenase deficiency

*Tends to present later in infancy.

oxidation defects, organic acidemias, and ketosis. Such an elevation in the esterified fraction may be a clue to the diagnosis of an underlying inborn error.

Acylcarnitine Profile

The plasma acylcarnitine profile is determined by fast-atom bombardment (FAB) or electrospray ionization tandem mass spectrometry (MS/MS). Whereas free and esterified carnitine levels may offer a clue to the presence of a fatty acid oxidation defect or organic acidemia, the acylcarnitine profile is a diagnostic tool that allows one to determine the biochemical composition of the elevated esterified fraction. Because of its potential for rapid sample processing and detection of multiple disorders virtually simultaneously, MS/MS is being used increasingly in newborn screening programs. MS/MS newborn screening can detect an additional 15 to 25 metabolic disorders and has the potential to detect these conditions presymptomatically or at least to provide physicians caring for acutely ill neonates with crucial diagnostic information.

Very Long-Chain Fatty Acids, Phytanic Acid, Pipecolic Acid, Bile Acid Intermediates, and Plasmalogens

Plasma very long-chain fatty acid, plasma or urine phytanic acid, pipecolic acid, or bile acid intermediates, and erythrocyte plasmalogen analyses are useful tests for the investigation of suspected peroxisomal disorders. These disorders might not show abnormalities that are apparent on routine biochemical testing. Abnormal bile acid levels are also seen in bile acid synthesis defects. Testing by GC-MS or fast atom bombardment–liquid secondary ion mass spectrometry (FAB-LSIMS) is performed only in highly specialized centers.

Mucopolysaccharides, Oligosaccharides, and Sialic Acid

Urine thin layer chromatography (TLC) is a useful screen for the detection of certain lysosomal storage diseases. This is a qualitative method for evaluating patients with

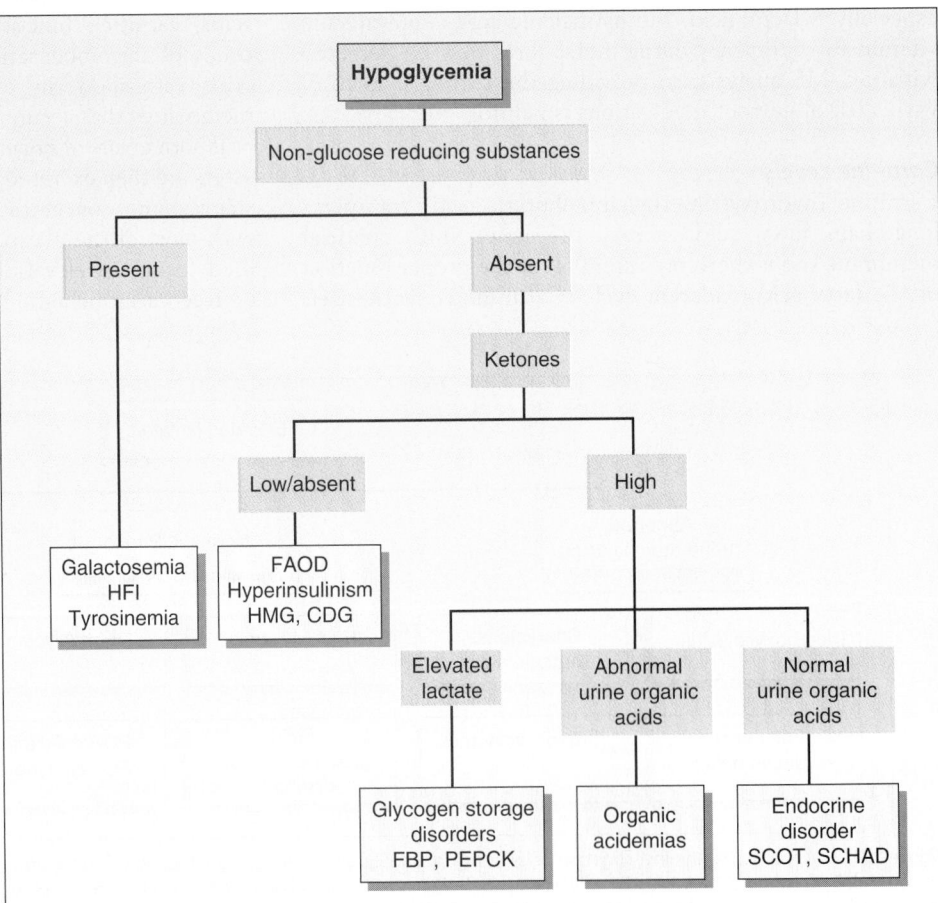

Figure 291-3. Approach to the investigation of hypoglycemia. CDG, congenital disorders of glycosylation (formerly carbohydrate-deficient glycoprotein syndrome); FAOD, fatty acid oxidation disorders; FBP, fructose-1,6-bisphosphatase deficiency; HFI, hereditary fructose intolerance; HMG, 3-hydroxy-3-methylglutaryl-CoA lyase deficiency; PEPCK, phosphoenolpyruvate carboxykinase deficiency; SCHAD, short-chain 3-hydroxyacyl-CoA dehydrogenase deficiency; SCOT, succinyl-CoA:3-oxoacid-CoA transferase deficiency. (*Note:* SCHAD deficiency may also be associated with hypoketotic hypoglycemia, and abnormal urine organic acids suggestive of an FAOD may be present.)

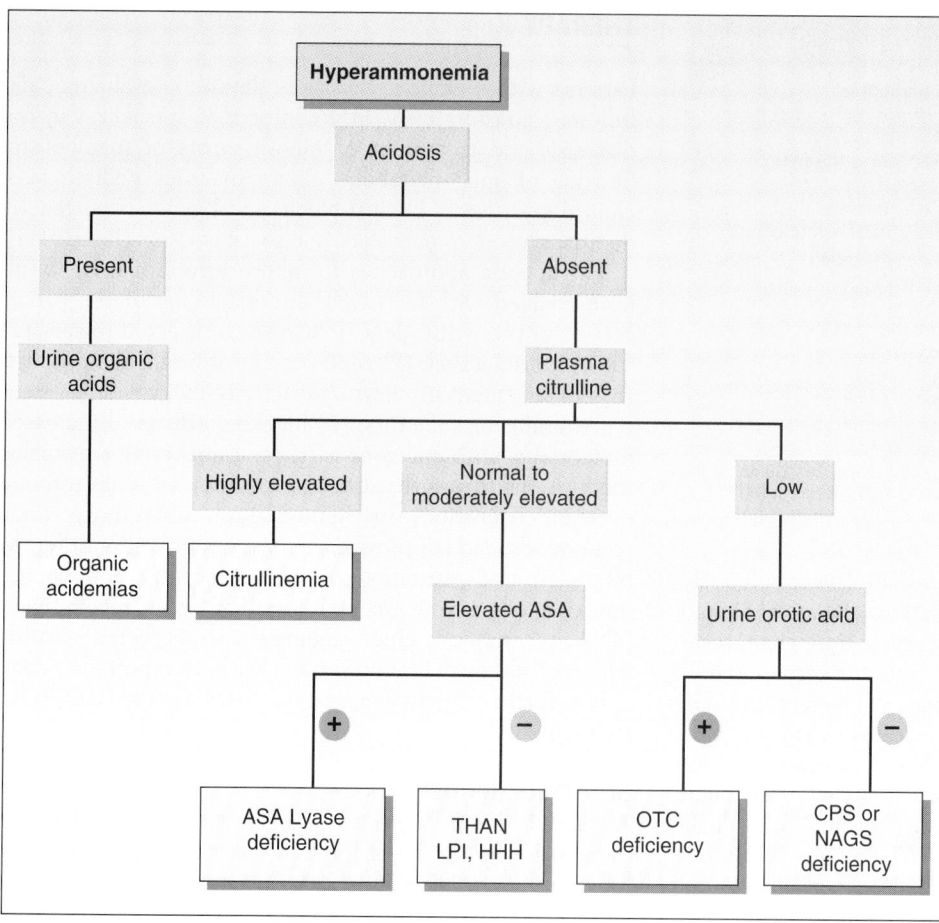

Figure 291-4. Approach to the investigation of hyperammonemia. ASA, argininosuccinic acid; CPS, carbamyl phosphate synthetase; HHH, hyperammonemia-hyperornithinemia-homocitrullinuria syndrome; LPI, lysinuric protein intolerance; NAGS, N-acetylglutamate synthetase; OTC, ornithine transcarbamylase; THAN, transient hyperammonemia of the newborn. (*Note:* Urine orotic acid also tends to be elevated in LPI and HHH, but citrulline concentration is normal.)

nonspecific features of lysosomal disorders, including coarseness, developmental regression, cataracts, hepatosplenomegaly, and dysostosis multiplex. Similar patterns of mucopolysaccharide elevation may be present in different disorders (e.g., Hurler and Hunter syndromes), so enzymology or DNA testing is needed to establish the diagnosis with certainty. Enzymology may be indicated even in the face of normal screening TLC or other analysis (e.g., urine spot testing), since those methods may lack sensitivity. Other disorders, including skeletal dysplasias and rheumatologic disease, also may be associated with abnormal elevation of mucopolysaccharides. Recently, the detection of lysosomal-associated membrane proteins 1 and 2 (LAMP1 and LAMP2) has been used as an initial test in newborn screening studies for lysosomal disorders. Although there is no proven effective therapy for most of these conditions, screening could at least provide the family with a diagnosis and potentially prevent the birth of a second affected sibling.

Additional Analyses

Final confirmation of the presence of an inborn error of metabolism may require molecular genetic (DNA) analysis or enzymology on leukocytes, fibroblasts, liver, or muscle. For further discussion on enzymology, please refer to the CD-ROM supplement.

Table 291-5. Urine Odors Associated with Inborn Errors of Metabolism

Odor	Compound	Disorder
Musty, mousy	Phenylacetate	Classical phenylketonuria
Maple syrup	2-Oxoisocaproic acid	Maple syrup urine disease
Sweaty feet	Isovaleric acid	Isovaleric acidemia
		Multiple acyl-CoA dehydrogenase deficiency (glutaric aciduria type II)
Cat urine	3-Hydroxyisovaleric acid	3-Methylcrotonylglycinuria
		Multiple carboxylase deficiency
Cabbage-like	2-Hydroxybutyric acid	Tyrosinemia type 1
		Methionine malabsorption
Rancid butter	2-Oxo-4-methiolbutyric acid	Tyrosinemia type 1
Acid smell	Methylmalonic acid	Methylmalonic acidemia
Sulfurous	Hydrogen sulfide	Cystinuria
Fish market	Trimethylamine	Trimethylaminuria

Adapted from Blau N, Duran M, Blaskovics ME (eds): Physician's Guide to the Laboratory Diagnosis of Metabolic Diseases. London, Chapman & Hall, 1996.

Table 291-6. Causes of Urine Reducing Substances

Compound	Disorders/Source
Glucose	Diabetes mellitus
	Renal Fanconi syndrome
Galactose	Galactosemia
	Severe liver disease
Fructose	Hereditary fructose intolerance
	Essential fructosuria
Xylose	Pentosuria
4-Hydroxyphenylpyruvic acid	Tyrosinemia
Homogentisic acid	Alkaptonuria
Oxalic acid	Hyperoxaluria
Uric acid	Hyperuricosuria
Ascorbic acid	Exogenous administration
Salicylates	Exogenous administration

Adapted from Blau N, Duran M, Blaskovics ME, (eds): Physician's Guide to the Laboratory Diagnosis of Metabolic Diseases. London, Chapman & Hall, 1996.

Some metabolic disorders are associated with relatively common mutations in some populations. Relatively rapid DNA diagnostic testing, often using polymerase chain reaction (PCR) technology, may be available for certain conditions. However, most inborn errors of metabolism are caused by a number of different mutations in a given gene. Therefore, the interpretation of DNA data must be done with caution. The absence of a detected mutation might simply mean that a limited screen excluded a given patient's mutant allele(s) by default. The picture is complicated further in the analysis of children with suspected mitochondrial disease, because a mutation might not necessarily be detected in all tissues; in general, it is easier to detect an mtDNA mutation in a muscle sample than in leukocytes. If an mtDNA mutation is detected in blood, the diagnosis has been established. On the other hand, if blood analysis is negative, other tissues need to be studied.

Enzymology and DNA studies are best performed by, or in conjunction with, metabolic centers that specialize in the diagnosis and treatment of children with inborn errors of metabolism. If one or more specific DNA mutations are found, there is also the possibility of performing prenatal diagnosis on a chorionic villus sample or amniocytes in any future pregnancy. DNA microchip technology offers the possibility of screening for a large number of mutations rapidly at low cost and will likely be more widely available in the near future (Box 291-2).

Box 291-2. Postmortem Diagnosis

Appropriate specimens should be collected from all children who die unexpectedly from unknown causes. Premortem and perimortem blood and urine samples should be sent for metabolic investigations as outlined in Table 291-2. The neonatal blood spot may also be retrieved for tandem mass spectrometry analysis. If consent is given for an autopsy, portions of muscle, heart, and liver should be snap frozen immediately for possible future analysis. A skin, diaphragm, Achilles tendon, or lung biopsy should also be obtained for establishing a fibroblast cell line. Only by making a diagnosis can the family be provided with accurate genetic counseling for future pregnancy and for evaluations of additional family members at risk.

THERAPY

Patients with metabolic disorders should be evaluated, and followed consultatively, in a center that specializes in the diagnosis and treatment of inborn errors of metabolism. Staffing of such metabolic clinics includes pediatricians, clinical geneticists, clinical biochemical geneticists, genetic dietitians, genetic counselors, and social workers (Box 291-3).

Therapeutic approaches to inborn errors of metabolism have evolved with increasing understanding of the pathogenesis of these disorders. Treatment is directed toward (1) substrate reduction, (2) replacement of metabolic product, (3) enhancement of enzymatic activity by providing essential vitamins or cofactors, (4) blocking effects of increased metabolites with antagonists, (5) administering scavenging medications (drugs that bind to specific metabolites to aid in their excretion) or hemodialysis to remove toxic compounds, and (6) providing enzyme replacement therapy by organ transplantation or, more recently, intravenous injection of enzyme manufactured by using recombinant DNA techniques. Gene therapy also is being actively explored, although limited success has been reported to date.

For further discussion, please refer to the CD-ROM supplement.

Substrate Reduction

A partial dietary restriction of carbohydrates, fats, or protein forms the basis for treating most small molecule metabolic disorders (Table 291-7). Complete restriction of certain foods may be necessary in some conditions.

In addition, a variety of medical food products have been formulated to address the specific requirements of individual inborn errors of metabolism. Formulas and special food products that are low in phenylalanine and supplemented with tyrosine, vitamins, and minerals are extremely effective in controlling the hyperphenylalaninemia associated with PKU; if the special diet is adhered to with care, mental retardation, which is nearly universal in untreated PKU, is prevented. Similarly, medical food products that are low in branched-chain amino acids have been very useful in managing patients with maple syrup urine disease (MSUD), propionic acidemia, and methylmalonic acidemia, although children with these disorders tend to have a less benign course than do those with PKU. Other examples of dietary therapy for metabolic disorders are shown in Table 291-8.

Although great strides have been made in improving the palatability of medical food products, children with inborn errors often must endure dietary restrictions that result in relatively monotonous meals. Therefore, adherence to the

---

Box 291-3. Services Offered in a Biochemical Genetics Clinic

Evaluation by a specialist in biochemical genetics
Complete dietary evaluation by a metabolic nutritionist
Genetic counseling, including prenatal counseling
Coordination of specialized diagnostic testing
Social work evaluation
Education of the patient and family

Table 291-7. Dietary Therapy of Inborn Errors of Metabolism

Type of Dietary Modification	Disorder
Low carbohydrate	Mitochondrial disorders
Low fructose/sucrose	Fructose-1,6-bisphosphatase deficiency
No fructose	Hereditary fructose intolerance
No galactose	Galactosemia
High carbohydrate	Gluconeogenesis disorders
	Glycogen storage disease
	HMG-CoA lyase deficiency
Low fat/cholesterol	Familial hypercholesterolemia
	Lipoprotein lipase deficiency
	SCAD deficiency
	SCHAD deficiency
Low long-chain fats	CPT-1 deficiency, LCAD deficiency, LCHAD deficiency, VLCAD deficiency
High fat (≥50%), low carbohydrate (20%)	Pyruvate dehydrogenase deficiency
Low protein	Urea cycle defects
	Lysinuric protein intolerance
	HHH syndrome
Low phenylalanine	Phenylketonuria
Low tyrosine, phenylalanine	Tyrosinemia, types I and II
Low isoleucine, threonine, methionine, valine	MMA, PA
Low leucine, isoleucine, valine	MSUD
Low leucine	IVA, multiple carboxylase deficiency
Low valine	3-Hydroxyisobutyric aciduria
Low tryptophan, lysine	Glutaric acidemia, type I
High protein	Glycogen storage disease, type III
Low purine	APRT deficiency
High fluid intake	APRT deficiency, cystinuria, XDH deficiency

APRT, adenosine phosphoribosyltransferase deficiency; CPT, carnitine palmitoyltransferase; HHH, hyperammonemia-hyperornithinemia-homocitrullinuria; HMG, 3-hydroxy-3-methylglutaryl; IVA, isovaleric acidemia; LCAD, long-chain acyl-CoA dehydrogenase; LCHAD, long-chain 3-hydroxyacyl-CoA dehydrogenase; MMA, methylmalonic acidemia; MSUD, maple syrup urine disease; PA, propionic acidemia; SCAD, short-chain acyl-CoA dehydrogenase; SCHAD, short-chain 3-hydroxyacyl-CoA dehydrogenase; VLCAD, very long-chain acyl-CoA dehydrogenase; XDH, xanthine dehydrogenase deficiency.

dietary regimen represents a challenge for parents and health care providers who care for these children. Some children may actually self-restrict the intake of a specific food, leading to a clue to the presence of an inborn error or metabolism.

Supplementation of Product
When a block in a biochemical pathway leads to a deficiency of products distal to the defective enzyme, the provision of the deficient metabolite may form an important part of therapy (see Table 291-8).

Cofactor Therapy
Many enzymes in biochemical pathways require vitamins, minerals, or other cofactors for proper functioning. Administering pharmacologic doses of vitamins can overcome a metabolic block if a given enzyme has residual activity. Patients with vitamin-responsive forms of inborn errors often show a dramatic recovery once vitamin therapy is started; vitamin therapy may be lifesaving in some patients who present with a severe metabolic decompensation. On the other hand, some conditions show only a partial response to cofactor therapy, though supplementation might help to improve symptoms in individual

patients. Examples of vitamin and cofactor therapy for inborn errors are listed in the CD-ROM supplement.

Pharmacologic Therapy
The many drugs that are used to treat inborn errors have limited effectiveness. Examples of the wide array of pharmacologic agents used to treat metabolic diseases are listed in the supplemental CD-ROM.

Other Therapies
Enzyme Replacement Therapy
Some lysosomal storage disorders have started to be treated with intermittent (e.g., every 1 to 4 weeks) infusion of enzyme manufactured by recombinant DNA techniques. The enzymes have full biologic activity and are tagged with specific mannose residues that enable them to be targeted to the lysosomes. Although success has been reported in treating Gaucher disease type I and Fabry disease, these disorders are not characterized by neurologic involvement. Enzyme replacement therapy (ERT) for other lysosomal disorders, including Hurler and Hunter syndromes, is being studied in clinical trials. ERT would be expected to work for the peripheral manifestations of these lysosomal storage disorders, but the neurologic features will likely be difficult to treat because of the inability of enzymes to cross the blood-brain barrier.

Organ Transplantation
Organ transplantation may cure the underlying metabolic defect in some inborn errors of metabolism but is also associated with considerable risks. Examples of successful organ transplantation for inborn errors of metabolism include liver transplantation for ornithine transcarbamylase

Table 291-8. Dietary Supplement Therapy of Inborn Errors of Metabolism

Compound	Disorder
Medium-chain triglycerides	CPT-1 deficiency, LCAD deficiency, LCHAD deficiency, VLCAD deficiency
Cornstarch	Fatty acid oxidation defects
	Gluconeogenesis disorders
	Glycogen storage disease
	HMG-CoA lyase deficiency
Mannose	Congenital disorder of glycosylation Ib
Glycine	IVA, MADD
Carnitine	Fatty acid oxidation defects
	MMA, PA, IVA, 3-MCC deficiency, HMG-CoA lyase deficiency
Citrulline	Lysinuric protein intolerance
	Ornithine transcarbamylase deficiency
Arginine	Urea cycle defects*
Trioleate:trierucate 4:1 (Lorenzo's oil)†	X-linked adrenoleukodystrophy
Docosahexanoic acid (DHA)	LCHAD deficiency

*Except arginase deficiency.
†Corrects blood very long chain fatty acid levels but does not halt CNS manifestations or disease progression.
CPT, carnitine palmitoyltransferase; HMG, 3-hydroxy-3-methylglutaryl; IVA, isovaleric acidemia; LCAD, long-chain acyl-CoA dehydrogenase; LCHAD, long-chain 3-hydroxyacyl-CoA dehydrogenase; MADD, multiple acyl-CoA dehydrogenase deficiency (glutaric acidemia, type II); MCC, 3-methylcrotonyl-CoA carboxylase; MMA, methylmalonic acidemia; PA, propionic acidemia; VLCAD, very long-chain acyl-CoA dehydrogenase.

deficiency and carbamyl phosphate synthetase deficiency, combined liver/kidney transplantation for vitamin B_{12}-unresponsive methylmalonic acidemia and primary hyperoxaluria type 1, and bone marrow transplantation for adenosine deaminase deficiency. Bone marrow transplantation has also been attempted in patients with lysosomal storage disorders and X-linked adrenoleukodystrophy with some encouraging results.

Gene Therapy

Gene therapy for inborn errors of metabolism is still in its early stages. Disorders primarily affecting bone marrow or liver are especially attractive candidates for gene therapy because of the relative accessibility to treatment (peripheral intravenous injection would be possible in theory). In addition, a correction of only a few percent of affected cells would potentially result in a cure or at least a significant clinical improvement.

THE METABOLIC CRISIS

Patients with inborn errors of metabolism may present with a severe illness characterized by various combinations of neurologic compromise (lethargy, coma, seizures), multiorgan system failure, metabolic acidosis, hypoglycemia, and hyperammonemia. Unless appropriate therapy is initiated without delay, there is a high risk of morbidity or mortality. The clinical presentation of a child with an inborn error of metabolism may be triggered by weaning, fasting, illness severe enough to cause catabolism, an excess intake of certain foods, or drugs. Common provocative factors in inborn errors of metabolism and associated disorders are listed in Table 291-9.

Management of patients who have or are suspected of having an inborn error of metabolism should be undertaken in consultation with an expert in biochemical genetics

Table 291-9. Provocative Factors in Inborn Errors of Metabolism

Symptoms Triggered by	Disorder
Weaning	Hereditary fructose intolerance
	Fructose-1,6-biphosphatase deficiency
	Maple syrup urine disease
	Organic acidemias
	Urea cycle defects
Catabolism (fever, fasting, infection)	Aminoacidemias
	Organic acidemias
	Fatty acid oxidation disorders
	Urea cycle defects
	Glycogen storage disease
	Gluconeogenesis disorders
Protein	Urea cycle defects
	Maple syrup urine disease
	Organic acidemias
Carbohydrate	Pyruvate dehydrogenase deficiency
	Mitochondrial disease
	Hereditary fructose intolerance
	Fructose-1,6-bisphosphatase deficiency
Medications/drugs	Porphyrias
	Glucose-6-phosphate dehydrogenase deficiency

Adapted from Saudubray J-M, Charpentier C: Clinical phenotypes: diagnosis/algorithms. In Scriver CR, Beaudet AL, Sly WS, Valle D (eds): New York, McGraw-Hill, 2001, p 1330.

Box 291-4. Preventive Care of Patients with Inborn Errors

If a patient with an inborn error has a history of poor fluid intake or gastrointestinal illness, it might be prudent to administer appropriate intravenous fluids with dextrose and observe until symptoms subside.

and metabolic diseases. *If a patient with an inborn error* (especially organic acidemia, urea cycle defect, gluconeogenic disorder, glycogen storage disease, or fatty acid oxidation defect) *has a history of poor fluid intake or gastrointestinal illness, it may be prudent to administer appropriate intravenous fluids with dextrose and observe until symptoms subside, rather than letting the vicious spiral of metabolic decompensation gain full force* (Box 291-4).

If a patient with an organic acidemia has an acute episode of ketoacidosis, intravenous fluids with dextrose should be started immediately. Typically, 10% dextrose plus electrolytes and sodium chloride or sodium bicarbonate are given, the total fluid volume being 150 to 200 mL/kg/day. Most often, the acidosis will resolve with treatment without resorting to bicarbonate use, and bicarbonate use may mask a metabolic crisis that is not optimally treated. A 5% dextrose solution may be adequate in some instances. Care should be taken to avoid fluid overload and the potential complication of cerebral edema. Intravenous carnitine (75 mg/kg/dose every 6 hours) is therapeutic in many organic acidemias and fatty acid oxidation defects. If a patient has a vitamin-responsive form of metabolic disease, the appropriate vitamin should be administered, intravenously if possible. It might be necessary to provide vitamins to comatose patients enterally by feeding tube. In the case of an initial presentation in a previously normal child in whom metabolic disease is suspected, a "vitamin cocktail" may be lifesaving (Table 291-10). Unfortunately, only a small proportion of inborn errors are vitamin responsive, although a dramatic improvement can occur in such cases with the initiation of appropriate therapy.

Hyperammonemia secondary to urea cycle defects may be possible to control with intravenous hydration and dextrose if the elevation in blood ammonia is relatively mild (<200 μmol/L). In more severe cases, intravenous administration of ammonia-scavenging medicines (sodium benzoate and sodium phenylbutyrate) is often necessary. These medications decrease the total body nitrogen load by conjugating with glycine (benzoate) or glutamine (phenylacetate) to form hippuric acid and phenylacetylglutamine, respectively, compounds that can then be

Table 291-10. Empiric Vitamin and Cofactor Therapy for Suspected Inborn Errors of Metabolism

Medication	Route	Dose
Carnitine	IV	100–300 mg/kg/day
Biotin	IV/IM/PO	5–20 mg/day
Riboflavin	IV/PO	50–200 mg/day
Hydroxocobalamin	IM	1000 μg/day
Thiamine	IV	100–400 mg/day

Note: Except for carnitine, doses are not per kilogram.

excreted by the kidneys. Intravenous supplementation of arginine (10% arginine HCl solution) can cause a rapid normalization of blood ammonia levels in argininosuccinic acid lyase deficiency and is also used to treat the acute decompensation associated with other urea cycle disorders (with the exclusion of arginase deficiency). In comatose patients with very elevated, or rapidly rising, plasma ammonia levels, the above measures are usually inadequate to correct the severe hyperammonemia (>500 μmol/L and often >2000 μmol/L). Such a presentation is often encountered in neonates with urea cycle disorders but may also be seen in older children with a catabolic illness. In cases of severe hyperammonemia, the treatment of choice is hemodialysis, sometimes followed by continuous venovenous hemofiltration. Intravenous boluses of sodium benzoate, sodium phenylacetate, and arginine HCl are given concurrently, followed by continuous infusion of these medications. Protein intake is stopped for 24 to 48 hours and is then reintroduced gradually. Peritoneal dialysis is far less effective and, in general, should not be used in the treatment of severe hyperammonemia. Exchange transfusions have no place in the therapy of these disorders today.

Hemodialysis may also be required for the rapid removal of elevated amino acids, for example, branched-chain amino acids in patients with MSUD, though this is falling out of favor and is usually avoided in MSUD owing to the catabolic effects of hemodialysis. Patients with organic acidemias (e.g., propionic, isovaleric, and methylmalonic acidemias) and those with some fatty acid oxidation defects (e.g., carnitine uptake defect, carnitine palmitoyltransferase 1 deficiency, and carnitine-acylcarnitine translocase deficiency) may have ammonia elevations similar to those encountered in urea cycle disorders caused by a secondary inhibition of the urea cycle by toxic metabolites. Measurement of blood gases, electrolytes, and urine ketones may help in distinguishing hyperammonemia secondary to a urea cycle defect from that caused by an organic acidemia. Unlike organic acidemias, urea cycle defects usually are not associated with significant metabolic acidosis or ketosis. However, tissue hypoxia may supervene in the critically ill child, making a distinction difficult in practice.

Preventing or correcting catabolism is an essential part of treating most inborn errors of metabolism. During periods of stress, the body breaks down its stores, releasing glucose, amino acids, and fatty acids in response to the insufficient exogenous energy intake. Tissue breakdown will continue until adequate calories are provided to prevent catabolism. Such breakdown results in further biochemical imbalance as more precursors are provided to a given pathway that is already overloaded. The importance of caloric supplementation is illustrated by the therapy of severe hyperammonemia. Although hemodialysis effectively lowers blood ammonia levels in patients with urea cycle disorders, there tends to be a rebound after dialysis is stopped unless adequate calories are provided (usually 80 to 120 kcal/kg/day) so that further muscle breakdown and endogenous protein release are halted.

CONCLUSIONS

By obtaining appropriate laboratory investigations, the clinician can provide the family with the best chance of arriving at a diagnosis for their child during an extremely stressful time. Establishing a diagnosis permits not only optimal management of the child, but also accurate genetic counseling. Tandem-mass spectrometry testing for a wide variety of aminoacidemias, organic acidemias, and fatty acid oxidation defects is currently being integrated into newborn screening programs throughout the world. Such technology provides new hope for presymptomatic diagnosis and treatment of inborn errors of metabolism, which collectively account for significant morbidity and mortality. The therapy of a patient presenting in an acute metabolic crisis remains particularly challenging. However, considering inborn errors of metabolism in the differential diagnosis and rapidly instituting simple therapy, such as intravenous fluids with dextrose, may be lifesaving.

Additional Resources, CD-ROM

Urine screening tests	Text
Initial laboratory investigation for inborn errors of metabolism	Text
Specialized laboratory examinations	Text
Enzymology	Text
Therapy for inborn errors of metabolism	Text
Bibliography	

SUGGESTED READINGS

Blau N, Duran M, Blaskovics ME (eds): Physician's Guide to the Laboratory Diagnosis of Metabolic Diseases. London, Chapman & Hall, 1996.

Clarke JTR: Acute metabolic illness in the newborn. In A Clinical Guide to Inherited Metabolic Diseases. New York, Cambridge University Press, 1996, pp 176–204.

Pass KA, Lane PA, Fernhoff PM, et al: US newborn screening system guidelines. II: Follow-up of children, diagnosis, management, and evaluation. Statement of the Council of Regional Networks for Genetic Services (CORN). J Pediatr 2000;137(4 suppl):S1–S46.

Saudubray J-M, Charpentier C: Clinical phenotypes: Diagnosis/algorithms. In Scriver CR, Beaudet AL, Sly WS, Valle D (eds): The Metabolic and Molecular Bases of Inherited Disease. New York, McGraw-Hill, 2001, pp 1327–1403.

Steiner RD, Cederbaum SD: Laboratory evaluation of urea cycle disorders. J Pediatr 2001;138:S21–S29.

292 Fluids and Electrolytes

Ann P. Guillot

A distinguishing feature of mammalian physiology is the ability to maintain a balance of water and salts within the body, necessary for a complex multicellular, multiorgan body to exist outside a saltwater environment. Survival depends on maintenance of the following:

- Adequate intravascular volume to ensure delivery of oxygen and nutrients to capillary beds
- Electrolyte intracellular/extracellular gradients (especially Na^+, K^+, and Ca^{++}), crucial for cellular function
- Range-specific osmolality to ensure normal cellular function and cell size

The human body has meticulous and sometimes redundant methods for maintaining fluid and electrolyte balance:

- The brain induces thirst if there is need for free water.
- The gut absorbs water.
- The kidneys reclaim or excrete water and/or electrolytes as necessary.
- Skin acts as an evaporative barrier.
- Lungs and skin together adjust body heat and consequent water loss.
- Lungs, kidneys, and bones help to buffer changes in the acid-base balance.

Diagnosis of the most common problems and abnormalities of fluids and electrolytes, based on an understanding of the previously discussed physiological mechanisms, can be straightforward, since the majority of clinical fluid and electrolyte problems fall within a fairly short list of categories:

- Volume depletion
  - Isotonic
  - Hypertonic
  - Hypotonic
- Water overload
  - Edema
  - Hyponatremia
- Excess water loss
- Excess sodium loss
- Sodium overload
- Potassium overload
- Potassium wasting

This chapter discusses fluid and electrolyte replacement for typical situations seen in children. When clinical attempts to correct fluid and electrolyte problems fail or produce unexpected results, consultation with a specialist or further clinical investigation is recommended.

VOLUME DEPLETION: DEHYDRATION AND LOSS OF ELECTROLYTES

Assessing volume adequacy, deficit, or excess is key to repairing fluid and electrolyte imbalance, to make sure there is adequate volume to ensure delivery of oxygen and nutrients to tissues and to optimize pump efficiency of the heart.

Basic steps for providing fluids and electrolytes to volume depleted patients are as follows:

- If the patient is showing signs of shock or compensated shock, rapidly infuse isotonic fluid to restore intravascular volume. (The patient has clinical findings noted in Table 292-1 for more than 10% severe volume depletion.)
- Provide fluids to replace calculated/observed volume deficit.
- Provide fluid and electrolytes to replace the amounts lost in normal daily metabolism ("maintenance fluids").

Table 292-1. Estimating Fluid Losses by Physical Examination as Percentage of Total Body Weight Lost

	3–6% Volume Depletion (Mild)	6–9% Volume Depletion (Moderate)	10+% Volume Depletion (Severe)
Blood pressure	Normal	Normal	Normal to reduced
Quality of pulses	Normal	Normal or slightly decreased	Moderately decreased
Heart rate	Normal	Increased	Increased
Skin turgor	Normal	Decreased	Decreased
Fontanelle	Normal	Sunken	Sunken
Mucous membranes	Slightly dry	Moderately dry	Very dry
Eyes	Mildly sunken	Moderately sunken	Very sunken
Extremities	Warm, normal capillary refill	Delayed capillary refill	Cool, mottled
Mental status	Normal	Normal to passive	Normal to obtunded
Urine output	Slightly decreased	Decreased (<1 mL/kg/hr)	Very decreased (<<1 mL/kg/hr)
Thirst	Increased	Very increased	Very strong or too obtunded

Table 292-2. How Can the Physical Examination Assessment of Fluid Losses Be Altered?

Hypertonicity/hypernatremia	Decreases the severity of physical exam changes	Sodium stays out of cells Pulls water out of cells Maintains extracellular volume
Hypotonicity/hyponatremia	May increase the severity of physical exam changes	Less osmolar force to keep water in the interstitium

Table 292-3. Distribution of Daily Metabolism Fluid Losses

"Insensible":	Respiratory	15% of total daily losses
	Skin/evaporative	30% of total daily losses
Urinary losses		55% of total daily losses

- Provide enough fluid to replace any ongoing losses that might not have been calculated as part of the "maintenance fluid" volume.

The most common fluid volume abnormality in childhood is volume depletion, since children are prone to illnesses that cause fluid loss. The degree of volume depletion can be assessed by physical examination. Table 292-1 describes physical signs associated with varying degrees of volume depletion, and Table 292-2 lists factors that may influence these physical signs.

Volume depletion may be due to direct fluid loss (diarrhea and vomiting), failure to replace fluids lost in daily metabolism (sweating, respiratory loss, or abnormal urinary losses), or both. All fluid losses must be replaced daily to maintain the body's euvolemic state.

The distribution of normal daily fluid losses is as follows: (1) insensible losses, including respiratory and skin, and (2) urinary losses (Table 292-3). Table 292-4 describes a simple method for determining daily maintenance fluid requirements based on the Holliday-Segar calculation of metabolic rate. Table 292-5 lists factors that can alter daily fluid requirements and ways to calculate fluid replacement on the basis of these alterations.

PROVIDING FLUIDS FOR "MAINTENANCE" OF THE EUVOLEMIC STATE

Assessing the patient's volume status (see Table 292-1) is essential before fluid is provided to maintain a euvolemic state. If the patient appears to be in normal fluid balance, provide fluids as noted for "maintenance" (see Table 292-4). If the patient is unable to take all of the required fluid by the oral route, then fluids must be administered intravenously or by an alternate enteral route, such as a nasogastric tube.

Whenever parenteral fluids are to be provided, it is practical to check the patient's serum electrolytes before beginning, or soon thereafter, to correct for any possible electrolyte imbalance. If the patient's history or physical examination suggests possible impaired renal function, checking the patient's serum creatinine is crucial to avoid fluid overload. When maintenance fluids are administered over time, either intravenously or via enteral/tube feedings, the patient's volume status must be regularly monitored by physical examination, weight, and blood pressure to ensure that the patient does not become overhydrated or remain dehydrated.

Table 292-4. Normal Fluid Losses and Therefore "Maintenance Fluid" Total per Kilogram Body Weight in Healthy People at Rest

Body Weight	Per Day	Per Hour if Evenly Distributed over 24 Hours
0–10 kg total body weight	100 cc/kg/24 hours	4 cc/kg/hr
10–20 kg total body weight	100 cc/kg for the 1st 10 kg + 50 cc/kg for each kg >10 kg	4 cc/kg/hr for the 1st 10 kg + 2 cc/kg/hr for the next 10 kg
>20 kg total body weight	100 cc/kg for the 1st 10 kg + 50 cc/kg for the next 10 kg + 20 cc/kg for each kg >20	4 cc/kg/hr for the 1st 10 kg + 2 cc kg/hr for the next 10 kg + 1 cc/kg/hr for each kg >20 kg

From Holliday Ma: Gamble and Darrow: Pathfinders in body fluid physiology and fluid therapy for children 1914–1964. Pediatric Nephrology 2002;15:317–324.

Table 292-5. Conditions That Can Alter Maintenance Fluid Needs by Altering the Rate of Fluid Loss

Condition	Amount of Change from
Fever	10–12% per degree > 38°C increase
Motor activity	5–30% increase
Tachypnea, hyperpnea (any increase in minute ventilation)	Variable 10–20% increase
Anuria	55–60% decrease
Obligate polyuria or inability to concentrate urine normally (e.g., obstructive uropathy or diabetes insipidus)	Variable increase
Very low-birth-weight babies (large surface area and poor vapor barrier)	50–300% increase

Table 292-6. Recommended Fluids for Maintenance (or Replacement of Normal Daily Fluid Losses) in Otherwise Healthy Patients

Route of Administration	Type of Fluid	Speed of Administration	Other Considerations
Intravenous	D5/normal saline with 40 mEq KCl/L	Evenly divided over 24 hours	
Enteral/PO	Any fluids providing water, Na and K as above	Divided over 24 hours or by bolus	If high osmolality fluids are used, increase extra water.

Note: Usual requirements are 2–4 mEq Na and 2–3 mEq K per 100 cc water per day. Provide volume as noted in Table 292-1 if the patient is euvolemic, healthy, and at rest.

Table 292-7. Recommended Fluids for Maintenance in Patients with No Urinary Losses (i.e., Anuria)

Route of Administration	Type of Fluid	Speed of Administration	Other Considerations
IV, PO, or enteral	Free H_2O only IV—D5W, or TPN with *no* Na or K Give 40% of volume calculated by weight as in Table 292-1	As evenly divided as possible over 24 hours	1. Volume must be decreased to 40% of that noted in Table 292-1 to replace only insensible losses 2. No Na or K will be lost via kidneys, and very little is lost via any other route

Table 292-6 lists the type of fluids that are recommended for replacing normal daily fluid losses and how best to administer these fluids. Table 292-7 lists the type of fluids that are recommended for the patient who has no urinary output. Table 292-8 lists the type of fluids and electrolytes that are recommended for replacing normal daily fluid losses for patients with various conditions that increase daily maintenance fluid loss (see Table 292-5).

PRECAUTIONS DURING PARENTERAL OR NONVOLUNTARY ENTERAL FLUID DELIVERY

In providing fluids to the hospitalized patient, care must be taken to account for conditions that could predispose to the patient to inappropriate retention of free water, such as the syndrome of inappropriate antidiuretic hormone secretion (SIADH), or to excessive salt wasting. Such conditions can be transient in children and may lead to severe hypona-

tremia and consequent seizures, thereby risking central nervous system damage. Table 292-9 lists conditions that may predispose children to SIADH. Table 292-10 lists conditions that may cause salt wasting in childhood.

Since SIADH and salt-wasting conditions are not extremely rare in sick children, whenever intravenous or enteral tube fed maintenance fluids are administered for more than a few hours, the patient's electrolyte status should be monitored, especially when the patient appears ill.

REPLACING VOLUME DEFICIT

Frequently, fluids must be given to return the sick patient to the euvolemic state. When the physical examination (detailed in Tables 292-1 and 292-2) indicates a volume deficit, attention must be focused on rapid volume repletion. The sicker the child, the more likely it is that there will be an electrolyte abnormality accompanying the

Table 292-8. Recommended Fluids for Maintenance of Patients Who Have Had Additional Losses (in Excess of Volume Noted in Table 292-4)

Start with amounts and types of fluids as in Table 292-4 and Table 292-6. Then Add as in this table.

	Examples	Volume to Estimate in Addition to Amounts as in Table 292-2	Content of Extra Fluids in Addition to Those as in Table 292-2	Type of Fluids to Choose for the Additional Increment
Patients with increased insensible losses	Fever	12% for every degree fever > 38°C.	Fluids as noted Free water	IV—D5W PO/enteral—water
	Increased motor activity, tachypnea	Estimate based on degree	Free water	IV—D5W PO/enteral—water
	VLBW infants	May be as high as 300% of amounts estimated by weight alone	Free water	IV—D5W or additional H_2O in TPN (Also, use vapor barrier when possible)
Patients with increased urinary losses	Diabetes insipidus (both central and nephrogenic)	Varies widely—use patient history (prior fluid needs) and assess output continuously to replace appropriately	Free water	IV—D5W or additional water in TPN —Free water ad lib or as necessary to match output
	Obstructive uropathy	Varies widely—use patient history (prior fluid needs) and assess output continuously to replace appropriately	Varies—there may be sodium, bicarbonate, and potassium wasting as well. Check urinary electrolyte content to plan replacement	Depends on urinary losses

Table 292-9. Conditions That Can Predispose Children to SIADH

With Decreased Intravascular Volume, with or without Edema	Without Intravascular Volume Derangement
Nephrotic syndrome	Inflammatory CNS disease (meningitis, encephalitis)
Congestive heart failure	CNS tumors
Liver disease	Pulmonary diseases (severe asthma)
Other forms of hypoalbuminemia	Drugs: cyclophosphamide, vincristine
Severe hypovolemia	Nausea
	Postanesthesia
	Post spinal fusion

Table 292-10. Conditions That Cause Salt Wasting in Childhood

Renal Urine Sodium Content >25 mEq/L	Gut Urine Sodium Content <25 mEq/L
Mineralocorticoid deficiency	Secretory diarrhea
Salt wasting nephropathies	
Cerebral salt wasting	

Box 292-1. Steps for Volume Repletion

- Assess the patient for shock.
- Decreased alertness: poor central nervous system perfusion
- Decreased urine flow: poor renal perfusion
- Decreased bowel sounds: poor gut perfusion
- Capillary refill time > 2 seconds: poor peripheral perfusion
- Restore peripheral perfusion rapidly using *only isotonic fluids* (see Table 292-11).
- Replace the remainder of an estimated volume deficit based on physical examination (see Table 292-1).
- Provide the day's maintenance fluids as well.
- Estimate and replace any ongoing fluid losses.

volume depletion, especially if the volume depletion occurred during hospitalization. If the volume depletion occurred outside the hospital as a result of gastroenteritis, the risk of electrolyte imbalance is considerably lower. Box 292-1 lists steps for volume repletion.

Table 292-11 lists fluids appropriate for rapid volume expansion and methods for administering the fluid. Table 292-12 lists how best to deliver the remaining deficit fluid after rapid fluid expansion. Table 292-13 lists commercially available intravenous fluids, and Table 292-14 suggests uses for the different types of available intravenous fluids.

PRECAUTIONS DURING VOLUME REPLETION

If the patient is initially hyperosmolar (owing to hypernatremia or hyperglycemia), rapid restoration of the entire volume deficit can cause cerebral edema. If hyperosmolarity is present, the rate of deficit replacement must be reduced to allow serum osmolality to decrease at a rate not in excess of 0.5 mEq/L/hour. (Therefore, proper volume repletion for hyperosmolar patients may take much longer than volume repletion for the dehydrated patient who presents with normal serum sodium and glucose.)

ORAL REHYDRATION FOR MILD TO MODERATE VOLUME DEPLETION CAUSED BY GUT LOSSES

When possible, oral rehydration should be attempted; not all fluids must be replenished intravenously. Oral rehydration is best used under the following circumstances:

- When volume depletion is due to only fluid loss from the gut
- When the patient is otherwise well
- When volume depletion is mild to moderate on presentation
- When perfusion has already been restored with intravenous fluids and the patient appears well

Oral rehydration works well when glucose and sodium are provided in equimolar concentrations so that cotransport of sodium and glucose can occur. Higher glucose concentration can exacerbate diarrhea. Table 292-15 lists commercially available oral rehydration fluids. Table 292-16 list fluids commonly used in households for rehydration that are not as effective as oral rehydration solutions.

See Box 292-2 for sample of fluid repletion in infants with moderate dehydration.

Table 292-11. Fluids Appropriate for Rapid Volume Expansion

Type of Fluid	Volume to Administer	Rate of Administration
Crystalloid		
Lactated Ringer	20 cc/kg body weight	As rapidly as IV access will allow
0.9% NaCl	Reassess PE findings	Follow PALS/APLS recommendations on establishing IV access.
Colloid		
Blood products	Repeat 20 cc/kg if symptoms of shock persist	
5% albumin		
Fresh frozen plasma		
Whole blood	Reassess	
Hetastarch	Repeat as necessary	

Note: Fluids less than isotonic will not stay in the intravascular space long enough to reverse shock.

Table 292-12. Replacement fluids for Remaining Deficit When Intravenous Route Is to Be Used

Choose a fluid.	If history of gut losses, try 0.45% NaCl.
	If history of acute bleeding, give blood products.
	If history of excessive insensible losses, check serum electrolytes and consider more free water.
Add KCl (and/or other electrolytes).	After gut losses, replace 60–120 mEq/L or replacement fluids.
Note: KCl can be added to maximum 40 mEq/L.	*Note:* It might take longer to replace the K deficit than it takes to replace volume deficit. Do not slow down the volume replacement to match the K replacement.
Choose a rate of administration.	The deficit can be replaced over 4–8 hours, after which the rest of the day's maintenance can be provided.
Provide the day's maintenance fluids.	Give IV or enterally along with, or following, the deficit replacement.
Replace any ongoing losses.	Examples: diarrhea, NG tube drainage

Table 292-13. Available IV Fluids

	Glucose (g/L)	Na (mEq/L)	Cl (mEq/L)	K (mEq/L)	Osmolality (mOs/L)
Isotonic Fluids					
Normal saline	0	154	154	0	308
Lactated Ringer	0	130	109	4	272
5% albumin	0	100–160	<120	0	
Other Fluids					
D5W	50	0	0	0	278
D5W/¼NS	50	34	34	0	355
¼NS	0	38.5	38.5	0	77
D5W/½NS	50	77	77	0	432
½NS	0	77	77	0	154
25% albumin	0	100–160	<120	0	
5% NaHCO₃	0	595	0	0	1190
8.4% NaHCO₃	0	1000	0	0	2000
Hypertonic saline					
3% NaCl	0	513	513	0	1026
5% NaCl	0	855	855	0	1710

Table 292-14. Suggested Uses for Available IV Fluids

Isotonic fluids	Rapid volume expansion
Lactated Ringer	Trauma, acute volume depletion in previously well patients
Normal saline	Rapid volume expansion in hyperosmolar patients, DKA, hypernatremic dehydration
0.2 and 0.45% saline	Provision of maintenance fluids to most people
Hypertonic saline	Correction of severe hyponatremia—only when severe CNS symptoms are occurring
NaHCO₃ (5% or 8.4%)	Correction of severe metabolic acidosis—Must be administered slowly (over 2–4 hours)

Table 292-15. Content of Available Oral Rehydration Solutions

	Na (mEq/L)	K (mEq/L)	Base (mEq/L)	Glucose (g/dL)	Osmolality (mOs/L)
WHO-ORS	90	20	30	2.0	310
Pedialyte	45	20	30	2.5	270
Ricelyte	50	25		3.0	290
Lytren	50	25	30	2.0	

Table 292-16. Content of Frequently Used Oral Fluids

	Na (mEq/L)	K (mEq/L)	Base (mEq/L)	Glucose (g/dL)	Osmolality (mOs/L)
Ginger ale	3	1	4	5–15	540
Apple juice	3	28	0	10–15	700
Gatorade	20	3	3	4.6	330
Tea	0	5	0	0	5

Box 292-2. Sample Strategy for Volume Repletion in 10-kg Infant with Moderately Severe Fluid Loss from a 3-Day History of Gastroenteritis*

A. Physical Exam

Heart rate: 160
Respiratory rate: 20
Blood pressure: 100/50
SaO$_2$ 93% in room air, afebrile
Pale, lethargic
Capillary refill time 3 seconds
Estimated volume deficit about 10% of total body weight

B. Treatment

Establish intravenous access, and draw serum sodium level.
Give IV fluids to reestablish peripheral perfusion.
  200 cc normal saline as a rapid infusion.
  Recheck physical findings: capillary refill 2 seconds.
Calculate total deficit based on initial physical examination.
  Total deficit = 1000 cc (including 200 cc given as bolus)
  Remaining to be given = 800 cc
Calculate "maintenance" needs for the day based on weight.
  Review any reasons for alteration of the maintenance rate.
  Maintenance rate = 1000 cc/day
Calculate any ongoing losses.
  No diarrhea noted in past several hours
  Ongoing losses = none (at least at present).
Check serum electrolytes to confirm that serum Na is normal:
  Serum Na = 140
Give 800 cc IV as 0.45% NaCl with 40 mEq/L KCl over 8 hours at 100 cc/hour.
Then give 1000 cc 0.2% NaCl with 40 mEq/L KCl over the next 16 hours at 62.5 cc/hour to complete the day's fluid needs.

C. Alternative Treatment

Establish IV access and draw serum sodium level.
Give IV fluid bolus to establish peripheral perfusion.
  200 cc 0.9% NaCl as a rapid infusion
  Recheck of PE: capillary refill now 2 seconds
  Infant more alert, heart rate down to 120/minute
Start 0.45% NaCl with 40 mEq/L KCl at 100 cc/hour, and do the following:
  Simultaneously start oral rehydration solution (ORS).
  When the infant is taking ORS well, discontinue the IV fluids.
Complete the volume repletion with ORS to total 1000 cc.
Give an additional 1000 cc breast milk or infant formula in the same day.

*Weight 3 days ago 10 kg, admission weight 9 kg.

COMMON ELECTROLYTE ABNORMALITIES

The following protocols describe steps for correcting hypernatremia, hyponatremia, hypokalemia, and hyperkalemia.

SODIUM IMBALANCE

Abnormalities of the serum sodium concentration are a signal of abnormalities of total body water and osmolality. There might be no actual deficit or excess of sodium.

Serum osmolality can be estimated by using the serum sodium, blood urea nitrogen (BUN), and glucose as follows:

$$\text{Serum Osm} = (2 \times [\text{Na}]) + \text{glucose}/18 + \text{BUN}/2.6$$

Hypernatremia

When serum sodium is greater than 150, hyperosmolality must be considered in planning treatment, and serum osmolality must be confirmed either directly or indirectly. When serum sodium is greater than 170, appropriate fluids must be provided slowly to avoid cerebral edema. Box 292-3 lists a pathway for treating hypernatremia of 175 mEq/L or more.

Hyponatremia

Understanding the cause of a patient's hyponatremia requires that the patient's volume status be assessed (Table 292-17). In addition, the urine osmolality, urine Na concentration, and serum creatinine can be helpful (Box 292-4). Box 292-5 lists pathways for treating hyponatremia.

Box 292-3. Patient with Serum Sodium of 175 mEq/L

1. Calculate water deficit.
   a. Assume that the volume deficit is all free water.
   b. Assume that the total body water = 0.6 × weight (kg)
   c. Water deficit (liters) = TBW × [(measured S$_{Na}$/135) − 1]
2. Check for other factors that may elevate serum osmolality.
   a. Measure osmolality directly.
   b. Calculate osmolality = 2 × [Na] + glucose/18 + BUN/2.8.
3. Hypernatremia is frequently discovered after the initial bolus has already been given to establish perfusion.
4. Subsequent fluid repletion should be administered as 0.2% NaCl, and the rate should be slowed to achieve a drop in serum Na no greater than 0.5 to 1.0 mEq/L/hour.

Table 292-17. Reasons for Hyponatremia

Serum sodium may be depressed because of the following:	
Actual total body water excess	SIADH
	Congestive heart failure
	Renal failure or nephrotic syndrome
	Water intoxication
Osmotic shift of water out of cells	Hyperglycemia
Spurious elevation (where serum space is occupied by large molecules)	Hyperlipidemia
	Hyperproteinemia
Actual sodium deficit (with volume deficit)	Salt-wasting nephropathies
	Mineralocorticoid deficit
	Secretory diarrhea

POTASSIUM IMBALANCE

When measuring serum potassium, keep in mind that most body potassium (K^+) is intracellular and is balanced by extracellular sodium. If hydrogen cations [H^+] are elevated (i.e., acidosis), K^+ will shift out of cells. As acidosis resolves, K^+ will shift back into cells. This phenomenon often occurs during treatment of diabetic ketoacidosis.

Also, blood collection technique is important, as spurious hyperkalemia is associated with red blood cell lysis, especially when blood specimens are obtained by heel stick or by venipuncture with a tiny needle.

True hyperkalemia occurs when K^+ enters the serum more rapidly than it can be excreted. The source of K^+ excess can be endogenous (the breakdown of cells and the release of intracellular K^+) or exogenous (either dietary or a parenteral source).

Hyperkalemia

Table 292-18 lists causes and consequences of hyperkalemia. Box 292-6 lists pathway for treating hyperkalemia.

Box 292-4. Hyponatremia Cause Based on Urine Sodium Content, Osmolality

If the patient appears dry and the following occurs:
Urine Na is low and urine osmolality is high, consider these:
  GI losses
  Cystic fibrosis with increased insensible losses
Urine Na is high and urine osmolality is low or isotonic, consider these:
  Obstructive uropathy with salt wasting
  Other forms of renal salt wasting
  Adrenal insufficiency or congenital adrenal hyperplasia
  If the patient appears euvolemic or edematous and the following occurs:
Urine Na is high and urine osmolality is also high, consider this:
  SIADH
Urine Na is low and urine osmolality is low, consider this:
  Psychogenic polydipsia or water intoxication
Urine Na is low and urine osmolality is high, consider these:
  Congestive heart failure
  Nephrotic syndrome
  Cirrhosis
Urine Na is high and urine osmolality is isotonic, consider these:
  Diuretic use
  Renal failure

Box 292-5. Treatment for Hyponatremia

If the patient has serum sodium of 118 mEq/L, the patient appears too dry by physical examination, and neurologic examination is normal, follow these guidelines:
1. Suspect that the physical examination assessment of volume depletion overestimates total body deficit.
2. Suspect the presence of mild cerebral edema.
3. Replace deficit slowly (allow serum [Na^+] to rise at a rate of 0.5 mEq/L per hour.
4. Use 0.9% NaCl for the deficit replacement fluid, given over 48 hours.
5. Use 0.45% NaCl for the maintenance fluid.
6. Check serum electrolytes regularly to avoid too rapid correction.
7. Monitor oxygenation and supplement O_2 as needed to keep SaO_2 > 95%.
   If the patient has serum sodium 118 and is having seizures, follow these guidelines:
1. Estimate volume depletion by physical examination.
2. Give 3% NaCl to increase serum sodium by a small increment (~3 mEq/L).
   a. Give 3% NaCl (513 mEq/L) or 5% NaCl (85 5mEq/L) to provide
      mEq = patient's weight (in kg) × 0.6 × desired increment change in serum Na, or
   b. Give 3% NaCl at 2 cc/kg total body weight.

Hypokalemia

To produce hypokalemia, there must be potassium wasting or decreased intake over a prolonged period, since there is a large intracellular store of potassium within the body, and the kidney has a large capacity to conserve potassium. Table 292-19 lists causes and consequences of hypokalemia. Box 292-7 lists treatment for hypokalemia.

SUMMARY

For most children who require fluid replacement, deciding how much and which fluid to administer is reasonably simple and straightforward based on the patient's history and physical examination findings and the patient's electrolyte and renal function status. In general, the sicker the patient, the sooner and more frequently the patient should be assessed, by both clinical and laboratory examination, to determine whether clinical estimates made at the start of fluid and electrolyte therapy were accurate and that current

Table 292-18. Hyperkalemia Causes and Consequences

Causes	Increased load	Catabolism
		Dietary or iatrogenic
	Decreased excretion	Renal failure
		Renal tubular abnormalities
		Adrenal insufficiency
		K^+-sparing diuretics
Consequences	Cardiac and neuromuscular	Severity directly related to ratio: extra/intracellular [K^+]

Box 292-6. Treatment of Severe Hyperkalemia: A Three-Phase Approach

Note: Treatment of hyperkalemia is aimed at restoring the balance of intracellular to extracellular K^+, since ratio imbalance can cause cardiac arrhythmias.

1. Stabilize the membrane effects of high extracellular/ intracellular $[K^+]$ ratio.
   a. Ca gluconate 10% 0.5 to 1.0 mg/kg IV slow push, or
   b. CaCl 100 mg/mL 0.2 cc/kg/dose: can be used only in a central vein
   c. Effect: immediate
   d. Duration: 10 to 15 minutes; therefore might need to be repeated
2. Shift K^+ into cells to decrease the extracellular/intracellular $[K^+]$ ratio.
   a. $NaHCO_3$ 1 to 2 mEq/kg IV over 30 to 60 minutes (more might be needed if there is a large deficit)
      i. Effect: within 30 minutes
      ii. Duration: up to 2 hours
      iii. *Note:* Cannot be mixed with calcium-containing solutions.
   b. Glucose (to induce an endogenous insulin surge) 0.5 to 1.0 g/kg IV over 15 minutes
      i. Effect: in 15 to 30 minutes
      ii. Duration: 4 to 6 hours

   iii. If insulin is needed, use 0.3 unit regular insulin per gram of glucose given; administer insulin as a drip over 2 hours.
   c. Beta agonists: albuterol nebulizer or MDI
      i. Effect: within 1 to 5 minutes
      ii. Duration: 1 to 2 hours
      iii. Does not require IV access
      iv. May increase heart rate
3. Remove K^+ from the body.
   a. Increase the glomerular filtration rate and tubular flow rate if possible.
      i. Expand intravascular volume if the patient's cardiovascular system will tolerate it and if the patient has renal function that will allow diuresis.
   b. Diuretics: furosemide 1 mg/kg IV
      i. Effect: depends on renal function
   c. Sodium polystyrene (Kayexelate): 1 g/kg
      i. Onset (when used as an enema): >2 hours
      ii. Onset (when used PO): 6 to 12 hours
      iii. Has caused bowel perforations when used as PR in postoperative patients
   d. Dialysis
      i. When the previously mentioned modalities are ineffective

Table 292-19. Hypokalemia Causes and Consequences

Causes	Decreased intake	Dietary
	Renal losses	Intrinsic defects
		Diuretics
		Renal response to gastrointestinal H^+ loss and volume depletion
		Hyperaldosteronism
Consequences	Muscle weakness	
	Loss of renal concentrating ability	Vacuolization of tubular cells
	Myocardial conduction abnormalities	Exacerbation of digoxin toxicity
Treatment	Total deficit cannot be known until:	Acid-base abnormalities are corrected and results of attempts at correction are known

Box 292-7. Treatment of Hypokalemia

1. When an acidemic patient is being treated, anticipate the need for potassium supplementation, especially in the setting of diabetic ketoacidosis, as those patients have been experiencing an osmotic diuresis for a few days at least and often for longer.
2. In a conscious patient who has mild symptoms and who is on oral therapies, PO supplementation with KCl or Kphos may suffice.
3. When K^+ deficiency has been caused by a reversible problem (e.g., K-wasting diuretics, DKA), reverse it as soon as possible.
4. In order for the provider to watch for arrhythmias, which may be caused by overly rapid infusion, patients experiencing severe symptoms must be on a cardiac monitor if they are to receive bolus KCl therapy.
5. If KCl can be added to other IV fluids so that the concentration is < 40 mEq/L, a cardiac monitor is not necessary.

patient response matches expectations. When the planned fluid and electrolyte treatment does not result in the expected resolution, the patient must be reassessed, and consultation should be considered.

SUGGESTED READINGS

Holliday MA: Gamble and Darrow: Pathfinders in body fluid physiology and fluid therapy for children 1914–1964. Pediatr Nephrol 2000;15:317–324.

Manz F, Wentz A, Sichert-Hellert W: The most essential nutrient: Defining the adequate intake of water. J Pediatr 2002;141:587–592.

Moritz ML, Ayus JC: The changing pattern of hypernatremia in hospitalized children. Pediatrics 1999;104:435–439.

Moritz ML, Ayus JC: Disorders of water metabolism in children: Hyponatremia and hypernatremia. Pediatr Rev 2002;23:371–379.

Sarnaik AP, Meert K, Hackbarth R, Fleishmann L: Management of hyponatremic seizures in children with hypertonic saline: A safe and effective strategy. Crit Care Med 1994;19:758–762.

293

Blood Product Transfusion

F. Leonard Johnson and Jason Lang

"Approximately 32,000 pints of blood are used in the USA every day."

National Volunteer Blood Donor Statistic

This chapter describes the indications, administration, benefits, and risks of available blood products. Fractionation of a unit of whole blood can provide packed red blood cells (PRBCs), platelets, granulocytes, fresh frozen plasma, and cryoprecipitate and allows for transfusion of the most specific component necessary. The indications, dosage, and effects of blood components used for transfusions in pediatric patients are shown in Table 293-1. Blood product transfusions in pediatric patients are also associated with special considerations, which are summarized in Box 293-1.

Although blood product transfusion has become increasingly safer with the recognition and prevention of hemolytic reactions and transmission of infectious agents, blood products should be transfused only on the basis of strict clinical and laboratory criteria, when no other alternative therapy is available and the benefits clearly outweigh the risks. For example, children with iron deficiency anemia can have extremely low hemoglobin levels (e.g., <5 mg/dL) but respond to iron replacement and do not need a red blood cell transfusion.

PACKED RED BLOOD CELLS

PRBC transfusions increase the oxygen-carrying capacity in anemic patients and help to ensure adequate tissue oxygenation. One unit of PRBCs derived from a routine blood donation is equivalent to 250 to 300 mL of red cells, with a hematocrit of 50% to 80% and, depending on the preservatives used, a shelf life of 35 to 42 days. Fresh

PRBCs have better oxygen-carrying capacity and are preferable in patients with cardiopulmonary disease. The longer storage time increases extracellular potassium, producing an increased risk for symptomatic hyperkalemia in large-volume transfusions.

Indications

Children and Adolescents

Guidelines for the transfusion of PRBCs are summarized in Table 293-2. The decision to transfuse PRBCs should be based on the patient's clinical condition, the cause and expected course of the underlying anemia, and whether other therapies such as iron or recombinant human erythropoietin therapy would be just as effective.

Generally, PRBCs are transfused in patients whose hemoglobin has fallen to 7 g/dL or less or to 8 g/dL or less in patients with cardiopulmonary compromise or active bleeding. In acutely ill children on assisted ventilation, it is a common practice to maintain the hemoglobin level even closer to the normal range. With anemias that develop slowly, the decision to transfuse red cells should not be based purely on the hemoglobin level. Children with chronic anemia may be asymptomatic despite very low hemoglobin levels and might not require transfusion until the hemoglobin level drops to less than 7 g/dL.

Premature Infants

All infants experience a decline in circulating red blood cell volume during the first week in life. This decline is more rapid and the hemoglobin level falls to lower levels in prematurely born infants because they are slow to produce and respond to appropriate levels of erythropoietin when compared to full-term infants. In addition, these infants with the smallest circulating red blood cell volumes are subject to significant phlebotomy blood loss associated with

Table 293-1. Blood Components for Transfusions in Pediatric Patients

Component	Indication	Dosage	Expected Increment
Red blood cells	Increase oxygen-carrying capacity	10–15 mL/kg	2–3 g/dL rise in hemoglobin (depends on anticoagulant/preservative)
Platelets	Correct/prevent bleeding due to thrombocytopenia or platelet dysfunction	10–15 mL/kg or 1 unit/10 kg (patients >10 kg)	50,000/mm³ rise in platelet count (ideal)
Fresh frozen plasma	Factor deficiency	10–15 mL/kg	15–20% rise in factor level
Cryoprecipitate	Deficiency of factor XIII or fibrinogen	1–2 units/10 kg (volume of a unit will vary: maximum of 15 mL)	60–100 mg/dL rise in fibrinogen

Modified from Pisciotto P (ed): Pediatric Hemotherapy Data Card. Bethesda, Md, American Association of Blood Banks, 2002.

laboratory testing. Additional factors contributing to the risk of tissue hypoxia include the diminished capacity of neonatal red cells to offload oxygen owing to the diminished interaction between fetal hemoglobin and 2,3 diphosphoglycerate and the impairment of neonatal hepatic and neurologic function. As a result, these infants often require PRBC transfusions. In neonates who require multiple small-volume transfusions, the blood bank divides a compatible regular unit into multiple small aliquots. These products should be irradiated to prevent graft-versus-host disease (GVHD) and should be leukodepleted to prevent cytomegalovirus (CMV) infection.

Practices vary, but in general, PRBCs should be transfused to maintain a higher hemoglobin level than for older children and one that is appropriate for the infant's clinical condition. For example, neonates with severe respiratory disease requiring ventilator support are usually transfused to maintain a hemoglobin level of 13.0 g/dL on the basis that red cells containing adult hemoglobin provide optimal oxygen delivery in the setting of diminished pulmonary function. For those facing surgery, a level of 10.0 g/dL is indicated because of the limited ability of the infant heart, lungs, and vasculature to compensate for the anemia. Premature infants who are not critically ill but develop moderate anemia do not necessarily require red blood cell transfusions.

Table 293-2. Indication Guidelines for Packed Red Blood Cell Transfusions

Condition	Hemoglobin	
	Children	Infants*
Surgery	<8.0 g/dL	<10.0 g/dL
Significant Cardiopulmonary disease	<13.0 g/dL	<13.0 g/dL
Symptomatic chronic anemia	<7.0 g/dL	<8.0 g/dL
Marrow failure	<7.0 g/dL	<8.0 g/dL

*First 4 months of life.

Administration

The usual volume of PRBCs administered is 10 to 15 mL/kg of PRBCs over 3 to 4 hours. This usually raises the hemoglobin level by 2 to 3 g/dL. Patients who are profoundly anemic (hemoglobin <5 g/dL) or at risk for heart failure or fluid overload should be transfused at a slower rate (e.g., 3 to 5 mL/kg over 3 to 4 hours) with careful monitoring of vital signs. Ideally, PRBCs should be infused within 4 hours of leaving the blood bank.

Special red blood cell products are indicated in certain situations. *Leukodepleted PRBCs*, produced by specialized filtering of freshly donated PRBCs prior to storage, are indicated for patients with a history of previous transfusion-associated febrile reactions, for decreasing the risk of CMV transmission, and for reducing exposure to HLA antigens. *Washed PRBCs* are given to prevent recurrent allergic reactions. *Frozen PRBCs* are used in the setting of autologous transfusion support or to store rare red blood cell phenotypes.

Special Situations
Acute Autoimmune Hemolytic Anemias
The acute autoimmune hemolytic anemias that are susceptible to transfusion-related complications are the warm and cold autoimmune hemolytic anemias. IgG antibodies that are reactive at 37°C cause warm autoimmune hemolytic anemias. Prednisone is the first line of therapy, but transfusion may be necessary for a life-threatening anemia (hemoglobin < 5 g/dL). The antibody usually reacts with Rh-like antigens on the red cells, and an incompatible cross-match is common. In this setting, small volumes of the most compatible PRBC units are transfused after pretreatment with corticosteroids. The cause of cold autoimmune hemolytic anemia is usually IgM antibodies that are reactive at 0°C to 30°C. They cause hemolysis even after the blood warms centrally to 37°C. In this situation, a servo-temperature blood warmer is used to reduce hemolysis of transfused cells.

Chronic Hereditary Anemias
Patients with hereditary anemias such as the thalassemias and, in certain clinical settings, sickle cell disease often benefit from a chronic red blood cell transfusion program. Finding compatible red blood cells, however, may become difficult over time. For example, patients of African descent have different rates of expression of common red cell antigens, and 30% may become alloimmunized from routinely typed multiple PRBC transfusions. This risk can be decreased in children with sickle cell disease by obtaining a full red blood cell phenotype and administering PRBCs matched for certain antigens (e.g., C, D, E, and Kell antigens) and any other specific antigen for which the patient has preexisting antibodies.

PLATELET TRANSFUSIONS

Platelet concentrates are used to prevent or stop bleeding from thrombocytopenia or abnormalities of platelet function. Platelets are collected from units of routinely donated whole blood and pooled (random donor platelets) or collected from a single donor by the technique of platelet apheresis. One unit of random donor platelets contains more than 5.5×10^{10} platelets, and one unit of single-donor apheresis platelets has over 3×10^{11} platelets (equivalent to 6 units of random donor platelets). Platelet concentrates are stored at room temperature and have a maximum shelf life of 5 days.

Indications

Children and Adolescents

Serious or spontaneous bleeding is rare until the platelet count drops below 50,000/mm³. Platelet transfusions are indicated when active bleeding is occurring or an invasive surgical procedure is planned and the platelet count is below 50,000/mm³.

The most common indication for prophylactic platelet transfusion is thrombocytopenia secondary to marrow failure associated with aplastic anemia, cancer, particularly acute leukemia, or chemotherapy. Traditionally, platelet transfusions in this setting have been given to maintain a platelet count of 20,000/mm³ or greater. Recent studies, however, suggest that this threshold is too high and that 10,000/mm³ should be the trigger level for a prophylactic platelet transfusion in the stable patient who is not bleeding. This lower level decreases the exposure to platelet transfusions and lowers the risk of the development of resistance to transfused platelets (platelet refractoriness). Maintaining a platelet level of at least 20,000/mm³ is prudent in children with hepatic, renal, or pulmonary complications (Table 293-3).

Transfusion with platelets is indicated for children who have inherited or acquired disorders of platelet function who are actively bleeding or who are undergoing an invasive surgical procedure.

There is no indication for platelet transfusions in patients with idiopathic thrombocytopenic purpura regardless of the platelet count, except in the extremely rare event of life-threatening hemorrhage (when platelets are transfused together with intravenous immunoglobulin).

Premature Infants

Premature infants are at greater risk for life-threatening hemorrhage, particularly intraventricular bleeding, because they have low numbers of bone marrow megakaryocytes, low thrombopoietin levels, and accelerated platelet destruction. For these reasons, the platelet count is usually kept at

higher levels than in older children. The decision to transfuse platelets is based on the clinical condition of the infant, the presence or absence of bleeding, or whether an invasive surgical procedure is necessary.

Prophylactic platelet transfusions are usually given in a stable neonate to maintain a platelet count of 20,000/mm³ or above. In extremely preterm infants or those being treated with medications that may affect platelet function, prophylactic platelet transfusions are given to maintain a platelet count of at least 50,000/mm³. The threshold rises to 100,000/mm³ for the critically ill infant.

Administration

One unit /10 kg of random donor platelets given over 15 to 30 minutes or one unit of single-donor apheresis platelets ideally raises the platelet count by 50,000/mm³. In neonates, 5 to 10 mL/kg of a standard platelet concentrate is infused as quickly as the clinical condition allows. Just as for PRBCs, platelet units, given to neonates and all immunosuppressed patients, should be irradiated and leukodepleted.

Platelet concentrates do contain less than 1 mL/unit of red blood cells, and so ABO- and Rh-compatible units should be used when possible. This is done to prevent isoagglutin-caused hemolysis caused by passive anti-A or anti-B antibodies in recipients who are type A, B, or AB when the platelet donor is type O. Patients receiving chronic platelet transfusions should receive leukocyte-depleted and type-specific platelets to try to prevent platelet refractoriness. Rh-immune globulin should be administered to prevent Rh-sensitization when Rh-positive platelets are given to an Rh-negative female patient. Neonates with alloimmune thrombocytopenia should receive washed maternal platelets.

Risks

Platelet Refractoriness

Refractoriness to platelet transfusions can be a major clinical problem. Patients requiring multiple platelet transfusions are at risk from alloimmunization caused by alloantibodies to HLA antigens on the platelet surface. When this occurs, there is no, or a less than expected, rise in the platelet count following a platelet transfusion. Although an increasing number of platelet transfusions predisposes a patient to refractoriness, some patients develop this complication more rapidly than others. To determine why a patient has become refractory to platelet transfusions, the platelet count is checked at 1 hour and then at 24 hours following the platelet transfusion. No rise in the platelet count 1 hour after infusion suggests antibody-mediated destruction. An initial rise followed by a greater than expected fall in the platelet count at 24 hours occurs when platelet survival is decreased by sepsis, disseminated intravascular consumption (DIC), or splenic sequestration.

Platelet survival can be increased by the use of leukocyte-depleted, HLA-matched, single-donor apheresis platelets in patients who have developed platelet refractoriness. Other interventions include giving intravenous immune globulin or corticosteroids before the transfusion or transfusing large amounts of random donor platelets to absorb antibody followed by transfusing single-donor matched platelets.

Table 293-3. Indication Guidelines for Platelet Transfusions

Condition	Platelet Count	
	Children	Infants*
Bleeding	<50,000/mm³	<100,000/mm³
Prior to surgery	<50,000/mm³	<50,000/mm³
Marrow Failure		
Other risk factors	<20,000/mm³	<100,000/mm³
No other risk factors	<10,000/mm³	<50,000/mm³
Stable	<10,000/mm³†	<20,000/mm³
Unstable	<20,000/mm³	<100,000/mm³
Platelet dysfunction and bleeding	Any	Any

*First four months of life.
†Excluding idiopathic thrombocytopenic purpura.

GRANULOCYTE TRANSFUSIONS

Indications

Cytokines (e.g., granulocyte-colony stimulating factor), which stimulate the production of granulocytes in the marrow, have enabled large numbers of granulocytes to be mobilized in donors. This development has recently rekindled interest in, and studies of, the role and effectiveness of granulocyte transfusions in preventing or treating infections. To date, however, no study has clearly defined the indications for granulocyte transfusions in pediatrics. Preparation of granulocyte concentrates by leukopheresis of a donor is difficult and expensive, and the collection and transfusion of granulocytes pose potential risks for both donor and recipient.

The one indication that is generally agreed upon is the neonate or infant with prolonged neutropenia and life-threatening sepsis who has not responded to intensive broad-spectrum antibiotics and the administration of granulocyte-colony stimulating factor.

Administration

A standard concentrate contains 1×10^{10} granulocytes in 200 to 300 mL of plasma. Storage is at room temperature, and the granulocytes are administered through a standard filter within 24 hours of collection. Granulocytes are given in a dose of 1 to 1.5×10^{10} granulocytes/M^2/day, and transfusions are repeated daily until there is clinical improvement or the absolute neutrophil count rises above 500/mm^3.

Risks

The risks of granulocyte infusions include fever, alloimmunization, fluid overload, and pulmonary leukostasis.

WHOLE BLOOD

The transfusion of whole blood is now rarely used except during exchange transfusions in neonates and when autologous whole-blood storage is performed prior to elective surgery. Two other occasional indications are massive, acute hemorrhage of greater than 25% of the patient's total blood volume and following cardiac surgery in early infancy. Crystalloid/colloid support and PRBC transfusions, however, are just as effective in treating significant, acute hemorrhage. Children undergoing open-heart surgery can experience postoperative bleeding for several reasons, including platelet dysfunction. Fresh whole blood to treat bleeding for the first 48 hours following surgery was, in the past, favored by some surgeons. This is now done less frequently because practical blood banking practices limit provision of whole blood for this indication, and there are other, readily available blood products that may be appropriate for treating the cause of bleeding.

AUTOLOGOUS STORAGE

The role of autologous storage in pediatrics is limited because of volume issues. It is occasionally used in otherwise healthy children and adolescents undergoing elective surgery, most commonly orthopedic procedures.

FRESH FROZEN PLASMA AND CRYOPRECIPITATE

Fresh frozen plasma (FFP) contains all of the clotting factors and is used predominantly in the following:

1. Preventing or stopping bleeding in children who have significant coagulation factor deficiencies for which purified concentrates are not available (e.g., deficiencies of factors V, XI, and XII, in which it is the only available therapy)
2. Stopping bleeding in the setting of DIC and infection or liver failure
3. Stopping bleeding in patients who are actively bleeding or who require emergency surgery and in whom functional deficiencies of factors II, VII, IX, and X cannot be rapidly reversed by vitamin K
4. Reversing rapidly the effect of warfarin therapy

Because FFP is obtained from single-donor units, its use decreases the risk of infectious complications. The dose is usually 15 mL/kg, producing a 20% to 30% rise in clotting factor activity.

Cryoprecipitate is the protein that precipitates in FFP thawed at 4°C. It is rich in factors VIII and XIII and fibrinogen. It is used as a source of fibrinogen and to treat factor XIII deficiency. The dose is 1 to 2 units/10 kg, providing the advantage over FFP of a small-volume infusion and a decreased risk of circulatory overload.

RISKS AND COMPLICATIONS OF BLOOD PRODUCT ADMINISTRATION

The most common transfusion reactions, in order of frequency, are allergic reactions, fever, hemolytic reactions, transmission of infectious agents, and GVHD.

Allergic Reactions

Allergic reactions occur in 1% to 2% of PRBC transfusions and are thought to be due to a reaction between preformed antibodies and plasma proteins. Pruritus, rash, and urticaria typically begin minutes after the infusion is started. The transfusion should be paused, and antihistamines should be administered. Antihistamine premedication can prevent this problem from occurring in subsequent transfusions.

Febrile Reactions

Febrile reactions are due to preformed antibodies to incompatible leukocytes present in PRBC and platelet transfusions. Febrile reactions usually occur within 30 to 60 minutes after the transfusion has started and can be associated with rigors, headache, nausea, and emesis. The transfusion should be paused, a blood bank transfusion work-up should be initiated, and antipyretics should be administered. Subsequent febrile reactions can be prevented by the use of leukocyte-depleted blood products and premedication of the recipient with acetaminophen and diphenhydramine.

Hemolytic Reactions

The most common cause of hemolytic reactions following red blood cell transfusions is clerical error involving misidentification of the patient or blood sample. In the venous pressure monitoring. PICC lines are frequently used for preterm neonates in the neonatal intensive care unit. Trained nursing personnel usually insert the catheters.

PICC lines are most commonly placed in the antecubital fossa; however, the saphenous vein, external jugular vein, axillary vein, and scalp veins can be used. The precise method for placement is dependent on the particular manufacturer. Some catheters utilize a guidewire and some do not. In general, the catheters are placed through a peel-away introducer needle. Prior to placement the operator is dressed in a sterile gown, gloves, cap, and mask, and the site is cleaned with an antibacterial solution and draped with sterile drapes. Local anesthesia is provided by 1% lidocaine, EMLA (eutectic mixture of local anesthetics), and general sedation is administered if necessary. After the catheter is placed through the needle, the needle is removed, the site is dressed with a sterile dressing, and line placement is confirmed with a radiograph.

Complications of PICC line placement include immediate and long-term complications. Immediate complications include bleeding or bruising at the site, local tendon or nerve damage, cardiac arrhythmias, and catheter embolism. Long-term complications include infection, thrombus formation, and occlusion. Rates of infection are generally lower than that reported for percutaneously inserted central venous catheters. Catheter occlusion requiring catheter removal is more common in smaller catheters.

The use of PICC lines to allow completion of medical therapy in the home or outpatient setting is increasing. With proper education, the catheters can be safely and effectively cared for by home caregivers. Because they last longer than peripheral intravenous lines, they are also frequently used in the hospital setting and decrease the number of venipunctures. Because of the relatively small diameter and long length, they are not suitable for infusions of large volumes of fluid or blood products quickly.

Umbilical Venous Catheter

The umbilical vessels of neonates can be cannulated in the first few days of life. Either the umbilical arteries or the umbilical vein can be cannulated and used for blood sampling; infusion of medications, blood products, fluids, or parenteral nutrition; and monitoring of arterial blood pressure of central venous pressure. The umbilical vein is preferred during newborn resuscitation because it is more easily accessed than the artery. The umbilical vein can be used in an emergency setting outside the delivery room if the umbilical cord is of sufficient length.

The infant is placed supine and the cord is cleaned with an antiseptic solution and draped with sterile drapes. The cord should be cut with a sterile blade approximately 1 cm above the skin and held with a ligature to stabilize it and prevent bleeding. The 3.5F or 5F umbilical catheter is flushed with saline and attached to a stopcock and syringe. The catheter is inserted in the vein until there is free flow of blood when the syringe is gently aspirated. Forceps to grip the end of the catheter can aid in placement. For emergency use the catheter should be inserted only until blood is first aspirated to avoid infusing solutions into the liver. For longer-term use the catheter can be inserted to the junction of the inferior vena cava and the right atrium.

Confirmation of proper positioning by radiograph is essential if the line is placed in this position in order to avoid infusion into the liver. The catheter is secured in place with a suture or umbilical tape tie around the cord and adhesive tape to the abdomen.

Complications of umbilical venous catheters include blood loss, air embolism, infection, and liver injury caused by improper placement. The catheters should be removed as soon as they are no longer needed.

Implanted Devices

Tunneled Silastic catheters (Broviac or Hickman) placed into a central vein are commonly used for long-term vascular access for delivery of chemotherapy, antibiotics, or parenteral nutrition. They are made of Silastic, which is relatively inert and pliable, and they have a cuff at the proximal end that adheres to the subcutaneous tract, anchoring the catheter in place and preventing infection. Patients who require long-term access that is more intermittent, such as monthly chemotherapy, are often managed with totally implanted venous access devices known as "ports" (Port-A-Cath, Mediport). These devices consist of a port made of a durable shell with an overlying Silastic diaphragm, with a Silastic catheter than enters the vein. A specially designed needle is used to puncture the diaphragm for access to the resevoir. The advantages of the port system over external central catheters include lower rate of infection, less frequent flushes and care, and less restriction of activity.

Complications of placement of either type of access device are similar to that of percutaneous central venous catheters and include bleeding, arrhythmias, pneumothorax, arterial puncture or vein laceration, and air embolism. The rate of serious complications is highly dependent on patient selection and operator experience. Long-term complications include infection, thrombosis in the vessel or right atrium, pulmonary embolus, thrombotic occlusion of the catheter tip or vessel, and catheter migration. The most common long-term complication necessitating catheter removal is infection. The incidence and clinical importance of thrombus formation is not well studied.

CONTROVERSIES REGARDING VASCULAR ACCESS

Controversies regarding vascular access primarily pertain to choice of access device and methods of preventing complications (Table 295-3). As with all medical procedures, each method of vascular access has risks as well as benefits, and each device or method will have risks that pertain to it specifically. Although all methods have risks, there are also risks for patients who have inadequate vascular access, which must be considered. One relatively new issue regarding vascular access is operator safety. Needleless systems are available that reduce the potential for the spread of communicable diseases such as human immunodeficiency virus (HIV) and hepatitis, but many are difficult to use and often are unavailable for use in small pediatric patients. As advances are made in the design of these catheters, they will become more widely used in the pediatric population.

Table 295-3. Features of Vascular Access Devices

Access Method	Indications	Advantages	Disadvantages
Peripheral catheter	Short-term medications or fluids, initial resuscitation	Easy to insert, low cost, low risk of infection	Easy to dislodge, high rate of occlusion, extravasation of medications or fluids
Intraosseous needle	Rapid access for resuscitation, medications, or fluids	Rapid insertion, ease or insertion	Not for long-term use, pain on insertion if patient conscious, leakage at site
Percutaneous central venous catheter	Central venous pressure monitoring, inotropic or pressor medications, parenteral nutrition, irritant medications	Stable access, difficult to dislodge, safe delivery of irritant medications or fluids	Mechanical risk to tissue during insertion, need for sedation for placement, infection, and thrombosis
Peripherally inserted central venous catheters	Intermediate-term for fluids, medications (e.g., antibiotics), or parenteral nutrition	Stable access, difficult to dislodge, safe delivery or irritant medications or fluids	Easily occluded, may be difficult to advance into central location
Umbilical venous catheter	Newborn resuscitation, fluids, or medications	Ease of insertion	Risk of infection
Tunneled central catheter	Long-term access for medication (chemotherapy) or parenteral nutrition	Less risk of infection, less thrombogenic	Requires surgical insertion, altered body image
Central port	Long-term access for intermittent use (chemotherapy)	Low visibility, low risk of infection	Requires surgical insertion

Additional Resources, CD-ROM

Bibliography

SUGGESTED READINGS

Abe KK, Blum GT, Yamamoto LG: Intraosseous is faster and easier than umbilical venous catheterization in newborn emergency vascular access models. Am J Emerg Med 2000;18(2):126–129.

Dolcourt JL, Bose CL: Percutaneous insertion of Silastic central venous catheters in newborn infants. Pediatrics 1980;70:484–486.

Massicote MP, Dix D, Monage P, et al: Central venous catheter related thrombosis in children: Analysis of the Canadian registry of venous thromboembolic complications. J Pediatr 1998;133:770–776.

Niermeyer S, Kattwinkel J, Van Reempts P, et al: International guidelines for neonatal resuscitation: An excerpt from the guidelines 2000 for cardiopulmonary resuscitation and emergency cardiovascular care: International consensus on science. Pediatrics 2000;106:E29.

Weiner ES, McGuire P, Stolar CJH, et al: The CCSG prospective study of venous access devices: An analysis of insertions and cause for removal. J Pediatr Surg 1992;27:155.

SECTION 9   DIAGNOSTICS AND THERAPEUTICS: *Procedural Medicine*

296   Wound Care and Suturing

Craig R. Warden

GENERAL WOUND MANAGEMENT

Clinicians caring for children should be able to recognize wounds that can be repaired effectively in the office or clinic versus wounds that need to need to be referred to an emergency department (ED) or specialist. Referral may be based on sedation requirements, time requirement to repair, or lack of experience with repairing difficult or cosmetically sensitive wounds (Table 296-1). In addition, clinicians need to recognize wounds that have injuries to underlying structures (including tendons, ligaments, joint capsules, bone, nerves, and arteries) that require special treatment. Wounds over mobile structures such as tendons have to be examined closely with full active and passive range of motion of the affected joints tested to make sure there is no hidden injury proximal or distal to the wound. Ligaments and tendons may appear to have full function despite a significant injury and risk delayed rupture or functionally impaired scarring if the injury is initially missed and not repaired. The possibility of a retained foreign body needs to be assessed because presence of a foreign body is associated with a much higher complication rate. Radiographic imaging may detect some foreign bodies (glass, metal) but most will be found only on close visual

Table 296-1. Categorization of Wound Types and Recommended Management

Wound Type	Features	Indication for Closure	Benefits	Risks	Controversies	Closure Options in Office
Facial						
Simple	Small (<3–4 cm) Little tension Epidermal and dermal only	Any with slightest amount of noticeable gaping	Cosmetic appearance Decrease infection risk	Infection: extremely low Dehiscence	Type of closure Absorbable vs. nonabsorbable sutures	Suture (tape and glue for low tension wounds)
Complex	Large Increased tension Involvement of fascia, muscle of expression, parotid or tear duct involvement Eyelid	All	Cosmetic appearance Decrease infection risk Maintain function	Infection: extremely low Poor cosmetic outcome Unrecognized neurovascular or muscular impairment Laceration of parotid or tear ducts Dehiscence	Depending on age: sedation options (ED, OR)	Most should be referred Suture at least deep layers Epidermal closure as above Nonsuture closure discouraged for wounds with residual tension
Scalp						
Simple	<8 cm in length Galea intact	Gaping, bleeding <12 hours old	Control bleeding Decrease risk of infection	Infection: extremely low Dehiscence	What size to leave alone	Staples, single-layer suture closure
Complex	Large (>8 cm) Galea lacerated Skull fracture	All	Control bleeding Decrease risk of infection Speed healing	Infection: extremely low Dehiscence	Depending on age: sedation options (ED, OR)	Most should be referred Galea with absorbable gut or synthetic Skin as above
Hand						
Simple	Small (<2 cm) No NV, tendon or joint involvement	<8 hours old Any gaping	Faster healing and return to activities	High risk for infection Dehiscence with activity	Allowable time Allowable contamination Primary or delayed repair to minimize infection risk	Suture or tape No glue or staples
Complex	Large NV, tendon, or joint involvement	<8 hours old Any gaping	Faster healing and return to activities Maintain function	High risk for infection Dehiscence with activity Tendon, NV disruption	Allowable time Allowable contamination Primary or delayed repair to minimize infection risk	Most should be referred Suture, layered closure with excellent hemostasis and visualization of structures
Extremity, nonhand						
Simple	Small (<6 cm)	<8 hours old Any gaping	Faster healing and return to activities Maintain function	Moderate risk for infection Dehiscence with activity	Allowable time Allowable contamination Primary or delayed repair to minimize infection risk	Suture (or tape for low tension wounds) Staples acceptable
Complex	Large Deeper than SQ	All <8 hours	Faster healing and return to activities Maintain function	Moderate risk for infection Dehiscence with activity Less risk of tendon, NV disruption than hand	Allowable time Allowable contamination Primary or delayed repair to minimize infection risk	Most should be referred Less meticulous closure than hand Only close fascia of large muscle groups Can use vertical mattress for high-tension wounds
Trunk						
Simple	Small (<6 cm)	All <10–12 hours old	Faster healing and return to activities Dehiscence with activity	Moderate risk for infection	Primary, delayed, or no repair to minimize infection risk	Suture (or tape for low-tension wounds) Staples acceptable in noncosmetic areas
Complex	Large Deeper than SQ Penetration of abdominal or thoracic cavities	All <10–12 hours old	Faster healing and return to activities Explore for penetration	Moderate risk for infection Dehiscence with activity Unrecognized penetration	Local exploration to exclude body cavity penetration	Most should be referred

ED, emergency department; NV, nerve; OR, operating room; SQ, subcutaneous.

and tactile evaluation. Some foreign bodies that are inert (glass, most metals) may be left in if not easily extractable, but other foreign bodies (wood, other plant material) have a surface that is usually irritating or contaminated with pathogenic organisms so that they have to be removed.

On occasion, seriously injured patients may present unexpectedly to an office or clinic. Office personnel should notify the clinician and initiate emergency transport when such patients with significant blood loss from the primary wound or who have other significant injuries (head injury, long bone fractures, or truncal injuries) appear. The office clinician should be able to stabilize and expeditiously transfer these patients. Large wounds should be dressed with saline-soaked gauze pads to prevent desiccation and heat loss and to decrease subsequent risk of infection. Effective phone triage of patients may minimize the number of patients with complicated severe wounds arriving to the clinic versus being referred initially to an ED or specialist for definitive care.

As for wounds that can be managed in the office setting, the primary care provider (PCP) must recognize which wounds are at risk for infection. Wounds that are extensively contaminated or aged should not be closed. Wounds exposed to wet environments (swamps, marshes) or to farm soil are also at high risk for infection owing to likely exposure to high organism counts. Other high-risk wounds include perioral wounds caused by teeth protruding through oral mucosa and wounds over metacarpal-phalangeal joints produced by "fight bites." Plantar puncture wounds may lead to osteochondritis or osteomyelitis, and it is unclear whether débridement and deep irrigation of these wounds or use of prophylactic antibiotics (Table 296-2) will change the natural history of these wounds. Wounds with a high risk of infection may be managed either by secondary intention, if there is minimal cosmetic or functional risk, or by delayed primary closure, a much underutilized procedure in both the office and ED setting. Discussion of complicated wounds that require significant débridement, extensive search for foreign bodies, or excision of tissue in order to close the wound is beyond the scope of this chapter.

To minimize the risk of infection, the PCP needs to adequately clean and débride wounds prior to exploring for foreign bodies and closing the wound. Equipment and assistants readily available minimize patient anxiety and time requirement for wound treatment. The provider should follow universal precautions throughout the procedure, wearing, at a minimum, gloves, goggles, and mask.

Irrigation with normal saline (NS), without any anti-infective additive, is the most important component of cleansing. Increased fluid volume and applied pressure (8 psi or more) during irrigation is associated with lower infection rates. Typical materials for irrigation include normal saline intravenous (IV) solution, large-bore tubing, a three-way stopcock, large syringe (60 mL) and 18-gauge IV catheter. At least 200 to 300 mL of fluid is necessary for cleaning the smallest, cleanest wounds, going up to several liters of fluid for the larger, more contaminated wounds. When using high-pressure irrigation, a splash guard (e.g., Zerowet) attached to the end of the syringe or tubing may help minimize exposure to body fluids. Topical antiseptics, such as povidone-iodine without detergents (e.g., Betadine), should be applied to the intact skin around the wound when the skin will be punctured by the skin closure technique (i.e., stapling or suturing). Topical antiseptics should not be placed directly into the wound. In highly contaminated wounds, gentle scrubbing with a surgical sponge may facilitate removal of dirt and pathogens. Hair removal is generally not necessary. Eyebrows should never be clipped or shaved. Shaving may nick the skin, thereby increasing infection risk, so any necessary hair removal should be by clipping only.

Primary care providers who elect to close wounds in the office will need to choose an appropriate closure method that is cosmetically acceptable, cost-effective, and expeditious (Table 296-3). Suture closure usually results in the best cosmetic and functional outcomes but can be technically challenging if not done often, particularly with an uncooperative, nonsedated young child. Wound closure using less technically challenging techniques has become more common both in the office and in the ED setting. These techniques include using tissue glues, tape, and skin staples. Tissue glue closure for low-tension facial lacerations is especially popular because of speedy application without the need for anesthesia or sedation while achieving cosmetic equivalence to suturing for selected lacerations.

For wounds that are either closed or left open, proper dressing is important to promote rapid healing and to prevent infections. Wounds heal best when kept in a moist environment. For simple wounds, the daily application of water-resistant antibiotic-containing ointments (e.g., Bacitracin, Polysporin) to the wound will maintain moisture and keep bacterial counts down. For larger wounds including burns, specialized nonwoven, microporous polypropylene dressings (e.g., OpSite) can be applied and left on until

Table 296-2. Recommendations for Wound Prophylaxis with Antibiotics

Type of Wound	Controversy	Recommended Regimen
Facial human or animal bite	Low risk for infection in general Assess for risk of rabies	Amoxicillin/clavulanic acid 45 mg/kg/d bid 5–7 d for all Alternate: Cat: cefuroxime, doxycycline Dogs and human: clindamycin + TMP/SMX
Human/animal bite: nonfacial	Risk of dog bite wound infection approximately 5% Assess for risk of rabies	Amoxicillin/clavulanic acid 45 mg/kg/d bid 5–7 d for all Alternate: cat: cefuroxime, doxycycline Dogs and human: clindamycin + TMP/SMX
Contaminated wounds Plantar puncture wounds	Actual risk of infection and efficacy of prophylaxis Efficacy of prophylactic antibiotics Amount of débridement	First-generation cephalosporins First-generation cephalosporins Fluoroquinolones (for skeletally mature)

TMP-SMX, trimethoprim-sulfamethoxazole.

Table 296-3. Comparison of Techniques of Wound Closure

Technique	Indications	Benefits	Risks	Controversies/Evidence-based Effectiveness
Tape	Low tension Small (<2–4 cm)	Painless, cheap, fast, easy, no anesthesia	Contact dermatitis, dehiscence	
Tissue glue	Low tension Small (<2–4 cm)	Painless, fast, easy, no anesthesia	Dehiscence	Increased infection rate? Equivalent to suturing for appropriate wounds
Staples	Noncosmetic wounds	Fast, low tissue reaction	Need staple remover	Parents may find unesthetic
Suturing	Any wound appropriate for closure	Most flexible, best cosmetic results	Tissue reaction Needs skill and time	Glue may be equivalent for small facial wounds

full healing occurs. For cosmetically important wounds, protection from the sun for 6 months is important for minimizing scar formation.

Office equipment necessary for wound management is listed in Table 296-4.

Before the patient leaves the office, his or her tetanus immune status needs to be updated based on current CDC (Centers for Disease Control) recommendations. For animal bites, rabies risk needs to be evaluated. Finally, appropriate follow-up should be arranged to make sure complications including evolving wound infections, retained foreign bodies, and damage to underlying structures do not develop.

ACUTE MANAGEMENT

Preparation of Patient

The patient and family should be advised before starting general wound management. What is said to the child should be developmentally appropriate and discussed as

Table 296-4. Equipment Needed for Wound Suturing

Irrigation and Cleaning Equipment
60-mL syringe
Three-way stopcock (if using IV tubing)
Large IV catheter (>18 gauge) or combination splashguard/catheter (e.g., Zerowet)
Normal saline in bowel or via IV tubing
Soft scrubbing sponge ± embedded antiseptic
Cotton-tip applicators

Standard Suture Tray
Sterile drapes and/or fenestrated drape
Adson forceps, serrated
Cotton-tip applicators
Gauze sponges, 4 × 4 inches
Iris scissors, straight
Curved mosquito clamp
Needles: 18 gauge for drawing up local anesthetic, 27 gauge (1¼ and ⅝ inches) for infiltration
Syringe, 10 mL
Webster needle holder
Medicine cups or other container for normal saline and topical antiseptic

Suture Material
Needles ½ circle, reverse cutting points
Absorbable synthetic suture (polyglycolic acid and polygalactin 910): 3-0 to 6-0
Absorbable natural sutures (fast-absorbing gut): 6-0 for facial lacerations
Nonabsorbable synthetic sutures (nylon and polypropylene): 2-0 to 6-0

close as possible to the actual time of the procedure in order to lessen anxiety. Techniques such as play therapy and distraction are as important as actual sedation or analgesia in the ultimate experience of the child. It is also important to proceed as expeditiously as possible once the procedure is initiated in order to minimize the anxiety and distress of the patient, the family, the staff, and the physician.

Sedation and Analgesia

Appropriate sedation and analgesia include topical and local anesthetic application. Although most patients who require sedation or systemic analgesia for laceration repair need to go to the ED or specialist, some sedation and analgesia can be achieved in the office. For a simple laceration repair in an otherwise uncooperative or anxious toddler or preschooler, oral midazolam administered as a 0.5-mg/kg oral dose (either as the proprietary suspension or with the IV solution mixed in a palatable syrup) about 20 minutes prior to the procedure may help sedate the patient. No monitoring is required. Some physical restraint may be necessary, yet one can reassure caretakers that midazolam induces some amnesia of the procedure. Occasionally, midazolam causes paradoxic agitation in some patients. Midazolam's effects peak about 20 minutes after application.

Local anesthesia for simple lacerations may be accomplished by either topical or injectable medications. The most currently used topical anesthetic is LET (lidocaine, epinephrine, and tetracaine) gel. LET is equivalent in efficacy to the more expensive and potentially toxic schedule II formulation of TAC (tetracaine, adrenaline, and cocaine). LET gel, once applied to the wound, preferably under a waterproof dressing, reaches peak effects in about 20 minutes, making the combination of LET and midazolam a very effective strategy in repair of simple lacerations in small children. Blanching of the skin at the wound edges demonstrates adequate tissue penetration. Testing the skin with a sharp object risks increasing the anxiety of an uncooperative young child. If adequate topical anesthesia is unobtainable, local anesthetics may need to be injected. Studies consistently show that alkalinization of the anesthetic solution (adding 1 mL of sodium bicarbonate solution to each 9 mL of local anesthetic) and slow injection with the smallest possible needle are the two most important factors in minimizing the pain of infiltration.

Adequate hemostasis is important for visualization of potential foreign bodies or injury to underlying structures. Adding epinephrine to local or topical anesthetics helps provide hemostasis. A sphygmomanometer provides a makeshift pneumatic tourniquet for complicated extremity wounds. Proprietary "donut" tourniquets or short lengths of latex drains can maintain hemostasis in digits prior to tourniquet application.

Method of Closure

Appropriate methods of closure include tape, glue, staples, and deep and superficial sutures (see Table 296-3). Most wounds selected for closure in the primary care physician's office or clinic may be amenable to taping, tissue gluing, or stapling. These methods require minimal experience, time to completion, analgesia, and sedation. Taping (Steri-Strips, Shur-Strips, Clearon tapes) may be used for superficial lacerations that are under minimal tension when closed. Taping induces less inflammation and infection because it does not seal the wound. However, a small child may try to pull the tape off. Tissue glue (e.g., Dermabond) is especially ideal for smaller (<4 cm) facial lacerations that are not under tension. Both taping and gluing techniques do not require any anesthesia, but tissue glue does require adequate hemostasis in order for the glue to polymerize appropriately to its maximum tensile strength. Brief exposure (5 to 10 minutes) of the wound to *topical* injectable 1% lidocaine with epinephrine or 1:1000 epinephrine usually maintains adequate hemostasis.

Staples are especially useful in noncosmetically important areas such as the scalp and extremities (not hands or feet) but do require good topical or local anesthesia. Staple technique is rapid but requires a special disposable instrument for staple removal. Suture closure allows the most cosmetically acceptable and strongest repair for all lacerations but this procedure requires the most expertise, time, and equipment.

Tape Closure

After appropriate cleansing, the skin adjacent to the laceration is prepped with tincture of benzoin to maximize adhesion of the tape strips. After the benzoin has dried (several minutes), the skin edges are approximated manually, and tape strips are laid across the laceration with firm pressure to make sure they adhere to the skin.

Tissue Glue Closure

After the wound is cleansed and hemostasis obtained with a topical epinephrine application, the wound edges are approximated either manually or with forceps. The tissue glue covers and seals the wound edges and should not enter the wound itself. It is important to take care not to glue objects (or subjects) to the patient and to avoid glue solution coating the eye or other mucosal surfaces. The tissue glue is applied in thin layers (at least three) allowing adequate drying in between applications, about 20 seconds. If excess fluid (blood or perspiration) interferes with the glue "setting" or if one is not satisfied with the approximation, the glue needs to be wiped away within 15 seconds of application. If left longer, dissolving the glue requires acetone use. Once the laceration is closed, it needs no dressing unless the caretaker believes the patient will pick at the glue over the ensuing 5 to 6 days. Tissue glue should not be used in hairy areas or on hands and feet because of increased infection risk.

Staple Closure

Older children and caretakers will need some explanation of the stapling procedure. Once the laceration is cleansed and satisfactory topical or local anesthesia is obtained, the skin edges are prepped with an appropriate antiseptic. The skin edges are approximated manually or with forceps. The stapler is firmly pressed onto the skin, centering the staple over the approximated skin edges. The stapler trigger is squeezed firmly and then released (Fig. 296-1). One staple is needed for approximately each centimeter of laceration length. Upon completing wound closure, the wound can be dressed with an antibiotic ointment and gauze. Staples in the scalp and extremities are usually removed in 7 to 10 days.

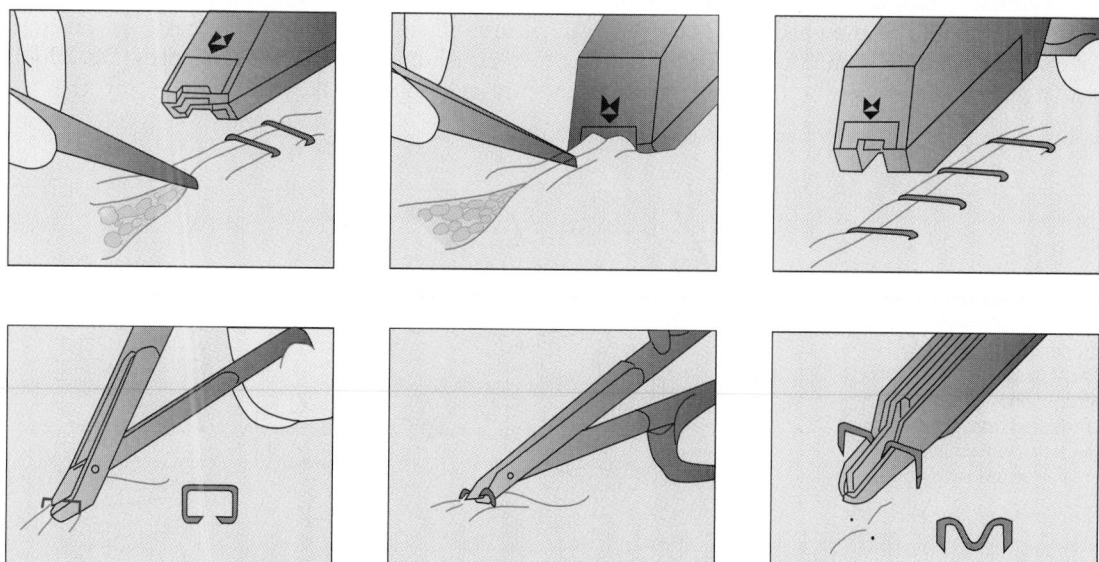

Figure 296-1. Use of a skin stapler. (Adapted from http://www.sino-sourcing.com/MedicalEquipment/Instrument/large.html)

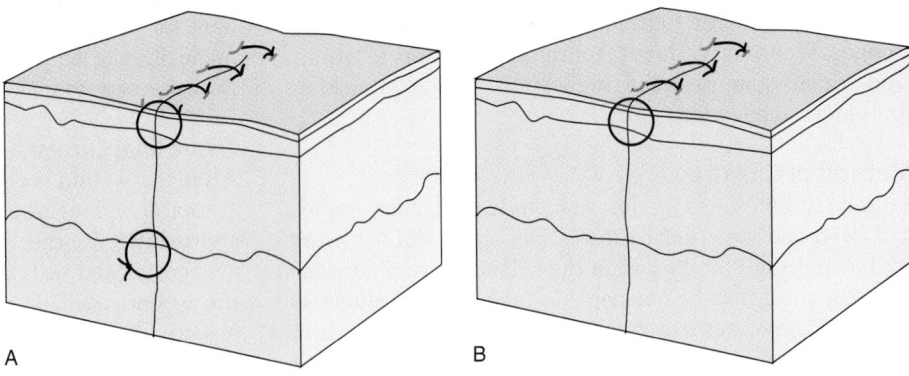

Figure 296-2. Proper tissue apposition (**A**) versus improper apposition and inappropriate excess tightness (**B**). (Adapted from Goepp JG, Hostetler MA (eds): Procedures for Primary Care Pediatricians. St. Louis, Mosby, 2001, p 138.)

A   B

Suture Closure

Suture closure may be accomplished with deep, vertical mattress, simple interrupted, or continuous sutures. Suturing requires sterile instruments, a sterile field, a variety of suture materials, good anesthesia, and a nearly motionless patient. Absorbable and nonabsorbable suture material and a reverse cutting needle are the best choices for general wound closure. In younger patients, one or more assistants may be needed to help restrain the patient.

The most common suturing technique used in both the ED and clinic setting is simple interrupted sutures. Simple interrupted suturing is adequate for most wounds that are not deeper than the subcutaneous layer of the skin and do not have excessive tension upon closure. For facial wounds, deeper sutures are necessary to maintain wound strength during the acute healing process because superficial sutures require removal in 3 to 5 days for best cosmetic results. It is important that the wound edges are apposed properly during suturing (Fig. 296-2).

Simple Interrupted Suture Closure

After opening the sterile suture kit, place appropriate suture material in a sterile fashion onto the tray. Facial wounds generally require 5-0 or 6-0 suture with rapidly absorbable material (chromic "gut") suited to minimize tissue reaction and eliminate the need for suture removal. For scalp and nonhand or nonfoot extremity wounds, generally a larger suture size can be used (3-0 to 4-0) for

more wound strength. Commonly used nonabsorbable sutures are a monofilament nylon (Dermalon, Ethilon) or polypropylene (Prolene). For simple interrupted suturing, evert the wound edges by placing the suture needle slightly deeper in the skin than the distance from suture entrance to wound edge (Fig. 296-3). Place the sutures equidistant from each other and equal to the total width of each suture. For the face, place percutaneous sutures generally closer together and take smaller "bites" of skin to minimize scarring. Each apposing wound edge should have separate "bites" with each suture to allow accurate placement of suture and to prevent inadvertently including deeper structures into the suture. Sutures are tied using a "surgeon's knot," with a total of four "throws" needed to secure monofilament material. Suture tension should just be enough to appose the wound edges. Additional tension may increase wound ischemia, delay healing, and increase the risk of wound infection. The ends of the suture should be cut long enough to discourage unraveling and facilitate removal.

Vertical Mattress Suture Closure

This suturing technique is especially useful for extremity wounds that are under a lot of tension but risk infection from deep suture placement. This technique is similar to simple interrupted suturing except that bigger initial "bites" are taken and a second "pass" is taken through the epithelium to appose the skin edges (Fig. 296-4). The initial bigger "bites" take the tension off the wound edges,

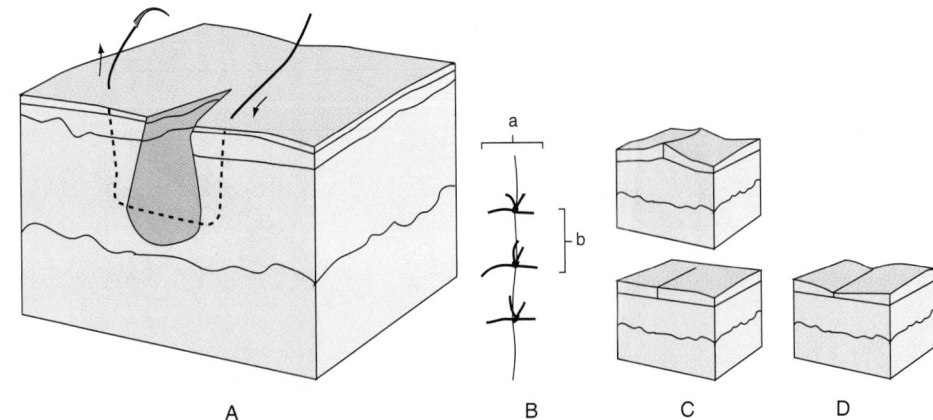

Figure 296-3. Features of the simple interrupted dermal suture. **A,** Proper depth. **B,** Proper spacing (*a* = *b*). **C,** Proper final appearance (everted or flat). **D,** Improper final appearance (inverted). (Adapted from Goepp JG, Hostetler MA (eds): Procedures for Primary Care Pediatricians. St. Louis, Mosby, 2001, p 138.)

A   B   C   D

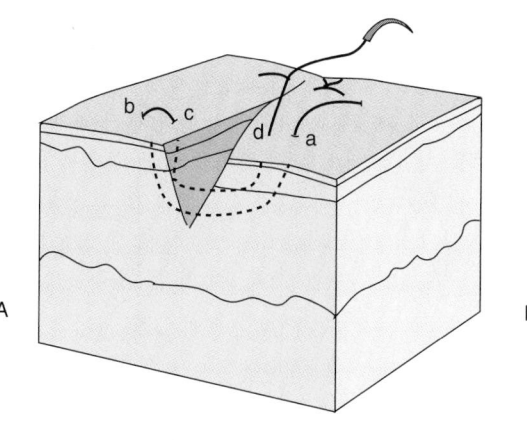

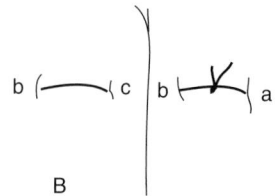

Figure 296-4. Vertical mattress suture. **A,** Cross section. **B,** Overhead view. Begin at *a* and go under skin to *b;* come out from *b,* go in at *c,* and exit at *d.* (Adapted from Goepp JG, Hostetler MA (eds): Procedures for Primary Care Pediatricians. St. Louis, Mosby, 2001, p 140.)

allowing the smaller skin "bites" to appose the skin with minimal tension. Vertical mattress suturing generally uses 3-0 monofilament suture.

Deep Sutures

Deep sutures help eliminate dead space and alleviate suture tension of the skin edges by approximating the dermis and fascial planes. However, deep sutures increase the risk of infection because they act as foreign bodies for the weeks they remain in the wound. Large sutures (2-0 and 3-0) of synthetic absorbable sutures (Vicryl, Dexon) are used to close muscle fascia in the nonhand and nonfoot parts of the extremities and the galea in the scalp. Deep suture placement is by simple interrupted suture technique (Fig. 296-5). A variation of this technique *(buried subcutaneous suturing)* helps close the dermis of the skin in facial lacerations when skin tension and wound gaping are not amenable to simple percutaneous closure (Fig. 296-6).

Simple Continuous Percutaneous Suture Closure

This technique is especially useful for long, linear lacerations and avoids tying multiple knots. One does a simple interrupted suture tie at one end of the wound followed by multiple passes of the suture needle for the rest of the wound length. As in interrupted suturing, the depth of the suture should be slightly greater than the distance from suture entry to wound edge and distance apart of each suture pass should be equal to the total width of the suture. To tie the opposite end of the suture line, one creates a loop with one pass of the suture and does a surgeon's knot instrument tie.

Antibiotic Prophylaxis

Except for bite wounds, controversy exists over which wounds require systemic antibiotic prophylaxis (see Table 296-2). Generally, if a wound is sufficiently contaminated to warrant antibiotic use, then one should consider not closing that wound and instead allow delayed primary or secondary intention closure. Contaminated wounds that may have significant cosmetic effect may be closed primarily followed by antibiotic therapy. Simple fresh dog bite wounds to the extremity without a significant crush injury may be sutured followed by appropriate antibiotic therapy. Human and cat bite wounds should rarely be closed unless they may have a significant cosmetic effect. Very contaminated wounds (dirt, barnyard debris, feces) should be left open and treated with either a first-generation cephalosporin or a penicillinase-resistant semisynthetic penicillin (e.g., dicloxacillin). Bite wounds from all species are covered adequately by amoxicillin-clavulanic acid.

Follow-up

Patient follow-up is necessary to make sure there are no wound infections, missed foreign bodies, or overlooked injury to other structures as well as to remove sutures or staples. All patients should receive general instructions on signs and symptoms of wound infection and loss of function. Severe wounds and wounds that significantly risk infection mandate re-evaluation in 24 to 48 hours. Prescribing antibiotic medications does not replace the need for rechecking the wound.

In general, facial wounds should have nonabsorbable sutures removed in 3 to 5 days. Absorbable sutures in the

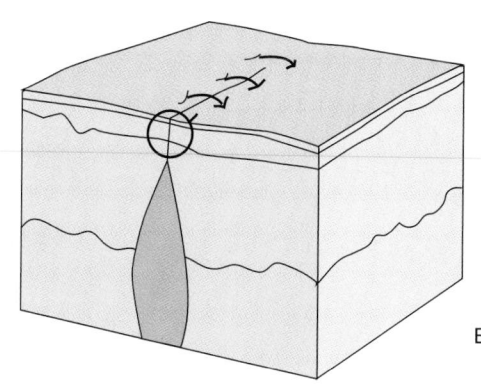

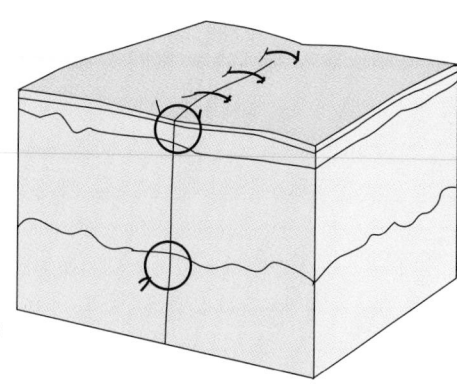

Figure 296-5. A, Improper wound closure. **B,** Proper subcutaneous and dermal wound closure using deep and superficial sutures. (Adapted from Goepp JG, Hostetler MA (eds): Procedures for Primary Care Pediatricians. St. Louis, Mosby, 2001, p 138.)

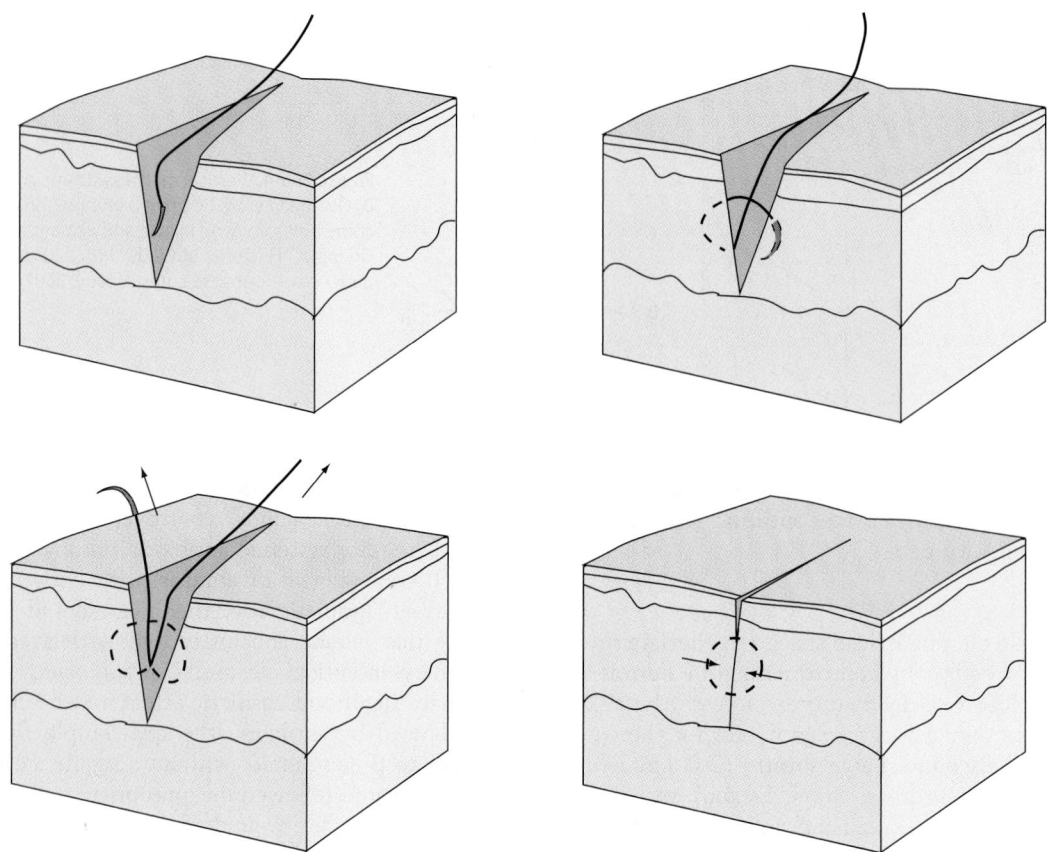

Figure 296-6. Buried subcutaneous suture. (Adapted from Goepp JG, Hostetler MA (eds): Procedures for Primary Care Pediatricians. St. Louis, Mosby, 2001, p 139.)

face do not need follow-up suture removal unless they remain in place after 5 days. Scalp, truncal, and extremity sutures and staples should generally be removed in 7 to 10 days. Sutures of high-tension wounds over extensor surfaces of the joints should come out 2 weeks after placement.

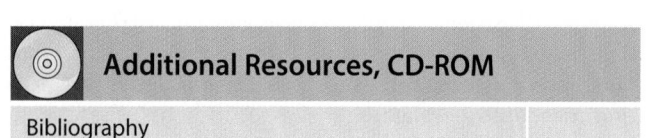

Additional Resources, CD-ROM

Bibliography

SUGGESTED READINGS

Bruns TB, Worthington JM: Using tissue adhesive for wound repair: A practical guide to dermabond. Am Fam Physician 2000; 61(5):1383–1388.

Chen E, Hornig S, Shepherd SM, Hollander JE: Primary closure of mammalian bites. Acad Emerg Med 2000;7(2):157–161.

Gouin S, Patel H: Office management of minor wounds. Can Fam Physician 2001;47:769-774.

Howard R: The appropriate use of topical antimicrobials and antiseptics in children. Pediatr Ann 2001;30(4): 219–224.

Kanegaye JT: A rational approach to the outpatient management of lacerations in pediatric patients. Curr Probl Pediatr 1998; 28(7):205–234.

297 Burn Care

Dennis Vane

DEFINITIONS

A *burn* is defined as cutaneous or deeper tissue damage caused by some mechanism of energy applied to the skin. Burns occur from a variety of causes, most commonly from extreme heat or extreme cold. Burns can also be caused by electricity or chemical substances. Physicians are often called on to treat burns caused by extreme heat or cold. Burns caused by heat are the most frequently occurring burns, generally caused by a hot liquid (scald) or hot surface (flame, stove, or even hot gas). Cold injuries are referred to as "frostbite."

Frostbite usually occurs at temperatures below 19°F or −7°C in a moist environment. The "burn" lesion is due to actual freezing of the skin layers, with tissue destruction secondary to the formation of ice crystals. Frostbite can be described in "degrees," much the same way a hot thermal burn is described. Digits, ears, and other protuberances some distance away from the central thermal core of the body are often affected because of their exposure, but any skin surface is at risk. The amount of damage depends on the complex relationship of the thickness of skin, the temperature, and time during which the skin is exposed. Thinner skin can be injured at lower temperatures and at lesser exposure times than thicker skin. Simple, brief skin discoloration with a minimum of blister formation may be treated by the generalist. Prolonged skin discoloration with significant blister formation requires the attention of a physician specialist. Frostbite can cause skin sloughing, underlying blood vessel damage, and even deep tissue sloughing after injury. Small vessels may clot, thereby causing necrosis of skin, digits, ears, and even entire extremities.

In general, electrical and chemical burns require the attention of a physician specialist. Electrical burns almost always cause significant deep tissue damage as well as other systemic problems including cardiac arrhythmias. Skin exposed to electrical arcs may reach temperatures of 3000 to 4000°F. Chemical burns may cause continued tissue destruction long after the initial exposure unless the chemicals are properly neutralized. Chemical neutralization may require surgical débridement.

ASSESSMENT OF THE BURN

Appropriate treatment of a burn wound depends on accurate assessment of the amount of tissue area involved and the depth of the burn wound. Burn assessment, coupled with the physician's expertise, resources, and the social situation of the child determine the best course of action for the physician.

Burn Depth

Initial assessment of burn depth is not often easy. The physician should never be concerned about changing the burn management of a child over time as burn depth becomes more evident. Today, burn depths are basically classified into four categories instead of the traditional three levels (Box 297-1).

First-degree burns describe simple redness of the skin. The skin is always intact, similar to minor sunburn. There are no blisters present and the burn is often quite painful.

Second-degree burns are divided today into two levels, superficial and deep. Superficial second-degree burns are usually red with blisters present. The burns are very tender, particularly when the blisters are broken and the underlying skin is exposed. The underlying dermis is red and weepy. Deep second-degree burns often, but not always, have blisters present. The underlying tissue usually produces an exudate early in the history of the burn, and skin sensation may range from normal to slightly diminished. The surface dermis is destroyed at varying levels. The hair follicles are intact and often appear as small red dots in the midst of a whitish eschar. Deep second-degree burns are often slow to heal and may require skin grafting for best results. Deep second-degree burns may not become evident until 24 to 48 hours after the initial burning incident.

Third-degree burns are the most difficult to treat. The dermis, including the hair follicles, is entirely destroyed. The burned skin is insensate and wooden in appearance. The skin is toughened and usually hard to palpation. Some skin may actually be turned to ash. These burns usually require skin grafts and should not be treated by the generalist. Even small third-degree burns left to heal by secondary intention will form a difficult scar, which often requires other therapies such as contracture release and ulcer excision.

Burn Size

Burn size has traditionally been determined by the "rule of nines," which is extremely inaccurate when applied to children. Today burns are determined by one of six distinct body shapes related to age development as described by Lund and Brower. Essentially the six body shapes include infants younger than 1 year of age, infants at 1 year of

Box 297-1. Categories of Burns

First degree
  Simple redness of intact skin
Second degree, superficial
  Red with blisters present
  Very tender, particularly when blisters are broken
  Underlying dermis red and weepy
Second degree, deep
  Dermis destroyed at varying levels
  Exposed dermis produces exudate early in the history of the burn
  Blisters may be present
  Sensation may range from normal to slightly diminished
  Hair follicles intact, appear as small red dots in white eschar
Third degree
  Dermis, including hair follicles, entirely destroyed
  Skin insensate
  Skin toughened, hard to palpation, "wooden" in appearance
  Some skin may be ash

age, children at preschool age (about age 5), children at school age (around age 10), teenagers (15 years), and adults.

Children with burns covering 7% to 15% of their total body surface should be hospitalized for initial resuscitation and treatment. Additionally, children with any burns to the face, hands, feet, and genitalia and any children with third-degree burns should also be hospitalized for initial care. All children with suspected inhalation burns or electrical burns must be admitted for burn treatment and for observation for possible later respiratory or cardiac abnormalities.

TREATMENT OPTIONS FOR BURNS (BOX 297-2)

The primary rule for the initial treatment of burns is to stop the burning. Causative material should be immediately removed from the skin. This includes all clothing, liquids, chemicals, and, of course, heat or cold.

Water is most often used to "flush" the offending agent from the burn site. Frostbite is usually warmed with 100°F water. Cool water is used to "flush" most other burn types. Water applied to alkali burns may cause the burn to progress further. Water cleansing of the burn past 20 minutes may cause hypothermia. In no case should a burn be cleansed with water for more than 20 minutes.

After the offending agent is cleansed from the wound, the burn is assessed for depth and size. Children with burns that cover over 7% to 15% of the total body surface area; involve the face, genitalia, hands, or feet; or appear to be third degree should be hospitalized and treated by a physician who specializes in burn therapy.

For lesser burns, outpatient therapy is usually sufficient. Very superficial burns of the face, hands, and feet may also be treated safely on an outpatient basis.

First-degree burns are cleansed with an antimicrobial soap and covered with any available soothing lotion such as aloe. Lotions with perfumes should be avoided as they often cause pain upon application to damaged epidermis.

Treatment of blisters in second-degree burns is controversial. Thick, intact blisters allow a more comfortable dressing. The fluid inside the blisters is sterile. The devitalized skin of a broken blister may serve as a nidus of infection. Infected second-degree burns may evolve into third-degree burns because unprotected, exposed dermis is easily destroyed by bacteria. In general, if the blisters are thick and intact, they can be left intact as long as the treating physician closely follows burn healing. If the blisters are thin, or the physician is concerned that normal activity of the child will cause them to break, the blisters should be opened, débrided, and appropriately bandaged. If the blisters are broken, the dead skin should be débrided prior to dressing the burn.

Superficial burns of the face are best treated with triple antibiotic ointment application without dressings. The ointment is applied three to four times daily, and the burn is washed with a dilute antimicrobial soap at least twice a day. It is crucial to remove the eschar or caked material with the washings. Any areas of necrotic skin are removed as they appear.

Burn dressings keep the burn clean and free of tissue necrosis and infection (Box 297-3). The wound is cleansed thoroughly with antimicrobial soap, patted dry, and an antibiotic cream is applied. Silver sulfadiazine (Sulfadine) is the most common agent of choice for burn dressing because it has excellent antibacterial coverage and good penetration of the burn and is painless when applied. Other antibiotic creams may be used such as mafenide acetate or nitrofurazone, but they have the disadvantage of having less adequate antimicrobial coverage, poorer penetration, or causing pain when applied. The burned area is then covered with a nonadherent dressing such as Telfa. Dressings can be changed once or twice a day depending on the physician's concern about healing and infection. When the dressing is changed all the antimicrobial cream must be removed and any eschar

Box 297-2. Burn Treatment

1. Stop the burning.
2. "Flush" the offending agent from burn site.
3. Assess burn depth and size.
4. Refer to specialist the following:
   Total body surface area burns that are 7% to 15% or more
   Burns to face, genitalia, hands, or feet
   Any third-degree burns
5. First-degree burns
   Cleanse with antimicrobial soap and cover with soothing lotion (aloe).
6. Second-degree burns
   If blister is thick and intact, leave intact and follow closely.
   If blister is broken, débride dead skin and apply dressing.
   If blister is thin, open blister, débride, and apply dressing.
7. Treat superficial facial burns with triple antibiotic ointment without dressing.
   Wash and apply ointment three or four times daily.
   Remove eschar, caked material with each washing.
   Remove areas of necrotic skin.
8. Refer to specialist any 14-day-old, unhealed burn.

Box 297-3. Burn Dressings

1. Antibiotic ointment
   Silver sulfadiazine (Sulfadine)
   Mafenide acetate
   Nitrofurazone
2. Nonadherent bandage
   Telfa
3. Semiporous membrane
   OpSite
   Omniderm
4. Bioactive membrane
   Biobran

or necrotic skin removed. The cream is then replaced and the occlusive dressing reapplied.

Larger burns that do not require treatment by a specialist can be cleaned, débrided, and covered with a semiporous membrane such as OpSite or Omniderm. It is essential that the OpSite or Omniderm adhere to undamaged skin around the burn. The dressing may often be left intact until the wound is entirely healed. Burn wounds should heal within 9 to 14 days. If not, the child should be referred to a burn wound specialist.

Second-degree burns may also be treated with bioactive dressings as well such as Biobran. Again the wound is débrided and cleaned and the bioactive dressing is applied. The dressing is covered with an occlusive gauze dressing. The wound is examined every day or two with debriding of the bioactive dressing so that the wound should be entirely epithelialized where the dressing has separated. Systemic antibiotics are administered when there is documented sepsis in burn patients. Some physicians will treat scald burns prophylactically with an antistaphylococcus antibiotic, even though there are inadequate data to support this.

As stated earlier, burns not healed by 14 days should be referred to a specialist for care. Any signs of systemic inflammatory reaction, fever, or sepsis merits consideration for hospital admission.

Third-degree burns require immediate medical attention. Third-degree burns that restrict blood flow to the extremities or chest wall excursion must undergo immediate escarotomy. The burns are excised (usually immediately) and the remaining beds are prepared for grafting. The affected area is grafted with homologous or autologous dermis as soon as the patient is stable for surgery and the true burn depth has been ascertained. Fluid resuscitation is crucial and is adjusted to maintain urine output in children.

PAIN MANAGEMENT

First-degree burns are often adequately treated with a soothing lotion such as aloe. Ibuprofen or acetaminophen may help. Rarely is other analgesia required. Second-degree burns can be extremely painful, particularly during dressing changes. Administration of codeine, meperidine (Demerol),

or oral diazepam (Valium) may be necessary for the first few days after the burn, particularly during dressing changes. Later, ibuprofen or acetaminophen often suffices. Topical analgesics are not used because absorption through the damaged skin is increased and may rapidly cause systemic effects. The administration of narcotics or other analgesics that can act as respiratory depressants must be used with caution in the outpatient setting. See Chapter 285 for a more detailed description of analgesic medications and their administration.

RECOGNIZING POTENTIAL CHILD ABUSE

Burns are a common manifestation of child abuse. Any burn whose age or appearance does not coincide with the history presented to the physician should raise the suspicion of child abuse. Children are as sensitive to pain as adults, and if a child encounters a burning surface, the child usually will rapidly pull away without exposing any other part of the body to the offending surface. Unusual burns are often associated with an intentional injury and should be thoroughly investigated. Burns of the genitalia and perineum and burns that demonstrate "patterns" such as the shape of a radiator, iron, or stove top should also raise the suspicion for abuse. Immersion burns of the buttocks with sparing of the feet, or immersion burns of the buttocks and one foot cannot be explained by an accident without forced immersion occurring. Burns to the back of the hand, which is not a common exploring surface, should also be investigated for the possibility of abuse.

PREVENTION STRATEGIES

Preventing burns is by far the most effective treatment. Often parents are not aware of the potential causes of burn injury and physicians should take the opportunity to add this information to their new parent counseling. New parents should adjust the regulators on hot water heaters to 120°F. Parents should be warned about electric shock exposure, cooking surfaces (pot or pan handles) within a child's reach, and the danger of easy access to such devices as matches and lighters. Steam radiators should be covered, as should space heaters, fireplaces, and wood stoves. Children's clothing should be labeled as flame retardant or nonflammable. Physicians should inquire about the presence of working smoke detectors in the home at every initial baby visit.

SUGGESTED READINGS

American Academy of Pediatrics. Available at: www.aap.org/family/1to2yrs.htm.

Bull MJ, Katcher ML, Palmer SD, et a:, Office-based counseling for injury prevention. Pediatrics 1994;94:566–567.

Davey RB, Wallis KA, Perkins K, et al: Thermal and electrical injuries. In Buntain WL (ed): Management of Pediatric Trauma. Philadelphia, WB Saunders, 1995, pp 431–449.

Herndon DN, Rutan RL, Allison WE, et al: Management of burn injuries. In Eichelberger MR (ed): Pediatric Trauma Prevention, Acute Care, Rehabilitation. St Louis, Mosby–YearBook, 1993, pp 568–590.

298

Incision and Drainage/Needle Aspiration of Cutaneous Abscesses

Craig R. Warden

Simple needle aspiration or incision and drainage (I&D) of superficial cutaneous abscesses can be accomplished in the primary care setting. Large abscesses, abscesses located in cosmetically significant areas, or abscesses that may be contiguous to important structures may require a specialist for proper drainage. Depending on time commitment and necessity for sedation and analgesia, the emergency department (ED) may be the best setting for abscess drainage. Table 298-1 lists management strategies for cutaneous abscesses.

PATIENT AND FAMILY PREPARATION

It is necessary to assess the patient's and family's ability to cooperate with a painful procedure. In general, achieving adequate local anesthesia of the skin overlying a cutaneous abscess is difficult. The patient and family should be aware that antibiotic medications alone would not heal most abscesses.

SEDATION AND ANALGESIA

Except for the smallest abscess amenable to a small incision or needle aspiration, most abscesses frequently require systemic analgesia or sedation to make drainage tolerable. The tissue pH overlying the abscess cavity is relatively acidotic, which may render local anesthetics less effective. Most abscesses require blunt dissection during drainage.

Local anesthesia frequently does not effectively reduce the discomfort of dissection. Sufficient analgesia and sedation may not be obtainable in the primary setting, thereby requiring referral of the patient to an emergency department or specialist. Table 298-2 lists choices for anesthetic agents.

NEEDLE ASPIRATION

Before initiating drainage, the health care provider should explain the procedure to the patient and family. Local anesthetics are injected into the skin where the incision or needle will be applied. Usually a simple local anesthetic such as 1% or 2% lidocaine is sufficient. Anesthetic solutions containing epinephrine are not necessary for hemostasis. Transcutaneous anesthetics may be applied provided sufficient time is given. EMLA cream (eutectic mixture of lidocaine and adrenaline) may be applied to intact skin with an occlusive dressing prior to local infiltration. EMLA must be applied at least 1 hour prior to the procedure to have any efficacy. An iontophoretic device (Numby) may also be used and needs only 10 minutes prior to the procedure to be effective. Before penetrating the skin, the abscessed area should be prepped with an antiseptic solution (usually a povidone-iodine solution, such as Betadine). Gauze or towels should be available to soak up any drained purulent material.

Small abscesses (especially ones on the face or neck) may be drained using a large-bore needle (18 gauge or larger).

Table 298-1. Selection of Management Strategies for Cutaneous Abscesses

Type of Drainage	Indications	Benefits	Risks	Controversies
No drainage	Small, superficial, not adjacent to significant anatomic structures	Minimal scarring No iatrogenic pain	Further expansion of abscess and cellulitis	Appropriate prospective selection
Needle aspiration	Small, superficial, cosmetically important areas, difficult to anesthetize adequately	Minimal scarring Minimal anesthesia required	Further expansion of abscess and cellulitis	Appropriate prospective selection
Incision and drainage	Larger abscesses	Complete drainage Break up loculations Find extent of abscess	Incomplete drainage Scarring, poor pain control	Need for endocarditis prophylaxis
Surgical/emergency department referral	Requiring significant time and/or sedation/analgesia Abscesses in cosmetically sensitive areas or areas with complex anatomy (perineum, face)	Surgical expertise and experience Adequate sedation/analgesia	Time and travel constraints Risks of sedation	Selection of sedation agents

Table 298-2. Choice of Anesthetic Agents*

Type of Anesthesia	Indications	Benefits	Risks	Controversies
EMLA cream	Initial topical anesthesia	Painless, lessen pain for injected anesthesia	Methemoglobinemia if used in large amounts Inadequate anesthesia	Time consuming
Numby iontophoretic	Initial topical anesthesia	Painless, lessen pain for injected anesthesia	Uncomfortable tingling sensation for some patients Inadequate anesthesia	Less time than EMLA
Local anesthesia	For needle aspiration or incision and drainage	Skin anesthesia	Neurologic complications with large amount Inadequate anesthesia	Most local anesthetics are partially inactivated in acidotic environment of abscesses
Regional anesthesia (nerve blocks)	Inadequate local anesthesia, large area to be anesthetized	More thorough anesthesia	Neurovascular injury possibly	Requires expertise
Parenteral sedation/analgesia	Uncooperative patient Inability to anesthetize otherwise Large abscess, prolonged procedure	Total pain control possible Cooperation ensured	Risks of sedation	What setting is appropriate?

*See Chapter 285 for detail on specific anesthetic agents.

This procedure causes less pain and anxiety than making an incision. The disadvantages are the inability to perform blunt dissection to break up loculations and the inability to pack the wound to maintain drainage. Serial needle aspirations may be necessary to maintain drainage. Needle aspiration also allows exploration of an indurated area of the skin to see if an abscess cavity requiring drainage is present. Initial decompression of "tense" abscesses with needle aspiration may give immediate pain relief and decrease the spread of purulent material upon incision.

INCISION AND DRAINAGE

For a more extensive incision and drainage, open the skin with a No. 11 or No. 15 surgical blade with an incision large enough to allow hemostat entry and dissection of the whole abscess cavity and sufficient packing of the cavity. Usually a 1- to 2-cm incision is sufficient to drain most cutaneous abscesses (Fig. 298-1). A hemostat is a good instrument for blunt dissection of the abscess cavity and breaking loculations by placing the closed hemostat into the cavity, opening the hemostat, and withdrawing the open hemostat from the wound. Application of gentle pressure on the periphery of the abscess cavity and gentle irrigation of the cavity with

normal saline encourages drainage. Removal of all purulent material is unnecessary as long as the wound is sufficiently packed after the incision and drainage procedure.

PACKING

Packing the abscess cavity helps prevent premature collapse of the cavity and reaccumulation of pus (see Fig. 298-1). The packing acts as a wick, allowing drainage while maintaining an open incision. Pushing the sterile gauze packing (available in widths from ¼ to 1 inch) into all recesses within the abscess cavity ensures complete drainage. The cavity does not need to be packed tightly, just enough to prevent collapse.

DRESSING AND ANTIBIOTICS

Dry, bulky gauze dressings allow further wicking of drainage. The patient or family may change this dressing if the dressing surface becomes damp, dirty, or saturated with drainage. During dressing change care must be taken not to pull out the packing material. Antibiotic medications are indicated if there is significant surrounding cellulitis or if the patient has immunocompromising conditions such as

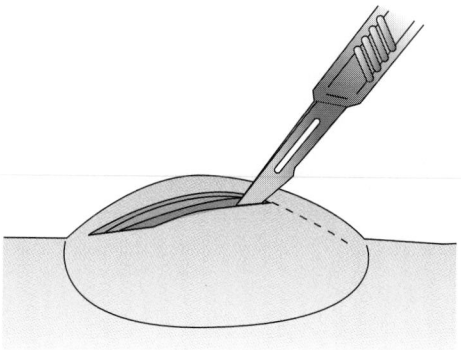

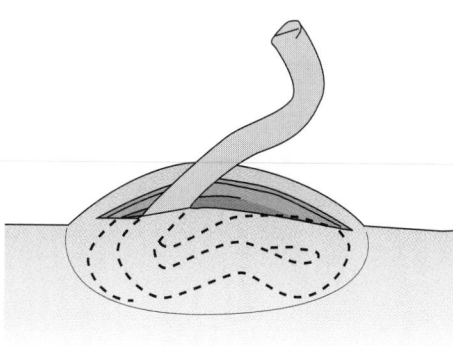

Figure 298-1. Incision and drainage of a cutaneous abscess and subsequent packing. Prepare and drape the area. After appropriate anesthesia, make an incision the length of the abscess (**A**). After allowing the abscess to drain, loosely pack the abscess cavity to prevent premature closure and recurrence (**B**). (From Goepp JG, Hostetler MA (eds): Procedures for Primary Care Pediatricians. St. Louis, Mosby, 2001, p 146.)

A

B

Table 298-3. Recommendations for Antibiotic Coverage for Cutaneous Abscesses

Type of Abscess	Controversies	Recommended Regimen
Simple abscess without cellulitis, normal host	Will usually resolve after adequate drainage	None 1st-generation cephalosporin or PRSP Clindamycin for PCN allergic patients
Surrounding cellulitis	What degree of cellulitis mandates antibiotics	1st-generation cephalosporin or PRSP Clindamycin for PCN allergic patients
Perineal abscesses ± cellulitis	Add anaerobic coverage, hospitalization indications	Amoxicillin/clavulanate 1st generation cephalosporin or PRSP + clindamycin or metronidazole
Diabetic patient Other immunocompromised patients	Broader spectrum coverage, hospitalization indications	Fluoroquinolone APSP

APSP, antipseudomonal synthetic penicillin; PCN, penicillin; PRSP, penicillinase-resistant synthetic penicillin.

diabetes, human immunodeficiency virus (HIV) infection, or therapy-induced immunosuppression (Table 298-3). The dominant bacteriology of cutaneous abscesses of children and adults is *Staphylococcus aureus* along with streptococcal species. Abscesses in perirectal, head, finger, and nailbed areas are often due to anaerobic bacteria. Culturing of abscesses is generally not indicated for simple abscesses in immunocompetent patients.

FOLLOW-UP

The clinician should re-evaluate the abscess 24 to 48 hours after incision and drainage to assess response and the need for repacking. Persisting signs or symptoms should prompt evaluation for a retained foreign body, undrained loculations, worsening cellulitis, or developing septic fasciitis or myositis. Depending on the extent of cavity and speed of healing, serial packing may be necessary to accomplish complete abscess drainage. Packing is removed when drainage resolves.

OUTCOME

The expected outcome in an otherwise healthy pediatric patient with a simple abscess is a relatively painless drainage procedure, rapid collapse of the abscess cavity, and successful healing by secondary intention. Except for needle drainage, scarring is an unavoidable outcome of abscess incision and drainage.

Table 298-4 lists typical equipment required for abscess drainage.

Table 298-4. Minimum Equipment Required for Drainage Procedures

Type of Procedure	Equipment Needed
Needle aspiration	Topical and/or local anesthetic Antiseptic 18- or 20-gauge needle with appropriate syringe or Vacutainer needle and collection tube Dressing with 2 × 2 or 4 × 4 inch gauze and tape
Incision and drainage	Topical and/or local anesthetic Sedation/analgesia as necessary Antiseptic and drapes Optional initial needle drainage (as above) Scalpel (No. 11 or 15 most commonly) Absorbent sponges (4 × 4 most commonly) Curved hemostats Packing (usually ¼- or ½-inch gauze) Scissors Dressing with 4 × 4 gauze and tape

SUGGESTED READINGS

Brook I, Finegold SM: Aerobic and anaerobic bacteriology of cutaneous abscesses in children. Pediatrics 1981;67(6):891–895.

Brook I, Frazier EH: Aerobic and anaerobic bacteriology of wounds and cutaneous abscesses. Arch Surg 1990;125(11):1445–1451.

Llera JL, Levy RC: Treatment of cutaneous abscess: A double-blind clinical study. Ann Emerg Med 1985:14(1):15–19.

Llera JL, Levy RC, Staneck JL: Cutaneous abscesses: Natural history and management in an outpatient facility. J Emerg Med 1984; 1(6):489–493.

Meislin HW: Pathogen identification of abscesses and cellulitis. Ann Emerg Med 1986;15(3):329–332.

299 Splinting and Casting

Ronald Turker

Immobilizing an injured extremity is one of the oldest forms of medical intervention and the simple act of putting an injured extremity at rest can be lifesaving. Immobilization of a fracture decreases blood loss, pain, and the potential for further injury to muscle, nerves, and blood vessels. Improper placement of a splint or cast may cause greater injury. Iatrogenic injuries range from mild skin abrasions and stiffness to complete neurovascular compromise and possible loss of an otherwise viable limb (Fig. 299-1). A thoughtful approach to the care of an injured extremity reduces risks while increasing benefits to the patient. See Chapter 50 for more detailed information on fractures and dislocations.

Splints and casts are employed for a variety of maladies. Fractures and dislocations are the most obvious indications but other common uses include soft tissue stretching to treat joint contractures and the placement of an infected limb at rest during recovery.

The main focus of this chapter will be on splinting. Many fractures can and should be treated initially, and sometimes completely, with a well-applied splint. The plaster or fiberglass splint should not cover more than two thirds of the

---

Box 299-1. Splinting Materials

Prefabricated fiberglass padding (e.g., Orthoglass), sizes 2, 3, 4 inches
Other padding: sizes 2 to 4 inches (e.g., Synthetic Webril, Specialist Padding)
Plaster splint slabs: 2, 3, 4, 5 inches
Ace bandage wraps: 2 to 6 inches
    Velcro tip is easier to use for children.
    Use nonlatex wrap for patients with myelomeningocele.
Towel

---

circumference of the affected limb in order to avoid neurovascular compromise during the period of acute swelling that frequently occurs 48 hours after injury.

Circumferential casts have a higher potential for morbidity and should be applied with caution. Circular cast placement requires hands-on training and is beyond the scope of this chapter.

Many objects at hand may serve to temporarily splint an injured limb. Scraps of wood, rolled magazines, and pillows are commonly used objects. Commercially available items such as vacuum and pneumatic splints are suitable for temporary use in the prehospital setting. The pneumatic splints theoretically control for internal blood loss, but have a potential to cause compartment syndrome when used for peripheral fractures. Pneumatic splints are best suited for fractures of the femur and pelvis. Temporary splints should be removed and replaced with a more appropriate long-term splint or cast as soon as feasible. Box 299-1 lists materials necessary for making splints.

In the clinical setting, splints are made of aesthetically pleasing and effective materials. The two most common materials available are the inexpensive (and well proved to be effective) plaster of paris and the new, innovative (and more expensive) prefabricated fiberglass and padding combination splints. The modern fiberglass and synthetic padding splints require little water to apply, are less exothermic than plaster, and allow placement of particular splints not possible to make with plaster. Both products work well when applied with care, but steps must be taken to avoid splint or cast burns with either material. Padding for splints or casts should be wrinkle-free. Wrinkles in hardened casts and splints can become quite uncomfortable, especially over a bony prominence.

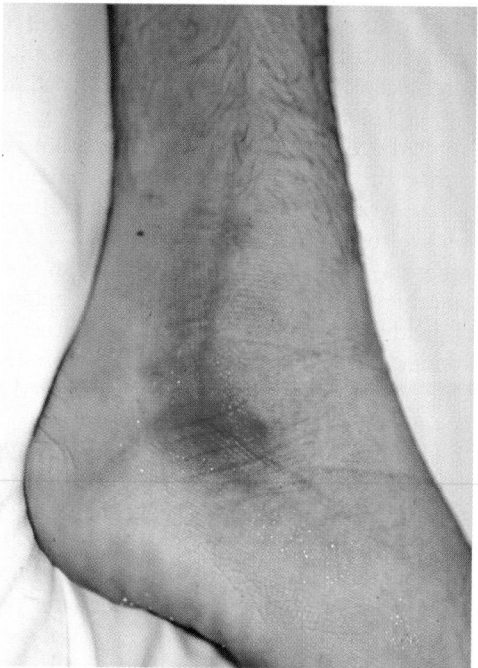

Figure 299-1. Pressure sore over lateral malleolus.

APPLICATION GUIDELINES

Box 299-2 lists the general guidelines for splinting. Immobilize a joint above and below the injured portion of the extremity whenever possible. Keep in mind that a splint applied to the leg and thigh for a midshaft femur fracture increases force of leverage on the fracture site more than it immobilizes the injured bone; traction splinting is more appropriate for injuries of the femur. Some injuries to the distal humerus, distal femur, and distal tibia can be treated without immobilizing the joint proximal to the injury.

Body habitus should be taken into account when applying a splint or cast. Thinner patients have less soft tissue between the splint or cast and the bone, thereby allowing better fixation of the fracture. The heavier the patient, the longer the splint or cast should be. A longer splint on the lever portion of the affected limb is more comfortable for the patient and provides better fixation (Fig. 299-2A–C).

Anticipate swelling of the affected limb. A poorly applied cast or splint may exacerbate limb swelling by impeding venous and lymphatic return. Edema of the affected limb may lead to a compartment syndrome within the first 2 days of injury. The degree of swelling depends on the anatomic location and severity of the injury. Injuries that cause extensive soft tissue injury can produce remarkable amounts of swelling. Comminuted fractures (multiple fragments) and fractures of the foot and ankle tend to cause considerable swelling.

All jewelry, including rings, medical alert bracelets, and hospital identification bands, should be removed from the injured limb before splint or cast placement (Fig. 299-3).

The padding of a splint or cast should be applied with as few wrinkles as possible. Circumferential rolling of the padding is a good way to decrease the number and size of wrinkles. Cotton padding is gently rolled onto the contours of the affected limb. Discreet incomplete tearing of the padding edge allows for changing the angle and direction of padding without leaving wrinkles or gaps. Three layers of padding are appropriate for most splint applications. However, more padding is neccessary for osseous prominences such as the malleoli or fibular head. When a splint involves a flexed joint (e.g., elbow or ankle), care must be taken to place equal amounts of padding and cast material over both flexor and extensor surfaces. Excess material in

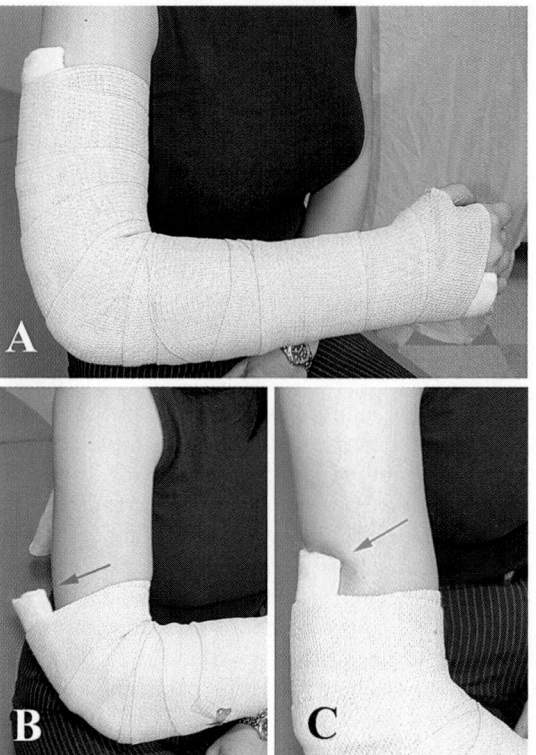

Figure 299-2. A, Longer proximal limb of arm splint provides comfort and stability. Shorter proximal limb splint allows more movement **(B)** and discomfort **(C).**

the flexed side of the joint (e.g., the anterior aspect of the ankle) may cause a pressure sore. Placing ripped pieces of cotton padding along the surface that needs extra padding instead of continuing to circumferentially roll the padding avoids placing too much unnecessary material on the concave side. The distal tips of the fingers and toes must be visible after splint or cast placement to allow neurovascular examination of the injured limb. If the fingers are included in the splint or cast, cotton is placed between the digits to avoid skin maceration from sweating. After padding placement, a fiberglass or plaster covering of appropriate thickness is applied over the padding. Casts or splints should be contoured to the extremity with a neat, smooth external surface. No wrinkles and fingertip indentations should appear on the surface.

Preparing the total splint before applying to the affected limb is another way to achieve wrinkle-free splinting. Four layers of padding are rolled on top of each other, making a slightly wider and longer spread than the intended plaster splint. One layer is peeled back, the plaster is laid on top of the three remaining layers of padding, and the single peeled layer is folded back onto the plaster. The combined plaster/padding splint is applied to the limb with the thicker padding toward the patient. An elastic wrap (Ace bandage) or muslin wrap is placed around the limb, holding the splint in place. The outside extra layer of padding keeps the plaster from sticking to the wrap, making later removal of the wrap easy.

Avoid splint or cast burns. Tepid, not hot, water should be used to cure the plaster or fiberglass material. The more

---

Box 299-2. Splinting Guidelines

1. Always immobilize a joint above and below the injured portion of the extremity if possible.
2. Consider body habitus for deciding splint size when applying a splint or cast.
3. Anticipate swelling of the affected limb.
4. Remove all jewelry, including rings, medical alert bracelets, and hospital identification from the injured limb before splint or cast placement.
5. Apply padding for splint or cast with as few wrinkles as possible.
6. Avoid splint or cast burns.
7. Make sure both patient and provider are comfortable during cast or splint application.

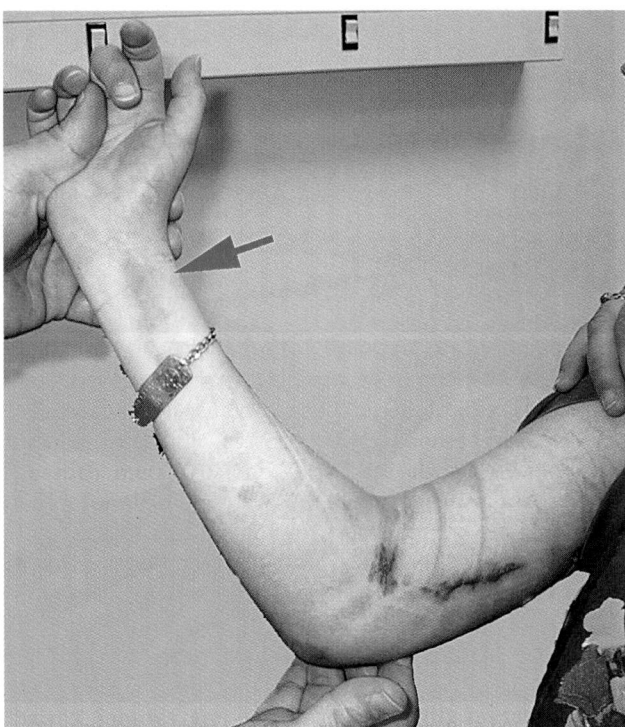

Figure 299-3. Wrist bruising *(red arrow)* caused by bracelet under splint. Turned-in edges of splint caused pressure sore on the proximal arm.

layers of plaster added, the hotter the splint becomes during the curing. After splint or cast application, the limb should rest in a position that allows maximal loss of exothermic heat as the plaster/fiberglass hardens. Resting a splinted limb on a pillow or plastic mattress prevents shedding of excess heat and may lead to burns.

Both patient and provider should be comfortable during cast or splint application. For upper extremity splinting, the patient should sit while resting the affected elbow on a nearby gurney or table. For lower extremity splinting, the patient should rest in either a supine or a seated position on the gurney with the lower leg hanging over the edge. Flexing the knee makes it easier for the patient to dorsiflex the ankle toward a neutral position.

Table 299-1. Splinting Techniques and Indications

Splint Type	Indication
Long leg splint	Knee immobilization (knee positioned in extension)
	Distal femur, proximal and midshaft tibia/fibula fractures (knee positioned in flexion)
Short leg posterior splint	Distal leg, foot, and ankle fractures
Sling and swathe	Upper extremity injuries between sternoclavicular joint and elbow
Long arm splint	Forearm and distal radius fractures
Posterior arm splint	Elbow and forearm injuries
	Wrist injuries requiring no forearm rotation or elbow flexion
Sugar tong splint	Humerus, forearm, elbow, and wrist injuries
Ulnar gutter splint	Nondisplaced fractures of 4th and 5th fingers
Thumb spica splint	Thumb injuries and scaphoid fractures

SPLINT VERSUS CAST

Splinting alone may be sufficient to treat an injured limb. In the upper extremity where weight bearing is not a concern, splints work well. In the case of a stable fracture (such as a torus or buckle fracture of the distal radius) a well-applied splint is as good as a cast. Many orthopedic surgeons prefer to use splints for both stable and unstable fractures for the entire treatment course. A well-applied, carefully molded splint can be as comfortable as a cast. In the lower extremity, if the patient is going to bear weight on the affected limb, a splint is not sufficient to withstand the force of ambulation. The stronger circular cast is the better therapeutic choice. However, a well-applied splint to the injured upper or lower body is an effective temporary measure before definitive treatment is possible.

Table 299-1 lists the indications for specific types of splints.

UPPER EXTREMITY SPLINTING

A good, neutral resting position of the hand is achieved by placing a rolled Ace bandage or roll of cotton padding in the palm and gently flexing the splinted fingers around the roll. When including the fingers in a splint (e.g., a metacarpal fracture) it is best to *flex* the metacarpophalangeal joint as much as possible. Mistakenly placing the fingers in extension relaxes the collateral ligaments. After 3 to 4 weeks in extension, the collateral ligaments may become tight, making flexion of the fingers difficult after the splint is removed. The wrist should be slightly extended. For distal radius fractures, a neutral pronation-supination position of the hand is probably best with the splint extending past the elbow.

There are many different splints for upper extremity injuries. This chapter outlines the more frequently used static splints for the acutely injured limb rather than the more complicated dynamic splints used in extremity rehabilitation.

Shoulder and Clavicle Injuries

The sling is one of the simplest methods for putting the injured arm at rest. Slings place an injured shoulder or clavicle at rest and are often used with other immobilization devices. Midshaft clavicle fractures usually heal well with minimal intervention. A sling is the only treatment needed for a straightforward clavicle fracture. A swathe may be added to the sling when rotation of the shoulder needs to be limited, as in the case of a freshly reduced anterior shoulder dislocation. To avoid skin maceration and poor hygiene, it is always important to place a cotton pad in the axilla when the shoulder is completely immobilized. Of note, the figure-eight harness for a clavicle fracture is infrequently recommended because it is difficult to wear, works effectively only when the patient is upright, and tends to press on the skin directly over the fracture site.

Humeral Fractures

Fractures in the humeral diaphysis are often treated with a coaptation splint, characterized by a plaster or fiberglass slab wrapped around the arm from medial to lateral aspect.

roller bandage. Another method is alternating three layers of cotton cast padding with a layer of kling roll twice, followed by an Ace wrap. Either method allows placement of a posterior slab of plaster if additional support is necessary.

Foot Fractures

Metatarsal shaft fractures are also treated with short leg splints. Metatarsal neck and phalangeal fractures often do well with just a hard-soled shoe.

CONCLUSION

Many fractures and soft tissue injuries are treated with a well-fitting splint or cast. The haphazard placement of an ill-fitting splint or cast may have devastating long-term consequences. Different types of casts and splints may be used for similar injuries, and the care provider should choose the splint or cast that works best for the injury, patient comfort, and physician expertise. Patients should be informed of the signs and symptoms of potential limb injuries associated with splints and casts.

SUGGESTED READINGS

Chan D, Goldberg RM, Mason J, Chan L: Backboard versus mattress splint immobilization: A comparison of symptoms generated. J Emerg Med 1996;14(3):293–298.

Harkess JW, Ramsey WC: Principles of fractures and dislocations. In Rockwood CA (ed): Fractures in Adults, 4th ed. Vol. 1. Philadelphia, Lippincott-Raven, 1996.

Howes DS, Kaufman JJ: Plaster splints: Techniques and indications. Am Fam Physician 1984;30(3):215–221.

Shakespeare DT, Henderson NJ, Sherman KP: Transmission of pressure into the human limb from pneumatic splints. Injury 1984;16:38–40.

Shaw DC, Heckman JD: Principles and techniques of splinting musculocutaneous injuries. Emerg Med Clin North Am 1984;2:391–407.

SECTION 9   DIAGNOSTICS AND THERAPEUTICS: *Procedural Medicine*

300 General Surgical Interventions and Techniques

Ann K. Seltman, Charles J. Smithers, and Mark L. Silen

Primary care physicians frequently encounter pediatric patients who require surgical intervention. The combination of a careful history and physical examination most often suggests the correct diagnosis, or a discrete number of differential diagnoses. Further evaluation through carefully selected laboratory tests and radiographic studies usually establishes the diagnosis and determines the correct therapy. The challenge for the primary care provider is balancing a thorough workup with prompt referral to a pediatric surgeon for definitive therapy. Early consultation with a pediatric surgeon may facilitate both timely evaluation and definitive therapy.

Most general surgical procedures involve exploration of the abdominal, pelvic, and retroperitoneal areas. Other procedures include noncardiac thoracic surgery and removal of airway and esophageal foreign bodies. This chapter describes commonly used surgical techniques.

SURGICAL EMERGENCIES

True pediatric surgical emergencies are generally diseases that threaten tissue viability by loss of blood supply, acute blood loss, or airway obstruction. Preparation of patients for surgery includes adequate volume resuscitation and the placement of urinary catheters or nasogastric tubes as indicated by the particular clinical situation. Family and patient education about possible resection of devitalized tissue is also crucial. Surgical illnesses tend to be acute in onset and may be emotionally difficult for families to handle, especially if family members are not adequately counseled preoperatively about the possibility of loss of tissue or the need for the creation of a temporary intestinal stoma.

Surgical emergencies need prompt referral to or consultation with a pediatric surgical specialist. Typical examples of ischemic emergencies include intussusception, malrotation of the intestine with midgut volvulus, acute torsion of a gonad, and strangulation of a viscus within a hernia. Airway compromise and significant major trauma should also be considered as surgical emergencies.

PREOPERATIVE EVALUATION AND PREPARATION

The preparation of an otherwise healthy child for an elective surgical procedure may not require any adjunctive laboratory or radiographic examinations. In contrast, if a previously healthy child with a reducible inguinal hernia has a history or physical examination that indicates the possibility of a bleeding disorder, then a complete blood cell count, including a platelet count, and coagulation panel (prothrombin time, partial thromboplastin time) are indicated. Routine imaging, such as a chest radiograph, is not recommended, or necessary, in the preoperative workup unless specifically indicated by the disease state. Other laboratory imaging is determined on an individual case basis.

The risk of aspiration following the induction of general anesthesia is minimized by protocols directed at having the stomach empty at the time of the planned elective procedure. The small size and large body surface area of children make them more susceptible to dehydration than adults. The traditional rule of nothing to eat or drink 6 hours prior to a general anesthetic is impractical, and potentially harmful, in children. Increased anxiety and agitation prior to surgery are also encountered in infants and children not allowed to eat or drink for prolonged periods of time. Children have a rapid gastric emptying time, especially for clear liquids. Most pediatric anesthesiologists allow milk and solids up to 6 hours prior to operation, and clear liquids up to 3 hours prior to an elective general anesthetic. These guidelines are often age- and procedure-specific and should be confirmed with the anesthesiologist.

Upper respiratory illnesses, especially those associated with fever and productive cough, are not uncommon in childhood. Children with upper respiratory illnesses, particularly neonates and younger children, who undergo general anesthesia are at greater risk for respiratory complications, and most pediatric surgeons and pediatric anesthesiologists recommend postponing truly elective procedures until the respiratory illness has resolved.

Premature infants subjected to general anesthesia are at risk for postoperative apnea and bradycardia. Infants younger than 44 to 60 weeks postconception age should be monitored in the hospital for 24 hours following surgery.

Exact guidelines for anesthesia should be confirmed with the anesthesiologist prior to surgery.

INCISION COMPLICATIONS

The creation and subsequent closure of any surgical wound must address several concerns. Sterile technique decreases the risk of wound infection. During the initial creation of a wound, careful attention should be paid to minimizing tissue injury. Devitalization of the skin, subcutaneous tissue, muscle, and fascia may have deleterious effects on the eventual healing and outcome of the wound. Lack of attention to hemostasis, especially in the subcutaneous tissues, may result in either a wound hematoma or a subsequent wound infection. Any failure of fascial closure may result in either an acute dehiscence of the wound or a postoperative hernia.

Acute wound cellulitis is rare, but may occur within the first 12 to 24 hours following surgery. Hallmarks of cellulitis are high fever and erythema around the wound. Common pathogens include *Clostridium* species, *Staphylococcus, Streptococcus,* and *Peptostreptococcus.* Early aggressive antibiotic therapy (usually with a semisynthetic

penicillin active against staphylococci and streptococci) is generally successful. See Chapter 284 for discussion of appropriate choice of antibiotic medications.

A more serious wound infection is gas gangrene. Early gas gangrene presents with severe wound pain and surrounding erythema. A dusky, brown, necrotic wound with crepitance appears in the later stages of infection. Systemic signs of gas gangrene include a general toxic appearance with fever, tachycardia, and shock. The usual pathogens are again *Clostridium* species, *Streptococcus,* or *Peptostreptococcus.* Gangrenous wounds should be emergently opened, irrigated, and surgically debrided. High-dose penicillin is the drug of choice for treatment with clindamycin, metronidazole, imipenem, cilastin, meropenem, and chloramphenicol as alternatives for patients with penicillin allergy (see Chapter 284). Some evidence supports hyperbaric oxygen therapy in the treatment of clostridial infection.

Late wound infections usually occur 5 days after surgery with infection presenting again as cellulitis or abscess. Antibiotic therapy to cover gram-positive organisms, such as *Staphylococcus* and *Streptococcus,* is the treatment of choice. In the event of abscess formation, opening the wound allows drainage of the abscess and speeds recovery.

Noninfectious wound complications include hematomas, skin and fascial wound dehiscence, and incisional hernias. Hematomas occur in about 2% of incisions and are due to inadequate hemostasis within the tissues of the abdominal wall. Pain and low-grade fever are frequently noted. Small hematomas usually resolve spontaneously. Larger hematomas may require percutaneous drainage or evacuation in the operating room.

Wound dehiscence is very uncommon in pediatric surgery and occurs in less than 1% of patients. Dehiscence is most frequently due to a technical error during closure. Malnutrition, diabetes, and parenteral steroid use may contribute to a higher rate of dehiscence. Fascial dehiscence usually presents on the *seventh* postoperative day with serosanguineous drainage from the wound, acute hernia, or evisceration. Early fascial dehiscence requires immediate surgical correction. Incisional hernias may develop at the incision site within weeks to several years postoperatively. Incisional hernias are not usually life threatening, but may cause discomfort and cosmetic deformity. These hernias should be electively repaired.

TYPES OF SURGERY

In general, there are two types of surgery: "open surgery" and "minimally invasive surgery." "Open surgery" involves making an incision large enough to provide easy access and exposure of the underlying tissues and organs to undergo surgery. "Minimally invasive surgery" generally refers to video-assisted surgery (laparoscopy), a technique prominently used by surgeons nowadays. "Minimal access surgery" may be a more applicable term because laparoscopy is still considered quite invasive. Despite the overall popularity for video-assisted surgery, obvious indications for open operations still exist. Other surgical procedures include percutaneous drainage and biopsy.

What follows is a description of the various surgical procedures performed on different body regions. Table 300-1

Table 300-1. Open versus Laparoscopic Surgery: Comparative Advantages and Disadvantages

Features	Open Surgery	Laparoscopic Surgery
Time	Shorter operative time	Longer operative time
Cost	Lower intraoperative costs	Higher equipment costs
Length of hospital stay	Longer hospital stay	Shorter length of stay
Equipment	Less reliance on equipment	Good visualization with improved optics/cameras
Postoperative course	Longer time to ambulate, resume oral intake	Laparoscopic specific complications (e.g., bowel injury upon trocar placement)
Pain	More postoperative pain	Less postoperative pain
Appearance	Larger incisional scar	Better cosmetic results
Experience	Long history of success	New, experimental techniques
Performance requirements	Training already in place	Technically challenging, steep learning curve

lists advantages and disadvantages of open versus laparoscopic surgery.

ABDOMINAL, PELVIC, AND RETROPERITONEAL SURGERY

Open Surgery

A variety of abdominal incisions expose intraperitoneal, pelvic, and retroperitoneal structures. Upper midline incisions provide access to the liver, diaphragm, stomach, duodenum, gallbladder, pancreas, esophageal hiatus, and the small and large intestine. Lower midline incisions expose the colon, rectum, small intestine, and pelvis. Right paramedian, muscle-sparing incisions, an alternative to right subcostal incisions, are excellent for surgical procedures involving the biliary tract, duodenum, and porta hepatis. Left paramedian incisions, or left subcostal incisions, are useful for total colectomy and splenectomy and allow placement of a right-sided ileostomy. Muscle-splitting right iliac fossa incisions are ideal for open appendectomy. Flank incisions may be used for exposure of retroperitoneal structures including the kidney and the great vessels. For newborns and infants, a transverse supraumbilical incision provides excellent access to most intraperitoneal structures.

Minimal Access Surgery

Minimal access surgical techniques are routinely used in a variety of operations of the abdomen in children including cholecystectomy, appendectomy, location of a nonpalpable testis, and exploratory laparoscopy. More advanced laparoscopic procedures include splenectomy, bowel resection, and antireflux procedures. Minimal access surgical techniques involve placement of one or more hollow ports through the abdominal wall into the peritoneal cavity and subsequent insufflation of the peritoneal cavity with carbon dioxide. The number and location of ports necessary depends on the planned operation. Fiberoptic telescopes and a variety of instruments and retractors can be introduced into the peritoneal cavity through these ports. Attaching a camera to the operating telescope allows image display of the procedure for other attendants in the operating room. (See the CD-ROM for a video showing a laparoscopic appendectomy.)

Surgeons performing minimal access surgery must be prepared to convert to an open operation. Indications for conversion include damage to major blood vessels, intestines, or solid organs during initial port placement, uncontrolled bleeding despite laparoscopic instrumentation, and inability to complete the planned operation using minimal access techniques. Although minimal access surgery incisions are smaller, these wounds are subject to the same complications of "open surgery" incisions.

Percutaneous Drainage and Biopsy

Recently, ultrasound- and computed tomography–guided procedures have taken an increasingly greater role in the diagnosis and management of disease within the abdomen and pelvis. Percutaneous biopsy of mass lesions and drainage of abscesses and fluid collections is safe and effective in the hands of experienced radiologists. These procedures should be considered in consultation with an experienced radiologist and pediatric surgeon.

NONCARDIAC THORACIC SURGERY

Pediatric surgeons treat a variety of diseases involving the contents of the thorax, thoracic wall, and mediastinum. Surgical approaches to the thorax include both standard "open" and "minimal access" techniques, and a discussion of different options for surgical access to the chest, along with anesthetic techniques specific to thoracic surgery, follows. Indications for the various thoracic incisions, expected outcomes, and common complications of thoracic surgery also follow.

Most thoracic surgical procedures for children require general anesthesia. Monitoring of the patient during a procedure utilizing a general anesthetic usually includes noninvasive methods of monitoring blood pressure, oxygen saturation, end-tidal CO_2 levels, temperature, and heart rate and rhythm. Invasive methods of monitoring arterial and venous pressures are used at the discretion of the pediatric anesthesiologist and pediatric surgeon.

Lung isolation techniques or "one lung" anesthesia are unique forms of anesthesia for thoracic surgery. Indications for "one lung" anesthesia include avoidance of tracheobronchial soilage from a lung abscess or need for more complete visualization of a pleural cavity. Three primary methods can be used to provide lung isolation: unilateral endobronchial blockers, unilateral main stem bronchus intubation with a single-lumen endotracheal tube, and double-lumen endotracheal tubes. Double-lumen endotracheal tubes are the most commonly used tubes for lung isolation. These tubes have one lumen for the trachea and a second lumen for one main stem bronchus. Both left- and right-sided bronchus versions are available. Flexible bronchoscopy helps ensure correct placement of these specialized endotracheal tubes. Each lumen of the double-lumen endotracheal tube may be used for either ventilation or suction of the lung. Endobronchial blockers have a balloon tip catheter that is advanced either through or adjacent to an endotracheal tube into the main stem bronchus to block ventilation of the desired lung. Complications lung isolation techniques include airway damage, tube malposition, and hypoxemia. Damage to the larynx may result from the larger diameter of the double lumen endotracheal tubes. Damage to the wall of the tracheobronchial tree, though rare, may be devastating.

Open Thoracotomy Incisions

Open thoracotomy may be accomplished by a variety of incisions. Choice of incision is dictated by required area of exposure necessary for the particular operation to be performed while preserving chest wall function and ensuring good cosmetic outcome.

Median sternotomy involves placing a vertical midline skin incision in the chest with division of the sternum for exposure of the anterior mediastinum. Median sternotomy provides access to the distal cervical and mediastinal trachea, mediastinal tumors, the thymus gland, the heart and great vessels, both lungs, and pulmonary hila. Advantages of this approach include safe, fast access; quick wound healing; and less postoperative pain compared to standard lateral thoracotomies. Disadvantages include possible brachial plexus injuries, unstable sternum, sternal osteomyelitis, and mediastinitis.

The different types of "lateral" thoracotomy are generally defined by their anterior, anterolateral, lateral, posterolateral, and posterior relationship to the latissimus dorsi muscle. These incisions provide a wide range of exposure to the thoracic cavity and its contents, including the lungs, pleura, aorta, trachea, esophagus, and other anterior and posterior mediastinal structures. The posterolateral thoracotomy is the most frequently used incision and is often inferred by the generic term *thoracotomy*. The pleural cavity is usually entered through the fourth or fifth intercostal space for most procedures, but other intercostal spaces may be chosen depending on the surgical target. A variation of the standard thoracotomy is the "muscle sparing" thoracotomy, which avoids division of the latissimus dorsi muscle, the serratus anterior muscle, or both. Instead, these muscles are isolated and retracted for adequate exposure. Muscle sparing thoracotomy may decrease the postoperative pain, immobility, and disability that accompany division of these muscles. Muscle sparing thoracotomy may also help preserve chest wall function and shoulder girdle strength and, in children, may decrease development of chest wall deformity during growth. Disadvantages of the muscle sparing techniques include less surgical exposure and increased incidence of wound seromas and infections (2% to 3%) compared to a standard thoracotomy.

Other options for open thoracotomy are worthy of mention. Vertical axillary incision provides exposure for lung apex operations, first rib resections, and thoracic sympathectomies. The anterior mediastinotomy incision, or Chamberlain procedure, is used mainly for biopsy of mass lesions in the anterior mediastinum. This procedure utilizes a lateral parasternal incision at the second or third rib with resection of the costal cartilage and division of the internal mammary artery. Open vertical axillary and anterior mediastinotomy approaches have largely been supplanted by thoracoscopy. Thoracoabdominal incisions may be utilized for exposure of the upper abdomen and lower thorax (e.g., to excise large Wilms' tumor, neuroblastoma) but are uncommon in general practice.

Minimal Access Thoracic Surgery

Virtually all open thoracotomy procedures performed may be achieved by "minimally invasive" techniques. The indications for thoracoscopy or video-assisted thoracic surgery (VATS) are expanding as surgeons gain more experience. VATS utilizes small incisions to access the thoracic cavity with a thoracoscope and other specialized instruments. Anesthesia for VATS is similar to that for open thoracotomies with single-lung ventilation most often utilized to improve visualization. Insufflation of the pleural cavity with carbon dioxide may be used to help collapse the ipsilateral lung. Processes that obliterate or obscure the pleural cavity such as adhesions from prior thoracotomies or extensive pleural inflammation may limit VATS's feasibility.

The most common indications for thoracoscopy are evaluation and treatment of pleural disorders such as effusions or empyema. Diagnostically, thoracoscopy may help obtain pleural fluid for laboratory evaluation and cytologic examination. For drainage of parapneumonic effusions or empyema, VATS is often superior to chest tube drainage alone because it may provide more complete drainage in a shorter time period. Thoracoscopy used for apical bleb resection for pneumothorax provides the chance to perform pleurodesis or apical pleurectomy at the same time, thereby decreasing pneumothorax recurrence rates. In the stable trauma patient, drainage of subacute or chronic hemothoraces by VATS helps prevent the development of fibrothorax or empyema.

VATS figures prominently in the diagnosis of various tumors of the thoracic cavity and mediastinum. It affords excellent visualization for biopsy of tumors of the anterior or posterior mediastinum, lung, and pleural surfaces with minimal morbidity. VATS resection of tumors is becoming feasible as technical skills and tools develop. However, lobectomies or complete pneumonectomies for small children are still best handled by open thoracotomy because these surgical procedures risk excessive and rapid blood loss.

Tube Thoracostomy

A chest tube may be required to drain air or fluid from a pleural cavity. In general, these tubes can be safely placed using sedation and local anesthesia. The intersection of the midaxillary line and fifth intercostal space is the most common location for placement, though placement may vary, depending on the location of the fluid or air to be drained. The use of intraluminal trocars is strongly discouraged because of the potential for organ damage. Most thoracic procedures, either by open thoracotomy or VATS, require chest tube placement for drainage of air or fluid from the pleural space afterward. These catheters are placed utilizing small incisions that allow tunneling over the rib, accessing the pleural cavity while avoiding the intercostal neurovascular bundle that resides on the undersurface of the corresponding rib. Chest tubes are directed posteriorly to drain fluid as a rule and anteriorly to drain air (pneumothoraces). Larger-diameter tubes are required for drainage of thicker or more viscous fluids such as blood or pus.

AIRWAY AND ESOPHAGEAL FOREIGN BODIES

Foreign bodies in the trachea, bronchus, or esophagus can present as a surgical emergency if the child's airway is compromised. Rigid endoscopy is the most common method of retrieval for both airway and esophageal foreign bodies. Use of a rigid ventilating bronchoscope maintains the airway and ventilation during the procedure better than flexible bronchoscopy and allows for insertion of forceps and other instruments useful in extracting the foreign body. Rigid esophagoscopy should be employed for patients with a prolonged history of esophageal foreign body, or certainly in those patients with any element of associated airway symptoms. The main risk for both of these procedures is perforation of the airway or esophagus.

An experienced pediatric radiologist using a Foley catheter extraction technique can safely remove some esophageal foreign bodies (e.g., coins). This procedure should be selected in consultation with an experienced pediatric radiologist and pediatric surgeon.

FUTURE TRENDS

The future of pediatric surgery will be shaped by attempts of physicians, patients, and their families to find safer, more efficient, and economical methods for surgical and medical therapy. As laparoscopic surgery techniques develop and more surgeons gain experience and comfort with these advances, laparoscopy may increasingly replace traditional open pediatric operations, such as pyloromyotomy, splenectomy, antireflux procedures, and bowel resections. In addition, open surgical procedures may utilize smaller and more cosmetically placed incisions.

The continuous improvement of imaging modalities will also have a significant impact on pediatric surgical procedures, allowing more outpatient percutaneous biopsy, drainage, and vascular procedures. Such augmentation of surgical evaluation and therapy will reduce patient morbidity and time in the hospital.

◎ **Additional Resources, CD-ROM**	
Laparoscopic appendectomy	Video
Bibliography	

SUGGESTED READINGS

Baue AE, Geha AS, Laks H, et al (eds): Glenn's Thoracic and Cardiovascular Surgery, 6th ed. Stamford, Conn, Appleton & Lange, 1996.

Ellis H: Incisions, closures, and management of the wound. In Zinner MJ, Schwartz SI, Ellis H (eds): Maingot's Abdominal Operations, 10th ed. Stamford, Conn, Appleton & Lange, 1997, pp 395–426.

Firilas AM, Jackson RJ, Smith SD: Minimally invasive surgery: The pediatric surgery experience. J Am Coll Surg 1998;186:542–544.

Lobe TE, Schropp KP: Pediatric Laparoscopy and Thoracoscopy, Philadelphia, WB Saunders, 1994.

O'Neill JA, et al (eds): Pediatric Surgery, 5th ed. St. Louis, Mosby-YearBook, 1998.

SECTION 9   DIAGNOSTICS AND THERAPEUTICS: *Procedural Medicine*

301 Circumcision

Dennis Vane

HISTORY

Circumcision is the most commonly performed surgical procedure in the United States. The procedure has cultural roots in the Mideast and Africa and has become commonplace in North America today, yet is rarely practiced in Europe, Asia, and South America. Even within areas of North America rates for circumcision vary greatly. Circumcision is an integral part of the Jewish and Islamic religions.

The medical community is historically divided regarding counseling parents on the benefits or risks of routine circumcision. During the 1960s neonatal circumcision was a generally accepted practice in the United States. However, in the 1970s and even into the 1980s major organizations such as the American Academy of Pediatrics (AAP) recommended against the procedure, citing no medical evidence supporting routine neonatal circumcision. Since that time the AAP has modified its policy based on multiple studies indicating that uncircumcised boys and men have a higher risk of penile problems, penile cancer, urinary tract infections, and sexually transmitted diseases including human immunodeficiency virus (HIV) infection (Box 301-1). Collected data demonstrate some, but not entirely conclusive (Box 301-2), medical benefits from circumcision, but more studies are clearly necessary before any definitive endorsement of routine circumcision can be issued.

There are definite medical indications for circumcision in infants and children (Box 301-3). Recurrent infection under the foreskin including balanitis and true phimosis and paraphimosis generally requires circumcision; however, assessing the risk of recurrent infection requires an understanding of the natural history of the foreskin in infancy. In general it is accepted that in about 46% of male newborns the foreskin is not retractable. By 3 years of age approximately 10% of boys still cannot reveal the urethral meatus, but by 17 years of age the foreskin should be retractable. Inability to easily retract the foreskin at an early age is not necessarily an indication for circumcision. There are conditions in infancy and early childhood that make circumcision advisable. Development of a phimosis or paraphimosis (usually secondary to infection or trauma from trying to reduce a tight foreskin) is one such indication. The presence or development of a circumferential scar in the foreskin indicates developing phimosis or paraphimosis. Circumferential scarring of the foreskin is not a normal condition and will generally not resolve. Circumcision is also indicated if the foreskin is so tight that the child develops a bulging or ballooning of the penile skin during urination.

THE PROCEDURE

Circumcision in the newborn and infant younger than 6 months of age can usually be performed as an outpatient with regional or local anesthesia. Under no circumstances should circumcision be entertained by anyone other than a qualified surgeon or urologist in infants older than 1 month of age because the procedure is usually more complex in those children. There is no place today for this procedure to be performed without appropriate pain management (Box 301-4). Recommendations include cutaneous application of a 2.5% lidocaine and 2.5% prilocaine mixture (EMLA cream) 45 to 60 minutes prior to the procedure, 0.8 to 1.2 mL of 1% lidocaine without epinephrine (3–4 mg/kg) administered as a penile block, or appropriate caudal block. The application of the cutaneous anesthetic has been associated with the development of methemoglobin in certain infants, and the analgesia is far inferior to the penile or caudal block. For this reason and because of its simplicity, a penile block is the recommended analgesic. Oral acetaminophen administration may provide adjunctive analgesia for postoperative pain, but it is not effective as a sole analgesic agent during circumcision. Studies have also shown that placing a pacifier dipped in sucrose solution into the infant's mouth may significantly diminish crying.

Circumcision in newborns is generally carried out with the assistance of a device such as the Plastibel, Gomco clamp, or Mogen clamp. These devices all function on the same principle of crushing tissue to obtain hemostasis and a fusion line for the circumcision (Box 301-5). The Gomco clamp is the most widely utilized and appears to give the most consistent and best results. The Plastibel, although easier to place, has more complications including the retention of nonviable tissue and more inflammation. The Mogen clamp takes the least time to apply, but its use may result in less foreskin removal than that provided by the other two devices. A dorsal slit may be required to place the devices in order to prevent tearing of the foreskin and later complications. Care must be taken in the placement of the dorsal slit to prevent bleeding and an incorrect circumcision. Occasionally fine sutures may be needed for hemostasis or perhaps utilization of a chemical or mechanical cauterant or hemostatic material. It is crucial that practitioners who perform circumcisions be facile with the procedure and can recognize and treat any potential complications.

Circumcision performed after the newborn period should generally be referred to an appropriate specialist. At an older age, circumcision requires more formal surgical procedures, hemostasis, and suturing and often requires general anesthesia.

COMPLICATIONS OF CIRCUMCISION

The reported complication rate for circumcision is below 1%. The most common reported complication is bleeding after the procedure. Bleeding is usually local and easily treated with local pressure, a suture, or perhaps a hemostatic agent. Infection is extremely rare and usually minor, consisting of local redness and purulence. Immediate postoperative swelling around the surgical site as well as redness are common and are often confused for infection. The shaft of the penis should not be tender, however, and there should be no erythematous streaking down the shaft. Streaking indicates an infection and should be treated aggressively with systemic antibiotics. There may be a small amount of exudate at the circumcision site. This exudate will usually disengage when the penis is bathed 3 to 4 days after surgery. Rarely are antibiotics necessary as long as the surgical wound is properly treated. Most physicians performing circumcision treat the fresh surgical site with a topical antibiotic cream for the first few days, applied with each diaper change. This method has the additional soothing advantage of protecting the fresh surgical site from urine. Meatal stenosis has been perceived as a common surgical complication of circumcision. In fact, it is extremely rare and perhaps no more common than in the uncircumcised population. Although the meatus may "appear" narrow, studies indicate that the majority of these children have a normal-caliber meatus and a normal urine flow. Unless the urine stream is significantly reduced in caliber and is deflected cephalad, stenosis is probably not present. The diagnosis of meatal stenosis requires calibration and measurement of the meatal opening for confirmation.

Other more serious, yet rare, complications include necrotizing fasciitis, penile degloving, resection of the glans, and creation of a chordee or urethral fistula. Circumcision, like any other surgical procedure, carries with it the potential risk for serious harm to the patient if done incorrectly. If a serious complication occurs, referral to an appropriately trained pediatric surgeon or pediatric urologist is recommended.

CONTRAINDICATIONS TO CIRCUMCISION

Thorough examination of the penis is necessary before performing a circumcision to make sure no anatomic abnormalities exist. Chordee, hypo- or epispadias, and micropenis (whether anatomic or morphologic) are all contraindications to the procedure. In many cases the surgeon repairing these abnormalities will require the redundant foreskin for surgical repair. Frequently anatomic abnormalities of the penis are identifiable by the presence of an abnormal foreskin. Clefts in the foreskin (creating an elephant ear foreskin) or in the scrotum are indications of potential anatomic abnormalities. When penile abnormalities are suspected, the practitioner should consult a pediatric surgeon or pediatric urologist.

RECOMMENDATIONS

The current policy of the AAP states that, although there may be potential medical benefits, data are insufficient to support routine male circumcision. Studies appear to indicate some reduction of penile medical problems in circumcised boys and men, but many of these problems are the result of poor hygiene. Parents must be informed about the proper care of the penis in circumcised as well as uncircumcised male infants. The physician should counsel parents that circumcision is not by itself essential to the child's well-being and that appropriate care and hygiene can prevent many of the potential medical problems of the uncircumcised penis. Discussion regarding the pros and cons of circumcision should be unbiased. The physician should also accept the cultural and religious background of the parents while discussing the procedure and support whatever parental decision is made. In all circumstances safe, adequate, and appropriate analgesia must be provided to the infant. Finally, only a stable healthy male infant should undergo routine circumcision.

SUGGESTED READINGS

American Academy of Pediatrics, Task Force on Circumcision: Circumcision Policy Statement. Pediatrics 1999;103: 686–693.

Castellsague X, Bosch FX, Munoz N, et al: Male circumcision, penile human papillomavirus, and cervical cancer in female partners. N Engl J Med 2002;34:1105–1112.

Ellis DG, Mann CM: Abnormalities of the urethra, penis and scrotum. In O'Neil JA, Rowe, MI, Grosfeld JL, et al (eds): Pediatric Surgery. St. Louis, Mosby, 1998, pp 1783–1795.

Gonzales ET, Guerriero WG: Genitourinary trauma in children. In Kelalis PP, King LR, Belman AB (eds): Clinical Pediatric Urology. Philadelphia, WB Saunders, 1985, pp 1125–1156.

Klauber GT, Grannum RS: Disorders of the external male genitalia. In Kelalis PP, King LR, Belman AB (eds): Clinical Pediatric Urology. Philadelphia, WB Saunders, 1985, pp 825–863.

302 Behavior Modification

Lisa D. Burrows-MacLean and William E. Pelham, Jr.

THE RATIONALE FOR A BEHAVIORAL APPROACH

One third of patient visits to a pediatrician's office are for behavioral concerns, not health-related issues. Behavior modification is the only evidence-based psychosocial intervention for producing behavior change in childhood mental health and behavioral health. Behavioral techniques can be applied to problems related to disease management, compliance with medical regimens, common behavior problems of childhood (e.g., the "terrible twos"), and mental health problems. Behavior modification is appropriate to use in the treatment of enuresis, obesity, diabetes management, and asthma management as well as internalizing mental health problems (e.g., depression) and externalizing behavior problems (e.g., attention deficit hyperactivity disorder, aggression, conduct problems). See Section 7 for further discussion of mental health care. Refer to the CD-ROM for examples of application of behavior modification principles

Behavior modification has been used to treat a wide variety of childhood difficulties for more than 30 years. The field was initially based on the work of psychologists such as B. F. Skinner, who studied the effects of environmental modifications on animal behavior. Studies documenting the effects of behavioral interventions with adults and children began to appear in the 1960s, and by the 1970s, it was clear that behavioral approaches to changing human behavior were more effective than most other psychological approaches. The techniques that have been developed by those working in the field of behavior modification with children, including time-out, praising and ignoring, and star charts, have been so widely adopted by parents and teachers in their daily interactions with children that it is difficult to find settings in which behavior modification is *not* used. Nevertheless, even though behavior modification techniques have become part of standard child-rearing practices, parents and teachers often struggle with implementing these techniques in a systematic way.

The purpose of this chapter is to provide the general practitioner with a framework for understanding the basic principles of behavior modification. This understanding allows the practitioner to better assist parents in developing solutions to their children's problems, ranging from establishing home-based interventions for attention deficit hyperactivity disorder (ADHD) to developing strategies that promote children's adherence to medical regimens prescribed for chronic health disorders.

SOCIAL LEARNING THEORY: A MODEL FOR UNDERSTANDING BEHAVIOR

What Is a Behavior?

Broadly, any action, thought, or feeling can be characterized as a behavior. When it comes to changing behavior in children, behaviors, even thoughts and emotions, need to be defined in observable and quantifiable terms in order to attempt to change them using behavior modification principles. In considering possible behaviors for change, it is essential that these behaviors be clearly defined so that the parent, the child, and other educators and professionals involved in the child's care understand exactly what is being targeted for change, what the goals are, and what has been determined as the criterion for improvement.

ABCs: Behavior (B) Is Controlled by Antecedents (A) and Consequences (C)

Social learning theory postulates that important components of what controls behavior are the events that happen immediately before and immediately after a behavior. In social learning theory, any event that happens before a behavior occurs is referred to as an antecedent and any event that happens immediately following a behavior is referred to as a consequence. Thus, social learning theorists use the *ABC model* in conceptualizing factors that control behavior. The A in the model stands for *antecedent*, the B in the model stands for the *behavior* itself, and the C in the model stands for the *consequences* of the behavior. Behavior can be modified by intervening at the antecedent or consequence level. Thus, if we change the precursors to a behavior, the behavior will change, and if we change or modify the results or consequences of a behavior, the behavior will change. In social learning theory, the consequences of a behavior may be positive or negative. For example, if 8-year-old Johnny refuses to eat his dinner and his mother makes him his favorite food, a peanut butter and jelly sandwich, to eat for dinner instead of the meal he refused to eat, the consequence of Johnny's refusal is positive. He will be *more likely* to eat less-preferred foods in the future if he learns that if he refuses for a long enough period of time, his mother will eventually give in and make him his favorite food. If, on the other hand, Johnny's mother refuses to fix him anything else to eat and Johnny goes to bed hungry, the consequence of Johnny's refusal is negative. He will be *less likely* to refuse to eat the meal prepared by his mother in the future. At the antecedent level, Johnny's refusal might have been avoided entirely if his mother had given him a choice of dinner entrees.

It should be noted that behavior modification can work regardless of the original cause of the behavior. The antecedents and consequences that are modified in a behavior program control the behavior, even though they might not have originally caused the behavior. For example, Johnny might have refused to eat his dinner because it was ham, and the last time Johnny ate ham, he got a stomach virus shortly afterward. Thus, the true cause of Johnny's refusal to eat his ham dinner was that he had developed an aversion to ham owing to previously being ill after eating that particular food. Nevertheless, changing the antecedents and consequences as described previously would still solve the problem of Johnny's refusing to eat his ham dinner.

When a child has a difficult behavior that a parent, teacher, or physician would like to change, the first thing to do is to clearly define the behavior. Good behaviors to target for change are behaviors that, if changed, would result in improved functioning in a key domain of the child's life. Key domains include physical health; social relationships with parents, teachers, and peers; and academic functioning. Examples of good versus bad targets for change can be seen in the case of a diabetic or obese child. In this case, a good behavior for change might be increasing the amount of physical activity the child gets each day. Another illustration is in the case of ADHD, in which one of the symptoms is fidgeting. Fidgeting is annoying to parents and teachers; however, fidgeting itself does not cause major problems for the child with ADHD. Thus, instead of trying to get the child to fidget less often while seated, parents and teachers should target a behavior that is causing problems in a key domain of functioning for the child, such as completing school assignments accurately, which will improve academic achievement.

Functional Behavior Analysis

Once the behavior that is targeted for change is clearly defined, a careful examination of the antecedents and consequences maintaining the behavior provides clues for ways in which to intervene and modify the behavior. This kind of careful examination is called a *functional behavior analysis*. A worksheet for conducting a functional behavioral analysis is presented in Figure 302-1.

Conducting a functional behavior analysis accomplishes several goals that are important to behavior change. First, it forces the parent or teacher to carefully define what the behavior is that he or she would like to change. Next, it

ABC Tracking Sheet

Operational definition of behavior being tracked: ______________________

Date/Time	Antecedents/Settings	Target behaviors	Consequences	Possible function	My thoughts/ emotions

The behaviors to be tracked should be those that are under consideration as target behaviors for change. The target behavior needs to be precisely defined (a different tracking sheet for each behavior) so that two different people could agree that the behavior has occurred. Antecedents are events or settings that precede or are associated with the behavior (e.g. whether a command was given prior to the behavior, whether the behavior occurs in one versus another setting), while consequences are events that follow the behavior (e.g., whether a tantrum enabled a child to avoid doing something that he had been directed to do). The function column should be used to make notes about what possible functions the behavior could have (e.g., got the child a positive outcome, avoided an undesired activity).

Figure 302-1. Functional behavior analysis.

forces the parent or teacher to observe and measure how often the behavior occurs and how severe the behavior is. It also requires parents and teachers to identify environmental triggers to the behavior that, if changed, would decrease the behavior. Similarly, functional behavior analysis requires the parent or teacher to determine the function of the behavior, including whether there are environmental consequences that may be maintaining the behavior. A behavior could be occurring for several reasons. Perhaps it results in a positive, tangible outcome for the child (e.g., a child throws a tantrum at the grocery store because his mother buys him candy to quiet him down when he does that). A behavior might be maintained by the peer or adult attention that the behavior elicits. A behavior can also be reinforced when it serves the function of avoiding activities or tasks that the child does not like (e.g., a child has a tantrum when told to perform chores because the parent removes the demand when the child has a tantrum). An added bonus of functional behavior analysis is that once the parents or teachers know how to monitor the frequency or severity of the behavior, they can determine whether or not the strategies they are using to elicit behavior change are effective. They can then adopt or modify these strategies accordingly. A brief example of a functional behavioral analysis is presented in Table 302-1.

Most children have tantrums at one time or another, and most parents would like to change this behavior in their children. However, parents often feel helpless in managing this behavior. By conducting a functional behavior analysis, the parent can determine how often the child is having tantrums and how long they typically last, what usually precedes the tantrum, and what happens after the tantrum that makes it more likely that a future tantrum will occur. As a simple example, consider a 7-year-old girl named Jane who frequently throws temper tantrums. Her parents tracked this behavior over the course of 2 weeks and found out that Jane had about four tantrums per week. The tantrums usually lasted about 15 minutes. The tantrums typically occurred in the morning and were related to getting ready for school. The tantrums typically resulted in Jane's missing the bus and having to be driven to school by her mother.

This information suggests that one function of Jane's tantrums has been to avoid the bus and have her mother drive her to school. There are several ways in which Jane's parents could intervene to decrease Jane's tantrums: (1) They could get more information about Jane's experiences while riding the bus to make sure she is not avoiding the bus ride for some reason (e.g., she is being teased on the bus), or (2) if Jane is not avoiding the bus ride itself, her parents could find out whether Jane is purposely missing the bus for other reasons (e.g., to spend more time with her mother

while being driven to school, to avoid having to wait at the bus stop in inclement weather). At the antecedent level, they could (1) have Jane pack her school bag and select her clothes the night before school so that she has less to do in the morning, (2) give her a checklist of the steps she needs to complete in her morning routine, or (3) wake her up earlier so that she has more time to get ready in the morning. At the consequence level, (1) they could reward her for completing the steps in her morning routine by allowing her to do something she likes for a few minutes if she finishes the steps in time, such as watching cartoons; (2) if feasible, they could make her walk to school on days she misses the bus; (3) they could reward Jane when she gets home from school every day she makes the school bus; or (4) if Jane is old enough to understand the value of money, they could charge her for "taxi service" every time she misses the school bus and has to be driven to school. The next step would be for Jane's parents to implement the aforementioned strategies and see how they work. If Jane's tantrums decrease, then her parents have found a solution. If her tantrums do not decrease, then her parents should do another functional behavior analysis to figure out why their original solution(s) did not work.

Reinforcement and Punishment

Once a behavior has been identified for change and the agent of change (e.g., parent, teacher, physician, social worker) has determined the typical antecedents and consequences controlling the behavior, numerous behavior modification techniques can be employed to change what happens before the behavior is emitted, immediately following the behavior, or at both the antecedent and consequence levels. In addition to changing what happens before the behavior occurs, at the antecedent level, behavior modification techniques also include *reinforcement* and *punishment*, which operate at the consequence level. Reinforcement refers to anything that *increases* the likelihood that the behavior will occur. Reinforcement can be positive and tangible, such as rewards and privileges, or it can involve social reinforcement such as praise. An example of positive social reinforcement is telling a child, "Good job!" for completing his homework. Another example of reinforcement is when a child is allowed to finish doing something she dislikes earlier in order to do something that she likes if she behaves appropriately while doing the thing she dislikes. For example, if parents want to make it more likely that their children perform chores without complaining and having to be nagged, they might try allowing their children to earn time off from doing chores if they do them well without complaining. Thus, the child is reinforced for doing chores without having to be nagged and without complaining by having to do fewer chores overall.

Table 302-1. Functional Behavior Analysis Example

A = Antecedent >	B = Behavior >	C = Consequence	Result
1. Parent gives command to child.	Child complies.	Parent praises child.	Child is *more* likely to comply in the future.
2. Parent gives command to child.	Child is defiant.	Parent withdraws request.	Child is *more* likely to be defiant in the future.
3. Parent gives command to child.	Child is defiant.	Parent sends child to time-out.	Child is *less* likely to be defiant in the future.

Punishment is any action that *decreases* the likelihood of a behavior's occurrence. An example of punishment that is used by many parents is putting a child in *time-out* for hitting his or her sibling. If time-out is consistently employed as a negative consequence for hitting, the child will, in time, stop hitting his or her sibling, and the aggression will be eliminated. Thus, behavior can be managed by environmental contingencies.

A key component in changing behavior is reinforcing the child for positive behavior change. Intuitively, almost all adults understand this. That is, children are more likely to change their behavior if they are rewarded for behavior change. However, what many adults fail to appreciate, and hence what causes many behavior change plans to fail, is that in getting a child to emit a new or different behavior response, reinforcement for that behavior response must be almost immediate. The younger the child, the more difficult it is for him or her to see the relationship between the behavior and the positive or negative consequence if there is a delay in the consequence. Parents and teachers understand that if a child misbehaves, the punishment needs to be immediate; they would think it absurd to wait until Friday to punish a child for pushing another child on Monday. However, parents and teachers routinely expect children to wait until the end of the day or week to get a reward for good behavior at the beginning of the day or week. Except for older children who have the ability to delay gratification, this is simply too long for a child to wait to earn a reward, and the promised reward thus loses its potency. Particularly when embarking on a behavior change program, children need very frequent rewards to motivate them to produce the desired behavior change. For children with severe behavior problems, young children, or developmentally delayed children, a tangible reward might need to be given immediately every time the desired behavior occurs. All children benefit from immediate positive verbal feedback for showing the desired behavior. Appropriate rewards and reward schedules is discussed in more detail later in this chapter.

Shaping

In attempting to change a behavior, the concept of *shaping* is important. As the word implies, shaping means slowly changing a behavior until the behavior reaches acceptable levels or stops completely. As an example, consider the case of Eric, who is obese, never exercises, and eats junk food and drinks soda for most of his meals and snacks. In this case, it would be unreasonable to expect that his eating and exercise habits could be completely changed simultaneously. Simply punishing him for eating junk food or rewarding him for eating vegetables would be unlikely to lead him to immediately adopt healthy eating habits. Instead, a behavior modification program could be started by requiring Eric to substitute one glass of water for one of his sodas or give up his afternoon snack of potato chips in favor of a piece of fruit, thereby reducing his overall daily consumption of fat and calories. If Eric makes these modifications to his diet, his parents would then reward him with an appropriate (nonfood) reward. The next step might be to shape Eric down to one soda per day and increase his fruit consumption to two or three servings per day. Once this criterion is reached, a new goal could be established in which Eric is taught to monitor his calories, dietary exchanges, or fat grams in an attempt to shape him down to a marginally acceptable level of fat and calorie consumption per day.

The next step would be to address Eric's exercise habits. Since Eric is not exercising at all, exercise is a new behavior that he will have to learn. Again, it would be unreasonable to expect Eric to go from not exercising at all to exercising for 30 minutes every day simply by punishing him for not exercising and rewarding him for exercising. Instead, the next step might be to add 10 minutes of exercise into Eric's daily routine. Adding a modest amount of exercise into Eric's daily routine is an example of *successive approximation*. Successive approximation refers to a good attempt at producing the desired behavior, and Eric's parents could help him start this process by rewarding him each day that he exercises for 10 minutes. Once Eric is consistently exercising for 10 minutes per day on most days (e.g., 5 out of 7 days), the next step might be to shape Eric up to 15 minutes and then eventually 20 minutes of exercise on 5 out of 7 days per week. Eventually, Eric's goals would be to minimize the amount of unhealthy food Eric consumes and maximize the amount of exercise Eric gets, but in the beginning, simply reducing the amount of fat and calories consumed daily by 20% and increasing his physical activity by even 10 or 15 minutes per day would represent a significant improvement in his eating and exercise behavior.

The preceding example illustrates several key components in effectively shaping a behavior:

1. Specific behaviors were targeted for change (e.g., drink one less soda and exercise for 10 minutes per day) instead of general behaviors (e.g., eat less and exercise more).
2. Appropriate rewards were provided for positive behavior change.
3. Both the eating and exercising shaping plans included several steps in order to help the child eventually reach the ultimate goal for each plan.

Modeling and Reinforced Practice

Other techniques can also be useful in modifying behavior. These techniques are usually used in conjunction with appropriate rewards and consequences. *Modeling and reinforced practice* is one such technique. Modeling and reinforced practice is useful in teaching a child a new way of behaving in a certain situation. A simple example of this might be teaching a child who is afraid of the dark, or has a phobia of the dark, to learn to sleep in the dark. This might be important if the child refuses to attend slumber parties or have friends sleep over because of this fear. In this case, the parent might model lying on a bed in a semidarkened room and then have the child practice lying in the bed in the darkened room for longer and longer periods of time. At first, the child might be given a reward for lying in the dark for 1 minute. Gradually, the time would be increased, and the amount of light in the room would be decreased. Eventually, through reinforced practice, the child would be rewarded for lying in the dark until she falls asleep. The final step might be to then reward the child for attending slumber parties. Modeling and reinforced practice can be very useful in treating most specific phobias because the child is taught a new behavioral response to a feared situation. Such situations might include anything from a fear of needles to a fear of dogs or spiders. Modeling and reinforced practice might also be very useful in teaching a child to become more independent in managing a chronic illness such as diabetes or practicing a clean intermittent catheterization program. Through modeling and reinforced practice, children can learn to test their blood glucose levels and administer medication or reliably adhere to a clean intermittent catheterization program or other complicated medical regimen.

BEHAVIOR MANAGEMENT TECHNIQUES

Positive Attending and Planned Ignoring

Important behavior management techniques for parents and teachers include *positive attending* and *planned ignoring*. Positive attending is the same thing as "catching the child being good," and many parents are familiar with this principle. Many studies show that in home, school, and other situations, children are motivated by the attention of parents, teachers, and other adults. Praise and other positive attention can be a very powerful motivator for almost all children. However, when children have a history of noncompliance with adult requests and rules, parents and teachers often spend a great deal of time issuing commands and reprimanding the child for misbehavior. When the child does comply, parents are often too tired to remember to praise the child or feel that the child does not deserve praise because the child is doing something that he or she should have been doing all along. When children have a history of noncompliance or behavior problems, it is highly important to praise them frequently whenever they are behaving appropriately in order to increase the likelihood that they will continue to behave appropriately. It is also important to look for opportunities to give the child positive feedback so that the child has an opportunity to enjoy a positive experience with an adult. In general, parents and teachers should try to find many more positive things to say to the child for every instance of a reprimand or command. Giving parents a yardstick of a 5:1 positive-to-negative ratio helps them become more aware of the degree to which they are providing positive reinforcement to their child and helps them to look for opportunities to give positive reinforcement.

Just as positive attention can increase a child's good behavior, ignoring certain behaviors can cause them to decrease or go away simply because they are not being reinforced by parental or teacher attention (see Table 302-1). Parents and teachers can be taught to ignore inappropriate behaviors. This is basically an issue of picking your battles. Children often do things that adults don't like, such as whining, complaining, making faces, rolling their eyes, and fidgeting in their seats. Parents and teachers find these behaviors to be irritating and disrespectful. Nevertheless, often the most effective way to decrease these kinds of behaviors is simply to ignore them. Children often whine and complain to get a reaction out of an adult. The adult's reaction reinforces the complaining and thus makes it more likely that the child will complain again in the future. If the parent or teacher does not respond to these kinds of behaviors, the child will derive no pleasure from showing them and over time will become less likely to whine and complain. Adult attention can increase a child's negative behavior even when the adult's reaction to the child is negative. One study of aggression in preschoolers showed that teacher attention to spats between children actually *increased* the number of arguments between the children in the classroom.

Using Effective Commands

Many studies have demonstrated that giving effective commands to a child will goes a long way toward changing oppositional or noncompliant behavior. Giving a good command is one way to help change a negative behavior at the antecedent level. Good commands are brief, specific, and appropriate to the child's developmental level. When a good command is given to a child, the child is more likely to comply with the adult's request because the child understands what the adult wants and is capable of performing the request. Box 302-1 lists the steps for giving good commands to children.

When working with parents of children with a history of noncompliance with adults' commands, it may be useful to have the parent keep track of the kind of commands they typically give to their children in order to help them become more aware of the ways in which they could give more effective commands and how they follow through with consistent consequences for compliance/noncompliance. A command tracking sheet for parents to use is presented in Figure 302-2. In treatment, the emphasis on the antecedents of noncompliance would go along with a focus on having parents provide consistent consequences for compliance with commands (see Table 302-1).

Transitional Warnings and When-Then Contingencies

Many children have trouble transitioning from one activity to the next, particularly when the transition involves stopping a fun activity and starting a less fun activity. One example of this might be when a child is asked to stop watching television and get ready for bed. Thinking again about the antecedents in an ABC analysis, we see that a child is more likely to cooperate with this type of request if the child is given a warning or two prior to being given an actual command. This gives the child time to mentally prepare for the transition and helps the child to feel more able to predict what is going to happen in the environment.

Box 302-1. Steps for Giving Good Commands

1. Obtain the child's attention.
2. Use command language, not question language.
3. Be specific about what you want the child to do.
4. A good command is brief and appropriate to the child's developmental level.
5. State consequences, and follow through.
6. Use a firm but neutral tone of voice.
7. Use neutral affect.
8. When possible, give the child a full 10 seconds to comply before issuing another command.
9. Reward compliance.

Time of day	Good commands	Bad commands	Comments

Instructions: Select times of the day when compliance is problematic and use this form to record good commands (those that meet criteria) and bad commands. Use a hash mark ("I") to indicate a command. If the child complies with the command, add a horizontal line to make the hash mark into a plus sign (+). Please describe additional information in the comments section (e.g., what you did when the child did comply).

Figure 302-2. Command compliance tracking sheet.

Transitional warnings are particularly important to use with younger children, as they are less likely to have internalized daily routines. An example of a sequence of transitional warnings is "Johnny, in 5 minutes, it will be time to get ready for bed." And then 3 minutes later, "Johnny, in 2 minutes, it will be time to get ready for bed." And finally, "Johnny, it's time to get ready for bed. Turn off the television and go upstairs." The timing of transitional warnings should vary according to the age of the child. Young children do well with shorter periods of time in between the warning and the final command.

Another strategy for improving a child's compliance with adult requests is to employ a *when-then* contingency. Simply put, this is setting up a condition in which the child gets to do what he or she wants once the child does what the parent wants. A basic format for this type of contingency statement is "When you do_____, then you can do_____." For example, "When you finish your homework, then you can play on the computer." "When you finish your dinner, then you can have dessert." Most parents use these kinds of contingencies to some degree. However, many parents would benefit from using them more frequently and systematically. Often children try to negotiate with their parents to change the contingency, and parents frequently give in to these pleas. Every time a parent gives in to the child after a contingency has been set up or stated, it makes it more difficult for the parent to enforce future contingencies because the child learns that if he or she negotiates long enough, the parent is likely to back down. Thus, when parents use when-then contingencies, transitional warnings, and commands, they must make sure they mean what they say and stick by it.

House Rules

All children benefit from rules and structure in the home. It is often the case that a child's behavior would improve considerably if a few modifications to the child's home were made. First, it is recommended that parents develop a schedule or daily routine for their children that includes homework time, meal time, chore time, recreational time, and bed time and that the family stick to this routine as much as possible. This helps the child to know what to expect each day. Naturally, deviations from routine will arise out of necessity from time to time, but having a general routine in place is an essential building block for changing problematic behavior. It is also recommended that daily routines be posted in the house. It is often a good idea to break up the day into segments and post routines for each part of the day separately. For example, parents might find it useful to post separate chore lists, a morning routine checklist, and an after-school/evening routine checklist.

Once the daily routine has been decided, it is recommended that parents choose behaviors that will become house rules. The number of house rules chosen should be fewer for households with young children. Examples might include no hitting, no swearing, no yelling, no eating outside of the kitchen/dining area, beginning homework when the child gets home from school, completing chores by 7:00 P.M., not taking food without asking, and telling a parent before leaving the yard. In establishing house rules, parents should be reminded that the rules should apply to every member of the family, not just the child or identified patient. Therefore, if no eating outside of the kitchen/dining area is a house rule, parents must heed this rule as well as children. If no yelling or swearing is a house rule, then parents must refrain from yelling and swearing. Parents should select only rules that, if broken, they are willing to enforce by administering a negative consequence to the child. They should keep the number of rules to a minimum and make sure that the child understands each rule. The rules should be posted in at least one location in the house (the refrigerator is a popular spot), and children should frequently be reminded of the rules.

Time-Out from Positive Reinforcement

In order for most discipline systems to be effective in managing behavior, it is usually essential to use negative consequences or punishment for more serious negative behaviors. It is widely recommended in most parenting programs for parents of nonproblematic children and is almost always employed in treatment programs for children with disruptive behavior problems (e.g., ADHD or conduct problems). Time-out from positive reinforcement ("time-out" for short) is a very effective negative consequence for most children when it is implemented correctly. Time-out from positive reinforcement means just that: removing the child from an enjoyable situation or activity and putting him or her in a less enjoyable situation or activity. Time-out works only if it is in fact a time-out from something the child would rather be doing. Parents often make the mistake of putting the child in time-out in his or her bedroom, which gives the child access to many enjoyable toys and activities. This defeats the power of time-out. Time-out should be implemented immediately on the exhibition of a few key behaviors that the parent finds intolerable. Examples of such behaviors might include intentional aggression, intentional destruction of property, breaking house rules, and repeated noncompliance with an adult's command.

Once the parent establishes which behaviors will result in time-out, he or she should decide the following in order to maximize the likelihood of compliance and effectiveness:

1. The location of the time-out
2. Rules for serving the time-out appropriately
3. The length of the time-out
4. How much the time-out will increase if the child breaks one of the time-out rules

Parents should select a safe place in their home to be used as a time-out area. Ideally, this area is out of sight of the television and other enjoyable items as well as away from anything that could be damaged if the child is angry or has trouble serving the time-out appropriately. Once this area is selected, parents should establish rules for serving a time-out. Such rules might include the following: (1) Go quickly to your time-out area; (2) stay in your time-out area until it is over; and (3) do not exhibit any negative behaviors during the time-out. The behaviors for which the child will receive a time-out, the location of the time-out area, and the rules for time-out should be explained to the child in advance. The child should also be reminded of the rules of the time-out and the location of the time-out area each time he is assigned a time-out.

The next step is for the parent to decide on the length of the time-out. For some children, especially children who are compliant with time-out, a flat 5-, 10-, or 15-minute time-out, depending on the child's age, might be effective (shorter time-outs are recommended for younger children and children with developmental delays). For children who do not comply with going to time-out or staying in their time-out area or who exhibit negative behavior while in time-out, a time-out system in which the child is able to earn time off of the time-out for serving it appropriately and have time added for inappropriate time-out behavior is likely to produce better results (Fig. 302-3). The way this system works is that the child is assigned an initial time-out of either 5, 10, or 20 minutes. Children ages 3 to 6 start with a 5-minute time out, children ages 7 to 10 start with a 10-minute time-out, and children ages 11 and up start with a 20-minute time-out. Once the time-out is assigned, the child is immediately informed that he or she can earn half the time off by serving the time-out appropriately. This means that the child goes to the time-out area immediately

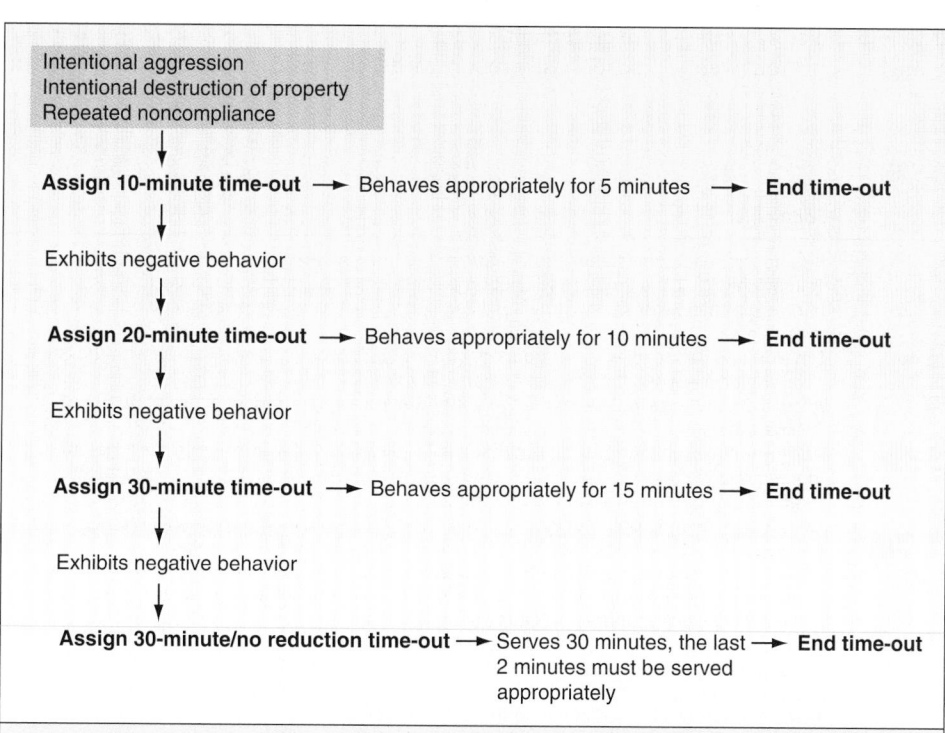

Figure 302-3. Schedule for escalating/deescalating time-out.

and follows the rules of time-out. Thus, the parent of an 8-year-old might say, "Johnny, you broke one our house rules, and you now have a 10-minute time-out. If you serve your time-out appropriately, you can earn 5 minutes off." If the child refuses to go to the time-out area or does not serve the time-out appropriately, the time is doubled. The parent should inform the child that the time has been doubled for breaking one of the time-out rules. For example, the parent might say, "Johnny, you broke one of the time-out rules because you left the time-out area. You now have a 20-minute time-out, but you can still earn half your time off if you follow the rules for the rest of your time-out." If Johnny serves the next 10 minutes appropriately, he should be released from the time-out. If he does not serve the time-out appropriately, the time-out is increased one more time, and he is given one more chance to earn half his time off. If Johnny continues to misbehave in time-out, he is given feedback only one more time, and no additional chances to earn time off. The parent might say, "Johnny, you broke the time-out rule because you are not in your time-out area. You now have a 30-minute time-out." At that point, the parent should ignore all misbehavior unless it is dangerous to the child, other people in the house, or property. Once the time-out time has elapsed, criteria for releasing the child from time-out should be invoked. We recommend telling the child that the time-out will not end until he or she serves the last 1 or 2 minutes appropriately. That is, the child must follow the time-out rules for 1 or 2 minutes, depending on age and developmental capabilities, before the time-out is over. Once the time-out is over, the parent should inform the child that the time is over and ask the child whether he or she knows why he or she was in time-out. If the child does not answer or says that he or she does not know (which is common), the parent should state in a matter-of-fact and neutral tone of voice why the child was in time-out. The parent might say, "You were in time-out because you broke one of our house rules by cursing."

When using time-out, parents should consider the following points: Time-out times and the amount of time required to be served appropriately should be determined on the basis of the child's age and developmental capabilities. Shorter time-outs are often as effective in reducing negative behavior as longer time-outs are. Parents should also have realistic expectations about behavior in time-out. Younger children in particular might be unable to sit or stand in one place for the entire time-out. If this seems to be the case, the parent should enlarge the time-out area so that the child has some room to move around in. Parents should give younger children timers and older children a clock or watch so that they can monitor the time of the time-out. Timers and clocks should be placed outside of the time-out area but in a place that the child can see them. It might also be the case that just as parents are instructed to ignore children while in time-out, siblings and other household members might need to be taught to do this. If a child is getting attention from parents, siblings, or other household members, the child is being reinforced, and the time-out will be less effective. As always, if a behavioral program is ineffective, a functional analysis of the antecedents and consequences should be conducted to determine how to modify the program. If parents are using this time-out system and still having trouble, Table 302-2 can help.

Home and School Daily Report Card

The techniques discussed so far in this chapter have been basic strategies that most parents would find useful in managing any child's behavior, whether or not the child is showing behavior problems or struggling with disease management issues. The next two techniques, home and school daily report cards, are designed to remediate specific

Table 302-2. Troubleshooting a Time-Out

Problem	Solution(s)
The child does not go to the time-out area.	Be sure the child understands the location of the time-out area.
	Tell the child that the time-out will not begin until he or she goes to the area.
	Inform the child he or she will lose a privilege (e.g., TV) if he or she does not comply with the time-out.
The child exhibits negative behavior in time-out.	Develop and define rules for appropriate time-out behavior, and review these with the child during a time when the child and parent are calm.
	Allow the child to earn time off the time-out duration for appropriate behavior during time-out.
	Add extra time to the total time-out duration for negative behaviors during the time-out.
	Ignore negative behaviors during time-out (and make sure other family members such as siblings ignore the child during time-out).
	Do not end the time-out until the child behaves appropriately for a specified time.
Time-out does not seem to decrease the occurrence of the target behavior (e.g., noncompliance) during an activity.	Ensure that the child understands the behaviors that will result in a time-out.
	Ensure that time-outs are assigned during reinforcing times. For example, receiving a time-out during homework time permits a child to escape from an aversive activity; therefore, a child may receive more time-outs during this time.
	Ensure that reinforcing activities are not available during time-out (e.g., TV in view of time-out area, toys in room).
	Postpone time-outs until an enjoyable time (e.g., free time, during a favorite TV show).
	Remove privileges instead of giving the child a time-out.
The child has difficulty behaving appropriately at the end of time-out.	If the time-out duration is too long, shorten the duration next time.
	Remind the child that he or she must serve the specified time appropriately to end the time-out.
	Set a timer for the specified time so that the child can observe the amount of time remaining.

areas of impairment that a child might face. These tools are individualized behavior programs that can be implemented in the home setting, the school setting, or both, as needed. They are widely used in interventions with children with ADHD, aggression, and oppositional behavior and conduct problems. They are made up of individualized targets or goals that are set up for the child and that allow the child to receive frequent feedback on progress toward these goals as well as frequent rewards for attaining these goals. A daily report card (DRC) program can be implemented at home or school, and these programs have been shown to be extremely effective in producing positive behavior change.

Examples of home and school DRCs are presented in Box 302-2.

The first step in setting up a DRC is to select the goals to be achieved. The goals selected should reflect the child's greatest areas of impairment—areas that, if changed, would improve the child's major problems in daily life functioning and, if left unchanged, would have long-term negative consequences. In considering goals, parents should consider the following key domains in which a child may be impaired: physical health, peer relations (particularly decreasing aggression and other negative interactions), academic work (task completion and accuracy), and relationships with

---

Box 302-2. School and Home Daily Report Card Samples

Sample School Daily Report Card

Child's Name: _____ Date: _____

	Special	Language Arts	Math	Reading	SS/Science
Follows class rules (no more than 3 rule violations per period).	Y N	Y N	Y N	Y N	Y N
Completes assignments within the designated time.	Y N	Y N	Y N	Y N	Y N
Completes assignments at 80% accuracy.	Y N	Y N	Y N	Y N	Y N
Complies with teacher requests (no more than 3 instances of noncompliance per period).	Y N	Y N	Y N	Y N	Y N
Gets along with peers (no more than 3 instances of teasing per period).	Y N	Y N	Y N	Y N	Y N

OTHER

Follows lunch rules (2 or fewer violations).   Y   N
Follows recess rules (2 or fewer violations).   Y   N
Total Number of Yeses   _____
Teacher's Initials: _____
Comments:

Sample Home Daily Report Card

Child's Name: _____ Date: _____

	Morning	After School	Dinner	Evening	Bedtime
Completes morning routine according to checklist with 2 or fewer reminders.	Y N	NA	NA	NA	NA
Takes medication with 1 or fewer reminders.	Y N	Y N	NA	NA	Y N
Teases siblings fewer than 3 times.	Y N	Y N	Y N	Y N	Y N
Completes homework assignments by 6:00 P.M. with 80% accuracy.					
Follows house rules (no more than 1 violation per time period).	Y N	Y N	Y N	Y N	Y N

OTHER

Brings home school DRC   Y   N
Total Number of Yeses on home DRC _____
Total Number of Yeses on School DRC _____
Total Yeses for the day: _____

Rewards for more Yeses than Nos (from after dinner the night before to through dinner today):	Choose 1 Watch 30 minutes of TV or play 30 minutes on computer or have special dessert.
Rewards for twice as many Yeses as Nos:	Choose 2 Watch 30 minutes of TV, play 30 minutes on computer/video game, have special dessert, stay up 15 minutes later, have friend over after school tomorrow.
Rewards for almost all Yeses (90% or better):	Choose 3 Watch 30 minutes of TV, play 30 minutes on computer/video game, have special dessert, stay up 15 minutes later, have friend over after school tomorrow.

adults (e.g., rule following, compliance with adult commands or requests); and once the goals have been selected, the next step is for the parent to clearly define a target behavior for change. It is important to remember that target behaviors, if changed, should improve the child's functioning in one of the aforementioned key domains. Target behaviors must be very clearly defined in a way that the child and parents or teachers understand. Target behaviors must be able to be observed and counted or measured by the parent or teacher and child. A list of sample target behaviors is presented in Table 302-3.

When a child is showing impairment in his or her daily life functioning, it is often because of many things. Frequently, parents and teachers want to change everything at once. However, behavior change requires a great deal of effort on the part of the child and the agents of change—parents and teachers. Thus, it is not reasonable to expend effort on changing behaviors that might be somewhat annoying or bothersome to the parent if the behavior is not causing problems in the child's ability to experience academic or social success. An example of such a behavior might be the state of the child's room. Many parents are dismayed when their child's room is a mess. If a messy room is the child's biggest problem, it makes sense to set up a behavior program to encourage the child to keep his or her room neater. However, if the child is also experiencing social rejection because he or she is obese or has ADHD or if the child is failing classes at school because the child is not completing school work and homework, it makes more sense for the parent and child to focus all their energy on addressing those problems and wait to address the messy room situation until the child's other areas of impairment have improved. A good DRC contains between three and eight target behaviors, depending on the child's age and ability.

Steps for Creating a Daily Report Card

1. *Decide on behaviors and criteria for the DRC.* Estimate about how often a child is doing the target behaviors (e.g., how many assignments the child completes, how often the child turns in homework, exercises, watches television). Next, parents can use these guesses to determine which behaviors need to be included on the DRC as well as how difficult to make the goal for the child to achieve. Target behaviors need to be evaluated several times throughout the day (e.g., in school, after each class or at least around lunchtime and the end of the day; at home, in the morning, after school, and evening; see the sample DRCs in Table 302-3), and the child should be given feedback each time the target is evaluated. The DRC should include only targets that are significant to the child's improvement; for example, if records show that the child does not forget to turn in assignments as often as was previously thought, this should not be included on the child's DRC. Once the behaviors have been chosen, parents or teacher must set a reasonable criterion for each target behavior. A criterion is a target level the child must meet to receive a positive mark for that behavior. A good criterion is one that the child can earn 75% to 90% of the time. The initial criterion should be set at a rate that is slightly better than what the child currently is doing to encourage improvement (e.g., 20% improvement). The 20% improvement rate refers back to the concept of shaping. It would be unrealistic to expect the child to go from turning in almost no homework assignments or engaging in virtually no physical activity to turning in all homework assignments or exercising every day. However, once the child consistently shows an improvement rate of about 20%, the goals can be revised again

---

Table 302-3. Example Targets for Home and School Daily Report Cards

Sample Home Targets	Sample School Targets
Follows house rules with X or fewer violations	Completes X assignments within the specified time
Follows direction or commands with X or fewer reminders	Completes X assignments with X% accuracy
Teases siblings fewer than X times per day/interval	Starts work with X or fewer reminders
Uses materials and possessions appropriately (as defined by parent and made clear to child)	Follows class/school rules with X or fewer violations
Follows rules at mall, store, in car, church, etc. with X or fewer rule violations	Follows direction with X or fewer repetitions
Serves time-outs appropriately (as defined by parent and made clear to child)	Stays on task with X or fewer reminders
Does not leave the yard (to go to friends) without permission	Sits appropriately in assigned area with X or fewer reminders
Completes homework assignments within the specified time	Uses material and possessions appropriately
Completes homework with X% accuracy	Teases peers X or fewer times per period
Responsible for own belongings (has belongings at appropriate times according to checklist or chart)	Fewer than X arguments with peers
Morning/bedtime routine completed according to checklist/chart	Fewer than X negative self comments
Completes chores by X o'clock	Accepts feedback appropriately
Uses good manners at dinner/breakfast/lunch (e.g., no more than XX times of bad manners)	Follows bus rules with X or fewer violations
Maintains appropriate eye contact when talking to an adult with X or fewer prompts	Serves time-outs appropriately
Stays in bed/bedroom after bedtime with XX reminders	Brings DRC to teacher before going to the next class/period/activity
Takes morning/afternoon medication with X or fewer reminders	Has materials necessary for class/subject
Exercises for X minutes	Brings completed homework to class
Completes glucose testing with X or fewer reminders	Takes medication at school/visits nurse with X or fewer reminders
Brings school DRC home to parent	Writes homework in assignment book with X or fewer reminders

until the desired amount of improvement has been achieved. Remember that the goals need to be feasible and within reach as perceived by both the child and the parent or teacher.

2. *Explain the DRC to the child.* The person setting up the DRC should explain the DRC to the child. If the DRC is for problems at school, this meeting should include both the parents and the teacher. The DRC should be explained to the child in a positive manner, and the child should be told that he or she will be able to earn rewards for good performance on the DRC.

3. *Establish a reward program.* Parents should establish a home-based reward system to provide the child with the motivation to work toward the goals on the DRC. Rewards are a necessary component of the program. A sample of home rewards is presented in Table 302-4. Some children need rewards more immediately than end-of-the-day rewards at home. In that case, a reward system can also be set up at school. See Box 302-3 for a list of classroom-based rewards.

Table 302-4. Possible Home Rewards List

Reward	Likely Frequency (Daily, Weekly)
Eating snacks	D
Staying up beyond bedtime	D
Visiting a friend's house	D, W
Having friend come over	D, W
Bike riding	D, W
Receiving allowance	D, W
Going fishing	W
Going shopping	W
Skating	D, W
Going to the movies	W
Doing a special activity with Mom or Dad	D, W
Earning day off from chores	D, W
Going to the park	W
Getting ice cream	W
Bowling, playing miniature golf	W
Playing a game of choice with parent/family	D, W
Going to the mall	W
Being read to	D
Choosing radio station in car	D
Selecting something special at the store	W
Making popcorn	W
Having friend over to spend night	W
Going to friend's to spend night	W
Having television time	D, W (for Sat/Sun)
Having video game time	D at home, W at mall
Listening to radio/stereo	D, W (for Sat/Sun)
Playing outside	D, W (for Sat/Sun)
Having extra bathtub time	D
Playing educational games on computer	D
Talking on phone	D (for friends), W (for long distance calls to relatives)
Choosing family TV show	D
Choosing family movie	W
Renting movie video	W
Going to a fast-food restaurant with parent and/or family	W
Watching taped TV shows	W

Note: Older children could save over weeks to get a monthly (or longer) reward as long as visuals (e.g., pieces of picture of activity) are used; for example, camping trip with parent, trip to baseball game, purchase of a video game cartridge. Rewards for an individual child need to be established as a *menu*.

4. *Monitor and modify the DRC.* Once the program has been established, parents and teachers need to monitor and modify the program as needed to gradually shape the child into increasing his or her appropriate behavior. This is done by making the child's criterion for earning a positive mark harder once he or she has begun to meet the criterion regularly (e.g., if the child is able to meet a target of "three or fewer rule violations per period" 90% of the time over a period of days, reduce the number to two or fewer rule violations per period), or if the child regularly fails to meet the criterion, it would be appropriate to make his or her criterion easier so that the child does not give up. Table 302-5 lists suggestions for troubleshooting DRCs.

Once the criterion for a target is at an acceptable level and the child is consistently reaching it, that target can be dropped from the DRC and replaced with another target if necessary. If the point is reached at which the child is doing so well that daily reports are unnecessary, parents or teachers might move to a weekly report/reward system. If and when the child is functioning within an appropriate range, the report card can be stopped and reinstated if problems reoccur. Parent and teachers should remember to *always* combine the report with lots of praise to the child for good days and good efforts and respond matter-of-factly (*not* negatively) to missed targets and not-so-good days with an encouraging statement about the next day.

IMPLEMENTATION OF BEHAVIOR MODIFICATION PROGRAMS

As was previously discussed, parents and teachers have a tremendous amount of control over the antecedents and consequences in a child's life. Because of this, they have the opportunity to be the *agents of change* for the child's behavior. If the parents are unable to successfully implement a behavior modification program with guidance from the child's primary care physician, they might need to seek out additional services from a mental health professional with experience in behavior modification. Most children with more severe behavior problems and many children with physical problems benefit from a combined approach to therapy that involves both the parents and school personnel. The first step in working with parents is to have them attend a behavioral parent-training class. These classes are often conducted in a group format, which is the most economical vehicle of service delivery. Most behavior modification programs also involve teacher training. Less often, behavior modification programs are conducted in established settings in which behavior modification can be implemented by professionals and paraprofessionals who are trained to deal with child behavior or health problems (e.g., in summer treatment programs). If the parents have attended a group parent-training class and are still struggling to address their child's behavioral issues or if the child's condition is atypical or severe, individual parent-training sessions can be useful in tailoring the behavior intervention to more keenly address the child's impairment.

Many studies have shown that behavioral parent training is a very effective way to teach parents the techniques necessary to produce behavior changes in their children.

Box 302-3. Suggested Rewards for Use in Classroom Interventions

Remember that these items are usually reinforcing to most children. However, what is reinforcing to one child might not be reinforcing to another. Before using a reinforcer in a program, teachers should make sure that a child wants it and will work for it.

1. Have free time.
2. Talk to best friend.
3. Listen to a tape player (with headphones).
4. Read a book.
5. Help clean up the classroom.
6. Clean the erasers.
7. Wash the chalkboard.
8. Be the teacher's helper.
9. Eat lunch outside on a nice day.
10. Have extra time at recess.
11. Write on the chalkboard.
12. Use magic markers.
13. Draw a picture.
14. Choose a book to read to the class.
15. Read to a friend.
16. Read with a friend.
17. Care for class animals.
18. Play "teacher."
19. See a movie or filmstrip.
20. Decorate the bulletin board.
21. Be a messenger for the office.
22. Grade papers.
23. Have treats.
24. Earn a class party.
25. Go on a class field trip.
26. Be student of the day/month.
27. Pop popcorn.
28. Be a line leader.
29. Visit the janitor.
30. Use the computer.
31. Make ice cream sundaes.
32. Teach a classmate.
33. Choose stickers.
34. Take a congratulatory note home.
35. Receive a positive phone call.
36. Receive lots of praise.
37. Find a special note in the desk.
38. Choose a seat for a specific time.
39. Play card games.
40. Receive an award certificate.
41. Take Polaroid pictures.
42. Draw from a "grab bag."
43. Eat at a special table.
44. Visit the principal.

Specific examples of conditions that parents can often learn to better manage through behavior parenting classes or individual behavior therapy include adherence to medical regimens to manage chronic illnesses, enuresis (bedwetting), obesity, asthma, diabetes, anxiety disorders, ADHD, and conduct problems. Many structured behavioral parenting courses have been developed that cover all topics of behavior management referred to in this chapter and could easily be offered by a nurse practitioner in the general practitioner's office. Once such program is the Community Parent Education Program (COPE), which meets all the requirements of what to look for in a comprehensive behavior parent training program (Box 302-4).

When problems exist at school, whether the problem involves acting out at school or fear of going to school, a comprehensive behavior management program needs to include school personnel. If the parents have been unable to successfully establish a DRC or other effective intervention at school, a mental health professional should be consulted. The mental health professional can assist school personnel in structuring the classroom environment to maximize the child's potential for success. The techniques for intervening with teachers are identical to the skills taught to parents in behavior parent training. In helping school personnel to increase the level of structure in the classroom and/or school, the following areas are often targeted for intervention:

1. *Establishing classroom rules and structure.* Typical classroom rules might include (a) being respectful of others, (b) obeying adults, (c) working quietly, (d) staying in one's assigned seat or area, (e) using materials appropriately. (f) raising one's hand to speak or ask for help, and (g) staying on task or completing assignments. The number of classroom rules depends on the children's developmental level. In generating classroom rules, it might be useful to allow the children to come up with some or all of the rules. Once the rules are decided on, the teacher should review the rules and have children recite them before each class until learned. The teacher should continue to review the rules frequently even after they are learned. Teachers can increase the overall level of structure in their classrooms by posting prompts (e.g., morning routine), keeping a predictable schedule, and helping all the children in the class with organization by giving them folders for each subject or assignment charts.

2. *Positive attending and planned ignoring.* The teacher is taught to praise appropriate behaviors and ignore mild inappropriate behaviors that are not reinforced by peer attention. Just as parents are taught when they learn to attend to their child's appropriate behavior positively, teachers are taught that praises should outnumber reprimands or commands by at least a 2- or 3-to-1 ratio and ideally by a 5-to-1 ratio. It is easier for a teacher to achieve this positive-to-negative ratio if he or she uses each command or reprimand as a cue to give two positive comments for children who are behaving appropriately; that is, find two children who can be praised each time a reprimand or command is given to a child who is misbehaving. Teachers should also be instructed to look for any opportunity to praise a child who is receiving a lot of reprimands. Teachers can also be instructed to shape appropriate behavior by working within the target

Table 302-5. Troubleshooting Home and School DRCs

Problem	Quick Fix Tip
Does the child understand the system?	Use a visual device, if possible (e.g., dry-erase board) to explain system to the child. Have the child explain system to the parent and teacher. Practice this several times a day until child understands the system.
Does the child bring the DRC home from school?	Give the child a special folder or backpack to transport the DRC. Have the teacher for the last class prompt child to bring the DRC home. Assume that the child received "all Nos" if the DRC is not brought home. Add "Brings DRC home from school" as a target on the home DRC.
Are the target behaviors appropriate, clearly defined, socially valid, and able to be attained by the child?	Redefine the behaviors for the child and/or modify the targets.
Does the child remember his goals?	Make up a task sheet to remind the child of his or her goals. Use pictures and numbers if necessary. Put the chart in a visible place (e.g., the refrigerator).
Can the child accurately monitor his progress throughout the day?	Have the child write down on the chart every time he or she receives feedback about performing a negative behavior.
Is something interfering with the child's reaching his or her goals (e.g., messy closet prohibiting him or her from being ready on time)?	Work on the interference first. In this example, have the child clean his or her closet thoroughly to avoid further problems.
Are the parent and teacher providing the child with accurate feedback so that the child knows how close he or she is to making his or her goals?	Provide feedback exactly when the behavior occurs, informing the child of his exact behavior. Write it on a chart if necessary.
Are rewards motivating for the child?	Ask the child what he or she would like to work for instead. Rearrange the ordering of the rewards so that the most motivating ones are for best behavior. Add new rewards to the menu and drop ones that the child no longer wants.
Are rewards given consistently?	Provide the child with the reward every time (but only when) the goal is met.
Are rewards given when they should be given?	Provide the child with the reward for meeting the goals as soon as possible. Spouses and teachers should communicate with each other to ensure that everyone is following the same reward schedule. Make sure that rewards are given every time they are earned. Always praise the child for doing well and combine that praise with the rewards to make them even more rewarding.

child's ability or skill level and praise and reward children for successively approximating the behavior the teacher is trying to improve in the child.

3. *Commands and reprimands.* In working with the target child or other problematic children in the classroom, the teacher can be instructed to give private reprimands (at the child's desk as much as possible) and appropriate commands (clear, specific, manageable) to these children. Steps for giving appropriate commands are identical to the instructions given to parents (see Box 302-1).

4. *Daily report card.* A daily report card or notebook can be established as discussed previously. The DRC can be modified if necessary and its effectiveness evaluated.

Box 302-4. Elements of a Good Behavioral Parenting Program

1. Positive attending
2. Planned ignoring
3. Transitional warnings
4. When-then contingencies
5. Effective commands
6. Daily report cards or token economies
7. Time out and loss of privileges

APPLICATION OF BEHAVIOR MODIFICATION PRINCIPLES: EXAMPLES

The accompanying CD-ROM contains examples that demonstrate the application of behavior modification principles to common behavioral and health problems such as diabetes (Chapter 155), ADHD (Chapter 244), and enuresis (Chapter 253).

 Additional Resources, CD-ROM

Application of behavior modification principles: examples	Text

SUGGESTED READINGS

Center for Children and Families: Available at: http://wings.buffalo.edu/adhd.

Cunningham CE, Bremner R, Secord M: Cope: The Community Parent Education Program. Hamilton, Ontario, Copeworks, 1998.

Kazdin AE: Behavior Modification in Applied Settings, 6th ed. Belmont, Calif, Wadsworth/Thomson Learning, 2001.

Martin G, Pear J: Behavior Modification: What It Is and How to Do It, 5th ed. Upper Saddle River, NJ, Simon & Schuster, 1996.

Sloane H: The Good Kid Book: How to Solve the 16 Most Common Behavior Problems. Champaign, Ill, Research Press, 1988.

303 Mental Health Interventions: Evidence-Based Approaches

William E. Pelham, Jr., and Lisa D. Burrows-MacLean

Box 303-1. Role of the Generalist

1. Screen for disorders using DSM criteria.
2. Focus on problems in daily life functioning/impairment in key domains of peer relationships, parenting skills/parent-child relationships, and school/academic functioning.
3. Use parents and teachers as primary informants.
4. Educate the family about suspected disorders.
5. Treat or refer for further assessment and treatment if problems in daily life functioning are viewed by parents and teachers as warranting intervention.
6. Utilize or refer to professionals who use evidence-based treatments.
7. Follow up to ensure that intervention provided is the EBT for which referral was made.
8. Establish plan in the practice and with the family to monitor ongoing response to treatment and target outcomes.

The primary care provider should be able to screen for mental health problems and know when to intervene or refer for treatment. This chapter briefly reviews the guidelines for recognizing the most common and some of the most severe mental health problems of childhood and describes the evidence-based treatments available for treating these disorders. Detailed understanding of the rules and procedures for formal diagnosis, as codified in the *Diagnostic and Statistical Manual of Mental Disorders* (DSM-IV) or the DSM-PC (see Section 7), is not necessary to recognize mental health problems or to *make referrals* for appropriate treatment. The role of the generalist is summarized in Box 303-1.

FOCUS ON IMPAIRMENT

Instead of making DSM-based diagnoses in cases of suspected mental health problems, the primary care provider should focus on whether the child's general symptoms of a mental health problem are associated with *problems in daily life functioning*—that is, *impairment*. For all childhood mental health problems, diagnoses are not made unless the child suffers significant impairment in daily life functioning. Indeed, it is for impairment, not DSM symptoms of the underlying disorder, that parents

bring most children for assessment and treatment. The generalist needs to recognize whether a child is having problems in key domains of daily life functioning and whether these problems are severe enough to warrant some form of intervention.

Studies of long-term outcome of children with behavior problems and mental health disorders show that continued difficulty into adulthood is best predicted by impairment in daily life functioning rather than by symptoms of disorders. Outcomes are best predicted by three factors: (1) the nature of the children's peer relationships (the degree to which they are rejected by other children in elementary school), (2) their parents' parenting skills and interactions with their children (e.g., overly harsh discipline, inconsistent monitoring, negative parent-child interactions), and (3) the children's academic adjustment at school (failure and dropout). The primary care clinician must therefore evaluate these three domains as well as initiate treatment.

The argument that a DSM diagnosis is necessary for treatment does not apply in the field of childhood mental health. The following evidence-based therapies (EBTs) involve general principles and procedures that cut across diagnosis and focus on treating problems in the common domains of impairment. Knowing a child's DSM diagnosis does not generally provide guidance regarding proper psychosocial treatment, but knowing a child's problems in daily life functioning helps in treatment planning. For example, the knowledge that a child has no friends and is rejected by classmates and neighborhood peers should prompt a referral for a behavioral social skills program regardless of whether that child meets formal diagnostic criteria for social anxiety, depression, attention deficit hyperactivity disorder (ADHD), conduct problems, or disorders commonly associated with difficulties in peer relationships.

There are no hard-and-fast rules about the degree of concern required before the generalist makes a referral for treatment, except to note that most childhood mental health problems are chronic and fail to resolve spontaneously with the passage of time. Furthermore, the nature of children's problems in all three key domains—relationships with peers, academic functioning at school, and parent-child relationships—worsens over time without appropriate intervention. The earlier the intervention, the better the outcome (Box 303-2).

The generalist must determine whether the child has significant problems in daily life functioning, that is, (1) peer relationships, (2) parent and family relationships, and (3) academic and social functioning at school. If these key problems exist, then appropriate referrals for a more detailed diagnostic workup and treatment are indicated.

Determination of impairment is made primarily through discussions with parents and the child's teacher. For some disorders, such as autism, observation of the child's behavior and interaction with the child in the clinic can be useful. For other disorders, such as depression, conversation with the child might reveal the degree to which the child is impaired. However, for the most common childhood disorders, the typical child does not show evidence of impairment in the office setting. Furthermore, most children do not report their impairment (or their symptoms) accurately in a conversation with the physician.

There are several standardized instruments that can be used to measure impairment, such as the Impairment Rating Scale (IRS) (Box 303-3). This scale asks teachers, parents, and others working with the child to judge whether or not the child has impairment in key parts of daily life functioning, sufficient to cause concern and warrant intervention. On the IRS, marks on the deviant half of the line indicate a level of perceived impairment, so a quick glance can tell whether a child may be experiencing impairment in any key domain. This simple rating scale may also target behaviors requiring intervention. The IRS can be downloaded without charge from www.summertreatmentprogram.com.

INITIATING TREATMENT OR REFERRAL

When the primary care physician decides that a child's problems in daily life functioning are sufficient to warrant treatment and perhaps a referral, the next step is to provide information to the parents about the suspected problem or diagnosis. Brief fact sheets and brochures are available from professional associations such as the American Academy of Pediatrics, the American Academy of Child and Adolescent Psychiatry, and the American Psychological Association, as well as from numerous parent advocate groups. Family education is a crucial component of a chronic care model for chronic conditions, and it should begin early in the process of evaluation and referral.

Not all methods of mental health therapy are equal. Referral for a suspected mental health problem should never be for generic "counseling" or "therapy." Over the past decade, extensive research in community mental health settings has shown that up to 80% of treatment for children's mental health problems is non-evidence-based and therefore ineffective. The most commonly provided therapeutic interventions—individual one-on-one talk therapy (between a therapist and a child) and one-on-one clinic-based play therapy (between a therapist and a child)—have no evidence for effectiveness and are not indicated for any childhood mental health disorder. In contrast, there is a group of interventions for most childhood mental health problems that have solid evidence for effectiveness. Box 303-4 lists features of evidenced-based mental health interventions. The primary care physician has key responsibility for making sure that the referral to a mental health professional is for appropriate treatment. To identify mental health practitioners who provide EBTs in their communities, primary care physicians should survey mental health practitioners in their communities to find out who is delivering these services.

The primary care provider must make sure the child undergoes referral to a mental health specialist. A recent study shows that nearly two thirds of families referred to mental health care providers by primary care physicians never follow through with the referral, and of those that do, more than half see the mental health care provider only once. The primary care provider must establish procedures in his or her practice that provide for follow-up to check on whether the patient is following through with the referral.

In summary, in cases of suspected mental health problems, the primary care clinician should follow the sequence in Box 303-1. This sequence covers initial evaluation through referral and follow-up.

CONDITIONS THAT REQUIRE MENTAL HEALTH INTERVENTION

The major mental health problems for childhood requiring treatment or referrals are divided into four broad categories: externalizing disorders, internalizing disorders, autism and other pervasive disorders, and disorders of behavioral health. Externalizing disorders, which include ADHD, oppositional defiant disorder (ODD), and conduct disorder (CD), are so labeled because behaviors are "external" to the child. Internalizing disorders, including anxiety and depression, do not have such obvious external manifestations, and the focus is on the internal, emotional aspects of the child's difficulties (hence the term *internalizing* disorders). A major difference between externalizing disorders and internalizing disorders is that the former are chronic, while the latter are generally transitory or episodic. Both externalizing and internalizing disorders in childhood have very negative impacts on children's daily life functioning. However, despite these negative effects, children with these disorders function in family settings and regular school settings rather than institutional settings. In contrast, children with autism and other pervasive developmental disorders are often dealt with in intensive special educational programs in schools or in institutional settings. Behavioral health disorders include a wide variety of disorders that involve mental health and physical health, including obesity, enuresis and encopresis, tic disorders, asthma, and diabetes.

Externalizing Disorders
ADHD, ODD, and CD are the most common mental health disorders of childhood, affecting up to 10% of the population and accounting for more than half of referrals to child mental health facilities. Furthermore, these disorders are frequently comorbid, commonly co-occurring with one another. For example, as many as 50% to 75% of ADHD

Box 303-3. Impairment Rating Scale

Narrative Description of Child—Parent

Child's Name: _____ Form completed by: _____ Date: _____

Instructions: In the space below, please describe what you see as your child's primary problems, both at home and at school. Also, please describe how your child's problems have affected the following areas and complete the rating at the end of each: (1) his or her relationships with playmates and brothers or sisters, (2) his or her relationship with you (and your spouse if present), (3) his or her academic progress at school, (4) his or her self-esteem, and (5) your family in general. Continue on a separate sheet if necessary. *For the ratings, please mark an "X" on the lines at the points that you believe reflect the impact of the child's problems on this area and whether he or she needs treatment or special services for the problems.* PLEASE COMPLETE BOTH SIDES OF THIS FORM.

---

(1) How your child's problems affect his or her relationship with playmates

No Problem _____ Extreme Problem
Definitely does not need treatment or special services   Definitely needs treatment or special services

---

Regardless of whether this child is popular or unpopular with peers, does he or she have a special, close "best friend" that he or she has kept for more than a few months? (Please circle)

YES   NO

How your child's problems affect his or her relationship with brothers or sisters
(If has no brothers or sisters, check here and skip to #2 _____)

No Problem _____ Extreme Problem
Definitely does not need treatment or special services   Definitely needs treatment or special services

---

(2) How your child's problems affect his or her relationship with you (and your spouse if present)

No Problem _____ Extreme Problem
Definitely does not need treatment or special services   Definitely needs treatment or special services

---

(3) How your child's problems affect his or her academic progress at school

No Problem _____ Extreme Problem
Definitely does not need treatment or special services   Definitely needs treatment or special services

---

(4) How your child's problems affect his or her self-esteem

No Problem _____ Extreme Problem
Definitely does not need treatment or special services   Definitely needs treatment or special services

---

(5) How your child's problems affect your family in general

No Problem _____ Extreme Problem
Definitely does not need treatment or special services   Definitely needs treatment or special services

---

Please mark an "X" on the following line at the point that you believe reflects the overall severity of this child's problem in functioning and *overall* need for treatment.

No Problem _____ Extreme Problem
Definitely does not need treatment or special services   Definitely needs treatment or special services

Box 303-4. Common Features of Evidence-Based Treatments for Childhood Mental Health Disorders

Extensively studied, efficacy documented, and listed in professional association guidelines

Based on a behavioral or cognitive-behavioral framework

Precisely described in treatment manuals

Focused on clearly described behaviors that are targeted for change, reducing impairments, building adaptive skills, and improving functional outcomes

Specific therapeutic activities tied to specific target behaviors/outcomes

Parents and often teachers involved as implementers or facilitators of treatment

MA and BA clinicians utilized to reduce costs and maximize transportability

Treatment response monitored

Functional analytic approach employed to develop and modify intervention as necessary

Procedures for generalization, maintenance, and relapse prevention included

children also have ODD, and up to 25% of ADHD children also meet criteria for CD. These disorders have many common features: chronicity, poor long-term prognosis, more common occurrence in boys than in girls, and severe problems in daily life functioning: peer relationships, parenting and family relationships, and academic functioning. ADHD is defined as developmentally inappropriate levels of the abilities to sustain attention, inhibit impulses, and modulate activity level, whereas ODD is characterized by developmentally inappropriate levels of oppositional and defiant behavior directed toward adults and other authority figures. Conduct disorder is characterized by violations of societal norms such as aggression toward other people and animals, theft, and lying. Both ODD and CD can be identified in toddlerhood, while CD typically does not manifest itself until middle to late elementary school. Across the life span, it is thought that ADHD reliably precedes ODD. As children develop into the elementary school years, ODD often develops into CD. Children with childhood histories of both ADHD and ODD are more likely to develop CD compared to children with either diagnosis alone, and children with lifetime histories of both ADHD and CD are far more likely to develop into adults with criminal justice problems—life-course-persistent delinquency and antisocial behavior—than are children with either diagnosis alone.

The core symptoms of the externalizing disorders are defined in DSM-IV and DSM-PC according to a number of specific descriptors. Specific descriptors can be evaluated in primary care settings by using one of the commonly available and free parent and teacher rating scales. These can be downloaded without cost from numerous websites, including www.summertreatmentprogram.com, www.ADHD.net, and www.NICHQ.org.

ADHD, ODD, and CD are commonly diagnosed during elementary school. Primary care practitioners have been reluctant to make a mental health diagnosis in young children, so problems go *unidentified* and, most important, *untreated* until the child comes to the attention of school

personnel. This situation frequently places school personnel (specifically kindergarten teachers) in the position of screening for mental health problems in children. It is incumbent on primary care professionals to be more proactive in screening for externalizing problems in preschool children.

Internalizing Disorders

The second most common type of mental health disorders of childhood are problems in anxiety and depression, anxiety being far more common than depression. Anxiety disorders include difficulties ranging from separation anxiety to specific phobias. Anxiety is expressed through physiological, cognitive, and behavioral manifestations. Inappropriate worry and distress may be about many things (generalized anxiety), a specific situation (separation anxiety or social phobia), or specific stimuli (specific phobias). In phobias, the anxiety is expressed with anticipation or experience of the feared stimulus and is accompanied by attempts to avoid the feared object or situation. Anxieties and fears are common and normative at some ages in children. When making a diagnosis, care must be taken to ensure that the described anxieties are developmentally inappropriate and are maladaptive. Nine anxiety disorders are described in the DSM-IV, and they are highly comorbid with one another. Generalized anxiety disorder and social anxiety have a later onset (latter elementary school) than specific phobias, but anxiety disorders can occur at any age.

Depression occurs far less commonly in children than in adults but has received increasing interest in recent years. The key features of depression are depressed mood and marked loss of interest or pleasure in activities. Additional symptoms are sleep difficulties, fatigue, and feelings of worthlessness. The symptoms must be sufficient to cause impairment in daily life activities. Depression is relatively rare in early childhood (with a prevalence of 1% to 2%), being diagnosed with increasing frequency as children grow into adolescence, in which lifetime diagnostic rates approximate those of adults. Depressive disorders are commonly comorbid with anxiety disorders and less so with externalizing disorders. In cases of comorbidity, it is important to determine whether the depression is in reaction to some of the difficulties of the other disorders (e.g., the peer relationship problems of ADHD children leading to depression over lack of friendships) and would therefore remit if the other disorders were effectively treated.

Many children experience anxiety problems and problems in depression that remit without intervention.

Autism and Other Pervasive Developmental Disorders

These are the most debilitating of childhood mental health disorders. Pervasive developmental disorders are characterized by severe impairment in multiple domains of functioning and are manifested by inability to engage in reciprocal social relationships, impaired communication skills, and idiosyncratic or bizarre behavior. Children with pervasive developmental disorders show atypical or unusual patterns of development. This is in contrast to a developmentally delayed or mentally retarded child who shows a normal developmental progression but at a much slower rate than a "normal" child. Autism is the most common of the pervasive developmental disorders and it is relatively rare, occurring in two to five cases per 10,000 individuals. (Other pervasive developmental disorders include Asperger disorder, Rett syndrome, and childhood disintegrative disorder.) All pervasive developmental disorders except childhood disintegrative disorder are evident during the first few years of life.

Autistic children, by definition, must show delays or abnormal functioning in social interaction, functional language (as used in social communication), or symbolic or imaginative play before age 3. Autism and other pervasive developmental disorders are recognized as biologically based, chronic, lifelong disabilities. Most children with pervasive developmental disorders also show mental retardation. The best predictors of long-term outcome in children with autism are IQ and language development. Children with moderate to severe mental retardation and autism have the poorest long-term outcomes, as do those children who do not develop language skills by age 5. Without treatment, autistic children may show some gradual improvement in symptoms over time but continue to display unusual or bizarre behavior and broad impairment in their social functioning and communication skills. The majority spend their adulthood in various levels of assisted living facilities, but intensive early behavioral interventions reduce the impairment and improve the outcomes of a portion of autistic individuals.

Problems in Behavioral Health

The primary care provider is likely to encounter health issues that have both physical and behavioral components. Enuresis, encopresis, and obesity in childhood are relatively common examples. Many parents try to solve behavioral health problems on their own and, in doing so, often use methods that have been shown to be ineffective. Evidence-based therapies may be of some help.

EVIDENCE-BASED TREATMENTS

Tables 303-1 through 303-4 list evidence-based treatments for childhood mental health disorders. Some of these can be provided by the primary care provider and office personnel, others are conducted exclusively by mental health clinicians (e.g., school-based programs for aggressive, CD children), and still others are comanaged by the primary care provider and a mental health or educational professional (e.g., multimodal treatment for ADHD).

Common Features of the Evidence-Based Treatments

The therapeutic interventions listed in Tables 303-1 through 303-4 share several features that distinguish them from widely used but ineffective psychotherapeutic programs. All evidence-based treatments (EBTs) are behavioral or cognitive-behavioral interventions with proven efficacy. Components of EBT intervention are specific and tied to targeted behaviors or goals of treatment.

The EBTs listed in Tables 303-1 through 303-4 include reward programs *both* during sessions in which children are being taught new skills *and* in the home and school settings to motivate the children to demonstrate changes in these settings. Even when the child-based intervention is primarily cognitive-behavioral (e.g., for depression), reward programs are employed.

Unlike traditional approaches to therapy, EBTs typically involve parents and often teachers and other adults as the facilitators of treatment. As shown in Tables 303-1 through 303-4, all EBTs involve teaching parents the skills that they need to eliminate the problems their children exhibit and adaptive skills the children need to acquire. The reason for this is that a therapist could have only a small impact on a child in a weekly 50-minute session, but the parents and teachers who spend every waking minute with the child have multiple opportunities to work on the target behaviors in the settings in which they occur.

A key characteristic of these behaviorally based EBTs is that they all employ a functional analytic approach to develop, monitor, and modify treatment. Following the ABC (antecedent, behavior, consequence) approach, therapists (and parents or teachers) keep systematic data tracking the specifically defined target behaviors in the settings in which they occur, evaluating the functions of the behavior, and tracking improvement. Treatment plans are modified on the basis of the results of ongoing functional analyses.

Finally, when the disorder in question is a chronic one or the possibility of recurrence exists, the EBTs include specific procedures designed to produce generalization (i.e., across settings) and maintenance (i.e., across time) of the changes the child has made. For example, if parents have taught an ODD child to comply with their commands, they teach other adults in the child's life (e.g., relatives, babysitters, sports coaches) how to employ the same effective procedures. They also develop procedures for ensuring that they and others are consistently employing the procedures to ensure long-term maintenance of the child's improvement. Therapists also develop plans to prevent relapse. For example, if a child's behavior problems have been well controlled through a behavior management plan implemented by his or her teacher at school, the teacher and parents establish a plan to train the next year's teacher to implement the same plan.

Evidence-Based Treatments for Externalizing Disorders

There are many EBTs for children with externalizing disorders. Table 303-1 lists the components of evidence-based treatments for ADHD, ODD, and CD (see the CD-ROM for lists of articles for these and the other EBTs listed later). The backbone of EBTs for externalizing disorders is behavioral parent training. In a series of sessions or classes, parents (either in individual pairs or in a group) are taught the skills in behavior modification. Parents learn programs in sessions and implement them during the week, reporting back each week to the therapist about progress and problems. After a course of parent training, booster sessions are planned so that parents can check back with therapists as they maintain their programs over time.

Similar plans are implemented with the child's teachers. The setting is the classroom, but the procedures that are

Table 303-1. Components of Evidence-Based Psychosocial Treatment for ADHD, ODD, and CD

Parent Training

Behavioral approach; therapist teaches parents contingency management techniques and other parenting skills to use with the child, and the parents implement the treatment. Focus on specific target behaviors that reflect impairment in key domains of functioning (e.g., peer relationships, parenting skills and family relationships, academic and school functioning); maladaptive behaviors are targeted for reduction, and adaptive skills are targeted for development.

Typical model is group-based, weekly session with therapist (8 to 16 sessions) initially, then contact is faded.

Adherence to treatment components is regularly checked, and treatment goals are continually added, deleted, or modified on the basis of an ongoing functional analysis of behavior.

Continued support and contact are maintained as long as necessary as determined through ongoing monitoring.

Program for maintenance and relapse prevention (e.g., develop plans for dealing with backsliding/concurrent cyclic parental problems, such as maternal depression, parental substance abuse, and divorce).

Re-establish contact for major developmental transitions (e.g., adolescence).

School Intervention

Behavioral approach; the therapist teaches teacher contingency management techniques to use with the child, and the teacher implements the treatment.

Focus on specific target behaviors that reflect impairment in key domains of functioning (e.g., peer relationships, interactions with adults/rule following, academic progress); maladaptive behaviors are targeted for reduction, and adaptive skills are targeted for development. The consultant works with the teacher: initial weekly face-to-face or phone sessions (3 to 8 contacts), then contact is faded.

Adherence to treatment components is regularly checked, and treatment goals are continually added, deleted, or modified on the basis of an ongoing functional analysis of behavior. Continued support and contact are maintained as long as necessary as determined through ongoing monitoring.

Program for maintenance and relapse prevention (e.g., schoolwide programs, inservice training of all school staff, including administrators; parent is eventually trained to work with the teacher and monitor/modify intervention).

Re-establish contact for major developmental transitions (e.g., the move from elementary school to middle school).

Child Intervention

A behavioral and developmental approach involves direct work in natural or analogue settings, *not* clinic settings.

Focus on specific target behaviors that reflect impairment in multiple domains of functioning (e.g., peer relationships, interactions with adults, sibling relationships, academic skills, classroom and family functioning, self-esteem); maladaptive behaviors are targeted for reduction, and adaptive skills (e.g., social skills, sports skills, academic skills) are targeted for development.

Often paraprofessional help is implemented.

Intensive treatment settings include summer treatment programs (9 hours daily for 8 weeks), and/or school-year, after-school, and Saturday (6 hours) sessions.

Behavioral (contingent rewards and negative consequences) and cognitive behavioral (e.g., social skills training, problem solving training) are integrated in the context of recreational activities.

Adherence to treatment components is regularly checked, and treatment goals are continually added, deleted, or modified on the basis of a current functional analysis of behavior. Treatment is provided as long as necessary (e.g., 2 or 3 years after initial contact).

A program for generalization and relapse prevention is instituted (e.g., integrate with school and parent treatments).

Re-establish contact for major developmental transitions (e.g., move from elementary to middle school).

taught are the same as those taught to parents. This is often accomplished by consultants or school personnel who work with the referred child's teacher. This form of intervention—individual programs for referred children—is labeled *targeted or indicated intervention*. Also common in school settings are classwide and schoolwide programs, labeled *universal intervention*. Universal interventions for ADHD, CD, and ODD follow the principles shown in Table 303-1. However, they are implemented at the systems level as prevention or early intervention programs, for example, violence prevention programs in elementary schools.

Finally, EBTs for the externalizing disorders include components of intervention focused on the children themselves. However, these child-based interventions are never implemented without the parent- and teacher-focused programs. These interventions typically focus on (1) reducing disruptive behavior and behaviors that interfere with peer relationships and (2) teaching skills that improve peer relationships and academic performance. Years of research have shown that these goals typically cannot be reached with interventions conducted in an office-based setting (except tutoring for improving academic skills). Instead, these interventions are usually conducted in group settings in which the behaviors to be reduced or increased can be worked on directly. Thus, in-school, after-school, weekend, or summer programs are used. Children are treated in groups, and the activities that form the context of the group are the recreational activities in which children engage daily. The two broad approaches utilized in EBTs are problem-solving training and social skills training, and many programs include both approaches. Problem-solving programs teach children to use a structured approach to evaluate problems in their interpersonal interactions and develop plans for solving them (e.g., identifying the problem, brainstorming for solutions, evaluating solutions, implementing a plan, and evaluating the plan). Social skills training involves teaching the key concepts of social interaction (e.g., cooperation, communication, participation, and validation). Both approaches involve teaching these skills to children and then having the children practice applying them in supervised interactions with other children, during which behavioral strategies are used to prompt and reward problem solving and social skills. Problem-solving and social skills programs are almost always taught in group settings.

Evidence-Based Treatments for Internalizing Disorders

Table 303-2 lists the components of evidence-based treatments for the internalizing disorders of anxiety and depression. In contrast to treatment for externalizing disorders, internalizing disorders require treating the child, with behavioral parent training becoming an adjunctive intervention designed to support the treatment offered the child, helping the child practice skills and maintain behavior change at home and school.

Notably, the child-based treatments for internalizing disorders are very similar to those employed for externalizing disorders: behavioral and cognitive-behavioral. The

Table 303-2. Components of Evidence-Based Treatments for Internalizing Disorders

Child Intervention

A behavioral and cognitive-behavioral approach in which therapist works with child to reduce depression/anxiety/fears and to increase adaptive skills can be done in office, school, and other settings.

Focus on specific target behaviors that reflect the depression/fears/anxieties that are causing impairment in key domains of functioning; maladaptive behaviors (withdrawal, depression, fears, and anxieties) are targeted for reduction, and adaptive skills (e.g., social skills, coping skills, increasing positive activities) are targeted for development.

Focus on specific cognitions that underlie the child's anxiety/fears/depression, teaching the child a new set of cognitions that will help him or her cope with anxiety and depression. Employ modeling, shaping, prompting, and role play to teach these skills, and practice with rewards within session to master them; employ acronyms and charts to help child learn and remember skills.

Expose the child to the situation that produces the anxiety/fears or depression so that the child learns mastery over the anxiety or depression.

Give homework assignments that involve exposure to the target situations and practice of the coping skills acquired in the training sessions.

Treatment can be individual or group sessions (12 to 16 sessions once or twice weekly), though group-based treatment is more effective.

Adherence to treatment components is regularly checked, and treatment goals are continually added, deleted, or modified on the basis of a current functional analysis of behavior.

Program for generalization, maintenance, and relapse prevention is instituted (e.g., integrate with parent training, develop plans with the child for what to do if the problem re-emerges).

Parent Training

In a behavioral approach, therapist teaches parents contingency management techniques and other parenting skills to use with the child, and the parents implement the treatment. Focus on specific target behaviors that reflect the depression/fears/anxieties that are causing impairment in key domains of functioning; teach parents behavioral skills to reinforce what the child is learning in child sessions—that is, to reduce the child's maladaptive behaviors (anxiety/fears/depression) and to reinforce the child's adaptive skills (e.g., social skills, coping skills).

Treatment involves dyadic or group-based, weekly sessions with therapist (8 to 10 sessions) initially, then contact is faded.

Adherence to treatment components is regularly checked, and treatment goals are continually added, deleted, or modified on the basis of an ongoing functional analysis of behavior.

Program for generalization, maintenance, and relapse prevention is instituted (e.g., parents work to reward the child for continuing his or her coping plans over time and with the teacher when necessary to ensure that the teacher backs up what the child and parent are doing; plan for what parents will do if the problem re-emerges).

social skills training programs and problem-solving approaches are identical, and reward programs are used to encourage the children to learn, practice, and display the social and problem-solving strategies that they learn to cope with their depression or anxiety. With respect to depression, children and adolescents are taught to monitor their moods, increase involvement in pleasant and fun activities, learn social skills, challenge their depressive cognitive styles and adopt positive thinking, and improve communication and conflict resolution skills. The same components are employed in the programs for generalized and social anxiety. In addition, anxious or phobic children are encouraged to expose themselves to the feared or anxiety-provoking situation, both in therapy sessions and in the natural setting. Exposure is typically gradual—as much as the child can

tolerate at one time—and children are rewarded with praise and tangible rewards for working to approach and engage in the feared situation.

As is the case with externalizing disorders, many of these interventions have been developed or adapted for universal use in school settings. For example, studies have shown that depression can be reduced in at-risk children and adolescents by implementing schoolwide EBTs that include the components shown in Table 303-2.

Of note, there is little evidence of any studies looking to see whether pharmacologic approaches are effective for treating internalizing disorders of childhood. This stands in stark contrast to the many studies undertaken that prove the effectiveness of pharmacologic agents in treatment of depression and anxiety in adults, as well as the effectiveness of psychostimulant medication in short-term treatment of ADHD.

Evidence-Based Treatments for Autism

Table 303-3 lists the components of evidence-based treatments for autism. These treatments are likely to apply to other forms of pervasive developmental disorders, although they have not been studied in children with the more rare pervasive developmental disorders. In general, effective treatments for autism involve an intensive one-on-one behavioral intervention that is carried out in the home and school settings. Early intervention in the treatment of autism is essential, and most children begin receiving intervention in the home and specialized preschools by the time they are 3 or 4 years old. EBTs for autism involve written protocols implemented by paraprofessional therapists and overseen by psychologists. Parents are included in treatment and receive training in working with their children. As the child progresses to school age, classroom peers may be included in treatments to help the child learn more appropriate social skills. In the most successful intensive treatment models, autistic children receive 15 to 40 hours of therapy per week. The effectiveness of treatment and treatment goals depends on the child's degree of language impairment and the child's level of intellectual functioning. Children who receive intensive early intervention, achieve language skills by age 5, and have IQs in the moderately retarded to normal range have the best long-term prognosis. They can often learn sufficient adaptive skills to enable eventual independent living or minimal assisted living.

EBTs for autism involve using behavior modification techniques to eliminate self-destructive and disruptive behaviors and teach the child appropriate communication and social skills. Treatments are individualized to address the child's specific impairments in the key domains of cognitive functioning, communication skills, social skills, and disruptive or abnormal behavior. Children with low cognitive abilities are taught skills of daily living, such as proper toileting behavior, and appropriate self-help skills. Children who show disruptive behavior receive EBTs described in the section on disruptive behavior disorders. Appropriate social behavior is taught through intensive modeling and reinforced practice. Initially, the focus of treatment may be on teaching children to show appropriate facial expressions and express affection. As children advance, treatment may

Table 303-3. Components of Evidence-Based Treatments for Autism

Child Intervention

An intensive behavioral approach has the goal of maximizing independent functioning.

The typical model is intensive training daily for multiple hours at school and home.

Conduct functional behavioral analysis to design interventions.

Focus on specific target behaviors that reflect key domains of functioning (social interactions and communication) and behaviors that interfere with adaptive functioning (disruptive behavior).

Social behavior

Focus on social skills, social play, and expressing affection.

Employ modeling, shaping, and prompting to teach these skills.

Normal or mildly handicapped peers may be utilized in teaching social interaction skills.

Communication skills

Focus on verbal imitation, receptive language skills, and expressive verbal language skill. Employ modeling, shaping, and prompting to teach these skills.

Adherence to treatment components is regularly checked, and treatment goals are continually added, deleted, or modified on the basis of an ongoing functional analysis of behavior

Intervention is continued for as long as necessary.

Program for generalization, maintenance, and relapse prevention is instituted.

Parent Training

In a behavioral approach, the therapist teaches the parents contingency management techniques and other parenting skills to use with the child, and the parents implement the treatment; work with parents is more intensive than for most other disorders.

Reinforce what the child is learning in child sessions—that is, to reduce the child's disruptive behaviors and to develop the child's adaptive skills (social behavior and communication skills).

Treatment involves dyadic or group-based sessions with a therapist (16 to 20 sessions) initially, then ongoing contact and support typically for very long periods of time.

Training involves modeling procedures with the parents and child and then observing and giving feedback to the parents while they implement the program with the child.

Adherence to treatment components is regularly checked, and treatment goals are continually added, deleted, or modified on the basis of an ongoing functional analysis of behavior.

Program for generalization, maintenance, and relapse prevention is instituted (e.g., periodic respite care for parents to avoid burn out).

---

involve teaching children appropriate play behaviors and initiating and engaging in appropriate social interactions. Communication skills are taught by using behavior modification principles. Children begin by learning to increase their vocalizations and progress to imitating sounds and words. They are then taught expressive language skills and progress toward learning to speak spontaneously and communicate with others.

Evidence-Based Treatments for Behavioral Health Disorders

Table 303-4 lists the components of evidence-based treatments for several health disorders (i.e., enuresis, encopresis, and obesity). One evidence-based treatment for enuresis is having the child go to bed wearing an alarm with a moisture sensor attached to the child's underwear or to the bedsheet. The alarm sounds at the first drop of moisture, which then awakens the child to get up and go to the bathroom before wetting the bed. This alarm system is commonly referred to as a *bell and pad alarm*. This

program is typically combined with a reward system for the child for having a dry bed. In a matter of weeks, the child becomes conditioned to awaken when he or she feels the sensation of bladder fullness and ceases to wet the bed. Most children treated with the bell and pad alarm system stop wetting the bed completely after 12 weeks. If a child relapses, a repeat use of the bell and pad system is typically

Table 303-4. Components of Evidence-Based Treatments for Behavioral Health Problems

Enuresis

In a behavioral approach, parents are taught contingency management skills and other interventions to implement the procedures with the child in the home setting.

Skills are typically taught by a psychologist or primary care physician in several sessions, with additional sessions as necessary.

Bell and pad conditioning procedures may be necessary.

In retention control training, the child is taught to inhibit urination for progressively longer time periods.

In dry bed training, for 1 or 2 nights, child is awakened hourly and sent to the bathroom to urinate. The child is rewarded for having a dry bed.

In cleanliness training, when accidents occur, the child is required to change clothes, remove wet sheets, and remake the bed; older children will also launder the sheets.

Functional analysis is performed, and treatment is modified as appropriate if standard interventions are insufficient.

Encopresis

In a behavioral approach, the parents are taught contingency management skills and other interventions to implement the procedures with the child in the home setting.

Skills are typically taught by a psychologist or primary care physician in several sessions, with additional sessions as necessary.

A high-fiber diet is used in conjunction with other medical and behavioral treatments.

Medical interventions (cathartics to treat megacolon) are used in conjunction with behavioral treatments.

The child is rewarded for not soiling and for having bowel movements on the toilet without suppositories.

In cleanliness training, the child is required to cleanse self, change underwear, and place soiled underwear with dirty laundry; older children will also launder soiled garments.

Biofeedback may be used as an adjunct, targeted at training external anal sphincter relaxation when attempting to have a bowel movement.

If associated with ODD or CD, behavioral treatments are given to address those symptoms (see Table 304-3). Functional analysis is performed and treatment is modified as appropriate if standard interventions are insufficient.

Obesity

The parent and patient are educated about nutrition and exercise.

In sessions with child and parents, contingency management programs are taught to the parents and child to have the entire family change eating and exercise habits and model health habits and healthy exercise habits for the target child.

Parents are taught the principles of social learning theory (see Chapter 302) to maximize behavior change in children and promote long-term maintenance.

Parents and children are taught to decrease sedentary behaviors and to increase physical activities.

Children are taught self-monitoring and eating control strategies.

Parents and children are taught a nutritional plan in which fat and calories are reduced to arrest weight gain in the child.

Adherence to treatment components is regularly checked, and treatment goals are continually added, deleted, or modified on the basis of an ongoing functional analysis of behavior.

Ongoing monitoring is conducted with continued intervention for as long as necessary.

Program for generalization, maintenance, and relapse prevention is instituted.

effective. Long-term effects of this approach are very positive and lasting.

Other EBTs for enuresis include dry bed training, urinary retention control training, and cleanliness training. These three methods are most often used in conjunction with each other and involve parents' having their children drink more fluids than usual and then progressively delaying urination for longer and longer periods of time, up to an hour (i.e., retention control training). Children are also awakened hourly during the night and sent to the bathroom (i.e., dry bed training). Children are rewarded the next day for dry nights and made to change clothes, remove wet sheets, and remake the bed when they have accidents (i.e., cleanliness training). The intensive components of training—retention control and dry bed training—usually take place over a 2-day period. These behavioral methods are most successful when used in conjunction with a bell and pad alarm system. Most parents can be instructed in the use of the bell and pad alarm system and other behavioral procedures in one or two office visits. Bell and pad alarm systems are widely available.

EBTs for encopresis involve dietary modifications used in conjunction with behavioral treatments and cathartics to treat megacolon. Encopretic children often develop a pattern of avoiding bowel movements and ignoring physiologic sensations. This leads to a buildup of hard stool in the colon, which causes future bowel movements to be painful and leads to further avoidance and suppression of bowel movements. Over time, the child receives fewer physiologic signals about the need to have a bowel movement owing to stretched muscles and nerves. Therefore, the first step in treating encopresis involves having the child adapt a high-fiber diet and using cathartics to clear the colon. Next, behavioral procedures are employed in which the child practices correct toileting behavior at the same time every day. The child is rewarded for having bowel movements on the toilet and practices cleanliness training—changing soiled clothes, washing the body—every time the child has an accident. If the child does not have a bowel movement in the allotted toileting time, he or she may be given a suppository in order to avoid stool buildup but is not given a reward. Most children who are treated with this approach show significant improvements within 2 weeks of initiating treatment, and the vast majority maintains these gains. Biofeedback has also been shown to be helpful in teaching children to relax rather than contract their external anal sphincter when attempting to have a bowel movement. Biofeedback should be used in conjunction with other behavioral treatment methods.

EBTs for the treatment of childhood obesity involve nutritional counseling and dietary changes with the goal of arresting the child's weight gain and helping the child to adopt a more active lifestyle. As is noted in Table 303-4, these changes are taught in a series of sessions with the children and their parents. These lifestyle changes are much more likely to occur and be maintained in the child if the child's parents are involved in treatment and are taught behavior modification techniques to facilitate these lifestyle changes in both the child and themselves. In children younger than age 12, treatment usually involves parent and patient education regarding proper nutrition and exercise—both decreasing sedentary activities and increasing activity, both lifestyle (e.g., walking) and active exercise. Children whose parents who are taught basic principles of behavior modification, such as social learning theory (see Chapter 302), have been shown to have the most success in reaching short-term weight control goals and in maintaining lifestyle changes over time. This is because parents who are taught about behavior modification are more likely to model good eating habits, to decrease sedentary behavior, and to appropriately monitor and reward their children for making similar lifestyle changes. These approaches have been shown to be very effective in long-term management of childhood obesity.

One feature that enuresis, encopresis, and obesity share is that parents and health care providers often assume that if a child suffers from one of these conditions, the condition is caused by an underlying mental health problem such as depression, repressed anger, or low self-esteem. However, this is rarely the case. The child may develop symptoms of depression or low self-esteem because of the underlying condition.

SUMMARY

The primary care clinician has an important role in the identification, treatment, and referral of the child with mental health problems. The primary care clinician should identify problems in daily life functioning, select appropriate referrals for EBTs, follow up with patients to ensure that appropriate EBTs are being implemented by the mental health specialist, and monitor patients over time using a chronic care model of treatment.

 Additional Resources, CD-ROM

Bibliography

SUGGESTED READINGS

Clarke GN, Rhode P, Lewinsohn PM, et al: Cognitive-behavioral treatment of adolescent depression: Efficacy of acute group treatment and booster sessions. J Am Acad Child Adolesc Psychiatry 1999;38:272–279.

Kendall PC, Southam-Gerow M: Long-term follow up of a cognitive-behavioral therapy for anxiety-disordered youth. J Consult Clin Psychol 1996;64:724–730.

Lonigan C, Elbert J: Special issue on empirically supported psychosocial interventions for children. J Clin Child Psychol 1998;26:138–145.

Pelham WE Jr, Fabiano GA: Behavior modification. Child Adolesc Psychiatr Clin N Am 2000;9:671–688.

Weiss B, Carton T, Harris V, Phung TM: The effectiveness of traditional child psychotherapy. J Consult Clin Psychol 1999;67:82–94.

304 Physical Therapy

Joshua Alexander and Darlene Sekerak

TYPES OF TREATMENTS

Pediatric physical therapy is based on scientific principles for the diagnosis and management of a wide array of movement-related impairments associated with developmental disability, injury, or disease. Collaboration between the pediatrician and pediatric physical therapist can facilitate optimal recovery, improve developmental outcomes, and promote overall physical fitness for the children they serve. By learning more about the principles and practices of this profession, the pediatrician can judiciously make referrals for physical therapy. This chapter provides pediatricians with information about the educational background of physical therapists, the physical therapy patient management model, and benefits gained from physical therapy consultation or referral.

HOW THE THERAPY IS ADMINISTERED

Personnel

Pediatric physical therapy is the delivery of any service by a licensed physical therapist (PT) that helps to restore, maintain, or promote the movement and physical function of a child or adolescent. All 50 states, the District of Columbia, and Puerto Rico license and regulate the practice of physical therapy. National licensure examination for physical therapists requires completion of a postgraduate masters (MS, MPT) or doctoral program (DPT) at a college or university accredited by the Commission on Accreditation in Physical Therapy Education. Training programs at these institutions include both didactic coursework and supervised clinical rotations in a variety of health care settings. PTs may also become board certified as a Pediatric Certified Specialist (PCS) by meeting stringent criteria set forth by the American Board of Physical Therapy Specialties and passing a specialty examination. This certification has only recently been introduced and should not be used as the sole criterion for evaluating the competency of a pediatric physical therapist. In any situation, the pediatrician should attempt to refer children to PTs with significant pediatric specialty training, experience, and professional reputation.

Limited aspects of physical therapy intervention may be delegated to a physical therapist assistant (PTA). PTAs obtain an associate's degree from a 2-year program, usually at a community or junior college, pass a state administered national examination, and must practice under the direction and supervision of a physical therapist. PTAs are licensed in many but not all jurisdictions.

Practice Settings

Pediatric physical therapists practice in a variety of settings, supporting the continuum of health care needs from infancy through childhood and adolescence (Box 304-1). Practice settings and the child's age may influence the PT's choice of intervention and the approach to care.

Treatment Process

When the pediatrician has identified a child who would benefit from physical therapy, a referral should be made to begin collaboration with the therapist. A sample referral is shown in Box 304-2.

On receiving a referral, the PT begins by obtaining a complete history; measuring components of movement such as range of motion, strength, sensation, and cardiovascular fitness; and assessing developmental or functional abilities using either norm-referenced or criterion-referenced testing instruments. The needs of the child and indications inherent in the referral guide the examination (Box 304-3).

The therapist uses the examination to evaluate the child's current level of functional impairment and establishes a working diagnosis and prognosis. A proposed plan of care, with available treatment options, is reviewed with the child, the family, and, when possible, other people who are involved in the child's care. Box 304-4 lists common interventions.

Therapy may incorporate the use of aquatics, therapeutic horseback riding, or other leisure or play-based activities. The therapist may offer services in one-on-one sessions, collaborative sessions with a provider from another discipline, or group sessions with several children and caregivers.

Box 304-1. Common Physical Therapy Practice Settings

1. Private practice
2. Medical institutions
   a. Neonatal intensive care
   b. Acute care
   c. Rehabilitation units/centers
3. Schools
4. Home health care agencies and home-based early intervention programs
5. Child care and developmental day care centers
6. Group homes
7. State agencies (e.g., developmental evaluation centers)

305 Occupational Therapy

Joshua Alexander and Linn Wakeford

TYPE OF TREATMENT

Pediatric occupational therapy is a health and rehabilitation profession that helps children develop or regain skills that are important for independent functioning, health, well-being, security, and happiness. Occupational therapists work with children who, because of illness, injury, or developmental disability, need specialized assistance in learning skills to enable them to lead independent, productive, and satisfying lives. Occupational therapy is based on the scientific study of humans as occupational beings. Practice is guided by overarching concepts and theories related to the role of occupation in human experience, and interventions incorporate specific biomechanical, neurodevelopmental, sensory integration, cognitive, motor control, and psychosocial treatments. The pediatrician can best collaborate with occupational therapists by learning more about the principles and practices of occupational therapy and the need for an interdisciplinary team approach to care of a child with special needs.

HOW THE THERAPY IS ADMINISTERED

Personnel

Occupational therapy is provided by practitioners who have been educated in the study of human growth, development, and engagement in life activities, with specific emphasis on the social, emotional, and physiologic effects of illness, injury, and developmental or psychological impairments. Like medical students, occupational therapy students are educated with a combination of classroom and laboratory learning experiences followed by supervised clinical rotations in a variety of settings. Occupational therapists (OTs) must pass a national certification examination prior to graduation and enter the field with a bachelor's or master's degree. Some therapists pursue postprofessional degrees, including doctoral studies in occupational science or other related disciplines. All 50 states, the District of Columbia, and Puerto Rico regulate the practice of occupational therapy, and many of these jurisdictions mandate periodic continuing education requirements. Occupational therapy assistants must earn an associate's degree, pass a national certification examination, and become licensed in their state to practice under the supervision of a certified occupational therapist. The pediatrician should keep in mind that although these practitioners are exposed to pediatric patients and settings during their training, efforts should be made to refer children to providers who have pediatric expertise.

Practice Settings

Pediatric OTs practice their profession in a wide variety of clinical settings that influence the practitioner's approach to care (Box 305-1).

Treatment Process

When the pediatrician has identified a child who could benefit from occupational therapy services, a referral should be made to begin the collaborative process with the therapist. For maximum benefit, referrals should include background medical information (diagnosis or condition), functional deficits, precautions (e.g., fall, seizure, range of motion), type of therapy requested, and plans for medical follow-up. Depending on the physician-therapist relationship and local managed care guidelines, other information provided in the referral may include frequency of therapy, length of treatment, anticipated goals, and expected outcomes.

Once a referral is received, the OT obtains a history and assesses occupational performance issues, specific performance components, and environmental or contextual factors that enhance or limit the child's abilities (Box 305-2).

Following the initial evaluation, the OT designs a personalized intervention plan for meeting the child's and family's identified needs. This plan may include one or several combined available interventions that focus on improving the child's abilities to engage in age-appropriate activities of daily living (e.g., bathing, toileting, feeding, dressing), play, school-related tasks, and, for adolescents, prevocational and vocational activities.

Occupational therapy interventions are provided through a variety of service delivery models (direct, consultative, integrated), either alone or in combination. Direct interventions designed and implemented by the OT may be

---

Box 305-1. Occupational Therapy Practice Settings

1. Private practice
2. Medical institutions
   a. Neonatal intensive care
   b. Acute care
   c. Rehabilitation
3. Schools
4. Home health care
5. Child care and developmental day programs
6. Group homes
7. State agencies (e.g., developmental evaluation centers)

Box 305-2. Occupational Performance Issues

Performance Areas

Broad categories of human activity that are typically part of daily life, including activities of daily living, work and productive activities, and play/leisure activities.

Performance Components

Elements of performance required for successful engagement in performance areas, including sensorimotor, cognitive, social, and psychological aspects.

Performance Contexts

Temporal (chronological, developmental, life cycle, disability status) and environmental (physical, social, political, cultural) situations or factors that influence an individual's engagement in desired or required performance areas.

Box 305-3. Common Conditions That May Benefit from Occupational Therapy Interventions

1. Orthopedic, neurologic, and neuromuscular disorders (e.g., arthrogryposis, cerebral palsy, spina bifida, rheumatic conditions)
2. Cognitive delays or learning problems
3. Genetic syndromes or hereditary disorders (e.g., Down syndrome, sickle-cell disorders)
4. Traumatic injuries (e.g., acquired brain injury, burns)
5. Sensory or sensory processing impairments (e.g., visual impairment, sensory neuropathies)
6. Social, emotional, or behavioral problems (e.g., attention deficit/hyperactivity disorders, pervasive developmental disorders)

provided during individual or group sessions. These interventions include the use of specified purposeful activities or therapeutic methods that are meaningful to the client and enhance the client's occupational performance. In the service delivery model, the OT may evaluate the benefits of splinting, adapted equipment, assistive technology devices, and environmental and task modifications that enhance and increase the child's functional mobility, communication, self-care skills, or participation in play or school-related or work-related activities.

The OT may also provide consultative (or indirect) services that help others to modify their interactions and the child's social and physical environment to promote optimal participation. Consultations include instructing care providers (e.g., parents, day care and school personnel) on appropriate teaching strategies, altering tasks to address physical, sensory processing, cognitive, or psychosocial impairments, and implementing therapeutic feeding, handling, and positioning techniques.

Throughout the intervention, the OT evaluates outcomes and determines whether to continue the current intervention, modify interventions to achieve current goals, establish new goals or objectives, refer to other professionals or services, or discharge the child from occupational therapy treatments. Best practice in pediatric occupational therapy dictates that services are evidence-based family- and child-centered interventions provided within an interdisciplinary context. However, practice setting and reimbursement issues may limit successful implementation of best practice.

INDICATIONS

The occupational therapy treatment process starts with the identification of a child with a disability, injury, or chronic illness that limits the child's ability to engage in self-care, school-related activities, work activities, or play activities (Box 305-3).

BENEFITS

Occupational therapy interventions should enable the child to engage in socially acceptable daily activities that are meaningful and satisfying. Although these benefits are age- and child-specific (Box 305-4), the overall goal of occupa-

tional therapy remains constant throughout the patient's life span. Through meaningful activities, adaptive equipment and assistive technology, and environmental modifications, the OT helps the child achieve an optimal level of independence and quality of life (see Box 305-4).

EVIDENCE-BASED EFFECTIVENESS

It is difficult to assess the effectiveness of occupational therapy on the basis of individual or small-group OT practices. In the field of occupational therapy, as in many

Box 305-4. Benefits of Occupational Therapy at Different Ages

Infants/Toddlers

Exploration of and learning about their environment
Improving space management (understanding and getting from one place to another)
Obtaining and manipulating toys and other items for play
Interacting with adults and developing relationships with peers
Improving independence in self-care skills (feeding)

Preschoolers

Continued interaction with and learning about environment but with more sophisticated skills in the following:
Space management
Manipulative and constructive play
Tool use (e.g., markers, crayons, glue, scissors)
Pretend and dramatic play
Social engagement
Self-care (feeding, dressing, bathing, toileting)

School-Age Children

Activities of daily living, including age-appropriate personal care (grooming, bathing, dressing)
Productivity, including school-related skills such as managing handwriting/written expression, computer use, and organizational and task completion skills
Play/leisure (recreation, sports, hobbies)

Adolescents/Young Adults

Independence in daily living skills
Participation in school-related activities
Prevocational and work activities
Enjoyment of leisure activities

other professional fields, research supports some portions of practice and equivocally confirms or questions other portions of practice. In occupational therapy, some research applies to more specific practice models (e.g., motor learning, biomechanical, coping/psychosocial), while some is directed at the more overarching constructs of occupation, occupation as a medium of change, and humans as occupational beings.

CONTROVERSIES

Current controversies within the profession revolve around (1) the need for more scientifically sound research and (2) the resurgent focus on the core philosophies of occupational therapy (occupation, humans as occupational beings, and occupation as a medium of change) rather than on component-level practice. Sensory integration and neuro-developmental treatment may be considered controversial owing to significant lack of evidence supporting these treatments as efficacious methods of intervention. Other approaches that seek to remediate components (e.g., strength, range of motion, or visual perception) may be controversial, since research indicates that improvements in these components do not necessarily improve functional performance of tasks and activities. Some controversial alternative therapies (e.g., cranial-sacral, myofascial release) have no evidence for effectiveness in the scientific literature and do not incorporate the core concepts of occupation and the use of occupation as a therapeutic medium.

FUTURE TRENDS

Future trends in pediatric occupational therapy include these:
- Increasing the numbers of therapists working in community-based and nontraditional practice settings
- Increasing the use of consultation as a method of service delivery using the child's natural environments or contexts as settings for service delivery
- Increasing the use of research evidence to support the occupational therapy intervention process
- Increasing the influence of occupational science to support the practice of occupational therapy
- Increasing the number of therapists providing population-based services and expanding the definition of "client" to include community groups, service agencies, and other organizations
- Increasing the involvement of occupational therapy practitioners in health-care- and education-related legislative and reimbursement issues

SUGGESTED READINGS

American Academy of Pediatrics Committee on Children with Disabilities: The role of the pediatrician in prescribing therapy services for children with motor disabilities. Pediatrics 1996;98(2):308–310.
American Occupational Therapy Association Commission on Practice: Standards of Practice for Occupational Therapy. Bethesda, Md, American Occupational Therapy Association, 1998. Available at: http://www.aota.org/general/about.asp.
Case-Smith J (ed): Occupational Therapy for Children, 4th ed. St Louis, Mosby, 2001.
Dunn W: Best Practice Occupational Therapy: In Community Service with Children and Families. Thorofare, NJ, Slack, 2000.

SECTION 9   DIAGNOSTICS AND THERAPEUTICS: *Rehabilitation Medicine*

306   Special Education

Stephen H. Contompasis

BACKGROUND

Prior to 1975, the special educational needs of children with disabilities were not being fully met, and more than one half of the children with disabilities in the United States did not receive appropriate educational services. Over 1 million children with disabilities in the United States were excluded entirely from the public school system, forcing families to find services outside the public school system, often at great distance from their residence and at their own expense. Furthermore, there were many children with disabilities throughout the United States participating in regular school programs whose disabilities prevented them from having successful educational experiences because their disabilities were undetected.

In 1975, a federal law was enacted (P.L. 94-142, the Education of All Handicapped Children Act of 1975) to support educational opportunities for children with disabilities. Now reauthorized and recently amended as the Individuals with Disabilities Education Act (IDEA '97), it ensures that all children with disabilities have available to them a free appropriate public education and protects the rights of children with disabilities and their parents within the special education process. Federal data suggest that more than 6 million children ages 3 to 21 with disabilities in the United States are served under IDEA '97. In the reauthorization, it is stated that improving educational results for children with disabilities is an essential element of our national policy of ensuring equality of opportunity, full participation, independent living, and economic self-sufficiency for individuals with disabilities.

INDICATIONS (FOR REFERRAL FOR SPECIAL EDUCATION)

The process by which children are referred for special education is only generally mentioned in the federal law or related guidelines. Each state, however, is required to have in effect policies and procedures to ensure that all children in need of special education and related services are identified, located, and evaluated. It is imperative that all people who are involved in the care or education of children are aware of the disability categories under special education law, and appropriately refer suspected children for evaluation.

For special education purposes, the term *child with a disability* means a child with mental retardation, hearing impairments (including deafness), speech or language impairments, visual impairments (including blindness), serious emotional disturbance, orthopedic impairments, autism, traumatic brain injury, other health impairments (such as attention deficit hyperactivity disorder), or specific learning disabilities. The health care provider may play a unique role in determining certain "other health impairments" or other medical conditions that make children eligible for special education (see Table 306-1 for categories and definitions of disability).

Once a child has been identified, the health care provider may provide other supports to the child, family, and educational team. These may include the following:

1. Documentation of the child's condition and its impact to help in the eligibility process and determine education and related service needs
2. Referral for other developmental services, for instance, respite, case management, mental health supports, family support, and other community supports
3. Referrals for vision and hearing evaluations if a child cannot perform either office-based or school-based evaluations
4. Referrals for other health issues, for example, seizure management or management of self-injurious behaviors
5. Child and family support, encouragement, anticipatory guidance, "demystification" of the disorder, linking to support groups
6. Coordination of mental health information and medication prescriptions as appropriate

Children who fail to meet criteria for special education services yet have a medical condition or disability that affects their access to school may qualify for accommodations or special services under section 504 of P.L. 101-476, the Rehabilitation Act of 1973. Children from low-income families who are experiencing learning difficulties can be provided learning supports under Title I, Part A of the Elementary and Secondary Education Act (ESEA).

DIAGNOSTICS

Tests to Determine a Disability and Need for Special Education and How They Work

IDEA '97 requires that state or local educational agencies conduct a full and individual initial evaluation before providing special education and related services. Typically, evaluations are carried out by a team of individuals under the direction of a special education teacher or administrator within the child's school or local school district. The initial evaluation determines whether a child has a disability and also should determine the child's educational needs.

On consent of the parents, the evaluation is planned; it must include the use of a variety of assessment tools and strategies to gather relevant functional and developmental information, including information provided by the parents. IDEA '97 requires that single procedures or evaluations (e.g., an IQ test alone) not be used as the sole criterion for determining a disability or determining an appropriate educational program. It also requires that technically sound instruments are selected and administered by trained and knowledgeable personnel and that evaluation methods are not discriminatory on a racial or cultural basis. A team of interdisciplinary professionals usually carries out evaluations. Typically, this might include the following:

- A licensed school psychologist or special educator to administer tests of intelligence and academic achievement
- A certified speech-language provider to administer specific tests of language ability or language use
- A registered physical or occupational therapist to administer specific tests of physical movement or ability, fine motor and adaptive skills, and visual perceptual or visual motor skills
- Other related service providers (e.g., the child's health care provider, a psychiatrist, an audiologist, a school nurse, a registered dietitian or nutritionist) who may be called on to provide testing or information relevant to the child and the suspected disability

INTERPRETATIONS (TABLES OF NORMAL/ABNORMAL)

The following case studies illustrate how a special education evaluation might be carried out, the types of tests used, and possible results.

Child with Cognitive Impairment (Mental Retardation, Learning Impairment)

Lewis was referred for a special education evaluation by his kindergarten teacher. This was Lewis's first educational experience, and despite some extra time and support from his teacher, he has had difficulty mastering some of the basic skills. Because of this concern, an evaluation was planned. Table 306-2 shows some of the testing that was performed as part of the evaluation and the child's results on those measures.

The team interpreted the results and found Lewis eligible for special education under the category of Mental

Table 306-1. Categories for eligibility

Mental retardation

Significantly subaverage general intellectual functioning, existing concurrently with deficits in adaptive behavior and manifested during the developmental period, that adversely affects a child's educational performance

[*Author's note:* States may vary. For instance, Vermont uses the terminology *learning impairment* and interprets significantly subaverage as an IQ 1.5 standard deviations below the mean.]

Specific Learning Disability

A disorder in one or more of the basic psychological processes involved in understanding or in using language, spoken or written, that may manifest itself in an imperfect ability to listen, thin, speak, read, write, spell, or to do mathematical calculations, including conditions such as perceptual disabilities, brain injury, minimal brain dysfunction, dyslexia, and developmental aphasia; the term does not include learning problems that are primarily the result of visual, hearing, or motor disabilities, of mental retardation, of emotional disturbance, or of environmental, cultural, or economic disadvantage

Speech or Language Impairment

A communication disorder, such as stuttering, impaired articulation, a language impairment, or a voice impairment, that adversely affects a child's educational performance

Deafness

A hearing impairment that is so severe that the child is impaired in processing linguistic information through hearing, with or without amplification, that adversely affects a child's educational performance

Visual Impairment

An impairment in vision that, even with correction, adversely affects a child's educational performance; the term includes both partial sight and blindness

Deaf-Blindness

Concomitant hearing and visual impairments, the combination of which causes such severe communication and other developmental and educational needs that they cannot be accommodated in special education programs solely for children with deafness or children with blindness

Autism

A developmental disability significantly affecting verbal and nonverbal communication and social interaction, generally evident before age 3, that adversely affects a child's educational performance; other characteristics often associated with autism are engagement in repetitive activities and stereotyped movements, resistance to environmental change or change in daily routines, and unusual responses to sensory experiences

[*Author's note:* The language in IDEA '97 does not match the commonly used diagnostic tools (DSM-IV and ICD-10).]

Emotional Disturbance

A condition exhibiting one or more of the following characteristics over a long period of time, and to a marked degree that adversely affects a child's educational performance:
1. An inability to learn that cannot be explained by intellectual, sensory, or health factors
2. An inability to build or maintain satisfactory interpersonal relationships with peers and teachers
3. Inappropriate types of behavior or feelings under normal circumstances
4. A general pervasive mood of unhappiness or depression
5. A tendency to develop physical symptoms or fears associated with personal or school problems

The term includes schizophrenia. The term does not apply to children who are socially maladjusted unless it is determined that they have an emotional disturbance.

Other Health Impairment

Having limited strength, vitality, or alertness, including a heightened alertness to environmental stimuli, that results in limited alertness with respect to the educational environment, that is due to chronic or acute health problems such as asthma, attention deficit disorder or attention deficit hyperactivity disorder, diabetes, epilepsy, a heart condition, hemophilia, lead poisoning, leukemia, nephritis, rheumatic fever, or sickle-cell anemia; and adversely affects a child's educational performance

Orthopedic Impairment

A severe orthopedic impairment that adversely affects a child's educational performance; the term includes impairments caused by congenital anomaly (e.g., clubfoot, absence of some member), impairments caused by disease (e.g., poliomyelitis, bone tuberculosis, and impairments from other causes (e.g., cerebral palsy, amputations, and fractures or burns that cause contractures)

Multiple Disabilities

Concomitant impairments (e.g., mental retardation-blindness, mental retardation-orthopedic impairment), the combination of which causes such severe educational needs that they cannot be accommodated in special education programs solely for one of the impairments. The term does not include deaf-blindness

Traumatic Brain Injury

An acquired injury to the brain caused by an external physical force, resulting in total or partial functional disability or psychosocial impairment, or both, that adversely affects a child's educational performance; the term applies to open or closed head injuries resulting in impairments in one or more areas (e.g., cognition; language; memory; attention; reasoning; abstract thinking; judgment; problem solving; sensory, perceptual, and motor abilities; psychosocial behavior; physical functions; information processing; and speech); the term does not apply to brain injuries that are congenital or degenerative or to brain injuries induced by birth trauma

From The Individuals With Disabilities Education Act (IDEA). 20 USC 1400 et seq, June 4, 1997.

Retardation, and plans were made to develop an individualized education plan (IEP).

Child with a Learning Disability

Jillian was referred for a special education evaluation by her second grade teacher. Despite some additional reading help over the past 2 years, Jillian is falling behind her classmates in her ability to read. She does well with math problems and other subjects. She has no apparent difficulty with physical activities and is experiencing some sadness that might be related to her difficulty keeping up in reading. On the basis of intake information, an evaluation was planned. Table 306-3 shows some of the testing that was performed

as part of the evaluation and the child's results on those measures.

Evaluations revealed a significant gap in Jillian's measure of intelligence and her reading ability (−28 points). She was found eligible for special education under the category of Learning Disability, and an IEP was developed.

THERAPEUTICS: TYPE(S) OF TREATMENTS

Special education services under IDEA are developed by a team and planned for utilizing an IEP. The IEP must state the category of disability and its impact on the child and must outline the special education (in measurable goals),

Table 306-2. Test Results for Lewis

Intelligence	Language Ability	Academic Achievement	Motor Ability
Wechsler Preschool Primary Scale of Intelligence–Revised (WPPSI–R) Verbal IQ: 64 Performance IQ: 61 Full Scale IQ: 62	Test of Language Development–Primary, Third Edition (TOLD–P:3) SS: 65	Wide Range Achievement Test (WRAT–R) Reading SS: 58 Arithmetic SS: 71 Spelling SS: 63	Peabody Scales of Motor Development SS: 72 The Beery-Buktenica Developmental Test of Visual-Motor Integration SS: 62

Note: Standard scores (SS) are a common form of reporting and are usually based on a mean score of 100 and standard deviation of ±15.

related services, supplementary aids, program modifications, and supports for school personnel that will be provided for the child. The IEP must be reviewed and, if necessary, revised on an annual basis, and a comprehensive re-evaluation of the child must be done every 3 years.

The *IEP Team*, as defined by IDEA '97, includes the parents, whenever appropriate the child with a disability, the regular education teacher (if the child is, or may be, participating in the regular education environment), the special education teacher, a representative of the local educational agency, an individual who can interpret the instructional implications of evaluation results, and other individuals who have knowledge or special expertise regarding the child, including related services personnel. In this role, the child's health care provider may attend or provide relevant information.

THE INDIVIDUALIZED EDUCATION PLAN

Child with Multiple Disabilities

Jason is a boy with multiple health issues related to premature birth, including spastic quadriparesis, severe dysarthria, and bilateral moderate sensorineural hearing deficits. A special education evaluation found him eligible for an IEP under the category of Multiple Disabilities. His team developed and began to implement an IEP. See Table 306-4 for examples of some of Jason's IEP goals, related services, and assistive technology supports.

Indications, Evidence-Based Effectiveness, Benefits, and Risks (Complications)

Since 1975, children in the United States have benefited from IEPs geared to their unique abilities and challenges. However, parents and children may experience emotional stress during the process if information related to the child's disability is not handled in a sensitive, empathetic, and family-centered way. The child's primary care provider, who has experience in presenting difficult diagnostic information and an established relationship with the family, may be a useful team member in this regard.

There are also risks that children may be inappropriately identified within the special education process. For example, a child with autism might be inappropriately assigned to a disability category of Mental Retardation or Language Impairment when, owing, to a lack of experience, the evaluation team fails to recognize features of autism and its impact on standardized testing.

Although special education has gained access to education for children with disability, it has not fully ensured that all children with disabilities are prepared for employment and independent living. In November 2000, the National Council on Disability and the Social Security Administration reported that students receiving special education had the following:

- Poor graduation rates from high school (only 27% received a diploma)
- Low employment rates after high school (only 59% were competitively employed 3 to 5 years after graduation)
- Low postsecondary education participation
- An increasing participation in Social Security benefits

To address these shortfalls, IDEA '97 requires transition planning toward greater independence on graduation. One purpose of transition planning is to identify the necessary services for students with disabilities prior to graduation and to connect students with those services.

CONTROVERSIES: HOW THE THERAPIES ARE ADMINISTERED, MAINSTREAMING OR INCLUSIVE EDUCATION

There is variability in how states and local educational districts provide special education services. For example, IDEA '97 requires that an IEP must show how it is meeting

Table 306-3. Test Results for Jillian

Intelligence	Language	Achievement	Motor Ability
Wechsler Intelligence Scale for Children–III Revised (WISC III–R) Verbal IQ: 104 Performance IQ: 98 Full Scale IQ: 100	Test of Language Test of Language Development Primary, Third Edition (TOLD–P:3) SS: 98	Wide Range Achievement Test (WRAT–R) Reading SS: 72 Arithmetic SS: 95 Spelling SS: 77	Peabody Scales of Motor Development SS: 106 The Beery-Buktenica Developmental Test of Visual-Motor Integration SS: 98

Note: Standard scores (SS) are a common form of reporting and are usually based on a mean score of 100 and standard deviation of ±15.

Table 306-4. IEP Goals, Related Services, and Assistive Technology Supports for Jason

IEP Entry	Definition	Examples
Goals	A statement of measurable annual goals, including benchmarks or short-term objectives	Jason will recognize all uppercase letters of the alphabet by November 1, 2002. Jason will recognize the letter sounds for B, P, T, M, and S by December 1, 2002.
Related services	The term *related services* means transportation and such developmental, corrective, and other supportive services, including speech-language pathology and audiology services, psychological services, physical and occupation therapy, recreation, including therapeutic recreation, social work services, counseling services, including rehabilitation counseling, orientation and mobility services, and medical services, (for diagnostic and evaluation purposes only), as may be required to assist a child with a disability to benefit from special education.	Jason will be provided specialized bus transportation to safely accommodate for his wheelchair. Jason will receive counseling that helps him with emotions related to his disability. Jason will have a special diet of soft-textured foods, determined by a speech-language provider (SLP) with experience in dysphagia, and is fed by personnel trained by the SLP.
Assistive technology devices	The term *assistive technology device* means any item, piece of equipment, or product system, whether acquired commercial off the shelf, modified, or customized, that is used to increase, maintain, or improve functional capabilities of a child with a disability.	Jason will have access to a communication device with a touch screen and voice output. Jason will have an FM sound system to enhance voice transmission from his teacher.
Assistive technology services	The term *assistive technology service* means any service that directly assists a child with a disability in the selection, acquisition, or use of an assistive technology device.	Jason's school team and parents will receive training in the programming and use of his communication device.

the child's needs to be involved in and progress in the general curriculum, to participate in extracurricular and other nonacademic activities, and to participate with other children with and without disabilities. It does, however, allow for an explanation of the extent, if any, to which the child will not participate with nondisabled children in the regular class and in other school activities. It also makes provisions for providing a range of educational placements to serve the unique needs of a child. Placement options that are available include instruction in regular classes, special classes, special schools, home instruction, and instruction in hospitals and institutions. Advocates of "mainstreaming" children with disabilities accurately point out that nondisabled children benefit from their increased awareness of the needs of individuals with disabilities and their role in supporting their peers.

States and regions differ in their interpretation of the least restrictive environment provision for special education services. For instance, in the author's home state of Vermont, most IEP services are carried out in the child's neighborhood or town school in the regular education classroom, while in other states, more children are served in special education classrooms designed and attended on the basis of disability category. However, as unique needs of the child are considered and because of appropriate pressures from families as active IEP team members, changes are occurring. In Vermont, the pendulum is shifting toward more specialized classes and programs, and in other states, parents are advocating for children to have more access to regular education settings. It seems that as children grow older and the gaps between their abilities and those of children in mainstream settings widen, many school systems utilize alternative classroom settings. The benefits and drawbacks of mainstream settings versus alternative

settings or combinations of both are matters best addressed by open and honest team communication around the IEP process and the child's unique needs.

CHALLENGES AND FUTURE TRENDS

Although special education as a continuum of the right to a free and public education is likely to exist under current and future federal mandates, areas of controversy and challenge are likely. Future trends might include the following:

1. Advances in understanding the neurobiology of certain disabilities that may enhance our ability to better detect and serve those children's needs
2. Increased involvement of families and children on IEP teams as active participants in decision making providing a more family centered versus child centered focus and increasing parent participation in interpreting special education law and devising policy and practice
3. Research leading to better understanding of the environment that provides maximal education and social benefit to children with disabilities and their nondisabled educational and future community peers
4. Increased efforts in the transition process to enable more students with disability to achieve greater independence in their communities
5. Finding new ways for the "Medical Home" to collaborate with the special education process and services

Additional Resources, CD-ROM

Bibliography

SUGGESTED READINGS

American Academy of Pediatrics: The pediatrician's role in development and implementation of an Individual Education Plan (IEP) and/or an Individual Family Service Plan (IFSP): Policy statement. Pediatrics 1999;104(1):124–127. Available at: http://www.aap.org/policy/re9823.html.

American Academy of Pediatrics, Committee on Children with Disabilities: Provision of educationally-related services for children and adolescents with chronic diseases and disabling conditions: Policy statement (RE9929). Pediatrics 2000;105(2):448–445. Available at: http://www.aap.org/policy/re9929.html.

Bateman B: The physician and the world of special education. J Child Neurol 1995;10(suppl 1):S114–S120.

Individuals with Disabilities Education Act (IDEA). 20 USC 1400 et seq, June 4, 1997.

McInerny TK: Children who have difficulty in school: A primary pediatrician's approach. Pediatr Rev 1995;16:325–332.

SECTION 9   DIAGNOSTICS AND THERAPEUTICS: *Complementary Health Care*

307 Principles of Integrative Pediatrics

Kathi J. Kemper and Cassandra Walcott

More and more parents are asking their clinicians a variety of questions about complementary and alternative medical therapies (CAM) for their children. While clinicians do not need to be experts in all forms of complementary and alternative therapies, they should be aware of the epidemiology, practice theories, evidence-based information about commonly used therapies, and changing definitions of CAM so that they can integrate this knowledge into their practices. Clinicians should be able to elicit a complete history of the different CAM therapies parents may be using for their children. Numerous resources to learn more about CAM are listed at the end of this chapter.

DEFINITIONS

The National Institutes of Health National Center for Complementary and Alternative Medicine defines CAM as a broad range of healing philosophies, approaches, and therapies that conventional medicine does not commonly use, accept, study, understand, or make available. CAM therapies include acupuncture, herbs, and therapeutic massage. CAM systems of health care include traditional Chinese medicine, Ayurveda (the traditional medicine of India), Native American healing practices, and homeopathy.

Alternative therapies initially referred to those that were not provided in hospitals, were not taught at U.S. medical schools, were not traditionally reimbursed by third-party payers, and for which there were limited efficacy data. However, in the 1990s, most American medical schools instituted curricula on CAM, and more recently, third-party payers have started to reimburse some CAM practitioners for their services.

A therapy is considered to be *complementary* if it is used together with mainstream medical therapies. Some therapies, such as massage, guided imagery, and biofeedback, are now being provided by mainstream clinics and hospitals. They are offered for patient and family support and do not replace traditional medical regimens.

Holistic means taking care of the whole person (body, mind, emotions, spirit, and relationships) in the context of the person's family, culture, and community. Holistic medicine describes an approach to the patient rather than a specific set of therapeutic techniques. Holistic may also mean patient-focused care or contextual pediatrics.

A practitioner of *integrative* pediatrics considers a wide range of therapies, examines the scientific evidence on a given therapy, and then, in collaboration with families, determines which one of these therapies is most appropriate for a particular patient. Integrative pediatrics is comprehensive, evidence-based medicine.

HISTORY AND EPIDEMIOLOGY OF CAM

Substantial and increasing numbers of children and adults use CAM. The percentage of American adults who reported using CAM in 1997 was 42% in contrast to the 34% in 1990. During this 7-year period, out-of pocket expenditures increased by 45% so that by 1997, the amount of money spent out-of-pocket for CAM use exceeded the amount spent out-of-pocket for all U.S. hospitalizations. By 1997, the annual number of outpatient visits to mainstream physicians was less than the number of outpatient visits to CAM providers.

Despite the increased CAM use and the significant out-of-pocket expenditures, patients were no more likely to discuss their use of CAM in 1997 than they were in 1990. In fact, the majority of adult patients do not talk to their physicians about their use of CAM therapies. However, parents are likely to be more conservative with CAM use for their children; hence, the increase in questions about CAM use in children with which pediatricians are faced.

The percentage of general pediatric patients using CAM in 1997 was approximately 20%. The prevalence is significantly higher among children with chronic, recurrent, or fatal conditions such as asthma, attention deficit disorder, cystic fibrosis, and cancer. The prevalence of CAM use among children and adolescents with these illnesses and even those with psychosocial risks alone (such as homeless teens) range from 30% to more than 70% depending on age and access to services.

Given these statistics, many physicians fear that patients will abandon mainstream medical care in favor of CAM therapies, but data do not support these concerns. The families who seek out complementary and alternative practitioners rarely abandon their physician but often are uncomfortable discussing these therapies if they perceive their provider to be judgmental or antagonistic toward them. The majority of families seek therapies that are consistent with their values, worldview, and culture, and they seek care from providers, whether mainstream or unconventional, who offer them respect, time, and attention.

GOALS OF HEALING

While mainstream and CAM providers have similar goals of healing (Table 307-1), many CAM healing practices and systems focus primarily on the more philosophical components of wellness, such as enhancing harmony and promoting inner peace. For example, the recent focus on patient-centered, culturally sensitive care has made prayer and other spiritual practices to achieve inner peace a more prominent feature of medical treatment. Individual families and patients under different circumstances may pursue multiple philosophical, spiritual, and medical goals simultaneously.

INTEGRATIVE MODEL

The integrative model provides a framework for understanding the similarities and differences between conventional, complementary, and alternative therapies. In Table 307-2, these therapies are grouped according to their func-

Table 307-1. Goals of Healing

Goal	Example of Therapy
Cure disease	Penicillin for strep throat
Manage or mitigate symptoms	Acetaminophen or massage to reduce pain
Prevent disease or disability	Immunize to prevent specific illnesses
Promote health and vitality	Exercise to enhance fitness
Eliminate toxins and minimize stress	Avoid tobacco smoke; meditate regularly
Enhance harmony, connections to family and community	Social support, church attendance, doctor-patient relationship
Promote inner peace	Prayer, ritual, spiritual practices

Table 307-2. Integrative Model

1. Biochemical therapies: medications, herbs, dietary supplements
2. Lifestyle therapies: diet, exercise, environment, mind-body therapies
3. Biomechanical therapies: massage, spinal adjustment, surgery
4. Bioenergetic therapies: acupuncture, Therapeutic Touch/Reiki and other healing touch therapies, prayer and ritual, homeopathy

tional similarities. A discussion of each of the major domains follows in further detail.

Biochemical Therapies: Medications, Herbs, and Dietary Supplements
Medications
Medications are discussed elsewhere in this text and therefore are not covered here. Many parents are concerned about overreliance on medications, which may be perceived as unnatural, laden with undesirable side effects and the potential for addiction. Some view medications as a cover-up rather than a cure of an underlying problem.

Herbs and Dietary Supplements
Herbs and other dietary supplements have biochemical effects; in fact, approximately 20% to 30% of modern medications are derived from herbs. Clinicians routinely advise families about supplements such as iron and calcium and may caution patients about tobacco. Parents often use herbal folk remedies such as chamomile to treat infant colic or echinacea to ward off the common cold. Teenage athletes frequently use creatine and other supplements to boost their athletic performance.

Many families assume that all herbs and dietary supplements are safe because they are natural. However, a major concern about using these products is the lack of quality control because of the 1994 U.S. Dietary Supplement Health Education Act (DSHEA). This act allows supplements to be sold without proof of either safety or efficacy prior to marketing. There is substantial product variability for commonly used herbs such as ginseng, Saint John's wort, echinacea, and ephedra. In addition, the purity of many herbs is questionable; for example, between 30% and 45% of Chinese (or Asian) patent medications contain conventional medications that are not listed on the label, which have resulted in serious toxicity to children. Herbal products can also be contaminated with the wrong herb, pesticides, herbicides, organic matter from animal fertilizers, and heavy metals.

Physicians should caution patients about the potential toxicities of some herbs and dietary supplements and should routinely recommend avoiding tobacco, ephedra, and Chinese patent medications and herbal products imported from other developing countries in which manufacturing standards might not be as rigorous as they are in Europe or the United States. Herbs that are generally considered safe for children include chamomile, ginger (as an antiemetic), and aloe vera (as a vulnerary). Since popular herb use changes rapidly each year, physicians who question the use of a particular herb or dietary supplement should consult with toxicologists, pharmacists, and dietitians. Additional references are included at the end of chapter.

Lifestyle Therapies: Diet, Exercise, Environment, and Mind-Body Therapies

Diet

Families who pursue CAM therapies are often interested in optimal diets for their children. During routine health supervision visits, physicians typically discuss diet with patients and families. Pediatric expertise in nutritional therapies range from promoting breast-feeding to managing diabetic diets and patients with gluten-sensitive enteropathy or milk allergy. Yet families often turn to CAM practitioners such as naturopaths, chiropractors, and licensed acupuncturists for advice about certain foods and food allergies. Many parents choose to have their children follow a vegetarian or macrobiotic diet for religious, ethical, or health reasons. Others choose to put their children on elimination diets in an attempt to omit possible allergens such as wheat, dairy, corn, and soy. Physicians should be aware of their patients' diets so as to avoid potential nutritional deficiencies.

Exercise

Exercise improves cardiovascular fitness, flexibility, and strength and should enhance the patient's general sense of well-being. Few studies have evaluated different therapeutic benefits for different types of exercise aimed at specific pediatric conditions, but all recognize that regular exercise is health promoting. Studies suggest that regular yoga practice might reduce symptoms in asthmatic children.

Environment

Clinicians and, in particular, pediatricians are well-known advocates for safe physical and psychosocial environments for children, that is, free from lead and mercury poisoning, poverty, racism, sexism, domestic violence, drug and alcohol use, maternal depression, unemployment, abuse, and media (especially television) violence. Physicians may also offer individualized environmental advice, for example, white noise and vibration for colic, phototherapy for jaundice, music therapy for stress reduction, and ice for sprains. Other therapies that are environmentally based, such as crystals, magnets, and aromatherapies, are widely marketed as being safe, effective treatments. There are few data investigating these claims, but most appear to be safe, and lavender aromatherapy has been shown to be helpful to patients with insomnia.

Mind-Body

Mind-body therapies, such as peer counseling, social support, and psychotherapy, have long been part of mainstream medicine. Hypnosis, guided imagery, and biofeedback are now often part of mainstream medical practice. Many physicians, psychologists, social workers, and other mainstream health professionals use them. Many studies have now proven that these techniques are useful in treating a variety of pediatric conditions that range from pain management to constipation.

Biomechanical Therapies: Massage, Adjustment (Chiropractic, Osteopathy), and Surgery

Massage

Massage therapy was part of conventional health care practices worldwide well into the 20th century. Following its virtual disappearance from U.S. medicine in the 1940s, it is again increasing in popularity. There are many different kinds of massage techniques (e.g., deep tissue massage, manual lymph drainage massage, myofascial release, neuromuscular massage, and Swedish massage) and movement integration (e.g., Feldenkrais and Alexander techniques).

Therapeutic massage is typically provided by professional massage therapists but can also be provided under a nurse's scope of practice or as part of physical therapy. Massage therapists focus primarily on muscles and connective tissues and do not perform spinal adjustments. The American Massage Therapy Association is the largest professional national organization of bodyworkers in the United States. To be a member of this association, a massage therapist must receive training from an accredited school and must have 500 hours of supervised practice. Most massage schools provide very little pediatric training, and most massage therapists rarely treat children.

Most hospitals do not provide therapeutic massage for pediatric patients despite its proven benefits. Massage enhances the growth rate of premature infants, reduces the severity of asthma in school-age children, and eases suffering from anxiety and depression in adolescents who are hospitalized for psychiatric disorders. Massage can also be helpful for relieving pain, improving circulation, reducing edema, loosening tight joints, increasing endogenous levels of serotonin, decreasing levels of stress hormones, and improving an overall sense of relaxation and well-being.

Spinal Adjustment

Two types of licensed practitioners—chiropractors and osteopaths—most often provide spinal adjustments.

Chiropractic

In the United States and Canada, chiropractors are the most common CAM therapists. They believe that proper alignment of the vertebrae is essential for optimal health. In 1998, there were more than 50,000 doctors of chiropractic in the United States, and numbers are expected to double by 2010. Chiropractors are licensed in all 50 states; Medicare and most major insurance carriers cover professional chiropractic care. Third-party payers cover almost 50% of chiropractor fees for pediatric care.

The number of pediatric visits to chiropractors has increased from an estimated 20 million visits in 1993 to 30 million in 1998. When treating children, chiropractors tend to take fewer radiographs and use lighter force during chiropractic adjustments than when treating adults. They sometimes use special pediatric tables or treat the child in a parent's laps. However, in contrast to conventional pediatricians, only one third of chiropractors actively recommend childhood immunizations.

Osteopath

Doctors of Osteopathy (DOs) are fully licensed and trained physicians and surgeons like MDs, but they have additional training in osteopathic manipulation. They are considered mainstream physician practitioners. In 1998, there were approximately 35,000 DOs in the United States, and this number is expected to increase to approximately 45,000 by the year 2000. In the United States, a DO must graduate from one of 16 accredited osteopathic medical schools to be considered a licensed practitioner. Training is similar to that of MDs in that osteopathy school is 4 years long, followed by a 1- to 6-year residency-training program in general or subspecialty areas. Like MDs, DOs have the right to prescribe drugs and perform surgery and usually practice in fully accredited, licensed hospitals and medical centers.

Osteopaths believe in a synergistic model of human functioning in which the whole is greater than the sum of the parts. They practice a holistic philosophy, which considers the human mind and spirit to be just as important as the human body. They also place a strong emphasis on health promotion and disease prevention while focusing on maintaining and promoting coping skills to combat stress. Many traditional MDs also practice a holistic philosophy.

Surgery

Surgery is discussed elsewhere in this text and therefore is not covered here.

Bioenergetic Therapies: Acupuncture, Therapeutic Touch/Reiki, and Homeopathy

Acupuncture

Acupuncture, commonly used by both adults and children, is the CAM therapy most frequently recommended by physicians. A National Institutes of Health consensus conference concluded that acupuncture is effective in reducing adult postoperative and chemotherapy-associated nausea and vomiting and postoperative dental pain. Acupuncture may be useful in treating headache, dysmenorrhea, and neck pain. By late 1998, approximately one third of North American pediatric pain clinics offered acupuncture services for pain management.

The number of graduates from American acupuncture schools doubled between 1992 and 1997. In 1998, there were approximately 11,000 practicing acupuncturists in the United States, and that number is expected to reach 21,000 by 2005. Patients receiving acupuncture treatments for acute conditions usually receive two or three treatments weekly for 2 to 3 weeks. If the treatments are effective, most patients note the benefits within the first five treatment sessions. Most insurance companies do not cover acupuncture treatments, so the majority of patients pay out of pocket for acupuncture services unless a physician acupuncturist administers the therapy.

Reports of serious adverse effects from acupuncture are rare. The reported incidence of serious side effects such as pneumothorax from acupuncture therapy when performed by a licensed acupuncturist are 1:10,000 to 1:100,000, which is comparable to the risk of a serious adverse event from taking penicillin.

Therapeutic Touch/Reiki

Therapeutic Touch and Reiki are considered bioenergetic therapies in which the practitioner transmits an invisible healing energy through his or her hands in the attempt to balance the patient's own energy fields. These therapies can also be described as nonreligious forms of "laying on of hands" healing.

Therapeutic Touch can be performed without touching the patient. It was invented in the 1970s by a nursing professor at New York University, Dolores Krieger, and a lay healer, Dora Kunz, and was based on their observations of numerous religious healers. In the following five steps, they described the technique so that it did not require a specific religious faith or belief:

1. Having a clear and conscious *intent* to be helpful and heal
2. Being *centered* in a peaceful state of mind
3. Using the hands to assess the patient's energy (typically, the hands are held 1 to 3 inches away from the patient's body and are moved in a slow downward motion from the head to the toes)
4. Using the hands to help *restore* the patient's energy to a balanced, peaceful, harmonious state
5. Releasing the patient to complete his or her healing process while the healer returns to his or her own centered, peaceful state of mind

Therapeutic Touch is currently taught in nursing schools across the United States and Canada and in over 80 other countries around the world. There are currently no certifying examinations, and no states currently license Therapeutic Touch.

There are limited data on the effectiveness of Therapeutic Touch in treating children. In adults, some studies report that Therapeutic Touch helps to enhance sleep and a sense of well-being and helps to reduce pain and anxiety. The cost varies depending on whether the therapy is provided as a part of routine nursing care or through an independent practice.

Reiki grew out of a Japanese tradition and is similar to Therapeutic Touch. Reiki practitioners believe in an invisible energy that may be transmitted from healer to patient through intention and focus via hands placed on particular parts of the patient's body. They are trained by a Reiki master through an apprenticeship and spiritual/energetic initiation. There are no certifying examinations, no state licensure, and no studies evaluating its effectiveness in treating children.

Homeopathy

Homeopathy was founded by a 19th-century German physician, Samuel Hahnemann, and is based on two major principles: (1) *similis similibus curentur*—"like is cured by like" (i.e., an illness, such as an allergic conjunctivitis, can be treated by a substance, such as red onions, that produces watery eyes in a healthy person)—and (2) *doses minimae*—"potentiation through dilution" (i.e., the more dilute a concoction is, the more powerful and therapeutic it is). Homeopathic remedies are prepared by serial dilutions and vigorous shaking and contain little or no measurable active ingredient. However, the homeopathic philosophy suggests that homeopathic remedies impart an energetic imprint that enables the patient's own body to fight the underlying cause of the disease.

Insurance coverage for homeopathic care varies according to state, insurance carrier, and the professional status of the homeopath. Homeopathic services provided by physicians and chiropractors are more likely to be covered than are services provided by nonphysicians. Many homeopaths also recommend dietary therapies, dietary supplements, and relaxation techniques. Pediatric and adolescent visits typically account for 20% to 30% of all visits to homeopaths.

Randomized controlled trials have shown that homeopathic medicine is more effective than placebo for treating otitis media and acute childhood diarrhea. In addition, two recent meta-analyses of controlled trials of homeopathy demonstrated positive trends for homeopathy compared with placebo. As mainstream doctors and nurses become uncomfortable with the side effects of modern medications, increasingly they are turning toward homeopathy as a safe alternative therapy. Homeopathic remedies are available over the counter and through mail-order catalogues and the Internet without a prescription, so almost anyone can claim to be a homeopathic practitioner.

SYSTEMS OF HEALING

Many medical systems incorporate numerous therapies from different domains in this integrative model. Although mainstream medicine is frequently identified with prescrip-

tion medications, physicians also provide expert advice and counsel about various lifestyle therapies. Traditional Chinese medicine, while providing acupuncture, also attends to diet, exercise, meditation, and massage. Ayurvedic medicine, which is native to India, promotes yoga, meditation, diet, and herbs. Naturopathy emphasizes a healthy diet, ample exercise, rest, and a positive mental and emotional state that is enhanced by meditation, imagery, and counseling. Naturopaths also recommend herbs and dietary supplements, massage, elements of chiropractic, acupuncture, and homeopathy.

SUMMARY

Clinicians increasingly encounter families who ask about CAM therapies. CAM use is even more common among children with chronic diseases or incurable conditions. Physicians need to be sensitive to families' values and cultural practices that highly esteem CAM therapies (see Table 307-1). They also need to be knowledgeable in answering families' questions about the safety and effectiveness about different CAM therapies. The integrative model may provide a useful way to discuss these issues with families (see Table 307-2). An additional number of books and publications are available as reliable resources (Table 307-3).

Table 307-3. Resources to Learn More	
Recent articles	*General Overviews:* Kemper KJ: Integrative Medicine: Talking with families about complementary, alternative and mainstream medical therapies in acute care settings. Emerg Office Pediatr 2000;13(2):45–49. Kemper KJ: Integrative medicine: Does it work? Arch Dis Child 2001;84:6–9. Kemper KJ, Wornham WL: Consultations for holistic pediatric services for inpatients and outpatient oncology patients at a children's hospital. Arch Pediatr Adolesc Med 2001;155:449–454. *Specific Conditions:* Chan E, Gardiner P, Kemper KJ: At least it's natural … Herbs and dietary supplements in ADHD. Contemp Pediatr 2000;17(9):116. Kemper KJ, Lester MR: Alternative asthma therapies: An evidence-based review. Contemp Pediatr 1999;16(3):162–195. Kemper KJ, Longwood Herbal Task Force: Shark cartilage, cat's claw and other complementary cancer therapies. Contemp Pediatr 1999;16(11):101–126. Gardiner P, Conboy LA, Kemper KJ. Herbs and adolescent girls: Avoiding the hazards of self-treatment. Contemp Pediatr 2000;17(3):133–154. *Specific Therapies:* Gardiner P, Kemper KJ: Peripheral brain: Herbs in pediatric and adolescent medicine. Pediatr Rev 2000;21(2):44–57. Kemper KJ, Sarah R, Silver-Highfield E, et al: On pins and needles: Pediatric pain patients' experience with acupuncture. Pediatrics 2000;105(4):941–947. Lee A, Highfield ES, Berde CB, Kemper KJ: Acupuncturists: Practice characteristics and pediatric care. West J Med 1999;171:153–157. Lee A, Kemper KJ: Homeopathy and naturopathy: Practice characteristics and pediatric care. Arch Pediatr Adolesc Med 2000;154:75–80. Lee A, Li DH, Berde CB, Kemper KJ: Practice characteristics of chiropractors who treat children. Arch Pediatr Adolesc Med 2000;154:401–407.
Books	■ Dillard J, Ziporyn T: Alternative Medicine for Dummies. New York, IDG Books, 1998. ■ Fugh-Berman A: Alternative Medicine: What Works. Baltimore, Williams & Wilkins, 1997. ■ Kemper KJ: The Holistic Pediatrician, 2nd ed. New York, HarperCollins, 2002. ■ Sierpina V: Integrative Healthcare: Complementary and Alternative Therapies for the Whole Person, Philadelphia, FA Davis, 2001.
Periodicals	■ Nutrition Action Newsletter. Washington, DC, Center for Science in the Public Interest.
Human	■ Pharmacists, nurses, physical therapists, chaplains, dietitians, poison control center, Center for Holistic Pediatric Education and Research, Center for Alternative and Complementary Medicine Research, New England School of Acupuncture, Massachusetts College of Pharmacy.
Websites	■ Comprehensive Natural Products Database (commercial): Available at: www.naturaldatabase.com. ■ Holistic Kids (Children's and Massachusetts College of Pharmacy collaborative database): Available at: http://www.holistickids.org. ■ Longwood Herbal Task Force: Available at: http://www.mcp.edu/herbal/. ■ NIH Center for Alternative Medicine: Available at: http://nccam.nih.gov. ■ Rosenthal Center for Complementary and Alternative Medicine: Available at: http://cpmcnet.columbia.edu/dept/rosenthal/.

Additional Resources, CD-ROM

Bibliography

SUGGESTED READINGS

Barnes J: Complementary medicine: Aromatherapy. Pharm J 1998;260:862–867.

Ernst E, Pittler MH: The effectiveness of acupuncture in treating acute dental pain. Br Dent J 1998;184:443–447.

Field T: Massage therapy for infants and children. J Dev Behav Pediatr 1995;16:105–111.

King CR: Nonpharmacologic management of chemotherapy-induced nausea and vomiting. Oncol Nurs Forum 1997;24:41–48.

Spence JE, Olson MA: Quantitative research on therapeutic touch: An integrative review of the literature 1985–1995. Scand J Caring Sci 1997;11:183–190.

INDEX

Note: Page numbers followed by the letter f refer to figures, those followed by t refer to tables, and those followed by b refer to boxes.

A

Abandonment
  avoidance of, in end-of-life care of child, 892–893
  defined, 1270
  inadequate, as child neglect, 1713–1714
ABC(s)
  in basic life support, 241
  in respiratory distress, 788
  in shock management, 250
  in sports injuries, 352
ABC model, of behavior, 1927–1928
  tracking sheet for, 1928f
ABCDE(s), of injury, 280, 280t
Abdomen
  accumulation of fluid in. See Ascites.
  examination of
    acute pain and, 623
    in newborns, 17–18
    in toddlers, 23, 24f
Abdominal distention, in newborns, 1258t, 1259
Abdominal injury, 282
Abdominal mass
  differential diagnosis of, 1349t
  in neonate, 1349–1350
  solid, evaluation of, 1100–1101, 1100b, 1101b
Abdominal pain
  acute
    causes of, 623t
    diagnostic approach to, 623–624, 624b
    location and structures involved in, 623t
    management of, 624
  chronic (recurrent)
    clinical presentation of, 625, 625t
    defined, 625
    diagnostic approach to, 625–626, 626b
    management of, 626
    outcome of, 627
    referral for, 626–627
  classification of, 623
  in HIV-infected patient, 1138
  in immunocompromised patient, 1096
  onset of, characteristics at, 623t
  sensory pathways involved in, 622–623
Abdominal surgery, 1922
Abdominal thrust technique, foreign object removal by, 244f
Abdominal wall defects, in newborns, 1258t, 1260, 1348–1349, 1348f
Abducens nerve palsy, 498
Abendazole, for pinworm infestation, 857t
ABO blood group compatibility, for renal transplantation, 1158, 1158t
Abortion, legally induced, 1493
Abscess
  deep neck, 462, 464, 466f
    follow-up for, 470
    management of, 469
  periapical, 485, 485f
  peritonsillar, 789–790

Abscess (Continued)
  retropharyngeal, 789–790
  skin. See Skin abscess.
Absence seizures (petit mal epilepsy), 753, 753t, 1772–1773, 1773f
  treatment of, 755t
Absorption, of drugs, 1805
Abstinence syndrome, defined, 308
Abuse. See also Child abuse.
  drug. See also Substance abuse; under specific drug.
    in adolescents, agitation due to, 309
  physical, 1716–1720, 1717b
  sexual, 750, 1716–1720, 1717b
Academic achievement tests, for oppositional defiant disorder and conduct disorder, 1585t
Acanthosis nigricans, 608, 608f, 609b, 1045
Acarus scabiei, 586. See also Scabies.
Acceptance stage, in homosexual identity development, 1636t
Accessibility, for special needs children in medical home, 871
Accommodative esotropia, acquired, 496, 497
Acculturation, 1648
Ace bandage, in splinting, 1915b, 1917
Acetaminophen
  for congenital muscular torticollis, 477
  for fever, 302
  for pain, 1830
    dosage of, 1830t
  for salivary gland inflammatory disease, 477
Acetaminophen poisoning
  causing liver disease, 966
  management of, 290
  symptoms of, 287t
  threshold dose and expected toxicity by serum level in, 288, 288t
N-Aceyl cysteine, for acetaminophen poisoning, 290
Achalasia, of esophagus, 621, 621t
Achilles tendinitis, 357
Achondroplasia, 33, 89f, 90, 203t, 902t, 903
Achromatopsia, diagnosis of, 978
Achromic nevus (nevus depigmentosus), 567, 568f
Acid suppressors, for gastroesophageal reflux disease, 664, 664t
Acid-base regulation, renal, 725, 735f, 736f
Acidemia
  associated with erythroderma or dermatitis, 610t
  hyperlactic, 999–1000
  organic, 1006, 1867t
    management of, 1874
Acid-fast bacillus, 812
Acid-fast staining, of microorganisms, 131, 131f

Acidosis
  lactic, in inborn errors of metabolism, 1869f
  metabolic, 138
    in inborn errors of metabolism, 1868f
    renal tubular, 734–737. See also Renal tubular acidosis.
Acne, 527–528, 528f, 1439–1445
  antibiotic treatment of, 1826t
  cystic, 1440, 1441f
  diagnosis of, 1440, 1440f
  infantile, 529, 529f
  inflammatory, 1439, 1440f
  management of, 1441–1445
    combination therapy in, 1444
    hormonal therapy in, 1444
    isotretinoin in, 1444–1445
    surgical, 1445
    systemic antibiotics in, 1443–1444, 1443t
    topical preparations in, 1441–1443, 1441t, 1442t, 1443t
  neonatal, 528–529, 529f
  noninflammatory, 1439–1440
  outcome and follow-up for, 1445
  patient education about, 1445
  physiologic factors associated with, 1439–1440
  prepubertal, 529
Acne conglobata, 529, 1440
Acne keloidalis, 530, 530f
Acne vulgaris, 529
Acneiform eruptions, drug-induced, 530, 530f
Acquired immunodeficiency syndrome (AIDS), 1132. See also Human immunodeficiency virus (HIV) infection.
  superinfections associated with, 126
Acrodermatitis, papular (Gianotti-Crosti syndrome), 523–524, 524f
  infectious agents and immunizations associated with, 524b
Acrodermatitis enteropathica, 610–611, 611f
Acromioclavicular joint, sports-related injury to, 355t
Acropustulosis, in infants, 558, 559f
Actinomycin-D, 1865
Activated charcoal, for poisonings, 289, 289t
Activated partial thromboplastin time (aPTT), for hemophilia, 709
Active listening, in clinical interview, 7, 7b
Activity, decreased, in ill newborn, 1287t
Acupuncture, 1962
Acute lymphoblastic leukemia (ALL), 1081–1082, 1081t, 1082f
  diagnosis of, 1083–1084
  NCI definition of risk and survival for, 1088t
  treatment of, 1085, 1110–1111
Acute myeloid leukemia (AML), 1081t, 1082, 1082f
  diagnosis of, 1084
  treatment of, 1085–1086, 1110t